KAPLAN & SADOCK'S

Synopsis of Psychiatry

Behavioral Sciences/Clinical Psychiatry

Tenth 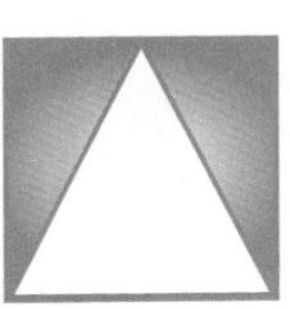 Edition

ABOUT THE AUTHORS

BENJAMIN JAMES SADOCK, M.D., is the Menas S. Gregory Professor of Psychiatry and Vice Chairman of the Department of Psychiatry at the New York University (NYU) School of Medicine, New York, New York. He is a graduate of Union College, received his M.D. degree from New York Medical College, and completed his internship at Albany Hospital. After finishing his residency at Bellevue Psychiatric Hospital, he entered military service, serving as Acting Chief of Neuropsychiatry at Sheppard Air Force Base, Wichita Falls, Texas. He has held faculty and teaching appointments at Southwestern Medical School and Parkland Hospital in Dallas and at New York Medical College, St. Luke's Hospital, the New York State Psychiatric Institute, and Metropolitan Hospital in New York. Dr. Sadock joined the faculty of the NYU School of Medicine in 1980 and served in various positions: Director of Medical Student Education in Psychiatry, Co-Director of the Residency Training Program in Psychiatry, and Director of Graduate Medical Education. Currently, Dr. Sadock is Co-Director of Student Mental Health Services, Psychiatric Consultant to the Admissions Committee, and Co-Director of Continuing Education in Psychiatry at the NYU School of Medicine. He is on the staff of Bellevue Hospital and Tisch Hospital and is a consulting psychiatrist at Lenox Hill Hospital. Dr. Sadock is a Diplomate of the American Board of Psychiatry and Neurology and served as Associate Examiner for the Board for more than a decade. He is a Distinguished Life Fellow of the American Psychiatric Association, a Fellow of the American College of Physicians, a Fellow of the New York Academy of Medicine, and a member of Alpha Omega Alpha Honor Society. He is active in numerous psychiatric organizations and is founder and president of the NYU-Bellevue Psychiatric Society. Dr. Sadock was a member of the National Committee in Continuing Education in Psychiatry of the American Psychiatric Association; he served on the Ad Hoc Committee on Sex Therapy Clinics of the American Medical Association, was a delegate to the conference on Recertification of the American Board of Medical Specialists, and was a representative of the American Psychiatric Association Task Force on the National Board of Medical Examiners and the American Board of Psychiatry and Neurology. In 1985, he received the Academic Achievement Award from New York Medical College and was appointed Faculty Scholar at NYU School of Medicine in 2000. He is the author or editor of more than 100 publications, a book reviewer for psychiatric journals, and he lectures on a broad range of topics in general psychiatry. Dr. Sadock maintains a private practice for diagnostic consultations and psychiatric treatment. He has been married to Virginia Alcott Sadock, M.D., Professor of Psychiatry at NYU School of Medicine, since completing his residency. Dr. Sadock enjoys opera, golf, skiing, and traveling, and is an enthusiastic fly fisherman.

VIRGINIA ALCOTT SADOCK, M.D., joined the faculty of the New York University (NYU) School of Medicine in 1980, where she is currently Professor of Psychiatry and Attending Psychiatrist at the Tisch Hospital and Bellevue Hospital. She is Director of the Program in Human Sexuality at the NYU Medical Center, one of the largest treatment and training programs of its kind in the United States. Dr. Sadock is the author of more than 50 articles and chapters on sexual behavior and was the developmental editor of *The Sexual Experience*, one of the first major textbooks on human sexuality, published by Williams & Wilkins. She serves as a referee and book reviewer for several medical journals, including the *American Journal of Psychiatry* and the *Journal of the American Medical Association*. She has long been interested in the role of women in medicine and psychiatry and was a founder of the Committee on Women in Psychiatry of the New York County District Branch of the American Psychiatric Association. She is active in academic matters, has served as Assistant and Associate Examiner for the American Board of Psychiatry and Neurology for more than 15 years; she was a member of the Test Committee in Psychiatry for both the American Board of Psychiatry and the Psychiatric Knowledge and Self-Assessment Program (PKSAP) of the American Psychiatric Association. She has chaired the Committee on Public Relations of the New York County District Branch of the American Psychiatric Association and has participated in the National Medical Television Network series *Women in Medicine* and the Emmy Award-winning PBS television documentary *Women and Depression*. She has been Vice-President of the Society of Sex Therapy and Research and a regional council member of the American Association of Sex Education Counselors and Therapists; she is currently President of the Alumni Association of Sex Therapists. She lectures extensively in the United States and abroad on sexual dysfunction, relational problems, and depression and anxiety disorders. She is a Distinguished Fellow of the American Psychiatric Association, a Fellow of the New York Academy of Medicine, and a Diplomate of the American Board of Psychiatry and Neurology. Dr. Sadock is a graduate of Bennington College; she received her M.D. degree from New York Medical College, and trained in psychiatry at Metropolitan Hospital. She maintains an active practice that includes individual psychotherapy, couples and marital therapy, sex therapy, psychiatric consultation, and pharmacotherapy. She lives in Manhattan with her husband Dr. Benjamin Sadock. They have two children, James William Sadock, M.D., and Victoria Anne Gregg, M.D., both emergency physicians, and two grandchildren, Emily Alcott and Celia Anne. In her leisure time, Dr. Sadock enjoys theater, film, golf, reading fiction, and traveling.

Drugs Used in Psychiatry

This guide contains color reproductions of some commonly prescribed psychotherapeutic drugs. This guide illustrates proprietary forms of tablets and capsules. A † symbol preceding the name of a drug indicates that other doses are available. Check directly with the manufacturer. (*Although the photos are intended as accurate reproductions of the drug, this guide should be used only as a quick identification aid.)*

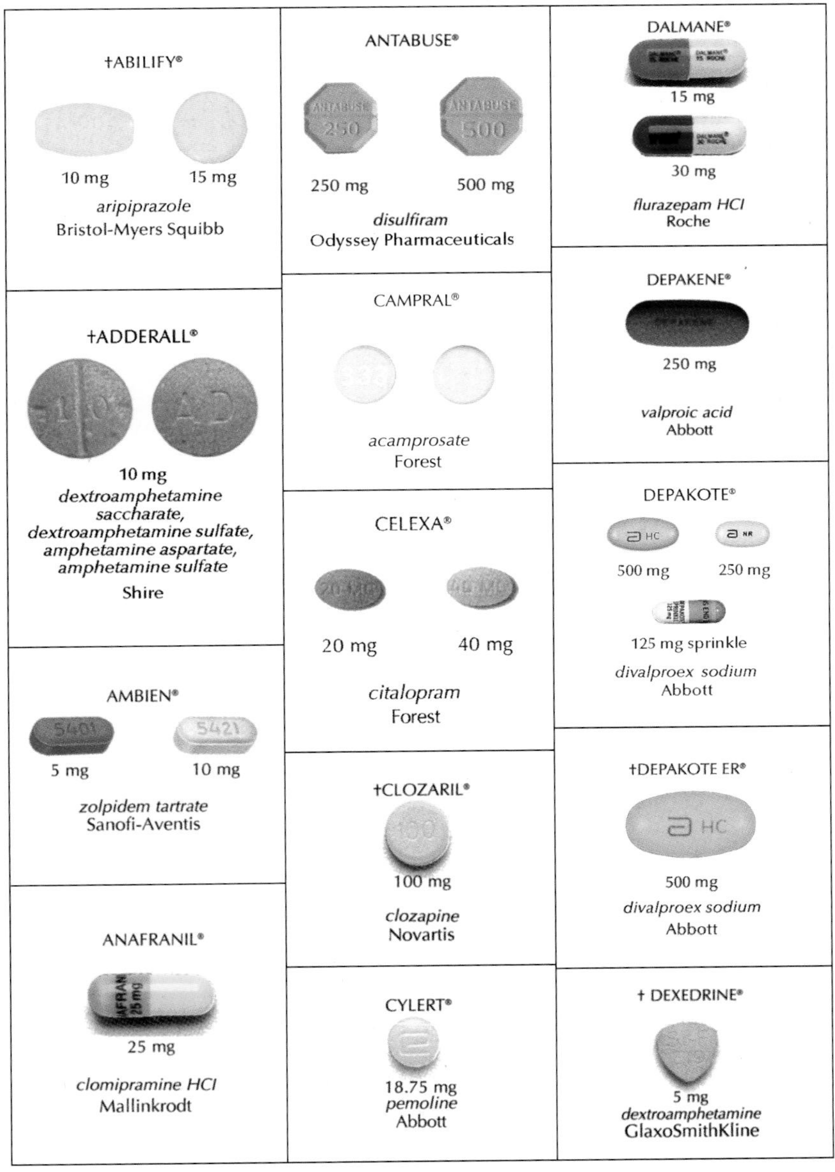

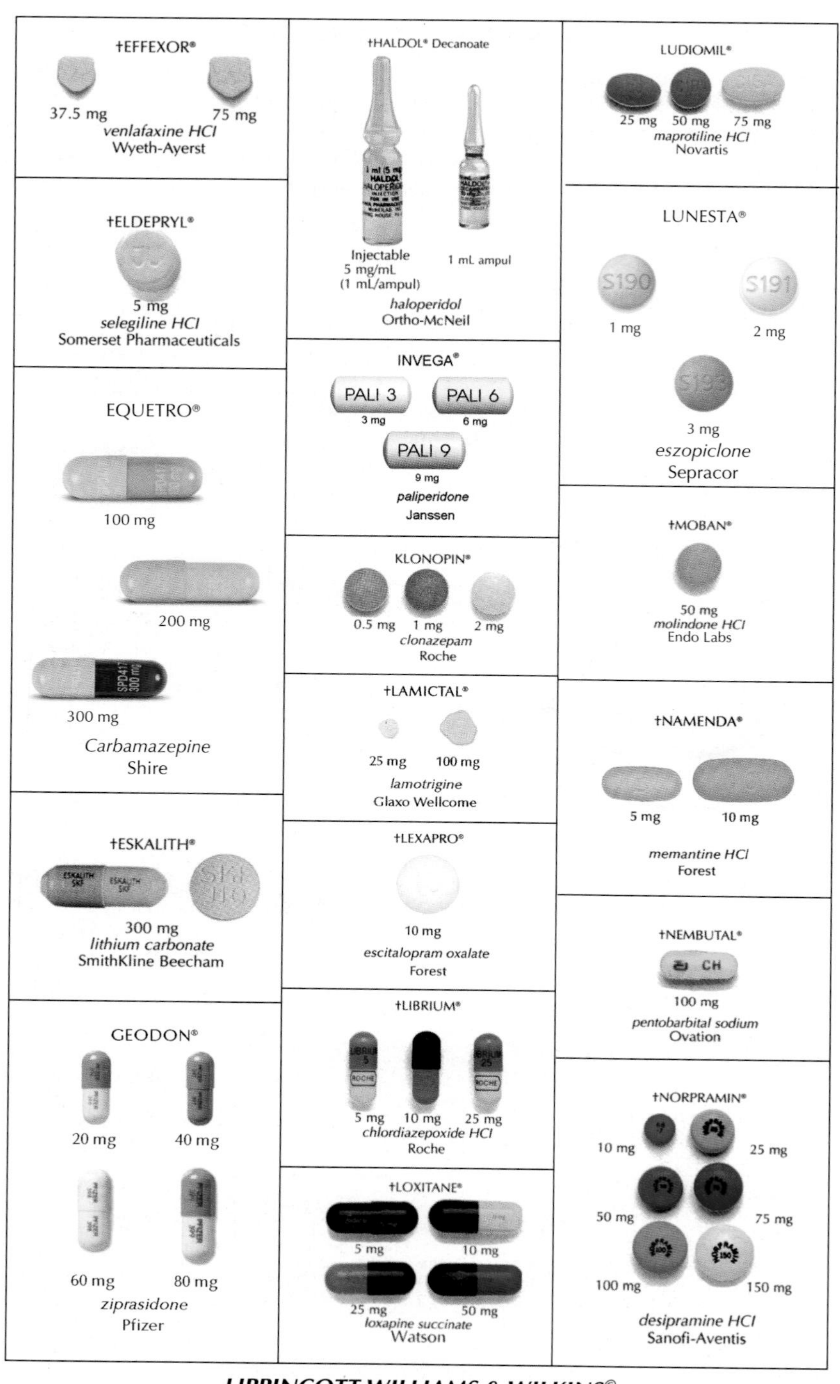
†EFFEXOR®
37.5 mg
75 mg
venlafaxine HCl
Wyeth-Ayerst
†ELDEPRYL®
5 mg
selegiline HCl
Somerset Pharmaceuticals
EQUETRO®
100 mg
200 mg
SPD417 300 mg
300 mg
Carbamazepine
Shire
†ESKALITH®
ESKALITH SKF
300 mg
lithium carbonate
SmithKline Beecham
GEODON®
20 mg
40 mg
60 mg
80 mg
ziprasidone
Pfizer
†HALDOL® Decanoate
Injectable
5 mg/mL
(1 mL/ampul)
1 mL ampul
haloperidol
Ortho-McNeil
INVEGA®
PALI 3
3 mg
PALI 6
6 mg
PALI 9
9 mg
paliperidone
Janssen
KLONOPIN®
0.5 mg
1 mg
2 mg
clonazepam
Roche
†LAMICTAL®
25 mg
100 mg
lamotrigine
Glaxo Wellcome
†LEXAPRO®
10 mg
escitalopram oxalate
Forest
†LIBRIUM®
LIBRIUM 5
ROCHE
LIBRIUM 25
5 mg
10 mg
25 mg
chlordiazepoxide HCl
Roche
†LOXITANE®
5 mg
10 mg
25 mg
50 mg
loxapine succinate
Watson
LUDIOMIL®
25 mg
50 mg
75 mg
maprotiline HCl
Novartis
LUNESTA®
S190
S191
1 mg
2 mg
S193
3 mg
eszopiclone
Sepracor
†MOBAN®
50 mg
molindone HCl
Endo Labs
†NAMENDA®
5 mg
10 mg
memantine HCl
Forest
†NEMBUTAL®
CH
100 mg
pentobarbital sodium
Ovation
†NORPRAMIN®
10 mg
25 mg
50 mg
75 mg
100 mg
150 mg
desipramine HCl
Sanofi-Aventis

LIPPINCOTT WILLIAMS & WILKINS©

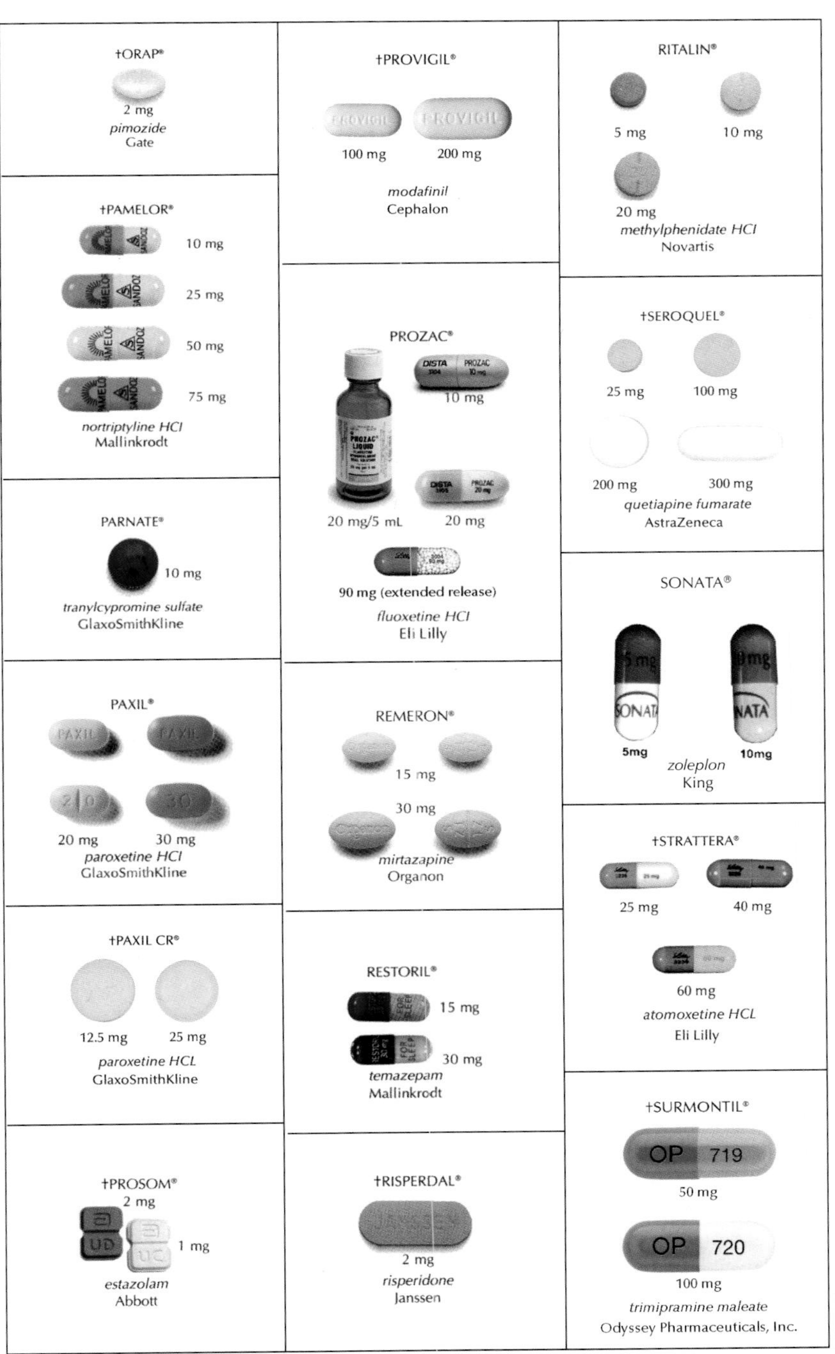

†ORAP®
2 mg
pimozide
Gate
†PAMELOR®
10 mg
25 mg
50 mg
75 mg
nortriptyline HCl
Mallinkrodt
PARNATE®
10 mg
tranylcypromine sulfate
GlaxoSmithKline
PAXIL®
20 mg
30 mg
paroxetine HCl
GlaxoSmithKline
†PAXIL CR®
12.5 mg
25 mg
paroxetine HCL
GlaxoSmithKline
†PROSOM®
2 mg
1 mg
estazolam
Abbott
†PROVIGIL®
100 mg
200 mg
modafinil
Cephalon
PROZAC®
10 mg
20 mg/5 mL
20 mg
90 mg (extended release)
fluoxetine HCl
Eli Lilly
REMERON®
15 mg
30 mg
mirtazapine
Organon
RESTORIL®
15 mg
30 mg
temazepam
Mallinkrodt
†RISPERDAL®
2 mg
risperidone
Janssen
RITALIN®
5 mg
10 mg
20 mg
methylphenidate HCl
Novartis
†SEROQUEL®
25 mg
100 mg
200 mg
300 mg
quetiapine fumarate
AstraZeneca
SONATA®
5mg
10mg
zoleplon
King
†STRATTERA®
25 mg
40 mg
60 mg
atomoxetine HCL
Eli Lilly
†SURMONTIL®
OP 719
50 mg
OP 720
100 mg
trimipramine maleate
Odyssey Pharmaceuticals, Inc.

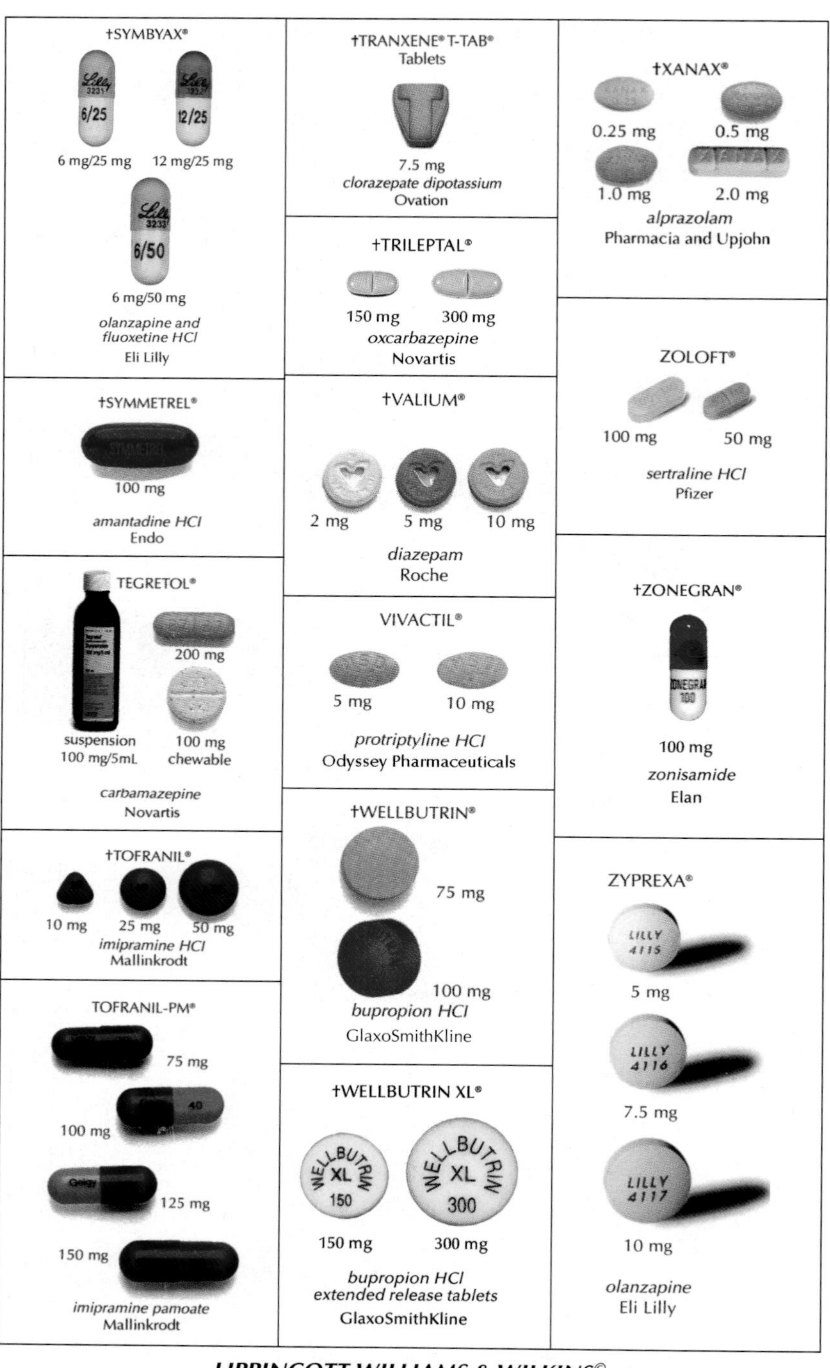

†SYMBYAX®
6/25
12/25
6 mg/25 mg
12 mg/25 mg
6/50
6 mg/50 mg
olanzapine and fluoxetine HCl
Eli Lilly
†SYMMETREL®
100 mg
amantadine HCl
Endo
TEGRETOL®
200 mg
suspension 100 mg/5mL
100 mg chewable
carbamazepine
Novartis
†TOFRANIL®
10 mg
25 mg
50 mg
imipramine HCl
Mallinkrodt
TOFRANIL-PM®
75 mg
100 mg
125 mg
150 mg
imipramine pamoate
Mallinkrodt
†TRANXENE® T-TAB®
Tablets
7.5 mg
clorazepate dipotassium
Ovation
†TRILEPTAL®
150 mg
300 mg
oxcarbazepine
Novartis
†VALIUM®
2 mg
5 mg
10 mg
diazepam
Roche
VIVACTIL®
5 mg
10 mg
protriptyline HCl
Odyssey Pharmaceuticals
†WELLBUTRIN®
75 mg
100 mg
bupropion HCl
GlaxoSmithKline
†WELLBUTRIN XL®
WELLBUTRIN XL 150
WELLBUTRIN XL 300
150 mg
300 mg
bupropion HCl extended release tablets
GlaxoSmithKline
†XANAX®
0.25 mg
0.5 mg
1.0 mg
2.0 mg
alprazolam
Pharmacia and Upjohn
ZOLOFT®
100 mg
50 mg
sertraline HCl
Pfizer
†ZONEGRAN®
ZONEGRAN 100
100 mg
zonisamide
Elan
ZYPREXA®
LILLY 4115
5 mg
LILLY 4116
7.5 mg
LILLY 4117
10 mg
olanzapine
Eli Lilly

KAPLAN & SADOCK'S

Synopsis of Psychiatry

Behavioral Sciences/Clinical Psychiatry

Tenth 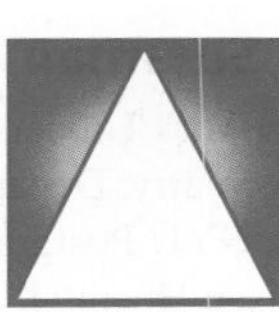 Edition

Contributing Editors

Jack A. Grebb, M.D.

Professor of Psychiatry, Department of Psychiatry, New York University School of Medicine, New York, New York; Vice President, Clinical Design and Evaluations, Neuroscience, Bristol-Myers Squibb, Walingford, Connecticut

Caroly S. Pataki, M.D.

Clinical Professor of Psychiatry and the Biobehavioral Sciences, Keck School of Medicine at the University of Southern California; Director, Child and Adolescent Psychiatry Residency Training Program, University of Southern California, Los Angeles, California

Norman Sussman, M.D.

Professor of Psychiatry, New York University School of Medicine; Co-director, Continuing Education in Psychiatry, Department of Psychiatry; Associate Dean for Postgraduate Programs, NYU Postgraduate Medical School; Attending Psychiatrist, Tisch Hospital, New York, New York

KAPLAN & SADOCK'S

Synopsis of Psychiatry

Behavioral Sciences/Clinical Psychiatry

TENTH 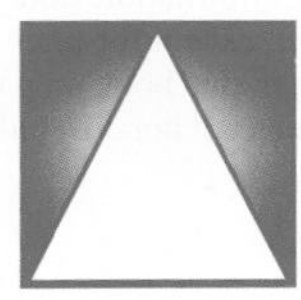 EDITION

Benjamin James Sadock, M.D.

Menas S. Gregory Professor of Psychiatry and Vice Chairman,
Department of Psychiatry, New York University School of Medicine;
Attending Psychiatrist, Tisch Hospital;
Attending Psychiatrist, Bellevue Hospital Center;
Consulting Psychiatrist, Lenox Hill Hospital,
New York, New York

Virginia Alcott Sadock, M.D.

Professor of Psychiatry, Department of Psychiatry,
New York University School of Medicine;
Attending Psychiatrist, Tisch Hospital;
Attending Psychiatrist, Bellevue Hospital Center,
New York, New York

Wolters Kluwer | Lippincott Williams & Wilkins
Health

Philadelphia • Baltimore • New York • London
Buenos Aires • Hong Kong • Sydney • Tokyo

Acquisitions Editor: Charles W. Mitchell
Managing Editor: Joyce A. Murphy
Developmental Editor: Katey Millet
Associate Director of Marketing: Adam Glazer
Production Editor: Bridgett Dougherty
Senior Manufacturing Manager: Benjamin Rivera
Design Coordinator: Stephen Druding
Compositor: Aptara, Inc.
Printer: Quebecor World-Taunton

530 Walnut Street
Philadelphia, PA 19106 USA
LWW.com

Printed in China

Previous Editions
First Edition 1972
Second Edition 1976
Third Edition 1981
Fourth Edition 1985
Fifth Edition 1988
Sixth Edition 1991
Seventh Edition 1994
Eighth Edition 1998
Ninth Edition 2003

Library of Congress Cataloging-in-Publication Data

Sadock, Benjamin J., 1933–
Kaplan & Sadock's synopsis of psychiatry : behavioral sciences/clinical psychiatry. —10th ed. / Benjamin James Sadock, Virginia Alcott Sadock.
p. ; cm.
Includes bibliographical references and index.
ISBN 978-0-7817-7327-0 (alk. paper)
1. Mental illness. 2. Psychiatry. I. Kaplan, Harold I., 1927- II. Sadock, Virginia A. III. Title. IV. Title: Kaplan and Sadock's synopsis of psychiatry. V. Title: Synopsis of psychiatry.
[DNLM: 1. Mental Disorders. WM 140 S126k 2007]
RC454.K35 2007
616.89—dc22

2007010597

---

10 9 8 7 6 5 4 3 2

Cover Illustration: *Melancholy* by Edvard Munch (1863–1943) © 2007 The Munch Museum/The Munch-Elligsen group/Artists Right Society (ARS) New York

To
Celia and Emily

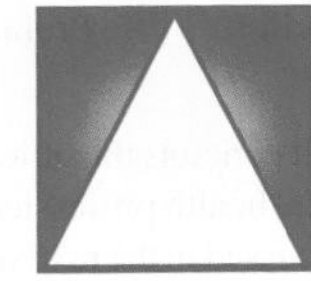

Preface

This is the tenth edition of *Kaplan & Sadock's Synopsis of Psychiatry* to appear since its founding over 35 years ago and the second edition to be published in the 21st century. Since its beginning, the goal of this book has been to foster professional competence and ensure the highest quality care to those with mental illness. An eclectic, multidisciplinary approach has been its hallmark; thus, biological, psychological, and sociological factors are equitably presented as they affect the person in health and disease. Each edition is thoroughly updated and the textbook has the reputation of being an independent, consistent, accurate, objective, and reliable compendium of new events in the field of psychiatry.

Synopsis serves the needs of diverse professional groups: psychiatrists and nonpsychiatric physicians, medical students, psychologists, social workers, psychiatric nurses, and other mental health professionals, such as occupational and art therapists, among others. *Synopsis* is also used by nonprofessionals as an authoritative guide to help them collaborate in the care of a family member or friend with mental illness. As authors and editors, we have been extremely gratified by the *Synopsis*' wide acceptance and use, both in the United States and around the world.

HISTORY

This textbook evolved from our experience editing the *Comprehensive Textbook of Psychiatry*. That book is nearly 4,000 double-column pages long, with more than 400 contributions by outstanding psychiatrists and behavioral scientists. It serves the needs of those who require an exhaustive, detailed, and encyclopedic survey of the entire field. In an effort to be as comprehensive as possible, the textbook spans two volumes to cover the material, clearly rendering it unwieldy for some groups, especially medical students, who need a brief and more condensed statement of the field of psychiatry. To accomplish this, sections of the *Comprehensive Textbook of Psychiatry* were deleted or condensed, new subjects were introduced, and all sections were brought up to date, especially certain key areas, such as psychopharmacology. We wish to acknowledge our great and obvious debt to more than 2,000 contributors to the current and previous editions of the *Comprehensive Textbook of Psychiatry*, all of whom have allowed us to synopsize their work. At the same time, we must accept responsibility for the modifications and changes in the new work.

COMPREHENSIVE TEACHING SYSTEM

The textbook forms one part of a comprehensive system developed by us to facilitate the teaching of psychiatry and the behavioral sciences. At the head of the system is the *Comprehensive Textbook of Psychiatry*, which is global in depth and scope; it is designed for and used by psychiatrists, behavioral scientists, and all workers in the mental health field. *Synopsis of Psychiatry* is a relatively brief, highly modified, and current version useful for medical students, psychiatric residents, practicing psychiatrists, and mental health professionals. A special edition of *Synopsis, Concise Textbook of Clinical Psychiatry* contains descriptions of all psychiatric disorders, including their diagnosis and treatment. It will be useful for clinical clerks and psychiatric residents who need a succinct overview of the management of clinical problems. Another part of the system, *Study Guide and Self-Examination Review of Psychiatry*, consists of multiple-choice questions and answers; it is designed for students of psychiatry and for clinical psychiatrists who require a review of the behavioral sciences and general psychiatry in preparation for a variety of examinations. The questions are modeled after and consistent with the format used by the American Board of Psychiatry and Neurology (ABPN), the National Board of Medical Examiners (NBME), and the United States Medical Licensing Examination (USMLE). Other parts of the system are the pocket handbooks: *Pocket Handbook of Clinical Psychiatry, Pocket Handbook of Psychiatric Drug Treatment, Pocket Handbook of Emergency Psychiatric Medicine,* and *Pocket Handbook of Primary Care Psychiatry*. Those books cover the diagnosis and treatment of psychiatric disorders, psychopharmacology, psychiatric emergencies, and primary care psychiatry, respectively, and are designed and written to be carried in the pocket by clinical clerks and practicing physicians, whatever their specialty, to provide a quick reference. Finally, *Comprehensive Glossary of Psychiatry and Psychology* provides simply written definitions for psychiatrists and other physicians, psychologists, students, other mental health professionals, and the general public. Together, these books create a multiple approach to the teaching, study, and learning of psychiatry.

CLASSIFICATION OF DISORDERS

DSM-IV-TR

A revision of the fourth edition of the *American Psychiatric Association Diagnostic and Statistical Manual of Mental Disorders* (DSM-IV), called DSM-IV-TR (TR stands for text revision), was published in 2000.

It contains the official nomenclature used by psychiatrists and other mental health professionals in the United States; the psychiatric disorders discussed in the textbook are consistent with and follow that nosology. Every section dealing with clinical disorders has been updated thoroughly and completely to include the revisions contained in DSM-IV-TR.

ICD-10

Synopsis was the first U.S. textbook to include the definitions and diagnostic criteria of mental disorders used in the tenth revision of the World Health Organization's *International Statistical Classification of Diseases and Related Health Problems* (ICD-10). There are textual differences between DSM and ICD, but according to treaties between the United States and the World Health Organization, the diagnostic code numbers must be identical to ensure uniform reporting of national and international psychiatric statistics. Currently, both DSM and ICD diagnoses and numerical codes are accepted by Medicare, Medicaid, and private insurance companies for reimbursement purposes in the United States. Readers can find the DSM-IV-TR classification with the equivalent ICD-10 classification listed in Chapter 9. Color cues differentiate DSM and ICD diagnostic tables as a further aid to the reader.

COVER ART AND ILLUSTRATIONS

Synopsis was one of the first modern psychiatric textbooks to use art and photographs to illustrate psychiatric subjects to enrich the learning experience.

The cover art is entitled *Melancholy* by the Norwegian artist, Edvard Munch (1863–1943). In this painting, the limp female figure with her hidden face is stooped over and unable to raise her eyes to view the beautiful landscape of the fjords which normally lighten the mood of those who gaze on them. To Munch, the inability to obtain pleasure coupled with withdrawal and introversion were the hallmarks of melancholic depression.

Color plates of all psychiatric drugs and their dosage forms, including all new drugs developed since the last edition was published, are also included, as in all *Kaplan & Sadock* books. New illustrations and color plates have been added to many sections.

CASE HISTORIES

Case histories, which make clinical disorders more vital for the student, are an integral part of *Synopsis.* All cases in this edition are new, derived from various sources: ICD-10 *Casebook, DSM-IV-TR Casebook, DSM-IV-TR Case Studies*, contributors to the *Comprehensive Textbook of Psychiatry*, and the authors' clinical experience at New York's Bellevue Hospital Center. We especially wish to thank the American Psychiatric Press and the World Health Organization for permission to use many of their cases. Cases appear in tinted type to help the reader find them easily.

NEW AND UPDATED SECTIONS

Chapter 1, *The Patient-Doctor Relationship*, has been rewritten to reflect new concepts in the complex relationship between the doctor and his or her patient. A discussion of the "narrative"—the story the patient tells—and its effect on that interaction is also included. Chapter 2 has been expanded to include a comprehensive survey of normality. Aging is covered in a new section that considers the process not as a disease but as an evolving part of the life cycle and includes a thorough survey of normal aging.

Chapter 3, *The Brain and Behavior*, has been reorganized, revised, updated, and extensively rewritten. The section, *Functional Neuroanatomy*, emphasizes the influence of function rather than structure on behavior. The sections, *Psychoneuroendocrinology,* and *Psychneuroimmunology and Chronobiology*, have been expanded to reflect the rapid advances in these fields. A newly written section, *Neurogenetics*, details the important and complex role of genetics in both normal and abnormal behavior.

The chapter *End-of-Life Care and Palliative Medicine* has been updated and reflects the important role that psychiatrists play in the clinical specialty of palliative care and pain control. Too little time—especially in medical school—is provided in training students to care for the dying patient with sensitivity and compassion. The chapter, *Psychiatry and Reproductive Medicine*, was extensively revised both to keep pace with advances in women's health issues and to clarify the confusion surrounding antepartum and postpartum events, contraception, abortion, and the role of hormone replacement therapy in women's mental health.

The chapter *Ethics in Psychiatry* was completely revised and updated and includes an extensive discussion of the role of euthanasia and physician-assisted suicide and their impact on the practice of medicine.

The section *Mental Disorders Due to a General Medical Condition* contains an updated discussion of prion disorders and "mad cow disease." In the last edition, the section *Posttraumatic Stress Disorder and Acute Stress Disorder* covered the tragic events of September 11, 2001, involving the World Trade Center in New York and the Pentagon in Washington. With the passage of time, we are now able to provide reliable data on the psychological sequelae of those events. Other disasters, however, have occurred since then, such as hurricane Katrina and the Pakistan earthquake in 2005. The psychological effects of those events are also covered. Two chapters, *Anthropology and Cross-Cultural Psychiatry*, and *Cross-Cultural Syndromes*, reflect the global scope of psychiatry and the need for clinicians to understand disorders that appear around the world. A new section called *Brain Stimulation Methods* describes many new advances in stimulating the brain in an effort to restore health to those patients who have not responded to conventional therapies and who are among the most severely mentally ill.

The sections on psychotherapy have been expanded with new, separate, and up-to-date discussions on *genetic counseling*, *cognitive therapy*, *interpersonal therapy*, *hypnosis*, and *dialectical behavior therapy.*

This edition continues the tradition of speaking out on sociopolitical issues that affect the delivery of health care. Practitioners have a special obligation to know about such issues that inform the physical and psychological well-being of their patients. Thus, discussions are included on the homeless mentally ill, deinstitutionalization, working conditions and number of hours medical house staff are on duty, the role of managed care in medicine and psychiatry, and the regulation of medicine by government agencies, among other areas of controversy.

Finally, every section on clinical psychiatry has been updated to include the latest information about diagnosing and treating mental disorders. The references are also completely up-to-date.

PSYCHOPHARMACOLOGY

The authors are committed to classifying drugs used to treat mental disorders according to their pharmacological activity and mechanism of action rather than using such broad categories as antidepressants, antipsychotics, anxiolytics, and mood stabilizers, which are overly broad and do not reflect, scientifically, the clinical use of psychotropic medication. For example, many antidepressant drugs are used to treat anxiety disorders; some anxiolytics are used to treat depression and bipolar disorders; and drugs from all categories are used to treat other clinical problems, such as eating disorders, panic disorders, and impulse-control disorders. Many drugs are also used to treat a variety of mental disorders that do not fit into any broad classification. Information about all pharmacological agents used in psychiatry, including pharmacodynamics, pharmacokinetics, dosages, adverse effects, and drug–drug interactions, was thoroughly updated and includes all drugs approved since publication of the previous edition.

CHILDHOOD DISORDERS

The chapters, *Adolescent Substance Abuse* and *Forensic Issues in Child Psychiatry*, were revised and expanded to reflect the epidemic of illicit drug use among youth and the problems of violence and delinquency. Data about posttraumatic stress disorders in children have been added, including the latest data on the psychological effects on children exposed to terrorist activities and natural disasters. The section *Anxiety Disorders* was reorganized and updated thoroughly. Every clinical disorder section was updated and revised, especially those that deal with the use of pharmacological agents in children.

ACKNOWLEDGMENTS

We deeply appreciate the work of our distinguished group of contributing editors, who gave generously of their time and expertise. Caroly Pataki, M.D., was responsible for updating and revising the section on childhood and adolescent disorders. We thank her for her tremendous help in this area. Norman Sussman, M.D., updated the section on psychopharmacology, enabling us to provide the reader with the current material in this ever-changing and rapidly expanding field. We thank Jack Grebb, M.D., who guided us in the neural sciences and who was coauthor of the seventh edition of *Synopsis*. He has an encyclopedic knowledge of the field from which we benefited immensely. We thank Dorice Viera, Associate Curator of the Frederick L. Ehrman Medical Library at the New York University School of Medicine, for her valuable assistance in the preparation of this and previous editions in which she was so very helpful.

Nitza Jones played a key and invaluable role as Project Editor, as she has for many of our other books. Her vast knowledge of every aspect of book publishing was indispensable and she contributed heavily to editing the text. She was ably assisted by Regina Furner who also performed an invaluable service as Picture Editor. Both worked with enthusiasm, alacrity, and intelligence. Among the many others to thank are René Robinson, M.D., Caroline Press, M.D., Michael Stanger, M.D., Rajan Bahl, M.D., Samoon Ahmad, M.D., and Jay K. Kantor, Ph.D., all of whom contributed to the text. Seeba Anam, M.D., deserves special mention for her help in the section on *Reproductive Psychiatry*.

We also wish to acknowledge the contributions of James Sadock, M.D., and Victoria Gregg, M.D., for their help in their areas of expertise: emergency adult and emergency pediatric medicine, respectively.

We want to take this opportunity to acknowledge those who have translated this and other *Kaplan & Sadock* books into foreign languages, including Chinese, Croation, French, German, Greek, Indonesian, Italian, Japanese, Polish, Portuguese, Romanian, Russian, Spanish, and Turkish, in addition to a special Asian and international student edition.

The staff at Lippincott Williams & Wilkins was most efficient. We wish to thank Katey Millet for her prodigious efforts. We have been fortunate to have worked with her for many years on many projects and her help and support have been invaluable. Bridgett Dougherty at LW&W and Judi Rohrbaugh and Chris Miller at Aptara also deserve our thanks. Joyce Murphy, Managing Editor, and Charley Mitchell, Executive Editor, have been loyal friends over the years and their help and enthusiasm for our projects have been most welcome.

We especially want to acknowledge and thank Alan and Marilyn Zublatt for their generous support of this and other *Kaplan & Sadock* textbooks. Over the years they have been unselfish benefactors to many educational, clinical and research projects at the NYU Medical Center. We are deeply grateful for their help. We thank them not only for ourselves but on behalf of all those at NYU—students, clinicians, and researchers—who have benefited from their extraordinary humanitarian vision.

Finally, we want to express our deep thanks to Robert Cancro, M.D., who retired after 28 years serving as Chairman of Psychiatry at New York University School of Medicine and who gave us his full support. He was succeeded as Chair in 2006 by Dolores Malaspina, M.D., to whom we extend a warm welcome as she leads the Department of Psychiatry at NYU into the 21st century.

B.J.S.
V.A.S.
New York University School of Medicine
New York, New York

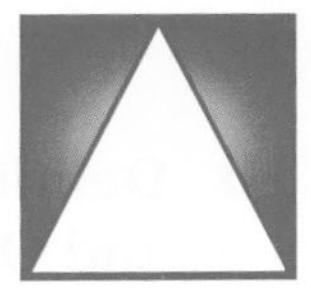

Contents

1

The Patient–Doctor Relationship

The quality of patient–doctor or patient–therapist relationship is crucial to the practice of medicine and psychiatry. The capacity to develop an effective relationship requires a solid appreciation of the complexities of human behavior and a rigorous education in the techniques of talking and listening to people. To diagnose, manage, and treat an ill person, doctors and therapists must learn to listen. They need the skills of active listening, which means listening both to what they and the patient are saying and to the undercurrents of the unspoken feelings between them (Fig. 1–1). A physician who monitors both the content of the interaction (what the patient and the doctor *actually* say) and the process (what the patient or the doctor *mean* to say) realizes that communication between two people occurs on several levels at once: what the person believes about himself or herself; what he or she wants others to believe about them; and finally who the person really is.

An effective relationship is characterized by good rapport. Rapport is the spontaneous, conscious feeling of harmonious responsiveness that promotes the development of a constructive therapeutic alliance. It implies an understanding and trust between the doctor and the patient. Frequently, the doctor is the only person to whom the patients can talk about things that they cannot tell anyone else. Most patients trust their doctors to keep secrets, and this confidence must not be betrayed. Patients who feel that someone knows them, understands them, and accepts them find that a source of strength. In his essay, "Caring for the Patient" Francis Peabody, M.D. (1881–1927), a talented teacher and clinician (Fig. 1–2), wrote:

> The good physician knows his patients through and through, and his knowledge is bought dearly. Time, sympathy, and understanding must be lavishly dispensed, but the reward is to be found in that personal bond which forms the greatest satisfaction of the practice of medicine. One of the essential qualities of the clinician is interest in humanity, for the secret of the care of the patient is in caring for the patient.

Establishing Rapport

Ekkehard Othmer and Sieglinde Othmer defined the development of rapport as encompassing six strategies: (1) putting patients and interviewers at ease; (2) finding patients' pain and expressing compassion; (3) evaluating patients' insight and becoming an ally; (4) showing expertise; (5) establishing authority as physicians and therapists; and (6) balancing the roles of empathic listener, expert, and authority. As part of a strategy for increasing rapport, they developed a checklist (Table 1–1) that enables interviewers to recognize problems and refine their skills in establishing rapport.

In one survey of 700 patients, patients substantially agreed that many physicians do not have the time or inclination to listen and consider their feelings, that physicians do not have enough knowledge of the emotional problems and socioeconomic background of their families, and that physicians increase their fear by giving explanations in technical language.

Evaluating the pressures in patients' early lives helps psychiatrists better understand patients. Emotional reactions, healthy or unhealthy, are the result of a constant interplay of biological, sociological, and psychological forces. Each stress leaves behind a trace of its influence and continues to manifest itself throughout life in proportion to the intensity of its effects and the susceptibility of the human being involved. Past and current stresses should be determined to the fullest extent possible.

Empathy. Empathy is a way of increasing rapport. It is an essential characteristic of psychiatrists, but it is not a universal human capacity. An incapacity for normal understanding of what other people are feeling appears to be central to certain personality disturbances, such as antisocial and narcissistic personality disorders. Although empathy probably cannot be created, it can be focused and deepened through training, observation, and self-reflection. It manifests in clinical work in a variety of ways. An empathic psychiatrist may anticipate what is felt before it is spoken and can often help patients articulate what they are feeling. Nonverbal cues, such as body posture and facial expression, are noted. Patients' reactions to the psychiatrist can be understood and clarified.

Patients sometimes say, "How can you understand me if you haven't gone through what I'm going through?" Clinical psychiatry, however, is predicated on the belief that it is not necessary to have other people's literal experiences to understand them. The shared experience of being human is often sufficient. Whether in an initial diagnostic setting or in ongoing therapy, patients draw comfort from knowing that psychiatrists are not mystified by their suffering.

Transference. *Transference* is generally defined as the set of expectations, beliefs, and emotional responses that a patient brings to the patient–doctor relationship. They are based not necessarily on who the doctor is or how the doctor acts in reality but, rather, on repeated experiences the patient has had with other important authority figures throughout life.

TRANSFERENTIAL ATTITUDES. The patient's attitude toward the physician is apt to be a repetition of the attitude he or she has had toward authority figures. The patient's attitude can range from one of realistic basic trust, with an expectation that the doctor has

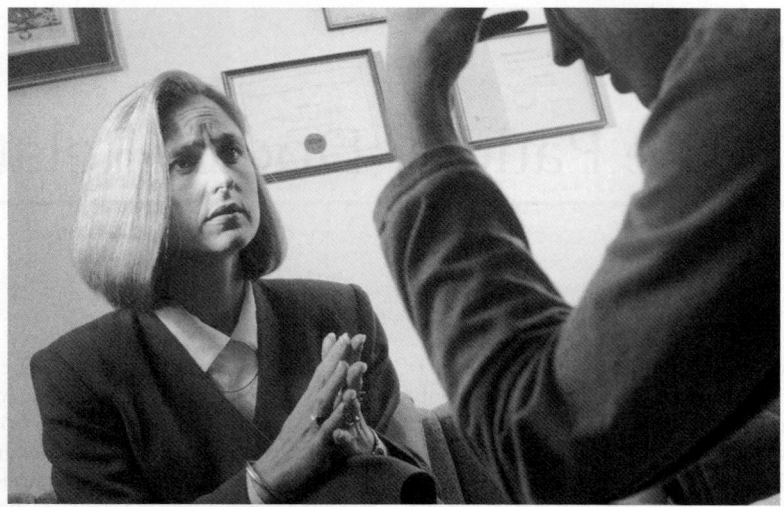

FIGURE 1–1
The active listening described in the text is illustrated by the therapist's expression of concern for what the patient is experiencing. The psychiatrist Harry Stack Sullivan referred to the therapist as a participant observer in the patient's life. (Courtesy of Corbis).

the patient's best interest at heart, through one of overidealization and even eroticized fantasy to one of basic mistrust, with an expectation that the doctor will be contemptuous and potentially abusive.

ROLE OF THE PSYCHIATRIST VERSUS THE NONPSYCHIATRIC PHYSICIAN. In many respects, the role of a psychiatrist differs from that of a nonpsychiatric physician, yet many patients expect

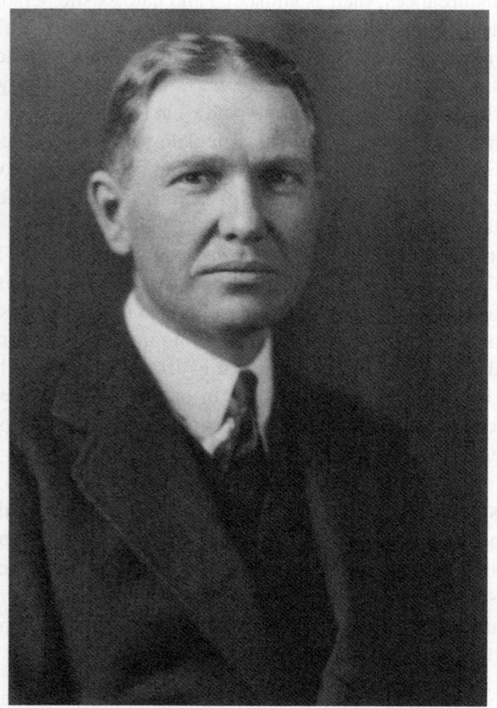

FIGURE 1–2
Francis W. Peabody, M.D. (1881–1927). (Courtesy of the National Library of Medicine.)

the same from the psychiatrist as they do from other physicians. If they expect a doctor to take action, give advice, and prescribe medication to cure an illness, they may well expect the same interaction with a psychiatrist and be disappointed or angry if it does not occur. Transferential reactions can be strongest with psychiatrists for a number of reasons. For example, in intensive insight-oriented psychotherapy the encouragement of transference feelings is an integral part of treatment. In some types of therapy, a psychiatrist is more or less neutral. The more neutral or less known the psychiatrist is, the more a patient's transferential fantasies and concerns are mobilized and projected onto the doctor. Once the fantasies are stimulated and projected, the psychiatrist can help patients gain insight into how those fantasies and concerns affect all the important relationships in their lives. Although a nonpsychiatrist does not use or even need to understand transference attitudes in that intensive way, a solid understanding of the power and the manifestations of transference is necessary for optimal treatment results in any patient–doctor relationship.

The doctor's words and deeds have a power far beyond the commonplace because of his or her unique authority and the patient's dependence on the doctor. How a particular physician behaves has a direct bearing on the patient's emotional and even physical reactions.

One patient repeatedly had high blood pressure readings when examined by a physician he considered cold, aloof, and stern. He had normal blood pressure readings, however, when seen by a doctor he regarded as warm, understanding, and sympathetic.

Countertransference. Just as the patient brings transferential attitudes to the patient–doctor relationship, doctors themselves often have countertransferential reactions to their patients. Countertransference can take the form of negative feelings that are disruptive to the patient–doctor relationship, but it can also encompass disproportionately positive, idealizing, or even eroticized reactions to patients. Just as patients have expectations for physicians—for example, competence, lack of exploitation,

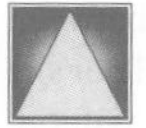

Table 1–1
Checklist for Clinicians

The following checklist allows clinicians to rate their skills in establishing and maintaining rapport. It helps them detect and eliminate weaknesses in interviews that failed in some significant way. Each item is rated "yes," "no," or "not applicable."

	Yes	No	N/A
1. I put the patient at ease.	—	—	—
2. I recognized the patient's state of mind.	—	—	—
3. I addressed the patient's distress.	—	—	—
4. I helped the patient warm up.	—	—	—
5. I helped the patient overcome suspiciousness.	—	—	—
6. I curbed the patient's intrusiveness.	—	—	—
7. I stimulated the patient's verbal production.	—	—	—
8. I curbed the patient's rambling.	—	—	—
9. I understood the patient's suffering.	—	—	—
10. I expressed empathy for the patient's suffering.	—	—	—
11. I tuned in on the patient's affect.	—	—	—
12. I addressed the patient's affect.	—	—	—
13. I became aware of the patient's level of insight.	—	—	—
14. I assumed the patient's view of the disorder.	—	—	—
15. I had a clear perception of the overt and the therapeutic goals of treatment.	—	—	—
16. I stated the overt goal of treatment to the patient.	—	—	—
17. I communicated to the patient that I am familiar with the illness.	—	—	—
18. My questions convinced the patient that I am familiar with the symptoms of the disorder.	—	—	—
19. I let the patient know that he or she is not alone with the illness.	—	—	—
20. I expressed my intent to help the patient.	—	—	—
21. The patient recognized my expertise.	—	—	—
22. The patient respected my authority.	—	—	—
23. The patient appeared fully cooperative.	—	—	—
24. I recognized the patient's attitude toward the illness.	—	—	—
25. The patient viewed the illness with distance.	—	—	—
26. The patient presented as a sympathy-craving sufferer.	—	—	—
27. The patient presented as a very important patient.	—	—	—
28. The patient competed with me for authority.	—	—	—
29. The patient was submissive.	—	—	—
30. I adjusted my role to the patient's role.	—	—	—
31. The patient thanked me and made another appointment.	—	—	—

Reprinted with permission from Othmer E, Othmer SC. *The Clinical Interview Using DSM-IV.* Washington, DC: American Psychiatric Press; 1994.

objectivity, comfort, and relief—physicians often have unconscious or unspoken expectations of patients. Most commonly, patients are thought of as good patients if their expressed severity of symptoms correlates with an overtly diagnosable biological disorder, if they are compliant with treatment, if they are emotionally controlled, and if they are grateful. If those expectations are not met, the patient may be disapproved of and experienced as unlikable, unworkable, or bad.

DISLIKING A PATIENT. A physician who actively dislikes a patient is apt to be ineffective in dealing with him or her. Emotion breeds counteremotion. For example, if the physician is hostile, the patient becomes hostile; the physician then becomes even angrier than before, and the relationship deteriorates rapidly. If the physician can rise above such emotions and handle a difficult patient with equanimity, the interpersonal relationship may shift from one of mutual overt antagonism to one of at least increased acceptance and grudging respect. Rising above such emotions involves being able to step back from the intense countertransferential reactions and dispassionately explore why the patient is reacting to the doctor in such an apparently self-defeating way. The patient needs the doctor, and hostility ensures that the needed help will occur in a less effective context. If the doctor can understand that the patient's antagonism is in some ways defensive or self-protective and most likely reflects transferential fears of disrespect, abuse, and disappointment, the doctor may be less angry and more empathic than otherwise.

Doctors who have strong unconscious needs to be all-knowing and all-powerful may have particular problems with certain types of patients. These patients may be difficult for most physicians to handle, but—if the physician is as aware as possible of his or her own needs, capabilities, and limitations—the patients will not be threatening. Such patients include the following: those who repeatedly appear to defeat attempts to help themselves (for example, patients with severe heart disease who continue to smoke or drink); those who are perceived as uncooperative (for example, patients who question or refuse treatment); those who request a second opinion; those who fail to recover in response to treatment; those who use physical or somatic complaints to mask emotional problems (for example, patients with somatization disorder, pain disorder, hypochondriasis, or factitious disorders); those with chronic cognitive disorders (for example, patients with dementia of the Alzheimer's type); and patients who represent a professional failure and, thus, are a threat to the physician's identity and self-esteem (for example, those who are dying or in chronic pain).

SEXUALITY AND THE PHYSICIAN. Physicians are bound to like some patients more than others. However, if the physician feels a strong attraction to a patient and is tempted to act on the attraction, stepping back and assessing the situation are essential. In some medical specialties in which the patient–doctor relationship is not particularly intimate or intense, the prohibition against romantic involvement with patients may not be strong.

In other specialties, however, especially psychiatry, the ethical and even legal prohibition is important. The doctor is a powerful figure in the United States culture and may trigger many unconscious fantasies of being rescued, taken care of, and loved. Doctors themselves may have their own unconscious fantasies of being and needing to be all-powerful, rescuing, and loving. Those fantasies are inherently unrealistic and are inevitably disappointed. The disappointments, if realized in a romantic relationship between the doctor and the patient, can be destructive, especially for the patient. Patient–therapist sex is discussed further in Chapter 59.

Another aspect of sexuality as it pertains to countertransference issues relates to asking patients about sexual issues and obtaining a sexual history. A reluctance to do so may reflect the physician's own anxiety about sexuality or even an unconscious attraction toward the patient. Moreover, the omission of those questions generally tells patients that the doctor is uncomfortable with the subject, thus leading to an inhibition about discussing any number of other sensitive subjects.

SELF-MONITORING OF COUNTERTRANSFERENCE FEELINGS. Countertransference feelings do not always have to be perceived in negative terms. They also have the potential, if recognized and analyzed, to help the doctor better understand the patient who has stimulated the feelings. For instance, if a doctor feels bored and restless when with a particular patient and has ascertained that the boredom is not secondary to his or her own preoccupations, the doctor may surmise that the patient is speaking about trivial or insignificant concerns to avoid real and potentially disturbing concerns.

PHYSICIANS AS PATIENTS. A special example of countertransference issues occurs when the patient being treated is a physician. Problems that can arise in that situation include an expectation that the physician-patient will take care of his or her own medications and treatment and the treating physician's fear of criticism of his or her skills or competence. Physicians are notoriously poor patients, most likely because physicians are trained to be in control of medical situations and to be the masters of the patient–doctor relationship. For a physician, being a patient may mean giving up control, becoming dependent, and appearing vulnerable and frightened—behaviors that most physicians are professionally trained to suppress. Physician-patients may be reluctant to become what they perceive as burdens to overworked colleagues, or they may be embarrassed to ask pertinent questions for fear of appearing ignorant or incompetent. Physician-patients may stimulate fear in the treating physicians who see themselves in the patient, an attitude that can lead to denial and avoidance on the part of the treating physician.

MODELS OF INTERACTION BETWEEN DOCTOR AND PATIENT

The interactions between a doctor and patient—the questions a patient asks, the way in which news is conveyed and treatment recommendations are made—can take different shapes. It is helpful in thinking about the relationship to formulate "models" of interaction. These are fluid concepts, however. A talented, sensitive physician will have different approaches with different patients and indeed may have different approaches with the same patient as time and medical circumstances vary.

1. *The paternalistic model.* In a paternalistic relationship between the doctor and patient, it is assumed that the doctor knows best. He or she will prescribe treatment, and the patient is expected to comply without questioning. Moreover, the doctor may decide to withhold information when it is believed to be in the patient's best interests. In this model, also called the "autocratic model," the physician asks most of the questions and generally dominates the interview.

Circumstances arise in which a paternalistic approach is desirable. In emergency situations the doctor needs to take control and make potentially life-saving decisions without long deliberation. In addition, some patients feel overwhelmed by their illness and are comforted by a doctor who can take charge. In general, however, the paternalistic approach risks a clash of values. A paternalistic obstetrician, for example, might insist on spinal anesthesia for delivery when the patient wants to experience natural childbirth.

2. *The informative model.* The doctor in this model dispenses information. All available data are freely given, but the choice is left wholly up to the patient. For example, doctors may quote 5-year survival statistics for various treatments of breast cancer and expect women to make up their own minds without suggestion or interference from them. This model may be appropriate for certain one-time consultations where no established relationship exists and the patient will be returning to the regular care of a known physician. At other times, the informative model places the patient in an unrealistically autonomous role and leaves him or her feeling the doctor is cold and uncaring.

3. *The interpretive model.* Doctors who have come to know their patients better and understand something of the circumstances of their lives, their families, their values, and their hopes and aspirations, are better able to make recommendations that take into account the unique characteristics of an individual patient. A sense of shared decision-making is established as the doctor presents and discusses alternatives, with the patient's participation, to find the one that is best for that particular person. The doctor in this model does not abrogate the responsibility for making decisions, but is flexible, and is willing to consider question and alternative suggestions.

4. *The deliberative model.* The physician in this model acts as a friend or counselor to the patient, not just by presenting information, but in actively advocating a particular course of action. The deliberative approach is commonly used by doctors hoping to modify injurious behavior, for example, in trying to get their patients to stop smoking or lose weight.

These models are only guides for thinking about the doctor–patient relationship. One is not intrinsically superior to any other, and a physician may use all four approaches with a patient during a single visit. Difficulties are most likely to arise not from the use of one or another of the models, but with the physician who is rigidly fixed in one approach and cannot switch strategies, even when indicated and desirable. The models do not, moreover, describe the presence or absence of interpersonal warmth. It is entirely possible for patients to see a paternalistic or autocratic physician as personable, caring, and concerned. In fact, a common image of the small town or country doctor in the early part of the 20th century was a man (seldom a woman) totally committed to the welfare of his patients, who would come in the middle of the night and sit at the bedside holding the patient's hand, who would be invited to Sunday dinner, and who expected his instructions to be followed exactly and without question.

ILLNESS BEHAVIOR

The term *illness behavior* describes patients' reactions to the experience of being sick. Aspects of illness behavior have sometimes been termed the *sick role*, the role that society ascribes to people when they are ill. The sick role can include being excused from responsibilities and the expectation of wanting to

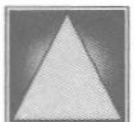

Table 1–2
Assessment of Individual Illness Behavior

Prior illness episodes, especially illnesses of standard severity (childbirth, renal stones, surgery)
Cultural degree of stoicism
Cultural beliefs concerning the specific problem
Personal meaning of or beliefs about the specific problem
Particular questions to ask to elicit the patient's explanatory model:

1. What do you call your problem? What name does it have?
2. What do you think caused your problem?
3. Why do you think it started when it did?
4. What does your sickness do to you?
5. What do you fear most about your sickness?
6. What are the chief problems that your sickness has caused you?
7. What are the most important results you hope to receive from treatment?
8. What have you done so far to treat your illness?

Courtesy of Mack Lipkin, Jr., M.D.

obtain help to get well. Illness behavior and the sick role are affected by people's previous experiences with illness and by their cultural beliefs about disease. The influence of culture on reporting and manifestation of symptoms must be evaluated. For some disorders, this varies little among cultures, whereas for others, the cultural mores may strongly shape the way the patient presents the condition. The relation of illness to family processes, class status, and ethnic identity is also important. The attitudes of peoples and cultures about dependency and helplessness greatly influence whether and how a person asks for help, as do such psychological factors as personality type and the personal meaning the person attributes to being ill. Some people experience illness as overwhelming loss; others see in the same illness a challenge they must overcome or a punishment they deserve. Table 1–2 lists essential areas to be addressed in assessing illness behavior and helpful questions for making the assessment.

Psychiatric versus Medical-Surgical Interviews. Mack Lipkin, Jr., described three functions of medical interviews: to assess the nature of the problem, to develop and maintain a therapeutic relationship, and to communicate information and implement a treatment plan (Table 1–3). These functions are exactly the same in psychiatric and surgical interviews. Also universal are the predominant coping mechanisms used in illness, both adaptive and maladaptive. These mechanisms include such reactions as anxiety, depression, regression, denial, anger, and dependency (Table 1–4). Physicians must anticipate, recognize, and address such reactions if treatment and intervention are to be effective.

Psychiatric interviews have two major technical goals: (1) recognition of the psychological determinants of behavior and (2) symptom classification. These goals are reflected in two styles of interviewing: the insight-oriented, or psychodynamic, style and the symptom-oriented, or descriptive, style. *Insight-oriented* interviewing attempts to elicit unconscious conflicts, anxieties, and defenses. The *symptom-oriented* approach emphasizes the classification of patients' complaints and dysfunctions as defined by specific diagnostic categories. The approaches are not mutually exclusive and, in fact, can be compatible. A diagnosis can be described as precisely as possible by eliciting such details as symptoms, course of illness, and family history and by understanding a patient's personality, developmental history, and unconscious conflicts.

Psychiatric patients often contend with stresses and pressures that differ from those of patients who do not have a psychiatric disorder. These stresses include the stigma attached to being a psychiatric patient (it is more acceptable to have a medical or surgical problem than a mental problem); communication difficulty because of disorders of thinking; oddities of behavior; and impairments of insight and judgment that might make compliance with treatment difficult. Because psychiatric patients often find it difficult to describe fully what is going on in their lives, physicians must be prepared to obtain information from other sources. Family members, friends, and spouses can provide critical data such as previous psychiatric history, responses to medication, and precipitating stresses that patients may not be able to describe themselves.

Psychiatric patients may not be able to tolerate a traditional interview format, especially in the acute stages of a disorder. For instance, a patient who has increased agitation or depression may not be able to sit for 30 to 45 minutes of discussion or questioning. In such cases, physicians must be prepared to conduct multiple brief interactions over time, for as long as the patient is able, stopping and returning when the patient appears able to tolerate more.

Studies show that about 60 percent of all patients with mental disorders visit a nonpsychiatric physician during any 6-month period and that patients with mental disorders are twice as likely to visit a primary care physician as are other patients. Nonpsychiatric physicians should be knowledgeable about the special problems of psychiatric patients and the specific techniques used to treat them.

Biopsychosocial Model

In 1977, George Engel at the University of Rochester, published a seminal paper that described the biopsychosocial model of disease, which stressed an integrated systems approach to human behavior and disease. The biopsychosocial model is derived from general systems theory. The *biological system* emphasizes the anatomical, structural, and molecular substrate of disease and its effects on the patient's biological functioning; the *psychological system* emphasizes the effects of psychodynamic factors, motivation, and personality on the experience of illness and the reaction to it; and the *social system* emphasizes cultural, environmental, and familial influences on the expression and the experience of illness. Engel postulated that each system affects, and is affected by, every other system. Engel's model does not assert that medical illness is a direct result of a person's psychological or sociocultural makeup but, rather, encourages a comprehensive understanding of disease and treatment.

A dramatic example of Engel's conception of the biopsychosocial model was a 1971 study of the relation between sudden death and psychological factors. After investigating 170 sudden deaths over about 6 years, he observed that serious illness or even death can be associated with psychological stress or trauma. Among the potential triggering events Engel listed are the following: the death of a close friend, grief, anniversary reactions, loss of self-esteem, personal danger or threat and the letdown after the threat has passed, and reunion or triumphs.

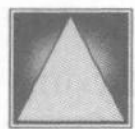

Table 1–3
Three Functions of the Medical Interview

Functions	Objectives	Skills
I. Determining the nature of the problem	1. To enable the clinician to establish a diagnosis or recommend further diagnostic procedures, suggest a course of treatment, and predict the nature of the illness	1. Knowledge base of diseases, disorders, problems, and clinical hypotheses from multiple conceptual domains: biomedical, sociocultural, psychodynamic, and behavioral 2. Ability to elicit data for the above conceptual domains (encouraging the patient to tell his or her story: organizing the flow of the interview, the form of questions, the characterization of symptoms, the mental status examination) 3. Ability to perceive data from multiple sources (history, mental status examination, physician's subjective response to the patient, nonverbal cues, listening at multiple levels) 4. Hypothesis generation and testing 5. Developing a therapeutic relationship (function II)
II. Developing and maintaining a therapeutic relationship	1. The patient's willingness to provide diagnostic information 2. Relief of physical and psychological distress 3. Willingness to accept a treatment plan or a process of negotiation 4. Patient satisfaction 5. Physician satisfaction	1. Defining the nature of the relationship 2. Allowing the patient to tell his or her story 3. Hearing, bearing, and tolerating the patient's expression of painful feelings 4. Appropriate and genuine interest, empathy, support, and cognitive understanding 5. Attending to common patient concerns over embarrassment, shame, and humiliation 6. Eliciting the patient's perspective 7. Determining the nature of the problem 8. Communicating information and recommending treatment (function III)
III. Communicating information and implementing a treatment plan	1. Patient's understanding of the illness 2. Patient's understanding of the suggested diagnostic procedures 3. Patient's understanding of the treatment possibilities 4. Consensus between physician and patient about the above items 1 to 3 5. Informed consent 6. Improve coping mechanisms 7. Lifestyle changes	1. Determining the nature of the problem (function I) 2. Developing a therapeutic relationship (function II) 3. Establishing the differences in perspective between physician and patient 4. Educational strategies 5. Clinical negotiations for conflict resolution

Reprinted with permission from Lazare A, Bird J, Lipkin M Jr, Putnam S. Three functions of the medical interview: An integrative conceptual framework. In: Lipkin Jr M, Putnam S, Lazare A, eds. *The Medical Interview.* New York: Springer; 1989:103.

The patient–doctor relationship is a critical component of the biopsychosocial model. Physicians must have both a working knowledge of the patient's medical status and be familiar with how the patient's individual psychology and sociocultural milieu affect the medical condition.

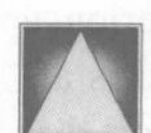

Table 1–4
Predictable Reactions to Illness

Intrapsychic	Clinical
Lowered self image → loss → grief	Anxiety or depression
Threat to homeostasis → fear	Denial or anxiety
Failure of (self) care → helplessness, hopelessness	Depression
	Bargaining and blaming
Sense of loss of control → shame (guilt)	Regression
	Isolation
	Dependency
	Anger
	Acceptance

Courtesy of Mack Lipkin, Jr, M.D.

Spirituality

The role of spirituality and religion in sickness and health has gained ascendancy in recent years, with some suggesting that it become part of the biopsychosocial model. Some evidence suggests that strong religious beliefs, spiritual yearnings, prayer, and devotional acts have positive influences on a person's mental and physical health. These issues are better attended to by theologians than by physicians; however, doctors need to be aware of spirituality in their patients' lives and sensitive to their patients' religious beliefs. In some instances, beliefs can impede medical care, such as the refusal of some religious groups to accept blood transfusions. In most cases, however, when treating patients with strong religious beliefs, the wise physician will welcome the collaboration of the pastoral counselor.

INTERVIEWING EFFECTIVELY

One of the physician's most important tools is the ability to interview effectively. Through a skilled interview, physicians can gather the data necessary to understand and treat patients and, in the process, to increase patients' understanding of, and compliance with, the physicians' advice.

Many factors influence both the content and the process of interviews. Patients' personalities and character styles significantly influence reactions as well as the emotional context in which interviews unfold. Various clinical situations—including whether patients are seen on a general hospital ward, on a psychiatric ward, in an emergency room, or as outpatients—shape the questions asked and the recommendations offered. Technical factors such as telephone interruptions, the use of an interpreter, note taking, and the patient's illness itself—whether in an acute stage or in remission—influence the content and process of the interview. Interviewers' styles, experiences, and theoretical orientations also have a significant impact. Even the timing of interjections such as "uh huh" can influence when patients speak and what they do or do not say as they unconsciously try to follow the subtle leads and cues provided by the doctor.

Beginning the Interview

How a physician begins an interview provides a powerful first impression to patients, which can affect the way the remainder of the interview proceeds. Patients are often anxious on first encounters with physicians and feel both vulnerable and intimidated. A physician who can establish rapport quickly, put the patient at ease, and show respect is well on the way to conducting a productive exchange of information. This exchange is critical to making a correct diagnosis and to establishing treatment goals.

Physicians should initially make sure that they know a patient's name and that the patient knows the physician's name. Physicians should introduce themselves to other people who have come with the patient and should find out if the patient wants another person present during the initial interview. The request for the presence of another person should be granted, but the physician should also attempt to speak with patients privately to determine if there is anything that they want the doctor to know but would be reluctant to say in front of someone else.

Patients have a right to know the position and professional status of persons involved in their care. For example, medical students should introduce themselves as such and not as doctors, and physicians should make it clear whether they are consultants (called in by another physician to see the patient), are covering for another physician, or are involved in the interview to teach students rather than to treat the patient.

After the introductions and other initial assessments have been made, useful and appropriate opening remarks are as follows: "Can you tell me about the troubles that bring you in today?" or "Tell me about the problems you have been having." Following up with a second one such as "What other problems have you been experiencing?" often elicits information that patients were reluctant to give initially. It also indicates to the patient that the doctor is interested in hearing as much as a patient wants to say.

A less directive approach is to ask a patient "Where shall we start?" or "Where would you prefer to begin?" If a patient has been referred by another doctor for consultation, the initial remarks can indicate that the consulting doctor already knows something about the patient. For instance, the consulting doctor might say, "Your doctor has told me something about what has been troubling you but I'd like to hear from you in your own words what you've been experiencing."

Most patients do not speak freely unless they have privacy and are sure that their conversations cannot be overheard. Physicians who have attended to such factors as privacy, quiet, and a lack of interruptions before the interview convey to patients that what they say is important and worthy of serious consideration.

Sometimes a patient will appear frightened at the beginning of an interview and may not want to answer questions. If this seems to be the case, the physician may comment on this impression directly in a gentle and supportive way and encourage the patient to talk about his or her feelings about the interview itself. Acknowledging a patient's anxiety is the first step in understanding and reducing it. An example of what could be said is "I notice that you seem to be feeling anxious about talking with me. Is there anything I can do or any questions I can answer that will make it easier?" or "I know it can be frightening to talk to a doctor, especially one you've never met before, but I'd like to make it as comfortable for you as possible. Is there anything you can put your finger on that's making it tough for you to talk with me?"

Another important initial question is "Why now?" A physician should be clear about why a patient has chosen that particular time to ask for help. The reason may be as simple as that it was the first available appointment hour. Very often, however, people seek out doctors as the result of particular events that have increased stress. These stressful events may be thought of as precipitants, and they often contribute significantly to patients' current problems. Examples of stressful precipitants include real or symbolic losses, such as deaths or separations; milestone events (for example, birthdays or anniversaries); and physical changes, such as the presence or intensification of symptoms.

The Interview Proper

In the interview proper, physicians discover in detail what is troubling patients. They must do so in a systematic way that facilitates the identification of relevant problems in the context of an ongoing empathic working alliance with patients.

The *content* of an interview is literally what is said between doctor and patient: the topics discussed, the subjects mentioned. The *process* of the interview is what occurs nonverbally between doctor and patient, that is, what is happening in the interview beneath the surface. Process involves feelings and reactions that are unacknowledged or unconscious. Patients may use body language to express feelings they cannot express verbally, for example, a clenched fist or nervous tearing at a tissue by a patient with an apparently calm outward demeanor. Patients may shift the interview away from an anxiety-provoking subject onto a neutral topic without realizing that they are doing so. Patients may return again and again to a particular topic, regardless of what direction the interview appears to be taking. Trivial remarks and apparently casual asides can reveal serious underlying concerns, for example, "Oh, by the way, a neighbor of mine tells me that he knows someone with the same symptoms as my son, and that person has cancer."

Specific Techniques. Table 1–5 lists some common interview techniques. Others are discussed below with examples.

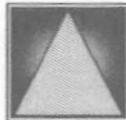

Table 1–5
Common Interview Techniques

1. Establish rapport as early in the interview as possible.
2. Determine the patient's chief complaint.
3. Use the chief complaint to develop a provisional differential diagnosis.
4. Rule the various diagnostic possibilities out or in by using focused and detailed questions.
5. Follow up on vague or obscure replies with enough persistence to accurately determine the answer to the question.
6. Let the patient talk freely enough to observe how tightly the thoughts are connected.
7. Use a mixture of open-ended and closed-ended questions.
8. Don't be afraid to ask about topics that you or the patient may find difficult or embarrassing.
9. Ask about suicidal thoughts.
10. Give the patient a chance to ask questions at the end of the interview.
11. Conclude the initial interview by conveying a sense of confidence and, if possible, of hope.

Reprinted with permission from Andreasen NC, Black DW. *Introduction Textbook of Psychiatry.* Washington, DC: American Psychiatric Association, 1991.

OPEN-ENDED VERSUS CLOSED-ENDED QUESTIONS. Interviewing any patient involves a fine balance between allowing the patient's story to unfold at will and obtaining the necessary data for diagnosis and treatment. Most experts agree that an ideal interview begins with broad, open-ended questioning, continues by becoming specific, and closes with detailed direct questioning.

An example of an open-ended question is "Can you tell me more about that?" A closed-ended question would be "How long have you been taking the medication?" Closed-ended questions can be effective in generating specific and quick responses about a clearly delineated topic. Closed-ended questions have also been found effective in assessing such factors as the presence or absence, frequency, severity, and duration of symptoms. Table 1–6 summarizes some of the pros and cons of open- and closed-ended questions.

REFLECTION. In the technique of reflection, a doctor repeats to a patient, in a supportive manner, something that the patient has said. The goal of reflection is twofold: to assure the doctor that he or she has correctly understood what the patient is trying to say and to let the patient know that the doctor is perceiving what is being said. The response is meant to let the patient know that the doctor is both listening to the patient's concerns and understanding them. For example, if a patient is speaking about fears of dying and the effects of talking about these fears with his or her family, the doctor might say, "It seems that you are concerned with becoming a burden to your family." This reflection is not an exact repetition of what the patient has said, but rather a paraphrase that indicates the doctor has perceived the essential meaning.

FACILITATION. Doctors help patients continue in the interview by providing both verbal and nonverbal cues that encourage patients to keep talking. Nodding one's head, leaning forward in the chair, and saying, "Yes, and then . . . ?" or "Uh-huh, go on," are all examples of facilitation.

SILENCE. Silence can be used in many ways in normal conversations, even to indicate disapproval or disinterest. In the doctor–patient relationship, however, silence can be constructive and, in certain situations, allow patients to contemplate, to cry, or just to sit in an accepting, supportive environment in which the doctor makes it clear that not every moment must be filled with talk.

CONFRONTATION. The technique of confrontation is meant to point out to a patient something to which the doctor thinks the patient is not paying attention, is missing, or is in some way denying. The confrontation is meant to help patients face whatever needs to be faced in a direct but respectful way. For example, a patient who has just made a suicidal gesture but is telling the doctor that it was not serious may be confronted with the following statement: "What you have done may not have killed you, but it's telling me that you are in serious trouble right now and that you need help so that you don't try suicide again."

CLARIFICATION. In clarification, doctors attempt to get details from patients about what they have already said. For example, a doctor may say, "You are feeling depressed. When do you feel most depressed?"

INTERPRETATION. The technique of interpretation is most often used when a doctor states something about a patient's behavior or thinking of which the patient may not be aware. The technique requires the doctor's careful listening for underlying themes and patterns in the patient's story. Interpretations usually help clarify interrelationships that the patient may not see. It is a sophisticated technique and should generally be used only after the doctor has established some rapport with the patient and has a reasonably good idea of what some interrelationships are. For example, a doctor may say, "When you talk about how angry you are that your family has not been supportive, I think you're also telling me how worried you are that I won't be there for you either. What do you think?"

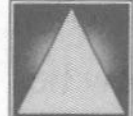

Table 1–6
Pros and Cons of Open-Ended and Closed-Ended Questions

Aspect	Broad, Open-Ended Questions	Narrow, Closed-Ended Questions
Genuineness	High They produce spontaneous formulations.	Low They lead the patient.
Reliability	Low They may lead to nonreproducible answers.	High Narrow focus, but they may suggest answers.
Precision	Low Intent of question is vague.	High Intent of question is clear.
Time efficiency	Low Circumstantial elaborations.	High May invite yes or no answers.
Completeness of diagnostic coverage	Low Patient selects topic.	High Interviewer selects topic.
Acceptance by patient	Varies Most patients prefer expressing themselves freely; others feel guarded and insecure.	Varies Some patients enjoy clear-cut checks; others hate to be pressed into a yes or no format.

Reprinted with permission from Othmer E, Othmer SC. *The Clinical Interview Using DSM-IV.* Washington, DC: American Psychiatric Press; 1994.

SUMMATION. Periodically during the interview, a doctor can take a moment and briefly summarize what a patient has said thus far. Doing so assures both the patient and doctor that the doctor has heard the same information that the patient has actually conveyed. For example, the doctor may say, "OK, I just want to make sure that I've got everything right up to this point."

EXPLANATION. Doctors explain treatment plans to patients in easily understandable language and allow patients to respond and ask questions. For example, a doctor may say, "It is essential that you come into the hospital now because of the seriousness of your condition. You will be admitted tonight through the emergency room, and I will be there to make all the arrangements. You will be given a small dose of medication that will make you sleepy. The medication is called lorazepam, and the dose you will be getting is 0.25 mg. I will see you again first thing in the morning, and we'll go over all the procedures that will be required before anything else happens. Now, what are your questions? I know you must have some." Note that when prescribing medication, the patient should be advised of common adverse effects.

TRANSITION. The technique of transition allows doctors to convey the idea that sufficient information has been obtained on one subject; the doctor's words encourage patients to continue on to another subject. For example, a doctor may say, "You've given me a good sense of that particular time in your life. Perhaps now you could tell me a bit more about an even earlier time in your life."

SELF-REVELATION. Limited, discreet self-disclosure by physicians may be useful in certain situations if physicians feel at ease and can communicate a sense of self-comfort. Conveying this sense may involve answering a patient's questions about whether a physician is married and where he or she comes from. A doctor who practices self-revelation excessively, however, is using a patient to gratify unfulfilled needs in his or her own life and is abusing the role of physician. If a doctor thinks that a piece of information will help a particular patient be more comfortable, the doctor can decide to be self-revealing. The decision depends on whether the information will further a patient's care or if it will provide nothing useful. Even if the doctor decides that self-revelation is not warranted, he or she should be careful not to make the patient feel embarrassed for asking a question. For example, the doctor may say, "I will be happy to tell you whether or not I am married, but first let's talk a little about why it is important for you to know that. If we talk about it, I'll have a bit more information about who you are and what your concerns are regarding me and my involvement in your care." Do not take patients' questions at face value alone. Many questions, especially personal ones, convey not just natural curiosity but also hidden concerns about the doctor that should not be ignored.

POSITIVE REINFORCEMENT. The technique of positive reinforcement allows patients to feel comfortable telling a doctor anything, even about such things as noncompliance with treatment. Encouraging a patient to feel that the doctor is not upset by whatever the patient has to say facilitates an open exchange. For example, a doctor might say, "I appreciate your telling me that you have stopped taking your medication. Can you tell me what the problem was?" An experienced psychiatrist, in response to patients who were afraid of revealing "shocking" material in the initial interview, may respond in the following manner: "After all these years in practice I don't think I have heard anything that could shock me." The implied acceptance of all things human usually puts patients at ease.

REASSURANCE. Truthful reassurance of a patient can lead to increased trust and compliance and can be experienced as an empathic response of a concerned physician. False reassurance, however, is essentially lying to a patient and can badly impair the patient's trust and compliance. False reassurance is often given from a desire to make a patient feel better, but once a patient knows that a doctor has not told the truth, the patient is unlikely to accept or believe truthful reassurance. In an example of false reassurance, a patient with a terminal illness asks, "Am I going to be all right, Doctor?" and the doctor responds, "Of course you're going to be all right. Everything's fine." An example of truthful reassurance is "I'm going to do everything possible to make you comfortable, and part of being comfortable is for you to know as much as I know about what is going on with you. We both know that what you have is serious. I'd like to know exactly what you think is happening to you and to clarify any questions you have." The patient may then be able to talk openly about his or her fear of dying.

ADVICE. In many situations it is not only acceptable but desirable for doctors to give patients advice. To be effective and to be perceived as empathic rather than inappropriate or intrusive, the advice should be given only after patients are allowed to talk freely about their problems so that physicians have an adequate information base from which to make suggestions. At times, after a doctor has listened carefully to a patient, it becomes clear that the patient does not, in fact, want advice as much as an objective, caring, nonjudgmental ear. Giving advice too quickly can lead a patient to feel that the doctor is not really listening but, rather, is responding, either out of anxiety or from the belief that the doctor inherently knows better than the patient what should be done in a particular situation. In an example of advice given too quickly, a patient says, "I can't take this medication. It's bothering me," and the physician responds, "Fine. I think you should stop taking it, and I'll prescribe something different." A more appropriate response is "I'm sorry to hear that. Tell me what about the medication has been bothering you, and I'll have a better idea what we should do to make you more comfortable." In another example, the patient says, "I've really been feeling down lately," and the doctor replies, "Well in that case, I think it's important that you go out and do some things that are fun, such as going to a movie or taking a walk in the park." In this case, a more appropriate and helpful response could be "Tell me more about what you mean by 'feeling down'."

ENDING THE INTERVIEW. Physicians want patients to leave an interview feeling understood and respected and believing that all the pertinent and important information has been conveyed to an informed, empathic listener. To this end, doctors should give patients a chance to ask questions and should let patients know as much as possible about future plans. Doctors should thank patients for sharing the necessary information and let patients know that the information conveyed has been helpful in clarifying the next steps. Any prescription of medication should be spelled out clearly and simply, and doctors should ascertain whether patients understand the prescription and how to take it. Doctors should make another appointment or give a referral and some indication about how patients can reach help quickly if it is necessary before the next appointment.

SPECIFIC ISSUES IN PSYCHIATRY

Fees

Before clinicians can establish an ongoing relationship with patients, they must address certain issues. For instance, they must openly discuss payment of fees. Discussing these issues and any other questions about fees from the beginning of the relationship can minimize misunderstanding later. Most patients have medical insurance through health maintenance organizations (HMOs) or Medicare. HMOs pay for doctors' visits in whole or in part, but only if the doctor is a member (or provider) in the patient's plan. Some plans (called point of service plans) offer partial payments even if the doctor is not a member (i.e., he or she is called "out-of-network"). That should be clarified; otherwise, the patient may have to pay out-of-pocket, which he or she may be unwilling or unable to do.

Confidentiality

Psychiatrists and mental health professionals should discuss the extent and limitations of confidentiality with patients, so that patients are clear about what can and cannot remain confidential. As much as physicians must legally and ethically respect patients' confidentiality, it may be wholly or partially broken in some specific situations. For example, if a patient makes clear that he or she intends to harm someone, the doctor has a responsibility to notify the intended victim. Other issues related to confidentiality include who has access to the patient's medical record, information required by insurance companies (which may be extensive), and the degree to which the patient's case will be used for teaching purposes. In all such situations, the patient must give permission for the use of medical records. (See Chapter 58 for a discussion of confidentiality.)

Supervision

It is both commonplace and necessary for doctors in training to receive supervision from experienced physicians. This practice is the norm in large teaching hospitals, and most patients are aware of it. When young doctors are receiving supervision from senior physicians, patients should know from the beginning. Informing patients is particularly important in psychiatry, in which the supervision of individual psychotherapy cases is a routine and established practice and in which the psychiatric resident is required to present verbatim accounts of an entire therapy session (process notes) to a senior supervisor. If a patient is curious about the level of the treating doctor's experience, the doctor or medical student should respond honestly and not mislead the patient. If the doctor is less than truthful and the patient later discovers this, the relationship between doctor and patient may become untenable.

Missed Appointments and Length of Sessions

Patients need to be informed about a doctor's policies for missed appointments and length of sessions. Psychiatrists generally see patients in regularly scheduled blocks of time ranging from 15 to 45 minutes. At the end of this time, psychiatrists expect patients to accept the fact that the session is over. Nonpsychiatric physicians may schedule somewhat differently, by putting aside 30 minutes to an hour for an initial visit and then perhaps scheduling patient visits every 15 to 20 minutes for follow-up appointments. Psychiatrists who are treating psychotic inpatients may determine that a patient cannot tolerate a lengthy session and may decide to see the patient in a series of 10-minute sessions throughout the week. Whatever the policies, patients must be made aware of them to prevent misunderstandings.

The same can be said about policies for missed appointments. Some doctors ask patients to give 24 hours' notice to avoid being billed for a missed session. Others bill for missed sessions regardless of advance notification. Still others decide on a case-by-case basis or perhaps state a 24-hour rule, but make exceptions when warranted. Some doctors state that if they receive advance notice and can fill the appointment time, they will not charge for missed sessions; others do not charge for missed appointments at all. The choice is up to the individual physician, but patients must know in advance to make an informed decision about whether to accept the doctor's policy or to choose another doctor.

Availability of Doctor

What are a doctor's obligations to be available between scheduled appointments? Is it incumbent on physicians to be available 24 hours a day? Once a patient enters into a contract to receive care from a particular physician, the doctor is responsible for having a mechanism in place for providing emergency service outside scheduled appointment times. Patients should be told what the mechanism is, whether it is an emergency phone number or a covering physician. If the physician is going to be away for a period of time, coverage by another physician is necessary, and patients must be informed how to reach the covering doctor. They should know that their doctor will be available between appointments to answer pressing questions and that extra appointments can be scheduled if necessary.

Within these general parameters, however, physicians must make their own decisions about their availability to specific patients. In some cases, doctors may have to place firm limits on availability between sessions. For instance, patients who repeatedly call at all hours with concerns that are best addressed during scheduled appointments should be respectfully but firmly discouraged from calling unnecessarily. They can be reassured that all concerns will be addressed and if insufficient time exists during the regular appointment, another appointment can be made, but they should be told that all nonemergency concerns will be postponed until the next session.

Follow-Up

Many events can disrupt the continuity of the patient–doctor relationship. Some of these events are routine, such as residents ending their training and moving on to another hospital; others are out of the ordinary and thus unpredictable, for example, when physicians become ill and can no longer take care of their patients. Patients must be assured that regardless of what occurs in the course of a particular patient–doctor relationship, their care will be ongoing.

A complex situation arises when physicians become ill and are unable to continue caring for patients. When they know in advance that they will have to interrupt therapy, clear arrangements for referral to other doctors can be made. Although arguments exist both for and against physicians revealing their illnesses to patients, it seems best to err on the side of truth. The information should be conveyed in as calm and nonthreatening a way as possible. The reason for telling the truth is that patients will fantasize reasons about why the doctor has stopped seeing them and may fear that something about them has made the doctor leave. Untruthfulness in this situation also encourages the view that being ill is shameful or frightening. It is not the role of patients, however, to take care of their doctors; informing patients should not carry with it any sense that a doctor's illness is a patient's burden.

QUALITIES OF THE PHYSICIAN

Physicians are drawn to the field of medicine for many reasons. These include a desire to help people, to cure illness, to

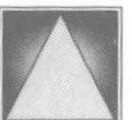

Table 1–7
Character and Qualities of the Physician*

Imperturbability	The ability to maintain extreme calm and steadiness
Presence of mind	Self-control in an emergency or embarrassing situation so that one can say or do the right thing
Clear judgment	The ability to make an informed opinion that is intelligible and free of ambiguity
Ability to endure frustration	The capacity to remain firm and deal with insecurity and dissatisfaction
Infinite patience	The unlimited ability to hear pain or trial calmly
Charity toward others	To be generous and helpful, especially toward the needy and suffering
The search for absolute truth	To investigate facts and pursue reality
Composure	Calmness of mind, bearing, and appearance
Bravery	The capacity to face or endure events with courage
Tenacity	To be persistent in attaining a goal or adhering to something valued
Idealism	Forming standards and ideals and living under their influence
Equanimity	The ability to handle stressful situations with an undisturbed, even temper

*After William Osler, M.D.

be part of a respected profession or to hold a position of authority, and to exert some control over life and death. Many people who choose to become physicians are perfectionistic, demanding of themselves, and attentive to details. These qualities can be adaptive—in fact, are probably necessary—but need to be balanced with healthy doses of self-knowledge, humility, humor, and kindness. William Osler, M.D. (1814–1919), physician and teacher, discussed the characteristics and quality of the physician in his book *Aequanimitas*, which are summarized in Table 1–7. They are ideals to be strived for, but they are rarely reached. Physicians (and other health care providers) must be tolerant about the limits on what they can realistically and honestly accomplish.

The demands on a physician can be daunting. In addition to the vast amount of knowledge and the skills required to practice medicine, the doctor must also develop the capacity of balancing compassionate concern with dispassionate objectivity, the wish to relieve pain with the ability to make painful decisions, and the desire to cure and control with an acceptance of one's human limitations. The lack of these capacities can lead a physician to feel overwhelmed and depressed. Learning to balance these interrelated aspects of the physician's role allows the doctor to cope productively within daily work that involves illness, pain, sadness, suffering, and death.

References

Alexander GC, Lantos JD. The doctor-patient relationship in the post-managed care era. *American Journal of Bioethics*. 2006;6(1):29–32.

Balint J. Should confidentiality in medicine be absolute? *American Journal of Bioethics*. 2006;6(2):19–20.

Brody H. Family medicine, the physician–patient relationship, and patient-centered care. *American Journal of Bioethics*. 2006;6(1):38–39.

Broom A. Medical specialists' accounts of the impact of the Internet on the doctor/patient relationship. *Health*. 2005;9(3):319–338.

Fadlon J, Pessach I, Toker A. Teaching medical students what they think they already know. *Education for Health*. 2004;17(1):35–41.

Fan VS, Burman M, McDonell MB, Fihn SD. Continuity of care and other determinants of patient satisfaction with primary care. *J Gen Intern Med*. 2005; 20(3):226–233.

Fredericks M, Odiet JA, Miller SI, Fredericks J. Toward a conceptual reexamination of the patient-physician relationship in the healthcare institution for the new millennium. *J Natl Med Assoc*. 2006;98(3):378–385.

Hsu J, Huang J, Fung V, Robertson N, Jimison H, Frankel R. Health information technology and physician-patient interactions: Impact of computers on communication during outpatient primary care visits. *J Am Med Inform Assoc*. 2005; 12:474–480.

Jotkowitz AB, Clarfield M. The physician as comforter. *Eur J Intern Med*. 2005; 16(2):95–96.

Larson EB, Yao X. Clinical empathy as emotional labor in the patient-physician relationship. *JAMA*. 2005;293:1100–1106.

Maynard DW, Heritage J. Conversation analysis, doctor-patient interaction and medical communication. *Med Educ*. 2005;39(4):428–435.

Piette JD, Heisler M, Krein S, Kerr EA. The role of patient-physician trust in moderating medication nonadherence due to cost pressures. *Arch Intern Med*. 2005;165:1749–1755.

Travaline JM, Ruchinskas R, D'Alonzo GE Jr. Patient-physician communication: Why and how. *J Am Osteopath Assoc*. 2005;105(1):13–18.

Weiner M, Biondich P. The influence of information technology on patient-physician relationships. *J Gen Intern Med*. 2006; 21(s1):S35.

Werner A, Malterud K. It is hard work behaving as a credible patient: Encounters between women with chronic pain and their doctors. *Social Science & Medicine*. 2003;57(8):1409–1419.

2 Human Development Throughout the Life Cycle

▲ 2.1 Normality

The World Health Organization (WHO) considers normality to be a state of complete physical, mental, and social well-being. Mental well-being presumes the absence of mental disorder defined in the text revision of the fourth edition of *Diagnostic and Statistical Manual of Mental Disorders* (DSM-IV-TR) as follows:

> A mental disorder is a behavioral or psychological syndrome or pattern associated with distress (e.g., a painful symptom), or with a significantly increased risk of suffering, death, pain, disability, or an important loss of freedom. In addition, the syndrome or pattern must not be merely an expected and culturally sanctioned response to a particular event, such as the death of a loved one.

Historically, the two broad categories of mental disorder are psychosis and neurosis. Psychosis is defined as grossly impaired reality testing. With gross impairment in reality testing, persons incorrectly evaluate the accuracy of their perceptions and thoughts and make incorrect inferences about external reality, even in the face of contrary evidence. The term *psychotic* does not apply to minor distortions of reality that involve matters of relative judgment. For example, depressed persons who underestimate their achievements are not described as psychotic, whereas those who believe that they have caused natural disasters are so described.

Neurosis is defined as a chronic or recurrent disorder that is characterized mainly by anxiety, which appears alone or as a symptom such as an obsession, compulsion, phobia, or a sexual dysfunction. Psychosis is synonymous with severe impairment of social and personal functioning characterized by social withdrawal and inability to perform the usual household and occupational roles. Neurosis implies that reality testing and personality organization is intact but the person is distressed by a variety of disturbing symptoms.

NORMALITY

Normality has been defined as patterns of behavior or personality traits that are typical or that conform to some standard of proper and acceptable ways of behaving and being. The use of terms such as *typical* or *acceptable*, however, has been criticized because they are ambiguous, involve value judgments, and vary from one culture to another. To overcome this objection, psychiatrist and historian George Mora, M.D. devised a system to describe behavioral manifestations that are normal in one context but not in another, depending on how the person is viewed by the society (Table 2.1–1). This paradigm, however, may give too much weight to peer group observations and judgments.

In *Mental Health: A Report of the Surgeon General*, mental health is defined as "the successful performance of mental functions, in terms of thought, mood, and behavior that results in productive activities, fulfilling relationships with others, and the ability to adapt to change and to cope with adversity."

A controversial view is held by the psychiatrist Thomas Szasz, who believes that the concept of mental illness should be abandoned entirely. In his book, *The Myth of Mental Illness*, Szasz states that normality can be measured only in terms of what persons do or do not do and that defining normality is beyond the realm of psychiatry. He claims that a belief in mental illness is akin to believing in witchcraft or demonology.

Psychiatry has been criticized over the years by certain groups for its portrayal of normality. The psychology of women, for example, has been criticized as sexist because it was formulated initially by men; similar criticism comes from other groups who believe the portrayal of their psychological issues is biased by placing undue emphasis on psychopathology rather than healthy attributes. A much discussed issue is the change in psychiatry's view of homosexuality from abnormal to normal that took place in 1973, an evolution shaped by cultural norms, society's expectations and values, professional biases, individual differences, and the political climate of the time.

FUNCTIONAL PERSPECTIVES OF NORMALITY

The many theoretical and clinical concepts of normality seem to fall into four functional perspectives. Although each perspective is unique and has its own definition and description, the perspectives complement each other, and together they represent the totality of the behavioral science and social science approaches to the subject. The four perspectives of normality as described by Daniel Offer and Melvin Sabshin are (1) normality as health, (2) normality as utopia, (3) normality as average, and (4) normality as process.

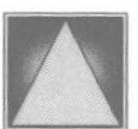

Table 2.1–1
Normality in Context

Term	Concept
Autonormal	Person seen as normal by his or her own society
Autopathological	Person seen as abnormal by his or her own society
Heteronormal	Person seen as normal by members of another society observing him or her
Heteropathological	Person seen as unusual or pathological by members of another society observing him or her

Data from George Mora, M.D.

Normality as Health

The first perspective is basically the traditional medical psychiatric approach to health and illness. Most physicians equate normality with health and view health as an almost universal phenomenon. As a result, behavior is assumed to be within normal limits when no manifest psychopathology is present. If all behavior were to be put on a scale, normality would encompass the major portion of the continuum, and abnormality would be the small remainder.

This definition of normality correlates with the traditional model of the doctor who attempts to free his or her patient from grossly observable signs and symptoms. To this physician, the lack of signs or symptoms indicates health. Health in this context refers to a reasonable, rather than an optimal, state of functioning. In its simplest form, this perspective described by John Romano views a healthy person as one who is reasonably free of undue pain, discomfort, and disability.

Normality as Utopia

The second perspective conceives of normality as that harmonious and optimal blending of the diverse elements of the mental apparatus that culminates in optimal functioning. Such a definition emerges when psychiatrists or psychoanalysts talk about the ideal person, when they grapple with a complex problem, or when they discuss their criteria for a successful treatment. This approach can be traced back to Sigmund Freud, who when discussing normality stated, "A normal ego is like normality in general, an ideal fiction."

Although this approach is characteristic of many psychoanalysts, it is by no means unique to them. It can also be found among other psychotherapists in the field of psychiatry and among psychologists of quite different persuasions.

Normality as Average

The third perspective, commonly used in normative studies of behavior, is based on a mathematical principle of the bell-shaped curve. This approach considers the middle range normal and both extremes deviant. The normative approach based on this statistical principle describes each individual in terms of general assessment and total score. Variability is described only within the context of groups, not within the context of the individual.

Although this approach is more commonly used in psychology than in psychiatry, psychiatrists have been relying on normative pencil-and-paper tests to a much larger extent than in the past. Not only do psychiatrists use instruments such as the Minnesota Multiple Personality Inventory (MMPI), they also construct their own tests and questionnaires. (Psychiatric rating scales are discussed in Section 9.2.)

Normality as Process

The fourth perspective stresses that normal behavior is the end result of interacting systems. Based on this definition, temporal changes are essential to a complete definition of normality. In other words, the normality-as-process perspective stresses changes or processes rather than a cross-sectional definition of normality.

Investigators who subscribe to this approach can be found in all the behavioral and social sciences. A typical example of the concepts in this perspective is Erik Erikson's conceptualization of the epigenesis of personality development and the seven developmental stages essential in the attainment of mature adult functioning. (Erikson's theories are discussed in Section 6.2.)

PSYCHOANALYTIC THEORIES OF NORMALITY

Some psychoanalysts base their concepts of normality on the absence of symptoms; but whereas the disappearance of symptoms is necessary for cure or improvement, the absence of symptoms alone does not suffice for a comprehensive definition of normality. Accordingly, most psychoanalysts view a capacity for work and enjoyment as indicating normality or, as Freud put it, the ability "to love and to work."

The psychoanalyst Heinz Hartmann, M.D. conceptualized normality by describing the "autonomous functions of the ego" (Fig. 2.1–1). These are psychological capacities present at birth that are conflict free, that is, uninfluenced by the internal psychic world. They include perception, intuition, comprehension, thinking, language, and certain aspects of motor development, learning, and intelligence. The concept of autonomous and conflict-free functions of the ego helps explain the mechanisms whereby some persons lead relatively normal lives in the presence of extraordinary external experiential traumas—the so-called invulnerable child, that is, a child who is invulnerable to the "slings and arrows of outrageous fortune" by virtue of autonomous ego strengths. A summary of some psychoanalytic views of normality is given in Table 2.1–2.

Karl Jaspers

Karl Jaspers (1883–1969), the German psychiatrist and philosopher, described a "personal world"—the way a person thinks or feels—that could be either normal or abnormal (Fig. 2.1–2). According to Jaspers, the personal world is abnormal when it (1) springs from a condition that is recognized universally as abnormal, such as schizophrenia; (2) separates the person from others emotionally; and (3) does not provide the person with a sense of "spiritual and material" security.

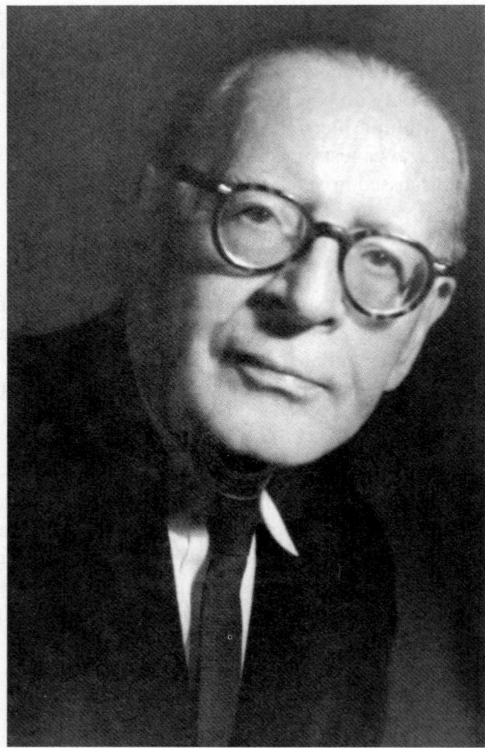

FIGURE 2.1–1
Heinz Hartmann, M.D. (Courtesy of New York Academy of Medicine, New York.)

Jaspers was a proponent of phenomenology, in which the clinician studies psychological signs and symptoms with the goal of understanding the internal experience of the patient. By listening carefully to the patient, the psychiatrist temporarily enters the mental life of the patient. Jaspers believed that to understand fully the signs and symptoms observed in the patient, the clinician must have no prior assumptions. A person who reports a hallucinatory experience, for example, must not be judged thereby as being abnormal or psychotic. To be used diagnostically, the phenomenon must occur repeatedly and be characteristic of a known disorder.

Some investigators are developing a research strategy that defines normality by examining a person's mental state at various times during the day in different life settings. What is abnormal in one setting or at one time of day may be normal in another.

Robert Campbell

Finally, the commonly accepted and widely used definition of mental health adapted from *Campbell's Psychiatric Dictionary* is as follows:

> Psychically normal persons are those who are in harmony with themselves and with their environment. They conform with the cultural requirements or injunctions of their community. They may possess medical deviation or disease, but as long as this does not impair their reasoning, judgment, intellectual capacity, and ability to make a harmonious personal and social adaptation, they may be regarded as psychically sound or normal.

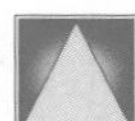

Table 2.1–2
Psychoanalytic Concepts of Normality

Theorist	Concept
Sigmund Freud	Normality is an idealized fiction.
Kurt Eissler	Absolute normality cannot be obtained because the normal person must be totally aware of his or her thoughts and feelings.
Melanie Klein	Normality is characterized by strength of character, the capacity to deal with conflicting emotions, the ability to experience pleasure without conflict, and the ability to love.
Erik Erikson	Normality is the ability to master the periods of life: trust vs. mistrust; autonomy vs. shame and doubt; initiative vs. guilt; industry vs. inferiority; identity vs. role confusion; intimacy vs. isolation; generativity vs. stagnation; and ego integrity vs. despair.
Laurence Kubie	Normality is the ability to learn by experience, to be flexible, and to adapt to a changing environment.
Heinz Hartmann	Conflict-free ego functions represent the person's potential for normality; the degree the ego can adapt to reality and be autonomous is related to mental health.
Karl Menninger	Normality is the ability to adjust to the external world with contentment and to master the task of acculturation.
Alfred Adler	The person's capacity to develop social feeling and to be productive is related to mental health; the ability to work heightens self-esteem and makes one capable of adaptation.
R. E. Money-Kryle	Normality is the ability to achieve insight into one's self, an ability that is never fully accomplished.
Otto Rank	Normality is the capacity to live without fear, guilt, or anxiety and to take responsibility for one's own actions.
W. Somerset Maughn	The normal is an ideal. It is a picture that one fabricates . . . and to find them all in a single man is hardly to be expected.

INCIDENCE OF MENTAL ILLNESS

In 2005, the National Institute of Mental Health (NIMH) completed a nationwide survey of how many Americans will develop a mental illness at some point in their lives. The findings indicated that more than 50 percent would do so, up from 20 percent in a similar survey done in 1984. The most common mental disorder was depression, which had a lifetime prevalence of 17 percent; followed by alcohol abuse, affecting 13 percent; and phobias, affecting 12 percent. Table 2.1–3 lists the findings in the mental health epidemiological survey. Of those people who had had a mental illness at some point in their lives, most developed the problem at a young age. Mood disorders were most prevalent in persons between the ages of 20 and 30. When treatment

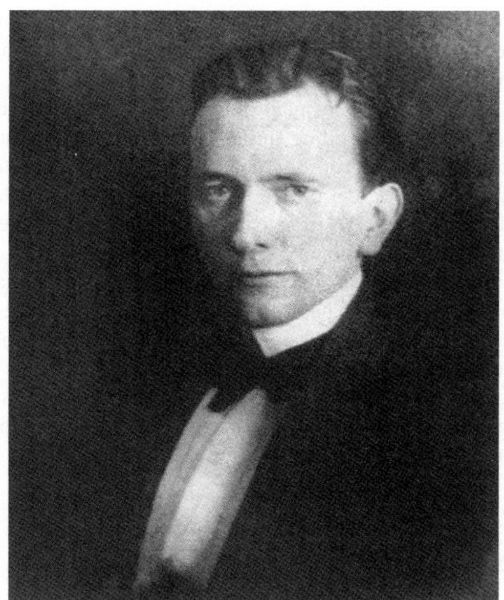

FIGURE 2.1–2
Karl Jaspers, M.D. (Courtesy of New York Academy of Medicine, New York.)

was factored into the study results, most persons did not receive treatment or, if they did, it was inadequate or ineffective according to the researchers.

The report generated controversy among several groups. Some medical anthropologists said the report reflected political and cultural shifts about how illness was defined in America over recent decades rather than a true increase in mental illness. They cited the example of homosexuality being declassified as a mental illness to support the view that culture affects the definition of illness. Other critics pointed out that the number of diagnostic disorders listed in the DSM, which increased from about 60 in 1952, to more than 300 in the current edition, accounted for the change. Behaviors, once seen as normal, were being medicalized. Some sociologists explained the increase as caused by modern western life, particularly urban life, which is more stressful than ever before and which more easily causes persons to break down. Advocates for the study cited historical precedent which, at one point, attributed mental illness to demonic possession. As science advances, mental illness is seen as a medical disease that can be distinguished, one from the other, on the basis of pathophysiological causes.

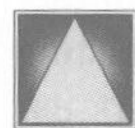

Table 2.1–3
Mental Health Census

Disorder	Lifetime Prevalence (%)
Any anxiety disorder	**28.8**
Panic disorder	4.7
Agoraphobia without panic	1.4
Specific phobia	12.5
Social phobia	12.1
Generalized anxiety disorder	5.7
Posttraumatic stress disorder	6.8
Obsessive-compulsive	1.6
Separation anxiety	5.2
Mood disorder	**20.8**
Major depression	16.6
Dysthymia	2.5
Bipolar I or II	3.9
Impulse-control disorder	**24.8**
Oppositional-defiant disorder	8.5
Conduct disorder	9.5
Attention-deficit hyperactivity	8.1
Intermittent explosive	5.2
Substance disorder	**14.6**
Alcohol abuse	13.2
Alcohol dependence	5.4
Drug abuse	7.9
Drug dependence	3.0

Ronald C. Kessler, M.D., Harvard University.

Cross-Cultural Issues

Certain mental illnesses are found throughout the world and in every culture; others are culture-bound or culture-specific. Schizophrenia, for example, has the same prevalence universally, whereas anorexia nervosa is seen mainly in western industrialized countries. That some psychiatric disorders appear to be relatively or largely culture-specific adds a further complication in determining normal from abnormal.

In China, for example, there is a stigma to being labeled mentally ill and depression is relatively unknown. But the Chinese are not immune from complaints of feelings of exhaustion, sleep disturbances, inability to relax, and other signs that in the west would be part of the depressive syndrome. In China, however, the condition is diagnosed as neurasthenia, a medical diagnosis attributed to a depletion of nervous energy. In Japan, too, reported levels of depression are low, in part because of the culture of stoicism in which one does not complain about vague signs or symptoms that might be diagnosed as depression.

LIFE CYCLE THEORY

The life cycle represents the stages through which all humans pass from birth to death. The fundamental assumption of all life cycle theories is that development occurs in successive, clearly defined stages. This sequence is invariant; that is, it occurs in a particular order in every person's life, whether or not all stages are completed. A second assumption of life cycle theory is the epigenetic principle, which maintains that each stage is characterized by events or crises that must be resolved satisfactorily for development to proceed smoothly. According to the epigenetic model, if resolution is not achieved within a given life period, all subsequent stages reflect that failure in the form of physical, cognitive, social, or emotional maladjustment. A third assumption is that each phase of the life cycle contains a dominant feature, complex of features, or a crisis point that distinguishes it from phases that either preceded or will follow it.

Charting of the life cycle lies within the study of developmental psychology and involves such diverse elements as biological maturity, psychological capacity, adaptive techniques, defense mechanisms, symptom complexes, role demands, social behavior, cognition, perception, language development, and interpersonal relationships. Various models of the life cycle describe the major developmental phases, but emphasize different elements.

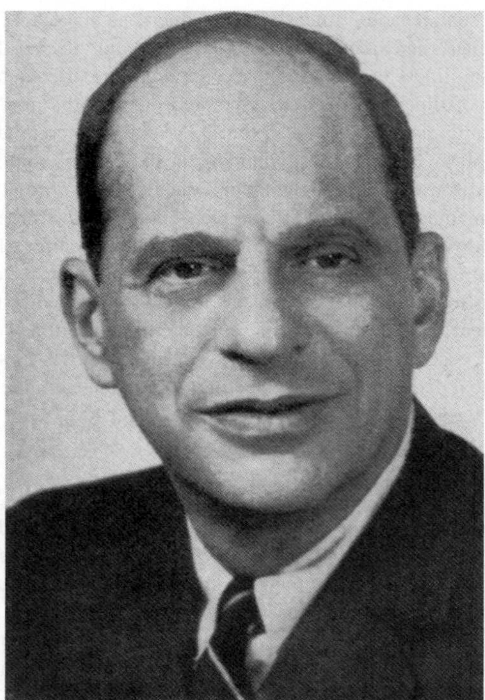

FIGURE 2.1–3
Theodore Lidz, M.D. (Courtesy of New York Academy of Medicine, New York.)

Taken together however, they demonstrate that an order to human life exists, despite that each person is unique.

Theodore Lidz, M.D. (Fig 2.1–3), a major exponent of life cycle theory, describes several factors that account for the phasic nature of the life cycle.

1. The acquisition of many abilities must wait for the physical maturation of the organism. For example, the infant cannot become a toddler until the pyramidal nerve tracts that permit voluntary discrete movements of the lower limbs become functional. Then, after such maturation occurs, it takes considerable practice to gain the skills needed to master a function, but the function becomes amenable to training and education. Adequate mastery of simple skills must precede their incorporation into more complex activities. In a somewhat different way, shifts in the physiological equilibrium can initiate a new phase in the life cycle, as when the new inner forces that come with puberty require changes in personality functioning, whatever the preparation in prior phases of childhood.
2. Cognitive development plays a significant role in creating phasic shifts. The ability to communicate needs and desires verbally and to understand what parents say is a major factor in ending the period of infancy, and children's ability to attend school depends to a great extent on their gaining the ability to form concrete categories at the age of 5 or 6. Cognitive development does not progress at an even pace, because qualitatively different capacities emerge in discrete stages.
3. Society establishes roles and sets of expectations for persons of different ages and statuses. At 5 or 6, a child becomes a schoolchild with new demands and opportunities. As adults, interpersonal relationships, such as marriage, require that the person attend to the needs of the other.
4. Children attain many attributes and capacities for directing the self and controlling impulses by internalizing parental characteristics to overcome gradually the need for surrogate egos to direct their lives and provide security. Such internalizations take place in stages in relation to the child's physical, intellectual, and emotional development.
5. Finally, time itself is a determinant of phasic changes, not only because of the need to move into age-appropriate roles, but because changes in physical make-up at puberty and old age require changes in self-concepts and attitudes. Awareness of the passage of time also fosters entry into new stages of life, as when persons realize that more time lies behind than ahead of them as they enter late middle age.

CONTEMPORARY DEVELOPMENTALISTS

The study of childhood preceded the study of adulthood because of social and psychological factors such as the spread of compulsory education and Freud's discovery of the influence of childhood experiences on adult psychopathology. The recent shift of interest to the adult years builds on this knowledge and can be traced to the increased life span and the need to understand and to accommodate the rapidly growing number of middle-aged and elderly individuals. Among the most influential current theoreticians are the following.

Daniel Levinson

Daniel Levinson and his associates devised a psychosocial theory of male development that proposes a life cycle consisting of distinctive, identifiable eras of approximately 20 years extending from birth to death. Within these eras are alternating periods of 6 to 7 years of stability followed by 4- to 5-year intervals of transition, each with its own tasks to be mastered. These concepts are clinically useful, because many patients, particularly the healthier ones, tend to present themselves during periods of transition when internal and external conflicts are increased.

Levinson's theory is currently being used as a framework for the study of various groups, such as aging gay men, and in gender-oriented research which has begun to question whether adult transitions are the same for men and women.

George Vaillant

George Vaillant, M.D. and his group studied a cohort of men for almost 50 years, starting when they were freshmen at Harvard University. A happy childhood manifested by few oral-dependent traits, little psychopathology, the capacity to play, and good object relationships was found to correlate significantly with positive traits in middle life.

Vaillant noted that a hierarchy of ego mechanisms was constructed as the men advanced in age. Defenses were organized

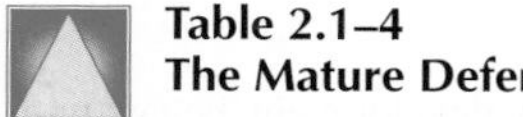

Table 2.1–4
The Mature Defenses

Altruism. The vicarious but constructive and instinctually gratifying service to others. This must be distinguished from altruistic surrender, which involves a surrender of direct gratification, or of instinctual needs, in favor of fulfilling the needs of others to the detriment of the self, with vicarious satisfaction only being gained through introjection.

Anticipation. The realistic anticipation of, or planning for, future inner discomfort; implies overly concerned planning, worrying, and anticipation of dire and dreadful possible outcomes.

Asceticism. The elimination of directly pleasurable affects attributable to an experience. The moral element is implicit in setting values on specific pleasures. Asceticism is directed against all "base" pleasures perceived consciously, and gratification is derived from the renunciation.

Humor. The overt expression of feelings without personal discomfort or immobilization and without unpleasant effect on others. Humor allows one to bear, and yet focus on, what is too terrible to be borne, in contrast to wit, which always involves distraction or displacement away from the affective issue.

Sublimation. The gratification of an impulse whose goal is retained, but whose aim or object is changed from a socially objectionable one to a socially valued one. Libidinal sublimation involves desexualization of drive impulses and placing a value judgment that substitutes what is valued by the superego or society. Sublimation of aggressive impulses takes place through pleasurable games and sports. Unlike neurotic defenses, sublimation allows instincts to be channeled rather than to be dammed up or diverted. Thus, in sublimation, feelings are acknowledged, modified, and directed toward a relatively significant person or goal so that modest instinctual satisfaction results.

Suppression. The conscious or semiconscious decision to postpone attention to a conscious impulse or conflict.

Courtesy of William W. Meissner, M.D.

along a continuum that reflected two aspects of the personality: (1) immaturity versus maturity and (2) psychopathology versus objective adaptation to the external environment. Moreover, the defensive style shifted as a person matured. Vaillant concluded that adaptive styles mature over the years and that the maturation depends more on development from within than on changes in the interpersonal environment. He also corroborated Erikson's model of the life cycle.

Vaillant described a scheme for a positive psychology that focuses on the normal, or positive, aspects of thinking, feeling, and behavior rather than on its negative, or pathological, aspects. He identified a group of adaptive or mature defense mechanisms that enable a person to cope with the stresses of life. Persons who use them are likely to have a normal adjustment in life as measured by economic stability, joy in living, marital satisfaction, and both a subjective sense and objective evidence of physical health. The mature, adaptive defenses, according to Vaillant, are altruism, sublimation, anticipation, and humor. Some also consider asceticism and suppression mature defenses (Table 2.1–4).

Adaptive defenses occur equally in men and women and are seen in all socioeconomic groups. Persons who used the most adaptive defenses were less likely to become depressed after stressful life events than those who did not. An incidental finding among men who had been in combat was that adaptive defenses were protective against posttraumatic stress disorders (PTSD).

More recently, because the subjects of the Grant Study are now in the developmental phase of late adulthood, Vaillant has used a modified version of Erikson's stage model to organize the process of psychosocial maturation in the latter third of life, focusing on the eriksonian tasks of generativity and integrity by rating longitudinal case histories of the Grant Study subjects. Success or failure to engage and to master these developmental themes was closely correlated with patterns established earlier in development in this select group of men who were originally chosen for their emotional and physical health and who have now been followed for more than half a century (18 to 65 years of age).

Bernice Neugarten

Through the study of adults in nonclinical settings, Bernice Neugarten and her colleagues have emphasized the psychological importance of an increased awareness of aging and the personalization of death, as expressed in body monitoring and a tendency to view time in terms of time left to live, rather than time since birth. Middle-aged adults develop a sense of competence that was unrealized earlier in life and have a unique perspective on the younger and older generations. As middle age progresses, people become more introspective and develop an increased sense of interiority.

Calvin Colarusso and Robert Nemiroff

On the basis of their experience as clinicians and psychoanalysts, Calvin Colarusso, M.D. and Robert Nemiroff, M.D. propose a broad theoretical foundation for adult development (Table 2.1–5) by suggesting that the developmental process is basically the same in the adult as in the child, because, as with the child, the adult is always in the midst of an ongoing dynamic process, continually influenced by a constantly changing environment, body, and mind. Whereas child development focuses primarily on the formation of psychic structure, adult development is concerned with the continuing evolution of existing psychic structure and with its use. Although the fundamental issues of childhood continue in altered form as central aspects of adult life, attempts to explain all adult behavior and pathology in terms of the experiences of childhood are considered reductionistic. The adult past must be taken into account in understanding adult behavior in the same way that the childhood past is considered. The aging body is understood to have a profound influence on psychological

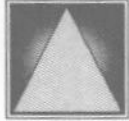

Table 2.1–5
Hypotheses about Development in Adulthood

Development is a lifelong, dynamic process that is basically the same in childhood and adulthood. Basic themes from childhood continue to affect psychic development in adulthood, but adult functioning and symptomatology are an amalgam of childhood and adult experiences. Recognition and acceptance of the finiteness of time and the inevitability of personal death are major psychic organizers in adulthood, in the promotion of normal development and in the formation of symptomatology.

development in adulthood, as is the growing midlife recognition and acceptance of the finiteness of time and the inevitability of personal death.

The eight conventional stages of development are as follows: (1) the prenatal period (from conception to birth), (2) infancy (from birth to about 15 months), (3) the toddler period (15 months to $2^1/_2$ years), (4) the preschool period ($2^1/_2$ to 6 years), (5) the middle years (6 to 12 years), (6) adolescence (12 to 19 years), (7) adulthood (20 to 65), and (8) late adulthood (old age). These stages form a continuum along which development proceeds, and rarely exists a clear-cut division between them. These stages will be discussed in detail in the following sections.

References

Alwin DF, Wray LA. A life-span developmental perspective on social status and health. *J Gernotol.* 2005;2:7–14.
Austrian SG, ed. *Developmental Theories through the Life Cycle.* New York: Columbia University Press; 2002.
Campbell AV. Mental health practice: Can philosophy help? *Aust N Z J Psychiatry.* 2005;39:1008–1010.
Colarusso CA. Adulthood. In: Sadock BJ, Sadock VA, eds. *Comprehensive Textbook of Psychiatry.* 8th ed. Vol. 2. Baltimore: Lippincott Williams & Wilkins; 2005:3565–3587.
de Winter AF, Oldehinkel AJ, Veenstra R, Brunnekreef JA, Verhulst FC, Ormel J. Evaluation of non-response bias in mental health determinants and outcomes in a large sample of pre-adolescents. *Eur J Epidemiol.* 2005;20(2):173–181.
Erikson E. *Childhood and Society.* New York: WW Norton; 1950.
Freud A. *The Ego and the Mechanisms of Defense.* New York: International Universities Press; 1966.
Kessler RC, Demler O, Frank RG, Olfson M, Pincus HA, Walters EE, Wang P, Wells KB, Zaslavsky AM. Prevalence and treatment of mental disorders, 1990 to 2003. *N Engl J Med.* 2005;24:2515.
Lidz T. *The Person: His and Her Development throughout the Life Cycle.* New York: Basic Books; 1976.
Vaillant GE, Valliant CO. Normality and mental health. In: Sadock BJ, Sadock VA, eds. *Kaplan & Sadock's Comprehensive Textbook of Psychiatry.* 8th ed. Vol. 1. Baltimore: Lippincott Williams & Wilkins; 2005:583–598.
Ziersch AM, Baum FE, MacDougall C, Putland C. Neighborhood life and social capital: The implication for health. *Soc Sci Med.* 2005;60 (1):71–86.

▲ 2.2 Embryo, Fetus, Infant, and Child

This section covers the embryo (conception to 8 weeks); the fetus (8 weeks to birth); infancy (birth to 15 months); the toddler period (15 months to $2^1/_2$ years); the preschool period ($2^1/_2$ to 6 years); and the middle years (6 to 12 years).

EMBRYO AND FETUS

Historically, the analysis of human development began with birth. The influence of endogenous and exogenous in utero factors, however, now requires that developmental schemes take intrauterine events into consideration. The infant is not a *tabula rasa*, a smooth slate upon which outside influences etch patterns. To the contrary, the newborn has already been influenced by myriad factors that have occurred in the *safety of the womb*, the result of which has produced wide individual differences among infants. For example, the studies of Stella Chess, M.D. and Alexander Thomas M.D. (described below) have demonstrated a wide range of temperamental differences among newborns. Maternal stress, through the production of adrenal hormones, also influences behavioral characteristics of newborns.

The time frame in which the development of the embryo and fetus occurs is known as the *prenatal period*. After implantation, the egg begins to divide and is known as an *embryo*. Growth and development occur at a rapid pace; by the end of 8 weeks, the shape is recognizably human, and the embryo has become a fetus. Figure 2.2–1 illustrates a sonogram of a 9- and 15-week fetus in utero.

The fetus maintains an internal equilibrium that, with variable effects, interacts continuously with the intrauterine environment. In general, most disorders that occur are multifactorial—the result of a combination of effects, some of which can be additive. Damage at the fetal stage usually has a more global impact than damage after birth, because rapidly growing organs are the most vulnerable. Boys are more vulnerable to developmental damage than girls; geneticists recognize that in humans and animals, girls show a propensity for greater biological vigor than boys, possibly because of the girls' second X chromosome.

Fetal Life

Much biological activity occurs in utero. A fetus is involved in a variety of behaviors that are necessary for adaptation outside the womb. For example, a fetus sucks on thumb and fingers; it folds and unfolds its body and eventually assumes a position in which its occiput is in an anterior vertex position, which is the position in which fetuses usually exit the uterus.

Behavior. Pregnant women are extraordinarily sensitive to prenatal movements. They describe their unborn babies as active or passive, as kicking vigorously or rolling around, as quiet when the mothers are active but as kicking as soon as the mothers try to rest.

Women usually detect fetal movements 16 to 20 weeks into the pregnancy; the fetus can be artificially set into total body motion by in utero stimulation of its ventral skin surfaces by the 14th week. The fetus may be able to hear by the 18th week, and it responds to loud noises with muscle contractions, movements, and an increased heart rate. Bright light flashed on the abdominal wall of the 20-week pregnant woman causes changes in fetal heart rate and position. The retinal structures begin to function at that time. Eyelids open at 7 months. Smell and taste are also developed at this time, and the fetus responds to substances that may be injected into the amniotic sac, such as contrast medium. Some reflexes present at birth exist in utero: the grasp reflex, which

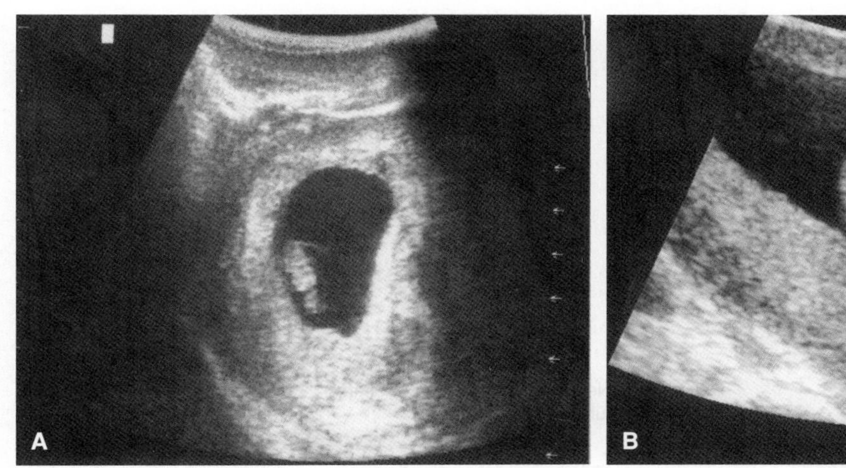

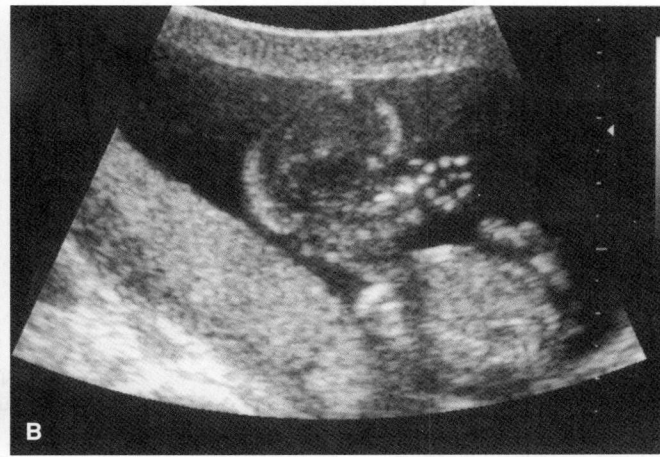

FIGURE 2.2–1
A. Sonogram of fetus at 9 weeks. **B.** Same fetus at 15 weeks. (Courtesy K.C. Attwell, M.D.)

appears at 17 weeks; the Moro (startle) reflex, which appears at 25 weeks; and the sucking reflex, which appears at about 28 weeks.

Nervous System. The nervous system arises from the neural plate, which is a dorsal ectodermal thickening that appears on about the 16th day of gestation. By the sixth week, part of the neural tube becomes the cerebral vesicle, which later becomes the cerebral hemispheres (Fig. 2.2–2).

The cerebral cortex begins to develop by the 10th week, but layers do not appear until the sixth month of pregnancy; the sensory cortex and the motor cortex are formed before the association cortex. Some brain function has been detected in utero by fetal encephalographic responses to sound. The human brain weighs about 350 g at birth and 1,450 g at full adult development, a fourfold increase, mainly in the neocortex. This increase is almost entirely because of the growth in the number and branching of dendrites establishing new connections. After birth, the number of new neurons is negligible. Uterine contractions can contribute to fetal neural development by causing the developing neural network to receive and transmit sensory impulses.

Pruning

Pruning refers to the programmed elimination during development of neurons, synapses, axons, and other brain structures from the original number, present at birth, to a lesser number. Thus, the developing brain contains structures and cellular elements that are absent in the older brain. The fetal brain generates more neurons than it will need for adult life. For example, in the visual cortex neurons increase from birth to 3 years of age, at which point they diminish in number. Another example is that the adult brain contains fewer neural connections than were present during the early and middle years of childhood. Approximately twice as many synapses are present in certain parts of the cerebral cortex during early postnatal life than during adulthood.

Pruning occurs to rid the nervous system of cells that have served their function in the development of the brain. Some neurons, for example, exist to produce neurotrophic or growth factors and are programmed to die—a process called apoptosis—when that function is fulfilled.

The implication of these observations is that the immature brain can be vulnerable in locations that lack sensitivity to injury later on. The developing white matter of the human brain before 32 weeks of gestation is especially sensitive to damage from hypoxic and ischemic injury and metabolic insults. Neurotransmitter receptors located on synaptic terminals are subject to injury from excessive stimulation by excitatory amino acids, (e.g., glutamate, aspartate), a process referred to as *excitotoxicity*. Research is proceeding on the implications of such events in the etiology of child and adult neuropsychiatric disorders such as schizophrenia.

Maternal Stress

Maternal stress correlates with high levels of stress hormones (epinephrine, norepinephrine, and adrenocorticotropic hormone) in the fetal bloodstream, which act directly on the fetal neuronal network to increase blood pressure, heart rate, and activity level. Mothers with high levels of anxiety are more likely to have babies who are hyperactive, irritable, and of low birthweight and who have problems feeding and sleeping than are mothers with low anxiety levels. A fever in the mother causes the fetus's temperature to rise.

Genetic Disorders

In many cases, genetic counseling depends on prenatal diagnosis. The diagnostic techniques used include amniocentesis (transabdominal aspiration of fluid from the amniotic sac), ultrasound examinations, X-ray studies, fetoscopy (direct visualization of the fetus), fetal blood and skin sampling, chorionic villus sampling, and α-fetoprotein screening. In about 2 percent of women tested, the results are positive for some abnormality, including X-linked disorders, neural tube defects (detected by high levels of α-fetoprotein), chromosomal disorders (e.g., trisomy 21), and various inborn errors of metabolism (e.g., Tay-Sachs disease

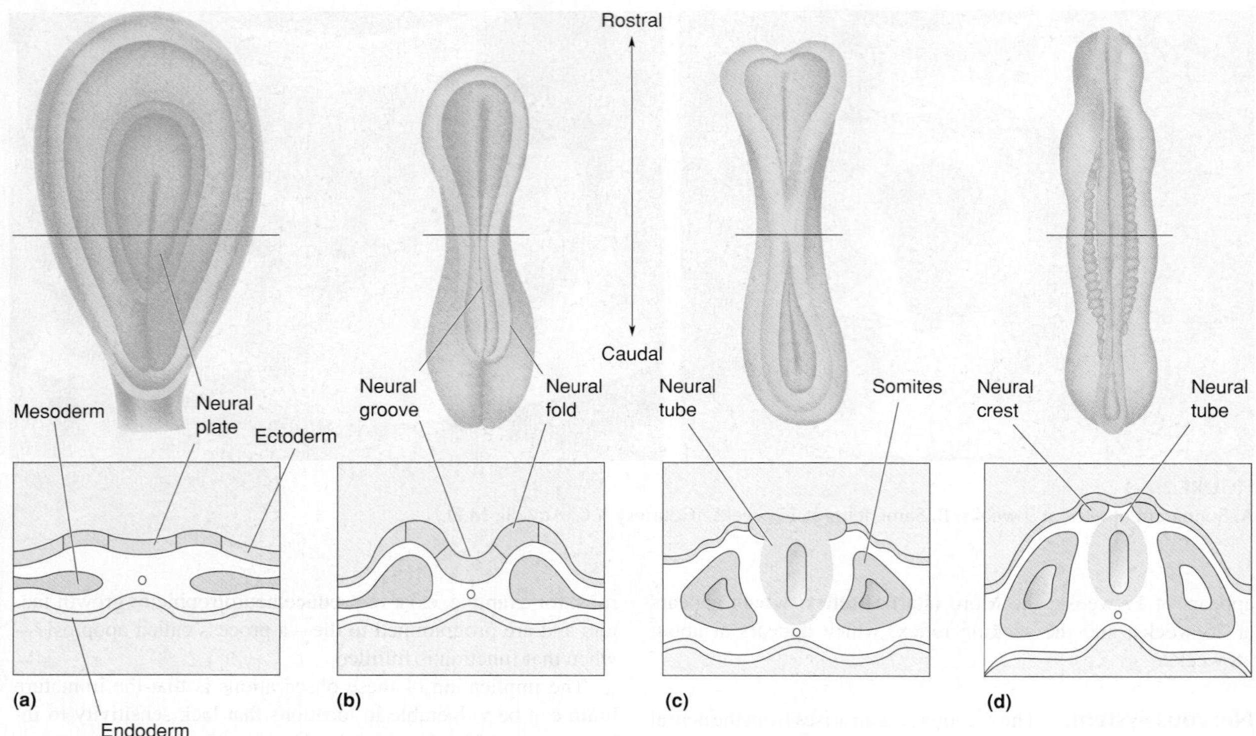

FIGURE 2.2–2

Formation of the neural tube and neural crest. These schematic illustrations follow the early development of the nervous system in the embryo. The drawings above are dorsal views of the embryo; those below are cross sections. **A.** The primitive embryonic central nervous system (CNS) begins as a thin sheet of ectoderm. **B.** The first important step in the development of the nervous system is the formation of the neural groove. **C.** The walls of the groove, called neural folds, come together and fuse, forming the neural tub. **D.** The bits of neural ectoderm that are pinched off when the tube rolls up are called the neural crest, from which the peripheral nervous system (PNS) will develop. The somites are mesoderm that will give rise to much of the skeletal system and the muscles. (Reprinted with permission from Bear MF, Conners BW, Paradiso MA, eds. *Neuroscience: Exploring the Brain.* 2nd ed. Baltimore: Lippincott Williams & Wilkins. 2001:179.)

and lipoidoses). Figure 2.2–3 illustrates hypertelorism of the eyes.

Some diagnostic tests carry a risk; for instance, about 5 percent of women who undergo fetoscopy miscarry. Amniocentesis, which is usually performed between the 14th and 16th weeks of pregnancy, causes fetal damage or miscarriage in less than 1 percent of women tested. Fully 98 percent of all prenatal tests in pregnant women reveal no abnormality in the fetus. Prenatal testing is recommended for women over 35 years of age and for those with a family history of a congenital defect.

Parental reactions to birth defects can include feelings of guilt, anxiety, or anger as their worst fears during the pregnancy are realized. Some degree of depression over the loss of the fantasized perfect child may be observed before the parents develop more active coping strategies. Termination of a pregnancy because of a known or suspected birth defect is an option chosen by some women.

Maternal Drug Use

Alcohol. Alcohol use in pregnancy is a major cause of serious physical and mental birth defects in children. Each year, up to 40,000 babies are born with some degree of alcohol-related damage. The National Institute on Drug Abuse (NIDA) reports that 19 percent of pregnant women used alcohol during their pregnancy, the highest rate being among white women.

Fetal alcohol syndrome (Fig. 2.2–4) affects about one third of all infants born to alcoholic women. The syndrome is characterized by growth retardation of prenatal origin (height, weight); minor anomalies, including microphthalmia (small eyeballs), short palpebral fissures, midface hypoplasia (underdevelopment), a smooth or short philtrum, and a thin upper lip; and central nervous system (CNS) manifestations, including microcephaly (head circumference below the third percentile), a history of delayed development, hyperactivity, attention deficits, learning disabilities, intellectual deficits, and seizures. The incidence of infants born with fetal alcohol syndrome is about 0.5 per 1,000 live births.

Some studies suggest that alcohol use during pregnancy may contribute to attention-deficit hyperactivity disorder (ADHD). Animal experiments have shown that alcohol reduces the number of active dopamine neurons in the midbrain area and ADHD is associated with reduced dopaminergic activity in the brain.

Smoking. At some point during their pregnancy, about 20 percent of women smoked, the highest rate being among white women. Smoking during pregnancy is associated with both

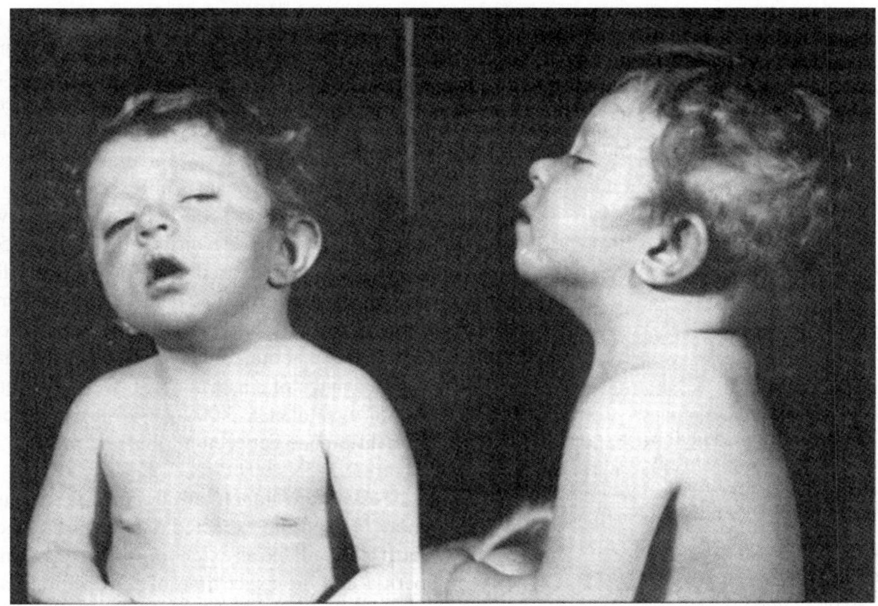

FIGURE 2.2–3

Hypertetorism. Note the wide distance between the eyes, flat nasal bridge, and external strabismus. (Courtesy of Michael Malone, M.D. Children's Hospital, Washington, D.C.)

premature births and below-average infant birthweight. Some reports have associated sudden infant death syndrome (SIDS) to be associated with mothers who smoke.

Other Substances. Marijuana (used by 3 percent of all pregnant women) and cocaine (used by 1 percent) are the two most commonly abused illegal drugs, followed by heroin. The use of illegal drugs is higher among African-American women than among white women. Marijuana is associated with low infant birthweight, prematurity, and withdrawal-like symptoms, including excessive crying, tremors, and hyperemesis (severe and chronic vomiting). Crack cocaine use by women during pregnancy has been correlated with behavioral abnormalities such as increased irritability and crying and decreased desire for human contact. Infants born to mothers dependent on narcotics go through a withdrawal syndrome at birth.

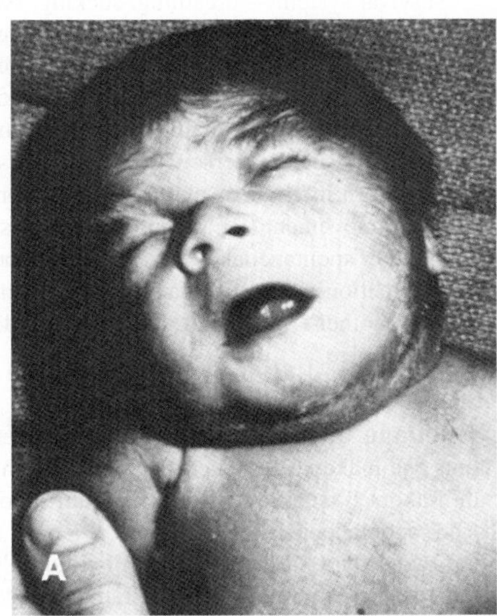

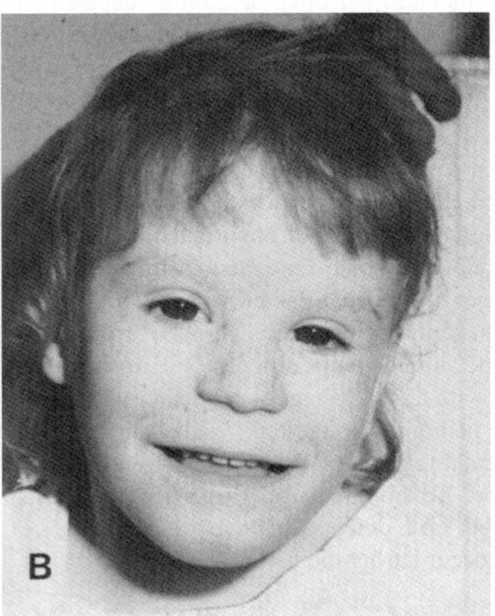

FIGURE 2.2–4

Photographs of children with "fetal-alcohol syndrome." **A.** Severe case. **B.** Slightly affected child. Note in both children the short palpebral fissures and hypoplasia of the maxilla. Usually, the defect includes other craniofacial abnormalities. Cardiovascular defects and limb deformities are also common symptoms of the fetal alcohol syndrome. (From Langman J. *Medical Embryology.* 7th ed. Baltimore: Williams & Wilkins; 1995:108, with permission.)

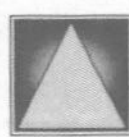

Table 2.2–1
Causes of Human Malformations Observed During the First Year of Life

Suspected Cause	% of Total
Genetic	
Autosomal genetic disease	15–20
Cytogenic (chromosomal abnormalities)	5
Unknown	
Polygenic	
Multifactorial (genetic-environmental interactions)	
Spontaneous error of development	
Synergistic interactions of teratogens	
Environmental	
Maternal conditions: diabetes; endocrinopathies; nutritional deficiencies, starvation; drug and substance addictions	4
Maternal infections: rubella, toxoplasmosis, syphilis, herpes, cytomegalic inclusion disease, varicella, Venezuelan equine encephalitis, parvovirus B19	3
Mechanical problems (deformations): abnormal cord constrictions, disparity in uterine size and uterine contents	1–2
Chemicals, drugs, radiation, hyperthermia	<1
Preconception exposures (excluding mutagens and infectious agents)	<1

Reprinted with permission from Brent RL, Beckman DA. Environmental teratogens. *Bull NY Acad Med.* 1990;66:125.

Prenatal exposure to various medications can also result in abnormalities. Common drugs with teratogenic effects include antibiotics (tetracyclines), anticonvulsants (valproate [Depakene], carbamazepine [Tegretol], phenytoin [Dilantin]), progesterone-estrogens, lithium (Eskalith), and warfarin (Coumadin).

Recently, a neonatal behavioral syndrome was described that was linked to in utero selective serotonin reuptake inhibitor (SSRI) exposure during the mother's last month of pregnancy. The CNS was affected with seizures occurring in severe cases.

Radiation. When a woman is exposed to severe radiation between weeks 2 and 15 of her pregnancy, the baby will be born with gross deformities, stunted growth, abnormal brain function, or cancer that may develop some time later in life. Estimates are that 3 to 6 percent of all newborns have some sort of birth defect that is fatal at birth or that causes permanent disability. Babies exposed to the atomic bombs dropped on Hiroshima and Nagasaki during the 8- to 15-week stage of pregnancy were found to have a high rate of brain damage that resulted in lower IQ and even severe mental retardation. They also suffered stunted growth (up to 4 percent shorter than average people) and an increased risk of other birth defects. Table 2.2–1 lists causes of malformations that occur during the first year of life.

INFANCY

The delivery of the fetus marks the start of infancy. The average newborn weighs about 3,400 g (7.5 lb). Small fetuses, defined as those with a birthweight below the 10th percentile for their gestational age, occur in about 7 percent of all pregnancies. At the 26th to the 28th week of gestation, the prematurely born fetus has a good chance of survival. Arnold Gesell, M.D. described developmental schedules that are widely used in both pediatrics and child psychiatry. These schedules outline the qualitative sequence of children's motor, adaptive, and personal-social behavior from birth to 6 years (Table 2.2–2).

Premature infants are defined as those with a gestation of less than 34 weeks or a birthweight under 2,500 g (5.5 lb). Such infants are at increased risk for learning disabilities, such as dyslexia, emotional and behavioral problems, mental retardation, and child abuse. With each 100-g increment of weight, beginning at about 1,000 g (2.2 lb), infants have a progressively better chance of survival. A 36-week-old fetus has less chance of survival than a 3,000-g (6.6-lb) fetus born close to term. The difference between normal and preterm infants is shown in Figure 2.2–5.

Postmature infants are defined as infants born 2 weeks or more beyond the expected date of birth. Because pregnancy at term is calculated as extending 40 weeks from the last menstrual period and the exact time of fertilization varies, the incidence of postmaturity is high if based on menstrual history alone. The postmature baby typically has long nails, scanty lanugo hair, more scalp hair than usual, and increased alertness.

Developmental Landmarks

Reflexes and Survival Systems at Birth. Reflexes are present at birth. They include the rooting reflex (puckering of the lips in response to perioral stimulation), the grasp reflex, the plantar (Babinski) reflex, the knee reflex, the abdominal reflexes, the startle (Moro) reflex (Fig. 2.2–6), and the tonic neck reflex. In normal children, the grasp reflex, the startle reflex, and the tonic neck reflex disappear by the fourth month. The Babinski reflex usually disappears by the 12th month.

Survival systems—breathing, sucking, swallowing, and circulatory and temperature homeostasis—are relatively functional at birth, but the sensory organs are incompletely developed. Further differentiation of neurophysiological functions depends on an active process of stimulatory reinforcement from the external environment, such as persons touching and stroking the infant. The newborn infant is awake for only a short period each day; rapid eye movement (REM) and non-REM sleep are present at birth. Other spontaneous behaviors include crying, smiling, and penile erection in males. Infants 1 day old can detect the smell of their mother's milk, and those 3 days old distinguish their mother's voice.

Language and Cognitive Development. At birth, infants can make noises, such as crying, but they do not vocalize until about 8 weeks. At that time, guttural or babbling sounds occur spontaneously, especially in response to the mother. The persistence and further evolution of children's vocalizations depend on parental reinforcement. Language development occurs in well-delineated stages as outlined in Table 2.2–3.

By the end of infancy (about 2 years), infants have transformed reflexes into voluntary actions that are the building blocks of cognition. They begin to interact with the environment, to experience feedback from their own bodies, and to become

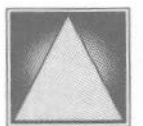

Table 2.2–2
Landmarks of Normal Behavioral Development

Age	Motor and Sensory Behavior	Adaptive Behavior	Personal and Social Behavior
Birth to 4 wks	Hand-to-mouth reflex, grasping reflex Rooting reflex (puckering lips in response to perioral stimulation), Moro reflex (digital extension when startled), sucking reflex, Babinski reflex (toes spread when sole of foot is touched) Differentiates sounds (orients to human voice) and sweet and sour tastes Visual tracking Fixed focal distance of 8 inches Makes alternating crawling movements Moves head laterally when placed in prone position	Anticipatory feeding-approach behavior at 4 days Responds to sound of rattle and bell Regards moving objects momentarily	Responsiveness to mother's face, eyes, and voice within first few hours of life Endogenous smile Independent play (until 2 years) Quiets when picked up Impassive face
4 wks	Tonic neck reflex positions predominate Hands fisted Head sags but can hold head erect for a few seconds Visual fixation, stereoscopic vision (12 weeks)	Follows moving objects to the midline Shows no interest and drops object immediately	Regards face and diminishes activity Responds to speech Smiles preferentially to mother
16 wks	Symmetrical postures predominate Holds head balanced Head lifted 90° when prone on forearm Visual accommodation	Follows a slowly moving object well Arms activate on sight of dangling object	Spontaneous social smile (exogenous) Aware of strange situations
28 wks	Sits steadily, leaning forward on hands Bounces actively when placed in standing position	One-hand approach and grasp of toy Bangs and shakes rattle Transfers toys	Takes feet to mouth Pats mirror image Starts to imitate mother's sounds and actions
40 wks	Sits alone with good coordination Creeps Pulls self to standing position Points with index finger	Matches two objects at midline Attempts to imitate scribble	Separation anxiety manifest when taken away from mother Responds to social play, such as pat-a-cake and peekaboo Feeds self cracker and holds own bottle
52 wks	Walks with one hand held Stands alone briefly	Seeks novelty	Cooperates in dressing
15 mos	Toddles Creeps up stairs		Points or vocalizes wants Throws objects in play or refusal
18 mos	Coordinated walking, seldom falls Hurls ball Walks up stairs with one hand held	Builds a tower of three or four cubes Scribbles spontaneously and imitates a writing stroke	Feeds self in part, spills Pulls toy on string Carries or hugs a special toy, such as a doll Imitates some behavioral patterns with slight delay
2 yrs	Runs well, no falling Kicks large ball Goes up and down stairs alone Fine motor skills increase	Builds a tower of six or seven cubes Aligns cubes, imitating train Imitates vertical and circular strokes Develops original behaviors	Pulls on simple garment Domestic mimicry Refers to self by name Says "no" to mother Separation anxiety begins to diminish Organized demonstrations of love and protest Parallel play (plays side by side but does not interact with other children)
3 yrs	Rides tricycle Jumps from bottom steps Alternates feet going up stairs	Builds tower of 9 or 10 cubes Imitates a three-cube bridge Copies a circle and a cross	Puts on shoes Unbuttons buttons Feeds self well Understands taking turns
4 yrs	Walks down stairs one step to a tread Stands on one foot for 5 to 8 seconds	Copies a cross Repeats four digits Counts three objects with correct pointing	Washes and dries own face Brushes teeth Associative or joint play (plays cooperatively with other children)
5 yrs	Skips, using feet alternately Usually has complete sphincter control Fine coordination improves	Copies a square Draws a recognizable person with a head, a body, and limbs Counts 10 objects accurately	Dresses and undresses self Prints a few letters Plays competitive exercise games
6 yrs	Rides two-wheel bicycle	Prints name Copies triangle	Ties shoelaces

Adapted from Arnold Gessell, M.D., and Stella Chess, M.D.

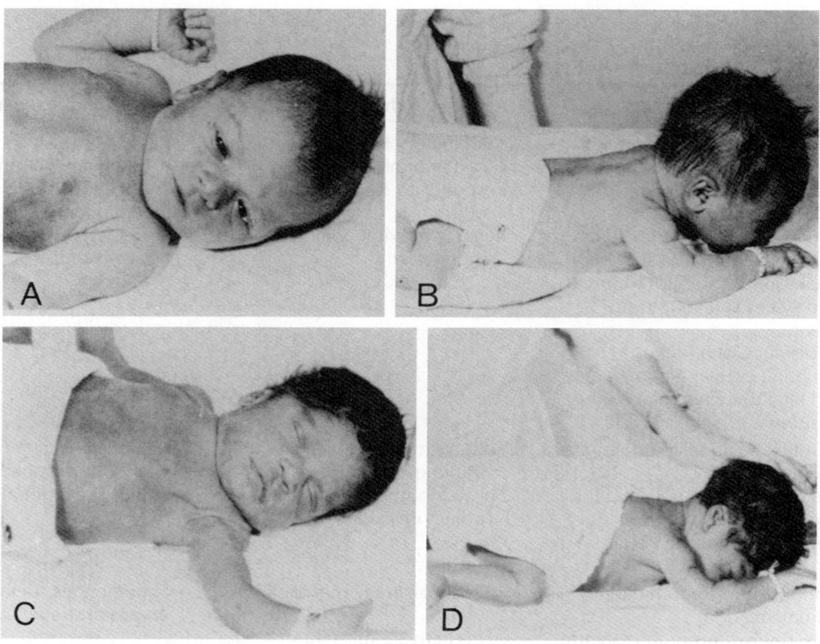

FIGURE 2.2–5
Contrast between full-term (**A** and **B**) and premature (**C** and **D**) infants. Note the limp sprawl of the baby in **C** and the difficulty in raising the head to clear the nose and mouth in **D**. (Reprinted with permission from Stone LJ, Church J. *Childhood and Adolescence.* 4th ed. New York: Random House; 1979:7.)

intentional in their actions. By the end of the second year of life, children begin to use symbolic play and language.

Jean Piaget (1896–1980), a Swiss psychologist, observed the growing capacity of young children (including his own) to think and to reason. An outline of the main stages of his theory of cognitive development is presented in Table 2.2–4, and his work is discussed extensively in Section 4.1.

Emotional and Social Development. By the age of 3 weeks, infants imitate the facial movements of adult caregivers. They open their mouths and thrust out their tongues in response to adults who do the same. By the third and fourth months of life, these behaviors are easily elicited. These imitative behaviors are believed to be the precursors of infants' emotional life. The smiling response occurs in two phases: the first phase is endogenous smiling, which occurs spontaneously within the first 2 months and is unrelated to external stimulation; the second phase is exogenous smiling, which is stimulated from the outside, usually by the mother, and occurs by the 16th week.

The stages of emotional development parallel those of cognitive development. Indeed, the caregiving person provides the major stimulus for both aspects of mental growth. Human infants

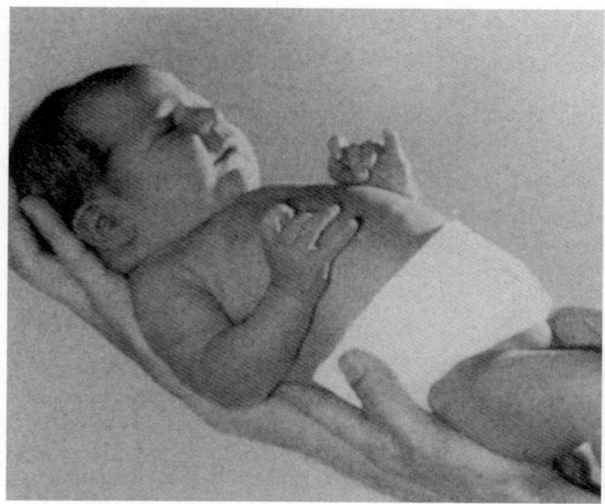

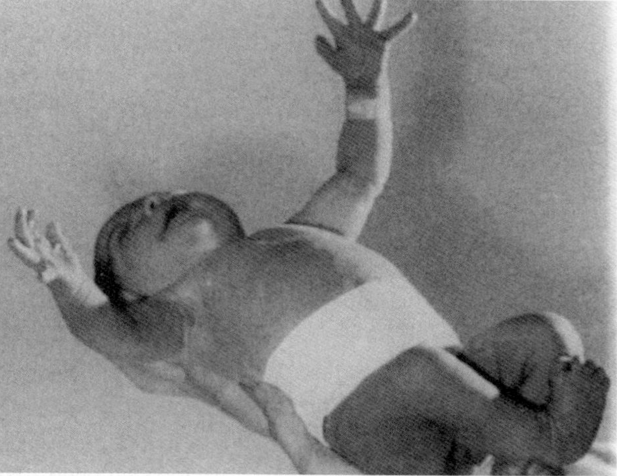

FIGURE 2.2–6
Moro reflex. (Reprinted with permission from Stone LJ, Church J. *Childhood and Adolescence.* 4th ed. New York: Random House; 1979:14.)

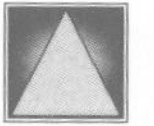

Table 2.2–3
Language Development

Age and Stage of Development	Mastery of Comprehension	Mastery of Expression
0–6 mos	Shows startle response to loud or sudden sounds Attempts to localize sounds, turning eyes or head Appears to listen to speakers, may respond with smile Recognizes warning, angry, and friendly voices Responds to hearing own name	Has vocalizations other than crying Has differential cries for hunger, pain Makes vocalizations to show pleasure Plays at making sounds Babbles (a repeated series of sounds)
7–11 mos Attending-to-Language	Shows listening selectivity (voluntary control over responses to sounds) Listens to music or singing with interest Recognizes "no," "hot," own name Looks at pictures being named for up to 1 minute Listens to speech without being distracted by other sounds	Responds to own name with vocalizations Imitates the melody of utterances Uses jargon (own language) Has gestures (shakes head for no) Has exclamation ("oh-oh") Plays language games (pat-a-cake, peekaboo)
12–18 mos Single-Word	Shows gross discriminations between dissimilar sounds (bells vs. dog vs. horn vs. mother's or father's voice) Understands basic body parts, names of common objects Acquires understanding of some new words each week Can identify simple objects (baby, ball, etc.) from a group of objects or pictures Understands up to 150 words by age 18 mos	Uses single words (mean age of first word is 11 months; by age 18 months, child is using up to 20 words) "Talks" to toys, self, or others using long patterns of jargon and occasional words Approximately 25% of utterances are intelligible All vowels articulated correctly Initial and final consonants often omitted
12–24 mos Two-Word Messages	Responds to simple directions ("Give me the ball") Responds to action commands ("Come here," "Sit down") Understands pronouns (me, him, her, you) Begins to understand complex sentences ("When we go to the store, I'll buy you some candy")	Uses two-word utterances ("Mommy sock," "all gone," "ball here") Imitates environmental sounds in play ("moo," "mmm, mmm," etc.) Refers to self by name, begins to use pronouns Echoes two or more last words of sentences Begins to use three-word telegraphic utterances ("all gone ball," "me go now") Utterances 26% to 50% intelligible Uses language to ask for needs
24–36 mos Grammar Formation	Understands small body parts (elbow, chin, eyebrow) Understands family name categories (grandma, baby) Understands size (little one, big one) Understands most adjectives Understands functions (why do we eat, why do we sleep)	Uses real sentences with grammatical function words (can, will, the, a) Usually announces intentions before acting "Conversations" with other children, usually just monologues Jargon and echolalia gradually drop from speech Increased vocabulary (up to 270 words at 2 years, 895 words at 3 years) Speech 50% to 80% intelligible *P, b, m* articulated correctly Speech may show rhythmic disturbances
36–54 mos Grammar Development	Understands prepositions (under, behind, between) Understands many words (up to 3,500 at 3 yrs, 5,500 at 4 yrs) Understands cause and effect (What do you do when you're hungry?, cold?) Understands analogies (Food is to eat, milk is to ____)	Correct articulation of *n, w, ng, h, t, d, k, g* Uses language to relate incidents from the past Uses wide range of grammatical forms: plurals, past tense, negatives, questions Plays with language: rhymes, exaggerates Speech 90% intelligible, occasional errors in the ordering of sounds within words Able to define words Egocentric use of language rare Can repeat a 12-syllable sentence correctly Some grammatical errors still occur
55 mos on True Communication	Understands concepts of number, speed, time, space Understands left and right Understands abstract terms Is able to categorize items into semantic classes	Uses language to tell stories, share ideas, and discuss alternatives Increasing use of varied grammar; spontaneous self-correction of grammatical errors Stabilizing of articulation *f, v, s, z, l, r, th,* and consonant clusters Speech 100% intelligible

(Reprinted from Rulter M, Hersov L, eds. *Child and Adolescent Psychiatry.* London: Blackwell; 1985, with permission.)

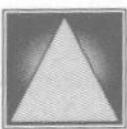

Table 2.2–4
Piaget's Stages of Cognitive Development

Period of Development	Cognitive Spatial Stages	Cognitive Achievements
Gestational		Fetus can "learn" sounds and respond differentially to them after birth
Infancy: Birth–2 yrs	Sensorimotor Includes concepts:	Infants "think" with their eyes, ears, and senses
Birth–1 mo	Reflective; egocentric (newer research refutes this)	Newborns can learn to associate stroking with sucking
4–8 mos	Secondary circular: looks for objects partially hidden	Newborns can learn to suck to produce certain visual displays or music
8–12 mos	Secondary circulation coordinated: peek-a-boo, finds hidden objects	Can remember for 1-mo periods Can play with parent by looking for partially hidden objects
12–18 mos	Tertiary circular: explores properties and drops objects	Memory improves
18 mos–2 yrs	Mental representation, make-believe play; memory of objects	Body parts used as objects Can stack one object within another Remembers hidden objects Drops objects over crib Knows animal sounds; names objects Knows body parts and familiar pictures Can understand causes not visible
Early Childhood: 2–5 yrs		
2–7 yrs	Preoperational Includes concepts:	Preschoolers use symbols Development of language and makebelieve
	Egocentrism: "I want you to eat this too." Animistic: "I'm afraid of the moon." Lack of hierarchy: "Where do these blocks go?" Centration: "I want it now, not after dinner." Irreversibility: "I don't know how to go back to that room."	No sign of logic 3-yr-olds can count 2–3 objects; know colors and age 4-yr-olds can fantasize without concrete props
2–5 yrs	Transductive reasoning: "We have to go this way because that's the way Daddy goes."	5- to 6-yr-olds get humor; understand good and bad; can do some chores 7- to 11-yr-olds have good memory; recall; can solve problems
Middle Childhood: 6–11 yrs		
6 yrs onward		Children begin to think logically
7–11 yrs	Concrete operational Includes concepts:	Understand conservation of matter
	Hierarchical classification—arranges cars by types	Frozen milk same amount as melted
	Reversibility—can play games backward and forward (e.g., checkers, triple kings)	Can organize objects into hierarchies
	Conservation—lose two dimes and look for same	Children seem rational and organized
	Decentration—worry about small details, obsessive Spatial operations—likes models for directions Horizontal decalage—conservation of weight, logic Transitive inference—syllogisms; compare everything, brand names important	
Adolescence: 11–19 yrs	Formal operational	
11 yrs onward	Includes concepts:	Abstraction and reason
	Hypothetical-deductive reasoning; adolescent quick thinking or excuses Imaginary audience—everyone is looking at them Personal fable—inflated opinion of themselves Propositional thinking—logic	Can think of all possibilities

depend totally on adults for survival. Through regular and predictable interaction, an infant's behavioral repertoire expands as a consequence of caregivers' social responses (Table 2.2–5).

In the first year, infants' moods are highly variable and intimately related to internal states such as hunger. Toward the second two thirds of the first year, infants' moods grow increasingly related to external social cues; a parent can get even a hungry infant to smile. When the infant is internally comfortable, a sense of interest and pleasure in the world and in its primary caregivers should prevail. Prolonged separation from the mother (or other primary caregiver) during the second 6 months of life can lead to depression that may persist into adulthood as part of an individual's character.

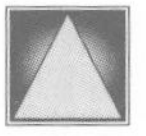

Table 2.2–5
Emotional Development

Stages First Seen	Emotional Skills	Emotional Behavior
Gestational–Infancy: 0–2 yrs		
0–2 mos onward	Love, evoked by touching Fear, evoked by loud noise Rage, evoked by body restrictions Brain pathways for emotion forming	Social smile and joy shown Responds to emotions of others All emotions there
3–4 mos onward	Self-regulation of emotions starts Brain pathways of emotion growing	Laughter possible and more control over smiles; anger shown
7–12 mos	Self-regulation of emotion grows Increased intensity of basic three	Able to elicit more responsiveness Denies to cope with stress
1–2 yrs	Shame and pride appear; envy, embarrassment appear Displaces onto other children	Some indications of empathy starting; expressions of feeling: "I like you, Daddy" "I'm sorry" Likes attention and approval; enjoys play alone or next to peers
Early Childhood: 2–5 yrs		
3–6 yrs	Can understand causes of many emotions Can begin to find ways for regulating emotions and for expressing them Identifies with adult to cope	Empathy increases with understanding More response and less reaction; self-regulation: "Use your words to say that you are angry with him" Aggression becomes competition By age 5, shows sensitivity to criticism and cares about feelings of others
Middle Childhood: 5–11 yrs		Ego rules until age 6
7–11 yrs	Can react to the feelings of others More aware of other's feelings	Empathy becomes altruism: "I feel so bad about their fire, I'm going to give them some of my things" Superego dominates

Temperamental Differences

There are strong suggestions of inborn differences and wide variability in autonomic reactivity and temperament among individual infants. Chess and Thomas identified nine behavioral dimensions, in which reliable differences among infants can be observed (Table 2.2–6).

The ratings of individual children showed considerable stability over a 25-year follow-up period, but some temperamental traits did not persist. This finding was attributed to genetic effects on personality; that is, some gene actions were discontinuous. A complex interplay exists among the initial characteristics of infants, the mode of parental management, children's subsequent behavior, and even the appearance of symptoms. These connections support the concept of the importance of both genetic endowment (nature) and environmental experience (nurture) in behavior.

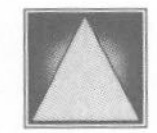

Table 2.2–6
Temperament—Newborn to 6 Years

Dimension	Description
Activity level	Percent of time spent in activities
Distractibility	Degree to which stimuli are allowed to alter behavior
Adaptability	Ease moving into change
Attention span	Amount of time spent on attending
Intensity	Energy level
Threshold of responsiveness	Intensity required for response
Quality of mood	Amount positive compared to amount negative behavior
Rhythmicity	Regulation of functions
Approach/withdrawal	Response to new situations

Attachment

Bonding is the term used to describe the intense emotional and psychological relationship a mother develops for her baby. Attachment is the relationship the baby develops with its caregivers. Infants in the first months after birth become attuned to social and interpersonal interaction. They show a rapidly increasing responsivity to the external environment and an ability to form a special relationship with significant primary caregivers—that is, to form an attachment. Table 2.2–7 lists the common attachment styles.

Harry Harlow. Harry Harlow, M.D. studied social learning and the effects of social isolation in monkeys. Harlow placed newborn rhesus monkeys with two types of surrogate mothers—one a wire-mesh surrogate with a feeding bottle and the other a wire-mesh surrogate covered with terry cloth. The monkeys preferred the terry-cloth surrogates, which provided contact and comfort, to the feeding surrogate. (When hungry, the infant monkeys would go to the feeding bottle but then would quickly return to the terry-cloth surrogate.) When frightened, monkeys raised with terry-cloth surrogates showed intense clinging behavior and appeared to be comforted, whereas those raised with wire-mesh surrogates gained no comfort and appeared to be disorganized. The results of Harlow's experiments were widely interpreted as indicating that infant attachment is not simply the result of feeding.

Both types of surrogate-reared monkeys were subsequently unable to adjust to life in a monkey colony and had extraordinary

Table 2.2–7
Types of Attachment

Secure Attachment	Children show fewer adjustment problems; however, these children have typically received more consistent and developmentally appropriate parenting for most of their life. The parents of securely attached children are likely better able to maintain these aspects of parenting through a divorce. Given that the family factors that lead to divorce also impact the children, there could be fewer securely attached children in divorcing families.
Insecure/Avoidant Attachment	Children become anxious, clinging, and angry with the parent. These children typically come from families with adults who were also insecurely attached to their families and, thus, were unable to provide the kind of consistency, emotional responsiveness, and care that securely attached parents could offer. Such parents have a more difficult time with divorce, and are more likely to become rejecting.
Insecure/Ambivalent Attachment	Children generally are raised with disorganized, neglecting, and inattentive parenting. The parents are even less able to provide stability and psychological strength for them after a divorce and, as a result, the children are even more likely to become clinging but unconsolable in their distress, as well as to act out, suffer mood swings, and become oversensitive to stress.

difficulty learning to mate. When impregnated, the females failed to mother their young. These behavioral peculiarities were attributed to the isolates' lack of mothering in infancy.

John Bowlby. John Bowlby studied the attachment of infants to mothers and concluded that early separation of infants from their mothers had severe negative effects on children's emotional and intellectual development. He described attachment behavior, which develops during the first year of life, as the maintenance of physical contact between the mother and child when the child is hungry, frightened, or in distress. (Section 4.2 discusses attachment theory.)

Mary Ainsworth. Mary Ainsworth expanded on Bowlby's observations and found that the interaction between mother and baby during the attachment period influences the baby's current and future behavior significantly. Many observers believe that patterns of infant attachment affect future adult emotional relationships. Patterns of attachment vary among babies; for example, some babies signal or cry less than others. Sensitive responsiveness to infant signals, such as cuddling the baby when it cries, causes infants to cry less in later months. Close bodily contact with the mother when the baby signals for her is also associated with the growth of self-reliance, rather than clinging dependence, as the baby grows older. Unresponsive mothers produce anxious babies.

Ainsworth also confirmed that attachment serves to reduce anxiety. What she called the *secured base effect* enables a child to move away from the attachment figure and explore the environment. Inanimate objects, such as a teddy bear or a blanket (called the *transitional object* by Donald Winnicott), also serve as a secure base, one that often accompanies children as they investigate the world. A growing body of literature derived from direct observation of mother–infant interactions and longitudinal studies has expanded on, and refined, Ainsworth's original descriptions. Maternal sensitivity and responsiveness are the main determinants of secure attachment. But when the attachment is insecure, the type of insecurity (avoidant, anxious, ambivalent) is determined by infant temperament. Overall, male infants are less likely to have secure attachments and are more vulnerable to changes in maternal sensitivity than are female infants.

The attachment of the firstborn child is decreased by the birth of a second, but it is decreased much more when the firstborn is 2 to 5 years of age when the younger sibling is born than when the firstborn is under 24 months. Not surprisingly, the extent of the decrease also depends on the mother's own sense of security, confidence, and mental health.

Social Deprivation Syndromes and Maternal Neglect. Investigators, especially René Spitz, have long documented the severe developmental retardation that accompanies maternal rejection and neglect. Infants in institutions characterized by low staff-to-infant ratios and frequent turnover of personnel tend to display marked developmental retardation, even with adequate physical care and freedom from infection. The same infants, placed in adequate foster or adoptive care, exhibit marked acceleration in development.

Fathers and Attachment. Babies become attached to fathers as well as to mothers, but the attachment is different. Generally, mothers hold babies for caregiving, and fathers hold babies for purposes of play. Given a choice of either parent after separation infants usually go to the mother, but if the mother is unavailable they turn to the father for comfort. Babies raised in extended families or with multiple caregivers are able to establish many attachments.

Stranger Anxiety. A fear of strangers is first noted in infants at about 26 weeks of age, but is not fully developed until about 32 weeks (8 months). At the approach of a stranger, infants cry and cling to their mothers. Babies exposed to only one caregiver are more likely to have stranger anxiety than are those exposed to a variety of caregivers. Stranger anxiety is believed to result from a baby's growing ability to distinguish caregivers from all other persons.

Separation anxiety, which occurs between 10 and 18 months of age, is related to stranger anxiety but is not identical to it. Separation from the person to whom the infant is attached precipitates separation anxiety. Stranger anxiety, however, occurs even when the infant is in the mother's arms. The infant learns to separate as it starts to crawl and move away from the mother, but the infant constantly looks back and frequently returns to the mother for reassurance.

Margaret Mahler (1897–1985) (Fig. 2.2–7) proposed a theory to describe how young children acquire a sense of identity separate from their mothers'. Her theory of separation-individuation was based on observations of the interactions of children and their mothers. This theory is outlined in Table 2.2–8.

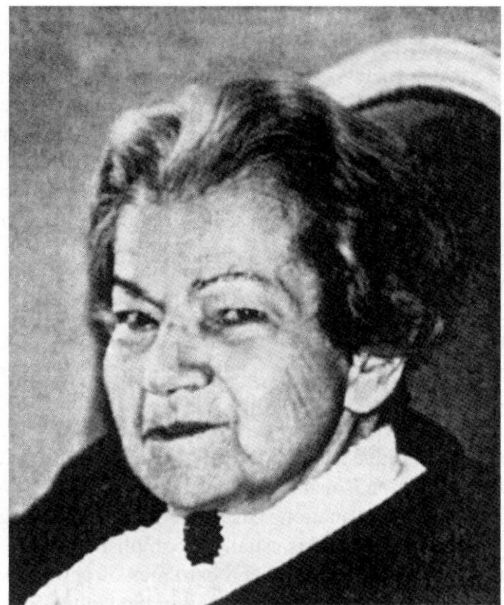

FIGURE 2.2–7
Margaret Mahler (1897–1985) elaborated the objects–relations approach, which many see as the main focus of contemporary psychoanalysis. (Reprinted with permission from Carson RC, Butcher JN, Coleman JC. Eds. *Abnormal Psychology and Modern Life.* 8th Ed. Illinois: Scott, Foresman and Company; 1988:66.)

Infant Care

Clinicians are now beginning to view infants as important actors in the family drama, ones who partly determine its course. Infants' behavior controls mothers' behavior, just as mothers' behavior modulates infants' behavior. A calm, smiling, predictable infant is a powerful reward for tender maternal care. A jittery, irregular, irritable infant tries a mother's patience. When a mother's capacity for giving is marginal, such infant traits may cause her to turn away from her child and thus complicate the child's already-troubled beginnings.

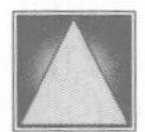

Table 2.2–8
Stages of Separation-Individuation Proposed by Mahler

1. Normal autism (birth–2 mos)
   Periods of sleep outweigh periods of arousal in a state reminiscent of intrauterine life.
2. Symbiosis (2–5 mos)
   Developing perceptual abilities gradually enable infants to distinguish the inner from the outer world; mother–infant is perceived as a single fused entity.
3. Differentiation (5–10 mos)
   Progressive neurological development and increased alertness draw infants' attention away from self to the outer world. Physical and psychological distinctiveness from the mother is gradually appreciated.
4. Practicing (10–18 mos)
   The ability to move autonomously increases children's exploration of the outer world.
5. Rapprochement (18–24 mos)
   As children slowly realize their helplessness and dependence, the need for independence alternates with the need for closeness. Children move away from their mothers and come back for reassurance.
6. Object constancy (2–5 yrs)
   Children gradually comprehend and are reassured by the permanence of mother and other important people, even when not in their presence.

Parental Fit. Parental fit describes how well the mother or father relates to the newborn or developing infant; the idea takes into account temperamental characteristics of both parent and child. Each newborn has innate psychophysiological characteristics, which are known collectively as *temperament.* Chess and Thomas identified a range of normal temperamental patterns, from the difficult child at one end of the spectrum to the easy child at the other end.

Difficult children, who make up 10 percent of all children, have a hyperalert physiological makeup. They react intensely to stimuli (cry easily at loud noises), sleep poorly, eat at unpredictable times, and are difficult to comfort. *Easy children,* who make up 40 percent of all children, are regular in eating, eliminating, and sleeping; they are flexible, can adapt to change and new stimuli with a minimum of distress, and are easily comforted when they cry. The other 50 percent of children are mixtures of these two types. The difficult child is harder to raise and places greater demands on the parent than the easy child. Chess and Thomas used the term *goodness of fit* to characterize the harmonious and consonant interaction between a mother and a child in their motivations, capacities, and styles of behavior. Poor fit is likely to lead to distorted development and maladaptive functioning. A difficult child must be recognized, because parents of such infants often have feelings of inadequacy and believe that they are doing something wrong to account for the child's difficulty in sleeping and eating and their problems comforting the child. In addition, most difficult children have emotional disturbances later in life.

Good-Enough Mothering. Winnicott believed that infants begin life in a state of nonintegration, with unconnected and diffuse experiences, and that mothers provide the relationship that enables infants' incipient selves to emerge. Mothers supply a holding environment in which infants are contained and experienced. During the last trimester of pregnancy and for the first few months of a baby's life, the mother is in a state of primary maternal preoccupation, absorbed in fantasies about, and experiences with, her baby. The mother need not be perfect, but she must provide good-enough mothering. She plays a vital role in bringing the world to the child and offering empathic anticipation of the infant's needs. If the mother can resonate with the infant's needs, the baby can become attuned to its own bodily functions and drives that are the basis for the gradually evolving sense of self.

TODDLER PERIOD

The second year of life is marked by accelerated motor and intellectual development. The ability to walk gives toddlers some control over their own actions; this mobility enables children to determine when to approach and when to withdraw. The acquisition of speech profoundly extends their horizons. Typically, children learn to say "no" before they learn to say "yes."

Toddlers' negativism is vital to the development of independence, but if it persists, oppositional behavior connotes a problem.

Learning language is a crucial task in the toddler period. Vocalizations become distinct, and toddlers can name a few objects and make needs known in one or two words. Near the end of the second year and into the third year toddlers sometimes use short sentences. The pace of language development varies considerably from child to child, and although a small number of children are truly late developers, most child experts recommend a hearing test if the child is not making two-word sentences by age 2.

Developmental Landmarks

Language and Cognitive Development. Toddlers begin to listen to explanations that can help them tolerate delay. They create new behaviors from old ones (originality) and engage in symbolic activities, for instance, using words and playing with dolls when the dolls represent something, such as a feeding sequence. Toddlers have varied capacities for concentration and self-regulation.

Emotional and Social Development. In the second year, pleasure and displeasure become further differentiated. *Social referencing* is often apparent at this age; the child looks to parents and others for emotional cues about how to respond to novel events. Toddlers show exploratory excitement, assertive pleasure, and pleasure in discovery and in developing new behavior (e.g., new games), including teasing and surprising or fooling the parent (e.g., hiding). The toddler has capacities for an organized demonstration of love as when the toddler runs up and hugs, smiles, and kisses the parent at the same time, and of protest when the toddler turns away, cries, bangs, bites, hits, yells, and kicks. Comfort with family and apprehension with strangers may increase. Anxiety appears to be related to disapproval and the loss of a loved caregiver and can be disorganizing.

Sexual Development. Sexual differentiation is evident from birth, when parents start dressing and treating infants differently because of the expectations evoked by sex typing. Through imitation, reward, and coercion, children assume the behaviors that their cultures define as appropriate for their sexual roles. Children exhibit curiosity about anatomical sex. When their curiosity is recognized as healthy and is met with honest, age-appropriate replies, children acquire a sense of the wonder of life and are comfortable with their own roles. If the subject of sex is taboo and children's questions are rebuffed, shame and discomfort may result.

Gender identity, the unshakable conviction of being male or female, begins to manifest at 18 months of age and is often fixed by 24 to 30 months. It was once widely believed that gender identity was primarily a function of social learning. John Money reported on children with ambiguous or damaged external genitalia who were raised as the sex opposite to their chromosomal sex. Long-term follow-up of those individuals suggests that the major part of gender identity is innate and that rearing may not affect the genetic diathesis.

Gender role describes the behavior that society deems appropriate for one sex or another, and it is not surprising that significant cultural differences exist. There may be different expectations for boys and girls in what and with whom they play, their tone of voice, the expression of emotions, and how they dress. Nevertheless, some generalizations are possible. Boys are more likely than girls to engage in rough and tumble play. Mothers talk more to girls than to boys, and by the time the child is 2 years of age, fathers generally pay more attention to boys. Many educated, middle-class parents determined to raise nonsexist children are startled to see their children's determined preference for sex-stereotyped toys: girls want to play with dolls, boys with guns.

Sphincter Control and Sleep. The second year of life is a period of increasing social demands on children. Toilet training serves as a paradigm of the family's general training practices; that is, the parent who is overly severe in the area of toilet training is likely to be punitive and restrictive in other areas also. Control of daytime urination is usually complete by the age of $2^1/_2$, and control of nighttime urination is usually complete by the age of 4 years, when bowel control is usually accomplished. Since 1900, the pendulum has swung between extremes of permissiveness and control in toilet training. The trend in the United States has been toward delayed training, but in the last few years this trend appears to be shifting back to early training.

Toddlers may have sleep difficulties related to fear of the dark, which can often be managed by using a nightlight. Most toddlers generally sleep about 12 hours a day, including a 2-hour nap. Parents must be aware that children of this age may need reassurance before going to bed and that the average 2-year-old takes about 30 minutes to fall asleep.

Parenting

Paralleling the changing tasks for children are changing tasks for parents. In infancy, the major responsibility for parents is to meet the infant's needs in a sensitive and consistent fashion. The parental task in the toddler stage requires firmness about the boundaries of acceptable behavior and encouragement of the child's progressive emancipation. Parents must be careful not to be too authoritarian at this stage; children must be allowed to operate for themselves and to learn from their mistakes and must be protected and assisted when challenges are beyond their abilities.

During the toddler period, children are likely to struggle for the exclusive affection and attention of their parents. This struggle includes rivalry, both with siblings and with one or another parent for the star role in the family. Although children are beginning to be able to share, they do so reluctantly. When the demands for exclusive possession are not resolved effectively, the result is likely to be jealous competitiveness in relationships with peers and lovers. The fantasies aroused by the struggle lead to fear of retaliation and to displacement of fear onto external objects. In an equitable, loving family a child elaborates a moral system of ethical rights. Parents need to balance between punishment and permissiveness and set realistic limits on a toddler's behavior.

PRESCHOOL PERIOD

The preschool period is characterized by marked physical and emotional growth. Generally, between 2 and 3 years of age, children reach half their adult height. The 20 baby teeth are in place at the beginning of the stage, and by the end they begin to fall out. Children are ready to enter school by the time the stage ends at age 5 or 6. They have mastered the tasks of primary socialization—to control their bowels and urine, to dress and feed themselves, and to control their tears and temper outbursts, at least most of the time.

The term preschool for the age group of $2^1/_2$ to 6 years may be a misnomer; many children are already in school-like settings, such as preschool nurseries and day care centers, where working mothers must often place their children. Preschool education can be valuable, but stressing academic advancement too far beyond a child's capabilities can be counterproductive.

Developmental Landmarks

Language and Cognitive Development. In the preschool period, children's use of language expands, and they use sentences. Individual words have regular and consistent meanings at the beginning of the period, and children begin to think symbolically. In general, however, their thinking is egocentric; they cannot place themselves in the position of another child and are incapable of empathy. Children think intuitively and prelogically and do not understand causal relations.

Emotional and Social Behavior. At the start of the preschool period, children can express such complex emotions as love, unhappiness, jealousy, and envy, both preverbally and verbally. Their emotions are still easily influenced by somatic events, such as tiredness and hunger. Although they still think mostly egocentrically, children's capacity for cooperation and sharing is emerging. Anxiety is related to loss of a person who was loved and depended on and to loss of approval and acceptance. Although still potentially disorganizing, anxiety can be tolerated better than in the past. Four-year-olds are learning to share and to have concern for others. Feelings of tenderness are sometimes expressed. Anxiety over bodily injury and the loss of a loved person's approval is sometimes disruptive.

By the end of the preschool period, children have many relatively stable emotions. Expansiveness, curiosity, pride, and gleeful excitement related to the self and the family are balanced with coyness, shyness, fearfulness, jealousy, and envy. Shame and humiliation are evident. Capacities for empathy and love are developed but fragile and easily lost if competitive or jealous strivings intervene. Anxiety and fears are related to bodily injury and loss of respect, love, and emerging self-esteem. Guilt feelings are possible.

Children between the ages of 3 and 6 years are aware of their bodies, of the genitalia, and of differences between the sexes. In their play, doctor–nurse games allow children to act out their sexual fantasies. Their awareness of their bodies extends beyond the genitalia; they show a preoccupation with illness or injury, so much so that the period has been called "the Band-Aid phase." Every injury must be examined and taken care of by a parent.

Children develop a division between what they want and what they are told to do. The division increases until a gap grows between their set of expanded desires, their exuberance at unlimited growth, and their parents' restrictions; they gradually turn parental values into self-obedience, self-guidance, and self-punishment.

At the end of the preschool stage, the child's conscience is established. The development of a conscience sets the tone for the moral sense of right and wrong. Until about 7 years of age, children experience rules as absolute and as existing for their own sake. They do not understand that more than one point of view to a moral issue may exist; a violation of the rules calls for absolute retribution—that is, children have the notion of immanent justice.

SIBLING RIVALRY. In the preschool period children relate to others in new ways. The birth of a sibling (a common occurrence during this time) tests a preschool child's capacity for further cooperation and sharing but may also evoke sibling rivalry, which is most likely to occur at this time. Sibling rivalry depends on child-rearing practice. Favoritism for any reason commonly aggravates such rivalry. Children who get special treatment because they are gifted, are defective in some way, or have a preferred gender are likely to receive angry feelings from their siblings. Experiences with siblings can influence growing children's relationships with peers and authority; for example, a problem may result if the needs of a new baby prevent the mother from attending to a firstborn child's needs. If not handled properly, the displacement of the firstborn can be a traumatic event.

PLAY. In the preschool years, children begin to distinguish reality from fantasy, and play reflects this growing awareness. Pretend games are popular and help test real-life situations in a playful manner. Dramatic play in which children act out a role, such as a housewife or a truck driver, is common. One-to-one play relationships advance to complicated patterns with rivalries, secrets, and two-against-one intrigues. Children's play behavior reflects their level of social development.

Between $2^1/_2$ and 3 years, children commonly engage in parallel play, solitary play alongside another child with no interaction between them. By age 3, play is often associative, that is, playing with the same toys in pairs or in small groups, but still with no real interaction among them. By age 4, children are usually able to share and engage in cooperative play. Real interactions and taking turns become possible.

Between 3 and 6 years of age, growth can be traced through drawings. A child's first drawing of a human being is a circular line with marks for the mouth, nose, and eyes; ears and hair are added later; arms and stick-like fingers appear next; and then legs appear. Last to appear is a torso in proportion to the rest of the body. Intelligent children can deal with details in their art. Drawings express creativity throughout a child's development: They are representational and formal in early childhood, make use of perspective in middle childhood, and become abstract and affect laden in adolescence. Drawings also reflect children's body image concepts and sexual and aggressive impulses.

IMAGINARY COMPANIONS. Imaginary companions most often appear during preschool years, usually in children with above-average intelligence and usually in the form of persons. Imaginary companions may also be things, such as toys that are anthropomorphized. Some studies indicate that up to 50 percent of children between the ages of 3 and 10 years have imaginary companions at one time or another. Their significance is not clear, but these figures are usually friendly, relieve loneliness, and reduce anxiety. In most instances, imaginary companions disappear by age 12, but they can occasionally persist into adulthood.

TELEVISION. Most children in the United States grow up watching an extraordinary amount of television. Preschoolers watch, on average, 3 to 4 hours per day, most of it unsupervised. Recent studies have confirmed a correlation between children watching a lot of violence on television and exhibiting more aggressiveness. Heavy television watching also appears to interfere with a child's learning to read.

MIDDLE YEARS

The period between age 6 and puberty is often called the middle years. During this time, children enter elementary school. The formal demands for academic learning and accomplishment become major determinants of further personality development.

Developmental Landmarks

Language and Cognitive Development. In the middle years, language expresses complex ideas with relations among several elements. Logical exploration tends to dominate fantasy, and children show an increased interest in rules and orderliness and an increased capacity for self-regulation. During this period, children's conceptual skills develop, and thinking becomes organized and logical. The ability to concentrate is well established by age 9 or 10, and by the end of the period, children begin to think in abstract terms. Improved gross motor coordination and muscle strength enable children to write fluently and draw artistically. They are also capable of complex motor tasks and activities, such as tennis, gymnastics, golf, baseball, and skateboarding.

Recent evidence has shown that changes in thinking and reasoning during the middle years result from maturational changes in the brain. Children are now capable of increased independence, learning, and socialization. Theorists consider moral development a gradual, stepwise process spanning childhood, adolescence, and young adulthood.

In the middle years, both girls and boys make new identifications with other adults, such as teachers and counselors. These identifications may so influence girls that their goals of wanting to marry and have babies, as their mothers did, may be combined with a desire for a career or may be postponed or abandoned entirely.

Girls who cannot identify with their mothers or whose fathers are overly attached may become fixated at about a 6-year-old level; as a result, they may fear men or women or both or become seductively close to them. In either case, such girls may not be seen as normal during the school-age years. A similar situation can occur in boys who have been unable to identify successfully with fathers who were aloof, brutal, or absent. Perhaps his mother prevented a boy from identifying with his father by being overprotective or by binding the son too closely to her. As a result, boys may enter this period with a variety of problems. They may be fearful of men, unsure of their sense of masculinity, or unwilling to leave their mothers (sometimes manifested by a school phobia); they may lack initiative and be unable to master school tasks, thus incurring academic problems.

The school-age period is a time when peer interaction assumes major importance. Interest in relationships outside the family takes precedence over those within the family. Nevertheless, a special relationship exists with the same-sex parent, with whom children identify and who is now an ideal and a role model.

Empathy and concern for others begin to emerge early in the middle years; by the time children are 9 or 10, they have well-developed capacities for love, compassion, and sharing. They have a capacity for long-term, stable relationships with family, peers, and friends, including best friends. Emotions about sexual differences begin to emerge as either excitement or shyness with the opposite sex. School-age children prefer to interact with children of the same sex. Although the middle years have sometimes been referred to as a *latency period*—a moratorium on psychosexual exploration and play until the eruption of sexual impulses with puberty—it is now recognized that a considerable amount of sexual interest continues through these years. Sex play and curiosity are common, especially among boys, but also among girls. Boys compare genitals and sometimes engage in group or mutual masturbation. An interest in anal humor and toilet jokes is often seen. Children this age often start using sexual and excretory words as expletives.

CHUM PERIOD. Harry Stack Sullivan postulated that a chum, or buddy, is an important phenomenon during the school years. By about 10 years of age, children develop a close same-sex relationship, which Sullivan believed is necessary for further healthy psychological growth. Moreover, Sullivan believed that the absence of a chum during the middle years of childhood is an early harbinger of schizophrenia.

SCHOOL REFUSAL. Some children refuse to go to school at this time, generally because of separation anxiety. A fearful mother may transmit her own fear of separation to a child, or a child who has not resolved dependence needs panics at the idea of separation. School refusal is usually not an isolated problem; children with the problem typically avoid many other social situations.

OTHER ISSUES IN CHILDHOOD

Sex Role Development

Persons' sex roles are similar to their gender identity; persons see themselves as male or female. The sex role also involves identification with culturally acceptable masculine or feminine ways of behaving; but changing expectations in society (particularly in the United States) of what constitutes masculine and feminine behavior can create ambiguity.

Parents react differently to their male and female children. Independence, physical play, and aggressiveness are encouraged in boys; dependence, verbalization, and physical intimacy are encouraged in girls. Nowadays, however, boys are encouraged to verbalize their feelings and to pursue interests traditionally associated with girls, whereas girls are encouraged to pursue careers traditionally dominated by men and to participate in competitive sports. As society grows more tolerant in its expectations of the sexes, roles become less rigid, and opportunities for boys and girls enlarge and broaden.

Biologically, boys are more physically aggressive than girls; and parental expectations, particularly the expectations of fathers, reinforce this trait. Differences also exist between boys and girls in the influence of persons outside the family. Girls tend to respond to the expectations and opinions of girls and of teachers of either sex, but to ignore boys. Boys, on the other hand, tend to respond to other boys, but to ignore girls and teachers.

Dreams and Sleep

Children's dreams can have a profound effect on behavior. During the first year of life, when reality and fantasy are not yet fully differentiated, dreams may be experienced as if they were, or could be, true. At age 3, many children believe dreams are shared directly by more than one person, but most 4-year-olds understand that dreams are unique to each person. Children view dreams either with pleasure or, as is most often reported, with fear. The dream content should be seen in connection with children's life experience, developmental stage, mechanisms used during dreaming, and sex.

Disturbing dreams peak when children are 3, 6, and 10 years of age. Two-year-old children may dream about being bitten or chased; at the age of 4, they may have many animal dreams and also dream of persons who either protect or destroy. At age 5 or 6, dreams of being killed or injured, of flying and being in cars, and of ghosts become prominent; the role of conscience, moral values, and increasing conflicts are concerned with these themes. In early childhood, aggressive dreams rarely seem to occur; instead, dreamers are in danger, a state that perhaps reflects children's dependent position. By about the age of 5, children realize that their dreams are not real; before then, they believed them to be real events. By age 7, children know that they create their dreams themselves.

Between the ages of 3 and 6 years, children normally want to keep their bedroom door open or to have a nightlight, so that they can either maintain contact with their parents or view the room in a realistic, nonfearful way. At times, children resist going to sleep to avoid dreaming. Disorders associated with falling asleep, therefore, are often connected with dreaming. Children often create rituals to protect themselves in the withdrawal from the world of reality into the world of sleep. Parasomnias, such as sleepwalking, sleep talking, enuresis (bed-wetting), and night terrors, are common at this age. They usually occur during stage 4 sleep when dreaming is minimal, and they do not indicate emotional trouble or underlying psychopathology. Most children grow out of parasomnias by adolescence.

Periods of REM occur about 60 percent of the time during the first few weeks of life, a period when infants sleep two thirds of the time. Premature babies sleep even longer than full-term babies, and a greater proportion of their sleep is REM sleep. The sleep–wake cycle of newborns is about 3 hours long. Among adults, the dream-to-sleep ratio is stable: 20 percent of sleeping time is spent dreaming. Even newborns have brain activity similar to that of the dreaming state.

Birth Spacing

For women in the United States, 10 percent of conceptions that lead to live births are considered unwanted, and 20 percent are wanted but considered ill timed. The implications of these figures are that some couples may be poorly prepared or may feel guilty about not wanting to be parents. It is desirable to plan pregnancies and to have mutual agreement on the spacing of children. The typical number of children in a present-day family is two, half the typical number at the beginning of the century. Repeated childbearing prevents adequate recuperation from the birth process and places mothers at risk for complications and injury. New mothers require time to adapt; the period of adaptation can range from a few weeks to several months. The demands of other children at home can be taxing, and if these children are also young, the family may be stressed beyond its capacity.

Children born close together have higher rates of premature or underweight births, and malnutrition; they develop more slowly and are at increased risk of contracting and dying from childhood infectious diseases. Studies have shown when a child is born 3 to 5 years after a previous birth, health risks are reduced for both mother and child. Compared with 24- to 29-month intervals, children born in 36- to 41-month intervals are associated with a 28 percent reduction in stunting and a 29 percent reduction of low birthweight. Women who have children at 27- to 32-month intervals are 1.3 times more likely to avoid anemia, 1.7 times more likely to avoid third-trimester bleeding, and 2.5 times more likely to survive childbirth.

Studies of children from large families (of four or five children) show that they are more likely to have conduct disorder and to have a slightly lower level of verbal intelligence than children from small families. Decreased parental interaction and discipline may account for these findings.

Birth Order

The effects of birth order vary. Firstborn children are often more highly valued than subsequent children, particularly if the firstborn is male, especially in non-Western cultures, but also sometimes in the United States. Firstborns have been found to have higher intelligence quotients (IQ) than their younger siblings, a finding that may reflect parents' having more time to interact with a firstborn child. Firstborn children appear to be more achievement oriented than subsequent children born to the same parents. Some studies show that people in certain occupational areas, such as architecture, accounting, and engineering, tend to be firstborn children. As more children enter the family, parental time for each child diminishes; prenatal stress may also increase as more children require care.

Second and third children have the advantage of their parents' previous experience. Younger children also learn from their older siblings. For example, they may show more sophisticated use of pronouns at an earlier age than firstborns did. When children are spaced too closely, however, there may not be enough lap time for each child. The arrival of new children in the family affects not only the parents but also the siblings. Firstborn children may resent the birth of a new sibling, who threatens their sole claim on parental attention. In some cases, regressive behavior, such as enuresis or thumb sucking, occurs.

In general, the oldest children achieve the most and are the most authoritarian; middle children usually receive the least attention in the home and may develop strong peer relationships to compensate; and the youngest children may receive too much attention and be spoiled. According to Frank Sulloway, firstborn children tend to be conservative and conformists; by contrast, youngest children tend to be independent and rebellious in regard to family and cultural norms. Sulloway found that a high proportion of prominent persons were lastborn children. He ascribes these differences to birth order and suggests that each child develops personality traits to fit an unfilled slot in the family. His findings need to be replicated.

Children and Divorce

Many children live in homes in which divorce has occurred. Approximately 30 percent of all children in the United States live in homes in which one parent (usually the mother) is the sole head of the household, and 61 percent of all children born in any given year can expect to live with only one parent before they reach the age of 18 years. A child's age at the time of the parents' divorce affects the child's reaction to the divorce. Immediately after a divorce, an increase in behavioral and emotional disorders appears in all age groups. Infants do not understand anything about separation or divorce; however, they do notice changes in their parents' responses to them and may experience changes in their eating or sleeping patterns, have bowel problems, and seem more fretful, fearful, or anxious. Children 3- to 6-years of age do not understand what is happening, and those who do understand often assume that they are somehow responsible for the divorce. If divorce occurs when a child is between 7 and 12 years, school performance generally declines. Older children, especially adolescents, comprehend the situation and believe that they could have prevented the divorce had they intervened in some way—had they, in effect, served as surrogate marriage therapists—but they are still hurt, angry, and critical of their parents' behavior.

Some children harbor the fantasy that their parents will be reunited in the future. Such children show animosity toward a parent's real or potential new mate because they are forced to recognize that no reconciliation is taking place. Recovery from, and adaptation to, the effects of divorce usually take 3 to 5 years, but about one third of all children from divorced homes have lasting psychological trauma. Among boys, physical aggression is a common sign of distress. Adolescents tend to spend more time away from the parental home after the divorce. Suicide attempts may occur as a direct result of the divorce; one of the predictors of suicide in adolescence is the recent divorce or separation of the parents. Children who adapt well to divorce do so if each parent makes an effort to continue to relate to the child despite the child's anger. To facilitate recovery, the divorced couple must avoid arguing with one another and must show consistent behavior toward the child. Table 2.2–9 lists some of the psychological effects of divorce on children.

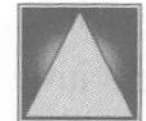

Table 2.2–9
Effects of Divorce on Children

- Children in homes with absent fathers are more likely to suffer from antisocial personality disorder, child conduct disorder, and attention-deficit hyperactivity disorder.
- The divorce rate of children of divorced parents doubles that of children from stable families.
- Children of divorce are far more likely to be delinquent, engage in premarital sex, and bear children out of wedlock during adolescence and young adulthood.
- Children from divorced homes function more poorly than children from continuously married parents across a variety of domains, including academic achievement, social relations, and conduct problems.
- Children from divorced homes have more psychological problems than those from homes disrupted by the death of a parent.
- Children from disrupted marriages experience greater risk of injury, asthma, headaches, and speech defects than children from intact families.
- Children of divorce tend to be impulsive, irritable, socially withdrawn, lonely, unhappy, anxious, and insecure.
- Children of divorce, especially boys, are more aggressive than children whose parents stayed married.
- Suicide rates for children of divorce are much higher than for children from intact families.
- Twenty to 25 percent have significant adjustment problems as teenagers

(Data adapted from Americans for Divorce Reform, Arlington, Virginia. Table by Nitza Jones.)

Stepparents. There are three types of step-families: (1) Neo-Traditional, (2) Romantic, and (3) Matriarchal (Table 2.2–10). When remarriage occurs, children must learn to adapt to the stepparent and to the so-called reconstituted family. Such adaptation is usually difficult, especially when the stepparent is nonsupportive, resents the stepchild, or favors his or her own natural children. Of step-families, 25 percent dissolve within the first 2 years, whereas 75 percent grow to find a new balance in their homes. A natural child born to the new couple—a stepsibling—sometimes receives more attention than a stepchild and, as a result, is the object of sibling rivalry. After 5 years, about 20 percent of adolescents in step-families want to move out and live with the other biological parent.

Adoption

Adoption is defined as the process by which a child is taken into a family by one or more adults who are not the biological parents but are recognized by law as the child's parents. About 2.5 million persons under 18 years of age are adopted each year. Of children adopted, 25 percent are adopted by persons not related to them by birth or marriage, and the remainder are adopted by relatives or stepparents. Most adopted children are born out of wedlock, and 40 percent of all such children are born to mothers between 15 and 19 years of age.

Adoptive parents most often tell their children of their status between the ages of 2 and 4 years. Informing children about their adoption reduces the possibility that the children learn of it from extrafamilial sources and then feel betrayed by their adoptive parents and abandoned by their biological parents.

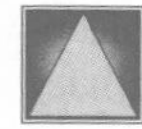

Table 2.2–10
Types of Step-Families

Neo-Traditional Families	▸ Resembles "traditional" families ▸ Absent biological parent is included at times. ▸ Discipline, boundaries and limits, and expectations are discussed openly. ▸ Family coalitions and "side-taking" are better avoided.
Romantic Families	▸ Expect to be a "traditional family" immediately ▸ The absent biological parent is expected to disappear and is often criticized. ▸ Stepparent/stepchild difficulties are common. ▸ Stress is unbearable. ▸ Few open and frank discussions about problems
Matriarchal Families	▸ Run by a highly competent mom and her companion follows ▸ Companion is a "buddy" to the children, not to the parent. ▸ Birth of a step-sibling causes problems.

Emotional and behavioral disorders, such as aggressive behavior, stealing, and learning disturbances, have been reported to be higher among adopted than nonadopted children. The later the age of adoption, the higher the incidence and the more severe the behavior problems.

Throughout childhood and adolescence, children may be preoccupied with fantasies of two sets of parents. An adopted child may split the two sets of parents into good and bad parents. Adopted children usually have a strong desire to know their biological parents; some children pattern themselves after their fantasies of their absent biological parents and create a conflict with their adoptive parents. In most cases in which adopted children have sought out and met their biological parents (and vice versa), the experience has been generally positive, especially if the child is in late adolescence or early adulthood.

Family Factors in Child Development

Family Stability. Parents and children living under the same roof in harmonious interaction is the expected cultural norm in Western society. Within this framework, childhood development presumably proceeds most expeditiously. Deviations from the norm, such as divorced- and single-parent families, are associated with a broad range of problems in children, including low self-esteem, increased risk of child abuse, increased incidence of divorce when they eventually marry, and increased incidence of mental disorders, particularly depressive disorders and antisocial personality disorder as adults. Why some children from unstable homes are less affected than others (or even immune to these deleterious effects) is of great interest. Michael Rutter has postulated that vulnerability is influenced by sex (boys are more affected than girls), age (older children are less vulnerable than younger ones), and inborn personality characteristics. For example, children who have a placid temperament are less likely to be victims of abuse within a family than are hyperactive children; by virtue of their placidity, they may be less affected by the emotional turmoil surrounding them.

Other Family Factors. In childhood and adolescence, the death of a parent is associated with adverse effects, such as an increase in later emotional problems, particularly a susceptibility to depression and divorce. This finding contrasts sharply to the results of separations caused by less traumatic events. For example, no evidence indicates that working mothers raise children who are less healthy than those brought up by mothers who stay at home. Home caregivers can act as surrogate mothers and, in such cases, the children do not become more attached to the caregiver than to the parent.

Day Care Centers. The role of day care centers for children is under continuous investigation and various studies have come up with different results. One study found that children placed in day care centers before the age of 5 are less assertive and less effectively toilet trained than home-reared children. Another study found children in day care to be more advanced in social and cognitive development than children who were not in day care. The National Institute of Child Health and Human Development reported 4 1/2 year olds who had spent more than 30 hours a week in child care were more demanding, more aggressive, and more noncompliant than those raised at home and showed higher cognitive skills, particularly in math and reading. These same children who were tracked through the third grade continued to score higher in math and reading skills but had poorer work habits and social skills. The researchers were careful to note that this behavior was within the normal range, however.

All studies of day care must take into account the quality of both the day care center and the homes from which children come. For example, a child from a disadvantaged home may be better off at a day care center than a child from an advantaged home. Similarly, a woman who wishes to leave the home to work for financial or other reasons and cannot do so may resent being forced to remain in the home in a child-rearing role, which may adversely affect the child.

Parenting Styles. The ways in which children are raised vary considerably between and within cultures. Rutter has clustered the diversity into four general styles. Subsequent research has confirmed that certain styles tend to correlate with certain behavior in the children, although the outcomes are by no means absolute. The *authoritarian style*, characterized by strict, inflexible rules, can lead to low self-esteem, unhappiness, and social withdrawal. The *indulgent-permissive style*, which includes little or no limit setting coupled with unpredictable parental harshness, can lead to low self-reliance, poor impulse control, and aggression. The *indulgent-neglectful style*, one of noninvolvement in the child's life and rearing, puts the child at risk for low self-esteem, impaired self-control, and increased aggression. The *authoritative-reciprocal style*, marked by firm rules and shared decision-making in a warm, loving environment, is believed to be the style most likely to result in self-reliance, self-esteem, and a sense of social responsibility.

Development and Expression of Psychopathology

The expression of psychopathology in children can be related to both age and developmental level. Specific developmental disorders, particularly developmental language disorders, often are diagnosed in the preschool years. Delayed development of language is a common parental concern. Children who do not use words by 18 months or phrases by 2 1/2 to 3 years may need assessment, particularly if they do not appear to understand normal verbal cues or much language at all. Mild mental retardation or specific learning problems often are not diagnosed until after the child begins elementary school. Disruptive behavior disorder will become apparent at that time as the child begins to interact with peers. Similarly, attention-deficit disorders are only diagnosed when the demands for sustained attention are made in school. Other conditions, particularly schizophrenia and bipolar disorder, are rare in preschool and school-aged children.

References

Briggs GG. *Drugs in Pregnancy and Lactation: A Reference Guide to Fetal and Neonatal Risk.* Baltimore: Lippincott Williams & Wilkins. 2005.

Gordon MF. Normal child development. In: Sadock BJ, Sadock VA, eds. *Kaplan & Sadock's Comprehensive Textbook of Psychiatry.* 8th ed. Vol. 2. Baltimore: Lippincott Williams & Wilkins; 2005:3018.

Moses-Kolko EL. Neonatal signs after later in utero exposure to serotonin reuptake inhibitors. *JAMA.* 2005;23:2372.

Nickman SL, Rosenfeld AA, Fine P, MacIntyre JC, Pilowsky DJ, Howe RA, Derdeyn A, Gonzales MB, Forsythe L, Sveda SA. Children in adoptive families:

Overview and update. *J Am Acad Child Adolesc Psychiatry*. 2005;44(10):987–995.
Norton M. New evidence on birth spacing: promising findings for improving newborn, infant, child, and maternal health. *Int J Gynaecol Obstet*. 2005;89(suppl 1):S1–S6.
Strauss B, ed. *Involuntary Childlessness: Psychological Assessment, Counseling, and Psychotherapy*. Kirkland, WA: Hogrefe & Huber Publishers; 2002.
Van den Bergh BR, Mulder EJ, Mennes M, Glover V. Antenatal maternal anxiety and stress and the neurobehavioural development of the fetus and child: links and possible mechanisms. A review. *Neurosci Biobehav Rev*. 2005;29(2):237–258.
Weinstock M. The potential influence of maternal stress hormones on development and mental health of the offspring. *Brain Behav Immun*. 2005;19(4):296–308.
Wolfinger NH. *Understanding the Divorce Cycle: The Children of Divorce in Their Own Marriages*. New York: Cambridge University Press. 2005.

▲ 2.3 Adolescence

Adolescence, marked by the physiological signs and surging sexual hormones of puberty, is the period of maturation between childhood and adulthood. Adolescence is a transitional period in which peer relationships deepen, autonomy in decision-making grows, and intellectual pursuits and social belonging are sought. Adolescence is largely a time of exploration and making choices, a gradual process of working toward an integrated concept of self. Adolescents can best be described as "works in progress," characterized by increasing ability for mastery over complex challenges of academic, interpersonal, and emotional tasks, while searching for new interests, talents, and social identities.

WHAT IS NORMAL ADOLESCENCE?

The concept of *normality* in adolescent development refers to the degree of psychological adaptation that is achieved while navigating the hurdles and meeting the milestones characteristic of this period of growth. For up to approximately 75 percent of youth, adolescence is a period of successful adaptation to physical, cognitive, and emotional changes, largely continuous with their previous functioning. Psychological maladjustment, self-loathing, disturbance of conduct, substance abuse, affective disorders, and other impairing psychiatric disorders emerge in approximately 20 percent of the adolescent population.

Adolescent adjustment is continuous with previous psychological function; thus, psychologically disturbed children are at greater risk for psychiatric disorders during adolescence. Adolescents with psychiatric disorders are at increased risk for greater conflicts with families and for feeling alienated from their families. Although up to 60 percent of adolescents endorse occasional distress, or a psychiatric symptom, this group of adolescents functions well academically and with peers and describes themselves as generally satisfied with their lives.

The psychoanalytic developmentalist Erik Erikson characterizes the normative task of adolescence as *identity versus role confusion*. The integration of past experiences with current changes takes place in what Erikson terms *ego identity*. Adolescents explore various aspects of their psychological selves by becoming fans of heroes, or other well-known musical or political idols. Some adolescents appear consumed by their identification with a particular idol, whereas others are more moderate in their expression. Adolescents who feel accepted by a peer group and are involved in a variety of activities are less likely to become consumed by adoration of an idol. Adolescents who are socially isolated, feel socially rejected, and become overly identified with an idol to the exclusion of all other activities are at greater risk for serious emotional problems and require psychiatric intervention.

Erickson uses the term *moratorium* to describe that interim period between the concrete thinking of childhood and a more evolved complex ethical development. Erikson defines *identity crisis* as a normative part of adolescence in which adolescents pursue alternative behaviors and styles and, then, successfully mold these different experiences into a solid identity. A failure to do so would result in *identity diffusion*, or role confusion, in which the adolescent lacks a cohesive or confident sense of identity. Adolescence is the time to bond with peers, experiment with new beliefs and styles, fall in love for the first time, and explore creative ideas for future endeavors.

Most adolescents go through this developmental process with optimism, develop good self-esteem, maintain good peer relationships, and sustain basically harmonious relationships with their families.

STAGES OF ADOLESCENCE

Early Adolescence

Early adolescence, from 12 to 14 years of age, is the period in which the most striking initial changes are noticed—physically, attitudinally, and behaviorally. Growth spurts often begin in these years for boys, whereas girls may have already had rapid growth for 1 to 2 years. At this stage, boys and girls begin to criticize usual family habits, insist on spending time with peers with less supervision, have a greater awareness of style and appearance, and may question previously accepted family values. A new awareness of sexuality may be displayed by increased modesty and embarrassment with their current physical development or may exhibit itself in an increased interest in the opposite sex.

Early adolescents engage in subtle or overt displays of their growing desire for autonomy, sometimes with challenging behaviors toward authority figures, including teachers and school administrators, and exhibit disdain for rules themselves. At this age, some adolescents begin to experiment with cigarettes, alcohol, and marijuana.

During early adolescence, there is normal variation in when new defining behaviors are acquired. Overall, although many early adolescents make new friends and modify their public image, most maintain positive connections to family members, old friends, and their family's values. However, early adolescence has been viewed as a time of overwhelming turmoil, during which there is a dramatic rejection of family, friends, and lifestyle, resulting in a powerful alienation of the adolescent.

Michael, a 13-year-old adolescent, had just started the 8th grade. He had been in middle school since 6th grade, but this year he found the school rules increasingly irritating and felt that his teachers were too strict. He had always been a good student and had been able to keep his grades up doing a minimum of work. His older brother Tim, now in 9th grade, had established himself as an outgoing, well-liked, and well-behaved student who always put maximal effort into school projects in the same school, so Michael was compared with his brother on a regular basis by most of his teachers. Michael resented these comparisons, because, unlike his brother, who he felt was a "nerd," Michael was more rebellious, took more risks, and made friends with more popular peers. To distinguish himself from his older brother in school and at home, Michael began to challenge the rules at school, stating that they were "stupid" and "meaningless." Michael began to cut classes, to stay out later than allowed, and started to experiment with alcohol and marijuana. He decided that his best friends from 6th and 7th grade no longer interested him and began to hang out with peers who liked to do the same things that he liked. When Michael was at home, he continued to get along with his older brother, with whom he played basketball and video games and occasionally went with to the movies, except when his friends came over, and then he acted like "a totally different person," according to Tim.

Michael's grades remained high, but his parents noticed that on his report cards, his effort and behavior were consistently considered problematic. During the second month of school, Michael's parents received a phone call that Michael was going to be suspended because of being found with marijuana on the school grounds during recess. When his parents went to the school to discuss this with the assistant principal and the school counselor, Michael insisted that the suspension was unfair and that he was doing just fine in school, so his marijuana smoking should not be held against him. When he was confronted with the fact that his behavior had not only broken the school rules, but also violated the law, he became angry and continued to insist that it was not his problem that marijuana was illegal and that it did not affect his school performance and, thus, there should be no school action. He also went on to blurt out his perception that his parents loved his older brother more than they loved him and that he would always feel like a second-class citizen because he could not be like Tim. Michael was suspended for several days, but the incident was not reported to the police by the school, who requested that Michael receive counseling.

Michael begrudgingly started to see a counselor and entered into a weekly therapy group for teens. Michael's parents also went to a therapist to work on becoming more unified in their parenting styles. Michael remained in counseling for the next 1½ years, during which time his attitude and reasoning style changed considerably. At age 15, Michael was able to understand why his school had taken action when he was found with marijuana. He was able to admit the dangers of using drugs, and he was able to take responsibility for his ill-advised behaviors. Alcohol and drug use continued to be actively discussed throughout his therapy and, at age 15, Michael had completely lost interest in alcohol and admitted to smoking marijuana rarely at parties. Michael was more open to making friends with a variety of peers, and he was able to say that he liked himself better now than he did when he was 13. He now treated his brother respectfully when alone or with friends, and he felt that his parents appreciated him for "who he was." (Courtesy of Caroly S. Pataki, M.D.).

Middle Adolescence

During the middle phase of adolescence (roughly between the ages of 14 and 16), adolescents' lifestyles may reflect their efforts to pursue their own stated goals of being independent. Their abilities to combine abstract reasoning with realistic decision-making and the application of social judgment is put to the test in this phase of adolescent development. In this phase, sexual behavior intensifies, making romantic relationships more complicated, and self-esteem becomes a pivotal influence on positive and negative risk-taking behaviors.

In this phase of development, adolescents tend to identify with a group of peers who become highly influential in their choices of activities, styles, music, idols, and role models. Adolescents' underestimation of the risks associated with a variety of recreational behaviors and their sense of "omnipotence," mixed with their drive to be autonomous, frequently cause some conflict with parental requests and expectations. For most teens, the process of defining themselves as unique and different from their families can be achieved while still maintaining alliances with family members.

Linda, a 16-year-old junior in high school, had just gotten her driver's license. She realized that she was lucky to have received her parents' old car as soon as she had turned age 16, but because many of her friends did not yet have cars, she was constantly being called on to drive them places. Linda was an attractive and well-liked adolescent who had always been an "A" and "B" student, and she and her family were satisfied that she tried her best in school. She played the flute in the school's orchestra and was considered to be a good athlete, although she was not on any varsity teams. Linda had been "going out" with a boy in her grade at school, Rob, who was also 16 years old, for 6 months, and she felt that they had a close relationship. Because he did not yet have a car, she was also the "identified driver" whenever they went to parties. Linda was relieved about this, because she did not drink alcohol and was glad that she would never have to be a passenger in a car with Rob after he would drink a few beers at a party. Linda got along well with her parents, who were considered fairly "easy-going" by her friends, and she felt that she and her parents had similar values and ideas.

Things were going well with her until Rob began to repeatedly tell her how much he wanted them to go further in their sexual relationship. When she said that she needed some time to think it over, Rob hounded her more. When this subject had come up with her parents hypothetically in the past, they had always told her that she would know when it was the right time for her to engage in sex. Linda felt that she was not ready to have sex, although she knew of many classmates who were sexually active within the first few months of a relationship. Linda had never been an impulsive person and liked to plan things carefully so that they would feel right to her. Linda realized that she would not be able to go along with Rob's request until she felt ready, which could be several months or even years, but she was confident that he would understand, despite being disappointed. One of Linda's friends pointed out to her that Rob might break up with her if she was not ready to be sexually active with him, and she responded that this was a possibility that she had considered, but, if that happened, then he was not the right boyfriend for her. Linda told Rob that she loved him but was not yet ready to be sexually active and found that he was accepting of that; in fact, it seemed to her that he was a little relieved.

Linda and Rob continued their relationship into their senior year of high school, and, toward the end of her senior year, Linda felt ready to be fully sexually active with him. They decided to go to a community clinic that was known for its positive attitude toward adolescents who want to learn about birth control methods and obtain a method of birth control without informing their parents. Linda and Rob took the time to learn about a variety of birth control methods and chose the use of condoms. When they left the clinic, Linda and Rob felt closer than they had before, and both felt good about their knowledge of safe sexual practice. Linda and Rob both felt that they were making a choice that was right for them. (Courtesy of Caroly S. Pataki, M.D.).

Late Adolescence

Late adolescence (between the ages of 17 and 19) is a time when continued exploration of academic pursuits, musical and artistic tastes, athletic participation, and social bonds leads a teen toward greater definition of self and a sense of belonging to certain groups or subcultures within mainstream society. Well-adjusted adolescents can be comfortable with current choices of activities, tastes, hobbies, and friendships, yet remain aware that their "identities" will continue to be refined during young adulthood.

Andy was in his second semester of his first year of college, living away from home, and had just turned 18 years of age. He reflected on the fact that he was no longer a "minor" and could make most decisions regarding his own fate without his parents being at all involved. This was a liberating feeling, yet, now that he had his freedom, he was not really sure what he wanted to do with his life. Since 10th grade, Andy had felt sure that he wanted to pursue a career in medicine like his father, and he had taken a heavy load of science courses in the first semester, all of which he had despised. So, this semester, he had signed up only for liberal arts classes. He was now enrolled in classes that ranged from art history to architectural drafting to sociology, philosophy, and music. He had been influenced in a positive way, he believed, by his roommate Will, who was in the architecture program, and by his girlfriend, Tina, who was majoring in studio art.

As the semester progressed, he found that his favorite course, similar to Will, was the drafting class. Although Will was in a more advanced class, having started the first semester, Andy pondered the question of whether he liked the drafting class so much because of how much his friendship with Will meant or because he really liked the field. He talked this over with Tina, who challenged his goal to figure out the rest of his life right now. She suggested that he take at least two more semesters of classes in the architecture curriculum before making a decision about which career was the best match for him. Andy realized that Tina's approach to life was very different than the one in which he had grown up, in which his parents had always pressed him to plan ahead, make choices and commitments early, and then see them through, even if they did not feel quite right. Tina's approach left more room for basing decisions on her experiences, rather than on what she felt she was "supposed" to do. Andy took her advice and allowed himself another year to decide on a major and what career to pursue. After taking more courses in architecture, Andy decided that he did truly enjoy it and switched his focus from premed to architecture. (Courtesy of Caroly S. Pataki M.D.)

COMPONENTS OF ADOLESCENCE

Physical Development

Puberty is the process by which adolescents develop physical and sexual maturity, along with reproductive ability. The first signs of the pubertal process are an increased rate of growth in both height and weight. This process begins in girls by approximately 10 years of age. By the age of 11 or 12, many girls noticeably tower over their male classmates, who do not experience a growth spurt, on average, until they reach 13 years of age. By age 13, many girls have experienced menarche, and most have developed breasts and pubic hair.

Wide variation exists in the normal range of onset and timing of pubertal development and its components. A set sequence occurs, however, in the order in which pubertal development proceeds. Thus, secondary sexual characteristics in boys, such as increased length and width of the penis, for example, will occur after the release of androgens from developed enlarged testes.

Sexual maturity rating (SMR), also referred to as *Tanner Stages*, range from SMR 1 (prepuberty) to SMR 5 (adult). The SMR ratings include stages of genital maturity in boys and breast development in girls, as well as pubic hair development. Table 2.3–1 outlines sexual maturity ratings for boys and girls.

The primary female sex characteristic is ovulation, the release of eggs from ovarian follicles, approximately once every 28 days. When adolescent girls reach SMR 3 to 4, ovarian follicles are producing enough estrogen to result in menarche, the onset of menstruation. When adolescent girls reach SMR 4 to 5, an ovarian follicle matures on a monthly basis and ovulation occurs. Estrogen and progesterone promote sexual maturation, including further development of fallopian tubes and breasts.

For adolescent boys, the primary sex characteristic is the development of sperm by the testes. In boys, sperm development

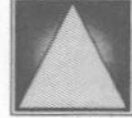

Table 2.3–1
Sexual Maturity Ratings for Male and Female Adolescents

Sexual Maturity Rating	Girls	Boys
Stage 1	Preadolescent, papilla elevated No pubic hair	Penis, testes, scrotum preadolescent No pubic hair
Stage 2	Breast bud, small mound; areola diameter increased Sparse long pubic hair, mainly along labia	Penis size same, testes and scrotum enlarged, with scrotal skin reddened Sparse long pubic hair, mainly at the base of penis
Stage 3	Breast and areola larger; no separation of contours Pubic hair darker and coarser; spread over pubic area	Penis elongated, with increased size of testes and scrotum Pubic hair darker and coarser; spread over pubic area
Stage 4	Breast size increased Areola and papilla raised Pubic hair coarse and thickened; covers less area than in adults, does not extend to thighs	Penis increased in length and width Testes and scrotum larger Pubic hair coarse and thickened; covers less area than in adults, does not extend to thighs
Stage 5	Breasts resemble adult female breast; areola has recessed to breast contour Pubic hair increased in density; area extends to thighs	Penis, testes, scrotum appear mature Pubic hair increased in density; area extends to thighs

occurs in response to follicle-stimulating hormone acting on the seminiferous tubules within the testes. The pubertal process in boys is marked by the growth of the testes stimulated by luteinizing hormone. An adolescent boy's ability to ejaculate generally emerges within 1 year of reaching SMR 2. Secondary sexual characteristics in boys include thickening of skin, broadening of the shoulders, and the development of facial hair.

Cognitive Maturation

Cognitive maturation in adolescence encompasses a wide range of expanded abilities that fall within the global category of executive functions of the brain. These include the transition from concrete thinking to more abstract thinking; an increased ability to draw logical conclusions in scientific pursuits, with peer interactions and in social situations; and new abilities for self-observation and self-regulation. Adolescents acquire increased awareness of their own intellectual, artistic, and athletic gifts and talents, yet it often takes many more years into young adulthood to establish a practical application for these abilities.

The central cognitive change that occurs gradually during adolescence is the shift from concrete thinking (*concrete operational thinking*, according to Jean Piaget) to the ability to think abstractly (*formal operational thinking*, in Piaget's terminology). This evolution occurs as an adaptation to stimuli that demand an adolescent to produce hypothetical responses, as well as in response to the adolescent's expanded abilities to provide generalizations from specific situations. The development of abstract thinking is not a sudden epiphany but, rather, a gradual process of expanding logical deductions beyond concrete experiences and achieving the capacity for idealistic and hypothetical thinking based on everyday life.

Adolescents often use an omnipotent belief system that reinforces their sense of immunity from danger, even when confronted with logical risks. Some degree of child-like magical thinking continues to coexist with more mature abstract thinking in many adolescents. Despite the persistence of magical thinking into adolescence, adolescent cognition departs from that of younger children insofar as the increased ability for self-observation and development of strategies to promote strengths and compensate for weaknesses.

One of the important cognitive tasks in adolescence is to identify and gravitate toward those pursuits that seem to match the adolescent's cognitive strengths, in academic courses and in thinking about future aspirations. Piaget believed that cognitive adaptation in adolescence is profoundly influenced by social relationships and the dialogue between adolescents and peers, making social cognition an integral part of cognitive development in adolescence.

Socialization

Socialization in adolescence encompasses the ability to find acceptance in peer relationships, as well as the development of more mature social cognition. The skills to develop a sense of belonging to a peer group, along with the ability to conform with the activities of that group are of central importance to a sense of well-being. Being viewed as socially competent by peers is a critical component in building good self-esteem for most early adolescents. Peer influences are powerful and can foster positive social interactions, as well as apply a pressure in less socially accepted behaviors or even high-risk behavior. Belonging to a peer group is, in general, a sign of adaptation and a developmentally appropriate step in separating from parents and turning the focus of loyalty toward friends. Children between the ages of 6 and 12 are able to engage in exchanges of ideas and opinions and acknowledge feelings of peers, but the relationships often wax and wane in a discontinuous way on the basis of altercations and good times. Friendships deepen with repeated good times but, for some school-aged children, a variety of peers are often interchangeable—that is, a companion is sought when a given child has free time, rather than out of a desire to spend time with a specific friend. As adolescence ensues, friendships become more individualized, and personal secrets are likely shared with a friend rather than a family member. A comfort level is achieved with one or several early adolescent peers, and the group may "stick together," spending most free time together. In early adolescence, a blend of the above two social modes may emerge, small "cliques" arise, and, even within the cliques, competition and jealousies regarding which dyads are "preferred" or higher ranked within the clique may result in some discontinuities in the relationships. In later adolescence, the peer group solidifies, leading to increased stability in the friendships and a greater mutuality in the quality of the interactions.

Moral Development

Morality is a set of values and beliefs about codes of behavior that conform to those shared by others in society. Adolescents, as do younger children, tend to develop patterns of behaviors characteristic of their family and educational environments and by imitation of specific peers and adults whom they admire. Moral development is not strictly tied to chronological age but, rather, is an outgrowth from cognitive development.

Piaget described moral development as a gradual process parallel to cognitive development, with expanded abilities in differentiating the best interests for society from those of individuals occurring during late adolescence. Preschool children simply follow rules set forth by the parents; in the middle years, children accept rules but show an inability to allow for exceptions; and during adolescence, young persons recognize rules in terms of what is good for the society at large.

Lawrence Kohlberg integrated Piaget's concepts and described three major levels of morality. The first level is preconventional morality, in which punishment and obedience to the parent are the determining factors. The second level is morality of conventional role-conformity, in which children try to conform to gain approval and to maintain good relationships with others. The third and highest level is morality of self-accepted moral principles, in which children voluntarily comply with rules on the basis of a concept of ethical principles and make exceptions to rules in certain circumstances.

Although Kohlberg's and Piaget's notions of moral development focus on a unified theory of cognitive maturation for both sexes, Carol Gilligan emphasizes the social context of moral development leading to divergent patterns in moral development. Gilligan points out that, in women, compassion and the ethics of caring are dominant features of moral decision-making, whereas, for men, predominant features of moral judgments are related more to a perception of justice, rationality, and a sense of fairness.

Self-Esteem

Self-esteem is a measure of one's sense of self-worth based on perceived success and achievements, as well as a perception of how much one is valued by peers, family members, teachers, and society in general. The most important correlates of good self-esteem are one's perception of positive physical appearance and high value to peers and family. Secondary features of self-esteem relate to academic achievement, athletic abilities, and special talents. Adolescent self-esteem is mediated, to a significant degree, by positive feedback received from a peer group and family members, and adolescents often seek out a peer group that offers acceptance, regardless of negative behaviors associated with that group. Adolescent girls have more of a problem maintaining self-esteem than do boys. Girls continued to rate themselves with generally lower self-esteem into adulthood.

CURRENT ENVIRONMENTAL INFLUENCES AND ADOLESCENCE

Adolescent Sexual Behavior

Sexual experimentation in adolescents often begins with fantasy and masturbation in early adolescence followed by noncoital genital touching with the opposite sex or, in some cases, same-sex partners, oral sex with partners, and initiation of sexual intercourse at a later point in development. By high school, most male adolescents report experience with masturbation, and more than half of adolescent girls report masturbation. The balance between healthy adolescent sexual experimentation and emotionally and physically safe sexual practices is one of the major challenges for society.

In 2003, 47 percent of 9th to 12th grade students reported having sexual intercourse, a decline from 53 percent in 1993. The median age at first intercourse is 16.9 years for boys and 17.4 years for girls. Boys generally have more sexual partners than do girls, and boys are less likely than girls to seek emotional attachments with their sexual partners. The prevalence of multiple sexual partners (four or greater) declined by 24 percent.

Factors that Influence Adolescent Sexual Behavior. Factors impacting sexual behavior in adolescents include personality traits, gender, cultural and religious background, racial factors, family attitudes, and sexual education and prevention programs.

Personality factors have been found to be associated with sexual behavior, as well as sexual risk-taking. Higher levels of impulsivity are associated with a younger age at first experience of sexual intercourse; higher number of sexual partners; sexual intercourse without the use of contraception, including condoms; and a history of sexually transmitted disease (chlamydia).

Historically, male adolescents have initiated sexual intercourse at a younger age than female adolescents. The younger a teenaged girl is when she has sex for the first time, the more likely she is to have had unwanted or nonvoluntary sex. Close to four of ten girls who had first intercourse at 13 or 14 years of age report it was either not voluntary or unwanted. Three of four girls and over half of boys report that girls who have sex do so because their boyfriends want them to. In general, adolescents who initiate sexual intercourse at younger ages are also more likely to have a greater number of sexual partners.

The additive effects of more highly educated families, social and religious youth groups, and school-based educational programs can be credited with a decline in high-risk sexual behavior among adolescents. Responsible sexual behavior among adolescents has been determined as one of the ten leading health indicators for the next decade. The primary reason that teenage girls who have never had intercourse give for abstaining from sex is that having sex would be against their religious or moral values. Other reasons include desire to avoid pregnancy, fear of contracting a sexually transmitted disease (STD), and not having met the appropriate partner.

Contraceptives. Currently, 98 percent of teenagers ages 15 to 19 years are using at least one method of birth control. The two most common methods are condoms and birth control pills. Sexually transmitted diseases (STDs) are still high among teenagers. Approximately one in four sexually active teens contracts an STD every year and half of all new human immunodeficiency virus (HIV) infections occur in people under the age of 25.

Pregnancy. Each year 750,000 to 850,000 teenage girls under the age of 19 become pregnant. Of this number, 432,000 give birth, a 19 percent decline from 532,000 in 1991; the rest (418,000) obtain abortions. The largest decline in teen pregnancy by race is for black women, with a decline of 42 percent between 1991 and 2002. Hispanic teen births have declined 20 percent, but continue to have the highest teen birth rates compared with other races.

Teenage pregnancy creates a plethora of health risks for both mother and child. Children born to teenage mothers have a greater chance of dying before the age of 5 years. Those who survive are more likely to perform poorly in school and are at greater risk of abuse and neglect. Teenage mothers are less likely to gain adequate weight during pregnancy, increasing the risk of premature births and low-birthweight infant. Low-birthweight babies are more likely to have organs that are not fully developed, resulting in bleeding in the brain, respiratory distress syndrome, and intestinal problems. Teenage mothers are also less likely to seek regular prenatal care, to take recommended daily multivitamins, and they are more likely to smoke, drink, or use drugs during pregnancy. Only one third of teenage mothers obtain high school diplomas and only 1.5 percent have a college degree by the age of 30.

The average adolescent mother who cannot care for her child, has the child either placed in foster care or raised by the teenager's already overburdened parents or other relatives. Few teenage mothers marry the fathers of their children; the fathers, usually teenagers, cannot care for themselves, much less the mothers of their children. If the two do marry, they usually divorce. Many are more likely to end up on welfare.

Abortion. Nearly four of ten teen pregnancies end in abortion. Almost all the girls are unwed mothers from low socioeconomic groups; their pregnancies result from sex with boys to whom they felt emotionally attached. Most (61 percent) teenagers elect to have abortions with their parents' consent, but laws of mandatory parental consent put two rights into competition: a girl's claim to privacy and a parent's need to know. Most adults believe that teenagers should have parental permission for an abortion; but when parents refuse to give their consent, most states prohibit parents from vetoing the teenager's decision.

The abortion rate in many European countries tends to be far lower than that in the United States. In the United States, the rate of abortion among girls between the ages of 15 and 19 is about 30 per 1,000 girls, according to the Centers for Disease Control and Prevention. In France, for instance, about 10.5 of every 1,000 girls under the age of 20 had an abortion in 2000, according to World Health Organization statistics. The rate of abortion in Germany was 6.8; in Italy, 6.3; and in Spain, 4.5. Britain has a higher rate, 18.5. Family planning experts believe that more sex education and availability of contraceptive devices help keep the number of abortions down. In Holland, where contraceptives are freely available in schools, the teenage pregnancy rate is among the lowest in the world.

Risk-Taking Behavior

Reasonable risk-taking is a necessary endeavor in adolescence, leading to confidence both in forming new relationships and in sports and social situations. High-risk behaviors among adolescents are associated with serious negative consequences, however, and can take many forms, including drug and alcohol use, unsafe sexual practices, self-injurious behaviors, and reckless driving.

Drug Use

Alcohol. In 2004, 29.2 percent of 12th graders reported having five or more drinks in a row within a 2-week period. The average age when youths first try alcohol is 11 years for boys and 13 years for girls. The national average age at which Americans begin drinking regularly is 15.9 years of age (Fig. 2.3–1). People ages 18 to 25 show the highest prevalence of binge and heavy drinking. Drunk driving has declined since 2002. Alcohol dependence, along with other drugs, is associated with depression, anxiety, oppositional defiant disorder, antisocial personality disorder, and an increased rate of suicide.

Nicotine. The number of younger Americans who smoke has declined since 1990; however, the rate of smoking among teenagers is still as high as or higher than those of adults. According to the American Cancer Society, on average in 2003, more than one of five students (22 percent) smoked cigarettes. Each day, more than 4,000 teenagers try their first cigarette and another 2,000 become regular, daily smokers. Cigarette smokers are more likely to get into fights, carry weapons, attempt suicide, suffer from mental health problems such as depression, and engage in high-risk sexual behaviors. One of three will eventually die from smoking-related diseases. Cigarettes are the most common type of tobacco used among middle-school students followed by cigars, smokeless tobacco, and pipes.

Cannabis. Marijuana is the most popular illicit drug, with 14.6 million people using it (6.2 percent of the population), two thirds being under the age of 18. Its use, however, is slowly declining. As of 2004, 5.6 percent of 12th graders reported daily use of marijuana, as compared with 6 percent in 1999. Among 8th graders, there has been a one-third (36 percent) decline from 18.3 in 1996 to 11.8 in 2004.

One of the major reasons for such prevalence of marijuana use among teenagers is because many find that marijuana is easier to get than alcohol or cigarettes. This belief has declined in recent years. Once teenagers are dependant on marijuana, they often tumble into truancy, crime, and depression.

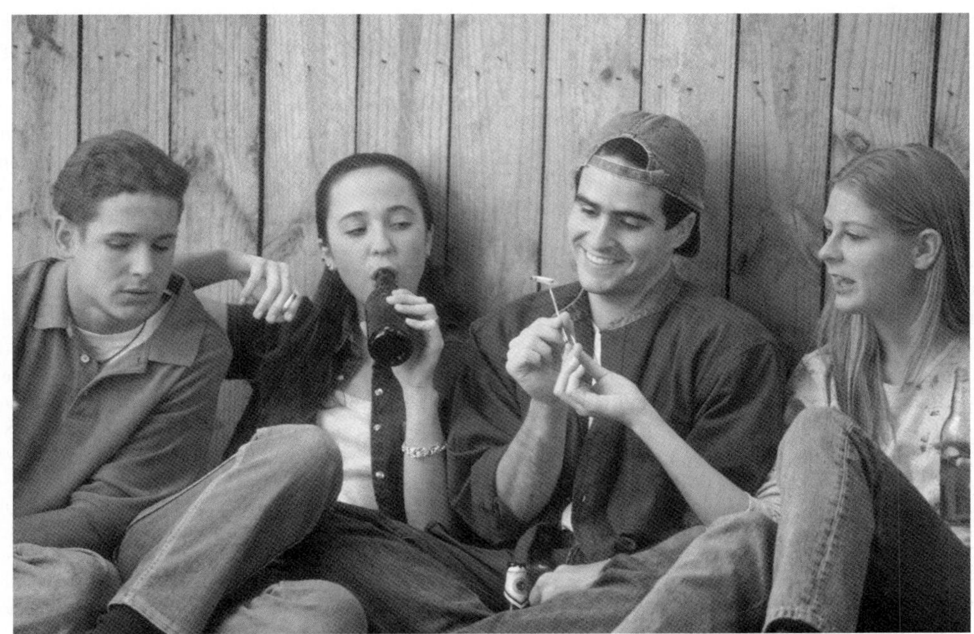

FIGURE 2.3–1
Adolescents remain one of the largest groups of abusers of alcohol, nicotine, cannabis, and opioids. (Courtesy of Corbis.)

Cocaine. In 2004, 13.1 percent of high school seniors used cocaine, a slight drop from 2003's figure of 14 percent, but still exceeding the national average of 3.6 percent. Also in 2004, 0.7 percent of 12th graders admitted to using phencyclidine (PCP). Crystal methamphetamine (ice) had an annual prevalence in 12th graders at 2.1 percent in 2004.

Opioids. In recent years, the number of teens using prescription pain relievers for nonmedical reasons has increased. Prescription drug abuse by people ages 18 to 25 has increased 15 percent. Drugs of specific concern are the pain relievers OxyContin and Vicodin. OxyContin has gained ground among high school students since its emergence in 2001, with 5 percent of 12th graders, 3.5 percent of 10th graders, and 1.7 percent of 8th graders reporting use in 2004. Vicodin was used by 9.3 percent of 12th graders, 6.2 percent of 10th graders, and 2.5 percent of 8th graders in 2004.

Heroin. Heroin use is prevalent among adolescents, although less so than cocaine. The average age of use is 19, but it is used by almost 2 percent of 12th graders, the nasal route (snorting) being the most common method of use.

Violence. Although rates of violent crime have decreased throughout the United States in the past 5 years—for example, the homicide rate in New York City fell by almost 50 percent between 1998 and 2000—violent crimes by young offenders are on the increase. Homicides are the second leading cause of death among persons aged 15 to 25. (Accidents are first; suicides, third.) Black male teenagers are far more likely to be murder victims than are boys from any other racial or ethnic group or girls of any race. The factor most strongly associated with violence among adolescent boys is growing up in a household without a father or father surrogate; this factor aside, race, socioeconomic status, and education show no effect on the propensity toward violence.

BULLYING. *Bullying* is defined as the use of one's strength or status to intimidate, injure, or humiliate another person of lesser strength or status. It can be categorized as physical, verbal, or social. *Physical* bullying involves physical injury or threat of injury to someone. *Verbal* bullying refers to teasing or insulting someone. *Social* bullying refers to the use of peer rejection or exclusion to humiliate or isolate a victim.

Approximately 30 percent of 6th through 10th grade students are involved in some aspect of moderate-to-frequent bullying, either as a bully, the target of bullying, or both. Approximately 1.7 million children within this age group can be identified as bullies. Boys are more likely to be involved in bullying and violent behavior than girls. Girls tend to use verbal bullying rather than physical.

Bullies are moving towards e-mail, websites, chat rooms, and text messaging to harass other students. In 2000, 1 of 17 children ages 10 to 17 years had been threatened or harassed online, one third of whom found the incidents extremely distressing.

An estimated 160,000 students miss school each day because of fear of attack or intimidation from peers; some are forced to drop out. Stresses of "victimization" can interfere with student's engagement and learning in school. Children who bully other children are at risk for engaging in more serious violent behaviors, such as frequent fighting and carrying a weapon. A correlation also exists between bullying and school shootings.

GANGS. Gang violence is a problem in various communities throughout the United States. There are 2,000 different youth gangs around the country with more than 200,000 teens and young adults as members. Most members are between the ages of 12 and 24 years with an average of 17 to 18 years. Gang membership is a brief phase for many teenagers; one half to two thirds leave the gang by the 1-year mark. Boys are more likely to join gangs than girls; however, the female gang membership may be underrepresented. Female gang members are more likely to be found in small cities and rural areas and tend to be younger than male gang members. Female gang members are also involved in less delinquent or criminal activity than males and commit fewer violent crimes.

WEAPONS. Each day, on average, nearly ten American children under the age of 18 years are killed in handgun suicides, homicides, and accidents. Many more are wounded. One in five youths in grades 9 to 12 carries a weapon: knife, gun, or club.

By law, firearms cannot be sold to anyone under the age of 18 years. Two thirds of students in grades 6 to 12 say that they can get a firearm within 24 hours, however. More than 22 million children live in a home with a firearm. In 40 percent of these homes, at least one gun is kept unlocked and 13 percent are kept unlocked and loaded. Two of three students involved in school shootings acquired their guns from their own home or that of a relative. At least 60 percent of suicide deaths in teens involve the use of a handgun.

SCHOOL VIOLENCE. In the 2003–2004 school year, 49 violent deaths (i.e., homicides, suicides) were reported in schools nationwide. Guns or knives were involved in most of these deaths. Much of school violence occurs in middle school and high school, but there have been instances as early as kindergarten.

Many factors can lead to violent acts in teenagers. Some inherited traits include impulsivity, learning difficulties, low IQ, or fearlessness. A correlation also exists between witnessing violent acts and involvement in violence. Children who witness violent acts are more aggressive and grow up more likely to become involved in violence—either as a victimizer or as a victim. Table 2.3–2 lists some of the early and imminent warning signs of school violence.

On April 20, 1999, two teenage boys, ages 17 and 18 years, went on a shooting rampage through Columbine High School of Littleton, Colorado. Armed with shotguns, a semiautomatic rifle, and a pistol, they laughed and hollered as they shot classmates and teachers at point-blank range while hurling homemade explosives. Fifteen were killed, including the two gunmen, and twenty-five were injured in the deadliest school shooting in U.S. history.

The gunmen were members of the "trench coat mafia" at the high school, a clique of social misfits who stood out at the school for their gothic style of dress and nihilistic attitude. The two gunmen were obsessed with violent video games and intrigued with Nazi culture, even though one was part Jewish. The date of the attack was picked because it was Adolf Hitler's birthday.

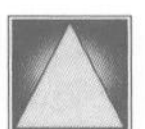

Table 2.3–2
Warning Signs of School Violence

Early Warning Signs
- Social withdrawal
- Excessive feelings of isolation and being alone
- Excessive feelings of rejection
- Being a victim of violence
- Feelings of being picked on and persecuted
- Expression of violence in writings and drawings
- Uncontrolled anger
- Patterns of impulsive and chronic hitting, intimidating, and bullying behaviors
- History of discipline problems
- History of violent and aggressive behavior
- Intolerance for differences and prejudicial attitudes
- Drug and alcohol use
- Affiliation with gangs
- Inappropriate access to, possession of, and use of firearms
- Serious threats of violence

Imminent Warning Signs
- Serious physical fighting with peers or family members
- Severe destruction of property
- Severe rage for seemingly minor reasons
- Detailed threats of lethal violence
- Possession and/or use of firearms and other weapons
- Other self-injurious behaviors or threats of suicide

On March 21, 2005, a 16-year-old boy went on a shooting rampage at Red Lake High School on the Red Lake Indian Reservation in far northern Minnesota. He began his shooting spree by killing his grandfather and the grandfather's companion. He then donned his grandfather's police-issue gunbelt and bulletproof vest before heading to the school, where he killed a security guard, a teacher, five students, and then himself. About 15 others were injured.

The gunman had a troubled childhood; his father committed suicide in 1997 and his mother suffered head injuries in an auto accident. He expressed an admiration of Adolf Hitler on a neo-Nazi website, using the handle "Todesengel," which is German for "Angel of Death." He had bouts of depression, suicide ideation, and was taking fluoxetine (Prozac). He was a member of a clique of about five students known as "The Darkers," who wore black clothes and chains, spiked or dyed their hair, and loved heavy-metal music. The gunman was usually seen in a long black trench coat, eyeliner, and combat boots, and was described as a quiet teenager.

SEXUAL OFFENSE. Adolescents under the age of 18 years account for 20 percent of arrests for all sexual offenses (excluding prostitution), 20 to 30 percent of rape cases, 14 percent of aggravated sexual assault offenses, and 27 percent of child sexual homicides. These adolescent offenders account for the victimization of approximately one half of boys and one quarter of girls who are molested or sexually abused. Most instances involved adolescent male perpetrators.

There appear to be two types of juvenile sex offenders: those who target children, and those who offend against peers or adults. The main distinction between the two groups is based on the age difference between the victim and the offender. Table 2.3–3 lists the differences and similarities of these two groups.

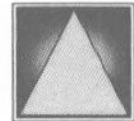

Table 2.3–3
Juvenile Sex Offender Subtypes

Juvenile Offenders Who Sexually Offend against Peers or Adults
- Predominantly assault females and strangers or casual acquaintances
- Sexual assaults occur in association with other types of criminal activity (e.g., burglary).
- Have histories of nonsexual criminal offenses, and appear more generally delinquent and conduct disordered
- Commit their offenses in public areas
- Display higher levels of aggression and violence in the commission of their sexual crimes
- More likely to use weapons and to cause injuries to their victims

Juvenile Offenders Who Sexually Offend against Children
- Most victims are male and are related to them, either siblings or other relatives.
- Almost half of the offenders have had at least one male victim.
- The sexual crimes tend to reflect a greater reliance on opportunity and guile than injurious force. This appears to be particularly true when their victim is related to them. These youths may "trick" the child into complying with the molestation, use bribes, or threaten the child with loss of the relationship.
- Within the overall population of juveniles who sexually assault children are certain youths who display high levels of aggression and violence. Generally, these are youths who display more severe levels of personality and/or psychosexual disturbances, such as psychopathy, sexual sadism, and so on.
- Suffer from deficits in self-esteem and social competency
- Many show evidence of depression.

Characteristics Common to Both Groups
- High rates of learning disabilities and academic dysfunction (30 to 60 percent)
- The presence of other behavioral health problems, including substance abuse, and disorders of conduct (up to 80 percent have some diagnosable psychiatric disorder)
- Observed difficulties with impulse control and judgment

Etiological factors of juvenile sex offending include maltreatment experiences, exposure to pornography, substance abuse, and exposure to aggressive role models. A significant number of offending adolescents have a childhood history of physical abuse (25 to 50 percent) or sexual abuse (10 to 80 percent). Half of adolescent offenders lived with both parents and one other juvenile at the time of their offending. Evidence also suggests that most juvenile sex offenders are likely to become adult sex offenders. The most common psychosocial deficits of adolescent sexual offenders include low self-esteem, few social skills, minimal assertive skills, and poor academic performance. The most common psychiatric diagnoses are conduct disorder, substance abuse disorder, adjustment disorder, attention-deficit/hyperactivity disorder, specific phobia, and mood disorders. Male offenders are more often diagnosed with paraphilias and antisocial behavior, whereas female offenders are more likely to be diagnosed with mood disorders and engage in self-mutilation.

PROSTITUTION. Teenagers constitute a large portion of all prostitutes, with estimates ranging up to 1 million teenagers involved in prostitution. The average age of a new recruit is 13 years; however, some are as young as 9 years of age. Most adolescent prostitutes are girls, but boys are involved as homosexual prostitutes. Most teenagers who enter a life of prostitution come from broken homes; however, a growing number of teenage prostitutes come from middle- to upper middle-class

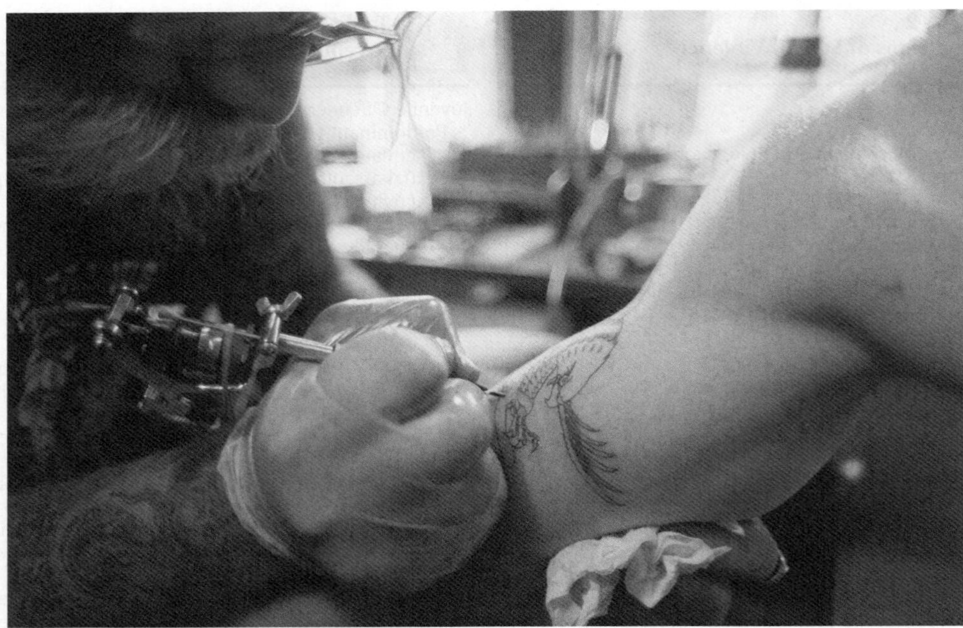

FIGURE 2.3–2
A person getting an eagle tattoo at a mobile tattoo parlor. (Courtesy of Corbis.)

homes. Many were victims of rape, or were abused as children. Most teenagers ran away from home and were taken in by pimps and substance abusers; the adolescents themselves then became substance abusers. Of teenage prostitution, 27 percent occurs in large cities and incidents usually take place at an outside location, such as highways, roads, alleys, fields, woods, or parking lots. They are at high risk for acquired immunodeficiency syndrome (AIDS), and many (up to 70 percent in some studies) are infected with HIV.

As many as 17,500 sex slaves are smuggled into the United States each year. They are brought under the pretences of a better life and job opportunities, but once they are in the United States, they are forced into prostitution, making little money while traffickers make thousands of dollars from their services. Many times they are raped and abused.

TATTOOS AND BODY PIERCING. Body piercing and tattoos have become more prevalent among adolescents since the 1980s. In the general population, approximately 10 to 13 percent of adolescents have tattoos. Of the more than 500 adolescents surveyed in a study, 13.2 percent report at least one tattoo, and 26.9 percent report at least one body piercing, other than in their ear lobe, at some point in their lives. Both tattoos and body piercing are more common in girls than in boys. Adolescents who endorsed possession of at least one tattoo or body piercing are more likely to endorse use of gateway drugs (cigarettes, alcohol, marijuana), as well as experience with hard drugs (cocaine, crystal methamphetamine, and ecstasy). Female adolescents who had tattoos or body piercings, especially younger adolescents, are more likely to endorse a history of suicidal ideation or behaviors. Male adolescents with tattoos and female adolescents with body piercings are more likely to report a history of involvement in physical fights, carrying a weapon, or bodily injury as a result of physical fighting. Adolescents with tattoos or piercings are more frequently sexually active than are adolescents without them, and at greater risk for unsafe sexual behavior (Fig. 2.3–2).

References

Burgess AW, Garbarino C, Carlson MI. Pathological teasing and bullying turned deadly: Shooters and suicide. *Victims & Offenders*. 2006;1:1–14.

Dishion TJ, Nelson SE, Yasui M. Predicting early adolescent gang involvement from middle school adaptation. *Journal of Clinical Child & Adolescent Psychology*. 2005;34(1):62–73.

Doyle AB, Markiewicz D. Parenting, marital conflict and adjustment from early- to mid-adolescence: Mediated by adolescent attachment style? *Journal of Youth and Adolescence*. 2005;34(2):97–110.

Gutgesell ME, Payne N. Issues of adolescent psychological development in the 21st century. *Pediatr Rev*. 2004;25:79.

Harris S. Bullying at school among older adolescents. *School Nurse News*. 2005; 22(3):18–21.

King CA, Knox MS, Henninger N, Nguyen TA, Ghaziuddin N, Maker A, Hanna GL. Major depressive disorder in adolescents: Family psychiatry history predicts severe behavioral disinhibition. *J Affect Disord.* 2006;90:111–121.

Monk CS, McClure EB, Nelson EE, Sarahn E, Bilder RM, Lienbenloft E, Charney DS, Ernst M, Pine DS. Adolescent immaturity in attention-related brain engagement to emotional facial expressions. *Neuroimage*. 2003;20:420.

Niederhiser JM, Reiss D, Pedersen NL, Lichtenstein P, Spotts EL, Hansson K, Cederblad M, Elhammer D. Genetic and environmental influences on mothering of adolescents: A comparison of two samples. *Dev Psychol*. 2004;40: 335.

Ozer EJ. The impact of violence on urban adolescents: Longitudinal effects of perceived school connection and family support. *Journal of Adolescent Research*. 2005; 20(2):167–192.

Pataki CS. Normal adolescence. In: Sadock BJ, Sadock VA, eds. *Kaplan & Sadock's Comprehensive Textbook of Psychiatry.* 8th ed. Vol. 2. Baltimore: Lippincott Williams & Wilkins; 2005:3035.

Robins RW, Trzesniewski KH. Self-esteem development across the lifespan. *Current Directions in Psychological Science*. 2005;14(3):158–162.

Spear LP, Varlinskaya EI. Adolescence. Alcohol sensitivity, tolerance, and intake. *Recent Dev Alcohol*. 2005;17:143–159.

Steinberg L, Scott ES. Less guilty by reason of adolescence: Developmental immaturity, diminished responsibility, and the juvenile death penalty. *Am Psychol*. 2003;58:1009.

Trzesniewski KH, Donnellan MB, Moffitt TE, Robins RW, Poulton R, Caspi A. Low self-esteem during adolescence predicts poor health, criminal behavior, and limited economic prospects during adulthood. *Dev Psychol*. 2006;42(2): 381–390.

▲ 2.4 Adulthood

Development in adulthood, as in childhood, is always the result of the interaction among body, mind, and environment, never exclusively the result of any one of the three variables. Most adults are forced to confront and adapt to similar circumstances: establishing an independent identity, forming a marriage or other partnership, raising children, building and maintaining careers, and accepting the disability and death of one's parents.

In modern Western societies, adulthood is the longest phase of human life. Although the exact age of consent varies from person to person, adulthood can be divided into three main parts: young or early adulthood (ages 20 to 40), middle adulthood (ages 40 to 65), and late adulthood or old age.

YOUNG ADULTHOOD (20 TO 40 YEARS OF AGE)

Usually considered to begin at the end of adolescence (about age 20) and to end at age 40, early adulthood is characterized by peaking biological development, the assumption of major social roles, and the evolution of an adult self and life structure. The successful passage into adulthood depends on satisfactory resolution of childhood and adolescent crises.

During late adolescence, young persons generally leave home and begin to function independently. Sexual relationships become serious, and the quest for intimacy begins. The 20s are spent, for the most part, exploring options for occupation and marriage or alternative relationships, and making commitments in various areas.

Early adulthood requires choosing new roles (e.g., husband, father) and establishing an identity congruent with those new roles. It involves asking and answering the questions "Who am I?" and "Where am I going?" The choices made during this time may be tentative; young adults may make several false starts.

Transition from Adolescence to Young Adulthood

The transition from adolescence to young adulthood is characterized by real and intrapsychic separation from the family of origin and the engagement of new, phase-specific tasks (Table 2.4–1). It involves many important events: graduating from high school, starting a job or entering college, and living independently. During these years, the individual resolves the issue of childhood dependency sufficiently to establish self-reliance and begins to formulate new, young-adult goals that eventually result in creation of new life structures that promote stability and continuity.

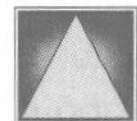

Table 2.4–1
Development Tasks of Young Adulthood

- To develop a young-adult sense of self and other: the third individuation
- To develop adult friendships
- To develop the capacity for intimacy; to become a spouse
- To become a biological and psychological parent
- To develop a relationship of mutuality and equality with parents while facilitating their midlife development
- To establish an adult work identity
- To develop adult forms of play
- To integrate new attitudes toward time

Developmental Tasks

Establishing a self that is separate from parents is a major task of young adulthood. For most individuals, the emotional detachment from parents that takes place in adolescence and young adulthood is followed by a new inner definition of themselves as comfortably alone and competent, able to care for themselves in the real world. This shift away from the parents continues long after marriage, and parenthood results in the formation of new relationships that replace the progenitors as the most important individuals in the young adult's life.

Psychological separation from the parents is followed by synthesis of mental representations from the childhood past and the young-adult present. The psychological separation from parents in adolescence has been called the *second individuation*, and the continued elaboration of these themes in young adulthood has been called the *third individuation*. The continuous process of elaboration of self and differentiation from others that occurs in the developmental phases of young (20 to 40 years of age) and middle (40 to 60 years of age) adulthood is influenced by all important adult relationships.

A number of different models have been proposed for understanding adult development. They are all theoretical and somewhat idealized. They all use metaphors to describe complex social, psychological, and interpersonal interactions. The models are heuristic: They provide a conceptual framework for thinking about common important experiences. They are descriptive rather than prescriptive; that is, they provide a useful way of looking at what many persons do, not a formula for what all persons should do. Some of the terms and concepts commonly used are explained in Table 2.4–2. These periods involve individuation, that is, leaving the family of origin and becoming one's own man or woman, passing through midlife, and preparing in middle adulthood for the transition into late adulthood.

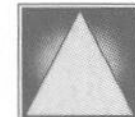

Table 2.4–2
Psychological Development Concepts

Concept	Definition	Example
Transition	The bridge between two successive stages	Late adolescence
Normative crisis	A period of rapid change or turmoil that strains a person's adaptive capacities	Midlife crisis
Stage	Period of consolidation of skills and capacities	Mature adulthood
Plateau	Period of developmental stability	Adulthood up to midlife
Rite of passage	Social ritual that facilitates a transition	Graduation; marriage

(Adapted from Wolman T, Thompson T. Adult and later-life development. In: Stoudemire A, ed. *Human Behavior.* Philadelphia: Lippincott-Raven; 1998, with permission.)

Work Identity. The transition from learning and play to work may be gradual or abrupt. Socioeconomic group, gender, and race affect the pursuit and development of particular occupational choices. Blue-collar workers generally enter the work force directly after high school; white-collar workers and professionals usually enter the work force after college or professional school. Depending on choice of career and opportunity, work may become a source of ongoing frustration or an activity that enhances self-esteem. Symptoms of job dissatisfaction are a high rate of job changes, absenteeism, mistakes at work, accident proneness, and even sabotage.

WOMEN AND WORK. Since the 1970s, women have become a significant economic force in the United States. Women's wages have steadily increased relative to men's, although the typical hourly wage for women is still less than that for men. More women have been entering the workplace. The proportion of working-age women with jobs has increased from 35 percent in 1960 to more than 70 percent in 2000. Even more impressive is that women now own one third of all businesses.

In general, families whose income is below $50,000 per year are more likely to include a working mother. Most nonworking mothers are found in families with an annual income over $100,000 per year. Despite this, however, the greatest increase in working wives has occurred toward the top of the income scale.

Women's increasing economic power has been accompanied by increasing political power. The political gender gap (men and women voting for different parties) has widened; women disproportionately favor Democrats. Political observers noted numerous instances in which presidential and other campaigns appeal specifically to women.

UNEMPLOYMENT. The effects of unemployment transcend those of loss of income; the psychological and physical tolls are enormous. The incidence of alcohol dependence, homicide, violence, suicide, and mental illness rises with unemployment. One's core identity, which is often tied to occupation and work, is seriously damaged when a job is lost, whether through firing, attrition, or early or sometimes even regular retirement. Seventy percent of married women with children under the age of 6 have paid employment. For many of these women, work enhances their self-esteem in addition to providing needed income.

A young-adult female patient had greatly enjoyed her 5 years in college and only reluctantly accepted a job with a large real estate firm. During college, she had had limited interest in her appearance, and she began work in clothing borrowed from family and friends. She scoffed when her boss began to criticize her dress and gave her an advance to buy an upscale wardrobe, but she began to enjoy the fine clothing and the respect engendered by her appearance and position. As her income began to rise, work became a source of pleasure and self-esteem and the way to acquire some of the trappings of adulthood. (Courtesy of Calvin Colarusso, M.D.)

Developing Adult Friendships. In late adolescence and young adulthood, before marriage and parenthood, friendships are often the primary source of emotional sustenance. Roommates, apartment mates, sorority sisters, and fraternity brothers, as indicated by the names used to describe them, are substitutes for parents and siblings, temporary stand-ins until more permanent replacements are found.

The emotional needs for closeness and confidentiality are largely met by friendships. All major developmental issues are discussed with friends, particularly those in similar circumstances. As marriages occur and children are born, the central emotional importance of friendships diminishes. Some friendships are abandoned at this point, because the spouse objects to the friend, recognizing at some level that they are competitors. Gradually, there is movement toward a new form of friendship, couples friendships. They reflect the newly committed status but are more difficult to form and to maintain, because four individuals must be compatible, not just two.

As children begin to move out of the family into the community, parents follow. Dance classes and Little League games provide the progenitors with a new focus and the opportunity to make friends with others who are at the same point developmentally and who are receptive to the formation of relationships that help explain, and cushion, the pressures of young-adult life.

Sexuality and Marriage. The developmental shift from sexual experimentation to the desire for intimacy is experienced in young adulthood as an intense loneliness, resulting from the awareness of an absence of committed love similar to that experienced in childhood with the parents. Brief sexual encounters in short-lived relationships no longer significantly boost self-esteem. Increasingly, the desire is for emotional involvement in a sexual context. The young adult who fails to develop the capacity for intimate relationships runs the risk of living in isolation and self-absorption in midlife.

For most individuals in Western culture, the experience of intimacy increases the desire for marriage. Most persons in the United States marry for the first time in their mid- to late 20s. The median age of first marriage has been rising steadily since 1950 for both men and women, and the number of persons who never marry has been increasing. By 2000, the proportion of 30- to 34-year-olds who never married almost tripled, and the proportion of never-married 35- to 39-year-olds doubled. The rate of divorce has also been declining. In 1998, it reached the lowest level in almost 20 years. Most divorced persons marry again—in most cases more successfully than the first time—an indication that the marital unit still provides a means for sustained intimacy, perpetuates the culture, and gratifies interpersonal needs.

INTERRACIAL MARRIAGE. Mixed-race marriages were banned in 19 states until a Supreme Court decision in 1967. In 1970, such marriages accounted for only 2 percent of all marriages involving at least one black partner. The trend has been steadily upward. Currently, interracial marriages account for about 1.5 million marriages in the United States.

Despite the trend toward more interracial marriages, they still remain a small proportion of all marriages. Most persons are more likely to marry someone from the same racial and ethnic background. Marriages between Hispanic whites and non-Hispanic whites and between Asians and whites are more common than those between blacks and whites.

MARITAL PROBLEMS. Although marriage tends to be regarded as a permanent tie, unsuccessful unions can be terminated, as indeed they are in most societies. Nevertheless, many marriages that do not end in separation or divorce are disturbed. In considering marital problems, clinicians are concerned with both the persons involved and with the marital unit itself. How any marriage works out relates to the partners selected, the personality organization or disorganization of each, the interaction between them, and the original reasons for the union. Persons marry for a variety of reasons—emotional, social, economic, and political, among others. One person may look to the spouse to meet unfulfilled childhood needs for good parenting. Another may see the spouse as someone to be saved from an otherwise unhappy life. Irrational expectations between spouses increase the risk of marital problems.

MARRIAGE AND COUPLES THERAPY. When families consist of grandparents, parents, children, and other relatives living under the same roof, assistance for marital problems can sometimes be obtained from a member of the extended family with whom one or both partners have rapport. With the contraction of the extended family in recent times, however, this source of informal help is no longer as accessible as it once was. Similarly, religion once played a more important role than now in the maintenance of family stability. Wise religious leaders are available to provide counseling, but they are not sought out to the extent that they once were, which reflects the decline in religious influence among large segments of the population. Formerly, both the extended family and religion provided guidance for couples in distress and also prevented dissolution of marriages by virtue of the social pressures that the extended family and religion exerted on couples to stay together. As family, religious, and societal pressures have relaxed, legal procedures for relatively easy separation and divorce have expanded. Concurrently, the need for formalized marriage counseling services has developed.

Marital therapy is a form of psychotherapy for married persons in conflict with each other. A trained person establishes a professional contract with the patient-couple and, through definite types of communication, attempts to alleviate the disturbance, to reverse or change maladaptive patterns of behavior, and to encourage personality growth and development.

In *marriage counseling*, only a particular conflict related to the immediate concerns of the family is discussed; marriage counseling is conducted much more superficially by persons with less psychotherapeutic training than is marital therapy. *Marital therapy* places greater emphasis on restructuring the interaction between the couple, including, at times, exploration of the psychodynamics of each partner. Both therapy and counseling emphasize helping marital partners cope effectively with their problems.

Parenthood. Parenthood intensifies the relationship between the new parents. Through their physical and emotional union, the couple has produced a fragile, dependent being that needs them in the interlocking roles of father and mother. This recognition expands their internal images of each other to include thoughts and feelings emanating from the role of parent. As they live together as a family, the lovers' relationship to each other changes. They become parents relating to one another and to their children.

Parent–child problems do arise, however. In addition to the economic burden of raising a child (estimated to be $250,000 for a middle-class family whose child goes to college), are emotional costs. Children may reawaken conflicts that parents themselves had as children, or children may have chronic illnesses that challenge families' emotional resources. In general, men have been more concerned with their work and occupational advancement than with child rearing, and women have been more concerned about their role as mothers than with advancement in their occupation, but this emphasis is changing dramatically for both sexes. A small, but growing, number of couples are choosing to split a job (or work at two part-time jobs) and share child-rearing duties.

For persons in their 20s and 30s, parenting has been described as a continuing process of letting go. Children must be allowed to separate from parents and, in some cases, must be encouraged to do so. When parents are in their 20s, letting go involves separation from children who are starting school. School phobias and school refusal syndromes that are accompanied by extreme separation anxiety may have to be dealt with. Often, a parent who cannot let go of a child accounts for this situation; some parents want their children to remain tightly bound to them emotionally. Family therapy that explores these dynamics may be needed to resolve such problems.

As children get older and enter adolescence, the process of establishing identity assumes great importance. Peer relationships become crucial to a child's development, and overprotective parents who keep a child from developing friendships or having the freedom to experiment with friends that the parents disapprove of can interfere with the child's passage through adolescence. Parents need not try to refrain from exerting influence over their children; guidance and involvement are crucial. But they must recognize that adolescents, especially, need parental approval; although rebellious on the surface, adolescents are much more tractable than they appear, provided parents are not overbearing or generally punitive.

SINGLE-PARENT FAMILIES. More than 10 million single-parent families exist with one or more children under the age of 18; of these families, 20 percent are single-parent homes in which a woman is the sole head of the household. Although most of these children were left in the custody of their mothers by the courts in divorce proceedings, other children have been abandoned by their fathers. The increase in number of single-parent families has risen almost 200 percent since 1980.

ALTERNATIVE LIFESTYLE PARENTING. Both single and married homosexual men and women are choosing to raise children (Fig. 2.4–1). In most cases, such children are obtained through adoption. Some, however, may be born to a lesbian woman through artificial insemination or obtained from a willing mother surrogate. The number of such family units is increasing. The data about the development of children in these homes indicate that they are at no greater risk for emotional problems (or for a homosexual orientation) than children raised in conventional households.

ADOPTION. Since the turn of the century, adoption or foster placement has replaced institutional care as the preferred way to raise children who are neglected, unwanted, or abandoned. Many couples who are unable to conceive (and some couples who already have children) turn to adoption.

In addition to the full range of normal parent–child developmental issues, adoptive parents face special problems. They

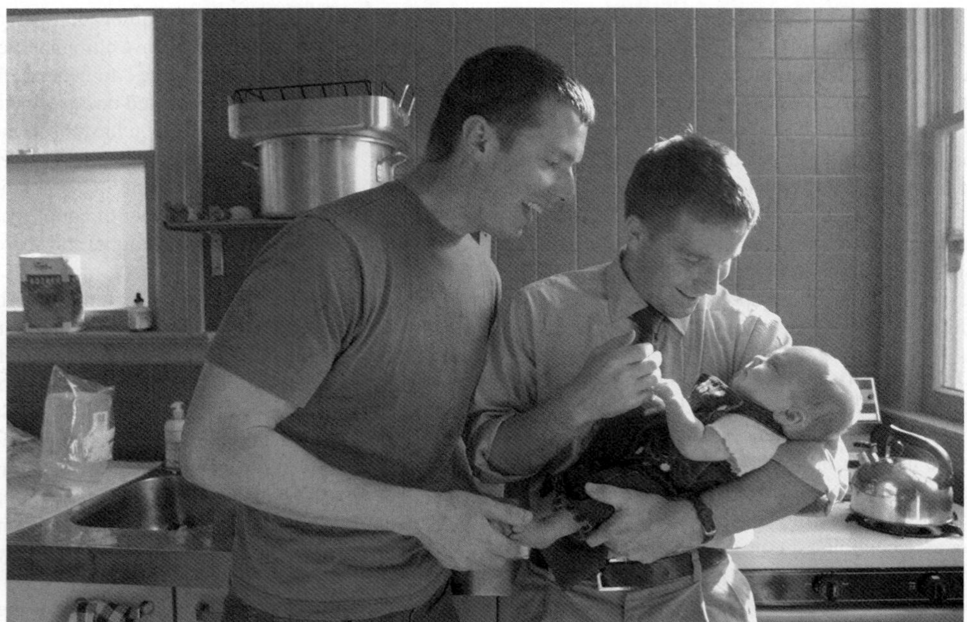

FIGURE 2.4–1
Gay fathers hold their 2-month-old adopted daughter. (Courtesy of Corbis.)

must decide how and when to tell the child about the adoption. They must deal with the child's possible desire for information about his or her biological parents. Adopted children are more likely to develop conduct disorders, problems with drug abuse, and antisocial personality traits. It is unclear whether these problems result from the process of adoption or whether parents who give up children for adoption are more likely to pass along a genetic predisposition for these behaviors.

With widespread use of birth control and access to abortions, the number of infants available for adoption has declined steeply. Wealthy parents may prefer to arrange for private adoption rather than wait many uncertain years for an institutional adoption. (In private adoptions, a biological mother is paid for her legal and medical expenses but not for the baby. Baby selling is a felony in all states.) International adoptions (especially from Bosnia, Latin America, eastern Europe, and China) have also become more common. Questionable regulation in these countries has raised concern that some infants put up for adoption in poor countries may not be orphans but are being sold by destitute mothers.

MIDDLE ADULTHOOD (40 TO 60 YEARS OF AGE)

Middle adulthood is the golden age of adulthood, similar to the latency years in childhood, but much longer. Physical health, emotional maturity, competence and power in the work situation, and gratifying relationships with spouse, children, parents, friends, and colleagues all contribute to a normative sense of satisfaction and well-being. With regard to occupation, many persons begin to experience the gap between early aspirations and current achievements. They may wonder whether the lifestyle and the commitments they chose in early adulthood are worth continuing; they may feel that they would like to live their remaining years in a different, more satisfying way, without knowing exactly how. As children grow up and leave home, parental roles change, and persons redefine their roles as husbands and wives.

Important gender changes occur in middle adulthood. Many women who no longer need to nurture young children can release their energy into independent pursuits that require assertiveness and a competitive spirit, traits that were traditionally considered masculine. Alternatively, men in middle adulthood may develop qualities that enable them to express their emotions and recognize their dependency needs, traits that were traditionally considered feminine. With the new balance of the masculine and the feminine, a person may now be able to relate more effectively to someone of the other sex than in the past.

Transition from Young to Middle Adulthood

The transition from young adulthood to middle adulthood is slow and gradual, with no sharp physical or psychological demarcation. The aging process picks up speed and becomes a powerful organizing influence on intrapsychic life, but the change is gradual, unlike during adolescence. Mental change is experienced in a similar fashion, slow and imperceptible, without a sense of disruption.

Development in young adulthood is embedded in close relationships. Intimacy, love, and commitment are related to the mastery of the relationships most immediate to personal experience. The transition from young adulthood to middle age includes widening concern for the larger social system and differentiation of one's own social, political, and historical system from others. Authors have described middle adulthood in terms of generativity, self-actualization, and wisdom.

Developmental Tasks

Robert Butler described several underlying themes in middle adulthood that appear to be present regardless of marital and

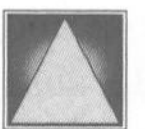

Table 2.4–3
Features Salient to Middle Adulthood

Issues	Positive Features	Negative Features
Prime of life	Responsible use of power; maturity; productivity	Winner-loser view; competitiveness
Stock taking: what to do with the rest of one's life	Possibility; alternatives; organization of commitments; redirection	Closure; fatalism
Fidelity and commitments	Commitment to self, others, career, society; filial maturity	Hypocrisy; self-deception
Growth-death (to grow is to die); juvenescence and rejuvenation fantasies	Naturality regarding body, time	Obscene or frenetic efforts (e.g., to be youthful); hostility and envy of youth and progeny; longing
Communication and socialization	Matters understood; continuity; picking up where left off; large social network; rootedness of relationships, places, and ideas	Repetitiveness; boredom; impatience; isolation; conservatism; confusion; rigidity

(Adapted from Robert N. Butler, M.D.)

family status, gender, or economic level (Table 2.4–3). These themes include aging (as changes in bodily functions are noticed in middle adulthood); taking stock of accomplishments and setting goals for the future; reassessing commitments to family, work, and marriage; dealing with parental illness and death; and attending to all the developmental tasks without losing the capacity to experience pleasure or to engage in playful activity.

Erik Erikson. Erikson described middle adulthood as characterized either by generativity or by stagnation. Erikson defined *generativity* as the process by which persons guide the oncoming generation or improve society. This stage includes having and raising children, but wanting or having children does not ensure generativity. A childless person can be generative by (1) helping others, (2) being creative, and (3) contributing to society. Parents must be secure in their own identities to raise children successfully: They cannot be preoccupied with themselves and act as if they were, or wished to be, the child in the family.

To be *stagnant* means that a person stops developing. For Erikson, stagnation was anathema, and he referred to adults without any impulses to guide the new generation or to those who produce children without caring for them as being "within a cocoon of self-concern and isolation." Such persons are in great danger. Because they are unable to negotiate the developmental tasks of middle adulthood, they are unprepared for the next stage of the life cycle, old age, which places more demands on the psychological and physical capacities than all the preceding stages.

George Vaillant. In his longitudinal study of 173 men who were interviewed at 5-year intervals after they graduated from Harvard, Vaillant found a strong correlation between physical and emotional health in middle age. In addition, those with the poorest psychological adjustment during college years had a high incidence of physical illness in middle age. No single factor in childhood accounted for adult mental health, but an overall sense of stability in the parental home predicted a well-adjusted adulthood. A close sibling relationship during college years was correlated with emotional and physical well-being in middle age. In another study, Vaillant found that childhood and adult work habits were correlated and that adult mental health and good interpersonal relationships were associated with the capacity to work in childhood. Vaillant's studies are ongoing and represent the longest continuous study of adulthood ever performed.

Developing Midlife Friendships. Unlike friendships in latency and adolescence and, to some extent, in young adulthood, midlife friendships do not usually have the sense of urgency or the need for frequent or nearly constant physical presence of the friend. Midlife individuals have neither the need to build new psychic structure (as do latency-age children and adolescents) nor the pressing need to find new relationships (as do young adults). They may have many sources of gratification available through relationships with spouse, children, and colleagues.

As their firstborn sons progressed through high school, two women in their mid-40s became fast friends. In addition to raising money for the school activities in which their sons were involved, thus maintaining a close involvement with the boys, they spent many hours talking about the boys' activities, girlfriends, and plans for college. Their husbands, who liked each other, became acquaintances, not friends. They directed their own feelings about their sons into other relationships. After the boys left for college, the intensity of the friendship diminished, tending to peak again during vacation periods. (Courtesy of Calvin Colarusso, M.D.)

Because of their unique position in the life cycle, midlife adults are easily able to initiate and to sustain friendships with individuals of different ages, as well as chronological peers. In the face of a disrupted marriage or intimacy or the pressure of other midlife developmental themes, friendships may quickly become vehicles for the direct expression of impulses.

Reappraising Relationships. Midlife is a time of serious reappraisal of marriage and committed relationships. In the process, individuals struggle with the question of whether to settle for what they have or to search for greater perfection with a new partner. For some, the conflict rages internally and is kept from others; others express it through actions that take the form of affairs, trial separations, and divorce.

Recent research on happy marriage indicates that these couples, despite internal and real conflict, have found or achieved a special *goodness-of-fit* between their individual needs, wishes, and expectations. In the eyes of these couples, marital success is based on the ongoing, successful engagement of a number of psychological tasks. Among the most important are providing a safe place for conflict and difference, holding a double vision of the other, and maintaining a satisfying sexual life.

The decision to leave a long-standing, committed relationship has great consequences, not only for the two individuals involved, but also for their friends and loved ones. The effect on children, in particular, is especially profound, extending far beyond childhood. The effects on the abandoned spouse, parents, and close relatives may be nearly as severe.

Various forms of therapeutic intervention, such as marital counseling, individual psychotherapy, and psychoanalysis, can be extremely effective in helping uncertain individuals decide what to do or in helping those who leave deal with the consequences of their decision on the abandoned partner, children, and other loved ones. Problems relating to intimacy, love, and sex can occupy a prominent position in an outpatient practice.

> Fifty-year-old Mrs. T. left her "wonderful" husband, because "I've missed something. I just have to get out on my own." Married at 18 years of age, "after going from my parent's home to his home," she recognized that her rage at her husband for "not being all the other men I could have married, for closing off all the living I could have done," was irrational but uncontrollable. "I have to live on my own for awhile, to see if I can do it, before it's too late." Fully intending to return to her husband, she continued exploring the infantile and adult issues that precipitated the separation, leaving the future of the marriage in doubt. (Courtesy of Calvin Colarusso, M.D.)

Sexuality

Whereas the young adult is preoccupied with developing the capacity for intimacy, the midlife individual is focused on maintaining intimacy in the face of deterring physical, psychological, and environmental pressures. In a long-standing relationship, these pressures include real and imaginary concerns about diminished sexual capability, emotional withdrawal because of preoccupation with developmental tasks, and the realistic pressures related to work and providing for dependent children and, sometimes, elderly parents as well. In relationships that begin in midlife, the maintenance of intimacy can be compromised by the absence of a common past, age and generational differences in interests and activities, and the difficulties involved in forming a stepfamily.

For sexual intimacy to continue, the participants must (1) accept the appearance of the partner's middle-aged body, (2) continue to find it sexually stimulating, and (3) accept the normative changes that occur in sexual functioning. For those who master these developmental issues, the partner's body remains sexually stimulating. Diminished sexual ability is compensated for by feelings of love and tenderness generated over the years by a satisfying relationship. Those who cannot accept the changes in the partner's body or their own stop having sex, begin affairs, or leave the relationship, usually in search of a younger partner.

Normative changes in midlife sexual functioning include diminished sexual drive and an increase in mechanical problems. Men have greater difficulty getting and sustaining erections and experience a longer refractory period after ejaculation. Because of diminished estrogen production, women experience a thinning of the vaginal mucosa, a decrease in secretions, and fewer contractions at the time of orgasm. Women do not reach their sexual prime until their mid-30s; consequently, they have a greater capacity for orgasm in middle adulthood than in young adulthood. Women, however, are more vulnerable than men to narcissistic blows to their self-esteem as they lose their youthful appearance, which is overvalued in today's society. During middle adulthood, they may feel less sexually desirable than in early adulthood and, thus, feel less entitled to an adequate sex life. An inability to deal with changes in body image prompts many women and men to undergo cosmetic surgery in an effort to maintain their youthful appearance.

The demands of raising children interfere with the privacy and emotional equilibrium required for intimacy, as do the pressures and responsibilities of work. Fatigue and diminished interest are common denominators in these circumstances. Patients with deeply rooted problems with sexuality or relationships may use aging, work, and relationships with children or elderly parents as a means of rationalizing their conflicts and refusing to analyze them.

Climacterium

Middle adulthood is the time of the male and female climacterium, the period in life characterized by decreased biological and physiological functioning. For women, the menopausal period is considered the climacterium, and it may start anywhere from the 40s to the early 50s. Bernice Neugarten studied this period and found that more than 50 percent of women described menopause as an unpleasant experience, but a significant portion believed that their lives had not changed in any significant way, and many women experienced no adverse effects. Because they no longer had to worry about becoming pregnant, some women report feeling sexually freer after menopause than before its onset. Generally, the female climacterium has been stereotyped as a sudden or radical psychophysiological experience, but it is more often a gradual experience as estrogen secretion decreases with changes in the flow, timing, and eventual cessation of the menses. Vasomotor instability (hot flashes) can occur, and menopause can extend over several years. Some women experience anxiety and depression, but usually women who have a history of poor adaptation to stress are predisposed to the menopausal syndrome. (Chapter 30 on reproductive medicine provides further discussion of menopause and its management.)

For men, the climacterium has no clear demarcation; male hormones stay fairly constant through the 40s and 50s and then begin to decline. Nevertheless, men must adapt to a decline in biological functioning and overall physical vigor. About age 50, a slight decrease in healthy sperm and seminal fluid occurs; not sufficient, however, to preclude insemination. Coincident with the decreased testosterone level, may be fewer and less firm erections and decreased sexual activity generally. Some men experience a so-called midlife crisis during this period. The crisis can be mild or severe, characterized by a sudden drastic change in work or marital relationships, severe depression, increased use of alcohol or drugs, or a shift to an alternate lifestyle.

MIDLIFE TRANSITION AND CRISIS

The *midlife transition* has been defined as an intense reappraisal of all aspects of life precipitated by the growing recognition that life is finite and approaching an end. It is characterized by mental turmoil, not action. For most people, the reappraisal results in decisions to keep most life structures, such as marriages and careers, which have been painstakingly built over time. When major changes are made, they are thoughtful and considered, even when they include major shifts, such as divorce or a job change. The developmentally aware clinician recognizes that every patient in this age group is engaged in a midlife transition (whether the patient is talking about it or not) and facilitates the process by making it conscious and verbal.

A true *midlife crisis* is a major, revolutionary turning point in life, involving changes in commitments to career or spouse, or both, and accompanied by significant, ongoing emotional turmoil for the individual and others. It is an upheaval of major proportions. A period of internal agitation is followed by a flurry of impulsive actions; for example, leaving spouse and children, becoming involved with a new sexual partner, and quitting a job, all within days or weeks of each other. Although unrecognized warning signs may have existed, those who are left behind are often shocked by the suddenness and abruptness of the change.

Efforts by family members or therapists to get the individual to stop and to reconsider usually fall on deaf ears. The overwhelming need is to avoid anyone who counsels restraint and to ignore therapists who recommend examining motivations and feelings before making such major decisions. Usually, in the midst of the crisis, the therapist is left with the painful job of helping those who have been left to deal with their shock and grief.

Empty-Nest Syndrome. Another phenomenon described in middle adulthood has been called the *empty-nest syndrome*, a depression that occurs in some men and women when their youngest child is about to leave home. Most parents, however, perceive the departure of the youngest child as a relief rather than a stress. If no compensating activities have been developed, particularly by the mother, some parents become depressed. This is especially true of women whose predominant role in life has been mothering or of couples who decided to stay in an otherwise unhappy marriage "for the sake of the children."

Other Tasks of Middle Adulthood

As persons approach the age of 50, they clearly define what they want from work, family, and leisure. Men who have reached their highest level of advancement in work may experience disillusionment or frustration when they realize that they can no longer anticipate new work challenges. For women who have invested themselves completely in mothering, this period leaves them with no suitable identity after the children leave home. Sometimes, social rules become rigidly established; lack of freedom in lifestyle and a sense of entrapment can lead to depression and a loss of confidence. Also unique financial burdens can occur in middle age, produced by pressures to care for aged parents at one end of the spectrum and children at the other end.

Daniel Levinson described a transitional period between the ages of 50 and 55 during which a developmental crisis may occur when persons feel incapable of changing an intolerable life structure. Although no single event characterizes the transition, the physiological changes that begin to appear may have a dramatic effect on a person's sense of self. For example, a person may experience a decrease in cardiovascular efficiency that accompanies aging. Chronological age and physical infirmity are not linear, however; those who exercise regularly, who do not smoke, and who eat and drink in moderation can maintain their physical health and emotional well-being.

Middle adulthood is when persons frequently feel overwhelmed by too many obligations and duties, but it is also a time of great satisfaction for most persons. They have developed a wide array of acquaintances, friendships, and relationships, and the satisfaction they express about their network of friends predicts positive mental health. Some social ties, however, may be a source of stress when demands either cannot be met or assault a person's self-esteem. Power, leadership, wisdom, and understanding are most generally possessed by persons who are middle aged, and if their health and vitality remain intact, it is truly the prime of life.

DIVORCE

Divorce is a major crisis of life. Spouses often grow, develop, and change at different rates; one spouse may discover that the other is not the same as when they first married. In truth, both partners have changed and evolved, not necessarily in complementary directions. Frequently, one spouse blames a third person for alienation of affections and refuses to examine his or her own role in the marital problems. Certain aspects of marital deterioration and divorce seem to be related to specific qualities of middle life—need for change, weariness with acting responsibly, fear of facing up to oneself.

Types of Separation

Paul Bohannan, an anthropologist with expertise in marriage and divorce, described the types of separations that take place at the time of divorce.

Psychic Divorce. In psychic divorce, the love object is given up, and a grief reaction about the death of the relationship occurs. Sometimes a period of anticipatory mourning sets in before the divorce. Separating from a spouse forces a person to become autonomous, to change from a position of dependence. The separation may be difficult to achieve, especially if both are used to being dependent on each other (as normally happens in marriage) or if one was so dependent as to be afraid or incapable of becoming independent. Most persons report such feelings as depression, ambivalence, and mood swings at the time of divorce. Studies indicate that recovery from divorce takes about 2 years; by then, the ex-spouse may be viewed neutrally, and each spouse accepts his or her new identity as a single person.

Legal Divorce. Legal divorce involves going through the courts so that each of the parties is remarriageable. Of divorced women and divorced men, 75 percent and 80 percent, respectively, remarry within 3 years of divorce. No-fault divorce, in which neither person is judged to be the guilty party, has become the most widely used legal mechanism for divorce.

Economic Divorce. Economic divorce involves major concerns to the division of the couple's property between them and economic support for the wife. Many men who are ordered by the courts to pay alimony or child support flout the law and create a major social problem.

Community Divorce. The social network of the divorced couple changes markedly. A few relatives and friends are retained from the community, and new ones are added. The task of meeting new friends is often difficult for divorced persons, who may realize how dependent they were on their spouses for social exchanges.

Coparental Divorce. Coparental divorce is the separation of a parent from the child's other parent. Being a single parent differs from being a married parent.

Custody

The parental right doctrine is a legal concept that awards custody to the more fit natural parent and attempts to ensure that the best interest of the child is served. In the past, mothers were almost always awarded custody, but custody is now given to fathers in about 15 percent of cases. Custodial fathers are likely to be white, married, older, and better educated than custodial mothers. Women who are granted custody have a better chance of being awarded child support and of actually receiving payment than do men who are granted custody. Nevertheless, women who receive payments still have lower incomes than men who receive payment.

The types of custody include *joint custody*, in which a child spends equal time with each parent, an increasingly common practice; *split custody*, in which siblings are separated and each parent has custody of one or more of the children; and *single custody*, in which the children live solely with one parent and the other parent has rights of visitation that may be limited in some way by the court. Child support payments are more likely to be made when parents have joint custody or when the noncustodial parent is given visitation rights.

Problems can surface in the parent–child relationship with the custodial or the noncustodial parent. The absence of the noncustodial parent in the home represents the reality of the divorce, and the custodial parent may become the target of the child's anger about the divorce. The parent under such stress may not be able to deal with the child's increased needs and emotional demands.

The noncustodial parent must cope with limits placed on time spent with the child. This parent loses the day-to-day gratification and the responsibilities involved with parenting. Emotional distress is common in parent and child. Joint custody offers a solution with some advantages, but it requires substantial maturity on the part of the parents and can present some problems. Parents must separate their child-rearing practices from their postdivorce resentments, and they must develop a spirit of cooperation about rearing the child. They must also be able to tolerate frequent communication with the ex-spouse.

Reasons for Divorce

Divorce tends to run in families and rates are highest in couples who marry as teenagers or come from different socioeconomic backgrounds. Every marriage is psychologically unique and so is each divorce. If a person's parents were divorced, he or she may choose to resolve a marital problem in the same way, through divorce. Expectations of the spouse may be unrealistic: One partner may expect the other to act as an all-giving mother or a magically protective father. The parenting experience places the greatest strain on a marriage. In surveys of couples with and without children, those without children reported getting more pleasure from the spouse than those with children. Illness in the child creates the greatest strain of all, and more than 50 percent of marriages in which a child has died through illness or accident end in divorce.

Other causes of marital distress are problems about sex and money. Both areas may be used as a means of control, and withholding sex or money is a means of expressing aggression. Also less social pressure to remain married currently exists. As discussed above, the easing of divorce laws and the declining influence of religion and the extended family make divorce an acceptable course of action today.

Intercourse Outside of Marriage. Adultery is defined as voluntary sexual intercourse between a married person and someone other than his or her spouse. For men, the first extramarital affair is often associated with the wife's pregnancy, when coitus may be interdicted. Most of these incidents are kept secret from the spouse and, if known, rarely account for divorce. Nevertheless, the infidelity can serve as the catalyst for basic dissatisfactions in the marriage to surface, and these problems may then lead to its dissolution. Adultery may decline, as potentially fatal sexually transmitted diseases such as acquired immune deficiency syndrome (AIDS) serve as sobering deterrents.

Adult Maturity

Success and happiness in adulthood are made possible by achieving a modicum of maturity—a mental state, not an age. The capacity for maturity, however, is a direct outgrowth of the engagement and mastery of the developmental tasks of young and middle adulthood. From a developmental perspective, maturity can be defined as a mental state found in healthy adults that is characterized by detailed knowledge of the parameters of human existence, a sophisticated level of self-awareness based on an honest appraisal of one's own experience within those basic parameters, and the ability to use this intellectual and emotional knowledge and insight caringly in relation to one's self and others.

The achievement of maturity in midlife leads to emergence of the capacity for wisdom. Those who possess wisdom have learned from the past and are fully engaged in life in the present. Just as important, they anticipate the future and make the necessary decisions to enhance prospects for health and happiness. In other words, a philosophy of life has been developed that includes understanding and acceptance of the person's place in the order of human existence.

References

Colarusso CA. Adulthood. In: Sadock BJ, Sadock VA, eds. *Kaplan & Sadock's Comprehensive Textbook of Psychiatry*. 8th ed. Vol. 2. Baltimore: Lippincott Williams & Wilkins; 2005:3565.

Goldberg AE, Sayer A. Lesbian couples' relationship quality across the transition to parenthood. *Journal of Marriage and Family.* 2006;68(1):87–100.
Joyner K, Kao G. Interracial relationships and the transition to adulthood. *American Sociological Review.* 2005;70:563–581.
Krueger RF, Markon KE, Patrick CJ, Iacono WG. Externalizing psychopathology in adulthood: A dimensional-spectrum conceptualization and its implications for DSM-V. *J Abnorm Psychol.* 2005;114(4):537–550.
Nelson LJ, Barry CM. Distinguishing features of emerging adulthood: The role of self-classification as an adult. *Journal of Adolescent Research.* 2005;20(2): 242–262.
Perrig-Chiello P, Perren S. Biographical transitions from a midlife perspective. *Journal of Adult Development.* 2005;12(4):169–181.
Qian Z. Breaking the last taboo: Interracial marriage in America. *Contexts.* 2005; 4(4):33–37.
Schwartz SJ, Côté JE, Arnett J. Identity and agency in emerging adulthood: Two developmental routes in the individualization process. *Youth & Society.* 2005; 37(2):201–229.
Tasker F. Lesbian mothers, gay fathers, and their children: A review. *J Dev Behav Pediatr.* 2005;26(3):224–240.
Vrdang E. *Human Behavior in the Social Environment.* New York: The Haworth Social Work Practice Press; 2002.

▲ 2.5 Late Adulthood (Old Age)

For many individuals, the passage from youth to old age is mirrored by a shift from the pursuit of wealth to the maintenance of health. In late adulthood, the aging body increasingly becomes a central concern, replacing the midlife preoccupations with career and relationships. This is so because of normal diminution in function, altered physical appearance, and the increased incidence of physical illness. Despite these occurrences, the body in late adulthood can still be a source of considerable pleasure and can convey a sense of competence, particularly if attention is paid to regular exercise, healthy diet, adequate rest, and preventive maintenance medical care. The normal state in late adulthood is physical and mental health, not illness and debilitation (Table 2.5–1).

Late adulthood, or old age, usually refers to the stage of the life cycle that begins at age 65. Gerontologists—those who study the aging process—divide older adults into two groups: young-old, ages 65 to 74; and old-old, ages 75 and beyond. Some use the term *oldest old* to refer to those over 85. Older adults can also be described as *well-old* (persons who are healthy) and *sick-old* (persons who have an infirmity that interferes with functioning and requires medical or psychiatric attention). The health needs of older adults have grown enormously as the population ages, and geriatric physicians and psychiatrists play major roles in treating this population.

Table 2.5–1
Developmental Tasks of Late Adulthood

To maintain the body image and physical integrity
To conduct the life review
To maintain sexual interests and activities
To deal with the death of significant loved ones
To accept the implications of retirement
To accept the genetically programmed failure of organ systems
To divest oneself of the attachment to possessions
To accept changes in the relationship with grandchildren

DEMOGRAPHICS

The number of individuals over age 65 is rapidly expanding. In 1900, for example, 4 percent of the U.S. population was older than 65 years. By 2003 it was 12.4 percent, and by 2030, it is projected to be 20 percent. That increase far exceeds the general population growth—10-fold compared with just over 3-fold between 1900 and 2000—and is projected to continue (e.g., $2^1/_2$ times vs. just over $1^1/_2$ times between 1990 and 2050) (Table 2.5–2).

The life expectancy for women at birth is projected to continue to exceed that for men by 7 years until the year 2050. By 2050, the composition of the U.S. population by age and sex is estimated to differ markedly from that today. Such changes are bound to influence income and marital statistics, the percentage of elderly persons living alone or in long-term care facilities, and other aspects of the social network.

The accuracy of the above projections, however, depends on the accuracy of other predications such as birth rates, immigration, and emigration—all of which are more difficult to gauge for the future than the remaining variables, death rates or life expectancies. Projections concerning life expectancy, for example, can change substantially within a single decade.

BIOLOGY OF AGING

The aging process, or senescence (from the Latin senescere, "to grow old"), is characterized by a gradual decline in the functioning of all the body's systems—cardiovascular, respiratory, genitourinary, endocrine, and immune, among others. But the belief that old age is invariably associated with profound intellectual and physical infirmity is a myth. Many older persons retain their cognitive abilities and physical capacities to a remarkable degree.

An overview of the biological changes that accompany old age is given in Table 2.5–3. The various decrements listed do not occur in a linear fashion in all systems. Not all organ systems deteriorate at the same rate, nor do they follow a similar pattern of decline for all persons. Each person is genetically endowed with one or more vulnerable systems, or a system may become vulnerable because of environmental stressors or intentional misuse, such as excessive ultraviolet exposure, smoking, or alcohol use. Moreover, not all organ systems deteriorate at the same time. Any one of a number of organ systems begins to deteriorate, and this deterioration then leads to illness or death.

Aging generally means the aging of cells. In the most commonly held theory, each cell has a genetically determined life span during which it can replicate itself a limited number of times before it dies. Structural changes occur in cells with age. In the central nervous system, for example, age-related cell changes occur in neurons, which show signs of degeneration. In senility (characterized by severe memory loss and a loss of intellectual functioning), signs of degeneration are much more severe. An example is the neurofibrillary degeneration seen most commonly in dementia of the Alzheimer's type.

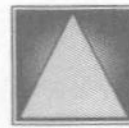

Table 2.5–2
Aging Population of the United States: 1900–2050

			Population, in Millions and as a Percentage of Total Population				
			All Ages	65 and Over		85 and Over	
Year	Median Age	Mean Age	(N)	(N)	(%)	(N)	(%)
1900			76.0	3.1	4.1	0.1	0.1
1950			150.1	12.3	8.2	0.6	0.4
1990			248.7	31.1	12.5	3.0	1.2
2000	35.7	36.5	276.2	35.3	12.8	4.3	1.6
2010	37.2	37.8	300.4	40.1	13.3	6.0	2.0
2030	38.5	39.9	350.0	70.2	20.1	8.8	2.5
2050	38.1	40.3	392.0	80.1	20.4	18.9	4.8

Population: U.S. Bureau of the Census. Current Population Reports, Special Studies, P23-190, 65+ in the United States. Washington, DC: U.S. Government Printing Office; 1996.
Mean/Median Age, 2000–2050: Day JC. Population projections of the United States by age, sex, race and Hispanic origin: 1995 to 2050. In: U.S. Bureau of the Census, Current Population Reports, P25-1130. Washington, DC: U.S. Government Printing Office; 1996.

Structural changes and mutations in deoxyribonucleic acid (DNA) and ribonucleic acid (RNA) are also found in aging cells; these have been attributed to genotypic programming, X-rays, chemicals, and food products, among others. Probably no single cause of aging exists, and all areas of the body are affected to some degree. Genetic factors have been implicated in disorders that commonly occur in older persons, such as hypertension, coronary artery disease, arteriosclerosis, and neoplastic disease. Family studies indicate inheritance factors for breast and stomach cancer, colon polyps, and certain mental disorders of old age. Huntington's disease shows an autosomal dominant mode of inheritance with complete penetrance. The average age of onset is between 35 and 40 years, but cases have occurred as late as 70 years.

Longevity

Longevity has been studied since the beginning of recorded history and has always been a topic of great interest. The research about longevity reveals that a family history of longevity is the best indicator of a long life; of persons who live past 80, half of their fathers also lived past 80. Nevertheless, many conditions leading to a shortened life can be prevented, ameliorated, or delayed with effective intervention. Heredity is but one factor—one beyond a person's control. Predictors of longevity that are within a person's control include regular medical checkups, minimal or no caffeine or alcohol consumption, work gratification, and a perceived sense of the self as being socially useful in an altruistic role, such as spouse, teacher, mentor, parent, or grandparent. Healthy eating and adequate exercise are also associated with health and longevity.

Life Expectancy

In the United States, the average life expectancy of both sexes has increased in every decade—from 48 years in 1900 to 73.5 years for men and 80.4 years for women in 2000. The projected life expectancy at birth and at age 65 is indicated in Table 2.5–4. Changes in morbidity and mortality have also occurred. Over the past 30 years, for example, a 60 percent decline has occurred in mortality from cerebrovascular disease and a 30 percent decline in mortality from coronary artery disease. In contrast, mortality from cancer, which rises steeply with age, has increased, especially cancer of the lung, colon, stomach, skin, and prostate.

The oldest old, persons over 85 years of age, is the most rapidly growing segment of the older population. Over the last 25 years, the population of all older persons increased by 100 percent, compared with 45 percent for the entire U.S. population, but the increase for the 85 and older group exceeded 275 percent. It is expected that by 2050, the oldest old will make up about 25 percent of the elderly population and 5 percent of the total population in the United States. Figure 2.5–1 gives projected percentages for the average annual growth rate of the elderly population to the year 2050.

The leading causes of death among older persons are heart disease, cancer, and stroke. Accidents are among the leading causes of death of persons over 65. Most fatal accidents are caused by falls, pedestrian incidents, and burns. Falls are most commonly the result of cardiac arrhythmias and hypotensive episodes.

Some gerontologists consider death in very old persons (over 85) to result from an aging syndrome characterized by diminished elastic-mechanical properties of the heart, arteries, lungs, and other organs. Death results from trivial tissue injuries that would not be fatal to a younger person; accordingly, senescence is viewed as the cause of death.

Ethnicity and Race

The proportion of older persons in the black, Hispanic, and Asian populations is smaller than that in the white population, but it is increasing rapidly. By 2050, 20 percent of older persons will be nonwhite. The proportion of older persons who are Hispanic will increase from 4 to approximately 14 percent over the same period. According to the U.S. Census Bureau, Hispanic refers to persons "whose origins are Mexican, Puerto Rican, Cuban, Central or South American, and other Hispanic or Latino, regardless of race" (Fig. 2.5–2).

Sex Ratios

On average, women live longer than men and are more likely than men to live alone. The number of men per 100 women decreases sharply from age 65 to 85 (Fig. 2.5–3).

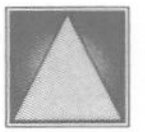

Table 2.5–3
Biological Changes Associated with Aging

Cellular Level
- Change in cellular DNA and RNA structures: intracellular organelle degeneration
- Neuronal degeneration in central nervous system, primarily in superior temporal precentral and inferior temporal gyri; no loss in brainstem nuclei
- Receptor sites and sensitivity altered
- Decreased anabolism and catabolism of cellular transmitter substances
- Intercellular collagen and elastin increase

Immune System
- Impaired T-cell response to antigen
- Increase in function of autoimmune bodies
- Increased susceptibility to infection and neoplasia
- Leukocytes unchanged, T lymphocytes reduced
- Increased erythrocyte sedimentation (nonspecific)

Musculoskeletal
- Decrease in height because of shortening of spinal column (2-inch loss in both men and women from the second to the seventh decade)
- Reduction in lean muscle mass and muscle strength; deepening of thoracic cage
- Increase in body fat
- Elongation of nose and ears
- Loss of bone matrix, leading to osteoporosis
- Degeneration of joint surfaces may produce osteoarthritis
- Risk of hip fracture is 10% to 25% by age 90
- Continual closing of cranial sutures (parietomastoid suture does not attain complete closure until age 80)
- Men gain weight until about age 60, then lose; women gain weight until age 70, then lose

Integument
- Graying of hair results from decreased melanin production in hair follicles (by age 50, 50% of all persons male and female are at least 50% gray; pubic hair is last to turn gray)
- General wrinkling of skin
- Less active sweat glands
- Decrease in melanin
- Loss of subcutaneous fat
- Nail growth slowed

Genitourinary and Reproductive
- Decreased glomerular filtration rate and renal blood flow
- Decreased hardness of erection, diminished ejaculatory spurt
- Decreased vaginal lubrication
- Enlargement of prostate
- Incontinence

Special Senses
- Thickening of optic lens, reduced peripheral vision
- Inability to accommodate (presbyopia)
- High-frequency sound hearing loss (presbyacusis)—25% show loss by age 60, 65% by age 80
- Yellowing of optic lens
- Reduced acuity of taste, smell, and touch
- Decreased light-dark adaption

Neuropsychiatric
- Takes longer to learn new material, but complete learning still occurs
- Intelligence quotient (IQ) remains stable until age 80
- Verbal ability maintained with age
- Psychomotor speed declines

Memory
- Tasks requiring shifting attentions performed with difficulty
- Encoding ability diminishes (transfer of short-term to long-term memory and vice versa)
- Recognition of right answer on multiple-choice tests remains intact
- Simple recall declines

Neurotransmitters
- Norepinephrine decreases in central nervous system
- Increased monoamine oxidase and serotonin in brain

Brain
- Decrease in gross brainweight, about 17% by age 80 in both sexes
- Widened sulci, smaller convolutions, gyral atrophy
- Ventricles enlarge
- Increased transport across blood–brain barrier
- Decreased cerebral blood flow and oxygenation

Cardiovascular
- Increase in size and weight of heart (contains lipofuscin pigment derived from lipids)
- Decreased elasticity of heart valves
- Increased collagen in blood vessels
- Increased susceptibility to arrhythmias
- Altered homeostasis of blood pressure
- Cardiac output maintained in absence of coronary heart disease

Gastrointestinal (GI) System
- At risk for atrophic gastritis, hiatal hernia, diverticulosis
- Decreased blood flow to gut, liver
- Diminished saliva flow
- Altered absorption from GI tract (at risk for malabsorption syndrome and avitaminosis)
- Constipation

Endocrine
- Estrogen levels decrease in women
- Adrenal androgen decreases
- Testosterone production declines in men
- Increase in follicle-stimulating hormone (FSH) and luteinizing hormone (LH) in postmenopausal women
- Serum thyroxine (T_4) and thyroid-stimulating hormone (TSH) normal, triiodothyronine (T_3) reduced
- Glucose tolerance test result decreases

Respiratory
- Decreased vital capacity
- Diminished cough reflex
- Decreased bronchial epithelium ciliary action

Geographic Distribution

The most populous states have the largest number of older persons. California has the most (3.3 million), followed by New York, Pennsylvania, Texas, Michigan, Illinois, Florida, and Ohio, each with more than 1 million. States with high proportions of older persons include Pennsylvania, Florida, Nebraska, and North Dakota. The high proportion in Florida is owing to those who move into the state for retirement; in the others, because of young persons moving out.

Exercise, Diet, and Health

Diet and exercise play a role in preventing or ameliorating chronic diseases of older persons, such as arteriosclerosis and hypertension. Hyperlipidemia, which correlates with coronary artery disease, can be controlled by reducing body weight, decreasing the intake of saturated fat, and limiting the intake of cholesterol. Increasing the daily intake of dietary fiber can also help decrease serum lipoprotein levels. A daily intake of 1 ounce (about 30 mL) of alcohol has been correlated with longevity

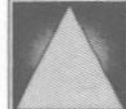

Table 2.5–4
Projected Life Expectancy at Birth and Age 65, by Sex: 1990–2050 (in Years)

	At Birth			At Age 65		
Year	Men	Women	Difference	Men	Women	Difference
1990	72.1	79.0	6.9	15.0	19.4	4.4
2000	73.5	80.4	6.9	15.7	20.3	4.6
2010	74.4	81.3	6.9	16.2	21.0	4.8
2020	74.9	81.8	6.9	16.6	21.4	4.8
2030	75.4	82.3	6.9	17.0	21.8	4.8
2040	75.9	82.8	6.9	17.3	22.3	5.0
2050	76.4	83.3	6.9	17.7	22.7	5.0

(Data from U.S. Bureau of the Census, Washington, DC.)

and elevated high-density lipoproteins (HDL). Studies have also clearly demonstrated that statin drugs that reduce cholesterol have a dramatic effect on reducing cardiovascular disease in persons with diet- or exercise-resistant hyperlipidemia.

Low salt intake (less than 3 g a day) is associated with a lowered risk of hypertension. Hypertensive geriatric patients can often correct their condition by moderate exercise and decreased salt intake without the addition of drugs.

A regimen of daily moderate exercise (walking for 30 minutes a day) has been associated with a reduction in cardiovascular disease, decreased incidence of osteoporosis, improved respiratory function, the maintenance of ideal weight, and a general sense of well-being. Exercise has been shown to improve strength and function even among the very old. In many cases, a disease process has been reversed and even cured by diet and exercise, without additional medical or surgical intervention.

Table 2.5–5 lists the biological changes associated with diet and exercise. A comparison with Table 2.5–2 reveals that almost every biological change associated with aging is positively affected by diet and exercise.

Stage Theories of Personality Development

Early personality theorists proposed that development was completed by the end of childhood or adolescence. One of the first development theorists to propose that personality continues to develop and grow over the life span was Erik Erikson (Table 2.5–6). Erikson believed that development proceeded through a series of psychosocial stages, each with its own conflict that is resolved by the individual with greater or lesser success. Erikson termed the crisis of the last epoch of life *integrity versus despair* and believed that successful resolution of this crisis involved a process of life review and achieved a sense of peace and wisdom through coming to terms with how one's life was lived. For example, Erikson proposed that successful resolution of this crisis would be characterized by a sense of having lived one's life well, whereas a less successful resolution would be characterized by feeling that life was too short, that one did not choose wisely, and bitterness that one will not have a chance to live life over.

Several studies have attempted to validate aspects of Erikson's theory. In one study, a sample of more than 400 men was studied prospectively, and the highest eriksonian life stage each achieved was rated

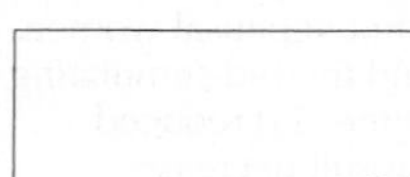

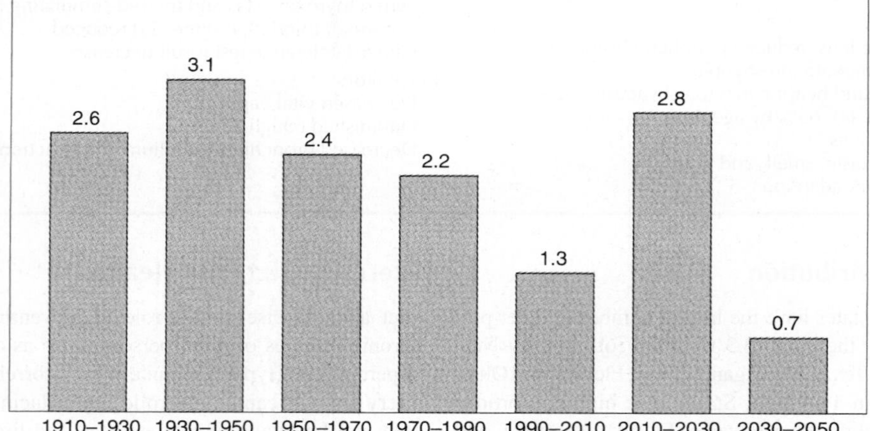

FIGURE 2.5–1
Average annual growth rate of the elderly population. (Data from U.S. Bureau of the Census.)

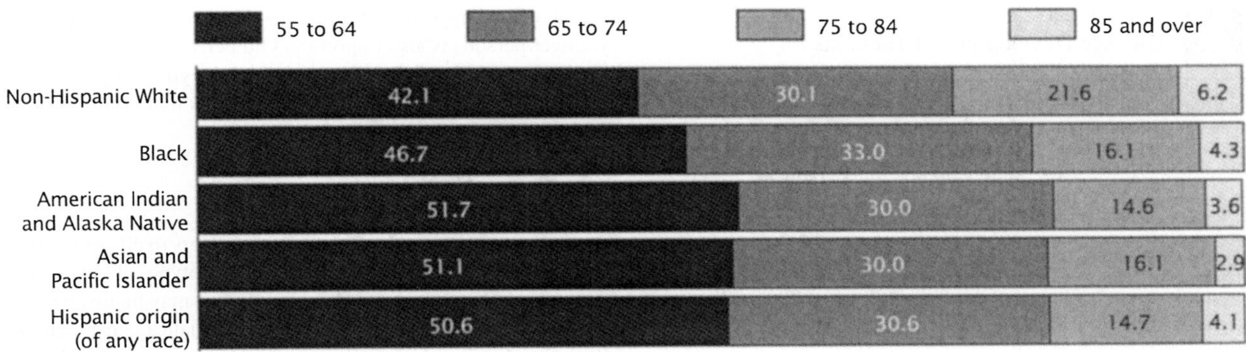

FIGURE 2.5–2
Percent distribution of people 55 years and over by race, Hispanic origin, and age: 2002. (Data from U.S. Bureau of the Census.)

according to data gathered on the circumstances of his life. For example, if a man had achieved independence from his family of origin and was self-sufficient but was unable to develop an intimate relationship, the highest life stage achieved would be the identity stage, not the intimacy stage. This study found that eriksonian stages are passed through in sequential order, although often not at the same age for every individual, and that the stages are surprisingly universal in populations that are ethnically and socioeconomically diverse.

A longitudinal study of approximately 500 subjects from two age cohorts found that the earlier age cohort scored significantly higher on integrity than the later age cohort, and scores for both age cohorts on integrity had declined significantly by the final time of testing. These data suggest that the conflict of integrity versus despair may have a more favorable outcome in earlier age cohorts than in later ones, raising the possibility that changing societal values have had a negative impact on the struggle for integrity. Another study found that wisdom, a construct related to integrity, bore a stronger relation to life satisfaction in elderly adults than other variables, including finances, health, and living situation.

Personality over the Life Span: Stability or Change?

While Erikson and other stage theorists focused on unique developmental tasks and stages central to each phase of life, other theorists focused on defining core personality traits within the individual and determining their course over the life span. For example, do those who are gregarious or extraverted during early childhood and adolescence remain extraverted through midlife and old age? Several well-designed longitudinal studies that have followed individuals over periods ranging from 10 to 50 years have found strong evidence for stability in five basic personality traits: extraversion, neuroticism, agreeableness, openness to experience, and conscientiousness. Some studies found slight decreases in extraversion and slight increases in agreeableness as individuals move into the oldest-old category, which contrasts

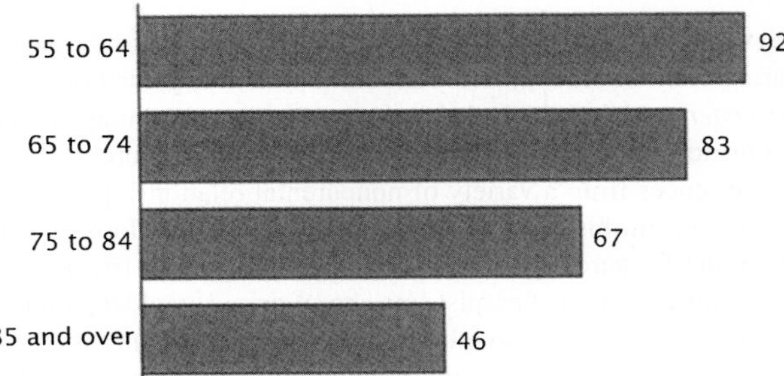

FIGURE 2.5–3
Sex ratio of people 55 years and over by age: 2002. (Data from U.S. Bureau of the Census.)

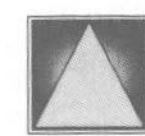

Table 2.5–5
Positive and Healthy Physiological Effects of Exercise and Nutrition

Increases
Strength of bones, ligaments, and muscles
Muscle mass and body density
Articular cartilage thickness
Skeletal muscle ATP, CRP, K+, and myoglobin
Skeletal muscle oxidative enzyme content and mitochondria
Skeletal muscle arterial collaterals and capillary density
Heart volume and weight
Blood volume and total circulating hemoglobin
Cardiac stroke volume
Myocardial contractility
Maximal CO_2(A-V)
Maximal blood lactate concentration
Maximal pulmonary ventilation
Maximal respiratory work
Maximal oxygen diffusing capacity
Maximal exercise capacity as measured by the maximal oxygen intake, exercise time, and distance
Serum high-density lipoprotein concentration
Anaerobic threshold
Plasma insulin concentration with submaximal exercise
Decreases
Heart rate at rest and during submaximal exercise
Blood lactate concentration during submaximal exercise
Pulmonary ventilation during submaximal work
Respiratory quotient during submaximal work
Serum triglyceride concentration
Body fatness
Serum low-density lipoprotein concentration
Systolic blood pressure
Core temperature threshold for initiation of sweating
Sweat sodium and chloride content
Plasma epinephrine and norepinephrine with submaximal exercise
Plasma glucagon and growth hormone concentrations with submaximal exercise
Relative hemoconcentration with submaximal exercise in the heat

(Reprinted from Buskirk ER. In: White PL, Monderka T, eds. *Diet and Exercise: Synergism in Health Maintenance*. Chicago: American Medical Association; 1982:133, with permission.)

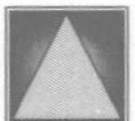

Table 2.5–6
Old Age Developmental Theorists

Sigmund Freud	Increasing control of the ego and id with aging results in increased autonomy. Regression may permit primitive modes of functioning to reappear.
Erik Erikson	The central conflict in old age is between integrity, the sense of satisfaction people feel reflecting on a life lived productively, and despair, the sense that life has little purpose or meaning. Contentment in old age comes only with getting beyond narcissism and into intimacy and generativity.
Heinz Kohut	Old people must continually cope with narcissistic injury as they attempt to adapt to the biological, psychological, and social losses associated with the aging process. The maintenance of self-esteem is a major task of old age.
Bernice Neugarten	The major conflict of old age relates to giving up the position of authority and evaluating achievements and former competence. It is a time of reconciliation with others and resolution of grief over the death of others and the approaching death of self.
Daniel Levinson	Ages 60 to 65 is a transition period ("the late adult transition"). People who are narcissistic and too heavily invested in body appearance are liable to become preoccupied with death. Creative mental activity is a normal and healthy substitute for reduced physical activity.

with early theories that proposed that personality rigidifies as individuals age.

Is the fact that personality appears to have considerable stability over time inconsistent with the basic tenets of stage theories? Perhaps not. It may be that although individuals are consistent over time in their basic personality structure, the themes and conflicts with which they struggle change considerably over the life span, from concerns about developing identity and a stable sense of self, to finding a life partner, to issues related to life review, as hypothesized by the stage theories. In addition, in developing theories about personality change, few studies have examined the impact of significant historical events on personality; thus, the ways in which these events may result in personality change have not been studied systematically.

PSYCHOSOCIAL ASPECTS OF AGING

Social Activity

Healthy older persons usually maintain a level of social activity that is only slightly changed from that of earlier years. For many, old age is a period of continued intellectual, emotional, and psychological growth. In some cases, however, physical illness or the death of friends and relatives may preclude continued social interaction. Moreover, as persons experience an increased sense of isolation, they may become vulnerable to depression. Growing evidence indicates that maintaining social activities is valuable for physical and emotional well-being. Contact with younger persons is also important. Old persons can pass on cultural values and provide care services to the younger generation and thereby maintain a sense of usefulness that contributes to self-esteem.

Ageism

Ageism, a term coined by Robert Butler, refers to discrimination toward old persons and to the negative stereotypes about old age that are held by younger adults. Old persons may themselves resent and fear other old persons and discriminate against them. In Butler's scheme, persons often associate old age with loneliness, poor health, senility, and general weakness or infirmity. The experience of older persons, however, does not consistently support this attitude. For example, although 50 percent of young adults expect poor health to be a problem for those over 65 years old, 75 percent of persons 65 to 74 years of age describe their health as good. Two thirds of persons 75 and older feel the same way. Health problems, when they do exist, more often involve chronic than acute conditions. More than four of five persons over the age of 65 have at least one chronic condition (Table 2.5–7).

Good health, however, is not the sole determinant of a good quality of life in old age. Surveys of old persons show that social contacts are at least as highly valued. In fact, the factors affecting good aging appear to be multidimensional. Aging "robustly" means considering aging in terms of productive involvement, affective status, functional status, and cognitive status. These four indicators are only minimally correlated. The most robustly aging individuals report greater social contact, better health and vision, and fewer significant life events in the past 3 years than their less robustly aging counterparts. A linear, age-related decrease occurs in robustness, but it can still be found among the oldest old.

George Vaillant followed up a group of Harvard freshmen into old age and found the following about emotional health at age 65: Having been close to brothers and sisters during college correlated with emotional well-being; undergoing early traumatic life experiences, such as the death of a parent or parental divorce, did not correlate with poor adaptation in old age; being depressed at some point between ages 21 and 50 predicted emotional problems at age 65; and possessing the personality traits of pragmatism and dependability as a young adult was associated with a sense of well-being at age 65.

Transference

Several forms of transference, some of them unique to adulthood, are present in older adults. First is the well-recognized *parental transference*, in which the patient reacts to the therapist as a child to a parent. *Peer* or *sibling transference*, expressions of experiences from a variety of nonparental relationships, is also common. In this form of transference, the patient looks to the therapist to share experiences with siblings, spouses, friends, and associates. At first, therapists may be surprised by older patients' ability to ignore their age in creating such transferences.

In *son* or *daughter transference*, quite common in middle-aged individuals and the elderly, the therapist is cast in the role of the patient's child, grandchild, or son-in-law or daughter-in-law.

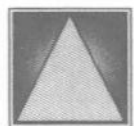

Table 2.5–7
Top 10 Chronic Conditions for People 65+, by Age and Race (Number Per 1,000 People)

	Age				Race (65+)		
Condition	**65+**	**45 to 64**	**65 to 74**	**75+**	**White**	**Black**	**Black as % of White**
Arthritis	483.0	253.8	437.3	554.5	483.2	522.6	108
Hypertension	380.6	229.1	383.8	375.6	367.4	517.7	141
Hearing impairment	286.5	127.7	239.4	360.3	297.4	174.5	59
Heart disease	278.9	118.9	231.6	353.0	286.5	220.5	77
Cataracts	156.8	16.1	107.4	234.3	160.7	139.8	87
Deformity or orthopedic impairment	155.2	155.5	141.4	177.0	156.2	150.8	97
Chronic sinusitis	153.4	173.5	151.8	155.8	157.1	125.2	80
Diabetes	88.2	58.2	89.7	85.7	80.2	165.9	207
Visual impairment	81.9	45.1	69.3	101.7	81.1	77.0	95
Varicose veins	78.1	57.8	72.6	86.6	80.3	64.0	80

(Data from National Center for Health Statistics, Washington, DC.)

The themes expressed in this form of transference are multiple and often center on defenses against dependency feelings, activity and dominance versus passivity and submission, and attempts to rework unsatisfying aspects of relationships with children before time runs out. Last, *sexual transferences* in older individuals are frequent, intense, and the therapist needs to be able to accept them and manage his or her countertransference responses.

Countertransference

Older individuals are dealing with illness and signs of aging, the loss of spouses and friends, and the constant awareness of time limitation and the nearness of death. These are painful issues that are just beginning to come into focus for younger therapists who would prefer not to confront them with great intensity on a daily basis.

A second source of countertransference responses centers on the older patient's sexuality. The presence of a vivid fantasy life, masturbation, and intercourse are disconcerting in and of themselves if the therapist has not had much experience in working with individuals who are the same age as their parents and grandparents. Consider the experience of this 31-year-old female therapist who was treating a 62-year-old man.

Early in the treatment process, Mr. E.'s sexual feelings emerged. His well-groomed appearance and adolescent-like nervousness caused the therapist discomfort. Her concern was how to engender respect and to develop a therapeutic alliance with a patient who approached each session as a date, particularly because he was old enough to be her grandfather. At first shocked by his open expression of sexual interest in her, with the help of supervision and her own therapy, she was able to recognize that she and the patient had similar conflicts to resolve, despite the 30-year age difference between them. She had hoped that Mr. E. would be "all grown up," devoid of issues that she was grappling with also. She came to recognize that failure to help him understand the relationship between his past and still vibrant sexuality would do the patient a great disservice and would spring from her lack of understanding of late-life sexual development and her countertransference reaction to him based on her conflicted attitudes toward the sexuality of her parents and grandparents. (Courtesy of Calvin A. Colarusso, M.D.)

Socioeconomics

The economics of old age is of paramount importance to older persons themselves and to society at large. The past 30 years has seen a dramatic decline in the proportion of the U.S. elderly population who are poor, primarily as a result of Medicare, Social Security, and private pensions. In 1959, 35.2 percent of persons over 65 lived below the poverty line, but by 2001 this figure had declined to 10.1 percent. Persons over age 65 make up 12 percent of the population, but they include only 9 percent of those living at low socioeconomic levels. Women are more likely than men to be poor. Income sources vary for persons age 65 and older. Despite overall economic gains, many older persons are so preoccupied by money worries that their enjoyment of life is lessened. Obtaining proper medical care may be especially difficult when personal funds are not available or are insufficient.

Medicare (Title 18) provides both hospital and medical insurance for those over age 65. About 150 million medical bills are reimbursed under the Medicare program each year; but only about 40 percent of all medical expenses incurred by older persons are covered under Medicare. The rest is paid by private insurance, state insurance, or personal funds. Some services—such as outpatient psychiatric treatment, skilled nursing care, physical rehabilitation, and preventive physical examinations—are covered minimally or not at all.

In addition to Medicare, the Social Security program pays benefits to persons over age 65 (over age 66 in the year 2009 and age 67 in 2027) and pays benefits at reduced rates from age 62 on. To qualify for benefits, a person must have worked long enough to become insured: A worker must have worked for 10 years to be eligible for benefits. Benefits are also paid to widows, widowers, and dependent children if those receiving benefits or contributing to Social Security die (survivor benefits). Social Security is not a pension scheme but a pay-as-you-go income supplement to prevent mass destitution among older persons. Benefits are paid

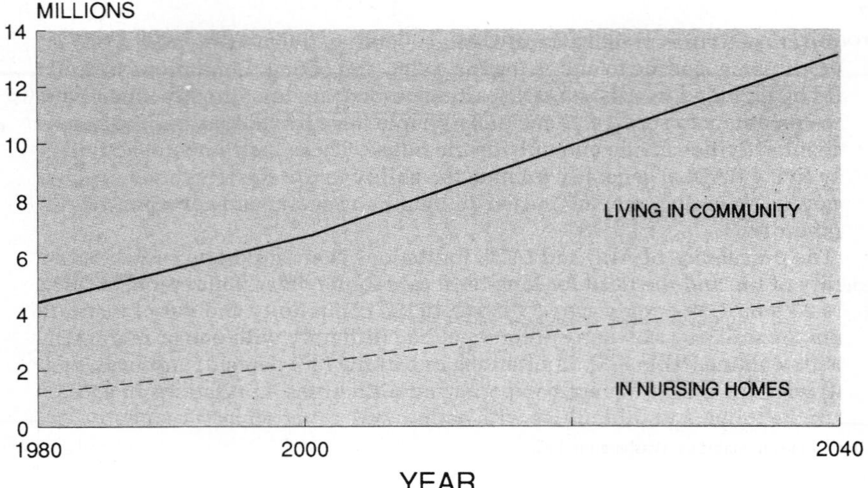

FIGURE 2.5–4

People age 65+ in need of long-term care: 1980–2040. (Reprinted from Manton B, Saldo J. Dynamics of health changes in the oldest old: New perspectives and evidence. *Milbank Q.* 1985;63:12, with permission.)

by those currently working to those retired. Serious difficulties for Social Security are forecast for the next three decades, when the number of baby boomers reaching old age will greatly exceed the number of younger workers paying into the plan.

Retirement

For many older persons, retirement is a time for the pursuit of leisure and for freedom from the responsibility of previous working commitments. For others, it is a time of stress, especially when retirement results in economic problems or a loss of self-esteem. Ideally, employment after age 65 should be a matter of choice. With the passage of the Age Discrimination in Employment Act of 1967 and its amendments, forced retirement at age 70 has been virtually eliminated in the private sector, and it is not legal in federal employment.

Most of those who retire voluntarily reenter the work force within 2 years, for a variety of reasons, including negative reactions to being retired, feelings of being unproductive, economic hardship, and loneliness. The amount of time spent in retirement has increased as the life span has nearly doubled since 1900. Currently, the number of years spent in retirement is almost equal to the number of years spent working.

Sexual Activity

The frequency of orgasm, from coitus or masturbation, decreases with age in men and women. The most important factors in determining the level of sexual activity with age are the health and survival of the spouse, one's own health, and the level of past sexual activity. Although some degree of declining sexual interest and function is inevitable with age, social and cultural factors appear to be more responsible for the sexual changes observed than the psychological changes of aging per se. Although satisfying sexual activity is possible for the reasonably healthy elderly, many do not actualize this potential. The widely held notion that the elderly are essentially asexual is often a self-fulfilling prophecy.

Long-Term Care

Many older persons who are infirm require institutional care. Although only 5 percent are institutionalized in nursing homes at any one time, about 35 percent of older persons require care in a long-term facility at some time during their lives (Fig. 2.5–4). Older nursing home residents are mainly widowed women, and about 50 percent are over age 85.

Nursing home care costs are not covered by Medicare; they range from $20,000 to $50,000 a year. About 20,000 long-term nursing care institutions are available in the United States—not enough to meet the need. Those older persons who do not require skilled nursing care can be managed in other types of health-related facilities, such as centers they attend during the daytime hours, but the need for care far exceeds the availability of such centers.

Outside institutions, care for older persons is provided by their children (primarily their daughters and daughters-in-law), their wives, and other women (Fig. 2.5–5). More than 50 percent

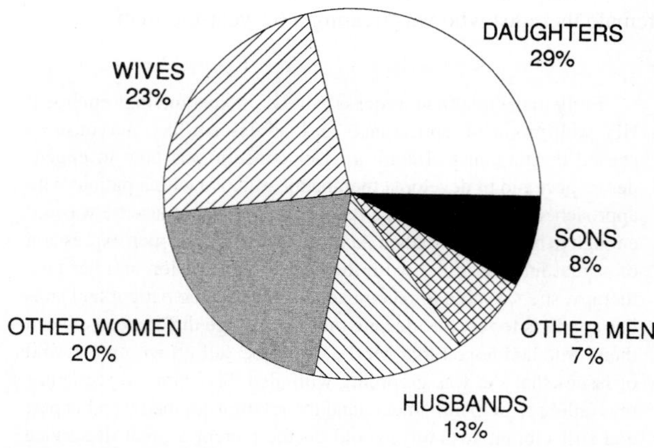

FIGURE 2.5–5

Caretakers and their relationship to the elderly care recipient. (Data from Select Committee on Aging, U.S. House of Representatives.)

of these women caregivers also work in jobs outside the home, and about 40 percent also care for their own children. In general, women end up as caregivers more often than men because of cultural and societal expectations. According to the American Association of Retired Persons, daughters with jobs spend an average of 12 hours a week providing care and currently spend about $150 a month for travel, telephone calls, special foods, and medication for older persons.

PSYCHIATRIC PROBLEMS OF OLDER PERSONS

Despite the ubiquity of loss in old age, the prevalence of major depressive disorder and dysthymia is actually less than in younger age groups. Several explanations for this phenomenon have been proposed: rarity of late-onset depression, higher mortality among persons with depression, and a general decrease in disorders caused by emotional upheavals or substance abuse in older persons. Depression in old persons is often accompanied by physical symptoms or cognitive changes that may mimic dementia.

The incidence of suicide among older persons is high (40 per 100,000 population) and is highest for older white men. The suicide of older persons is perceived differently by surviving friends and family members on the basis of gender: Men are thought to have been physically ill, and women are thought to have been mentally ill.

The relation between good mental and good physical health is clear in older persons. Adverse effects on the course of chronic medical illness are correlated with emotional problems. (An extensive discussion of psychiatric problems in older persons appears in Chapter 56.)

References

Angus J, Reeve P. Ageism: A threat to "aging well" in the 21st century. *Journal of Applied Gerontology*. 2006;25(2):137–152.

Benetos A, Thomas F, Bean KE, Pannier B, Guize L. Role of modifiable risk factors in life expectancy in the elderly. *J Hyperten*. 2005;23(10):1803–1808.

Bytheway B. Ageism and age categorization. *Journal of Social Issues*. 2005;61(2): 361.

Colarusso CA. Adulthood. In: Sadock BJ, Sadock VA, eds. *Kaplan & Sadock's Comprehensive Textbook of Psychiatry*. 8th ed. Vol. 2. Baltimore: Lippincott Williams & Wilkins; 2005:3565.

Ginsberg TB, Pomerantz SC, Kramer-Feeley V. Sexuality in older adults: Behaviours and preferences. *Age Ageing*. 2005;34(5):475–480.

Hagestad GO, Uhlenberg P. The social separation of old and young: A root of ageism. *Journal of Social Issues*. 2005;61(2):343.

Johnson W, McGue M, Krueger RF. Personality stability in late adulthood: A behavioral genetic analysis. *J Pers*. 2005;73(2):523.

Kaasinen V, Maguire RP, Kurki T, Bruck A, Rinne JO. Mapping brain structure and personality in late adulthood. *Neuroimage*. 2005;24(2):315–322.

King DA, Wynne LC. The emergence of "family integrity" in later life. *Family Process*. 2004;43(1):7–21.

Kunitz SJ, Pesis-Katz I. Mortality of white Americans, African Americans, and Canadians: The causes and consequences for health of welfare state institutions and policies. *Milbank Q*. 2005;83(1):5–39.

Moody HR. *Aging: Concepts and Controversies*. Thousand Oaks, CA: Pine Forge Press; 2006.

Nelson TD. Ageism: Prejudice against our feared future self. *Journal of Social Issues*. 2005;61(2):207.

Smith DP, Bradshaw BS. Rethinking the Hispanic paradox: Death rates and life expectancy for US non-Hispanic white and Hispanic populations. *Am J Public Health*. 2006;96(2):1–7.

Vrdang E. *Human Behavior in the Social Environment*. New York: The Hawthorn Social Work Practice Press; 2002.

Wilson RS, Barnes LL, Krueger KR, Hoganson G, Bienias JL, Bennett DA. Early and late life cognitive activity and cognitive systems in old age. *Journal of the International Neuropsychological Society*. 2005;11:400–407.

▲ 2.6 Death, Dying, and Bereavement

DEATH AND DYING

Definitions

The terms *death* and *dying* require definition: *Death* may be considered the absolute cessation of vital functions, whereas *dying* is the process of losing these functions. Dying may also be seen as a developmental concomitant of living, a part of the birth-to-death continuum. Living may entail numerous mini-deaths—the end of growth and its potential, health-compromising illnesses, multiple losses, decreasing vitality and growing dependency with aging, and dying. Dying, and the individual's awareness of it, imbues humans with values, passions, wishes, and the impetus to make the most of time.

Two terms that have been used with increased frequency in recent years refer to the quality of living as death comes near. A *good death* is one that is free from avoidable distress and suffering for patients, families, and caregivers and is reasonably consistent with clinical, cultural, and ethical standards. A *bad death*, in contrast, is characterized by needless suffering, a dishonoring of patient or family wishes or values, and a sense among participants or observers that norms of decency have been offended.

Uniform Determination of Death Act. The President's Commission for the Study of Ethical Problems in Medicine and Biomedical and Behavioral Research published its definition of death in 1981. Working with the American Bar Association, the American Medical Association (AMA), and the National Conference of Commissioners on Uniform State Laws, the Commission established that one who has sustained either (1) irretrievable cessation of circulatory and respiratory functions or (2) irretrievable cessation of all functions of the entire brain, including the brainstem, is dead. Determination of death must be in accordance with accepted medical standards.

Generally accepted criteria for determining brain death require a series of neurological and other assessments. For children, special guidelines apply. They generally specify two assessments separated by an interval of at least 48 hours for those between the ages of 1 week and 2 months, 24 hours for those between the ages of 2 months and 1 year, and 12 hours for older children; additional confirmatory tests may also be advisable under some circumstances. Brain death criteria are normally not applied to infants younger than 7 days. Table 2.6–1 lists the clinical criteria for brain death in adults and children.

Legal Aspects of Death

According to law, physicians must sign the death certificate, which attests to the cause of death (e.g., congestive heart failure or pneumonia). They must also attribute the death to natural, accidental, suicidal, homicidal, or unknown causes. A medical examiner, coroner, or pathologist must examine anyone who dies unattended by a physician and perform an autopsy to determine the cause of death. In some cases, a psychological autopsy is

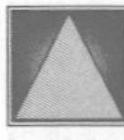

Table 2.6–1
Clinical Criteria for Brain Death in Adults and Children

Coma
Absence of motor responses
Absence of pupillary responses to light and pupils at midposition with respect to dilatation (4–6 mm)
Absence of corneal reflexes
Absence of caloric responses
Absence of gag reflex
Absence of coughing in response to tracheal suctioning
Absence of sucking and rooting reflexes
Absence of respiratory drive at a Pa_{CO_2} that is 60 mm Hg or 20 mm Hg above normal base-line values[a]
Interval between two evaluations, according to patient's age
- Term to 2 mos old, 48 hr
- >2 mos to 1 yr old, 24 hr
- >1 yr to <18 yr old, 12 hr
- ≥18 yr old, interval optional

Confirmatory tests
- Term to 2 mos old, two confirmatory tests
- >2 mos to 1 yr old, one confirmatory test
- >1 yr to <18 yr old, optional
- ≥18 yr old, optional

[a] Pa_{CO_2} denotes the partial pressure of arterial carbon dioxide.
(Reprinted from Wijdicks EFM. The diagnosis of brain death. *N Engl J Med.* 2001;344:1216, with permission.)

performed: A person's sociocultural and psychological background is examined retrospectively by interviewing friends, relatives, and doctors to determine whether a mental illness, such as a depressive disorder, was present. For example, a determination can be made that a person died because he or she was pushed (murder) or because he or she jumped (suicide) from a high building. Each situation has clear medical and legal implications.

Stages of Death and Dying

Elisabeth Kübler-Ross (Fig. 2.6–1), a psychiatrist and thanatologist, made a comprehensive and useful organization of reactions to impending death. A dying patient seldom follows a regular series of responses that can be clearly identified; no established sequence is applicable to all patients. Nevertheless, the following five stages proposed by Kübler-Ross are widely encountered.

Stage 1: Shock and Denial. On being told that they are dying, persons initially react with shock. They may appear dazed at first and then may refuse to believe the diagnosis; they may deny that anything is wrong. Some persons never pass beyond this stage and may go from doctor to doctor until they find one who supports their position. The degree to which denial is adaptive or maladaptive appears to depend on whether a patient continues to obtain treatment even while denying the prognosis. In such cases, physicians must communicate to patients and their families, respectfully and directly, basic information about the illness, its prognosis, and the options for treatment. For effective communication, physicians must allow for patients' emotional responses and reassure them that they will not be abandoned.

Stage 2: Anger. Persons become frustrated, irritable, and angry at being ill. They commonly ask, "Why me?" They may

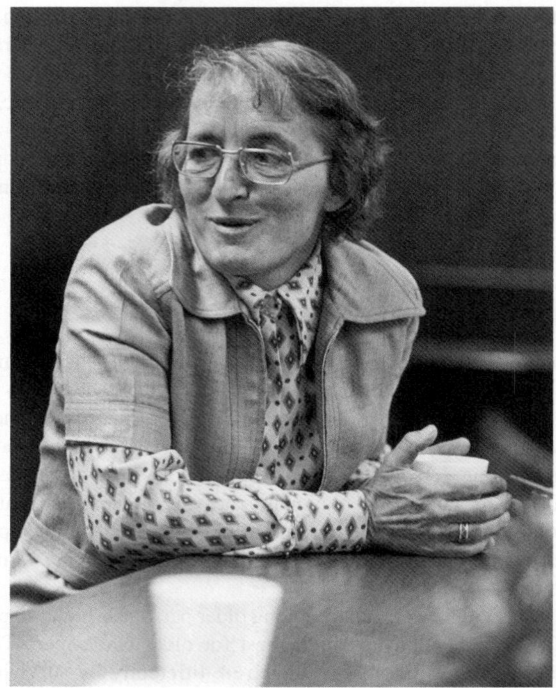

FIGURE 2.6–1
Elisabeth Kübler-Ross, M.D. (1926–2004), eminent Swiss-born U.S. psychiatrist, is shown in this close-up. Her 1969 best selling book, *On Death and Dying*, described the five stages experienced by the dying. (Courtesy of Corbis.)

become angry at God, their fate, a friend, or a family member; they may even blame themselves. They may displace their anger onto the hospital staff members and the doctor, whom they blame for the illness. Patients in the stage of anger are difficult to treat. Doctors who have difficulty understanding that anger is a predictable reaction and is really a displacement may withdraw from patients or transfer them to other doctors' care.

Physicians treating angry patients must realize that the anger being expressed cannot be taken personally. An empathic, nondefensive response can help defuse patients' anger and can help them refocus on their own deep feelings (e.g., grief, fear, loneliness) that underlie the anger. Physicians should also recognize that anger may represent patients' desire for control in a situation in which they feel completely out of control.

Stage 3: Bargaining. Patients may attempt to negotiate with physicians, friends, or even God; in return for a cure, they promise to fulfill one or many pledges, such as giving to charity and attending church regularly. Some patients believe that if they are good (compliant, nonquestioning, cheerful), the doctor will make them better. The treatment of such patients involves making it clear that they will be taken care of to the best of the doctor's abilities and that everything that can be done will be done, regardless of any action or behavior on the patients' part. Patients must also be encouraged to participate as partners in their treatment and to understand that being a good patient means being as honest and straightforward as possible.

Stage 4: Depression. In the fourth stage, patients show clinical signs of depression—withdrawal, psychomotor retardation, sleep disturbances, hopelessness, and, possibly, suicidal ideation. The depression may be a reaction to the effects of the illness on their lives (e.g., loss of a job, economic hardship, helplessness, hopelessness, and isolation from friends and family), or it may be in anticipation of the loss of life that will eventually occur. A major depressive disorder with vegetative signs and suicidal ideation may require treatment with antidepressant medication or electroconvulsive therapy (ECT). All persons feel some sadness at the prospect of their own death, and normal sadness does not require biological intervention. But major depressive disorder and active suicidal ideation can be alleviated and should not be accepted as normal reactions to impending death. A person who suffers from major depressive disorder may be unable to sustain hope, which can enhance the dignity and quality of life and even prolong longevity. Studies have shown that some terminally ill patients can delay their death until after a loved one's significant event, such as graduation of a grandson from college.

Stage 5: Acceptance. In the stage of acceptance, patients realize that death is inevitable, and they accept the universality of the experience. Their feelings can range from a neutral to a euphoric mood. Under ideal circumstances, patients resolve their feelings about the inevitability of death and can talk about facing the unknown. Those with strong religious beliefs and a conviction of life after death sometimes find comfort in the ecclesiastical maxim, "Fear not death; remember those who have gone before you and those who will come after."

Near-Death Experiences

Near-death descriptions are often strikingly similar, involving an out-of-body experience of viewing one's body and overhearing conversations, feelings of peace and quiet, hearing a distant noise, entering a dark tunnel, leaving the body behind, meeting dead loved ones, witnessing beings of light, returning to life to complete unfinished business, and a deep sadness on leaving this new dimension. This pattern of sensations and perceptions is usually described as peaceful and loving; it feels real to participants, who distinguish it from dreams or hallucinations. These experiences provoke sweeping lifestyle changes, such as fewer material concerns, heightened sense of purpose, belief in God, joy of life, compassion, less fear of death, enhanced approach to life, and intense feelings of love. In a similar vein, hospice nurses have described experiences among the terminally ill of visions that may include a sense of presence of departed loved ones, of spiritual beings, of a bright light, or of being in a particular place, often described with a sense of warmth and love. Although such "visions" do not readily lend themselves to scientific investigation and, thus, are not legitimized, patients may benefit from discussing them with clinicians. A term to describe this experience is *unio mystica*, which refers to an oceanic feeling of mystic unity with an infinite power.

Life Cycle Considerations about Death and Dying

The clinical diversity of death-related attitudes and behaviors between children and adults has its roots in developmental factors and age-dependent differences in causes of death. As opposed to adults, who usually die from chronic illness, children are apt to die from sudden, unexpected causes. Almost half of the children who die between the ages of 1 and 14 and nearly 75 percent of those who die in late adolescence and early adulthood die from accidents, homicides, and suicides. With their characteristics of violence, suddenness, and mutilation, such unnatural causes of death are special stressors for grieving survivors. Bereaved parents and siblings of dead young children and teenagers often feel victimized and traumatized by their losses; their grief reactions resemble posttraumatic stress disorder (PTSD). Devastating family disruptions can occur, and surviving siblings risk having their emotional needs put on the back burner, ignored, or completely unnoticed.

Children. Children's attitudes toward death mirror their attitudes toward life. Although they share with adolescents, adults, and the elderly similar fears, anxieties, beliefs, and attitudes about dying, some of their interpretations and reactions are age-specific. None welcome it without ambivalence, and all temper their acceptance with healthy doses of denial and avoidance. Dying children are often aware of their condition and want to discuss it. They often have more sophisticated views about dying than their medically well counterparts, engendered by their own failing health, separations from parents, subjection to painful procedures, and the deaths of hospital chums.

At the preschool, preoperational stage of cognitive development, death is seen as a temporary absence, incomplete and reversible, like departure or sleep. Separation from the primary caretaker(s) is the main fear of preschool-age children. This fear surfaces as an increase in nightmares, more aggressive play, or concern about the deaths of others, rather than in direct discourse. Terminally ill children may assume responsibility for their death, feeling guilty for dying. Preschool children may be unable to relate the treatment to the illness, instead viewing treatment as punishment and family separation as rejection. They need reassurance that they are loved, have done nothing wrong, are not responsible for their illness, and will not be abandoned.

School-age children manifest concrete-operational thinking and recognize death as a final reality. They, however, view death as something that happens to old people, not to them. Between the ages of 6 and 12, children have active fantasies of violence and aggression, often dominated by themes of death and killing. School-age children ask questions about serious illness and death if encouraged to do so; however, if they receive cues that the subject is taboo, they may withdraw and participate less fully in their care. Facilitating open discussion and updating children with important information, including prognostic changes, can be very helpful. In addition, children may need help coping with peers and school demands. Teachers should be informed and updated. Classmates may need education and assistance to help them understand the situation and respond appropriately.

Adolescents. Capable of formal cognitive operations, adolescents understand that death is inevitable and final but may not accept that their own death is possible. The major fears of dying teenagers parallel those of all teenagers—losing control, being imperfect, and being different. Concerns about body image, hair loss, or loss of bodily control can generate great resistance to continuing treatment. Alternating emotions of despair, rage, grief, bitterness, numbness, terror, and joy are common. The potential for withdrawal and isolation is great, as teenagers may equate parental support with loss of independence or may deny their fears of abandonment by actually repulsing friendly gestures. Teenagers must be included in all decision-making processes surrounding their deaths. Many are capable of great courage, grace, and dignity in facing death.

Adults. Some of the most often expressed fears of adult patients entering hospice care, listed in the approximate order of frequency, include fears of (1) separation from loved ones, homes, and jobs; (2) becoming a burden to others; (3) losing control; (4) what will happen to dependents; (5) pain or other worsening symptoms; (6) being unable to complete life tasks or responsibilities; (7) dying; (8) being dead; (9) the fears of others (reflected fears); (10) the fate of the body; and (11) the afterlife. Problems in communication arise out of trepidation, making it important for those involved in health care to provide environments of trust and safety in which people can begin to talk about uncertainties, anxieties, and concerns.

Late-age adults often accept that their time has come. Their main fears include long, painful, and disfiguring deaths; prolonged vegetative states; isolation; and loss of control or dignity. Elderly patients may talk or joke openly about dying and, sometimes, welcome it. In their 70s and beyond, they rarely harbor illusions of indestructibility—most have already had several close calls: their parents have died and they have gone to funerals for friends and relatives. Although they may not be happy to die, they can be reconciled to it.

According to Erik Erikson, the eighth and final stage in the life cycle brings a sense of either integrity or despair. As the elderly enter the last phase of their lives, they reflect on their pasts. When they have taken care of their affairs, have been relatively successful, and have adapted to the triumphs and disappointments of life, they can look back with satisfaction and only a few regrets. Integrity of the self allows people to accept inevitable disease and death without fear of succumbing helplessly. If elderly individuals look back on life as a series of missed opportunities or personal misfortunes, however, they feel a sense of bitter despair, a preoccupation with what might have been if only this or that had happened. Then, death is fearsome because it symbolizes emptiness and failure.

Management

Caring for a dying patient is highly individual. Caretakers need to deal with death honestly, tolerate wide ranges of affects, connect with suffering patients and bereaved loved ones, and resolve routine issues as they arise. Although each therapeutic relationship between a patient and health provider has a uniqueness derived from the patient's and health provider's gender, constitution, life experience, age, stage of life, resources, faith, culture, and other considerations, major themes confront all health providers caring for dying patients. End-of-life care and palliative medicine, including physician-assisted suicide, is discussed in Chapter 57.

BEREAVEMENT, GRIEF, AND MOURNING

Bereavement, grief, and mourning are terms that apply to the psychological reactions of those who survive a significant loss. Grief is the subjective feeling precipitated by the death of a loved one. The term is used synonymously with mourning, although, in the strictest sense, mourning is the process by which grief is resolved; it is the societal expression of postbereavement behavior and practices. Bereavement literally means the state of being deprived of someone by death and refers to being in the state of mourning. Regardless of the fine points that differentiate these terms, the experiences of grief and bereavement have sufficient similarities to warrant a syndrome that has signs, symptoms, a demonstrable course, and an expected resolution. Figure 2.6–2 summarizes one concept of some recognizable and predictable manifestations of the phases of uncomplicated grief.

Normal Bereavement Reactions

The first response to loss, *protest*, is followed by a longer period of *searching* behavior. As hope to reestablish the attachment bond diminishes, searching behaviors give way to *despair* and *detachment* before bereaved individuals eventually *reorganize* themselves around the recognition that the lost person will not return. Although the bereaved ultimately learn to accept the reality of the death, they also find psychological and symbolic ways of keeping the memory of the deceased person very much alive. Grief work allows the survivor to redefine his or her relationship to the deceased and to form new but enduring ties.

Duration of Grief

Most societies mandate modes of bereavement and time for grieving. In contemporary America, the bereaved is expected to return to work or school in a few weeks, to establish equilibrium within a few months, and to be capable of pursuing new relationships within 6 months to 1 year. Ample evidence suggests that the bereavement process does not end within a prescribed interval; certain aspects persist indefinitely for many otherwise high-functioning, normal individuals.

The most lasting manifestation of grief, especially after spousal bereavement, is loneliness. Often present for years after the death of a spouse, loneliness may, for some, be a daily reminder of the loss. Other common manifestations of protracted grief occur intermittently. For example, a man who has lost his wife may experience elements of acute grief every time he hears her name or sees her picture on the nightstand. Usually, these reactions become increasingly short-lived over time, dissipating within minutes, and become tinged with positive and pleasant affects. Such bittersweet memories may last a lifetime. Thus, most grief does not fully resolve or permanently disappear; rather, grief becomes circumscribed and submerged only to reemerge in response to certain triggers.

Anticipatory Grief

In *anticipatory grief*, grief reactions are brought on by the slow dying process of a loved one through injury, illness, or high-risk activity. Although anticipatory grief may soften the blow of the eventual death, it can also lead to premature separation and withdrawal, while not necessarily mitigating later bereavement. At times, the intensification of intimacy during

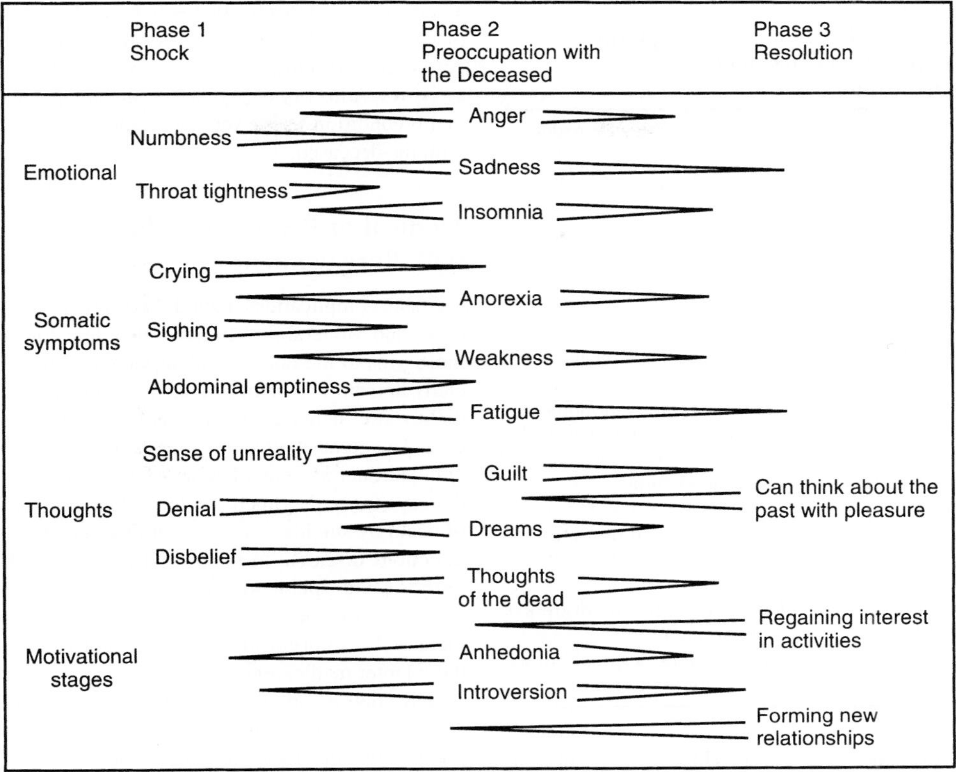

FIGURE 2.6–2
Phases of uncomplicated grief. (Reprinted from Brown JT, Soudemire A. Normal and pathological grief. *JAMA* 1983;250:378, with permission.)

this period may heighten the actual sense of loss, even though it prepares the survivor in other ways.

Anniversary Reactions. When the trigger for an acute grief reaction is a special occasion, such as a holiday or birthday, the rekindled grief is called an *anniversary reaction*. It is not unusual for anniversary reactions to occur each year on the same day the person died or, in some cases, when the bereaved individual becomes the same age the deceased was at the time of death. Although these anniversary reactions tend to become relatively mild and brief over time, they can be experienced as the reliving of one's original grief and prevail for hours or days.

Mourning

From earliest history, every culture records its own beliefs, customs, and behaviors related to bereavement. Specific patterns include rituals for mourning (e.g., wakes or Shiva), for disposing of the body, for invocation of religious ceremonies, and for periodic official remembrances. The funeral is the prevailing public display of bereavement in contemporary North America. The funeral and burial service acknowledge the real and final nature of the death, countering denial; they also garner support for the bereaved, encouraging tribute to the dead, uniting families, and facilitating community expressions of sorrow. If cremation replaces burial, ceremonies associated with dissemination of the ashes perform similar functions. Visits, prayers, and other ceremonies allow for continuing support, coming to terms with reality, remembering, emotional expression, and concluding unfinished business with the deceased. Several cultural and religious rituals provide purpose and meaning, protect the survivors from isolation and vulnerability, and set limits on grieving. Subsequent holidays, birthdays, and anniversaries serve to remind the living of the dead and may elicit grief as real and fresh as the original experience; over time, these anniversary grievings become attenuated but often remain in some form.

Bereavement

Because bereavement often evokes depressive symptoms, it may be necessary to demarcate normal grief reactions from major depressive disorder (Table 2.6–2). According to DSM-IV-TR, if the symptoms of a major depressive episode begin within 2 months of the loss of a loved one and do not persist beyond those 2 months, they are generally considered to result from bereavement, unless they are associated with marked functional impairment or include morbid preoccupation with worthlessness, suicidal ideation, psychotic symptoms, or psychomotor retardation. This is discussed further below.

Complicated Bereavement

Complicated bereavement has a confusing array of terms to describe it—*abnormal, atypical, distorted, morbid, traumatic,*

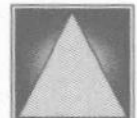

Table 2.6–2
Differentiating the Depressive Symptoms Associated with Bereavement from Major Depression

Bereavement	Major Depressive Disorder
Symptoms may meet syndromal criteria for major depressive episode, but survivor rarely has morbid feelings of guilt and worthlessness, suicidal ideation, or psychomotor retardation.	Any symptoms as defined by DSM-IV-TR
Considers self bereaved	May consider self weak, defective, bad
Dysphoria often triggered by thoughts or reminders of the deceased.	Dysphoria often autonomous and independent of thoughts or reminders of the deceased
Onset is within the first 2 mos of bereavement.	Onset at any time
Duration of depressive symptoms is less than 2 mos.	Depression often becomes chronic, intermittent, or episodic.
Functional impairment is transient and mild	Clinically significant distress or impairment
No family or personal history of major depression.	Family and/or personal history of major depression.

and *unresolved*, to name a few types. Three patterns of complicated, dysfunctional grief syndromes have been identified—chronic, hypertrophic, and delayed grief.

Chronic Grief. The most common type of complicated grief is chronic grief, often highlighted by bitterness and idealization of the dead. Chronic grief is most likely to occur when the relationship between the bereaved and the deceased had been extremely close, ambivalent, or dependent or when social supports are lacking and friends and relatives are not available to share the sorrow over the extended period of time needed for most mourners.

Hypertrophic Grief. Most often seen after a sudden and unexpected death, bereavement reactions are extraordinarily intense in hypertrophic grief. Customary coping strategies are ineffectual to mitigate anxiety, and withdrawal is frequent. When one family member is experiencing a hypertrophic grief reaction, disruption of family stability can occur. Hypertrophic grief frequently takes on a long-term course, albeit one attenuated over time.

Delayed Grief. Absent or inhibited grief when one normally expects to find overt signs and symptoms of acute mourning is referred to as delayed grief. This pattern is marked by prolonged denial; anger and guilt may complicate its course.

Traumatic Bereavement. Traumatic bereavement refers to grief that is both chronic and hypertrophic. This syndrome is characterized by recurrent, intense pangs of grief with persistent yearning, pining, and longing for the deceased; recurrent intrusive images of the death; and a distressing admixture of avoidance and preoccupation with reminders of the loss. Positive memories are often blocked or excessively sad, or they are experienced in prolonged states of reverie that interfere with daily activities. A history of psychiatric illness appears to be common in this condition, as is a very close, identity-defining relationship with the deceased.

Medical or Psychiatric Illnesses Associated with Bereavement

Medical complications include exacerbations of existing diseases and vulnerability to new ones; fear for one's health and more trips to the doctor; and an increased mortality rate, especially in men. The highest relative mortality risk is found immediately after bereavement, particularly from ischemic heart disease. The greatest effect of bereavement on mortality is for men younger than 65 years. Higher mortality rates in bereaved men than in bereaved women are due to increases in the relative risk of death by suicide, accident, cardiovascular disease, and some infectious diseases. In widows, the relative risk of death from cirrhosis and suicide may increase. In both sexes, bereavement appears to exacerbate health-compromising behaviors, such as increased alcohol consumption, smoking, and the use of the over-the-counter medications.

Psychiatric complications of bereavement include increased risk for major depressive disorder, prolonged anxiety, panic, and a posttraumatic stress–like syndrome; increased alcohol, drug, and cigarette consumption; and increased risk of suicide. Because of their psychosocial, emotional, and cognitive immaturity, bereaved children may be especially vulnerable to psychopathology.

Bereavement and Depression. Although symptoms overlap, grief can be distinguished from a full depressive episode. Most bereaved individuals experience intense sadness, but only a few meet DSM-IV-TR criteria for major depressive episode. Grief is a complex experience in which positive emotions take their place beside the negative ones. Grief is fluid and changing, an evolving state in which emotional intensity gradually lessens and positive, comforting aspects of the lost relationship come to the fore. Pangs of grief are stimulus bound, related to internal and external reminders of the deceased. This differs from depression, which is more pervasive and characterized by much difficulty experiencing self-validating, positive feelings. Grief is a fluctuating state with individual variability, in which cognitive and behavioral adjustments are progressively made until the bereaved can hold the deceased in a comfortable place in memory and a satisfying life can be resumed. By contrast, major depressive episode is comprised of a recognizable and stable cluster of debilitating symptoms, accompanied by a protracted, enduring low mood. Major depressive episode tends to be persistent and associated with poor work and social functioning, pathological psychoneuroimmunological function, and other neurobiological changes, unless treated.

Bereavement and Posttraumatic Stress Disorder. Unnatural and violent deaths, such as homicide, suicide, or death in the context of terrorism, are much more likely to precipitate

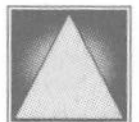

Table 2.6–3
Phases of Grief

Shock and denial (minutes, days, weeks)
  Disbelief and numbness
  Searching behaviors: pining, yearning, and protest
Acute anguish (weeks, months)
  Waves of somatic distress
  Withdrawal
  Preoccupation
  Anger
  Guilt
Lost patterns of conduct
  Restless and agitated
  Aimless and amotivational
  Identification with the bereaved
Resolution (months, years)
  Have grieved
  Return to work
  Resume old roles
  Acquire new roles
  Reexperience pleasure
  Seek companionship and love of others

PTSD in surviving loved ones than are natural deaths. In such circumstances, themes of violence, victimization, and volition (i.e., the choice of death over life, as in the case of suicide) are intermixed with other aspects of grief, and traumatic distress marked by fear, horror, vulnerability, and disintegration of cognitive assumptions ensues. Disbelief, despair, anxiety symptoms, preoccupation with the deceased and the circumstances of the death, withdrawal, hyperarousal, and dysphoria are more intense and more prolonged than they are under nontraumatic circumstances, and an increased risk may exist for other complications. Although treatment studies in survivors of sudden death are few and far between, most experts agree that initial attention should be focused on traumatic distress, that a role is seen for both pharmacotherapy and psychotherapy, and that self-help support groups can be enormously beneficial.

Biological Perspectives

Grief is both a physiological and an emotional response. During acute grief (as with other stressful events), persons may suffer disruption of biological rhythms. Grief is also accompanied by impaired immune functioning: decreased lymphocyte proliferation and impaired functioning of natural killer cells. Whether the immune changes are clinically significant has not been established, but the mortality rate for widows and widowers following the death of a spouse is higher than that in the general population. Widowers appear to be at risk longer than widows.

Phenomenology of Grief. Bereavement reactions include intense feeling states, invoke a variety of coping strategies, and lead to alterations in interpersonal relationships, biopsychosocial functioning, self-esteem, and world view that can last indefinitely. Manifestations of grief reflect the individual's personality, previous life experiences, and past psychological history; the significance of the loss; the nature of the bereaved's relationship with the deceased; the existing social network; intercurrent life events; health; and other resources. Despite individual variations in the bereavement process, investigators have proposed grieving process models, which include at least three partially overlapping phases or states: (1) initial shock, disbelief, and denial; (2) an intermediate period of acute discomfort and social withdrawal; and (3) a culminating period of restitution and reorganization. As with Kübler-Ross' stages of dying, the grieving stages do not prescribe a correct course of grief; rather, they are general guidelines describing an overlapping and fluid process that varies with the survivors (Table 2.6–3).

LIFE CYCLE PERSPECTIVES ABOUT BEREAVEMENT

Bereavement during Childhood and Adolescence

Approximately 4 percent of North American children lose one or both parents by the age of 15; sibling death is the second most commonly experienced bereavement. Grief reactions are colored by developmental levels and concepts of death and may not resemble adult reactions. Children may display minimal grief at time of death and experience the full effect of the loss later. Grieving children may not withdraw and dwell on the person who died but, instead, may throw themselves into activities. Indifference, anger, or misbehavior may be displayed rather than sadness; behaviors can be erratic and labile. Strong feelings of anger and fears of abandonment or death may show up in the behavior of grieving children. Children often play death games as a way of working out their feelings and anxieties. These games are familiar to the children and provide safe opportunities to express their feelings. Although they may seem to show grief only occasionally and briefly, in reality, a child's grief often lasts longer than that of an adult.

Mourning in children may need to be addressed again and again as the child gets older. Children will think about the loss repeatedly, especially during important times in their life, such as going to camp, graduating from school, getting married, or giving birth to their own children. A child's grief can be influenced by his or her age, personality, developmental stage, earlier experiences with death, and his or her relationship with the deceased. The surroundings, cause of death, and family members' ability to communicate with one another and to continue as a family after the death can also affect grief. The child's ongoing need for care, his or her opportunity to share feelings and memories, the parent's ability to cope with stress, and the child's steady relationships with other adults are other factors that may influence grief. Even older children frequently feel abandoned or rejected when a parent dies and may show hostility toward the deceased or the surviving parent, now perceived as one who might also "abandon" them. They may feel responsible because of earlier misbehavior or because they said or wished that that person would die at some time.

Children younger than 2 years may show loss of speech or diffuse distress. Children younger than 5 years are apt to respond with eating, sleeping, bowel, and bladder dysfunctions. Strong feelings of sadness, fear, and anxiety can occur, but these feelings are not persistent and tend to alternate between longer-lasting normal states. School-age children may become phobic or hypochondriacal, withdrawn, or pseudomature, and school performance and peer relations often suffer. Adolescents, as with adults, run the gamut in expressing bereavement, ranging from behavioral problems, somatic symptoms, and erratic moods to stoicism. Adolescent boys losing a parent may become delinquent, whereas girls may turn to a sexual pattern for comfort and reassurance. Behavioral disturbances and depressions are common at all ages. Rates of depressive episodes in bereaved children and adolescents are as high as in bereaved adults.

Bereaved children must be treated with respect to their own levels of emotional and cognitive maturity. They need to be told that the death is real and irreversible and that they are blameless. Feelings and concerns should be expressed, and questions should be invited and answered with simplicity, candor, and clarity. Children, as with adults, need rituals to commemorate their loved ones; attendance at the funeral and participation in mourning may be beneficial first steps.

Bereavement during Adulthood

No consensus exists on which type of loss is associated with the most severe reactions. Although the death of a spouse is often ranked as the most stressful life event, some have argued that losing a child is even more profound. The death of a child is a special sorrow, a lifelong loss for surviving mothers, fathers, brothers, sisters, grandparents, and other family members. A child's death is a life-altering experience. The deaths of parents and siblings in adult life have not achieved much systematic study, but they are generally considered relatively mild compared with the loss of a spouse or child.

Grief appears most intense for the mother in late perinatal losses (stillbirths or neonatal deaths rather than miscarriages) and often is reexperienced during subsequent pregnancies. Sudden infant death syndrome is particularly problematic in that the death is sudden and unexpected. Parents may experience extra guilt or blame each other, often resulting in subsequent marital difficulties.

The surviving family members, friends, or lovers of individuals who have died from acquired immunodeficiency syndrome (AIDS) are uniquely challenged. The illness carries with it the stigmata of the illness itself and of the gay community in general; it carries with it caretakers' fears of contracting the illness; and it is most prevalent in people who are in the prime of life. Asymptomatic infection may permit the infected person and those close to him or her time to adapt to the diagnosis. When a person who is human immunodeficiency virus (HIV) positive begins to manifest symptoms of opportunistic infection or associated cancer, however, the illness again becomes a threat. Coping with the emotional reality is arduous and complex. Often caretakers, as well as HIV-positive patients, wish for death, which can evoke feelings of guilt. For bereaved lovers, their own HIV status, multiple losses, and other concurrent stressors can complicate recovery. Gay men who have lost lovers to AIDS may be more depressed, consider suicide more often, and be more vulnerable to illicit drug use than are other bereaved individuals.

The elderly face more losses than individuals at other phases of the life cycle, and intense loneliness may be a lasting memorial to those who have died. For highly impaired elders who lose a spouse they depended on for daily functions or who was their sole source of companionship, bereavement reactions are profound.

Grief Therapy

Persons in normal grief seldom seek psychiatric help because they accept their reactions and behavior as appropriate. Accordingly, a bereaved person should not routinely see a psychiatrist or psychologist unless a markedly divergent reaction to the loss is noted. For example, under usual circumstances a bereaved person does not make a suicide attempt; if someone seriously contemplates suicide, psychiatric intervention is indicated.

When professional assistance is sought, it usually involves a request for sleeping medication from a family physician. A mild sedative to induce sleep may be useful in some situations, but antidepressant medication or antianxiety agents are rarely indicated in normal grief. Bereaved persons may have to go through the mourning process, however painful it is, for successful resolution to occur. Narcotizing patients with drugs interferes with the normal process that ultimately can lead to a favorable outcome.

Because grief reactions can develop into a depressive disorder or pathological mourning, specific counseling sessions for those bereaved are often valuable. Grief therapy is an increasingly important skill. In regularly scheduled sessions, grieving persons are encouraged to talk about feelings of loss and about the person who has died. Many bereaved persons have difficulty recognizing and expressing angry or ambivalent feelings toward a deceased person, and they must be reassured that these feelings are normal.

Grief therapy need not be conducted only on a one-to-one basis; group counseling is also effective. Self-help groups also have great value in certain cases. About 30 percent of widows and widowers report that they become isolated from friends, withdraw from social life, and thus experience feelings of isolation and loneliness. Self-help groups offer companionship, social contacts, and emotional support; they eventually enable their members to reenter society in a meaningful way. Bereavement care and grief therapy have been most effective with widows and widowers. The necessity for this therapy stems, in part, from the contraction of the family unit; extended family members are no longer available to provide the needed emotional support and guidance during the mourning period.

References

Beale EA, Baile WF, Aaron J. Silence is not golden: Communicating with children dying from cancer. *J Clin Oncol*. 2005;23(15):3629–3631.

Carter JH. Death and dying among African-Americans: Cultural characteristics and coping tidbits. *J Nerv Ment Dis*. 2003;290:820.

Carter PA. Bereaved caregivers' descriptions of sleep: impact on daily life and the bereavement process. *Oncol Nurs Forum*. 2005;32(4):741.

Field NP, Gao B, Paderna L. Continuing bonds in bereavement: An attachment theory based perspective. *Death Studies*. 2005;29(4):277–299.

Freud S. Mourning and melancholia. In: *Standard Edition of the Complete Psychological Works of Sigmund Freud*. London: Hogarth Press; 1953.

Gundel H, O'Connor MF, Littrell L, Fort C, Lane RD. Functional neuroanatomy of grief: An fMRI study. *Am J Psychiatry*. 2003;160:1946.

Hayslip B. *Cultural Changes in Attitudes toward Death, Dying and Bereavement*. New York: Springer Publishing Company Inc., 2005.

Jordan JR, Neimeyer RA. Does grief counseling work? *Death Studies*. 2003;27:765.

Kleespies PK. *Life and Death Decisions: Psychological and Ethical Consideration in End-of-Life Care*. Washington, DC: American Psychological Association; 2004.

Kirwin KM, Hamrin V. Decreasing the risk of complicated bereavement and future psychiatric disorders in children. *J of Child Adolesc Psychiatr Nurs*. 2005;18(2):62–78.

Materstvedt LJ, Clark D, Ellershaw J, Forde R, Gravgaard AMB, Mueller-Busch HC, Porta I, Sales J, Rapin CH. Euthanasia and physician assisted suicide: A view from an EAPC Ethics Task Force. *Palliat Med.* 2003; 17:97.

Moskowitz TJ, Folkman JS, Acree SM. Do positive psychological states shed light on recovery from bereavement? Finding from a 3-year longitudinal study. *Death Studies.* 2003;27:471.

Rynearson EK, Balk DE. The synergism of trauma and bereavement. *Death Studies.* 2004;28:80.

Shear K, Frank E, Houck PR, Reynolds CF 3rd. Treatment of complicated grief: A randomized controlled trial. *JAMA.* 2005;293(21):2601–2608.

Stroebe W, Schut H, Stroebe MS. Grief work, disclosure and counseling: Do they help the bereaved? *Clin Psychol Rev.* 2005;25(4):395–414.

Tate FB, Longo DA. Death and dying: Implications for inpatient, psychiatric care. *Palliative & Supportive Care.* 2005;3:239–243.

Zisook S, Zisook SA. Death, dying, and bereavement. In: Sadock BJ, Sadock VA, eds. *The Comprehensive Textbook of Psychiatry.* 8th ed. Baltimore: Lippincott Williams & Wilkins; 2005:2367.

3 The Brain and Behavior

▲ 3.1 Functional and Behavioral Neuroanatomy

The human brain is the organ that is the basis of what persons sense, do, feel, and think; or put in more formal terms, our sensory, behavioral, affective, and cognitive experiences and attributes. It is the organ that perceives and affects the environment and integrates past and present.

By processing external stimuli into neuronal impulses, *sensory systems* create an internal representation of the external world. A separate map is formed for each sensory modality. *Motor systems* enable persons to manipulate their environment and to influence others' behavior through communication. In the brain, sensory input, representing the external world, is integrated with internal drivers, memories, and emotional stimuli in *association units*, which in turn drive the actions of motor units. Although psychiatry is primarily concerned with the brain's association function, an appreciation of the sensory and motor systems' information processing is essential for sorting logical thought from the distortions introduced by psychopathology.

BRAIN ORGANIZATION

The human brain contains approximately 10^{11} *neurons* (nerve cells) and approximately 10^{12} *glial cells*. Neurons most classically consist of a *soma*, or cell body, which contains the nucleus; usually multiple *dendrites*, which are processes that extend from the cell body and receive signals from other neurons; and a single *axon*, which extends from the cell body and transmits signals to other neurons. Connections between neurons are made at *axon terminals*; there the axons of one neuron generally contact the dendrite or cell body of another neuron. Neurotransmitter release occurs within axon terminals and is one of the major mechanisms for intraneuronal communications, and also for the effects of psychotropic drugs.

There are three types of glial cells, and although they have often been thought of as having only a supportive role for neuronal functioning, they have been increasingly appreciated as potentially involved in brain functions that may contribute more directly to both normal and disease mental conditions. The most common type of glial cells are the *astrocytes*, which have a number of functions, including nutrition of neurons, deactivation of some neurotransmitters, and integration with the blood-brain barrier. The *oliogodendrocytes* in the central nervous system and the *Schwann cells* in the peripheral nervous system wrap their processes around neuronal axons, resulting in *myeline sheaths* that facilitate the conduction of electrical signals. The third type of glial cells, the *microglia*, which derived from macrophages, are involved in removing cellular debris following neuronal death.

The neurons and glial cells of the brain are arranged in regionally distinct patterns within the brain. Korbinian Brodmann divided the hemispheres into 47 areas (Fig. 3.1–1) based on differences in cellular arrangements. The cortex can contain multiple layers of cells that differ in the types of neurons contained, the degree of myelination, and the types of neurotransmitters present.

SENSORY SYSTEMS

The external world offers an infinite amount of potentially relevant information. In this overwhelming volume of sensory information in the environment, the sensory systems must both detect and discriminate stimuli; they winnow relevant information from the mass of confounding input by applying filtration at all levels. Sensory systems first transform external stimuli into neural impulses and then filter out irrelevant information to create an internal image of the environment, which serves as a basis for reasoned thought. Feature extraction is the quintessential role of sensory systems, which achieve this goal with their hierarchical organizations, which first transform physical stimuli into neural activity in the primary sense organs and then refine and narrow the neural activity in a series of higher cortical processing areas. This neural processing eliminates irrelevant data from higher representations and reinforces crucial features. At the highest levels of sensory processing, neural images are transmitted to the association areas to be acted on in the light of emotions, memories, and drives.

Somatosensory System

The *somatosensory system*, an intricate array of parallel point-to-point connections from the body surface to the brain, was the first sensory system to be understood in anatomical detail. The six somatosensory modalities are light touch, pressure, pain, temperature, vibration, and proprioception (position sense). The organization of nerve bundles and synaptic connections in the somatosensory system encodes spatial relationships at all levels, so that the organization is strictly *somatotopic* (Fig. 3.1–2).

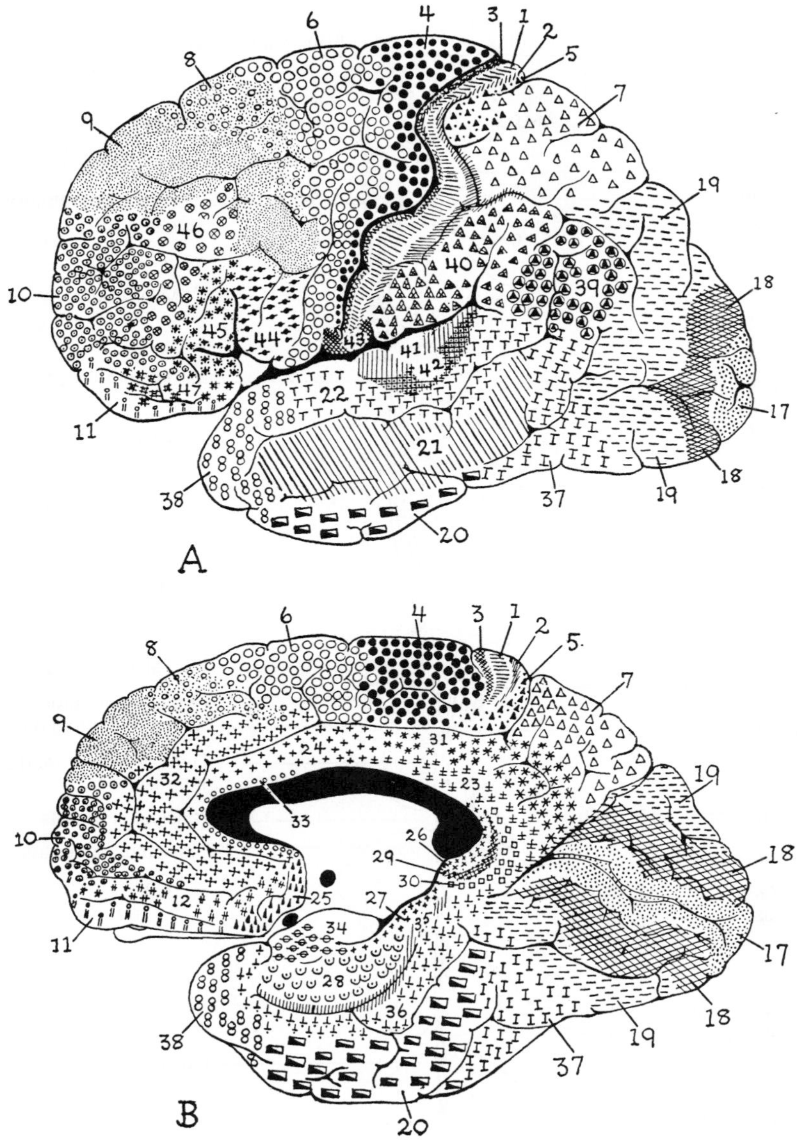

FIGURE 3.1–1

Cytoarchitectonic regions of the brain according to Brodmann. **A.** Lateral surface. **B.** Medial surface. (From Carpenter MD. *Core Text of Neuranatomy,* 4th ed. Baltimore: Williams & Wilkins; 1991:399, with permission.)

Within a given patch of skin, various receptor nerve terminals act in concert to mediate distinct modalities. The mechanical properties of the skin's mechanoreceptors and thermoreceptors generate neural impulses in response to dynamic variations in the environment while they suppress static input. Nerve endings are either fast or slow responders; their depth in the skin also determines their sensitivity to sharp or blunt stimuli. Thus, the representation of the external world is significantly refined at the level of the primary sensory organs.

The receptor organs generate coded neural impulses that travel proximally along the sensory nerve axons to the spinal cord. These far-flung routes are susceptible to varying systemic medical conditions and to pressure palsies. Pain, tingling, and numbness are the typical presenting symptoms of peripheral neuropathies.

All somatosensory fibers project to, and synapse in, the thalamus. The thalamic neurons preserve the somatotopic representation by projecting fibers to the somatosensory cortex, located immediately posterior to the sylvian fissure in the parietal lobe. Despite considerable overlap, several bands of cortex roughly parallel to the sylvian fissure are segregated by a somatosensory modality. Within each band is the sensory "homunculus" (Fig. 3.1–1, Brodmann areas 1, 2, and 3), the culmination of the careful somatotopic segregation of the sensory fibers at the lower levels. The clinical syndrome of *tactile agnosia* (*astereognosis*) is defined by the inability to recognize objects based on touch, although the primary somatosensory modalities—light touch, pressure, pain, temperature,

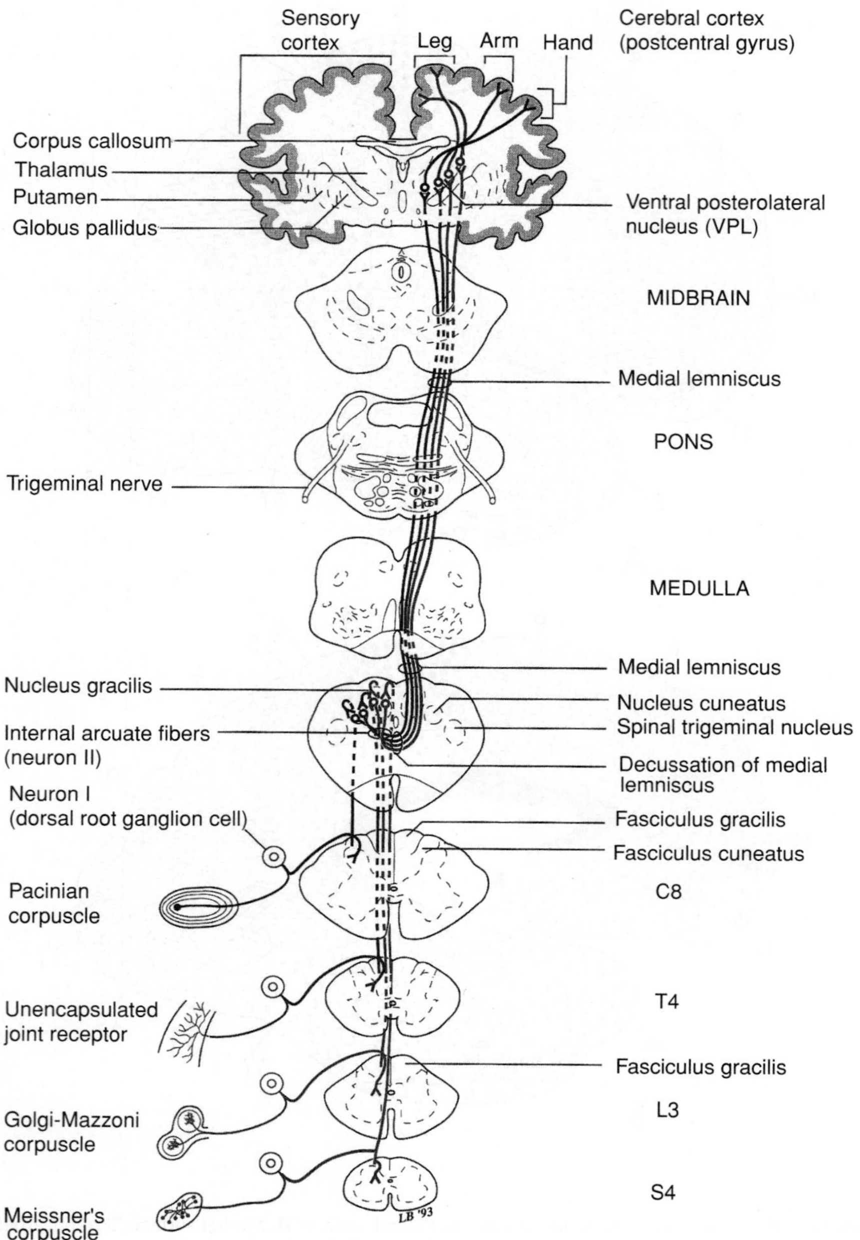

FIGURE 3.1–2

Somatotopic organization of the somatosensory system. Each somatosensory modality is carefully segregated from the other modalities, and the fibers of different spinal levels are segregated as they ascend to the somatosensory cortex. (From Parent A. *Carpenter's Human Neuranatomy,* 9th ed. Baltimore: Williams & Wilkins; 1996:369, with permission.)

vibration, and proprioception—are intact. This syndrome, localized at the border of the somatosensory and association areas in the posterior parietal lobe, appears to represent an isolated failure of only the highest order of feature extraction, with preservation of the more basic levels of the somatosensory pathway.

Reciprocal connections are a key anatomical feature of crucial importance to conscious perception—as many fibers project down from the cortex to the thalamus as project up from the thalamus to the cortex. These reciprocal fibers play a critical role in filtering sensory input. In normal states, they facilitate the sharpening of internal representations, but in pathological states, they can generate false signals or inappropriately suppress sensation. Such cortical interference with sensory perception is thought to underlie many psychosomatic syndromes, such as the hemisensory loss that characterizes conversion disorder.

The prenatal development of the strict point-to-point pattern that characterizes the somatosensory system remains an area of active study. Patterns of sensory innervation result from a combination of axonal guidance by particular molecular cues and pruning of exuberant synaptogenesis on the basis of an organism's experience. Leading hypotheses weigh contributions from

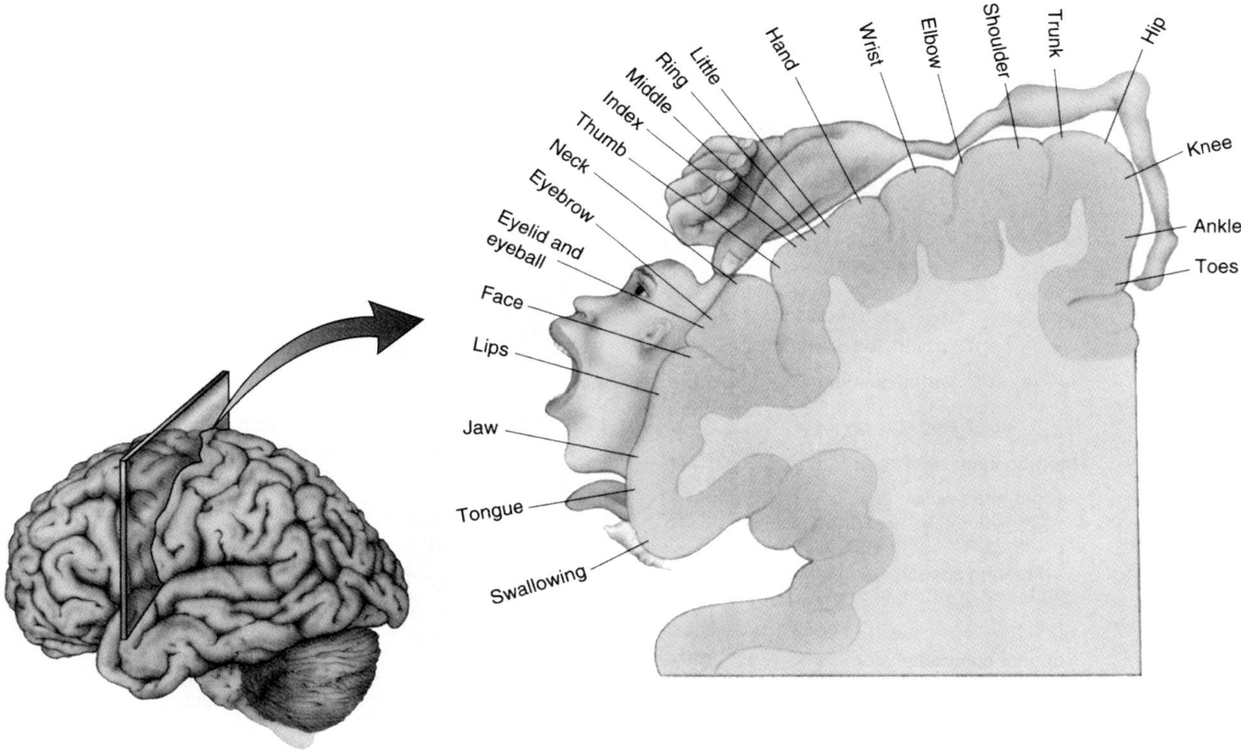

FIGURE 3.1–3
Somatopic map of the human precentral gyrus. (From Bear MF, Conors BW, Paradiso MA. *Neuroscience: Exploring the Brain.* Baltimore: Williams & Wilkins; 1996:383, with permission.)

a genetically determined molecular map, in which the arrangement of fiber projections is organized by fixed and diffusible chemical cues, against contributions from the modeling and remodeling of projections on the basis of coordinated neural activity. Thumbnail calculations suggest that the 30,000 to 40,000 genes in human DNA are far too few to encode completely the position of all the trillions of synapses in the brain. In fact, genetically determined positional cues probably steer growing fibers toward the general target, and the pattern of projections is fine-tuned by activity-dependent mechanisms. Recent data suggest that well-established adult thalamocortical sensory projections can be gradually remodeled as a result of a reorientation of coordinated sensory input or in response to loss of part of the somatosensory cortex, for instance, in stroke.

Development of the Somatosensory System. A strict somatotopic representation exists at each level of the somatosensory system. During development, neurons extend axons to connect to distant brain regions; after arriving at the destination, a set of axons must therefore sort itself to preserve the somatotopic organization. A classic experimental paradigm for this developmental process is the representation of a mouse's whiskers in the somatosensory cortex. The murine somatosensory cortex contains a barrel field of cortical columns, each of which corresponds to one whisker. When mice are inbred to produce fewer whiskers, fewer somatosensory cortex barrels appear. Each barrel is expanded in area, and the entire barrel field covers the same area of the somatosensory cortex as it does in normal animals. This experiment demonstrates that certain higher cortical structures can form in response to peripheral input and that different input complexities determine different patterns of synaptic connectivity. Although the mechanisms by which peripheral input molds cortical architecture are largely unknown, animal model paradigms are beginning to yield clues. For example, in a mutant mouse that lacks monoamine oxidase A and, thus, has extremely high cortical levels of serotonin, barrels fail to form in the somatosensory cortex. This result indirectly implicates serotonin in the mechanism of barrel field development.

In adults, the classic mapping studies of Wilder Penfield suggested the existence of a homunculus, an immutable cortical representation of the body surface. More recent experimental evidence from primate studies and from stroke patients, however, has promoted a more plastic conception than Penfield's. Minor variations exist in the cortical pattern of normal individuals, yet dramatic shifts in the map can occur in response to loss of cortex from stroke or injury. When a stroke ablates a significant fraction of the somatosensory homunculus, the homuncular representation begins to contract and shift proportionately to fill the remaining intact cortex.

Moreover, the cortical map can be rearranged solely in response to a change in the pattern of tactile stimulation of the fingers. The somatotopic representation of the proximal and distal segments of each finger normally forms a contiguous map, presumably because both segments contact surfaces simultaneously. But under experimental conditions in which the distal segments of all fingers are simultaneously stimulated while contact of the distal and proximal parts of each finger is separated, the cortical map gradually shifts 90 degrees to reflect the new sensory experience. In the revised map, the cortical representation of the

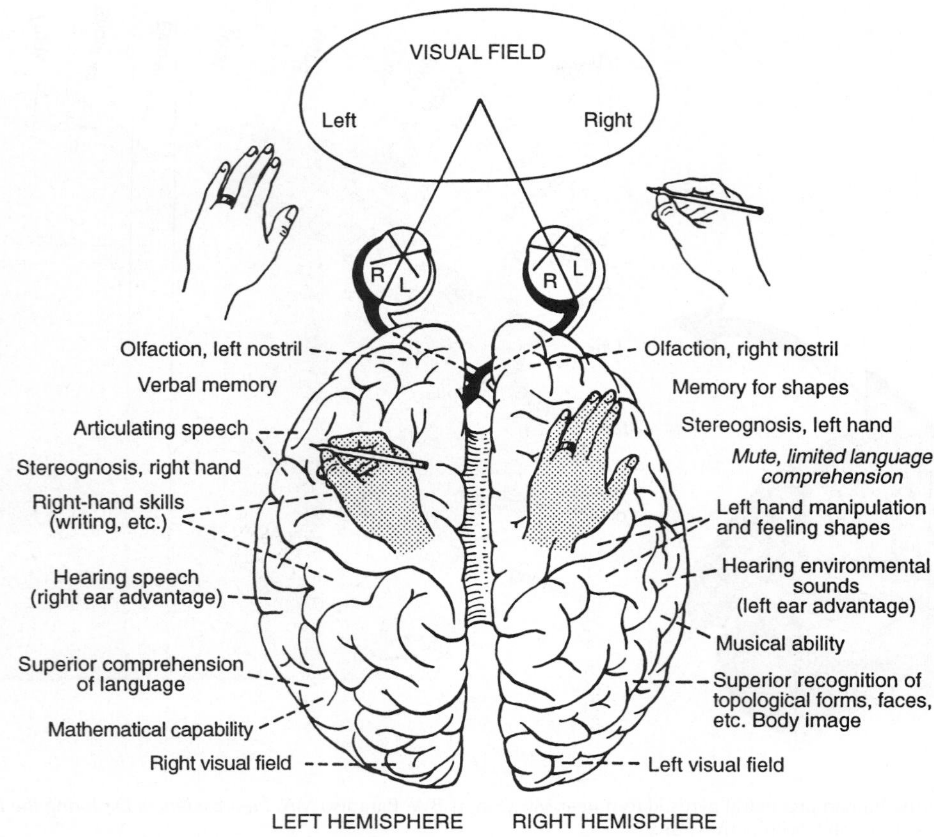

FIGURE 3.1–4

Drawing of the dorsal surface of the human brain showing the tendency for certain functions to be preferentially localized to one hemisphere. The intact brain, however, may not be as lateralized as some studies (e.g., of patients with commissurotomies) suggest, the degree of lateralization differs across individuals, and in the intact brain it is rare that one hemisphere can mediate a function that the other hemisphere is completely unable to perform. (From Fuchs AF, Phillips JO. Association cortex. In: Patton HD, et al. *Textbook of Physiology,* 21st ed. Vol. 1. Philadelphia:WB Saunders; 1989, with permission.)

proximal segment of each finger is no longer contiguous with that of the distal segment.

These data support the notion that the internal representation of the external world, although static in gross structure, can be continuously modified at the level of synaptic connectivity to reflect relevant sensory experiences. The cortical representation also tends to shift to fit entirely into the available amount of cortex.

These results also support the notion that cortical representations of sensory input, or of memories, may be holographic rather than spatially fixed: The pattern of activity, rather than the physical structure, may encode information. In sensory systems, this plasticity of cortical representation allows recovery from brain lesions; the phenomenon may also underlie learning. Figure 3.1–4 depicts localized functional areas of the brain.

Visual System

Visual images are transduced into neural activity within the retina and are processed through a series of brain cells, which respond to increasingly complex features, from the eye to the higher visual cortex. The neurobiological basis of feature extraction is best understood in finest detail in the visual system. Beginning with classic work in the 1960s, research in the visual pathway has produced two main paradigms for all sensory systems. The first paradigm, mentioned above with respect to the somatosensory system, weighs the contributions of genetics and experience—or nature and nurture—to the formation of the final synaptic arrangement. Transplantation experiments, resulting in an accurate point-to-point pattern of connectivity even when the eye was surgically inverted, suggested an innate, genetically determined mechanism of synaptic pattern formation. The crucial role of early visual experience in establishing the adult pattern of visual connections, on the other hand, crystallized the hypothesis of activity-dependent formation of synaptic connectivity. The final adult pattern is the result of both factors.

The second main paradigm, most clearly revealed in the visual system, is that of highly specialized brain cells that respond exclusively to extremely specific stimuli. Recent work, for example, has defined cells in the inferior temporal cortex that respond only to faces viewed at a specific angle. An individual's response to a particular face requires the activity of large neural networks and may not be limited to a single neuron. Nevertheless, the cellular localization of specific feature extraction is of critical importance in defining the boundary between sensory and association systems, but only in the visual system has this significant question been posed experimentally.

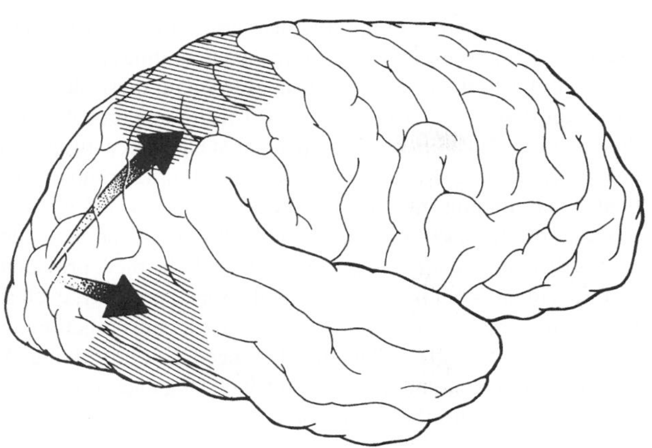

FIGURE 3.1–5

Visual association areas. At the far left pole of the cortex, impulses from the primary visual cortex spread both to the parietal lobe (*upper shaded area*), which tracks where the image is in space, and to the temporal lobe (*lower shaded area*), which determines what the image is. (From Filly CM. *Neurobehavioral Anatomy.* Niwot, CO: University Press of Colorado; 1995, with permission.)

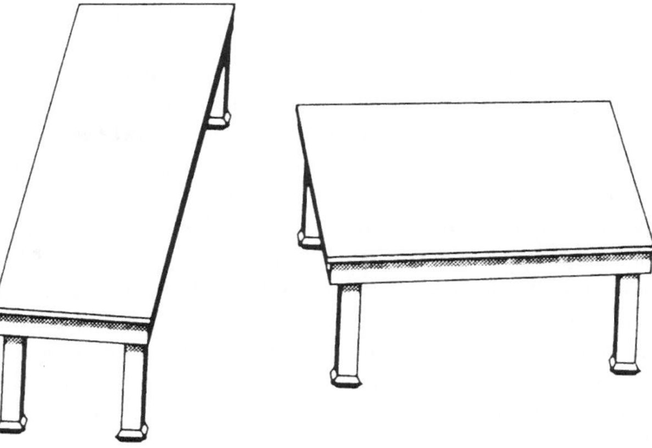

FIGURE 3.1–6

Optical illusion: perspective. Two tables are drawn in a perspective view. The *left table* appears to be long and narrow, whereas the *right table* appears to be short and wide. In fact, both tabletops are drawn exactly the same size on the page (the reader can measure them). Closest attention is paid to those feature recognition modules that identify items that can be used best. Unlike the brain's very familiar ideal of a table top, the two-dimensional shapes depicted by the actual printed lines on the paper are so unfamiliar that we find it almost impossible to see them as abstract drawings. This is because the ability to draw a perspectival image such as this one is evolutionarily extremely recent—at most a few thousand years—whereas the ability to recognize a "raised, flat surface on which to prepare food" is probably 100 million years old or older. (Modified from Gazzaniga MS. *The Mind's Past.* Berkeley: University of California Press; 1988:88, with permission.)

In the primary visual cortex, columns of cells respond specifically to lines of a specific orientation. The cells of the primary visual cortex project to the secondary visual cortex, where cells respond specifically to particular movements of lines and to angles. In turn, these cells project to two association areas, where additional features are extracted and conscious awareness of images forms (Fig. 3.1–5). The inferior temporal lobe detects the shape, form, and color of the object—the *what* questions; the posterior parietal lobe tracks the location, motion, and distance—the *where* questions. The posterior parietal lobe contains distinct sets of neurons that signal the intention either to look into a certain part of visual space or to reach for a particular object. In the inferior temporal cortices (ITCs), adjacent cortical columns respond to complex forms. Responses to facial features tend to occur in the left ITC, and responses to complex shapes tend to occur in the right ITC. The brain devotes specific cells to the recognition of facial expressions and to the aspect and position of faces of others with respect to the individual. Other body parts have a less complete representation among feature-specific cells, and inanimate objects occupy another set of cellular addresses.

The crucial connections between the feature-specific cells and the association areas involved in memory and conscious thought remain to be delineated. Much elucidation of feature recognition is based on invasive animal studies. In humans, the clinical syndrome of *prosopagnosia* describes the inability to recognize faces, in the presence of preserved recognition of other environmental objects. On the basis of pathological and radiological examination of individual patients, prosopagnosia is thought to result from disconnection of the left ITC from the visual association area in the left parietal lobe. Such lesional studies are useful in identifying necessary components of a mental pathway, but they may be inadequate to define the entire pathway. One noninvasive technique that is still being perfected and is beginning to reveal the full anatomical relation of the human visual system to conscious thought and memory is functional neuroimaging (Section 3.3).

As is true for language, there appears to be a hemispheric asymmetry for certain components of visuospatial orientation. Although both hemispheres cooperate in perceiving and drawing complex images, the right hemisphere, especially the parietal lobe, contributes the overall contour, perspective, and right-left orientation, and the left hemisphere adds internal detail, embellishment, and complexity. The brain can be fooled in optical illusions (Fig. 3.1–6).

Neurological conditions such as strokes and other focal lesions have permitted the definition of several disorders of visual perception. *Apperceptive visual agnosia* is the inability to identify and draw items using visual cues, with preservation of other sensory modalities. It represents a failure of transmission of information from the higher visual sensory pathway to the association areas and is caused by bilateral lesions in the visual association areas. *Associative visual agnosia* is the inability to name or use objects despite the ability to draw them. It is caused by bilateral medial occipitotemporal lesions and can occur along with other visual impairments. Color perception may be ablated in lesions of the dominant occipital lobe that include the splenium of the corpus callosum. *Color agnosia* is the inability to recognize a color despite being able to match it. *Color anomia* is the inability to name a color despite being able to point to it. *Central achromatopsia* is a complete inability to perceive color. *Anton's syndrome* is a failure to acknowledge blindness, possibly owing to interruption of fibers involved in self-assessment. It is seen with bilateral occipital lobe lesions. The most common causes are hypoxic injury, stroke, metabolic encephalopathy, migraine, herniation resulting from mass lesions, trauma, and leukodystrophy. *Balint's syndrome* consists of a triad of optic ataxia (the inability to direct optically guided movements), *oculomotor apraxia* (inability to direct gaze rapidly), and *simultanagnosia* (inability to integrate a visual scene to perceive it as a whole). Balint's syndrome is seen in bilateral parieto-occipital lesions. *Gerstmann syndrome* includes agraphia, calculation difficulties (acalculia), right-left disorientation, and finger agnosia. It has been attributed to lesions of the dominant parietal lobe.

Development of the Visual System. In humans, the initial projections from both eyes intermingle in the cortex. During the development of visual connections in the early postnatal period, there is a window of time during which binocular visual input is required for development of ocular dominance columns in the primary visual cortex. Ocular dominance columns are stripes of cortex that receive input from only one eye, separated by stripes innervated only by fibers from the other eye. Occlusion of one eye during this critical period completely eliminates the persistence of its fibers in the cortex and allows the fibers of the active eye to innervate the entire visual cortex. In contrast, when normal binocular vision is allowed during the critical development window, the usual dominance columns form; occluding one eye after the completion of innervation of the cortex produces no subsequent alteration of the ocular dominance columns. This paradigm crystallizes the importance of early childhood experience on the formation of adult brain circuitry.

Auditory System

Sounds are instantaneous, incremental changes in ambient air pressure. The pressure changes cause the ear's tympanic membrane to vibrate; the vibration is then transmitted to the ossicles (malleus, incus, and stapes) and thereby to the endolymph or fluid of the cochlear spiral. Vibrations of the endolymph move cilia on hair cells, which generate neural impulses. The hair cells respond to sounds of different frequency in a tonotopic manner within the cochlea, like a long, spiral piano keyboard. Neural impulses from the hair cells travel in a tonotopic arrangement to the brain in the fibers of the cochlear nerve. They enter the brainstem cochlear nuclei, are relayed through the lateral lemniscus to the inferior colliculi, and then to the medial geniculate nucleus (MGN) of the thalamus. MGN neurons project to the primary auditory cortex in the posterior temporal lobe. Dichotic listening tests, in which different stimuli are presented to each ear simultaneously, demonstrate that most of the input from one ear activates the contralateral auditory cortex and that the left hemisphere tends to be dominant for auditory processing.

Sonic features are extracted through a combination of mechanical and neural filters. The representation of sound is roughly tonotopic in the primary auditory cortex, whereas *lexical processing* (i.e., the extraction of vowels, consonants, and words from the auditory input) occurs in higher language association areas, especially in the left temporal lobe. The syndrome of *word deafness*, characterized by intact hearing for voices but an inability to recognize speech, may reflect damage to the left parietal cortex. This syndrome is thought to result from disconnection of the auditory cortex from Wernicke's area. A rare, complementary syndrome, *auditory sound agnosia*, is defined as the inability to recognize nonverbal sounds, such as a horn or a cat's meow, in the presence of intact hearing and speech recognition. Researchers consider this syndrome the right hemisphere correlate of pure word deafness.

Development of the Auditory System. Certain children are unable to process auditory input clearly and therefore have impaired speech and comprehension of spoken language. Studies on some of these children have determined that, in fact, they can discriminate speech if the consonants and vowels—the phonemes—are slowed two- to fivefold by a computer. Based on this observation, a tutorial computer program was designed that initially asked questions in a slowed voice and, as subjects answered questions correctly, gradually increased the rate of phoneme presentation to approximate normal rates of speech. Subjects gained some ability to discriminate routine speech over a period of 2 to 6 weeks and appeared to retain these skills after the tutoring period was completed. This finding probably has therapeutic applicability to 5 to 8 percent of children with speech delay, but ongoing studies may expand the eligible group of students. This finding, moreover, suggests that neuronal circuits required for auditory processing can be recruited and be made more efficient long after language is normally learned, provided that the circuits are allowed to finish their task properly, even if this requires slowing the rate of input. Circuits thus functioning with high fidelity can then be trained to speed their processing. A recent report has extended the age at which language acquisition may be acquired for the first time.

A boy who had intractable epilepsy of one hemisphere was mute because the uncontrolled seizure activity precluded the development of organized language functions. At the age of 9 years he had the abnormal hemisphere removed to cure the epilepsy. Although he had not spoken to that point of his life, he initiated an accelerated acquisition of language milestones beginning at that age and ultimately gained language abilities only a few years delayed relative to his chronological age.

Researchers cannot place an absolute upper limit on the age at which language abilities can be learned, although acquisition at ages beyond the usual childhood period is usually incomplete. Anecdotal reports document acquisition of reading skills after the age of 80 years.

Olfaction

Odorants, or volatile chemical cues, enter the nose, are solubilized in the nasal mucus, and bind to odorant receptors displayed on the surface of the sensory neurons of the olfactory epithelium. Each neuron in the epithelium displays a unique odorant receptor, and cells displaying a given receptor are randomly arranged within the olfactory epithelium. Humans possess several hundred distinct receptor molecules that bind the huge variety of environmental odorants; workers estimate that humans can discriminate 10,000 different odors. Odorant binding generates neural impulses, which travel along the axons of the sensory nerves through the cribriform plate to the olfactory bulb. Within the bulb, all axons corresponding to a given receptor converge onto only 1 or 2 of 3,000 processing units called *glomeruli*. Because each odorant activates several receptors that activate a characteristic pattern of glomeruli, the identity of external chemical molecules is represented internally by a spatial pattern of neural activity in the olfactory bulb.

Each glomerulus projects to a unique set of 20 to 50 separate columns in the olfactory cortex. In turn, each olfactory cortical column receives projections from a unique combination of glomeruli. The connectivity of the olfactory system is genetically determined. Because each odorant activates a unique set of several receptors and thus a unique set of olfactory bulb glomeruli, each olfactory cortical column is tuned to detect a different odorant of some evolutionary significance to the species. Unlike the signals of the somatosensory, visual, and auditory systems, olfactory signals do not pass through the thalamus but project directly to the frontal lobe and the limbic system, especially the pyriform cortex.

The connections to the limbic system (amygdala, hippocampus, pyriform cortex) are significant. Olfactory cues stimulate strong emotional responses and can evoke powerful memories.

Olfaction, the most ancient sense in evolutionary terms, is tightly associated with sexual and reproductive responses. A related chemosensory structure, the vomeronasal organ, is thought to detect *pheromones*, chemical cues that trigger unconscious, stereotyped responses. In some animals, ablation of the vomeronasal organ in early life may prevent the onset of puberty. Recent studies have suggested that humans also respond to pheromones in a manner that varies according to the menstrual cycle. The structures of higher olfactory processing in phylogenetically more primitive animals have evolved in humans into the limbic system, the center of the emotional brain and the gate through which experience is admitted into memory according to emotional significance. The elusive basic animal drives with which clinical psychiatry constantly grapples may therefore, in fact, originate from the ancient centers of higher olfactory processing.

Development of the Olfactory System. During normal development, axons from the nasal olfactory epithelium project to the olfactory bulb and segregate into about 3,000 equivalent glomeruli. If an animal is exposed to a single dominant scent in the early postnatal period, then one glomerulus expands massively within the bulb at the expense of the surrounding glomeruli. Thus, as discussed above with reference to the barrel fields of the somatosensory cortex, the size of brain structures may reflect the environmental input.

Taste

Soluble chemical cues in the mouth bind to receptors in the tongue and stimulate the gustatory nerves, which project to the nucleus solitarius in the brainstem. The sense of taste is believed to discriminate only broad classes of stimuli: sweet, sour, bitter, and salty. Each modality is mediated through a unique set of cellular receptors and channels, of which several may be expressed in each taste neuron. The detection and the discrimination of foods, for example, involve a combination of the senses of taste, olfaction, touch, vision, and hearing. Taste fibers activate the medial temporal lobe, but the higher cortical localization of taste is only poorly understood.

Autonomic Sensory System

The autonomic nervous system (ANS) monitors the basic functions necessary for life. The activity of visceral organs, blood pressure, cardiac output, blood glucose levels, and body temperature are all transmitted to the brain by autonomic fibers. Most autonomic sensory information remains unconscious; if such information rises to conscious levels, it is only as a vague sensation, in contrast to the capacity of the primary senses to transmit sensations rapidly and exactly.

Alteration of Conscious Sensory Perception through Hypnosis

Hypnosis is a state of heightened suggestibility attainable by a certain proportion of the population. Under a state of hypnosis, gross distortions of perception in any sensory modality and changes in the ANS can be achieved instantaneously. The anatomy of the sensory system does not change, yet the same specific stimuli may be perceived with diametrically opposed emotional value before and after induction of the hypnotic state. For example, under hypnosis a person may savor an onion as if it were a luscious chocolate truffle, only to reject the onion as abhorrently pungent seconds later, when the hypnotic suggestion is reversed. The localization of the hypnotic switch has not been determined, but it presumably involves both sensory and association areas of the brain. Experiments tracing neural pathways in human volunteers via functional neuroimaging have demonstrated that shifts in attention in an environmental setting determine changes in the regions of the brain that are activated, on an instantaneous time scale. Thus, the organizing centers of the brain may route conscious and unconscious thoughts through different sequences of neural processing centers, depending on a person's ultimate goals and emotional state. These attention-mediated variations in synaptic utilization can occur instantaneously, much like the alteration in the routing of associational processing that may occur in hypnotic states.

MOTOR SYSTEMS

Body muscles movements are controlled by the lower motor neurons, which extend axons—some as long as 1 meter—to the muscle fibers. Lower motor neuron firing is regulated by the summation of upper motor neuron activity. In the brainstem, primitive systems produce gross coordinated movements of the entire body. Activation of the rubrospinal tract stimulates flexion of all limbs, whereas activation of the vestibulospinal tract causes all limbs to extend. Newborn infants, for example, have all limbs tightly flexed, presumably through the dominance of the rubrospinal system. In fact, the movements of an anencephalic infant, who completely lacks a cerebral cortex, may be indistinguishable from the movements of a normal newborn. In the first few months of life, the flexor spasticity is gradually mitigated by the opposite actions of the vestibulospinal fibers, and more limb mobility occurs.

At the top of the motor hierarchy is the corticospinal tract, which controls fine movements and which eventually dominates the brainstem system during the first years of life. The upper motor neurons of the corticospinal tract reside in the posterior frontal lobe, in a section of cortex known as the *motor strip* (Fig. 3.1–1, Brodmann area 4). Planned movements are conceived in the association areas of the brain and, in consultation with the basal ganglia and cerebellum, the motor cortex directs their smooth execution. The importance of the corticospinal system becomes immediately evident in strokes, in which spasticity returns as the cortical influence is ablated and the actions of the brainstem motor systems are released from cortical modulation.

Basal Ganglia

The *basal ganglia*, a subcortical group of gray matter nuclei, appear to mediate postural tone. The four functionally distinct ganglia are the striatum, the pallidum, the substantia nigra, and the subthalamic nucleus. Collectively known as the corpus striatum, the caudate and putamen harbor components of both motor and association systems. The caudate nucleus plays an important role in the modulation of motor acts. Anatomical and functional neuroimaging studies have correlated decreased activation of the caudate with obsessive–compulsive behavior. When functioning properly, the caudate nucleus acts as a gatekeeper to allow the motor system to perform only those acts that are goal directed. When it fails to perform its gatekeeper function, extraneous acts are performed as in obsessive–compulsive disorder or in the tic disorders, such as Tourette's disorder. Overactivity of the striatum owing to lack of dopaminergic inhibition (e.g., in parkinsonian conditions) results in *bradykinesia*, an inability to initiate movements. The caudate, in particular, shrinks dramatically in Huntington's disease. This disorder is characterized by rigidity, on which is gradually superimposed choreiform, or "dancing," movements. Psychosis may be a prominent feature of Huntington's disease, and suicide is not uncommon. The caudate is also thought to influence associative, or cognitive, processes. Figure 3.1–7 is a schematic drawing of the basal ganglia.

The globus pallidus contains two parts linked in series. In a cross section of the brain, the internal and external parts of the globus pallidus are nested within the concavity of the putamen. The globus pallidus receives input from the corpus striatum and projects fibers to the thalamus. This structure may be severely damaged in Wilson's disease and in carbon monoxide poisoning, which are characterized by dystonic posturing and flapping movements of the arms and legs.

The substantia nigra is named the black substance because the presence of melanin pigment causes it to appear black to the naked eye. It has two parts, one of which is functionally equivalent to the globus pallidus interna. The other part degenerates in Parkinson's disease. Parkinsonism is characterized by rigidity and tremor and is associated with depression in more than 30 percent of cases.

Finally, lesions in the subthalamic nucleus yield ballistic movements, sudden limb jerks of such velocity that they are compared to projectile movement.

Together, the nuclei of the basal ganglia appear capable of initiating and maintaining the full range of useful movements. Workers have speculated that the nuclei serve to configure the activity of the overlying motor cortex to fit the purpose of the association areas. In addition, they appear to integrate proprioceptive feedback to maintain an intended movement.

Cerebellum

The cerebellum consists of a simple six-cell pattern of circuitry that is replicated roughly 10 million times. Simultaneous recordings of the cerebral cortex and the cerebellum have shown that the cerebellum is activated several milliseconds before a planned movement. Moreover, ablation of the cerebellum renders intentional movements coarse and tremulous. These data suggest that the cerebellum carefully modulates the tone of agonistic and antagonistic muscles by predicting the relative contraction needed for smooth motion. This prepared motor plan is used to ensure that exactly the right amount of flexor and extensor stimuli is sent to the muscles. Recent functional imaging data have shown that the cerebellum is active even during the mere imagination of motor acts, when no movements ultimately result from its calculations. The cerebellum harbors two, and possibly more, distinct "homunculi" or cortical representations of the body plan. Figure 3.1–8 depicts the cerebellar nuclei.

Motor Cortex

Penfield's groundbreaking work defined a motor homunculus in the precentral gyrus, Brodmann area 4 (Fig. 3.1–1), where a somatotopic map of the motor neurons is found. Individual cells within the motor strip cause contraction of single muscles. The brain region immediately anterior to the motor strip is called the *supplementary motor area*, Brodmann area 6. This region contains cells that when individually stimulated can trigger more complex movements, by influencing a firing sequence of motor strip cells. Recent studies have demonstrated wide representation of motor movements in the brain (see Color Plate 3.1–9 on p. 81).

The skillful use of the hands is called *praxis*, and deficits in skilled movements are termed *apraxias*. The three levels of apraxia are limb-kinetic, ideomotor, and ideational. *Limb-kinetic apraxia* is the inability to use the contralateral hand in the presence of preserved strength; it results from isolated lesions in the supplementary motor area, which contains neurons that stimulate functional sequences of neurons in the motor strip.

Ideomotor apraxia is the inability to perform an isolated motor act on command, despite preserved comprehension, strength, and spontaneous performance of the same act. Ideomotor apraxia simultaneously affects both limbs and involves functions so specialized that they are localized to only one hemisphere. Conditions in two separate areas can produce this apraxia. Disconnection of the language comprehension area, Wernicke's area, from the motor regions causes an inability to follow spoken commands, and lesions to the left premotor area may impair the actual motor program as it is generated by the higher-order motor neurons. This program is transmitted across the corpus callosum to the right premotor area, which directs the movements of the left hand. A lesion in this callosal projection can also cause an isolated ideomotor apraxia in the left hand. This syndrome implies the representation of specific motor acts within discrete sections of the left premotor cortex. Thus, just as some cells respond selectively to specific environmental features in the higher sensory cortices, some cells in the premotor cortex direct specific complex motor tasks.

Ideational apraxia occurs when the individual components of a sequence of skilled acts can be performed in isolation, but the entire series cannot be organized and executed as a whole. For example, the sequence of opening an envelope, removing the letter, unfolding it, and placing it on the table cannot be performed in order, even though the individual acts can be performed in isolation. The representation of the concept of a motor sequence may involve several areas, specifically the left parietal cortex, but it likely also relies on the sequencing and executive functions of the prefrontal cortex. This apraxia is a typical finding of diffuse cortical degeneration, such as Alzheimer's disease.

Autonomic Motor System

The *autonomic system* is divided into a sensory component (described above) and a motor component. The *autonomic motor system* is divided into two branches, the sympathetic and the parasympathetic. As a rule, organs are innervated by both types of fibers, which often serve antagonistic roles. The *parasympathetic system* slows the heart rate and begins the process of digestion. In contrast, the *sympathetic system* mediates the fight or flight response, with increased heart rate, shunting of blood away from the viscera, and increased respiration. The sympathetic system is highly activated by sympathomimetic drugs, such as amphetamine and cocaine, and may also be activated by withdrawal from sedating drugs such as alcohol, benzodiazepines, and opioids. Investigators who have found an increased risk of heart attacks in persons with high levels of hostility have

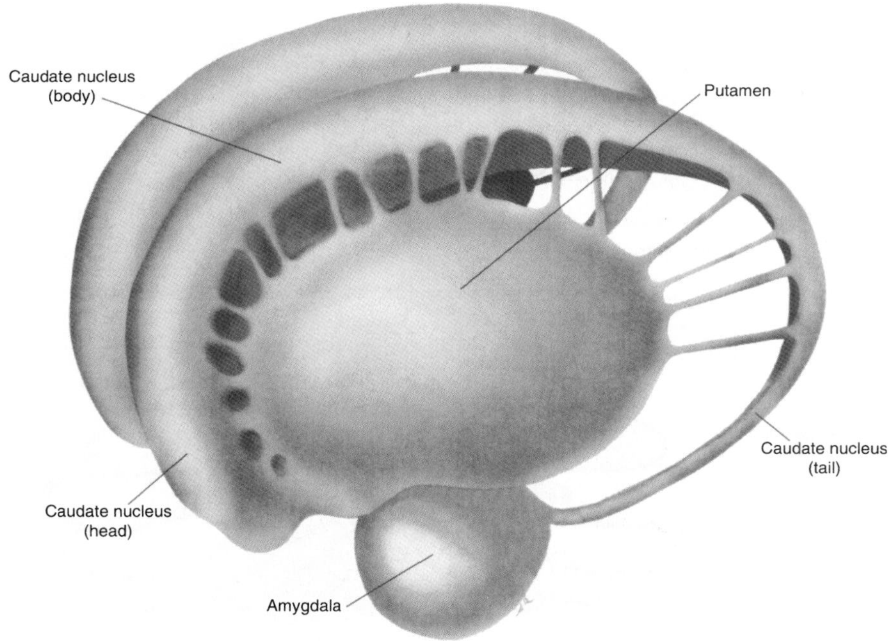

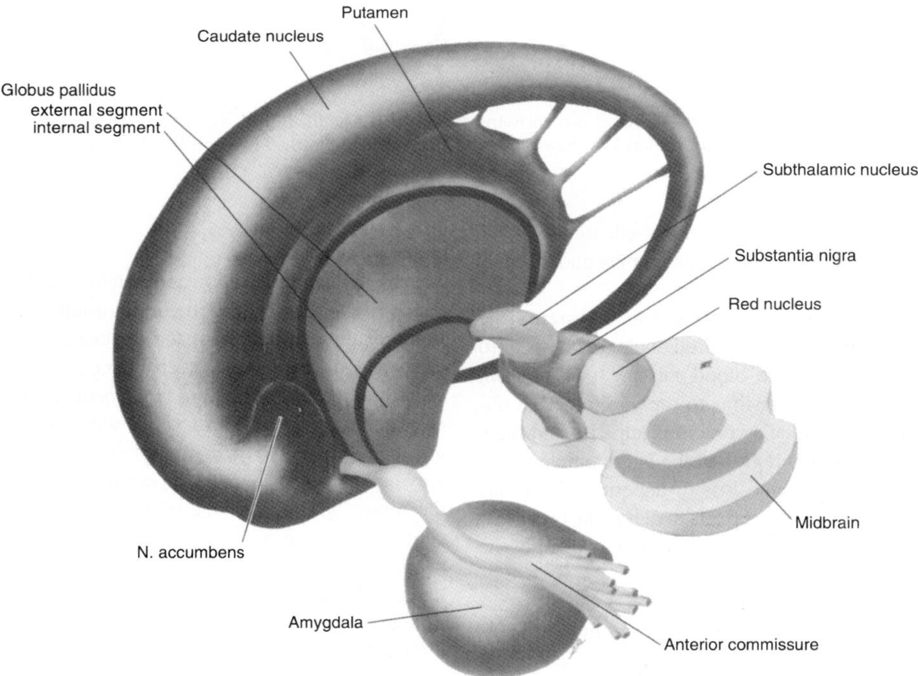

FIGURE 3.1–7

Schematic drawing of the isolated basal ganglia as seen from the dorsolateral perspective, so that the caudate nucleus is apparent bilaterally. In the *bottom panel,* the basal ganglia from the left hemisphere have been removed, exposing the medial surface of the right putamena and globus pallidus, as well as the subthalmic nucleus and substantia nigra. (Adapted from Hendleman WF. *Student's Atlas of Neuroanatomy.* Philadelphia: WB Saunders; 1994.)

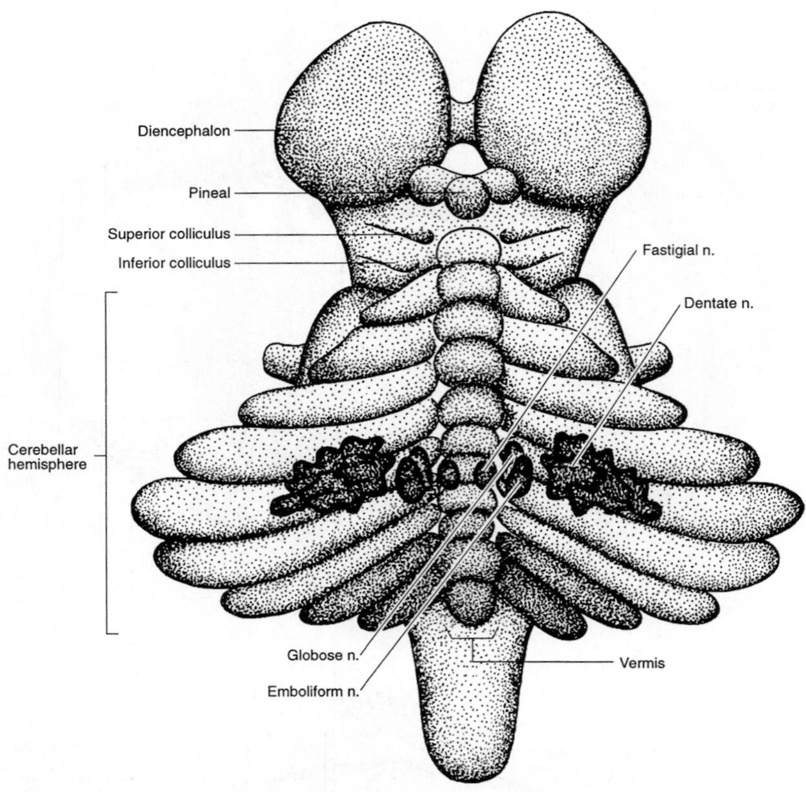

FIGURE 3.1–8
Schematic drawing of the dorsal view of the cerebellum showing the relative location and size of the cerebullar nuclei situated deep within the cerebellum. (Adapted from Hendleman WF. *Student's Atlas of Neuroanatomy.* Philadelphia: WB Saunders; 1994.)

suggested that chronic activation of the sympathetic fight or flight response, with elevated secretion of adrenaline, may underlie this association.

The brain center that drives the autonomic motor system is the *hypothalamus*, which houses a set of paired nuclei that appear to control appetite, rage, temperature, blood pressure, perspiration, and sexual drive. For example, lesions to the ventromedial nucleus, the satiety center, produce a voracious appetite and rage. In contrast, lesions to the upper region of the lateral nucleus, the hunger center, produce a profound loss of appetite. Numerous research groups are making intense efforts to define the biochemical regulation of appetite and obesity and frequently target the role of the hypothalamus.

In the regulation of sexual attraction, the role of the hypothalamus has also become an area of active research. In the 1990s, three groups independently reported neuroanatomical differences between certain of the hypothalamic nuclei of heterosexual and homosexual men. Researchers interpreted this finding to suggest that human sexual orientation has a neuroanatomical basis, and this result has stimulated several follow-up studies of the biological basis of sexual orientation. At present, however, these controversial findings are not accepted without question, and no clear consensus has emerged about whether the structure of the hypothalamus consistently correlates with sexual orientation. In animal studies, early nurturing and sexual experiences consistently alter the size of specific hypothalamic nuclei.

Primitive Reflex Circuit

Sensory pathways function as extractors of specific features from the overwhelming multitude of environmental stimuli, whereas motor pathways carry out the wishes of the organism. These pathways may be linked directly, for example, in the spinal cord, where a primitive reflex arc may mediate the brisk withdrawal of a limb from a painful stimulus, without immediate conscious awareness. In this loop, the peripheral stimulus activates the sensory nerve, the sensory neuron synapses on and directly activates the motor neuron, and the motor neuron drives the muscle to contract. This response is strictly local and all-or-none. Such primitive reflex arcs, however, rarely generate an organism's behaviors. In most behaviors, sensory systems project to association areas, where sensory information is interpreted in terms of internally determined memories, motivations, and drives. The exhibited behavior results from a plan of action determined by the association components and carried out by the motor systems.

Localization of Brain Functions

Many theorists have subdivided the brain into functional systems. Brodmann defined 47 areas on the basis of cytoarchitectonic distinctions, a cataloguing that has been remarkably durable as the functional anatomy of the brain has been elucidated (Fig. 3.1–1). A separate function, based on data from lesion

(Text continues on page 85.)

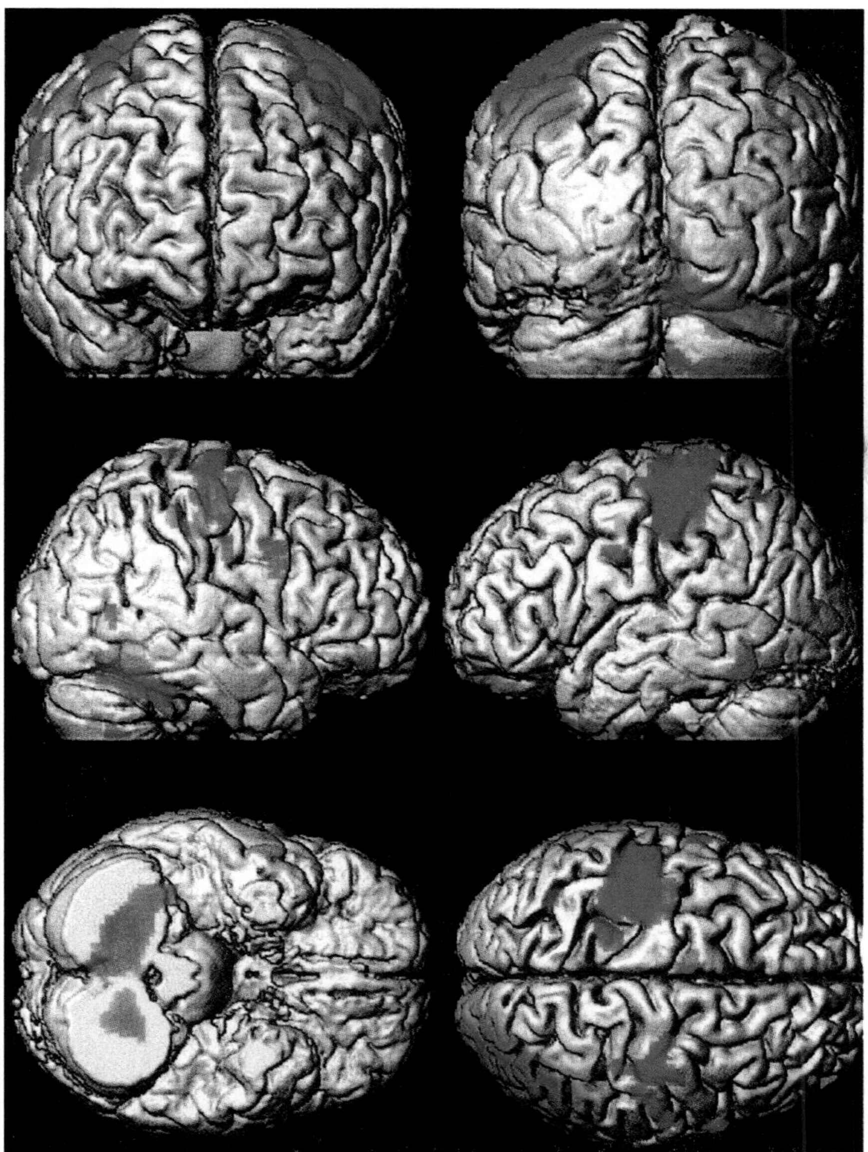

COLOR PLATE 3.1–9

Wide distribution of brain activity during repeated movement of the right hand. Areas of increased neuronal activity, shown in red, are superimposed on a computer-reconstructed 3-dimensional MRI of the human brain projected in six views: *(top left)* front coronal view, *(top right)* back coronal view, *(middle left)* right sagittal view, *(middle right)* left sagittal view, *(bottom left)* bottom axial view, and *(bottom right)* top axial view. The patterns of neuronal activity are defined using functional MRI neuroimaging. Activity is seen in widely distributed, discrete areas, most strongly in the left cerebral hemisphere and the right cerebellum. Most higher-order functional brain modules, such as that for hand movements, are widely distributed among local networks in the brain. (Modified from Lawler A. New brain institute struggles for traction. *Science.* 2001;293:1421, with permission.)

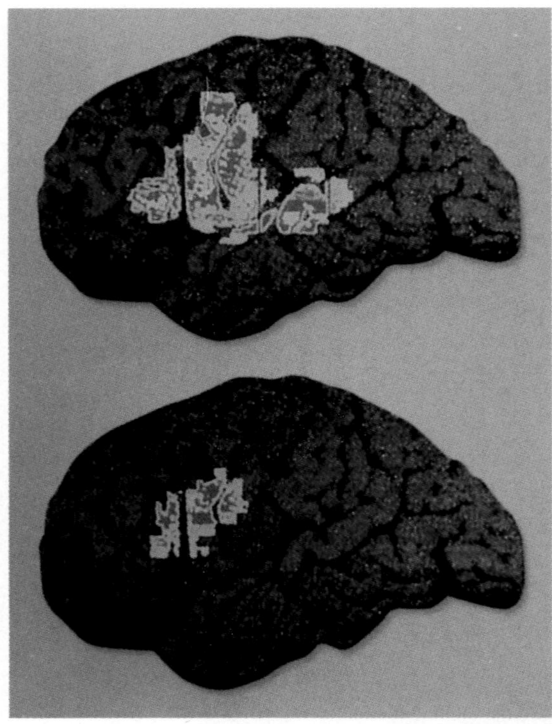

COLOR PLATE 3.3–4

Functional MRI during rhyming tasks in normal people and people with dyslexia. The left hemisphere is depicted in green. Normal (*top*) and dyslexic (*bottom*) subjects were shown two letters and asked to determine whether the letters rhymed (B-T) or not (B-K). To perform the task, the subjects had to translate the letters into sounds, or phonemes, (/bee/,/lee/), then compare only the rhyming part of the phonemes (/ee/). In normals, three contiguous areas were activated, including Broca's area, Wernicke's area, and the intervening insula. In those with dyslexia, only Broca's area was activated. Dyslexic patients required much more time to complete the task and were more prone to make errors. (Reprinted with permission from Frith C, Frith U. A biological marker for dyslexia. *Nature*. 1996;382:19.)

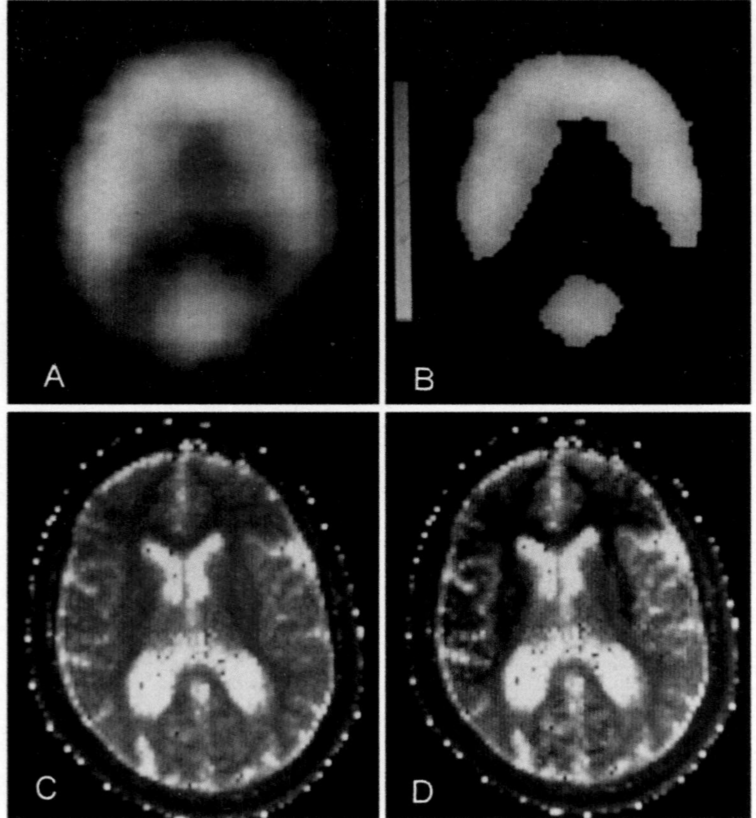

COLOR PLATE 3.3–5

Stages of the superimposition of a SPECT cerebral blood-flow image (**A**), which has been redefined (**B**), and an MRIT1-weighted image (**C**), to produce a combination (**D**). (Reprinted with permission from Besson JAO. Magnetic resonance imaging and its application in neuropsychiatry. *Br J Psychiatry*. 1990;25(9 Suppl):157.)

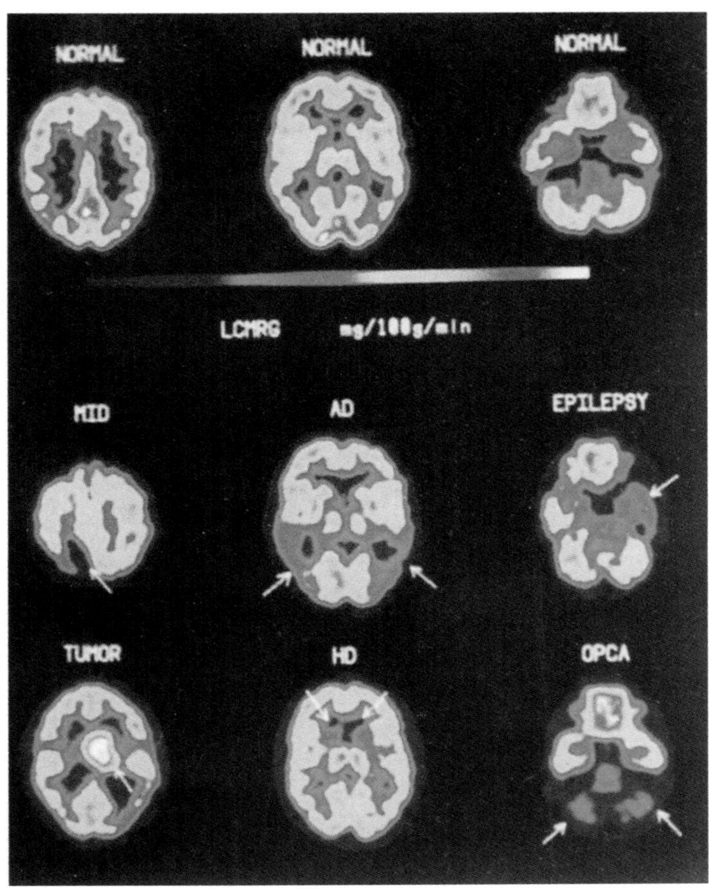

COLOR PLATE 3.3–6

PET scans with [^{18}F]fluorodeoxyglucose in a control (*top*) and six patients with neurological disorders. The three images from the control show transverse sections of the brain at a high level through the parietal lobes (*left*), an intermediate level through the basal ganglia and the thalamus (*center*), and a low level through the base of the frontal lobes, the temporal lobes, and the cerebellum (*right*). The level of each image corresponds approximately to the level of the scans below. The *bar* indicates the level of glucose metabolic activity in the images, with colors on the left indicating low levels of metabolism and colors on the right indicating high levels. The middle and bottom scans are from patients with multi-infarct dementia (*MID*) (also known as vascular dementia), Alzheimer's disease (*AD*), temporal lobe epilepsy, brain tumor (primitive neuroectodermal tumor), Huntington's disease (*HD*), and olivopontocerebellar atrophy (*OPCA*). A small region of absent glucose metabolism is seen in the patient with multi-infarct dementia (*arrow*); PET scans at other levels in the patient revealed a number of similar areas, which represent small focal infarctions. The scan in the patient with Alzheimer's disease shows hypometabolism in both parietal lobes (*arrows*). The image in the patient with epilepsy shows hypometabolism in the right temporal lobe (*arrow*), which is the site of origin of the seizure disorder. The scan in the patient with a tumor shows a region of hypermetabolism in the thalamus, which is the location of the tumor (*arrow*). The image in the patient with Huntington's disease shows hypometabolism in the caudate nuclei bilaterally (*arrows*). The scan in the patient with olivopontocerebellar atrophy shows hypometabolism in the cerebellum (*arrows*) and the brainstem. (Reprinted with permission from Gilman S. Advanced in neurology. *N Engl J Med.* 1992;326:1610.)

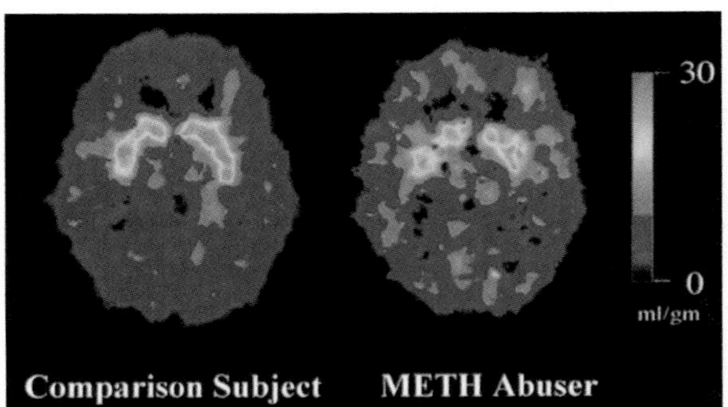

COLOR PLATE 3.3–7

Positron emission tomography scan showing striatal dopamine transporter density in a 33-year-old male methamphetamine (METH) abuser 30 days after detoxification, compared to a 33-year-old male control subject. (See Color Plate). (From Volkow ND, Chang L, Wang GJ, et al. Association of dopamine transporter reduction with psychomotor impairment in methamphetamine abusers. *Am J Psychiatry.* 2001:158;377, with permission.)

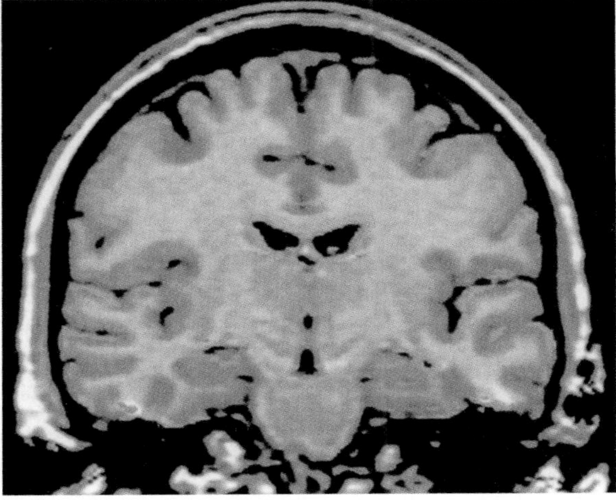

COLOR PLATE 3.3–8

Whole-brain atrophy in a patient with probable Alzheimer's dementia, computed by the digital subtraction of a baseline magnetic resonance image (MRI) from an MRI acquired 1 year later. Areas in red reflect 1-year reductions in tissue volume and areas in green reflect 1-year gains (e.g., displacement in tissue volume). (Courtesy of N. Fox and colleagues.)

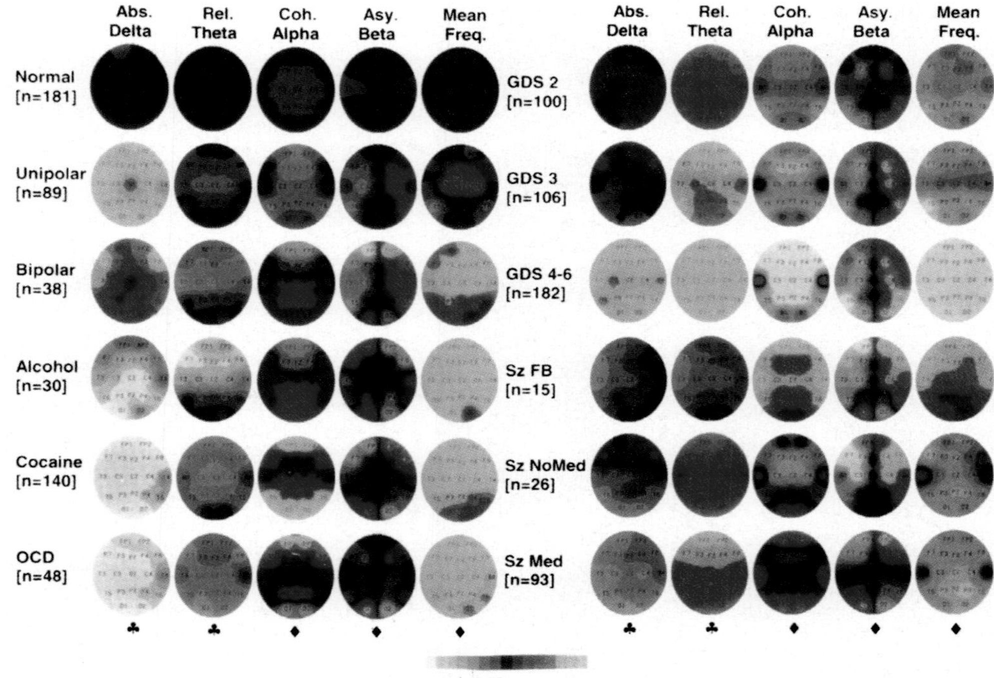

COLOR PLATE 3.4–3

Baseline group average topographic images of z scores for selected quantitative electroencephalography (QEEG) features in different *Diagnostic and Statistical Manual of Mental Disorders*, 4th edition, text revision, psychiatric populations. Successive columns in the left and right panels include absolute (Abs) power delta, relative (Rel.) power theta, interhemispheric coherence (Coh.) alpha, interhemispheric power asymmetry (Asy.) beta, and total power mean frequency (Freq.). Populations include normal adults; unipolar depressions; bipolar depressions; alcoholics (in withdrawl); cocaine-dependent subjects (5 to 14 days after last drug use); obsessive-compulsive disorder (OCD); global deterioration scale (GDS) 2, which are normal elderly with only subjective congnitive complaints; GDS 3 which meet criteria for mild cognitive impairment; GDS 4 through 6, which meet criteria for dementia; first-break schizophrenics (Sz FB); schizophrenics off medication (5z NoMed); and schizophrenics on medication (Sz Med). The color scale of each z image is in standard deviation units, with a range of +0.75, indicated with a diamond, or +1.25, indicated with a club. To estimate the significant of any regional z score for this group average data, the z score should be multiplied by the square root of the number of patients in the group. For a group with 100 subjects, the z value imaged should be multiplied by 10 to get the estimate of the significance of that z. (See Color Plate.) (Courtesy of Dr. E. Roy John, Director, Brain Research Laboratories, Department of Psychiarty, New York University, School of Medicine, New York, NY, and Nathan S. Kline Institute for Psychiatric Research, Orangeburg, NY.)

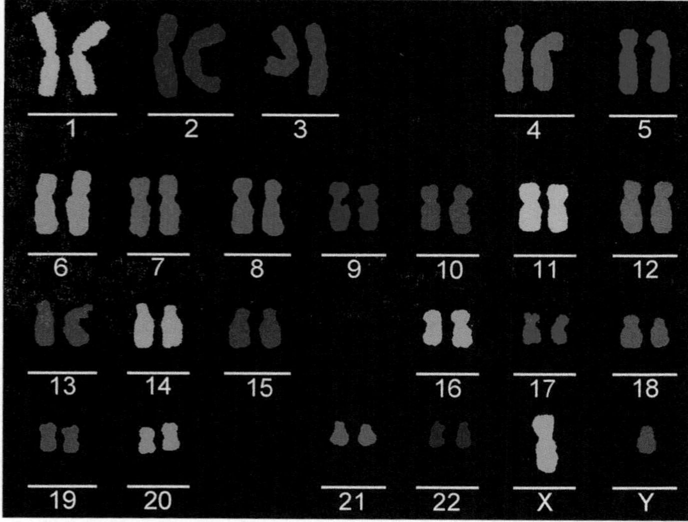

COLOR PLATE 3.6–4

The Human Karyotype. The normal human genetic material contains two copies of the 3,000,000,000 DNA-base genomic sequence packaged into 22 matched pairs of autosomes and X and Y sex chromosomes. Here the human karyotype has been stained using different colored chromosome-specific probes. Identical twins share identical copies of genomic DNA. (Adapted from Bentley D. *The Geography of Our Genome.* Supplement to *Nature,* 2001, with permission.)

studies and from functional neuroimaging, has been assigned to nearly all Brodmann areas. At the other extreme, certain experts have distinguished only three processing blocks: The brainstem and the thalamic reticular activating system provide arousal and set up attention; the posterior cortex integrates perceptions and generates language; and, at the highest level, the frontal cortex generates programs and executes plans like an orchestra conductor.

Hemispheric lateralization of function is a key feature of higher cortical processing. The primary sensory cortices for touch, vision, hearing, smell, and taste are represented bilaterally, and the first level of abstraction for these modalities is also usually represented bilaterally. The highest levels of feature extraction, however, are generally unified in one brain hemisphere only. For example, recognition of familiar and unfamiliar faces seems localized to the left inferior temporal cortex, and cortical processing of olfaction occurs in the right frontal lobe.

Hypotheses about the flow of thought in the brain are based on few experimental data, although this scarcity of findings has not impeded numerous theoreticians from speculating about functional neuroanatomy. Several roles have been tentatively assigned to specific lobes of the brain, on the basis of the functional deficits resulting from localized injury. These data indicate that certain regions of cortex may be necessary for a specific function, but they do not define the complete set of structures that suffices for a complex task. Anecdotal evidence from surface electrocorticography for the study of epilepsy, for example, suggests that a right parietal seizure impulse may shoot immediately to the left frontal lobe and then to the right temporal lobe before spreading locally to the remainder of the parietal lobe. This evidence illustrates the limitations of naively assigning a mental function to a single brain region. Functional neuroimaging studies frequently reveal simultaneous activation of disparate brain regions during the performance of even a simple cognitive task. Nevertheless, particularly in the processing of vision and language, fairly well-defined lobar syndromes have been confirmed (Table 3.1–1).

Language. The clearest known example of hemispheric lateralization is the localization of language functions to the left hemisphere. Starting with the work of Pierre Broca and Karl Wernicke in the 19th century, researchers have drawn a detailed map of language comprehension and expression (Color Plate 3.1–9 on p. 81). At least eight types of aphasias in which one or more components of the language pathway are inured have been defined (Table 3.1–2). *Prosody*, the emotional and affective components of language, or "body language," appears to be localized in a mirror set of brain units in the right hemisphere.

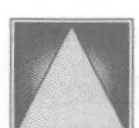

Table 3.1–1
Regional Functions of the Human Brain

Frontal lobes
- Voluntary movement
- Language production (left)
- Motor prosody (right)
- Comportment
- Executive function
- Motivation

Temporal lobes
- Audition
- Language comprehension (left)
- Sensory prosody (right)
- Memory
- Emotion

Parietal lobes
- Tactile sensation
- Visuospatial function (right)
- Reading (left)
- Calculation (left)

Occipital lobes
- Vision
- Visual perception

(Reprinted from Filley CM. *Neurobehavioral Anatomy*. Niwot, CO: University Press of Colorado; 1995:6, with permission.)

Because of the major role of verbal and written language in human communication, the neuroanatomical basis of language is the most completely understood association function. Language disorders, also called *aphasias*, are readily diagnosed in routine conversation, whereas perceptual disorders may escape notice, except during detailed neuropsychological testing, although these disorders may be caused by injury of an equal volume of cortex. Among the earliest models of cortical localization of function were Broca's 1865 description of a loss of fluent speech caused by a lesion in the left inferior frontal lobe and Wernicke's 1874 localization of language comprehension to the left superior temporal lobe. Subsequent analyses of patients rendered aphasic by strokes, trauma, or tumors have led to the definition of the entire language association pathway from sensory input through the motor output (Fig. 3.1–10).

Language most clearly demonstrates hemispheric localization of function. In most persons, the hemisphere dominant for language also directs the dominant hand. Ninety percent of the population is right-handed, and 99 percent of right-handers have left hemispheric dominance for language. Of the 10 percent who are left-handers, 67 percent also have left hemispheric language

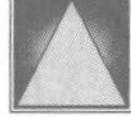

Table 3.1–2
Localization of Aphasia Syndromes

Aphasia Type	Spontaneous Speech	Auditory Comprehension	Repetition	Naming	Localization (Left Hemisphere)
Broca's	Nonfluent	Good	Poor	Poor	Broca's area
Wernicke's	Fluent	Poor	Poor	Poor	Wernicke's area
Conduction	Fluent	Good	Poor	Poor	Arcuate fasciculus
Global	Nonfluent	Poor	Poor	Poor	Perisylvian region
Transcortical motor	Nonfluent	Good	Good	Poor	Anterior border zone
Transcortical sensory	Fluent	Poor	Good	Poor	Posterior border zone
Anomic	Fluent	Good	Good	Poor	Angular gyrus
Mixed transcortical	Nonfluent	Poor	Good	Poor	Anterior and posterior border zone

(Reprinted from Filley CM. *Neurobehavioral Anatomy*. Niwot, CO: University Press of Colorado; 1995:80, with permission.)

dominance; the other 33 percent have either mixed or right hemispheric language dominance. This innate tendency to lateralization of language in the left hemisphere is highly associated with an asymmetry of the planum temporale, a triangular cortical patch on the superior surface of the temporal lobe that appears to harbor Wernicke's area. Patients with mixed hemispheric dominance for language lack the expected asymmetry of the planum temporale. That asymmetry has been observed in prenatal brains suggests a genetic determinant. Indeed, the absence of asymmetry runs in families, although both genetic and intrauterine influences probably contribute to the final pattern.

Language comprehension is processed at three levels. First, in *phonological processing*, individual sounds, such as vowels or consonants, are recognized in the inferior gyrus of the frontal lobes. Phonological processing improves if lip reading is allowed, if speech is slowed, or if contextual clues are provided. Second, *lexical processing* matches the phonological input with recognized words or sounds in the individual's memory. Lexical processing determines whether a sound is a word or not. Recent evidence has localized lexical processing to the left temporal lobe, where the representations of lexical data are organized according to semantic category. Third, *semantic processing* connects the words to their meaning. Persons with an isolated defect in semantic processing may retain the ability to repeat words in the absence of an ability to understand or spontaneously generate speech. Semantic processing activates the middle and superior gyri of the left temporal lobe, whereas the representation of the conceptual content of words is widely distributed in the cortex. Language production proceeds in the opposite direction, from the cortical semantic representations through the left temporal lexical nodes to either the oromotor phonological processing area (for speech) or the graphomotor system (for writing). Each of these areas can be independently or simultaneously damaged by stroke, trauma, infection, or tumor, resulting in a specific type of aphasia.

The garbled word salad or illogical utterances of an aphasic patient leave little uncertainty about the diagnosis of left-sided cortical injury, but the right hemisphere contributes a somewhat more subtle, but equally important, affective quality to language. For example, the phrase "I feel good" may be spoken with an infinite variety of shadings, each of which is understood differently. The perception of prosody and the appreciation of the associated gestures, or "body language," appear to require an intact right hemisphere. Behavioral neurologists have mapped an entire pathway for prosody association in the right hemisphere that mirrors the language pathway of the left hemisphere. Patients with right hemisphere lesions, who have impaired comprehension or expression of prosody, may find it difficult to function in society despite their intact language skills.

Developmental dyslexia is defined as an unexpected difficulty with learning in the context of adequate intelligence, motivation, and education. Whereas speech consists of the logical combination of 44 basic phonemes of sounds, reading requires a broader set of brain functions and, thus, is more susceptible to disruption. The awareness of specific phonemes develops about the age of 4 to 6 years and appears to be prerequisite to acquisition of reading skills. Inability to recognize distinct phonemes is the best predictor of a reading disability. Functional neuroimaging studies have localized the identification of letters to the occipital lobe adjacent to the primary visual cortex. Phonological processing occurs in the inferior frontal lobe, and semantic processing requires the superior and middle gyri of the left temporal lobe. A recent finding of uncertain significance is that phonological processing in men activates only the left inferior frontal gyrus, whereas phonological processing in women activates the inferior frontal gyrus bilaterally. Careful analysis of an individual's particular reading deficits can guide remedial tutoring efforts that can focus on weaknesses and thus attempt to bring the reading skills up to the general level of intelligence and verbal skills.

In children, developmental nonverbal learning disorder is postulated to result from right hemisphere dysfunction. Nonverbal learning disorder is characterized by poor fine-motor control in the left hand, deficits in visuoperceptual organization, problems with mathematics, and incomplete or disturbed socialization.

Patients with nonfluent aphasia, who cannot complete a simple sentence, may be able to sing an entire song, apparently because many aspects of music production are localized to the right hemisphere. Music is represented predominantly in the right hemisphere, but the full complexity of musical ability seems to involve both hemispheres. Trained musicians appear to transfer many musical skills from the right hemisphere to the left as they gain proficiency in musical analysis and performance.

Arousal and Attention. Arousal, or the establishment and maintenance of an awake state, appears to require at least three brain regions. Within the brainstem, the ascending reticular activating system (ARAS), a diffuse set of neurons, appears to set the level of consciousness. The ARAS projects to the intralaminar nuclei of the thalamus, and these nuclei in turn project widely throughout the cortex. Electrophysiological studies show that both the thalamus and the cortex fire rhythmical bursts of neuronal activity at the rates of 20 to 40 cycles per second. During sleep, these bursts are not synchronized. During wakefulness, the ARAS stimulates the thalamic intralaminar nuclei, which in turn coordinate the oscillations of different cortical regions. The greater the synchronization, the higher the level of wakefulness. The absence of arousal produces stupor and coma. In general, small discrete lesions of the ARAS can produce a stuporous state, whereas at the hemispheric level, large bilateral lesions are required to cause the same depression in alertness.

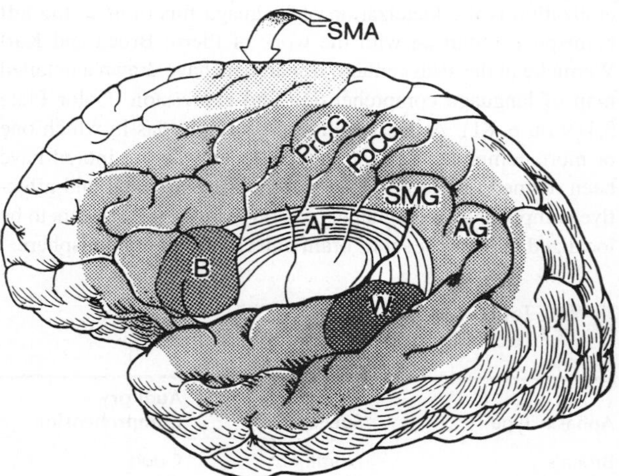

FIGURE 3.1–10

Language areas of the left hemisphere: *B*, Broca's area; *W*, Wernicke's area; *AF*, arcuate fasciculus; *SMA*, supplementary motor area; *PrCG*, precentral gyrus; *PoCG*, postcentral gyrus; *SMG*, supramarginal gyrus; and *AG*, angular gyrus. Language comprehension occurs in Wernicke's area, which is connected to Broca's area by the arcuate fasciculus. Generation of speech occurs in Broca's area. (From Filly CM. *Neurobehavioral Anatomy*. Niwot, CO: University of Colorado Press; 1995:76, with permission.)

Table 3.1–3
Derivatives of the Neural Tube

Primary Vesicles	Secondary Vesicles	Brain Components
Prosencephalon	Telencephalon	Cerebral cortex Hippocampus Amygdala Striatum
	Diencephalon	Thalamus Hypothalamus Epithalamus
Mesencephalon	Mesencephalon	Midbrain
Rhombencephalon	Metencephalon	Pons Cerebellum
	Myelencephalon	Medulla

(Modified from Nolte J. *The Human Brain: An Introduction to Its Functional Anatomy.* 3rd ed. St. Louis: Mosby; 1993:9.)

One particularly unfortunate but instructive condition involving extensive, permanent, bilateral cortical dysfunction is the persistent vegetative state. Sleep–wake cycles may be preserved, and the eyes may appear to gaze; but the external world does not register and no evidence of conscious thought exists. This condition represents the expression of the isolated actions of the ARAS and the thalamus.

The maintenance of attention appears to require an intact right frontal lobe. For example, a widely used test of persistence requires scanning and identifying only the letter A from a long list of random letters. Healthy persons can usually maintain performance of such a task for several minutes, but in patients with right frontal lobe dysfunction, this capacity is severely curtailed. Lesions of similar size in other regions of the cortex usually do not affect persistence tasks. In contrast, the more generally adaptive skill of maintaining a coherent line of thought is diffusely distributed throughout the cortex. Many medical conditions can affect this skill and may produce acute confusion or delirium (Table 3.1–3).

One widely diagnosed disorder of attention is attention-deficit/hyperactivity disorder (ADHD). No pathological findings have been consistently associated with this disorder. Functional neuroimaging studies, however, have variously documented either frontal lobe or right hemisphere hypometabolism in patients with ADHD, compared with normal controls. These findings strengthen the notion that the frontal lobes—especially the right frontal lobe—are essential to the maintenance of attention.

Memory. The clinical assessment of memory should test three periods, which have distinct anatomical correlates. *Immediate memory* functions over a period of seconds; *recent memory* applies on the scale of minutes to days; and *remote memory* encompasses months to years. Immediate memory is implicit in the concept of attention and the ability to follow a train of thought. This ability has been divided into phonological and visuospatial components, and functional imaging has localized them to the left and right hemispheres, respectively. A related concept, incorporating immediate and recent memory, is *working memory*, which is the ability to store information for several seconds, whereas other, related cognitive operations take place on this information. Recent studies have shown that single neurons in the dorsolateral prefrontal cortex not only record features necessary for working memory, but also record the certainty with which the information is known and the degree of expectation assigned to the permanence of a particular environmental feature. Some neurons fire rapidly for an item that is eagerly awaited, but may cease firing if hopes are dashed unexpectedly. The encoding of the emotional value of an item contained in the working memory may be of great usefulness in determining goal-directed behavior. Some researchers localize working memory predominantly to the left frontal cortex. Clinically, however, bilateral prefrontal cortex lesions are required for severe impairment of working memory. Other types of memory have been described: episodic, semantic, and procedural (Table 3.1–4).

Three brain structures are critical to the formation of memories: the medial temporal lobe, certain diencephalic nuclei, and the basal forebrain. The *medial temporal lobe* houses the *hippocampus*, an elongated, highly repetitive network. The *amygdala* is adjacent to the anterior end of the hippocampus. The amygdala has been suggested to rate the emotional importance of an experience and to activate the level of hippocampal activity accordingly. Thus, an emotionally intense experience is indelibly etched in memory, but indifferent stimuli are quickly disregarded.

Animal studies have defined a hippocampal place code, a pattern of cellular activation in the hippocampus that corresponds to the animal's location in space. When the animal is introduced to

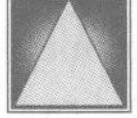

Table 3.1–4
Categories of Memory

Memory System	Major Anatomical Structures	Length of Storage of Memory	Type of Awareness	Examples
Episodic memory	Medial temporal lobes, anterior thalamic nucleus, mamillary body, fornix, prefrontal cortex	Minutes to years	Explicit, declarative	Remembering a short story, what you had for dinner last night, and what you did on your last birthday
Semantic memory	Inferolateral temporal lobes	Minutes to years	Explicit, declarative	Knowing who was the first president of the United States, the color of a lion, and how a fork differs from a comb
Procedural memory	Basal ganglia, cerebellum, supplementary motor area	Minutes to years	Explicit or implicit, nondeclarative	Driving a car with a standard transmission (explicit) and learning the sequence of numbers on a touch tone phone without trying (implicit)

(Data from Budson AE, Price BH. Memory dysfunction. *N Engl J Med.* 2005;352:7.)

a novel environment, the hippocampus is broadly activated. As the animal explores and roams, the firing of certain hippocampal regions begins to correspond to specific locations in the environment. In about 1 hour, a highly detailed internal representation of the external space (a "cognitive map") appears in the form of specific firing patterns of the hippocampal cells. These patterns of neuronal firing may bear little spatial resemblance to the environment they represent; rather, they may seem randomly arranged in the hippocampus. If the animal is manually placed in a certain part of a familiar space, only the corresponding hippocampal regions show intense neural activity. When recording continues into sleep periods, firing sequences of hippocampal cells outlining a coherent path of navigation through the environment are registered, even though the animal is motionless. If the animal is removed from the environment for several days and then returned, the previously registered hippocampal place code is immediately reactivated. A series of animal experiments has dissociated the formation of the hippocampal place code from either visual, auditory, or olfactory cues, although each of these modalities may contribute to place code generation. Other factors may include internal calculations of distances based on counting footsteps or other proprioceptive information. Data from targeted genetic mutations in mice have implicated both the *N*-methyl-D-aspartate (NMDA) glutamate receptors and the calcium-calmodulin kinase II (CaMKII) in the proper formation of hippocampal place fields. These data suggest that the hippocampus is a significant site for formation and storage of immediate and recent memories. Although no data yet support the notion, it is conceivable that the hippocampal cognitive map is inappropriately reactivated during a *déjà vu* experience.

The most famous human subject in the study of memory is H. M., a man with intractable epilepsy, who had both his hippocampi and amygdalae surgically removed to alleviate his condition. The epilepsy was controlled, but he was left with a complete inability to form and recall memories of facts. H. M.'s learning and memory skills were relatively preserved, which led to the suggestion that declarative or factual memory may be separate within the brain from procedural or skill-related memory. A complementary deficit in procedural memory with preservation of declarative memory may be seen in persons with Parkinson's disease, in whom dopaminergic neurons of the nigrostriatal tract degenerate. Because this deficit in procedural memory can be ameliorated with treatment with levodopa (Larodopa), which is thought to potentiate dopaminergic neurotransmission in the nigrostriatal pathway, a role has been postulated for dopamine in procedural memory. Additional case reports have further implicated the amygdala and the afferent and efferent fiber tracts of the hippocampus as essential to the formation of memories. Lesional studies have also suggested a mild lateralization of hippocampal function in which the left hippocampus is more efficient at forming verbal memories and the right hippocampus tends to form nonverbal memories. After unilateral lesions in humans, however, the remaining hippocampus may compensate to a large extent. Medical causes of amnesia include alcoholism, seizures, migraine, drugs, vitamin deficiencies, trauma, strokes, tumors, infections, and degenerative diseases.

The motor system within the cortex receives directives from the association areas. The performance of a novel act requires constant feedback from the sensory and association areas for completion, and functional neuroimaging studies have demonstrated widespread activation of the cortex during unskilled acts. Memorized motor acts initially require activation of the medial temporal lobe. With practice, however, the performance of ever-larger segments of an act necessary to achieve a goal become encoded within discrete areas of the premotor and parietal cortices, particularly the left parietal cortex, with the result that a much more limited activation of the cortex is seen during highly skilled acts, and the medial temporal lobe is bypassed. This process is called the *corticalization of motor commands*. In lay terms, the process suggests a neuroanatomical basis for the adage "practice makes perfect."

Within the diencephalon, the dorsal medial nucleus of the thalamus and the mamillary bodies appear necessary for memory formation. These two structures are damaged in thiamine deficiency states usually seen in chronic alcoholics, and their inactivation is associated with Korsakoff's syndrome. This syndrome is characterized by severe inability to form new memories and a variable inability to recall remote memories.

The most common clinical disorder of memory is Alzheimer's disease. Alzheimer's disease is characterized pathologically by the degeneration of neurons and their replacement by senile plaques and neurofibrillary tangles. Clinicopathological studies have suggested that the cognitive decline is best correlated with the loss of synapses. Initially, the parietal and temporal lobes are affected, with relative sparing of the frontal lobes. This pattern of degeneration correlates with the early loss of memory, which is largely a temporal lobe function. Also, syntactical language comprehension and visuospatial organization, functions that rely heavily on the parietal lobe, are impaired early in the course of Alzheimer's disease. In contrast, personality changes, which reflect frontal lobe function, are relatively late consequences of Alzheimer's disease. Alzheimer's disease is discussed in Chapter 10. A rarer, complementary cortical degeneration syndrome, Pick's disease, first affects the frontal lobes while sparing the temporal and parietal lobes. In Pick's disease, disinhibition and impaired language expression, which are signs of frontal dysfunction, appear early, with relatively preserved language comprehension and memory.

Memory loss can also result from disorders of the subcortical gray matter structures, specifically the basal ganglia and the brainstem nuclei, from disease of the white matter, or from disorders that affect both gray and white matter.

Emotion. Persons' emotional experiences occupy the attention of all mental health professionals. Emotion derives from basic drives, such as feeding, sex, reproduction, pleasure, pain, fear, and aggression, which all animals share. The neuroanatomical basis for these drives appears to be centered in the limbic system. Distinctly human emotions, such as affection, pride, guilt, pity, envy, and resentment, are largely learned and most likely are represented in the cortex. The regulation of drives appears to require an intact frontal cortex. The complex interplay of the emotions, however, is far beyond the understanding of functional neuroanatomists. Where, for example, are the representations of the id, the ego, and the superego? Through what pathway are ethical and moral judgments shepherded? What processes allow beauty to be in the eye of the beholder? These philosophical questions represent a true frontier of human discovery.

Several studies have suggested that within the cortex exists a hemispheric dichotomy of emotional representation. The left hemisphere houses the analytical mind but may have a limited emotional repertoire. For example, lesions to the right hemisphere, which cause profound functional deficits, may be noted with indifference by the intact left hemisphere. The denial of illness and of the inability to move the left hand in cases of right hemisphere injury is called *anosognosia*. In contrast, left hemisphere lesions, which cause profound aphasia, can trigger a catastrophic depression, as the intact right hemisphere struggles with the realization of the loss. The right hemisphere also appears dominant for affect, socialization, and body image.

Damage to the left hemisphere produces intellectual disorder and loss of the narrative aspect of dreams. Damage to the right hemisphere produces affective disorders, loss of the visual aspects of dreams, and a failure to respond to humor, shadings of metaphor, and connotations. In dichotic vision experiments, two scenes of varied emotional content were displayed simultaneously to each half of the visual field and were perceived separately by each hemisphere. A more intense emotional response attended the scenes displayed to the left visual field that were processed by the right hemisphere. Moreover, hemisensory changes representing conversion disorders have been repeatedly noted to involve the left half of the body more often than the right, an observation that suggests an origin in the right hemisphere.

Within the hemispheres, the temporal and frontal lobes play a prominent role in emotion. The temporal lobe exhibits a high frequency of epileptic foci, and temporal lobe epilepsy (TLE) presents an interesting model for the role of the temporal lobe in behavior. In studies of epilepsy, abnormal brain activation is analyzed, rather than the deficits in activity analyzed in classic lesional studies. TLE is of particular interest in psychiatry because patients with temporal lobe seizures often manifest bizarre behavior without the classic grand mal shaking movements caused by seizures in the motor cortex. A proposed TLE personality is characterized by hyposexuality, emotional intensity, and a perseverative approach to interactions, termed *viscosity*. Patients with left TLE may generate references to personal destiny and philosophical themes and display a humorless approach to life. In contrast, patients with right TLE may display excessive emotionality, ranging from elation to sadness. Although patients with TLE may display excessive aggression between seizures, the seizure itself may evoke fear.

The inverse of a TLE personality appears in persons with bilateral injury to the temporal lobes after head trauma, cardiac arrest, herpes simplex encephalitis, or Pick's disease. This lesion resembles the one described in the Klüver-Bucy syndrome, an experimental model of temporal lobe ablation in monkeys. Behavior in this syndrome is characterized by hypersexuality, placidity, a tendency to explore the environment with the mouth, inability to recognize the emotional significance of visual stimuli, and constantly shifting attention, called *hypermetamorphosis*. In contrast to the aggression–fear spectrum sometimes seen in patients with TLE, complete experimental ablation of the temporal lobes appears to produce a uniform, bland reaction to the environment, possibly because of an inability to access memories.

The prefrontal cortices influence mood in a complementary way. Whereas activation of the left prefrontal cortex appears to lift the mood, activation of the right prefrontal cortex causes depression. A lesion to the left prefrontal area, at either the cortical or the subcortical level, abolishes the normal mood-elevating influences and produces depression and uncontrollable crying. In contrast, a comparable lesion to the right prefrontal area may produce laughter, euphoria, and *witzelsucht*, a tendency to joke and make puns. Effects opposite to those caused by lesions appear during seizures, in which occurs abnormal, excessive activation of either prefrontal cortex. A seizure focus within the left prefrontal cortex can cause gelastic seizures, for example, in which the ictal event is laughter. Functional neuroimaging has documented left prefrontal hypoperfusion during depressive states, which normalized after the depression was treated successfully.

Limbic System Function

The limbic system was delineated by James Papez in 1937. The Papez circuit consists of the hippocampus, the fornix, the mamillary bodies, the anterior nucleus of the thalamus, and the cingulate gyrus (Fig. 3.1–11). The boundaries of the limbic system were subsequently expanded to include the amygdala, septum, basal forebrain, nucleus accumbens, and orbitofrontal cortex. Although this schema creates an anatomical loop for emotional processing, the specific contributions of the individual components other than the hippocampus or even whether a given train of neural impulses actually travels along the entire pathway is unknown.

The amygdala appears to be a critically important gate through which internal and external stimuli are integrated. Information from the primary senses is interwoven with internal drives, such as hunger and thirst, to assign emotional significance to sensory experiences. The amygdala may mediate learned fear responses, such as anxiety and panic, and may direct the expression of certain emotions by producing a particular affect. Neuroanatomical data suggest that the amygdala exerts a more powerful influence on the cortex, to stimulate or suppress cortical activity, than the cortex exerts on the amygdala. Pathways from the sensory thalamic relay stations separately send sensory data to the amygdala and the cortex, but the subsequent effect of the amygdala on the cortex is the more potent of the two reciprocal connections. In contrast, damage to the amygdala has been reported to ablate the ability to distinguish fear and anger in other persons' voices and facial expressions. Persons with such injuries may have a preserved ability to recognize happiness, sadness, or disgust. The limbic system appears to house the emotional association areas, which direct the hypothalamus to express the motor and endocrine components of the emotional state.

Fear and Aggression. Electrical stimulation of animals throughout the subcortical area involving the limbic system produces rage reactions (e.g., growling, spitting, arching of the back). Whether the animal flees or attacks depends on the intensity of the stimulation.

Limbic System and Schizophrenia. The limbic system has been particularly implicated in neuropathological studies of schizophrenia. Eugen Bleuler's well-known four As of schizophrenia—affect, associations, ambivalence, and autism—refer to brain functions served in part by limbic structures. Several clinicopathological studies have found a reduction in the brain weight of the gray matter but not of the white matter in persons with schizophrenia. In pathological as well as in magnetic resonance imaging (MRI) reports, persons with schizophrenia may have reduced volume of the hippocampus, amygdala, and parahippocampal gyrus. Schizophrenia may be a late sequela of a temporal epileptic focus, with some studies reporting an association in 7 percent of patients with TLE.

Functional neuroimaging studies have demonstrated decreased activation of the frontal lobes in many patients with schizophrenia, particularly during tasks requiring willed action. A reciprocal increase in activation of the temporal lobe can occur during willed actions, such as finger movements or speaking, in persons with schizophrenia. Neuropathological studies have shown a decreased density of neuropil, the intertwined axons

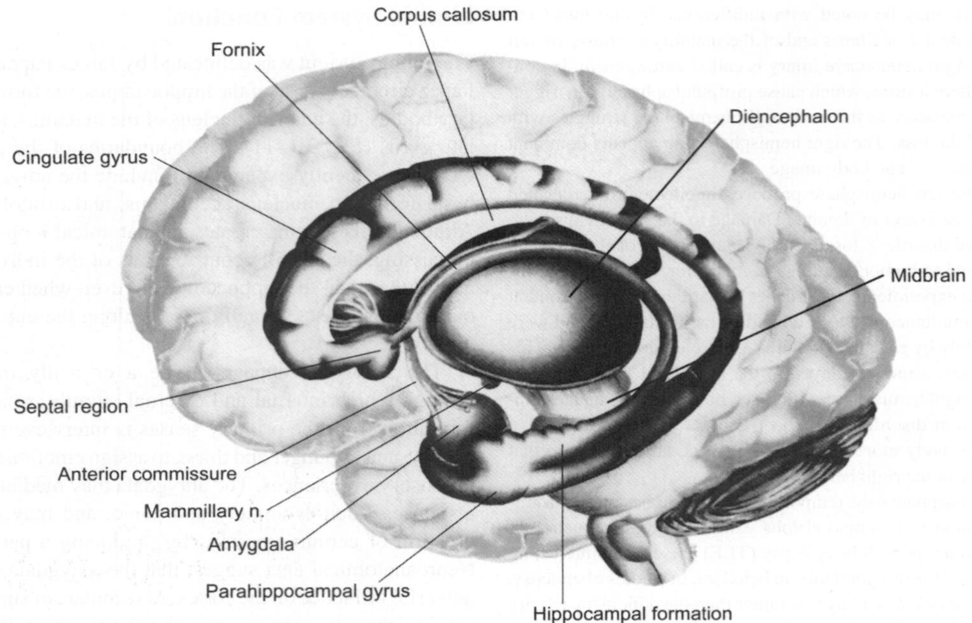

FIGURE 3.1–11

Schematic drawing of the major anatomical structures of the limbic system. Note: The cingulated and parahippocampal gyri form the *limbic lobe,* a rim of tissue located along the junction of the diencephalons and the cerebral hemispheres. *n,* nucleus. (Adapted from Handelman WJ. *Student's Atlas of Neuroanatomy.* Philadelphia: WB Saunders; 1994:179.)

and dendrites of the neurons, in the frontal lobes of these patients. During development, the density of neuropil is highest around age 1 year and then is reduced somewhat through synaptic pruning; the density plateaus throughout childhood and is further reduced to adult levels in adolescence. One hypothesis of the appearance of schizophrenia in the late teenage years is that excessive adolescent synaptic pruning occurs and results in too little frontolimbic activity. Some experts have suggested that hypometabolism and paucity of interneuronal connections in the prefrontal cortex may reflect inefficiencies in working memory, which permits the disjointed discourse and loosening of associations that characterize schizophrenia. At present, the molecular basis for the regulation of the density of synapses within the neuropil is unknown. Other lines of investigation aimed at understanding the biological basis of schizophrenia have documented inefficiencies in the formation of cortical synaptic connections in the middle of the second trimester of gestation, which may result from a viral infection or malnutrition. Neurodevelopmental surveys administered during childhood have found an increased incidence of subtle neurological abnormalities before the appearance of the thought disorder in persons who subsequently exhibited signs of schizophrenia.

In one intriguing study, positron emission tomography (PET) scanning was used to identify the brain regions that are activated when a person hears spoken language. A consistent set of cortical and subcortical structures demonstrated increased metabolism when speech was processed. The researchers then studied a group of patients with schizophrenia who were experiencing active auditory hallucinations. During the hallucinations, the same cortical and subcortical structures were activated as were activated by the actual sounds, including the primary auditory cortex. At the same time, decreased activation was seen of areas thought to monitor speech, including the left middle temporal gyrus and the supplementary motor area. This study raises the questions of what brain structure is activating the hallucinations and by what mechanism do neuroleptic drugs suppress the hallucinations. Clearly, functional imaging has much to tell about the neuroanatomical basis of schizophrenia.

Frontal Lobe Function

The *frontal lobes*, the region that determines how the brain acts on its knowledge, constitute a category unto themselves. In comparative neuroanatomical studies, the massive size of the frontal lobes is the main feature that distinguishes the human brain from that of other primates and that lends it uniquely human qualities. There are four subdivisions of the frontal lobes. The first three—the motor strip, the supplemental motor area, and Broca's area—are mentioned above in the discussion of the motor system and language. The fourth, most anterior, division is the prefrontal cortex. The prefrontal cortex contains three regions in which lesions produce distinct syndromes: the *orbitofrontal*, the *dorsolateral*, and the *medial*. Dye-tracing studies have defined dense reciprocal connections between the prefrontal cortex and all other brain regions. Therefore, to the extent that anatomy can predict function, the prefrontal cortex is ideally connected to allow sequential use of the entire palette of brain functions in executing goal-directed activity. Indeed, frontal lobe injury usually impairs the executive functions: motivation, attention, and sequencing of actions.

Bilateral lesions of the frontal lobes are characterized by changes in personality—how persons interact with the world. The *frontal lobe syndrome*, which is most commonly produced by trauma, infarcts, tumors, lobotomy, multiple sclerosis, or Pick's disease, consists of slowed thinking, poor judgment, decreased curiosity, social withdrawal, and irritability. Patients typically display apathetic indifference to experience that can suddenly explode into impulsive disinhibition. Unilateral frontal lobe lesions may be largely unnoticed because the intact lobe can compensate with high efficiency.

Frontal lobe dysfunction may be difficult to detect by means of highly structured, formal neuropsychological tests. Intelligence, as reflected in the intelligence quotient (IQ), may be normal, and functional neuroimaging studies have shown that the IQ seems to require mostly parietal lobe activation. For example, during administration of the Wechsler Adult Intelligence Scale-Revised (WAIS-R), the highest levels of increased metabolic activity during verbal tasks occurred in the left parietal lobe, whereas the highest levels of increased metabolic activity during performance skills occurred in the right parietal lobe. In contrast, frontal lobe pathology may become apparent only under unstructured, stressful, real-life situations.

A famous case illustrating the result of frontal lobe damage involves Phineas Gage, a 25-year-old railroad worker. While he was working with explosives, an accident drove an iron rod through Gage's head. He survived, but both frontal lobes were severely damaged (Fig. 3.1–12). After the accident, his behavior changed dramatically. The case was written up by J. M. Harlow, M.D., in 1868, as follows:

[George] is fitfull, irreverent, indulging at times in the grossest profanity (which was not previously his custom), manifesting but little deference for his fellows, impatient of restraint or advice when it conflicts with his desires . . . His mind was radically changed, so decidedly that his friends and acquaintances said he was "no longer Gage."

In one study of right-handed males, lesions of the right prefrontal cortex eliminated the tendency to use internal, associative memory cues and led to an extreme tendency to interpret the task at hand in terms of its immediate context. In contrast, right-handed males who had lesions of the left prefrontal cortex produced no context-dependent interpretations and interpreted the tasks entirely in terms of their own internal drives. A mirror image of the functional lateralization appeared in left-handed subjects. This test thus revealed the clearest known association of higher cortical functional lateralization with the subjects' dominant hand. Future experiments in this vein will attempt to reproduce these findings with functional neuroimaging. If corroborated, these studies suggest a remarkable complexity of functional localization within the prefrontal cortex and may also have implications for the understanding of psychiatric diseases in which prefrontal pathology has been postulated, such as schizophrenia and mood disorders.

The heavy innervation of the frontal lobes by dopamine-containing nerve fibers is of interest because of the action of antipsychotic medications. At the clinical level, antipsychotic medications may help to organize the rambling associations of a patient with schizophrenia. At the neurochemical level, most typical antipsychotic medications block the actions of dopamine at the dopamine D_2 receptors. The frontal lobes, therefore, may be a major therapeutic site of action for antipsychotic medications.

DEVELOPMENT

The nervous system is divided into the central and peripheral nervous systems (CNS and PNS). The CNS consists of the brain and spinal cord; the PNS refers to all the sensory, motor, and autonomic fibers and ganglia outside the CNS. During development, both divisions arise from a common precursor, the neural tube, which in turn is formed through folding of the neural plate, a

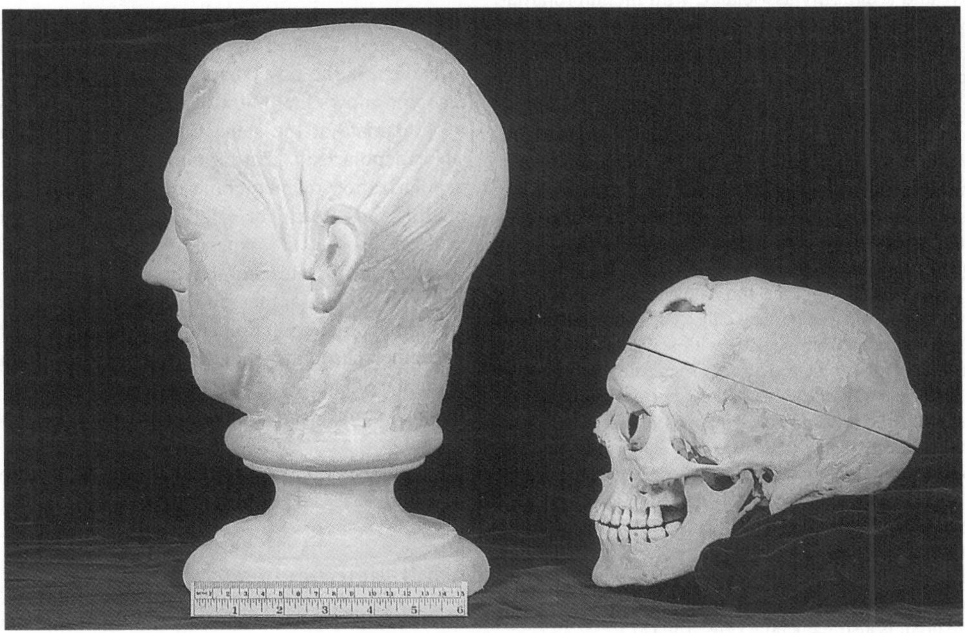

FIGURE 3.1–12

Death Mask of Phineas Gage with his skull. Note the defect in the frontal area of the skull and eye orbit, through which the metal rod lodged. (Courtesy of Anthony A. Walsh, Ph.D.)

specialization of the ectoderm, the outermost of the three layers of the primitive embryo. During embryonic development, the neural tube itself becomes the CNS (Table 3.1–3); the ectoderm immediately superficial to the neural tube becomes the neural crest, which gives rise to the PNS. The formation of these structures requires chemical communication between the neighboring tissues in the form of cell surface molecules and diffusible chemical signals. In many cases, an earlier-formed structure, such as the notochord, is said to *induce* the surrounding ectoderm to form a later structure, in this case the neural plate. Identification of the chemical mediators of tissue induction is an active area of research. Investigators have begun to examine whether failures of the interactions of these mediators and their receptors could underlie errors in brain development that cause psychopathology.

Neuronal Migration and Connections

The life cycle of a neuron consists of cell birth, migration to the adult position, extension of an axon, elaboration of dendrites, synaptogenesis, and, finally, the onset of chemical neurotransmission. Individual neurons are born in proliferative zones generally located along the inner surface of the neural tube. At the peak of neuronal proliferation in the middle of the second trimester, 250,000 neurons are born each minute. Postmitotic neurons migrate outward to their adult locations in the cortex, guided by radially oriented astrocytic glial fibers. Glial-guided neuronal migration in the cerebral cortex occupies much of the first 6 months of gestation. For some neurons in the prefrontal cortex, migration occurs over a distance 5,000 times the diameter of the neuronal cell body. Neuronal migration requires a complex set of cell–cell interactions and is susceptible to errors in which neurons fail to reach the cortex and instead reside in ectopic positions. A group of such incorrectly placed neurons is called a *heterotopia*. Neuronal heterotopias have been shown to cause epilepsy and are highly associated with mental retardation. In a neuropathological study of the planum temporale of four consecutive patients with dyslexia, heterotopias were a common finding. Recently, heterotopic neurons within the frontal lobe have been postulated to play a causal role in some cases of schizophrenia.

Many neurons lay an axon down as they migrate, whereas others do not initiate axon outgrowth until they have reached their cortical targets. Thalamic axons that project to the cortex initially synapse on a transient layer of neurons called the *subplate neurons*. In normal development, the axons subsequently detach from the subplate neurons and proceed superficially to synapse on the true cortical cells. The subplate neurons then degenerate. Some brains from persons with schizophrenia reveal an abnormal persistence of subplate neurons, suggesting a failure to complete axonal pathfinding in the brains of these persons. This finding does not correlate with the presence of schizophrenia in every case, however. A characteristic branched dendritic tree elaborates once the neuron has completed migration. Synaptogenesis occurs at a furious rate from the second trimester through the first 10 years or so of life. The peak of synaptogenesis occurs within the first 2 postnatal years, when as many as 30 million synapses form each second. Ensheathment of axons by myelin begins prenatally; it is largely complete in early childhood, but does not reach its full extent until late in the third decade of life. Myelination of the brain is also sequential (Fig. 3.1–13).

Neuroscientists are tremendously interested in the effect of experience on the formation of brain circuitry in the first years

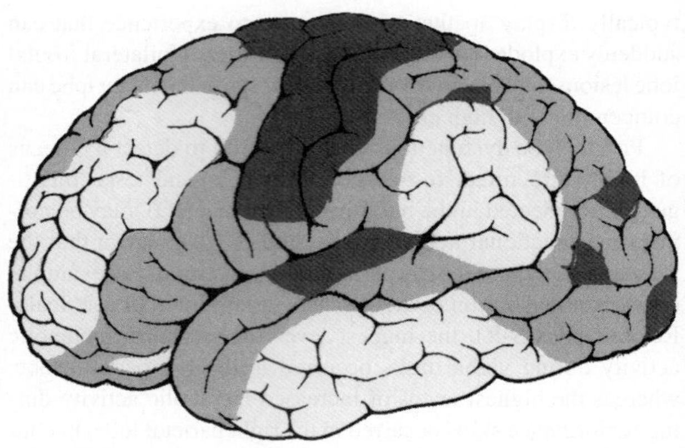

FIGURE 3.1–13
Sequence of myelination of the brain. Myelination occurs first in brain areas involved with leg movements, primitive vision, and primitive hearing, shown in *dark gray*. Next, shown in *light gray*, are the brain areas involved in arm movements, the supplementary motor areas, the higher visual and auditory areas, and the lower association areas. Finally, the frontal executive cortex, the parieto-occipital association area, the temporal object recognition areas, shown in *white*, do not complete their myelination until the time of puberty. (Modified from Spitzer M. *The Mind within the Net: Models of Learning, Thinking, and Acting*. Cambridge, MA: Bradford; 1991:179, with permission.)

of life. As noted above, many examples are seen of the impact of early sensory experience on the wiring of cortical sensory processing areas. Similarly, early movement patterns are known to reinforce neural connections in the supplemental motor area that drive specific motor acts. Neurons rapidly form a fivefold excess of synaptic connections; then, through a darwinian process of elimination, only those synapses that serve a relevant function persist. This synaptic pruning appears to preserve input in which the presynaptic cell fires in synchrony with the postsynaptic cell, a process that reinforces repeatedly activated neural circuits. One molecular component that is thought to mediate synaptic reinforcement is the postsynaptic NMDA glutamate receptor. This receptor allows the influx of calcium ions only when activated by glutamate at the same time as the membrane in which it sits is depolarized. Thus, glutamate binding without membrane depolarization or membrane depolarization without glutamate binding fails to trigger calcium influx. NMDA receptors open in dendrites that are exposed to repeated activation, and their activation stimulates stabilization of the synapse. Calcium is a crucial intracellular messenger that initiates a cascade of events, including gene regulation and the release of trophic factors that strengthen particular synaptic connections. Although less experimental evidence exists for the role of experience in modulating synaptic connectivity of association areas than has been demonstrated in sensory and motor areas, neuroscientists assume that similar activity-dependent mechanisms may apply in all areas of the brain.

Adult Neurogenesis

A remarkable recent discovery has been that new neurons can be generated in certain brain regions (particularly the dentate gyrus of the hippocampus) in adult animals, including humans. This is in marked contrast to the previous belief that no neurons were produced after birth in most species. This discovery has a potentially profound impact on our understanding of normal development, incorporation of experiences, as well as the ability of the brain to repair itself after various types of injuries.

Neurological Basis of Development Theories

In the realm of emotion, early childhood experiences have been suspected to be at the root of psychopathology since the earliest theories of Sigmund Freud. Freud's psychoanalytic method aimed at tracing the threads of a patient's earliest childhood memories. Franz Alexander added the goal of allowing the patient to relive them in a less pathological environment, a process known as a *corrective emotional experience.* Although neuroscientists have no data demonstrating that this method operates at the level of neurons and circuits, emerging results reveal a profound effect of early caregivers on an adult individual's emotional repertoire. For example, the concept of attunement is defined as the process by which caregivers "play back a child's inner feelings." If a baby's emotional expressions are reciprocated in a consistent and sensitive manner, certain emotional circuits are reinforced. These circuits likely include the limbic system, in particular, the amygdala, which serves as a gate to the hippocampal memory circuits for emotional stimuli. In one anecdote, for example, a baby whose mother repeatedly failed to mirror her level of excitement emerged from childhood an extremely passive girl, who was unable to experience a thrill or a feeling of joy.

The relative contributions of nature and nurture are perhaps nowhere more indistinct than in the maturation of emotional responses, partly because the localization of emotion within the adult brain is only poorly understood. It is reasonable to assume, however, that the reactions of caregivers during a child's first 2 years of life are eventually internalized as distinct neural circuits, which may be only incompletely subject to modification through subsequent experience. For example, axonal connections between the prefrontal cortex and the limbic system, which probably play a role in modulating basic drives, are established between the ages of 10 and 18 months. Recent work suggests that a pattern of terrifying experiences in infancy may flood the amygdala and drive memory circuits to be specifically alert to threatening stimuli, at the expense of circuits for language and other academic skills. Thus, infants raised in a chaotic and frightening home may be neurologically disadvantaged for the acquisition of complex cognitive skills in school.

An adult correlate to this cascade of detrimental overactivity of the fear response is found in posttraumatic stress disorder (PTSD), in which persons exposed to an intense trauma involving death or injury may have feelings of fear and helplessness for years after the event. A PET scanning study of patients with PTSD revealed abnormally high activity in the right amygdala while the patients were reliving their traumatic memories. The researchers hypothesized that the stressful hormonal milieu present during the registration of the memories may have served to burn the memories into the brain and to prevent their erasure by the usual memory modulation circuits. As a result, the traumatic memories exerted a pervasive influence and led to a state of constant vigilance, even in safe, familiar settings.

Workers in the related realms of mathematics have produced results documenting the organizing effects of early experiences on internal representations of the external world. Since the time of Pythagoras, music has been considered a branch of mathematics. A series of recent studies has shown that groups of children who were given 8 months of intensive classical music lessons during preschool years later had significantly better spatial and mathematical reasoning in school than a control group. Nonmusical tasks, such as navigating mazes, drawing geometric figures, and copying patterns of two-color blocks, were performed significantly more skillfully by the musical children. Early exposure to music, thus, may be ideal preparation for later acquisition of complex mathematical and engineering skills.

These tantalizing observations suggest a neurological basis for the developmental theories of Jean Piaget, Erik Erikson, Margaret Mahler, John Bowlby, Freud, and others. Erikson's epigenetic theory states that normal adult behavior results from the successful, sequential completion of each of several infantile and childhood stages (see Chapter 6, Section 6.3). According to the epigenetic model, failure to complete an early stage is reflected in subsequent physical, cognitive, social, or emotional maladjustment. By analogy, the experimental data just discussed suggest that early experience, particularly during the critical window of opportunity for establishing neural connections, primes the basic circuitry for language, emotions, and other advanced behaviors. Clearly, miswiring of an infant's brain may lead to severe handicaps later when the person attempts to relate to the world as an adult. These findings support the vital need for adequate public financing of Early Intervention and Head Start programs, programs that may be the most cost-effective means of improving persons' mental health.

References

Aleman A, Formisano E, Koppenhagen H, Hagoort P, de Haan EHF, Kahn RS. The functional neuroanatomy of metrical stress evaluation of perceived and imagined spoken words. *Cerebral Cortex.* 2005;15(2):221–228.

Bedwell JS, Horner MD, Yamanaka K, Li X, Myrick H, Nahas Z, George MS. Functional neuroanatomy of subcomponent cognitive processes involved in verbal working memory. *Int J Neurosci.* 2005;115(7):1017–1032.

Clark D, Boutros N, Mendez M. *The Brain and Behavior: An Introduction to Behavioral Neuroanatomy.* Cambridge, NY: Cambridge University Press; 2005.

Gallese V, Lakoff G. The brain's concepts: The role of the sensory-motor system in conceptual knowledge. *Cognitive Neuropsychology.* 2005;22(3–4):455–479.

Gould RL, Brown RG, Owen AM, Bullmore ET, Williams SCR, Howard RJ. Functional neuroanatomy of successful paired associate learning in Alzheimer's disease. *Am J Psychiatry.* 2005;162:2049–2060.

Gruber O, Goschke T. Executive control emerging from dynamic interactions between brain systems mediating language, working memory and attentional processes. *Acta Psychologicia.* 2004;115(2–3):105–121.

Hashimoto T, Volk DW, Eggan SM, Mirnics K, Pierri JN, Sun Z, Sampson AR, Lewis DA. Gene expression deficits in a subclass of GABA neurons in the prefrontal cortex of subjects with schizophrenia. *J Neurosci.* 2003;23:6315–6350.

Koechlin E, Ody C, Kounelher F. The architecture of cognitive control in human prefrontal cortex. *Science.* 2003;302:1181–1185.

Piefke M, Weiss PH, Markowitsch HJ, Fink GR. Gender differences in the functional neuroanatomy of emotional episodic autobiographical memory. *Human Brain Mapping.* 2005;24(4):313–324.

Pierri JN, Lewis DA. Functional Neuroanatomy. In: Sadock BJ, Sadock VA, eds. *Kaplan & Sadock's Comprehensive Textbook of Psychiatry.* 8th ed. Vol. 1. Baltimore: Lippincott Williams & Wilkins; 2005:3.

Simó LS, Krisky CM, Sweeney JA. Functional neuroanatomy of anticipatory behavior: Dissociation between sensory-driven and memory-driven systems. *Cerebral Cortex.* 2005;15(12):1982–1991.

Simons JS, Spiers HJ. Prefrontal and medial temporal lobe interactions in long-term memory. *Nat Rev Neurosci.* 2003;4:637–649.

Strakowski SM, DelBello DP, Adler CM. The functional neuroanatomy of bipolar disorder: A review of neuroimaging findings. *Mol Psychiatry.* 2005;10:105–116.

Taber KH, Hurley RA. Functional neuroanatomy of sleep and sleep deprivation. *Neuropsychiatry Clin Neurosci.* 2006;18:1–5.

Toga AW, Thompson PM. Mapping brain asymmetry. *Nat Rev Neurosci.* 2003; 4:37–48.

▲ 3.2 Neurophysiology and Neurochemistry

The complexity of our thoughts, feelings, and behaviors mirrors the complexity and heterogeneity within the brain. The previous chapter on neuroanatomy described the different regions of the brain, the different types of neurons and glial cells, and some of the many different neuronal circuits or pathways within the brain. This chapter focuses on neurophysiological and neurochemical heterogeneity within the brain. It is, in fact, within each neuron that multiple inputs are integrated to affect processes including gene expression, synapse formation, and neuronal firing rates and patterns.

Single neurons communicate by interpreting their chemical environment, by instantly changing the chemical cues to electrical activity for transport down axons, and, finally, by efficiently translating the electrical data into finely modulated chemical emissions that can be secreted to influence other neuronal or nonneuronal cells. Thus, electrical impulses facilitate instantaneous responses, and the chemical milieu is of paramount importance in maintaining the fidelity of the brain's image of the world.

HISTORY

The study of chemical interneuronal communication is called *neurochemistry*. With the acceptance in the late 19th century of the neuronal theory of Wilhelm His and Santiago Ramon y Cajal, which stated that the brain consists of individual cells rather than a syncytium of cytoplasm, a search was initiated for the mediators of intercellular communication. At the turn of the century, the effects of extracts of the adrenal gland on sympathetic nerve tissue were elucidated, and soon scientists discovered chemicals in the brain—neurotransmitters—with similar stimulatory actions. Postulating that cells also contained inhibitory and excitatory "receptive substances," Karl Lashley envisioned the entire basic apparatus of chemical neurotransmission: neurotransmitters and specific receptor molecules. In the first half of the 20th century, the major biogenic amine neurotransmitters were characterized; the more abundant amino acid neurotransmitters were not recognized as transmitters until much more recently. Recent years have seen a massive proliferation in known peptide neurotransmitters and receptors, and novel classes of neurotransmitters have been identified, including nucleotides, prostaglandins, lipids, and gases. Through advanced molecular cloning techniques, dozens of orphan receptor genes have been sequenced, for which no known ligand exists. Moreover, in addition to their role in modulating cellular electrical excitability, molecules identified initially as neurotransmitters (e.g., serotonin) have been found to influence gene expression and synapse formation.

In psychopharmacology, the major available therapeutic interventions center on modification of biogenic amine neurotransmission and, to a lesser extent, amino acid neurotransmission. Although these systems are discussed in detail below, students of psychiatry must be aware of the entire range of neurochemistry, because many new classes of psychopharmacological agents that act on more recently defined neurotransmitter systems are likely to emerge. Moreover, neuronal electrical activity is continuously modulated by excitatory and inhibitory neurotransmitters, by circulating hormones, by immune surveillance, by general medical homeostasis, and by chronobiological rhythms, each of which may be influenced with existing therapeutic methods. Neuronal electrical activity, along with the chemical factors, simultaneously modifies the abundance and phosphorylation status of cellular proteins, the level of expression of certain genes, and the connectivity of a neuron to thousands of neighboring neurons. Each of these avenues of therapeutic influence may open in the future.

BASIC ELECTROPHYSIOLOGY

Membranes and Charge

In the resting state, the intracellular compartment of a neuron is more negatively charged than the extracellular compartment. The charge gradient is maintained across the hydrophobic plasma membrane, which consists of a lipid bilayer containing embedded cholesterol molecules that modify membrane rigidity, and numerous proteins, including ion pumps, ion channels, and neurotransmitter receptors. Ion pumps and ion channels maintain a gradient of cations; potassium ions are 15 to 20 times more concentrated inside neurons, and sodium ions are 8 to 15 times less concentrated inside neurons than in the extracellular space (Fig. 3.2–1). The principal ion pump is the energy-requiring sodium-potassium-adenosine triphosphatase (ATPase) exchange pump, which maintains an electrical gradient by pumping sodium out and potassium in. The principal ion channels are the sodium, potassium, calcium, and chloride ion channels. The membrane is described as *semipermeable* because it is selective regarding which ions can pass through it.

Ion Channels

The rapid transmission of information along neuronal axons, which can exceed a velocity of 60 meters per second, is mediated by instantaneous changes in membrane potential called *action potentials*. These changes in membrane potential occur when the charge gradients maintained by the insulator function of the membrane are allowed to flow unimpeded through protein pores called *ion channels*. Ion channels are selective for specific ions, such as sodium channels that may not allow passage of potassium ions. In the resting state, ion channels are closed. Ion channels open in response to binding of ligands to receptors—*ligand-gated ion channels*—or in response to changes in membrane potential—*voltage-gated ion channels*. Among ligand-gated ion channels, certain ligands, called *excitatory neurotransmitters*, open cation channels that depolarize the membrane and increase the likelihood of the generation of an action potential. These ligands are said to elicit excitatory postsynaptic potentials (EPSPs). Other ligands, called *inhibitory neurotransmitters*, open chloride channels that hyperpolarize the membrane and decrease the likelihood of the generation of an action potential. These ligands are said to elicit inhibitory postsynaptic potentials (IPSPs). In the central nervous system (CNS), the binding of a single ligand to a ligand-gated ion channel may change the neuronal membrane potential by 1 mV. Therefore, the combined activation of several ligand-gated channels is needed to trigger an action potential.

The ion channels themselves are glycoproteins (proteins with sugar moieties) that span the neuronal membrane and contain a pore that can be opened and closed, through which specific ions can flow.

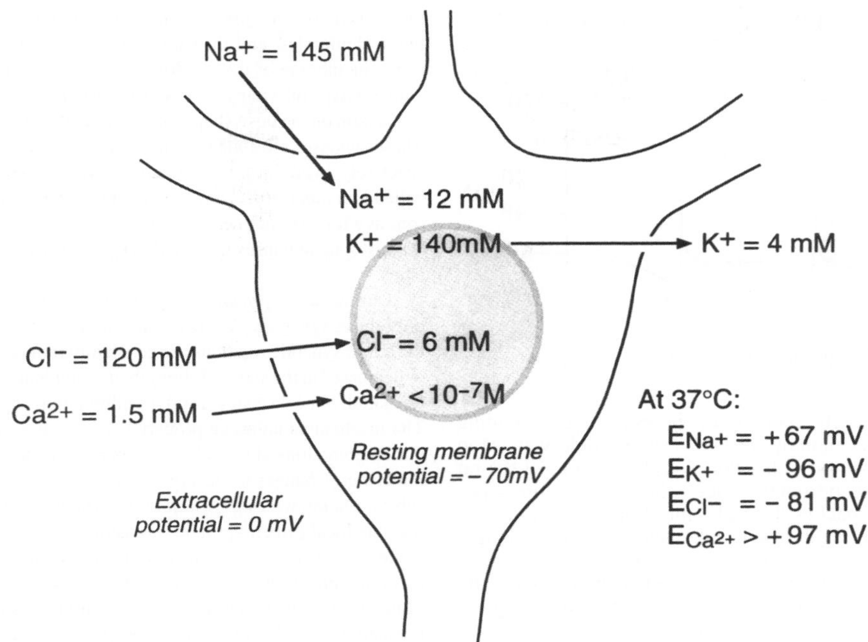

FIGURE 3.2–1
The distribution of Na^+, K^+, Ca^{2+}, and Cl^- across the membrane of a typical neuron; the *arrows* show the direction of current flow down the chemical gradient. Using the indicated ion concentrations, the equilibrium (Nemst) potentials (E) for these ions at 37°C are shown at the lower right.

Clinical Relevance. Many drugs used in psychiatry affect ion channel activity. Also, pathology in ion channel activity or regulation is hypothesized to be involved in the pathogenesis of many neuropsychiatric disorders. Anticonvulsant drugs used to treat epilepsy, bipolar disorders, and other psychiatric conditions have their major effects on ion channel regulation. Benzodiazepines act by modulating the activity of receptor-modulated chloride ion channels. Examples of drugs of abuse that have their effects through ion channels include phencyclidine (PCP), which affects glutamate-regulated calcium channels, and nicotine, which acts at acetylcholine-regulated sodium or potassium channels. In other branches of medicine, sodium channel blockers are used as local anesthetics, and potassium channel blockers are used as antiarrhythmics. Dantrolene (Dantrium), a blocker of calcium channels in skeletal muscle, is used to treat neuroleptic malignant syndrome.

Action Potentials

In the resting state, the intracellular compartment of the neuron is negatively charged at a potential of −70 to −80 mV; during an action potential, however, this membrane potential reverses in a thin zone immediately adjacent to the membrane. For an action potential to be generated by a neuron, ligand-gated ion channels open, and sodium ions begin to enter the cell and gradually make the inner surface of the membrane less negatively charged relative to the outside. The point at which the negative charge on the interior of the membrane is sufficiently low to open adjacent voltage-gated sodium channels is called the *spike threshold*, characteristically approximately −55 mV. The inward flow of sodium ions then rapidly depolarizes the membrane and initiates an action potential, which propagates itself along the membrane by sequentially triggering adjacent voltage-gated sodium channels. The action potential itself is a brief (0.1 to 2 msec) wave of reversal of membrane potential that moves along an axon (Fig. 3.2–2). During the action potential, the interior of the membrane is positively charged with respect to the outside of the membrane. The initial ion channel involved in the action potential is the Na^+ channel, which, when opened, allows positively charged sodium ions to enter the neuron. The Ca^{2+} channels open next, allowing the positively charged calcium ions to enter the neuron and further contribute to the spike of the action potential. Not only does the entry of calcium ions affect the membrane potential, but also the calcium ion is an important second-messenger molecule that is involved in initiating protein–protein interactions and gene regulation. Entry of the calcium ion into the synaptic terminal is also critical for the release of neurotransmitter molecules, and calcium ion entry activates ion channels that carry an outflow of potassium ions that are involved in arresting the action potential. Activation of those K^+ channels results in afterhyperpolarization of the membrane after an action potential. During the afterhyperpolarization, the inside of the membrane is even more negatively charged than it was at baseline. Afterhyperpolarization contributes to the refractory period of a neuron after an action potential; during this period, no other action potential can be generated.

Translation of the Action Potential into Chemical Neurotransmission

At the synaptic terminus of the axon, action potentials trigger the release of neurotransmitters (Fig. 3.2–3) into the synaptic cleft, where they may

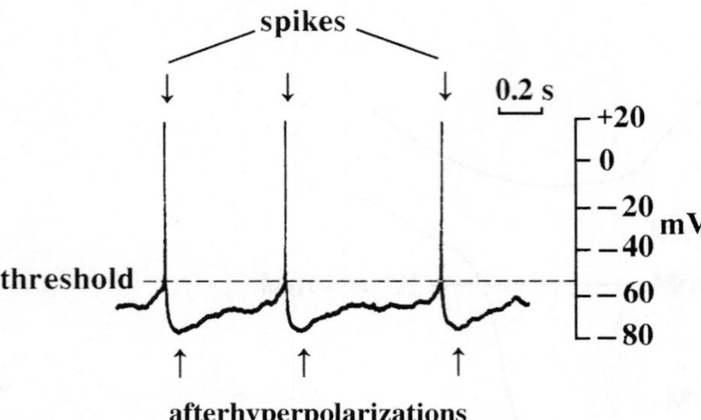

FIGURE 3.2–2

Action potentials. An oscilloscope trace shows a repetitively firing neuron recorded intracellularly *in vivo.* This example was taken from a serotonergic neuron in the dorsal raphe nucleus of the rat midbrain. As can be seen from the trace, when the membrane potential, in millivolts, reaches the spike threshold (−55 mV), and all-or-none spike occurs. After each spike, and afterhyperpolarization moves the cell away from the threshold into a more negative potential (near −80 mV). As the afterhyperpolarization decays, the cell again approaches the spike threshold. (Courtesy of George K. Aghajanian, M.D., and Meenakshi Alreja, Ph.D.)

act on other neurons or muscles. The presynaptic nerve terminals contain voltage-gated calcium channels that locally raise the intracellular calcium concentration. This initiates a cascade of protein–protein and protein–lipid interactions in which neurotransmitter-containing synaptic vesicles fuse with the presynaptic membrane and release their contents into the synaptic cleft. In muscles, voltage-gated calcium channels that are opened by the arriving action potentials trigger the movement of myosin on actin fibers, a process called *excitation-contraction coupling*. In each of these instances, the electrical impulse causes changes in local calcium concentrations, which in turn rapidly trigger physical changes in the ultrastructure of the cell (Fig. 3.2–4). (Specific neurotransmitters are discussed below.)

SYNAPSES

The propagation of an action potential along an axon is described as an *all-or-none phenomenon*; that is, once an action potential has been triggered, it is propagated at full strength for the entire length of the axon. Subtleties of neuronal processing are thus generally not represented by modulation of the intensity of the action potential, although an exception to this rule may occur at axoaxonal synapses. In most neurons, however, the essence of neuronal processing occurs in the regulation of whether an action potential is generated. This determination is the summation of excitatory and inhibitory chemical influences that act on the *axon hillock*, which originates the action potential. The synapse is the site at which stimuli are given and received and where the finest shadings of neuronal activity are negotiated.

The components of the synapse are the axon terminal of the presynaptic neuron, the synaptic cleft, and the dendrite of the postsynaptic neuron. When an action potential develops in the presynaptic neuron, it moves down the axon to the axon terminal or to other, functionally similar regions of the axons called *axonal varicosities*. The action potential causes the release of neurotransmitter molecules discussed below into the *synaptic cleft*, the small space between the presynaptic neuron and the postsynaptic neuron. The neurotransmitter molecules diffuse across the synaptic cleft and then bind to their specific receptors on the external membrane of the dendrite of the postsynaptic neuron. The most common type of synapse involves the termination of the presynaptic neuronal axon on the postsynaptic neuronal cell body, an axon, or a dendrite. These synapses are called *axosomatic*, *axoaxonic*, and *axodendritic*, respectively. In addition to the chemical synapses, electrical synapses, also called *gap junctions*, allow the direct transfer of ions between two neurons as a form of interneuronal neurochemical communication. *Conjoint synapses* are synapses that have both electrical and chemical characteristics.

During development, a severalfold excess of synapses forms, and only those synapses of functional relevance survive into adulthood. In the adult, synaptic relations are constantly remodeled through increases or decreases in the size and strength of individual synapses, as well as the formation of new synapses and the elimination of unnecessary synapses. The mechanical adhesive properties of synapses are mediated by various combinations of the calcium-dependent cadherin family of adhesion molecules. Changes in the structure of synapses are mediated by trophic substances known as *growth factors*, which act on specific receptors to regulate local protein–protein interactions and to modify levels of gene expression. Thus, not only neurotransmitters subtly modulate intercellular communication, trophic substances constantly remodel the synaptic channels through which chemical neurotransmission occurs. *N*-Methyl-D-aspartate (NMDA) glutamate receptors are particularly important to the process of synaptic remodeling. NMDA receptors are essential to certain forms of long-term potentiation (LTP) in which coordinated neuronal activity strengthens certain synapses. On the basis of much electrophysiological data, LTP has been proposed to be the cellular correlate of long-term memory, although molecular biological experiments suggest that other systems must also contribute.

Presynaptic Components

The presynaptic terminals contain the synthetic machinery responsible for the synthesis of all neurotransmitters, except peptide neurotransmitters, which are synthesized in the cell body. Neurotransmitter synthesis can be stimulated by an influx of calcium ions, variations in levels of the second-messenger cyclic adenosine monophosphate (cAMP), or changes in levels of circulating hormones. Once synthesized, neurotransmitters are packaged into synaptic vesicles, which may store a mixture of amine and peptide neurotransmitters. Data indicate that all termini of a single neuron secrete the same combination of neurotransmitters. In practice, however, probably a few neurons have more than one axonal terminus, and newer techniques suggest a possible heterogeneity of neurotransmitter composition among different vesicles in a single neuron. Energy for the synthesis, storage, release, and degradation of neurotransmitters is provided by mitochondria. (The life cycle of specific neurotransmitters is discussed below.) The presynaptic membrane contains ion channels, neurotransmitter receptors, and neurotransmitter transporters. Voltage-gated calcium channels trigger vesicle release. Presynaptic neurotransmitter receptors mediate feedback inhibition of neurotransmitter synthesis and release. For example, many norepinephrine-releasing neurons have presynaptic α_2-adrenergic receptors that, when occupied by the released norepinephrine, cause the releasing neuron to decrease or stop the release of norepinephrine. Transporters take neurotransmitters up from the synaptic cleft for recycling or degradation. Additional transporters in the membranes of storage vesicles load the vesicles with neurotransmitters.

BIOGENIC AMINE NEUROTRANSMITTERS

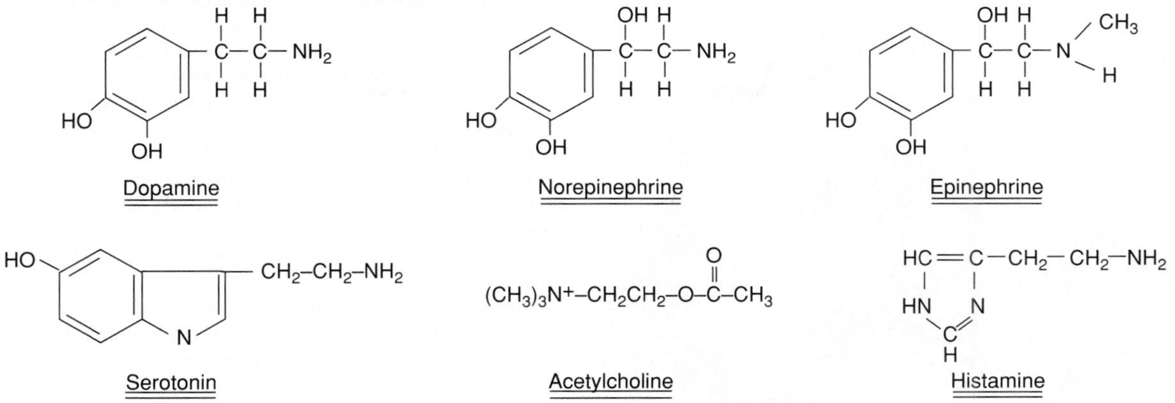

Dopamine

Norepinephrine

Epinephrine

Serotonin

$(CH_3)_3N^+–CH_2CH_2–O–C(=O)–CH_3$

Acetylcholine

Histamine

AMINO ACID NEUROTRANSMITTERS (examples)

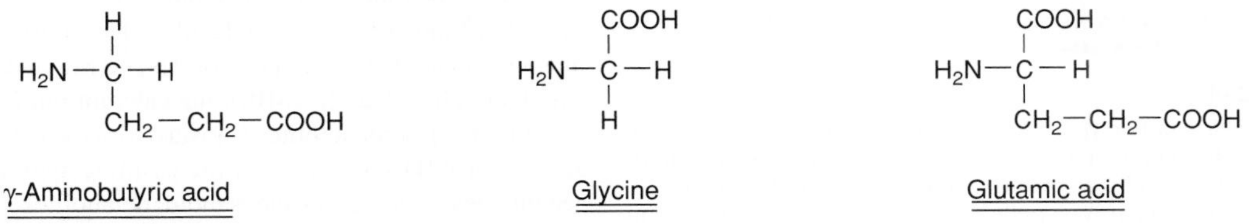

γ-Aminobutyric acid

Glycine

Glutamic acid

PEPTIDE NEUROTRANSMITTERS

NEUROTENSIN:

Glu – Leu – Tyr – Glu – Asn – Lys – Pro – Arg – Arg – Pro – Tyr – Ile – Leu

THYROTROPIN – RELEASING HORMONE (TRH):

Glu – His – Pro

CHOLECYSTOKININ OCTAPEPTIDE (CCK-8):

Asp – Tyr – Met – Gly – Trp – Met – Asp – Phe

FIGURE 3.2–3
Three major classes of neurotransmitters.

Synapse

Although it makes up less than 1 percent of the total volume of the brain, the *synaptic compartment*—the space between the presynaptic and postsynaptic membranes—contains the mixture of neurotransmitters with the greatest influence on thought and behavior. These molecules are available to act on specific receptors and to initiate or inhibit the generation of action potentials in the postsynaptic cell. The list of neurotransmitters includes amino acids (e.g., glutamate, γ-aminobutyric acid [GABA], glycine, aspartate, homocystine), biogenic amines (e.g., norepinephrine, serotonin, dopamine, epinephrine, acetylcholine, histamine), neuropeptides (e.g., vasopressin, oxytocin, enkephalins, endorphins, substance P, neurotensin, and several hundred others), nucleotides (adenosine, cAMP), gases (e.g., nitric oxide [NO], carbon monoxide [CO], ammonia [NH_3]), and prostaglandins. The concentrations of various neurotransmitters in the synaptic cleft are carefully regulated by feedback inhibition of transmitter release and by reuptake into the presynaptic terminal by transporter molecules. This regulation is critically important because the concentration of each neurotransmitter determines the degree to which it activates its specific receptors.

Postsynaptic Components

Receptors. Neurotransmitter receptors are the sites of action for many of the psychotherapeutic and psychoactive drugs used today. The techniques of molecular biology have led to the identification and sequencing of many new subtypes of receptors. The importance of those advances lies in the long-standing hypothesis that the ability to subtype receptors would refine both the hunt for pathology in disease states and the design of specifically acting drugs.

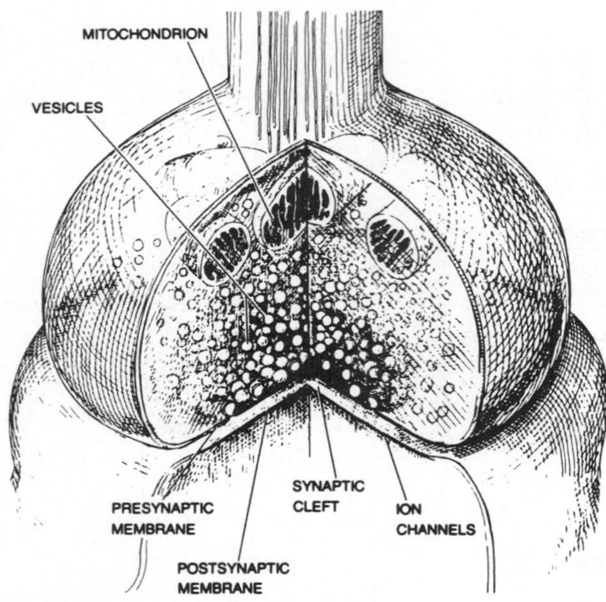

FIGURE 3.2–4
Synapse consists of two parts: the knoblike tip of an axon terminal and the receptor region on the surface of another neuron. The membranes are separated by a synaptic cleft some 20 to 30 nm across. Molecules of chemical transmitter, stored in vesicles in the axon terminal, are released into the cleft by arriving nerve impulses and change the electrical state of the receiving neuron, making it either more likely or less likely to fire an impulse. (From Stevens CF. The neuron. In: Llinas RD, ed. *The Biology of the Brain from Neurons to Networks.* New York: Freedman; 1988:3, with permission.)

Two terms often used in conjunction with receptors are *supersensitivity* and *subsensitivity*. These terms refer, respectively, to a greater than usual response and a less than usual response of the receptor to a constant amount of neurotransmitter. The sensitivity of receptor activity may be owing to the number of receptors present, the affinity of the receptor for the neurotransmitter, and the efficiency with which binding of the neurotransmitter to the receptor is translated into an intraneuronal message. All these steps in receptor function are variable and subject to regulation.

Fundamentally, two major types of neurotransmitter receptors exist: seven-transmembrane-domain receptors, which require G proteins, and ligand-gated ion channels, in which the channel is an integral part of the complex that binds the ligand. Many of the biogenic amine receptors, regardless of whether they are associated with G proteins or directly with ion channels, are listed in Table 3.2–1.

Another type of postsynaptic membrane receptor, which does not cause changes in membrane potential, is the family of tyrosine kinase receptors, which triggers a cascade of intracellular phosphorylations that ultimately lead to changes in gene expression. A vast diversity is seen of tyrosine kinase receptors, much of which is owing to various combinations of modular segments of the receptor genes that have arisen during evolution. Tyrosine kinase receptors bind growth factors and mediate the plasticity of synaptic associations. Two such factors are nerve growth factor (NGF) and brain-derived neurotropic factor (BDNF), which have opposite effects on the size of developing cortical somatosensory receptive fields and, thus, may collaborate in the remodeling of neuronal circuits that underlies synaptic plasticity during development and in adults.

Another group of tyrosine kinases exists within the cytoplasm of neurons and, thus, do not have membrane-bound receptors. These nonreceptor tyrosine kinases include molecules, such as *fyn*, *src*, and *yes*, and although their regulation is poorly understood, this cytoplasmic class of tyrosine kinases is likely very important to intraneuronal function.

Whereas tyrosine kinase receptors (called the *JAK/STAT-coupled receptors*) have the kinase activity within their own protein, another class of receptors requires the association of a separate intracellular protein with kinase activity. This is the type of receptor utilized by several neurotrophic factors, hormones (including prolactin), interferon, and cytokines. They also regulate gene expression.

The G proteins are a family of guanosine triphosphate (GTP)-binding proteins, which interact with members of the very large family of seven-transmembrane-domain receptors. When an intact G protein binds to a receptor, the receptor assumes a state with a high affinity for the neurotransmitter molecule.

Another class of G proteins includes Ras, which is involved in neurotrophin receptor actions, and Rho, which may be involved in the guidance of axonal migration during development.

Second Messengers. The neurotransmitters themselves are conceptualized as the first messengers that bring a signal to a neuron. For the neuron to act on the signal, the first-messenger signal must be translated into an intraneuronal signal via formation of second-messenger molecules. The most classic second messengers are the cyclic nucleotides (cAMP and cyclic guanosine monophosphate [cGMP]), the calcium ion (Ca^{2+}), and the phosphoinositol metabolites (inositol triphosphate [IP3] and diacylglycerol [DAG]). Another increasingly appreciated class of second messengers is the eicosanoid metabolites. Gases, such as NO and CO, not only mediate interneuronal communication but also serve as intraneuronal second-messenger molecules.

One of the primary activities of the second-messenger molecules is to activate a class of molecules known as the protein kinases. *Protein kinases* catalyze the transfer of the terminal phosphate group of ATP onto protein molecules (Fig. 3.2–5). Tyrosine kinases are activated by growth factors binding to specific transmembrane receptors. Kinases also play an important role in the regulation of cellular proliferation—many oncogenes are kinases—and the regulation of numerous other genes. In psychiatry, lithium therapy has been shown to reduce the activity of protein kinase in concert with its salutary effects on bipolar disorder. Likely, ongoing investigations will implicate kinases in the etiology of other psychiatric disorders.

NEUROTRANSMITTERS

A molecule must meet a number of criteria to be classified as a neurotransmitter (Table 3.2–2). These criteria must usually be met through a variety of basic science and clinical research studies. Substances that have only been shown to meet a few of the criteria are referred to as *putative neurotransmitters*, meaning they have not been shown experimentally to meet all of the criteria.

Chemical Neurotransmission

Chemical neurotransmission is the process involving the release of a neurotransmitter by one neuron and the binding of the neurotransmitter molecule to a receptor on another neuron. The process of chemical neurotransmission is affected by most drugs used in psychiatry. Older antipsychotics, but not the serotonin-dopamine antagonists, are believed to exert their effects mainly by blocking dopamine type 2 (D_2) receptors; virtually all antidepressants are believed to exert their effects by increasing the amount of

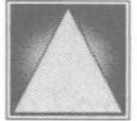

Table 3.2–1
Monoamine Receptors: Overview

Transmitter	Subtype	Primary Effector	Proposed Clinical Relevance
Serotonin	5-HT_{1A}	↓ AC	Antidepressant action; partial agonist; anxiolytic
	5-HT_{1B}	↓ AC	Possible role in locomotor activity, aggression
	5-HT_{1D}	↓ AC	Target of antimigraine drug sumatriptan
	5-HT_{1E}	↓ AC	Unknown
	5-HT_{1F}	↓ AC	Target of antimigraine drug sumatriptan
	5-HT_{2A}	↑ PI turnover	Target of hallucinogens, atypical antipsychotics
	5-HT_{2B}	↑ PI turnover	Regulation of stomach contraction
	5-HT_{2C}	↑ PI turnover	Regulation of appetite, anxiety, seizures; target of hallucinogens, antipsychotics
	5-HT_{3}	Cation selective Ion channel	Antagonists antiemetic, anxiolytic, cognitive enhancement
	5-HT_{4}	↑ AC	Modulation of cognition, anxiety
	$5\text{-HT}_{5\alpha}$	Unknown	Unknown
	$5\text{-HT}_{5\beta}$	Unknown	Unknown
	5-HT_{6}	↑ AC	Target of hallucinogens, atypical antipsychotics
	5-HT_{7}	↑ AC	Possible regulation of circadian rhythms
Histamine	H_1	↑ PI turnover	Antagonists produce sedation, weight gain
	H_2	↑ AC	Antagonists for peptic ulcer disease
	H_3	Unknown	Antagonists produce arousal, appetite suppression
Dopamine	D_1	↑ AC	D_1 and D_2 receptor stimulation synergistic; required for stimulant effects of cocaine
	D_2	↓ AC	Target of therapeutic and extrapyramidal effects of dopamine receptor antagonists ("typical antipsychotics")
	D_3	↓ AC	Unknown
	D_4	↓ AC	Target of serotonin-dopamine antagonists ("atypical antipsychotics")
	D_5	↑ AC	Unknown
Adrenergic	$\alpha_{1A,B,D}$	↑ PI turnover	Antagonists antihypertensive
	$\alpha_{2A,B,C}$	↓ AC	Agonists sedative and antihypertensive
	β_1	↑ AC	Regulation of cardiac function
	β_2	↑ AC	Regulation of bronchial muscle contraction
	β_3	↑ AC	Regulation of adipose tissue function
Cholinergic	M1	↑ PI turnover	Regulation of cognition, seizures
	M2	↓ AC	Regulation of cardiac function
	M3	↑ PI turnover	Regulation of smooth muscle contraction
	M4	↓ AC	Target of antiparkinsonian anticholinergic drugs
	M5	↑ PI turnover	Unknown
	NAChR	Cation selective Ion channel	Regulation of tobacco use, seizures; possible cognitive enhancement

↑ AC, increases activity of adenylate cyclase; ↓ AC, decreases activity of adenylate cyclase; ↑ PI turnover, increases turnover of phosphoinositides.

serotonin or norepinephrine, or both, in the synaptic cleft; and almost all benzodiazepine anxiolytics are believed to exert their effects on the $GABA_A$ receptors that are linked to chloride ion channels.

Neuromodulators and Neurohormones. The word used most commonly to denote the chemical signals that flow between neurons is *neurotransmitter*, although the words *neuromodulators* and *neurohormones* are also used in some cases to emphasize specific characteristics. In contrast to the characteristically immediate and short-lived effects of a neurotransmitter, a neuromodulator, as the name implies, modulates the response of a neuron to a neurotransmitter. The modulatory effect may be present for a longer time than is usual for a neurotransmitter molecule to be present. Thus, a neuromodulating substance may have an effect on a neuron over a long period of time, and that effect may be more involved with fine tuning than with activating or directly inhibiting the generation of an action potential. A neurohormone is distinguished by the fact that it is released into the bloodstream rather than into the extraneuronal space in the brain. Once in the bloodstream, the neurohormone can then diffuse into the extraneuronal space and have its effects on neurons.

Classification. The three major types of neurotransmitters in the brain are the biogenic amines, the amino acids, and the peptides (Fig. 3.2–3). The biogenic amines are the best known and most understood neurotransmitters because they were the first to be discovered. They constitute the neurotransmitter substance in only a small percentage of neurons, however. The amino acid neurotransmitters were late to be discovered, principally because of the difficulty in differentiating amino acids present in most proteins from the same amino acids acting separately as neurotransmitters. The amino acid neurotransmitters are present in upward of 70 percent of neurons. The peptide neurotransmitters are intermediate in terms of the percentage of neurons that contain a neurotransmitter of that type, but they far surpass the other two categories in the sheer number (about 200 to 300 of neurotransmitters of that type have been putatively identified). The full neurotransmitter criteria have been met for only

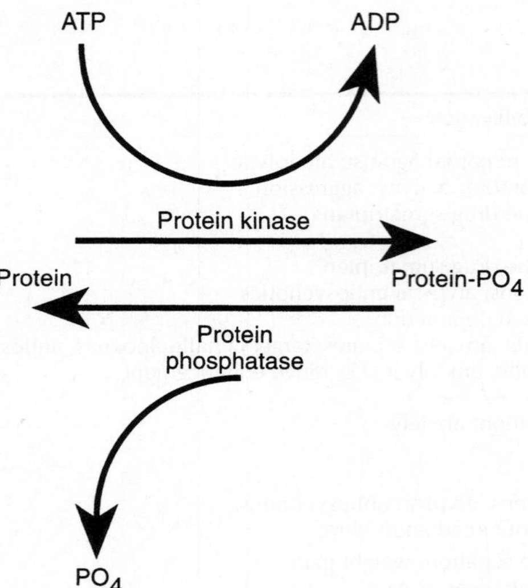

FIGURE 3.2–5
Regulation of protein function by phosphorylation. Numerous cellular proteins are activated or inactivated by the addition of a phosphate group (PO_4) from adenosine triphosphate (ATP). Addition of the phosphate is catalyzed by specific protein kinases, whereas removal of the phosphate is catalyzed by protein phosphates. (Courtesy of Jack A. Grebb, M.D.)

a few of these peptides at this time (Table 3.2–2). Nevertheless, the evidence indicating that the putative peptide neurotransmitters are, in fact, neurotransmitters is generally robust. Recent data have led to the identification of at least four other classes of neurotransmitters—nucleotides, gases, eicosanoids, and anandamides—and have hinted at receptors for others, including so-called sigma (Σ) receptors.

Thus, the current psychopharmacological agents influence only a small fraction of the neurons in the brain. This may represent a fortunate coincidence, because drugs that influence amino acid neurotransmitters generally have adverse effects at low doses, and relatively few drugs have been found to act on peptide receptors, most notably the opiates. The small number of biogenic amine-containing neurons belies their significant functional importance, because they project widely throughout the brain and modulate activity in practically every brain region.

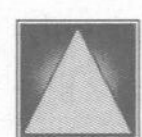

Table 3.2–2
Criteria for a Neurotransmitter

1. The molecule is synthesized in the neuron.
2. The molecule is present in the presynaptic neuron and is released on depolarization in physiologically significant amounts.
3. When administered exogenously as a drug, the exogenous molecule mimics the effects of the endogenous neurotransmitter.
4. A mechanism in the neurons or the synaptic cleft acts to remove or deactivate the neurotransmitter.

BIOGENIC AMINES

Each of these biogenic amine neurotransmitters is synthesized in a discrete nucleus of neurons from which axons project widely throughout the brain and spinal cord. They therefore exert a disproportionate influence on the activity of the brain, and they are of central importance to the pharmacological therapy of thought, mood, and anxiety disorders. Dopamine, norepinephrine, and epinephrine are products of the catecholamine synthetic pathway, whereas serotonin, acetylcholine, and histamine are derived from distinct precursors. A full understanding of the role of these neurotransmitters in psychiatry includes knowledge of their anatomy, their life cycle (synthesis, secretion, reuptake, and degradation), receptors, and the drugs that modify their activity.

Dopamine

CNS Dopaminergic Tracts. The three most important dopaminergic tracts for psychiatry are the nigrostriatal tract, the mesolimbic–mesocortical tract, and the tuberoinfundibular tract (Fig. 3.2–6). The nigrostriatal tract projects from its cell bodies in the substantia nigra to the corpus striatum. When the D_2 receptors at the end of this tract are blocked by classic antipsychotic drugs, parkinsonian side effects emerge. In Parkinson's disease the nigrostriatal tract degenerates, resulting in the motor symptoms of the disease. Because of the significant association between Parkinson's disease and depression, the nigrostriatal tract may somehow be involved with the control of mood, in addition to its classic role in motor control.

D_2 receptors in the caudate nucleus suppress the activity of the caudate nucleus. The caudate neurons regulate motor acts by gating, in which intended acts are actually carried out. The absence of D_2 receptor activity allows the caudate to dampen motor activity excessively, resulting in the bradykinesia that typifies parkinsonism. At the other extreme, excess dopamine activity in the caudate removes the gating control and may result in extraneous motor acts, such as tics. A recent study of patients with obsessive–compulsive disorder, for example, correlated increased caudate dopamine analogue binding, which reflects increased numbers of the D_2 receptors, with more prominent clinical tics.

The mesolimbic-mesocortical tract projects from its cell bodies in the ventral tegmental area (VTA), which lies adjacent to the substantia nigra, to most areas of the cerebral cortex, and to the limbic system. Because the tract projects to the limbic system and the neocortex, the tract may be involved in mediating the antipsychotic effects of antipsychotic drugs.

The cell bodies of the tuberoinfundibular tract, which are in the arcuate nucleus and the periventricular area of the hypothalamus, project to the infundibulum and the anterior pituitary. Dopamine acts as a release-inhibiting factor in the tract by inhibiting the release of prolactin from the anterior pituitary. Patients who take dopamine receptor antagonists often have roughly threefold elevated prolactin levels because the blockade of dopamine receptors in the tract eliminates the inhibitory effect of dopamine.

Dopamine Life Cycle. The dopaminergic axon terminal is the site of synthesis for dopamine. Dopamine is one of the three catecholamine neurotransmitters that are synthesized, starting with the amino acid tyrosine. The other two catecholamine neurotransmitters are norepinephrine and epinephrine (Fig. 3.2–7). The rate-limiting enzymatic step in the synthesis of any of the catecholamines is catalyzed by tyrosine hydroxylase. Dietary changes in tyrosine levels, therefore, do not

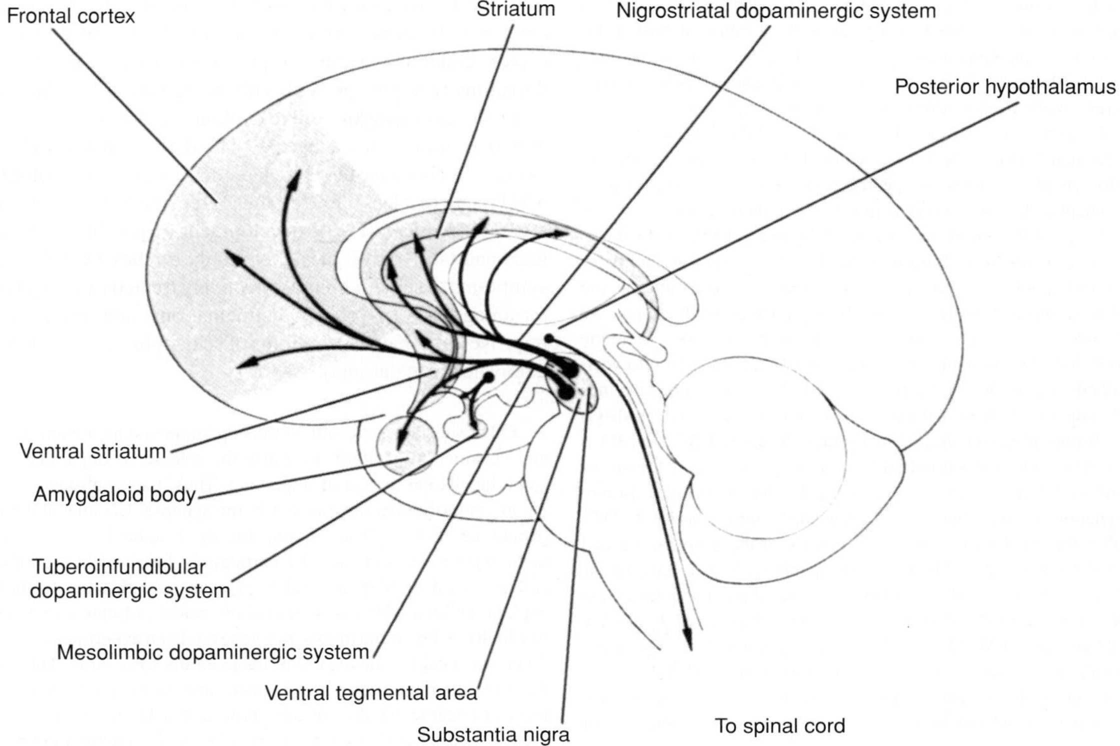

FIGURE 3.2–6

Dopaminergic (DA) pathways. The nigrostriatal DA system originates in the substantia nigra and terminates in the main dorsal part of the striatum. The ventral tegmental area gives rise to the mesolimbic DA system, which terminates in the ventral striatum, the amygdaloid body, the frontal lobe, and some other basal forebrain areas. The tuberoinfundibular system innervates the median eminence and the posterior and intermediate lobes of the pituitary, and dopamine neurons in the posterior hypothalamus project to the spinal cord. (Reprinted from Heimer L. *The Human Brain and Spinal Cord.* New York: Springer; 1983, with permission.)

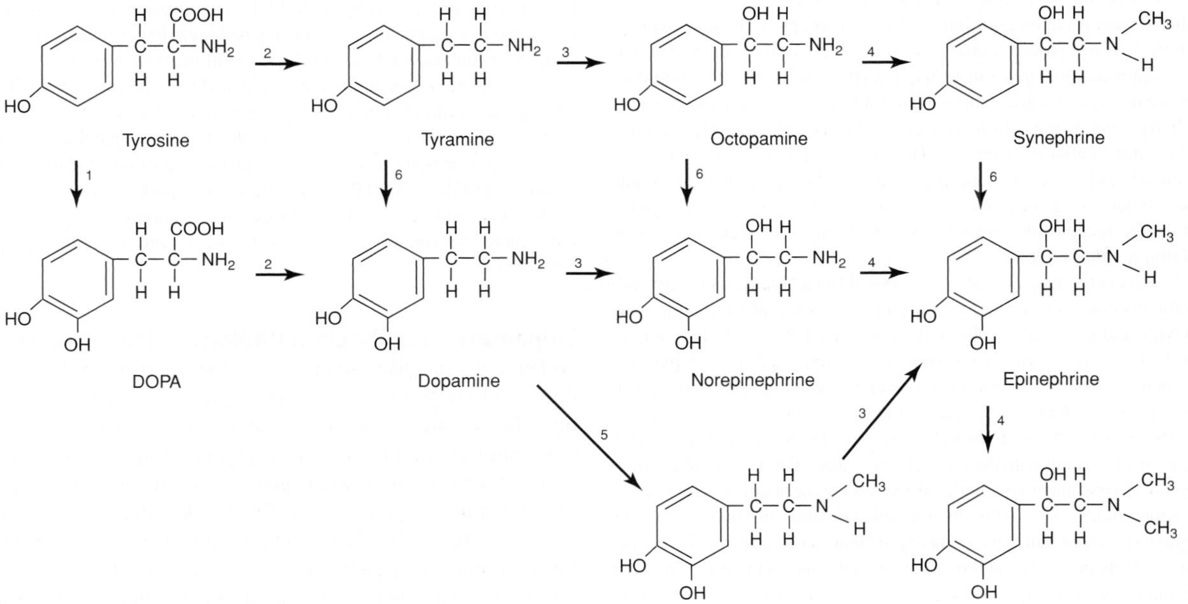

FIGURE 3.2–7

Primary and alternative pathways for the formation of catecholamines: (1) tyrosine hydroxylase; (2) aromatic amino acid decarboxylase; (3) dopamine-β-hydroxylase; (4) phenylethanolamine-*N*-methyltransferase; (5) nonspecific *N*-methyltransferase in lung and folate-dependent *N*-methyltransferase in brain; and (6) catechol-forming enzyme. (Reprinted from Cooper JR, Bloom FE, Roth RH. *The Biochemical Basis of Neuropharmacology.* 7th ed. New York: Oxford University Press; 1996:232, with permission.)

influence the synthesis of catecholamines. Tyrosine hydroxylase is a phosphoprotein that is subject to regulation by a range of protein kinases and protein phosphatases. Tyrosine hydroxylase transforms tyrosine into 3,4-dihydroxyphenylalanine (DOPA). Because it is beyond the rate-limiting synthetic step, dopa can be administered orally to increase the rate of synthesis of its product, dopamine, and dopa is used for this purpose to treat Parkinson's disease. Once dopamine is produced, it is taken into synaptic vesicles by specific transporters and then released into the synaptic cleft on depolarization of the axon terminal.

The actions of dopamine are terminated by two general routes. First, dopamine can be taken back up into the presynaptic neuron and recycled as a neurotransmitter; this pathway is generally referred to as the *reuptake mechanism*. Reuptake occurs by the passage of the dopamine molecule from the synaptic space, through the presynaptic dopamine transporter, into the intracellular space, where it is packaged into vesicles. Second, dopamine can be metabolized. The two major enzymes involved in the metabolism of dopamine are monoamine oxidase (MAO) and, less importantly, catechol-*O*-methyltransferase (COMT). MAO is localized on the outer mitochondrial membrane, principally in the presynaptic terminal, where it acts on dopamine that has been taken up into the presynaptic terminal but not yet repackaged into vesicles. COMT is a soluble enzyme localized in the cytoplasm of the postsynaptic cell and of glial cells and, possibly also, extracellularly. When dopamine is metabolized extraneuronally by COMT, the resulting metabolites are then taken back into the neuron and further metabolized by MAO. There are two types of MAOs. MAO_B selectively metabolizes dopamine. The primary metabolite of dopamine is homovanillic acid (HVA), and many research studies of cerebrospinal fluid, urine, and serum attempt to assess dopamine activity in the CNS by measuring concentrations of HVA.

Dopamine Receptors. The five subtypes of dopamine receptors (Table 3.2–1) can be put into two groups. In the first group, the D_1 and D_5 receptors stimulate the formulation of cAMP by activating the stimulatory G protein, Gs. The D_5 receptor has only recently been discovered, and less is known about it than about the D_1 receptor. One difference between these two receptors is that the D_5 receptor has a much higher affinity for dopamine than does the D_1 receptor. The second group of dopamine receptors is made up of the D_2, D_3, and D_4 receptors. The D_2 receptor inhibits the formation of cAMP by activating the inhibitory G protein, Gi, and some data indicate that the D_3 and D_4 receptors act similarly. One of the differences among the D_2, D_3, and D_4 receptors is their differential distribution. The D_2 receptor is prominent in the striatum (caudate nucleus and putamen); the D_3 receptor is especially concentrated in the nucleus accumbens, in addition to other regions; and the D_4 receptor is especially concentrated in the frontal cortex, in addition to other regions.

In a recent study, a scale of emotional detachment, with high values for aloofness and vindictiveness and low values for overly nurturing behavior and excessive exploitability, was used to rate 24 individuals, and then the density of D_2 receptors was determined in each person's putamen. A strong correlation was found between high levels of detachment and a low density of putaminal D_2 receptors, whereas low levels of detachment correlated strongly with high D_2 receptor density. This finding is in keeping with the clinical observation that D_2 receptor antagonists (i.e., typical antipsychotic drugs) reduce the positive symptoms of schizophrenia, such as hallucinations and delusions, but may worsen the negative symptoms, such as social ambivalence and catatonia. In another study, experts postulate that dopamine activity may act in the medial left prefrontal cortex to suppress signals of emotional distress. A recent report supporting this hypothesis correlated a genetic polymorphism in the D_4 receptor with differences in subjective reports of mood.

Dopamine and Drugs. In the past, the potency of antipsychotic compounds has been correlated with their affinity for the D_2 receptor. Because blockade of dopamine receptors, particularly the D_2 receptor, has been associated with the efficacy of antipsychotic drugs, long-term administration of dopamine receptor antagonists results in an upregulation in the number of dopamine receptors present. This upregulation may be involved in the development of tardive dyskinesia. A new class of highly effective antipsychotic agents, called the *serotonin-dopamine antagonists* because they block predominantly the serotonin type 5-HT_2 and, to a lesser extent, the D_2 receptors, is associated with a greatly reduced risk of development of parkinsonian side effects and tardive dyskinesia. Not only do they treat the positive symptoms of schizophrenia, effectively treated by pure D_2 receptor antagonists (psychosis, hallucinations, agitation), they also improve the negative symptoms of schizophrenia (blunted affect, ambivalence, catatonia).

Other substances that affect the dopamine system are amphetamines and cocaine. Amphetamines cause the release of dopamine, and cocaine blocks the uptake of dopamine. Thus, these substances increase the amount of dopamine present in the synapse. Cocaine and methamphetamine (Desoxyn) are among the most addicting substances. The dopaminergic systems may be particularly involved in the brain's so-called reward or pleasure-seeking system, and this involvement may explain the high addiction potential of cocaine. Mutant knockout mice, in which the dopamine transporter gene has been experimentally deleted, do not respond biochemically or behaviorally to cocaine. This suggests that the dopamine transporter is necessary for the pharmacological effects of cocaine. Studies in rats showed that D_2 receptor agonists increased cocaine self-administration, whereas D_1 receptor agonists lowered the desire for cocaine. Nicotine, the most psychoactive ingredient in cigarette smoke, stimulates the release of dopamine and glutamate. Epidemiological studies have found that smokers have a reduced risk of developing Parkinson's disease, Alzheimer's disease, and ulcerative colitis. A nicotine analogue that stimulates dopamine release is under study for treatment of Parkinson's disease, and the nicotine transdermal patch is being studied to counteract the cognitive impairment caused by treatment with haloperidol (Haldol). The nicotine-stained fingers of many patients with schizophrenia may be a sign that they are medicating themselves unknowingly with this powerful neurotransmitter.

The dopamine transporter can be blocked by bupropion (Wellbutrin), although it is unlikely that sufficient CNS concentrations of this drug are routinely obtained to have an appreciable effect on dopamine transport. The transporter is the portal of entry of the neurotoxin methylphenyltetrahydropyridine (MPTP), which may cause parkinsonism by killing the nigral dopaminergic neurons. Dopamine-containing storage vesicles are depleted irreversibly by reserpine (Serpasil) and reversibly by tetrabenazine.

Dopamine and Psychopathology. The *dopamine hypothesis of schizophrenia* grew from the observations that drugs that block dopamine receptors (e.g., haloperidol) have antipsychotic activity and drugs that stimulate dopamine activity (e.g., amphetamine) can induce psychotic symptoms in nonschizophrenic persons when given in sufficiently high doses. The dopamine hypothesis remains the leading neurochemical hypothesis for schizophrenia, but room is being made for a role for serotonin, based on the therapeutic success of the serotonin-dopamine antagonists. A recent series of studies showed that plasma concentrations of HVA, in fact, are reduced in many patients with schizophrenia who respond to antipsychotic drugs. A major problem with the hypothesis is that blockade of dopamine receptors reduces psychotic symptoms in virtually any disorder, such as psychosis associated with a brain tumor and psychosis associated with mania. Thus, some as yet unrecognized neurochemical abnormality in schizophrenia may be unique to the condition.

Dopamine may also be involved in the pathophysiology of mood disorders. Dopamine activity may be low in depression and high in mania. Amphetamines, which potentiate dopamine activity, are highly effective antidepressants. The observation that levodopa (Larodopa) can cause mania and psychosis in some patients with parkinsonian side effects also supports the hypothesis. Some studies have found low levels of dopamine metabolites in depressed patients.

Norepinephrine and Epinephrine

Although norepinephrine and epinephrine are discussed together, norepinephrine is the more important and more abundant of the two related neurotransmitters in the brain, although adrenally derived epinephrine is more abundant than norepinephrine in the serum. The norepinephrine system and the epinephrine system are also referred to as the *noradrenergic system* and the *adrenergic system*, respectively. The receptors are referred to simply as adrenergic receptors, however, because they are receptors for both epinephrine and norepinephrine.

CNS Noradrenergic Tracts. The major concentration of noradrenergic (and adrenergic) cell bodies that project upward in the brain is in the compact locus ceruleus in the pons (Fig. 3.2–8). The axons of these neurons project through the medial forebrain bundle to the cerebral cortex, the limbic system, the thalamus, and the hypothalamus.

Norepinephrine and Epinephrine Life Cycle. Norepinephrine and epinephrine, along with dopamine, constitute the catecholamines. As discussed above, the catecholamines are synthesized from tyrosine, and the rate-limiting enzyme is tyrosine hydroxylase (Fig. 3.2–7). In neurons that release norepinephrine, the enzyme dopamine β-hydroxylase converts dopamine to norepinephrine; neurons that release dopamine lack this enzyme. In neurons that release epinephrine, the enzyme phenylethanolamine-*N*-methyltransferase (PNMT) converts norepinephrine into epinephrine. Neurons that release either dopamine or norepinephrine do not have PNMT.

Once norepinephrine or epinephrine is formed, it is taken through specific transporter proteins into synaptic vesicles, from which it is released on depolarization of the axonal terminal. As with dopamine, the two major routes of deactivation are uptake back into the presynaptic neuron and metabolism by MAO and COMT. The MAO_A subtype preferentially metabolizes norepinephrine and epinephrine, as well as serotonin.

Noradrenergic and Adrenergic Receptors. The two broad groups of adrenergic and noradrenergic receptors, often just

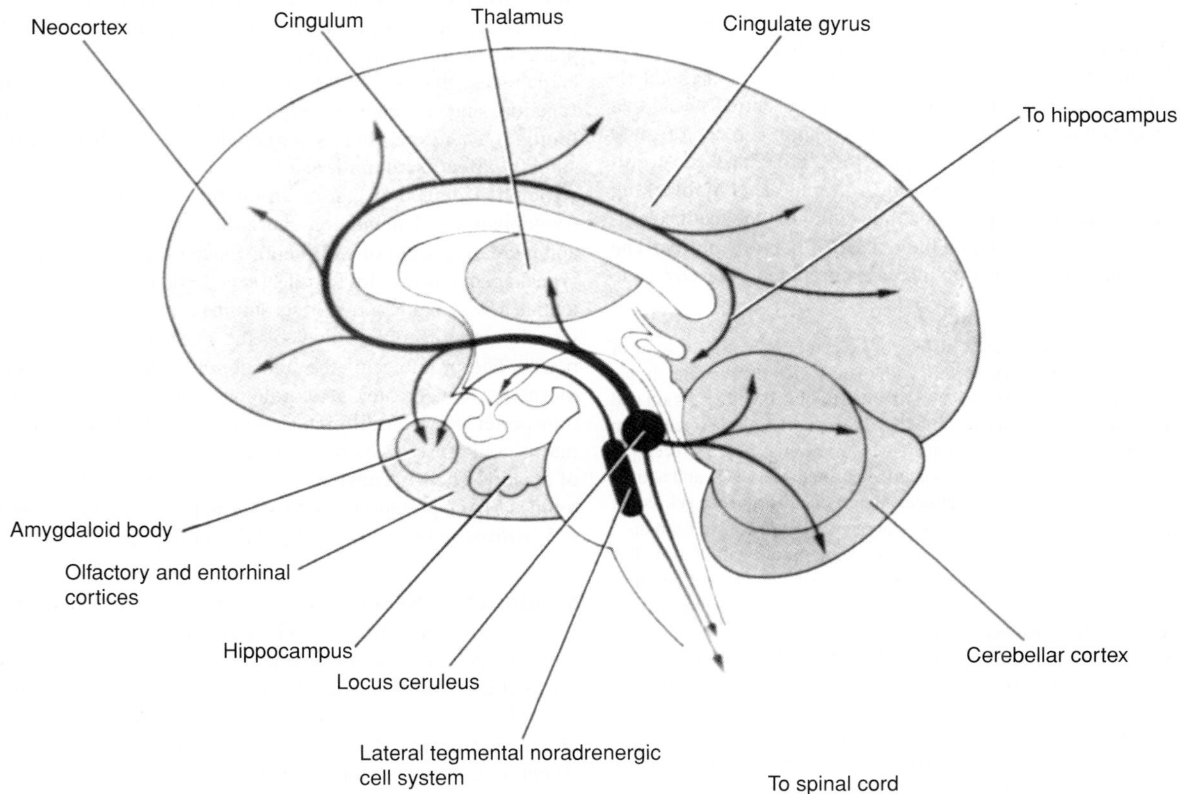

FIGURE 3.2–8

Noradrenergic pathways. The locus ceruleus, which is located immediately underneath the floor of the fourth ventricle in the rostrolateral part of the pons, is the most important noradrenergic nucleus in the brain. The projections reach many areas in the forebrain, the cerebellum, and the spinal cord. Noradrenergic neurons in the lateral brainstem tegmentum innervate several structures in the basal forebrain, including the hypothalamus and the amygdaloid body. (Reprinted from Heimer L. *The Human Brain and Spinal Cord.* New York: Springer; 1983, with permission.)

referred to as adrenergic receptors, are the α-adrenergic receptors and the β-adrenergic receptors (Table 3.2–1). The advances of molecular biology have now subtyped these receptors into three types of α_1-receptors (α_{1A}, α_{1B}, and α_{1D}), three types of α_2-receptors (α_{2A}, α_{2B}, α_{2C}), and three types of β-receptors (β_1, β_2, and β_3). Although the field is changing rapidly, all α_1-receptors seem to be linked to the phosphoinositol turnover system, α-receptors seem to inhibit the formation of cAMP, and β-receptors seem to stimulate the formation of cAMP. The surface availability and the efficiency of signal transduction of the adrenergic receptors are constantly regulated by phosphorylations and changes in protein–protein interactions. Significant data have long been available on the β_1- and β_2-receptors, which regulate the function of nearly every organ in the body, often in antagonism to the effects of the α-receptors. The β_3-receptors have recently been found to regulate energy metabolism. They are expressed in adipocytes, and their activation by agonists reduces the amount of body fat. They, therefore, are a target for the development of antiobesity drugs.

Norepinephrine and Drugs. The psychiatric drugs that are most associated with norepinephrine are the classic antidepressant drugs, the tricyclic drugs and the MAO inhibitors (MAOIs), and, more recently, venlafaxine (Effexor), mirtazapine (Remeron), bupropion, and nefazodone (Serzone). The tricyclic drugs, venlafaxine, bupropion, and nefazodone, block the reuptake of norepinephrine (and serotonin) into the presynaptic neuron, and the MAOIs block the catabolism of norepinephrine (and serotonin). Thus, the immediate effect of tricyclic drugs and MAOIs is to increase the concentrations of norepinephrine (and serotonin) in the synaptic cleft. Because antidepressants take 2 to 4 weeks to exert their therapeutic effects, it is obviously not the immediate effect alone that results in their beneficial effects. The immediate effects, however, may eventually lead to a downregulation of the number of postsynaptic β-receptors, and this downregulation of postsynaptic β-receptors has been correlated with clinical improvement. Mirtazapine acts by blocking the presynaptic α_2-receptors and thus removing the feedback inhibition normally exerted on the release of norepinephrine. The net effect of mirtazapine is to increase norepinephrine secretion.

The α-adrenergic system is also involved in the production of some of the adverse events that can be seen with many psychotherapeutic drugs. Blockade of the α_1-receptors is commonly associated with sedation and postural hypotension. Another drug that affects the α-adrenergic system is clonidine (Catapres), which is an α-receptor agonist. The α_2-receptors are generally located on the presynaptic neuron in the CNS, and activation of these receptors downregulates the production and the release of norepinephrine. The sympatholytic actions of clonidine have been used for a variety of psychiatric disorders, including opioid withdrawal. The antihypertensive agent methyldopa (Aldomet) is a competitive inhibitor of L-aromatic amino acid decarboxylase, which transforms methyldopa to methyldopamine and eventually to methylnorepinephrine, which displaces norepinephrine from storage vesicles. Methylnorepinephrine acts as an α_2-receptor agonist to lower blood pressure. The α_2-receptor antagonist yohimbine (Yocon) is used to reverse the antisexual effects of antidepressants, especially those of the serotonergic class.

The β-adrenergic receptor antagonists, such as propranolol (Inderal), have also been used in psychiatry. In general, β-receptors are located postsynaptically, and inhibition of their activity results in a decrease in cAMP formation in the postsynaptic neuron. The β-adrenergic antagonists have been used to treat social phobia (e.g., performance anxiety), akathisia (a movement disorder associated with antipsychotic compounds), and lithium-induced tremor.

Norepinephrine and Psychopathology. The *biogenic amine hypothesis of mood disorders* was based on the observation that the tricyclic drugs and the MAOIs are effective in alleviating the symptoms of depression. What the relative roles of serotonin and norepinephrine are in the pathophysiology of depression is still unclear. Drugs that affect both neurotransmitters are effective, and drugs that affect primarily norepinephrine—for example, desipramine (Norpramin)—and drugs that affect primarily serotonin—for example, fluoxetine—are also effective. When noradrenergic neurons are destroyed in experimental animal models, however, drugs that affect serotonin do not have their usual effects; and when serotonergic neurons are destroyed, drugs that affect norepinephrine do not have their usual effects. These experimental results indicate that the interrelationships between serotonergic and noradrenergic neurons are incompletely understood.

Serotonin

CNS Serotonergic Tracts. The major site of serotonergic cell bodies is in the upper pons and the midbrain—specifically, the median and dorsal raphe nuclei and, to a lesser extent, the caudal locus ceruleus, the area postrema, and the interpeduncular area (Fig. 3.2–9). These neurons project to the basal ganglia, the limbic system, and the cerebral cortex.

Serotonin Life Cycle. As with the catecholamines, serotonin is synthesized in the axonal terminal (Fig. 3.2–10). The precursor amino acid is tryptophan. In contrast to the catecholamines, the availability of tryptophan is the rate-limiting function, and the enzyme tryptophan hydroxylase is not rate limiting. Therefore, dietary variations in tryptophan can measurably affect serotonin levels in the brain. For example, tryptophan depletion causes irritability and hunger, whereas tryptophan supplementation can induce sleep, relieve anxiety, and increase a sense of well-being. Once synthesized, serotonin is packaged into vesicles for release on the arrival of an action potential. The synaptic action of serotonin is terminated by reuptake into the presynaptic terminal by the plasma membrane transporter. The promoter of the transporter gene contains a polymorphism that creates a twofold variation in the amount of transporter between different individuals, which in some way may account for 3 to 4 percent of the biological variation in levels of anxiety. The key enzyme involved in the metabolism of serotonin is MAO, preferentially MAO_A, and the primary metabolite is 5-hydroxyindoleacetic acid (5-HIAA) (Fig. 3.2–10).

Serotonergic Receptors. Seven types of serotonin receptors are now recognized: 5-HT_1 through 5-HT_7, with numerous subtypes, totaling 14 distinct receptors. The various functional effector mechanisms of some of these receptors are listed in Table 3.2–1. The diversity of serotonin receptors has initiated a significant effort to study the distribution of serotonin receptor subtypes in pathological states and to design subtype-specific drugs that may be of particular therapeutic benefit in specific conditions. For example, buspirone (BuSpar), a clinically effective anxiolytic, is a potent 5-HT_{1A} agonist, and other 5-HT_{1A} agonists are being developed for the treatment of anxiety and depression. Clozapine, the prototypical serotonin-dopamine

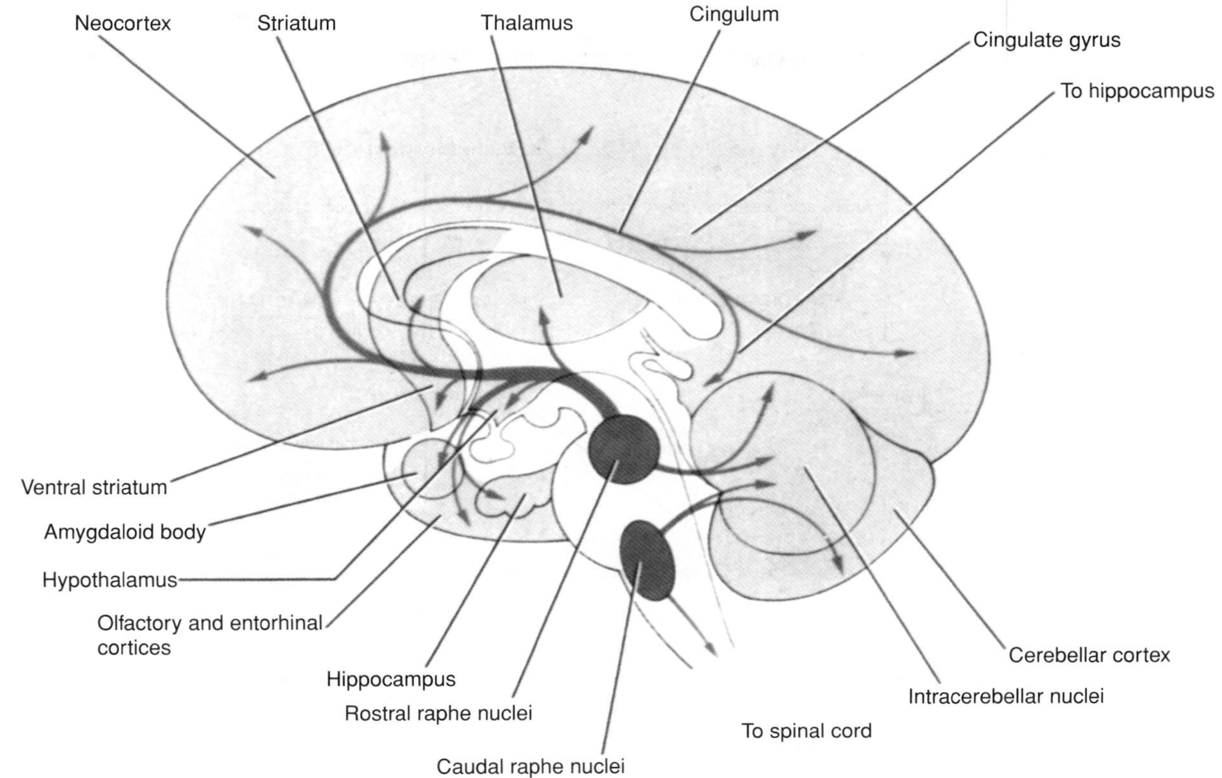

FIGURE 3.2–9

Serotenergic (5-HT) pathways. The raphe nuclei form a more or less continuous collection of cell groups close to the midline throughout the brainstem; for simplicity, they have been subdivided into a rostral group and a caudal group in the drawing. The rostral raphe nuclei project to a large number of forebrain structures. The fibers that project laterally through the internal and external capsules to widespread areas of the neocortex are not indicated in this highly schematic drawing. (Reprinted from Heimer L. *The Human Brain and Spinal Cord.* New York: Springer; 1983, with permission.)

antagonist antipsychotic agent, has significant activity as an antagonist of 5-HT_2 receptors, and this observation has initiated a major effort to study the role of this serotonin receptor subtype and to develop drugs that are 5-HT_2 antagonists for the treatment of schizophrenia.

Antagonists of the 5-HT_3 receptor are also under study as potential antianxiety and antipsychotic compounds. The distributed serotonin receptors are sometimes responsible for the side effects of serotonergic drugs, many of which nonspecifically raise serotonin levels and thus indiscriminately increase receptor activation. Serotonin receptors in the basal ganglia may be responsible for akathisia and agitation; 5-HT_3 receptors in the brainstem vomiting center (area postrema) or the hypothalamus may cause nausea and vomiting; receptors in the limbic system may cause an initial increase in anxiety; receptors in various parts of the brainstem sleep centers may produce either insomnia or somnolence; spinal cord pathways may produce sexual dysfunction; receptors in the intestines (where 90 percent of the body's serotonin is found) may cause gastrointestinal upset and diarrhea; and receptors in the cranial blood vessel may cause headache. Which, if any, of these adverse effects will occur in a particular patient cannot be predicted.

Serotonin and Drugs. Some of the new relations between serotonin and drugs under development are discussed above; however, the historical association of serotonin and psychotropic drugs was first made with the tricyclic drugs and the MAOIs, as described for norepinephrine and epinephrine. The tricyclic drugs and the MAOIs, respectively, block the uptake and the metabolism of serotonin and norepinephrine, thus increasing the concentration of both neurotransmitters in the synaptic cleft. Fluoxetine is one of the selective serotonin reuptake inhibitors (SSRIs) that are used in the treatment of depression. Other drugs in that class include paroxetine (Paxil), sertraline (Zoloft), fluvoxamine (Luvox), and citalopram (Celexa), all of which are usually associated with minimal adverse effects, especially in comparison with the tricyclic drugs and the MAOIs.

Venlafaxine blocks the reuptake of both serotonin and norepinephrine. With respect to serotonin, both trazodone (Desyrel) and nefazodone block the reuptake of serotonin and directly antagonize 5-HT_2 receptors, with the net effect stimulating 5-HT_1 receptors. Trazodone and nefazodone and the 5-HT_1 receptor agonist buspirone are the first of what will likely be a series of drugs that target subtypes of serotonin receptors.

Another serotonergic drug that has been used in psychiatry is L-tryptophan. Because the concentration of L-tryptophan is the rate-limiting function in the synthesis of serotonin, ingestion of L-tryptophan can increase the concentration of serotonin in the CNS. L-tryptophan was withdrawn from the market in 1990 in the United States by the Food and Drug Administration (FDA) because a contaminant from the production process at one particular manufacturing site caused an eosinophilia-myalgia syndrome in some patients taking the drug. Recent data suggest

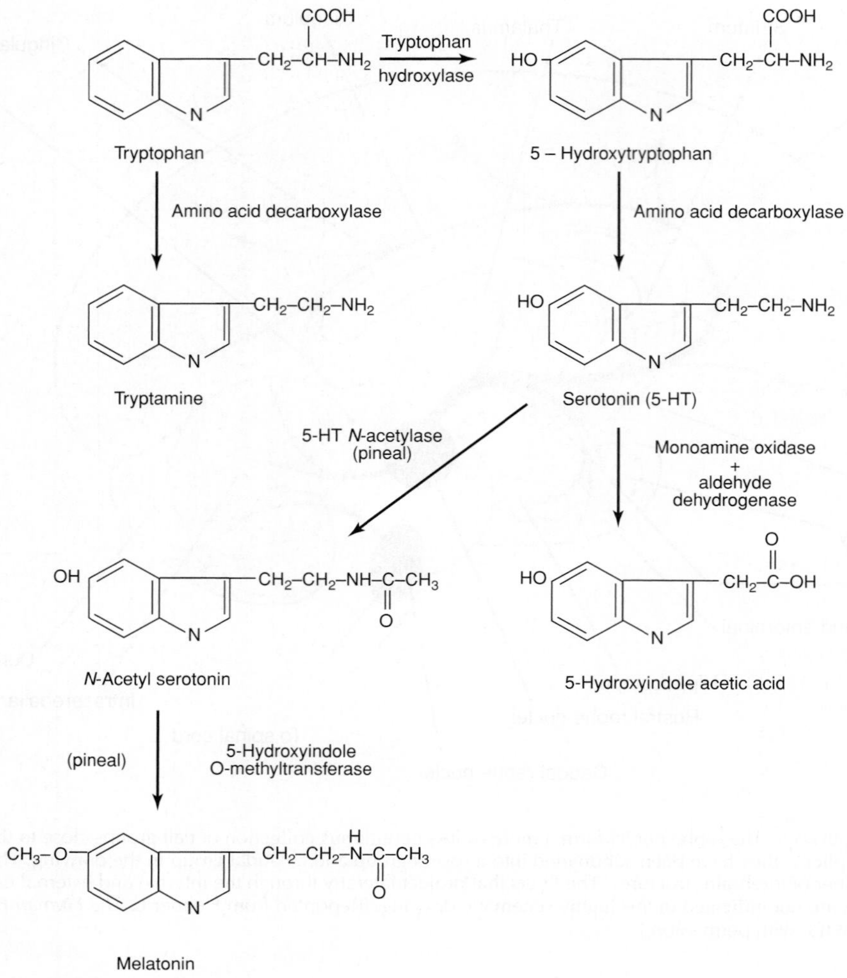

FIGURE 3.2–10
Synthetic and metabolic pathways of serotonin. (From Cooper JR, Bloom FE, Roth RH. *The Biochemical Basis of Neuropharmacology.* 7th ed. New York: Oxford University Press; 1996:355, with permission.)

that L-tryptophan itself may cause the eosinophilia-myalgia syndrome.

Serotonin is also involved in the mechanism of at least two major substances of abuse, lysergic acid diethylamide (LSD) and 3,4-methylenedioxymethamphetamine (MDMA), also known as "ecstasy." The serotonin system is the major site of action for LSD, but exactly how LSD exerts its effects remains unclear. MDMA has dual effects: blocking the uptake of serotonin and inducing the massive release of the serotonin contents of serotonergic neurons.

Serotonin and Psychopathology. The principal association of serotonin with a psychopathological condition is with depression, as suggested in the biogenic amine hypothesis of mood disorders. This hypothesis is simply that depression is associated with too little serotonin and that mania is associated with too much serotonin. As explained above for norepinephrine, that simplified view is undoubtedly not entirely accurate. The *permissive hypothesis* postulates that low levels of serotonin permit abnormal levels of norepinephrine to cause depression or mania. With the introduction of a variety of new drugs, serotonin is one of the most exciting areas for research in the anxiety disorders and schizophrenia, in addition to its role in depression. For example, early theories about the causes of anxiety focused on the GABA system because the first effective anxiolytics were the benzodiazepines, which potentiate GABAergic neurotransmission. With the success of SSRIs and buspirone, which are effective antianxiety agents, the theory of anxiety needed room for a role for serotonin. Similarly, schizophrenia was previously thought to result from an imbalance of dopamine, but since the therapeutic success of the serotonin-dopamine antagonists, schizophrenia is now thought to result from misregulation of both dopamine and serotonin function. It is likely that theories will need to be revised several times over in the near future as agents become available for modification of particular receptor subtypes.

Histamine

Neurons that release histamine as their neurotransmitter are located in the hypothalamus and project to the cerebral cortex, the limbic system, and the thalamus. There are three types of histamine receptors (Table 3.2–1): H_1-receptor stimulation increases the production of IP_3 and DAG; H_2 stimulation increases the production of cAMP; and the H_3 receptor may regulate vascular tone. Blockade of H_1 receptors is the mechanism of action for allergy medications and is partly the mechanism for commonly observed side effects (e.g., sedation, weight gain, and hypotension) of some psychotropic drugs.

Acetylcholine

CNS Cholinergic Tracts. A group of cholinergic neurons in the nucleus basalis of Meynert projects to the cerebral cortex and the limbic system. Additional cholinergic neurons in the reticular system project to the cerebral cortex, the limbic system, the hypothalamus, and the thalamus. Some patients with dementia of the Alzheimer's type or Down syndrome appear to have specific degeneration of the neurons in the nucleus basalis of Meynert.

Acetylcholine Life Cycle. Acetylcholine is synthesized in the cholinergic axon terminal from acetylcoenzyme A (acetyl-CoA) and choline by the enzyme choline acetyltransferase. Once made, acetylcholine is packaged into storage vesicles for release when triggered by an action potential. Acetylcholine is metabolized in the synaptic cleft by acetylcholinesterase, and the resulting choline is taken back up into the presynaptic neuron and is recycled to make new acetylcholine molecules. Acetylcholinesterase is affected by the drugs currently in use for the treatment of Alzheimer's disease.

Cholinergic Receptors. The two major subtypes of cholinergic receptors are muscarinic and nicotinic (Table 3.2–1). There are five recognized types of muscarinic receptors with various effects on phosphoinositol turnover, cAMP and cGMP production, and potassium ion channel activity. Muscarinic receptors are antagonized by atropine and by the anticholinergic drugs. The nicotinic receptors are ligand-gated ion channels that have the receptor site directly on the ion channel itself. The nicotinic receptor is actually made up of four subunits (α, β, γ, and δ). Nicotinic receptors can vary in the number of each of those subunits; thus, a multitude of subtypes of nicotinic receptors exist, based on the specific configuration of the subunits.

Acetylcholine and Drugs. The most common use of anticholinergic drugs in psychiatry is in treatment of the motor abnormalities caused by the use of classic antipsychotic drugs (e.g., haloperidol). The efficacy of the drugs for that indication is determined by the balance between acetylcholine activity and dopamine activity in the basal ganglia. In healthy people, the activity of the nigrostriatal dopamine pathway is partially balanced by the activity of cholinergic pathways in the basal ganglia. Blockade of D_2 receptors in the striatum upsets this balance, but the balance can be partially restored, albeit at a lower set point, by antagonism of muscarinic receptors. Blockade of muscarinic cholinergic receptors is a common pharmacodynamic effect of many psychotropic drugs. Blockade of those receptors leads to the commonly seen adverse effects of blurred vision, dry mouth, constipation, and difficulty in initiating urination. Excessive blockade of CNS cholinergic receptors causes confusion and delirium. Drugs that increase cholinergic activity by blocking breakdown by acetylcholinesterase (e.g., donepezil [Aricept]) have been shown to be effective in the treatment of dementia of the Alzheimer's type.

When bound by nicotine, CNS presynaptic nicotinic receptors mediate a large influx of calcium and, therefore, cause neurotransmitter release in many types of neurons. Recent evidence has shown that nicotine increases the strength of synaptic connections in the hippocampus, the brain region that supports short-term memory. Several nicotine-like compounds that stimulate acetylcholine release are under study as cognitive enhancers for treatment of Alzheimer's disease.

Acetylcholine and Psychopathology. The most common association with acetylcholine is dementia of the Alzheimer's type and other dementias. Anticholinergic agents can impair learning and memory in healthy people. With the recent identification of the protein structures of the various muscarinic and nicotinic receptors, many researchers are working on specific muscarinic and nicotinic agonists that may have some benefit in the treatment of dementia of the Alzheimer's type. Acetylcholine may also be involved in mood and sleep disorders.

PEPTIDE NEUROTRANSMITTERS

As many as 300 peptide neurotransmitters may be in the human brain (Table 3.2–3). A peptide is a short protein consisting of fewer than 100 amino acids. Peptides are made in the neuronal cell body by the transcription and translation of a genetic message. Peptides are stored in synaptic vesicles and are released from the axon terminals. The activity of peptides is terminated by the action of enzymes, peptidases, which cleave the peptides between specific amino acid residues. In addition to the regulatory mechanisms shared with other neurotransmitters, neuroactive peptides are subject to additional refinements in regulation. Differential ribonucleic acid (RNA) processing of the RNA first transcribed from the deoxyribonucleic acid (DNA) (heterogeneous nuclear RNA [hnRNA]) can result in different messenger RNAs (mRNAs). Most of these initial mRNAs for peptide neurotransmitters actually code for much longer peptides, called *preprohormones*, which are cleaved in the cell body before they are packaged as prohormones into vesicles for transport to the axon terminals. During the transport phase, the prohormone is usually further cleaved to form the final form of the peptide, which can then be subject to additional posttranslational modifications. Peptide receptors are members of the seven-transmembrane-domain, G protein-linked receptor family. In addition, most, if not all, peptide neurotransmitters coexist in storage vesicles with other neurotransmitters.

Selected Peptide Neurotransmitters

Endogenous Opioids. The remarkable analgesic and psychological effects of opium have been recognized since biblical times. The isolation of the alkaloid morphine in 1806 led in this century to the development of extensive pharmacological assays for opiate agents and raised the question of whether there were endogenous opiate-like compounds. In the mid-1970s, peptides isolated from brain extracts were shown to interact with opioid receptors and were called *opioids*. The endogenous opioids act on three major receptors, μ, κ, and δ, and are believed to be involved in the regulation of stress, pain, and mood. Three classes of

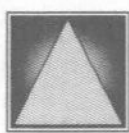

Table 3.2–3
Selected Neuropeptide Transmitters

Adrenocorticotropin hormone (ACTH)
Angiotensin
Atrial natriuretic peptide
Bombesin
Calcitonin
Calcitonin gene-related peptide (CGRP)
Cholecystokinin (CCK)
Cocaine and amphetamine regulated transcript (CART)
Corticotropin-releasing factor (CRF)
Dynorphin
β-Endorphin
Leu-enkephalin
Met-enkephalin
Galanin
Gastrin
Gonadotropin-releasing hormone (GnRH)
Growth hormone
Growth hormone-releasing hormone (GHRH; GRF)
Insulin
Motilin
Neuropeptide Y (NPY)
Neuromedin N
Neurotensin (NT)
Orexin
Orphanin FQ/Nociceptin
Oxytocin (OT)
Pancreatic polypeptide
Prolactin
Secretin
Somatostatin (SS; SRIF)
Substance K
Substance P
Thyrotropin-releasing hormone (TRH)
Urocortin
Vasoactive intestinal polypeptide (VIP)
Vasopressin (AVP; ADH)

endogenous opioids were recognized, the enkephalins, endorphins, and dynorphins, and recently, the endomorphins, which at last rival morphine itself in potency. Although evidence of opioids as true neurotransmitters has been difficult to distinguish from their potentiating effects on glutamatergic or adrenergic neurotransmission, a true role for endogenous opioid neurotransmission has been established in the hippocampus, where associative learning may contribute to addiction. Endogenous opioid-containing neurons are found in several brain regions, including the medial hypothalamus, diencephalon, pons, hippocampus, and midbrain, and their axons project both locally and widely. Emerging data on endomorphins and other, so far unknown ligands, may yet unlock the mystery of addiction.

Corticotropin-Releasing Factor (CRF). CRF was first isolated and characterized in 1981 as the hypothalamic messenger molecule that stimulated the release of adrenocorticoid hormone (ACTH) from the anterior pituitary. Although originally identified in this narrow role, CRF is located throughout the nervous system, as are its two receptors, CRF_1 and CRF_2, thus suggesting a much broader role for CRF in brain functioning. The most common hypotheses have involved a general role for CRF in modulating the organism's response to internal and external stress. The long-standing observation that a subpopulation of depressed patients has elevated cortisol levels, sometimes evidenced by nonsuppression on a dexamethasone suppression test, has led to the hypothesis that a CRF antagonist might be useful in the treatment of depression. Indeed, a number of pharmaceutical companies have such drugs in early development.

Substance P. Substance P is the primary neurotransmitter in most primary afferent sensory neurons and in the striatonigral pathway, which are most prominently associated with mediation of the perception of pain. Abnormalities affecting substance P have been hypothesized for Huntington's disease, dementia of the Alzheimer's type, and mood disorders.

Neurotensin. Neurotensin has been hypothesized to be involved in the pathophysiology of schizophrenia, mostly because of its coexistence with dopamine in some axon terminals. Some preliminary reports suggest that neurotensin-related peptides or drugs have beneficial effects for some psychotic symptoms.

Cholecystokinin. As with neurotensin and for the same reasons, cholecystokinin (CCK) has been hypothesized to be involved in the pathophysiology of schizophrenia. CCK has also been implicated in the pathophysiologies of eating disorders and movement disorders. It causes anxiety and triggers panic attacks in people with panic disorder. CCK antagonists are under study as possible anxiolytic agents.

Somatostatin. Somatostatin is also known as growth hormone-inhibiting factor. Postmortem studies have implicated somatostatin in Huntington's disease and dementia of the Alzheimer's type.

Vasopressin and Oxytocin. Vasopressin and oxytocin, two related peptides, have been postulated to be involved in the regulation of mood and most recently, social behavior. They are both synthesized in the hypothalamus and are released in the posterior pituitary.

Neuropeptide Y. Neuropeptide Y has been shown to stimulate the appetite, and development of neuropeptide Y receptor antagonists is an active area of interest for obesity researchers.

AMINO ACID NEUROTRANSMITTERS

Amino acids are the building blocks of proteins. Because of their abundance, it has long been assumed that they could not also serve as neurotransmitters. Their roles as neurotransmitters have now been broadly accepted, however. The two major amino acid neurotransmitters are GABA and glutamate. GABA is an inhibitory amino acid, and glutamate is an excitatory amino acid. It is occasionally suggested that a simplified way to look at the brain is as a balance between just those two neurotransmitters, with all the biogenic amine and peptide neurotransmitters simply involved in modulating that balance. Recent discoveries have further increased the importance of the study of amino acid neurotransmitters. These discoveries include the observations that the benzodiazepines, barbiturates, and several anticonvulsants act primarily through GABAergic mechanisms and that an important substance of abuse, phencyclidine (PCP), acts at glutamate receptors. One of the most active areas of recent neuroscience research is the role of NMDA glutamate receptors in learning and memory. These observations have led to an intensive study of these receptors with regard to major psychiatric disorders, such as anxiety disorders and schizophrenia.

Inhibitory Amino Acid Neurotransmitters

γ-Aminobutyric Acid (GABA). GABA is found almost exclusively in the CNS, and it does not cross the blood-brain barrier. The highest concentrations are in the midbrain and diencephalon, with lower amounts in the cerebral hemispheres, the pons, and the medulla. GABA is synthesized from glutamate by the rate-limiting enzyme glutamic acid decarboxylase (GAD), which requires pyridoxine (vitamin B_6) as a cofactor. GABA is the primary neurotransmitter in intrinsic neurons that function as local mediators for the inhibitory feedback loops. GABA commonly coexists with biogenic amine neurotransmitters, glycine, and peptide neurotransmitters, including somatostatin, NPY, CCK, substance P, and vasoactive intestinal peptide (VIP).

Because GABA is thought to suppress seizure activity, anxiety, and mania, considerable effort has been devoted to synthesizing drugs that potentiate GABA activity. One such drug, progabide, is a hydrophobic GABA receptor agonist with good brain penetration, which has anticonvulsant activity. Tiagabine (Gabitril), which inhibits the GABA transporter, and vigabatrin (Sabril), which inhibits GABA-T, raise the effective synaptic levels of GABA and exhibit anticonvulsant activity. The anticonvulsant topiramate (Topamax) potentiates GABA receptor activity by unclear mechanisms. Gabapentin (Neurontin), a GABA derivative, is an effective anticonvulsant with good brain penetration; yet, curiously, it has no activity at GABA receptors or the GABA transporter. The GABA receptor has binding sites for the benzodiazepines, and the barbiturates. The benzodiazepines increase the affinity of the $_A$-receptor for GABA. The β-carbolines are a class of drugs that are inverse agonists of the benzodiazepine receptors; thus, their activity results in anxiety and convulsions. Flumazenil (Romazicon) is a benzodiazepine antagonist that is currently being used in hospital emergency rooms as a treatment for benzodiazepine overdose.

GABA AND PSYCHOPATHOLOGY. Clinical research on the GABAergic system, because it is associated with benzodiazepines, has focused on its potential role in the pathophysiology of anxiety disorders. Many of the standard anticonvulsants also have their effects on the GABA system; therefore, researchers in epilepsy also are actively studying the GABA system. The success of the anticonvulsants carbamazepine (Tegretol) and valproic acid (Depakote) for the treatment of rapid cycling bipolar I disorder has stimulated trials of the GABAergic anticonvulsants listed above for this indication.

Glycine.

Glycine is synthesized primarily from serine by the actions of serine *trans*-hydroxymethylase and β-glycerate dehydrogenase, both of which are rate limiting. Glycine does double duty as a mandatory adjunctive neurotransmitter for glutamate activity and an independent inhibitory neurotransmitter at its own receptors. The excitatory amino acid-binding site for glycine on the NMDA glutamate receptor is referred to as the *non–strychnine-sensitive glycine receptor*, and it contrasts with the strychnine-sensitive glycine receptor, which is an inhibitory receptor. Improvement of NMDA receptor activity by occupancy of the glycine-binding site has been hypothesized to present an adjunctive mode for the treatment of schizophrenia. Some, but not all, clinical trials of this hypothesis have shown a reduction in the negative symptoms of schizophrenia by glycine.

Excitatory Amino Acid Neurotransmitters

Glutamate.

Glutamate is synthesized from glucose and glutamine in presynaptic neuron terminals and is stored in synaptic vesicles. Once released into the synaptic cleft, it acts on receptors, and its action is terminated by highly efficient uptake into the presynaptic neuron or adjacent glia. Glutamate is the primary neurotransmitter in cerebellar granule cells, the striatum, the cells of the hippocampal molecular layer and entorhinal cortex, the pyramidal cells of the cortex, and the thalamocortical and corticostriatal projections. Glutamate release is stimulated by nicotine. Of the five major types of glutamate receptors, the NMDA receptor is the best understood and most complex of the receptors, because it may play an essential role in learning and memory, as well as psychopathology.

GLUTAMATE AND PSYCHOPATHOLOGY. The major pathophysiological conditions currently associated with the glutamate systems are excitotoxicity and schizophrenia. *Excitotoxicity* relates to the hypothesis that excessive stimulation of glutamate receptors leads to prolonged and excessive intraneuronal concentrations of calcium and NO. Such conditions activate many enzymes (especially proteases) that are destructive to neuronal integrity. The association with schizophrenia is partly owing to the psychotomimetic effects observed with PCP. In this model, a reduction in NMDA receptor activity is thought to cause psychotic symptoms. Attempts to reduce excitotoxicity during strokes with the NMDA receptor blocker MK-801 were terminated because of precipitation of psychosis. It seems, therefore, that the glutamate neurotransmitter-receptor system is poorly suited to be a target for psychotherapeutic drugs; too much NMDA receptor activity kills neurons, and too little NMDA receptor activity induces psychosis. Memantine (Namenda), an NMDA antagonist, however, was recently approved for the treatment of Alzheimer's disease. Some basic science studies show that dopamine and glutamate have opposing effects. Because of that association or because of the sensitivity of nigral dopamine-containing neurons to excitotoxicity, glutamate may be involved in the pathophysiology of Parkinson's disease.

Other Neurotransmitters

NUCLEOTIDES. Of the four nucleotides in DNA, the purine adenosine and its high-energy phosphorylated form, ATP, have also been shown to be neurotransmitters. Receptors for purines have been found in the brain. P_1 receptors have a high affinity for adenosine, and P_2 receptors have a high affinity for ATP. Two subtypes of the P_1 receptor are the adenosine A_1 and A_2 receptors, both of which are G protein-linked receptors. Binding of adenosine to A_1 receptors results in cellular responses opposite to those of binding of adenosine to A_2 receptors in some systems. The P_1 receptors are blocked by xanthines, such as caffeine and theophylline. Adenosine is concentrated in specific cellular layers of discrete regions of the brain and appears to have the general effect of inhibiting the release of most other neurotransmitters. During a seizure, it is released from cells and appears to act to terminate the seizure. The actions of adenosine, which are opposite to those of caffeine, have led to various research efforts to study adenosine analogues for use as anticonvulsants or sedatives. In clinical use as a cardiac antiarrhythmic agent, intravenous adenosine has a half-life on the order of less than 5 minutes. ATP itself may also serve as a neurotransmitter. It is stored in synaptic vesicles along with catecholamines and is released when the catecholamines are released.

NEUROTROPHIC FACTORS. The neurotrophic factors are a diverse class of protein molecules that bind to the tyrosine kinase receptors that were discussed previously. A number of families of neurotrophic factors exist, including the neurotrophins, the glial-derived neurotrophic factor family, the insulin family, and the cytokines. The neurotrophins are currently the most interesting to psychiatric research and include brain-derived neurotrophic factor (BDNF), nerve growth factor (NGF), and neurotrophin-3 and -4.

Neurotrophic factor release appears to happen during unstimulated resting conditions, and it is also increased in some studies by neuronal stimulation. The regulation of neurotrophic factors is a focus of research.

A major role for neurotrophic factors is in long-term effects such as neuronal growth, development, and survival. Increasing evidence, however, suggests that neurotrophic factors may also serve more short-term roles that more closely resemble the activities of classic neurotransmitters.

EICOSANOIDS. The metabolites of arachidonic acid, prostaglandins, prostacyclins, thromboxane, and leukotrienes, also called eicosanoids or prostanoids, are all present in the brain. Although these substances have not yet fulfilled all the criteria for neurotransmitters, efforts are being made to explore this possible role.

ENDOCANNABINOIDS. A novel compound formed from arachidonic acid and ethanolamine, N-arachidonoylethanolamine (anadamide), and 2-arachnidonylglycerol are now recognized as weak and strong endogenous ligands, respectively, for the cannabinoid receptor family. Cannabinoids are the active ingredients in marijuana. The two types of cannabinoid receptors, central (CB_1) and peripheral (CB_2), bind tetrahydrocannabinol (THC), the active ingredient of marijuana. Anandamides generally exhibit pharmacological effects that are less potent, but similar to those of THC, including lowering intraocular pressure, decreasing activity level, and relieving pain. The colocalization of anandamides and cannabinoid receptors in the thalamus suggests that anandamides may act as neurotransmitters.

SIGMA RECEPTORS. The Σ-receptor site has been defined pharmacologically but has not yet been purified or cloned, and the endogenous ligand for the receptors has not been identified. Only recently has the site now known as the Σ *receptor* been distinguished from the PCP receptor. It is now clear that the principal site of action for PCP is the NMDA glutamate receptor, where PCP binding results in an indirect inhibition of calcium ion influx. The Σ site binds pentazocine (Talwin) and haloperidol, which belong to distinct drug classes. Although the study of the Σ-binding characteristic remains an area of active research, consistent results from efforts to purify the receptor have been elusive.

References

Anagnostaras SG, Murphy GG, Hamilton SE, Mitchell SL, Rahnama NP, Nathanson NM, Silva AJ. Selective cognitive dysfunction in acetylcholine M1 muscarinic receptor mutant mice. *Nat Neuroscience*. 2003;6:51.

Anguelova M, Benkelfat C, Turecki G. A systematic review of association studies investigating genes coding for serotonin receptors and the serotonin transporter: II. Suicidal behavior. *Mol Psychiatry*. 2003;8:646.

Bortolozzi A, Artigas F. Control of 5-hydroxytryptamine release in the dorsal raphe nucleus by the noradrenergic system in rat brain. Role of α-adrenoceptors. *Neuropsychopharmacology*. 2003;28:421.

Bymaster FP, McKinzie DL, Felder CC, Wess J. Use of M_1-M_5 muscarinic receptor knockout mice as novel tools to delineate the physiological roles of the muscarinic cholinergic system. *Neurochem Res*. 2003;28:437.

Dunn AJ, Swiergiel AH, de Beaurepaire R. Cytokines as mediators of depression: What can we learn from animal studies? *Neuroscience & Biobehavioral Reviews*. 2005;29(4–5):891–909.

Fritschy J, Horesh L, Holder D, Bayford R. Applications of GRID in clinical neurophysiology and electrical impedance tomography of brain function. *Studies in Health Technology and Informatics*. 2005;112:138–145.

Givre SJ. Essentials of clinical neurophysiology, third edition. *J Neuroophthalmol*. 2005;25(1):61–62.

Heyman K. Neurophysiology: Dust clearing on the long-term potentiation debate. *The Scientist*. 2005;19(10):14.

Morillo CA, Baranchuk A. Deductive electrophysiology in the modern device technology era: The quest for the prevention of inappropriate ICD shocks. *J Cardiovasc Electrophysiol*. 2005;16(6):606.

Praamstra P, Seiss E. The neurophysiology of response competition: Motor cortex activation and inhibition following subliminal response priming. *J Cogn Neurosci*. 2005;17:483–493.

Phillips C. Electrophysiology in the study of developmental language impairments: Prospects and challenges for a top-down approach. *Applied Psycholinguistics*. 2005;26:79–96.

Siegel GJ, Albers RW, Brady ST, Price DL, eds. *Basic Neurochemistry: Molecular, Cellular and Medical Aspects*. 7th ed. Boston: Elsevier Academic Press. 2006.

Sourkes TL. Social and medical origins of neurochemistry. *Prog Neuropsychopharmacol Biol Psychiatry*. 2004;28(5):885–890.

Tecott LH, Smart SL. Monoamine neurotransmitters. In: Sadock BJ, Sadock VA, eds. *Kaplan & Sadock's Comprehensive Textbook of Psychiatry*. 8th ed. Vol. 1. Baltimore: Lippincott Williams & Wilkins; 2005:49.

Torres GE, Gainetdinov RR, Caron MG. Plasma membrane monoamine transporters: structure, regulation and function. *Nat Rev Neurosci*. 2003;4:13.

▲ 3.3 Neuroimaging

Neuroimaging methodologies allow measurement of the structure, function, and chemistry of the living human brain. Over the past decade, studies using these methods have provided new information about the pathophysiology of psychiatric disorders that may prove to be useful for diagnosing illness and for developing new treatments. Computer tomographic (CT) scanners, the first widely used neuroimaging devices, allowed assessment of structural brain lesions such as tumors or strokes. Magnetic resonance imaging (MRI) scans, developed next, distinguish gray and white matter better than CT scans do and allow visualizations of smaller brain lesions as well as white matter abnormalities. In addition to structural neuroimaging with CT and MRI, a revolution in functional neuroimaging has enabled clinical scientists to obtain unprecedented insights into the diseased human brain. The foremost techniques for functional neuroimaging include positron emission tomography (PET) and single photon emission computer tomography (SPECT).

Primary observation of structural and functional brain imaging in neuropsychiatric disorders such as dementia, movement disorders, demyelinating disorders, and epilepsy has contributed to a greater understanding of the pathophysiology of neurological and psychiatric illnesses and helps practicing clinicians in difficult diagnostic situations.

USES OF NEUROIMAGING

Indications for Ordering Neuroimaging in Clinical Practice

Neurological Deficits. In a neurological examination, any change that can be localized to the brain or spinal cord requires neuroimaging. Neurological examination includes mental status, cranial nerves, motor system, coordination, sensory system, and reflex components. The mental status examination assesses arousal, attention, and motivation; memory; language; visuospatial function; complex cognition; and mood and affect. Consultant psychiatrists should consider a workup including neuroimaging for patients with new-onset psychosis and acute changes in mental status. The clinical examination always assumes priority, and neuroimaging is ordered on the basis of clinical suspicion of a central nervous system (CNS) disorder.

Dementia. Loss of memory and cognitive abilities affects more than 10 million persons in the United States and will affect an increasing number as the population ages. Reduced mortality from cancer and heart disease has increased life expectancy and has allowed persons to survive to the age of onset of degenerative brain disorders, which have proved more difficult to treat. Depression, anxiety, and psychosis are common in patients with dementia. The most common cause of dementia is Alzheimer's disease, which does not have a characteristic appearance on routine neuroimaging but, rather, is associated with diffuse loss of brain volume.

One treatable cause of dementia that requires neuroimaging for diagnosis is *normal pressure hydrocephalus*, a disorder of the drainage of cerebrospinal fluid (CSF). This condition does not progress to the point of acutely increased intracranial pressure but stabilizes at a pressure at the upper end of the normal range. The dilated ventricles, which may be readily visualized with CT or MRI, exert pressure on the frontal lobes. A gait disorder is almost uniformly present; dementia, which may be indistinguishable from that of Alzheimer's disease, appears less consistently. Relief of the increased CSF pressure may completely restore gait and mental function.

Infarction of the cortical or subcortical areas, or stroke, can produce focal neurological deficits, including cognitive and emotional changes. Strokes are easily seen on MRI scans. Depression is common among stroke patients, either because of direct damage to the emotional centers of the brain or because of the patient's reaction to the disability. Depression, in turn, can cause pseudodementia. In addition to major strokes, extensive atherosclerosis in brain capillaries can cause countless tiny infarctions of brain tissue; patients with this phenomenon may develop dementia as fewer and fewer neural pathways participate in cognition. This state, called *vascular dementia*, is characterized on MRI scans by patches of increased signal in the white matter.

Certain degenerative disorders of basal ganglia structures, associated with dementia, may have a characteristic appearance on MRI scans. Huntington's disease typically produces atrophy of the caudate nucleus; thalamic degeneration can interrupt the neural links to the cortex (Fig. 3.3–1).

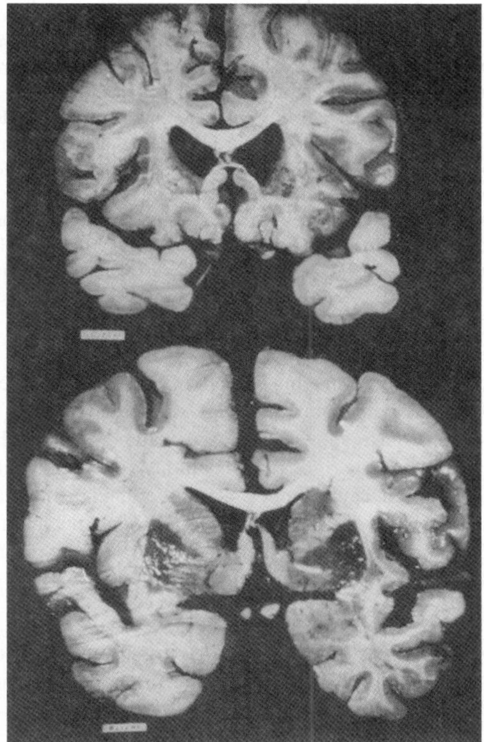

FIGURE 3.3–1
Brain slices. **Top:** Huntington disease. Atrophy of caudate nucleus and lentiform nuclei with dilatation of lateral ventricle. **Bottom:** Normal brain. (From Fahn S. Huntington disease. In: Rowland LP, ed. *Merritt's Textbook of Neurology.* 10th ed. Philadelphia: Lippincott Williams & Wilkins; 2000:659, with permission.)

Space-occupying lesions can cause dementia. Chronic subdural hematomas and cerebral contusions, caused by head trauma, can produce focal neurological deficits or may only produce dementia. Brain tumors can affect cognition in several ways. Skull-based meningiomas can compress the underlying cortex and impair its processing. Infiltrative glial cell tumors, such as astrocytoma or glioblastoma multiforme, can cut off communication between brain centers by interrupting white matter tracts. Tumors located near the ventricular system can obstruct the flow of CSF and gradually increase the intracranial pressure.

Chronic infections, including neurosyphilis, cryptococcosis, tuberculosis, and Lyme disease, can cause symptoms of dementia and may produce a characteristic enhancement of the meninges, especially at the base of the brain. Serological studies are needed to complete the diagnosis. Human immunodeficiency virus (HIV) infection can cause dementia directly, in which case is seen a diffuse loss of brain volume, or it can allow proliferation of the Creutzfeldt-Jakob virus to yield progressive multifocal leukoencephalopathy, which affects white matter tracts and appears as increased white matter signal on MRI scans.

Chronic demyelinating diseases, such as multiple sclerosis, can affect cognition because of white matter disruption. Multiple sclerosis plaques are easily seen on MRI scans as periventricular patches of increased signal intensity.

Any evaluation of dementia should consider medication effects, metabolic derangements, infections, and nutritional causes that may not produce abnormalities on neuroimaging.

Indications for Neuroimaging in Clinical Research

Analysis of Clinically Defined Groups of Patients. Psychiatric research aims to categorize patients with psychiatric disorders to facilitate the discovery of neuroanatomical and neurochemical bases of mental illness. Researchers have used functional neuroimaging to study groups of patients with such psychiatric conditions as schizophrenia, affective disorders, and anxiety disorders, among others. In schizophrenia, for example, neuropathological volumetric analyses have suggested a loss of brain weight, specifically of gray matter. A paucity of axons and dendrites appears present in the cortex, and CT and MRI may show compensatory enlargement of the lateral and third ventricles. Specifically, the temporal lobes of persons with schizophrenia appear to lose the most volume relative to healthy persons. Recent studies have found that the left temporal lobe is generally more affected than the right. The frontal lobe may also have abnormalities, not in the volume of the lobe, but in the level of activity detected by functional neuroimaging. Persons with schizophrenia consistently exhibit decreased metabolic activity in the frontal lobes, especially during tasks that require the prefrontal cortex. As a group, patients with schizophrenia are also more likely to have an increase in ventricular size than are healthy controls.

Disorders of mood and affect can also be associated with loss of brain volume and decreased metabolic activity in the frontal lobes. Inactivation of the left prefrontal cortex appears to depress mood; inactivation of the right prefrontal cortex elevates it. Among anxiety disorders, studies of obsessive–compulsive disorder with conventional CT and MRI have shown either no specific abnormalities or a smaller caudate nucleus. Functional PET and SPECT studies suggest abnormalities in the corticolimbic, basal ganglial, and thalamic structures in the disorder. When patients are experiencing obsessive–compulsive disorder symptoms, the orbital prefrontal cortex shows abnormal activity. A partial normalization of caudate glucose metabolism appears in patients taking medications such as fluoxetine (Prozac) or clomipramine (Anafranil) or undergoing behavior modification.

Functional neuroimaging studies of persons with attention-deficit/hyperactivity disorder (ADHD) either have shown no abnormalities or have shown decreased volume of the right prefrontal cortex and the right globus pallidus. In addition, whereas normally the right caudate nucleus is larger than the left caudate nucleus, persons with ADHD may have caudate nuclei of equal size. These findings suggest dysfunction of the right prefrontal-striatal pathway for control of attention.

Analysis of Brain Activity during Performance of Specific Tasks. Many original conceptions of different brain region functions emerged from observing deficits caused by local injuries, tumors, or strokes. Functional neuroimaging allows researchers to review and reassess classic teachings in the intact brain. Most work, to date, has been aimed at language and vision. Although many technical peculiarities and limitations of SPECT, PET, and functional MRI (fMRI) have been overcome, none of these techniques has demonstrated clear superiority. Studies require carefully controlled conditions, which subjects may find arduous. Nonetheless, functional neuroimaging has contributed major conceptual advances, and the methods are now limited mainly by the creativity of the investigative protocols.

Studies have been designed to reveal the functional neuroanatomy of all sensory modalities, gross and fine motor skills, language, memory, calculations, learning, and disorders of thought, mood, and anxiety. Unconscious sensations transmitted by the autonomic nervous system have been localized to specific brain regions. These analyses provide a basis for comparison with results of studies of clinically defined patient groups and may lead to improved therapies for mental illnesses.

SPECIFIC TECHNIQUES

Computed Tomography (CT) Scans

In 1972, CT scanning revolutionized diagnostic neuroradiology by permitting imaging of the brain tissue in live patients. CT scanners are currently the most widely available and convenient imaging tools available in clinical practice; practically every hospital emergency room has immediate access to a CT scanner at all times. CT scanners effectively take a series of head X-ray pictures from all vantage points, 360 degrees around a patient's head. The amount of radiation that passes through, or is not absorbed from, each angle is digitized and entered into a computer. The computer uses matrix algebra calculations to assign a specific density to each point within the head and displays these data as a set of two-dimensional images. When viewed in sequence, the images allow mental reconstruction of the shape of the brain.

The CT image is determined only by the degree to which tissues absorb X-irradiation. The bony structures absorb high amounts of irradiation and tend to obscure details of neighboring structures, an especially troublesome problem in the brainstem, which is surrounded by a thick skull base. Within the brain itself, there is relatively little difference in the attenuation between gray matter and white matter in X-ray images. Although the gray–white border is usually distinguishable, details of the gyral pattern may be difficult to appreciate in CT scans. Certain tumors may be invisible on CT because they absorb as much irradiation as the surrounding normal brain.

Appreciation of tumors and areas of inflammation, which can cause changes in behavior, can be increased by intravenous infusion of iodine-containing contrast agents. Iodinated compounds, which absorb much more irradiation than the brain, appear white. The intact brain is separated from the bloodstream by the blood-brain barrier, which normally prevents the passage of the highly charged contrast agents. The blood-brain barrier, however, breaks down in the presence of inflammation or fails to form within tumors and thus allows accumulation of contrast agents. These sites appear whiter than the surrounding brain. Iodinated contrast agents must be used with caution in patients who are allergic to these agents or to shellfish.

With the introduction of MRI scanning, CT scans have been supplanted as the nonemergency neuroimaging study of choice (Fig. 3.3–2). The increased resolution and delineation of detail afforded by MRI scanning is often required for diagnosis in psychiatry. In addition, performing the most detailed study available inspires the most confidence in the analysis. The only component of the brain better seen on CT scanning is calcification, which may be invisible on MRI.

Magnetic Resonance Imaging (MRI) Scans

MRI scanning entered clinical practice in 1982 and soon became the test of choice for clinical psychiatrists and neurologists. The technique does not rely on the absorption of X-rays but is based on nuclear magnetic resonance (NMR). The principle of NMR is that the nuclei of all atoms are thought to spin about an axis, which is randomly oriented in space. When atoms are placed in a magnetic field, the axes of all odd-numbered nuclei align with the magnetic field. The axis of a nucleus deviates away from the magnetic field when exposed to a pulse of radiofrequency electromagnetic radiation oriented at 90 or 180 degrees to the magnetic field. When the pulse terminates, the axis of the spinning nucleus realigns itself with the magnetic field, and during this realignment, it emits its own radiofrequency signal. MRI scanners collect the emissions of individual, realigning nuclei and use computer analysis to generate a series of two-dimensional images that represent the brain. The images can be in the axial, coronal, or sagittal planes.

By far the most abundant odd-numbered nucleus in the brain belongs to hydrogen. The rate of realignment of the hydrogen axis is determined by its immediate environment, a combination of both the nature of the molecule of which it is a part and the degree to which it is surrounded by water. Hydrogen nuclei within fat realign rapidly, and hydrogen nuclei within water realign slowly. Hydrogen nuclei in proteins and carbohydrates realign at intermediate rates.

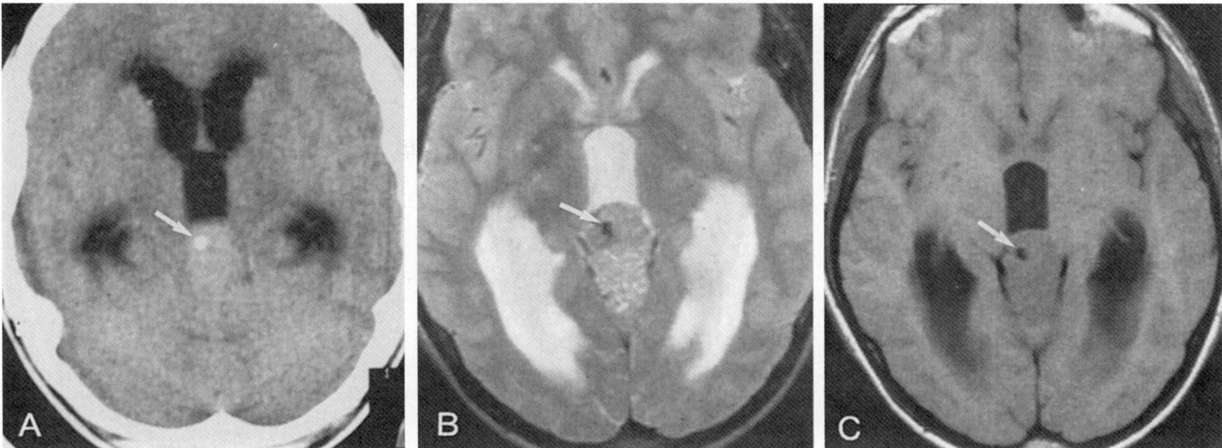

FIGURE 3.3–2

Comparison of CT and MRI. **A.** Computed tomography (CT) scan in the axial plane at the level of the third ventricle. The cerebrospinal fluid (CSF) within the ventricles appears black, the brain tissue appears gray, and the skull appears white. There is very poor discrimination between the gray and white matter of the brain. The *arrow* indicates a small calcified lesion in a tumor of the pineal gland. Detection of calcification is one role in which CT is superior to magnetic resonance imaging (MRI). **B.** T2-weighted image of the same patient at roughly the same level. With T2, the CSF appears white, the gray matter appears gray, the white matter is clearly distinguished from the gray matter; the skull and indicated calcification appear black. Much more detail of the brain is visible than with CT. **C.** T1-weighted image of the same patient at roughly the same level. With T1, the CSF appears dark, the brain appears more uniformly gray; the skull and indicated calcification appear black. T1 MRI images are the most similar to CT images. (Reprinted from Grossman CB. *Magnetic Resonance Imaging and Computed Tomography of the Head and Spine,* 2nd ed. Baltimore: Williams & Wilkins; 1996:101, with permission.)

Routine MRI studies use three different radiofrequency pulse sequences. The two parameters that are varied are the duration of the radiofrequency excitation pulse and the length of the time that data are collected from the realigning nuclei. Because T1 pulses are brief and data collection is brief, hydrogen nuclei in hydrophobic environments are emphasized. Thus, fat is bright on T1, and CSF is dark. The T1 image most closely resembles that of CT scans and is most useful for assessing overall brain structure. T1 is also the only sequence that allows contrast enhancement with the contrast agent gadolinium-diethylenetriamine pentaacetic acid (gadolinium-DTPA). As with the iodinated contrast agents used in CT scanning, gadolinium remains excluded from the brain by the blood-brain barrier, except in areas where this barrier breaks down, such as inflammation or tumor. On T1 images, gadolinium-enhanced structures appear white.

T2 pulses last four times as long as T1 pulses, and the collection times are also extended, to emphasize the signal from hydrogen nuclei surrounded by water. Thus, brain tissue is dark, and CSF is white on T2 images. Areas within the brain tissue that have abnormally high water content, such as tumors, inflammation, or strokes, appear brighter on T2 images. T2 images reveal brain pathology most clearly. The third routine pulse sequence is the proton density, or balanced, sequence. In this sequence, a short radio pulse is followed by a prolonged period of data collection, which equalizes the density of the CSF and the brain and allows distinction of tissue changes immediately adjacent to the ventricles.

An additional technique, sometimes used in clinical practice for specific indications, is fluid-attenuated inversion recovery (FLAIR). In this method, the T1 image is inverted and added to the T2 image to double the contrast between gray matter and white matter. Inversion recovery imaging is useful for detecting sclerosis of the hippocampus caused by temporal lobe epilepsy and for localizing areas of abnormal metabolism in degenerative neurological disorders.

MRI magnets are rated in teslas (T), units of magnetic field strength. MRI scanners in clinical use range from 0.3 to 2.0 T. Higher field-strength scanners produce images of markedly higher resolution. In research settings for humans, magnets as powerful as 4.7 T are used; for animals, magnets up to 12 T are used. Unlike the well-known hazards of X-irradiation, exposure to electromagnetic fields of the strength used in MRI machines has not been shown to damage biological tissues.

MRI scans cannot be used for patients with pacemakers or implants of ferromagnetic metals. MRI involves enclosing a patient in a narrow tube, in which the patient must remain motionless for up to 20 minutes. The radiofrequency pulses create a loud banging noise that may be obscured by music played in headphones. A significant number of patients cannot tolerate the claustrophobic conditions of routine MRI scanners and may need an open MRI scanner, which has less power and thus produces images of lower resolution. The resolution of brain tissue of even the lowest power MRI scan, however, exceeds that of CT scanning. Figure 3.3–3 reveals that a brain tumor is the cause of a patient's depression.

Magnetic Resonance Spectroscopy (MRS)

Whereas routine MRI detects hydrogen nuclei to determine brain structure, MRS can detect several odd-numbered nuclei (Table 3.3–1). The ability of MRS to detect a wide range of biologically important nuclei permits the use of the technique to study many metabolic processes. Although the resolution and sensitivity of MRS machines are poor compared with those of currently available PET and SPECT devices, the use of stronger magnetic fields will improve this feature to some extent in the future.

MRS can image nuclei with an odd number of protons and neutrons. The unpaired protons and neutrons (nucleons) appear naturally and are nonradioactive. As in MRI, the nuclei align themselves in the strong magnetic field produced by an MRS device. A radiofrequency pulse causes the nuclei of interest to absorb and then emit energy. The readout of an MRS device is

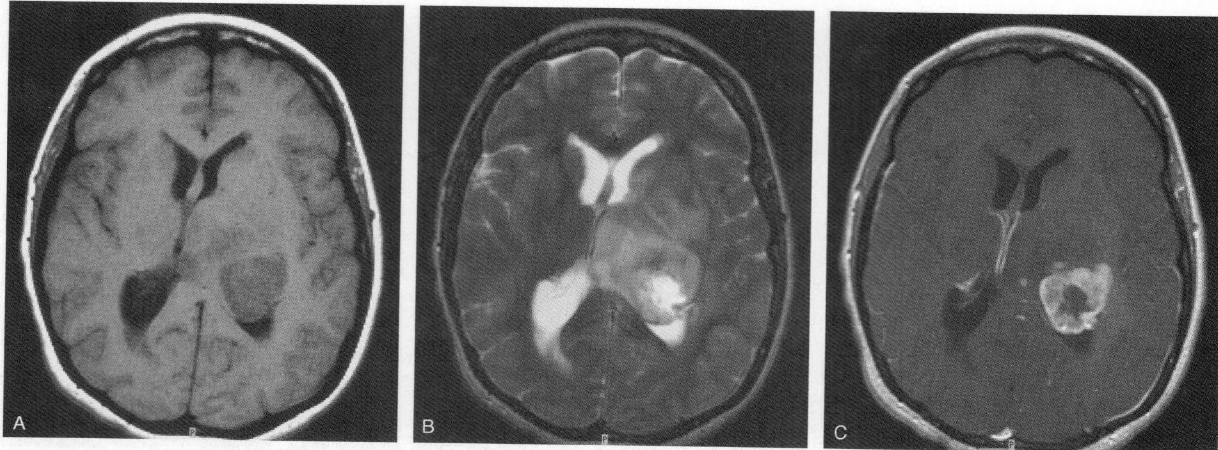

FIGURE 3.3–3

Three axial images from a 46-year-old woman who was hospitalized for the first time for depression and suicidality following the end of a long-standing relationship. A malignant neoplasm extending into the posterior aspect of the left lateral ventricle is clearly seen in all three images. Images **A** and **B** are T1- and T2-weighted, respectively. Image **C** demonstrates the effects of postcontrast enhancement. (Courtesy of Craig N. Carson, M.D., and Perry F. Renshaw, M.D.)

usually in the form of a spectrum, such as those for phosphorus-31 and hydrogen-1 nuclei, although the spectrum can also be converted into a pictorial image of the brain. The multiple peaks for each nucleus reflect that the same nucleus is exposed to different electron environments (electron clouds) in different molecules. The hydrogen-1 nuclei in a molecule of creatine, therefore, have a different chemical shift (position in the spectrum) than the hydrogen-1 nuclei in a choline molecule, for example. Thus, the position in the spectrum (the chemical shift) indicates the identity of the molecule in which the nuclei are present. The height of the peak with respect to a reference standard of the molecule indicates the amount of the molecule present.

The MRS of the hydrogen-1 nuclei is best at measuring N-acetylaspartate (NAA), creatine, and choline-containing molecules; but MRS can also detect glutamate, glutamine, lactate, and myo-inositol. Although glutamate and γ-aminobutyric acid (GABA), the major amino acid neurotransmitters, can be detected by MRS, the biogenic amine neurotransmitters (e.g., dopamine) are present in concentrations too low to be detected with the technique. MRS of phosphorus-31 can be used to determine the pH of brain regions and the concentrations of phosphorus-containing compounds (e.g., adenosine triphosphate [ATP] and guanosine triphosphate [GTP]), which are important in the energy metabolism of the brain.

MRS has revealed decreased concentrations of NAA in the temporal lobes and increased concentrations of inositol in the occipital lobes of persons with dementia of the Alzheimer's type. In a series of subjects with schizophrenia, decreased NAA concentrations were found in the temporal and frontal lobes. MRS has been used to trace the levels of ethanol in various brain regions. In panic disorder, MRS has been used to record the levels of lactate, whose intravenous infusion can precipitate panic episodes in about three fourths of patients with either panic disorder or major depression. Brain lactate concentrations were found to be elevated during panic attacks, even without provocative infusion.

Additional indications include the use of MRS to measure concentrations of psychotherapeutic drugs in the brain. One study used MRS to measure lithium concentrations in the brains of patients with bipolar disorder and found that lithium concentrations in the brain were half those in the plasma during depressed and euthymic periods but exceeded those in the plasma during manic episodes. Some compounds, such as fluoxetine and trifluoperazine (Stelazine), contain fluorine-19, which can also be detected in the brain and measured by MRS. For example, MRS has demonstrated that it takes 6 months of steady use for fluoxetine to reach maximal concentrations in the brain, which equilibrate at about 20 times the serum concentrations.

Functional Magnetic Resonance Imaging (fMRI)

Recent advances in data collection and computer data processing have reduced the acquisition time for an MRI image to less than 1 second. A new sequence of particular interest to psychiatrists is the T2, or blood oxygen level-dependent (BOLD) sequence, which detects levels of oxygenated hemoglobin in the blood. Neuronal activity within the brain causes a local increase in blood flow, which in turn increases the local hemoglobin concentration. Although neuronal metabolism extracts more oxygen in active areas of the brain, the net effect of neuronal activity is to increase the local amount of oxygenated hemoglobin. This change can be detected essentially in real time with the T2 sequence, which thus detects the functionally active brain regions. This process is the basis for the technique of fMRI.

What fMRI detects is not brain activity per se, but blood flow. The volume of brain in which blood flow increases exceeds the volume of activated neurons by about 1 to 2 cm and limits the resolution of the technique. Sensitivity and resolution can be improved with the use of nontoxic, ultrasmall iron oxide particles. Thus, two tasks that activate clusters of neurons 5 mm apart, such as recognizing two different faces, yield overlapping signals on fMRI and so are usually indistinguishable by this technique. Functional MRI is useful to localize neuronal activity to a particular lobe or subcortical nucleus and has even been able to localize activity to a single gyrus. The method detects tissue perfusion, not neuronal metabolism. In contrast, PET scanning may give information specifically about neuronal metabolism.

No radioactive isotopes are administered in fMRI, a great advantage over PET and SPECT. A subject can perform a variety of tasks, both experimental and control, in the same imaging session. First, a routine T1

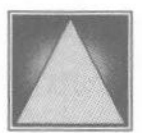

Table 3.3–1
Nuclei Available for In Vivo Magnetic Resonance Spectroscopy (MRS)[a]

Nucleus	Natural Abundance	Relative Sensitivity	Potential Clinical Uses
^{1}H	99.99	1.00	Magnetic resonance imaging (MRI) Analysis of metabolism Identification of unusual metabolites Characterization of hypoxia
^{19}F	100.00	0.83	Measurement of pO_2 Analysis of glucose metabolism Measurement of pH Noninvasive pharmacokinetics
^{7}Li	92.58	0.27	Pharmacokinetics
^{23}Na	100.00	0.09	MRI
^{31}P	100.00	0.07	Analysis of bioenergetics Identification of unusual metabolites Characterization of hypoxia Measurement of pH
^{14}N	93.08	0.001	Measurement of glutamate, urea, ammonia
^{39}K	93.08	0.0005	?
^{13}C	1.11	0.0002	Analysis of metabolite turnover rate Pharmacokinetics of labeled drugs
^{17}O	0.04	0.00001	Measurement of metabolic rate
^{2}H	0.02	0.000002	Measurement of perfusion

[a] Natural abundance is given as percentage abundance of the isotope of interest. Nuclei are tabulated in order of decreasing relative sensitivity; relative sensitivity is calculated by multiplying the relative sensitivity for equal numbers of nuclei (at a given field strength) by the natural abundance of that nucleus. A considerable gain in relative sensitivity can be obtained by isotopic enrichment of the nucleus of choice or by the use of novel pulse sequences.

(Reprinted from Dager SR, Steen RG. Applications of magnetic resonance spectroscopy to the investigation of neuropsychiatric disorders. *Neuropsychopharmacology.* 1992;6:249, with permission.)

MRI image is obtained; then the T2 images are superimposed to allow more precise localization. Acquisition of sufficient images for study can require 20 minutes to 3 hours, during which time the subject's head must remain in exactly the same position. Several methods, including a frame around the head and a special mouthpiece, have been used. Although realignments of images can correct for some head movement, small changes in head position may lead to erroneous interpretations of brain activation.

Functional MRI has recently revealed unexpected details about the organization of language within the brain. Using a series of language tasks requiring semantic, phonemic, and rhyming discrimination, one study found that rhyming (but not other types of language processing) produced a different pattern of activation in men and women. Rhyming activated the inferior frontal gyrus bilaterally in women, but only on the left in men. In another study, fMRI revealed a previously suspected, but unproved, neural circuit for lexical categories, interpolated between the representations for concepts and those for phonemes. This novel circuit was located in the left anterior temporal lobe. Data from patients with dyslexia (reading disorder) doing simple rhyming tasks demonstrated a failure to activate Wernicke's area and the insula, which were active in normal subjects doing the same task (*see* Color Plate 3.3–4 on p. 82).

Sensory functions have also been mapped in detail with fMRI. The activation of the visual and auditory cortices has been visualized in real time. In a recent intriguing study, the areas that were activated while a subject with schizophrenia listened to speech were also activated during auditory hallucinations. These areas included the primary auditory cortex as well as higher-order auditory processing regions. fMRI is the imaging technique most widely used to study brain abnormality related to cognitive dysfunction.

Single Photon Emission Computed Tomography (SPECT) Scanning

Manufactured radioactive compounds are used in SPECT to study regional differences in cerebral blood flow within the brain. This high-resolution imaging technique records the pattern of photon emission from the bloodstream according to the level of perfusion in different regions of the brain. As with fMRI, it provides information on the cerebral blood flow, which is highly correlated with the rate of glucose metabolism, but does not measure neuronal metabolism directly.

SPECT uses compounds labeled with single photon-emitting isotopes: iodine-123, technetium-99m, and xenon-133. Xenon-133 is a noble gas that is inhaled directly. The xenon quickly enters the blood and is distributed to areas of the brain as a function of regional blood flow. Xenon-SPECT is thus referred to as the *regional cerebral blood flow* (*rCBF*) *technique*. For technical reasons, xenon-SPECT can measure blood flow only on the surface of the brain, which is an important limitation. Many mental tasks require communication between the cortex and subcortical structures, and this activity is poorly measured by xenon-SPECT.

Assessment of blood flow over the whole brain with SPECT requires the injectable tracers, technetium-99m-*d*,*l*-hexamethylpropyleneamine oxime (HMPAO [Ceretec]) or iodoamphetamine [Spectamine]). These isotopes are attached to molecules that are highly lipophilic and rapidly cross the blood-brain barrier and enter cells. Once inside the cell, the ligands are enzymatically converted to charged ions, which remain trapped in the cell. Thus, over time, the tracers are concentrated in areas of relatively higher blood flow. Although blood flow is usually assumed to be the major variable tested in HMPAO SPECT, local variations in the permeability of the blood-brain barrier and in the enzymatic conversion of the ligands within cells also contribute to regional differences in signal levels.

In addition to these compounds used for measuring blood flow, iodine-123 (^{123}I)-labeled ligands for the muscarinic, dopaminergic, and serotonergic receptors, for example, can be used to study these receptors by SPECT technology. Once photon-emitting compounds reach the brain, detectors surrounding the patient's head pick up their light emissions. This information is relayed to a computer, which constructs a two-dimensional image of the isotope's distribution within a slice of the brain. A key difference between SPECT and PET is that in SPECT a single particle is emitted, whereas in PET two particles are emitted; the latter reaction gives a more precise location for the event and better resolution of the image. Increasingly, for both SPECT and PET studies, investigators are performing prestudy MRI or CT studies, then superimposing the SPECT or PET image on the MRI or CT image to obtain a more accurate anatomical location for the functional information (*see* Color Plate 3.3–5 on p. 82). SPECT is useful in diagnosing decreased or blocked cerebral blood flow in stroke victims. Some workers have described abnormal flow patterns in the early stage of Alzheimer's disease that may aid in early diagnosis.

Positron Emission Tomography (PET) Scanning

The isotopes used in PET decay by emitting positrons, antimatter particles that bind with and annihilate electrons, thereby giving off photons that travel in 180-degree opposite directions. Because detectors have twice as much signal from which to generate an image as SPECT scanners have, the resolution of the PET image is higher. A wide range of compounds can be used in PET studies, and the resolution of PET continues to be refined closer to its theoretical minimum of 3 mm, which is the distance positrons move before colliding with an electron. Relatively few PET scanners are available because they require an on-site cyclotron to make the isotopes.

The most commonly used isotopes in PET are fluorine-18, nitrogen-13, and oxygen-15. These isotopes are usually linked to another molecule, except in the case of oxygen-15 (^{15}O). The most commonly reported ligand has been [^{18}F]fluorodeoxyglucose (FDG), an analogue of glucose that the brain cannot metabolize. Thus, the brain regions with the highest metabolic rate and the highest blood flow take up the most FDG but cannot metabolize and excrete the usual metabolic products. The concentration of ^{18}F builds up in these neurons and is detected by the PET camera. Water-15 ($H_2{}^{15}O$) and nitrogen-13 (^{13}N) are used to measure blood flow, and oxygen-15 (^{15}O) can be used to determine metabolic rate. Glucose is by far the predominant energy source available to brain cells, and its use is thus a highly sensitive indicator of the rate of brain metabolism. [^{18}F]-labeled 3,4-dihydroxyphenylalanine (DOPA), the fluorinated precursor to dopamine, has been used to localize dopaminergic neurons.

PET has been used increasingly to study normal brain development and function as well as to study neuropsychiatric disorders. With regard to brain development, PET studies have found that glucose use is greatest in the sensorimotor cortex, thalamus, brainstem, and cerebellar vermis when an infant is 5 weeks of age or younger. By 3 months of age, most areas of the cortex show increased use, except for the frontal and association cortices, which do not begin to exhibit an increase until the infant is 8 months of age. An adult pattern of glucose metabolism is achieved by the age of 1 year, but use in the cortex continues to rise above adult levels until the child is about 9 years of age, when use in the cortex begins to decrease and reaches its final adult level in the late teen years. In another study, subjects listened to a rapidly presented list of thematically related words. When asked to recall words in the thematic category that may or may not have been on the list, some subjects falsely recalled that they had heard words that were actually not on the list. By PET scanning, the hippocampus was active during both true and false recollections, whereas the auditory cortex was only active during recollection of words that were actually heard. When pressed to determine whether memories were true or false, subjects activated the frontal lobes. FDG studies have also investigated pathology in neurological disorders and psychiatric disorders (*see* Color Plate 3.3–6 on p. 83). Two other types of studies use precursor molecules and receptor ligands. The dopamine precursor dopa has been used to visualize pathology in patients with Parkinson's disease, and radiolabeled ligands for receptors have been useful in determining the occupancy of receptors by specific psychotherapeutic drugs (*see* Color Plate 3.3–7 on p. 83). Neurochemical findings from PET radiotracer scan are listed in Table 3.3–2.

For example, dopamine receptor antagonists such as haloperidol (Haldol) block almost 100 percent of D_2 receptors. The atypical antipsychotic drugs block serotonin 5-HT_2 receptors in addition to D_2 receptors; hence they are referred to as *serotonin-dopamine receptor antagonists*.

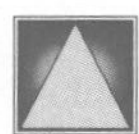

Table 3.3–2
Neurochemical Findings from PET Radiotracer Scans

Dopamine	Decreased uptake of dopamine in striatum in parkinsonian patients Dopamine release is higher in patients with schizophrenia than in controls. High dopamine release associated with positive symptoms in schizophrenia.
Receptors	
▸ D_1 receptor	Lower D_1 receptor binding in prefrontal cortex of patients with schizophrenia compared with controls; correlates with negative symptoms
▸ D_2 receptor	Schizophrenia associated with small elevations of binding at D_2 receptor
▸ Serotonin Type 1A (5-HT_{1A})	Reduction in receptor binding in patients with unipolar major depression
Transporters	
▸ Dopamine	Amphetamine and cocaine cause increase in dopamine. Tourette's syndrome shows increase in dopamine transporter system (may account for success of dopamine blocking therapies).
▸ Serotonin	Serotonin binding is low in depression, alcoholism, cocainism, binge eating, and impulse control disorders.
Metabolism	
▸ Nicotine	Cigarette smoking inhibits MAO activity in brain.
▸ Amyloid-β Deposits	Can be visualized in vivo with PET.
Pharmacology	Plasma levels of cocaine peak at 2 min. D_2 receptor occupancy lasts for several weeks after discontinuation of antipsychotic medication. D_2 receptor occupancy is lower for atypical antipsychotics than typical antipsychotics (may account for decrease in extrapyramidal side effects). Low doses (10–20 mg) of selective serotonin reuptake inhibitors (SSRIs) cause occupancy of up to 90 percent of serotonin receptors.

The following case illustrates the potential diagnostic value of three-dimensional PET imaging.

> Patient A is a 70-year-old man who had gotten more forgetful, to the point that his family was worried about him. The patient's family was interested in getting a diagnostic workup to evaluate the possible causes for his memory disorder. His PET scan showed that he had functional parietotemporal decrease (*see* Color Plate 3.3–8 on p. 83), which corroborated other neurological evaluations suggesting that he had Alzheimer's disease. The patient was treated with tacrine (Cognex) and benefited from some stabilization of his symptoms. (Courtesy of Joseph C. Wu, M.D., Daniel G. Amen, M.D., and H. Stefan Bracha, M.D.)

Pharmacological and Neuropsychological Probes

With both PET and SPECT and eventually with MRS, more studies and possibly more diagnostic procedures will use pharmacological and neuropsychological probes. The purpose of such probes is to stimulate particular regions of brain activity, so that, when compared with a baseline, workers can reach conclusions about the functional correspondence to particular brain regions. One example of the approach is the use of PET to detect regions of the brain involved in the processing of shape, color, and velocity in the visual system. Another example is the use of cognitive activation tasks (e.g., the Wisconsin Card Sorting Test) to study frontal blood flow in patients with schizophrenia. A key consideration in the evaluation of reports that measure blood flow is the establishment of a true baseline value in the study design. Typically, the reports use an awake, resting state, but there is variability in whether the patients have their eyes closed or their ears blocked; both conditions can affect brain function. There is also variability in such baseline brain function factors as gender, age, anxiety about the test, nonpsychiatric drug treatment, vasoactive medications, and time of day.

References

Boguski MS, McIntosh MW. Biomedical informatics for proteomics. *Nature*. 2003;422:233.

Botstein D, Risch N. Discovering genotypes underlying human phenotypes: past successes for mendelian disease, future approaches for complex disease. *Nat Genet*. 2003;33[Suppl]:228.

Carlson CS, Eberle MA, Rieder MJ, Smith JD, Kruglyak L, Nickerson DA. Additional SNPs and linkage-disequilibrium analyses are necessary for whole-genome association studies in humans. *Nat Genet*. 2003;33:518.

Démonet JF, Thierry G, Cardebat D. Renewal of the neurophysiology of language: Functional neuroimaging. *Physiol Rev*. 2005;85:49–95.

Friston KJ. Models of brain function in neuroimaging. *Annual Review of Psychology*. 2005;56:57–87.

Henson R. What can functional neuroimaging tell the experimental psychologist? *The Quarterly Journal of Experimental Psychology: Section A*. 2005;58(2): 193–233.

Kelly AMC, Garavan H. Human functional neuroimaging of brain changes associated with practice. *Cereb Cortex*. 2005;15(8):1089–1102.

Mathews CA, Freimer NB. Genetic linkage analysis of the psychiatric disorders. In: Sadock BJ, Sadock VA, eds. *Kaplan & Sadock's Comprehensive Textbook of Psychiatry*. 8th ed. Vol. 1. Baltimore: Lippincott Williams & Wilkins; 2005:252.

Matise TC, Sachidanandam R, Clark AG, Kruglyak L, Wijsman E, Kakol J, Buyske S, Chui B, Cohen P, de Toma C, Ehm M, Glanowski S, He C, Heil J, Markianos K, McMullen I, Pericak-Vance MA, Silbergleit A, Stein L, Wagner M, Wilson AF, Winick JD, Winn-Deen ES, Yamashiro CT, Cann HM, Lai E, Holden AL. A 3.9-centimorgan-resolution human single-nucleotide polymorphism linkage map and screening set. *Am J Hum Genet*. 2003;73:271.

Moldin SO. Population genetics and genetic epidemiology. In: Sadock BJ, Sadock VA, eds. *Kaplan & Sadock's Comprehensive Textbook of Psychiatry*. 8th ed. Vol. 1. Baltimore: Lippincott Williams & Wilkins; 2005:236.

Moldin SO, Hyman SE. Genome, transcriptome, and proteome. In: Sadock BJ, Sadock VA, eds. *Kaplan & Sadock's Comprehensive Textbook of Psychiatry*. 8th ed. Vol. 1. Baltimore: Lippincott Williams & Wilkins; 2005:115.

Muñoz-Cespedes JM, Rios-Lago M, Paul N, Maestu F. Functional neuroimaging studies of cognitive recovery after acquired brain damage in adults. *Neuropsychol Rev*. 2005;15(4):169–183.

Pike B. What does fMRI measure: Bold and beyond. *J Clin Neurophysiol*. 2005; 22(5):372.

Strangman G, O'Neil-Pirozzi TM, Burke D, Cristina D, Goldstein R, Rauch SL, Savage CR, Glenn MB. Functional neuroimaging and cognitive rehabilitation for people with traumatic brain injury. *Am J Phys Med Rehabil*. 2005;84:62–75.

Zivadinov R, Leist TP. Clinical–magnetic resonance imaging correlations in Multiple Sclerosis. *J Neuroimaging*. 2005;15[4 Suppl]:10S–21S.

▲ 3.4 Electrophysiology

Electroencephalography (EEG) is the recording of the electrical activity of the brain. It is used in clinical psychiatry principally to evaluate the presence of seizures, particularly temporal lobe, frontal lobe, and petit mal seizures which can produce complex behaviors. The EEG is also used during electroconvulsive therapy (ECT) to monitor the success of the stimulus in producing seizure activity, and as a key component of the polysomnogram used in the evaluation of sleep disorders. Quantitative electroencephalography (QEEG) and cerebral evoked potentials (EP) represent newer EEG-based methods that provide improved research and clinical insights into brain functioning.

ELECTROENCEPHALOGRAPHY

A brain wave is the transient difference in electrical potential (greatly amplified) between any two points on the scalp or between some electrode placed on the scalp and a reference electrode located elsewhere on the head (i.e., ear lobe or nose). The difference in electrical potential measured between any two EEG electrodes fluctuates or oscillates rapidly, usually many times per second. It is this oscillation that produces the characteristic "squiggly line" that is recognized as the appearance of "brain waves."

Brain waves reflect change by becoming faster or slower in frequency or lower or higher in voltage, or perhaps some combination of these two responses. A normal EEG can never constitute positive proof of absence of brain dysfunction. Even in diseases with established brain pathophysiology, such as multiple sclerosis, deep subcortical neoplasm, some seizure disorders, and Parkinson's disease and other movement disorders, a substantial incidence of patients with normal EEGs may be encountered. Nonetheless, a normal EEG can often provide convincing evidence for excluding certain types of brain pathology that may present with behavioral or psychiatric symptoms. More often, information from the patient's symptoms, clinical course and history, and other laboratory results identifies a probable cause for the EEG findings. EEGs are often ordered when a pathophysiological process is already suspected or a patient experiences a sudden, unexplained change in mental status.

Electrode Placement

The electrodes normally used to record the EEG are attached to the scalp with a conductive paste. A standard array consists of 21 electrodes. Placement of the electrodes is based on the 10/20 International System of Electrode Placement. This system measures the distance between readily identifiable landmarks on the head and then locates electrode positions at 10 percent or 20 percent of that distance in an anterior-posterior or transverse direction. Electrodes are then designated by an uppercase letter denoting the brain region beneath that electrode and a number, with odd numbers used for the left hemisphere and with even numbers signifying the right hemisphere (the subscript Z denotes midline electrodes). Thus, the O_2 electrode is placed over the right occipital region, and the P_3 lead is found over the left parietal area.

In special circumstances, other electrodes may be used. Nasopharyngeal (NP) electrodes can be inserted into the NP space through the nostrils and can be closer to the temporal lobe than scalp electrodes. No actual penetration of tissue occurs. These electrodes may be contraindicated with many psychiatric patients displaying behaviors, such as confusion, agitation, or belligerence, which could pull the leads out, possibly lacerating the nasal passage. Sphenoidal electrodes use a hollow needle through which a fine electrode that is insulated, except at the tip, is inserted between the zygoma and the sigmoid notch in the mandible, until it is in contact with the base of the skull lateral to the foramen ovale.

Activated EEG

Certain activating procedures are used to increase the probability that abnormal discharges, particularly spike or spike-wave seizure discharges, will occur. Strenuous hyperventilation is one of the most frequently used activation procedures. While remaining reclined with the eyes closed, the patient is asked to overbreathe through the open mouth with deep breaths for 1 to 4 minutes, depending on the laboratory (3 minutes is common). In general, hyperventilation is one of the safest EEG activating procedures, and, for most of the population, it presents no physical risk. It can pose a risk for patients with cardiopulmonary disease or risk factors for cerebral vascular pathophysiology, however. Photic stimulation (PS) generally involves placing an intense strobe light approximately 12 inches in front of the subject's closed eyes and flashing at frequencies that can range from 1 to 50 Hz, depending on how the procedure is carried out. Retinal damage does not occur, because each strobe flash, although intense, is extremely brief in duration. When the resting EEG is normal, and a seizure disorder or behavior that is suspected to be a manifestation of a paroxysmal EEG dysrhythmia is suspected, PS can be a valuable activation to use. EEG recording during sleep, natural or sedated, is now widely accepted as an essential technique for eliciting a variety of paroxysmal discharges, when the wake tracing is normal, or for increasing the number of abnormal discharges to permit a more definitive interpretation to be made. It has been shown that the central nervous system (CNS) stress produced by 24 hours of sleep deprivation alone can lead to the activation of paroxysmal EEG discharges in some cases.

NORMAL EEG TRACING

The normal EEG tracing (Fig. 3.4–1) is composed of a complex mixture of many different frequencies. Discrete frequency bands within the broad EEG frequency spectrum are designated with Greek letters.

Awake EEG

The four basic wave forms are alpha, beta, delta, and theta. Highly rhythmic *alpha waves* with a frequency range of 8 to 13 Hz constitute the dominant brain wave frequency of the normal eyes-closed wake EEG. Alpha frequency can be increased or decreased by a wide variety of pharmacological, metabolic, or endocrine variables. Frequencies that are faster than the upper 13 Hz limit of the alpha rhythm are termed *beta waves*, and they are not uncommon in normal adult waking EEGs, particularly over frontal-central regions. *Delta waves* ($\leq$3.5 Hz) are not present in the normal waking EEG but are a prominent feature of deeper stages of sleep. The presence of significant generalized or focal delta waves in the wake EEG is strongly indicative of a pathophysiological process. Waves with a frequency of 4.0 to

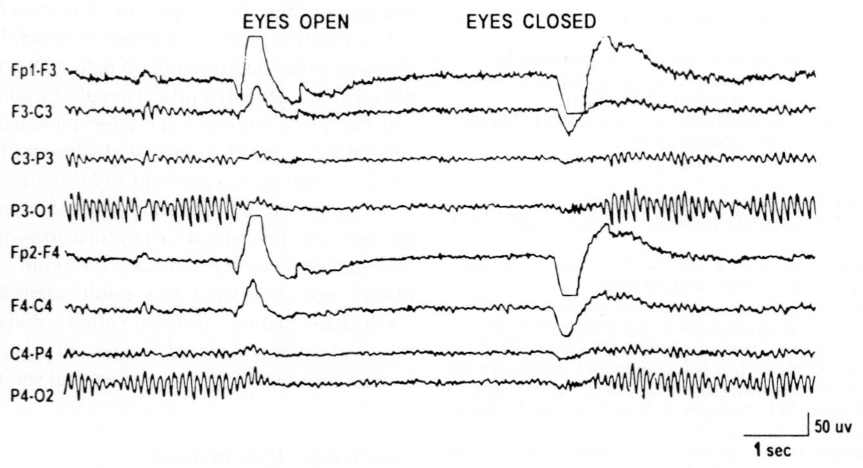

FIGURE 3.4–1

Normal electroencephalogram (EEG) tracings in an awake 28-year-old man. (Reprinted from Emerson RG, Walesak TS, Turner CA. EEG and evoked potentials. In: Rowland LP, ed. *Merritt's Textbook of Neurology*. 9th ed. Baltimore: Lippincott Williams & Wilkins; 1995:68, with permission.)

7.5 Hz are collectively referred to as *theta waves*. A small amount of sporadic, arrhythmic, and isolated theta activity can be seen in many normal waking EEGs, particularly in frontal-temporal regions. Although theta activity is limited in the waking EEG, it is a prominent feature of the drowsy and sleep tracing. Excessive theta in wake, generalized or focal in nature, suggests the operation of a pathological process.

With maturation, EEG activity gradually goes from a preponderance of irregular medium- to high-voltage delta activity in the tracing of the infant, to greater frequency and more rhythmic pattern. Rhythmic activity in the upper theta–lower alpha range (7 to 8 Hz) can be seen in posterior areas by early childhood, and, by the time mid-adolescence is reached, the EEG essentially has the appearance of an adult tracing.

Sleep EEG

The EEG patterns that characterize drowsy and sleep states are different from the patterns seen during wake state. The rhythmic posterior alpha activity of the waking state subsides during drowsiness and is replaced by irregular low-voltage theta activity. As drowsiness deepens, slower frequencies emerge, and sporadic vertex sharp waves may appear at central electrode sites, particularly among younger persons. Finally, the progression into sleep is marked by the appearance of 14-Hz sleep spindles (also called *sigma waves*), which, in turn, gradually become replaced by high-voltage delta waves as deep sleep stages are reached.

EEG Abnormalities

Apart from some of the obvious indications for an EEG study (i.e., suspected seizures), EEGs are not routinely performed as part of a diagnostic work-up in psychiatry. EEG, however, is a valuable assessment tool in clinical situations in which the initial presentation or the clinical course appear to be unusual or atypical (Table 3.4–1). Table 3.4–2 summarizes some common types of EEG abnormalities.

Some psychotropic medications and recreational or abused drugs produce EEG changes, yet, with the exception of the benzodiazepines and some compounds with a propensity to induce paroxysmal EEG discharges, little, if any, clinically relevant effect is noted when the medication is not causing any toxicity. Benzodiazepines, which always generate a significant amount of diffuse beta activity, have EEG-protective effects, so that they can mask alterations caused by concomitant medications (Table 3.4–3).

Medical and neurological conditions produce a wide range of abnormal EEG findings. EEGs, thus, can contribute to the detection of unsuspected organic pathophysiology influencing a psychiatric presentation (Fig. 3.4–2). Table 3.4–4 lists EEG

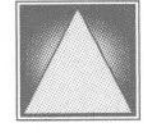

Table 3.4–1
Warning Signs of the Presence of Covert Medical or Organic Factors Causing or Contributing to Psychiatric Presentation

Atypical age of onset (i.e., anorexia nervosa beginning at mid-adulthood)
Complete lack of positive family history of the disorder when a positive family history is expected
Any focal or localized symptoms (i.e., unilateral hallucinations)
Focal neurological abnormalities
Catatonia
Presence of any difficulty with orientation or memory (in general, Mini Mental State Examination should be normal)
Atypical response to treatment
Atypical clinical course

Note: Clinicians should have a high index of suspicion for underlying medical conditions and a low threshold for initiating appropriate workups.

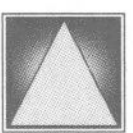

Table 3.4–2
Common Electroencephalogram (EEG) Abnormalities

Diffuse slowing of background rhythms	Most common EEG abnormality; nonspecific and is present in patients with diffuse encephalopathies of diverse causes
Focal slowing	Suggests localized parenchymal dysfunction and focal seizure disorder; seen with focal fluid collection, such hematomas
Triphasic waves	Typically consist of generalized synchronous waves occurring in brief runs; approximately one half the patients with triphasic waves have hepatic encephalopathy, and the remainder have other toxic-metabolic encephalopathies
Epileptiform discharges	Interictal hallmark of epilepsy; strongly associated with seizure disorders
Periodic lateralizing epilptiform discharges	Suggest the presence of an acute destructive cerebral lesion; associated with seizures, obtundation, and focal neurological signs
Generalized periodic sharp waves	Most commonly seen following cerebral anoxia; recorded in about 90% of patients with Creutzfeldt-Jakob disease

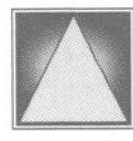

Table 3.4–3
Electroencephalogram (EEG) Alterations Associated with Medication and Drugs

Drug	Alterations
Benzodiazepines	Increased beta activity
Clozapine (Clozaril)	Nonspecific change
Olanzapine (Zyprexa)	Nonspecific change
Risperidone (Risperdal)	Nonspecific change
Quetiapine (Seroquel)	No significant changes
Aripiprazole (Abilify)	No significant changes
Lithium	Slowing or paroxysmal activity
Alcohol	Decreased alpha activity; increased theta activity
Opioids	Decreased alpha activity; increased voltage of theta and delta waves; in overdose, slow waves
Barbiturates	Increased beta activity; in withdrawal states, generalized paroxysmal activity and spike discharges
Marijuana	Increased alpha activity in frontal area of brain; overall slow alpha activity
Cocaine	Similar to marijuana
Inhalants	Diffuse slowing of delta and theta waves
Nicotine	Increased alpha activity; in withdrawal, marked decrease in alpha activity
Caffeine	In withdrawal, increase in amplitude or voltage of theta activity

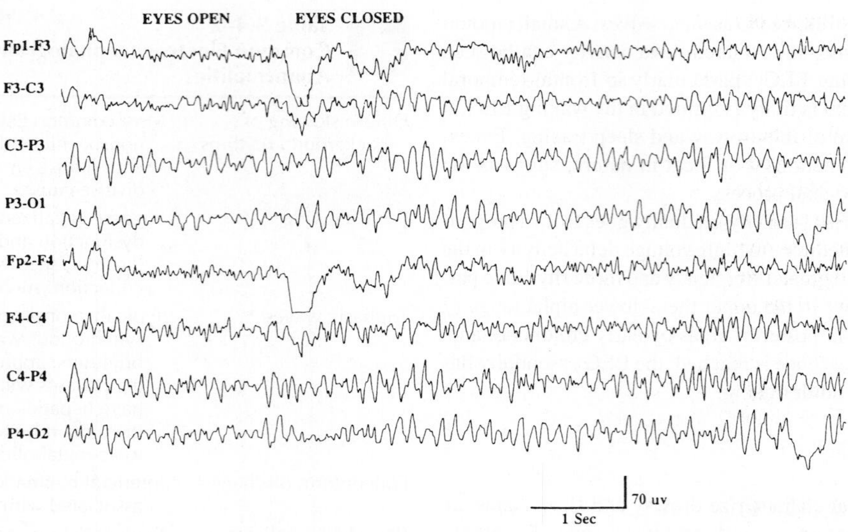

FIGURE 3.4–2
Diffuse slowing in a 67-year-old patient with dementia. Six- to seven-cps activity predominates over the parieto-occipital regions. Although reactive to eye closure, the frequency of this rhythm is abnormally slow. (Reprinted from Emerson RG, Walesak TS, Turner CA. EEG and evoked potentials. In: Rowland LP, ed. *Merritt's Textbook of Neurology*. 9th ed. Baltimore: Lippincott Williams & Wilkins. 1995:68, with permission.)

alterations in medical disorders and Table 3.4–5 lists EEG alterations associated with psychiatric disorders.

TOPOGRAPHIC QUANTITATIVE ELECTROENCEPHALOGRAPHY (QEEG)

Unlike standard EEG interpretation, which relies on waveform recognition, QEEG involves a computer analysis of data extracted from the EEG. Findings are compared with a large population database of subjects without any known neurological or psychiatric disorder as well as QEEG profiles that may be characteristic of some defined diagnostic group. In QEEG, the analogue-based electrical signals are processed digitally and converted to graphic, colored topographical displays. These images are sometimes called "brain maps." Figure 3.4–3 illustrates topographic QEEG images of patients with psychiatric disorders (see Color Plate 3.4–3 on p. 84).

QEEG remains primarily a research method, but it holds considerable clinical potential for psychiatry, mainly in establishing

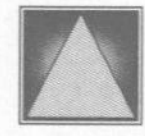

Table 3.4–4
Electroencephalogram (EEG) Alterations Associated with Medical Disorders

Seizures	Generalized, hemispheric, or focal spike, spike-wave discharge, or both
Structural lesions	Focal slowing, with possible focal spike activity
Closed head injuries	Focal slowing (sharply focal head trauma)
	Focal delta slowing or more widespread slowing (subdural hematomas)
Infectious disorders	Diffuse, often synchronous, high voltage slowing (acute phase of encephalitis)
Metabolic and endocrine disorders	Diffuse generalized slowing of wake frequencies
	Triphasic waves: 1.5 to 3.0 per second high-voltage slow-waves, with each slow wave initiated by a blunt or rounded spike-like transient (hepatic encephalopathy)
Vascular pathophysiology	Slowed alpha frequency and increased generalized theta slowing (diffuse atherosclerosis)
	Focal or regional delta activity (cerebrovascular accidents)

Table 3.4–5
Electroencephalogram (EEG) Alterations Associated with Psychiatric Disorders

Panic disorder	Paroxysmal EEG changes consistent with partial seizure activity during attack in one third of patients; focal slowing in about 25% of patients
Catatonia	Usually normal, but EEG indicated in new patient presenting with catatonia to rule out other causes
Attention-deficit/hyperactivity disorder (ADHD)	High prevalence (up to 60%) of EEG abnormalities versus normal controls; spike or spike-wave discharges
Antisocial personality disorder	Increased incidence of EEG abnormalities in those with aggressive behavior
Borderline personality disorder	Positive spikes: 14- and 6 per second seen in 25% of patients
Chronic alcoholism	Prominent slowing and periodic lateralized paroxysmal discharges
Alcohol withdrawal	May be normal in patients who are not delirious; excessive fast activity in patients with delirium
Dementia	Rarely normal in advanced dementia; may be helpful in differentiating pseudodementia from dementia

neurophysiological subtypes of specific disorders and for identifying electrophysiological predictors of response. Examples of some of the more promising results of QEEG research include the identification of subtypes of cocaine dependence and the subtype most likely to be associated with sustained abstinence; identification of subtypes of obsessive–compulsive disorder (OCD) that predict clinical responsiveness or lack of responsiveness to selective serotonin reuptake inhibitors (SSRIs); and the differentiation between normals, attention–deficit disorder and attention-deficit/hyperactivity disorder (ADHD), and learning disability subpopulations. QEEG findings in ADHD show that increased theta abnormality frontally may be a strong predictor of response to methylphenidate and other psychostimulants and that favorable clinical responses may be associated with a normalization of the EEG abnormality.

CEREBRAL EVOKED POTENTIALS

Cerebral EPs are a series of surface (scalp) recordable waves that result from brain visual, auditory, somatosensory, and cognitive stimulation. They have been shown to be abnormal in many psychiatric conditions, including schizophrenia and Alzheimer's disease, thus creating difficulty in using cerebral EPs for differential diagnosis purposes.

References

Boutros NN, Mirolo HA, Struve FA. Normal analog EEG in neuropsychiatry: Examination of adequacy for neuropsychiatric research. *J Neuropsychiatry Clin Neurosci.* 2005;17:84.

Boutros NN, Struve FA. Applied electrophysiology. In: Sadock BJ, Sadock VA, eds. *Kaplan & Sadock's Comprehensive Textbook of Psychiatry.* 8th ed. Vol. 1. Baltimore: Lippincott Williams & Wilkins; 2005:171.

Hanson ES, Prichep LS, Bolwig TG, John ER. Quantitative electroencephalography in OCD patients treated with Paroxetine. *Clin Electroencephalogr.* 2003; 34:70.

Jevtovic-Todorovic V, Hartman RE, Izumi Y, Benshoff ND, Dikranian K, Zorumski CF, Olney JW, Wozniak DW. Early exposure to common anesthetic agents causes widespread neurodegeneration in the developing rat brain and persistent learning deficits. *J Neurosci.* 2003;23:876–882.

Jiang Y, Lee A, Chen J, Ruta V, Cadene M, Chait BT, MacKinnon R. X-ray structure of a voltage-dependent K^+ channel. *Nature.* 2003;423:33–41.

Jiang Y, Ruta V, Chen J, Lee A, MacKinnon R. The principle of gating charge movement in a voltage-dependent K^+ channel. *Nature.* 2003;423:42–48.

Jorgensen PL, Hakansson KO, Karlish SJD. Structure and mechanism of Na, K-ATPase: functional sites and their interactions. *Annu Rev Physiol.* 2003;65:817–849.

Karlin A. Emerging structure of the nicotinic acetylcholine receptors. *Nat Rev Neurosci.* 2002;3:102–114.

Noebels JL. The biology of epilepsy genes. *Annu Rev Neurosci.* 2003;26:599–625.

Reid MS, Prichep LS, Ciplet D, O'Leary S, Tom ML, Howard B, Rotrosen J, John ER. Quantitative electroencephalographic studies of cue-induced cocaine craving. *Clin Electroencephalogr.* 2003;34:110.

Sadja R, Alagem N, Reuveny E. Gating of GIRK channels: Details of an intricate, membrane-delimited signaling complex. *Neuron.* 2003;39:9–12.

Sather WA, McClesky EW. Permeation and selectivity in calcium channels. *Annu Rev Physiol.* 2003;65:133–159.

Smirnow BW, Holloway HC. The neuroscience of psychotherapy: Building and rebuilding the human brain. *Psychiatry.* 2005;68(2):187–192.

Struve FA, Manno BR, Kemp P, Patrick G, Manno JE. Acute marijuana (THC) exposure produces a "transient" topographic quantitative EEG profile identical to the "persistent" profile seen in chronic heavy users. *Clin Electroencephalogr.* 2003;34:75.

Umbricht D, Koller R, Schmid L, Skrabo A, Grubel C, Huber T, Stassen H. How specific are deficits in mismatch negativity generation to schizophrenia? *Biol Psychiatry.* 2003;53:1120.

Yang-Whan J, Polich J. Meta-analysis of P300 and schizophrenia: Patients, paradigms, and practical implications. *Psychophysiology.* 2003;40:684.

Zorumski CF, Isenberg KE, Mennerick SJ. Basic electrophysiology. In: Sadock BJ, Sadock VA, eds. *Kaplan & Sadock's Comprehensive Textbook of Psychiatry.* 8th ed. Vol. 1. Baltimore: Lippincott Williams & Wilkins; 2005:99.

▲ 3.5 Psychoneuroendocrinology, Psychoneuroimmunology, and Chronobiology

Just as the central and peripheral nervous system extend their cells and synapses throughout the body, the endocrine and immune systems also extend their components throughout the body, utilizing hormones, immune-modulating molecules, and immune system cells (e.g., B cells and T cells). These three communicating systems—the nervous, endocrine, and immune systems—also communicate among themselves. This is evident from the observations that psychiatric disorders can have endocrinologic and immunologic manifestations and symptoms, and that the endocrine and immune disorders can have psychiatric and neurological symptoms.

PSYCHONEUROENDOCRINOLOGY

The term *psychoneuroendocrinology* refers to the structural and functional relations between the hormonal system and the central nervous system (CNS) and the behaviors that modulate and arise from both. In previous sections, a number of peptide neurotransmitters were discussed. Some of these peptide neurotransmitters (e.g., corticotrophin-releasing hormone [CRH]) are also hormones within the endocrine system. This reflects a certain amount of "efficiency" in how the body can use the same molecules; for example, CRH, both as a neurotransmitter between synapsing neurons in the nervous system, and as a circulating hormone in the periphery regulating growth and development as part of the endocrine system. This chapter is focused on the endocrine roles of these molecules.

Hormone Secretion

Hormones are divided into two general classes: (1) proteins, polypeptides, and glycoproteins and (2) steroids and steroid-like compounds (Table 3.5–1) that are secreted by an endocrine gland into the bloodstream and are transported to their sites of action.

Hormone secretion is stimulated by the action of a neurohormone, a neuronal secretory product of neuroendocrine transducer cells of the hypothalamus. Neurohormones (Table 3.5–2) include CRH, which stimulates adrenocorticotropin (adrenocorticotropic hormone [ACTH]); thyrotropin-releasing hormone (TRH), which stimulates release of thyroid-stimulating hormone (TSH); gonadotropin-releasing hormone (GnRH), which stimulates release of luteinizing hormone (LH) and follicle-stimulating hormone (FSH); and somatostatin (somatotropin release-inhibiting factor [SRIF]) and growth-hormone-releasing hormone (GHRH), both of which stimulate growth hormone (GH) release. Chemical signals cause the release of these neurohormones from the median eminence of the hypothalamus into the portal hypophyseal bloodstream and coordinate their transport to the anterior pituitary to regulate the release of target hormones. Pituitary hormones, in turn, act directly on target cells (e.g., ACTH on the adrenal gland) or stimulate release of other hormones from peripheral endocrine organs. In addition, these hormones have feedback actions that regulate neurohormone secretion

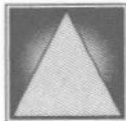

Table 3.5–1
Classifications of Hormones

Structure	Examples	Storage	Lipid Soluble
Proteins, polypeptides, glycoproteins	ACTH, β-endorphin, TRH, LH, FSH	Vesicles	No
Steroids, steroid-like compounds	Cortisol, estrogen, thyroxine	Diffusion after synthesis	Yes
Functions			
Autocrine	Self-regulatory effects		
Paracrine	Local or adjacent cellular action		
Endocrine	Distant target site		

ACTH, adrenocorticotropin; TRH, thyrotropin-releasing hormone; LH, luteinizing hormone; FSH, follicle-stimulating hormone.
(Courtesy of Victor I Reus, M.D., and Sydney Frederick-Osborne, Ph.D.)

and effects in the brain itself, both directly and as modulators of neurotransmitter action (neuromodulation).

Developmental Psychoneuroendocrinology

Hormones can have both organizational and activational effects. Exposure to gonadal hormones during critical stages of neural development directs changes in brain morphology and function (e.g., sex-specific behavior in adulthood). Similarly, thyroid hormones are essential for the normal development of the CNS, and thyroid deficiency during critical stages of postnatal life will severely impair growth and development of the brain, resulting in behavioral disturbances that may be permanent if replacement therapy is not instituted.

Endocrine Assessment

Neuroendocrine function can be studied by assessing baseline measures and by measuring the response of the axis to some neurochemical or hormonal challenge. The first method has two approaches. One approach is to measure a single time point—for example, morning levels of growth hormone; this approach is subject to significant error because of the pulsatile nature of the release of most hormones. The second approach is to collect blood samples at multiple points or to collect 24-hour urine samples; these measurements are less susceptible to major errors. The best approach, however, is to perform a neuroendocrine challenge test, in which the person is given a drug or a hormone that perturbs the endocrine axis in some standard way. Persons with no disease show much less variation in their responses to such challenge studies than in their baseline measurements.

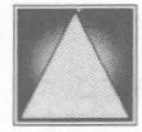

Table 3.5–2
Neurohormones

Neurohormone	Hormone Stimulated
Corticotropin-releasing hormone (CRH)	Adrenocorticotropic hormone (ACTH)
Thyrotropin-releasing hormone (TRH)	Thyroid-stimulating hormone (TSH)
Gonadotropin-releasing hormone (GnRH)	Luteinizing hormone (LH) Follicle-stimulating hormone (FSH)
Somatostatin (somatotropin release-inhibiting factor [SRIF])	Growth hormone (GH)
Growth-hormone-releasing hormone (GHRH)	GH
Oxytocin	Prolactin
Arginine vasopressin (AVP)	ACTH

(Courtesy of Victor I Reus, M.D., and Sydney Frederick-Osborne, Ph.D.)

Hypothalamic-Pituitary-Adrenal Axis

Since the earliest conceptions of the stress response, by Hans Selye and others, investigation of hypothalamic-pituitary-adrenal function has occupied a central position in psychoendocrine research. CRH, ACTH, and cortisol levels all rise in response to a variety of physical and psychic stresses and serve as prime factors in maintaining homeostasis and developing adaptive responses to novel or challenging stimuli. The hormonal response depends both on the characteristics of the stressor itself and on how the individual assesses and is able to cope with it. Aside from generalized effects on arousal, distinct effects on sensory processing, stimulus habituation and sensitization, pain, sleep, and memory storage and retrieval have been documented. In primates, social status can influence adrenocortical profiles and, in turn, be affected by exogenously induced changes in hormone concentration.

Pathological alterations in hypothalamic-pituitary-adrenal function have been associated primarily with mood disorders, posttraumatic stress disorder, and dementia of the Alzheimer's type, although recent animal evidence points toward a role of this system in substance use disorders as well. Disturbances of mood are found in more than 50 percent of patients with Cushing's syndrome (characterized by elevated cortisol concentrations), with psychosis or suicidal thought apparent in more than 10 percent of patients studied. Cognitive impairments similar to those seen in major depressive disorder (principally in visual memory and higher cortical functions) are common and relate to the severity of the hypercortisolemia and possible reduction in hippocampal size. In general, reduced cortisol levels normalize mood and mental status. Conversely, in Addison's disease (characterized by adrenal insufficiency), apathy, social withdrawal, impaired sleep, and decreased concentration frequently accompany prominent fatigue. Replacement of glucocorticoid (but not of electrolyte) resolves behavioral symptomatology. Similarly, hypothalamic-pituitary-adrenal abnormalities are reversed in persons who are treated successfully with antidepressant medications. Failure to normalize hypothalamic-pituitary-adrenal abnormalities is a poor prognostic sign. Alterations in hypothalamic-pituitary-adrenal function associated with depression include elevated cortisol concentrations, failure to suppress cortisol in response to dexamethasone, increased adrenal size and sensitivity to ACTH, a blunted ACTH response to CRH, and, possibly, elevated CRH concentrations in the brain.

Hypothalamic-Pituitary-Gonadal Axis

The gonadal hormones (progesterone, androstenedione, testosterone, estradiol, and others) are steroids that are secreted principally by the ovary and testes, but significant amounts of androgens arise from the adrenal cortex as well. The prostate gland and adipose tissue, also involved in the synthesis and storage of dihydrotestosterone, contribute to individual variance in sexual function and behavior.

The timing and presence of gonadal hormones play a critical role in the development of sexual dimorphisms in the brain. Developmentally, these hormones direct the organization of many sexually dimorphic CNS structures and functions, such as the size of the hypothalamic nuclei and corpus callosum, neuronal density in the temporal cortex, the organization of language ability, and responsivity in Broca's motor speech area. Women with congenital adrenal hyperplasia, a deficiency of the enzyme 21-hydroxylase, which leads to high exposure to adrenal androgens in prenatal and postnatal life, in some studies, have been found to be more aggressive and assertive and less interested in traditional female roles than control female subjects. Sexual dimorphisms may also reflect acute and reversible actions of relative steroid concentrations (e.g., higher estrogen levels transiently increase CNS sensitivity to serotonin).

Testosterone. Testosterone is the primary androgenic steroid, with both androgenic (i.e., facilitating linear body growth) and somatic growth functions. Testosterone is associated with increased violence and aggression in animals and in correlation studies in humans, but anecdotal reports of increased aggression with testosterone treatment have not been substantiated in investigations in humans. In hypogonadal men, testosterone improves mood and decreases irritability. Varying effects of anabolic-androgenic steroids on mood have been noted anecdotally. A prospective, placebo-controlled study of anabolic-androgenic steroid administration in normal subjects reported positive mood symptoms, including euphoria, increased energy, and sexual arousal, in addition to increases in the negative mood symptoms of irritability, mood swings, violent feelings, anger, and hostility.

Testosterone is important for sexual desire in both men and women. In males, muscle mass and strength, sexual activity, desire, thoughts, and intensity of sexual feelings depend on normal testosterone levels, but these functions are not clearly augmented by supplemental testosterone in those with normal androgen levels. Adding small amounts of testosterone to normal hormonal replacement in postmenopausal women has proved, however, to be as beneficial as its use in hypogonadal men.

Dihydroepiandrosterone (DHEA), an adrenal androgen, is the most abundant circulating steroid. It has many physiological effects, but behavioral interest has centered on its steady decrement over the life span in humans, and its possible involvement in memory. Several controlled trials of DHEA administration point to improved well-being and functional status in both depressed and normal individuals. Its effects may result from its transformation into estrogen or testosterone or from its antiglucocorticoid activity.

Estrogen and Progesterone. Estrogens can influence neural activity in the hypothalamus and limbic system directly through modulation of neuronal excitability, and they have complex multiphasic effects on nigrostriatal dopamine receptor sensitivity. Accordingly, evidence indicates that the antipsychotic effect of psychiatric drugs can change over the menstrual cycle and that the risk of tardive dyskinesia depends partly on estrogen concentrations. Several studies have suggested that gonadal steroids modulate spatial cognition and verbal memory and are involved in impeding age-related neuronal degeneration. Increasing evidence also suggests that estrogen administration decreases the risk and severity of dementia of the Alzheimer's type in postmenopausal women. Estrogen has mood-enhancing properties and can also increase sensitivity to serotonin, possibly by inhibiting monoamine oxidase. In animal studies, long-term estrogen treatment results in a decrease in serotonin 5-HT_1 receptors and an increase in 5-HT_2 receptors. In oophorectomized women, significant reductions in tritiated imipramine binding sites (which indirectly measures presynaptic serotonin uptake) were restored with estrogen treatment.

The association of these hormones with serotonin is hypothetically relevant to mood change in premenstrual and postpartum mood disturbances. In premenstrual dysphoric disorder, a constellation of symptoms resembling major depressive disorder occurs in most menstrual cycles, appearing in the luteal phase and disappearing within a few days of the onset of menses. No definitive abnormalities in estrogen or progesterone levels have been demonstrated in women with premenstrual dysphoric disorder, but decreased serotonin uptake with premenstrual reductions in steroid levels has been correlated with the severity of some symptoms.

Most psychological symptoms associated with the menopause are actually reported during perimenopause rather than after complete cessation of menses. Although studies suggest no increased incidence of major depressive disorder, reported symptoms include worry, fatigue, crying spells, mood swings, diminished ability to cope, and diminished libido or intensity of orgasm. Hormone replacement therapy (HRT) is effective in preventing osteoporosis and reinstating energy, a sense of well-being, and libido; however, its use is extremely controversial. A 2002 National Institutes of Health study found that combined estrogen-progestin drugs (e.g., Premarin) caused small increases in breast cancer, heart attack, strokes, and blood clots among menopausal women. Studies of the effects of estrogen alone in women who have had hysterectomies (because estrogen alone increases the risk for uterine cancer) are ongoing.

Hypothalamic-Pituitary-Thyroid Axis

Thyroid hormones are involved in the regulation of nearly every organ system, particularly those integral to the metabolism of food and the regulation of temperature, and are responsible for optimal development and function of all body tissues. In addition to its prime endocrine function, TRH has direct effects on neuronal excitability, behavior, and neurotransmitter regulation.

Thyroid disorders can induce virtually any psychiatric symptom or syndrome, although no consistent associations of specific syndromes and thyroid conditions are found. Hyperthyroidism is commonly associated with fatigue, irritability, insomnia, anxiety, restlessness, weight loss, and emotional lability; marked impairment in concentration and memory may also be evident. Such states can progress into delirium or mania or they can be episodic. On occasion, a true psychosis develops, with paranoia as a particularly common presenting feature. In some cases, psychomotor retardation, apathy, and withdrawal are the presenting features rather than agitation and anxiety. Symptoms of mania have also been reported following rapid normalization of thyroid status in hypothyroid individuals and may covary with thyroid level in individuals with episodic endocrine dysfunction. In general, behavioral abnormalities resolve with normalization of thyroid function and respond symptomatically to traditional psychopharmacological regimens.

The psychiatric symptoms of chronic hypothyroidism are generally well recognized (Fig. 3.5–1). Classically, fatigue, decreased libido, memory impairment, and irritability are noted, but a true secondary psychotic disorder or dementia-like state can also develop. Suicidal ideation is common, and the lethality of actual attempts is profound. In milder, subclinical states of hypothyroidism, the absence of gross signs accompanying endocrine dysfunction can result in its being overlooked as a possible cause of a mental disorder.

Growth Hormone

Growth hormone deficiencies interfere with growth and delay the onset of puberty. Low GH levels can result from a

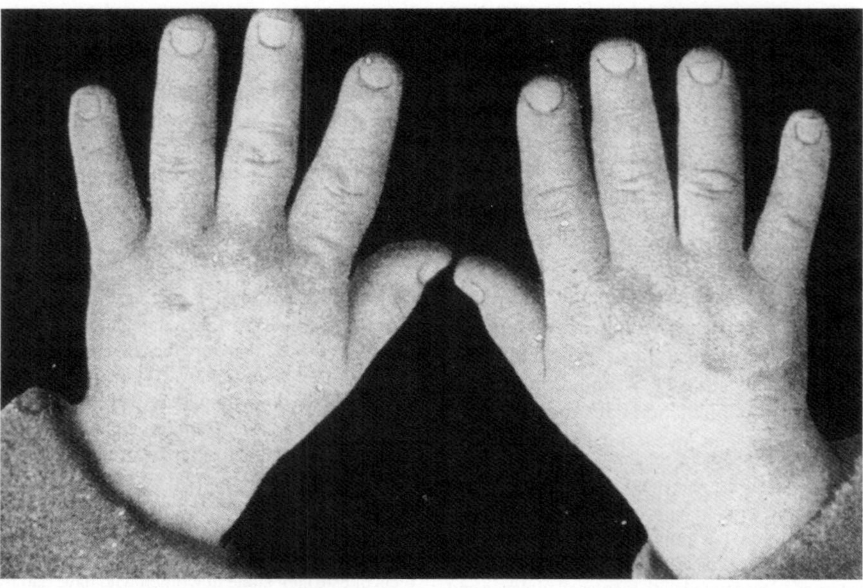

FIGURE 3.5–1
Hands of a patient with hypothyroidism (myxedema), illustrating the swelling of the soft parts, the broadening of the fingers, and their consequent stumpy or pudgy appearance. (Reprinted from Waterfield RL. Anæmia. In: *French's Index of Differential Diagnosis,* 7th ed. AH Douthwaite, ed. Baltimore: Williams & Wilkins, 1954, with permission.)

stressful experience. Administration of GH to individuals with GH deficiency benefits cognitive function in addition to its more obvious somatic effects, but evidence indicates poor psychosocial adaptation in adulthood for children who were treated for GH deficiency. A significant percentage of patients with major depressive disorder and dysthymic disorder may have a GH deficiency. Some prepubertal and adult patients with diagnoses of major depressive disorder exhibit hyposecretion of GHRH during an insulin tolerance test, a deficit that has been interpreted as reflecting alterations in both cholinergic and serotonergic mechanisms. A number of GH abnormalities have been noted in patients with anorexia nervosa. Secondary factors, such as weight loss, however, in both major depressive disorder and eating disorders, may be responsible for alterations in endocrine release. Nonetheless, at least one study has reported that GHRH stimulates food consumption in patients with anorexia nervosa and lowers food consumption in patients with bulimia. Administration of GH to elderly men increases lean body mass and improves vigor. GH is released in pulses throughout the day, but the pulses are closer together during the first hours of sleep than at other times.

Prolactin

Prolactin is primarily involved in reproductive functions. During maturation, prolactin secretion is important in gonadal development. In adults, prolactin contributes to the regulation of the behavioral aspects of reproduction and infant care, including estrogen-dependent sexual receptivity and breastfeeding.

Prolactin release is normally inhibited by the presence of dopamine in the brain. When patients are treated with dopamine receptor antagonists, such as antipsychotic agents, these patients have an elevation in prolactin levels because the normal inhibition of dopamine on prolactin release is blocked by the receptor antagonist drugs. Another cause of increased prolactin levels is prolactin-secreting tumors.

Patients with hyperprolactinemia sometimes experience depression, decreased libido, stress intolerance, anxiety, and increased irritability. These behavioral symptoms usually resolve in parallel with a decrease in prolactin levels following surgical treatment of tumors or changes in pharmacological treatment.

Melatonin

Melatonin, a pineal hormone, is derived from the serotonin molecule and it controls photoperiodically mediated endocrine events (particularly those of the hypothalamic-pituitary-gonadal axis). It also modulates immune function, mood, and reproductive performance and is a potent antioxidant and free-radical scavenger. Melatonin has a depressive effect on CNS excitability, is an analgesic, and has seizure-inhibiting effects in animal studies. Melatonin can be a useful therapeutic agent in the treatment of circadian phase disorders such as jet lag. Intake of melatonin increases the speed of falling asleep, as well as its duration and quality.

Oxytocin

Oxytocin, also a posterior pituitary hormone, is involved in osmoregulation, the milk ejection reflex, food intake, and female maternal and sexual behaviors. Oxytocin is theorized to be released during orgasm, more so in women than in men, and is presumed to promote bonding between the sexes. It has been used in autistic children experimentally in an attempt to increase socialization.

Insulin

Increasing evidence indicates that insulin may be integrally involved in learning and memory. Insulin receptors occur in high density in the hippocampus and are thought to help neurons metabolize glucose. Patients with Alzheimer's disease have lower insulin concentrations in the cerebrospinal fluid (CSF) than controls, and both insulin and glucose dramatically improve verbal memory. Depression is frequent in patients with diabetes, as are indexes of impaired hormonal response to stress. It is not known whether these findings represent direct effects of the disease or are secondary, nonspecific effects. Some antipsychotics are known to dysregulate insulin metabolism.

PSYCHONEUROIMMUNOLOGY

The nervous system and the immune system represent two networks within the body. Each contains a massive diversity of cell types and uses a large pharmacopoeia of chemical signals. Until about 20 years ago, these two systems were considered to act as parallel but independent entities. Since the 1980s, however, a small but growing number of elegant studies has revealed a set of direct interactions between the two systems and has spawned the field of psychoneuroimmunology.

Behavioral Conditioning

Demonstration that learning processes can influence immunological function is another example of interactions between the immune system and the nervous system. Several classical conditioning paradigms have been associated with suppression or enhancement of the immune response in various experimental designs.

In an effort to condition rats to avoid saccharine-flavored water, the flavored water was presented simultaneously with an injection of cyclophosphamide (Cytoxan), to induce nausea. Although the method engendered an aversion to saccharine, the immunosuppressive effect of cyclophosphamide also became a conditioned response. Thus, conditioned rats, when given saccharine-flavored water, suppressed their T cells, contracted infectious diseases, and died unexpectedly.

Stress and the Immune Response

Experiments conducted on laboratory animals in the late 1950s and the early 1960s indicated that a wide variety of stressors, including isolation, rotation, crowding, exposure to a predator, and electric shock, increased morbidity and mortality in response to several types of tumors and infectious diseases caused by viruses and parasites. Evidence indicates that stressful life events can increase the susceptibility to infectious diseases in humans. For example, investigators have found that infection rates by five separate rhinoviruses administered intranasally are significantly higher in persons under high psychological stress than in those under low stress. Some studies have indicated a relation between depressive symptoms (presumably secondary to increased stress and inability to cope) and cancer development; others have been unable to replicate these findings. Once cancer has developed, however, data on women with metastatic breast cancer indicate that supportive group therapy may increase the time of survival and reduce pain episodes. Other studies report that quality of life, rather than survival, is improved, but even that is significant.

Studies on academic stress among medical students found less natural killer cell activity during the final examination period than during a preexamination baseline. Examination stress has also been associated with decreased numbers of T cells, mitogen responses, interferon production, and antibody responses to recombinant hepatitis B vaccine. In addition, increased antibody titers to latent herpes viruses, presumably secondary to impaired cellular immunity, have been observed. Investigators have also reported decreases in measures of immune function in persons exposed to chronic life stressors, such as divorce and taking care of patients with Alzheimer's disease. For example, caregivers to patients with Alzheimer's disease showed alterations in lymphocyte subpopulations, increased antibody titers to herpes simplex virus, decreased proliferative response to mitogens, more days of illness from infectious disease, impaired antibody responses to an influenza virus vaccine, and longer latency for wound healing. Conjugal bereavement, one of the most stressful commonly occurring life events, has been associated with increased medical morbidity and mortality.

Finally, much attention has been directed to the notion that stress and depression may influence immunocompetence in seropositive persons with human immunodeficiency virus (HIV), thereby serving as cofactors in the progression of HIV infection to acquired immune deficiency syndrome (AIDS). Studies found that HIV-positive subjects who experienced severe stress had relevant changes in immune parameters, including lower CD8+ and lower natural killer cell counts. Ongoing studies are examining psychosocial variables and immunological and clinical endpoints in persons with HIV infection.

Psychiatric Disorders and Manifestations

The idea that altered CNS function results from a combination of the direct effects of an injurious event on various cell types and the effects of inflammatory mediators on neurons and supporting cells is a cornerstone of neuroimmunology. The idea that infectious agents can lead to psychiatric disorders is well established. Obvious examples include the mental retardation that may develop after congenital infection with rubella or cytomegalovirus, the delirium that accompanies acute meningoencephalitis after CNS infection by herpes simplex virus type I, dementias caused by slow viruses (e.g., kuru and Creutzfeldt-Jakob disease), and the neuropsychiatric manifestations that occur during neurosyphilis.

Schizophrenia. Several lines of evidence suggest that virus infection during neural development may be involved in the pathogenesis of some cases of schizophrenia. The data include (1) an excess number of patient births in the late winter and early spring, suggesting possible exposure to viral infection in utero during the fall and winter peak of viral illnesses; (2) an association between exposure to viral epidemics in utero and later development of schizophrenia; (3) an increased likelihood for patients with schizophrenia to have had older siblings in the household (a potential source of viral infections) compared with controls; and (4) geographical variation in prevalence, with schizophrenia being more common at greater distance from the equator. Investigators have also reported various alterations in immune markers in patients with schizophrenia, including increased levels of interferon, lower interleukin-2 (IL-2) production, and increased numbers of IL-2 receptors. Some studies have found an increase in immunoglobulin levels in the CSF.

Neural cells are the targets for autoantibodies in many syndromes. For example, autoantibodies to cytoplasmic proteins of Purkinje cells are associated with subacute cortical cerebellar degeneration, which is a rare complication of breast or ovarian cancers. Autoantibodies to γ-aminobutyric acid (GABA)-ergic neurons in the serum and the CSF appear to be the mechanism behind the stiff-man syndrome, a rare disorder characterized by progressive rigidity accompanied by recurrent painful muscle spasms. Antineuronal antibodies can also arise following infection with group A β-hemolytic streptococci, as exemplified by Sydenham's chorea. Considering that children with Sydenham's chorea frequently exhibit obsessive–compulsive symptoms, emotional lability, and hyperactivity, a spectrum may be seen of pediatric autoimmune neuropsychiatric disorders associated with streptococcal infections (pediatric autoimmune neuropsychiatric disorders associated with streptococcus [PANDAS]). In particular, sudden onset of obsessive–compulsive disorder, tics, attention-deficit/hyperactivity disorder (ADHD), and other psychiatric syndromes have been characterized in children following infection with group A β-hemolytic streptococci.

Major Depressive Disorder. Increasing interest exists in the possibility that immune activation may contribute to the pathophysiology of depression. For example, elevated serum concentrations of the proinflammatory cytokines IL-1 and IL-6, as well as increased acute-phase proteins, including C-reactive protein, haptoglobin, and α_1-acid glycoprotein, have been found in patients with major depressive disorder. In addition, cellular markers of immune activation have been described. The source of immune activation in major depressive disorder is unknown, although studies have shown that both stress and CRH can induce proinflammatory cytokines in the absence of a formal immune challenge. Administration of a variety of cytokines in clinical trials also has been associated with the development of depressive syndromes (sickness behavior).

Alzheimer's Disease. Although Alzheimer's disease is not considered primarily an inflammatory disease, emerging evidence indicates that the immune system may contribute to its pathogenesis. The discovery that amyloid plaques are associated with acute-phase proteins, such as complement proteins and C-reactive protein, suggests the possibility of an ongoing immune response. The idea that inflammatory processes are involved in Alzheimer's disease has been bolstered by recent studies showing that long-term use of nonsteroidal anti-inflammatory drugs (NSAIDs) is negatively correlated with the development of Alzheimer's disease.

HIV Infection. Infection with HIV is an immunological disease associated with a variety of neurological manifestations, including dementia. HIV encephalitis results in synaptic abnormalities and loss of neurons in the limbic system, basal ganglia, and neocortex. A thorough discussion of HIV is provided in Chapter 11.

Multiple Sclerosis. Multiple sclerosis is a demyelinating disease characterized by disseminated inflammatory lesions of white matter. Considerable progress has been made in elucidating the immunopathology of myelin destruction that occurs in multiple sclerosis and in the animal model for the disease, experimental allergic encephalomyelitis. Although the initial step in lesion formation has not been determined, disruption of the blood-brain barrier and infiltration of T cells, B cells, plasma cells, and macrophages appear to be associated with lesion formation.

Other Disorders. Finally, several disorders are seen in which neural-immune interactions are suspected but not well documented. *Chronic fatigue syndrome* is an illness with a controversial etiology and pathogenesis. Besides persistent fatigue, symptoms frequently include depression and sleep disturbances. Tests of immune function have found indications of both immune activation and immunosuppression. Neuroendocrine assessments indicate that patients with chronic fatigue syndrome may be hypocortisolemic because of impaired activation of the hypothalamic-pituitary-adrenal axis. Although an acute viral infection frequently precedes the onset of chronic fatigue syndrome, no infectious agent has been causally associated with it. In contrast, *Lyme disease*, in which sleep disturbances and depression are also common, is clearly caused by infection with the tick-borne spirochete *Borrelia burgdorferi*, which can invade the CNS and cause encephalitis and neurological symptoms. Lyme disease is remarkable because it appears to produce a spectrum of neuropsychiatric disorders, including anxiety, irritability, obsessions, compulsions, hallucinations, and cognitive deficits. Immunopathology of the CNS may be involved, because symptoms can persist or reappear even after a lengthy course of antibiotic treatment, and the spirochete is frequently difficult to isolate from the brain. *Gulf War syndrome* is a controversial condition with inflammatory and neuropsychiatric features. The condition has been attributed variously to combat stress, chemical weapons (e.g., cholinesterase inhibitors), infections, and vaccines. Given the impact of stress on neurochemistry and immune responses, these pathogenic mechanisms are not mutually exclusive.

CHRONOBIOLOGY AND BIOLOGICAL RHYTHMS

Biological systems constantly oscillate between different states at different rates. The obvious physical cycles to which a person's biological rhythms conform include the day–night cycle, the lunar month, the solar year, and biophysical constraints, such as the rate of pulmonary gas diffusion that determines the respiratory rate and the cardiac contractile parameters that dictate the heart rate. Patterned mealtimes and the 9-to-5 workday are examples of other exogenous influences. The brain is filled with oscillations, some of which provide a constant drone over which others weave an elaborate melody. Theorists of higher perception and thought, such as Rudolfo Llinas, are increasingly interested in how the brain may use rhythmical patterns of neuronal firing to encode information, in addition to using different spatial combinations of synaptic connections. Thus, biological rhythms range from the monthly menstrual cycle to brain oscillations occurring at the rate of 30 to 60 times per second.

Sleep is one of several biological rhythms within the body. Circadian biological rhythms are set by both internal and external forces, generally called *zeitgebers* (time givers, time clues, synchronizers), which constitute a widely distributed set of nuclei. The principal circadian influences emanate from the pontine reticular formation as well as from the suprachiasmatic nuclei of the hypothalamus. Recent evidence has shown that the suprachiasmatic nucleus can entrain circadian rhythms even in the absence of physical synaptic connections with the remainder of the hypothalamus, suggesting that this zeitgeber can act through elaboration of diffusible substances. In the absence of exogenous clues, the period of human circadian rhythms is a bit longer than a day (24.5 hours).

The sleep–wake cycle, hormonal levels, body temperature, and the menstrual cycle are all examples of biological rhythms in the human body that can be measured. When a person is in a healthy state, all the rhythms have a natural relation, and they are said to be *in phase*. When the system is perturbed (e.g., by staying up all night), certain biological rhythms are thrown off (e.g., those for growth hormone and cortisol), and the rhythms are then considered *out of phase*. The state of having one's biological rhythms out of phase contributes to the ill effects experienced by the person. Some disorders have phase perturbations as part of their symptoms. When rhythms are disordered, a particular rhythm may have an *abnormal phase advance*, in which it begins earlier than usual, or a *phase delay*, in which it begins later than usual. Under experimental conditions, a phase-responsive curve for a biological rhythm may show that a particular stimulus (e.g., light) can cause either a phase advance or a phase delay, depending on when it is delivered in a cycle (e.g., the sleep-wake cycle). Lithium (Eskalith) and many of the tricyclic drugs and monamine oxidase inhibitors (MAOIs) delay rhythms in experimental animal models, supporting the hypothesis that at least some forms of depression represent phase-advance disorders.

Sleep is an essential phase of human daily existence in which much mental activity occurs. While most of the period of sleep remains unconscious, dream states can engrave vivid and bizarre memories. Freud, in *The Interpretation of Dreams*, called dreams the "royal road to the unconscious." The sleep-wake cycle is synchronized with cyclic changes in the levels of several circulating hormones. Serum cortisol levels are lowest at the onset of sleep and highest in morning. TSH secretion is suppressed by the onset of sleep, whereas melatonin is secreted at night and terminates on retinal stimulation by sunlight. GH levels surge during deep sleep, and this stimulus for growth gradually ceases by late adult life as deep sleep disappears. Prolactin and LH also reach their highest levels during sleep. Other hormones, such as testosterone, vary markedly throughout the day (thus, a single reading does not measure testosterone accurately).

The necessity for sleep is demonstrated by experiments in which animals deprived of sleep die within a few weeks. Humans deprived of sleep for 60 to 200 hours begin to exhibit a breakdown in concentration, motor skills, self-care, attention, judgment, and eventually communication. Hallucinations and illusions can appear. A wide variation, however, exists in the requirement for sleep, which is determined by genetic factors, habits formed early in life, and particular physical and emotional states. The circadian (24-hour) rhythm appears in the first few months of life and remains intact until old age, when it may begin to fragment.

Depression is the psychiatric symptom that has been most associated with disruptions in biological rhythms. Early morning awakening, decreased latency of rapid eye movement (REM) sleep, and neuroendocrine perturbations seen in depression can all be conceptualized as reflecting a disorder of coordination of biological rhythms. One hypothesis is that depression occurs in some persons when the sleep-sensitive phase of the circadian system advances from the first hours of awakening to the last hours of sleep. Research indicates that alterations in the light–dark cycle (by exposing the patient to artificial light or by changing the patient's sleep–wake cycle) (Fig. 3.5–2) can relieve the symptoms.

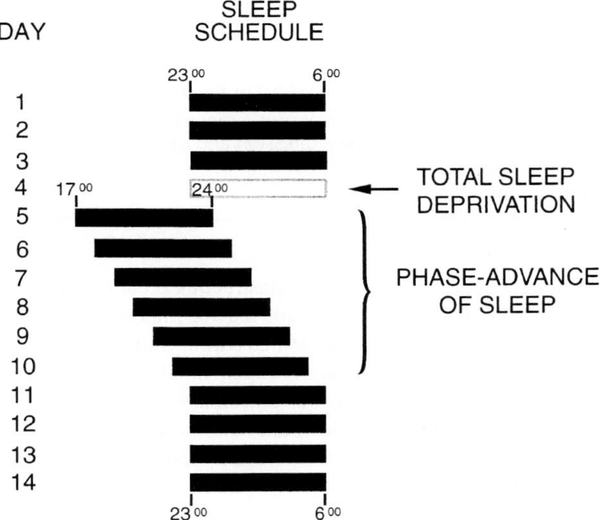

FIGURE 3.5–2

Treatment of depression by shifting the sleep–wake cycle earlier (phase advancing it), relative to other circadian rhythms, then gradually shifting it back to a normal schedule. The phase-advance treatment is based on experimental observations that sleep is depressant when it coincides with late night and early morning circadian phases, but not when it coincides with late afternoon and early evening circadian phases. (See Wehr TA, Wirz-Justice A, Duncan WC, Gillin JC, Goodwin FK. Phase-advance of the circadian sleep-wake cycle as an antidepressant. *Science* 206:710; Berger M, Vollmann J, Hohagen F, et al. Sleep deprivation combined with consecutive sleep phase advance as a fast-acting therapy in depression: An open pilot trial in medicated and unmedicated patients. *Am J Psychiatry*. 1997;154:870.)

References

Bailer UF, Kaye WH. A review of neuropeptide and neuroendocrine dysregulation in anorexia and bulimia nervosa. *Curr Drug Target CNS Neurol Disord.* 2003;2:53.

Dantzer R. Innate immunity at the forefront of psychoneuroimmunology. *Brain, Behavior, & Immunity*. 2004;18(1):1–6.

Halbreich U, Kahn LS. Hormonal aspects of schizophrenias: An overview. *Psychoneuroendocrinology.* 2003;28[Suppl 2]:1.

Harris DS, Wolkowitz OM, Reus VI. Psychoneuroendocrinology. In: Sadock BJ, Sadock VA, eds. *Kaplan & Sadock's Comprehensive Textbook of Psychiatry*. 8th ed. Vol 1. Baltimore: Lippincott Williams & Wilkins; 2005:126.

Holsboer F. The role of peptides in treatment of psychiatric disorders. *J Neural Transm Suppl.* 2003;64:17.

Losel RM, Falkenstein E, Feuring M, Schultz A, Tillmann HC, Rossol-Haseroth K, Wehling M. Nongenomic steroid action: Controversies, questions, and answers. *Physiol Rev.* 2003;83:965.

McEwan BS. Mood disorders and allostatic load. *Biol Psychiatry.* 2003;54:200.

Muscat L, Huberman AD, Jordan CL, Morin LP. Crossed and uncrossed retinal projections to the hamster circadian system. *J Comp Neurol.* 2003;466:513.

Panda S, Provencio I, Tu DC, Pires SS, Rollag MD, Castrucci AM, Pletcher MT, Sato TK, Wiltshire T, Andahazy M, Kay SA, Van Gelder RN, Hogenesch JB. Melanopsin is required for non-image-forming photic responses in blind mice. *Science*. 2003;301:525.

Provencio I. Chronobiology. In: Sadock BJ, Sadock VA, eds. *Kaplan & Sadock's Comprehensive Textbook of Psychiatry*. 8th ed. Vol. 1. Baltimore: Lippincott Williams & Wilkins; 2005:161.

Quintero JE, Kuhlman SJ, McMahon DG. The biological clock nucleus: A multiphasic oscillator network regulated by light. *J Neurosci.* 2003;23:8070.

Rohan KJ, Tierney LK, Roecklein KA, Lacy TA. Cognitive-behavioral therapy, light therapy, and their combination in treating seasonal affective disorder: A pilot study. *J Affect Disord.* 2004:80;273.

Rupprecht R. Neuroactive steroids: Mechanisms of action and neuropsychopharmacological properties. *Psychoneuroendocrinology.* 2003;28:139.

Seidman SN. Testosterone deficiency and mood in aging men: Pathogenic and therapeutic interactions. *World J Biol Psychiatry.* 2003;4:14.

Steiner M, Dunn E, Born L. Hormones and mood: From menarche to menopause and beyond. *J Affect Disord.* 2003;74:67.

Wolkowitz OM, Rothschild AJ, eds. *Psychoneuroendocrinology: The Scientific Basis of Clinical Practice*. Washington, DC: American Psychiatric Press, Inc.; 2003.

▲ 3.6 Neurogenetics

Many major psychiatric disorders have been shown to have a strong hereditary predisposition. In the case of schizophrenia, for example, a first-degree relative of an affected patient has about a 10 percent chance of having the illness, far in excess of the 1 percent risk in the general population. Monozygotic twins display nearly 50 percent concordance for schizophrenia. Bipolar I disorder and major depressive disorder exhibit similar familial clustering, in that first-degree relatives are 8 to 18 times more likely to have a mood disorder than is the general population, and monozygotic twins show a 33 to 90 percent concordance rate. Tourette's syndrome shows an even more convincing genetic association. Several family pedigrees have been constructed in which transmission of the syndrome is consistent with an autosomal-dominant mode, with penetrance of 99 percent in males and 70 percent in females. Only 10 percent of patients with Tourette's syndrome do not have an affected family member. These facts stimulate the expectation that a specific genetic basis will emerge for certain psychiatric diseases.

Traits are clinically defined features, such as sickle crises in sickle cell anemia or blue eyes. Some traits are determined by a single gene, whereas others emerge from the interactions of the products of (in some cases) hundreds of genes. Behavior likely is the expression of the products of thousands of genes, although specific single-gene mutations may influence certain behaviors in consistent ways. Studies of animal behavior, especially that of the fruit fly and the laboratory mouse, have documented many behaviors inherited as single-gene traits. These heritable behaviors have often been traced to a specific gene, whereas others are only known to be heritable. The former category, however, is rapidly expanding at the expense of the latter. A glossary of genetic terms is given in Table 3.6–1.

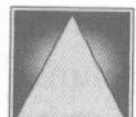

Table 3.6–1
Glossary of Genetic Terms

Allele: One of the variant forms of a gene at a particular locus, or location, on a chromosome. Different alleles produce variation in inherited characteristics, such as hair color or blood type.

Codon: In DNA or RNA, a sequence of three nucleotides that codes for a certain amino acid or signals the termination of translation (stop or termination codon).

Epigenetics: Any heritable influence (in the progeny of cells or of individuals) on gene activity, unaccompanied by a change in DNA sequence.

Genome: The complete DNA sequence, containing all genetic information and supporting proteins, in the chromosomes of an individual or species.

Genotype: The genetic constitution of an organism or cell; also refers to the specific set of alleles inherited at a locus.

Linkage analysis: A statistical method that examines pedigree data to determine whether a trait cosegregates with a genetic marker.

Multifactorial: The combined contribution of one or more often unspecified genes and environmental factors, often unknown, in the causation of a particular trait or disease.

Phenotype: Observable characteristics of an organism produced by the organism's genotype interacting with the environment.

Polygenic: Genetic disorder resulting from the combined action of alleles of more than one gene. Although such disorders are inherited, they depend on the simultaneous presence of several alleles; thus, the hereditary patterns usually are more complex than those of single-gene disorders.

Polymorphism: Natural variations in a gene, DNA sequence, or chromosome that have no adverse effects on the individual and occur with fairly high frequency in the general population.

Positional cloning: The process of correlating a specific gene to a clinical trait.

Proband: The individual in a pedigree who causes the pedigree to come to the attention of medical or research personnel.

Proteomics: A research area that uses a range of bioinformatics approaches to analyze the expression and function of proteins within specific systems, cells, or organisms.

Trait: An inherited characteristic.

For traits determined by single genes, three common inheritance patterns are recognized: *autosomal dominant*, *autosomal recessive*, and *X-linked recessive* transmission. In autosomal dominant transmission of disease only one of the two copies of the gene in the cell nucleus needs to be inherited to produce the clinical trait. A parent with one copy of a dominant mutation has a 50 percent chance of passing the trait to his or her child. In autosomal recessive transmission, the trait can be passed on only when both copies are inherited. Thus, a parent with an autosomal recessive trait can transmit it to a child only when the other parent also passes on the mutant gene. In X-linked recessive transmission, the gene is found on an unpaired X chromosome and, thus, is the only copy of the gene in the nucleus. An X-linked recessive trait, therefore, occurs in males, who have only one X chromosome; females are carriers, but they do not display the clinical traits because they have a second, normal X chromosome (Fig. 3.6–1).

In psychiatry, the largest hurdle in the process of assigning behavioral traits to specific genes is the rigorous clinical definition of psychiatric traits. The text revision of the fourth edition of *Diagnostic and Statistical Manual of Mental Disorders* (DSM-IV-TR), which provides exact categorization for most psychiatric disorders, nonetheless probably includes a genetically heterogeneous population of patients under each diagnostic category. The situation is further muddled by the lack of objective, quantifiable tests for psychiatric disorders. Moreover, because familial clustering of certain behavioral traits can result from either genetics (nature) or upbringing (nurture), constructing accurate pedigrees strictly according to genetic criteria may be impossible. Finally, the multigenic determination of behavioral traits serves to increase the complexity of analysis exponentially.

At this writing, pedigrees have been assembled for each of the main psychiatric disorders, and chromosomal linkage has been sought with the tools of molecular genetics. Even in the apparently straightforward case of Tourette's syndrome, screening of almost all chromosomes has failed to identify a specific genetic locus always inherited with the clinical behavior. This finding suggests that Tourette's syndrome is a multigenic trait, that is, a disorder that may be caused by the combined influences of several genes. Screening for mutations in genes that regulate the dopamine pathway in patients with Tourette's syndrome, as well as neurotransmitters in other disorders, is ongoing.

Genetic causes are being sought for other psychiatric disorders. Based on an analysis of 22 pedigrees, a locus that confers an increased risk of bipolar disorder has been identified on chromosome 18. The correlation is not robust, which indicates a need for further investigation. For the personality trait of anxiety, a genetic variant of the serotonin transporter gene has been

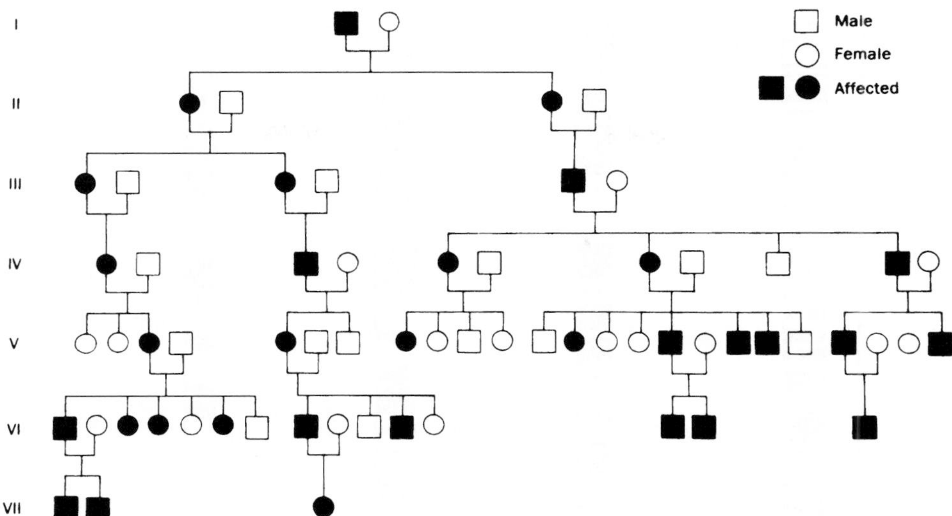

FIGURE 3.6–1

Transmission of traits through sexual reproduction. Sexual reproduction permits the propagation of novel advantageous mutations through a population. This pedigree shows seven generations in which a dominant trait (*dark circles and squares*) is transmitted from generation to generation. From a single trait-bearing individual in generation I, the trait is transmitted to roughly half of the offspring of 17 unaffected individuals (*open circles and squares*): one in generation I, two in generation II, three in generation III, five in generation IV, four in generation V, and two VI. (Modified from Jones S, Martin R, Pilbeam D. *The Cambridge Encyclopedia of Human Evolution.* Cambridge, UK: Cambridge University Press, 1992:258, with permission.)

described that alters the number of transporter molecules in the presynaptic membrane of serotonergic neurons. This alternative version of the transporter has been calculated to account for less than 5 percent of the genetic variance for anxiety in the general population.

Persons with schizophrenia may have difficulty filtering auditory input to screen out extraneous sounds. A carefully performed positional cloning project has identified a locus on chromosome 15 that encodes the a1 nicotinic acetylcholine receptor and appears to account for the abnormality in auditory processing in several pedigrees of patients with schizophrenia. Another study, examining the previously described negative association between schizophrenia and rheumatoid arthritis, found that the human lymphocyte antigen (HLA) DRB1*04 allele was significantly associated with a reduced risk of rheumatoid arthritis in 94 unrelated patients with schizophrenia. A study of 265 Irish families with a high incidence of schizophrenia found two loci, one on chromosome 8 and the other on chromosome 6, each of which accounted for the vulnerability to schizophrenia in 10 to 30 percent of the families. These findings should be viewed as preliminary, and each will require further work.

Alzheimer's disease can be definitively diagnosed only by pathological examination of brain tissue, either at autopsy or from brain biopsy. Whereas shrinkage of neuronal volume without loss of neurons is a feature of normal aging, loss of neurons is typical of Alzheimer's disease. The two characteristic neuropathological features are senile plaques and neurofibrillary tangles. A recent clinicopathological study found that elderly nuns with senile plaques and neurofibrillary tangles do not always have dementia, but the risk is greatly increased (from 57 to 93 percent) if they also have had strokes. A separate study of nuns showed that writing style at age 20 years predicted the onset of dementia (presumably Alzheimer's) over the age of 70 years. Nuns with a simple writing style in their youth were more likely to develop dementia than nuns with a complex command of written language. These two studies illustrate that dementia of the Alzheimer's type likely results from a combination of genetically determined and acquired factors.

Of cases of Alzheimer's disease, 10 percent are hereditary, and the remaining 90 percent are sporadic, but even sporadic cases seem to associate with certain genetic predispositions. Of the hereditary cases, 70 to 80 percent are attributable to mutations in the presenilin 1 gene, located on chromosome 14, which causes onset of symptoms at age 40 to 50 years. Another 20 to 30 percent are attributable to mutations in a related gene, presenilin 2, located on chromosome 1, which causes onset of symptoms at age 50 years. A final 2 to 3 percent of the familial cases are attributable to mutations in the β-amyloid precursor protein (APP) gene, located on chromosome 21, which causes onset of symptoms at age 50 years. APP and a cytoskeletal protein called *tau* are prominent components of senile plaques and neurofibrillary tangles in both familial and sporadic cases of Alzheimer's disease. Tau protein polymerizes into the paired helical filaments that are the main components of neurofibrillary tangles if it is not protected from phosphorylation. This protection is afforded by apolipoprotein E (Apo E), encoded by a gene on chromosome 19 that has three alleles. The e2 allele protects tau, whereas the e3 and (especially) the e4 alleles do not associate as strongly with tau and leave it susceptible to phosphorylation and eventual polymerization. Presence of the e3/e4 or the e4/e4 alleles has been claimed to account for 10 to 50 percent of the risk of sporadic Alzheimer's disease with onset of symptoms about age 60 years. Such individuals seem to have a particular loss of acetylcholine-containing neurons and, thus, may be less likely to respond to acetylcholinesterase inhibitors, such as donepezil (Aricept). The known genetic risk factors for Alzheimer's

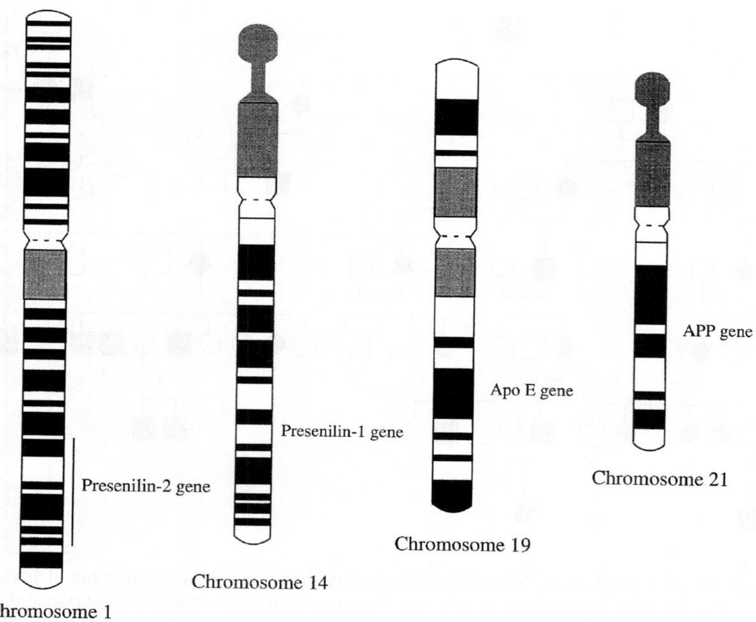

FIGURE 3.6–2
Chromosomal location of the genes implicated in Alzheimer's disease. Apo E, apolipoprotein E; APP, amyloid precursor protein. (Courtesy of Carol A. Matthews, M.D. and Nelson B. Freimer, M.D.)

disease so far account for less than 50 percent of cases (Fig. 3.6–2).

GENOME

The human genome consists of between 30,000 and 50,000 genes, of which more than 20,000 have been identified. More than 5,000 genetic disorders, each transmitted through a single mutant gene, have been characterized. The application of more powerful quantitative methods of analysis, new molecular technologies, and more detailed maps of the human genome have permitted localization to chromosomal regions of more than 400 of these disease genes, with precise identification of more than 80.

Major public health implications exist to identifying genes that influence an individual's risk of developing the more common familiar mental disorders such as schizophrenia, bipolar I disorder, alcoholism (alcohol abuse or dependence), and obsessive–compulsive disorder. Such findings may ultimately have relevance for many affected individuals and their relatives, given the potential for developing a genetic test to identify individuals at risk, and equally important, provide the pharmaceutical industry with new drug therapy targets. Clinicians and researchers must understand the basic principles of genetics and genetic epidemiology so that they can appreciate the relevance of new data derived from the genetic analysis of mental disorders.

Basic Molecular Biology

The central dogma of molecular biology is "DNA makes RNA makes protein." Deoxyribonucleic acid (DNA) is a genetic code consisting of a series of bases, adenine (A), cytosine (C), guanine (G), and thymine (T), which are covalently linked to form extremely long molecules (Fig. 3.6–3). Genes consist of strings of DNA that serve as templates for messenger ribonucleic acid (mRNA) molecules, which in turn specify a sequence of amino acids, the building blocks of proteins. mRNA is assembled according to the DNA code by the stepwise addition of bases according to a complementation algorithm. Ribonucleic adenine (rA) is complementary to deoxyribonucleic thymine (T), rG to C, rC to G, and ribonucleic uracil (rU) to adenine (A). Thus, the DNA string ATGTCTTAG would encode the mRNA string UACAGAAUC. mRNA has stretches of protein-coding sequences, called *exons*, which are interrupted by noncoding sequences, called *introns*. Soon after the mRNA is transcribed from the DNA, the exons are spliced together to form a continuous stretch of coding sequence. The mRNA moves into the cytoplasm and binds to ribosomes, which read it as a series of base triplets, called *codons*. Each codon specifies an amino acid, and the amino acids are strung together to form a specific protein. There are 20 amino acids, each with a common core atomic structure, but unique side chains. Depending on the primary amino acid sequence, the protein folds into a three-dimensional molecule that interacts specifically with other proteins, carbohydrates, nucleic acids, or lipids to carry out the functions of the cell.

The relative abundance of various proteins in the cell may be regulated by the rate of mRNA transcription, at the level of mRNA translation into protein, or at the level of the degradation of the protein molecules. mRNA transcriptional control is the most common type of specific gene regulation. Initiation of mRNA transcription involves general factors, called *transcription factors*, common to all genes, but it is regulated by specific transcription factors that bind only to certain genes and are themselves regulated by intracellular and extracellular signals. Thus, thyroid hormones diffuse into the cell and bind to the thyroid receptors, and the hormone-receptor complex, which

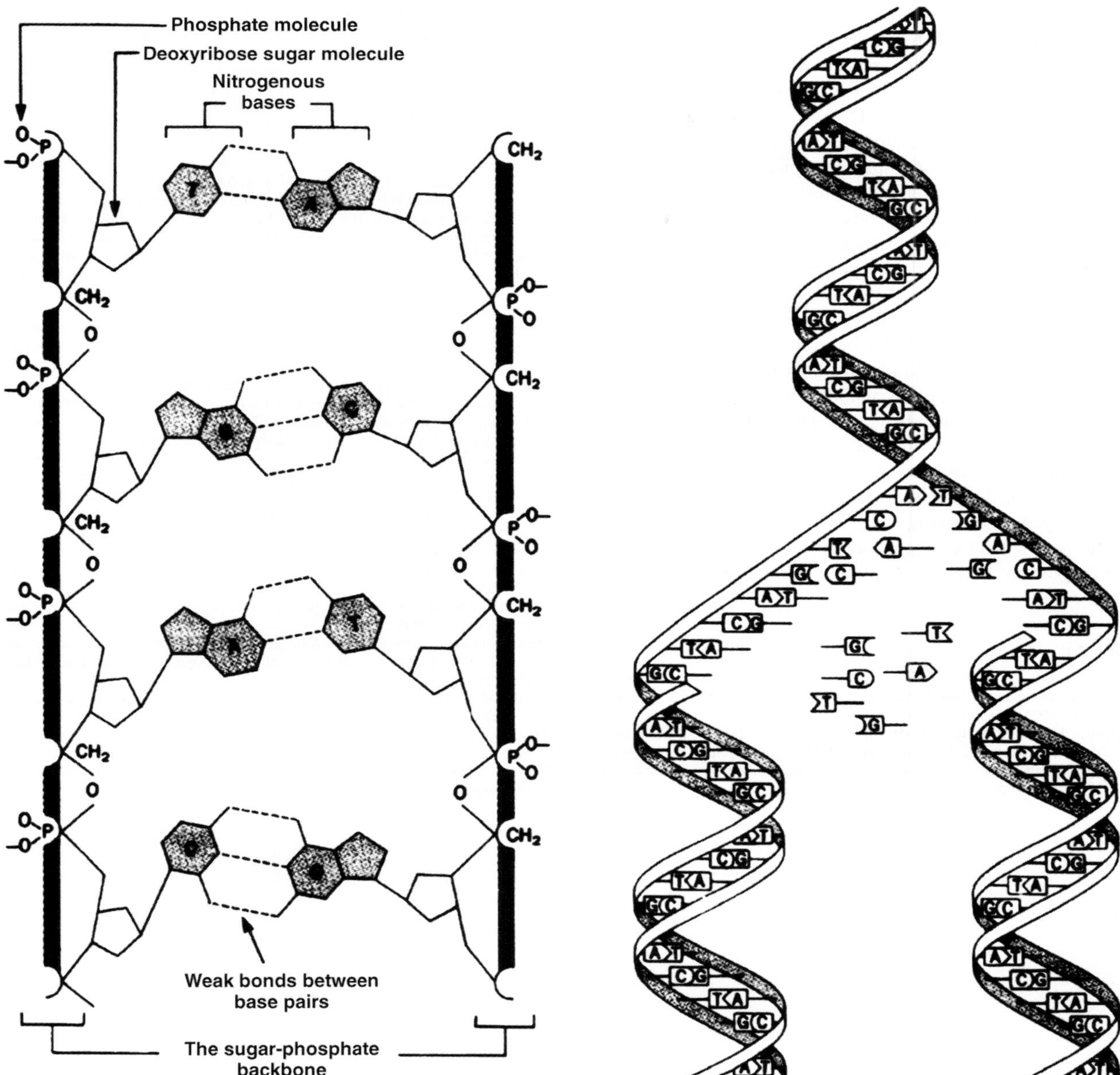

FIGURE 3.6–3

The chemical structure of a DNA molecule. (**Left**) A short segment of DNA showing the sugar and phosphate backbone of each strand, together with the four different DNA bases: adenine, guanine, cytosine, and thymine. The complementary pairing of A with T and G with C is what holds the strands together and permits the molecule to make copies of itself of almost infinite length. (**Right**) Replication of DNA, showing how the molecule unwinds and, by pairing of the complementary bases with each other, makes two identical copies of the original DNA sequence. (Modified from Jones S, Martin R, Pilbeam D. *The Cambridge Encyclopedia of Human Evolution*. Cambridge, UK: Cambridge University Press, 1992:11, with permission.)

acts as a transcription factor, enters the nucleus and activates certain genes by binding to specific DNA sequences immediately adjacent to these genes. Psychiatry is very interested in gene regulation by neurotransmitters and in the regulation of the synaptic neurochemical milieu by variations in the levels of gene transcription.

The human genetic material consists of 3 billion bases of DNA, which are divided into units of roughly 60 million bases, called *chromosomes*. The normal cell nucleus contains 23 pairs of chromosomes: 22 matched pairs of autosomes and the X and Y sex chromosomes (*see* Color Plate 3.6–4 on p. 84). Chromosomes are bound by a variety of structural and regulatory proteins. The most important structural proteins are *histones,* which are small, positively charged proteins that serve to package DNA into structures that fit into the cell nucleus. The DNA helix is wrapped around core histones to form a simple "beads on a string" structure that is then folded into a higher-order structure called *chromatin*. Modification of chromatin structure by transcription proteins serves as one important mechanism of activating or repressing mRNA transcription initiation.

Humans are estimated to have about 30,000 to 40,000 distinct genes, and of these, the function of only a few thousand is known at this time. Only about 1 percent of the total DNA encodes genes that may be translated into proteins; and the remaining 99 percent is noncoding, "junk" DNA. Complexity arises because most proteins seem to be modified in complex ways and can be the products of differential splicing. Consequently, the relatively low number of human genes has a very high potential to generate an enormous proteome of great complexity.

Some genes encode proteins that play housekeeping roles within the cell; that is, they are present in all cells and are essential to the survival of the cell. Other genes play specific regulatory roles and are cell-type specific. Among these latter genes are those of particular interest to psychiatrists. Intense research is under way to identify both those genes that, when altered, may cause psychiatric illness and those that may determine normal emotional behaviors and responses. At this time, these goals tax, and in most cases exceed, the data-processing capabilities of even the most sophisticated investigators, but major technical advances are appearing at a rapid rate. With the complete sequencing of the human genome, most gene experts now anticipate significant advances in the identification of the genetic basis of complex human behaviors early in the 21st century.

References

Botstein D, Risch N. Discovering genotypes underlying human phenotypes: Past successes for mendelian disease, future approaches for complex disease. *Nat Genet.* 2003;33[Suppl]:228

Bunney WE, Bunney BG, Vawter MP, Tomita H, Li J, Evans SJ, Choudary PV, Myers RM, Jones EG, Watson SJ, Akil H. Microarray technology: A review of new strategies to discover candidate vulnerability genes in psychiatric disorders. *Am J Psychiatry.* 2003;160:657.

Carlson CS, Eberle MA, Rieder MJ, Smith JD, Kruglyak L, Nickerson DA. Additional SNPs and linkage-disequilibrium analyses are necessary for whole-genome association studies in humans. *Nat Genet.* 2003;33:518.

Chakravarti A, Little P. Nature, nurture, and human disease. *Nature.* 2003;421:412.

Flouris AD, Faugth BE, Hay J, Cairney J. Exploring the origins of the developmental disorders. *Dev Med Child Neurol.* 2005;47(7):436.

Harnson PJ, Owen MJ. Genes for schizophrenia? Recent findings and their pathophysiological implications. *Lancet.* 2003;361:417.

Mathews CA, Freimer NB. Genetic linkage analysis of psychiatric disorders. In: Sadock BJ, Sadock VA, eds. *Kaplan & Sadock's Comprehensive Textbook of Psychiatry.* 8th ed. Vol. 1. Baltimore: Lippincott Williams & Wilkins; 2005:252.

Matise TC, Sachidanandam R, Clark AG, Kruglyak L, Wijsman E, Kakol J, Buyske S, Chui B, Cohen P, de Toma C, Ehm M, Glanowski S, He C, Heil J, Markianos K, McMullen I, Pericak-Vance MA, Silbergleit A, Stein L, Wagner M, Wilson AF, Winick JD, Winn-Deen ES, Yamashiro CT, Cann HM, Lai E, Holden AL. A 3.9-centimorgan-resolution human single-nucleotide polymorphism linkage map and screening set. *Am J Hum Genet.* 2003;73:271.

Mitchell AA, Cutler DJ, Chakravarti A. Undetected genotyping errors cause apparent overtransmission of common alleles in the transmission/disequilibrium test. *Am J Hum Genet.* 2003;72:598.

Moldin SO. Population genetics and genetic epidemiology. In: Sadock BJ, Sadock VA, eds. *Kaplan & Sadock's Comprehensive Textbook of Psychiatry.* 8th ed. Vol. 1. Baltimore: Lippincott Williams & Wilkins; 2005:236.

Moldin SO, Hyman SE. Genome, transcriptome, and proteome. In: Sadock BJ, Sadock VA, eds. *Kaplan & Sadock's Comprehensive Textbook of Psychiatry.* 8th ed. Vol. 1. Baltimore: Lippincott Williams & Wilkins; 2005:115.

O'Donovan MC, Williams NM, Owen MJ. Recent advances in the genetics of schizophrenia. *Hum Mol Genet.* 2003;12:125.

Patterson SD, Aebersold RH. Proteomics: The first decade and beyond. *Nat Genet.* 2003;33[Suppl]:311.

Pauls DL. An update on the genetics of Gilles de la Tourette syndrome. *J Psychosom Res.* 2003;55:7.

Plomin R, McGuffin P. Psychopathology in the postgenomic era. *Annual Review of Psychology.* 2003;54:205.

Reiss Al, Dant CC. The behavioral neurogenetics of fragile X syndrome: Analyzing gene-brain-behavior relationships in child developmental psychopathologies. *Dev Psychopathol.* 2003;15(4):927–968.

Snyder M, Gerstein M. Genomics. Defining genes in the genomics era. *Science.* 2003;300:258.

Venter JC, Levy S, Stockwell T, Remington K, Halpern A. Massive parallelism, randomness and genomic advances. *Nat Genet.* 2003;33[Suppl]:219.

Wang S, Kidd KK, Zhao H. On the use of DNA pooling to estimate haplotype frequencies. *Genet Epidemiol.* 2003;24:74.

4 Contributions of the Psychosocial Sciences

▲ 4.1 Jean Piaget

Jean Piaget (1896–1980) was born in Neuchatel, Switzerland, where he studied at the university and received a doctorate in biology at the age of 22 (Fig. 4.1–1). Interested in psychology, he studied and carried out research at several centers, including the Sorbonne in Paris, and worked with Eugen Bleuler at the Burghöltzli Psychiatric Hospital.

Widely renowned as a child (or developmental) psychologist, Piaget referred to himself primarily as a *genetic epistemologist*, which he defined as the study of the development of abstract thought on the basis of a biological or innate substrate. That self-designation reveals that Piaget's central project was more than the articulation of a *developmental child psychology*, as this term is generally understood, but rather an account of the progressive development of human knowledge.

Piaget created a broad theoretical system for the development of cognitive abilities; in this sense, his work was similar to that of Sigmund Freud, but Piaget emphasized the ways that children think and acquire knowledge.

COGNITIVE DEVELOPMENT STAGES

Piaget described four major stages leading to the capacity for adult thought (Table 4.1–1). Each stage is a prerequisite for the following one, but the rate at which different children move through different stages varies with their native endowment and environmental circumstances. Piaget's four stages are (1) sensorimotor, (2) preoperational thought, (3) concrete operations, and (4) formal operations.

Sensorimotor Stage (Birth to 2 Years)

Piaget used the term *sensorimotor* to describe the first stage: Infants begin to learn through sensory observation, and they gain control of their motor functions through activity, exploration, and manipulation of the environment. Piaget divided this stage into six substages, listed in Table 4.1–2.

From the outset, biology and experience blend to produce learned behavior. For example, infants are born with a sucking reflex, but a type of learning occurs when infants discover the location of the nipple and alter the shape of their mouths. A stimulus is received, and a response results, accompanied by a sense of awareness that is the first schema, or elementary concept. As infants become more mobile, one schema is built on another, and new and more complex schemata are developed. Infants' spatial, visual, and tactile worlds expand during this period; children interact actively with the environment and use previously learned behavior patterns. For example, having learned to use a rattle, infants shake a new toy as they did the rattle they had already learned to use. Infants also use the rattle in new ways.

The critical achievement of this period is the development of *object permanence* or the *schema of the permanent object*. This phrase relates to a child's ability to understand that objects have an existence independent of the child's involvement with them. Infants learn to differentiate themselves from the world and are able to maintain a mental image of an object, even when it is not present and visible. When an object is dropped in front of infants, they look down to the ground to search for the object; that is, they behave for the first time as though the object has a reality outside themselves.

At about 18 months, infants begin to develop mental symbols and to use words, a process known as *symbolization*. Infants are able to create a visual image of a ball or a mental symbol of the word *ball* to stand for, or signify, the real object. Such mental representations allow children to operate on new conceptual levels. The attainment of object permanence marks the transition from the sensorimotor stage to the preoperational stage of development.

Stage of Preoperational Thought (2 to 7 Years)

During the stage of preoperational thought, children use symbols and language more extensively than in the sensorimotor stage. Thinking and reasoning are intuitive; children learn without the use of reasoning. They are unable to think logically or deductively, and their concepts are primitive; they can name objects but not classes of objects. Preoperational thought is midway between socialized adult thought and the completely autistic freudian unconscious. Events are not linked by logic. Early in this stage, if children drop a glass that then breaks, they have no sense of cause and effect. They believe that the glass was ready to break, not that they broke the glass. Children in this stage also cannot grasp the sameness of an object in different circumstances: The same doll in a carriage, a crib, or a chair is perceived to be three different objects. During this time, things are represented in terms of their function. For example, a child defines a bike as "to ride" and a hole as "to dig."

In this stage, children begin to use language and drawings in more elaborate ways. From one-word utterances, two-word phrases, made up of either a noun and a verb or a noun and an objective, develop. A child may say, "Bobby eat," or "Bobby up."

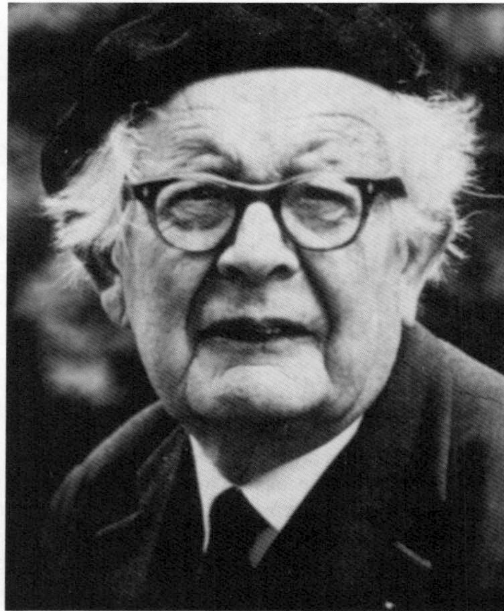

FIGURE 4.1–1
Jean Piaget (1896–1980). (Reprinted from the Jean Piaget Society, Temple University, Philadelphia, PA, with permission.)

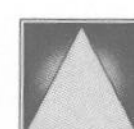

Table 4.1–2
Piaget's Sensorimotor Period of Cognitive Development

Age	Characteristics
Birth–2 mos	Uses inborn motor and sensory reflexes (sucking, grasping, looking) to interact and accommodate to the external world
2–5 mos	Primary circular reaction: Coordinates activities of own body and five senses (e.g., sucking thumb); reality remains subjective—does not seek stimuli outside of its visual field; displays curiosity
5–9 mos	Secondary circular reaction: Seeks out new stimuli in the environment; starts both to anticipate consequences of own behavior and to act purposefully to change the environment; beginning of intentional behavior
9 mos–1 yr	Shows preliminary signs of object permanence; has a vague concept that objects exist apart from itself; plays peek-a-boo; imitates novel behaviors
1 yr–18 mos	Tertiary circular reaction: Seeks out new experiences; produces novel behaviors
18 mos–2 yrs	Symbolic thought: Uses symbolic representations of events and objects; shows signs of reasoning (e.g., uses one toy to reach for and get another); attains object permanence

Children in the preoperational stage cannot deal with moral dilemmas, although they have a sense of what is good and bad. For example, when asked, "Who is more guilty, the person who breaks one dish on purpose or the person who breaks 10 dishes by accident?" a young child usually answers that the person who breaks 10 dishes by accident is more guilty because more dishes are broken. Children in this stage have a sense of *immanent justice*, the belief that punishment for bad deeds is inevitable.

Children in this developmental stage are *egocentric*: They see themselves as the center of the universe; they have a limited point of view; and they are unable to take the role of another person. Children are unable to modify their behavior for someone else; for example, children are not being negativistic when they do not listen to a command to be quiet because their brother has to study. Instead, egocentric thinking prevents an understanding of their brother's point of view.

During this stage, children also use a type of magical thinking, called *phenomenalistic causality*, in which events that occur together are thought to cause one another (e.g., thunder causes lightning, and bad thoughts cause accidents). In addition, children use *animistic thinking*, which is the tendency to endow physical events and objects with life-like psychological attributes, such as feelings and intentions.

Semiotic Function. The semiotic function emerges during the preoperational period. With this new ability, children can represent something—such as an object, an event, or a conceptual scheme—with a signifier, which serves a representative function (e.g., language, mental image, symbolic gesture). That is, children use a symbol or sign to stand for something else. Drawing is a semiotic function initially done as a playful exercise but eventually signifying something else in the real world.

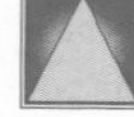

Table 4.1–1
Stages of Intellectual Development Postulated by Piaget

Age (Yr)	Period	Cognitive Developmental Characteristics
0–1.5 (to 2)	Sensorimotor	Divided into six stages, characterized by: 1. Inborn motor and sensory reflexes 2. Primary circular reaction 3. Secondary circular reaction 4. Use of familiar means to obtain ends 5. Tertiary circular reaction and discovery through active experimentation 6. Insight and object permanence
2–7	Preoperations subperiod[a]	Deferred imitation, symbolic play, graphic imagery (drawing), mental imagery, and language
7–11	Concrete operations	Conservation of quantity, weight, volume, length, and time based on reversibility by inversion or reciprocity; operations; class inclusion and seriation
11–end of adolescence	Formal operations	Combinatorial system, whereby variables are isolated and all possible combinations are examined; hypothetical-deductive thinking

[a] This subperiod is considered by some authors to be a separate developmental period.

Stage of Concrete Operations (7 to 11 Years)

The stage of concrete operations is so named because in this period children operate and act on the concrete, real, and perceivable world of objects and events. Egocentric thought is replaced by *operational thought*, which involves dealing with a wide array of information outside the child. Therefore, children can now see things from someone else's perspective.

Children in this stage begin to use limited logical thought processes and can serialize, order, and group things into classes on the basis of common characteristics. *Syllogistic reasoning*, in which a logical conclusion is formed from two premises, appears during this stage; for example, all horses are mammals (premise); all mammals are warm blooded (premise); therefore, all horses are warm blooded (conclusion). Children are able to reason and to follow rules and regulations. They can regulate themselves, and they begin to develop a moral sense and a code of values.

Children who become overly invested in rules may show obsessive–compulsive behavior; children who resist a code of values often seem willful and reactive. The most desirable developmental outcome in this stage is that a child attains a healthy respect for rules and understands that there are legitimate exceptions to rules.

Conservation is the ability to recognize that, although the shape of objects may change, the objects still maintain or conserve other characteristics that enable them to be recognized as the same. For example, if a ball of clay is rolled into a long, thin sausage shape, children recognize that each form contains the same amount of clay. An inability to conserve (which is characteristic of the preoperational stage) is observed when a child declares that there is more clay in the sausage-shaped piece because it is longer. *Reversibility* is the capacity to understand the relation between things, to realize that one thing can turn into another and back again—for example, ice and water.

The most important sign that children are still in the preoperational stage is that they have not achieved conservation or reversibility. The ability of children to understand concepts of quantity is one of Piaget's most important cognitive developmental theories. Measures of quantity include measures of substance, length, number, liquids, and area (Fig. 4.1–2).

The 7- to 11-year-old child must organize and order occurrences in the real world. Dealing with the future and its possibilities occurs in the formal operational stage.

Stage of Formal Operations (11 through the End of Adolescence)

The stage of formal operations is so named because young persons' thinking operates in a formal, highly logical, systematic, and symbolic manner. This stage is characterized by the ability to think abstractly, to reason deductively, and to define concepts and also by the emergence of skills for dealing with permutations and combinations; young persons can grasp the concept of probabilities. Adolescents attempt to deal with all possible relations and hypotheses to explain data and events during this stage. Language

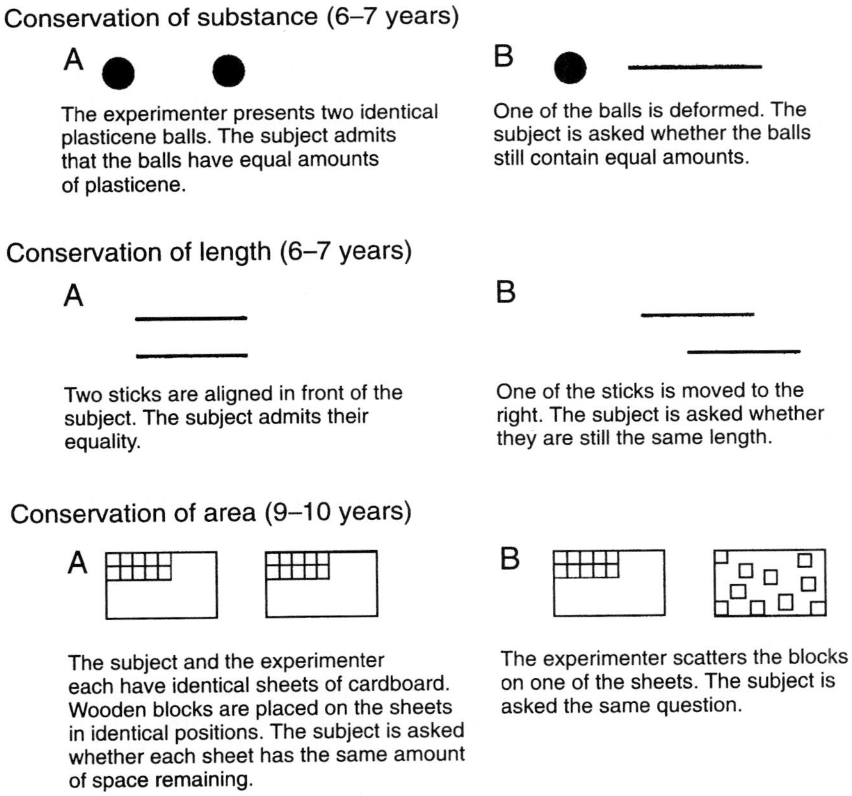

Conservation of substance (6–7 years)

A — The experimenter presents two identical plasticene balls. The subject admits that the balls have equal amounts of plasticene.

B — One of the balls is deformed. The subject is asked whether the balls still contain equal amounts.

Conservation of length (6–7 years)

A — Two sticks are aligned in front of the subject. The subject admits their equality.

B — One of the sticks is moved to the right. The subject is asked whether they are still the same length.

Conservation of area (9–10 years)

A — The subject and the experimenter each have identical sheets of cardboard. Wooden blocks are placed on the sheets in identical positions. The subject is asked whether each sheet has the same amount of space remaining.

B — The experimenter scatters the blocks on one of the sheets. The subject is asked the same question.

FIGURE 4.1–2

Some simple tests for conservation, with approximate ages of attainment. When the sense of conservation is achieved, the child answers that **B** contains the same quantity as **A.** (Modified from Lefrancois GR. *Of Children: An Introduction to Child Development.* Wadsworth: Belmont, CA; 1973:305, with permission.)

use is complex; it follows formal rules of logic and is grammatically correct. Abstract thinking is shown by adolescents' interest in a variety of issues—philosophy, religion, ethics, and politics.

Hypotheticodeductive Thinking. Hypotheticodeductive thinking, the highest organization of cognition, enables persons to make a hypothesis or proposition and to test it against reality. *Deductive reasoning* moves from the general to the particular and is a more complicated process than *inductive reasoning*, which moves from the particular to the general.

Because young persons can reflect on their own and other persons' thinking, they are susceptible to self-conscious behavior. As adolescents attempt to master new cognitive tasks, they may return to egocentric thought, but on a higher level than in the past. For example, adolescents may think that they can accomplish everything or can change events by thought alone. Not all adolescents enter the stage of formal operations at the same time or to the same degree. Depending on individual capacity and intervening experience, some may not reach the stage of formal operational thought at all and may remain in the concrete operational mode throughout life.

PSYCHIATRIC APPLICATIONS

Piaget's theories have many psychiatric implications. Hospitalized children who are in the sensorimotor stage have not achieved object permanence and, therefore, suffer from separation anxiety. They are best off if their mothers are allowed to stay with them overnight. Children at the preoperational stage, who are unable to deal with concepts and abstractions, benefit more from role-playing proposed medical procedures and situations than by having them verbally described in detail. For example, a child who is to receive intravenous therapy is helped by acting out the procedure with a toy intravenous set and dolls.

Because children at the preoperational stage do not understand cause and effect, they may interpret physical illness as punishment for bad thoughts or deeds; and because they have not yet mastered the capacity to conserve and do not understand the concept of reversibility (which normally occurs during the concrete operational stage), they cannot understand that a broken bone mends or that blood lost in an accident is replaced.

Adolescents' thinking, during the stage of formal operations, may appear overly abstract when it is, in fact, a normal developmental stage. Adolescent turmoil may not herald a psychotic process but may well result from a normal adolescent's coming to grips with newly acquired abilities to deal with the unlimited possibilities of the surrounding world.

Adults under stress may regress cognitively as well as emotionally. Their thinking can become preoperational, egocentric, and sometimes animistic.

Implications for Psychotherapy

Piaget was not an applied psychologist and did not develop the implications of his cognitive model for psychotherapeutic intervention. Nevertheless, his work formed one of the foundations of the "cognitive revolution" in psychology. One aspect of this revolution was an increasing emphasis on the cognitive components of the therapeutic endeavor. In contrast to classic psychodynamic therapy, which focused primarily on drives and affects, and in contrast to behavior therapy, which focused on overt actions, cognitive approaches to therapy focused on thoughts, including automatic assumptions, beliefs, plans, and intentions.

Aaron Beck, M.D., for example, developed an entire school of cognitive therapy that focuses on the role of cognitions in causing or maintaining psychopathology. Cognitive therapy has been shown to be an effective treatment for problems as diverse as depression, anxiety disorders, and substance abuse.

A core idea in cognitive therapy is that the patient can be assisted to identify the negative automatic thoughts and underlying dysfunctional attitudes or beliefs that contribute to emotional distress or addictive behavior. The cognitive component of the therapy begins with identification of automatic thoughts, so designated because they are rapid, overlearned responses that instantaneously mediate between an event and an affective reaction. The key therapeutic process after identification of the maladaptive thoughts is to help the patient view these thoughts more objectively rather than accepting them unquestioningly as valid.

Developmentally Based Psychotherapy

Developmentally based psychotherapy, developed by Stanley Greenspan, M.D., integrates cognitive, affective, drive, and relationship-based approaches with new understanding of the stages of human development. The clinician first determines the level of the patient's ego or personality development and the presence or absence of deficits or constrictions. For example, can the person regulate activity and sensations, relate to others, read nonverbal affective symbols, represent experience, build bridges between representations, integrate emotional polarities, abstract feelings, and reflect on internal wishes and feelings?

From a developmental point of view, the integral parts of the therapeutic process include learning how to regulate experience; to engage more fully and deeply in relationships; to perceive, comprehend, and respond to complex behaviors, and interactive patterns; and to be able to engage in the ever-changing opportunities, tasks, and challenges during the course of life (e.g., adulthood and aging) and, throughout, to observe and reflect on one's own and others' experiences. These processes are the foundation of the ego, and more broadly, the personality. Their presence constitutes emotional health and their absence, emotional disorder. The developmental approach describes how to harness these core processes and so assist the patients in mobilizing their own growth.

EXTENSIONS OF PIAGET'S THEORY

The first and, perhaps, best-known attempt to extend Piaget's theory in this way was made by Lawrence Kohlberg, who studied the moral reasoning of children. Kohlberg developed a stage model of moral reasoning in which the child's stage of moral reasoning depended on the child's stage of (Piagetian) cognitive development. The three major stages included the morality of the preschool period (based on notions of avoiding punishment and striving for reward), conventional morality (based on notions of authority or mutual benefit), and principled morality (based on general internalized moral principles). Kohlberg investigated the moral reasoning of individuals by presenting them with moral dilemmas and then observing their thinking as they attempted to resolve the dilemmas. The theory of development pertained to the form of their thinking and not to the content of their solution.

The second type of extension of Piaget's work into the interpersonal domain abandoned the position that stages of social cognition depended on broad structures of intellectual development in favor of the position that the active abstracting processes discovered by Piaget were operative across both types of cognition. James Youniss then developed a theory of children's concepts of other people that appropriated a different key element from Piaget's work. Rather than attempting to layer stages of social cognition on stages of intellectual development, Youniss proposed that social cognition has its own process of development, but that these are based on abstractions from interpersonal interactions. Youniss proposed two major categories of children's social cognition: schemas about peers and schemas about authority figures. Each of these develops as a function of repeated interactions with peers or elders.

A third type of extension of Piaget's work is less direct but also involves his key concepts of egocentrism and perspective taking. Perspective taking implies a certain degree of *thinking about thinking*, in that the perceptions, thoughts, and emotions of the self are seen as only one among two or more possible perceptions, thoughts, and emotions. Implicit in this process is what contemporary psychologists term a *theory of mind*, an awareness that others have internal states and mental representations.

Finally, increased attention is now being directed toward the child's acquisition of social knowledge. To the extent that Piaget neglected or underemphasized the acquisition of knowledge through social transmission, his theory would be deficient in accounting for children's knowledge of social and cultural material that is passed on rather than actively constructed by the individual. Such material would range from the obvious (socially and culturally acceptable behavior) to the subtle (mathematical inventions, such as the current number system). The implications for education are significant. Discovery methods of education, including experimentation and peer discussion, may be more appropriate when the goal is to assist children in formulating the most general principles of reasoning, but other methods, including lecture, assigned reading, and modeling, may be more appropriate when the goal is to convey specific socially constructed content.

References

Brainerd CJ. Jean Piaget, learning research, and American education. In: Zimmerman BJ, ed. *Educational Psychology: A Century of Contributions*. Mahwah, NJ: L. Erlbaum Associates; 2003:251–287.

Costall A, Leudar I. Where is the 'theory' in theory of mind? *Theory & Psychology*. 2004;14(5):623–646.

Cozolino LJ, Siegel DJ. Sensation, perception, and cognition. In: Sadock BJ, Sadock VA, eds. *Kaplan & Sadock's Comprehensive Textbook of Psychiatry*. 8th ed. Vol. 1. Baltimore: Lippincott Williams & Wilkins; 2005:512.

Cunningham P. Early years teachers and the influence of Piaget: Evidence from oral history. *Early Years: An International Journal of Research and Development*. 2006;26:5–16.

Ferrari M, Okamoto CM. Moral development as the personal education of feeling and reason: From James to Piaget. *Journal of Moral Education*. 2003;32(4):341–355.

Greenspan SI, Curry JF. Extending Jean Piaget's approach to intellectual functioning. In: Sadock BJ, Sadock VA, eds. *Kaplan & Sadock's Comprehensive Textbook of Psychiatry*. 8th ed. Vol. 1. Baltimore: Lippincott Williams & Wilkins; 2005:528.

Greenspan SI, Shanker S. *The Evolution of Intelligence: How Language, Consciousness, and Social Groups Come About*. Reading, MA: Perseus Books; 2003.

Hsueh Y. "He sees the development of children's concepts upon a background of sociology": Jean Piaget's honorary degree at Harvard University in 1936. *History of Psychology*. 2004;7(1):20–44.

Lourenço O. Children's appraisals of antisocial acts: A Piagetian perspective. *British Journal of Developmental Psychology*. 2003;21(1):19–31.

Mayer SJ. The early evolution of Jean Piaget's clinical method. *History of Psychology*. 2005;8:362–382.

McInerney DM. Educational psychology—theory, research, and teaching: A 25-year retrospective. *Educational Psychology*. 2005;25(6):585–599.

Mooney CG. *Theories of Childhood: An Introduction to Dewey, Montessori, Erickson, Piaget & Vygotsky*. Upper Saddle River, NJ: Pearson/Merrill Prentice Hall; 2006.

Ortega R. Play, activity, and thought: Reflections on Piaget's and Vygotsky's theories. In: Lytle DE, ed. *Play and Educational Theory and Practice*. Play and Culture Studies. Vol. 5. Westport, CT: Praeger Publishers; 2003:99–115.

Reginensi L. On the status of logic in Piaget. *International Social Science Journal*. 2004;56:439–454.

Shayer M. Not just Piaget, not just Vygotsky, and certainly not Vygotsky as alternative to Piaget. *Learning and Instruction*. 2003;13:465–485.

▲ 4.2 Attachment Theory

ATTACHMENT AND DEVELOPMENT

Attachment theory originated in the work of John Bowlby, a British psychoanalyst (1907–1990) (Fig. 4.2–1). In his studies of infant attachment and separation, Bowlby pointed out that attachment constituted a central motivational force and that mother–child attachment was an essential medium of human interaction that had important consequences for later development and personality functioning. Being monotropic, infants tend to attach to one person; but they can form attachments to several persons,

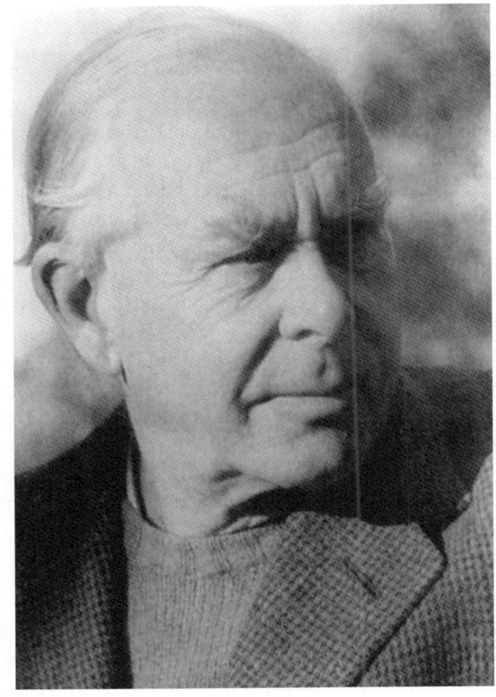

FIGURE 4.2–1
John Bowlby (1907–1990).

such as the father or a surrogate. Attachment develops gradually; it results in an infant's wanting to be with a preferred person, who is perceived as stronger, wiser, and able to reduce anxiety or distress. Attachment thus gives infants feelings of security. The process is facilitated by interaction between mother and infant; the amount of time together is less important than the amount of activity between the two.

Attachment can be defined as the emotional tone between children and their caregivers and is evidenced by an infant's seeking and clinging to the caregiving person, usually the mother. By their first month, infants usually have begun to show such behavior, which is designed to promote proximity to the desired person.

The term *bonding* is sometimes used synonymously with attachment, but the two are different phenomena. Bonding concerns the mother's feelings for her infant and differs from attachment. Mothers do not normally rely on their infants as a source of security, as is the case in attachment behavior. Much research reveals that the bonding of mother to infant occurs when there is skin-to-skin contact between the two or when other types of contact, such as voice and eye contact, are made. Some workers have concluded that a mother who has skin-to-skin contact with her baby immediately after birth shows a stronger bonding pattern and may provide more attentive care than a mother who does not have this experience. Some researchers have even proposed a critical period immediately after birth, during which such skin-to-skin contact must occur if bonding is to take place. This concept is much disputed: Many mothers are clearly bonded to their infants and display excellent maternal care even though they did not have skin-to-skin contact immediately postpartum. Because human beings can develop representational models of their babies in utero and even before conception, this representational thinking may be as important to the bonding process as skin, voice, or eye contact.

Ethological Studies

Bowlby suggested a darwinian evolutionary basis for attachment behavior; namely, such behavior ensures that adults protect their young. Ethological studies show that nonhuman primates and other animals exhibit attachment behavior patterns that are presumably instinctual and are governed by inborn tendencies. An example of an instinctual attachment system is *imprinting*, in which certain stimuli can elicit innate behavior patterns during the first few hours of an animal's behavioral development; thus, the animal offspring becomes attached to its mother at a critical period early in its development. A similar sensitive or critical period during which attachment occurs has been postulated for human infants. The presence of imprinting behavior in humans is highly controversial, but bonding and attachment behavior during the first year of life closely approximate the critical period; in humans, however, this period occurs over a span of years rather than hours.

Harry Harlow. Harry Harlow's work with monkeys is relevant to attachment theory. Harlow demonstrated the emotional and behavioral effects of isolating monkeys from birth and keeping them from forming attachments. The isolates were withdrawn, unable to relate to peers, unable to mate, and incapable of caring for their offspring. (Harlow's work is discussed further in Section 4.5.)

PHASES OF ATTACHMENT

In the first attachment phase, sometimes called the *preattachment stage* (birth to 8 or 12 weeks), babies orient to their mothers, follow them with their eyes over a 180-degree range, and turn toward and move rhythmically with their mother's voice. In the second phase, sometimes called *attachment in the making* (8 to 12 weeks to 6 months), infants become attached to one or more persons in the environment. In the third phase, sometimes called *clear-cut attachment* (6 through 24 months), infants cry and show other signs of distress when separated from the caretaker or mother; this phase can occur as early as 3 months in some infants. On being returned to the mother, the infant stops crying and clings, as if to gain further assurance of the mother's return. Sometimes, seeing the mother after a separation is sufficient for crying to stop. In the fourth phase (25 months and beyond), the mother figure is seen as independent, and a more complex relationship between the mother and the child develops. Table 4.2–1 summarizes the development of normal attachment from birth through 3 years.

MARY AINSWORTH

Mary Ainsworth expanded on Bowlby's observations and found that the interaction between the mother and her baby during the attachment period significantly influences the baby's current and future behavior. Patterns of attachments vary among babies; for example, some babies signal or cry less than others. Sensitive responsiveness to infant signals, such as cuddling a crying baby, causes infants to cry less in later months, rather than reinforcing crying behavior. Close bodily contact with the mother when the baby signals for her is also associated with the growth of self-reliance, rather than a clinging dependence, as the baby grows older. Unresponsive mothers produce anxious babies; these mothers often have lower intelligence quotients (IQs) and are emotionally more immature and younger than responsive mothers.

Ainsworth described three main types of insecure attachment: insecure–avoidant, insecure–ambivalent, and insecure–disorganized. The insecure–avoidant child, having experienced brusque or aggressive parenting, tends to avoid close contact with people and lingers near caregivers rather than approaching them directly when faced with a threat. The insecure–ambivalent child finds exploratory play difficult, even in the absence of danger, and clings to his or her inconsistent parents. Insecure–disorganized children have parents who are emotionally absent with a parental history of abuse in their childhood. These children tend to behave in bizarre ways when threatened. According to Ainsworth, disorganization is a severe form of insecure attachment and a possible precursor of severe personality disorder and dissociative phenomena in adolescence and early adulthood.

Ainsworth also confirmed that attachment serves to reduce anxiety. What she called the *secure base effect* enables children to move away from attachment figures and to explore the environment. Inanimate objects, such as a teddy bear and a blanket

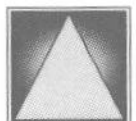

Table 4.2–1
Normal Attachment

Birth to 30 days
- Reflexes at birth
  - Rooting
  - Head turning
  - Sucking
  - Swallowing
  - Hand-mouth
  - Grasp
  - Digital extension
  - Crying—signal for particular kind of distress
  - Responsiveness and orientation to mother's face, eyes, and voice
- 4 days—anticipatory approach behavior at feeding
- 3 to 4 wks—infant smiles preferentially to mother's voice

Age 30 days through 3 mos
- Vocalization and gaze reciprocity further elaborated from 1 to 3 mos; babbling at 2 mos, more with the mother than with a stranger
- Social smile
- In strange situation, increased clinging response to mother

Age 4 through 6 mos
- Briefly soothed and comforted by sound of mother's voice
- Spontaneous, voluntary reaching for mother
- Anticipatory posturing to be picked up
- Differential preference for mother intensifies
- Subtle integration of responses to mother

Age 7 through 9 mos
- Attachment behaviors further differentiated and focused specifically on mother
- Separation distress, stranger distress, strange-place distress

Age 10 through 15 mos
- Crawls or walks toward mother
- Subtle facial expressions (coyness, attentiveness)
- Responsive dialogue with mother clearly established
- Early imitation of mother (vocal inflections, facial expression)
- More fully developed separation distress and mother preference
- Pointing gesture
- Walking to and from mother
- Affectively positive reunion responses to mother after separation or, paradoxically, short-lived, active avoidance or delayed protest

Age 16 mos through 2 yrs
- Involvement in imitative jargon with mother (12 to 14 mos)
- Head-shaking "no" (15 to 16 mos)
- Transitional object used during the absence of mother
- Separation anxiety diminishes
- Mastery of strange situations and persons when mother is near
- Evidence of delayed imitation
- Object permanence
- Microcosmic symbolic play

Age 25 mos through 3 yrs
- Able to tolerate separations from mother without distress when familiar with surroundings and given reassurances about mother's return
- Two- and three-word speech
- Stranger anxiety much reduced
- Object consistency achieved—maintains composure and psychosocial functioning without regression in absence of mother
- Microcosmic play and social play; cooperation with others begins

Based on material by Justin Call, M.D.

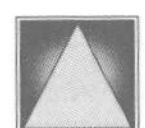

Table 4.2–2
The Strange Situation

Episode[a]	Persons Present	Change
1	Parent, infant	Enter room
2	Parent, infant, stranger	Unfamiliar adult joins the dyad
3	Infant, stranger	Parent leaves
4	Parent, infant	Parent returns, stranger leaves
5	Infant	Parent leaves
6	Infant, stranger	Stranger returns
7	Parent, infant	Parent returns, stranger leaves

[a] All episodes are usually 3 minutes long, but episodes 3, 5, and 6 can be curtailed if the infant becomes too distressed, and episodes 4 and 7 are sometimes extended.

(Reprinted from Lamb ME, Nash A, Teti DM, Bornstein MH. Infancy. In: Lewis M, ed. *Child and Adolescent Psychiatry: A Comprehensive Textbook*. 2nd ed. Baltimore: Williams & Wilkins; 1996:256, with permission.)

(called the transitional object by Donald Winnicott), also serve as a secure base, one that often accompanies them as they investigate the world.

Strange Situation. Ainsworth developed strange situation, the research protocol for assessing the quality and security of an infant's attachment. In this procedure, the infant is exposed to escalating amounts of stress; for example, the infant and the parent enter an unfamiliar room, an unfamiliar adult then enters the room, and the parent leaves the room. The protocol has seven steps (Table 4.2–2). According to Ainsworth's studies, about 65 percent of infants are securely attached by the age of 24 months.

ANXIETY

Bowlby's theory of anxiety holds that a child's sense of distress during separation is perceived and experienced as anxiety and is the prototype of anxiety. Any stimuli that alarm children and cause fear (e.g., loud noises, falling, and cold blasts of air) mobilize signal indicators (e.g., crying) that cause the mother to respond in a caring way by cuddling and reassuring the child. The mother's ability to relieve the infant's anxiety or fear is fundamental to the growth of attachment in the infant. When the mother is close to the child and the child experiences no fear, the child gains a sense of security, the opposite of anxiety. When the mother is unavailable to the infant because of physical absence (e.g., if the mother is in prison) or because of psychological impairment (e.g., severe depression), anxiety develops in the infant.

Expressed as tearfulness or irritability, separation anxiety is the response of a child who is isolated or separated from its mother or caretaker. It is most common at 10 to 18 months of age and disappears generally by the end of the third year. Somewhat earlier (at about 8 months) stranger anxiety, an anxiety response to someone other than the caregiver, appears.

Signal Indicators

Signal indicators are infants' signs of distress that prompt or elicit a behavioral response in the mother. The primary signal is crying.

The three types of signal indicators are hunger (the most common), anger, and pain. Some mothers can distinguish between them, but most mothers generalize the hunger cry to represent distress from pain, frustration, or anger. Other signal indicators that reinforce attachment are smiling, cooing, and looking. The sound of an adult human voice can prompt these indicators.

Losing Attachments

Persons' reactions to the death of a parent or a spouse can be traced to the nature of their past and present attachment to the lost figure. An absence of demonstrable grief may be owing to real experiences of rejection and to the lack of closeness in the relationship. The person may even consciously offer an idealized picture of the deceased. Persons who show no grief usually try to present themselves as independent and as disinterested in closeness and attachment.

Sometimes, however, the severing of attachments is traumatic. The death of a parent or a spouse can precipitate a depressive disorder, and even suicide, in some persons. The death of a spouse increases the chance that the surviving spouse will experience a physical or mental disorder during the next year. The onset of depression and other dysphoric states often involves having been rejected by a significant figure in a person's life.

DISORDERS OF ATTACHMENT

Attachment disorders are characterized by biopsychosocial pathology that results from maternal deprivation, a lack of care by, and interaction with, the mother or caregiver. Failure-to-thrive syndromes, psychosocial dwarfism, separation anxiety disorder, avoidant personality disorder, depressive disorders, delinquency, academic problems, and borderline intelligence have been traced to negative attachment experiences. When maternal care is deficient because (1) a mother is mentally ill, (2) a child is institutionalized for a long time, or (3) the primary object of attachment dies, children suffer emotional damage. Bowlby originally thought that the damage was permanent and invariable, but he revised his theories to take into account the time at which the separation occurred, the type and degree of separation, and the level of security that the child experienced before the separation.

Bowlby described a predictable set and sequence of behavior patterns in children who are separated from their mothers for long periods (more than 3 months): protest, in which the child protests the separation by crying, calling out, and searching for the lost person; despair, in which the child appears to lose hope that the mother will return; and detachment, in which the child emotionally separates himself or herself from the mother. Bowlby believed that this sequence involves ambivalent feelings toward the mother; the child both wants her and is angry with her for her desertion.

Children in the detachment stage respond in an indifferent manner when the mother returns; the mother has not been forgotten, but the child is angry at her for having gone away in the first place and fears that she will go away again. Some children have affectionless personalities characterized by emotional withdrawal, little or no feeling, and a limited ability to form affectionate relationships.

Anaclitic Depression

Anaclitic depression, also known as hospitalism, was first described by René Spitz in infants who had made normal attachments but were then suddenly separated from their mothers for varying times and placed in institutions or hospitals. The children became depressed, withdrawn, nonresponsive, and vulnerable to physical illness but recovered when their mothers returned or when surrogate mothering was available.

CHILD MALTREATMENT

Abused children often maintain their attachments to abusive parents. Studies of dogs have shown that severe punishment and maltreatment increase attachment behavior. When children are hungry, sick, or in pain, they too show clinging attachment behavior. Similarly, when children are rejected by their parents or are afraid of them, their attachment may increase; some children want to remain with an abusive parent. Nevertheless, when a choice must be made between a punishing and a nonpunishing figure, the nonpunishing person is the preferable choice, especially if the person is sensitive to the child's needs. (Child abuse is discussed at length in Chapter 32.)

PSYCHIATRIC APPLICATIONS

The applications of attachment theory in psychotherapy are numerous. When a patient is able to attach to a therapist, a secure base effect is seen. The patient may then be able to take risks, mask anxiety, and practice new patterns of behavior that otherwise might not have been attempted. Patients whose impairments can be traced to never having made an attachment in early life may do so for the first time in therapy, with salutary effects.

Patients whose pathology stems from exaggerated early attachments may attempt to replicate them in therapy. Therapists must enable such patients to recognize the ways their early experiences have interfered with their ability to achieve independence.

For patients who are children and whose attachment difficulties may be more apparent than those of adults, therapists represent consistent and trusted figures who can engender a sense of warmth and self-esteem in children, often for the first time.

Relationship Disorders

A person's psychological health and sense of well-being depend significantly on the quality of his or her relationships and attachment to others, and a core issue in all close personal relationships is establishing and regulating that connection. In a typical attachment interaction, one person seeks more proximity and affection, and the other either reciprocates, rejects, or disqualifies the request. A pattern is shaped through repeated exchanges. Distinct attachment styles have been observed. Adults with an anxious–ambivalent attachment style tend to be obsessed with romantic partners, suffer from extreme jealousy, and have a high divorce rate. Persons with an avoidant attachment style are relatively uninvested in close relationships, although they often feel lonely. They seem afraid of intimacy and tend to withdraw when there is stress or conflict in the relationship. Break-up rates are high.

Persons with a secure attachment style are highly invested in relationships and tend to behave without much possessiveness or fear of rejection.

References

Ainsworth MS. Attachments across the life span. *Bull N Y Acad Med*. 1985;61:792.

Akister J, Reibstein J. Links between attachment theory and systemic practice: some proposals. *Journal of Family Therapy*. 2004;26(1):2.

Berlin LJ, Amaya-Jackson L, Greenberg MT, Ziv Y. *Enhancing Early Attachments: Theory, Research, Intervention, and Policy*. New York: Guilford Press; 2005.

Blum HP. Separation-individuation theory and attachment theory. *J Am Psychoanal Assoc*. 2004;52:535–553.

Bowlby J. *Attachment and Loss*. Vols. 1, 2, 3. New York: Basic Books; 1969, 1973, 1980.

Carlson EA. Sampson MC, Sroufe LA. Implications of attachment theory and research for developmental-behavioral pediatrics. *J Dev Behav Pediatr*. 2003; 24:364–379.

Gordon MF. Normal Child Development. In: Sadock BJ, Sadock VA, eds. *Kaplan & Sadock's Comprehensive Textbook of Psychiatry*. 8th ed. Vol. 2. Baltimore: Lippincott Williams & Wilkins; 2005:3018.

Grossman KE, Grossman K, Waters E. *Attachment from Infancy to Adulthood: The Major Longitudinal Studies*. New York: Guilford Press; 2005.

Gullestad SE. Attachment theory and psychoanalysis: controversial issues. *Scandinavian Psychoanalytic Review*. 2001;24:3.

Kennedy JH, Kennedy CE. Attachment theory: Implications for school psychology. *Psychology in the Schools*. 2004;41(2):247–259.

Kerns KA, Richardson RA. *Attachment in Middle Childhood*. New York: Guildford Press; 2005.

MacDonald SG. The real and the researchable: A brief review of the contribution of John Bowlby (1907–1990). *Perspectives in Psychiatric Care*. 2001; 37:60.

Park LE, Crocker J, Mickelson KD. Attachment styles and contingencies of self-worth. *Personality and Social Psychology Bulletin*. 2004;30(10):1243–1254.

Shilkret CJ. Some clinical applications of attachment theory in adult psychotherapy. *Clinical Social Work Journal*. 2005;33:55–68.

Thompson RA, Raikes HA. Toward the next quarter-century: Conceptual and methodological challenges for attachment theory. *Dev Psychopathol*. 2003;15: 691–718.

▲ 4.3 Learning Theory

Learning plays a central role in the development of human behavior, including voluntary and involuntary motor behaviors, thinking, and emotion. *Learning* is defined as a change in behavior resulting from repeated practice, and both the environment and the behavior interact to produce the learned change. To assess learning, an aspect of performance, such as the accuracy of a motor skill or the ability to recognize and repeat words, is measured. Learning and performance are related but should not be confused; when performance is adversely affected by insufficient motivation or by anxiety, learning that has occurred may not be demonstrable.

Learning can be state dependent, that is, it may occur when the person is in a special internal state (e.g., under the influence of a drug) or in a special environment. Such learning is best recalled when the person is in the same internal state or external environment in which the information was first acquired. For example, when a behavior is acquired under the influence of a pharmacological agent and tests for learning are carried out in the absence of the drug, little or no evidence may exist of acquisition. When the learning test is carried out under the influence of the drug, however, performance may change, and learning may then be demonstrated. Some common terms used in learning theory are listed and defined in Table 4.3–1.

TYPES OF LEARNING

The three types of learning are as follows: (1) In classic conditioning, learning is thought to take place as a result of the contiguity of environmental events; when events occur closely together in time, persons will probably come to associate the two. (2) In operant conditioning, learning is thought to result from the consequences of a person's actions. (3) Social learning theory incorporates both classic and operant models of learning, but also considers a reciprocal interaction between the person and the environment. Cognitive processes are viewed as important factors in modulating a person's responses to environmental events.

Psychoanalytic theory and practice developed concurrently with learning theory, and attempts have been made over the last 50 years to integrate the two theoretical approaches. For example, in 1950 John Dollard and Neal Miller reformulated many psychoanalytic concepts in terms of learning theory. Such attempts, however, have had little lasting influence on psychoanalytic thought or therapy.

Classic Conditioning

Classic (also called *respondent*) *conditioning* results from the repeated pairing of a neutral (conditioned) stimulus with one that evokes a response (unconditioned stimulus), such that the neutral stimulus eventually comes to evoke the response. The time relation between the presentation of the conditioned and unconditioned stimuli is important and varies for optimal learning from a fraction of a second to several seconds.

The Russian physiologist and Nobel Prize winner Ivan Petrovich Pavlov (1849–1936) (Fig. 4.3–1), observed in his work on gastric secretion that a dog salivated not only when food was placed in its mouth but also at the sound of the footsteps of the person coming to feed it, even though the dog could not see or smell the food. Pavlov analyzed these events and called the saliva flow that occurred with the sound of footsteps a *conditioned response* (CR)—a response elicited under certain conditions by a particular stimulus.

In a typical pavlovian experiment, a *stimulus* (S) that had no capacity to evoke a particular response before training did so after consistent association with another stimulus. For example, under normal circumstances, a dog does not salivate at the sound of a bell, but when the bell sound is always followed by the presentation of food, the dog ultimately pairs the bell and the food. Eventually, the bell sound alone elicits salivation (CR).

Because the food naturally produces salivation, it is referred to as an *unconditioned stimulus* (UCS). Salivation, a response that is reliably elicited by food (UCS), is referred to as an *unconditioned response* (UCR). The bell, which was originally unable to evoke salivation but came to do so when paired with food, is referred to as a *conditioned stimulus* (CS). Classic conditioning is most often applied to responses mediated by the autonomic nervous system.

Classic conditioning is diagramed as follows:

Before conditioning

Food (UCS) → Salivation (UCR)

Bell (CS) paired with food (UCS) → Salivation (UCR)

After conditioning

Bell (CS) → Salivation (CR)

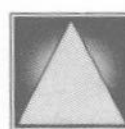

Table 4.3–1
Common Terms Used in Learning Theory

Aversive conditioning: a procedure in which punishment or aversive stimulation is used to reduce the frequency of a target behavior

Avoidance learning: a form of operant learning in which an organism learns to avoid certain responses or situations

Classic conditioning: the association of a neutral stimulus with an unconditioned stimulus, such that the neutral stimulus comes to bring about a response similar to that originally elicited by the unconditioned stimulus

Conditioned response: in classic conditioning, the response elicited by the conditioned stimulus

Conditioned stimulus: in classic conditioning, the originally neutral stimulus that comes to be associated with the unconditioned stimulus and eventually elicits a conditioned response

Continuous reinforcement: a schedule of reinforcement in which a reward is administered every time a response is emitted

Covert reinforcement: a method of increasing behavioral frequency by using the imagination of pleasant events as a reinforcement

Covert sensitization: a method of reducing the frequency of behavior by associating it with the imagination of unpleasant consequences

Discrimination learning: a process in which the tendency toward stimulus generalization is counteracted and responses are made only to specific stimuli

Experimental neurosis: an abnormal behavior pattern produced in animals through the application of classic or operant conditioning techniques

Extinction: the reduction of frequency of a learned response as a result of the cessation of reinforcement

Fixed-interval schedule: a reinforcement schedule in which a reward is given after a specific amount of time has passed

Fixed-ratio schedule: a reinforcement schedule in which a reward is given after a specific number of responses have been emitted

Habituation: a simple form of learning in which the response to a repeated stimulus lessens over time

Higher-order conditioning: in classic conditioning, the establishment of a new conditioned stimulus through association with an established conditioned stimulus

Instrumental learning: operant conditioning

Law of effect: the principle that behaviors followed by pleasant consequences are strengthened and that those followed by negative consequences are weakened

Modeling: observational learning

Negative practice: a method for reducing the frequency of a behavior by the intense repetition of the response

Observational learning: learning new behaviors by observing others responding and receiving some form of consequence; vicarious learning

Operant conditioning: a form of learning in which behavioral frequency is altered through the application of positive and negative consequences

Partial reinforcement: a schedule of reinforcement in which rewards are not given each time a response is made, rendering a learned response highly resistant to extinction

Primary reinforcer: a stimulus affecting a biological process (e.g., food that increases the probability of behaviors it follows)

Reinforcer: a stimulus that increases the frequency of responses it follows

Respondent learning: classic conditioning

Secondary reinforcers: stimuli that gain the power to reinforce a behavior through association with primary reinforcers

Shaping: an operant procedure in which a desirable behavior pattern is learned by the successive reinforcement of approximations to that behavior

Spontaneous recovery: the increase in the strength of an extinguished behavior after the passage of a period of time

Successive approximation: see the term *shaping*

Unconditioned response: in classic conditioning, a response that occurs spontaneously to the unconditioned stimulus

Unconditioned stimulus: a stimulus that, without any training, produces a specific response

Variable-interval schedule: a reinforcement schedule in which a reward is given after varying periods of time have passed

Variable-ratio schedule: a reinforcement schedule in which a reward is given after a varying number of responses have been emitted

(Courtesy of Marshall P. Duke, Ph.D., and Stephen Nowicki, Jr., Ph.D.)

Extinction. Extinction occurs when the conditioned stimulus is constantly repeated without the unconditioned stimulus until the response evoked by the conditioned stimulus gradually weakens and eventually disappears. In the previous example, extinction would occur if the bell (CS) is rung repeatedly without the food (UCS) being given. Eventually, salivation (CR) does not occur when the bell sounds, and extinction occurs. Extinction, however, does not completely destroy a conditioned response. If an animal is rested after extinction, the conditioned response returns, although less strong than originally, a phenomenon known as *partial recovery*.

The American psychologist John B. Watson (1878–1958) (Fig. 4.3–2) used Pavlov's theory of classic conditioning to explain certain aspects of human behavior. In 1920, Watson described producing a phobia in an 11-month-old boy called Little Albert. At the same time that the boy was shown a white rat that he initially did not fear, he was exposed to a loud, frightening noise. After several such pairings, Albert became fearful of the white rat, even when he heard no loud noise. Watson and his colleagues obtained the same results using a white rabbit and eventually managed to generalize the response to any furry object. Many theorists believe that this process accounts for the development of childhood phobias, which are considered learned responses based on classic conditioning.

Stimulus Generalization. *Stimulus generalization* describes a process whereby a conditioned response is transferred from one stimulus to another. Animals respond to stimuli similar to the original conditioned stimulus: A dog conditioned to respond to a bell also responds to the sound of a tuning fork. The theory of stimulus generalization is sometimes used to explain higher learning by showing how persons learn similarities. For example, a street sign is recognized whether it is on a pole, a building, or a curb, because there is sufficient stimulus similarity for generalization to occur.

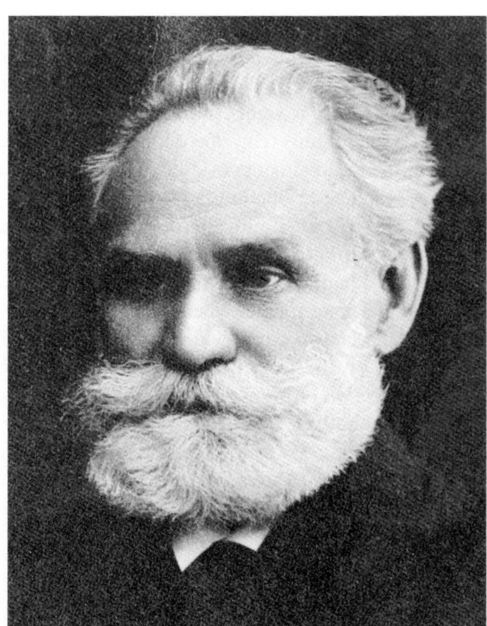

FIGURE 4.3–1
Ivan Pavlov (1849–1936). (Courtesy of the National Library of Medicine.)

Discrimination. *Discrimination* is the process of recognizing and responding to differences between similar stimuli. If the two stimuli are sufficiently different, an animal can learn to respond to one and not to the other; for example, an animal can learn to respond differentially to similar bells. A child learns to discriminate four-legged animals (the common stimulus) into dogs, cats, cows, and other quadrupeds.

When learning is viewed as a balance of generalization and discrimination, some disorders of thinking can be considered to stem from difficulties with these two processes. A person who had a traumatic childhood experience with a person who wore a moustache may transfer these negative feelings to all men with moustaches; this example shows both faulty discrimination and stimulus generalization.

Operant Conditioning

B. F. Skinner (1904–1990) developed a theory of learning and behavior known as *operant conditioning* (Fig. 4.3–3). Whereas in classic conditioning an animal is passive or restrained and behavior is reinforced by the experimenter, in operant conditioning the animal is active and behaves in a way that produces a reward; thus learning occurs as a consequence of action. For example, a rat receives a reinforcing stimulus (food) only when it correctly responds by pressing a lever. Food, approval, praise, good grades, or any other response that satisfies a need in an animal or a person can serve as a reward.

Operant conditioning is related to trial-and-error learning, as described by the American psychologist Edward L. Thorndike (1874–1949) (Fig. 4.3–4). In trial-and-error learning, a person or animal attempts to solve a problem by trying different actions until one proves successful. A freely moving organism behaves in a way that is instrumental in producing a reward. For example, a cat in a Thorndike puzzle box must learn to lift a latch to escape from the box. For this reason, operant conditioning is sometimes called *instrumental conditioning*. Thorndike's law of

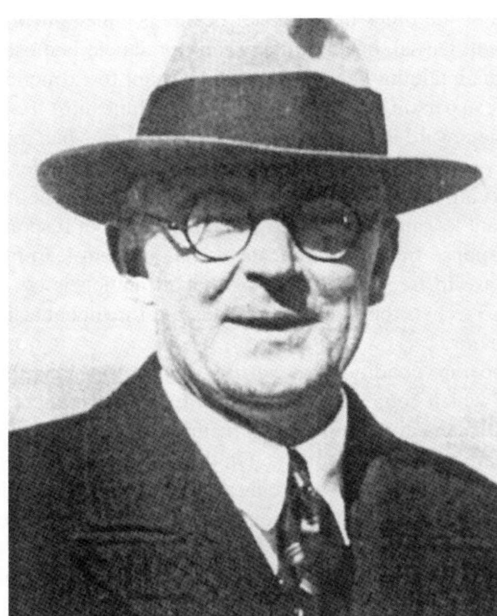

FIGURE 4.3–2
J. B. Watson (1878–1958) changed the focus of psychology from the study of inner sensations to the study of outer behavior, an approach called behaviorism. (From Carson RC, Butcher JN, Coleman JC, eds. *Abnormal Psychology and Modern Life*, 8th ed. Glenview, IL: Scott, Foresman and Company; 1988:69, with permission.)

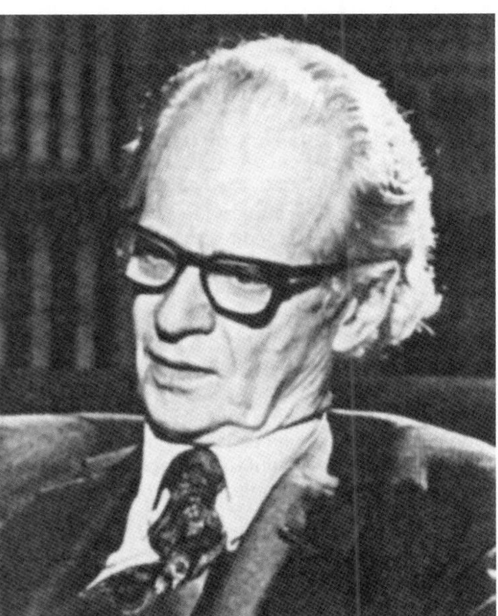

FIGURE 4.3–3
B. F. Skinner (1904–1990) formulated the concept of operant conditioning as a kind of conditioning in which reinforcers could be used to make a response more less probable and frequent. (From Carson RC, Butcher JN, Coleman JC, eds. *Abnormal Psychology and Modern Life*, 8th ed. Glenview, IL: Scott, Foresman and Company; 1988:69, with permission.)

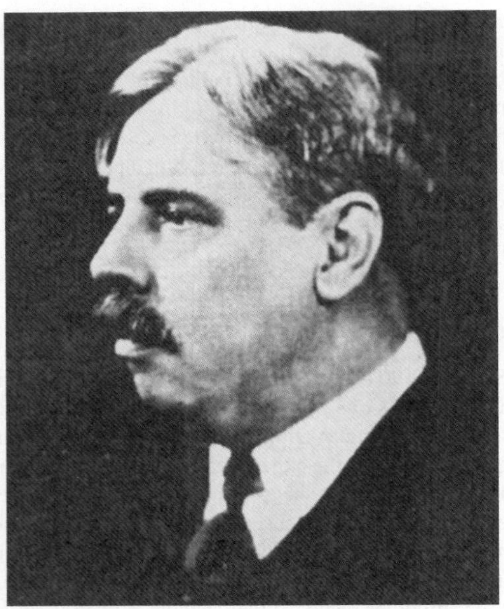

FIGURE 4.3–4

E. L. Thorndike (1874–1949) formulated the law of effect—seemingly simple observation that rewarded responses are strengthened and unrewarded responses are weakened—which laid the foundations of understanding learning and suggested means for the control of human behavior. (From Carson RC, Butcher JN, Coleman JC, eds. *Abnormal Psychology and Modern Life*, 8th ed. Glenview, IL: Scott, Foresman and Company; 1988:69, with permission.)

effect states that certain responses are reinforced by reward, and the organism learns from these experiences. Four kinds of operant conditioning are described in Table 4.3–2: primary reward conditioning, escape conditioning, avoidance conditioning, and secondary reward conditioning.

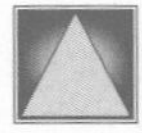

Table 4.3–2
Four Kinds of Operant or Instrumental Conditioning

Primary reward conditioning	The simplest kind of conditioning. The learned response is instrumental in obtaining a biologically significant reward, such as a pellet of food or a drink of water.
Escape conditioning	The organism learns a response that is instrumental in getting out of some place where it prefers not to be.
Avoidance conditioning	The kind of learning in which a response to a cue is instrumental in avoiding a painful experience. A rat on a grid, for example, may avoid a shock if it quickly pushes a lever when a light signal goes on.
Secondary reward conditioning	The kind of learning in which instrumental behavior to get at a stimulus has no biological usefulness itself but has in the past been associated with a biologically significant stimulus. For example, chimpanzees learn to press a lever to obtain poker chips, which they insert into a slot to secure grapes. Later, they work to accumulate poker chips even when they are not interested in grapes.

Respondent and Operant Behavior. Skinner described two types of behavior: *respondent behavior*, which results from known stimuli (e.g., the knee jerk reflex to patellar stimulation or the pupillary constriction to light), and *operant behavior*, which is independent of a stimulus (e.g., the random movements of an infant or the aimless movements of a laboratory rat in a cage). Skinner took advantage of operant behavior by placing a rat in a Skinner box (named after him, its developer). The rat was deprived of food; in the course of moving around the box, it randomly pressed a bar. At some point in the experiment, food was released by the experimenter when the bar was pressed. The food reinforced the bar pressing, which increased or decreased in rate depending on the level of reinforcement given by the experimenter. A *reinforcer* is anything that maintains a response or increases its strength; the term is used synonymously with reward. Some workers, however, distinguish between the two and point out that responses are reinforced, whereas subjects are rewarded.

Reinforcement Schedule (Programming). Reinforcers are described as *primary* when they are independent of previous learning (e.g., the need for food or water) and *secondary* when they are based on previously rewarded learning (e.g., giving money to a child with good grades). In operant conditioning, the schedule of reward or reinforcement for a behavioral pattern can vary in a process known as *programming*. The intervals between reinforcements may be *fixed* (e.g., every third response is rewarded) or *variable* (e.g., sometimes the third response is rewarded; at other times, the sixth response is rewarded).

A *continuous reinforcement* (also called *contingency reinforcement* or *management*) schedule, in which every response is reinforced, leads to the most rapid acquisition of a behavior, not the maintenance of behavior. Reinforcing a response only a fraction of the times the behavior occurs is called *partial reinforcement*. Partial, or intermittent, reinforcement is most effective in maintaining behavior that is resistant to extinction. For example, a person uses a gambling slot machine most frequently when the reward is partially reinforced—that is, when money is won at variable times. This procedure keeps the gambler guessing or trying to anticipate when a payoff will occur. The strength of operant learning is reflected in the frequency of responses: A high response frequency indicates strong operant learning, and a decrease in frequency indicates that extinction is occurring. Table 4.3–3 lists the effects of various reinforcement schedules on behavior.

In operant conditioning, *positive reinforcement* is the process by which certain consequences of a response increase the probability that the response will recur. Food, water, praise, and money are positive reinforcers. On the other hand, events aversive to some may be reinforcing for others. For example, the behavior of some children is reinforced by scolding, which, after all, is a form of attention. Many substances also appear to be positive reinforcers, including opium, cocaine, nicotine, and barbiturates.

Positive reinforcement is a useful therapeutic method for severely ill psychiatric patients, as in the following case.

A young woman had developed agoraphobia during adolescence. Agoraphobic avoidance had progressed over the subsequent decade

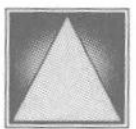

Table 4.3–3
Reinforcement Schedules in Operant Conditioning

Reinforcement Schedule	Example	Behavioral Effect
Fixed-ratio (FR) schedule	Reinforcement occurs after every ten responses (10:1 ratio); ten bar presses release a food pellet; workers are paid for every ten items they make.	Rapid rate of response to obtain the greatest number of rewards. Animal knows that the next reinforcement depends on a certain number of responses being made.
Variable-ratio (VR) schedule	Variable reinforcement occurs (e.g., after the third, sixth, then second response, and so on).	Generates a fairly constant rate of response because the probability of reinforcement at any given time remains relatively stable.
Fixed-interval (FI) schedule	Reinforcement occurs at regular intervals (e.g., every 10 minutes or every third hr).	Animal keeps track of time. Rate of responding drops to near 0 after reinforcement and then increases at about the expected time of reward.
Variable-interval (VI) schedule	Reinforcement occurs after variable intervals (e.g., every 3, 6, and then 2 hrs), similar to VR schedule.	Response rate does not change between reinforcements. Animal responds at a steady rate to get the reward when it is available; common in trout fishing, use of slot machines, checking mailbox.

until she was essentially housebound. She could only leave home accompanied by her mother or husband and, even in that circumstance, with considerable anxiety. Leaving home alone had, in the past, often precipitated a panic attack. She had been treated with various medications and with psychotherapy without significant improvement. She was admitted to a clinical research center as part of a study examining the use of social reinforcement in various phobic conditions. A therapist with whom she had developed a good relationship delivered reinforcement in the form of praise contingent on progress. In the baseline period, the patient was encouraged to walk as far away from the clinical research unit as she could. Reinforcement for staying outside the unit resulted in only a small increase in distance walked away from the unit. Positive reinforcement was then introduced. In this phase, praise for progress was given on a shaping schedule. For example, if the patient had been reinforced at a criterion of 100-yards distance on one trial and walked 150 yards on the next trial, the criterion would become 125 yards. She would be praised on the next trial only if she walked 125 yards or more. In this phase, distance walked began to increase. When reinforcement was stopped, distance walked increased dramatically and then decreased, an example of an extinction burst. This phenomenon is well known in animal experiments. Finally, when reinforcement was reintroduced, the patient was able to walk long distances away from the unit. This was then generalized to the patient's home environment. In theory, further natural reinforcement would continue to strengthen the patient's new freedom, because being free to move around allows contact with many reinforcing activities. (Courtesy of W. Stewart Agras, M.D., and G. Terence Wilson, Ph.D.)

Negative reinforcement is a process by which a response that leads to the removal of an aversive event is increased. For example, a teenager mows the lawn to avoid parental complaints, or an animal jumps off a grid to escape a painful shock. Any behavior that enables a person or animal to avoid or escape a punishing consequence is strengthened.

Negative reinforcement is not punishment. *Punishment* is an aversive stimulus (e.g., a slap) that is presented specifically to weaken or suppress an undesired response; punishment reduces the probability that a response will recur. The usual use of the term punishment must be distinguished from the technical use of the term. In learning theory, the punishing event delivered is always contingent on performance and demonstrably reduces the frequency of the behavior being punished. This meaning differs from the use of the term to denote imprisonment, for example, because the prison sentence follows long after the crime has been committed and may not affect future criminal behavior. Punishment is less useful as a therapeutic procedure than reinforcement or extinction, because it can produce unwanted effects, such as aggressive behavior, and the possibility of inflicting physical damage is always present. For the most part, punishment is used only in situations in which the behavior to be changed is injurious to the patient.

A clinical example of such a condition is rumination disorder in which infants regurgitate their food mouthful by mouthful, which leads to malnutrition and dehydration and is frequently life threatening. One treatment is to use the principle of punishment, making an unpleasant event contingent on each episode of regurgitation. A drop of lemon juice applied to the infant's tongue can be used as the unpleasant event. During the baseline period before treatment, the infant ruminated between 40 and 70 percent of the time that he was awake. Once lemon juice was presented contingent on spitting up food, the frequency of rumination steadily declined. Punishment was then briefly removed, and rumination returned to baseline levels, demonstrating the efficacy of punishment. The reintroduction of punishment eventually led to the virtual elimination of the behavior and a return to normal weight, with no relapse at 1-year follow-up. (Courtesy of W. Stewart Agras, M.D., and G. Terence Wilson, Ph.D.)

Aversive Control. In aversive control or conditioning, an organism changes its behavior to avoid a painful, noxious, or aversive stimulus. Electric shocks are common aversive stimuli used in laboratory experiments. Any behavior that avoids an aversive stimulus is reinforced as a result.

Escape Learning and Avoidance Learning. Negative reinforcement is related to two types of learning, escape learning and avoidance learning. In *escape learning*, an animal learns a response to get out of a place where it does not want to be (e.g., an animal jumps off an electric grid whenever the grid is charged). *Avoidance learning* requires an additional response. The rat on the grid learns to avoid a shock if it quickly pushes a lever when a light signal goes on. To move from escape learning to avoidance learning, an animal must make an *anticipatory response* to prevent the punishment. Escape learning and avoidance learning are two forms of aversive control; behavior that terminates the source of aversive stimuli is strengthened and maintained.

Shaping Behavior. Shaping involves changing behavior in a deliberate and predetermined way. By reinforcing those responses that are in the desired direction, an experimenter shapes an animal's behavior. An experimenter who wants to train a seal to ring a bell with its nose can give a food reinforcement as the animal's random behavior brings its nose near the bell. To teach a mute schizophrenic patient to talk, a therapist may first reward the patient for simply looking at the therapist; later, the therapist reinforces any vocalizations and then simple speech. The closer the time of the reinforcement is to the operant behavior, the better the learning. Shaping is also called *successive approximation*.

Adventitious Reinforcement. Responses accidentally reinforced by coincidental pairing of response and reinforcement are adventitious. Such events may have clinical implications in the development of phobias and other behavior.

Premack's Principle. A concept developed by David Premack states that a behavior engaged in with high frequency can be used to reinforce a low-frequency behavior. In one experiment, Premack observed that children spent more time playing with a pinball machine than eating candy when both were freely available. When he made playing with the pinball machine contingent on eating a certain amount of candy, the children increased the amount of candy they ate. In a therapeutic application of this principle, patients with schizophrenia were observed to spend more time in a rehabilitation center sitting down doing nothing than they did working at a simple task. When 5 minutes of sitting down was made contingent on a certain amount of work, the work output was considerably increased, as was skill acquisition. This principle is also known as *Grandma's rule* ("If you eat your spinach, you can have dessert").

SOCIAL LEARNING THEORY

Social learning theory relies on role modeling, identification, and human interactions. A person can learn by imitating the behavior of another person, but personal factors are involved. When a person dislikes a role model, imitative behavior is unlikely. Social learning theorists combine operant and classic conditioning theories. For example, although the observation of models may be a major factor in the learning process, imitation of the model must be reinforced or rewarded if the behaviors are to become part of the person's repertoire.

Albert Bandura is a major proponent of the social learning school. According to Bandura, behavior results from the interplay between cognitive and environmental factors, a concept known as *reciprocal determinism*. Persons learn by observing others, intentionally or accidentally; this process is described as modeling, or learning through imitation. A person's choice of model is influenced by a variety of factors, such as age, sex, status, and similarity. If a chosen model reflects healthy norms and values, the person develops *self-efficacy*, the capacity to adapt to normal, everyday life as well as to threatening situations. It is possible to eliminate negative behavior patterns by having a person learn alternative techniques from other role models. For example, fearful children become less fearful when they watch other children acting fearlessly in the same situation. Similarly, demonstrating a fearless approach to a phobic situation may be useful to motivate a patient's approach to the feared object or situation.

Modeling has also been used in weight reduction and smoking cessation programs. It is an important component of group treatment plans in which members of the group learn from one another.

COGNITIVE LEARNING

Cognition is the process of obtaining, organizing, and using intellectual knowledge. Persons perform mental operations and store bits of information in memory to be retrieved later. Cognitive learning theories focus on the role of understanding: Cognition implies understanding the connection between cause and effect, between action and the consequences of the action. *Cognitive strategies* are mental plans that persons use to understand themselves and the environment.

The cognitive strategy of patients with depression focuses on what is wrong rather than what is right. A form of cognitive therapy developed by Aaron Beck for the treatment of depression teaches patients to recognize and value their assets and alerts them to the cognitive pattern that causes their depression. Beck described the cognitive triad that exists in depression as consisting of a person's negative view of self, negative interpretation of experience, and negative expectation of the future.

Many theorists, such as Jean Piaget, have defined a series of stages in cognitive growth. Another approach toward cognition is *information processing*, a sequence of mental operations involving input, storage, and output of information. Cognition involves calling up and processing relevant information from stored memory.

Behavior can change through techniques in which persons learn by listening to or reading instructions. Therapeutic instructions modify both a person's outcome and efficacy expectations. For example, patients told that their blood pressure readings would drop if they followed certain relaxation procedures showed a decline in blood pressure. To learn new patterns of behavior, persons can monitor their behavior by charting events, such as when they eat or smoke. Self-monitoring also reduces the rate of relapse. If a therapist helps patients define and set realistic and well-specified goals, they have a greater likelihood of achieving them than if goals are poorly defined or unrealistic. Goal attainment enhances self-efficacy, which in turn affects future performance positively.

Piaget was a major theorist of cognitive development. His work is discussed in Section 4.1.

Cognitive Dissonance

Cognitive dissonance means incongruity or disharmony among a person's beliefs, knowledge, and behavior. When dissonance becomes too great, persons change their ways of thinking or behaving to lessen the disharmony. An example of cognitive dissonance is a person's unwillingness to believe that a very expensive car or one that is considered a status symbol could have anything wrong with it or could be defective in any way. Another example is believing strongly in a decision after it has been made. Dissonance generally occurs when a palpable disparity exists between two experimental or behavioral elements. Cognitive dissonance apparently produces an uncomfortable tension state (e.g., hunger) that persons are motivated to change.

Attribution Theory

Attribution theory is a cognitive approach concerned with how persons perceive the causes of behavior. According to attribution theory, persons are likely to attribute their own behavior to situational causes but are likely to attribute others' behavior to stable internal dispositions (personality traits); the particular cause that a person attributes to a given event influences subsequent feelings and behavior. In psychiatry, attribution theory may help explain why some persons attribute a change in behavior to an external event (situation) or to a change in internal state (disposition or ability). Similarly, behavioral change can be attributed to the effects of taking a drug or to interpersonal events. Research on drug effects by attribution theorists has shown that it may be unwise to describe a drug as very strong or as very effective because, if it does have the desired effect, patients may believe that is the only reason they got better.

NEUROPHYSIOLOGY OF LEARNING

One of the first theorists to explore the neurophysiological aspects of learning was Clark L. Hull (1884–1952), who developed a drive reduction theory of learning. Hull postulated that neurophysiological connections established in the central nervous system reduce the level of a drive (e.g., obtaining food reduces hunger). An external stimulus stimulates an efferent system and elicits a motor impulse. The critical connection is between the stimulus and the motor response, which is a neurophysiological reaction that leads to what Hull called a *habit*. Habits are strengthened when a response further reduces the drive associated with the aroused need.

By exploring the human brain, researchers such as Pierre Broca and Karl Wernicke identified specific areas of the brain involved in the development and retention of speech and language. Electrical stimulation of certain brain sites evoked vivid mental imagery in patients, and lesions of the amygdaloid nucleus in animals interfered with learning. Learning produces changes in the structure and function of nerve cells. In one study, monkeys that were trained to use a particular finger to obtain food showed hypertrophy of the area of the brain responsible for finger control.

Habituation and Sensitization

In the study of the snail *Aplysia*, Eric Kandel showed how simple forms of learning, such as habituation and sensitization, can occur. Kandel studied a defensive reflex involving the withdrawal of the snail's siphon when the animal is tactually stimulated. If the snail is touched repeatedly, it is subject to habituation and learns not to withdraw its siphon and gill. Habituation causes the organism to stop responding reflexively as a result of the repeated stimulus.

Aplysia can also be sensitized; that is, a reflex response can be made more sensitive, so that a subthreshold stimulus elicits a response. If the snail receives a strong stimulus (e.g., an electric shock), it becomes sensitized; then, even a previously subthreshold stimulation causes the animal to withdraw its gill and siphon. Experimental work with *Aplysia* has also shown that habituation develops before sensitization. Kandel's research with simple organisms, such as *Aplysia*, revealed that learning avoidance behavior alters the chemical structure of cells in the nervous system. When the avoidance is unlearned, these chemical changes are reversed. Such research provides a foundation for understanding the neurochemistry of learning and for exploring reciprocal interactions between ongoing biological processes in the central nervous system and behavior changes resulting from environmental influences. Kandel received the Nobel Prize for his work in 2000.

Memory Formation and Storage

The neurobiological basis of learning is located in the structures of the brain involved in forming and storing information, which include the hippocampus, the cortex, and the cerebellum. One hundred billion neurons in the brain are involved in forming memories, including a layer of 4.6 million cells in the hippocampus.

Learning begins with the senses taking in an environmental stimulus that is eventually transformed into a memory trace or memory link. An electrical or chemical impulse, passing through a neuron when the brain receives information, triggers the formation of connections between synapses. Animal experiments have shown an increase in synaptic connections when learning occurs.

Long-term memories have increased time to link with many locations in the cortex and, thus, are retained longer than short-term memories. The more connections, the better the chance of contacting a neural pathway leading to the memory; repeated reliving of a memory enhances its permanence.

Storage is the key to a good memory. Relating material to something that is already known creates more pathways and increases the storage power. Processing information at a semantic level involves more of the mind than does rote memorization. Semantic information decays at a slower rate than information superficially memorized, without meaning and comprehension.

Memory is divided into short-term and long-term types; long-term memory is also known as *recent memory*, *recent past memory*, *remote memory*, and *secondary memory*. Short-term memory—also called *immediate memory*, *working memory*, *primary memory*, and *buffer memory*—is adversely affected by chronic emotional stress, psychological exhaustion, or too much input. Short-term and long-term memory differ in the amount of information that can be stored. The capacity of short-term memory is limited (five to nine bits of information).

Smell and emotion may underlie long-term memories. Scent conveys information through the olfactory nerve to the hippocampus, which plays a role in the control of emotion. Learning and memory are affected by stress. The increase in adrenaline resulting from stress can enhance learning, but if stress is too great, learning is inhibited. A person's mood affects learning and the recall of material; a person learning material in a happy mood enhances his or her memory and has better recall. Those childhood memories that survive are memories associated with the time the child learned to speak, between the ages of 3 and 5 years. Before then, only memories associated with traumatic events or with smell are likely to be remembered.

MOTIVATION

Motivation is a state of being that produces a tendency toward action. The state may be one of deprivation (e.g., hunger), a value system, or a strongly held belief (e.g., religion). In the mediation of learning and perception, biological mechanisms play an important role in motivating behavior. An organism tries to maintain homeostasis or internal balance against any disturbance of equilibrium (e.g., a thirsty animal is motivated to find water and drink). Social motives, such as the need for recognition and achievement, also account for behavioral patterns (e.g., studying hard to get good grades). But the intensity of motivation to master any task in a particular situation is determined by at least two factors: the achievement motive (desire to achieve) and the likelihood of success.

Persons show marked individual differences in the values placed on objects and goals. Some students strive for As; others depreciate the importance of grades and place higher value on intellectual satisfaction or on extracurricular activities. The expectancy factor refers to the subjective probability that by expending sufficient effort, the object can be acquired or the goal reached.

Psychiatric Applications

In 1950, Joseph Wolpe defined *anxious behavior* as persistent habits of learned or conditioned responses acquired in anxiety-generating situations. If a response inhibitory to anxiety can occur in the presence of anxiety-evoking stimuli, it weakens the connection between the stimuli and the anxiety response. Wolpe referred to this process as *reciprocal inhibition*. Relaxation, for instance, is considered incompatible with anxiety and, therefore, inhibits it. Wolpe was a pioneer in the development of behavior therapy.

Anxiety Hierarchy. In Wolpe's method of therapy, known as *systematic desensitization*, the goal is to eliminate maladaptive anxiety and behavior. To accomplish this goal, Wolpe asked his patients to imagine the least disturbing item on a list of potentially anxiety-evoking stimuli and then to proceed step by step up the list to the most disturbing stimulus. For example, a patient with a fear of heights ranked the sight of a tall building lower in the anxiety hierarchy than standing on a high ledge; being on the 10th floor of a building fell somewhere in between. In a relaxed state (usually induced by hypnosis but sometimes induced by drugs), the patient was instructed to visualize the least anxiety-producing situation; if this visualization did not produce anxiety, the person moved up the hierarchy. Eventually, the patient was desensitized to the source of anxiety.

Tension Reduction Theory. Dollard and Miller attempted to reconcile behavioral theory and freudian psychodynamics by stressing the commonalities between the two. Subscribing to the tension reduction theory of behavior, they considered behavior to be motivated by an organism's attempt to reduce tension produced by unsatisfied or unconscious drives. Similarly, Sigmund Freud's pleasure principle is a tension-reducing force and, consequently, a strong motivator. When a drive is repressed, anxiety occurs and acts as an acquired drive; a person's behavior may be motivated by an attempt to reduce that anxiety. Adults may avoid situations that are likely to stimulate anxiety, but they may be completely unaware of their avoidance patterns. Therapy, in part, is an unlearning process. The patient learns that certain behaviors can reduce anxiety, and avoidance patterns are replaced by approach patterns. (Table 4.3–4 gives a comparison of the behavioral and psychoanalytic models.)

Learned Helplessness Model of Depression. A laboratory animal may be classically conditioned to accept a painful stimulus when restrained. Such restraint eventually teaches the animal that it has no way to avoid the aversive stimulus. A condition known as *learned helplessness* develops when an organism learns that no behavioral pattern can influence the environment. The learned helplessness paradigm has been used to explain depression in humans who feel helpless, without options, and unable to control events.

Brain Stimulation and Reinforcement. When certain areas of the hypothalamus are electrically stimulated, intense pleasure is experienced by both humans and other animals. When nonhuman primates were provided with a way to stimulate pleasure centers in their brains, they preferred stimulating themselves

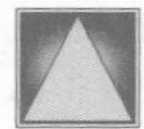

Table 4.3–4
Behavioral and Psychoanalytic Models

Behavioral Model	Psychoanalytic Model
Behavior is determined by current contingencies, reinforcement history, and genetic endowment.	Behavior is determined by intrapsychic processes.
Problem behavior is the focus of study and treatment.	Behavior is but a symbol of intrapsychic processes and a symptom of unconscious conflict; the underlying conflict is the focus of treatment.
Contemporary variables, such as contingencies of reinforcement, are the focus of the analysis.	Historical variables, such as childhood experiences, are the focus of the analysis.
Treatment entails the application of the principles of operant or classical conditioning.	Treatment consists of bringing unconscious conflicts into consciousness.
Objective observation, measurement, and experimentation are the methods used; the focus is on observable behavior and environmental events (antecedents and consequences).	Subjective methods of interpretation of behavior and inference regarding unobservable events (e.g., intrapsychic processes) are used.
Theory is based on experimentation.	Theory is predominantly based on case histories.
Tenets can be formulated into testable hypotheses and evaluated through experimentation.	Many tenets cannot be formulated into testable hypotheses to be evaluated through experimentation.

(Reprinted from Dorsett PC. Behavioral and social learning psychology. In: Stoudemire A, ed. *Human Behavior: An Introduction for Medical Students.* Philadelphia: JB Lippincott; 1990:105, with permission.)

to eating or drinking. In human beings, similar phenomena occur; in one case, a patient stimulated his brain 1,000 times in a 6-hour period until he was forced to stop.

References

Agras WS, Wilson GT. Learning theory. In: Sadock BJ, Sadock VA, eds. *Kaplan & Sadock's Comprehensive Textbook of Psychiatry*. 8th ed. Vol. 1. Baltimore: Lippincott Williams & Wilkins; 2005:541.

Buehner MJ, May J. Rethinking temporal contiguity and the judgment of causality: Effects of prior knowledge, experience, and reinforcement. *J Exp Psychol.* 2003;56:865.

Clark RE. The classical origins of Pavlov's conditioning. *Integr Physiol Behav Sci.* 2004;39(4):279–294.

Domjan M. Pavlovian conditioning: A functional perspective. *Annual Review of Psychology*. 2005;56:179–206.

Donahoe JW, Vegas R. Pavlovian conditioning: The CS-UR relation. *J Exp Psychol Anim Behav Process*. 2004;30(1):17–33.

Dygdon JA, Conger AJ, Strahan EY. Multimodal classical conditioning of fear: Contributions of direct, observational, and verbal experiences to current fears. *Psychol Rep*. 2004;95(1):133–153.

Havermans RC, Jansen AT. Increasing the efficacy of cue exposure treatment in preventing relapse of addictive behavior. *Addict Behav.* 2003;28:989.

Jones MB. Two early studies of learning theory and genetics. *Behav Genet.* 2003;33:669.

Kirsch I, Lynn SJ, Vigorito M, Miller RR. The role of cognition in classical and operant conditioning. *J Clin Psychol*. 2004;60(4):369–392.

Lidz J, Waxman S, Freedman J. What infants know about syntax but couldn't have learned: Experimental evidence for syntactic structure at 18 months. *Cognition.* 2003;89:65.

Newman BM, Newman PR. *Development through Life: A Psychosocial Approach.* 9th ed. Belmont, CA: Thomson Wadsworth; 2006.

Reinhard G, Lachnit H, König S. Tracking stimulus processing in Pavlovian pupillary conditioning. *Psychophysiology*. 2006;43(1):73.

Schmajuk NA, Larrauri JA. Experimental challenges to theories of classical conditioning: Application of an attentional model of storage and retrieval. *J Exp Psychol Anim Behav Process*. 2006;32(1):1–20.

Schultz W. Behavioral theories and the neurophysiology of reward. *Annual Review of Psychology*. 2006;57:87–115.

Sigelman CK, Rider EA. *Life Span Human Development*. 5th ed. Belmont, CA: Thomson Wadsworth; 2005.

▲ 4.4 Aggression

In humans, aggressive behavior assumes the form of violent actions against others, who may avoid such treatment or may fight back. Aggression implies the intent to harm or otherwise injure another person, an implication inferred from events preceding or following the act of aggression.

A classification system of aggression has been organized around behavior patterns; that is, behavior patterns similar in form are assigned to the same category. For example, one category of aggression behavior might include physical attacks against the self, and another, physical attacks against objects or others.

The term *aggression* is not specifically defined in the text revision of the fourth edition of the American Psychiatric Association's *Diagnostic and Statistical Manual of Mental Disorders* (DSM-IV-TR). The definition used in this section, which refers to behavior intended to cause physical injury to others, is descriptive by virtue of its short-term consequence, harm to others. Many behaviors are aggressive even though they do not involve physical injury. Verbal aggression is one example. Others include coercion, intimidation, managerial styles that result in harmful psychological consequences to others, and premeditated social ostracism of others. The importance of these behaviors in day-to-day living should not be underestimated, nor should their effects on recipients' self-esteem, social status, and happiness.

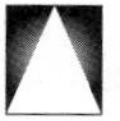

Table 4.4–1
Some DSM-IV-TR Disorders Associated with Aggression

Mental retardation
Attention-deficit/hyperactivity disorder
Conduct disorder
Cognitive disorders
Delirium
Dementia
Psychotic disorders
Schizophrenia
Psychotic disorder not otherwise specified
Mood disorders
Mood disorder because of a general medical condition
Substance-induced mood disorder
Intermittent explosive disorder
Adjustment disorder with disturbance of conduct
Personality disorders
Paranoid personality disorder
Antisocial personality disorder
Borderline personality disorder
Narcissistic personality disorder
Axis V conditions
Childhood, adolescent, or adult antisocial behavior

FANTASIES VERSUS ACTS

Persons may have violent thoughts or fantasies, but unless they lose control, thoughts do not become acts. Any set of conditions that produce increased aggressive impulses in the context of diminished control may produce violent acts, however. Situations with combinations of factors include toxic and organic states, developmental disabilities, florid psychosis, conduct disorder, and overwhelming psychological and environmental stress. Table 4.4–1 outlines some of the disorders listed in DSM-IV-TR that have been associated with violent and aggressive behavior.

Distinguishing fantasies from the threat of a real act is extremely important, because certain laws require psychiatrists to warn both legal authorities and potential victims when they suspect one of their patients will actually commit foul play. Fantasies, however—even the most violent, murderous, or sadistic—are not subject to such reporting requirements. (Chapter 58 on forensic psychiatry discusses these issues further.)

PREDICTORS OF AGGRESSION

Most adults with and without mental disorders who commit aggressive acts are likely to do so against persons they know, usually family members. This fact indicates that aggression is not directed indiscriminately. A possible exception to the familiar-person generalization is reported among male adolescents, who often behave aggressively toward casual acquaintances or strangers.

Generally, the probability of aggressive behavior increases when persons become psychologically decompensated and perhaps also when the onset of a mental disorder is rapid. Otherwise, little is known about the relation between the course of illness

Table 4.4–2
Commonly Cited Predictors of Dangerousness to Others

High degree of intent to harm
Presence of a victim
Frequent and open threats
Concrete plan
Access to instruments of violence
History of loss of control
Chronic anger, hostility, or resentment
Enjoyment in watching or inflicting harm
Lack of compassion
Self-view as victim
Resentful of authority
Childhood brutality or deprivation
Decreased warmth and affection in home
Early loss of parent
Fire-setting, bed-wetting, and cruelty to animals
Prior violent acts
Reckless driving

and aggression. Episodic decompensation may occur in those who ingest large quantities of alcohol; more than 50 percent of persons who commit criminal homicides and who engage in assaultive behavior are reported to have imbibed significant amounts of alcohol immediately beforehand.

Researchers have recently turned their attention to sex differences in the predisposition to, and frequency of, aggression. For aggression classified as homicide, battery, assault with a weapon, or rape, the frequency among males clearly exceeds that among females. In domestic violence, when one marital partner acts to hurt another, the frequency among men and women is about equal. Studies of persons who are hospitalized in psychiatric facilities for long periods indicate that the prevalence of male and female aggression is about equal. Tables 4.4–2 and 4.4–3 summarize predictors of violence. Among all factors, the best predictor of violence is a history of violent behavior.

ETIOLOGY

Psychological Factors

Instinctive Behavior

FREUD'S VIEW. In his early writings, Sigmund Freud held that all human behavior stems either directly or indirectly from Eros—the life instinct—whose energy, or libido, is directed toward the enhancement or reproduction of life. In this framework, aggression was viewed simply as a reaction to the blocking or thwarting of libidinal impulses and was neither an automatic nor an inevitable part of life.

After the tragic events of World War I, Freud gradually came to adopt a gloomier position about the nature of human aggression. He proposed the existence of a second major instinct—*Thanatos*, the death force—whose energy is directed toward the destruction or termination of life. According to Freud, all human behavior stems from the complex interplay of Thanatos and Eros and the constant tension between them.

Because the death instinct, if unrestrained, soon results in self-destruction, Freud hypothesized that through mechanisms, such as displacement, the energy of Thanatos is redirected outward and serves as the basis for aggression against others. Thus, in Freud's latter view, aggression stems primarily from the redirection of the self-destructive death instinct away from the self and toward others.

LORENZ'S VIEW. According to Konrad Lorenz, aggression that causes physical harm to others springs from a fighting instinct that humans share with other organisms. The energy associated with this instinct is produced spontaneously in organisms at a more or less constant rate. The probability of aggression increases as a function of the amount of stored energy and the presence and strength of aggression-releasing stimuli. Aggression is inevitable, and, at times, spontaneous eruptions occur.

Learned Behavior. From another perspective, aggression is primarily a learned form of social behavior—one that is acquired and maintained in much the same manner as other forms of activity. According to Albert Bandura, neither innate urges toward violence nor aggressive drives aroused by frustration are the roots of human aggression. Rather, persons acquire aggression, much like other forms of social behavior, through either personal experience or by observation of others. These learned behaviors vary between cultures, depending on experience. At the same time, people also learn through experience which persons or groups, behaviors, and situation warrant aggression. In contrast to instinct and drive theories (the psychological representation of a need that impels an organism to seek a goal), the social learning perspective does not attribute aggression to one or a few potential causes but suggests that the roots of such behavior are varied and involve an aggressor's previous experience, learning, and a wide range of external situational factors. For example, soldiers receive medals for killing enemy troops during times of war, and professional athletes earn widespread admiration and large financial rewards by competing aggressively (Table 4.4–4).

Social Factors

Frustration. The single most potent means of inciting human beings to aggression is frustration. Widespread acceptance of this view stems mainly from John Dollard's frustration-aggression hypothesis. In its original form, the hypothesis indicated that frustration always leads to a form of aggression and that aggression always stems from frustration.

Frustrated persons, however, do not always respond with aggressive thoughts, words, or deeds. They may show a wide variety of reactions, ranging from resignation, depression, and despair to attempts to overcome the sources of their frustration. And not all aggression results from frustration. Persons (e.g., boxers and football players) act aggressively for many reasons and in response to many stimuli.

Examination of the evidence indicates that whether frustration increases or fails to enhance overt aggression depends largely on two factors. First, frustration appears to increase aggression only when the frustration is intense. When it is mild or moderate, aggression may not be enhanced. Second, frustration is likely to facilitate aggression when it is perceived as arbitrary or illegitimate, rather than when it is viewed as deserved or legitimate.

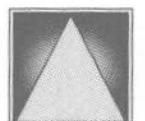

Table 4.4–3
Assessing the Risk of Committing a Homicide[a]

Clinical Characteristics	Low Risk	Medium Risk	High Risk
Hostility indicators (history)			
Family life	Wanted child, good loving family	Some family disruption, loss of a parent or one-parent family	Early violence, battered child, poor parent model
Significant others	Several reliable family members or friends available	Few or one available	None available
Daily functioning	Good in most activities	Moderately good in some activities	Not good in any activities
Lifestyle	Stable	Moderately stable	Unstable
Socioeconomic	Upper	Middle	Lower
Employment	Employed	Employment history fairly stable	Unemployed
Education	High school graduate or more (university or technical training)	High school dropout, can read and write	School dropout, semiliterate to illiterate
Housing	Lives in adequate housing, clean environment and space	Fair housing, some overcrowding	Poor housing, crowded, slums
Isolation or withdrawal	Able to relate well to others, outgoing	Mild, some withdrawal and feelings of hopelessness	Long history of being a loner, antisocial, withdrawn, hopeless and helpless feelings
Alcohol or other substance use	Nondrinker, occasional social use	Social drinker or user to occasional abuse	Chronic abuse
Psychological help	No history of need for, or use of, psychiatric hospitalization	Some outpatient psychiatric help, moderately satisfied with self	History of psychiatric hospitalization, negative view of help
Personal history	No history of violence or impulsive behavior	Occasional history of violence or impulsive behavior	Frequent history of violence or impulsive behavior
Perturbation (negative emotional states)			
Anxiety	Low, good emotional control	Occasional feelings of anxiety	Easily aroused to anxiety, high or panic state
Depression	Low	Occasional depression	Severe, chronically moody
Self-esteem	Good, has reinforcements from others	Usually good	Chronically poor self-image
Hostility	Low	Some	Marked, aggressive
Impulse control	Controlled	Some impulsive acting out; not physically violent	Feels need for violence
Constriction (narrowing of vision)			
Coping strategies and devices being used	Able to cope with stress and outside irritating influences; well-developed defense mechanisms	Usually can cope under most pressures; sometimes becomes constrictive in thinking and acts out	Becomes constrictive under most stress; acts out in destructive, socially unacceptable ways
Disorientation and disorganization	None, is in good contact with what is happening	Little to moderate	Marked, losing contact with reality
Resources	Able to make good use of resources available	Some use of resources; aware of most resources	Unable either to use resources available or to recognize that help is available
Cessation (stop the person causing the problem)			
Previous arrests	None	Has been arrested, has not served time	Multiple arrest history, served time in prison, would murder to avoid going back to prison
Previous homicide	None	Has exhibited aggressive behavior; been in fights but no attempt to kill another	Yes, looks at the killing of another as a feasible act
Homicide plan	None	Has held fleeting thoughts of killing another; no definite plan	Frequent or constant thoughts with a specific plan
Weapon available	None that person thinks of	Yes, person aware of weapons in immediate environment but not seriously considering use	Yes, and planning on use (a loaded gun should be considered highly lethal)

[a] No one clinical characteristic predicts homicide. However, the greater the number of clinical characteristics in the medium-risk and high-risk categories, the greater is the risk.
(Adapted from Allen N. *Homicide: Perspectives on Prevention.* New York: Human Sciences; 1979, with permission.)

Table 4.4–4
Theoretical Perspectives on Aggression

Theory	Assumed Source of Aggression	Possibility of Preventing or Controlling Aggression
Instinct	Innate tendencies or instincts	Low: Aggressive impulses are constantly generated and impossible to avoid.
Drive	Externally elicited aggressive drive	Low: External sources of aggressive drive are common (e.g., frustration) and impossible to eliminate.
Social learning	Present social or environmental conditions plus past social learning	Moderate to high: Appropriate changes in current social and environmental conditions or in reinforcement contingencies can reduce or prevent overt aggressive actions.

(Courtesy of Robert A. Baron, Ph.D.)

Direct Provocation. Evidence indicates that physical abuse and verbal taunts from others often elicit aggressive actions. Once aggression begins, it often shows an unsettling pattern of escalation; as a result, even mild verbal slurs or glancing blows may initiate a process in which stronger and stronger provocations are exchanged.

Media Violence. Media may influence behavior through modeling, disinhibition, desensitization, the arousal of aggressive feelings, and the encouragement of risk taking. Exposure to violent material reportedly increases violent fantasies, especially in men; youth are very vulnerable to such exposure. Whereas young children may persist in acting aggressively despite a victim's pain and young abused children seem to have special difficulties empathizing, older children and adults are usually more inhibited by the victim's suffering. An extensive review of violence and television reported a concomitant rise in violence and in television viewing in the United States and noted that American children spend more time watching television than they spend in school. The influence of television violence on societal violence is reportedly less in countries in which societies are more "rigid" (e.g., Japan, Singapore). Television violence is thought to contribute to violence in children and adults in the following ways:

- It has a short-term stimulating effect on aggressive behaviors in all ages.
- It portrays the world as a more hostile place than it is.
- It justifies violence (e.g., 40 percent of violent television acts are performed by heroes).
- It cues aggressive ideas in children.

The processes that account for the effects of filmed and televised violence on the behavior of viewers are outlined in Table 4.4–5.

Another source of entertainment containing violent themes is video games. It has been estimated that more than 90 percent of children in the United States between the ages of 2 and 17 now play video games and spend, on average, 20 to 33 minutes per day in this activity. Recent studies indicate that 89 percent of the top-selling games contain violence. Boys spend substantially more time than girls playing violent video games, and some reports indicate that minority youngsters from low- and middle-income communities play more of the time than do white children from higher-income communities. Some studies indicate that adolescents become desensitized to homicidal activities after repeated exposure, especially if the game involves their killing virtual opponents, which is common in many computer programs.

Environmental Factors

Air Pollution. Exposure to noxious odors, such as those produced by chemical plants and other industries, may increase personal irritability and, therefore, aggression, although this effect appears to be true only up to a point. If the odors in question are truly foul, aggression appears to decrease—perhaps because escaping from the unpleasant environment becomes a dominant goal for those involved.

Noise. Several studies have reported that persons exposed to loud, irritating noise direct stronger assaults against others than those not exposed to such environmental conditions.

Crowding. Some studies indicate that overcrowding may produce elevated levels of aggression, but other investigations have failed to obtain evidence of such a link. Crowding may enhance the likelihood of aggressive outbursts when typical reactions are negative (e.g., annoyance, irritation, and frustration). The crowding of airline passengers in coach class has been suggested as contributing to violent incidents among passengers.

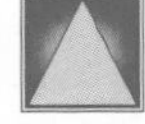

Table 4.4–5
Mechanisms Underlying the Effects of Televised and Filmed Violence on the Behavior of Viewers

Mechanism	Effects
Observational learning	Viewers acquire new means of harming others not previously present in their behavior repertoires.
Disinhibition	Viewers' restraints or inhibitions against performing aggressive actions are weakened as a result of observing others engaging in such behavior.
Desensitization	Viewers' emotional responsivity to aggressive actions and their consequences—signs of suffering on the part of victims—is reduced. As a result, they show little, if any, emotional arousal in response to such stimuli.

(Courtesy of Robert A. Baron, Ph.D.)

Situational Factors

Heightened Physiological Arousal. Some research indicates that heightened arousal stemming from such diverse sources as participation in competitive activities, vigorous exercise, and exposure to provocative films enhances overt aggression.

Sexual Arousal. Recent investigations indicate that the effects of sexual arousal on aggression depend strongly on the erotic materials used to induce such reactions and on the precise nature of the reactions themselves. When the erotica viewed are mild, such as photos of attractive nudes, aggression is reduced. When they are explicit, such as films of couples engaged in various sex acts, aggression is enhanced.

Pain. Physical pain may arouse an aggressive drive—the motive to harm or injure others. This drive, in turn, may find expression against any available target, including those not in any way responsible for the aggressor's discomfort. This hypothesis may partly explain why persons exposed to aggression act aggressively toward others.

Biological Factors

Aggression has been linked in animals with testosterone, progesterone, luteinizing hormone, renin, β-endorphin, prolactin, melatonin, norepinephrine, dopamine, epinephrine, acetylcholine, serotonin, 5-hydroxyindoleacetic acid (5-HIAA), and phenylacetic acid, among others. Some studies have related the level of aggression to androgen levels. These studies point to the androgen insensitivity syndrome (in which there is defective binding of androgens to proteins, resulting in male offspring with a feminine appearance and a decreased propensity for rough-and-tumble play) and to the adrenogenital syndrome (in which the mother's adrenal cortex exposes the fetus to elevated adrenal androgens, resulting in masculinization, partly evidenced by increased rough-and-tumble play in masculinized girls).

In regard to drugs and substances of abuse, several generalizations appear to hold. Small doses of alcohol inhibit aggression, and large doses facilitate it. Barbiturate effects are similar to the effects of alcohol, as are the effects of aerosols and commercial solvents. Anxiolytics generally inhibit aggression, although paradoxical aggression is sometimes observed. Opioid dependence (but not opioid intoxication) is associated with increased aggression, as is the use of stimulants, cocaine, hallucinogens, and, in some cases, variable doses of marijuana.

Neuroanatomical Damage. Increasingly, several investigators are hypothesizing that the root of the aggressive behavior of certain chronically aggressive persons is organic brain damage. This perspective is an elaboration of the theory that aggression is a learned social behavior, in that persons who have been the victims of severe physical abuse may suffer neurological sequelae secondary to the abuse, and the sequelae biologically predispose them to violent behavior. In 1986, Dorothy Lewis reported that every death-row inmate studied by her team of researchers had a history of head injury, often inflicted by abusive parents. This study concluded that death-row inmates constitute an especially neuropsychiatrically impaired prison population. Researchers investigating the association between head injury and violent behavior have been careful to point out that the linkage of physical abuse, head injury, and violence is uncertain, although most studies do show an association between early physical abuse and later aggressive behavior. Some researchers speculate that the combination of brain injury and a history of undergoing and observing chronic severe abuse is particularly lethal.

Neurotransmitters. Generally, cholinergic and catecholaminergic mechanisms seem to be involved in the induction and enhancement of predatory aggression, whereas serotonergic systems and γ-aminobutyric acid (GABA) seem to inhibit such behavior. The catecholaminergic and serotonergic systems evidently modulate affective aggression. Dopamine seems to facilitate aggression, whereas norepinephrine and serotonin appear to inhibit it. Recently, serotonin has again gained attention as a potentially important mediating factor in aggression. Rapid declines in serotonin levels or function are associated with increased irritability and, in nonhuman primates, with increased aggression. Some human studies have indicated that 5-HIAA levels in cerebrospinal fluid inversely correlate with the frequency of aggression, particularly among persons who commit suicide.

Genetic Factors

Twin Studies. Research involving monozygotic twins indicates a hereditary component to aggressive behavior. Thus far, most studies have focused on nonpsychiatric populations, in which the concordance rates for monozygotic twins exceed the rates for dizygotic twins.

Pedigree Studies. Several studies show that persons with family histories of mental disorders are more susceptible to mental disorders and engage in more aggressive behavior than those without such histories. Those with low intelligence quotient (IQ) scores appear to have a higher frequency of delinquency and aggression than those with normal IQ scores. Observed correlations between aggressive behavior and other atypical behaviors indicate that genetic predispositions to atypical behavior, including behaviors associated with mental disorders, are associated with atypical physiological functions, one consequence of which is an increase in the probability of aggression.

Chromosomal Influences. Behavior research involving the influence of chromosomes has concentrated primarily on abnormalities in X and Y chromosomes, particularly the 47-chromosome XYY syndrome. Early studies indicated that persons with the syndrome could be characterized as tall, of below-average intelligence, and likely to be apprehended and in prison for engaging in criminal behavior. Subsequent studies indicated, however, that, at most, the XYY syndrome contributes to aggressive behavior in only a small percentage of cases. Studies of the androgen and gonadotropin characteristics of persons with XYY syndrome have been inconclusive. A famous case of an "XYY" insanity defense is illustrated in Figure 4.4–1.

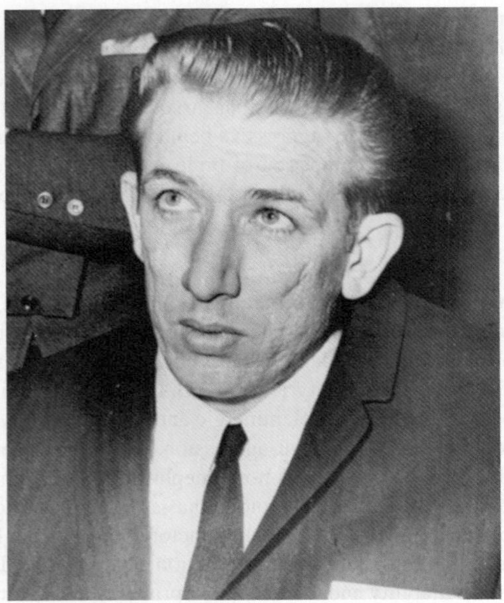

FIGURE 4.4–1
Richard Speck. He was convicted in 1966 of slaying eight nurses in Chicago by stabbing and strangulation. His legal defense was based on his genetic makeup, which was "XYY." Individuals with these genes have been reported to be tall, mentally retarded, have acne, and show aggressive behavior. A jury found him guilty, and he was sentenced to death in the electric chair. (Courtesy of Wide World Photos.)

EPIDEMIOLOGY

According to the Federal Bureau of Investigation (FBI) Uniform Crime Reports, about 1.5 million violent crimes (murder, rape, forcible robbery, and aggravated assault) are committed in the United States each year. Of this number, about 90,000 are rapes, and about 15,000 are homicides. These statistics have decreased by 25.5 percent since 1991. Violent crime rates are highest in large metropolitan areas and lowest in rural areas.

Violent acts are most often committed by persons who know or knew each other. Homicides are most prevalent among strangers (55 percent); more than 65 percent of homicides are committed with handguns. In the United States, homicide is the second leading cause of death among persons 15 to 24 years of age. Furthermore, a young black man is eight times more likely to be murdered than a white man of the same age. Much lower homicide rates have been reported in such countries as England, Sweden, Japan, and Canada, which all have strict handgun-control laws. Homicide is most prevalent in low socioeconomic groups and is more commonly committed by men than by women.

One national survey of high school students reported that 28 percent of the boys and 7 percent of the girls had been in a physical fight in the previous month. Nearly 35 percent of those surveyed reported having been in at least one physical fight that resulted in an injury requiring medical attention.

Studies estimate that 4 to 6 percent of elderly persons experience forms of abuse within their homes. One study of nursing home staff found that 10 percent of staff members admitted to at least one act of physical abuse toward elderly patients within the previous year. The number of helpless elderly patients tied to beds and chairs for lack of sufficient caretakers attest to the type of care (or lack thereof) available to the elderly indigent who cannot afford even the simplest of private care.

PREVENTION AND CONTROL

For physicians, the prevention of death and disability resulting from aggressive, violent, or homicidal behavior begins at the individual level. For instance, violence within a family (such as sexual and physical abuse of children, wife beating, and self-destructive behavior) is often revealed through sensitive questioning and a high index of suspicion on the clinician's part. Preventive interventions include psychiatric referral, notification of the proper legal or other authorities (mandatory in such cases as child abuse and specific threats of harm to persons), and skilled counseling by appropriately trained therapists. Many experts advocate limiting exposure to violence on television and in movies and computer games as way to decrease violence.

Punishment

Punishment is sometimes an effective deterrent to overt aggression. Research findings indicate that the frequency or intensity of such behavior can be reduced by even mild forms of punishment, such as social disapproval; but punishment does not always, or even usually, produce such effects.

The recipients of punishment often interpret it as an attack against them. To the extent that it is, aggressors may respond even more aggressively. Strong punishment is more likely to provoke desires for revenge or retribution than to instill lasting restraints against violence. Persons who administer punishment may serve as aggressive models for those on the receiving end of such discipline, and as noted above, exposure to such models can potentiate violent acts. Because of the conditions under which it is usually administered (a long time after the aggression is committed), punishment may only temporarily reduce the strength or frequency of aggressive behavior. Once the punishment is discontinued, the aggressive acts quickly reappear. For these reasons, certain punishments may backfire and actually encourage, rather than inhibit, the dangerous actions they are designed to prevent.

Catharsis

The *catharsis hypothesis* is the belief that the participation in activities, such as running or kickboxing, allows persons to vent their anger and hostility and therefore reduces aggressive behavior. Although Freud accepted the existence of such catharsis, he was relatively pessimistic about its usefulness in preventing overt aggression. At present, catharsis is thought to help some persons discharge aggression. Other persons, however, may become more aggressive as a result of the expressive behaviors. Catharsis, therefore, may not be effective for long-term reduction of aggression.

Training in Social Skills

A major reason why many persons become involved in repeated aggressive encounters is their lack of basic social skills. These persons do not know how to communicate effectively, and thus they adopt an abrasive style of self-expression. Their ineptness in performing such basic tasks as making requests, engaging in negotiations, and lodging complaints often irritates friends, acquaintances, and strangers. Their severe social deficits seem to ensure that they experience repeated frustration and frequently anger those with whom they have direct contact. A technique for reducing the frequency of such behavior involves providing these persons with the social skills that they sorely lack. Social skills training has been applied to diverse groups, including highly aggressive teenagers, police, and even child-abusing parents. In many cases, dramatic changes in the targeted behaviors have been produced (e.g., enhanced interpersonal communication and improved ability to handle rejection and stress), and reduced aggressive behavior related to these shifts is frequently observed. The results are encouraging and indicate that training in appropriate social skills can offer a promising approach to the reduction of human violence.

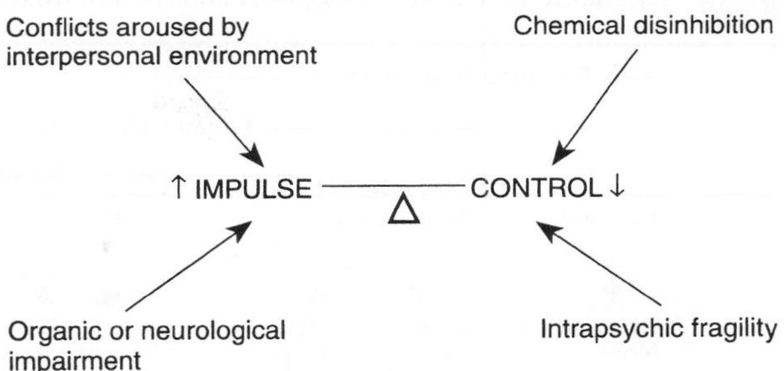

FIGURE 4.4–2
Mechanisms of violence.

Induction of Incompatible Responses

Empathy. When aggressors attack other persons in face-to-face confrontations, the aggressors may block out, ignore, or deny signs of pain and suffering on the part of their victims. If aggressors are exposed to such feedback, they may feel empathy and subsequently reduce further aggression. In several experiments, exposure to signs of pain or discomfort on the victim's part has inhibited further aggression.

Humor. Informal observation indicates that anger can often be reduced through exposure to humorous material, and some laboratory studies support this hypothesis. Several types of humor, presented in various formats, can induce reactions or emotions incompatible with aggression among the persons who observe the humor.

Other Factors. Many other reactions may also be incompatible with anger or overt aggression. As noted, mild sexual arousal sometimes operates in this fashion. Similarly, feelings of guilt about the performance of aggressive actions often reduce such behavior. Participation in absorbing cognitive tasks, such as solving mathematics problems, may induce reactions incompatible with anger and aggressive actions. A summary of mechanisms of violence is given in Figure 4.4–2.

Pharmacotherapy

Several types of drugs and clinical monitoring—for example, blood pressure and electroencephalogram (EEG)—are essential for the optimal treatment of specific aggressive persons. Lithium (Eskalith) appears to be a drug of major promise for some violent patients, especially delinquent adolescent boys. Anticonvulsants occasionally reduce seizure-induced forms of aggression, and they may have the same effect on persons who do not have epilepsy. Antipsychotic medications seem to reduce aggression in both psychotic and nonpsychotic violent patients. Antidepressants may be effective in reducing violence in some depressed patients. Antianxiety agents appear to have a limited role in reducing aggression. Anticonvulsant agents, such as gabapentin (Neurontin), have been of use in reducing aggressive outbursts. Antiandrogenic agents may be effective in the treatment of aggressive sex offenders. β-adrenergic receptor antagonists (beta-blockers) and stimulants may be effective in aggressive children. And electroconvulsive therapy may be effective in a small group of selected patients. Table 4.4–6 outlines some possible psychopharmacological interventions for aggression.

VICTIMS

An estimated 18 million persons in the United States at some time have suffered psychiatric disturbance as a result of crime. At any given moment, up to 5 million persons in the United States may suffer from crime-related symptoms. The National Institute of Justice estimates that a 12-year-old American has an 80 percent chance of being the victim of a serious crime at some point in his or her life. Recent research indicates that many victims of violent crimes are at increased risk for major psychiatric problems. Long-term depressive disorders and phobias are two mental disorders reported to occur more frequently in victims of crime than in the general population. Many researchers believe that distinct, characteristic emotional effects are associated with being the victim of a crime and that these effects are related to the fact that victims are the targets of another person's intentional aggression. Table 4.4–7 lists the main emotional aftereffects of crime.

ACCIDENTS

An accident is an event that occurs by chance or unexpectedly, without conscious planning. Studies of accidents show that causes can sometimes be determined and possibly corrected, but they are often multiple and require a multifaceted approach to the problem. For instance, both behavioral and psychological characteristics can be related to the occurrence of accidents. These characteristics include anxiety, boredom, fatigue, and the ingestion of substances that alter concentration and motor coordination. According to the Centers for Disease Control and Prevention (CDC), in 2002 accidents were the leading cause of death for persons under the age of 35 years. In 2002 a total of about 107,000 deaths and more than 20 million disabling injuries resulted from accidents. Nearly 40 percent of self-reported injuries occurred during sports or leisure activities and 40 percent occurred within or around the home.

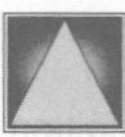

Table 4.4–6
Schematic Differential Diagnosis and the Pharmacological Treatment of Violence

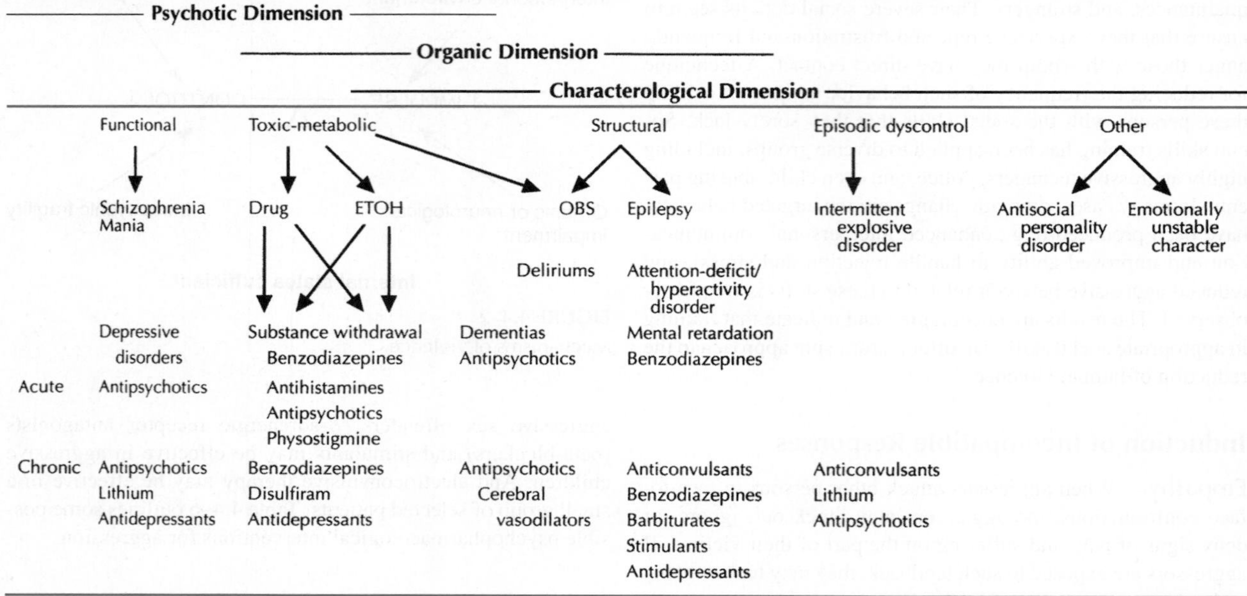

ETOH, ethanol; OBS, organic brain syndrome.
(Adapted from Skodol A. Emergency management of potentially violent patients. In: Bassul E, Birk A, eds. *Emergency Psychiatry: Concepts, Methods and Practice.* New York: Plenum; 1984.)

Accidents are the fifth most common cause of death overall in the United States. The most recent national data on the cost of injuries reported that, for the noninstitutionalized population, accidents were the second leading cause of direct medical costs (second only to heart disease and exceeding cancer) and also accounted for major indirect costs, such as work loss and disability.

Vehicular accidents, industrial accidents, and home accidents were the most frequent types of injuries. One third of all injury deaths are secondary to automobile accidents, and one third are secondary to other accidents; the remaining one third are evenly divided between suicide and homicide. After motor vehicle accidents, the most common causes of accidental death are firearms, followed by poisoning, falls, and suffocation.

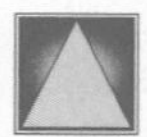

Table 4.4–7
Aftermath of Crime: Main Emotional Effects

Sense of helplessness: The world seems unsafe; victims lack confidence in their judgment and competence to deal with the world.

Rage at being a victim: Intense anger is usually expressed toward family members and those who try to help; conversely, sometimes the victim is unable to express any anger at anything.

Sense of being permanently damaged: Rape victims, for example, may feel that they will never be attractive again.

Inability to trust or to be intimate with others: The effect can include a loss of faith in institutions such as the police and the courts.

Persistent preoccupation with the crime: Excessive concern with the crime and its details may reach the point of obsession.

Loss of belief that the world is just: The effect may include self-blame and a sense of having done something to deserve being a victim.

(Courtesy of Stuart Kleinman, M.D.)

Psychophysiological Considerations

Victims' psychophysiological states must be considered in all injuries and accidents. A physical condition such as fatigue can lead to either distraction or an inability to respond sufficiently quickly to avoid an accident. Intake of such toxic substances as barbiturates, antihistamines, marijuana, and particularly alcohol is an important consideration. About one half of reported automobile accidents occur in conjunction with alcohol intake. Persons with diabetes, epilepsy, cardiovascular disease, and mental disorders are involved in more than twice as many accidents per 1,000 miles of driving as are those who do not have these illnesses. Age-related impairments, both motor and cerebral function deficits, can lead to potentially impaired judgment, which contributes to fatal accidents among persons aged 65 and older.

Motivations

From a motivational point of view, the first writings on the subject of an accident-prone personality date to Freud's *The Psychopathology of Everyday Life* (1904):

> Many apparently accidental injuries that happen to such patients are really instances of self-injuries. What happens is an impulse to self-punishment, which is constantly on the watch and which normally finds expression in self-reproach or contributes to the formation of a symptom, takes ingenious advantage of an external situation that chance happens to offer, or lends assistance to that situation until the desired injurious effect is brought about.

Many retrospective studies have explored the personality characteristics of persons who have had severe or frequent accidents. In these studies, workers have speculated that persons repeatedly involved in accidents may have an underlying self-destructive tendency that suggests the existence of depression, poor control of hostility, a tendency to be more action oriented and less reflective than the general population, and a propensity for intrapsychic or interpersonal difficulties at least partially resolved by the occurrence of the accident. The concept of an unconscious sense of guilt and a need to atone or to be punished for such guilt feelings may provide the motivation for many accidents. Motivations other than an unconscious sense of guilt may be found by examining the life situations of persons involved in accidents. An unconscious wish to escape or to avoid something is often apparent. The desire to escape may be related to external situations in which an accident provides a convenient way of avoiding a possibly humiliating experience. One such example is the man who has an accident on his way to a job interview and thereby avoids the possible humiliation of not obtaining the position he was seeking. Accidents help a person avoid new responsibilities by providing a convenient and acceptable rationale for not entering into the new situation without losing self-esteem or the esteem of others.

References

Bartholow BD, Anderson CA, Carnagey NL, Benjamin AJ Jr. Interactive effects of life experience and situational cues on aggression: The weapons priming effect in hunters and nonhunters. *Journal of Experimental Social Psychology*. 2005;41:48–60.

Bond MH. Culture and aggression—From context to coercion. *Personality and Social Psychology Review*. 2004;8(1):62–78.

Burnett DM, Kolakowsky-Hayner SA, Slater D, Stringer A, Bushnik T, Zafonte R, Cifu DX. Ethnographic analysis of traumatic brain injury patients in the national Model Systems database. *Arch Phys Med Rehabil*. 2003;84:263–267.

Coyne SM, Archer J. The relationship between indirect and physical aggression on television and in real life. *Social Development*. 2005;14(2):324.

Kindlundh AM, Lundblom J, Bergstrom L, Nyberg F. The anabolic-androgenic steroid nandrolone induces alterations in the density of serotonergic 5HT1B and 5HT2 receptors in the male rat brain. *Neuroscience*. 2003;119:113–120.

Lewis DO. Adult antisocial behavior, criminality, and violence. In: Sadock BJ, Sadock VA, eds. *Kaplan & Sadock's Comprehensive Textbook of Psychiatry*. 8th ed. Vol. 2. Baltimore: Lippincott Williams & Wilkins; 2005:2258.

Nelson HD, Nygren P, McInerney Y, Klein J. Screening women and elderly adults for family and intimate partner violence: A review of the evidence for the U.S. Preventive Services Task Force. *Ann Intern Med*. 2004;140:387–396.

Perez M, Vohs KD, Joiner TE Jr. Discrepancies between self- and other-esteem as correlates of aggression. *Journal of Social and Clinical Psychology*. 2005;24(5):607–620.

Ramírez JM, Bonniot-Cabanac MC, Cabanac M. Can aggression provide pleasure? *European Psychologist*. 2005;10(2):136–145.

Serper MR, Goldberg BR, Herman KG, Richarme D, Chou J, Dill CA, Cancro R. Predictors of aggression on the psychiatric inpatient service. *Compr Psychiatry*. 2005;46:121–127.

Soderstrom H, Blennow K, Sjodin AK, Forsman A. New evidence for an association between the CSF HVA:5-HIAA ratio and psychopathic traits. *J Neurol Neurosurg Psychiatry*. 2003;74:918–921.

Tardiff K. Adult antisocial behavior and criminality. In: Sadock BJ, Sadock VA, eds. *Kaplan & Sadock's Comprehensive Textbook of Psychiatry*. 7th ed. Vol. 2. Baltimore: Lippincott Williams & Wilkins; 2000:1908.

Teicher MH, Andersen SL, Polcari A, Anderson CM, Navalta CP, Kim DM. The neurobiological consequences of early stress and childhood maltreatment. *Neurosci Behav Rev*. 2003;27:33–44.

Tremblay RE, Hartup WW, Archer J. *Developmental Origins of Aggression*. New York: Guilford Press; 2005.

Turkstra L, Jones D, Toler HL. Brain injury and violent crime. *Brain Inj*. 2003;17:39–47.

▲ 4.5 Sociobiology and Ethology

SOCIOBIOLOGY

Sociobiology, also called *evolutionary psychology*, is the study of human behavior based on the transmission and modification of genetically influenced behavioral traits. A major thinker in the field is E. O. Wilson, whose book *Sociobiology* emphasized the role of evolution in shaping behavior.

Evolution

Evolution is described as any change in the genetic makeup of a population. Evolution occurs through natural selection, as formulated by Charles Darwin, which is the reproduction of those genes produced by mutation that account for the most successful offspring. Lamarckian evolution, which occurs through the inheritance of acquired characteristics, describes the evolution of culture.

Competition. Animals vie with one another for resources and territory, the area that is defended for the exclusive use of the animal and that ensures access to food and reproduction. The ability of one animal to defend a disputed territory or resource is called *resource holding potential*, and the greater this potential, the more successful the animal.

Aggression. Aggression serves both to increase territory and to eliminate competitors. Defeated animals can emigrate, disperse, or remain in the social group as subordinate animals. A dominance hierarchy in which animals are associated with one another in subtle but well-defined ways is part of every social pattern.

Reproduction. Because behavior is influenced by heredity, those behaviors that promote reproduction and survival of the species are among the most important. Men tend to have a higher variance in reproductive success than do women, thus, inclining men to be competitive with other men. Male–male competition can take various forms; for example, sperm can be thought of as competing for access to the ovum. Competition among women, although genuine, typically involves social undermining rather than overt violence. Sexual dimorphism, or different behavioral patterns for males and females, evolves to ensure the maintenance of resources and reproduction.

Altruism. *Altruism* is defined by sociobiologists as a behavior that reduces the personal reproductive success of the initiator while increasing that of the recipient. According to traditional Darwinian theory, altruism should not occur in nature because, by definition, selection acts against any trait whose effect is to decrease its representation in future generations; and yet, an array of altruistic behaviors occurs among free-living mammals as well as humans. In a sense, altruism is selfishness at the level of the gene rather than at the level of the individual animal. A classic case of altruism is the female worker classes of certain wasps, bees, and ants. These workers are sterile and do not reproduce but labor altruistically for the reproductive success of the queen.

Another possible mechanism for the evolution of altruism is group selection. If groups containing altruists are more successful than those composed entirely of selfish members, the altruistic groups succeed at the expense of the selfish ones, and altruism evolves. But within each group, altruists are at a severe disadvantage relative to selfish members, however well the group as a whole does.

Implications for Psychiatry. Evolutionary theory provides possible explanations for some disorders. Some may be manifestations of adaptive strategies. For example, cases of anorexia nervosa may be partially understood as a strategy ultimately caused to delay mate selection, reproduction, and maturation in situations where males are perceived as scarce. Persons who take risks may do so to obtain resources and gain social influence. An erotomanic delusion in a postmenopausal single woman may represent an attempt to compensate for the painful recognition of reproductive failure.

Studies of Identical Twins Reared Apart: Nature versus Nurture

Studies in sociobiology have stimulated one of the oldest debates in psychology. Does human behavior owe more to nature or to nurture? Curiously, humans readily accept the fact that genes determine most of the behaviors of nonhumans, but tend to attribute their own behavior almost exclusively to nurture. In fact, however, recent data unequivocally identify our genetic endowment as an equally important, if not more important, factor.

The best "experiments of nature" permitting an assessment of the relative influences of nature and nurture are cases of genetically identical twins separated in infancy and raised in different social environments. If nurture is the most important determinant of behavior, they should behave differently. On the other hand, if nature dominates, each will closely resemble the other, despite their never having met. Several hundred pairs of twins separated in infancy, raised in separate environments, then reunited in adulthood have been rigorously analyzed. Nature has emerged as a key determinant of human behavior.

Jim L. and Jim S. were first reunited at age 39. They were genetically identical twins, reared apart since infancy by different adoptive families in Ohio and unaware of each other's existence. As children, each twin had had a dog named Toy. Each bit his fingernails and, since age 18, had suffered from mixed headache syndrome, a combined tension and migraine headache. Each had been married twice, first to a Linda and then to a Betty. One twin had named his son James Alan, and the other, James Allen. Each had put a circular bench around a tree in his garden. Each had worked at a gas station and later part-time in law enforcement as a sheriff. Each chain-smoked Salems and preferred an occasional Miller Lite beer. Each scattered love notes to his wife around the house. Every summer, unbeknownst to the other, each had driven his family in a light blue Chevrolet from Ohio to the Pas-Grille Beach in St. Petersburg, Florida, for their summer vacation. They had similar voices, hand gestures, and mannerisms.

Jerry L. and Mark N., identical twins separated in infancy, were first reunited at age 30. Each was nearly bald and had a bushy mustache. Each was a volunteer firefighter and made his living installing safety equipment. Each wore aviator glasses, big belt buckles, and big key rings. Each drank Budweiser with his pinky hooked on the bottom of the can and crushed the can when he was finished.

Jack Y. and Oskar S., identical twins born in Trinidad in 1933 and separated in infancy by their parents' divorce, were first reunited at age 46. Oskar was raised by his Catholic mother and grandmother in Nazi-occupied Sudetenland, Czechoslovakia. Jack was raised by his Orthodox Jewish father in Trinidad and spent time on an Israeli kibbutz. Each wore aviator glasses and a blue sport shirt with shoulder plackets, had a trim mustache, liked sweet liqueurs, stored rubber bands on his wrists, read books and magazines from back to front, dipped buttered toast in his coffee, flushed the toilet before and after using it, enjoyed sneezing loudly in crowded elevators to frighten other passengers, and routinely fell asleep at night while watching television. Each was impatient, squeamish about germs, and gregarious.

Bessie and Jessie, identical twins separated at 8 months of age after their mother's death, were first reunited at age 18. Each had had a bout of tuberculosis, and they had similar voices, energy levels, administrative talents, and decision-making styles. Each had had her hair cut short in early adolescence. Jessie had a college-level education, whereas Bessie had had only 4 years of formal education; yet Bessie scored 156 on intelligence quotient testing and Jessie scored 153. Each read avidly, which may have compensated for Bessie's sparse education; she created an environment compatible with her inherited potential.

Neuropsychological Testing Results

A dominant influence of genetics on behavior has been documented in several sets of identical twins on the Minnesota Multiphasic Personality Inventory (MMPI). Twins reared apart generally showed the same degree of genetic influence across the different scales as twins reared together. Two particularly fascinating identical twin pairs, despite being reared on different continents, in countries with different political systems and different languages, generated scores more closely correlated across 13 MMPI scales than the already tight correlation noted among all tested identical twin pairs, most of whom had shared similar rearing.

Reared-apart twin studies report a high correlation ($r = 0.75$) for intelligence quotient (IQ) similarity. In contrast, the IQ correlation for reared-apart nonidentical twin siblings is 0.38, and for sibling pairs in general, is in the 0.45 to 0.50 range. Strikingly, IQ similarities are not influenced by similarities in access to dictionaries, telescopes, and original artwork; in parental education and socioeconomic status; or in characteristic parenting practices. These data overall suggest that tested intelligence is determined roughly two thirds by genes and one third by environment.

Studies of reared-apart identical twins reveal a genetic influence on alcohol use, substance abuse, childhood antisocial behavior, adult antisocial behavior, risk aversion, and visuomotor skills, as well as on psychophysiological reactions to music, voices, sudden noises, and other stimulation, as revealed by brain wave patterns and skin conductance tests. Moreover, reared-apart identical twins show that genetic influence is pervasive, affecting virtually every measured behavioral trait. For example, many individual preferences previously assumed to be due to nurture (e.g., religious interests, social attitudes, vocational interests, job satisfaction, and work values) are strongly determined by nature.

A selected glossary of some terms used in this section and other ethological terms is given in Table 4.5–1.

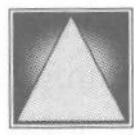

Table 4.5–1
Selected Glossary of Ethological Terms

Action-specific energy	Energy associated with the innate releasing mechanism and specific to a particular behavior pattern, which builds up if the releasing stimulus is not present to activate the behavior pattern; conversely, it is depleted by repetition.
Aggression	Intraspecific conflict manifested by physical attack or social signaling.
Appetitive behavior	Phase of behavior involving the active seeking of sign stimuli and thought to be driven by action-specific energy accumulating through inactivity of the specific behavior pattern.
Consummatory response	Phase of behavior whereby the energy driving the appetitive phase is released. Involves the perception of sign stimuli, the activation of the innate releasing mechanism (IRM), and the performance of the fixed action pattern (FAP).
Critical period	The time during which imprinting must occur, usually shortly after birth or early in life. Also known as "sensitive period."
Displacement activity	A set of behavior patterns occurring alongside an unrelated set of behavior patterns. Originally, irrelevant movements from one behavioral system occurring in the presence of powerful but thwarted drive from another behavior system.
Ethology	The biological study of behavior. From the Greek ethos, meaning custom, usage, manner, habit. The modern usage is attributed to Oskar Heinroth, Konrad Lorenz's teacher.
Fixed action pattern (FAP)	A genetically determined behavior pattern that is initiated by stimuli particular to the pattern and that consists of species-specific, stereotyped movements.
Imprinting	A specialized form of learning occurring early in life and often influencing behavior later in life. The exposure to the stimulus situation must occur during a particular period, the critical period, and the exposure can be of short duration and without obvious reward. The learning is particularly resistant to change.
Innate	Genetically determined behavior patterns; in theory not influenced by experience.
Innate releasing mechanism (IRM)	Sensory mechanism selectively responsive to specific external stimuli and responsible for triggering the stereotyped motor response.
Instinct	A developmental process resulting in species-typical behavior.
Redirection activity	The venting of one drive from two or more incompatible, but simultaneously activated, drives on some third animal or object.
Ritualization	Process of a behavior pattern being incorporated through evolution into a primary signaling function, frequently with exaggeration and embellishment of some of the movements.

(Courtesy of William T. McKinney, Jr., M.D.)

ETHOLOGY

Ethology is the systematic study of animal behavior. Its roots lie in the natural science of biology, in particular, in zoology. In 1973 the Nobel Prize in psychiatry and medicine was awarded to three ethologists, Karl von Frisch, Konrad Lorenz, and Nikolaas Tinbergen. Those awards highlighted the special relevance of ethology, not only for medicine, but also for psychiatry.

Konrad Lorenz

Born in Austria, Konrad Lorenz (1903–1989) is best known for his studies of imprinting. Imprinting implies that, during a certain short period of development, a young animal is highly sensitive to a certain stimulus that then, but not at other times, provokes a specific behavior pattern. Lorenz described newly hatched goslings that are programmed to follow a moving object and thereby become imprinted rapidly to follow it and, possibly, similar objects. Typically, the mother is the first moving object the gosling sees, but should it see something else first, the gosling follows it. For instance, a gosling imprinted by Lorenz followed him and refused to follow a goose (Fig. 4.5–1). Imprinting is an important concept for psychiatrists to understand in their effort to link early developmental experiences with later behaviors.

Lorenz also studied the behaviors that function as sign stimuli—that is, social releasers—in communications between individual animals of the same species. Many signals have the character of fixed motor patterns that appear automatically; the reaction of other members of the species to the signals is equally automatic.

Lorenz is also well known for his study of aggression. He wrote about the practical function of aggression, such as territorial defense by fish and birds. Aggression among members of the same species is common, but Lorenz pointed out that in normal conditions, it seldom leads to killing or even to serious injury. Although animals attack one another, a certain balance appears between tendencies to fight and flight, with the tendency to fight being strongest in the center of the territory and the tendency to flight strongest at a distance from the center.

In many works, Lorenz tried to draw conclusions from his ethological studies of animals that could also be applied to human problems. The postulation of a primary need for aggression in humans, cultivated by the pressure for selection of the best territory, is a primary example. Such a need may have served a practical purpose at an early time, when humans lived in small groups that had to defend themselves from other groups. Competition with neighboring groups could become an important factor in selection. Lorenz pointed out, however, that this need has survived the advent of weapons that can be used not merely to kill individuals but to wipe out all humans.

Nikolaas Tinbergen

Born in the Netherlands, Nikolaas Tinbergen (1907–1988), a British zoologist, conducted a series of experiments to analyze various aspects of animals' behavior. He was also successful in quantifying behavior and in measuring the power or strength of various stimuli in eliciting specific behavior. Tinbergen described displacement activities, which have been studied mainly in birds. For example, in a conflict situation, when the needs for fight and for flight are of roughly equal strength, birds sometimes do neither. Rather, they display behavior that appears to be

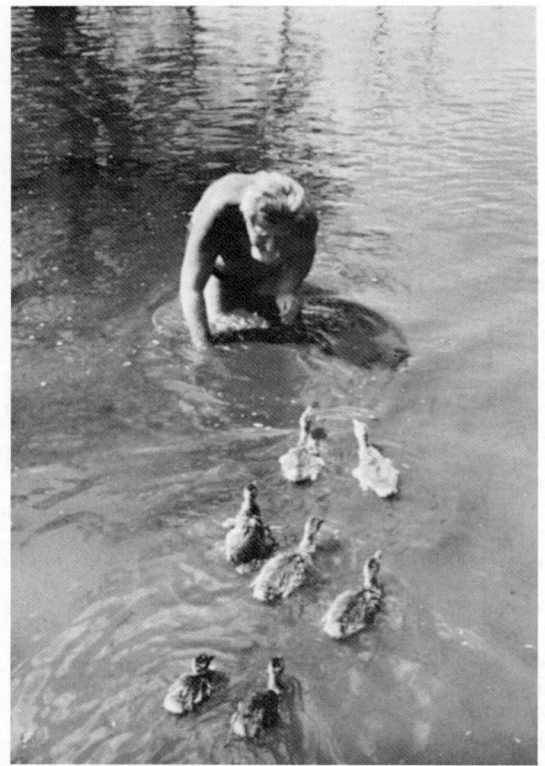

FIGURE 4.5–1
In a famous experiment, Konrad Lorenz demonstrated that goslings responded to him as if he were the natural mother. (Reprinted from Hess EH: Imprinting: An effect of an early experience. *Science.* 130:133, 1959, with permission.)

irrelevant to the situation (e.g., a herring gull defending its territory can start to pick grass). Displacement activities of this kind vary according to the situation and the species concerned. Humans can engage in displacement activities when under stress.

Lorenz and Tinbergen described innate releasing mechanisms, animals' responses triggered by releasers, which are specific environmental stimuli. Releasers (including shapes, colors, and sounds) evoke sexual, aggressive, or other responses. For example, big eyes in human infants evoke more caretaking behavior than do small eyes.

In his later work, Tinbergen, along with his wife, studied early childhood autistic disorder. They began by observing the behavior of autistic and normal children when they meet strangers, analogous to the techniques used in observing animal behavior. In particular, they observed in animals the conflict that arises between fear and the need for contact and noted that the conflict can lead to behavior similar to that of autistic children. They hypothesized that, in certain predisposed children, fear can greatly predominate and can also be provoked by stimuli that normally have a positive social value for most children. This innovative approach to studying infantile autistic disorder opened up new avenues of inquiry. Although their conclusions about preventive measures and treatment must be considered tentative, their method shows another way in which ethology and clinical psychiatry can relate to each other.

Karl Von Frisch

Born in Austria, Karl von Frisch (1886–1982) conducted studies on changes of color in fish and demonstrated that fish could learn to distinguish among several colors and that their sense of color was fairly congruent with that of humans. He later went on to study the color vision and behavior of bees and is most widely known for his analysis of how bees communicate with one another—that is, their language, or what is known as their dances. His description of the exceedingly complex behavior of bees prompted an investigation of communication systems in other animal species, including humans.

Characteristics of Human Communication

A human's communicative operations are based on two fundamentally different symbolization systems: nonverbal communication rests on the analogue principle, and verbal codification rests on the digital principle. The inner experience of what is going on at any moment involves nonverbal images that in some way reflect the total situation. Bodily movements and spontaneous, immediate reactions require an analogical appreciation of events. Persons, thus, develop within themselves a small-scale model of the world based on the recognition of similarities or differences. This method is used for gaining a bird's-eye view of events and for implementing quick reactions necessary for survival. But when persons have time to analyze a situation, they use words or numbers, which can detail aspects of events without recourse to analogies. In the digital-verbal system, numbers or letters are arbitrarily assigned to events, and a legend indicates to what these symbols refer. In complex human encounters, verbal and nonverbal communication is used together. The object-oriented parts of the message are expressed in words, and the subject- or participant-oriented parts are expressed nonverbally.

SUBHUMAN PRIMATE DEVELOPMENT

An area of animal research that has relevance to human behavior and psychopathology is the longitudinal study of nonhuman primates. Monkeys have been observed from birth to maturity, not only in their natural habitats and laboratory facsimiles but also in laboratory settings that involve various degrees of social deprivation early in life. Social deprivation has been produced

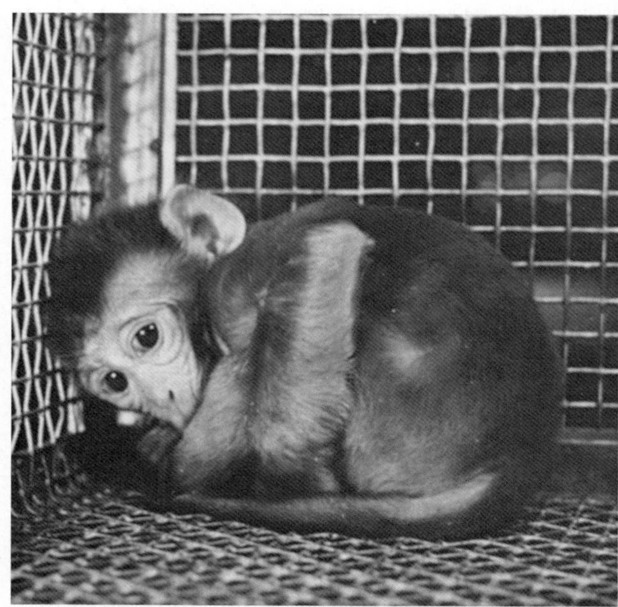

FIGURE 4.5–2
Social isolate after removal of isolation screen.

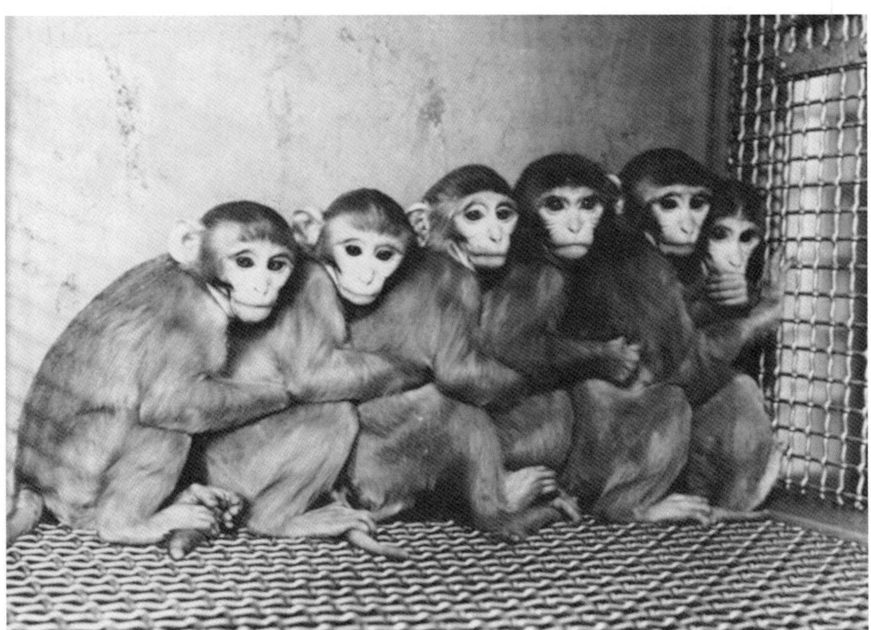

FIGURE 4.5–3
Choo-choo phenomenon in peer-only-reared infant rhesus monkeys.

through two predominant conditions: social isolation and separation. Socially isolated monkeys are raised in varying degrees of isolation and are not permitted to develop normal attachment bonds. Monkeys separated from their primary caretakers thereby experience disruption of an already developed bond. Social isolation techniques illustrate the effects of an infant's early social environment on subsequent development (Figs. 4.5–2 and 4.5–3), and separation techniques illustrate the effects of loss of a significant attachment figure. The name most associated with isolation and separation studies is Harry Harlow. A summary of Harlow's work is presented in Table 4.5–2.

In a series of experiments, Harlow separated rhesus monkeys from their mothers during their first weeks of life. During this time, the monkey infant depends on its mother for nourishment and protection, as well as for physical warmth and emotional security—*contact comfort*, as Harlow first termed it in 1958. Harlow substituted a surrogate mother made from wire or cloth for the real mother. The infants preferred the cloth-covered surrogate mother, which provided contact comfort, to the wire-covered surrogate, which provided food but no contact comfort (Fig. 4.5–4).

Treatment of Abnormal Behavior

Stephen Suomi demonstrated that monkey isolates can be rehabilitated if they are exposed to monkeys that promote physical contact without threatening the isolates with aggression or overly complex play interactions. These monkeys were called therapist monkeys. To fill such a therapeutic role, Suomi chose young normal monkeys that would play gently with the isolates and approach and cling to them. Within 2 weeks, the isolates were reciprocating the social contact, and their incidence of abnormal self-directed behaviors began to decline significantly. By the end of the 6-month therapy period, the isolates were actively initiating play bouts with both the therapists and each other, and most of their self-directed behaviors had disappeared. The isolates were observed closely for the next 2 years, and their improved behavioral repertoires did not regress over time. The results of this and subsequent monkey-therapist studies underscored the potential reversibility of early cognitive and social deficits at the human level. The studies also served as a model for developing therapeutic treatments for socially retarded and withdrawn children.

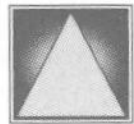

Table 4.5–2
Social Deprivation in Nonhuman Primates

Type of Social Deprivation	Effects
Total isolation (not allowed to develop caretaker or peer bond)	Self-orality, self-clasping, very fearful when placed with peers, unable to copulate. If impregnated, female is unable to nurture young (motherless mothers). If isolation goes beyond 6 months, no recovery is possible.
Mother-only reared	Fails to leave mother and explore. Terrified when finally exposed to peers. Unable to play or to copulate.
Peer-only reared	Engages in self-orality, grasps others in clinging manner, easily frightened, reluctant to explore, timid as adult, play is minimal.
Partial isolation (can see, hear, and smell other monkeys)	Stares vacantly into space, engages in self-mutilation, stereotyped behavior patterns.
Separation (taken from caretaker after bond has developed)	Initial protest stage changing to despair 48 hours after separation; refuses to play. Rapid reattachment when returned to mother.

(Adapted from work of Harry Harlow, M.D.)

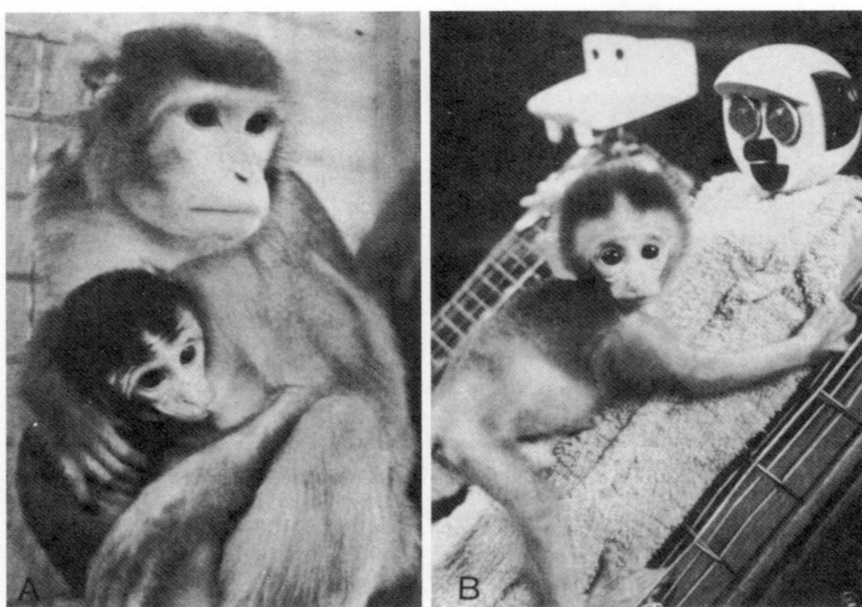

FIGURE 4.5–4
Monkey infant with mother (**left**) and with cloth-covered surrogate (**right**).

Several investigators have argued that social separation manipulations with nonhuman primates provide a compelling basis for animal models of depression and anxiety. Some monkeys react to separations with behavioral and physiological symptoms similar to those seen in depressed human patients; both electroconvulsive therapy (ECT) and tricyclic drugs are effective in reversing the symptoms in monkeys. Not all separations produce depressive reactions in monkeys, just as separation does not always precipitate depression in humans, young and old.

Individual Differences

Recent research has revealed that some rhesus monkey infants consistently display fearfulness and anxiety in situations in which similarly reared peers show normal exploratory behavior and play. These situations generally involve exposure to a novel object or situation. Once the object or situation has become familiar, any behavioral differences between the anxiety-prone, or timid, infants and their outgoing peers disappear, but the individual differences appear to be stable during development. Infant monkeys at 3 to 6 months of age that are at high risk for fearful or anxious reactions tend to remain at high risk for such reactions, at least until adolescence.

Long-term follow-up study of these monkeys has revealed some behavioral differences between fearful and nonfearful female monkeys when they become adults and have their first infants. Fearful female monkeys who grow up in socially benign and stable environments typically become fine mothers, but fearful female monkeys who have reacted with depression to frequent social separations during childhood are at high risk for maternal dysfunction; more than 80 percent of these mothers either neglect or abuse their first offspring. Yet nonfearful female monkeys that encounter the same number of social separations but do not react to any of these separations with depression turn out to be good mothers.

EXPERIMENTAL DISORDERS

Stress Syndromes

Several researchers, including Ivan Petrovich Pavlov in Russia and W. Horsley Gantt and Howard Scott Liddell in the United States, studied the effects of stressful environments on animals, such as dogs and sheep. Pavlov produced a phenomenon in dogs, which he labeled *experimental neurosis*, by the use of a conditioning technique that led to symptoms of extreme and persistent agitation. The technique involved teaching dogs to discriminate between a circle and an ellipse and then progressively diminishing the difference between the two. Gantt used the term *behavior disorders* to describe the reactions he elicited from dogs forced into similar conflictual learning situations. Liddell described the stress response he obtained in sheep, goats, and dogs as *experimental neurasthenia*, which was produced in some cases by merely doubling the number of daily test trials in an unscheduled manner.

Learned Helplessness

The learned helplessness model of depression, developed by Martin Seligman, is a good example of an experimental disorder. Dogs were exposed to electric shocks from which they could not escape. The dogs eventually gave up and made no attempt to escape new shocks. The apparent giving up generalized to other situations, and eventually the dogs always appeared to be helpless and apathetic. Because the cognitive, motivational, and affective deficits displayed by the dogs resembled symptoms common to human depressive disorders, learned helplessness, although controversial, was proposed as an animal model of human depression. In connection with learned helplessness and the expectation of inescapable punishment, research on subjects has revealed brain release of endogenous opiates, destructive effects on the immune system, and elevation of the pain threshold.

A social application of this concept involves school children who have learned that they fail in school no matter what they do; they view themselves as helpless losers, and this self-concept causes them to stop trying. Teaching them to persist may reverse the process, with excellent results in self-respect and school performance.

Unpredictable Stress

Rats subjected to chronic unpredictable stress (crowding, shocks, irregular feeding, and interrupted sleep time) show decreases in movement and exploratory behavior; this finding illustrates the roles of unpredictability and lack of environmental control in producing stress. These behavioral changes can be reversed by antidepressant medication. Animals under experimental stress (Fig. 4.5–5) become tense, restless, hyperirritable, or inhibited in certain conflict situations.

Dominance

Animals in a dominant position in a hierarchy have certain advantages (e.g., in mating and feeding). Being more dominant than peers is associated with elation, and a fall in position in the hierarchy is associated with depression. When persons lose jobs, are replaced in organizations, or otherwise have their dominance or hierarchical status changed, they can experience depression.

Temperament

Temperament mediated by genetics plays a role in behavior. For example, one group of pointer dogs was bred for fearfulness and a lack of friendliness toward persons, and another group was bred for the opposite characteristics. The phobic dogs were extremely timid and fearful and showed decreased exploratory capacity, increased startle response, and cardiac arrhythmias. Benzodiazepines diminished these fearful, anxious responses. Amphetamines and cocaine aggravated the responses of genetically nervous dogs to a greater extent than they did the responses of the stable dogs.

Brain Stimulation

Pleasurable sensations have been produced in both humans and animals through self-stimulation of certain brain areas, such as the medial forebrain bundle, the septal area, and the lateral hypothalamus. Rats have engaged in repeated self-stimulation (2,000 stimulations per hour) to gain rewards. Catecholamine production increases with self-stimulation of the brain area, and drugs that decrease catecholamines decrease the process. The centers for sexual pleasure and opioid reception are closely related anatomically. Heroin addicts report that the so-called rush after intravenous injection of heroin is akin to an intense sexual orgasm.

Pharmacological Syndromes

With the emergence of biological psychiatry, many researchers have used pharmacological means to produce syndrome analogues in animal subjects. Two classic examples are the reserpine (Serpasil) model of depression and the amphetamine psychosis model of paranoid schizophrenia. In the depression studies, animals given the norepinephrine-depleting drug reserpine exhibited behavioral abnormalities analogous to those of major depressive disorder in humans. The behavioral abnormalities produced were generally reversed by antidepressant drugs. These studies tended to corroborate the theory that depression in humans is, in part, the result of diminished levels of norepinephrine. Similarly, animals given amphetamines acted in a stereotypical, inappropriately aggressive, and apparently frightened manner that resembled paranoid psychotic symptoms in humans. Both of these models are considered too simplistic in their concepts of cause, but they remain as early paradigms for this type of research.

Studies have also been done on the effects of catecholamine-depleting drugs on monkeys during separation and reunion periods. These studies showed that catecholamine depletion and social separation can interact in a highly synergistic fashion and can yield depressive symptoms in subjects for whom mere separation or low-dosage treatment by itself does not suffice to produce depression.

Reserpine has produced severe depression in humans and, as a result, is rarely used as either an antihypertensive (its original indication) or an antipsychotic. Similarly, amphetamine and its congeners (including cocaine) can induce psychotic behavior in persons who use it in overdose or over long periods of time.

SENSORY DEPRIVATION

The history of sensory deprivation and its potentially deleterious effects evolved from instances of aberrant mental behavior in explorers, shipwrecked sailors, and prisoners in solitary confinement. Toward the end of World War II, startling confessions, induced by brainwashing prisoners of war, caused a rise of interest in this psychological phenomenon brought about by the deliberate diminution of sensory input.

To test the hypothesis that an important element in brainwashing is prolonged exposure to sensory isolation, D. O. Hebb and his coworkers brought solitary confinement into the laboratory and demonstrated that volunteer subjects—under conditions of visual, auditory, and tactile deprivation for periods of up to 7 days—reacted with increased suggestibility. Some subjects also showed characteristic symptoms of the sensory deprivation state: anxiety, tension, inability to concentrate or organize thoughts, increased suggestibility, body illusions, somatic complaints, intense subjective emotional distress, and vivid sensory imagery—usually visual and sometimes reaching the proportions of hallucinations with a delusionary quality.

Psychological Theories

Anticipating psychological explanation, Sigmund Freud wrote: "It is interesting to speculate what could happen to ego function if the excitations or stimuli from the external world were either drastically diminished or repetitive. Would there be an alteration in the unconscious mental processes and an effect upon the conceptualization of time?"

Indeed, under conditions of sensory deprivation, the abrogation of such ego functions as perceptual contact with reality

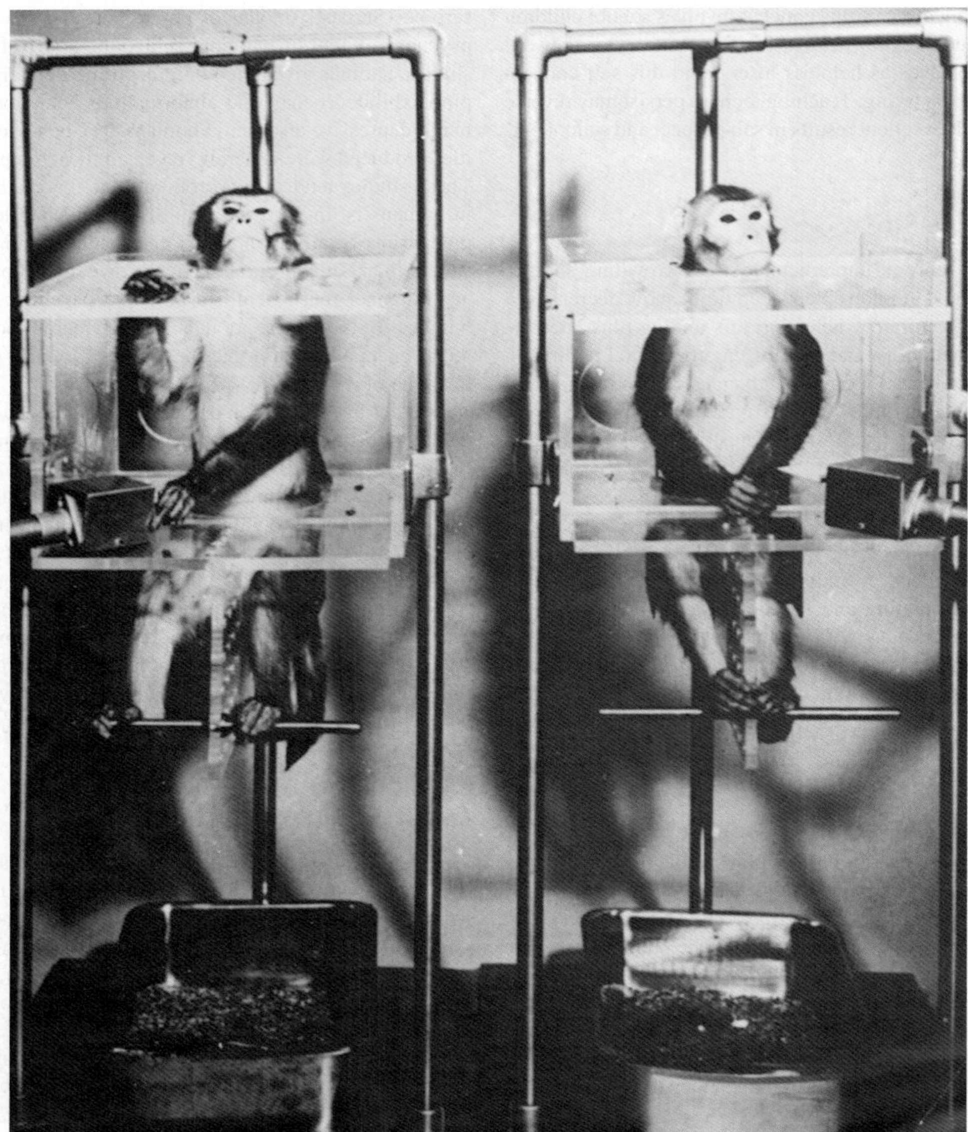

FIGURE 4.5–5
The monkey on the **left**, known as the executive monkey, controls whether or not both will receive an electric shock. The decision-making task produces a state of chronic tension. Note the more relaxed attitude of the monkey on the **right**. (From U.S. Army photographs, with permission.)

and logical thinking brings about confusion, irrationality, fantasy formation, hallucinatory activity, and wish-dominated mental reactions. In the sensory-deprivation situation, the subject becomes dependent on the experimenter and must trust the experimenter for the satisfaction of such basic needs as feeding, toileting, and physical safety. A patient undergoing psychoanalysis may be in a kind of sensory deprivation room (e.g., a soundproof room with dim lights and a couch) in which primary-process mental activity is encouraged through free association.

Cognitive. Cognitive theories stress that the organism is an information-processing machine, whose purpose is optimal adaptation to the perceived environment. Lacking sufficient information, the machine cannot form a cognitive map against which current experience is matched. Disorganization and maladaptation then result. To monitor their own behavior and to attain optimal responsiveness, persons must receive continuous feedback; otherwise, they are forced to project outward idiosyncratic themes that have little relation to reality. This situation is similar to that of many psychotic patients.

Physiological Theories

The maintenance of optimal conscious awareness and accurate reality testing depends on a necessary state of alertness. This alert state, in turn, depends on a constant stream of changing stimuli from the external world, mediated through the ascending reticular activating system in the brainstem. In the absence or impairment of such a stream, as occurs in sensory deprivation, alertness drops away, direct contact with the outside world diminishes, and impulses from the inner body and the central nervous system may gain prominence. For example, idioretinal phenomena, inner ear noise, and somatic illusions may take on a hallucinatory character.

References

Barash DP. *The Survival Game: How Game Theory Explains the Biology of Cooperation and Competition*. New York: Times/Holt; 2003.

Buller DJ. *Adapting Minds: Evolutionary Psychology & the Persistent Quest for Human Nature*. Cambridge, MA: MIT Press; 2005.

Buller DJ. Evolutionary psychology: The emperor's new paradigm. *Trends in Cognitive Sciences*. 2005;9(6):277–283.

Burns JK. An evolutionary theory of schizophrenia: Cortical connectivity, metarepresentation, and the social brain. *Behav Brain Sci.* 2004;27:831–855.

Buss DM. *The Handbook of Evolutionary Psychology*. New York: John Wiley & Sons; 2005.

Foerster K, Delhey K, Johnsen A, Lifjeld JT, Kempenaers B. Females increase offspring heterozygosity and fitness through extra-pair matings. *Nature.* 2003;425:714.

Giaccio RG. The dual origin hypothesis: An evolutionary brain-behavior framework for analyzing psychiatric disorders. *Neurosci Biobehav Rev.* 2006;30(4):526–550.

Hariharan IK, Haber DA. Yeast, flies, worms, and fish in the study of human disease. *N Engl J Med.* 2003;348:2457.

Lipton JE, Barash DP. Sociobiology. In: Sadock BJ, Sadock VA, eds. *Kaplan & Sadock's Comprehensive Textbook of Psychiatry*. 8th ed. Vol. 1. Baltimore: Lippincott Williams & Wilkins; 2005:634.

Pinker S. *The Blank Slate*. New York: Viking; 2002.

Potkin H. *Evolutionary Thought in Psychology: A Brief History*. Malden, MA: Blackwell; 2004.

Sable P. Attachment, ethology and adult psychotherapy. *Attachment & Human Development*. 2004;6(1):3–19.

Workman L, Reader W. *Evolutionary Psychology: An Introduction*. New York: Cambridge University Press; 2004.

Young A. Remembering the evolutionary Freud. *Science in Context*. 2006;19:175–189.

▲ 4.6 Anthropology and Cross-Cultural Psychiatry

Anthropology is the study of human beings. The relationship between anthropology and psychiatry are mainly limited to *cultural psychiatry*: the definition of culture, interaction between it and the individual, culture-specific syndromes, and cross-cultural differences in definitions of health, illness, and healing.

Researchers in human behavior often turn to anthropology for examples of normal and maladaptive behavior in various cultures. Because psychiatric theorists have long predicted that cultural variables influence behavior, these variables may help further the understanding of the nature–nurture controversy; namely, which aspects of human beings are innate and biological, which aspects are shaped by the environment, and how the constant feedback between these two aspects affects human beings.

In psychiatry, the increasingly acknowledged evidence of biological factors has altered the view of persons as largely determined by the outcome of relationships shaping children's earliest years. And, although anthropological cross-cultural studies have focused on differences as well as similarities in human beings, some anthropologists have emphasized that people cannot be independent of their cultures and that even the attempt to study cross-cultural behavior is a culturally bound viewpoint.

PSYCHOANALYTICAL THEORY

Beginning with Sigmund Freud, psychoanalysts have applied their insights to cultural data. In his 1913 work *Totem and Taboo*, Freud described the earliest humans as a group of brothers who killed and devoured their violent primal father. This criminal act and the so-called totem meal made the brothers feel guilty. Consequently, they formulated rules to prevent similar acts from occurring, and these rules were the beginning of social organization. Carl Gustav Jung's writings include many anthropological references, especially to archaeology and mythology. In *Symbols and Transformations*, written in 1912, Jung traced patients' fantasies back to earliest human artifacts. Neither Freud nor Jung had field experience, but Erik Erikson did. Erikson is best known for his psychocultural biographies of Mohandas Gandhi and Martin Luther and for his 1950 book *Childhood and Society*, in which he attempted to integrate individual psychosexual development with cultural influences. Many of his conclusions were based on his experiences with the Pine Ridge Indians in the Dakotas and the Yurok Indians in Oregon.

George Devereux studied American Plains Native Americans and provided insights into the problems that arise in dealing with patients from diverse ethnic backgrounds. In the 1930s and the 1940s, Abraham Kardiner worked with the concept of national character and suggested that each culture is associated with a common (or at least widely shared) personality structure. Kardiner believed that the adult Russian personality, for example, is characterized by depressive and manic traits. Other such generalities about national character were set forth by various workers, but these descriptions were often used to foster political, ideological, or discriminatory attitudes and so have fallen out of favor. The current consensus is that a clinically meaningful prediction about personality cannot be made on the basis of nationality alone. But as Ruth Benedict wrote in *Patterns of Culture*, personality types may reflect a culture's configuration because people are malleable and they assume a society's expected behavior pattern.

Bronislaw Malinowski and Margaret Mead were among the anthropologists who examined the psychoanalytic concept that adult personality and mental functioning are largely determined during childhood. Malinowski examined childhood and adult sexuality in the Trobriand Islanders and claimed that he found no evidence of the Oedipus complex, which at the time was believed to be universal. Margaret Mead examined gender and sex-role behavior. She observed three tribes in New Guinea and found different patterns of sex-role behavior for men and women in each tribe. According to Mead, behavior is relative, and a society can create deviance by either condoning or condemning certain behavior patterns. Mead considered the Oedipus complex a useful concept in its widest meaning, which is that in all societies adults are involved in the growing child's sexual attitudes, especially those toward the parent of the opposite sex.

MARGARET MEAD

In her *Coming of Age in Samoa*, published in 1928, Mead (Fig. 4.6–1) described a society in the South Pacific in which adolescent turmoil—widely believed at the time to be universal—appeared not to exist. This was the result, she argued, of the unusual Samoan culture that nurtured open, nonpossessive sexual relationships among adolescents, encouraged communal child rearing, and denigrated aggressiveness and competitiveness. Growing up was "so easy," she stated, because of "the general casualness of the whole society."

Widely publicized and discussed, Mead's observations helped to entrench a belief in cultural determinism that persisted for decades. Research has shown, however, that Mead's methodology was seriously flawed, and her conclusions were questionable. When Mead went to Samoa at the age of 23, she spoke no Samoan language, and her data were based, not on direct observation, but on the hearsay reports of adolescent and preadolescent girls from nearby villages.

Rather than an idyllic paradise of free love among gentle people, most observers, including Samoans themselves, describe a competitive society marked by interfamily and intervillage networks in which female virginity is highly prized at the time of marriage. Ample evidence (e.g., teenage delinquency and suicide rates) shows that during the 1920s, "adolescent turmoil" was not only present, but pronounced. One critic has described Mead's Samoan study as an example of how "as evidence is sought to substantiate a cherished doctrine, the deeply held beliefs of those involved may lead them unwillingly into error."

The absolute cultural determinism advocated by Mead arose in response to the absolute biological determinism of an earlier generation. Neither extreme is believed credible by behavioral researchers today.

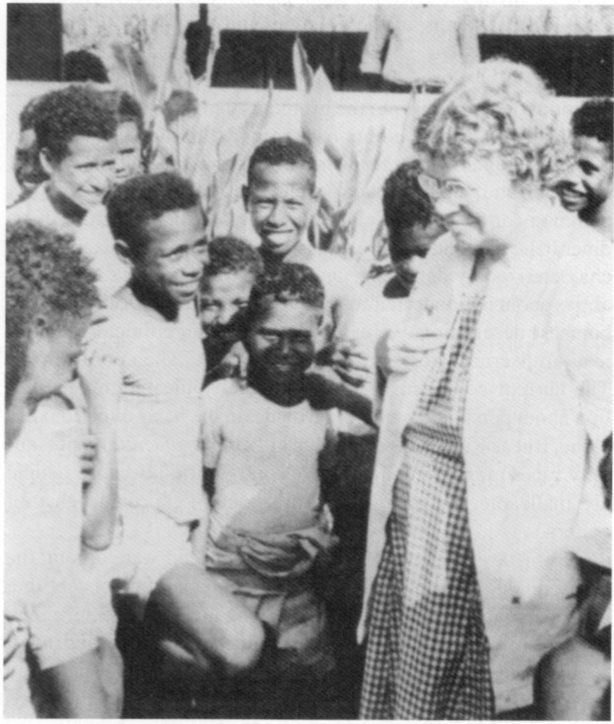

FIGURE 4.6–1
Margaret Mead (1901–1978), the world-famous anthropologist, spent years studying other societies and amassing cross-cultural data. Her *Coming of Age in Samoa* (published in 1928) gave a favorable picture of many aspects of life in a "primitive" society and was influential in establishing an attitude of cultural relativism among many scientists and thinkers. Here she is pictured meeting with schoolchildren in New Guinea. (From Carson RC, Butcher JN, Coleman JC. *Abnormal Psychology and Modern Life*, 8th ed. Boston: Scott, Foresman; 1988:83. Institute for Cultural Studies, Inc., with permission.)

Psychosocial Growth

The effects of early life experiences on adult mental health and the explanations for deviance or maladaptive behavior are still controversial issues. Psychodynamic psychiatrists and theorists rely on historical data about adverse experiences to explain later behavior; but new work shows that few experiences are irreversible. Some affection-deprived children described by John Bowlby were able to grow up capable of forming attachments if other experiences later in life were favorable. Similarly, many successful adults come from deprived or otherwise toxic homes and appear to be, or are, invulnerable to these stressors.

Freud postulated a universal sequence of emotional development. Beyond some very general elements (the existence of infantile sexuality, the formation of an attachment to a primary caretaker who is usually the mother, the ubiquity of conflicts and jealousies within the family), this allegedly universal sequence has never found empirical support in cross-cultural studies of human behavioral psychological development. Such studies, however, have produced extensive evidence supporting empirically grounded putative universals of psychosocial growth.

Among the well-established cross-cultural universals of psychosocial development, the best supported and most plausibly related to underlying neural or neuroendocrine maturational events are the emergence of sociality, as heralded by social smiling, during the first 4 months of life, in parallel with the maturation of basal ganglia and cortical motor circuits; the emergence of strong attachments, awareness of separation, and recognition of strangers, in the second half of the first year of life, in parallel with the maturation of the major fiber tracts of the limbic system; the emergence of language during the second year and after, in parallel with the maturation of the thalamic projection to the auditory cortex among other circuits; the emergence of a sex difference in physical aggressiveness in early and middle childhood, with male children on average more aggressive than female children, a consequence in part of prenatal androgenization of the hypothalamus; the emergence of adult sexual motivation and functioning in adolescence, in parallel with and following the maturation of the hypothalamic-pituitary-gonadal axis at puberty, against the background of the previously mentioned prenatal androgenization of the hypothalamus in males.

As for the effect of early life experiences on psychological development, recent work has established an extraordinary fact. In rigorous twin, adoption, and family studies, variance in personality as well as in mental ability can be statistically apportioned among various sources. The results routinely accord a large proportion of the variance to environmental influence (roughly half in numerous studies). The effect of family relationships on personality and mental ability, however, appears to be minimal.

The portion of the variance in outcome measures (e.g., behavior and questionnaire results) attributable to environment is composed almost entirely of within-family variance, such as sibling differences. Identical twins reared together are routinely found to be no more similar in personality than identical twins reared in separate families; sometimes, the separately reared twins are found to be more similar. (See the discussion in Section 4.5 on identical twins.) To the extent that children in different families differ in personality, the difference can be explained almost entirely by their genetic differences. Differences between non-identical twin siblings, however, cannot be explained by their genetic differences alone but require environmental explanations as well, such as birth order.

This conclusion seems to indicate that parents' attempts to treat their children similarly (rules, religion, schooling, toys, television) do not make their offspring more similar in personality, or more different from their counterparts in other families, than they would be on the basis of genes alone. No one understands the reason for this phenomenon. Whatever the explanation, the challenge posed by the extremely small measurable between-family variance poses a major challenge to the explanatory paradigms of child psychiatry, psychodynamic theory, and developmental psychology.

Although cultural anthropologists have described and analyzed cross-cultural variation, they have also studied the features of human behavior that do not vary. The concept of universals has several different meanings. Behaviors such as coordinated bipedal walking or smiling in social greeting are exhibited by all normal members of every known society. Behaviors are universal within an age or sex class, such as the Moro reflex in all normal neonates or the ejaculatory motor action pattern in all postpubertal males. Population characteristics apply to all populations but not to all individual members of the populations, such as the sex difference in physical aggressiveness. Universal features of culture rather than of behavior exist, such as the taboos against incest and homicide, or the highly variable but always present institution of marriage, or the social construction of illness and attempts at healing (Fig. 4.6–2). Characteristics, although unusual or even rare, are found at some low level in every population, such as homicidal violence, thought disorder, depression, suicide, and incest.

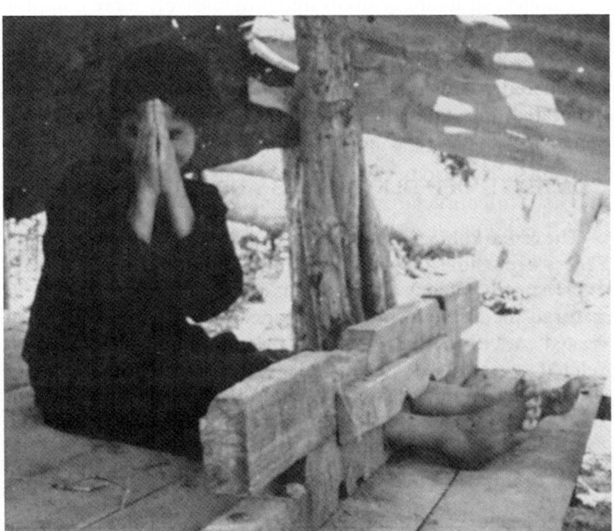

FIGURE 4.6–2
Psychotic woman in Laos. She was kept in stocks for several months to prevent her from running off into the forest, a well-known fatal outcome of psychosis in the area. (Courtesy of Joseph Westermeyer, M.D.)

Cross-Cultural Diagnosis. Jane Murphy and Alexander Leighton studied the incidence of psychiatric disorders cross-culturally. Certain conclusions emerged: (1) both the general category of psychological deviance and at least several major syndromes appear to be characteristic of all cultures for which information is available; (2) some psychiatric disorders appear to be relatively or largely culture-specific; and (3) it is extremely difficult, if not impossible, to compare incidence or prevalence of most disorders cross-culturally.

Medical Anthropology. The sick role, whether in relation to psychological or physical illness, occurs in all cultures, but carries many different meanings and expectations. The same ailment, even what is apparently the same degree of physical pain, varies greatly in designation and interpretation, to the extent that some cultures recognize diseases unrecognized as abnormalities in others, and some encourage the expression of pain, whereas others discourage it.

CROSS-CULTURAL PSYCHIATRY

Cross-cultural psychiatry as practiced by both anthropologists and psychiatrists has consisted of three closely related enterprises: (1) *psychological anthropology*, using psychodynamic and other psychological theory to interpret the relationship among elements of society and culture; (2) *comparative psychiatry*, using formal epidemiological or less formal observational and clinical methods to describe and analyze cross-cultural variations in incidence or prevalence of syndromes and symptoms; and (3) *medical anthropology*, using traditional anthropological methods to elucidate cross-cultural variation in the social and cultural construction of illness from disease, and in the elaboration of healing or care-taking roles and relationships.

The role of culture often becomes apparent only when psychiatrists assess and treat patients whose cultural backgrounds differ from theirs. The special problems that arise in such situations can be resolved only if psychiatrists can adapt their standard procedures. From a cultural perspective, no one biological, psychological, or social approach can fulfill the needs of all patients. The text revision of the fourth edition of *Diagnostic and Statistical Manual of Mental Disorders* (DSM-IV-TR) provides an outline for a cultural formulation designed to assist in the systematic evolution and treatment of patients. The formulation calls for data on (1) the cultural identity of the patients, including ethnicity, involvement with original and host cultures, and language abilities; (2) the cultural explanations and idioms of distress used by patients and their community concerning their illness or situation; (3) the cultural factors impacting patients' social situations, including work, religion, and kin networks; (4) the cultural and social status differences between the patient and clinician that may affect assessment and treatment, including problems with communicating, negotiating a patient–clinician relationship, and distinguishing between normal and pathological behaviors; and (5) the formulation of an overall cultural assessment for diagnosis and care.

Definitions and Key Concepts

Culture. *Culture* is a vast, complex concept that is used to encompass the behavior patterns and lifestyle of a society—a group of persons sharing a self-sufficient system of action that is capable of existing longer than the life span of an individual and whose adherents are recruited, at least in part, by the sexual reproduction of the group members. Culture consists of shared symbols, artifacts, beliefs, values, and attitudes. It is manifested in rituals, customs, and laws and is perpetuated and reflected in shared sayings, legends, literature, art, diet, costume, religion, mating preferences, child-rearing practices, entertainment, recreation, philosophical thought, and government. Culture serves many purposes. It provides an overall consistency to a society's patterns and components over the generations. It helps organize diversity and mediate between the forces of stability and conformity and those of new ideas and actions. By classifying phenomena into good and bad, right and wrong, healthy and sick, desirable and undesirable, people are provided with behavioral guidelines and an interpretation of life's events. Culture is learned through contact with family, friends, classmates, teachers, significant persons, and the media; the term for this process is *enculturation*. It results in a personal sense of belonging to one's own society and in a native identity.

No pure cultures exist. Societies are not static. Access to printed media, radio, telephone, television, and easy travel, as well as geopolitical changes, has resulted in much cultural blending. Adults, such as migrants or refugees, who only in part adopt the culture of a host society are said to be *assimilated*, whereas those who assume a new cultural identity consonant with that of the host culture are said to be *acculturated*. Persons who, voluntarily or by force, abandon their native culture but fail to be assimilated or acculturated usually lose their sense of identity or purpose in life and are at high risk for suicide, substance abuse, and alcoholism.

The holistic and functional concept of culture also allows for the existence of smaller subcultural groups and patterns within the larger society. Native Americans, for example, have distinct cultures, especially in tribal groups that live on reservations. On a smaller, less comprehensive scale, many subcultural groups and units exist in which feelings, ideas, and behaviors are shared; for example, cults, neighborhood associations, institutional inmates, athletic teams, students and teachers at a school, and unions. Many subcultural patterns serve to preserve and to integrate the general society, but some may be socially disruptive (organized criminal groups) or truly destructive (terrorist organizations). Each family may be said to have its own microculture. Although the term *culture* is a grand abstraction that implies stability, homogeneity, and coherence, social life is often replete with change, heterogeneity, and inconsistencies.

Scope of Culture. Although the manifestations of culture are sufficiently broad to be considered almost infinite, the noted American anthropologist George P. Murdock described a long list of features considered to be universally present in the hundreds of societies studied by contemporary anthropologists. In alphabetical order, they are "age-grading, athletic sports, bodily adornment, calendar, cleanliness training, community organization, cooking, cooperative labor, cosmology, courtship, dancing, decorative art, divination, division of labor, dream interpretation, education, eschatology, ethics, ethnobotany, etiquette, faith healing, family feasting, fire-making, folklore, food taboos, funeral rites, games, gestures, gift-giving, government, greetings, hair styles, hospitality, housing, hygiene, incest taboos, inheritance rules, joking, kin groups, kinship nomenclature, language, law, luck, magic, marriage, mealtimes, medicine, obstetrics, penal sanction, personal names, population policy, postnatal care, pregnancy usages, property rights, propitiation of supernatural beings, puberty customs, religious ritual, residence rules, sexual restrictions, soul concepts, status differentiation, superstition, surgery, tool-making, trade, visiting, weather control, and weaving." Obviously some of these dimensions are more central than others to the relation of culture to psychology and psychopathology. Among these are rules related to sexuality and reproduction (incest taboo and rules of marriage), community and social organizations (kinship, kin groups, power relations, and division of labor), and cosmological visions (magic, superstition, and creational myths).

Race and Ethnicity. Traditionally, race denotes human groupings that are biologically (and, in theory, genetically) determined. In fact, other contemporary biologists consider race to be poorly correlated with any measurable biological or cultural phenomenon. Although some characteristics of a given "racial" group (e.g., skin color) may appear phenotypically compelling, the use of the race to aggregate individuals displaying that characteristic may convey a false sense of distinctiveness and may imply the existence of a biological basis for such classification systems. Such is not the case for any of the phenotypic characteristics used to establish race. On the other hand, ethnicity, a term increasingly preferred by cross-cultural researchers, connotes groups of individuals sharing a sense of common identity, a common ancestry, and shared beliefs and history. A given patient's ethnicity can be assessed by focusing the clinical history-taking on key ethnically shaped developmental experiences, such as special rituals and rites of passage, and adherence to ethnically prescribed family roles, religious observances, food preferences, and the like. Cultural identity denotes the internalized self-definition resulting from the person's selective, developmentally mediated incorporation of values, beliefs, history, and customs from those available in that person's native environment. Typically, it contains many dimensions of self-experience, including age, gender, race, sexual orientation, ethnicity, language, class, and religious and spiritual beliefs.

CULTURE AND PSYCHOPATHOLOGY

Culture is an all-pervasive medium for humans. It is driven by the human brain's unique ability to create images and symbols and structure them into complex wholes that, in turn, can drive brain function to produce defined behaviors and modulate instinctually driven ones. The ability to mediate biological functions via symbolic (and image) representation and manipulation is dramatically expanded in humans by the function of awareness or consciousness leading to the notion of the self.

Humans structure symbols into progressively more complex sequences, ranging from basic, simple ideas to complex holistic beliefs, values, and ideals. These, in turn, are codified by language, images, and other means and shared with others to constitute the building blocks of common culture. Culture, thus, becomes a hierarchical array of complex symbols that affect the individual's emotions and behaviors and, when communicated to others, affect social and group function.

All cultures develop both processes that facilitate adjustment and conflict resolution and pressures that foster conflict, deviance, and maladjustment. These pressures can act broadly on large social groups and selectively on specific cultural subgroups. All cultures define a spectrum of "normal behaviors" as well as thresholds of tolerance for diverse "abnormalities," imposing different social consequences on different patterns of deviance.

Each culture provides its own unique stresses as well as beliefs and rituals to reduce psychological tension. Ashley Montagu has indicated, for example, that cultures that provide adaptive channels for the expression of aggression and the satisfaction of dependency needs can significantly reduce personal and interpersonal conflict. In the modern era, cultures and subcultures change at increasing rates in response to the adaptive demands represented by a global world in increasing economic, political,

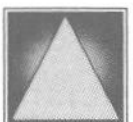

Table 4.6–1
Aspects of Cultural Identity Development

Ethnicity	Gender
Race	Age
Country of origin	Sexual orientation
Language	Religious and spiritual beliefs
Acculturation	Socioeconomic class and education

(From Lu FG, Russell FL, Mezzich JE. Issues in the assessment and diagnosis of culturally diverse individuals. In: Oldham J, Riba M, eds. *Ann Rev Psychiatry.* 1995;14. Washington, DC: American Psychiatric Press, with permission.)

and social competition. This progressive globalization imposes additional adaptive stresses on individuals and cultural groups.

Cultural Identity. DSM-IV-TR recommends that in assessing an individual's cultural identity, clinicians should "note the individual's ethnic or cultural reference group. For immigrants and ethnic minorities, they should assess the degree of involvement with both culture of origin and host culture." Frances G. Lu and coworkers summarized the essential components of cultural identity (Table 4.6–1).

To these factors must be added migration history, which is commonly left out of the clinical evaluation of cross-cultural patients. Culturally uninformed clinicians often treat their immigrant patients as if their lives began when they arrived in the United States, and their clinical narratives often lack key data from the patients' preimmigration experience. Careful attention must be paid to the traumas and losses encountered by refugees in their country of origin, often including exposure (as witnesses or victims) to physical or emotional torture or both. The process of acculturation is once again key to understanding the psychological distress and psychopathology of immigrants. The three major sources of stress in the migration experience are (1) entry into the host society, frequently at lower occupational and social levels; (2) disruption of interpersonal relationships; and (3) the acculturation process. The clinician can assess the degree of acculturation and the nature of the acculturation process through many indirect means. Age at immigration, number of years in the United States, occupational status, language proficiency, and participation in the host culture social networks give the clinician some idea of the rate and ease of acculturation for a given patient.

Families can also be classified by degree of acculturation. From this perspective, immigrant families may be described along a continuum of acculturation as traditional, transitional bicultural, and Americanized. Each of these family structures presents different assets and vulnerabilities in relation to the immigration experience.

CULTURE-BOUND SYNDROMES

Extreme diversity is seen among the peoples of the world concerning the recognition, classification, and understanding of mental behavior symptoms. Western psychiatrists classify mental diseases according to the DSM-IV-TR and the tenth edition of the *International Classification of Diseases* (ICD-10), which are thought to reflect scientific categories. The DSM-IV-TR and ICD-10 are not universally applicable; psychopathological syndromes exist, especially in non-Western cultures that do not fit the scientific nomenclature unless they are placed into the "atypical" category. These syndromes are perceived to be more influenced by culture than are most Western syndromes and, therefore, have been labeled *culture-bound*. Some syndromes are found in distinct cultural groups, whereas others are found in large cultural regions. The reader is referred to Section 14.5 for an extensive discussion of culture-bound syndromes.

REFERENCES

Bains J. Race, culture and psychiatry: A history of transcultural psychiatry. *History of Psychiatry*. 2005;16(2):139–154.

Belkin GS. Hard questions in court: Culture and psychiatry on trial. *Cult Med Psychiatry.* 2003;27:157–159.

Bhugra D, Mastrogianni A, Maharajh H, Harvey S. Prevalence of bulimic behaviours and eating attitudes in schoolgirls from Trinidad and Barbados. *Transcultural Psychiatry.* 2003;40:408–428.

Faison WE, Armstrong D. Cultural aspects of psychosis in the elderly. *J Geriatr Psychiatry Neurol.* 2003;16:225–231.

Favazza A. Anthropology and psychiatry. In: Sadock BJ, Sadock VA, eds. *Kaplan & Sadock's Comprehensive Textbook of Psychiatry*. 8th ed. Vol. 1. Baltimore: Lippincott Williams & Wilkins; 2005:598.

Favazza A. *PsychoBible: Behavior, Religion, and the Holy Book.* Charlottesville, VA: Pitchstone Publishing; 2004.

Frank E, Shear MK, Rucci P, Banti S, Mauri M, Maser JD, Kupfer DJ, Miniati M, Fagiolini A, Cassano GB. Cross-cultural validity of the structured clinical interview for panic-agoraphobic spectrum. *Soc Psychiatry Psychiatr Epidemiol.* 2005;40(4):283–290.

Hollifield M, Geppert C, Johnson Y, Fryer C. A Vietnamese man with selective mutism: The relevance of multiple interacting "cultures" in clinical psychiatry. *Transcultural Psychiatry*. 2003;40:329.

Keel PK, Klump KL. Are eating disorders culture-bound syndromes? Implications for conceptualizing their etiology. *Psychological Bull.* 2003;129:747–769.

Kirmayer LJ. Asklepian dreams: The ethos of the wounded healer in the clinical encounter. *Transcultural Psychiatry*. 2003;40:248–277.

Kleinman A, Eisenberg L, Good B. Culture, illness, and care: Clinical lessons from anthropologic and cross-cultural research. *Focus*. 2006;4:140.

Parzen MD. Towards a culture-bound syndrome-based insanity defense? *Cult Med Psychiatry.* 2003;27:131–155.

Skultans V. Psychiatry through the ethnographic lens. *Int J Soc Psychiatry*. 2006;52:73–83.

Trujillo M. Culture-bound syndromes. In: Sadock BJ, Sadock VA, eds. *Kaplan & Sadock's Comprehensive Textbook of Psychiatry*. 8th ed. Vol. 2. Baltimore: Lippincott Williams & Wilkins; 2005:2282.

Tseng WS, Streltzer J, eds. *Cultural Competence in Clinical Psychiatry*. Washington, DC: American Psychiatric Publishing; 2004.

▲ 4.7 Epidemiology and Biostatistics

EPIDEMIOLOGY

Epidemiology is one of the fundamental sciences of public health and a major approach to the understanding and advancement of medicine and health care. Epidemiology is a useful tool for clinicians to link their work to populations and complete the clinical picture. It provides a perspective about the health of the general population, including the causes and courses of these illnesses.

Results from epidemiological studies are routinely included in the *Diagnostic and Statistical Manual of Mental Disorders* (DSM) to describe the frequency and correlates of mental disorders. In developing the diagnostic criteria themselves, secondary analyses of many epidemiological studies assessed the frequency with which discrete symptoms appeared together, to define syndromes in large community and clinical populations. Epidemiological studies that demonstrate the significance of depression as a risk factor for death in persons with cardiovascular disease have engendered new interest in pathophysiological mechanisms that might account for the relation between these two disorders.

One of the most visible indicators of the policy use of epidemiological data is found in the joint publication by the World Bank and the World Health Organization (WHO) entitled *The Global Burden of Disease*. Based on data developed over the past two decades, mental disorders have been found to be among the leading causes of disability worldwide, with major depression currently the fourth leading cause of disability.

DEFINITION

Epidemiology is the study of the distribution, incidence, prevalence, and duration of disease. *Psychiatric epidemiology* can be defined as the study of the distribution of mental illness and positive mental health and related factors in human populations. Among the principal positive mental health variables to be considered are individual strengths, social functioning and participation, social supports, and quality of life. These positive health aspects are, of course, not only relevant to mental health, but also to general health. Among related factors could be included contributing etiological factors, associated general health conditions, phenomenological and course characteristics, mental health services, and mental health policies. Evidence-based medicine enhanced by experience and wisdom is a basic methodological approach for epidemiological study.

Epidemiological surveys reveal that about one third of all Americans have had or will have a mental disorder at some time in their lives. The most common mental disorders are anxiety disorders, and the next most common are depressive disorders and alcohol or other substance abuse. In addition, surveys have found that about 15 percent—if not more—of all patients seen for a medical or surgical problem by nonpsychiatric physicians have an associated emotional disorder, most often depression, alcohol abuse, or both.

Epidemiology advances psychiatric research by correlating clinical findings with such sociodemographic variables as age, gender, and socioeconomic status. For example, higher rates of almost every mental disorder are found in persons under age 45 than in those over 45. In general, women have significantly higher rates than men for all disorders, particularly depressive and anxiety disorders. Men, however, have significantly higher rates of substance-related disorders and antisocial personality disorder. Schizophrenia, which affects about 1 percent of the population, shows similar rates for men and women.

Epidemiological studies are also used to compare the incidence and the prevalence of diseases internationally and cross-culturally. In general, the prevalence of mental disorders appears to be fairly constant, regardless of nationality or cultural background; however, schizophrenia has a better prognosis and outcome in less developed third-world countries than it does in better developed societies such as the United States and the United Kingdom. Table 4.7–1 describes the four eras in the evolution of epidemiology.

Types of Clinical and Epidemiological Studies

Clinical and epidemiological studies in psychiatry attempt to answer questions relating to the causes, treatment, course, prognosis, and prevention of various disorders. The two main types of studies are (1) *observational,* in which the natural course of an illness is followed without any intervention, and (2) *experimental*, in which some or all factors under study are controlled by the investigator. Most studies are experimental; however, because of

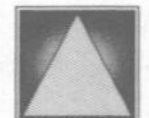

Table 4.7–1
Four Eras in the Evolution of Modern Epidemiology

Era	Paradigm	Analytical Approach	Preventive Approach
Sanitary statistics (first half of 19th century)	Miasma: poisoning by foul emanations from soil, air, and water	Demonstrate clustering of morbidity and mortality	Draining, sewage, sanitation
Infectious disease epidemiology (late 19th century through first half of 20th century)	Germ theory: single agents relate one to one to specific diseases	Laboratory isolation and culture from disease sites, experimental transmission, and reproduction of lesions	Interrupt transmission (vaccines, isolation of the affected through quarantine and fever hospitals, and, ultimately, antibiotics)
Chronic disease epidemiology (second half of 20th century)	Black box: exposure related to outcome without necessity for intervening factors or pathogenesis	Risk ratio of exposure to outcome at individual level in populations	Control risk factors by modifying lifestyle (e.g., diet, exercise) or agent (e.g., guns, food) or environment (e.g., pollution, passive smoking)
Ecological epidemiology (emerging)	Chinese boxes: relations within and between localized structures organized in a hierarchy of levels	Analysis of determinants and outcomes at different levels of organization: within and across contexts (using new information systems) and in depth (using new biomedical techniques)	Apply both information and biomedical technology to find leverage at efficacious levels, from contextual to molecular

(From Susser M, Susser E: Choosing a future for epidemiology. II. From black box to Chinese boxes and eco-epidemiology. *Am J Public Health.* 1996;86:674–677, with permission.)

the many variables involved in mental disorders, it is difficult to design well-controlled experimental studies. The most common types of experimental designs used in psychiatry are described below.

Cohort Study. A *cohort* is a group chosen from a well-defined population and studied over a long period of time. Cohort studies are also known as longitudinal studies. An example is the study by Stella Chess and Alexander Thomas of temperamental characteristics of the same group of infants at ages 3 months, 2 years, 5 years, and 20 years. The researchers detected a relation between the initial characteristics of the infant and a subgroup of children who eventually had clinical psychiatric problems. In that study, the cohort was the group born and studied in the year the study began.

Cohort studies provide direct estimates of risk associated with a suspected causal factor. They are more time-consuming and expensive to perform than case history studies, which are usually quick and inexpensive. Cohort studies are usually conducted when ample evidence from case-history studies indicates that a relation exists between a risk factor and a disorder. For example, in the relation between lung cancer and smoking, many case-history studies had been published before the first cohort study was reported.

Retrospective and Prospective Studies. Prospective studies, also called longitudinal studies, are based on observing events as they occur. A major problem in psychiatric longitudinal studies is that some persons are lost to follow-up over time. Retrospective studies are based on past data or past events.

Cross-Sectional Study. Cross-sectional studies provide information about the prevalence of disease in a representative study population at a particular point in time. For that reason, they are also known as *prevalence studies*.

Case-History Study. A case-history study is a retrospective study that examines persons with a particular disease.

Case-Control Study. A case-control study is a retrospective study that examines persons without a particular disease.

Clinical Trial. In a clinical trial, specially selected patients receive a course of treatment, and another group does not. Eligible patients are randomly assigned to the treatment group or to the control group. The goal of the study is to determine the effects of a given treatment.

Double-Blind Study. A double-blind study helps eliminate bias because neither the patient nor the persons involved in the study know which, if any, treatment is being given to the patient. In drug studies, a control group of patients may receive a placebo (i.e., an inert substance prepared to resemble the active drug being tested in the experiment). A response to the placebo may represent the psychological effect of taking a pill, a response not caused by any psychopharmacological property (so-called placebo effect). In addition, the investigators do not know the treatment given because drugs are identified by special codes unknown to them. The outcome may be assessed by persons other than those administering the treatment (so-called blind evaluators). Control subjects may receive an alternative comparison treatment, rather than just a placebo.

Crossover Study. A crossover study is a variation of the double-blind study. The treatment group and the control or placebo group change places at some point, so that the placebo group gets the treatment and the treatment group now receives the placebo. That procedure eliminates bias because, if the treatment group improves in both instances and the placebo group does not, the conclusion is that the makeup of the two groups was truly random. Each group serves as the control for the other.

Psychiatric Case Register. A case register maintains a longitudinal record of psychiatric contacts for each person receiving care in a geographically defined community. Not all areas lend themselves to a register because persons may leave the area for treatment or the population may be highly mobile. A well-maintained register is of great value in determining accurate treated-incidence rates, lifetime- or period-treated prevalence rates, comparative rates for different time periods for the same population, and information regarding the use of services over time, as well as in identifying high-risk groups for further study.

Major Epidemiological Studies

Major psychiatric epidemiological research studies have been conducted over the years. The goal of each study was to determine the prevalence of psychopathology in a defined community. Persons in a particular community were interviewed directly (usually using a structured interview protocol) to determine the presence or absence of psychological symptoms. The major studies are described below.

Chicago Study. A team under the direction of Robert E. L. Faris and Henry Warren Dunham examined about 35,000 admissions to mental hospitals in Chicago between 1922 and 1934. The survey found that first hospital admissions for schizophrenia were highest among persons from the central sections of Chicago, members of the city's lowest socioeconomic group. Rates of admission decreased as one moved away from the central areas and into more affluent communities. Faris and Dunham developed a *drift hypothesis*, which holds that impaired persons slide down the social scale because of their illness. By contrast, a *segregation hypothesis* holds that instead of helplessly drifting downward, schizophrenic persons actively seek city areas where anonymity and isolation protect them from the demands that more organized societies make on them. That study helped conceptualize two additional hypotheses about mental illness: (1) the *social causation theory*, which holds that being a member of a low socioeconomic group is significant in causing illness, and (2) the *social selection theory*, which holds that having a mental disorder leads a person to become a member of the low socioeconomic group as a secondary phenomenon. In other words, the disorder is caused by genetic or psychological factors, and the drift downward results.

Midtown Manhattan Study. In 1954, a team directed by Thomas Rennie and Leo Srole designed and conducted a survey involving 1,660 adults sampled from a specific section of New York City. The objective of the study was to determine the effects of demographic, social, and personal factors on mental health and illness by use of a structured interview conducted by nonpsychiatrists. Mental disorder was rated not present, mild, moderate, or marked. The main objective was to test the association between life stress and psychological symptoms, and some of the findings follow. The incidence of mental disorders rose as age increased; 81 percent of persons from 20 to 59 years of age had symptoms that were mild to severely incapacitating, and 23.4 percent of persons in that age group were substantially impaired. Socioeconomic status was the single most significant variable affecting mental illness; persons in the low socioeconomic group had six times as many symptoms as those in the high groups.

New Haven Study. In 1950, August De Belmont Hollingshead and Fredrick Carl Redlich studied the relation of social class to the prevalence of treated mental disorders in New Haven, Connecticut. Their studies included a census of psychiatric patients, a survey of the population

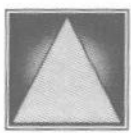

Table 4.7–2
Class Status and Cultural Characteristics of Subjects in the New Haven Study

Class	Class Status and Cultural Characteristics
I	Class I, containing the community's business and professional leaders, has two segments: a long-established core group of interrelated families and a smaller, upwardly mobile group of new people. Members of the core group usually inherit money, along with group values that stress tradition, stability, and social responsibility. Those in the new group are highly educated, self-made, able, and aggressive. Their family relationships often are not cohesive or stable. Socially, they are rejected by the core group, to whom they are, however, a threat by the vigor of their leadership in community affairs.
II	Class II is marked by at least some education beyond high school and occupations as managers or in the lower ranking professions. Four of five are upwardly mobile. They are joiners at all ages and tend to have stable families, but they have usually gone apart from parental families and often from their home communities. Tensions arise generally from striving for educational, economic, and social success.
III	Class III men for the most part are in salaried administrative and clerical jobs (51 percent) or own small businesses (24 percent); many of the women also have jobs. Typically, they are high school graduates. They usually have economic security but little opportunity for advancement. Families tend to be less stable than those in class II. Family members of all ages tend to join organizations and to be active in them. They have less satisfaction with present living conditions and less optimism than in class II.
IV	In class IV, 53 percent say they belong to the working class. Seven of 10 show no generational mobility. Most are content and make no sacrifices to get ahead. Most of the men are semiskilled (53 percent) or skilled (35 percent) manual employees. Practically all the women who are able to hold jobs do so. Education usually stops shortly after graduation from grammar school for both parents and children. Families are much different from those in class III. Families are larger, and they are more likely to include three generations. Households are more likely to include boarders and roomers. Homes are more likely to be broken.
V	Class V adults usually have not completed elementary school. Most are semiskilled factory workers or unskilled laborers. They are concentrated in tenement and cold water flat areas of New Haven or in suburban slums. Generally, family ties are brittle. Very few participate in organized community institutions. Leisure activities in the household and on the street are informal and spontaneous. Adolescent boys frequently have contact with the law in their search for adventure. There is a struggle for existence; much resentment, expressed freely in primary groups, about how they are treated by those in authority; and much acting out of hostility.

at large, a study of psychiatrists, and a controlled-case study. Analysis of the data revealed a definite relation between social class and mental disorders. Neurosis was most prevalent among persons in the high socioeconomic groups; psychosis was most prevalent among persons in the low socioeconomic groups. The poor were more often seen in mental health clinics than by private psychiatrists. In addition, low socioeconomic status, occupational instability, and downward mobility were associated with the highest frequency of psychiatric disability. Hollingshead and Redlich devised a subgrouping of class structure in the county based on education, occupation, and income. Their class distinctions, described in Table 4.7–2, are used by sociologists and epidemiologists. Another New Haven study used a structured diagnostic interview to make specific diagnoses. A major finding of that study was that 15.1 percent of the adult population over age 26 showed evidence of a mental disorder, and a probable mental disorder was present in an additional 2.7 percent.

Stirling County Study. In 1952, Alexander H. Leighton conducted a psychiatric epidemiological study of Stirling County, a Nova Scotian county of 20,000 persons. Information was recorded by nonclinician interviewers using structured interviews. The information was later rated by a psychiatrist. Unlike the New Haven and Midtown Manhattan surveys, the subjects of the Stirling County study lived in rural areas—small villages, one small town, and many isolated farms. Male and female household heads were interviewed. The major findings were that 57 percent of the persons interviewed had experienced some mental disorder, 24 percent had a notable impairment, and 20 percent needed psychiatric attention. Women exhibited considerably more psychiatric disorders than men, and mental disorders were found to increase in number with age and degree of poverty.

National Institute of Mental Health Epidemiologic Catchment Area (NIMH-ECA) Survey. The NIMH-ECA project evolved from the report of the 1977 President's Commission on Mental Health, which highlighted the need to identify the mentally ill and indicate how they are treated and by whom. Darrel Regier and his associates at the Division of Biometry and Epidemiology of the NIMH sought to identify the percentage of the population with mental disorders. The objective was to determine the percentages of the population with mental disorders that were receiving treatment in mental health settings (such as psychiatric clinics), private psychiatrists' offices, and such nonpsychiatric settings as general medical treatment centers and internists' offices. Estimates indicated that at least 15 percent of the population of the United States is affected by mental disorders in 1 year, and only one fifth of those persons received care from mental health specialists. Three fifths of persons with identified mental disorders were treated by primary care physicians. Various sites around the country are being studied to assess mental disorder prevalence, incidence, and service use in geographically defined community populations of at least 200,000 residents. Random samples are drawn to obtain completed interviews on at least 20,000 community and institutional residents. The *Diagnostic Interview Schedule* (DIS), which assesses the presence, duration, and severity of symptoms, is the major instrument that the trained lay interviewer uses to interview each subject. Compared with all previous studies, the NIMH-ECA study uses better diagnostic tools and more specific criteria to make a reliable diagnosis, including careful clinical descriptions and follow-up studies. Much larger samples are used than in the previously described studies. In general, findings of the ECA survey show the following: rates of depression are twice as high for females as for males, males are more likely than females to have alcohol dependence, and substance abuse is more common

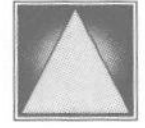

Table 4.7–3
Comparison of One-Year and Lifetime Prevalence Rates Limited to Common Age Range of 18–54 Years

Disorder	Prevalence (%)
Any 12-mo disorder	29.8 (0.6)
Any lifetime disorder	46.9 (0.7)
Any substance use or dependence	
12 mo	10.5 (0.4)
Lifetime	24.3 (0.6)
Alcohol dependence	
12 mo	4.4 (0.2)
Lifetime	11.3 (0.4)
Drug dependence	
12 mo	2.4 (0.2)
Lifetime	6.4 (0.3)
Any affective (mood) disorder	
12 mo	10.1 (0.4)
Lifetime	14.9 (0.4)
Major depressive episode	
12 mo	6.4 (0.3)
Lifetime	12.5 (0.4)
Dysthymia—lifetime	5.5 (0.3)
Any anxiety disorder	
12 mo	11.8 (0.4)
Lifetime	19.2 (0.5)
Panic disorder	
12 mo	1.5 (0.1)
Lifetime	2.8 (0.2)
Social phobia	
12 mo	2.1 (0.2)
Lifetime	3.7 (0.3)
Schizophrenia	
12 mo	0.9 (0.1)
Lifetime	1.5 (0.1)
Somatization	
12 mo	0.1 (0.0)
Lifetime	0.1 (0.0)

(Adapted from Regier DA, Kaelber CT, Rae DS, et al. Limitations of diagnostic criteria and assessment instruments for mental disorders: implications for research and policy. *Arch Gen Psychiatry.* 1998;55:109, with permission.)

in persons under age 30 than in older persons. The epidemiological findings of 1-year and lifetime prevalence rates for specific mental disorders in the five ECA sites are listed in Table 4.7–3. More specific data about each disorder are found in the chapter that discusses the disorder in depth.

Assessment Instruments

The major obstacle to the identification of cases has been the lack of an explicit set of criteria for diagnostic classification. Over the years, a variety of diagnostic procedures and assessment instruments has been developed. Information about a subject can be collected in several ways. Medical records are often used for patients in clinical settings. Records in central data banks called *case registers* can be used. In Scandinavian countries, particularly Sweden, control data banks are extensive. An important source of information about a subject is the *direct interview*, which is a person-to-person interaction. *Indirect surveys* using a structured self-report form may be used, but they lack the clinical judgment of an experienced practitioner that is necessary in some instances. The most common assessment approach is an interview format, which can be *structured* (the same questions asked of all subjects) or *unstructured* (interviewers use their own clinical judgment in choosing their questions). Several structured instruments with acceptable interrater reliability are outlined in Table 4.7–4. An effective assessment instrument must be reliable, valid, and free of bias. *Reliability* concerns whether or not the findings of the assessment instrument or diagnostic procedure are reproducible and can be replicated when the instrument is used by different examiners (*interrater reliability*) or on different occasions (*test-retest reliability*). *Validity* concerns whether the test measures what it is supposed to measure. Does the assessment instrument identify the cases it is designed to identify? Validity can be broken down further into the following categories: *criterion validity*, in which results from one test instrument are compared with the results of another test whose validity has already been established; *face validity*, which concerns whether the test makes sense to the investigator using it; *content validity*, which concerns whether the test covers specific types of information that can be interpreted or scored at a later date; *concurrent validity*, which concerns whether the results correspond to the results of another test with the same variable; and *construct validity*, which concerns whether the test instrument is in fact measuring what it was designed to measure. The two properties of validity and reliability are extremely important in psychiatric epidemiology, especially if attempting to identify a specific disorder or syndrome. Analytic studies can also be flawed by *bias*, an error in construction that favors one outcome over another. Bias can occur if examiners know something about the status of the case that influences their judgment (e.g., they know that one group is receiving medication). These potential flaws can affect the validity of a study's findings. To eliminate this kind of bias, researchers developed the double-blind method. Bias is also diminished by randomizing the sample so that each member of the total group studied has an equal chance of being selected—for example, by assigning each person a number from a table of random numbers.

Assessment instruments must be sensitive; that is, they must be able to detect the thing being evaluated (e.g., to diagnose a disorder when it is present). If an instrument detects a disorder in a person who does not have the disorder, the result is called *false positive*, rather than *true positive*. Tests must also be specific; that is, they must not detect things not being evaluated. For example, tests must be able to determine the absence of a disorder in a person who does not have the disorder, which is called a *true-negative* result. A disorder reported to be absent in a person when it is present is a *false-negative* result. Assessment instruments should also have good *predictive value*, which is the proportion of true-positive or true-negative results. Predictive values indicate what percentage of test outcomes are expected to coincide with assigned diagnoses. Table 4.7–5 summarizes the interpretation of sensitivity, specificity, and predictive value.

BIOSTATISTICS

Biostatistics is the mathematical science of describing, organizing, and interpreting data related to medicine. Epidemiology relies on statistics to enable investigators to examine possible causes of disease and to evaluate treatment strategies. The principles of statistics are beyond the scope of this book, but a glossary of statistical terms used in most elementary textbooks of

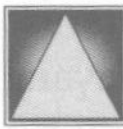

Table 4.7–4
Commonly Used Assessment Instruments

Instrument	Condition	Interviewer	Comments
Present State Examination (PSE)	Psychotic disorders, schizophrenia	Psychiatrists	Limited to 1-mo period before interview; can be used with computer program CATEGO
Schedule for Affective Disorders and Schizophrenia (SADS)	Schizophrenia and mood disorders	Psychiatrists or specially trained interviewer	Variations: SADS-C measures current disorder, and SADS-L measures lifetime disorders
General Health Questionnaire (GHQ)	Medical patients with psychiatric symptoms of anxiety or depression	Self-report	Does not identify specific mental disorders
Diagnostic Interview Schedule (DIS)	Covers more than 30 mental disorders, including schizophrenia, mood disorders, anxiety disorders, substance abuse, cognitive disorders	Self-report combined with specially trained interviewers	Correlates with range of DSM-III diagnostic classification; assesses symptoms over lifetime; used in the NIMH-ECA program
Iowa Structured Psychiatric Interview (ISPI)	Major mental disorders	Trained interviewer	Provides detailed psychosocial and family history; covers lifetime prevalence

DSM-III, *Diagnostic and Statistical Manual of Mental Disorders,* 3rd ed; NIMH-ECA, National Institute of Mental Health Epidemiologic Catchment Area.

statistics is presented here. Knowledge of such terms is necessary both for understanding epidemiological concepts and for accurately assessing statistical methods that appear in scientific publications.

The two major types of statistics are descriptive and inferential. *Descriptive statistics* are numerical values that summarize, organize, and describe observations (e.g., the average number of symptoms associated with an anxiety disorder). Examples include mean, standard deviation, and variance. *Inferential statistics* are numerical values used to generalize about probabilities on the basis of a sample (e.g., comparing the effect of drug A with that of drug B in the treatment of a group of depressed patients). Examples include the analysis of variance, probability, and probability (*P*) value.

Data (factual information) are derived from a population or a sample. A *population* is the entire collection of a set of objects, persons, or events in a particular context (e.g., all patients with schizophrenia in a particular hospital). A *sample* is a subset selected from this population (e.g., one half of the patients with schizophrenia in a particular hospital). Data can be *nominal* (organized into categories), *ordinal* (ranked in order), or *organized into interval ratios* (measured on a scale, graph, or table).

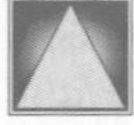

Table 4.7–5
Definitions and Calculations for Interpreting Performance of Diagnostic Tests

Term	Definition	Calculation
True positive (TP)	Diseased person with abnormal test results	
True negative (TN)	Nondiseased person with normal test results	
False positive (FP)	Nondiseased person with abnormal test results	
False negative (FN)	Diseased person with normal test results	
Referent value	A value to which laboratory results can be referred and from which the probability of disease or predictive value can be calculated	
Sensitivity	True-positive rate	$\frac{TP}{TP + FN} \times 100$
Specificity	True-negative rate	$\frac{TN}{TN + FP} \times 100$
Predictive value of abnormal test results (PV +)	Proportion of abnormal test results that are true positive	$\frac{TP}{TP + FP} \times 100$
Predictive value of normal test results (PV −)	Proportion of normal test results that are true negative	$\frac{TN}{TN + FN} \times 100$
Efficiency	Percentage of all results that are true results, whether positive or negative	$\frac{TP + TN}{\text{Grand total}} \times 100$

Table by John F. Greden, M.D.

Glossary of Statistical Terms

Analysis of Variance (ANOVA). A set of statistical procedures designed to compare two or more groups of observations. It determines whether the differences between groups are owing to experimental influence or to chance alone.

Chi-Square Test. A set of statistical procedures used to evaluate the relative frequency or proportion of events in a population that fall into well-defined categories.

Confidence Interval. An interval that is likely to capture the population mean with a specified level of confidence. For the 95 percent confidence interval, the chances are estimated to be 95 in 100 that the true mean falls within that interval.

Control Group. A group that does not receive treatment and is used as a standard of comparison.

Correlation Coefficient. A measurement of the direction and strength of the relation between two variables. Two of the most commonly used are the Spearman rank order coefficient for ordinal data and the Pearson correlation coefficient for nominal data. The Pearson correlation coefficient (r) takes any value between -1 and $+1$. A*positive correlation* means that as one variable increases (or decreases) the other moves in the same direction. A negative r indicates that the variables move in opposite directions. A correlation approaching -1 or $+1$ indicates a strong relationship; a correlation approaching 0 indicates a weak relationship. Correlation coefficients indicate only the degree of relationship; they say nothing about cause and effect.

Dependent Variable. The phenomenon of interest in a research study, often called the *outcome variable*.

Descriptive Statistics. Methods used to summarize, organize, and describe observations. Examples include the mean, standard deviation, and variance.

Discriminant Analysis. A multivariate method for finding the relation between a single discrete outcome and a linear combination of two or more predictors.

Distribution. A series or range of values that can be organized according to their frequency of occurrence (*frequency distribution*). A symmetrical, bell-shaped frequency distribution of scores is called a *normal distribution* (the bell curve). Distribution can be normal or skewed in a positive or negative direction (Fig. 4.7–1).

Incidence. The number of new cases occurring over a specified time. The most common period used is 1 year, which produces an annual incidence calculated as follows:

$$\text{Incidence} = \frac{\text{Number of new cases of a disease (over a 1-year period)}}{\text{Total number of persons in the population (over 1-year period)}}$$

A study of incidence is more difficult to do than a study of prevalence cases because those who already have the disease must be excluded from the incidence numerator; they cannot be considered new cases. Because those who have had the disease are no longer at risk for it, they also must be excluded from the denominator. A broader concept of total incidence includes those with a new episode of illness, regardless of whether they have had previous episodes.

Lifetime Expectancy. The total probability of a person's having a disorder during his or her lifetime. Prevalence and incidence vary for sex and age; thus, sex-specific and age-specific rates are used to express the relative frequency of cases in each category.

Measure of Central Tendency. A central value in a distribution around which other values are distributed. Three measures of central tendency are the mean, the median, and the mode.

MEAN. A statistical measurement derived from adding a set of scores and then dividing by the number of scores. The mean is the average score.

Multivariate Analysis. Method of considering the relation of three or more variables. Multivariate methods include multiple regression, discriminant analysis, canonical correlation, and factor analysis.

Multivariate Analysis of Variance. A multivariate technique that uses an analysis of variance design but includes a dependent variable that is a linear combination of variables.

Null Hypothesis. The assumption that no significant difference exists between two random samples of a population. When the null hypothesis is rejected, observed differences between groups are deemed improbable by chance alone.

Percentile Rank. The percentage of scores in a distribution exceeded by any particular score. For example, a percentile rank of 80 for a given score means that this score exceeds 80 percent of all scores in the distribution.

Population. The entire collection of a set of objects or persons with the same definition.

Power Analysis. Analytical method for estimating the sample size required to detect statistical effects of a defined size for variables with known variances.

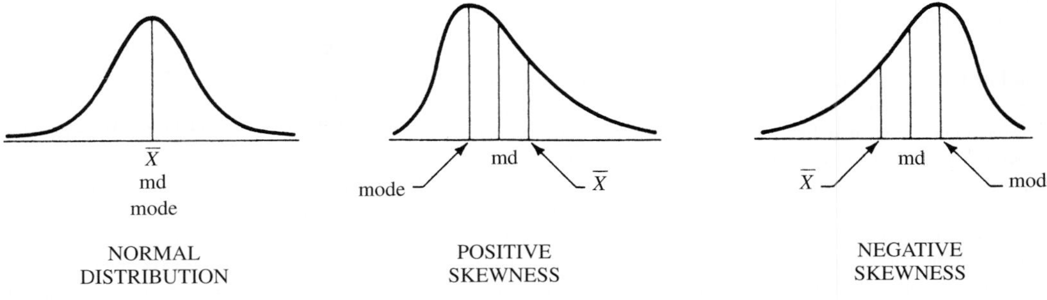

FIGURE 4.7–1
Examples of normal distribution, positive skewness, and negative skewness.

Prevalence.

The number of existing cases of a disorder. Several types of prevalence exist.

POINT PREVALENCE. The number of persons who have a disorder at a specified point in time. The point can be a certain calendar day (e.g., April 1, 1993) or any day during a particular study (e.g., the fourth day of the study), regardless of the calendar day. It is calculated as follows:

$$\text{Point prevalence} = \frac{\text{Number of persons with a disorder at a specific point in time}}{\text{Total population at a specific point in time}}$$

PERIOD PREVALENCE. The number of persons who have a disorder at any time during a specified period (longer than a calendar day or a point in time). It is calculated as follows:

$$\text{Period prevalence} = \frac{\text{Number of persons with a disorder during a period of time}}{\text{Total population during a period of time}}$$

The numerator includes any existing cases at the start of the period and any new cases that develop during the period. Period prevalence can be used to determine the number of persons with a disorder, the number of those in treatment, and the duration of an illness.

LIFETIME PREVALENCE. A measure at a point in time of the number of persons who had a disorder at some time during their lives. A potential problem with determining lifetime prevalence is that it is almost always based on subject recall, which can be inaccurate.

TREATED PREVALENCE. The number of persons being treated for a disorder, determined by counting all those in a defined geographic area who are receiving treatment. Treated point prevalence (e.g., the number of patients being treated for a disorder in a clinic on a certain day) or treated period prevalence (e.g., the number of patients being treated for a disorder at a clinic over the past year) can be measured.

Probability.

A quantitative statement of the likelihood that an event will occur. A probability of 0 means that the event is certain not to occur; a probability of 1 means that the event will occur with certainty.

P Value.

The probability of obtaining a result by chance alone. A *P* value of 0.01 means that the probability of obtaining a result by chance alone is 1 in 100; a value of 0.05 means that the result will occur 5 times out of every 100 times by chance alone.

Randomization.

The process allowing each patient in a clinical trial to have an equal chance to be assigned to a control or experimental treatment group. It protects against selection bias and guarantees the validity of statistical tests of significance.

Regression Analysis.

A method for obtaining a prediction from observed data to predict the value of one variable (x) in relation to the value of another variable (y).

Risk Factor.

A disorder-associated factor that may support a causal connection. A risk may be factor specific (e.g., it occurs in only one sex) or factor related (e.g., it is likely to occur in a certain environment). A causal connection between a risk factor and a disorder is shown by temporality, in which a factor precedes the disorder being studied; the repeated appearance of the same risk factor in multiple studies; specificity, in which a risk factor is associated with one disorder only; and a determination that the experimental intervention eliminating the risk factor also eliminates the disorder. Determining what factor or factors account for the increased risk of a disorder is one of the challenges of psychiatric epidemiology

RELATIVE RISK. The ratio of the incidence of the disease among persons exposed to the risk factor to the incidence among those not exposed. For example, the relative risk of lung cancer is much greater for heavy smokers than for nonsmokers.

ATTRIBUTABLE RISK. The absolute incidence of the disease in exposed persons that can be attributed to the exposure. The measure is derived by subtracting the incidence of the disease in question among unexposed persons from its total incidence among those exposed. For example, the lung cancer death rate for nonsmokers may be subtracted from the total community lung cancer death rate. The results are the attributable community risk for lung cancer. Attributable risk is a useful concept that shows what may be expected if the risk is removed. For example, on the basis of available data, the attributable risk for deaths from lung cancer could be avoided if smoking were eliminated.

Sample.

A subset of observations selected from a population.

Sensitivity.

The number of true-positive results divided by the sum of the number of true-positive and false-negative findings. It is the proportion of patients with the condition in question that the test can detect.

Specificity.

The number of true-negative results divided by the sum of the number of true-negative and false-positive findings. It is the proportion of patients without the condition that the test finds to be negative.

Standard Deviation (SD).

A measure of variation derived by squaring each deviation in a set of scores, taking the average of these squares, and then taking the square root of the result. The standard deviation is represented by the Greek letter sigma (σ). In a normal distribution, ± 1 SD includes 68 percent of the population; ± 2 SD includes 95 percent of the population; and ± 3 SD includes 99 percent of the population.

Standardized or Z-Score.

The deviation of a score from its group mean expressed in standard deviation units.

Survival Analysis.

Method for evaluating the timing of events. These methods can be used to evaluate life expectancy, age of onset of psychological illness, time to relapse for those in treatment, or the timing of developmental milestones such as first word, age of initiation of smoking, or age at marriage or any other time-dependent variable.

t-Test.

A statistical procedure designed to compare two sets of observations.

Type I Error.

The error that occurs when the null hypothesis is rejected when it should have been retained; the false claim of a true difference because the observed difference is entirely by chance.

Type II Error.

The error that occurs when the null hypothesis is retained when it should have been rejected; the false acceptance of the null hypothesis when, in fact, there is a true difference, but the difference is so small that it falls within the acceptance region of the null hypothesis.

Variable.

A characteristic that can assume different values in different experimental situations. In research, independent variables are those qualities that the experimenter systematically varies (e.g., time, age, sex, type of drug) in the experiment. Dependent variables are those qualities that measure the influence of the independent variable or the outcome of the experiment (e.g., the measurement of a person's specific physiological reactions to a drug).

References

Berganza CE. Broadening the international base for the development of an integrated diagnostic system in psychiatry. *World Psychiatry*. 2003;1:38–40.

Costello EJ, Mustillo S, Erkanli A, Keeler G, Angold A. Prevalence and development of psychiatric disorders in childhood and adolescence. *Arch Gen Psychiatry*. 2003;60:837–844.

Laska EM, Meisner M, Siegel C. Statistics and experimental design. In: Sadock BJ, Sadock VA, eds. *Kaplan & Sadock's Comprehensive Textbook of Psychiatry*. 8th ed. Vol. 1. Baltimore: Lippincott Williams & Wilkins; 2005:672.

Laska EM, Meisner M, Siegel C, Wanderling J. Statistical determination of cost-effectiveness frontier based on net health benefits. *Health Econ*. 2002;11:249–264.

Merikangas KR. Bridging genetics and epidemiology of mental disorders. In: Zorumski CF, Rubin EH, ed. *Psychopathology in the Genome and Neuroscience Era*. Washington: American Psychiatric Publishing, Inc; 2005:3–16.

Mezzich JE. From financial analysis to policy development in mental health care: the need for broader conceptual models and partnerships. *J Ment Health Policy Econ*. 2003;6:156–158.

Mezzich JE, Berganza CE, von Cranach M, Jorge MR, Kastrup MC, Murthy RS, Okasha A, Pull C, Sartorius N, Skodol A, Zaudig M, eds. Essentials of the World Psychiatric Association's International Guidelines for Diagnostic Assessment (IGDA). *Br J Psychiatry*. 2003;182[Suppl 45]:S37–S66.

Mezzich JE, Üstün TB. Epidemiology. In: Sadock BJ, Sadock VA, eds. *Kaplan & Sadock's Comprehensive Textbook of Psychiatry*. 8th ed. Vol. 1. Baltimore: Lippincott Williams & Wilkins; 2005:656.

Rosenbaum PR. *Observational Studies*. New York: Springer Verlag; 2002.

Rosenberger WF, Lachin JM. *Randomization in Clinical Trials: Theory and Practice*. New York: Wiley; 2002.

Schmolke MM, Lecic-Tosevski D, eds. Health promotion as an integral component of clinical care. *Dynamic Psychiatry*. 2003;36(special issue).

Üstün TB, Ayuso-Mateos JL, Chatterji S, Mathers C, Murray CJR. Global burden of depressive disorders in the year 2000. *Br J Psychiatry*. 2004;184:386–392.

Üstün TB, Chatterji S, Bickenbach J, Kostanjsek N, Schneider M. The international classification of functioning, disability and health: A new tool for understanding disability and health. *Disabil Rehabil*. 2003;25:565–571.

Whitehead A. *Meta-Analysis of Controlled Clinical Trials*. New York: Wiley; 2002.

WHO World Mental Health Survey Consortium. Prevalence, severity, and unmet need for treatment of mental disorders in the World Health Organization. World Mental Health (WMH) Surveys. *JAMA*. 2004;291:2581–2590.

5 Clinical Neuropsychological Testing

▲ 5.1 Clinical Neuropsychological Testing of Intelligence and Personality

Clinical neuropsychology is a specialty in psychology that examines the relationship between behavior and brain functioning in the realms of cognitive, motor, sensory, and emotional functioning. In general, the clinical neuropsychologist integrates the medical and psychosocial history with the reported complaints and the pattern of performance on neuropsychological procedures to determine whether results are consistent with a particular area of brain damage or a particular diagnosis. Although neurological syndromes are often the focus of referrals, the neuropsychological examination also has a valuable place in diagnosing and treating behavioral symptoms that are associated with other medical, psychological, and psychiatric conditions.

Most commonly used assessment instruments are standardized against normal control subjects, who are required to respond to the same stimuli or set of questions. Their responses are tabulated into a normal distribution pattern against which new subjects are compared. With standardization, test administration and scoring are invariant across time and examiners. Related to the standardization of any test are the available data that presumably show whether the test is valid and reliable. *Reliability* assesses the reproducibility of results; *validity* assesses whether the test measures what it purports to measure (see Chapter 4, Section 4.7, which discusses biostatistics).

The two types of tests are as follows: *Objective tests*, which are typically pencil-and-paper tests based on specific items and questions. They yield numerical scores and profiles easily subjected to mathematical or statistical analysis. An example is the Minnesota Multiphasic Personality Inventory (MMPI). (2) *Projective tests*, which present stimuli whose meanings are not immediately obvious; some ambiguity forces persons to project their own needs into the test situation. Projective tests presumably have no right or wrong answers. Those being tested impute meanings to the stimulus, apparently based on psychological and emotional factors. Examples include the Thematic Apperception Test (TAT), the Draw-a-Person test, the Rorschach test, and the Sentence Completion Test.

INTELLIGENCE TESTING

Intelligence can be defined as the ability to assimilate factual knowledge, to recall either recent or remote events, to reason logically, to manipulate concepts (either numbers or words), to translate the abstract to the literal and the literal to the abstract, to analyze and synthesize forms, and to deal meaningfully and accurately with problems and priorities deemed important in a particular setting. Intelligence varies tremendously from person to person.

In 1905, Alfred Binet introduced the concept of the mental age (MA), which is the average intellectual level of a particular age. The intelligence quotient (IQ) is the ratio of MA to CA (chronological age), multiplied by 100 to eliminate the decimal point; it is represented by the following equation:

$$IQ = \frac{MA}{CA} \times 100$$

An IQ of 100, or average, results when chronological and mental ages are equal. Because it is impossible to measure age-associated changes in intellectual power after the age of 15 with available intelligence tests, the highest divisor in the IQ formula is 15. One way of expressing a person's relative standing within a group is by using percentile. The higher the percentile, the higher the rank within a group. An IQ of 100 corresponds to the 50th percentile in intellectual ability for the general population.

As measured by most intelligence tests, IQ is an interpretation or classification of a total test score in relation to norms established by a group. IQ is a measure of present functioning ability, not necessarily of future potential. Although under ordinary circumstances the IQ is stable throughout life, there is no absolute certainty about its predictive properties. A person's IQ must be examined in the light of past experiences and future opportunities.

The IQ itself does not indicate the origins of its reflected capacities—genetic (innate) or environmental. The most useful intelligence test must measure a variety of skills and abilities, including verbal and performance, early learned and recently learned, timed and not timed, culture free, and culture bound. No intelligence test is totally culture free, although tests do differ significantly in degree.

Wechsler Adult Intelligence Scale (WAIS)

The Wechsler Adult Intelligence Scale (WAIS) is the best standardized and most widely used intelligence test in clinical practice today. It was constructed by David Wechsler at New York University Medical Center and Bellevue Psychiatric Hospital. Designed in 1939, the original WAIS has gone through several revisions. The latest revision, the WAIS-III, is designed for persons 16 to 89 years of age. A scale for children ages

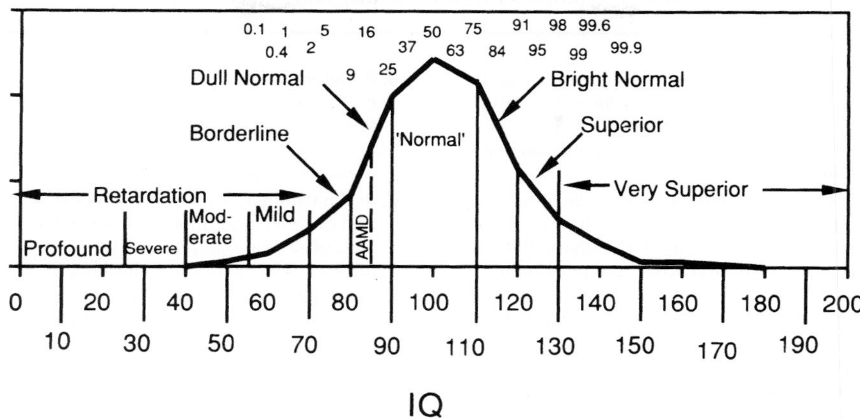

FIGURE 5.1–1
The distribution of Wechsler Adult Intelligence Scale IQ categories. (Adapted from Matarazzo JD. *Wechsler's Measurement and Appraisal of Adult Intelligence,* 5th ed. New York: Oxford University Press; 1972:124, with permission.)

5 through 15 years has been devised (Wechsler Intelligence Scale for Children-III [WISC-III]) as has a scale for children ages 4 to $6^1/_2$ years (Wechsler Preschool and Primary Scale of Intelligence-Revised [WPPSI-R]).

The WAIS is composed of 11 subtests made up of six verbal subtests and five performance subtests, which yield a verbal IQ, a performance IQ, and a combined or full-scale IQ. Intelligence levels are based on the assumption that intellectual abilities are normally distributed (in a bell-shaped curve) throughout the population (Fig. 5.1–1). Verbal and performance IQs and the full-scale IQ are determined by the use of separate tables for each of the seven age groups (from 16 to 64 years) on which the test was standardized. Variability in functioning is revealed through discrepancies between verbal and performance IQs and by the scatter pattern between subtests.

Distribution of IQ Scores. The average, or normal, range of IQ is 90 to 110; IQ scores of at least 120 are considered superior (Table 5.1–1). According to the American Association of Mental Deficiency (AAMD) and the text revision of the fourth edition of *Diagnostic and Statistical Manual of Mental Disorders* (DSM-IV-TR), mental retardation is defined as an IQ below 70, which corresponds to the lowest 2.2 percent of the population. Consequently, 2 of every 100 persons have IQ scores consistent with mental deficiency, which can range from mild to profound.

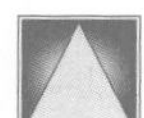

Table 5.1–1
Classification of Intelligence by IQ Range

Classification	IQ Range
Profound mental retardation (MR)[a]	Below 20 or 25
Severe MR[a]	20–25 to 35–40
Moderate MR[a]	35–40 to 50–55
Mild MR[a]	50–55 to about 70
Borderline	70–79
Dull normal	80 to 90
Normal	90 to 110
Bright normal	110 to 120
Superior	120 to 130
Very superior	130 and above

[a] According to the text revision of the fourth edition of *Diagnostic and Statistical Manual of Mental Disorders* (DSM-IV-TR).

ADULT PERSONALITY ASSESSMENT

Objective Personality Assessment

The objective approach to personality assessment is characterized by the reliance on structured, standardized measurement devices, which typically have a self-report nature. A structured approach reflects the tendency to use straightforward test stimuli, such as direct questions about persons' opinions of themselves and unambiguous instructions about completing the test.

Minnesota Multiphasic Personality Inventory (MMPI). The MMPI, a self-report inventory, is the most widely used and most thoroughly researched objective personality assessment instrument. The MMPI was developed in 1937 by Starke Hathaway, a psychologist, and J. Charnley McKinley, a psychiatrist. The test was eventually updated and is now called the MMPI-2. The test consists of more than 500 statements, such as, "I worry about sex matters"; "I sometimes tease animals"; "I believe I am being plotted against," to which subjects must respond with "true," "false," or "cannot say." The test may be used in card or booklet form, and several computer programs exist to process responses.

The MMPI gives scores on 10 standard clinical scales, each of which was derived empirically (i.e., homogeneous criterion groups of psychiatric patients were used in developing the scales). The items for each scale were selected for their ability to separate medical and psychiatric patients from normal control subjects. The scales are listed in Table 5.1–2.

Structured Clinical Diagnostic Assessments. Several structured and semistructured interviews based on DSM-IV-TR

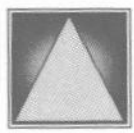

Table 5.1–2
Minnesota Multiphasic Personality Inventory (MMPI) Validity and Clinical Scales

Validity

L: Lie Scale. A nonempirically derived social desirability scale. Items tend to reflect behaviors that are considered socially desirable but rarely practiced. The score can suggest defensiveness, illiteracy, psychosis, or personality processes, depending on various factors.

F: Infrequency Scale. Measures a tendency to endorse selected items that are statistically rare responses (less than 10 percent of the original normal sample). Useful in identifying illiteracy, malingering, panic, confusion, psychosis, and personality processes.

K: Suppressor Scale. Used to adjust mathematically certain clinical scales to decrease false positives and false negatives. The scale is also useful in determining overall test-taking attitude and is an indication of personality variables.

Clinical

1: Hypochondriasis. Reflects somatic concerns and preoccupation with bodily functioning. Interpretation needs to take into account such factors as age and actual health status. As with all MMPI scales, interpretation is furthered by looking at its relation to other scales.

2: Depression. Tends to reflect depression as a mood disorder. The fact that the scale is sensitive to situational variables suggests that it may be a good index of state personality status.

3: Hysteria. Involves the identification of classic histrionic symptoms, including the presence of physical symptoms coupled with indifference, denial, repression, and inhibition. The scale does not necessarily measure other popularly conceived traits, such as liability and melodramatic attitude.

4: Psychopathic Deviance. Developed to assess the amorality and asociality aspects of psychopathy, rather than the criminal or antisocial. Its meaning depends on other scale configurations. The scale provides good information on the quality of interpersonal relationships.

5: Masculinity-Femininity. Originally developed to identify homosexuality but rarely used for that purpose, although it does provide information on gender identity. The scale reflects a variety of personality and interest areas, such as dependence, sensitivity, intellectuality, and tendencies toward introspection.

6: Paranoia. Developed by the empirical identification of classic paranoiacs, assesses vigilance, sensitivity, delusional thought, distrust, and suspicion. Except for the paranoid areas, the members of the original criterion group were considered functional in their lives.

7: Psychasthenia. A diverse scale designed to measure anxiety and obsessive-compulsive traits. Endorsed items can reflect fear, obsessive-compulsive symptoms, interpersonal hostility, tension, specific phobias, and impaired concentration.

8: Schizophrenia. Reflects the acute positive symptoms of psychotic breaks with reality, rather than the chronic negative symptoms. The scale also assesses alienation, impaired self-identity, and isolation.

9: Hypomania. Measures the classic symptoms of mania, including elated and unstable mood, psychomotor excitement, and flight of ideas. It also appears to reflect narcissistic personality traits. In general, the scale provides information on the degree of drivenness of the person's personality characteristics. It has a strong age component.

10: Social Introversion. Provides information on social withdrawal, shyness, leadership, talkativeness, levels of gregariousness, and, to a small degree, self-concept and neurotic tendencies. It is more two-dimensional and bipolar (introversion versus extroversion) than the other scales.

Special

A: Anxiety. The first general factor extracted from factor analytic studies on the MMPI. It is thought to reflect generalized endorsement of psychopathology.

R: Repression. The second factor that is found on factor analytic studies of the MMPI. It can be conceptualized as measuring the tendency to engage in denial.

ES: Ego Strength. Provides an index of how functional the patient may be in terms of work and other social areas regardless of level of psychopathology.

MAS: *McAndrews Alcoholism Scale* Estimates the person's degree of addiction proneness, especially with alcohol, opiates, and opioids. It is especially sensitive to daily substance abuse, rather than episodic abuse.

(Courtesy of Robert W. Butler, Ph.D., and Paul Satz, Ph.D., with the assistance of Alex Caldwell, Ph.D.)

criteria have been designed to provide numerical scores on diagnostic scales. The scales are useful in establishing the severity of illness and in monitoring recovery. Although used clinically, their greatest use is as research instruments; they help to standardize a subject cohort and provide objective outcome measures for assessing treatment response. Among these instruments are the Hamilton Rating Scale for Depression, the Hamilton Anxiety Rating Scale, the Yale-Brown Obsessive-Compulsive Scale (YBOCS), and the Structural Clinical Interview for DSM-IV Dissociative Disorders (SCID-D). A list of tests is given in Table 5.1–3.

Projective Personality Assessment

The projective approach to personality assessment is defined by the use of unstructured, often ambiguous test stimuli. A basic assumption is that when confronted with a vague stimulus and required to respond to it in some manner, persons cannot help but reveal information about themselves, not only in the way the ambiguity is confronted but also in the content of their responses.

Several semistructured situations and projective-type stimuli have been developed, including perceiving inkblots, drawing pictures, and telling stories on the basis of presented pictures. Various projective personality measures are listed in Table 5.1–4.

Rorschach Test. The Rorschach test was devised by Hermann Rorschach, a Swiss psychiatrist (Fig. 5.1–2), who in about 1910 began to experiment with ambiguous inkblots. A standard set of ten inkblots serves as a stimulus for associations; one inkblot is shown in Figure 5.1–3. In the standard series, the blots are reproduced on cards 7 by $9^1/_2$ inches and are numbered from I to X. Five of the blots are black and white; the other five include colors. The cards are shown to a patient in a particular order, and the psychologist keeps a record of the patient's verbatim responses, along with initial reaction times and total time spent on each card. After completion of what is called the *free-association phase*, the examiner conducts an inquiry phase

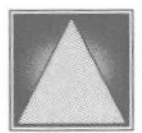

Table 5.1–3
Objective Measures of Personality in Adults

Name	Description	Strengths	Weaknesses
Minnesota-Multiphasic Personality Inventory (MMPI)	566 items, true-false; self-report format; 17 primary scales (numerous special scales)	Provides wide range of data on numerous personality variables; strong research base	Tends to emphasize major psychopathology; needs revision with current normative data
Minnesota Multiphasic Personality Inventory-2 (MMPI-2)	567 items; true-false; self-report format; 20 primary scales	Current revision of MMPI with updated response booklet; revised scaling methods, and new validity scores; new normative data	Preliminary data indicate that the MMPI-2 and the MMPI can provide discrepant results; normative sample biased toward upper socioeconomic status; no normative data for adolescents
Million Clinical Multiaxial Inventory (MCMI)	175 items; true-false; self-report format; 20 primary scales	Brief administration time; corresponds well with DSM-III diagnostic classifications	Needs more validation research; no information on disorder severity; needs revision for DSM-IV
Million Clinical Multiaxial Inventory-II (MCMI-II)	175 items; true-false; self-report format; 25 primary scales	Brief administration time; corresponds well with DSM-III-R	High degree of item overlap in various scales; no information on disorder or trait severity
16 Personality Factor Questionnaire (16 PF)	True-false; self-report format; 16 personality dimensions	Sophisticated psychometric instrument with considerable research conducted on nonclinical populations	Limited usefulness with clinical populations
Personality Assessment Inventory (PAI)	344 items; Likert-type format; self-report; 22 scales	Includes measures of psychopathology, personality dimensions, validity scales, and specific concerns to psychotherapeutic treatment	Inventory is new and has not yet generated a supportive research base
California Personality Inventory (CPI)	True-false; self-report format; 17 scales	Well-accepted method of assessing patients who do not exhibit major psychopathology	Limited usefulness with clinical populations
Jackson Personality Inventory (JPI)	True-false; self-report format; 15 personality scales	Constructed in accord with sophisticated psychometric techniques; controls for response sets	Unproved usefulness in clinical settings
Edwards Personal Preference Schedule (EPPS)	Forced choice; self-report format	Follows Murray's theory of personology; accounts for social desirability	Not widely used clinically because restricted information obtained
Psychological Screening Inventory (PSI)	103 items; true-false; self-report format	Yields four scores that can be used as screening measures for the possibility of a need for psychological help	Scales are short and have correspondingly low reliability
Eysenck Personality Questionnaire (EPQ)	True-false; self-report format	Useful as a screening device; test has a theoretical basis with research support	Scales are short, and items are transparent as to purpose; not recommended for other than a screening device
Adjective Checklist (ACL)	True-false; self-report or informant report	Can be used for self-rating or other rating	Scores rarely correlate highly with conventional personality inventories
Comrey Personality Scales (CPS)	True-false; self-report format; eight scales	Factor-analytical techniques used with a high degree of sophistication in test constructed	Not widely used; factor-analytical interpretation problems
Tennessee Self-Concept Scale (TSCS)	100 items; true-false; self-report format; 14 scales	Brief administration time yields considerable information	Brevity is also a disadvantage, lowering reliability and validity; useful as a screening device only

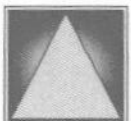

Table 5.1–4
Projective Measures of Personality

Name	Description	Strengths	Weaknesses
Rorschach test	10 stimulus cards of inkblots, some colored, others achromatic	Most widely used projective device and certainly the best researched; considerable interpretative data available	Some Rorschach interpretive systems have unproved validity
Thematic Apperception Test (TAT)	20 stimulus cards depicting a number of scenes of varying ambiguity	A widely used method that, in the hands of a well-trained person, provides valuable information	No generally accepted scoring system results in poor consistency in interpretation; time-consuming administration
Sentence Completion Test	A number of different devices available, all sharing the same format with more similarities than differences	Brief administration time; can be a useful adjunct to clinical interviews if supplied beforehand	Stimuli are obvious in intent and subject to easy falsification
Holtzman Inkblot Technique (HIT)	Two parallel forms of inkblot cards with 45 cards per form	Only one response is allowed per card, making research less troublesome	Not widely accepted and rarely used; not directly comparable to Rorschach interpretive strategies
Figure drawing	Typically human forms but can involve houses or other forms	Quick administration	Interpretive strategies have typically been unsupported by research
Make-a-Picture Story (MAPS)	Similar to TAT; however, stimuli can be manipulated by the patient	Provides idiographic personality information through thematic analysis	Minimal research support; not widely used

(Courtesy of Robert W. Butler, Ph.D., and Paul Satz, Ph.D.)

to determine important aspects of each response that are crucial to its scoring. Table 5.1–5 contains examples of responses to Rorschach stimuli.

Thematic Apperception Test (TAT). The TAT was designed by Henry Murray and Christiana Morgan as part of a normal personality study conducted at the Harvard Psychological Clinic in 1943. The TAT consists of a series of 30 pictures and a blank card. Typically, a patient is shown ten TAT cards and asked to make up stories about them. The patient is asked to tell what is going on in the picture, what was going on before the picture was taken, what the individuals in the picture are thinking and feeling, and what is likely to happen in the future. An example of a TAT card is presented in Figure 5.1-4.

Sentence Completion Test (SCT). The SCT is designed to tap patients' conscious associations to areas of functioning in which clinicians may be interested. The SCT is composed of a series of sentence stems (usually 75 to 100), such as, "I like . . . ," "Sometimes I wish . . . ," that patients are asked to complete in their own words.

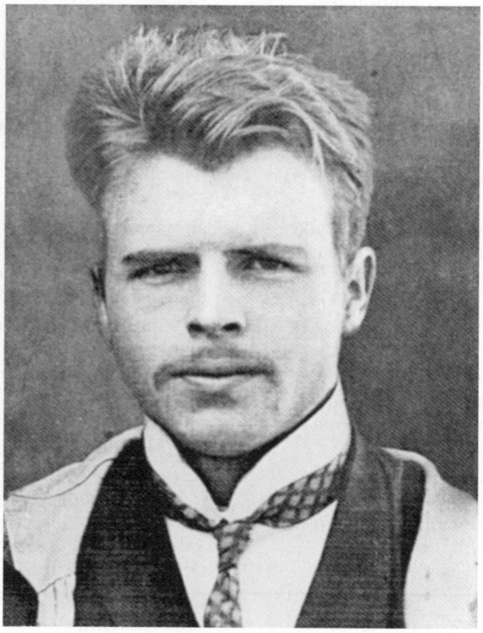

FIGURE 5.1–2
Herman Rorschach. (Courtesy of New York Academy of Medicine, New York, NY.)

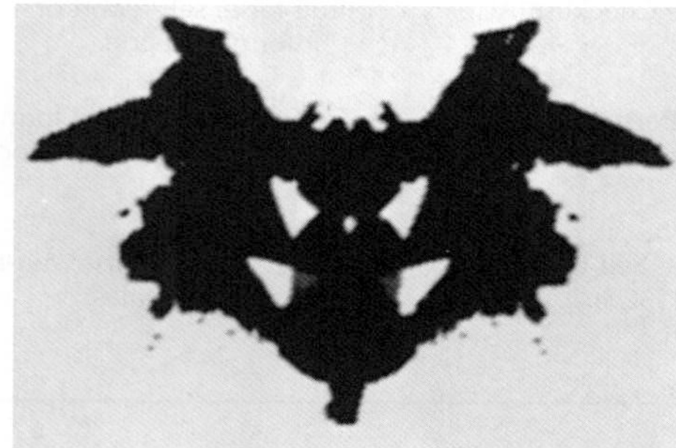

FIGURE 5.1–3
Plate 1 of the Rorschach test. (Reprinted from Huber Medical Publisher, Bern, with permission.)

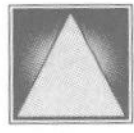

Table 5.1–5
Sample Rorschach Responses and Interpretation to Card I by Diagnostic Category

Diagnostic Category	Patient's Response Proper	Patient's Response on Inquiry	Interpretation
Nonpatient	Well the first impression is of a wolf's head, ears here and eyes.	"Overall the head, nose, eyes, ears, the whole thing."	Common response using the white space as the eyes, responding to the whole blot
Schizophrenic patient	I will say the first thing that comes to mind, it would be a predator on the movie, lots of ink, predator, have you seen that movie?	"The whole picture all the way, and I liked the movie and the reason why is because you said the first thing that comes to mind. I've seen the movie over and over again, ten times. The whole picture, something that looks at me mean. (Looks at you mean?) Because it's a person that kills without any feeling, that's why I thought the movie was good."	The response shows difficulty staying focused on the task at hand, tangential thought process, some paranoia and distortion of the form of the card
Depression	Could be a leaf.	"Could be a leaf that has fallen off the tree and started to decay, leaves have jagged edges. (You said decayed?) Because if it was a perfect leaf all this would be part of the blot, and here parts of it that have fallen off. That would have been the stem. Also you have the main vein running down the middle, this is more prevalent because it's biggest, if it was on a tree it would get nutrients to the leaf like our blood system."	The response shows morbid content (decay) that indicates a poor view of self and the world; leaf responses also weigh on the isolation index
Anxiety	I don't know, I'd have to think about it. It could be trees.	"Like if you are in the forest, stalks you know, when trees blend together they are nondescript. I'm a real outdoor person, I like to go to the forest and spend time there. (Can you help me see the trees?) Just this little Christmas tree here and here, the outline."	The response shows discomfort in committing to a response, and discomfort in beginning the task; some anxiety is also seen in the rambling personalization used to justify the response

(Courtesy of Dana Foley, Ph.D.)

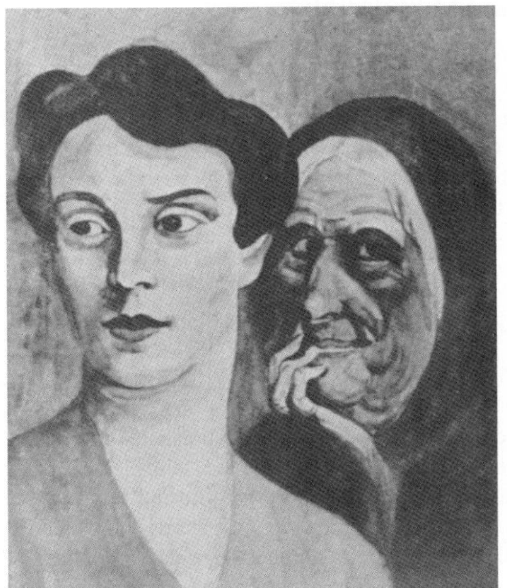

FIGURE 5.1–4
Card 12F of the Thematic Apperception Test. (Courtesy of Harvard University Press, Cambridge, MA.)

Time pressure is usually applied; patients are instructed to write down the first thing that comes to mind. In other instances, the test is administered orally by the examiner, as in the word-association technique. Sentence stems vary in their ambiguity; hence, some items serve as projective test stimuli ("Sometimes I . . . "). Others closely resemble direct-response questionnaires ("My greatest fear is . . . ").

With the individual protocol, most clinicians use an inspection technique and note particularly those responses that express strong affects, that tend to be given repetitively, or that are unusual or particularly informative in any way. Areas in which denial operates are often revealed through omissions, bland expressions, or factual reports ("My mother is a woman."). Humor may also reflect an attempt to deny anxiety about a particular issue, person, or event. Important historical material is sometimes revealed directly ("I feel guilty about the way my sister was drowned.").

Word-Association Technique. Carl Gustav Jung devised the word-association technique. Jung presented stimulus words to patients and had them respond with the first word that came to mind. After the initial administration of the list, some clinicians today repeat the list and ask the patient to respond with the same words that he or she used previously; discrepancies between the two administrations may reveal associational difficulties. Complex indicators include long reaction times, blocking difficulties in making responses, unusual responses, repetition of the stimulus word, apparent misunderstanding of the word, slang associations, perseveration of earlier responses, and ideas or unusual mannerisms or movements accompanying a response. Because it is easily quantified, the test continues to be used as a research instrument, although its popularity has diminished greatly over the years.

Draw-a-Person Test. This test was first used as a measure of intelligence in children. Detail was correlated with intelligence and developmental level. It has since become useful as an adult test. The Draw-a-Person test is easily administered, usually with the instructions, "I'd like you to draw a picture of a person; draw the best person you can." After completion of the first drawing, the patient is asked to draw a picture of a person of the sex opposite that of the figure in the drawing. Some clinicians use an interrogation procedure in which the patient is questioned about his or her drawings. ("What is he doing?" "What are her best qualities?") Modifications include asking for a drawing of a house and a tree (House-Tree-Person test), of the patient's family, and of an animal.

A general assumption is that the drawing of a person represents the expression of the self or of the body in the environment. Interpretive principles rest largely on the assumed functional significance of each body part. Most clinicians use drawings primarily as a screening technique, particularly to detect brain damage.

INTEGRATION OF TEST FINDINGS

The integration of test findings into a comprehensive, meaningful report is probably the most difficult aspect of psychological evaluation. Inferences from various tests must be related to one another in terms of clinicians' confidence in them and of a patient's presumed level of awareness that consciousness is being tapped.

Most clinicians follow some general outline in preparing a psychological report, such as test behavior, intellectual functioning, personality functioning (reality-testing ability, impulse control, manifest depression and guilt, manifestations of major dysfunction, major defenses, overt symptoms, interpersonal conflicts, self-concept, affects), inferred diagnosis, degree of present overt disturbance, prognosis for social recovery, motivation for personality change, primary assets and weaknesses, recommendations, and summary.

REFERENCES

Adams RL, Culbertson JL. Personality Assessment: Adults and Children. In: Sadock BJ, Sadock VA, eds. *Kaplan & Sadock's Comprehensive Textbook of Psychiatry*. 8th ed. Vol. 1. Baltimore: Lippincott Williams & Wilkins; 2005:874.

Beck JG, Novy DM, Diefenbach GJ, Stanley MA, Averill PM, Swann AC. Differentiating anxiety and depression in older adults with generalized anxiety disorder. *Psychol Assess*. 2003;15:184.

Cummings J, Mega MS. *Neuropsychiatry and Behavioral Neuroscience*. New York: Oxford University Press; 2003.

Devinsky O, D'Esposito M. *Neurology of Cognitive and Behavioral Disorders*. New York: Oxford University Press; 2004.

Gomez R, Burns GL, Walsh JA, Alves de Moura M. A multitrait-multisource confirmatory factor analytic approach to the construct validity of ADHD rating scales. *Psychol Assess*. 2003;15:3.

Groth-Marnot G. *Handbook of Psychological Assessment*. 4th ed. New York: John Wiley & Sons; 2003.

Heilman KM, Valenstein E. *Clinical Neuropsychology*. 4th ed. New York: Oxford University Press; 2003.

Hunsley J, Meyer GJ. The incremental validity of psychological testing and assessment: Conceptual, methodological, and statistical issues. *Psychol Assess*. 2003;15:446.

Lopez SJ, Snyder CR, eds. *Positive Psychological Assessment, A Handbook of Models and Measures*. Washington, DC: American Psychological Association; 2003.

Petersen RC. *Mild Cognitive Impairment: Aging to Alzheimer's Disease*. New York: Oxford University Press; 2003.

Price KJ, Joschko M, Kerns K. The ecological validity of pediatric neuropsychological tests of attention. *Clinical Neuropsychologist*. 2003; 71:170–181.

Spirito A, Overholser J. *Evaluating and Treating Adolescent Suicide Attempter: From Research to Practice*. San Diego: Elsevier; 2003.

Swanda RM, Haaland KY. Clinical neuropsychology and intellectual assessment of adults. In: Sadock BJ, Sadock VA, eds. *Kaplan & Sadock's Comprehensive Textbook of Psychiatry*. 8th ed. Vol. 1. Baltimore: Lippincott Williams & Wilkins; 2005:860.

Vittengl JR, Clark LA, Jarrett RB. Interpersonal problems, personality psychopathology, and social adjustment after cognitive therapy for depression. *Psychol Assess*. 2003;15:29.

▲ 5.2 Clinical Neuropsychological Assessment of Adults

Clinical assessment of adults examines the relationship between behavior and brain functioning in the realms of cognitive, motor, sensory, and emotional functioning. Neuropsychological assessment is indicated to identify cognitive defects, to differentiate incipient depression from dementia, to determine the course of an illness, to assess neurotoxic effects (such as memory impairment by substance abuse), to evaluate the effects of treatment (e.g., surgery for epilepsy, pharmacotherapy), and to evaluate learning disorders.

REASONING, CONCEPT FORMATION, AND PROBLEM SOLVING

Patients with cerebral disease are likely to lose the capacity to reason abstractly and to lack flexibility in problem solving or adapting to changed situations. Frontal lobe disease is often associated with impaired abstract reasoning, although other areas of the brain can also be involved. Workers can use many tests to assess the capacity for concept formation.

Wisconsin Card Sorting Test (WCST)

The Wisconsin Card Sorting Test (WCST) assesses abstract reasoning and flexibility in problem solving. Stimulus cards of different color, form, and number are presented to patients to sort into groups according to a principle established by the examiner (e.g., to sort by color, ignoring form and number). The procedure, repeated several times, measures the capacity for abstract thinking (i.e., the number of trials required to achieve a solution) and flexibility (perseverative errors on successive sorting trials). Persons with damage to the frontal lobes or to the caudate and some persons with schizophrenia give abnormal responses.

MEMORY

Impairment of various types of memory, most notably short-term and recent memory, is a prominent behavioral deficit in patients with brain damage. In addition, it is often the first sign of cerebral disease and of aging. *Memory* is a comprehensive term that covers the retention of all types of material over various times and involves diverse forms of response. Consequently, a neuropsychological examiner is more inclined to give specific memory tests and evaluate them separately than to use an omnibus battery that provides a brief assessment of a large variety of performances and yields a single score.

Types of Memory

Immediate (or *short-term*) *memory* can be defined as the reproduction, recognition, or recall of perceived material within a period up to 30 seconds after presentation. It is most often assessed by digit repetition and reversal (auditory) and memory-for-designs (visual) tests. Both an auditory-verbal task, such as digit span or memory for words or sentences, and a nonverbal visual task, such as memory for designs or for objects or faces, should be given to assess a patient's immediate memory. Patients can also be asked to listen to a standardized story and then repeat it as accurately as possible. Patients with lesions of the right hemisphere are likely to show more severe defects on visual nonverbal tasks than on auditory verbal tasks. Conversely, patients with left hemisphere disease, including those who are not aphasic, are likely to show severe deficits on the auditory verbal tests, with variable performance on the visual nonverbal tasks.

Recent memory concerns events over the past few hours or days and can be tested by asking patients what they had for breakfast and who visited with them in the hospital.

Recent past memory concerns the retention of information over the past few months. Patients can be asked questions about current events.

Remote memory is the ability to remember events in the distant past. It is commonly believed that remote memory is well preserved in patients who show pronounced defects in recent memory, but the remote memory of senile and amnestic patients is usually significantly inferior to that of normal persons of comparable age and education. Even patients who appear able to recount their past fairly accurately show gaps and inconsistencies in their recitals on close examination.

Memory theorists have described three other types of memories: episodic, for specific events (e.g., a telephone message); semantic, for knowledge and facts (e.g., the first president of the United States); and implicit, for automatic skills (e.g., speaking grammatically or driving a car). Semantic and implicit memories do not decline with age, and persons continue to accumulate information over a lifetime. A minimal decline in episodic memory with aging may relate to impaired frontal lobe functioning.

Testing Memory

Wechsler Memory Scale. The Wechsler Memory Scale-Revised (WMS-R) is the most widely used memory test battery for adults. It is a composite of verbal paired associate and paragraph retention, visual memory for designs, orientation, digit span, rote recall of the alphabet, and counting backward. The scale yields a memory quotient (MQ), which is corrected for age and generally approximates the Wechsler Adult Intelligence Scale intelligence quotient (WAIS IQ); amnestic conditions, such as Korsakoff's syndrome, are characterized by a disproportionately low MQ but a relatively preserved IQ.

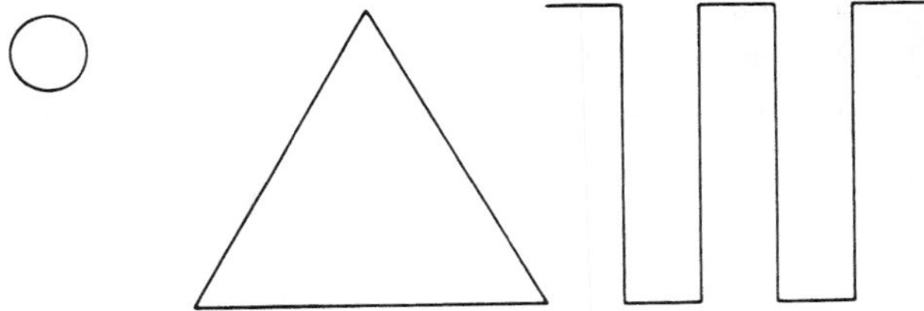

FIGURE 5.2–1
Test item from the Benton Visual Retention Test. The most frequently used testing condition involves the presentation of each geometric figure for 10 seconds, after which the patient attempts to draw the figure from memory. (Reprinted from Benton AL: *The Revised Visual Retention Test: Clinical and Experimental Applications,* 4th ed. New York: Psychological Corporation; 1974:32, with permission.)

Benton Visual Retention Test. The Benton Visual Retention Test is sensitive to short-term memory loss (Fig. 5.2–1).

ORIENTATION

Orientation for person or place is rarely disturbed in patients who are brain damaged and who are not psychotic or severely demented, although defects in temporal orientation, which can reflect the integrity of recent memory, are common. Clinical examiners often miss these defects because of the tendency to regard as inconsequential slight inaccuracies in giving the day of the week or the date of the month. About 25 percent of patients who are not psychotic with hemispheric cerebral disease, however, are likely to show significantly decreased performance with respect to the precision of temporal orientation. A simple test for orientation is outlined in Table 5.2–1.

PERCEPTUAL AND PERCEPTUOMOTOR PERFORMANCE

Many patients with brain disease show an impaired ability to analyze complex stimulus constellations or an inability to translate their perception into appropriate motor action. Unless the impairment is gross (e.g., as in visual object agnosia or dressing apraxia) or it interferes with a specific occupation skill, these deficits are not likely to be the subject of spontaneous complaint. Appropriate testing, however, discloses a remarkably high incidence of impaired performance on visuoanalytic, visuospatial, and visuoconstructive tasks in patients who are brain damaged, particularly in persons with disease involving the right hemisphere. This type of impairment also extends to tactile and auditory perceptual task performances.

Visuoperceptive and visuoconstructive capacity and somatoperceptual defects can be assessed by tests. Double simultaneous stimulation is tested by lightly touching one of the patient's cheeks with one hand and simultaneously touching the back of one of the patient's hands with the other. A patient with brain dysfunction is unable to recognize one or both of the stimuli.

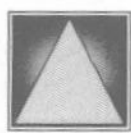

Table 5.2–1
Temporal Orientation Schedule

Administration
What is today's date? (The patient is required to give month, day, and year.)
What day of the week is it?
What time is it now? (Examiner makes sure that the patient cannot look at a watch or clock.)

Scoring
Day of week: 1 error point for each day removed from the correct day to a maximum of 3 points
Day of month: 1 error point for each day removed from the correct day to a maximum of 15 points
Month: 5 error points for each month removed from the correct month, with the qualification that, if the stated date is within 15 days of the correct date, no points are scored for the incorrect month (e.g., May 29 for June 2 = 4 points off)
Year: 10 error points for each year removed from the correct year to a maximum of 60 points, with the qualification that, if the stated date is within 15 days of the correct date, no points are scored for the incorrect year (e.g., December 26, 1982, for January 2, 1983 = 7 points off)
Time of day: 1 error point for each 30 minutes removed from the correct time to a maximum of 5 points

(Courtesy of Arthur L. Benton, Ph.D.)

The double simultaneous stimulation is a general test of defective capacity for perceptual integration.

Perceptuomotor tests often help localize cerebral lesions. A significant portion of patients with lesions of the right hemisphere who do not show obvious impairment in language functions perform poorly on perceptual tests.

HEMISPHERIC DOMINANCE AND INTRAHEMISPHERIC LOCALIZATION

Many functions are mediated by both the right and left cerebral hemispheres. Important qualitative differences between the two hemispheres can be demonstrated, however, in the presence of lateralized brain injury. Various cognitive skills that have been linked to the left or right hemisphere in right-handed people are listed in Table 5.2–2. Although language is the most obvious area that is largely controlled by the left hemisphere, the left hemisphere is also generally considered to be dominant for limb praxis (i.e., performing complex movements, such as brushing teeth, to command or to imitate) and has been associated with the cluster of deficits identified as Gerstmann syndrome (i.e., finger agnosia, dyscalculia, dysgraphia, and right-left disorientation). In contrast, the right hemisphere is thought to play a more important role in controlling visuospatial abilities and hemispatial attention, which are associated with the clinical presentations of constructional apraxia and neglect, respectively.

Table 5.2–2
Selected Neuropsychological Deficits Associated with Left or Right Hemisphere Damage

Left Hemisphere	Right Hemisphere
Aphasia	Visuospatial deficits
Right-left disorientation	Impaired visual perception
Finger agnosia	Neglect
Dysgraphia (aphasic)	Dysgraphia (spatial, neglect)
Dyscalculia (number alexia)	Dyscalculia (spatial)
Constructional apraxia (details)	Constructional apraxia (Gestalt)
Limb apraxia	Dressing apraxia
	Anosognosia

Although lateralized deficits such as these are typically characterized in terms of damage to the right or left hemisphere, the patient's performance can also be characterized in terms of preserved brain functions. In other words, it is the remaining intact brain tissue that drives many behavioral responses following injury to the brain—not only the absence of critical brain tissue.

Bender Visual Motor Gestalt Test

The Bender Visual Motor Gestalt Test is a test of visuomotor coordination that is useful for both children and adults. It was designed in 1938 by Lauretta Bender of New York University Medical Center and Bellevue Psychiatric Hospital, who used it to evaluate maturational levels in children. Developmentally, a child younger than 3 years of age is generally unable to reproduce any of the test's designs meaningfully. About 4 years of age, a child may be able to copy several designs but does so poorly. At about age 6, a child should produce some recognizable, although still uneven, representations of all the designs. By age 10 and certainly by age 12, a child's copies should be reasonably accurate and well organized. Bender also presented studies of adults with cognitive disorders, mental retardation, aphasias, psychoses, neuroses, and malingering.

The test material consists of nine separate designs, adapted from those used by Max Wertheimer in his studies in gestalt psychology. Each design is printed against a white background on a separate card (Fig. 5.2–2). Presented with unlined paper,

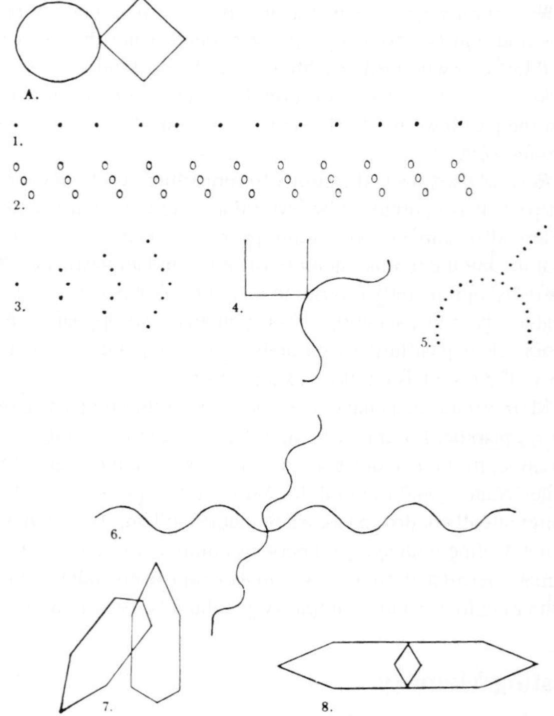

FIGURE 5.2–2
Text figures from the Bender Visual Motor Gestalt test, adapted from Max Wertheimer. (Reprinted from Bender L: *A Visual Motor Gestalt Test and Its Clinical Use.* New York: American Orthopsychiatric Association, 1938:33, with permission.)

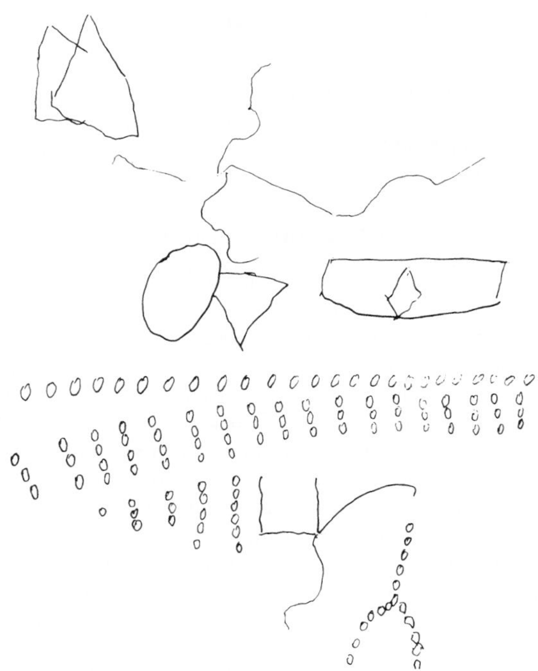

FIGURE 5.2–3
Bender gestalt drawing of a 57-year-old woman with brain damage.

patients are asked to copy each design with the card in front of them. There is no time limit. This phase of the test is highly structured and does not investigate memory function, because the cards remain in front of patients while they copy them. Many clinicians include a subsequent recall phase, in which (after an interval of 45 to 60 seconds) patients are asked to reproduce as many of the designs as they can from memory. This phase not only investigates visual memory, but also presents a less structured situation, in which patients must rely essentially on their own resources. It is often particularly helpful to compare the patient's functioning under the two conditions.

The Bender Gestalt Test is probably used most frequently with adults as a screening device for signs of organic dysfunction. Evaluation of the protocol depends on the form of the reproduced figures and on their relation to one another and to the whole spatial background (Figs. 5.2–3 and 5.2–4).

Complex Visual Discrimination

Although the inability to recognize familiar faces (prosopagnosia) is an uncommon disorder, defective discrimination of unfamiliar faces is a common finding in patients with right-hemisphere or bilateral lesions. The Facial Recognition Test, in which a patient is required to identify a photograph of a face originally presented in a front view when it is included in various displays (e.g., side view and a front view with shadows), produces a high frequency of failure in patients with posterior right hemisphere lesions. Performance is generally intact in patients with left hemisphere lesions (provided that receptive language is not seriously limited) and in patients with schizophrenia.

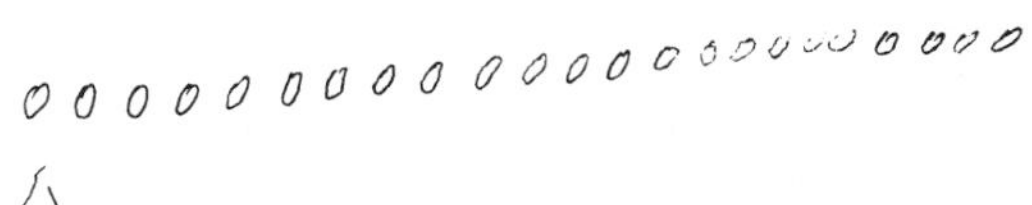

FIGURE 5.2–4
Bender gestalt recall of the 57-year-old woman with brain damage shown in Figure 5.2–3.

LANGUAGE

Relatively minor defects in the use of language may be valid indicators of the presence of brain disease. The dominant hemisphere controls language function. The affective part of speech that conveys mood, *prosody*, is controlled by the nondominant hemisphere. Fluency is tested by asking patients to give all the words they can think of beginning with a given letter of the alphabet. Aphasic patients with left hemisphere disease fail this task. Variables influencing language tests are educational background, sex, and age. Reading and writing are also associated with the dominant hemisphere and are tested by asking patients to read aloud from prepared material and to write their names or a brief passage. Dyslexia and dysgraphia are suspected if patients have difficulties in performing these tasks.

The Boston Diagnostic Aphasia Examination includes a speech rating scale that is useful for comparing with test scores and a brief schedule of items for assessing ideomotor praxis—that is, symbolic buccofacial and limb movements to exhibit gestures and to demonstrate the use of imagined or real objects.

ATTENTION AND CONCENTRATION

The capacity to sustain a maximal level of attention over a period is sometimes impaired in patients who are brain damaged, and this impairment is reflected in an oscillation in performance level for a continuous or repeated activity. Some evidence indicates that the instability in performance is related to an electroencephalographic abnormality and that an inexplicable decline in performance is related temporally to the occurrence of certain types of abnormal electrical activity. Simple reaction time provides a convenient measure of the variability and speed of simple responses.

The reaction time needed to respond to a stimulus is impaired in 40 to 45 percent of patients who are brain damaged and it is a sensitive indicator of overall cerebral integrity. Comparison of the reaction times of the right and left hands often provides an indication of the site of the lesion in a patient and of unilateral cerebral disease.

Mini-Mental State Examination (MMSE)

Although formal evaluation of cognitive impairment requires time-consuming consultation with an expert in psychological testing, one practical and clinically useful test for practitioners is the Mini-Mental State Examination (MMSE). The MMSE is a screening test that can be used during a patient's clinical examination. It is also a practical test to track the changes in a patient's cognitive state. Of a possible 30 points, a score below 25 suggests possible impairment, and a score below 20 indicates definite impairment.

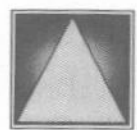

Table 5.2–3
Neuropsychiatric Mental Status Examination

A. General Description
1. General appearance, dress, sensory aids (glasses, hearing aid)
2. Level of consciousness and arousal
3. Attention to environment
4. Posture (standing and seated)
5. Gait
6. Movements of limbs, trunk, and face (spontaneous, resting, and after instruction)
7. General demeanor (including evidence of responses to internal stimuli)
8. Response to examiner (eye contact, cooperation, ability to focus on interview process)
9. Native or primary language

B. Language and Speech
1. Comprehension (words, sentences, simple and complex commands, and concepts)
2. Output (spontaneity, rate, fluency, melody or prosody, volume, coherence, vocabulary, paraphasic errors, complexity of usage)
3. Repetition
4. Other aspects
   a. Object naming
   b. Color naming
   c. Body part identification
   d. Ideomotor praxis to command

C. Thought
1. Form (coherence and connectedness)
2. Content
   a. Ideational (preoccupations, overvalued ideas, delusions)
   b. Perceptual (hallucinations)

D. Mood and Affect
1. Internal mood state (spontaneous and elicited; sense of humor)
2. Future outlook
3. Suicidal ideas and plans
4. Demonstrated emotional status (congruence with mood)

E. Insight and Judgment
1. Insight
   a. Self-appraisal and self-esteem
   b. Understanding of current circumstances
   c. Ability to describe personal psychological and physical status
2. Judgment
   a. Appraisal of major social relationships
   b. Understanding of personal roles and responsibilities

F. Cognition
1. Memory
   a. Spontaneous (as evidenced during interview)
   b. Tested (incidental, immediate repetition, delayed recall, cued recall, recognition; verbal, nonverbal; explicit, implicit)
2. Visuospatial skills
3. Constructional ability
4. Mathematics
5. Reading
6. Writing
7. Fine sensory function (stereognosis, graphesthesia, two-point discrimination)
8. Finger gnosis
9. Right-left orientation
10. "Executive functions"
11. Abstraction

Courtesy of Eric D. Caine, M.D., and Jeffrey M. Lyness, M.D.

COMPREHENSIVE TESTING

Several test batteries have been developed to help in neuropsychological and neuropsychiatric evaluation. Among them are the Luria-Nebraska and the Halstead-Reitan neuropsychological test batteries and the Caine-Lyness Neuropsychiatric Mental Status Examination (Table 5.2-3).

Luria-Nebraska Neuropsychological Battery

Based on the work of the Russian neuropsychologist Alexander Luria, the Luria-Nebraska Neuropsychological Battery was developed at the University of Nebraska. The test assesses a wide range of cognitive functions: memory; motor functions; rhythm; tactile, auditory, and visual functions; receptive and expressive speech; writing; spelling; reading; and arithmetic. The test is designed for persons who are at least 15 years of age, and a children's version can be used with 8- to 12-year-olds. The test is extremely sensitive for identifying specific types of problems (e.g., dyslexia and dyscalculia), rather than being limited to global impressions of brain dysfunction. It also helps localize the various cortical zones that are involved in a particular function and is useful in establishing left or right cerebral dominance.

Halstead-Reitan Battery of Neuropsychological Tests

In the early 1940s, Ward Halstead and his student Ralph Reitan developed a battery of tests that was used to determine the location and the effects of specific brain lesions. The battery is composed of ten tests.

1. Category test: Patients must discover the common element in a set of pictures; the test measures concept function, abstraction, and visual acuity.
2. Tactual performance test: Patients place shapes in a form board while blindfolded and then must recall the arrangement of the board; the performance tests dexterity, spatial memory, and tactual discrimination.
3. Rhythm test: Patients identify 30 pairs of rhythmic beats as either the same or different to test auditory perception, attention, and concentration.
4. Finger-oscillation test: Patients tap the index finger of each hand in a measured 10-second period; the test measures dexterity and motor speed.
5. Speech-sounds perception test: Patients match 60 nonsense syllables that they hear with several printed alternatives; the test measures auditory discrimination and phonetic skills.
6. Trail-making test: Patients first connect 25 numbered circles in order and then connect 25 lettered and numbered circles in order, alternating between numbered and alphabetical circles; the procedure tests visuomotor perception and motor speed.
7. Critical flicker frequency: Patients note when a flickering light becomes steady for a test of visual perception.
8. Time sense test: Patients judge, without looking, the time it takes for the second hand of a watch to make several revolutions as a test of memory and spatial perception.
9. Aphasia screening test: Patients must name objects, read, write, calculate, draw shapes, identify body parts, perform acts, and differentiate between left and right as a means of testing a wide range of verbal and nonverbal brain functions.
10. Sensory-perceptual tests: Patients perform several tasks with eyes closed—such as identifying where they are touched simultaneously on the hand and the face (simultaneous sensory stimulation test),

which finger is touched (finger localization), what coins are placed in the hand (stereognosis), and what numbers are written on the skin (tactile perception).

The Halstead-Reitan Battery has the advantage of providing a uniform profile of scores that must be weighed against the considerable time required for administration. The test can differentiate those who are brain damaged from neurologically intact persons. Persons with schizophrenia tend to perform above the level of patients who are subacutely brain damaged but not differently from those with chronic brain damage. Moreover, the pattern of deficits on the Halstead-Reitan Battery is similar in patients with brain damage and with schizophrenia.

THERAPEUTIC DISCUSSION OF RESULTS

A key component of the neuropsychological examination process is the opportunity to discuss results of the examination with the patient and family or other caregivers. This meeting can be a powerful therapeutic opportunity to educate them and clarify individual and relationship issues that can affect the patient's functioning. If the patient's active cooperation in the initial examination was enlisted appropriately, the patient will be optimally prepared to invest value and confidence in the findings of the examination. When the results are discussed, it is useful to review the goals of the examination with the patient and supportive family or caregivers and to clarify the expectations of those who are present. Typically, these sessions include information about the patient's diagnosis, with emphasis on the natural course and prognosis as well as compensation and coping strategies for the patient and family. If findings show evidence of chronic or progressive neurological disease, these issues must be explicitly discussed, including rehabilitative sources. It is equally important to relate the impact of the results to the patient's current living circumstances, future goals, and course of adjustment. Strong emotions and underlying tensions within family relationships frequently come to light in the context of honest discussion, and so the results discussion can be an important therapeutic opportunity to model effective communication and problem-solving techniques.

References

Beck JG, Novy DM, Diefenbach GJ, Stanley MA, Averill PM, Swann AC. Differentiating anxiety and depression in older adults with generalized anxiety disorder. *Psychol Assess.* 2003;15:184.

Binder LM, Campbell KA. Medically unexplained symptoms and neuropsychological assessment. *J Clin Exp Neuropsychol.* 2004;26(3):369–392.

Groth-Marnot G. *Handbook of Psychological Assessment*. 4th ed. New York: John Wiley & Sons; 2003.

Hunsley J, Meyer GJ. The incremental validity of psychological testing and assessment: Conceptual, methodological, and statistical issues. *Psychol Assess.* 2003;15:446.

Jones JE, Hermann BP, Barry JJ, Gilliam F, Kanner AM, Meador KJ. Clinical assessment of Axis I psychiatric morbidity in chronic epilepsy: A multicenter investigation. *J Neuropsychiatry Clin Neurosci.* 2005;17: 172–179.

Lopez SJ, Snyder CR, eds. *Positive Psychological Assessment, A Handbook of Models and Measures*. Washington, DC: American Psychological Association; 2003.

Rabin LA, Barr WB, Burton LA. Assessment practices of clinical neuropsychologists in the United States and Canada: A survey of INS, NAN, and APA Division 40 members. *Arch Clin Neuropsychol.* 2005;20(1):33–65.

Ricker JH, ed. *Differential Diagnosis in Adult Neuropsychological Assessment.* New York: Springer Publishing Co.; 2004.

Spirito A, Overholser J. *Evaluating and Treating Adolescent Suicide Attempter: From Research to Practice*. San Diego: Elsevier; 2003.

Swanda RM, Haaland KY. Clinical neuropsychology and intellectual assessment of adults. In: Sadock BJ, Sadock VA, eds. *Kaplan & Sadock's Comprehensive Textbook of Psychiatry*. 8th ed. Vol. 1. Baltimore: Lippincott Williams & Wilkins; 2005:860.

Vittengl JR, Clark LA, Jarrett RB. Interpersonal problems, personality psychopathology, and social adjustment after cognitive therapy for depression. *Psychol Assess.* 2003;15:29.

6 Theories of Personality and Psychopathology

▲ 6.1 Sigmund Freud: Founder of Classic Psychoanalysis

Psychoanalysis has existed since before the turn of the 20th century and, in that span of years, has established itself as one of the fundamental disciplines within psychiatry. The science of psychoanalysis is the bedrock of psychodynamic understanding and forms the fundamental theoretical frame of reference for a variety of forms of therapeutic intervention, embracing not only psychoanalysis itself but also various forms of psychoanalytically oriented psychotherapy and related forms of therapy using psychodynamic concepts. Likewise, current efforts are being directed to connecting psychoanalytic understandings of human behavior and emotional experience with emerging findings of neuroscientific research.

Psychoanalysis was the child of Sigmund Freud's genius. He put his stamp on it from the very beginning, and it can be fairly said that, although the science of psychoanalysis has advanced far beyond Freud's wildest dreams, his influence is still strong and pervasive. In understanding the origins of psychoanalytic thinking, it is useful to keep in mind that Freud himself was an outstanding product of the scientific training and thinking of his era.

Certain basic tenets of Freud's thinking have remained central to psychiatric and psychotherapeutic practice. Among these are the notion of psychic determination, unconscious mental activity, and the role of childhood experience in shaping the adult personality.

The role of meaning was also central to Freud's vision of psychoanalysis. In his view, symptoms, thoughts, feelings, and behavior could all be viewed as the final common pathways of meaningful psychological processes, many of which were unconscious. Even when biological factors influence the pathogenesis of a disorder, the symptoms nevertheless have psychological meaning to the person. For example, in auditory hallucinations, biological mechanisms may produce the symptom, but the content of that symptom and its meaning to the patient relate to specific psychological characteristics unique to that patient. The role of unconscious factors in determining the shape of symptoms and their meaning is crucial to a psychoanalytic point of view.

In addition, as William Wordsworth noted, "The child is father of the man." In other words, childhood experiences are repeated throughout life and are critical in determining one's adult relationships. It is now known that childhood experience is pivotal in creating neural networks that shape the personality and persons' expectations of how others will respond to them.

Certain principles of technique, such as resistance, transference, and countertransference, are also at the core of psychoanalysis as a treatment. Freud recognized that patients often *resist* the physician's efforts to heal. For example, when he asked patients to say whatever came to mind, a technique known as *free association*, some patients either became silent or were unable to follow his suggestion. Freud ultimately had the insight that patients are often unconsciously ambivalent about getting better, so they oppose the efforts of the physician to help them. Freud developed the idea while working with psychoanalytic patients, but the contemporary psychiatrist will see resistance with most patients in everyday practice. Mundane behaviors, such as forgetting medication, missing a scheduled appointment, and neglecting to fill a prescription, may all reflect unconscious resistance to getting better.

The other cornerstones of technique in psychoanalysis involve transference and countertransference. *Transference* is the patient's displacement onto the analyst of early wishes and feelings toward persons from the past. Some resistances may emerge because patients experience the psychiatrist as a parental figure from the past, and they seek to defy the perceived parental control. A contemporary view of transference would acknowledge that the analyst or physician's real characteristics always influence the transference. That is, transference could be described as an admixture of figures from the patient's past and the *real relationship* with the clinician in the present. *Countertransference* is the flip side of transference—the clinician's feelings toward the patient, based on a mixture of the real characteristics of the patient and qualities associated with figures from the clinician's past.

Freud was convinced that the unconscious could be directly observed in the psychoanalyst's consulting room. Slips of the tongue, which he called *parapraxes*, often reveal unconscious intent that is outside the individual's awareness. One woman who was asked about her religion responded, "Prostitute, I mean, Protestant." Her guilt feelings about her sexuality had overridden her conscious intent to identify her religious views. Unconscious mental activity is also seen in dreams and many nonverbal behaviors. As more and more knowledge about implicit and explicit memory has accumulated in neuroscience investigations, the fact that much of mental life is unconscious is no longer controversial.

Psychoanalysis today is recognized as having three crucial aspects: it is a therapeutic technique, a body of scientific and theoretical knowledge, and a method of investigation. This section focuses on psychoanalysis as both a theory and a treatment, but the basic tenets elaborated here have wide applications to nonpsychoanalytic settings in clinical psychiatry.

LIFE OF FREUD

Freud was born on May 6, 1856, in Freiburg, a small town in Moravia, which is now part of the Czech Republic. When Freud was 4 years old, his father, a Jewish wool merchant, moved the family to Vienna, where Freud spent most of his life. Following medical school, he specialized in neurology and studied for a year in Paris with Jean-Martin Charcot. He was also influenced by Ambroise-August Liebault and Hippolyte-Marie Bernheim, both of whom taught him hypnosis while he was in France. After his education in France, he returned to Vienna and began clinical work with hysterical patients. Between 1887 and 1897, his work with these patients led him to develop psychoanalysis. Figures 6.1–1 and 6.1–2 show Freud at age 47 and 79, respectively. He died in London in 1939.

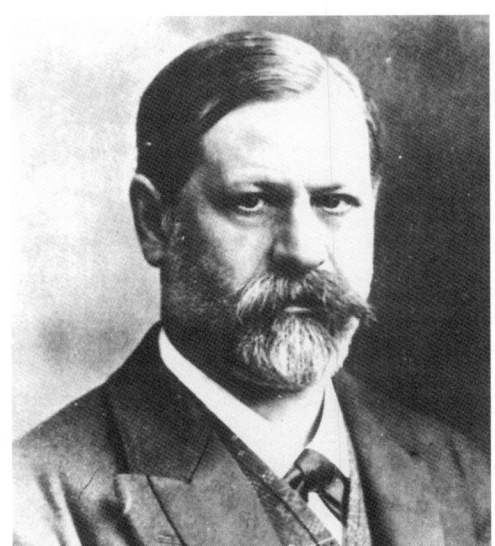

FIGURE 6.1–1
Sigmund Freud at age 47. (Courtesy of Menninger Foundation Archives, Topeka, KS.)

BEGINNINGS OF PSYCHOANALYSIS

In the decade from 1887 to 1897, Freud turned his attention to the serious study of the disturbances of his hysterical patients, and, in this period, the beginnings of psychoanalysis took root. These slender beginnings had a threefold aspect: emergence of psychoanalysis as a (1) method of investigation, (2) therapeutic technique, and (3) body of scientific knowledge based on an increasing fund of information and basic theoretical propositions. In conjunction with his colleague Joseph Breuer (Fig. 6.1–3), he treated a series of female patients suffering from hysterical symptoms that defied neurological explanation. One particular patient, Bertha Pappenheim, who was treated by Breuer as Anna O., intrigued Freud and led him to investigate the use of hypnosis as a routine part of his clinical practice. In 1889, Freud turned to the cathartic method, which he used in conjunction

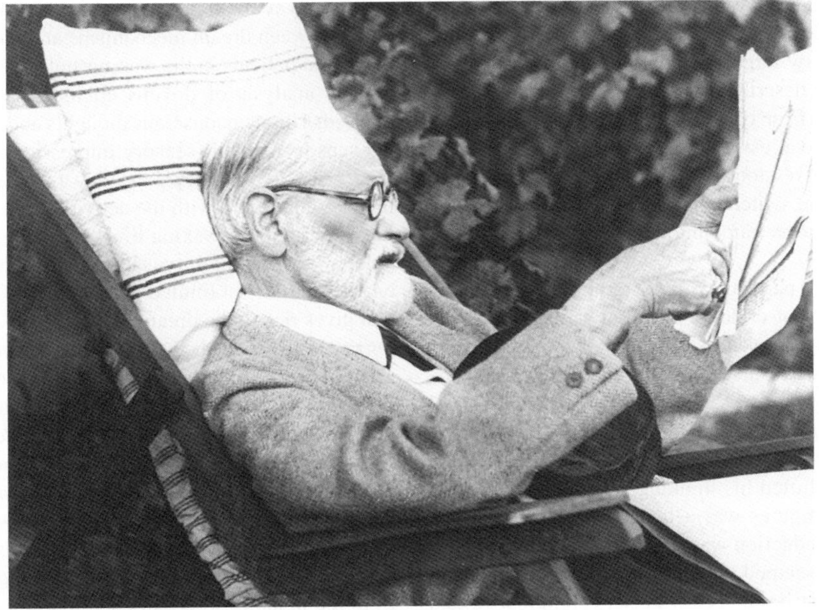

FIGURE 6.1–2
Sigmund Freud at age 79. (Courtesy of Menninger Foundation Archives, Topeka, KS.)

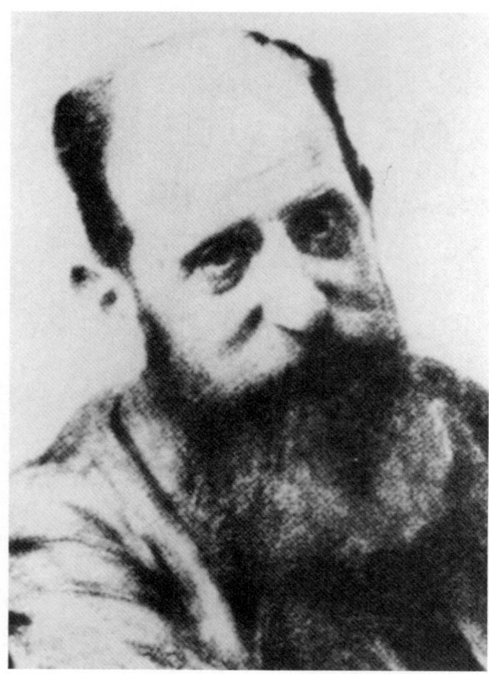

FIGURE 6.1–3
Joseph Breuer (1842–1925). (From Carson RC, Butcher JN, Coleman JC. *Abnormal Psychology and Modern Life,* 8th ed. Boston: Scott, Foresman; 1988:61, with permission. Copyright Culver Pictures.)

with hypnosis. Using this approach, Freud attempted to remove symptoms through a process of recovering and verbalizing suppressed feelings with which the symptoms were associated. This method came to be known as *abreaction.*

Through his experiments with abreaction and catharsis, Freud learned that his patients were often unable or unwilling to recount memories that subsequently proved very significant. Freud referred to this reluctance as *resistance*, and later determined that resistance was caused by largely unconscious, active forces in patients' minds. Freud described this active process of excluding distressing material from conscious awareness as *repression*, which he came to regard as essential to symptom formation. Because of the forces of repression and resistance, Freud abandoned his cathartic method and switched to *free association*—inviting his patients to say whatever came into their minds without censoring their thoughts.

Freud's treatment of patients with hysteria during the early 1890s convinced him that childhood sexual seduction played a major role in causing the neuroses. Many of his patients reported such seductions by nursemaids, fathers, and caretakers, and Freud believed that repressed memories of actual sexual trauma created neurotic symptoms.

In the later 1890s, however, he began to reconsider these views; ultimately, he shifted his thinking. The idea that sexual seduction by parental figures was a fantasy began to displace his theory that actual seduction was a pivotal pathogenic factor in neuroses. This shift seemed to be influenced by Freud's own self-analysis, in which he became convinced of childhood sexual fantasies in himself as well as in his patients. Moreover, some patients' reports of abuse sounded so fantastic that it became difficult for Freud to distinguish truth from fiction in such accounts. Contrary to recent reports by Freud's critics, however, he never actually abandoned his belief that real incest was a factor contributing to psychopathology in adults, and throughout his career he reasserted that he was convinced of actual sexual seductions of children by parents. Nevertheless, he placed much greater emphasis on childhood sexual fantasies as the core of neuroses. Freud's self-analysis also was instrumental in his deciphering of dreams and led to the appearance in 1900 of perhaps his most monumental work, *The Interpretation of Dreams.*

THE INTERPRETATION OF DREAMS

Freud became aware of the significance of dreams when he noted that patients frequently reported their dreams in the process of free association. Through their further associations to the dream content, he learned that dreams were definitely meaningful, even though meanings were often hidden or disguised. Most of all, Freud was struck by the intimate connection between dream content and unconscious memories or fantasies that were long repressed. This observation led Freud to declare that the interpretation of dreams was the royal road to understanding the unconscious.

In *The Interpretation of Dreams*, Freud asserted that a dream is the disguised fulfillment of an unconscious childhood wish that is not readily accessible to conscious awareness in waking life. In attempting to characterize the psychology of dreaming, Freud laid the foundations for ego psychology. He suggested that unconscious childhood wishes can be transformed into disguised conscious manifestations only if a censor exists in the mind. The censor, acting in the service of the ego, functions to preserve sleep. By disguising disturbing thoughts and feelings, the censor makes sure that the dreamer's sleep is not disturbed. Moreover, early forms of defense mechanisms in the ego were delineated by Freud's investigation of the different methods of disguise used by the ego—for example, displacement, condensation, and symbolic representation. Freud drew beginning parallels between dream mechanisms and pathological thoughts of psychotic patients in the waking state.

The analysis of dreams elicits material that has been repressed. These unconscious thoughts and wishes include nocturnal sensory stimuli (sensory impressions such as pain, hunger, thirst, urinary urgency), the day residue (thoughts and ideas that are connected with the activities and preoccupations of the dreamer's current waking life), and repressed unacceptable impulses. Because motility is blocked by the sleep state, the dream enables partial but limited gratification of the repressed impulse that gives rise to the dream.

Freud distinguished between two layers of dream content. The *manifest* content refers to what is recalled by the dreamer; the *latent* content involves the unconscious thoughts and wishes that threaten to awaken the dreamer. Freud described the unconscious mental operations by which latent dream content is transformed into manifest dream as the *dream work.* Repressed wishes and impulses must attach themselves to innocent or neutral images to pass the scrutiny of the dream censor. This process involves selection of apparently meaningless or trivial images from the dreamer's current experience, images that are dynamically associated with the latent images that they resemble in some respect.

Condensation

Condensation is the mechanism by which several unconscious wishes, impulses, or attitudes can be combined into a single image in the manifest dream content. Thus, in a child's nightmare, an attacking monster may come to represent not only the dreamer's father but may also represent some aspects of the mother and even some of the child's own primitive hostile impulses as well. The converse of condensation can also occur in the dream work, namely, an irradiation or diffusion of a single latent wish or impulse that is distributed through multiple representations in the manifest dream content. The combination of mechanisms of condensation and diffusion provides the dreamer with a highly flexible and economic device for facilitating, compressing, and diffusing or expanding the manifest dream content, which is derived from latent or unconscious wishes and impulses.

Displacement

The mechanism of *displacement* refers to the transfer of amounts of energy (cathexis) from an original object to a substitute or symbolic representation of the object. Because the substitute object is relatively neutral—that is, less invested with affective energy—it is more acceptable to the dream censor and can pass the borders of repression more easily. Thus, whereas symbolism can be taken to refer to the substitution of one object for another, displacement facilitates distortion of unconscious wishes through transfer of affective energy from one object to another. Despite the transfer of cathectic energy, the aim of the unconscious impulse remains unchanged. For example, in a dream, the mother may be represented visually by an unknown female figure (at least one who has less emotional significance for the dreamer), but the naked content of the dream nonetheless continues to derive from the dreamer's unconscious instinctual impulses toward the mother.

Symbolic Representation

Freud noted that the dreamer would often represent highly charged ideas or objects by using innocent images that were in some way connected with the idea or object being represented. In this manner, an abstract concept or a complex set of feelings toward a person could be symbolized by a simple, concrete, or sensory image. Freud noted that symbols have unconscious meanings that can be discerned through the patient's associations to the symbol, but he also believed that certain symbols have universal meanings.

Secondary Revision

The mechanisms of condensation, displacement, and symbolic representation are characteristic of a type of thinking that Freud referred to as *primary process*. This primitive mode of cognitive activity is characterized by illogical, bizarre, and absurd images that seem incoherent. Freud believed that a more mature and reasonable aspect of the ego works during dreams to organize primitive aspects of dreams into a more coherent form. *Secondary revision* is Freud's name for this process, in which dreams become somewhat more rational. The process is related to mature activity characteristic of waking life, which Freud termed *secondary process*.

Affects in Dreams

Secondary emotions may not appear in the dream at all, or they may be experienced in somewhat altered form. For example, repressed rage toward a person's father may take the form of mild annoyance. Feelings may also appear as their opposites.

Anxiety Dreams

Freud's dream theory preceded his development of a comprehensive theory of the ego. Hence, his understanding of dreams stresses the importance of discharging drives or wishes through the hallucinatory contents of the dream. He viewed such mechanisms as condensation, displacement, symbolic representation, projection, and secondary revision primarily as facilitating the discharge of latent impulses, rather than as protecting dreamers from anxiety and pain. Freud understood anxiety dreams as reflecting a failure in the protective function of the dream-work mechanisms. The repressed impulses succeed in working their way into the manifest content in a more or less recognizable manner.

Punishment Dreams

Dreams in which dreamers experience punishment represented a special challenge for Freud because they appear to represent an exception to his wish fulfillment theory of dreams. He came to understand such dreams as reflecting a compromise between the repressed wish and the repressing agency or conscience. In a punishment dream, the ego anticipates condemnation on the part of the dreamer's conscience if the latent unacceptable impulses are allowed direct expression in the manifest dream content. Hence, the wish for punishment on the part of the patient's conscience is satisfied by giving expression to punishment fantasies.

TOPOGRAPHICAL MODEL OF THE MIND

The publication of *The Interpretation of Dreams* in 1900 heralded the arrival of Freud's topographical model of the mind, in which he divided the mind into three regions: the conscious system, the preconscious system, and the unconscious system. Each system has its own unique characteristics.

The Conscious

The conscious system in Freud's topographical model is the part of the mind in which perceptions coming from the outside world or from within the body or mind are brought into awareness. Consciousness is a subjective phenomenon whose content can be communicated only by means of language or behavior. Freud assumed that consciousness used a form of neutralized psychic energy that he referred to as *attention cathexis*, whereby persons were aware of a particular idea or feeling as a result of investing a discrete amount of psychic energy in the idea or feeling.

The Preconscious

The preconscious system is composed of those mental events, processes, and contents that can be brought into conscious awareness by the act of focusing attention. Although most persons are not consciously aware of the appearance of their first-grade teacher, they ordinarily can bring this image to mind by deliberately focusing attention on the memory. Conceptually, the preconscious interfaces with both unconscious and conscious regions of the mind. To reach conscious awareness, contents of the unconscious must become linked with words and thus become preconscious. The preconscious system also serves to maintain the repressive barrier and to censor unacceptable wishes and desires.

The Unconscious

The unconscious system is dynamic. Its mental contents and processes are kept from conscious awareness through the force of censorship or repression and it is closely related to instinctual drives. At this point in Freud's theory of development, instincts were thought to consist of sexual and self-preservative drives, and the unconscious was thought to contain primarily the mental representations and derivatives of the sexual instinct.

The content of the unconscious is limited to wishes seeking fulfillment. These wishes provide the motivation for dream and neurotic symptom formation. This view is now considered reductionist.

The unconscious system is characterized by *primary process thinking*, which is principally aimed at facilitating wish fulfillment and instinctual discharge. It is governed by the pleasure principle and, therefore, disregards logical connections; it has no concept of time, represents wishes as fulfillments, permits contradictions to exist simultaneously, and denies the existence of negatives. The primary process is also characterized by extreme mobility of drive cathexis; the investment of psychic energy can shift from object to object without opposition. Memories in the unconscious have been divorced from their connection with verbal symbols. Hence, when words are reapplied to forgotten memory traits, as in psychoanalytic treatment, the verbal recathexis allows the memories to reach consciousness again.

The contents of the unconscious can become conscious only by passing through the preconscious. When censors are overpowered, the elements can enter consciousness.

Limitations of the Topographical Theory

Freud soon realized that two main deficiencies in the topographical theory limited its usefulness. First, many patients' defense mechanisms that guard against distressing wishes, feelings, or thoughts were themselves not initially accessible to consciousness. Thus, repression cannot be identical with preconscious, because by definition this region of the mind is accessible to consciousness. Second, Freud's patients frequently demonstrated an unconscious need for punishment. This clinical observation made it unlikely that the moral agency making the demand for punishment could be allied with anti-instinctual forces that were available to conscious awareness in the preconscious. These difficulties led Freud to discard the topographical theory, but certain concepts derived from the theory continue to be useful, particularly, primary and secondary thought processes, the fundamental importance of wish fulfillment, the existence of a dynamic unconscious, and a tendency toward regression under frustrating conditions.

INSTINCT OR DRIVE THEORY

After the development of the topographical model, Freud turned his attention to the complexities of instinct theory. Freud was determined to anchor his psychological theory in biology. His choice led to terminological and conceptual difficulties when he used terms derived from biology to denote psychological constructs. *Instinct*, for example, refers to a pattern of species-specific behavior that is genetically derived and, therefore, is more or less independent of learning. Modern research demonstrating that instinctual patterns are modified through experiential learning, however, has made Freud's instinctual theory problematic. Further confusion has stemmed from the ambiguity inherent in a concept on the borderland between the biological and the psychological: Should the mental representation aspect of the term and the physiological component be integrated or separated? Although *drive* may have been closer than instinct to Freud's meaning, in contemporary usage, the two terms are often used interchangeably.

In Freud's view, an instinct has four principal characteristics: source, impetus, aim, and object. The *source* refers to the part of the body from which the instinct arises. The *impetus* is the amount of force or intensity associated with the instinct. The *aim* refers to any action directed toward tension discharge or satisfaction, and the *object* is the target (often a person) for this action.

Instincts

Libido. The ambiguity in the term *instinctual drive* is reflected also in use of the term *libido*. Briefly, Freud regarded the sexual instinct as a psychophysiological process that had both mental and physiological manifestations. Essentially, he used the term *libido* to refer to "the force by which the sexual instinct is represented in the mind." Thus, in its accepted sense, *libido* refers specifically to the mental manifestations of the sexual instinct. Freud recognized early that the sexual instinct did not originate in a finished or final form, as represented by the stage of genital primacy. Rather, it underwent a complex process of development at each phase of which the libido had specific aims and objects that diverged in varying degrees from the simple aim of genital union. The libido theory thus came to include all of these manifestations and the complicated paths they followed in the course of psychosexual development.

Ego Instincts. From 1905 on, Freud maintained a dual instinct theory, subsuming sexual instincts and ego instincts connected with self-preservation. Until 1914, with the publication of *On Narcissism*, Freud had paid little attention to ego instincts; in this communication, however, Freud invested ego instinct with libido for the first time by postulating an ego libido and an object libido. Freud thus viewed narcissistic investment as an essentially libidinal instinct and called the remaining nonsexual components the *ego instincts*.

Aggression. When psychoanalysts today discuss the dual instinct theory, they are generally referring to libido and aggression. Freud, however, originally conceptualized aggression as a component of the sexual instincts in the form of sadism. As he became aware that sadism had nonsexual aspects to it, he made finer gradations, which enabled him to categorize aggression and hate as part of the ego instincts and the libidinal aspects of sadism as components of the sexual instincts. Finally, in 1923, to account for the clinical data he was observing, he was compelled to conceive of aggression as a separate instinct in its own right. The source of this instinct, according to Freud, was largely in skeletal muscles, and the aim of the aggressive instincts was destruction.

Life and Death Instincts. Before designating aggression as a separate instinct, Freud, in 1920, subsumed the ego instincts under a broader category of life instincts. These were juxtaposed with death instincts and were referred to as *Eros* and *Thanatos* in *Beyond the Pleasure Principle*. The life and death instincts were regarded as forces underlying the sexual and aggressive instincts. Although Freud could not provide clinical data that directly verified the death instinct, he thought the instinct could be inferred by observing *repetition compulsion*, a person's tendency to repeat past traumatic behavior. Freud thought that the dominant force in biological organisms had to be the death instinct. In contrast to the death instinct, Eros (the life instinct) refers to the tendency of particles to reunite or bind to one another, as in sexual reproduction. The prevalent view today is that the dual instincts of sexuality and aggression suffice to explain most clinical phenomena without recourse to a death instinct.

Pleasure and Reality Principles

In 1911, Freud described two basic tenets of mental functioning, the pleasure principle and the reality principle. He essentially recast the primary process and secondary process dichotomy into the pleasure and reality principles and thus took an important step toward solidifying the notion of the ego. Both principles, in Freud's view, are aspects of ego functioning. The *pleasure principle* is defined as an inborn tendency of the organism to avoid pain and to seek pleasure through the discharge of tension. The *reality principle*, on the other hand, is considered to be a learned function closely related to the maturation of the ego; this principle modifies the pleasure principle and requires delay or postponement of immediate gratification.

Infantile Sexuality

Freud set forth the three major tenets of psychoanalytic theory when he published *Three Essays on the Theory of Sexuality*. First, he broadened the definition of sexuality to include forms of pleasure that transcend genital sexuality. Second, he established a developmental theory of childhood sexuality that delineated the vicissitudes of erotic activity from birth through puberty. Third, he forged a conceptual linkage between neuroses and perversions.

Freud's notion that children are influenced by sexual drives has made some persons reluctant to accept psychoanalysis. Freud noted that infants are capable of erotic activity from birth, but the earliest manifestations of infantile sexuality are basically nonsexual and are associated with such bodily functions as feeding and bowel-bladder control. As libidinal energy shifts from the oral zone to the anal zone to the phallic zone, each stage of development is thought to build on and to subsume the accomplishments of the preceding stage. The *oral stage*, which occupies the first 12 to 18 months of life, centers on the mouth and lips, and is manifested in chewing, biting, and sucking. The dominant erotic activity of the anal stage, from 18 to 36 months of age, involves bowel function and control. The *phallic stage*, from 3 to 5 years of life, initially focuses on urination as the source of erotic activity. Freud suggested that phallic erotic activity in boys is a preliminary stage leading to adult genital activity. Whereas the penis remains the principal sexual organ throughout male psychosexual development, Freud postulated that females have two principal erotogenic zones, the vagina and the clitoris. He thought that the clitoris was the chief erotogenic focus during the infantile genital period but that erotic primacy shifted to the vagina after puberty. Studies of human sexuality have subsequently questioned the validity of this distinction.

Freud discovered that in the psychoneuroses, only a limited number of the sexual impulses that had undergone repression and were responsible for creating and maintaining the neurotic symptoms were normal. For the most part, these were the same impulses that were given overt expression in the perversions. The neuroses, then, were the negative of perversions.

Object Relationships in Instinct Theory

Freud suggested that the choice of a love object in adult life, the love relationship itself, and the nature of all other object relationships depend primarily on the nature and quality of children's relationships during the early years of life. In describing the libidinal phases of psychosexual development, Freud repeatedly referred to the significance of a child's relationships with parents and other significant persons in the environment.

The awareness of the external world of objects develops gradually in infants. Soon after birth, they are primarily aware of physical sensations, such as hunger, cold, and pain, which give rise to tension, and caregivers are regarded primarily as persons who relieve their tension or remove painful stimuli. Recent infant research, however, suggests that awareness of others begins much sooner than Freud originally thought. Table 6.1–1 provides a summary of the stages of psychosexual development and the object relationships associated with each stage. Although the table goes only as far as young adulthood, development is now recognized as continuing throughout adult life.

Concept of Narcissism

According to Greek myth, Narcissus, a beautiful youth, fell in love with his reflection in the water of a pool and drowned in his attempt to embrace his beloved image. Freud used the term *narcissism* to describe situations in which an individual's libido was invested in the ego itself rather than in other persons. This concept of narcissism presented him with vexing problems for his instinct theory and essentially violated his distinction between libidinal instincts and ego or self-preservative instincts. Freud's understanding of narcissism led him to use the term to describe a wide array of psychiatric disorders, very much in contrast to the

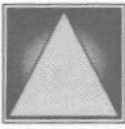

Table 6.1–1
Stages of Psychosexual Development

Oral Stage			
Definition	The earliest stage of development in which the infant's needs, perceptions, and modes of expression are primarily centered in the mouth, lips, tongue, and other organs related to the oral zone.	Objectives	To establish a trusting dependence on nursing and sustaining objects, to establish comfortable expression and gratification of oral libidinal needs without excessive conflict or ambivalence from oral sadistic wishes.
Description	The oral zone maintains its dominant role in the organization of the psyche through approximately the first 18 months of life. Oral sensations include thirst, hunger, pleasurable tactile stimulations evoked by the nipple or its substitute, sensations related to swallowing, and satiation. Oral drives consist of two separate components: libidinal and aggressive. States of oral tension lead to a seeking for oral gratification, typified by quiescence at the end of nursing. The oral triad consists of the wish to eat, to sleep, and to reach that relaxation that occurs at the end of sucking just before the onset of sleep. Libidinal needs (oral erotism) are thought to predominate in the early parts of the oral phase, whereas they are mixed with more aggressive components later (oral sadism). Oral aggression may express itself in biting, chewing, spitting, or crying. Oral aggression is connected with primitive wishes and fantasies of biting, devouring, and destroying.	Pathological traits	Excessive oral gratifications or deprivation can result in libidinal fixations that contribute to pathological traits. Such traits can include excessive optimism, narcissism, pessimism (often seen in depressive states), and demandingness. Oral characters are often excessively dependent and require others to give to them and to look after them. Such persons want to be fed but may be exceptionally giving to elicit a return of being given to. Oral characters are often extremely dependent on objects for the maintenance of their self-esteem. Envy and jealousy are often associated with oral traits.
		Character traits	Successful resolution of the oral phase provides a basis in character structure for capacities to give to and receive from others without excessive dependence or envy and a capacity to rely on others with a sense of trust, as well as with a sense of self-reliance and self-trust.
Anal Stage			
Definition	The stage of psychosexual development that is prompted by maturation of neuromuscular control over sphincters, particularly the anal sphincters, thus permitting more voluntary control over retention or expulsion of feces.	Objectives	The anal period is essentially a period of striving for independence and separation from the dependence on and control by the parent. The objectives of sphincter control without overcontrol (fecal retention) or loss of control (messing) are matched by the child's attempts to achieve autonomy and independence without excessive shame or self-doubt from loss of control.
Description	This period, which extends roughly from 1 to 3 years of age, is marked by a recognizable intensification of aggressive drives mixed with libidinal components and in sadistic impulses. Acquisition of voluntary sphincter control is associated with an increasing shift from passivity to activity. The conflicts over anal control and the struggle with the parent over retaining or expelling feces in toilet training give rise to increased ambivalence, together with a struggle over separation, individuation, and independence. Anal erotism refers to the sexual pleasure in anal functioning, both in retaining the precious feces and in presenting them as a precious gift to the parent. Anal sadism refers to the expression of aggressive wishes connected with discharging feces as powerful and destructive weapons. These wishes are often displayed in such children's fantasies as bombing and explosions.	Pathological traits	Maladaptive character traits, often apparently inconsistent, are derived from anal erotism and the defenses against it. Orderliness, obstinacy, stubbornness, willfulness, frugality, and parsimony are features of the anal character derived from a fixation on anal functions. When defenses against anal traits are less effective, the anal character reveals traits of heightened ambivalence, lack of tidiness, messiness, defiance, rage, and sadomasochistic tendencies. Anal characteristics and defenses are most typically seen in obsessive-compulsive neuroses.
		Character traits	Successful resolution of the anal phase provides the basis for the development of personal autonomy, a capacity for independence and personal initiative without guilt, a capacity for self-determining behavior without a sense of shame or self-doubt, a lack of ambivalence and a capacity for willing cooperation without either excessive willfulness or sense of self-diminution or defeat.

(continued)

Table 6.1–1 (Continued)

	Urethral Stage		
Definition	This stage was not explicitly treated by Freud but is envisioned as a transitional stage between the anal and the phallic stages of development. It shares some of the characteristics of the preceding anal stage and some from the subsequent phallic stage.	Objectives	Issues of control and urethral performance and loss of control. It is not clear whether or to what extent the objectives of urethral functioning differ from those of the anal period.
Description	The characteristics of the urethral stage are often subsumed under those of the phallic stage. Urethral erotism, however, is used to refer to the pleasure in urination, as well as the pleasure in urethral retention analogous to anal retention. Similar issues of performance and control are related to urethral functioning. Urethral functioning may also be invested with a sadistic quality, often reflecting the persistence of anal sadistic urges. Loss of urethral control, as in enuresis, may frequently have regressive significance that reactivates anal conflicts.	Pathological traits	The predominant urethral trait is that of competitiveness and ambition, probably related to the compensation for shame due to loss of urethral control. In control this may be the start for the development of penis envy, related to the feminine sense of shame and inadequacy in being unable to match the male urethral performance. This is also related to issues of control and shaming.
		Character traits	Besides the healthy effects analogous to those from the anal period, urethral competence provides a sense of pride and self-competence derived from performance. Urethral performance is an area in which the small boy can imitate and match his father's more adult performance. The resolution of urethral conflicts sets the stage for budding gender identity and subsequent identifications.
	Phallic Stage		
Definition	The phallic stage of sexual development begins sometime during the third year of life and continues until approximately the end of the fifth year.	Pathological traits	The derivation of pathological traits from the phallic-oedipal involvement is sufficiently complex and subject to such a variety of modifications that it encompasses nearly the whole of neurotic development. The issues, however, focus on castration in males and on penis envy in females. The other important focus of developmental distortions in this period derives from the patterns of identification that are developed out of the resolution of the oedipal complex. The influence of castration anxiety and penis envy, the defenses against both, and the patterns of identification that emerge from the phallic phase are the primary determinants of the development of human character. They also subsume and integrate the residues of previous psychosexual stages, so that fixations or conflicts that derive from any of the preceding stages can contaminate and modify the oedipal resolution.
Description	The phallic phase is characterized by a primary focus of sexual interests, stimulation, and excitement in the genital area. The penis becomes the organ of principal interest to children of both sexes, with the lack of a penis in the female being considered evidence of castration. The phallic phase is associated with an increase in genital masturbation accompanied by predominantly unconscious fantasies of sexual involvement with the opposite-sex parent. The threat of castration and its related castration anxiety arise in connection with guilt over masturbation and oedipal wishes. During this phase the oedipal involvement and conflict are established and consolidated.		
Objectives	The objective of this phase is to focus erotic interest in the genital area and genital functions. This focusing lays the foundation for gender identity and serves to integrate the residues of previous stages of psychosexual development into a predominantly genital-sexual orientation. The establishing of the oedipal situation is essential for the furtherance of subsequent identifications that will serve as the basis for important and enduring dimensions of character organization.	Character traits	The phallic stage provides the foundations for an emerging sense of sexual identity, a sense of curiosity without embarrassment, initiative without guilt, as well as a sense of mastery not only over objects and persons in the environment but also over internal processes and impulses. The resolution of the oedipal conflict at the end of the phallic period gives rise to powerful internal resources for regulation of drive impulses and their direction to constructive ends. This internal source of regulation is the superego, and it is based on identifications derived primarily from parental figures.
	Latency Stage		
Definition	The stage of relative quiescence or inactivity of the sexual drive during the period from the resolution of the Oedipus complex until pubescence (from about 5–6 years until about 11–13 years).	Pathological traits	The danger in the latency period can arise from either a lack of development of inner controls or an excess of them. The lack of control can lead to a failure of the child to sufficiently sublimate energies in the interests of learning and development of skills; an excess of inner control, however, can lead to premature closure of personality development and the precocious elaboration of obsessive character traits.

(continued)

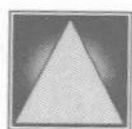

Table 6.1–1 (Continued)

Description	The institution of the superego at the close of the oedipal period and the further maturation of ego functions allow considerably greater control of instinctual impulses. Sexual interests during this period are generally thought to be quiescent. This is a period of primarily homosexual affiliations for both boys and girls, as well as a sublimation of libidinal and aggressive energies into energetic learning and play activities, exploring the environment, and becoming more proficient in dealing with the world of things and persons around them. It is a period for the development of important skills. The relative strength of regulatory elements often gives rise to patterns of behavior that are somewhat obsessive and hypercontrolling.
Objectives	The primary objective in this period is the further integration of oedipal identifications and a consolidation of sex-role identity and sex roles. The relative quiescence and control of instinctual impulses allow for the development of ego apparatuses and mastery skills. Further identificatory components may be added to the oedipal ones on the basis of broadening contacts with other significant figures outside the family, such as teachers, coaches, and other adults.
Character traits	The latency period has frequently been regarded as a period of relatively unimportant inactivity in the developmental scheme. Recently, great respect has been gained for the developmental processes that take place in this period. Important consolidations and additions are made to the basic postoedipal identifications. It is a period of integrating and consolidating previous attainments in psychosexual development and establishing decisive patterns of adaptive functioning. The child can develop a sense of industry and a capacity for mastery of objects and concepts that allows autonomous function with a sense of initiative without running the risk of failure or defeat or a sense of inferiority. These important attainments need to be further integrated, ultimately as the essential basis for a mature adult life of satisfaction in work and love.
Genital Stage	
Definition	The genital or adolescent phase of psychosexual development extends from the onset of puberty from ages 11–13 until the person reaches young adulthood. In current thinking, there is a tendency to subdivide this stage into preadolescent, early adolescent, middle adolescent, late adolescent, and even postadolescent periods.
Description	The physiological maturation of systems of genital (sexual) functioning and attendant hormonal systems leads to an intensification of drives, particularly libidinal drives. This produces a regression in personality organization, which reopens conflicts of previous stages of psychosexual development and provides the opportunity for a reresolution of these conflicts in the context of achieving a mature sexual and adult identity.
Objectives	The primary objectives of this period are the ultimate separation from dependence on and attachment to the parents and the establishment of mature, nonincestuous object relations. Related to this are the achievement of a mature sense of personal identity and acceptance and the integration of a set of adult roles and functions that permit new adaptive integrations with social expectations and cultural values.
Pathological traits	The pathological deviations due to a failure to achieve successful resolution of this stage of development are multiple and complex. Defects can arise from the whole spectrum of psychosexual residues, since the developmental task of the adolescent period is in a sense a partial reopening and reworking and reintegrating of all those aspects of development. Previous unsuccessful resolutions and fixations in various phases or aspects of psychosexual development will produce pathological defects in the emerging adult personality. A more specific defect from a failure to resolve adolescent issues has been described by Erikson as identity diffusion.
Character traits	The successful resolution and reintegration of previous psychosexual stages in the adolescent, fully genital phase sets the stage normally for a fully mature personality with a capacity for full and satisfying genital potency and a self-integrated and consistent sense of identity. Such a person has reached a satisfying capacity for self-realization and meaningful participation in the areas of work and love and in the creative and productive application to satisfying and meaningful goals and values. Only in the last few years has the presumed relationship between psychosexual genitality and maturity of personality functioning been put in question.

(Adapted by Glen O. Gabbard, M.D., from Meissner WW. Theories of personality and psychopathology. In: Kaplan HI, Sadock BJ, eds. *Comprehensive Textbook of Psychiatry.* 4th ed. Vol. 1. Baltimore: Williams & Wilkins; 1985:360, with permission.)

term's contemporary use to describe a specific personality disorder. Freud grouped several disorders together as the narcissistic neuroses, in which a person's libido is withdrawn from objects and turned inward. He believed that this withdrawal of libidinal attachment to objects accounted for the loss of reality testing in patients who were psychotic; grandiosity and omnipotence in such patients reflected excessive libidinal investment in the ego.

Freud did not limit his use of narcissism to psychoses. In states of physical illness and hypochondriasis, he observed that libidinal investment was frequently withdrawn from external objects and from outside activities and interests. Similarly, he suggested that in normal sleep, libido was also withdrawn and reinvested in a sleeper's own body. Freud regarded homosexuality as an instance of a narcissistic form of object choice, in which persons fall in love with an idealized version of themselves projected onto another person. He also found narcissistic manifestations in the beliefs and myths of primitive people, especially those involving the ability to influence external events through the magical omnipotence of thought processes. In the course of normal development, children also exhibit this belief in their own omnipotence.

Freud postulated a state of primary narcissism at birth in which the libido is stored in the ego. He viewed the neonate as completely narcissistic, with the entire libidinal investment in physiological needs and their satisfaction. He referred to this self-investment as *ego libido*. The infantile state of self-absorption changes only gradually, according to Freud, with the dawning awareness that a separate person—the mothering figure—is responsible for gratifying an infant's needs. This realization leads to the gradual withdrawal of the libido from the self and its redirection toward the external object. Hence, the development of object relations in infants parallels the shift from primary narcissism to object attachment. The libidinal investment in the object is referred to as *object libido*. If a developing child suffers rebuffs or trauma from the caretaking figure, object libido may be withdrawn and reinvested in the ego. Freud called this regressive posture *secondary narcissism*.

Freud used the term *narcissism* to describe many different dimensions of human experience. At times, he used it to describe a perversion in which persons used their own bodies or body parts as objects of sexual arousal. At other times, he used the term to describe a developmental phase, as in the state of primary narcissism. In still other instances, the term referred to a particular object choice. Freud distinguished love objects who are chosen "according to the narcissistic type," in which case the object resembles the subject's idealized or fantasied self-image, from objects chosen according to the "anaclitic," in which the love object resembles a caretaker from early in life. Finally, Freud also used the word *narcissism* interchangeably and synonymously with *self-esteem*.

EGO PSYCHOLOGY

Although Freud had used the construct of the ego throughout the evolution of psychoanalytic theory, ego psychology as it is known today really began with the publication in 1923 of *The Ego and the Id*. This landmark publication also represented a transition in Freud's thinking from the topographical model of the mind to the tripartite structural model of ego, id, and superego. He had observed repeatedly that not all unconscious processes can be relegated to a person's instinctual life. Elements of the conscience, as well as functions of the ego, are clearly also unconscious.

Structural Theory of the Mind

The structural model of the psychic apparatus is the cornerstone of ego psychology. The three provinces—id, ego, and superego—are distinguished by their different functions (Fig. 6.1–4).

Id. Freud used the term *id* to refer to a reservoir of unorganized instinctual drives. Operating under the domination of the primary process, the id lacks the capacity to delay or modify the instinctual drives with which an infant is born. The id, however, should not be viewed as synonymous with the unconscious, because both the ego and the superego have unconscious components.

Ego. The ego spans all three topographical dimensions of conscious, preconscious, and unconscious. Logical and abstract thinking and verbal expression are associated with conscious and preconscious functions of the ego. Defense mechanisms reside in the unconscious domain of the ego. The ego, the executive organ of the psyche, controls motility, perception, contact with reality, and, through the defense mechanisms available to it, the delay and modulation of drive expression.

Freud believed that the id is modified as a result of the impact of the external world on the drives. The pressures of external reality enable the ego to appropriate the energies of the id to do its work. As the ego brings influences from the external world to bear on the id, it simultaneously substitutes the reality principle for the pleasure principle. Freud emphasized the role of conflict within the structural model and observed that conflict occurs initially between the id and the outside world, only to be transformed later to conflict between the id and the ego.

The third component of the tripartite structural model is the superego. The superego establishes and maintains an individual's moral conscience on the basis of a complex system of ideals and values internalized from parents. Freud viewed the superego as the heir to the Oedipus complex. Children internalize parental values and standards at about the age of 5 or 6 years. The superego then serves as an agency that provides ongoing scrutiny of a person's behavior, thoughts, and feelings; it makes comparisons

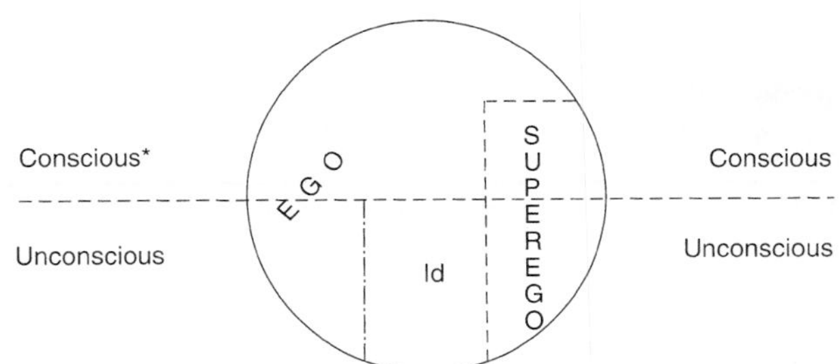

*The preconscious has been deleted for the sake of simplicity.

FIGURE 6.1–4

Freud's structural model. (Reprinted from Gabbard GO. *Psychodynamic Psychiatry in Clinical Practice: The DSM-IV Edition.* Washington, DC: American Psychiatric Press; 1994:31, with permission.)

with expected standards of behavior and offers approval or disapproval. These activities occur largely unconsciously.

The ego ideal is often regarded as a component of the superego. It is an agency that prescribes what a person should do according to internalized standards and values. The superego, by contrast, is an agency of moral conscience that *proscribes*—that is, dictates what a person should not do. Throughout the latency period and thereafter, persons continue to build on early identifications through their contact with admired figures who contribute to the formation of moral standards, aspirations, and ideals.

Functions of the Ego

Modern ego psychologists have identified a set of basic ego functions that characterizes the operations of the ego. These descriptions reflect the ego activities that are generally regarded as fundamental.

Control and Regulation of Instinctual Drives. The development of the capacity to delay or postpone drive discharge, like the capacity to test reality, is closely related to the early childhood progression from the pleasure principle to the reality principle. This capacity is also an essential aspect of the ego's role as mediator between the id and the outside world. Part of infants' socialization to the external world is the acquisition of language and secondary process or logical thinking.

Judgment. A closely related ego function is judgment, which involves the ability to anticipate the consequences of actions. As with control and regulation of instinctual drives, judgment develops in parallel with the growth of *secondary process thinking*. The ability to think logically allows assessment of how contemplated behavior may affect others.

Relation to Reality. The mediation between the internal world and external reality is a crucial function of the ego. Relations with the outside world can be divided into three aspects: the sense of reality, reality testing, and adaptation to reality. The *sense of reality* develops in concert with an infant's dawning awareness of bodily sensations. The ability to distinguish what is outside the body from what is inside is an essential aspect of the sense of reality, and disturbances of body boundaries, such as depersonalization, reflect impairment in this ego function. *Reality testing*, an ego function of paramount importance, refers to the capacity to distinguish internal fantasy from external reality. This function differentiates persons who are psychotic from those who are not. *Adaptation to reality* involves persons' ability to use their resources to develop effective responses to changing circumstances on the basis of previous experience with reality.

Object Relationships. The capacity to form mutually satisfying relationships is related in part to patterns of internalization stemming from early interactions with parents and other significant figures. This ability is also a fundamental function of the ego, in that satisfying relatedness depends on the ability to integrate positive and negative aspects of others and self and to maintain an internal sense of others even in their absence. Similarly, mastery of drive derivatives is also crucial to the achievement of satisfying relationships. Although Freud did not develop an extensive object relations theory, British psychoanalysts, such as Ronald Fairbairn (1889–1964) and Michael Balint (1886–1970), elaborated greatly on the early stages in infants' relationships with need-satisfying objects and on the gradual development of a sense of separateness from the mother. Another of their British colleagues, Donald W. Winnicott (1897–1971), described the *transitional object* (e.g., a blanket, teddy bear, or pacifier) as the link between developing children and their mothers. A child can separate from the mother because a transitional object provides feelings of security in her absence. The stages of human development and object relations theory are summarized in Table 6.1–2.

Synthetic Function of the Ego. First described by Herman Nunberg in 1931, the *synthetic function* refers to the ego's capacity to integrate diverse elements into an overall unity. Different aspects of self and others, for example, are synthesized into a consistent representation that endures over time. The function also involves organizing, coordinating, and generalizing or simplifying large amounts of data.

Primary Autonomous Ego Functions. Heinz Hartmann described the so-called primary autonomous functions of the ego as rudimentary apparatuses present at birth that develop independently of intrapsychic conflict between drives and defenses. These functions include perception, learning, intelligence, intuition, language, thinking, comprehension, and motility. In the course of development, some of these conflict-free aspects of the ego may eventually become involved in conflict. They will

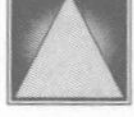

Table 6.1–2
Parallel Lines of Development

Instinctual Phases	Separation–Individuation	Object Relations	Psychosocial Crises
Oral	Autism, symbiosis	Primary narcissism, need-satisfying	Trust or mistrust
Anal	Differentiation, practicing, rapprochement	Need-satisfying, object constancy	Autonomy or shame, self-doubt
Phallic	Object constancy, Oedipal complex	Object constancy, ambivalence	Initiative or guilt
Latency	—	—	Industry or inferiority
Adolescence	Genitality, secondary individuation	Object love	Identity or identity confusion
Adulthood	Mature genitality	—	Intimacy or isolation, generativity or stagnation, integrity or despair

develop normally if the infant is raised in what Hartmann referred to as *an average expectable environment*.

Secondary Autonomous Ego Functions. Once the sphere where primary autononomous function develops becomes involved with conflict, so-called *secondary autonomous ego functions* arise in the defense against drives. For example, a child may develop caretaking functions as a reaction formation against murderous wishes during the first few years of life. Later, the defensive functions may be neutralized or deinstinctualized when the child grows up to be a social worker and cares for homeless persons.

Defense Mechanisms

At each phase of libidinal development, specific drive components evoke characteristic ego defenses. The anal phase, for example, is associated with reaction formation, as manifested by the development of shame and disgust in relation to anal impulses and pleasures.

Defenses can be grouped hierarchically according to the relative degree of maturity associated with them. Narcissistic defenses are the most primitive and appear in children and persons who are psychotically disturbed. Immature defenses are seen in adolescents and some nonpsychotic patients. Neurotic defenses are encountered in obsessive–compulsive and hysterical patients as well as in adults under stress. Table 6.1–3 lists the defense mechanisms according to George Valliant's classification of the four types.

Theory of Anxiety

Freud initially conceptualized anxiety as "dammed up libido." Essentially, a physiological increase in sexual tension leads to a corresponding increase in libido, the mental representation of the physiological event. (See Chapter 18 for a discussion of neurasthenia.) The *actual neuroses* are caused by this buildup. Later, with the development of the structural model, Freud developed a new theory of a second type of anxiety that he referred to as *signal anxiety*. In this model, anxiety operates at an unconscious level and serves to mobilize the ego's resources to avert danger. Either external or internal sources of danger can produce a signal that leads the ego to marshal specific defense mechanisms to guard against, or reduce, instinctual excitation.

Freud's later theory of anxiety explains neurotic symptoms as the ego's partial failure to cope with distressing stimuli. The drive derivatives associated with danger may not have been adequately contained by the defense mechanisms used by the ego. In phobias, for example, Freud explained that fear of an external threat (e.g., dogs or snakes) is an externalization of an internal danger.

Danger situations can also be linked to developmental stages and, thus, can create a developmental hierarchy of anxiety. The earliest danger situation is a fear of disintegration or annihilation, often associated with concerns about fusion with an external object. As infants mature and recognize the mothering figure as a separate person, separation anxiety, or fear of the loss of an object, becomes more prominent. During the oedipal psychosexual stage, girls are most concerned about losing the love of the most important figure in their lives, their mother. Boys are primarily anxious about bodily injury or castration. After resolution of the oedipal conflict, a more mature form of anxiety occurs, often termed *superego anxiety*. This latency-age concern involves the fear that internalized parental representations, contained in the superego, will cease to love, or will angrily punish, the child.

Character

In 1913, Freud distinguished between neurotic symptoms and personality or character traits. *Neurotic symptoms* develop as a result of the failure of repression; *character traits* owe their existence to the success of repression, that is, to the defense system that achieves its aim through a persistent pattern of reaction formation and sublimation. In 1923, Freud also observed that the ego can only give up important objects by identifying with them or introjecting them. This accumulated pattern of identifications and introjections also contributes to character formation. Freud specifically emphasized the importance of superego formation in the character construction.

Contemporary psychoanalysts regard character as a person's habitual or typical pattern of adaptation to internal drive forces and to external environmental forces. *Character* and *personality* are used interchangeably and are distinguished from the ego in that they largely refer to styles of defense and of directly observable behavior rather than to feeling and thinking.

Character is also influenced by constitutional temperament; the interaction of drive forces with early ego defenses and with environmental influences; and various identifications with, and internalizations of, other persons throughout life. The extent to which the ego has developed a capacity to tolerate the delay of impulse discharge and to neutralize instinctual energy determines the degree to which such character traits emerge in later life. Exaggerated development of certain character traits at the expense of others can lead to personality disorders or produce a vulnerability or predisposition to psychosis.

CLASSIC PSYCHOANALYTIC THEORY OF NEUROSES

The classic view of the genesis of neuroses regards conflict as essential. The conflict can arise between instinctual drives and external reality or between internal agencies, such as the id and the superego or the id and the ego. Moreover, because the conflict has not been worked through to a realistic solution, the drives or wishes that seek discharge have been expelled from consciousness through repression or another defense mechanism. Their expulsion from conscious awareness, however, does not make the drives any less powerful or influential. As a result, the unconscious tendencies (e.g., the disguised neurotic symptoms) fight their way back into consciousness. This theory of the development of neurosis assumes that a rudimentary neurosis based on the same type of conflict existed in early childhood.

Deprivation during the first few months of life because of absent or impaired caretaking figures can adversely affect ego development. This impairment, in turn, can result in failure to make appropriate identifications. The resulting ego difficulties create problems in mediating between the drives and the environment. Lack of capacity for constructive expression of drives, especially aggression, can lead some children to turn their

Text continues on page 206.

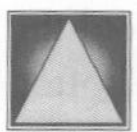

Table 6.1–3
Classification of Defense Mechanisms

	Narcissistic Defenses[a]		
Denial	Avoiding the awareness of some painful aspect of reality by negating sensory data. Although repression defends against affects and drive derivatives, denial abolishes external reality. Denial may be used in both normal and pathological states.	Projection	Perceiving and reacting to unacceptable inner impulses and their derivatives as though they were outside the self. On a psychotic level, this defense mechanism takes the form of frank delusions about external reality (usually persecutory) and includes both perception of one's own feelings in another and subsequent acting on the perception (psychotic paranoid delusions). The impulses may derive from the id or the superego (hallucinated recriminations) but may undergo transformation in the process. Thus, according to Freud's analysis of paranoid projections, homosexual libidinal impulses are transformed into hatred and then projected onto the object of the unacceptable homosexual impulse.
Distortion	Grossly reshaping external reality to suit inner needs (including unrealistic megalomania beliefs, hallucinations, wish-fulfilling delusions) and using sustained feelings of delusional superiority or entitlement.		
	Immature Defenses		
Acting out	Expressing an unconscious wish or impulse through action to avoid being conscious of an accompanying affect. The unconscious fantasy is lived out impulsively in behavior, thereby gratifying the impulse, rather than the prohibition against it. Acting out involves chronically giving in to an impulse to avoid the tension that would result from the postponement of expression.	Passive-aggressive behavior	Expressing aggression toward others indirectly through passivity, masochism, and turning against the self. Manifestations of passive-aggressive behavior include failure, procrastination, and illnesses that affect others more than oneself.
Blocking	Temporarily or transiently inhibiting thinking. Affects and impulses may also be involved. Blocking closely resembles repression but differs in that tension arises when the impulse, affect, or thought is inhibited.	Regression	Attempting to return to an earlier libidinal phase of functioning to avoid the tension and conflict evoked at the present level of development. It reflects the basic tendency to gain instinctual gratification at a less-developed period. Regression is a normal phenomenon as well, as a certain amount of regression is essential for relaxation, sleep, and orgasm in sexual intercourse. Regression is also considered an essential concomitant of the creative process.
Hypochondriasis	Exaggerating or overemphasizing an illness for the purpose of evasion and regression. Reproach arising from bereavement, loneliness, or unacceptable aggressive impulses toward others is transformed into self-reproach and complaints of pain, somatic illness, and neurasthenia. In hypochondriasis, responsibility can be avoided, guilt may be circumvented, and instinctual impulses are warded off. Because hypochondriacal introjects are ego-alien, the afflicted person experiences dysphoria and a sense of affliction.	Schizoid fantasy	Indulging in autistic retreat to resolve conflict and to obtain gratification. Interpersonal intimacy is avoided, and eccentricity serves to repel others. The person does not fully believe in the fantasies and does not insist on acting them out.
		Somatization	Converting psychic derivatives into bodily symptoms and tending to react with somatic manifestations, rather than psychic manifestations. In desomatization, infantile somatic responses are replaced by thought and affect; in resomatization, the person regresses to earlier somatic forms in the face of unresolved conflicts.
Introjection	Internalizing the qualities of an object. Although vital to development, introjection also serves specific defensive functions. When used as a defense, it can obliterate the distinction between the subject and the object. Through the introjection of a loved object, the painful awareness of separateness or the threat of loss may be avoided. Introjection of a feared object serves to avoid anxiety when the aggressive characteristics of the object are internalized, thus placing the aggression under one's own control. A classic example is identification with the aggressor. An identification with the victim may also take place, whereby the self-punitive qualities of the objects are taken over and established within one's self as a symptom or character trait.		

(continued)

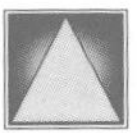

Table 6.1–3
(Continued)

Neurotic Defenses			
Controlling	Attempting to manage or regulate events or objects in the environment to minimize anxiety and to resolve inner conflicts.	Dissociation	Temporarily but drastically modifying a person's character or one's sense of personal identity to avoid emotional distress. Fugue states and hysterical conversion reactions are common manifestations of dissociation. Dissociation may also be found in counter-phobic behavior, dissociative identity disorder, the use of pharmacological highs or religious joy.
Displacement	Shifting an emotion or drive cathexis from one idea or object to another that resembles the original in some aspect or quality. Displacement permits the symbolic representation of the original idea or object by one that is less highly cathected or evokes less distress.	Reaction formation	Transforming an unacceptable impulse into its opposite. Reaction formation is characteristic of obsessional neurosis, but it may occur in other forms of neuroses as well. If this mechanism is frequently used at any early stage of ego development, it can become a permanent character trait, as in an obsessional character.
Externalization	Tending to perceive in the external world and in external objects elements of one's own personality, including instinctual impulses, conflicts, moods, attitudes, and styles of thinking. Externalization is a more general term than projection.	Repression	Expelling or withholding from consciousness an idea or feeling. Primary repression refers to the curbing of ideas and feelings before they have attained consciousness: secondary repression excludes from awareness what was once experienced at a conscious level. The repressed is not really forgotten in that symbolic behavior may be present. This defense differs from suppression by effecting conscious inhibition of impulses to the point of losing and not just postponing cherished goals. Conscious perception of instincts and feelings is blocked in repression.
Inhibition	Consciously limiting or renouncing some ego functions, alone or in combination, to evade anxiety arising out of conflict with instinctual impulses, the superego, or environmental forces or figures.	Sexualization	Endowing an object or function with sexual significance that it did not previously have or possessed to a smaller degree to ward off anxieties associated with prohibited impulses or their derivatives.
Intellectualization	Excessively using intellectual processes to avoid affective expression or experience. Undue emphasis is focused on the inanimate to avoid intimacy with people, attention is paid to external reality to avoid the expression of inner feelings, and stress is excessively placed on irrelevant details to avoid perceiving the whole. Intellectualization is closely allied to rationalization.		
Isolation	Splitting or separating an idea from the affect that accompanies it but is repressed. Social isolation refers to the absence of object relationships.		
Rationalization	Offering rational explanations in an attempt to justify attitudes, beliefs, or behavior that may otherwise be unacceptable. Such underlying motives are usually instinctually determined.		
Mature Defenses			
Altruism	Using constructive and instinctually gratifying service to others to undergo a vicarious experience. It includes benign and constructive reaction formation. Altruism is distinguished from altruistic surrender, in which a surrender of direct gratification or of instinctual needs takes place in favor of fulfilling the needs of others to the detriment of the self, and the satisfaction can only be enjoyed vicariously through introjection.	Humor	Using comedy to overtly express feelings and thoughts without personal discomfort or immobilization and without producing an unpleasant effect on others. It allows the person to tolerate and yet focus on what is too terrible to be borne; it is different from wit, a form of displacement that involves distraction from the affective issue.
Anticipation	Realistically anticipating or planning for future inner discomfort. The mechanism is goal-directed and implies careful planning or worrying and premature but realistic affective anticipation of dire and potentially dreadful outcomes.	Sublimation	Achieving impulse gratification and the retention of goals but altering a socially objectionable aim or object to a socially acceptable one. Sublimation allows instincts to be channeled, rather than blocked or diverted. Feelings are acknowledged, modified, and directed toward a significant object or goal, and modest instinctual satisfaction occurs.
Asceticism	Eliminating the pleasurable effects of experiences. There is a moral element in assigning values to specific pleasures. Gratification is derived from renunciation, and asceticism is directed against all base pleasures perceived consciously.	Suppression	Consciously or semiconsciously postponing attention to a conscious impulse or conflict. Issues may be deliberately cut off, but they are not avoided. Discomfort is acknowledged but minimized.

[a]The categorization of these defenses as narcissistic is controversial. Many psychoanalysts would subsume them under "Immature Defenses."

(Adapted by Glen O. Gabbard, M.D., from Vaillant GE. *Adaptation to Life.* Boston: Little, Brown; 1977; Semrad E. The operation of ego defenses in object loss. In: Moriarily DM, ed. *The Loss of Loved Ones.* Springfield, IL: Charles C Thomas; 1967; and Bibring GL, Dwyer TF, Huntington DS, Valenstein AA. A study of the psychological process in pregnancy and of the earliest mother-child relationship: methodological considerations. *Psychoanal Stud Child.* 1961;16:25, with permission.)

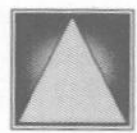

Table 6.1–4
Classic Psychoneurotic Reactions of Childhood

	Conversion Reaction (Dora)	Phobic Reaction (Hans)	Obsessive–Compulsive Reaction (Rat Man)	Mixed Neurotic Reaction (Wolf Man)
Family history	Striking family history of psychiatric and physical illness	Both parents treated for neurotic conflict but not severe	No family history of mental illness	Striking family history of psychiatric and physical illness
Symptoms	Enuresis and masturbation, 6–8 yr; onset of neurosis at 8; migraine, nervous cough, and hoarseness at 12; aphonia at 16; "appendicitis" at 16; convulsions at 16; facial neuralgia at 19; change of personality at 8 from "wild creature" to quiet child	Compulsive questions at 3 to 3 1/2 yr in regard to sex difference; jealous reaction to sibling birth at 3 1/2; overt castration threat; overt masturbation at 3 1/2; overeating and constipation at 4 to 5; phobic reaction at 4 to 5; attack of flu at 5 worsens phobia; tonsillectomy at 5 worsens phobia	Naughty period at 3 to 4 yr; marked timidity after beating by father at 4; recognizing people by their smells as a child (Renifleur); precocious ego development; onset of obsessive ideas at 6 to 7	Tractable and quiet up to 3 1/4 yr; "naughty" period at 3 1/4 to 4 yr; phobias at 4 to 5 with nightmares; obsessional reaction at 6 to 7 (pious ceremonials). Disappearance of neuroses at 8
Causes	Seduction by older man; father's illness; father's affair	Seductive care by mother; sibling birth at 3 1/2	Seduction by governess at 4; death of sibling at 4; beating by father at 4	Seduction by older sister at 3 1/4; mother's illness; conflict between maid and governess

(Courtesy of E. James Anthony, M.D.)

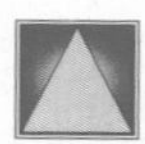

Table 6.1–5
Transference Variants

Libidinal transferences

Follow the classic model and usually in milder forms as positive *transference reactions* but can take the form of more intense and disturbing *erotic transferences*. They are derivatives of phallic-oedipal, libidinal impulses and may be permeated variously by pregenital influences. They can occur with varying degrees of intensity, and in mild forms, may not even require interpretation if they contribute to and support the therapeutic relation. Sigmund Freud recommended that they call for interpretation only when they begin to serve as a resistance.

Aggressive transferences

Take the form either of negative or more pathological paranoid transferences. *Negative transferences* are seen at all levels of psychopathology, but can predominate in some borderline patients who tend to see the therapeutic relationship in terms of power and victimization, regarding the therapist as omnipotent and powerful, whereas the patient experiences him- or herself as helpless, weak, and vulnerable. Negative transferences are identifiable in varying degrees in all analyses and usually require specific intervention and interpretation.

Transferences of defense

Opposed to *transferences of impulse*; defense against impulses finds its way into the transference rather than the impulses themselves. In this form of transference, attention shifts from drives to the ego's defensive functioning so that transference is no longer merely repetition of instinctual cathexes but includes aspects of ego functioning as well.

Transference neurosis

Involves the re-creation or more ample expression of the patient's neurosis enacted anew within the analytical relation and at least theoretically mirroring aspects of the infantile neurosis. The transference neurosis usually develops in the middle phase of analysis, when the patient, at first eager for improved mental health, no longer consistently displays such motivation but engages in a continuing battle with the analyst over the desire to attain some kind of emotional satisfaction from the analyst so that this becomes the most compelling reason for continuing analysis. At this point of the treatment, the transference emotions become more important to the patient than alleviation of distress sought initially, and the major, unresolved, unconscious problems of childhood begin to dominate the patient's behavior. They are now reproduced in the transference, with all their pent-up emotion.

The transference neurosis is governed by three outstanding characteristics of instinctual life in early childhood: the pleasure principle (before effective reality testing), ambivalence, and repetition compulsion. Emergence of the transference neurosis is usually a slow and gradual process, although in certain patients with a propensity for *transference regression*, particularly more hysterical patients, elements of transference and transference neurosis may manifest themselves relatively early in the analytical process. One situation after another in the life of the patient is analyzed and progressively interpreted until the original infantile conflict is sufficiently revealed. Only then does the transference neurosis begin to subside. At that point, termination begins to emerge as a more central concern.

Contemporary opinion is divided to its importance and centrality, whether it forms to the extent Freud believed, and whether it is necessary for successful analysis—for some, it remains an essential vehicle for analytical interpretation and therapeutic effectiveness; for others, it may never develop or, to the extent that it does, may play a less central role in the process of cure.

(*continued*)

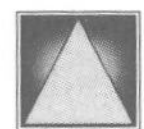

Table 6.1–5 (Continued)

Transference psychosis

Occurs when failure of reality testing leads to loss of self–object differentiation and diffusion of self and object boundaries. This may reflect an attempt to re-fuse with an omnipotent object, investing the self with omnipotent powers as defense against underlying fears of vulnerability and powerlessness. Transference psychosis can also include negative transference elements in which fusion carries the threat of engulfment and loss of self that may precipitate a *paranoid transference reaction.*

Narcissistic transferences

Clarified by Heinz Kohut (1971) as variations of patterns of projection of archaic narcissistic configurations onto the therapist. They are based on projections of narcissistic introjective configurations, both superior and inferior—the superior form reflecting narcissistic superiority, grandiosity, and enhanced self-esteem, and the inferior opposite qualities of inferiority, self-depletion, and diminished self-esteem. The therapist comes to represent, in Kohut's terms, either the grandiose self in *mirror transferences* or the idealized parental imago in *idealizing transferences.* In idealizing transferences, all power and strength are attributed to the idealized object, leaving the subject feeling empty and powerless when separated from that object. Union with the idealized object enables the subject to regain narcissistic equilibrium. Idealizing transferences may reflect developmental disturbances in the idealized parent imago, particularly at the time of formation of the ego ideal by introjection of the idealized object. In some individuals, narcissistic fixation leads to development of the grandiose self. Reactivation in analysis of the grandiose self provides the basis of mirror transferences formation, which occur in three forms: *archaic merger transference,* a less archaic *alter-ego* or *twinship transference,* and *mirror transference in the narrow sense.* In the most primitive merger transference, the analyst is experienced only as an extension of the subject's grandiose self and, thus, becomes the repository of the patient's grandiosity and exhibitionism. In the alter-ego or twinship transference, activation of the grandiose self leads to experience of the narcissistic object as similar to the grandiose self. In the most mature form of mirror transference, the analyst is experienced as a separate person but, nonetheless, one who becomes important to the patient and is accepted by him or her only to the degree that he or she is responsive to the narcissistic needs of the reactivated grandiose self.

Self-object transferences

Represent extensions of the self-psychology paradigm beyond merely narcissistic configurations. The self-object involves investment of the self in the object so that the object comes to serve a self-sustaining function that the self cannot perform for itself—either in maintaining fragile self-cohesion or in regulating self-esteem. The other, thus, is not experienced as an autonomous and separate object or agency in its own right but as present only to serve the needs of the self. Transference in this sense reflects a continuing developmental need that seeks satisfaction in the analytical relation.

Self-object transferences reflect the underlying need structure the patient brings to the therapeutic relationship based on the predominant pattern of self-object deprivation or frustration and the corresponding seeking for the appropriate form of self-object involvement. These configurations have been described as the *understimulated self,* the *overstimulated self,* the *overburdened self,* and the *fragmenting self.* Other descriptions of self-object need translate patterns of transference interaction based on narcissistic dynamics into the perspective of the relationship between self and self-object, as in mirror-hungry personalities and ideal-hungry personalities. Variations on the mirroring transference theme include the alter-ego–hungry personality, the merger-hungry personality, and, in contrast, the contact-shunning personality. In transferences derived from such personality configurations, the classic meaning of transference has undergone radical modification. Rather than displacements or projections from earlier object relational contexts, the patient brings to bear a need based in his or her own currently deficient capacity and defective character structure—a need to involve the object in a dependent relationship to complete or stabilize his or her own psychic integration.

Transitional relatedness

This transference model is based on Donald Winnicott's notion of the transitional object. Transference in more primitive character structures is regarded as a form of *transitional object relation* in which the therapist is perceived as outside the self but is invested with qualities from the patient's own archaic self-image. The transference field in this view is envisioned as a transitional space in which the transference illusion is allowed to play itself out.

Transference as psychic reality

Reflects the need of each participant in analysis to draw the other into a stance corresponding to his or her own intrapsychic configuration and needs as a reflection of the individual subject's psychic reality. This regards the classic view of transference, based on displacement or projection from past objects, as inadequate, resulting in further diffusion of meaning of transference as equivalent to the individual's capacity to create a meaningful world or to inform the world with meaning. In this rendition, transference becomes equivalent to the patient's psychic reality so that any distinction between the meanings given to reality and the meanings inherent in transference are lost. Transference in these terms becomes all-encompassing, and whatever distinguishing and dynamic significance it may have had fades into obscurity. In this form of transference, no definable mechanism seems to be at work other than whatever is involved in the subject's psychic reality. The subject's view of his or her environment and impression of objects of his or her experience, including the analytical object, are indistinguishable from ordinary cognitive and affective processes characterizing personal involvement and responsiveness to the world about him or her.

Transference as relational or intersubjective

The relational or intersubjective view of transference as emerging from or cocreated by the subjective interaction between analyst and analysand transforms transference into an interactive phenomenon in which individual intrapsychic contributions from either participant are obscured. Transference in this sense is not anything individual to, or intrapsychically derived from, the patient but is based on the present ongoing interaction between analyst and patient coconstructing transference. On these terms, analysis of transference has little to do with past derivatives and everything to do with the ongoing relation with the analyst, primarily in the form of interpersonal enactments. Transference in this sense is no longer a one-person phenomenon but reflects a two-person transference–countertransference interaction. The supposition is that no such thing as transference exists without countertransference and no such thing as countertransference without transference. The patient is thus relieved of any burden of a personal dynamic unconscious reflecting developmental vicissitudes and residues of a life history. Transference is created anew in the immediacy of present analytical interaction as the product of mutual influence and communication between analyst and analysand, probably relying on some form of mutual projective identification to sustain the interactive connotation.

aggression on themselves and become overtly self-destructive. Parents who are inconsistent, excessively harsh, or overly indulgent can influence children to develop disordered superego functioning. Severe conflict that cannot be managed through symptom formation can lead to extreme restrictions in ego functioning and fundamentally impair the capacity to learn and develop new skills.

Traumatic events that seem to threaten survival can break through defenses when the ego has been weakened. More libidinal energy is then required to master the excitation that results. The libido thus mobilized, however, is withdrawn from the supply that is normally applied to external objects. This withdrawal further diminishes the strength of the ego and produces a sense of inadequacy. Frustrations or disappointments in adults may revive infantile longings that are then dealt with through symptom formation or further regression.

In his classic studies, Freud described four different types of childhood neuroses, three of which had later neurotic developments in adult life. This well-known series of cases shown in tabulated form in Table 6.1–4 exemplifies some of Freud's important conclusions: (1) neurotic reactions in the adult are associated frequently with neurotic reactions in childhood; (2) the connection is sometimes continuous but more often is separated by a latent period of nonneurosis; and (3) infantile sexuality, both fantasized and real, occupies a memorable place in the early history of the patient.

Certain differences are worth noting in the four cases shown in Table 6.1–4. First, the phobic reactions tend to start at about 4 or 5 years of age, the obsessional reactions between 6 and 7, and the conversion reactions at 8. The degree of background disturbance is greatest in the conversion reaction and the mixed neurosis, and it seems only slight in the phobic and obsessional reactions. The course of the phobic reaction seems little influenced by severe traumatic factors, whereas traumatic factors, such as sexual seductions, play an important role in the three other subgroups. It was during this period that Freud elaborated

Table 6.1–6
Transference Mechanisms

Displacement

The basic mechanism of classic transference paradigms in which an object representation derived from any level or combination of levels of the subject's developmental experience is displaced to the representation of the new object, namely, the analyst, in the therapeutic relationship. Displacement is the basic mechanism for libidinally based transferences, both positive and erotic, as well as for aggressive and especially negative transferences. By and large, displacement transferences tend to play a more dominant role in neurotic disorders in which phallic-oedipal (and to a lesser degree pre-oedipal) dynamics tend to play a dominant, although not exclusive, role.

Projection

Process by which qualities or characteristics of the self-as-object, usually involving introjections or self-representations, are attributed to an external object, and the subsequent interaction with the object is determined by the projected characteristics. Thus, the analyst or object may be seen as sadistic—that is, as possessing the sadistic character of the analysand or subject, an aspect of the subject's self that is denied or disowned by the subject. Projection tends to play a more prominent, although again not exclusive, role in formation of transferences in more primitive character disorders but can be found in variously modified forms throughout the spectrum of neuroses. Because projections derive primarily from the configuration of introjects constituting the patient's self-as-object, the effect of projective or externalizing transferences is that the image of the therapist comes to represent part of the patient's own self-organization rather than simply an object representation.

Projections derived from destructive introjects can provide the basis for both negative and paranoid transference reactions. Those based on the victim or introject result in the patient relating to the therapist as his or her victim and him- or herself assuming a hostile or sadistic position as a destructive aggressor or victimizer to the therapist's victim. Then again, projection based on the aggressor or introject results in the patient relating to the therapist as an aggressor and him- or herself assuming a weak, vulnerable, or masochistic position in which he or she becomes a passive and vulnerable victim to the therapist's destructive aggression. Similar patterns can take place around narcissistic issues involving introjective configurations of narcissistic superiority and inferiority.

Projective dynamics in self-object transferences, however, seem to involve more than narcissistic projections because these forms of transference tend to draw the analyst into meeting the pathological needs of the self. If anything is projected, it is an infantile wished-for imago, one lacking earlier in the patient's experience, as, for example, an empathic and idealized parental figure. On the other hand, transitional transferences, despite their considerable overlap with self-object phenomena, tend to involve a more explicit projective element as the self-related contribution to the transitional experience.

Projective identification

The concept of projective identification was first proposed by Melanie Klein, arguing that the projection of impulses or feelings into another person brought about an identification with that person based on attribution of one's own qualities to that other. This attribution served as the basis for a sense of empathy and connection with the other. On these terms, projective identification was a fantasy taking place solely in the mind of the one projecting.

Projective identification is often appealed to as a mechanism of transference, or more exactly transference–countertransference interactions, particularly in Kleinian usage. Confusion arises from the failure to clearly distinguish between projection and projective identification. The notion of projective identification added to the basic concept of projection of the notes of diffusion of ego boundaries, a loss or diminishing of self–object differentiation, and inclusion of the object as part of the self.

Later elaborations of the notion of projective identification transformed it from a one-body to a two-body phenomenon, describing interaction between two subjects, one of whom projects something onto or into the other, whereon the other introjects or internalizes what has been projected. Instead of the projection and introjection taking place in the same subject, the projection now takes place in one and the internalization in the other. This latter usage has led to extensive extrapolation of the concept of projective identification to apply to all sorts of object relations, including transference. The emphasis in Kleinian transference is less on the influence of the past on the present but rather the influence of the internal world on the external in the here-and-now interaction with the analyst.

his seduction hypothesis for the cause of the neuroses, in terms of which the obsessive–compulsive and hysterical reactions were alleged to originate in active and passive sexual experiences.

TREATMENT AND TECHNIQUE

The cornerstone of psychoanalytic technique is free association, in which patients say whatever comes to mind. Free association does more than provide content for the analysis: It also induces the necessary regression and dependency connected with establishing and working through the transference neurosis. When this development occurs, all the original wishes, drives, and defenses associated with the infantile neurosis are transferred to the person of the analyst.

As patients attempt to free associate, they soon learn that they have difficulty saying whatever comes to mind, without censoring certain thoughts. They develop conflicts about their wishes and feelings toward the analyst that reflect childhood conflicts. The *transference* that develops toward the analyst may also serve as resistance to the process of free association. Freud discovered that *resistance* was not simply a stoppage of a patient's associations, but also an important revelation of the patient's internal object relations as they were externalized and manifested in the transference relationship with the analyst. The systematic analysis of transference and resistance is the essence of psychoanalysis. Freud was also aware that the analyst might have transferences to the patient, which he called *countertransference*. Countertransference, in Freud's view, was an obstacle that the analyst needed to understand so that it did not interfere with treatment. In this spirit, he recognized the need for all analysts to have been analyzed themselves. Variations in transference and their descriptions are contained in Table 6.1–5. The basic mechanisms by which transferences are effected—displacement, projection, and projective identification—are described in Table 6.1–6.

Analysts after Freud began to recognize that countertransference was not only an obstacle, but also a source of useful information about the patient. In other words, the analyst's feelings in response to the patient reflect how other persons respond to the patient and provide some indication of the patient's own internal object relations. By understanding the intense feelings that occur in the analytic relationship, the analyst can help the patient broaden understanding of past and current relationships outside the analysis. The development of insight into neurotic conflicts also expands the ego and provides an increased sense of mastery. (Psychoanalysis and other techniques derived from it are discussed in greater detail in Chapter 35, Section 35.1.)

REFERENCES

Biran MW. Between science and art: Freud on the couch. *Psychocrtiques*. 2004; 49[Suppl 11].

Blum HP. Beneath and beyond the "formulations on the two principles of mental functioning". Freud and Jung. *Psychoanal Study Child*. 2004;59:240–257.

Buhler KE. Existential analysis and psychoanalysis. Specific differences and personal relationship between Ludwig Binswanger and Sigmund Freud. *Am J Psychother.* 2004;58.34–50.

Clewell T. Mourning beyond melancholia. Freud's psychoanalysis of loss. *J Am Psychoanal Assoc*. 2004;52:43–67.

Ekstrom SR. The mind beyond our immediate awareness. Freudian, Jungian, and cognitive models of the unconscious. *J Anal Psychol*. 2004;49(5):657.

Franklin PA. Dreaming by the book. Freud's "The Interpretation of Dreams" and the history of the psychoanalytic movement. *J Nerv Ment Dis*. 2005;193(1):74–75.

Freud S. *The Standard Edition of the Complete Psychological Works of Sigmund Freud*. 24 Vols. London. Hogarth Press; 1953–1974.

Geller J. The psychopathology of everyday Vienna. Psychoanalysis and Freud's familiars. *Int J Psychoanal*. 2004;85(5):1209–1224.

Hartocollis P. Origins and evolution of the Oedipus complex as conceptualized by Freud. *Psychoanal Rev*. 2005;92(3):315–334.

Levin FM. *Psyche and Brain. The Biology of Talking Cures*. Madison, CT: International Universities Press; 2003.

Meissner WW. Classic psychoanalysis. In: Sadock BJ, Sadock VA, eds. *Kaplan & Sadock's Comprehensive Textbook of Psychiatry*. 8th ed. Vol. 1. Baltimore: Lippincott Williams & Wilkins; 2005:7.

Meissner WW. *The Ethical Dilemma of Psychoanalysis—A Dialogue*. Albany, NY: State University of New York Press; 2003.

Person ES. As the wheel turns: a centennial reflection on Freud's three essays on the theory of sexuality. *J Am Psychoanal Assoc*. 2005;53(4):1257–1282.

Rizzuto AM, Meissner WW, Buie DH. *The Dynamics of Human Aggression: Theoretical Foundations, Clinical Applications*. New York: Brunner-Routledge; 2004.

Wulff D. Freud and Freudians on religion: A reader. *Int J Psychol Rel*. 2003;13:223.

▲ 6.2 Erik Erikson

Erik Erikson was a psychoanalyst who created an original and highly influential theory of psychological development and crisis occurring in periods that extended across the entire life cycle. His theory grew out of his work first as a teacher, then as a child psychoanalyst, next as an anthropological field worker, and, finally, as a biographer. Rather than starting within the nervous system of the individual, as Sigmund Freud had done, Erikson focused on the boundary between the child and the environment and then graphed the evolution of the maturing ego's relations with an expanding social world. Erikson identified dilemmas or polarities in the ego's relations with the family and larger social institutions at nodal points in childhood, adolescence, and early, middle, and late adulthood.

Erik Homburger Erikson (Fig. 6.2–1) was born June 15, 1902, in Karlsruhe, Germany. He died in 1994. His father, a Danish Protestant, and his mother, a Danish Jew, separated before he was born, and he grew up in the home of his mother and German-Jewish stepfather, Theodore Homburger, a pediatrician. Erikson was never able to learn the identity of his biological father; his mother withheld that information from him all her life.

Erikson immigrated to the United States in 1933. He worked at the Austen Riggs Center in Stockbridge, Massachusetts, and conducted research at Harvard, Yale, and the University of California at Berkeley. He became interested in the influence of culture on child development, and as a result of his studies in the 1930s and the 1940s, including anthropological work with the Sioux in South Dakota and the Yurok in northern California, his book *Childhood and Society* was published in 1950. In this publication, he presented a psychosocial theory of development that describes crucial steps in persons' relationships with the social world, based on the interplay between biology and society.

EPIGENETIC PRINCIPLE

Erikson's formulations were based on the concept of *epigenesis*, a term borrowed from embryology. His *epigenetic principle* holds that development occurs in sequential, clearly defined stages, and that each stage must be satisfactorily resolved for development to proceed smoothly. According to the epigenetic model, if successful resolution of a particular stage does not

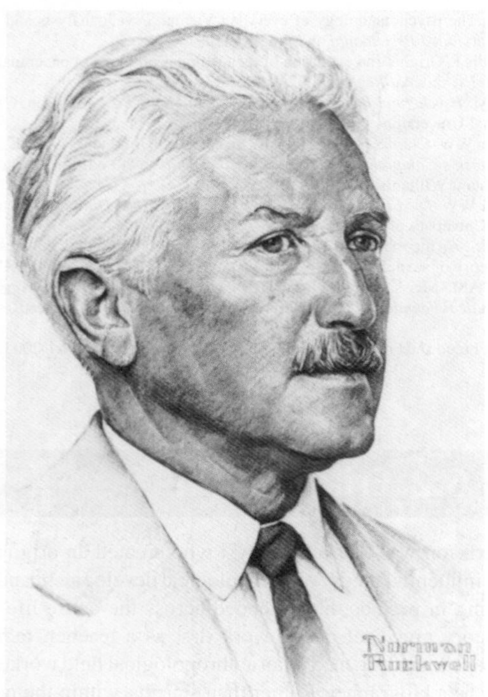

FIGURE 6.2–1
Painting of Erikson (by Norman Rockwell, Courtesy of Edward R. Shapiro, M.D.).

occur, all subsequent stages reflect that failure in the form of physical, cognitive, social, or emotional maladjustment.

Relation to Freudian Theory

Erikson accepted Freud's concepts of instinctual development and infantile sexuality. For each of Freud's psychosexual stages (e.g., oral, anal, and phallic), Erikson described a corresponding zone with a specific pattern or mode of behavior. Thus, the oral zone is associated with sucking or taking-in behavior; the anal zone is associated with holding on and letting go. Erikson emphasized that the development of the ego is more than the result of intrapsychic wants or inner psychic energies. It is also a matter of mutual regulation between growing children and a society's culture and traditions.

Eight Stages of the Life Cycle

Erikson's conception of the eight stages of ego development across the life cycle is the centerpiece of his life's work, and he elaborated the conception throughout his subsequent writings (Table 6.2–1). The eight stages represent points along a continuum of development in which physical, cognitive, instinctual, and sexual changes combine to trigger an internal crisis whose resolution results in either psychosocial regression or growth and the development of specific virtues. In *Insight and Responsibility* Erikson defined virtue as "inherent strength," as in the active quality of a medicine or liquor. He wrote in *Identity: Youth and Crisis* that "crisis' refers not to a "threat of catastrophe, but to a turning point, a crucial period of increased vulnerability and heightened potential, and therefore, the ontogenetic source of generational strength and maladjustment."

Stage 1: Trust versus Mistrust (Birth to about 18 Months). In *Identity: Youth and Crisis*, Erikson noted that the infant "lives through and loves with" its mouth. Indeed, the mouth forms the basis of its first mode or pattern of behavior, that of incorporation. The infant is taking the world in through the mouth, eyes, ears, and sense of touch. The baby is learning a cultural modality that Erikson termed *to get*, that is, to receive what is offered and elicit what is desired. As the infant's teeth develop and it discovers the pleasure of biting, it enters the second oral stage, the active-incorporative mode. The infant is no longer passively receptive to stimuli; it reaches out for sensation and grasps at its surroundings. The social modality shifts to that of *taking and holding* on to things.

The infant's development of basic trust in the world stems from its earliest experiences with its mother or primary caretaker. In *Childhood and Society* Erikson asserts that trust depends not on "absolute quantities of food or demonstrations of love, but rather on the quality of maternal relationship." A baby whose mother can anticipate and respond to its needs in a consistent and timely manner despite its oral aggression will learn to tolerate the inevitable moments of frustration and deprivation. The defense mechanisms of introjection and projection provide the infant with the means to internalize pleasure and externalize pain such that "consistency, continuity, and sameness of experience provide a rudimentary sense of ego identity." Trust will predominate over mistrust, and hope will crystallize. For Erikson, the element of society corresponding to this stage of ego identity is religion, as both are founded on "trust born of care."

In keeping with his emphasis on the epigenetic character of psychosocial change, Erikson conceived of many forms of psychopathology as examples of what he termed *aggravated development crisis*, development, which having gone awry at one point, affects subsequent psychosocial change. A person who, as a result of severe disturbances in the earliest dyadic relationships, fails to develop a basic sense of trust or the virtue of hope may be predisposed as an adult to the profound withdrawal and regression characteristic of schizophrenia. Erikson hypothesized that the depressed patient's experience of being empty and of being no good is an outgrowth of a developmental derailment that causes oral pessimism to predominate. Addictions may also be traced to the mode of oral incorporation.

Stage 2: Autonomy versus Shame and Doubt (about 18 Months to about 3 Years). In the development of speech and sphincter and muscular control, the toddler practices the social modalities of *holding on and letting go*, and experiences the first stirrings of the virtue that Erikson termed *will*. Much depends on the amount and type of control exercised by adults over the child. Control that is exerted too rigidly or too early defeats the toddler's attempts to develop its own internal controls, and regression or false progression results. Parental control that fails to protect the toddler from the consequences of his or her own lack of self-control or judgment can be equally disastrous to the child's development of a healthy sense of autonomy. In *Identity: Youth and Crisis*, Erikson asserted: "This stage, therefore, becomes decisive for the ratio between loving good will and hateful self-insistence, between cooperation and

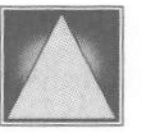

Table 6.2–1
Erikson's Psychosocial Stages

Psychosocial Stage	Associated Virtue	Related Forms of Psychopathology	Positive and Negative Forerunners of Identity Formation	Enduring Aspects of Identity Formation
Trust vs. mistrust (birth—)	Hope	Psychosis Addictions Depression	Mutual recognition vs. autistic isolation	Temporal perspective vs. time confusion
Autonomy vs. shame and doubt (~18 months—)	Will	Paranoia Obsessions Compulsions Impulsivity	Will to be oneself vs. self-doubt	Self-certainty vs. self-consciousness
Initiative vs. guilt (~3 years—)	Purpose	Conversion disorder Phobia Psychosomatic disorder Inhibition	Anticipation of roles vs. role inhibition	Role experimentation vs. role fixation
Industry vs. inferiority (~5 years—)	Competence	Creative inhibition Inertia	Task identification vs. sense of futility	Apprenticeship vs. work paralysis
Identity vs. role confusion (~13 years—)	Fidelity	Delinquent behavior Gender-related identity disorders Borderline psychotic episodes		Identity vs. identity confusion
Intimacy vs. isolation (~20s—)	Love	Schizoid personality disorder Distantiation		Sexual polarization vs. bisexual confusion
Generativity vs. stagnation (~40s—)	Care	Mid-life crisis Premature invalidism		Leadership and followership vs. abdication of responsibility
Integrity vs. despair (~60s—)	Wisdom	Extreme alienation Despair		Ideological commitment vs. confusion of values

(Adapted from Erikson E. *Insight and Responsibility*. New York: WW Norton; 1964; Erikson E. *Identity: Youth and Crisis*. New York: WW Norton; 1968, with permission.)

willfulness, and between self-expression and compulsive self-restraint or meek compliance."

Where that ratio is favorable, the child develops an appropriate sense of autonomy and the capacity to "have and to hold"; where it is unfavorable, doubt and shame will undermine free will. According to Erikson, the principle of law and order has at its roots this early preoccupation with the protection and regulation of will. In *Childhood and Society*, he concluded, "The sense of autonomy fostered in the child and modified as life progresses, serves (and is served by) the preservation in economic and political life of a sense of justice."

A person who becomes fixated at the transition between the development of hope and autonomous will, with its residue of mistrust and doubt, may develop paranoiac fears of persecution. When psychosocial development is derailed in the second stage, other forms of pathology may emerge. The perfectionism, inflexibility, and stinginess of the person with an obsessive–compulsive personality disorder may stem from conflicting tendencies to hold on and to let go. The ruminative and ritualistic behavior of the person who suffers from an obsessive–compulsive disorder may be an outcome of the triumph of doubt over autonomy and the subsequent development of a primitively harsh conscience.

Stage 3: Initiative versus Guilt (about 3 Years to about 5 Years). The child's increasing mastery of locomotor and language skills expands its participation in the outside world and stimulates omnipotent fantasies of wider exploration and conquest. Here the youngster's mode of participation is active and intrusive; its social modality is that of being on the make. The intrusiveness is manifested in the child's fervent curiosity and genital preoccupations, competitiveness, and physical aggression. The Oedipus complex is in ascendance as the child competes with the same-sex parent for the fantasized possession of the other parent. In *Identity: Youth and Crisis*, Erikson wrote that "jealousy and rivalry now come to a climax in a final contest for a favored position with one of the parents: the inevitable and necessary failure leads to guilt and anxiety."

Guilt over the drive for conquest and anxiety over the anticipated punishment are both assuaged in the child through repression of the forbidden wishes and development of a superego to regulate its initiative. This conscience, the faculty of self-observation, self-regulation, and self-punishment, is an internalized version of parental and societal authority. Initially, the conscience is harsh and uncompromising; however, it constitutes the foundation for the subsequent development of morality. Having renounced oedipal ambitions, the child begins to look outside the family for arenas in which it can compete with less conflict and guilt. This is the stage that highlights the child's expanding initiative and forms the basis for the subsequent development of realistic ambition and the virtue of *purpose*. As Erikson noted in *Childhood and Society*, "The 'oedipal' stage sets the direction toward the possible and the tangible which permits the dreams of early childhood to be attached to the goals of an active adult life." Toward this end, social institutions provide the youngster with an economic ethos in the form of adult heroes who begin to take the place of their storybook counterparts.

When there has been an inadequate resolution of the conflict between initiative and guilt, the person may ultimately develop a conversion disorder, inhibition, or phobia. Those who overcompensate for the conflict by driving themselves too hard may experience sufficient stress to produce psychosomatic symptoms.

Stage 4: Industry versus Inferiority (about 5 Years to about 13 Years). With the onset of latency, the child discovers the pleasures of production. He or she develops industry by learning new skills and takes pride in the things made. Erikson wrote in *Childhood and Society* that the child's "ego boundaries include his tools and skills: the work principle teaches him the pleasure of work completion by steady attention and persevering diligence." Across cultures, this is a time when the child receives systematic instruction and learns the fundamentals of technology as they pertain to the use of basic utensils and tools. As children work, they identify with their teachers and imagine themselves in various occupational roles.

A child who is unprepared for this stage of psychosocial development, either through insufficient resolution of previous stages or by current interference, may develop a sense of inferiority and inadequacy. In the form of teachers and other role models, society becomes crucially important in the child's ability to overcome that sense of inferiority and to achieve the virtue known as competence. In *Identity: Youth and Crisis*, Erikson noted: "This is socially a most decisive stage. Since industry involves doing things beside and with others, a first sense of division of labor and of differential opportunity, that is, a sense of the technological ethos of a culture, develops at this time."

The pathological outcome of a poorly navigated stage of industry versus inferiority is less well defined than in previous stages, but it may concern the emergence of a conformist immersion into the world of production in which creativity is stifled and identity is subsumed under the worker's role.

Stage 5: Identity versus Role Confusion (about 13 Years to about 21 Years). With the onset of puberty and its myriad social and physiological changes, the adolescent becomes preoccupied with the question of identity. Erikson noted in *Childhood and Society* that youth are now "primarily concerned with what they appear to be in the eyes of others as compared to what they feel they are, and with the question of how to connect the roles and skills cultivated earlier with the occupational prototypes of the day." Childhood roles and fantasies are no longer appropriate, yet the adolescent is far from equipped to become an adult. In *Childhood and Society* Erikson writes that the integration that occurs in the formation of ego identity encompasses far more than the summation of childhood identifications. "It is the accrued experience of the ego's ability to integrate these identifications with the vicissitudes of the libido, with the aptitudes developed out of endowment, and with the opportunities offered in social roles."

The formation of cliques and an identity crisis occur at the end of adolescence. Erikson calls the crisis normative because it is a normal event. Failure to negotiate this stage leaves adolescents without a solid identity; they suffer from identity diffusion or role confusion, characterized by not having a sense of self and by confusion about their place in the world. Role confusion can manifest in such behavioral abnormalities as running away, criminality, and overt psychosis. Problems in gender identity and sexual role may manifest at this time. Adolescents may defend against role diffusion by joining cliques or cults or by identifying with folk heroes. Intolerance of individual differences is a way in which the young person attempts to ward off a sense of identity loss. Falling in love, a process by which the adolescent may clarify a sense of identity by projecting a diffused self-image onto the partner and seeing it gradually assume a more distinctive shape, and an overidentification with idealized figures are means by which the adolescent seeks self-definition. With the attainment of a more sharply focused identity, the youth develops the virtue of *fidelity*—faithfulness not only to the nascent self-definition but also to an ideology that provides a version of self-in-world. As Erikson, Joan Erikson, and Helen Kivnick wrote in *Vital Involvement in Old Age*, "Fidelity is the ability to sustain loyalties freely pledged in spite of the inevitable contradictions of value systems. It is the cornerstone of identity and receives inspiration from confirming ideologies and affirming companionships." Role confusion ensues when the youth is unable to formulate a sense of identity and belonging. Erikson held that delinquency, gender-related identity disorders, and borderline psychotic episodes can result from such confusion.

Stage 6: Intimacy versus Isolation (about 21 Years to about 40 Years). Freud's famous response to the question of what a normal person should be able to do well, "Lieben und arbeiten" (to love and to work), is one that Erikson often cited in his discussion of this psychosocial stage, and it emphasizes the importance he placed on the virtue of love within a balanced identity. Erikson asserted in *Identity: Youth and Crisis* that Freud's use of the term love referred to "the generosity of intimacy as well as genital love; when he said love and work, he meant a general work productiveness which would not preoccupy the individual to the extent that he might lose his right or capacity to be a sexual and a loving being."

Intimacy in the young adult is closely tied to fidelity; it is the ability to make and honor commitments to concrete affiliations and partnerships even when that requires sacrifice and compromise. The person who cannot tolerate the fear of ego loss arising out of experiences of self-abandonment (e.g., sexual orgasm, moments of intensity in friendships, aggression, inspiration, and intuition) is apt to become deeply isolated and self-absorbed. *Distantiation*, an awkward term coined by Erikson to mean "the readiness to repudiate, isolate, and, if necessary, destroy those forces and persons whose essence seems dangerous to one's own," is the pathological outcome of conflicts surrounding intimacy and, in the absence of an ethical sense where intimate, competitive, and combative relationships are differentiated, forms the basis for various forms of prejudice, persecution, and psychopathology.

Erikson's separation of the psychosocial task of achieving identity from that of achieving intimacy, and his assertion that substantial progress on the former task must precede development on the latter have engendered much criticism and debate. Critics have argued that Erikson's emphasis on separation and occupationally based identity formation fails to take into account the importance for women of continued attachment and the formation of an identity based on relationships.

Stage 7: Generativity versus Stagnation (about 40 Years to about 60 Years). Erikson asserted in *Identity: Youth and Crisis* that "generativity is primarily the concern for establishing and guiding the next generation." The term *generativity* applies not so much to rearing and teaching one's offspring as it does to a protective concern for all the generations and for social institutions. It encompasses productivity and creativity as well. Having previously achieved the capacity to form intimate relationships, the person now broadens the investment of ego and libidinal energy to include groups, organizations, and society. *Care* is the virtue that coalesces at this stage. In *Childhood and Society* Erikson emphasized the importance to the mature person of feeling needed. "Maturity needs guidance as well as encouragement from what has been produced and must be taken care of." Through generative behavior, the individual can pass on knowledge and skills while obtaining a measure of satisfaction in having achieved a role with senior authority and responsibility in the tribe.

When persons cannot develop true generativity, they may settle for pseudoengagement in occupation. Often, such persons restrict their focus to the technical aspects of their roles, at which they may now have become highly skilled, eschewing greater responsibility for the organization or profession. This failure of generativity can lead to profound personal stagnation, masked by a variety of escapisms, such as alcohol and drug abuse, and sexual and other infidelities. Mid-life crisis or premature invalidism (physical and psychological) can occur. In this case, pathology appears not only in middle-aged persons but also in the organizations that depend on them for leadership. Thus, the failure to develop at mid life can lead to sick, withered, or destructive organizations that spread the effects of failed generativity throughout society; examples of such failures have become so common that they constitute a defining feature of modernity.

Stage 8: Integrity versus Despair (about 60 Years to Death). In *Identity: Youth and Crisis*, Erikson defined integrity as "the acceptance of one's one and only life cycle and of the persons who have become significant to it as something that had to be and that, by necessity, permitted of no substitutions." From the vantage point of this stage of psychosocial development, the individual relinquishes the wish that important persons in his life had been different and is able to love in a more meaningful way—one that reflects accepting responsibility for one's own life. The individual in possession of the virtue of wisdom and a sense of integrity has room to tolerate the proximity of death and to achieve what Erikson termed in *Identity: Youth and Crisis* a "detached yet active concern with life."

Erikson underlined the social context for this final stage of growth. In *Childhood and Society*, he wrote, "The style of integrity developed by his culture or civilization thus becomes the 'patrimony' of his soul.... In such final consolidation, death loses its sting."

When the attempt to attain integrity has failed, the individual may become deeply disgusted with the external world and contemptuous of persons as well as institutions. Erikson wrote in *Childhood and Society* that such disgust masks a fear of death and a sense of despair that "time is now short, too short for the attempt to start another life and to try out alternate roads to integrity." Looking back on the eight ages of man, he noted the relation between adult integrity and infantile trust, "Healthy children will not fear life if their elders have integrity enough not to fear death."

PSYCHOPATHOLOGY

Each stage of the life cycle has its own psychopathological outcome if it is not mastered successfully.

Basic Trust

An impairment of basic trust leads to basic mistrust. In infants, social trust is characterized by ease of feeding, depth of sleep, smiling, and general physiological homeostasis. Prolonged separation during infancy can lead to hospitalism or anaclitic depression (see Chapter 4, Section 4.2). In later life, this lack of trust may be manifested by dysthymic disorder, a depressive disorder, or a sense of hopelessness. Persons who develop and rely on the defense of projection—in which, according to Erikson, "we endow significant persons with the evil which actually is in us"—experienced a sense of social mistrust in the first years of life and are likely to develop paranoid or delusional disorders. Basic mistrust is a major contributor to the development of schizoid personality disorder and, in most severe cases, to the development of schizophrenia. Substance-related disorders can also be traced to social mistrust; substance-dependent personalities have strong oral-dependency needs and use chemical substances to satisfy themselves because of their belief that human beings are unreliable and, at worst, dangerous. If not nurtured properly, infants may feel empty, starved not just for food but also for sensual and visual stimulation. As adults, they may become seekers after stimulating thrills that do not involve intimacy and that help ward off feelings of depression.

Autonomy

The stage in which children attempt to develop into autonomous beings is often called the *terrible twos*, referring to toddlers' willfulness at this period of development. If shame and doubt dominate over autonomy, compulsive doubting can occur. The inflexibility of the obsessive personality also results from an overabundance of doubt. Too rigorous toilet training, commonplace in today's society, which requires a clean, punctual, and deodorized body, can produce an overly compulsive personality that is stingy, meticulous, and selfish. Known as anal personalities, such persons are parsimonious, punctual, and perfectionistic (the three Ps).

Too much shaming causes children to feel evil or dirty and may pave the way for delinquent behavior. In effect, children say, "If that's what they think of me, that's the way I'll behave." Paranoid personalities feel that others are trying to control them, a feeling that may have its origin during the stage of autonomy versus shame and doubt. When coupled with mistrust, the seeds are planted for persecutory delusions. Impulsive disorder may be explained as a person's refusing to be inhibited or controlled.

Initiative

Erikson stated: "In pathology, the conflict over initiative is expressed either in hysterical denial, which causes the repression of the wish or the abrogation of its executive organ by paralysis or impotence; or in overcompensatory showing off, in which the scared individual, so eager to 'duck,' instead 'sticks his neck out.'" In the past, hysteria was the usual form of pathological regression in this area, but a plunge into psychosomatic disease is now common.

Excessive guilt can lead to a variety of conditions, such as generalized anxiety disorder and phobias. Patients feel guilty because of normal impulses, and they repress these impulses, with resulting symptom formation. Punishment or severe prohibitions during the stage of initiative versus guilt can produce sexual inhibitions. Conversion disorder or specific phobia can result when the oedipal conflict is not resolved. As sexual fantasies are accepted as unrealizable, children may punish themselves for these fantasies by fearing harm to their genitals. Under the brutal assault of the developing superego, they may repress their wishes and begin to deny them. If this pattern is carried forward, paralysis, inhibition, or impotence can result. Sometimes, in fear of not being able to live up to what others expect, children may develop psychosomatic disease.

Industry

Erikson described industry as a "sense of being able to make things and make them well and even perfectly." When children's efforts are thwarted, they are made to feel that personal goals cannot be accomplished or are not worthwhile, and a sense of inferiority develops. In adults, this sense of inferiority can result in severe work inhibitions and a character structure marked by feelings of inadequacy. For some persons, the feelings may result in a compensatory drive for money, power, and prestige. Work can become the main focus of life, at the expense of intimacy.

Identity

Many disorders of adolescence can be traced to identity confusion. The danger is role diffusion. Erikson stated:

> Where this is based on a strong previous doubt to one's sexual identity, delinquent and outright psychotic incidents are not uncommon. If diagnosed and treated correctly, those incidents do not have the same fatal significance that they have at other ages. It is primarily the inability to settle on an occupational identity that disturbs young persons. Keeping themselves together, they temporarily overidentify, to the point of apparent complete loss of identity, with the heroes of cliques and crowds.

Other disorders during the stage of identity versus role diffusion include conduct disorder, disruptive behavior disorder, gender identity disorder, schizophreniform disorder, and other psychotic disorders. The ability to leave home and live independently is an important task during this period. An inability to separate from the parent and prolonged dependence may occur.

Intimacy

The successful formation of a stable marriage and family depends on the capacity to become intimate. The years of early adulthood are crucial for deciding whether to get married and to whom. Gender identity determines object choice, either heterosexual or homosexual, but making an intimate connection with another person is a major task. Persons with schizoid personality disorder remain isolated from others because of fear, suspicion, the inability to take risks, or the lack of a capacity to love.

Generativity. From about 40 to 65 years, the period of middle adulthood, specific disorders are less clearly defined than in the other stages described by Erikson. Persons who are middle aged show a higher incidence of depression than younger adults, which may be related to middle-aged persons' disappointments and failed expectations as they review the past, consider their lives, and contemplate the future. The increased use of alcohol and other psychoactive substances also occurs during this time.

Integrity. Anxiety disorders often develop in older persons. In Erikson's formulation, this development may be related to persons' looking back on their lives with a sense of panic. Time has run out, and chances are used up. The decline in physical functions can contribute to psychosomatic illness, hypochondriasis, and depression. The suicide rate is highest in persons over the age of 65. Persons facing dying and death may find it intolerable not to have been generative or able to make significant attachments in life. Integrity, for Erikson, is characterized by an acceptance of life. Without acceptance, persons feel despair and hopelessness that can result in severe depressive disorders.

TREATMENT

Although no independent eriksonian psychoanalytic school exists in the same way that freudian and jungian schools do, Erikson made many important contributions to the therapeutic process. Among his most important contributions is his belief that establishing a state of trust between doctor and patient is the basic requirement for successful therapy. When psychopathology stems from basic mistrust (e.g., depression), a patient must reestablish trust with the therapist, whose task, as that of the good mother, is to be sensitive to the patient's needs. The therapist must have a sense of personal trustworthiness that can be transmitted to the patient.

Techniques

For Erikson, a psychoanalyst is not a blank slate in the therapeutic process, as he or she commonly is in freudian psychoanalysis. To the contrary, effective therapy requires that therapists actively convey to patients the belief that they are understood. This is done through both empathetic listening and by verbal assurances, which enable a positive transference built on mutual trust to develop.

Beginning as an analyst for children, Erikson tried to provide this mutuality and trust while he observed children recreating their own worlds by structuring dolls, blocks, vehicles, and miniature furniture into the dramatic situations that were bothering them. Then, Erikson correlated his observations with statements by the children and their family members. He began treatment of a child only after eating an evening meal with the entire family, and his therapy was usually conducted with much cooperation from the family. After each regressive episode in the treatment of a schizophrenic child, for instance, Erikson discussed with every member of the family what had been going on with them before the episode. Only when he was thoroughly satisfied that he had identified the problem did treatment begin. Erikson sometimes provided corrective information to the child—for instance, telling a boy who could not release his feces and had made himself ill from constipation that food is not an unborn infant.

Erikson often turned to play, which, along with specific recommendations to parents, proved fruitful as a treatment modality. Play, for Erikson, is diagnostically revealing and thus helpful for a therapist who seeks to promote a cure, but it is also curative in its own right. Play is a function of the ego and gives children a chance to synchronize social and bodily processes with the self. Children playing with blocks or adults playing out an imagined dramatic situation can manipulate the environment and develop the sense of control that the ego needs. Play therapy is not the same for children and adults, however. Children create models in an effort to gain control of reality; they look ahead to new areas of mastery. Adults use play to correct the past and to redeem their failures.

Mutuality, which is important in Erikson's system of health, is also vital to a cure. Erikson applauded Freud for the moral choice of abandoning hypnosis, because hypnosis heightens both the demarcation between the healer and the sick and the inequality that Erikson compares with the inequality of child and adult. Erikson urged that the relationship of the healer to the sick person be one of equals "in which the observer who has learned to observe himself teaches the observed to become self-observant."

Dreams and Free Association

As with Freud, Erikson worked with the patient's associations to the dream as the "best leads" to understanding the dream's meaning. He valued the first association to the dream, which he believed to be powerful and important. Ultimately, Erikson listened for "a central theme which, once found, gives added meaning to all the associated material."

Erikson believed that interpretation was the primary therapeutic agent, sought as much by the patient as by the therapist. He emphasized free-floating attention as the method that enabled discovery to occur. Erikson once described this attentional stance by commenting that in clinical work, "You need a history and you need a theory, and then you must forget them both and let each hour stand for itself." This frees both parties from counterproductive pressures to advance in the therapy and allows them both to notice the gaps in the patient's narrative that signal the unconscious.

Goals

Erikson discussed four dimensions of the psychoanalyst's job. The patient's desire to be cured and the analyst's desire to cure is the first dimension. Mutuality exists in that patient and therapist are motivated by cure, and labor is divided. The goal is always to help the patient's ego get stronger and cure itself. The second dimension Erikson called objectivity-participation. Therapists must keep their minds open. "Neuroses change," wrote Erikson. New generalizations must be made and arranged in new configurations. The third dimension runs along the axis of knowledge-participation. The therapist "applies selected insights to more strictly experimental approaches." The fourth dimension is tolerance-indignation. Erikson stated: "Identities based on Talmudic argument, on messianic zeal, on punitive orthodoxy, on faddist sensationalism, on professional and social ambition" are harmful and tend to control patients. Control widens the gap of inequality between the doctor and the patient and makes realization of the recurrent idea in Erikson's thought—mutuality—difficult.

According to Erikson, therapists have the opportunity to work through past unresolved conflicts in the therapeutic relationship. Erikson encouraged therapists not to shy away from guiding patients; he believes that therapists must offer patients both prohibitions and permissions. Nor should therapists be so engrossed in patients' past life experiences that current conflicts are overlooked.

The goal of therapy is to recognize how patients have passed through the various stages of the life cycle and how the various crises in each stage have or have not been mastered. Equally important, future stages and crises must be anticipated, so that they can be negotiated and mastered appropriately. Unlike Freud, Erikson does not believe that the personality is so inflexible that change cannot occur in middle and late adulthood. For Erikson, psychological growth and development occur throughout the entire span of the life cycle.

The Austen Riggs Center in Stockbridge, Massachusetts, is a repository of Erikson's work and many of his theories are put into practice there. Erik's wife, Joan, developed an activities program at the Austen Riggs Center as an "interpretation-free zone" where patients could take up work roles or function as students with artists and craftspersons, without the burden of the patient role. This workspace encouraged the play and creativity required for the patients' work development to parallel the process of their therapy.

References

Brown C, Lowis MJ. Psychosocial development in the elderly: An investigation into Erikson's ninth stage. *J Aging Stud.* 2003;17:415–426.

Capps D. The decades of life: Relocating Erikson's stages. *Pastoral Psychology.* 2004;53:3–32.

Chodorow NJ. The American independent tradition: Loweward Erikson, and the (possible) rise of intersubjective ego psychology. *Psychoanal Dialogues.* 2004;14:207–232.

Crawford TN, Cohen P, Johnson JG, Sneed JR, Brook JS. The course and psychosocial correlates of personality disorder symptoms in adolescence: Erikson's developmental theory revisited. *J Youth Adolesc.* 2004;33(5):373–387.

Friedman LJ. Erik Erikson on identity, generativity, and pseudospeciation: A biographer's perspective. *Psychoanalytic History.* 2001;3:179.

Hoare CH. Erikson's general and adult developmental revisions of Freudian thought: "Outward, forward, upward". *Journal of Adult Development.* 2005;12:19–31.

Newton DS. Erik H. Erikson. In: Sadock BJ, Sadock VA, eds. *Kaplan & Sadock's Comprehensive Textbook of Psychiatry.* 8th ed. Vol. 1. Baltimore: Lippincott Williams & Wilkins; 2005:746.

Pietikainen P, Ihanus J. On the origins of psychoanalytic psychohistory. *Historical Psychology.* 2003;6:171.

Shapiro ER, Fromm MG. Eriksonian clinical theory and psychiatric treatment. In: Sadock BJ, Sadock VA, eds. *Comprehensive Textbook of Psychiatry.* Ed. 7. New York: Lippincott Williams & Wilkins; 2000.

Slater C. Generativity versus stagnation: An elaboration of Erikson's adult stage of human development. *Journal of Adult Development.* 2003;10:53.

Van Hiel A, Mervielde I, De Fruyt F. Stagnation and generativity: Structure, validity, and differential relationships with adaptive and maladaptive personality. *J Pers.* 2006;74(2):543.

Westermeyer JF. Predictors and characteristics of Erikson's life cycle model among men: A 32-year longitudinal study. *Int J Aging Hum Dev.* 2004;58:29–48.

Wulff D. Freud and Freudians on religion: A reader. *Int. J. of Psychol and Rel.* 2003;13:223.

▲ 6.3 Schools Derived from Psychoanalysis and Psychology

At various stages in the evolution of psychoanalysis, several of Freud's colleagues expanded or revised his formulations. At times, these modifications were subsequently incorporated into the body of psychoanalytic theory. Other innovations produced schisms within the Freudian movement, however, and, in some instances, led to the establishment of new schools of psychoanalysis.

Among the most prominent of these early "dissenters" were Alfred Adler and Carl Jung, both of whom rejected Freud's belief that sexuality plays a unique role in normal and pathological human behavior. Jung's rejection of Freud's libido theory led to the elaboration of a rather mystical psychoanalytic system. Adler turned to the sociocultural determinants of behavior. Social, cultural, and interpersonal behavioral determinants were also emphasized in the so-called "culturalist" theories of Sandor Rado, Karen Horney, Harry Sack Sullivan, and Eric Fromm. And concomitantly, these workers deemphasized the biological instinctual drives, particularly sexuality, as dominant determinants of behavior.

Other theories of psychopathology did not evolve as direct offshoots of freudian psychoanalysis. Among these is the theory of Adolf Meyer, who conceived of normal as well as abnormal behavior as deriving from a series of adaptive reactions to the environment.

Other theories of personality derive from various aspects of psychology, such as learning theory and the quantitative methods of personality assessment. No attempt has been made to present a comprehensive survey of this field. Rather, those theories selected for discussion are those considered most relevant for psychiatry.

Brief synopses of the theories that exert the greatest influence on current psychiatric thought are listed below in alphabetical order of their proponent. Each of these theories contains insights that merit consideration because they enhance our understanding of the complexities of human behavior. They also illustrate the diversity of theoretical orientation that characterizes psychiatry today.

KARL ABRAHAM (1877–1925)

Karl Abraham, one of Sigmund Freud's earliest disciples, was the first psychoanalyst in Germany. He is best known for his explication of depression from a psychoanalytic perspective and for his elaboration of Freud's stages of psychosexual development. Abraham divided the oral stage into a biting phase and a sucking phase; the anal stage into a destructive-expulsive (anal-sadistic) phase and a mastering-retentive (anal-erotic) phase; and the phallic stage into an early phase of partial genital love (true phallic phase) and a later mature genital phase. Abraham also linked the psychosexual stages to specific syndromes. For example, he postulated that obsessional neurosis resulted from fixation at the anal-sadistic phase, and depression from fixation at the oral stage.

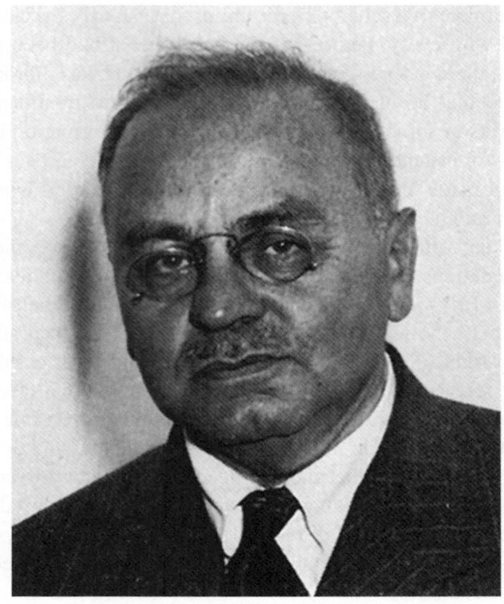

FIGURE 6.3–1
Alfred Adler. (Reprinted from Carson RC, Butcher JN, Coleman JC. Eds. *Abnormal Psychology and Modern Life*. 8th ed. Illinois: Scott, Foresman and Company; 1988:78, with permission.)

ALFRED ADLER (1870–1937)

Alfred Adler (Fig. 6.3–1) was born in Vienna, Austria, where he spent most of his life. A general physician, he became one of the original four members of Freud's circle in 1902. Adler never accepted the primacy of the libido theory, the sexual origin of neurosis, or the importance of infantile wishes. Adler thought that aggression was far more important, specifically in its manifestation as a striving for power, which he believed to be a masculine trait. He introduced the term *masculine protest* to describe the tendency to move from a passive, feminine role to a masculine, active role. Adler's theories are collectively known as *individual psychology*.

Adler coined the term *inferiority complex* to refer to a sense of inadequacy and weakness that is universal and inborn. A developing child's self-esteem is compromised by a physical defect, and Adler referred to this phenomenon as *organ inferiority*. He also thought that a basic inferiority tied to children's oedipal longings could never be gratified.

Adler was one of the first developmental theorists to recognize the importance of children's birth order in their families of origin. The firstborn child reacts with anger to the birth of siblings and struggles against giving up the powerful position of only child. The second-born child must constantly strive to compete with the firstborn. Adler thought that a child's sibling position results in lifelong influences on character and lifestyle.

The primary therapeutic approach in adlerian therapy is encouragement, through which Adler believed his patients could overcome feelings of inferiority. Consistent human relatedness, in his view, leads to greater hope, less isolation, and greater affiliation with society. He believed that patients needed to develop a greater sense of their own dignity and worth and renewed appreciation of their abilities and strengths.

FRANZ ALEXANDER (1891–1964)

Franz Alexander (Fig. 6.3–2) emigrated from his native Germany to the United States, where he settled in Chicago and founded

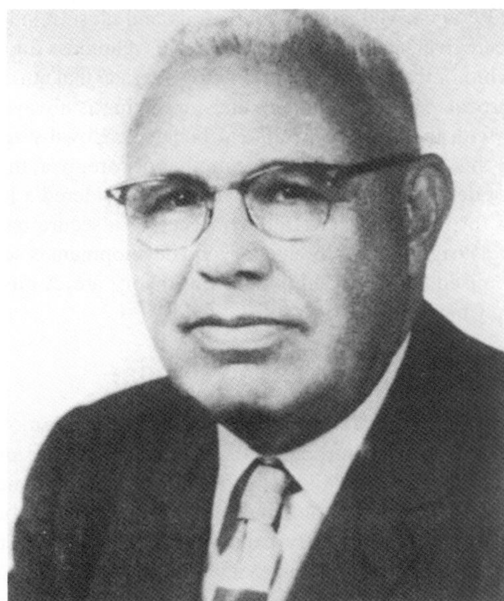

FIGURE 6.3–2
Franz Alexander. (Courtesy of Franz Alexander.)

the Chicago Institute for Psychoanalysis. He wrote extensively about the association between specific personality traits and certain psychosomatic ailments, a point of view that came to be known as the *specificity hypothesis*. Alexander fell out of favor with classic analysts for advocating the *corrective emotional experience* as part of analytic technique. In this approach, Alexander suggested that an analyst must deliberately adopt a particular mode of relatedness with a patient to counteract noxious childhood influences from the patient's parents. He believed that the trusting, supportive relationship between patient and analyst enabled the patient to master childhood traumas and to grow from the experience.

GORDON ALLPORT (1897–1967)

Gordon Allport (Fig. 6.3–3), a psychologist in the United States, is known as the founder of the humanistic school of psychology, which holds that each person has an inherent potential for autonomous function and growth. At Harvard University, he taught the first course in the psychology of personality offered at a college in the United States.

Allport believed that a person's only real guarantee of personal existence is a sense of self. Selfhood develops through a series of stages, from awareness of the body to self-identity. Allport used the term *propriem* to describe strivings related to maintenance of self-identity and self-esteem. He used the term *traits* to refer to the chief units of personality structure. *Personal dispositions* are individual traits that represent the essence of an individual's unique personality. Maturity is characterized by a capacity to relate to others with warmth and intimacy and an expanded sense of self. In Allport's view, mature persons have security, humor, insight, enthusiasm, and zest. Psychotherapy is geared to helping patients realize these characteristics.

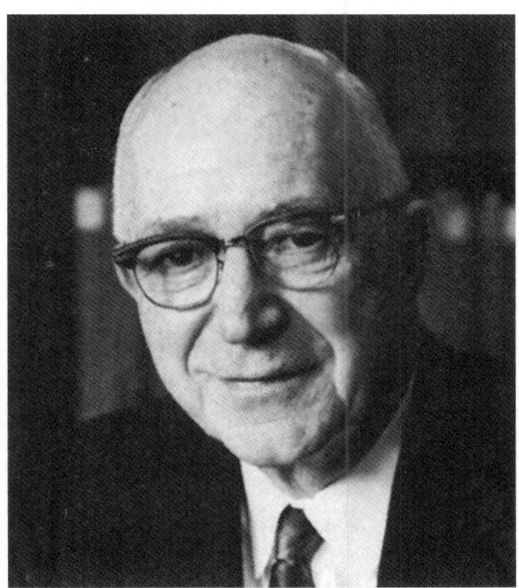

FIGURE 6.3–3
Gordon Allport. (Reprinted from Carson RC, Butcher JN, Coleman JC. Eds. *Abnormal Psychology and Modern Life*. 8th ed. Illinois: Scott, Foresman and Company; 1988:74, with permission.)

MICHAEL BALINT (1896–1970)

Michael Balint was considered a member of the independent or middle group of object relations theorists in the United Kingdom. Balint believed that the urge for the primary love object underlies virtually all psychological phenomena. Infants wish to be loved totally and unconditionally, and when a mother is not forthcoming with appropriate nurturance, a child devotes his or her life to a search for the love missed in childhood. According to Balint, the *basic fault* is the feeling of many patients that something is missing. As with Ronald Fairbairn and Donald W. Winnicott, Balint understood this deficit in internal structure to result from maternal failures. He viewed all psychological motivations as stemming from the failure to receive adequate maternal love.

Unlike Fairbairn, however, Balint did not entirely abandon drive theory. He suggested that libido, for example, is both pleasure seeking and object seeking. He also worked with seriously disturbed patients, and like Winnicott, he thought that certain aspects of psychoanalytic treatment occur at a more profound level than that of the ordinary verbal explanatory interpretations. Although some material involving genital psychosexual stages of development can be interpreted from the perspective of intrapsychic conflict, Balint believed that certain preverbal phenomena are reexperienced in analysis and that the relationship itself is decisive in dealing with this realm of early experience.

ERIC BERNE (1910–1970)

Eric Berne (Fig. 6.3–4) began his professional life as a training and supervising analyst in classic psychoanalytic theory and technique, but ultimately developed his own school, known as *transactional analysis*. A *transaction* is a stimulus presented by one person that evokes a corresponding response in another. Berne defined psychological games as stereotyped and predictable transactions that persons learn in childhood and continue to play throughout their lives. *Strokes*, the basic motivating factors of human behavior, consist of specific rewards, such as

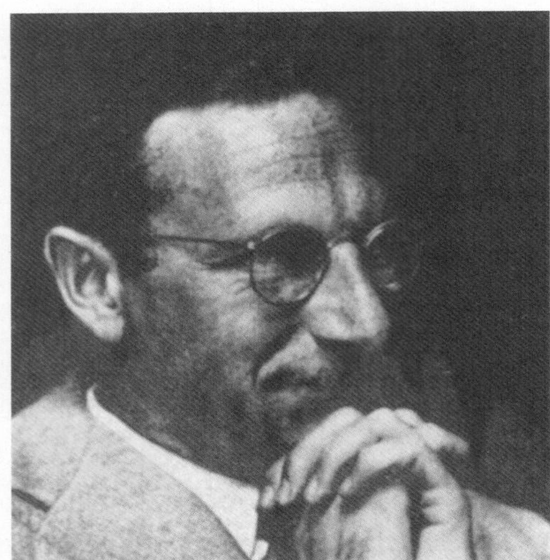

FIGURE 6.3–4
Eric Berne. (Courtesy of Wide World Photos.)

approval and love. All persons have three ego states that exist within them: the *child*, which represents primitive elements that become fixed in early childhood; the *adult*, which is the part of the personality capable of objective appraisals of reality; and the *parent*, which is an introject of the values of a person's actual parents. The therapeutic process is geared toward helping patients understand whether they are functioning in the child, adult, or parent mode in their interactions with others. As patients learn to recognize characteristic games played again and again throughout life, they can ultimately function in the adult mode as much as possible in interpersonal relationships.

WILFRED BION (1897–1979)

Wilfred Bion expanded Melanie Klein's concept of *projective identification* to include an interpersonal process in which a therapist feels coerced by a patient into playing a particular role in the patient's internal world. He also developed the notion that the therapist must contain what the patient has projected so that it is processed and returned to the patient in modified form. Bion believed that a similar process occurs between mother and infant. He also observed that "psychotic" and "nonpsychotic" aspects of the mind function simultaneously as suborganizations. Bion is probably best known for his application of psychoanalytic ideas to groups. Whenever a group gets derailed from its task, it deteriorates into one of three basic states: dependency, pairing, or fight-flight.

JOHN BOWLBY (1907–1990)

John Bowlby is generally considered the founder of attachment theory. He formed his ideas about attachment in the 1950s while he was consulting with the World Health Organization (WHO) on the problems of homelessness in children. He stressed that the essence of attachment is *proximity* (i.e., the tendency of a child to stay close to the mother or caregiver). His theory of the mother–infant bond was firmly rooted in biology and drew extensively from ethology and evolutionary theory. A basic sense of security and safety is derived from a continuous and close relationship with a caregiver, according to Bowlby. This readiness for attachment is biologically driven, and Bowlby stressed that attachment is reciprocal. Maternal bonding and caregiving is always intertwined with the child's attachment behavior. Bowlby felt that without this early proximity to the mother or caregiver, the child does not develop a *secure base*, which he considered a launching pad for independence. In the absence of a secure base, the child feels frightened or threatened, and development is severely compromised. Bowlby and attachment theory are discussed in detail in Chapter 4, Section 4.2.

RAYMOND CATTELL (1905–1998)

Raymond Cattell obtained his Ph.D. in England before moving to the United States. He introduced the use of *multivariate analysis* and *factor analysis*—statistical procedures that simultaneously examine the relations among multiple variables and factors—to the study of personality. By examining a person's life record objectively, using personal interviewing and questionnaire data, Cattell described a variety of traits that represent the building blocks of personality.

Traits are both biologically based and environmentally determined or learned. Biological traits include sex, gregariousness, aggression, and parental protectiveness. Environmentally learned traits include cultural ideas, such as work, religion, intimacy, romance, and identity. An important concept is the *law of coercion* to the biosocial mean, which holds that society exerts pressure on genetically different persons to conform to social norms. For example, a person with a strong genetic tendency toward dominance is likely to receive social encouragement for restraint, whereas the naturally submissive person will be encouraged toward self-assertion.

RONALD FAIRBAIRN (1889–1964)

Ronald Fairbairn, a Scottish analyst who worked most of his life in relative isolation, was one of the major psychoanalytic theorists in the British school of object relations. He suggested that infants are not primarily motivated by the drives of libido and aggression but are by an object-seeking instinct. Fairbairn replaced the freudian ideas of energy, ego, and id with the notion of *dynamic structures*. When an infant encounters frustration, a portion of the ego is defensively split off in the course of development and functions as an entity in relation to internal objects and to other subdivisions of the ego. He also stressed that both an object and an object *relationship* are internalized during development, so that a self is always in relationship to an object, and the two are connected with an affect.

SÁNDOR FERENCZI (1873–1933)

Although Sándor Ferenczi, a Hungarian analyst, had been analyzed by Freud and was influenced by him, he later discarded Freud's techniques and introduced his own method of analysis. He understood the symptoms of his patients as related to sexual and physical abuse in childhood and proposed that analysts need to love their patients in a way that compensates them for the love they did not receive as children. He developed a procedure known as *active therapy*, in which he encouraged patients to develop an awareness of reality through active confrontation by the therapist. He also experimented with *mutual analysis*, in

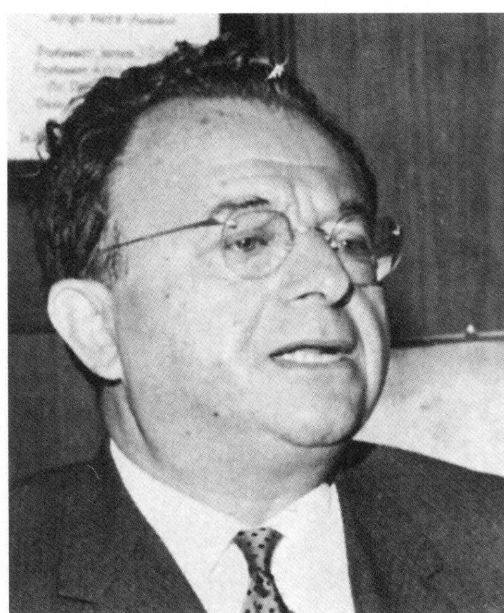

FIGURE 6.3–5
Erich Fromm. (Reprinted from Carson RC, Butcher JN, Coleman JC. Eds. *Abnormal Psychology and Modern Life.* 8th ed. Illinois: Scott, Foresman and Company; 1988:78, with permission.)

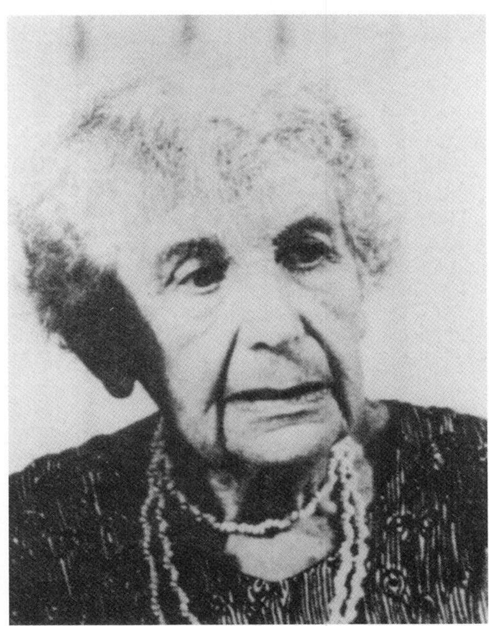

FIGURE 6.3–6
Anna Freud. (From Carson RC, Butcher JN, Coleman JC. *Abnormal Psychology and Modern Life.* 8th ed. Illinois: Scott, Foresman; 1988:66, with permission.)

which he would analyze his patient for a session and then allow the patient to analyze him for a session.

ERICH FROMM (1900–1980)

Erich Fromm (Fig. 6.3–5) came to the United States in 1933 from Germany, where he had received his Ph.D. He was instrumental in founding the William Alanson White Institute for Psychiatry in New York. Fromm identified five character types that are common to, and determined by, Western culture; each person may possess qualities from one or more types. The types are (1) the *receptive personality* is passive; (2) the *exploitative personality* is manipulative; (3) the *marketing personality* is opportunistic and changeable; (4) the *hoarding personality* saves and stores; and (5) the *productive personality* is mature and enjoys love and work. The therapeutic process involves strengthening the person's sense of ethical behavior toward others and developing productive love, which is characterized by care, responsibility, and respect for other persons.

ANNA FREUD (1895–1982)

Anna Freud (Fig. 6.3–6), the daughter of Sigmund Freud, ultimately made her own set of unique contributions to psychoanalysis. While her father focused primarily on repression as the central defense mechanism, Anna Freud greatly elaborated on individual defense mechanisms, including reaction formation, regression, undoing, introjection, identification, projection, turning against the self, reversal, and sublimation. She was also a key figure in the development of modern ego psychology in that she emphasized that there was "depth in the surface." The defenses marshaled by the ego to avoid unacceptable wishes from the id were in and of themselves complex and worthy of attention. Up to that point, the primary focus had been on uncovering unconscious sexual and aggressive wishes. She also made seminal contributions to the field of child psychoanalysis and studied the function of the ego in personality development. She founded the Hampstead child therapy course and clinic in London in 1947 and served as its director.

KURT GOLDSTEIN (1878–1965)

Kurt Goldstein (Fig. 6.3–7) was born in Germany and received his M.D. from the University of Breslau. He was influenced by existentialism and Gestalt psychology—every organism has dynamic properties, which are energy supplies that are relatively constant and evenly distributed. When states of tension-disequilibrium occur, an organism automatically attempts to return to its normal state. What happens in one part of the organism affects every other part, a phenomenon known as *holocoenosis.*

Self-actualization was a concept Goldstein used to describe persons' creative powers to fulfill their potentialities. Because each person has a different set of innate potentialities, persons strive for self-actualization along different paths. Sickness severely disrupts self-actualization. Responses to disruption of an organism's integrity may be rigid and compulsive; regression to more primitive modes of behavior is characteristic. One of Goldstein's major contributions was his identification of the *catastrophic reaction* to brain damage, in which a person becomes fearful and agitated and refuses to perform simple tasks because of the fear of possible failure.

KAREN HORNEY (1885–1952)

Born and educated in Germany, Karen Horney (Fig. 6.3–8) taught at the Institute of Psychoanalysis in Berlin before immigrating to the United States. Horney believed that a person's current personality attributes result from the interaction between the person and the environment and are not solely based on infantile

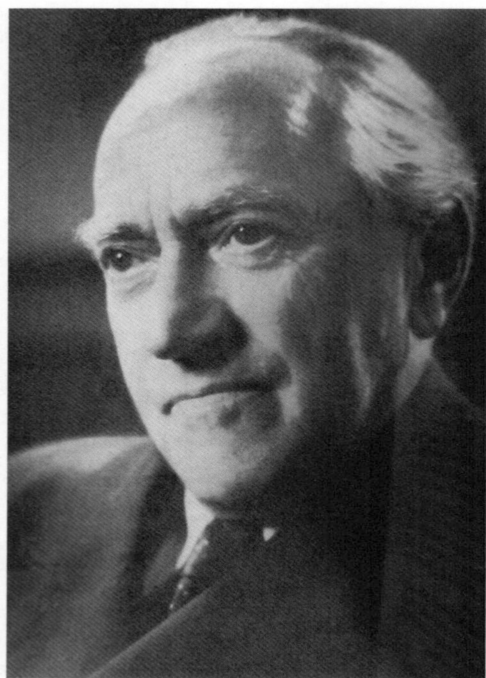

FIGURE 6.3–7
Kurt Goldstein. (Courtesy of New York Academy of Medicine, New York.)

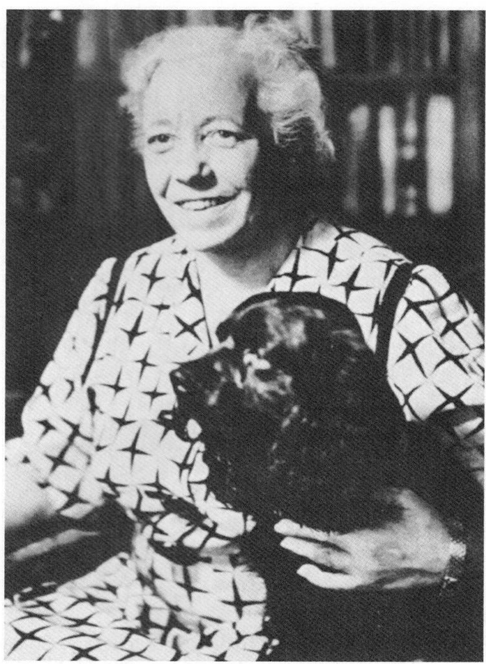

FIGURE 6.3–8
Karen Horney. (Courtesy of the Association for the Advancement of Psychoanalysis, New York.)

libidinal strivings carried over from childhood. Her theory, known as *holistic psychology*, maintains that a person needs to be seen as a unitary whole who influences, and is influenced by, the environment. She thought that the Oedipus complex was overvalued in terms of its contribution to adult psychopathology, but she also believed that rigid parental attitudes about sexuality led to excessive concern with the genitals.

She proposed three separate concepts of the self: the *actual self*, the sum total of a person's experience; the *real self*, the harmonious, healthy person; and the *idealized self*, the neurotic expectation or glorified image that a person feels he or she should be. A person's *pride system* alienates him or her from the real self by overemphasizing prestige, intellect, power, strength, appearance, sexual prowess, and other qualities that can lead to self-effacement and self-hatred. Horney also established the concepts of *basic anxiety* and *basic trust*. The therapeutic process, in her view, aims for *self-realization* by exploring distorting influences that prevent the personality from growing.

EDITH JACOBSON (1897–1978)

Edith Jacobson, a psychiatrist in the United States, believed that the structural model and an emphasis on object relations are not fundamentally incompatible. She thought that the ego, self-images, and object images exert reciprocal influences on each other's development. She also stressed that the infant's disappointment with the maternal object is not necessarily related to the mother's actual failure. In Jacobson's view, disappointment is related to a specific, drive-determined demand, rather than to a global striving for contact or engagement. She viewed an infant's experience of pleasure or "unpleasure" as the core of the early mother–infant relationship. Satisfactory experiences lead to the formation of good or gratifying images, whereas unsatisfactory experiences create bad or frustrating images. Normal and pathological development is based on the evolution of these self-images and object images. Jacobson believed that the concept of *fixation* refers to modes of object relatedness, rather than to modes of gratification.

CARL GUSTAV JUNG (1875–1961)

Carl Gustav Jung (Fig. 6.3–9), a Swiss psychiatrist, formed a psychoanalytic school known as *analytic psychology*, which includes basic ideas related to, but going beyond, Freud's theories. After initially being Freud's disciple, Jung broke with Freud over the latter's emphasis on infantile sexuality. He expanded on Freud's concept of the unconscious by describing the *collective unconscious* as consisting of all humankind's common, shared mythological and symbolic past. The collective unconscious includes *archetypes*—representational images and configurations with universal symbolic meanings. Archetypal figures exist for the mother, father, child, and hero, among others. Archetypes contribute to *complexes*, feeling-toned ideas that develop as a result of personal experience interacting with archetypal imagery. Thus, a mother complex is determined not only by the mother–child interaction but also by the conflict between archetypal expectation and actual experience with the real woman who functions in a motherly role.

Jung noted that there are two types of personality organizations: introversion and extroversion. *Introverts* focus on their inner world of thoughts, intuitions, emotions, and sensations; *extroverts* are more oriented toward the outer world, other persons, and material goods. Each person has a mixture of both components. The *persona*, the mask covering the personality, is the face a person presents to the outside world. The persona may become fixed, and the real person hidden from himself or

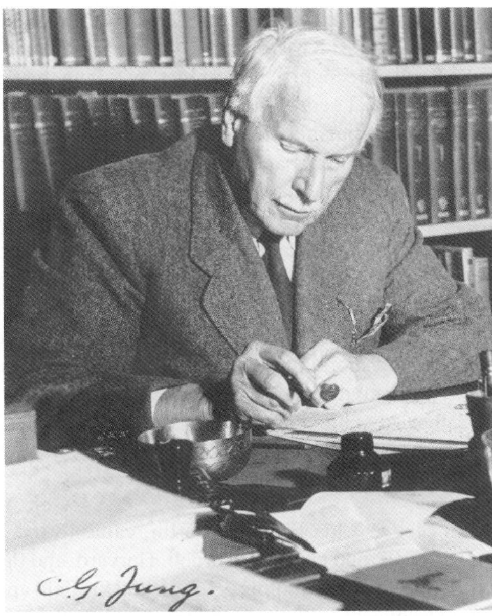

FIGURE 6.3–9
Carl Gustave Jung (print includes signature). (Courtesy of National Library of Medicine, Bethesda, MD.)

herself. *Anima* and *animus* are unconscious traits possessed by men and women, respectively, and are contrasted with the persona. *Anima* refers to a man's undeveloped femininity, whereas *animus* refers to a woman's undeveloped masculinity.

The aim of jungian treatment is to bring about an adequate adaptation to reality, which involves a person's fulfilling his or her creative potentialities. The ultimate goal is to achieve *individuation*, a process continuing throughout life whereby persons develop a unique sense of their own identity. This developmental process may lead them down new paths away from their previous directions in life.

OTTO KERNBERG (B. 1928)

Otto Kernberg is perhaps the most influential object relations theorist in the United States. Influenced by both Klein and Jacobson, much of his theory is derived from his clinical work with patients who have borderline personality disorder. Kernberg places great emphasis on the splitting of the ego and the elaboration of good and bad self-configurations and object configurations. Although he has continued to use the structural model, he views the id as composed of self-images, object images, and their associated affects. Drives appear to manifest themselves only in the context of internalized interpersonal experience. Good and bad self-representations and object relations become associated, respectively, with libido and aggression. Object relations constitute the building blocks of both structure and drives. Goodness and badness in relational experiences precede drive cathexis. The dual instincts of libido and aggression arise from object-directed affective states of love and hate.

Kernberg proposed the term *borderline personality organization* for a broad spectrum of patients characterized by a lack of an integrated sense of identity, ego weakness, absence of superego integration, reliance on primitive defense mechanisms such as splitting and projective identification, and a tendency to shift into primary process thinking. He suggested a specific type of psychoanalytic psychotherapy for such patients in which transference issues are interpreted early in the process.

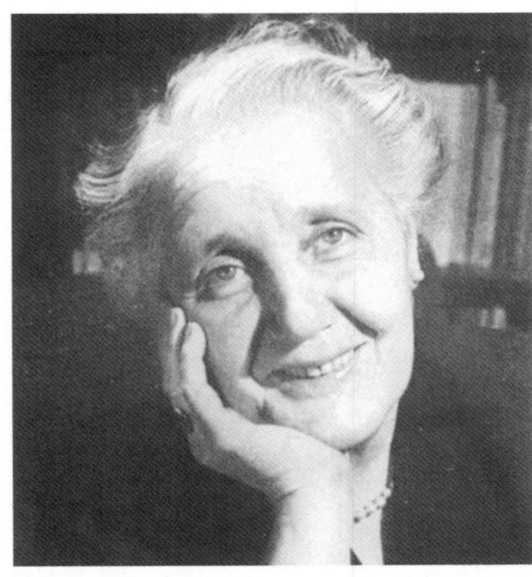

FIGURE 6.3–10
Melanie Klein. (Courtesy of Melanie Klein and Douglas Glass.)

MELANIE KLEIN (1882–1960)

Melanie Klein (Fig. 6.3–10) was born in Vienna, worked with Abraham and Ferenczi, and later moved to London. Klein evolved a theory of internal object relations that was intimately linked to drives. Her unique perspective grew largely from her psychoanalytic work with children, in which she became impressed with the role of unconscious intrapsychic fantasy. She postulated that the ego undergoes a splitting process to deal with the terror of annihilation. She also thought that Freud's concept of the death instinct was central to understanding aggression, hatred, sadism, and other forms of "badness," all of which she viewed as derivatives of the death instinct.

Klein viewed projection and introjection as the primary defensive operations in the first months of life. Infants project derivatives of the death instinct into the mother and then fear attack from the "bad mother," a phenomenon that Klein referred to as *persecutory anxiety*. This anxiety is intimately associated with the *paranoid-schizoid position*, infants' mode of organizing experience in which all aspects of infant and mother are split into good and bad elements. As the disparate views are integrated, infants become concerned that they may have harmed or destroyed the mother through the hostile and sadistic fantasies directed toward her. At this developmental point, children have arrived at the *depressive position*, in which the mother is viewed ambivalently as having both positive and negative aspects and as the target of a mixture of loving and hateful feelings. Klein was also instrumental in the development of child analysis, which evolved from an analytic play technique in which children used toys and played in a symbolic fashion that allowed analysts to interpret the play.

HEINZ KOHUT (1913–1981)

Heinz Kohut (Fig. 6.3–11) is best known for his writings on narcissism and the development of self-psychology. He viewed the development and maintenance of self-esteem and self-cohesion as more important than sexuality or aggression. Kohut described Freud's concept of narcissism as judgmental, in that development was supposed to proceed toward object relatedness and away from narcissism. He conceived of two separate lines of

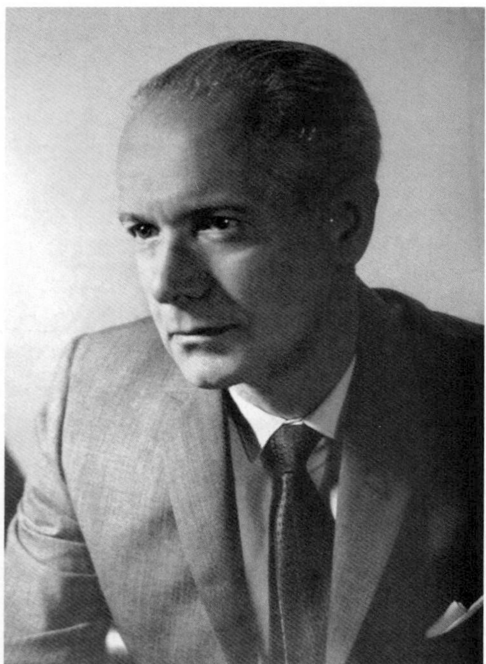

FIGURE 6.3–11
Heinz Kohut. (Courtesy of New York Academy of Medicine, New York.)

development, one moving in the direction of object relatedness and the other in the direction of greater enhancement of the self.

In infancy, children fear losing the protection of the early mother–infant bliss and resort to one of three pathways to save the lost perfection: the grandiose self, the alter ego or twinship, and the idealized parental image. These three poles of the self manifest themselves in psychoanalytic treatment in terms of characteristic transferences, known as *self-object transferences*. The *grandiose self* leads to a *mirror transference*, in which patients attempt to capture the gleam in the analyst's eye through exhibitionistic self-display. The *alter ego* leads to the *twinship transference*, in which patients perceive the analyst as a twin. The *idealized parental image* leads to an *idealizing transference*, in which patients feel enhanced self-esteem by being in the presence of the exalted figure of the analyst.

Kohut suggested that empathic failures in the mother lead to a developmental arrest at a particular stage when children need to use others to perform self-object functions. Although Kohut originally applied this formulation to narcissistic personality disorder, he later expanded it to apply to all psychopathology.

JACQUES LACAN (1901–1981)

Born in Paris and trained as a psychiatrist, Jacques Lacan founded his own institute, the Freudian School of Paris. He attempted to integrate the intrapsychic concepts of Freud with concepts related to linguistics and semiotics (the study of language and symbols). Whereas Freud saw the unconscious as a seething cauldron of needs, wishes, and instincts, Lacan saw it as a sort of language that helps to structure the world. His two principal concepts are that the unconscious is structured as a language and the unconscious is a discourse. Primary process thoughts are actually uncontrolled free-flowing sequences of meaning. Symptoms are signs or symbols of underlying processes. The role of the therapist is to interpret the semiotic text of the personality structure. Lacan's most basic phase is the mirror stage; it is here that infants learn to recognize themselves by taking the perspective of others. In that sense, the ego is not part of the self but, rather, is something outside of, and viewed by, the self. The ego comes to represent parents and society more than it represents the actual self of the person.

Lacan's therapeutic approach involves the need to become less alienated from the self and more involved with others. Relationships are often fantasized, which distorts reality and must be corrected. Among his most controversial beliefs was that the resistance to understanding the real relationship with the therapist can be reduced by shortening the length of the therapy session and that psychoanalytic sessions need to be standardized not to time but, rather, to content and process.

KURT LEWIN (1890–1947)

Kurt Lewin received his Ph.D. in Berlin, came to the United States in the 1930s, and taught at Cornell, Harvard, and the Massachusetts Institute of Technology. He adapted the field approach of physics to a concept called *field theory*. A *field* is the totality of coexisting, mutually interdependent parts. Behavior becomes a function of persons and their environment, which together make up the *life space*. The life space represents a field in constant flux, with *valences* or needs that require satisfaction. A hungry person is more aware of restaurants than someone who has just eaten, and a person who wants to mail a letter is aware of mailboxes.

Lewin applied field theory to groups. *Group dynamics* refers to the interaction among members of a group, each of whom depends on the others. The group can exert pressure on a person to change behavior, but the person also influences the group when change occurs.

ABRAHAM MASLOW (1908–1970)

Abraham Maslow (Fig. 6.3–12) was born in Brooklyn, New York, and completed both his undergraduate and graduate work at the University of Wisconsin. Along with Goldstein, Maslow believed in *self-actualization theory*—the need to understand the totality of a person. A leader in humanistic psychology, Maslow described a hierarchical organization of needs present in everyone. As the more primitive needs, such as hunger and thirst, are satisfied, more advanced psychological needs, such as affection and self-esteem, become the primary motivators. Self-actualization is the highest need.

A peak experience, frequently occurring in self-actualizers, is an episodic, brief occurrence in which a person suddenly experiences a powerful transcendental state of consciousness—a sense of heightened understanding, an intense euphoria, an integrated nature, unity with the universe, and an altered perception of time and space. This powerful experience tends to occur most often in the psychologically healthy and can produce long-lasting beneficial effects.

KARL A. MENNINGER (1893–1990)

Karl A. Menninger was one of the first physicians in the United States to receive psychiatric training. With his brother, Will, he pioneered the concept of a psychiatric hospital based on psychoanalytic principles and founded the Menninger Clinic

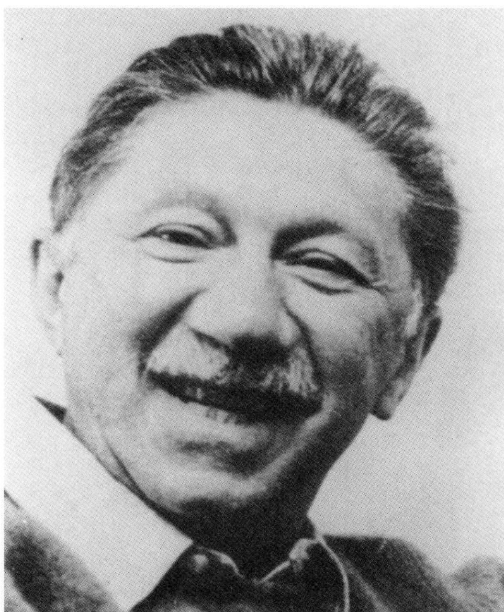

FIGURE 6.3–12
Abraham H. Maslow. (From Carson RC, Butcher JN, Coleman JC. *Abnormal Psychology and Modern Life*, 8th ed. Boston: Scott, Foresman; 1988:74, with permission. Copyright The Bettman Archive.)

in Topeka, Kansas. He also was a prolific writer; *The Human Mind*, one of his most popular books, brought psychoanalytic understanding to the lay public. He made a compelling case for the validity of Freud's death instinct in *Man Against Himself*. In *The Vital Balance*, his magnum opus, he formulated a unique theory of psychopathology. Menninger maintained a lifelong interest in the criminal justice system and argued in *The Crime of Punishment* that many convicted criminals needed treatment rather than punishment. Finally, his volume entitled *Theory of Psychoanalytic Technique* was one of the few books to examine the theoretical underpinnings of psychoanalysts' interventions.

ADOLPH MEYER (1866–1950)

Adolph Meyer (Fig. 6.3–13) came to the United States from Switzerland in 1892 and eventually became director of the psychiatric Henry Phipps Clinic of the Johns Hopkins Medical School. Not interested in metapsychology, he espoused a common sense psychobiological methodology for the study of mental disorder, emphasizing the interrelationship of symptoms and individual psychological and biological functioning. His approach to the study of personality was biographical; he attempted to bring psychiatric patients and their treatment out of isolated state hospitals and into communities and was also a strong advocate of social action for mental health. Meyer introduced the concept of *common sense psychiatry*, and focused on ways in which a patient's current life situation could be realistically improved. He coined the concept of *ergasia*, the action of the total organism. His goal in therapy was to aid patients' adjustment by helping them modify unhealthy adaptations. One of Meyer's tools was an autobiographical life chart constructed by the patient during therapy.

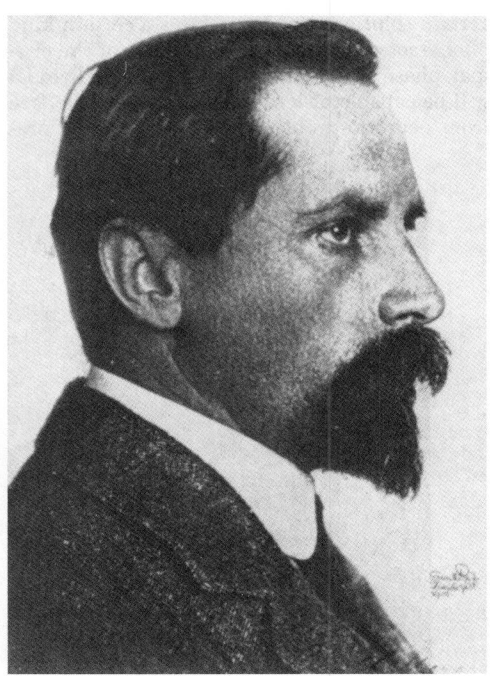

FIGURE 6.3–13
Adolf Meyer. (From the National Library of Medicine, Bethesda, MD.)

GARDNER MURPHY (1895–1979)

Gardner Murphy (Fig. 6.3–14) was born in Ohio and received his Ph.D. from Columbia University. He was among the first to publish a comprehensive history of psychology and made major contributions to social, general, and educational psychology. According to Murphy, three essential stages of personality development are the stage of undifferentiated wholeness, the stage of differentiation, and the stage of integration. This development is frequently uneven, with both regression and progression occurring along the way. The four inborn human needs are visceral, motor, sensory, and emergency-related. These needs become increasingly specific in time as they are molded by a person's experiences in various social and environmental contexts. *Canalization* brings about these changes by establishing a connection between a need and a specific way of satisfying the need.

Murphy was interested in parapsychology. States such as sleep, drowsiness, certain drug and toxic conditions, hypnosis, and delirium tend to be favorable to paranormal experiences. Impediments to paranormal awareness include various intrapsychic barriers, conditions in the general social environment, and a heavy investment in ordinary sensory experiences.

HENRY MURRAY (1893–1988)

Henry Murray (Fig. 6.3–15) was born in New York City, attended medical school at Columbia University, and was a founder of the Boston Psychoanalytic Institute. He proposed the term *personology* to describe the study of human behavior. He focused on *motivation*, a need that is aroused by internal or external stimulation; once aroused, motivation produces continued activity until the need is reduced

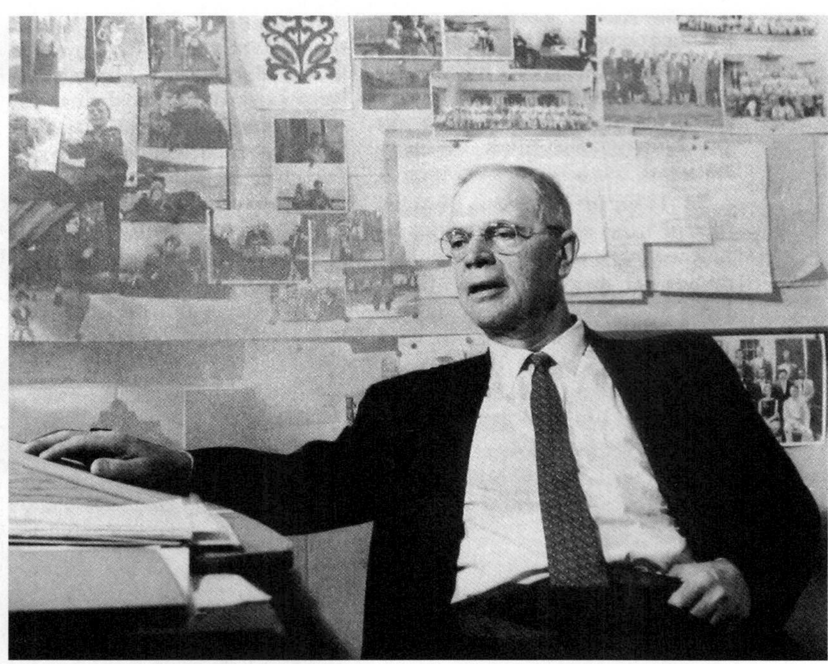

FIGURE 6.3–14
Gardner Murphy. (Courtesy of New York Academy of Medicine, New York.)

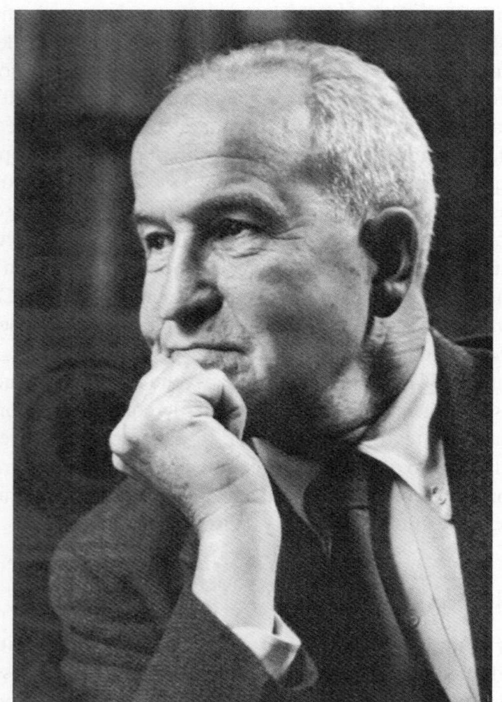

FIGURE 6.3–15
Henry Murray. (Courtesy of New York Academy of Medicine, New York.)

or satisfied. He developed the *Thematic Apperception Test* (TAT), a projective technique used to reveal both unconscious and conscious mental processes and problem areas.

FREDERICK S. PERLS (1893–1970)

Gestalt theory developed in Germany under the influence of several men: Max Wertheimer (1880–1943), Wolfgang Köhler (1887–1967), and Lewin. Frederick "Fritz" Perls (Fig. 6.3–16) applied Gestalt theory to a therapy that emphasizes the current experiences of the patient in the here and now, as contrasted to the there and then of psychoanalytic schools. In terms of motivation, patients learn to recognize their needs at any given time and the ways that the drive to satisfy these needs may influence their current behavior. According to the Gestalt point of view, behavior represents more than the sum of its parts. A *gestalt*, or a whole, both includes, and goes beyond, the sum of smaller, independent events; it deals with essential characteristics of actual experience, such as value, meaning, and form.

SANDOR RADO (1890–1972)

Sandor Rado (Fig. 6.3–17) came to the United States from Hungary in 1945 and founded the Columbia Psychoanalytic Institute in New York. His theories of *adaptational dynamics* hold that the organism is a biological system operating under hedonic control, which is somewhat similar to Freud's pleasure principle. Cultural factors often cause excessive hedonic control and disordered behavior by interfering with the organism's ability

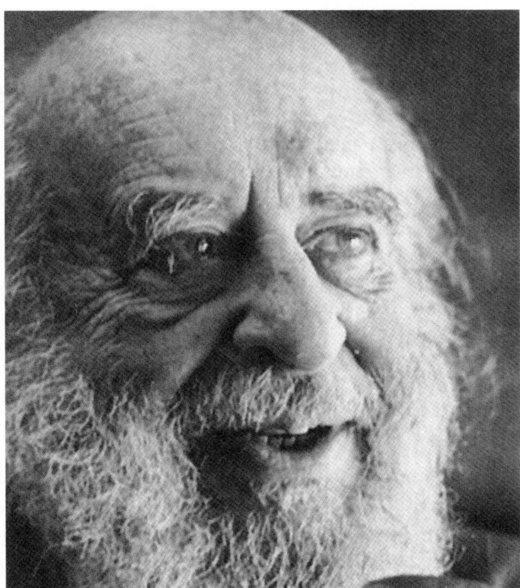

FIGURE 6.3–16
Fritz Perls. (Reprinted from Carson RC, Butcher JN, Coleman JC. Eds. *Abnormal Psychology and Modern Life.* 8th ed. Illinois: Scott, Foresman and Company; 1988:75, with permission.)

for *self-regulation*. In therapy, the patient needs to relearn how to experience pleasurable feelings.

OTTO RANK (1884–1939)

An Austrian psychologist and a protégé of Sigmund Freud, Otto Rank (Fig. 6.3–18) broke with Freud in his 1924 publication, *The Trauma of the Birth*, and developed a new theory, which he called *birth trauma*. Anxiety is correlated with separation from the mother—specifically, with separation from the womb, the source of effortless gratification. This painful experience results in primal anxiety. Sleep and dreams symbolize the return to the womb.

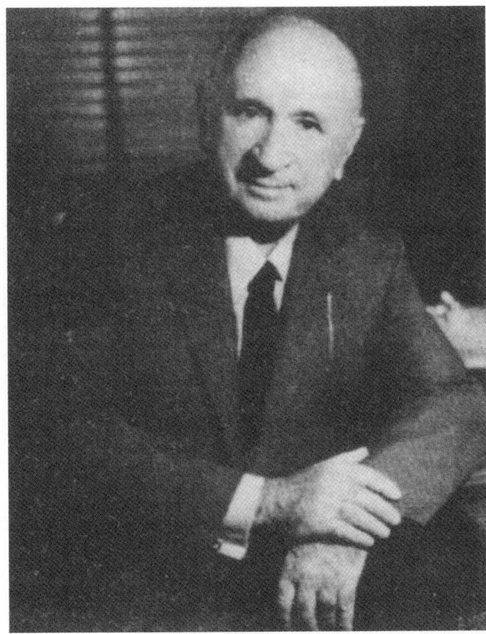

FIGURE 6.3–17
Sandor Rado. (Courtesy of New York Academy of Medicine.)

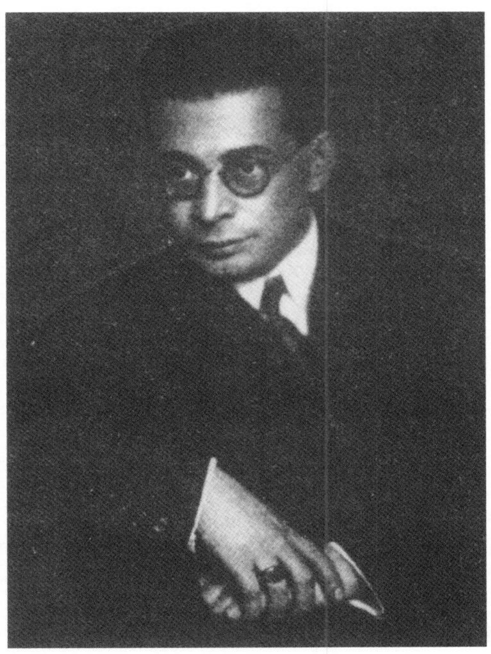

FIGURE 6.3–18
Otto Rank. (Courtesy of New York Academy of Medicine.)

The personality is divided into impulses, emotions, and will. Children's impulses seek immediate discharge and gratification. As impulses are mastered, as in toilet training, children begin the process of will development. If will is carried too far, pathological traits (e.g., stubbornness, disobedience, and inhibitions) may develop.

WILHELM REICH (1897–1957)

Wilhelm Reich (Fig. 6.3–19), an Austrian psychoanalyst, made major contributions to psychoanalysis in the area of character formation and character types. The term *character armor* refers to the personality's defenses that serve as resistance to self-understanding and change. The four major character types are as follows: the *hysterical character* is sexually seductive, anxious, and fixated at the phallic phase of libido development; the *compulsive character* is controlled, distrustful, indecisive, and fixated at the anal phase; the *narcissistic character* is fixated at the phallic state of development, and if the person is male, he has contempt for women; and the *masochistic character* is long-suffering, complaining, and self-deprecatory, with an excessive demand for love.

The therapeutic process, called *will therapy*, emphasizes the relationship between patient and therapist; the goal of treatment is to help patients accept their separateness. A definite termination date for therapy is used to protect against excessive dependence on the therapist.

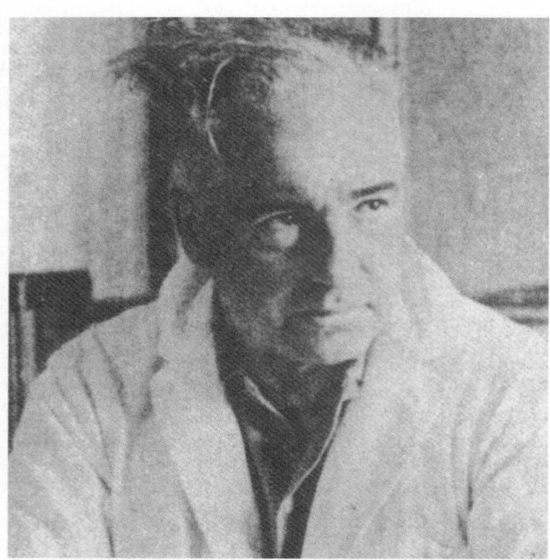

FIGURE 6.3–19
Wilhelm Reich. (Courtesy of New York Academy of Medicine.)

CARL ROGERS (1902–1987)

Carl Rogers (Fig. 6.3–20) received his Ph.D. in psychology from Columbia University. After attending Union Theological Seminary in New York, Rogers studied for the ministry. His name is most clearly associated with the *person-centered theory* of personality and psychotherapy, in which the major concepts are self-actualization and self-direction. Specifically, persons are born with a capacity to direct themselves in the healthiest way toward a level of completeness called self-actualization. From his person-centered approach, Rogers viewed personality not as a static entity composed of traits and patterns but as a dynamic phenomenon involving ever-changing communications, relationships, and self-concepts.

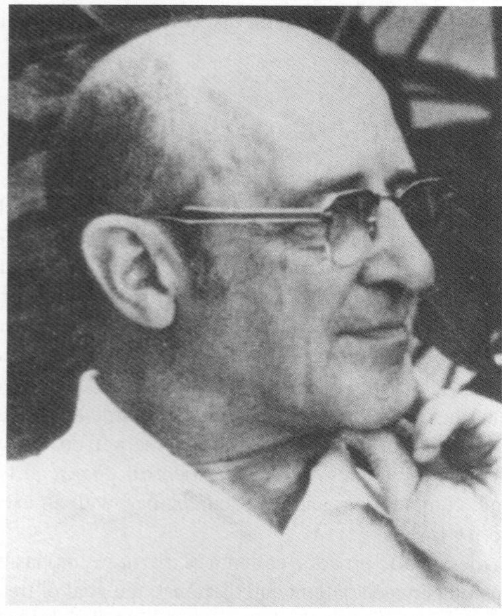

FIGURE 6.3–20
Carl Rogers. (From Carson RC, Butcher JN, Coleman JC. *Abnormal Psychology and Modern Life,* 8th ed. Illinois: Scott, Foresman;1988:75, with permission. Copyright Hugh L. Wilkerson.)

Rogers developed a treatment program called *client-centered psychotherapy*. Therapists attempt to produce an atmosphere in which clients can reconstruct their strivings for self-actualization. Therapists hold clients in unconditional positive regard, which is the total nonjudgmental acceptance of clients as they are. Other therapeutic practices include attention to the present, focus on clients' feelings, emphasis on process, trust in the potential and self-responsibility of clients, and a philosophy grounded in a positive attitude toward them, rather than a preconceived structure of treatment.

JEAN-PAUL SARTRE (1905–1980)

Born in Paris, Jean-Paul Sartre wrote plays and novels before turning to psychology. He was a German prisoner of war from 1940 to 1941 during World War II. Influenced by the ideas of Martin Heidegger, he developed what he called *existential psychoanalysis*. The reflective self was a key concept in Sartre's psychology. He recognized that humans alone could reflect on themselves as objects, so that the experience of "being" in humans is unique in the natural world. This capacity to reflect leads humans to impose a meaning on existence. For Sartre, this meaning allows a human being to create his or her own essence.

Sartre denied the realm of the unconscious; he thought that human beings were condemned to be free and to face the fundamental existential dilemma—their aloneness without a god to provide meaning. As a result, each individual creates values and meanings. Neurosis is an escape from freedom, which is the key to maintaining psychological health. Sartre made no distinction between philosophy and psychology. Psychologists, as with philosophers, search for the truth about the world. Part of this truth, in Sartre's view, was the dialectic between consciousness and *being*. Consciousness introduces nothingness and is a negation of being-in-itself. Ideals are revealed in actions, not in professed beliefs.

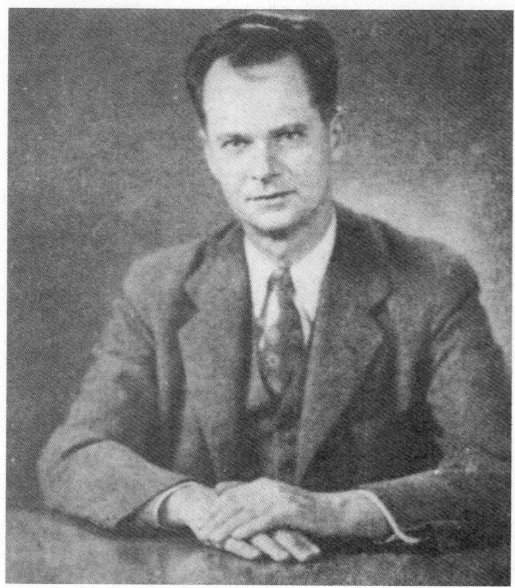

FIGURE 6.3–21
B.F. Skinner. (Courtesy of New York Academy of Medicine, New York)

B. F. SKINNER (1904–1990)

Burrhus Frederic Skinner (Fig. 6.3–21), commonly known as B. F. Skinner, received his Ph.D. in psychology from Harvard University, where he taught for many years. Skinner's seminal work in operant learning laid much of the groundwork for many current methods of behavior modification, programmed instruction, and general education. His global beliefs about the nature of behavior have been applied more widely, it can be argued, than those of any other theorist except, perhaps, Freud. His impact has been impressive in scope and magnitude.

Skinner's approach to personality was derived more from his basic beliefs about behavior than from a specific theory of personality per se. To Skinner, personality did not differ from other behaviors or sets of behaviors; it is acquired, maintained, and strengthened or weakened according to the same rules of reward and punishment that alter any other form of behavior. *Behaviorism*, as Skinner's basic theory is most commonly known, is concerned only with observable, measurable behavior that can be operationalized. Many abstract and mentalistic hallmarks of other dominant personality theories have little place in Skinner's framework. Concepts such as self, ideas, and ego are considered unnecessary for understanding behavior and are shunned. Through the process of operant conditioning and the application of basic principles of learning, persons are believed to develop sets of behavior that characterize their responses to the world of stimuli that they face in their lives. Such a set of responses is called *personality*.

HARRY STACK SULLIVAN (1892–1949)

Harry Stack Sullivan (Fig. 6.3–22) received his training in psychiatry in the United States in the 1920s and 1930s, during the early years of Freud's profound influence on American psychiatry. As with Meyer, under whom he studied, Sullivan, however, insisted on formulating his concepts on observable data.

Sullivan described three modes of experiencing and thinking about the world. The *prototaxic mode* is undifferentiated thought that cannot separate the whole into parts or use symbols. It occurs normally in infancy and also appears in patients with schizophrenia. In the *parataxic mode*, events are causally related because of temporal or serial connections. Logical relationships, however, are not perceived. The *syntaxic mode* is the logical, rational, and most mature type of cognitive functioning of which a person is capable. These three types of thinking and experiencing occur side by side in all persons; it is the rare person who functions exclusively in the syntaxic mode.

The total configuration of personality traits is known as the *self-system*, which develops in various stages and is the outgrowth of interpersonal experiences, rather than an unfolding of intrapsychic forces. During infancy, anxiety occurs for the first time when infants' primary needs are not satisfied. During childhood, from 2 to 5 years, a child's main tasks are to learn the requirements of the culture and how to deal with powerful adults. As a juvenile, from 5 to 8 years, a child has a need for peers and must learn how to deal with them. In preadolescence, from 8 to 12 years, the capacity for love and for collaboration with another person of the same sex develops. This so-called *chum period* is the prototype for a sense of intimacy. In the history of patients with schizophrenia, this experience of chums is often missing. During adolescence, major tasks include the separation from the family, the development of standards and values, and the transition to heterosexuality.

The therapy process requires the active participation of the therapist, who is known as a *participant observer*. Modes of experience, particularly the parataxic, need to be clarified, and new patterns of behavior need to be implemented. Ultimately, persons need to see themselves as they really are, instead of as they think they are or as they want others to think they are.

Sullivan is best known for his creative psychotherapeutic work with severely disturbed patients. He believed that even the most psychotic

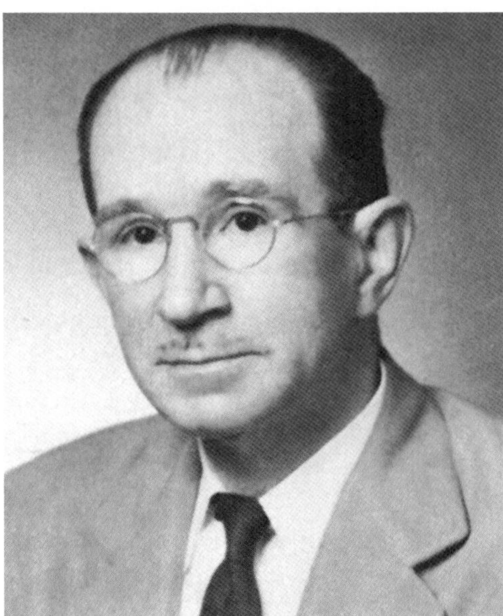

FIGURE 6.3–22
Harry Stack Sullivan. (Reprinted from Carson RC, Butcher JN, Coleman JC. Eds. *Abnormal Psychology and Modern Life.* 8th ed. Illinois: Scott, Foresman and Company; 1988:79, with permission.)

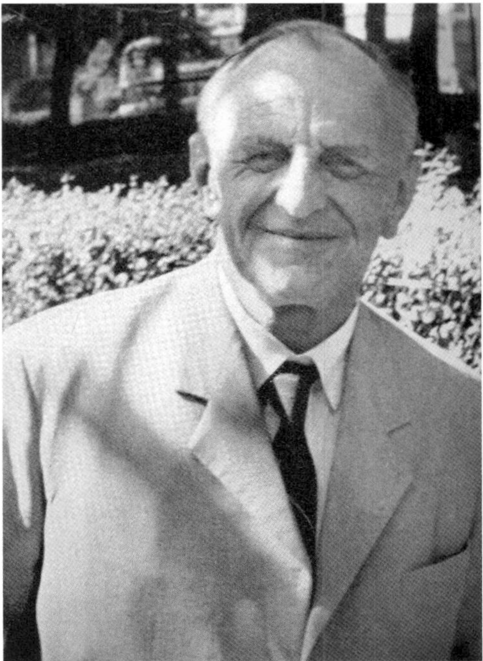

FIGURE 6.3–23
Donald Winnicott. (Courtesy of New York Academy of Medicine, New York.)

patients with schizophrenia could be reached through the human relationship of psychotherapy.

DONALD W. WINNICOTT (1897–1971)

Donald W. Winnicott (Fig. 6.3–23) was one of the central figures in the British school of object relations theory. His theory of *multiple self-organizations* included a *true self*, which develops in the context of a responsive *holding environment* provided by a *good-enough mother*. When infants experience a traumatic disruption of their developing sense of self, however, a false self emerges and monitors and adapts to the conscious and unconscious needs of the mother; it thus provides a protected exterior behind which the true self is afforded a privacy that it requires to maintain its integrity.

Winnicott also developed the notion of the *transitional object*. Ordinarily a pacifier, blanket, or teddy bear, this object serves as a substitute for the mother during infants' efforts to separate and become independent. It provides a soothing sense of security in the absence of the mother.

References

Caspi A, Sugden K, Moffitt TE, Taylor A, Craig IW, Harrington HL, McClay J, Mill J, Martin J, Braithwaite A, Poulton R. Influence of life stress on depression: Moderation by a polymorphism in the 5-HTT gene. *Science*. 2003;301:386.

Conger JC. *Jung & Reich: The Body as Shadow*. Berkeley, CA: North Atlantic Books; 2005.

Costa PT, McCrae RR. Approaches derived from philosophy and psychology. In: Sadock BJ, Sadock VA, eds. *Kaplan & Sadock's Comprehensive Textbook of Psychiatry*. 8th ed. Vol. 1. Baltimore: Lippincott Williams & Wilkins; 2005:778.

Elms AC. Jung's lives. *J Hist Behav Sci*. 2005;41(4):331–346.

Haynal AE. In the shadow of a controversy: Freud and Ferenczi 1925–33. *Int J Psychoanal*. 2005;86:457–466.

Hirsch P. Apostle of freedom: Alfred Adler and his British disciples. *Hist Educ*. 2005;34(5):473–481.

Lakasing E. Reflection—Michael Balint—An outstanding medical life. *Br J Gen Pract*. 2005;55(518):724–725.

McCrae RR, Costa PT Jr. *Personality in Adulthood: A Five-Factor Theory Perspective*. New York: Guilford; 2003.

Mohl PC. Other psychodynamic schools. In: Sadock BJ, Sadock VA, eds. *Kaplan & Sadock's Comprehensive Textbook of Psychiatry*. 8th ed. Vol. 1. Baltimore: Lippincott Williams & Wilkins; 2005:755.

Robertson R. Jung and the making of modern psychology. *Psychological Perspectives: A Semiannual Journal of Jungian Thought*. 2005;48:48–67.

Wiggins JS. *Paradigms of Personality Assessment*. New York: Guilford; 2003.

Wilke G. Beyond Balint. A group-analytic support model for traumatized doctors. *Group Analysis*. 2005;38(2):265–280.

7 Clinical Examination of the Psychiatric Patient

▲ 7.1 Psychiatric History and Mental Status Examination

PSYCHIATRIC HISTORY

The psychiatric history is the record of the patient's life; it allows a psychiatrist to understand who the patient is, where the patient has come from, and where the patient is likely to go in the future. The history is the patient's life story told to the psychiatrist in the patient's own words from his or her own point of view. Many times, the history also includes information about the patient obtained from other sources, such as a parent or spouse. Obtaining a comprehensive history from a patient and, if necessary, from informed sources is essential to making a correct diagnosis and formulating a specific and effective treatment plan. A psychiatric history differs slightly from histories taken in medicine or surgery. In addition to gathering the concrete and factual data related to the chronology of symptom formation and to the psychiatric and medical history, a psychiatrist strives to derive from the history the elusive picture of a patient's individual personality characteristics, including both strengths and weaknesses. The psychiatric history provides insight into the nature of relationships with those closest to the patient and includes all the important persons in his or her life. Usually, a reasonably comprehensive picture can be elicited of the patient's development from the earliest formative years until the present.

The most important technique for obtaining a psychiatric history is to allow patients to tell their stories in their own words in the order that they consider most important. As patients relate their stories, skillful interviewers recognize the points at which they can introduce relevant questions about the areas described in the outline of the history and mental status examination.

The structure of the history and mental status examination presented in this section is not intended to be a rigid plan for interviewing a patient; it is meant to be a guide in organizing the patient's history prior to its being written. A standard format for a psychiatric history is presented in Table 7.1–1. Each topic is discussed below.

Identifying Data

The identifying data provide a succinct demographic summary of the patient by name, age, marital status, sex, occupation, language (if other than English), ethnic background, and religion, insofar as they are pertinent, and the patient's current living circumstances. The information can also include the place or situation in which the current interview took place, the source(s) of the information, the reliability of the source(s), and whether the current disorder is the first episode for the patient. The psychiatrist should indicate whether the patient came in on his or her own, was referred by someone else, or was brought in by someone else. The identifying data are meant to provide a thumbnail sketch of potentially important patient characteristics that may affect diagnosis, prognosis, treatment, and compliance. An example of the written report of the identifying data follows:

> Mr. John Jones is a 25-year-old single, white, Protestant male who works as a department store clerk. He is a college graduate living with his parents. He was referred by his internist for psychiatric evaluation.

Chief Complaint

The chief complaint, in the patient's own words, states why he or she has come or been brought in for help. It should be recorded even if the patient is unable to speak, and the patient's explanation, regardless of how bizarre or irrelevant it is, should be recorded verbatim in the section on the chief complaint. The other individuals present as sources of information can then give their versions of the presenting events in the section on the history of the present illness.

If the patient is comatose or mute that should be noted in the chief complaint as such. Examples of chief complaints follow:

> "I am having thoughts of wanting to harm myself."
> "People are trying to drive me insane."
> "I feel I am going mad."
> "I am angry all the time."

History of Present Illness

The history of present illness provides a comprehensive and chronological picture of the events leading up to the current moment in the patient's life. This part of the psychiatric history is probably the most helpful in making a diagnosis: When was the onset of the current episode, and what were the immediate

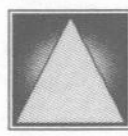

Table 7.1–1
Outline of Psychiatric History

I. Identifying data
II. Chief complaint
III. History of present illness
  A. Onset
  B. Precipitating factors
IV. Past illnesses
  A. Psychiatric
  B. Medical
  C. Alcohol and other substance history
V. Family history
VI. Personal history (anamnesis)
  A. Prenatal and perinatal
  B. Early childhood (Birth through age 3)
  C. Middle childhood (ages 3–11)
  D. Late childhood (puberty through adolescence)
  E. Adulthood
    1. Occupational history
    2. Marital and relationship history
    3. Military history
    4. Educational history
    5. Religion
    6. Social activity
    7. Current living situation
    8. Legal history
  F. Sexual history
  G. Fantasies and dreams
  H. Values

precipitating events or triggers? An understanding of the history of the present illness helps answer the question, Why now? Why did the patient come to the doctor at this time? What were the patient's life circumstances at the onset of the symptoms or behavioral changes, and how did they affect the patient so that the presenting disorder became manifest? Knowing the previously well patient's personality also helps give perspective on the currently ill patient.

The evolution of the patient's symptoms should be determined and summarized in an organized and systematic way. Symptoms not present should also be delineated. The more detailed the history of the present illness, the more likely the clinician is to make an accurate diagnosis. What past precipitating events were part of the chain leading up to the immediate events? In what ways has the patient's illness affected his or her life activities (e.g., work, important relationships)? What is the nature of the dysfunction (e.g., details about changes in such factors as personality, memory, speech)? Are there psychophysiological symptoms? If so, they should be described in terms of location, intensity, and fluctuation. Any relation between physical and psychological symptoms should be noted. A description of the patient's current anxieties, whether they are generalized and nonspecific (free floating) or are specifically related to particular situations, is helpful. How does the patient handle these anxieties? Frequently, a relatively open-ended question such as "How did this all begin?" leads to an adequate unfolding of the history of the present illness. A well-organized patient is generally able to present a chronological account of the history, but a disorganized patient is difficult to interview, as the chronology of events is confused. In such cases, contacting other informants, such as family members and friends, can be a valuable aid in clarifying the patient's story.

Past Illnesses

The past illnesses section of the psychiatric history is a transition between the story of the present illness and the patient's personal history (also called the *anamnesis*). Past episodes of both psychiatric and medical illnesses are described. Ideally, a detailed account of the patient's preexisting and underlying psychological and biological substrates is given at this point, and important clues to, and evidence of, vulnerable areas in the patient's functioning are provided. The patient's symptoms, extent of incapacity, type of treatment received, names of hospitals, length of each illness, effects of previous treatments, and degree of compliance should all be explored and recorded chronologically. Particular attention should be paid to the first episodes that signaled the onset of illness, because first episodes can often provide crucial data about precipitating events, diagnostic possibilities, and coping capabilities.

With regard to medical history, the psychiatrist should obtain a medical review of symptoms and note any major medical or surgical illnesses and major traumas, particularly those requiring hospitalization. Episodes of craniocerebral trauma, neurological illness, tumors, and seizure disorders are especially relevant to psychiatric histories, as is a history of testing positive for the human immunodeficiency virus (HIV) or having acquired immune deficiency syndrome (AIDS). Specific questions need to be asked about the presence of a seizure disorder, episodes of loss of consciousness, changes in usual headache patterns, changes in vision, and episodes of confusion and disorientation. A history of infection with syphilis is critical and relevant.

Causes, complications, and treatment of any illness and the effects of the illness on the patient should be noted. Specific questions about psychosomatic disorders should be asked and the answers noted. Included in this category are hay fever, rheumatoid arthritis, ulcerative colitis, asthma, hyperthyroidism, gastrointestinal upsets, recurrent colds, and skin conditions. All patients must be asked about alcohol and other substances used, including details about the quantity and frequency of use. It is often advisable to frame questions in the form of an assumption of use, such as, "How much alcohol would you say you drink in a day?" rather than "Do you drink?" The latter question may put the patient on the defensive, concerned about what the physician will think if the answer is yes. If the physician assumes that drinking is a fact, the patient is likely to feel comfortable admitting use.

The importance of a thorough, accurate medical history cannot be overstated. Many medical conditions and their treatments cause psychiatric symptoms that without an attentive medical history may be mistaken for a primary psychiatric disorder. Endocrinopathies such as hypothyroidism or Addison's disease may manifest with depression. Treatment with corticosteroids can precipitate manic and psychotic symptoms. In addition, the coexistence of physical disease may result in secondary psychiatric symptoms. A middle-aged man in the aftermath of a heart attack may suffer from anxiety and depression. A patient's medical status will also guide psychiatric treatment decisions. A depressed patient with cardiac conduction abnormalities will not be treated (at least initially) with a tricyclic antidepressant. A bipolar disorder patient with kidney disease will receive an anticonvulsant mood stabilizer rather than lithium. The names and dosing schedules for all currently prescribed nonpsychiatric drugs should be obtained to avoid adverse interactions with prescribed psychiatric medication.

Family History

A brief statement about any psychiatric illness, hospitalization, and treatment of the patient's immediate family members should be placed in the family history part of the report. Does the family have a history of alcohol and other substance abuse or of antisocial behavior? In addition, the family history should provide a description of the personalities and intelligence of the various persons living in the patient's home from childhood to the present as well as a description of the various households in which the patient lived. The psychiatrist should also define the role each person played in the patient's upbringing and this person's current relationship with the patient. What were and are the family ethnic, national, and religious traditions? Informants other than the patient may be available to contribute to the family history, and the source should be cited in the written record. Various members of the family often give different descriptions of the same persons and events. The psychiatrist should determine the family's attitude toward, and insight into, the patient's illness. Does the patient feel that the family members are supportive, indifferent, or destructive? What is the role of illness in the family?

Other questions that provide useful information in this section include the following: What is the patient's attitude toward his or her parents and siblings? The psychiatrist should ask the patient to describe each family member. Who is mentioned first? Who is left out? What does each parent do for a living? What do the siblings do? How do the siblings' occupations compare with the patient's work, and how does the patient feel about it? Who does the patient feel most similar to in the family and why?

Personal History (Anamnesis)

In addition to studying the patient's present illness and current life situation, the psychiatrist needs a thorough understanding of the patient's past and its relation to the present emotional problem. The anamnesis, or personal history, is usually divided into perinatal, early childhood, late childhood, and adulthood (Table 7.1–2). The predominant emotions associated with the different life periods (e.g., painful, stressful, conflictual) should be noted. Depending on time and situation, the psychiatrist may go into detail with regard to each of the following.

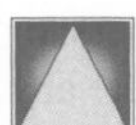

Table 7.1–2
Outline of a Developmental History

A. Prenatal and perinatal
  1. Full-term pregnancy or premature
  2. Vaginal delivery or caesarian
  3. Drugs taken by mother during pregnancy (prescription and recreational)
  4. Birth complications
  5. Defects at birth
B. Infancy and early childhood
  1. Infant–mother relationship
  2. Problems with feeding and sleep
  3. Significant milestones
    a. Standing/walking
    b. First words/two-word sentences
    c. Bowel and bladder control
  4. Other caregivers
  5. Unusual behaviors (e.g., head-banging)
C. Middle childhood
  1. Preschool and school experiences
  2. Separations from caregivers
  3. Friendships/play
  4. Methods of discipline
  5. Illness, surgery, or trauma
D. Adolescence
  1. Onset of puberty
  2. Academic achievement
  3. Organized activities (sports, clubs)
  4. Areas of special interest
  5. Romantic involvements and sexual experience
  6. Work experience
  7. Drug/alcohol use
  8. Symptoms (moodiness, irregularity of sleeping or eating, fights and arguments)
E. Young adulthood
  1. Meaningful long-term relationship
  2. Academic and career decisions
  3. Military experience
  4. Work history
  5. Prison experience
  6. Intellectual pursuits and leisure activities
F. Middle adulthood and old age
  1. Changing family constellation
  2. Social activities
  3. Work and career changes
  4. Aspirations
  5. Major losses
  6. Retirement and aging

Perinatal History. The psychiatrist considers the home situation into which the patient was born and whether the patient was planned and wanted. Were there any problems with the mother's pregnancy and delivery? What was the mother's emotional and physical state at the time of the patient's birth? Were there any maternal health problems during pregnancy? Was the mother abusing alcohol or other substances during her pregnancy?

Early Childhood (Birth through Age 3 Years). The early childhood period consists of the first 3 years of the patient's life. The quality of the mother–child interaction during feeding and toilet training is important. Frequently, one can learn whether the child presented problems in these areas. Early disturbances in sleep patterns, including episodes of head banging and body rocking, provide clues about possible maternal deprivation or developmental disability. In addition, the psychiatrist should obtain a history of human constancy and attachments during the first 3 years. Were any psychiatric or medical illnesses present in the parents that may have interfered with parent–child interactions? Did persons other than the mother care for the patient? Did the patient exhibit problems at an early period such as severe stranger anxiety or separation anxiety? Explore the patient's siblings and the details of his or her relationship with them. The emerging personality of the child is a topic of crucial importance. Was the child shy, restless, overactive, withdrawn, studious, outgoing, timid, athletic, friendly? Seek data about the child's ability to concentrate, to tolerate frustration, and to postpone gratification. Also note the child's preference for active or passive roles in physical play. What were the child's favorite games or toys? Did the child prefer to play alone, with others, or not at all? What is the patient's earliest memory? Were there any recurrent dreams or fantasies during this period? A summary of the important areas to be covered follows.

FEEDING HABITS. Breast-fed or bottle-fed, eating problems

EARLY DEVELOPMENT. Walking, talking, teething, language development, motor development, signs of unmet needs, sleep pattern, object constancy, stranger anxiety, maternal deprivation, separation anxiety, other caretakers in the home

TOILET TRAINING. Age, attitude of parents, feelings about it

SYMPTOMS OF BEHAVIOR PROBLEMS. Thumb-sucking, temper tantrums, tics, head-bumping, rocking, night terrors, fears, bed-wetting or bed-soiling, nail-biting, excessive masturbation

PERSONALITY AS A CHILD. Shy, restless, overactive, withdrawn, persistent, outgoing, timid, athletic, friendly, patterns of play

Middle Childhood (Ages 3 to 11 Years).

In addressing the middle childhood, the psychiatrist focuses on such important subjects as gender identification, punishments used in the home, and the persons who provided the discipline and influenced early conscience formation. The psychiatrist must inquire about the patient's early school experiences, especially how the patient first tolerated being separated from his or her mother. Data about the patient's earliest friendships and personal relationships are valuable. The psychiatrist should determine the number and the closeness of the patient's friends, describe whether the patient took the role of a leader or a follower, and describe the patient's social popularity and participation in group or gang activities. Was the child able to cooperate with peers, to be fair, to understand and comply with rules, and to develop an early conscience? Early patterns of assertion, impulsiveness, aggression, passivity, anxiety, or antisocial behavior emerge in the context of school relationships. A history of the patient's learning to read and developing other intellectual and motor skills is important. A history of learning disabilities, their management, and their effects on the child is of particular significance. The presence of nightmares, phobias, bed-wetting, fire-setting, cruelty to animals, and excessive masturbation should also be explored.

Late Childhood (Puberty through Adolescence).

During late childhood, persons begin to develop independence from their parents through relationships with peers and group activities. The psychiatrist should attempt to ascertain the values of the patient's social groups and to determine who were the patient's idealized figures. This information provides useful clues about the patient's emerging self-image.

It is helpful to explore the patient's school history, relationships with teachers, and favorite studies and interests, both in school and in extracurricular areas. Ask about the patient's participation in sports and hobbies and inquire about any emotional or physical problems that may have first appeared during this phase. Examples of the types of questions that are commonly asked include the following: What was the patient's sense of personal identity? How extensive was the use of alcohol and other substances? Was the patient sexually active, and what was the quality of the sexual relationships? Was the patient interactive and involved with school and peers, or was he or she isolated, withdrawn, and perceived as odd by others? Did the patient have a generally intact self-esteem, or was there evidence of an inferiority complex? What was the patient's body image? Were there suicidal episodes? Were there problems in school, including excessive truancy? How did the patient use private time? What was the relationship with the parents? What were the feelings about the development of secondary sex characteristics? What was the response to menarche? What were the attitudes about dating, petting, crushes, parties, and sex games? One way to organize the diverse and large amount of information is to break late childhood into subsets of behavior (e.g., social relationships, school history, cognitive and motor development, emotional and physical problems, and sexuality), as described next.

SOCIAL RELATIONSHIPS. Attitudes toward sibling(s) and playmates, number and closeness of friends, leader or follower, social popularity, participation in group or gang activities, idealized figures, patterns of aggression, passivity, anxiety, antisocial behavior

SCHOOL HISTORY. How far the patient progressed, adjustment to school, relationships with teachers—teacher's pet versus rebel—favorite studies or interests, particular abilities or assets, extracurricular activities, sports, hobbies, relations of problems or symptoms to any social period

COGNITIVE AND MOTOR DEVELOPMENT. Learning to read and other intellectual and motor skills, minimal cerebral dysfunction, learning disabilities—their management and effects on the child

EMOTIONAL AND PHYSICAL PROBLEMS. Nightmares, phobias, bed-wetting, running away, delinquency, smoking, alcohol or other substance use, anorexia, bulimia, weight problems, feelings of inferiority, depression, suicidal ideas and acts

Adulthood

OCCUPATIONAL HISTORY. The psychiatrist should describe the patient's choice of occupation, the requisite training and preparation, any work-related conflicts, and the long-term ambitions and goals. Also explore the patient's feelings about his or her current job and relationships at work (with authorities, peers, and, if applicable, subordinates) and describe the job history (e.g., number and duration of jobs, reasons for job changes, and changes in job status). What would the patient do for work if he or she could choose freely?

> A 40-year-old physician in a successful general practice also had many business ventures in which he invested a great deal of the money he had earned from property development. The ventures frequently entangled him in legal disputes. He spent 12 to 14 hours in his medical office each day seeing patients, completed his charting and paperwork on weekends, and snatched odd moments to conduct complicated business transactions with his attorney. He was snappy and irritable with his family; he expected them to be at his beck and call and to notice his "self-sacrificing" on their behalf. Reducing his practice, taking on an associate, and limiting his business activities were all unacceptable to him.

MARITAL AND RELATIONSHIP HISTORY. The psychiatrist elicits a history of each marriage, legal or common law. Significant relationships with persons with whom the patient has lived for a protracted period are also included. The story of the marriage or long-term relationship should describe the evolution of the relationship, including the age of the patient at the beginning of the relationship. The areas of agreement and disagreement—including money management, housing difficulties, the roles of in-laws, and attitudes toward raising children—should be described. Other questions include: Is the patient currently in a long-term relationship? How long is the longest relationship that the patient has had? What is the quality of the patient's sexual relationship (e.g., is the patient's sexual life experienced as satisfactory or inadequate)? What does the patient look for in a partner? Can the patient initiate a relationship or approach someone with whom he or she feels attracted? How does the patient describe the current relationship in terms of its positive and negative qualities? How does the patient perceive failures of past relationships in terms of understanding what went wrong and who was or was not to blame?

A 32-year-old woman had a series of relationships in which she was ultimately abused, always emotionally and often physically and sexually. Despite her conscious intent to find a caring man with whom she could have a less abusive relationship, the pattern repeated itself. Her mother had been chronically beaten by her abusive father. She recalled that her mother warned her repeatedly, "A woman's role is to give in to her husband and put up with the crap as best we can."

MILITARY HISTORY. The psychiatrist should inquire about the patient's general adjustment to the military, whether he or she saw combat or sustained an injury, and the nature of the discharge. Was the patient ever referred for psychiatric consultation, and did he or she incur any disciplinary action during the period of service?

A 22-year-old soldier returning from Vietnam claimed to have no memory of his last month in combat. He had been assigned to a squad conducting a long-range patrol; only three of eight soldiers returned alive. Through repeated amobarbital interviews conducted in a supportive setting, gradually and with much emotion he recalled that his squad had been ambushed, that early in the firefight he had killed two or three 12- or 13-year-old Vietnamese boys who were in the attacking group, and that at a certain point he turned and ran away, leaving one or two of his wounded buddies behind, who were pleading with him to help them.

EDUCATION HISTORY. The psychiatrist needs to have a clear picture of the patient's educational background. This information can provide clues about the patient's social and cultural background, intelligence, motivation, and any obstacles to achievement. For instance, a patient from an economically deprived background who never had the opportunity to attend the best schools and whose parents never graduated from high school shows strength of character, intelligence, and tremendous motivation by graduating from college. A patient who dropped out of high school because of violence and substance use displays creativity and determination by going to school at night to obtain a high school diploma while working during the day as a drug counselor. How far did the patient go in school? What was the highest grade or graduate level attained? What did the patient like to study, and what was the level of academic performance? How far did the other members of the patient's family go in school, and how do they compare with the patient's progress? What is the patient's attitude toward academic achievement?

RELIGION. The psychiatrist determines the religious background of both parents and the details of the patient's religious instruction. Was the family's attitude toward religion strict or permissive, and were there any conflicts between the parents over the child's religious education? The psychiatrist should trace the evolution of the patient's adolescent religious practices to present beliefs and activities. Does the patient have a strong religious affiliation, and, if so, how does this affiliation affect the patient's life? What does the patient's religion say about the treatment of psychiatric or medical illness? What is the religious attitude toward suicide?

SOCIAL ACTIVITY. The psychiatrist elicits information about the patient's social life and the nature of friendships, with an emphasis on the depth, duration, and quality of human relationships. What social, intellectual, and physical interests does the patient share with friends? What relationships does the patient have with persons of the same sex and the opposite sex? Is the patient essentially isolated and asocial? Does the patient prefer isolation, or is the patient isolated because of anxieties and fears about other people? Who visits the patient in the hospital and how frequently?

An attractive, successful 32-year-old woman reported having a long string of admiring suitors and a series of intimate sexual relationships since the age of 17. Although several of the suitors to whom she was strongly attracted had proposed marriage, she felt unable to commit herself; she was never sufficiently in love with any of them and hoped that she would someday meet "Mr. Perfect."

CURRENT LIVING SITUATION. Ask the patient to describe where he or she lives in terms of the neighborhood and the residence as well as the number of rooms, the number of family members living in the home, and the sleeping arrangements. Inquire how issues of privacy are handled, with particular emphasis on parental and sibling nudity and bathroom arrangements. Also ask about the sources of family income and any financial hardships. If applicable, inquire about public assistance and the patient's feelings about it. If the patient has been hospitalized, have provisions been made so that he or she will not lose a job or an apartment? Ask who is caring for the children at home, who visits the patient in the hospital, and how frequently.

LEGAL HISTORY. Has the patient ever been arrested and, if so, for what? How many times? Was the patient ever in jail? For how long? Is the patient on probation, or are charges pending? Is the patient mandated to be in treatment as part of a stipulation of probation? Does the patient have a history of assault or violence? Against whom? Were weapons used? What is the patient's attitude toward the arrests or prison terms? An extensive legal history, as well as the patient's attitude toward it, may indicate antisocial trends or a litigious personality. An extensive history of violence may alert the psychiatrist to the potential for violence in the future.

Sexual History

Much of the history of infantile sexuality is not recoverable, although many patients can recall curiosities and sexual games played from the ages of 3 to 6 years. The psychiatrist should ask how the patient learned about sex and what he or she felt were parents' attitudes about sexual development. Also inquire whether the patient was sexually abused in childhood. Some material discussed in this section may also be covered in the section on adolescent sexuality. It is not important where in the history it is covered, as long as it is included.

The onset of puberty and the patient's feelings about this milestone are important. Adolescent masturbatory history, including the nature of the patient's fantasies and feelings about them, is of significance. Attitudes toward sex should be described in detail. Is the patient shy, timid, aggressive? Does the patient need to impress others and boast of sexual conquests? Did the patient experience anxiety in the sexual setting? Was there promiscuity? What is the patient's sexual orientation?

The sexual history (Table 7.1–3) should include any sexual symptoms, such as anorgasmia, vaginismus, erectile disorder (impotence), premature or retarded ejaculation, lack of sexual desire, and paraphillias (e.g., sexual sadism, fetishism, voyeurism). Attitudes toward fellatio, cunnilingus, and coital techniques may be discussed. The topic of sexual adjustment should include a

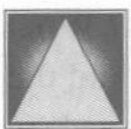

Table 7.1–3
Sexual History

1. Screening questions
   a. Are you sexually active?
   b. Have you noticed any changes or problems with sex recently?
2. Developmental
   a. Acquisition of sexual knowledge
   b. Onset of puberty/menarche
   c. Development of sexual identity and orientation
   d. First sexual experiences
   e. Sex in romantic relationship
   f. Changing experiences or preferences over time
   g. Sex and advancing age
3. Clarification of sexual problems
   a. Desire phase
      Presence of sexual thoughts or fantasies
      When do they occur and what is their object?
      Who initiates sex and how?
   b. Excitement phase
      Difficulty in sexual arousal (achieving or maintaining erections, lubrication), during foreplay and preceding orgasm
   c. Orgasm phase
      Does orgasm occur?
      Does it occur too soon or too late?
      How often and under what circumstances does orgasm occur?
      If orgasm does not occur, is it because of not being excited or lack of orgasm despite being aroused?
   d. Resolution phase
      What happens after sex is over (e.g., contentment, frustration, continued arousal)?

description of how sexual activity is usually initiated, the frequency of sexual relations, and sexual preferences, variations, and techniques. It is usually appropriate to inquire whether the patient has engaged in extramarital relationships and, if so, under what circumstances and whether the spouse knew of the affair. If the spouse did learn of the affair, the psychiatrist should ask the patient to describe what happened. The reasons underlying an extramarital affair are just as important as understanding its effect on the marriage. Attitudes toward contraception and family planning are important. What form of contraception does the patient use? The psychiatrist, however, should not assume that the patient uses birth control. If an interviewer asks a lesbian patient to describe what type of birth control she uses (on the assumption that she is heterosexual), the patient may surmise that the interviewer will not understand or accept her sexual orientation. A more helpful question is, "Do you need to use birth control?" or "Is contraception something that is part of your sexuality?"

The psychiatrist should ask whether the patient wants to mention other areas of sexual functioning and sexuality. Is the patient aware of the issues involved in safe sex? Does the patient have a sexually transmitted disease, such as herpes or AIDS? Does the patient worry about being HIV positive?

A woman reported that she was addicted to using perfume and that her coworkers began to comment on her excessive use. Analysis revealed that she believed she exuded an odor after she masturbated. She masturbated daily and used the perfume to mask the smell that she believed was apparent to others. The basis of her belief could be traced to severe guilt over her masturbatory practices. (Otto Fenichel, M.D.)

Fantasies and Dreams. Freud stated that dreams are the royal road to the unconscious. Repetitive dreams have particular value. If the patient has nightmares, what are their repetitive themes? Some of the most common dream themes are food, examinations, sex, helplessness, and feelings of impotence. Can the patient describe a recent dream and discuss its possible meanings? Fantasies and daydreams are another valuable source of unconscious material. As with dreams, the psychiatrist can explore and record details of the fantasy and attendant feelings.

What are the patient's fantasies about the future? If the patient could make any change in his or her life, what would it be? What are the patient's most common or favorite current fantasies? Does the patient experience daydreams? Are the patient's fantasies grounded in reality, or is the patient unable to tell the difference between fantasy and reality?

Values. The psychiatrist may inquire about the patient's system of values—both social and moral—including values about work, money, play, children, parents, friends, sex, community concerns, and cultural issues. For instance, are children a burden or a joy? Is work a necessary evil, an unavoidable chore, or an opportunity? What is the patient's concept of right and wrong?

MENTAL STATUS EXAMINATION

The mental status examination is the part of the clinical assessment that describes the sum total of the examiner's observations and impressions of the psychiatric patient at the time of the interview. Whereas the patient's history remains stable, the patient's mental status can change from day to day or hour to hour. The mental status examination is the description of the patient's appearance, speech, actions, and thoughts during the interview. Even when a patient is mute, is incoherent, or refuses to answer questions, the clinician can obtain a wealth of information through careful observation. A mental status format is outlined in Table 7.1–4.

General Description

Appearance. In this category, the psychiatrist describes the patient's appearance and overall physical impression, as reflected by posture, poise, clothing, and grooming. If the patient appears particularly bizarre, the clinician may ask, "Has anyone ever commented on how you look?" "How would you describe how you look?" "Can you help me understand some of the choices you make in how you look?"

Examples of items in the appearance category include body type, posture, poise, clothes, grooming, hair, and nails. Common terms used to describe appearance are healthy, sickly, ill at ease, poised, old looking, young looking, disheveled, childlike, and bizarre. Signs of anxiety are noted: moist hands, perspiring forehead, tense posture, wide eyes.

Table 7.1–4
Outline for the Mental Status Examination

1. Appearance
2. Overt behavior
3. Attitude
4. Speech
5. Mood and affect
6. Thinking
   a. Form
   b. Content
7. Perceptions
8. Sensorium
   a. Alertness
   b. Orientation (person, place, time)
   c. Concentration
   d. Memory (immediate, recent, long term)
   e. Calculations
   f. Fund of knowledge
   g. Abstract reasoning
9. Insight
10. Judgment

Attitude Toward Examiner. The patient's attitude toward the examiner can be described as cooperative, friendly, attentive, interested, frank, seductive, defensive, contemptuous, perplexed, apathetic, hostile, playful, ingratiating, evasive, or guarded; any number of other adjectives can be used. Record the level of rapport established.

Speech Characteristics. This part of the report describes the physical characteristics of speech. Speech can be described in terms of its quantity, rate of production, and quality. The patient may be described as talkative, garrulous, voluble, taciturn, unspontaneous, or normally responsive to cues from the interviewer. Speech can be rapid or slow, pressured, hesitant, emotional, dramatic, monotonous, loud, whispered, slurred, staccato, or mumbled. Speech impairments, such as stuttering, are included in this section. Any unusual rhythms (termed *dysprosody*) or accent should be noted. The patient's speech may be spontaneous.

Overt Behavior and Psychomotor Activity. Here is described both the quantitative and qualitative aspects of the patient's motor behavior. Included are mannerisms, tics, gestures, twitches, stereotyped behavior, echopraxia, hyperactivity, agitation, combativeness, flexibility, rigidity, gait, and agility. Describe restlessness, wringing of hands, pacing, and other physical manifestations. Note psychomotor retardation or generalized slowing of body movements. Describe any aimless, purposeless activity.

Mood and Affect

Mood. *Mood* is defined as a pervasive and sustained emotion that colors the person's perception of the world. The psychiatrist is interested in whether the patient remarks voluntarily about feelings or whether it is necessary to ask the patient how he or she feels. Statements about the patient's mood should include depth, intensity, duration, and fluctuations. Common adjectives used to describe mood include depressed, despairing, irritable, anxious, angry, expansive, euphoric, empty, guilty, hopeless, futile, self-contemptuous, frightened, and perplexed. Mood can be labile, fluctuating or alternating rapidly between extremes (e.g., laughing loudly and expansively one moment, tearful and despairing the next).

Affect. *Affect* can be defined as the patient's present emotional responsiveness, inferred from the patient's facial expression, including the amount and the range of expressive behavior. Affect may or may not be congruent with mood. Affect can be described as within normal range, constricted, blunted, or flat. In the normal range of affect can be variation in facial expression, tone of voice, use of hands, and body movements. When affect is constricted, the range and intensity of expression are reduced. In blunted affect, emotional expression is further reduced. To diagnose flat affect, virtually no signs of affective expression should be present; the patient's voice should be monotonous and the face should be immobile. Note the patient's difficulty in initiating, sustaining, or terminating an emotional response.

Appropriateness of Affect. The psychiatrist can consider the appropriateness of the patient's emotional responses in the context of the subject the patient is discussing. Delusional patients who are describing a delusion of persecution should be angry or frightened about the experiences they believe are happening to them. Anger or fear in this context is an appropriate expression. Psychiatrists use the term *inappropriate affect* for a quality of response found in some schizophrenia patients, in which the patient's affect is incongruent with what the patient is saying (e.g., flattened affect when speaking about murderous impulses).

Perception

Perceptual disturbances, such as hallucinations and illusions, can be experienced in reference to the self or the environment. The sensory system involved (e.g., auditory, visual, taste, olfactory, or tactile) and the content of the illusion or the hallucinatory experience should be described. The circumstances of the occurrence of any hallucinatory experience are important; hypnagogic hallucinations (occurring as a person falls asleep) and hypnopompic hallucinations (occurring as a person awakens) have much less serious significance than other types of hallucinations. Hallucinations can also occur in particular times of stress for individual patients. Feelings of depersonalization and derealization (extreme feelings of detachment from the self or the environment) are other examples of perceptual disturbance. Formication, the feeling of bugs crawling on or under the skin, is seen in cocainism.

Examples of questions used to elicit the experience of hallucinations include the following: Have you ever heard voices or other sounds that no one else could hear or when no one else was around? Have you experienced any strange sensations in your body that others do not seem to see?

A young man with schizophrenia heard an insistent voice repeatedly telling him to stop his antipsychotic medication. After resisting the command for many weeks, the patient felt that he could no longer fight the voice, and he discontinued treatment. Two months later, he was hospitalized involuntarily and near cardiovascular collapse. He later said that once he stopped the medication, the voice further insisted that he should stop eating and drinking to purify himself.

A terrified 37-year-old man in acute delirium tremens glanced agitatedly about the room. He pointed out the window and said: "My God, the Spanish armada is on the lawn. They're about to attack." He experienced the hallucination as real, and it persisted intermittently for 3 days before abating. Subsequently, the patient had no memory of the experience.

Thought Content and Mental Trends. Thought can be divided into process (or form) and content. *Process* refers to the way in which a person puts together ideas and associations, the form in which a person thinks. Process or form of thought can be logical and coherent or completely illogical and even incomprehensible. *Content* refers to what a person is actually thinking about: ideas, beliefs, preoccupations, obsessions. Table 7.1–5 lists common thought disorders.

THOUGHT PROCESS (FORM OF THINKING). The patient may have either an overabundance or a poverty of ideas. There may be rapid thinking, which, if carried to the extreme, is called a *flight of ideas*. A patient may exhibit slow or hesitant thinking.

Thought can be vague or empty. Do the patient's replies really answer the questions asked, and does the patient have the capacity for goal-directed thinking? Are the responses relevant or irrelevant? Is there a clear cause-and-effect relation in the patient's explanations? Does the patient have *loose associations* (e.g., do the ideas expressed seem unrelated and idiosyncratically connected)? Disturbances of thought continuity include statements that are tangential, circumstantial, rambling, evasive, or perseverative.

Blocking is interruption of the train of thought before an idea has been completed; the patient may indicate an inability to recall what was being said or intended to be said. *Circumstantiality* indicates the loss of capacity for goal-directed thinking; in the process of explaining an idea, the patient brings in many irrelevant details and parenthetical comments but eventually does get back to the original point. *Tangentiality* is a disturbance in which the patient loses the thread of the conversation, pursues divergent thoughts stimulated by various external or internal irrelevant stimuli, and never returns to the original point. Thought process impairments may be reflected by incoherent or incomprehensible connections of thoughts (*word salad*), *clang associations* (association by rhyming), *punning* (association by double meaning), and *neologisms* (new words created by the patient by combining or condensing other words).

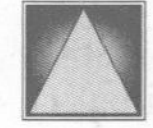

Table 7.1–5
Formal Thought Disorders

Circumstantiality. Overinclusion of trivial or irrelevant details that impede the sense of getting to the point.

Clang associations. Thoughts are associated by the sound of words rather than by their meaning (e.g., through rhyming or assonance).

Derailment. (Synonymous with loose associations.) A breakdown in both the logical connection between ideas and the overall sense of goal-directedness. The words make sentences, but the sentences do not make sense.

Flight of ideas. A succession of multiple associations so that thoughts seem to move abruptly from idea to idea; often (but not invariably) expressed through rapid, pressured speech.

Neologism. The invention of new words or phrases or the use of conventional words in idiosyncratic ways.

Perseveration. Repetition of out of context of words, phrases, or ideas.

Tangentiality. In response to a question, the patient gives a reply that is appropriate to the general topic without actually answering the question. Example:
Doctor: "Have you had any trouble sleeping lately?"
Patient: "I usually sleep in my bed, but now I'm sleeping on the sofa."

Thought blocking. A sudden disruption of thought or a break in the flow of ideas.

THOUGHT CONTENT. Disturbances in content of thought include delusions, preoccupations (which may involve the patient's illness), obsessions ("Do you have ideas that are intrusive and repetitive?"), compulsions ("Are there things you do over and over, in a repetitive manner?" "Are there things you must do in a particular way or order?" "If you do not do them that way, must you repeat them?" "Do you know why you do things that way?"), phobias, plans, intentions, recurrent ideas about suicide or homicide, hypochondriacal symptoms, and specific antisocial urges.

A patient had the compulsion to do everything eight times, which permeated all his behavior whether it was brushing his teeth or locking the door to his house each of which he had to do eight times. He knew his behavior was irrational but could not stop himself from this activity.

Does the patient have thoughts of doing self-harm? Is there a plan? A major category of disturbances of thought content involves delusions. Delusions—fixed, false beliefs out of keeping with the patient's cultural background—may be mood congruent (thoughts that are in keeping with a depressed or elated mood, e.g., a depressed patient thinks he is dying or an elated patient thinks she is the Virgin Mary) or mood incongruent (e.g., an elated patient thinks he has a brain tumor). The psychiatrist should describe the content of any delusional system and attempt to evaluate its organization and the patient's conviction about its validity. The manner in which it affects the patient's life is appropriately described in the history of the present illness. Delusions can be bizarre and may involve beliefs about external control. Delusions can have themes that are persecutory or paranoid, grandiose, jealous, somatic, guilty, nihilistic, or erotic. The clinician should describe ideas of reference and of influence. Examples of *ideas of reference* include a person's belief that the television or radio is speaking to or about him or her. Examples of *ideas of influence* are beliefs about another person or force controlling some aspect of one's behavior.

A young man with schizophrenia, a college dropout who could work only part time at low-level jobs and who lived with his high-achieving family, believed he was the Messiah. He was fully convinced that his struggles and lack of occupational success were merely God's tests until the patient's true identity would be revealed. As he improved, he would, if asked, say that he was God's chosen but, when questioned further, would admit the slight possibility that he was wrong. On reaching his best clinical state, he would muse on the possibility that he was the Messiah but state that he was not sure.

Sensorium and Cognition

The sensorium and cognition portion of the mental status examination seeks to assess brain function, including intelligence, capacity for abstract thought, and level of insight and judgment. Questions that test cognitive function are listed in Table 7.1–6.

Consciousness. Disturbances of consciousness usually indicate organic brain impairment. Clouding of consciousness is an overall reduced awareness of the environment. A patient may be unable to sustain attention to environmental stimuli or to maintain goal-directed thinking or behavior. Clouding or obtunding of consciousness is frequently not a fixed mental state. A patient typically exhibits fluctuations in the level of awareness of the surrounding environment. The patient who has an altered state of consciousness often shows some impairment of orientation as well, although the reverse is not necessarily true. Some terms used to describe the patient's level of consciousness are *clouding*, *somnolence*, *stupor*, *coma*, *lethargy*, or *alert*.

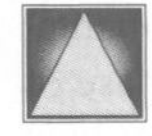

Table 7.1–6
Questions Used to Test Cognitive Functions in the Sensorium Section of the Mental Status Examination

1. Alertness	(Observation)
2. Orientation	What is your name? Who am I? What place is this? Where is it located? What city are we in?
3. Concentration	Starting at 100, count backward by 7 (or 3). Say the letters of the alphabet backward starting with Z. Name the months of the year backward starting with December.
4. Memory	
Immediate	Repeat these numbers after me: 1, 4, 9, 2, 5.
Recent	What did you have for breakfast? What were you doing before we started talking this morning? I want you to remember these three things: a yellow pencil, a cocker spaniel, and Cincinnati. After a few minutes I'll ask you to repeat them.
Long term	What was your address when you were in the third grade? Who was your teacher? What did you do during the summer between high school and college?
5. Calculations	If you buy something that costs $3.75 and you pay with a $5 bill, how much change should you get? What is the cost of three oranges if a dozen oranges cost $4.00?
6. Fund of knowledge	What is the distance between New York and Los Angeles? What body of water lies between South America and Africa?
7. Abstract reasoning	Which one does not belong in this group: a pair of scissors, a canary, and a spider? Why? How are an apple and an orange alike?

Orientation and Memory. Disorders of orientation are traditionally separated according to time, place, and person. Any impairment usually appears in this order (i.e., sense of time is impaired before sense of place); similarly, as the patient improves, the impairment clears in the reverse order. The psychiatrist must determine whether a patient can give the approximate date and time of day. In addition, if hospitalized, does the patient know how long he or she has been there? Does the patient seem to be oriented to the present? In questions about orientation to place, patients should be able to state the name and the location of the hospital correctly and to behave as though they know where they are. In assessing orientation for person, the psychiatrist asks patients whether they know the names of the people around them and whether they understand their roles in relationship to them. Do they know who the examiner is? Only in the most severe instances do patients not know who they themselves are.

A 42-year-old alcoholic man in delirium tremens, examined in a California hospital in 1995, was asked the date and where he was. He replied: "I'm standing on a street corner in Kansas City in 1966 minding my own business. Why don't you mind yours?"

Memory functions have traditionally been divided into four areas: remote memory, recent past memory, recent memory, and immediate retention and recall. Recent memory can be checked by asking patients about their appetite and then about what they had for breakfast or for dinner the previous evening. Patients can be asked at this point if they recall the interviewer's name. Asking patients to repeat six digits forward and then backward is a test of immediate retention. Remote memory can be tested by asking patients for information about their childhood that can be verified later. Asking patients to recall important news events from the past few months checks recent past memory. Often in cognitive disorders, recent or short-term memory is impaired first, and remote or long-term memory is impaired later. If there is impairment, what efforts are made to cope with it or to conceal it? Is denial, confabulation, or circumstantiality used to conceal a deficit? Reactions to the loss of memory can give important clues to underlying disorders and coping mechanisms. For instance, a patient who appears to have memory impairment but, in fact, is depressed is more likely to be concerned about memory loss than is someone with memory loss secondary to dementia. The clinician must also determine whether a catastrophic reaction is present (anxious crying when unable to remember).

A 40-year-old chronically alcoholic man, whose memory on the mental status examination was markedly impaired, frantically demanded to be released from the hospital, saying that his wife had just been in an automobile accident and that he had to rush to another hospital to see her. He said it with sincere conviction and appropriate fearful concern; for the patient, at least, the story was real. In

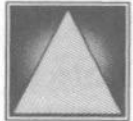

Table 7.1–7
Summary of Memory Tests

Try to assess whether the process of registration, retention, or recollection of material is involved.

Remote memory: Childhood data, important events known to have occurred when the patient was younger or free of illness, personal matters, neutral material

Recent past memory: The past few months

Recent memory: The past few days, what the patient did yesterday, the day before, what the patient had for breakfast, lunch, dinner

Immediate retention and recall: Digit-span measures; ability to repeat six figures after examiner dictates them—first forward, then backward (patients with unimpaired memory can usually repeat six digits backward); ability to repeat three words immediately and 3 to 5 minutes later

fact, his wife had been dead for 15 years. The patient told the same story over and over again, always with evident conviction, despite that staff members confronted him with the reality that his wife had been dead for years. The patient was never influenced by their assertions, because he could not register new memories. Although his past memory was patchy at best, he could repeatedly recall the story of his wife's emergency.

Confabulation (unconsciously making up false answers when memory is impaired) is most closely associated with cognitive disorders. Table 7.1–7 gives a summary of memory tests.

Concentration and Attention. A patient's concentration can be impaired for many reasons. A cognitive disorder, anxiety, depression, and internal stimuli, such as auditory hallucinations, can all contribute to impaired concentration. Subtracting serial 7s from 100 is a simple task that requires intact concentration and cognitive capacities. Could the patient subtract 7 from 100 and keep subtracting 7s? If the patient could not subtract 7s, could 3s be subtracted? Were easier tasks accomplished: 4×9, 5×4? The examiner must always assess whether anxiety, some disturbance of mood or consciousness, or a learning deficit (dyscalculia) is responsible for the difficulty.

Attention is assessed by calculations or by asking the patient to spell the word *world* (or others) backward. The patient can also be asked to name five things that start with a particular letter.

During his most recent manic episode, a 48-year-old man with bipolar disorder had intense, grandiose, psychotic ideas. He was convinced that he could control the traffic in Los Angeles by driving on certain freeways at specified times and willing others to leave the road. After the manic episode ended and during the depressive episode that immediately followed, he could recall virtually no details of his previous thought content while he was manic. Later, when euthymic, he remembered only a few hazy images. A year later, the beginning of a new hypomanic period was heralded by the patient's spontaneously remembering and describing in great detail the psychotic plans of the previous episode.

Reading and Writing. The psychiatrist should ask the patient to read a sentence. The patient should also be asked to write a simple but complete sentence.

Visuospatial Ability. The patient should be asked to copy a figure, such as a clock face or interlocking pentagons.

Abstract Thought. Abstract thinking is the ability to deal with concepts. Patients can have disturbances in the manner in which they conceptualize or handle ideas. Can the patient explain similarities, such as those between an apple and a pear or between truth and beauty? Are the meanings of simple proverbs, such as "A rolling stone gathers no moss," understood? Answers can be concrete (giving specific examples to illustrate the meaning) or overly abstract (giving too generalized an explanation). The appropriateness of answers and the manner in which they are given should be noted. In a catastrophic reaction, brain-damaged patients become extremely emotional and cannot think abstractly.

When asked to explain the proverb "People in glass houses should not throw stones" a schizophrenic patient replied, "That's easy, you can break the glass."

Information and Intelligence. If a possible cognitive impairment is suspected, does the patient have trouble with mental tasks, such as counting the change from $10 after a purchase of $6.37? If this task is too difficult, are easy problems (such as how many nickels are in $1.35) solved? The patient's intelligence is related to vocabulary and general fund of knowledge (e.g., the distance from New York to Paris, presidents of the United States). The patient's educational level (both formal and self-education) and socioeconomic status must be taken into account. Handling difficult or sophisticated concepts can reflect intelligence, even in the absence of formal education or an extensive fund of information. Ultimately, the psychiatrist estimates the patient's intellectual capability and capacity to function at the level of basic endowment.

Impulsivity

Is the patient capable of controlling sexual, aggressive, and other impulses? An assessment of impulse control is critical in ascertaining the patient's awareness of socially appropriate behavior and is a measure of the patient's potential danger to self and others. Patients may be unable to control impulses secondary to cognitive and psychotic disorders or because of chronic characterological defects, as observed in the personality disorders. Impulse control can be estimated from information in the patient's recent history and from behavior observed during the interview.

Judgment and Insight

Judgment. During the course of history taking, the psychiatrist should be able to assess many aspects of the patient's capability for social judgment. Does the patient understand the likely outcome of his or her behavior, and is he or she influenced by this understanding? Can the patient predict what he or she would do in imaginary situations (e.g., smelling smoke in a crowded movie theater)?

When asked what she would do if she found a stamped addressed envelope on the street, the patient replied, "Well, I would open it of course and read what it said. Maybe there would be money in it."

Insight. Insight is a patient's degree of awareness and understanding about being ill. Patients may exhibit complete denial of their illness or may show some awareness that they are ill but place the blame on others, on external factors, or even on organic factors. They may acknowledge that they have an illness but ascribe it to something unknown or mysterious in themselves.

An 18-year-old man went to an emergency room with the belief that he was controlled by a computer on an Enterprise-like starship, an elaboration from the television series Star Trek. He was convinced that all his thoughts, actions, and feelings were being programmed onboard the starship, which was located light years away and, therefore, could never be detected by anyone else.

Intellectual insight is present when patients can admit that they are ill and acknowledge that their failures to adapt are partly because of their own irrational feelings. Patients' inability to apply their knowledge to alter future experiences, however, is the major limitation to intellectual insight. True emotional insight is present when patients' awareness of their own motives and deep feelings leads to a change in their personality or behavior patterns.

A summary of six levels of insight follows:

1. Complete denial of illness
2. Slight awareness of being sick and needing help, but denying it at the same time
3. Awareness of being sick but blaming it on others, on external factors, or on organic factors
4. Awareness that illness is caused by something unknown in the patient
5. Intellectual insight: admission that the patient is ill and that symptoms or failures in social adjustment are caused by the patient's own particular irrational feelings or disturbances without applying this knowledge to future experiences
6. True emotional insight: emotional awareness of the motives and feelings within the patient and the important persons in his or her life, which can lead to basic changes in behavior.

Reliability

The mental status part of the report concludes with the psychiatrist's impressions of the patient's reliability and capacity to report his or her situation accurately. It includes an estimate of the psychiatrist's impression of the patient's truthfulness or veracity. For instance, if the patient is open about significant active substance abuse or about circumstances that the patient knows may reflect badly (e.g., trouble with the law), the psychiatrist may estimate the patient's reliability to be good.

PSYCHIATRIC REPORT

The psychiatric report is a written document that details the findings obtained from the psychiatric history and mental status examination. A detailed outline of the psychiatric report is found in Table 7.1–8. It includes a final summary of both positive and negative findings and an interpretation of the data. It has more than descriptive value; it has meaning that helps provide an understanding of the case. The examiner addresses critical questions in the report: Are future diagnostic studies needed and, if so, which ones? Is a consultant needed? Is a comprehensive neurological workup needed, including an electroencephalogram or computerized tomography scan? Are psychological tests indicated? Are psychodynamic factors relevant? The report includes a diagnosis made according to the revised fourth edition of the *Diagnostic and Statistical Manual of Mental Disorders* (DSM-IV-TR), which uses a multiaxial classification scheme consisting of five axes, each of which should be covered (see Table 9.1–7 in Section 9.1). A prognosis is also discussed in the report, with both good and bad prognostic factors listed. Finally, a treatment plan discusses, and makes firm recommendations about, management issues.

PRACTICAL ASPECTS OF THE PSYCHIATRIC INTERVIEW

Session Length

The initial consultation lasts for 30 minutes to 1 hour, depending on the circumstances. Interviews with patients who are psychotic or medically ill are brief because patients may find the interview stressful. Similarly, emergency room interviews vary in length. Initial interviews to evaluate patients for pharmacotherapy or psychotherapy tend to be longer; second visits and ongoing therapeutic interviews vary in length. The American Board of Psychiatry and Neurology, in its clinical oral examination in psychiatry, allows 30 minutes for candidates to conduct a psychiatric examination.

Patients' management of appointment times reveals important aspects of personality and coping. Most often, patients arrive a few minutes before their appointments. An anxious patient may arrive as much as 30 minutes early. When a patient arrives very early, the clinician may want to explore the reasons. The patient who arrives significantly late for an appointment also poses potential questions. The first time a patient is late, the clinician can listen to the explanation offered and respond sympathetically if the lateness is because of circumstances beyond the patient's control. A patient who states, "I forgot all about the appointment," however, is offering a clue that there is something about going to the doctor that makes that patient anxious or uncomfortable. This reaction needs to be explored further. The psychiatrist may ask, "Did you feel reluctant to come in today?" If the answer is, "Yes," the psychiatrist can begin to explore the possible reasons for the patient's reluctance. If the answer is, "No," it is probably best to drop the direct questioning about the lateness and just listen to the patient. By listening carefully, the psychiatrist can usually detect themes that the patient may not recognize. These themes can then be explored by both the patient and the psychiatrist in an attempt to understand better what the patient is experiencing.

Text continues on page 241.

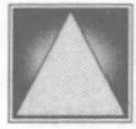

Table 7.1–8
Psychiatric Report

I. Psychiatric History
   A. Identification: Name, age, marital status, sex, occupation, language if other than English, race, nationality, and religion if pertinent; previous admissions to a hospital for the same or a different condition; with whom the patient lives
   B. Chief complaint: Exactly why the patient came to the psychiatrist, preferably in the patient's own words; if that information does not come from the patient, note who supplied it
   C. History of present illness: Chronological background and development of the symptoms or behavioral changes that culminated in the patient's seeking assistance; patient's life circumstances at the time of onset; personality when well; how illness has affected life activities and personal relations—changes in personality, interests, mood, attitudes toward others, dress, habits, level of tenseness, irritability, activity, attention, concentration, memory, speech; psychophysiological symptoms—nature and details of dysfunction; pain—location, intensity, fluctuation; level of anxiety—generalized and nonspecific (free floating) or specifically related to particular situations, activities, or objects; how anxieties are handled—avoidance, repetition of feared situation, use of drugs or other activities for alleviation
   D. Past psychiatric and medical history: (1) Emotional or mental disturbances—extent of incapacity, type of treatment, names of hospitals, length of illness, effect of treatment; (2) psychosomatic disorders: hay fever, arthritis, colitis, rheumatoid arthritis, recurrent colds, skin conditions; (3) medical conditions: follow customary review of systems—sexually transmitted diseases, alcohol or other substance abuse, at risk for acquired immunodeficiency syndrome (AIDS); (4) neurological disorders: headache, craniocerebral trauma, loss of consciousness, seizures or tumors
   E. Family history: Elicited from patient and from someone else, since quite different descriptions may be given of the same persons and events; ethnic, national, and religious traditions; other persons in the home, descriptions of them—personality and intelligence—and what has become of them since patient's childhood; descriptions of different households lived in; present relationships between patient and those who were in family; role of illness in the family; family history of mental illness; where does patient live—neighborhood and particular residence of the patient; is home crowded; privacy of family members from each other and from other families; sources of family income and difficulties in obtaining it; public assistance (if any) and attitude about it; will patient lose job or apartment by remaining in the hospital; who is caring for children
   F. Personal history (anamnesis): History of the patient's life from infancy to the present to the extent it can be recalled; gaps in history as spontaneously related by the patient; emotions associated with different life periods (painful, stressful, conflictual) or with phases of life cycle
      1. Early childhood (Birth through age 3)
         a. Prenatal history and mother's pregnancy and delivery: Length of pregnancy, spontaneity and normality of delivery, birth trauma, whether patient was planned and wanted, birth defects
         b. Feeding habits: Breast-fed or bottle-fed, eating problems
         c. Early development: Maternal deprivation, language development, motor development, signs of unmet needs, sleep pattern, object constancy, stranger anxiety, separation anxiety
         d. Toilet training: Age, attitude of parents, feelings about it
         e. Symptoms of behavior problems: Thumb sucking, temper tantrums, tics, head bumping, rocking, night terrors, fears, bed-wetting or bed soiling, nail biting, masturbation
         f. Personality and temperament as a child: Shy, restless, overactive, withdrawn, studious, outgoing, timid, athletic, friendly patterns of play, reactions to siblings
      2. Middle childhood (ages 3 to 11): Early school history—feelings about going to school, early adjustment, gender identification, conscience development, punishment; social relationships, attitudes toward siblings and playmates
      3. Later childhood (prepuberty through adolescence)
         a. Peer relationships: Number and closeness of friends, leader or follower, social popularity, participation in group or gang activities, idealized figures; patterns of aggression, passivity, anxiety, antisocial behavior
         b. School history: How far the patient went, adjustment to school, relationships with teachers—teacher's pet or rebellious—favorite studies or interests, particular abilities or assets, extracurricular activities, sports, hobbies, relationships of problems or symptoms to any school period
         c. Cognitive and motor development: Learning to read and other intellectual and motor skills, minimal cerebral dysfunction, learning disabilities—their management and effects on the child
         d. Particular adolescent emotional or physical problems: Nightmares, phobias, masturbation, bed-wetting, running away, delinquency, smoking, drug or alcohol use, weight problems, feeling of inferiority
         e. Psychosexual history
            i. Early curiosity, infantile masturbation, sex play
            ii. Acquiring of sexual knowledge, attitude of parents toward sex, sexual abuse
            iii. Onset of puberty, feelings about it, kind of preparation, feelings about menstruation, development of secondary sexual characteristics
            iv. Adolescent sexual activity: Crushes, parties, dating, petting, masturbation, wet dreams and attitudes toward them
            v. Attitudes toward same and opposite sex: Timid, shy, aggressive, need to impress, seductive, sexual conquests, anxiety
            vi. Sexual practices: Sexual problems, homosexual and heterosexual experiences, paraphilias, promiscuity
         f. Religious background: Strict, liberal, mixed (possible conflicts), relation of background to current religious practices

(*continued*)

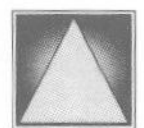

Table 7.1–8 (Continued)

4. Adulthood
    a. Occupational history: Choice of occupation, training, ambitions, conflicts; relations with authority, peers, and subordinates; number of jobs and duration; changes in job status; current job and feelings about it
    b. Social activity: Whether patient has friends or not; is patient withdrawn or socializing well; social, intellectual, and physical interests; relationships with same sex and opposite sex; depth, duration, and quality of human relations
    c. Adult sexuality
        i. Premarital sexual relationships, age of first coitus, sexual orientation
        ii. Marital history: Common-law marriages, legal marriages, description of courtship and role played by each partner, age at marriage, family planning and contraception, names and ages of children, attitudes toward raising children, problems of any family members, housing difficulties if important to the marriage, sexual adjustment, extramarital affairs, areas of agreement and disagreement, management of money, role of in-laws
        iii. Sexual symptoms: Anorgasmia, impotence, premature ejaculation, lack of desire
        iv. Attitudes toward pregnancy and having children; contraceptive practices and feelings about them
        v. Sexual practices: Paraphilias such as sadism, fetishes, voyeurism; attitude toward fellation, cunnilingus; coital techniques, frequency
    d. Military history: General adjustment, combat, injuries, referral to psychiatrists, type of discharge, veteran status
    e. Value systems: Whether children are seen as a burden or a joy; whether work is seen as a necessary evil, an avoidable chore, or an opportunity; current attitude about religion; belief in heaven and hell

Summation of the examiner's observations and impressions derived from the initial interview

II. Mental Status
- A. Appearance
    1. Personal identification: May include a brief nontechnical description of the patient's appearance and behavior as a novelist might write it; attitude toward examiner can be described here—cooperative, attentive, interested, frank, seductive, defensive, hostile, playful, ingratiating, evasive, guarded
    2. Behavior and psychomotor activity: Gait, mannerisms, tics, gestures, twitches, stereotypes, picking, touching examiner, echopraxia, clumsy, agile, limp, rigid, retarded, hyperactive, agitated, combative, waxy
    3. General description: Posture, bearing, clothes, grooming, hair, nails; healthy, sickly, angry, frightened, apathetic, perplexed, contemptuous, ill at ease, poised, old looking, young looking, effeminate, masculine; signs of anxiety—moist hands, perspiring forehead, restlessness, tense posture, strained voice, wide eyes; shifts in level of anxiety during interview or with particular topic
- B. Speech: Rapid, slow, pressured, hesitant, emotional, monotonous, loud, whispered, slurred, mumbled, stuttering, echolalia, intensity, pitch, ease, spontaneity, productivity, manner, reaction time, vocabulary, prosody
- C. Mood and affect
    1. Mood (a pervasive and sustained emotion that colors the person's perception of the world): How does patient say he or she feels; depth, intensity, duration, and fluctuations of mood—depressed, despairing, irritable, anxious, terrified, angry, expansive, euphoric, empty, guilty, awed, futile, self-contemptuous, anhedonic, alexithymic
    2. Affect (the outward expression of the patient's inner experiences): How examiner evaluates patient's affects—broad, restricted, blunted or flat, shallow, amount and range of expression; difficulty in initiating, sustaining, or terminating an emotional response; is the emotional expression appropriate to the thought content, culture, and setting of the examination; give examples if emotional expression is not appropriate
- D. Thinking and perception
    1. Form of thinking
        a. Productivity: Overabundance of ideas, paucity of ideas, flight of ideas, rapid thinking, slow thinking, hesitant thinking; does patient speak spontaneously or only when questions are asked, stream of thought, quotations from patient
        b. Continuity of thought: Whether patient's replies really answer questions and are goal directed, relevant, or irrelevant; loose associations; lack of causal relations in patient's explanations; illogical, tangential, circumstantial, rambling, evasive, perseverative statements, blocking or distractibility
        c. Language impairments: Impairments that reflect disordered mentation, such as incoherent or incomprehensible speech (word salad), clang associations, neologisms
    2. Content of thinking
        a. Preoccupations: About the illness, environmental problems; obsessions, compulsions, phobias; obsessions or plans about suicide, homicide; hypochondriacal symptoms, specific antisocial urges or impulses
    3. Thought disturbances
        a. Delusions: Content of any delusional system, its organization, the patient's convictions as to its validity, how it affects his or her life: persecutory delusions—isolated or associated with pervasive suspiciousness; mood-congruent or mood-incongruent
        b. Ideas of reference and ideas of influence: How ideas began, their content, and the meaning the patient attributes to them
    4. Perceptual disturbances
        a. Hallucinations and illusions: Whether patient hears voices or sees visions; content, sensory system involvement, circumstances of the occurrence; hypnagogic or hypnopompic hallucinations; thought broadcasting
        b. Depersonalization and derealization: Extreme feelings of detachment from self or from the environment

(*continued*)

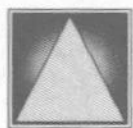

Table 7.1–8
(Continued)

5. Dreams and fantasies
   a. Dreams: Prominent ones, if patient will tell them; nightmares
   b. Fantasies: Recurrent, favorite, or unshakable daydreams

E. Sensorium
1. Alertness: Awareness of environment, attention span, clouding of consciousness, fluctuations in levels of awareness, somnolence, stupor, lethargy, fugue state, coma
2. Orientation
   a. Time: Whether patient identifies the day correctly; or approximate date, time of day; if in a hospital, knows how long he or she has been there; behaves as though oriented to the present
   b. Place: Whether patient knows where he or she is
   c. Person: Whether patient knows who the examiner is and the roles or names of the persons with whom in contact
3. Concentration and calculation: Subtracting 7 from 100 and keep subtracting 7s; if patient cannot subtract 7s, can easier tasks be accomplished—4 × 9; 5 × 4; how many nickels are in $1.35; whether anxiety or some disturbance of mood or concentration seems to be responsible for difficulty
4. Memory: Impairment, efforts made to cope with impairment—denial, confabulation, catastrophic reaction, circumstantiality used to conceal deficit: whether the process of registration, retention, or recollection of material is involved
   a. Remote memory: Childhood data, important events known to have occurred when the patient was younger or free of illness, personal matters, neutral material
   b. Recent past memory: Past few months
   c. Recent memory: Past few days, what did patient do yesterday, the day before, have for breakfast, lunch, dinner
   d. Immediate retention and recall: Ability to repeat six figures after examiner dictates them—first forward, then backward, then after a few minutes' interruption; other test questions; did same questions, if repeated, call forth different answers at different times
   e. Effect of defect on patient: Mechanisms patient has developed to cope with defect
5. Fund of knowledge: Level of formal education and self-education; estimate of the patient's intellectual capability and whether capable of functioning at the level of his or her basic endowment; counting, calculation, general knowledge; questions should have relevance to the patient's educational and cultural background
6. Abstract thinking: Disturbances in concept formation; manner in which the patient conceptualizes or handles his or her ideas; similarities (e.g., between apples and pears), differences, absurdities; meanings of simple proverbs (e.g., "A rolling stone gathers no moss") answers may be concrete (giving specific examples to illustrate the meaning) or overly abstract (giving generalized explanation); appropriateness of answers

F. Insight: Degree of personal awareness and understanding of illness
1. Complete denial of illness
2. Slight awareness of being sick and needing help but denying it at the same time
3. Awareness of being sick but blaming it on others, on external factors, on medical or unknown organic factors
4. Intellectual insight: Admission of illness and recognition that symptoms or failures in social adjustment are due to irrational feelings or disturbances, without applying that knowledge to future experiences
5. True emotional insight: Emotional awareness of the motives and feelings within, of the underlying meaning of symptoms; does the awareness lead to changes in personality and future behavior; openness to new ideas and concepts about self and the important persons in his or her life

G. Judgment
1. Social judgment: Subtle manifestations of behavior that are harmful to the patient and contrary to acceptable behavior in the culture; does the patient understand the likely outcome of personal behavior and is patient influenced by that understanding; examples of impairment
2. Test judgment: Patient's prediction of what he or she would do in imaginary situations (e.g., what patient would do with a stamped, addressed letter found in the street)

III. Further Diagnostic Studies
A. Physical examination
B. Neurological examination
C. Additional psychiatric diagnostic
D. Interviews with family members, friends, or neighbors by a social worker
E. Psychological, neurological, or laboratory tests as indicated: Electroencephalogram, computed tomography scan, magnetic resonance imaging, tests of other medical conditions, reading comprehension and writing tests, test for aphasia, projective or objective psychological tests, dexamethasone-suppression test, 24-hour urine test for heavy metal intoxication, urine screen for drugs of abuse

IV. Summary of Findings

Summarize mental symptoms, medical and laboratory findings, and psychological and neurological test results, if available; include medications patient has been taking, dosage, duration. Clarity of thinking is reflected in clarity of writing. When summarizing the mental status (e.g., the phrase "Patient denies hallucinations and delusions" is not as precise as "Patient denies hearing voices or thinking that he is being followed."). The latter indicates the specific question asked and the specific response given. Similarly, in the conclusion of the report one would write "Hallucinations and delusions were not elicited."

(*continued*)

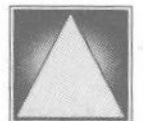

Table 7.1–8
(Continued)

V. Diagnosis

Diagnostic classification is made according to DSM-IV-TR, which uses a multiaxial classification scheme consisting of five axes, each of which should be covered in the diagnosis

Axis I: Clinical syndromes (e.g., mood disorders, schizophrenia, generalized anxiety disorder) and other conditions that may be a focus of clinical attention

Axis II: Personality disorders, mental retardation, and defense mechanisms

Axis III: Any general medical conditions (e.g., epilepsy, cardiovascular disease, endocrine disorders)

Axis IV: Psychosocial and environmental problems (e.g., divorce, injury, death of a loved one) relevant to the illness

Axis V: Global assessment of functioning exhibited by the patient during the interview (e.g., social, occupational, and psychological functioning); a rating scale with a continuum from 100 (superior functioning) to 1 (grossly impaired functioning) is used

VI. Prognosis

Opinion about the probable future course, extent, and outcome of the disorder; good and bad prognostic factors; specific goals of therapy

VII. Psychodynamic Formulation

Causes of the patient's psychodynamic breakdown—influences in the patient's life that contributed to present disorder; environmental, genetic, and personality factors relevant to determining patient's symptoms; primary and secondary gains; outline of the major defense mechanism used by the patient

VIII. Comprehensive Treatment Plan

Modalities of treatment recommended, role of medication, inpatient or outpatient treatment, frequency of sessions, probable duration of therapy; type of psychotherapy; individual, group, or family therapy; symptoms or problems to be treated. Initially, treatment must be directed toward any life-threatening situations such as suicidal risk or risk of danger to others that require psychiatric hospitalization. Danger to self or others is an acceptable reason (both legally and medically) for involuntary hospitalization. In the absence of the need for confinement, a variety of outpatient treatment alternatives are available: day hospitals, supervised residences, outpatient psychotherapy or pharmacotherapy, among others. In some cases, treatment planning must attend to vocational and psychosocial skills training and even legal or forensic issues.

Comprehensive treatment planning requires a therapeutic team approach using the skills of psychologists, social workers, nurses, activity and occupational therapists, and a variety of other mental health professionals, with referral to self-help groups (e.g., Alcoholics Anonymous [AA]) if needed. If either the patient or family members are unwilling to accept the recommendations of treatment and the clinician thinks that the refusal of the recommendations may have serious consequences, the patient, parent, or guardian should sign a statement to the effect that the recommended treatment was refused.

A psychiatrist's handling of time is also an important factor in the interview. Carelessness about time indicates a lack of concern for the patient. If a psychiatrist is unavoidably detained for an interview, it is appropriate to express regret at having kept the patient waiting.

Seating and Arrangement of Office

The arrangement of chairs in the psychiatrist's office affects the interview. Both chairs should be of approximately equal height, so that neither person looks down on the other. Most psychiatrists think that it is desirable to place the chairs without any furniture between the clinician and the patient. If the room contains several chairs, the psychiatrist indicates his or her own chair and then allows the patient to choose the chair in which he or she will feel most comfortable.

The evaluation should be conducted in a comfortable room with pleasant lighting. Better rapport can be established and fuller observations made if the psychiatrist is not sitting behind a desk. Although no reason exists to make the room impersonal, dramatic paintings, spectacular, panoramic views, or expensive antiques may distract the patient. A comfortable waiting area should be provided for patients who arrive early.

A psychiatrist can never remain entirely unknown to patients, and the office can tell patients a good deal about the doctor's personality. The colors in the office, paintings and diplomas on the wall, the furniture, plants, books, and personal photographs all describe the psychiatrist in ways that are not directly verbalized. Patients often have reactions to their doctors' offices that may or may not be distortions, and carefully listening to any comments can help a psychiatrist understand the patient. Studies have shown that patients respond more positively to male physicians who wear jackets and ties than to those who do not. No studies have been done on the dress of female physicians, but, by extrapolation, professional attire would probably elicit a positive response.

Types of Interventions

Psychiatrists do much more during an interview than ask questions. They provide feedback and information, offer reassurances, and respond emotionally to what the patient is saying. The psychiatrist's facial expression and body posture also convey information to the patient. Interventions are described as "supportive" or "obstructive," depending on the extent to which they increase the flow of information and enhance or diminish rapport. Table 7.1–9 contains examples of both.

The concept of supportive and obstructive interventions has broad, general use, but it cannot be applied rigidly. The psychiatric interview is a complex, multifaceted task that is shaped by the personalities and circumstances of the interview. Above all, it is a human endeavor. The personality of the interviewer

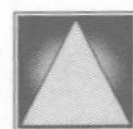

Table 7.1–9
Supportive and Obstructive Interventions

Supportive

Acknowledging emotion

Doctor: "Even after all these years, talking about your mother brings tears to your eyes."

Encouragement

Patient: "I've never been very good at putting things into words."

Doctor: "I think you've described the situation well—in a way that helps me understand what you have been going through."

Reassurance

Doctor: "The hopelessness you feel right now seems overwhelming. I think it is very likely with the proper treatment you can get back to feeling yourself."

Nonverbal

Facial expression and body posture that convey interest, concern, and attentiveness.

Obstructive

Compound questions

Doctor: "Do you take a vacation every year, and are you able to relax?"

Trapping the patient in his or her own words

Doctor: "When I asked you before, you said nothing had gone well over the last year, and now you are telling me you got a raise and have been exercising more."

Why questions

Doctor: "Why do you keep waking up so early in the morning?"

Dismissal or minimization

Patient: "Over the last month I have had trouble with sex."

Doctor: "That happens from time to time."

Premature advice

Patient: "Ever since my girlfriend and I split up last year, I cannot seem to meet anyone new."

Doctor: "Why not try spending time in bookstores and coffee houses? There are usually lots of single people in those places."

Not following the patient's lead

Doctor: "How long have you been feeling so sad?"

Patient: "Over 6 months. Nothing is getting better. I am starting to wonder if it is worth it."

Doctor: "Do you have trouble sleeping through the night?"

Judgmental

Doctor: "Have you been using any drugs?"

Patient: "Well besides drinking, I smoke a little grass on weekends."

Doctor: "Do you not know that marijuana can cause serious problems with motivation over the long term?"

Nonverbal

Facial expression, body posture, and behavior that indicate lack of interest or inattentiveness, such as yawning, or checking one's watch. The doctor who shows no emotional reaction to what a patient is saying usually conveys a sense of not listening or being uninterested.

is an inevitable and desirable component of the interview and it need not to be veiled behind a mask of austerity or indifference. The concept of "neutrality" as proposed in psychoanalytic psychiatry means that the psychiatrist does not take sides in the patient's intrapsychic conflicts. It does not mean the clinician is a nonresponding robot.

Ending the Interview

At the end of the evaluation, the psychiatrist must give the patient his or her impressions and suggestions, even if they are preliminary. Patients seeing a psychiatrist for the first time are often apprehensive. They wonder if they are "crazy," if their problems can be understood, if they will be judged, and most importantly whether they can be helped. Although patients can experience significant relief just in talking with another person about their concerns, these fears should be explicitly addressed and realistic reassurance offered about available treatments. The concluding moments of the initial interview prepare the patient for follow-up, and handling them well increases the likelihood of helping the patient. It is especially important to give persons who have become emotionally distraught a few minutes to collect themselves before they are asked to leave the office. For example, a psychiatrist might say to a patient who is sobbing heavily near the end of the interview, "It's clear these things are still very painful to talk about. We have to finish in a few minutes, but let me take a moment to give you my impressions and tell you what I think is best to do next."

Note Taking

For legal and medical reasons, an adequate written record of each patient's treatment must be maintained. The patient's record also aids the psychiatrist's memory. Each clinician must establish a system of record keeping and decide which information to record. Many psychiatrists make complete notes during the first few sessions while eliciting historical data. Afterward, most psychiatrists record only new historical information, important events in the patient's life, medications prescribed, dreams, and general comments about the patient's progress. Some psychiatrists maintain detailed process notes (verbatim record of a session) for specific patients by writing out immediately after a session as much of the session as they can remember. Process notes make it much easier to determine trends in the treatment (with regard to transference and countertransference issues) and to go back over the session to pick up ideas that may have been missed. Process notes are also helpful if a psychiatrist is working with a supervisor or a consultant who needs an accurate presentation of a particular session.

Most psychiatrists do not recommend taking extensive notes during a session; writing can cut down on the ability to listen. Some patients, however, may express resentment if a psychiatrist does not write notes during an interview; they may fear that their comments were not important enough to record or that the psychiatrist was not interested in them. Because not taking notes during a session presumably has no relation to the psychiatrist's listening, this feeling on a patient's part can be further explored to understand the fear of not being taken seriously.

An increasing number of psychiatrists are communicating with patients through e-mail. E-mail has the advantages of being quick, usually brief, and often less disruptive than telephone calls. As a result, e-mail communication often feels more spontaneous and casual than a telephone call or letter. For all their apparent casualness, e-mail messages, however, constitute a formal part of the treatment record and are subject to review in court proceedings.

Stress Interview

A stress interview has its advocates and has a minor place in the armamentarium of interview techniques. Most patients feel some anxiety or other emotion when talking to a psychiatrist. Through his or her manner or a word of reassurance or praise the psychiatrist can often decrease this emotion so that the patient can continue to tell his or her story. Certain patients, however, are monotonously repetitious or show insufficient emotion for motivation. Apathy, indifference, and emotional blunting are not conducive to discussion of personality problems. In patients with such reactions, stimulation of emotions can be constructive. These patients may require probing, challenging, or confrontation to arouse feelings that will promote progress in furthering understanding. For example, the *la belle indifférence* of the hysteric may be converted into anxiety so that the patient can experience sufficient discomfort to talk about his or her conflicts.

Follow-Up Interviews

Interviews after the initial one allow patients to correct any misinformation provided in the first meeting. It is often helpful to start the second interview by asking a patient whether he or she has thought about the first interview and what his or her reactions to the experience were. Another variation is to say, "Frequently, people think of additional things they wanted to discuss after they leave. What thoughts have you had?"

Psychiatrists often learn something of value when they ask patients whether they have discussed the interview with anyone else. If the patient has done so, the details of the conversation and the person with whom the patient spoke are enlightening. No set rules exist about which topics are best deferred until the second interview. In general, as patients' comfort and familiarity with the psychiatrist increase, they become increasingly able to reveal the intimate details of their lives.

References

Benazzi F. Bipolar II disorder family history using the family history screen: Findings and clinical implications. *Compr Psychiatry*. 2004;45(2):77–82.

First MB, Frances A, Pincus HA. *DSM-IV-TR Handbook of Differential Diagnosis*. Washington DC: American Psychiatric Publishing, Inc.; 2002.

International Guidelines for Diagnostic Assessment (IGDA). Workgroup, WPA (World Psychiatric Association). *Br J Psychiatry*. 2003;182[Suppl 45]:S40–S59.

Kendell RE. Five criteria for an improved taxonomy of mental disorders. In: Helzer JE, Hudziak JJ, eds. *Defining Psychopathology in the 21st Century. DSM-V and Beyond*. Washington DC: American Psychiatric Publishing, Inc.; 2002:3–17.

King CA, Knox MS, Henninger N, Nguyen TA, Ghaziuddin N, Maker A, Hanna GL. Major depressive disorder in adolescents: Family psychiatric history predicts severe behavioral disinhibition. *J Affect Disord*. 2006;90(2–3):111–121.

Kraemer HC, Measelle JR, Ablow JC, Essex MJ, Boyce T, Kupfer DJ. A new approach to integrating data from multiple informants in psychiatric assessment and research: Mixing and matching contexts and perspectives. *Am J Psychiatry*. 2003;160:1566–1577.

Larsson HJ, Eaton WW, Madsen KM, Vestergaard M, Olesen AV, Agerbo E, Schende D, Thorsen P, Mortensen PB. Risk factors for autism: Perinatal factors, parental psychiatric history, and socioeconomic status. *Am J Epidemiol*. 2005; 161(10):916–925.

Moran P, Leese M, Lee T, Walters P, Thornicroft G, Mann A. Standardised Assessment of Personality—Abbreviated Scale (SAPAS): Preliminary validation of a brief screen for personality disorder. *Br J Psychiatry*. 2003;183:228–232.

Othmer E, Othmer SC, Othmer JP. Psychiatric interview, history, and mental status examination. In: Sadock BJ, Sadock VA, eds. *Kaplan & Sadock's Comprehensive Textbook of Psychiatry*. 8th ed. Vol. 1. Baltimore: Lippincott Williams & Wilkins; 2005:794.

Trémeau F, Staner L, Duval F, Corrêa H, Crocq MA, Darreye A, Czobor P, Dessoubrais C, Macher JP. Suicide attempts and family history of suicide in three psychiatric populations. *Suicide Life Threat Behav*. 2005;35(6):702–713.

Zimmerman M. What should the standard of care for psychiatric diagnostic evaluations be? *J Nerv Ment Disord*. 2003;191:281–286.

Zun LS. Evidence-based evaluation of psychiatric patients. *J Emerg Med*. 2005; 28:35–39.

▲ 7.2 Interviewing Techniques with Special Patient Populations

Various types of patients fall under the rubric of special patient populations. They include patients with urgent issues, the severely mentally ill, patients from different cultural backgrounds who are unassimilated, those who cannot communicate well because of difficulties with the English language, and patients whose personality problems make them, difficult, demanding, uncooperative, or likely to engage in power struggles.

Inherent in the management of all such cases is the doctor's understanding of the emotions, fears, and conflicts that the patient's behavior represents. Different patient types and special situations and guidelines for handling them are discussed below.

PSYCHOTIC PATIENTS

By definition, psychotic patients have poor or absent reality testing abilities. Therefore, the evaluation of a patient with psychotic symptoms needs to be more focused and structured than that of other patients. Open-ended questions and long periods of silence are apt to be disorganizing. Short questions are easier to follow than long ones. Questions calling for abstract responses or hypothetical conjectures may be unanswerable.

Thought Disorders

Disorders of thought can seriously impair effective communications. The evaluating psychiatrist should note formal thought disorders while minimizing their adverse impact on the interview. When derailment is evident, the psychiatrist typically proceeds with questions calling for short responses. For a patient experiencing thought blocking, the psychiatrist needs to repeat questions, to remind the patient of what was already said, and, in general, to provide an organization for thinking that the patient is unable to provide.

For example, in response to the question, "Why did you come to the clinic?" a patient responded: "When I got up this morning, I showered and dressed. I was angry at my landlord for not fixing the faucet in my bathroom. I tried to get him on the phone. He wouldn't talk to me. I'll call my lawyer. You see, my rent is supposed to be paid by the Department of Welfare, but they're so nasty. [But why did you come to the clinic?] I'm coming to that, Doctor. You see, they don't care about an upright citizen. I did so much for my community. No one can say I wasn't a hard worker, etc." After repeated questioning, she finally stated she was worried about being constipated.

Hallucinations

Hallucinations are false sensory perceptions. For patients with hallucinations, the full phenomenology of the hallucination should be explored. The patient is asked to describe the sensory misperception as fully as possible. For auditory hallucinations, this includes content, volume, clarity, and circumstances; for visual hallucinations, this includes content, intensity, the situations in which they occur, and the patient's response. The evaluator should distinguish between true hallucinations, on the one hand, and illusions, hypnagogic and hypnopompic hallucinations, and vivid imaginings, on the other. Hallucinations are perceived as real sensory stimuli and should not be dismissed as fanciful; however, the psychiatrist should ask questions about their fixity and the patient's level of insight: "Does it ever seem that the voices are coming from your own thoughts?" or "What do you think is causing the voices?"

Delusions

Delusions are fixed, false beliefs not in keeping with the culture. Delusional patients often come to psychiatric evaluation having had their beliefs dismissed or belittled by friends and family. They are on guard for similar reactions from the examiner. It is possible to ask questions about delusions without revealing belief or disbelief (e.g., "Does it seem that people are intent on hurting you?" rather than "Do you believe there is a plot to hurt you?"). Careless use of psychiatric jargon should be avoided, particularly in evaluating delusions. Many psychiatrists have found that patients can speak more freely when asked to talk about the accompanying emotions rather than the belief itself ("It must be frightening to think there are people you do not know who are plotting against you"). Although the psychiatrist does not attempt to reason them away, a gentle probe may determine how tenaciously the beliefs are held ("Do you ever wonder whether those things might not be true?").

The following case illustrates ideas of reference and paranoid delusions. A married man, aged 58, with a life history of dependable, conscientious work as a bookkeeper, became sleepless, anxious, and unable to concentrate. He developed the belief that his vision was failing because of poisons secretly placed in his food by former neighbors. He found a misprint in a newspaper that he felt was placed there by the editor to shame him publicly. Admitted to the psychiatric service of a general hospital, he said that cars passing up and down the street contained agents who were spying on him. He believed that the electric light bulbs in his room were emanating a purifying radiation to counteract syphilitic germs, which he was supposedly breathing into the atmosphere, although a physical examination was negative for syphilis.

SUSPICIOUS PATIENTS

Some persons, usually those with a paranoid personality, have a chronic, deeply ingrained suspicion that other people want to cause them harm. Although their suspiciousness does not crystallize into a delusion, they misinterpret neutral events as evidence of a conspiracy against them. They are critical and evasive, and are sometimes called "grievance collectors" because they tend to blame other people for everything bad in their lives. They are extremely mistrustful and may question everything the doctor says or does. The physician should try to maintain a respectful but somewhat formal and distant approach with these patients. Expressions of warmth often heighten their suspicions. The doctor should explain in detail every decision and planned procedure and should try to respond nondefensively to the patient's suspiciousness.

DEPRESSED AND POTENTIALLY SUICIDAL PATIENTS

Severely depressed patients may have difficulty concentrating, thinking clearly, and speaking spontaneously. The psychiatrist evaluating a depressed patient may need to be more forceful and directive than usual. Although depressed patients should not be badgered, long silences are seldom useful, and the examiner may need to repeat questions more than once. Ruminative patients—for example, those who continually repeat how worthless or guilty they are—need to be interrupted and redirected.

A 52-year-old man began to experience insomnia, weight loss, and feelings of worthlessness that began after his wife had died 6 months previously. He was unable to work effectively and told his daughter that he felt "life is hopeless." He agreed to a psychiatric consultation at her request.

All patients must be asked about suicidal thoughts; however, depressed patients may need to be questioned more fully. A thorough assessment of suicide potential addresses intent, plans, means, and perceived consequences, as well as history of attempts and family history of suicide. The examiner must feel sufficiently comfortable to ask simple, straightforward, noneuphemistic questions. Asking about suicide does not increase the risk. The psychiatrist is not raising a topic that the patient has not already contemplated. Specific, detailed questions are essential for prevention.

Intent

The examiner must determine the seriousness of the wish to die. Some patients report that they wish that they were dead, but would never intentionally do anything to take their own lives. This level of intent is sometimes referred to as *passive suicidal ideation*. Other patients express greater degrees of determination. At the most extreme level of determination are the patients who are the most difficult to help, those who tell no one about their suicidal plans and proceed in a deliberate, systematic manner. It is useful to ask about restraining influences, internal and external (e.g., "Do you worry that you might not be able to resist those impulses?" or "How have you been able to keep from hurting yourself so far?"). Patients with auditory hallucinations commanding them to kill themselves often describe the hallucinations as irresistible despite not having any real desire to die.

Plans

Patients with well-formulated plans are generally at greater risk than patients who do not know what they would do, but the method of suicide is not always a reliable indication of the risk. The psychiatrist should also ask about preparatory actions, such as giving away goods and putting one's estate in order.

Means

Asking patients about the intended means of suicide is helpful in two ways. First, it clarifies the urgency of the situation. Second, the understanding of intent is sharpened by knowing whether a patient has thought through the steps necessary to carry out the action.

Perceived Consequences

Patients who see something desirable resulting from their deaths are at increased risk for suicide (e.g., reunion fantasy, the belief that a person will be reunited with a deceased loved one). On the other hand, some potentially suicidal patients are restrained by what they see as negative consequences (e.g., "My children need me too much; they'd never be able to get along without me"). The psychiatric history and the family history for all patients, even those not currently suicidal, should mention any previous suicide attempt or suicides by family members. Both circumstances are recognized to increase the current risk, even if previous attempts were thought to be superficial.

In rare circumstances, the threat of suicide is so imminent that immediate action must be taken to hospitalize the patient. Even during a first evaluation session, the psychiatrist must be prepared to make whatever professional response is necessary to safeguard the well-being of the patient.

SOMATIZING PATIENTS

Some patients experience and describe emotional distress in terms of physical symptoms. Somatizing patients pose a number of difficulties for the consulting and the treating psychiatrist because they may be reluctant to engage in self-reflection and psychological exploration. Moreover, somatic distress without physical findings can lead to diagnostic uncertainty, which, in turn, makes treatment less certain.

Many somatizing patients live with the fear that their symptoms are not being taken seriously and the parallel fear that something medically serious may be overlooked. Psychiatrists' main task in dealing with these patients is to acknowledge the suffering conveyed by the symptoms without necessarily accepting the patient's explanation for the symptoms. Clinicians should be curious about both the nature of the physical complaints and the impact of those complaints on the patient's life.

It is essential that somatizing patients feel that their physical complaints are not being dismissed. Rather than limiting the scope of inquiry to psychological issues, the psychiatrist wants to expand discussion to include all aspects of the patient's well-being and emotional and physical health. It is often helpful for the physician to propose a purely pragmatic approach—one that stresses a willingness to use whatever works to relieve the patient's suffering without causing harm. At times, this may include nonstandard approaches, such as meditation, yoga, or acupuncture, in addition to psychotherapy.

It is especially important for the psychiatrist working with a somatizing patient to form a collaborative relationship with the primary medical doctor; to obtain thorough copies of medical records and evaluations; and for them to consult freely with one another about the patient's health and symptoms. An important goal of treatment is to minimize the harm caused by aggressive and unwarranted medical interventions.

It is foolhardy for the psychiatrist to assume with absolute conviction that a patient's physical complaints have no real medical basis. The psychiatrist's task is not to close the door on medical investigation, but to invite patients to consider an even larger range of factors, including emotional and psychological issues, all of which can affect their health.

A 45-year-old man was convinced he had acquired immune deficiency syndrome (AIDS), despite having no risk factors. He repeatedly sought out human immunodeficiency virus (HIV) testing and blood cell counts. When tests reported that he was not HIV positive, he felt considerable, but short-lived, relief. He soon began to doubt the accuracy of the tests and reporting. "Can you tell me with certainty, that there is 100 percent no chance of error?" he asked his medical doctor. Over several months, his anxiety and depression increased, and he accepted referral to a psychiatrist.

The psychiatrist reframed the issue by saying that the major cause of the patient's distress was not AIDS, but the fear of AIDS. He observed that frequent testing had not provided reassurance but, in fact, had increased the patient's anxiety. The psychiatrist stressed that he would not ignore the patient's physical health. The patient agreed to scheduled medical consultations every 6 months and, in the course of psychotherapy, became more open in discussing considerable nonsomatic concerns. He also benefited from antidepressant medication.

AGITATED AND POTENTIALLY VIOLENT PATIENTS

When interviewing potentially violent patients, the task is to conduct an assessment and to contain behavior and limit the potential for harm.

Most unpremeditated violence is preceded by a prodrome of accelerating psychomotor agitation. Researchers and clinicians in emergency psychiatry suggest that the prodrome lasts from 30 to 60 minutes before erupting into physical violence. Thus, the psychiatric evaluator has early signals of impending violence and a period of time in which the agitation may be quieted.

Several steps can be taken to minimize the agitation and potential risk. The interview should be conducted in a quiet, nonstimulating environment. Sufficient space should be available for the comfort of the patient and the psychiatrist, with no physical barrier to leaving the examination room for either of them. During the interview, the psychiatrist should avoid any behavior that could be misconstrued as menacing: standing over the patient, staring, or touching.

The psychiatrist should ask whether the patient is carrying weapons and may ask the patient to leave the weapon with a guard or in a holding area. The psychiatrist should not request that the patient hand over any weapons. If the patient's agitation continues to increase, the psychiatrist may need to terminate the interview. Depending on the setting, assistance from security personnel or physical or chemical restraints may be appropriate. The physician's own subjective sense of comfort or fear should be heeded.

A 35-year-old man is brought to the emergency room by the police shouting that he plans "to kill anyone I can get my hands on." He is in restraints and both pleading and shouting that he be released. There is a strong odor of alcohol on his breath. The examining doctor insists that the restraints remain in place during the preliminary medical evaluation, which included taking blood specimens. Not until the patient was calm were the restraints removed.

SEDUCTIVE PATIENTS

Seductiveness can be manifested in a patient's dress, behavior, and speech. It runs the gamut from gentle suggestion to explicit proposition.

Of course, sex is not the only enticement with which psychiatrists can be seduced. Patients may offer insider information for profitable trading in the stock market, may promise an introduction to a movie star friend, or may suggest that they will dedicate their next novel to the psychiatrist.

Whatever the offer, the psychiatrist's response is the same. In the course of ongoing psychotherapy and in the context of an established relationship, seductive behavior is discussed and examined in an effort to understand its meaning. The psychiatrist should make it clear that what is being offered will not be accepted, in a way that preserves good rapport and does not unnecessarily assault the patient's self-esteem.

Seductive behavior during an initial psychiatric assessment must be handled somewhat differently. When the behavior is mild and indirect, it may be best to ignore it. More explicit propositions call for more direct responses and may afford the psychiatrist the chance to explain the nature of the therapeutic relationship and the need to establish boundaries. The psychiatrist should also make clear that it is the violation of those boundaries that is being rejected and not the patient.

A woman who was pregnant and in her late trimester began acting seductively toward her obstetrician. She would rub against him whenever possible and constantly asked him questions about his personal life. Recognizing this behavior as unusual, the obstetrician decided to explore the possible underlying reasons for the change. He began by asking what prompted her and her husband to have a child at this time and how each of them was feeling about becoming a parent. The patient quickly told how difficult it was to think about becoming a mother, because she was afraid that her husband would no longer find her sexually attractive. Further discussions about her past revealed that the patient's parents did not seem interested in each other as a husband and wife once they became parents. There was even a strong suspicion that, after the birth of the patient's younger sister, the patient's father had an affair. She now began to recognize that she was afraid that her husband would react in exactly the same way as her father did. In this transference reaction, the patient was responding to her husband as though he were her father. After discussing the problem further, the obstetrician suggested to the patient that she share her concerns with her husband. As she did, the marital relationship improved considerably, and the patient's sexual interest in her obstetrician disappeared.

DEPENDENT PATIENTS

Some patients seem to need an inordinate amount of attention and yet never seem reassured. They are the patients who are likely to make repeated urgent calls between scheduled appointments and to demand special consideration. The doctor needs to be firm in establishing limits when reassuring the patient that his or her needs are taken seriously and are treated professionally.

DEMANDING PATIENTS

Some patients have a difficult time delaying gratification and demand that their discomfort be eliminated immediately. They are easily frustrated and can become petulant or even angry and hostile if they do not get what they want when they want it. They may impulsively do something self-destructive if they feel thwarted, and they appear manipulative and attention seeking. Beneath their surface behavior, they may fear that they will never get what they need from others and, thus, must act in that inappropriately aggressive way. The doctor must be firm with these patients from the outset and must clearly define acceptable and unacceptable behavior. These patients must be treated with respect and care, but they must also be confronted with their behavior.

A cardiologist complained that many patients exhausted him with trivial details about minor noncardiac complaints whenever he queried them about their heart conditions. He found this behavior particularly exasperating because he was unable to influence it by cajolery or stern remonstrations. It was explained to him that these patients are fearful and are seeking to postpone as long as possible confronting what they fear most, namely, the possibility of cardiac invalidism or death. By prefacing his crisp inquiry about the patient's cardiac symptoms with a few words of reassurance, he found that such patients quickly became more cooperative.

NARCISSISTIC PATIENTS

Narcissistic patients act as though they are superior to everyone around them, including the doctor. They have a tremendous need to appear perfect and are contemptuous of others whom they perceive to be imperfect. They can be rude, abrupt, arrogant, and demanding. They may initially idealize a doctor out of a need to have their doctor be as perfect as they are, but the idealization can quickly turn to disdain when they realize that the doctor is only human after all. Underneath their surface arrogance, narcissistic patients feel desperately inadequate and fear that others will see through them.

ISOLATED PATIENTS

Isolated and solitary patients do not appear to need or to want much contact with other people. Intimate contact with the doctor is viewed with distaste, and such patients would prefer to take care of themselves entirely without the doctor's help if it were possible. Some isolated patients would receive a diagnosis of schizoid personality disorder. They are withdrawn, absorbed in a world of fantasy, and are unable to talk about their feelings. The doctor should treat these patients with as much respect for their privacy as possible and should not expect them to respond to the doctor's concern with openness.

OBSESSIVE PATIENTS

Obsessive patients are orderly, punctual, and so concerned with detail that they often do not see the larger picture. They may appear unemotional, even aloof, especially when confronted with anything disturbing or frightening. They have a strong need to be in control of everything in their lives and may struggle with their doctor whenever they feel that decisions are being imposed. Underneath, obsessive patients are often frightened of losing control and of becoming helpless and dependent. Their physicians should try to include them in their own care and treatment as much as possible. Doctors should explain in detail what is going on and what is being planned, allowing the patient to make choices on his or her own behalf.

PATIENTS WHO LIE

A fundamental stance in psychiatric interviewing is recognizing that what is being heard may not be the literal truth. The unreliability of memory and the vagaries of psychopathology through which a patient's narrative is processed distort and falsify. At times, patients lie consciously with the explicit intent of deceiving the therapist. The purpose may be secondary gain (e.g., exemption from jury duty, a supply of psychoactive drugs, or leave of absence from graduate school), in which case the person is malingering. Malingering is not a mental disorder in the revised fourth edition of the *Diagnostic and Statistical Manual of Mental Disorders* (DSM-IV-TR). More rarely, a patient explicitly lies not for any obvious external advantage, but simply for whatever psychological advantage is conferred by assuming the sick role, in which case the person has a factitious disorder that is a DSM-IV-TR diagnosis.

Because psychiatrists do not have recourse to biological markers or other external validating criteria, the patient's report must be accepted as an honest statement of experience. No way exists to establish whether a person is experiencing auditory hallucinations other than through self-report. Nevertheless, an experienced clinician may detect subtle discrepancies, internal inconsistencies, or suspiciously atypical symptoms; these can certainly be queried without necessarily assuming that the patient is lying.

A 29-year-old woman describes an almost unremitting migraine headache and is asking for narcotic pain medication.

Patient: I really need your help. The pain is unbearable. I can't do anything anymore. I just want to lie in bed in a dark room with the cover pulled up over my head.

Doctor: That does sound miserable. I am struck by the fact that you obviously care about your appearance and have given some time and attention to your hair, makeup, and the way you are dressed. Was that despite the pain that you have been describing?

It may be difficult to catch a practiced liar in an initial session. Arguably, the interviewer should not try to do so. Psychiatrists are trained to detect, to understand, and to treat psychopathology, not to function as lie detectors. Although a certain level of suspicion is essential to the practice of psychiatry, a clinician who is determined never to be taken in by deceitful patients approaches patients with such exaggerated suspiciousness that therapeutic work is not possible.

Patients with somatoform disorders, such as conversion disorder or pain disorder, are presumably unaware of the emotional bases of their physical complaints. In describing their somatic symptoms, they are stating psychological reality, not attempting to deceive the interviewer.

PATIENTS WHO DO NOT COOPERATE

Lack of patient cooperation can take many forms: failure to keep appointments, refusal to talk or to take the session seriously, failure to pay for services. Causes of noncooperation include manifestations of the patient's underlying pathology, anger at the psychiatrist, feelings of being coerced into an evaluation or treatment against one's will, or manifestations of transference. How the psychiatrist responds depends on the setting and context.

The evaluation of an uncooperative patient during an emergency necessarily proceeds differently from that during nonemergencies; an emergency psychiatric evaluation must often proceed without full cooperation or even against the patient's will. In such situations, sedation or restraint is sometimes necessary to complete even a basic triage assessment. The patient's refusal to cooperate is superseded by concern for the patient's life and the safety of others.

The patient who has been engaged in a meaningful therapy for some time and then becomes uncooperative is sending a powerful signal to the psychiatrist, the meaning of which must be explored. The change in behavior may be a manifestation of resistance to upsetting material that is beginning to emerge in therapy or of transference. It may also be in response to real life interactions between doctor and patient.

A 52-year-old man who had been in psychotherapy for 1.5 years following difficulties in his marriage began missing sessions and arriving late. This followed several last-minute cancellations by the psychiatrist who offered neither explanation nor apology. When asked about his absences, the man quickly acknowledged how angry he was at the therapist for standing him up. "I see no reason why I should have to be more responsible than you," he said. The lateness and absences in therapy were motivated by anger at the psychiatrist's unprofessional behavior.

Although transference and countertransference are important concepts in psychoanalytic psychotherapies, their use in other modalities, such as cognitive-behavioral therapy, may be inappropriate and counterproductive.

Little basis exists for pursuing the meaning of uncooperative behavior when a psychiatrist is meeting with a patient for the first time. The psychiatrist may need to insist on change in the patient's behavior as a precondition for proceeding. This can be done in a nonjudgmental and nonpunitive manner. For patients who cannot or will not cooperate, the treatment contract may need to be renegotiated, for example, by changing the frequency of sessions, switching to a different psychotherapeutic modality, or focusing on medication management rather than psychotherapy. In certain circumstances however, the initial assessment or therapy has to be terminated because of a patient's uncooperative behavior.

A third-year psychiatry resident working in the outpatient clinic of a large hospital was assigned, for twice-a-week psychodynamic psychotherapy, a 26-year-old man with mild anxiety and depression and career difficulties. From the start of treatment, however, the patient came no more than three or four times per month, usually calling in advance to cancel, but sometimes simply not showing up. The resident struggled to build a treatment alliance and to interpret the man's behavior by using the little that she knew about him, but the pattern of noninvolvement continued. After 3 months, a new supervisor pointed out to the resident that therapy had never really started and that her first task was to create a situation in which therapy could occur. The resident explained to her patient that meaningful therapy was possible only with his full cooperation and that they needed to decide on what level of involvement he could commit. The patient agreed to come once a week. He was able to keep that schedule for the most part and, over the next 6 months, engaged in a beneficial supportive therapy.

PATIENTS FROM DIFFERENT CULTURES AND BACKGROUNDS

Differences in race, nationality, and religion and other significant cultural differences between patient and interviewer can impair communication and can lead to misunderstandings. In addition, it may be difficult for a culturally naïve psychiatrist to evaluate symptoms that are relative rather than absolute. There is usually no difficulty in documenting the presence of auditory hallucinations regardless of cultural differences. Assessing whether a delusion is *bizarre* (as required by DSM-IV-TR for delusional disorder) is more difficult, however, because the term *bizarre* has meaning only in reference to cultural norms.

Apart from diagnostic categories, the vocabulary used to describe emotional distress varies from culture to culture. Sometimes, symptoms that are commonplace within a culture are unheard of to outsiders.

Additional problems are encountered when doctor and patient speak different languages. When an interpreter is needed, the person should be a disinterested third party, unknown to the patient. Translators must be instructed to translate verbatim what the patient says—a difficult task for even the most experienced professional translators. Some words and expressions are simply untranslatable. It may be impossible to convey a formal thought disorder through translation.

An additional difficulty can arise in establishing rapport between doctor and patient of different ethnic or cultural groups. Patients from minority groups may be guarded in speaking with a doctor from the majority group. The evaluating psychiatrist must proceed with humility and respect. Rather than offer reassurances of understanding and acceptance, it is usually better to ask, "Have I understood this in the way that you meant it?"

EMPATHIC LISTENING

Listening to the patient is a critical skill in psychiatry, but listening is more than just hearing what the patient is saying. Listening must be empathic; the empathic listener is affected by the sorrow or suffering of the person being interviewed. It is characterized by placing oneself in the patient's shoes and differs slightly from sympathy. The sympathetic listener says, "I know how you feel but I don't feel the same way," whereas the empathic listener says, "I know how you feel and I feel the same way." Empathy enables the listener to understand emotionally the experiences of his or her patients. It is important, however, that empathic listening not be carried too far—the therapist must be able to step out of the patient's shoes. There are cases on record of psychiatrists who empathized to such a degree that they began to accept the delusional beliefs of their patients as their own.

Empathy is an essential characteristic of psychiatrists, but it is not a universal human capacity. An incapacity for normal understanding of what other people are feeling appears to be central to certain personality disturbances, such as antisocial and narcissistic personality disorders. Although empathy can probably not be created, it can be focused and deepened through training, observation, and self-reflection. It manifests in clinical work in a variety of ways. An empathic psychiatrist may anticipate what is felt before it is spoken and can often help patients articulate what they are feeling. Nonverbal cues, such as body posture and facial expression, are noted. Patients' reactions to the psychiatrist can be understood and clarified.

Patients sometimes say, "How can you understand me if you haven't gone through what I'm going through?" Clinical psychiatry, however, is predicated on the belief that it is not necessary to have other people's literal experiences to understand them. The shared experience of being human is often sufficient. Whether in an initial diagnostic setting or in an ongoing therapy, patients draw comfort from knowing that psychiatrists are not mystified by their suffering.

References

Cohen BJ. *Theory and Practice of Psychiatry*. New York: Oxford University Press; 2003.

Essary AC, Symington SL. How to make the "difficult" patient encounter less difficult. *JAAPA*. 2005;18(5):49–54.

Fadem B. *Behavioral Science Medicine*. Philadelphia: Lippincott Williams & Wilkins; 2004.

Kirk HW, Weisbrod JA, Ericson KA. *Psychosocial and Behavioral Aspects of Medicine*. Philadelphia: Lippincott Williams & Wilkins; 2003.

Manley M. Interviewing techniques with the difficult patient. In: Sadock BJ, Sadock VA, eds. *Comprehensive Textbook of Psychiatry*. 8th ed. Baltimore: Lippincott Williams & Wilkins; 2005:827.

Manley M. *Psychiatry Clerkship Guide*. New York: Elsevier; 2003.

Othner E, Othner S. *The Clinical Interview Using DSM-IV-TR: The Difficult Patient*. Vol. 2. Washington, DC: American Psychiatric Association Press; 2002.

Platt FW, Gordon GH. *Field Guide to the Difficult Patient Interview*. Philadelphia: Lippincott Williams & Wilkins; 2004.

Sadock BJ, Sadock VA. *Kaplan and Sadock's Synopsis of Psychiatry*. 9th ed. Baltimore: Lippincott Williams & Wilkins; 2003.

Shaw I. Doctors, "Dirty work" patients, and "revolving doors". *Qualitative Health Research*. 2004;14(8):1032–1045.

Simon RI. *Assessing and Managing Suicide Risk*. Washington, DC: American Psychiatric Publishing, Inc.; 2004.

▲ 7.3 Physical Examination of the Psychiatric Patient

Confronted with a patient who has a mental disorder, the psychiatrist must decide whether or not a medical, surgical, or neurological condition may be the cause. Once satisfied that no disease process can be held accountable, then the diagnosis of mental disorder not attributable to a medical illness can be made. Although psychiatrists do not perform routine physical examinations of their patients, a knowledge and understanding of physical signs and symptoms is part of their training, which enables them to recognize signs and symptoms that may indicate possible medical or surgical illness. For example, palpitations can be associated with mitral valve prolapse, which is diagnosed by cardiac auscultation. Psychiatrists are also able to recognize and treat the adverse effects of psychotropic medications, which are used by an increasing number of patients seen by psychiatrists and nonpsychiatric physicians.

Some psychiatrists insist that every patient have a complete medical workup; others may not. Whatever their policy, psychiatrists should consider patients' medical status at the outset of a psychiatric evaluation. Psychiatrists must often decide whether a patient needs a medical examination and, if so, what it should include—most commonly, a thorough medical history, including a review of systems, a physical examination, and relevant diagnostic laboratory studies. A recent study of 1,000 medical patients found that in 75 percent of cases no cause of symptoms (i.e., subjective complaints) could be found, and a psychological basis was assumed in 10 percent of those cases.

HISTORY OF MEDICAL ILLNESS

In the course of conducting a psychiatric evaluation, information should be gathered about known bodily diseases or dysfunctions, hospitalizations and operative procedures, medications taken recently or at present, personal habits and occupational history, family history of illnesses, and specific physical complaints. Information about medical illnesses should be gathered from the patient, the referring physician, and the family, if necessary.

Information about previous episodes of illness may provide valuable clues about the nature of the present disorder. For example, a distinctly delusional disorder in a patient with a history of several similar episodes that responded promptly to diverse forms of treatment strongly suggests the possibility of substance-induced psychotic disorder. To pursue this lead, the psychiatrist should order a drug screen. The history of a surgical procedure may also be useful; for instance, a thyroidectomy suggests hypothyroidism as the cause of depression.

Depression is an adverse effect of several medications prescribed for hypertension. Medication taken in a therapeutic dosage occasionally reaches high concentrations in the blood. Digitalis intoxication, for example, can occur under such circumstances and result in impaired mental functioning. Proprietary drugs can cause or contribute to an anticholinergic delirium. The psychiatrist, therefore, must inquire about over-the-counter remedies as well as prescribed medications. A history of herbal intake and alternative therapy is essential in view of their increased use.

An occupational history may also provide essential information. Exposure to mercury can result in complaints suggesting a psychosis, and exposure to lead, as in smelting, can produce a cognitive disorder. The latter clinical picture can also result from imbibing moonshine whiskey with a high lead content.

In eliciting information about specific symptoms, the psychiatrist brings medical and psychological knowledge into full play. For example, the psychiatrist should elicit sufficient information from the patient complaining of headache to predict whether the pain results from intracranial disease that requires neurological testing. Also, the psychiatrist should be able to recognize that the pain in the right shoulder of a hypochondriacal patient with abdominal discomfort may be the classic referred pain of gallbladder disease.

REVIEW OF SYSTEMS

An inventory by systems should follow the open-ended inquiry. The review can be organized according to organ systems (e.g., liver, pancreas), functional systems (e.g., gastrointestinal), or a combination of the two, as in the following outline. In all cases, the review should be comprehensive and thorough. Even if a psychiatric component is suspected, a complete workup is still indicated.

Head

Many patients give a history of headache; its duration, frequency, character, location, and severity should be ascertained. Headaches often result from substance abuse, including alcohol, nicotine, and caffeine. Vascular (migraine) headaches are precipitated by stress. Temporal arteritis causes unilateral throbbing headaches and can lead to blindness. Brain tumors are associated with headaches as a result of increased intracranial pressure; but some may be silent, the first signs being a change in personality or cognition. A head injury can result in subdural hematoma and in boxers can cause progressive dementia with extrapyramidal symptoms. The headache of subarachnoid hemorrhage is sudden, severe, and associated with changes in the sensorium. Normal pressure hydrocephalus can follow a head injury or encephalitis and be associated with dementia, shuffling gait, and urinary incontinence. Dizziness occurs in up to 30 percent of persons and determining its cause is challenging (Table 7.3–1) and often difficult. A change in the size or shape of the head may be indicative of Paget's disease.

Eye, Ear, Nose, and Throat

Visual acuity, diplopia, hearing problems, tinnitus, glossitis, and bad taste are covered in this area. A patient taking antipsychotics who gives a history of twitching about the mouth or disturbing movements of the tongue may be in the early and potentially reversible stage of tardive dyskinesia. Impaired vision can occur with thioridazine (Mellaril) in high dosages (over 800 mg a day). A history of glaucoma contraindicates drugs with anticholinergic effects. Aphonia may be hysterical in nature. The late stage of cocaine abuse can result in perforations of the nasal septum and difficulty breathing. A transitory episode of diplopia may herald multiple sclerosis. Delusional disorder is more common in hearing-impaired persons than in those with normal hearing. Complaints of bad odors may be a symptom of temporal lobe epilepsy rather than schizophrenia. Blue-tinged vision can occur transiently when using sildenafil (Viagra) or similar drugs.

Respiratory System

Cough, asthma, pleurisy, hemoptysis, dyspnea, and orthopnea are considered in this section. Hyperventilation is suggested if the patient's symptoms include all or a few of the following: onset at rest, sighing respirations, apprehension, anxiety, depersonalization, palpitations, inability to swallow, numbness of the feet and hands, and carpopedal spasm. Dyspnea and breathlessness can occur in depression. In pulmonary or obstructive airway

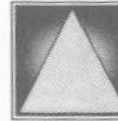

Table 7.3–1
Approach to the Differentiation of Dizziness Subtypes

Dizziness Subtype	Type of Sensation	Temporal Characteristics	Other Specifications
Vertigo	A feeling that one or one's surroundings are moving (typically, spinning)	Episodic vertigo occurs in attacks that last seconds to days Continuous vertigo is present all or most of the time for at least a week	Descriptions of episodic vertigo should include the characteristics, duration, and date of the first episode; length of episodes; and exacerbating factors
Presyncope	A lightheaded, faint feeling as though one were about to pass out	Typically occurs in episodes lasting seconds to hours	The following questions should be answered: (1) Has syncope ever occurred during an episode? (2) Do episodes occur only when the patient is upright, or do they occur in other positions? (3) Are episodes associated with palpitations, medication, meals, bathing, dyspnea, or chest discomfort?
Disequilibrium	A sense of unsteadiness that is (1) primarily felt in the lower extremities, (2) most prominent when standing or walking, and (3) relieved by sitting or lying down	Usually present, although it may fluctuate in intensity	Identify whether symptom occurs in isolation or accompanies another dizziness subtype; describe exacerbating factors
Other dizziness: anxiety-related, ocular, tilting environment, other	A feeling not covered by the above definitions. May include swimming or floating sensations, vague lightheadedness, or feelings of dissociation. May be difficult for the patient to describe	Usually present all or most of the time for days or weeks, sometimes years	The following questions should be answered: (1) Is dizziness associated with anxiety or hyperventilation? (2) Was change in vision connected with dizziness onset? (3) Is dizziness a sensation that the environment is tilting sideways (suggests an otolith problem)?

(From Sloane PD, Coeytaux RR, Beck RS, Dallara J. Dizziness. State of the science. *Ann Intern Med.* 2001;134:825, with permission.)

disease, the onset of symptoms is usually insidious, whereas in depression, it is sudden. In depression, breathlessness is experienced at rest, shows little change with exertion, and can fluctuate within a matter of minutes; the onset of breathlessness coincides with the onset of a mood disorder and is often accompanied by attacks of dizziness, sweating, palpitations, and paresthesias.

In obstructive airway disease, patients with the most advanced respiratory incapacity experience breathlessness at rest. Most striking and of greatest assistance in making a differential diagnosis is the emphasis placed on the difficulty in inspiration experienced by patients with depression and on the difficulty in expiration experienced by patients with pulmonary disease. Bronchial asthma has sometimes been associated with a childhood history of extreme dependence on the mother. Patients with bronchospasm should not receive propranolol (Inderal) because it can block catecholamine-induced bronchodilation; propranolol is specifically contraindicated for patients with bronchial asthma because epinephrine given to such patients in an emergency will not be effective. Patients taking angiotensin-converting enzyme (ACE) inhibitors can develop a dry cough as an adverse effect of the drug.

Cardiovascular System

Tachycardia, palpitations, and cardiac arrhythmia are among the most common signs of anxiety about which the patient may complain. Pheochromocytoma usually produces symptoms that mimic anxiety disorders, such as rapid heartbeat, tremors, and pallor. Increased urinary catecholamines are diagnostic of pheochromocytoma. Patients taking guanethidine (Ismelin) for hypertension should not receive tricyclic drugs, which reduce or eliminate the antihypertensive effect of guanethidine. A history of hypertension can preclude the use of monoamine oxidase inhibitors (MAOIs) because of the risk of a hypertensive crisis if such patients with hypertension inadvertently ingest foods high in tyramine. Patients with a suspected cardiac disease should have an electrocardiogram before tricyclics or lithium (Eskalith) is prescribed. A history of substernal pain should be evaluated, and the clinician should keep in mind that psychological stress can precipitate angina-type chest pain in the presence of normal coronary arteries. Patients taking opioids should never receive MAOIs; the combination can cause cardiovascular collapse.

Gastrointestinal System

Such topics as appetite, distress before or after meals, food preferences, diarrhea, vomiting, constipation, laxative use, and abdominal pain relate to the gastrointestinal system. A history of weight loss is common in depressive disorders, but depression can accompany the weight loss caused by ulcerative colitis, regional enteritis, and cancer. Atypical depression is accompanied by hyperphagia and weight gain. Anorexia nervosa is accompanied by severe weight loss in the presence of normal appetite. Avoidance of certain foods may be a phobic phenomenon or part of an obsessive ritual. Laxative abuse and induced vomiting are common in bulimia nervosa. Constipation can be caused by

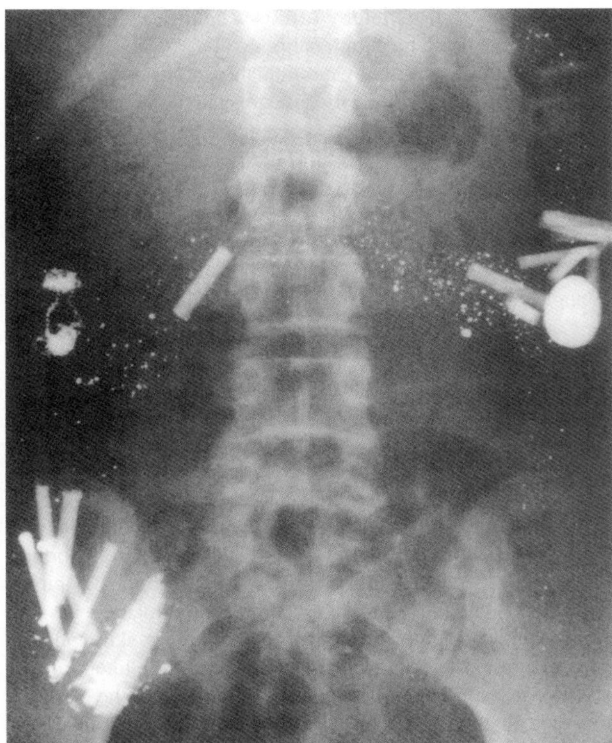

FIGURE 7.3–1
A mentally ill patient who is a habitual swallower of foreign objects. Included in his colonic lumen are 13 thermometers and 8 pennies. The dense, round, almost punctate densities are globules of liberated liquid mercury. (Courtesy of Stephen R. Baker, M.D., and Kyunghee C. Cho, M.D.)

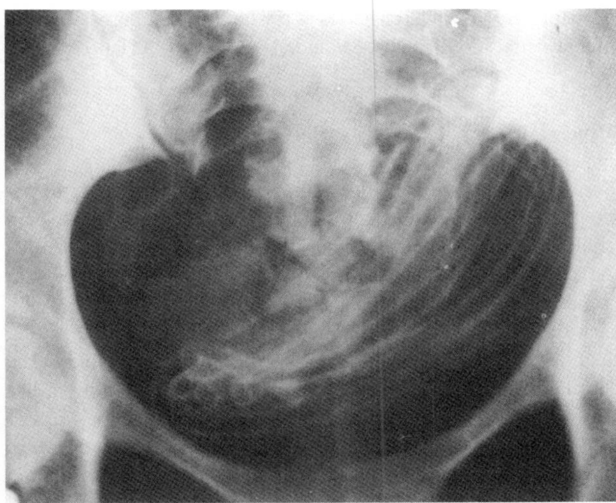

FIGURE 7.3–2
A patient brought to the emergency room with lower abdominal pain. X-ray shows a nasogastric tube folded into the bladder. The patient would insert the tube into his urethra as part of a masturbatory ritual (urethral eroticism). (Courtesy of Stephen R. Baker, M.D., and Kyunghee C. Cho, M.D.)

opioid dependence and by psychotropic drugs with anticholinergic side effects. Cocaine or amphetamine abuse causes a loss of appetite and weight loss. Weight gain can occur under stress or in association with atypical depression. Polyphagia, polyuria, and polydipsia are the triad of diabetes mellitus. Polyuria, polydipsia, and diarrhea are signs of lithium toxicity. Some patients take enemas routinely as part of paraphilic behavior and anal fissures or recurrent hemmorhoids may indicate anal penetration by foreign objects. Some patients may ingest foreign objects that produce symptoms that can be diagnosed only by X-ray (Fig. 7.3–1).

Genitourinary System

Urinary frequency, nocturia, pain or burning on urination, and changes in the size and the force of the stream are some of the signs and symptoms emanating from the genitourinary system. Anticholinergic adverse effects associated with antipsychotics and tricyclic drugs can cause urinary retention in men with prostate hypertrophy. Erectile difficulty and retarded ejaculation are also common adverse effects of these drugs, and retrograde ejaculation occurs with thioridazine. A baseline level of sexual responsiveness before using pharmacological agents should be obtained. A history of sexually transmitted diseases—for example, gonorrheal discharge, chancre, herpes, and pubic lice—may indicate sexual promiscuity or unsafe sexual practices. In some cases, the first symptom of acquired immune deficiency syndrome (AIDS) is the gradual onset of mental confusion leading to dementia. Incontinence should be evaluated carefully, and if it persists, further investigation for more extensive disease should include a workup for human immunodeficiency virus (HIV) infection. Drugs with anticholinergic adverse effects should be avoided in men with prostatism. Urethral eroticism in which catheters or other objects are inserted into the urethra can cause infection or laceration (Fig. 7.3–2).

Orgasm causes prostatic contractions which may artificially raise Prostate Specific Antigen (PSA) and give a false positive test for prostatic cancer. Men scheduled to have a PSA test should avoid masturbation or coitus for 7 to 10 days prior to the test.

Menstrual History

A menstrual history should include the age of the onset of menarche and menopause; the interval, regularity, duration, and amount of flow of periods; irregular bleeding; dysmenorrhea; and abortions. Amenorrhea is characteristic of anorexia nervosa and also occurs in women who are psychologically stressed. Women who are afraid of becoming pregnant or who have a wish to be pregnant may have delayed periods. *Pseudocyesis* is false pregnancy with complete cessation of the menses. Perimenstrual mood changes (e.g., irritability, depression, and dysphoria) should be noted. Painful menstruation can result from uterine disease (e.g., myomata), from psychological conflicts about the menses, or from a combination of the two. Some women report a perimenstrual increase in sexual desire. The emotional reaction associated with abortion should be explored, because it can be mild or severe.

GENERAL OBSERVATION

An important part of the medical examination is subsumed under the broad heading of general observation—visual, auditory, and olfactory. Such nonverbal clues as posture, facial expression, and mannerisms should also be noted.

Visual Inspection

Scrutiny of the patient begins at the first encounter. When the patient goes from the waiting room to the interview room, the psychiatrist should observe the patient's gait. Is the patient unsteady? Ataxia suggests diffuse brain disease, alcohol or other substance intoxication, chorea, spinocerebellar degeneration, weakness based on a debilitating process, and an underlying disorder, such as myotonic dystrophy. Does the patient walk without the usual associated arm movements and turn in a rigid fashion, as a toy soldier, as is seen in early Parkinson's disease? Does the patient have asymmetry of gait, such as turning one foot outward, dragging a leg, or not swinging one arm, suggesting a focal brain lesion?

As soon as the patient is seated, the psychiatrist should direct attention to grooming. Is the patient's hair combed, are the nails clean, and are the teeth brushed? Has clothing been chosen with care, and is it appropriate? Although inattention to dress and hygiene is common in mental disorders—in particular, depressive disorders—it is also a hallmark of cognitive disorders. Lapses, such as mismatching socks, stockings, or shoes, may suggest a cognitive disorder.

The patient's posture and automatic movements or the lack of them should be noted. A stooped, flexed posture with a paucity of automatic movements may be caused by Parkinson's disease or diffuse cerebral hemispheric disease or be an adverse effect of antipsychotics. An unusual tilt of the head may be adopted to avoid eye contact, but it can also result from diplopia, a visual field defect, or focal cerebellar dysfunction. Frequent quick, purposeless movements are characteristic of anxiety disorders, but they are equally characteristic of chorea and hyperthyroidism. Tremors, although commonly seen in anxiety disorders, may point to Parkinson's disease, essential tremor, or adverse effects of psychotropic medication. Patients with essential tremor sometimes seek psychiatric treatment because they believe the tremor must be caused by unrecognized fear or anxiety, as others often suggest. Unilateral paucity or excess of movement suggests focal brain disease.

The patient's appearance is then scrutinized to assess general health. Does the patient appear to be robust, or is there a sense of ill health? Does looseness of clothing indicate recent weight loss? Is the patient short of breath or coughing? Does the patient's general physiognomy suggest a specific disease? Men with Klinefelter's syndrome have a feminine fat distribution and lack the development of secondary male sex characteristics. Acromegaly is usually immediately recognizable by the large head and jaw.

What is the patient's nutritional status? Recent weight loss, although often seen in depressive disorders and schizophrenia, may be caused by gastrointestinal disease, diffuse carcinomatosis, Addison's disease, hyperthyroidism, and many other somatic disorders. Obesity can result from either emotional distress or organic disease. Moon facies, truncal obesity, and buffalo hump are striking findings in Cushing's syndrome. The puffy, bloated appearance seen in hypothyroidism and the massive obesity and periodic respiration seen in Pickwickian syndrome are easily recognized in patients referred for psychiatric help. Hyperthyroidism is indicated by exophthalmos.

The skin frequently provides valuable information. The yellow discoloration of hepatic dysfunction and the pallor of anemia are reasonably distinctive. Intense reddening may be caused by carbon monoxide poisoning or by photosensitivity resulting from porphyria or phenothiazines. Eruptions can be manifestations of such disorders as systemic lupus erythematosus (e.g., the butterfly on the face), tuberous sclerosis with adenoma sebaceum, and sensitivity to drugs. A dusky purplish cast to the face, plus telangiectasia, is almost pathognomonic of alcohol abuse.

Careful observation may reveal clues that lead to the correct diagnosis in patients who create their own skin lesions. For example, the location and shape of the lesions and the time of their appearance may be characteristic of dermatitis factitia.

The patient's face and head should be scanned for evidence of disease. Premature whitening of the hair occurs in pernicious anemia, and thinning and coarseness of the hair occur in myxedema. In alopecia areata, patches of hair are lost, leaving bald spots; trichotillomania presents a similar picture. Pupillary changes are produced by various drugs—constriction by opioids and dilation by anticholinergic agents and hallucinogens. The combination of dilated and fixed pupils and dry skin and mucous membranes should immediately suggest the likelihood of atropine use or atropine-like toxicity. Diffusion of the conjunctiva suggests alcohol abuse, cannabis abuse, or obstruction of the superior vena cava. Flattening of the nasolabial fold on one side or weakness of one side of the face—as manifested in speaking, smiling, and grimacing—may be the result of focal dysfunction of the contralateral cerebral hemisphere or of Bell's palsy. A drooping eyelid may be an early sign of myasthenia gravis.

The patient's state of alertness and responsiveness should be evaluated carefully. Drowsiness and inattentiveness may be caused by a psychological problem, but they are more likely to result from organic brain dysfunction, whether secondary to an intrinsic brain disease or to an exogenous factor, such as substance intoxication.

Listening

Listening intently is just as important as looking intently for evidence of somatic disorders. Slowed speech is characteristic not only of depression but also of diffuse brain dysfunction and subcortical dysfunction; unusually rapid speech is characteristic of manic episodes and anxiety disorders, and also of hyperthyroidism. A weak voice with monotonous tone may be a clue to Parkinson's disease in patients who complain mainly of depression. A slow, low-pitched, hoarse voice should suggest the possibility of hypothyroidism; this voice quality has been described as sounding like a drowsy, slightly intoxicated person with a bad cold and a plum in the mouth. A soft or tremulous voice accompanies anxiety.

Difficulty initiating speech may be owing to anxiety or stuttering or may indicate Parkinson's disease or aphasia. Easy fatigability of speech is sometimes a manifestation of an emotional problem, but it is also characteristic of myasthenia gravis. Patients with these complaints are likely to be seen by a psychiatrist before the correct diagnosis is made.

Word production, as well as the quality of speech, is important. Mispronounced or incorrectly used words suggest a possibility of aphasia caused by a lesion of the dominant hemisphere. The same possibility exists when the patient perseverates, has trouble finding a name or a word, or describes an object or an event in an indirect fashion (paraphasia). When not consonant with patients' socioeconomic and educational levels, coarseness, profanity, or inappropriate disclosures may indicate loss of inhibition caused by dementia.

Smell

Smell may also provide useful information. The unpleasant odor of a patient who fails to bathe suggests a cognitive or a depressive disorder. The odor of alcohol or of substances used to hide it is revealing in a patient who attempts to conceal a drinking problem. Occasionally, a uriniferous odor calls attention to bladder dysfunction secondary to a nervous system disease. Characteristic odors are also noted in patients with diabetic acidosis, flatulence, uremia, and hepatic coma. Precocious puberty can be associated with the smell of adult sweat produced by mature apocrine glands.

PHYSICAL EXAMINATION

Patient Selection

The nature of the patient's complaints is critical in determining whether a complete physical examination is required. Complaints fall into the three categories of body, mind, and social interactions. Bodily symptoms (e.g., headaches and palpitations) call for a thorough medical examination to determine what part, if any, somatic processes play in causing the distress. The same can be said for mental symptoms such as depression, anxiety, hallucinations, and persecutory delusions, which can be expressions of somatic processes. If the problem is clearly limited to the social sphere (e.g., long-standing difficulties in interactions with teachers, employers, parents, or a spouse), there may be no special indication for a physical examination. Personality changes, however, can result from a medical disorder (e.g., early Alzheimer's disease) and cause interpersonal conflicts.

Psychological Factors

Even a routine physical examination may evoke adverse reactions; instruments, procedures, and the examining room may be frightening. A simple running account of what is being done can prevent much needless anxiety. Moreover, if the patient is consistently forewarned of what will be done, the dread of being suddenly and painfully surprised recedes. Comments such as "There's nothing to this" and "You don't have to be afraid because this won't hurt" leave the patient in the dark and are much less reassuring than a few words about what actually will be done.

Although the physical examination is likely to engender or intensify a reaction of anxiety, it can also stir up sexual feelings. Some women with fears or fantasies of being seduced may misinterpret an ordinary movement in the physical examination as a sexual advance. Similarly, a delusional man with homosexual fears may perceive a rectal examination as a sexual attack. Lingering over the examination of a particular organ because an unusual but normal variation has aroused the physician's scientific curiosity is likely to raise concern in the patient that a serious pathological process has been discovered. Such a reaction may be profound in an anxious or hypochondriacal patient.

The physical examination occasionally serves a psychotherapeutic function. Anxious patients may be relieved to learn that, despite troublesome symptoms, no evidence is found of the serious illness that they fear. The young person who complains of chest pain and is certain that the pain heralds a heart attack can usually be reassured by the report of normal findings after a physical examination and electrocardiogram. The reassurance relieves only the worry occasioned by the immediate episode, however. Unless psychiatric treatment succeeds in dealing with the determinants of the reaction, recurrent episodes are likely.

Sending a patient who has a deeply rooted fear of malignancy for still another test that is intended to be reassuring is usually unrewarding. Some patients may have a false fixed belief that a disorder is present.

During the performance of the physical examination, an observant physician may note indications of emotional distress. For instance, during genital examinations, a patient's behavior may reveal information about sexual attitudes and problems, and these reactions can be used later to open this area for exploration.

Timing of the Physical Examination

Circumstances occasionally make it desirable or necessary to defer a complete medical assessment. For example, a delusional or manic patient may be combative or resistive or both. In this instance, a medical history should be elicited from a family member, if possible, but unless a pressing reason exists to proceed with the examination, it should be deferred until the patient is tractable.

For psychological reasons, it may be ill advised to recommend a medical assessment at the time of an initial office visit. In view of today's increased sensitivity and openness about sexual matters and a tendency to turn quickly to psychiatric help, young men may complain about their failure to consummate their first coital attempt. After taking a detailed history, the psychiatrist may conclude that the failure was because of situational anxiety. If so, neither a physical examination nor psychotherapy should be recommended; they would have the undesirable effect of reinforcing the notion of pathology. Should the problem be recurrent, further evaluation would be warranted.

Neurological Examination

If the psychiatrist suspects that the patient has an underlying somatic disorder, such as diabetes mellitus or Cushing's syndrome, referral is usually made to a medical physician for diagnosis and treatment. The situation is different when a cognitive disorder is suspected. The psychiatrist often chooses to assume responsibility in these cases. At some point, however, a thorough neurological evaluation may be indicated.

During the history-taking process in such cases, the patient's level of awareness, attentiveness to the details of the examination, understanding, facial expression, speech, posture, and gait are noted. It is also assumed that a thorough mental status examination will be performed. The neurological examination is carried out with two objectives in mind: to elicit (1) signs pointing to focal, circumscribed cerebral dysfunction and (2) signs suggesting diffuse, bilateral cerebral disease. The first objective is met by the routine neurological examination, which is designed primarily to reveal asymmetries in the motor, perceptual, and reflex functions of the two sides of the body, caused by focal hemispheric disease. The second objective is met by seeking to elicit signs that have been attributed to diffuse brain dysfunction and to frontal lobe disease. These signs include the sucking, snout, palmomental, and grasp reflexes and the persistence of the glabella tap response. Regrettably, with the exception of the grasp reflex, such signs do not correlate strongly with the presence of underlying brain pathology.

Other Findings

Psychiatrists should be able to evaluate the significance of findings uncovered by consultants. With a patient who complains of a lump in the throat (globus hystericus) and who is found on examination to have hypertrophied lymphoid tissue, it is tempting to wonder about a causal relation. How can a clinician be sure that the finding is not incidental? Has the patient been known to have hypertrophied lymphoid tissue at a time when no complaint was made? Do many persons with hypertrophied lymphoid tissue never experience the sensation of a lump in the throat?

With a patient with multiple sclerosis who complains of an inability to walk but, on neurological examination, has only mild spasticity and a unilateral Babinski sign, it is tempting to ascribe the symptom to the neurological disorder; but the complaint may be aggravated by emotional distress. The same holds true for a patient with profound dementia in whom a small frontal meningioma is seen on a computed tomography (CT) scan. Dementia is not always correlated with the findings. Significant brain atrophy could cause very mild dementia, and minimal brain atrophy could cause significant dementia.

A lesion is often found that can account for a symptom, but the psychiatrist should make every effort to separate an incidental finding from a causative one and to distinguish a lesion merely found in the area of the symptom from a lesion producing the symptom.

PATIENTS UNDERGOING PSYCHIATRIC TREATMENT

While patients are being treated for psychiatric disorders, psychiatrists should be alert to the possibility of intercurrent illnesses that call for diagnostic studies. Patients in psychotherapy, particularly those in psychoanalysis, may be all too willing to ascribe their new symptoms to emotional causes. Attention should be given to the possible use of denial, especially if the symptoms seem to be unrelated to the conflicts currently in focus.

Not only may patients in psychotherapy be likely to attribute new symptoms to emotional causes, but sometimes their therapists do so as well. The danger of providing psychodynamic explanations for physical symptoms is ever present.

Symptoms such as drowsiness and dizziness and signs such as a skin eruption and a gait disturbance, common adverse effects of psychotropic medication, call for a medical reevaluation if the patient fails to respond in a reasonable time to changes in the dosage or the kind of medication prescribed. If patients who are receiving tricyclic or antipsychotic drugs complain of blurred vision (usually an anticholinergic adverse effect) and the condition does not recede with a reduction in dosage or a change in medication, they should be evaluated to rule out other causes. In one case, the diagnosis proved to be *Toxoplasma* chorioretinitis. The absence of other anticholinergic adverse effects, such as a dry mouth and constipation, is an additional clue alerting the psychiatrist to the possibility of a concomitant medical illness.

Early in an illness, there may be few if any positive physical or laboratory results. In such instances, especially if the evidence of psychic trauma or emotional conflicts is glaring, all symptoms are likely to be regarded as psychosocial in origin, and new symptoms also seen in this light. Indications for repeating portions of the medical workup may be missed unless the psychiatrist is alert to clues suggesting that some symptoms do not fit the original diagnosis and, instead, point to a medical illness. Occasionally, a patient with an acute illness, such as encephalitis, is hospitalized with the diagnosis of schizophrenia, or a patient with a subacute illness, such as carcinoma of the pancreas, is treated in a private office or clinic with the diagnosis of a depressive disorder. Although it may not be possible to make the correct diagnosis at the time of the initial psychiatric evaluation, continued surveillance and attention to clinical details usually provide clues leading to the recognition of the cause.

The likelihood of intercurrent illness is greater with some psychiatric disorders than with others. Substance abusers, for example, because of their life patterns, are susceptible to infection and are likely to suffer from the adverse effects of trauma, dietary deficiencies, and poor hygiene. Depression decreases the immune response.

When somatic and psychological dysfunctions are known to coexist, the psychiatrist should be thoroughly conversant with the patient's medical status. In cases of cardiac decompensation, peripheral neuropathy, and other disabling disorders, the nature and degree of impairment that can be attributed to the physical disorder should be assessed. It is important to answer the question: Does the patient exploit a disability, or is it ignored or denied with resultant overexertion? To answer this question, the psychiatrist must assess the patient's capabilities and limitations, rather than make sweeping judgments based on a diagnostic label.

Special vigilance about medical status is required for some patients in treatment for somatoform and eating disorders. Such is the case for patients with ulcerative colitis who are bleeding profusely and for patients with anorexia nervosa who are losing appreciable weight. These disorders can become life threatening.

Importance of Medical Screening

Numerous articles have called attention to the need for thorough medical screening of patients seen in psychiatric inpatient services and clinics. (A similar need has been demonstrated for the psychiatric evaluation of patients seen in medical inpatient services and clinics.) The concept of *medical clearance* remains ambiguous and has meaning in the context of psychiatric admission or clearance for transfers from different settings or institutions. It implies that no medical condition exists to account for the patient's condition.

Among identified psychiatric patients, from 24 to 60 percent have been shown to suffer from associated physical disorders. In a survey of 2,090 psychiatric clinic patients, 43 percent were found to have associated physical disorders; of these, almost half the physical disorders had not been diagnosed by the referring sources. (In this study, 69 patients were found to have diabetes mellitus, but only 12 of these cases had been diagnosed before referral.)

Expecting all psychiatrists to be experts in internal medicine is unrealistic, but expecting them to recognize or have high suspicion of physical disorders that are present is realistic. Moreover, they should make appropriate referrals and collaborate in treating patients who have both physical and mental disorders.

Psychiatric symptoms are nonspecific; they can herald medical as well as psychiatric illness. They often precede the appearance of definitive medical symptoms. Some psychiatric symptoms (e.g., visual hallucinations, distortions, and illusions) should evoke a high level of suspicion of a medical toxicity.

The medical literature abounds with case reports of patients whose disorders were initially considered emotional but ultimately proved to be secondary to medical conditions. The data in most of the reports revealed features pointing toward organicity. Diagnostic errors arose because such features were accorded too little weight.

References

Aronne LJ, Segal KR. Weight gain in the treatment of mood disorders. *J Clin Psychiatry.* 2003;64[Suppl 8]:22–29.

Chue P, Kovacs CS. Safety and tolerability of atypical antipsychotics in patients with bipolar disorder: Prevalence, monitoring, and management. *Bipolar Disord.* 2003;5[Suppl 2]:62–79.

Cormac I, Ferriter M, Benning R, Saul C. Physical health and health risk factors in a population of long-stay psychiatric patients. *Psychol Bull.* 2005;29:18-20.

Foster NL. Validating FDG-PET as a biomarker for frontotemporal dementia. *Exp Neurol.* 2003;184[Suppl 1]:S2–S8.

Garden G. Physical examination in psychiatric practice. *Advances in Psychiatric Treatment.* 2005;11:142–149.

Guze BH, Love MJ. Medical assessment and laboratory testing in psychiatry. In: Sadock BJ, Sadock VA, eds. *Kaplan & Sadock's Comprehensive Textbook of Psychiatry.* 8th ed. Vol. 1. Baltimore: Lippincott Williams & Wilkins; 2005: 916.

Hodgson R, Adeyamo O. Physical examination performed by psychiatrists. *International J of Psych in Clin Practice.* 2004;8:57–60.

Lambert TJ, Velakoulis D, Pantelis C. Medical comorbidity in schizophrenia. *Med J Aust.* 2003;178[Suppl]:S67–S70.

Lyndenmayer JP, Czobor P, Volavka J, Sheitman B, McEvoy JP, Cooper TB, Chakos M, Lieberman JA. Changes in glucose and cholesterol levels in patients with schizophrenia treated with typical or atypical antipsychotics. *Am J Psychiatry.* 2003;160:290–296.

Marder SR, Essock SM, Miller AL, Buchanan RW, Casey DE, Davis JM, Kane JM, Lieberman J, Schooler NR, Covell N, Stroup S, Weissman EM, Wirshing DA, Hall CS, Pogach L, Xavier P, Bigger JT, Friedman A, Kleinber D, Yevich S, Davis B, Shon S. Health monitoring of patients with schizophrenia. *Am J Psychiatry.* 2004; 161:1334-1349.

Rosse RB, Deutsch LH, Deutsch SI. Medical assessment and laboratory testing in psychiatry. In: Sadock BJ, Sadock VA, eds. *Kaplan & Sadock's Comprehensive Textbook of Psychiatry.* 7th ed. Vol. 1. Baltimore: Lippincott Williams & Wilkins; 2000:732.

Saunders RD, Keshavan MS. Physical and neurologic examinations in neuropsychiatry. *Semin Clin Neuropsychiatry.* 2002;7:18–29.

Schulte P. What is an adequate trial with clozapine? Therapeutic drug monitoring and time to response in treatment refractory schizophrenia. *Clin Pharmacokinet.* 2003;42:607–618.

▲ 7.4 Laboratory Tests in Psychiatry

Psychiatrists depend more on the clinical examination and the patient's signs and symptoms to make a diagnosis than do other medical specialists. No laboratory tests in psychiatry can confirm or rule out diagnoses such as schizophrenia, bipolar I disorder, and major depressive disorder. With the continuing advances in biological psychiatry and neuropsychiatry, however, laboratory tests have become increasingly valuable, both to the clinical psychiatrist and to the biological researcher.

In clinical psychiatry, laboratory tests can help rule out potential underlying organic causes of psychiatric symptoms—for example, impaired copper metabolism in Wilson's disease and a positive result on an antinuclear antibody (ANA) test in systematic lupus erythematosus (SLE). Laboratory work is then used to monitor treatment, such as measuring the blood levels of antidepressant medications and assessing the effects of lithium on electrolytes, thyroid metabolism, and renal function. Laboratory data, however, can serve only as an underlying support for the essential skill of clinical assessment.

BASIC SCREENING TESTS

Before initiating psychiatric treatment, a clinician should undertake a routine medical evaluation for the purposes of screening for concurrent disease, ruling out organicity, and establishing baseline values of functions to be monitored. Such an evaluation includes a medical history and routine medical laboratory tests, such as a complete blood count (CBC); hematocrit and hemoglobin; renal, liver, and thyroid function; electrolytes; and blood sugar.

Thyroid disease and other endocrinopathies can present as a mood disorder or a psychotic disorder; cancer or infectious disease can present as depression; infection and connective tissue diseases can present as short-term changes in mental status. In addition, a range of medical and neurological conditions may present initially to the psychiatrist. Those conditions include multiple sclerosis, Parkinson's disease, dementia of the Alzheimer's type, Huntington's disease, dementia caused by human immunodeficiency virus (HIV) disease, and temporal lobe epilepsy. Any suspected medical or neurological condition should be thoroughly evaluated with appropriate laboratory tests and consultation (Table 7.4–1).

NEUROENDOCRINE TESTS

Thyroid Function Tests

Several thyroid function tests are available, including tests for thyroxine (T_4) by competitive protein binding (T_4D) and by radioimmunoassay (T_4RIA) involving a specific antigen-antibody reaction. More than 90 percent of T_4 is bound to serum protein and is responsible for thyroid-stimulating hormone (TSH) secretion and cellular metabolism. Other thyroid measures include the free T_4 index (FT_4I), triiodothyronine uptake, and total serum triiodothyronine measured by radioimmunoassay (T_3RIA). These tests are used to rule out hypothyroidism, which can appear with symptoms of depression. In some studies, up to 10 percent of patients complaining of depression and associated fatigue had incipient hypothyroid disease. Other associated signs and symptoms common to both depression and hypothyroidism include weakness, stiffness, poor appetite, constipation, menstrual irregularities, slowed speech, apathy, impaired memory, and even hallucinations and delusions. Lithium can cause hypothyroidism and, more rarely, hyperthyroidism. Table 7.4–2 outlines the suggested monitoring of thyroid function for patients taking lithium. Neonatal hypothyroidism results in mental retardation and is preventable if the diagnosis is made at birth.

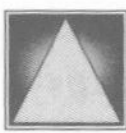

Table 7.4–1
Some Medical Conditions That May Manifest with Neuropsychiatric Symptoms

Neurological	Toxic
Cerebrovascular disorders (hemorrhage, infarction) Head trauma (concussion, posttraumatic hematoma) Epilepsy (especially complex partial seizures) Narcolepsy Brain neoplasms (primary or metastatic) Normal-pressure hydrocephalus Parkinson's disease Multiple sclerosis Huntington's disease Dementia of the Alzheimer's type Metachromatic leukodystrophy Migraine	Intoxication or withdrawal associated with drug or alcohol abuse Adverse effects of prescribed and over-the-counter medications Environmental toxins (volatile hydrocarbons, heavy metals, carbon monoxide, organophosphates)

Neurological
- Cerebrovascular disorders (hemorrhage, infarction)
- Head trauma (concussion, posttraumatic hematoma)
- Epilepsy (especially complex partial seizures)
- Narcolepsy
- Brain neoplasms (primary or metastatic)
- Normal-pressure hydrocephalus
- Parkinson's disease
- Multiple sclerosis
- Huntington's disease
- Dementia of the Alzheimer's type
- Metachromatic leukodystrophy
- Migraine

Endocrine
- Hypothyroidism
- Hyperthyroidism
- Hypoadrenalism
- Hyperadrenalism
- Hypoparathyroidism
- Hyperparathyroidism
- Hypoglycemia
- Hyperglycemia
- Diabetes mellitus
- Panhypopituitarism
- Pheochromocytoma
- Gonadotropic hormonal disturbances
- Pregnancy

Metabolic and systemic
- Fluid and electrolyte disturbances (e.g., syndrome of inappropriate antidiuretic hormone secretion [SIADH])
- Hepatic encephalopathy
- Uremia
- Porphyria
- Hepatolenticular degeneration (Wilson's disease)
- Hypoxemia (chronic pulmonary disease)
- Hypotension
- Hypertensive encephalopathy

Toxic
- Intoxication or withdrawal associated with drug or alcohol abuse
- Adverse effects of prescribed and over-the-counter medications
- Environmental toxins (volatile hydrocarbons, heavy metals, carbon monoxide, organophosphates)

Nutritional
- Vitamin B_{12} deficiency (pernicious anemia)
- Nicotinic acid deficiency (pellagra)
- Folate deficiency (megaloblastic anemia)
- Thiamine deficiency (Wernicke-Korsakoff syndrome)
- Trace metal deficiency (zinc, magnesium)
- Nonspecific malnutrition and dehydration

Infectious
- Acquired immunodeficiency syndrome (AIDS)
- Neurosyphilis
- Viral meningitides and encephalitides (e.g., herpes simplex)
- Brain abscess
- Viral hepatitis
- Infectious mononucleosis
- Tuberculosis
- Systemic bacterial infections (especially pneumonia) and viremia
- Streptococcal infections
- Pediatric infection-triggered, autoimmune neuropsychiatric disorders

Autoimmune
- Systemic lupus erythematosus

Neoplastic
- Central nervous system (CNS) primary and metastatic tumors
- Endocrine tumors
- Pancreatic carcinoma
- Paraneoplastic syndromes

(Table adapted from Darrell G. Kirch, M.D.)

Table 7.4–3 lists the thyroid function test changes associated with hypothyroidism.

The thyrotropin-releasing hormone (TRH) stimulation test is indicated for patients whose marginally abnormal thyroid test results suggest subclinical hypothyroidism, which can account for clinical depression. The test is also used for patients with possible lithium-induced hypothyroidism. The procedure entails an intravenous (IV) injection of 500 mg of TRH, which produces a sharp rise in serum TSH when measured at 15, 30, 60, and 90 minutes. An increase in serum TSH from 5 to 25 international units per milliliter (IU/mL) above baseline is normal. An increase of less than 7 IU/mL is considered a blunted response, which may correlate with a diagnosis of a depressive disorder. Eight percent of all patients with depressive disorders have some thyroid illness.

Dexamethasone-Suppression Test

The dexamethasone suppression test (DST) is used to help confirm a diagnostic impression of major depressive disorder.

The patient is given 1 mg of dexamethasone (a long-acting synthetic glucocorticoid) by mouth at 11 PM, and the plasma cortisol level is measured at 8 AM, 4 PM, and 11 PM. Plasma cortisol concentrations above 5 mg/dL (known as nonsuppression) are considered abnormal (i.e., a positive result). Suppression of cortisol indicates that the hypothalamic-adrenal-pituitary axis is functioning properly. Since the 1930s, dysfunction of this axis has been known to be associated with stress.

The problems associated with the DST include varying reports of sensitivity and specificity. False-positive and false-negative results are common and many medical conditions and pharmacological agents can interfere with results. Some evidence indicates that patients with a positive DST result (especially, 10 mg/dL) will have a good response to somatic treatment, such as electroconvulsive therapy (ECT) or cyclic antidepressant therapy.

Other Endocrine Tests

Many other hormones affect behavior. Exogenous hormonal administration has been shown to affect behavior, and known endocrine diseases have associated mental disorders. In addition to thyroid hormones, these hormones include the anterior pituitary hormone prolactin, growth hormone, somatostatin, gonadotrophin-releasing hormone (GnRH), the sex steroids, luteinizing hormone (LH), follicle-stimulating hormone (FSH), testosterone, and estrogen. Melatonin from the pineal gland has been implicated in seasonal affective disorder. Symptoms

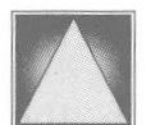

Table 7.4–2
Thyroid Monitoring for Patients Taking Lithium

Evaluation	Before Treatment	Repeat at 6 Months	Repeat Yearly
Medical			
1. Careful medical and family history to detect family history of thyroid disease	x		
2. Review of symptoms of hyperthyroidism and hypothyroidism	x	x	x
3. Physical examination, including palpation of thyroid	x		x
Laboratory			
T_3RU (triiodothyronine resin uptake)	x		x
T_4RIA (triiodothyronine measured by radioimmunoassay)	x		x
T_2I (free thyroxine index)	x		x
TSH (thyroid-stimulating hormone)	x	x	x
Antithyroid antibodies	x		x

(Reprinted from MacKinnon RA, Yudofsky SC. *Principles of the Psychiatric Evaluation.* Philadelphia: JB Lippincott; 1991:104, with permission.)

of anxiety or depression in some patients may be explained on the basis of unspecified changes in endocrine function or homeostasis.

Prolactin. Prolactin levels can become elevated in response to the administration of antipsychotic agents. Elevations in serum prolactin result from blockade of dopamine receptors in the pituitary. This blockade produces an increase in prolactin synthesis and release. Elevated prolactin levels are associated with galactorrhea, menstrual abnormalities, and alterations in libido and bone calcium concentrations.

Prolactin can briefly rise after a seizure. For this reason, prompt measurement of a prolactin level after possible seizure activity may assist in differentiating a seizure from a pseudoseizure.

Catecholamines

The level of serotonin metabolite 5-hydroxyindoleacetic acid (5-HIAA) is elevated in the urine of patients with carcinoid tumors. Elevated levels are noted at times in patients who take phenothiazine medication and in those who eat foods high in serotonin (e.g., walnuts, bananas, and avocados). The concentration of 5-HIAA in cerebrospinal fluid is low in some persons who are in a suicidal depression and in postmortem studies of those who have committed suicide in particularly violent ways. Low 5-HIAA levels in cerebrospinal fluid are associated with violence in general. Norepinephrine and its metabolic products—metanephrine, normetanephrine, and vanillylmandelic acid (VMA)—can be measured in urine, blood, and plasma. Plasma catecholamine levels are markedly elevated in pheochromocytoma, which is associated with anxiety, agitation, and hypertension. Some patients with chronic anxiety may exhibit elevated blood norepinephrine and epinephrine levels. Some depressed patients have a low urinary norepinephrine-to-epinephrine ratio (NE:E).

High levels of urinary norepinephrine and epinephrine have been found in some patients with posttraumatic stress disorder. The norepinephrine metabolite 3-methoxy-4-hydroxyphenylglycol (MHPG) concentration is decreased in patients with severe depressive disorders, especially those patients who attempt suicide.

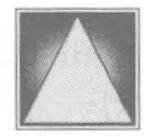

Table 7.4–3
Thyroid Function Test Changes in Patients with Hypothyroidism

1. Serum T_4 concentration is decreased.
2. Serum-free thyroxine is decreased.
3. Serum T_3 concentration is decreased.
4. Serum T_3 uptake is decreased.
5. Serum protein-bound iodine (PBI) is decreased.
6. Serum thyroxine-binding globulin is normal.
7. Serum T_3-to-T_4 ratio is increased.
8. Serum TSH is increased.

(Reprinted from MacKinnon RA, Yudofsky SC. *Principles of the Psychiatric Evaluation.* Philadelphia: JB Lippincott; 1991:97, with permission.)

Kidney Function Tests

Creatinine clearance detects early kidney damage and can be serially monitored to follow the course of renal disease. Blood urea nitrogen (BUN) is also elevated in renal disease and is excreted via the kidneys; serum BUN and creatinine levels are monitored in patients taking lithium. If the serum BUN or creatinine level is abnormal, the patient's 2-hour creatinine clearance and ultimately the 24-hour creatinine clearance are tested. Table 7.4–4 outlines a suggested protocol for monitoring renal function in patients taking lithium. Table 7.4–5 summarizes other laboratory testing for patients taking lithium.

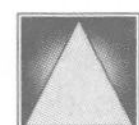

Table 7.4–4
Renal Monitoring for Patients Taking Lithium

Evaluation	Before Treatment	Repeat at 6 Months	Repeat Yearly
Medical			
1. Careful medical and family history to detect presence of familial kidney disease or predisposition to kidney disease (diabetes, hypertension)	x		
2. Specific comprehensive review of genitourinary system symptoms	x	x	x
3. Physical examination	x		x
Laboratory			
BUN (blood, urea, nitrogen)	x		x
Creatinine	x	x	x
Creatinine clearance (24-hour urine) urinalysis	x		x
24-hour urine volume	x		x
12-hour fluid deprivation test	x		

(Reprinted from MacKinnon RA, Yudofsky SC. *Principles of the Psychiatric Evaluation.* Philadelphia: JB Lippincott; 1991:103, with permission.)

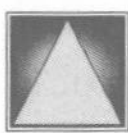

Table 7.4–5
Other Laboratory Testing for Patients Taking Lithium

Test	Frequency
1. Complete blood count	Before treatment and yearly
2. Serum electrolytes	Before treatment and yearly
3. Fasting blood glucose	Before treatment and yearly
4. Electrocardiogram	Before treatment and yearly
5. Pregnancy testing for women of childbearing age[a]	Before treatment

[a] Test more frequently when compliance with treatment plan is uncertain. (Reprinted from MacKinnon RA, Yudofsky SC. *Principles of the Psychiatric Evaluation.* Philadelphia: JB Lippincott; 1991:106, with permission.)

Liver Function Tests

Total bilirubin and direct bilirubin values are elevated in hepatocellular injury and intrahepatic bile stasis, which can occur with phenothiazine or tricyclic medication and with alcohol and other substance abuse. Certain drugs (e.g., phenobarbital [Luminal]) can lower the serum bilirubin concentration. Liver damage or disease, which is reflected by abnormal findings in liver function tests (LFTs), can manifest with signs and symptoms of a cognitive disorder, including disorientation and delirium. Impaired hepatic function can increase the elimination half-lives of certain drugs, including some benzodiazepines, so that the drug may stay in a patient's system longer than it would under normal circumstances. LFTs must be monitored routinely when using certain drugs, such as carbamazepine (Tegretol) and valproate (Depakene).

Lipids, Fasting Blood Sugar and Glycosylated Hemoglobin. Some atypical antipsychotic agents have been associated with abnormalities in lipid and serum glucose levels, including the development of diabetes mellitus. Patients who take atypical antipsychotic agents should be monitored for the development of hyperglycemia by obtaining fasting blood glucose levels and glycosylated hemoglobin levels on a quarterly or semiannual basis. In addition, extremes in serum glucose concentrations have been associated with delirium. Hypoglycemia has also been associated with agitation and anxiety. Evaluation for diabetes or other abnormalities in glucose metabolism is usually best done by specialists.

BLOOD TEST FOR SEXUALLY TRANSMITTED DISEASES

The Venereal Disease Research Laboratory (VDRL) is a screening test for syphilis. If positive, the result is confirmed by using the specific fluorescent treponemal antibody-absorption (FTA-ABS) test, in which the spirochete *Treponema pallidum* is used as the antigen. A central nervous system (CNS) VDRL test is performed in patients with suspected neurosyphilis. A positive HIV test result indicates that a person has been exposed to infection with the virus that causes acquired immune deficiency syndrome (AIDS).

TESTS RELATED TO PSYCHOTROPIC DRUGS

In caring for patients receiving psychotropic medication, the trend is to measure regularly the concentration of the prescribed drug in plasma. For some drugs, such as lithium, the monitoring is essential; for other drugs, such as antipsychotics, it is mainly of academic or research interest. A clinician need not practice defensive medicine by insisting that all patients receiving psychotropic drugs have blood levels determined for medicolegal purposes. The current status of psychopharmacological treatment is such that a psychiatrist's clinical judgment and experience, except in rare instances, are better indications of a drug's therapeutic efficacy than determining its level in plasma. The reliance on plasma levels cannot replace clinical skills.

The major classes of drugs and the suggested guidelines for their use are outlined below.

Benzodiazepines

No special tests are needed for patients taking benzodiazepines. Among the benzodiazepines metabolized in the liver by oxidation, impaired hepatic function increases the half-life. Baseline LFTs are indicated for patients with suspected liver damage. Urine is tested routinely for benzodiazepines in patients being treated for substance abuse.

Antipsychotics

No special tests are needed for patients taking antipsychotics, although it is a good idea to obtain baseline values for liver function and a complete blood cell count. Antipsychotics are metabolized primarily in the liver, with metabolites excreted primarily in urine. Many metabolites are active. Peak plasma concentration usually is reached 2 to 3 hours after an oral dose. Elimination half-life is 12 to 30 hours, but can be much longer. Steady state requires at least 1 week at a constant dose (months at a constant dose of depot antipsychotics). With the exception of clozapine (Clozaril), all antipsychotics cause a short-term elevation in serum prolactin concentration (secondary to tuberoinfundibular activity). A normal prolactin level often indicates either noncompliance or nonabsorption. Adverse effects include leukocytosis, leukopenia, impaired platelet function, mild anemia (both aplastic and hemolytic), and agranulocytosis. Bone marrow and blood element adverse effects can occur abruptly, even when the dosage has remained constant. Low-potency antipsychotics are most likely to cause agranulocytosis, which is the most common bone marrow adverse effect. These agents can cause hepatocellular injury and intrahepatic biliary stasis (indicated by elevated total and direct bilirubin and elevated transaminases). They also can cause electrocardiographic changes (not as frequently as with tricyclic antidepressants), including a prolonged QT interval; flattened, inverted, or bifid T waves; and U waves. The relation of dose to plasma concentration differs widely among patients.

Clozapine. Clozapine levels are determined in the morning before administration of the morning dose of medication. Weekly CBCs are required during the first 6 months of treatment with clozapine because of the risk of agranulocytosis. After the first 6 months of treatment, CBCs are checked every 2 weeks.

Table 7.4–6
Clinical Management of Reduced White Blood Cell Count (WBC), Leukopenia, and Agranulocytosis

Problem Phase	WBC Findings	Clinical Findings	Treatment Plan
Reduced WBC count	WBC count reveals a significant drop (even if WBC count is still in normal range). "Significant drop" is (1) drop of more than 3,000 cells from prior test or (2) three or more consecutive drops in WBC counts	No symptoms of infection	1. Monitor patient closely 2. Institute twice-weekly CBC tests with differentials if deemed appropriate by attending physician 3. Clozapine therapy may continue
Mild leukopenia	WBC = 3,000 to 3,500	Patient may or may not show clinical symptoms, such as lethargy, fever, sore throat, weakness	1. Monitor patient closely 2. Institute a minimum of twice-weekly complete blood count (CBC) tests with differentials 3. Clozapine therapy may continue
Leukopenia or granulocytopenia	WBC = 2,000 to 3,000 or granulocytes = 1,000 to 1,500	Patient may or may not show clinical symptoms, such as fever, sore throat, lethargy, weakness	1. Interrupt clozapine at once 2. Institute daily CBC tests with differentials 3. Increase surveillance, consider hospitalization 4. Clozapine therapy may be reinstituted after normalization of WBC
Agranulocytosis (uncomplicated)	WBC count less than 2,000 or granulocytes less than 1,000	The patient may or may not show clinical symptoms, such as fever, sore throat, lethargy, weakness	1. Discontinue clozapine at once 2. Place patient in protective isolation in a medical unit with modern facilities 3. Consider a bone marrow specimen to determine if progenitor cells are being suppressed 4. Monitor patient every 2 days until WBC and differential counts return to normal (about 2 weeks) 5. Avoid use of concomitant medications with bone marrow-suppressing potential
Agranulocytosis (with complications)	WBC count less than 2,000 or granulocytes less than 1,000	Definite evidence of infection, such as fever, sore throat, lethargy, weakness, malaise, skin ulcerations, and so on.	1. Consult with hematologist or other specialist to determine appropriate antibiotic regimen 2. Start appropriate therapy; monitor closely
Recovery	WBC count more than 4,000 and granulocytes more than 2,000	No symptoms of infection	1. Once-weekly CBC with differential counts for four consecutive normal values 2. Clozapine must not be restarted

(Reprinted from Sandoz Pharmaceuticals Corporation and MacKinnon RA, Yudofsky SC. *Principles of the Psychiatric Evaluation.* Philadelphia: JB Lippincott; 1991:118, with permission.)

Results must be sent to a pharmacy for the patient to receive his or her medication. Clozapine should be held for a WBC of less than 3,000 per mm^3 or a neutrophil count of less than 1,500 per mm^3.

A therapeutic range for clozapine has not been established; however, a level of 100 nanograms per milliliter (ng/mL) is widely considered to be a minimal therapeutic threshold. Although concentrations between 200 and 700 ng/mL correlate more with response, nonresponse does occur within this range. At least 350 ng/mL of clozapine is considered to be necessary to achieve a therapeutic response in patients with refractory schizophrenia. The likelihood of seizures and other side effects increases with clozapine levels greater than 1,200 ng/mL or dosages greater than 600 mg per day, or both.

Physicians and pharmacists who provide clozapine must be registered through the Clozaril National Registry (1-800-448-5938). Table 7.4–6 summarizes the clinical management of reduced WBC, leukopenia, and agranulocytosis in patients treated with clozapine.

Tricyclic and Tetracyclic Drugs

An electrocardiogram (ECG) can be taken before starting a regimen of cyclic drugs to assess for conduction delays, which may lead to heart block at therapeutic levels. Some clinicians believe that all patients receiving prolonged cyclic drug therapy should have an annual ECG. At therapeutic levels, the drugs suppress arrhythmias through a quinidine-like effect.

Blood levels should be determined routinely when using imipramine (Tofranil), desipramine (Norpramin), or nortriptyline (Pamelor) in the treatment of depressive disorders. Blood level determinations can also be useful for patients with a poor response at normal dosage ranges and with high-risk patients for whom there is an urgent need to know whether a therapeutic or toxic plasma level of the drug has been reached. Blood level determinations should also include the measurement of active metabolites (e.g., imipramine is converted to desipramine, amitriptyline [Elavil] to nortriptyline). Some characteristics of tricyclic drug plasma levels are described as follows.

Imipramine. The percentage of favorable responses correlates with plasma levels in a linear manner between 200 and 250 ng/mL, but some patients respond at a lower level. Levels above 250 ng/mL yield no improved favorable response, and adverse effects increase.

Nortriptyline. The therapeutic window (the range within which a drug is most effective) is between 50 and 150 ng/mL. The response rate decreases at levels above 150 ng/mL.

Desipramine. Levels above 125 ng/mL correlate with a higher percentage of favorable responses.

Amitriptyline. Different studies have produced conflicting results with regard to blood levels, but they range from 75 to 175 ng/mL.

Procedure for Determining Blood Concentrations. The blood specimen should be drawn 10 to 14 hours after the last dose, usually in the morning after a bedtime dose. Patients must have received a stable daily dose for at least 5 days for the test to be valid. Some patients who metabolize cyclic drugs unusually poorly may have levels as high as 2,000 ng/mL while taking normal dosages and before showing a favorable clinical response. Such patients must be monitored closely for cardiac adverse effects. Patients with levels above 1,000 ng/mL are generally at risk for cardiotoxicity.

Monoamine Oxidase Inhibitors

Patients taking monoamine oxidase inhibitors (MAOIs) are instructed to avoid tyramine-containing foods because of the danger of a hypertensive crisis. A baseline normal blood pressure (BP) must be recorded, and the BP must be monitored during treatment. MAOIs can also cause orthostatic hypotension as a direct drug adverse effect unrelated to diet. Other than their potential for elevating BP when taken with certain foods, MAOIs are relatively free of other adverse effects. A test used both in a research setting and in current clinical practice involves correlating the therapeutic response with the degree of platelet MAO inhibition.

Lithium

Patients receiving lithium should have baseline thyroid function tests, electrolyte monitoring, a WBC, renal function tests (specific gravity, BUN, and creatinine), and a baseline ECG. The rationale for these tests is that lithium can cause renal concentrating defects, hypothyroidism, and leukocytosis; sodium depletion can cause toxic lithium levels; and about 95 percent of lithium is excreted in the urine. Lithium has also been shown to cause ECG changes, including various conduction defects.

Lithium is most clearly indicated in the prophylactic treatment of manic episodes (its direct antimanic effect can take up to 2 weeks), and it is commonly coupled with antipsychotics for the treatment of acute manic episodes. Lithium itself may also have antipsychotic activity. The maintenance level is 0.6 to 1.2 mEq/L, although acutely manic patients can tolerate up to 1.5 to 1.8 mEq/L. Some patients respond at lower levels; others require higher levels. A response below 0.4 mEq/L is probably a placebo effect. Toxic reactions can occur with levels above 2.0 mEq/L. Regular lithium monitoring is essential; a narrow therapeutic range exists beyond which cardiac problems and CNS effects can occur.

Blood for lithium level determination is drawn 8 to 12 hours after the last dose, usually in the morning after the bedtime dose. The level should be measured at least twice a week while stabilizing the patient's condition and can be determined monthly thereafter.

Carbamazepine

A pretreatment CBC, including a platelet count should be done. Reticulocyte count and serum iron tests are also desirable. These tests should be repeated weekly during the first 3 months of treatment and monthly thereafter. Carbamazepine can cause aplastic anemia, agranulocytosis, thrombocytopenia, and leukopenia. Because of the minor risk of hepatotoxicity, LFTs should be done every 3 to 6 months. The medication should be discontinued if the patient shows any signs of bone marrow suppression as measured with periodic CBC. The therapeutic level of carbamazepine is 8 to 12 ng/mL, with toxicity most often reached at levels of 15 ng/mL. Most clinicians report that levels as high as 12 ng/mL are hard to achieve. Table 7.4–7 summarizes one

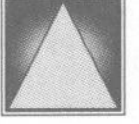

Table 7.4–7
Laboratory Monitoring of Patients Taking Carbamazepine

Test	Frequency
1. Complete blood count (CBC)	Before treatment and every 2 weeks for the first 2 months of treatment; thereafter, once every 3 months
2. Platelet count and reticulocyte count	Before treatment and yearly
3. Serum electrolytes	Before treatment and yearly
4. Electrocardiogram	Before treatment and yearly
5. Aspartate aminotransferase (SGOT), alanine aminotransferase (SGPT), lactate dehydrogenase (LDH) alkaline phosphatase	Before treatment and every month for the first 2 months of treatment; thereafter, every 3 months
6. Pregnancy test for women of childbearing age	Before treatment and as frequently as monthly in noncompliant patients

(Reprinted from MacKinnon RA, Yudofsky SC. *Principles of the Psychiatric Evaluation.* Philadelphia: JB Lippincott; 1991:108, with permission.)

suggested protocol for laboratory monitoring of patients taking carbamazepine.

Valproate

Serum levels of valproic acid and divalproex (Depakote) are therapeutic in the range of 45 to 50 ng/mL. Above 125 ng/mL, adverse effects occur, including thrombocytopenia. Serum levels should be determined periodically, and LFTs should be run every 6 to 12 months.

Tacrine

Tacrine (Cognex) can cause liver damage. A baseline of liver function should be established, and follow-up serum transaminase levels should be determined every other week for about 5 months. Patients who develop jaundice or who have bilirubin levels above 3 mg/dL must be withdrawn from the drug.

PROVOCATION OF PANIC ATTACKS WITH SODIUM LACTATE

Up to 72 percent of patients with panic disorder have a panic attack when administered IV injection of sodium lactate. Therefore, lactate provocation is used to confirm a diagnosis of panic disorder. Lactate provocation has also been used to trigger flashbacks in patients with posttraumatic stress disorder. Hyperventilation, another known trigger of panic attacks in predisposed persons, is not as sensitive as lactate provocation in inducing panic attacks. Carbon dioxide (CO_2) inhalation also precipitates panic attacks in those so predisposed. Panic attacks triggered by sodium lactate are not inhibited by peripherally acting β-adrenergic receptor antagonists (beta-blockers), but are inhibited by alprazolam (Xanax) and tricyclic drugs.

DRUG-ASSISTED INTERVIEW

Interviews with amobarbital (Amytal) have both diagnostic and therapeutic indications. Diagnostically, the interviews are helpful in differentiating nonorganic and organic conditions, particularly in patients with symptoms of catatonia, stupor, and muteness. Organic conditions tend to worsen with infusions of amobarbital, but nonorganic or psychogenic conditions tend to get better because of disinhibition, decreased anxiety, or increased relaxation. Therapeutically, amobarbital interviews are useful in disorders of repression and dissociation—for example, in the recovery of memory in psychogenic amnestic disorders and fugue, in the recovery of function in conversion disorder, and in facilitation of emotional expression in posttraumatic stress disorder. Benzodiazepines can be substituted for amobarbital in the infusion. The procedure is outlined in Table 7.4–8.

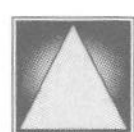

Table 7.4–8
Drug-Assisted Interview Procedure

1. Have patient recline in an environment in which cardiopulmonary resuscitation is readily available should hypotension or respiratory depression develop.
2. Explain to patient that medication should help him or her relax and feel like talking.
3. Insert a narrow-bore needle into a peripheral vein.
4. Inject a 5% solution of sodium amobarbital (500 mg dissolved in 10 mL of sterile water) at a rate no faster than 1 mL/min (50 mg/min).
5. Begin interview by discussing neutral topics: often, it is helpful to prompt the patient with known facts about his or her life.
6. Continue infusion until either sustained lateral nystagmus or drowsiness is noted.
7. To maintain the level of narcosis, continue infusion at a rate of 0.5 to 1.0 mL/5 minutes (25 to 50 mg/5 minutes)
8. Have the patient recline for at least 15 minutes after the interview is terminated, until the patient can walk without supervision.
9. Use the same method every time to avoid dosage errors.

LUMBAR PUNCTURE

Lumbar puncture is useful in patients who have a sudden manifestation of new psychiatric symptoms, especially changes in cognition. The clinician should be especially vigilant when fever or neurological symptoms, such as seizures are present. Lumbar puncture is of use in diagnosing CNS infection (e.g., meningitis).

URINE TESTING FOR SUBSTANCE ABUSE

A number of substances may be detected in a patient's urine if the urine is tested within a specific (and variable) period after ingestion of the substance. Knowledge of urine substance testing is becoming crucial for practicing physicians in view of the controversial issue of mandatory or random substance testing. Table 7.4–9 provides a summary of substances of abuse that can be detected in urine.

Laboratory tests are also used to detect substances that may be contributing to cognitive disorders. Table 7.4–10 is an outline of therapeutic, toxic, and lethal levels of substances most commonly implicated in cognitive disorders.

OTHER LABORATORY TESTS

Laboratory tests not already discussed are covered in Table 7.4–11 in terms of their indications and significance in medical conditions that affect behavior. See Chapter 11 for information about testing for HIV.

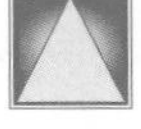

Table 7.4–9
Substances of Abuse That Can Be Tested in Urine

Substance	Length of Time Detected in Urine
Alcohol	7–12 hours
Amphetamine	48 hours
Barbiturate	24 hours (short-acting) 3 weeks (long-acting)
Benzodiazepine	3 days
Cannabis	3 days to 4 weeks (depending on use)
Cocaine	6–8 hours (metabolites 2–4 days)
Codeine	48 hours
Heroin	36–72 hours
Methadone	3 days
Methaqualone	7 days
Morphine	48–72 hours
Phencyclidine (PCP)	8 days
Propoxyphene	6–48 hours

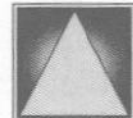

Table 7.4–10
Blood Level Data for Clinical Assessment

Substance	Therapeutic or Normal (%)	Blood Levels	
		Toxic (%)	Lethal (%)
Acetaminophen (Tylenol)	1.0–2.0 mg	15.0 mg	150.0 mg
Acetylsalicylic acid (salicylate)	10–30.0 mg	>39.0 mg	50.0 mg
Aminophylline (theophylline)	1.0–2.0 mg	3.0–4.0 mg	21.0–25.0 mg
Amitriptyline (Elavil)	5.0–20.0 μg	>50.0 μg	1.0–2.0 mg
Amphetamines	2.0–3.0 μg	50.0 μg	200.0 μg
Arsenic	0.0–2.0 μg	0.10 mg	1.5 mg
Barbiturates			
Short-acting	0.1 mg	0.7 mg	1.0 mg
Intermediate-acting	0.1–0.5 mg	1.0–3.0 mg	>3.0 mg
Phenobarbital	1.5–3.9 mg	4.0–6.0 mg	8.0–>15 mg
Barbital	1.0 mg	6.0–8.0 mg	>10.0 mg
Bromide	5.0–30 mg	50–150 mg	200 mg
Carbamazepine (Tegretol)	0.8–1.2 mg	>1.5 mg	—
Chloral hydrate	0.2–1.0 mg	10.0 mg	25.0 mg
Chlordiazepoxide (Librium)	0.1–0.3 mg	0.55 mg	2.0 mg
Chlorpromazine (Thorazine)	0.05 mg	0.1–0.2 mg	0.3–1.2 mg
Cocaine	—	90.0 μg	0.1–2.0 mg
Codeine	2.5–12.0 μg	—	20.0–60.0 μg
Desipramine (Norpramin)	15.0–30.0 μg	>50.0 μg	1.0–2.0 mg
Diazepam (Valium)	0.05–0.25 mg	0.5–2.0 mg	>2.0 mg
Digoxin	0.06–0.20 μg	0.21–0.90 μg	1.5 μg
Diphenhydramine (Benadryl)	1.0–10.0 μg	0.5 mg	>1.0 mg
Doxepin (Sinequan)	10.0–25.0 μg	50.0–200.0 μg	>1.0 mg
Ethanol	—	100.0 mg (legal intoxication)	350.0 mg
Glutethimide (Doriden)	0.02–0.08 mg	1.0–8.0 mg	3.0–10.0 mg
Haloperidol (Haldol)	0.05–0.9 μg	1.0–4.0 mg	—
Imipramine (Tofranil)	15.0–25.0 μg	50.0–150.0 μg	0.2 mg
Lead	0.0–30.0 μg	130 μg	110.0–350.0 μg
Lithium	0.42–0.83 mg (0.6–1.2 mEq/L)	1.39 mg (2.0 mEq/L)	>3.47 mg (>4.0 mEq/L)
Lysergic acid diethylamide (LSD)	—	0.1–0.4 μg	—
Meperidine (Demerol)	0.03–0.10 mg	0.5 mg	3.0 mg
Meprobamate	0.8–2.4 mg	6.0–10.0 mg	14.0–35.0 mg
Mercury	0.0–8 μg	100 μg	600.0 μg
Methadone (Dolophine)	30.0–110.0 μg	0.2 mg	>0.4 mg
Methamphetamine	0.02–0.06 mg	0.06–0.5 mg	1.0–4.0 mg
Methanol	—	20.0 mg	>89.0 mg
Methaqualone (Quaalude)	0.3–0.6 mg	1.0–3.0 mg	>3.0 mg
Methylphenidate (Ritalin)	1.0–6.0 μg	80.0 μg	230.0 μg
Morphine	10.0 μg	—	5.0–400 μg (free morphine from heroin)
Nortriptyline (Pamelor)	12.0–16.0 μg	0.05 mg	1.3 mg
Oxycodone (Percodan)	1.7–3.6 μg	20.0–500.0 μg	—
Paraldehyde	2.0–11.0 mg	20.0–40.0 mg	>50.0 mg
Pentazocine (Talwin)	0.01–0.06 mg	0.2–0.5 mg	1.0–2.0 mg
Perphenazine (Trilafon)	0.5 μg	100.0 μg	—
Phencyclidine (PCP)	—	0.7–24.0 μg	100.0–500.0 μg
Phenytoin (Dilantin)	1.0–2.0 mg	2.0–5.0 mg	>10 mg
Primidone (Mysoline)	0.5–1.2 mg	5.0–8.0 mg	10.0 mg
Propoxyphene (Darvon)	5.0–20.0 μg	30.0–60.0 μg	80.0–200.0 μg
Propranolol (Inderal)	2.5–20.0 μg	—	0.8–1.2 mg
Quinidine	0.03–0.6 mg	1.0 mg	3.0–5.0 mg
Quinine	0.18 mg	—	1.2 mg
Thioridazine (Mellaril)	0.10–0.15 mg	1.0 mg	2.0–8.0 mg
Trifluoperazine (Stelazine)	0.08 mg	0.12–0.3 mg	0.3–0.8 mg

(Reprinted from Winek L. *Drug and Chemical Blood-Level Data*. Pittsburgh: Fisher Scientific; 1985, with permission.)

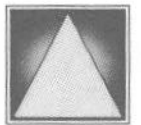

Table 7.4–11
Other Laboratory Tests

Test	Major Psychiatric Indications	Comments
Acid phosphatase	Organic workup for cognitive disorders	Increased in prostate cancer, benign prostatic hypertrophy, excessive platelet destruction, bone disease
Adrenocorticotropic hormone (ACTH)	Organic workup	Increased in steroid abuse; may be increased in seizures, psychotic disorders, Cushing's disease, and in response to stress Decreased in Addison's disease
Alanine aminotransferase (ALT) (formerly called serum glutamic-pyruvic transaminase [SGPT])	Organic workup	Increased in hepatitis, cirrhosis, liver metastases Decreased in pyridoxine (vitamin B_6) deficiency
Albumin	Organic workup	Increased in dehydration Decreased in malnutrition, hepatic failure, burns, multiple myeloma, carcinomas
Aldolase	Eating disorders Schizophrenia	Increased in patients who abuse ipecac (e.g., bulimic patients), schizophrenia (60%–80%)
Alkaline phosphatase	Organic workup Use of psychotropic medications	Increased in Paget's disease, hyperparathyroidism, hepatic disease, hepatic metastases, heart failure, phenothiazine use Decreased in pernicious anemia (vitamin B_{12} deficiency)
Ammonia, serum	Organic workup	Increased in hepatic encephalopathy
Amylase, serum	Eating disorders	May be increased in bulimia nervosa
Antinuclear antibodies	Organic workup	Found in systemic lupus erythematosus (SLE) and drug-induced lupus (e.g., secondary to phenothiazines, anticonvulsants); SLE can be associated with delirium, psychotic disorders, mood disorders
Aspartate aminotransferase (AST) (formerly SGOT)	Organic workup	Increased in heart failure, hepatic disease, pancreatitis, eclampsia, cerebral damage, alcohol dependence Decreased in pyridoxine (vitamin B_6) deficiency, terminal stages of liver disease
Bicarbonate, serum	Panic disorder Eating disorders	Decreased in hyperventilation syndrome, panic disorder, anabolic steroid abuse May be elevated in patients with bulimia nervosa, in laxative abuse, in psychogenic vomiting
Bilirubin	Organic workup	Increased in hepatic disease
Blood urea nitrogen (BUN)	Delirium Use of psychotropic medications	Elevated in renal disease, dehydration Elevations associated with lethargy, delirium If elevated, can increase toxic potential of psychiatric medications, especially lithium and amantadine (Symmetrel)
Bromide, serum	Dementia Psychosis	Bromide intoxication can cause psychosis, hallucinations, delirium Part of dementia workup, especially when serum chloride is elevated
Caffeine level, serum	Anxiety	Evaluation of patients with suspected caffeinism
Calcium (Ca), serum	Organic workup Mood disorders Psychosis Eating disorders	Increased in hyperparathyroidism, bone metastases Increase associated with delirium, depression, psychosis Decreased in hypoparathyroidism, renal failure Decrease associated with depression, irritability, delirium, long-term laxative abuse
Carotid ultrasound	Dementia	Occasionally included in dementia workup, especially to rule out multi-infarct dementia Primary value is in search for possible infarct causes
Catecholamines, urinary and plasma	Panic attacks Anxiety disorders	Elevated in pheochromocytoma
Cerebrospinal fluid (CSF)	Organic workup	Increased protein and cells in infection, positive VDRL result in neurosyphilis, bloody CSF in hemorrhagic conditions
Ceruloplasmin, serum; copper, serum	Organic workup	Low in Wilson's disease (hepatolenticular disease)
Chloride (Cl), serum	Eating disorders Panic disorder	Decreased in patients with bulimia nervosa and psychogenic vomiting Mild elevation in hyperventilation syndrome, panic disorder
Cholecystokinin (CCK)	Eating disorders	Compared with controls, blunted in bulimic patients after eating meal (may normalize after treatment with antidepressants)

(*continued*)

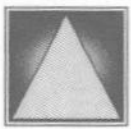

Table 7.4–11 (Continued)

Test	Major Psychiatric Indications	Comments
CO_2 inhalation; sodium bicarbonate infusion	Anxiety	Panic attacks produced in subgroup of patients
Coombs test, direct and indirect	Hemolytic anemias secondary to psychotropic medications	Evaluation of drug-induced hemolytic anemias, such as those secondary to chlorpromazine, phenytoin, levodopa, and methyldopa
Copper, urine	Organic workup	Elevated in Wilson's disease
Cortisol (hydrocortisone)	Organic workup Mood disorders	Excessive level may indicate Cushing's disease associated with anxiety, depression, and a variety of other conditions
Creatine phosphokinase (CPK)	Use of antipsychotics Use of restraints Substance abuse	Increased in neuroleptic malignant syndrome, intramuscular injection, rhabdomyolysis (secondary to substance abuse), patients in restraints, patients experiencing dystonic reactions; asymptomatic elevations seen with use of antipsychotics
Creatinine, serum	Organic workup	Elevated in renal disease Inhibits prolactin
Dopamine (DA) (L-dopa stimulation of dopamine)	Depression	Test used to assess functional integrity of dopaminergic system, which is impaired in Parkinson's disease, depression
Doppler ultrasound	Impotence Organic workup	Carotid occlusion, transient ischemic attack (TIA), reduced penile blood flow in impotence
Echocardiogram	Panic disorder	10%–40% of patients with panic disorder show mitral valve prolapse
Electroencephalogram (EEG)	Organic workup	Seizures, brain death, lesions; shortened rapid eye movement (REM) latency in depression High-voltage activity in stupor; low-voltage fast activity in excitement; in functional nonorganic cases (e.g., dissociative disorders), alpha activity is present in the background, which responds to auditory and visual stimuli Biphasic or triphasic slow bursts seen in dementia of Creutzfeldt-Jakob disease
Epstein-Barr virus (EBV); cytomegalovirus (CMV)	Organic workup Chronic fatigue Mood disorders	Part of herpesvirus group EBV is causative agent for infectious mononucleosis, which can manifest with depression and personality change CMV can produce anxiety, confusion, mood disorders EBV associated with chronic mononucleosislike syndrome associated with chronic depression and fatigue; may be association between EBV and major depressive disorder
Erythrocyte sedimentation rate (ESR)	Organic workup	An increase in ESR represents a nonspecific test of infectious, inflammatory, autoimmune, or malignant disease; sometimes recommended in the evaluation of anorexia nervosa
Estrogen	Mood disorder	Decreased in menopausal depression and premenstrual syndrome; variable changes in anxiety
Ferritin, serum	Organic workup	Most sensitive test for iron deficiency
Folate (folic acid), serum	Alcohol abuse Use of specific medications	Usually measured with vitamin B_{12} deficiencies associated with psychotic disorders, paranora, fatigue, agitation, dementia, delirium Associated with alcohol dependence, use of phenytoin, oral contraceptives, estrogen
Follicle-stimulating hormone (FSH)	Depression	High normal in anorexia nervosa, higher values in postmenopausal women; low levels in patients with panhypopituitarism
Glucose, fasting blood (FBS)	Panic attacks Anxiety Delirium Depression	Very high FBS associated with delirium Very low FBS associated with delirium, agitation, panic attacks, anxiety, depression
Glutamyl transaminase, serum	Alcohol abuse Organic workup	Increased in alcohol abuse, cirrhosis, liver disease
Gonadotropin-releasing hormone (GnRH)	Depression Anxiety Schizophrenia	Decreased in schizophrenia; increased in anorexia nervosa; variable in depression, anxiety
Growth hormone (GH)	Depression Schizophrenia	Blunted GH responses to insulin-induced hypoglycemia in depressed patients; increased GH responses to dopamine agonist challenge in schizophrenic patients; increased in some patients with anorexia nervosa

(continued)

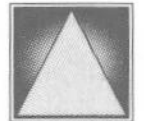

Table 7.4–11
(Continued)

Test	Major Psychiatric Indications	Comments
Hematocrit (Hct); hemoglobin (Hb)	Organic workup	Assessment of anemia (anemia may be associated with depressive and psychotic disorders)
Hepatitis A viral antigen (HAAg)	Mood disorders Organic workup	Less severe, better prognosis than hepatitis B; may present with anorexia nervosa, depression
Hepatitis B surface antigen (HBsAg); hepatitis Bc antigen (HBcAg)	Mood disorders Organic workup	Active hepatitis B infection indicates greater infectivity and progression to chronic liver disease May present with depression
Holter monitor	Panic disorder	Evaluation of panic-disordered patients with palpitations and other cardiac symptoms
Human immunodeficiency virus (HIV)	Organic workup	CNS involvement: acquired immune deficiency syndrome (AIDS) dementia, personality change due to a general medical condition, mood disorder due to a general medical condition, acute psychotic disorders
17-Hydroxycorticosteroid	Depression	Deviations detect hyperadrenocorticalism, which can be associated with major depressive disorder Increased in steroid abuse
5-Hydroxyindoleacetic acid (5-HIAA)	Depression Suicide Violence	Decreased in CSF in aggressive or violent patients with suicidal or homicidal impulses May indicate decreased impulse control and predict suicide
Iron, serum	Organic workup	Iron-deficiency anemia
Lactate dehydrogenase (LDH)	Organic workup	Increased in myocardial infarction, pulmonary infarction, hepatic disease, renal infarction, seizures, cerebral damage, megaloblastic (pernicious) anemia, factitious elevations secondary to rough handling of blood specimen tube
Lupus anticoagulant (LA)	Use of phenothiazines	An antiphospholipid antibody, which has been described in some patients using phenothiazines, especially chlorpromazine
Lupus erythematosus (LE) test	Depression Psychosis Delirium Dementia	Positive test result associated with SLE, which may manifest with various psychiatric disturbances, such as psychotic disorders, depressive disorders, delirium, dementia; also tested for with antinuclear antibody (ANA) and anti-DNA antibody tests
Luteinizing hormone (LH)	Depression	Low in patients with panhypopituitarism; decrease associated with depression
Magnesium, serum	Alcohol abuse Organic workup	Decreased in alcohol dependence; low levels associated with agitation, delirium, seizures
MAO, platelet	Depression	Low in depression
MCV (mean corpuscular volume) (average volume of a red blood cell)	Alcohol abuse	Elevated in alcohol dependence, vitamin B_{12}, folate deficiency
Melatonin	Mood disorder with seasonal pattern	Produced by light and pineal gland and decreased in mood disorder with seasonal pattern
Metal (heavy) intoxication (serum or urinary)	Organic workup	Lead—apathy, irritability, anorexia nervosa, confusion Mercury—psychosis, fatigue, apathy, decreased memory, emotional lability, "mad hatter" Manganese—manganese madness, Parkinsonlike syndrome Aluminum—dementia Arsenic—fatigue, blackouts, hair loss
3-Methoxy-4-hydroxyphenylglycol (MHPG)	Depression Anxiety	Most useful in research; decreases in urine may indicate decreases centrally
Myoglobin, urine	Phenothiazine use Substance abuse Use of restraints	Increased in neuroleptic malignant syndrome; in phencyclyine (PCP) cocaine, or lysergic acid diethylamide (LSD) intoxication; in patients in restraints
Nicotine	Anxiety Nicotine addiction	Anxiety, smoking
Nocturnal penile tumescence	Erectile disorder	Quantification of penile circumference changes, penile rigidity, frequency of penile tumescence Evaluation of erectile function during sleep Erections associated with rapid eye movement (REM) sleep Helpful in differentiation between organic and functional causes of impotence
Parathyroid (parathormone) hormone	Anxiety Organic workup	Low level causes hypocalcemia and anxiety Dysregulation associated with wide variety of cognitive disorders

(*continued*)

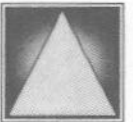

Table 7.4–11 (Continued)

Test	Major Psychiatric Indications	Comments
Phosphorus, serum	Organic workup Panic disorder	Increased in renal failure, diabetic acidosis, hypoparathyroidism, hypervitamin D Decreased in cirrhosis, hypokalemia, hyperparathyroidism, panic attack, hyperventilation syndrome
Platelet count	Use of psychotropic medications	Decreased by certain psychotropic medications (carbamazepine, clozapine, phenothiazines)
Porphobilinogen (PBG)	Organic workup	Increased in acute porphyria
Porphyria-synthesizing enzyme	Psychosis Organic workup	Acute panic attack or a cognitive disorder can occur in acute porphyria attack, which may be precipitated by barbiturates, imipramine
Potassium (K), serum	Organic workup Eating disorders	Increased in hyperkalemic acidosis; increase is associated with anxiety in cardiac arrhythmia Decreased in cirrhosis, metabolic alkalosis, laxative abuse, diuretic abuse; decrease is common in bulimic patients and in psychogenic vomiting, anabolic steroid abuse
Prolactin, serum	Use of antipsychotic medication Cocaine use Pseudoseizures	Antipsychotics, by decreasing dopamine, increase prolactin synthesis and release, especially in women Elevated prolactin levels may be seen secondary to cocaine withdrawal Lack of prolactin rise after seizure suggests pseudoseizure
Protein, total serum	Organic workup Use of psychotropic medications	Increased in multiple myeloma, myxedema, lupus Decreased in cirrhosis, malnutrition, overhydration Low serum protein can result in greater sensitivity to conventional doses of protein-bound medications (lithium is not protein bound)
Prothrombin time (PT)	Organic workup	Elevated in significant liver damage (cirrhosis), patients with lupus anticoagulant, which can be found in certain patients receiving antipsychotic medications, especially chlorpromazine
Reticulocyte count (estimate of red blood cell production in bone marrow)	Organic workup Use of carbamazepine	Low in megaloblastic or iron deficiency anemia and anemia of chronic disease Must be monitored in patient taking carbamazepine
Salicylate, serum	Psychotic disorder due to a general medical condition with hallucinations Suicide attempts	Toxic levels may be seen in suicide attempts and may cause psychotic disorder due to a general medical condition with hallucinations
Sodium (Na), serum	Organic workup	Decreased with water intoxication syndrome of inappropriate antidiuretic hormone secretion (SIADH) Increased with excessive salt intake; diabetes Decreased in hypoadrenalism, myxedema, congestive heart failure, diarrhea, polydipsia, use of carbamazepine, anabolic steroids Low levels associated with greater sensitivity to conventional dose of lithium
Testosterone, serum	Impotence Hypoactive sexual desire disorder	Increased in anabolic steroid abuse Follow-up of sex offenders treated with medroxyprogesterone May be decreased in organic workup of impotence Decrease may be seen in hypoactive sexual desire disorder Decreased with medroxyprogesterone treatment
Thyroid function tests	Organic workup Depression	Detection of hypothyroidism or hyperthyroidism Abnormalities can be associated with depression, anxiety, psychosis, dementia, delirium
Urinalysis	Organic workup Pretreatment workup of lithium Drug screening	Provides clues to cause of various cognitive disorders (assessing general appearance, pH, specific gravity, bilirubin, glucose, blood, ketones, protein, etc.); specific gravity may be affected by lithium
Urinary creatinine	Organic workup Substance abuse Lithium use	Increased in renal failure, dehydration Part of pretreatment workup for lithium
Venereal Disease Research Laboratory (VDRL)	Syphilis	Positive (high titers) in secondary syphilis (may be positive or negative in primary syphilis) Low titers (or negative) in tertiary syphilis
Vitamin A, serum	Depression Delirium	Hypervitaminosis A is associated with a variety of mental status changes

(*continued*)

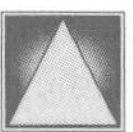

Table 7.4–11 (Continued)

Test	Major Psychiatric Indications	Comments
Vitamin B_{12}, serum	Organic workup Dementia	Part of workup of megaloblastic anemia and dementia B_{12} deficiency associated with psychosis, paranoia, fatigue, agitation, dementia, delirium Often associated with chronic alcohol abuse
White blood cell (WBC)	Use of psychotropic medications	Leukopenia and agranulocytosis associated with certain psychotropic medications, such as phenothiazines, carbamazepine, clozapine Leukocytosis associated with lithium and neuroleptic malignant syndrome

REFERENCES

Aronne LJ, Segal KR. Weight gain in the treatment of mood disorders. *J Clin Psychiatry.* 2003;64[Suppl 8]:22–29.

Chue P, Kovacs CS. Safety and tolerability of atypical antipsychotics in patients with bipolar disorder: Prevalence, monitoring, and management. *Bipolar Disord.* 2003;5[Suppl 2]:62–79.

Foster NL. Validating FDG-PET as a biomarker for frontotemporal dementia. *Exp Neurol.* 2003;184[Suppl 1]:S2–S8.

Guze BH, Love MJ. Medical assessment and laboratory testing in psychiatry. In: Sadock BJ, Sadock VA, eds. *Kaplan & Sadock's Comprehensive Textbook of Psychiatry*. 8th ed. Vol. 1. Baltimore: Lippincott Williams & Wilkins; 2005:916.

Kantarci K, Jack CR Jr. Neuroimaging in Alzheimer's disease: An evidence-based review. *Neuroimaging Clin N Am.* 2003;13:197–209.

Lyndenmayer JP, Czobor P, Volavka J, Sheitman B, McEvoy JP, Cooper TB, Chakos M, Lieberman JA. Changes in glucose and cholesterol levels in patients with schizophrenia treated with typical or atypical antipsychotics. *Am J Psychiatry.* 2003;160:290–296.

Marder SR, Essock SM, Miller AL, Buchanan RW, Casey DE, Davis JM, Kane JM, Lieberman J, Schooler NR, Covell N, Stroup S, Weissman EM, Wirshing DA, Hall CS, Pogach L, Xavier P, Bigger JT, Friedman A, Kleinber D, Yevich S, Davis B, Shon S. Health monitoring of patients with schizophrenia. *Am J Psychiatry.* 2004;161:1334–1349.

Rosse RB, Deutsch LH, Deutsch SI. Medical assessment and laboratory testing in psychiatry. In: Sadock BJ, Sadock VA, eds. *Kaplan & Sadock's Comprehensive Textbook of Psychiatry*. 7th ed. Vol. 2. Baltimore: Lippincott Williams & Wilkins; 2000:2329.

Schulte P. What is an adequate trial with clozapine? Therapeutic drug monitoring and time to response in treatment refractory schizophrenia. *Clin Pharmacokinet.* 2003;42:607–618.

▲ 7.5 Medical Record and Medical Error

MEDICAL RECORD

The medical record is used by physicians, by regulatory agencies, and by managed care companies to determine length of stay, quality of care, and reimbursement to doctors and hospitals. In theory, the inpatient medical record is accessible to authorized persons only and is safeguarded for confidentiality. In practice, however, absolute confidentiality cannot be guaranteed. Guidelines for what material needs to be incorporated into the medical record are given in Table 7.5–1.

The medical record is also crucial in malpractice litigation. Robert I. Simon summarized the liability issues as follows:

Properly kept medical records can be the psychiatrist's best ally in malpractice litigation. If no record is kept, numerous questions will be raised regarding the psychiatrist's competence and credibility. This failure to keep medical records may also violate state statutes or licensing provisions. Failure to keep medical records may arise out of the psychiatrist's concern that patient treatment information be totally protected. Although this is an admirable ideal, in real life the psychiatrist may be legally compelled under certain circumstances to testify directly about confidential treatment matters.

Outpatient records are also subject to scrutiny by third parties under certain circumstances, and psychiatrists in private practice are under the same obligation to maintain a record of the patient in treatment as the hospital psychiatrist. Table 7.5–2 lists documentation issues of concern to third-party payers.

Personal Notes and Observations

According to laws relating to access to medical records, some jurisdictions (such as in the Public Health Law of New York State) have a provision that applies to a physician's personal notes and observations. *Personal notes* are defined as "a

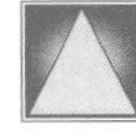

Table 7.5–1 Medical Record

There shall be an individual record for each person admitted to the psychiatric inpatient unit. Patient records shall be safeguarded for confidentiality and should be accessible only to authorized persons. Each case record shall include:

- Legal admission documents
- Identifying information on the individual and family
- Source of referral, date of commencement of service, and name of staff member carrying overall responsibility for treatment and care
- Initial, intercurrent, and final diagnoses, including psychiatric or mental retardation diagnoses in official terminology
- Reports of all diagnostic examinations and evaluations, including findings and conclusions
- Reports of all special studies performed, including X-rays, clinical laboratory tests, clinical psychological testing, electroencephalograms, and psychometric tests
- The individual written plan of care, treatment, and rehabilitation
- Progress notes written and signed by all staff members having significant participation in the program of treatment and care
- Summaries of case conferences and special consultations
- Dated and signed prescriptions or orders for all medications, with notation of termination dates
- Closing summary of the course of treatment and care
- Documentation of any referrals to another agency

(Adapted from the 1995 guidelines of the New York State Office of Mental Health, with permission.)

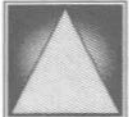

Table 7.5–2
Documentation Issues

Are patient's areas of dysfunction described? From the biological, psychological, and social points of view?
Is alcohol or substance abuse addressed?
Do clinical activities happen at the expected time? If too late or never, why?
Are issues identified in the treatment plan and followed in progress notes?
When a variance occurs in the patient's outcome, is such noted in the progress notes? Is there also a note in the progress notes reflecting the clinical strategies recommended to overcome the impediments to the patient's improvement?
If new clinical strategies are implemented, how is their impact evaluated? When?
Is there a sense of multidisciplinary input and coordination of treatment in the progress notes?
Do progress notes indicate the patient's functioning in the therapeutic community and its relationship to their discharge criteria?
Can one extrapolate from the patient's behavior in the therapeutic community how he or she will function in the community at large?
Are notes included depicting the patient's understanding of his or her discharge planning? Family participation in discharge planning must be entered in the progress notes with their reaction to the plan.
Do attending progress notes bridge the differences in thinking of other disciplines?
Are the patient's needs addressed in the treatment plan?
Are the patient's family needs evaluated and implemented?
Is patient and family satisfaction evaluated in any way?
Is alcohol and substance abuse addressed as a possible contributor to readmission?
If the patient was readmitted, are there indications that previous records were reviewed, and, if the patient is on medication other than that prescribed on discharge, is there a rationale for this change?
Do the progress notes identify the type of medication used and the rationale for its increase, decrease, discontinuation, or augmentation?
Are medication effects documented, including dosages, response, and adverse or other side effects?

Note: Documentation issues are of concern to third-party payers, such as insurance companies and health maintenance organizations who examine patients' charts to see if the areas listed above are covered. In many cases, however, the review is conducted by persons with little or no background in psychiatry or psychology who do not recognize the complexities of psychiatric diagnosis and treatment. Payments to hospitals, doctors, and patients are often denied because of what such reviewers consider to be so-called inadequate documentation.

practitioner's speculations, impressions (other than tentative or actual diagnosis) and reminders." The data are maintained only by the clinician and cannot be disclosed to any other person, including the patient. Psychiatrists concerned about material that may prove damaging or otherwise hurtful to the patient if released to a third party may consider using this provision to maintain doctor–patient confidentiality.

Psychotherapy Notes

Psychotherapy notes include details of transference, fantasies, dreams, personal information about persons with whom the patient interacts, and other intimate details of the patient's life. They can also include the psychiatrist's comments on his or her countertransference and feelings toward the patient. Psychotherapy notes should be kept separate from the rest of the medical records.

Patient Access to Records

Patients have a legal right to access their medical records. This right represents society's belief that the responsibility for medical care has become a collaborative process between doctor and patient. Patients see many different physicians, and they can be more effective historians and coordinators of their own care with such information.

Psychiatrists must be careful in releasing their records to the patient if, in their judgment, the patient can be harmed emotionally as a result. Under these circumstances, the psychiatrist may choose to prepare a summary of the patient's course of treatment, holding back material that might be hurtful—especially if it were to get into the hands of third parties. In malpractice cases, however, it may not be possible to do so.

When litigation occurs, the entire medical record is subject to discovery. Psychotherapy notes are usually protected, but not always. If psychotherapy notes are ordered to be produced, the judge would probably review them privately and select what is relevant to the case in question.

E-Mail

E-mail is increasingly being used by physicians as a quick and efficient way to communicate with patients and with other doctors about their patients; however, it is a public document and should be treated as such. The dictum of not diagnosing or prescribing medication over the telephone to a patient one has not examined should also apply to e-mail. It is not only dangerous but also unethical. All e-mail messages should be printed out for the paper chart unless electronic archives are regularly backed up and secure.

Ethical Issues and the Medical Record

Psychiatrists continually make judgments about what is appropriate material to include in the psychiatric report, the medical record, the case report, and other written communications about the patient. Such judgments often involve ethical issues. In a case report, for example, the patient should not be identifiable, a position made clear in the American Psychiatric Association's (APA's) *Principles of Medical Ethics with Annotations Especially Applicable to Psychiatry*, which states that published case reports must be suitably disguised to safeguard patient confidentiality without altering material to provide a less-than-complete portrayal of the patient's actual condition. In some instances, obtaining a written release from the patient that allows the psychiatrist to publish the case may also be advisable, even if the patient is appropriately disguised.

Psychiatrists sometimes include material in the medical record that is specifically directed toward warding off future culpability if liability issues are ever raised. This may include having advised the patient about specific adverse effects of medication to be prescribed.

MEDICAL ERROR

In 2000, the public was warned about medical errors as a significant cause of patient mortality by the Institute of Medicine, which reported that more than 90,000 Americans may die each year as a result of such mistakes. A number of congressional actions followed that led eventually to legislation requiring mandatory national or state reporting by hospitals of medical errors. The result of such documentation is not yet known: Issues to contend with are the need to protect doctors and hospitals from frivolous lawsuits resulting from public disclosure and failure to maintain confidential information about patients. Additionally, a clear description of what constitutes a medical error is needed. Did the error occur because the physician departed from an accepted standard of treatment? Was the error avoidable, or the result of poor training? Or, was it unintentional—an accident—and better considered a close call or a borderline case? The term "never event" has come into recent use to refer to medical error, derived from the concept that it is an event that never should have happened. The authors of *Synopsis* believe the term to be diingenuous and prefer the more accurate term medical error.

In 2006, Hillary Clinton and Barack Obama introduced legislation, the National Medical Error Disclosure and Compensation (MEDiC) Bill (S.1784) to improve patient safety. It would force doctors and other providers of health care, including hospitals, to disclose medical error to patients. At the time of disclosure, which would be kept confidential, compensation for the patient or family would be negotiated by a neutral third-party mediator. Any apology offered during negotiations would not be admissible in any subsequent legal proceedings as an expression of guilt if those negotiations ended without mutually acceptable compensation. The federal government would develop grant programs to encourage participation in the MEDiC program and to analyze outcomes.

Psychiatric Errors

Medication. Most mistakes in psychiatry occur in two major areas: medication errors and suicide. A wrong prescription may be written; for example, the wrong medication for a disorder or the wrong dosage of a drug. A common cause of medication error is poor handwriting by physicians, which is then misread by a pharmacist or nurse. A remedy is to insist that all prescriptions be typed or transmitted via computer. Similar-sounding drug names have also been to blame for medication mistakes; for example, citalopram (Celexa) and celecoxib (Celebrex) and buspirone (BuSpar) and bupropion (Wellbutrin) (Table 7.5–3).

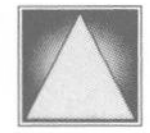

Table 7.5–3
Examples of Drug Name Confusion

Psychoactive Medication	Confused with
Metadate CD (methylphenidate)	Methadone (Dolophine)
Levoxine[a] (levothyroxine) (thyroid preparation)	Lanoxin (digoxin)
Serzone (nefazodone)	Seroquel (quetiapine)
Lamictal (lamotrigine)	Lamisil (terbinafine) (for nail infection)
Zyprexa (olanzapine)	Zyrtec (cetirizine) (for allergies)
Celexa (citalopram)	Celebrex (celecoxib) (for arthritis)

[a] Name changed to Levoxyl after US Food and Drug Administration report in 1994.

Drugs with similar phonemes lend themselves to miscommunication in writing or in speech. To reduce the number of medication errors in hospitals, the US Food and Drug Administration (FDA) will require bar codes—similar to those found on consumer goods—on most prescriptions and over-the-counter drugs.

Not to be confused with error are the side effects and possible adverse reactions to psychotropic or other medications. In general, most drug side effects are annoying and do not lead to serious complications, but patients must be advised if and when to expect them. Generally, litigation is rare even if the drug effect was severe, provided that informed consent is obtained beforehand, a legal requirement. A medication error would be to prescribe drugs that should not be given concomitantly, for example, imipramine (Tofranil) and meperidine (Demerol), which may be fatal.

Suicide. Unlike most physicians, psychiatrists rarely have to deal with the death of patients. Exceptions may be made for geriatric psychiatrists who deal with the aged or for consultation-liaison psychiatrists who deal with the seriously medically ill; however, when death occurs in those instances, it is often expected and part of the disease progress.

Suicide is unexpected. It is also viewed by many persons as preventable. Based on that expectation, family members may sue for malpractice after the event. Suicide is not always preventable, however. Some persons who have a strong desire to kill themselves will do so despite the many advances that have been made in the treatment and management of suicidal patients. When mistakes occur, they are usually the result of the psychiatrist having underestimated the suicidal risk or, if the psychiatrist has appraised it accurately, the nurses and attendants not taking the necessary steps to ensure the patient's safety (e.g., constant observation). Litigation is more common for suicides that occur in a hospital than for those that occur in an outpatient setting, presumably because one-to-one coverage is the standard of care in the actively suicidal hospitalized patient.

Courts have not penalized psychiatrists for honest errors of judgment in clinical practice. One court stated: "The accurate predication of dangerous behavior, and particularly suicide and homicide, are almost never possible. Thus, an error of prediction or even of judgment does not necessarily establish negligence." Despite this, however, psychiatrists are expected to evaluate patients properly for suicide risk and to establish a rational treatment plan to ensure that the risk of a patient successfully killing himself or herself is minimized as much as possible.

In the following case, the psychiatrist and hospital were held to be guilty of negligence at trial and the patient's family was awarded $950,000.

A 33-year-old woman was admitted to the hospital for suicidal risk and psychosis. When she was admitted, the locked ward had no empty beds. To lower her risk of suicide, she was sedated but placed in an open ward with no special suicidal precautions. On awakening, she jumped to her death.

Preventing Medical Error

Practice Guidelines. Practice guidelines have been developed by the APA for a variety of disorders. These include delirium, dementia, substance use disorder, depressive disorder, panic disorder, borderline personality disorder, suicide, and schizophrenia, among others. According to the APA, the term *practice guideline* refers to a "set of patient care strategies developed to assist physicians in clinical decisions." They are careful to point out that guidelines are not meant to be standards of care:

> The APA practice guidelines are not intended to be construed or to serve as a standard of medical care. Standards of medical care are determined on the basis of all clinical data available for an individual case and are subject to change as scientific knowledge and technology advance and patterns evolve. These parameters of practice should be considered guidelines only. Adherence to them will not ensure a successful outcome in every case, nor should they be construed as including all proper methods of care or excluding other acceptable methods of care aimed at the same results. The ultimate judgment regarding a particular clinical procedure or treatment plan must be made by the psychiatrist in light of the clinical data presented by the patient and the diagnosis and treatment options available.

No indication suggests an increase in malpractice suits against psychiatrists has occurred since guideline introduction; however, published guidelines are often brought forward in litigation as standards of care. Psychiatrists and other physicians should not be intimidated by this practice. Psychiatrists may legally and ethically deviate from guidelines; however, the decision to do so and its rationale should be documented in the chart.

The APA guidelines do not include all proper methods of care for a particular disorder, nor do they allow for ambiguity, controversy, or dissent. For this, the practitioner must turn to a textbook, such as the *Comprehensive Textbook of Psychiatry*, in which such differences are discussed.

Regulating Work Hours of Interns and Residents

Teaching hospitals often rely on interns and residents to perform services such as phlebotomies and intravenous (IV) therapy and to serve as messengers and transporters, tasks that are more appropriately performed by ancillary personnel. In addition, house staff are often required to work long hours, and sleep deprivation can impair their judgment and clinical skills. The average resident works more than 80 hours per week, with a shift of 30 hours every third or fourth night. Because of this, in 1988, a limit on the number of hours interns and residents may work was set forth by the US Health Care Financing Administration (HCFA), now officially known as the Center for Medicare and Medicaid Services (CMS). Their work rules are (1) residents are limited to no more than 12 consecutive hours per assignment in emergency services; (2) residents may not work more than 80 hours per week over a 4-week period and cannot be scheduled to work more than 24 consecutive hours; and (3) scheduled rotations must be separated by not less than 8 hours of nonworking time, provided for each week. Nonworking time is time away from training and patient care activities.

Many medical educators believe that the current CMS rules do not go far enough and that interns and residents are not used properly by many teaching hospitals. It is not uncommon for a resident in cardiac surgery to assist at an operation for 14 hours and then to stay on duty for an additional 10 hours. Similarly, a pediatric resident may be in the emergency room for 24 hours without sleep. Although their hours fall within the CMS guidelines, they are not conducive to the resident's education in view of the inevitable fatigue when a person is without sleep for 24 hours. For residents with families, especially those who are mothers, current work schedules disrupt marital harmony and child rearing. This added stress interferes with optimal functioning. It has been suggested that chronic sleep deprivation may put residents at increased risk for motor vehicle crashes, medication errors, and decreased mental clarity. No easy answers exist to these problems, but the current situation clearly requires resolution.

Ethics of Disclosure

It is an ethical duty of physicians to disclose medical errors, accidents, injury, or bad results to their patients who have an absolute right to understand what occurred during their course of treatment. An explanation is mandatory, and an apology is appropriate, if an error was made. If, as a result of disclosure, legal proceedings ensue, the physician has the opportunity to offer an explanation—but appropriate compensation for harm suffered as a result of malpractice is a patient's legal right.

Doctor–Patient Relationship

A good doctor–patient relationship is characterized by a sense of trust, respect, and honesty between the two parties. The better the doctor–patient relationship, the less chance for misunderstanding leading to litigation. Studies have shown that, when a medical error or adverse event occurs within the context of a good doctor–patient relationship, litigation is rare. In surveys of patients, almost 100 percent desire that doctors report and discuss medical errors with them. Acknowledging medical error, minor or major, may actually reduce the risk of malpractice action.

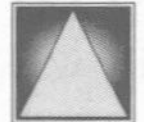

Table 7.5–4
Confusing Medical Notations

Prohibited Abbreviation	Potential Problem	Preferred Term
U (for unit)	Read as a zero (0) or a four (4), causing a tenfold overdose or greater (4 U seen as "40" or 4 u seen as "44").	Write "unit."
IU (for international unit)	Misread as "IV" (intravenous) or 10.	Write "international unit."
Q.D. and Q.O.D. (Latin for once daily and every other day)	Mistaken for each other. Also, the period after the Q can be mistaken for an I and the O can be mistaken for an I.	Write "daily" or "every other day."
Trailing zero (X.0 mg) and lack of leading zero (.X mg)	Decimal point is missed.	Never write a zero by itself after a decimal point (X mg) and always use a zero before a decimal point (0.X mg).
MS, MSO_4, and $MgSO_4$	Confused for one another. Can mean morphine sulfate or magnesium sulfate.	Write "morphine sulfate" or "magnesium sulfate."

Regulation of the Quality of Health Care

A group of agencies, such as the Joint Commission of Accreditation of Healthcare Organizations (JCAHO) and the Liaison Committee on Medical Education (LCME), influence the standards of hospital care and performance. In addition, hospitals must comply with government regulations (city and state health rules). The JCAHO inspects hospitals every 2 years and is also responsible for determining the requirements for hospital accreditation. Hospital reimbursements from Medicare and Medicaid are contingent on meeting these standards, but the accreditation is done on a voluntary basis. The LCME and the Liaison Committee on Graduate Education are charged with accrediting medical schools and residency training programs, respectively. The two accrediting committees review education and training programs every 4 years; the procedure is voluntary.

The JCAHO, which is also involved in preventing medical errors, developed guidelines to help surgical teams standardize safety systems. The guidelines, called "The Universal Protocol for Preventing Wrong Site, Wrong Procedure, Wrong Person Surgery," address the verification of documents, marking operative sites, and other issues related to patient safety.

The JCAHO issued a list of dangerous, unapproved abbreviations, acronyms, and symbols that accredited organizations must discontinue using as part of their National Patient Safety Goal requirements. The list of unapproved abbreviations pertains to all handwritten, patient-specific communication (Table 7.5–4).

References

Berlinger N. *After Harm: Medical Error and the Ethics of Forgiveness*. Baltimore: John Hopkins University Press; 2005.

Clinton HR, Obama B. Making patient safety the centerpiece of medical liability reform. *N Engl J Med.* 2006; 354(21):2205.

Engel KG, Rosenthal M, Sutcliffe KM. Residents' responses to medical error: Coping, learning, and change. *Acad Med.* 2006;81(1):86–93.

Fischer CB, Fried AL. Internet-mediated psychological services and the American Psychological Association Ethics Code. *Psychother Theor Res Pract Train.* 2003;40:103.

Groth-Marnat G. *Handbook of Psychological Assessment.* 4th ed. New York: John Wiley & Sons, Inc.; 2003.

Koppel R, Metlay JP, Cohen A, Abaluck B, Localio AR, Kimmel SE, Strom BL. Role of computerized physician order entry systems in facilitating medication errors. *JAMA*. 2005;293:1197–1203.

Krauss JB. A matter of privacy. *Arch Pract Nurs.* 2003;17:99.

Lysaker PH, Wickett AM, Campbell K, Buck KD. Movement toward coherence in the psychotherapy of schizophrenia: A method for assessing narrative transformation. *J Nerv Ment Dis.* 2003;191:538.

Maio JE. HIPAA and the special status of psychotherapy notes. *Lippincott Case Manage.* 2003;8:24.

Pierluissi E, Fischer MA, Campbell AR, Landefeld CS. Discussion of medical errors in morbidity and mortality conferences. *JAMA.* 2003;290:2838.

Ross SE, Todd J, Moore LA, Beaty BL, Wittevrongel L, Lin CT. Expectations of patients and physicians regarding patient-accessible medical records. *J Med Internet Res.* 2005;7(2):e13.

Sadock BJ. Psychiatric report, medical record, and medical error. In: Sadock BJ, Sadock VA, eds. *Kaplan & Sadock's Comprehensive Textbook of Psychiatry.* 8th ed. Vol. 1. Baltimore: Lippincott Williams & Wilkins; 2005:834.

Weber B, Schneider B, Fritze J, Gille B, Hornung S, Kuehner T, Maurer K. Acceptance of computerized compared to pencil-and-paper assessment in psychiatric inpatients. *Comput Hum Behav.* 2003;19:81.

8 Signs and Symptoms in Psychiatry

Signs are objective; symptoms are subjective. Signs are the clinician's observations, such as noting a patient's agitation; symptoms are subjective experiences, such as a person's complaint of feeling depressed. In psychiatry, signs and symptoms are not as clearly demarcated as in other fields of medicine; they often overlap. Because of this, disorders in psychiatry are often described as syndromes—a constellation of signs and symptoms that together make up a recognizable condition. Schizophrenia, for example, is more often viewed as a syndrome than as a specific disorder. This concept is expressed in the use of the terms *schizophrenic spectrum* or *the group of schizophrenias*.

DESCRIPTIVE TERMS

Descriptions of signs and symptoms in psychiatry have remained fairly constant over the years; however, some terms fall in and out of favor. In the various editions of the *Diagnostic and Statistical Manual of Mental Disorders* (DSM), for example, some terms have been retained and others omitted, and some terms are not common to DSM and the *International Classification of Diseases* (ICD).

The fourth edition of DSM (DSM-IV) eliminated the diagnosis of organic mental disorder in an attempt to indicate that all mental disorders may have a biological basis, or medical cause. Thus, the diagnosis of organic mental disorder is now called "delirium, dementia, and amnestic and other cognitive disorders." The 10th revision of the *International Statistical Classification of Diseases and Related Health Problems* (ICD-10), however, retains the diagnostic category organic mental disorders to refer to these conditions.

In a further effort to emphasize the biological aspects of mental illness, DSM-IV and the text revision of DSM-IV (DSM-IV-TR) eschew the term *psychogenic*. Nevertheless, it still appears in ICD-10 to refer to the fact that life events or difficulties play an important role in the genesis of many psychiatric disorders. Similarly, DSM has eliminated the term *neurosis,* which is also used in ICD-10. Both terms—*organic* and *neurosis*—remain in common parlance among health professionals, however.

Neurosis

A neurosis is a chronic or recurrent nonpsychotic disorder characterized mainly by anxiety, which is experienced or expressed directly or is altered through defense mechanisms; it appears as a symptom, such as an obsession, a compulsion, a phobia, or a sexual dysfunction. In the third edition of DSM (DSM-III), a neurotic disorder was defined as follows:

> A mental disorder in which the predominant disturbance is a symptom or group of symptoms that is distressing to the individual and is recognized by him or her as unacceptable and alien (ego-dystonic); reality testing is grossly intact. Behavior does not actively violate gross social norms (though it may be quite disabling). The disturbance is relatively enduring or recurrent without treatment, and is not limited to a transitory reaction to stressors. There is no demonstrable organic etiology or factor.

The term *neuroses* encompasses a broad range of disorders of various signs and symptoms. As such, it has lost precision, except to signify that the person's gross reality testing and personality organization are intact. However, a neurosis can be, and usually is, sufficient to impair the person's functioning in a number of areas. It remains a useful term, especially when compared to the term *psychosis,* described below, still used in DSM-IV-TR.

Psychosis

The traditional meaning of the term *psychotic* emphasized loss of reality testing and impairment of mental functioning—manifested by delusions, hallucinations, confusion, and impaired memory. In the most common psychiatric use of the term, *psychotic* became synonymous with severe impairment of social and personal functioning characterized by social withdrawal and an inability to perform the usual household and occupational roles. Another use of the term—based on psychoanalytic concepts—specifies the degree of ego regression as the criterion for psychotic illness. As a consequence of those multiple meanings, the term has lost its precision in current clinical and research practice.

According to the *American Psychiatric Glossary* of the American Psychiatric Association, the term *psychotic* means grossly impaired reality testing. The term can be used to describe the behavior of a person at a given time or a mental disorder in which at some time during its course all persons with the disorder have grossly impaired reality testing. With gross impairment in reality testing, persons incorrectly evaluate the accuracy of their perceptions and thoughts and make incorrect inferences about external reality, even in the face of contrary evidence. The term *psychotic* does not apply to minor distortions of reality that involve matters of relative judgment. For example, depressed persons who underestimate their achievements are not described as psychotic; those who believe that they have caused natural catastrophes are so described.

Patients are more than a collection of signs and symptoms. The trend toward collecting symptoms and its possible dehumanizing effects was described by Karl Menninger over 35 years ago. As if anticipating the mathematical device currently in use in

DSM-IV-TR, he wrote: "If the patient has, let us say, five symptoms, one can look up each of these symptoms and find which disease is so characterized under all five headings. Then, *voilà!* The diagnosis!" Menninger suggested that the trend toward tabulating disease states was antithetical to understanding the person experiencing the illness and deemphasized the compassionate approach toward the patient that is the hallmark of psychiatry. The algorithms and decision trees used in DSM-IV-TR and in the various computer programs that record signs and symptoms to provide a diagnosis are useful; however, Menninger's cautionary note must not be forgotten. A description of signs and symptoms is the science of psychiatry; the skill of the observers and their creative imaginations and ability to empathize is the art of psychiatry.

Finally, as the physician–philosopher William Osler (1898–1919) said of medicine in general, "It is learned only by experience; it is not an inheritance; it cannot be revealed. Learn to see, learn to hear, learn to feel, learn to smell, and know that by practice alone can you become expert." So it is with psychiatry. One sees the posture of depression, hears the neologisms in schizophrenia, smells the odor of alcoholism, and feels the violent patient's anger. Eventually, with practice, the psychiatrist learns the full range of signs and symptoms. It is the rare psychiatrist, however, who encounters them all.

The glossary that follows is a comprehensive list of signs and symptoms, each of which has a definition or description. Most psychiatric signs and symptoms are rooted in normal behavior and can be understood as various points on a spectrum of behavior ranging from normal to pathological. They are listed alphabetically.

Glossary of Signs and Symptoms

abreaction A process by which repressed material, particularly a painful experience or a conflict, is brought back to consciousness; in this process, the person not only recalls, but also relives the repressed material, which is accompanied by the appropriate affective response.

abstract thinking Thinking characterized by the ability to grasp the essentials of a whole, to break a whole into its parts, and to discern common properties. To think symbolically.

abulia Reduced impulse to act and to think, associated with indifference about consequences of action. Occurs as a result of neurological deficit, depression, and schizophrenia.

acalculia Loss of ability to do calculations; not caused by anxiety or impairment in concentration. Occurs with neurological deficit and learning disorder.

acataphasia Disordered speech in which statements are incorrectly formulated. Patients may express themselves with words that sound like the ones intended, but are not appropriate to the thoughts, or they may use totally inappropriate expressions.

acathexis Lack of feeling associated with an ordinarily emotionally charged subject; in psychoanalysis, it denotes the patient's detaching or transferring of emotion from thoughts and ideas. Also called *decathexis.* Occurs in anxiety, dissociative, schizophrenic, and bipolar disorders.

acenesthesia Loss of sensation of physical existence.

acrophobia Dread of high places.

acting out Behavioral response to an unconscious drive or impulse that brings about temporary partial relief of inner tension; relief is attained by reacting to a present situation as if it were the situation that originally gave rise to the drive or impulse. Common in borderline states.

aculalia Nonsense speech associated with marked impairment of comprehension. Occurs in mania, schizophrenia, and neurological deficit.

adiadochokinesia Inability to perform rapid alternating movements. Occurs with neurological deficit and cerebellar lesions.

adynamia Weakness and fatigability, characteristic of neurasthenia and depression.

aerophagia Excessive swallowing of air. Seen in anxiety disorder.

affect The subjective and immediate experience of emotion attached to ideas or mental representations of objects. Affect has outward manifestations that can be classified as restricted, blunted, flattened, broad, labile, appropriate, or inappropriate. *See also* **mood.**

ageusia Lack or impairment of the sense of taste. Seen in depression and neurological deficit.

aggression Forceful, goal-directed action that can be verbal or physical; the motor counterpart of the affect of rage, anger, or hostility. Seen in neurological deficit, temporal lobe disorder, impulse-control disorders, mania, and schizophrenia.

agitation Severe anxiety associated with motor restlessness.

agnosia Inability to understand the importance or significance of sensory stimuli; cannot be explained by a defect in sensory pathways or cerebral lesion; the term has also been used to refer to the selective loss or disuse of knowledge of specific objects because of emotional circumstances, as seen in certain schizophrenic, anxious, and depressed patients. Occurs with neurological deficit.

agoraphobia Morbid fear of open places or leaving the familiar setting of the home. May be present with or without panic attacks.

agraphia Loss or impairment of a previously possessed ability to write.

ailurophobia Dread of cats.

akathisia Subjective feeling of motor restlessness manifested by a compelling need to be in constant movement; may be seen as an extrapyramidal adverse effect of antipsychotic medication. May be mistaken for psychotic agitation.

akinesia Lack of physical movement, as in the extreme immobility of catatonic schizophrenia; can also occur as an extrapyramidal effect of antipsychotic medication.

akinetic mutism Absence of voluntary motor movement or speech in a patient who is apparently alert (as evidenced by eye movements). Seen in psychotic depression and catatonic states.

alexia Loss of a previously possessed reading facility; not explained by defective visual acuity. *Compare with* **Dyslexia.**

alexithymia Inability or difficulty in describing or being aware of one's emotions or moods; elaboration of fantasies associated with depression, substance abuse, and posttraumatic stress disorder (PTSD).

algophobia Dread of pain.

alogia Inability to speak because of a mental deficiency or an episode of dementia.

ambivalence Coexistence of two opposing impulses toward the same thing in the same person at the same time. Seen in schizophrenia, borderline states, and obsessive-compulsive disorders (OCDs).

amimia Lack of the ability to make gestures or to comprehend those made by others.

amnesia Partial or total inability to recall past experiences; may be organic (*amnestic disorder*) or emotional (*dissociative amnesia*) in origin.

amnestic aphasia Disturbed capacity to name objects, even though they are known to the patient. Also called *anomic aphasia.*

anaclitic Depending on others, especially as the infant on the mother; anaclitic depression in children results from an absence of mothering.

analgesia State in which one feels little or no pain. Can occur under hypnosis and in dissociative disorder.

anancasm Repetitious or stereotyped behavior or thought usually used as a tension-relieving device; used as a synonym for obsession and seen in obsessive-compulsive (anankastic) personality.

androgyny Combination of culturally determined female and male characteristics in one person.

anergia Lack of energy.

anhedonia Loss of interest in, and withdrawal from, all regular and pleasurable activities. Often associated with depression.

anomia Inability to recall the names of objects.

anorexia Loss or decrease in appetite. In *anorexia nervosa*, appetite may be preserved, but the patient refuses to eat.

anosognosia Inability to recognize a physical deficit in oneself (e.g., patient denies paralyzed limb).

anterograde amnesia Loss of memory for events subsequent to the onset of the amnesia; common after trauma. *Compare with* **retrograde amnesia.**

anxiety Feeling of apprehension caused by anticipation of danger, which may be internal or external.

apathy Dulled emotional tone associated with detachment or indifference; observed in certain types of schizophrenia and depression.

aphasia Any disturbance in the comprehension or expression of language caused by a brain lesion.

aphonia Loss of voice. Seen in conversion disorder.

apperception Awareness of the meaning and significance of a particular sensory stimulus as modified by one's own experiences, knowledge, thoughts, and emotions. *See also* **perception.**

appropriate affect Emotional tone in harmony with the accompanying idea, thought, or speech.

apraxia Inability to perform a voluntary purposeful motor activity; cannot be explained by paralysis or other motor or sensory impairment. In *constructional apraxia*, a patient cannot draw two- or three-dimensional forms.

astasia abasia Inability to stand or to walk in a normal manner, even though normal leg movements can be performed in a sitting or lying down position. Seen in conversion disorder.

astereognosis Inability to identify familiar objects by touch. Seen with neurological deficit. *See also* **neurological amnesia.**

asyndesis Disorder of language in which the patient combines unconnected ideas and images. Commonly seen in schizophrenia.

ataxia Lack of coordination, physical or mental. (1) In neurology, refers to loss of muscular coordination. (2) In psychiatry, the term *intrapsychic ataxia* refers to lack of coordination between feelings and thoughts; seen in schizophrenia and in severe OCD.

atonia Lack of muscle tone. *See* **waxy flexibility.**

attention Concentration; the aspect of consciousness that relates to the amount of effort exerted in focusing on certain aspects of an experience, activity, or task. Usually impaired in anxiety and depressive disorders.

auditory hallucination False perception of sound, usually voices, but also other noises, such as music. Most common hallucination in psychiatric disorders.

aura (1) Warning sensations, such as automatisms, fullness in the stomach, blushing, and changes in respiration; cognitive sensations, and mood states usually experienced before a seizure. (2) A sensory prodrome that precedes a classic migraine headache.

autistic thinking Thinking in which the thoughts are largely narcissistic and egocentric, with emphasis on subjectivity rather than objectivity, and without regard for reality; used interchangeably with autism and dereism. Seen in schizophrenia and autistic disorder.

behavior Sum total of the psyche that includes impulses, motivations, wishes, drives, instincts, and cravings, as expressed by a person's behavior or motor activity. Also called *conation.*

bereavement Feeling of grief or desolation, especially at the death or loss of a loved one.

bizarre delusion False belief that is patently absurd or fantastic (e.g., invaders from space have implanted electrodes in a person's brain). Common in schizophrenia. In nonbizarre delusion, content is usually within the range of possibility.

blackout Amnesia experienced by alcoholics about behavior during drinking bouts; usually indicates reversible brain damage.

blocking Abrupt interruption in train of thinking before a thought or idea is finished; after a brief pause, the person indicates no recall of what was being said or was going to be said (also known as *thought deprivation* or *increased thought latency*). Common in schizophrenia and severe anxiety.

blunted affect Disturbance of affect manifested by a severe reduction in the intensity of externalized feeling tone; one of the fundamental symptoms of schizophrenia, as outlined by Eugen Bleuler.

bradykinesia Slowness of motor activity, with a decrease in normal spontaneous movement.

bradylalia Abnormally slow speech. Common in depression.

bradylexia Inability to read at normal speed.

bruxism Grinding or gnashing of the teeth, typically occurring during sleep. Seen in anxiety disorder.

carebaria Sensation of discomfort or pressure in the head.

catalepsy Condition in which persons maintain the body position into which they are placed; observed in severe cases of catatonic schizophrenia. Also called *waxy flexibility* and *cerea flexibilitas. See also* **command automatism.**

cataplexy Temporary sudden loss of muscle tone, causing weakness and immobilization; can be precipitated by a variety of emotional states and is often followed by sleep. Commonly seen in narcolepsy.

catatonic excitement Excited, uncontrolled motor activity seen in catatonic schizophrenia. Patients in catatonic state may suddenly erupt into an excited state and may be violent.

catatonic posturing Voluntary assumption of an inappropriate or bizarre posture, generally maintained for long periods of time. May switch unexpectedly with catatonic excitement.

catatonic rigidity Fixed and sustained motoric position that is resistant to change.

catatonic stupor Stupor in which patients ordinarily are well aware of their surroundings.
cathexis In psychoanalysis, a conscious or unconscious investment of psychic energy in an idea, concept, object, or person. *Compare with* **acathexis.**
causalgia Burning pain that can be organic or psychic in origin.
cenesthesia Change in the normal quality of feeling tone in a part of the body.
cephalagia Headache.
cerea flexibilitas Condition of a person who can be molded into a position that is then maintained; when an examiner moves the person's limb, the limb feels as if it were made of wax. Also called *catalepsy* or *waxy flexibility.* Seen in schizophrenia.
chorea Movement disorder characterized by random and involuntary quick, jerky, purposeless movements. Seen in Huntington's disease.
circumstantiality Disturbance in the associative thought and speech processes in which a patient digresses into unnecessary details and inappropriate thoughts before communicating the central idea. Observed in schizophrenia, obsessional disturbances, and certain cases of dementia. *See also* **tangentiality.**
clang association Association or speech directed by the sound of a word rather than by its meaning; words have no logical connection; punning and rhyming may dominate the verbal behavior. Seen most frequently in schizophrenia or mania.
claustrophobia Abnormal fear of closed or confining spaces.
clonic convulsion An involuntary, violent muscular contraction or spasm in which the muscles alternately contract and relax. Characteristic phase in grand mal epileptic seizure.
clouding of consciousness Any disturbance of consciousness in which the person is not fully awake, alert, and oriented. Occurs in delirium, dementia, and cognitive disorder.
cluttering Disturbance of fluency involving an abnormally rapid rate and erratic rhythm of speech that impedes intelligibility; the affected individual is usually unaware of communicative impairment.
cognition Mental process of knowing and becoming aware; function is closely associated with judgment.
coma State of profound unconsciousness from which a person cannot be roused, with minimal or no detectable responsiveness to stimuli; seen in injury or disease of the brain, in systemic conditions, such as diabetic ketoacidosis and uremia; and in intoxications with alcohol and other drugs. Coma can also occur in severe catatonic states and in conversion disorder.
coma vigil Coma in which a patient appears to be asleep, but can be aroused (also known as *akinetic mutism*).
command automatism Condition associated with catalepsy in which suggestions are followed automatically.
command hallucination False perception of orders that a person may feel obliged to obey or unable to resist.
complex A feeling-toned idea.
complex partial seizure A seizure characterized by alterations in consciousness that may be accompanied by complex hallucinations (sometimes olfactory) or illusions. During the seizure, a state of impaired consciousness resembling a dream-like state may occur, and the patient may exhibit repetitive, automatic, or semipurposeful behavior.
compulsion Pathological need to act on an impulse that, if resisted, produces anxiety; repetitive behavior in response to an obsession or performed according to certain rules, with no true end in itself other than to prevent something from occurring in the future.
conation That part of a person's mental life concerned with cravings, strivings, motivations, drives, and wishes as expressed through behavior or motor activity.
concrete thinking Thinking characterized by actual things, events, and immediate experience, rather than by abstractions; seen in young children, in those who have lost or never developed the ability to generalize (as in certain cognitive mental disorders), and in schizophrenic persons. *Compare with* **abstract thinking.**
condensation Mental process in which one symbol stands for a number of components.
confabulation Unconscious filling of gaps in memory by imagining experiences or events that have no basis in fact, commonly seen in amnestic syndromes; should be differentiated from lying. *See also* **paramnesia.**
confusion Disturbances of consciousness manifested by a disordered orientation in relation to time, place, or person.
consciousness State of awareness, with response to external stimuli.
constipation Inability to defecate or difficulty in defecating.
constricted affect Reduction in intensity of feeling tone that is less severe than that of blunted affect.
constructional apraxia Inability to copy a drawing, such as a cube, clock, or pentagon, as a result of a brain lesion.
conversion phenomena The development of symbolic physical symptoms and distortions involving the voluntary muscles or special sense organs; not under voluntary control and not explained by any physical disorder. Most common in conversion disorder, but also seen in a variety of mental disorders.
convulsion An involuntary, violent muscular contraction or spasm. *See also* **clonic convulsion** *and* **tonic convulsion.**
coprolalia Involuntary use of vulgar or obscene language. Observed in some cases of schizophrenia and in Tourette's syndrome.
coprophagia Eating of filth or feces.
cryptographia A private written language.
cryptolalia A private spoken language.
cycloplegia Paralysis of the muscles of accommodation in the eye; observed, at times, as an autonomic adverse effect (anticholinergic effect) of antipsychotic or antidepressant medication.
Decompensation Deterioration of psychic functioning caused by a breakdown of defense mechanisms. Seen in psychotic states.
déjà entendu Illusion that what one is hearing one has heard previously. *See also* **paramnesia.**
déjà pensé Condition in which a thought never entertained before is incorrectly regarded as a repetition of a previous thought. *See also* **paramnesia.**
déjà vu Illusion of visual recognition in which a new situation is incorrectly regarded as a repetition of a previous experience. *See also* **paramnesia.**
delirium Acute reversible mental disorder characterized by confusion and some impairment of consciousness; generally associated with emotional lability, hallucinations or illusions, and inappropriate, impulsive, irrational, or violent behavior.
delirium tremens Acute and sometimes fatal reaction to withdrawal from alcohol, usually occurring 72 to 96 hours after

the cessation of heavy drinking; distinctive characteristics are marked autonomic hyperactivity (tachycardia, fever, hyperhidrosis, and dilated pupils), usually accompanied by tremulousness, hallucinations, illusions, and delusions. Called *alcohol withdrawal delirium* in DSM-IV-TR. *See also* **formication.**

delusion False belief, based on incorrect inference about external reality, that is firmly held despite objective and obvious contradictory proof or evidence and despite the fact that other members of the culture do not share the belief.

delusion of control False belief that a person's will, thoughts, or feelings are being controlled by external forces.

delusion of grandeur Exaggerated conception of one's importance, power, or identity.

delusion of infidelity False belief that one's lover is unfaithful. Sometimes called *pathological jealousy.*

delusion of persecution False belief of being harassed or persecuted; often found in litigious patients who have a pathological tendency to take legal action because of imagined mistreatment. Most common delusion.

delusion of poverty False belief that one is bereft or will be deprived of all material possessions.

delusion of reference False belief that the behavior of others refers to oneself or that events, objects, or other people have a particular and unusual significance, usually of a negative nature; derived from idea of reference, in which persons falsely feel that others are talking about them (e.g., belief that people on television or radio are talking to or about the person). *See also* **thought broadcasting.**

delusion of self-accusation False feeling of remorse and guilt. Seen in depression with psychotic features.

dementia Mental disorder characterized by general impairment in intellectual functioning without clouding of consciousness; characterized by failing memory, difficulty with calculations, distractibility, alterations in mood and affect, impaired judgment and abstraction, reduced facility with language, and disturbance of orientation. Although irreversible because of underlying progressive degenerative brain disease, dementia may be reversible if the cause can be treated.

denial Defense mechanism in which the existence of unpleasant realities is disavowed; refers to keeping out of conscious awareness any aspects of external reality that, if acknowledged, would produce anxiety.

depersonalization Sensation of unreality concerning oneself, parts of oneself, or one's environment that occurs under extreme stress or fatigue. Seen in schizophrenia, depersonalization disorder, and schizotypal personality disorder.

depression Mental state characterized by feelings of sadness, loneliness, despair, low self-esteem, and self-reproach; accompanying signs include psychomotor retardation or, at times, agitation, withdrawal from interpersonal contact, and vegetative symptoms, such as insomnia and anorexia. The term refers to a mood that is so characterized or to a mood disorder.

derailment Gradual or sudden deviation in train of thought without blocking; sometimes used synonymously with *loosening of association.*

derealization Sensation of changed reality or that one's surroundings have altered. Usually seen in schizophrenia, panic attacks, and dissociative disorders.

dereism Mental activity that follows a totally subjective and idiosyncratic system of logic and fails to take the facts of reality or experience into consideration. Characteristic of schizophrenia. *See also* **autistic thinking.**

detachment Characterized by distant interpersonal relationships and lack of emotional involvement.

devaluation Defense mechanism in which a person attributes excessively negative qualities to self or others. Seen in depression and paranoid personality disorder.

diminished libido Decreased sexual interest and drive. (Increased libido is often associated with mania.)

dipsomania Compulsion to drink alcoholic beverages.

disinhibition (1) Removal of an inhibitory effect, as in the reduction of the inhibitory function of the cerebral cortex by alcohol. (2) In psychiatry, a greater freedom to act in accordance with inner drives or feelings and with less regard for restraints dictated by cultural norms or one's superego.

disorientation Confusion; impairment of awareness of time, place, and person (the position of the self in relation to other persons). Characteristic of cognitive disorders.

displacement Unconscious defense mechanism by which the emotional component of an unacceptable idea or object is transferred to a more acceptable one. Seen in phobias.

dissociation Unconscious defense mechanism involving the segregation of any group of mental or behavioral processes from the rest of the person's psychic activity; may entail the separation of an idea from its accompanying emotional tone, as seen in dissociative and conversion disorders. Seen in dissociative disorders.

distractibility Inability to focus one's attention; the patient does not respond to the task at hand but attends to irrelevant phenomena in the environment.

dread Massive or pervasive anxiety, usually related to a specific danger.

dreamy state Altered state of consciousness, likened to a dream situation, which develops suddenly and usually lasts a few minutes; accompanied by visual, auditory, and olfactory hallucinations. Commonly associated with temporal lobe lesions.

drowsiness State of impaired awareness associated with a desire or inclination to sleep.

dysarthria Difficulty in articulation, the motor activity of shaping phonated sounds into speech, not in word finding or in grammar.

dyscalculia Difficulty in performing calculations.

dysgeusia Impaired sense of taste.

dysgraphia Difficulty in writing.

dyskinesia Difficulty in performing movements. Seen in extrapyramidal disorders.

dyslalia Faulty articulation caused by structural abnormalities of the articulatory organs or impaired hearing.

dyslexia Specific learning disability syndrome involving an impairment of the previously acquired ability to read; unrelated to the person's intelligence. *Compare with* **alexia.**

dysmetria Impaired ability to gauge distance relative to movements. Seen in neurological deficit.

dysmnesia Impaired memory.

dyspareunia Physical pain in sexual intercourse, usually emotionally caused and more commonly experienced by women; can also result from cystitis, urethritis, or other medical conditions.

dysphagia Difficulty in swallowing.

dysphasia Difficulty in comprehending oral language (*reception dysphasia*) or in trying to express verbal language (*expressive dysphasia*).

dysphonia Difficulty or pain in speaking.
dysphoria Feeling of unpleasantness or discomfort; a mood of general dissatisfaction and restlessness. Occurs in depression and anxiety.
dysprosody Loss of normal speech melody (*prosody*). Common in depression.
dystonia Extrapyramidal motor disturbance consisting of slow, sustained contractions of the axial or appendicular musculature; one movement often predominates, leading to relatively sustained postural deviations; acute dystonic reactions (facial grimacing and torticollis) are occasionally seen with the initiation of antipsychotic drug therapy.
echolalia Psychopathological repeating of words or phrases of one person by another; tends to be repetitive and persistent. Seen in certain kinds of schizophrenia, particularly the catatonic types.
ego-alien Denoting aspects of a person's personality that are viewed as repugnant, unacceptable, or inconsistent with the rest of the personality. Also called *ego-dystonia. Compare with* **ego-syntonic.**
egocentric Self-centered; selfishly preoccupied with one's own needs; lacking interest in others.
ego-dystonic *See* **ego-alien.**
egomania Morbid self-preoccupation or self-centeredness. *See also* **narcissism.**
ego-syntonic Denoting aspects of a personality that are viewed as acceptable and consistent with that person's total personality. Personality traits are usually ego-syntonic. *Compare with* **ego-alien.**
eidetic image Unusually vivid or exact mental image of objects previously seen or imagined.
elation Mood consisting of feelings of joy, euphoria, triumph, and intense self-satisfaction or optimism. Occurs in mania when not grounded in reality.
elevated mood Air of confidence and enjoyment; a mood more cheerful than normal but not necessarily pathological.
emotion Complex feeling state with psychic, somatic, and behavioral components; external manifestation of emotion is *affect.*
emotional insight A level of understanding or awareness that one has emotional problems. It facilitates positive changes in personality and behavior when present.
emotional lability Excessive emotional responsiveness characterized by unstable and rapidly changing emotions.
encopresis Involuntary passage of feces, usually occurring at night or during sleep.
enuresis Incontinence of urine during sleep.
erotomania Delusional belief, more common in women than in men, that someone is deeply in love with them (also known as *de Clérambault syndrome*).
erythrophobia Abnormal fear of blushing.
euphoria Exaggerated feeling of well-being that is inappropriate to real events. Can occur with drugs such as opiates, amphetamines, and alcohol.
euthymia Normal range of mood, implying absence of depressed or elevated mood.
evasion Act of not facing up to, or strategically eluding, something; consists of suppressing an idea that is next in a thought series and replacing it with another idea closely related to it. Also called *paralogia* and *perverted logic.*
exaltation Feeling of intense elation and grandeur.
excited Agitated, purposeless motor activity uninfluenced by external stimuli.
expansive mood Expression of feelings without restraint, frequently with an overestimation of their significance or importance. Seen in mania and grandiose delusional disorder.
expressive aphasia Disturbance of speech in which understanding remains, but ability to speak is grossly impaired; halting, laborious, and inaccurate speech (also known as *Broca's*, *nonfluent*, and *motor aphasias*).
expressive dysphasia Difficulty in expressing verbal language; the ability to understand language is intact.
externalization More general term than *projection* that refers to the tendency to perceive in the external world and in external objects elements of one's own personality, including instinctual impulses, conflicts, moods, attitudes, and styles of thinking.
extroversion State of one's energies being directed outside oneself. *Compare with* **introversion.**
false memory A person's recollection and belief of an event that did not actually occur. In *false memory syndrome*, persons erroneously believe that they sustained an emotional or physical (e.g., sexual) trauma in early life.
fantasy Daydream; fabricated mental picture of a situation or chain of events. A normal form of thinking dominated by unconsciousness material that seeks wish fulfillment and solutions to conflicts; may serve as the matrix for creativity. The content of the fantasy may indicate mental illness.
fatigue A feeling of weariness, sleepiness, or irritability after a period of mental or bodily activity. Seen in depression, anxiety, neurasthenia, and somatoform disorders.
fausse reconnaissance False recognition, a feature of paramnesia. Can occur in delusional disorders.
fear Unpleasurable emotional state consisting of psychophysiological changes in response to a realistic threat or danger. *Compare with* **anxiety.**
flat affect Absence or near absence of any signs of affective expression.
flight of ideas Rapid succession of fragmentary thoughts or speech in which content changes abruptly and speech may be incoherent. Seen in mania.
floccillation Aimless plucking or picking, usually at bedclothes or clothing, commonly seen in dementia and delirium.
fluent aphasia Aphasia characterized by inability to understand the spoken word; fluent but incoherent speech is present. Also called *Wernicke's*, *sensory*, and *receptive aphasias.*
folie à deux Mental illness shared by two persons, usually involving a common delusional system; if it involves three persons, it is referred to as *folie à trois*, and so on. Also called *shared psychotic disorder.*
formal thought disorder Disturbance in the form rather than the content of thought; thinking characterized by loosened associations, neologisms, and illogical constructs; thought process is disordered, and the person is defined as psychotic. Characteristic of schizophrenia.
formication Tactile hallucination involving the sensation that tiny insects are crawling over the skin. Seen in cocaine addiction and delirium tremens.
free-floating anxiety Severe, pervasive, generalized anxiety that is not attached to any particular idea, object, or event. Observed particularly in anxiety disorders, although it may be seen in some cases of schizophrenia.

fugue Dissociative disorder characterized by a period of almost complete amnesia, during which a person actually flees from an immediate life situation and begins a different life pattern; apart from the amnesia, mental faculties and skills are usually unimpaired.

galactorrhea Abnormal discharge of milk from the breast; may result from the endocrine influence (e.g., prolactin) of dopamine receptor antagonists, such as phenothiazines.

generalized tonic-clonic seizure Generalized onset of tonic-clonic movements of the limbs, tongue-biting, and incontinence followed by slow, gradual recovery of consciousness and cognition; also called *grand mal seizure.*

global aphasia Combination of grossly nonfluent aphasia and severe fluent aphasia.

glossolalia Unintelligible jargon that has meaning to the speaker but not to the listener. Occurs in schizophrenia.

grandiosity Exaggerated feelings of one's importance, power, knowledge, or identity. Occurs in delusional disorder and manic states.

grief Alteration in mood and affect consisting of sadness appropriate to a real loss; normally, it is self-limited. *See also* **depression** *and* **mourning.**

guilt Emotional state associated with self-reproach and the need for punishment. In psychoanalysis, refers to a feeling of culpability that stems from a conflict between the ego and the superego (conscience). Guilt has normal psychological and social functions, but special intensity or absence of guilt characterizes many mental disorders, such as depression and antisocial personality disorder, respectively. Psychiatrists distinguish shame as a less internalized form of guilt that relates more to others than to the self. *See also* **shame.**

gustatory hallucination Hallucination primarily involving taste.

gynecomastia Female-like development of the male breasts; can occur as an adverse effect of antipsychotic and antidepressant drugs because of increased prolactin levels or anabolic-androgenic steroid abuse.

hallucination False sensory perception occurring in the absence of any relevant external stimulation of the sensory modality involved. For types of hallucinations, see the specific term.

hallucinosis State in which a person experiences hallucinations without any impairment of consciousness.

haptic hallucination Hallucination of touch.

hebephrenia Complex of symptoms, considered a form of schizophrenia, characterized by wild or silly behavior or mannerisms, inappropriate affect, and delusions and hallucinations that are transient and unsystematized. Hebephrenic schizophrenia is now called *disorganized schizophrenia.*

holophrastic Using a single word to express a combination of ideas. Seen in schizophrenia.

hyperactivity Increased muscular activity. The term is commonly used to describe a disturbance found in children that is manifested by constant restlessness, overactivity, distractibility, and difficulties in learning. Seen in *attention-deficit/hyperactivity disorder* (ADHD).

hyperalgesia Excessive sensitivity to pain. Seen in somatoform disorder.

hyperesthesia Increased sensitivity to tactile stimulation.

hypermnesia Exaggerated degree of retention and recall. It can be elicited by hypnosis and may be seen in certain prodigies; also can be a feature of OCD, some cases of schizophrenia, and manic episodes of bipolar I disorder.

hyperphagia Increase in appetite and intake of food.

hyperpragia Excessive thinking and mental activity. Generally associated with manic episodes of bipolar I disorder.

hypersomnia Excessive time spent asleep. Can be associated with underlying medical or psychiatric disorder or narcolepsy, can be part of the Kleine-Levin syndrome, or may be primary.

hyperventilation Excessive breathing, generally associated with anxiety, which can reduce blood carbon dioxide concentration and can produce lightheadedness, palpitations, numbness, tingling periorally and in the extremities, and, occasionally, syncope.

hypervigilance Excessive attention to, and focus on, all internal and external stimuli; usually seen in delusional or paranoid states.

hypesthesia Diminished sensitivity to tactile stimulation.

hypnagogic hallucination Hallucination occurring while falling asleep, not ordinarily considered pathological.

hypnopompic hallucination Hallucination occurring while awakening from sleep, not ordinarily considered pathological.

hypnosis Artificially induced alteration of consciousness characterized by increased suggestibility and receptivity to direction.

hypoactivity Decreased motor and cognitive activity, as in psychomotor retardation; visible slowing of thought, speech, and movements. Also called *hypokinesis.*

hypochondria Exaggerated concern about health that is based not on real medical pathology, but on unrealistic interpretations of physical signs or sensations as abnormal.

hypomania Mood abnormality with the qualitative characteristics of mania, but somewhat less intense. Seen in cyclothymic disorder.

idea of reference Misinterpretation of incidents and events in the outside world as having direct personal reference to oneself; occasionally observed in normal persons, but frequently seen in paranoid patients. If present with sufficient frequency or intensity or if organized and systematized, they constitute delusions of reference.

illogical thinking Thinking containing erroneous conclusions or internal contradictions; psychopathological only when it is marked and not caused by cultural values or intellectual deficit.

illusion Perceptual misinterpretation of a real external stimulus. *Compare with* **hallucination.**

immediate memory Reproduction, recognition, or recall of perceived material within seconds after presentation. *Compare with* **long-term memory** *and* **short-term memory.**

impaired insight Diminished ability to understand the objective reality of a situation.

impaired judgment Diminished ability to understand a situation correctly and to act appropriately.

impulse control Ability to resist an impulse, drive, or temptation to perform some action.

inappropriate affect Emotional tone out of harmony with the idea, thought, or speech accompanying it. Seen in schizophrenia.

incoherence Communication that is disconnected, disorganized, or incomprehensible. *See also* **word salad**.

incorporation Primitive unconscious defense mechanism in which the psychic representation of another person or aspects of another person are assimilated into oneself through a figurative process of symbolic oral ingestion; represents a special form of introjection and is the earliest mechanism of identification.

increased libido Increase in sexual interest and drive.
ineffability Ecstatic state in which persons insist that their experience is inexpressible and indescribable and that it is impossible to convey what it is like to one who has never experienced it.
initial insomnia Falling asleep with difficulty; usually seen in anxiety disorder. *Compare with* **middle insomnia** *and* **terminal insomnia.**
insight Conscious recognition of one's own condition. In psychiatry, it refers to the conscious awareness and understanding of one's own psychodynamics and symptoms of maladaptive behavior; highly important in effecting changes in the personality and behavior of a person.
insomnia Difficulty in falling asleep or difficulty in staying asleep. It can be related to a mental disorder, a physical disorder, or an adverse effect of medication; or it can be primary (not related to a known medical factor or another mental disorder). *See also* **initial insomnia, middle insomnia,** *and* **terminal insomnia.**
intellectual insight Knowledge of the reality of a situation without the ability to use that knowledge successfully to effect an adaptive change in behavior or to master the situation. *Compare with* **true insight.**
intelligence Capacity for learning and ability to recall, integrate constructively, and apply what one has learned; the capacity to understand and to think rationally.
intoxication Mental disorder caused by recent ingestion or presence in the body of an exogenous substance producing maladaptive behavior by virtue of its effects on the central nervous system (CNS). The most common psychiatric changes involve disturbances of perception, wakefulness, attention, thinking, judgment, emotional control, and psychomotor behavior; the specific clinical picture depends on the substance ingested.
intropunitive Turning anger inward toward oneself. Commonly observed in depressed patients.
introspection Contemplating one's own mental processes to achieve insight.
introversion State in which a person's energies are directed inward toward the self, with little or no interest in the external world.
irrelevant answer Answer that is not responsive to the question.
irritability Abnormal or excessive excitability, with easily triggered anger, annoyance, or impatience.
irritable mood State in which one is easily annoyed and provoked to anger. *See also* **irritability.**
jamais vu Paramnestic phenomenon characterized by a false feeling of unfamiliarity with a real situation that one has previously experienced.
jargon aphasia Aphasia in which the words produced are neologistic; that is, nonsense words created by the patient.
judgment Mental act of comparing or evaluating choices within the framework of a given set of values for the purpose of electing a course of action. If the course of action chosen is consonant with reality or with mature adult standards of behavior, judgment is said to be *intact* or *normal*; judgment is said to be *impaired* if the chosen course of action is frankly maladaptive, results from impulsive decisions based on the need for immediate gratification, or is otherwise not consistent with reality as measured by mature adult standards.
kleptomania Pathological compulsion to steal.
la belle indifférence Inappropriate attitude of calm or lack of concern about one's disability. May be seen in patients with conversion disorder.
labile affect Affective expression characterized by rapid and abrupt changes, unrelated to external stimuli.
labile mood Oscillations in mood between euphoria and depression or anxiety.
laconic speech Condition characterized by a reduction in the quantity of spontaneous speech; replies to questions are brief and unelaborated, and little or no unprompted additional information is provided. Occurs in major depression, schizophrenia, and organic mental disorders. Also called *poverty of speech.*
lethologica Momentary forgetting of a name or proper noun. *See* **blocking.**
lilliputian hallucination Visual sensation that persons or objects are reduced in size; more properly regarded as an illusion. *See also* **micropsia.**
localized amnesia Partial loss of memory; amnesia restricted to specific or isolated experiences. Also called *lacunar amnesia* and *patch amnesia.*
logorrhea Copious, pressured, coherent speech; uncontrollable, excessive talking; observed in manic episodes of bipolar disorder. Also called *tachylogia,verbomania*, and *volubility.*
long-term memory Reproduction, recognition, or recall of experiences or information that was experienced in the distant past. Also called *remote memory*. *Compare with* **immediate memory** *and* **short-term memory.**
loosening of associations Characteristic schizophrenic thinking or speech disturbance involving a disorder in the logical progression of thoughts, manifested as a failure to communicate verbally adequately; unrelated and unconnected ideas shift from one subject to another. *See also* **tangentiality.**
macropsia False perception that objects are larger than they really are. *Compare with* **micropsia.**
magical thinking A form of dereistic thought; thinking similar to that of the preoperational phase in children (Jean Piaget), in which thoughts, words, or actions assume power (e.g., to cause or to prevent events).
malingering Feigning disease to achieve a specific goal, for example, to avoid an unpleasant responsibility.
mania Mood state characterized by elation, agitation, hyperactivity, hypersexuality, and accelerated thinking and speaking (flight of ideas). Seen in bipolar I disorder. *See also* **hypomania.**
manipulation Maneuvering by patients to get their own way; characteristic of antisocial personalities.
mannerism Ingrained, habitual involuntary movement.
melancholia Severe depressive state. Used in the term *involutional melancholia* as a descriptive term and also in reference to a distinct diagnostic entity.
memory Process whereby what is experienced or learned is established as a record in the CNS (registration), where it persists with a variable degree of permanence (retention) and can be recollected or retrieved from storage at will (recall). For types of memory, see **immediate memory, long-term memory,** and **short-term memory.**
mental disorder Psychiatric illness or disease whose manifestations are primarily characterized by behavioral or psychological impairment of function, measured in terms of deviation from some normative concept; associated with distress or disease, not

just an expected response to a particular event or limited to relations between a person and society.

mental retardation Subaverage general intellectual functioning that originates in the developmental period and is associated with impaired maturation and learning, and social maladjustment. Retardation is commonly defined in terms of intelligent quotient (IQ): mild (between 50 and 55 to 70), moderate (between 35 and 40 to between 50 and 55), severe (between 20 and 25 to between 35 and 40), and profound (below 20 to 25).

metonymy Speech disturbance common in schizophrenia in which the affected person uses a word or phrase that is related to the proper one but is not the one ordinarily used; for example, the patient speaks of consuming a *menu* rather than a *meal*, or refers to losing the *piece of string* of the conversation, rather than the *thread* of the conversation. *See also* **paraphasia** *and* **word approximation.**

microcephaly Condition in which the head is unusually small as a result of defective brain development and premature ossification of the skull.

micropsia False perception that objects are smaller than they really are. Sometimes called *lilliputian hallucination. Compare with* **macropsia.**

middle insomnia Waking up after falling asleep without difficulty and then having difficulty in falling asleep again. *Compare with* **initial insomnia** *and* **terminal insomnia.**

mimicry Simple, imitative motion activity of childhood.

monomania Mental state characterized by preoccupation with one subject.

mood Pervasive and sustained feeling tone that is experienced internally and that, in the extreme, can markedly influence virtually all aspects of a person's behavior and perception of the world. Distinguished from affect, the external expression of the internal feeling tone.

mood-congruent delusion Delusion with content that is mood appropriate (e.g., depressed patients who believe that they are responsible for the destruction of the world).

mood-congruent hallucination Hallucination with content that is consistent with a depressed or manic mood (e.g., depressed patients hearing voices telling them that they are bad persons and manic patients hearing voices telling them that they have inflated worth, power, or knowledge).

mood-incongruent delusion Delusion based on incorrect reference about external reality, with content that has no association to mood or is mood inappropriate (e.g., depressed patients who believe that they are the new Messiah).

mood-incongruent hallucination Hallucination not associated with real external stimuli, with content that is not consistent with depressed or manic mood (e.g., in depression, hallucinations not involving such themes as guilt, deserved punishment, or inadequacy; in mania, not involving such themes as inflated worth or power).

mood swings Oscillation of a person's emotional feeling tone between periods of elation and periods of depression.

motor aphasia Aphasia in which understanding is intact, but the ability to speak is lost. Also called *Broca's, expressive,* or *nonfluent aphasias.*

mourning Syndrome following loss of a loved one, consisting of preoccupation with the lost individual, weeping, sadness, and repeated reliving of memories. *See also* **bereavement** *and* **grief.**

muscle rigidity State in which the muscles remain immovable; seen in schizophrenia.

mutism Organic or functional absence of the faculty of speech. *See also* **stupor.**

mydriasis Dilation of the pupil; sometimes occurs as an autonomic (anticholinergic) or atropine-like adverse effect of some antipsychotic and antidepressant drugs.

narcissism In psychoanalytic theory, divided into primary and secondary types: primary narcissism, the early infantile phase of object relationship development, when the child has not differentiated the self from the outside world, and all sources of pleasure are unrealistically recognized as coming from within the self, giving the child a false sense of omnipotence; secondary narcissism, when the libido, once attached to external love objects, is redirected back to the self. *See also* **autistic thinking.**

needle phobia The persistent, intense, pathological fear of receiving an injection.

negative signs In schizophrenia: flat affect, alogia, abulia, and apathy.

negativism Verbal or nonverbal opposition or resistance to outside suggestions and advice; commonly seen in catatonic schizophrenia in which the patient resists any effort to be moved or does the opposite of what is asked.

neologism New word or phrase whose derivation cannot be understood; often seen in schizophrenia. It has also been used to mean a word that has been incorrectly constructed but whose origins are nonetheless understandable (e.g., *headshoe* to mean *hat*), but such constructions are more properly referred to as *word approximations.*

neurological amnesia (1) Auditory amnesia: loss of ability to comprehend sounds or speech. (2) Tactile amnesia: loss of ability to judge the shape of objects by touch. *See also* **astereognosis.** (3) Verbal amnesia: loss of ability to remember words. (4) Visual amnesia: loss of ability to recall or to recognize familiar objects or printed words.

nihilism Delusion of the nonexistence of the self or part of the self; also refers to an attitude of total rejection of established values or extreme skepticism regarding moral and value judgments.

nihilistic delusion Depressive delusion that the world and everything related to it have ceased to exist.

noeisis Revelation in which immense illumination occurs in association with a sense that one has been chosen to lead and command. Can occur in manic or dissociative states.

nominal aphasia Aphasia characterized by difficulty in giving the correct name of an object. *See also* **anomia** *and* **amnestic aphasia.**

nymphomania Abnormal, excessive, insatiable desire in a woman for sexual intercourse. *Compare with* **satyriasis.**

obsession Persistent and recurrent idea, thought, or impulse that cannot be eliminated from consciousness by logic or reasoning; obsessions are involuntary and ego-dystonic. *See also* **compulsion.**

olfactory hallucination Hallucination primarily involving smell or odors; most common in medical disorders, especially in the temporal lobe.

orientation State of awareness of oneself and one's surroundings in terms of time, place, and person.

overactivity Abnormality in motor behavior that can manifest itself as psychomotor agitation, hyperactivity (hyperkinesis), tics, sleepwalking, or compulsions.

overvalued idea False or unreasonable belief or idea that is sustained beyond the bounds of reason. It is held with less intensity or duration than a delusion, but is usually associated with mental illness.

panic Acute, intense attack of anxiety associated with personality disorganization; the anxiety is overwhelming and accompanied by feelings of impending doom.

panphobia Overwhelming fear of everything.

pantomime Gesticulation; psychodrama without the use of words.

paramnesia Disturbance of memory in which reality and fantasy are confused. It is observed in dreams and in certain types of schizophrenia and organic mental disorders; it includes phenomena such as *déjà vu* and *déjà entendu*, which can occur occasionally in normal persons.

paranoia Rare psychiatric syndrome marked by the gradual development of a highly elaborate and complex delusional system, generally involving persecutory or grandiose delusions, with few other signs of personality disorganization or thought disorder.

paranoid delusions Includes persecutory delusions and delusions of reference, control, and grandeur.

paranoid ideation Thinking dominated by suspicious, persecutory, or grandiose content of less than delusional proportions.

paraphasia Abnormal speech in which one word is substituted for another, the irrelevant word generally resembling the required one in morphology, meaning, or phonetic composition; the inappropriate word may be a legitimate one used incorrectly, such as *clover* instead of *hand*, or a bizarre nonsense expression, such as *treen* instead of *train*. Paraphasic speech may be seen in organic aphasias and in mental disorders such as schizophrenia. *See also* **metonymy** *and* **word approximation.**

parapraxis Faulty act, such as a slip of the tongue or the misplacement of an article. Freud ascribed parapraxes to unconscious motives.

paresis Weakness or partial paralysis of organic origin.

paresthesia Abnormal spontaneous tactile sensation, such as a burning, tingling, or pins-and-needles sensation.

perception Conscious awareness of elements in the environment by the mental processing of sensory stimuli; sometimes used in a broader sense to refer to the mental process by which all kinds of data, intellectual, emotional, and sensory, are meaningfully organized. *See also* **apperception.**

perseveration (1) Pathological repetition of the same response to different stimuli, as in a repetition of the same verbal response to different questions. (2) Persistent repetition of specific words or concepts in the process of speaking. Seen in cognitive disorders, schizophrenia, and other mental illness. *See also* **verbigeration.**

phantom limb False sensation that an extremity that has been lost is, in fact, present.

phobia Persistent, pathological, unrealistic, intense fear of an object or situation; the phobic person may realize that the fear is irrational but, nonetheless, cannot dispel it.

pica Craving and eating of nonfood substances, such as paint and clay.

polyphagia Pathological overeating.

positive signs In schizophrenia: hallucinations, delusions, and thought disorder.

posturing Strange, fixed, and bizarre bodily positions held by a patient for an extended time. *See also* **catatonia.**

poverty of speech content Speech that is adequate in amount, but conveys little information because of vagueness, emptiness, or stereotyped phrases.

poverty of speech Restriction in the amount of speech used; replies may be monosyllabic. *See also* **laconic speech.**

preoccupation of thought Centering of thought content on a particular idea, associated with a strong affective tone, such as a paranoid trend or a suicidal or homicidal preoccupation.

pressured speech Increase in the amount of spontaneous speech; rapid, loud, accelerated speech, as occurs in mania, schizophrenia, and cognitive disorders.

primary process thinking In psychoanalysis, the mental activity directly related to the functions of the id and characteristic of unconscious mental processes; marked by primitive, prelogical thinking and by the tendency to seek immediate discharge and gratification of instinctual demands. Includes thinking that is dereistic, illogical, magical; normally found in dreams, abnormally in psychosis. *Compare with* **secondary process thinking.**

projection Unconscious defense mechanism in which persons attribute to another those generally unconscious ideas, thoughts, feelings, and impulses that are in themselves undesirable or unacceptable as a form of protection from anxiety arising from an inner conflict; by externalizing whatever is unacceptable, they deal with it as a situation apart from themselves.

prosopagnosia Inability to recognize familiar faces that is not caused by impaired visual acuity or level of consciousness.

pseudocyesis Rare condition in which a nonpregnant patient has the signs and symptoms of pregnancy, such as abdominal distention, breast enlargement, pigmentation, cessation of menses, and morning sickness.

pseudodementia (1) Dementia-like disorder that can be reversed by appropriate treatment and is not caused by organic brain disease. (2) Condition in which patients show exaggerated indifference to their surroundings in the absence of a mental disorder; also occurs in depression and factitious disorders.

pseudologia phantastica Disorder characterized by uncontrollable lying in which patients elaborate extensive fantasies that they freely communicate and act on.

psychomotor agitation Physical and mental overactivity that is usually nonproductive and is associated with a feeling of inner turmoil, as seen in agitated depression.

psychosis Mental disorder in which the thoughts, affective response, ability to recognize reality, and ability to communicate and relate to others are sufficiently impaired to interfere grossly with the capacity to deal with reality; the classic characteristics of psychosis are impaired reality testing, hallucinations, delusions, and illusions.

psychotic (1) Person experiencing psychosis. (2) Denoting or characteristic of psychosis.

rationalization An unconscious defense mechanism in which irrational or unacceptable behavior, motives, or feelings are logically justified or made consciously tolerable by plausible means.

reaction formation Unconscious defense mechanism in which a person develops a socialized attitude or interest that is the direct antithesis of some infantile wish or impulse that is harbored consciously or unconsciously. One of the earliest and most unstable defense mechanisms, closely related to repression; both are defenses against impulses or urges that are unacceptable to the ego.

reality testing Fundamental ego function that consists of tentative actions that test and objectively evaluate the nature and limits of the environment; includes the ability to differentiate between the external world and the internal world and to accurately judge the relation between the self and the environment.

recall Process of bringing stored memories into consciousness. *See also* **memory.**

recent memory Recall of events over the past few days.

recent past memory Recall of events over the past few months.

receptive aphasia Organic loss of ability to comprehend the meaning of words; fluid and spontaneous, but incoherent and nonsensical, speech. *See also* **fluent aphasia** *and* **sensory aphasia.**

receptive dysphasia Difficulty in comprehending oral language; the impairment involves comprehension and production of language.

regression Unconscious defense mechanism in which a person undergoes a partial or total return to earlier patterns of adaptation; observed in many psychiatric conditions, particularly schizophrenia.

remote memory Recall of events from the distant past.

repression Freud's term for an unconscious defense mechanism in which unacceptable mental contents are banished or kept out of consciousness; important in normal psychological development and in neurotic and psychotic symptom formation. Freud recognized two kinds of repression: (1) repression proper, in which the repressed material was once in the conscious domain, and (2) primal repression, in which the repressed material was never in the conscious realm. *Compare with* **suppression.**

restricted affect Reduction in intensity of feeling tone, which is less severe than in blunted affect, but clearly reduced. *See also* **constricted affect.**

retrograde amnesia Loss of memory for events preceding the onset of the amnesia. *Compare with* **anterograde amnesia.**

retrospective falsification Memory becomes unintentionally (unconsciously) distorted by being filtered through a person's present emotional, cognitive, and experiential state.

rigidity In psychiatry, a person's resistance to change, a personality trait.

ritual (1) Formalized activity practiced by a person to reduce anxiety, as in OCD. (2) Ceremonial activity of cultural origin.

rumination Constant preoccupation with thinking about a single idea or theme, as in OCD.

satyriasis Morbid, insatiable sexual need or desire in a man. *Compare with* **nymphomania.**

scotoma (1) In psychiatry, a figurative blind spot in a person's psychological awareness. (2) In neurology, a localized visual field defect.

secondary process thinking In psychoanalysis, the form of thinking that is logical, organized, reality oriented, and influenced by the demands of the environment; characterizes the mental activity of the ego. *Compare with* **primary process thinking.**

seizure An attack or sudden onset of certain symptoms, such as convulsions, loss of consciousness, and psychic or sensory disturbances; seen in epilepsy and can be substance induced.

sensorium Hypothetical sensory center in the brain that is involved with clarity of awareness about oneself and one's surroundings, including the ability to perceive and to process ongoing events in light of past experiences, future options, and current circumstances; sometimes used interchangeably with *consciousness.*

sensory aphasia Organic loss of ability to comprehend the meaning of words; fluid and spontaneous, but incoherent and nonsensical, speech. *See also* **fluent aphasia** *and* **receptive aphasia.**

sensory extinction Neurological sign operationally defined as failure to report one of two simultaneously presented sensory stimuli, despite that either stimulus alone is correctly reported. Also called *sensory inattention.*

shame Failure to live up to self-expectations; often associated with fantasy of how person will be seen by others. *See also* **guilt.**

short-term memory Reproduction, recognition, or recall of perceived material within minutes after the initial presentation. *Compare with* **immediate memory** and **long-term memory.**

simultanagnosia Impairment in the perception or integration of visual stimuli appearing simultaneously.

somatic delusion Delusion pertaining to the functioning of one's body.

somatic hallucination Hallucination involving the perception of a physical experience localized within the body.

somatopagnosia Inability to recognize a part of one's body as one's own (also called *ignorance of the body* and *autotopagnosia*).

somnolence Pathological sleepiness or drowsiness from which one can be aroused to a normal state of consciousness.

spatial agnosia Inability to recognize spatial relations.

speaking in tongues Expression of a revelatory message through unintelligible words; not considered a disorder of thought if associated with practices of specific Pentecostal religions. *See also* **glossolalia.**

stereotypy Continuous mechanical repetition of speech or physical activities; observed in catatonic schizophrenia.

stupor (1) State of decreased reactivity to stimuli and less than full awareness of one's surroundings; as a disturbance of consciousness, it indicates a condition of partial coma or semicoma. (2) In psychiatry, used synonymously with *mutism* and does not necessarily imply a disturbance of consciousness; in *catatonic stupor,* patients are ordinarily aware of their surroundings.

stuttering Frequent repetition or prolongation of a sound or syllable, leading to markedly impaired speech fluency.

sublimation Unconscious defense mechanism in which the energy associated with unacceptable impulses or drives is diverted into personally and socially acceptable channels; unlike other defense mechanisms, it offers some minimal gratification of the instinctual drive or impulse.

substitution Unconscious defense mechanism in which a person replaces an unacceptable wish, drive, emotion, or goal with one that is more acceptable.

suggestibility State of uncritical compliance with influence or of uncritical acceptance of an idea, belief, or attitude; commonly observed among persons with hysterical traits.

suicidal ideation Thoughts or act of taking one's own life.

suppression Conscious act of controlling and inhibiting an unacceptable impulse, emotion, or idea; differentiated from repression in that repression is an unconscious process.

symbolization Unconscious defense mechanism in which one idea or object comes to stand for another because of some common aspect or quality in both; based on similarity and association; the symbols formed protect the person from the anxiety that may be attached to the original idea or object.

synesthesia Condition in which the stimulation of one sensory modality is perceived as sensation in a different modality, as when a sound produces a sensation of color.

syntactical aphasia Aphasia characterized by difficulty in understanding spoken speech; associated with gross disorder of thought and expression.
systematized delusion Group of elaborate delusions related to a single event or theme.
tactile hallucination Hallucination primarily involving the sense of touch. Also called *haptic hallucination.*
tangentiality Oblique, digressive, or even irrelevant manner of speech in which the central idea is not communicated.
tension Physiological or psychic arousal, uneasiness, or pressure toward action; an unpleasurable alteration in mental or physical state that seeks relief through action.
terminal insomnia Early morning awakening or waking up at least 2 hours before planning to wake up. *Compare with* **initial insomnia** *and* **middle insomnia.**
thought broadcasting Feeling that one's thoughts are being broadcast or projected into the environment. *See also* **thought withdrawal.**
thought disorder Any disturbance of thinking that affects language, communication, or thought content; the hallmark feature of schizophrenia. Manifestations range from simple blocking and mild circumstantiality to profound loosening of associations, incoherence, and delusions; characterized by a failure to follow semantic and syntactic rules that is inconsistent with the person's education, intelligence, or cultural background.
thought insertion Delusion that thoughts are being implanted in one's mind by other people or forces.
thought latency The period of time between a thought and its verbal expression. Increased in schizophrenia (*see* **blocking**) and decreased in mania (*see* **pressured speech**).
thought withdrawal Delusion that one's thoughts are being removed from one's mind by other people or forces. *See also* **thought broadcasting.**
tic disorders Predominantly psychogenic disorders characterized by involuntary, spasmodic, stereotyped movement of small groups of muscles; seen most predominantly in moments of stress or anxiety, rarely as a result of organic disease.
tinnitus Noises in one or both ears, such as ringing, buzzing, or clicking; an adverse effect of some psychotropic drugs.
tonic convulsion Convulsion in which the muscle contraction is sustained.
trailing phenomenon Perceptual abnormality associated with hallucinogenic drugs in which moving objects are seen as a series of discrete and discontinuous images.
trance Sleep-like state of reduced consciousness and activity.
tremor Rhythmical alteration in movement, which is usually faster than one beat a second; typically, tremors decrease during periods of relaxation and sleep and increase during periods of anger and increased tension.
true insight Understanding of the objective reality of a situation coupled with the motivational and emotional impetus to master the situation or change behavior.
twilight state Disturbed consciousness with hallucinations.
twirling Sign present in autistic children who continually rotate in the direction in which their head is turned.
unconscious (1) One of three divisions of Freud's topographic theory of the mind (the others being the conscious and the preconscious) in which the psychic material is not readily accessible to conscious awareness by ordinary means; its existence may be manifest in symptom formation, in dreams, or under the influence of drugs. (2) In popular (but more ambiguous) usage, any mental material not in the immediate field of awareness. (3) Denoting a state of unawareness, with lack of response to external stimuli, as in a coma.
undoing Unconscious primitive defense mechanism, repetitive in nature, by which a person symbolically acts out in reverse something unacceptable that has already been done or against which the ego must defend itself; a form of magical expiatory action, commonly observed in OCD.
unio mystica Feeling of mystic unity with an infinite power.
vegetative signs In depression, denoting characteristic symptoms such as sleep disturbance (especially early morning awakening), decreased appetite, constipation, weight loss, and loss of sexual response.
verbigeration Meaningless and stereotyped repetition of words or phrases, as seen in schizophrenia. Also called *cataphasia. See also* **perseveration.**
vertigo Sensation that one or the world around one is spinning or revolving; a hallmark of vestibular dysfunction, not to be confused with dizziness.
visual agnosia Inability to recognize objects or persons.
visual amnesia *See* **neurological amnesia.**
visual hallucination Hallucination primarily involving the sense of sight.
waxy flexibility Condition in which a person maintains the body position into which they are placed. Also called *catalepsy*.
word approximation Use of conventional words in an unconventional or inappropriate way (metonymy or of new words that are developed by conventional rules of word formation) (e.g., *handshoes* for *gloves* and *time measure* for *clock*); distinguished from a *neologism,* which is a new word whose derivation cannot be understood. *See also* **paraphasia.**
word salad Incoherent, essentially incomprehensible, mixture of words and phrases commonly seen in far-advanced cases of schizophrenia. *See also* **incoherence.**
xenophobia Abnormal fear of strangers.
zoophobia Abnormal fear of animals.

References

Baethge C, Salvatore P, Baldessarini RJ. "On cyclic insanity" by Karl Ludwig Kahlbaum, MD: A translation and commentary. *Harv Rev Psychiatry.* 2003;11:78.

Erhart SM, Young AS, Marder SR, Mintz J. Clinical utility of magnetic resonance imaging radiographs for suspected organic syndromes in adult psychiatry. *J Clin Psychol.* 2005;66:968–973.

Gonzalez-Pinto A, Ballesteros J, Aldama A, Perez de Heredia JL, Gutierrez M, Mosquera F. Principal components of mania. *J Affect Disord.* 2003;76:95.

Hemmings CP, Gravestock S, Pickard M, Bouras N. Psychiatric symptoms and problem behaviours in people with intellectual disabilities. *J Intellect Disabil Res.* 2006;50(4):269.

Moise D, Madhusoodanan S. Psychiatric symptoms associated with brain tumors: A clinical enigma. *CNS Spectr.* 2006;11:28–31.

Reichborn-Kjennerud T, Bulik CM, Sullivan PF, Tambs K, Harris JR. Psychiatric and medical symptoms in binge eating in the absence of compensatory behaviors. *Obes Res.* 2004;12:1445–1454.

Sadock BJ. Signs and Symptoms in Psychiatry. In: Sadock BJ, Sadock VA, eds. *Kaplan & Sadock's Comprehensive Textbook of Psychiatry*. 8th ed. Vol. 1. Baltimore: Lippincott Williams & Wilkins; 2005:847.

Segal DL, Coolidge FL. Structured interviewing and DSM classification. In: Hersen M, Turner SM, eds. *Adult Psychopathology and Diagnosis.* 4th ed. New York: John Wiley & Sons, Inc.; 2003:72.

Woods BT. Utility of soft and hard signs in psychiatric research. *Psychiatr Ann.* 2003;33:181.

Zisselman MH, Smith RV, Smith SA, Daskalakis C, Sanchez F. Racial and socioeconomic differences in psychiatric symptoms in nursing home residents: A minimum data set-based pilot study. *J Assoc. Am Med Dir* 2006;7(1): 17–22.

9 Classification in Psychiatry and Psychiatric Rating Scales

▲ 9.1 Classification in Psychiatry

Systems of classification for psychiatric diagnoses have several purposes: to distinguish one psychiatric diagnosis from another, so that clinicians can offer the most effective treatment; to provide a common language among health care professionals; and to explore the still unknown causes of many mental disorders. The two most important psychiatric classifications are the *Diagnostic and Statistical Manual of Mental Disorders* (DSM) developed by the American Psychiatric Association in collaboration with other groups of mental health professionals, and the *International Classification of Diseases* (ICD), developed by the World Health Organization.

HISTORY

The various classification systems used in psychiatry date back to Hippocrates, who introduced the terms *mania* and *hysteria* as forms of mental illness in the fifth century BC. Since then, each era has introduced its own psychiatric classification. The first US classification was introduced in 1869 at the annual meeting of the American Medico-Psychological Association, which later became the American Psychiatric Association. In 1952, the American Psychiatric Association's Committee on Nomenclature and Statistics published the first edition of DSM (DSM-I). Five editions have been published since then: DSM-II (1968); DSM-III (1980); a revised DSM-III, DSM-III-R (1987); DSM-IV (1994); and DSM-IV-TR (TR stands for Text Revision) (2000).

DSM-IV-TR's Relation to ICD-10. DSM-IV-TR was designed to correspond to the 10th revision of ICD (ICD-10), developed in 1992. This was done to ensure uniform reporting of national and international health statistics. In addition, Medicare requires that billing codes for reimbursement follow ICD. ICD-10 is the official classification system used in Europe and many other parts of the world. All categories used in DSM-IV-TR are found in ICD-10, but not all ICD-10 categories are in DSM-IV-TR.

DSM-IV-TR

The DSM-IV-TR is the official psychiatric coding system used in the United States. Although some psychiatrists have been critical of the many versions of DSM that have appeared since 1952, DSM-IV-TR is the official US nomenclature. All terminology used in this textbook conforms to DSM-IV-TR nomenclature.

Three tables are listed in this section that relate to DSM and ICD classification. Table 9.1-1 lists the DSM diagnostic categories and the corresponding ICD numerical codes (all codes begin with F). Table 9.1-2 lists the DSM diagnostic categories and the corresponding DSM numerical codes and Table 9.1-3 lists the ICD diagnostic categories and the corresponding ICD code. Either DSM or ICD codes may be used for insurance purposes and medical reporting.

Basic Features

Descriptive Approach. The approach to DSM-IV-TR is atheoretical with regard to causes. Thus, DSM-IV-TR attempts to describe the manifestations of the mental disorders and only rarely attempts to account for how the disturbances come about. The definitions of the disorders usually consist of descriptions of clinical features.

Diagnostic Criteria. Specified diagnostic criteria are provided for each specific mental disorder. These criteria include a list of features that must be present for the diagnosis to be made. Such criteria increase the reliability of the diagnostic process.

Systematic Description. DSM-IV-TR also systematically describes each disorder in terms of its associated features: specific age-, culture-, and gender-related features; prevalence, incidence, and risk; course; complications; predisposing factors; familial pattern; and differential diagnosis. In some instances, when many specific disorders share common features, this information is included in the introduction to the entire section. Laboratory findings and associated physical examination signs and symptoms are described when relevant. DSM-IV-TR is not, and does not purport to be, a textbook: No mention is made of theories of causes, management, or treatment, and the controversial issues surrounding a particular diagnostic category are not discussed.

DSM-IV-TR Classification

The DSM-IV-TR lists 365 disorders in 17 sections (Table 9.1–4), plus some diagnostic criteria proposed for further study are included in the appendix. Each disorder is described in detail in

Table 9.1–1
DSM-IV-TR Classification of Mental Disorders (With *International Statistical Classification of Diseases, Tenth Revision*, Codes)

Disorders usually first diagnosed in infancy, childhood, or adolescence (39)	
Mental retardation (41)	
	Note: These are coded on Axis II.
F70.9	Mild mental retardation (43)
F71.9	Moderate mental retardation (43)
F72.9	Severe mental retardation (43)
F73.9	Profound mental retardation (44)
F79.9	Mental retardation, severity unspecified (44)
Learning disorders (49)	
F81.0	Reading disorder (51)
F81.2	Mathematics disorder (53)
F81.8	Disorder of written expression (54)
F81.9	Learning disorder NOS (56)
Motor skills disorder (56)	
F82	Developmental coordination disorder (56)
Communication disorders (58)	
F80.1	Expressive language disorder (58)
F80.2	Mixed receptive-expressive language disorder (62)
F80.0	Phonological disorder (65)
F98.5	Stuttering (67)
F80.9	Communication disorder NOS (69)
Pervasive developmental disorders (69)	
F84.0	Autistic disorder (70)
F84.2	Rett's syndrome (76)
F84.3	Childhood disintegrative disorder (77)
F84.5	Asperger syndrome (80)
F84.9	Pervasive developmental disorder NOS (84)
Attention-deficit and disruptive behavior disorders (85)	
—.–	Attention-deficit/hyperactivity disorder (85)
F90.0	Combined type
F98.8	Predominantly inattentive type
F90.0	Predominantly hyperactive-impulsive type
F90.9	Attention-deficit/hyperactivity disorder NOS (93)
F91.8	Conduct Disorder (93)
	Specify type: childhood-onset type or adolescent-onset type
F91.3	Oppositional defiant disorder (100)
F91.9	Disruptive behavior disorder NOS (103)
Feeding and eating disorders of infancy or early childhood (103)	
F98.3	Pica (103)
F98.2	Rumination disorder (105)
F98.2	Feeding disorder of infancy or early childhood (107)
Tic disorders (108)	
F95.2	Tourette syndrome (111)
F95.1	Chronic motor or vocal tic disorder (114)
F95.0	Transient tic disorder (115)
	Specify if: single episode or recurrent
F95.9	Tic disorder NOS (116)
Elimination disorders (116)	
—.–	Encopresis (116)
R15	With constipation and overflow incontinence (*also code K59.0 constipation on Axis III*)
F98.1	Without constipation and overflow incontinence
F98.0	Enuresis (not due to a general medical condition) (118)
	Specify type: nocturnal only, diurnal only, or nocturnal and diurnal
Other disorders of infancy, childhood, or adolescence (121)	
F93.0	Separation anxiety disorder (121)
	Specify if: early onset
F94.0	Selective mutism (125)
F94.x	Reactive attachment disorder of infancy or early childhood (127)
.1	Inhibited type
.2	Disinhibited type
F98.4	Stereotypic movement disorder (131)
	Specify if: with self-injurious behavior
F98.9	Disorder of infancy, childhood, or adolescence NOS (134)
Delirium, dementia, and amnestic and other cognitive disorders (135)	
Delirium (136)	
F05.0	Delirium due to . . . *[indicate the general medical condition] (code F05.1 if superimposed on dementia)* (141)
—.–	Substance intoxication delirium *(refer to substance-related disorders for substance-specific codes)* (143)
—.–	Substance withdrawal delirium *(refer to substance-related disorders for substance-specific codes)* (143)
—.–	Delirium due to multiple etiologies *(code each of the specific etiologies)* (146)
F05.9	Delirium NOS (147)
Dementia (147)	
F00.xx	Dementia of the Alzheimer's type, with early onset *(also code G30.0 Alzheimer's disease, with early onset, on Axis III)* (154)
.00	Uncomplicated
.01	With delusions
.03	With depressed mood
	Specify if: with behavioral disturbance
F00.xx	Dementia of the Alzheimer's type, with late onset *(also code G30.1 Alzheimer's disease, with late onset, on Axis III)* (154)
.10	Uncomplicated
.11	With delusions
.13	With depressed mood
	Specify if: with behavioral disturbance
F01.xx	Vascular dementia (158)
.80	Uncomplicated
.81	With delusions
.83	With depressed mood
	Specify if: with behavioral disturbance
F02.4	Dementia due to HIV disease *(also code B22.0 HIV disease resulting in encephalopathy on Axis III)* (163)
F02.8	Dementia due to head trauma *(also code S06.9 intracranial injury on Axis III)* (164)
F02.3	Dementia due to Parkinson's disease *(also code G20 Parkinson's disease on Axis III)* (164)
F02.2	Dementia due to Huntington's disease *(also code G10 Huntington's disease on Axis III)* (165)
F02.0	Dementia due to Pick's disease *(also code G31.0 Pick's disease on Axis III)* (165)
F02.1	Dementia due to Creutzfeldt-Jakob disease *(also code A81.0 Creutzfeldt-Jakob disease on Axis III)* (166)
F02.8	Dementia due to . . . *[indicate the general medical condition not listed above] (also code the general medical condition on Axis III)* (167)
—.–	Substance-induced persisting dementia *(refer to substance-related disorders for substance-specific codes)* (168)

(*continued*)

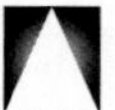

Table 9.1–1
(Continued)

F02.8 Dementia due to multiple etiologies *(instead code F00.2 for mixed Alzheimer's and vascular dementia)* (170)
F03 Dementia NOS (171)
Amnestic disorders (172)
F04 Amnestic disorder due to . . . *[indicate the general medical condition]* (175)
Specify if: transient or chronic
—.– Substance-induced persisting amnestic disorder *(refer to substance-related disorders for substance-specific codes)* (177)
R41.3 Amnestic disorder NOS (179)
Other cognitive disorders (179)
F06.9 Cognitive disorders NOS (179)

Mental disorders due to a general medical condition not elsewhere classified (181)
F06.1 Catatonic disorder due to . . . *[indicate the general medical condition]* (185)
F07.0 Personality change due to . . . *[indicate the general medical condition]* (187)
Specify type: labile type, disinhibited type, aggressive type, apathetic type, paranoid type, other type, combined type, or unspecified type
F09 Mental disorder NOS due to . . . *[indicate the general medical condition]* (190)

Substance-related disorders (191)
[a] *The following specifiers may be applied to substance dependence:*
Specify if: with physiological dependence or without physiological dependence
Code course of dependence in fifth character:
0 = Early full remission or early partial remission
0 = Sustained full remission or sustained partial remission
1 = In a controlled environment
2 = On agonist therapy
4 = Mild, moderate, or severe
The following specifiers apply to substance-induced disorders as noted:
[I]With onset during intoxication
[W]With onset during withdrawal
Alcohol-related disorders (212)
Alcohol use disorders (213)
F10.2x Alcohol dependence[a] (213)
F10.1 Alcohol abuse (214)
Alcohol-induced disorders (214)
F10.00 Alcohol intoxication (214)
F10.3 Alcohol withdrawal (215)
Specify if: with perceptual disturbances
F10.03 Alcohol intoxication delirium (143)
F10.4 Alcohol withdrawal delirium (143)
F10.73 Alcohol-induced persisting dementia (168)
F10.6 Alcohol-induced persisting amnestic disorder (177)
F10.xx Alcohol-induced psychotic disorder (338)
.51 With delusions[I,W]
.52 With hallucinations[I,W]
F10.8 Alcohol-induced mood disorder[I,W] (405)
F10.8 Alcohol-induced anxiety disorder[I,W] (479)
F10.8 Alcohol-induced sexual dysfunction[I] (562)
F10.8 Alcohol-induced sleep disorder[I,W] (655)
F10.9 Alcohol-related disorder NOS (223)
Amphetamine (or amphetamine-like)–related disorders (223)
Amphetamine use disorders (224)
F15.2x Amphetamine dependence[a] (224)
F15.1 Amphetamine abuse (225)
Amphetamine-induced disorders (226)
F15.00 Amphetamine intoxication (226)
F15.04 Amphetamine intoxication, with perceptual disturbances (226)
F15.3 Amphetamine withdrawal (227)
F15.03 Amphetamine intoxication delirium (143)
F15.xx Amphetamine-induced psychotic disorder (338)
.51 With delusions[I]
.52 With hallucinations[I]
F15.8 Amphetamine-induced mood disorder[I,W] (405)
F15.8 Amphetamine-induced anxiety disorder[I] (479)
F15.8 Amphetamine-induced sexual dysfunction[I] (562)
F15.8 Amphetamine-induced sleep disorder[I,W] (655)
F15.9 Amphetamine-related disorder NOS (231)
Caffeine-related disorders (231)
Caffeine-induced disorders (232)
F15.00 Caffeine intoxication (232)
F15.8 Caffeine-induced anxiety disorder[I] (479)
F15.8 Caffeine-induced sleep disorder[I] (655)
F15.9 Caffeine-related disorder NOS (234)
Cannabis-related disorders (234)
Cannabis use disorders (236)
F12.2x Cannabis dependence[a] (236)
F12.1 Cannabis abuse (236)
Cannabis-induced disorders (237)
F12.00 Cannabis intoxication (237)
F12.04 Cannabis intoxication, with perceptual disturbances (237)
F12.03 Cannabis intoxication delirium (143)
F12.xx Cannabis-induced psychotic disorder (338)
.51 With delusions[I]
.52 With hallucinations[I]
F12.8 Cannabis-induced anxiety disorder[I] (479)
F12.9 Cannabis-related disorder NOS (241)
Cocaine-related disorders (241)
Cocaine use disorders (242)
F14.2x Cocaine dependence[a] (242)
F14.1 Cocaine abuse (243)
Cocaine-induced disorders (244)
F14.00 Cocaine intoxication (244)
F14.04 Cocaine intoxication, with perceptual disturbances (244)
F14.3 Cocaine withdrawal (245)
F14.03 Cocaine intoxication delirium (143)
F14.xx Cocaine-induced psychotic disorder (338)
.51 With delusions[I]
.52 With hallucinations[I]
F14.8 Cocaine-induced mood disorder[I,W] (405)
F14.8 Cocaine-induced anxiety disorder[I,W] (479)
F14.8 Cocaine-induced sexual dysfunction[I] (562)
F14.8 Cocaine-induced sleep disorder[I,W] (655)
F14.9 Cocaine-related disorder NOS (250)
Hallucinogen-related disorders (250)
Hallucinogen use disorders (251)
F16.2x Hallucinogen dependence[a] (251)
F16.1 Hallucinogen abuse (252)
Hallucinogen-induced disorders (252)
F16.00 Hallucinogen intoxication (252)
F16.70 Hallucinogen persisting perception disorder (flashbacks) (253)
F16.03 Hallucinogen intoxication delirium (143)
F16.xx Hallucinogen-induced psychotic disorder (338)
.51 With delusions[I]
.52 With hallucinations[I]

(continued)

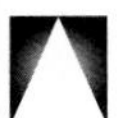

Table 9.1–1
(Continued)

F16.8 Hallucinogen-induced mood disorder[I] (405)
F16.8 Hallucinogen-induced anxiety disorder[I] (479)
F16.9 Hallucinogen-related disorder NOS (256)
Inhalant-related disorders (257)
Inhalant use disorders (258)
F18.2x Inhalant dependence[a] (258)
F18.1 Inhalant abuse (259)
Inhalant-induced disorders (259)
F18.00 Inhalant intoxication (259)
F18.03 Inhalant intoxication delirium (143)
F18.73 Inhalant-induced persisting dementia (168)
F18.xx Inhalant-induced psychotic disorder (338)
.51 With delusions[I]
.52 With hallucinations[I]
F18.8 Inhalant-induced mood disorder[I] (405)
F18.8 Inhalant-induced anxiety disorder[I] (479)
F18.9 Inhalant-related disorder NOS (263)
Nicotine-related disorders (264)
Nicotine use disorder (264)
F17.2x Nicotine dependence[a] (264)
Nicotine-induced disorders (265)
F17.3 Nicotine withdrawal (265)
F17.9 Nicotine-related disorders NOS (269)
Opioid-related disorders (269)
Opioid use disorders (270)
F11.2x Opioid dependence[a] (270)
F11.1 Opioid abuse (271)
Opioid-induced disorders (271)
F11.00 Opioid intoxication (271)
F11.04 Opioid intoxication, with perceptual disturbances (272)
F11.3 Opioid withdrawal (272)
F11.03 Opioid intoxication delirium (143)
F11.xx Opioid-induced psychotic disorder (338)
.51 With delusions[I]
.52 With hallucinations[I]
F11.8 Opioid-induced mood disorder[I] (405)
F11.8 Opioid-induced sexual dysfunction[I] (562)
F11.8 Opioid-induced sleep disorder[I,W] (655)
F11.9 Opioid-related disorder NOS (277)
Phencyclidine (or phencyclidine-like)–related disorders (278)
Phencyclidine use disorders (279)
F19.2x Phencyclidine dependence[a] (279)
F19.1 Phencyclidine abuse (279)
Phencyclidine-induced disorders (280)
F19.00 Phencyclidine intoxication (280)
F19.04 Phencyclidine intoxication, with perceptual disturbances (280)
F19.03 Phencyclidine intoxication delirium (143)
F19.xx Phencyclidine-induced psychotic disorder (338)
.51 With delusions[I]
.52 With hallucinations[I]
F19.8 Phencyclidine-induced mood disorder[I] (405)
F19.8 Phencyclidine-induced anxiety disorder[I] (479)
F19.9 Phencyclidine-related disorder NOS (283)
Sedative-, hypnotic-, or anxiolytic-related disorders (284)
Sedative, hypnotic, or anxiolytic use disorders (285)
F13.2x Sedative, hypnotic, or anxiolytic dependence[a] (285)
F13.1 Sedative, hypnotic, or anxiolytic abuse (286)
Sedative-, hypnotic-, or anxiolytic-induced disorders (286)
F13.00 Sedative, hypnotic, or anxiolytic intoxication (286)
F13.3 Sedative, hypnotic, or anxiolytic withdrawal (287)
Specify if: with perceptual disturbances
F13.03 Sedative, hypnotic, or anxiolytic intoxication delirium (143)
F13.4 Sedative, hypnotic, or anxiolytic withdrawal delirium (143)
F13.73 Sedative-, hypnotic-, or anxiolytic-induced persisting dementia (168)
F13.6 Sedative-, hypnotic-, or anxiolytic-induced persisting amnestic disorder (177)
F13.xx Sedative-, hypnotic-, or anxiolytic-induced psychotic disorder (338)
.51 With delusions[I,W]
.52 With hallucinations[I,W]
F13.8 Sedative-, hypnotic-, or anxiolytic-induced mood disorder[I,W] (405)
F13.8 Sedative-, hypnotic-, or anxiolytic-induced anxiety disorder[W] (479)
F13.8 Sedative-, hypnotic-, or anxiolytic-induced sexual dysfunction[I] (562)
F13.8 Sedative-, hypnotic-, or anxiolytic-induced sleep disorder[I,W] (655)
F13.9 Sedative-, hypnotic-, or anxiolytic-related disorder NOS (293)
Polysubstance-related disorder (293)
F19.2x Polysubstance dependence[a] (293)
Other (or unknown) substance-related disorders (294)
Other (or unknown) substance use disorders (294)
F19.2x Other (or unknown) substance dependence[a] (192)
F19.1 Other (or unknown) substance abuse (198)
Other (or unknown) substance-induced disorders (295)
F19.00 Other (or unknown) substance intoxication (199)
F19.04 Other (or unknown) substance intoxication, with perceptual disturbances (199)
F19.3 Other (or unknown) substance withdrawal (201)
Specify if: with perceptual disturbances
F19.03 Other (or unknown) substance-induced delirium *(code F19.4 if onset during withdrawal)* (143)
F19.73 Other (or unknown) substance-induced persisting dementia (168)
F19.6 Other (or unknown) substance-induced persisting amnestic disorder (177)
F19.xx Other (or unknown) substance-induced psychotic disorder (338)
.51 With delusions[I,W]
.52 With hallucinations[I,W]
F19.8 Other (or unknown) substance-induced mood disorder[I,W] (405)
F19.8 Other (or unknown) substance-induced anxiety disorder[I,W] (479)
F19.8 Other (or unknown) substance-induced sexual dysfunction[I] (562)
F19.8 Other (or unknown) substance-induced sleep disorder[I,W] (655)
F19.9 Other (or unknown) substance-related disorder NOS (295)
Schizophrenia and other psychotic disorders (297)
F20.xx Schizophrenia (298)
.0x Paranoid type (313)
.1x Disorganized type (314)
.2x Catatonic type (315)
.3x Undifferentiated type (316)
.5x Residual type (316)

(*continued*)

Table 9.1–1 (Continued)

Code course of schizophrenia in fifth character:
2 = Episodic with interepisode residual symptoms (*specify* if: with prominent negative symptoms)
3 = Episodic with no interepisode residual symptoms
0 = Continuous (*specify* if: with prominent negative symptoms)
4 = Single episode in partial remission (*specify* if: with prominent negative symptoms)
5 = Single episode in full remission
8 = Other or unspecified pattern
9 = Less than 1 year since onset of initial active-phase symptoms

F20.8 Schizophreniform disorder (317)
Specify if: without good prognostic features/ with good prognostic features
F25.x Schizoaffective disorder (319)
.0 Bipolar type
.1 Depressive type
F22.0 Delusional disorder (323)
Specify type: erotomanic type, grandiose type, jealous type, persecutory type, somatic type, mixed type, or unspecified type
F23.xx Brief psychotic disorder (329)
.81 With marked stressor(s)
.80 Without marked stressor(s)
Specify if: with postpartum onset
F24 Shared psychotic disorder (332)
F06.x Psychotic disorder due to . . . *[indicate the general medical condition]* (334)
.2 With delusions
.0 With hallucinations
—.– Substance-induced psychotic disorder *(refer to substance-related disorders for substance-specific codes)* (338)
Specify if: with onset during intoxication/with onset during withdrawal
F29 Psychotic disorder NOS (343)

Mood disorders (345)

The following specifiers apply (for current or most recent episode) to mood disorders as noted:
[a]Severity, psychotic, and remission specifiers
[b]Chronic
[c]With catatonic features
[d]With melancholic features
[e]With atypical features
[f]With postpartum onset
The following specifiers apply to mood disorders as noted:
[g]With or without full interepisode recovery
[h]With seasonal pattern
[i]With rapid cycling

Depressive disorders (369)
F32.x Major depressive disorder, single episode[a,b,c,d,e,f] (369)
F33.x Major depressive disorder, recurrent[a,b,c,d,e,f,g,h] (369)
Code current state of major depressive episode in fourth character:
0 = Mild
1 = Moderate
2 = Severe without psychotic features
3 = Severe with psychotic features
Specify: mood-congruent psychotic features or mood-incongruent psychotic features
4 = In partial remission
5 = In full remission
9 = Unspecified
F34.1 Dysthymic disorder (376)
Specify if: early onset or late onset
Specify: with atypical features
F32.9 Depressive disorder NOS (381)

Bipolar disorders (382)
F30.x Bipolar I disorder, single manic episode[a,c,f] (382)
Specify if: mixed
Code current state of manic episode in fourth character:
1 = Mild, moderate, or severe without psychotic features
2 = Severe with psychotic features
8 = In partial or full remission
F31.0 Bipolar I disorder, most recent episode hypomanic[g,h,i] (382)
F31.x Bipolar I disorder, most recent episode manic[a,c,f,g,h,i] (382)
Code current state of manic episode in fourth character:
1 = Mild, moderate, or severe without psychotic features
2 = Severe with psychotic features
7 = In partial or full remission
F31.6 Bipolar I disorder, most recent episode mixed[a,c,f,g,h,i] (382)
F31.x Bipolar I disorder, most recent episode depressed[a,b,c,d,e,f,g,h,i] (382)
Code current state of major depressive episode in fourth character:
3 = Mild or moderate
4 = Severe without psychotic features
5 = Severe with psychotic features
7 = In partial or full remission
F31.9 Bipolar I disorder, most recent episode unspecified[g,h,i] (382)
F31.8 Bipolar II disorder[a,b,c,d,e,f,g,h,i] (392)
Specify (current or most recent episode): hypomanic or depressed
F34.0 Cyclothymic disorder (398)
F31.9 Bipolar disorder NOS (400)
F06.xx Mood disorder due to . . . *[indicate the general medical condition]* (401)
.32 With depressive features
.32 With major depressive–like episode
.30 With manic features
.33 With mixed features
—.– Substance-induced mood disorder *(refer to substance-related disorders for substance-specific codes)* (405)
Specify type: with depressive features, with manic features, or with mixed features
Specify if: with onset during intoxication or with onset during withdrawal
F39 Mood disorder NOS (410)

Anxiety disorders (429)
F41.0 Panic disorder without agoraphobia (433)
F40.01 Panic disorder with agoraphobia (433)
F40.00 Agoraphobia without history of panic disorder (441)
F40.2 Specific phobia (443)
Specify type: animal type, natural environment type, blood-injection-injury type, situational type, or other type
F40.1 Social phobia (450)
Specify if: generalized
F42.8 Obsessive-compulsive disorder (456)
Specify if: with poor insight

(continued)

Table 9.1–1 (Continued)

F43.1	Posttraumatic stress disorder (463)
	Specify if: acute or chronic
	Specify if: with delayed onset
F43.0	Acute stress disorder (469)
F41.1	Generalized anxiety disorder (472)
F06.4	Anxiety disorder due to ... *[indicate the general medical condition]* (476)
	Specify if: with generalized anxiety, with panic attacks, or with obsessive-compulsive symptoms
—.–	Substance-induced anxiety disorder *(refer to substance-related disorders for substance-specific codes)* (479)
	Specify if: with generalized anxiety, with panic attacks, with obsessive-compulsive symptoms, or with phobic symptoms
	Specify if: with onset during intoxication or with onset during withdrawal
F41.9	Anxiety disorder NOS (484)
Somatoform disorders (485)	
F45.0	Somatization disorder (486)
F45.1	Undifferentiated somatoform disorder (490)
F44.x	Conversion disorder (492)
.4	With motor symptom or deficit
.5	With seizures or convulsions
.6	With sensory symptom or deficit
.7	With mixed presentation
F45.4	Pain disorder (498)
	Specify type: associated with psychological factors or associated with psychological factors and a general medical condition
	Specify if: acute or chronic
F45.2	Hypochondriasis (504)
	Specify if: with poor insight
F45.2	Body dysmorphic disorder (507)
F45.9	Somatoform disorder NOS (511)
Factitious disorders (513)	
F68.1	Factitious disorder (513)
	Specify type: with predominantly psychological signs and symptoms, with predominantly physical signs and symptoms, or with combined psychological and physical signs and symptoms
F68.1	Factitious disorder NOS (517)
Dissociative disorders (519)	
F44.0	Dissociative amnesia (520)
F44.1	Dissociative fugue (523)
F44.81	Dissociative identity disorder (526)
F48.1	Depersonalization disorder (530)
F44.9	Dissociative disorder NOS (532)
Sexual and gender identity disorders (535)	
Sexual dysfunctions (535)	
The following specifiers apply to all primary sexual dysfunctions:	
Lifelong type, acquired type, generalized type, situational type, due to psychological factors, or due to combined factors	
Sexual desire disorders (539)	
F52.0	Hypoactive sexual desire disorder (539)
F52.10	Sexual aversion disorder (541)
Sexual arousal disorders (543)	
F52.2	Female sexual arousal disorder (543)
F52.2	Male erectile disorder (545)
Orgasmic disorders (547)	
F52.3	Female orgasmic disorder (547)
F52.3	Male orgasmic disorder (550)
F52.4	Premature ejaculation (552)
Sexual pain disorders (554)	
F52.6	Dyspareunia (not due to a general medical condition) (554)
F52.5	Vaginismus (not due to a general medical condition) (556)
Sexual dysfunction due to a general medical condition (558)	
N94.8	Female hypoactive sexual desire disorder due to ... *[indicate the general medical condition]* (558)
N50.8	Male hypoactive sexual desire disorder due to ... *[indicate the general medical condition]* (558)
N48.4	Male erectile disorder due to ... *[indicate the general medical condition]* (558)
N94.1	Female dyspareunia due to ... *[indicate the general medical condition]* (558)
N50.8	Male dyspareunia due to ... *[indicate the general medical condition]* (558)
N94.8	Other female sexual dysfunction due to ... *[indicate the general medical condition]* (558)
N50.8	Other male sexual dysfunction due to ... *[indicate the general medical condition]* (558)
—.–	Substance-induced sexual dysfunction *(refer to substance-related disorders for substance-specific codes)* (562)
	Specify if: with impaired desire, with impaired arousal, with impaired orgasm, or with sexual pain
	Specify if: with onset during intoxication
F52.9	Sexual dysfunction NOS (565)
Paraphilias (566)	
F65.2	Exhibitionism (569)
F65.0	Fetishism (569)
F65.8	Frotteurism (570)
F65.4	Pedophilia (571)
	Specify if: sexually attracted to males, sexually attracted to females, or sexually attracted to both
	Specify if: limited to incest
	Specify type: exclusive type or nonexclusive type
F65.5	Sexual masochism (572)
F65.5	Sexual sadism (573)
F65.1	Transvestic fetishism (574)
	Specify if: with gender dysphoria
F65.3	Voyeurism (575)
F65.9	Paraphilia NOS (576)
Gender identity disorders (576)	
F64.x	Gender identity disorder (576)
.2	In children
.0	In adolescents or adults
	Specify if: sexually attracted to males, sexually attracted to females, sexually attracted to both, or sexually attracted to neither
F64.9	Gender identity disorder NOS (582)
F52.9	Sexual disorder NOS (582)
Eating disorders (583)	
F50.0	Anorexia nervosa (583)
	Specify type: restricting type or binge-eating and purging type
F50.2	Bulimia nervosa (589)
	Specify type: purging type or nonpurging type
F50.9	Eating disorder NOS (594)
Sleep disorders (597)	
Primary sleep disorders (598)	
Dyssomnias (598)	
F51.0	Primary insomnia (599)
F51.1	Primary hypersomnia (604)
	Specify if: recurrent
G47.4	Narcolepsy (609)
G47.3	Breathing-related sleep disorder (615)

(continued)

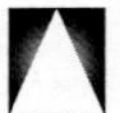

Table 9.1–1
(Continued)

F51.2 Circadian rhythm sleep disorder (622)
Specify type: delayed sleep phase type, jet lag type, shift work type, or unspecified type
F51.9 Dyssomnia NOS (629)
Parasomnias (630)
F51.5 Nightmare disorder (631)
F51.4 Sleep terror disorder (634)
F51.3 Sleepwalking disorder (639)
F51.8 Parasomnia NOS (644)
Sleep disorders related to another mental disorder (645)
F51.0 Insomnia related to . . . *[indicate the Axis I or Axis II disorder]* (645)
F51.1 Hypersomnia related to . . . *[indicate the Axis I or Axis II disorder]* (645)
Other sleep disorders (651)
G47.x Sleep disorder due to . . . *[indicate the general medical condition]* (651)
.0 Insomnia type
.1 Hypersomnia type
.8 Parasomnia type
.8 Mixed type
—.– Substance-induced sleep disorder *(refer to substance-related disorders for substance-specific codes)* (655)
Specify type: insomnia type, hypersomnia type, or parasomnia type/mixed type
Specify if: with onset during intoxication or with onset during withdrawal

Impulse-control disorders not elsewhere classified (663)
F63.8 Intermittent explosive disorder (663)
F63.2 Kleptomania (667)
F63.1 Pyromania (669)
F63.0 Pathological gambling (671)
F63.3 Trichotillomania (674)
F63.9 Impulse-control disorder NOS (677)

Adjustment disorders (679)
F43.x Adjustment disorder (679)
.20 With depressed mood
.28 With anxiety
.22 With mixed anxiety and depressed mood
.24 With disturbance of conduct
.25 With mixed disturbance of emotions and conduct
.9 Unspecified
Specify if: acute or chronic

Personality disorders (685)
Note: These are coded on Axis II.
F60.0 Paranoid personality disorder (690)
F60.1 Schizoid personality disorder (694)
F21 Schizotypal personality disorder (697)
F60.2 Antisocial personality disorder (701)
F60.31 Borderline personality disorder (706)
F60.4 Histrionic personality disorder (711)
F60.8 Narcissistic personality disorder (714)
F60.6 Avoidant personality disorder (718)
F60.7 Dependent personality disorder (721)
F60.5 Obsessive-compulsive personality disorder (725)
F60.9 Personality disorder NOS (729)

Other conditions that may be a focus of clinical attention (731)
Psychological factors affecting medical condition (731)
F54 . . . *[Specified psychological factor]* affecting . . . *[indicate the general medical condition]*
Choose name based on nature of factors: (731)
Mental disorder affecting medical condition
Psychological symptoms affecting medical condition
Personality traits or coping style affecting medical condition
Maladaptive health behaviors affecting medical condition
Stress-related physiological response affecting medical condition
Other or unspecified psychological factors affecting medical condition
Medication-induced movement disorders (734)
G21.0 Neuroleptic-induced parkinsonism (735)
G21.0 Neuroleptic malignant syndrome (735)
G24.0 Neuroleptic-induced acute dystonia (735)
G21.1 Neuroleptic-induced acute akathisia (735)
G24.0 Neuroleptic-induced tardive dyskinesia (736)
G25.1 Medication-induced postural tremor (736)
G25.9 Medication-induced movement disorder NOS (736)
Other medication-induced disorder (736)
T88.7 Adverse effects of medication NOS (736)
Relational problems (736)
Z63.7 Relational problem related to a mental disorder or general medical condition (737)
Z63.8 Parent–child relational problem (*code Z63.1 if focus of attention is on child*) (737)
Z63.0 Partner relational problem (737)
F93.3 Sibling relational problem (737)
Z63.9 Relational problem NOS (737)
Problems related to abuse or neglect (738)
T74.1 Physical abuse of child (738)
T74.2 Sexual abuse of child (738)
T74.0 Neglect of child (738)
T74.1 Physical abuse of adult (738)
T74.2 Sexual abuse of adult (738)
Additional conditions that may be a focus of clinical attention (739)
Z91.1 Noncompliance with treatment (739)
Z76.5 Malingering (739)
Z72.8 Adult antisocial behavior (740)
Z72.8 Child or adolescent antisocial behavior (740)
R41.8 Borderline intellectual functioning (740)
R41.8 Age-related cognitive decline (740)
Z63.4 Bereavement (740)
Z55.8 Academic problem (741)
Z56.7 Occupational problem (741)
F93.8 Identity problem (741)
Z71.8 Religious or spiritual problem (741)
Z60.3 Acculturation problem (741)
Z60.0 Phase of life problem (742)

Additional codes (743)
F99 Unspecified mental disorder (nonpsychotic) (743)
Z03.2 No diagnosis or condition on Axis I (743)
R69 Diagnosis or condition deferred on Axis I (743)
Z03.2 No diagnosis on Axis II (743)
R46.8 Diagnosis deferred on Axis II, (743)

Note: An x appearing in a diagnostic code indicates that a specific code number is required. An ellipsis (. . .) is used in the names of certain disorders to indicate that the name of a specific mental disorder or general medical condition should be inserted when recording the name (e.g., F05.0 Delirium Due to Hypothyroidism). Numbers in parentheses are page numbers. If criteria are currently met, one of the following severity specifiers may be noted after the diagnosis: *mild, moderate,* or *severe.* If criteria are no longer met, one of the following specifiers may be noted: *in partial remission, in full remission,* or *prior history.*
HIV, human immunodeficiency virus; NOS, not otherwise specified.
(From American Psychiatric Association. *Diagnostic and Statistical Manual of Mental Disorders.* 4th ed. Text rev. Washington, DC: American Psychiatric Association; 2000, with permission.)

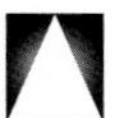

Table 9.1–2
Alphabetical Listing of DSM-IV-TR Diagnoses and DSM-IV-TR Codes

NOS = Not Otherwise Specified.

V62.3	Academic Problem
V62.4	Acculturation Problem
308.3	Acute Stress Disorder
	Adjustment Disorders
309.9	Unspecified
309.24	With Anxiety
309.0	With Depressed Mood
309.3	With Disturbance of Conduct
309.28	With Mixed Anxiety and Depressed Mood
309.4	With Mixed Disturbance of Emotions and Conduct
V71.01	Adult Antisocial Behavior
995.2	Adverse Effects of Medication NOS
780.9	Age-Related Cognitive Decline
300.22	Agoraphobia Without History of Panic Disorder
	Alcohol
305.00	Abuse
303.90	Dependence
291.89	-Induced Anxiety Disorder
291.89	-Induced Mood Disorder
291.1	-Induced Persisting Amnestic Disorder
291.2	-Induced Persisting Dementia
	-Induced Psychotic Disorder
291.5	With Delusions
291.3	With Hallucinations
291.89	-Induced Sexual Dysfunction
291.89	-Induced Sleep Disorder
303.00	Intoxication
291.0	Intoxication Delirium
291.9	-Related Disorder NOS
291.81	Withdrawal
291.0	Withdrawal Delirium
294.0	Amnestic Disorder Due to . . . *[Indicate the General Medical Condition]*
294.8	Amnestic Disorder NOS
	Amphetamine (or Amphetamine-Like)
305.70	Abuse
304.40	Dependence
292.89	-Induced Anxiety Disorder
292.84	-Induced Mood Disorder
	-Induced Psychotic Disorder
292.11	With Delusions
292.12	With Hallucinations
292.89	-Induced Sexual Dysfunction
292.89	-Induced Sleep Disorder
292.89	Intoxication
292.81	Intoxication Delirium
292.9	-Related Disorder NOS
292.0	Withdrawal
307.1	Anorexia Nervosa
301.7	Antisocial Personality Disorder
293.84	Anxiety Disorder Due to . . . *[Indicate the General Medical Condition]*
300.00	Anxiety Disorder NOS
299.80	Asperger's Disorder
	Attention-Deficit/Hyperactivity Disorder
314.01	Combined Type
314.01	Predominantly Hyperactive-Impulsive Type
314.00	Predominantly Inattentive Type
314.9	Attention-Deficit/Hyperacrivity Disorder NOS
299.00	Autistic Disorder
301.82	Avoidant Personality Disorder
V62.82	Bereavement
296.80	Bipolar Disorder NOS
	Bipolar I Disorder, Most Recent Episode Depressed
296.56	In Full Remission
296.55	In Partial Remission
296.51	Mild
296.52	Moderate
296.53	Severe Without Psychotic Features
296.54	Severe With Psychotic Features
296.50	Unspecified
296.40	Bipolar I Disorder, Most Recent Episode Hypomanic
	Bipolar I Disorder, Most Recent Episode Manic
296.46	In Full Remission
296.45	In Partial Remission
296.41	Mild
296.42	Moderate
296.43	Severe Without Psychotic Features
296.44	Severe With Psychotic Features
296.40	Unspecified
	Bipolar I Disorder, Most Recent Episode Mixed
296.66	In Full Remission
296.65	In Partial Remission
296.61	Mild
296.62	Moderate
296.63	Severe Without Psychotic Features
296.64	Severe With Psychotic Features
296.60	Unspecified
296.7	Bipolar I Disorder, Most Recent Episode Unspecified
	Bipolar I Disorder, Single Manic Episode
296.06	In Full Remission
296.05	In Partial Remission
296.01	Mild
296.02	Moderate
296.03	Severe Without Psychotic Features
296.04	Severe With Psychotic Features
296.00	Unspecified
296.89	Bipolar II Disorder
300.7	Body Dysmorphic Disorder
V62.89	Borderline Intellectual Functioning
301.83	Borderline Personality Disorder
780.59	Breathing-Related Sleep Disorder
298.8	Brief Psychotic Disorder
307.51	Bulimia Nervosa
	Caffeine
292.89	-Induced Anxiety Disorder
292.89	-Induced Sleep Disorder
305.90	Intoxication
292.9	-Related Disorder NOS
	Cannabis
305.20	Abuse
304.30	Dependence
292.89	-Induced Anxiety Disorder
	-Induced Psychotic Disorder
292.11	With Delusions
292.12	With Hallucinations
292.89	Intoxication
292.81	Intoxication Delirium
292.9	-Related Disorder NOS
293.89	Catatonic Disorder Due to . . . *[Indicate the General Medical Condition]*
299.10	Childhood Disintegrative Disorder
V71.02	Child or Adolescent Antisocial Behavior
307.22	Chronic Motor or Vocal Tic Disorder
307.45	Circadian Rhythm Sleep Disorder
	Cocaine
305.60	Abuse
304.20	Dependence
292.89	-Induced Anxiety Disorder
292.84	-Induced Mood Disorder
	-Induced Psychotic Disorder
292.11	With Delusions
292.12	With Hallucinations
292.89	-Induced Sexual Dysfunction
292.89	-Induced Sleep Disorder

(continued)

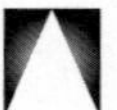

Table 9.1–2 (Continued)

292.89	Intoxication
292.81	Intoxication Delirium
292.9	-Related Disorder NOS
292.0	Withdrawal
294.9	Cognitive Disorder NOS
307.9	Communication Disorder NOS
	Conduct Disorder
312.81	Childhood-Onset Type
312.82	Adolescent-Onset Type
312.89	Unspecified Type
300.11	Conversion Disorder
301.13	Cyclothymic Disorder
293.0	Delirium Due to ... *[Indicate the General Medical Condition]*
780.09	Delirium NOS
297.1	Delusional Disorder
	Dementia Due to Creutzfeldt-Jakob Disease
294.10*	Without Behavioral Disturbance
294.11*	With Behavioral Disturbance
	Dementia Due to Head Trauma
294.10*	Without Behavioral Disturbance
294.11*	With Behavioral Disturbance
	Dementia Due to HIV Disease
294.10*	Without Behavioral Disturbance
294.11*	With Behavioral Disturbance
	Dementia Due to Huntington's Disease
294.10*	Without Behavioral Disturbance
294.11*	With Behavioral Disturbance
	Dementia Due to Parkinson's Disease
294.10*	Without Behavioral Disturbance
294.11*	With Behavioral Disturbance
	Dementia Due to Pick's Disease
294.10*	Without Behavioral Disturbance
294.11*	With Behavioral Disturbance
	Dementia Due to . . . *[Indicate Other General Medical Condition]*
294.10*	Without Behavioral Disturbance
294.11*	With Behavioral Disturbance
294.8	Dementia NOS
	Dementia of the Alzheimer's Type, With Early Onset
294.10*	Without Behavioral Disturbance
294.11*	With Behavioral Disturbance
	Dementia of the Alzheimer's Type, With Late Onset
294.10*	Without Behavioral Disturbance
294.11*	With Behavioral Disturbance
301.6	Dependent Personality Disorder
300.6	Depersonalization Disorder
311	Depressive Disorder NOS
315.4	Developmental Coordination Disorder
799.9	Diagnosis Deferred on Axis II
799.9	Diagnosis or Condition Deferred on Axis I
313.9	Disorder of Infancy, Childhood, or Adolescence NOS
315.2	Disorder of Written Expression
312.9	Disruptive Behavior Disorder NOS
300.12	Dissociative Amnesia
300.15	Dissociative Disorder NOS
300.13	Dissociative Fugue
300.14	Dissociative Identity Disorder
302.76	Dyspareunia (Not Due to a General Medical Condition)
307.47	Dyssomnia NOS
300.4	Dysthymic Disorder
307.50	Eating Disorder NOS
787.6	Encopresis, With Constipation and Overflow Incontinence
307.7	Encopresis, Without Constipation and Overflow Incontinence
307.6	Enuresis (Not Due to a General Medical Condition)
302.4	Exhibitionism
315.31	Expressive Language Disorder
	Factitious Disorder
300.19	With Combined Psychological and Physical Signs and Symptoms
300.19	With Predominantly Physical Signs and Symptoms
300.16	With Predominantly Psychological Signs and Symptoms
300.19	Factitious Disorder NOS
307.59	Feeding Disorder of Infancy or Early Childhood
625.0	Female Dyspareunia Due to... *[Indicate the General Medical Condition]*
625.8	Female Hypoactive Sexual Desire Disorder Due to ... *[Indicate the General Medical Condition]*
302.73	Female Orgasmic Disorder
302.72	Female Sexual Arousal Disorder
302.81	Fetishism
302.89	Frotteurism
	Gender Identity Disorder
302.85	in Adolescents or Adults
302.6	in Children
302.6	Gender Identity Disorder NOS
300.02	Generalized Anxiety Disorder
	Hallucinogen
305.30	Abuse
304.50	Dependence
292.89	-Induced Anxiety Disorder
292.84	-Induced Mood Disorder
	-Induced Psychotic Disorder
292.11	With Delusions
292.12	With Hallucinations
292.89	Intoxication
292.81	Intoxication Delirium
292.89	Persisting Perception Disorder
292.9	-Related Disorder NOS
301.50	Histrionic Personality Disorder
307.44	Hypersomnia Related to ... *[Indicate the Axis I or Axis II Disorder]*
302.71	Hypoactive Sexual Desire Disorder
300.7	Hypochondriasis
313.82	Identity Problem
312.30	Impulse-Control Disorder NOS
	Inhalant
305.90	Abuse
304.60	Dependence
292.89	-Induced Anxiety Disorder
292.84	-Induced Mood Disorder
292.82	-Induced Persisting Dementia
	-Induced Psychotic Disorder
292.11	With Delusions
292.12	With Hallucinations
292.89	Intoxication
292.81	Intoxication Delirium
292.9	-Related Disorder NOS
307.42	Insomnia Related to ... *[Indicate the Axis I or Axis II Disorder]*
312.34	Intermittent Explosive Disorder
312.32	Kleptomania
315.9	Learning Disorder NOS
	Major Depressive Disorder, Recurrent
296.36	In Full Remission
296.35	In Partial Remission
296.31	Mild
296.32	Moderate
296.33	Severe Without Psychotic Features
296.34	Severe With Psychotic Features
296.30	Unspecified
	Major Depressive Disorder, Single Episode
296.26	In Full Remission
296.25	In Partial Remission
296.21	Mild

(continued)

Table 9.1–2 (Continued)

Code	Diagnosis
296.22	Moderate
296.23	Severe Without Psychotic Features
296.24	Severe With Psychotic Features
296.20	Unspecified
608.89	Male Dyspareunia Due to ...*[Indicate the General Medical Condition]*
302.72	Male Erectile Disorder
607.84	Male Erectile Disorder Due to ... *[Indicate the General Medical Condition]*
608.89	Male Hypoactive Sexual Desire Disorder Due to ... *[Indicate the General Medical Condition]*
302.74	Male Orgasmic Disorder
V65.2	Malingering
315.1	Mathematics Disorder
	Medication-Induced
333.90	Movement Disorder NOS
333.1	Postural Tremor
293.9	Mental Disorder NOS Due to ... *[Indicate the General Medical Condition]*
319	Mental Retardation, Severity Unspecified
317	Mild Mental Retardation
315.32	Mixed Receptive-Expressive Language Disorder
318.0	Moderate Mental Retardation
293.83	Mood Disorder Due to ... *[Indicate the General Medical Condition]*
296.90	Mood Disorder NOS
301.81	Narcissistic Personality Disorder
347	Narcolepsy
V61.21	Neglect of Child
995.52	Neglect of Child *(if focus of attention is on victim)*
	Neuroleptic-Induced
333.99	Acute Akathisia
333.7	Acute Dystonia
332.1	Parkinsonism
333.82	Tardive Dyskinesia
333.92	Neuroleptic Malignant Syndrome
	Nicotine
305.1	Dependence
292.9	-Related Disorder NOS
292.0	Withdrawal
307.47	Nightmare Disorder
V71.09	No Diagnosis on Axis II
V71.09	No Diagnosis or Condition on Axis I
V15.81	Noncompliance With Treatment
300.3	Obsessive-Compulsive Disorder
301.4	Obsessive-Compulsive Personality Disorder
V62.2	Occupational Problem
	Opioid
305.50	Abuse
304.00	Dependence
292.84	-Induced Mood Disorder
	-Induced Psychotic Disorder
292.11	With Delusions
292.12	With Hallucinations
292.89	-Induced Sexual Dysfunction
292.89	-Induced Sleep Disorder
292.89	Intoxication
292.81	Intoxication Delirium
292.9	-Related Disorder NOS
292.0	Withdrawal
313.81	Oppositional Defiant Disorder
625.8	Other Female Sexual Dysfunction Due to ... *[Indicate the General Medical Condition]*
608.89	Other Male Sexual Dysfunction Due to ... *[Indicate the General Medical Condition]*
	Other (or Unknown) Substance
305.90	Abuse
304.90	Dependence
292.89	-Induced Anxiety Disorder
292.81	-Induced Delirium
292.84	-Induced Mood Disorder
292.83	-Induced Persisting Amnestic Disorder
292.82	-Induced Persisting Dementia
	-Induced Psychotic Disorder
292.11	With Delusions
292.12	With Hallucinations
292.89	-Induced Sexual Dysfunction
292.89	-Induced Sleep Disorder
292.89	Intoxication
292.9	-Related Disorder NOS
292.0	Withdrawal
	Pain Disorder
307.89	Associated With Both Psychological Factors and a General Medical Condition
307.80	Associated With Psychological Factors
	Panic Disorder
300.21	With Agoraphobia
300.01	Without Agoraphobia
301.0	Paranoid Personality Disorder
302.9	Paraphilia NOS
307.47	Parasomnia NOS
V61.20	Parent-Child Relational Problem
V61.10	Partner Relational Problem
312.31	Pathological Gambling
302.2	Pedophilia
310.1	Personality Change Due to ... *[Indicate the General Medical Condition]*
301.9	Personality Disorder NOS
299.80	Pervasive Developmental Disorder NOS
V62.89	Phase of Life Problem
	Phencyclidine (or Phencyclidine-Like)
305.90	Abuse
304.60	Dependence
292.89	-Induced Anxiety Disorder
292.84	-Induced Mood Disorder
	-Induced Psychotic Disorder
292.11	With Delusions
292.12	With Hallucinations
292.89	Intoxication
292.81	Intoxication Delirium
292.9	-Related Disorder NOS
315.39	Phonological Disorder
V61.12	Physical Abuse of Adult (if by partner)
V62.83	Physical Abuse of Adult (if by person other than partner)
995.81	Physical Abuse of Adult *(if focus of attention is on victim)*
V61.21	Physical Abuse of Child
995.54	Physical Abuse of Child *(if focus of attention is on victim)*
307.52	Pica
304.80	Polysubstance Dependence
309.81	Posttraumatic Stress Disorder
302.75	Premature Ejaculation
307.44	Primary Hypersomnia
307.42	Primary Insomnia
318.2	Profound Mental Retardation
316	Psychological Factor Affecting Medical Condition
	Psychotic Disorder Due to ... *[Indicate the General Medical Condition]*
293.81	With Delusions
293.82	With Hallucinations
298.9	Psychotic Disorder NOS
312.33	Pyromania
313.89	Reactive Attachment Disorder of Infancy or Early Childhood
315.00	Reading Disorder
V62.81	Relational Problem NOS
V61.9	Relational Problem Related to a Mental Disorder or General Medical Condition
V62.89	Religious or Spiritual Problem
299.80	Rett's Disorder

(continued)

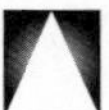

Table 9.1–2
(Continued)

307.53	Rumination Disorder	302.79	Sexual Aversion Disorder
295.70	Schizoaffective Disorder	302.9	Sexual Disorder NOS
301.20	Schizoid Personality Disorder Schizophrenia	302.70	Sexual Dysfunction NOS
295.20	Catatonic Type	302.83	Sexual Masochism
295.10	Disorganized Type	302.84	Sexual Sadism
295.30	Paranoid Type	297.3	Shared Psychotic Disorder
295.60	Residual Type	V61.8	Sibling Relational Problem
295.90	Undifferentiated Type		Sleep Disorder Due to . . . *[Indicate the General Medical Condition]*
295.40	Schizophreniform Disorder		
301.22	Schizotypal Personality Disorder	780.54	Hypersomnia Type
	Sedative, Hypnotic, or Anxiolytic	780.52	Insomnia Type
305.40	Abuse	780.59	Mixed Type
304.10	Dependence	780.59	Parasomnia Type
292.89	-Induced Anxiety Disorder	307.46	Sleep Terror Disorder
292.84	-Induced Mood Disorder	307.46	Sleepwalking Disorder
292.83	-Induced Persisting Amnestic Disorder	300.23	Social Phobia
292.82	-Induced Persisting Dementia	300.81	Somatization Disorder
	-Induced Psychotic Disorder	300.82	Somatoform Disorder NOS
292.11	With Delusions	300.29	Specific Phobia
292.12	With Hallucinations	307.3	Stereotypic Movement Disorder
292.89	-Induced Sexual Dysfunction	307.0	Stuttering
292.89	-Induced Sleep Disorder	307.20	Tic Disorder NOS
292.89	Intoxication	307.23	Tourette's Disorder
292.81	Intoxication Delirium	307.21	Transient Tic Disorder
292.9	-Related Disorder NOS	302.3	Transvestic Fetishism
292.0	Withdrawal	312.39	Trichotillomania
292.81	Withdrawal Delirium	300.82	Undifferentiated Somatoform Disorder
313.23	Selective Mutism	300.9	Unspecified Mental Disorder (nonpsychotic)
309.21	Separation Anxiety Disorder	306.51	Vaginismus (Not Due to a General Medical Condition)
318.1	Severe Mental Retardation		
V61.12	Sexual Abuse of Adult (if by partner)		Vascular Dementia
V62.83	Sexual Abuse of Adult (if by person other than partner)	290.40	Uncomplicated
995.83	Sexual Abuse of Adult *(if focus of attention is on victim)*	290.41	With Delirium
		290.42	With Delusions
V61.21	Sexual Abuse of Child	290.43	With Depressed Mood
995.53	Sexual Abuse of Child *(if focus of attention is on victim)*	302.82	Voyeurism

*ICD-9-CM code valid after October 1, 2000.

the sections of the book that follow and include discussion, epidemiology, etiology, diagnosis, comorbidity, differential diagnosis, clinical features, and treatment. In this section, only a brief description of the disorder is provided to give the reader an overview of psychiatric classification.

Disorders Usually First Diagnosed in Infancy, Childhood, or Adolescence

The section of disorders grouped here are included based on the age that they are usually first diagnosed rather than shared phenomenological features. DSM-IV-TR notes that this separation is for convenience only, and it does not indicate a clear distinction between these disorders and the others in the manual.

Mental Retardation. Mental retardation is characterized by significant, below average intelligence (as demonstrated by a score below 70 on a standardized, individually administered, intelligence test) and impairment in adaptive functioning in at least two areas. *Adaptive functioning* refers to how effective individuals are in achieving age-appropriate common demands of life in areas such as communication, self-care, and interpersonal skills.

Learning Disorders. The three specific learning disorders (reading, mathematics, and written expression) are diagnosed when performance on standardized achievement tests are substantially below expectations based on age, education, and intelligence, and these learning problems cause significant impairment in functioning. Learning disorders can be comorbid with mild mental retardation if the achievement is below that expected based on intelligence level.

Motor Skills Disorder. Analogous to learning disorders, developmental coordination disorder is diagnosed when motor coordination is substantially below expectations based on age and intelligence, and when the coordination problem significantly interferes with functioning. Examples include delays in achieving developmental milestones, such as crawling or walking; dropping things; and poor sports performance.

Communication Disorders. The four specific communication disorders (expressive language disorder, mixed receptive-expressive language disorder, phonological disorder, and stuttering) are characterized by speech or language difficulties. The diagnosis of expressive and mixed receptive-expressive language disorders depends on standardized testing (similar to mental retardation and learning disorders), whereas the two articulation disorders do not.

Pervasive Developmental Disorders. The four specific pervasive developmental disorders (autistic disorder, Rett syndrome, childhood disintegrative disorder, and Asperger syndrome) are characterized by severe difficulties in multiple developmental areas, including social relatedness, communication, and range of activity and interests. The diagnostic criteria for the social interaction deficits and repetitive

Table 9.1–3
ICD-10 Classification of Mental Disorders with ICD Codes

F00 to F09	**Organic, including symptomatic, mental disorders**
F00	Dementia in Alzheimer's disease
F00.0	Dementia in Alzheimer's disease with early onset
F00. 1	Dementia in Alzheimer's disease with late onset
F00.2	Dementia in Alzheimer's disease, atypical or mixed type
F00.9	Dementia in Alzheimer's disease, unspecified
F01	Vascular dementia
F01.0	Vascular dementia of acute onset
F01.1	Multiinfarct dementia
F01.2	Subcortical vascular dementia
F01.3	Mixed cortical and subcortical vascular dementia
F01 .8	Other vascular dementia
F01 .9	Vascular dementia, unspecified
F02	Dementia in other diseases classified elsewhere
F02.0	Dementia in Pick's disease
F02.1	Dementia in Creutzfeldt-Jakob disease
F02.2	Dementia in Huntington's disease
F02.3	Dementia in Parkinson's disease
F02.4	Dementia in human immunodeficiency virus (HIV) disease
F02.8	Dementia in other specified diseases classified elsewhere
F03	Unspecified dementia
A fifth character may be added to specify dementia in F00 to F03, as follows:	
.x0	Without additional symptoms
.x1	Other symptoms, predominantly delusional
.x2	Other symptoms, predominantly hallucinatory
.x3	Other symptoms, predominantly depressive
.x4	Other mixed symptoms
F04	Organic amnestic, syndrome, not induced by alcohol and other psychoactive substances
F05	Delirium, not induced by alcohol and other psychoactive substances
F05.0	Delirium, not superimposed on dementia, so described
F05.1	Delirium, superimposed on dementia
F05.8	Other delirium
F05.9	Delirium, unspecified
F06	Other mental disorders due to brain damage and dysfunction and to physical disease
F06.0	Organic hallucinosis
F06.1	Organic catatonic disorder
F06.2	Organic delusional (schizophrenia-like) disorder
F06.3	Organic mood (affective) disorders
.30	Organic manic disorder
.31	Organic bipolar disorder
.32	Organic depressive disorder
.33	Organic mixed affective disorder
F06.4	Organic anxiety disorder
F06.5	Organic dissociative disorder
F06.6	Organic emotionally labile (asthenic) disorder
F06.7	Mild cognitive disorder
F06.8	Other specified mental disorders due to brain damage and dysfunction and to physical disease
F06.9	Unspecified mental disorder due to brain damage and dysfunction and to physical disease
F07	Personality and behavioral disorders due to brain disease, damage, and dysfunction
F07.0	Organic personality disorder
F07.1	Postencephalitic syndrome
F07.2	Postconcussional syndrome
F07.8	Other organic personality and behavioral disorders due to brain disease, damage, and dysfunction
F07.9	Unspecified organic personality and behavioral disorder due to brain disease, damage, and dysfunction
F09	Unspecified organic or symptomatic mental disorder
F10 to F19	**Mental and behavioral disorders due to psychoactivc substance use**
F10.—	Mental and behavioral disorders due to use of alcohol
F11.—	Mental and behavioral disorders due to use of opioids
F12.—	Mental and behavioral disorders due to use of cannabinoids
F13.—	Mental and behavioral disorders due to use of sedatives or hypnotics
F14.—	Mental and behavioral disorders due to use of cocaine
F15.—	Mental and behavioral disorders due to use of other stimulants, including caffeine
F16.—	Mental and behavioral disorders due to use of hallucinogens
F17.—	Mental and behavioral disorders due to use of tobacco
F18.—	Mental and behavioral disorders due to use of volatile solvents
F19.—	Mental and behavioral disorders due to multiple drug use and use of other psychoactive substances
Four- and five-character categories may be used to specify the clinical conditions, as follows:	
F1x.0	Acute intoxication
.00	Uncomplicated
.01	With trauma or other bodily injury
.02	With other medical complications
.03	With delirium
.04	With perceptual distortions
.05	With coma
.06	With convulsions
.07	Pathological intoxication
F1x.1	Harmful use
F1x.2	Dependence syndrome
.20	Currently abstinent
.21	Currently abstinent, but in a protected environment
.22	Currently on a clinically supervised maintenance or replacement regime (controlled dependence)
.23	Currently abstinent, but receiving treatment with aversive or blocking drugs
.24	Currently using the substance (active dependence)
.25	Continuous use
.26	Episodic use (dipsomania)
F1x.3	Withdrawal state
.30	Uncomplicated
.31	Convulsions
F1x.4	Withdrawal state with delirium
.40	Without convulsions
.41	With convulsions

(*continued*)

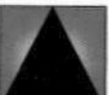

Table 9.1–3 (Continued)

Code	Description
F1x.5	Psychotic disorder
.50	Schizophrenia-like
.51	Predominantly delusional
.52	Predominantly hallucinatory
.53	Predominantly polymorphic
.54	Predominantly depressive symptoms
.55	Predominantly manic symptoms
.56	Mixed
F1x.6	Amnestic syndrome
F1x.7	Residual and late-onset psychotic disorder
.70	Flashbacks
.71	Personality or behavior disorder
.72	Residual affective disorder
.73	Dementia
.74	Other persisting cognitive impairment
.75	Late-onset psychotic disorder
F1x.8	Other mental and behavioral disorders
F1x.9	Unspecified mental and behavioral disorder
F20 to F29	**Schizophrenia and schizotypal and delusional disorders**
F20	Schizophrenia
F20.0	Paranoid schizophrenia
F20.1	Hebephrenic schizophrenia
F20.2	Catatonic schizophrenia
F20.3	Undifferentiated schizophrenia
F20.4	Postschizophrenic depression
F20.5	Residual schizophrenia
F20.6	Simple schizophrenia
F20.8	Other schizophrenia
F20.9	Schizophrenia, unspecified
A fifth character may be used to classify course:	
.x0	Continuous
.x1	Episodic with progressive deficit
.x2	Episodic with stable deficit
.x3	Episodic remittent
.x4	Incomplete remission
.x5	Complete remission
.x8	Other
.x9	Period of observation less than 1 year
F21	Schiztotypal disorder
F22	Persistent delusional disorders
F22.0	Delusional disorder
F22.8	Other persistent delusional disorders
F22.9	Persistent delusional disorder, unspecified
F23	Acute and transient psychotic disorders
F23.0	Acule polymorphic psychotic disorder without symptoms of schizophrenia
F23.1	Acute polymorphic psychotic disorder with symptoms of schizophrenia
F23.2	Acute schizophrenia-like psychotic disorder
F23.3	Other acute predominantly delusional psychotic disorders
F23.8	Other acute transient psychotic disorders
F23.9	Acute and transient psychotic disorders unspecified
A fifth character may be used to identify the presence or absence of associated acute stress:	
.x0	Without associated acute stress
.x1	With associated acute stress
F24	Induced delusional disorder
F25	Schizoaffective disorders
F25.0	Schizoaffective disorder, manic type
F25.1	Schizoaffective disorder, depressive type
F25.2	Schizoaffective disorder, mixed type
F25.8	Other Schizoaffective disorders
F25.9	Schizoaffective disorder, unspecified
F28	Other nonorganic psychotic disorders
F29	Unspecified nonorganic psychosis
F30 to F39	**Mood (affective) disorders**
F30	Manic episode
F30.0	Hypomania
F30.1	Mania without psychotic symptoms
F30.2	Mania with psychotic symptoms
F30.8	Other manic episodes
F30.9	Manic episode, unspecified
F31	Bipolar affective disorder
F31.0	Bipolar affective disorder, current episode hypomanic
F31.1	Bipolar affective disorder, current episode manic without psychotic symptoms
F31.2	Bipolar affective disorder, current episode manic with psychotic symptoms
F31.3	Bipolar affective disorder, current episode mild or moderate depression
.30	Without somatic symptoms
.31	With somatic symptoms
F31.4	Bipolar affective disorder, current episode severe depression without psychotic symptoms
F31.5	Bipolar affective disorder, current episode severe depression with psychotic symptoms
F31.6	Bipolar affective disorder, current episode mixed
F31.7	Bipolar affective disorder, currently in remission
F31.8	Other bipolar affective disorders
F31.9	Bipolar affective disorder, unspecified
F32	Depressive episode
F32.0	Mild depressive episode
.00	Without somatic symptoms
.01	With somatic symptoms
F32.1	Moderate depressive episode
.10	Without somatic symptoms
.11	With somatic symptoms
F32.2	Severe depressive episode without psychotic symptoms
F32.3	Severe depressive episode with psychotic symptoms
F32.8	Other depressive episodes
F32.9	Depressive episode, unspecified
F33	Recurrent depressive disorder
F33.0	Recurrent depressive disorder, current episode mild
.00	Without somatic symptoms
.00	With somatic symptoms
F33.1	Recurrent depressive disorder, current episode moderate
.10	Without somatic symptoms
.11	With somatic symptoms
F33.2	Recurrent depressive disorder, current episode severe without psychotic symptoms
F33.3	Recurrent depressive disorder, current episode severe with psychotic symptoms

(continued)

Table 9.1–3
(Continued)

F33.4	Recurrent depressive disorder, currently in remission
F33.8	Other recurrent depressive disorders
F33 9	Recurrent depressive disorder, unspecified
F34	Persistent mood (affective) disorders
F34.0	Cyclothymia
F34.1	Dysthymia
F34.8	Other persistent mood (affective) disorders
F34.9	Persistent mood (affective) disorder, unspecified
F38	Older mood (affective) disorders
F38.0	Other single mood (affective) disorders
.00	Mixed affective episode
F38.1	Other recurrent mood (affective) disorders
.10	Recurrent brief depressive disorder
F38.8	Other specified mood (affective) disorders
F39	Unspecified mood (affective) disorder
F40 to F48	**Neurotic stress-related and somatoform disorders**
F40	Phobic anxiety disorders
F40.0	Agoraphobia
.00	Without panic disorder
.01	With panic disorder
F40.1	Social phobias
F40.2	Specific (isolated) phobias
F40.8	Other phobic anxiety disorders
F40.9	Phohic anxiety disorder, unspecified
F41	Other anxiety disorders
F41.0	Panic disorder (episodic paroxysmal anxiety)
F41.1	Generalized anxiety disorder
F41.2	Mixed anxiety and depressive disorder
F41.3	Other mixed anxiety disorders
F41.8	Other specified anxiety disorders
F41.9	Anxiety disorder, unspecified
F42	Obsessive-compulsive disorder
F42.0	Predominantly obsessional thoughts or ruminations
F42.1	Predominantly compulsive acts (obsessional rituals)
F42.2	Mixed obsessional thoughts and acts
F42.8	Other obsessive-compulsive disorders
F42.9	Obsessive-compulsive disorder, unspecified
F43	Reaction to severe stress, and adjustment disorders
F43.0	Acute stress reaction
F43.1	Posttraumatic stress disorder
F43.2	Adjustment disorders
.20	Brief depressive reaction
.21	Prolonged depressive reaction
.22	Mixed anxiety and depressive reaction
.23	With predominant disturbance of other emotions
.24	With predominant disturbance of conduct
.25	With mixed disturbance of emotions and conduct
.28	With other specified predominant symptoms
F43.8	Other reactions to severe stress
F43.9	Reaction to severe stress, unspecified
F44	Dissociative (conversion) disorders
F44.0	Dissociative amnesia
F44.1	Dissociative fugue
F44.2	Dissociative stupor
F44.3	Trance and possession disorders
F44.4	Dissociative motor disorders
F44.5	Dissociative convulsions
F44.6	Dissociative anesthesia and sensory loss
F44.7	Mixed dissociative (conversion) disorders
F44.8	Other dissociative (conversion) disorders
.80	Ganser syndrome
.81	Multiple personality disorder
.82	Transient dissociative (conversion) disorders occurring in childhood and adolescence
.88	Other specified dissociative (conversion) disorders
F44.9	Dissociative (conversion) disorder, unspecified
F45	Somatoform disorders
F45.0	Somatization disorder
F45.1	Undifferentiated somatoform disorder
F45.2	Hypochondriacal disorder
F45.3	Somatoform autonomic dysfunction
.30	Heart and cardiovascular system
.31	Upper gastrointestinal tract
.32	Lower gastrointestinal tract
.33	Respiratory system
.34	Genitourinary system
.38	Other organ or system
F45.4	Persistent somatoform pain disorder
F45.8	Other somatoform disorders
F45.9	Somatoform disorder, unspecified
F48	Other neurotic disorders
F48.0	Neurasthenia
F48.1	Depersonalization-derealization syndrome
F48.8	Other specified neurotic disorders
F48.9	Neurotic disorder, unspecified
F50 to F59	**Behavioral syndromes associated with physiological disturbances and physical factors**
F50	Eating disorders
F50.0	Anorexia nervosa
F50.l	Atypical anorexia nervosa
F50.2	Bulimia nervosa
F50.3	Atypical bulimia nervosa
F50.4	Overeating associated with other psychological disturbances
F50.5	Vomiting associated with other psychological disturbances
F50.8	Other eating disorders
F50.9	Eating disorder, unspecified
F51	Nonorganic sleep disorders
F51.0	Nonorganic insomnia
F51.1	Nonorganic hypersomnia
F51.2	Nonorganic disorder of the sleep-wake schedule
F51.3	Sleepwalking (somnambulism)
F51.4	Sleep terrors (night terrors)
F51.5	Nightmares
F51.8	Other nonorganic sleep disorders
F51.9	Nonorganic sleep disorder, unspecified
F52	Sexual dysfunction, not caused by organic, disorder or disease
F52.0	Lack or loss of sexual desire
F52.1	Sexual aversion and lack of sexual enjoyment
.10	Sexual aversion
.11	Lack of sexual enjoyment
F52.2	Failure of genital response

(*continued*)

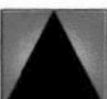

Table 9.1–3 (Continued)

Code	Description
F52.3	Orgasmic dysfunction
F52.4	Premature ejaculation
F52.5	Nonorganic vaginismus
F52.6	Nonorganic dyspareunia
F52.7	Excessive sexual drive
F52.8	Other sexual dysfunction, not caused by organic disorder or disease
F52.9	Unspecified sexual dysfunction, not caused by organic disorder or disease
F53	Mental and behavioral disorders associated with the puerperium, not elsewhere classified
F53.0	Mild mental and behavioral disorders associated with the puerperium, not elsewhere classified
F53.1	Severe mental and behavioral disorders associated with the puerperium, not elsewhere classified
F53.8	Other mental and behavioral disorders associated with the puerperium, not elsewhere classified
F53.9	Puerperal mental disorder, unspecified
F54	Psychological and behavioral factors associated with disorders or diseases classified elsewhere
F55	Abuse of non-dependence-producing substances
F55.0	Antidepressants
F55.1	Laxatives
F55.2	Analgesics
F55.3	Antacids
F55.4	Vitamins
F55.5	Steroids or hormones
F55.6	Specific herbal or folk remedies
F55.8	Other substances that do not produce dependence
F55.9	Unspecified
F59	Unspecified behavioral syndromes associated with physiological disturbances and physical factors
F60 to F69	**Disorders of adult personality and behavior**
F60	Specific personality disorders
F60.0	Paranoid personality disoider
F60.1	Schizoid personality disorder
F60.2	Dissocial personality disorder
F60.3	Emotionally unstable personality disorder
.30	Impulsive type
.31	Borderline type
F60.4	Histrionic personality disorder
F60.5	Anankastic personality disorder
F60.6	Anxious (avoidant) personality disorder
F60.7	Dependent personality disorder
F60.8	Other specific personality disorders
F60.9	Personality disorder, unspecified
F61	Mixed and other personality disorders
F61.0	Mixed personality disorders
F61.1	Troublesome personality changes
F62	Enduring personality changes, not attributable to brain damage and disease
F62.0	Enduring personality change after catastrophic experience
F62.1	Enduring personality change after psychiatric illness
F62.8	Other enduring personality changes
F62.9	Enduring personality change, unspecified
F63	Habit and impulse disorders
F63.0	Pathological gambling
F63.1	Pathological fire-setting (pyromania)
F63.2	Pathological stealing (kleptomania)
F63.3	Trichotillomania
F63.8	Other habit and impulse disorders
F63.9	Habit and impulse disorder, unspecified
F64	Gender identity disorders
F64.0	Transsexualism
F64.1	Dual-role transvestism
F64.2	Gender identity disorder of childhood
F64.8	Other gender identity disorders
F64.9	Gender identity disorder, unspecified
F65	Disorders of sexual preference
F65.0	Fetishism
F65.1	Fetishistic transvestism
F65.2	Exhibitionism
F65.3	Voyeurism
F65.4	Pedophilia
F65.5	Sadomasochism
F65.6	Multiple disorders or sexual preference
F65.8	Other disorders of sexual preference
F65.9	Disorder of sexual preference, unspecified
F66	Psychological and behavioral disorders associated with sexual development and orientation
F66.0	Sexual maturation disorder
F66.1	Ego-dystonic sexual orientation
F66.2	Sexual relationship disorder
F66.8	Other psychosexual development disorders
F66.9	Psychosexual development disorder, unspecified
A fifth character may be used to indicate association with:	
.x0	Heterosexuality
.x1	Homosexuality
.x2	Bisexuality
.x8	Other, including, prepubertal
F68	Other disorders of adult personality and behavior
F68.0	Elaboration of physical symptoms for psychological reasons
F68.1	Intentional production or feigning of symptoms or disabilities, physical or psychological (factitious disorder)
F68.8	Other specified disorders of adult personality and behavior
F69	Unspecified disorder of adult personality and behavior
F70 to F79	**Mental retardation**
F70	Mild mental retardation
F71	Moderate mental retardation
F72	Severe mental retardation
F73	Profound mental retardation
F78	Other mental retardation
F79	Unspecified mental retardation
A fourth character may be used to specify the extent of associated behavioral impairment:	
F7x.0	No, or minimal, impairment of behavior
F7x.1	Significant impairment of behavior requiring attention or treatment
F7X.8	Other impairments of behavior
F7x.9	Without mention of impairment of behavior
F80 to F89	**Disorders of psychological development**
F80	Specific development disorders of speech and language

(continued)

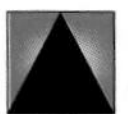

Table 9.1–3 (Continued)

Code	Disorder
F80.0	Specific speech articulation disorder
F80.1	Expressive language disorder
F80.2	Receptive language disorder
F80.3	Acquired aphasia with epilepsy (Landau-Kleffner syndrome)
F80.8	Other developmental disorders of speech and language
F80.9	Developmental disorder of speech and language, unspecified
F81	Specific developmental disorders of scholastic skills
F81.0	Specific reading disorder
F81.1	Specific spelling disorder
F81.2	Specific disorder of arithmetic skills
F81.3	Mixed disorder of scholastic skills
F81.8	Other developmental disorders of scholastic skills
F81.9	Developmental disorder of scholastic skills, unspecified
F82	Specific developmental disorder of motor function
F83	Mixed specific developmental disorders
F84	Pervasive developmental disorders
F84.0	Childhood autism
F84.1	Atypical autism
F84.2	Rett's syndrome
F84.3	Other childhood disintegrative disorder
F84.4	Overactive disorder associated with mental retardation and stereotyped movements
F84.5	Asperger's syndrome
F84.8	Other pervasive developmental disorders
F84.9	Pervasive developmental disorder, unspecified
F88	Other disorders of psychological development
F89	Unspecified disorder of psychological development
F90 to F98	**Behavioral and emotional disorders with onset usually occurring in childhood and adolescence**
F90	Hyperkinetic disorders
F90.0	Disturbance of activity and attention
F90.1	Hyperkinetic conduct disorder
F90.8	Other hyperkinetic disorders
F90.9	Hyperkinetic disorder, unspecified
F91	Conduct disorders
F91.0	Conduct disorder confined to the family context
F91.1	Unsocialized conduct disorder
F91.2	Socialized conduct disorder
F91.3	Oppositional defiant disorder
F91.8	Other conduct disorders
F91.9	Conduct disorder, unspecified
F92	Mixed disorders of conduct and emotions
F92.0	Depressive conduct disorder
F92.8	Other mixed disorders of conduct and emotions
F92.9	Mixed disorder of conduct and emotions, unspecified
F93	Emotional disorders with onset specific to childhood
F93.0	Separation anxiety disorder of childhood
F93.1	Phobic anxiety disorder of childhood
F93.2	Social anxiety disorder of childhood
F93.3	Sibling rivalry disorder
F93.8	Other chilhood emotional disorders
F93.9	Childhood emotional disorder, unspecified
F94	Disorders of social functioning with onset specific to childhood and adolescence
F94.0	Elective mutism
F94.1	Reactive attachment disorder of childhood
F94.2	Disinhibited attachment disorder of childhood
F94.8	Other childhood disorders of social functioning
F94.9	Childhood disorders of social functioning, unspecified
F95	Tic disorders
F95.0	Transient tic disorder
F95.1	Chronic motor or vocal tic disorder
F95.2	Combined vocal and multiple motor tic disorder (Tourette's syndrome)
F95.8	Other tic disorders
F95.9	Tic disorder, unspecified
F98	Other behavioral and emotional disorders with onset usually occurring in childhood and adolescence
F98.0	Nonorganic enuresis
F98.1	Nonorganic encopresis
F98.2	Feeding disorder of infancy and childhood
F98.3	Pica of infancy and childhood
F98.4	Stereotyped movement disorders
F98.5	Stuttering (stammering)
F98.6	Cluttering
F98.8	Other specified behavioral and emotional disorders with onset usually occurring in childhood and adolescence
F98.9	Unspecified behavioral and emotional disorders with onset usually occurring in childhood and adolescence
F99	Unspecified mental disorder

From World Health Organization: *The ICD-10 Classification of Mental and Behavioral Disorders; Clinical Descriptions and Diagnostic Guidelines.* Geneva: World Health Organization; 1992, with permission.

and stereotypical patterns of behavior and interests are identical for autistic disorder and Asperger syndrome. They differ in that communication deficits are required to diagnose autistic disorder and are absent in Asperger syndrome.

Attention-Deficit/Hyperactivity Disorder (ADHD).

Since the 1990s, ADHD has been one of the most frequently discussed psychiatric disorders in the lay media because of the sometimes unclear line between age-appropriate normal and disordered behavior and because of the concern that children without the disorder are being so diagnosed and treated with medication. The central feature of the disorder is persistent inattention or hyperactivity and impulsivity, or both, that cause clinically significant impairment in functioning.

Conduct Disorder. Conduct disorder, the childhood precursor of antisocial personality disorder, is characterized by a behavior pattern in which age-appropriate societal norms and rules are violated (e.g., aggression toward people and animals, destruction of property, deceitfulness or theft, serious violation of rules).

Oppositional Defiant Disorder. Oppositional defiant disorder is characterized by an ongoing pattern of negativistic, defiant, disobedient, and hostile behavior toward authority figures. Because many of the features of oppositional defiant disorder occur in children who do not have the disorder (e.g., deliberate annoyance of others and refusal to comply with adults' requests), DSM-IV-TR includes a note in the diagnostic criteria that a criterion is met only when the behavior occurs more

Table 9.1–4
Groups of Conditions in DSM-IV-TR

Disorders usually first diagnosed in infancy, childhood, or adolescence
Delirium, dementia, amnestic, and other cognitive disorders
Mental disorders due to a general medical condition
Substance-related disorders
Schizophrenia and other psychotic disorders
Mood disorders
Anxiety disorders
Somatoform disorders
Factitious disorders
Dissociative disorders
Sexual and gender identity disorders
Eating disorders
Sleep disorders
Impulse-control disorders not elsewhere classified
Adjustment disorders
Personality disorders
Other conditions that may be a focus of clinical attention

Diagnostic and Statistical Manual of Mental Disorders, 4th ed., text rev.

frequently than that of other children of the same age and developmental level.

Pica. *Pica* refers to persistent eating of nonnutritive substances, such as dirt, paint, plaster, sand, and pebbles, that is inappropriate to developmental level and cultural practice.

Rumination Disorder. The core feature of rumination disorder is the repeated regurgitation and rechewing of food after a period of normal food consumption. The diagnosis is excluded if a specific general medical condition, such as pyloric stenosis or esophageal reflux, accounts for the symptoms.

Feeding Disorder of Infancy or Early Childhood. Feeding disorder of infancy or early childhood, sometimes referred to as *failure to thrive*, is characterized by weight loss or a failure to make expected weight gain in an infant or young child because of inadequate food intake.

Tic Disorders. The three specific tic disorders (Tourette syndrome, chronic motor or vocal tic disorder, and transient tic disorder) are characterized by "sudden, rapid, recurrent, nonrhythmic, stereotyped motor movements or vocalization." The three disorders are distinguished in terms of chronicity (Tourette syndrome and chronic tic disorder are of at least 12 months in duration; transient tic disorder is of at least 1 month in duration but less than 12 months in duration) and range of tics (Tourette syndrome has motor and vocal tics; chronic tic disorder has motor or vocal tics; and transient tic disorder has motor or vocal tics, or both).

Elimination Disorders. The two specific elimination disorders (encopresis and enuresis) are characterized by repeated inappropriate passing of feces or urine, whether voluntary or involuntary.

Separation Anxiety Disorder. Separation anxiety disorder is characterized by excessive anxiety about separation from home or attachment figures beyond that expected for the child's developmental level.

Selective Mutism. Selective mutism is characterized by persistent refusal to speak in specific situations in which speaking is expected, despite the demonstration of speaking ability in other situations.

Reactive Attachment Disorder of Infancy or Early Childhood. Reactive attachment disorder of infancy or early childhood is characterized by one of two patterns of developmentally inappropriate social relatedness—excessively inhibited or disinhibited attachments—because of grossly pathological caregiving.

Stereotypic Movement Disorder. The core feature of stereotypic movement disorder is "repetitive, seemingly driven, nonfunctional motor behavior," such as body rocking, hand-waving, head-banging, self-biting, and other self-mutilating behaviors.

Delirium, Dementia, and Amnestic and Other Cognitive Disorders

The disorders in this section previously were included in a section entitled "Organic Mental Syndromes and Disorders." The term *organic mental disorder* is not used in DSM-IV-TR, because it incorrectly implies that other disorders in other sections of the manual do not have an organic basis.

Delirium. Delirium is characterized by a relatively rapid onset of problems in attention associated with memory impairment, disorientation, language impairment, hallucinations, or illusions. DSM-IV-TR presents separate discussions and criteria for delirium caused by a general medical condition, substance intoxication, or substance withdrawal, although the core features of impaired attention and cognitive deficits are the same across disorders. Delirium superimposed on a preexisting vascular dementia is classified as dementia with delirium.

Dementia. Dementia is characterized by memory impairment and one or more other cognitive impairments (aphasia, apraxia, agnosia, and executive functioning dysfunction). DSM-IV-TR distinguishes between five types (Alzheimer's disease, vascular, caused by other general medical condition, substance-induced, and towing to multiple etiologies). Alzheimer's dementia and dementia caused by a general medical condition are subtyped according to the presence or absence of clinically significant behavioral disturbances.

Amnestic Disorder. Amnestic disorder is characterized by clinically significant memory impairment, similar to dementia, but without the other cognitive impairments that define dementia. Two specific amnestic disorders are defined—amnestic disorder caused by a general medical condition (which is subtyped as transient or chronic) and substance-induced persisting amnestic disorder.

Mental Disorders Due to a General Medical Condition Not Elsewhere Classified

This section of mental disorders due to a general medical condition not elsewhere classified includes ten disorders are listed (delirium, dementia, amnestic disorder, psychotic disorder, mood disorder, anxiety disorder, sexual dysfunction, sleep disorder, catatonic disorder, and personality change).

Substance-Related Disorders

The term *substance* in DSM-IV-TR includes what are commonly thought of as substances of abuse (alcohol, street drugs), as well as medications and toxins. The disorders described are: dependence, abuse, intoxication with or without delirium, withdrawal with or without delirium, dementia, amnestic disorder, psychosis, mood disorder, anxiety, sexual dysfunction, and sleep disorder. The section is organized according to the 11 specific classes of substances that can cause these disorders (alcohol, amphetamines, caffeine, cannabis, cocaine, hallucinogen, inhalant, nicotine, opioid, phencyclidine [PCP], and sedative-hypnotics). In addition, a group of *other* substances is included for substances such as anabolic steroids, nitrite inhalants, nitrous oxide, and over-the-counter and prescription drugs that are not covered by the 11 specific classes.

There is also a category for polysubstance dependence, which is diagnosed when dependence criteria are met during a 1-year period during which three or more groups of substances are used.

Substance Dependence Disorders. Each of the specific substances, except caffeine, can manifest a dependence syndrome. The criteria for substance dependence cover three major constructs: withdrawal, tolerance, and loss of control over use.

Substance Abuse Disorders. Substance abuse can be diagnosed for each of the specific substances, except caffeine and nicotine. Substance abuse is characterized by a maladaptive pattern of use that results in recurrent psychosocial problems.

Substance-Induced Disorders. The symptoms of many disorders can be produced by substance use; consequently, the differential diagnosis of many psychiatric disorders includes ruling out that it is substance induced. The criteria for diagnosing substance-induced disorders, therefore, are placed in the phenomenologically relevant section to facilitate differential diagnosis, although these disorders are also listed in the substance-related disorders section. For example, the diagnostic criteria for substance-induced mood disorder are included in the mood disorders section to ensure that the clinician considers this potential cause of the presenting symptoms.

Schizophrenia and Other Psychotic Disorders

The section on schizophrenia and other psychotic disorders includes eight specific disorders (schizophrenia, schizophreniform disorder, schizoaffective disorder, delusional disorder, brief psychotic disorder, shared psychotic disorder, psychotic disorder due to a general medical condition, and substance-induced psychotic disorder) in which psychotic symptoms are a prominent feature of the clinical picture. The grouping of disorders in this section was made to facilitate differential diagnosis and not to imply etiological links among those disorders included.

Schizophrenia. Schizophrenia is a chronic disorder in which prominent hallucinations or delusions are usually present. The individual must be ill for at least 6 months, although he or she need not be actively psychotic during all of that time. Three phases of the disorder are defined. The *prodrome phase* refers to deterioration in function before the onset of the active psychotic phase. The *active phase* symptoms (delusions, hallucinations, disorganized speech, grossly disorganized behavior, or negative symptoms such as flat affect, avolition, and alogia) must be present for at least 1 month. The residual phase follows the active phase. The features of the residual and prodromal phases include functional impairment and abnormalities of affect, cognition, and communication. Schizophrenia is subtyped according to the most prominent symptoms present at the time of the evaluation (paranoid, disorganized, catatonic, undifferentiated, and residual types).

Schizophreniform Disorder. Schizophreniform disorder is characterized by the same active phase symptoms of schizophrenia (delusions, hallucinations, disorganized speech, grossly disorganized behavior, or negative symptoms), but it lasts between 1 and 6 months and has no prodromal or residual phase features of social or occupational impairment.

Schizoaffective Disorder. Schizoaffective disorder is also characterized by the same active phase symptoms of schizophrenia (delusions, hallucinations, disorganized speech, grossly disorganized behavior, or negative symptoms), as well as the presence of a manic or depressive syndrome that is not brief relative to the duration of the psychosis. Individuals with schizoaffective disorder, in contrast to a mood disorder with psychotic features, have delusions or hallucinations for at least 2 weeks without coexisting prominent mood symptoms.

Delusional Disorder. Delusional disorder is characterized by nonbizarre delusions (i.e., delusions about situations that could occur in real life, such as infidelity, being followed, or having an illness). The presence of bizarre delusions or the other active phase psychotic symptoms of schizophrenia excludes the diagnosis of delusional disorder.

Brief Psychotic Disorder. Brief psychotic disorder requires the presence of delusions, hallucinations, disorganized speech, grossly disorganized behavior, or catatonic behavior for at least 1 day but less than 1 month. The individual returns to his or her usual level of functioning.

Shared Psychotic Disorder. Shared psychotic disorder, also called *folie à deux*, is characterized by a delusional belief that develops in an individual involved in a close relationship with someone who has an established delusion. The content of the delusion is similar to the content in the person with the established delusion.

Psychotic Disorder Due to a General Medical Condition. Psychotic disorder due to a general medical condition is diagnosed when evidence exists of hallucinations or delusions that are the direct consequence of a general medical condition other than delirium or dementia.

Substance-Induced Psychotic Disorder. Substance-induced psychotic disorder is analogous to psychotic disorder caused by a general medical condition, except the cause of the hallucinations or delusions is substance intoxication, substance withdrawal, or a medication.

Mood Disorders

The section on mood disorders describes the seven specific mood disorders: major depressive disorder; bipolar I disorder; bipolar II disorder; dysthymic disorder; cyclothymic disorder; and mood disorder caused by a general medical condition or by an induced substance.

Major Depressive Disorder. The necessary feature of major depressive disorder is depressed mood or loss of interest or pleasure in usual activities. All symptoms must be present nearly every day, except suicidal ideation or thoughts of death, which need only be recurrent. The diagnosis is excluded if the symptoms are the result of a normal bereavement and if psychotic symptoms are present in the absence of mood symptoms.

Dysthymic Disorder. Dysthymic disorder is a mild, chronic form of depression that lasts at least 2 years, during which, on most days, the individual experiences depressed mood for most of the day and at least two other symptoms of depression.

Bipolar I Disorder. The necessary feature of bipolar I disorder is a history of a manic or mixed manic and depressive episode. Bipolar I disorder is subtyped in many ways: type of current episode (manic, hypomanic depressed, or mixed), severity and remission status (mild, moderate, severe without psychosis, severe with psychotic features, partial remission, or full remission), and whether the recent course is characterized by rapid cycling (at least four episodes in 12 months).

Bipolar II Disorder. Bipolar II disorder is characterized by a history of hypomanic and major depressive episodes. The symptom criteria for a hypomanic episode are the same as those for a manic episode, although hypomania only requires a minimal duration of 4 days. The major difference between mania and hypomania is the severity of the impairment associated with the syndrome.

Cyclothymic Disorder. The bipolar equivalent to dysthymic disorder, cyclothymic disorder is a mild, chronic mood disorder with numerous depressive and hypomanic episodes over the course of at least 2 years.

Mood Disorder Due to a General Medical Condition. Mood disorder caused by a general medical condition is diagnosed when evidence indicates that a significant mood disturbance is the direct consequence of a general medical condition other than delirium.

Substance-Induced Mood Disorder. Substance-induced mood disorder is diagnosed when the cause of the mood disturbance is substance intoxication, withdrawal, or a medication.

Anxiety Disorders

The section on anxiety disorders includes ten specific disorders (panic disorder, agoraphobia, specific phobia, social phobia, obsessive–compulsive disorder [OCD], posttraumatic stress disorder [PTSD], acute stress disorder, generalized anxiety disorder, anxiety disorder caused by a general medical condition, and substance-induced anxiety disorder) in which anxious symptoms are a prominent feature of the clinical picture. The grouping of disorders in this section was made to facilitate differential diagnosis and not to imply etiological links among the disorders in this section. Because separation anxiety disorder occurs in childhood, it is included in the childhood disorders section.

Panic Disorder. A panic attack is characterized by feelings of intense fear or terror that come on out of the blue in situations in which there is nothing to fear and that is accompanied by heart racing or pounding, chest pain, shortness of breath or choking, dizziness, trembling or shaking, feeling faint or lightheaded, sweating, and nausea. Panic disorder is subtyped according to the presence or absence of agoraphobia.

Agoraphobia. Agoraphobia is a frequent consequence of panic disorder, although it can occur in the absence of panic attacks. Individuals with agoraphobia avoid (or try to avoid) situations that they think might trigger a panic attack (or panic-like symptoms) or situations from which they think escape might be difficult if they have a panic attack.

Specific Phobia. Specific phobia is characterized by an excessive, unreasonable fear of specific objects or situations that occurs almost always on exposure to the feared stimulus. The phobic stimulus is avoided, or, when not avoided, the individual feels severely anxious or uncomfortable.

Social Phobia. Social phobia is characterized by the fear of being embarrassed or humiliated in front of others. Similar to specific phobia, and the phobic stimuli are avoided, or, when not avoided, the individual feels severely anxious or uncomfortable. When the phobic stimuli include most social situations, then it is specified as generalized social phobia.

Obsessive–Compulsive Disorder. OCD is characterized by repetitive and intrusive thoughts or images that are unwelcome (obsessions) or repetitive behaviors that the person feels compelled to do (compulsions), or both. Most often, the compulsions are done to reduce the anxiety associated with the obsessive thought.

Posttraumatic Stress Disorder. PTSD occurs after a traumatic event in which the individual believes that he or she is in physical danger or that his or her life is in jeopardy. PTSD can also occur after witnessing a violent or life-threatening event happening to someone else. The symptoms of PTSD usually occur soon after the traumatic event, although, in some cases, the symptoms develop months or even years after the trauma. PTSD is diagnosed when a person reacts to the traumatic event with fear and experiences at least one reexperiencing symptom, three or more symptoms of avoidance, and two or more symptoms of hyperarousal. The symptoms must persist for at least 1 month and cause clinically significant impairment in functioning or distress.

Acute Stress Disorder. Acute stress disorder occurs after the same type of stressors that precipitate PTSD. Acute stress disorder is not diagnosed if the symptoms last beyond 1 month.

Generalized Anxiety Disorder. Generalized anxiety disorder is characterized by chronic excessive worry that occurs more days than not and is difficult to control. The worry is associated with symptoms, such as concentration problems, insomnia, muscle tension, irritability, and physical restlessness, and causes clinically significant distress or impairment.

Anxiety Disorder Due to a General Medical Condition. Anxiety disorder caused by a general medical condition is diagnosed when evidence indicates that significant anxiety is the direct consequence of a general medical condition other than delirium or dementia.

Substance-Induced Anxiety Disorder. Substance-induced anxiety disorder is diagnosed when the cause of the anxiety is substance intoxication, substance withdrawal, or a medication.

Somatoform Disorders

The section on somatoform disorders includes six specific disorders (somatization disorder, undifferentiated somatoform disorder, conversion disorder, pain disorder, hypochondriasis, and body dysmorphic disorder) in which physical symptoms suggestive of a general medical condition, but not accounted for by such a condition, are a prominent feature of the clinical picture.

Somatization Disorder. Somatization disorder is characterized by multiple unexplained medical symptoms in diverse organ systems occurring over several years that are not explained by general medical conditions. The symptoms are grouped into four categories: pain, gastrointestinal (GI), sexual, and pseudoneurological. Symptoms from each group must be present, resulting in functional impairment or treatment, beginning before 30 years of age.

Undifferentiated Somatoform Disorder. Undifferentiated somatoform disorder is a residual category for conditions characterized by unexplained medical symptoms that are not as pervasive and long-lasting as those of somatization disorder.

Conversion Disorder. Conversion disorder is characterized by unexplained voluntary motor or sensory deficits that suggest the presence of a neurological or other general medical condition. Psychological conflict is determined to be responsible for the symptoms.

Pain Disorder. The core feature of pain disorder is impairing or distressing pain that is the primary focus of attention. Psychological factors are determined to have an important role in the onset, severity, or maintenance of the pain.

Hypochondriasis. Hypochondriasis is a distressing and impairing preoccupation with the belief of having a serious illness based on a misinterpretation of physical symptoms. After a thorough medical evaluation rules out the medical illness, the preoccupation remains.

Body Dysmorphic Disorder. Body dysmorphic disorder is a distressing and impairing preoccupation with an imagined or slight defect in appearance. If the belief is held with delusional intensity, then delusional disorder, somatic type, might also be diagnosed.

Factitious Disorder

Factitious disorder refers to the deliberate feigning of physical or psychological symptoms to assume the sick role. Factitious disorder is distinguished from malingering in which symptoms are also falsely reported;

however, the motivation in malingering is external incentives, such as avoidance of responsibility, obtaining financial compensation, or obtaining substances. Factitious disorder is subtyped according to whether the predominant symptoms are psychological, physical, or a mixture of the two.

Dissociative Disorders

The section on dissociative disorders includes four specific disorders (dissociative amnesia, dissociative fugue, dissociative identity disorder, and depersonalization disorder) characterized by a "disruption in the usually integrated functions of consciousness, memory, identity, or perception."

Dissociative Amnesia. Dissociative amnesia is characterized by memory loss of important personal information that is usually traumatic in nature.

Dissociative Fugue. Dissociative fugue is characterized by sudden travel away from home associated with partial or complete memory loss about one's identity.

Dissociative Identity Disorder (Formerly, Multiple Personality Disorder). The essential feature of dissociative identity disorder is the presence of two or more distinct identities that assume control of the individual's behavior.

Depersonalization Disorder. The essential feature of depersonalization disorder is persistent or recurrent episodes of depersonalization (an altered sense of one's physical being, including feeling that one is outside of one's body, physically cut off or distanced from people, floating, observing oneself from a distance, as though in a dream, or that one's body is physically changed in shape or size).

Sexual and Gender Identity Disorders

The section on sexual and gender identity disorders includes three groups of disorders: sexual dysfunctions, paraphilias, and gender identity disorder.

Sexual Dysfunctions. The group of sexual dysfunction disorders is organized on the basis of the phase of sexual response that is affected. Sexual pain disorders are also included in this category. The sexual dysfunction disorders are diagnosed only when they cause marked distress or interpersonal difficulty. The two sexual desire disorders are hypoactive sexual desire disorder (lack of desire for sexual activity) and sexual aversion disorder (active avoidance of sexual contact). The two sexual arousal disorders are female sexual arousal disorder (inability to attain or maintain adequate lubrication until completion of sexual activity) and male erectile disorder (inability to attain or maintain adequate erection until completion of sexual activity). The three orgasmic disorders are female orgasmic disorder, male orgasmic disorder, and premature ejaculation. The two sexual pain disorders are dyspareunia (pain during sexual intercourse) and vaginismus (vaginal spasm interfering with sexual intercourse). Sexual dysfunction caused by a general medical condition and substance-induced sexual dysfunction are also included.

Paraphilias. The characteristic features of paraphilias are recurrent, sexually arousing fantasies, urges, or behaviors lasting at least 6 months and involving nonhuman objects, suffering or humiliation of oneself or one's partner, or children or other nonconsenting partners. DSM-IV-TR includes eight specific paraphilias: exhibitionism (exposure of genitals to strangers), fetishism (use of nonliving objects), frotteurism (touching and rubbing against a nonconsenting person), pedophilia (attraction to children), sexual masochism (suffering pain or humiliation), sexual sadism (causing pain or humiliation to someone else), transvestic fetishism (cross-dressing), and voyeurism (observing unsuspecting individuals).

Gender Identity Disorder. The characteristic feature of gender identity disorder is a persistent discomfort with one's own gender and strong cross-gender identification. Gender identity disorder is subtyped according to the individual's current age, and the subtypes are distinguished by different diagnostic codes.

Eating Disorders

The section on eating disorders includes two specific disorders—anorexia nervosa and bulimia nervosa—that are characterized by abnormal eating behavior. Other disorders of eating that usually are diagnosed in infancy and childhood (i.e., pica, rumination disorder, and feeding disorder of infancy or early childhood) are included in the *Disorders Usually First Diagnosed in Infancy, Childhood, or Adolescence* section.

Anorexia Nervosa. The core feature of anorexia nervosa is a strong fear of gaining weight or becoming fat, resulting in deliberate maintenance of low body weight. Individuals are preoccupied with their weight and body image, and their weight and perceived body shape markedly influence their self-image. Anorexia is subtyped based on whether the individual engages in binge eating or purging behavior (binge eating or purging type) or maintains low weight through restricting food intake or excessive exercise (restricting type).

Bulimia Nervosa. Individuals with bulimia nervosa engage in recurrent binge eating during which they eat an abnormally large amount of food over a short period of time. During the binge, the person feels like he or she cannot control his or her eating. To prevent weight gain from the overeating, the individual engages in compensatory behavior, such as self-induced vomiting, excessive exercise, laxative use, or going on strict diets.

Sleep Disorders

The sleep disorders are divided into four groups based on the presumed cause: primary, or caused by another mental disorder, a general medical condition, or substance use. The sleep disorders are diagnosed only when they cause marked distress or interpersonal difficulty. The primary sleep disorders are subdivided into five dyssomnias (primary insomnia, primary hypersomnia, narcolepsy, breathing-related sleep disorder, and circadian rhythm sleep disorder) and three parasomnias (nightmare disorder, sleep terror disorder, and sleepwalking disorder).

Impulse-Control Disorders Not Elsewhere Classified

Impulse-control disorders not classified elsewhere are characterized by the failure to resist urges to engage in behaviors that are harmful to the individual or to others.

Intermittent Explosive Disorder. Intermittent explosive disorder is characterized by recurrent, discrete, episodes of assaultive and violent behavior that is out of proportion to possible precipitating factors.

Kleptomania. Kleptomania is characterized by repeated stealing of items that are not needed for personal use or for their monetary value. The stealing is not done for the purpose of expressing anger or revenge.

Pyromania. Pyromania is characterized by recurrent setting of fires because of a preoccupation or fascination with fire rather than being done for other purposes such as financial gain, political expression, revenge, or hiding of criminal behavior, which is known as arson.

Pathological Gambling. Pathological gambling is characterized by a maladaptive pattern of gambling behavior. Although classified as an impulse-control disorder, many experts draw parallels between pathological gambling and addictive disorders (i.e., substance use disorders).

Trichotillomania. Trichotillomania is characterized by repeated hair pulling causing noticeable hair loss.

Adjustment Disorders

Adjustment disorders are diagnosed when the person's distress in response to an event is in excess of a normative reaction to the stressor or when the symptoms cause significant impairment in functioning. The adjustment disorders are subtyped according to the predominant symptom picture (depressed mood, anxiety, mixed anxiety and depression, disturbance of conduct, mixed disturbance of emotions and conduct, unspecified).

Personality Disorders

Personality refers to an individual's characteristic pattern of affect, emotional regulation, behavior, motivation, cognition about self, and interactions with others that are long-standing, present since adolescence or early adulthood. Aspects of personality include the way people tend to think about themselves (e.g., self-confident or lacking confidence), how they relate to people (e.g., shy vs. friendly), how they interpret and deal with events in the environment (e.g., paranoid people believe that others are out to get them and may try to attack first before being attacked), and how an individual reacts emotionally to this situation. It is not easy to define a *healthy personality*; in general, however, it allows one to cope with the normal stress of life and to develop and maintain satisfying friendships and intimate relationships. When long-standing patterns of thinking, behaving, and emotional response are rigid, inflexible, and cause significant distress or impairment in functioning, then a DSM-IV-TR personality disorder may be present. DSM-IV-TR includes ten specific personality disorders that are listed below.

Paranoid Personality Disorder. Individuals with paranoid personality disorder are suspicious and distrustful of others. They may think that others do things just to annoy or to hurt them, and they often read hidden threats or put-downs in the comments of others. They may worry that friends or coworkers are not really loyal or trustworthy and are often reluctant to confide in others, because they believe "there is a price to pay" when something personal is shared. Persons with paranoid personality disorder may have problems with anger management. When involved in a relationship, they often worry that their partner is unfaithful.

Schizoid Personality Disorder. Schizoid personality disorder is characterized by lack of emotionality and social relationships. Individuals with schizoid personality disorder are socially isolated, but this does not bother them. They usually prefer to work and do things alone. They are emotionally cold and are neither bothered by criticism from others nor joyful when complimented. Individuals with schizoid personality disorder usually do not get pleasure from many activities and often have little interest in sexual experiences with another person.

Schizotypal Personality Disorder. Individuals with schizotypal personality disorder are odd and eccentric. They may dress, act, or speak in a peculiar manner. They are often suspicious and paranoid and feel anxious in social situations because of their distrust. Because of these beliefs, they have few friends. People with schizotypal personality disorder frequently feel that others are talking about them behind their back and that strangers are taking special notice of them. They may believe in extrasensory perception (ESP), hexes, telepathy, and superstitions more strongly than most people, and their behavior may be influenced by these beliefs.

Antisocial Personality Disorder. Antisocial personality disorder, the adult manifestation of childhood conduct disorder, is characterized by selfish, irresponsible, unlawful, and impulsive behavior that shows a lack of regard for the rights of others. Individuals with antisocial personality disorder often find it easy to lie if it serves their purpose. They lack a conscience and usually do not feel remorseful at having hurt others but instead justify or rationalize their behavior.

Borderline Personality Disorder. Borderline personality disorder is characterized by emotional dysregulation, unstable interpersonal relationships, and unstable self-image. Individuals with borderline personality disorder have strong and intense emotions, often in reaction to how they perceive and believe others are treating them, and these emotions are difficult to control. The moods of the individual with borderline personality disorder are strong and frequently change. Often, they have problems with controlling anger, and anger outbursts are common. Self-destructive behavior is common. Individuals with borderline personality disorder make recurrent suicide attempts, suicide threats, or engage in self-damaging behavior, such as cutting or burning.

Histrionic Personality Disorder. Individuals with histrionic personality disorder are loud, overly emotionally expressive, and attention seeking. They act as if they are on stage and tend not to feel comfortable unless they are the center of attention. They may be flirtatious and sexually seductive and may use physical appearance to get people's attention. They often feel a close bond to someone they have just met and are quick to share personal details of their life with new acquaintances.

Narcissistic Personality Disorder. Individuals with narcissistic personality disorder have too high of an opinion of themselves and little regard for others, except as how others meet their needs. They see themselves as accomplishing great things that establish their superiority over others. They view themselves as special and unique and that only similarly special people could understand them. They have a sense of entitlement, and they often feel that they have earned the right to special treatment or consideration because of who they are or what they have done.

Avoidant Personality Disorder. Avoidant personality disorder is characterized by social inhibition related to low self-esteem and sensitivity to rejection and criticism from others. Individuals with avoidant personality disorder have difficulty making friends and feel uncomfortable in social situations.

Dependent Personality Disorder. Individuals with dependent personality disorder have difficulty with self-sufficiency and have a strong need to be taken care of by others. They often believe that they cannot care for themselves, and, if a close relationship ends, they may be desperate to get into another relationship right away, even if it is not the best person for them.

Obsessive–Compulsive Personality Disorder. Obsessive–compulsive personality disorder is characterized by a pattern of perfectionism, stinginess, stubbornness, orderliness, and inflexibility. Individuals with this disorder frequently are workaholics, who spend so much time working that they have little time for family activities, friendships, or entertainment. Individuals with obsessive–compulsive personality disorder frequently find it difficult to throw things away, even when the object is old and worn and has no sentimental value. They have been called the three "ps": parsimonious, perfectionistic, and punctual.

Other Conditions That May Be a Focus of Clinical Attention

The conditions included in the section are not considered mental disorders, but they may become the focus of clinical attention. There are six major groups: psychological factors affecting medical conditions, medication-induced movement disorders, other medication-induced disorders, relational problems, problems related to abuse or neglect, and other miscellaneous conditions.

Psychological Problems Affecting Medical Conditions. The category of psychological problems affecting medical conditions refers to those situations in which psychological factors negatively affect the course or outcome of a general medical condition or significantly increase the risk of an adverse outcome.

Medication-Induced Movement Disorders. The category of medication-induced movement disorders is included because of its clinical importance in treatment and differential diagnosis. Five of the six specific movement disorders described are related to the use of neuroleptics (neuroleptic-induced parkinsonism, acute dystonia, acute akathisia, tardive dyskinesia, and neuroleptic malignant syndrome). The sixth disorder is medication-induced postural tremor, which is most often associated with antidepressants and mood stabilizers.

Other Medication-Induced Disorders. The category of other medication-induced disorders is included so that clinicians could code medication side effects that are a focus of clinical attention (e.g., severe hypotension, priapism, weight gain, and sexual dysfunction).

Relational Problems. Relational problems that cause significant symptoms or functional impairment are frequently the focus of clinical attention. These problems can be associated with a mental or general medical disorder in one of the members of the relational unit.

Problems Related to Abuse or Neglect. The category of problems related to abuse or neglect includes five problems (physical abuse of child, sexual abuse of child, neglect of child, physical abuse of adult, and sexual abuse of adult) that frequently are the focus of clinical attention.

Other Conditions That May Be a Focus of Clinical Attention. The last group in this class of problems includes a heterogeneous collection of 13 problems that may be the focus of treatment (noncompliance with treatment, malingering, adult antisocial behavior, child or adolescent antisocial behavior, borderline intellectual functioning, age-related cognitive decline, bereavement, academic problem, occupational problem, identity problem, religious or spiritual problem, acculturation problem, and phase of life problem).

Appendix Diagnoses

The DSM-IV-TR contains proposed criteria for 20 specific disorders that were not included in the official classification but are included in an appendix, so that research can be conducted on their reliability, validity, and potential clinical usefulness. Many of these disorders are currently captured by a classification under "not-otherwise-specified (NOS) designations" (e.g., depressive disorder NOS for minor depressive disorder or premenstrual dysphoric disorder). In addition, a separate section on culture-bound syndromes is categorized in DSM-IV-TR.

Postconcussional Disorder. Postconcussional disorder is discussed in Chapter 10, Section 10.5. In ICD-10, it is referred to as *postconcussional syndrome*, which occurs after head trauma that usually is sufficiently severe to result in loss of consciousness. Symptoms include headache, dizziness (usually lacking the features of true vertigo), fatigue, irritability, difficulty concentrating and performing mental tasks, memory impairment, insomnia, and reduced tolerance for stress, emotional excitement, and alcohol abuse.

Mild Neurocognitive Disorder. This condition is discussed in Chapter 10, Section 10.1.

Caffeine Withdrawal. This disorder is covered in Chapter 12, Section 12.4.

Postpsychotic Depressive Disorder of Schizophrenia. This disorder is discussed in Chapter 15, Section 15.3. In ICD-10, postschizophrenic depression is described as follows:

> A depressive episode, which may be prolonged, arising in the aftermath of a schizophrenic illness. Some schizophrenic symptoms must still be present but no longer dominate the clinical picture. These persisting schizophrenic symptoms may be "positive" or "negative," though the latter are more common. It is uncertain, and immaterial to the diagnosis, to what extent the depressive symptoms have merely been uncovered by the resolution of earlier psychotic symptoms (rather than being a new development) or are an intrinsic part of schizophrenia rather than a psychological reaction to it. They are rarely sufficiently severe or extensive to meet criteria for a severe depressive episode, and it is often difficult to decide which of the patient's symptoms are due to depression and which to neuroleptic medication or to the impaired volition and affective flattening of schizophrenia itself. This depressive disorder is associated with an increased risk of suicide.

Simple Deteriorative Disorder. This disorder is covered in Chapter 13 and Chapter 14, Section 14.4. In ICD-10, it is described as an uncommon disorder characterized by oddities of conduct, inability to meet the demands of society, blunting of affect, loss of volition, and social impoverishment. Delusions and hallucinations are not evident.

Minor Depressive Disorder, Recurrent Brief Depressive Disorder, and Premenstrual Dysphoric Disorder. These disorders are covered in Chapter 15, Section 15.3. Minor depressive disorder is associated with comparatively mild symptoms, such as worry and over concern with minor autonomic symptoms (e.g., tremor and palpitations). Most cases never come to medical or psychiatric attention. In ICD-10, recurrent brief depressive disorder is characterized by recurrent episodes of depression, each of which lasts less than 2 weeks (typically 2 to 3 days) and ends with complete recovery.

Mixed Anxiety–Depressive Disorder. This disorder is covered in Chapter 16, Section 16.7. Mixed anxiety and depressive disorder is listed in ICD-10, where it is described as encompassing symptoms of both anxiety and depression, neither of which predominates.

Factitious Disorder by Proxy. This disorder, also known as Munchausen syndrome by proxy, is discussed in Chapter 19. In the disorder, parents feign illness in their children.

Dissociative Trance Disorder. The dissociative disorders are discussed in Chapter 20. ICD-10 lists trance and possession disorders, in which a patient experiences temporary loss of both the sense of personal identity and full awareness of the surroundings. The disorders are involuntary or unwanted. In some cases, patients act as if taken over by another personality, spirit, or force.

Binge-Eating Disorder. This disorder is a variant of bulimia nervosa, which is discussed in Chapter 23, Section 23.2. It consists of recurrent episodes of binge eating without compensatory behavior, such as self-induced vomiting and laxative abuse.

Depressive Personality Disorder and Passive-Aggressive Personality Disorder. These personality disorders are classified in the NOS category of personality disorders. Each is described in Chapter 27.

Culture-Bound Syndromes. An appendix of culturally related syndromes includes the name of each condition, the culture in which it was first described, a brief description of its psychopathology, and a list of possibly related DSM-IV-TR categories. Chapter 14, Section 14.5 includes a discussion of culture-bound syndromes.

The implication of culture and its relation to diagnosis is set forth in DSM-IV-TR as follows:

Diagnostic assessment can be especially challenging when a clinician from one ethnic or cultural group uses the DSM-IV Classification to evaluate an individual from a different ethnic or cultural group. A clinician who is unfamiliar with the nuances of an individual's cultural frame of reference may incorrectly judge as psychopathology those normal variations in behavior, belief, or experience that are particular to the individual's culture. For example, certain religious practices or beliefs (e.g., hearing or seeing a deceased relative during bereavement) may be misdiagnosed as manifestations of a Psychotic Disorder. Applying Personality Disorder criteria across cultural settings may be especially difficult because of the wide cultural variation in concepts of self, styles of communication, and coping mechanisms.

Multiaxial Evaluation

The DSM-IV-TR is a multiaxial system that evaluates patients along several variables and contains five axes. Axis I and Axis II make up the entire classification of mental disorder: 17 major classifications (Tables 9.1–1 and 9.1–4) and more than 300 specific disorders. In many instances, patients have a disorder on both axes. For example, a patient may have major depressive disorder noted on Axis I and obsessive–compulsive personality disorder on Axis II.

Axis I. Axis I consists of clinical disorders and other conditions that may be a focus of clinical attention (Table 9.1–5).

Axis II. Axis II consists of personality disorders and mental retardation (Table 9.1–6). The habitual use of a particular defense mechanism can be indicated on Axis II.

Axis III. Axis III lists any physical disorder or general medical condition that is present in addition to the mental disorder. The physical condition may be causative (e.g., kidney failure causing delirium), the result of a mental disorder (e.g., alcohol gastritis secondary to alcohol dependence), or unrelated to the mental disorder. When a medical condition is causative or causally related to a mental disorder, a mental disorder caused by a general condition is listed on Axis I, and the general medical condition is listed on both Axis I and Axis III. In DSM-IV-TR's example—a case in which hypothyroidism is a direct cause of major depressive disorder—the designation on Axis I is mood disorder due to hypothyroidism with depressive features, and hypothyroidism is listed again on Axis III (Table 9.1–7).

Axis IV. Axis IV is used to code the psychosocial and environmental problems that contribute significantly to the development or exacerbation of the current disorder (Table 9.1–8). The evaluation of stressors is based on a clinician's assessment of the stress that an average person with similar sociocultural values and circumstances would experience from the psychosocial stressors. This judgment is based on the degree of change that the stressor causes in the person's life, the degree to which the event is desired and under the person's control, and the number of stressors. Stressors can be positive (e.g., a job promotion) or negative (e.g., the loss of a loved one). Information about stressors may be important in formulating a treatment plan that includes attempts to remove the psychosocial stressors or to help the patient cope with them.

Axis V. Axis V is a global assessment of functioning (GAF) scale in which clinicians judge patients' overall levels of functioning during a particular time (e.g., at the time of the evaluation or the patient's highest level of functioning for at least a few months during the past year). Functioning is considered a composite of three major areas: social functioning,

Table 9.1–5
DSM-IV-TR Axis I: Clinical Disorders and Other Disorders That May Be a Focus of Clinical Attention

- Disorders usually first diagnosed in infancy, childhood, or adolescence (excluding mental retardation)
- Delirium, dementia, and amnestic and other cognitive disorders
- Mental disorders due to a general medical condition not elsewhere classified
- Substance-related disorders
- Schizophrenia and other psychotic disorders
- Mood disorders
- Anxiety disorders
- Somatoform disorders
- Factitious disorders
- Dissociative disorders
- Sexual and gender identity disorders
- Eating disorders
- Sleep disorders
- Impulse-control disorders not elsewhere classified
- Adjustment disorders
- Other conditions that may be a focus of clinical attention

(From American Psychiatric Association. *Diagnostic and Statistical Manual of Mental Disorders.* 4th ed. Text rev. Washington; DC: American Psychiatric Association; copyright 2000, with permission.)

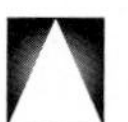

Table 9.1–6
DSM-IV-TR Axis II: Personality Disorders and Mental Retardation

- Paranoid personality disorder
- Schizoid personality disorder
- Schizotypal personality disorder
- Antisocial personality disorder
- Borderline personality disorder
- Histrionic personality disorder
- Narcissistic personality disorder
- Avoidant personality disorder
- Dependent personality disorder
- Obsessive–compulsive personality disorder
- Personality disorder not otherwise specified
- Mental retardation

(From American Psychiatric Association. *Diagnostic and Statistical Manual of Mental Disorders.* 4th ed. Text rev. Washington, DC: American Psychiatric Association; copyright 2000, with permission.)

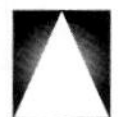

Table 9.1–7
DSM-IV-TR Axis III: ICD-9-CM General Medical Conditions

Infectious and parasitic diseases (001–139)
Neoplasms (140–239)
Endocrine, nutritional, and metabolic diseases and immunity disorders (240–279)
Diseases of the blood and blood-forming organs (280–289)
Diseases of the nervous system and sense organs (320–389)
Diseases of the circulatory system (390–459)
Diseases of the respiratory system (460–519)
Diseases of the digestive system (520–579)
Diseases of the genitourinary system (580–629)
Complications of pregnancy, childbirth, and the puerperium (630–676)
Diseases of the skin and subcutaneous tissue (680–709)
Diseases of the musculoskeletal system and connective tissue (710–739)
Congenital anomalies (740–759)
Certain conditions originating in the perinatal period (760–779)
Symptoms, signs, and ill-defined conditions (780–799)
Injury and poisoning (800–999)

(From American Psychiatric Association. *Diagnostic and Statistical Manual of Mental Disorders.* 4th ed. Text rev. Washington, DC: American Psychiatric Association; copyright 2000, with permission.)

occupational functioning, and psychological functioning. The GAF scale, based on a continuum of mental health and mental illness, is a 100-point scale, 100 representing the highest level of functioning in all areas. Persons who had a high level of functioning before an episode of illness generally have a better prognosis than do those who had a low level of functioning.

Multiaxial Evaluation Report Form. Table 9.1–9 shows the DSM-IV-TR Multiaxial Evaluation Report form. Examples of how to record the results of a DSM-IV-TR multiaxial evaluation are given in Table 9.1–10.

Nonaxial Format. DSM-IV-TR also allows clinicians who do not wish to use the multiaxial format to list the diagnoses serially, with the principal diagnosis listed first (Table 9.1–11).

Severity of Disorder. Depending on the clinical picture and the presence or absence of signs and symptoms and their intensity, a disorder can be mild, moderate, or severe, and it may be in partial or full remission. The following guidelines are used by DSM-IV-TR.

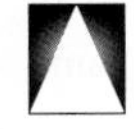

Table 9.1–8
DSM-IV-TR Axis IV: Psychosocial and Environmental Problems

Problems with primary support group
Problems related to the social environment
Educational problems
Occupational problems
Housing problems
Economic problems
Problems with access to health care services
Problems related to interaction with the legal system/crime
Other psychosocial and environmental problems

(From American Psychiatric Association. *Diagnostic and Statistical Manual of Mental Disorders.* 4th ed. Text rev. Washington, DC: American Psychiatric Association; copyright 2000, with permission.)

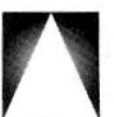

Table 9.1–9
DSM-IV-TR Multiaxial Evaluation Report Form

The following form is offered as one possibility for reporting multiaxial evaluations. In some settings, this form may be used exactly as is; in other settings, the form may be adapted to satisfy special needs.

AXIS I: Clinical Disorders
Other Conditions That May Be a Focus of Clinical Attention
Diagnostic code DSM-IV name
__ __ __.__ __ ____________________
__ __ __.__ __ ____________________
__ __ __.__ __ ____________________

AXIS II: Personality Disorders
Mental Retardation
Diagnostic code DSM-IV name
__ __ __.__ __ ____________________
__ __ __.__ __ ____________________

AXIS III: General Medical Conditions
ICD-9-CM code ICD-9-CM name
__ __ __.__ __ ____________________
__ __ __.__ __ ____________________
__ __ __.__ __ ____________________

AXIS IV: Psychosocial and Environmental Problems
Check:
❑ Problems with primary support group *Specify:* __________
❑ Problems related to the social environment *Specify:* __________
❑ Educational problems *Specify:* __________
❑ Occupational problems *Specify:* __________
❑ Housing problems *Specify:* __________
❑ Economic problems *Specify:* __________
❑ Problems with access to health care services *Specify:* __________
❑ Problems related to interaction with the legal system/crime *Specify:* __________
❑ Other psychosocial and environmental problems *Specify:* __________

AXIS V: Global Assessment of Functioning Scale
Score: __________
Time Frame: __________

(From American Psychiatric Association. *Diagnostic and Statistical Manual of Mental Disorders.* 4th ed. Text rev. Washington, DC: American Psychiatric Association; copyright 2000, with permission.)

MILD. Few, if any, symptoms are present in excess of those required to make the diagnosis and symptoms result in no more than minor impairment in social or occupational functioning.

MODERATE. Symptoms or functional impairment between "mild" and "severe" are present.

SEVERE. Many symptoms are present in excess of those required to make the diagnosis, or several symptoms that are particularly severe are present, or the symptoms result in marked impairment in social or occupational functioning.

IN PARTIAL REMISSION. The full criteria for the disorder were previously met, but currently only some of the symptoms or signs of the disorder remain.

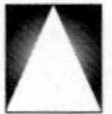

Table 9.1–10
DSM-IV Examples of How to Record the Results of a DSM-IV Multiaxial Evaluation

Example 1:		
Axis I	296.23	Major depressive disorder, single episode, severe without psychotic features
	305.00	Alcohol abuse
Axis II	301.6	Dependent personality disorder Frequent use of denial
Axis III		None
Axis IV		Threat of job loss
Axis V	GAF = 35	(current)
Example 2:		
Axis I	300.4	Dysthymic disorder
	315.00	Reading disorder
Axis II	V71.09	No diagnosis
Axis III	382.9	Otitis media, recurrent
Axis IV		Victim of child neglect
Axis V	GAF = 53	(current)
Example 3:		
Axis I	293.83	Mood disorder due to hypothyroidism, with depressive features
Axis II	V71.09	No diagnosis, histrionic personality features
Axis III	244.9	Hypothyroidism
	365.23	Chronic angle-closure glaucoma
Axis IV		None
Axis V	GAF = 45	(on admission)
	GAF = 65	(at discharge)
Example 4:		
Axis I	V61.1	Partner relational problem
Axis II	V71.09	No diagnosis
Axis III		None
Axis IV		Unemployment
Axis V	GAF = 83	(highest level past year)

(From American Psychiatric Association. *Diagnostic and Statistical Manual of Mental Disorders.* 4th ed. Text rev. Washington, DC: American Psychiatric Association; copyright 2000, with permission.)

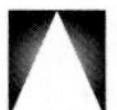

Table 9.1–11
DSM-IV-TR Nonaxial Format

Clinicians who do not wish to use the multiaxial format may simply list the appropriate diagnoses. Those choosing this option should follow the general rule of recording as many coexisting mental disorders, general medical conditions, and other factors that are relevant to the care and treatment of the individual. The principal diagnosis or the reason for visit should be listed first.

The examples below illustrate the reporting of diagnoses in a format that does not use the multiaxial system.

Example 1:	
296.23	Major depressive disorder, single episode, severe without psychotic features
305.00	Alcohol abuse
301.6	Dependent personality disorder Frequent use of denial
Example 2:	
300.4	Dysthymic disorder
315.00	Reading disorder
382.9	Otitis media, recurrent
Example 3:	
293.83	Mood disorder due to hypothyroidism with depressive features
244.9	Hypothyroidism
365.23	Chronic angle-closure glaucoma Histrionic personality features
Example 4:	
V61.1	Partner relational problem

(From American Psychiatric Association. *Diagnostic and Statistical Manual of Mental Disorders.* 4th ed. Text rev. Washington, DC: American Psychiatric Association; copyright 2000, with permission.)

IN FULL REMISSION. No longer are any symptoms or signs of the disorder present, but it is still clinically relevant to note the disorder. The differentiation of *in full remission* from *recovered* requires consideration of many factors, including the characteristic course of the disorder, the length of time since the last period of disturbance, the total duration of the disturbance, and the need for continued evaluation or prophylactic treatment.

Other Criteria

Multiple Diagnoses. When a person has more than one Axis I disorder, the principal diagnosis is indicated by listing it first. According to DSM-IV-TR, the *principal diagnosis* is the condition chiefly responsible for the signs and symptoms of the individual's disorder. It may be difficult in situations of "dual diagnosis" (a substance-related diagnosis such as amphetamine dependence accompanied by a non–substance-related diagnosis such as schizophrenia), which is the principal diagnosis. DSM-IV-TR states: "For example, it may be unclear which diagnosis should be considered 'principal' for an individual hospitalized with both Schizophrenia and Amphetamine Intoxication, because each condition may have contributed equally to the need for admission and treatment."

Provisional Diagnosis. If diagnosis is uncertain, the clinician can write "(Provisional)" following the diagnosis. A person may appear to have major depressive disorder but be unable to give an adequate history to establish that the full criteria are met. The differential diagnosis depends on the duration of illness. For example, DSM-IV-TR states, "a diagnosis of Schizophreniform Disorder requires a duration of less than 6 months and can only be given provisionally if assigned before remission has occurred."

Prior History. For some purposes, noting a prior history of a disorder may be useful. DSM states that a past diagnosis of mental disorder can "be indicated by using the specifier Prior History (e.g., Separation Anxiety Disorder, Prior History, for an individual with a history of Separation Anxiety Disorder who has no current disorder or who currently meets criteria for Panic Disorder)."

Not Otherwise Specified Categories. Each diagnosis has a "not otherwise specified" (NOS) category. According to DSM-IV-TR, an NOS diagnosis may be appropriate (1) either when the symptoms are below the diagnostic threshold for one of the specific disorders or when there is an atypical or mixed presentation, (2) the symptom pattern has not been included in the DSM-IV-TR classification but it causes clinically significant distress or impairment (research criteria for some of these symptom patterns have been included in an appendix), or (3) the cause is uncertain (i.e., whether it is primary or secondary).

References

Cooper R. *Classifying Madness: A Philosophical Examination of the Diagnostic and Statistical Manual of Mental Disorders.* Berlin: Springer; 2005.
Eriksen K, Kress VE. *Beyond the DSM Story: Ethical Quandaries, Challenges, and Best Practices.* Thousand Oaks, CA: Sage Publications, Inc.; 2005.
Gottesman II, Gould TD. The endophenotype concept in psychiatry: Etymology and strategic intentions. *Am J Psychiatry.* 2003;160:636–645.
Jäger M, Bottlender R, Strauss A, Möller HJ. Classification of functional psychoses and its implication for prognosis: Comparison between ICD-10 and DSM-IV. *Psychopathology.* 2004;37:110–117.
Kendell R, Jablensky A. Distinguishing between the validity and utility of psychiatric diagnoses. *Am J Psychiatry.* 2003;160:4–12.
Mayes R, Horwitz AV. DSM-III and the revolution in the classification of mental illness. *J Hist Behav Sci.* 2005;41(3):249–267.
Merikangas KR, Risch N. Will the genomics revolution revolutionize psychiatry? *Am J Psychiatry.* 2003;160:625–635.
Möller HJ. Problems associated with the classification and diagnosis of psychiatric disorders. *World J Biol Psychiatry.* 2005;6:45–56.
Mundt C, Backenstrass M. Psychotherapy and classification: Psychological, psychodynamic, and cognitive aspects. *Psychopathology.* 2005;38: 219–222.
Saules KK. Advancing DSM: Dilemmas in psychiatric diagnosis. *J Nerv Ment Dis.* 2004;192(2):167–169.
Svanborg P, Ekseli L. Self-assessment of DSM-IV criteria for major depression in psychiatric out- and inpatients. *Nordic J Psychiatry.* 2003;57:291–296.
Zimmerman M, Spitzer RL. Psychiatric classification. In: Sadock BJ, Sadock VA, eds. *Kaplan & Sadock's Comprehensive Textbook of Psychiatry.* 8th ed. Vol. 1. Baltimore: Lippincott Williams & Wilkins; 2005:1003.

▲ 9.2 Psychiatric Rating Scales

Many different questionnaires, interviews, checklists, outcome assessments, and other instruments are used by psychiatrists and mental health professionals to aid in treatment planning by helping to establish a diagnosis, identify comorbid conditions, and assess levels of functioning. They are collectively called *psychiatric rating scales* or *rating instruments* and hundreds of them have been developed, some better than others.

It is important to realize that rating scales are not a panacea. They can provide erroneous measurements because of difficulties in administration or limitations in the construct of the scale itself. Ideally, they aid clinicians by helping them to confirm their diagnoses or clarify their thinking in ambiguous situations. They also can provide a baseline for follow-up of the progress of an illness over time or in response to specific interventions. This is particularly useful in the conduct of psychiatric research.

Characteristics of Rating Scales

Rating scales can be specific or comprehensive, and they can measure both internally experienced variables (e.g., mood) and externally observable variables (e.g., behavior). Specific scales measure discrete thoughts, moods, or behaviors, such as obsessive thoughts and temper tantrums; comprehensive scales measure broad abstractions, such as depression and anxiety.

Signs and Symptoms. Classic items from the mental status examination are the most frequently assessed items on rating scales. These items include thought disorders, mood disturbances, and gross behaviors. Rating scales also cover the assessment of adverse effects from psychotherapeutic drugs. Social adjustments (e.g., occupational success and quality of relationships) and psychoanalytic concepts (e.g., ego strength and defense mechanisms) are also measured by some rating scales, although the reliability and the validity of such scales are lowered by the absence of agreed-on norms, the high level of inference required on some items, and the lack of independence between measures.

Other Characteristics. Other characteristics of rating scales include the time covered, the level of judgment required, and the method of recording answers. The time covered by a rating scale must be specified, and the rate must adhere to this period. For example, a particular rating scale may rate a 5-minute observation period, a week-long period, or a patient's entire life.

The most reliable rating scales require a limited amount of judgment or inference on the part of the rater. Whatever the level of judgment required, clear definitions of the answer scale, preferable with clinical examples, should be provided by the developer of the scale and should be read by the rater.

The actual answer given can be recorded as either a dichotomous variable (e.g., true or false, present or absent) or a continuous variable. Continuous items may ask the rater to choose a term to describe the severity (absent, slight, mild, moderate, severe, or extreme) or frequency (never, rarely, occasionally, often, very often, or always). Although many psychiatric symptoms are thought of as existing in dichotomous states—for example, the presence or absence of delusions—most experienced clinicians know that the world is not so simple. Most psychiatric signs and symptoms can occur in normal persons under certain conditions (e.g., hallucinations can occur in normal persons who are sleep deprived).

Rating Scales Used in DSM-IV-TR

Rating scales form an integral part of *Diagnostic and Statistical Manual of Mental Disorders*, 4th ed, text revision (DSM-IV-TR). The rating scales used are broad and measure the overall severity of a patient's illness.

Global Assessment of Functioning (GAF) Scale. Axis V in DSM-IV-TR uses the GAF scale (Table 9.2–1). This axis is used to report a clinician's judgment of a patient's overall level of functioning. The information is used to decide on a treatment plan and later to measure the plan's effect.

Social and Occupational Functioning Assessment Scale (SOFAS). This scale can be used to track a patient's progress in social and occupational areas (Table 9.2–2). It is independent of the psychiatric diagnosis and the severity of the patient's psychological symptoms.

Global Assessment of Relational Functioning (GARF). This scale measures the overall functioning of a family or other ongoing relationship. It is an important measurement because the development of mental illness is higher in dysfunctional families and recovery is slower in the absence of a supportive social network (Table 9.2–3).

Defensive Functioning Scale (DFS). This scale covers the defense mechanisms used by the patient to cope with stressors. Humor, suppression, anticipation, and sublimation are

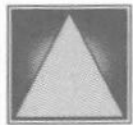

Table 9.2–1
Global Assessment of Functioning (GAF) Scale

Consider psychological, social, and occupational functioning on a hypothetical continuum of mental health–illness. Do not include impairment in functioning due to physical (or environmental) limitations.

Code	(**Note:** Use intermediate codes when appropriate, e.g., 45, 68, 72.)
100–91	Superior functioning in a wide range of activities, life's problems never seem to get out of hand, is sought out by others because of his or her many positive qualities. No symptoms.
90–81	Absent or minimal symptoms (e.g., mild anxiety before an exam), good functioning in all areas, interested and involved in a wide range of activities, socially effective, generally satisfied with life, no more than everyday problems or concerns (e.g., an occasional argument with family members).
80–71	If symptoms are present, they are transient and expectable reactions to psychosocial stressors (e.g., difficulty concentrating after family argument): no more than slight impairment in social, occupational, or school functioning (e.g., temporarily falling behind in schoolwork).
70–61	Some mild symptoms (e.g., depressed mood and mild insomnia) OR some difficulty in social, occupational, or school functioning (e.g., occasional truancy, or theft within the household), but generally functioning pretty well, has some meaningful interpersonal relationships.
60–51	Moderate symptoms (e.g., flat affect and circumstantial speech, occasional panic attacks) OR moderate difficulty in social, occupational, or school functioning (e.g., few friends, conflicts with peers or coworkers).
50–41	Serious symptoms (e.g., suicidal ideation, severe obsessional rituals, frequent shoplifting) OR any serious impairment in social, occupational, or school functioning (e.g., no friends, unable to keep a job).
40–31	Some impairment in reality testing or communication (e.g., speech is at times illogical, obscure, or irrelevant) OR major impairment in several areas, such as work or school, family relations, judgment, thinking, or mood (e.g., depressed man avoids friends, neglects family, and is unable to work; child frequently beats up younger children, is defiant at home, and is failing at school).
30–21	Behavior is considerably influenced by delusions or hallucinations OR serious impairment in communication or judgment (e.g., sometimes incoherent, acts grossly inappropriately, suicidal preoccupation) OR inability to function in almost all areas (e.g., stays in bed all day; no job, home, or friends).
20–11	Some danger of hurting self or others (e.g., suicide attempts without clear expectation of death, frequently violent, manic excitement) OR occasionally fails to maintain minimal personal hygiene (e.g., smears feces) OR gross impairment in communication (e.g., largely incoherent or mute).
10–1	Persistent danger of severely hurting self or others (e.g., recurrent violence) OR persistent inability to maintain minimal personal hygiene OR serious suicidal act with clear expectation of death.
0	Inadequate information.

The GAF Scale is a revision of the GAS (Endicott J, Spitzer RL, Fleiss JL, Cohen I. The Global Assessment Scale: a procedure for measuring overall severity of psychiatric disturbance. *Arch Gen Psychiatry.* 1976;33:766) and CGAS (Shaffer D, Gould MS, Brasio J, et al. Children's Global Assessment Scale (CGAS). *Arch Gen Psychiatry.* 1983;40:1228). They are revisions of the Global Scale of the Health-Sickness Rating Scale (Luborsky I. Clinicians' judgments of mental health. *Arch Gen Psychiatry.* 1962;7:407).

(From American Psychiatric Association. *Diagnostic and Statistical Manual of Mental Disorders,* 4th ed. Text rev. Washington, DC: American Psychiatric Association; copyright 2000, with permission.)

among the healthiest defense mechanisms. Denial, acting-out, projection, and projective identification are some of the most pathological (Table 9.2–4).

Other Scales

Brief Psychiatric Rating Scale (BPRS). This is a short scale used to measure the severity of psychiatric symptomotology. It has been used for decades as an outcome measure in treatment studies of schizophrenia. It is most useful for patients with fairly significant impairment. See Table 9.2–5.

Hamilton Rating Scales for Depression and Anxiety (HAM-D and HAM-A). These rating scales are used to monitor the severity of depression and anxiety and are scored from 0 to 4 with total scored of above 9 considered the borderline of pathology. The scales are useful to measure the effects of treatment, particularly with pharmacologic agents (Tables 9.2–6 and 9.2–7).

Scales for the Assessment of Positive Symptoms (SAPS) and Assessment of Negative Symptoms (SANS). These scales are designed to measure negative and positive symptoms in schizophrenia. They are primarily used in research to measure change induced by psychopharmacologic agents over the course of treatment (Tables 9.2–8 and 9.2–9).

Positive and Negative Syndrome Scale (PANSS). This scale also measures negative and positive symptoms of schizophrenia and other psychotic disorders. It has become the standard tool of assessing clinical outcome in treatment studies of schizophrenia.

Table 9.2–2
Social and Occupational Functioning Assessment Scale (SOFAS)

Consider social and occupational functioning on a continuum from excellent functioning to grossly impaired functioning. Include impairments in functioning due to physical limitations, as well as those due to mental impairments. To be counted, impairment must be a direct consequence of mental and physical health problems; the effects of lack of opportunity and other environmental limitations are not to be considered.

Code	(**Note:** Use intermediate codes when appropriate, e.g., 45, 68, 72.)
100–91	Superior functioning in a wide range of activities.
90–81	Good functioning in all areas, occupationally and socially effective.
80–71	No more than a slight impairment in social, occupational, or school functioning (e.g., infrequent interpersonal conflict, temporarily falling behind in schoolwork).
70–61	Some difficulty in social, occupational, or school functioning, but generally functioning well, has some meaningful interpersonal relationships.
60–51	Moderate difficulty in social, occupational, or school functioning (e.g., few friends, conflicts with peers or coworkers).
50–41	Serious impairment in social, occupational, or school functioning (e.g., no friends, unable to keep a job).
40–31	Major impairment in several areas, such as work or school, family relations (e.g., depressed man avoids friends, neglects family, and is unable to work; child frequently beats up younger children, is defiant at home, and is failing at school).
30–21	Inability to function in almost all areas (e.g., stays in bed all day; no job, home, or friends).
20–11	Occasionally fails to maintain minimal personal hygiene; unable to function independently.
10–1	Persistent inability to maintain minimal personal hygiene. Unable to function without harming self or others or without considerable external support (e.g., nursing care and supervision).
0	Inadequate information.

Note: The rating of overall psychological functioning on a scale of 0–100 was operationalized by Luborsky in the Health-Sickness Rating Scale. (Luborsky L. Clinicians' judgments of mental health. *Arch Gen Psychiatry*. 1962;7:407). Spitzer and colleagues developed a revision of the Health-Sickness Rating Scale called the Global Assessment Scale (GAS) (Endicott J, Spitzer RL, Fleiss JL, et al. The Global Assessment Scale: a procedure for measuring overall severity of psychiatric disturbance. *Arch Gen Psychiatry*. 1976;33:766). The SOFAS is derived from the GAS and its development is described in Goldman HH, Skodol AE, Lave TR. Revising Axis V for DSM-IV: a review of measures of social functioning. *Am J Psychiatry*. 1992;149:1148.

(From American Psychiatric Association. *Diagnostic and Statistical Manual of Mental Disorders*. 4th ed. Text rev. Washington, DC: American Psychiatric Association; copyright 2000, with permission.)

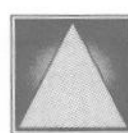

Table 9.2–3
Global Assessment of Relational Functioning (GARF)

INSTRUCTIONS: The GARF Scale can be used to indicate an overall judgment of the functioning of a family or other ongoing relationship on a hypothetical continuum ranging from competent, optimal relational functioning to a disrupted, dysfunctional relationship. It is analogous to Axis V (Global Assessment of Functioning Scale) provided for individuals in DSM-IV. The GARF Scale permits the clinician to rate the degree to which a family or other ongoing relational unit meets the affective and/or instrumental needs of its members in the following areas:

A. *Problem solving*—skills in negotiating goals, rules, and routines: adaptability to stress; communication skills; ability to resolve conflict.

B. *Organization*—maintenance of interpersonal roles and subsystem boundaries; hierarchical functioning, coalitions and distribution of power, control and responsibility.

C. *Emotional climate*—tone and range of feelings; quality of caring, empathy, involvement and attachment/commitment; sharing of values; mutual affective responsiveness, respect, and regard; quality of sexual functioning.

In most instances, the GARF Scale should be used to rate functioning during the current period (i.e., the level of relational functioning at the time of the evaluation). In some settings, the GARF Scale may also be used to rate functioning for other time periods (i.e., the highest level of relational functioning for at least a few months during the past year). **Note:** Use specific, intermediate codes when possible, for example, 45, 68, 72. If detailed information is not adequate to make specific ratings, use midpoints of the five ranges, that is, 90, 70, 50, 30, or 10. **(81–100) Overall:** Relational unit is functioning satisfactorily from self-report of participants and from perspectives of observers.

Agreed-on patterns or routines exist that help meet the usual needs of each family/couple member; there is flexibility for change in response to unusual demands or events; occasional conflicts and stressful transitions are resolved through problem-solving communication and negotiation.

There is a shared understanding and agreement about roles and appropriate tasks; decision making is established for each functional area, and there is recognition of the unique characteristics and merit of each subsystem (e.g., parents/spouses, siblings, and individuals).

There is a situationally appropriate, optimistic atmosphere in the family; a wide range of feelings is freely expressed and managed within the family; there is a general atmosphere of warmth, caring, and sharing of values among all family members. Sexual relations of adult members are satisfactory.

(61–80) Overall: Functioning of relational unit is somewhat unsatisfactory. Over a period of time, many but not all difficulties are resolved without complaints.

Daily routines are present but there is some pain and difficulty in responding to the unusual. Some conflicts remain unresolved, but do not disrupt family functioning.

(*continued*)

Table 9.2–3 (Continued)

Decision making is usually competent, but efforts at control of one another quite often are greater than necessary or are ineffective. Individuals and relationships are clearly demarcated but sometimes a specific subsystem is depreciated or scapegoated.

A range of feeling is expressed, but instances of emotional blocking or tension are evident. Warmth and caring are present but are marred by a family member's irritability and frustrations. Sexual activity of adult members may be reduced or problematic.

(41–60) Overall: Relational unit has occasional times of satisfying and competent functioning together, but clearly dysfunctional, unsatisfying relationships tend to predominate.

Communication is frequently inhibited by unresolved conflicts that often interfere with daily routines; there is significant difficulty in adapting to family stress and transitional change.

Decision making is only intermittently competent and effective; either excessive rigidity or significant lack of structure is evident at these times. Individual needs are quite often submerged by a partner or coalition.

Pain or ineffective anger or emotional deadness interferes with family enjoyment. Although there is some warmth and support for members, it is usually unequally distributed. Troublesome sexual difficulties between adults are often present.

(21–40) Overall: Relational unit is obviously and seriously dysfunctional; forms and time periods of satisfactory relating are rare.

Family/couple routines do not meet the needs of members; they are grimly adhered to or blithely ignored. Life cycle changes, such as departures or entries into the relational unit, generate painful conflict and obviously frustrating failures of problem solving.

Decision making is tyrannical or quite ineffective. The unique characteristics of individuals are unappreciated or ignored by either rigid or confusingly fluid coalitions.

There are infrequent periods of enjoyment of life together; frequent distancing or open hostility reflect significant conflicts that remain unresolved and quite painful. Sexual dysfunction among adult members is commonplace.

(1–20) Overall: Relational unit has become too dysfunctional to retain continuity of contact and attachment.

Family/couple routines are negligible (e.g., no mealtime, sleeping, or waking schedule); family members often do not know where others are or when they will be in or out; there is little effective communication among family members.

Family/couple members are not organized in such a way that personal or generational responsibilities are recognized. Boundaries of relational unit as a whole and subsystems cannot be identified or agreed upon. Family members are physically endangered or injured or sexually attacked.

Despair and cynicism are pervasive; there is little attention to the emotional needs of others; there is almost no sense of attachment, commitment, or concern about one another's welfare.

0 Inadequate information.

(From American Psychiatric Association. *Diagnostic and Statistical Manual of Mental Disorders.* 4th ed. Text rev. Washington, DC: American Psychiatric Association; copyright 2000, with permission.)

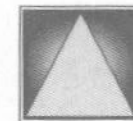

Table 9.2–4 Defensive Functioning Scale

High adaptive level. This level of defensive functioning results in optimal adaptation in the handling of stressors. These defenses usually maximize gratification and allow the conscious awareness of feelings, ideas, and their consequences. They also promote an optimum balance among conflicting motives. Examples of defenses characteristically at this level are

- anticipation
- affiliation
- altruism
- humor
- self-assertion
- self-observation
- sublimation
- suppression

Mental inhibitions (compromise formation) level. Defensive functioning at this level keeps potentially threatening ideas, feelings, memories, wishes, or fears out of awareness. Examples are

- displacement
- dissociation
- intellectualization
- isolation of affect
- reaction formation
- repression
- undoing

Minor image-distorting level. This level is characterized by distortions in the image of the self, body, or others that may be employed to regulate self-esteem. Examples are

- devaluation
- idealization
- omnipotence

Disavowal level. This level is characterized by keeping unpleasant or unacceptable stressors, impulses, ideas, affect, or responsibility out of awareness with or without a misattribution of these to external causes. Examples are

- denial
- projection
- rationalization

Major image-distorting level. This level is characterized by gross distortion or misattribution of the image of self or others. Examples are

- autistic fantasy
- projective identification
- splitting of self-image or image of others

Action level. This level is characterized by defensive functioning that deals with internal or external stressors by action or withdrawal. Examples are

- acting out
- apathetic withdrawal
- help-rejecting complaining
- passive aggression

Level of defensive dysregulation. This level is characterized by failure of defensive regulation to contain the individual's reaction to stressors, leading to a pronounced break with objective reality. Examples are

- delusional projection
- psychotic denial
- psychotic distortion

(From American Psychiatric Association. *Diagnostic and Statistical Manual of Mental Disorders.* 4th ed. Text rev. Washington, DC: American Psychiatric Association; copyright 2000, with permission.)

Table 9.2–5
Brief Psychiatric Rating Scale

DIRECTIONS: Place an X in the appropriate box to represent the level of severity of each symptom.
PATIENT ______________________
RATER ______________________
NO. ______________________
DATE ______________________

	Not present = 0 0	Very mild = 1 1	Mild = 2 2	Moderate = 3 3	Mod. severe = 4 4	Severe = 5 5	Extremely severe = 6 6
1. Somatic concern—preoccupation with physical health, fear of physical illness, hypochondriases	❑	❑	❑	❑	❑	❑	❑
2. Anxiety—worry, fear, overconcern for present or future	❑	❑	❑	❑	❑	❑	❑
3. Emotional withdrawal—lack of spontaneous interaction, isolation, deficiency in relating to others	❑	❑	❑	❑	❑	❑	❑
4. Conceptual disorganization—thought processes confused, disconnected, disorganized, disrupted	❑	❑	❑	❑	❑	❑	❑
5. Guilt feelings—self-blame, shame, remorse for past behavior	❑	❑	❑	❑	❑	❑	❑
6. Tension—physical and motor manifestations or nervousness, overactivation, tension	❑	❑	❑	❑	❑	❑	❑
7. Mannerisms and posturing—peculiar, bizarre, unnatural motor behavior (not including tic)	❑	❑	❑	❑	❑	❑	❑
8. Grandiosity—exaggerated self-opinion, arrogance, conviction of unusual power or abilities	❑	❑	❑	❑	❑	❑	❑
9. Depressive mood—sorrow, sadness, despondency, pessimism	❑	❑	❑	❑	❑	❑	❑
10. Hostility—animosity, contempt, belligerence, disdain for others	❑	❑	❑	❑	❑	❑	❑
11. Suspiciousness—mistrust, belief that others harbor malicious or discriminatory intent	❑	❑	❑	❑	❑	❑	❑
12. Hallucinatory behavior—perceptions without normal external stimulus correspondence	❑	❑	❑	❑	❑	❑	❑
13. Motor retardation—slowed, weakened movements or speech, reduced body tone	❑	❑	❑	❑	❑	❑	❑
14. Uncooperativeness—resistance, guardedness, rejection of authority	❑	❑	❑	❑	❑	❑	❑
15. Unusual thought content—unusual, odd, strange, bizarre thought content	❑	❑	❑	❑	❑	❑	❑
16. Blunted affect—reduced emotional tone, reduction in normal intensity of feelings, flatness	❑	❑	❑	❑	❑	❑	❑
17. Excitement—heightened emotional tone, agitation, increased reactivity	❑	❑	❑	❑	❑	❑	❑
18. Disorientation—confusion or lack of proper association for person, place, or time	❑	❑	❑	❑	❑	❑	❑

(Courtesy of John E. Overall, Ph.D.)

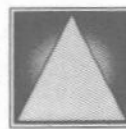

Table 9.2–6
Hamilton Anxiety Rating Scale

Instructions: This checklist is to assist the physician or psychiatrist in evaluating each patient as to his degree of anxiety and pathological condition. Please fill in the appropriate rating:

NONE = 0 MILD = 1 MODERATE = 2 SEVERE = 3 SEVERE, GROSSLY DISABLING = 4

Item		Rating	Item		Rating
Anxious	Worries, anticipation of the worst, fearful anticipation, irritability	______	Somatic (sensory)	Tinnitus, blurring of vision, hot and cold flushes, feelings of weakness, picking sensation	______
Tension	Feelings of tension, fatigability, startle response, moved to tears easily, trembling, feelings of restlessness, inability to relax	______	Cardiovascular symptoms	Tachycardia, palpitations, pain in chest, throbbing of vessels, fainting feelings, missing beat	______
Fears	Of dark, of strangers, of being left alone, of animals, of traffic, of crowds	______	Respiratory symptoms	Pressure or constriction in chest, choking feelings, sighing, dyspnea	______
Insomnia	Difficulty in falling asleep, broken sleep, unsatisfying sleep and fatigue on waking, dreams, nightmares, night-terrors	______	Gastrointestinal symptoms	Difficulty in swallowing, wind, abdominal pain, burning sensations, abdominal fullness, nausea, vomiting, borborygmi, looseness of bowels, loss of weight, constipation	______
Intellectual (cognitive)	Difficulty in concentration, poor memory	______	Genitourinary symptoms	Frequency of micturition, urgency of micturition, amenorrhea, menorrhagia, development of frigidity, premature ejaculation, loss of libido, impotence	______
Depressed mood	Loss of interest, lack of pleasure in hobbies, depression, early waking, diurnal swing	______	Autonomic symptoms	Dry mouth, flushing, pallor, tendency to sweat, giddiness, tension headache, raising of hair	______
Somatic (muscular)	Pains and aches, twitching, stiffness, myoclonic jerks, grinding of teeth, unsteady voice, increased muscular tone	______	Behavior at interview	Fidgeting, restlessness or pacing, tremor of hands, furrowed brow, strained face, sighing or rapid respiration, facial pallor, swallowing, belching, brisk tendon jerks, dilated pupils, exophthalmos	______

ADDITIONAL COMMENTS

Investigator's signature:

(From Hamilton M. The assessment of anxiety states by rating. *Br J Psychiatry.* 1959;32:50, with permission.)

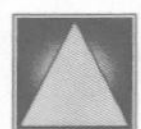

Table 9.2–7
Hamilton Rating Scale for Depression

For each item select the "cue" which best characterizes the patient.

1: Depressed mood (Sadness, hopeless, helpless, worthless)
- 0 Absent
- 1 These feeling states indicated only on questioning
- 2 These feeling states spontaneously reported verbally
- 3 Communicates feeling states nonverbally—i.e., through facial expression, posture, voice, and tendency to weep
- 4 Patient reports VIRTUALLY ONLY these feeling states in his spontaneous verbal and nonverbal communication

2: Feelings of guilt
- 0 Absent
- 1 Self-reproach, feels he has let people down
- 2 Ideas of guilt or rumination over past errors or sinful deeds
- 3 Present illness is a punishment. Delusions of guilt
- 4 Hears accusatory or denunciatory voices and/or experiences threatening visual hallucinations

3: Suicide
- 0 Absent
- 1 Feels life is not worth living
- 2 Wishes he were dead or any thoughts of possible death to self
- 3 Suicide ideas or gesture
- 4 Attempts at suicide (any serious attempt rates 4)

4: Insomnia early
- 0 No difficulty falling asleep
- 1 Complains of occasional difficulty falling asleep—i.e., more than $^1/_4$ hour
- 2 Complains of nightly difficulty falling asleep

5: Insomnia middle
- 0 No difficulty
- 1 Patient complains of being restless and disturbed during the night
- 2 Waking during the night—any getting out of bed rates 2 (except for purpose of voiding)

(*continued*)

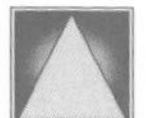

Table 9.2–7
(Continued)

6: Insomnia late
- 0 No difficulty
- 1 Waking in early hours of the morning but goes back to sleep
- 2 Unable to fall asleep again if gets out of bed

7: Work and activities
- 0 No difficulty
- 1 Thoughts and feelings of incapacity, fatigue, or weakness related to activities, work, or hobbies
- 2 Loss of interest in activity, hobbies, or work—either directly reported by patient, or indirect in listlessness, indecision, and vacillation (feels he has to push self to work or activities)
- 3 Decrease in actual time spent in activities or decrease in productivity. In hospital, rate 3 if patient does not spend at least three hours a day in activities (hospital job or hobbies) exclusive of ward chores
- 4 Stopped working because of present illness. In hospital, rate 4 if patient engages in no activities except ward chores, or if patient fails to perform ward chores unassisted

8: Retardation (Slowness of thought and speech; impaired ability to concentrate; decreased motor activity)
- 0 Normal speech and thought
- 1 Slight retardation at interview
- 2 Obvious retardation at interview
- 3 Interview difficult
- 4 Complete stupor

9: Agitation
- 0 None
- 1 "Playing with" hands, hair, etc.
- 2 Hand-wringing, nail biting, hair pulling, biting of lips

10: Anxiety psychic
- 0 No difficulty
- 1 Subjective tension and irritability
- 2 Worrying about minor matters
- 3 Apprehensive attitude apparent in face or speech
- 4 Fears expressed without questioning

11: Anxiety somatic

0 Absent	Physiological concomitants of anxiety, such as:
1 Mild	
2 Moderate	Gastrointestinal—dry mouth, wind, indigestion, diarrhea, cramps, belching
3 Severe	
4 Incapacitating	Cardiovascular—palpitations, headaches
	Respiratory—hyperventilation, sighing
	Urinary frequency
	Sweating

12: Somatic symptoms gastrointestinal
- 0 None
- 1 Loss of appetite but eating without staff encouragement. Heavy feelings in abdomen
- 2 Difficulty eating without staff urging; requests or requires laxatives or medication for bowels or medication for G.I. symptoms

13: Somatic symptoms general
- 0 None
- 1 Heaviness in limbs, back or head. Backaches, headache, muscle aches. Loss of energy and fatigability
- 2 Any clear-cut symptom rates 2

14: Genital symptoms

0 Absent	Symptoms such as:
1 Mild	Loss of libido
2 Severe	Menstrual disturbances

15: Hypochondriasis
- 0 Not present
- 1 Self-absorption (bodily)
- 2 Preoccupation with health
- 3 Frequent complaints, requests for help, etc.
- 4 Hypochondriacal delusions

16: Loss of weight
- A: When rating by history
- 0 No weight loss
- 1 Probable weight loss associated with present illness
- 2 Definite (according to patient) weight loss
- B: On weekly ratings by ward psychiatrist, when actual weight changes are measured
- 0 Less than 1 lb weight loss in week
- 1 Greater than 1 lb weight loss in week
- 2 Greater than 2 lb weight loss in week

17: Insight
- 0 Acknowledges being depressed and ill
- 1 Acknowledges illness but attributes cause to bad food, climate, overwork, virus, need for rest, etc.
- 2 Denies being ill at all

18: Diurnal variation

AM	PM		
0	0	Absent	If symptoms are worse in the morning or evening, note which it is and rate severity of variation
1	1	Mild	
2	2	Severe	

19: Depersonalization and derealization

0 Absent	
1 Mild	Such as:
2 Moderate	Feeling of unreality
3 Severe	Nihilistic ideas
4 Incapacitating	

20: Paranoid symptoms
- 0 None
- 1, 2 Suspiciousness
- 3 Ideas of reference
- 4 Delusions of reference and persecution

21: Obsessional and compulsive symptoms
- 0 Absent
- 1 Mild
- 2 Severe

22: Helplessness
- 0 Not present
- 1 Subjective feelings which are elicited only by inquiry
- 2 Patient volunteers his helpless feelings
- 3 Requires urging, guidance, and reassurance to accomplish ward chores or personal hygiene
- 4 Requires physical assistance for dress, grooming, eating, bedside tasks, or personal hygiene

23: Hopelessness
- 0 Not present
- 1 Intermittently doubts that "things will improve" but can be reassured
- 2 Consistently feels "hopeless" but accepts reassurances
- 3 Expresses feelings of discouragement, despair, pessimism about future, which cannot be dispelled
- 4 Spontaneously and inappropriately perseverates: "I'll never get well" or its equivalent

24: Worthlessness (Ranges from mild loss of esteem, feelings of inferiority, self-deprecation to delusional notions of worthlessness)
- 0 Not present
- 1 Indicates feelings of worthlessness (loss of self-esteem) only on questioning
- 2 Spontaneously indicates feelings of worthlessness (loss of self-esteem)
- 3 Different from 2 by degree. Patient volunteers that he is "no good," "inferior," etc.
- 4 Delusional notions of worthlessness—i.e., "I am a heap of garbage" or its equivalent

(From Hamilton M. A rating scale for depression. *J Neurol Neurosurg Psychiatry*. 1960;23:56, with permission.)

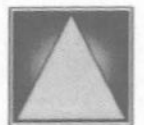

Table 9.2–8
Scale for the Assessment of Negative Symptoms (SANS)

0 = None 1 = Questionable 2 = Mild 3 = Moderate 4 = Marked 5 = Severe

Affective flattening or blunting	
1 *Unchanging facial expression* The patient's face appears wooden, changes less than expected as emotional content of discourse changes.	0 1 2 3 4 5
2 *Decreased spontaneous movements* The patient shows few or no spontaneous movements, does not shift position, move extremities, etc.	0 1 2 3 4 5
3 *Paucity of expressive gestures* The patient does not use hand gestures, body position, etc., as an aid to expressing his ideas.	0 1 2 3 4 5
4 *Poor eye contact* The patient avoids eye contact or "stares through" interviewer even when speaking.	0 1 2 3 4 5
5 *Affective nonresponsivity* The patient fails to smile or laugh when prompted.	0 1 2 3 4 5
6 *Lack of vocal inflections* The patient fails to show normal vocal emphasis patterns, is often monotonic.	0 1 2 3 4 5
7 *Global rating of affective flattening* This rating should focus on overall severity of symptoms, especially unresponsiveness, eye contact, facial expression, and vocal inflections.	0 1 2 3 4 5
Alogia	
8 *Poverty of speech* The patient's replies to questions are restricted in *amount* tend to be brief, concrete, and unelaborated.	0 1 2 3 4 5
9 *Poverty of content of speech* The patient's replies are adequate in amount but tend to be vague, overconcrete, or over-generalized, and convey little information.	0 1 2 3 4 5
10 *Blocking* The patient indicates, either spontaneously or with prompting, that his [her] train of thought was interrupted.	0 1 2 3 4 5
11 *Increased latency of response* The patient takes a long time to reply to questions; prompting indicates the patient is aware of the question.	0 1 2 3 4 5
12 *Global rating of alogia* The core features of alogia are poverty of speech and poverty of content.	0 1 2 3 4 5
Avolition-apathy	
13 *Grooming and hygiene* The patient's clothes may be sloppy or soiled, and he [she] may have greasy hair, body odor, etc.	0 1 2 3 4 5
14 *Impersistence at work or school* The patient has difficulty seeking or maintaining employment, completing school work, keeping house, etc. If an inpatient, cannot persist at ward activities, such as occupational therapy, playing cards, etc.	0 1 2 3 4 5
15 *Physical anergia* The patient tends to be physically inert. He [she] may sit for hours and does not initiate spontaneous activity.	0 1 2 3 4 5
16 *Global rating of avolition-apathy* Strong weight may be given to one or two prominent symptoms if particularly striking.	0 1 2 3 4 5
Anhedonia-asociality	
17 *Recreational interests and activities* The patient may have few or no interests. Both the quality and quantity of interests should be taken into account.	0 1 2 3 4 5
18 *Sexual activity* The patient may show a decrease in sexual interest and activity, or enjoyment when active.	0 1 2 3 4 5
19 *Ability to feel intimacy and closeness* The patient may display an inability to form close or intimate relationships, especially with the opposite sex and family.	0 1 2 3 4 5
20 *Relationships with friends and peers* The patient may have few or no friends and may prefer to spend all of his [her] time isolated.	0 1 2 3 4 5
21 *Global rating of anhedonia-asociality* This rating should reflect overall severity, taking into account the patient's age, family status, etc.	0 1 2 3 4 5
Attention	
22 *Social inattentiveness* The patient appears uninvolved or unengaged. He [she] may seem spacey.	0 1 2 3 4 5
23 *Inattentiveness during mental status testing* Tests of "serial 7s" (at least five subtractions) and spelling *world* backwards: Score: 2 = 1 error; 3 = 2 errors; 4 = 3 errors.	0 1 2 3 4 5
24 *Global rating of attention* This rating should assess the patient's overall concentration, clinically and on tests.	0 1 2 3 4 5

(From Nancy C. Andreasen, M.D., Ph.D., Department of Psychiatry, College of Medicine, The University of Iowa, Iowa City, 1A 52242. with permission.)

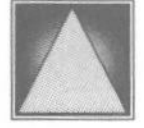

Table 9.2–9
Scale for the Assessment of Positive Symptoms (SAPS)

0 = None 1 = Questionable 2 = Mild 3 = Moderate 4 = Marked 5 = Severe

Hallucinations	
1 *Auditory hallucinations* The patient reports voices, noises, or other sounds that no one else hears.	0 1 2 3 4 5
2 *Voices commenting* The patient reports a voice which makes a running commentary on his [her] behavior or thoughts.	0 1 2 3 4 5
3 *Voices conversing* The patient reports hearing two or more voices conversing.	0 1 2 3 4 5
4 *Somatic or tactile hallucinations* The patient reports experiencing peculiar physical sensations in the body.	0 1 2 3 4 5
5 *Olfactory hallucinations* The patient reports experiencing unusual smells which no one else notices.	0 1 2 3 4 5
6 *Visual hallucinations* The patient sees shapes or people that are not actually present.	0 1 2 3 4 5
7 *Global rating of hallucinations* This rating should be based on the duration and severity of the hallucinations and their effects on the patient's life.	0 1 2 3 4 5
Delusions	
8 *Persecutory delusions* The patient believes he [she] is being conspired against or persecuted in some way.	0 1 2 3 4 5
9 *Delusions of jealousy* The patient believes his [her] spouse is having an affair with someone.	0 1 2 3 4 5
10 *Delusions of guilt or sin* The patient believes that he [she] has committed some terrible sin or done something unforgivable.	0 1 2 3 4 5
11 *Grandiose delusions* The patient believes he [she] has special powers or abilities.	0 1 2 3 4 5
12 *Religious delusions* The patient is preoccupied with false beliefs of a religious nature.	0 1 2 3 4 5
13 *Somatic delusions* The patient believes that somehow his [her] body is diseased, abnormal, or changed.	0 1 2 3 4 5
14 *Delusions of reference* The patient believes that insignificant remarks or events refer to him [her] or have some special meaning.	0 1 2 3 4 5
15 *Delusions of being controlled* The patient feels that his [her] feelings or actions are controlled by some outside force.	0 1 2 3 4 5
16 *Delusions of mind reading* The patient feels that people can read his [her] mind or know his [her] thoughts.	0 1 2 3 4 5
17 *Thought broadcasting* The patient believes that his [her] thoughts are broadcast so that he himself [she herself] or others can hear them.	0 1 2 3 4 5
18 *Thought insertion* The patient believes that thoughts that are not his [her] own have been inserted into his [her] mind.	0 1 2 3 4 5
19 *Thought withdrawal* The patient believes that thoughts have been taken away from his [her] mind.	0 1 2 3 4 5
20 *Global rating of delusions* This rating should be based on the duration and persistence of the delusions and their effect on the patient's life.	0 1 2 3 4 5
Bizarre behavior	
21 *Clothing and appearance* The patient dresses in an unusual manner or does other strange things to alter his [her] appearance.	0 1 2 3 4 5
22 *Social and sexual behavior* The patient may do things considered inappropriate according to usual social norms (e.g., masturbating in public).	0 1 2 3 4 5
23 *Aggressive and agitated behavior* The patient may behave in an aggressive, agitated manner, often unpredictably.	0 1 2 3 4 5
24 *Repetitive or stereotyped behavior* The patient develops a set of repetitive actions or rituals that he [she] must perform over and over.	0 1 2 3 4 5
25 *Global rating of bizarre behavior* This rating should reflect the type of behavior and the extent to which it deviates from social norms.	0 1 2 3 4 5
Positive formal thought disorder	
26 *Derailment* A pattern of speech in which ideas slip off track onto ideas obliquely related or unrelated.	0 1 2 3 4 5
27 *Tangentiality* Replying to a question in an oblique or irrelevant manner.	0 1 2 3 4 5
28 *Incoherence* A pattern of speech which is essentially incomprehensible at times.	0 1 2 3 4 5
29 *Illogicality* A pattern of speech in which conclusions are reached which do not follow logically.	0 1 2 3 4 5
30 *Circumstantiality* A pattern of speech which is very indirect and delayed in reaching its goal idea.	0 1 2 3 4 5
31 *Pressure of speech* The patient's speech is rapid and difficult to interrupt; the amount of speech produced is greater than that considered normal.	0 1 2 3 4 5
32 *Distractible speech* The patient is distracted by nearby stimuli which interrupt his [her] flow of speech.	0 1 2 3 4 5
33 *Clanging* A pattern of speech in which sounds rather than meaningful relationships govern word choice.	0 1 2 3 4 5
34 *Global rating of positive formal thought disorder* This rating should reflect the frequency of abnormality and degree to which it affects the patient's ability to communicate.	0 1 2 3 4 5
Inappropriate affect	
35 *Inappropriate affect* The patient's affect is inappropriate or incongruous, not simply flat or blunted.	0 1 2 3 4 5

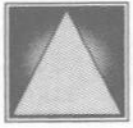

Table 9.2–10
Psychiatric Rating Scales

Scale	Source
Rating scales used for schizophrenia and psychosis	
Brief Psychiatric Rating Scale	*Psychological Reports* 1962; 10:799.
Schedule for Affective Disorders and Schizophrenia (SADS)	*Archives of General Psychiatry* 1978;35:837.
Scale for the Assessment of Negative Symptoms (SANS)	University of Iowa Press, 1983.
Scale for the Assessment of Thought, Language, and Communication (TLC)	University of Iowa Press, 1978.
Thought Disorder Index (TDI)	*Archives of General Psychiatry* 1983;40:1281.
Quality of Life Scale (QLS)	*Schizophrenia Bulletin* 1984; 10:383.
Chestnut Lodge Prognostic Scale for Chronic Schizophrenia	*Schizophrenia Bulletin* 1987; 13:277.
Rating scales used for mood disorders	
Beck Depression Inventory	*Archives of General Psychiatry* 1961;4:561.
Standard Assessment of Depressive Disorders (SADD)	*Psychological Medicine* 1979;10:743.
Zung Self-Rating Scale for Depression	*Archives of General Psychiatry* 1965;12:63.
Carroll Rating Scale for Depression	*British Journal of Psychiatry* 1981;138:194.
Montgomery-Asberg Scale	*British Journal of Psychiatry* 1979;134:382.
Raskin Depression Rating Scale	*Journal of Nervous and Mental Disease* 1969;148:87.
Inventory to Diagnose Depression	*Archives of General Psychiatry* 1986;43:1976.
Mania Rating Scale	*Journal of Clinical Psychiatry* 1983;44:98.
Manic State Rating Scale	*Archives of General Psychiatry* 1971;25:256.
Rating scales used for anxiety disorders	
Brief Outpatient Psychopathology Scale	*Journal of Clinical Pharmacology* 1969;9:187.
Physicians Questionnaire	*Psychopharmacologia* 1970;17:338.
Covi Anxiety Scale	*Psychopharmacology Bulletin* 1982;18:69.
Anxiety States Inventory	*Psychosomatics* 1971;12:371.
Fear Questionnaire	*Behavioral Research and Therapeutics* 1979;17:263.
Mobility Inventory for Agoraphobia	*Behavioral Research and Therapeutics* 1985;23:35.
Social Avoidance and Distress Scale	*Journal of Consulting and Clinical Psychology* 1969;33:448.
Acute Panic Inventory	*Archives of General Psychiatry* 1984;41:764.
Leyton Obsessional Inventory	*Psychological Medicine* 1970;1:48.
Maudsley Obsessional–Compulsive Inventory	*Behavioral Research and Therapeutics* 1977;15:389.
Fear Thermometer	*Journal of Consulting and Clinical Psychiatry* 1983;15:488.
Impact of Events Scale	*Psychosomatic Medicine* 1979;41:209.
Other rating scales	
Child and adolescent patients	
General reference for adult scales that have been modified for children	*Psychopharmacology Bulletin* 1985;21:737.
Adverse effects of drugs	
Systematic Assessment for Treatment of Emergent Events (SAFTEE):	*Psychopharmacology Bulletin* 1986;22:343.
General Inquiry (GI)	
Systematic Inquiry (SI)	
Quality of life	
Patterns of Individual Change Scale (PICS)	*Archives of General Psychiatry* 1985;42:703.
Dissociative disorders	
Structured Clinical Interview for DSM-IV Dissociative Disorders (SCID-IV)	*American Journal of Psychiatry* 1993;150:1011.
Obsessive–Compulsive Disorder	
Yale Brown Obsessive–Compulsive Scale	*Archives of General Psychiatry* 1989;46:1006.

Rating scales have been developed for almost every diagnostic group and are central to psychiatric research, but they can also be used in clinical practice. They tend to be rather long, however, especially with individuals reporting many symptoms. Table 9.2–10 lists references for a variety of scales used in psychiatry. Access to instruments via the World Wide Web is increasing rapidly and many of these tests are available for purchase or download by using a search engine such as Google scholar.

References

Blacker D. Psychiatric Rating Scales. In: Sadock BJ, Sadock VA, eds. *Kaplan & Sadock's Comprehensive Textbook of Psychiatry*. 8th ed. Vol. 1. Baltimore: Lippincott Williams & Wilkins; 2005:929.

Buka SL, Monuteaux M, Earls F. Epidemiology of childhoodspsychiatric disorders. In: Tsuang MT, Tohen M, eds. *Textbook in Psychiatric Epidemiology*. 2nd ed. New York: Wiley; 2002.

Burt T, Sederer L, Isgak WW, eds. *Outcome Measurement in Psychiatry, A Critical Review*. Washington, DC: American Psychiatric Press; 2002.

Cooper JE. Measuring psychopathology. *Psychol Med*. 2003;33:749–750.

DeFife JA, Hilsenroth MJ. Clinical utility of the Defensive Functioning Scale in the assessment of depression. *J Nerv Ment Dis*. 2005;193(3): 176–182.

Keller J, Gomez RG, Kenna HA, Poesner J, DeBattista C, Flores B, Schatzberg AF. Detecting psychotic major depression using psychiatric rating scales. *J Psychiatr Res*. 2006;40(1):22–29.

Kessler RC. The categorical versus dimensional assessment controversy in the sociology of mental illness. *J Health Soc Behav*. 2002;43:171.

Mossbarger B. A modified Global Assessment of Functioning (GAF) Scale for use in long-term care settings. *Educ Gerontol*. 2005;31(9):715–725.

Myers K, Winters NC. Ten-year review of rating scales. I: overview of scale functioning, psychometric properties, and selection. *J Am Acad Child Adolesc Psychiatry*. 2002;41:114–122.

Tyson EH. Ethnic differences using behavior rating scales to assess the mental health of children: A conceptual and psychometric critique. *Child Psychiatry Hum Devt*. 2004;34:167–201.

10 Delirium, Dementia, and Amnestic and Other Cognitive Disorders

▲ 10.1 Overview

Cognition includes memory, language, orientation, judgment, conducting interpersonal relationships, performing actions (praxis), and problem solving. Cognitive disorders reflect disruption in one or more of the above domains, and are also frequently complicated by behavioral symptoms. Cognitive disorders exemplify the complex interface between neurology, medicine, and psychiatry in that medical or neurological conditions often lead to cognitive disorders that, in turn, are associated with behavioral symptoms. It can be argued that of all psychiatric conditions, cognitive disorders best demonstrate how biological insults result in behavioral symptomatology. The clinician must carefully assess the history and context of the presentation of these disorders before arriving at a diagnosis and treatment plan. Advances in molecular biology, diagnostic techniques, and medication management have significantly improved the ability to recognize and to treat cognitive disorders.

In the text revision of the fourth edition of *Diagnostic Statistical Manual of Mental Disorders* (DSM-IV-TR), three groups of disorders—delirium, dementia, and the amnestic disorders—are characterized by the primary symptom common to all the disorders, which is an impairment in cognition (as in memory, language, or attention). Although DSM-IV-TR acknowledges that other psychiatric disorders can exhibit some cognitive impairment as a symptom, cognitive impairment is the cardinal symptom in delirium, dementia, and the amnestic disorders. Within each of these diagnostic categories, DSM-IV-TR delimits specific types (Table 10.1–1).

In the past, these conditions were classified under the heading "organic mental disorders" or "organic brain disorders." Traditionally, those disorders had an identifiable pathological condition such as brain tumor, cerebrovascular disease, or drug intoxication. Those brain disorders with no generally accepted organic basis (e.g., depression) were called *functional disorders*.

This century-old distinction between organic and functional disorders is outdated and has been deleted from the nomenclature. Every psychiatric disorder has an organic (i.e., biological or chemical) component. Because of this reassessment, the concept of functional disorders has been determined to be misleading, and the term *functional* and its historical opposite, *organic*, are not used in DSM-IV-TR.

A further indication that the dichotomy is no longer valid is the revival of the term *neuropsychiatry* which emphasizes the somatic substructure on which mental operations and emotions are based; it is concerned with the psychopathological accompaniments of brain dysfunction as observed in seizure disorders, for example. Neuropsychiatry focuses on the psychiatric aspects of neurological disorders and the role of brain dysfunction in psychiatric disorders.

CLASSIFICATION

For each of the three major groups—delirium, dementia, and amnestic disorders—there are subcategories based on etiology. They are defined and summarized as follows.

Delirium

Delirium is marked by short-term confusion and changes in cognition. There are four subcategories based on several causes: (1) general medical condition (e.g., infection); (2) substance induced (e.g., cocaine, opioids, phencyclidine [PCP]); (3) multiple causes (e.g., head trauma and kidney disease); and (4) delirium not otherwise specified (e.g., sleep deprivation).

Dementia

Dementia is marked by severe impairment in memory, judgment, orientation, and cognition. The six subcategories are (1) dementia of the Alzheimer's type, which usually occurs in persons over 65 years of age and is manifested by progressive intellectual disorientation and dementia, delusions, or depression; (2) vascular dementia, caused by vessel thrombosis or hemorrhage; (3) other medical conditions (e.g., human immunodeficiency virus [HIV] disease, head trauma, Pick's disease, Creutzfeldt-Jakob disease, which is caused by a slow-growing transmittable virus); (4) substance induced, caused by toxin or medication (e.g., gasoline fumes, atropine); (5) multiple etiologies; and (6) not otherwise specified (if cause is unknown).

Amnestic Disorder

Amnestic disorder is marked by memory impairment and forgetfulness. The three subcategories are (1) caused by medical condition (hypoxia); (2) caused by toxin or medication (e.g., marijuana, diazepam); and (3) not otherwise specified.

Table 10.1–1
DSM-IV-TR Cognitive Disorders

- Delirium
  - Caused by a general medical condition
  - Substance-induced
  - From multiple etiologies
  - Not otherwise specified
- Dementia
  - Of the Alzheimer's type
  - Vascular
  - Dementia due to other general medical conditions
    - Human immunodeficiency virus (HIV) disease
    - Head trauma
    - Parkinson's disease
    - Huntington's disease
    - Pick's disease
    - Creutzfeldt-Jakob disease
    - Other general medical conditions
  - Substance-induced persisting dementia
  - Multiple etiologies
  - Dementia not otherwise specified
- Amnestic Disorders
  - Caused by a general medical condition
  - Substance-induced persisting amnestic disorder
  - Not otherwise specified
- Cognitive disorder not otherwise specified

Cognitive Disorder Not Otherwise Specified

Cognitive disorder not otherwise specified is a DSM-IV-TR category that allows for the diagnosis of a cognitive disorder that does not meet the criteria for delirium, dementia, or amnestic disorders (Table 10.1–2). The cause of these syndromes is presumed to involve a specific general medical condition, a pharmacologically active agent, or possibly both.

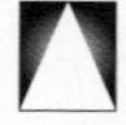

Table 10.1–2
DSM-IV-TR Diagnostic Criteria for Cognitive Disorder Not Otherwise Specified

This category is for disorders that are characterized by cognitive dysfunction presumed to result from the direct physiological effect of a general medical condition that does not meet criteria for any of the specific deliriums, dementias, or amnestic disorders listed in this section and that are not better classified as delirium not otherwise specified, dementia not otherwise specified, or amnestic disorder not otherwise specified. For cognitive dysfunction caused by a specific or unknown substance, the specific substance-related disorder not otherwise specified category should be used.

Examples include

1. Mild neurocognitive disorder: impairment in cognitive functioning as evidenced by neuropsychological testing or quantified clinical assessment, accompanied by objective evidence of a systemic general medical condition or central nervous system dysfunction
2. Postconcussional disorder: following a head trauma, impairment in memory or attention with associated symptoms

(From American Psychiatric Association. *Diagnostic and Statistical Manual of Mental Disorders.* 4th ed. Text rev. Washington, DC: American Psychiatric Association; copyright 2000, with permission.)

CLINICAL EVALUATION

During the history taking, the clinician seeks to elicit the development of the illness. Subtle cognitive disorders, fluctuating symptoms, and progressing disease processes may be tracked effectively. The clinician should obtain a detailed rendition of changes in the patient's daily routine involving such factors as self-care, job responsibilities, and work habits; meal preparation; shopping and personal support; interactions with friends; hobbies and sports; reading interests; religious, social, and recreational activities; and ability to maintain personal finances. Understanding the past life of each patient provides an invaluable source of baseline data regarding changes in function, such as attention and concentration, intellectual abilities, personality, motor skills, and mood and perception. The examiner seeks to find the particular pursuits that the patient considers most important, or central, to his or her lifestyle and attempts to discern how those pursuits have been affected by the emerging clinical condition. Such a method provides the opportunity to appraise both the impact of the illness and the patient-specific baseline for monitoring the effects of future therapies.

Mental Status Examination

After taking a thorough history, the clinician's primary tool is the assessment of the patient's mental status. As with the physical examination, the mental status examination is a means of surveying functions and abilities, to allow a definition of personal strengths and weakness. It is a repeatable, structured assessment of symptoms and signs that promotes effective communication between clinicians. It also establishes the basis for future comparison, essential for documenting therapeutic effectiveness, and it allows comparisons between different patients, with a generalization of findings from one patient to another. Table 10.1–3 lists the components of a comprehensive neuropsychiatric mental status examination.

Cognition

When testing cognitive functions, the clinician should evaluate memory; visuospatial and constructional abilities; and reading, writing, and mathematical abilities. Assessment of abstraction ability is also valuable, although a patient's performance on tasks such as proverb interpretation may be a useful bedside projective test in some patients, the specific interpretation may result from a variety of factors, such as poor education, low intelligence, and failure to understand the concept of proverbs, as well as from a broad array of primary and secondary psychopathological disturbances.

PATHOLOGY AND LABORATORY EXAMINATION

As with all medical tests, psychiatric evaluations such as the mental status examination must be interpreted in the overall context of thorough clinical and laboratory assessment. Psychiatric and neuropsychiatric patients require careful physical examination especially when issues exist that involve etiologically related or comorbid medical conditions. When consulting internists and other medical specialists, the clinician must ask specific

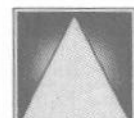

Table 10.1–3
Neuropsychiatric Mental Status Examination

A. General Description
  1. General appearance, dress, sensory aids (glasses, hearing aid)
  2. Level of consciousness and arousal
  3. Attention to environment
  4. Posture (standing and seated)
  5. Gait
  6. Movements of limbs, trunk, and face (spontaneous, resting, and after instruction)
  7. General demeanor (including evidence of responses to internal stimuli)
  8. Response to examiner (eye contact, cooperation, ability to focus on interview process)
  9. Native or primary language

B. Language and Speech
  1. Comprehension (words, sentences, simple and complex commands, and concepts)
  2. Output (spontaneity, rate, fluency, melody or prosody, volume, coherence, vocabulary, paraphasic errors, complexity of usage)
  3. Repetition
  4. Other aspects
    a. Object naming
    b. Color naming
    c. Body part identification
    d. Ideomotor praxis to command

C. Thought
  1. Form (coherence and connectedness)
  2. Content
    a. Ideational (preoccupations, overvalued ideas, delusions)
    b. Perceptual (hallucinations)

D. Mood and Affect
  1. Internal mood state (spontaneous and elicited; sense of humor)
  2. Future outlook
  3. Suicidal ideas and plans
  4. Demonstrated emotional status (congruence with mood)

E. Insight and Judgment
  1. Insight
    a. Self-appraisal and self-esteem
    b. Understanding of current circumstances
    c. Ability to describe personal psychological and physical status
  2. Judgment
    a. Appraisal of major social relationships
    b. Understanding of personal roles and responsibilities

F. Cognition
  1. Memory
    a. Spontaneous (as evidenced during interview)
    b. Tested (incidental, immediate repetition, delayed recall, cued recall, recognition; verbal, nonverbal; explicit, implicit)
  2. Visuospatial skills
  3. Constructional ability
  4. Mathematics
  5. Reading
  6. Writing
  7. Fine sensory function (stereognosis, graphesthesia, two-point discrimination)
  8. Finger gnosis
  9. Right-left orientation
  10. "Executive functions"
  11. Abstraction

(Courtesy of Eric D. Caine, M.D., and Jeffrey M. Lyness, M.D.)

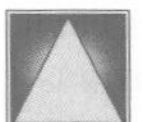

Table 10.1–4
Screening Laboratory Tests

General Tests
Complete blood cell count
Erythrocyte sedimentation rate
Electrolytes
Glucose
Blood urea nitrogen and serum creatinine
Liver function tests
Serum calcium and phosphorus
Thyroid function tests
Serum protein
Levels of all drugs
Urinalysis
Pregnancy test for women of childbearing age
Electrocardiography

Ancillary Laboratory Tests
Blood
  Blood cultures
  Rapid plasma reagin test
  Human immunodeficiency virus (HIV) testing (enzyme-linked immunosorbent assay [ELISA] and Western blot)
  Serum heavy metals
  Serum copper
  Ceruloplasmin
  Serum B_{12}, red blood cell (RBC) folate levels
Urine
  Culture
  Toxicology
  Heavy metal screen
Electrography
  Electroencephalography
  Evoked potentials
  Polysomnography
  Nocturnal penile tumescence
Cerebrospinal fluid
  Glucose, protein
  Cell count
  Cultures (bacterial, viral, fungal)
  Cryptococcal antigen
  Venereal Disease Research Laboratory test
Radiography
  Computed tomography
  Magnetic resonance imaging
  Positron emission tomography
  Single photon emission computed tomography

(Courtesy of Eric D. Caine, M.D., and Jeffrey M. Lyness, M.D.)

questions to focus the differential diagnostic process and use the consultation most effectively. In particular, most systemic medical or primary cerebral diseases that lead to psychopathological disturbances also manifest with a variety of peripheral or central abnormalities.

A screening laboratory evaluation is sought initially and may be followed by a variety of ancillary tests to increase the diagnostic specificity. Table 10.1–4 lists such procedures, some of which are described below.

ELECTROENCEPHALOGRAPHY

Electroencephalography (EEG) is an easily accessible, noninvasive test of brain dysfunction that has high sensitivity for many disorders, but relatively low specificity. Beyond its recognized uses in epilepsy, EEG's greatest utility is in detecting altered electrical rhythms associated with mild delirium, space-occupying lesions, and continuing complex partial seizures (in which the patient remains conscious, although behaviorally impaired). EEG is also sensitive to metabolic and toxic states, often showing a diffuse slowing of brain activity. The EEG is discussed in Section 3.4, Electrophysiology.

COMPUTED TOMOGRAPHY AND MAGNETIC RESONANCE IMAGING

Computed tomography (CT) and magnetic resonance imaging (MRI) have proved to be powerful neuropsychiatric research tools. Recent developments in MRI allow the direct measurement of structures such as the thalamus, basal ganglia, hippocampus, and amygdala, as well as temporal and apical areas of the brain and the structures of the posterior fossa. MRI has largely replaced CT as the most utilitarian and cost-effective method of imaging in neuropsychiatry. Patients with acute cerebral hemorrhages or hematomas must continue to be assessed using CT, but these patients present infrequently in psychiatric settings. MRI better discriminates the interface between gray and white matter and is useful in detecting a variety of white matter lesions in the periventricular and subcortical regions. The pathophysiological significance of such findings remains to be defined. White matter abnormalities are detected in younger patients with multiple sclerosis or human immunodeficiency virus (HIV) infection and in older patients with hypertension, vascular dementia, or dementia of the Alzheimer's type. The prevalence of these abnormalities is also increased in healthy, aging individuals who have no defined disease process. As with CT, the greatest utility of MRI in the evaluation of patients with dementia arises from what it may exclude (tumors, vascular disease) rather than what it can demonstrate specifically. These and other imaging techniques, such as positron emission tomography (PET), are discussed in Section 3.3, Neuroimaging.

NEUROPSYCHOLOGICAL TESTING

Neuropsychological testing provides a standardized, quantitative, reproducible evaluation of a patient's cognitive abilities. Such procedures may be useful for initial evaluation and periodic assessment. Tests are available that assess abilities across the broad array of cognitive domains, and many offer comparative normative groups or adjusted scores based on normative samples. The clinician seeking neuropsychological consultation should understand enough about the strengths and weaknesses of selected procedures to benefit fully from the results obtained. (Chapter 5 includes a complete survey of neuropsychological tests.)

ICD-10

Unlike in DSM-IV-TR, organic (including symptomatic) mental disorders are organized in the 10th revision of the *International Statistical Classification of Disease and Related Health Problems* (ICD-10) on the basis of "their common, demonstrable etiology in cerebral disease, brain injury, or other insult leading to cerebral dysfunction." In the ICD-10, rather than being deleted, the term *organic* implies only that "the syndrome . . . can be attributed to an independently diagnosable cerebral or systemic disease or disorder." Primary dysfunction affects the brain directly; secondary dysfunctions occur as a result of diseases or disorders attacking several organs or body systems, including the brain. According to ICD-10, all the disorders can be divided into two groups: one in which the invariable and most prominent features are disturbances of cognitive functions or of the sensorium and one in which the most conspicuous manifestations are in the areas of perception, thought contents, mood and emotion, or in the overall pattern of personality and behavior.

Consequently, categories included as organic mental disorders, including symptomatic ones, in ICD-10 are dementia in Alzheimer's disease; vascular dementia; dementia in other diseases classified elsewhere (e.g., dementia in Pick's disease); unspecified dementia; organic amnesia syndrome, not induced by alcohol and other psychoactive substances; delirium, not induced by alcohol and other psychoactive substances; other mental disorders from brain damage and dysfunction and caused by physical disease (e.g., organic mood disorders caused by brain disease, damage, and dysfunction); and unspecified organic or symptomatic mental disorder.

REFERENCES

Albert MS, Blacker D. Mild cognitive impairment and dementia. *Annual Review of Clinical Psychology*. 2006;2:379–388.

Clark R. Disease overview: Alzheimer's disease. *Drugs in Context*. 2005;1:5–16.

Davis KL. Cognitive disorders: Introduction and overview. In: Sadock BJ, Sadock VA, eds. *Kaplan & Sadock's Comprehensive Textbook of Psychiatry*. 8th ed. Vol. 1. Baltimore: Lippincott Williams & Wilkins; 2005:1053.

Helmes E, Bowler JV, Merskey H, Munoz DG, Hachinski VC. Rates of cognitive decline in Alzheimer's disease and dementia with Lewy bodies. *Dement Geriatr Cogn Disord*. 2003;15:67–71.

Morita T, Tei Y, Inoue S. Agitated terminal delirium and associations with partial opioid substitution and hydration. *J Palliat Med*. 2003;6:557–563.

Rubey RN. Treatment of chronic pain in persons with dementia: An overview. *Am J Alzheimers Dis Other Demen*. 2005;20(1):12–20.

Serby M, Almiron N. Dementia with Lewy bodies: An overview. *Annals of Long-Term Care*. 2005;13(2):20–22.

Wild R, Pettit T, Burns A. Cholinesterase inhibitors for dementia with Lewy bodies. *Cochrane Database Syst Rev*. 2003;3:CD003672.

▲ 10.2 Delirium

Delirium is defined by the acute onset of fluctuating cognitive impairment and a disturbance of consciousness. Delirium is a syndrome, not a disease, and it has many causes, all of which result in a similar pattern of signs and symptoms relating to the patient's level of consciousness and cognitive impairment. Delirium is underrecognized by health care workers. Part of the problem is that the syndrome has a variety of other names (Table 10.2–1). The intent of the text revision of the fourth edition of the *Diagnostic and Statistical Manual of Mental Disorders* (DSM-IV-TR) was to help consolidate the myriad of terms into a single diagnostic label.

In DSM-IV-TR, delirium is "characterized by a disturbance of consciousness and a change in cognition that develop over a short . . . time." The hallmark symptom of delirium is an

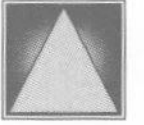

Table 10.2–1
Delirium by Other Names

Intensive care unit psychosis
Acute confusional state
Acute brain failure
Encephalitis
Encephalopathy
Toxic metabolic state
Central nervous system toxicity
Paraneoplastic limbic encephalitis
Sundowning
Cerebral insufficiency
Organic brain syndrome

impairment of consciousness, usually occurring in association with global impairments of cognitive functions. Abnormalities of mood, perception, and behavior are common psychiatric symptoms; tremor, asterixis, nystagmus, incoordination, and urinary incontinence are common neurological symptoms. Classically, delirium has a sudden onset (hours or days), a brief and fluctuating course, and rapid improvement when the causative factor is identified and eliminated, but each of these characteristic features can vary in individual patients. Physicians must recognize delirium to identify and treat the underlying cause and to avert the development of delirium-related complications such as accidental injury because of the patient's clouded consciousness.

EPIDEMIOLOGY

Delirium is a common disorder. According to DSM-IV-TR, the point prevalence of delirium in the general population is 0.4 percent for people 18 years of age and older and 1.1 percent for people 55 and older. Approximately 10 to 30 percent of medically ill patients who are hospitalized exhibit delirium. Approximately 30 percent of patients in surgical intensive care units and cardiac intensive care units and 40 to 50 percent of patients who are recovering from surgery for hip fractures have an episode of delirium. The highest rate of delirium is found in postcardiotomy patients, more than 90 percent in some studies. An estimated 20 percent of patients with severe burns and 30 to 40 percent of patients with acquired immune deficiency syndrome (AIDS) have episodes of delirium while they are hospitalized. Delirium develops in 80 percent of terminally ill patients. The causes of postoperative delirium include the stress of surgery, postoperative pain, insomnia, pain medication, electrolyte imbalances, infection, fever, and blood loss. The incidence and prevalence rates for delirium across settings are shown in Table 10.2–2.

Numerous factors can increase a patient's risk for delirium (Table 10.2–3). These range from extremes of age to the number of medications taken. Advanced age is a major risk factor for the development of delirium. Approximately 30 to 40 percent of hospitalized patients older than age 65 have an episode of delirium, and another 10 to 15 percent of elderly persons exhibit delirium on admission to the hospital. Of nursing home residents over age 75, 60 percent have repeated episodes of delirium. Other predisposing factors for the development of delirium are preexisting brain damage (e.g., dementia, cerebrovascular disease, tumor), a history of delirium, alcohol dependence, diabetes, cancer, sensory impairment (e.g., blindness), and malnutrition. Male gender is an independent risk factor for delirium according to DSM-IV-TR.

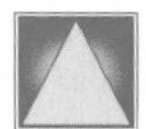

Table 10.2–2
Delirium Incidence and Prevalence in Multiple Settings

Population	Prevalence Range (%)	Incidence Range (%)
General medical inpatients	10–30	3–16
Medical *and* surgical inpatients	5–15	10–55
General surgical inpatients	N/A	9–15 postoperatively
Critical care unit patients	16	16–83
Cardiac surgery inpatients	16–34	7–34
Orthopedic surgery patients	33	18–50
Emergency department	7–10	N/A
Terminally ill cancer patients	23–28	83
Institutionalized elderly	44	33

N/A, not available.

Delirium is a poor prognostic sign. Rates of institutionalization are increased threefold for patients 65 years and older who exhibit delirium while in the hospital. The 3-month mortality rate of patients who have an episode of delirium is estimated to be 23 to 33 percent. The 1-year mortality rate for patients who have an episode of delirium may be as high as 50 percent. Elderly patients who experience delirium while hospitalized have a 20 to 75 percent mortality rate during that hospitalization. After discharge, up to 15 percent of these persons die within a 1-month period, and 25 percent die within 6 months.

ETIOLOGY

The major causes of delirium are central nervous system disease (e.g., epilepsy), systemic disease (e.g., cardiac failure), and either intoxication or withdrawal from pharmacological or toxic agents (Table 10.2–4). When evaluating patients with delirium, clinicians should assume that any drug that a patient has taken may be etiologically relevant to the delirium.

DIAGNOSIS AND CLINICAL FEATURES

The syndrome of delirium is almost always caused by one or more systemic or cerebral derangements that affect brain function.

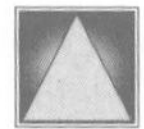

Table 10.2–3
Factors that Predispose Patients to Delirium

Vision impairment	Hypertension	Use of bladder catheter
Medical illnesses (severity and quantity)	Chronic obstructive pulmonary disease	Preoperative cognitive impairment
Cognitive impairment	Alcohol abuse	Functional limitations
Older than 70 years	Smoking history	History of delirium
Any iatrogenic event	Abnormal sodium level	Abnormal potassium, sodium, or glucose test
Use of physical restraints	Abnormal glucose level	Preoperative use of benzodiazepines
Malnutrition	Abnormal bilirubin level	Preoperative use of narcotic analgesics
More than three medications added	Blood urea nitrogen to creatinine ratio >18	Epidural use

Table 10.2–4
Common Causes of Delirium

Central nervous system disorder	Seizure (postictal, nonconvulsive status, status) Migraine Head trauma, brain tumor, subarachnoid hemorrhage, subdural, epidural hematoma, abscess, intracerebral hemorrhage, cerebellar hemorrhage, nonhemorrhagic stroke, transient ischemia
Metabolic disorder	Electrolyte abnormalities Diabetes, hypoglycemia, hyperglycemia, or insulin resistance
Systemic illness	Infection (e.g., sepsis, malaria, erysipelas, viral, plague, Lyme disease, syphilis, or abscess) Trauma Change in fluid status (dehydration or volume overload) Nutritional deficiency Burns Uncontrolled pain Heat stroke High altitude (usually >5,000 m)
Medications	Pain medications (e.g., postoperative meperidine [Demerol] or morphine [Duramorph]) Antibiotics, antivirals, and antifungals Steroids Anesthesia Cardiac medications Antihypertensives Antineoplastic agents Anticholinergic agents Neuroleptic malignant syndrome Serotonin syndrome
Over-the-counter preparations	Herbals, teas, and nutritional supplements
Botanicals	Jimsonweed, oleander, foxglove, hemlock, dieffenbachia, and *Amanita phalloides*
Cardiac	Cardiac failure, arrhythmia, myocardial infarction, cardiac assist device, cardiac surgery
Pulmonary	Chronic obstructive pulmonary disease, hypoxia, SIADH, acid base disturbance
Endocrine	Adrenal crisis or adrenal failure, thyroid abnormality, parathyroid abnormality
Hematological	Anemia, leukemia, blood dyscrasia, stem cell transplant
Renal	Renal failure, uremia, SIADH
Hepatic	Hepatitis, cirrhosis, hepatic failure
Neoplasm	Neoplasm (primary brain, metastases, paraneoplastic syndrome)
Drugs of abuse	Intoxication and withdrawal
Toxins	Intoxication and withdrawal Heavy metals and aluminum

SIADH, syndrome of inappropriate secretion of antidiuretic hormone.

Mrs. T is a 79-year-old retired schoolteacher who was brought to the emergency room after being found wandering around her neighborhood in a confused and disoriented state. She seemed to be in good health until a few months ago when her husband was hospitalized for 10 days for relatively minor surgery. About a month after her husband returned home, he and their two married daughters, who do not live at home, reported a noticeable change in Mrs. T's mental status. She became somewhat hyperactive and seemed to have excessive energy, was irritable and agitated, had difficulty getting to sleep at night, and became preoccupied with concerns that she was going to die. She began to prepare for death and wanted to visit relatives in the Midwest to see them for the last time.

After Mrs. T's confused and depressive symptoms had gone on for about a week, she was taken to see a psychiatrist, who made a diagnosis of depression and started her on imipramine and haloperidol (Haldol). Shortly after beginning these medications, her agitation decreased slightly, but she began to have difficulty remembering recent events and seemed even more confused and disoriented. These difficulties continued, and one day Mrs. T called the police telling them she was being poisoned by the pills she was being given. She became disoriented to time and place, markedly confused, incontinent, and began wandering away from home. When she encountered anyone, she became verbally and physically abusive.

When Mrs. T was brought in for an evaluation, the initial diagnostic impression was of a psychotic depression superimposed on a dementing illness. The consultant also noted that Mrs. T was experiencing a number of anticholinergic side effects, such as dry mouth, constipation, and racing heart, and suggested that she be removed from all medications. After she discontinued all medications, Mrs. T's condition improved rapidly; her psychotic thinking and assaultiveness disappeared, and her agitation and confusion decreased.

During the next several weeks, however, Mrs. T continued to have intermittent episodes of clouding of consciousness during which she became confused and disoriented. She was found wandering around her neighborhood in a confused state and was brought to the emergency room for evaluation.

Mrs. T's mental status examination on admission showed her to be disoriented to time and place, agitated, and confused. During an interview with the patient's husband, an important piece of information about Mrs. T's recent history was brought to light for the first time. Mrs. T had suffered for many years from dizziness and lightheadedness on standing and has had occasional falls, none of which have caused any lasting damage. Shortly before her depressive and confused symptoms began, Mrs. T apparently suffered a fall during the night and was found by her husband in the morning lying next to her bed in a confused state. Because they were accustomed to such falls, neither Mr. nor Mrs. T made much to this experience, nor did they report it to any of Mrs. T's physicians. A computed tomography (CT) scan revealed the presence of a subdural hematoma, which was then evacuated. After this procedure Mrs. T's confusion and disorientation cleared completely and she returned to her previous level of functioning. (Reprinted with permission from *DSM-IV-TR Case Studies.*)

The DSM-IV-TR gives separate diagnostic criteria for each type of delirium: (1) delirium due to a general medical condition (Table 10.2–5), (2) substance intoxication delirium (Table 10.2–6), (3) substance withdrawal delirium (Table 10.2–7), (4) delirium due to multiple etiologies (Table 10.2–8), and (5) delirium not otherwise specified (Table 10.2–9) for a delirium of unknown cause or of causes not listed, such as sensory deprivation. The syndrome, however, is the same, regardless of cause.

The core features of delirium include altered consciousness, such as decreased level of consciousness; altered attention, which can include diminished ability to focus, sustain, or shift attention; impairment in other realms of cognitive function, which can manifest as disorientation (especially to time and space)

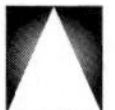

Table 10.2–5
DSM-IV-TR Diagnostic Criteria for Delirium Due to General Medical Condition

A. Disturbance of consciousness (i.e., reduced clarity of awareness of the environment) with reduced ability to focus, sustain, or shift attention.
B. A change in cognition (such as memory deficit, disorientation, language disturbance) or the development of a perceptual disturbance that is not better accounted for by a preexisting, established, or evolving dementia.
C. The disturbance develops over a short period of time (usually hours to days) and tends to fluctuate during the course of the day.
D. There is evidence from the history, physical examination, or laboratory findings that the disturbance is caused by the direct physiological consequences of a general medical condition.

Coding note: If delirium is superimposed on a preexisting vascular dementia, indicate the delirium by coding vascular dementia, with delirium.

Coding note: Include the name of the general medical condition on Axis I, e.g., Delirium due to hepatic encephalopathy; also code the general medical condition on Axis III.

(From American Psychiatric Association. *Diagnostic and Statistical Manual of Mental Disorders.* 4th ed. Text rev. Washington, DC: American Psychiatric Association; copyright 2000, with permission.)

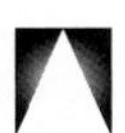

Table 10.2–6
DSM-IV-TR Diagnostic Criteria for Substance Intoxication Delirium

A. Disturbance of consciousness (i.e., reduced clarity of awareness of the environment) with reduced ability to focus, sustain, or shift attention.
B. A change in cognition (such as memory deficit, disorientation, language disturbance) or the development of a perceptual disturbance that is not better accounted for by a preexisting, established, or evolving dementia.
C. The disturbance develops over a short period of time (usually hours to days) and tends to fluctuate during the course of the day.
D. There is evidence from the history, physical examination, or laboratory findings of either (1) or (2):
   (1) the symptoms in Criteria A and B developed during substance intoxication
   (2) medication use is etiologically related to the disturbance*

   Note: This diagnosis should be made instead of a diagnosis of substance intoxication only when the cognitive symptoms are in excess of those usually associated with the intoxication syndrome and when the symptoms are sufficiently severe to warrant independent clinical attention.

   ***Note**: The diagnosis should be recorded as substance-induced delirium if related to medication use.

Code (Specific substance) intoxication delirium:

(Alcohol; Amphetamine [or amphetaminelike substance]; Cannabis; Cocaine; Hallucinogen; Inhalant; Opioid; Phencyclidine [or phencyclidinelike substance]; Sedative, hypnotic, or anxiolytic; Other [or unknown] substance [e.g., cimetidine, digitalis, benztropine])

(From American Psychiatric Association. *Diagnostic and Statistical Manual of Mental Disorders.* 4th ed. Text rev. Washington, DC: American Psychiatric Association; copyright 2000, with permission.)

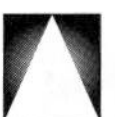

Table 10.2–7
DSM-IV-TR Diagnostic Criteria for Substance Withdrawal Delirium

A. Disturbance of consciousness (i.e., reduced clarity of awareness of the environment) with reduced ability to focus, sustain, or shift attention.
B. A change in cognition (such as memory deficit, disorientation, language disturbance) or the development of a perceptual disturbance that is not better accounted for by a preexisting, established, or evolving dementia.
C. The disturbance develops over a short period of time (usually hours to days) and tends to fluctuate during the course of the day.
D. There is evidence from the history, physical examination, or laboratory findings that the symptoms in Criteria A and B developed during, or shortly after, a withdrawal syndrome.

Note: This diagnosis should be made instead of a diagnosis of substance withdrawal only when the cognitive symptoms are in excess of those usually associated with the withdrawal syndrome and when the symptoms are sufficiently severe to warrant independent clinical attention.

Code (Specific substance) withdrawal delirium:

(Alcohol; Sedative, hypnotic, or anxiolytic; Other [or unknown] substance)

(From American Psychiatric Association. *Diagnostic and Statistical Manual of Mental Disorders.* 4th ed. Text rev. Washington, DC: American Psychiatric Association; copyright 2000, with permission.)

and decreased memory; relatively rapid onset (usually hours to days); brief duration (usually days to weeks); and often marked, unpredictable fluctuations in severity and other clinical manifestations during the course of the day, sometimes worse at night (sundowning), which may range from periods of lucidity to severe cognitive impairment and disorganization.

Associated clinical features are often present and may be prominent. They can include disorganization of thought processes (ranging from mild tangentiality to frank incoherence),

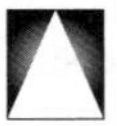

Table 10.2–8
DSM-IV-TR Diagnostic Criteria for Delirium Due to Multiple Etiologies

A. Disturbance of consciousness (i.e., reduced clarity of awareness of the environment) with reduced ability to focus, sustain, or shift attention.
B. A change in cognition (such as memory deficit, disorientation, language disturbance) or the development of a perceptual disturbance that is not better accounted for by a preexisting, established, or evolving dementia.
C. The disturbance develops over a short period of time (usually hours to days) and tends to fluctuate during the course of the day.
D. There is evidence from the history, physical examination, or laboratory findings that the delirium has more than one etiology (e.g., more than one etiological general medical condition, a general medical condition plus substance intoxication or medication side effect).

Coding note: Use multiple codes reflecting specific delirium and specific etiologies, e.g., Delirium due to viral encephalitis; Alcohol withdrawal delirium.

(From American Psychiatric Association. *Diagnostic and Statistical Manual of Mental Disorders.* 4th ed. Text rev. Washington, DC: American Psychiatric Association; copyright 2000, with permission.)

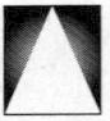

Table 10.2–9
DSM-IV-TR Diagnostic Criteria for Delirium Not Otherwise Specified

This category should be used to diagnose a delirium that does not meet criteria for any of the specific types of delirium described in this section.

Examples include

1. A clinical presentation of delirium that is suspected to be due to a general medical condition or substance use but for which there is insufficient evidence to establish a specific etiology
2. Delirium due to causes not listed in this section (e.g., sensory deprivation)

(From American Psychiatric Association. *Diagnostic and Statistical Manual of Mental Disorders.* 4th ed. Text rev. Washington, DC: American Psychiatric Association; copyright 2000, with permission.)

perceptual disturbances such as illusions and hallucinations, psychomotor hyperactivity and hypoactivity, disruption of the sleep–wake cycle (often manifested as fragmented sleep at night, with or without daytime drowsiness), mood alterations (from subtle irritability to obvious dysphoria, anxiety, or even euphoria), and other manifestations of altered neurological function (e.g., autonomic hyperactivity or instability, myoclonic jerking, and dysarthria). The electroencephalogram (EEG) usually shows diffuse slowing of background activity, although patients with delirium caused by alcohol or sedative-hypnotic withdrawal have low-voltage fast activity.

The major neurotransmitter hypothesized to be involved in delirium is acetylcholine, and the major neuroanatomical area is the reticular formation. The reticular formation of the brainstem is the principal area regulating attention and arousal; the major pathway implicated in delirium is the dorsal tegmental pathway, which projects from the mesencephalic reticular formation to the tectum and thalamus. Several studies have reported that a variety of delirium-inducing factors result in decreased acetylcholine activity in the brain. One of the most common causes of delirium is toxicity from too many prescribed medications with anticholinergic activity. In addition to the anticholinergic drugs themselves, many drugs used in psychiatry have similar effects (e.g., atropine, amitriptyline [Elavil], doxepin [Sinequan], nortriptyline [Aventyl], imipramine [Tofranil], and the phenothiazine class). Researchers have suggested other pathophysiological mechanisms for delirium. In particular, the delirium associated with alcohol withdrawal has been associated with hyperactivity of the locus ceruleus and its noradrenergic neurons. Other neurotransmitters that have been implicated are serotonin and glutamate.

PHYSICAL AND LABORATORY EXAMINATIONS

Delirium is usually diagnosed at the bedside and is characterized by the sudden onset of symptoms. A bedside mental status examination—such as the Mini-Mental State Examination, the mental status examination, or neurological signs—can be used to document the cognitive impairment and to provide a baseline from which to measure the patient's clinical course. The physical examination often reveals clues to the cause of the delirium (Table 10.2–10). The presence of a known physical illness or a history of head trauma or alcohol or other substance dependence increases the likelihood of the diagnosis.

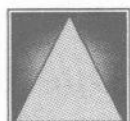

Table 10.2–10
Physical Examination of the Delirious Patient

Parameter	Finding	Clinical Implication
1. Pulse	Bradycardia	Hypothyroidism Stokes-Adams syndrome Increased intracranial pressure
	Tachycardia	Hyperthyroidism Infection Heart failure
2. Temperature	Fever	Sepsis Thyroid storm Vasculitis
3. Blood pressure	Hypotension	Shock Hypothyroidism Addison's disease
	Hypertension	Encephalopathy Intracranial mass
4. Respiration	Tachypnea	Diabetes Pneumonia Cardiac failure Fever Acidosis (metabolic)
	Shallow	Alcohol or other substance intoxication
5. Carotid vessels	Bruits or decreased pulse	Transient cerebral ischemia
6. Scalp and face	Evidence of trauma	
7. Neck	Evidence of nuchal rigidity	Meningitis Subarachnoid hemorrhage
8. Eyes	Papilledema	Tumor Hypertensive encephalopathy
	Pupillary dilatation	Anxiety Autonomic overactivity (e.g., delirium tremens)
9. Mouth	Tongue or cheek lacerations	Evidence of generalized tonic-clonic seizures
10. Thyroid	Enlarged	Hyperthyroidism
11. Heart	Arrhythmia	Inadequate cardiac output, possibility of emboli
	Cardiomegaly	Heart failure Hypertensive disease
12. Lungs	Congestion	Primary pulmonary failure Pulmonary edema Pneumonia
13. Breath	Alcohol	
	Ketones	Diabetes
14. Liver	Enlargement	Cirrhosis Liver failure
15. Nervous system		
a. Reflexes—muscle stretch	Asymmetry with Babinski's signs	Mass lesion Cerebrovascular disease Preexisting dementia
	Snout	Frontal mass Bilateral posterior cerebral artery occlusion
b. Abducent nerve (sixth cranial nerve)	Weakness in lateral gaze	Increased intracranial pressure
c. Limb strength	Asymmetrical	Mass lesion Cerebrovascular disease
d. Autonomic	Hyperactivity	Anxiety Delirium

(From Strub RL, Black FW. *Neurobehavioral Disorders: A Clinical Approach.* Philadelphia; FA Davis; 1981:120, with permission.)

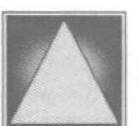

Table 10.2–11
Laboratory Workup of the Patient with Delirium

Standard studies
- Blood chemistries (including electrolytes, renal and hepatic indexes, and glucose)
- Complete blood count with white cell differential
- Thyroid function tests
- Serologic tests for syphilis
- Human immunodeficiency virus (HIV) antibody test
- Urinalysis
- Electrocardiogram
- Electroencephalogram
- Chest radiograph
- Blood and urine drug screens

Additional tests when indicated
- Blood, urine, and cerebrospinal fluid (CSF) cultures
- B_{12}, folic acid concentrations
- Computed tomography or magnetic resonance imaging brain scan
- Lumbar puncture and CSF examination

The laboratory workup of a patient with delirium should include standard tests and additional studies indicated by the clinical situation (Table 10.2–11). In delirium, the EEG characteristically shows a generalized slowing of activity and may be useful in differentiating delirium from depression or psychosis. The EEG of a delirious patient sometimes shows focal areas of hyperactivity. In rare cases, it may be difficult to differentiate delirium related to epilepsy from delirium related to other causes.

DIFFERENTIAL DIAGNOSIS

Delirium versus Dementia

A number of clinical features help distinguish delirium from dementia (Table 10.2–12). The major differential points between dementia and delirium are the time to development of the condition and the fluctuation in level of attention in delirium compared with relatively consistent attention in dementia. The time to development of symptoms is usually short in delirium and, except for vascular dementia caused by stroke, it is usually gradual and insidious in dementia. Although both conditions include cognitive impairment, the changes in dementia are more stable over time and, for example, usually do not fluctuate over the course of a day. A patient with dementia is usually alert; a patient with delirium has episodes of decreased consciousness. Occasionally, delirium occurs in a patient with dementia, a condition known as *beclouded dementia.* A dual diagnosis of delirium can be made when there is a definite history of preexisting dementia.

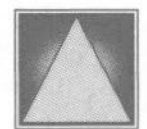

Table 10.2–12
Frequency of Clinical Features of Delirium Contrasted with Dementia

Feature	Dementia	Delirium
Onset	Slow	Rapid
Duration	Months to years	Hours to weeks
Attention	Preserved	Fluctuates
Memory	Impaired remote memory	Impaired recent and immediate memory
Speech	Word-finding difficulty	Incoherent (slow or rapid)
Sleep–wake cycle	Fragmented sleep	Frequent disruption (e.g., day–night reversal)
Thoughts	Impoverished	Disorganized
Awareness	Unchanged	Reduced
Alertness	Usually normal	Hypervigilant or reduced vigilance

(Adapted from Lipowski ZJ. *Delirium: Acute Confusional States.* Oxford: Oxford University Press; 1990, with permission.)

Delirium versus Schizophrenia or Depression

Delirium must also be differentiated from schizophrenia and depressive disorder. Some patients with psychotic disorders, usually schizophrenia or manic episodes, can have periods of extremely disorganized behavior difficult to distinguish from delirium. In general, however, the hallucinations and delusions of patients with schizophrenia are more constant and better organized than those of patients with delirium. Patients with schizophrenia usually experience no change in their level of consciousness or in their orientation. Patients with hypoactive symptoms of delirium may appear somewhat similar to severely depressed patients, but they can be distinguished on the basis of an EEG. Other psychiatric diagnoses to consider in the differential diagnosis of delirium are brief psychotic disorder, schizophreniform disorder, and dissociative disorders. Patients with factitious disorders may attempt to simulate the symptoms of delirium, but usually reveal the factitious nature of their symptoms by inconsistencies on their mental status examinations, and an EEG can easily separate the two diagnoses.

COURSE AND PROGNOSIS

Although the onset of delirium is usually sudden, prodromal symptoms (e.g., restlessness and fearfulness) can occur in the days preceding the onset of florid symptoms. The symptoms of delirium usually persist as long as the causally relevant factors are present, although delirium generally lasts less than a week. After identification and removal of the causative factors, the symptoms of delirium usually recede over a 3- to 7-day period, although some symptoms may take up to 2 weeks to resolve completely. The older the patient and the longer the patient has been delirious, the longer the delirium takes to resolve. Recall of what transpired during a delirium, once it is over, is characteristically spotty; a patient may refer to the episode as a bad dream or a nightmare only vaguely remembered. As stated in the discussion on epidemiology, the occurrence of delirium is associated with a high mortality rate in the ensuing year, primarily because of the serious nature of the associated medical conditions that lead to delirium.

Whether delirium progresses to dementia has not been demonstrated in carefully controlled studies, although many clinicians believe that they have seen such a progression. A clinical observation that has been validated by some studies, however, is that periods of delirium are sometimes followed by depression or posttraumatic stress disorder.

TREATMENT

In treating delirium, the primary goal is to treat the underlying cause. When the underlying condition is anticholinergic toxicity, the use of physostigmine salicylate (Antilirium), 1 to 2 mg intravenously or intramuscularly, with repeated doses in 15 to

30 minutes may be indicated. The other important goal of treatment is to provide physical, sensory, and environmental support. Physical support is necessary so that delirious patients do not get into situations in which they may have accidents. Patients with delirium should be neither sensory deprived nor overly stimulated by the environment. They are usually helped by having a friend or relative in the room or by the presence of a regular sitter. Familiar pictures and decorations, the presence of a clock or a calendar, and regular orientations to person, place, and time help make patients with delirium comfortable. Delirium can sometimes occur in older patients wearing eye patches after cataract surgery ("black-patch delirium"). Such patients can be helped by placing pinholes in the patches to let in some stimuli or by occasionally removing one patch at a time during recovery.

Pharmacotherapy

The two major symptoms of delirium that may require pharmacological treatment are psychosis and insomnia. A commonly used drug for psychosis is haloperidol (Haldol), a butyrophenone antipsychotic drug. Depending on a patient's age, weight, and physical condition, the initial dose may range from 2 to 6 mg intramuscularly, repeated in an hour if the patient remains agitated. As soon as the patient is calm, oral medication in liquid concentrate or tablet form should begin. Two daily oral doses should suffice, with two thirds of the dose being given at bedtime. To achieve the same therapeutic effect, the oral dose should be approximately 1.5 times the parenteral dose. The effective total daily dose of haloperidol may range from 5 to 40 mg for most patients with delirium. Droperidol (Inapsine) is a butyrophenone available as an alternative intravenous formulation, although careful monitoring of the electrocardiogram may be prudent with this treatment. Phenothiazines should be avoided in delirious patients because these drugs are associated with significant anticholinergic activity.

Use of second-generation antipsychotics, such as risperidone (Risperdal), clozapine, olanzapine (Zyprexa), quetiapine (Seroquel), ziprasidone (Geodon), and aripiprazole (Abilify), may be considered for delirium management, but clinical trial experience with these agents for delirium is limited. Ziprasidone appears to have an activating effect and may not be appropriate in delirium management. Olanzapine is available for intramuscular (IM) use and as a rapidly disintegrating oral preparation. These routes of administration may be preferable for some patients with delirium who are poorly compliant with medications or who are too sedated to safely swallow medications. For patients with Parkinson's disease and delirium who require antipsychotic medications, clozapine or quetiapine have some support in the literature and are less likely to exacerbate parkinsonian symptoms.

Insomnia is best treated with benzodiazepines with short or intermediate half-lives (e.g., lorazepam [Ativan] 1 to 2 mg at bedtime). Benzodiazepines with long half-lives and barbiturates should be avoided unless they are being used as part of the treatment for the underlying disorder (e.g., alcohol withdrawal). There have been case reports of improvement in or remission of delirious states caused by intractable medical illnesses with electroconvulsive therapy (ECT); however, routine consideration of ECT for delirium is not advised. If delirium is caused by severe pain or dyspnea, a physician should not hesitate to prescribe opioids for both their analgesic and sedative effects.

Treatment in Special Populations

Parkinson's Disease. In Parkinson's disease, the antiparkinsonian agents are frequently implicated in causing a delirium. If a coexistent dementia is present, delirium is twice as likely to develop in patients with Parkinson's disease with dementia receiving antiparkinsonian agents than in those without dementia. Decreasing the dosage of the antiparkinsonian agent has to be weighed against a worsening of motor symptoms. If the antiparkinsonian agents cannot be further reduced, or if the delirium persists after attenuation of the antiparkinsonian agents, clozapine is recommended. If a patient is not able to tolerate clozapine or the required blood monitoring, alternative antipsychotic agents should be considered. Quetiapine has not been as rigorously studied as clozapine and may have parkinsonian side

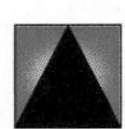

Table 10.2–13
ICD-10 Diagnostic Criteria for Delirium, Not Induced by Alcohol and Other Psychoactive Substances

A. There is clouding of consciousness, i.e., reduced clarity of awareness of the environment, with reduced ability to focus, sustain, or shift attention.

B. Disturbance of cognition is manifest by both:
(1) impairment of immediate recall and recent memory, with relatively intact remote memory;
(2) disorientation in time, place, or person.

C. At least one of the following psychomotor disturbances is present:
(1) rapid, unpredictable shifts from hypoactivity to hyperactivity;
(2) increased reaction time;
(3) increased or decreased flow of speech;
(4) enhanced startle reaction.

D. There is disturbance of sleep or of the sleep-wake cycle, manifest by at least one of the following:
(1) insomnia, which in severe cases may involve total sleep loss, with or without daytime drowsiness, or reversal of the sleep-wake cycle;
(2) nocturnal worsening of symptoms;
(3) disturbing dreams and nightmares, which may continue as hallucinations or illusions after awakening.

E. Symptoms have rapid onset and show fluctuations over the course of the day.

F. There is objective evidence from history, physical and neurological examination, or laboratory tests of an underlying cerebral or systemic disease (other than psychoactive substance-related) that can be presumed to be responsible for the clinical manifestations in Criteria A–D.

Comments

Emotional disturbances such as depression, anxiety or fear, irritability, euphoria, apathy, or wondering perplexity, disturbances of perception (illusions or hallucinations, often visual), and transient delusions are typical but are not specific indications for the diagnosis. A fourth character may be used to indicate whether or not the delirium is superimposed on dementia:

Delirium, not superimposed on dementia
Delirium, superimposed on dementia
Other delirium
Delirium, unspecified

(Reprinted with permission from World Health Organization. *The ICD-10 Classification of Mental and Behavioural Disorders: Diagnostic Criteria for Research.* Copyright, World Health Organization, Geneva, 1993.)

effects, but it is used in clinical practice to treat psychosis in Parkinson's disease.

Terminally Ill Patients. When delirium occurs in the context of a terminal illness, issues about advanced directives and the existence of a health care proxy become more significant. This scenario emphasizes the importance of early development of advance directives for health care decision-making while a person has the capacity to communicate the wishes regarding the extent of aggressive diagnostic tests at life's end. The focus may change from an aggressive search for the etiology of the delirium to one of palliation, comfort, and assistance with dying.

ICD-10

The 10th revision of *International Statistical Classification of Diseases and Related Health Problems* (ICD-10) criteria for delirium, not induced by alcohol and other psychoactive substances, are presented in Table 10.2–13.

References

Bogardus ST Jr, Desai MM, Williams CS, Leo-Summers L, Acampora D, Inouye SK. The effects of a targeted multicomponent delirium intervention on postdischarge outcomes for hospitalized older adults. *Am J Med.* 2003;114:383–390.

Centeno C, Sanz Á, Bruera E. Delirium in advanced cancer patients. *Palliat Med.* 2004;18(3):184–194.

Engel GL, Romano J. Delirium, a syndrome of cerebral insufficiency. *J Neuropsychiatry Clin Neurosci.* 2004;16:526–538.

Inouye SK, Bogardus ST Jr, Williams CS, Leo-Summers L, Agostini JV. The role of adherence on the effectiveness of nonpharmacologic interventions: Evidence from the delirium prevention trial. *Arch Intern Med.* 2003;163:958–964.

Kales HC, Kamholz BA, Visnic SG, Blow FC. Recorded delirium in a national sample of elderly inpatients: Potential implications for recognition. *J Geriatr Psychiatry Neurol.* 2003;16:32–38.

Leslie DL, Zhang Y, Holford TR, Bogardus ST, Leo-Summers LS, Inouye SK. Premature death associated with delirium at 1-year follow-up. *Arch Intern Med.* 2005;165:1657–1662.

Minden SL, Carbone LA, Barsky A, Borus JF, Fife A, Fricchione GL, Orav EJ. Predictors and outcomes of delirium. *Gen Hosp Psychiatry.* 2005;27(3):209–214.

Samuels SC, Neugroschl JA. Delirium. In: Sadock BJ, Sadock VA, eds. *Kaplan & Sadock's Comprehensive Textbook of Psychiatry.* 8th ed. Vol. 1. Baltimore: Lippincott Williams & Wilkins; 2005:1054.

Tancredi DN, Shannon MW. Case records of the Massachusetts General Hospital. Weekly clinicopathological exercises. Case 30-2003. A 21-year-old man with sudden alteration of mental status. *N Engl J Med.* 2003;349:1267–1275.

Young LJ, George J. Do guidelines improve the process and outcomes of care in delirium? *Age Aging.* 2003;32:525–528.

▲ 10.3 Dementia

Dementia is defined as a progressive impairment of cognitive functions occurring in clear consciousness (i.e., in the absence of delirium). Dementia consists of a variety of symptoms that suggest chronic and widespread dysfunction. Global impairment of intellect is the essential feature, manifested as difficulty with memory, attention, thinking, and comprehension. Other mental functions can often be affected, including mood, personality, judgment, and social behavior. Although specific diagnostic criteria are found for various dementias, such as Alzheimer's disease or vascular dementia, all dementias have certain common elements that result in significant impairment in social or occupational functioning and cause a significant decline from a previous level of functioning.

The critical clinical points of dementia are the identification of the syndrome and the clinical workup of its cause. The disorder can be progressive or static, permanent or reversible. An underlying cause is always assumed, although, in rare cases, it is impossible to determine a specific cause. The potential reversibility of dementia is related to the underlying pathological condition and to the availability and application of effective treatment. Approximately 15 percent of people with dementia have reversible illnesses if treatment is initiated before irreversible damage takes place.

EPIDEMIOLOGY

With the aging population, the prevalence of dementia is rising. The prevalence of moderate to severe dementia in different population groups is approximately 5 percent in the general population older than 65 years of age, 20 to 40 percent in the general population older than 85 years of age, 15 to 20 percent in outpatient general medical practices, and 50 percent in chronic care facilities.

Of all patients with dementia, 50 to 60 percent have the most common type of dementia, dementia of the Alzheimer's type (Alzheimer's disease). Dementia of the Alzheimer's type increases in prevalence with increasing age. For persons aged 65 years, men have a prevalence rate of 0.6 percent and women of 0.8 percent. At age 90, rates are 21 percent. For all these figures, 40 to 60 percent of cases are moderate to severe. The rates of prevalence (males to females) are 11 and 14 percent at age 85, 21 and 25 percent at age 90, and 36 and 41 percent at age 95. Patients with dementia of the Alzheimer's type occupy more than 50 percent of nursing home beds. More than 2 million persons with dementia are cared for in these homes. By 2050, current predictions suggest that there will be 14 million Americans with Alzheimer's disease and, therefore, more than 18 million people with dementia.

The second most common type of dementia is vascular dementia, which is causally related to cerebrovascular diseases. Hypertension predisposes a person to the disease. Vascular dementias account for 15 to 30 percent of all dementia cases. Vascular dementia is most common in persons between the ages of 60 and 70 and is more common in men than in women. Approximately 10 to 15 percent of patients have coexisting vascular dementia and dementia of the Alzheimer's type.

Other common causes of dementia, each representing 1 to 5 percent of all cases, include head trauma, alcohol-related dementias, and various movement disorder-related dementias, such as Huntington's disease and Parkinson's disease. Because dementia is a fairly general syndrome, it has many causes, and clinicians must embark on a careful clinical workup of a patient with dementia to establish its cause.

ETIOLOGY

The most common causes of dementia in individuals older than 65 years of age are (1) Alzheimer's disease; (2) vascular dementia and, (3) mixed vascular and Alzheimer's dementia. Other illnesses that account for approximately 10 percent include Lewy body dementia; Pick's disease; frontotemporal dementias;

Table 10.3–1
Possible Etiologies of Dementia

Degenerative dementias
- Alzheimer's disease
- Frontotemporal dementias (e.g., Pick's disease)
- Parkinson's disease
- Lewy body dementia
- Idiopathic cerebral ferrocalcinosis (Fahr's disease)
- Progressive supranuclear palsy

Miscellaneous
- Huntington's disease
- Wilson's disease
- Metachromatic leukodystrophy
- Neuroacanthocytosis

Psychiatric
- Pseudodementia of depression
- Cognitive decline in late-life schizophrenia

Physiologic
- Normal pressure hydrocephalus

Metabolic
- Vitamin deficiencies (e.g., vitamin B_{12}, folate)
- Endocrinopathies (e.g., hypothyroidism)
- Chronic metabolic disturbances (e.g., uremia)

Tumor
- Primary or metastatic (e.g., meningioma or metastatic breast or lung cancer)

Traumatic
- Dementia pugilistica, posttraumatic dementia
- Subdural hematoma

Infection
- Prion diseases (e.g., Creutzfeldt-Jakob disease, bovine spongiform encephalitis, Gerstmann-Sträussler syndrome)
- Acquired immune deficiency syndrome (AIDS)
- Syphilis

Cardiac, vascular, and anoxia
- Infarction (single or multiple or strategic lacunar)
- Binswanger's disease (subcortical arteriosclerotic encephalopathy)
- Hemodynamic insufficiency (e.g., hypoperfusion or hypoxia)

Demyelinating diseases
- Multiple sclerosis

Drugs and toxins
- Alcohol
- Heavy metals
- Irradiation
- Pseudodementia due to medications (e.g., anticholinergics)
- Carbon monoxide

normal pressure hydrocephalus (NPH); alcoholic dementia; infectious dementia, such as human immunodeficiency virus (HIV) or syphilis; and Parkinson's disease. Many types of dementias evaluated in clinical settings can be attributable to reversible causes, such as metabolic abnormalities (e.g., hypothyroidism), nutritional deficiencies (e.g., vitamin B_{12} or folate deficiencies), or dementia syndrome caused by depression. See Table 10.3–1 for a review of possible etiologies of dementia.

Dementia of the Alzheimer's Type

In 1907, Alois Alzheimer first described the condition that later assumed his name. He described a 51-year-old woman with a $4^1/_2$-year course of progressive dementia. The final diagnosis of Alzheimer's disease requires a neuropathological examination of the brain; nevertheless, dementia of the Alzheimer's type is commonly diagnosed in the clinical setting after other causes of dementia have been excluded from diagnostic consideration.

Genetic Factors. Although the cause of dementia of the Alzheimer's type remains unknown, progress has been made in understanding the molecular basis of the amyloid deposits that are a hallmark of the disorder's neuropathology. Some studies have indicated that as many as 40 percent of patients have a family history of dementia of the Alzheimer's type; thus, genetic factors are presumed to play a part in the development of the disorder, at least in some cases. Additional support for a genetic influence is the concordance rate for monozygotic twins, which is higher than the rate for dizygotic twins (43 percent vs. 8 percent, respectively). In several well-documented cases, the disorder has been transmitted in families through an autosomal dominant gene, although such transmission is rare. Alzheimer's type dementia has shown linkage to chromosomes 1, 14, and 21.

AMYLOID PRECURSOR PROTEIN. The gene for amyloid precursor protein is on the long arm of chromosome 21. The process of differential splicing yields four forms of amyloid precursor protein. The β/A4 protein, the major constituent of senile plaques, is a 42-amino acid peptide that is a breakdown product of amyloid precursor protein. In Down syndrome (trisomy 21) are found three copies of the amyloid precursor protein gene, and in a disease in which a mutation is found at codon 717 in the amyloid precursor protein gene, a pathological process results in the excessive deposition of β/A4 protein. Whether the processing of abnormal amyloid precursor protein is of primary causative significance in Alzheimer's disease is unknown, but many research groups are studying both the normal metabolic processing of amyloid precursor protein and its processing in patients with dementia of the Alzheimer's type in an attempt to answer this question.

MULTIPLE E4 GENES. One study implicated gene E4 in the origin of Alzheimer's disease. People with one copy of the gene have Alzheimer's disease three times more frequently than do those with no E4 gene, and people with two E4 genes have the disease eight times more frequently than do those with no E4 gene. Diagnostic testing for this gene is not currently recommended because it is found in persons without dementia and not found in all cases of dementia.

Neuropathology. The classic gross neuroanatomical observation of a brain from a patient with Alzheimer's disease is diffuse atrophy with flattened cortical sulci and enlarged cerebral ventricles. The classic and pathognomonic microscopic findings are senile plaques, neurofibrillary tangles, neuronal loss (particularly in the cortex and the hippocampus), synaptic loss (perhaps as much as 50 percent in the cortex), and granulovascular degeneration of the neurons. Neurofibrillary tangles (Fig. 10.3–1) are composed of cytoskeletal elements, primarily phosphorylated tau protein, although other cytoskeletal proteins are also present. Neurofibrillary tangles are not unique to Alzheimer's disease; they also occur in Down syndrome, dementia pugilistica (punch-drunk syndrome), Parkinson-dementia complex of Guam, Hallervorden-Spatz disease, and the brains of normal people as they age. Neurofibrillary tangles are commonly found in the cortex, the hippocampus, the substantia nigra, and the locus ceruleus.

Senile plaques, also referred to as *amyloid plaques*, more strongly indicate Alzheimer's disease, although they are also

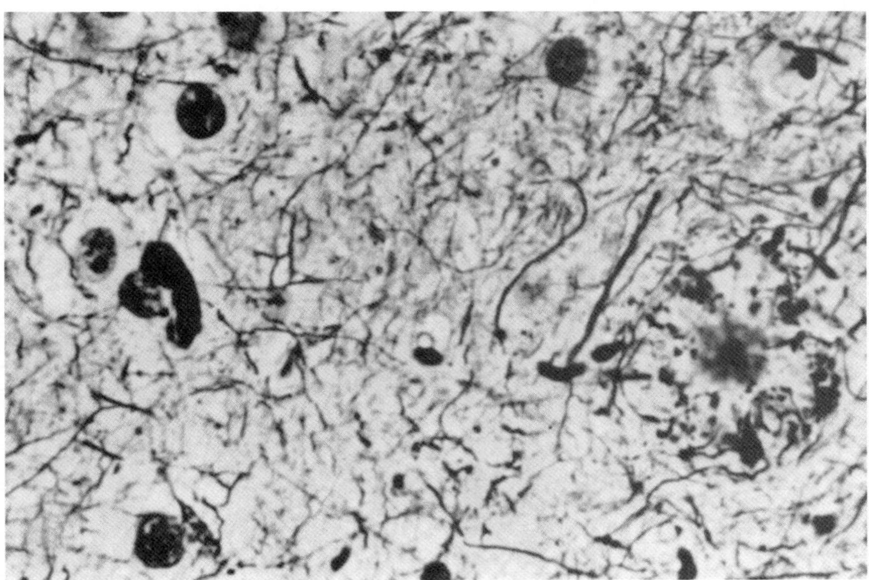

FIGURE 10.3–1
Alzheimer's disease. Prominent senile plaques on **left**. Several neurons with neurofibrillary tangles on **right**. Note also disruption of cortical organization. (From Mayeux R, Chun MR. Acquired and hereditary dementias. In: Rowland LP, ed. *Merritt's Textbook of Neurology*, 10th ed. Philadelphia: Lippincott Williams & Wilkins; 2000:636, with permission.)

seen in Down syndrome and, to some extent, in normal aging. Senile plaques are composed of a particular protein, β/A4, and astrocytes, dystrophic neuronal processes, and microglia. The number and the density of senile plaques present in postmortem brains have been correlated with the severity of the disease that affected the persons.

Neurotransmitters. The neurotransmitters that are most often implicated in the pathophysiological condition of Alzheimer's disease are acetylcholine and norepinephrine, both of which are hypothesized to be hypoactive in Alzheimer's disease. Several studies have reported data consistent with the hypothesis that specific degeneration of cholinergic neurons is present in the nucleus basalis of Meynert in persons with Alzheimer's disease. Other data supporting a cholinergic deficit in Alzheimer's disease demonstrate decreased acetylcholine and choline acetyltransferase concentrations in the brain. Choline acetyltransferase is the key enzyme for the synthesis of acetylcholine, and a reduction in choline acetyltransferase concentration suggests a decrease in the number of cholinergic neurons present. Additional support for the cholinergic deficit hypothesis comes from the observation that cholinergic antagonists, such as scopolamine and atropine, impair cognitive abilities, whereas cholinergic agonists, such as physostigmine and arecoline, enhance cognitive abilities. Decreased norepinephrine activity in Alzheimer's disease is suggested by the decrease in norepinephrine-containing neurons in the locus ceruleus found in some pathological examinations of brains from persons with Alzheimer's disease. Two other neurotransmitters implicated in the pathophysiological condition of Alzheimer's disease are the neuroactive peptides somatostatin and corticotropin; decreased concentrations of both have been reported in persons with Alzheimer's disease.

Other Causes. Another theory to explain the development of Alzheimer's disease is that an abnormality in the regulation of membrane phospholipid metabolism results in membranes that are less fluid—that is, more rigid—than normal. Several investigators are using molecular resonance spectroscopic imaging to assess this hypothesis directly in patients with dementia of the Alzheimer's type. Aluminum toxicity has also been hypothesized to be a causative factor, because high levels of aluminum have been found in the brains of some patients with Alzheimer's disease; but this is no longer considered a significant etiological factor. Excessive stimulation by the transmitter glutamate that may damage neurons is another theory of causation.

Familial Multiple System Taupathy with Presenile Dementia. A recently discovered type of dementia, familial multiple system taupathy, shares some brain abnormalities found in people with Alzheimer's disease. The gene that causes the disorder is thought to be carried on chromosome 17. The symptoms of the disorder include short-term memory problems and difficulty maintaining balance and walking. The onset of disease occurs in the 40s and 50s, and persons with the disease live an average of 11 years after the onset of symptoms.

As in patients with Alzheimer's disease, tau protein builds up in neurons and glial cells of persons with familial multiple system taupathy. Eventually, the protein buildup kills brain cells. The disorder is not associated with the senile plaques seen with Alzheimer's disease.

Vascular Dementia

The primary cause of vascular dementia, formerly referred to as *multi-infarct dementia*, is presumed to be multiple areas of cerebral vascular disease, resulting in a symptom pattern of

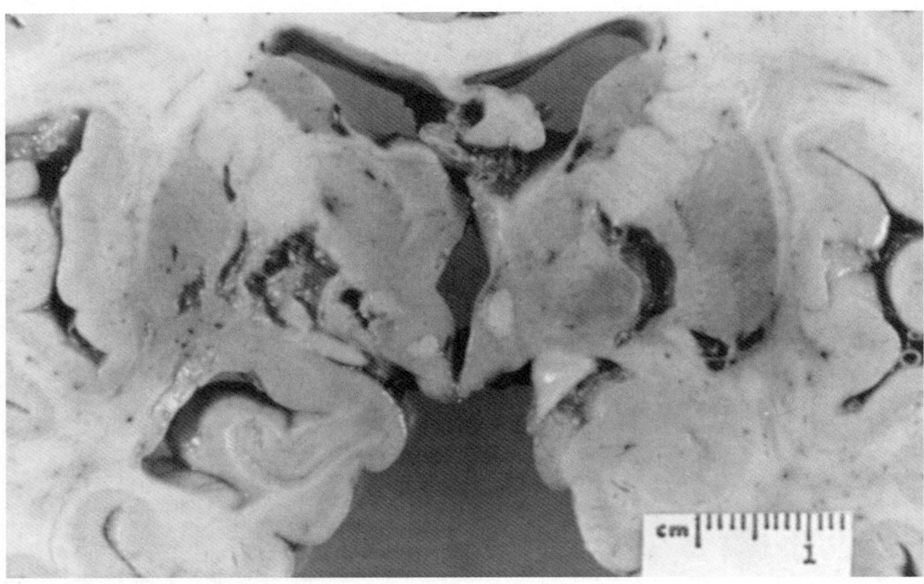

FIGURE 10.3–2
Gross appearance of the cerebral cortex on coronal section from a case of vascular dementia. The multiple bilateral lacunar infarcts involve the thalamus, the internal capsule, and the globus pallidus. (Courtesy of Daniel P. Perl, M.D.)

dementia. Vascular dementia most commonly is seen in men, especially those with preexisting hypertension or other cardiovascular risk factors. The disorder affects primarily small- and medium-sized cerebral vessels, which undergo infarction and produce multiple parenchymal lesions spread over wide areas of the brain (Fig. 10.3–2). The causes of the infarctions can include occlusion of the vessels by arteriosclerotic plaques or thromboemboli from distant origins (e.g., heart valves). An examination of a patient may reveal carotid bruits, fundoscopic abnormalities, or enlarged cardiac chambers (Fig. 10.3–3).

Binswanger's Disease. Binswanger's disease, also known as *subcortical arteriosclerotic encephalopathy*, is characterized by the presence of many small infarctions of the white matter that spare the cortical regions (Fig. 10.3–4). Although Binswanger's disease was previously considered a rare condition, the advent of sophisticated and powerful imaging techniques, such as magnetic resonance imaging (MRI), has revealed that the condition is more common than previously thought.

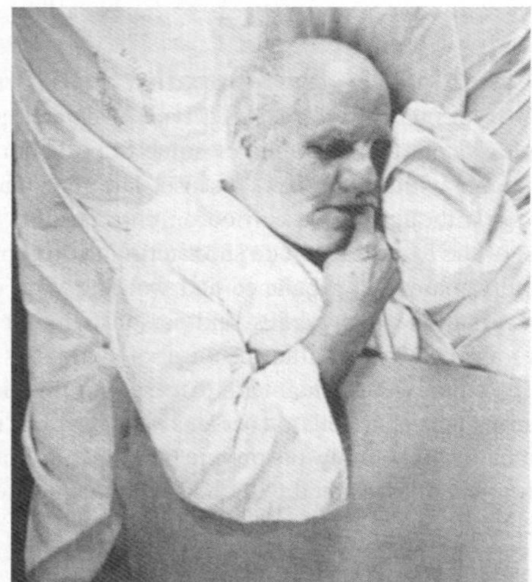

FIGURE 10.3–3
The patient with chronic dementia usually requires custodial care in his declining years. Regressive behavior, such as finger-sucking, is typical in this state. (Courtesy of Bill Stanton for Magnum Photos, Inc.)

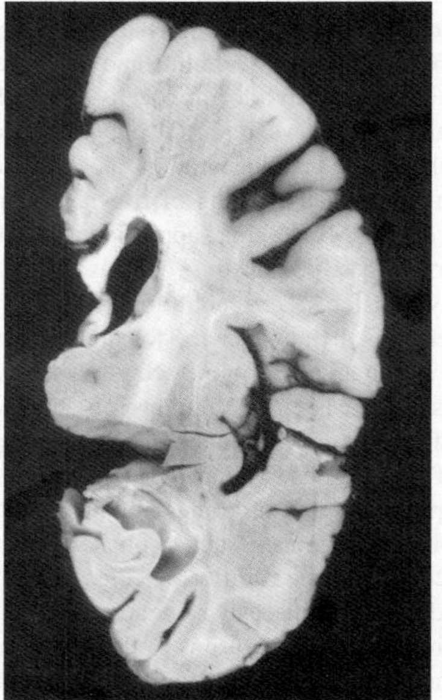

FIGURE 10.3–4
Binswanger's disease. Cross section demonstrating extensive subcortical white matter infarction, with sparing of the overlying gray matter. (Courtesy of Dushyant Purohit, M.D., Neuropathology Division, Mount Sinai School of Medicine, New York, NY.)

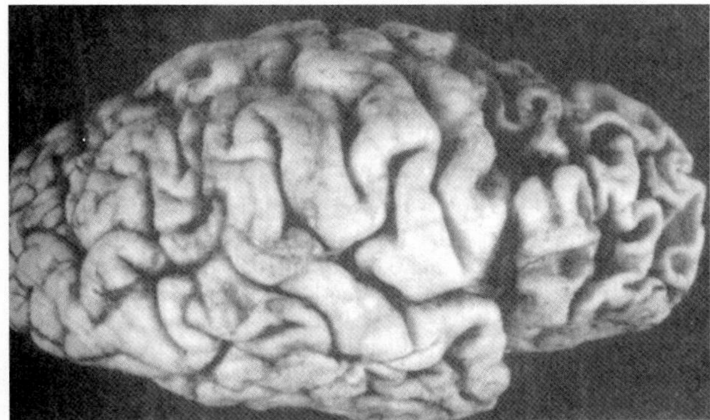

FIGURE 10.3–5

Pick's disease gross pathology. This demonstrates the marked frontal and temporal atrophy seen in frontotemporal dementias, such as Pick's disease. (Courtesy of Dushyant Purohit, M.D., Neuropathology Division, Mount Sinai School of Medicine, New York, NY.)

Pick's Disease

In contrast to the parietal-temporal distribution of pathological findings in Alzheimer's disease, Pick's disease is characterized by a preponderance of atrophy in the frontotemporal regions. These regions also have neuronal loss, gliosis, and neuronal Pick's bodies, which are masses of cytoskeletal elements. Pick's bodies are seen in some postmortem specimens but are not necessary for the diagnosis. The cause of Pick's disease is unknown, but the disease constitutes approximately 5 percent of all irreversible dementias. It is most common in men, especially those who have a first-degree relative with the condition. Pick's disease is difficult to distinguish from dementia of the Alzheimer's type, although the early stages of Pick's disease are more often characterized by personality and behavioral changes, with relative preservation of other cognitive functions, and it typically begins before 75 years of age. Familial cases may have an earlier onset, and some studies have shown that approximately one half of the cases of Pick's disease are familial (Fig. 10.3–5). Features of Klüver-Bucy syndrome (e.g., hypersexuality, placidity, and hyperorality) are much more common in Pick's disease than in Alzheimer's disease.

Lewy Body Disease

Lewy body disease is a dementia clinically similar to Alzheimer's disease and often characterized by hallucinations, parkinsonian features, and extrapyramidal signs (Table 10.3–2). Lewy inclusion bodies are found in the cerebral cortex (Fig. 10.3–6). The exact incidence is unknown. These patients show marked adverse effects when given antipsychotic medications.

Huntington's Disease

Huntington's disease is classically associated with the development of dementia. The dementia seen in this disease is the subcortical type of dementia, characterized by more motor abnormalities and fewer language abnormalities than in the cortical type of dementia (Table 10.3–3). The dementia of Huntington's disease exhibits psychomotor slowing and difficulty with complex tasks, but memory, language, and insight remain relatively intact in the early and middle stages of the illness. As the disease progresses, however, the dementia becomes complete; the features distinguishing it from dementia of the Alzheimer's type are the high incidence of depression and psychosis, in addition to the classic choreoathetoid movement disorder.

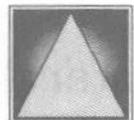

Table 10.3–2
Clinical Criteria for Dementia with Lewy Bodies (DLB)

The patient must have sufficient cognitive decline to interfere with social or occupational functioning. Of note early in the illness, memory symptoms may not be as prominent as attention, frontosubcortical skills, and visuospatial ability. Probable DLB requires two or more core symptoms, whereas possible DLB only requires one core symptom.

Core features
Fluctuating levels of attention and alertness
Recurrent visual hallucinations
Parkinsonian features (cogwheeling, bradykinesia, and resting tremor)

Supporting features
Repeated falls
Syncope
Sensitivity to neuroleptics
Systematized delusions
Hallucinations in other modalities (e.g. auditory, tactile)

(Adapted from McKeith LG, Galasko D, Kosaka K. Consensus guidelines for the clinical and pathologic diagnosis of dementia with Lewy bodies (DLB): Report of the consortium on DLB international workshop. *Neurology.* 1996;47:1113–1124, with permission.)

Parkinson's Disease

As with Huntington's disease, parkinsonism is a disease of the basal ganglia, commonly associated with dementia and depression. An estimated 20 to 30 percent of patients with Parkinson's disease have dementia, and an additional 30 to 40 percent have measurable impairment in cognitive abilities. The slow movements of persons with Parkinson's disease are paralleled in the slow thinking of some affected patients, a feature that clinicians may refer to as *bradyphrenia*.

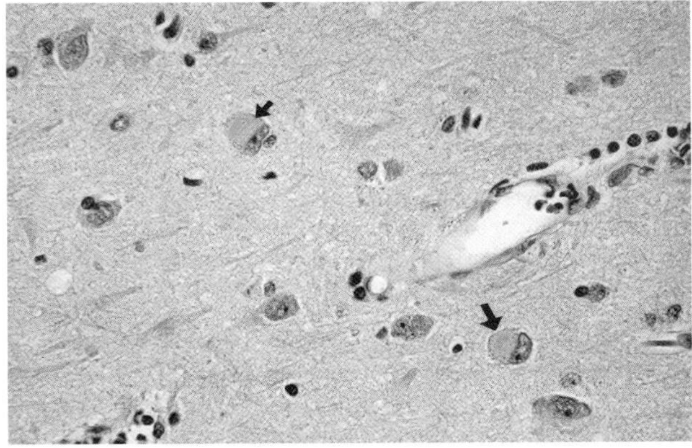

FIGURE 10.3–6

Cortical Lewy bodies (*arrows*), seen with hematoxylin and eosin staining. Lewy bodies are weakly eosinophilic, spherical, cytoplasmic inclusions. (Courtesy of Dushyant Purohit, M.D., Neuropathology Division, Mount Sinai School of Medicine, New York, NY.)

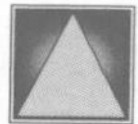

Table 10.3–3
Distinguishing Features of Subcortical and Cortical Dementias

Characteristic	Subcortical Dementia	Cortical Dementia	Recommended Tests
Language	No aphasia (anomia, if severe)	Aphasia early	FAS test Boston Naming test WAIS-R vocabulary test
Memory	Impaired recall (retrieval) > recognition (encoding)	Recall and recognition impaired	Wechsler memory scale; Symbol Digit Paired Associate Learning (Brandt)
Attention and immediate recall	Impaired	Impaired	WAIS-R digit span
Visuospatial skills	Impaired	Impaired	Picture arrangement, object assembly and block design; WAIS subtests
Calculation	Preserved until late	Involved early	Mini-Mental State
Frontal system abilities (executive function)	Disproportionately affected	Degree of impairment consistent with other involvement	Wisconsin Card Sorting Test; Odd Man Out test; Picture Absurdities
Speed of cognitive processing	Slowed early	Normal until late in disease	Trail making A and B: Paced Auditory Serial Addition Test (PASAT)
Personality	Apathetic, inert	Unconcerned	MMPI
Mood	Depressed	Euthymic	Beck and Hamilton depression scales
Speech	Dysarthric	Articulate until late	Verbal fluency (Rosen, 1980)
Posture	Bowed or extended	Upright	
Coordination	Impaired	Normal until late	
Motor speed and control	Slowed	Normal	Finger-tap; grooved pegboard
Adventitious movements	Chorea,tremor tics, dystonia	Absent (Alzheimer's dementia—some myoclonus)	
Abstraction	Impaired	Impaired	Category test (Halstead Battery)

(From Pajeau AK, Román GC. HIV encephalopathy and dementia. In: J Biller, RG Kathol, eds. *The Psychiatric Clinics of North America: The Interface of Psychiatry and Neurolgy.* Vol. 15. Philadelphia: WB Saunders; 1992:457, with permission.)

HIV-Related Dementia

Encephalopathy in HIV infection is associated with dementia and is termed *acquired immune deficiency syndrome* (AIDS) *dementia complex,* or *HIV dementia.* Patients infected with HIV experience dementia at an annual rate of approximately 14 percent. An estimated 75 percent of patients with AIDS have involvement of the central nervous system (CNS) at the time of autopsy. The development of dementia in people infected with HIV is often paralleled by the appearance of parenchymal abnormalities in MRI scans. Other infectious dementias are caused by *Cryptococcus* or *Treponema pallidum.*

The diagnosis of AIDS dementia complex is made by confirmation of HIV infection and exclusion of alternative pathology to explain cognitive impairment. The American Academy of Neurology AIDS Task Force developed research criteria for the clinical diagnosis of CNS disorders in adults and adolescents (Table 10.3–4). The AIDS Task Force criteria for AIDS dementia complex require laboratory evidence for systemic HIV, at least two cognitive deficits, and the presence of motor abnormalities or personality changes. Personality changes may be manifested by apathy, emotional lability, or behavioral disinhibition. As with the DSM-IV-TR, the AIDS Task Force criteria also require the absence of clouding of consciousness or evidence of another etiology that could produce the cognitive impairment. Cognitive, motor, and behavioral changes are assessed using physical, neurological, and psychiatric examinations, in addition to neuropsychological testing.

Head Trauma-Related Dementia

Dementia can be a sequela of head trauma. The so-called punch-drunk syndrome (dementia pugilistica) occurs in boxers after repeated head trauma over many years. It is characterized by emotional lability, dysarthria, and impulsivity.

DIAGNOSIS AND CLINICAL FEATURES

The dementia diagnoses in DSM-IV-TR are dementia of the Alzheimer's type (Table 10.3–5), vascular dementia (Table 10.3–6), dementia due to other general medical conditions (Table 10.3–7), substance-induced persisting dementia (Table 10.3–8), dementia due to multiple etiologies (Table 10.3–9), and dementia not otherwise specified (Table 10.3–10).

The diagnosis of dementia is based on the clinical examination, including a mental status examination, and on information from the patient's family, friends, and employers. Complaints of a personality change in a patient older than age 40 suggest that a diagnosis of dementia should be carefully considered.

Clinicians should note patients' complaints about intellectual impairment and forgetfulness as well as evidence of patients' evasion, denial, or rationalization aimed at concealing cognitive deficits. Excessive orderliness, social withdrawal, or a tendency to relate events in minute detail can be characteristic, and sudden outbursts of anger or sarcasm can occur. Patients' appearance and behavior should be observed. Lability of emotions, sloppy grooming, uninhibited remarks, silly jokes, or a dull, apathetic, or vacuous facial expression and manner suggest the presence of dementia, especially when coupled with memory impairment.

Memory impairment is typically an early and prominent feature in dementia, especially in dementias involving the cortex, such as dementia of the Alzheimer's type. Early in the course of dementia, memory impairment is mild and usually most marked for recent events; people forget telephone numbers, conversations, and events of the day. As the course of dementia progresses, memory impairment becomes severe, and only the earliest learned information (e.g., a person's place of birth) is retained.

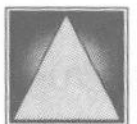

Table 10.3–4
Criteria for Clinical Diagnosis of HIV Type 1-Associated Dementia Complex

Laboratory evidence for systemic human immunodeficiency virus (HIV) type 1 infection with confirmation by Western blot, polymerase chain reaction, or culture.
Acquired abnormality in at least *two* of cognitive abilities for a period of at least 1 month: attention and concentration, speed of processing information, abstraction and reasoning, visuospatial skills, memory and learning, and speech and language. The decline should be verified by reliable history and mental status examination. History should be obtained from an informant, and examination should be supplemented by neuropsychological testing.
Cognitive dysfunction causes impairment in social or occupational functioning. Impairment should not be attributable solely to severe systemic illness.
At least *one* of the following:
  Acquired abnormality in motor function verified by clinical examination (e.g., slowed rapid movements, abnormal gait, incoordination, hyperreflexia, hypertonia, or weakness), neuropsychological tests (e.g., fine motor speed, manual dexterity, or perceptual motor skills), or both.
  Decline in motivation or emotional control or a change in social behavior. This may be characterized by a change in personality with apathy, inertia, irritability, emotional lability, or a new onset of impaired judgment or disinhibition.
This does not exclusively occur in the context of a delirium.
Evidence of another etiology, including active central nervous system opportunistic infection, malignancy, psychiatric disorders (e.g., major depression), or substance abuse, if present, is *not* the cause of the previously mentioned symptoms and signs.

(Adapted from Working Group of the American Academy of Neurology AIDS Task Force: Nomenclature and research case definitions for neurologic manifestations of human immunodeficiency virus–type 1 (HIV-1) infection. *Neurology.* 1991;41:778–785, with permission.)

Inasmuch as memory is important for orientation to person, place, and time, orientation can be progressively affected during the course of a dementing illness. For example, patients with dementia may forget how to get back to their rooms after going to the bathroom. No matter how severe the disorientation seems, however, patients show no impairment in their level of consciousness.

Dementing processes that affect the cortex, primarily dementia of the Alzheimer's type and vascular dementia, can affect patients' language abilities. DSM-IV-TR includes aphasia as one of the diagnostic criteria. The language difficulty may be characterized by a vague, stereotyped, imprecise, or circumstantial locution, and patients may also have difficulty naming objects.

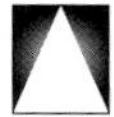

Table 10.3–5
DSM-IV-TR Diagnostic Criteria for Dementia of the Alzheimer's Type

A. The development of multiple cognitive deficits manifested by both
  (1) memory impairment (impaired ability to learn new information or to recall previously learned information)
  (2) one (or more) of the following cognitive disturbances:
    (a) aphasia (language disturbance)
    (b) apraxia (impaired ability to carry out motor activities despite intact motor function)
    (c) agnosia (failure to recognize or identify objects despite intact sensory function)
    (d) disturbance in executive functioning (i.e., planning, organizing, sequencing, abstracting)
B. The cognitive deficits in Criteria A1 and A2 each cause significant impairment in social or occupational functioning and represent a significant decline from a previous level of functioning.
C. The course is characterized by gradual onset and continuing cognitive decline.
D. The cognitive deficits in Criteria A1 and A2 are not due to any of the following:
  (1) other central nervous system conditions that cause progressive deficits in memory and cognition (e.g., cerebrovascular disease, Parkinson's disease, Huntington's disease, subdural hematoma, normal-pressure hydrocephalus, brain tumor)
  (2) systemic conditions that are known to cause dementia (e.g., hypothyroidism, vitamin B_{12} or folic acid deficiency, niacin deficiency, hypercalcemia, neurosyphilis, HIV infection)
  (3) substance-induced conditions
E. The deficits do not occur exclusively during the course of a delirium.
F. The disturbance is not better accounted for by another Axis I disorder (e.g., major depressive disorder, schizophrenia).

Code based on presence or absence of a clinically significant behavioral disturbance:
  Without behavioral disturbance: if the cognitive disturbance is not accompanied by any clinically significant behavioral disturbance.
  With behavioral disturbance: if the cognitive disturbance is accompanied by a clinically significant behavioral disturbance (e.g., wandering, agitation).
Specify subtype:
  With early onset: if onset is at age 65 years or below
  With late onset: if onset is after age 65 years
Coding note: Also code Alzheimer's disease on Axis III. Indicate other prominent clinical features related to the Alzheimer's disease on Axis I (e.g., Mood disorder due to Alzheimer's disease, with depressive features, and Personality change due to Alzheimer's disease, aggressive type).

(From American Psychiatric Association. *Diagnostic and Statistical Manual of Mental Disorders.* 4th ed. Text rev. Washington, DC: American Psychiatric Association; copyright 2000, with permission.)

Psychiatric and Neurological Changes

Personality. Changes in the personality of a person with dementia are especially disturbing for their families. Preexisting personality traits may be accentuated during the development of a dementia. Patients with dementia may also become introverted and seem to be less concerned than they previously were about the effects of their behavior on others. Persons with dementia who have paranoid delusions are generally hostile to family members and caretakers. Patients with frontal and temporal involvement are likely to have marked personality changes and may be irritable and explosive.

Hallucinations and Delusions. An estimated 20 to 30 percent of patients with dementia (primarily patients with dementia of the Alzheimer's type) have hallucinations, and 30 to 40 percent have delusions, primarily of a paranoid or persecutory and unsystematized nature, although complex, sustained, and well-systematized delusions are also reported by these patients. Physical aggression and other forms of violence are common in demented patients who also have psychotic symptoms.

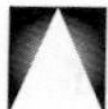

Table 10.3–6
DSM-IV-TR Diagnostic Criteria for Vascular Dementia

A. The development of multiple cognitive deficits manifested by both
  (1) memory impairment (impaired ability to learn new information or to recall previously learned information)
  (2) one (or more) of the following cognitive disturbances:
    (a) aphasia (language disturbance)
    (b) apraxia (impaired ability to carry out motor activities despite intact motor function)
    (c) agnosia (failure to recognize or identify objects despite intact sensory function)
    (d) disturbance in executive functioning (i.e., planning, organizing, sequencing, abstracting)

B. The cognitive deficits in Criteria A1 and A2 each cause significant impairment in social or occupational functioning and represent a significant decline from a previous level of functioning.

C. Focal neurological signs and symptoms (e.g., exaggeration of deep tendon reflexes, extensor plantar response, pseudobulbar palsy, gait abnormalities, weakness of an extremity) or laboratory evidence indicative of cerebrovascular disease (e.g., multiple infarctions involving cortex and underlying white matter) that are judged to be etiologically related to the disturbance.

D. The deficits do not occur exclusively during the course of a delirium.

Code based on predominant features:
  With delirium: if delirium is superimposed on the dementia
  With delusions: if delusions are the predominant feature
  With depressed mood: if depressed mood (including presentations that meet full symptom criteria for a major depressive episode) is the predominant feature. A separate diagnosis of mood disorder due to a general medical condition is not given.
  Uncomplicated: if none of the above predominates in the current clinical presentation

Specify if:
  With behavioral disturbance

Coding note: Also code cerebrovascular condition on Axis III.

(From American Psychiatric Association. *Diagnostic and Statistical Manual of Mental Disorders*. 4th ed. Text rev. Washington, DC: American Psychiatric Association; copyright 2000, with permission.)

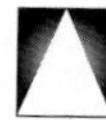

Table 10.3–7
DSM-IV-TR Diagnostic Criteria for Dementia Due to Other General Medical Conditions

A. The development of multiple cognitive deficits manifested by both
  (1) memory impairment (impaired ability to learn new information or to recall previously learned information)
  (2) one (or more) of the following cognitive disturbances:
    (a) aphasia (language disturbance)
    (b) apraxia (impaired ability to carry out motor activities despite intact motor function)
    (c) agnosia (failure to recognize or identify objects despite intact sensory function)
    (d) disturbance in executive functioning (i.e., planning, organizing, sequencing, abstracting)

B. The cognitive deficits in Criteria A1 and A2 each cause significant impairment in social or occupational functioning and represent a significant decline from a previous level of functioning.

C. There is evidence from the history, physical examination, or laboratory findings that the disturbance is the direct physiological consequence of a general medical condition other than Alzheimer's disease or cerebrovascular disease (e.g., HIV infection, traumatic brain injury, Parkinson's disease, Huntington's disease, Pick's disease, Creutzfeldt-Jakob disease, normal-pressure hydrocephalus, hypothyroidism, brain tumor, or vitamin B_{12} deficiency).

D. The deficits do not occur exclusively during the course of a delirium.

Code based on presence or absence of a clinically significant behavioral disturbance:
  Without behavioral disturbance: if the cognitive disturbance is not accompanied by any clinically significant behavioral disturbance.
  With behavioral disturbance: if the cognitive disturbance is accompanied by a clinically significant behavioral disturbance (e.g., wandering, agitation).

Coding note: Also code the general medical condition on Axis III (e.g., HIV infection, head injury, Parkinson's disease, Huntington's disease, Pick's disease, Creutzfeldt-Jakob disease).

(From American Psychiatric Association. *Diagnostic and Statistical Manual of Mental Disorders*. 4th ed. Text rev. Washington, DC: American Psychiatric Association; copyright 2000, with permission.)

Mood. In addition to psychosis and personality changes, depression and anxiety are major symptoms in an estimated 40 to 50 percent of patients with dementia, although the full syndrome of depressive disorder may be present in only 10 to 20 percent. Patients with dementia also may exhibit pathological laughter or crying—that is, extremes of emotions—with no apparent provocation.

Cognitive Change. In addition to the aphasias in patients with dementia, apraxias and agnosias are common, and they are included as potential diagnostic criteria in DSM-IV-TR. Other neurological signs that can be associated with dementia are seizures, seen in approximately 10 percent of patients with dementia of the Alzheimer's type and in 20 percent of patients with vascular dementia, and atypical neurological presentations, such as nondominant parietal lobe syndromes. Primitive reflexes, such as the grasp, snout, suck, tonic-foot, and palmomental reflexes, may be present on neurological examination, and myoclonic jerks are present in 5 to 10 percent of patients.

Patients with vascular dementia may have additional neurological symptoms, such as headaches, dizziness, faintness, weakness, focal neurological signs, and sleep disturbances, possibly attributable to the location of the cerebrovascular disease. Pseudobulbar palsy, dysarthria, and dysphagia are also more common in vascular dementia than in other dementing conditions.

Catastrophic Reaction. Patients with dementia also exhibit a reduced ability to apply what Kurt Goldstein called the "abstract attitude." Patients have difficulty generalizing from a single instance, forming concepts, and grasping similarities and differences among concepts. Furthermore, the ability to solve problems, to reason logically, and to make sound judgments is compromised. Goldstein also described a catastrophic reaction marked by agitation secondary to the subjective awareness of intellectual deficits under stressful circumstances. Persons usually attempt to compensate for defects by using strategies to avoid demonstrating failures in intellectual performance; they may change the subject, make jokes, or otherwise divert the

Table 10.3–8
DSM-IV-TR Diagnostic Criteria for Substance-Induced Persisting Dementia

A. The development of multiple cognitive deficits manifested by both
 (1) memory impairment (impaired ability to learn new information or to recall previously learned information)
 (2) one (or more) of the following cognitive disturbances:
  (a) aphasia (language disturbance)
  (b) apraxia (impaired ability to carry out motor activities despite intact motor function)
  (c) agnosia (failure to recognize or identify objects despite intact sensory function)
  (d) disturbance in executive functioning (i.e., planning, organizing, sequencing, abstracting)

B. The cognitive deficits in Criteria A1 and A2 each cause significant impairment in social or occupational functioning and represent a significant decline from a previous level of functioning.

C. The deficits do not occur exclusively during the course of a delirium and persist beyond the usual duration of substance intoxication or withdrawal.

D. There is evidence from the history, physical examination, or laboratory findings that the deficits are etiologically related to the persisting effects of substance use (e.g., a drug of abuse, a medication).

Code (Specific substance)-induced persisting dementia:
 (Alcohol; Inhalant; Sedative, hypnotic, or anxiolytic; Other [or unknown] substance)

(From American Psychiatric Association. *Diagnostic and Statistical Manual of Mental Disorders.* 4th ed. Text rev. Washington, DC: American Psychiatric Association; copyright 2000, with permission.)

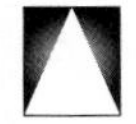

Table 10.3–9
DSM-IV-TR Diagnostic Criteria for Dementia Due to Multiple Etiologies

A. The development of multiple cognitive deficits manifested by both
 (1) memory impairment (impaired ability to learn new information or to recall previously learned information)
 (2) one (or more) of the following cognitive disturbances:
  (a) aphasia (language disturbance)
  (b) apraxia (impaired ability to carry out motor activities despite intact motor function)
  (c) agnosia (failure to recognize or identify objects despite intact sensory function)
  (d) disturbance in executive functioning (i.e., planning, organizing, sequencing, abstracting)

B. The cognitive deficits in Criteria A1 and A2 each cause significant impairment in social or occupational functioning and represent a significant decline from a previous level of functioning.

C. There is evidence from the history, physical examination, or laboratory findings that the disturbance has more than one etiology (e.g., head trauma plus chronic alcohol use, dementia of the Alzheimer's type with the subsequent development of vascular dementia).

D. The deficits do not occur exclusively during the course of a delirium.

Coding note: Use multiple codes based on specific dementias and specific etiologies e.g., Dementia of the Alzheimer's type, with late onset, without behavioral disturbance; Vascular dementia, uncomplicated.

(From American Psychiatric Association. *Diagnostic and Statistical Manual of Mental Disorders.* 4th ed. Text rev. Washington, DC: American Psychiatric Association; copyright 2000, with permission.)

Table 10.3–10
DSM-IV-TR Diagnostic Criteria for Dementia Not Otherwise Specified

This category should be used to diagnose a dementia that does not meet criteria for any of the specific types described in this section.

An example is a clinical presentation of dementia for which there is insufficient evidence to establish a specific etiology.

(From American Psychiatric Association. *Diagnostic and Statistical Manual of Mental Disorders.* 4th ed. Text rev. Washington, DC: American Psychiatric Association; copyright 2000, with permission.)

interviewer. Lack of judgment and poor impulse control appear commonly, particularly in dementias that primarily affect the frontal lobes. Examples of these impairments include coarse language, inappropriate jokes, neglect of personal appearance and hygiene, and a general disregard for the conventional rules of social conduct.

Sundowner Syndrome. Sundowner syndrome is characterized by drowsiness, confusion, ataxia, and accidental falls. It occurs in older people who are overly sedated and in patients with dementia who react adversely to even a small dose of a psychoactive drug. The syndrome also occurs in demented patients when external stimuli, such as light and interpersonal orienting cues, are diminished.

Dementia of the Alzheimer's Type

The DSM-IV-TR diagnostic criteria for dementia of the Alzheimer's type emphasize the presence of memory impairment and the associated presence of at least one other symptom of cognitive decline (aphasia, apraxia, agnosia, or abnormal executive functioning). The diagnostic criteria also require a continuing and gradual decline in functioning, impairment in social or occupational functioning, and the exclusion of other causes of dementia. According to DSM-IV-TR, the age of onset can be characterized as early (at age 65 or younger) or late (after age 65) and any predominant behavioral symptom should be coded with the diagnosis, if appropriate.

A 61-year-old high-school science department head, an experienced and enthusiastic camper and hiker, became extremely fearful while on a trek in the mountains. Gradually, over the next few months, he lost interest in his usual hobbies. Formerly a voracious reader, he stopped reading. He had difficulty doing computations and made gross errors in home financial management. On several occasions, he became lost while driving in areas that were formerly familiar to him. He began to write notes to himself so that he would not forget to do errands. Very abruptly, and in uncharacteristic fashion, he decided to retire from work, without discussing his plans with his wife. Intellectual deterioration gradually progressed. He spent most of the day piling miscellaneous objects in one place and then transporting them to another spot in the house. He became stubborn and querulous. Eventually, he required assistance in shaving and dressing.

When examined 6 years after the first symptoms had developed, the patient was alert and cooperative. He was disoriented with respect to place and time. He could not recall the names of four or five objects after a 5-minute interval of distraction. He could not remember the names of his college and graduate school or the subject in which he had majored. He could describe his job by title only. In 1978, he thought that Kennedy was president of the United States. He did not know Stalin's nationality. His speech was fluent and well articulated, but he had considerable difficulty finding words and used many long, essentially meaningless phrases. He called a cup a vase and identified the rims of his glasses as the "the holders." He did simple calculations poorly. He could not copy a cube or draw a house. His interpretation of proverbs was concrete, and he had no insight into the nature of his disturbance.

An elementary neurological examination revealed nothing abnormal, and routine laboratory tests were also negative. A computed tomography scan, however, showed marked cortical atrophy. (From *DSM-IV-TR Casebook.*)

Vascular Dementia

The general symptoms of vascular dementia are the same as those for dementia of the Alzheimer's type, but the diagnosis of vascular dementia requires either clinical or laboratory evidence in support of a vascular cause of the dementia. Vascular dementia is more likely to show a decremental, stepwise deterioration than is Alzheimer's disease.

Dementia Due to Other General Medical Conditions

The DSM-IV-TR lists six specific causes of dementia that can be coded directly: HIV disease, head trauma, Parkinson's disease, Huntington's disease, Pick's disease, and Creutzfeldt-Jakob disease. A seventh category allows clinicians to specify other nonpsychiatric medical conditions associated with dementia.

Substance-Induced Persisting Dementia

To facilitate the clinician's thinking about differential diagnosis, substance-induced persisting dementia is listed in two places in the DSM-IV-TR, with the dementias and with the substance-related disorders. The specific substances that DSM-IV-TR cross references are alcohol, inhalants, sedatives, hypnotics, or anxiolytics, and other or unknown substances.

Alcohol-Induced Persisting Dementia. To make the diagnosis of alcohol-induced persisting dementia, the criteria for dementia must be met. Because amnesia can also occur in the context Korsakoff's psychosis, it is important to distinguish between memory impairment accompanied by other cognitive deficits (i.e., dementia) and amnesia caused by thiamine deficiency. To complicate matters, however, evidence also suggests that other cognitive functions, such as attention and concentration, may also be impaired in Wernicke-Korsakoff syndrome. In addition, alcohol abuse is frequently associated with mood changes, so poor concentration and other cognitive symptoms often observed in the context of a major depression must also be ruled out. Prevalence rates differ considerably according to the population studied and the diagnostic criteria used, although alcohol-related dementia has been estimated to account for approximately 4 percent of dementias.

PATHOLOGY, PHYSICAL FINDINGS, AND LABORATORY EXAMINATION

A comprehensive laboratory workup must be performed when evaluating a patient with dementia. The purposes of the workup are to detect reversible causes of dementia and to provide the patient and family with a definitive diagnosis. The range of possible causes of dementia mandates selective use of laboratory tests. The evaluation should follow informed clinical suspicion, based on the history and physical and mental status examination results. Table 10.1–5 in Section 10.1 lists a number of laboratory tests that are useful in evaluating specific diseases presenting as dementia. The continued improvements in brain imaging techniques, particularly MRI, have made differentiation between dementia of the Alzheimer's type and vascular dementia, in some cases, somewhat more straightforward than in the past. An active area of research is the use of single photon emission computed tomography (SPECT) to detect patterns of brain metabolism in various types of dementias; the use of SPECT images may soon help in the clinical differential diagnosis of dementing illnesses.

A general physical examination is a routine component of the workup for dementia. It may reveal evidence of systemic disease causing brain dysfunction, such as an enlarged liver and hepatic encephalopathy, or it may demonstrate systemic disease related to particular CNS processes. The detection of Kaposi's sarcoma, for example, should alert the clinician to the probable presence of AIDS and the associated possibility of AIDS dementia complex. Focal neurological findings, such as asymmetrical hyperreflexia or weakness, are seen more often in vascular than in degenerative disease. Frontal lobe signs and primitive reflexes occur in many disorders and often point to greater progression.

DIFFERENTIAL DIAGNOSIS

Dementia of the Alzheimer's Type versus Vascular Dementia

Classically, vascular dementia has been distinguished from dementia of the Alzheimer's type by the decremental deterioration that can accompany cerebrovascular disease over time. Although the discrete, stepwise deterioration may not be apparent in all cases, focal neurological symptoms are more common in vascular dementia than in dementia of the Alzheimer's type, as are the standard risk factors for cerebrovascular disease.

Vascular Dementia versus Transient Ischemic Attacks

Transient ischemic attacks (TIAs) are brief episodes of focal neurological dysfunction lasting less than 24 hours (usually 5 to 15 minutes). Although a variety of mechanisms may be responsible, the episodes are frequently the result of microembolization from a proximal intracranial arterial lesion that produces transient brain ischemia, and the episodes usually resolve without significant pathological alteration of the parenchymal tissue. Approximately one third of persons with untreated TIAs experience a brain infarction later; therefore, recognition of TIAs is an important clinical strategy to prevent brain infarction.

Clinicians should distinguish episodes involving the vertebrobasilar system from those involving the carotid arterial system. In general, symptoms of vertebrobasilar disease reflect a transient functional disturbance in either the brainstem or the occipital lobe; carotid distribution symptoms reflect unilateral retinal or hemispheric abnormality. Anticoagulant therapy, antiplatelet agglutinating drugs such as aspirin, and extracranial and intracranial reconstructive vascular surgery are effective in reducing the risk of infarction in patients with TIAs.

Delirium

Differentiating between delirium and dementia can be more difficult than the DSM-IV-TR classification indicates. In general, delirium is distinguished by rapid onset, brief duration, cognitive impairment fluctuation during the course of the day, nocturnal exacerbation of symptoms, marked disturbance of the sleep–wake cycle, and prominent disturbances in attention and perception.

Depression

Some patients with depression have symptoms of cognitive impairment difficult to distinguish from symptoms of dementia. The clinical picture is sometimes referred to as *pseudodementia*, although the term *depression-related cognitive dysfunction* is preferable and more descriptive (Table 10.3–11). Patients with depression-related cognitive dysfunction generally have prominent depressive symptoms, more insight into their symptoms than do demented patients, and often a history of depressive episodes.

Factitious Disorder

Persons who attempt to simulate memory loss, as in factitious disorder, do so in an erratic and inconsistent manner. In true dementia, memory for time and place is lost before memory for person, and recent memory is lost before remote memory.

Schizophrenia

Although schizophrenia can be associated with some acquired intellectual impairment, its symptoms are much less severe than are the related symptoms of psychosis and thought disorder seen in dementia.

Normal Aging

Aging is not necessarily associated with any significant cognitive decline, but minor memory problems can occur as a normal part of aging. These normal occurrences are sometimes referred to as *benign senescent forgetfulness* or *age-associated memory impairment*. They are distinguished from dementia by their minor severity and because they do not interfere significantly with a person's social or occupational behavior.

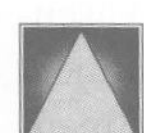

Table 10.3–11
Major Clinical Features Differentiating Pseudodementia from Dementia

Pseudodementia	Dementia
Clinical course and history	
Family always aware of dysfunction and its severity	Family often unaware of dysfunction and its severity
Onset can be dated with some precision	Onset can be dated only within broad limits
Symptoms of short duration before medical help is sought	Symptoms usually of long duration before medical help is sought
Rapid progression of symptoms after onset	Slow progression of symptoms throughout course
History of previous psychiatric dysfunction common	History of previous psychiatric dysfunction unusual
Complaints and clinical behavior	
Patients usually complain much of cognitive loss	Patients usually complain little of cognitive loss
Patients' complaints of cognitive dysfunction usually detailed	Patients' complaints of cognitive dysfunction usually vague
Patients emphasize disability	Patients conceal disability
Patients highlight failures	Patients delight in accomplishments, however trivial
Patients make little effort to perform even simple tasks	Patients struggle to perform tasks
	Patients rely on notes, calendars, etc., to keep up
Patients usually communicate strong sense of distress	Patients often appear unconcerned
Affective change often pervasive	Affect labile and shallow
Loss of social skills often early and prominent	Social skills often retained
Behavior often incongruent with severity of cognitive dysfunction	Behavior usually compatible with severity of cognitive dysfunction
Nocturnal accentuation of dysfunction uncommon	Nocturnal accentuation of dysfunction common
Clinical features related to memory, cognitive, and intellectual dysfunctions	
Attention and concentration often well preserved	Attention and concentration usually faulty
"Don't know" answers typical	Near-miss answers frequent
On tests of orientation, patients often give "don't know" answers	On tests of orientation, patients often mistake unusual for usual
Memory loss for recent and remote events usually severe	Memory loss for recent events usually more severe than for remote events
Memory gaps for specific periods or events common	Memory gaps for specific periods unusual[a]
Marked variability in performance on tasks of similar difficulty	Consistently poor performance on tasks of similar difficulty

[a]Except when caused by delirium, trauma, seizures, etc.
(Reprinted with permission from Wells CE. Pseudodementia. *Am J Psychiatry*. 1979;36:898.)

Other Disorders

Mental retardation, which does not include memory impairment, occurs in childhood. Amnestic disorder is characterized by circumscribed loss of memory and no deterioration. Major depression in which memory is impaired responds to antidepressant medication. Malingering and pituitary disorder must be ruled out, but they are unlikely.

COURSE AND PROGNOSIS

The classic course of dementia is an onset in the patient's 50s or 60s, with gradual deterioration over 5 to 10 years, leading eventually to death. The age of onset and the rapidity of deterioration vary among different types of dementia and within individual diagnostic categories. The average survival expectation for patients with dementia of the Alzheimer's type is approximately 8 years, with a range of 1 to 20 years. Data suggest that in persons with an early onset of dementia or with a family history of dementia the disease is likely to have a rapid course. In a recent study of 821 persons with Alzheimer's disease, the median survival time was 3.5 years. Once dementia is diagnosed, patients must have a complete medical and neurological workup, because 10 to 15 percent of all patients with dementia have a potentially reversible condition if treatment is initiated before permanent brain damage occurs.

The most common course of dementia begins with a number of subtle signs that may, at first, be ignored by both the patient and the people closest to the patient. A gradual onset of symptoms is most commonly associated with dementia of the Alzheimer's type, vascular dementia, endocrinopathies, brain tumors, and metabolic disorders. Conversely, the onset of dementia resulting from head trauma, cardiac arrest with cerebral hypoxia, or encephalitis can be sudden. Although the symptoms of the early phase of dementia are subtle, they become conspicuous as the dementia progresses, and family members may then bring a patient to a physician's attention. People with dementia may be sensitive to the use of benzodiazepines or alcohol, which can precipitate agitated, aggressive, or psychotic behavior. In the terminal stages of dementia, patients become empty shells of their former selves—profoundly disoriented, incoherent, amnestic, and incontinent of urine and feces.

With psychosocial and pharmacological treatment and possibly because of the self-healing properties of the brain, the symptoms of dementia may progress slowly for a time or may even recede somewhat. Symptom regression is certainly a possibility in reversible dementias (dementias caused by hypothyroidism, normal pressure hydrocephalus, and brain tumors) once treatment is initiated. The course of the dementia varies from a steady progression (commonly seen with dementia of the Alzheimer's type) to an incrementally worsening dementia (commonly seen with vascular dementia) to a stable dementia (as may be seen in dementia related to head trauma).

Psychosocial Determinants

The severity and course of dementia can be affected by psychosocial factors. The greater a person's premorbid intelligence and education, the better the ability to compensate for intellectual deficits. People who have a rapid onset of dementia use fewer defenses than do those who experience an insidious onset. Anxiety and depression can intensify and aggravate the symptoms. Pseudodementia occurs in depressed people who complain of impaired memory but, in fact, are suffering from a depressive disorder. When the depression is treated, the cognitive defects disappear.

TREATMENT

The first step in the treatment of dementia is verification of the diagnosis. Accurate diagnosis is imperative, for the progression may be halted or even reversed if appropriate therapy is provided. Preventive measures are important, particularly in vascular dementia. Such measures might include changes in diet, exercise, and control of diabetes and hypertension. Pharmacological agents might include antihypertensive, anticoagulant, or antiplatelet agents. Blood pressure control should aim for the higher end of the normal range, because that has been demonstrated to improve cognitive function in patients with vascular dementia. Blood pressure below the normal range has been demonstrated to further impair cognitive function in the patient with dementia. The choice of antihypertensive agent can be significant in that β-adrenergic receptor antagonists have been associated with exaggeration of cognitive impairment. Angiotensin-converting enzyme (ACE) inhibitors and diuretics have not been linked to exaggeration of cognitive impairment and are thought to lower blood pressure without affecting cerebral blood flow, which is presumed to be correlated with cognitive function. Surgical removal of carotid plaques may prevent subsequent vascular events in carefully selected patients. The general treatment approach to patients with dementia is to provide supportive medical care, emotional support for the patients and their families, and pharmacological treatment for specific symptoms, including disruptive behavior.

Psychosocial Therapies

The deterioration of mental faculties has significant psychological meaning for patients with dementia. The experience of a sense of continuity over time depends on memory. Recent memory is lost before remote memory in most cases of dementia, and many patients are highly distressed by clearly recalling how they used to function while observing their obvious deterioration. At the most fundamental level, the self is a product of brain functioning. Patients' identities begin to fade as the illness progresses, and they can recall less and less of their past. Emotional reactions ranging from depression to severe anxiety to catastrophic terror can stem from the realization that the sense of self is disappearing.

Patients often benefit from a supportive and educational psychotherapy in which the nature and course of their illness are clearly explained. They may also benefit from assistance in grieving and accepting the extent of their disability and from attention to self-esteem issues. Any areas of intact functioning should be maximized by helping patients identify activities in which successful functioning is possible. A psychodynamic assessment of defective ego functions and cognitive limitations can also be useful. Clinicians can help patients find ways to deal with the defective ego functions, such as keeping calendars for

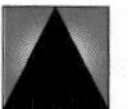

Table 10.3–12
ICD-10 Diagnostic Criteria for Dementia

G1. There is evidence of each of the following:

(1) A decline in memory, which is most evident in the learning of new information, although, in more severe cases, the recall of previously learned information may also be affected. The impairment applies to both verbal and nonverbal material. The decline should be objectively verified by obtaining a reliable history from an informant, supplemented, if possible, by neuropsychological tests or quantified cognitive assessments. The severity of the decline, with mild impairment as the threshold for diagnosis, should be assessed as follows:

Mild. The degree of memory loss is sufficient to interfere with everyday activities, though not so severe as to be incompatible with independent living. The main function affected is the learing of new material. For example, the individual has difficulty in registering, storing, and recalling elements involved in daily living, such as where belongings have been put, social arrangements, or information recently imparted by family members.

Moderate. The degree of memory loss represents a serious handicap to independent living. Only highly learned or very familiar material is retained. New information is retained only occasionally and very briefly. Individuals are unable to recall basic information about their own local geography, what they have recently been doing, or the names of familiar people.

Severe. The degree of memory loss is characterized by the complete inability to retain new information. Only fragments of previously learned information remain. The individual fails to recognize even close relatives.

(2) A decline in other cognitive abilities characterized by deterioration in judgment and thinking, such as planning and organizing, and in the general processing of information. Evidence for this should ideally be obtained from an informant and supplemented, if possible, by neuropsychological tests or quantified objective assessments. Deterioration from a previously higher level of performance should be established. The severity of the decline, with mild impairment as the threshold for diagnosis, should be assessed as follows:

Mild. The decline in cognitive abilities causes impaired performance in daily living, but not to a degree that makes the individual dependent on others. Complicated daily tasks or recreational activities cannot be undertaken.

Moderate. The decline in cognitive abilities makes the individual unable to function without the assistance of another in daily living, including shopping and handling money. Within the home, only simple chores can be performed. Activities are increasingly restricted and poorly sustained.

Severe. The decline is characterized by an absence, or virtual absence, of intelligible ideation.

The overall severity of the dementia is best expressed as the level of decline in memory *or* other cognitive abilities, whichever is the more severe (e.g., mild decline in memory *and* moderate decline in cognitive abilities indicate a dementia of moderate severity).

G2. Awareness of the environment (i.e., absence of clouding of consciousness [as defined in delirium, not induced by alcohol and other psychoactive substances. Criterion A]) is preserved during a period sufficiently long to allow the unequivocal demonstration of the symptoms in Criterion G1. When there are superimposed episodes of delirium, the diagnosis of dementia should be deferred.

G3. There is a decline in emotional control or motivation, or a change in social behavior manifest as at least one of the following:

(1) emotional lability
(2) irritability
(3) apathy
(4) coarsening of social behavior

G4. For a confident clinical diagnosis, the symptoms in criterion G1 should have been present for at least 6 months; if the period since the manifest onset is shorter, the diagnosis can be only tentative.

Comments

The diagnosis is further supported by evidence of damage to other higher cortical functions, such as aphasia, agnosia, apraxia.

Judgment about independent living or the development of dependence (upon others) should take account of the cultural expectation and context.

Dementia is specified here as having a minimum duration of 6 months to avoid confusion with reversible states with identical behavioral syndromes, such as traumatic subdural hemorrhage, normal pressure hydrocephalus, and diffuse or focal brain injury.

A fifth character may be used to indicate the presence of additional symptoms: Dementia in Alzheimer's disease, vascular dementia, dementia in diseases classified elsewhere, unspecified dementia, as follows:

Without additional symptoms
With other symptoms, predominantly delusional
With other symptoms, predominantly hallucinatory
With other symptoms, predominantly depressive
With other mixed symptoms

A sixth character may be used to indicate the severity of the dementia:

Mild
Moderate
Severe

As mentioned above, the overall severity of the dementia depends on the level of memory *or* intellectual impairment, whichever is the more severe.

ICD, International Classification of Diseases.
(From Wolrd Health Organization. *The ICD-10 Classification of Mental and Behavioural Disorders: Diagnostic Criteria for Research*. Copyright, World Health Organization, Geneva, 1993, with permission.)

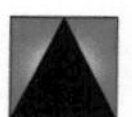

Table 10.3–13
ICD-10 Diagnostic Criteria for Dementia in Alzheimer's Disease

A. The general criteria for dementia G1–G4 must be met.
B. There is no evidence from the history, physical examination, or special investigations for any other possible cause of dementia (e.g., cerebrovascular disease, HIV disease, Parkinson's disease, Huntington's disease, normal pressure hydrocephalus), a systemic disorder (e.g., hypothyroidism, vitamin B_{12} or folic acid deficiency, hypercalcemia), or alcohol or drug abuse.

Comments

The diagnosis is confirmed by postmortem evidence of neurofibrillary tangles and neuritic plaques in excess of those found in normal aging of the brain.

The following features support the diagnosis, but are not necessary elements: involvement of cortical functions as evidenced by aphasia, agnosia, or apraxia; decrease of motivation and drive, leading to apathy and lack of spontaneity; irritability and disinhibition of social behavior; evidence from special investigations that there is cerebral atrophy, particularly if this can be shown to be increasing over time. In severe cases there may be Parkinson-like extrapyramidal changes, logoclonia, and epileptic fits.

Specification of features for possible subtypes

Because of the possibility that subtypes exist, it is recommended that the following characteristics be ascertained as a basis for a further classification age at onset; rate of progression; configuration of the clinical features, particularly the relative prominence (or lack) of temporal, parietal or frontal lobe signs; any neuropathological or neurochemical abnormalities, and their pattern.

The division of Alzheimer's disease into subtypes can at present be accomplished in two ways: first by taking only the age of onset and labeling the disease as either early or late, with an approximate cutoff point at 65 years; or second, by assessing how well the individual conforms to one of the two putative syndromes, early- or late- onset type.

It should be noted that a sharp distinction between early- and late-onset types is unlikely. Early-onset type may occur in late life, just as late-onset type may occasionally have an onset before the age of 65. The following criteria may be used to differentiate dementia in Alzheimer's disease with early and late onset, but it should be remembered that the status of this subdivision is still controversial.

Dementia in Alzheimer's disease with early onset

1. The criteria for dementia in Alzheimer's disease must be met, and the age at onset must be below 65 years.
2. In addition, at least one of the following requirements must be met:
   (a) evidence of a relatively rapid onset and progression;
   (b) in addition to memory impairment, there must be aphasia (amnesic or sensory), agraphia, alexia, acalculia, or apraxia (indicating the presence of temporal, parietal, and/or frontal lobe involvement).

Dementia in Alzheimer's disease with late onset

1. The criteria for dementia in Alzheimer's disease must be met and the age at onset must be 65 years or more.
2. In addition, at least one of the following requirements must be met:
   (a) evidence of a very slow, gradual onset and progression (the rate of the latter may be known only retrospectively after a course of 3 years or more);
   (b) predominance of memory impairment G1(1), over intellectual impairment G1(2) (see general criteria for dementia).

Dementia in Alzheimer's disease, atypical or mixed type

This term and code should be used for dementias that have important atypical features or that fulfill criteria for both early- and late-onset types of Alzheimer's disease. Mixed Alzheimer's and vascular dementia are also included here.

Dementia in Alzheimer's disease, unspecified

ICD, International Classification of Diseases.

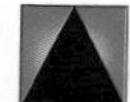

Table 10.3–14
ICD-10 Diagnostic Criteria for Vascular Dementia

G1. The general criteria for dementia (G1–G4) must be met.
G2. Deficits in higher cognitive functions are unevenly distributed, with some functions affected and others relatively spared. Thus, memory may be markedly affected while thinking, reasoning, and information processing may show only mild decline.
G3. There is clinical evidence of focal brain damage, manifest as at least one of the following:
(1) lateral spastic weakness of the limbs;
(2) unilaterally increased tendon reflexes;
(3) extensor plantar response;
(4) pseudobulbar palsy.
G4. There is evidence from the history, examination, or tests of a significant cerebrovascular disease, which may reasonably be judged to be etiologically related to the dementia (e.g., a history of stroke, evidence of cerebral infarction).

The following criteria may be used to differentiate subtypes of vascular dementia, but it should be remembered that the usefulness of this subdivision may not be generally accepted.

Vascular dementia of acute onset

A. The general criteria for vascular dementia must be met.
B. The dementia develops rapidly (i.e., usually within 1 month, but within no longer than 3 months) after succession of strokes or (rarely) after a single large infarction.

Multi-infarct dementia

A. The general criteria for vascular dementia must be met.
B. The onset of the dementia is gradual (i.e., within 3–6 months), following a number of minor ischemic episodes.

Comments

It is presumed that there is an accumulation of infarcts in the cerebral parenchyma. Between the ischemic episodes there may be period of actual clinical improvement.

Subcortical vascular dementia

A. The general criteria for vascular dementia must be met.
B. There is a history of hypertension.
C. There is evidence from clinical examination and special investigation of vascular disease located in the deep white matter of the cerebral hemispheres, with preservation of the cerebral cortex.

Mixed cortical and subcortical vascular dementia

Mixed cortical and subcortical components of the vascular dementia may be suspected from the clinical features, the results of investigation (including autopsy), or both.

Other vascular dementia

Vascular dementia, unspecified

ICD, International Classification of Diseases.

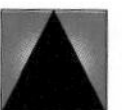

Table 10.3–15
ICD-10 Diagnostic Criteria for Dementia in Other Diseases

Classified elsewhere

Dementia in Pick's disease

A. The general criteria for dementia (G1–G4) must be met.
B. Onset is slow with steady deterioration.
C. Predominance of frontal lobe involvement is evidenced by two or more of the following:
 (1) emotional blunting;
 (2) coarsening of social behavior;
 (3) disinhibition;
 (4) apathy or restlessness;
 (5) aphasia
D. In the early stages, memory and parietal lobe functions are relatively preserved.

Dementia in Creutzfeldt-Jakob disease

A. The general criteria for dementia (G1–G4) must be met.
B. There is very rapid progression of the dementia, with disintegration of virtually all higher cerebral functions.
C. One or more of the following types of neurological symptoms and signs emerge, usually after or simultaneously with the dementia.
 (1) pyramidal symptoms;
 (2) extrapyramidal symptoms;
 (3) cerebellar symptoms;
 (4) aphasia;
 (5) visual impairment.

Comments

An akinetic and mute state is the typical terminal stage. An amyotrophic variant may be seen, where the neurological signs precede the onset of the dementia. A characteristic electroencephalogram (periodic spikes against a slow and low voltage background), if present in association with the above clinical signs, increases the probability of the diagnosis. However, the diagnosis can be confirmed only by neuropathological examination (neuronal loss, astrocytosis, and spongiform changes). Because of the risk of infection, this should be carried out only under special protective conditions.

Dementia in Huntington's disease

A. The general criteria for dementia (G1–G4) must be met.
B. Subcortical functions are affected first and dominate the picture of dementia throughout; subcortical involvement is manifested by slowness of thinking or movement and personality alteration with apathy or depression.
C. There are involuntary choreiform movements, typically of the face, hands, or shoulders, or in the gait. The patient may attempt to conceal them by converting them into a voluntary action.
D. There is a history of Huntington's disease in one parent or a sibling, or a family history that suggests the disorder.
E. There are no clinical features that otherwise account for the abnormal movements.

Comments

In addition to involuntary choreiform movements, there may be development of extrapyramidal rigidity or of spasticity with pyramidal signs.

Dementia in Parkinson's disease

A. The general criteria for dementia (G1–G4) must be met.
B. A diagnosis of Parkinson's disease has been established.
C. None of the cognitive impairment is attributable to antiparkinsonian medication.
D. There is no evidence from the history, physical examination, or special investigations for any other possible cause of dementia, including other forms of brain disease, damage, or dysfunction (e.g., cerebrovascular disease, HIV disease, Huntington's disease, normal pressure hydrocephalus), a systemic disorder (e.g., hypothyroidism, vitamin B_{12} or folic acid deficiency, hypercalcemia), or alcohol or drug abuse.

If criteria are also fulfilled for dementia in Alzheimer's disease with late onset, that category should be used in combination with Parkinson's disease.

Dementia in human immunodeficiency virus (HIV) disease

A. The general criteria for dementia (G1–G4) must be met.
B. A diagnosis of HIV infection has been established.
C. There is no evidence from the history, physical examination, or special investigations for any other possible cause of dementia, including other forms of brain disease, damage, or dysfunction (e.g., Alzheimer's disease, cerebrovascular disease, Parkinson's disease, Huntington's disease, normal pressure hydrocephalus), a systemic disorder (e.g., hypothyroidism, vitamin B_{12} or folic acid deficiency, hypercalcemia), or alcohol or drug abuse.

Dementia in other specified diseases classified elsewhere

Dementia can occur as a manifestation or consequence of a variety of cerebral and somatic conditions. To specify the etiology the ICD-10 code for the underlying condition should be added.

ICD, International Classification of Diseases.
(From World Health Organization. *The ICD-10 Classification of Mental and Behavioural Disorders: Diagnostic Criteria for Research.* Copyright, World Health Organization, Geneva, 1993, with permission.)

orientation problems, making schedules to help structure activities, and taking notes for memory problems.

Psychodynamic interventions with family members of patients with dementia may be of great assistance. Those who take care of a patient struggle with feelings of guilt, grief, anger, and exhaustion as they watch a family member gradually deteriorate. A common problem that develops among caregivers involves their self-sacrifice in caring for a patient. The gradually developing resentment from this self-sacrifice is often suppressed because of the guilt feelings it produces. Clinicians can help caregivers understand the complex mixture of feelings associated with seeing a loved one decline and can provide understanding as well as permission to express these feelings. Clinicians must also be aware of the caregivers' tendencies to blame themselves or others for patients' illnesses and must appreciate the role that patients with dementia play in the lives of family members.

Pharmacotherapy

Clinicians may prescribe benzodiazepines for insomnia and anxiety, antidepressants for depression, and antipsychotic drugs for delusions and hallucinations, but they should be aware of possible idiosyncratic drug effects in older people (e.g., paradoxical excitement, confusion, and increased sedation). In general, drugs with high anticholinergic activity should be avoided.

Donepezil (Aricept), rivastigmine (Exelon), galantamine (Remiryl), and tacrine (Cognex) are cholinesterase inhibitors used to treat mild to moderate cognitive impairment in Alzheimer's disease. They reduce the inactivation of the neurotransmitter acetylcholine and, thus, potentiate the cholinergic neurotransmitter, which in turn produces a modest improvement in memory and goal-directed thought. These drugs are most useful for persons with mild to moderate memory loss who have sufficient preservation of their basal forebrain cholinergic neurons to benefit from augmentation of cholinergic neurotransmission.

Donepezil is well tolerated and widely used. Tacrine is rarely used, because of its potential for hepatotoxicity. Fewer clinical data are available for rivastigmine and galantamine, which appear more likely to cause gastrointestinal (GI) and neuropsychiatric adverse effects than does donepezil. None of these medications prevents the progressive neuronal degeneration of the disorder. Prescribing information for anticholinesterase inhibitors can be found in Section 36.14.

Memantine (Namenda) protects neurons from excessive amounts of glutamate, which may be neurotoxic. The drug is sometimes combined with donepezil. It has been known to improve dementia.

Other Treatment Approaches. Other drugs being tested for cognitive-enhancing activity include general cerebral metabolic enhancers, calcium channel inhibitors, and serotonergic agents. Some studies have shown that selegiline (Eldepryl), a selective type B monoamine oxidase (MAO_B) inhibitor, may slow the advance of this disease. Ondansetron (Zofran), a 5-HT_3 receptor antagonist, is under investigation.

Estrogen replacement therapy may reduce the risk of cognitive decline in postmenopausal women; however, more studies are needed to confirm this effect. Complementary and alternative medicine studies of ginkgo biloba and other phytomedicinals to see if they have a positive effect on cognition. Reports have appeared of patients using nonsteroidal antiinflammatory agents having a lower risk of developing Alzheimer's disease. Vitamin E has not been shown to be of value in preventing the disease.

ICD-10

Except for dementia due to head trauma, all the dementias included in DSM-IV-TR are also in the tenth revision of the *International Statistical Classification of Diseases and Related Health Problems* (ICD-10). ICD-10 also includes general criteria for dementia (Table 10.3–12). Dementia in Alzheimer's disease is divided into four types (Table 10.3–13). ICD-10 divides vascular dementia into nine types based on the nature of the vascular disease (Table 10.3–14). ICD-10 includes two residual categories: dementia in other diseases classified elsewhere (e.g., dementia in Pick's disease) (Table 10.3–15) and unspecified dementia (dementia with an unknown cause).

References

Ferris SH, Yan B. Differential diagnosis and clinical assessment of patients with severe Alzheimer's disease. *Alzheimer Dis Assoc Disord.* 2003;17[Suppl 3]:S92–S93.

Helmes E, Bowler JV, Merskey H, Munoz DG, Hachinski VC. Rates of cognitive decline in Alzheimer's disease and dementia with Lewy bodies. *Dement Geriatr Cogn Disord.* 2003;15:67–71.

Lyketsos CG, Toone L, Tschanz J, Rabins PV, Steinberg M, Onyike CU, Corcoran C, Norton M, Zandi P, Breitner JCS, Welsh-Bohmer K. Population-based study of medical comorbidity in early dementia and "Cognitive impairment, no dementia (CIND)": Association with functional and cognitive impairment: The Cache County Study. *Am J Geriatric Psychiatry.* 2005;13:656–664.

Misciagna S, Masullo C, Giordano A, Silveri MC. Vascular dementia and Alzheimer's disease: The unsolved problem of clinical and neuropsychological differential diagnosis. *Int J Neurosci.* 2005;115:1657–1667.

Mosimann UP, Rowan EN, Partington CE, Collerton D, Littlewood E, O'Brien JT, Burn DJ, McKeith IG. Characteristics of visual hallucinations in Parkinson disease dementia and dementia with Lewy bodies. *Am J Geriatr Psychiatry.* 2006;14:153–160.

Neugroschl JA, Kolevzon A, Samuels SC, Marin DB. Dementia. In: Sadock BJ, Sadock VA, eds. *Kaplan & Sadock's Comprehensive Textbook of Psychiatry.* 8th ed. Vol. 1. Baltimore: Lippincott Williams & Wilkins; 2005:1068.

Reisberg B, Doody R, Stoffler A, Schmitt F, Ferris S, Mobius HJ. Memantine Study Group: Memantine in moderate-to-severe Alzheimer's disease. *N Engl J Med.* 2003;348:1333–1341.

Sano M, Wilcock GK, van Baelen B, Kavanagh S. The effects of galantamine treatment on caregiver time in Alzheimer's disease. *Int J Geriatr Psychiatry.* 2003;18:942–950.

Shumaker SA, Legault C, Rapp SR, Thal L, Wallace RB, Ockene JK, Hendrix SL, Jones BN 3rd, Assaf AR, Jackson RD, Kotchen JM, Wassertheil-Smoller S, Wactawski-Wende J; WHIMS Investigators. Estrogen plus progestin and the incidence of dementia and mild cognitive impairment in postmenopausal women: The Women's Health Initiative Memory Study: A randomized controlled trial. *JAMA.* 2003;289:2651–2662.

Wancata J, Musalek M, Alexandrowicz R, Krautgartner M. Number of dementia sufferers in Europe between the years 2000 and 2050. *Eur Psychiatry.* 2003;18:306–313.

Zandi PP, Sparks DL, Khachaturian AS, Tschanz JA, Norton M, Steinberg M, Welsh-Bohmer KA, Breitner JCS. Do statins reduce risk of incident dementia and Alzheimer disease? *Arch Gen Psychiatry.* 2005;62:217–224.

▲ 10.4 Amnestic Disorders

The amnestic disorders are a broad category that includes a variety of diseases and conditions that present with an amnestic syndrome. The syndrome is defined primarily by impairment in the ability to create new memories. Three variations of the amnestic disorder diagnosis, differing in etiology, are offered: amnestic disorder caused by a general medical condition (e.g., head trauma), substance-induced persisting amnestic disorder (e.g., caused by carbon monoxide poisoning or chronic alcohol consumption), and amnestic disorder not otherwise specified for cases in which the etiology is unclear. The two modifiers are (1) transient, for duration less than 1 month, and (2) chronic, for conditions extending beyond 1 month.

EPIDEMIOLOGY

No adequate studies have reported on the incidence or prevalence of amnestic disorders. Amnesia is most commonly found in alcohol use disorders and in head injury. In general practice and hospital settings, the frequency of amnesia related to chronic alcohol abuse has decreased, and the frequency of amnesia related to head trauma has increased.

ETIOLOGY

The major neuroanatomical structures involved in memory and in the development of an amnestic disorder are particular diencephalic structures such as the dorsomedial and midline nuclei of the thalamus and midtemporal lobe structures such as the hippocampus, the mamillary bodies, and the amygdala. Although amnesia is usually the result of bilateral damage to these structures, some cases of unilateral damage result in an amnestic disorder, and evidence indicates that the left hemisphere may be more critical than the right hemisphere in the development of memory disorders. Many studies of memory and amnesia in animals have suggested that other brain areas may also be involved in the symptoms accompanying amnesia. Frontal lobe involvement can result in such symptoms as confabulation and apathy, which can be seen in patients with amnestic disorders.

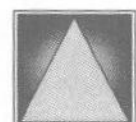

Table 10.4–1
Major Causes of Amnestic Disorders

Systemic medical conditions
  Thiamine deficiency (Korsakoff's syndrome)
Hypoglycemia
Primary brain conditions
  Seizures
  Head trauma (closed and penetrating)
  Cerebral tumors (especially thalamic and temporal lobe)
  Cerebrovascular diseases (especially thalamic and temporal lobe)
  Surgical procedures on the brain
  Encephalitis due to herpes simplex
  Hypoxia (including nonfatal hanging attempts and carbon monoxide poisoning)
  Transient global amnesia
  Electroconvulsive therapy
  Multiple sclerosis
Substance-related causes
  Alcohol use disorders
  Neurotoxins
  Benzodiazepines (and other sedative-hypnotics)
  Many over-the-counter preparations

Amnestic disorders have many potential causes (Table 10.4–1). Thiamine deficiency, hypoglycemia, hypoxia (including carbon monoxide poisoning), and herpes simplex encephalitis all have a predilection to damage the temporal lobes, particularly the hippocampi, and thus can be associated with the development of amnestic disorders. Similarly, when tumors, cerebrovascular diseases, surgical procedures, or multiple sclerosis plaques involve the diencephalic or temporal regions of the brain, the symptoms of an amnestic disorder may develop. General insults to the brain, such as seizures, electroconvulsive therapy (ECT), and head trauma, can also result in memory impairment. Transient global amnesia is presumed to be a cerebrovascular disorder involving transient impairment in blood flow through the vertebrobasilar arteries.

Many drugs have been associated with the development of amnesia, and clinicians should review all drugs taken, including nonprescription drugs, in the diagnostic workup of a patient with amnesia. The benzodiazepines are the most commonly used prescription drugs associated with amnesia. All benzodiazepines can be associated with amnesia, especially if combined with alcohol. When triazolam (Halcion) is used in doses of 0.25 mg or less, which are generally equivalent to standard doses of other benzodiazepines, amnesia is no more often associated with triazolam than with other benzodiazepines. With alcohol and higher doses, anterograde amnesia has been reported.

DIAGNOSIS

For the diagnosis of amnestic disorder, the text revision of the fourth edition of *Diagnostic and Statistical Manual of Mental Disorders* (DSM-IV-TR) requires the "development of memory impairment as manifested by impairment in the ability to learn new information or the inability to recall previously learned information," and the "memory disturbance [must cause] . . . significant impairment in social or occupational functioning." A diagnosis of amnestic disorder caused by a general medical condition (Table 10.4–2) is made when evidence exists of a causatively relevant specific medical condition (including physical trauma). DSM-IV-TR further categorizes the diagnosis as transient or chronic. A diagnosis of substance-induced persisting amnestic disorder is made when evidence suggests that the symptoms are causatively related to the use of a substance (Table 10.4–3). DSM-IV-TR refers clinicians to specific diagnoses within substance-related disorders: alcohol-induced persisting amnestic disorder; sedative, hypnotic, or anxiolytic-induced persisting amnestic disorder; and other (or unknown) substance-induced persisting amnestic disorder. DSM-IV-TR also provides the diagnosis of amnestic disorder not otherwise specified (Table 10.4–4).

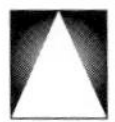

Table 10.4–2
DSM-IV-TR Diagnostic Criteria for Amnestic Disorder Due to a General Medical Condition

A. The development of memory impairment as manifested by impairment in the ability to learn new information or the inability to recall previously learned information.
B. The memory disturbance causes significant impairment in social or occupational functioning and represents a significant decline from a previous level of functioning.
C. The memory disturbance does not occur exclusively during the course of a delirium or a dementia.
D. There is evidence from the history, physical examination, or laboratory findings that the disturbance is the direct physiological consequence of a general medical condition (including physical trauma).

Specify if:
  Transient: if memory impairment lasts for 1 month or less
  Chronic: if memory impairment lasts for more than 1 month

Coding note: Include the name of the general medical condition on Axis I, e.g., Amnestic disorder due to head trauma; also code the general medical condition on Axis III.

(From American Psychiatric Association. *Diagnostic and Statistical Manual of Mental Disorders.* 4th ed. Text rev. Washington, DC: American Psychiatric Association; copyright 2000, with permission.)

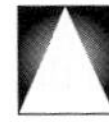

Table 10.4–3
DSM-IV-TR Diagnostic Criteria for Substance-Induced Persisting Amnestic Disorder

A. The development of memory impairment as manifested by impairment in the ability to learn new information or the inability to recall previously learned information.
B. The memory disturbance causes significant impairment in social or occupational functioning and represents a significant decline from a previous level of functioning.
C. The memory disturbance does not occur exclusively during the course of a delirium or a dementia and persists beyond the usual duration of substance intoxication or withdrawal.
D. There is evidence from the history, physical examination, or laboratory findings that the memory disturbance is etiologically related to the persisting effects of substance use (e.g., a drug of abuse, a medication).

Code (Specific substance)-induced persisting amnestic disorder: (Alcohol; Sedative, hypnotic, or anxiolytic; Other [or unknown] substance)

(From American Psychiatric Association. *Diagnostic and Statistical Manual of Mental Disorders.* 4th ed. Text rev. Washington, DC: American Psychiatric Association; copyright 2000, with permission.)

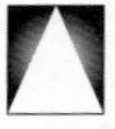

Table 10.4–4
DSM-IV-TR Diagnostic Criteria for Amnestic Disorder Not Otherwise Specified

This category should be used to diagnose an amnestic disorder that does not meet criteria for any of the specific types described in this section.

An example is a clinical presentation of amnesia for which there is insufficient evidence to establish a specific etiology (i.e., dissociative, substance induced, or due to a general medical condition).

(From American Psychiatric Association. *Diagnostic and Statistical Manual of Mental Disorders.* 4th ed. Text rev. Washington, DC: American Psychiatric Association; copyright 2000, with permission.)

CLINICAL FEATURES AND SUBTYPES

The central symptom of amnestic disorders is the development of a memory disorder characterized by impairment in the ability to learn new information (anterograde amnesia) and the inability to recall previously remembered knowledge (retrograde amnesia). The symptom must result in significant problems for patients in their social or occupational functioning. The time in which a patient is amnestic can begin directly at the point of trauma or include a period before the trauma. Memory for the time during the physical insult (e.g., during a cerebrovascular event) may also be lost.

Short-term and recent memory are usually impaired. Patients cannot remember what they had for breakfast or lunch, the name of the hospital, or their doctors. In some patients, the amnesia is so profound that the patient cannot orient him-or-herself to city and time, although orientation to person is seldom lost in amnestic disorders. Memory for overlearned information or events from the remote past, such as childhood experiences, is good; but memory for events from the less remote past (over the past decade) is impaired. Immediate memory (tested, for example, by asking a patient to repeat six numbers) remains intact. With improvement, patients may experience a gradual shrinking of the time for which memory has been lost, although some patients experience a gradual improvement in memory for the entire period.

The onset of symptoms can be sudden, as in trauma, cerebrovascular events, and neurotoxic chemical assaults, or gradual, as in nutritional deficiency and cerebral tumors. The amnesia can be of short duration (specified by DSM-IV-TR as transient if lasting 1 month or less) or of long duration (specified by DSM-IV-TR as persistent if lasting more than 1 month).

A variety of other symptoms can be associated with amnestic disorders. For patients with other cognitive impairments, a diagnosis of dementia or delirium is more appropriate than a diagnosis of an amnestic disorder. Both subtle and gross changes in personality can accompany the symptoms of memory impairment in amnestic disorders. Patients may be apathetic, lack initiative, have unprovoked episodes of agitation, or appear to be overly friendly or agreeable. Patients with amnestic disorders can also appear bewildered and confused and may attempt to cover their confusion with confabulatory answers to questions. Characteristically, patients with amnestic disorders do not have good insight into their neuropsychiatric conditions.

A 73-year-old survivor of the Holocaust was admitted to the psychiatric unit from a local nursing home. She was born in Germany to a middle-class family. Her education was truncated because of internment in a concentration camp. She immigrated to Israel after liberation from the concentration camp and later to the United States, where she married and raised a family. Premorbidly, she was described as a quiet, intelligent, and loving woman who spoke several languages. At 55 years of age, she had a significant carbon monoxide exposure when a gas line leaked while she and her husband slept. Her husband died of carbon monoxide poisoning, but the patient survived after a period of coma. Once stabilized, she displayed significant cognitive and behavioral problems. She had difficulty with learning new information and making appropriate plans. She retained the ability to perform activities of daily living, but could not be relied on to pay bills, buy food, cook, or clean, despite appearing to have retained the intellectual ability to do these tasks. She was admitted to a nursing home after several difficult years at home or in the homes of relatives. In the nursing home, she was able to learn her way about the facility. She displayed little interest in scheduled group activities, hobbies, reading, or television. She had frequent behavioral problems. She repeatedly pressed staff to get her sweets and snacks and cursed them vociferously with racial epithets and disparaging comments on their weight and dress. On one occasion, she scratched the cars of several staff with a key. Neuropsychological testing demonstrated severe deficits in delayed recall, intact performance on language and general knowledge measures, and moderate deficits on domains of executive function, such as concept formation and cognitive flexibility. She was noted to respond immediately to firmly set limits and rewards, but deficits in memory prevented long-term incorporation of these boundaries. Management involved development of a behavioral plan that could be implemented at the nursing home and empirical trials of medications aimed at amelioration of irritability.

Cerebrovascular Diseases

Cerebrovascular diseases affecting the hippocampus involve the posterior cerebral and basilar arteries and their branches. Infarctions are rarely limited to the hippocampus; they often involve the occipital or parietal lobes. Thus, common accompanying symptoms of cerebrovascular diseases in this region are focal neurological signs involving vision or sensory modalities. Cerebrovascular diseases affecting the bilateral medial thalamus, particularly the anterior portions, are often associated with symptoms of amnestic disorders. A few case studies report amnestic disorders from rupture of an aneurysm of the anterior communicating artery, resulting in infarction of the basal forebrain region.

Multiple Sclerosis

The pathophysiological process of multiple sclerosis involves the seemingly random formation of plaques within the brain parenchyma. When the plaques occur in the temporal lobe and the diencephalic regions, symptoms of memory impairment can occur. In fact, the most common cognitive complaints in patients with multiple sclerosis involve impaired memory, which occurs in 40 to 60 percent of patients. Characteristically, digit span memory is normal, but immediate recall and delayed recall of information are impaired. The memory impairment can affect both verbal and nonverbal material.

Korsakoff's Syndrome

Korsakoff's syndrome is an amnestic syndrome caused by thiamine deficiency, most commonly associated with the poor nutritional habits of people with chronic alcohol abuse. Other causes of poor nutrition (e.g., starvation), gastric carcinoma, hemodialysis, hyperemesis gravidarum, prolonged intravenous hyperalimentation, and gastric plication can also result in thiamine deficiency. Korsakoff's syndrome is often associated with Wernicke's encephalopathy, which is the associated syndrome of confusion, ataxia, and ophthalmoplegia. In patients with these thiamine deficiency-related symptoms, the neuropathological findings include hyperplasia of the small blood vessels with occasional hemorrhages, hypertrophy of astrocytes, and subtle changes in neuronal axons. Although the delirium clears up within a month or so, the amnestic syndrome either accompanies or follows untreated Wernicke's encephalopathy in approximately 85 percent of all cases.

Patients with Korsakoff's syndrome typically demonstrate a change in personality as well, such that they display a lack of initiative, diminished spontaneity, and a lack of interest or concern. These changes appear frontal lobe-like, similar to the personality change ascribed to patients with frontal lobe lesions or degeneration. Indeed, such patients often demonstrate *executive function* deficits on neuropsychological tasks involving attention, planning, set shifting, and inferential reasoning consistent with frontal pattern injuries. For this reason, Korsakoff's syndrome is not a pure memory disorder, although it certainly is a good paradigm of the more common clinical presentations for the amnestic syndrome.

The onset of Korsakoff's syndrome can be gradual. Recent memory tends to be affected more than is remote memory, but this feature is variable. Confabulation, apathy, and passivity are often prominent symptoms in the syndrome. With treatment, patients may remain amnestic for up to 3 months and then gradually improve over the ensuing year. Administration of thiamine may prevent the development of additional amnestic symptoms, but the treatment seldom reverses severe amnestic symptoms once they are present. Approximately one third to one fourth of all patients recover completely, and approximately one fourth of all patients have no improvement of their symptoms.

Alcoholic Blackouts

Some persons with severe alcohol abuse may exhibit the syndrome commonly referred to as an alcoholic blackout. Characteristically, these persons awake in the morning with a conscious awareness of being unable to remember a period the night before during which they were intoxicated. Sometimes, specific behaviors (hiding money in a secret place and provoking fights) are associated with the blackouts.

Electroconvulsive Therapy

Electroconvulsive therapy (ECT) treatments are usually associated with retrograde amnesia for a period of several minutes before the treatment and anterograde amnesia after the treatment. The anterograde amnesia usually resolves within 5 hours. Mild memory deficits may remain for 1 to 2 months after a course of ECT treatments, but the symptoms are completely resolved 6 to 9 months after treatment.

Head Injury

Head injuries (both closed and penetrating) can result in a wide range of neuropsychiatric symptoms, including dementia, depression, personality changes, and amnestic disorders. Amnestic disorders caused by head injuries are commonly associated with a period of retrograde amnesia leading up to the traumatic incident and amnesia for the traumatic incident itself. The severity of the brain injury correlates somewhat with the duration and severity of the amnestic syndrome, but the best correlate of eventual improvement is the degree of clinical improvement in the amnesia during the first week after the patient regains consciousness.

Transient Global Amnesia

Transient global amnesia is characterized by the abrupt loss of the ability to recall recent events or to remember new information. The syndrome is often characterized by mild confusion and a lack of insight into the problem, a clear sensorium, and, occasionally, the inability to perform some well-learned complex tasks. Episodes last from 6 to 24 hours. Studies suggest that transient global amnesia occurs in 5 to 10 cases per 100,000 persons per year; although, for patients older than age 50, the rate may be as high as 30 cases per 100,000 persons per year. The pathophysiology is unknown, but it likely involves ischemia of the temporal lobe and the diencephalic brain regions. Several studies of patients with single photon emission computed tomography (SPECT) have shown decreased blood flow in the temporal and parietotemporal regions, particularly in the left hemisphere (Fig. 10.4–1). Patients with transient global amnesia almost universally experience complete improvement, although one study found that approximately 20 percent of patients may have recurrence of the episode, and another study found that approximately 7 percent of patients may have epilepsy. Patients with transient global amnesia have been differentiated from patients with transient ischemic attacks in that fewer patients have diabetes, hypercholesterolemia, and hypertriglyceridemia, but more have hypertension and migrainous episodes.

PATHOLOGY AND LABORATORY EXAMINATION

Laboratory findings diagnostic of anmestic disorder may be obtained using quantitative neuropsychological testing. Standardized tests also are available to assess recall of well-known historical events or public figures, to characterize an individual's inability to remember previously learned information. Performance on such tests varies among individuals with amnestic disorder. Subtle deficits in other cognitive functions may be noted in individuals with amnestic disorder. Memory deficits, however, constitute the predominant feature of the mental status examination and account largely for any functional deficits. No specific or diagnostic features are detectable on imaging studies such as magnetic resonance imagery (MRI) or computed tomography (CT). Damage of midtemporal lobe structures is common, however, and may be reflected in enlargement of third ventricle or temporal horns or in structural atrophy detected by MRI.

DIFFERENTIAL DIAGNOSIS

Table 10.4–1 lists the major causes of amnestic disorders. To make the diagnosis, clinicians must obtain a patient's history, conduct a complete physical examination, and order all appropriate laboratory tests. Other diagnoses, however, can be confused with the amnestic disorders.

Dementia and Delirium

Amnestic disorders can be distinguished from delirium, because they occur in the absence of a disturbance of consciousness and are striking for the relative preservation of other cognitive domains.

Table 10.4–5 outlines the key distinctions between Alzheimer's dementia and the amnestic disorders. Both disorders

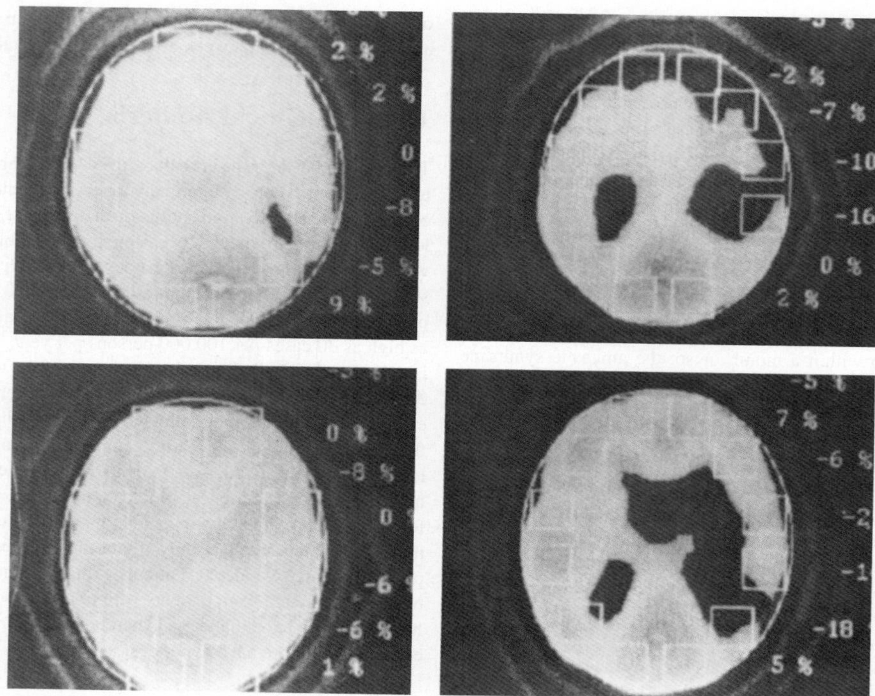

FIGURE 10.4–1
Technetium-99m HP-PAO single photon emission computed tomography scans. Left-sided temporal hypoperfusion is seen in **patients 2** (*top left*), **3** (*top right*), **4** (*bottom left*), and **5** (*bottom right*), 18 months, 4 days, 1 day, and 4 days, respectively, after the transient global amnestic attack. The right side of the patient is at the left side of the figure. (From Laloux P, Brichant C, Cauwe F, Decoster P. Technetium-99m HM-PAO single photon emission computed tomography imaging in transient global amnesia. *Arch Neurol.* 1992;49:545, with permission.)

can have an insidious onset with slow progression, as in a Korsakoff's psychosis in a chronic drinker. Amnestic disorders, however, can also develop precipitously, as in Wernicke's encephalopathy, transient global amnesia, or anoxic insults. Although Alzheimer's dementia progresses relentlessly, amnestic disorders tend to remain static or even improve once the offending cause has been removed. In terms of the actual memory deficits, the amnestic disorder and Alzheimer's disease still differ. Alzheimer's disease has an impact on retrieval, in addition to encoding and consolidation. The deficits in Alzheimer's disease extend beyond memory to general knowledge (semantic memory), language, praxis, and general function. These are spared in amnestic disorders. The dementias associated with Parkinson's disease, acquired immune deficiency syndrome (AIDS), and other subcortical disorders demonstrate disproportionate impairment of retrieval, but relatively intact encoding and consolidation and, thus, can be distinguished from amnestic disorders. The subcortical pattern dementias are also likely to display motor symptoms, such as bradykinesia, chorea, or tremor, that are not components of the amnestic disorders.

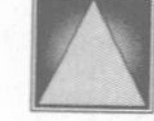

Table 10.4–5
Comparison of Syndrome Characteristics in Alzheimer's Disease and Amnestic Disorder

Characteristic	Alzheimer's Dementia	Amnestic Disorder
Onset	Insidious	Can be abrupt
Course	Progressive deterioration	Static or improvement
Anterograde memory	Impaired	Impaired
Retrograde memory	Impaired	Temporal gradient
Episodic memory	Impaired	Impaired
Semantic memory	Impaired	Intact
Language	Impaired	Intact
Praxis or function	Impaired	Intact

Normal Aging

Some minor impairment in memory may accompany normal aging, but the DSM-IV-TR requirement that the memory impairment cause significant impairment in social or occupational functioning should exclude normal aging from the diagnosis.

Dissociative Disorders

The dissociative disorders can sometimes be difficult to differentiate from the amnestic disorders. Patients with dissociative disorders, however, are more likely to have lost their orientation to self and may have more selective memory deficits than do patients with amnestic disorders. For example, patients with dissociative disorders may not know their names or home addresses, but they are still able to learn new information and remember selected past memories. Dissociative disorders are also often associated with emotionally stressful life events involving money, the legal system, or troubled relationships.

Factitious Disorders

Patients with factitious disorders who are mimicking an amnestic disorder often have inconsistent results on memory tests and have no evidence of an identifiable cause. These findings, coupled with evidence of primary or secondary gain for a patient, should suggest a factitious disorder.

COURSE AND PROGNOSIS

The course of an amnestic disorder depends on its etiology and treatment, particularly acute treatment. Generally, the amnestic disorder has a static course. Little improvement is seen over time, but also no progression of the disorder occurs. The exceptions are the acute amnesias, such as transient global amnesia, which resolves entirely over hours to days, and the amnestic disorder associated with head trauma, which improves steadily in the months subsequent to the trauma. Amnesia secondary to processes that destroy brain tissue, such as stroke, tumor, and infection, are irreversible, although, again, static, once the acute infection or ischemia has been staunched.

TREATMENT

The primary approach to treating amnestic disorders is to treat the underlying cause. Although a patient is amnestic, supportive prompts about the date, the time, and the patient's location can be helpful and can reduce the patient's anxiety. After resolution of the amnestic episode, psychotherapy of some type (cognitive, psychodynamic, or supportive) may help patients incorporate the amnestic experience into their lives.

Psychotherapy

Psychodynamic interventions may be of considerable value for patients who have amnestic disorders that result from insults to the brain. Understanding the course of recovery in such patients helps clinicians to be sensitive to the narcissistic injury inherent in damage to the central nervous system.

The first phase of recovery, in which patients are incapable of processing what happened because the ego defenses are overwhelmed, requires clinicians to serve as a supportive auxiliary ego who explains to a patient what is happening and provides missing ego functions. In the second phase of recovery, as the realization of the injury sets in, patients may become angry and feel victimized by the malevolent hand of fate. They may view others, including the clinician, as bad or destructive, and clinicians must contain these projections without becoming punitive or retaliatory. Clinicians can build a therapeutic alliance with patients by explaining slowly and clearly what happened and by offering an explanation for a patient's internal experience. The third phase of recovery is integrative. As a patient accepts what has happened, a clinician can help the patient form a new identity by connecting current experiences of the self with past experiences. Grieving over the lost faculties may be an important feature of the third phase.

Most patients who are amnestic because of brain injury engage in denial. Clinicians must respect and empathize with the patient's need to deny the reality of what has happened. Insensitive and blunt confrontations destroy any developing therapeutic alliance and can cause patients to feel attacked. In a sensitive approach, clinicians help patients accept their cognitive limitations by exposing them to these deficits bit by bit over time. When patients fully accept what has happened, they may need assistance in forgiving themselves and any others involved, so that they can get on with their lives. Clinicians must also be wary of being seduced into thinking that all of the patient's symptoms are directly related to the brain insult. An evaluation of preexisting personality disorders, such as borderline, antisocial, and narcissistic personality disorders, must be part of the overall assessment; many patients with personality disorders place themselves in situations that predispose them to injuries. These personality features may become a crucial part of the psychodynamic psychotherapy.

Recently, centers for cognitive rehabilitation have been established whose rehabilitation-oriented therapeutic milieu is intended to promote recovery from brain injury, especially that from traumatic causes. Despite the high cost of extended care at these sites, which provide both long-term institutional and daytime services, no data have been developed to define therapeutic effectiveness for the heterogeneous groups of patients who participate in such tasks as memory retaining.

ICD-10

The criteria for organic amnesic syndrome, not induced by alcohol and other psychoactive substances, in the 10th revision of *International Statistical Classification of Diseases and Related Health Problems* (ICD-10) are presented in Table 10.4–6. In ICD-10, deliriums associated with the use of a substance are classified under the category of mental and

Table 10.4–6
ICD-10 Diagnostic Criteria for Organic Amnesic Syndrome, Not Induced by Alcohol and Other Psychoactive Substances

A. There is memory impairment, manifest in both
   1. A defect of recent memory (impaired learning of new material) to a degree sufficient to interfere with daily living
   2. A reduced ability to recall past experiences

B. There is no
   1. Defect in immediate recall (as tested, for example, by the digit span)
   2. Clouding of consciousness and disturbance of attention. Delirium, not induced by alcohol and other psychoactive substances
   3. Global intellectual decline (dementia)

C. There is objective evidence (from physical and neurological examination, laboratory tests) and/or history of an insult to, or a disease of, the brain (especially involving bilaterally the diencephalic and medial temporal structures but other than alcohol encephalopathy) that can reasonably be presumed to be responsible for the clinical manifestations

Comments

Associated features, including confabulations, emotional changes (apathy, lack of initiative), and lack of insight are useful additional pointers to the diagnosis but are not invariably present.

(Adapted from World Health Organization. The *ICD-10 Classification of Mental and Behavioural Disorders: Diagnostic Criteria for Research.* Copyright, World Health Organization, Geneva, 1993, with permission.)

behavioral disorders due to psychoactive substance use as a withdrawal state with delirium, as a subtype of acute intoxication (e.g., acute intoxication due to the use of alcohol with delirium), and as an additional specifier to alcohol withdrawal state and sedative or hypnotic withdrawal state.

References

Candel I, Jelicic M, Merckelbach H, Wester A. Korsakoff patients' memories of September 11, 2001. *J Nerv Ment Dis.* 2003;191:262–265.

Carlesimo GA, Bonanni R, Caltagirone C. Memory for the perceptual and semantic attributes of information in pure amnestic and severe closed-head injured patients. *J Clin Exp Neuropsychol.* 2003;25:391–406.

Griffith HR, Netson KL, Harrell LE, Zamrini EY, Brockington JC, Marson DC. Amnestic mild cognitive impairment: Diagnostic outcomes and clinical prediction over a two-year time period. *J Int Neuropsychol Soc.* 2006;12(2):166–175.

Grossman H. Amnestic Disorders. In: Sadock BJ, Sadock VA, eds. *Kaplan & Sadock's Comprehensive Textbook of Psychiatry.* 8th ed. Vol. 1. Baltimore: Lippincott Williams & Wilkins; 2005:1093.

Kensinger EA, Clarke RJ, Corkin S. What neural correlates underlie successful encoding and retrieval? A functional magnetic resonance imaging study using a divided attention paradigm. *J Neurosci.* 2003;23:2407–2415.

Kryscio RJ, Schmitt FA, Salazar JC, Mendiondo MS, Markesbery WR. Risk factors for transitions from normal to mild cognitive impairment and dementia. *Neurology.* 2006;66(6):828–832.

Levin LI, Munger KL, Rubertone MV, Peck CA, Lennette ET, Spiegelman D, Ascherio A. Temporal relationship between elevation of Epstein-Barr virus antibody titers and initial onset of neurological symptoms in multiple sclerosis. *JAMA.* 2005;293:2496–2500.

Manns JR, Hopkins RO, Reed JM, Kitchener EG, Squire LR. Recognition memory and the human hippocampus. *Neuron.* 2003;37:171–180.

Manns JR, Hopkins RO, Squire LR. Semantic memory and the human hippocampus. *Neuron.* 2003;38:127–133.

Meulemans T, Van der Linden M. Implicit learning of complex information in amnesia. *Brain Cogn.* 2003;52:250–257.

Oscar-Berman M, Kirkley SM, Gansler DA, Couture A. Comparisons of Korsakoff and non-Korsakoff alcoholics on neuropsychological tests of prefrontal brain functioning. *Alcohol Clin Exp Res.* 2004;28(4):667–675.

Petersen RC, Parisi JE, Dickson DW, Johnson KA, Knopman DS, Boeve BF, Jicha GA, Ivnik RJ, Smith GE, Tangalos EG, Braak H, Kokmen E. Neuropathologic features of amnestic mild cognitive impairment. *Arch Neurol.* 2006;63(5):665–672.

Quinette P, Guillery B, Desgranges B, de la Sayette V, Viader F, Eustache F. Working memory and executive functions in transient global amnesia. *Brain.* 2003;126:1917–1934.

▲ 10.5 Mental Disorders Due to a General Medical Condition

Increasingly, scientific views of mental illness recognize that, whether caused by an identifiable anomaly (e.g., brain tumor), a neurotransmitter disturbance of unclear origin (e.g., schizophrenia), or a consequence of deranged upbringing or environment (e.g., personality disorder), all mental disorders ultimately share one common underlying theme: aberration in brain function. Treatments for those conditions, whether psychological or biological, attempt to restore normal brain chemistry. The differential diagnosis for a mental syndrome in a patient should always include consideration of (1) any general medical condition that a patient may have and (2) any prescription, nonprescription, or illegal substances that a patient may be taking. Although some specific medical conditions have classically been associated with mental syndromes, a much larger number of general medical conditions have been associated with mental syndromes in case reports and small studies.

In the text revision of the fourth edition of *Diagnostic and Statistical Manual of Mental Disorders* (DSM-IV-TR), each mental disorder due to a general medical condition is classified within the category that most resembles the symptoms (Table 10.5–1). For example, the diagnosis of psychotic disorder due to general medical condition is found in the DSM-IV-TR section on schizophrenia and other psychotic disorders. A clinician evaluating a patient with depression can refer to the DSM-IV-TR section on mood disorders and find mood disorder due to a general medical condition as one of the diagnoses.

MOOD DISORDER DUE TO A GENERAL MEDICAL CONDITION

Mood disorders, particularly depression, accompany a range of medical problems. Also known as *secondary mood disorders*, these conditions are characterized by a prominent mood alteration thought to be the direct physiological effect of a specific medical illness or agent. These disorders are often difficult to define and have not been extensively researched; however, the key feature is prominent, persistent, distressing, or functionally impairing depressed mood (anhedonia) or elevated, expansive, or irritable mood, judged to be caused either by medical or surgical illness or by substance intoxication or withdrawal. Cognitive impairment is not the predominant clinical feature; otherwise, the mood disturbance would be viewed as part of delirium, dementia, or other cognitive deficit disorder. The diagnostician is asked to specify if the mood syndrome is manic, depressed, or mixed, and if criteria for a fully symptomatic major depressive or manic syndromic are fulfilled.

Epidemiology

Mood disorder caused by a general medical condition, with depressive features, appears to affect men and women equally, in contrast to major depressive disorder, which predominates in women. As much as 50 percent of all poststroke patients experience depressive illness. A similar prevalence pertains to individuals with pancreatic cancer. Forty percent of patients with Parkinson's disease are depressed. Major and minor depressive episodes are common after certain illnesses such as Huntington's disease, human immunodeficiency virus (HIV) infection, and multiple sclerosis (MS). Secondary mania is less prevalent in neurological disease than is depression; however, many experienced clinicians report a high rate of euphoria in patients with MS. Depressive disorders associated with terminal or painful conditions carry the greatest risk of suicide.

Etiology

The list of potential causes for both depressive and manic syndromes is long. Table 10.5–2 lists some of the causes most commonly considered.

Diagnosis and Clinical Features

Patients with depression may experience psychological symptoms (e.g., sad mood, lack of pleasure or interest in usual activities, tearfulness, concentration disturbance, and suicidal ideation) or somatic symptoms (e.g., fatigue, sleep disturbance, and appetite disturbance), or both psychological and somatic

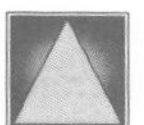

Table 10.5–1
Mental Disorders Due to a General Medical Condition

DSM-IV-TR Category	Mental Disorders Due to a General Medical Condition	Section
Delirium, dementia, amnestic and other cognitive disorders	Delirium due to a general medical condition	10.2
	Dementia due to other general medical conditions	10.3
	Amnestic disorder due to a general medical condition	10.4
Schizophrenia and other psychotic disorders	Psychotic disorder due to a general medical condition	14.1
Mood disorders	Mood disorder due to a general medical condition	15.3
Anxiety disorders	Anxiety disorder due to a general medical condition	16.7
Sexual disorders	Sexual dysfunction due to a general medical condition	21.2
Sleep disorders	Sleep disorder due to a general medical condition	24.2
Mental disorders due to a general medical condition not elsewhere classified	Catatonic disorder due to a general medical condition	10.5
	Personality change due to a general medical condition	10.5
	Mental disorder not otherwise specified due to a general medical condition	10.5

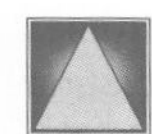

Table 10.5–2
Causes of Secondary Mood Disorders

Drug Intoxication
- Alcohol or sedative-hypnotics
- Antipsychotics
- Antidepressants
- Metoclopramide, H_2-receptor blockers
- Antihypertensives (especially centrally acting agents, e.g., methyldopa, clonidine, reserpine)
- Sex steroids (e.g., oral contraceptives, anabolic steroids)
- Glucocorticoids
- Levodopa
- Bromocriptine

Drug Withdrawal
- Nicotine, caffeine, alcohol or sedative-hypnotics, cocaine, amphetamines

Tumor
- Primary cerebral
- Systemic neoplasm

Trauma
- Cerebral contusion
- Subdural hematoma

Infection
- Cerebral (e.g., meningitis, encephalitis, HIV, syphilis)
- Systemic (e.g., sepsis, urinary tract infection, pneumonia)

Cardiac and Vascular
- Cerebrovascular (e.g., infarcts, hemorrhage, vasculitis)
- Cardiovascular (e.g., low-output states, congestive heart failure, shock)

Physiological or Metabolic
- Hypoxemia, electrolyte disturbances, renal or hepatic failure, hypo- or hyperglycemia, postictal states

Endocrine
- Thyroid or glucocorticoid disturbances

Nutritional
- Vitamin B_{12}, folate deficiency

Demyelinating
- Multiple sclerosis

Neurodegenerative
- Parkinson's disease, Huntington's disease

HIV, human immunodeficiency virus.
(Courtesy of Eric D. Caine, M.D., and Jeffrey M. Lyness, M.D.)

symptoms. Diagnosis in the medically ill can be confounded by the presence of somatic symptoms related purely to medical illness, not to depression. In an effort to overcome the underdiagnosis of depression in the medically ill, most practitioners favor including somatic symptoms in identifying mood syndromes.

The DSM-IV-TR provides diagnostic criteria for mood disorder due to a general medical condition *with* (1) *depressive features*, (2) *major depressive-like episode*, (3) *manic features*, or (4) *mixed features*. In general, these criteria are less strict than for corresponding primary mood disorders. The subtype *with major depressive-like episode* is not available for substance-induced mood disorder (Table 10.5–3).

A 45-year-old toy designer was admitted to the hospital after a series of suicidal gestures culminating in an attempt to strangle himself with a piece of wire. Four months before admission, his family had observed that he was becoming depressed: when at home, he spent long periods sitting in a chair; he slept more than usual; and he had given up his habits of reading the evening paper and puttering around the house. Within 1 month, he was unable to get out of bed in the morning to go to work. He expressed considerable guilt but could not make up his mind to seek help until forced to do so by his family. He had not responded to 2 months of outpatient antidepressant drug therapy and had made several half-hearted attempts to cut his wrists before the serious attempt that precipitated the admission.

Physical examination revealed signs of increased intracranial pressure, and a CT scan showed a large frontal-lobe tumor. (Reprinted with permission from *DSM-IV-TR Casebook*.)

Differential Diagnosis

Mood changes occurring during the course of delirium are acute and fluctuating and should be attributed to that disorder, not to mood disorder due to a general medical condition or to substance-induced mood disorder. Pain syndromes can depress mood, but do so through psychological, not physiological means, and may appropriately lead to a diagnosis of primary mood disorder. In the medically ill, somatic complaints, such as sleep disturbance, anorexia, and fatigue, may be counted toward a diagnosis of major depressive episode or mood disorder due to a general medical condition, unless those complaints are purely attributable to the medical illness.

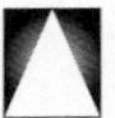

Table 10.5–3
DSM-IV-TR Criteria for Mood Disorder Due to a General Medical Condition

A. A prominent and persistent disturbance in mood predominates in the clinical picture and is characterized by either (or both) of the following:
  (1) Depressed mood or markedly diminished pleasure in all, or almost all, activities
  (2) Elevated, expansive, or irritable mood.
B. There is evidence from the history, physical examination, or laboratory findings that the disturbance is the direct physiological consequence of a general medical condition.
C. The disturbance is not better accounted for by another mental disorder (e.g., adjustment disorder with depressed mood in response to the stress of having a general medical condition).
D. The disturbance does not occur exclusively during the course of a delirium.
E. The symptoms cause clinically significant distress or impairment in social, occupational, or other important areas of functioning.

Specify:
With depressive features: if the predominant mood is depressed, but the full criteria are not met for a major depressive disorder
With major depressive-like episode: if all criteria for major depressive episode are met, except, clearly, for the criterion that the symptoms are not due to the physiological effects of a substance or a general medical condition
With manic features: if the predominant mood is elevated, euphoric, or irritable
With mixed features: if the symptoms of mania and depression are present, but neither predominates

(From American Psychiatric Association. *Diagnostic and Statistical Manual of Mental Disorders.* 4th ed. Text rev. Washington, DC; American Psychiatric Association; 2000, with permission.)

Mood disorder due to a general medical condition can be distinguished from substance-induced mood disorder by examination of time course of symptoms, response to correction of suspect medical conditions or discontinuation of substances, and, occasionally, by urine or blood toxicology results.

Course and Prognosis

The course of mood disorder due to a general medical condition largely depends on the course of the underlying medical state, as well as the extent of concurrent psychiatric intervention. Similar considerations apply to substance-induced mood disorder. Prognosis for mood symptoms is best when etiological medical illnesses or medications are most susceptible to correction (e.g., treatment of hypothyroidism and cessation of alcohol use).

When such intervention is not possible (e.g., halting immunosuppressant use in an individual after kidney transplant) or fails to lead to prompt remission of mood symptoms, formal psychiatric treatment is indicated.

Treatment

Standard antidepressant medications, including tricyclic drugs, monoamine oxidase inhibitors (MAOIs), selective serotonin reuptake inhibitors (SSRIs), and psychostimulants, are effective in many depressed patients with medical and neurological illnesses or substance use disorders. Electroconvulsive therapy (ECT) may be useful in patients who do not respond to medication.

The clinician treating a patient with a secondary mood disorder should treat the underlying medical cause as effectively as possible. Standard treatment approaches for the corresponding primary mood disorder should be used, although the risk of toxic effects from psychotropic drugs may require more gradual dosage increases. At a minimum, psychotherapy should focus on psychoeducational issues. The concept of a behavioral disturbance secondary to medical illness may be new or difficult for many patients and families to understand. Specific intrapsychic, interpersonal, and family issues are addressed as indicated in psychotherapy.

PSYCHOTIC DISORDER DUE TO A GENERAL MEDICAL CONDITION

To establish the diagnosis of psychotic disorder due to a general medical condition, the clinician first must exclude syndromes in which psychotic symptoms may be present in association with cognitive impairment (e.g., delirium and dementia of the Alzheimer's type). Disorders in this category usually are not associated with changes in the sensorium.

Epidemiology

The incidence and prevalence of secondary psychotic disorders in the general population are unknown. As much as 40 percent of individuals with temporal lobe epilepsy experience psychosis. The prevalence of psychotic symptoms is increased in selected clinical populations, such as nursing home residents, but it is unclear how to extrapolate these findings to other patient groups.

Etiology

Virtually any cerebral or systemic disease that affects brain function can produce psychotic symptoms. Degenerative disorders, such as Alzheimer's disease or Huntington's disease, can present initially with new-onset psychosis, with minimal evidence of cognitive impairment at the earliest stages.

Diagnosis and Clinical Features

Two DSM-IV-TR subtypes exist for psychotic disorder due to a general medical condition: *with delusions*, to be used if the predominant psychotic symptoms are delusional, and *with hallucinations*, to be used if hallucinations of any form comprise the primary psychotic symptoms (Table 10.5–4).

To establish the diagnosis of a secondary psychotic syndrome, the clinician first determines that the patient is not delirious, as evidenced by a stable level of consciousness. A careful mental status assessment is conducted to exclude significant cognitive impairments, such as those encountered in dementia or amnestic disorder. The next step is to search for systemic or cerebral diseases that might be causally related to the psychosis. Psychotic symptomatology per se is not helpful in distinguishing a secondary from a primary (idiopathic) cause.

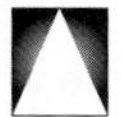

Table 10.5–4
DSM-IV-TR Criteria for Psychotic Disorder Due to a General Medical Condition

A. Prominent hallucinations or delusions.
B. There is evidence from the history, physical examination, or laboratory findings that the disturbance is the direct physiological consequence of a general medical condition.
C. The disturbance is not better accounted for by another mental disorder.
D. The disturbance does not occur exclusively during the course of a delirium.

Specify:
With delusions: if delusions are the predominant symptom
With hallucinations: if hallucinations are the predominant symptom

(From American Psychiatric Association. *Diagnostic and Statistical Manual of Mental Disorders.* 4th ed. Text rev. Washington, DC; American Psychiatric Association; 2000, with permission.)

A systematic physical and neurological examination should be performed. The examiner should bear in mind, however, that nonlocalizing, soft neurological signs and a variety of dyskinesias can be present in schizophrenia. An evaluation with magnetic resonance imaging (MRI) for any new-onset psychosis is recommended, irrespective of patient age. The detection of a systemic or cerebral abnormality (e.g., a brain tumor) may lead to the determination of secondary psychosis; however, establishing a diagnosis of secondary psychotic syndrome requires thoughtful clinical reasoning. Table 10.5–5 lists a number of specific psychotic symptoms that have been consistently associated with disease in particular brain regions.

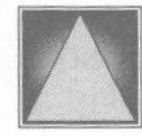

Table 10.5–5
Psychotic Symptoms Associated with Abnormality of Specific Brain Regions

Symptoms	Site	Laterality
First-rank symptoms	Temporal lobe	Dominant hemisphere
Thoughts spoken aloud		
Voices commenting		
Third-person voices arguing		
Made actions		
Made feelings		
Thought withdrawal		
Thought diffusion		
Delusional perception		
Complex delusions	Subcortical or limbic	
Anton syndrome	Occipital lobe, optic tract	Bilateral
Anosognosia	Parietal lobe	Nondominant hemisphere
Misidentification syndromes	Parietal, temporal, frontal lobes	Nondominant hemisphere, bilateral
Capgras syndrome		
Reduplicative paramnesia		
Fregoli syndrome		
Intermetamorphosis syndrome		

(Courtesy of Eric D. Caine, M.D., and Jeffrey M. Lyness, M.D.)

Differential Diagnosis

Primary psychotic disorders, such as schizophrenia, and primary mood disorders with psychotic features may present with symptoms identical or similar to psychotic disorder due to a general medical condition; however, in primary disorders, no medical or substance cause is identifiable, despite laboratory workup. Delirium may present with psychotic symptoms, but, in contrast to psychotic disorder due to a general medical condition, delirium-related psychosis is acute and fluctuating, commonly associated with disturbance in consciousness and cognitive defects. Psychosis resulting from dementia may be diagnosed as psychotic disorder due to a general medical condition, except in the case of vascular dementia, which, according the International Classification of Diseases (ICD) coding requirements, should be diagnosed as vascular dementia with delusions.

Unique characteristics may assist in differentiating primary from induced psychoses. Most cases of nonauditory hallucinosis are due to medical conditions, substances, or both. The converse is not true: Auditory hallucinations can occur in primary and induced psychoses. Stimulant (e.g., amphetamine and cocaine) intoxication psychosis may involve a perception of bugs crawling under the skin (formication). Temporal lobe epilepsy often is associated with olfactory hallucinations and religious delusions. Right parietal lobe lesions can induce a contralateral neglect state of delusional nature in which individuals disown parts of their bodies. Occipital lesions, whether caused by tumor or cerebrovascular accident, can produce visual hallucinations.

When the clinician is considering the relative roles of medical conditions and substances in a patient with psychosis, diagnosis may be assisted by chronology of symptoms, response to removal of suspect substances or alleviation of medical illnesses, and toxicology results.

Course and Prognosis

The course of the underlying medical illness or substance use commonly dictates the course of psychosis due to a general medical condition or substance, with several notable exceptions. Psychosis caused by certain medications (e.g., immunosuppressants) gradually may subside even when use of those medications is continued. Minimizing dosages of such medications consistent with therapeutic efficacy often facilitates resolution of psychosis. Certain degenerative brain disorders (e.g., Parkinson's disease) can be characterized by episodic lapses into psychosis, even as the underlying medical condition advances. If abuse of substances persists over a lengthy period, psychosis (e.g., hallucinations from alcohol) may fail to remit even during extended intervals of abstinence.

Treatment

The principles of treatment for a secondary psychotic disorder are similar to those for any secondary neuropsychiatric disorder, namely, rapid identification of the etiological agent and treatment of the underlying cause. Antipsychotic medication may provide symptomatic relief.

ANXIETY DISORDER DUE TO A GENERAL MEDICAL CONDITION

Definition

In *anxiety disorder due to a general medical condition*, the individual experiences anxiety that causes clinically significant distress or impairment in functioning. This anxiety must represent a direct physiological, not emotional, consequence of a general medical condition. In *substance-induced anxiety disorder*, the anxiety symptoms are the product of a prescribed medication or stem from intoxication or withdrawal from a nonprescribed substance, typically a drug of abuse.

Epidemiology

Little data exist by which to estimate the prevalence of anxiety disorder due to a general medical condition. It is believed that medically ill individuals generally have higher rates of anxiety disorder than do the general population. Rates of panic and generalized anxiety are especially high in neurological, endocrine, and cardiology patients, although this finding does not necessarily prove a physiological link. Approximately one third of patients with hypothyroidism and two thirds of patients with hyperthyroidism may experience anxiety symptoms. As much as 40 percent of patients with Parkinson's disease have anxiety disorders. Prevalence of most anxiety disorders is higher in women than in men.

Etiology

Causes most commonly described in anxiety syndromes include substance-related states (intoxication with caffeine, cocaine, amphetamines, and other sympathomimetic agents; withdrawal from nicotine, sedative-hypnotics, and alcohol), endocrinopathies (especially pheochromocytoma, hyperthyroidism, hypercortisolemic states, and hyperparathyroidism), metabolic derangements (e.g., hypoxemia, hypercalcemia, and hypoglycemia), and neurological disorders (including vascular, trauma, and degenerative types). Many of these conditions are either inherently transient or easily remediable. Whether that reflects the pathophysiology of secondary anxiety or is an artifact of reporting (e.g., anxiety with subacute onset and complete resolution after removal of a pheochromocytoma is more likely to be reported as an example of anxiety due to a medical illness than is chronic anxiety in the context of chronic obstructive pulmonary disease) is not known. Much attention has been paid to the association of panic attacks and mitral valve prolapse. The nature of that association is unknown, and therefore the diagnosis of panic attacks secondary to mitral valve prolapse currently is premature. Interestingly, several recent reports have sought to tie obsessive–compulsive symptoms to the development of pathology in the basal ganglia.

Diagnosis and Clinical Features

Anxiety stemming from a general medical condition or substance may present with physical complaints (e.g., chest pain, palpitation, abdominal distress, diaphoresis, dizziness, tremulousness, and urinary frequency), generalized symptoms of fear and excessive worry, outright panic attacks associated with fear of dying or losing control, recurrent obsessive thoughts or ritualistic compulsive behaviors, or phobia with associated avoidant behavior (Table 10.5–6).

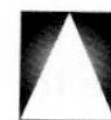

Table 10.5–6
DSM-IV-TR Criteria for Anxiety Disorder Due to a General Medical Condition

A. Prominent anxiety, panic attacks, or obsessions or compulsions predominate in the clinical picture.
B. There is evidence from the history, physical examination, or laboratory findings that the disturbance is the direct physiological consequence of a general medical condition.
C. The disturbance is not better accounted for by another mental disorder (e.g., adjustment disorder with anxiety in which the stressor is a serious general medical condition).
D. The disturbance does not occur exclusively during the course of a delirium.
E. The disturbance causes clinical significant distress or impairment in social, occupational, or other important areas of functioning.

Specify:
- **With generalized anxiety:** if excessive anxiety or worry about a number of events or activities predominates in the clinical presentation
- **With panic attacks:** if panic attacks predominate in the clinical presentation
- **With obsessive–compulsive symptoms:** if obsessions or compulsions predominate in the clinical presentation

(From American Psychiatric Association. *Diagnostic and Statistical Manual of Mental Disorders*. 4th ed. Text rev. Washington, DC; American Psychiatric Association; 2000, with permission.)

A 78-year-old retired lumber-company president sought help for the onset of a series of attacks in which he experienced marked apprehension, restlessness, and the need to be outdoors to relieve his sense of discomfort. He described the most recent event as having occurred at 3:00 AM a week earlier: He awoke from sleep and felt "the walls were caving in" on him. He denied that this was related to dreaming and said that he was fully awake at the time. He arose, dressed, and went outside in subzero weather; once outside, he noted gradual improvement (but not full resolution) of his symptoms. Complete resolution took a full day.

In response to pointed questioning, the patient denied dyspnea, palpitations, choking sensations, paresthesias, or nausea. He reported trembling and some sweating, together with intermittent dizziness. He imagined that he would die (or lose consciousness) if he could not "escape" from his house. He spoke of a need "to be active."

On questioning, the patient recalled a similar series of attacks almost 30 years earlier after eye surgery for an injury. He described bilateral patching of his eyes and being confined to bed for days, with his head sandbagged to preclude movement. Once ambulatory, he had experienced these attacks for more than 1 year.

The patient denied recent sleep dysfunction, change in appetite or weight, crying spells, or decreased energy. He had been taking diazepam for approximately 2 months for feelings of increased nervousness and tension. He had noted mild memory problems of late.

Further inquiry established a problem with balance and intermittent pain in the right arm and a complaint of indigestion and intermittent diarrhea. The patient had stopped gardening the past summer because of his balance problem. On examination, he was found to have a "beefy" red tongue (which he said was painful), difficulty with tandem gait and rapid alternating motion, and a mild intention tremor. He denied urinary incontinence.

Laboratory studies revealed a macrocytic anemia and vitamin B_{12} deficiency. The patient was given vitamin B_{12} replacement, and his attacks did not recur. (Reprinted with permission from *DSM-IV-TR Casebook.*)

Differential Diagnosis

Anxiety disorder due to a general medical condition symptomatically can resemble corresponding primary anxiety disorders. Acute onset, lack of family history, and occurrence within the context of acute medical illness or introduction of new medications or substances suggest a nonprimary cause.

Individuals with delirium commonly experience anxiety and panic symptoms, but these fluctuate and are accompanied by other delirium symptoms such as cognitive loss and inattentiveness; furthermore, anxiety symptoms diminish as delirium subsides. Patients with psychosis of any origin can experience anxiety commonly related to delusions or hallucinations. Depressive disorders often present with anxiety symptoms, mandating that the clinician inquire broadly about depressive symptoms in any patient whose primary complaint is anxiety. Dementia often is associated with agitation or anxiety, especially at night (called *sundowning*), but an independent anxiety diagnosis is warranted only if it becomes a source of prominent clinical attention. Adjustment disorders with anxiety arising within the context of reaction to medical or other life stressors should not be diagnosed as anxiety disorder due to a general medical condition.

Course and Prognosis

Anxiety disorder due to a general medical condition usually fluctuates in direct relation to the course of the provoking factor. Medical conditions responsive to treatment or cure (e.g., correction of hypothyroidism and reduction in caffeine consumption) often provide concomitant relief of anxiety symptoms, although such relief may lag the rate or extent of improvement in the underlying medical condition. Chronic, incurable medical conditions associated with persistent physiological insult (e.g., chronic obstructive pulmonary disease) or recurrent relapse to substance use can contribute to seeming refractoriness of associated anxiety symptoms. In medication-induced anxiety, if complete cessation of the offending factor (e.g., immunosuppressant therapy) is not possible, dose reduction, when clinically feasible, often brings substantial relief.

Treatment

Aside from treating the underlying causes, clinicians have found benzodiazepines helpful in decreasing anxiety symptoms; supportive psychotherapy (including psychoeducational issues focusing on the diagnosis and prognosis) may also be useful. The efficacy of other, more specific therapies in secondary syndromes (e.g., antidepressant medications for panic attacks, SSRIs for obsessive–compulsive symptoms, behavior therapy for simple phobias) is unknown, but they may be of use.

SLEEP DISORDER DUE TO A GENERAL MEDICAL CONDITION

Diagnosis

Sleep disorders can manifest in four ways: by an excess of sleep (hypersomnia), by a deficiency of sleep (insomnia), by abnormal behavior or activity during sleep (parasomnia), and by a disturbance in the timing of sleep (circadian rhythm sleep disorders). Primary sleep disorders occur unrelated to any other medical or psychiatric illness (Table 10.5–7).

Mr. Thompson, a 62-year-old married man, has diabetic neuropathy, which contributes to bilateral leg pain and resultant middle-of-the-night awakening. Recently, after having surgical resection of pancreatic cancer, Mr. Thompson began to experience difficulty falling asleep as well.

At the time of interview, Mr. Thompson reported that he was depressed and worried about his cancer diagnosis. He had concentration difficulties and loss of pleasure in usual activities. Furthermore, as bedtime approached, he acknowledged becoming extremely anxious in anticipation of sleep difficulties. Mr. Thompson slept into the late morning hours and took daytime naps to compensate for nocturnal sleep difficulties. To promote sleep, his general practitioner had prescribed diazepam, and then temazepam (Restoril), with limited success.

A trial of nortriptyline, 25 mg at bedtime, was initiated to foster pain relief and to promote sleep. When this proved only partially efficacious, trazodone, 50 mg at bedtime, was added. Mr. Thompson was instructed to establish a standard time for lying down at night and arising in the morning. Evening relaxation strategies also

Table 10.5–7 DSM-IV-TR Criteria for Sleep Disorder Due to a General Medical Condition

A. A prominent disturbance in sleep that is sufficiently severe to warrant independent clinical attention.

B. There is evidence from the history, physical examination, or laboratory findings that the sleep disturbance is the direct physiological consequence of a general medical condition.

C. The disturbance is not better accounted for by another mental disorder (e.g., an adjustment disorder in which the stressor is a serious medical illness).

D. The disturbance does not occur exclusively during the course of a delirium.

E. The disturbance does not meet the criteria for breathing-related sleep disorder or narcolepsy.

F. The sleep disturbance causes clinically significant distress or impairment in social, occupational, or other important areas of functioning.

Specify type:

Insomnia type: if the predominant sleep disturbance is insomnia

Hypersomnia type: if the predominant sleep disturbance is hypersomnia

Parasomnia type: if the predominant sleep disturbance is a parasomnia

Mixed type: if more than one sleep disturbance is present and none predominate of comparable sexual dysfunction that was not substance-induced

(From American Psychiatric Association. *Diagnostic and Statistical Manual of Mental Disorders.* 4th ed. Text rev. Washington, DC; American Psychiatric Association; 2000, with permission.)

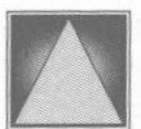

Table 10.5–8
Medical Conditions Commonly Associated with a Secondary Sleep Disorder

Condition	Sleep Symptoms
Parkinsonism	Frequent awakenings, disturbance of circadian rhythms
Dementia	Sundowning, frequent awakenings
Epilepsy	Difficulty initiating sleep, frequent awakenings, parasomnias
Cerebrovascular disease	Difficulty initiating sleep, frequent awakenings
Huntington's disease	Frequent awakening
Kleine-Levin syndrome	Hypersomnia
Uremia	Restless legs, nocturnal myoclonus

(Courtesy of Eric D. Caine, M.D., and Jeffrey M. Lyness, M.D.)

were identified. Nortriptyline dosing was gradually raised until an antidepressant therapeutic blood level was achieved. Psychotherapy was used to assist Mr. Thompson in coping with his medical problems and his fears of death related to his cancer diagnosis. With this regimen, pain, mood, and sleep symptoms gradually subsided.

Etiology and Differential Diagnosis

Table 10.5–8 lists a number of medical conditions in which a sleep disturbance has been frequently described.

Treatment

The diagnosis of a secondary sleep disorder hinges on the identification of an active disease process known to exert the observed effect on sleep. Treatment first addresses the underlying neurological or medical disease. Symptomatic treatments focus on behavior modification, such as improvement of sleep hygiene. Pharmacological options can also be used, such as benzodiazepines for restless legs syndrome or nocturnal myoclonus, stimulants for hypersomnia, and tricyclic antidepressant medications for manipulation of rapid eye movement (REM) sleep.

SEXUAL DYSFUNCTION DUE TO A GENERAL MEDICAL CONDITION

Sexual dysfunction often has psychological and physical underpinnings. *Sexual dysfunction due to a general medical condition* subsumes multiple forms of medically induced sexual disturbance, including erectile dysfunction, pain during sexual intercourse, low sexual desire, and orgasmic disorders. The DSM-IV-TR criteria for sexual dysfunction are listed in Table 10.5–9.

Epidemiology

Little is known regarding the prevalence of sexual dysfunction due to general medical illness. In general, prevalence rates for sexual complaints are highest for female hypoactive sexual desire and orgasm problems and for premature ejaculation in men. High rates of sexual dysfunction are described in patients with cardiac conditions, cancer, diabetes, and HIV. Forty to 50 percent of individuals with MS describe sexual dysfunction. Cerebrovascular accident impairs sexual functioning, with the possibility that, in men, greater impairment follows right-hemispheric cerebrovascular injury than left-hemispheric injury. Delayed orgasm can affect as much as 50 percent of individuals taking SSRIs.

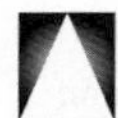

Table 10.5–9
DSM-IV-TR Criteria for Sexual Dysfunction Due to a General Medical Condition

A. Clinically significant sexual dysfunction that results in marked distress or interpersonal difficulty predominates in the clinical picture.
B. There is evidence from the history, physical examination, or laboratory findings that the sexual dysfunction is fully explained by the direct physiological effects of a general medical condition.
C. The disturbance is not better accounted for by another mental disorder (e.g., major depressive disorder).

Select code and term based on the predominant sexual dysfunction:

- Female hypoactive sexual desire disorder due to . . . [insert general medical condition here]: if deficient or absent sexual desire is the predominant feature.
- Male hypoactive sexual desire disorder due to . . . [insert general medical condition here]: if deficient or absent sexual desire is the predominant feature.
- Male erectile disorder due to . . . [insert general medical condition here]: if male erectile dysfunction is the predominant feature.
- Female dyspareunia due to . . . [insert general medical condition here]: if pain associated with intercourse is the predominant feature.
- Male dyspareunia due to . . . [insert general medical condition here]: if pain associated with intercourse is the predominant feature.
- Other female sexual dysfunction due to . . . [insert general medical condition here]: if some other feature is predominant (e.g., orgasmic disorder) or if no feature predominates.
- Other male sexual dysfunction due to . . . [insert general medical condition here]: if some other feature is predominant (e.g., orgasmic disorder) or if no feature predominates.

(From American Psychiatric Association. *Diagnostic and Statistical Manual of Mental Disorders.* 4th ed. Text rev. Washington, DC; American Psychiatric Association; 2000, with permission.)

Etiology

Potential causes of sexual dysfunctions are listed in Table 10.5–10. The type of sexual dysfunction is affected by the cause, but specificity is rare; that is, a given cause can manifest as one (or more than one) of several syndromes. General categories include medications and drugs of abuse, local disease processes that affect the primary or secondary sexual organs, and systemic illnesses that affect sexual organs via neurological, vascular, or endocrinological routes.

Course and Prognosis

The course and prognosis of secondary sexual dysfunctions vary widely, depending on the cause. Drug-induced syndromes generally remit with discontinuation (or dosage reduction) of the offending agent. Endocrine-based dysfunctions also generally

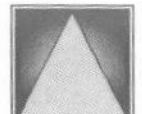

Table 10.5–10
Causes of Secondary Sexual Dysfunctions

Medications
- Cardiac drugs, antihypertensives (e.g., reserpine, β-adrenergic receptor antagonists, clonidine, α-methyldopa, diuretics)
- H_2-receptor blockers
- Carbonic anhydrase inhibitors
- Anticholinergics
- Anticonvulsants (e.g., carbamazepine, phenytoin, primidone)
- Antipsychotics
- Antidepressants (e.g., tricyclic drugs, MAO inhibitors, trazodone, SSRIs)
- Sedative-hypnotics

Substances of abuse
- Alcohol
- Opioids
- Stimulants
- Cannabis
- Sedative-hypnotics

Local disease processes that affect primary or secondary sexual organs
- Congenital anomalies or malformations
- Trauma
- Tumor
- Infection
- Postsurgical or postirradiation local neurological and vascular pathology

Systemic disease processes
- Neurological
  - Central nervous system (e.g., strokes, multiple sclerosis)
  - Peripheral nervous system (e.g., peripheral neuropathy)
- Vascular
  - Atherosclerosis, vasculitis (as examples)
- Endocrine
  - Diabetes mellitus, alterations in function of thyroid, adrenal cortex, gonadotropins, gonadal hormones (as examples)

MAO, monoamine oxidase; SSRI, selective serotonin reuptake inhibitor.
(Courtesy of Eric D. Caine, M.D., and Jeffrey M. Lyness, M.D.)

improve with restoration of normal physiology. By contrast, dysfunctions caused by neurological disease can run protracted, even progressive, courses.

Treatment

The treatment approach varies widely, depending on the etiology. When reversal of the underlying cause is not possible, supportive and behaviorally oriented psychotherapy with the patient (and perhaps the partner) may minimize distress and increase sexual satisfaction (e.g., by developing sexual interactions that are not limited by the specific dysfunction). Support groups for people with specific types of dysfunctions are available. Other symptom-based treatments can be used in certain conditions; for example, sildenafil (Viagra) administration or surgical implantation of a penile prosthesis may be used in the treatment of male erectile dysfunction.

MENTAL DISORDERS DUE TO A GENERAL MEDICAL CONDITION NOT ELSEWHERE CLASSIFIED

The DSM-IV-TR has three additional diagnostic categories for clinical presentations of mental disorders due to a general medical condition that do not meet the diagnostic criteria for specific diagnoses. The first of the diagnoses is catatonic disorder due to a general medical condition (Table 10.5–11). The second is personality change due to a general medical condition. The third diagnosis is mental disorder not otherwise specified due to a general medical condition (Table 10.5–12).

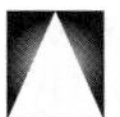

Table 10.5–11
DSM-IV-TR Diagnostic Criteria for Catatonic Disorder Due to a General Medical Condition

A. The presence of catatonia as manifested by motoric immobility, excessive motor activity (that is apparently purposeless and not influenced by external stimuli), extreme negativism or mutism, peculiarities of voluntary movement, or echolalia or echopraxia.
B. There is evidence from the history, physical examination, or laboratory findings that the disturbance is the direct physiological consequence of a general medical condition.
C. The disturbance is not better accounted for by another mental disorder (e.g., a manic episode).
D. The disturbance does not occur exclusively during the course of a delirium.

Coding note: Include the name of the general medical condition on Axis I, e.g., Catatonic disorder due to hepatic encephalopathy; also code the general medical condition on Axis III.

(From American Psychiatric Association. *Diagnostic and Statistical Manual of Mental Disorders.* 4th ed. Text rev. Washington, DC: American Psychiatric Association; copyright 2000, with permission.)

Catatonia Due to a Medical Condition

Catatonia can be caused by a variety of medical or surgical conditions. It is characterized usually by fixed posture and waxy flexibility. Mutism, negativism, and echolalia may be associated features.

Epidemiology. Catatonia is an uncommon condition. It is mostly seen in advanced primary mood or psychotic illnesses. Among inpatients with catatonia, 25 to 50 percent are related to mood disorders (e.g., major depressive episode, recurrent, with catatonic features), and approximately 10 percent are associated with schizophrenia. Data are scant as to catatonia's rate of occurrence due to medical conditions or substances.

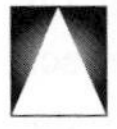

Table 10.5–12
DSM-IV-TR Diagnostic Criteria for Mental Disorder Not Otherwise Specified Due to a General Medical Condition

This residual category should be used for situations in which it has been established that the disturbance is caused by the direct physiological effects of a general medical condition, but the criteria are not met for a specific mental disorder due to a general medical condition (e.g., dissociative symptoms due to complex partial seizures).

Coding note: Include the name of the general medical condition on Axis I, e.g., Mental disorder not otherwise specified due to HIV disease; also code the general medical condition on Axis III.

(From American Psychiatric Association. *Diagnostic and Statistical Manual of Mental Disorders.* 4th ed. Text rev. Washington, DC: American Psychiatric Association; copyright 2000, with permission.)

Diagnosis and Clinical Features. Peculiarities of movement are the most characteristic feature, usually rigidity. Hyperactivity and psychomotor agitation can also occur (Table 10.5–11). A thorough medical workup is necessary to confirm the diagnosis.

Course and Prognosis. The course and prognosis are intimately related to the cause. Neoplasms, encephalitis, head trauma, diabetes, and other metabolic disorders can manifest with catatonic features. If the underlying disorder is treatable, the catatonic syndrome will resolve.

Treatment. Treatment must be directed to the underlying cause. Antipsychotic medications may improve postural abnormalities even though they have no effect on the underlying disorder. Schizophrenia must always be ruled out in patients who present with catatonic symptoms.

Personality Change Due to a General Medical Condition

Personality change means that the person's fundamental means of interacting and behaving have been altered. When a true personality change occurs in adulthood, the clinician should always suspect brain injury. Almost every medical disorder can be accompanied by personality change, however.

Epidemiology. No reliable epidemiological data exist on personality trait changes in medical conditions. Specific personality trait changes for particular brain diseases—for example, passive and self-centered behaviors in patients with dementia of the Alzheimer's type—have been reported. Similarly, apathy has been described in patients with frontal lobe lesions.

Etiology. Diseases that preferentially affect the frontal lobes or subcortical structures are more likely to manifest with prominent personality change. Head trauma is a common cause. Frontal lobe tumors, such as meningiomas and gliomas, can grow to considerable size before coming to medical attention, because they can be neurologically silent (i.e., without focal signs). Progressive dementia syndromes, especially those with a subcortical pattern of degeneration, such as acquired immune deficiency syndrome (AIDS) dementia complex, Huntington's disease, or progressive supranuclear palsy, often cause significant personality disturbance. MS can impinge on the personality, reflecting subcortical white matter degeneration. Exposure to toxins with a predilection for white matter, such as irradiation, can also produce significant personality change disproportionate to the cognitive or motor impairment.

Diagnosis and Clinical Features. The DSM-IV-TR diagnostic criteria for personality change due to a general medical condition are listed in Table 10.5–13.

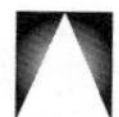

Table 10.5–13
DSM-IV-TR Diagnostic Criteria for Personality Change Due to General Medical Condition

A. A persistent personality disturbance that represents a change from the individual's previous characteristic personality pattern. (In children, the disturbance involves a marked deviation from normal development or a significant change in the child's usual behavior patterns lasting at least 1 year.)

B. There is evidence from the history, physical examination, or laboratory findings that the disturbance is the direct physiological consequence of a general medical condition.

C. The disturbance is not better accounted for by another mental disorder (including other mental disorders due to a general medical condition).

D. The disturbance does not occur exclusively during the course of a delirium.

E. The disturbance causes clinically significant distress or impairment in social, occupational, or other important areas of functioning.

Specify type:
- **Labile type:** if the predominant feature is affective lability
- **Disinhibited type:** if the predominant feature is poor impulse control as evidenced by sexual indiscretions, etc.
- **Aggressive type:** if the predominant feature is aggressive behavior
- **Apathetic type:** if the predominant feature is marked apathy and indifference
- **Paranoid type:** if the predominant feature is suspiciousness or paranoid ideation
- **Other type:** if the presentation is not characterized by any of the above subtypes
- **Combined type:** if more than one feature predominates in the clinical picture
- **Unspecified type**

Coding note: Include the name of the general medical condition on Axis I, e.g., Personality change due to temporal lobe epilepsy; also code the general medical condition on Axis III.

(From American Psychiatric Association. *Diagnostic and Statistical Manual of Mental Disorders.* 4th ed. Text rev. Washington, DC: American Psychiatric Association; copyright 2000, with permission.)

Mr. Davis is a 49-year-old married man without a psychiatric history who was admitted to the hospital with sudden onset of severe headache. Workup revealed subarachnoid hemorrhage caused by the rupture of an intracranial aneurysm. Cerebral vasospasm, obstructive hydrocephalus, and coma ensued. Neurosurgical intervention was undertaken to clip the aneurysm and to install a ventriculoperitoneal shunt.

After a lengthy course of inpatient rehabilitation, Mr. Davis experienced outbursts of anger, episodic depressed mood, off-color remarks that verged on offensive, and impairment in his appreciation for subtlety in humor and conversation. No evidence of psychosis was observed. Family members reported that Mr. Davis always had been one to "speak his mind" and to react defensively when he felt criticized.

Brain imaging demonstrated encephalomalacia in the right frontal lobe. Mild cognitive dysfunction not rising to the level of dementia was diagnosed on neuropsychological testing.

Course and Prognosis. Course depends on the nature of the medical or neurological insult. Personality changes resulting from medical conditions likely to yield to intervention (e.g., correction of hypothyroidism) are more amenable to improvement than are personality changes due to medical conditions that are static (e.g., brain injury after head trauma) or progressive in nature (e.g., Huntington's disease).

Treatment. Treatment of secondary personality syndromes is first directed toward correcting the underlying cause. Lithium carbonate (Eskalith), carbamazepine (Tegretol), and valproic acid (Depakote) have been used to control affective lability and impulsivity. Aggression or explosiveness can be treated with lithium, anticonvulsant medications, or a combination of lithium and an anticonvulsant agent. Centrally active β-adrenergic receptor antagonists, such as propranolol (Inderal), have some efficacy as well. Apathy and inertia have occasionally improved with psychostimulant agents. Because cognition and verbal skills may be preserved in patients with secondary personality changes, they may be candidates for psychotherapy. Families should be involved in the therapy process, with a focus on education and understanding the origins of the patient's inappropriate behaviors. Issues such as competency, disability, and advocacy are frequently of clinical concern with these patients in light of the unpredictable and pervasive behavior change.

SPECIFIC DISORDERS

Epilepsy

Epilepsy is the most common chronic neurological disease in the general population and affects approximately 1 percent of the population in the United States. For psychiatrists, the major concerns about epilepsy are consideration of an epileptic diagnosis in psychiatric patients, the psychosocial ramifications of a diagnosis of epilepsy for a patient, and the psychological and cognitive effects of commonly used anticonvulsant drugs. With regard to the first of these concerns, 30 to 50 percent of all persons with epilepsy have psychiatric difficulties sometime during the course of their illness. The most common behavioral symptom of epilepsy is a change in personality. Psychosis and violence occur much less commonly than was previously believed.

Definitions. A seizure is a transient paroxysmal pathophysiological disturbance of cerebral function caused by a spontaneous, excessive discharge of neurons. Patients are said to have epilepsy if they have a chronic condition characterized by recurrent seizure. The ictus, or ictal event, is the seizure itself. The nonictal periods are categorized as preictal, postictal, and interictal. The symptoms during the ictal event are determined primarily by the site of origin in the brain for the seizure and by the pattern of the spread of seizure activity through the brain. Interictal symptoms are influenced by the ictal event and other neuropsychiatric and psychosocial factors, such as coexisting psychiatric or neurological disorders, the presence of psychosocial stressors, and premorbid personality traits.

Classification. The two major categories of seizures are partial and generalized. Partial seizures involve epileptiform activity in localized brain regions. Generalized seizures involve the entire brain (Fig. 10.5–1). A classification system for seizures is outlined in Table 10.5–14.

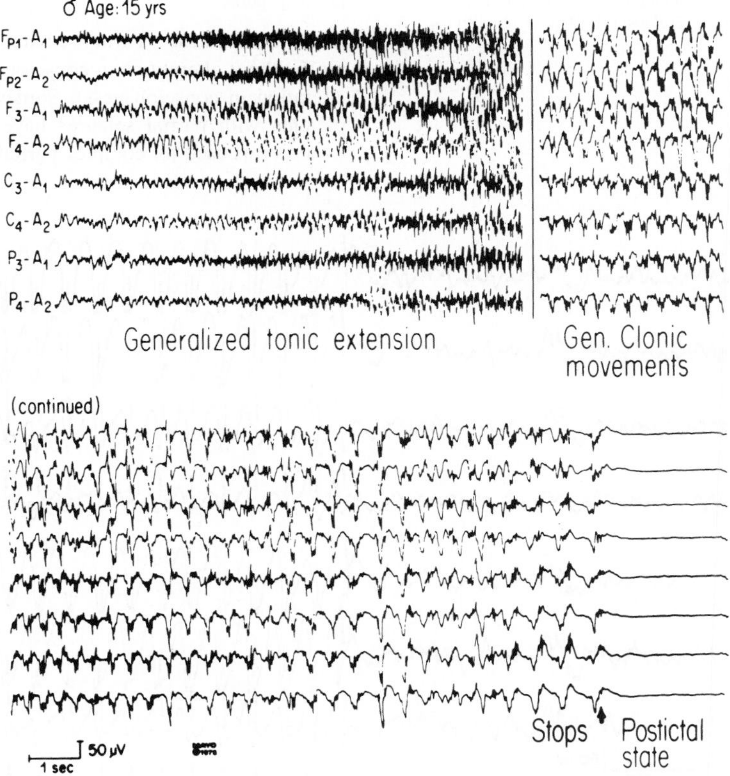

FIGURE 10.5–1

Electroencephalographic recording during generalized tonic-clonic seizure, showing rhythmic sharp waves and muscles artifact during tonic phase; spike and wave discharges during clonic phase; and attenuation of activity during postictal state. (Courtesy of Barbara F. Westmoreland, M.D.)

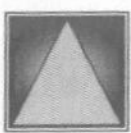

Table 10.5–14
International Classification of Epileptic Seizures

I. Partial seizures (seizures beginning locally)
  A. Partial seizures with elementary symptoms (generally without impairment of consciousness)
    1. With motor symptoms
    2. With sensory symptoms
    3. With autonomic symptoms
    4. Compound forms
  B. Partial seizures with complex symptoms (generally with impairment of consciousness; temporal lobe or psychomotor seizures)
    1. With impairment of consciousness only
    2. With cognitive symptoms
    3. With affective symptoms
    4. With psychosensory symptoms
    5. With psychosensory symptoms (automatisms)
    6. Compound forms
  C. Partial seizures secondarily generalized
II. Generalized seizures (bilaterally symmetrical and without local onset)
  A. Absences (petit mal)
  B. Myoclonus
  C. Infantile spasms
  D. Clonic seizures
  E. Tonic seizures
  F. Tonic-clonic seizures (grand mal)
  G. Atonic seizures
  H. Akinetic seizures
III. Unilateral seizures
IV. Unclassified seizures (because of incomplete data)

(Adapted from Gastaut H. Clinical and electroencephalographical classification of epileptic seizures. *Epilepsia.* 1970;11:102, with permission.)

GENERALIZED SEIZURES. Generalized tonic-clonic seizures exhibit the classic symptoms of loss of consciousness, generalized tonic-clonic movements of the limbs, tongue biting, and incontinence. Although the diagnosis of the ictal events of the seizure is relatively straightforward, the postictal state, characterized by a slow, gradual recovery of consciousness and cognition, occasionally presents a diagnostic dilemma for a psychiatrist in an emergency room. The recovery period from a generalized tonic-clonic seizure ranges from a few minutes to many hours, and the clinical picture is that of a gradually clearing delirium. The most common psychiatric problems associated with generalized seizures involve helping patients adjust to a chronic neurological disorder and assessing the cognitive or behavioral effects of anticonvulsant drugs.

Absence Seizure (Petit Mal). A difficult type of generalized seizure for a psychiatrist to diagnose is an absence, or petit mal, seizure. The epileptic nature of the episodes may go unrecognized, because the characteristic motor or sensory manifestations of epilepsy may be absent or so slight that they do not arouse suspicion. Petit mal epilepsy usually begins in childhood between the ages of 5 and 7 years and ceases by puberty. Brief disruptions of consciousness, during which the patient suddenly loses contact with the environment, are characteristic of petit mal epilepsy, but the patient has no true loss of consciousness and no convulsive movements during the episodes. The electroencephalogram (EEG) produces a characteristic pattern of three-per-second spike-and-wave activity (Fig. 10.5–2). In rare instances, petit mal epilepsy begins in adulthood. Adult-onset petit mal epilepsy can be characterized by sudden, recurrent psychotic episodes or deliriums that appear and disappear abruptly. The symptoms may be accompanied by a history of falling or fainting spells.

PARTIAL SEIZURES. Partial seizures are classified as either simple (without alterations in consciousness) or complex (with an alteration in consciousness). Somewhat more than half of all patients with partial seizures have complex partial seizures. Other terms used for complex partial seizures are temporal lobe

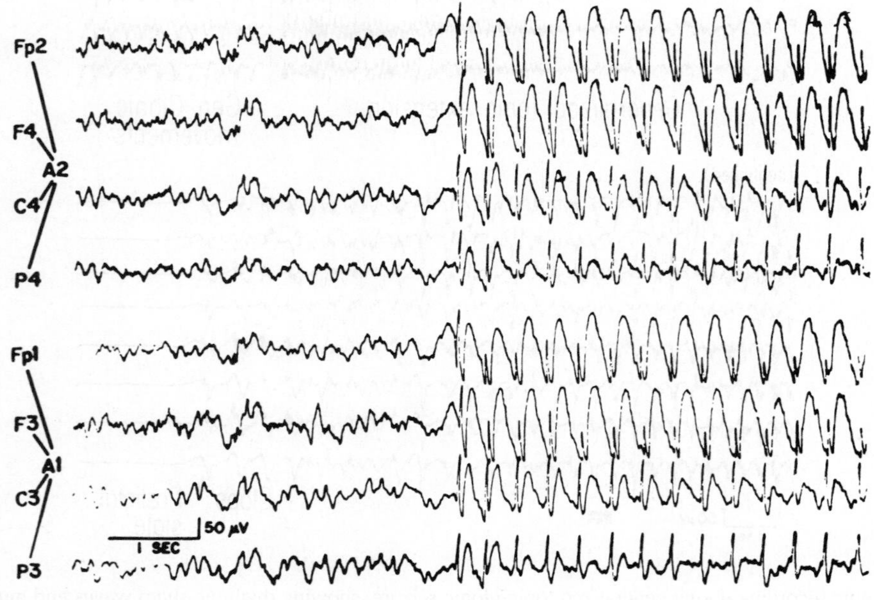

FIGURE 10.5–2
Petit mal epilepsy characterized by bilaterally synchronous, 3-Hz spike and slow-wave activity.

epilepsy, psychomotor seizures, and limbic epilepsy; these terms, however, are not accurate descriptions of the clinical situation. Complex partial epilepsy, the most common form of epilepsy in adults, affects approximately 3 of 1,000 persons. About 30 percent of patients with complex partial seizures have major mental illness such as depression.

Symptoms

PREICTAL SYMPTOMS. Preictal events (auras) in complex partial epilepsy include autonomic sensations (e.g., fullness in the stomach, blushing, and changes in respiration), cognitive sensations (e.g., *déjà vu*, *jamais vu*, forced thinking, dreamy states), affective states (e.g., fear, panic, depression, elation), and, classically, automatisms (e.g., lip smacking, rubbing, chewing).

ICTAL SYMPTOMS. Brief, disorganized, and uninhibited behavior characterizes the ictal event. Although some defense attorneys may claim otherwise, rarely does a person exhibit organized, directed violent behavior during an epileptic episode. The cognitive symptoms include amnesia for the time during the seizure and a period of resolving delirium after the seizure. A seizure focus can be found on an EEG in 25 to 50 percent of all patients with complex partial epilepsy (Fig. 10.5–3). The use of sphenoidal or anterior temporal electrodes and sleep-deprived EEGs may increase the likelihood of finding an EEG abnormality. Multiple normal EEGs are often obtained for a patient with complex partial epilepsy; therefore, normal EEGs cannot be used to exclude a diagnosis of complex partial epilepsy. The use of long-term EEG recordings (usually 24 to 72 hours) can help clinicians detect a seizure focus in some patients. Most studies show that the use of nasopharyngeal leads does not add much to the sensitivity of an EEG, but they do add to the discomfort of the procedure for the patient.

INTERICTAL SYMPTOMS

Personality Disturbances. The most frequent psychiatric abnormalities reported in patients with epilepsy are personality disorders, and they are especially likely to occur in patients with epilepsy of temporal lobe origin. The most common features are religiosity, a heightened experience of emotions—a quality usually called *viscosity of personality*—and changes in sexual behavior. The syndrome in its complete form is relatively rare, even in those with complex partial seizures of temporal lobe origin. Many patients are not affected by personality disturbances; others suffer from a variety of disturbances that differ strikingly from the classic syndrome.

A striking religiosity may be manifested not only by increased participation in overtly religious activities but also by unusual concern for moral and ethical issues, preoccupation with right and wrong, and heightened interest in global and philosophical concerns. The hyperreligious features can sometimes seem like the prodromal symptoms of schizophrenia and can result in a diagnostic problem in an adolescent or a young adult.

The symptom of viscosity of personality is usually most noticeable in a patient's conversation, which is likely to be slow, serious, ponderous, pedantic, overly replete with nonessential details, and often circumstantial. The listener may grow bored but be unable to find a courteous and successful way to disengage from the conversation. The speech tendencies, often mirrored in the patient's writing, result in a symptom known as *hypergraphia*, which some clinicians consider virtually pathognomonic for complex partial epilepsy.

Changes in sexual behavior may be manifested by hypersexuality; deviations in sexual interest, such as fetishism and transvestism; and, most commonly, hyposexuality. The hyposexuality is characterized both

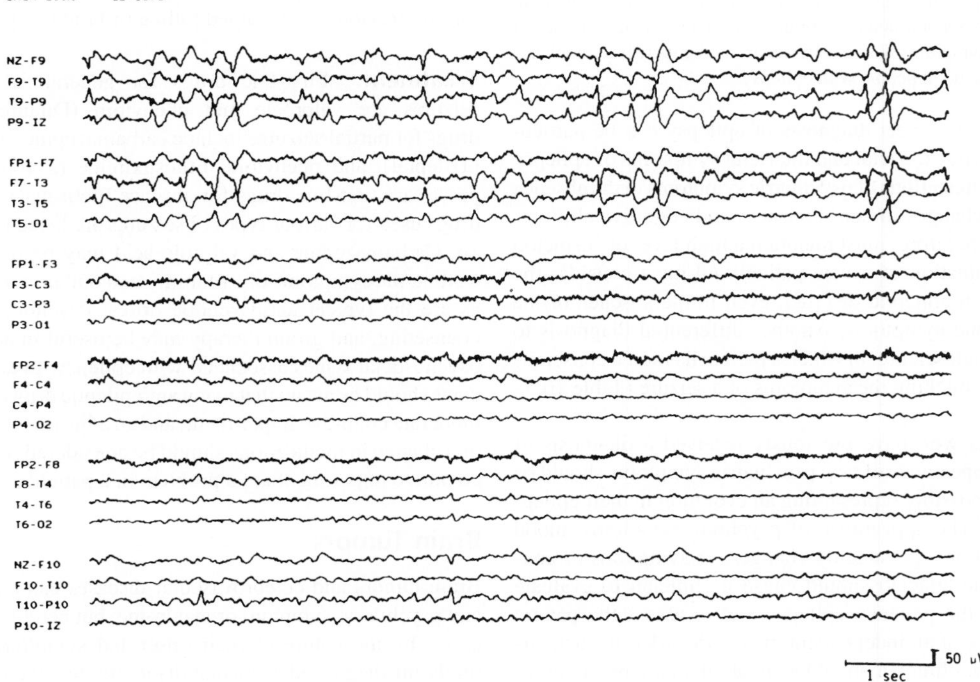

FIGURE 10.5–3
An interictal encephalograph in a patient with complex partial seizures reveals frequent left-temporal spike discharges and rare, independent right-temporal sharp-wave activity. (From Cascino GD. Complex partial seizures: clinical features and differential diagnosis. *Psychiatr Clin North Am.* 1992;15:377, with permission.)

by a lack of interest in sexual matters and by reduced sexual arousal. Some patients with the onset of complex partial epilepsy before puberty may fail to reach a normal level of sexual interest after puberty, although this characteristic may not disturb the patient. For patients with the onset of complex partial epilepsy after puberty, the change in sexual interest may be bothersome and worrisome.

Psychotic Symptoms. Interictal psychotic states are more common than ictal psychoses. Schizophrenia-like interictal episodes can occur in patients with epilepsy, particularly those with temporal lobe origins. An estimated 10 percent of all patients with complex partial epilepsy have psychotic symptoms. Risk factors for the symptoms include female gender, left-handedness, the onset of seizures during puberty, and a left-sided lesion.

The onset of psychotic symptoms in epilepsy is variable. Classically, psychotic symptoms appear in patients who have had epilepsy for a long time, and the onset of psychotic symptoms is preceded by the development of personality changes related to the epileptic brain activity. The most characteristic symptoms of the psychoses are hallucinations and paranoid delusions. Patients usually remain warm and appropriate in affect, in contrast to the abnormalities of affect commonly seen in patients with schizophrenia. The thought disorder symptoms in patients with psychotic epilepsy are most commonly those involving conceptualization and circumstantiality, rather than the classic schizophrenic symptoms of blocking and looseness.

Violence. Episodic violence has been a problem in some patients with epilepsy, especially epilepsy of temporal and frontal lobe origin. Whether the violence is a manifestation of the seizure itself or is of interictal psychopathological origin is uncertain. Most evidence points to the extreme rarity of violence as an ictal phenomenon. Only in rare cases should violence in the patient with epilepsy be attributed to the seizure itself.

Mood Disorder Symptoms. Mood disorder symptoms, such as depression and mania, are seen less often in epilepsy than are schizophrenia-like symptoms. The mood disorder symptoms that do occur tend to be episodic and appear most often when the epileptic foci affect the temporal lobe of the nondominant cerebral hemisphere. The importance of mood disorder symptoms may be attested to by the increased incidence of attempted suicide in people with epilepsy.

Diagnosis. A correct diagnosis of epilepsy can be particularly difficult when the ictal and interictal symptoms of epilepsy are severe manifestations of psychiatric symptoms in the absence of significant changes in consciousness and cognitive abilities. Psychiatrists, therefore, must maintain a high level of suspicion during the evaluation of a new patient and must consider the possibility of an epileptic disorder, even in the absence of the classic signs and symptoms. Another differential diagnosis to consider is pseudoseizure, in which a patient has some conscious control over mimicking the symptoms of a seizure (Table 10.5–15).

For patients who have previously received a diagnosis of epilepsy, the appearance of new psychiatric symptoms should be considered as possibly representing an evolution in their epileptic symptoms. The appearance of psychotic symptoms, mood disorder symptoms, personality changes, or symptoms of anxiety (e.g., panic attacks) should cause a clinician to evaluate the control of the patient's epilepsy and to assess the patient for the presence of an independent mental disorder. In such circumstances, the clinician should evaluate the patient's compliance with the anticonvulsant drug regimen and should consider whether the psychiatric symptoms could be adverse effects from the antiepileptic drugs themselves. When psychiatric symptoms appear in a patient who has had epilepsy diagnosed or considered

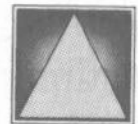

Table 10.5–15
Differentiating Features of Pseudoseizures and Epileptic Seizures

Feature	Epileptic Seizures	Pseudoseizure
Clinical features		
Nocturnal seizure	Common	Uncommon
Stereotyped aura	Usually	None
Cyanotic skin changes during seizures	Common	None
Self-injury	Common	Rare
Incontinence	Common	Rare
Postictal confusion	Present	None
Body movements	Tonic or clonic or both	Nonstereotyped and asynchronous
Affected by suggestion	No	Yes
EEG features		
Spike and waveforms	Present	Absent
Postictal slowing	Present	Absent
Interictal abnormalities	Variable	Variable

EEG, electroencephalogram.
(From Stevenson JM, King JH. Neuropsychiatric aspects of epilepsy and epileptic seizures. In: Hales RE, Yodofsky SC, eds. *American Psychiatric Press Textbook of Neuropsychiatry.* Washington, DC: American Psychiatric Press; 1987:220, with permission.)

as a diagnosis in the past, the clinician should obtain results of one or more EEG examinations.

In patients who have not previously received a diagnosis of epilepsy, four characteristics should cause a clinician to be suspicious of the possibility: the abrupt onset of psychosis in a person previously regarded as psychologically healthy, the abrupt onset of delirium without a recognized cause, a history of similar episodes with abrupt onset and spontaneous recovery, and a history of previous unexplained falling or fainting spells.

Treatment. First-line drugs for generalized tonic-clonic seizures are valproate and phenytoin (Dilantin). First-line drugs for partial seizures include carbamazepine, oxcarbazepine (Trileptal), and phenytoin. Ethosuximide (Zarontin) and valproate are first-line drugs for absence (petit mal) seizures. The drugs used for various types of seizures are listed in Table 10.5–16. Carbamazepine and valproic acid may be helpful in controlling the symptoms of irritability and outbursts of aggression, as are the typical antipsychotic drugs. Psychotherapy, family counseling, and group therapy may be useful in addressing the psychosocial issues associated with epilepsy. In addition, clinicians should be aware that many antiepileptic drugs cause mild to moderate cognitive impairment, and an adjustment of the dosage or a change in medications should be considered if symptoms of cognitive impairment are a problem in a patient.

Brain Tumors

Brain tumors and cerebrovascular diseases can cause virtually any psychiatric symptom or syndrome, but cerebrovascular diseases, by the nature of their onset and symptom pattern, are rarely misdiagnosed as mental disorders. In general, tumors are associated with fewer psychopathological signs and symptoms than are cerebrovascular diseases affecting a similar volume of brain tissue. The two key approaches to the diagnosis of either condition are a comprehensive clinical history and a complete

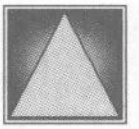

Table 10.5–16
Commonly Used Anticonvulsant Drugs

Drug	Use	Maintenance Dosage (mg/day)
Carbamazepine (Tegretol, Carbatrol)	Generalized tonic-clonic, partial	600–1,200
Clonazepam (Klonopin)	Absence, atypical myoclonic	2–12
Ethosuximide (Zarontin)	Absence	1,000–2,000
Gabapentin (Neurontin)	Complex partial seizures (augmentation)	900–3,600
Lamotrigine (Lamictal)	Complex partial seizures, generalized (augmentation)	300–500
Oxcarbazepine (Trileptal)	Partial	600–2,400
Phenobarbital	Generalized tonic-clonic	100–200
Phenytoin (Dilantin)	Generalized tonic-clonic, partial, status epilepticus	300–500
Primidone (Mysoline)	Partial	750–1,000
Tiagabine (Gabitril)	Generalized	32–56
Topiramate (Topamax)	Complex partial seizures (augmentation)	200–400
Valproate	Absence, myoclonic generalized tonic-clonic akinetic, partial seizures	750–1,000
Zonisamide (Zonegran)	Generalized	400–600

neurological examination. Performance of the appropriate brain imaging technique is usually the final diagnostic procedure; the imaging should confirm the clinical diagnosis.

Clinical Features, Course, and Prognosis. Mental symptoms are experienced at some time during the course of illness in approximately 50 percent of patients with brain tumors. In approximately 80 percent of these patients with mental symptoms, the tumors are located in frontal or limbic brain regions rather than in parietal or temporal regions. Meningiomas are likely to cause focal symptoms by compressing a limited region of the cortex, whereas gliomas are likely to cause diffuse symptoms. Delirium is most often a component of rapidly growing, large, or metastatic tumors. If a patient's history and a physical examination reveal bowel or bladder incontinence, a frontal lobe tumor should be suspected; if the history and examination reveal abnormalities in memory and speech, a temporal lobe tumor should be suspected.

COGNITION. Impaired intellectual functioning often accompanies the presence of a brain tumor, regardless of its type or location.

LANGUAGE SKILLS. Disorders of language function may be severe, particularly if tumor growth is rapid. In fact, defects of language function often obscure all other mental symptoms.

MEMORY. Loss of memory is a frequent symptom of brain tumors. Patients with brain tumors exhibit Korsakoff's syndrome and retain no memory of events that occurred since the illness began. Events of the immediate past, even painful ones, are lost. Patients, however, retain old memories and are unaware of their loss of recent memory.

PERCEPTION. Prominent perceptual defects are often associated with behavioral disorders, especially because patients must integrate tactile, auditory, and visual perceptions to function normally.

AWARENESS. Alterations of consciousness are common late symptoms of increased intracranial pressure caused by a brain tumor. Tumors arising in the upper part of the brainstem can produce a unique symptom called *akinetic mutism*, or *vigilant coma*. The patient is immobile and mute, yet alert.

Colloid Cysts. Although they are not brain tumors, colloid cysts located in the third ventricle can exert physical pressure on structures within the diencephalon and produce such mental symptoms as depression, emotional lability, psychotic symptoms, and personality changes. The classic associated neurological symptoms are position-dependent intermittent headaches.

Head Trauma

Head trauma can result in an array of mental symptoms and lead to a diagnosis of dementia due to head trauma or to mental disorder not otherwise specified due to a general medical condition (e.g., postconcussional disorder). The postconcussive syndrome remains controversial, because it focuses on the wide range of psychiatric symptoms, some serious, that can follow what seems to be minor head trauma. DSM-IV-TR includes a set of research criteria for postconcussional disorder in an appendix (Table 10.5–17).

Pathophysiology. Head trauma is a common clinical situation; an estimated 2 million incidents involve head trauma each year. Head trauma most commonly occurs in people 15 to 25 years of age and has a male-to-female predominance of approximately 3 to 1. Gross estimates based on the severity of the head trauma suggest that virtually all patients with serious head trauma, more than half of patients with moderate head trauma, and about 10 percent of patients with mild head trauma have ongoing neuropsychiatric sequelae resulting from the head trauma. Head trauma can be divided grossly into penetrating head trauma (e.g., trauma produced by a bullet) and blunt trauma, in which there is no physical penetration of the skull. Blunt trauma is far more common than penetrating head trauma. Motor vehicle accidents account for more than half of all the incidents of blunt central nervous system (CNS) trauma; falls, violence, and sports-related head trauma account for most of the remaining cases (Fig. 10.5–4).

Whereas brain injury from penetrating wounds is usually localized to the areas directly affected by the missile, brain injury from blunt trauma involves several mechanisms. During the actual head trauma, the head usually moves back and forth violently, so that the brain hits repeatedly against the skull as it and the skull are mismatched in their rapid deceleration and acceleration. This crashing results in focal contusions, and the stretching

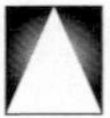

Table 10.5–17
DSM-IV-TR Research Criteria for Postconcussional Disorder

A. A history of head trauma that has caused significant cerebral concussion.
Note: The manifestations of concussion include loss of consciousness, posttraumatic amnesia, and, less commonly, posttraumatic onset of seizures. The specific method of defining this criterion needs to be established by further research.

B. Evidence from neuropsychological testing or quantified cognitive assessment of difficulty in attention (concentrating, shifting focus of attention, performing simultaneous cognitive tasks) or memory (learning or recalling information).

C. Three (or more) of the following occur shortly after the trauma and last at least 3 months:
(1) becoming fatigued easily
(2) disordered sleep
(3) headache
(4) vertigo or dizziness
(5) irritability or aggression on little or no provocation
(6) anxiety, depression, or affective lability
(7) changes in personality (e.g., social or sexual inappropriateness)
(8) apathy or lack of spontaneity

D. The symptoms in Criteria B and C have their onset following head trauma or else represent a substantial worsening of preexisting symptoms.

E. The disturbance causes significant impairment in social or occupational functioning and represents a significant decline from a previous level of functioning. In school-age children, the impairment may be manifested by a significant worsening in school or academic performance dating from the trauma.

F. The symptoms do not meet criteria for dementia due to head trauma and are not better accounted for by another mental disorder (e.g., amnestic disorder due to head trauma, personality change due to head trauma).

(From American Psychiatric Association. *Diagnostic and Statistical Manual of Mental Disorders*. 4th ed. Text rev. Washington, DC: American Psychiatric Association; copyright 2000, with permission.)

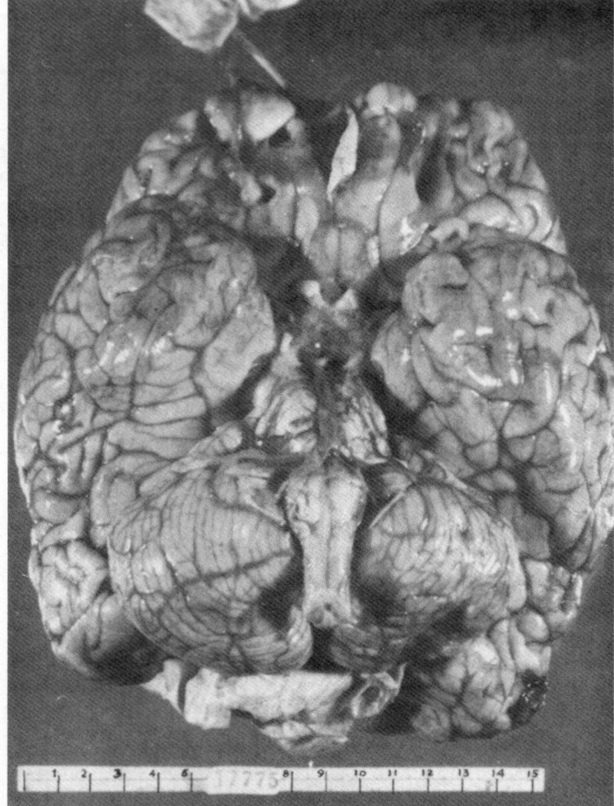

FIGURE 10.5–4
Severe contusion of the frontal poles has resulted in their atrophy and distortion. (Courtesy of Dr. H. M. Zimmerman.)

of the brain parenchyma produces diffuse axonal injury. Later-developing processes, such as edema and hemorrhaging, can result in further damage to the brain.

Symptoms. The two major clusters of symptoms related to head trauma are those of cognitive impairment and of behavioral sequelae. After a period of posttraumatic amnesia, there is usually a 6- to 12-month period of recovery, after which the remaining symptoms are likely to be permanent. The most common cognitive problems are decreased speed in information processing, decreased attention, increased distractibility, deficits in problem-solving and in the ability to sustain effort, and problems with memory and learning new information. A variety of language disabilities can also occur.

Behaviorally, the major symptoms involve depression, increased impulsivity, increased aggression, and changes in personality. These symptoms can be further exacerbated by the use of alcohol, which is often involved in the head trauma event itself. A debate has ensued about how preexisting character and personality traits affect the development of behavioral symptoms after head trauma. The critical studies needed to answer the question definitively have not yet been done, but the weight of opinion is leaning toward a biologically and neuroanatomically based association between the head trauma and the behavioral sequelae.

Treatment. The treatment of the cognitive and behavioral disorders in patients with head trauma is basically similar to the treatment approaches used in other patients with these symptoms. One difference is that patients with head trauma may be particularly susceptible to the side effects associated with psychotropic drugs; therefore, treatment with these agents should be initiated in lower dosages than usual, and they should be titrated upward more slowly than usual. Standard antidepressants can be used to treat depression, and either anticonvulsants or antipsychotics can be used to treat aggression and impulsivity. Other approaches to the symptoms include lithium, calcium channel blockers, and β-adrenergic receptor antagonists.

Clinicians must support patients through individual or group psychotherapy and should support the major caretakers through couples and family therapy. Patients with minor and moderate head trauma often rejoin their families and restart their jobs; therefore, all involved parties need help to adjust to any changes in the patient's personality and mental abilities.

Demyelinating Disorders

Multiple sclerosis is the major demyelinating disorder. Other demyelinating disorders include amyotrophic lateral sclerosis (ALS), metachromatic leukodystrophy, adrenoleukodystrophy, gangliosidoses, subacute sclerosing panencephalitis, and Kufs' disease. All these disorders can be associated with neurological, cognitive, and behavioral symptoms.

Multiple Sclerosis. MS is characterized by multiple episodes of symptoms, pathophysiologically related to multifocal lesions in the white matter of the CNS (Fig. 10.5–5). The cause remains unknown, but studies have focused on slow viral infections and disturbances in the immune system. The estimated prevalence of MS in the Western Hemisphere is 50 per 100,000 people. The disease is much more frequent in cold and temperate climates than in the tropics and subtropics and more common in women than in men; it is predominantly a disease of young adults. In most patients, the onset occurs between the ages of 20 and 40 years.

The neuropsychiatric symptoms of MS can be divided into cognitive and behavioral types. Research reports have found that 30 to 50 percent of patients with MS have mild cognitive impairment and that 20 to 30 percent of them have serious cognitive impairments. Although evidence indicates that patients with MS experience a decline in their general intelligence, memory is the most commonly affected cognitive function. The severity of the memory impairment does not seem to be correlated with the severity of the neurological symptoms or the duration of the illness.

The behavioral symptoms associated with MS are varied and can include euphoria, depression, and personality changes. Psychosis is a rare complication. Approximately 25 percent of persons with MS exhibit a euphoric mood that is not hypomanic, but somewhat more cheerful than their situation warrants and not necessarily in character with their disposition before the onset of MS. Only 10 percent of patients with MS have a sustained and elevated mood, although it is still not truly hypomanic. Depression, however, is common; it affects 25 to 50 percent of patients with MS and results in a higher rate of suicide than is seen in the general population. Risk factors for suicide in patients with MS are male sex, onset of MS before age 30, and a relatively recent diagnosis of the disorder. Personality changes are also common in patients with MS; they affect 20 to 40 percent of patients and are often characterized by increased irritability or apathy.

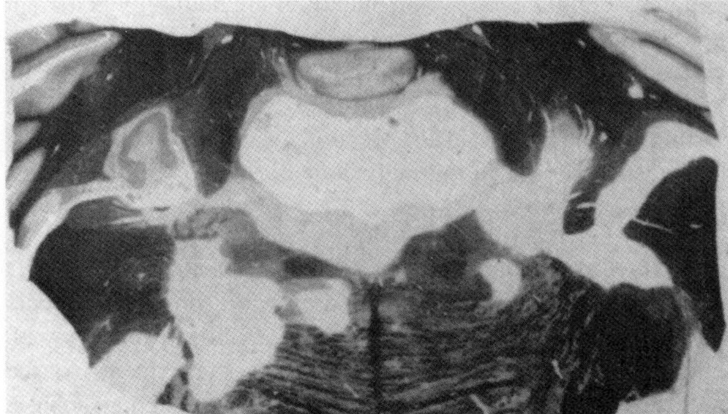

FIGURE 10.5–5
Multiple sclerosis. Irregular, seemingly punched out zones of demyelination are evident in this section through the level of the fourth ventricle. Myelin stain. 2.6×. (Courtesy of Dr. H. M. Zimmerman.)

Amyotrophic Lateral Sclerosis. ALS is a progressive, noninherited disease of asymmetrical muscle atrophy. It begins in adult life and progresses over months or years to involve all the striated muscles except the cardiac and ocular muscles. In addition to muscle atrophy, patients have signs of pyramidal tract involvement. The illness is rare and occurs in approximately 1.6 persons per 100,000 annually. A few patients have concomitant dementia. The disease progresses rapidly, and death generally occurs within 4 years of onset.

Infectious Diseases

Herpes Simplex Encephalitis. Herpes simplex encephalitis, the most common type of focal encephalitis, most commonly affects the frontal and temporal lobes. The symptoms often include anosmia, olfactory and gustatory hallucinations, and personality changes and can also involve bizarre or psychotic behaviors. Complex partial epilepsy may also develop in patients with herpes simplex encephalitis. Although the mortality rate for the infection has decreased, many patients exhibit personality changes, symptoms of memory loss, and psychotic symptoms.

Rabies Encephalitis. The incubation period for rabies ranges from 10 days to 1 year, after which symptoms of restlessness, overactivity, and agitation can develop. Hydrophobia, present in up to 50 percent of patients, is characterized by an intense fear of drinking water. The fear develops from the severe laryngeal and diaphragmatic spasms that the patients experience when they drink water. Once rabies encephalitis develops, the disease is fatal within days or weeks.

Neurosyphilis. Neurosyphilis (also known as general paresis) appears 10 to 15 years after the primary *Treponema* infection. Since the advent of penicillin, neurosyphilis has become a rare disorder, although AIDS is associated with reintroducing neurosyphilis into medical practice in some urban settings. Neurosyphilis generally affects the frontal lobes and results in personality changes, development of poor judgment, irritability, and decreased care for self. Delusions of grandeur develop in 10 to 20 percent of affected patients. The disease progresses with the development of dementia and tremor, until patients are paretic. The neurological symptoms include Argyll-Robertson pupils, which are small, irregular, and unequal and have light-near reflex dissociation, tremor, dysarthria, and hyperreflexia. Cerebrospinal fluid (CSF) examination shows lymphocytosis, increased protein, and a positive result on a Venereal Disease Research Laboratory (VDRL) test.

Chronic Meningitis. Chronic meningitis is now seen more often than in the recent past because of the immunocompromised condition of people with AIDS. The usual causative agents are *Mycobacterium tuberculosis*, *Cryptococcus*, and *Coccidioides*. The usual symptoms are headache, memory impairment, confusion, and fever.

Subacute Sclerosing Panencephalitis. Subacute sclerosing panencephalitis is a disease of childhood and early adolescence, with a 3-to-1 male-to-female ratio. The onset usually follows either an infection with measles or a vaccination for measles. The initial symptoms may be behavioral change, temper tantrums, sleepiness, and hallucinations, but the classic symptoms of myoclonus, ataxia, seizures, and intellectual deterioration eventually develop. The disease progresses relentlessly to coma and death in 1 to 2 years.

Lyme Disease. Lyme disease is caused by infection with the spirochete *Borrelia burgdorferi* transmitted through the bite of the deer tick (*Ixodes scapularis*), which feeds on infected deer and mice. About 16,000 cases are reported annually in the United States.

A characteristic bull's-eye rash (Fig. 10.5–6) is found at the site of the tick bite, followed shortly thereafter by flu-like symptoms. Impaired cognitive functioning and mood changes are associated with the illness and may be the presenting complaint. These include memory lapses, difficulty concentrating, irritability, and depression.

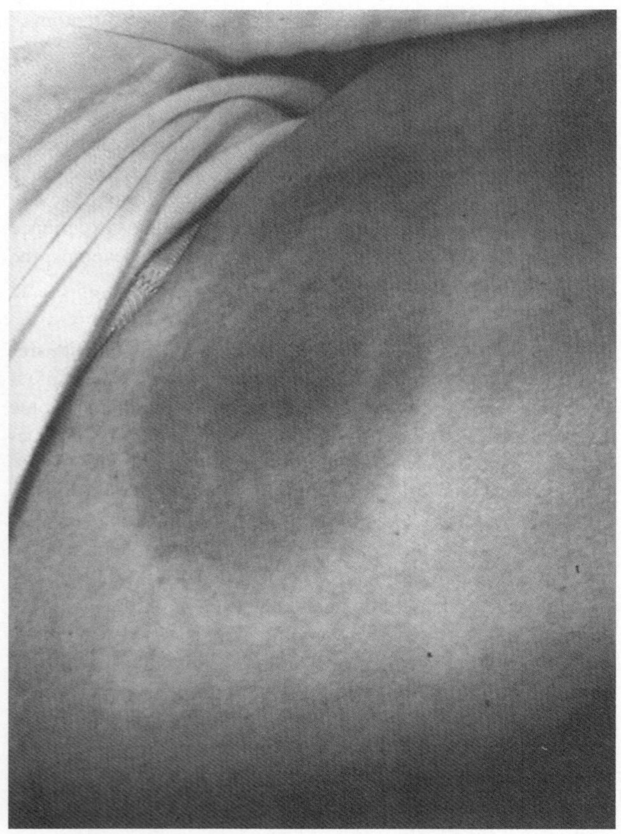

FIGURE 10.5–6

Erythema migrans ("bull's-eye" rash) on the thigh. (From Barbour R. Lyme disease. In: Hoeprich PD, Jordan MC, Ronald AR, eds. *Infectious Diseases: A Treatise of Infectious Processes*. Philadelphia: JB Lippincott; 1994:1329, with permission.)

No clear-cut diagnostic test is available. About 50 percent of patients become seropositive to *B. burgdorferi*. Prophylaxis vaccine is not always effective and is controversial. Treatment consists of a 14- to 21-day course of doxycycline (Vibramycin), which results in a 90 percent cure rate. Specific psychotropic drugs can be targeted to treat the psychiatric sign or symptom (e.g., diazepam [Valium] for anxiety). Left untreated, about 60 percent of persons develop a chronic condition. Such patients may be given an erroneous diagnosis of a primary depression rather than one secondary to the medical condition. Support groups for patients with chronic Lyme disease are important. Group members provide each other with emotional support that helps improve their quality of life.

Prion Disease. Prion disease is a group of related disorders caused by a transmissible infectious protein known as a *prion*. Included in this group are Creutzfeldt-Jakob disease (CJD), Gerstmann-Straussler-Scheinker disorder (GSS), fatal familial insomnia (FFI), and kuru. A variant of CJD (vCJD), also called "mad cow disease," appeared in 1995 in the United Kingdom and is attributed to the transmission of bovine spongiform encephalopathy (BSE) from cattle to humans. Collectively, these disorders are also known as *subacute spongiform encephalopathy* because of shared neuropathological changes that consist of (1) spongiform vacuolization, (2) neuronal loss, and (3) astrocyte proliferation in the cerebral cortex. Amyloid plaques may or may not be present.

ETIOLOGY. Prions are transmissible agents, but differ from viruses in that they lack nucleic acid. Prions are mutated proteins generated from the human prion protein gene (PrP), which is located on the short arm of chromosome 20. No direct link exists between prion disease and Alzheimer's disease, which has been traced to chromosome 21.

The PrP mutates into a disease-related isoform PrP-Super-C (PrP^{Sc}) that can replicate and is infectious. The neuropathological changes that occur in prion disease are presumed to be caused by direct neurotoxic effects of PrP^{Sc}.

The specific prion disease that develops depends on the mutation of PrP that occurs. Mutations at PrP 178N/129V cause CJD; mutations at 178N/129M cause FFI; and mutations at 102L/129M cause GSS and kuru. Other mutations of PrP have been described, and research continues in this important area of genomic identification. Some mutations are both fully penetrant and autosomal dominant and account for inherited forms of prion disease. For example, both GSS and FFI are inherited disorders, and about 10 percent of cases of CJD are also inherited. Prenatal testing for the abnormal PrP gene is available; whether or not such testing should be routinely done is open to question at this time.

CREUTZFELDT-JAKOB DISEASE. First described in 1920, CJD is an invariably fatal, rapidly progressive disorder that occurs mainly in middle-aged or older adults. It manifests initially with fatigue, flu-like symptoms, and cognitive impairment. As the disease progresses, focal neurological findings such as aphasia and apraxia occur. Psychiatric manifestations are protean and include emotional lability, anxiety, euphoria, depression, delusions, hallucinations, or marked personality changes. The disease progresses over months, leading to dementia, akinetic mutism, coma, and death.

The rates of CJD range from 1 to 2 cases per 1 million persons a year, worldwide. The infectious agent self-replicates and can be transmitted to humans by inoculation with infected tissue and sometimes by ingestion of contaminated food. Iatrogenic transmission has been reported via transplantation of contaminated cornea or dura mater or to children via contaminated supplies of human growth hormone derived from infected persons. Neurosurgical transmission has also been reported. Household contacts are not at greater risk for developing the disease than the general population, unless there is direct inoculation.

Diagnosis requires pathological examination of the cortex, which reveals the classic triad of spongiform vacuolation, loss of neurons, and astrocyte cell proliferation. The cortex and basal ganglia are most affected. An immunoassay test for CJD in the CSF shows promise in supporting the diagnosis; however, this needs to be tested more extensively. Although not specific for CJD, EEG abnormalities are present in nearly all patients, consisting of a slow and irregular background rhythm with periodic complex discharges. Computed tomography (CT) and MRI studies may reveal cortical atrophy later in the course of disease. Single photon emission computed tomography (SPECT) and positron emission tomography (PET) reveal heterogeneously decreased uptake throughout the cortex.

No known treatment exists for Creutzfeldt-Jakob disease. Death usually occurs within 6 months after diagnosis.

VARIANT CJD. In 1995 a variant of CJD (vCJD) appeared in the United Kingdom. The patients affected all died; they were young (under age 40 years), and none had risk factors of CJD. At autopsy, prion disease was found. The disease was attributed to the transmission in the United Kingdom of BSE between cattle and from cattle to humans in the 1980s. BSE appears to have originated from sheep scrapie-contaminated feed given to cattle. Scrapie is a spongiform encephalopathy found in sheep and goats that has not been shown to cause human disease; however, it is transmissible to other animal species.

The mean age of onset is 29 years and about 150 people worldwide had been infected as of 2006. Clinicians must be alert to the diagnosis in young people with behavioral and psychiatric abnormalities in association with cerebellar signs such as ataxia or myoclonus. The psychiatric presentation of vCJD is not specific. Most patients have reported depression, withdrawal, anxiety, and sleep disturbance. Paranoid delusions have occurred. Neuropathological changes are similar to those in vCJD, with the addition of amyloid plaques.

Epidemiological data are still being gathered. The incubation period for vCJD and the amount of infected meat product required to cause infection are unknown. One patient was reported to have been a vegetarian for 5 years before his disease was diagnosed. vCJD can be diagnosed antemortem by examining the tonsils with Western blot immunostains to detect PrP^{Sc} in lymphoid tissue. Diagnosis relies on the development of progressive neurodegenerative features in persons who have ingested contaminated meat or brains. No cure exists, and death usually occurs within 2 to 3 years after diagnosis. Prevention is dependent on careful monitoring of cattle for disease and feeding them grain instead of meat by-products.

KURU. Kuru is an epidemic prion disease found in New Guinea that is caused by cannibalistic funeral rituals in which the brains of the deceased are eaten. Women are more affected by the disorder than men, presumably because they participate in the ceremony to a greater extent. Death usually occurs within 2 years after symptoms develop. Neuropsychiatric signs and symptoms consist of ataxia, chorea, strabismus, delirium, and dementia. Pathological changes are similar to those with other prion disease: neuronal loss, spongiform lesions, and astrocytic proliferation. The cerebellum is most affected. Iatrogenic transmission of kuru has occurred when cadaveric material such as dura mater and cornea was transplanted into normal recipients. Since the cessation of cannibalism in New Guinea, the incidence of the disease has decreased drastically.

GERSTMANN-STRAUSSLER-SCHEINKER DISEASE. First described in 1928, GSS is a neurodegenerative syndrome characterized by ataxia, chorea, and cognitive decline leading to dementia. It is caused by a mutation in the PrP gene that is fully penetrant and autosomal dominant; thus the disease is inherited, and affected families have been identified over several generations. Genetic testing can confirm the presence of the abnormal genes before onset. Pathological changes characteristic of prion disease are present: spongiform lesions, neuronal loss, and astrocyte proliferation. Amyloid plaques have been found in the cerebellum. Onset of the disease occurs between 30 and 40 years of age. The disease is fatal within 5 years of onset.

FATAL FAMILIAL INSOMNIA. FFI is an inherited prion disease that primarily affects the thalamus. A syndrome of insomnia and autonomic nervous system dysfunction consisting of fever, sweating, labile blood pressure, and tachycardia occurs that is debilitating. Onset is in middle adulthood, and death usually occurs in 1 year. No treatment currently exists.

FUTURE DIRECTIONS. Determining how prions mutate to produce disease phenotypes and determining how they are transmitted between different mammalian species are major areas of research. Public health measures to prevent transmission of animal disease to humans are ongoing and must be relentless, especially because these disorders are invariably fatal within a few years of onset. Developing genetic interventions that prevent or repair damage to the normal prion gene offers the best hope of cure. Psychiatrists are faced with having to manage cases of persons who actually have the disease and those with hypochondriacal fears of having contracted the disease. In some patients, such fears can reach delusional proportions. Treatment is symptomatic and involves anxiolytics, antidepressants, and psychostimulants, depending on symptoms. Supportive psychotherapy may be of use in early stages to help patients and family cope with the illness.

Preventing unintentional human-to-human or animal-to-human transmission of prions remains the best way to limit the scope of these diseases. Sporadic cases of CJD will still appear, however, because of the rare spontaneous mutation of the normal prion protein into the abnormal form. At present, little exists to offer patients with prion disease other than supportive treatment and emotional support.

Immune Disorders

The major immune disorder in contemporary society is AIDS, but other immune disorders can also present diagnostic and treatment challenges to mental health clinicians.

Systemic Lupus Erythematosus. Systemic lupus erythematosus (SLE) is an autoimmune disease that involves inflammation of multiple organ systems. The officially accepted diagnosis of SLE requires a patient to have 4 of 11 criteria that have been defined by the American Rheumatism Association. Between 5 and 50 percent of patients with SLE have mental symptoms at the initial presentation, and approximately 50 percent eventually show neuropsychiatric manifestations. The major symptoms are depression, insomnia, emotional lability, nervousness, and confusion. Treatment with steroids commonly induces further psychiatric complications, including mania and psychosis.

Endocrine Disorders

Thyroid Disorders. Hyperthyroidism is characterized by confusion, anxiety, and an agitated, depressive syndrome. Patients may also complain of being easily fatigued and of feeling generally weak. Insomnia, weight loss despite increased appetite, tremulousness, palpitations, and increased perspiration are also common symptoms. Serious psychiatric symptoms include impairments in memory, orientation, and judgment; manic excitement; delusions; and hallucinations.

In 1949, Irvin Asher named hypothyroidism "myxedema madness." In its most severe form, hypothyroidism is characterized by paranoia, depression, hypomania, and hallucinations. Slowed thinking and delirium can also be symptoms. The physical symptoms include weight gain, a deep voice, thin and dry hair, loss of the lateral eyebrow, facial puffiness, cold intolerance, and impaired hearing. Approximately 10 percent of all patients have residual neuropsychiatric symptoms after hormone replacement therapy.

Parathyroid Disorders. Dysfunction of the parathyroid gland results in the abnormal regulation of calcium metabolism. Excessive secretion of parathyroid hormone causes hypercalcemia, which can result in delirium, personality changes, and apathy in 50 to 60 percent of patients and cognitive impairments in approximately 25 percent of patients. Neuromuscular excitability, which depends on proper calcium ion concentration, is reduced, and muscle weakness may appear.

Hypocalcemia can occur with hypoparathyroid disorders and can result in neuropsychiatric symptoms of delirium and personality changes. If the calcium level decreases gradually, clinicians may see the psychiatric symptoms without the characteristic tetany of hypocalcemia. Other symptoms of hypocalcemia are cataract formation, seizures, extrapyramidal symptoms, and increased intracranial pressure.

Adrenal Disorders. Adrenal disorders disturb the normal secretion of hormones from the adrenal cortex and produce significant neurological and psychological changes. Patients with chronic adrenocortical insufficiency (Addison's disease), which is most frequently the result of adrenocortical atrophy or granulomatous invasion caused by tuberculous or fungal infection, exhibit mild mental symptoms, such as apathy, easy fatigability, irritability, and depression. Occasionally, confusion or psychotic reactions develop. Cortisone or one of its synthetic derivatives is effective in correcting such abnormalities.

Excessive quantities of cortisol produced endogenously by an adrenocortical tumor or hyperplasia (Cushing's syndrome) lead to a secondary mood disorder, a syndrome of agitated depression, and often suicide. Decreased concentration and memory deficits may also be present. Psychotic reactions, with schizophrenia-like symptoms, are seen in a few patients. The administration of high doses of exogenous corticosteroids typically leads to a secondary mood disorder similar to mania. Severe depression can follow the termination of steroid therapy.

Pituitary Disorders. Patients with total pituitary failure can exhibit psychiatric symptoms, particularly postpartum women who have hemorrhaged into the pituitary, a condition known as *Sheehan's syndrome*. Patients have a combination of symptoms, especially of thyroid and adrenal disorders, and can show virtually any psychiatric symptom.

Metabolic Disorders

A common cause of organic brain dysfunction, metabolic encephalopathy can produce alterations in mental processes, behavior, and neurological functions. The diagnosis should be considered whenever recent and rapid changes in behavior, thinking, and consciousness have occurred. The earliest signals are likely to be impairment of memory, particularly recent memory, and impairment of orientation. Some patients become agitated, anxious, and hyperactive; others become quiet, withdrawn, and inactive. As metabolic encephalopathies progress, confusion or delirium gives way to decreased responsiveness, stupor, and, eventually, death.

Hepatic Encephalopathy. Severe hepatic failure can result in hepatic encephalopathy, characterized by asterixis, hyperventilation, EEG abnormalities, and alterations in consciousness. The alterations in consciousness can range from apathy to drowsiness to coma. Associated psychiatric symptoms are changes in memory, general intellectual skills, and personality.

Uremic Encephalopathy. Renal failure is associated with alterations in memory, orientation, and consciousness. Restlessness, crawling sensations on the limbs, muscle twitching, and persistent hiccups are associated symptoms. In young people with brief episodes of uremia, the neuropsychiatric symptoms tend to be reversible; in elderly people with long episodes of uremia, the neuropsychiatric symptoms can be irreversible.

Hypoglycemic Encephalopathy. Hypoglycemic encephalopathy can be caused either by excessive endogenous production of insulin or by excessive exogenous insulin administration. The premonitory symptoms, which do not occur in every patient, include nausea, sweating, tachycardia, and feelings of hunger, apprehension, and restlessness. As the disorder progresses, disorientation, confusion, and hallucinations, as well as other neurological and medical symptoms, can develop. Stupor and coma can occur, and a residual and persistent dementia can sometimes be a serious neuropsychiatric sequela of the disorder.

Diabetic Ketoacidosis. Diabetic ketoacidosis begins with feelings of weakness, easy fatigability, and listlessness and increasing polyuria and polydipsia. Headache and sometimes nausea and vomiting appear. Patients with diabetes mellitus have an increased likelihood of chronic dementia with general arteriosclerosis.

Acute Intermittent Porphyria. The porphyrias are disorders of heme biosynthesis that result in excessive accumulation of porphyrins.

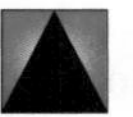

Table 10.5–18
ICD-10 Diagnostic Criteria for Personality and Behavioral Disorders Due to Brain Disease, Damage, and Dysfunction

G1. There must be objective evidence (from physical and neurological examination and laboratory tests) and/or history of cerebral disease, damage, or dysfunction.

G2. There is no clouding of consciousness or significant memory deficit.

G3. There is insufficient evidence for an alternative causation of the personality or behavior disorder that would justify its placement in disorders of adult personality and behavior category.

Organic personality disorder

A. The general criteria for personality and behavioral disorders due to brain disease, damage, and dysfunction must be met.

B. At least three of the following features must be present over a period of 6 months or more:
  (1) consistently reduced ability to persevere with goal-directed activities, especially those involving relatively long periods and postponed gratification;
  (2) one or more of the following emotional changes:
    (a) emotional lability (uncontrolled, unstable, and fluctuating expression of emotions):
    (b) euphoria and shallow, inappropriate jocularity, unwarranted by the circumstances;
    (c) irritability and/or outbursts of anger and aggression;
    (d) apathy;
  (3) disinhibited expression of needs or impulses without consideration of consequences or of social conventions (the individual may engage in dissocial acts such as stealing, inappropriate sexual advances, or voracious eating, or exhibit extreme disregard for personal hygiene);
  (4) cognitive disturbances, typically in the form of:
    (a) excessive suspiciousness and paranoid ideas;
    (b) excessive preoccupation with a single theme such as religion, or rigid categorization of other people's behavior in terms of "right" and "wrong";
  (5) marked alteration of the rate and flow of language production, with features such as circumstantiality, overinclusiveness, viscosity, and hypergraphia;
  (6) altered sexual behavior (hyposexuality or change in sexual preference).

Specification of features for possible subtypes

Option 1. A marked predominance of the symptoms in criteria (1) and (2) (d) is thought to define a pseudoretarded or apathetic type; a predominance of (1), (2) (c), and (3) is considered a pseudopsychopathic type; and a combination of (4), (5), and (6) is regarded as characteristic of the limbic epilepsy personality syndrome. None of these entities has yet been sufficiently validated to warrant a separate description.

Option 2. If desired, the following types may be specified: labile type, disinhibited type, aggressive type, apathetic type, paranoid type, mixed type, and other.

Postencephalitic syndrome

A. The general criteria for personality and behavioral disorders due to brain disease, damage, and dysfunction must be met.

B. At least one of the following residual neurological dysfunctions must be present:
  (1) paralysis;
  (2) deafness;
  (3) aphasia;
  (4) constructional apraxia;
  (5) acalculia.

C. The syndrome is reversible, and its duration rarely exceeds 24 months.

Comments

Criterion C constitutes the main difference between this disorder and organic personality disorder.

Residual symptoms and behavioral change following either viral or bacterial encephalitis are nonspecific and do not provide a sufficient basis for a clinical diagnosis. They may include: general malaise, apathy, or irritability; some lowering of cognitive functioning (learning difficulties); disturbances in the sleep–wake pattern; or altered sexual behavior.

Postconcussional syndrome

Note: The nosological status of this syndrome is uncertain, and criterion G1 of the introduction to this rubric is not always ascertainable. However, for those undertaking research into this condition, the following criteria are recommended:

A. The general criteria of personality and behavioral disorders due to brain disease, damage, and dysfunction must be met.

B. There must be a history of head trauma with loss of consciousness, preceding the onset of symptoms by a period of up to 4 weeks. (Objective EEG, brain imaging, or oculonystagmographic evidence for brain damage may be lacking.)

C. At least three of the following features must be present:
  (1) complaints of unpleasant sensations and pains, such as headache, dizziness (usually lacking the features of true vertigo), general malaise, and excessive fatigue, or noise intolerance;
  (2) emotional changes, such as irritability, emotional lability (both easily provoked or exacerbated by emotional excitement or stress), or some degree of depression and/or anxiety:
  (3) subjective complaints of difficulty in concentration and in performing mental tasks, and of memory problems (without clear objective evidence, e.g., psychological tests, of marked impairment):
  (4) insomnia;
  (5) reduced tolerance to alcohol;
  (6) preoccupation with the above symptoms and fear of permanent brain damage, to the extent of hypochondriacal, overvalued ideas and adoption of a sick role.

Other organic personality and behavioral disorders due to brain disease, damage, and dysfunction

Brain disease, damage, or dysfunction may produce a variety of cognitive, emotional, personality, and behavioral disorders, some of which may not be classifiable under organic personality disorder, postencephalitic syndrome, postconcussional syndrome. However, since the nosological status of the tentative syndromes in this area is uncertain, they should be coded as "other." A fifth character may be added, if necessary, to identify presumptive individual entities.

Unspecified organic personality and behavioral disorder due to brain disease, damage, and dysfunction

ICD, International Classification of Diseases.
(From World Health Organization. *The ICD-10 Classification of Mental and Behavioural Disorders: Diagnostic Criteria for Research*, Copyright, World Health Organization, Geneva, 1993, with permission.)

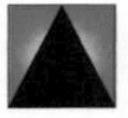

Table 10.5–19
ICD-10 Diagnostic Criteria for Other Mental Disorders Due to Brain Damage and Dysfunction and Due to Physical Disease

G1. There is objective evidence (from physical and neurological examination and laboratory tests) and/or history of cerebral disease, damage, or dysfuction, or of systemic physical disorder known to cause cerebral dysfunction, including hormonal disturbances (other than alcohol- or other psychoactive substance-related) and nonpsychoactive drug effects.

G2. There is a presumed relationship between the development (or marked exacerbation) of the underlying disease, damage, or dysfunction, and the mental disorder, the symptoms of which may have immedite onset or may be delayed.

G3. There is recovery from or significant improvement in the mental disorder following removal or improvement of the underlying presumed cause.

G4. There is insufficient evidence for an alternative causation of the mental disorder, e.g., a strong family history of a clinically similar or related disorder.

If criteria G1, G2, and G4 are met, a provisional diagnosis is justified; if, in addition, there is evidence of G3, the diagnosis can be regarded as certain.

Organic hallucinosis

A. The general criteria for other mental disorders due to brain damage and dysfunction and to physical disease must be met.

B. The clinical picture is dominated by persistent or recurrent hallucinations (usually visual or auditory).

C. Hallucinations occur in clear consciousness.

Comments

Delusional elaboration of the hallucinations, as well as full or partial insight, may or may not be present: these features are not essential for the diagnosis.

Organic catatonic disorder

A. The general criteria for other mental disorders due to brain damage and dysfunction and to physical diseases must be met.

B. One of the following must be present:
(1) stupor, i.e., profound diminution or absence of voluntary movements and speech, and of normal responsiveness to light, noise, and touch, but with normal muscle tone, static posture, and breathing maintained (and often limited coordinated eye movements);
(2) negativism (positive resistance to passive movement of limbs or body or rigid posturing).

C. There is catatonic excitement (gross hypermotility of a chaotic quality, with or without a tendency to assaultiveness).

D. There is rapid and unpredictable alternation of stupor and excitement.

Comments

Confidence in the diagnosis is increased if additional catatonic phenomena are present, e.g., stereotypies, waxy flexibility, and impulsive acts. Care should be taken to exclude delirium; however, it is not known whether an organic catatonic state always occurs in clear consciousness, or whether it represents an atypical manifestation of a delirium in which criteria A, B, and D are only marginally met, whereas criterion C is prominent.

Organic delusional (schizophrenialike) disorder

A. The general criteria for other mental disorders due to brain damage and dysfunction and to physical disease must be met.

B. The clinical picture is dominated by delusions (of persecution, bodily change, disease, death, jealousy), which may exhibit a varying degree of systematization.

C. Consciousness is clear and memory is intact.

Comments

Further features that complete the clinical picture but that are not invariably present include: hallucinations (in any modality); schizophrenic-type thought disorder, isolated catatonic phenomena such as stereotypies, negativism, or impulsive acts. The clinical picture may meet the symptomatic criteria for schizophrenia, persistent delusional disorder, or acute and transient psychotic disorders. However, if the state also meets the general criteria for a presumptive organic etiology laid down in the introduction to other mental disorders due to brain damage and dysfunction and to physical disease, it should be classified here. Marginal or nonspecific findings such as enlarged cerebral ventricles or "soft" neurological signs do not qualify as evidence for criterion G1 of other mental disorders due to brain damage and dysfunction and to physical disease.

Organic mood (affective) disorder

A. The general criteria for other medical disorders due to brain damage and dysfunction and to physical disease must be met.

B. The condition must meet the criteria for one of the affective disorders.

The diagnosis of the affective disorder may be specified by using a fifth character:

Organic manic disorder

Organic bipolar disorder

Organic depressive disorder

Organic mixed affective disorder

Organic anxiety disorder

A. The general criteria for other medical disorders due to brain damage and dysfunction and to physical disease must be met.

B. The condition must meet the criteria for either panic disorder or generalized anxiety disorder.

Organic dissociative disorder

A. The general criteria for other mental disorders due to brain damage and dysfunction and to physical disease must be met.

B. The condition must meet the criteria for one of the dissociative (conversion) disorders categories.

Organic emotionally labile (asthenic) disorder

A. The general criteria for other mental disorders due to brain damage and dysfunction and to physical disease must be met.

B. The clinical picture is dominated by emotional lability (uncontrolled, unstable, and fluctuating expression of emotions).

C. There is a variety of unpleasant physical sensations such as dizziness or pains and aches.

Comments

Fatigability and listlessness (asthenia) are often present but are not essential for the diagnosis.

Mild cognitive disorder

Note: The status of this construct is being examined. Specific research criteria must be viewed as tentative. One of the principal reasons for its inclusion is to obtain further evidence allowing its differentiation from disorders such as dementia organic amnestic syndrome, delirium, and several disorders in personality and behavioral disorders due to brain disease, damage, and dysfunction.

A. The general criteria for other mental disorders due to brain damage and dysfunction and to physical disease must be met.

(continued)

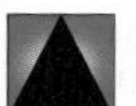

Table 10.5–19
(Continued)

	Comments
B. There is a disorder in cognitive function for most of the time over a period of at least 2 weeks as reported by the individual or a reliable informant. The disorder is exemplified by difficulties in any of the following areas: (1) memory (particularly recall) or new learning; (2) attention or concentration; (3) thinking (e.g., slowing in problem solving or abstraction); (4) language (e.g., comprehension, word finding); (5) visual-spatial functioning. C. There is an abnormality or decline in performance in quantified cognitive assessments (e.g., neuropsychological tests or mental status examination). D. None of the difficulties listed in criterion B(1)–(5) is such that a diagnosis made of dementia, organic amnesic syndrome, delirium, postencephalitic syndrome, postconcussional syndrome, or other persisting cognitive impairment due to psychoactive substance use.	If criterion G1 for other mental disorders due to brain damage and dysfunction and to physical disease is fulfilled by the presence of central nervous system dysfunction, it is usually presumed that this is the cause of the mild cognitive disorder. If criterion G1 is fulfilled by the presence of a systemic physical disorder, it is often unjustified to assume that there is a direct causative relationship. Nevertheless, it may be useful in such instances to record the presence of the systemic physical disorder as "associated," without implying a necessary causation. An additional fifth character may be used for this: **Not associated with a systemic physical disorder** **Associated with a systemic physical disorder** The systemic physical disorder should be recorded separately by its appropriate ICD-10 code. **Other specified mental disorders due to brain damage and dysfunction and to physical disease** Examples of this category are transient or mild abnormal mood states occurring during treatment with steroids or antidepressants which do not meet the criteria for organic mood disorder. **Unspecified mental disorder due to brain damage and dysfunction and to physical disease**

ICD, International Classification of Diseases.
(From World Health Organization. *The ICD-10 Classification of Mental and Behavioural Disorders: Diagnostic Criteria for Research.* Copyright, World Health Organization, Geneva, 1993, with permission.)

The triad of symptoms is acute, colicky abdominal pain, motor polyneuropathy, and psychosis. Acute intermittent porphyria is an autosomal dominant disorder that affects more women than men and has its onset between ages 20 and 50. The psychiatric symptoms include anxiety, insomnia, lability of mood, depression, and psychosis. Some studies have found that between 0.2 and 0.5 percent of chronic psychiatric patients may have undiagnosed porphyrias. Barbiturates precipitate or aggravate the attacks of acute porphyria, and the use of barbiturates for any reason is absolutely contraindicated in a person with acute intermittent porphyria and in anyone who has a relative with the disease.

Nutritional Disorders

Niacin Deficiency. Dietary insufficiency of niacin (nicotinic acid) and its precursor tryptophan is associated with pellagra, a globally occurring nutritional deficiency disease seen in association with alcohol abuse, vegetarian diets, and extreme poverty and starvation. The neuropsychiatric symptoms of pellagra include apathy, irritability, insomnia, depression, and delirium; the medical symptoms include dermatitis, peripheral neuropathies, and diarrhea. The course of pellagra has traditionally been described as "five Ds": dermatitis, diarrhea, delirium, dementia, and death. The response to treatment with nicotinic acid is rapid, but dementia from prolonged illness may improve only slowly and incompletely.

Thiamine Deficiency. Thiamine (vitamin B_1) deficiency leads to beriberi, characterized chiefly by cardiovascular and neurological changes, and to Wernicke-Korsakoff syndrome, which is most often associated with chronic alcohol abuse. Beriberi occurs primarily in Asia and in areas of famine and poverty. The psychiatric symptoms include apathy, depression, irritability, nervousness, and poor concentration; severe memory disorders can develop with prolonged deficiencies.

Cobalamin Deficiency. Deficiencies in cobalamin (vitamin B_{12}) arise because of the failure of the gastric mucosal cells to secrete a specific substance, intrinsic factor, required for the normal absorption of vitamin B_{12} in the ileum. The deficiency state is characterized by the development of a chronic macrocytic megaloblastic anemia (pernicious anemia) and by neurological manifestations resulting from degenerative changes in the peripheral nerves, the spinal cord, and the brain. Neurological changes are seen in approximately 80 percent of all patients. These changes are commonly associated with megaloblastic anemia, but they occasionally precede the onset of hematological abnormalities.

Mental changes, such as apathy, depression, irritability, and moodiness, are common. In a few patients, encephalopathy and its associated delirium, delusions, hallucinations, dementia, and, sometimes, paranoid features are prominent and are sometimes called *megaloblastic madness*. The neurological manifestations of vitamin B_{12} deficiency can be rapidly and completely arrested by early and continued administration of parenteral vitamin therapy.

Toxins

Environmental toxins are becoming an increasingly serious threat to physical and mental health in contemporary society.

Mercury. Mercury poisoning can be caused by either inorganic or organic mercury. Inorganic mercury poisoning results in the "mad hatter" syndrome (previously seen in workers in the hat industry who softened felt by putting it in their mouths), with depression, irritability, and psychosis. Associated neurological symptoms are headache, tremor, and weakness. Organic mercury poisoning can be caused by contaminated fish or grain and can result in depression, irritability, and cognitive impairment. Associated symptoms are sensory neuropathies, cerebellar ataxia, dysarthria, paresthesias, and visual field defects. Mercury poisoning in pregnant women causes abnormal fetal development. No specific therapy is available, although chelation therapy with dimercaprol has been used in acute poisoning.

Lead. Lead poisoning occurs when the amount of lead ingested exceeds the body's ability to eliminate it. It takes several months for toxic symptoms to appear.

The signs and symptoms of lead poisoning depend on the level of lead in the blood. When lead reaches levels above 200 milligrams per liter, symptoms of severe lead encephalopathy occur, with dizziness, clumsiness, ataxia, irritability, restlessness, headache, and insomnia. Later, an excited delirium occurs, with associated vomiting and visual disturbances, and progresses to convulsions, lethargy, and coma.

Treatment of lead encephalopathy should be instituted as rapidly as possible, even without laboratory confirmation, because of the high mortality. The treatment of choice to facilitate lead excretion is intravenous administration of calcium disodium edetate (calcium disodium versenate) daily for 5 days.

Manganese. Early manganese poisoning (sometimes called *manganese madness*) causes symptoms of headache, irritability, joint pains, and somnolence. An eventual picture appears of emotional lability, pathological laughter, nightmares, hallucinations, and compulsive and impulsive acts associated with periods of confusion and aggressiveness. Lesions involving the basal ganglia and pyramidal system result in gait impairment, rigidity, monotonous or whispering speech, tremors of the extremities and tongue, masked facies (manganese mask), micrographia, dystonia, dysarthria, and loss of equilibrium. The psychological effects tend to clear 3 or 4 months after the patient's removal from the site of exposure, but neurological symptoms tend to remain stationary or to progress. No specific treatment exists for manganese poisoning, other than removal from the source of poisoning. The disorder is found in persons working in refining ore, brick workers, and those making steel casings.

Arsenic. Chronic arsenic poisoning most commonly results from prolonged exposure to herbicides containing arsenic or from drinking water contaminated with arsenic. Arsenic is also used in the manufacture of silicon-based computer chips. Early signs of toxicity are skin pigmentation, gastrointestinal complaints, renal and hepatic dysfunction, hair loss, and a characteristic garlic odor to the breath. Encephalopathy eventually occurs, with generalized sensory and motor loss. Chelation therapy with dimercaprol has been used successfully to treat arsenic poisoning.

ICD-10

In the 10th revision of *International Statistical Classification of Disease and Related Health Problems* (ICD-10), mental disorders related to medical conditions are covered by two categories: personality and behavioral disorders due to brain disease, damage, and dysfunction (Table 10.5–18) and other mental disorders due to brain damage and dysfunction and to physical disease (Table 10.5–19).

References

Chapman DP, Perry GS, Strine TW. The vital link between chronic disease and depressive disorders. *Prev Chronic Dis.* 2005;2:A14.

Drooker MA. Other cognitive disorders and mental disorders due to a general medical condition. In: Sadock BJ, Sadock VA, eds. *Kaplan & Sadock's Comprehensive Textbook of Psychiatry.* 8th ed. Vol. 1. Baltimore: Lippincott Williams & Wilkins; 2005:1106.

Greenloe BA, Ferrell RB, Kauffman CI, McAllister TW. Complex partial seizures and depression. *Curr Psychiatry Rep.* 2003;5:410.

Ketterer MW, Wulsin L, Cao JJ, Schairer J, Hakim A, Hudson M, Keteyian SJ, Khanal S, Clark V, Weaver WD. "Major" depressive disorder, coronary heart disease, and the DSM–IV threshold problem. *Psychosomatics.* 2006;47: 50–55

Kilbourne AM, Cornelius JR, Han X, Haas GL, Salloum I, Conigliaro J, Pincus HA. General-medical conditions in older patients with serious mental illness. *Am J Geriatr Psychiatry.* 2005;13:250–254.

Kilbourne AM, Cornelius JR, Han X, Pincus HA, Shad M, Salloum I, Conigliaro J, Haas GL. Burden of general medical conditions among individuals with bipolar disorder. *BipolarDisorder.* 2004:6:368–373.

Lin MY, Gutierrez PR, Stone KL, Yaffe K, Ensrud KE, Fink HA, Sarkisian CA, Coleman AL, Mangione CM. *J Am Geriatr Soc.* 2004;52:1996–2002.

Nilsson FM. Psychiatric and cognitive disorders in Parkinson's disease. *Curr Opin Psychiatry.* 2004;17:197–202.

Poggi G, Liscio M, Galbiati S, Adduci A, Massimino M, Gandola L, Spreafico F, Clerici CA, Fossati-Bellani F, Sommovigo M, Castelli E. *Psycho-Oncology.* 2005;14:386–395.

Raymont V, Bingley W, Buchanan A, David AS, Hayward P, Wessely S, Hotopf M. Prevalence of mental incapacity in medical inpatients and associated risk factors: Cross-sectional study. *Lancet.* 2004;364:1421–1427.

Riello R, Geoldi C, Zanetti O, Vergani C, Frisoni GB. Differential associations of head and body symptoms with depression and physical comorbidity in patients with cognitive impairment. *Int J Geriatr Psychiatry.* 2004;19: 209–215.

Soares CN, Poitras JR, Prouty J. Effect of reproductive hormones and selective estrogen receptor modulators on mood during menopause. *Drugs Aging.* 2003;20:85.

Sokal J, Messias E, Dickerson FB, Kreyenbuhl J, Brown CH, Goldberg RW, Dixon LB. Comorbidity of medical illnesses among adults with serious mental illness who are receiving community psychiatric services. *J Nerv Ment Dis.* 2004;192(6):421–427.

Strassnig M, Stowell KR, First MB, Pincus HA. General medical and psychiatric perspectives on somatoform disorders: Separated by an uncommon language. *Curr Opin Psychiatry.* 2006;19(2):194–200.

Taylor WD, Steffens DC, MacFall JR, McQuoid DR, Payne ME, Provenzale JM, Krishnan KR. White matter hyperdensity progression and late-life depression outcomes. *Arch Gen Psychiatry.* 2003;60:1090.

11 Neuropsychiatric Aspects of HIV Infection and AIDS

The human immunodeficiency virus (HIV) epidemic was identified in the 1980s and neurologists described several HIV-related central nervous system (CNS) syndromes within the first several years of the epidemic. Mental health professionals from nursing, social work, psychology, and psychiatry followed the plight of patients of the epidemic and helped to mobilize interest and galvanize a response. Initially, much of the work focused on grief and loss issues, as well as supportive psychotherapy, but quickly broadened to recognize a number of specific psychiatric conditions, including acquired immune deficiency syndrome (AIDS) dementia, the associated AIDS mania, increased rates of major depression, and psychiatric consequences of CNS injuries.

The first case of AIDS was reported in 1981. Analysis of specimens retained from persons who died before 1981, however, has shown that HIV infections were present as early as 1959. This suggests that in the 1960s and 1970s, HIV-related disorders and AIDS were increasingly common but unrecognized, particularly in Africa and North America. According to the Centers for Disease Control and Prevention (CDC), in 2005 almost 950,000 persons in Americas were diagnosed with full-blown AIDS since 1981. There were about 43,000 new infections, in 2004 with about 15,000 deaths. The CDC estimates that approximately 460,000 person are living with AIDS in the United States. The World Health Organization (WHO) estimates that, worldwide, 2.5 million adults and 1 million children have AIDS and about 30 million persons are infected with HIV. The CDC statistics on epidemiological data on AIDS in the United States is listed in Table 11–1.

OVERVIEW OF HIV TRANSMISSION

Human immunodeficiency virus is a retrovirus related to the human T-cell leukemia viruses (HTLV) and to retroviruses that infect animals, including nonhuman primates. At least two types of HIV have been identified, HIV-1 and HIV-2. HIV-1 is the causative agent for most HIV-related diseases; HIV-2, however, seems to be causing an increasing number of infections in Africa. Other subtypes of HIV may exist, which are now classified as HIV-O. HIV is present in blood, semen, cervical and vaginal secretions, and, to a lesser extent, in saliva, tears, breast milk, and the cerebrospinal fluid of those who are infected. HIV is most often transmitted through sexual intercourse or the transfer of contaminated blood from one person to another. Unprotected anal and vaginal sex are the sexual activities most likely to transmit the virus. Oral sex has also been implicated, but rarely. Health providers should be aware of the guidelines for safe sexual practices and should advise their patients to practice safe sex (Table 11–2).

The chance of becoming infected after a single exposure to an HIV-infected person is relatively low: 0.8 to 3.2 percent for unprotected receptive anal intercourse, 0.05 to 0.15 percent with unprotected vaginal sex, 0.32 percent after puncture with an HIV-contaminated needle, and 0.67 percent after using a contaminated needle to inject drugs. The probability of transmission, however, could be higher, depending on the viral load of the contact person (which tends to be higher at the beginning and end of the course of the illness) or other factors, such as sexually transmitted diseases. The presence of sexually transmitted diseases, such as herpes or syphilis, or other lesions that compromise the integrity of skin or mucosa, further increases the risk of transmission. Transmission also occurs through exposure to contaminated needles, thus accounting for the high incidence of HIV infection among drug users. HIV is also transmitted by infusions of whole blood, plasma, and clotting factors, but not immune serum globulin or hepatitis B vaccine.

Although male-to-male transmission has been the most common route of sexual transmission in North America, male-to-female and female-to-male transmissions are increasing, and they represent most transmission worldwide. Some studies have shown that about 50 percent of the regular sex partners of persons with HIV infection become infected themselves, a statistic suggesting that some persons do not yet understand immunity or resistance to HIV infection.

Transmission by contaminated blood most often occurs when those abusing a substance intravenously (IV) share hypodermic needles without proper sterilization techniques. Transmission of HIV through blood transfusions, organ transplantation, and artificial insemination is no longer a problem now that donors are tested for HIV infection. Many hemophilia patients, however, received transfusions of HIV-infected blood products before HIV was identified as the causative agent. The risk of infection of health care workers after a needlestick is rare, about 1 in 300 incidents.

Children can be infected in utero or through breast-feeding when their mothers are infected with HIV. Zidovudine (Retrovir) and protease inhibitors taken by the HIV-infected pregnant woman prevent perinatal transmission in more than 95 percent of cases. Health workers are theoretically at risk because of potential contact with bodily fluids from HIV-infected patients. In practice, however, the incidence of such transmission is very low, and almost all reported cases have been traced to accidental punctures with contaminated hypodermic needles. No evidence has been found that HIV can be contracted through casual contact, such as by sharing a living space or a classroom with a person who is infected, although direct and indirect contact with an infected person's bodily fluids, such as blood and semen, should be avoided (Table 11–3).

After infection with HIV, AIDS is estimated to develop in 8 to 11 years, although this time is gradually increasing because

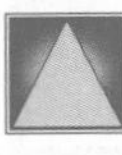

Table 11–1
The Centers for Disease Control and Prevention (CDC) Statistics on Epidemiological Data on Acquired Immunodeficiency Syndrome (AIDS) in the United States

- 35% were white
- 43% were black
- 20% were Hispanic
- 1% was of other race/ethnicity

Of the adults and adolescents with AIDS, 77% were men. Of these men,

- 58% were men who had sex with men (MSM)
- 21% were injection drug users (IDU)
- 11% were exposed through heterosexual contact
- 8% were both MSM and IDU.

Of the 93,566 adult and adolescent women with AIDS,

- 64% were exposed through heterosexual contact
- 34% were exposed through injection drug use

An estimated 3,927 children were living with AIDS at the end of 2004, of whom 97% probably acquired the infection from their mothers.

People with AIDS are surviving longer and are contributing to a steady increase in the number of people living with AIDS. This trend will continue as long as the number of new diagnoses exceeds the number of people dying each year.

of early treatment. Once a person is infected with HIV, the virus primarily targets T4 (helper) lymphocytes, also called CD4+ lymphocytes, to which the virus binds because a glycoprotein (gp120) on the viral surface has a high affinity for the CD4 receptor on T4 lymphocytes. After binding, the virus can inject its RNA into the infected lymphocyte, where the RNA is transcribed into DNA by the action of reverse transcriptase. The resultant DNA can then be incorporated into the host cell's genome and translated and eventually transcribed, once the lymphocyte is stimulated to divide. After viral proteins have been produced by lymphocytes, the various components of the virus assemble, and new mature viruses bud off from the host cell. Although the process of budding may cause lysis of the lymphocyte, other HIV pathophysiological mechanisms can gradually disable a patient's entire complement of T4 lymphocytes.

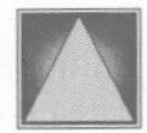

Table 11–2
AIDS Safe-Sex Guidelines

Remember: Any activity that allows for the exchange of body fluids of one person through the mouth, anus, vagina, bloodstream, cuts, or sores of another person is considered unsafe at this time.

Safe-sex practices
- Massage, hugging, body-to-body rubbing
- Dry social kissing
- Masturbation
- Acting out sexual fantasies (that do not include any unsafe-sex practices)
- Using vibrators or other instruments (provided they are not shared)

Low-risk sex practices

These activities are not considered completely safe:
- French (wet) kissing (without mouth sores)
- Mutual masturbation
- Vaginal and anal intercourse while using a condom
- Oral sex, male (fellatio), while using a condom
- Oral sex, female (cunnilingus), while using a barrier
- External contact with semen or urine, provided there are no breaks in the skin

Unsafe-sex practices
- Vaginal or anal intercourse without a condom
- Semen, urine, or feces in the mouth or the vagina
- Unprotected oral sex (fellatio or cunnilingus)
- Blood contact of any kind
- Sharing sex instruments or needles

AIDS, acquired immunodeficiency syndrome.
(From Moffatt B, Spiegel J, Parrish S, Helquist M. *AIDS: A Self-Care Manual.* Santa Monica, CA: IBS Press; 1987:125, with permission.)

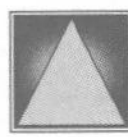

Table 11–3
Centers for Disease Control and Prevention (CDC) Guidelines for the Prevention of HIV Transmission from Infected to Uninfected Persons

Infected persons should be counseled to prevent the further transmission of HIV by:

1. Informing prospective sex partners of their infection with HIV, so they can take appropriate precautions. Abstention from sexual activity with another person is one option that would eliminate any risk of sexually transmitted HIV infection.
2. Protecting a partner during any sexual activity by taking appropriate precautions to prevent that person's coming into contact with the infected person's blood, semen, urine, feces, saliva, cervical secretions, or vaginal secretions. Although the efficacy of using condoms to prevent infections with HIV is still under study, the consistent use of condoms should reduce the transmission of HIV by preventing exposure to semen and infected lymphocytes.
3. Informing previous sex partners and any persons with whom needles were shared of their potential exposure to HIV and encouraging them to seek counseling and testing.
4. For IV drug abusers, enrolling or continuing in programs to eliminate the abuse of IV substances. Needles, other apparatus and drugs must never be shared.
5. Never sharing toothbrushes, razors, or other items that could become contaminated with blood.
6. Refraining from donating blood, plasma, body organs, other tissue, or semen.
7. Avoiding pregnancy until more is known about the risks of transmitting HIV from the mother to the fetus or newborn.
8. Cleaning and disinfecting surfaces on which blood or other body fluids have spilled, in accordance with previous recommendations.
9. Informing physicians, dentists, and other appropriate health professionals of antibody status when seeking medical care, so that the patient can be appropriately evaluated.

HIV, human immunodeficiency virus; IV, intravenous.
(From *MMWR Morb Mortal Wkly Rep.* 1986;35:152, with permission.)

Diagnosis

Serum Testing. Techniques are now widely available to detect the presence of anti-HIV antibodies in human serum. The conventional test uses blood (time to result, 3 to 10 days) and the rapid test uses an oral swab (time to result, 20 minutes). Both tests are 99.9 percent sensitive and specific. Health care workers and their patients must understand that the presence of HIV antibodies indicates infection, not immunity to infection. Those with a positive finding on an HIV test have been exposed to the virus, have the virus within their bodies, have the potential to transmit the virus to another person, and will almost certainly eventually develop AIDS. Those with a negative HIV test result have either

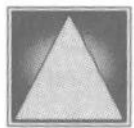

Table 11–4
Possible Indications for Human Immunodeficiency Virus (HIV) Testing

1. Patients who belong to a high-risk group: (1) men who have had sex with another man since 1977; (2) intravenous drug abusers since 1977; (3) hemophiliacs and other patients who have received since 1977 blood or blood product transfusions not screened for HIV; (4) sexual partners of people from any of those groups; (5) sexual partners of people with known HIV exposure—people with cuts, wounds, sores, or needlesticks whose lesions have had direct contact with HIV-infected blood.
2. Patients who request testing. Not all patients admit to the presence of risk factors (e.g., because of shame, fear).
3. Patients with symptoms or acquired immunodeficiency syndrome (AIDS).
4. Women belonging to a high-risk group who are planning pregnancy or who are pregnant.
5. Blood, semen, or organ donors.

(Adapted from Rosse RB, Giese AA, Deutsch S, Morihisa JM. *Laboratory and Diagnostic Testing in Psychiatry*. Washington, DC: American Psychiatric Press; 1989:54, with permission.)

not been exposed to the HIV virus and are not infected or were exposed to the HIV virus but have not yet developed antibodies, a possibility if the exposure occurred less than a year before the testing. Seroconversion most commonly occurs 6 to 12 weeks after infection, although in rare cases seroconversion can take 6 to 12 months.

Counseling. The major issues in counseling persons about HIV serum testing are who should be tested; why a particular person should or should not be tested; what the test results signify; and what the implications are. Although specific groups of persons are at high risk for contracting HIV and should be tested (Table 11–4), any person who wants to be tested should probably be tested. The reasons for requesting a test should be ascertained to detect unspoken concerns and motivations that may merit psychotherapeutic intervention.

Past practices that may have put the testee at risk for HIV infection and safe sexual practices should be discussed (Table 11–5). During posttest counseling (Table 11–6), counselors should explain that a negative test finding implies that safe sexual behavior and the avoidance of shared hypodermic needles are recommended for the person to remain free of HIV infection. A positive test result indicates that the person is infected with HIV and can spread the disease. Those with positive results must receive counseling about safe practices and potential treatment options. They may need additional psychotherapeutic interventions if anxiety or depressive disorders develop after they discover that they are infected. Common issues and concerns are fear of disclosure, relationships with friends and family, employment and financial security, medical condition, and such psychological issues as self-esteem and self-blame. A person may react to a positive HIV test finding with a syndrome similar to posttraumatic stress disorder. Concern about minor physical symptoms, insomnia, and dependence on health care workers commonly arise. Adjustment disorder with anxiety or depressed mood may develop in as many as 25 percent of those informed of a positive HIV test result. Clinical interactions with patients should emphasize the meaning of a positive test result and should encourage reestablishment of emotional and functional stability.

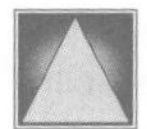

Table 11–5
Pretest HIV Counseling

1. Discuss meaning of a positive result and clarify distortions (e.g., the test detects exposure to the AIDS virus; it is not a test for AIDS).
2. Discuss the meaning of a negative result (e.g., seroconversion requires time, recent high-risk behavior may require follow-up testing).
3. Be available to discuss the patient's fears and concerns (unrealistic fears may require appropriate psychological intervention).
4. Discuss why the test is necessary. (Not all patients will admit to high-risk behaviors.)
5. Explore the patient's potential reactions to a positive result (e.g. "I'll kill myself if I'm positive"). Take appropriate necessary steps to intervene in a potentially catastrophic reaction.
6. Explore past reactions to severe stresses.
7. Discuss the confidentiality issues relevant to the testing situation (e.g., is it an anonymous or nonanonymous setting?). Inform the patient of other possible testing options where the counseling and testing can be done completely anonymously (e.g., where the result is not made a permanent part of a hospital chart). Discuss who has access to the test results.
8. Discuss with the patient how being seropositive can potentially affect social status (e.g., health and life insurance coverage, employment, housing).
9. Explore high-risk behaviors and recommend risk-reducing interventions.
10. Document discussions in chart.
11. Allow the patient time to ask questions.

HIV, human immunodeficiency virus; AIDS, acquired immunodeficiency syndrome.
(Reprinted with permission from Rosse RB, Giese AA, Deutsch SI, Morihisa JM. *Laboratory and Diagnostic Testing in Psychiatry*. Washington, DC: American Psychiatric Press; 1989:55, with permission.)

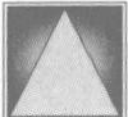

Table 11–6
Posttest HIV Counseling

1. Interpretation of test result:
   Clarify distortion (e.g., "a negative test still means you could contract the virus at a future time; it does not mean you are immune from AIDS").
   Ask questions about the patient's understanding and emotional reaction to the test result.
2. Recommendations for prevention of transmission (careful discussion of high-risk behaviors and guidelines for prevention of transmission).
3. Recommendations on the follow-up of sexual partners and needle contacts.
4. If test result is positive, recommendations against donating blood, sperm, or organs and against sharing razors, toothbrushes, and anything else that may have blood on it.
5. Referral for appropriate psychological support: HIV-positive patients often need access to a mental health team (assess need for inpatient versus outpatient care; consider individual or group supportive therapy). Common themes include the shock of the diagnosis, the fear of death, and social consequences, grief over potential losses, and dashed hopes for good news.
   Also look for depression, hopelessness, anger, frustration, guilt, and obsessional themes. Activate supports available to patient (e.g., family, friends, community services).

HIV, human immunodeficiency virus; AIDS, acquired immunodeficiency syndrome.
(From Rosse RB, Giese AA, Deutsch SI, Morihisa JM. *Laboratory and Diagnostic Testing in Psychiatry*. Washington, DC: American Psychiatric Press; 1989:58, with permission.)

Couples who are considering taking the HIV antibody test must decide who will be tested and whether to go alone or together. The therapist should ask why they are considering taking the test; partners often for the first time discuss issues of commitment, honesty, and trust, such as sexual contacts outside the relationship. They need to be prepared for the possibility that one or both are infected and must discuss what effect this will have on their relationship.

Confidentiality. Confidentiality is a key issue in serum testing. No one should be given an HIV test without previous knowledge and consent, although various jurisdictions and organizations, such as the military, now require HIV testing for all inhabitants or members. The results of an HIV test can be shared with other members of a medical team, although the information should be provided to no one else except in the special circumstances discussed below. The patient should be advised against disclosing the results of HIV testing too readily to employers, friends, and family members; the information could result in discrimination in employment, housing, and insurance.

The major exception to restriction of disclosure is the need to notify potential and past sexual or IV substance use partners. Most patients who are HIV positive act responsibly. If, however, a treating physician knows that a patient who is HIV infected is putting another person at risk of becoming infected, the physician may try either to hospitalize the infected person involuntarily (to prevent danger to others) or to notify the potential victim. Clinicians should be aware of the laws about such issues, which vary among the states. These guidelines also apply to inpatient psychiatric wards when a patient who is HIV infected is believed to be sexually active with other patients.

CLINICAL FEATURES

Nonneurological Factors

About 30 percent of persons infected with HIV experience a flulike syndrome 3 to 6 weeks after becoming infected; most never notice any symptoms immediately or shortly after their infection. When symptoms do appear, the flulike syndrome includes fever, myalgia, headaches, fatigue, gastrointestinal symptoms, and sometimes a rash. The syndrome may be accompanied by splenomegaly and lymphadenopathy. Rarely, acute aseptic meningitis develops shortly after infection, as does encephalopathy or Guillain-Barré syndrome.

In the United States, the median duration of the asymptomatic stages is 10 years, although nonspecific symptoms—lymphadenopathy, chronic diarrhea, weight loss, malaise, fatigue, fevers, night sweats—may variably appear. During the asymptomatic period, however, the T4 cell count almost always declines from normal values (>1,000/mm^3) to grossly abnormal values (<200/mm^3).

The most common infection in persons infected with HIV who have AIDS is *Pneumocystis carinii* pneumonia, which is characterized by a chronic, nonproductive cough, and dyspnea, sometimes sufficiently severe to result in hypoxemia and its resultant cognitive effects. Diagnosis is made with fiberoptic bronchoscopy and alveolar lavage. The pneumonia is usually treatable with trimethoprim and sulfamethoxazole (Bactrim, Septra) or pentamidine isethionate (Pentam), which can also be used for prophylaxis against the pneumonia. The other disease that was initially associated with the development of AIDS is Kaposi's sarcoma, a previously rare, blue-purple-tinted skin lesion. For unknown reasons, Kaposi's sarcoma is less commonly associated with cases of recently diagnosed AIDS.

Although *Pneumocystis carinii* pneumonia and Kaposi's sarcoma are the two classic AIDS-related infectious and neoplastic disorders, the severely disabled cellular immune system of patients infected with HIV permits the development of a staggering array of infections and neoplasms. The most common infections are from protozoa such as *Toxoplasma gondii*; fungi such as *Cryptococcus neoformans* and *Candida albicans*; bacteria such as *Mycobacterium avium-intracellulare*; and viruses such as cytomegalovirus and herpes simplex virus.

For psychiatrists, the importance of these nonneurological, nonpsychiatric complications lies in their biological effects on patients' brain functions (e.g., hypoxia with *Pneumocystis carinii* pneumonia) and their psychological effects on patients' moods and anxiety states. Further, because each of the conditions is usually treated by an additional drug, psychiatrists need to be aware of the adverse CNS effects of many medications.

Neurological Factors

An extensive array of disease processes can affect the brain of a patient infected with HIV (Table 11–7). The most important diseases for mental health workers to be aware of are *HIV mild neurocognitive disorder* and

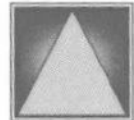

Table 11–7
Conditions Associated with Human Immunodeficiency Virus (HIV) Infection

Bacterial infections, multiple or recurrent[a]
Candidiasis of bronchi, trachea, or lungs
Candidiasis, esophageal
Cervical cancer, invasive[b]
Coccidioidomycosis, disseminated or extrapulmonary
Cryptococcosis, extrapulmonary
Cryptosporidiosis, chronic intestinal (>1 month's duration)
Cytomegalovirus disease (other than liver, spleen, or nodes)
Cytomegalovirus retinitis (with loss of vision)
Encephalopathy, HIV-related
Herpes simplex, chronic ulcers (>1 month's duration); or bronchitis, pulmonitis, or esophagitis
Histoplasmosis, disseminated or extrapulmonary
Isosporiasis, chronic intestinal (>1 month's duration)
Kaposi's sarcoma
Lymphoid interstitial pneumonia and/or pulmonary lymphoid hyperplasia[a]
Lymphoma, Burkitt's (or equivalent term)
Lymphoma, immunoblastic (or equivalent term)
Lymphoma, primary, of brain
Mycobacterium avium complex or *M. kansasii*, disseminated or extrapulmonary
Mycobacterium tuberculosis, any site (pulmonary[b] or extrapulmonary)
Mycobacterium, other species or unidentified species, disseminated or extrapulmonary
Pneumocystis carinii pneumonia
Pneumonia, recurrent[b]
Progressive multifocal leukoencephalopathy
Salmonella septicemia, recurrent
Toxoplasmosis of brain
Wasting syndrome due to HIV

[a]Children <13 years old.
[b]Added in the 1993 expansion of the AIDS surveillance case definition for adolescents and adults.
(Adapted from 1993 revised classification system for HIV infection and expanded surveillance, case definition for AIDS among adolescents and adults. *MMWR Morb Mortal Wkly Rep.* 1992:41, with permission.)

HIV-associated dementia. The latter is a cortical or subcortical type of dementia that can affect 50 percent of patients infected with HIV to some degree. Other diseases and complications of treatment must also be considered in the differential diagnosis of a patient who is HIV infected with neuropsychiatric symptoms. Symptoms such as photophobia, headache, stiff neck, motor weakness, sensory loss, and changes in level of consciousness should alert a mental health worker that the patient should be examined for possible development of a CNS opportunistic infection or a CNS neoplasm. HIV infection can also result in a variety of peripheral neuropathies that should prompt mental health clinicians to reconsider the extent of CNS involvement.

Psychiatric Syndromes

HIV-Associated Dementia. The text revision of the fourth edition of the *Diagnostic and Statistical Manual of Mental Disorders* (DSM-IV-TR) allows the diagnosis of dementia due to HIV disease in "the presence of a dementia that is judged to be the direct pathophysiological consequence of human immunodeficiency virus (HIV) disease." (*See* Table 10.3–7.)

Although HIV-associated dementia is found in a large proportion of patients infected with HIV, other causes of dementia in these patients must be considered. These causes include CNS infections, CNS neoplasms, CNS abnormalities caused by systemic disorders and endocrinopathies, and adverse CNS responses to drugs. The development of dementia is generally a poor prognostic sign, and 50 to 75 percent of patients with dementia die within 6 months.

Mild Neurocognitive Disorder. A less severe form of brain involvement is called *HIV-associated neurocognitive disorder*, also known as *HIV encephalopathy*. It is characterized by impaired cognitive functioning and reduced mental activity that interferes with work, homemaking, or social functioning. No laboratory findings are specific to the disorder, and it occurs independently of depression and anxiety. Progression to HIV-associated dementia usually occurs but may be prevented by early treatment.

Delirium. Delirium can result from the same causes that lead to dementia in patients infected with HIV (Table 11–7). Clinicians have classified delirious states characterized by both increased and decreased activity. Delirium in patients infected with HIV is probably underdiagnosed, but it should always precipitate a medical workup of a patient infected with HIV to determine whether a new CNS-related process has begun.

Anxiety Disorders. Patients with HIV infection may have any of the anxiety disorders, but generalized anxiety disorder, posttraumatic stress disorder, and obsessive–compulsive disorder are particularly common.

Adjustment Disorder. Adjustment disorder with anxiety or depressed mood has been reported to occur in 5 to 20 percent of patients infected with HIV. The incidence of adjustment disorder in persons infected with HIV is higher than usual in some special populations, such as military recruits and prison inmates.

Depressive Disorders. A range of 4 to 40 percent of those infected with HIV have been reported to meet the diagnostic criteria for depressive disorders. The pre-HIV infection prevalence of depressive disorders may be higher than usual in some groups who are at risk for contracting HIV. Another reason for the reported variation in prevalence rates is the variable application of the diagnostic criteria; some of the criteria for depressive disorders (poor sleep and weight loss) can also be caused by the HIV infection itself. Depression is higher in women than in men.

Mania. Mood disorder with manic features, with or without hallucinations, delusions, or a disorder of thought process, can complicate any stage of HIV infection, but most commonly occurs in late-stage disease complicated by neurocognitive impairment.

Substance Abuse. Substance abuse is a problem both for IV substance abusers who contract HIV-related diseases and for other patients with HIV, who may have used illegal substances only occasionally in the past but may now be tempted to use them regularly to deal with depression or anxiety.

Suicide. Suicidal ideation and suicide attempts may increase in patients with HIV infection and AIDS. The risk factors for suicide among persons infected with HIV are having friends who died from AIDS, recent notification of HIV seropositivity, relapses, difficult social issues relating to homosexuality, inadequate social and financial support, and the presence of dementia or delirium.

Psychotic Disorder. Psychotic symptoms are usually later stage complications of HIV infection. They require immediate medical and neurological evaluation and often require management with antipsychotic medications.

Worried Well. The so-called worried well are those in high-risk groups who, although they are seronegative and disease free, are anxious about contracting the virus. Some are reassured by repeated negative serum test results, but others cannot be reassured. Their worried well status can progress quickly to generalized anxiety disorder, panic attacks, obsessive–compulsive disorder, and hypochondriasis.

TREATMENT

Prevention is the primary approach to HIV infection. Primary prevention involves protecting persons from getting the disease; secondary prevention involves modification of the disease's course. All persons with any risk of HIV infection should be informed about safe-sex practices and about the necessity to avoid sharing contaminated hypodermic needles. Preventive strategies, however, are complicated by the complex societal values surrounding sexual acts, sexual orientation, birth control, and substance abuse. Many public health officials have advocated condom distribution in schools and the distribution of clean needles to drug addicts. These issues remain controversial, although condom use has been shown to be a fairly (although not completely) safe and effective preventive strategy against HIV infection. Those who are conservative and religious argue that the educational message should be sexual abstinence. Many university laboratories and pharmaceutical companies are attempting to develop a vaccine to protect persons from infection by HIV. The development of such a vaccine, however, is probably at least a decade away.

The assessment of patients infected with HIV should include a complete sexual and substance-abuse history, a psychiatric history, and an evaluation of the support systems available to them. Clinicians must understand a patient's history with regard to sexual orientation and substance abuse, and the patient must feel that the therapist is not judging past or present behaviors. A therapist can often encourage a sense of trust and empathy in the patient by asking specific, well-informed, straightforward questions about the homosexual or substance-using culture. The therapist must also determine the patient's knowledge about HIV and AIDS.

The homosexual community has provided a significant support system for those infected with HIV, particularly for persons who are gay and bisexual. Public education campaigns within this community have resulted in significant (more than 50 percent) reductions in the highest risk sexual practices, although some gay men still practice high-risk sex. Homosexual men are likely to practice safe sex if they know the safe-sex guidelines, have access to a support group, are in a steady relationship, and have a close relationship with a person with AIDS. Partly because of the many biases against them, IV substance users with AIDS have received little support, and little progress has been made in educating these persons who are a major reservoir for spread of the virus to women, heterosexual men, and children.

Pharmacotherapy

A growing list of agents that act at different points in viral replication has raised for the first time the hope that HIV might be permanently suppressed or actually eradicated from the body. At the time of this writing, the active agents were in two general classes: reverse transcriptase inhibitors and protease inhibitors. The reverse transcriptase inhibitors are further subdivided into the nucleoside reverse transcriptase inhibitor group and the nonnucleoside reverse transcriptase inhibitors. In addition to the new nucleoside reverse transcriptase inhibitors, nonnucleoside reverse transcriptase inhibitors, and protease inhibitors, other classes of drugs are under investigation. These include agents that interfere with HIV cell binding and fusion inhibitors (e.g., enfurvitide [Fuzeon]), the action of HIV integrase, and certain HIV genes such as *gag*, among others. Table 11–8 lists some of the available agents in each of these four categories.

The antiretroviral agents have many adverse effects. Of importance to psychiatrists is that protease inhibitors are metabolized by the hepatic cytochrome P450 oxidase system and, therefore, can increase levels of certain psychotropic drugs that are similarly metabolized. These include bupropion (Wellbutrin), meperidine (Demerol), various benzodiazepines, and selective serotonin reuptake inhibitors (SSRIs). Therefore, caution must be exercised in prescribing psychotropic drugs to persons taking protease inhibitors.

Table 11–8
Antiretroviral Agents

Generic Name	Trade Name	Usual Abbreviation
Nucleoside reverse transcriptase inhibitors		
Zidovudine	Retrovir	AZT or ZDV
Didanosine	Videx	ddl
Zalcitabine	Hivid	ddC
Stavudine	Zerit	d4T
Lamivudine	Epivir	3TC
Abacavir	Ziagen	
Nonnucleoside reverse transcriptase inhibitors		
Nevirapine	Viramune	
Delavirdine	Rescriptor	
Efavirenz	Sustiva	
Protease inhibitors		
Saquinavir	Invirase	
Ritonavir	Norvir	
Indinavir	Crixivan	
Nelfinavir	Viracept	
Fusion inhibitors		
Enfurvitide	Fuzeon	

Beyond treatment directed specifically against HIV, many interventions are available to prevent and treat various complications of immunodeficiency caused by opportunistic viral, bacterial, fungal, and protozoan infections. Both survival and quality of life have improved substantially because of early diagnosis and treatment of these opportunistic conditions.

The use of combination antiretroviral regimens in conjunction with more specific treatments of complications has prolonged the survival of persons, both asymptomatic and symptomatic HIV infected. Despite progress in maintaining patients longer and in better states of health, the ultimate outcome, however, is still uncertain; that is, it is unclear at present whether any person who is HIV infected can expect to escape developing AIDS and ultimately dying. Those who are HIV infected are keenly aware of this prognosis, and their concern sometimes takes the form of psychiatric disturbances.

Novel treatments may also be useful. Neuronal excitotoxicity, mediated through the activation of glutamatergic receptors by the HIV envelope protein gp120, is a potentially important mechanism by which brain dysfunction might occur in HIV infection. Memantine is an open-channel antagonist of N-methyl-d-aspartate (NMDA)-type glutamate receptors that is generally well tolerated. It is currently being used as a treatment for dementia of the Alzheimer's type in Europe. On the assumption that an agent that could dislodge gp120 from neural receptor sites might be useful, an octapeptide called d-ala-peptide-t-amide (peptide t) has been used in phase II clinical trials. Compared with placebo, peptide t was associated with neuropsychological improvement in cognitively impaired individuals (with CD4 counts <200) and a reduced likelihood of progression of impairment on 6-month follow-up. Calcium channel inhibitors, which theoretically seemed potentially useful, have not proved successful.

The remaining forms of treatment are principally supportive. The most important step is to exclude other potentially treatable conditions, such as secondary infections or neoplasia, metabolic abnormalities with low-grade delirium, or other psychiatric disorders (e.g., major depressive disorder). Once the diagnosis is clear, then the usual supportive measures for neurocognitively impaired persons should be used. These include identifying areas of cognitive strength and deficit, reducing emphasis on areas that are now impaired (e.g., divided attention, speeded processing), emphasizing efforts to maintain good orientation and reality testing, and avoiding medications that might further compromise cognitive function, in particular, benzodiazepine drugs. If they must be used, such medications should be given at lower than usual doses. Antidepressant and antipsychotic agents, if indicated, may also have to be prescribed in much lower dosages (e.g., 25 percent of the usual recommended dosage).

Psychotherapy

Approaches. Major psychodynamic themes for patients infected with HIV involve self-blame, self-esteem, and issues regarding death. The psychiatrist can help patients deal with feelings of guilt regarding behaviors that contributed to infection or AIDS. Some patients with HIV and AIDS feel that they are being punished. Difficult health care decisions, such as whether to initiate or continue taking antiretroviral medication and terminal care and life-support systems, should be explored, and here denial of illness may be evident. Major practical themes involve employment, medical benefits, life insurance, career plans, dating and sex, and relationships with families and friends. The entire range of psychotherapeutic approaches may be appropriate for patients with HIV-related disorders. Both individual and group therapy can be effective. Individual therapy may be either short term or long term and may be supportive, cognitive, behavioral, or psychodynamic. Group therapy techniques can range from psychodynamic to completely supportive in nature.

Among the fears that must be confronted is the concern that once the individual's serostatus has been revealed, he or she has lost control of who next learns of the seroconversion. In deciding whether or not to tell others, patients must also address their sense of betrayal if they are not told. The same issues apply to the person's work environment. As a practical matter, the individual may need to decide whether to tell a trusted colleague in case of a job-related accident that might put others at risk of infection. Similarly, parents must decide when or whether to tell their children. Some parents want to tell very young children as soon as possible, whereas other parents prefer to withhold this information until their child's teenage years, for fear of "taking away their childhood." The question of custody of children after the parent's death must be considered. The same question of timing will arise about when to tell children that they are seropositive. The parent must balance fears that telling the child's school will lead to discrimination while guarding their child's and others' safety in case of an accident.

The psychiatrist may have a special role regarding HIV treatment. The advent of protease inhibitors and the promise of additional increasingly effective therapies have brought hopes of a "cure" to patients and physicians alike. Even patients who have failed one or more rounds of combination therapies may find that family, friends, and physicians continue to be optimistic. The psychiatrist may be the only "safe" person to whom the patient can express discouragement, weariness, fear of treatment failure, and fury or guilt for not being able to tolerate successful therapy or for not responding to regimens that have benefited others. The psychiatrist also may be the only one confronting unrealistic expectations of cure or the assumption that safe sex practices are no longer relevant. Paradoxically, the therapeutic task also may be to examine the patient's reaction to a reprieve from certain death—the so-called second-life agenda.

Direct counseling regarding substance use and its potential adverse effects on health of the patient who is HIV infected is indicated. Specific treatments for particular substance-related disorders should be initiated if necessary for the total well-being of the patient.

Therapist-Related Issues. Countertransference issues and burnout of therapists who treat many patients infected with HIV must be evaluated regularly. Therapists must acknowledge to themselves their predetermined attitudes toward sexual orientation and substance use so that those attitudes do not interfere with the treatment of the patient. Issues regarding the therapist's own sexual identity, past behaviors, and eventual death may also give rise to countertransference issues. Psychotherapists who have practices with many patients infected with HIV can begin to have their effectiveness impaired by professional burnout. Some studies have found that seeing many such patients in a short time seems to be more stressful to therapists than seeing a smaller number of those infected with HIV over a longer period.

Involvement of Significant Others. The patient's family, lover, and close friends are often important allies in treatment. The patient's spouse or lover may have guilt feelings about possibly having infected the patient or may experience anger at the patient for possibly infecting him or her. The involvement of members of the patient's support group can help the therapist assess the patient's cognitive function and can also aid in planning financial and living arrangements for the patient. The patient's significant others may themselves benefit from the attention of the therapist in helping them cope with the illness and the impending loss of a friend or family member.

Partner Notification. Although no clear consensus has been reached, recommendations are that patients who are sexually active and infected with HIV should be counseled about potential risk to their sexual partners. Additionally, known partners should be notified of exposure risk and potential infection as well. Partner notification has been an extremely hotly debated topic; however, many states have developed legislation requiring or allowing either physicians or health department officials to notify partners of patients who are HIV infected of their risk. The current standard, despite the controversy, appears to be an obligation on the part of health care professionals to notify anyone who could be construed as clearly at risk and clearly identifiable and who may be unaware of their risk.

A particularly difficult situation is that of sex-industry workers known to be HIV infected and known to be working actively as prostitutes. Public health issues exist that pose a risk both for these patients and, depending on the politics of the circumstances, for their potential partners, clients, customers, victims, or victimizers. The response to this problem has ranged from a sense that sex-industry workers and their clients can make their own decisions and should be responsible for their own behavior all the way to the sentiment that such people should be arrested and jailed for attempted murder. It has additionally been noted that some sex-industry workers are impaired by a variety of psychiatric conditions, including cognitive impairment, major mental illness, personality disorder, and substance abuse disorders. These may further contribute to the sense that some sex-industry workers may be less than fully responsible for their behavior. Recommendations have been made for voluntary and involuntary interventions regarding these patients. Specific psychiatric interventions regarding competency, ability to consent, capacity, and, most importantly, treatment for the conditions that impair such people are critical to the mental health needs of patients with HIV.

References

Becker JT, Lopez OL, Dew MA, Aizenstein HJ. Prevalence of cognitive disorders differs as a function of age in HIV virus infection. *AIDS.* 2004;18[Suppl 1]: S11–S18.

Castellon SA, Hardy DJ, Hinkin CH, Satz P, Stenquist PK, van Gorp WG, Myers HF, Moore L. Components of depression in HIV-1 infection: Their differential relationship to neurocognitive performance. *J Clin Exp Neuropsychol.* 2006;28(3):420–437.

Davis HF, Skolasky RL Jr, Selnes OA, Burgess DM, McArthur JC. Assessing HIV-associated dementia: Modified HIV dementia scale versus the grooved pegboard. *AIDS Reader* 2002;12:29–31, 38.

Grant I, Atkinson JH Jr. Neuropsychiatric aspects of HIV infection and AIDS. In: Sadock BJ, Sadock VA, eds. *Kaplan & Sadock's Comprehensive Textbook of Psychiatry*. 7th ed. Vol. 2. Baltimore: Lippincott Williams & Wilkins; 2000:308.

Hilsabeck RC, Castellon SA, Hinkin CH. Neuropsychological aspects of coinfection with HIV and hepatitis C virus. *Clin Infect Dis.* 2005;41:S38–S44.

Maldonado JL, Fernandez F, Levy JK. Acquired immunodeficiency syndrome. In: Lauterbach EC, ed. *Psychiatric Management in Neurological Disease*. Washington, DC: American Psychiatric Press; 2000:271.

Martin L, Tummala R, Fernandez F. Psychiatric management of HIV infection and AIDS. *Psychiatr Ann.* 2002;32:133.

Olley BO, Zeier MD, Seedat S, Stein DJ. Post-traumatic stress disorder among recently diagnosed patients with HIV/AIDS in South Africa. *AIDS Care*. 2005;17:550–557.

Paul RH, Brickman AM, Navia B, Hinkin C, Malloy PF, Jefferson AL, Cohen RA, Tate DE, Flanigan TP. Apathy is associated with volume of the nucleus accumbens in patients infected with HIV. *J Neuropsychiatry Clin Neurosci*. 2005;17:167–171.

Paul RH, Flanigan TP, Tashima K, Cohen R, Lawrence J, Alt E, Tate D, Ritchie C, Hinkin C. Apathy correlates with cognitive function but not CD4 status in patients with human immunodeficiency virus. *J Neuropsychiatry Clin Neurosci*. 2005;17:114–118.

Pieper AA, Treisman GJ. Drug treatment of depression in HIV-positive patients: Safety considerations. *Drug Saf*. 2005;28(9):753–762.

Roseengarten M, Imrie J, Flowers P, Davis MD, Hart GJ. After euphoria: HIV medical technologies from the perspective of their prescribers. *Sociol Health Illn*. 2004;26(5):575–596.

Stoff DM, Mitnick L, Kalichman S. Research issues in the multiple diagnosis of HIV/AIDS, mental illness and substance abuse. *AIDS Care*. 2004;16[Suppl 1]:S1–S5.

Treisman GJ, Angelino AF, Hsu J, Lyketsos CG. Neuropsychiatric aspects of HIV infection and AIDS. In: Sadock BJ, Sadock VA, eds. *Kaplan & Sadock's Comprehensive Textbook of Psychiatry*. 8th ed. Vol. 1. Baltimore: Lippincott Williams & Wilkins; 2005:426.

von Giesen HJ, Haslinger BA, Rohe S, Roller H, Arendt G. HIV Dementia scale and psychomotor slowing—The best methods in screening for neuro-AIDS. *J Neuropsychiatry Clin Neurosci*. 2005;17:185–191.

12 Substance-Related Disorders

▲ 12.1 Introduction and Overview

This section covers substance dependence and substance abuse with descriptions of the clinical phenomena associated with the use of 11 designated classes of pharmacological agents: alcohol; amphetamines or similarly acting agents; caffeine; cannabis; cocaine; hallucinogens; inhalants; nicotine; opioids; phencyclidine (PCP) or similar agents; and a group that includes sedatives, hypnotics, and anxiolytics. A residual 12th category includes a variety of agents not in the 11 designated classes, such as anabolic steroids and nitrous oxide.

A perennial debate in the United States relates to the most effective way to handle drug problems. In the past few years, a small but growing number of government officials, commentators, and academics have argued that the present policy of aggressively prosecuting drug sellers and users should be reconsidered. They have compared the current drug policy with the prohibition of alcohol from 1920 to 1934 and have argued that abolishing drug laws would eliminate the profit motive, the gangs, and the drug dealers. Although stopping short of endorsing such a radical reversal of the nation's drug policy, a former US Surgeon General, Joycelyn Elders, M.D. (from 1993 to 1994), recommended that the government study the possibility of legalizing drugs of abuse and suggested that doing so might reduce the incidence of violent crimes.

TERMINOLOGY

The concept of substance dependence has had many officially recognized and commonly used meanings over the decades. Two concepts have been used to define aspects of dependence: behavioral and physical. In *behavioral dependence*, substance-seeking activities and related evidence of pathological use patterns are emphasized, whereas *physical dependence* refers to the physical (physiological) effects of multiple episodes of substance use. In definitions stressing physical dependence, ideas of tolerance or withdrawal appear in the classification criteria (Table 12.1–1). The term *intoxication* is used for a reversible nondependent experience with a substance that produces impairment (Table 12.1–2)

Somewhat related to dependence are the related words addiction and addict. The word *addict* has acquired a distinctive, unseemly, and pejorative connotation that ignores the concept of substance abuse as a medical disorder. Addiction has also been trivialized in popular usage, as in the terms *TV addiction* and *money addiction*. Although these connotations have helped the officially sanctioned nomenclature to avoid use of the word addiction, common neurochemical and neuroanatomical substrates may be found among all addictions, whether to substances or to gambling, sex, stealing, or eating. These various addictions may have similar effects on the activities of specific reward areas of the brain, such as the ventral tegmental area, the locus ceruleus, and the nucleus accumbens.

Psychological dependence, also referred to as habituation, is characterized by a continuous or intermittent craving for the substance to avoid a dysphoric state.

When making a diagnosis, clinicians should specify whether symptoms of physiological abuse or dependence are present (Tables 12.1–3 and 12.1–4) and also determine whether the disorder is in full or partial remission. The fourth edition, text revision of the *Diagnosis and Statistical Manual of Mental Disorders* (DSM-IV-TR) allows clinicians to record the current state of the substance dependence by providing a list of course modifiers (Table 12.1–5). A summary of key terms related to dependence and abuse are provided in Table 12.1–6.

Other Terms

Codependence. The terms *coaddiction*, *coalcoholism*, and, more commonly, *codependency* or *codependence* are used to designate the behavioral patterns of family members who have been significantly affected by another family member's substance use or addiction. The terms have been used in various ways and no established criteria for codependence exist.

Enabling. Enabling was one of the first, and more agreed on, characteristics of codependence or coaddiction. Sometimes, family members feel that they have little or no control over the enabling acts. Either because of the social pressures for protecting and supporting family members or because of pathological interdependencies, or both, enabling behavior often resists modification. Other characteristics of codependence include unwillingness to accept the notion of addiction as a disease. The family members continue to behave as if the substance-using behavior were voluntary and willful (if not actually spiteful) and the user cares more for alcohol and drugs than for family members. This results in feelings of anger, rejection, and failure. In addition to those feelings, family members may feel guilty and depressed because addicts, in an effort to deny loss of control over drugs and to shift the focus of concern away from their use, often try to place the responsibility for such use on other family members, who often seem willing to accept some or all of it.

Table 12.1–1
DSM-IV-TR Criteria for Substance Withdrawal

A. The development of a substance-specific syndrome due to the cessation of (or reduction in) substance use that has been heavy and prolonged.
B. The substance-specific syndrome causes clinically significant distress or impairment in social, occupational, or other important areas of functioning.
C. The symptoms are not due to a general medical condition and are not better accounted for by another mental disorder.

(From American Psychiatric Association. *Diagnostic and Statistical Manual of Mental Disorders.* 4th ed. Text rev. Washington, DC: American Psychiatric Association; copyright 2000, with permission.)

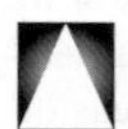

Table 12.1–2
DSM-IV-TR Criteria for Substance Intoxication

A. The development of a reversible substance-specific syndrome due to recent ingestion of (or exposure to) a substance. Note: Different substances may produce similar or identical syndromes.
B. Clinically significant maladaptive behavioral or psychological changes that are due to the effect of the substance on the central nervous system (e.g., belligerence, mood lability, cognitive impairment, impaired judgment, impaired social or occupational functioning) and develop during or shortly after use of the substance.
C. The symptoms are not due to a general medical condition and are not better accounted for by another mental disorder.

(From American Psychiatric Association. *Diagnostic and Statistical Manual of Mental Disorders.* 4th ed. Text rev. Washington, DC: American Psychiatric Association; copyright 2000, with permission.)

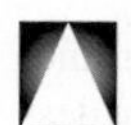

Table 12.1–3
DSM-IV-TR Criteria for Substance Abuse

A. A maladaptive pattern of substance use leading to clinically significant impairment or distress, as manifested by one (or more) of the following, occurring within a 12-month period:
(1) recurrent substance use resulting in a failure to fulfill major role obligations at work, school, or home (e.g., repeated absences or poor work performance related to substance use; substance-related absences, suspensions, or expulsions from school; neglect of children or household)
(2) recurrent substance use in situations in which it is physically hazardous (e.g., driving an automobile or operating a machine when impaired by substance use)
(3) recurrent substance-related legal problems (e.g., arrests for substance-related disorderly conduct)
(4) continued substance use despite having persistent or recurrent social or interpersonal problems caused or exacerbated by the effects of the substance (e.g., arguments with spouse about consequences of intoxication, physical fights)
B. The symptoms have never met the criteria for Substance Dependence for this class of substance.

(From American Psychiatric Association. *Diagnostic and Statistical Manual of Mental Disorders.* 4th ed. Text rev. Washington, DC: American Psychiatric Association; copyright 2000, with permission.)

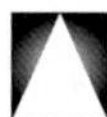

Table 12.1–4
DSM-IV-TR Diagnostic Criteria for Substance Dependence

A maladaptive pattern of substance use, leading to clinically significant impairment or distress, as manifested by three (or more) of the following, occurring at any time in the same 12-month period:
(1) tolerance, as defined by either of the following:
(a) a need for markedly increased amounts of the substance to achieve intoxication or desired effect
(b) markedly diminished effect with continued use of the same amount of the substance
(2) withdrawal, as manifested by either of the following:
(a) the characteristic withdrawal syndrome for the substance (refer to Criteria A and B of the criteria sets for Withdrawal from the specific substances)
(b) the same (or a closely related) substance is taken to relieve or avoid withdrawal symptoms
(3) the substance is often taken in larger amounts or over a longer period than was intended
(4) there is a persistent desire or unsuccessful efforts to cut down or control substance use
(5) a great deal of time is spent in activities necessary to obtain the substance (e.g., visiting multiple doctors or driving long distances), use the substance (e.g., chain-smoking), or recover from its effects
(6) important social, occupational, or recreational activities are given up or reduced because of substance use
(7) the substance use is continued despite knowledge of having a persistent or recurrent physical or psychological problem that is likely to have been caused or exacerbated by the substance (e.g., current cocaine use despite recognition of cocaine-induced depression, or continued drinking despite recognition that an ulcer was made worse by alcohol consumption)

Specify if:
With Physiological Dependence: evidence of tolerance or withdrawal (i.e., either Item 1 or 2 is present)
Without Physiological Dependence: no evidence of tolerance or withdrawal (i.e., neither Item 1 nor 2 is present)

Course specifiers (see Table 12.1–5 for definitions):
Early Full Remission
Early Partial Remission
Sustained Full Remission
Sustained Partial Remission
On Agonist Therapy
In a Controlled Environment

(From American Psychiatric Association. *Diagnostic and Statistical Manual of Mental Disorders.* 4th ed. Text rev. Washington, DC: American Psychiatric Association; copyright 2000, with permission.)

Denial. Family members, as with the substance users themselves, often behave as if the substance use that is causing obvious problems were not really a problem; that is, they engage in denial. The reasons for the unwillingness to accept the obvious vary. Sometimes denial is self-protecting, in that the family members believe that if a drug or alcohol problem exists, then they are responsible.

As with the addicts themselves, codependent family members seem unwilling to accept the notion that outside intervention is needed and, despite repeated failures, continue to believe that greater willpower and greater efforts at control can restore tranquility. When additional efforts at control fail, they often attribute the failure to themselves rather than to the addict or the disease

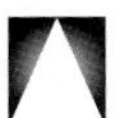

Table 12.1–5
DSM-IV Course Modifiers for Substance Dependence

Six course specifiers are available for substance dependence. The four remission specifiers can be applied only after none of the criteria for substance dependence or substance abuse has been present for at least 1 month. The definition of these four types of remission is based on the interval of time that has elapsed since the cessation of dependence (early versus sustained remission) and whether there is continued presence of one or more of the items included in the criteria sets for dependence or abuse (partial versus full remission). Because the first 12 months following dependence is a time of particularly high risk for relapse, this period is designated early remission. After 12 months of early remission have passed without relapse to dependence, the person enters into sustained remission. For both early remission and sustained remission, a further designation of full is given if no criteria for dependence or abuse have been met during the period of remission; a designation of partial is given if at least one of the criteria for dependence or abuse has been met intermittently or continuously, during the period of remission. The differentiation of sustained full remission from recovered (no current substance use disorder) requires consideration of the length of time since the last period of disturbance, the total duration of the disturbance, and the need for continued evaluation. If, after a period of remission or recovery, the individual again becomes dependent, the application of the early remission specifier requires that there again be at least 1 month in which no criteria for dependence or abuse are met. Two additional specifiers have been provided: on agonist therapy and in a controlled environment. For an individual to qualify for early remission after cessation of agonist therapy or release from a controlled environment, there must be a 1-month period in which none of the criteria for dependence or abuse is met.

The following remission specifiers can be applied only after no criteria for dependence or abuse have been met for at least 1 month. Note that these specifiers do not apply if the individual is on agonist therapy or in a controlled environment (see below).

Early full remission. This specifier is used if, for at least 1 month, but for less than 12 months, no criteria for dependence or abuse have been met.

Dependence — 1 month — 0-11 months

Early partial remission. This specifier is used if, for at least 1 month, but less than 12 months, one or more criteria for dependence or abuse have been met (but the full criteria for dependence have not been met).

Dependence — 1 month — 0-11 months

Sustained full remission. This specifier is used if none of the criteria for dependence or abuse has been met at any time during a period of 12 months or longer.

Dependence — 1 month — 11+ months

Sustained partial remission. This specifier is used if full criteria for dependence have not been met for a period of 12 months or longer; however, one or more criteria for dependence or abuse have been met.

Dependence — 1 month — 11+ months

The following specifiers apply if the individual is on agonist therapy or in a controlled environment:

On agonist therapy. This specifier is used if the individual is on a prescribed agonist medication, and no criteria for dependence or abuse have been met for the class of medication for at least the past month (except tolerance to, or withdrawal from, the agonist). This category also applies to those being treated for dependence using a partial agonist or an agonist/antagonist.

In a controlled environment. This specifier is used if the individual is in an environment where access to alcohol and controlled substances is restricted, and no criteria for dependence or abuse have been met for at least the past month. Examples of these environments are closely supervised and substance-free jails, therapeutic communities, or locked hospital units.

(From American Psychiatric Association. *Diagnostic and Statistical Manual of Mental Disorders.* 4th ed. Text rev. Washington, DC: American Psychiatric Association; copyright 2000, with permission.)

process, and along with failure come feelings of anger, lowered self-esteem, and depression.

EPIDEMIOLOGY

The National Institute of Drug Abuse (NIDA) and other agencies, such as the National Survey of Drug Use and Heath (NSDUH), conduct periodic surveys of the use of illicit drugs in the United States. As of 2004, an estimated 22.5 million persons over the age of 12 years (about 10 percent of the total US population) were classified as suffering from a substance-related disorder. Of this group, about 15 million were dependent on, or abused, alcohol (Fig. 12.1–1).

Figure 12.1–2 shows data from the NSDUH survey on the percentage of respondents who reported using various drugs. In 2004, 67.8 percent (0.3 million) persons were dependent on, or abused, heroin; 17.6 percent (4.5 million) abused marijuana; 27.8 percent (1.6 million) abused cocaine; and 12.3 percent (1.4 million) were classified as dependent on, or abuse of, pain relievers.

With regard to age at first use, those who started to use drugs at an earlier age (14 years or younger) were more likely to become addicted than those who started at a later age. This applied to all substances of abuse, but particularly to alcohol. Among adults aged 18 or older who first tried alcohol at age 14 or younger, 17.9 percent were classified as alcoholics compared with only 4.1 percent who first used alcohol at age 18 or older.

Rates of abuse also varied according to age (Table 12.1–7). The rate for dependence or abuse was 1.3 percent at age 12, and rates generally increased until the highest rate (25.4 percent) at age 21. After age 21, a general decline occurred with age. By age 65, only about 1 percent of persons have used an illicit substance within the past year, which lends credence to the clinical observation that addicts tend to "burn out" as they age.

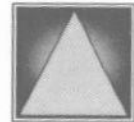

Table 12.1–6
Terms Used in Dependence and Abuse

Dependence The repeated use of a drug or chemical substance, with or without physical dependence. Physical dependence indicates an altered physiologic state caused by repeated administration of a drug, the cessation of which results in a specific syndrome.

Abuse Use of any drug, usually by self-administration, in a manner that deviates from approved social or medical patterns.

Misuse Similar to abuse, but usually applies to drugs prescribed by physicians that are not used properly.

Addiction The repeated and increased use of a substance, the deprivation of which gives rise to symptoms of distress and an irresistible urge to use the agent again and which leads also to physical and mental deterioration. The term is no longer included in the official nomenclature, having been replaced by the term *dependence*, but it is a useful term in common usage.

Intoxication A reversible syndrome caused by a specific substance (e.g., alcohol) that affects one or more of the following mental functions: memory, orientation, mood, judgment, and behavioral, social, or occupational functioning.

Withdrawal A substance-specific syndrome that occurs after stopping or reducing the amount of the drug or substance that has been used regularly over a prolonged period of time. The syndrome is characterized by physiologic signs and symptoms in addition to psychological changes, such as disturbances in thinking, feeling, and behavior. Also called *abstinence syndrome* or *discontinuation syndrome.*

Tolerance Phenomenon in which, after repeated administration, a given dose of drug produces a decreased effect or increasingly larger doses must be administered to obtain the effect observed with the original dose. *Behavioral tolerance* reflects the ability of the person to perform tasks despite the effects of the drug.

Cross-tolerance Refers to the ability of one drug to be substituted for another, each usually producing the same physiologic and psychological effect (e.g., diazepam and barbiturates). Also known as *cross-dependence.*

Neuroadaptation Neurochemical or neurophysiologic changes in the body that result from the repeated administration of a drug. Neuroadaptation accounts for the phenomenon of tolerance. *Pharmacokinetic adaptation* refers to adaptation of the metabolizing system in the body. *Cellular or pharmacodynamic adaptation* refers to the ability of the nervous system to function despite high blood levels of the offending substance.

Codependence Term used to refer to family members affected by or influencing the behavior of the substance abuser. Related to the term *enabler,* which is a person who facilitates the abuser's addictive behavior (e.g., providing drugs directly or money to buy drugs). Enabling also includes the unwillingness of a family member to accept addiction as a medical-psychiatric disorder or to deny that person is abusing a substance.

Table 12.1–8 summarizes data about the demographic characteristics of those who use illicit drugs. More men use drugs that do women; the highest lifetime rate is among American Indian or Alaska Natives; whites are more affected than blacks or African Americans; those with some college education use more substances than those with less education; and the unemployed have higher rates that those with either part-time or full-time employment.

Rates of substance dependence or abuse varied by region in the United States. Rates were higher in the Midwest and West

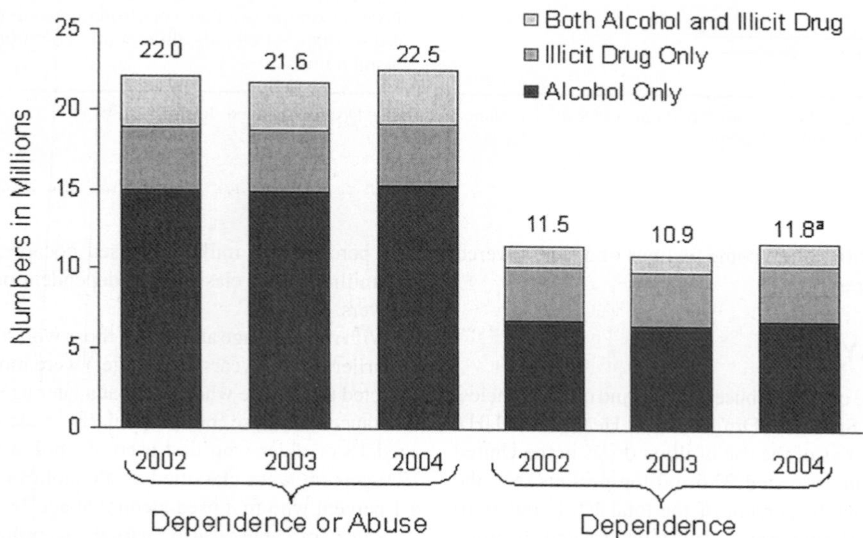

FIGURE 12.1–1

Substance dependence or abuse among persons age 12 or over: 2002–2004. (From National Survey on Drug Use and Health, with permission.)

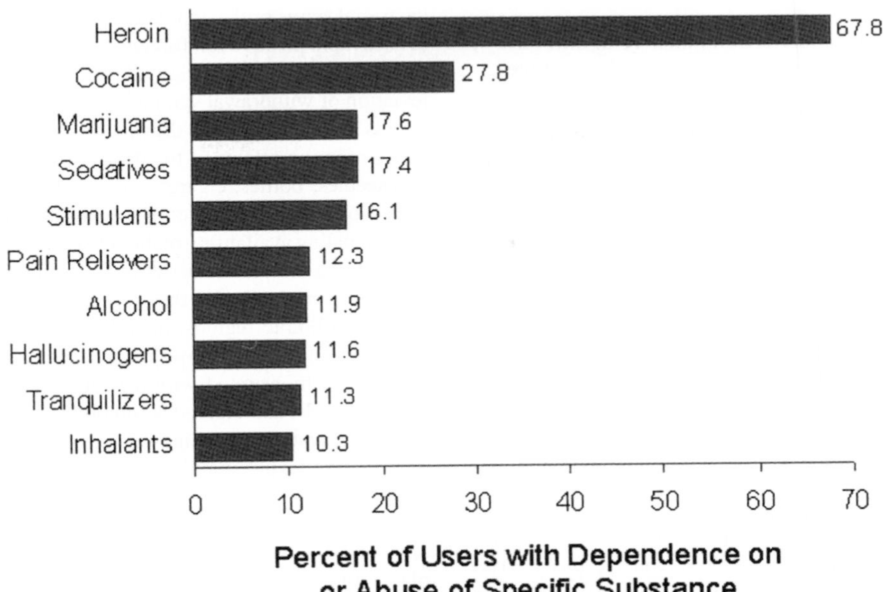

FIGURE 12.1–2
Dependence on, or abuse of, specific substances within the past year, 2004. (From National Survey on Drug Use and Abuse, with permission.)

than in the Northeast and South. Rates were also higher in large metropolitan counties compared with small metropolitan counties and were lowest in completely rural counties. Rates are also higher among persons on parole or on supervised release from jail (40.8 percent vs. 9.2 percent). A continued need exists for programs to reduce the number of persons driving while under the influence of drugs or alcohol. The percentage driving under the influence of alcohol increased from 10 percent in 2000 to 13.5 percent in 2004, and those driving under the influence of drugs increased from 3.1 percent to 6 percent during the same period. A comprehensive survey of drug use and trends in the United States is available at www.samhasa.gov.

ETIOLOGY

The model of drug dependence conceptualizes dependence as a result of a process in which multiple interacting factors influence drug-using behavior and the loss of flexibility with respect to decisions about using a given drug. Although the actions of a given drug are critical in the process, it is not assumed that all people who become dependent on the same drug experience its effects in the same way or are motivated by the same set of factors. Furthermore, it is postulated that different factors may be more or less important at different stages of the process. Thus, drug availability, social acceptability, and peer pressures may be the major determinants of initial experimentation with a drug, but other factors, such as personality and individual biology, probably are more important in how the effects of a given drug are perceived and the degree to which repeated drug use produces changes in the central nervous system (CNS). Still other factors, including the particular actions of the drug, may be primary determinants of whether drug use progresses to drug dependence, whereas still others may be important influences on the likelihood that drug use (1) leads to adverse effects or (2) to successful recovery from dependence.

It has been asserted that addiction is a "brain disease," that the critical processes that transform voluntary drug-using behavior to compulsive drug use are changes in the structure and neurochemistry of the brain of the drug user. Sufficient evidence now indicates that such changes in relevant parts of the brain do occur. The perplexing and unanswered question is whether these changes are both necessary and sufficient to account for the drug-using behavior. Many argue that they are not, that the capacity of drug-dependent individuals to modify their drug-using behavior in response to positive reinforcers or aversive contingencies indicates that the nature of addiction is more complex and requires the interaction of multiple factors.

Figure 12.1–3 illustrates how various factors might interact in the development of drug dependence. The central element is the drug-using behavior itself. The decision to use a drug is influenced by immediate social and psychological situations as well as by the person's more remote history. Use of the drug initiates a sequence of consequences that can be rewarding or aversive and which, through a process of learning, can result in a greater or lesser likelihood that the drug-using behavior will be repeated. For some drugs, use also initiates the biological processes associated with tolerance, physical dependence, and (not shown in the figure) sensitization. In turn, tolerance can reduce some of the adverse effects of the drug, permitting or requiring the use of larger doses, which then can accelerate or intensify the development of physical dependence. Above a certain threshold, the aversive qualities of a withdrawal syndrome provide a distinct recurrent motive for further drug use. Sensitization of motivational systems can increase the salience of drug-related stimuli.

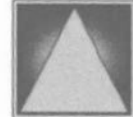

Table 12.1–7
Illicit Drug Use in Lifetime, Past Year, and Past Month, by Detailed Age Category: Percentages, 2003 and 2004

	Time Period					
	Lifetime		Past Year		Past Month	
Age Category	2003	2004	2003	2004	2003	2004
TOTAL	46.4	45.8	14.7	14.5	8.2	7.9
12	12.2	11.2	6.2	6.7	2.7	2.8
13	18.7	18.4	11.9	11.6	4.9	4.6
14	26.3	25.2	18.7	17.8	8.5	9.0
15	34.2	34.7	25.2	24.6	13.3	12.7
16	43.8	42.5	33.2	31.0	18.6[b]	15.5
17	48.4	48.4	36.1	34.9	19.7	19.1
18	53.5	53.4	38.2	38.8	22.6	21.2
19	58.3	56.6	39.9	38.6	23.5	22.8
20	62.0	59.0	40.3	38.1	24.0	21.3
21	61.6	62.3	35.0	36.6	20.7	21.7
22	64.0	62.9	33.5	35.1	19.6	20.5
23	63.4[a]	59.5	32.2[a]	28.3	18.0[a]	15.4
24	62.3	59.8	30.1	27.6	17.2	16.2
25	60.1	60.5	25.9	26.7	15.7	15.2
26–29	57.9	60.0	23.6	23.5	13.4	13.2
30–34	56.8	54.5	16.6	15.7	8.8	9.4
35–39	61.7	59.4	15.0	14.1	8.4	7.2
40–44	65.3	64.9	14.0	14.4	8.1	7.5
45–49	62.3	61.8	12.6	11.8	6.8	6.8
50–54	52.0	56.3	7.4	9.0	3.9	4.8
55–59	38.3	38.2	4.4	5.1	2.0	2.6
60–64	23.8	24.2	2.9	2.0	1.1	1.1
65 or Older	9.9	8.3	0.7	0.9	0.6	0.4

* Low precision; no estimate reported.
NOTE: Illicit Drugs include marijuana/hashish, cocaine (including crack), heroin, hallucinogens, inhalants, or prescription-type psychotherapeutics used nonmedically.
[a] Difference between estimate and 2004 estimate is statistically significant at the 0.05 level.
[b] Difference between estimate and 2004 estimate is statistically significant at the 0.01 level.
(From SAMHSA, Office of Applied Studies. National Survey on Drug Use and Health, 2003 and 2004, with permission.)

Psychodynamic Factors

The range of psychodynamic theories about substance abuse reflects the various popular theories during the past 100 years. According to classic theories, substance abuse is a masturbatory equivalent (some heroin users describe the initial "rush" as similar to a prolonged sexual orgasm), a defense against anxious impulses, or a manifestation of oral regression (i.e., dependency). Recent psychodynamic formulations relate substance use as a reflection of disturbed ego functions (i.e., the inability to deal with reality). As a form of self-medication, alcohol may be used to control panic, opioids to diminish anger, and amphetamines to alleviate depression. Some addicts have great difficulty recognizing their inner emotional states, a condition called *alexithymia* (i.e., being unable to find words to describe their feelings).

Learning and Conditioning. Drug use, whether occasional or compulsive, can be viewed as behavior maintained by its consequences. Drugs can reinforce antecedent behaviors by terminating some noxious or aversive state such as pain, anxiety, or depression. In some social situations, the drug use, apart from its pharmacological effects, can be reinforcing if it results in special status or the approval of friends. Each use of the drug evokes rapid positive reinforcement, either as a result of the rush (the drug-induced euphoria), alleviation of disturbed affects, alleviation of withdrawal symptoms, or any combination of these effects. In addition, some drugs may sensitize neural systems to the reinforcing effects of the drug. Eventually, the paraphernalia (needles, bottles, cigarette packs) and behaviors associated with substance use can become secondary reinforcers, as well as cues signaling availability of the substance, and in their presence, craving or a desire to experience the effects increases.

Drug users respond to the drug-related stimuli with increased activity in limbic regions, including the amygdala and the anterior cingulate. Such drug-related activation of limbic areas has been demonstrated with a variety of drugs, including cocaine, opioids, and cigarettes (nicotine). Interestingly, the same regions activated by cocaine-related stimuli in cocaine users are activated by sexual stimuli in both normal controls and cocaine users.

In addition to the operant reinforcement of drug-using and drug-seeking behaviors, other learning mechanisms probably play a role in dependence and relapse. Opioid and alcohol withdrawal phenomena can be conditioned (in the Pavlovian or classic sense) to environmental or interoceptive stimuli. For a long time after withdrawal (from opioids, nicotine, or alcohol), the addict exposed to environmental stimuli previously linked with substance use or withdrawal may experience conditioned withdrawal, conditioned craving, or both. The increased feelings of craving are not necessarily accompanied by symptoms of withdrawal. The most intense craving is elicited by conditions associated with the availability or use of the substance, such as watching someone else use heroin or light a cigarette or being offered some drug by a friend. Those learning and conditioning phenomena can be superimposed on any preexisting psychopathology, but preexisting difficulties are not required for the development of powerfully reinforced substance-seeking behavior.

Genetic Factors

Strong evidence from studies of twins, adoptees, and siblings brought up separately indicates that the cause of alcohol abuse has a genetic component. Many less conclusive data show that other types of substance abuse or substance dependence have a genetic pattern in their development. Researchers recently have used restriction fragment length polymorphism (RFLP) in the study of substance abuse and substance dependence, and associations to genes that affect dopamine production have been postulated.

Neurochemical Factors

Receptors and Receptor Systems. With the exception of alcohol, researchers have identified particular neurotransmitters or neurotransmitter receptors involved with most substances of abuse. Some researchers base their studies on such hypotheses. The opioids, for example, act on opioid receptors. A person with too little endogenous opioid activity (e.g., low concentrations of endorphins) or with too much activity of an endogenous opioid antagonist may be at risk for developing opioid dependence. Even in a person with completely normal endogenous receptor function and neurotransmitter concentration, the long-term use

Table 12.1–8
Illicit Drug Use in Lifetime, Past Year, and Past Month among Persons Aged 18 or Older, by Demographic Characteristics: Percentages, 2003 and 2004

	Time Period					
	Lifetime		Past Year		Past Month	
Demographic Characteristic	2003	2004	2003	2004	2003	2004
TOTAL	48.2	47.6	13.9	13.7	7.8	7.6
GENDER						
Male	53.7	53.2	16.7	16.4	9.8	9.8
Female	43.2	42.4	11.3	11.2	6.0	5.6
HISPANIC ORIGIN AND RACE						
Not Hispanic or Latino	49.7	49.2	13.9	14.0	7.9	7.7
White	51.1	51.0	14.1	14.2	8.0	7.8
Black or African American	46.8	45.7	14.7	14.0	8.6	8.6
American Indian or Alaska Native	65.7	*	16.6	24.0	10.9	10.3
Native Hawaiian or Other Pacific Islander	*	*	17.8	*	10.5	*
Asian	26.2	24.8	6.5	6.2	3.5	2.8
Two or More Races	65.1	58.4	19.4	20.3	11.4	13.6
Hispanic or Latino	37.9	36.2	13.6[a]	11.8	7.5	6.7
EDUCATION						
<High School	38.0	37.2	14.7	14.3	9.0	8.6
High School Graduate	46.5	44.7	14.2	13.7	8.3	7.8
Some College	54.8	53.8	16.5	15.9	9.2	8.7
College Graduate	51.1	51.8	10.4	11.1	5.2	5.6
CURRENT EMPLOYMENT						
Full-Time	56.6	56.4	14.8	14.6	7.9	8.0
Part-Time	51.5	50.2	18.5	18.5	10.7	10.3
Unemployed	62.1	64.1	28.7	28.8	18.2	19.2
Other[1]	28.2	27.3	7.8	8.0	4.8	4.3

* Low precision; no estimate reported.
NOTE: Illicit Drugs include marijuana/hashish, cocaine (including crack), heroin, hallucinogens, inhalants, or prescription-type psychotherapeutics used nonmedically.
[a] Difference between estimate and 2004 estimate is statistically significant at the 0.05 level.
[b] Difference between estimate and 2004 estimate is statistically significant at the 0.01 level.
[1] Retired persons, disabled persons, homemakers, students, or other persons not in the labor force are included in the Other Employment category.
(From SAMHSA, Office of Applied Studies. National Survey on Drug Use and Health, 2003 and 2004, with permission.)

of a particular substance of abuse may eventually modulate receptor systems in the brain so that the presence of the exogenous substance is needed to maintain homeostasis. Such a receptor-level process may be the mechanism for developing tolerance within the CNS. Demonstrating modulation of neurotransmitter release and neurotransmitter receptor function has proved difficult, however, and recent research focuses on the effects of substances on the second-messenger system and on gene regulation.

Pathways and Neurotransmitters

The major neurotransmitters possibly involved in developing substance abuse and substance dependence are the opioid, catecholamine (particularly dopamine), and γ-aminobutyric acid (GABA) systems. The dopaminergic neurons in the ventral tegmental area are particularly important. These neurons project to the cortical and limbic regions, especially the nucleus accumbens. This pathway is probably involved in the sensation of reward and may be the major mediator of the effects of such substances as amphetamine and cocaine. The locus ceruleus, the largest group of adrenergic neurons, probably mediates the effects of the opiates and the opioids. These pathways have collectively been called the *brain-reward circuitry*.

COMORBIDITY

Comorbidity is the occurrence of two or more psychiatric disorders in a single patient at the same time. A high prevalence of additional psychiatric disorders is found among persons seeking treatment for alcohol, cocaine, or opioid dependence; some studies have shown that up to 50 percent of addicts have a comorbid psychiatric disorder. Although opioid, cocaine, and alcohol abusers with current psychiatric problems are more likely to seek treatment, those who do not seek treatment are not necessarily free of comorbid psychiatric problems; such persons may have social supports that enable them to deny the impact that drug use is having on their lives. Two large epidemiological studies have shown that even among representative samples of the population, those who meet the criteria for alcohol or drug abuse and dependence (excluding tobacco dependence) are far more likely to meet the criteria for other psychiatric disorders also.

Antisocial Personality Disorder. In various studies, a range of 35 to 60 percent of patients with substance abuse or substance dependence also meets the diagnostic criteria for antisocial personality disorder. The range is even higher when investigators include persons who meet all the antisocial personality disorder diagnostic criteria, except the requirement that the symptoms started at an early age. That is, a high percentage of patients with substance abuse or substance dependence diagnoses have a pattern of antisocial behavior, whether it was present

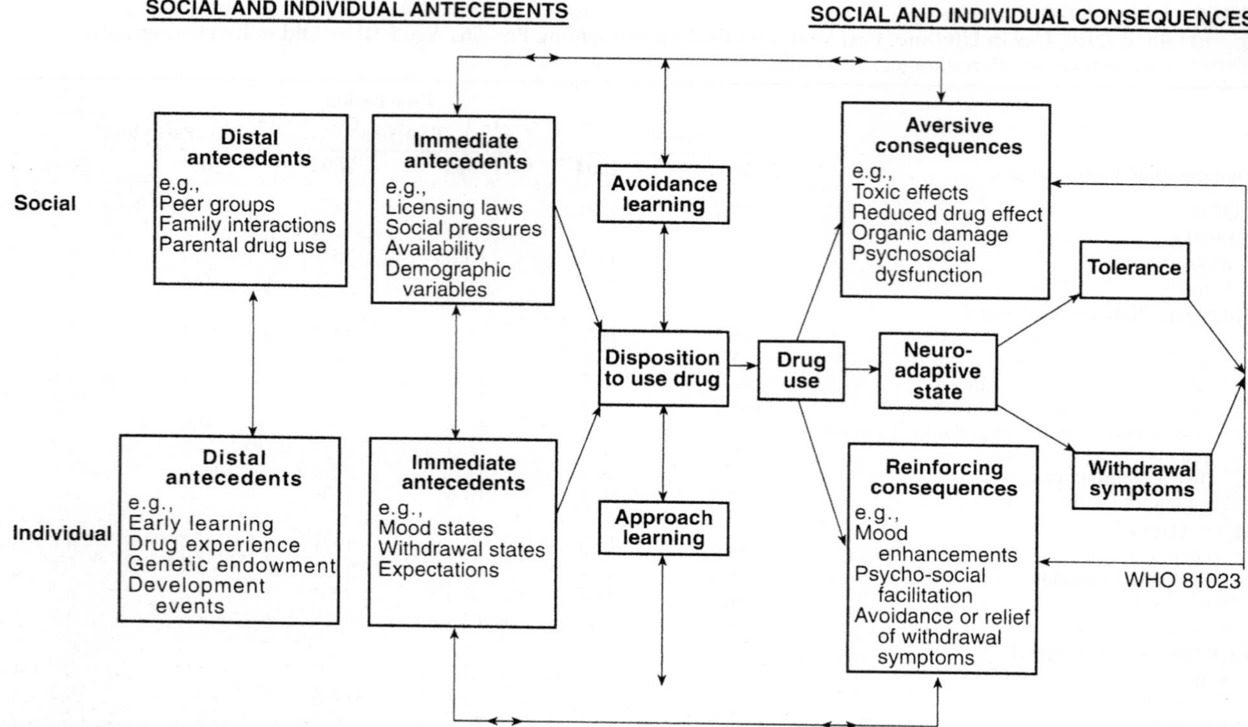

FIGURE 12.1–3
World Health Organization schematic model of drug use and dependence. (From Edwards G, Arif A, Hodgson R. Nemenclature and classification of drug-and alcohol-related problems. A WHO memorandum. *Bull WHO.* 1981;99:225, with permission.)

before the substance use started or developed during the course of the substance use. Patients with substance abuse or substance dependence diagnoses who have antisocial personality disorder are likely to use more illegal substances; to have more psychopathology; to be less satisfied with their lives; and to be more impulsive, isolated, and depressed than patients with antisocial personality disorders alone.

Depression and Suicide. Depressive symptoms are common among persons diagnosed with substance abuse or substance dependence. About one third to one half of all those with opioid abuse or opioid dependence and about 40 percent of those with alcohol abuse or alcohol dependence meet the criteria for major depressive disorder sometime during their lives. Substance use is also a major precipitating factor for suicide. Persons who abuse substances are about 20 times more likely to die by suicide than the general population. About 15 percent of persons with alcohol abuse or alcohol dependence have been reported to commit suicide. This frequency of suicide is second only to the frequency in patients with major depressive disorder.

TREATMENT AND REHABILITATION

Some persons who develop substance-related problems recover without formal treatment, especially as they age. For those patients with less severe disorders, such as nicotine addiction, relatively brief interventions are often as effective as more intensive treatments. Because these brief interventions do not change the environment, alter drug-induced brain changes, or provide new skills, a change in the patient's motivation (cognitive change) probably has the best impact on the drug-using behavior. For those individuals who do not respond or whose dependence is more severe, a variety of interventions appear to be effective.

It is useful to distinguish among specific procedures or techniques (e.g., individual therapy, family therapy, group therapy, relapse prevention, and pharmacotherapy) and treatment programs. Most programs use a number of specific procedures and involve several professional disciplines as well as nonprofessionals who have special skills or personal experience with the substance problem being treated. The best treatment programs combine specific procedures and disciplines to meet the needs of the individual patient after a careful assessment.

No classification is generally accepted for either the specific procedures used in treatment or programs using various combinations of procedures. This lack of standardized terminology for categorizing procedures and programs presents a problem, even when the field of interest is narrowed from substance problems in general to treatment for a single substance, such as alcohol, tobacco, or cocaine. Except in carefully monitored research projects, even the definitions of specific procedures (e.g., individual counseling, group therapy, and methadone maintenance) tend to be so imprecise that usually just what transactions are supposed to occur cannot be inferred. Nevertheless, for descriptive purposes, programs are often broadly grouped on the basis of one or more of their salient characteristics: whether the program is aimed at merely controlling acute withdrawal and consequences of recent drug use (detoxification) or is focused on longer-term behavioral change; whether the program makes extensive use of pharmacological interventions; and the degree to which the program is based on individual psychotherapy, Alcoholics Anonymous (AA) or other 12-step principles, or therapeutic community principles. For example, government agencies recently categorized publicly funded treatment programs for drug dependence as (1) methadone maintenance (mostly outpatient), (2) outpatient drug-free programs, (3) therapeutic communities, or (4) short-term inpatient programs.

Selecting a Treatment

Not all interventions are applicable to all varieties of substance use or dependence, and some of the more coercive interventions used for illicit drugs are not applicable to substances that are legally available, such as tobacco. Addictive behaviors do not change abruptly, but through a series of stages. Five stages in this gradual process have been proposed: precontemplation, contemplation, preparation, action, and maintenance. For some types of addictions the therapeutic alliance is enhanced when the treatment approach is tailored to the patient's stage of readiness to change. Interventions for some drug use disorders may have a specific pharmacological agent as an important component; for example, disulfiram, naltrexone (ReVia), or acamprosate for alcoholism; methadone (Dolophine), levomethadyl acetate (ORLAAM), or buprenorphine (Buprenex) for heroin addiction; and nicotine delivery devices or bupropion (Zyban) for tobacco dependence. Not all interventions are likely to be useful to health care professionals. For example, many youthful offenders with histories of drug use or dependence are now remanded to special facilities (boot camps); other programs for offenders (and sometimes for employees) rely almost exclusively on the deterrent effect of frequent urine testing; and a third group are built around religious conversion or rededication in a specific religious sect or denomination. In contrast to the numerous studies suggesting some value for brief interventions for smoking and for problem drinking, few controlled studies are conducted of brief interventions for those seeking treatment for dependence on illicit drugs.

In general, brief interventions (e.g., a few weeks of detoxification, whether in or out of a hospital) used for persons who are severely dependent on illicit opioids have limited effect on outcome measured a few months later. Substantial reductions in illicit drug use, antisocial behaviors, and psychiatric distress among patients dependent on cocaine or heroin are much more likely following treatment lasting at least 3 months. Such a time-in-treatment effect is seen across very different modalities, from residential therapeutic communities to ambulatory methadone maintenance programs. Although some patients appear to benefit from a few days or weeks of treatment, a substantial percentage of users of illicit drugs drop out (or are dropped) from treatment before they have achieved significant benefits.

Some of the variance in treatment outcomes can be attributed to differences in the characteristics of patients entering treatment and by events and conditions following treatment. Programs based on similar philosophical principles and using what seem to be similar therapeutic procedures vary greatly in effectiveness, however. Some of the differences among programs that seem to be similar reflect the range and intensity of services offered. Programs with professionally trained staffs that provide more comprehensive services to patients with more severe psychiatric difficulties are more likely able to retain those patients in treatment and help them make positive changes. Differences in the skills of individual counselors and professionals can strongly affect outcomes.

Such generalizations concerning programs serving illicit drug users may not hold for programs dealing with those seeking treatment for alcohol, tobacco, or even cannabis problems uncomplicated by heavy use of illicit drugs. In such cases, relatively brief periods of individual or group counseling can produce long-lasting reductions in drug use. The outcomes usually considered in programs dealing with illicit drugs have typically included measures of social functioning, employment, and criminal activity, as well as decreased drug-using behavior.

Treatment of Comorbidity—Integrated versus Concurrent

Treatment of the severely mentally ill (primarily those with schizophrenia and schizoaffective disorders) who are also drug dependent continues to pose problems for clinicians. Although some special facilities have been developed that use both antipsychotic drugs and therapeutic community principles, for the most part, specialized addiction agencies have difficulty treating these patients. Generally, integrated treatment in which the same staff can treat both the psychiatric disorder and the addiction is more effective than either parallel treatment (a mental health and a specialty addiction program providing care concurrently) or sequential treatment (treating either the addiction or the psychiatric disorder first and then dealing with the comorbid condition).

Services and Outcome

The extension of managed care into the public sector has produced a major reduction in the use of hospital-based detoxification and virtual disappearance of residential rehabilitation programs for alcoholics. Managed-care organizations, however, tend to assume that the relatively brief courses of outpatient counseling that are effective with private-sector alcoholic patients are also effective with patients who are dependent on illicit drugs and who have minimal social supports. For the present, the trend is to provide the care that costs least over the short term and to ignore studies showing that more services can produce better long-term outcomes.

Treatment is often a worthwhile social expenditure. For example, treatment of antisocial illicit drug users in outpatient settings can decrease antisocial behavior and reduce rates of human immunodeficiency virus (HIV) seroconversion that more than offset the treatment cost. Treatment in a prison setting can decrease postrelease costs associated with drug use and rearrests. Despite such evidence, problems exist in maintaining public support for treatment of substance dependence in both the public and private sectors. This lack of support suggests that these problems continue to be viewed, at least in part, as moral failings rather than as medical disorders.

ICD-10

The approach used in the 10th revision of *International Statistical Classification of Diseases and Related Health Problems* (ICD-10) differs somewhat from that in DSM-IV-TR. In the section titled "Mental and Behavioral Disorders Due to Psychoactive Substance Use," the term *psychoactive substance* refers to alcohol, opioids, cannabinoids, sedatives and hypnotics, cocaine, other stimulants such as caffeine, hallucinogens, tobacco, volatile solvents, multiple drugs, and other psychoactive substances. Thus, solvents are considered psychoactive, although their accidental ingestion is not mentioned. ICD-10 does not distinguish between legal and illegal substances but stipulates that the substances may or may not have been medically prescribed.

The disorders related to psychoactive substance use are described as mental and behavioral, with diagnostic guidelines provided for identifying the substance and for determining the specific nature of the disorder. When appropriate, references to other categories are given. For instance, under *psychotic disorder* in the substance use section, ICD-10 mentions schizophrenia, mood disorder, and paranoid or schizoid personality disorder as possible diagnoses for mental disorders "aggravated or precipitated by psychoactive substance use." In addition, ICD-10 includes a separate category for non–dependence-producing substances, including antidepressants, laxatives, analgesics, and vitamins, among others. DSM-IV-TR does not contain a similar category.

References

Anthony JC. Epidemiology of drug dependence. In: Galanter M, Kleber HD, eds. *Textbook of Substance Abuse Treatment*. 3rd ed. Washington, DC: The American Psychiatric Press, Inc.; 2003.

Farrell M, Howes S, Bebbington P, Brugha T, Jenkins R, Lewis G, Marsden J, Taylor C, Meltzer H. Nicotine, alcohol and drug dependence, and psychiatric comorbidity—Results of a national household survey. *International Review of Psychiatry*. 2003;15:50.

Farrell M, Howes S, Taylor C, Lewis G, Jenkins R, Bebbington P, Jarvis M, Brugha T, Gill B, Meltzer H. Substance misuse and psychiatric comorbidity: An overview of the OPCS National Psychiatric Morbidity Survey. *International Review Psychiatry*. 2003;15:43.

Hubbard RL, Craddock SG, Anderson J. Overview of 5-year follow-up outcomes in the Drug Abuse Treatment Outcome Studies (DATOS). *J Subst Abuse Treat*. 2003;25:125.

Humphreys K. *Circles of Recovery: Self-Help Organizations for Addictions*. Cambridge, UK: Cambridge University Press; 2004.

Jaffe JH. Substance-related disorders: introduction and overview. In: Sadock BJ, Sadock VA, eds. *Kaplan & Sadock's Comprehensive Textbook of Psychiatry*. 7th ed. Vol. 1. Baltimore: Lippincott Williams & Wilkins; 2000:924.

Jaffe JH, Anthony JC. Substance-related disorders: introduction and overview. In: Sadock BJ, Sadock VA, eds. *Kaplan & Sadock's Comprehensive Textbook of Psychiatry*. 8th ed. Vol. 1. Baltimore: Lippincott Williams & Wilkins; 2005:1137.

Jarvis TJ, Tebbutt J, Mattick RP, Shand F, Heather N. *Treatment Approaches for Alcohol and Drug Dependence : An Introductory Guide*. 2nd ed. Hoboken: John Wiley & Sons Inc.; 2005.

Johnston LD, O'Malley PM, Bachman JG. *Monitoring the Future National Results on Drug Use: Overview of Key Findings, 2002*. (NIH Publ. No. 03-5374). Bethesda, MD: National Institute on Drug Abuse; 2003.

Kendler KS, Jacobson KC, Prescott CA, Neale MC. Specificity of genetic and environmental risk factors for use and abuse/dependence of cannabis, cocaine, hallucinogens, sedatives, stimulants, and opiates in male twins. *Am J Psychiatry*. 2003;160:687.

McNiel DE, Binder RL, Robinson JC. Incarceration associated with homelessness, mental disorder, and co-occurring substance abuse. *Psychiatric Services*. 2005;56:840–846.

Pagnin D, de Queiroz V, Saggese EG. Predictors of attrition from day treatment of adolescents with substance-related disorders. *Addict Behav*. 2005;30:1065–1069.

Somers JM, Goldner EM, Waraich P, Hsu L. Prevalence studies of substance-related disorders: A systematic review of the literature. *Can J Psychiatry*. 2004;49.

Suelves JM. Preparing professionals to treat substance-related disorders. *PsychCRITIQUES*. 2005;50.

Weisner C, Matzger H, Kaskutas LA. How important is treatment? One-year outcomes of treated and untreated alcohol-dependent individuals. *Addiction*. 2003;98:901.

▲ 12.2 Alcohol-Related Disorders

Alcohol use disorders are common lethal conditions that often masquerade as other psychiatric syndromes. The average alcohol-dependent person decreases his or her life span by 10 to 15 years, and alcohol contributes to 22,000 deaths and 2 million nonfatal injuries each year. Recent years have witnessed a blossoming of clinically relevant research regarding alcohol abuse and dependence, including information on specific genetic influences, the clinical course of these conditions, and the development of new and helpful treatments.

An understanding of the effects of alcohol and the clinical importance of alcohol-related disorders is essential for the practice of psychiatry. Alcohol intoxication can cause irritability, violent behavior, feelings of depression, and, in rare instances, hallucinations and delusions. Long-term, escalating levels of alcohol consumption can produce tolerance as well as such intense adaptation of the body that cessation of use can precipitate a withdrawal syndrome usually marked by insomnia, evidence of hyperactivity of the autonomic nervous system, and feelings of anxiety. Thus, in an adequate evaluation of life problems and psychiatric symptoms in a patient, the clinician must consider the possibility that the clinical situation reflects the effects of alcohol.

Although alcohol abuse and dependency are commonly called alcoholism, the text revision of the fourth edition of the *Diagnostic and Statistical Manual of Mental Disorders* (DSM-IV-TR) does not use the term because it lacks a precise definition. The term remains in common use, however.

EPIDEMIOLOGY

Psychiatrists need to be concerned about alcoholism because this condition is common; intoxication and withdrawal mimic many major psychiatric disorders and the usual alcoholic person does not fit the common stereotype.

Prevalence of Drinking

At some time during life, 90 percent of the population in the United States drinks, with most people beginning their alcohol intake in the early to middle teens (Table 12.2–1). By the end of high school, 80 percent of students have consumed alcohol, and more than 60 percent have been intoxicated. At any time,

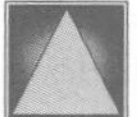

Table 12.2–1
Alcohol Epidemiology

Condition	Population (%)
Ever had a drink	90
Current drinker	60–70
Temporary problems	40+
Abuse[a]	Male: 10+ Female: 5+
Dependence[a]	Male: 10 Female: 3–5

[a]Twenty to 30 percent of psychiatric patients.

two of three men are drinkers, with a ratio of persisting alcohol intake of approximately 1.3 men to 1.0 women, and the highest prevalence of drinking is from the middle or late teens to the mid-20s.

Different groups in the United States have different rates of drinkers. Generally, groups with high education and high socioeconomic status have the highest proportion of people who currently imbibe. Among religious groups, Jews have the highest proportion of persons who consume alcohol, but the lowest number of people with alcohol dependence. Conservative Protestants and Catholics are less likely to use alcohol than liberal Protestants and Catholics. Other groups, such as the Irish, have higher rates of severe alcohol problems, but they also have significantly higher rates of abstention. Very high rates of alcohol problems are found among most, but not all, American Indian and Inuit tribes.

In the United States in the mid-1990s, the average person older than 14 years of age consumed 2.2 gallons of absolute alcohol a year. This amount sounds substantial, but it is considerably less than the more than 5 gallons of absolute ethanol consumed each year at the time of the American Revolution. The current figure also represents a significant decrease from the amounts consumed during the mid-1970s and the 2.7 gallons per capita in 1981.

Drinking alcohol-containing beverages is generally considered an acceptable and common habit in the United States. About 90 percent of all US residents have had an alcohol-containing drink at least once in their lives, and about 51 percent of all US adults are current users of alcohol. After heart disease and cancer, alcohol-related disorders constitute the third largest health problem in the United States today; beer accounts for about one half of all alcohol consumption, liquor for about one third, and wine for about one sixth. About 30 to 45 percent of all adults in the United States have had at least one transient episode of an alcohol-related problem, usually an alcohol-induced amnestic episode (e.g., a blackout), driving a motor vehicle while intoxicated, or missing school or work because of excessive drinking. About 10 percent of women and 20 percent of men have met the diagnostic criteria for alcohol abuse during their lifetimes, and 3 to 5 percent of women and 10 percent of men have met the diagnostic criteria for the more serious diagnosis of alcohol dependence during their lifetimes. About 200,000 deaths each year are directly related to alcohol abuse. The common causes of death among persons with the alcohol-related disorders are suicide, cancer, heart disease, and hepatic disease. Although persons involved in automotive fatalities do not always meet the diagnostic criteria for an alcohol-related disorder, drunken drivers are involved in about 50 percent of all automotive fatalities, and this percentage increases to about 75 percent when only accidents occurring in the late evening are considered. Alcohol use and alcohol-related disorders are also associated with about 50 percent of all homicides and 25 percent of all suicides. Alcohol abuse reduces life expectancy by about 10 years, and alcohol leads all other substances in substance-related deaths. Table 12.2–2 lists other epidemiological data about alcohol use.

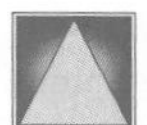

Table 12.2–2
Epidemiological Data for Alcohol-Related Disorders

Race and Ethnicity	▸ Whites have the highest rate of alcohol use ▸ Hispanics and blacks have similar rate of binge use, but is lower among blacks than among whites
Gender	▸ Men are much more likely than women to be binge drinkers and heavy drinkers
Region and Urbanicity	▸ Alcohol use is highest in western states and lowest in southern states ▸ North central and northeast regions are about the same ▸ The rate of past month alcohol use was 56 percent in large metropolitan areas, 52 percent in small metropolitan areas, and 46 percent in nonmetropolitan areas. ▸ Little variation seen in binge and heavy alcohol use rates by population density.
Education	▸ About 70 percent of adults with college degrees are current drinkers, compared with only 40 percent of those with less than a high school education. ▸ Binge alcohol use rates are similar across different levels of education.
Socioeconomic Class	▸ Alcohol-related disorders appear among persons of all socioeconomic classes. ▸ Persons who are stereotypical skid-row alcoholics constitute less than 5 percent of those with alcohol-related disorders.

COMORBIDITY

The psychiatric diagnoses most commonly associated with the alcohol-related disorders are other substance-related disorders, antisocial personality disorder, mood disorders, and anxiety disorders. Although the data are somewhat controversial, most suggest that persons with alcohol-related disorders have a markedly higher suicide rate than the general population.

Antisocial Personality Disorder

A relation between antisocial personality disorder and alcohol-related disorders has frequently been reported. Some studies suggest that antisocial personality disorder is particularly common in men with an alcohol-related disorder and can precede the development of the alcohol-related disorder. Other studies, however, suggest that antisocial personality disorder and alcohol-related disorders are completely distinct entities that are not causally related.

Mood Disorders

About 30 to 40 percent of persons with an alcohol-related disorder meet the diagnostic criteria for major depressive disorder sometime during their lifetimes. Depression is more common in women than in men with these disorders. Several studies reported that depression is likely to occur in patients with alcohol-related disorders who have a high daily consumption of alcohol and a family history of alcohol abuse. Persons with alcohol-related disorders and major depressive disorder are at great risk for attempting suicide and are likely to have other substance-related disorder diagnoses. Some clinicians recommend antidepressant drug therapy for depressive symptoms that remain after 2 to 3 weeks of sobriety. Patients with bipolar I disorder are thought to be at risk for developing an alcohol-related disorder; they may use alcohol to self-medicate their manic episodes. Some studies have shown that persons with both alcohol-related disorder and depressive disorder diagnoses have concentrations of dopamine metabolites (homovanillic acid) and γ-aminobutyric acid (GABA) in their cerebrospinal fluid (CSF).

Anxiety Disorders

Many persons use alcohol for its efficacy in alleviating anxiety. Although the comorbidity between alcohol-related disorders and mood disorders is fairly widely recognized, it is less well known that perhaps 25 to 50 percent of all persons with alcohol-related disorders also meet the diagnostic criteria for an anxiety disorder. Phobias and panic disorder are particularly frequent comorbid diagnoses in these patients. Some data indicate that alcohol may be used in an attempt to self-medicate symptoms of agoraphobia or social phobia, but an alcohol-related disorder is likely to precede the development of panic disorder or generalized anxiety disorder.

Suicide

Most estimates of the prevalence of suicide among persons with alcohol-related disorders range from 10 to 15 percent, although alcohol use itself may be involved in a much higher percentage of suicides. Some investigators have questioned whether the suicide rate among persons with alcohol-related disorders is as high as the numbers suggest. Factors that have been associated with suicide among persons with alcohol-related disorders include the presence of a major depressive episode, weak psychosocial support systems, a serious coexisting medical condition, unemployment, and living alone.

ETIOLOGY

Many factors affect the decision to drink, the development of temporary alcohol-related difficulties in the teenage years and the 20s, and the development of alcohol dependence. The initiation of alcohol intake probably depends largely on social, religious, and psychological factors, although genetic characteristics might also contribute. The factors that influence the decision to drink or those that contribute to temporary problems might differ, however, from those that add to the risk for the severe, recurring problems of alcohol dependence.

A similar interplay between genetic and environmental influences contributes to many medical and psychiatric conditions, and, thus, a review of these factors in alcoholism offers information about complex genetic disorders overall. Dominant or recessive genes, although important, only explain relatively rare conditions. Most disorders have some level of genetic predisposition that usually relates to a series of different genetically influenced characteristics, each of which increases or decreases the risk for the disorder.

It is likely that a series of genetic influences combine to explain approximately 60 percent of the proportion of risk for alcoholism, with environment responsible for the remaining proportion of the variance. The divisions offered in this section, therefore, are more heuristic than real, because it is the combination of a series of psychological, sociocultural, biological, and other factors that are responsible for the development of severe, repetitive alcohol-related life problems.

Psychological Theories

A variety of theories relate to the use of alcohol to reduce tension, increase feelings of power, and decrease the effects of psychological pain. Perhaps the greatest interest has been paid to the observation that people with alcohol-related problems often report that alcohol decreases their feelings of nervousness and helps them cope with the day-to-day stresses of life. The psychological theories are built, in part, on the observation among nonalcoholic people that the intake of low doses of alcohol in a tense social setting or after a difficult day can be associated with an enhanced feeling of well-being and an improved ease of interactions. In high doses, especially at falling blood alcohol levels, however, most measures of muscle tension and psychological feelings of nervousness and tension are increased. Thus, tension-reducing effects of this drug might have an impact most on light to moderate drinkers or add to the relief of withdrawal symptoms, but play a minor role in causing alcoholism. The theories that focus on alcohol's potential to enhance feelings of being powerful and sexually attractive and to decrease the effects of psychological pain are difficult to evaluate definitively.

Psychodynamic Theories

Perhaps related to the disinhibiting or anxiety-lowering effects of lower doses of alcohol is the hypothesis that some people may use this drug to help them deal with self-punitive harsh superegos and to decrease unconscious stress levels. Also, classic psychoanalytical theory hypothesizes that at least some alcoholic people may have become fixated at the oral stage of development and use alcohol to relieve their frustrations by taking the substance by mouth. Hypotheses regarding arrested phases of psychosexual development, although heuristically useful, have had little effect on the usual treatment approaches and are not the focus of extensive ongoing research. Similarly, most studies have not been able to document an "addictive personality" present in most alcoholics and associated with a propensity to lack control of intake of a wide range of substances and foods. Although pathological scores on personality tests are often seen during intoxication, withdrawal, and early recovery, many of these characteristics are not found to predate alcoholism, and most disappear with abstinence. Similarly, prospective studies of children of alcoholics who themselves have no co-occurring disorders usually document high risks mostly for alcoholism. As will be described below, one partial exception to these comments occurs with the extreme levels of impulsivity seen in the 15 to 20 percent of alcoholic men with antisocial personality disorder, because they have high risks for criminality, violence, and multiple substance dependencies.

Behavioral Theories

Expectations about the rewarding effects of drinking, cognitive attitudes toward responsibility for one's behavior, and subsequent reinforcement after alcohol intake all contribute to the decision to drink again after the first experience with alcohol and to continue to imbibe despite problems. These issues are important in efforts to modify drinking behaviors in the general population, and they contribute to some important aspects of alcoholic rehabilitation.

Sociocultural Theories

Sociocultural theories are often based on extrapolations from social groups that have high and low rates of alcoholism.

Theorists hypothesize that ethnic groups, such as Jews, who introduce children to modest levels of drinking in a family atmosphere and eschew drunkenness have low rates of alcoholism. Some other groups, such as Irish men or some American Indian tribes with high rates of abstention but a tradition of drinking to the point of drunkenness among drinkers, are believed to have high rates of alcoholism. These theories, however, often depend on stereotypes that tend to be erroneous, and prominent exceptions to these rules exist. For example, some theories based on observations of the Irish and the French have incorrectly predicted high rates of alcoholism among the Italians.

Yet, environmental events, presumably including cultural factors, account for as much as 40 percent of the alcoholism risk. Thus, although these are difficult to study, it is likely that cultural attitudes toward drinking, drunkenness, and personal responsibility for consequences are important contributors to the rates of alcohol-related problems in a society. In the final analysis, social and psychological theories are probably highly relevant, because they outline factors that contribute to the onset of drinking, the development of temporary alcohol-related life difficulties, and even alcoholism. The problem is how to gather relatively definitive data to support or refute the theories.

Childhood History

Researchers have identified several factors in the childhood histories of persons with later alcohol-related disorders and in children at high risk for having an alcohol-related disorder because one or both of their parents are affected. In experimental studies, children at high risk for alcohol-related disorders have been found to possess, on average, a range of deficits on neurocognitive testing, low amplitude of the P300 wave on evoked potential testing, and a variety of abnormalities on electroencephalogram (EEG) recordings. Studies of high-risk offspring in their 20s have also shown a generally blunted effect of alcohol compared with that seen in persons whose parents have not been diagnosed with alcohol-related disorder. These findings suggest that a heritable biological brain function may predispose a person to an alcohol-related disorder. A childhood history of attention-deficit/hyperactivity disorder, conduct disorder, or both, increases a child's risk for an alcohol-related disorder as an adult. Personality disorders, especially antisocial personality disorder, as noted above, also predispose a person to an alcohol-related disorder.

Genetic Theories

Importance of Genetic Influences. Four lines of evidence support the conclusion that alcoholism is genetically influenced. First, a three- to fourfold increased risk for severe alcohol problems is seen in close relatives of alcoholic people. The rate of alcohol problems increases with the number of alcoholic relatives, the severity of their illness, and the closeness of their genetic relationship to the person under study. The family investigations do little to separate the importance of genetics and environment, and the second approach, twin studies, takes the data a step further. The rate of similarity, or concordance, for severe alcohol-related problems is significantly higher in identical twins of alcoholic individuals than in fraternal twins in most investigations, which estimate that genes explain 60 percent of the variance, with the remainder relating to nonshared, probably adult environmental influences. Third, the adoption-type studies have all revealed a significantly enhanced risk for alcoholism in the offspring of alcoholic parents, even when the children had been separated from their biological parents close to birth and raised without any knowledge of the problems within the biological family. The risk for severe alcohol-related difficulties is not further enhanced by being raised by an alcoholic adoptive family. Finally, studies in animals support the importance of a variety of yet-to-be-identified genes in the free-choice use of alcohol, subsequent levels of intoxication, and some consequences.

EFFECTS OF ALCOHOL

The term *alcohol* refers to a large group of organic molecules that have a hydroxyl group (-OH) attached to a saturated carbon atom. Ethyl alcohol, also called *ethanol*, is the common form of alcohol; sometimes referred to as *beverage alcohol*, ethyl alcohol is used for drinking. The chemical formula for ethanol is CH_3-CH_2-OH.

The characteristic tastes and flavors of alcohol-containing beverages result from their methods of production, which produce various congeners in the final product, including methanol, butanol, aldehydes, phenols, tannins, and trace amounts of various metals. Although the congeners may confer some differential psychoactive effects on the various alcohol-containing beverages, these differences are minimal compared with the effects of ethanol itself. A single drink is usually considered to contain about 12 g of ethanol, which is the content of 12 ounces of beer (7.2 proof, 3.6 percent ethanol in the United States), one 4-ounce glass of nonfortified wine, or 1 to 1.5 ounces of an 80-proof (40 percent ethanol) liquor (e.g., whiskey or gin). In calculating patients' alcohol intake, however, clinicians should be aware that beers vary in their alcohol content, that beers are available in small and large cans and mugs, that glasses of wine range from 2 to 6 ounces, and that mixed drinks at some bars and in most homes contain 2 to 3 ounces of liquor. Nonetheless, using the moderate sizes of drinks, clinicians can estimate that a single drink increases the blood alcohol level of a 150-pound man by 15 to 20 mg/dL, which is about the concentration of alcohol that an average person can metabolize in 1 hour.

The possible beneficial effects of alcohol have been publicized, especially by the makers and the distributors of alcohol. Most attention has been focused on some epidemiological data that suggest that one or two glasses of red wine each day lower the incidence of cardiovascular disease; these findings, however, are highly controversial.

Absorption

About 10 percent of consumed alcohol is absorbed from the stomach, the remainder from the small intestine. Peak blood concentration of alcohol is reached in 30 to 90 minutes and usually in 45 to 60 minutes, depending on whether the alcohol was taken on an empty stomach (which enhances absorption) or with food (which delays absorption). The time to peak blood concentration also depends on the time during which the alcohol was consumed; rapid drinking reduces the time to peak concentration, slower drinking increases it. Absorption is most rapid with beverages containing 15 to 30 percent alcohol (30 to 60 proof). There is some dispute about whether carbonation (e.g., in champagne and in drinks mixed with seltzer) enhances the absorption of alcohol.

The body has protective devices against inundation by alcohol. For example, if the concentration of alcohol in the stomach becomes too high, mucus is secreted, and the pyloric valve closes. These actions slow the absorption and keep the alcohol from passing into the small intestine, where there are no significant restraints to absorption. Thus, a large amount of alcohol can remain unabsorbed in the stomach for hours. Furthermore, pylorospasm often results in nausea and vomiting.

Once alcohol is absorbed into the bloodstream, it is distributed to all body tissues. Because alcohol is uniformly dissolved in the body's water, tissues containing a high proportion of water receive a high concentration of alcohol. The intoxicating effects are greater when the blood alcohol concentration is rising than when it is falling (the Mellanby effects). For this reason, the rate of absorption bears directly on the intoxication response.

Metabolism

About 90 percent of absorbed alcohol is metabolized through oxidation in the liver; the remaining 10 percent is excreted unchanged by the kidneys and lungs. The rate of oxidation by the liver is constant and independent of the body's energy requirements. The body can metabolize about 15 mg/dL per hour, with a range of 10 to 34 mg/dL per hour. That is, the average person oxidizes three fourths of an ounce of 40 percent (80 proof) alcohol in an hour. In persons with a history of excessive alcohol consumption, upregulation of the necessary enzymes results in rapid alcohol metabolism.

Alcohol is metabolized by two enzymes: alcohol dehydrogenase (ADH) and aldehyde dehydrogenase. ADH catalyzes the conversion of alcohol into acetaldehyde, which is a toxic compound; aldehyde dehydrogenase catalyzes the conversion of acetaldehyde into acetic acid. Aldehyde dehydrogenase is inhibited by disulfiram (Antabuse), often used in the treatment of alcohol-related disorders. Some studies have shown that women have a lower ADH blood content than men; this fact may account for woman's tendency to become more intoxicated than men after drinking the same amount of alcohol. The decreased function of alcohol-metabolizing enzymes in some Asian persons can also lead to easy intoxication and toxic symptoms.

Effects on the Brain

Biochemistry. In contrast to most other substances of abuse with identified receptor targets—such as the N-methyl-d-aspartate (NMDA) receptor of phencyclidine (PCP)—no single molecular target has been identified as the mediator for the effects of alcohol. The long-standing theory about the biochemical effects of alcohol concerns its effects on the membranes of neurons. Data support the hypothesis that alcohol produces its effects by intercalating itself into membranes and, thus, increasing fluidity of the membranes with short-term use. With long-term use, however, the theory hypothesizes that the membranes become rigid or stiff. The fluidity of the membranes is critical to normal functioning of receptors, ion channels, and other membrane-bound functional proteins. In recent studies, researchers have attempted to identify specific molecular targets for the effects of alcohol. Most attention has been focused on the effects of alcohol at ion channels. Specifically, studies have found that alcohol ion channel activities associated with the nicotinic acetylcholine, serotonin 5-hydroxytryptamine3 (5-HT_3,) and GABA type A ($GABA_A$) receptors are enhanced by alcohol, whereas ion channel activities associated with glutamate receptors and voltage-gated calcium channels are inhibited.

Behavioral Effects. As the net result of the molecular activities, alcohol functions as a depressant much as do the barbiturates and the benzodiazepines, with which alcohol has some cross-tolerance and cross-dependence. At a level of 0.05 percent alcohol in the blood, thought, judgment, and restraint are loosened and sometimes disrupted. At a concentration of 0.1 percent, voluntary motor actions usually become perceptibly clumsy. In most states, legal intoxication ranges from 0.1 to 0.15 percent blood alcohol level. At 0.2 percent, the function of the entire motor area of the brain is measurably depressed, and the parts of the brain that control emotional behavior are also affected. At 0.3 percent, a person is commonly confused or may become stuporous; at 0.4 to 0.5 percent, the person falls into a coma. At higher levels, the primitive centers of the brain that control breathing and heart rate are affected, and death ensues secondary to direct respiratory depression or the aspiration of vomitus. Persons with long-term histories of alcohol abuse, however, can tolerate much higher concentrations of alcohol than can alcohol-naïve persons; their alcohol tolerance may cause them to falsely appear less intoxicated than they really are.

Sleep Effects. Although alcohol consumed in the evening usually increases the ease of falling asleep (decreased sleep latency), alcohol also has adverse effects on sleep architecture. Specifically, alcohol use is associated with a decrease in rapid eye movement sleep (REM or dream sleep) and deep sleep (stage 4) and more sleep fragmentation, with more and longer episodes of awakening. Therefore, the idea that drinking alcohol helps persons fall asleep is a myth.

Other Physiological Effects

Liver. The major adverse effects of alcohol use are related to liver damage. Alcohol use, even as short as week-long episodes of increased drinking, can result in an accumulation of fats and proteins, which produce the appearance of a fatty liver, sometimes found on physical examination as an enlarged liver. The association between fatty infiltration of the liver and serious liver damage remains unclear. Alcohol use, however, is associated with the development of alcoholic hepatitis and hepatic cirrhosis.

Gastrointestinal System. Long-term heavy drinking is associated with developing esophagitis, gastritis, achlorhydria, and gastric ulcers. The development of esophageal varices can accompany particularly heavy alcohol abuse; the rupture of the varices is a medical emergency often resulting in death by exsanguination. Disorders of the small intestine occasionally occur, and pancreatitis, pancreatic insufficiency, and pancreatic cancer are also associated with heavy alcohol use. Heavy alcohol intake can interfere with the normal processes of food digestion and absorption; as a result, consumed food is inadequately digested. Alcohol abuse also appears to inhibit the intestine's capacity to absorb various nutrients, such as vitamins and amino acids. This effect, coupled with the often poor dietary habits of those with alcohol-related disorders, can cause serious vitamin deficiencies, particularly of the B vitamins.

Other Bodily Systems. Significant intake of alcohol has been associated with increased blood pressure, dysregulation of lipoprotein and triglyceride metabolism, and increased risk for myocardial infarctions and cerebrovascular diseases. Alcohol has been shown to affect the hearts of nonalcoholic persons who do not usually drink, increasing the resting cardiac output, the heart rate, and the myocardial oxygen consumption. Evidence indicates that alcohol intake can adversely affect the hematopoietic system and can increase the incidence of cancer, particularly head, neck, esophageal, stomach, hepatic, colonic, and lung cancer. Acute intoxication may also be associated with hypoglycemia, which, when unrecognized, may be responsible for some of the sudden deaths of persons who are intoxicated. Muscle weakness is another side effect of alcoholism. Recent evidence shows that alcohol intake raises the blood concentration of estradiol in women. The increase in estradiol correlates with the blood alcohol level.

Laboratory Tests. The adverse effects of alcohol appear in common laboratory tests, which can be useful diagnostic aids in identifying persons with alcohol-related disorders. The γ-glutamyl transpeptidase levels are high in about 80 percent of those with alcohol-related disorders, and the mean corpuscular volume (MCV) is high in about 60 percent, more so in women than in men. Other laboratory test values that may be high in association with alcohol abuse are those of uric acid, triglycerides, aspartate aminotransferase (AST), and alanine aminotransferase (ALT).

Drug Interactions

The interaction between alcohol and other substances can be dangerous, even fatal. Certain substances, such as alcohol and phenobarbital (Luminal), are metabolized by the liver, and their prolonged use can lead to acceleration of their metabolism. When persons with alcohol-related disorders are sober, this accelerated metabolism makes them unusually tolerant to many drugs such as sedatives and hypnotics; when they are intoxicated, however, these drugs compete with the alcohol for the same detoxification mechanisms, and potentially toxic concentrations of all involved substances can accumulate in the blood.

The effects of alcohol and other central nervous system (CNS) depressants are usually synergistic. Sedatives, hypnotics, and drugs that relieve pain, motion sickness, head colds, and allergy symptoms must be used with caution by persons with alcohol-related disorders. Narcotics depress the sensory areas of the cerebral cortex and can produce pain relief, sedation, apathy, drowsiness, and sleep; high doses can result in respiratory failure and death. Increasing the dosages of sedative-hypnotic drugs, such as chloral hydrate (Noctec) and benzodiazepines, especially when they are combined with alcohol, produces a range of effects from sedation to motor and intellectual impairment to stupor, coma, and death. Because sedatives and other psychotropic drugs can potentiate the effects of alcohol, patients should be instructed about the dangers of combining CNS depressants and alcohol, particularly when they are driving or operating machinery.

DISORDERS

The DSM-IV-TR lists the alcohol-related disorders (Table 12.2–3) and specifies the diagnostic criteria for alcohol intoxication (Table 12.2–4) and alcohol withdrawal (Table 12.2–5). The diagnostic criteria for the other alcohol-related disorders are listed in DSM-IV-TR under the major symptom. For example, the diagnostic criteria for alcohol-induced anxiety disorder are found in the anxiety disorders category, under the heading "Substance-Induced Anxiety Disorder."

Alcohol Dependence and Alcohol Abuse

Diagnosis and Clinical Features. In DSM-IV-TR, all substance-related disorders use the same criteria for dependence and abuse (*see* Tables 12.1–3 and 12.1–4). A need for daily use of large amounts of alcohol for adequate functioning, a regular pattern of heavy drinking limited to weekends, and long periods of sobriety interspersed with binges of heavy alcohol intake lasting for weeks or months strongly suggest alcohol dependence and alcohol abuse. The drinking patterns are often associated with certain behaviors: the inability to cut down or stop

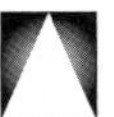

Table 12.2–3
DSM-IV-TR Alcohol-Related Disorders

Alcohol use disorders
Alcohol dependence
Alcohol abuse
Alcohol-induced disorders
Alcohol intoxication
Alcohol withdrawal
Specify if:
With perceptual disturbances
Alcohol intoxication delirium
Alcohol withdrawal delirium
Alcohol-induced persisting dementia
Alcohol-induced persisting amnestic disorder
Alcohol-induced psychotic disorder, with delusions
Specify if:
With onset during intoxication
With onset during withdrawal
Alcohol-induced psychotic disorder, with hallucinations
Specify if:
With onset during intoxication
With onset during withdrawal
Alcohol-induced mood disorder
Specify if:
With onset during intoxication
With onset during withdrawal
Alcohol-induced anxiety disorder
Specify if:
With onset during intoxication
With onset during withdrawal
Alcohol-induced sexual dysfunction
Specify if:
With onset during intoxication
Alcohol-induced sleep disorder
Specify if:
With onset during intoxication
With onset during withdrawal
Alcohol disorder not otherwise specified

(From American Psychiatric Association. *Diagnostic and Statistical Manual of Mental Disorders.* 4th ed. Text rev. Washington, DC: American Psychiatric Association; copyright 2000, with permission.)

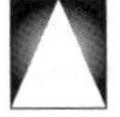

Table 12.2–4
DSM-IV-TR Diagnostic Criteria for Alcohol Intoxication

A. Recent ingestion of alcohol.
B. Clinically significant maladaptive behavioral or psychological changes (e.g., inappropriate sexual or aggressive behavior, mood lability, impaired judgment, impaired social or occupational functioning) that developed during, or shortly after, alcohol ingestion.
C. One (or more) of the following signs, developing during, or shortly after, alcohol use:
(1) slurred speech
(2) incoordination
(3) unsteady gait
(4) nystagmus
(5) impairment in attention or memory
(6) stupor or coma
D. The symptoms are not due to a general medical condition and are not better accounted for by another mental disorder.

(From American Psychiatric Association. *Diagnostic and Statistical Manual of Mental Disorders.* 4th ed. Text rev. Washington, DC: American Psychiatric Association; copyright 2000, with permission.)

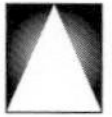

Table 12.2–5
DSM-IV-TR Diagnostic Criteria for Alcohol Withdrawal

A. Cessation of (or reduction in) alcohol use that has been heavy and prolonged.
B. Two (or more) of the following, developing within several hours to a few days after Criterion A:
   (1) autonomic hyperactivity (e.g., sweating or pulse rate greater than 100)
   (2) increased hand tremor
   (3) insomnia
   (4) nausea or vomiting
   (5) transient visual, tactile, or auditory hallucinations or illusions
   (6) psychomotor agitation
   (7) anxiety
   (8) grand mal seizures
C. The symptoms in Criterion B cause clinically significant distress or impairment in social, occupational, or other important areas of functioning.
D. The symptoms are not due to a general medical condition and are not better accounted for by another mental disorder.

Specify if:
With perceptual disturbances

(From American Psychiatric Association. *Diagnostic and Statistical Manual of Mental Disorders.* 4th ed. Text rev. Washington, DC: American Psychiatric Association; copyright 2000, with permission.)

drinking; repeated efforts to control or reduce excessive drinking by "going on the wagon" (periods of temporary abstinence) or by restricting drinking to certain times of the day; binges (remaining intoxicated throughout the day for at least 2 days); occasional consumption of a fifth of spirits (or its equivalent in wine or beer); amnestic periods for events occurring while intoxicated (blackouts); the continuation of drinking despite a serious physical disorder that the person knows is exacerbated by alcohol use; and drinking nonbeverage alcohol, such as fuel and commercial products containing alcohol. In addition, persons with alcohol dependence and alcohol abuse show impaired social or occupational functioning because of alcohol use (e.g., violence while intoxicated, absence from work, job loss), legal difficulties (e.g., arrest for intoxicated behavior and traffic accidents while intoxicated), and arguments or difficulties with family members or friends about excessive alcohol consumption. According to DSM-IV-TR, the current rate of alcohol dependence is 5 percent.

A 39-year-old prominent businessman, Mr. G, was referred for evaluation by a clinician who was concerned that he was making little progress with the patient's mood swings and somatic complaints. Therapy, primarily using a cognitive and behavioral approach, had been instituted 6 months previously for a condition that involved depressive symptoms and irritability present most, but not all, days for the prior several years. Mr. G had recently had a routine physical examination at work and was noted to have mild hypertension (blood pressure of 145/95) along with a blood test that revealed an MCV of 92.5 μm^3 and a γ-glutamyltransferase level of 43 U/L.

On interview, the patient admitted that his wife had been complaining for several years about his drinking pattern of one to two bottles of wine (i.e., 6 to 12 standard drinks) per day. She noted that the mornings after drinking he was more irritable than usual, and she complained about his restless sleep. Mr. G had recognized potential problems and tried on several occasions to cut back on his drinking. These efforts usually resulted in periods of abstinence of between 2 and 4 weeks, followed by several months of establishing clear rules that set limits on his intake that always gave way to increased drinking as part of a celebration, business trip, vacation, or in the context of daily stresses. Mr. G noted that once ad-lib drinking began, he slowly increased the amount consumed per day to maintain the desired effects. He denied ever experiencing full-blown alcohol withdrawal, although he did report "hangovers" lasting 6 to 12 hours but rarely going into the second day. (Courtesy of Marc A. Schuckit, M.D.)

Subtypes of Alcohol Dependence. Various researchers have attempted to divide alcohol dependence into subtypes based primarily on phenomenological characteristics. One recent classification notes that type A alcohol dependence is characterized by late onset, few childhood risk factors, relatively mild dependence, few alcohol-related problems, and little psychopathology. Type B alcohol dependence is characterized by many childhood risk factors, severe dependence, an early onset of alcohol-related problems, much psychopathology, a strong family history of alcohol abuse, frequent polysubstance abuse, a long history of alcohol treatment, and a lot of severe life stresses. Some researchers have found that type A persons who are alcohol dependent may respond to interactional psychotherapies, whereas type B persons who are alcohol dependent may respond to training in coping skills.

Other subtyping schemes of alcohol dependence have received fairly wide recognition in the literature. One group of investigators proposed three subtypes: early-stage problem drinkers, who do not yet have complete alcohol dependence syndromes; affiliative drinkers, who tend to drink daily in moderate amounts in social settings; and schizoid-isolated drinkers, who have severe dependence and tend to drink in binges and often alone.

Another investigator described gamma alcohol dependence, which is thought to be common in the United States and represents the alcohol dependence seen in those who are active in Alcoholics Anonymous (AA). This variant concerns control problems in which persons are unable to stop drinking once they start. When drinking is terminated as a result of ill health or lack of money, these persons can abstain for varying periods. In delta alcohol dependence, perhaps more common in Europe than in the United States, persons who are alcohol dependent must drink a certain amount each day but are unaware of a lack of control. The alcohol use disorder may not be discovered until a person who must stop drinking for some reason exhibits withdrawal symptoms.

Another researcher has suggested a *type I, male-limited* variety of alcohol dependence, characterized by late onset, more evidence of psychological than of physical dependence, and the presence of guilt feelings. *Type II, male-limited* alcohol dependence is characterized by onset at an early age, spontaneous seeking of alcohol for consumption, and a socially disruptive set of behaviors when intoxicated.

Four subtypes of alcoholism were postulated by still another investigator. The first is *antisocial alcoholism*, typically with a predominance in men, a poor prognosis, early onset of alcohol-related problems, and a close association with antisocial personality disorder. The second is *developmentally cumulative alcoholism*, with a primary tendency for alcohol abuse that is exacerbated with time as cultural expectations foster increased opportunities to drink. The third is *negative-affect alcoholism*, which is more common in women than in men; according to this hypothesis, women are likely to use alcohol for mood regulation and to help ease social relationships. The fourth is *developmentally limited alcoholism*, with frequent bouts of consuming large amounts of alcohol; the bouts become less frequent as persons age and respond to the increased expectations of society about their jobs and families.

Alcohol Intoxication

The DSM-IV-TR diagnostic criteria for alcohol intoxication are based on evidence of recent ingestion of ethanol, maladaptive behavior, and at least one of six possible physiological correlates of intoxication (Table 12.2–3). The tenth revision of the *International Statistical Classification of Diseases and Related Health Problems* (ICD-10) criteria for acute alcohol intoxication are generally similar to DSM-IV-TR, listing seven physiological signs of intoxication, some of which, such as conjunctival injection, are not seen in DSM-IV-TR.

As a conservative approach to identifying blood levels that are likely to have major effects on driving abilities, the legal definition of intoxication in most states in the United States requires a blood concentration of 80 or 100 mg ethanol per deciliter of blood (mg/dL), which is the same as 0.08 to 0.10 g/dL. For most people, a rough estimate of the levels of impairment likely to be seen at various blood alcohol concentrations can be outlined. Evidence of behavioral changes, a slowing in motor performance, and a decrease in the ability to think clearly occurs at doses as low as 20 to 30 mg/dL, as shown in Table 12.2–6. Blood concentrations between 100 and 200 mg/dL are likely to increase the impairment in coordination and judgment to severe problems with coordination (ataxia), increasing lability of mood, and progressively greater levels of cognitive deterioration. Anyone who does not show significant levels of impairment in motor and mental performance at approximately 150 mg/dL probably has significant pharmacodynamic tolerance. In that range, most people without significant tolerance also experience relatively severe nausea and vomiting. With blood alcohol concentrations in the 200 to 300 mg/dL range, the slurring of speech is likely to become more intense, and memory impairment (*anterograde amnesia* or *alcoholic blackouts*) becomes pronounced. Further increases in blood alcohol concentration result in the first level of anesthesia, and the nontolerant person who reaches 400 mg/dL or more risks respiratory failure, coma, and death.

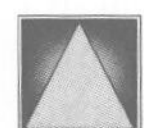

Table 12.2–6
Impairment Likely to be Seen at Different Blood Alcohol Concentrations

Level	Likely Impairment
20–30 mg/dL	Slowed motor performance and decreased thinking ability
30–80 mg/dL	Increases in motor and cognitive problems
80–200 mg/dL	Increases in incoordination and judgment errors Mood lability Deterioration in cognition
200–300 mg/dL	Nystagmus, marked slurring of speech, and alcoholic blackouts
>300 mg/dL	Impaired vital signs and possible death

Alcohol Withdrawal

Alcohol withdrawal, even without delirium, can be serious; it can include seizures and autonomic hyperactivity. Conditions that may predispose to, or aggravate, withdrawal symptoms include fatigue, malnutrition, physical illness, and depression. The DSM-IV-TR criteria for alcohol withdrawal (Table 12.2–5) require the cessation or reduction of alcohol use that was heavy and prolonged as well as the presence of specific physical or neuropsychiatric symptoms. The diagnosis also allows for the specification "with perceptual disturbances." One recent positron emission tomographic (PET) study of blood flow during alcohol withdrawal in otherwise healthy persons with alcohol dependence reported a globally low rate of metabolic activity (Fig. 12.2–1), although, with further inspection of the data, the authors concluded that activity was especially low in the left parietal and right frontal areas.

The classic sign of alcohol withdrawal is tremulousness, although the spectrum of symptoms can expand to include psychotic and perceptual symptoms (e.g., delusions and hallucinations), seizures, and the symptoms of delirium tremens (DTs), called alcohol withdrawal delirium in DSM-IV-TR. Tremulousness (commonly called the "shakes" or the "jitters") develops 6 to 8 hours after the cessation of drinking, the psychotic and perceptual symptoms begin in 8 to 12 hours, seizures in 12 to 24 hours, and DTs during 72 hours, although physicians should watch for the development of DTs for the first week of withdrawal. The syndrome of withdrawal sometimes skips the usual progression and, for example, goes directly to DTs.

The tremor of alcohol withdrawal can be similar to either physiological tremor, with a continuous tremor of great amplitude and of more than 8 Hz, or familial tremor, with bursts of tremor activity slower than 8 Hz. Other symptoms of withdrawal include general irritability, gastrointestinal symptoms (e.g., nausea and vomiting), and sympathetic autonomic hyperactivity, including anxiety, arousal, sweating, facial flushing, mydriasis, tachycardia, and mild hypertension. Patients experiencing alcohol withdrawal are generally alert but may startle easily.

Mr. T is a 64-year-old lawyer with a 35-year history of alcohol dependence. Alcohol-related problems have included tolerance, spending a great deal of time using alcohol (despite a relatively successful career), repeatedly giving up important business and family events because he was too intoxicated or hung over, and significant interference with his relationship with his wife. She complained about his sarcastic wit and lack of care about her areas of interest while drinking heavily.

Mr. T had been able to stop drinking on multiple occasions in the past, at which times he experienced a tremor, anxiety, and problems sleeping. He typically self-medicated these symptoms with five or more 10-mg capsules of chlordiazepoxide per day, using pills that had been prescribed for him by his general practitioner in response to his complaints of anxiety and insomnia. Recently, Mr. T was

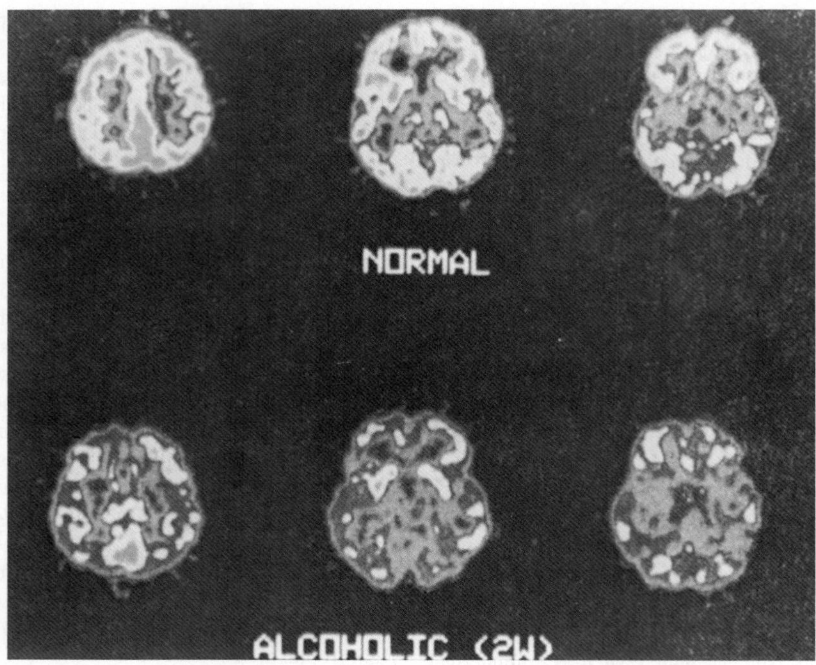

FIGURE 12.2–1

Brain PET metabolic images in a normal control subject and an alcoholic subject tested 2 weeks after the last use of alcohol. Notice the decreased cortical metabolic activity in the alcoholic person. (From Volkow ND, Hitzemann R, Wang G-J, et al. Decreased brain metabolism in neurologically intact healthy alcoholics. *Am J Psychiatry.* 1992;149:1019, with permission.)

diagnosed with moderate hypertension and adult-onset diabetes, with the result that his family practitioner urged him to stop drinking. In recognition of his age and his associated medical problems, it was believed that withdrawal would be best treated in a medical setting.

An examination confirmed the medical diagnoses along with a mildly decreased hematocrit (38 percent). The evaluation, carried out approximately 12 hours after his most recent drink, also revealed the smell of alcohol remaining on his breath, with a blood alcohol level of 50 mg/dL. The patient demonstrated a prominent tremor of both hands along with a pulse of 110 beats per minute, a respiratory rate of 25 breaths per minute, and a blood pressure of 150/96. Mr. T complained of feeling agitated, noted that he felt very tired but was unable to sleep, but was otherwise alert and oriented. (Courtesy of Marc A. Schuckit, M.D.)

Withdrawal Seizures. Seizures associated with alcohol withdrawal are stereotyped, generalized, and tonic-clonic in character. Patients often have more than one seizure 3 to 6 hours after the first seizure. Status epilepticus is relatively rare and occurs in less than 3 percent of patients. Although anticonvulsant medications are not required in the management of alcohol withdrawal seizures, the cause of the seizures is difficult to establish when a patient is first assessed in the emergency room; thus, many patients with withdrawal seizures receive anticonvulsant medications, which are then discontinued once the cause of the seizures is recognized. Seizure activity in patients with known alcohol abuse histories should still prompt clinicians to consider other causative factors, such as head injuries, CNS infections, CNS neoplasms, and other cerebrovascular diseases; long-term severe alcohol abuse can result in hypoglycemia, hyponatremia, and hypomagnesaemia—all of which can also be associated with seizures.

Treatment. The primary medications to control alcohol withdrawal symptoms are the benzodiazepines (Table 12.2–7). Many studies have found that benzodiazepines help control seizure activity, delirium, anxiety, tachycardia, hypertension, diaphoresis, and tremor associated with alcohol withdrawal. Benzodiazepines can be given either orally or parenterally; neither diazepam (Valium) nor chlordiazepoxide (Librium), however, should be given intramuscularly (IM) because of their erratic absorption by this route. Clinicians must titrate the dosage of the benzodiazepine, starting with a high dosage and lowering the dosage as the patient recovers. Sufficient benzodiazepines should be given to keep patients calm and sedated but not so sedated that they cannot be aroused for clinicians to perform appropriate procedures, including neurological examinations.

Although benzodiazepines are the standard treatment for alcohol withdrawal, studies have shown that carbamazepine (Tegretol) in daily doses of 800 mg is as effective as benzodiazepines and has the added benefit of minimal abuse liability. Carbamazepine use is gradually becoming common in the United States and Europe. The β-adrenergic receptor antagonists and clonidine (Catapres) have also been used to block the symptoms of sympathetic hyperactivity, but neither drug is an effective treatment for seizures or delirium.

Delirium

Diagnosis and Clinical Features. The DSM-IV-TR contains the diagnostic criteria for alcohol intoxication delirium in

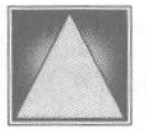

Table 12.2–7
Drug Therapy for Alcohol Intoxication and Withdrawal

Clinical Problem	Drug	Route	Dosage	Comment
Tremulousness and mild to moderate agitation	Chlordiazepoxide	Oral	25–100 mg every 4–6 hr	Initial dose can be repeated every 2 hr until patient is calm; subsequent doses must be individualized and titrated
	Diazepam	Oral	5–20 mg every 4–6 hr	
Hallucinosis	Lorazepam	Oral	2–10 mg every 4–6 hr	
Extreme agitation	Chlordiazepoxide	Intravenous	0.5 mg/kg at 12.5 mg/min	Give until patient is calm; subsequent doses must be individualized and titrated
Withdrawal seizures	Diazepam	Intravenous	0.15 mg/kg at 2.5 mg/min	
Delirium tremens	Lorazepam	Intravenous	0.1 mg/kg at 2.0 mg/min	

(Adapted from Koch-Weser J, Sellers EM, Kalant J. Alcohol intoxication and withdrawal. *N Engl J Med.* 1976;294:757.)

the category of substance intoxication delirium and the diagnostic criteria for alcohol withdrawal delirium in the category of substance withdrawal delirium (*see* Tables 10.2–6 and 10.2–7 in Chapter 10, Section 10.2). Patients with recognized alcohol withdrawal symptoms should be carefully monitored to prevent progression to alcohol withdrawal delirium, the most severe form of the withdrawal syndrome, also known as DTs. Alcohol withdrawal delirium is a medical emergency that can result in significant morbidity and mortality. Patients with delirium are a danger to themselves and to others. Because of the unpredictability of their behavior, patients with delirium may be assaultive or suicidal or may act on hallucinations or delusional thoughts as if they were genuine dangers. Untreated, DTs has a mortality rate of 20 percent, usually as a result of an intercurrent medical illness such as pneumonia, renal disease, hepatic insufficiency, or heart failure. Although withdrawal seizures commonly precede the development of alcohol withdrawal delirium, delirium can also appear unheralded. The essential feature of the syndrome is delirium occurring within 1 week after a person stops drinking or reduces the intake of alcohol. In addition to the symptoms of delirium, the features of alcohol intoxication delirium include autonomic hyperactivity such as tachycardia, diaphoresis, fever, anxiety, insomnia, and hypertension; perceptual distortions, most frequently visual or tactile hallucinations; and fluctuating levels of psychomotor activity, ranging from hyperexcitability to lethargy.

About 5 percent of persons with alcohol-related disorders who are hospitalized have DTs. Because the syndrome usually develops on the third hospital day, a patient admitted for an unrelated condition may unexpectedly have an episode of delirium, the first sign of a previously undiagnosed alcohol-related disorder. Episodes of DTs usually begin in a patient's 30s or 40s after 5 to 15 years of heavy drinking, typically of the binge type. Physical illness (e.g., hepatitis or pancreatitis) predisposes to the syndrome; a person in good physical health rarely has DTs during alcohol withdrawal.

A 73-year-old professor emeritus at a university was believed to be in good health when he entered the hospital for an elective hernia repair. Perhaps reflecting his status in the community, the relatively brief history contained no detailed notes of his drinking pattern and made no mention of his γ-glutamyltransferase value of 55 U/L along with the MCV of 93.5 μm^3. Eight hours postsurgery, the nursing staff noted a sharp increase in the pulse rate to 110, an increase in blood pressure to 150/100, prominent diaphoresis, and a tremor to both hands, after which the patient demonstrated a brief but intense grand mal convulsion. He awoke extremely agitated and disoriented to time, place, and person. A reevaluation of the history and an interview with the wife documented alcohol dependence with a consumption of approximately six standard drinks per night. Over the following 4 days, the patient's autonomic nervous system dysfunction decreased as his cognitive impairment disappeared. His condition is classified as alcohol withdrawal delirium in DSM-IV-TR.

Treatment. The best treatment for DTs is prevention. Patients withdrawing from alcohol who exhibit withdrawal phenomena should receive a benzodiazepine, such as 25 to 50 mg of chlordiazepoxide every 2 to 4 hours until they seem to be out of danger. Once the delirium appears, however, 50 to 100 mg of chlordiazepoxide should be given every 4 hours orally, or lorazepam (Ativan) should be given intravenously (IV) if oral medication is not possible (Table 12.2–7). Antipsychotic medications that may reduce the seizure threshold in patients should be avoided. A high-calorie, high-carbohydrate diet supplemented by multivitamins is also important.

Physically restraining patients with the DTs is risky; they may fight against the restraints to a dangerous level of exhaustion. When patients are disorderly and uncontrollable, a seclusion room can be used. Dehydration, often exacerbated by diaphoresis and fever, can be corrected with fluids given by mouth or IV. Anorexia, vomiting, and diarrhea often occur during withdrawal. Antipsychotic medications should be avoided because they can reduce the seizure threshold in the patient. The emergence of focal neurological symptoms, lateralizing seizures, increased intracranial pressure, or evidence of skull fractures or other indications of CNS pathology should prompt clinicians to examine a patient for additional neurological disease. Nonbenzodiazepine anticonvulsant medication is not useful in preventing or treating alcohol withdrawal convulsions, although benzodiazepines are generally effective.

Warm, supportive psychotherapy in the treatment of DTs is essential. Patients are often bewildered, frightened, and anxious because of their tumultuous symptoms, and skillful verbal support is imperative.

Alcohol-Induced Persisting Dementia

The legitimacy of the concept of alcohol-induced persisting dementia remains controversial; some clinicians and researchers believe that it is difficult to separate the toxic effects of alcohol abuse from the CNS damage done by poor nutrition and multiple trauma and that following the malfunctioning of other bodily organs such as the liver, the pancreas, and the kidneys. Although several studies have found enlarged ventricles and cortical atrophy in persons with dementia and a history of alcohol dependence, the studies do not help clarify the cause of the dementia. Nonetheless, DSM-IV-TR includes the diagnosis of alcohol-induced persisting dementia (*see* Table 10.3–8). The controversy about the diagnosis should encourage clinicians to complete a diagnostic assessment of the dementia before concluding that it was caused by alcohol.

Alcohol-Induced Persisting Amnestic Disorder

Diagnosis and Clinical Features. The diagnostic criteria of alcohol-induced persisting amnestic disorder are contained in the DSM-IV-TR category of substance-induced persisting amnestic disorder (*see* Table 10.4–3). The essential feature of alcohol-induced persisting amnestic disorder is a disturbance in short-term memory caused by prolonged heavy use of alcohol. Because the disorder usually occurs in persons who have been drinking heavily for many years, the disorder is rare in persons younger than age 35.

Wernicke-Korsakoff Syndrome. The classic names for alcohol-induced persisting amnestic disorder are Wernicke's encephalopathy (a set of acute symptoms) and Korsakoff's syndrome (a chronic condition). Whereas Wernicke's encephalopathy is completely reversible with treatment, only about 20 percent of patients with Korsakoff's syndrome recover. The pathophysiological connection between the two syndromes is thiamine deficiency, caused either by poor nutritional habits or by malabsorption problems. Thiamine is a cofactor for several important enzymes and may also be involved in conduction of the axon potential along the axon and in synaptic transmission. The neuropathological lesions are symmetrical and paraventricular, involving the mammillary bodies, the thalamus, the hypothalamus, the midbrain, the pons, the medulla, the fornix, and the cerebellum.

Wernicke's encephalopathy, also called *alcoholic encephalopathy*, is an acute neurological disorder characterized by ataxia (affecting primarily the gait), vestibular dysfunction, confusion, and a variety of ocular motility abnormalities, including horizontal nystagmus, lateral orbital palsy, and gaze palsy. These eye signs are usually bilateral but not necessarily symmetrical. Other eye signs may include a sluggish reaction to light and anisocoria. Wernicke's encephalopathy may clear spontaneously in a few days or weeks or may progress into Korsakoff's syndrome.

Treatment. In the early stages, Wernicke's encephalopathy responds rapidly to large doses of parenteral thiamine, which is believed to be effective in preventing the progression into Korsakoff's syndrome. The dosage of thiamine is usually initiated at 100 mg by mouth two to three times daily and is continued for 1 to 2 weeks. In patients with alcohol-related disorders who are receiving IV administration of glucose solution, it is good practice to include 100 mg of thiamine in each liter of the glucose solution.

Korsakoff's syndrome is the chronic amnestic syndrome that can follow Wernicke's encephalopathy, and the two syndromes are believed to be pathophysiologically related. The cardinal features of Korsakoff's syndrome are impaired mental syndrome (especially recent memory) and anterograde amnesia in an alert and responsive patient. The patient may or may not have the symptom of confabulation. Treatment of Korsakoff's syndrome is also thiamine given 100 mg by mouth two to three times daily; the treatment regimen should continue for 3 to 12 months. Few patients who progress to Korsakoff's syndrome ever fully recover, although many have some improvement in their cognitive abilities with thiamine and nutritional support.

Blackouts. Alcohol-related blackouts are not included in DSM-IV-TR's diagnostic classification, although the symptom of alcohol intoxication is common. Blackouts are similar to episodes of transient global amnesia (see Chapter 10, Section 10.4) in that they are discrete episodes of anterograde amnesia that occur in association with alcohol intoxication. The periods of amnesia can be particularly distressing when persons fear that they have unknowingly harmed someone or behaved imprudently while intoxicated. During a blackout, persons have relatively intact remote memory but experience a specific short-term memory deficit in which they are unable to recall events that happened in the previous 5 or 10 minutes. Because their other intellectual faculties are well preserved, they can perform complicated tasks and appear normal to casual observers. The neurobiological mechanisms for alcoholic blackouts are now known at the molecular level; alcohol blocks the consolidation of new memories into old memories, a process that is thought to involve the hippocampus and related temporal lobe structures.

Alcohol-Induced Psychotic Disorder

Diagnosis and Clinical Features. The diagnostic criteria for alcohol-induced psychotic disorders, such as delusions and hallucinations, are found in the DSM-IV-TR category of substance-induced psychotic disorder (*see* Table 14.4–7). DSM-IV-TR further allows the specification of onset (during intoxication or withdrawal) and whether hallucinations or delusions are present. The most common hallucinations are auditory, usually voices, but they are often unstructured. The voices are characteristically maligning, reproachful, or threatening, although some patients report that the voices are pleasant and nondisruptive. The hallucinations usually last less than a week, but during that week impaired reality testing is common. After the episode, most patients realize the hallucinatory nature of the symptoms.

Hallucinations after alcohol withdrawal are considered rare, and the syndrome is distinct from alcohol withdrawal delirium. The hallucinations can occur at any age, but usually appear in persons abusing alcohol for a long time. Although the hallucinations usually resolve within a week, some linger; in these cases, clinicians must consider other psychotic disorders in the differential diagnosis. Alcohol withdrawal-related hallucinations are differentiated from the hallucinations of schizophrenia by the temporal association with alcohol withdrawal, the absence of a classic history of schizophrenia, and their usually short-lived duration. Alcohol withdrawal-related hallucinations are differentiated from the DTs by the presence of a clear sensorium in patients.

A 39-year-old male letter carrier was brought to an emergency room by the police after he behaved in an unusual fashion at home and complained that his neighbors were trying to kill him. The history obtained from the patient and his wife revealed that his psychotic thinking developed slowly over the preceding 3 weeks; he began with feelings that persons were looking at him at work, progressed to vague feelings that persons were against him, and went on to frank auditory hallucinations that persons at work and in the neighboring houses were talking about their plans to kill him. He had no insight into those paranoid delusions and auditory hallucinations. The relatively abrupt onset of the syndrome—he was in his late 30s—pointed to a potential organic cause, and further probing documented that he had been drinking between 6 and 18 beers daily for at least the preceding 10 weeks. A diagnosis of alcohol-induced psychotic disorder with onset during intoxication was made, and both hallucinations and delusions disappeared after 3 weeks of abstinence. After alcohol treatment, the man stayed sober for the next 8 months. He later resumed heavy drinking, however, and had a recurrence of both hallucinations and delusions. (Courtesy of Marc A. Schuckit, M.D.)

Treatment. The treatment of alcohol withdrawal-related hallucinations is much like the treatment of DTs—benzodiazepines, adequate nutrition, and fluids, if necessary. If this regimen fails or for long-term cases, antipsychotics may be used.

Alcohol-Induced Mood Disorder

The DSM-IV-TR allows for the diagnosis of alcohol-induced mood disorder with manic, depressive, or mixed features (*see* Table 15.3–10) and also for the specification of onset during either intoxication or withdrawal. As with all the secondary and substance-induced disorders, clinicians must consider whether the abused substance and the symptoms have a causal relation.

A consultation was requested on a 42-year-old woman with alcohol dependence who complained of persisting severe depressive symptoms despite 5 days of abstinence. In the initial stage of the interview, she noted that she had "always been depressed" and felt that she "drank to cope with the depressive symptoms." Her current complaint included a prominent sadness that had persisted for several weeks, difficulties concentrating, initial and terminal insomnia, and a feeling of hopelessness and guilt. In an effort to distinguish between an alcohol-induced mood disorder and an independent major depressive episode, a time-line-based history was obtained. This focused on the age of onset of alcohol dependence, periods of abstinence that extended for several months or more since the onset of dependence, and the ages of occurrence of clear major depressive episodes lasting several weeks or more at a time. Despite this patient's original complaints, it became clear that there had been no major depressive episodes prior to her mid-20s when alcohol dependence began, and that during a 1-year period of abstinence related to the gestation and neonatal period of her son, her mood had significantly improved. A provisional diagnosis of an alcohol-induced mood disorder was made. The patient was offered education, reassurance, and cognitive therapy to help her to deal with the depressive symptoms, but no antidepressant medications were prescribed. The depressive symptoms remained at their original intensity for several additional days and then began to improve. By approximately 3 weeks abstinent the patient no longer met criteria for a major depressive episode, although she demonstrated mood swings similar to dysphemia for several additional weeks. This case is a fairly typical example of an alcohol-induced mood disorder in an individual with alcohol dependence. (Courtesy of Marc A. Shuckit, M.D.)

Alcohol-Induced Anxiety Disorder

The DSM-IV-TR allows for the diagnosis of alcohol-induced anxiety disorder (*see* Table 16.7–3) and suggests that the diagnosis specify whether the symptoms are those of generalized anxiety, panic attacks, obsessive–compulsive symptoms, or phobic symptoms and whether the onset was during intoxication or during withdrawal. The association between alcohol use and anxiety symptoms is discussed above; deciding whether the anxiety symptoms are primary or secondary can be difficult.

A 48-year-old woman was referred for evaluation and treatment of her recent onset of panic attacks. These episodes occurred two to three times per week over the past 6 months, with each lasting typically between 10 and 20 minutes. Panic symptoms occurred regardless of levels of life stress and could not be explained by current medications or medical conditions. The workup included an evaluation of her laboratory test values, which revealed a carbohydrate-deficient transferrin (CDT) level of 28 U/L, a uric acid level of 7.1 mg, and a γ-glutamyltransferase value of 47. All other blood tests were within normal limits.

The atypical age of onset of the panic attacks, along with the blood results, encouraged the clinician to probe further regarding the pattern of alcohol-related life problems with both the patient and, separately, her spouse. This step documented a history of alcohol dependence with an onset at approximately 35 years of age, with no evidence of panic disorder before that date. Nor did the patient have repetitive panic attacks beyond 2 weeks of abstinence during her frequent periods of nondrinking, which often lasted for 3 or 4 months. A working diagnosis of alcohol dependence with an alcohol-induced anxiety disorder characterized by panic attacks was made, and the patient was encouraged to abstain and was appropriately treated for possible withdrawal symptoms. Over the subsequent 3 weeks after a taper of benzodiazepines used for the treatment of withdrawal, the panic symptoms diminished in intensity and subsequently disappeared. (Courtesy of Marc A. Schuckit, M.D.)

Alcohol-Induced Sexual Dysfunction

In DSM-IV-TR, the formal diagnosis of symptoms of sexual dysfunction associated with alcohol intoxication is alcohol-induced sexual dysfunction (*see* Table 21.2–17).

Alcohol-Induced Sleep Disorder

In DSM-IV-TR, the diagnostic criteria for alcohol-induced sleep disorders with an onset during either alcohol intoxication or alcohol withdrawal are found in the sleep disorders section (*see* Table 24.2–21).

Alcohol-Related Use Disorder Not Otherwise Specified

The DSM-IV-TR allows for the diagnosis of alcohol-related disorder not otherwise specified for alcohol-related disorders that do not meet the diagnostic criteria for any of the other diagnoses (Table 12.2–8).

Idiosyncratic Alcohol Intoxication. Whether there is such a diagnostic entity as idiosyncratic alcohol intoxication is under debate; DSM-IV-TR does not recognize this category as an official diagnosis. Several well-controlled studies of persons who supposedly have the disorder have raised questions about the validity of the designation. The condition has been variously called pathologic, complicated, atypical, and paranoid alcohol intoxication; all these terms indicate that a severe behavioral syndrome develops rapidly after a person consumes a small amount of alcohol that would have minimal behavioral effects on most persons. The diagnosis is important in the forensic arena because alcohol intoxication is not generally accepted as a reason for judging persons not responsible for their activities. Idiosyncratic alcohol intoxication, however, can be used in a person's defense if a defense lawyer can argue successfully that the defendant has an unexpected, idiosyncratic, pathological reaction to a minimal amount of alcohol.

In anecdotal reports, persons with idiosyncratic alcohol intoxication have been described as confused and disoriented and as experiencing illusions, transitory delusions, and visual hallucinations. Persons may display greatly increased psychomotor activity and impulsive, aggressive behavior. They can be dangerous to others and may also exhibit suicidal ideation and make suicide attempts. The disorder, usually described as lasting for a few hours, terminates in prolonged sleep, and those affected cannot recall the episodes on awakening. The cause of the condition is unknown, but it is reported to be most common in persons with high levels of anxiety. According to one hypothesis, alcohol causes sufficient disorganization and loss of control to release aggressive impulses. Another suggestion is that brain damage, particularly encephalitic or traumatic damage, predisposes some persons to an intolerance for alcohol and thus to abnormal behavior after they ingest only small amounts. Other predisposing factors may include advancing age, using sedative-hypnotic drugs, and feeling fatigued. A person's behavior while intoxicated tends to be atypical; after one weak drink, a quiet, shy person becomes belligerent and aggressive.

In treating idiosyncratic alcohol intoxication, clinicians must help protect patients from harming themselves and others. Physical restraint may be necessary, but is difficult because of the abrupt onset of the condition. Once a patient has been restrained, injection of an antipsychotic drug, such as haloperidol (Haldol), is useful for controlling assaultiveness. This condition must be differentiated from other causes of abrupt behavioral change, such as complex partial epilepsy. Some persons with the disorder reportedly showed temporal lobe spiking on an EEG after ingesting small amounts of alcohol.

Table 12.2–8
DSM-IV-TR Diagnostic Criteria for Alcohol-Related Disorder Not Otherwise Specified

The alcohol-related disorder not otherwise specified category is for disorders associated with the use of alcohol that are not classifiable as alcohol dependence, alcohol abuse, alcohol intoxication, alcohol withdrawal, alcohol intoxication delirium, alcohol withdrawal delirium, alcohol-induced persisting dementia, alcohol-induced persisting amnestic disorder, alcohol-induced psychotic disorder, alcohol-induced mood disorder, alcohol-induced anxiety disorder, alcohol-induced sexual dysfunction, or alcohol-induced sleep disorder.

(From American Psychiatric Association. *Diagnostic and Statistical Manual of Mental Disorders.* 4th ed. Text rev. Washington, DC: American Psychiatric Association; copyright 2000, with permission.)

Other Alcohol-Related Neurological Disorders

Only the major neuropsychiatric syndromes associated with alcohol use have been discussed here. The complete list of neurological syndromes is lengthy (Table 12.2–9). Alcoholic pellagra encephalopathy is one diagnosis of potential interest to psychiatrists presented with a patient who appears to be afflicted with Wernicke-Korsakoff syndrome but does not respond to thiamine treatment. The symptoms of alcoholic pellagra encephalopathy include confusion, clouding of consciousness, myoclonus, oppositional hypertonias, fatigue, apathy, irritability, anorexia, insomnia, and sometimes delirium. Patients suffer from a deficiency of niacin (nicotinic acid), and the specific treatment is 50 mg of niacin by mouth four times daily or 25 mg parenterally two to three times daily.

Fetal Alcohol Syndrome

Data indicate that women who are pregnant or are breast-feeding should not drink alcohol. Fetal alcohol syndrome, the leading cause of mental retardation in the United States, occurs when mothers drinking alcohol expose fetuses to alcohol in utero. The alcohol inhibits intrauterine growth and postnatal development. Microcephaly, craniofacial malformations, and limb and heart defects are common in affected infants. Short adult stature and development of a range of adult maladaptive behaviors have also been associated with fetal alcohol syndrome.

Women with alcohol-related disorders have a 35 percent risk of having a child with defects. Although the precise mechanism of the damage to the fetus is unknown, the damage seems to result from exposure in utero to ethanol or to its metabolites; alcohol may also cause hormone imbalances that increase the risk of abnormalities.

PROGNOSIS

Between 10 and 40 percent of alcoholic persons enter some kind of formal treatment program during the course of their alcohol problems. A number of prognostic signs are favorable. First is the absence of preexisting antisocial personality disorder or a diagnosis of other substance abuse or dependence. Second, evidence of general life stability with a job, continuing close family contacts, and the absence of severe legal problems also bodes well for the patient. Third, if the patient stays for the full course of the initial rehabilitation (perhaps 2 to 4 weeks), the chances of maintaining abstinence are good. The combination

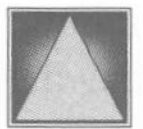

Table 12.2–9
Neurological and Medical Complications of Alcohol Use

- Alcohol intoxication
  - Acute intoxication
  - Pathological intoxication (atypical, complicated, unusual)
  - Blackouts
- Alcohol withdrawal syndromes
  - Tremulousness (the shakes or the jitters)
  - Alcoholic hallucinosis (horrors)
  - Withdrawal seizures (rum fits)
  - Delirium tremens (shakes)
- Nutritional diseases of the nervous system secondary to alcohol abuse
  - Wernicke-Korsakoff syndrome
  - Cerebellar degeneration
  - Peripheral neuropathy
  - Optic neuropathy (tobacco-alcohol amblyopia)
  - Pellagra
- Alcoholic diseases of uncertain pathogenesis
  - Central pontine myelinolysis
  - Marchiafava-Bignami disease
  - Fetal alcohol syndrome
  - Myopathy
  - Alcoholic dementia
  - Alcoholic cerebral atrophy
- Systemic diseases due to alcohol with secondary neurological complications
  - Liver disease
    - Hepatic encephalopathy
    - Acquired (non-Wilsonian) chronic hepatocerebral degeneration
  - Gastrointestinal diseases
    - Malabsorption syndromes
  - Postgastrectomy syndromes
  - Possible pancreatic encephalopathy
- Cardiovascular diseases
  - Cardiomyopathy with potential cardiogenic emboli and cerebrovascular disease
  - Arrhythmias and abnormal blood pressure leading to cerebrovascular disease
- Hematological disorders
  - Anemia, leukopenia, thrombocytopenia (could possibly lead to hemorrhagic cerebrovascular disease)
- Infectious disease, especially meningitis (especially pneumococcal and meningococcal)
- Hypothermia and hyperthermia
- Hypotension and hypertension
- Respiratory depression and associated hypoxia
- Toxic encephalopathies, including alcohol and other substances
- Electrolyte imbalances leading to acute confusional states and, rarely, local neurological signs and symptoms
  - Hypoglycemia
  - Hyperglycemia
  - Hyponatremia
  - Hypercalcemia
  - Hypomagnesemia
  - Hypophosphatemia
- Increased incidence of trauma
  - Epidural, subdural, and intracerebral hematoma
  - Spinal cord injury
  - Posttraumatic seizure disorders
  - Compressive neuropathies and brachial plexus injuries (Saturday night palsies)
  - Posttraumatic symptomatic hydrocephalus (normal pressure hydrocephalus)
  - Muscle crush injuries and compartmental syndromes

(From Rubino FA. Neurologic complications of alcoholism. *Psychiatr Clin North Am.* 1992;15:361, with permission.)

of these three attributes predicts at least a 60 percent chance for 1 or more years of abstinence. Few studies have documented the long-term course, but researchers agree that 1 year of abstinence is associated with a good chance for continued abstinence over an extended period. Alcoholic persons with severe drug problems (especially IV drug use or cocaine or amphetamine dependence) and those who are homeless may have only a 10 to 15 percent or so chance of achieving 1 year of abstinence, however.

Accurately predicting whether any specific person will achieve or maintain abstinence is impossible, but the prognostic factors listed above are associated with an increased likelihood of abstinence. The factors reflecting life stability, however, probably explain only 20 percent or less of the course of alcohol use disorders. Many forces that are difficult to measure affect the clinical course significantly; they are likely to include such intangibles as motivational level and the quality of the patient's social support system.

In general, alcoholic persons with preexisting independent major psychiatric disorders—such as antisocial personality disorder, schizophrenia, and bipolar I disorder—are likely to run the course of their independent psychiatric illness. Thus, for example, clinicians must treat the patient with bipolar I disorder who has secondary alcoholism with appropriate psychotherapy and lithium (Eskalith), use relevant psychological and behavioral techniques for the patient with antisocial personality disorder, and offer appropriate antipsychotic medications on a long-term basis to the patient with schizophrenia. The goal is to minimize the symptoms of the independent psychiatric disorder in the hope that greater life stability will be associated with a better prognosis for the patient's alcohol problems.

TREATMENT AND REHABILITATION

Three general steps are involved in treating the alcoholic person after the disorder has been diagnosed: intervention, detoxification, and rehabilitation. These approaches assume that all possible efforts have been made to optimize medical functioning and to address psychiatric emergencies. Thus, for example, an alcoholic person with symptoms of depression sufficiently severe to be suicidal requires inpatient hospitalization for at least several days until the suicidal ideation disappears. Similarly, a person presenting with cardiomyopathy, liver difficulties, or gastrointestinal bleeding first needs adequate treatment of the medical emergency.

The patient with alcohol abuse or dependence must then be brought face-to-face with the reality of the disorder (intervention), be detoxified if needed, and begin rehabilitation. The essentials of these three steps for an alcoholic person with independent psychiatric syndromes closely resemble the approaches used for the primary alcoholic person without independent psychiatric syndromes. In the former case, however, the treatments are applied after the psychiatric disorder has been stabilized as much as possible.

Intervention

The goal in the intervention step, which has also been called *confrontation*, is to break through feelings of denial and help the patient recognize the adverse consequences likely to occur if the disorder is not treated. Intervention is a process aimed at maximizing the motivation for treatment and continued abstinence.

This step often involves convincing patients that they are responsible for their own actions while reminding them of how alcohol has created significant life impairments. The psychiatrist often finds it useful to take advantage of the person's chief presenting complaint, whether it is insomnia, difficulties with sexual performance, an inability to cope with life stresses, depression, anxiety, or psychotic symptoms. The psychiatrist can then explain how alcohol has either created or contributed to these problems and can reassure the patient that abstinence can be achieved with a minimum of discomfort.

A physician was consulted by a 43-year-old businessman who was concerned about his wife. He had recently been confronted by their 21-year-old daughter, who felt that her mother was an alcoholic. The daughter noted her mother's slurred speech on several recent occasions when she had called home, noted times during the day when the mother was apparently home but did not answer the telephone, and observed high levels of alcohol consumption. A more detailed history revealed that the husband had been concerned about the wife's drinking pattern for at least 5 years; he related her practice of staying up after he went to bed and retiring later with alcohol on her breath. He also noted her consumption of 10 to 12 drinks at parties, with the resulting tendency to isolate herself from the remaining guests, her panic-like behavior regarding the need to pack liquor when they went on trips where alcohol might not be readily available, and what he observed to be a tremor of her hands some mornings during breakfast. The husband was given several potential courses of action, including the possibility of referring his wife for treatment with the physician. He was advised to share his concern with his wife when she was not actively intoxicated, emphasizing specific times and events when her impairment with alcohol was noted. He was also asked to consider whether a close friend of many years and the adult daughter might be included in this intervention, and it was suggested that a tentative appointment might be made with the clinician (or with an alcohol and drug treatment program) so that a next step could be established if the intervention was successful.

A physician intervening with a patient can use the same nonjudgmental but persistent approach each time an alcohol-related impairment is identified. It is the persistence rather than exceptional interpersonal skills that usually gets results. A single intervention is rarely sufficient. Most alcoholic persons need a series of reminders of how alcohol contributed to each developing crisis before they seriously consider abstinence as a long-term option.

Family

The family can be of great help in the intervention. Family members must learn not to protect the patient from the problems caused by alcohol; otherwise, the patient may not be able to gather the energy and the motivation necessary to stop drinking. During the intervention stage, the family can also suggest that the patient meet with persons who are recovering from alcoholism, perhaps through AA, and they can meet with groups, such as Al-Anon, that reach out to family members. Those support groups for families meet many times a week and help family members and friends see that they are not alone in their fears, worry, and feelings of guilt. Members share coping strategies and help each other find community resources. The groups can be most useful in helping family members rebuild their lives, even if the alcoholic person refuses to seek help.

Detoxification

Most persons with alcohol dependence have relatively mild symptoms when they stop drinking. If the patient is in relatively good health, is adequately nourished, and has a good social support system, the depressant withdrawal syndrome usually resembles a mild case of the flu. Even intense withdrawal syndromes rarely approach the severity of symptoms described by some early textbooks in the field.

The essential first step in detoxification is a thorough physical examination. In the absence of a serious medical disorder or combined drug abuse, severe alcohol withdrawal is unlikely. The second step is to offer rest, adequate nutrition, and multiple vitamins, especially those containing thiamine.

Mild or Moderate Withdrawal

Withdrawal develops because the brain has physically adapted to the presence of a brain depressant and cannot function adequately in the absence of the drug. Giving sufficient brain depressant on the first day to diminish symptoms and then weaning the patient off the drug over the next 5 days offers most patients optimal relief and minimizes the possibility that severe withdrawal will develop. Any depressant—including alcohol, barbiturates, or any of the benzodiazepines—can work, but most clinicians choose a benzodiazepine for its relative safety. Adequate treatment can be given with either short-acting drugs (e.g., lorazepam), or long-acting substances (e.g., chlordiazepoxide and diazepam).

An example of treatment is the administration of 25 mg of chlordiazepoxide by mouth three or four times a day on the first day, with a notation to skip a dose if the patient is asleep or feeling sleepy. An additional one or two 25-mg doses can be given during the first 24 hours if the patient is jittery or shows signs of increasing tremor or autonomic dysfunction. Whatever benzodiazepine dosage is required on the first day can be decreased by 20 percent each subsequent day, with a resulting need for no further medication after 4 or 5 days. When giving a long-acting agent, such as chlordiazepoxide, the clinician must avoid producing excessive sleepiness through overmedication; if the patient is sleepy, the next scheduled dose should be omitted. When taking a short-acting drug, such as lorazepam, the patient must not miss any dose because rapid changes in benzodiazepine concentrations in the blood can precipitate severe withdrawal.

A social model program of detoxification saves money by avoiding medications while using social supports. This less-expensive regimen can be helpful for mild or moderate withdrawal syndromes. Some clinicians have also recommended β-adrenergic receptor antagonists (e.g., propranolol [Inderal]) or α-adrenergic receptor agonists (e.g., clonidine), although these medications do not appear to be superior to the benzodiazepines. Unlike the brain depressants, these other agents do little to decrease the risk of seizures or delirium.

Severe Withdrawal

For the approximately 1 to 3 percent of alcoholic patients with extreme autonomic dysfunction, agitation, and confusion—that is, those with alcoholic withdrawal delirium, or DTs—no optimal treatment has yet been developed. The first step is to ask why such a severe and relatively uncommon withdrawal syndrome has occurred; the answer often relates to a severe concomitant medical problem that needs immediate treatment. The withdrawal symptoms can then be minimized through the use of either benzodiazepines (in which case high doses are sometimes required) or antipsychotic agents, such as haloperidol. Once again, on the first or second day doses are used to control behavior, and the patient can be weaned off the medication by about the fifth day.

Another 1 to 3 percent of patients may have a single grand mal convulsion; the rare person has multiple fits, with the peak incidence on the second day of withdrawal. Such patients require neurological evaluation, but in the absence of evidence of a seizure disorder, they do not benefit from anticonvulsant drugs.

Rehabilitation

For most patients, rehabilitation includes three major components: (1) continued efforts to increase and maintain high levels of motivation for abstinence; (2) work to help the patient readjust to a lifestyle free of alcohol; and (3) relapse prevention. Because these steps are carried out in the context of acute and protracted withdrawal syndromes and life crises, treatment requires repeated presentations of similar materials that remind the patient how important abstinence is and that help the patient develop new day-to-day support systems and coping styles.

No single major life event, traumatic life period, or identifiable psychiatric disorder is known to be a unique cause of alcoholism. In addition, the effects of any causes of alcoholism are likely to have been diluted by the effects of alcohol on the brain and the years of an altered lifestyle, so that the alcoholism has developed a life of its own. This is true even though many alcoholic persons believe that the cause was depression, anxiety, life stress, or pain syndromes. Research, data from records, and resource persons usually reveal that alcohol contributed to the mood disorder, accident, or life stress, not vice versa.

The same general treatment approach is used in inpatient and outpatient settings. Selection of the more expensive and intensive inpatient mode often depends on evidence of additional severe medical or psychiatric syndromes, the absence of appropriate nearby outpatient groups and facilities, and the patient's history of having failed in outpatient care. The treatment process in either setting involves intervention, optimizing physical and psychological functioning, enhancing motivation, reaching out to family, and using the first 2 to 4 weeks of care as an intensive period of help. Those efforts must be followed by at least 3 to 6 months of less frequent outpatient care. Outpatient care uses a combination of individual and group counseling, judicious avoidance of psychotropic medications unless needed for independent disorders, and involvement in such self-help groups as AA.

Counseling

Counseling efforts in the first several months should focus on day-to-day life issues to help patients maintain a high level of motivation for abstinence and to enhance their functioning. Psychotherapy techniques that provoke anxiety or that require deep insights have not been shown to be of benefit during the early months of recovery and, at least theoretically, may actually impair efforts at maintaining abstinence. Thus, this discussion focuses on the efforts likely to characterize the first 3 to 6 months of care.

Counseling or therapy can be carried out in an individual or group setting; few data indicate that either approach is superior. The technique used is not likely to matter greatly and usually boils down to simple day-to-day counseling or almost any behavioral or psychotherapeutic approach focusing on the here and now. To optimize motivation, treatment sessions should explore the consequences of drinking, the likely future course of alcohol-related life problems, and the marked improvement that can be expected with abstinence. Whether in an inpatient or an outpatient setting, individual or group counseling is usually offered a minimum of three times a week for the first 2 to 4 weeks, followed by less intense efforts, perhaps once a week, for the subsequent 3 to 6 months.

Much time in counseling deals with how to build a lifestyle free of alcohol. Discussions cover the need for a sober peer group, a plan for social and recreational events without drinking, and approaches for reestablishing communication with family members and friends.

The third major component, relapse prevention, first identifies situations in which the risk for relapse is high. The counselor must help the patient develop modes of coping to be used when the craving for alcohol increases or when any event or emotional state makes a return to drinking likely. An important part of relapse prevention is reminding the patient about the appropriate attitude toward slips. Short-term experiences with alcohol can never be used as an excuse for returning to regular drinking. The efforts to achieve and maintain a sober lifestyle are not a game in which all benefits are lost with that first sip. Rather, recovery is a process of trial and error; patients use slips that occur to identify high-risk situations and to develop more appropriate coping techniques.

Most treatment efforts recognize the effects that alcoholism has on the significant persons in the patient's life, and an important aspect of recovery involves helping family members and close friends understand alcoholism and realize that rehabilitation is an ongoing process that lasts for 6 to 12 or more months. Couples and family counseling and support groups for relatives and friends help the persons involved to rebuild relationships, to learn how to avoid protecting the patient from the consequences of any drinking in the future, and to be as supportive as possible of the alcoholic patient's recovery program.

Medications

If detoxification has been completed and the patient is not one of the 10 to 15 percent of alcoholic persons who have an independent mood disorder, schizophrenia, or anxiety disorder, little evidence favors prescribing psychotropic medications for the treatment of alcoholism. Lingering levels of anxiety and insomnia as part of a reaction to life stresses and protracted abstinence should be treated with behavior modification approaches and reassurance. Medications for these symptoms (including benzodiazepines) are likely to lose their effectiveness much faster than the insomnia disappears; thus, the patient may

Table 12.2–10
Medications for Treating Alcohol Dependence

	Disulfiram (Anatabuse)	Naltrexone (Re Via)	Acamprosate (Campral)
Action	Inhibits intermediate metabolism of alcohol, causing a build-up of acetaldehyde and a reaction of flushing, sweating, nausea, and tachycardia if a patient drinks alcohol	Blocks opioid receptors, resulting in reduced craving and reduced reward in response to drinking	Affects glutamate and GABA neurotransmitter systems, but its alcohol-related action is unclear
Contraindications	Concomitant use of alcohol or alcohol-containing preparations or metronidazole; coronary artery disease; severe myocardial disease	Currently using opioids or in acute opioid withdrawal; anticipated need for opioid analgesics; acute hepatitis or liver failure	Severe renal impairment (CrCl* $\leq$ 30 mL/min)
Precautions	High impulsivity—likely to drink while using it; psychoses (current or history); diabetes mellitus; epilepsy; hepatic dysfunction; hypothyroidism; renal impairment; rubber contact dermatitis	Other hepatic disease; renal impairment; history of suicide attempts. If opioid analgesia is required, larger doses may be required, and respiratory depression may be deeper and more prolonged.	Moderate renal impairment (dose adjustment for CrCl* between 30 and 50 mL/min); depression or suicidality
Serious Adverse Reactions	Hepatitis; optic neuritis; peripheral neuropathy; psychotic reactions. Pregnancy Category C.	Will precipitate severe withdrawal if patient is dependent on opioids; hepatoxicity (uncommon at usual doses). Pregnancy Category C.	Anxiety; depression. Rare events include the following: suicide attempt, acute kidney failure, heart failure, mesenteric arterial occlusion, cardiomyopathy, deep thrombophlebitits, and shock. Pregnancy Category C.
Common Side Effects	Metallic after-taste; dermatitis	Nausea; abdominal pain; constipation; dizziness; headache; anxiety; fatigue	Diarrhea; flatulence; nausea; abdominal pain; headache; back pain; infection; flu syndrome; chills; somnolence; decreased libido; amnesia; confusion
Examples of drug Interactions	Amitryptyline; anticoagulants such as warfarin; diazepam; isoniazid; metronidazole; phenytoin; theophylline; warfarin; any nonprescription drug containing alcohol	Opioid analgesics (blocks action); yohimbine (use with naltrexone increases negative drug effects)	No clinically relevant interactions known
Usual Adult Dosage	*Oral dose*: 250 mg daily (range 125–500 mg) *Before prescribing*: (1) warn that the patient should not take disulfiram for at least 12 hours after drinking and that a disulfiram-alcohol reaction can occur up to 2 weeks after the last dose; and (2) warn about alcohol in the diet (e.g., sauces and vinegars) and in medications and toiletries *Follow up*: Monitor liver function tests periodically	*Oral dose*: 50 mg daily *Before prescribing*: Evaluate for possible current opioid use; consider a urine toxicology screen for opioids, including synthetic opioids. Obtain liver function tests *Follow up*: Monitor liver function tests periodically	*Oral dose*: 666 mg (two 333-mg tablets) three times daily *or*, for patients with moderate renal impairment (CrCl* 30–50 mL/min), reduce to 333 mg (one tablet) three times daily *Before prescribing*: Establish abstinence

*CrCl, creatinine clearance; GABA, γ-aminobutyric acid.

increase the dose and have subsequent problems. Similarly, sadness and mood swings can linger at low levels for several months. Controlled clinical trials, however, indicate no benefit in prescribing antidepressant medications or lithium to treat the average alcoholic person who has no independent or long-lasting psychiatric disorder. The mood disorder will clear before the medications can take effect, and patients who resume drinking while on the medications face significant potential dangers. With little or no evidence that the medications are effective, the dangers significantly outweigh any potential benefits from their routine use.

One possible exception to the proscription against the use of medications is the alcohol-sensitizing agent disulfiram. Disulfiram is given in daily doses of 250 mg before the patient is discharged from the intensive first phase of outpatient rehabilitation or from inpatient care. The goal is to place the patient in a condition in which drinking alcohol precipitates an uncomfortable physical reaction, including nausea, vomiting, and a burning sensation in the face and stomach. Few data prove that disulfiram is more effective than a placebo, however, probably because most persons stop taking the disulfiram when they resume drinking. Many clinicians have stopped routinely prescribing the agent, partly in recognition of the dangers associated with the drug itself: mood swings, rare instances of psychosis, the possibility of increased peripheral neuropathies, the relatively rare occurrence of other significant neuropathies, and potentially fatal hepatitis. Moreover, patients with preexisting heart disease, cerebral thrombosis, diabetes, and a number of other conditions cannot be given disulfiram because an alcohol reaction to the disulfiram could be fatal.

Two additional promising pharmacological interventions have recently been studied. The first involves the opioid antagonist naltrexone (ReVia), which at least theoretically is believed possibly to decrease the craving for alcohol or blunt the rewarding effects of drinking. In any event, two relatively small (approximately 90 patients on the active drug across the studies) and short-term (3 months of active treatment) investigations using 50 mg per day of this drug had potentially promising results. Evaluating the full impact of this medication, however, will require longer-term studies of relatively large groups of more diverse patients.

The second medication of interest, acamprosate (Campral), has been tested in over 5,000 alcohol-dependent patients in Europe. This drug is not yet available in the United States. Used in dosages of approximately 2,000 mg per day, this medication was associated with approximately 10 to 20 percent more positive outcomes than placebo when used in the context of the usual psychological and behavioral treatment regimens for alcoholism. The mechanism of action of acamprosate is not known, but it may act directly or indirectly at GABA receptors or at NMDA sites, the effects of which alter the development of tolerance or physical dependence on alcohol. A summary of medications used for alcohol dependence is given in Table 12.2–10.

Another medication with potential promise in the treatment of alcoholism is the nonbenzodiazepine antianxiety drug buspirone (BuSpar), although the effect of this drug on alcohol rehabilitation is inconsistent between studies. No evidence exists that antidepressant medications, such as the selective serotonin reuptake inhibitors (SSRIs), lithium, or antipsychotic medications, are significantly effective in the treatment of alcoholism.

Alcoholics Anonymous

Clinicians must recognize the potential importance of self-help groups such as AA. Members of AA have help available 24 hours a day, associate with a sober peer group, learn that it is possible to participate in social functions without drinking, and are given a model of recovery by observing the accomplishments of sober members of the group.

Learning about AA usually begins during inpatient or outpatient rehabilitation. The clinician can play a major role in helping patients understand the differences between specific groups. Some are composed only of men or women, and others are mixed; some meetings are composed mostly of blue collar men and women, whereas others are mostly for professionals; some groups place great emphasis on religion, and others are eclectic. Patients with coexisting psychiatric disorders may need some additional education about AA. The clinician should remind them that some members of AA may not understand their special need for medications and should arm the patients with ways of coping when group members inappropriately suggest that the required medications be stopped. Although difficult to evaluate using double-blind controls, most studies indicate that participation in AA is associated with improved outcomes, and incorporation into treatment programs saves money.

References

Dawson DA, Grant BF, Stinson FS, Chou PS. Psychopathology associated with drinking and alcohol use disorders in the college and general adult populations. *Drug Alcohol Depend*. 2005;77(2):139–150.

Goodwin RD, Lipsitz JD, Chapman TF, Mannuzza S, Klein DF, Fyer AJ. Alcohol use disorders in relatives of patients with panic disorder. *Compr Psychiatry*. 2006;47(2):88–90.

Hasin DS, Schuckit MA, Martin CS, Grant BF, Buchalz KK, Helzer JE. The validity of DSM IV alcohol dependence. *Alcohol Clin Exp Res*. 2003;27:244.

Johnston LD, O'Malley PM, Backman JG. *Monitoring the Future: National Survey Results on Drug Use, 1975–2002*. Vols I and II. Washington, DC: National Institute on Drug Abuse (NIH Publication #03-5375); 2003.

Kiefer F, Holger J, Tarnaske T, Helwig H, Briken P, Holzbach R, Kempf P, Stracke R, Baehr M, Naber D, Wiedemann K. Comparing and combining naltrexone and acamprosate in relapse prevention of alcoholism. *Arch Gen Psychiatry*. 2003;60:92.

Preuss UW, Schuckit MA, Smith TL, Danko GP, Bucholz KK, Hesselbrock MN, Hesselbrock V, Kramer JR. Predictors and correlates of suicide attempts over five years in 1237 alcohol dependent men and women. *Am J Psychiatry*. 2003;160:56.

Schuckit MA. Alcohol-related disorders. In: Sadock, BJ, Sadock VA, eds. *Kaplan & Sadock's Comprehensive Textbook of Psychiatry*. 8th ed. Vol. 1. Baltimore: Lippincott Williams & Wilkins; 2005:1168.

Schuckit MA, Danko GP, Smith TL, Hesselbrock V, Kramer J, Bucholz K. A five-year prospective evaluation of DSM-IV alcohol dependence with and without a physiological component. *Alcohol Clin Exp Res*. 2003;27:818.

Slutske WS. Alcohol use disorders among US college students and their non–college-attending peers. *Arch Gen Psychiatry*. 2005;62:321–327

Zilberman M, Tavares H, el-Guebaly N. Gender similarities and difference: The prevalence and course of alcohol- and other substance-related disorders. *J Addict Dis*. 2003; 22:61–74.

▲ 12.3 Amphetamine (or Amphetamine-like)-Related Disorders

Amphetamines and amphetamine-like drugs are the most widely used illicit substances, second only to cannabis, in the United States, Asia, Great Britain, Australia, and several other western European countries. Methamphetamine, a congener of amphetamine, has become even more popular in recent years.

The racemate amphetamine sulfate (Benzedrine) was first synthesized in 1887 and was introduced to clinical practice in 1932 as an over-the-counter inhaler for the treatment of nasal congestion and asthma. In 1937, amphetamine sulfate tablets were introduced for the treatment of narcolepsy, postencephalitic parkinsonism, depression, and lethargy. In the 1970s, a variety of social and regulatory factors began to curb widespread amphetamine distribution. The current US Food and Drug Administration (FDA)-approved indications for amphetamine are limited to attention-deficit/hyperactivity disorder (ADHD) and narcolepsy; however, amphetamines are also used in the treatment of obesity, depression, dysthymia, chronic fatigue syndrome, acquired immune deficiency syndrome (AIDS), dementia, and neurasthenia.

PREPARATIONS

The major amphetamines currently available and used in the United States are dextroamphetamine (Dexedrine), methamphetamine (Desoxyn), a mixed dextroamphetamine-amphetamine salt (Adderall), and the amphetamine-like compound methylphenidate (Ritalin). These drugs go by such street names as ice, crystal, crystal meth, and speed. As a general class, the amphetamines are referred to as analeptics, sympathomimetics, stimulants, and psychostimulants. The typical amphetamines are used to increase performance and to induce a euphoric feeling, for example, by students studying for examinations, by long-distance truck drivers on trips, by business people with important deadlines, by athletes in competition, and by soldiers during wartime. Although not as addictive as cocaine, amphetamines are nonetheless addictive drugs.

Other amphetamine-like substances are ephedrine, pseudoephedrine, and phenylpropanolamine (PPA). These drugs, PPA in particular, can dangerously exacerbate hypertension, precipitate a toxic psychosis, cause intestinal infarction, or result in death. The safety margin for PPA is particularly narrow, and three to four times the normal dose can result in life-threatening hypertension. In 2005, medications containing PPA were recalled by the FDA, and in 2006, the FDA prohibited the sale of over-the-counter medications containing ephedrine and regulated the sale of over-the-counter medications containing pseudoephedrine, which was being used illegally to make methamphetamine.

Amphetamine-type drugs with abuse potential also include phendimetrazine (Preludin), which is included in Schedule II of the Controlled Substance Act (CSA), and diethylpropion (Tenuate), benzphetamine (Didrex), and phentermine (Ionamin), which are included in Schedules III or IV of the CSA. It is presumed that all of these drugs are capable of producing all of the listed amphetamine-induced disorders. Modafinil (Provigil), used in the treatment of narcolepsy, also has stimulant and euphorigenic effects in humans but its toxicity and likelihood of producing amphetamine-induced disorders are unknown.

Methamphetamine is a potent form of amphetamine that abusers of the substance inhale, smoke, or inject intravenously (IV). Its psychological effects last for hours and are described as particularly powerful. Unlike cocaine (see Section 12.6), which must be imported, methamphetamine is a synthetic drug that can be manufactured domestically in illicit laboratories.

Other agents called *substituted* or *designer amphetamines* are discussed separately later in this section.

EPIDEMIOLOGY

The National Household Survey on Drug Abuse (NHSDA) conducted in 2001 found that 7.1 percent of persons (12 years of age and older) reported lifetime nonmedical use of stimulants, a significant increase since the 4.5 percent found in the 1997 survey. The highest rates of use in the past year (1.5 percent) were among 18- to 25-year-olds, followed by 12- to 17-year-olds. The treatment admission rate for primary amphetamine abuse in the United States is about 30 per 100,000 people 12 years of age or older. Thirteen states had amphetamine admission rates of at least 55 per 100,000, and eight of these had rates of 100 per 100,000 or more. A strong association of methamphetamine abuse and crime exists.

Amphetamine use occurs in all socioeconomic groups, and is increasing among white professionals. Because amphetamines are available by prescription for specific indications, prescribing physicians must be aware of the risk of amphetamine abuse by others, including friends and family members of the patient receiving the amphetamine. No reliable data are available on the epidemiology of designer amphetamine use, but they are greatly abused. According to the text revision of the 4th edition of *Diagnostic and Statistical Manual of Mental Disorders* (DSM-IV-TR), the lifetime prevalence of amphetamine dependence and abuse is 1.5 percent, and the male to female ratio is 1.

According to NHSDA, methamphetamine abuse continues to spread geographically and to different populations. In addition to the "super labs" in California and trafficking from Mexico, a proliferation of small "mom and pop" laboratories has occurred throughout the country, especially in rural areas. Methamphetamine abuse and production levels are high in Hawaii, West Coast areas, and some Southwestern areas, and abuse and manufacture continue to move eastward. New populations of methamphetamine uses include Hispanics, young people in Denver, club goers in Boston, and African-Americans in Texas. One half of women arrested in Honolulu tested positive in 2002, as did nearly 42 percent in Phoenix and 37 percent in San Diego. Not only methamphetamine users, but also children exposed to methamphetamine laboratories are also in danger of serious health consequences.

NEUROPHARMACOLOGY

All the amphetamines are rapidly absorbed orally and have a rapid onset of action, usually within 1 hour when taken orally. The classic amphetamines are also taken IV and have an almost immediate effect by this route. Nonprescribed amphetamines and designer amphetamines are also inhaled ("snorting"). Tolerance develops with both classic and designer amphetamines, although amphetamine users often overcome the tolerance by taking more of the drug. Amphetamine is less addictive than cocaine, as evidenced by experiments on rats in which not all animals spontaneously self-administered low doses of amphetamine.

The classic amphetamines (i.e., dextroamphetamine, methamphetamine, and methylphenidate) produce their primary effects by causing the release of catecholamines, particularly dopamine, from presynaptic terminals (*see* Fig. 3.3–7). The effects are particularly potent for the dopaminergic neurons projecting from the ventral tegmental area to the cerebral cortex and the limbic areas. This pathway has been termed the *reward circuit pathway*, and its activation is probably the major addicting mechanism for the amphetamines. The designer amphetamines cause the release of catecholamines (dopamine and norepinephrine) and of serotonin, the neurotransmitter implicated as the major neurochemical pathway for hallucinogens. Therefore, the clinical effects of designer amphetamines are a blend of the effects of classic amphetamines and those of hallucinogens.

DIAGNOSIS

The DSM-IV-TR lists many amphetamine (or amphetamine-like)-related disorders (Table 12.3–1), but specifies diagnostic criteria only for amphetamine intoxication (Table 12.3–2), amphetamine withdrawal (Table 12.3–3), and amphetamine-related disorder not otherwise specified (Table 12.3–4) in the section on amphetamine (or amphetamine-like)-related disorders. The diagnostic criteria for the other amphetamine (or amphetamine-like)-related disorders are contained in the DSM-IV-TR sections dealing with the primary phenomenological symptom (e.g., psychosis).

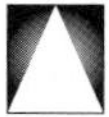

Table 12.3–1
DSM-IV-TR Amphetamine (or Amphetamine-like)-Related Disorders

Amphetamine use disorders
Amphetamine dependence
Amphetamine abuse
Amphetamine-induced disorders
Amphetamine intoxication
Specify if:
 With perceptual disturbances
Amphetamine withdrawal
Amphetamine intoxication delirium
Amphetamine-induced psychotic disorder, with delusions
Specify if:
 With onset during intoxication
Amphetamine-induced psychotic disorder, with hallucinations
Specify if:
 With onset during intoxication
Amphetamine-induced mood disorder
Specify if:
 With onset during intoxication
 With onset during withdrawal
Amphetamine-induced anxiety disorder
Specify if:
 With onset during intoxication
Amphetamine-induced sexual dysfunction
Specify if:
 With onset during intoxication
Amphetamine-induced sleep disorder
Specify if:
 With onset during intoxication
 With onset during withdrawal
Amphetamine-related disorder not otherwise specified

(From American Psychiatric Association. *Diagnostic and Statistical Manual of Mental Disorders.* 4th ed. Text rev. Washington, DC: American Psychiatric Association; copyright 2000, with permission.)

Amphetamine Dependence and Amphetamine Abuse

The DSM-IV-TR criteria for dependence and abuse are applied to amphetamine and its related substances (see Tables 12.1–3, 12.1–4, and 12.1–5 in Section 12.1). Amphetamine dependence can result in a rapid downward spiral of a person's abilities to cope with work- and family-related obligations and stresses. A person who abuses amphetamines requires increasingly high doses of amphetamine to obtain the usual high, and physical signs of amphetamine abuse (e.g., decreased weight and paranoid ideas) almost always develop with continued abuse.

Amphetamine Intoxication

The intoxication syndromes of cocaine (which blocks dopamine reuptake) and amphetamines (which cause the release of dopamine) are similar. Because more rigorous, in-depth research has been done on cocaine abuse and intoxication than on amphetamines, the clinical literature on amphetamines has been strongly influenced by the clinical findings of cocaine abuse. In DSM-IV-TR, the diagnostic criteria for amphetamine intoxication (Table 12.3–2) and cocaine intoxication (*see* Table 12.6–2) are separated, but are virtually the same. DSM-IV-TR specifies perceptual disturbances as a symptom of amphetamine

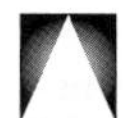

Table 12.3–2
DSM-IV-TR Diagnostic Criteria for Amphetamine Intoxication

A. Recent use of amphetamine or a related substance (e.g., methylphenidate).
B. Clinically significant maladaptive behavioral or psychological changes (e.g., euphoria or affective blunting; changes in sociability; hypervigilance; interpersonal sensitivity; anxiety, tension, or anger; stereotyped behaviors; impaired judgment; or impaired social or occupational functioning) that developed during, or shortly after, use of amphetamine or a related substance.
C. Two (or more) of the following, developing during, or shortly after, use of amphetamine or a related substance:
 (1) tachycardia or bradycardia
 (2) apillary dilation
 (3) elevated or lowered blood pressure
 (4) perspiration or chills
 (5) nausea or vomiting
 (6) evidence of weight loss
 (7) psychomotor agitation or retardation
 (8) muscular weakness, respiratory depression, chest pain, or cardiac arrhythmias
 (9) confusion, seizures, dyskinesias, dystonias, or coma
D. The symptoms are not due to a general medical condition and are not better accounted for by another mental disorder.

Specify if:
With perceptual disturbances

(From American Psychiatric Association. *Diagnostic and Statistical Manual of Mental Disorders.* 4th ed. Text rev. Washington, DC: American Psychiatric Association; copyright 2000, with permission.)

intoxication. If intact reality testing is absent, a diagnosis of amphetamine-induced psychotic disorder with onset during intoxication is indicated. The symptoms of amphetamine intoxication are mostly resolved after 24 hours and are generally completely resolved after 48 hours.

An 18-year-old high school senior was brought to the emergency room by police after being picked up wandering in traffic on the Triborough Bridge. He was angry, agitated, and aggressive and talked

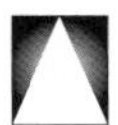

Table 12.3–3
DSM-IV-TR Diagnostic Criteria for Amphetamine Withdrawal

A. Cessation of (or reduction in) amphetamine (or a related substance) use that has been heavy and prolonged.
B. Dysphoric mood and two (or more) of the following physiological changes, developing within a few hours to several days after Criterion A:
 (1) fatigue
 (2) vivid, unpleasant dreams
 (3) insomnia or hypersomnia
 (4) increased appetite
 (5) psychomotor retardation or agitation
C. The symptoms in Criterion B cause clinically significant distress or impairment in social, occupational, or other important areas of functioning.
D. The symptoms are not due to a general medical condition and are not better accounted for by another mental disorder.

(From American Psychiatric Association. *Diagnostic and Statistical Manual of Mental Disorders.* 4th ed. Text rev. Washington, DC: American Psychiatric Association; copyright 2000, with permission.)

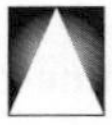

Table 12.3–4
DSM-IV-TR Diagnostic Criteria for Amphetamine-Related Disorder Not Otherwise Specified

The amphetamine-related disorder not otherwise specified category is for disorders associated with the use of amphetamine (or a related substance) that are not classifiable as amphetamine dependence, amphetamine abuse, amphetamine intoxication, amphetamine withdrawal, amphetamine intoxication delirium, amphetamine-induced psychotic disorder, amphetamine-induced mood disorder, amphetamine-induced anxiety disorder, amphetamine-induced sexual dysfunction, or amphetamine-induced sleep disorder.

(From American Psychiatric Association. *Diagnostic and Statistical Manual of Mental Disorders.* 4th ed. Text rev. Washington, DC: American Psychiatric Association; copyright 2000, with permission.)

of various people who were deliberately trying to "confuse" him by giving him misleading directions. His story was rambling and disjointed, but he admitted to the police officer that he had been using "speed." In the emergency room he had difficulty focusing his attention and had to ask that questions be repeated. He was disoriented as to time and place and was unable to repeat the names of three objects after five minutes. The family gave a history of the patient's regular use of "pep pills" over the past two years, during which time he was frequently "high" and did very poorly in school. (From *DSM-III-R Casebook.*)

Amphetamine Withdrawal

After amphetamine intoxication, a crash occurs with symptoms of anxiety, tremulousness, dysphoric mood, lethargy, fatigue, nightmares (accompanied by rebound rapid eye movement [REM] sleep), headache, profuse sweating, muscle cramps, stomach cramps, and insatiable hunger. The withdrawal symptoms generally peak in 2 to 4 days and are resolved in 1 week. The most serious withdrawal symptom is depression, which can be particularly severe after the sustained use of high doses of amphetamine and which can be associated with suicidal ideation or behavior. The DSM-IV-TR diagnostic criteria for amphetamine withdrawal (Table 12.3–3) specify that a dysphoric mood and physiological changes are necessary for the diagnosis.

Amphetamine Intoxication Delirium

Under substance-related disorder, DSM-IV-TR includes a diagnosis of amphetamine intoxication delirium (*see* Table 10.2–6). Delirium associated with amphetamine use generally results from high doses of amphetamine or from sustained use, and so sleep deprivation affects the clinical presentation. The combination of amphetamines with other substances and the use of amphetamines by a person with preexisting brain damage can also cause development of delirium. It is not uncommon for university students using amphetamines to cram for examinations to exhibit this type of delirium.

Amphetamine-Induced Psychotic Disorder

The clinical similarity of amphetamine-induced psychosis to paranoid schizophrenia has prompted extensive study of the neurochemistry of amphetamine-induced psychosis to elucidate the pathophysiology of paranoid schizophrenia. The hallmark of amphetamine-induced psychotic disorder is the presence of paranoia. Amphetamine-induced psychotic disorder can be distinguished from paranoid schizophrenia by several differentiating characteristics associated with the former, including a predominance of visual hallucinations, generally appropriate affects, hyperactivity, hypersexuality, confusion and incoherence, and little evidence of disordered thinking (e.g., looseness of associations). In several studies, investigators also noted that, although the positive symptoms of amphetamine-induced psychotic disorder and schizophrenia are similar, amphetamine-induced psychotic disorder generally lacks the affective flattening and alogia of schizophrenia. Clinically, however, acute amphetamine-induced psychotic disorder can be completely indistinguishable from schizophrenia, and only the resolution of the symptoms in a few days or a positive finding in a urine drug screen test eventually reveals the correct diagnosis.

The treatment of choice for amphetamine-induced psychotic disorder is the short-term use of an antipsychotic medication such as haloperidol (Haldol). DSM-IV-TR lists the diagnostic criteria for amphetamine-induced psychotic disorder with the other psychotic disorders (*see* Table 14.4–7) and allows clinicians to specify whether delusions or hallucinations are the predominant symptoms.

Amphetamine-Induced Mood Disorder

According to DSM-IV-TR, the onset of amphetamine-induced mood disorder can occur during intoxication or withdrawal (*see* Table 15.3–10). In general, intoxication is associated with manic or mixed mood features, whereas withdrawal is associated with depressive mood features.

Amphetamine-Induced Anxiety Disorder

In DSM-IV-TR, the onset of amphetamine-induced anxiety disorder can also occur during intoxication or withdrawal (*see* Table 16.7–3). Amphetamine, as with cocaine, can induce symptoms similar to those seen in obsessive-compulsive disorder, panic disorder, and phobic disorders, in particular.

Amphetamine-Induced Sexual Dysfunction

Amphetamines may be prescribed as an antidote to the sexual side effects of serotonergic agents such as fluoxetine (Prozac), but they are often misused by persons to enhance sexual experiences. High doses and long-term use are associated with erectile disorder and other sexual dysfunctions. These dysfunctions are classified in DSM-IV-TR as amphetamine-induced sexual dysfunction with onset during intoxication (*see* Table 21.2–17).

Amphetamine-Induced Sleep Disorder

The diagnostic criteria for amphetamine-induced sleep disorder with onset during intoxication or withdrawal are found in the DSM-IV-TR section on sleep disorders (*see* Table 24.2–21). Amphetamine intoxication can produce insomnia and sleep deprivation, whereas persons undergoing amphetamine withdrawal can experience hypersomnolence and nightmares.

Disorder Not Otherwise Specified

If an amphetamine (or amphetamine-like)-related disorder does not meet the criteria of one or more of the categories discussed above, it can be diagnosed as an amphetamine-related disorder not otherwise specified (Table 12.3–4).

CLINICAL FEATURES

In persons who have not previously used amphetamines, a single 5-mg dose increases the sense of well-being and induces elation, euphoria, and friendliness. Small doses generally improve attention and increase performance on written, oral, and performance tasks. An associated decrease in fatigue, induction of anorexia, and heightening of the pain threshold are also seen. Undesirable effects result from the use of high doses for long periods.

Adverse Effects

Amphetamines

PHYSICAL. Amphetamine abuse can produce adverse effects, the most serious of which include cerebrovascular, cardiac, and gastrointestinal effects. Among the specific life-threatening conditions are myocardial infarction, severe hypertension, cerebrovascular disease, and ischemic colitis. A continuum of neurological symptoms, from twitching to tetany to seizures to coma and death, is associated with increasingly high amphetamine doses. Intravenous use of amphetamines can transmit human immunodeficiency virus (HIV) and hepatitis and further the development of lung abscesses, endocarditis, and necrotizing angiitis. Several studies have shown that abusers of amphetamines knew little—or did not care—about safe-sex practices and the use of condoms. The non–life-threatening adverse effects of amphetamine abuse include flushing, pallor, cyanosis, fever, headache, tachycardia, palpitations, nausea, vomiting, bruxism (teeth grinding), shortness of breath, tremor, and ataxia. Pregnant women who use amphetamines often have babies with low birthweight, small head circumference, early gestational age, and growth retardation.

PSYCHOLOGICAL. The adverse psychological effects associated with amphetamine use include restlessness, dysphoria, insomnia, irritability, hostility, and confusion. Amphetamine use can also induce symptoms of anxiety disorders, such as generalized anxiety disorder and panic disorder, as well as ideas of reference, paranoid delusions, and hallucinations.

Other Agents

Substituted Amphetamines. MDMA (3,4-methylenedioxymethamphetamine) is one of a series of substituted amphetamines that also includes MDEA, MDA (3,4-methylenedioxyamphetamine), DOB (2,5-dimethoxy-4-bromoamphetamine), PMA (paramethoxyamphetamine), and others. These drugs produce subjective effects resembling those of amphetamine and LSD (lysergic acid diethylamide), and in that sense, MDMA and similar analogues may represent a distinct category of drugs.

A methamphetamine derivative that came into use in the 1980s, MDMA was not technically subject to legal regulation at the time. Although it has been labeled a "designer drug" in the belief that it was deliberately synthesized to evade legal regulation, it was actually synthesized and patented in 1914. Several psychiatrists used it as an adjunct to psychotherapy and concluded that it had value. At one time, it was advertised as legal and was used in psychotherapy for its subjective effects. It was never approved by the FDA, however. Its use raised questions of both safety and legality, because the related amphetamine derivatives MDA, DOB, and PMA had caused a number of overdose deaths, and MDA was known to cause extensive destruction of serotonergic nerve terminals in the central nervous system (CNS). Using emergency scheduling authority, the Drug Enforcement Agency made MDMA a Schedule I drug under the CSA, along with LSD, heroin, and marijuana. Despite its illegal status, MDMA continues to be manufactured, distributed, and used in the United States, Europe, and Australia. Its use is common in Australia and Great Britain at extended dances ("raves") popular with adolescents and young adults.

MECHANISMS OF ACTION. The unusual properties of the drugs may be a consequence of the different actions of the optical isomers: the $R(-)$ isomers produce LSD-like effects and the amphetamine-like properties are linked to $S(+)$ isomers. The LSD-like actions, in turn, may be linked to the capacity to release serotonin. The various derivatives may exhibit significant differences in subjective effects and toxicity. Animals in laboratory experiments will self-administer the drugs, suggesting prominent amphetamine-like effects.

SUBJECTIVE EFFECTS. After taking usual doses (100 to 150 mg), MDMA users experience elevated mood and, according to various reports, increased self-confidence and sensory sensitivity; peaceful feelings coupled with insight, empathy, and closeness to persons; and decreased appetite. Difficulty concentrating and an increased capacity to focus have both been reported. Dysphoric reactions, psychotomimetic effects, and psychosis have also been reported. Higher doses seem more likely to produce psychotomimetic effects. Sympathomimetic effects of tachycardia, palpitation, increased blood pressure, sweating, and bruxism are common. The subjective effects are reported to be prominent for about 4 to 8 hours, but they may not last as long or may last longer, depending on the dose and route of administration. The drug is usually taken orally but is also snorted and injected. Both tachyphylaxis and some tolerance are reported by users.

TOXICITY. Although it is not as toxic as MDA, various somatic toxicities have been attributed to MDMA use as well as fatal overdoses. It does not appear to be neurotoxic when injected into the brains of animals, but it is metabolized to MDA in both animals and humans. In animals, MDMA produces selective, long-lasting damage to serotonergic nerve terminals. It is not certain if the levels of the MDA metabolite reached in humans after the usual doses of MDMA suffice to produce lasting damage. Users of MDMA show differences in neuroendocrine responses to serotonergic probes, and studies of former MDMA users show global and regional decreases in serotonin transporter binding, as measured by positron emission tomography.

Currently, no established clinical uses exist for MDMA, although before its regulation, there were several reports of its beneficial effects as an adjunct to psychotherapy.

Khat. The fresh leaves of *Catha edulis*, a bush native to East Africa, have been used as a stimulant in the Middle East, Africa, and the Arabian Peninsula for at least 1,000 years. Khat is still widely used in Ethiopia, Kenya, Somalia, and Yemen. The amphetamine-like effects of khat have long been recognized, and although efforts to isolate the active ingredient were first undertaken in the 19th century, only since the 1970s has cathinone ($S[-]$ α-aminopropiophenone or $S[-]$2-amino-1-phenyl-1-propanone) been identified as the substance responsible. Cathinone is a precursor moiety that is normally enzymatically converted in the plant to the less-active entities norephedrine and cathine (norpseudoephedrine), which explains why only the fresh leaves of the plant are valued for their stimulant effects. Cathinone has most of the CNS and peripheral actions of amphetamine and appears to have the same mechanism of action. In humans, it elevates mood, decreases hunger, and alleviates fatigue. At high doses, it can induce an amphetamine-like psychosis in humans. Because it is typically absorbed buccally after chewing the leaf and because the alkaloid is metabolized relatively rapidly, high toxic blood levels are rarely reached. Concern about khat use is linked to its dependence-producing properties rather than to its acute toxicity. It is estimated that five million doses are consumed each day, despite prohibition of its use in a number of African and Arab countries.

In the 1990s, several clandestine laboratories began synthesizing methcathinone, a drug with actions similar to those of cathinone. Known by a number of street names (e.g., "CAT," "goob," and "crank"), its popularity is primarily owing to its ease of synthesis from ephedrine or pseudoephedrine, which were readily available until placed under special controls. Methcathinone has been moved to Schedule I of the CSA. The patterns of use, adverse effects, and complications closely resemble those reported for amphetamine.

"Club Drugs". The use of a certain group of substances popularly called *club drugs* is often associated with dance clubs, bars, and all-night dance parties (raves). The group includes LSD, γ-hydroxybutyrate (GHB), ketamine, methamphetamine, MDMA (ecstasy), and Rohypnol or "roofies" (flunitrazepam). These substances are not all in the same drug class, nor do they produce the same physical or subjective effects. GHB, ketamine, and Rohypnol have been called *date rape drugs* because they produce disorienting and sedating effects, and often users cannot recall what occurred during all or part of an episode under the influence of the drug. Hence, it is alleged that these drugs might be surreptitiously placed in a beverage, or a person might be convinced to take the drug and then not recall clearly what occurred after ingestion.

Emergency department mentions of GHB, ketamine, and Rohypnol are relatively few. Of the club drugs, methamphetamine is the substance that accounts for the largest share of treatment admissions.

TREATMENT AND REHABILITATION

The treatment of amphetamine (or amphetamine-like)-related disorders shares with cocaine-related disorders the difficulty of helping patients remain abstinent from the drug, which is powerfully reinforcing and induces craving. An inpatient setting and the use of multiple therapeutic methods (individual, family, and group psychotherapy) are usually necessary to achieve lasting abstinence. The treatment of specific amphetamine-induced disorders (e.g., amphetamine-induced psychotic disorder and amphetamine-induced anxiety disorder) with specific drugs (e.g., antipsychotic and anxiolytics) may be necessary on a short-term basis. Antipsychotics may be prescribed for the first few days. In the absence of psychosis, diazepam (Valium) is useful to treat patients' agitation and hyperactivity.

Physicians should establish a therapeutic alliance with patients to deal with the underlying depression, personality disorder, or both. Because many patients are heavily dependent on the drug, however, psychotherapy may be especially difficult.

Comorbid conditions, such as depression, may respond to antidepressant medication. Bupropion (Wellbutrin) may be of use after patients have withdrawn from amphetamine. It has the effect of producing feelings of well-being as these patients cope with the dysphoria that may accompany abstinence.

References

Ellis RJ, Childers ME, Cherner M, Lazzaretto D, Letendre S, Grant I. The HIV Neurobehavioral Research Center Group. Increased human immunodeficiency virus loads in active methamphetamine users are explained by reduced effectiveness of antiretroviral therapy. *J Infect Dis*. 2003;188:1820.

Gorelick DA. Pharmacologic interventions for cocaine, crack, and other stimulant addiction. In: Graham AW, Schultz TK, Mayo-Smith FM, Ries RK, Wilford BB, eds. *Principles of Addiction Medicine*. 3rd ed. Chevy Chase, MD: American Society of Addiction Medication, Inc.; 2003.

Gorelick DA, Cornish JL. The pharmacology of cocaine, amphetamines, and other stimulants. In: Graham AW, Schultz TK, Mayo-Smith FM, Ries RK, Wilford BB, eds. *Principles of Addiction Medicine*. 3rd ed. Chevy Chase, MD: American Society of Addiction Medication, Inc.; 2003.

Green AR, Mechan AO, Elliott JM, O'Shea E, Colado MI. The pharmacology and clinical pharmacology of 3,4-methylenedioxymethamphetamine (MDMA, "Ecstasy"). *Pharmacol Rev*. 2003;55:463.

Jaffe JH. Amphetamine (or amphetamine-like)-related disorders. In: Sadock BJ, Sadock VA, eds. *Kaplan & Sadock's Comprehensive Textbook of Psychiatry*. 7th ed. Vol. 1. Baltimore: Lippincott Williams & Wilkins; 2000:924.

Jaffe JH, Ling W, Rawson RA. Amphetamine (or amphetamine-like)-related disorders. In: Sadock BJ, Sadock VA, eds. *Kaplan & Sadock's Comprehensive Textbook of Psychiatry*. 8th ed. Vol. 1. Baltimore: Lippincott Williams & Wilkins; 2005:1188.

Jaworski JN, Kozel MA, Philpot KB, Kuhar MJ. Intra-accumbal injection of CART (cocaine-amphetamine regulated transcript) peptide reduces cocaine-induced locomotor activity. *J Pharmacol Exp Ther*. 2003;307:1038.

Kendler KS, Prescott CA, Myers J, Neale MC. The structure of genetic and environmental risk factors for common psychiatric and substance use disorders in men and women. *Arch Gen Psychiatry*. 2003;60:929.

London ED, Simon SL, Berman SM, Mandelkern MA, Lichtman AM, Bramen J, Shinn AK, Miotto K, Learn J, Dong Y, Matochik JA, Kurian V, Newton T, Woods R, Rawson R, Ling R. Regional cerebral dysfunction associated with mood disturbances in abstinent methamphetamine abusers. *Arch Gen Psychiatry*. 2004;61:73.

Rodriguez N, Katz C, Webb VJ, Schaefer DR. Examining the impact of individual, community, and market factors on methamphetamine use: A tale of two cities. *Journal of Drug Issues*. 2005;35:665–694.

Suto N, Tanabe LM, Austin JD, Creekmore E, Vezina P. Previous exposure to VTA amphetamine enhances cocaine self-administration under a progressive ratio schedule in an NMDA, AMPA/Kainate, and metabotropic glutamate receptor-dependent manner. *Neuropsychopharmacology*. 2003;28:629.

Sweeting M, Farrell M. Methamphetamine psychosis: How is it related to schizophrenia? A review of the literature. *Current Psychiatry Reviews*. 2005;1:115–122.

▲ 12.4 Caffeine-Related Disorders

Caffeine is the most widely consumed psychoactive substance in the world. Although numerous studies have documented the safety of caffeine when used in typical daily doses, psychiatric symptoms and disorders can be associated with its use. Although rates for these disorders are not well established, even a low prevalence could still result in a considerable number of people with these disorders because of the widespread use of caffeine.

Hence, it is important for the clinician to be familiar with caffeine, its effects, and problems that can be associated with its use.

The text revision of the 4th edition of the American Psychiatric Association's *Diagnostic and Statistical Manual of Mental Disorders* (DSM-IV-TR) recognizes several caffeine-related disorders (e.g., caffeine intoxication, caffeine-induced anxiety disorder, and caffeine-induced sleep disorder). Other caffeine-related disorders, such as caffeine withdrawal and caffeine dependence, are not official diagnoses in DSM-IV-TR, but they can also be of clinical interest.

EPIDEMIOLOGY

Caffeine is contained in drinks, foods, prescription medicines, and over-the-counter medicines (Table 12.4–1). An adult in the United States consumes about 200 mg of caffeine per day on average, although 20 to 30 percent of all adults consume more than 500 mg per day. The per capita use of coffee in the United States is 10.2 pounds per year. A cup of coffee generally contains 100 to 150 mg of caffeine; tea contains about one third as much. Many over-the-counter medications contain one third to one half as much caffeine as a cup of coffee, and some migraine medications and over-the-counter stimulants contain more caffeine than a cup of coffee. Cocoa, chocolate, and soft drinks contain significant amounts of caffeine, enough to cause some symptoms of caffeine intoxication in small children when they ingest a candy bar and a 12-ounce cola drink.

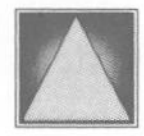

Table 12.4–1
Common Sources of Caffeine and Representative Decaffeinated Products

Source	Caffeine per Unit (mg)
Beverages and foods (5–6 oz)	
Fresh drip coffee, brewed coffee	90–140
Instant coffee	66–100
Tea (leaf or bagged)	30–100
Cocoa	5–50
Decaffeinated coffee	2–4
Chocolate bar or ounce of baking chocolate	25–35
Soft drinks (8–12 oz)	
Pepsi, Coke, Tab, Royal Crown Cola, Dr. Pepper, Mountain Dew	25–50
Canada Dry Ginger Ale, Caffeine-Free Coke, Caffeine-Free Pepsi, 7-Up, Sprite, Squirt, Caffeine-Free Tab	0
Prescription medications (1 tablet or capsule)	
Cafergot, Migralam	100
Anoquan, Aspir-code, BAC, Darvon, Fiorinal	32–50
Over-the-counter analgesics and cold preparations (1 tablet or capsule)	
Excedrin	60
Aspirin compound, Anacin, B-C powder, Capron, Cope, Dolor, Midol, Nilain, Norgesic, PAC, Trigesic, Vanquish	~30
Advil, aspirin, Empirin, Midol 200, Nuprin, Pamprin	0
Over-the-counter stimulants and appetite suppressants (1 tablet or capsule)	
Caffin-TD, Caffedrine	250
Vivarin, Ver	200
Quick-Pep	140–150
Amostant, Anorexin, Appedrine, Nodoz, Wakoz	100

(Adapted from table by Jerome H. Jaffe, M.D.)

Caffeine consumption also varies by age. The average daily caffeine consumption of caffeine consumers of all ages is 2.79 mg/kg of body weight in the United States. A substantial amount of caffeine is consumed even by young children (i.e., more than 1 mg/kg for children between the ages of 1 and 5 years). Worldwide, estimates place the average daily per capita caffeine consumption at about 70 mg. According to DSM-IV-TR, the actual prevalence of caffeine-related disorders is unknown, but up to 85 percent of adults consume caffeine in any given year.

COMORBIDITY

Persons with caffeine-related disorders are more likely to have additional substance-related disorders than are those without diagnoses of caffeine-related disorders. About two thirds of those who consume large amounts of caffeine daily also use sedative and hypnotic drugs.

ETIOLOGY

After exposure to caffeine, continued caffeine consumption can be influenced by several different factors, such as the pharmacological effects of caffeine, caffeine's reinforcing effects, genetic predispositions to caffeine use, and personal attributes of the consumer.

NEUROPHARMACOLOGY

Caffeine, a methylxanthine, is more potent than another commonly used methylxanthine, theophylline (Primatene). The half-life of caffeine in the human body is 3 to 10 hours, and the time of peak concentration is 30 to 60 minutes. Caffeine readily crosses the blood–brain barrier. Caffeine acts primarily as an antagonist of the adenosine receptors. Adenosine receptors activate an inhibitory G protein (Gi) and, thus, inhibit the formation of the second-messenger cyclic adenosine monophosphate (cAMP). Caffeine intake, therefore, results in an increase in intraneuronal cAMP concentrations in neurons with adenosine receptors. Three cups of coffee are estimated to deliver so much caffeine to the brain that about 50 percent of the adenosine receptors are occupied by caffeine. Several experiments indicate that caffeine, especially at high doses or concentrations, can affect dopamine and noradrenergic neurons. Specifically, dopamine activity may be enhanced by caffeine, a hypothesis that could explain clinical reports associating caffeine intake with an exacerbation of psychotic symptoms in patients with schizophrenia. Activation of noradrenergic neurons has been hypothesized to be involved in the mediation of some symptoms of caffeine withdrawal.

Subjective Effects and Reinforcement

Single low to moderate doses of caffeine (i.e., 20 to 200 mg) can produce a profile of subjective effects in humans that is generally identified as pleasurable. Thus, studies have shown that such doses of caffeine result in increased ratings on measures such as well-being, energy and concentration, and motivation to work. In addition, these doses of caffeine produce decreases in ratings of feeling sleepy or tired. Doses of caffeine in the range of 300 to 800 mg (the equivalent of several cups of brewed coffee ingested at once) produce effects that are often rated as being unpleasant, such as anxiety and nervousness. Although animal studies have generally found it difficult to demonstrate that caffeine functions as a reinforcer, well-controlled studies in humans have shown that people choose caffeine over placebo when given the choice under controlled experimental conditions. In habitual users, the reinforcing effects of caffeine are potentiated by the ability to suppress low-grade withdrawal symptoms after overnight abstinence. Thus, the profile of caffeine's subjective effects and its ability to function as a reinforcer contribute to the regular use of caffeine.

Genetics and Caffeine Use

Some genetic predisposition may exist to continued coffee use after exposure to coffee. Investigations comparing coffee or caffeine use in monozygotic and dizygotic twins have shown higher concordance rates for monozygotic twins for total caffeine consumption, heavy use, caffeine tolerance, caffeine withdrawal, and caffeine intoxication, with heritabilities ranging between 35 and 77 percent. Multivariate structural equation modeling of caffeine use, cigarette smoking, and alcohol use suggests that a common genetic factor—polysubstance use—underlines use of these three substances.

Age, Sex, and Race

The relationship between long-term chronic caffeine use and demographical features, such as age, sex, and race, has not been widely studied. Some evidence suggests middle-aged people may use more caffeine, although caffeine use in adolescents is not uncommon. No known evidence indicates that caffeine use differs between men and women, and no data specifically address caffeine use for different races. Some evidence suggests that, for both children and adults in the United States, whites consume more caffeine than blacks.

Special Populations

Cigarette smokers consume more caffeine than nonsmokers. This observation may reflect a common genetic vulnerability to caffeine use and cigarette smoking. It may also be related to increased rates of caffeine elimination in cigarette smokers. Preclinical and clinical studies indicate that regular caffeine use can potentiate the reinforcing effects of nicotine.

Heavy use and clinical dependence on alcohol is associated with heavy use and clinical dependence on caffeine as well. Individuals with anxiety disorders tend to report lower levels of caffeine use, although one study showed that a greater proportion of heavy caffeine consumers also use benzodiazepines. Several studies have also shown high daily amounts of caffeine use in psychiatric patients. For example, several studies have found that such patients consume the equivalent of an average of five or more cups of brewed coffee each day. Finally, high daily caffeine consumption has also been noted in prisoners.

Personality

Although attempts have been made to link preferential use of caffeine to particular personality types, results from these studies do not suggest that any particular personality type is especially linked to caffeine use.

Effects on Cerebral Blood Flow

Most studies have found that caffeine results in global cerebral vasoconstriction, with a resultant decrease in cerebral blood flow (CBF), although this effect may not occur in persons over 65 years of age. According to one recent study, tolerance does not develop to these vasoconstrictive effects, and the CBF shows a rebound increase after withdrawal from caffeine. Some clinicians believe that caffeine use can cause a similar constriction in the coronary arteries and produce angina in the absence of atherosclerosis.

DIAGNOSIS

The diagnosis of caffeine intoxication or other caffeine-related disorders depends primarily on a comprehensive history of a patient's intake of caffeine-containing products. The history should cover whether a patient has experienced any symptoms of caffeine withdrawal during periods when caffeine consumption was either stopped or severely reduced. The differential diagnosis for caffeine-related disorders should include the following psychiatric diagnoses: generalized anxiety disorder, panic disorder with or without agoraphobia, bipolar II disorder, attention-deficit/hyperactivity disorder, and sleep disorders. The differential diagnosis should include the abuse of caffeine-containing over-the-counter medications, anabolic steroids, and other stimulants, such as amphetamines and cocaine. A urine sample may be needed to screen for these substances. The differential diagnosis should also include hyperthyroidism and pheochromocytoma.

The DSM-IV-TR lists the caffeine-related disorders (Table 12.4–2) and provides diagnostic criteria for caffeine intoxication (Table 12.4–3), but does not formally recognize a diagnosis of caffeine withdrawal, which is classified as a caffeine-related disorder not otherwise specified (Table 12.4–4). The diagnostic criteria for other caffeine-related disorders are contained in the sections specific for the principal symptom (e.g., as a substance-induced anxiety disorder for caffeine-induced anxiety disorder).

Caffeine Intoxication

The DSM-IV-TR specifies the diagnostic criteria for caffeine intoxication (Table 12.4–3), including the recent consumption of caffeine, usually in excess of 250 mg. The annual incidence of caffeine intoxication is an estimated 10 percent, although some clinicians and investigators suspect that the actual incidence is much higher. The common symptoms associated with caffeine intoxication include anxiety, psychomotor agitation, restlessness, irritability, and psychophysiological complaints such as muscle twitching, flushed face, nausea, diuresis, gastrointestinal distress, excessive perspiration, tingling in the fingers and toes,

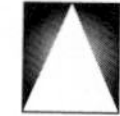

Table 12.4–2
DSM-IV-TR Caffeine-Related Disorders

Caffeine-induced disorders
- **Caffeine intoxication**
- **Caffeine-induced anxiety disorder**
  - *Specify* if:
    - With onset during intoxication
- **Caffeine-induced sleep disorder**
  - *Specify* if:
    - With onset during intoxication
- **Caffeine-related disorder not otherwise specified**

(From American Psychiatric Association. *Diagnostic and Statistical Manual of Mental Disorders.* 4th ed. Text rev. Washington, DC: American Psychiatric Association; copyright 2000, with permission.)

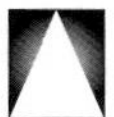

Table 12.4–3
DSM-IV-TR Diagnostic Criteria for Caffeine Intoxication

A. Recent consumption of caffeine, usually in excess of 250 mg (e.g., more than 2–3 cups of brewed coffee).
B. Five (or more) of the following signs, developing during, or shortly after, caffeine use:
 (1) restlessness
 (2) nervousness
 (3) excitement
 (4) insomnia
 (5) flushed face
 (6) diuresis
 (7) gastrointestinal disturbance
 (8) muscle twitching
 (9) rambling flow of thought and speech
 (10) tachycardia or cardiac arrhythmia
 (11) periods of inexhaustibility
 (12) psychomotor agitation
C. The symptoms in Criterion B cause clinically significant distress or impairment in social, occupational, or other important areas of functioning.
D. The symptoms are not due to a general medical condition and are not better accounted for by another mental disorder (e.g., an Anxiety Disorder).

(From American Psychiatric Association. *Diagnostic and Statistical Manual of Mental Disorders.* 4th ed. Text rev. Washington, DC: American Psychiatric Association; copyright 2000, with permission.)

and insomnia. Consumption of more than 1 g of caffeine can produce rambling speech, confused thinking, cardiac arrhythmias, inexhaustibleness, marked agitation, tinnitus, and mild visual hallucinations (light flashes). Consumption of more than 10 g of caffeine can cause generalized tonic-clonic seizures, respiratory failure, and death.

Caffeine Withdrawal

Despite that the DSM-IV-TR does not include a diagnosis of caffeine withdrawal, several well-controlled studies indicate that caffeine withdrawal is a real phenomenon, and DSM-IV-TR gives research criteria for caffeine withdrawal (Table 12.4–5). The appearance of withdrawal symptoms reflects the tolerance and physiological dependence that develop with continued caffeine use. Several epidemiological studies have reported symptoms of caffeine withdrawal in 50 to 75 percent of all caffeine users studied. The most common symptoms are headache and fatigue; other symptoms include anxiety, irritability, mild depressive symptoms, impaired psychomotor performance, nausea, vomiting, craving for caffeine, and muscle pain and stiffness.

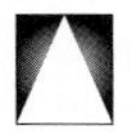

Table 12.4–4
DSM-IV-TR Diagnostic Criteria for Caffeine-Related Disorder Not Otherwise Specified

The caffeine-related disorder not otherwise specified category is for disorders associated with the use of caffeine that are not classifiable as caffeine intoxication, caffeine-induced anxiety disorder, or caffeine-induced sleep disorder. An example is caffeine withdrawal.

(From American Psychiatric Association. *Diagnostic and Statistical Manual of Mental Disorders.* 4th ed. Text rev. Washington, DC: American Psychiatric Association; copyright 2000, with permission.)

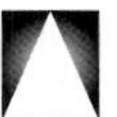

Table 12.4–5
DSM-IV-TR Research Criteria for Caffeine Withdrawal

A. Prolonged daily use of caffeine.
B. Abrupt cessation of caffeine use, or reduction in the amount of caffeine used, closely followed by headache and one (or more) of the following symptoms:
 (1) marked fatigue or drowsiness
 (2) marked anxiety or depression
 (3) nausea or vomiting
C. The symptoms in Criterion B cause clinically significant distress or impairment in social, occupational, or other important areas of functioning.
D. The symptoms are not due to the direct physiological effects of a general medical condition (e.g., migraine, viral illness) and are not better accounted for by another mental disorder.

(From American Psychiatric Association. *Diagnostic and Statistical Manual of Mental Disorders.* 4th ed. Text rev. Washington, DC: American Psychiatric Association; copyright 2000, with permission.)

The number and severity of the withdrawal symptoms are correlated with the amount of caffeine ingested and the abruptness of the withdrawal. Caffeine withdrawal symptoms have their onset 12 to 24 hours after the last dose; the symptoms peak in 24 to 48 hours and resolve within 1 week.

The induction of caffeine withdrawal can sometimes be iatrogenic. Physicians often ask their patients to discontinue caffeine intake before certain medical procedures, such as endoscopy, colonoscopy, and cardiac catheterization. Physicians also often recommend that patients with anxiety symptoms, cardiac arrhythmias, esophagitis, hiatal hernias, fibrocystic disease of the breast, and insomnia stop caffeine intake. Some persons simply decide that it would be good for them to stop using caffeine-containing products. In all these situations, caffeine users should taper the use of caffeine-containing products over a 7- to 14-day period rather than stop abruptly.

Caffeine-Induced Anxiety Disorder

Caffeine-induced anxiety disorder, which can occur during caffeine intoxication, is a DSM-IV-TR diagnosis (*see* Table 16.7–3). The anxiety related to caffeine use can resemble that of generalized anxiety disorder. Patients with the disorder may be perceived as "wired," overly talkative, and irritable; they may complain of not sleeping well and of having energy to burn. Caffeine can induce and exacerbate panic attacks in persons with a panic disorder and although a causative association between caffeine and a panic disorder has not yet been demonstrated, patients with panic disorder should avoid caffeine.

Caffeine-Induced Sleep Disorder

Caffeine-induced sleep disorder, which can occur during caffeine intoxication, is a DSM-IV-TR diagnosis (*see* Table 24.2–21). Caffeine is associated with delay in falling asleep, inability to remain asleep, and early morning awakening.

Caffeine Dependence

Caffeine dependence is not included in DSM-IV-TR, which explicitly states, "A diagnosis of Substance Dependence can be applied to every class of substance except caffeine." Despite the absence of caffeine dependence in DSM-IV-TR, evidence supports a diagnosis of caffeine dependence in some people with problematic caffeine consumption. No studies have examined the course and prognosis for patients with a diagnosis of caffeine dependence. Subjects with caffeine dependence have reported continued use of caffeine despite repeated efforts to discontinue their caffeine use. No studies have examined the course and prognosis for patients with a diagnosis of caffeine dependence. Subjects with caffeine dependence have reported continued use of caffeine despite repeated efforts to discontinue their caffeine use.

Ms. G was a 35-year-old married, white homemaker with three children, aged 8, 6, and 2. She took no prescription medications, took a multivitamin and vitamins C and E on a daily basis, did not smoke, and had no history of psychiatric problems. She drank moderate amounts of alcohol on the weekends, had smoked marijuana in college but had not used it since, and had no other history of illicit drug use.

She had started consuming caffeinated beverages while in college, and her current beverage of choice was caffeinated diet cola. Ms. G had her first soft drink early in the morning, shortly after getting out of bed, and she jokingly called it her "morning hit." She spaced out her bottles of soft drinks over the course of the day, with her last bottle at dinnertime. She typically drank four to five 20-oz bottles of caffeinated diet cola each day.

She and her husband had argued about her caffeinated soft drink use in the past, and her husband had believed she should not drink caffeinated soft drinks while pregnant. However, she had continued to do so during each of her pregnancies. Despite a desire to stop drinking caffeinated soft drinks, she was unable to do so. She described having a strong desire to drink caffeinated soft drinks, and if she resisted this desire, she found that she could not think of anything else. She drank caffeinated soft drinks in her car, which had a manual transmission, and noted that she fumbled while shifting and holding the soft drink and spilled it in the car. She also noted that her teeth had become yellowed, and she suspected this was related to her tendency to swish soft drink in her mouth before swallowing it. When asked to describe a time when she stopped using soft drinks, she reported that she had run out of it on the day one of her children was to have a birthday party, and she did not have time to leave her home to buy more. In the early afternoon of that day, a few hours before the scheduled start of the party, she felt extreme lethargy, a severe headache, irritability, and craving for a soft drink. She called her husband and told him she planned to cancel the party. She then went to the grocery store to buy soft drinks, and after drinking two bottles, she felt well enough to host the party.

Although initially expressing interest in decreasing or stopping her caffeinated soft drink use, Ms. G did not attend scheduled follow-up appointments after her first evaluation. When finally contacted at home, she reported she had only sought help initially at her husband's request, and she had decided to try to cut down on her caffeine use on her own. (Courtesy of Eric Stain, M.D.)

Caffeine-Related Disorder Not Otherwise Specified

The DSM-IV-TR contains a residual category for caffeine-related disorders that do not meet the criteria for caffeine intoxication, caffeine-induced anxiety disorder, or caffeine-induced sleep disorder (Table 12.4–4).

CLINICAL FEATURES

Signs and Symptoms

After the ingestion of 50 to 100 mg of caffeine, common symptoms include increased alertness, a mild sense of well-being, and a sense of improved verbal and motor performance. Caffeine ingestion is also associated with diuresis, cardiac muscle stimulation, increased intestinal peristalsis, increased gastric acid secretion, and (usually mildly) increased blood pressure.

Caffeine Use and Nonpsychiatric Illnesses. Despite numerous studies examining the relationship between caffeine use and physical illness, significant health risk from nonreversible pathological consequences of caffeine use, such as cancer, heart disease, and human reproduction, has not been conclusively demonstrated. Nonetheless, caffeine use is often considered to be contraindicated for various conditions, including generalized anxiety disorder, panic disorder, primary insomnia, gastroesophageal reflux, and pregnancy. In addition, the modest ability of caffeine to increase blood pressure and the documented cholesterol-elevating compounds of unfiltered coffee have raised the issue of the relationship of caffeine and coffee use to cardiovascular disease. Finally, there may be a mild association between higher daily caffeine use in women and delayed conception and slightly lower birth weight. Studies, however, have not found such associations, and effects, when found, are usually with relatively high daily dosages of caffeine (e.g., the equivalent of five cups of brewed coffee per day). For a woman who is considering pregnancy, especially if there is some difficulty in conceiving, it may be useful to counsel eliminating caffeine use. Similarly, for a woman who becomes pregnant and has moderate to high daily caffeine consumption, a discussion about decreasing her daily caffeine use may be warranted.

TREATMENT

Analgesics, such as aspirin, almost always can control the headaches and muscle aches that may accompany caffeine withdrawal. Rarely do patients require benzodiazepines to relieve withdrawal symptoms. If benzodiazepines are used for this purpose, they should be used in small dosages for a brief time, about 7 to 10 days at the longest.

The first step in reducing or eliminating caffeine use is to have patients determine their daily consumption of caffeine. This can best be accomplished by having the patient keep a daily food diary. The patient must recognize all sources of caffeine in the diet, including forms of caffeine (e.g., beverages, medications), and accurately record the amount consumed. After several days of keeping such a diary, the clinician can meet with the patient, review the diary, and determine the average daily caffeine dose in milligrams.

The patient and clinician should then decide on a fading schedule for caffeine consumption. Such a schedule could involve a decrease in increments of 10 percent every few days. Because caffeine is typically consumed in beverage form, the patient can use a substitution procedure in which a decaffeinated beverage is gradually used in place of the caffeinated beverage. The diary should be maintained during this time, so that the patient's progress can be monitored. The fading should be individualized for each patient so that the rate of decrease in caffeine consumption minimizes withdrawal symptoms. The patient should probably avoid stopping all caffeine use abruptly, because withdrawal symptoms are likely to develop with sudden discontinuation of all caffeine use.

References

Casas M, Ramos-Quiroga JA, Prat G, Qureshi A. Effects of coffee and caffeine on mood and mood disorders. In: Nehlig A, ed. *Coffee, Tea, Chocolate, and the Brain*. Boca Raton: CRC Press; 2004:73–83.

Cauli O, Pinna A, Valentini V, Morelli M. Subchronic caffeine exposure induces sensitization to caffeine and cross-sensitization to amphetamine ipsilateral turning behavior independent from dopamine release. *Neuropsychopharmacology*. 2003;28:1752–1759.

Griffiths RR, Juliano LM, Chausmer AL. Caffeine pharmacology and clinical effects. In: Graham AW, Schultz TK, Mayo-Smith M, Ries RK, Wilford BB, eds. *Principles of Addiction Medicine*. 3rd ed. Chevy Chase, MD: American Society of Addiction Medicine; 2003.

Kushner M. *The Truth About Caffeine: How Companies That Promote It Deceive Us and What We Can Do About It*. New York: SCR Books, LLC; 2006.

McCusker RR, Goldberger BA, Cone EJ. Caffeine content of specialty coffees. *J Anal Toxicol*. 2003;27:520–522.

Nawrot P, Jordan S, Eastwood J, Rotstein J, Hugenholtz A, Feeley M. Effects of caffeine on human health. *Food Addit Contam*. 2003;20:1–30.

Orbeta RL, Overpeck MD, Ramcharran D, Kogan MD, Ledsky R. High caffeine intake in adolescents: Associations with difficulty sleeping and feeling tired in the morning. *J Adolesc Health*. 2006;38(4):451–453.

Rogers PJ, Martin J, Smith C, Heatherley SV, Smit HJ. Absence of reinforcing, mood and psychomotor performance effects of caffeine in habitual non-consumers of caffeine. *Psychopharmacology (Berl)*. 2003;167:54–62.

Strain EC, Griffiths RR. In: Sadock BJ, Sadock VA, eds. *Kaplan & Sadock's Comprehensive Textbook of Psychiatry*. 8th ed. Vol. 1. Baltimore: Lippincott Williams & Wilkins; 2005:1201.

Striegel-Moore RH, Franko DL, Thompson D, Barton B, Schreiber GB, Daniels SR. Caffeine intake in eating disorders. *Int J Eat Disord*. 2006;39:162–165.

Tinley Em, Yeomans MR, Durlach PJ. Caffeine reinforces flavour preference in caffeine-dependent, but not long-term withdrawn, caffeine consumers. *Psychopharmacology (Berl)*. 2003;166:416–423.

▲ 12.5 Cannabis-Related Disorders

Cannabis preparations are obtained from the Indian hemp plant *Cannabis sativa*, a hardy, aromatic annual herb (Fig. 12.5–1). The cannabis plant has been used in China, India and the Middle East for approximately 8,000 years for its fiber and as a medicinal agent. It is the most commonly used illicit drug in the United States and, by most estimates, around the world as well.

CANNABIS PREPARATIONS

All parts of *Cannabis sativa* contain psychoactive cannabinoids, of which (−)-Δ9-tetrahydrocannabinol (Δ9-THC) is most abundant. The most potent forms of cannabis come from the flowering tops of the plants or from the dried, black-brown, resinous exudate from the leaves, which is referred to as hashish or hash. The cannabis plant is usually cut, dried, chopped, and rolled into cigarettes (commonly called "joints"), which are then smoked. The common names for cannabis are marijuana, grass, pot, weed, tea, and Mary Jane. Other names, which describe cannabis types of various strengths, are hemp, chasra, bhang, ganja, dagga, and sinsemilla. The potency of marijuana preparations has increased in recent years because of improved agricultural techniques used in cultivation so that plants may contain up to 15 or 20 percent THC.

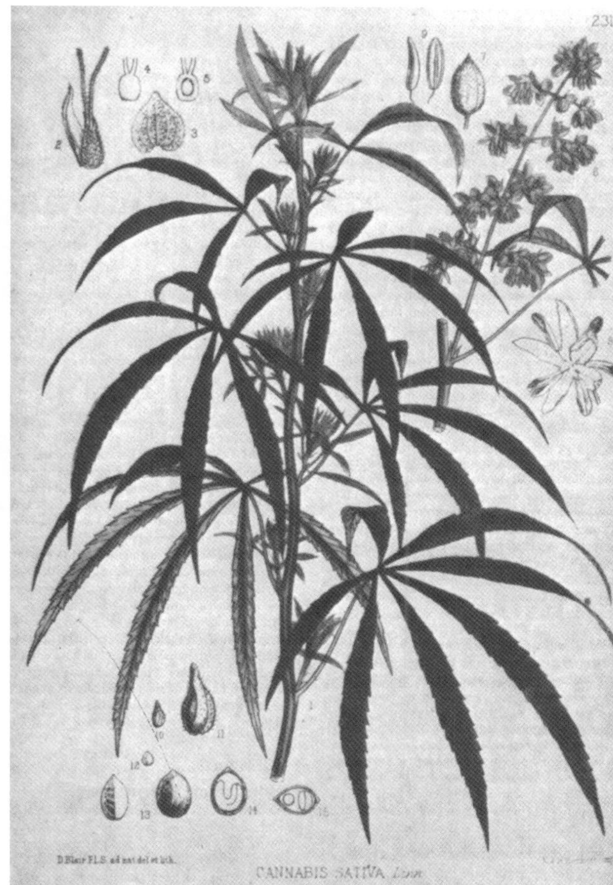

FIGURE 12.5–1
Marijuana (*Cannabis sataiva*).

EPIDEMIOLOGY

Prevalence and Recent Trends

Based on the 2003 National Surveys on Drug Use and Health (NSDUH), an estimated 90.8 million adults (42.9 percent) aged 18 years or older had used marijuana at least once in their lifetime. Among this group, about 2 percent used the drug before age 12, about 53 percent between 12 and 17 and about 45 percent after age 18.

The *Monitoring the Future* survey of adolescents in school indicates recent increases in lifetime, annual, current (within the past 30 days), and daily use of marijuana by eighth and tenth graders, continuing a trend that began in the early 1990s. In 1996, about 23 percent of eighth graders and about 40 percent of tenth graders reported having used marijuana and, in 1998 and 1999, more that a quarter of marijuana initiates were aged 14 years or younger. The average age was 17.

According to the text revision of the fourth edition of *Diagnostic and Statistical Manual of Mental Disorders* (DSM-IV-TR), there is a 5 percent lifetime rate of cannabis abuse or

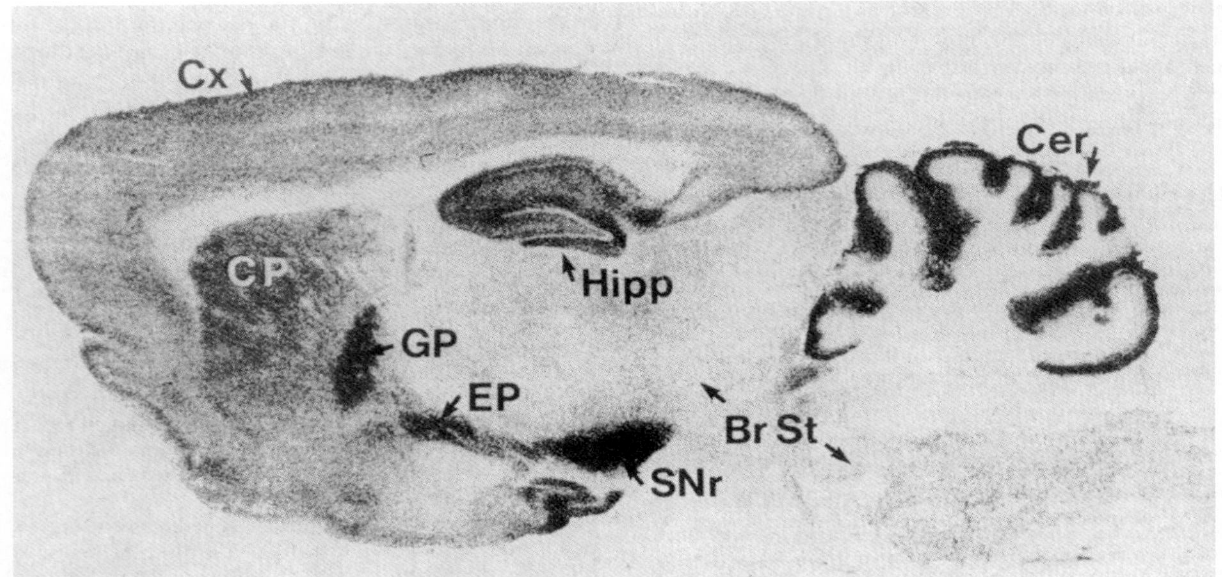

FIGURE 12.5–2
Autoradiography of cannabinoid receptor distribution in a sagittal section of rat brain. Binding of tritiated ligand is dense in the hippocampus (*Hipp*), the globus pallidus (*GP*), the entopeduncular nucleus (*EP*), the substantia nigra pars reticulata (*SNr*), and the cerebellum (*Cer*). Binding is moderate in the cerebral cortex (*Cx*) and the caudate putamen (*CP*) and sparse in the brainstem (*Br St*) and spinal cord. (From Howlett AC, Bidaut-Russell M, Devane WA, et al. The cannabinoid receptor: Biochemical anatomical, and behavioral characterization. *Trends Neurosci.* 1990;13:422, with permission.)

dependence, but that figure may be too low according to NSDUH surveys.

Demographic Correlates

The rate of past year and current marijuana use by males was almost twice the rate for females overall among those aged 26 and older. This gap between the sexes narrows with younger users; at ages 12 to 17, there are no significant differences.

Race and ethnicity were also related to marijuana use, but the relationships varied by age group. Among those aged 12 to 17, whites had higher rates of lifetime and past-year marijuana use than blacks. Among those 17 to 34 years of age, whites reported higher levels of lifetime use than blacks and Hispanics. But among those 35 and older, whites and blacks reported the same levels of use. The lifetime rates for black adults were significantly higher than those for Hispanics.

NEUROPHARMACOLOGY

As stated above, the principal component of cannabis is Δ9-THC; however, the cannabis plant contains more than 400 chemicals, of which about 60 are chemically related to Δ9-THC. In humans, Δ9-THC is rapidly converted into 11-hydroxy-Δ9-THC, the metabolite that is active in the central nervous system (CNS).

A specific receptor for the cannabinols has been identified, cloned, and characterized. The cannabinoid receptor, a member of the G protein-linked family of receptors, is linked to the inhibitory G protein (Gi), which is linked to adenylyl cyclase in an inhibitory fashion. The cannabinoid receptor is found in highest concentrations in the basal ganglia, the hippocampus, and the cerebellum, with lower concentrations in the cerebral cortex (Fig. 12.5–2). It is not found in the brainstem, a fact consistent with cannabis's minimal effects on respiratory and cardiac functions. Studies in animals have shown that the cannabinoids affect the monoamine and γ-aminobutyric acid (GABA) neurons.

According to most studies, animals do not self-administer cannabinoids as they do most other substances of abuse. Moreover, some debate questions whether the cannabinoids stimulate the so-called reward centers of the brain, such as the dopaminergic neurons of the ventral tegmental area. Tolerance to cannabis does develop, however, and psychological dependence has been found, although the evidence for physiological dependence is not strong. Withdrawal symptoms in humans are limited to modest increases in irritability, restlessness, insomnia, and anorexia and mild nausea; all these symptoms appear only when a person abruptly stops taking high doses of cannabis.

When cannabis is smoked, the euphoric effects appear within minutes, peak in about 30 minutes, and last 2 to 4 hours. Some motor and cognitive effects last 5 to 12 hours. Cannabis can also be taken orally when it is prepared in food, such as brownies and cakes. About two to three times as much cannabis must be taken orally to be as potent as cannabis taken by inhaling its smoke. Many variables affect the psychoactive properties of cannabis, including the potency of the cannabis used, the route of administration, the smoking technique, the effects of pyrolysis on the cannabinoid content, the dose, the setting, and the user's past experience, expectations, and unique biological vulnerability to the effects of cannabinoids.

DIAGNOSIS AND CLINICAL FEATURES

The most common physical effects of cannabis are dilation of the conjunctival blood vessels (red eye) and mild tachycardia.

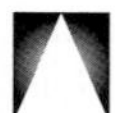

Table 12.5–1
DSM-IV-TR Cannabis-Related Disorders

Cannabis use disorders
Cannabis dependence
Cannabis abuse
Cannabis-induced disorders
Cannabis intoxication
Specify if:
With perceptual disturbances
Cannabis intoxication delirium
Cannabis-induced psychotic disorder, with delusions
Specify if:
With onset during intoxication
Cannabis-induced psychotic disorder, with hallucinations
Specify if:
With onset during intoxication
Cannabis-induced anxiety disorder
Specify if:
With onset during intoxication
Cannabis-related disorder not otherwise specified

(From American Psychiatric Association. *Diagnostic and Statistical Manual of Mental Disorders.* 4th ed. Text rev. Washington, DC: American Psychiatric Association; copyright 2000, with permission.)

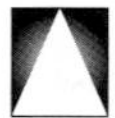

Table 12.5–2
DSM-IV-TR Diagnostic Criteria for Cannabis Intoxication

A. Recent use of cannabis.
B. Clinically significant maladaptive behavioral or psychological changes (e.g., impaired motor coordination, euphoria, anxiety, sensation of slowed time, impaired judgment, social withdrawal) that developed during, or shortly after, cannabis use.
C. Two (or more) of the following signs, developing within 2 hours of cannabis use:
(1) conjunctival injection
(2) increased appetite
(3) dry mouth
(4) tachycardia
D. The symptoms are not due to a general medical condition and are not better accounted for by another mental disorder.

Specify if:
With perceptual disturbances

(From American Psychiatric Association. *Diagnostic and Statistical Manual of Mental Disorders.* 4th ed. Text rev. Washington, DC: American Psychiatric Association; copyright 2000, with permission.)

At high doses, orthostatic hypotension may appear. Increased appetite—often referred to as "the munchies"—and dry mouth are common effects of cannabis intoxication. That no clearly documented case of death caused by cannabis intoxication alone reflects the substance's lack of effect on the respiratory rate. The most serious potential adverse effects of cannabis use are those caused by inhaling the same carcinogenic hydrocarbons present in conventional tobacco, and some data indicate that heavy cannabis users are at risk for chronic respiratory disease and lung cancer. The practice of smoking cannabis-containing cigarettes to their very ends, so-called "roaches," further increases the intake of tar (particulate matter). Many reports indicate that long-term cannabis use is associated with cerebral atrophy, seizure susceptibility, chromosomal damage, birth defects, impaired immune reactivity, alterations in testosterone concentrations, and dysregulation of menstrual cycles; these reports, however, have not been conclusively replicated, and the association between these findings and cannabis use is uncertain.

The DSM-IV-TR lists the cannabis-related disorders (Table 12.5–1), but has specific criteria within the cannabis-related disorders section only for cannabis intoxication (Table 12.5–2). The diagnostic criteria for the other cannabis-related disorders are contained in those DSM-IV-TR sections that focus on the major phenomenological symptom—for example, cannabis-induced psychotic disorder, with delusions, in the DSM-IV-TR section on substance-induced psychotic disorder (*see* Table 14.4–7).

Cannabis Dependence and Cannabis Abuse

The DSM-IV-TR includes the diagnoses of cannabis dependence and cannabis abuse (*see* Tables 12.1–3, 12.1–4, and 12.1–5). The experimental data clearly show tolerance to many of the effects of cannabis, but the data are less supportive of the existence of physical dependence. Psychological dependence on cannabis use does develop in long-term users.

Cannabis Intoxication

The DSM-IV-TR formalizes the diagnostic criteria for cannabis intoxication (Table 12.5–2). These criteria state that the diagnosis can be augmented with the phrase "with perceptual disturbances." If intact reality testing is not present, the diagnosis is cannabis-induced psychotic disorder.

Cannabis intoxication commonly heightens users' sensitivities to external stimuli, reveals new details, makes colors seem brighter and richer than in the past, and subjectively slows the appreciation of time. In high doses, users may experience depersonalization and derealization. Motor skills are impaired by cannabis use, and the impairment in motor skills remains after the subjective, euphoriant effects have resolved. For 8 to 12 hours after using cannabis, users' impaired motor skills interfere with the operation of motor vehicles and other heavy machinery. Moreover, these effects are additive to those of alcohol, which is commonly used in combination with cannabis.

Cannabis Intoxication Delirium

Cannabis intoxication delirium is a DSM-IV-TR diagnosis (*see* Table 10.2–6). The delirium associated with cannabis intoxication is characterized by marked impairment on cognition and performance tasks. Even modest doses of cannabis impair memory, reaction time, perception, motor coordination, and attention. High doses that also impair users' levels of consciousness have marked effects on cognitive measures.

Cannabis-Induced Psychotic Disorder

Cannabis-induced psychotic disorder (*see* Table 14.4–7) is diagnosed in the presence of a cannabis-induced psychosis. Cannabis-induced psychotic disorder is rare; transient paranoid ideation is more common.

A 35-year-old white married male who was naïve to cannabis use was given two "joints" by a friend. He smoked the first of the two in the same manner that he normally smoked a cigarette (in about 3 to 5 minutes). Noting no major effects, he proceeded immediately to smoke the second in the same amount of time. Within 30 minutes, he began to experience rapid heartbeat, dry mouth, mounting anxiety and the delusional belief that his throat was closing up and that he was going to die. That belief induced further panic and the patient was brought to the emergency room in the midst of a psychotic experience. Reassurance that he would not die had no effect. He was sedated with diazepam and some of his anxiety diminished. He eventually went to sleep and on awakening in about 5 hours he was asymptomatic with full recall of pervious events.

Florid psychosis is somewhat common in countries in which some persons have long-term access to cannabis of particularly high potency. The psychotic episodes are sometimes referred to as "hemp insanity." Cannabis use rarely causes a "bad-trip" experience, which is often associated with hallucinogen intoxication. When cannabis-induced psychotic disorder does occur, it may be correlated with a preexisting personality disorder in the affected person.

Cannabis-Induced Anxiety Disorder

Cannabis-induced anxiety disorder (*see* Table 16.7–3) is a common diagnosis for acute cannabis intoxication, which in many persons induces short-lived anxiety states often provoked by paranoid thoughts. In such circumstances, panic attacks may be induced, based on ill-defined and disorganized fears. The appearance of anxiety symptoms is correlated with the dose and is the most frequent adverse reaction to the moderate use of smoked cannabis. Inexperienced users are much more likely to experience anxiety symptoms than are experienced users.

Cannabis-Related Disorder Not Otherwise Specified

The DSM-IV-TR does not formally recognize cannabis-induced mood disorders; therefore, such disorders are classified as cannabis-related disorders not otherwise specified (Table 12.5–3). Cannabis intoxication can be associated with depressive symptoms, although such symptoms may suggest long-term cannabis use. Hypomania, however, is a common symptom in cannabis intoxication.

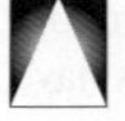

Table 12.5–3
DSM-IV-TR Diagnostic Criteria for Cannabis-Related Disorder Not Otherwise Specified

The cannabis-related disorder not otherwise specified category is for disorders associated with the use of cannabis that are not classifiable as cannabis dependence, cannabis abuse, cannabis intoxication, cannabis intoxication delirium, cannabis-induced psychotic disorder, or cannabis-induced anxiety disorder.

(From American Psychiatric Association. *Diagnostic and Statistical Manual of Mental Disorders.* 4th ed. Text rev. Washington, DC: American Psychiatric Association; copyright 2000, with permission.)

The DSM-IV-TR also does not formally recognize cannabis-induced sleep disorders or cannabis-induced sexual dysfunction; therefore, both are classified as cannabis-related disorders not otherwise specified. When either sleep disorder or sexual dysfunction symptoms are related to cannabis use, they almost always resolve within days or a week after cessation of cannabis use.

Flashbacks. Persisting perceptual abnormalities after cannabis use are not formally classified in DSM-IV-TR, although there are case reports of persons who have experienced—at times significantly—sensations related to cannabis intoxication after the short-term effects of the substance have disappeared. Continued debate concerns whether flashbacks are related to cannabis use alone or to the concomitant use of hallucinogens or of cannabis tainted with phencyclidine (PCP).

Cognitive Impairment. Clinical and experimental evidence indicates that the long-term use of cannabis may produce subtle forms of cognitive impairment in the higher cognitive functions of memory, attention, and organization and in the integration of complex information. This evidence suggests that the longer the period of heavy cannabis use, the more pronounced the cognitive impairment. Nonetheless, because the impairments in performance are subtle, it remains to be determined how significant they are for everyday functioning. It also remains to be investigated whether these impairments can be reversed after an extended period of abstinence from cannabis.

Amotivational Syndrome. A controversial cannabis-related syndrome is *amotivational syndrome*. Whether the syndrome is related to cannabis use or reflects characterological traits in a subgroup of persons regardless of cannabis use is under debate. Traditionally, the amotivational syndrome has been associated with long-term heavy use and has been characterized by a person's unwillingness to persist in a task—be it at school, at work, or in any setting that requires prolonged attention or tenacity. Persons are described as becoming apathetic and anergic, usually gaining weight, and appearing slothful.

TREATMENT AND REHABILITATION

Treatment of cannabis use rests on the same principles as treatment of other substances of abuse—abstinence and support. Abstinence can be achieved through direct interventions, such as hospitalization, or through careful monitoring on an outpatient basis by the use of urine drug screens, which can detect cannabis for up to 4 weeks after use. Support can be achieved through the use of individual, family, and group psychotherapies. Education should be a cornerstone for both abstinence and support programs. A patient who does not understand the intellectual reasons for addressing a substance-abuse problem has little motivation to stop. For some patients, an antianxiety drug may be useful for short-term relief of withdrawal symptoms. For other patients, cannabis use may be related to an underlying depressive disorder that may respond to specific antidepressant treatment.

Medical Use of Marijuana

Marijuana has been used as a medicinal herb for centuries, and cannabis was listed in the US Pharmacopeia until the end of the 19th century as a remedy for anxiety, depression, and gastrointestinal disorders, among others. Currently, cannabis is a controlled substance with a high potential for abuse and no medical use recognized by the Drug Enforcement Agency (DEA); however, it is used to treat various disorders, such as the nausea secondary to chemotherapy, multiple sclerosis (MS) chronic pain, acquired immune deficiency syndrome (AIDS), epilepsy, and glaucoma. In 1996, California residents approved the California Compensation Use Act that allowed state residents to grow and use marijuana for these disorders: in 2001, however, the US Supreme Court ruled 8 to 0 that the manufacture and distribution of marijuana are illegal under any circumstances. In addition, the Court held that patients using marijuana for medical purposes can be prosecuted; however, as of 2006, eleven states—Alaska, California, Colorado, Hawaii, Maine, Maryland, Montana, Nevada, Oregon, Vermont and Washington—have passed laws exempting patients who use cannabis under a physician's supervision from state criminal penalties.

In addition to the Supreme Court ruling, periodically the federal government attempts to prosecute doctors who prescribe the drug for medical use with the threat of loss of licensure or jail sentences. In a strongly worded editorial, the *New England Journal of Medicine* urged that "Federal authorities should rescind their prohibition of the medical use of marijuana for seriously ill patients and allow physicians to decide which patients to treat." The editorial concluded by commenting on the role of the physician: "Some physicians will have the courage to challenge the continued proscription of marijuana for the sick. Eventually, their actions will force the courts to adjudicate between the rights of those at death's door and the absolute power of bureaucrats whose decisions are based more on reflexive ideology and political correctness than on compassion."

Dronabinol, a synthetic form of THC, has been approved by the US Food and Drug Administration (FDA); some researchers believe, however, that when taken orally, it is not as effective as smoking the entire plant product. In 2006, regulatory officials authorized the first US clinical trial investigating the efficacy of Sativex, an oral spray consisting of natural cannabis extracts, for the treatment of cancer pain. Sativex is currently available by prescription in Canada and on a limited basis in Spain and Great Britain for patients suffering from neuropathic pain, multiple sclerosis, and other conditions.

References

Charuvastra A, Friedmann PD, Stein MD. Physician attitudes regarding the prescription of medical marijuana. *J Addict Dis*. 2005;24:87–94.

Coggans N, Dalgarno P, Johnson L, Shewan D. Long-term heavy cannabis use: Implications for health education. *Drugs: Education, Prevention & Policy*. 2004;11:299–313.

Fergusson DM, Horwood JL, Swain-Campbell NR. Cannabis dependence and psychotic symptoms in young people. *Psychol Med*. 2003;33:15–21.

Gerberich SG, Sidney S, Braun BL, Tekawa IS, Tolan KK, Quesenberry CP. Marijuana use and injury events resulting in hospitalization. *Ann Epidemiol*. 2003;13:230–237.

Hall W, Degenhardt L. Cannabis-related disorders. In: Sadock BJ, Sadock VA, eds. *Kaplan & Sadock's Comprehensive Textbook of Psychiatry*. 8th ed. Vol. 1. Baltimore: Lippincott Williams & Wilkins; 2005:1211.

Hall W, Pacula R. *Cannabis Use and Dependence: Public Health and Public Policy*. New York: Cambridge University Press; 2003.

Lynskey MT, Heath AC, Bucholz KK, Slutske WS. Escalation of drug use in early-onset cannabis users versus co-twin controls. *JAMA*. 2003;289:427–433.

Mura P, Kintz P, Ludes B, Gaulier JM, Marquet P, Martin-Dupont S, Vincent F, Kaddour A, Goulle JP, Nouveau J, Moulsma M, Tilhet-Coartet S, Pourrat O. Comparison of the prevalence of alcohol, cannabis, and other drugs between 900 injured drivers and 900 control subjects: Results of a French collaborative study. *Forensic Sci Int*. 2003;133:79–85.

ter Bogt T, Schmid H, Gabhainn SN, Fotiou A, Vollebergh W. Economic and cultural correlates of cannabis use among mid-adolescents in 31 countries. *Addiction*. 2006;101:241–251.

Vandrey RG, Budney AJ, Moore BA, Hughes JR. A cross-study comparison of cannabis and tobacco withdrawal. *Am J Addict*. 2005;14:54–63.

Zajicek J, Fox P, Sanders H, Wright D, Vickery J, Nunn AQ, Thompson A. Cannabinoids for treatment of spasticity and other symptoms related to multiple sclerosis (CAMS) study: Multicenter randomised placebo-controlled trial. *Lancet*. 2003;362:1517–1526.

▲ 12.6 Cocaine-Related Disorders

Few public health issues attracted as much media attention in the United States during the 1980s and early 1990s as the problems resulting from the use of cocaine and crack, a highly potent form of cocaine. Although the intranasal use of cocaine hydrochloride during that time was associated with high-income, "jet-set" users, since the beginning of the 21st century, smokable crack cocaine has become an endemic drug problem in the inner cities across the United States and around the world.

Cocaine is an alkaloid derived from the shrub *Erythroxylon coca*, which is indigenous to South America, where the leaves of the shrub are chewed by local inhabitants to obtain the stimulating effects (Fig. 12.6–1). The cocaine alkaloid was first isolated in 1860 and first used as a local anesthetic in 1880. It is still used as a local anesthetic, especially for eye, nose, and throat surgery, for which its vasoconstrictive and analgesic effects are helpful. In 1884, Sigmund Freud made a study of cocaine's general pharmacological effects and, for a period of time, according to his biographers, was addicted to the drug. In the 1880s and 1890s, cocaine was widely touted as a cure for many ills and was listed in the 1899 *Merck Manual*. It was the active ingredient in the beverage Coca-Cola until 1902. In 1914, however, once its addictive and adverse effects had been recognized, cocaine was classified as a narcotic, along with morphine and heroin.

DEFINITIONS

Substance use can be associated with a number of distinct disorders of which dependence and abuse are but two; the text revision of the fourth edition of *Diagnostic and Statistical Manual of Mental Disorders* (DSM-IV-TR) describes ten others for cocaine. Cocaine dependence is defined in DSM-IV-TR as a cluster of physiological, behavioral, and cognitive symptoms that, taken together, indicate that the person continues to use cocaine despite significant problems related to such use. It is defined in the 10th revision of *International Statistical Classification of Diseases and Related Health Problems* (ICD-10) as a cluster of physiological, behavioral, and cognitive phenomena in which a person gives much higher priority to cocaine use than to other

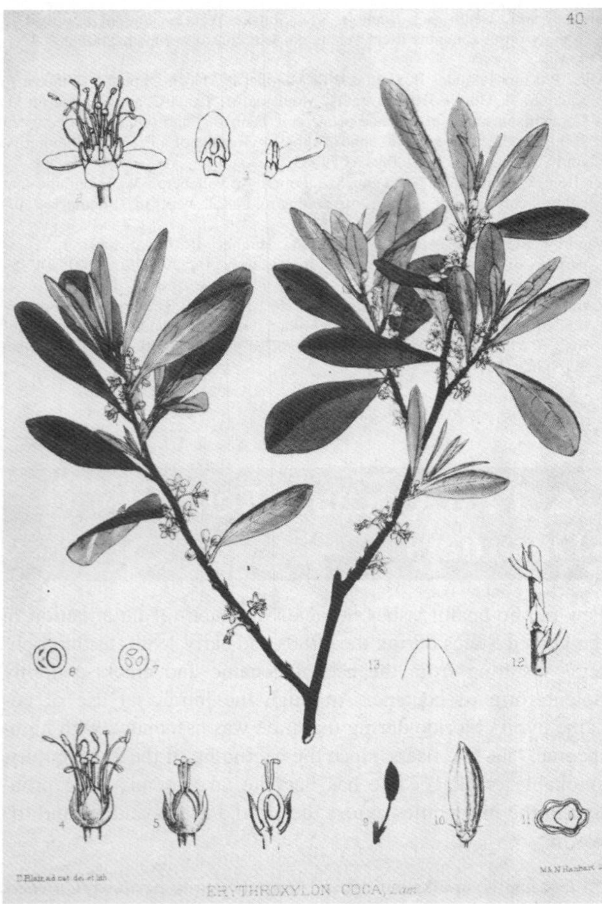

FIGURE 12.6–1
Cocaine is an alkaloid obtained from coca leaves.

behaviors that once had a greater value. Central to these definitions is the emphasis placed on the drug-using behavior, its maladaptive nature, and how over time the voluntary choice to engage in that behavior shifts and becomes constrained as a result of interactions with the drug.

The ICD-10 and DSM-IV-TR differ in their classification of what is called *substance abuse*. ICD-10 does not use the term *abuse* and includes instead the category of *harmful use*, which differs substantially from the concept of abuse used in DSM-IV-TR. Moreover, the concept of harm is limited to physical and mental health (e.g., hepatitis, cardiac damage, episodes of depression, or toxic psychosis). It specifically excludes social impairments, as follows: Harmful patterns of use are often criticized by others and frequently associated with adverse social consequences of various kinds. That a pattern of use of a particular substance is disapproved of by another person or by the culture, or may have led to socially negative consequences, such as arrest or marital arguments, is not in itself evidence of harmful use.

EPIDEMIOLOGY

Cocaine Use

In 2002 and 2003, 5.9 million (2.5 percent) persons aged 12 years or older used cocaine in the past year, and more than 2.1 million (0.9 percent) persons used cocaine in the past month. Persons aged 18 to 25 (6.7 percent) had a higher rate of past year cocaine use than persons aged 26 or older (1.9 percent) and youths aged 12 to 17 (1.9 percent). Males (3.4 percent) were more than twice as likely as females (1.6 percent) to have used cocaine in the past year. Asians had the lowest rate of past year cocaine use (0.7 percent) compared with other racial or ethnic groups.

Cocaine Abuse and Dependence

In 2002 and 2003, more than 1.5 million (0.6 percent) persons aged 12 or older met the criteria for abuse of, or dependence on, cocaine in the past year. Persons aged 18 to 25 (1.2 percent) had the highest rate of past year cocaine abuse or dependence, followed by persons aged 26 or older (0.6 percent) and youths aged 12 to 17 (0.4 percent). Males (0.9 percent) were more than twice as likely as females (0.4 percent) to have met the criteria for cocaine abuse or dependence. Blacks (1.1 percent) and Hispanics (0.9 percent) had higher rates of cocaine abuse or dependence than whites (0.5 percent), and the rate for Asians (0.1 percent) was lower than that for blacks, Hispanics, whites, American Indians or Alaskan Natives (1.2 percent), and non-Hispanic persons who identified themselves with two or more races (0.9 percent).

Crack Cocaine

An estimated 1.5 million (0.6 percent) persons aged 12 or older used crack cocaine in the past year, and 586,000 (0.2 percent) persons used crack cocaine in the past month. Persons aged 18 to 25 (0.9 percent) had the highest rate of past year crack use, followed by persons aged 26 or older (0.6 percent) and youths aged 12 to 17 (0.4 percent). Males (0.9 percent) were more than twice as likely as females (0.4 percent) to have used crack cocaine in the past year. Asians had the lowest rate of past year crack cocaine use (0.1 percent) compared with other racial or ethnic groups. Blacks (1.6 percent), American Indians or Alaska Natives (1.3 percent), Native Hawaiians or Other Pacific Islanders (1.2 percent), and persons who identified themselves with two or more non-Hispanic races (1.5 percent) had higher rates of past year crack cocaine use than whites (0.5 percent) and Hispanics or Latinos (0.5 percent).

Current cocaine use is on the decline, primarily because of increased awareness of cocaine's risks as well as a comprehensive public campaign about cocaine and its effects. The societal effects of the decrease in cocaine use, however, have been somewhat offset by the frequent use over the past years of crack.

COMORBIDITY

As with other substance-related disorders, cocaine-related disorders are often accompanied by additional psychiatric disorders. The development of mood disorders and alcohol-related disorders usually follows the onset of cocaine-related disorders, whereas anxiety disorders, antisocial personality disorder, and attention-deficit/hyperactivity disorder (ADHD) are thought to precede the development of cocaine-related disorders. Most studies of comorbidity in patients with cocaine-related disorders have shown that major depressive disorder, bipolar II disorder, cyclothymic disorder, anxiety disorders, and antisocial personality disorder are the most commonly associated psychiatric

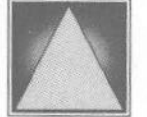

Table 12.6–1
Additional Psychiatric Diagnoses among Cocaine Users Seeking Treatment (New Haven Cocaine Diagnostic Study Results, Percentages)

Psychiatric Diagnosis	Current Disorder	Lifetime Disorder
Major depression	4.7	30.5
Cyclothymia/hyperthymia	19.9	19.9
Mania	0.0	3.7
Hypomania	2.0	7.4
Panic disorder	0.3	1.7
Generalized anxiety disorder	3.7	7.0
Phobia	11.7	13.4
Schizophrenia	0.0	0.3
Schizoaffective disorder	0.3	1.0
Alcoholism	28.9	61.7
Antisocial personality disorder—RDC	7.7	7.7
Antisocial personality disorder—DSM-III	32.9	32.9
Attention-deficit disorder		34.9

(Adapted from Rounsaville BJ, Anton SI, Caroll K, et al. Psychiatric diagnoses of treatment-seeking cocaine abusers. *Arch Gen Psychiatry.* 1991;48:43, with permission.)

diagnoses. The percentages of comorbidity in cocaine users are presented in Table 12.6–1.

ETIOLOGY

Genetic Factors

The most convincing evidence to date of a genetic influence on cocaine dependence comes from studies of twins. Monozygotic twins have higher concordance rates for stimulant dependence (cocaine, amphetamines, and amphetamine-like drugs) than dizygotic twins. The analyses indicate that genetic factors and unique (unshared) environmental factors contribute about equally to the development of stimulant dependence.

Sociocultural Factors

Social, cultural, and economic factors are powerful determinants of initial use, continuing use, and relapse. Excessive use is far more likely in countries where cocaine is readily available. Different economic opportunities may influence certain groups more than others to engage in selling illicit drugs, and selling is more likely to be carried out in familiar communities than in those where the seller runs a high risk of arrest.

Learning and Conditioning

Learning and conditioning are also considered important in perpetuating cocaine use. Each inhalation or injection of cocaine yields a "rush" and a euphoric experience that reinforce the antecedent drug-taking behavior. In addition, the environmental cues associated with substance use become associated with the euphoric state so that long after a period of cessation, such cues (e.g., white powder and paraphernalia) can elicit memories of the euphoric state and reawaken craving for cocaine.

In cocaine abusers (but not in normal controls), cocaine-related stimuli activate brain regions subserving episodic and working memory and produce electroencephalographic (EEG) arousal (desynchronization). Increased metabolic activity in the limbic-related regions, such as the amygdala, parahippocampal gyrus, and dorsolateral prefrontal cortex, reportedly correlates with reports of craving for cocaine, but the degree of EEG arousal does not.

Pharmacological Factors

As a result of actions in the central nervous system (CNS), cocaine can produce a sense of alertness, euphoria, and well-being. Users may experience decreased hunger and less need for sleep. Performance impaired by fatigue is usually improved. Some users believe that cocaine enhances sexual performance.

NEUROPHARMACOLOGY

Cocaine's primary pharmacodynamic action related to its behavioral effects is competitive blockade of dopamine reuptake by the dopamine transporter. This blockade increases the concentration of dopamine in the synaptic cleft and results in increased activation of both dopamine type 1 (D_1) and type 2 (D_2) receptors. The effects of cocaine on the activity mediated by D_3, D_4, and D_5 receptors are not yet well understood, but at least one preclinical study has implicated the D_3 receptor. Although the behavioral effects are attributed primarily to the blockade of dopamine reuptake, cocaine also blocks the reuptake of norepinephrine and serotonin. The behavioral effects related to these activities are receiving increased attention in the scientific literature. The effects of cocaine on cerebral blood flow and cerebral glucose use have also been studied. Results in most studies generally showed that cocaine is associated with decreased cerebral blood flow and possibly with the development of patchy areas of decreased glucose use.

The behavioral effects of cocaine are felt almost immediately and last for a relatively brief time (30 to 60 minutes); thus, users require repeated doses of the drug to maintain the feelings of intoxication. Despite the short-lived behavioral effects, metabolites of cocaine can be present in the blood and urine for up to 10 days.

Cocaine has powerful addictive qualities. Because of its potency as a positive reinforcer of behavior, psychological dependence on cocaine can develop after a single use. With repeated administration, both tolerance and sensitivity to various effects of cocaine can arise, although the development of tolerance or sensitivity is apparently caused by many factors and is not easily predicted. Physiological dependence on cocaine does occur, although cocaine withdrawal is mild compared with withdrawal from opiates and opioids.

Researchers recently reported that positron emission tomography (PET) scans of the brains of patients being treated for cocaine addiction show high activation in the mesolimbic dopamine system when addicts profoundly crave a drug. Researchers exposed patients to cues that had previously caused them to crave cocaine, and patients described feelings of intense cravings for the drug while PET scans showed activation in areas from the amygdala and the anterior cingulate to the tip of both temporal lobes. Some researchers claim that the mesolimbic dopamine system is also active in patients with nicotine addiction, and the same system has been linked to cravings for heroin, morphine, amphetamines, marijuana, and alcohol.

The D_2 receptors in the mesolimbic dopamine system have been held responsible for the heightened activity during periods of craving. PET scans of patients recovering from cocaine addiction are reported to show a drop in neuronal activity consistent with a lessened ability to receive dopamine, and the reduction in this ability, although it decreases over time, is apparent as long as a year and a half after withdrawal. The pattern of reduced brain activity reflects the course of the craving; between the third and fourth weeks of withdrawal, the activity is at its lowest level, and the risk of patient relapse is highest. After about 1 year, the brains of former addicts are almost back to normal, although whether the dopamine cells ever return to a completely normal state is debatable.

METHODS OF USE

Because drug dealers often dilute cocaine powder with sugar or procaine, street cocaine varies greatly in purity. Cocaine is sometimes cut with amphetamine. The most common method of using cocaine is inhaling the finely chopped powder into the nose, a practice referred to as "snorting" or "tooting." Other methods of ingesting cocaine are subcutaneous or intravenous (IV) injection and smoking (freebasing). Freebasing involves mixing street cocaine with chemically extracted pure cocaine alkaloid (the freebase) to get an increased effect. Smoking is also the method used to ingest crack cocaine. Inhaling is the least dangerous method of cocaine use; IV injection and smoking are the most dangerous. The most direct methods of ingestion are often associated with cerebrovascular diseases, cardiac abnormalities, and death. Although cocaine can be taken orally, it is rarely ingested via this, the least effective, route.

Crack

Crack, a freebase form of cocaine, is extremely potent. It is sold in small, ready-to-smoke amounts, often called "rocks." Crack cocaine is highly addictive; even one or two experiences with the drug can cause intense craving for more. Users have been known to resort to extremes of behavior to obtain the money to buy more crack. Reports from urban emergency rooms have also associated extremes of violence with crack abuse.

DIAGNOSIS AND CLINICAL FEATURES

The DSM-IV-TR lists many cocaine-related disorders (Table 12.6–2), but only specifies the diagnostic criteria for cocaine intoxication (Table 12.6–3) and cocaine withdrawal (Table 12.6–4) within the cocaine-related disorders section. The diagnostic criteria for the other cocaine-related disorders are in the DSM-IV-TR sections that focus on the principal symptom—for example, cocaine-induced mood disorder in the mood disorders section (*see* Table 15.3–10).

Cocaine Dependence and Abuse

The DSM-IV-TR uses the general guidelines for substance dependence and substance abuse to diagnose cocaine dependence and cocaine abuse (*see* Tables 12.1–3, 12.1–4, and 12.1–5). Clinically and practically, cocaine dependence or cocaine abuse can be suspected in patients who evidence unexplained changes in personality. Common changes associated with cocaine use are irritability, impaired ability to concentrate, compulsive behavior, severe insomnia, and weight loss. Colleagues at work and family members may notice a person's general and increasing inability to perform the expected tasks associated with work and family life. The patient may show new evidence of increased debt or inability to pay bills on time because of the large sums used to buy cocaine. Cocaine abusers often excuse themselves from work or social situations every 30 to 60 minutes to find a secluded place to inhale more cocaine. Because of the vasoconstricting effects of cocaine, users almost always develop nasal congestion, which they may attempt to self-medicate with decongestant sprays.

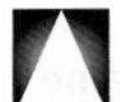

Table 12.6–2
DSM-IV-TR Cocaine-Related Disorders

Cocaine use disorders
Cocaine dependence
Cocaine abuse
Cocaine-induced disorders
Cocaine intoxication
Specify if:
With perceptual disturbances
Cocaine withdrawal
Cocaine intoxication delirium
Cocaine-induced psychotic disorder, with delusions
Specify if:
With onset during intoxication
Cocaine-induced psychotic disorder, with hallucinations
Specify if:
With onset during intoxication
Cocaine-induced mood disorder
Specify if:
With onset during intoxication
With onset during withdrawal
Cocaine-induced anxiety disorder
Specify if:
With onset during intoxication
With onset during withdrawal
Cocaine-induced sexual dysfunction
Specify if:
With onset during intoxication
Cocaine-induced sleep disorder
Specify if:
With onset during intoxication
With onset during withdrawal
Cocaine-related disorder not otherwise specified

(From American Psychiatric Association. *Diagnostic and Statistical Manual of Mental Disorders.* 4th ed. Text rev. Washington, DC: American Psychiatric Association; copyright 2000, with permission.)

T. Taylor was a separated, 39-year-old African American man who was admitted to a psychiatric day program in the shelter where he lived when he complained of sudden impulses to stab other residents. The staff in the shelter described him variously as "manipulative" and "charming." He gives a long history of abuse of alcohol, heroin, and cocaine, but says he has been "clean" for 3 weeks. He reports several arrests for felonies, including armed robbery and kidnapping, for which he always seems to have an explanation that minimizes his own responsibility.

Mr. Taylor entered the city shelter system 2 years earlier when the woman he was living with threw him out because she couldn't tolerate his temper and substance abuse. During his marriage to another woman 20 years ago, he was able to work briefly in blue-collar jobs in between prison and hospital stays. He has not worked for the past 7 years and has never paid child support to his wife.

Life did not begin easily for Mr. Taylor. His father left home before he was born, leaving behind a family scandal. The family story is that his father impregnated his wife's sister, causing Mr. Taylor to be treated like an outcast by the family. His mother had nine children, each with a different father. She had chronic depression and had received extensive psychiatric treatment. All of her children have psychiatric or substance abuse problems.

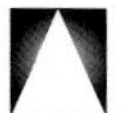

Table 12.6–3
DSM-IV-TR Diagnostic Criteria for Cocaine Intoxication

A. Recent use of cocaine.
B. Clinically significant maladaptive behavioral or psychological changes (e.g., euphoria or affective blunting; changes in sociability; hypervigilance; interpersonal sensitivity; anxiety, tension, or anger; stereotyped behaviors; impaired judgment; or impaired social or occupational functioning) that developed during, or shortly after, use of cocaine.
C. Two (or more) of the following, developing during, or shortly after, cocaine use:
(1) tachycardia or bradycardia
(2) pupillary dilation
(3) elevated or lowered blood pressure
(4) perspiration or chills
(5) nausea or vomiting
(6) evidence of weight loss
(7) psychomotor agitation or retardation
(8) muscular weakness, respiratory depression, chest pain, or cardiac arrhythmias
(9) confusion, seizures, dyskinesias, dystonias, or coma
D. The symptoms are not due to a general medical condition and are not better accounted for by another mental disorder.

Specify if:
With perceptual disturbances

(From American Psychiatric Association. *Diagnostic and Statistical Manual of Mental Disorders.* 4th ed. Text rev. Washington, DC: American Psychiatric Association; copyright 2000, with permission.)

When Mr. Taylor was 3, his mother turned him over to a succession of reluctant caregivers on both sides of the family. He was physically abused by some of his mother's boyfriends, being whipped with belts and electric cords. He dropped out of school in seventh grade because "a teacher embarrassed me." He began drinking when he entered the Job Corps at age 16. In his late teens and early 20s, he used nasal cocaine and heroin, then intravenous heroin for about a year. He stopped using drugs in his mid-20s, but continued to binge on alcohol every few weeks.

At age 19, after an argument with his wife, he cut his wrists and was hospitalized for 6 months. He was given an antidepressant, an unknown tranquilizer, and psychotherapy following his discharge, but stopped treatment when he felt better. Over the ensuing 20 years there were multiple hospitalizations when he was suicidal or had violent impulses. At one point he jumped off a bridge, sustaining multiple fractures. He has never exhibited manic symptoms, nor has he ever had delusions or hallucinations.

The one psychiatric chart that was available outlined an extensive criminal record and gives the patient the diagnosis of Antisocial Personality Disorder. His criminal history included charges for multiple armed robberies, desertion and neglect of a minor, and kidnapping of a 20-year-old man. With reference to the last crime, he said that he held the man at bay with a machete while his friends stole the man's car.

FOLLOW-UP

Over a 10-month treatment period, Mr. Taylor exhibited an intense attachment to his female caseworker. He often demanded immediate attention. When frustrated, he would occasionally become intoxicated and verbally abusive. This was especially the case when his caseworker left the program for another job. However, he did refrain from violent behavior and enrolled in a group for drug abusers who also have other psychiatric problems. An anticonvulsant drug helped him control his aggressive impulses. He also received individual and group counseling and social skills training and took part in a work and money-management program.

Mr. Taylor was accepted into a community residence and has been able to maintain his housing and his outpatient treatment in a day program during a 9-month period. He is monitored closely by his shelter caseworker, who intervenes when problems arise. (From *DSM-IV-TR Casebook.*)

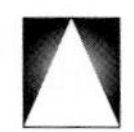

Table 12.6–4
DSM-IV-TR Diagnostic Criteria for Cocaine Withdrawal

A. Cessation of (or reduction in) cocaine use that has been heavy and prolonged.
B. Dysphoric mood and two (or more) of the following physiological changes, developing within a few hours to several days after Criterion A:
(1) fatigue
(2) vivid, unpleasant dreams
(3) insomnia or hypersomnia
(4) increased appetite
(5) psychomotor retardation or agitation
C. The symptoms in Criterion B cause clinically significant distress or impairment in social, occupational, or other important areas of functioning.
D. The symptoms are not due to a general medical condition and are not better accounted for by another mental disorder.

(From American Psychiatric Association. *Diagnostic and Statistical Manual of Mental Disorders.* 4th ed. Text rev. Washington, DC: American Psychiatric Association; copyright 2000, with permission.)

Cocaine Intoxication

The DSM-IV-TR specifies the diagnostic criteria for cocaine intoxication (Table 12.6–3), which emphasizes the behavioral and physical signs and symptoms of cocaine use. The DSM-IV-TR diagnostic criteria allow for specification of the presence of perceptual disturbances. If hallucinations are present in the absence of intact reality testing, the appropriate diagnosis is cocaine-induced psychotic disorder, with hallucinations.

Persons use cocaine for its characteristic effects of elation, euphoria, heightened self-esteem, and perceived improvement on mental and physical tasks. Some studies have indicated that low doses of cocaine can actually be associated with improved performance on some cognitive tasks. With high doses, however, the symptoms of intoxication include agitation, irritability, impaired judgment, impulsive and potentially dangerous sexual behavior, aggression, a generalized increase in psychomotor activity, and, potentially, symptoms of mania. The major associated physical symptoms are tachycardia, hypertension, and mydriasis.

Cocaine Withdrawal

After cessation of cocaine use or after acute intoxication, postintoxication depression ("crash") may be associated with symptoms of dysphoria, anhedonia, anxiety, irritability, fatigue, hypersomnolence, and sometimes agitation. With mild to moderate cocaine use, these withdrawal symptoms end within 18 hours. With heavy use, as in cocaine dependence, withdrawal symptoms can last up to a week, but usually peak in 2 to 4 days. Some patients and some anecdotal reports have described cocaine withdrawal syndromes that have lasted for weeks or months. The withdrawal symptoms can also be associated with suicidal ideation in affected persons. A person in the state of withdrawal can experience powerful and intense cravings for cocaine, especially because taking cocaine can eliminate the unpleasant withdrawal symptoms. Persons experiencing cocaine withdrawal often attempt to self-medicate with alcohol, sedatives, hypnotics, or antianxiety agents such as diazepam (Valium). The DSM-IV-TR diagnostic criteria for cocaine withdrawal are listed in Table 12.6–4.

Cocaine Intoxication Delirium

The DSM-IV-TR has specified a diagnosis for cocaine intoxication delirium (*see* Table 10.2–6). Cocaine intoxication delirium is most common when high doses of cocaine are used; when cocaine has been used over a short time, so that cocaine blood concentrations rapidly increase; or when cocaine is mixed with other psychoactive substances (e.g., amphetamine, opiates, opioids, and alcohol). Persons with preexisting brain damage (often resulting from previous episodes of cocaine intoxication) are also at increased risk for cocaine intoxication delirium.

Cocaine-Induced Psychotic Disorder

Paranoid delusions and hallucinations can occur in up to 50 percent of all persons who use cocaine. The occurrence of these psychotic symptoms depends on the dose, the duration of use, and the individual user's sensitivity to the substance. Cocaine-induced psychotic disorders are most common with IV and crack users. Men are much more likely to have psychotic symptoms than are women. Paranoid delusions are the most frequent psychotic symptoms. Auditory hallucinations are also common, but visual and tactile hallucinations may be less common than paranoid delusions. The sensation of bugs crawling just beneath the skin (formication) has been reported to be associated with cocaine use. Psychotic disorders can develop with grossly inappropriate sexual and generally bizarre behavior and homicidal or other violent actions related to the content of the paranoid delusions or hallucinations. The DSM-IV-TR diagnostic criteria of cocaine-induced psychotic disorders are listed in Table 14.4–7. Clinicians can further specify whether delusions or hallucinations are the predominant symptom.

Cocaine-Induced Mood Disorder

The DSM-IV-TR allows for the diagnosis of cocaine-induced mood disorder (*see* Table 15.3–10), which can begin during either intoxication or withdrawal. Classically, the mood disorder symptoms associated with intoxication are hypomanic or manic; the mood disorder symptoms associated with withdrawal are characteristic of depression.

Cocaine-Induced Anxiety Disorder

The DSM-IV-TR also allows for the diagnosis of cocaine-induced anxiety disorder (*see* Table 16.7–3). Common anxiety disorder symptoms associated with cocaine intoxication or withdrawal are those of obsessive–compulsive disorder, panic disorders, and phobias.

Cocaine-Induced Sexual Dysfunction

The DSM-IV-TR allows for the diagnosis of cocaine-induced sexual dysfunction (*see* Table 21.2–17), which can begin when a person is intoxicated with cocaine. Although cocaine is used as an aphrodisiac and as a way to delay orgasm, its repeated use can result in impotence.

Cocaine-Induced Sleep Disorder

Cocaine-induced sleep disorder, which can begin during either intoxication or withdrawal, is described under substance-induced sleep disorders (*see* Table 24.2–21). Cocaine intoxication is associated with the inability to sleep; cocaine withdrawal is associated with disrupted sleep or hypersomnolence.

Cocaine-Related Disorder Not Otherwise Specified

The DSM-IV-TR provides a diagnosis of cocaine-related disorder not otherwise specified for cocaine-related disorders that cannot be classified into one of the previously discussed diagnoses (Table 12.6–5).

Adverse Effects

A common adverse effect associated with cocaine use is nasal congestion; serious inflammation, swelling, bleeding, and ulceration of the nasal mucosa can also occur. Long-term use of cocaine can also lead to perforation of the nasal septa. Freebasing and smoking crack can damage the bronchial passages and the lungs. The IV use of cocaine can result in infection, embolisms, and the transmission of human immunodeficiency virus (HIV). Minor neurological complications with cocaine use include the development of acute dystonia, tics, and migraine-like headaches. The major complications of cocaine use, however, are cerebrovascular, epileptic, and cardiac. About two thirds of

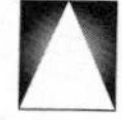

Table 12.6–5
DSM-IV-TR Diagnostic Criteria for Cocaine-Related Disorder Not Otherwise Specified

The cocaine-related disorder not otherwise specified category is for disorders associated with the use of cocaine that are not classifiable as cocaine dependence, cocaine abuse, cocaine intoxication, cocaine withdrawal, cocaine intoxication delirium, cocaine-induced psychotic disorder, cocaine-induced mood disorder, cocaine-induced anxiety disorder, cocaine-induced sexual dysfunction, or cocaine-induced sleep disorder.

(From American Psychiatric Association. *Diagnostic and Statistical Manual of Mental Disorders.* 4th ed. Text rev. Washington, DC: American Psychiatric Association; copyright 2000, with permission.)

these acute toxic effects occur within 1 hour of intoxication, about one fifth occur in 1 to 3 hours, and the remainder occurs up to several days later.

Cerebrovascular Effects. The most common cerebrovascular diseases associated with cocaine use are nonhemorrhagic cerebral infarctions. When hemorrhagic infarctions do occur, they can include subarachnoid, intraparenchymal, and intraventricular hemorrhages. Transient ischemic attacks have also been associated with cocaine use. Although these vascular disorders usually affect the brain, spinal cord hemorrhages have also been reported. The obvious pathophysiological mechanism for these vascular disorders is vasoconstriction, but other pathophysiological mechanisms have also been proposed.

Seizures. Seizures have been reported to account for 3 to 8 percent of cocaine-related emergency room visits. Cocaine is the substance of abuse most commonly associated with seizures; the second most common substance is amphetamine. Cocaine-induced seizures are usually single events, although multiple seizures and status epilepticus are also possible. A rare and easily misdiagnosed complication of cocaine use is partial complex status epilepticus, which should be considered as a diagnosis in a patient who seems to have cocaine-induced psychotic disorder with an unusually fluctuating course. The risk of having cocaine-induced seizures is highest in patients with a history of epilepsy who use high doses of cocaine as well as crack.

Cardiac Effects. Myocardial infarctions and arrhythmias are perhaps the most common cocaine-induced cardiac abnormalities. Cardiomyopathies can develop with long-term use of cocaine, and cardioembolic cerebral infarctions can be a further complication of cocaine-induced myocardial dysfunction.

Death. High doses of cocaine are associated with seizures, respiratory depression, cerebrovascular diseases, and myocardial infarctions—all of which can lead to death in persons who use cocaine. Users may experience warning signs of syncope or chest pain but may ignore these signs because of the irrepressible desire to take more cocaine. Deaths have also been reported with the ingestion of "speedballs," which are combinations of opioids and cocaine.

TREATMENT AND REHABILITATION

Detoxification

The cocaine withdrawal syndrome is distinct from that of opioids, alcohol, or sedative-hypnotic agents, because no physiological disturbances necessitate inpatient or residential drug withdrawal. Thus, it is generally possible to engage in a therapeutic trial of outpatient withdrawal before deciding whether a more intensive or controlled setting is required for patients unable to stop without help in limiting their access to cocaine. Patients withdrawing from cocaine typically experience fatigue, dysphoria, disturbed sleep, and some craving; some may experience depression. No pharmacological agents reliably reduce the intensity of withdrawal, but recovery over a week or two is generally uneventful. It may take longer, however, for sleep, mood, and cognitive function to recover fully.

Most cocaine users do not come to treatment voluntarily. Their experience with the substance is too positive, and the negative effects are perceived as too minimal, to warrant seeking treatment. Those who do not seek treatment often have polysubstance-related disorder, fewer negative consequences associated with cocaine use, fewer work- or family-related obligations, and increased contact with the legal system and with illegal activities.

The major hurdle to overcome in the treatment of cocaine-related disorders is the user's intense craving for the drug. Although animal studies have shown that cocaine is a powerful inducer of self-administration, these studies have also shown that animals limit their use of cocaine when negative reinforcers are experimentally linked to the cocaine intake. In humans, negative reinforcers may take the form of work and family-related problems brought on by cocaine use. Therefore, clinicians must take a broad treatment approach and include social, psychological, and perhaps biological strategies in the treatment program.

Attaining abstinence from cocaine in patients may require complete or partial hospitalization to remove them from the usual social settings in which they had obtained or used cocaine. Frequent, unscheduled urine testing is almost always necessary to monitor patients' continued abstinence, especially in the first weeks and months of treatment. Relapse prevention therapy (RPT) relies on cognitive and behavioral techniques in addition to hospitalization and outpatient therapy to achieve the goal of abstinence.

Psychosocial Therapies

Psychological intervention usually involves individual, group, and family modalities. In individual therapy, therapists should focus on the dynamics leading to cocaine use, the perceived positive effects of the cocaine, and other ways to achieve these effects. Group therapy and support groups, such as Narcotics Anonymous, often focus on discussions with other persons who use cocaine and on sharing experiences and effective coping methods. Family therapy is often an essential component of the treatment strategy. Common issues discussed in family therapy are the ways the patient's past behavior has harmed the family and the responses of family members to these behaviors. Therapy should also focus, however, on the future and on changes in the family's activities that may help the patient stay off the drug and direct energies in different directions. This approach can be used on an outpatient basis.

Network Therapy Network therapy was developed as a specialized type of combined individual and group therapy to ensure greater success in the office-based treatment of addicted patients. Network therapy uses both psychodynamic and cognitive-behavioral approaches to individual therapy while engaging the patient in a group support network. The group, composed of the patient's family and peers, is used as a therapeutic network joining the patient and therapist at intervals in therapy sessions. The approach promotes group cohesiveness as a vehicle for engaging patients in this treatment. This network is managed by the therapist to provide cohesiveness and support and to promote compliance with treatment. Although network therapy has not received systematic controlled evaluation, it is frequently applied in the psychiatric practice because it is one of the few manualized approaches that has been designed for use by individual practitioners in an office setting.

Pharmacological Adjuncts

Presently, no pharmacological treatments produce decreases in cocaine use comparable to the decreases in opioid use seen when heroin users are treated with methadone, levomethadyl acetate (ORLAAM) (commonly called L-a-acetylmethadol [LAAM]) or buprenorphine (Buprenex). A variety of pharmacological agents, most of which are approved for other uses, have been, and are being, tested clinically for the treatment of cocaine dependence and relapse.

Cocaine users presumed to have preexisting ADHD or mood disorders have been treated with methylphenidate (Ritalin) and lithium (Eskalith), respectively. Those drugs are of little or no benefit in patients without the disorders, and clinicians should adhere strictly to maximal diagnostic criteria before using either of them in the treatment of cocaine dependence. In patients with ADHD, slow-release forms of methylphenidate may be less likely to trigger cocaine craving, but the impact of such pharmacotherapy on cocaine use remains to be demonstrated.

Many pharmacological agents have been explored on the premise that chronic cocaine use alters the function of multiple neurotransmitter systems, especially the dopaminergic and serotonergic transmitters regulating hedonic tone, and that cocaine induces a state of relative dopaminergic deficiency. Although the evidence for such alterations in dopaminergic function has been growing, it has been difficult to demonstrate that agents theoretically capable of modifying dopamine function can alter the course of treatment.

Tricyclic antidepressant drugs yielded some positive results when used early in treatment with minimally drug-dependent patients; however, they are of little or no use inducing abstinence in moderate or severe cases.

Also tried but not confirmed effective in controlled studies are other antidepressants, such as bupropion, monoamine oxidase inhibitors (MAOIs), selective serotonin reuptake inhibitors (SSRIs), antipsychotics, lithium, several different calcium channel inhibitors, and anticonvulsants. One study found that 300 mg a day of phenytoin (Dilantin) reduced cocaine use; this study requires further replication.

Several agents are being developed that have not been tried in human studies. These include agents that would selectively block or stimulate dopamine receptor subtypes (e.g., selective D_1 agonists) and drugs that can selectively block the access of cocaine to the dopamine transporters but still permit the transporters to remove cocaine from the synapse. Another approach is aimed at preventing cocaine from reaching the brain by using antibodies to bind cocaine in the bloodstream (a so-called "cocaine vaccine"). Such cocaine-binding antibodies do reduce the reinforcing effects of cocaine in animal models. Also under study are catalytic antibodies that accelerate the hydrolysis of cocaine, and butyrylcholinesterase (pseudocholinesterase), which appears to hydrolyze cocaine selectively and is normally present in the body.

Vigabatrin is a drug that has been used as a treatment for refractory pediatric epilepsy, that appears to function by significantly elevating brain GABA levels. In animals, it was also noted to attenuate cocaine, nicotine, heroin, alcohol, and methamphetamine-induced increases in extracellular nucleus accumbens dopamine as well as drug-seeking behaviors associated with these biochemical changes. Preliminary clinical studies suggest efficacy for the treatment of cocaine and methamphetamine dependence. Large scale clinical trials for this indication are underway.

References

Flynn PM, Joe GW, Broome KM, Simpson DD, Brown BS. Looking back on cocaine dependence: Reasons for recovery. *Am J Addict*. 2003;12:398.

Gorelick DA. Pharmacologic interventions for cocaine, crack, and other stimulant addiction. In: Graham AW, Schultz TK, Mayo-Smith FM, Ries RK, Wilford BB, eds. *Principles of Addiction Medicine*. 3rd ed. Chevy Chase, MD: American Society of Addiction Medication, Inc.; 2003.

Gorelick DA, Cornish JL. The pharmacology of cocaine, amphetamines, and other stimulants. In: Graham AW, Schultz TK, Mayo-Smith FM, Ries RK, Wilford BB, eds. *Principles of Addiction Medicine*. 3rd ed. Chevy Chase, MD: American Society of Addiction Medication, Inc.; 2003.

Grella CE, Joshi V, Hser Y-I. Predictors of drug treatment re-entry following relapse to cocaine use in DATOS. *J Subst Abuse Treat*. 2003;25:145.

Higgins ST, Simon SC, Wong CJ, Heil SH, Badger GJ, Donham R, Dantona RL, Anthony S. Community reinforcement therapy for cocaine-dependent outpatients. *Arch Gen Psychiatry*. 2003;60:1043.

Jaffe JH. Cocaine-related disorders. In: Sadock BJ, Sadock VA, eds. *Kaplan & Sadock's Comprehensive Textbook of Psychiatry*. 7th ed. Vol. 1. Baltimore: Lippincott Williams & Wilkins; 2000:999.

Jaffe JH, Rawson RA, Ling W. Cocaine-related disorders. In: Sadock BJ, Sadock VA, eds. *Kaplan & Sadock's Comprehensive Textbook of Psychiatry*. 8th ed. Vol. 1. Baltimore: Lippincott Williams & Wilkins; 2005:1220.

Jaworski JN, Kozel MA, Philpot KB, Kuhar MJ. Intra-accumbal injection of CART (cocaine-amphetamine regulated transcript) peptide reduces cocaine-induced locomotor activity. *J Pharmacol Exp Ther*. 2003;307:1038.

Kendler KS, Jacobson KC, Prescott CA, Neale MC. Specificity of genetic and environmental risk factors for use and abuse/dependence of cannabis, cocaine, hallucinogens, sedatives, stimulants, and opiates in male twins. *Am J Psychiatry*. 2003;160:687.

Little KY, Krolewski DM, Zhang L, Cassin BJ. Loss of striatal vesicular monoamine transporter protein (VMAT2) in human cocaine users. *Am J Psychiatry*. 2003;160:47.

O'Brien MS, Anthony JC. Risk of becoming cocaine dependent: Epidemiological estimates for the United States, 2000–2001. *Neuropsychopharmacology*. 2005;30(5):1006–1018.

Shearer J, Wodak A, van Beek I, Mattick RP, Lewis J. Pilot randomized double blind placebo-controlled study of dexamphetamine for cocaine dependence. *Addiction*. 2003;98:1137.

Suto N, Tanabe LM, Austin JD, Creekmore E, Vezina P. Previous exposure to VTA amphetamine enhances cocaine self-administration under a progressive ratio schedule in an NMDA, AMPA/kainate, and metabotropic glutamate receptor-dependent manner. *Neuropsychopharmacology*. 2003;28:629.

▲ 12.7 Hallucinogen-Related Disorders

Hallucinogenic drugs have been used for thousands of years. Historically, drug-induced hallucinogenic states were usually part of social and religious rituals. Recognition of profound effects of lysergic acid diethylamide (LSD) on mental functioning in 1943 markedly changed things. Unlike plant-based hallucinogens, such as psilocybin mushrooms and peyote cacti, more potent chemically synthesized hallucinogenic compounds, such as LSD, could be more readily researched, distributed, and used, leading to continued fascination with this heterogeneous group of drugs and to many thousands of scientific reports of hallucinogenic drug effects, speculations about mechanisms of action, and discussions of medical and societal problems resulting from hallucinogen distribution, use, and consequences.

PREPARATIONS

Hallucinogens are natural and synthetic substances that are variously called *psychedelics* or *psychotomimetics* because, besides inducing hallucinations, they produce a loss of contact with reality and an experience of expanded and heightened consciousness. The hallucinogens are classified as Schedule I drugs; the US Food and Drug Administration (FDA) has decreed that they have no medical use and a high abuse potential.

The classic, naturally occurring hallucinogens are psilocybin (from some mushrooms) and mescaline (from peyote cactus); others are harmine, harmaline, ibogaine, and dimethyltryptamine (DMT). The classic synthetic hallucinogen is LSD, synthesized in 1938 by Albert Hoffman, who later accidentally ingested some of the drug and experienced the first LSD-induced hallucinogenic episode. Some researchers classify the substituted or so-called designer amphetamines, such as 3,4-methylenedioxyamphetamine (MDMA), as hallucinogens. Because these drugs are structurally related to amphetamines, this textbook classifies them as amphetamine-like substances, and they are covered in Section 12.3. Table 12.7–1 lists some representative hallucinogens.

EPIDEMIOLOGY

The incidence of hallucinogen use has exhibited two notable periods of increase. Between 1965 and 1969, there was a tenfold increase in the estimated annual number of initiates. This increase was driven primarily by the use of LSD. The second period of increase in first-time hallucinogen use occurred from around 1992 until 2000, fueled mainly by increases in use of ecstasy (i.e., MDMA). Decreases in initiation of both LSD and ecstasy were evident between 2001 and 2002, coinciding with an overall drop in hallucinogen incidence from 1.6 million to 1.1 million.

According to the text revision of the fourth edition of *Diagnostic and Statistical Manual of Mental Disorders* (DSM-IV-TR), 10 percent of persons in the United States had used a hallucinogen at least once. Hallucinogen use is most common among young (15 to 35 years of age) white men. The ratio of whites to blacks who have used a hallucinogen is 2 to 1, the white to Hispanic ratio is about 1.5 to 1. Men represent 62 percent of those who have used a hallucinogen at some time and 75 percent of those who have used a hallucinogen in the preceding month. Persons 26 to 34 years of age show the highest use of hallucinogens, with 15.5 percent having used a hallucinogen at least once. Persons 18 to 25 years of age have the highest recent use of a hallucinogen.

Cultural factors influence the use of hallucinogens; their use in the western United States is significantly higher than in the southern United States. Hallucinogen use is associated with less morbidity and less mortality than that of some other substances. For example, one study found that only 1 percent of substance-related emergency room visits were related to hallucinogens, compared with 40 percent for cocaine-related problems. Of persons visiting the emergency room for hallucinogen-related reasons, however, more than 50 percent were younger than 20 years of age. A resurgence in the popularity of hallucinogens has been reported. According to DSM-IV-TR, the lifetime rate of hallucinogen abuse is about 0.6 percent, with a 12-month prevalence of about 0.1 percent.

NEUROPHARMACOLOGY

Although most hallucinogenic substances vary in their pharmacological effects, LSD can serve as a hallucinogenic prototype. The pharmacodynamic effect of LSD remains controversial, although it is generally agreed that the drug acts on the serotonergic system, either as an antagonist or as an agonist. Data at this time suggest that LSD acts as a partial agonist at postsynaptic serotonin receptors.

Most hallucinogens are well absorbed after oral ingestion, although some are ingested by inhalation, smoking, or intravenous injection. Tolerance for LSD and other hallucinogens develops rapidly and is virtually complete after 3 or 4 days of continuous use. Tolerance also reverses quickly, usually in 4 to 7 days. Neither physical dependence nor withdrawal symptoms occur with hallucinogens, but a user can develop a psychological dependence on the insight-inducing experiences of episodes of hallucinogen use.

DIAGNOSIS

The DSM-IV-TR lists a number of hallucinogen-related disorders (Table 12.7–2), but contains specific diagnostic criteria only for hallucinogen intoxication (Table 12.7–3) and hallucinogen persisting perception disorder (flashbacks) (Table 12.7–4). The diagnostic criteria for the other hallucinogen use disorders are contained in the DSM-IV-TR sections that are specific to each symptom—for example, hallucinogen-induced mood disorder (*see* Table 15.3–10).

Hallucinogen Dependence and Hallucinogen Abuse

Long-term hallucinogen use is not common. As stated above, no physical addiction occurs. Although psychological dependence occurs, it is rare, in part because each LSD experience is different and in part because there is no reliable euphoria. Nonetheless, hallucinogen dependence and hallucinogen abuse are genuine syndromes, defined by DSM-IV-TR criteria (*see* Tables 12.1–3, 12.1–4, and 12.1–5).

Hallucinogen Intoxication

Intoxication with hallucinogens is defined in DSM-IV-TR as characterized by maladaptive behavioral and perceptual changes and by certain physiological signs (Table 12.7–3). The differential diagnosis for hallucinogen intoxication includes anticholinergic and amphetamine intoxication and alcohol withdrawal. The preferred treatment for hallucinogen intoxication is talking down the patient; during this process, guides can reassure patients that the symptoms are drug induced, that they are not going crazy, and that the symptoms will resolve shortly. In the most severe cases, dopaminergic antagonists—for example, haloperidol (Haldol)—or benzodiazepines—for example, diazepam (Valium)—can be used for a limited time. Hallucinogen intoxication usually lacks a withdrawal syndrome.

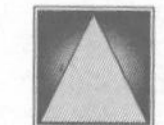

Table 12.7–1
Overview of Representative Hallucinogens

Agent	Locale	Chemical Classification	Biological Sources	Common Route	Typical Dose	Duration of Effects	Adverse Reactions
Lysergic acid diethylamide	Globally distributed, semisynthetic	Indolealkylamine	Fungus in rye yields lysergic acid	Oral	100 μg	6–12 hr	Extensive, including pandemic 1965–1975
Mescaline	Southwestern U.S.	Phenethylamine	Peyote cactus, *L. williamsii*	Oral	200–400 mg or 4–6 cactus buttons	10–12 hr	Little or none verified
Methylene-dioxyamphetamine (MDA)	U.S., synthetic	Phenethylamine	Synthetic	Oral	80–160 mg	8–12 hr	Documented
Methylenedioxymethamphetamine (MDMA)	U.S., synthetic	Phenethylamine	Synthetic	Oral	80–150 mg	4–6 hr	Documented
Psilocybin	Southern U.S., Mexico, South America	Phosphorylated hydroxylated DMT	Psilocybin mushrooms	Oral	4–6 mg or 5–10 g of dried mushroom	4–6 hr	Psychosis
Ibogaine	West Central Africa	Indolealkylamine	Tabernanthe iboga	Eating powdered root	200–400 mg	8–48 hr	CNS excitation, death?
Ayahuasca	S. American tropics	Harmine, other β-carbolines	Bark or leaves of *Banisteriopsis caapi*	As a tea	300–400 mg	4–8 hr	None reported
Dimethyltryptamine	S. America, synthetic	Substituted tryptamine	Leaves of *Virola calophylla*	As a snuff, IV	0.2 mg/kg I.V.	30 min	None reported
Morning glory	American tropics and warm zones	D-Lysergic acid alkaloids	Seeds of *I. violacea, T. corymbosa*	Orally as infusion	7–13 seeds	3 hr	Toxic delirium
Nutmeg and mace	Warm zones of Europe, Africa, Asia	Myristicin and aromatic ethers	Fruit of *M. fragrans*, commerical spcies	Orally or as a snuff	1 teaspoon, 5–15 g	Unknown	Similar to atropinism, with seizures, death
Yopo/Cohoba	Northern South America, Argentina	β-carbolines and tryptamines	Beans of *Anadenanthera peregrina*	Smoked or as a snuff	Unknown	Unknown	Ataxia, hallucinations, seizures?
Bufotenin	Northern South America, Argentina	5-OH-dimethyltryptamine	Skin glands of toads; seeds of *A. peregrina*	As a snuff or IV	Unknown	15 min	None reported

(Courtesy of Henry David Abraham, M.D.)

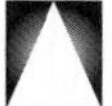

Table 12.7–2
DSM-IV-TR Hallucinogen-Related Disorders

Hallucinogen use disorders
Hallucinogen dependence
Hallucinogen abuse
Hallucinogen-induced disorders
Hallucinogen intoxication
Hallucinogen persisting perception disorder (flashbacks)
Hallucinogen intoxication delirium
Hallucinogen-induced psychotic disorder, with delusions
Specify if:
With onset during intoxication
Hallucinogen-induced psychotic disorder, with hallucinations
Specify if:
With onset during intoxication
Hallucinogen-induced mood disorder
Specify if:
With onset during intoxication
Hallucinogen-induced anxiety disorder
Specify if:
With onset during intoxication
Hallucinogen-related disorder not otherwise specified

(From American Psychiatric Association. *Diagnostic and Statistical Manual of Mental Disorders.* 4th ed. Text rev. Washington, DC: American Psychiatric Association; copyright 2000, with permission.)

Hallucinogen Persisting Perception Disorder

Long after ingesting a hallucinogen, a person can experience a flashback of hallucinogenic symptoms. This syndrome is diagnosed as *hallucinogen persisting perception disorder* (Table 12.7–4) in DSM-IV-TR. According to studies, from 15 to 80 percent of users of hallucinogens report having experienced flashbacks. The differential diagnosis for flashbacks includes migraine, seizures, visual system abnormalities, and posttraumatic stress disorder. The following can trigger a flashback: emotional stress; sensory deprivation, such as monotonous driving; or use of another psychoactive substance, such as alcohol or marijuana.

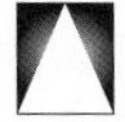

Table 12.7–3
DSM-IV-TR Diagnostic Criteria for Hallucinogen Intoxication

A. Recent use of a hallucinogen.
B. Clinically significant maladaptive behavioral or psychological changes (e.g., marked anxiety or depression, ideas of reference, fear of losing one's mind, paranoid ideation, impaired judgment, or impaired social or occupational functioning) that developed during, or shortly after, hallucinogen use.
C. Perceptual changes occurring in a state of full wakefulness and alertness (e.g., subjective intensification of perceptions, depersonalization, derealization, illusions, hallucinations, synesthesias) that developed during, or shortly after, hallucinogen use.
D. Two (or more) of the following signs, developing during, or shortly after, hallucinogen use:
(1) pupillary dilation
(2) tachycardia
(3) sweating
(4) palpitations
(5) blurring of vision
(6) tremors
(7) incoordination
E. The symptoms are not due to a general medical condition and are not better accounted for by another mental disorder.

(From American Psychiatric Association. *Diagnostic and Statistical Manual of Mental Disorders.* 4th ed. Text rev. Washington, DC: American Psychiatric Association; copyright 2000, with permission.)

Table 12.7–4
DSM-IV-TR Diagnostic Criteria for Hallucinogen Persisting Perception Disorder (Flashbacks)

A. The reexperiencing, following cessation of use of a hallucinogen, of one or more of the perceptual symptoms that were experienced while intoxicated with the hallucinogen (e.g., geometric hallucinations, false perceptions of movement in the peripheral visual fields, flashes of color, intensified colors, trails of images of moving objects, positive afterimages, halos around objects, macropsia, and micropsia).
B. The symptoms in Criterion A cause clinically significant distress or impairment in social, occupational, or other important areas of functioning.
C. The symptoms are not due to a general medical condition (e.g., anatomical lesions and infections of the brain, visual epilepsies) and are not better accounted for by another mental disorder (e.g., delirium, dementia, schizophrenia) or hypnopompic hallucinations.

(From American Psychiatric Association. *Diagnostic and Statistical Manual of Mental Disorders.* 4th ed. Text rev. Washington, DC: American Psychiatric Association; copyright 2000, with permission.)

Flashbacks are spontaneous, transitory recurrences of the substance-induced experience. Most flashbacks are episodes of visual distortion, geometric hallucinations, hallucinations of sounds or voices, false perceptions of movement in peripheral fields, flashes of color, trails of images from moving objects, positive afterimages and halos, macropsia, micropsia, time expansion, physical symptoms, or relived intense emotion. The episodes usually last a few seconds to a few minutes, but sometimes last longer. Most often, even in the presence of distinct perceptual disturbances, the person has insight into the pathological nature of the disturbance. Suicidal behavior, major depressive disorder, and panic disorders are potential complications.

A 20-year-old undergraduate presented with a chief complaint of seeing the air. The visual disturbance consisted of perception of white pinpoint specks in both the central and peripheral visual fields too numerous to count. They were constantly present and were accompanied by the perception of trails of moving objects left behind as they passed through the patient's visual field. Attending a hockey game was difficult, as the brightly dressed players left streaks of their own images against the white of the ice for seconds at a time. The patient also described the false perception of movement in stable objects, usually in his peripheral visual fields; halos around objects; and positive and negative afterimages. Other symptoms included mild depression, daily bitemporal headache, and a loss of concentration in the last year.

The visual syndrome had gradually emerged over the past 3 months following experimentation with the hallucinogenic drug LCD-25 on three separate occasions in the preceding 3 months. He feared he had sustained some kind of "brain damage" from the drug experience. He denied use of any other agents, including amphetamines, phencyclidine, narcotics, or alcohol, to excess. He had smoked marijuana twice a week for a period of 7 months at age 17.

The patient had consulted two ophthalmologists, both of whom confirmed that the white pinpoint specks were not vitreous floaters (diagnostically insignificant particulate matter floating in the vitreous humor of the eye that can cause the perception of "specks"). A neurologist's examination also proved negative. A therapeutic trial of an anticonvulsant medication resulted in a 50 percent improvement in the patient's visual symptoms and remission of his depression. (Courtesy of *DSM-IV-TR Casebook.*)

Hallucinogen Intoxication Delirium

The DSM-IV-TR allows for the diagnosis of hallucinogen intoxication delirium (*see* Table 10.2–6), a relatively rare disorder beginning during intoxication in those who have ingested pure hallucinogens. Hallucinogens are often mixed with other substances, however, and the other components or their interactions with the hallucinogens can produce clinical delirium.

Hallucinogen-Induced Psychotic Disorders

If psychotic symptoms are present in the absence of retained reality testing, a diagnosis of hallucinogen-induced psychotic disorder may be warranted (*see* Table 14.4–7). DSM-IV-TR also allows clinicians to specify whether hallucinations or delusions are the prominent symptoms. The most common adverse effect of LSD and related substances is a "bad trip," an experience resembling the acute panic reaction to cannabis but sometimes more severe; a bad trip can occasionally produce true psychotic symptoms. The bad trip generally ends when the immediate effects of the hallucinogen wear off, but its course is variable. Occasionally, a protracted psychotic episode is difficult to distinguish from a nonorganic psychotic disorder. Whether a chronic psychosis after drug ingestion is the result of the drug ingestion, is unrelated to the drug ingestion, or is a combination of both the drug ingestion and predisposing factors is currently unanswerable.

Occasionally, the psychotic disorder is prolonged, a reaction thought to be most common in persons with preexisting schizoid personality disorder and prepsychotic personalities, an unstable ego balance, or much anxiety. Such persons cannot cope with the perceptual changes, body-image distortions, and symbolic unconscious material stimulated by the hallucinogen. The rate of previous mental instability in persons hospitalized for LSD reactions is high. Adverse reactions occurred in the late 1960s when LSD was being promoted as a self-prescribed psychotherapy for emotional crises in the lives of seriously disturbed persons. Now that this practice is less frequent, prolonged adverse reactions are less common.

A 22-year-old female photography student presented to the hospital with inappropriate mood and bizarre thinking. She had no prior psychiatric history. Nine days before admission, she ingested one or two psilocybin mushrooms. Following the immediate ingestion, the patient began to giggle. She then described euphoria, which progressed to auditory hallucinations and belief in the ability to broadcast her thoughts on the media. Two days later she repeated the ingestion, and continued to exhibit psychotic symptoms to the day of admission. When examined she heard voices telling her she could be president, and reported the sounds of "lambs crying." She continued to giggle inappropriately, bizarrely turning her head from side to side ritualistically. She continued to describe euphoria, but with an intermittent sense of hopelessness in a context of thought blocking. Her self-description was "feeling lucky." She was given haloperidol, 10 mg twice a day, along with benztropine (Cogentin) 1 mg three times a day and lithium carbonate (Eskalith) 300 mg twice a day. On this regimen her psychosis abated after 5 days.

Hallucinogen-Induced Mood Disorder

The DSM-IV-TR provides a diagnostic category for hallucinogen-induced mood disorder (*see* Table 15.3–10). Unlike cocaine-induced mood disorder and amphetamine-induced mood disorder, in which the symptoms are somewhat predictable, mood disorder symptoms accompanying hallucinogen abuse can vary. Abusers may experience manic-like symptoms with grandiose delusions or depression-like feelings and ideas or mixed symptoms. As with the hallucinogen-induced psychotic disorder symptoms, the symptoms of hallucinogen-induced mood disorder usually resolve once the drug has been eliminated from the person's body.

Hallucinogen-Induced Anxiety Disorder

Hallucinogen-induced anxiety disorder (*see* Table 16.7–3) also varies in its symptom pattern, but few data about symptom patterns are available. Anecdotally, emergency room physicians who treat patients with hallucinogen-related disorders frequently report panic disorder with agoraphobia.

A 20-year-old man had a 7-year history of polysubstance abuse, including having used LSD an estimated 400 times. While driving with his girlfriend, he ingested an unknown quantity of LSD and became intoxicated; he reported using no other drugs at this time. Within minutes after ingestion, he began to experience visual hallucinations that intensified as he drove. When he attempted to speak to his girlfriend, he saw that she had become a giant lizard. He became terrified and attempted to kill her by crashing the car, injuring himself and his passenger. By the time of discharge from the hospital 3 days later, his panic had resolved.

Hallucinogen-Related Disorder Not Otherwise Specified

When a patient with a hallucinogen-related disorder does not meet the diagnostic criteria for any of the standard hallucinogen-related disorders, the patient may be classified as having hallucinogen-related disorder not otherwise specified (Table 12.7–5). DSM-IV-TR does not have a diagnostic category of hallucinogen withdrawal, but some clinicians anecdotally report a syndrome with depression and anxiety after cessation of frequent hallucinogen use. Such a syndrome may best fit the diagnosis of hallucinogen-related disorder not otherwise specified.

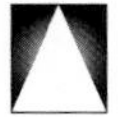

Table 12.7–5
DSM-IV-TR Diagnostic Criteria for Hallucinogen-Related Disorder Not Otherwise Specified

The hallucinogen-related disorder not otherwise specified category is for disorders associated with the use of hallucinogens that are not classifiable as hallucinogen dependence, hallucinogen abuse, hallucinogen intoxication, hallucinogen persisting perception disorder, hallucinogen intoxication delirium, hallucinogen-induced psychotic disorder, hallucinogen-induced mood disorder, or hallucinogen-induced anxiety disorder.

(From American Psychiatric Association. *Diagnostic and Statistical Manual of Mental Disorders.* 4th ed. Text rev. Washington, DC: American Psychiatric Association; copyright 2000, with permission.)

CLINICAL FEATURES

Lysergic Acid Diethylamide

A large class of hallucinogenic compounds with well-studied structure–activity relationships is represented by the prototype LSD. LSD is a synthetic base derived from the lysergic acid nucleus from the ergot alkaloids. That family of compounds was discovered in rye fungus and was responsible for lethal outbreaks of St. Anthony's fire in the Middle Ages. The compounds are also present in morning glory seeds in low concentrations. Many homologs and analogs of LSD have been studied. None of them has potency exceeding that of LSD.

Physiological symptoms from LSD are typically few and relatively mild. Dilated pupils, increased deep tendon motor reflexes and muscle tension, and mild motor incoordination and ataxia are common. Increased heart rate, respiration, and blood pressure are modest in degree and variable, as are nausea, decreased appetite, and salivation.

The usual sequence of changes follows a pattern of somatic symptoms appearing first, then mood and perceptual changes, and, finally, psychological changes, although effects overlap and, depending on the particular hallucinogen, the time of onset and offset varies. The intensity of LSD effects in a nontolerant user generally is proportional to dose, with 25 μg as an approximate threshold dose.

The syndrome produced by LSD resembles that produced by mescaline, psilocybin, and some of the amphetamine analogs. The major difference among LSD, psilocybin, and mescaline is potency. A 1.5 μg/kg dose of LSD is roughly equivalent to 225 μg/kg of psilocybin, which is equivalent to 5 mg/kg of mescaline. With mescaline, onset of symptoms is slower and more nausea and vomiting occurs, but in general, the perceptual effects are more similar than different.

Tolerance, particularly to the sensory and other psychological effects, is evident as soon as the second or third day of successive LSD use. Four to 6 days free of LSD is necessary to lose significant tolerance. Tolerance is associated with frequent use of any of the hallucinogens. Cross-tolerance among mescaline, psilocybin, and LSD occurs, but not between amphetamine and LSD, despite the chemical similarity of amphetamine and mescaline.

Previously distributed as tablets, liquid, powder, and gelatin squares, in recent years, LSD has been commonly distributed as "blotter acid." Sheets of paper are soaked with LSD, dried, and perforated into small squares. Popular designs are stamped on the paper. Each sheet contains as many as a few hundred squares; one square containing 30 to 75 μg of LSD is one chewed dose, more or less. Planned massive ingestion is uncommon but happens by accident.

The onset of action of LSD occurs within an hour, peaks in 2 to 4 hours, and lasts 8 to 12 hours. The sympathomimetic effects of LSD include tremors, tachycardia, hypertension, hyperthermia, sweating, blurring of vision, and mydriasis. Death caused by cardiac or cerebrovascular pathology related to hypertension or hyperthermia can occur with hallucinogenic use. A syndrome similar to neuroleptic malignant syndrome has reportedly been associated with LSD. Death can also be caused by a physical injury when LSD use impairs judgment about traffic or a person's ability to fly, for example. The psychological effects are usually well tolerated, but when persons cannot recall experiences or appreciate that the experiences are substance induced, they may fear the onset of insanity.

With hallucinogen use, perceptions become unusually brilliant and intense. Colors and textures seem to be richer than in the past, contours sharpened, music more emotionally profound, and smells and tastes heightened. Synesthesia is common; colors may be heard or sounds seen. Changes in body image and alterations of time and space perception also occur. Hallucinations are usually visual, often of geometric forms and figures, but auditory and tactile hallucinations are sometimes experienced. Emotions become unusually intense and may change abruptly and often; two seemingly incompatible feelings may be experienced at the same time. Suggestibility is greatly heightened, and sensitivity or detachment from other persons may arise. Other common features are a seeming awareness of internal organs, the recovery of lost early memories, the release of unconscious material in symbolic form, and regression and the apparent reliving of past events, including birth. Introspective reflection and feelings of religious and philosophical insight are common. The sense of self is greatly changed, sometimes to the point of depersonalization, merging with the external world, separation of self from body, or total dissolution of the ego in mystical ecstasy.

No clear evidence indicates a drastic personality change or chronic psychosis produced by long-term LSD use by moderate users not otherwise predisposed to these conditions. Some heavy users of hallucinogens, however, may experience chronic anxiety or depression and may benefit from a psychological or pharmacological approach that addresses the underlying problem.

Many persons maintain that a single experience with LSD has given them increased creative capacity, new psychological insight, relief from neurotic or psychosomatic symptoms, or a desirable change in personality. In the 1950s and 1960s, psychiatrists showed great interest in LSD and related substances, both as potential models for functional psychosis and as possible pharmacotherapeutic agents. The availability of these compounds to researchers in the basic neurosciences has led to many scientific advances.

Phenethylamines

Phenethylamines are compounds with simple chemical structures and structural similarity to the neurotransmitters dopamine and norepinephrine. Mescaline (3,4,5-trimethoxyphenethylamine), a classic hallucinogen in every sense of the term, was the first hallucinogen isolated from the peyote cactus that grows in the southwestern United States and northern Mexico. Mescaline human pharmacology was characterized in 1896 and its structure verified by synthesis 23 years later. Although many psychoactive plants have been recognized dating to before recorded history, mescaline was the only structurally identified hallucinogen until LSD was described in 1943.

Mescaline

Mescaline is usually consumed as peyote "buttons," picked from the small blue-green cacti *Lophophora williamsii* and *Lophophora diffusa*. The buttons are the dried, round, fleshy cacti tops. Mescaline is the active hallucinogenic alkaloid in the buttons. Use of peyote is legal for the Native American Church members in some states. Adverse reactions to peyote are rare during structured religious use. Peyote usually is not consumed casually because of its bitter taste and sometimes severe nausea and vomiting preceding the hallucinogenic effects.

Many structural variations of mescaline have been investigated and structural activity relationships fairly well characterized. One analog, 2,5-dimethoxy-4-methylamphetamine (DOM), also known as STP, an unusually potent amphetamine with hallucinogen properties, had a relatively brief period of illicit popularity and notoriety in the 1960s.

Another series of phenethylamine analogs with hallucinogenic properties is the 3,4-methylenedioxyamphetamine (MDA)–related amphetamines. The currently most popular and, to society, most troublesome member of this large family of drugs is MDMA, or ecstasy, more a relatively mild stimulant than hallucinogen. MDMA produces an altered state of consciousness with sensory changes and, most important for some users, a feeling of enhanced personal interactions. MDMA is discussed in more detail in Section 12.3 on amphetamine-related disorders.

Many plants contain N,N-dimethyltryptamine (DMT), which is also found normally in human biofluids at very low concentrations. When DMT is taken parenterally or by sniffing, a brief, intense hallucinogenic episode can result. As with mescaline in the phenethylamine group, DMT is one of the oldest, best documented, but least potent of the tryptamine hallucinogens. Synthesized homologs of DMT have been evaluated in humans and structure activity relationships reasonably well described.

Psilocybin Analogs

An unusual collection of tryptamines has its origin in the world of fungi. The natural prototype is psilocybin itself. That and related homologs have been found in as many as 100 species of mushroom, largely of the *Psilocybe* genus.

Psilocybin is usually ingested as mushrooms. Many species of psilocybin-containing mushrooms are found worldwide. In the United States, large *Psilocybe cubensis* (gold caps) grow in Florida and Texas and are easily grown with cultivation kits advertised in drug-oriented magazines and on the Internet. The tiny *Psilocybe semilanceata* (liberty cap) grows in lawns and pastures in the Pacific Northwest. Psilocybin remains active when the mushrooms are dried or cooked into omelets or other foods.

Psilocybin mushrooms are used in religious activities by Mexican Indians. They are valued in Western society by users who prefer to ingest a mushroom instead of a synthetic chemical. Of course, one danger of eating wild mushrooms is misidentification and ingestion of a poisonous variety. At a large American university, 24 percent of students reported using psychedelic mushrooms or mescaline, compared with 17 percent who reported LSD use. Psilocybin sold as pills or capsules usually contains phencyclidine (PCP) or LSD instead.

ADDITIONAL HALLUCINOGENS

Ibogaine

Ibogaine is a complex alkaloid found in the African shrub *Tabernanthe iboga*. Ibogaine is a hallucinogen at the 400-mg dose range. The plant originates in Africa and traditionally is used in sacramental initiation ceremonies. Although it has not been a popular hallucinogen because of its unpleasant somatic effects when taken at hallucinogenic doses, patients exposed to ibogaine may be encountered by a psychiatrist because of the therapeutic claims.

Ayahuasca

Ayahuasca, much discussed on Internet hallucinogen Web sites, originally referred to a decoction from one or more South American plants. The substance contains the alkaloids harmaline and harmine. Both of those β-carboline alkaloids have hallucinogenic properties, but the resulting visual sensory alterations are accompanied by considerable nausea.

Salvia Divinorum

American Indians in northern Oaxaca, Mexico, have used *Salvia divinorum* as a medicine and as a sacred sacrament, which is now widely discussed, advertised, and sold on the Internet. When the plant is chewed or dried leaves smoked, it produces hallucinogen effects. Salvinorin-A, an active component in the plant, is parenterally potent, active at 250-μg doses when smoked, and of scientific and potential medical interest because it binds to the opioid κ-receptor.

TREATMENT

Hallucinogen Intoxication

Persons have historically been treated for hallucinogen intoxication by psychological support for the remainder of the trip, so-called "talking down." This is a time-consuming and potentially hazardous undertaking, given the lability of a patient with hallucinogen-related delusions. Accordingly, treatment of hallucinogen intoxication is the oral administration of 20 mg of diazepam. This medication brings the LSD experience and any associated panic to a halt within 20 minutes and should be considered superior to "talking down" the patient over a period of hours or to administering antipsychotic agents. The marketing of lower doses of LSD and a more sophisticated approach to treatment of casualties by drug users themselves have combined to reduce the appearance of this once-common disorder in psychiatric treatment facilities.

Hallucinogen Persisting Disorder

Treatment for hallucinogen persisting perception disorder is palliative. The first step in the process is correct identification of the disorder; it is not uncommon for the patient to consult a number of specialists before the diagnosis is made. Pharmacological approaches include long-lasting benzodiazepines, such as clonazepam (Klonopin) and, to a lesser extent, anticonvulsants including valproic acid (Depakene) and carbamazepine (Tegretol). Currently, no drug is completely effective in ablating symptoms. Antipsychotic agents should only be used in the treatment of hallucinogen-induced psychoses, because they may have a paradoxical effect and exacerbate symptoms. A second dimension of treatment is behavioral. The patient must be instructed to avoid gratuitous stimulation in the form of over-the-counter drugs, caffeine, and alcohol, and avoidable physical and emotional stressors. Marijuana smoke is a particularly strong intensifier of the disorder, even when passively inhaled. Finally, three comorbid conditions are associated with hallucinogen persisting perception disorder: panic disorder, major depression, and alcohol dependence. All these conditions require primary prevention and early intervention.

Hallucinogen-Induced Psychosis

Treatment of hallucinogen-induced psychosis does not differ from conventional treatment for other psychoses. In addition to antipsychotic medications, a number of agents are reportedly effective, including lithium carbonate, carbamazepine, and electroconvulsive therapy. Antidepressant drugs, benzodiazepines, and anticonvulsant agents may each have a role in treatment as well. One hallmark of this disorder is that, as opposed to schizophrenia, in which negative symptoms and poor interpersonal relatedness may commonly be found, patients with hallucinogen-induced psychosis exhibit the positive symptoms of hallucinations and delusions while retaining the ability to relate to the psychiatrist. Medical therapies are best applied in a context of supportive, educational, and family therapies. The goals of treatment are the control of symptoms, a minimal use of hospitals, daily work, the development and preservation of social relationships, and the management of comorbid illnesses such as alcohol dependence.

References

Da Silveira DX, Grob CS, de Rios MD, Lopez E, Alonso LK, Tacia C, Doering-Silveir E. Ayahuasca in adolescence: A preliminary psychiatric assessment. *J Psychoactive Drugs*. 2005;37:129–133.

Halpern JH, Pope HG Jr. Hallucinogen persisting perception disorder: What do we know after 50 years? *Drug Alcohol Depend*. 2003;69:109.

Jones RT. Hallucinogen-related disorders. In: Sadock BJ, Sadock VA, eds. *Kaplan & Sadock's Comprehensive Textbook of Psychiatry*. 8th ed. Vol. 1. Baltimore: Lippincott Williams & Wilkins; 2005:1238.

Seeman P, Ko F, Tallerico T. Dopamine receptor contribution to the addiction of PCP, LSD, and ketamine psychotomimetics. *Mol Psychiatry*. 2005;10:877–883.

Sessa B. Can psychedelics have a role in psychiatry once again? *Br J Psychiatry*. 2005;186:457–458.

Sheffler DJ, Roth BL, Salvinorin A. The "magic mint" hallucinogen finds a molecular target in the kappa opioid receptor. *Trends Pharmacol Sci*. 2003;24:107.

Shulgin A. Basic pharmacology and effects. In: Laing R, ed. *Hallucinogens: A Forensic Handbook*. London: Academic Press; 2003.

Tacke U, Ebert MH. Hallucinogens and phecyclidine. In: Kranzler HR, Ciraulo DA, eds. *Clinical Manual of Addiction Psychopharmacology*. Washington DC: American Psychiatric Publishing, Inc.; 2005:211–241.

Wu LT, Schlenger WE, Ringwalt CL. Use of nitrite inhalants ("poppers") among American youth. *J Adolesc Health*. 2005;37:52–60.

Yacoubian GS, Green MK, Peters RJ. Identifying the prevalence and correlates of ecstasy and other club drug (EOCD) use among high school seniors. *J Ethn Subst Abuse*. 2003;2:53–66.

▲ 12.8 Inhalant-Related Disorders

Inhalant drugs (also called *inhalants* or *volatile substances*) are volatile hydrocarbons such as toluene, *n*-hexane, methyl butyl ketone, trichloroethylene, trichloroethane, dichloromethane, gasoline, and butane. These chemicals are sold in four commercial classes: (1) solvents for glues and adhesives; (2) propellants for aerosol paint sprays, hair sprays, frying pan sprays, and shaving cream; (3) thinners (e.g., for paint products and typing correction fluids); and (4) fuels. At room temperature, these compounds volatilize to gaseous fumes that can be inhaled through the nose or mouth, entering the bloodstream by the transpulmonary route. Despite their chemical differences, it is generally believed, although not proved, that these compounds share certain pharmacological properties.

The text revision of the fourth edition of *Diagnostic and Statistical Manual of Mental Disorders* (DSM-IV-TR) specifically excludes anesthetic gases (e.g., nitrous oxide and ether) and short-acting vasodilators (e.g., amyl nitrite) from the inhalant-related disorders, which are classified as other (or unknown) substance-related disorders and are discussed in Section 12.14.

EPIDEMIOLOGY

Inhalant substances are easily available, legal, and inexpensive. These three factors contribute to the high use of inhalants among poor persons and young persons. According to DSM-IV-TR, about 6 percent of persons in the United States had used inhalants at least once, and about 1 percent of persons are current users. Among young adults 18 to 25 years of age, 11 percent had used inhalants at least once, and 2 percent were current users. Among adolescents 12 to 17 years of age, 7 percent had used inhalants at least once, and 2 percent were current users. In one study of high school seniors, 18 percent reported having used inhalants at least once, and 2.7 percent reported having used inhalants within the preceding month. White users of inhalants are more common than either black or Hispanic users. Most users (up to 80 percent) are male. Some data suggest that inhalant use may be more common in suburban communities in the United States than in urban communities.

Inhalant use accounts for 1 percent of all substance-related deaths and less than 0.5 percent of all substance-related emergency room visits. About 20 percent of the emergency room visits for inhalant use involve persons younger than 18 years of age. Inhalant use among adolescents may be most common in those whose parents or older siblings use illegal substances. Inhalant use among adolescents is also associated with an increased likelihood of conduct disorder or antisocial personality disorder. Between 1994 and 2000, the number of new inhalant users increased more than 50 percent, from 618,000 new users in 1994 to 979,000 in 2000. These estimates were higher than a previous peak in 1978 (662,000 new users).

NEUROPHARMACOLOGY

Inhalants most used by American adolescents are (in descending order) gasoline, glue (which usually contains toluene), spray paint, solvents, cleaning fluids, and assorted other aerosols. Sniffing vapor through the nose or huffing (taking deep breaths) through the mouth leads to transpulmonary absorption with very rapid drug access to the brain. Breathing through a solvent-soaked cloth, inhaling fumes from a glue-containing bag, huffing vapor sprayed into a plastic bag, or breathing vapor from a gasoline can are common. Approximately 15 to 20 breaths of 1 percent gasoline vapor produce several hours of intoxication. Inhaled toluene concentrations from a glue-containing bag may reach 10,000 ppm, and vapors from several tubes of glue may be inhaled each day. By comparison, one study of just 100 ppm of toluene showed that a 6-hour exposure produced a temporary neuropsychological performance decrement of approximately 10 percent.

Inhalants generally act as a central nervous system (CNS) depressant. Tolerance for inhalants can develop, although withdrawal symptoms are usually fairly mild and are not classified as a disorder in DSM-IV-TR.

Inhalants are rapidly absorbed through the lungs and rapidly delivered to the brain. The effects appear within 5 minutes and can last for 30 minutes to several hours, depending on the inhalant substance and the dose. The concentrations of many inhalant substances in blood are increased when used in combination with alcohol, perhaps because of competition for hepatic enzymes. Although about one fifth of an inhalant substance is excreted unchanged by the lungs, the remainder is metabolized by the liver. Inhalants are detectable in the blood for 4 to 10 hours after use, and blood samples should be taken in the emergency room when inhalant use is suspected.

Much like alcohol, inhalants have specific pharmacodynamic effects that are not well understood. Because their effects are generally similar and additive to the effects of other CNS depressants (e.g., ethanol, barbiturates, and benzodiazepines), some investigators have suggested that inhalants operate by enhancing the γ-aminobutyric acid (GABA) system. Other investigators have suggested that inhalants work through membrane fluidization, which has also been hypothesized to be a pharmacodynamic effect of ethanol.

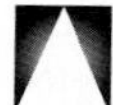

Table 12.8–1
DSM-IV-TR Inhalant-Related Disorders

Inhalant use disorders
Inhalant dependence
Inhalant abuse
Inhalant-induced disorders
Inhalant intoxication
Inhalant intoxication delirium
Inhalant-induced persisting dementia
Inhalant-induced psychotic disorder, with delusions
Specify if:
With onset during intoxication
Inhalant-induced psychotic disorder, with hallucinations
Specify if:
With onset during intoxication
Inhalant-induced mood disorder
Specify if:
With onset during intoxication
Inhalant-induced anxiety disorder
Specify if:
With onset during intoxication
Inhalant-related disorder not otherwise specified

(From American Psychiatric Association. *Diagnostic and Statistical Manual of Mental Disorders.* 4th ed. Text rev. Washington, DC: American Psychiatric Association; copyright 2000, with permission.)

DIAGNOSIS

The DSM-IV-TR lists a number of inhalant-related disorders (Table 12.8–1), but contains specific diagnostic criteria only for inhalant intoxication (Table 12.8–2) within the inhalant-related disorders section. The diagnostic criteria of other inhalant-related disorders are specified in the DSM-IV-TR sections that specifically address the major symptoms—for example, inhalant-induced psychotic disorders (*see* Table 14.4–7).

Inhalant Dependence and Inhalant Abuse

Most persons probably use inhalants for a short time without developing a pattern of long-term use resulting in dependence and abuse. Nonetheless, dependence and abuse of inhalants occur and are diagnosed according to the standard DSM-IV-TR criteria for substance abuse and dependence (*see* Tables 12.1–3, 12.1–4, and 12.1–5).

Inhalant Intoxication

The DSM-IV-TR diagnostic criteria for inhalant intoxication (Table 12.8–2) specify the presence of maladaptive behavioral changes and at least two physical symptoms. The intoxicated state is often characterized by apathy, diminished social and occupational functioning, impaired judgment, and impulsive or aggressive behavior, and it can be accompanied by nausea, anorexia, nystagmus, depressed reflexes, and diplopia. With high doses and long exposures, a user's neurological status can progress to stupor and unconsciousness, and a person may later be amnestic for the period of intoxication. Clinicians can sometimes identify a recent user of inhalants by rashes around the patient's nose and mouth; unusual breath odors; the residue of the inhalant substances on the patient's face, hands, or clothing; and irritation of the patient's eyes, throat, lungs, and nose. The disorder can be chronic as in the following case.

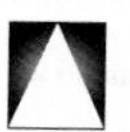

Table 12.8–2
DSM-IV-TR Diagnostic Criteria for Inhalant Intoxication

A. Recent intentional use or short-term, high-dose exposure to volatile inhalants (excluding anesthetic gases and short-acting vasodilators).
B. Clinically significant maladaptive behavioral or psychological changes (e.g., belligerence, assaultiveness, apathy, impaired judgment, impaired social or occupational functioning) that developed during, or shortly after, use of or exposure to volatile inhalants.
C. Two (or more) of the following signs, developing during, or shortly after, inhalant use or exposure:
 (1) dizziness
 (2) nystagmus
 (3) incoordination
 (4) slurred speech
 (5) unsteady gait
 (6) lethargy
 (7) depressed reflexes
 (8) psychomotor retardation
 (9) tremor
 (10) generalized muscle weakness
 (11) blurred vision or diplopia
 (12) stupor or coma
 (13) euphoria
D. The symptoms are not due to a general medical condition and are not better accounted for by another mental disorder.

(From American Psychiatric Association. *Diagnostic and Statistical Manual of Mental Disorders.* 4th ed. Text rev. Washington, DC: American Psychiatric Association; copyright 2000, with permission.)

A 16-year-old single Hispanic female was referred to a university substance-treatment program for evaluation. The patient had been convicted for auto theft, menacing with a weapon, and being out of control by her family. By age 15, she had regularly been using inhalants and drinking alcohol heavily. She had tried typewriter-erasing fluid, bleach, tile cleaner, hairspray, nail polish, glue, and gasoline, but preferred spray paint. She had sniffed paint many times each day for about 6 months at age 15, using a maximum of eight paint cans per day. The patient said, "It blacks out everything." Sometimes she had lost consciousness, and she believed that the paint had impaired her memory and made her "dumb." (Courtesy of Thomas J. Crowley, M.D.)

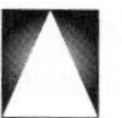

Table 12.8–3
DSM-IV-TR Diagnostic Criteria for Inhalant-Related Disorder Not Otherwise Specified

The inhalant-related disorder not otherwise specified category is for disorders associated with the use of inhalants that are not classifiable as inhalant dependence, inhalant abuse, inhalant intoxication, inhalant intoxication delirium, inhalant-induced persisting dementia, inhalant-induced psychotic disorder, inhalant-induced mood disorder, or inhalant-induced anxiety disorder.

(From American Psychiatric Association. *Diagnostic and Statistical Manual of Mental Disorders.* 4th ed. Text rev. Washington, DC: American Psychiatric Association; copyright 2000, with permission.)

Inhalant Intoxication Delirium

The DSM-IV-TR provides a diagnostic category for inhalant intoxication delirium (*see* Table 10.2–6). Delirium can be induced by the effects of the inhalants themselves, by pharmacodynamic interactions with other substances, and by the hypoxia that may be associated with either the inhalant or its method of inhalation. If the delirium results in severe behavioral disturbances, short-term treatment with a dopamine receptor antagonist, such as haloperidol (Haldol), may be necessary. Benzodiazepines should be avoided because of the possibility of increasing the patient's respiratory depression.

Inhalant-Induced Persisting Dementia

Inhalant-induced persisting dementia (*see* Table 10.3–8), as with delirium, may result from the neurotoxic effects of the inhalants themselves; the neurotoxic effects of the metals (e.g., lead) commonly used in inhalants; or the effects of frequent and prolonged periods of hypoxia. The dementia caused by inhalants is likely to be irreversible in all but the mildest cases.

Inhalant-Induced Psychotic Disorder

Inhalant-induced psychotic disorder is a DSM-IV-TR diagnosis (*see* Table 14.4–7). Clinicians can specify hallucinations or delusions as the predominant symptoms. Paranoid states are probably the most common psychotic syndromes during inhalant intoxication.

Inhalant-Induced Mood Disorder and Inhalant-Induced Anxiety Disorder

Inhalant-induced mood disorder (*see* Table 15.3–10) and inhalant-induced anxiety disorder (*see* Table 16.7–3) are DSM-IV-TR diagnoses that allow the classification of inhalant-related disorders characterized by prominent mood and anxiety symptoms. Depressive disorders are the most common mood disorders associated with inhalant use, and panic disorders and generalized anxiety disorder are the most common anxiety disorders.

Inhalant-Related Disorder Not Otherwise Specified

Inhalant-related disorder not otherwise specified is the recommended DSM-IV-TR diagnosis for inhalant-related disorders that do not fit into one of the diagnostic categories discussed above (Table 12.8–3).

CLINICAL FEATURES

In small initial doses, inhalants can be disinhibiting and produce feelings of euphoria and excitement and pleasant floating sensations, the effects for which persons presumably use the drugs. High doses of inhalants can cause psychological symptoms of fearfulness, sensory illusions, auditory and visual hallucinations, and distortions of body size. The neurological symptoms can include slurred speech, decreased speed of talking, and ataxia. Long-term use can be associated with irritability, emotional lability, and impaired memory.

Tolerance for the inhalants does develop; although not recognized by DSM-IV-TR, a withdrawal syndrome can accompany the cessation of inhalant use. The withdrawal syndrome does not occur frequently; when it does, it can be characterized by sleep disturbances, irritability, jitteriness, sweating, nausea, vomiting, tachycardia, and (sometimes) delusions and hallucinations.

Organ Pathology and Neurological Effects

Inhalants are associated with many potentially serious adverse effects. The most serious of these is death, which can result from respiratory depression, cardiac arrhythmias, asphyxiation, aspiration of vomitus, or accident or injury (e.g., driving while intoxicated with inhalants). Placing an inhalant-soaked rag and one's head into a plastic bag, a common procedure, can cause coma and suffocation.

Chronic inhalant users may have numerous neurological problems. Computed tomography (CT) and magnetic resonance imaging (MRI) reveal diffuse cerebral, cerebellar, and brainstem atrophy with white matter disease, a leukoencephalopathy. Single photon CT of former solvent-abusing adolescents showed both increases and decreases of blood flow in different cerebral areas. Several studies of house painters and factory workers who have been exposed to solvents for long periods also have found evidence of brain atrophy on CT scans, with decreased cerebral blood flow.

Neurological and behavioral signs and symptoms can include hearing loss, peripheral neuropathy, headache, paresthesias, cerebellar signs, persisting motor impairment, parkinsonism, apathy, poor concentration, memory loss, visual-spatial dysfunction, impaired processing of linguistic material, and lead encephalopathy. White matter changes, or pontine atrophy on MRI, have been associated with worse intelligence quotient (IQ) test results. The combination of organic solvents with high concentrations of copper, zinc, and heavy metals has been associated with the development of brain atrophy, temporal lobe epilepsy, decreased IQ, and a variety of electroencephalographic (EEG) changes.

Other serious adverse effects associated with long-term inhalant use include irreversible hepatic disease or renal damage (tubular acidosis) and permanent muscle damage associated with rhabdomyolysis. Additional adverse effects include cardiovascular and pulmonary symptoms (e.g., chest pain and bronchospasm) as well as gastrointestinal (GI) symptoms (e.g., pain, nausea, vomiting, and hematemesis). There are several clinical reports of toluene embryopathy, with signs such as those of fetal alcohol syndrome. These include low birth weight, microcephaly, shortened palpebral fissures, small face, low-set ears, and other dysmorphic signs. These babies reportedly develop slowly, show hyperactivity, and have cerebellar dysfunction. No convincing evidence indicates, however, that toluene, the best-studied inhalant, produces genetic damage in somatic cells.

TREATMENT

Inhalant intoxication, as with alcohol intoxication, usually requires no medical attention and resolves spontaneously. Effects of the intoxication, such as coma, bronchospasm, laryngospasm, cardiac arrhythmias, trauma, or burns, need treatment, however. Otherwise, care primarily involves reassurance, quiet support, and attention to vital signs and level of consciousness. Sedative drugs, including benzodiazepines, are contraindicated because they worsen inhalant intoxication.

No established treatment exists for the cognitive and memory problems of inhalant-induced persisting dementia. Street outreach and extensive social service support have been offered to severely deteriorated, inhalant-dependent, homeless adults. Patients may require extensive support within their families or in foster or domiciliary care.

The course and treatment of inhalant-induced psychotic disorder are like those of inhalant intoxication. The disorder is brief, lasting a few hours to (at most) a very few weeks beyond the intoxication. Appropriate is vigorous treatment of such life-threatening complications as respiratory or cardiac arrest, together with conservative management of the intoxication itself. Confusion, panic, and psychosis mandate special attention to patient safety. Severe agitation may require cautious control with haloperidol (5 mg intramuscularly per 70 kg body weight). Sedative drugs should be avoided because they may aggravate the psychosis. Inhalant-induced anxiety and mood disorders may precipitate suicidal ideation, and patients should be carefully evaluated for that possibility. Antianxiety medications and antidepressants are not useful in the acute phase of the disorder; they may be of use in cases of a coexisting anxiety or depressive illness.

Day Treatment and Residential Programs

Day treatment and residential programs have been used successfully, especially for adolescent abusers with combined substance dependence and other psychiatric disorders. Treatment addresses the comorbid state which, in most cases, is conduct disorder or, in other instances, may be attention-deficit/hyperactivity disorder (ADHD), major depressive disorder, dysthymic disorder, and posttraumatic stress disorder (PTSD). Attention is also directed to experiences of abuse or neglect, which is very common in these patients. Both group and individual therapy are used that are behaviorally oriented, with immediate rewards for progress toward objectively defined goals in treatment and punishments for lapses to previous behaviors. Patients attend on-site schools with special education teachers, together with planned recreational activities and the programs provide birth control consultations. The patients' families, often very chaotic, are engaged in modifications of structural family therapy or multisystemic therapy, both of which have good empirical support. Participation in 12-step programs is required. Treatment interventions are coordinated closely with interventions by community social workers and probation officers. Progress is monitored with urine and breath samples analyzed for alcohol and other drugs at intake and frequently during treatment.

Treatment usually lasts 3 to 12 months. Termination is considered successful if the youth has practiced a plan to stay abstinent; is showing fewer antisocial behaviors; has a plan to continue any needed psychiatric treatment (e.g., treatment for comorbid depression); has a plan to live in a supportive, drug-free environment; is interacting with the family in a more productive way; is working or attending school; and is associating with drug-free, nondelinquent peers.

References

Crowley TJ, Sakai J. Inhalant-related disorders. In: Sadock BJ, Sadock VA, eds. *Kaplan & Sadock's Comprehensive Textbook of Psychiatry*. 8th ed. Vol. 1. Baltimore: Lippincott Williams & Wilkins; 2005:1247.

Evren C, Barut T, Saatcioglu O, Cakmak D. Axis I psychiatric comorbidity among adult inhalant dependents seeking treatment. *J Psychoactive Drugs*. 2006;38(1):57–64.

Lopreato GF, Phelan R, Borghese CM, Beckstead MJ, Mihic SJ. Inhaled drugs of abuse enhance serotonin-3 receptor function. *Drug Alcohol Depend*. 2003;70:11.

Lorenc JD. Inhalant abuse in the pediatric population: A persistent challenge. *Curr Opin Pediatr*. 2003;15:204.

Pack R, Krishnamurthy G, Cottrell L, Stanton B, D'Alessandri D, Burns J. Caregiver predictors of adolescent inhalant abuse in rural Appalachia. *Am J Health Behav*. 2005;29(4): 331–341.

Riegel AC, Ali SF, French ED. Toluene-induced locomotor activity is blocked by 6-hydroxydopamine lesions of the nucleus accumbens and the mGluR2/3 agonist LY379268. *Neuropsychopharmacology*. 2003;28:1440.

Sakai JT, Hall SK, Mikulich-Gilbertson SK, Crowley TJ. Inhalant use, abuse, and dependence among adolescent patients: Commonly comorbid problems. *J Am Acad Child Adolesc Psychiatry*. 2004;43(9):1080–1088.

Sakai JT, Mikulich-Gilbertson SK, Crowley TJ. Adolescent inhalant use among male patients in treatment for substance and behavior problems: Two-year outcome. *Am J Drug Alcohol Abuse*. 2006;32:29–40.

Storr CL, Westergaard R, Anthony JC. Early onset inhalant use and risk for opiate initiation by young adulthood. *Drug Alcohol Depend*. 2005;78(3):253–261.

Wu LT, Pilowsky DJ, Schlenger WE. Inhalant abuse and dependence among adolescents in the United States. *J Am Acad Child Adolesc Psychiatry*. 2004;43(10):1206–1214.

Wu LT, Schlenger WE, Ringwalt CL. Use of nitrite inhalants ("poppers") among American youth. *J Adolesc Health*. 2005;37:52–60.

▲ 12.9 Nicotine-Related Disorders

Nicotine is one of the most highly addictive and heavily used drugs in the United States and around the world. It causes lung cancer, emphysema, and cardiovascular disease and secondhand smoke is associated with lung cancer in adults and respiratory illness in children.

The landmark 1988 publication called *The Surgeon General's Report on the Health Consequences of Smoking: Nicotine Addiction* increased the awareness of the hazards of smoking to the American public. However, the fact that about 30 percent continue to smoke despite the mountain of data showing how dangerous the habit is to their health is testament to the powerfully addictive properties of nicotine. The ill effects of cigarette and cigar smoking are reflected in the estimate that 60 percent of the direct health care costs in the United States go to treat tobacco-related illnesses and amount to an estimated $1 billion a day.

EPIDEMIOLOGY

The *2004 Monitoring the Future Survey* concluded that, despite the demonstrated health risk associated with cigarette smoking, young Americans continue to smoke. However, 30-day smoking rates among high school students declined from peaks reached in 1996 for eighth-graders (21.0 percent) and tenth-graders (30.4 percent) and in 1997 for seniors (36.5 percent). In 2004, 30-day rates reached the lowest levels ever reported by Monitoring the Future surveys for eighth-graders (9.2 percent) and tenth-graders (16.0 percent). Of high school seniors, 25 percent reported smoking during the month preceding their responses to the survey.

Lifetime cigarette use among tenth-graders decreased significantly, from 43.0 percent in 2003 to 40.7 percent in 2004. Among tenth-graders, a significantly decreased number of students reported that they smoke one-half pack or more cigarettes per day.

The decrease in smoking rates among young Americans corresponds to several years in which increased proportions of teens said they believe a "great" health risk is associated with cigarette smoking and expressed disapproval of smoking one or more packs of cigarettes a day. Students' personal disapproval of smoking had risen for some years, but showed no further increase in 2004. In 2004, 85.7 percent of eighth-graders, 82.7 percent of tenth-graders, and 76.2 percent of twelfth-graders stated that they "disapprove" or "strongly disapprove" of people smoking one or more packs of cigarettes per day. In addition, eighth- and tenth-graders reported significant increases in the perceived harmfulness of smoking one or more packs of cigarettes per day.

The World Health Organization (WHO) estimates there are 1 billion smokers worldwide, and they smoke 6 trillion cigarettes a year. The WHO also estimates that tobacco kills more than 3 million persons each year. Although the number of persons in the United States who smoke is decreasing, the number of persons smoking in developing countries is increasing. The rate of quitting smoking has been highest among well-educated white men and lowest among women, blacks, teenagers, and those with low levels of education.

Tobacco is the most common form of nicotine. It is smoked most commonly in cigarettes, then, in descending order, cigars, snuff, chewing tobacco, and in pipes. About 3 percent of all persons in the United States currently use snuff or chewing tobacco, and about 6 percent of young adults ages 18 to 25 use those forms of tobacco.

Currently, about 25 percent of Americans smoke, 25 percent are former smokers, and 50 percent have never smoked cigarettes. The mean age of onset of smoking is 16 years, and few persons start smoking after 20. Dependence features appear to develop quickly. Classroom and other programs to prevent initiation are only mildly effective, but increased taxation does decrease initiation.

More than 75 percent of smokers have tried to quit, and about 40 percent try to quit each year. On a given attempt, only 30 percent remain abstinent for even 2 days, and only 5 to 10 percent stop permanently. Most smokers make 5 to 10 attempts, however, so eventually 50 percent of "ever smokers" quit. In the past, 90 percent of successful attempts to quit involved no treatment. With the advent of over-the-counter (OTC) and nonnicotine medications in 1998, about one third of all attempts involved the use of medication.

In terms of the diagnosis of nicotine dependence per se, about 20 percent of the population develops nicotine dependence at some point, making it one of the most prevalent psychiatric disorders. According to the text revision of the fourth edition of *Diagnostic and Statistical Manual of Mental Disorders* (DSM-IV-TR), approximately 85 percent of current daily smokers are nicotine dependent. Nicotine withdrawal occurs in about 50 percent of smokers who try to quit.

According to the CDC, regional differences exist in smoking throughout the United States. The 12 areas with the highest prevalence of current smoking are Kentucky, Nevada, Missouri, Indiana, Ohio, West Virginia, North Carolina, Tennessee, New Hampshire, Alabama, Arkansas, and Alaska. The 12 areas with lowest prevalence are Utah, Puerto Rico, California, Arizona, Montana, Hawaii, Minnesota, Connecticut, Massachusetts, Colorado, Maryland, and Washington. Utah had the lowest prevalence for men (14.5 percent), and Puerto Rico had the lowest for women (9.9 percent).

Education

Level of education attainment correlated with tobacco usage. Of adults who had not completed high school, 37 percent smoked cigarettes, whereas only 17 percent of college graduates smoked.

Psychiatric Patients

Psychiatrists must be particularly concerned and knowledgeable about nicotine dependence because of the high proportion of psychiatric patients who smoke. Approximately 50 percent of all psychiatric outpatients, 70 percent of outpatients with bipolar I disorder, almost 90 percent of outpatients with schizophrenia, and 70 percent of substance use disorder patients smoke. Moreover, data indicate that patients with depressive disorders or anxiety disorders are less successful in their attempts to quit smoking than other persons; thus, a holistic health approach for these patients probably includes helping them address their smoking habits in addition to the primary mental disorder. The high percentage of patients with schizophrenia who smoke has been attributed to nicotine's ability to reduce their extraordinary sensitivity to outside sensory stimuli and to increase their concentration. In that sense, such patients are self-monitoring to relieve distress.

Death

Death is the primary adverse effect of cigarette smoking. Tobacco use is associated with approximately 400,000 premature deaths each year in the United States—25 percent of all deaths.

The causes of death include chronic bronchitis and emphysema (51,000 deaths), bronchogenic cancer (106,000 deaths), 35 percent of fatal myocardial infarctions (115,000 deaths), cerebrovascular disease, cardiovascular disease, and almost all cases of chronic obstructive pulmonary disease and lung cancer. The increased use of chewing tobacco and snuff (smokeless tobacco) has been associated with the development of oropharyngeal cancer, and the resurgence of cigar smoking is likely to lead to an increase in the occurrence of this type of cancer.

Researchers have found that 30 percent of cancer deaths in the United States are caused by tobacco smoke, the single most lethal carcinogen in the United States. Smoking (mainly cigarette smoking) causes cancer of the lung, upper respiratory tract, esophagus, bladder, and pancreas and probably of the stomach, liver, and kidney. Smokers are eight times more likely than nonsmokers to develop lung cancer, and lung cancer has surpassed breast cancer as the leading cause of cancer-related deaths in women. Even secondhand smoke (discussed below) causes a few thousand cancer deaths each year in the United States, about the same number as are caused by radon exposure. Despite these staggering statistics, smokers can dramatically lower their chances of developing smoke-related cancers simply by quitting.

NEUROPHARMACOLOGY

The psychoactive component of tobacco is nicotine, which affects the central nervous system (CNS) by acting as an agonist at the nicotinic subtype of acetylcholine receptors. About 25 percent of the nicotine inhaled during smoking reaches the bloodstream, through which nicotine reaches the brain within 15 seconds. The half-life of nicotine is about 2 hours. Nicotine is believed to produce its positive reinforcing and addictive properties by activating the dopaminergic pathway projecting from the ventral tegmental area to the cerebral cortex and the limbic system. In addition to activating this dopamine reward system, nicotine causes an increase in the concentrations of circulating norepinephrine and epinephrine and an increase in the release of vasopressin, β-endorphin, adrenocorticotropic hormone (ACTH), and cortisol. These hormones are thought to contribute to the basic stimulatory effects of nicotine on the CNS.

DIAGNOSIS

The DSM-IV-TR lists three nicotine-related disorders (Table 12.9–1), but contains specific diagnostic criteria for only nicotine withdrawal (Table 12.9–2) in the nicotine-related disorders section. The other nicotine-related disorders recognized by DSM-IV-TR are nicotine dependence and nicotine-related disorder not otherwise specified.

Table 12.9–1
DSM-IV-TR Nicotine-Related Disorders

Nicotine use disorder
Nicotine dependence
Nicotine-induced disorder
Nicotine withdrawal
Nicotine-related disorder not otherwise specified

(From American Psychiatric Association. *Diagnostic and Statistical Manual of Mental Disorders.* 4th ed. Text rev. Washington, DC: American Psychiatric Association; copyright 2000, with permission.)

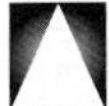

Table 12.9–2
DSM-IV-TR Diagnostic Criteria for Nicotine Withdrawal

A. Daily use of nicotine for at least several weeks.
B. Abrupt cessation of nicotine use, or reduction in the amount of nicotine used, followed within 24 hours by four (or more) of the following signs:
(1) dysphoric or depressed mood
(2) insomnia
(3) irritability, frustration, or anger
(4) anxiety
(5) difficulty concentrating
(6) restlessness
(7) decreased heart rate
(8) increased appetite or weight gain
C. The symptoms in Criterion B cause clinically significant distress or impairment in social, occupational, or other important areas of functioning.
D. The symptoms are not due to a general medical condition and are not better accounted for by another mental disorder.

(From American Psychiatric Association. *Diagnostic and Statistical Manual of Mental Disorders.* 4th ed. Text rev. Washington, DC: American Psychiatric Association; copyright 2000, with permission.)

Nicotine Dependence

The DSM-IV-TR does have a diagnosis of nicotine dependence (*see* Tables 12.1–4 and 12.1–5), but not nicotine abuse. Dependence on nicotine develops quickly, probably because nicotine activates the ventral tegmental area dopaminergic system, the same system affected by cocaine and amphetamine. The development of dependence is enhanced by strong social factors that encourage smoking in some settings and by the powerful effects of tobacco company advertising. Persons are likely to smoke if their parents or siblings smoke and serve as role models. Several recent studies have also suggested a genetic diathesis toward nicotine dependence. Most persons who smoke want to quit and have tried many times to quit but have been unsuccessful.

Nicotine Withdrawal

The DSM-IV-TR does not have a diagnostic category for nicotine intoxication, but does have a diagnostic category for nicotine withdrawal (Table 12.9–2). Withdrawal symptoms can develop within 2 hours of smoking the last cigarette; they generally peak in the first 24 to 48 hours and can last for weeks or months. The common symptoms include an intense craving for nicotine, tension, irritability, difficulty concentrating, drowsiness and paradoxical trouble sleeping, decreased heart rate and blood pressure, increased appetite and weight gain, decreased motor performance, and increased muscle tension. A mild syndrome of nicotine withdrawal can appear when a smoker switches from regular to low-nicotine cigarettes.

Nicotine-Related Disorder Not Otherwise Specified

Nicotine-related disorder not otherwise specified is a diagnostic category for nicotine-related disorders that do not fit into one of

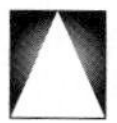

Table 12.9–3
DSM-IV-TR Diagnostic Criteria for Nicotine-Related Disorder Not Otherwise Specified

The nicotine-related disorder not otherwise specified category is for disorders associated with the use of nicotine that are not classifiable as nicotine dependence or nicotine withdrawal.

(From American Psychiatric Association. *Diagnostic and Statistical Manual of Mental Disorders.* 4th ed. Text rev. Washington, DC: American Psychiatric Association; copyright 2000, with permission.)

the categories discussed above (Table 12.9–3). Such diagnoses may include nicotine intoxication, nicotine abuse, and mood disorders and anxiety disorders associated with nicotine use.

CLINICAL FEATURES

Behaviorally, the stimulatory effects of nicotine produce improved attention, learning, reaction time, and problem-solving ability. Tobacco users also report that cigarette smoking lifts their mood, decreases tension, and lessens depressive feelings. Results of studies of the effects of nicotine on cerebral blood flow (CBF) suggest that short-term nicotine exposure increases CBF without changing cerebral oxygen metabolism, but long-term nicotine exposure decreases CBF. In contrast to its stimulatory CNS effects, nicotine acts as a skeletal muscle relaxant.

Adverse Effects

Nicotine is a highly toxic alkaloid. Doses of 60 mg in an adult are fatal secondary to respiratory paralysis; doses of 0.5 mg are delivered by smoking an average cigarette. In low doses the signs and symptoms of nicotine toxicity include nausea, vomiting, salivation, pallor (caused by peripheral vasoconstriction), weakness, abdominal pain (caused by increased peristalsis), diarrhea, dizziness, headache, increased blood pressure, tachycardia, tremor, and cold sweats. Toxicity is also associated with an inability to concentrate, confusion, and sensory disturbances. Nicotine is further associated with a decrease in the user's amount of rapid eye movement (REM) sleep. Tobacco use during pregnancy has been associated with an increased incidence of low birth weight babies and an increased incidence of newborns with persistent pulmonary hypertension.

Health Benefits of Smoking Cessation

Smoking cessation has major and immediate health benefits for persons of all ages and provides benefits for persons with and without smoking-related diseases. Former smokers live longer than those who continue to smoke. Smoking cessation decreases the risk for lung cancer and other cancers, myocardial infarction, cerebrovascular diseases, and chronic lung diseases. Women who stop smoking before pregnancy or during the first 3 to 4 months of pregnancy reduce their risk for having low birth weight infants to that of women who never smoked. The health benefits of smoking cessation substantially exceed any risks from the average 5-pound (2.3 kg) weight gain or any adverse psychological effects after quitting.

TREATMENT

Psychiatrists should advise all patients to quit smoking. For patients who are ready to stop smoking, it is best to set a "quit date." Most clinicians and smokers prefer abrupt cessation, but because no good data indicate that abrupt cessation is better than gradual cessation, patient preference for gradual cessation should be respected. Brief advice should focus on the need for medication or group therapy, weight gain concerns, high-risk situations, making cigarettes unavailable, and so forth. Because relapse is often rapid, the first follow-up phone call or visit should be 2 to 3 days after the quit date. These strategies have been shown to double self-initiated quit rates (Table 12.9–4).

Psychosocial Therapies

Behavior therapy is the most widely accepted and well-proved psychological therapy for smoking. Skills training and relapse prevention identify high-risk situations and plan and practice behavioral or cognitive coping skills for those situations in which smoking occurs. Stimulus control involves eliminating cues for smoking in the environment. Aversive therapy has smokers smoke repeatedly and rapidly to the point of nausea that associates smoking with unpleasant, rather than pleasant, sensations. Aversive therapy appears to be effective but requires a good therapeutic alliance and patient compliance.

Hypnosis. Some patients benefit from a series of hypnotic sessions. Suggestions about the benefits of not smoking are offered and assimilated into the patient's cognitive framework as a result. Posthypnotic suggestions that cause cigarettes to taste bad or to produce nausea when smoked are also used.

Psychopharmacological Therapies

Nicotine Replacement Therapies. All nicotine replacement therapies double cessation rates, presumably because they reduce nicotine withdrawal. These therapies can also be used to reduce withdrawal in patients on smoke-free wards. Replacement therapies use a short period of maintenance of 6 to 12 weeks often followed by a gradual reduction period of another 6 to 12 weeks.

Nicotine polacrilex gum (Nicorette) is an OTC product that releases nicotine via chewing and buccal absorption. A 2-mg variety for those who smoke fewer than 25 cigarettes a day and a 4-mg variety for those who smoke more than 25 cigarettes a day are available. Smokers are to use one to two pieces of gum per hour up to a maximum of 24 pieces per day after abrupt cessation.

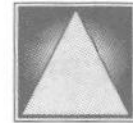

Table 12.9–4
Typical Quit Rates of Common Therapies

Therapy	Rate (%)
Self-quit	5
Self-help books	10
Physician advice	10
Over-the-counter patch or gum	15
Medication plus advice	20
Behavior therapy alone	20
Medication plus group therapy	30

Venous blood concentrations from the gum are one third to one half the between-cigarette levels. Acidic beverages (coffee, tea, soda, and juice) should not be used before, during, or after gum use because they decrease absorption. Compliance with the gum has often been a problem. Adverse effects are minor and include bad taste and sore jaws. About 20 percent of those who quit use the gum for long periods, but 2 percent use gum for longer than a year; long-term use does not appear to be harmful. The major advantage of nicotine gum is its ability to provide relief in high-risk situations.

Nicotine lozenges (Commit) deliver nicotine and are also available in 2-mg and 4-mg forms; they are useful especially for patients who smoke a cigarette immediately on awakening. Generally, 9 to 20 lozenges a day are used during the first 6 weeks with decrease in dosage thereafter. Lozenges offer the highest level of nicotine of all nicotine replacement products. Users must suck the lozenge until dissolved and not swallow it. Side effects include insomnia, nausea, heartburn, headache, and hiccups.

Nicotine patches, also sold OTC, are available in a 16-hour, no-taper preparation (Nicotrol) and a 24- or 16-hour tapering preparation (Nicoderm CQ). Patches are administered each morning and produce blood concentrations about half those of smoking. Compliance is high, and the only major adverse effects are rashes and, with 24-hour wear, insomnia. Using gum and patches in high-risk situations increases quit rates by another 5 to 10 percent. No studies have been done to determine the relative efficacies of 24- or 16-hour patches or of taper and no-taper patches. After 6 to 12 weeks, the patch is discontinued because it is not for long-term use.

Nicotine nasal spray (Nicotrol), available only by prescription, produces nicotine concentrations in the blood that are more similar to those from smoking a cigarette, and it appears to be especially helpful for heavily dependent smokers. The spray, however, causes rhinitis, watering eyes, and coughing in more than 70 percent of patients. Although initial data suggested abuse liability, further trials have not found this.

The nicotine inhaler, a prescription product, was designed to deliver nicotine to the lungs, but the nicotine is actually absorbed in the upper throat. It delivers 4 mg per cartridge and resultant nicotine levels are low. The major asset of the inhaler is that it provides a behavioral substitute for smoking. The inhaler doubles quit rates. These devices require frequent puffing—about 20 minutes to extract 4 mg of nicotine—and have minor adverse effects.

Non-nicotine Medications. Non-nicotine therapy may help smokers who object philosophically to the notion of replacement therapy and smokers who fail replacement therapy. Bupropion (Zyban) (marketed as Wellbutrin for depression) is an antidepressant medication that has both dopaminergic and adrenergic actions. Bupropion is started at 150 mg per day for 3 days and increased to 150 mg twice a day for 6 to 12 weeks. Daily dosages of 300 mg doubles quit rates in smokers with and without a history of depression. In one study, combined bupropion and nicotine patch had higher quit rates than either alone. Adverse effects include insomnia and nausea, but these are rarely significant. Seizures have not occurred in smoking trials. Interestingly, nortriptyline (Pamelor) appears to be effective for smoking cessation and is recommended as a second-line drug.

Clonidine (Catapres) decreases sympathetic activity from the locus ceruleus and, thus, is thought to abate withdrawal symptoms. Whether given as a patch or orally, 0.2 to 0.4 mg a day of clonidine appears to double quit rates; however, the scientific database for the efficacy of clonidine is neither as extensive nor as reliable as that for nicotine replacement; also, clonidine can cause drowsiness and hypotension. Some patients benefit from benzodiazepine therapy (10 to 30 mg per day) for the first 2 to 3 weeks of abstinence.

A nicotine vaccine that produces nicotine-specific antibodies in the brain is under investigation at the National Institute on Drug Abuse (NIDA).

Combined Psychosocial and Pharmacological Therapy

Several studies have shown that combining nicotine replacement and behavior therapy increases quit rates over either therapy alone.

Smoke-Free Environment

Secondhand smoke can contribute to lung cancer death and coronary heart disease in adult nonsmokers. Each year, an estimated 3,000 lung cancer deaths and 62,000 deaths from coronary artery disease in adult nonsmokers are attributed to secondhand smoke. Among children, secondhand smoke is implicated in sudden infant death syndrome, low birth weight, chronic middle ear infections, and respiratory illnesses (e.g., asthma, bronchitis, and pneumonia). Two national health objectives for 2010 are to reduce cigarette smoking among adults to 12 percent and the proportion of nonsmokers exposed to environment tobacco smoke to 45 percent.

Involuntary exposure to secondhand smoke remains a common public health hazard that is preventable by appropriate regulatory policies. Bans on smoking in public places reduce exposure to secondhand smoke and the number of cigarettes smoked by smokers. Support is nearly universal for bans in schools and day-care centers and strong support for bans in indoor work areas and restaurants. Clean indoor air policies are one way to change social norms about smoking and reduce tobacco consumption. Bans on outdoor smoking in areas, such as public parks, are increasing and in 2006 one municipality in California banned smoking entirely within city limits except in one's own home or car and windows had to remain closed.

References

Abrams DB, Niaura R, Brown RA, Emmons KM, Goldstein MG, Monti PM. *The Tobacco Dependence Treatment Handbook. A Guide to Best Practices.* Barlow DH, ed. New York: The Guilford Press; 2003.

Dudas MM, George TP. Non-nicotine pharmacotherapies for nicotine dependence. *Essential Psychopharmacol.* 2005;6(3):158–172.

Einarson A, Sarkar M, Djulus J, Koren G. Smoking habits, nicotine use, and congenital malformations. *Obstet Gynecol.* 2006;107:1167.

Giovino GA. Epidemiology of tobacco use in the United States. *Oncogene.* 2002;21:7326–7340.

Hughes JR. Nicotine-related disorders. In: Sadock BJ, Sadock VA, eds. *Kaplan & Sadock's Comprehensive Textbook of Psychiatry.* 8th ed. Vol. 1. Baltimore: Lippincott Williams & Wilkins; 2005:1257.

Montoya ID, Herbeck DM, Svikis DS, Pincus HA. Identification and treatment of patients with nicotine problems in routine clinical psychiatry. *Am J Addict.* 2005;14:441–454.

National Cancer Institute. *Those Who Continue to Smoke: Is Achieving Abstinence Harder and Do We Need to Change Our Interventions? Smoking and Tobacco Control Monograph No. 15.* Bethesda, MD: USDHHS, National Institutes of Health, National Cancer Institute; 2003.

Niaura R, Abrams DB. Smoking cessation: Progress, priorities, and prospects. *J Consult Clin Psychol.* 2002;70:494–509.

O'Malley SS, Cooney JL, Krishnan-Sarin S, Dubin JA, McKee SA, Cooney NL, Blakeslee A, Meandzija B, Romano-Dahlgard D, Wu R, Makuch R, Jatlow P. A controlled trial of naltrexone augmentation of nicotine replacement therapy for smoking cessation. *Arch Intern Med.* 2006;166:667–674.

Patton GC, Coffey C, Carlin JB, Sawyer SM, Lynskey M. Reverse gateways? Frequent cannabis use as a predictor of tobacco initiation and nicotine dependence. *Addiction.* 2005;100:1518–1525.

Piasecki M, Newhouse PA. *Nicotine in Psychiatry. Psychopathology and Emerging Therapeutics.* Washington, DC: American Psychiatric Press; 2002.

Rigotti NA. Clinical practice: Treatment of tobacco use and dependence. *N Engl J Med.* 2002;346:506.

Upadhyaya H, Deas D, Brady K. A practical clinical approach to the treatment of nicotine dependence in adolescents. *J Am Acad Child Adolesc Psychiatry.* 2005;44:942–946.

▲ 12.10 Opioid-Related Disorders

More than 20 chemically distinct opioid drugs are in clinical use throughout the world. In the developed countries, the opioid drug most frequently associated with abuse and dependence is heroin—a drug that is not approved for therapeutic purposes in the United States. These drugs are all prototypical μ-opioid receptor agonists and all produce similar subjective effects. The patterns of use and some aspects of opioid toxicity are powerfully influenced, however, by the route of administration and the metabolism of the specific opioid, as well as by the social conditions that determine its price and purity and the sanctions attached to nonmedical use.

Opioids have been used for at least 3,500 years, mostly in the form of crude opium or in alcoholic solutions of opium. Morphine was first isolated in 1806 and codeine in 1832. Over the next century, pure morphine and codeine gradually replaced crude opium for medicinal purposes, although nonmedical use of opium (as for smoking) still persists in some parts of the world.

Table 12.10–1 lists various opioids that are used therapeutically in the United States with the exception of heroin.

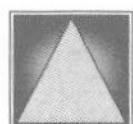

Table 12.10–1
Opioids

Proprietary Name	Trade Name
Morphine	
Heroin (diacetylmorphine)	
Hydromorphone (dihydromorphinone)	Dilaudid
Oxymorphone (dihydrohydroxymorphinone)	Numorphan
Levorphanol	Levo-Dromoran
Methadone	Dolophine
Meperidine (pethidine)	Demerol, Pethadol
Fentanyl	Sublimaze
Codeine	
Hydrocodone (dihydrocodeinone)	Hycodan, others
Drocode (dihydrocodeine)	Synalgos-DC, Compal
Oxycodone (dihydrohydroxycodeinone)	Roxicodone, OxyContin, Percodan, Percocet, Vicodin
Propoxyphene	Darvon, others
Buprenorphine	Buprenex
Pentazocine	Talwin
Nalbuphine	Nubain
Butorphanol	Stadol

The text revision of the fourth edition of *Diagnostic and Statistical Manual of Mental Disorders* (DSM-IV-TR) divides opioid-related disorders into opioid use disorders (opioid abuse and opioid dependence) and nine other opioid-induced disorders (e.g., intoxication, withdrawal).

Opioid dependence is a cluster of physiological, behavioral, and cognitive symptoms, which together indicates repeated and continuing use of opioid drugs, despite significant problems related to such use. Drug dependence, in general, has also been defined by the World Health Organization (WHO) as a syndrome in which the use of a drug or class of drugs takes on a much higher priority for a given person than other behaviors that once had a higher value. These brief definitions each have as their central features an emphasis on the drug-using behavior itself, its maladaptive nature, and how the choice to engage in that behavior shifts and becomes constrained as a result of interaction with the drug over time.

Opioid abuse is a term used to designate a pattern of maladaptive use of an opioid drug leading to clinically significant impairment or distress and occurring within a 12-month period, but one in which the symptoms have never met the criteria for opioid dependence.

The opioid-induced disorders as defined by DSM-IV-TR include such common phenomena as opioid intoxication, opioid withdrawal, opioid-induced sleep disorder, and opioid-induced sexual dysfunction. Opioid intoxication delirium is occasionally seen in hospitalized patients. Opioid-induced psychotic disorder, opioid-induced mood disorder, and opioid-induced anxiety disorder, by contrast, are quite uncommon with μ-agonist opioids, but have been seen with certain mixed agonist-antagonist opioids acting at other receptors. DSM-IV-TR also includes opioid-related disorder not otherwise specified for situations that do not meet the criteria for any of the other opioid-related disorders.

In addition to the morbidity and mortality associated directly with the opioid-related disorders, the association between the transmission of the human immunodeficiency virus (HIV) and intravenous opioid and opiate use is now recognized as a leading national health concern. The words *opiate* and *opioid* come from the word opium, the juice of the opium poppy, *Papaver somniferum*, which contains approximately 20 opium alkaloids, including morphine.

Many synthetic opioids have been manufactured, including meperidine (Demerol), methadone (Dolophine), pentazocine (Talwin), and propoxyphene (Darvon). Methadone is the current gold standard in the treatment of opioid dependence. Opioid antagonists have been synthesized to treat opioid overdose and opioid dependence. This class of drugs includes naloxone (Narcan), naltrexone (ReVia), nalorphine, levallorphan, and apomorphine. Compounds with mixed agonist and antagonist activity at opioid receptors have been synthesized and they include pentazocine, butorphanol (Stadol), and buprenorphine (Buprenex). Studies have found buprenorphine to be an effective treatment for opioid dependence.

EPIDEMIOLOGY

The use and dependence rates derived from national surveys do not accurately reflect fluctuations in drug use among opioid-dependent and previously opioid-dependent populations. When the supply of illicit heroin increases in purity or decreases in price, use among that vulnerable population tends to increase, with subsequent increases in adverse consequences (emergency room visits) and requests for treatment. The number of current heroin users in the United States has been estimated to be between 600,000 and 800,000. The number of people estimated to have used heroin at any time in their lives (lifetime users) is estimated at approximately 3 million.

In 2004, an estimated 118,000 persons had used heroin for the first time within the past 12 months. The average age of first use among recent initiates was 24.4 years in 2004. No significant changes were seen in the number of initiates or in the average age of first use from 2002 to 2004. Opioid use in the United States experienced a resurgence in the 1990s, with emergency department visits related to heroin abuse doubling between 1990 and 1995. This increase in heroin use was associated with an increase in heroin purity and a decrease in its street price. In the late 1990s, heroin use increased among people who were 18 to 25 years of age and a brief upsurge was seen in the use of oxycodone (OxyContin) from pharmaceutical sources. Methods of administration other than injecting, such as smoking and snorting, increased in popularity. In 2004, the number of new nonmedical users of OxyContin was 615,000, with an average age at first use of 24.5 years. Comparable data on past year OxyContin initiation are not available for prior years, but calendar year estimates of OxyContin initiation show a steady increase in the number of initiates from 1995, the year this drug was first available, through 2003. The male-to-female ratio of persons with heroin dependence is about 3 to 1. Users of opioids typically started to use substances in their teens and early 20s; currently, most persons with opioid dependence are in their 30s and 40s. According to DSM-IV-TR, the tendency for dependence to remit generally begins after age 40 years and has been called "maturing out." Many persons, however, have remained opioid dependent for 50 years or longer. In the United States, persons tend to experience their first opioid-induced experience in their early teens or even as young as 10 years of age. Early induction into the drug culture is likely in communities in which substance abuse is rampant and in families in which the parents are substance abusers. A heroin habit can cost a person hundreds of dollars a day; thus, a person with opioid dependence needs to obtain money through criminal activities and prostitution. The involvement of persons with opioid dependence in prostitution accounts for much of the spread of HIV. According to DSM-IV-TR, the lifetime prevalence for heroin use is about 1 percent, with 0.2 percent having taken the drug during the prior year.

NEUROPHARMACOLOGY

The primary effects of the opioids are mediated through the opioid receptors, which were discovered in the second half of the 1970s. The μ-opioid receptors are involved in the regulation and mediation of analgesia, respiratory depression, constipation, and dependence; the κ-opioid receptors, with analgesia, diuresis, and sedation; and the δ-opioid receptors, possibly with analgesia.

In 1974, enkephalin, an endogenous pentapeptide with opioid-like actions, was identified. This discovery led to the identification of three classes of endogenous opioids within the brain, including the endorphins and the enkephalins. Endorphins are involved in neural transmission and pain suppression. They are released naturally in the body when a person is physically hurt and account, in part, for the absence of pain during acute injuries.

The opioids also have significant effects on the dopaminergic and noradrenergic neurotransmitter systems. Several types of data indicate that the addictive rewarding properties of opioids are mediated through activation of the ventral tegmental area dopaminergic neurons that project to the cerebral cortex and the limbic system (Fig. 12.10–1).

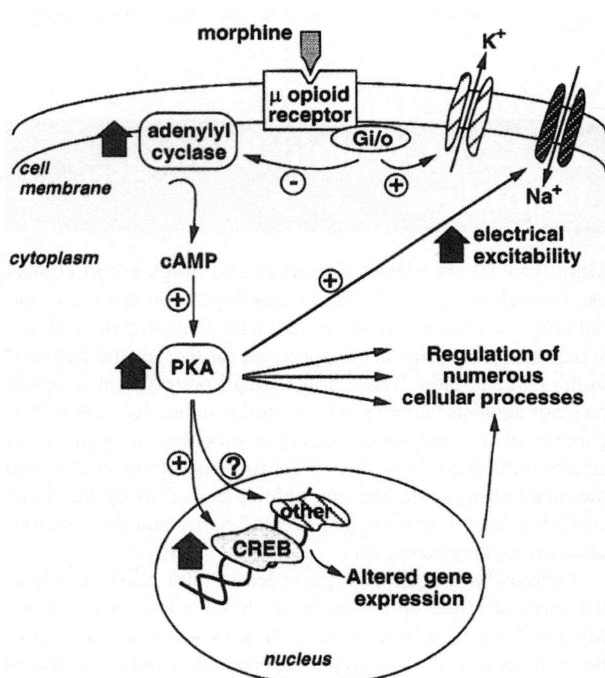

FIGURE 12.10–1

Scheme illustrating opioid actions in the locus ceruleus (LC). Opioids acutely inhibit LC neurons by increasing the conductance of a K^+ channel (*light cross-hatch*) via coupling with subtypes of G_i and/or G_o and by decreasing an Na^+-dependent inward current (*dark cross-hatch*) via coupling with $G_{i/o}$ and the consequent inhibition of adenylyl cyclase. Reduced levels of cAMP decrease PKA and the phosphorylation of the responsible channel or pump. Inhibition of the cyclic adenosine monophosphate (cAMP) pathway also decreases phosphorylation of numerous other proteins and thereby affects many additional processes in the neuron. For example, it reduces the phosphorylation state of CREB, which may initiate some of the longer-term changes in LC function. *Upper bold arrows* summarize effects of repeated morphine administration in the LC. Repeated morphine administration increases levels of adenylyl cyclase, PKA, and several phosphoproteins, including CREB. These changes contribute to the altered phenotype of the drug-addicted state. For example, the intrinsic excitability of LC neurons is increased via enhanced activity of the cAMP pathway and Na^+-dependent inward current, which contributes to the tolerance, dependence, and withdrawal exhibited by the these neurons. This altered phenotypic state appears to be maintained, in part, by upregulation of CREB expression. (From Nestler EJ. Molecular mechanisms underlying opiate addiction: Implications for medications development. *Semin Neurosci.* 1997;0:84, with permission.)

Heroin, the most commonly abused opioid, is more potent and lipid soluble than morphine. Because of those properties, heroin crosses the blood–brain barrier faster and has a more rapid onset than morphine. Heroin was first introduced as a treatment for morphine addiction, but heroin, in fact, is more dependence producing than morphine. Codeine, which occurs naturally as about 0.5 percent of the opiate alkaloids in opium, is absorbed easily through the gastrointestinal tract and is subsequently transformed into morphine in the body. Results of at least one study using positron emission tomography (PET) have suggested that one effect of all opioids is decreased cerebral blood flow in selected brain regions in persons with opioid dependence.

Tolerance and Dependence

Tolerance does not develop uniformly to all actions of opioid drugs. Tolerance to some actions of opioids can be so high that a hundredfold increase in dose is required to produce the original effect. For example, terminally ill cancer patients may need 200 to 300 mg a day of morphine, whereas a dose of 60 mg can easily be fatal to an opioid-naïve person. The symptoms of opioid withdrawal do not appear unless a person has been using opioids for a long time or when cessation is particularly abrupt, as occurs functionally when an opioid antagonist is given. The long-term use of opioids results in changes in the number and sensitivity of opioid receptors, which mediate at least some of the effects of tolerance and withdrawal. Although long-term use is associated with increased sensitivity of the dopaminergic, cholinergic, and serotonergic neurons, the effect of opioids on the noradrenergic neurons is probably the primary mediator of the symptoms of opioid withdrawal. Short-term use of opioids apparently decreases the activity of the noradrenergic neurons in the locus ceruleus; long-term use activates a compensatory homeostatic mechanism within the neurons and opioid withdrawal results in rebound hyperactivity. This hypothesis also provides an explanation for why clonidine (Catapres), an α_2-adrenergic receptor agonist that decreases the release of norepinephrine, is useful in the treatment of opioid withdrawal symptoms.

COMORBIDITY

About 90 percent of persons with opioid dependence have an additional psychiatric disorder. The most common comorbid psychiatric diagnoses are major depressive disorder, alcohol use disorders, antisocial personality disorder, and anxiety disorders. About 15 percent of persons with opioid dependence attempt to commit suicide at least once. The high prevalence of comorbidity with other psychiatric diagnoses highlights the need to develop a broad-based treatment program that also addresses patients' associated psychiatric disorders (Table 12.10–2).

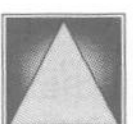

Table 12.10–2
Non–Substance-Related Axis I Psychiatric Disorders in Opioid Users

	Lifetime Rates % (Current Rates %)		
Diagnostic Category[a]	**Men ($N = 378$)**	**Women ($N = 338$)**	**Total**
Any Axis I disorder	15.6 (5.0)	33.4 (11.2)	24.0 (8.0)
Mood disorder	11.4 (2.1)	27.5 (5.3)	19.0 (3.6)
Major depressive disorder	8.7 (1.3)	23.7 (5.3)	15.8 (3.2)
Dysthymic disorder	2.4 (2.4)	4.4 (4.4)	3.4 (3.4)
Bipolar I disorder	0.8 (0.8)	0.0 (0.0)	0.4 (0.4)
Anxiety disorder	6.1 (3.4)	10.7 (6.8)	8.2 (5.0)
Simple phobia	1.9 (1.9)	5.3 (3.6)	3.5 (2.7)
Social phobia	1.9 (0.8)	3.6 (2.7)	2.7 (1.7)
Panic disorder	2.1 (0.3)	1.8 (0.9)	2.0 (0.6)
Agoraphobia	0.0 (0.0)	0.6 (0.3)	0.3 (0.1)
Obsessive-compulsive disorder	0.5 (0.5)	0.0 (0.0)	0.3 (0.3)
General anxiety disorder	0.8 (0.8)	0.0 (0.0)	0.1 (0.1)
Eating disorders	0.0 (0.0)	1.5 (0.0)	0.7 (0.0)
Bulimia nervosa	0.0 (0.0)	0.9 (0.0)	0.4 (0.0)
Anorexia nervosa	0.0 (0.0)	0.6 (0.0)	0.3 (0.0)
Schizophrenia	0.0 (0.0)	0.3 (0.3)	0.1 (0.1)

[a]Multiple disorders possible.
(Adapted from Brooner RK, King VL, Kidorf M, Schmidt CW, Bigelow GE. Psychiatric and substance use comorbidity among treatment-seeking opioid abusers. *Arch Gen Psychiatry*. 1997;54:71.)

ETIOLOGY

Psychosocial Factors

Opioid dependence is not limited to low socioeconomic classes, although the incidence of opioid dependence is greater in these groups than in higher socioeconomic classes. Social factors associated with urban poverty probably contribute to opioid dependence. About 50 percent of urban heroin users are children of single parents or divorced parents and are from families in which at least one other member has a substance-related disorder. Children from such settings are at high risk for opioid dependence, especially if they also evidence behavioral problems in school or other signs of conduct disorder.

Some consistent behavior patterns seem to be especially pronounced in adolescents with opioid dependence. These patterns have been called the *heroin behavior syndrome*: underlying depression, often of an agitated type and frequently accompanied by anxiety symptoms; impulsiveness expressed by a passive-aggressive orientation; fear of failure; use of heroin as an antianxiety agent to mask feelings of low self-esteem, hopelessness, and aggression; limited coping strategies and low frustration tolerance, accompanied by the need for immediate gratification; sensitivity to drug contingencies, with a keen awareness of the relation between good feelings and the act of drug taking; feelings of behavioral impotence counteracted by momentary control over the life situation by means of substances; disturbances in social and interpersonal relationships with peers maintained by mutual substance experiences.

Biological and Genetic Factors

Evidence now exists for common and drug-specific, genetically transmitted vulnerability factors that increase the likelihood of developing drug dependence. Individuals who abuse a substance from any category are more likely to abuse substances from other categories. Monozygotic twins are more likely than dizygotic twins to be concordant for opioid dependence. Multivariate modeling techniques indicated that not only was the genetic contribution high for heroin abuse in this group, but also a higher proportion of the variance because of genetic factors was not shared with the common vulnerability factor—that is, it was specific for opioids.

A person with an opioid-related disorder may have had genetically determined hypoactivity of the opiate system. Researchers are investigating the possibility that such hypoactivity may be caused by too few, or less-sensitive, opioid receptors, by release of too little endogenous opioid, or by overly high concentrations of a hypothesized endogenous opioid antagonist. A biological predisposition to an opioid-related disorder may also be associated with abnormal functioning in either the dopaminergic or the noradrenergic neurotransmitter system.

Psychodynamic Theory

In psychoanalytic literature, the behavior of persons addicted to narcotics has been described in terms of libidinal fixation, with regression to pregenital, oral, or even more archaic levels of psychosexual development. The need to explain the relation of drug abuse, defense mechanisms, impulse control, affective disturbances, and adaptive mechanisms led to the shift from psychosexual formulations to formulations emphasizing ego psychology. Serious ego pathology, often thought to be associated with substance abuse, is considered to indicate profound developmental disturbances. Problems of the relation between the ego and affects emerge as a key area of difficulty.

DIAGNOSIS

The DSM-IV-TR lists several opioid-related disorders (Table 12.10–3) but contains specific diagnostic criteria only for opioid intoxication (Table 12.10–4) and opioid withdrawal (Table 12.10–5) within the section on opioid-related disorders. The diagnostic criteria for the other opioid-related disorders are contained within the DSM-IV-TR sections that deal specifically with the predominant symptom—for example, opioid-induced mood disorder (*see* Table 15.3–10).

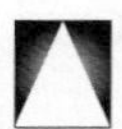

Table 12.10–3
DSM-IV-TR Opioid-Related Disorders

Opioid use disorders
Opioid dependence
Opioid abuse
Opioid-induced disorders
Opioid intoxication
Specify if:
  With perceptual disturbances
Opioid withdrawal
Opioid intoxication delirium
Opioid-induced psychotic disorder, with delusions
Specify if:
  With onset during intoxication
Opioid-induced psychotic disorder, with hallucinations
Specify if:
  With onset during intoxication
Opioid-induced mood disorder
Specify if:
  With onset during intoxication
Opioid-induced sexual dysfunction
Specify if:
  With onset during intoxication
Opioid-induced sleep disorder
Specify if:
  With onset during intoxication
  With onset during withdrawal
Opioid-related disorder not otherwise specified

(From American Psychiatric Association. *Diagnostic and Statistical Manual of Mental Disorders.* 4th ed. Text rev. Washington, DC: American Psychiatric Association; copyright 2000, with permission.)

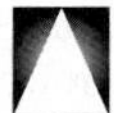

Table 12.10–4
DSM-IV-TR Diagnostic Criteria for Opioid Intoxication

A. Recent use of an opioid.
B. Clinically significant maladaptive behavioral or psychological changes (e.g., initial euphoria followed by apathy, dysphoria, psychomotor agitation or retardation, impaired judgment, or impaired social or occupational functioning) that developed during, or shortly after, opioid use.
C. Pupillary constriction (or pupillary dilation due to anoxia from severe overdose) and one (or more) of the following signs, developing during, or shortly after, opioid use:
   (1) drowsiness or coma
   (2) slurred speech
   (3) impairment in attention or memory
D. The symptoms are not due to a general medical condition and are not better accounted for by another mental disorder.

Specify if:
  With perceptual disturbances

(From American Psychiatric Association. *Diagnostic and Statistical Manual of Mental Disorders.* 4th ed. Text rev. Washington, DC: American Psychiatric Association; copyright 2000, with permission.)

Opioid Dependence and Opioid Abuse

Opioid dependence and opioid abuse are defined in DSM-IV-TR according to the general criteria for these disorders (*see* Tables 12.1–3, 12.1–4, and 12.1–5).

Table 12.10–5
DSM-IV-TR Diagnostic Criteria for Opioid Withdrawal

A. Either of the following:
   (1) cessation of (or reduction in) opioid use that has been heavy and prolonged (several weeks or longer)
   (2) administration of an opioid antagonist after a period of opioid use
B. Three (or more) of the following, developing within minutes to several days after Criterion A:
   (1) dysphoric mood
   (2) nausea or vomiting
   (3) muscle aches
   (4) lacrimation or rhinorrhea
   (5) pupillary dilation, piloerection, or sweating
   (6) diarrhea
   (7) yawning
   (8) fever
   (9) insomnia
C. The symptoms in Criterion B cause clinically significant distress or impairment in social, occupational, or other important areas of functioning.
D. The symptoms are not due to a general medical condition and are not better accounted for by another mental disorder.

(From American Psychiatric Association. *Diagnostic and Statistical Manual of Mental Disorders.* 4th ed. Text rev. Washington, DC: American Psychiatric Association; copyright 2000, with permission.)

A 42-year-old executive in a public relations firm was referred for psychiatric consultation by his surgeon, who discovered him sneaking large quantities of a codeine-containing cough medicine into the hospital. The patient had been a heavy cigarette smoker for 20 years and had a chronic, hacking cough. He had come into the hospital for a hernia repair and found the pain for the incision unbearable when he coughed.

An operation on his back 5 years previously had led his doctors to prescribe codeine to help relieve the incisional pain at that time. Over the intervening 5 years, however, the patient had continued to use codeine-containing tablets and had increased his intake to 60–90 mg tablets daily. He stated that he often "just took them by the handful—not to feel good, you understand, just to get by." He spent considerable time and effort developing a circle of physicians and pharmacists to whom he would "make the rounds" at least three times a week to obtain new supplies of pills. He had tried several times to stop using codeine, but had failed. During this period he lost two jobs because of lax work habits and was divorced by his wife of 11years. (Courtesy of *DSM-IV-TR Casebook*.)

Opioid Intoxication

The DSM-IV-TR defines opioid intoxication as including maladaptive behavioral changes and some specific physical symptoms of opioid use (Table 12.10–4). In general, altered mood, psychomotor retardation, drowsiness, slurred speech, and impaired memory and attention in the presence of other indicators of recent opioid use strongly suggest a diagnosis of opioid intoxication. DSM-IV-TR allows for the specification of "with perceptual disturbances."

Opioid Withdrawal

The general rule about the onset and duration of withdrawal symptoms is that substances with short durations of action tend to produce short, intense withdrawal syndromes and substances with long durations of action produce prolonged, but mild, withdrawal syndromes. An exception to the rule, narcotic antagonist-precipitated withdrawal after long-acting opioid dependence can be severe.

An abstinence syndrome can be precipitated by administration of an opioid antagonist. The symptoms can begin within seconds of such an intravenous injection and peak in about 1 hour. Opioid craving rarely occurs in the context of analgesic administration for pain from physical disorders or surgery. The full withdrawal syndrome, including intense craving for opioids, usually occurs only secondary to abrupt cessation of use in persons with opioid dependence.

Morphine and Heroin. The morphine and heroin withdrawal syndrome begins 6 to 8 hours after the last dose, usually after a 1- to 2-week period of continuous use or after the administration of a narcotic antagonist. The withdrawal syndrome reaches its peak intensity during the second or third day and subsides during the next 7 to 10 days, but some symptoms may persist for 6 months or longer.

Meperidine. The withdrawal syndrome from meperidine begins quickly, reaches a peak in 8 to 12 hours, and ends in 4 to 5 days.

Methadone. Methadone withdrawal usually begins 1 to 3 days after the last dose and ends in 10 to 14 days.

Symptoms. Opioid withdrawal (Table 12.10–5) consists of severe muscle cramps and bone aches, profuse diarrhea, abdominal cramps, rhinorrhea, lacrimation, piloerection or gooseflesh (from which comes the term *cold turkey* for the abstinence syndrome), yawning, fever, pupillary dilation, hypertension, tachycardia, and temperature dysregulation, including hypothermia and hyperthermia. Persons with opioid dependence seldom die from opioid withdrawal, unless they have a severe preexisting physical illness such as cardiac disease. Residual symptoms—such as insomnia, bradycardia, temperature dysregulation, and a craving for opioids—can persist for months after withdrawal. Associated features of opioid withdrawal include restlessness, irritability, depression, tremor, weakness, nausea, and vomiting. At any time during the abstinence syndrome, a single injection of morphine or heroin eliminates all the symptoms.

Opioid Intoxication Delirium

Opioid intoxication delirium (*see* Table 10.2–6) is most likely to happen when opioids are used in high doses, are mixed with other psychoactive compounds, or are used by a person with preexisting brain damage or a central nervous system (CNS) disorder (e.g., epilepsy).

Opioid-Induced Psychotic Disorder

Opioid-induced psychotic disorder can begin during opioid intoxication. The DSM-IV-TR diagnostic criteria are contained in the section on schizophrenia and other psychotic disorders (*see* Table 14.4–7). Clinicians can specify whether hallucinations or delusions are the predominant symptoms.

Opioid-Induced Mood Disorder

Opioid-induced mood disorder can begin during opioid intoxication (*see* Table 15.3–10). Opioid-induced mood disorder symptoms can have a manic, depressed, or mixed nature, depending on a person's response to opioids. A person coming to psychiatric attention with opioid-induced mood disorder usually has mixed symptoms, combining irritability, expansiveness, and depression.

Opioid-Induced Sleep Disorder and Opioid-Induced Sexual Dysfunction

Opioid-induced sleep disorder (*see* Table 24.2–21) and opioid-induced sexual dysfunction (*see* Table 21.2–17) are diagnostic categories in DSM-IV-TR. Hypersomnia is likely to be more common with opioids than insomnia. The most common sexual dysfunction is likely to be impotence.

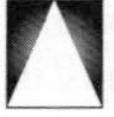

Table 12.10–6
DSM-IV-TR Diagnostic Criteria for Opioid-Related Disorder Not Otherwise Specified

The opioid-related disorder not otherwise specified category is for disorders associated with the use of opioids that are not classifiable as opioid dependence, opioid abuse, opioid intoxication, opioid withdrawal, opioid intoxication delirium, opioid-induced psychotic disorder, opioid-induced mood disorder, opioid-induced sexual dysfunction, or opioid-induced sleep disorder.

(From American Psychiatric Association. *Diagnostic and Statistical Manual of Mental Disorders.* 4th ed. Text rev. Washington, DC: American Psychiatric Association; copyright 2000, with permission.)

Opioid-Related Disorder Not Otherwise Specified

The DSM-IV-TR includes diagnoses for opioid-related disorders with symptoms of delirium, abnormal mood, psychosis, abnormal sleep, and sexual dysfunction. Clinical situations that do not fit into these categories exemplify appropriate cases for the use of the DSM-IV-TR diagnosis of opioid-related disorder not otherwise specified (Table 12.10–6).

CLINICAL FEATURES

Opioids can be taken orally, snorted intranasally, and injected intravenously (IV) or subcutaneously (Fig. 12.10–2). Opioids are subjectively addictive because of the euphoric high (the rush) that users experience, especially those who take the substances IV. The associated symptoms include a feeling of warmth, heaviness of the extremities, dry mouth, itchy face (especially the nose), and facial flushing. The initial euphoria is followed by a period of sedation, known in street parlance as "nodding off." Opioid use can induce dysphoria, nausea, and vomiting in opioid-naïve persons.

The physical effects of opioids include respiratory depression, pupillary constriction, smooth muscle contraction (including the ureters and the bile ducts), constipation, and changes in blood pressure, heart rate, and body temperature. The respiratory depressant effects are mediated at the level of the brainstem.

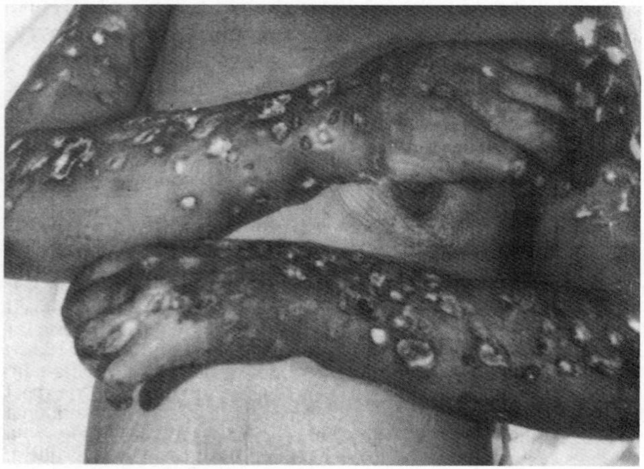

FIGURE 12.10–2
Skin popper. Circular depressed scars, often with underlying chronic abscesses, can result from skin popping. (Courtesy of Michael Baden, M.D.)

Adverse Effects

The most common and most serious adverse effect associated with the opioid-related disorders is the potential transmission of hepatitis and HIV through the use of contaminated needles by more than one person. Persons can experience idiosyncratic allergic reactions to opioids, which result in anaphylactic shock, pulmonary edema, and death if they do not receive prompt and adequate treatment. Another serious adverse effect is an idiosyncratic drug interaction between meperidine and monoamine oxidase inhibitors (MAOIs), which can produce gross autonomic instability, severe behavioral agitation, coma, seizures, and death. Opioids and MAOIs should not be given together for this reason.

Opioid Overdose

Death from an overdose of an opioid is usually attributable to respiratory arrest from the respiratory depressant effect of the drug. The symptoms of overdose include marked unresponsiveness, coma, slow respiration, hypothermia, hypotension, and bradycardia. When presented with the clinical triad of coma, pinpoint pupils, and respiratory depression, clinicians should consider opioid overdose as a primary diagnosis. They can also inspect the patient's body for needle tracks in the arms, legs, ankles, groin, and even the dorsal vein of the penis.

MPTP-Induced Parkinsonism

In 1976, after ingesting an opioid contaminated with methyl-phenyltetrahydropyridine (MPTP), several persons developed a syndrome of irreversible parkinsonism. The mechanism for the neurotoxic effect is as follows: MPTP is converted into 1-methyl-4-phenylpyridinium (MPP+) by the enzyme monoamine oxidase and is then taken up by dopaminergic neurons. Because MPP+ binds to melanin in substantia nigra neurons, MPP+ is concentrated in these neurons and eventually kills the cells. PET studies of persons who ingested MPTP but remained asymptomatic have shown a decreased number of dopamine-binding sites in the substantia nigra. This decrease reflects a loss in the number of dopaminergic neurons in that region.

TREATMENT AND REHABILITATION

Overdose Treatment

The first task in overdose treatment is to ensure an adequate airway. Tracheopharyngeal secretions should be aspirated; an airway may be inserted. The patient should be ventilated mechanically until naloxone, a specific opioid antagonist, can be given. Naloxone is administered IV at a slow rate—initially about 0.8 mg per 70 kg of body weight. Signs of improvement (increased respiratory rate and pupillary dilation) should occur promptly. In opioid-dependent patients, too much naloxone may produce signs of withdrawal as well as reversal of overdosage. If no response to the initial dosage occurs, naloxone administration may be repeated after intervals of a few minutes. Previously, it was thought that if no response was observed after 4 to 5 mg, the CNS depression was probably not caused solely by opioids. The duration of action of naloxone is short compared with that of many opioids, such as methadone and levomethadyl acetate, and repeated administration may be required to prevent recurrence of opioid toxicity.

Medically Supervised Withdrawal and Detoxification

Opioid Agents for Treating Opioid Withdrawal

METHADONE. Methadone is a synthetic narcotic (an opioid) that substitutes for heroin and can be taken orally. When given to addicts to replace their usual substance of abuse, the drug suppresses withdrawal symptoms. A daily dosage of 20 to 80 mg suffices to stabilize a patient, although daily doses of up to 120 mg have been used. The duration of action for methadone exceeds 24 hours; thus, once-daily dosing is adequate. Methadone maintenance is continued until the patient can be withdrawn from methadone, which itself causes dependence. An abstinence syndrome occurs with methadone withdrawal, but patients are detoxified from methadone more easily than from heroin. Clonidine (0.1 to 0.3 mg three to four times a day) is usually given during the detoxification period.

Methadone maintenance has several advantages. First, it frees persons with opioid dependence from using injectable heroin and, thus, reduces the chance of spreading HIV through contaminated needles. Second, methadone produces minimal euphoria and rarely causes drowsiness or depression when taken for a long time. Third, methadone allows patients to engage in gainful employment instead of criminal activity. The major disadvantage of methadone use is that patients remain dependent on a narcotic.

Other Opioid Substitutes

LEVOMETHADYL (LAAM). LAAM is an opioid agonist that suppresses opioid withdrawal. It is no longer used, however, because some patients developed prolonged QT intervals associated with potentially fatal arrhythmias (*torsades de pointes*).

BUPRENORPHINE. As with methadone and LAAM, buprenorphine is an opioid agonist approved for opioid dependence in 2002. It can be dispensed on an outpatient basis but prescribing physicians must demonstrate that they have revived special training in its use. Buprenorphine in a daily dose of 8 to 10 mg appears to reduce heroin use. Buprenorphine also is effective in thrice-weekly dosing because of its slow dissociation from opioid receptors. After repeated administration, it attenuates or blocks the subjective effects of parenterally administered opioids such as heroin or morphine. A mild opioid withdrawal syndrome occurs if the drug is abruptly discontinued after chronic administrations.

Opioid Antagonists. Opioid antagonists block or antagonize the effects of opioids. Unlike methadone, they do not exert narcotic effects and do not cause dependence. Opioid antagonists include naloxone, which is used in the treatment of opioid overdose because it reverses the effects of narcotics, and naltrexone, the longest-acting (72 hours) antagonist. The theory for using an antagonist for opioid-related disorders is that blocking opioid agonist effects, particularly euphoria, discourages persons with opioid dependence from substance-seeking behavior and, thus, deconditions this behavior. The major weakness of the antagonist treatment model is the lack of any mechanism that compels a person to continue to take the antagonist.

Pregnant Women with Opioid Dependence

Neonatal addiction is a significant problem. About three fourths of all infants born to addicted mothers experience the withdrawal syndrome.

Neonatal Withdrawal. Although opioid withdrawal rarely is fatal for the otherwise healthy adult, it is hazardous to the fetus and can lead to miscarriage or fetal death. Maintaining a pregnant woman with opioid dependence on a low dose of methadone (10 to 40 mg daily) may be the least hazardous course to follow. At this dose, neonatal withdrawal is usually mild and can be managed with low doses of paregoric. If pregnancy begins while a woman is taking high doses of methadone, the dosage should be reduced slowly (e.g., 1 mg every 3 days), and fetal movements should be monitored. If withdrawal is necessary or desired, it is least hazardous during the second trimester.

Fetal AIDS Transmission. Acquired immune deficiency syndrome (AIDS) is the other major risk to the fetus of a woman with opioid dependence. Pregnant women can pass HIV, the causative agent of AIDS, to the fetus through the placental circulation. An HIV-infected mother can also pass HIV to the infant through breast-feeding. The use of zidovudine (Retrovir) alone or in combination with other anti-HIV medication in infected women can decrease the incidence of HIV in newborns.

Psychotherapy

The entire range of psychotherapeutic modalities is appropriate for treating opioid-related disorders. Individual psychotherapy, behavioral therapy, cognitive-behavioral therapy, family therapy, support groups (e.g., Narcotics Anonymous [NA]), and social skills training may all prove effective for specific patients. Social skills training should be particularly emphasized for patients with few social skills. Family therapy is usually indicated when the patient lives with family members.

Therapeutic Communities

Therapeutic communities are residences in which all members have a substance abuse problem. Abstinence is the rule; to be admitted to such a community, a person must show a high level of motivation. The goals are to effect a complete change of lifestyle, including abstinence from substances; to develop personal honesty, responsibility, and useful social skills; and to eliminate antisocial attitudes and criminal behavior.

The staff members of most therapeutic communities are persons with former substance dependence who often put prospective candidates through a rigorous screening process to test their motivation. Self-help through the use of confrontational groups and isolation from the outside world and from friends associated with the drug life are emphasized. The prototypical community for persons with substance dependence is Phoenix House, where the residents live for long periods (usually 12 to 18 months) while receiving treatment. They are allowed to return to their old environments only when they have demonstrated their ability to handle increased responsibility within the therapeutic community. Therapeutic communities can be effective but require large staffs and extensive facilities. Moreover, dropout rates are high; up to 75 percent of those who enter therapeutic communities leave within the first month.

Education and Needle Exchange

Although the essential treatment of opioid use disorders is encouraging persons to abstain from opioids, education about the transmission of HIV must receive equal attention. Persons with opioid dependence who use IV or subcutaneous routes of administration must be taught available safe-sex practices. Free needle-exchange programs are often subject to intense political and societal pressures but, where allowed, should be made available to persons with opioid dependence. Several studies have indicated that unsafe needle sharing is common when it is difficult to obtain enough clean needles and is also common in persons with legal difficulties, severe substance problems, and psychiatric symptoms. These are just the persons most likely to be involved in transmitting HIV.

Narcotic Anonymous

Narcotics Anonymous is a self-help group of abstinent drug addicts modeled on the 12-step principles of Alcoholics Anonymous (AA). Such groups now exist in most large cities and can provide useful group support. The outcome for patients treated in 12-step programs is generally good, but the anonymity that is at the core of the 12-step model has made detailed evaluation of its efficacy in treating opioid dependence difficult.

REFERENCES

Bird SM, Hutchinson SJ. Male drugs-related deaths in the fortnight after release from prison: Scotland, 1996–99. *Addiction.* 2003;98:185.

Clarke C, Fitzpatrick C. Psychiatric problems of children exposed to opiates in utero—A descriptive study. *Irish Journal of Psychological Medicine.* 2005;22:121–123.

Donaher PA, Welsh C. Managing opioid addiction with buprenorphine. *Am Fam Physician.* 2006;73(9):1573–1582.

Jaffe JH. Opioid-related disorders. In: Sadock BJ, Sadock VA, eds. *Kaplan & Sadock's Comprehensive Textbook of Psychiatry.* 7th ed. Vol. 1. Baltimore: Lippincott Williams & Wilkins; 2000:1038.

Jaffe JH, Strain EC. Opioid-related disorders. In: Sadock BJ, Sadock VA, eds. *Kaplan & Sadock's Comprehensive Textbook of Psychiatry.* 8th ed. Vol. 1. Baltimore: Lippincott Williams & Wilkins; 2005:1265.

Johnson RE, Jones HE, Fischer G. Use of buprenorphine in pregnancy: Patient management and effects on the neonate. *Drug Alcohol Depend.* 2003;70[Suppl 1]:S87.

Kakko J, Svanborg KD, Kreek MJ, Heilig M. 1-Year retention and social function after buprenorphine-assisted relapse prevention treatment for heroin dependence in Sweden: A randomized, placebo-controlled trial. *Lancet.* 2003;361:662.

Kendler KS, Jacobson KC, Prescott CA, Neale MC. Specificity of genetic and environmental risk factors for use and abuse/dependence of cannabis, cocaine, hallucinogens, sedatives, stimulants, and opiates in male twins. *Am J Psychiatry.* 2003;160:687.

Krantz MJ, Jutinsky IB, Robertson AD, Mehler PS. Dose-related effects of methadone on QT prolongation in a series of patients with torsade de pointes. *Pharmacotherapy.* 2003;23:802.

Loxterkamp D. Helping 'them': Our role in recovery from opioid dependence. *Annals of Family Medicine.* 2006;4:168–171.

Popik P, Kozela E, Wrobel M, Wozniak KM, Slusher BS. Morphine tolerance and reward but not expression of morphine dependence are inhibited by the selective glutamate carboxypeptidase II (GCP II, NAALADasa) inhibitor, 2-PMPA. *Neuropsychopharmacology.* 2003;28:457.

Ritter AJ, Lintzeris N, Clark N, Kutin JJ, Bammer G, Manjari M. A randomized trial comparing levo-alpha acetylmethadol with methadone maintenance for patients in primary care settings in Australia. *Addiction.* 2003;98:1605.

Sigmon SC. Characterizing the emerging population of prescription opioid abusers. *American Journal on Addictions.* 2006;15(3): 208–212.

Sullivan MD, Edlund MJ, Steffick D, Unutzer J. Regular use of prescribed opioids: Association with common psychiatric disorders. *Pain.* 2005;119:95–103.

Tornay CB, Favrat B, Monnat M, Daeppen JB, Schnyder C, Bertschy G, Besson J. Ultra-rapid opiate detoxification using deep sedation and prior oral buprenorphine preparation: Long-term results. *Drug Alcohol Depend.* 2003;69:283.

▲ 12.11 Phencyclidine (or Phencyclidine-like)-Related Disorders

Phencyclidine (PCP; 1-1 [phenylcyclohexyl] piperidine), also known as *angel dust,* was first developed as a novel anesthetic in the late 1950s. This drug and the closely related compound ketamine were termed *dissociative anesthetics*, because they produced a condition in which subjects were awake but apparently insensitive to, or dissociated from, the environment. The symptoms induced by PCP and ketamine closely resemble those observed in schizophrenia. As early as 1959, therefore, it was proposed that PCP psychosis might serve as a heuristically valuable model for schizophrenia. PCP entered the illicit street market in 1965. In the late 1970s, it was one of the leading drugs of abuse in the United States. Although its popularity has subsequently declined, the popularity of ketamine has been steadily increasing.

Phencyclidine and ketamine exert their unique behavioral effects by blocking *N*-methyl-D-aspartate (NMDA)–type receptors for the excitatory neurotransmitter glutamate. PCP and ketamine intoxication can present with a variety of symptoms, from anxiety to psychosis. Treatment remains largely symptomatic and supportive. Few studies have assessed medication effects on PCP or ketamine intoxication effects directly. PCP and ketamine induce psychotic symptoms that closely resemble those of schizophrenia. As such, these drugs have been frequently used in challenge studies to investigate brain mechanisms in schizophrenia. Although PCP is no longer used in controlled human studies, ketamine challenge studies are ongoing and continue to provide critical insights into schizophrenia.

Phencyclidine was first used illicitly in San Francisco in the late 1960s. Since then, about 30 chemical analogues have been produced and are intermittently available on the streets of major US cities. The effects of PCP are similar to those of such hallucinogens as lysergic acid diethylamide (LSD). Because of differing pharmacology and some difference in clinical effects, however, the text revision of the fourth edition of *Diagnostic and Statistical Manual of Mental Disorders* (DSM-IV-TR) classifies the arylcyclohexylamines as a separate category. PCP has also been of interest to schizophrenia researchers, who have used PCP-induced chemical and behavioral changes in animals as a possible model of schizophrenia.

EPIDEMIOLOGY

Phencyclidine and some related substances are relatively easy to synthesize in illegal laboratories and relatively inexpensive to buy on the streets. The variable quality of the laboratories, however, results in a range of potency and purity. PCP use varies most markedly with geography. Most users of PCP also use other substances, particularly alcohol, but also opiates, opioids, marijuana, amphetamines, and cocaine. PCP is frequently added to marijuana, with severe untoward effects on users. According to DSM-IV-TR, the actual rate of PCP dependence and abuse is not known, but PCP is associated with 3 percent of substance abuse deaths and 32 percent of substance-related emergency room visits nationally.

Some areas of some cities have a tenfold higher usage rate of PCP than other areas. The highest PCP use in the United States is in Washington, DC, where PCP accounts for 18 percent of all substance-related deaths and more than 1,000 emergency room visits per year. In Los Angeles, Chicago, and Baltimore, the comparable figure is 6 percent. Overall, most users are between 18 and 25 years of age and they account for 50 percent of cases. Patients are more likely to be male rather than female, especially those who visit emergency rooms. Twice as many white as blacks are users, although blacks account for more visits to hospitals for PCP-related disorders than do whites. PCP use appears to be rising, with some reports showing a 50 percent increase, particularly in urban areas.

NEUROPHARMACOLOGY

Phencyclidine and its related compounds are variously sold as a crystalline powder, paste, liquid, or drug-soaked paper (blotter). PCP is most commonly used as an additive to a cannabis- or parsley-containing cigarette. Experienced users report that the effects of 2 to 3 mg of smoked PCP occur in about 5 minutes and plateau in 30 minutes. The bioavailability of PCP is about 75 percent when taken by intravenous administration and about 30 percent when smoked. The half-life of PCP in humans is about 20 hours, and the half-life of ketamine in humans is about 2 hours.

The primary pharmacodynamic effect of PCP and ketamine is as an antagonist at the NMDA subtype of glutamate receptors. PCP binds to a site within the NMDA-associated calcium channel and prevents the influx of calcium ions. PCP also activates the dopaminergic neurons of the ventral tegmental area, which project to the cerebral cortex and the limbic system. Activation of these neurons is usually involved in mediating the reinforcing qualities of PCP.

Tolerance for the effects of PCP occurs in humans, although physical dependence generally does not occur. In animals that are administered more PCP per pound for longer times than virtually any humans, PCP does induce physical dependence, however, with marked withdrawal symptoms of lethargy, depression, and craving. Physical symptoms of withdrawal in humans are rare, probably as a function of dose and duration of use. Although physical dependence on PCP is rare in humans, psychological dependence on both PCP and ketamine are common, and some users become psychologically dependent on the PCP-induced psychological state.

That PCP is made in illicit laboratories contributes to the increased likelihood of impurities in the final product. One such contaminant is 1-piperidenocyclohexane carbonitrite, which releases hydrogen cyanide in small quantities when ingested. Another contaminant is piperidine, which can be recognized by its strong, fishy odor.

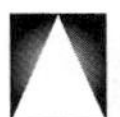

Table 12.11–1
DSM-IV-TR Phencyclidine-Related Disorders

Phencyclidine use disorders
Phencyclidine dependence
Phencyclidine abuse
Phencyclidine-induced disorders
Phencyclidine intoxication
Specify if:
With perceptual disturbances
Phencyclidine intoxication delirium
Phencyclidine-induced psychotic disorder, with delusions
Specify if:
With onset during intoxication
Phencyclidine-induced psychotic disorder, with hallucination
Specify if:
With onset during intoxication
Phencyclidine-induced mood disorder
Specify if:
With onset during intoxication
Phencyclidine-induced anxiety disorder
Specify if:
With onset during intoxication
Phencyclidine-related disorder not otherwise specified

(From American Psychiatric Association. *Diagnostic and Statistical Manual of Mental Disorders.* 4th ed. Text rev. Washington, DC: American Psychiatric Association; copyright 2000, with permission.)

DIAGNOSIS

The DSM-IV-TR lists a number of PCP (or PCP-like)-related disorders (Table 12.11–1), but outlines the specific diagnostic criteria for only PCP intoxication (Table 12.11–2) within the PCP (or PCP-like)-related disorders section. The diagnostic criteria for other PCP (or PCP-like)-related disorders are listed in the

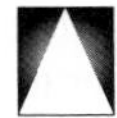

Table 12.11–2
DSM-IV-TR Diagnostic Criteria for Phencyclidine Intoxication

A. Recent use of phencyclidine (or a related substance).
B. Clinically significant maladaptive behavioral changes (e.g., belligerence, assaultiveness, impulsiveness, unpredictability, psychomotor agitation, impaired judgment, or impaired social or occupational functioning) that developed during, or shortly after, phencyclidine use.
C. Within an hour (less when smoked, "snorted," or used intravenously), two (or more) of the following signs:
(1) vertical or horizontal nystagmus
(2) hypertension or tachycardia
(3) numbness or diminished responsiveness to pain
(4) ataxia
(5) dysarthria
(6) muscle rigidity
(7) seizures or coma
(8) hyperacusis
D. The symptoms are not due to a general medical condition and are not better accounted for by another mental disorder.

Specify if:
With perceptual disturbances

(From American Psychiatric Association. *Diagnostic and Statistical Manual of Mental Disorders.* 4th ed. Text rev. Washington, DC: American Psychiatric Association; copyright 2000, with permission.)

sections that deal with specific symptoms—for example, PCP-induced anxiety disorder is in the anxiety disorders section.

PCP Dependence and PCP Abuse

The DSM-IV-TR uses the general criteria for PCP dependence and PCP abuse (*see* Tables 12.1–3, 12.1–4, and 12.1–5). Some long-term users of PCP are said to be "crystallized," a syndrome characterized by dulled thinking, decreased reflexes, loss of memory, loss of impulse control, depression, lethargy, and impaired concentration.

According to DSM-IV-TR, in the United States, more than 3 percent of those age 12 and older acknowledged ever using PCP, with 0.2 percent reporting use in the prior year. The highest lifetime prevalence was in those aged 26 to 34 years (4 percent), whereas the highest proportion using PCP in the prior year (0.7 percent) was in those aged 12 to 17 years.

PCP Intoxication

Short-term PCP intoxication can have potentially severe complications and must often be considered a psychiatric emergency. DSM-IV-TR gives specific criteria for PCP intoxication (Table 12.11–2). Clinicians can specify the presence of perceptual disturbances.

Some patients may be brought to psychiatric attention within hours of ingesting PCP, but often 2 to 3 days elapse before psychiatric help is sought. The long interval between drug ingestion and the appearance of the patient in a clinic usually reflects the attempts of friends to deal with the psychosis by "talking down." Persons who lose consciousness are brought for help earlier than those who remain conscious. Most patients recover completely within a day or two, but some remain psychotic for as long as 2 weeks. Patients who are first seen in a coma often exhibit disorientation, hallucinations, confusion, and difficulty communicating on regaining consciousness. These symptoms may also be seen in noncomatose patients, but their symptoms appear to be less severe than those of comatose patients. Behavioral disturbances sometimes are severe; they can include public masturbation, stripping off clothes, violence, urinary incontinence, crying, and inappropriate laughing. Patients frequently have amnesia for the entire period of the psychosis.

The patient was a 20-year-old man who was brought to the hospital, trussed in ropes, by his four brothers. This was his seventh hospitalization in the last 2 years, each for similar behavior. One of his brothers reported that he "came home crazy," threw a chair through a window, tore a gas heater off the wall, and ran into the street. The family called the police, who apprehended him shortly thereafter as he stood, naked, directing traffic at a busy intersection. He assaulted the arresting officers, escaped from them, and ran home screaming threats at his family. There, his brothers were able to subdue him.

On admission, the patient was observed to be agitated, with his mood fluctuating between anger and fear. He had slurred speech and staggered when he walked. He remained extremely violent and disorganized for the first several days of his hospitalization, then began having longer and longer lucid intervals, still interspersed with sudden, unpredictable periods in which he displayed great suspiciousness, a fierce expression, slurred speech, and clenched fists.

After calming down, the patient denied ever having been violent or acting in an unusual way ("I'm a peaceable man") and said he could not remember how he got to the hospital. He admitted using alcohol and marijuana socially, but denied phencyclidine (PCP) use except for once, experimentally, 3 years previously. Nevertheless, blood and urine tests were positive for phencyclidine, and his brother believed "he gets dusted every day."

According to his family, the patient was perfectly normal until about 3 years before. He made above-average grades in school, had a part-time job and a girlfriend, and was of a sunny and outgoing disposition. Then, at age 17 he had his first episode of emotional disturbance. This was of very sudden onset, with symptoms similar to the present episode. He quickly recovered entirely from that first episode, went back to school, and graduated from high school. From subsequent episodes, however, his improvement was less and less encouraging.

After 3 weeks of the recent hospitalization, the patient was sullen and watchful, and quick to remark sarcastically on the smallest infringement of the respect due him. He was mostly quiet and isolated from others, but was easily provoked to fury. His family reported that "this is as good as he gets" and that he had returned to his baseline functioning. When he was at home, he kept himself physically clean, but mostly lied around the house, did no housework, and had not held a job for nearly 2 years. The family does not know how he obtained spending money or how he spent his time outside the house. (Courtesy of DSM-IV-TR Casebook.)

PCP Intoxication Delirium

Phencyclidine intoxication delirium is included as a diagnostic category in DSM-IV-TR (*see* Table 10.2–6). An estimated 25 percent of all PCP-related emergency room patients may meet the criteria for the disorder, which can be characterized by agitated, violent, and bizarre behavior.

PCP-Induced Psychotic Disorder

Phencyclidine-induced psychotic disorder is included as a diagnostic category in DSM-IV-TR (*see* Table 14.4–7). Clinicians can further specify whether the predominant symptoms are delusions or hallucinations. An estimated 6 percent of PCP-related emergency room patients may meet the criteria for the disorder. About 40 percent of these patients have physical signs of hypertension and nystagmus, and 10 percent have been injured accidentally during the psychosis. The psychosis can last from 1 to 30 days, with an average of 4 to 5 days.

PCP-Induced Mood Disorder

Phencyclidine -induced mood disorder is included as a diagnostic category in DSM-IV-TR (*see* Table 15.3–10). An estimated 3 percent of PCP-related emergency room patients meet the criteria for the disorder, with most fitting the criteria for a manic-like episode. About 40 to 50 percent have been accidentally injured during the course of their manic symptoms.

PCP-Induced Anxiety Disorder

Phencyclidine-induced anxiety disorder is included as a diagnostic category in DSM-IV-TR (*see* Table 16.7–3). Anxiety is

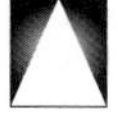

Table 12.11–3
DSM-IV-TR Diagnostic Criteria for Phencyclidine-Related Disorder Not Otherwise Specified

The phencyclidine-related disorder not otherwise specified category is for disorders associated with the use of phencyclidine that are not classifiable as phencyclidine dependence, phencyclidine abuse, phencyclidine intoxication, phencyclidine intoxication delirium, phencyclidine-induced psychotic disorder, phencyclidine-induced mood disorder, or phencyclidine-induced anxiety disorder.

(From American Psychiatric Association. *Diagnostic and Statistical Manual of Mental Disorders.* 4th ed. Text rev. Washington, DC: American Psychiatric Association; copyright 2000, with permission.)

probably the most common symptom causing a PCP-intoxicated person to seek help in an emergency room.

PCP-Related Disorder Not Otherwise Specified

The diagnosis of PCP-related disorder not otherwise specified is the appropriate diagnosis for a patient who does not fit into any of the previously described diagnoses (Table 12.11–3).

CLINICAL FEATURES

The amount of PCP varies greatly from PCP-laced cigarette to cigarette; 1 g may be used to make as few as four or as many as several dozen cigarettes. Less than 5 mg of PCP is considered a low dose, and doses above 10 mg are considered high. Dose variability makes it difficult to predict the effect, although smoking PCP is the easiest and most reliable way for users to titrate the dose.

Persons who have just taken PCP are frequently uncommunicative, appear to be oblivious, and report active fantasy production. They experience speedy feelings, euphoria, bodily warmth, tingling, peaceful floating sensations, and, occasionally, feelings of depersonalization, isolation, and estrangement. Sometimes, they have auditory and visual hallucinations. They often have striking alterations of body image, distortions of space and time perception, and delusions. They may experience intensified dependence feelings, confusion, and disorganization of thought. Users may be sympathetic, sociable, and talkative at one moment but hostile and negative at another. Anxiety is sometimes reported; it is often the most prominent presenting symptom during an adverse reaction. Nystagmus, hypertension, and hyperthermia are common effects of PCP. Head-rolling movements, stroking, grimacing, muscle rigidity on stimulation, repeated episodes of vomiting, and repetitive chanting speech are sometimes observed.

The short-term effects last 3 to 6 hours and sometimes give way to a mild depression in which the user becomes irritable, somewhat paranoid, and occasionally belligerent, irrationally assaultive, suicidal, or homicidal. The effects can last for several days. Users sometimes find that it takes 1 to 2 days to recover completely; laboratory tests show that PCP can remain in the patient's blood and urine for more than a week.

DIFFERENTIAL DIAGNOSIS

Depending on a patient's status at the time of admission, the differential diagnosis may include sedative or narcotic overdose, psychotic disorder as a consequence of the use of psychedelic drugs, and brief psychotic disorder. Laboratory analysis may help to establish the diagnosis, particularly in the many cases in which the substance history is unreliable or unattainable.

TREATMENT

Treatment of PCP intoxication aims to reduce systemic PCP levels and to address significant medical, behavioral, and psychiatric issues. For intoxication and PCP-induced psychotic disorder, although resolution of current symptoms and signs is paramount, the long-term goal of treatment is to prevent relapse to PCP use. PCP levels can fluctuate over many hours or even days, especially after oral administration. A prolonged period of clinical observation is therefore mandatory before concluding that no serious or life-threatening complications will ensue.

Trapping of ionized PCP in the stomach has led to the suggestion of continuous nasogastric suction as a treatment for PCP intoxication. This strategy, however, can be needlessly intrusive and can induce electrolyte imbalances. Administration of activated charcoal is safer, and it binds PCP and diminishes toxic effects of PCP in animals.

Trapping of ionized PCP in urine has led to the suggestion of urinary acidification as an aid to drug elimination. This strategy, however, may be ineffective and is potentially dangerous. Only a small portion of PCP is excreted in urine, metabolic acidosis itself carries significant risks, and acidic urine can increase the risk of renal failure secondary to rhabdomyolysis. Because of the extremely large volume of distribution of PCP, neither hemodialysis nor hemoperfusion can significantly promote drug clearance.

No drug is known to function as a direct PCP antagonist. Any compound binding to the PCP receptor, which is located within the ion channel of the NMDA receptor, would block NMDA receptor–mediated ion fluxes as does PCP itself. NMDA receptor mechanisms predict that pharmacological strategies promoting NMDA receptor activation (e.g., administration of a glycine site agonist drug) would promote rapid dissociation of PCP from its binding sites. No clinical trials of NMDA agonists for PCP or ketamine intoxication in humans have been carried out to date. Treatment must therefore be supportive and directed at specific symptoms and signs of toxicity. Classic measures should be used for medical crises, including seizures, hypothermia, and hypertensive crisis.

Because PCP disrupts sensory input, environmental stimuli can cause unpredictable, exaggerated, distorted, or violent reactions. A cornerstone of treatment, therefore, is minimization of sensory inputs to PCP-intoxicated patients. Patients should be evaluated and treated in as quiet and isolated an environment as possible. Precautionary physical restraint is recommended by some authorities, with the risk of rhabdomyolysis from struggle against the restraints balanced by the avoidance of violent or disruptive behavior. Pharmacological sedation can be accomplished with oral or intramuscular (IM) antipsychotics or benzodiazepines; no convincing evidence indicates that either class of compounds is clinically superior. Because of the anticholinergic actions of PCP at high doses, neuroleptics with potent intrinsic anticholinergic properties should be avoided.

COURSE AND PROGNOSIS

Complete recovery from PCP intoxication is the rule in the absence of major medical complications. Many patients, however, relapse to PCP use immediately after discharge from treatment, even for severe PCP-related complications. Intoxication usually occurs in the context of abuse, dependence, or both. No specific behavioral treatments for PCP abuse and dependence have been described, however. Case reports indicate successful responses to residential and intensive outpatient treatment regimens with long-term follow-up, including urine monitoring with or without contingency contracting.

Ketamine

Ketamine is a dissociative anesthetic agent, originally derived from PCP, that is available for use in human and veterinary medicine. It has become a drug of abuse, with sources exclusively from stolen supplies. It is available as a powder or in solution for intranasal, oral, inhalational, or (rarely) intravenous use. Ketamine functions by working at the NMDA receptor and, as with PCP, can cause hallucinations and a dissociated state in which the patient has an altered sense of the body and reality and little concern for the environment.

Ketamine causes cardiovascular stimulation and no respiratory depression. On physical examination, the patient may be hypertensive and tachycardic, have increased salivation and bidirectional or rotary nystagmus, or both. The onset of action is within seconds when used intravenously, and analgesia lasting 40 minutes and dissociative effects lasting for hours have been described. Cardiovascular status should be monitored and supportive care administered. A dystonic reaction has been described, as have flashbacks, but a more common complication is related to a lack of concern for the environment or personal safety.

Ketamine has a briefer duration of effect than PCP. Peak ketamine levels occur approximately 20 minutes after IM injection. After intranasal administration, the duration of effect is approximately 1 hour. Ketamine is *N*-demethylated by liver microsomal cytochrome P450, especially CYP3A, into norketamine. Ketamine, norketamine, and dehydronorketamine can be detected in urine, with half-lives of 3, 4, and 7 hours, respectively. Urinary ketamine and norketamine levels vary widely from individual to individual and can range from 10 to 7,000 ng/mL after intoxication. As of yet, the relationship between serum ketamine levels and clinical symptoms has not been formally studied. Ketamine is often used in combination with other drugs of abuse, especially cocaine. Ketamine does not appear to interfere with, and may enhance, cocaine metabolism.

REFERENCES

Balla A, Sershen H, Serra M, Koneru R, Javitt DC. Subchronic continuous phencyclidine administration potentiates amphetamine-induced frontal cortex dopamine release. *Neuropsychopharmacology.* 2003;28:34.

Copeland J, Dillon P. The health and psycho-social consequences of ketamine use. *International Journal of Drug Policy*. 2005;16(2):122–131.

Dix P, Martindale S, Stoddart PA. Double-blind randomized placebo-controlled trial of the effect of ketamine on postoperative morphine consumption in children following appendectomy. *Paediatr Anaesth.* 2003;13:422.

Hocking G, Cousins MJ. Ketamine in chronic pain management: An evidence-based review. *Anesth Analg.* 2003;97:1730.

Javitt D, Zukin SR. Phencyclidine (or phencyclidine-like)-related disorders. In: Sadock BJ, Sadock VA, eds. *Kaplan & Sadock's Comprehensive Textbook of Psychiatry*. 8th ed. Vol. 1. Baltimore: Lippincott Williams & Wilkins; 2005:1291.

Lankenau SE, Clatts MC. Drug injection practices among high-risk youths: The first shot of ketamine. *J Urban Health.* 2004;81(2):232–248.

Noda Y, Nabeshima T. Involvement of signal transduction cascade via dopamine-D_1 receptors in phencyclidine dependence. *Ann N Y Acad Sci.* 2004;1025:62–68.

Peters RJ Jr, Kelder SH, Meshack A, Yacoubian GS Jr, McCrimmons D, Ellis A. Beliefs and social norms about cigarettes or marijuana sticks laced with embalming fluid and phencyclidine (PCP): Why youth use "fry". *Subst Use Misuse.* 2005;40(4):563–571.

Yanagihara Y, Ohtani M, Kariya S, Uchino K, Hiraishi T, Ashizawa N, Aoyama T, Yamamura Y, Yamada Y, Iga T. Plasma concentration profiles of ketamine and norketamine after administration of various ketamine preparations to healthy Japanese volunteers. *Biopharm Drug Dispos.* 2003;24:37.

Zukin SR. Phencyclidine (or phencyclidine-like)-related disorders. In: Sadock BJ, Sadock VA, eds. *Kaplan & Sadock's Comprehensive Textbook of Psychiatry.* 7th ed. Vol. 1. Baltimore: Lippincott Williams & Wilkins; 2000:1063.

▲ 12.12 Sedative-, Hypnotic-, or Anxiolytic-Related Disorders

The drugs discussed in this section are referred to as *anxiolytic* or *sedative-hypnotic* drugs. The terminology is ambiguous for several reasons: (1) sedatives are drugs that reduce subjective tension and induce mental calmness; however, the same can be said of anxiolytics; (2) hypnotics are drugs used to induce sleep; but sedatives and anxiolytics given in sufficiently high doses also produce sleep; and (3) hypnotics in low doses, instead of inducing sleep, produce daytime sedation just as do sedatives and anxiolytics. Finally, in the older literature, all of these drugs are sometimes called *minor tranquillizers*, a term that is vague , poorly defined, and, therefore, best avoided.

The three groups of drugs associated with this class of substance-related disorders are benzodiazepines, barbiturates, and barbiturate-like substances. Each group is discussed below.

In addition to their psychiatric indications, these drugs are also used as antiepileptics, muscle relaxants, anesthetics, and anesthetic adjuvants. Alcohol and all drugs of this class are cross-tolerant, and their effects are additive. Physical and psychological dependence develops to these drugs, and all are associated with withdrawal symptoms.

Benzodiazepines

Many benzodiazepines, differing primarily in their half-lives, are available in the United States. Examples of benzodiazepines are diazepam, flurazepam (Dalmane), oxazepam (Serax), and chlordiazepoxide (Librium). Benzodiazepines are used primarily as anxiolytics, hypnotics, antiepileptics, and anesthetics, as well as for alcohol withdrawal. After their introduction in the United States in the 1960s, benzodiazepines rapidly became the most prescribed drugs; about 15 percent of all persons in the United States have had a benzodiazepine prescribed by a physician.

Increasing awareness of the risks for dependence on benzodiazepines and increased regulatory requirements, however, have decreased the number of benzodiazepine prescriptions. The Drug Enforcement Agency (DEA) classifies all benzodiazepines as Schedule IV controlled substances.

Flunitrazepam (Rohypnol), a benzodiazepine used in Mexico, South America, and Europe but not available in the United States, has become a drug of abuse. When taken with alcohol, it has been associated with promiscuous sexual behavior and rape. It is illegal to bring flunitrazepam into the United States. Although misused in the United States, it remains a standard anxiolytic in many countries.

Non-benzodiazepine sedatives such as zolpidem (Ambien) zalepon (Sonata) and esczopiclone (Lunesta)—the so called Z drugs—have clinical effects similar to the benzodiapines and are also subject to misuse and dependence.

Barbiturates

Before the introduction of benzodiazepines, barbiturates were frequently prescribed, but because of their high abuse potential, their use is much rarer today. Secobarbital (popularly known as "reds," "red devils," "seggies," and "downers"), pentobarbital (Nembutal) (known as "yellow jackets," "yellows," and "nembies"), and a secobarbital-amobarbital combination (known as "reds and blues," "rainbows," "double-trouble," and "tooies") are easily available on the street from drug dealers. Pentobarbital, secobarbital, and amobarbital (Amytal) are now under the same federal legal controls as morphine.

The first barbiturate, barbital (Veronal), was introduced in the United States in 1903. Barbital and phenobarbital (Solfoton, Luminal), which was introduced shortly thereafter, are long-acting drugs with half-lives of 12 to 24 hours. Amobarbital is an intermediate-acting barbiturate with a half-life of 6 to 12 hours. Pentobarbital and secobarbital are short-acting barbiturates with half-lives of 3 to 6 hours. Although barbiturates are useful and effective sedatives, they are highly lethal with only ten times the normal dose producing coma and death.

Barbiturate-like Substances

The most commonly abused barbiturate-like substance is methaqualone, which is no longer manufactured in the United States. It is often used by young persons who believe that the substance heightens the pleasure of sexual activity. Abusers of methaqualone commonly take one or two standard tablets (usually 300 mg per tablet) to obtain the desired effects. The street names for methaqualone include "mandrakes" (from the United Kingdom preparation Mandrax) and "soapers" (from the brand name Sopor). "Luding out" (from the brand name Quaalude) means getting high on methaqualone, which is often combined with excessive alcohol intake.

Other barbiturate-like substances include meprobamate (Equanil), a carbamate derivative that has weak efficacy as an antianxiety agent but has muscle-relaxant effects and is used for that purpose; chloral hydrate, a hypnotic which is highly toxic to the gastrointestinal (GI) system and, when combined with alcohol, is known as a "mickey finn"; and ethchlorvynol, a rapidly acting sedative agent with anticonvulsant and muscle relaxing properties. All are subject to abuse.

EPIDEMIOLOGY

According to DSM-IV-TR, about 6 percent of individuals have used either sedatives or tranquilizers illicitly, including 0.3 percent who reported illicit use of sedatives in the prior year and 0.1 percent who reported use of sedatives in the prior month. The age group with the highest lifetime prevalence of sedative (3 percent) or tranquilizer (6 percent) use was 26- to 34-years of age, and those aged 18 to 25 were most likely to have used them in the prior year. About one quarter to one third of all substance-related emergency room visits involve substances of this class. The patients have a female-to-male ratio of 3 to 1 and a white-to-black ratio of 2 to 1. Some persons use benzodiazepines alone, but persons who use cocaine often use benzodiazepines to reduce withdrawal symptoms, and opioid abusers use them to enhance the euphoric effects of opioids. Because they are easily obtained, benzodiazepines are also used by abusers of stimulants, hallucinogens, and phencyclidine (PCP) to help reduce the anxiety that can be caused by those substances.

Whereas barbiturate abuse is common among mature adults who have long histories of abuse of these substances, benzodiazepines are abused by a younger age group, usually those under 40 years of age. This group may have a slight male predominance and has a white-to-black ratio of about 2 to 1. Benzodiazepines are probably not abused as frequently as other substances for the purpose of getting "high," or inducing a euphoric feeling. Rather, they are used when a person wishes to experience a general relaxed feeling.

NEUROPHARMACOLOGY

The benzodiazepines, barbiturates, and barbiturate-like substances all have their primary effects on the γ-aminobutyric acid (GABA) type A ($GABA_A$) receptor complex, which contains a chloride ion channel, a binding site for GABA, and a well-defined binding site for benzodiazepines. The barbiturates and barbiturate-like substances are also believed to bind somewhere on the $GABA_A$ receptor complex. When a benzodiazepine, barbiturate, or barbiturate-like substance does bind to the complex, the effect is to increase the affinity of the receptor for its endogenous neurotransmitter, GABA, and to increase the flow of chloride ions through the channel into the neuron. The influx of negatively charged chloride ions into the neuron is inhibitory, and hyperpolarizes the neuron relative to the extracellular space.

Although all the substances in this class induce tolerance and physical dependence, the mechanisms behind these effects are best understood for the benzodiazepines. After long-term benzodiazepine use, the receptor effects caused by the agonist are attenuated. Specifically, GABA stimulation of the $GABA_A$ receptors results in less chloride influx than was caused by GABA stimulation before the benzodiazepine administration. This downregulation of receptor response is not caused by a decrease in receptor number or by decreased affinity of the receptor for GABA. The basis for the downregulation seems to be in the coupling between the GABA binding site and the activation of the chloride ion channel. This decreased efficiency in coupling may be regulated within the $GABA_A$ receptor complex itself or by other neuronal mechanisms.

DIAGNOSIS

The text revision of the fourth edition of *Diagnostic and Statistical Manual of Mental Disorders* (DSM-IV-TR) lists a number of sedative-, hypnotic-, or anxiolytic-related disorders (Table 12.12–1), but includes specific diagnostic criteria only for sedative, hypnotic, or anxiolytic intoxication (Table 12.12–2) and sedative, hypnotic, or anxiolytic withdrawal (Table 12.12–3). The diagnostic criteria for other sedative-, hypnotic-, or anxiolytic-related disorders are outlined in the DSM-IV-TR sections that are specific for the major symptom—for example, sedative-, hypnotic-, or anxiolytic-induced psychotic disorder (*see* Table 14.4–7).

Dependence and Abuse

Sedative, hypnotic, or anxiolytic dependence and sedative, hypnotic, or anxiolytic abuse are diagnosed according to the general criteria in DSM-IV-TR for substance dependence and substance abuse (*see* Tables 12.1–3, 12.1–4, and 12.1–5).

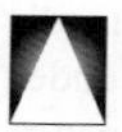

Table 12.12–1
DSM-IV-TR Sedative-, Hypnotic-, or Anxiolytic-Related Disorders

Sedative, hypnotic, or anxiolytic use disorders
Sedative, hypnotic, or anxiolytic dependence
Sedative, hypnotic, or anxiolytic abuse
Sedative-, hypnotic-, or anxiolytic-induced disorders
Sedative, hypnotic, or anxiolytic intoxication
Sedative, hypnotic, or anxiolytic withdrawal
Specify if:
With perceptual disturbances
Sedative, hypnotic, or anxiolytic intoxication delirium
Sedative, hypnotic, or anxiolytic withdrawal delirium
Sedative-, hypnotic-, or anxiolytic-induced persisting dementia
Sedative-, hypnotic-, or anxiolytic-induced psychotic disorder, with delusions
Specify if:
With onset during intoxication
With onset during withdrawal
Sedative-, hypnotic-, or anxiolytic-induced psychotic disorder, with hallucinations
Specify if:
With onset during intoxication
With onset during withdrawal
Sedative-, hypnotic-, or anxiolytic-induced mood disorder
Specify if:
With onset during intoxication
With onset during withdrawal
Sedative-, hypnotic-, or anxiolytic-induced anxiety disorder
Specify if:
With onset during withdrawal
Sedative-, hypnotic-, or anxiolytic-induced sexual dysfunction
Specify if:
With onset during intoxication
Sedative-, hypnotic-, or anxiolytic-induced sleep disorder
Specify if:
With onset during intoxication
With onset during withdrawal
Sedative-, hypnotic-, or anxiolytic-related disorder not otherwise specified

(From American Psychiatric Association. *Diagnostic and Statistical Manual of Mental Disorders.* 4th ed. Text rev. Washington, DC: American Psychiatric Association; copyright 2000, with permission.)

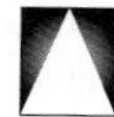

Table 12.12–2
DSM-IV-TR Diagnostic Criteria for Sedative, Hypnotic, or Anxiolytic Intoxication

A. Recent use of a sedative, hypnotic, or anxiolytic.
B. Clinically significant maladaptive behavioral or psychological changes (e.g., inappropriate sexual or aggressive behavior, mood lability, impaired judgment, impaired social or occupational functioning) that developed during, or shortly after, sedative, hypnotic, or anxiolytic use.
C. One (or more) of the following signs, developing during, or shortly after, sedative, hypnotic, or anxiolytic use:
(1) slurred speech
(2) incoordination
(3) unsteady gait
(4) nystagmus
(5) impairment in attention or memory
(6) stupor or coma
D. The symptoms are not due to a general medical condition and are not better accounted for by another mental disorder.

(From American Psychiatric Association. *Diagnostic and Statistical Manual of Mental Disorders.* 4th ed. Text rev. Washington, DC: American Psychiatric Association; copyright 2000, with permission.)

Intoxication

The DSM-IV-TR contains a single set of diagnostic criteria for intoxication by any sedative, hypnotic, or anxiolytic substance (Table 12.12–2). Although the intoxication syndromes induced by all these drugs are similar, subtle clinical differences are observable, especially with intoxications that involve low doses. The diagnosis of intoxication by one of this class of substances

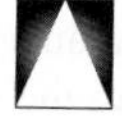

Table 12.12–3
DSM-IV-TR Diagnostic Criteria for Sedative, Hypnotic, or Anxiolytic Withdrawal

A. Cessation of (or reduction in) sedative, hypnotic, or anxiolytic use that has been heavy and prolonged.
B. Two (or more) of the following, developing within several hours to a few days after criterion A:
(1) autonomic hyperactivity (e.g., sweating or pulse rate greater than 100)
(2) increased hand tremor
(3) insomnia
(4) nausea or vomiting
(5) transient visual, tactile, or auditory hallucinations or illusions
(6) psychomotor agitation
(7) anxiety
(8) grand mal seizures
C. The symptoms in criterion B cause clinically significant distress or impairment in social, occupational, or other important areas of functioning.
D. The symptoms are not due to a general medical condition and are not better accounted for by another mental disorder.

Specify if:
With perceptual disturbances

(From American Psychiatric Association. *Diagnostic and Statistical Manual of Mental Disorders.* 4th ed. Text rev. Washington, DC: American Psychiatric Association; copyright 2000, with permission.)

is best confirmed by obtaining a blood sample for substance screening.

Benzodiazepines. Benzodiazepine intoxication can be associated with behavioral disinhibition, potentially resulting in hostile or aggressive behavior in some persons. The effect is perhaps most common when benzodiazepines are taken in combination with alcohol. Benzodiazepine intoxication is associated with less euphoria than is intoxication by other drugs in this class. This characteristic is the basis for the lower abuse and dependence potential of benzodiazepines than of barbiturates.

Barbiturates and Barbiturate-like Substances. When barbiturates and barbiturate-like substances are taken in relatively low doses, the clinical syndrome of intoxication is indistinguishable from that associated with alcohol intoxication. The symptoms include sluggishness, incoordination, difficulty thinking, poor memory, slow speech and comprehension, faulty judgment, disinhibited sexual aggressive impulses, narrowed range of attention, emotional lability, and exaggerated basic personality traits. The sluggishness usually resolves after a few hours, but depending primarily on the half-life of the abused substance, impaired judgment, distorted mood, and impaired motor skills may remain for 12 to 24 hours. Other potential symptoms are hostility, argumentativeness, moroseness, and, occasionally, paranoid and suicidal ideation. The neurological effects include nystagmus, diplopia, strabismus, ataxic gait, positive Romberg's sign, hypotonia, and decreased superficial reflexes.

Withdrawal

The DSM-IV-TR contains a single set of diagnostic criteria for withdrawal from any sedative, hypnotic, or anxiolytic substance (Table 12.12–3). Clinicians can specify "with perceptual disturbances" if illusions, altered perceptions, or hallucinations are present but accompanied by intact reality testing. Remember, benzodiazepines are associated with a withdrawal syndrome and that withdrawal from barbiturates can be life threatening. Withdrawal from benzodiazepines can also result in serious medical complications, such as seizures.

Benzodiazepines. The severity of the withdrawal syndrome associated with the benzodiazepines varies significantly depending on the average dose and the duration of use, but a mild withdrawal syndrome can follow even short-term use of relatively low doses of benzodiazepines. A significant withdrawal syndrome is likely to occur at cessation of dosages in the range of 40 mg a day for diazepam, for example, although 10 to 20 mg a day, taken for a month, can also result in a withdrawal syndrome when drug administration is stopped. The onset of withdrawal symptoms usually occurs 2 to 3 days after the cessation of use, but with long-acting drugs, such as diazepam, the latency before onset can be 5 or 6 days. The symptoms include anxiety, dysphoria, intolerance for bright lights and loud noises, nausea, sweating, muscle twitching, and sometimes seizures (generally at dosages of 50 mg a day or more of diazepam).

Barbiturates and Barbiturate-like Substances. The withdrawal syndrome for barbiturate and barbiturate-like substances ranges from mild symptoms (e.g., anxiety, weakness, sweating, and insomnia) to severe symptoms (e.g., seizures, delirium, cardiovascular collapse, and death). Persons who have been abusing phenobarbital in the range of 400 mg a day may experience mild withdrawal symptoms; those who have been abusing the substance in the range of 800 mg a day can experience orthostatic hypotension, weakness, tremor, and severe anxiety. About 75 percent of these persons have withdrawal-related seizures. Users of dosages higher than 800 mg a day may experience anorexia, delirium, hallucinations, and repeated seizures.

Most symptoms appear in the first 3 days of abstinence, and seizures generally occur on the second or third day, when the symptoms are worst. If seizures do occur, they always precede the development of delirium. The symptoms rarely occur more than a week after stopping the substance. A psychotic disorder, if it develops, starts on the third to eighth day. The various associated symptoms generally run their course within 2 to 3 days, but can last as long as 2 weeks. The first episode of the syndrome usually occurs after 5 to 15 years of heavy substance use.

Delirium

The DSM-IV-TR allows for the diagnosis of sedative, hypnotic, or anxiolytic intoxication delirium and sedative, hypnotic, or anxiolytic withdrawal delirium (*see* Tables 10.2–6 and 10.2–7). Delirium that is indistinguishable from delirium tremens associated with alcohol withdrawal is seen more commonly with barbiturate withdrawal than with benzodiazepine withdrawal. Delirium associated with intoxication can be seen with either barbiturates or benzodiazepines if the dosages are sufficiently high.

Persisting Dementia

The DSM-IV-TR allows for the diagnosis of sedative-, hypnotic-, or anxiolytic-induced persisting dementia (*see* Table 10.3–8). The existence of the disorder is controversial, because uncertainty exists whether a persisting dementia is caused by the substance use itself or by associated features of the substance use. The diagnosis must be further evaluated by using DSM-IV-TR criteria to ascertain validity.

Persisting Amnestic Disorder

The DSM-IV-TR allows for the diagnosis of sedative-, hypnotic-, or anxiolytic-induced persisting amnestic disorder (*see* Table 10.4–7). Amnestic disorders associated with sedatives, hypnotics, and anxiolytics may be underdiagnosed. One exception is the increased number of reports of amnestic episodes associated with short-term use of benzodiazepines with short half-lives (e.g., triazolam [Halcion]).

Psychotic Disorders

The psychotic symptoms of barbiturate withdrawal can be indistinguishable from those of alcohol-associated delirium tremens. Agitation, delusions, and hallucinations are usually visual, but sometimes tactile or auditory features develop after about 1 week of abstinence. Psychotic symptoms associated with intoxication or withdrawal are more common with barbiturates than with

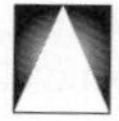

Table 12.12–4
DSM-IV-TR Diagnostic Criteria for Sedative-, Hypnotic-, or Anxiolytic-Related Disorder Not Otherwise Specified

The sedative-, hypnotic-, or anxiolytic-related disorder not otherwise specified category is for disorders associated with the use of sedatives, hypnotics, or anxiolytics that are not classifiable as sedative, hypnotic, or anxiolytic dependence; sedative, hypnotic, or anxiolytic abuse; sedative, hypnotic, or anxiolytic intoxication; sedative, hypnotic, or anxiolytic withdrawal; sedative, hypnotic, or anxiolytic intoxication delirium; sedative, hypnotic, or anxiolytic withdrawal delirium; sedative-, hypnotic-, or anxiolytic-induced persisting dementia; sedative-, hypnotic-, or anxiolytic-induced persisting amnestic disorder; sedative-, hypnotic-, or anxiolytic-induced psychotic disorder; sedative-, hypnotic-, or anxiolytic-induced mood disorder; sedative-, hypnotic-, or anxiolytic-induced anxiety disorder; sedative-, hypnotic-, or anxiolytic-induced sexual dysfunction; or sedative-, hypnotic-, or anxiolytic-induced sleep disorder.

(From American Psychiatric Association. *Diagnostic and Statistical Manual of Mental Disorders*. 4th ed. Text rev. Washington, DC: American Psychiatric Association; copyright 2000, with permission.)

benzodiazepines and are diagnosed as sedative-, hypnotic-, or anxiolytic-induced psychotic disorders (*see* Table 14.4–7). Clinicians can further specify whether delusions or hallucinations are the predominant symptoms.

Other Disorders

Sedative, hypnotic, and anxiolytic use has also been associated with mood disorders (*see* Table 15.3–10), anxiety disorders (*see* Table 16.7–3), sleep disorders (*see* Table 24.2–21), and sexual dysfunctions (*see* Table 21.2–17). When none of the previously discussed diagnostic categories is appropriate for a person with a sedative, hypnotic, or anxiolytic use disorder, the appropriate diagnosis is sedative-, hypnotic-, or anxiolytic-related disorder not otherwise specified (Table 12.12–4).

CLINICAL FEATURES

Patterns of Abuse

Oral Use. Sedatives, hypnotics, and anxiolytics can all be taken orally, either occasionally to achieve a time-limited specific effect or regularly to obtain a constant, usually mild, intoxication state. The occasional use pattern is associated with young persons who take the substance to achieve specific effects—relaxation for an evening, intensification of sexual activities, and a short-lived period of mild euphoria. The user's personality and expectations about the substance's effects and the setting in which the substance is taken also affect the substance-induced experience. The regular use pattern is associated with middle-aged, middle-class persons who usually obtain the substance from a family physician as a prescription for insomnia or anxiety. Abusers of this type may have prescriptions from several physicians, and the pattern of abuse may go undetected until obvious signs of abuse or dependence are noticed by the person's family, coworkers, or physicians.

Intravenous Use. A severe form of abuse involves the intravenous use of this class of substances. The users are mainly young adults intimately involved with illegal substances. Intravenous barbiturate use is associated with a pleasant, warm, drowsy feeling, and users may be inclined to use barbiturates more than opioids because barbiturates are less costly. The physical dangers of injection include transmission of the human immunodeficiency virus (HIV), cellulitis, vascular complications from accidental injection into an artery, infections, and allergic reactions to contaminants. Intravenous use is associated with rapid and profound tolerance and dependence and a severe withdrawal syndrome.

Overdose

Benzodiazepines. In contrast to the barbiturates and the barbiturate-like substances, the benzodiazepines have a large margin of safety when taken in overdoses, a feature that has contributed significantly to their rapid acceptance. The ratio of lethal dose to effective dose is about 200 to 1 or higher, because of the minimal degree of respiratory depression associated with the benzodiazepines. A list of equivalent therapeutic doses of benzodiazepines is given in Table 12.12–5. Even when grossly excessive amounts (more than 2 g) are taken in suicide attempts, the symptoms include only drowsiness, lethargy, ataxia, some confusion, and mild depression of the user's vital signs. A much more serious condition prevails when benzodiazepines are taken in overdose in combination with other sedative-hypnotic substances, such as alcohol. In such cases, small doses of benzodiazepines can cause death. The availability of flumazenil (Romazicon), a specific benzodiazepine antagonist, has reduced the lethality of the benzodiazepines. Flumazenil can be used in emergency rooms to reverse the effects of the benzodiazepines.

Barbiturates. Barbiturates are lethal when taken in overdose because they induce respiratory depression. In addition to intentional suicide attempts, accidental or unintentional overdoses are common. Barbiturates in home medicine cabinets are a common cause of fatal drug overdoses in children. As with benzodiazepines, the lethal effects of the barbiturates are additive to those of other sedatives or hypnotics, including alcohol

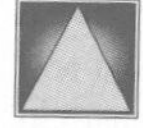

Table 12.12–5
Approximate Therapeutic Equivalent Doses of Benzodiazepines

Generic Name	Trade Name	Dose (mg)
Alprazolam	Xanax	1
Chlordiazepoxide	Librium	25
Clonazepam	Klonopin	0.5–1.0
Clorazepate	Tranxene	15
Diazepam	Valium	10
Estazolam	ProSom	1
Flurazepam	Dalmane	30
Lorazepam	Ativan	2
Oxazepam	Serax	30
Temazepam	Restoril	20
Triazolam	Halcion	0.25
Quazepam	Doral	15
Zolpidem	Ambien	10
Zaleplon	Sonata	10

and benzodiazepines. Barbiturate overdose is characterized by the induction of coma, respiratory arrest, cardiovascular failure, and death.

The lethal dose varies with the route of administration and the degree of tolerance for the substance after a history of long-term abuse. For the most commonly abused barbiturates, the ratio of lethal dose to effective dose ranges between 3 to 1 and 30 to 1. Dependent users often take an average daily dose of 1.5 g of a short-acting barbiturate, and some have been reported to take as much as 2.5 g a day for months.

The lethal dose is not much greater for the long-term abuser than for the neophyte. Tolerance develops quickly to the point at which withdrawal in a hospital becomes necessary to prevent accidental death from overdose.

Barbiturate-like Substances. The barbiturate-like substances vary in their lethality and are usually intermediate between the relative safety of the benzodiazepines and the high lethality of the barbiturates. An overdose of methaqualone, for example, can result in restlessness, delirium, hypertonia, muscle spasms, convulsions, and, in very high doses, death. Unlike barbiturates, methaqualone rarely causes severe cardiovascular or respiratory depression, and most fatalities result from combining methaqualone with alcohol.

TREATMENT AND REHABILITATION

Withdrawal

Benzodiazepines. Because some benzodiazepines are eliminated from the body slowly, symptoms of withdrawal can continue to develop for several weeks. To prevent seizures and other withdrawal symptoms, clinicians should gradually reduce the dosage. Several reports indicate that carbamazepine (Tegretol) may be useful in the treatment of benzodiazepine withdrawal. Table 12.12–6 lists guidelines for treating benzodiazepine withdrawal.

Barbiturates. To avoid sudden death during barbiturate withdrawal, clinicians must follow conservative clinical guidelines. Clinicians should not give barbiturates to a comatose or grossly intoxicated patient. A clinician should attempt to determine a patient's usual daily dose of barbiturates and then verify the dosage clinically. For example, a clinician can give a test dose of 200 mg of pentobarbital every hour until a mild intoxication occurs but withdrawal symptoms are absent (Table 12.12–7). The clinician can then taper the total daily dose at a rate of about 10 percent of the total daily dose. Once the correct dosage is determined, a long-acting barbiturate can be used for the detoxification period. During this process, the patient may begin to experience withdrawal symptoms, in which case the clinician should halve the daily decrement.

In the withdrawal procedure, phenobarbital can be substituted for the more commonly abused short-acting barbiturates. The effects of phenobarbital last longer, and because barbiturate blood levels fluctuate less, phenobarbital does not cause observable toxic signs or a serious overdose. An adequate dose is 30 mg of phenobarbital for every 100 mg of the short-acting substance. The user should be maintained for at least 2 days at that level

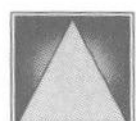

Table 12.12–6
Guidelines for Treatment of Benzodiazepine Withdrawal

1. Evaluate and treat concomitant medical and psychiatric conditions.
2. Obtain drug history and urine and blood sample for drug and ethanol assay.
3. Determine required dose of benzodiazepine or barbiturate for stabilization, guided by history, clinical presentation, drug-ethanol assay, and (in some cases) challenge dose.
4. Detoxification from supratherapeutic dosages:
   a. Hospitalize if there are medical or psychiatric indications, poor social supports, or polysubstance dependence or the patient is unreliable.
   b. Some clinicians recommend switching to longer-acting benzodiazepine for withdrawal (e.g., diazepam, clonazepam); others recommend stabilizing on the drug that patient was taking or on phenobarbital.
   c. After stabilization reduce dosage by 30 percent on the second or third day and evaluate the response, keeping in mind that symptoms that occur after decreases in benzodiazepines with short elimination half-lives (e.g., lorazepam) appear sooner than with those with longer elimination half-lives (e.g., diazepam)
   d. Reduce dosage further by 10 to 25 percent every few days if tolerated.
   e. Use adjunctive medications if necessary—carbamazepine, β-adrenergic receptor antagonists, valproate, clonidine, and sedative antidepressants have been used but their efficacy in the treatment of the benzodiazepine abstinence syndrome has not been established).
5. Detoxification from therapeutic dosages:
   a. Initiate 10 to 25 percent dose reduction and evaluate response.
   b. Dose, duration of therapy, and severity of anxiety influence the rate of taper and need for adjunctive medications.
   c. Most patients taking therapeutic doses have uncomplicated discontinuation.
6. Psychological interventions may assist patients in detoxification from benzodiazepines and in the long-term management of anxiety.

(Courtesy of Domenic A. Ciraulo, M.D., and Ofra Sarid-Segal, M.D.)

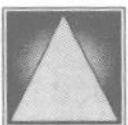

Table 12.12–7
Pentobarbital Test Dose Procedure for Barbiturate Withdrawal

Symptoms after Test Dose of 200 mg Oral Pentobarbital	Estimated 24-Hour Oral Pentobarbital Dose (mg)	Estimated 24-Hour Oral Phenobarbital Dose (mg)
Level I: Asleep but arousable; withdrawal symptoms not likely	0	0
Level II: Mild sedation; patient may have slurred speech, ataxia, nystagmus	500–600	150–200
Level III: Patient is comfortable: no evidence of sedation; may have nystagmus	800	250
Level IV: No drug effect	1,000–1,200	300–600

(Modified from Ciraulo DA, Shader RI, eds. *Clinical Manual of Chemical Dependence*. Washington, DC: American Psychiatric Press; 1991. From data in Ewing JA, Bakewell WE. Diagnosis and management of depressant drug dependence. *Am J Psychiatry* 1967;123:909.)

before the dose is reduced further. The regimen is analogous to the substitution of methadone for heroin.

After withdrawal is complete, the patient must overcome the desire to start taking the substance again. Although substitution of nonbarbiturate sedatives or hypnotics for barbiturates has been suggested as a preventive therapeutic measure, this often results in replacing one substance dependence with another. If a user is to remain substance free, follow-up treatment, usually with psychiatric help and community support, is vital. Otherwise, a patient will almost certainly return to barbiturates or a substance with similar hazards.

Overdose

The treatment of overdose of this class of substances involves gastric lavage, activated charcoal, and careful monitoring of vital signs and central nervous system (CNS) activity. Patients who overdose and come to medical attention while awake should be kept from slipping into unconsciousness. Vomiting should be induced, and activated charcoal should be administered to delay gastric absorption. If a patient is comatose, the clinician must establish an intravenous fluid line, monitor the patient's vital signs, insert an endotracheal tube to maintain a patent airway, and provide mechanical ventilation, if necessary. Hospitalization of a comatose patient in an intensive care unit is usually required during the early stages of recovery from such overdoses.

EXPERT OPINION

The International Study of Expert Judgment on Therapeutic Use of Benzodiazepines and Other Psychotherapeutic Medications was designed to gather systematic data on the opinions of leading clinicians concerning the benefits and risks of benzodiazepines and alternative treatments of anxiety. This survey study addressed the relative risks of benzodiazepines compared with other agents and comparative risks within the class. The expert panel assessed risk based on a drug's potential to produce tolerance, rebound symptoms, a withdrawal syndrome, and ease of discontinuation.

Two thirds of the expert panel reported that long-term use of benzodiazepines for the treatment of anxiety disorders does not pose a high risk of dependence and abuse. Although agreement was that the pharmacological properties of the medication may be the most important contributor to development of withdrawal symptoms, no consensus existed on whether benzodiazepines with shorter and longer half-lives have similar dependence potential. A clear consensus was that the differences in withdrawal symptoms are clinically negligible with gradual dose tapering. Because differences in abuse liability among the various benzodiazepines have not been demonstrated in humans, and because the benefits of benzodiazepine treatment clearly outweigh the risks, most physicians on the expert panel opposed increased restrictions on benzodiazepine prescribing.

Despite the expert opinion stated above, state and federal agencies have attempted to restrict the distribution of benzodiazepines by requiring special reporting forms. For example, through the use of New York State official prescription forms, the names of doctors and patients are kept on file in a data bank. Governments have taken such measures to stem the tide of abuse. But most abuse results from the illicit manufacture, sale, and diversion of substances, particularly to cocaine and opioid addicts, not from physicians' prescriptions or legitimate pharmaceutical companies. The attempt to curtail the use of substances with unquestionable, invaluable therapeutic benefits exemplifies increasing government interference in the practice of medicine and in the confidential relationship between doctor and patient. Such restrictions do little to curb cocaine, opioid, or benzodiazepine abuse.

References

Allison C, Pratt JA. Neuroadaptive processes in GABAergic and glutamatergic systems in benzodiazepine dependence. *Psychopharmacol Ther.* 2003;98:171.

Ashton H. The diagnosis and management of benzodiazepine dependence. *Curr Opin Psychiatry*. 2005;18(3):249–255.

Bruce SE, Vasile RG, Goisman RM, Salzman C, Spencer M, Machan JT, Keller MB. Are benzodiazepines still the medication of choice for patients with panic disorder with or without agoraphobia? *Am J Psychiatry.* 2003;160:1432.

Ciraulo DA, Ciraulo JA, Sands BF, Knapp CM, Sarid-Segal O. Sedative-hypnotics. In: Kranzler HR, Ciraulo DA, eds. *Clinical Manual of Addiction Psychopharmacology*. Washington DC: American Psychiatric Publishing, Inc.; 2005:111–162.

Ciraulo, DA, Sarid-Segal O. Sedative-, hypnotic-, or anxiolytic-related disorders. In: Sadock BJ, Sadock VA, eds. *Kaplan & Sadock's Comprehensive Textbook of Psychiatry*. 8th ed. Vol. 1. Baltimore: Lippincott Williams & Wilkins; 2005:1300.

de las Cuevas C, Sanz E, de la Fuente J. Benzodiazepines: More "behavioural" addiction than dependence. *Psychopharmacology.* 2003;167:297.

Griffiths RR, Johnson MW. Relative abuse liability of hypnotic drugs: A conceptual framework and algorithm for differentiating among compounds. *J Clin Psychiatry*. 2005;66[Suppl 9]:31–41.

Jaffe JH, Bloor R, Crome I, Carr M, Alam F, Simmons A, Meyer RE. A postmarketing study of relative abuse liability of hypnotic sedative drugs. *Addiction*. 2004;99(2):165.

Vorma H, Naukkarinen H, Sarna S, Kuoppsalami K. Long-term outcome after benzodiazepine withdrawal treatment in subjects with complicated dependence. *Drug Alcohol Abuse.* 2003;70:309.

Zawertailo LA, Busto UE, Kaplan HL, Greenblatt DJ, Sellers EM. Comparative abuse liability and pharmacological effects of meprobamate, triazolam, and butabarbital. *J Clin Psychopharmacol.* 2003;23:269.

▲ 12.13 Anabolic-Androgenic Steroid Abuse

Anabolic steroids are a family of drugs composed of the natural male hormone testosterone and a group of more than 50 synthetic analogs of testosterone, synthesized over the last 60 years (Table 12.13–1). These drugs all exhibit various degrees of anabolic (muscle building) and androgenic (masculinizing) effects. It is important not to confuse the anabolic-androgenic steroids (AAS) (testosterone-like hormones) with corticosteroids (cortisol-like hormones such as hydrocortisone and prednisone). Corticosteroids have no muscle-building properties and, hence, little abuse potential; they are widely prescribed to treat numerous inflammatory conditions such as poison ivy or asthma. AAS, by contrast, have only limited legitimate medical applications, such as in the treatment of hypogonadal men, the wasting syndrome associated with human immunodeficiency virus (HIV) infection, and a few specific diseases such as hereditary angioedema and Fanconi's anemia. AAS, however, are widely used illicitly, especially by boys and young men seeking to gain increased muscle mass and strength, either for athletic purposes or simply to improve personal appearance.

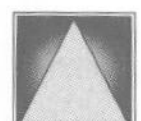

Table 12.13–1
Examples of Commonly Used Anabolic Steroids

Compounds usually administered orally
- Fluoxymesterone (Halotestin, Android-F, Ultandren)
- Methandienone (formerly called methandrostenolone; Dianabol)
- Methyltestosterone (Android, Testred, Virilon)
- Mibolerone (Cheque Drops[a])
- Oxandrolone (Anavar)
- Oxymetholone (Anadrol, Hemogenin)
- Mesterolone (Mestoranum, Proviron)
- Stanozolol (Winstrol)

Compounds usually administered intramuscularly
- Nandrolone decanoate (Deca-Durabolin)
- Nandrolone phenpropionate (Durabolin)
- Methenolone enanthate (Primobolan Depot)
- Boldenone undecylenate (Equipoise[a])
- Stanozolol (Winstrol-V[a])
- Testosterone esters blends (Sustanon, Sten)
- Testosterone cypionate
- Testosterone enanthate (Delatestryl)
- Testosterone propionate (Testoviron, Androlan)
- Testosterone undecanoate (Andriol, Restandol)
- Trenbolone acetate (Finajet, Finaplix[a])
- Trenbolone hexahydrobencylcarbonate (Parabolan)

Note: Many of the brand names listed above are foreign, but are included because of the widespread illicit use of foreign steroid preparations in the United States.

[a] Veterinary compound.

EPIDEMIOLOGY

Use of AAS is widespread among men in the United States, but is much less frequently used by women. Approximately 890,000 American men and approximately 190,000 American women reported having used AAS at some time during their lives. Approximately 286,000 men and 26,000 women are estimated to use steroids each year. Among this number, nearly one third, or 98,000, were between 12 and 17 years of age. Various studies of high school students in the United States have produced even higher estimates of the prevalence of anabolic steroid use among adolescents. Across studies of high school students, it is estimated that 3 to 12 percent of males and 0.5 to 2.0 percent of females have used AAS during their lifetimes.

The current high rates of steroid use among younger individuals appear to represent an important shift in the epidemiology of steroid use. In the 1970s, use of these drugs was largely confined to competition bodybuilders, other elite weight-training athletes, and elite athletes in other sports. Since then, however, it appears that an increasing number of young men, and occasionally even young women, may be using these drugs purely to enhance personal appearance rather than for any athletic purpose.

PHARMACOLOGY

All steroid drugs—including AAS, estrogens, and corticosteroids—are synthesized in vivo from cholesterol and resemble cholesterol in their chemical structure. Testosterone has a four-ring chemical structure containing 19 carbon atoms (Fig. 12.13–1).

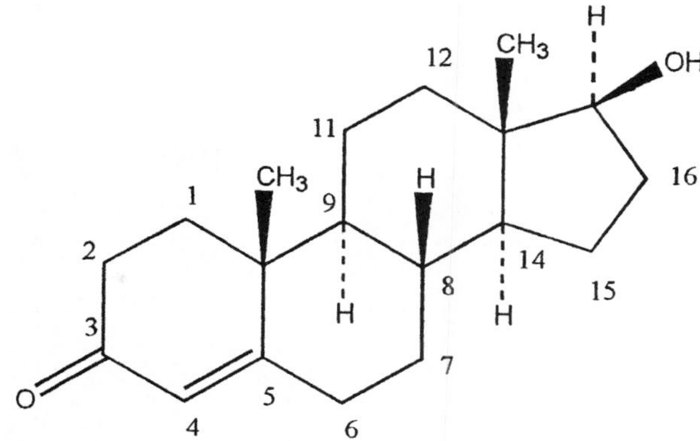

FIGURE 12.13–1
Molecular structure of testosterone.

Normal testosterone plasma concentrations for men range from 300 to 1,000 ng/dL. Generally, 200 mg of testosterone cypionate taken every 2 weeks restores physiological testosterone concentrations in a hypogonadal male. A eugonadal male who initiates physiological dosages of testosterone has no net gain in testosterone concentrations because exogenously administered AAS shut down endogenous testosterone production via feedback inhibition of the hypothalamic-pituitary-gonadal axis. Consequently, illicit users take higher than therapeutic dosages to achieve supraphysiological effects. The dose–response curve for anabolic effects may be logarithmic, which could explain why illicit users generally take 10 to 100 times the therapeutic dosages. Doses in this range are most easily achieved by taking combinations of oral and injected AAS, which illicit AAS users often do. Transdermal testosterone, available by prescription for testosterone replacement therapy, may also be used.

Therapeutic Indications

The AAS are primarily indicated for testosterone deficiency (male hypogonadism), hereditary angioedema (a congenital skin disorder), and some uncommon forms of anemia caused by bone marrow or renal failure. In women, they are given, although not as first-choice agents, for metastatic breast cancer, osteoporosis, endometriosis, and adjunctive treatment of menopausal symptoms. In men, they have been used experimentally as a male contraceptive and for treating major depressive disorder and sexual disorders in eugonadal men. Recently, they have been used to treat wasting syndromes associated with acquired immune deficiency syndrome (AIDS). Controlled studies have also suggested that testosterone has antidepressant effects in some men infected with HIV with major depressive disorder, and is also a supplementary (augmentation) treatment in some depressed men with low endogenous testosterone levels who are refractory to conventional antidepressants.

Adverse Reactions

The most common adverse medical effects of AAS involve the cardiovascular, hepatic, reproductive, and dermatological systems.

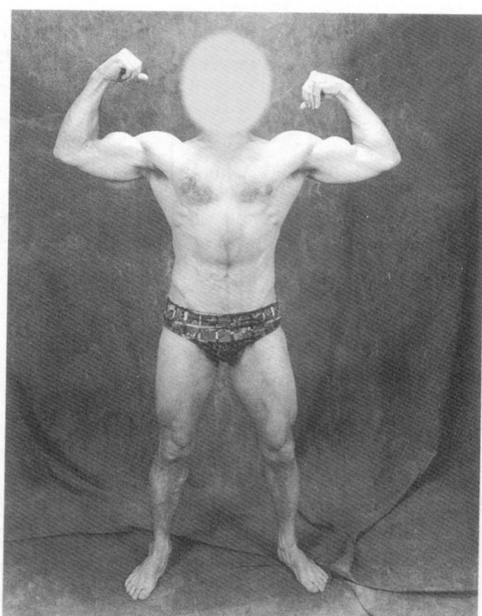

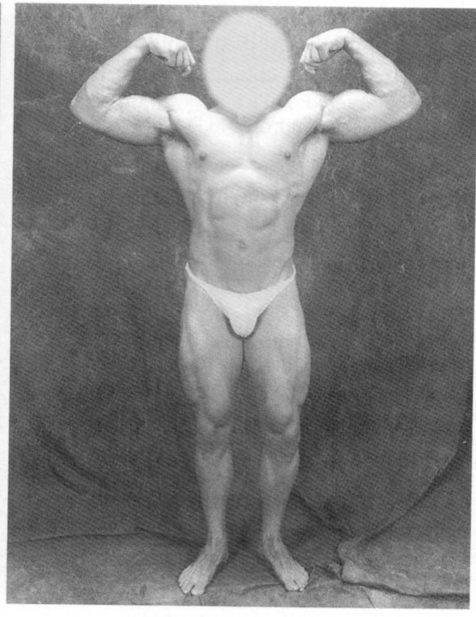

FIGURE 12.13–2

Physical effects of anabolic steroid use. The photographs compare a "natural" bodybuilder who has never used anabolic steroids (**left**) with a man who has used large doses of anabolic steroids over several years (**right**). Both men are 67 inches tall and have 7 percent body fat. The man on the left weighs 170 lbs and represents approximately the maximum degree of muscularity obtainable without drugs. His fat-free mass index is 25.4 kg/m^2 by the formula of Elana Kouri, et al. The man on the right weighs 213 lbs and has a fat-free mass index of 31.7 kg/m^2. Note the muscle hypertrophy from steroid use is particularly marked in the upper body in the pectoralis, deltoid, trapezius, and biceps muscles. Any man significantly more muscular than the man on the left has almost certainly abused anabolic steroids.

The AAS produce an adverse cholesterol profile by increasing levels of low-density lipoprotein cholesterol and decreasing levels of high-density lipoprotein cholesterol. High-dose use of AAS can also activate hemostasis and increase blood pressure. Isolated case reports of myocardial infarction, cardiomyopathy, left ventricular hypertrophy, and stroke among users of AAS, including fatalities, have appeared,

Among the AAS-induced endocrine effects in men are testicular atrophy and sterility, both usually reversible after discontinuing AAS, and gynecomastia, which may persist until surgical removal. In women, shrinkage of breast tissue, irregular menses (diminution or cessation), and masculinization (clitoral hypertrophy, hirsutism, and deepened voice) can occur. Masculinizing effects in women may be irreversible. Androgens taken during pregnancy could cause masculinization of a female fetus. Dermatological effects include acne and male pattern baldness. Abuse of AAS by children has led to concerns that AAS-induced premature closure of bony epiphyses could cause shortened stature. Other uncommon adverse effects include edema of the extremities caused by water retention, exacerbation of tic disorders, sleep apnea, and polycythemia.

ETIOLOGY

The major reason for taking illicit AAS is to enhance either athletic performance or physical appearance. Taking AAS is reinforced because they can produce the athletic and physical effects that users desire, especially when combined with proper diet and training. Further reinforcement derives from winning competitions and from social admiration for physical appearance. AAS users also perceive that they can train more intensively for longer durations with less fatigue and with decreased recovery times between workouts.

The dramatic effects of AAS on muscle growth are illustrated in Figure 12.13–2, which compares a "natural" bodybuilder who has never used these drugs with a bodybuilder of identical height and body fat who has used AAS extensively.

Although the anabolic or muscle-building properties of AAS are clearly important to those seeking to enhance athletic performance and physical appearance, psychoactive effects may also be important in the persistent and dependent use of AAS. Anecdotally, some AAS users report feelings of power, aggressiveness, and euphoria, which become associated with, and can, reinforce AAS taking.

In general, males are more likely to take AAS than females, and athletes are more likely to take AAS than nonathletes. Some male and female weight lifters may have muscle dysmorphia, a form of body dysmorphic disorder in which the individual feels that he or she is not sufficiently muscular and lean.

DIAGNOSIS AND CLINICAL FEATURES

Steroids may initially induce euphoria and hyperactivity. After relatively short periods, however, their use can become associated with increased anger, arousal, irritability, hostility, anxiety, somatization, and depression (especially during times when steroids are not used). Several studies have demonstrated that 2 to 15 percent of anabolic steroid abusers experience hypomanic or manic episodes, and a smaller percentage may have clearly psychotic symptoms. Also disturbing is a correlation between steroid abuse and violence ("roid rage" in the parlance of users).

Steroid abusers with no record of antisocial behavior or violence have committed murders and other violent crimes.

Steroids are addictive substances. When abusers stop taking steroids, they can become depressed, anxious, and concerned about their bodies' physical state. Some similarities have been noted between athletes' views of their muscles and the views of patients with anorexia nervosa about their bodies; to an observer, both groups seem to distort realistic assessment of the body.

Iatrogenic addiction is a consideration in view of the increasing number of geriatric patients who are receiving testosterone from their physicians in an attempt to increase libido and reverse some aspects of aging.

TREATMENT

Abstinence is the treatment goal of choice for patients manifesting AAS abuse or dependence. To the extent that users of AAS abuse other addictive substances (including alcohol), traditional treatment approaches for substance-related disorders may be used. Nevertheless, AAS users may differ from other addicted patients in several ways that have implications for treatment. First, the euphorigenic and reinforcing effects of AAS may only become apparent after weeks or months of use in conjunction with intensive exercising. When compared with immediately and passively reinforcing drugs, such as cocaine, heroin, and alcohol, AAS use may entail more delayed gratification. Second, AAS users may manifest greater commitment to culturally endorsed values of physical fitness, success, victory, and goal directness than users of other illicit drugs. Finally, AAS users are often preoccupied with their physical attributes and may rely excessively on these attributes for self-esteem. Treatment therefore depends on a therapeutic alliance that is based on a thorough and nonjudgmental understanding of the patient's values and motivations for using AAS.

AAS Withdrawal

Supportive therapy and monitoring are essential for treating AAS withdrawal because suicidal depressions can occur. Hospitalization may be required when suicidal ideation is severe. Patients should be educated about the possible course of withdrawal and reassured that symptoms are time limited and manageable. Antidepressant agents are best reserved for patients whose depressive symptomatology persists for several weeks after AAS discontinuation and who meet criteria for major depressive disorder. Selective serotonin reuptake inhibitors (SSRIs) are the preferred agents because of their favorable adverse effect profile and their effectiveness in the only reported case series of treated AAS users with major depressive disorder. Physical withdrawal symptoms are not life threatening and do not ordinarily require pharmacotherapy. Nonsteroidal anti-inflammatory drugs (NSAIDs) may be useful to treat musculoskeletal pain and headaches.

ANABOLIC STEROID–INDUCED MOOD DISORDERS

Irritability, aggressiveness, hypomania, and frank mania associated with anabolic steroid use probably represent one of the most important public health issues associated with these drugs. Although athletes using these drugs have long recognized that syndromes of anger and irritability could be associated with AAS use, these syndromes were little recognized in the scientific literature until the late 1980s and 1990s. Since then, a series of observational field studies of athletes has suggested that some AAS users develop prominent hypomanic or even manic symptoms during AAS use.

A possible serious consequence of AAS-induced mood disorders may be violent or even homicidal behavior. Several published reports have anecdotally described individuals with no apparent history of psychiatric disorder, no criminal record, and no history of violence, who committed violent crimes, including murder, while under the influence of AAS. In a number of cases, AAS use has been cited in criminal trials as a possible mitigating factor in the defense of such individuals. Although a causal link is difficult to establish in these cases, evidence of AAS use has frequently been presented in forensic settings as a possible mitigating factor in criminal behavior.

Depressive syndromes induced by AAS have occurred and suicide is a risk. A brief and self-limited syndrome of depression occurs on AAS withdrawal, probably as a result of the depression of the hypothalamic-pituitary-gonadal axis after exogenous AAS administration.

ANABOLIC STEROID–INDUCED PSYCHOTIC DISORDER

Psychotic symptoms are rare in association with anabolic steroid use, but they have been described in a few cases, primarily in individuals who were using the equivalent of more than 1,000 mg of testosterone a week. Usually, these symptoms have consisted of grandiose or paranoid delusions, generally occurring in the context of a manic episode, although occasionally occurring in the absence of a frank manic syndrome. In most cases reported, psychotic symptoms have disappeared promptly (within a few weeks) after the discontinuation of the offending agent, although temporary treatment with antipsychotic agents was sometimes required.

ANABOLIC STEROID–RELATED DISORDER NOT OTHERWISE SPECIFIED

Symptoms of anxiety disorders, such as panic disorder and social phobia can occur during AAS use. AAS use may serve as a "gateway to the use of opioid agonist or antagonists, such as nalbuphine, or to use of frank opioid agonists, such as heroin." A study of men admitted for substance dependence treatment in Massachusetts produced similar findings.

DEHYDROEPIANDROSTERONE AND ANDRO-STENEDIONE

Dehydroepiandrosterone (DHEA), a precursor hormone for both estrogens and androgens, is available over the counter. Recent years have seen an interest in DHEA for improving cognition, depression, sex drive, and general well-being in elderly adults. Some reports suggest that DHEA in dosages of 50 to 100 mg per day increases the sense of physical and social well-being in women aged 40 to 70 years. Reports also exist of androgenic effects, including irreversible hirsutism, hair loss, voice deepening, and other undesirable sequelae. In addition, DHEA has at least a theoretical potential of enhancing tumor growth in persons with latent, hormone-sensitive malignancies, such as prostate, cervical, and breast cancer. Despite its significant popularity, few controlled data exist on the safety or efficacy of DHEA.

References

Brower KJ. Anabolic steroid abuse and dependence. *Current Psychiatry Report*. 2002;4:377.

Hall RCW, Hall RCW, Chapman MJ. Psychiatric complications of anabolic steroid abuse. *Psychosomatics: Journal of Consultation Liaison Psychiatry*. 2005;46:285–290.

Kanayama G, Barry S, Hudson JI, Pope HG Jr. Body image and attitudes toward male roles in anabolic-androgenic steroid users. *Am J Psychiatry*. 2006;163(4):697–703.

Kanayama G, Cohane G, Weiss RD, Pope HG Jr. Past anabolic-androgenic steroid use among men admitted for substance abuse treatment—An underrecognized problem? *J Clin Psychiatry*. 2003;64:156.

Kanayama G, Pope HG Jr, Cochane G, Hudson JI. Risk factors for anabolic-androgenic steroid use among weightlifters: A case-control study. *Drug Alcohol Depend*. 2003;71:77–86.

Modlinski R, Fields KB. The effect of anabolic steroids on the gastrointestinal system, kidneys, and adrenal glands. *Curr Sports Med Rep*. 2006;5(2):104–109.

Nottin S, Nguyen LD, Terbah M, Obert P. Cardiovascular effects of androgenic anabolic steroids in male bodybuilders determined by tissue Doppler imaging. *Am J Cardiol*. 2006;97(6):912–915.

Pope Hg Jr, Brower KJ. Anabolic-androgenic steroid abuse. In: Sadock BJ, Sadock VA, eds. *Kaplan & Sadock's Comprehensive Textbook of Psychiatry*. 8th ed. Vol. 1. Baltimore: Lippincott Williams & Wilkins; 2005:1318.

Pope HG Jr, Katz DL. Psychiatric effects of exogenous anabolic-androgenic steroids. In: Wolkowitz OM, Rothschild AJ, eds. *Psychoneuroendocrinology for the Clinician*. Washington, DC: American Psychiatric Press; 2003:331–358.

Trenton AJ, Currier GW. Behavioural manifestations of anabolic steroid use. *CNS Drugs*. 2005;19(7):571–595.

▲ 12.14 Other Substance-Related Disorders

This section deals with a diverse group of drugs not covered in the previous section that cannot be easily grouped together. The text revision of the fourth edition of *Diagnostic and Statistical Manual of Mental Disorders* (DSM-IV-TR) includes a diagnostic category for these substances called other (or unknown) substance-related disorders (Table 12.14–1). Some of these substances are discussed below.

Gamma Hydroxybutyrate

Gamma hydroxybutyrate (GHB) is a naturally occurring transmitter in the brain that is related to sleep regulation. GHB increases dopamine levels in the brain. In general, GHB is a central nervous system (CNS) depressant with effects through the endogenous opioid system. It is used to induce anesthesia and long-term sedation, but its unpredictable duration of action limits its use. It has recently been studied for the treatment of alcohol and opioid withdrawal and narcolepsy.

Until 1990, GHB was sold in US health food stores, and body builders used it as a steroid alternative. Reports indicate, however, that GHB is abused for its intoxicating effects and consciousness-altering properties. It is variously referred to as "GBH" and "liquid ecstasy" and is sold illicitly in various forms (e.g., powder and liquid). Similar chemicals, which the body converts to GBH, include γ-butyrolactone (GBL) and 1,4-butanediol. Adverse effects include nausea, vomiting, respiratory problems, seizures, coma, and death. In some reports, GHB abuse has been linked to a syndrome similar to Wernicke-Korsakoff syndrome.

NITRITE INHALANTS

The nitrite inhalants include amyl, butyl, and isobutyl nitrites, all of which are called "poppers" in popular jargon. The intoxication syndromes seen with nitrites can differ markedly from the syndromes seen with the standard inhalant substances, such as lighter fluid and airplane glue. Nitrite inhalants are used by persons seeking the associated mild euphoria, altered sense of time, feeling of fullness in the head, and, possibly, increased sexual feelings. The nitrite compounds are used by some gay men and users of other drugs to heighten sexual stimulation during orgasm and, in some cases, to relax the anal sphincter for penile penetration. Under such circumstances, a person may use the substance for a few or a dozen times within several hours.

Adverse reactions include a toxic syndrome characterized by nausea, vomiting, headache, hypotension, drowsiness, and irritation of the respiratory tract. Some evidence indicates that nitrite inhalants can adversely affect immune function. Because sildenafil (Viagra) and its congeners are lethal when combined with nitrite compounds, persons at risk should be cautioned never to use the two together.

NITROUS OXIDE

Nitrous oxide, commonly known as "laughing gas," is a widely available anesthetic agent that is subject to abuse because of its ability to produce feelings of lightheadedness and of floating, sometimes experienced as pleasurable or specifically as sexual. With long-term abuse patterns, nitrous oxide use has been associated with delirium and paranoia. Female dental assistants exposed to high levels of nitrous oxide have reportedly experienced reduced fertility.

> A 35-year-old male dentist with no history of other substance problems complained of problems with nitrous oxide abuse for 10 years. This had begun as experimentation with what he had considered a harmless substance. His rate of use increased over several years, however, eventually becoming almost daily for months at a time. He felt a craving before sessions of use. Then, using the gas while alone in his office, he immediately felt numbness, a change in his temperature and heart rate, and alleviation of depressed feelings. "Things would go through my mind. Time was erased." He sometimes fell asleep. Sessions might last a few minutes or up to 8 hours. They ended when the craving and euphoria ended. He had often tried to stop or cut down, sometimes consulting a professional about the problem.

Other Substances

Nutmeg. Nutmeg can be ingested in a number of preparations. When nutmeg is taken in sufficiently high doses, it can induce depersonalization, derealization, and a feeling of heaviness in the limbs. In sufficiently high doses, morning glory seeds

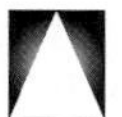

Table 12.14–1
DSM-IV-TR Criteria for Other (or Unknown) Substance-Related Disorders

The other or (unknown) substance-related disorders category is for classifying substance-related disorders associated with substances not listed above. Examples of these substances, which are described in more detail below, include anabolic steroids, nitrite inhalants ("poppers"), nitrous oxide, over-the-counter and prescription medications not otherwise covered by the 11 categories (e.g., cortisol, antihistamines, benztropine), and other substances that have psychoactive effects. In addition, this category may be used when the specific substance is unknown (e.g., an intoxication after taking a bottle of unlabeled pills).

Anabolic steroids sometimes produce an initial sense of enhanced well-being (or even euphoria), which is replaced after repeated use by lack of energy, irritability, and other forms of dysphoria. Continued use of these substances may lead to more severe symptoms (e.g., depressive symptomatology) and general medical conditions (liver disease).

Nitrite inhalants ("poppers" forms of amyl, butyl, and isobutyl nitrite) produce an intoxication that is characterized by a feeling of fullness in the head, mild euphoria, a change in the perception of time, relaxation of smooth muscles, and a possible increase in sexual feelings. In addition to possible compulsive use, these substances carry dangers of potential impairment of immune functioning, irritation of the respiratory system, a decrease in the oxygen-carrying capacity of the blood, and a toxic reaction that can include vomiting, severe headache, hypotension, and dizziness.

Nitrous Oxide ("laughing gas") causes rapid onset of an intoxication that is characterized by lightheadedness and a floating sensation that clears in a matter of minutes after administration is stopped. There are reports of temporary but clinically relevant confusion and reversible paranoid states when nitrous oxide is used regularly.

Other substances that are capable of producing mild intoxication include **catnip,** which can produce states similar to those observed with marijuana and which in high doses is reported to result in LSD-type perceptions; **betel nut,** which is chewed in many cultures to produce a mild euphoria and floating sensation; and **kava** (a substance derived from the South Pacific pepper plant), which produces sedation, incoordination, weight loss, mild forms of hepatitis, and lung abnormalities. In addition, individuals can develop dependence and impairment through repeated self-administration of **over-the-counter** and **prescription drugs,** including **cortisol, antiparkinsonian agents** that have anticholinergic properties, and **antihistamines.**

Texts and criteria sets have already been provided to define the generic aspects of substance dependence, substance abuse, substance intoxication, and substance withdrawal that are applicable across classes of substances. The other (or unknown) substance-induced disorders are described in the sections of the manual with disorders with which they share phenomenology (e.g., other for unknown); substance-induced mood disorder is included in the mood disorders section. Listed below are the other (or unknown) substance use disorders and the other (or unknown) substance-induced disorders.

Other (or unknown) substance use disorders

Other (or unknown) substance use dependence

Other (or unknown) substance abuse

Other (or unknown) substance-induced disorders

Other (or unknown) substance intoxication
Specify if:
With perceptual disturbances

Other (or unknown) substance withdrawal
Specify if:
With perceptual disturbances

Other (or unknown) substance-induced delirium

Other (or unknown) substance-induced persisting dementia

Other (or unknown) substance-induced persisting amnestic disorder

Other (or unknown) substance psychotic disorder, with delusions
Specify if:
With onset during intoxication
With onset during withdrawal

Other (or unknown) substance-induced psychotic disorder, with hallucinations
Specify if:
With onset during intoxication
With onset during withdrawal

Other (or unknown) substance-induced mood disorder
Specify if:
With onset during intoxication
With onset during withdrawal

Other (or unknown) substance-induced anxiety disorder
Specify if:
With onset during intoxication
With onset during withdrawal

Other (or unknown) substance-induced sexual dysfunction
Specify if:
With onset during intoxication

Other (or unknown) substance-induced sleep disorder
Specify if:
With onset during intoxication

Other (or unknown) substance-related disorder not otherwise specified

(From American Psychiatric Association. *Diagnostic and Statistical Manual of Mental Disorders.* 4th ed. Text rev. Washington, DC: American Psychiatric Association; copyright 2000, with permission.)

can produce a syndrome resembling that seen with lysergic acid diethylamide (LSD), characterized by altered sensory perceptions and mild visual hallucinations.

Catnip. Catnip can produce cannabis-like intoxication in low doses and LSD-like intoxication in high doses.

Betel Nuts. Betel nuts, when chewed, can produce a mild euphoria and a feeling of floating in space.

Kava. Kava, derived from a pepper plant native to the South Pacific, produces sedation and incoordination and is associated with hepatitis, lung abnormalities, and weight loss.

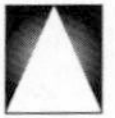

Table 12.14–2
DSM-IV-TR Criteria for Polysubstance Dependence

This diagnosis is reserved for behavior during the same 12-month period in which the person was repeatedly using at least three groups of substances (not including caffeine and nicotine), but no single substance has predominated. Further, during this period, the dependence criteria were met for substances as a group but not for any specific substance.

(From American Psychiatric Association. *Diagnostic and Statistical Manual of Mental Disorders.* 4th ed. Text rev. Washington, DC: American Psychiatric Association; copyright 2000, with permission.)

Over-the-Counter Drugs. Some persons abuse over-the-counter and prescription medications, such as cortisol, antiparkinsonian agents, and antihistamines.

Ephedra. Ephedra, a natural substance found in herbal tea, acts like epinephrine and, when abused, produces cardiac arrhythmia and fatalities.

Chocolate. A controversial possible substance of abuse is chocolate derived from the cacao bean. Anandamide, an ingredient in chocolate, stimulates the same receptors as marijuana. Other compounds in chocolate include tryptophan, the precursor of serotonin, and phenylalanine, an amphetamine-like substance, both of which improve mood. So-called chocoholics may be self-medicating because of a depressive diathesis.

POLYSUBSTANCE-RELATED DISORDER

Substance users often abuse more than one substance. In DSM-IV-TR, a diagnosis of polysubstance dependence is appropriate if, for a period of at least 12 months, a person has repeatedly used substances from at least three categories (not including nicotine and caffeine), even if the diagnostic criteria for a substance-related disorder are not met for any single substance, as long as, during this period, the criteria for substance dependence have been met for the substances considered as a group (Table 12.14–2).

TREATMENT AND REHABILITATION

Treatment approaches for the substances covered in this section vary according to substances, patterns of abuse, availability of psychosocial support systems, and patients' individual features. Two major treatment goals for substance abuse have been determined: the first is abstinence from the substance, and the second is the physical, psychiatric, and psychosocial well-being of the patient. Significant damage has often been done to a patient's support systems during prolonged periods of substance abuse. For a patient to stop a pattern of substance abuse successfully, adequate psychosocial supports must be in place to foster the difficult change in behavior.

In some rare cases, it may be necessary to initiate treatment on an inpatient unit. Although an outpatient setting is more desirable than an inpatient setting, the temptations available to an outpatient for repeated use may present too high a hurdle for the initiation of treatment. Inpatient treatment is also indicated in the case of severe medical or psychiatric symptoms, a history of failed outpatient treatments, a lack of psychosocial supports, or a particularly severe or long-term history of substance abuse. After an initial period of detoxification, patients need a sustained period of rehabilitation. Throughout treatment, individual, family, and group therapies can be effective. Education about substance abuse and support for patients' efforts are essential factors in treatment.

REFERENCES

Anderson IB, Kim SY, Dyer JE, Burkhardt CB, Iknoian JC, Walsh MJ, Blanc PD. Trends in gamma-hydroxybutyrate (GHB) and related drug intoxication: 1999 to 2003. *Ann Emerg Med.* 2006;47(2):177–183.

Camacho A, Matthews SC, Murray B, Dimsdale JE. Use of GHB compounds among college students. *Am J Drug Alcohol Abuse.* 2005;31(4):601–607.

Colfax G, Guzman R. Club drugs and HIV infection: A review. *Clin Infect Dis.* 2006;42:1463–1469.

Gahlinger PM. Club drugs: MDMA, gamma-hydroxybutyrate (GHB), Rohypnol, and ketamine. *Am Fam Physician.* 2004;69(11):2619–2626.

Haller C, Thai D, Manktelow TC, Wesnes K, Benowitz N. Cognitive and mood effects of GHB and ethanol in humans. *J Toxicol Clin Toxicol.* 2004;42(5):762.

Jaffe JH. Substance-related disorders: Introduction and overview. In: Sadock BJ, Sadock VA, eds. *Kaplan & Sadock's Comprehensive Textbook of Psychiatry.* 7th ed. Vol. 1. Baltimore: Lippincott Williams & Wilkins; 2000:924.

Jaffe JH, Anthony JC. Substance-related disorders: Introduction and overview. In: Sadock BJ, Sadock VA, eds. *Kaplan & Sadock's Comprehensive Textbook of Psychiatry.* 8th ed. Vol. 1. Baltimore: Lippincott Williams & Wilkins; 2005: 1137.

Medina KL, Shear PK, Schafer J, Armstrong TG, Dyer P. Cognitive functioning and length of abstinence in polysubstance dependent men. *Arch Clin Neuropsychol.* 2004;19(2):245–258.

Peters RJ, Adams LF, Barnes JB, Hines LA, Jones DE, Krebs KMA, Kelder SH. Beliefs and social norms about Ephedra onset and perceived addiction among college male and female athletes. *Subst Use Misuse.* 2005;40:125–135.

Wu LT, Schlenger WE, Ringwalt CL. Use of nitrite inhalants ("poppers") among American youth. *J Adolesc Health.* 2005;37:52–60.

13 Schizophrenia

Schizophrenia is a clinical syndrome of variable, but profoundly disruptive, psychopathology that involves cognition, emotion, perception, and other aspects of behavior. The expression of these manifestations varies across patients and over time, but the effect of the illness is always severe and is usually long lasting. The disorder usually begins before age 25, persists throughout life, and affects persons of all social classes. Both patients and their families often suffer from poor care and social ostracism because of widespread ignorance about the disorder. Although schizophrenia is discussed as if it is a single disease, it probably comprises a group of disorders with heterogeneous etiologies, and it includes patients whose clinical presentations, treatment response, and courses of illness vary. Clinicians should appreciate that the diagnosis of schizophrenia is based entirely on the psychiatric history and mental status examination. There is no laboratory test for schizophrenia.

HISTORY

Written descriptions of symptoms commonly observed today in patients with schizophrenia are found throughout history. Early Greek physicians described delusions of grandeur, paranoia, and deterioration in cognitive functions and personality. It was not until the 19th century, however, that schizophrenia emerged as a medical condition worthy of study and treatment. Two major figures in psychiatry and neurology who studied the disorder were Emil Kraepelin (1856–1926) and Eugene Bleuler (1857–1939). Earlier, Benedict Morel (1809–1873), a French psychiatrist, had used the term *démence précoce* to describe deteriorated patients whose illness began in adolescence.

Emil Kraepelin

Kraepelin (Fig. 13–1) translated Morel's *démence précoce* into dementia precox, a term that emphasized the change in cognition (dementia) and early onset (precox) of the disorder. Patients with dementia precox were described as having a long-term deteriorating course and the clinical symptoms of hallucinations and delusions. Kraepelin distinguished these patients from those who underwent distinct episodes of illness alternating with periods of normal functioning which he classified as having manic-depressive psychosis. Another separate condition called *paranoia* was characterized by persistent persecutory delusions. These patients lacked the deteriorating course of dementia precox and the intermittent symptoms of manic-depressive psychosis.

Eugene Bleuler

Bleuler (Fig. 13–2) coined the term *schizophrenia*, which replaced dementia precox in the literature. He chose the term to express the presence of schisms between thought, emotion, and behavior in patients with the disorder. Bleuler stressed that, unlike Kraepelin's concept of dementia precox, schizophrenia need not have a deteriorating course. This term is often misconstrued, especially by lay people, to mean split personality. Split personality, called dissociative identity disorder, in the text revision of the fourth edition of *Diagnostic and Statistical Manual of Mental Disorders* (DSM-IV-TR) differs completely from schizophrenia (see Chapter 20).

The Four As. Bleuler identified specific fundamental (or primary) symptoms of schizophrenia to develop his theory about the internal mental schisms of patients. These symptoms included associational disturbances of thought, especially looseness, affective disturbances, autism, and ambivalence, summarized as the four As: associations, affect, autism, and ambivalence. Bleuler also identified accessory (secondary) symptoms, which included those symptoms that Kraepelin saw as major indicators of dementia precox: hallucinations and delusions.

Other Theorists

Ernst Kretschmer (1888–1926). Kretschmer compiled data to support the idea that schizophrenia occurred more often among persons with asthenic (i.e., slender, lightly muscled physiques), athletic, or dysplastic body types rather than among persons with pyknic (i.e., short, stocky physiques) body types. He thought the latter were more likely to incur bipolar disorders. His observations may seem strange, but they are not inconsistent with a superficial impression of the body types in many persons with schizophrenia.

Kurt Schneider (1887–1967). Schneider contributed a description of first-rank symptoms, which, he stressed, were not specific for schizophrenia and were not to be rigidly applied but were useful for making diagnoses. He emphasized that in patients who showed no first-rank symptoms, the disorder could be diagnosed exclusively on the basis of second-rank symptoms and an otherwise typical clinical appearance. Clinicians frequently ignore his warnings and sometimes see the absence of first-rank symptoms during a single interview as evidence that a person does not have schizophrenia (Table 13–1).

Karl Jaspers (1883–1969). Jaspers, a psychiatrist and philosopher, played a major role in developing existential psychoanalysis. He was interested in the phenomenology of mental illness and the subjective feelings of patients with mental illness. His work paved the way toward

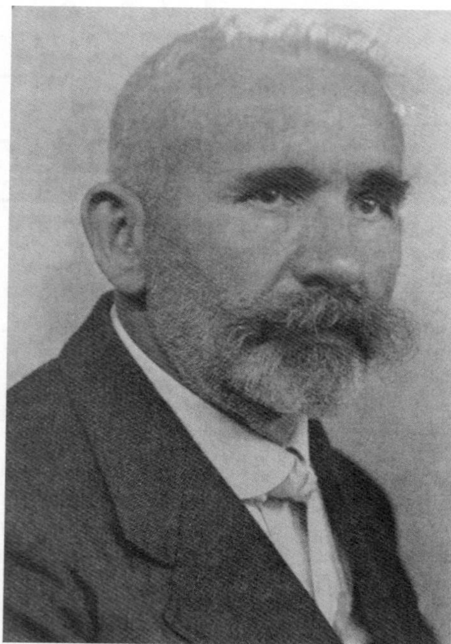

FIGURE 13–1
Emil Kraepelin, 1856–1926. (Courtesy of National Library of Medicine, Bethesda, MD.)

trying to understand the psychological meaning of schizophrenic signs and symptoms such as delusions and hallucinations.

Adolf Meyer (1866–1950). Meyer, the founder of psychobiology, saw schizophrenia as a reaction to life stresses. It was a maladaptation that was understandable in terms of the patient's life experiences. Meyer's view was represented in the nomenclature of the 1950s, which referred to the schizophrenic reaction. In later editions of DSM, the term reaction was dropped.

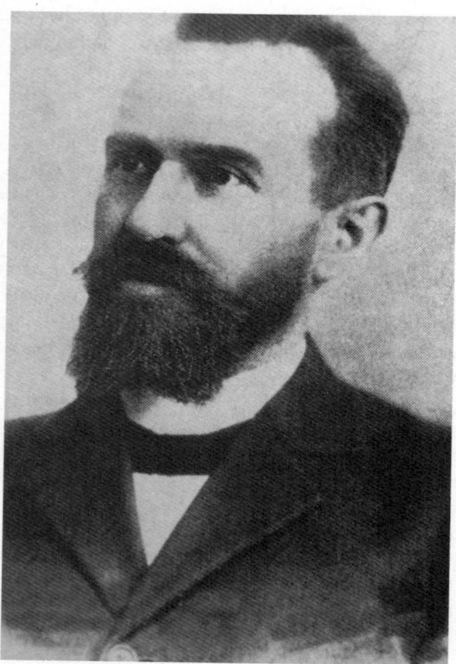

FIGURE 13–2
Eugene Bleuler, 1857–1939. (Courtesy of National Library of Medicine, Bethesda, MD.)

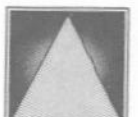

Table 13–1
Kurt Schneider Criteria for Schizophrenia

1. First-rank symptoms
   a. Audible thoughts
   b. Voices arguing or discussing or both
   c. Voices commenting
   d. Somatic passivity experiences
   e. Thought withdrawal and other experiences of influenced thought
   f. Thought broadcasting
   g. Delusional perceptions
   h. All other experiences involving volition made affects, and made impulses
2. Second-rank symptoms
   a. Other disorders of perception
   b. Sudden delusional ideas
   c. Perplexity
   d. Depressive and euphoric mood changes
   e. Feelings of emotional impoverishment
   f. "... and several others as well"

EPIDEMIOLOGY

In the United States, the lifetime prevalence of schizophrenia is about 1 percent, which means that about 1 person in 100 will develop schizophrenia during their lifetime. The Epidemiologic Catchment Area study sponsored by the National Institute of Mental Health reported a lifetime prevalence of 0.6 to 1.9 percent. According to DSM-IV-TR, the annual incidence of schizophrenia ranges from 0.5 to 5.0 per 10,000, with some geographic variation (e.g., the incidence is higher for persons born in urban areas of industrialized nations). Schizophrenia is found in all societies and geographical areas, and incidence and prevalence rates are roughly equal worldwide. In the United States, about 0.05 percent of the total population is treated for schizophrenia in any single year, and only about half of all patients with schizophrenia obtain treatment, despite the severity of the disorder.

Gender and Age

Schizophrenia is equally prevalent in men and women. The two genders differ, however, in the onset and course of illness. Onset is earlier in men than in women. More than half of all male schizophrenia patients, but only one-third of all female schizophrenia patients, are first admitted to a psychiatric hospital before age 25. The peak ages of onset are 10 to 25 years for men and 25 to 35 years for women. Unlike men, women display a bimodal age distribution, with a second peak occurring in middle age. Approximately 3 to 10 percent of women with schizophrenia present with disease onset after age 40. About 90 percent of patients in treatment for schizophrenia are between 15 and 55 years old. Onset of schizophrenia before age 10 or after age 60 is extremely rare. Some studies have indicated that men are more likely to be impaired by negative symptoms (described below) than are women and that women are more likely to have better social functioning than are men prior to disease onset. In general, the outcome for female schizophrenia patients is better than that for male schizophrenia patients. When onset occurs after age 45, the disorder is characterized as late-onset schizophrenia.

Reproductive Factors

The use of psychopharmacological drugs, the open-door policies in hospitals, the deinstitutionalization in state hospitals, and the emphasis on rehabilitation and community-based care for patients have all led to an increase in the marriage and fertility rates among persons with schizophrenia. Because of these factors, the number of children born to parents with schizophrenia is continually increasing. The fertility rate for persons with schizophrenia is close to that for the general population. First-degree biological relatives of persons with schizophrenia have a ten times greater risk for developing the disease than the general population.

Medical Illness

Persons with schizophrenia have a higher mortality rate from accidents and natural causes than the general population. Institution- or treatment-related variables do not explain the increased mortality rate, but the higher rate may be related to the fact that the diagnosis and treatment of medical and surgical conditions in schizophrenia patients can be clinical challenges. Several studies have shown that up to 80 percent of all schizophrenia patients have significant concurrent medical illnesses and that up to 50 percent of these conditions may be undiagnosed.

Infection and Birth Season

Persons who develop schizophrenia are more likely to have been born in the winter and early spring and less likely to have been born in late spring and summer. In the Northern Hemisphere, including the United States, persons with schizophrenia are more often born in the months from January to April. In the Southern Hemisphere, persons with schizophrenia are more often born in the months from July to September. Season-specific risk factors, such as a virus or a seasonal change in diet, may be operative. Another hypothesis is that persons with a genetic predisposition for schizophrenia have a decreased biological advantage to survive season-specific insults.

Studies have pointed to gestational and birth complications, exposure to influenza epidemics, or maternal starvation during pregnancy, Rhesus factor incompatibility, and an excess of winter births in the etiology of schizophrenia. The nature of these factors suggests a neurodevelopmental pathological process in schizophrenia, but the exact pathophysiological mechanism associated with these risk factors is not known.

Evidence that prenatal malnutrition may play a role in schizophrenia was derived from the studies of the Dutch Hunger Winter of 1944 to 1945. Severe caloric restriction in the western Netherlands was associated with substantially decreased fertility, increased mortality, and diminished birth weight. Unlike most other famines, it was time limited, and the extent and timing of caloric restriction and psychiatric outcomes were well documented. Exposure to the peak of the famine during the periconceptional period was associated with a significant, twofold increased risk of schizophrenia. In a subsequent study, this cohort exposed to famine in early gestation also showed an increase in risk of schizoid personality disorders.

Epidemiological data show a high incidence of schizophrenia after prenatal exposure to influenza during several epidemics of the disease. Some studies show that the frequency of schizophrenia is increased following exposure to influenza—which occurs in the winter—during the second trimester of pregnancy. Other data supporting a viral hypothesis are an increased number of physical anomalies at birth, an increased rate of pregnancy and birth complications, seasonality of birth consistent with viral infection, geographical clusters of adult cases, and seasonality of hospitalizations.

Viral theories stem from the fact that several specific viral theories have the power to explain the particular localization of pathology necessary to account for a range of manifestations in schizophrenia without overt febrile encephalitis. There are six hypothetical models of viral and immune pathophysiology relevant to schizophrenia (Table 13–2).

Substance Abuse

Substance abuse is common in schizophrenia. The lifetime prevalence of any drug abuse (other than tobacco) is often greater than 50 percent. For all drugs of abuse (other than tobacco), abuse is associated with poorer function. In one population-based study, the lifetime prevalence of alcohol within schizophrenia was 40 percent. Alcohol abuse increases risk of hospitalization and, in some patients, may increase psychotic symptoms. People with schizophrenia have an increased prevalence of abuse of common street drugs. There has been particular interest in the association between cannabis and schizophrenia. Those reporting high levels of cannabis use (more than 50 occasions) were at sixfold increased risk of schizophrenia compared to nonusers. The use of amphetamines, cocaine, and similar drugs should raise particular concern because of their marked ability to increase psychotic symptoms.

Nicotine. Up to 90 percent of schizophrenic patients may be dependent on nicotine. Apart from smoking-associated mortality, nicotine decreases the blood concentrations of some antipsychotics. There are suggestions that the increased prevalence in smoking is due, at least in part, to brain abnormalities in nicotinic receptors. A specific polymorphism in a nicotinic receptor has been linked to genetic risk for schizophrenia. Nicotine administration appears to improve some cognitive impairments and Parkinsonism in schizophrenia, possibly because of nicotine-dependent activation of dopamine neurons. Recent studies have also demonstrated that nicotine may decrease positive symptoms such as hallucinations in schizophrenia patients by its effect on nicotine receptors in the brain that reduce the perception of outside stimuli, especially noise. In that sense, smoking is a form of self-medication.

Population Density

The prevalence of schizophrenia has been correlated with local population density in cities with populations of more than 1 million people. The correlation is weaker in cities of 100,000 to 500,000 people and is absent in cities with fewer than 10,000 people. The effect of population density is consistent with the

Table 13–2
Models of Viral and Immune Causes of Schizophrenia

Retroviral infection	Altered expression of the host's own genes and the genes of the host's offspring toward the development of schizophrenia (the virogene hypothesis).
Current or active viral infection	Viruses with an affinity for the central nervous system can cause sustained alterations in the functioning and can infect the brain, with substantive disease manifestations only showing up many years later. The past viral infection hypothesis posits a virus infecting certain brain tissues early in life to create a vulnerability to schizophrenia or as a causal mechanism for the initial illness processes that later lead to the picture of classical schizophrenia.
Virus-activated immunopathology	In theory, viral reactivation might result in an induction of schizophrenic psychopathology. Alternatively, a virus may induce the host to fail to recognize its own tissues as "self" and, as a consequence, to mount a destructive immune response.
Autoimmune pathology	Schizophrenia has been hypothesized to be an idiopathic autoimmune disease, such as rheumatoid arthritis or systemic lupus erythematosus, wherein, for reasons not entirely clear but probably involving genetics, some tissues are not recognized as self and become the target of immune response.
Maternal infection	Exposure to influenza epidemics during the second trimester of pregnancy are more likely to give birth to offspring at increased risk for schizophrenia. Prenatal rubella infection may increase the risk for development of schizophrenia and other nonaffective psychotic disorders.

observation that the incidence of schizophrenia in children of either one or two parents with schizophrenia is twice as high in cities as in rural communities. These observations suggest that social stressors in urban settings may affect the development of schizophrenia in persons at risk.

Socioeconomic and Cultural Factors

Economics. Because schizophrenia begins early in life, causes significant and long-lasting impairments, makes heavy demands for hospital care, and requires ongoing clinical care, rehabilitation, and support services, the financial cost of the illness in the United States is estimated to exceed that of all cancers combined. The locus of care has shifted dramatically since the mid-1950s from long-term hospital-based care to acute hospital care and community-based services. In 1955, approximately 500,000 hospital beds in the United States were occupied by the mentally ill—the majority of those with a diagnosis of schizophrenia. The figure is now less than 250,000 hospital beds. Deinstitutionalization has dramatically reduced the number of beds in custodial facilities, but an overall evaluation of its consequences is disheartening. Many patients have simply been transferred to alternative forms of custodial care (in contrast to treatment or rehabilitative services), including nursing home care and poorly supervised shelter arrangements. Patients with a diagnosis of schizophrenia are reported to account for 15 to 45 percent of homeless Americans.

Hospitalization. As mentioned previously, the development of effective antipsychotic drugs and changes in political and popular attitudes toward the treatment and the rights of persons who are mentally ill have dramatically changed the patterns of hospitalization for schizophrenia patients since the mid-1950s. Even with antipsychotic medication, however, the probability of readmission within 2 years after discharge from the first hospitalization is about 40 to 60 percent. Patients with schizophrenia occupy about 50 percent of all mental hospital beds and account for about 16 percent of all psychiatric patients who receive any treatment.

ETIOLOGY

Genetic Factors

There is a genetic contribution to some, perhaps all, forms of schizophrenia, and a high proportion of the variance in liability to schizophrenia is due to additive genetic effects. For example, schizophrenia and schizophrenia-related disorders (e.g., schizotypal, schizoid, and paranoid personality disorders) occur at an increased rate among the biological relatives of patients with schizophrenia. The likelihood of a person having schizophrenia is correlated with the closeness of the relationship to an affected relative (e.g., first- or second-degree relative) (Table 13–3). In the case of monozygotic twins who have identical genetic endowment, there is an approximately 50 percent concordance rate for schizophrenia. This rate is four to five times the concordance rate in dizygotic twins or the rate of occurrence found in other first-degree relatives (i.e., siblings, parents, or offspring). The role of genetic factors is further reflected in the drop-off in the occurrence of schizophrenia among second- and third-degree relatives, in whom one would hypothesize a decreased genetic loading. The finding of a higher rate of schizophrenia among the biological relatives of an adopted-away person who develops

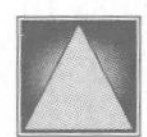

Table 13–3
Prevalence of Schizophrenia in Specific Populations

Population	Prevalence (%)
General population	1
Non-twin sibling of a schizophrenia patient	8
Child with one parent with schizophrenia	12
Dizygotic twin of a schizophrenia patient	12
Child of two parents with schizophrenia	40
Monozygotic twin of a schizophrenia patient	47

schizophrenia, as compared to the adoptive, nonbiological relatives who rear the patient, provides further support to the genetic contribution in the etiology of schizophrenia. Nevertheless, the monozygotic twin data clearly demonstrate the fact that individuals who are genetically vulnerable to schizophrenia do not inevitably develop schizophrenia; other factors (e.g., environment) must be involved in determining a schizophrenia outcome. If a vulnerability-liability model of schizophrenia is correct in its postulation of an environmental influence, then other biological or psychosocial environment factors may prevent or cause schizophrenia in the genetically vulnerable individual.

There is robust data indicating that the age of the father has a direct correlation with the development of schizophrenia. In studies of schizophrenic patients with no history of illness in either the maternal or paternal line, it was found that those born from fathers older than the age of 60 were vulnerable to developing the disorder. Presumably, spermatogenesis in older men is subject to greater epigenetic damage than in younger men.

The modes of genetic transmission in schizophrenia are unknown, but several genes appear to make a contribution to schizophrenia vulnerability. Linkage and association genetic studies have provided strong evidence for nine linkage sites: 1q, 5q, 6p, 6q, 8p, 10p, 13q, 15q, and 22q. Further analyses of these chromosomal sites have led to the identification of specific candidate genes, and the best current candidates are alpha-7 nicotinic receptor, *DISC 1*, *GRM 3*, *COMT*, *NRG 1*, *RGS 4*, and *G 72*. Recently, mutations of the genes dystrobrevin (DTNBP1) and neureglin 1 have been found to be associated with negative features of schizophrenia.

Biochemical Factors

Dopamine Hypothesis. The simplest formulation of the dopamine hypothesis of schizophrenia posits that schizophrenia results from too much dopaminergic activity. The theory evolved from two observations. First, the efficacy and the potency of many antipsychotic drugs (i.e., the dopamine receptor antagonists [DRAs]) are correlated with their ability to act as antagonists of the dopamine type 2 (D_2) receptor. Second, drugs that increase dopaminergic activity, notably cocaine and amphetamine, are psychotomimetic. The basic theory does not elaborate on whether the dopaminergic hyperactivity is due to too much release of dopamine, too many dopamine receptors, hypersensitivity of the dopamine receptors to dopamine, or a combination of these mechanisms. Which dopamine tracts in the brain are involved is also not specified in the theory, although the mesocortical and mesolimbic tracts are most often implicated. The dopaminergic neurons in these tracts project from their cell bodies in the midbrain to dopaminoceptive neurons in the limbic system and the cerebral cortex.

Excessive dopamine release in patients with schizophrenia has been linked to the severity of positive psychotic symptoms. Position emission tomography studies of dopamine receptors document an increase in D_2 receptors in the caudate nucleus of drug-free patients with schizophrenia. There have also been reports of increased dopamine concentration in the amygdala, decreased density of the dopamine transporter, and increased numbers of dopamine type 4 receptors in the entorhinal cortex.

Serotonin. Current hypotheses posit serotonin excess as a cause of both positive and negative symptoms in schizophrenia. The robust serotonin antagonist activity of clozapine and other second-generation antipsychotics, coupled with the effectiveness of clozapine to decrease positive symptoms in chronic patients has contributed to the validity of this proposition.

Norepinephrine. Anhedonia—the impaired capacity for emotional gratification and the decreased ability to experience pleasure—has long been noted to be a prominent feature of schizophrenia. A selective neuronal degeneration within the norepinephrine reward neural system could account for this aspect of schizophrenic symptomatology. However, biochemical and pharmacological data bearing on this proposal are inconclusive.

GABA. The inhibitory amino acid neurotransmitter γ-aminobutyric acid (GABA) has been implicated in the pathophysiology of schizophrenia based on the finding that some patients with schizophrenia have a loss of GABAergic neurons in the hippocampus. GABA has a regulatory effect on dopamine activity, and the loss of inhibitory GABAergic neurons could lead to the hyperactivity of dopaminergic neurons.

Neuropeptides. Neuropeptides, such as substance P and neurotensin, are localized with the catecholamine and indolamine neurotransmitters and influence the action of these neurotransmitters. Alteration in neuropeptide mechanisms could facilitate, inhibit, or otherwise alter the pattern of firing these neuronal systems.

Glutamate. Glutamate has been implicated because ingestion of phencyclidine, a glutamate antagonist, produces an acute syndrome similar to schizophrenia. The hypotheses proposed about glutamate include those of hyperactivity, hypoactivity, and glutamate-induced neurotoxicity.

Acetylcholine and Nicotine. Postmortem studies in schizophrenia have demonstrated decreased muscarinic and nicotinic receptors in the caudate-putamen, hippocampus, and selected regions of the prefrontal cortex. These receptors play a role in the regulation of neurotransmitter systems involved in cognition, which is impaired in schizophrenia.

Neuropathology

In the 19th century, neuropathologists failed to find a neuropathological basis for schizophrenia, and thus they classified schizophrenia as a functional disorder. By the end of the 20th century, however, researchers had made significant strides in revealing a potential neuropathological basis for schizophrenia, primarily in the limbic system and the basal ganglia, including neuropathological or neurochemical abnormalities in the cerebral cortex, the thalamus, and the brainstem. The loss of brain volume widely reported in schizophrenic brains appears to result from reduced density of the axons, dendrites, and synapses that mediate associative functions of the brain. Synaptic density is highest at age 1, then is pared down to adult values in early adolescence. One theory, based in part on the observation that patients often develop schizophrenic symptoms during adolescence, holds that schizophrenia results from excessive pruning of synapses during this phase of development.

Cerebral Ventricles. Computed tomography (CT) scans of patients with schizophrenia have consistently shown lateral and third ventricular enlargement and some reduction in cortical volume. Reduced volumes of cortical gray matter have been demonstrated during the earliest stages of the disease. Several investigators have attempted to determine whether the abnormalities detected by CT are progressive or static. Some studies have concluded that the lesions observed on CT scan are present at the onset of the illness and do not progress. Other studies, however, have concluded that the pathological process visualized on CT scan continues to progress during the illness. Thus, whether an active pathological process is continuing to evolve in schizophrenia patients is still uncertain.

Reduced Symmetry. There is a reduced symmetry in several brain areas in schizophrenia, including the temporal, frontal, and occipital lobes. This reduced symmetry is believed by some investigators to originate during fetal life and to be indicative of a disruption in brain lateralization during neurodevelopment.

Limbic System. Because of its role in controlling emotions, the limbic system has been hypothesized to be involved in the pathophysiology of schizophrenia. Studies of postmortem brain samples from schizophrenic patients have shown a decrease in the size of the region including the amygdala, the hippocampus, and the parahippocampal gyrus. This neuropathological finding agrees with the observation made by magnetic resonance imaging studies of patients with schizophrenia. The hippocampus is not only smaller in size in schizophrenia, but is also functionally abnormal as indicated by disturbances in glutamate transmission. Disorganization of the neurons within the hippocampus of schizophrenia patients has also been reported (Fig. 13–3).

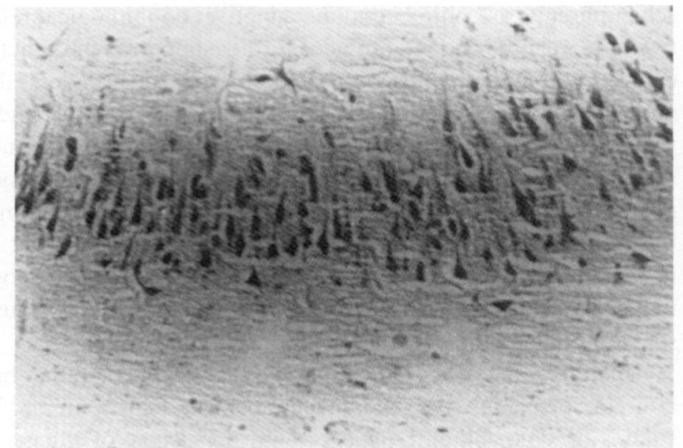

A

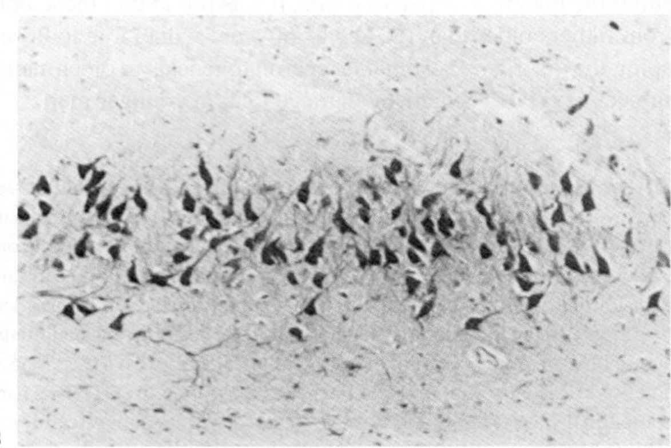

B

FIGURE 13–3

Comparison of cell orientation patterns of hippacampal pyramids at the CA1 to CA2 interface between nonschizophrenic control subjects **(top)** and schizophrenia patients **(bottom).** Cresolecht violet stain, original magnification ×250. Positives were overexposed to enhance contrast. (Reprinted with permission from Conrad AI, Abebe T, Austin R, Forsethe S, Scheibel AB. Hippocampal pyramidal cell disarray in schizophrenia as a bilateral phenomenon. *Arch Gen Psychiatric.* 1991;48:415.)

Prefrontal Cortex. There is considerable evidence from postmortem brain studies that supports anatomical abnormalities in the prefrontal cortex in schizophrenia. Functional deficits in the prefrontal brain imaging region have also been demonstrated. It has long been noted that several symptoms of schizophrenia mimic those found in persons with prefrontal lobotomies or *frontal lobe syndromes*.

Thalamus. Some studies of the thalamus show evidence of volume shrinkage or neuronal loss, in particular subnuclei. The medial dorsal nucleus of the thalamus, which has reciprocal connections with the prefrontal cortex, has been reported to contain a reduced number of neurons. The total number of neurons, oligodendrocytes, and astrocytes is reduced by 30 to 45 percent in schizophrenic patients. This putative finding does not appear to be due to the effects of antipsychotic drugs because the volume of the thalamus is similar in size between schizophrenics treated chronically with medication and neuroleptic-naive subjects.

Basal Ganglia and Cerebellum. The basal ganglia and cerebellum have been of theoretical interest in schizophrenia for at least two reasons. First, many patients with schizophrenia show odd movements, even in the absence of medication-induced movement disorders (e.g., tardive dyskinesia). The odd movements can include an awkward gait, facial grimacing, and stereotypies. Because the basal ganglia and cerebellum are involved in the control of movement, disease in these areas is implicated in the pathophysiology of schizophrenia. Second, the movement disorders involving the basal ganglia (e.g., Huntington's disease, Parkinson's disease) are the ones most commonly associated with psychosis. Neuropathological studies of the basal ganglia have produced variable and inconclusive reports about cell loss or the reduction of volume of the globus pallidus and the substantia nigra. Studies have also shown an increase in the number of D_2 receptors in the caudate, the putamen, and the nucleus accumbens. The question remains, however, whether the increase is secondary to the patient having received antipsychotic medications. Some investigators have begun to study the serotonergic system in the basal ganglia; a role for serotonin in psychotic disorder is suggested by the clinical usefulness of antipsychotic drugs that are serotonin antagonists (e.g., clozapine, risperidone).

Neural Circuits

There has been a gradual evolution from conceptualizing schizophrenia as a disorder that involves discrete areas of the brain to a perspective that views schizophrenia as a disorder of brain neural circuits. For example, as mentioned previously, the basal ganglia and cerebellum are reciprocally connected to the frontal lobes, and the abnormalities in frontal lobe function seen in some brain imaging studies may be due to disease in either area rather than in the frontal lobes themselves. It is also hypothesized that an early developmental lesion of the dopaminergic tracts to the prefrontal cortex results in the disturbance of prefrontal and limbic system function, and leads to the positive and negative symptoms and cognitive impairments observed in patients with schizophrenia.

Of particular interest in the context of neural circuit hypotheses linking the prefrontal cortex and limbic system are studies demonstrating a relationship between hippocampal morphological abnormalities and disturbances in prefrontal cortex metabolism or function, or both. Data from functional and structural imaging studies in humans suggest that dysfunction of the anterior cingulate basal ganglia thalamocortical circuit underlies the production of positive psychotic symptoms, whereas dysfunction of the dorsolateral prefrontal circuit underlies the production of primary, enduring, negative or deficit symptoms. There is a neural basis for cognitive functions that are impaired in patients with schizophrenia. The observation of the relationship among impaired working memory performance, disrupted prefrontal neuronal integrity, altered prefrontal, cingulate, and inferior parietal cortex, and altered hippocampal blood flow provides strong support for disruption of the normal working memory neural circuit in patients with schizophrenia. The involvement of this circuit, at least for auditory hallucinations, has been documented in a number of functional imaging studies that contrast hallucinating and nonhallucinating patients.

Brain Metabolism

Studies using magnetic resonance spectroscopy, a technique that measures the concentration of specific molecules in the brain, found that patients with schizophrenia had lower levels of phosphomonoester and inorganic phosphate and higher levels of phosphodiester than a control group. Furthermore, concentrations of N-acetyl aspartate, a marker of neurons, were lower in the hippocampus and frontal lobes of patients with schizophrenia.

Applied Electrophysiology

Electroencephalographic studies indicate that many schizophrenia patients have abnormal records, increased sensitivity to activation procedures (e.g., frequent spike activity after sleep deprivation), decreased alpha activity, increased theta and delta activity, possibly more epileptiform activity than usual, and possibly more left-sided abnormalities than usual. Schizophrenia patients also exhibit an inability to filter out irrelevant sounds and are extremely sensitive to background noise. The flooding of sound that results makes concentration difficult and may be a factor in the production of auditory hallucinations. This sound sensitivity may be associated with a genetic defect.

Complex Partial Epilepsy. Schizophrenia-like psychoses have been reported to occur more frequently than expected in patients with complex partial seizures, especially seizures involving the temporal lobes. Factors associated with the development of psychosis in these patients include a left-sided seizure focus, medial temporal location of the lesion, and early onset of seizures. The first-rank symptoms described by Schneider may be similar to symptoms of patients with complex partial epilepsy and may reflect the presence of a temporal lobe disorder when seen in patients with schizophrenia.

Evoked Potentials. A large number of abnormalities in evoked potential among patients with schizophrenia has been described. The P300 has been most studied and is defined as a large, positive evoked-potential wave that occurs about 300 milliseconds after a sensory stimulus is detected. The major source of the P300 wave may be located in the limbic system structures of the medial temporal lobes. In patients with schizophrenia, the P300 has been reported to be statistically smaller than that in comparison groups. Abnormalities in the P300 wave have also been reported to be more common in children who, because they have affected parents, are at high risk for schizophrenia. Whether the characteristics of the P300 represent a state or a trait phenomenon remains controversial. Other evoked potentials reported to be abnormal in patients with schizophrenia are the N100 and the contingent negative variation. The N100 is a negative wave that occurs about 100 milliseconds after a stimulus, and the contingent negative variation is a slowly developing, negative-voltage shift following the presentation of a sensory stimulus that is a warning for an upcoming stimulus. The evoked-potential data have been interpreted as indicating that although patients with schizophrenia are unusually sensitive to a sensory stimulus (larger early evoked potentials), they compensate for the increased sensitivity by blunting the processing of information at higher cortical levels (indicated by smaller late evoked potentials).

Eye Movement Dysfunction

The inability to follow a moving visual target accurately is the defining basis for the disorders of smooth visual pursuit and disinhibition of saccadic eye movements seen in patients with schizophrenia. Eye movement dysfunction may be a trait marker for schizophrenia; it is independent of drug treatment and clinical state and is also seen in first-degree relatives of probands with schizophrenia. Various studies have reported abnormal eye movements in 50 to 85 percent of patients with schizophrenia, compared with about 25 percent in psychiatric patients without schizophrenia and less than 10 percent in nonpsychiatrically ill control subjects.

Psychoneuroimmunology

Several immunological abnormalities have been associated with patients who have schizophrenia. The abnormalities include decreased T-cell interleukin-2 production, reduced number and responsiveness of peripheral lymphocytes, abnormal cellular and humoral reactivity to neurons, and the presence of brain-directed (antibrain) antibodies. The data can be interpreted variously as representing the effects of a neurotoxic virus or of an endogenous autoimmune disorder. Most carefully conducted investigations that have searched for evidence of neurotoxic viral infections in schizophrenia have had negative results, although epidemiological data show a high incidence of schizophrenia after prenatal exposure to influenza during several epidemics of the disease. Other data supporting a viral hypothesis are an increased number of physical anomalies at birth, an increased rate of pregnancy and birth complications, seasonality of birth consistent with viral infection, geographical clusters of adult cases, and seasonality of hospitalizations. Nonetheless, the inability to detect genetic evidence of viral infection reduces the significance of all circumstantial data. The possibility of autoimmune brain antibodies has some data to support it; the pathophysiological process, if it exists, however, probably explains only a subset of the population with schizophrenia.

Psychoneuroendocrinology

Many reports describe neuroendocrine differences between groups of patients with schizophrenia and groups of control subjects. For example, results of the dexamethasone-suppression test have been reported to be abnormal in various subgroups of patients with schizophrenia, although the practical or predictive value of the test in schizophrenia has been questioned. One carefully done report, however, has correlated persistent nonsuppression on the dexamethasone-suppression test in schizophrenia with a poor long-term outcome.

Some data suggest decreased concentrations of luteinizing hormone/follicle-stimulating hormone, perhaps correlated with age of onset and length of illness. Two additional reported abnormalities may be correlated with the presence of negative symptoms: a blunted release of prolactin and growth hormone on gonadotropin-releasing hormone or thyrotropin-releasing hormone stimulation, and a blunted release of growth hormone on apomorphine stimulation.

PSYCHOSOCIAL AND PSYCHOANALYTIC THEORIES

If schizophrenia is a disease of the brain, it is likely to parallel diseases of other organs (e.g., myocardial infarctions, diabetes) whose courses are affected by psychosocial stress. Thus, clinicians should consider both psychosocial and biological factors affecting schizophrenia.

The disorder affects individual patients, each of whom has a unique psychological makeup. Although many psychodynamic theories about the pathogenesis of schizophrenia seem outdated, perceptive clinical observations can help contemporary clinicians understand how the disease may affect a patient's psyche.

Psychoanalytic Theories

Sigmund Freud postulated that schizophrenia resulted from developmental fixations that occurred earlier than those culminating in the development of neuroses. These fixations produce defects in ego development and Freud postulated that such defects contributed to the symptoms of schizophrenia. Ego disintegration in schizophrenia represents a return to the time when the ego was not yet, or had just begun, to be established. Because the ego affects the interpretation of reality and the control of inner drives, such as sex and aggression, these ego functions are impaired. Thus, intrapsychic conflict arising from the early fixations and the ego defect, which may have resulted from poor early object relations, fuel the psychotic symptoms.

As described by Margaret Mahler, there are distortions in the reciprocal relationship between the infant and the mother. The child is unable to separate from, and progress beyond, the closeness and complete dependence that characterize the mother–child relationship in the oral phase of development. As a result, the person's identity never becomes secure.

Paul Federn hypothesized that the defect in ego functions permits intense hostility and aggression to distort the mother–infant relationship, which leads to eventual personality disorganization and vulnerability to stress. The onset of symptoms during adolescence occurs when teenagers need a strong ego to function independently, to separate from the parents, to identify tasks, to control increased internal drives, and to cope with intense external stimulation.

Harry Stack Sullivan viewed schizophrenia as a disturbance in interpersonal relatedness. The patient's massive anxiety creates a sense of unrelatedness that is transformed into parataxic distortions, which are usually, but not always, persecutory. To Sullivan, schizophrenia is an adaptive method used to avoid panic, terror, and disintegration of the sense of self. The source of pathological anxiety results from cumulative experiential traumas during development.

Psychoanalytic theory also postulates that the various symptoms of schizophrenia have symbolic meaning for individual patients. For example, fantasies of the world coming to an end may indicate a perception that a person's internal world has broken down. Feelings of inferiority are replaced by delusions of grandeur and omnipotence. Hallucinations may be substitutes for a patient's inability to deal with objective reality and may represent inner wishes or fears. Delusions, like hallucinations, are regressive, restitutive attempts to create a new reality or to express hidden fears or impulses (Fig. 13–4).

Regardless of the theoretical model, all psychodynamic approaches are founded on the premise that psychotic symptoms have meaning in schizophrenia. Patients, for example, may become grandiose after an injury to their self-esteem. Similarly, all theories recognize that human relatedness may be terrifying for persons with schizophrenia. Although research on the efficacy of psychotherapy with schizophrenia shows mixed results, concerned persons who offer compassion and a sanctuary in the confusing world of the schizophrenic must be a cornerstone of any overall treatment plan. Long-term follow-up studies show that some patients who bury psychotic episodes probably do not benefit from exploratory psychotherapy, but those who are able to integrate the psychotic experience into their lives may benefit from some insight-oriented approaches. There is renewed interest in the use of long-term individual

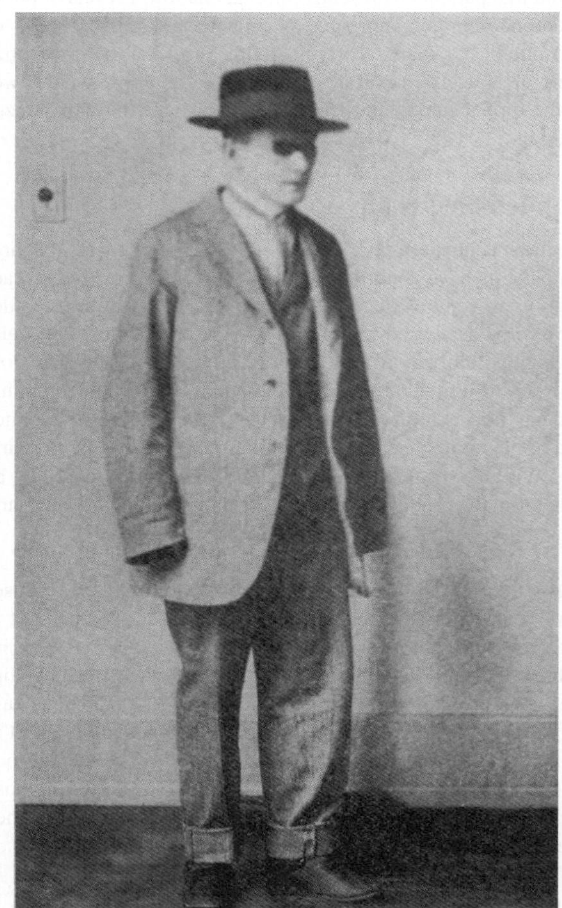

FIGURE 13–4
This patient wore suits too large for him in the delusional belief that he would appear taller to others. (Courtesy of Emil Kraepelin, M.D.)

psychotherapy in the treatment of schizophrenia, especially when combined with medication.

Learning Theories

According to learning theorists, children who later have schizophrenia learn irrational reactions and ways of thinking by imitating parents who have their own significant emotional problems. In learning theory, the poor interpersonal relationships of persons with schizophrenia develop because of poor models for learning during childhood.

Family Dynamics

In a study of British 4-year-old children, those who had a poor mother–child relationship had a sixfold increase in the risk of developing schizophrenia, and offspring from schizophrenic mothers who were adopted away at birth were more likely to develop the illness if they were reared in adverse circumstances compared to those raised in loving homes by stable adoptive parents. Nevertheless, no well-controlled evidence indicates that a specific family pattern plays a causative role in the development of schizophrenia. Some patients with schizophrenia do come from dysfunctional families, just as do many nonpsychiatrically ill persons. It is important, however, not to overlook pathological family behavior that can significantly increase the emotional stress with which a vulnerable patient with schizophrenia must cope.

Double Bind. The double-bind concept was formulated by Gregory Bateson and Donald Jackson to describe a hypothetical family in which children receive conflicting parental messages about their behavior, attitudes, and feelings. In Bateson's hypothesis, children withdraw into a psychotic state to escape the unsolvable confusion of the double bind. Unfortunately, the family studies that were conducted to validate the theory were seriously flawed methodologically. The theory has value only as a descriptive pattern, not as a causal explanation of schizophrenia. An example of a double bind is the parent who tells the child to provide cookies for his or her friends and then chastises the child for giving away too many cookies to playmates.

Schisms and Skewed Families. Theodore Lidz described two abnormal patterns of family behavior. In one family type, with a prominent schism between the parents, one parent is overly close to a child of the opposite gender. In the other family type, a skewed relationship between a child and one parent involves a power struggle between the parents and the resulting dominance of one parent. These dynamics stress the tenuous adaptive capacity of the schizophrenic person.

Pseudomutual and Pseudohostile Families. As described by Lyman Wynne, some families suppress emotional expression by consistently using pseudomutual or pseudohostile verbal communication. In such families, a unique verbal communication develops, and when a child leaves home and must relate to other persons, problems may arise. The child's verbal communication may be incomprehensible to outsiders.

Expressed Emotion. Parents or other caregivers may behave with overt criticism, hostility, and overinvolvement toward a person with schizophrenia. Many studies have indicated that in families with high levels of expressed emotion, the relapse rate for schizophrenia is high. The assessment of expressed emotion involves analyzing both what is said and the manner in which it is said.

DIAGNOSIS

The DSM-IV-TR diagnostic criteria include course specifiers (i.e., prognosis) that offer clinicians several options and describe actual clinical situations (Table 13–4). The presence of hallucinations or delusions is not necessary for a diagnosis of schizophrenia; a patient's disorder is diagnosed as schizophrenia

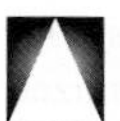

Table 13–4
DSM-IV-TR Diagnostic Criteria for Schizophrenia

A. Characteristic symptoms: Two (or more) of the following, each present for a significant portion of time during a 1-month period (or less if successfully treated):
   (1) delusions
   (2) hallucinations
   (3) disorganized speech (e.g., frequent derailment or incoherence)
   (4) grossly disorganized or catatonic behavior
   (5) negative symptoms, i.e., affective flattening, alogia, or avolition

Note: Only one Criterion A symptom is required if delusions are bizarre or hallucinations consist of a voice keeping up a running commentary on the person's behavior or thoughts, or two or more voices conversing with each other.

B. *Social/occupational dysfunction*: For a significant portion of the time since the onset of the disturbance, one or more major areas of functioning such as work, interpersonal relations, or self-care are markedly below the level achieved prior to the onset (or when the onset is in childhood or adolescence, failure to achieve expected level of interpersonal, academic, or occupational achievement).

C. *Duration*: Continuous signs of the disturbance persist for at least 6 months. This 6-month period must include at least 1 month of symptoms (or less if successfully treated) that meet Criterion A (i.e., active-phase symptoms) and may include periods of prodromal or residual symptoms. During these prodromal or residual periods, the signs of the disturbance may be manifested by only negative symptoms or two or more symptoms listed in Criterion A present in an attenuated form (e.g., odd beliefs, unusual perceptual experiences).

D. *Schizoaffective and mood disorder exclusion*: Schizoaffective disorder and mood disorder with psychotic features have been ruled out because either (1) no major depressive, manic, or mixed episodes have occurred concurrently with the active-phase symptoms; or (2) if mood episodes have occurred during active-phase symptoms, their total duration has been brief relative to the duration of the active and residual periods.

E. *Substance/general medical condition exclusion*: The disturbance is not due to the direct physiological effects of a substance (e.g., a drug of abuse, a medication) or a general medical condition.

F. *Relationship to a pervasive developmental disorder*: If there is a history of autistic disorder or another pervasive developmental disorder, the additional diagnosis of schizophrenia is made only if prominent delusions or hallucinations are also present for at least a month (or less if successfully treated).

Classification of longitudinal course (can be applied only after at least 1 year has elapsed since the initial onset of active-phase symptoms):

Episodic with interepisode residual symptoms (episodes are defined by the reemergence of prominent psychotic symptoms); also specify if: **with prominent negative symptoms**

Episodic with no interepisode residual symptoms

Continuous (prominent psychotic symptoms are present throughout the period of observation); also *specify* if: **with prominent negative symptoms**

Single episode in partial remission: also *specify* if: **with prominent negative symptoms**

Single episode in full remission

Other or unspecified pattern

(From American Psychiatric Association. *Diagnostic and Statistical Manual of Mental Disorders*. 4th ed. Text rev. Washington, DC: American Psychiatric Association; copyright 2000, with permission.)

when the patient exhibits two of the symptoms listed as symptoms 1 through 5 in Criterion A in Table 13–4 (e.g., disorganized speech). Criterion B requires that impaired functioning, although not deteriorations, be present during the active phase of the illness. Symptoms must persist for at least 6 months, and a diagnosis of schizoaffective disorder or mood disorder must be absent.

Subtypes

DSM-IV-TR classifies the subtypes of schizophrenia as paranoid, disorganized, catatonic, undifferentiated, and residual (Table 13–5), based predominantly on clinical presentation. These subtypes are not closely correlated with different prognoses; for such differentiation, specific predictors of prognosis are best consulted (Table 13–6). The 10th revision of the *International Statistical Classification of Diseases and Related Health Problems* (ICD-10), in contrast, uses nine subtypes: paranoid schizophrenia, hebephrenia, catatonic schizophrenia, undifferentiated schizophrenia, postschizophrenic depression, residual schizophrenia, simple schizophrenia, other schizophrenia, and schizophrenia, unspecified, with eight possibilities for classifying the course of the disorder, ranging from continuous to complete remission.

Table 13–5
DSM-IV-TR Diagnostic Criteria for Schizophrenia Subtypes

Paranoid type

A type of schizophrenia in which the following criteria are met:

A. Preoccupation with one or more delusions or frequent auditory hallucinations.

B. None of the following is prominent: disorganized speech, disorganized or catatonic behavior, or flat or inappropriate affect.

Disorganized type

A type of schizophrenia in which the following criteria are met:

A. All of the following are prominent:
   (1) disorganized speech
   (2) disorganized behavior
   (3) flat or inappropriate affect

B. The criteria are not met for catatonic type.

Catatonic type

A type of schizophrenia in which the clinical picture is dominated by at least two of the following:

(1) motoric immobility as evidenced by catalepsy (including waxy flexibility) or stupor

(2) excessive motor activity (that is apparently purposeless and not influenced by external stimuli)

(3) extreme negativism (an apparently motiveless resistance to all instructions or maintenance of a rigid posture against attempts to be moved) or mutism

(4) peculiarities of voluntary movement as evidenced by posturing (voluntary assumption of inappropriate or bizarre postures), stereotyped movements, prominent mannerisms, or prominent grimacing

(5) echolalia or echopraxia

Undifferentiated type

A type of schizophrenia in which symptoms that meet Criterion A are present, but the criteria are not met for the paranoid, disorganized, or catatonic type.

Residual type

A type of schizophrenia in which the following criteria are met:

A. Absence of prominent delusions, hallucinations, disorganized speech, and grossly disorganized or catatonic behavior.

B. There is continuing evidence of the disturbance, as indicated by the presence of negative symptoms or two or more symptoms listed in Criterion A for schizophrenia, present in an attenuated form (e.g., odd beliefs, unusual perceptual experiences).

(From American Psychiatric Association. *Diagnostic and Statistical Manual of Mental Disorders*. 4th ed. Text rev. Washington, DC: American Psychiatric Association; copyright 2000, with permission.)

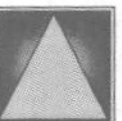

Table 13–6
Features Weighting Toward Good to Poor Prognosis in Schizophrenia

Good Prognosis	Poor Prognosis
Late onset	Young onset
Obvious precipitating factors	No precipitating factors
Acute onset	Insidious onset
Good premorbid social, sexual, and work histories	Poor premorbid social, sexual, and work histories
Mood disorder symptoms (especially depressive disorders)	Withdrawn, autistic behavior
Married	Single, divorced, or widowed
Family history of mood disorders	Family history of schizophrenia
Good support systems	Poor support systems
Positive symptoms	Negative symptoms
	Neurological signs and symptoms
	History of perinatal trauma
	No remissions in 3 years
	Many relapses
	History of assaultiveness

Paranoid Type. The paranoid type of schizophrenia is characterized by preoccupation with one or more delusions or frequent auditory hallucinations. Classically, the paranoid type of schizophrenia is characterized mainly by the presence of delusions of persecution or grandeur (Fig. 13–5). Patients with paranoid schizophrenia usually have their first episode of illness at an older age than do patients with catatonic or disorganized schizophrenia. Patients in whom schizophrenia occurs in the late 20s or 30s have usually established a social life that may help them through their illness, and the ego resources of paranoid patients tend to be greater than those of patients with catatonic and disorganized schizophrenia. Patients with the paranoid type of schizophrenia show less regression of their mental faculties, emotional responses, and behavior than do patients with other types of schizophrenia.

Patients with paranoid schizophrenia are typically tense, suspicious, guarded, reserved, and sometimes hostile or aggressive, but they can occasionally conduct themselves adequately in social situations. Their intelligence in areas not invaded by their psychosis tends to remain intact.

The following case illustrates ideas of reference and paranoid delusions. A married man, age 38, with a history of dependable, conscientious work as a bookkeeper, became sleepless, anxious, and unable to concentrate. He developed the belief that his vision was failing because of poisons secretly placed in his food by former neighbors. He found a misprint in a newspaper that he felt was placed there by the editor to shame him publicly. Admitted to the psychiatric

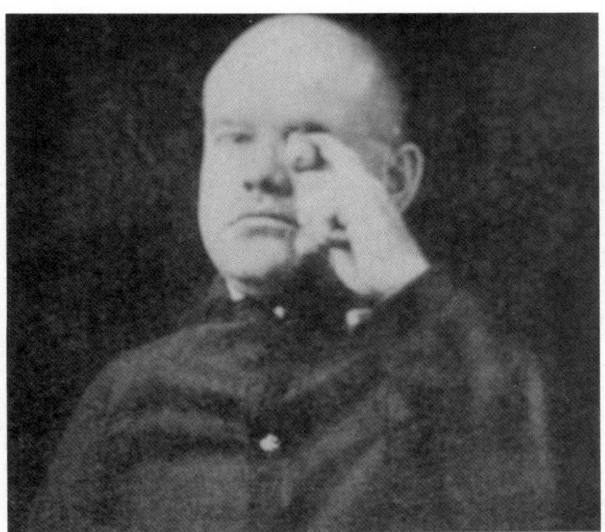

FIGURE 13–5
This patient had an artificial eye that he believed had special powers when removed from the socket. (Courtesy of Emil Kraepelin, M.D.)

service of a general hospital, he said that cars passing up and down the street contained agents who were spying on him. He believed that the electric light bulbs in his room were emanating a purifying radiation to counteract syphilitic germs, which he was supposedly breathing into the atmosphere, although a physical examination was negative for syphilis.

Disorganized Type. The disorganized (formerly called hebephrenic) type of schizophrenia is characterized by a marked regression to primitive, disinhibited, and unorganized behavior and by the absence of symptoms that meet the criteria for the catatonic type. The onset of this subtype is generally early, occurring before age 25. Disorganized patients are usually active but in an aimless, nonconstructive manner. Their thought disorder is pronounced, and their contact with reality is poor. Their personal appearance is disheveled, and their social behavior and their emotional responses are inappropriate. They often burst into laughter without any apparent reason. Incongruous grinning and grimacing are common in these patients, whose behavior is best described as silly or fatuous.

Patient AB, a 32-year-old woman, began to lose weight and became careless about her work, which deteriorated in quality and quantity. She believed that other women at her place of employment were circulating slanderous stories concerning her and complained that a young man employed in the same plant had put his arm around her and insulted her. Her family demanded that the charge be investigated, which showed not only that the charge was without foundation but also that the man in question had not spoken to her for months. One day she returned home from work, and as she entered the house, she laughed loudly, watched her sister-in-law suspiciously, refused to answer questions, and at the sight of her brother began to cry. She refused to go to the bathroom, saying that a man was looking in the windows at her. She ate no food, and the next day declared that her sisters were "bad women," that everyone was talking about her, and that someone had been having sexual relations with her, and although she could not see him, he was "always around."

The patient was admitted to a public psychiatric hospital. As she entered the admitting office, she laughed loudly and repeatedly screamed in a loud tone, "She cannot stay here; she's got to go home!" She grimaced and performed various stereotyped movements of her hands. When seen on the ward an hour later, she paid no attention to questions, although she talked to herself in a childish tone. She moved about constantly, walked on her toes in a dancing manner, pointed aimlessly about, and put out her tongue and sucked her lips in the manner of an infant. At times she moaned and cried like a child but shed no tears. As the months passed, she remained silly, childish, preoccupied, inaccessible, grimacing, gesturing, pointing at objects in a stereotyped way, and usually chattering to herself in a peculiar high-pitched voice, with little of what she said being understood. Her condition continued to deteriorate, she remained unkempt, and she presented a picture of extreme introversion and regression, with no interest either in the activities of the institution or in her relatives who visited her. (Adapted from case of Arthur P. Noyes, M.D., and Lawrence C. Kolb, M.D.)

Catatonic Type. The catatonic type of schizophrenia, which was common several decades ago, has become rare in Europe and North America. The classic feature of the catatonic type is a marked disturbance in motor function; this disturbance may involve stupor, negativism, rigidity, excitement, or posturing (Fig. 13–6). Sometimes, the patient shows rapid alteration between extremes of excitement and stupor. Associated features include stereotypies, mannerisms, and waxy flexibility. Mutism is particularly common. During catatonic excitement, patients need careful supervision to prevent them from hurting themselves or others. Medical care may be needed because of malnutrition, exhaustion, hyperpyrexia, or self-inflicted injury.

AC, age 32, was admitted to the hospital. On arrival, he was noted to be an asthenic, poorly nourished man with dilated pupils, hyperactive tendon reflexes, and a pulse rate of 120. He showed many mannerisms, laid down on the floor, pulled at his foot, made undirected violent striking movements, struck attendants, grimaced, assumed rigid and strange postures, refused to speak, and appeared to be having auditory hallucinations. When seen later in the day, he was found to be in a stuporous state. His face was without expression, he was mute and rigid, and he paid no attention to those about him or to their questions. His eyes were closed, and the lids could be separated only with effort. There was no response to pinpricks or other painful stimuli.

He gradually became accessible, and when asked concerning himself, he referred to his stuporous period as sleep and maintained that he had no recollection of any events occurring during it. He said, "I didn't know anything. Everything seemed to be dark as far as my mind is concerned. Then I began to see a little light, like the shape of a star. Then my head got through the star gradually. I saw more and more light until I saw everything in a perfect form a few days ago." He explained his mutism by saying that he had been afraid he would "say the wrong thing" and also that he "didn't know exactly what to talk about." From his obviously inadequate emotional response and his statement that he was "a scientist and an inventor of the most extraordinary genius of the twentieth century," it was plain that he was still far from well. (Adapted from case of Arthur P. Noyes, M.D., and Lawrence C. Kolb, M.D.)

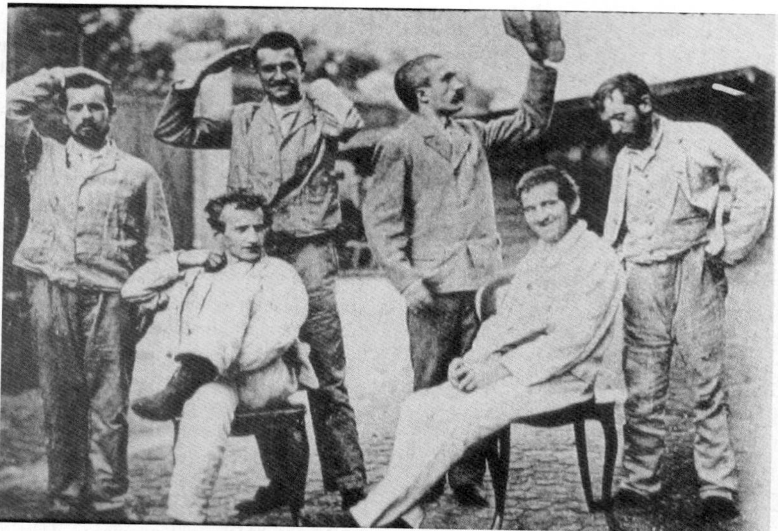

FIGURE 13–6
Photograph of a group of catatonic patients. This photograph appeared in the fifth edition of Emil Kraepelin's *Psychiatrie* (Leipzig Johann Ambrosius Barth, 1896).

Undifferentiated Type. Frequently, patients who are clearly schizophrenic cannot be easily fit into one type or another. DSM-IV-TR classifies these patients as having schizophrenia of the undifferentiated type.

A 15-year-old girl attended a summer camp, where she had difficulties getting along with the other children and developed animosity toward one of the counselors. On her return home, she refused to listen to her parents and said she heard the voice of a man talking to her, although she could not see him. She rapidly began to show bizarre behavior, characterized by grimacing, violent outbursts, and inability to take care of herself.

Her school record has always been good, and she was fluent in three languages. Her parents described her as having been a quiet, rather shut-in child with no abnormal traits in childhood. Family relations were reported as having been satisfactory.

On admission to a psychiatric hospital, the patient's speech was incoherent. She showed marked disturbances of formal thinking and blocking of thoughts. She was impulsive and appeared to be hallucinating. She stated that she heard voices in her right ear that a popular singer was running after her with a knife. She also thought that her father was intent on killing her. She thought that she was pregnant because she had hugged one of the residents.

She was often incontinent, and most of the time neglected her physical appearance. But occasionally she spent hours dressing herself, looking in the mirror, and putting on excessive makeup. At times, she was eating her feces. Occasionally, she adopted the roles of a singer or dancer. She made incoherent statements like: "Will I live forever? Nurse, I don't throw may love away. It is my stomach and it hurts." In the dining room, she attempted to grasp the genitals of male patients.

Two months of neuroleptic treatment brought no apparent improvement. She was given a course of electroconvulsive therapy (ECT). She remained in the hospital, where her behavior continued to be very distrubed.

Residual Type

According to DSM-IV-TR, the residual type of schizophrenia is characterized by continuing evidence of the schizophrenic disturbance in the absence of a complete set of active symptoms or of sufficient symptoms to meet the diagnosis of another type of schizophrenia. Emotional blunting, social withdrawal, eccentric behavior, illogical thinking, and mild loosening of associations commonly appear in the residual type. When delusions or hallucinations occur, they are neither prominent nor accompanied by strong affect (Fig. 13–7).

Other Subtypes

The subtyping of schizophrenia has had a long history; other subtyping schemes appear in the literature, especially literature from countries other than the United States.

***Bouffée Délirante* (Acute Delusional Psychosis).** This French diagnostic concept differs from a diagnosis of schizophrenia primarily on the basis of a symptom duration of less than 3 months. The diagnosis is similar to the DSM-IV-TR diagnosis of schizophreniform disorder. French clinicians report that about 40 percent of patients with a diagnosis of *bouffée délirante* progress in their illness and are eventually classified as having schizophrenia.

Latent. The concept of latent schizophrenia was developed during a time when theorists conceived of the disorder in broad diagnostic terms. Currently, patients must be very mentally ill to warrant a diagnosis of schizophrenia, but with a broad diagnostic concept of schizophrenia, the condition of patients who would not currently be thought of as severely ill could have received a diagnosis of schizophrenia. Latent schizophrenia, for example, was often the diagnosis used for what are now called borderline, schizoid, and schizotypal personality disorders. These patients

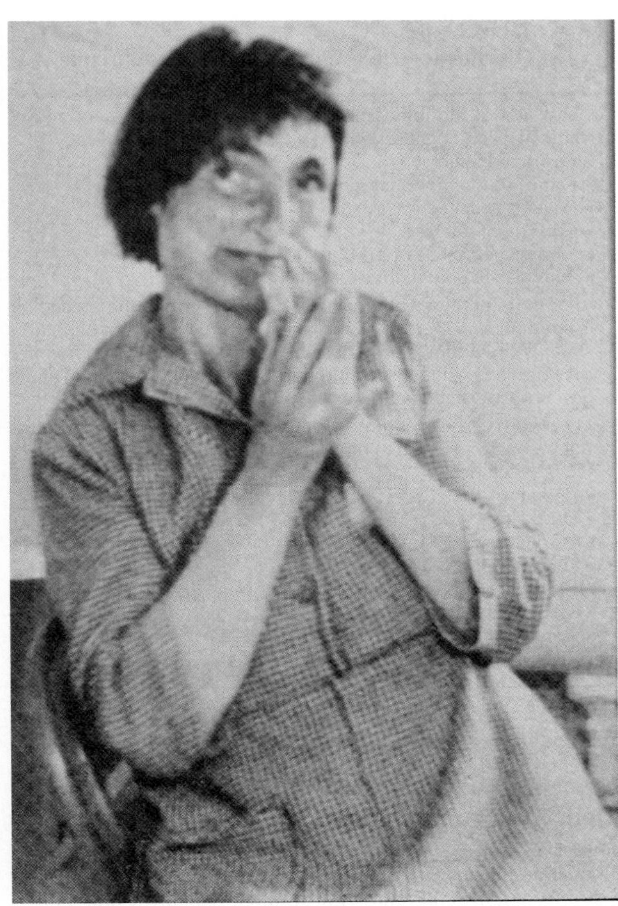

FIGURE 13–7
A 44-years-old chronic schizophrenic woman showing characteristic mannerism and facial grimacing. (Courtesy of New York Academy of Medicine.)

may occasionally show peculiar behaviors or thought disorders but do not consistently manifest psychotic symptoms. In the past, the syndrome was also termed borderline schizophrenia.

Oneiroid. The oneiroid state refers to a dream-like state in which patients may be deeply perplexed and not fully oriented in time and place. The term oneiroid schizophrenic has been used for patients who are engaged in their hallucinatory experiences to the exclusion of involvement in the real world. When an oneiroid state is present, clinicians should be particularly careful to examine patients for medical or neurological causes of the symptoms.

After a 20-year-old female college student had recovered from her schizophrenic breakdown, she wrote the following description of her experiences during the oneiroid phase:

This is how I remember it. The road has changed. It is twisted and it used to be straight. Nothing is constant—all is in motion. The trees are moving. They do not remain at rest. How is it my mother does not bump into the trees that are moving? I follow my mother. I am afraid, but I follow. I have to share my strange thoughts with someone. We are sitting on a bench. The bench seems low. It, too, has moved. "The bench is low," I say, "Yes," says my mother. "This isn't how it used to be. How come there are no people around? There are usually lots of people and it is Sunday and there are no people. This is strange." All these strange questions irritate my mother who then says she must be going soon. While I continue thinking I'm in a kind of nowhere...

There are no days; no nights; sometimes it is darker than other times—that's all. It is never quite black, just dark gray. There is no such thing as time—there is only eternity. There is no such thing as death—nor heaven and hell—there is only a timeless—hateful—spaceless—worsening of things. You can never go forward; you must always regress into this horrific mess...

The outside was moving rather swiftly, everything seemed topsy-turvy—things were flying about. It was very strange. I wanted to get back to the quiet very badly but when I got back I couldn't remember where anything was (e.g., the bathroom)... (Courtesy of Heinz E. Lehmann, M.D.)

Paraphrenia. The term paraphrenia is sometimes used as a synonym for paranoid schizophrenia, or for either a progressively deteriorating course of illness or the presence of a well-systemized delusional system. The multiple meanings of the term render it ineffectual in communicating information.

Pseudoneurotic Schizophrenia. Occasionally, patients who initially have such symptoms as anxiety, phobias, obsessions, and compulsions later reveal symptoms of thought disorder and psychosis. These patients are characterized by symptoms of pananxiety, panphobia, panambivalence, and sometimes chaotic sexuality. Unlike persons with anxiety disorders, pseudoneurotic patients have free-floating anxiety that rarely subsides. In clinical descriptions, the patients seldom become overtly and severely psychotic. This condition is currently diagnosed in DSM-IV-TR as borderline personality disorder.

Simple Deteriorative Disorder (Simple Schizophrenia). Simple deteriorative disorder is characterized by a gradual, insidious loss of drive and ambition. Patients with the disorder are usually not overtly psychotic and do not experience persistent hallucinations or delusions. Their primary symptom is withdrawal from social and work-related situations. The syndrome must be differentiated from depression, a phobia, a dementia, or an exacerbation of personality traits. Clinicians should be sure that patients truly meet the diagnostic criteria for schizophrenia before making the diagnosis. Simple deteriorative disorder appears as a diagnostic category in an appendix of DSM-IV-TR (Table 13–7).

An unmarried man, 27 years old, was brought to the mental hospital because he had on several occasions become violent toward his father. For a few weeks, he had hallucinations and heard voices. The voices eventually ceased, but he then adopted a strange way of life. He would sit up all night, sleep all day, and become very angry when his father tried to get him out of bed. He did not shave or wash for weeks, smoked continuously, ate very irregularly, and drank enormous quantities of tea.

In the hospital, he adjusted rapidly to the new environment and was found to be generally cooperative. He showed no marked abnormalities of mental state or behavior, except for his lack of concern for just about anything. He kept to himself as much as possible and conversed little with patients or staff. His personal hygiene had to be supervised by the nursing staff; otherwise, he would quickly become dirty and untidy.

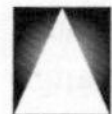

Table 13–7
DSM-IV-TR Research Criteria for Simple Deteriorative Disorder (Simple Schizophrenia)

A. Progressive development over a period of at least a year of all of the following:
  (1) marked decline in occupational or academic functioning
  (2) gradual appearance and deepening of negative symptoms such as affective flattening, alogia, and avolition
  (3) poor interpersonal rapport, social isolation, or social withdrawal
B. Criterion A for schizophrenia has never been met.
C. The symptoms are not better accounted for by schizotypal or schizoid personality disorder, a psychotic disorder, a mood disorder, an anxiety disorder, a dementia, or mental retardation and are not due to the direct physiological effects of a substance or a general medical condition.

(From American Psychiatric Association. *Diagnostic and Statistical Manual of Mental Disorders.* 4th ed. Text rev. Washington, DC: American Psychiatric Association; copyright 2000, with permission.)

Six years after his admission to the hospital, he is described as shiftless and careless, sullen and unreasonable. He lies on a couch all day long. Although many efforts have been made to get the patient to accept therapeutic work assignments, he refuses to consider any kind of regular occupation. In the summer, he wanders about the hospital grounds or lies under a tree. In the winter, he wanders through the tunnels connecting the various hospital buildings and is often seen stretched out for hours under the warm pipes that carry the steam through the tunnels. (Courtesy of Heinz E. Lehmann, M.D.)

Postpsychotic Depressive Disorder of Schizophrenia. Following an acute schizophrenia episode, some patients become depressed. The symptoms of postpsychotic depressive disorder of schizophrenia can closely resemble the symptoms of the residual phase of schizophrenia and the adverse effects of commonly used antipsychotic medications. The diagnosis should not be made if they are substance induced or part of a mood disorder due to a general medical condition. ICD-10 describes a category called postschizophrenia depression arising in the aftermath of a schizophrenic illness. These depressive states occur in up to 25 percent of patients with schizophrenia and are associated with an increased risk of suicide. (Further discussion of the disorder can be found in Section 15.3.)

Early-Onset Schizophrenia. A small minority of patients manifest schizophrenia in childhood. Such children may at first present diagnostic problems, particularly with differentiation from mental retardation and autistic disorder. Recent studies have established that the diagnosis of childhood schizophrenia may be based on the same symptoms used for adult schizophrenia. Its onset is usually insidious, its course tends to be chronic, and the prognosis is mostly unfavorable. (Chapter 51 contains further discussion of early-onset schizophrenia.)

Late-Onset Schizophrenia. Late-onset schizophrenia is clinically indistinguishable from schizophrenia but has an onset after age 45. This condition tends to appear more frequently in women and also tends to be characterized by a predominance of paranoid symptoms. The prognosis is favorable, and these patients usually do well on antipsychotic medication.

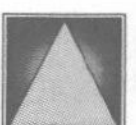

Table 13–8
Diagnostic Criteria for Deficit Schizophrenia

At least two of the following six features must be present and of clinically significant severity:
- Restricted affect
- Diminished emotional range
- Poverty of speech
- Curbing of interests
- Diminished sense of purpose
- Diminished social drive

Two or more of these features have been present for the preceding 12 months and were always present during periods of clinical stability (including chronic psychotic states). These symptoms may or may not be detectable during transient episodes of acute psychotic disorganization or decompensation.

Two or more of these enduring features are also idiopathic, that is, not secondary to factors other than the disease process. Such factors include
- Anxiety
- Drug effect
- Suspiciousness
- Formal thought disorder
- Hallucinations or delusions
- Mental retardation
- Depression

The patient meets DSM-IV-TR criteria for schizophrenia.

Deficit Schizophrenia. In the 1980s, criteria were promulgated for a subtype of schizophrenia characterized by enduring, idiopathic negative symptoms. These patients were said to exhibit the deficit syndrome. This group of patients is now said to have deficit schizophrenia (see the criteria for that putative disease diagnosis in Table 13–8). Patients with schizophrenia with positive symptoms are said to have nondeficit schizophrenia. The symptoms used to define deficit schizophrenia are strongly interrelated, although various combinations of the six negative symptoms in the criteria can be found.

Deficit patients have a more severe course of illness than nondeficit patients, with a higher prevalence of abnormal involuntary movements before administration of antipsychotic drugs and poorer social function before the onset of psychotic symptoms. The onset of the first psychotic episode is more often insidious, and these patients show less long-term recovery of function than do nondeficit patients. Deficit patients are also less likely to marry than are other patients with schizophrenia. However, despite their poorer level of function and greater social isolation, both of which should increase a patient's stress and, therefore, the risk of serious depression, deficit patients appear to have a decreased risk of major depression and probably have a decreased risk of suicide as well.

The risk factors of deficit patients differ from those of nondeficit patients; deficit schizophrenia is associated with an excess of summer births, whereas nondeficit patients have an excess of winter births. Deficit schizophrenia may also be associated with a greater familial risk of schizophrenia and of mild, deficit-like features in the nonpsychotic relatives of deficit probands. Within a family with multiply affected siblings, the deficit-nondeficit categorization tends to be uniform. The deficit group also has a higher prevalence of men.

The psychopathology of deficit patients impacts treatment; their lack of motivation, lack of distress, greater cognitive impairment, and asocial nature undermine the efficacy of psychosocial interventions, as well as their adherence to medication regimens. Their cognitive impairment, which is greater than that of nondeficit subjects, also contributes to this lack of efficacy.

PSYCHOLOGICAL TESTING. Patients with schizophrenia generally perform poorly on a wide range of neuropsychological tests. Vigilance, memory, and concept formation are most affected and consistent with pathological involvement in the frontotemporal cortex.

Objective measures of neuropsychological performance, such as the Halstead-Reitan battery and the Luria-Nebraska battery, often give abnormal findings, such as bilateral frontal and temporal lobe dysfunction, including impairments in attention, retention time, and problem-solving ability. Motor ability is also impaired, possibly related to brain asymmetry.

INTELLIGENCE TESTS. When groups of patients with schizophrenia are compared with groups of psychiatric patients without schizophrenia or with the general population, the schizophrenia patients tend to score lower on intelligence tests. Statistically, the evidence suggests that low intelligence is often present at the onset, and intelligence may continue to deteriorate with the progression of the disorder.

PROJECTIVE AND PERSONALITY TESTS. Projective tests, such as the Rorschach test and the Thematic Apperception Test, may indicate bizarre ideation. Personality inventories, such as the Minnesota Multiphasic Personality Inventory, often give abnormal results in schizophrenia, but the contribution to diagnosis and treatment planning is minimal.

CLINICAL FEATURES

A discussion of the clinical signs and symptoms of schizophrenia raises three key issues. First, no clinical sign or symptom is pathognomonic for schizophrenia; every sign or symptom seen in schizophrenia occurs in other psychiatric and neurological disorders. This observation is contrary to the often-heard clinical opinion that certain signs and symptoms are diagnostic of schizophrenia. Therefore, a patient's history is essential for the diagnosis of schizophrenia; clinicians cannot diagnose schizophrenia simply by results of a mental status examination, which may vary. Second, a patient's symptoms change with time. For example, a patient may have intermittent hallucinations and a varying ability to perform adequately in social situations, or significant symptoms of a mood disorder may come and go during the course of schizophrenia. Third, clinicians must take into account the patient's educational level, intellectual ability, and cultural and subcultural membership. An impaired ability to understand abstract concepts, for example, may reflect either the patient's education or his or her intelligence. Religious organizations and cults may have customs that seem strange to outsiders but are normal to those within the cultural setting.

Premorbid Signs and Symptoms

In theoretical formulations of the course of schizophrenia, premorbid signs and symptoms appear before the prodromal phase of the illness. The differentiation implies that premorbid signs and symptoms exist before the disease process evidences itself and that the prodromal signs and symptoms are parts of the evolving disorder. In the typical, but not invariable, premorbid history of schizophrenia, patients had schizoid or schizotypal personalities characterized as quiet, passive, and introverted; as children, they had few friends. Preschizophrenic adolescents may have no close friends and no dates and may avoid team sports. They may enjoy watching movies and television, listening to music, or playing computer games to the exclusion of social activities. Some adolescent patients may show a sudden onset of obsessive-compulsive behavior as part of the prodromal picture.

The validity of the prodromal signs and symptoms, almost invariably recognized after the diagnosis of schizophrenia has been made, is uncertain; once schizophrenia is diagnosed, the retrospective remembrance of early signs and symptoms is affected. Nevertheless, although the first hospitalization is often believed to mark the beginning of the disorder, signs and symptoms have often been present for months or even years. The signs may have started with complaints about somatic symptoms, such as headache, back and muscle pain, weakness, and digestive problems. The initial diagnosis may be malingering, chronic fatigue syndrome, or somatization disorder. Family and friends may eventually notice that the person has changed and is no longer functioning well in occupational, social, and personal activities. During this stage, a patient may begin to develop an interest in abstract ideas, philosophy, and the occult or religious questions (Fig. 13–8). Additional prodromal signs and symptoms

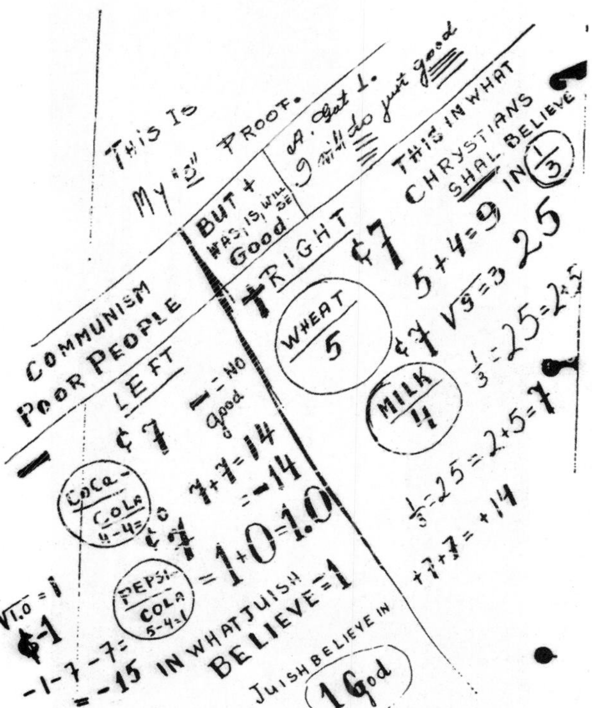

FIGURE 13–8

Schizophrenic patient schema. This illustrates his fragmented, abstract, and overly inclusive thinking and preoccupation with religious ideologies and mathematical proofs. (Courtesy of Heinz E. Lehmann.)

can include markedly peculiar behavior, abnormal affect, unusual speech, bizarre ideas, and strange perceptual experiences.

Mental Status Examination

General Description. The appearance of a patient with schizophrenia can range from that of a completely disheveled, screaming, agitated person to an obsessively groomed, completely silent, and immobile person. Between these two poles, patients may be talkative and may exhibit bizarre postures. Their behavior may become agitated or violent, apparently in an unprovoked manner, but usually in response to hallucinations. In contrast, in catatonic stupor, often referred to as catatonia, patients seem completely lifeless and may exhibit such signs as muteness, negativism, and automatic obedience. Waxy flexibility, once a common sign in catatonia, has become rare, as has manneristic behavior (Fig. 13–9). A person with a less extreme subtype of catatonia may show marked social withdrawal and egocentricity, lack of spontaneous speech or movement, and an absence of goal-directed behavior. Patients with catatonia may sit immobile and speechless in their chairs, respond to questions with only short answers, and move only when directed to move. Other obvious behavior may include odd clumsiness or stiffness in body movements, signs now seen as possibly indicating a disease process in the basal ganglia. Patients with schizophrenia are often poorly groomed, fail to bathe, and dress much too warmly for the prevailing temperatures. Other odd behaviors include tics, stereotypies, mannerisms, and, occasionally, echopraxia, in which patients imitate the posture or the behavior of the examiner.

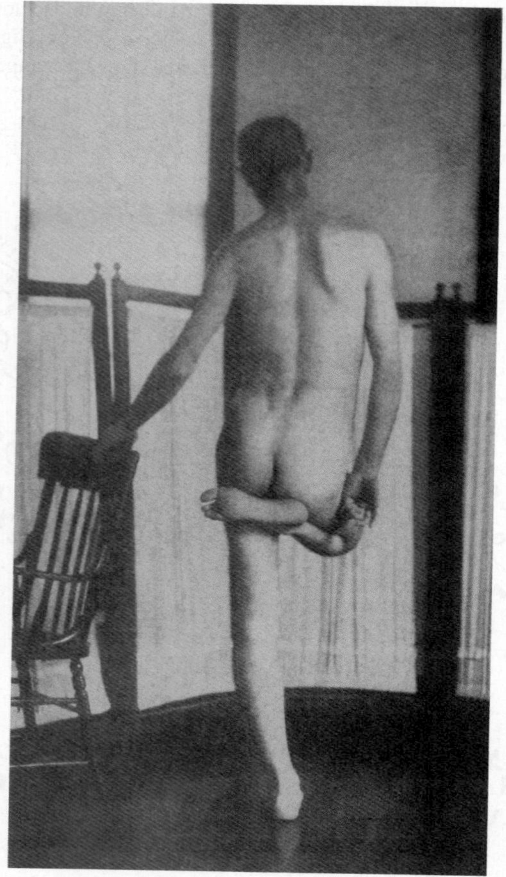

FIGURE 13–9
A chronic schizophrenic patient stands in a catatonic position. He maintained this uncomfortable position for hours. (Courtesy of Emil Kraepelin, M.D.)

PRECOX FEELING. Some experienced clinicians report a precox feeling, an intuitive experience of their inability to establish an emotional rapport with a patient. Although the experience is common, no data indicate that it is a valid or reliable criterion in the diagnosis of schizophrenia.

Mood, Feelings, and Affect

Two common affective symptoms in schizophrenia are reduced emotional responsiveness, sometimes severe enough to warrant the label of anhedonia, and overly active and inappropriate emotions such as extremes of rage, happiness, and anxiety. A flat or blunted affect can be a symptom of the illness itself, of the parkinsonian adverse effects of antipsychotic medications, or of depression, and differentiating these symptoms can be a clinical challenge. Overly emotional patients may describe exultant feelings of omnipotence, religious ecstasy, terror at the disintegration of their souls, or paralyzing anxiety about the destruction of the universe. Other feeling tones include perplexity, a sense of isolation, overwhelming ambivalence, and depression.

Perceptual Disturbances

HALLUCINATIONS. Any of the five senses may be affected by hallucinatory experiences in patients with schizophrenia. The most common hallucinations, however, are auditory, with voices that are often threatening, obscene, accusatory, or insulting. Two or more voices may converse among themselves, or a voice may comment on the patient's life or behavior. Visual hallucinations are common, but tactile, olfactory, and gustatory hallucinations are unusual; their presence should prompt the clinician to consider the possibility of an underlying medical or neurological disorder that is causing the entire syndrome (Fig. 13–10).

Cenesthetic Hallucinations. Cenesthetic hallucinations are unfounded sensations of altered states in bodily organs. Examples of cenesthetic hallucinations include a burning sensation in the brain, a pushing sensation in the blood vessels, and a cutting sensation in the bone marrow. Bodily distortions may also occur.

ILLUSIONS. As differentiated from hallucinations, illusions are distortions of real images or sensations, whereas hallucinations are not based on real images or sensations. Illusions can occur in schizophrenia patients during active phases, but they can also occur during the prodromal phases and during periods of remission. Whenever illusions or hallucinations occur, clinicians should consider the possibility of a substance-related cause for the symptoms, even when patients have already received a diagnosis of schizophrenia.

Thought. Disorders of thought are the most difficult symptoms for many clinicians and students to understand, but they may be the core symptoms of schizophrenia. Dividing the

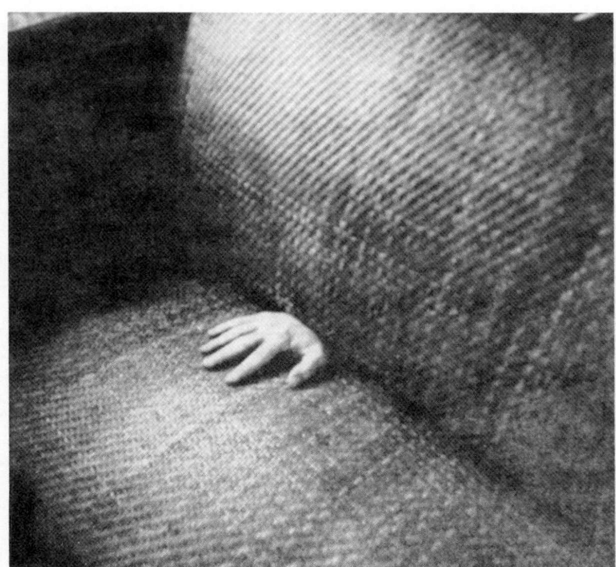

FIGURE 13–10
A symbolic representation of the strange perceptions of the schizophrenic patient. (Courtesy of Arther Tress.)

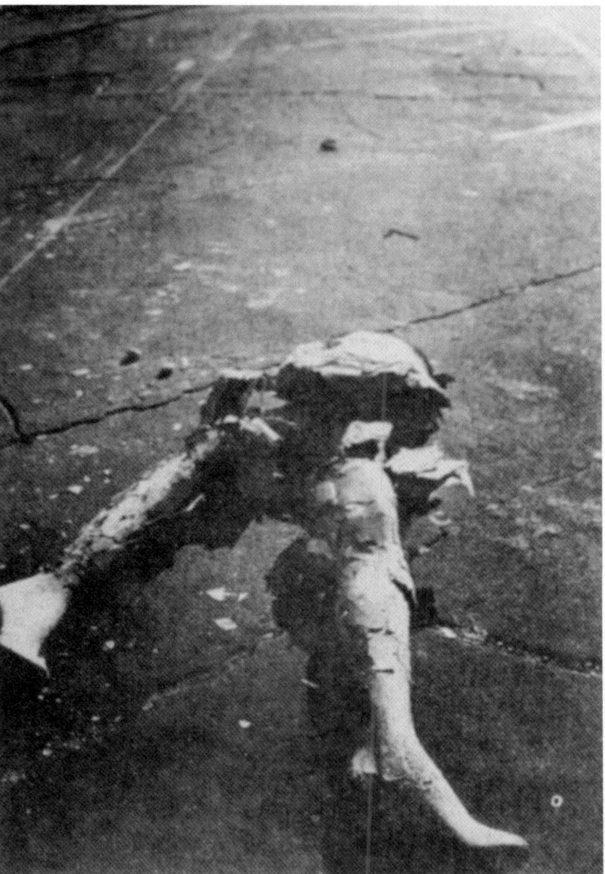

FIGURE 13–11
Patients often cannot separate the thought from the deed and fear that their angry impulses can kill others or themselves as symbolized in this photograph. (Courtesy of Arthur Tress.)

disorders of thought into disorders of thought content, form of thought, and thought process is one way to clarify them.

THOUGHT CONTENT. Disorders of thought content reflect the patient's ideas, beliefs, and interpretations of stimuli. Delusions, the most obvious example of a disorder of thought content, are varied in schizophrenia and may assume persecutory, grandiose, religious, or somatic forms.

Patients may believe that an outside entity controls their thoughts or behavior or, conversely, that they control outside events in an extraordinary fashion (such as causing the sun to rise and set or by preventing earthquakes [Fig. 13–11]). Patients may have an intense and consuming preoccupation with esoteric, abstract, symbolic, psychological, or philosophical ideas. Patients may also worry about allegedly life-threatening but bizarre and implausible somatic conditions, such as the presence of aliens inside the patient's testicles affecting his ability to father children.

The phrase *loss of ego boundaries* describes the lack of a clear sense of where the patient's own body, mind, and influence end and where those of other animate and inanimate objects begin. For example, patients may think that other persons, the television, or the newspapers are referring to them (*ideas of reference*). Other symptoms of the loss of ego boundaries include the sense that the patient has physically fused with an outside object (e.g., a tree or another person) or that the patient has disintegrated and fused with the entire universe (*cosmic identity*). With such a state of mind, some patients with schizophrenia doubt their gender or their sexual orientation. These symptoms should not be confused with transvestism, transsexuality, or other gender identity problems.

FORM OF THOUGHT. Disorders of the form of thought are objectively observable in patients' spoken and written language (Fig. 13–12). The disorders include looseness of associations, derailment, incoherence, tangentiality, circumstantiality, neologisms, echolalia, verbigeration, word salad, and mutism. Although looseness of associations was once described as pathognomonic for schizophrenia, the symptom is frequently seen in mania. Distinguishing between looseness of associations and tangentiality can be difficult for even the most experienced clinicians.

The following sample is taken from a memo typed by a schizophrenic secretary who was still able to work part time in an office. Note her preoccupation with the mind, the Trinity, and other esoteric matters. Also note that peculiar restructuring of concepts by hyphenating the words germ-any (the patient had a distinct fear of germs) and infer-no (inferring that there will be no salvation). The "chain reaction" is a reference to atomic piles.

> Mental health is the Blessed Trinity, and as man cannot be without God, it is futile to deny His Son. For the Creation understand germ-any in Voice New Order, not lie of chained reaction, spawning mark in temple Cain with Babel grave'n image to wanton V day "Israel."
>
> Lucifer fell Jew prostitute and lambeth walks by roam to sex ritual, in Bible six million of the Babylon woman, infer-no Salvation.

The one common factor in the thought process above is a preoccupation with invisible forces, radiation, witchcraft, religion, philosophy, psychology and a leaning toward the esoteric, the abstract, and the symbolic. Consequently, a

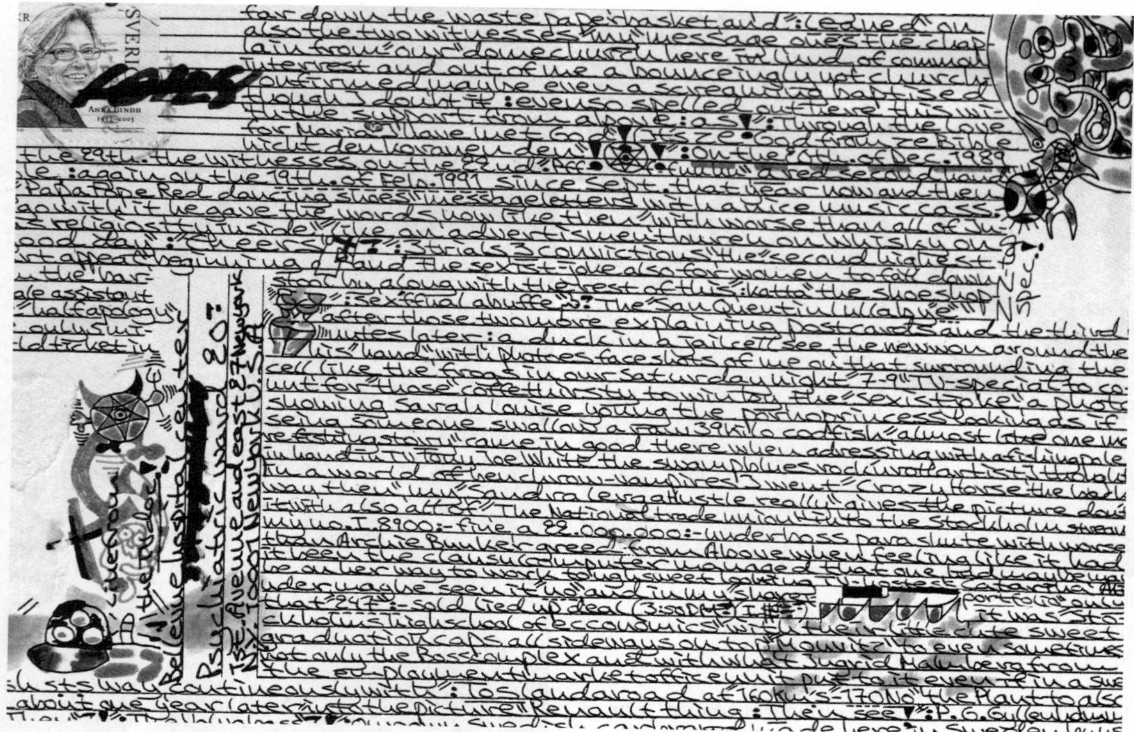

FIGURE 13–12

Sample of noncommunicative writing by a patient with chronic paranoid schizophrenia. This letter, written to the patient's psychiatrist, illustrates manneristic writing, verbigeration, and neologisms.

schizophrenic patient's thinking is characterized simultaneously by both an overly concrete and an overly symbolic nature.

THOUGHT PROCESS. Disorders in thought process concern the way ideas and languages are formulated. The examiner infers a disorder from what and how the patient speaks, writes, or draws. The examiner may also assess the patient's thought process by observing his or her behavior, especially in carrying out discrete tasks (e.g., in occupational therapy). Disorders of thought process include flight of ideas, thought blocking, impaired attention, poverty of thought content, poor abstraction abilities, perseveration, idiosyncratic associations (e.g., identical predicates, clang associations), over inclusion, and circumstantiality. *Thought control*, in which outside forces are controlling what the patient thinks or feels, is common, as is *thought broadcasting*, in which patients think others can read their minds or that their thoughts are broadcast through television sets or radios.

Impulsiveness, Violence, Suicide, and Homicide.

Patients with schizophrenia may be agitated and have little impulse control when ill. They may also have decreased social sensitivity and appear to be impulsive when, for example, they grab another patient's cigarettes, change television channels abruptly, or throw food on the floor. Some apparently impulsive behavior, including suicide and homicide attempts, may be in response to hallucinations commanding the patient to act.

VIOLENCE. Violent behavior (excluding homicide) is common among untreated schizophrenia patients. Delusions of a persecutory nature, previous episodes of violence, and neurological deficits are risk factors for violent or impulsive behavior. Management includes appropriate antipsychotic medication. Emergency treatment consists of restraints and seclusion. Acute sedation with lorazepam (Ativan), 1 to 2 mg intramuscularly, repeated every hour as needed, may be necessary to prevent the patient from harming others. If a clinician feels fearful in the presence of a schizophrenia patient, it should be taken as an internal clue that the patient may be on the verge of acting out violently. In such cases, the interview should be terminated or be conducted with an attendant at the ready.

SUICIDE. Suicide is the single leading cause of premature death among people with schizophrenia. Suicide attempts are made by 20 to 50 percent of the patients, with long-term rates of suicide estimated to be 10 to 13 percent. These numbers reflect an approximately 20-fold increase over the suicide rate in the general population. Often, suicide in schizophrenia seems to occur "out of the blue," without prior warnings or expressions of verbal intent. The most important factor is the presence of a major depressive episode. Epidemiological studies indicate that up to 80 percent of schizophrenia patients may have a major depressive episode at some time in their lives. Some data suggest that those patients with the best prognosis (few negative symptoms, preservation of capacity to experience affects, better abstract thinking) can paradoxically also be at highest risk for suicide. The profile of the patient at greatest risk is a young man who once had high expectations, declined from a higher level of functioning, realizes that his dreams are not likely to come true, and has lost faith in the effectiveness of treatment. Other possible contributors to the high rate of suicide include command hallucinations and drug abuse. Two-thirds or more of schizophrenic patients who commit suicide have seen an apparently unsuspecting clinician within 72 hours of death. A large pharmacological study suggests that clozapine (Clozaril) may have particular efficacy in reducing suicidal ideation in schizophrenia patients with prior hospitalizations for suicidality. Adjunctive antidepressant medications have been shown to be effective in alleviating co-occurring major depression in schizophrenia.

The following is an example of an unpredictable suicide in a schizophrenic who had been responding to psychiatric treatment:

The patient had been an autistic child and did not speak until he was 7 years old. He had responded well to psychiatric treatment, and at age 13 his IQ was reported as 122. At age 17 he became violent toward his parents, shaved all his hair off, and made such statements as, "I like bank robbers knocking people unconscious" and "I think tough gangs are funny because they beat down people." While saying this, he laughed loudly. He was admitted to a mental hospital, where he responded with definite improvement to pharmacotherapy and psychotherapy, and he went home regularly for weekends.

He left various notes on his desk before committing suicide. Among these notes was an eight-page list giving 211 "inexcusable mistakes throughout my life." Each one was dated, for example, "1952, 2nd of November: throwing up in my friend's house on a shoebox. 1953, 17th August: accidentally wearing a watch that wasn't water-proof in the bath-tub. 1956, 23rd of September: slamming back-door of Meteor after getting in."

He then proceeded in his notes to give "the causes of the mistakes:" "Montreal having a mountain; I have a receding hair-line; my height since I was nine years old; Canada having two languages . . ." He also wrote: "My feelings of tension since 1962 is getting worse most of the time. I planned the date of my death without the slightest trace of emotion . . ."

The boy hanged himself at age 18 in the family garage. An experienced psychiatrist who had repeatedly interviewed him noted no signs of depression only a week before. (Courtesy of Heinz E. Lehmann, M.D.)

HOMICIDE. Despite the sensational attention that the news media provides when a patient with schizophrenia murders someone, the available data indicate that these patients are no more likely to commit homicide than is a member of the general population. When a patient with schizophrenia does commit homicide, it may be for unpredictable or bizarre reasons based on hallucinations or delusions. Possible predictors of homicidal activity are a history of previous violence, dangerous behavior while hospitalized, and hallucinations or delusions involving such violence.

A schizophrenic man who had been going home on weekends for many months was told by his sister that she would not ask for permission any more to take him out of the hospital if he would not do his part with the housework in the future, for instance, help with the dishes. On the next weekend visit, the patient killed his sister and mother. He had shown no signs of disturbance whatsoever during the preceding week, had been sleeping well, and had been attending occupational therapy classes as usual.

A 19-year-old boy who had been discharged from a mental hospital, in what appeared to be a residual state of chronic schizophrenia of the undifferentiated type, stabbed his father to death when the latter, during a state of intoxication, told the patient that he was too much of a bother around the house and that he might as well return to the hospital.

Another schizophrenic, whose condition had not yet been diagnosed, complained to a general practitioner about various physical ailments. When the physician finally told him that he should not come anymore because there was nothing else he could do for him, the patient quickly left the office but returned a few hours later and killed the doctor. (Courtesy of Heinz E. Lehmann, M.D.)

Sensorium and Cognition

Orientation. Patients with schizophrenia are usually oriented to person, time, and place. The lack of such orientation should prompt clinicians to investigate the possibility of a medical or neurological brain disorder. Some patients with schizophrenia may give incorrect or bizarre answers to questions about orientation, for example, "I am Christ; this is heaven; and it is AD 35."

A schizophrenic patient asserted that he was in a prison elaborately disguised to look like a hospital with a staff of jailers disguised as doctors and nurses who were all engaged in a charade to elicit incriminating facts about the patient and his family. He made a severe suicidal attempt because he believed that only upon his death would the jailers spare the lives of his loved ones.

Memory. Memory, as tested in the mental status examination, is usually intact, but there can be minor cognitive deficiencies. It may not be possible, however, to get the patient to attend closely enough to the memory tests for the ability to be assessed adequately.

Cognitive Impairment. An important development in the understanding of the psychopathology of schizophrenia is an appreciation of the importance of cognitive impairment in the disorder. In outpatients, cognitive impairment is a better predictor of level of function than is the severity of psychotic symptoms. Patients with schizophrenia typically exhibit subtle cognitive dysfunction in the domains of attention, executive function, working memory, and episodic memory. Although a substantial percentage of patients have normal intelligence quotients, it is possible that every person who has schizophrenia has cognitive dysfunction compared to what he or she would be able to do without the disorder. Although these impairments cannot function as diagnostic tools, they are strongly related to the functional outcome of the illness and, for that reason, have clinical value as prognostic variables, as well as for treatment planning.

The cognitive impairment seems already to be present when patients have their first episode and appears largely to remain stable over the course of early illness. (There may be a small subgroup of patients who have a true dementia in late life that is not due to other cognitive disorders, such as Alzheimer's disease.) Cognitive impairments are also present in attenuated forms in nonpsychotic relatives of schizophrenia patients.

The cognitive impairments of schizophrenia have become the target of pharmacological and psychosocial treatment trials. It is likely that effective treatments will become widely available within a few years, and these are likely to lead to an improvement in the quality of life and level of functioning of people with schizophrenia.

Judgment and Insight. Classically, patients with schizophrenia are described as having poor insight into the nature and the severity of their disorder. The so-called lack of insight is associated with poor compliance with treatment. When examining schizophrenia patients, clinicians should carefully define various aspects of insight, such as awareness of symptoms, trouble getting along with people, and the reasons for these problems. Such information can be clinically useful in tailoring a treatment strategy and theoretically useful in postulating what areas of the brain contribute to the observed lack of insight (e.g., the parietal lobes).

Reliability. A patient with schizophrenia is no less reliable than any other psychiatric patient. The nature of the disorder, however, requires the examiner to verify important information through additional sources.

Somatic Comorbidity

Neurological Findings. Localizing and nonlocalizing neurological signs (also known as hard and soft signs, respectively) have been reported to be more common in patients with schizophrenia than in other psychiatric patients. Nonlocalizing signs include dysdiadochokinesia, astereognosis, primitive reflexes, and diminished dexterity. The presence of neurological signs and symptoms correlates with increased severity of illness, affective blunting, and a poor prognosis. Other abnormal neurological signs include tics, stereotypies, grimacing, impaired fine motor skills, abnormal motor tone, and abnormal movements. One study has found that only about 25 percent of patients with schizophrenia are aware of their own abnormal involuntary movements and that the lack of awareness is correlated with lack of insight about the primary psychiatric disorder and the duration of illness.

Eye Examination. In addition to the disorder of smooth ocular pursuit (saccadic movement), patients with schizophrenia have an elevated blink rate. The elevated blink rate is believed to reflect hyperdopaminergic activity. In primates, blinking can be increased by dopamine agonists and reduced by dopamine antagonists.

Speech. Although the disorders of speech in schizophrenia (e.g., looseness of associations) are classically considered to indicate a thought disorder, they may also indicate a *forme fruste* of aphasia, perhaps implicating the dominant parietal lobe. The inability of schizophrenia patients to perceive the prosody of speech or to inflect their own speech can be seen as a neurological symptom of a disorder in the nondominant parietal lobe. Other parietal lobe-like symptoms in schizophrenia include the inability to carry out tasks (i.e., apraxia), right-left disorientation, and lack of concern about the disorder.

Other Comorbidity

Obesity. Patients with schizophrenia appear to be more obese, with higher body mass indexes (BMIs) than age- and gender-matched cohorts in the general population. This is due, at least in part, to the effect of many antipsychotic medications, as well as poor nutritional balance and decreased motor activity. This weight gain, in turn, contributes to an increased risk of cardiovascular morbidity and mortality, an increased risk of diabetes, and other obesity-related conditions such as hyperlipidemia and obstructive sleep apnea.

Diabetes Mellitus. Schizophrenia is associated with an increased risk of type II diabetes mellitus. This is probably due, in part, to the association with obesity noted previously, but there is also evidence that some antipsychotic medications cause diabetes through a direct mechanism.

Cardiovascular Disease. Many antipsychotic medications have direct effects on cardiac electrophysiology. In addition, obesity, increased rates of smoking, diabetes, hyperlipidemia, and a sedentary lifestyle all independently increase the risk of cardiovascular morbidity and mortality.

HIV. Patients with schizophrenia appear to have a risk of HIV infection that is 1.5 to 2 times that of the general population. This association is thought to be due to increased risk behaviors, such as unprotected sex, multiple partners, and increased drug use.

Chronic Obstructive Pulmonary Disease. Rates of chronic obstructive pulmonary disease are reportedly increased in schizophrenia compared to the general population. The increased prevalence of smoking is an obvious contributor to this problem and may be the only cause.

Rheumatoid Arthritis. Patients with schizophrenia have approximately one-third the risk of rheumatoid arthritis that is found in the general population. This inverse association has been replicated several times, the significance of which is unknown.

DIFFERENTIAL DIAGNOSIS

Secondary Psychotic Disorders

A wide range of nonpsychiatric medical conditions and a variety of substances can induce symptoms of psychosis and catatonia (Table 13–9). The most appropriate diagnosis for such psychosis or catatonia is psychotic disorder due to a general medical condition, catatonic disorder due to a general medical condition, or substance-induced psychotic disorder.

When evaluating a patient with psychotic symptoms, clinicians should follow the general guidelines for assessing nonpsychiatric conditions. First, clinicians should aggressively pursue an undiagnosed nonpsychiatric medical condition when a

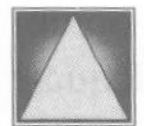

Table 13–9
Differential Diagnosis of Schizophrenia-Like Symptoms

Medical and Neurological
Substance induced—amphetamine, hallucinogens, belladonna alkaloids, alcohol hallucinosis, barbiturate withdrawal, cocaine, phencyclidine
Epilepsy—especially temporal lobe epilepsy
Neoplasm, cerebrovascular disease, or trauma—especially frontal or limbic
Other conditions
- Acute intermittent porphyria
- AIDS
- B_{12} deficiency
- Carbon monoxide poisoning
- Cerebral lipoidosis
- Creutzfeldt-Jakob disease
- Fabry's disease
- Fahr's disease
- Hallervorden-Spatz disease
- Heavy metal poisoning
- Herpes encephalitis
- Homocystinuria
- Huntington's disease
- Metachromatic leukodystrophy
- Neurosyphilis
- Normal pressure hydrocephalus
- Pellagra
- Systemic lupus erythematosus
- Wernicke-Korsakoff syndrome
- Wilson's disease

Psychiatric
Atypical psychosis
Autistic disorder
Brief psychotic disorder
Delusional disorder
Factitious disorder with predominantly psychological signs and symptoms
Malingering
Mood disorders
Normal adolescence
Obsessive-compulsive disorder
Personality disorders—schizotypal, schizoid, borderline, paranoid
Schizoaffective disorder
Schizophrenia
Schizophreniform disorder

patient exhibits any unusual or rare symptoms or any variation in the level of consciousness. Second, clinicians should attempt to obtain a complete family history, including a history of medical, neurological, and psychiatric disorders. Third, clinicians should consider the possibility of a nonpsychiatric medical condition, even in patients with previous diagnoses of schizophrenia. A patient with schizophrenia is just as likely to have a brain tumor that produces psychotic symptoms as is a patient without schizophrenia.

Other Psychotic Disorders

The psychotic symptoms of schizophrenia can be identical with those of schizophreniform disorder, brief psychotic disorder, schizoaffective disorder, and delusional disorders. *Schizophreniform disorder* differs from schizophrenia in that the symptoms have a duration of at least 1 month but less than 6 months. *Brief psychotic disorder* is the appropriate diagnosis when the symptoms have lasted at least 1 day but less than 1 month and when the patient has not returned to the premorbid state of functioning within that time. There may also be a precipitating traumatic event. When a manic or depressive syndrome develops concurrently with the major symptoms of schizophrenia, *schizoaffective disorder* is the appropriate diagnosis. Nonbizarre delusions present for at least 1 month without other symptoms of schizophrenia or a mood disorder warrant the diagnosis of *delusional disorder*.

Mood Disorders

A patient with a major depressive episode may present with delusions and hallucinations, whether the patient has unipolar or bipolar mood disorder. Delusions seen with psychotic depression are typically mood congruent and involve themes such as guilt, self-depreciation, deserved punishment, and incurable illnesses. In mood disorders, psychotic symptoms resolve completely with the resolution of depression. A depressive episode that is this severe may also result in loss of functioning, decline in self-care, and social isolation, but these are secondary to the depressive symptoms and should not be confused with the negative symptoms of schizophrenia.

A full-blown manic episode often presents with delusions and sometimes hallucinations. Delusions in mania are most often mood congruent and typically involve grandiose themes. The flight of ideas seen in mania may, at times, be confused with the thought disorder of schizophrenia. Special attention during mental status examination of a patient with a flight of ideas is required to note whether the associative links between topics are conserved, although the conversation is difficult for the observer to follow because of the patient's accelerated rate of thinking.

Personality Disorders

Various personality disorders may have some features of schizophrenia. Schizotypal, schizoid, and borderline personality disorders are the personality disorders with the most similar symptoms. Severe obsessive-compulsive personality disorder may mask an underlying schizophrenic process. Personality disorders, unlike schizophrenia, have mild symptoms and a history of occurring throughout a patient's life; they also lack an identifiable date of onset.

Malingering and Factitious Disorders

For a patient who imitates the symptoms of schizophrenia but does not actually have the disorder, either malingering or factitious disorder may be an appropriate diagnosis. Persons have faked schizophrenic symptoms and have been admitted into and treated at psychiatric hospitals. The condition of patients who are completely in control of their symptom production may qualify for a diagnosis of malingering; such patients usually have some obvious financial or legal reason to want to be considered mentally ill. The condition of patients who are less in control of their falsification of psychotic symptoms may qualify for a diagnosis of factitious disorder. Some patients with schizophrenia, however, may falsely complain of an exacerbation of psychotic symptoms to obtain increased assistance benefits or to gain admission to a hospital. (Factitious disorders are the subject of Chapter 19.)

COURSE AND PROGNOSIS

Course

A premorbid pattern of symptoms may be the first evidence of illness, although the importance of the symptoms is usually recognized only retrospectively. Characteristically, the symptoms begin in adolescence and are followed by the development of prodromal symptoms in days to a few months. Social or environmental changes, such as going away to college, using a substance, or a relative's death, may precipitate the disturbing symptoms, and the prodromal syndrome may last a year or more before the onset of overt psychotic symptoms.

The classic course of schizophrenia is one of exacerbations and remissions. After the first psychotic episode, a patient gradually recovers and may then function relatively normally for a long time. Patients usually relapse, however, and the pattern of illness during the first 5 years after the diagnosis generally indicates the patient's course. Further deterioration in the patient's baseline functioning follows each relapse of the psychosis. This failure to return to baseline functioning after each relapse is the major distinction between schizophrenia and the mood disorders. Sometimes, a clinically observable postpsychotic depression follows a psychotic episode, and the schizophrenia patient's vulnerability to stress is usually lifelong. Positive symptoms tend to become less severe with time, but the socially debilitating negative or deficit symptoms may increase in severity. Although about one-third of all schizophrenia patients have some marginal or integrated social existence, most have lives characterized by aimlessness, inactivity, frequent hospitalizations, and, in urban settings, homelessness and poverty.

Prognosis

Several studies have shown that over the 5- to 10-year period after the first psychiatric hospitalization for schizophrenia, only about 10 to 20 percent of patients can be described as having a good outcome. More than 50 percent of patients can be described as having a poor outcome, with repeated hospitalizations, exacerbations of symptoms, episodes of major mood disorders, and suicide attempts. Despite these glum figures, schizophrenia does not always run a deteriorating course, and several factors have been associated with a good prognosis (Table 13–6).

Reported remission rates range from 10 to 60 percent, and a reasonable estimate is that 20 to 30 percent of all schizophrenia patients are able to lead somewhat normal lives. About 20 to 30 percent of patients continue to experience moderate symptoms, and 40 to 60 percent of patients remain significantly impaired by their disorder for their entire lives. Patients with schizophrenia do much poorer than patients with mood disorders, although 20 to 25 percent of mood disorder patients are also severely disturbed at long-term follow-up.

TREATMENT

Although antipsychotic medications are the mainstay of the treatment for schizophrenia, research has found that psychosocial interventions, including psychotherapy, can augment the clinical improvement. Just as pharmacological agents are used to treat presumed chemical imbalances, nonpharmacological strategies must treat nonbiological issues. The complexity of schizophrenia usually renders any single therapeutic approach inadequate to deal with the multifaceted disorder. Psychosocial modalities should be integrated into the drug treatment regimen and should support it. Patients with schizophrenia benefit more from the combined use of antipsychotic drugs and psychosocial treatment than from either treatment used alone.

Hospitalization

Hospitalization is indicated for diagnostic purposes, for stabilization of medications, for patients' safety because of suicidal or homicidal ideation, and for grossly disorganized or inappropriate behavior, including the inability to take care of basic needs such as food, clothing, and shelter. Establishing an effective association between patients and community support systems is also a primary goal of hospitalization.

Short stays of 4 to 6 weeks are just as effective as long-term hospitalizations and those hospital settings with active behavioral approaches produce better results than do custodial institutions. Hospital treatment plans should be oriented toward practical issues of self-care, quality of life, employment, and social relationships. During hospitalization, patients should be coordinated with aftercare facilities, including their family homes, foster families, board-and-care homes, and halfway houses. Day care centers and home visits by therapists or nurses can help patients remain out of the hospital for long periods and can improve the quality of their daily lives.

Pharmacotherapy

The introduction of chlorpromazine (Thorazine) in 1952 may be the most important single contribution to the treatment of a psychiatric illness. Henri Laborit, a surgeon in Paris, noticed that administering chlorpromazine to patients before surgery resulted in an unusual state in which they seemed less anxious regarding the procedure. Chlorpromazine was subsequently shown to be effective at reducing hallucinations and delusions, as well as excitement. It was also noted that it caused side effects that appeared similar to Parkinsonism.

Antipsychotics diminish psychotic symptom expression and reduce relapse rates. Approximately 70 percent of patients treated with any antipsychotic achieve remission.

The drugs used to treat schizophrenia have a wide variety of pharmacological properties, but all share the capacity to antagonize postsynaptic dopamine receptors in the brain. Antipsychotics can be categorized into two main groups: the older conventional antipsychotics, which have also been called *first-generation antipsychotics* or dopamine receptor antagonists, and the newer drugs, which have been called *second-generation antipsychotics or serotonin dopamine antagonists (SDAs).*

Clozapine (Clozaril), the first effective antipsychotic with negligible extrapyramidal side effects, was discovered in 1958 and first studied during the 1960s. However, in 1976, it was noted that clozapine was associated with a substantial risk of agranulocytosis. This property resulted in delays in the introduction of clozapine. In 1990, clozapine finally became available in the United States, but its use was restricted to patients who responded poorly to other agents.

PHASES OF TREATMENT IN SCHIZOPHRENIA

Treatment of Acute Psychosis

Acute psychotic symptoms require immediate attention. Treatment during the acute phase focuses on alleviating the most severe psychotic symptoms. This phase usually lasts from 4 to 8 weeks. Acute schizophrenia is typically associated with severe agitation, which can result from such symptoms as frightening delusions, hallucinations, or suspiciousness, or from other causes, including stimulant abuse. Patients with akathisia can appear agitated when they experience a subjective feeling of motor restlessness. Differentiating akathisia from psychotic agitation can be difficult, particularly when patients are incapable of describing their internal experience. If patients are receiving an agent associated with extrapyramidal side effects, usually a first-generation antipsychotic, a trial with an anticholinergic anti-Parkinson medication, benzodiazepine, or propranolol (Inderal) may be helpful in making the discrimination.

Clinicians have a number of options for managing agitation that results from psychosis. Antipsychotics and benzodiazepines can result in relatively rapid calming of patients. With highly agitated patients, intramuscular administration of antipsychotics produces a more rapid effect. An advantage of an antipsychotic is that a single intramuscular injection of haloperidol (Haldol), fluphenazine (Prolixin, Permitil), olanzapine (Zyprexa), or ziprasidone (Geodon) will often result in calming without an excess of sedation. Low-potency antipsychotics are often associated with sedation and postural hypotension, particularly when they are administered intramuscularly. Intramuscular ziprasidone and olanzapine are similar to their oral counterparts in not causing substantial extrapyramidal side effects during acute treatment. This can be an important advantage over haloperidol or fluphenazine, which can cause frightening dystonias or akathisia in some patients. A rapidly dissolving oral formulation of olanzapine (Zydis) may also be helpful as an alternative to an intramuscular injection.

Benzodiazepines are also effective for agitation during acute psychosis. Lorazepam (Ativan) has the advantage of reliable absorption when it is administered either orally or intramuscularly. The use of benzodiazepines may also reduce the amount of antipsychotic that is needed to control psychotic patients.

Some studies suggest that a longer time between the first onset of psychosis and the initiation of treatment is related to a worse outcome. As a result, clinicians must consider the possibility that delayed treatment may worsen the patient's prognosis. However, these data do not mean that all patients need to be treated immediately. A brief delay may permit clinicians to develop a more thorough diagnostic evaluation and rule out causes of abnormal behavior, such as substance abuse, extreme stress, medical illnesses, and other psychiatric illnesses.

Treatment During Stabilization and Maintenance Phase

In the stable or maintenance phase, the illness is in a relative stage of remission. The goals during this phase are to prevent psychotic relapse and to assist patients in improving their level of functioning. As newer medications have been introduced with a substantively reduced risk of tardive dyskinesia, one of the major concerns about long-term treatment has been diminished. During this phase, patients are usually in a relative state of remission with only minimal psychotic symptoms. Stable patients who are maintained on an antipsychotic have a much lower relapse rate than patients who have their medications discontinued. Data suggest that 16 to 23 percent of patients receiving treatment will experience a relapse within a year and 53 to 72 percent will relapse without medications. Even patients who have had only one episode have a four in five chance of relapsing at least once over the following 5 years. Stopping medication increases this risk fivefold. Although published guidelines do not make definitive recommendations about the duration of maintenance treatment after the first episode, recent data suggest that 1 or 2 years might not be adequate. This is a particular concern when patients have achieved good employment status or are involved in educational programs because they have a lot to lose if they experience another psychotic decompensation.

It is generally recommended that multiepisode patients receive maintenance treatment for at least 5 years, and many experts recommend pharmacotherapy on an indefinite basis.

Noncompliance. Noncompliance with long-term antipsychotic treatment is very high. An estimated 40 to 50 percent of patients become noncompliant within 1 or 2 years. Compliance increases when long-acting medication is used instead of oral medication.

When beginning long-acting drugs, some oral supplementation is necessary while peak plasma levels are being achieved. Fluphenazine and haloperidol have been formulated as long-acting injectables. A long-acting form of risperidone is also available.

There are a number of advantages to using long-acting injectable medication. Clinicians know immediately when noncompliance occurs and have some time to initiate appropriate interventions before the medication effect dissipates; there is less day-to-day variability in blood levels, making it easier to establish a minimum effective dose; and finally, many patients prefer it to having to remember dosage schedules of daily oral preparations.

STRATEGIES FOR POOR RESPONDERS

When patients with acute schizophrenia are administered an antipsychotic medication, approximately 60 percent will improve to the extent that they will achieve a complete remission or experience only mild symptoms; the remaining 40 percent of patients will improve but still demonstrate variable levels of positive symptoms that are resistant to the medications. Rather than categorizing patients into responders and nonresponders, it is more accurate to consider the degree to which the illness is improved by medication. Some resistant patients are so severely ill that they require chronic institutionalization. Others will respond to an antipsychotic with substantial suppression of their psychotic symptoms but demonstrate persistent symptoms, such as hallucinations or delusions.

Before considering a patient a poor responder to a particular drug, it is important to assure that they received an adequate trial of the medication. A 4- to 6-week trial on an adequate dose of an antipsychotic represents a reasonable trial for most patients. Patients who demonstrate even a mild amount of improvement during this period may continue to improve at a steady rate for

3 to 6 months. It may be helpful to confirm that the patient is receiving an adequate amount of the drug by monitoring the plasma concentration. This information is available for a number of antipsychotics, including haloperidol, clozapine, fluphenazine, trifluoperazine (Stelazine), and perphenazine (Trilafon). A very low plasma concentration may indicate that the patient has been noncompliant or, more commonly, only partially compliant. It may also suggest that the patient is a rapid metabolizer of the antipsychotic or that the drug is not being adequately absorbed. Under these conditions, raising the dose may be helpful. If the level is relatively high, clinicians should consider whether side effects may be interfering with therapeutic response.

If the patient is responding poorly, one may increase the dose above the usual therapeutic level; however, higher doses are not usually associated with greater improvement than conventional doses. Changing to another drug is preferable to changing to a high dose.

If a patient has responded poorly to a conventional DRA, it is unlikely that this individual will do well on another DRA. Changing to an SDA is more likely to be helpful.

Clozapine is effective for patients who respond poorly to DRAs. Double-blind studies comparing clozapine to other antipsychotics indicated that clozapine had the clearest advantage over conventional drugs in patients with the most severe psychotic symptoms, as well as in those who had previously responded poorly to other antipsychotics. When clozapine was compared with chlorpromazine in a severely psychotic group of individuals who had failed in trials with at least three antipsychotics, clozapine was significantly more effective in nearly every dimension of psychopathology, including both positive symptoms and negative symptoms.

MANAGING SIDE EFFECTS

Patients will frequently experience side effects of an antipsychotic before they experience clinical improvement. Whereas a clinical response may be delayed for days or weeks after drugs are started, side effects may begin almost immediately. For low-potency drugs, these side effects are likely to include sedation, postural hypotension, and anticholinergic effects, whereas high-potency drugs are likely to cause extrapyramidal side effects.

Extrapyramidal Side Effects

Clinicians have a number of alternatives for treating extrapyramidal side effects. These include reducing the dose of the antipsychotic (which is most commonly a DRA), adding an anti-Parkinson medication, and changing the patient to an SDA that is less likely to cause extrapyramidal side effects. The most effective anti-Parkinson medications are the anticholinergic anti-Parkinson drugs. However, these medications have their own side effects, including dry mouth, constipation, blurred vision, and, often, memory loss. Also, these medications are often only partially effective, leaving patients with substantial amounts of lingering extrapyramidal side effects. Centrally acting β-blockers, such as propranolol, are also often effective for treating akathisia. Most patients respond to dosages between 30 and 90 mg per day.

If conventional antipsychotics are being prescribed, clinicians may consider prescribing prophylactic anti-Parkinson medications for patients who are likely to experience disturbing extrapyramidal side effects. These include patients who have a history of extrapyramidal side effect sensitivity and those who are being treated with relatively high doses of high-potency drugs. Prophylactic anti-Parkinson medications may also be indicated when high-potency drugs are prescribed for young men who tend to have an increased vulnerability for developing dystonias. Again, these patients should be candidates for newer drugs.

Some individuals are highly sensitive to extrapyramidal side effects at the dose that is necessary to control their psychosis. For many of these patients, medication side effects may seem worse than the illness itself. These patients should be treated routinely with an SDA because these agents result in substantially fewer extrapyramidal side effects than the DRAs. However, these highly sensitive individuals may even experience extrapyramidal side effects on an SDA. Risperidone may cause extrapyramidal side effects even at low doses—for example, 0.5 mg—but the severity and risk are increased at higher doses—for example, more than 6 mg. Olanzapine and ziprasidone are also associated with dose-related Parkinsonism and akathisia.

Tardive Dyskinesia

About 20 to 30 percent of patients on long-term treatment with a conventional DRA will exhibit symptoms of tardive dyskinesia. Three to five percent of young patients receiving a DRA develop tardive dyskinesia each year. The risk in elderly patients is much higher. Although seriously disabling dyskinesia is uncommon, it can affect walking, breathing, eating, and talking when it occurs. Individuals who are more sensitive to acute extrapyramidal side effects appear to be more vulnerable to developing tardive dyskinesia. Patients with comorbid cognitive or mood disorders may also be more vulnerable to tardive dyskinesia than those with only schizophrenia.

The onset of the abnormal movements usually occurs either while the patient is receiving an antipsychotic or within 4 weeks of discontinuing an oral antipsychotic or 8 weeks after the withdrawal of a depot antipsychotic. There is a slightly lower risk of tardive dyskinesia with new-generation drugs. However, the risk of tardive dyskinesia is not absent with SDAs.

Recommendations for preventing and managing tardive dyskinesia include (1) using the lowest effective dose of antipsychotic; (2) prescribing cautiously with children, elderly patients, and patients with mood disorders; (3) examining patients on a regular basis for evidence of tardive dyskinesia; (4) considering alternatives to the antipsychotic being used and considering dosage reduction when tardive dyskinesia is diagnosed; and (5) considering a number of options if the tardive dyskinesia worsens, including discontinuing the antipsychotic or switching to a different drug. Clozapine has been shown to be effective in reducing severe tardive dyskinesia or tardive dystonia. The reader is referred to Section 36.2 for an extensive discussion of medication-induced movement disorders.

Other Side Effects

Sedation and postural hypotension can be important side effects for patients who are being treated with low-potency DRAs, such as perphenazine. These effects are often most severe during the initial dosing with these medications. As a result, patients treated with these medications—particularly clozapine—may require weeks to reach a therapeutic dose. Although most patients develop tolerance to sedation and postural hypotension, sedation may continue to be a problem. In these patients, daytime drowsiness may interfere with a patient's attempts to return to community life.

All DRAs, as well as SDAs, elevate prolactin levels, which can result in galactorrhea and irregular menses. Long-term elevations in prolactin and the resultant suppression in gonadotropin-releasing hormone can cause suppression in gonadal hormones. These, in turn, may have effects on libido and sexual functioning. There is also concern that elevated prolactin may cause decreases in bone density and lead to osteoporosis. The concerns about hyperprolactinemia, sexual functioning, and bone density are based on experiences with prolactin elevations related to tumors and other causes. It is unclear if these risks are also associated with the lower elevations that occur with prolactin-elevating drugs.

Health Monitoring in Patients Receiving Antipsychotics

Because of the effects of the SDAs on insulin, metabolism psychiatrists should monitor a number of health indicators, including BMI, fasting blood glucose, and lipid profiles. Patients should be weighed and their BMI calculated for every visit for 6 months after a medication change.

Side Effects of Clozapine

Clozapine has a number of side effects that make it a difficult drug to administer. The most serious is a risk of agranulocytosis. This potentially fatal condition occurs in approximately 0.3 percent of patients treated with clozapine during the first year of exposure. Subsequently, the risk is substantially lower. As a result, patients who receive clozapine in the United States are required to be in a program of weekly blood monitoring for the first 6 months and biweekly monitoring for the next 6 months. After 1 year of treatment without hematological problems, monitoring can be performed monthly.

Clozapine is also associated with a higher risk of seizures than other antipsychotics. The risk reaches nearly 5 percent at doses of more than 600 mg. Patients who develop seizures with clozapine can usually be managed by reducing the dose and adding an anticonvulsant, usually valproate (Depakene). Myocarditis has been reported to occur in approximately 5 patients per 100,000 patient-years. Other side effects with clozapine include hypersalivation, sedation, tachycardia, weight gain, diabetes, fever, and postural hypotension.

OTHER BIOLOGICAL THERAPIES

ECT has been studied in both acute and chronic schizophrenia. Studies in recent-onset patients indicate that ECT is about as effective as antipsychotic medications and more effective than psychotherapy. Other studies suggest that supplementing antipsychotic medications with ECT is more effective than antipsychotic medications alone. Antipsychotic medications should be administered during and after ECT treatment. Although psychosurgery is no longer considered an appropriate treatment, it is practiced on a limited experimental basis for severe, intractable cases.

PSYCHOSOCIAL THERAPIES

Psychosocial therapies include a variety of methods to increase social abilities, self-sufficiency, practical skills, and interpersonal communication in schizophrenia patients. The goal is to enable persons who are severely ill to develop social and vocational skills for independent living. Such treatment is carried out at many sites: hospitals, outpatient clinics, mental health centers, day hospitals, and home or social clubs.

Social Skills Training

Social skills training is sometimes referred to as behavioral skills therapy (Table 13–10). Along with pharmacological therapy, this

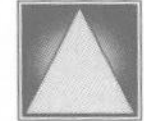

Table 13–10
Goals and Targeted Behaviors for Social Skills Therapy

Phase	Goals	Targeted Behaviors
Stabilization and assessment	Establish therapeutic alliance Assess social performance and perception skills Assess behaviors that provoke expressed emotion	Empathy and rapport Verbal and nonverbal communication
Social performance within family	Express positive feelings within family Teach effective strategies for coping with conflict	Compliments, appreciation, interest in others Avoidance response to criticism, stating preferences and refusals
Social perception in the family	Correctly identify content, context, and meaning of messages	Reading a message Labeling an idea Summarizing other's intent
Extrafamilial relationships	Enhance socialization skills Enhance prevocational and vocational skills	Conversational skills Dating Recreational activities Job interviewing, work habits
Maintenance	Generalize skills to new situations	

(Adapted with permission from Hogarty GE, Anderson CM, Reiss DJ, et al. Family psychoeducation, social skills training and maintenance chemotherapy in aftercare treatment of schizophrenia: I. One-year effects of a controlled study on relapse and expressed emotion. *Arch Gen Psychiatry.* 1986;43:633.)

therapy can be directly supportive and useful to the patient. In addition to the psychotic symptoms seen in patients with schizophrenia, other noticeable symptoms involve the way the person relates to others, including poor eye contact, unusual delays in response, odd facial expressions, lack of spontaneity in social situations, and inaccurate perception or lack of perception of emotions in other people. Behavioral skills training addresses these behaviors through the use of videotapes of others and of the patient, role playing in therapy, and homework assignments for the specific skills being practiced. Social skills training has been shown to reduce relapse rates as measured by the need for hospitalization.

Family-Oriented Therapies

Because patients with schizophrenia are often discharged in an only partially remitted state, a family to which a patient returns can often benefit from a brief but intensive (as often as daily) course of family therapy. The therapy should focus on the immediate situation and should include identifying and avoiding potentially troublesome situations. When problems do emerge with the patient in the family, the aim of the therapy should be to resolve the problem quickly.

In wanting to help, family members often encourage a relative with schizophrenia to resume regular activities too quickly, both from ignorance about the disorder and from denial of its severity. Without being overly discouraging, therapists must help both the family and the patient understand and learn about schizophrenia and must encourage discussion of the psychotic episode and the events leading up to it. Ignoring the psychotic episode, a common occurrence, often increases the shame associated with the event and does not exploit the freshness of the episode to understand it better. Psychotic symptoms often frighten family members, and talking openly with the psychiatrist and with the relative with schizophrenia often eases all parties. Therapists can direct later family therapy toward long-range application of stress-reducing and coping strategies and toward the patient's gradual reintegration into everyday life.

Therapists must control the emotional intensity of family sessions with patients with schizophrenia. The excessive expression of emotion during a session can damage a patient's recovery process and undermine potentially successful future family therapy. Several studies have shown that family therapy is especially effective in reducing relapses.

NATIONAL ALLIANCE FOR THE MENTALLY ILL. The National Alliance for the Mentally Ill (NAMI) and similar organizations offer support groups for family members and friends of patients who are mentally ill and for patients themselves. These organizations offer emotional and practical advice about obtaining care in the sometimes complex health care delivery system and are useful sources to which to refer family members. NAMI has also waged a campaign to destigmatize mental illness and to increase government awareness of the needs and rights of persons who are mentally ill and their families.

Case Management

Because a variety of professionals with specialized skills, such as psychiatrists, social workers, and occupational therapists, among others, are involved in a treatment program, it is helpful to have one person aware of all the forces acting on the patient. The case manager ensures that their efforts are coordinated and that the patient keeps appointments and complies with treatment plans; the case manager may make home visits and even accompany the patient to work. The success of the program depends on the educational background, training, and competence of the individual case manager, which varies. Case managers often have too many cases to manage effectively. The ultimate benefits of the program have yet to be demonstrated.

Assertive Community Treatment

The Assertive Community Treatment (ACT) program was originally developed by researchers in Madison, Wisconsin, in the 1970s, for the delivery of services for persons with chronic mental illness. Patients are assigned to one multidisciplinary team (case manager, psychiatrist, nurse, general physicians, etc.). The team has a fixed caseload of patients and delivers all services when and where needed by the patient, 24 hours a day, 7 days a week. This is mobile and intensive intervention that provides treatment, rehabilitation, and support activities. These include home delivery of medications, monitoring of mental and physical health, in vivo social skills, and frequent contact with family members. There is a high staff-to-patient ratio (1:12). ACT programs can effectively decrease the risk of rehospitalization for persons with schizophrenia, but they are labor-intensive and expensive programs to administer.

Group Therapy

Group therapy for persons with schizophrenia generally focuses on real-life plans, problems, and relationships. Groups may be behaviorally oriented, psychodynamically or insight oriented, or supportive. Some investigators doubt that dynamic interpretation and insight therapy are valuable for typical patients with schizophrenia. But group therapy is effective in reducing social isolation, increasing the sense of cohesiveness, and improving reality testing for patients with schizophrenia. Groups led in a supportive manner appear to be most helpful for schizophrenia patients.

Cognitive Behavioral Therapy

Cognitive behavioral therapy has been used in schizophrenia patients to improve cognitive distortions, reduce distractibility, and correct errors in judgment. There are reports of ameliorating delusions and hallucinations in some patients using this method. Patients who might benefit generally have some insight into their illness.

Individual Psychotherapy

Studies of the effects of individual psychotherapy in the treatment of schizophrenia have provided data that the therapy is helpful and that the effects are additive to those of pharmacological treatment. In psychotherapy with a schizophrenia patient, developing a therapeutic relationship that the patient experiences as safe is critical. The therapist's reliability, the emotional distance between the therapist and the patient, and the genuineness

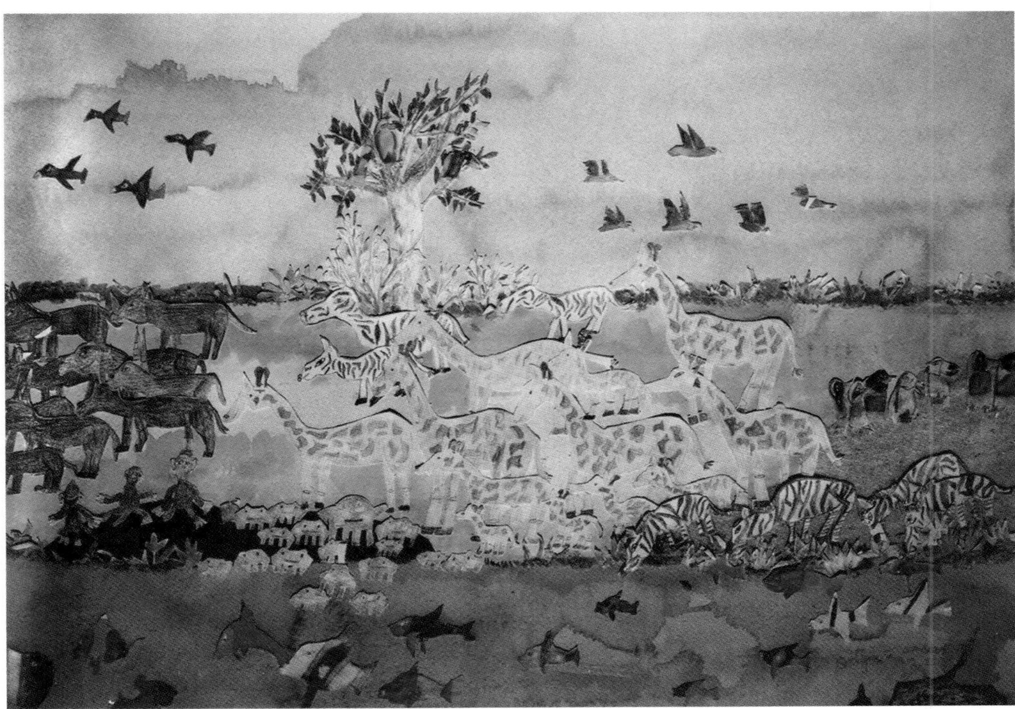

COLOR PLATE 13–14

A schizophrenic patient was unable to express himself, except in paintings. He constructed a collage called *Africa*, featuring dozens of tiny animals: fish, birds, giraffes, zebras, warthogs, monkeys, frogs. He had meticulously drawn them with colored pencils, and used a pair of tiny scissors to cut each one out. Then he painted a background and glued them on. Some of the animals were smiling, he explained, while others were angry. Pointing to the pack of zebras, he said, "They're all looking out for themselves, and they're happy to be by the water." (Courtesy of the artist and Roxanne Lanquetot.)

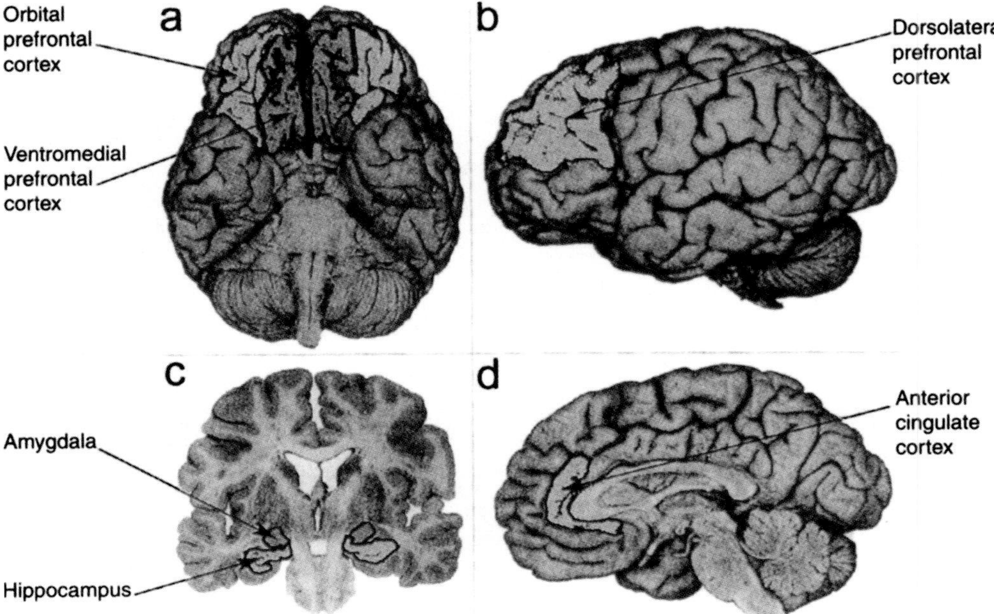

COLOR PLATE 15.1–2

Key brain regions involved in affect and mood disorders. **a:** Orbital prefrontal cortex and the ventromedial prefrontal cortex. **b:** corsolateral prefrontal cortex. **c:** Hippocampus and amygdala. **d:** Anterior cingulated cortex.

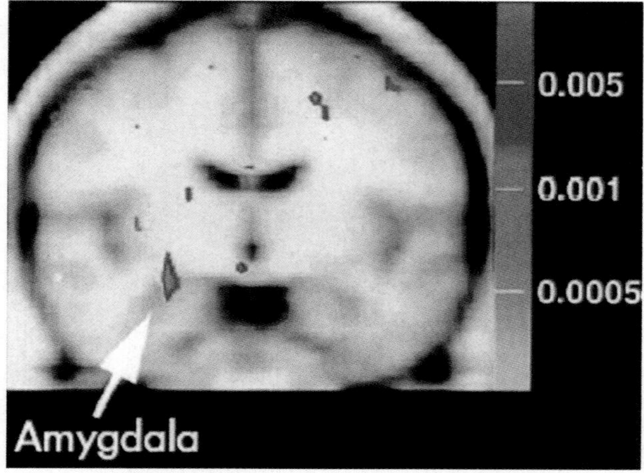

COLOR PLATE 16.1–1

Statistical map of functional magnetic resonance imaging (fMRI) blood oxygenation level-dependent signal intensity differences demonstrating significantly increased activity in the right amygdale in subjects with posttraumatic stress disorder (PTSD) compared with traumatized subjects without PTSD. The response to masked, fearful faces in PTSD and non-PTSD groups were compared after normalizing to masked, happy faces. fMRI data are displayed in Talairach template space and are co-registered with structural magnetic resonance imaging data.

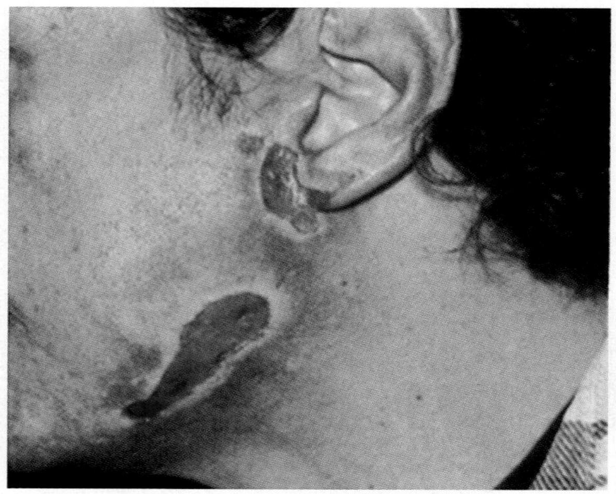

COLOR PLATE 19–2

Factitial ulcerations. These were created by the patient. Note their geometric appearance.

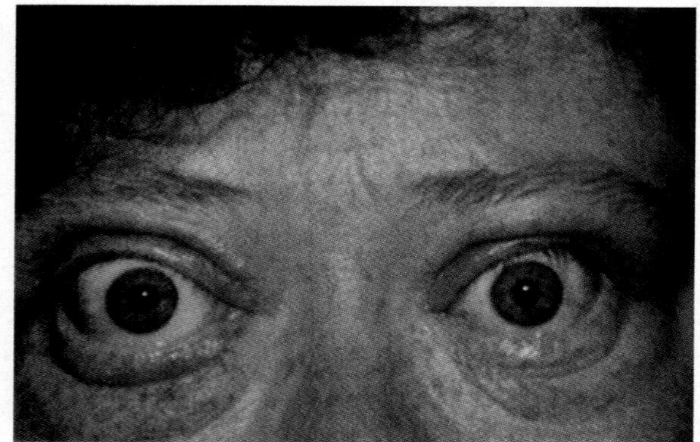

COLOR PLATE 16.7–1

Expohthalmos. This patient has Graves' disease. Note the lid retraction and proptosis.

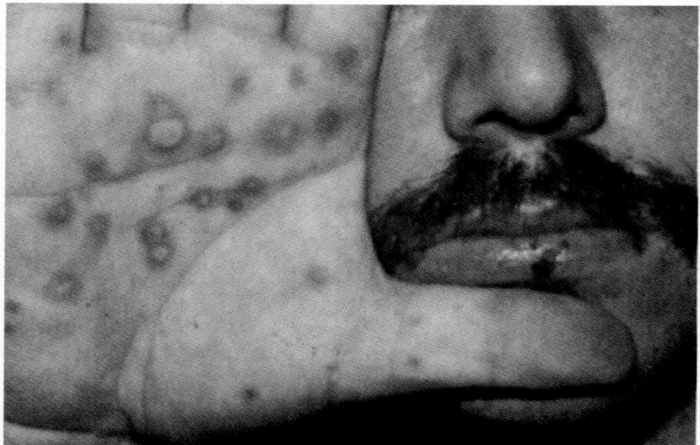

COLOR PLATE 36.19–2

Erythema multiforme minor caused by hypersensitivity to certain antiepileptic drugs used in psychiatry (i.e., lamictal).

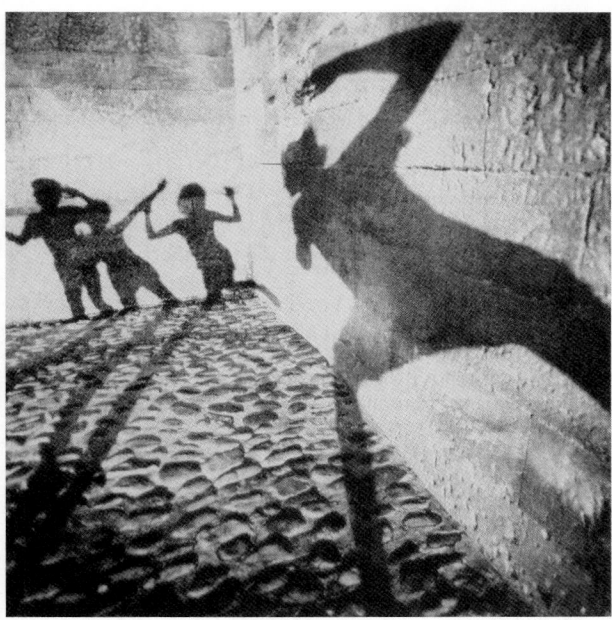

FIGURE 13–13
Patients with schizophrenia live in a state of chronic anxiety and fear. The environment is seen as hostile and threatening as symbolized in this illustration. (Courtesy of Arthur Tress.)

of the therapist as interpreted by the patient all affect the therapeutic experience. Psychotherapy for a schizophrenia patient should be thought of in terms of decades, rather than sessions, months, or even years.

Some clinicians and researchers have emphasized that the ability of a patient with schizophrenia to form a therapeutic alliance with a therapist is predictive of the outcome. Schizophrenia patients who are able to form a good therapeutic alliance are likely to remain in psychotherapy, to remain compliant with their medications, and to have good outcomes at 2-year follow-up evaluations.

The relationship between clinicians and patients differs from that encountered in the treatment of nonpsychotic patients. Establishing a relationship is often difficult. Persons with schizophrenia are desperately lonely, yet defend against closeness and trust; they are likely to become suspicious, anxious, or hostile or to regress when someone attempts to draw close (Fig. 13–13). Therapists should scrupulously respect a patient's distance and privacy, and should demonstrate simple directness, patience, sincerity, and sensitivity to social conventions in preference to premature informality and the condescending use of first names. The patient is likely to perceive exaggerated warmth or professions of friendship as attempts at bribery, manipulation, or exploitation.

In the context of a professional relationship, however, flexibility is essential in establishing a working alliance with the patient. A therapist may have meals with the patient, sit on the floor, go for a walk, eat at a restaurant, accept and give gifts, play table tennis, remember the patient's birthday, or just sit silently with the patient. The major aim is to convey the idea that the therapist is trustworthy, wants to understand the patient and tries to do so, and has faith in the patient's potential as a human, no matter how disturbed, hostile, or bizarre the patient may be at the moment.

Personal Therapy

A flexible type of psychotherapy called personal therapy is a recently developed form of individual treatment for schizophrenia patients. Its objective is to enhance personal and social adjustment and to forestall relapse. It is a select method using social skills and relaxation exercises, psychoeducation, self-reflection, self-awareness, and exploration of individual vulnerability to stress. The therapist provides a setting that stresses acceptance and empathy. Patients receiving personal therapy show improvement in social adjustment (a composite measure that includes work performance, leisure, and interpersonal relationships) and have a lower relapse rate after 3 years than patients not receiving personal therapy.

Dialectical Behavior Therapy

This form of therapy, which combines cognitive and behavioral theories in both individual and group settings, has proved useful in borderline states and may have benefit in schizophrenia. Emphasis is placed on improving interpersonal skills in the presence of an active and empathic therapist.

Vocational Therapy

A variety of methods and settings are used to help patients regain old skills or develop new ones. These include sheltered workshops, job clubs, and part-time or transitional employment programs. Enabling patients to become gainfully employed is both a means toward, and a sign of, recovery. Many schizophrenia patients are capable of performing high-quality work despite their illness. Others may exhibit exceptional skill or even brilliance in a limited field as a result of some idiosyncratic aspect of their disorder.

Art Therapy

Many schizophrenic patients benefit from art therapy, which provides them with an outlet for their constant bombardment of imagery. It helps them communicate with others and share their inner, often frightening world with others. In some circles, the art of the mentally ill is highly collectable; however, whether purchased or not, the production of a work that is appreciated by others can do much to raise self-esteem (*see* Color Plate 13–14 on page 493.)

Integrating Psychosocial and Medication Treatments

Antipsychotic medication has been established as the single most effective treatment for schizophrenia, but it is not sufficient for many patients who greatly benefit from the addition of psychosocial therapy. In fact, many studies show that combining both approaches produces the best results.

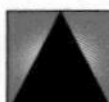

Table 13–11
ICD-10 Diagnostic Criteria for Schizophrenia

This overall category includes the common varieties of schizophrenia, together with some less common varieties and closely related disorders.

General criteria for paranoid, hebephrenic, catatonic, and undifferentiated schizophrenia

G1. Either *at least one* of the syndromes, symptoms, and signs listed under (1) below, *or* at least two of the symptoms and signs listed under (2) should be present for most of the time during an episode of psychotic illness lasting for at least 1 month (or at some time during most of the days).
- (1) At least one of the following must be present:
  - (a) thought echo, thought insertion or withdrawal, or thought broadcasting;
  - (b) delusions of control, influence, or passivity, clearly referred to body or limb movements or specific thoughts, actions, or sensations; delusional perception;
  - (c) hallucinatory voices giving a running commentary on the patient's behavior, or discussing the patient among themselves, or other types of hallucinatory voices coming from some part of the body;
  - (d) persistent delusions of other kinds that are culturally inappropriate and completely impossible (e.g., being able to control the weather, or being in communication with aliens from another world).
- (2) *Or* at least two of the following:
  - (a) persistent hallucinations in any modality, when occurring every day for at least 1 month, when accompanied by delusions (which may be fleeting or half-formed) without clear affective content, or when accompanied by persistent overvalued ideas;
  - (b) neologisms, breaks, or interpolations in the train of thought, resulting in incoherence or irrelevant speech;
  - (c) catatonic behavior, such as excitement, posturing or waxy flexibility, negativism, mutism, and stupor;
  - (d) "negative" symptoms, such as marked apathy, paucity of speech, and blunting or incongruity of emotional responses (it must be clear that these are not due to depression or to neuroleptic medication).

G2. *Most commonly used exclusion clauses*
- (1) If the patient also meets criteria for manic episode or depressive episode, the criteria listed under G1(1) and GI(2) above must have been met *before* the disturbance of mood developed.
- (2) The disorder is not attributable to organic brain disease or to alcohol- or drug-related intoxication, dependence, or withdrawal.

Comments

In evaluating the presence of these abnormal subjective experiences and behavior, special care should be taken to avoid false-positive assessments, especially where culturally or subculturally influenced modes of expression and behavior or a subnormal level of intelligence are involved.

Pattern of course

In view of the considerable variation of the course of schizophrenic disorders it may be desirable (especially for research) to specify the pattern *of course* by using a fifth character. Course should not usually be coded unless there has been a period of observation of at least 1 year.

Continuous

No remission of psychotic symptoms throughout the period of observation.

Episodic with progressive deficit

Progressive development of "negative" symptoms in the intervals between psychotic episodes.

Episodic with stable deficit

Persistent but nonprogressive "negative" symptoms in the intervals between psychotic episodes.

Episodic remittent

Complete or virtually complete remissions between psychotic episodes.

Incomplete remission

Complete remission

Other

Course uncertain, period of observation too short

Paranoid schizophrenia

A. The general criteria for schizophrenia must be met.

B. Delusions or hallucinations must be prominent (such as delusions of persecution, reference, exalted birth, special mission, bodily change, or jealousy; threatening or commanding voices, hallucinations of smell or taste, sexual or other bodily sensations).

C. Flattening or incongruity of affect, catatonic symptoms, or incoherent speech must not dominate the clinical picture, although they may be present to a mild degree.

Hebephrenic schizophrenia

A. The general criteria for schizophrenia must be met.

B. Either of the following must be present:
- (1) definite and sustained flattening or shallowness of affect;
- (2) definite and sustained incongruity or inappropriateness of affect.

C. Either of the following must be present:
- (1) behavior that is aimless and disjointed rather than goal-directed;
- (2) definite thought disorder, manifesting as speech that is disjointed, rambling, or incoherent.

D. Hallucinations or delusions must not dominate the clinical picture, although they may be present to a mild degree.

Catatonic schizophrenia

A. The general criteria for schizophrenia must eventually be met, although this may not be possible initially if the patient is uncommunicative.

B. For a period of at least 2 weeks one or more of the following catatonic behaviors must be prominent:
- (1) stupor (marked decrease in reactivity to the environment and reduction of spontaneous movements and activity) or mutism;
- (2) excitement (apparently purposeless motor activity, not influenced by external stimuli);
- (3) posturing (voluntary assumption and maintenance of inappropriate or bizarre postures);
- (4) negativism (an apparently motiveless resistance to all instructions or attempts to be moved, or movement in the opposite direction);
- (5) rigidity (maintenance of a rigid posture against efforts to be moved);
- (6) waxy flexibility (maintenance of limbs and body in externally imposed positions);
- (7) command automatism (automatic compliance with instruction).

Undifferentiated schizophrenia

A. The general criteria for schizophrenia must be met.

Either of the following must apply:
- (1) insufficient symptoms to meet the criteria for any of the subtypes
- (2) so many symptoms that the criteria for more than one of the subtypes listed above are met.

Postschizophrenic depression

A. The general criteria for schizophrenia must have been met within the past 12 months but are not met at the present time.

B. One of the conditions in Criterion G1(2) a, b, c, or d for general schizophrenia must still be present.

(*continued*)

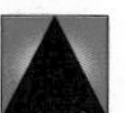

Table 13–11 (Continued)

C. The depressive symptoms must be sufficiently prolonged, severe, and extensive to meet criteria for at least a mild depressive episode.

Residual schizophrenia

A. The general criteria for schizophrenia must have been met at some time in the past but are not met at the present time.

B. At least four of the following "negative" symptoms have been present throughout the previous 12 months:
 (1) psychomotor slowing or underactivity;
 (2) definite blunting of affect;
 (3) passivity and lack of initiative;
 (4) poverty of either the quantity or the content of speech;
 (5) poor nonverbal communication by facial expression, eye contact, voice modulation, or posture;
 (6) poor social performance or self-care.

Simple schizophrenia

A. There is slow but progressive development, over a period of at least 1 year, of all three of the following:
 (1) a significant and consistent change in the overall quality of some aspects of personal behavior, manifest as loss of drive and interests, aimlessness, idleness, a selfabsorbed attitude, and social withdrawal;
 (2) gradual appearance and deepening of "negative" symptoms such as marked apathy, paucity of speech, underactivity, blunting of affect, passivity and lack of initiative, and poor nonverbal communication (by facial expression, eye contact, voice modulation, and posture);
 (3) marked decline in social, scholastic, or occupational performance.

B. At no time are there any of the symptoms referred to in criterion G1 for general schizophrenia, nor are there hallucinations or well-formed delusions of any kind; i.e., the individual must never have met the criteria for any other type of schizophrenia or for any other psychotic disorder.

C. There is no evidence of dementia or any other organic mental disorder.

Other schizophrenia

Schizophrenia, unspecified

(From World Health Organization. *The ICD-10 Classification of Mental and Behavioural Disorders: Diagnostic Criteria for Research.* Copyright, World Health Organization, Geneva, 1993.)

ICD-10

According to ICD-10, nine groups of symptoms are important for diagnosing schizophrenia: (1) thought echo, insertion, withdrawal, and broadcasting; (2) delusions of control, influence, or passivity; (3) hallucinatory voices; (4) other persistent delusions that are culturally inappropriate and impossible; (5) persistent hallucinations; (6) breaks or interpolation in thinking; (7) catatonic behavior; (8) "negative" symptoms resulting in social withdrawal and poor social performance but not caused by depression or medication; and (9) consistent, overall change in behavior. Unlike requirements in DSM-IV-TR for a diagnosis of schizophrenia, ICD-10 requires one clear symptom or two less clear symptoms from any one of groups 1 through 4 or symptoms from at least two of groups 5 through 8 to be present for most of the time during 1 month or more. Similar conditions lasting less than a month should be diagnosed as schizophrenia-like disorders. DSM-IV-TR defines schizophrenia as a disturbance of at least 6 months' duration, with two or more symptoms active for at least a month. A disorder diagnosed as schizophrenia under ICD-10 standards may be diagnosed as schizophreniform disorder under DSM-IV-TR standards. The latter disorder is, according to DSM-IV-TR, equivalent to schizophrenia, except for its duration, which is 1 to 6 months, and the absence of functional decline.

The ICD-10 general criteria for schizophrenia apply to all ICD-10 subtypes, except simple schizophrenia. The ICD-10 diagnostic criteria for the schizophrenia subtypes are presented in Table 13–11, and ICD-10 includes two residual categories: other schizophrenia (e.g., cenesthopathic schizophrenia [a disorder in which patients complain about or have delusions of a general sense of bodily existence]) and unspecified schizophrenia.

References

Angermeyer MC, Matchinger H. Labeling—stereotype—discrimination: An investigation of the stigma process. *Soc Psychiatry Psychiatr Epidemiol.* 2005;40:391.

Buchanan RW, Carpenter WT. Concept of schizophrenia. In: Sadock BJ, Sadock VA, eds. *Kaplan & Sadock's Comprehensive Textbook of Psychiatry.* 8th ed. Vol 1. Baltimore: Lippincott Williams & Wilkins; 2005:1329.

de Leon J, Diaz FJ. A meta-analysis of worldwide studies demonstrates an association between schizophrenia and tobacco smoking behaviors. *Schizophr Res.* 2005;76:135.

Hans SL, Auerbach JG, Auerbach AG, Marcus J. Development from birth to adolescence of children at-risk for schizophrenia. *J Child Adolesc Psychopharmacol.* 2005;15:384.

Hoff AL, Svetina C, Shields G, Stewart J, DeLisi LE. Ten year longitudinal study of neuropsychological functioning subsequent to a first episode of schizophrenia. *Schizophr Res.* 2005;78:2.

Keefe RSE, Young CA, Rock SL, Purdon SE, Gold JM, Breier A. One-year double-blind study of the neurocognitive efficacy of olanzapine, risperidone, and haloperidol in schizophrenia. *Schizophr Res.* 2006;81:1.

Krakowski M. Schizophrenia with aggressive and violent behaviors. *Psychiatr Ann.* 2005;35:45.

Mazeh D, Zemishlani C, Aizenberg D, Barak Y. Patients with very-late-onset schizophrenia-like psychosis: A follow-up study. *Am J Geriatr Psychol.* 2005;13:417.

Melle I, Johannesen JO, Friis S, Haahr U, Joa I, Larsen TK, Opjordsmoen S, Rond BK, Simonsen E, Vaglum P, McGlashan T. Early detection of the first episode of schizophrenia and suicidal behavior. *Am J of Psych.* 2006;163:800.

Vita A, De Peri L, Silenzi C, Dieci M. Brain morphology in first-episode schizophrenia: A meta-analysis of quantitative magnetic resonance imaging studies. *Schizophr Res.* 2006;82:75.

14 Other Psychotic Disorders

▲ 14.1 Schizophreniform Disorder

Gabriel Langfeldt (1895–1983) first used the term *schizophreniform* in 1939, at the University Psychiatric Clinic in Oslo, Norway, to describe a condition with sudden onset and benign course associated with mood symptoms and clouding of consciousness. The text revision of the fourth edition of the *Diagnostic and Statistical Manual of Mental Disorders* (DSM-IV-TR) describes schizophreniform disorder as similar to schizophrenia, except that its symptoms last at least 1 month but less than 6 months. Patients with schizophreniform disorder return to their baseline level of functioning once the disorder has resolved. In contrast, for a patient to meet the diagnostic criteria for schizophrenia, the symptoms must have been present for at least 6 months.

EPIDEMIOLOGY

Little is known about the incidence, prevalence, and sex ratio of schizophreniform disorder. The disorder is most common in adolescents and young adults and is less than half as common as schizophrenia. A lifetime prevalence rate of 0.2 percent and a 1-year prevalence rate of 0.1 percent have been reported.

Several studies have shown that the relatives of patients with schizophreniform disorder are at high risk of having other psychiatric disorders, but the distribution of the disorders differs from the distribution seen in the relatives of patients with schizophrenia and bipolar disorders. Specifically, the relatives of patients with schizophreniform disorders are more likely to have mood disorders than are the relatives of patients with schizophrenia. In addition, the relatives of patients with schizophreniform disorder are more likely to have a diagnosis of a psychotic mood disorder than are the relatives of patients with bipolar disorders.

ETIOLOGY

The cause of schizophreniform disorder is not known. As Langfeldt noted in 1939, patients with this diagnostic label are likely to be heterogeneous. In general, some patients have a disorder similar to schizophrenia, whereas others have a disorder similar to a mood disorder. Because of the generally good outcome, the disorder probably has similarities to the episodic nature of mood disorders. Some data, however, indicate a close relation to schizophrenia.

In support of the relation to mood disorders, several studies have shown that patients with schizophreniform disorder, as a group, have more affective symptoms (especially mania) and a better outcome than patients with schizophrenia. Also, the increased occurrence of mood disorders in the relatives of patients with schizophreniform disorder indicates a relation to mood disorders. Thus, the biological and epidemiological data are most consistent with the hypothesis that the current diagnostic category defines a group of patients, some of whom have a disorder similar to schizophrenia, whereas others have a disorder resembling a mood disorder.

Brain Imaging

A relative activation deficit in the inferior prefrontal region of the brain while the patient is performing a region-specific psychological task (the Wisconsin Card Sorting Test), as reported for patients with schizophrenia, has been reported in patients with schizophreniform disorder (Fig. 14.1–1). One study showed the deficit to be limited to the left hemisphere and also found impaired striatal activity suppression limited to the left hemisphere during the activation procedure. The data can be interpreted to indicate a physiological similarity between the psychosis of schizophrenia and the psychosis of schizophreniform disorder. Additional central nervous system (CNS) factors, as yet unidentified, may lead to either the long-term course of schizophrenia or the foreshortened course of schizophreniform disorder.

Although some data indicate that patients with schizophreniform disorder may have enlarged cerebral ventricles, as determined by computed tomography and magnetic resonance imaging, other data indicate that, unlike the enlargement seen in schizophrenia, the ventricular enlargement in schizophreniform disorder is not correlated with either outcome or other biological measures.

Other Biological Measures

Although brain imaging studies point to a similarity between schizophreniform disorder and schizophrenia, at least one study of electrodermal activity indicated a difference. Patients with schizophrenia who were born during the winter and spring months (a period of high risk for the birth of these patients) had hyporesponsive skin conductances, but this association was absent in patients with schizophreniform disorder. The significance and the meaning of this single study are difficult to interpret, but the results do suggest caution in assuming similarity between

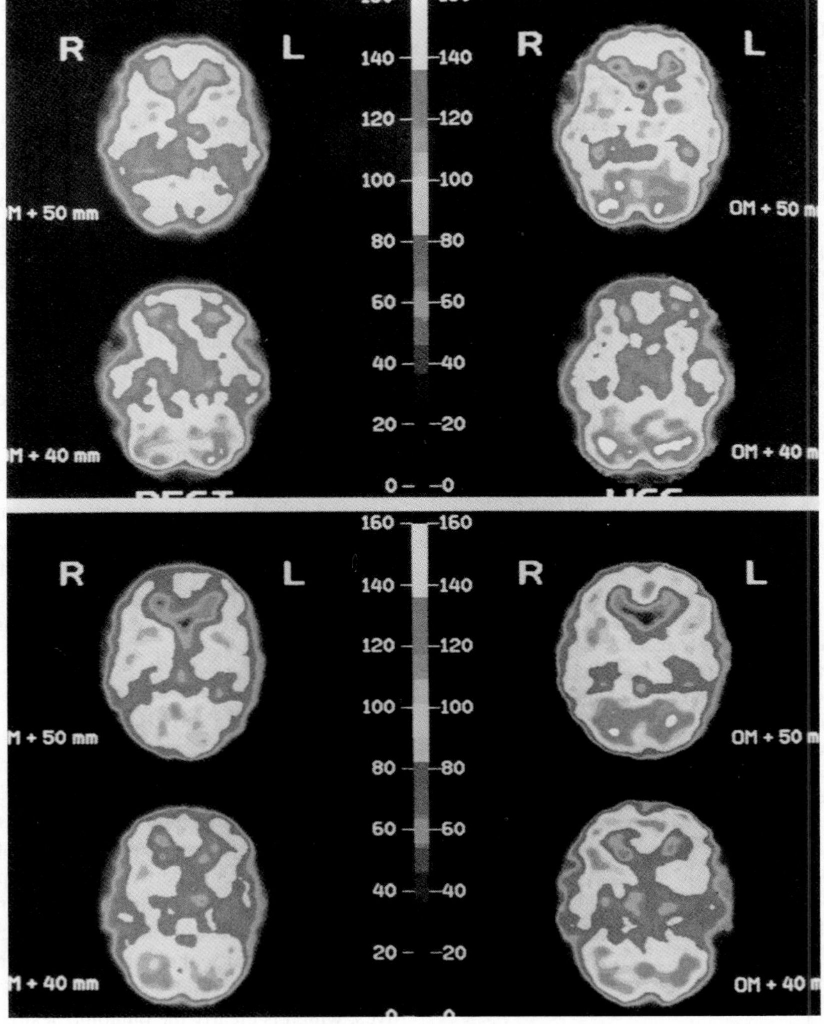

FIGURE 14.1–1

Regional cerebral blood flow distribution at rest (**left**) and during cerebral activation with the Wisconsin Card Sorting Test (**right**) in a patient with schizophreniform disorder (**top**) and a healthy volunteer (**bottom**). *OM* indicates orbitometeal line. (Reprinted from Rubin P, Holm S, Friberg L, et al. Altered modulation of prefrontal and subcortical brain activity in newly diagnosed schizophrenia and schizophreniform disorder. *Arch Gen Psychiatry*. 1991;48:992, with permission.)

patients with schizophrenia and those with schizophreniform disorder. Data from at least one study of eye tracking in the two groups also indicate that they may differ in some biological measures.

DIAGNOSTIC AND CLINICAL FEATURES

The DSM-IV-TR criteria for schizophreniform disorder are listed in Table 14.1–1. Schizophreniform disorder is an acute psychotic disorder that has a rapid onset and lacks a long prodromal phase. Although many patients with schizophreniform disorder may experience functional impairment at the time of an episode, they are unlikely to report a progressive decline in social and occupational functioning. The initial symptom profile is the same as that of schizophrenia in that two or more psychotic symptoms (hallucinations, delusions, disorganized speech and behavior, or negative symptoms) must be present. Schneiderian first-rank symptoms are frequently observed. Also an increased likelihood is found of emotional turmoil and confusion, the presence of which may indicate a good prognosis. Although negative symptoms may be present, they are relatively uncommon in schizophreniform disorder and are considered poor prognostic features. In a small series of first-admission patients with schizophreniform, one fourth had moderate to severe negative symptoms. Almost all were initially categorized as "schizophreniform disorder without good prognostic features," and 2 years later, 73 percent were rediagnosed with schizophrenia, compared with 38 percent of those with "good prognostic features."

By definition, patients with schizophreniform disorder return to their baseline state within 6 months. In some instances, the illness is episodic, with more than one episode occurring after long periods of full remission. If the combined duration of symptomatology exceeds 6 months, however, then schizophrenia should be considered.

Table 14.1–1
DSM-IV-TR Diagnostic Criteria for Schizophreniform Disorder

A. Criteria A, D, and E of schizophrenia are met.
B. An episode of the disorder (including prodromal, active, and residual phases) lasts at least 1 month but less than 6 months. (When the diagnosis must be made without waiting for recovery, it should be qualified as "provisional.")

Specify if:
Without good prognostic features
With good prognostic features: as evidenced by two (or more) of the following:
(1) onset of prominent psychotic symptoms within 4 weeks of the first noticeable change in usual behavior or functioning
(2) confusion or perplexity at the height of the psychotic episode
(3) good premorbid social and occupational functioning
(4) absence of blunted or flat affect

(From American Psychiatric Association. *Diagnostic and Statistical Manual of Mental Disorders*. 4th ed. Text rev. Washington, DC: American Psychiatric Association; copyright 2000, with permission.)

Ms. V was a 30-year-old white woman from a working-class family. She was born prematurely and as a toddler had a seizure disorder that was treated with phenobarbital (Luminal, Solfoton) for 1 year. She did well in school, but dropped out in the 12th grade, obtained a General Educational Development (GED) diploma, and began working at 18 years of age. She described her adolescence as a time when she was happy, outgoing, and had several friends. She married at 21 years of age and had two children, but 9 months before her initial hospitalization, she and her husband separated. Ms. V began working in a local factory, and she and her children moved in with her mother. About 6 weeks before her initial admission, Ms. V started feeling that drug dealers and gangsters were out to hurt her and that people were poisoning her food. She also did not let her children eat, fearing they would die from food poisoning. She was admitted to the hospital for 2 weeks but did not receive any medications at that time. Three weeks after discharge, she was readmitted with the same symptoms and also experienced thought broadcasting, thought insertion, and olfactory hallucinations. She was treated with haloperidol (Haldol) and was discharged after 1 month. She later moved to Florida with her mother and children, worked full time, and remained free of symptoms without treatment for 9 years. At that time, she again became psychotic, but after treatment with olanzapine (Zyprexa) for 1 month, she recovered fully and resumed her usual social and occupational functioning. (Courtesy of Bushra Naz, M.D., Laura J. Fochtmann, M.D., and Evelyn J. Bromet, M.D.)

DIFFERENTIAL DIAGNOSIS

It is important to first differentiate schizophreniform disorder from psychoses that can arise from medical conditions. This is accomplished by taking a detailed history and physical examination and, when indicated, performing laboratory tests or imaging studies. A detailed history of medication use, including over-the-counter medications and herbal products, is essential because many therapeutic agents can also produce an acute psychosis. Although it is not always possible to distinguish substance-induced psychosis from other psychotic disorders cross-sectionally, a rapid onset of psychotic symptoms in a patient with a significant substance history should raise the suspicion of a substance-induced psychosis. A detailed substance use history and toxicological screen are also important for treatment planning in an individual with a new onset of psychosis.

The duration of psychotic symptoms is one of the factors that distinguish schizophreniform disorder from other syndromes. Schizophrenia is diagnosed if the duration of the prodromal, active, and residual phases lasts for more than 6 months, whereas symptoms that occur for less than 1 month indicate a brief psychotic disorder. In DSM-IV-TR, a diagnosis of brief psychotic disorder does not require that a major stressor be present.

To distinguish mood disorders with psychotic features from schizophreniform disorder is sometimes difficult. Furthermore, schizophreniform disorder and schizophrenia can be highly comorbid with mood and anxiety disorders. Additional confounds are that mood symptoms, such as loss of interest and pleasure, may be difficult to distinguish from negative symptoms, avolition, and anhedonia. Some mood symptoms may also be present during the early course of schizophrenia. A thorough longitudinal history is important in elucidating the diagnosis because the presence of psychotic symptoms exclusively during periods of mood disturbance is an indication of a primary mood disorder.

COURSE AND PROGNOSIS

The course of schizophreniform disorder, for the most part, is defined in the criteria. It is a psychotic illness lasting more than 1 month and less than 6 months. The real issue is what happens to persons with this illness over time. Most estimates of progression to schizophrenia range between 60 and 80 percent. What happens to the other 20 to 40 percent is currently not known. Some will have a second or third episode during which they will deteriorate into a more chronic condition of schizophrenia. A few, however, may have only this single episode and then continue on with their lives, which is clearly the outcome desired by all clinicians and family members, although it is probably a rare occurrence and should not be held out as likely.

TREATMENT

Hospitalization, which is often necessary in treating patients with schizophreniform disorder, allows effective assessment, treatment, and supervision of a patient's behavior. The psychotic symptoms can usually be treated by a 3- to 6-month course of antipsychotic drugs (e.g., risperidone). Several studies have shown that patients with schizophreniform disorder respond to antipsychotic treatment much more rapidly than patients with schizophrenia. In one study, about 75 percent of patients with schizophreniform disorder and only 20 percent of the patients with schizophrenia responded to antipsychotic medications within 8 days. A trial of lithium (Eskalith), carbamazepine (Tegretol), or valproate (Depakene) may be warranted for treatment and prophylaxis if a patient has a recurrent episode. Psychotherapy is usually necessary to help patients integrate the psychotic experience into their understanding of their own minds and lives. Electroconvulsive therapy may be indicated for some patients, especially those with marked catatonic or depressed features.

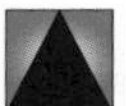

Table 14.1–2
ICD-10 Diagnostic Guidelines for Acute Schizophrenia-Like Psychotic Disorder

A. The onset of psychotic symptoms must be acute (2 weeks or less from a nonpsychotic to a clearly psychotic state).
B. Symptoms that fulfill the criteria of schizophrenia must have been present for the majority of time.
C. The criteria for acute polymorphic psychotic disorder are not fulfilled.

If the psychotic symptoms last for more than 1 month, then the diagnosis should be changed to schizophrenia.

(From World Health Organization. *The ICD-10 Classification of Mental and Behavioural Disorders: Diagnostic Criteria for Research*. Geneva: World Health Organization; 1992, with permission.)

Finally, most patients with schizophreniform disorder progress to full-blown schizophrenia despite treatment. In those cases, a course of management consistent with a chronic illness must be formulated.

ICD-10

The tenth revision of *International Statistical Classification of Diseases and Related Health Problems* (ICD-10) contains a conceptually similar category to schizophreniform disorder, namely, acute schizophrenia-like psychotic disorder. For this disorder, patients fulfill the ICD-10 criteria for schizophrenia, but the duration is less than 1 month. Most important, the onset of symptoms must be acute ("2 weeks or less from a nonpsychotic to a clearly psychotic state"). Thus, in contrast to the DSM-IV-TR, the ICD-10 is more specific about the nature of the onset of psychotic symptoms (Table 14.1–2).

References

Arseneault L, Cannon M, Murray R, Poulton R, Caspi A, Moffitt TE. Childhood origins of violent behaviour in adults with schizophreniform disorder. *Br J Psychiatry.* 2003;183:520–525.

Benazzi F. Outcome of schizophreniform disorder. *Curr Psychiatry Rep.* 2003; 5:192.

Bertolino A, Sciota D, Brudaglio F, Altamura M, Blasi G, Bellomo A, Antonucci N, Callicott JH, Goldberg TE, Scarabino T, Weinberger DR, Nardini M. Working memory deficits and levels of *N*-acetylaspartate in patients with schizophreniform disorder. *Am J Psychiatry.* 2003;160:483–489.

Keshavan MS, Duggal HS, Veeragandham G, McLaughlin NM, Montrose DM, Haas GL, Schooler NR. Personality dimensions in first-episode psychoses. *Am J Psychiatry.* 2005;162:102–109.

Kim-Cohen J, Caspi A, Moffitt TE, Harrington H, Milne BJ, Poulton R. Prior juvenile diagnoses in adults with mental disorder: Developmental follow-back of a prospective-longitudinal cohort. *Arch Gen Psychiatry.* 2003; 60:709.

Lauriello J, Erickson BR, Keith SJ. Schizoaffective disorder, schizophreniform disorder, and brief psychotic disorder. In: Sadock BJ, Sadock VA, eds. *Kaplan & Sadock's Comprehensive Textbook of Psychiatry.* 7th ed. Vol. 1. Baltimore: Lippincott Williams & Wilkins; 2000:1232.

Naz B, Bromet EJ, Mojtabai R. Distinguishing between first-admission schizophreniform disorder and schizophrenia. *Schizophren Res.* 2003; 62:51.

Naz B, Fochtmann LJ, Bromet EJ. Schizophreniform disorder. In: Sadock BJ, Sadock VA, eds. *Kaplan & Sadock's Comprehensive Textbook of Psychiatry.* 8th ed. Vol. 1. Baltimore: Lippincott Williams & Wilkins; 2005: 1522.

Norman RMG, Scholten DJ, Malla AK, Ballageer T. Early signs for schizophrenia spectrum disorders. *J Nerv Ment Dis.* 2005;193:17–23.

Perkins D, Lieberman J, Gu H, Tohen M, McEvoy J, Green A, Zipursky R, Strakowski S, Sharma T, Kahn R, Gur R, Tollefson G. Predictors of antipsychotic treatment response in patients with first-episode schizophrenia, schizoaffective and schizophreniform disorders. *Br J Psychiatry.* 2004;185: 18–24.

▲ 14.2 Schizoaffective Disorder

As the term implies, *schizoaffective disorder* has features of both schizophrenia and affective disorders (now called *mood disorders*). In current diagnostic systems, patients can receive the diagnosis of schizoaffective disorder if they fit into one of the following six categories: (1) patients with schizophrenia who have mood symptoms; (2) patients with mood disorder who have symptoms of schizophrenia; (3) patients with both mood disorder and schizophrenia; (4) patients with a third psychosis unrelated to schizophrenia and mood disorder; (5) patients whose disorder is on a continuum between schizophrenia and mood disorder; and (6) patients with some combination of the above. The revised fourth edition of the *Diagnostic and Statistical Manual of Mental Disorders* (DSM-IV-TR) incorporated the stricter time frame of 1 month's duration of schizophrenia symptoms and required an "uninterrupted period of illness during which at some time, either there is a Major Depressive Episode, a Manic Episode, or a Mixed Episode concurrent with symptoms that meet Criterion A for Schizophrenia." DSM-IV-TR also elaborated more on the criterion of duration of the mood symptoms relative to the psychotic symptoms. In the tenth revision of *International Statistical Classification of Diseases and Related Health Problems* (ICD-10), schizoaffective disorder is a distinct entity and can be applied to patients who have co-occurring mood symptoms and schizophrenic-like mood-incongruent psychosis.

George H. Kirby, in 1913, and August Hoch, in 1921, both described patients with mixed features of schizophrenia and affective (mood) disorders. Because their patients did not have the deteriorating course of dementia praecox, Kirby and Hoch classified them in Emil Kraepelin's manic-depressive psychosis group.

In 1933, Jacob Kasanin introduced the term *schizoaffective disorder* to refer to a disorder with symptoms of both schizophrenia and mood disorders. In patients with the disorder, the onset of symptoms was sudden and often occurred in adolescence. Patients tended to have a good premorbid level of functioning, and often a specific stressor preceded the onset of symptoms. The family histories of the patients often included a mood disorder. Because Eugen Bleuler's broad concept of schizophrenia had eclipsed Kraepelin's narrow concept, Kasanin believed that the patients had a type of schizophrenia. From 1933 to about 1970, patients whose symptoms were similar to those of Kasanin's patients were variously classified as having schizoaffective disorder, atypical schizophrenia, good-prognosis schizophrenia, remitting schizophrenia, and cycloid psychosis—terms that emphasized a relation to schizophrenia.

Around 1970, two sets of data shifted the view of schizoaffective disorder from a schizophrenic illness to a mood disorder. First, lithium carbonate (Eskalith) was shown to be an effective and specific treatment for both bipolar disorders and some cases of schizoaffective disorder. Second, the United States–United Kingdom study published in 1968 by John Cooper and his colleagues showed that the variation in the number of patients classified as schizophrenic in the United States and in the United Kingdom resulted from an overemphasis in the United States on the presence of psychotic symptoms as a diagnostic criterion for schizophrenia.

EPIDEMIOLOGY

The lifetime prevalence of schizoaffective disorder is less than 1 percent, possibly in the range of 0.5 to 0.8 percent. These figures, however, are estimates; various studies of schizoaffective disorder have used varying diagnostic criteria. In clinical practice, a preliminary diagnosis of schizoaffective disorder is frequently used when a clinician is uncertain of the diagnosis.

Gender and Age Differences

The literature describing gender and age differences among patients with schizoaffective disorder is limited. The depressive type of schizoaffective disorder may be more common in older persons than in younger persons, and the bipolar type may be more common in young adults than in older adults. The prevalence of the disorder has been reported to be lower in men than in women, particularly married women; the age of onset for women is later than that for men, as in schizophrenia. Men with schizoaffective disorder are likely to exhibit antisocial behavior and to have a markedly flat or inappropriate affect.

ETIOLOGY

The cause of schizoaffective disorder is unknown. The disorder may be a type of schizophrenia, a type of mood disorder, or the simultaneous expression of each. Schizoaffective disorder may also be a distinct third type of psychosis, one that is unrelated to either schizophrenia or a mood disorder. The most likely possibility is that schizoaffective disorder is a heterogeneous group of disorders encompassing all of these possibilities.

Studies designed to explore the etiology have examined family histories, biological markers, short-term treatment responses, and long-term outcomes. Most studies have considered patients with schizoaffective disorder to be a homogeneous group, but recent studies have examined the bipolar and depressive types of schizoaffective disorder separately, and DSM-IV-TR has a classification for each type.

Although much of the family and genetic research in schizoaffective disorder is based on the premise that schizophrenia and the mood disorders are completely separate entities, some data indicate that they may be genetically related. Studies of the relatives of patients with schizoaffective disorder have reported inconsistent results; however, according to DSM-IV-TR, an increased risk of schizophrenia exists among the relatives of probands with schizoaffective disorder.

As a group, patients with schizoaffective disorder have a better prognosis than patients with schizophrenia and a worse prognosis than patients with mood disorders. Also, as a group, patients with schizoaffective disorder tend to have a nondeteriorating course and respond better to lithium than do patients with schizophrenia.

Consolidation of Data

A reasonable conclusion from the available data is that patients with schizoaffective disorder are a heterogeneous group: some have schizophrenia with prominent affective symptoms, others have a mood disorder with prominent schizophrenic symptoms, and still others have a distinct clinical syndrome. The hypothesis that patients with schizoaffective disorder have both schizophrenia and a mood disorder is untenable, because the calculated co-occurrence of the two disorders is much lower than the incidence of schizoaffective disorder.

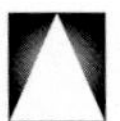

Table 14.2–1
DSM-IV-TR Diagnostic Criteria for Schizoaffective Disorder

A. An uninterrupted period of illness during which, at some time, there is either a major depressive episode, a manic episode, or a mixed episode concurrent with symptoms that meet Criterion A for schizophrenia.
Note: The major depressive episode must include Criterion A1: depressed mood.
B. During the same period of illness, there have been delusions or hallucinations for at least 2 weeks in the absence of prominent mood symptoms.
C. Symptoms that meet criteria for a mood episode are present for a substantial portion of the total duration of the active and residual periods of the illness.
D. The disturbance is not due to the direct physiological effects of a substance (e.g., a drug of abuse, a medication) or a general medical condition.

Specify type:
Bipolar type: if the disturbance includes a manic or a mixed episode (or a manic or a mixed episode and major depressive episodes)
Depressive type: if the disturbance only includes major depressive episodes

(From American Psychiatric Association. *Diagnostic and Statistical Manual of Mental Disorders.* 4th ed. Text rev. Washington, DC: American Psychiatric Association; copyright 2000, with permission.)

DIAGNOSIS AND CLINICAL FEATURES

The DSM-IV-TR diagnostic criteria are provided in Table 14.2–1. The diagnostic criteria, however, still leave much to interpretation. The clinician must accurately diagnose the affective illness, making sure it meets the criteria of either a manic or a depressive episode but also determining the exact length of each episode (not always easy or even possible).

The length of each episode is critical for two reasons. First, to meet the Criterion B (psychotic symptoms in the absence of the mood syndrome), it is important to know when the affective episode ends and the psychosis continues. Second, to meet Criterion C, the length of all mood episodes must be combined and compared with the total length of the illness. If the mood component is present for a substantial portion of the total illness, then that criterion is met. Calculating the total length of the episodes can be difficult, and the term "substantial portion" is not defined. In practice, most clinicians look for the mood component to be 15 to 20 percent of the total illness. Patients who have one full manic episode lasting 2 months, but who have had symptoms of schizophrenia for 10 years, do not meet the criteria for schizoaffective disorder. Instead, the diagnosis would be a mood episode superimposed on schizophrenia. Whether the bipolar or depressive type specifiers are helpful is unclear, but they may direct treatment options. These subtypes are often confused with earlier subtypes (schizophrenic versus affective type) thought to have implications in course and prognosis. As with most psychiatric diagnoses, schizoaffective disorder should not be used if the symptoms are caused by substance abuse or a secondary medical condition.

The ICD-10 diagnostic criteria for schizoaffective disorder are listed in Table 14.2–2.

Mrs. P was a 47-year-old, divorced, unemployed woman who lived alone and was chronically psychotic despite treatment with olanzapine, 20 mg per day, and citalopram (Celexa), 20 mg per day. She believed that she was getting messages from God and the police department to go on a mission to fight drug dealers. She also believed that the Mafia was trying to stop her in this pursuit. The onset of her illness began at 20 years of age, when she experienced the first of several depressive episodes. She also described periods when she felt more energetic, talkative, had decreased need for sleep, and was more active, sometimes cleaning her house the whole night. Approximately 4 years after the onset of her symptoms, she began to hear "voices" that became stronger when she got depressed, but were still present and continued to disturb her even when her mood was euthymic. Approximately 10 years after her illness began, she developed the belief that policemen were everywhere and that the neighbors were spying on her. She was hospitalized voluntarily. Two years later, she had another depressive episode, and the voices told her she could not live in her apartment. She was tried on lithium, antidepressants, and antipsychotic medications but continued to be chronically symptomatic with mood symptoms as well as psychosis. (Courtesy of Shmuel Fennig, M.D., Laura J. Fochtmann, M.D., and Gabrielle A. Carlson, M.D.)

DIFFERENTIAL DIAGNOSIS

The psychiatric differential diagnosis includes all the possibilities usually considered for mood disorders and for schizophrenia. In any differential diagnosis of psychotic disorders, a complete medical workup should be performed to rule out organic causes for the symptoms. A history of substance use (with or without positive results on a toxicology screening test) may indicate a substance-induced disorder. Preexisting medical conditions, their treatment, or both can cause psychotic and mood disorders. Any suspicion of a neurological abnormality warrants consideration of a brain scan to rule out anatomical pathology and an electroencephalogram (EEG) to determine any possible seizure disorders (e.g., temporal lobe epilepsy). Psychotic disorder caused by seizure disorder is more common than that seen in the general population. It tends to be characterized by paranoia, hallucinations, and ideas of reference. Patients with epilepsy with psychosis are believed to have a better level of function than patients with schizophrenic spectrum disorders. Better control of the seizures can reduce the psychosis.

COURSE AND PROGNOSIS

Considering the uncertainty and evolving diagnosis of schizoaffective disorder, it is difficult to determine the long-term course and prognosis. Given the definition of the diagnosis, patients with schizoaffective disorder might be expected to have a course similar to an episodic mood disorder, a chronic schizophrenic course, or some intermediate outcome. It has been presumed that an increasing presence of schizophrenic symptoms predicted worse

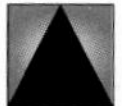

Table 14.2–2
ICD-10 Diagnostic Criteria for Schizoaffective Disorders

Note: This diagnosis depends upon an approximate "balance" between the number, severity, and duration of the schizophrenic and affective symptoms.

G1. The disorder meets the criteria for one of the affective disorders of moderate or severe degree, as specified for each category.

G2. Symptoms from at least one of the groups listed below must be clearly present for most of the time during a period of at least 2 weeks (these groups are almost the same as for schizophrenia):
  (1) Thought echo, thought insertion or withdrawal, thought broadcasting (Criterion G1[1]a for paranoid, hebephrenic, or catatonic schizophrenia);
  (2) Delusions of control, influence, or passivity, clearly referred to body or limb movements or specific thoughts, actions, or sensations (Criterion G1[1]b for paranoid, hebephrenic, or catatonic schizophrenia);
  (3) Hallucinatory voices giving a running commentary on the patient's behavior or discussing the patient among themselves, or other types of hallucinatory voices coming from some part of the body (Criterion G1[1]c for paranoid, hebephrenic, or catatonic schizophrenia);
  (4) Persistent delusions of other kinds that are culturally inappropriate and completely impossible, but not merely grandiose or persecutory (Criterion G1[1]d for paranoid, hebephrenic, or catatonic schizophrenia), e.g., has visited other worlds; can control the clouds by breathing in and out; can communicate with plants or animals without speaking;
  (5) Grossly irrelevant or incoherent speech, or frequent use of neologisms (a marked form of Criterion G1[2]b for paranoid, hebephrenic, or catatonic schizophrenia);
  (6) Intermittent but frequent appearance of some forms of catatonic behavior, such as posturing, waxy flexibility, and negativism (Criterion G1[2]c for paranoid, hebephrenic, or catatonic schizophrenia).

G3. Criteria G1 and G2 above must be met within the same episode of the disorder, and concurrently for at least part of the episode. Symptoms from both G1 and G2 must be prominent in the clinical picture.

G4. *Most commonly used exclusion clause.* The disorder is not attributable to organic mental disorder, or to psychoactive substance-related intoxication, dependence, or withdrawal.

Schizoaffective disorder, manic type

A. The general criteria for schizoaffective disorder must be met.

B. Criteria for a manic disorder must be met.

Other schizoaffective disorders

Schizoaffective disorder, unspecified

Comments

If desired, further subtypes of schizoaffective disorder may be specified, according to the longitudinal development of the disorder, as follows:

Concurrent affective and schizophrenic symptoms only

Symptoms as defined in Criterion G2 for schizoaffective disorders

Concurrent affective and schizophrenic symptoms beyond the duration of affective symptoms

(Reprinted with permission from World Health Organization. The *ICD-10 Classification of Mental and Behavioural Disorders: Diagnostic Criteria for Research.* Copyright, World Health Organization, Geneva, 1993.)

prognosis. After 1 year, patients with schizoaffective disorder had different outcomes, depending on whether their predominant symptoms were affective (better prognosis) or schizophrenic (worse prognosis). One study that followed patients diagnosed with schizoaffective disorder for 8 years found that the outcomes of these patients more closely resembled schizophrenia than a mood disorder with psychotic features.

TREATMENT

Mood stabilizers are a mainstay of treatment for bipolar disorders and would be expected to be important in the treatment of patients with schizoaffective disorder. One study that compared lithium with carbamazepine (Tegretol) found that carbamazepine was superior for schizoaffective disorder, depressive type, but found no difference in the two agents for the bipolar type. In practice, however, these medications are used extensively alone, in combination with each other, or with an antipsychotic agent. In manic episodes, patients who are schizoaffective should be treated aggressively with dosages of a mood stabilizer in the middle to high therapeutic blood concentration range. As the patient enters maintenance phase, the dosage can be reduced to low to middle range to avoid adverse effects and potential effects on organ systems (e.g., thyroid and kidney) and to improve ease of use and compliance. Laboratory monitoring of plasma drug concentrations and periodic screening of thyroid, kidney, and hematological functioning should be performed.

By definition many patients who are schizoaffective have major depressive episodes. Treatment with antidepressants mirrors treatment of bipolar depression. Care should be taken not to precipitate a cycle of rapid switches from depression to mania with the antidepressant. The choice of antidepressant should take into account previous antidepressant successes or failures. Selective serotonin reuptake inhibitors (e.g., fluoxetine [Prozac] and sertraline [Zoloft]) are often used as first-line agents because they have less effect on cardiac status and have a favorable overdose profile. Agitated or insomniac patients, however, may benefit from a tricyclic drug. As in all cases of intractable mania, the use of electroconvulsive therapy (ECT) should be considered. As mentioned, antipsychotic agents are important in the treatment of the psychotic symptoms of schizoaffective disorder.

Psychosocial Treatment

Patients benefit from a combination of family therapy, social skills training, and cognitive rehabilitation. Because the psychiatric field has had difficulty deciding on the exact diagnosis and prognosis of schizoaffective disorder, this uncertainty must be explained to the patient. The range of symptoms can be vast as patients contend with both ongoing psychosis and varying mood states. It can be very difficult for family members to keep up with the changing nature and needs of these patients. Medication regimens can be complicated, with multiple medications from all classes of drugs.

REFERENCES

Fennig S, Fochtmann LJ, Carlson GL. Schizoaffective disorder. In: Sadock BJ, Sadock VA, eds. *Kaplan & Sadock's Comprehensive Textbook of Psychiatry*. 8th ed. Vol. 1. Baltimore: Lippincott Williams & Wilkins; 2005:1533.

Hamshere ML, Bennett P, Williams N, Segurado R, Cardno A, Norton N, Lambert D, Williams H, Kirov G, Corvin A, Holmans P, Jones L, Jones I, Gill M, O'Donovan MC, Owen MJ, Craddock N. Genomewide linkage scan in schizoaffective disorder: Significant evidence for linkage at 1q42 close to DISC1, and suggestive evidence at 22q11 and 19p13. *Arch Gen Psychiatry*. 2005;62(10):1081–1088.

Ho BC, Black DW, Andreasen NC. Schizophrenia and other psychotic disorders. In: Hales RE, Yudofsky SC, eds. *The American Psychiatric Publishing Textbook of Clinical Psychiatry*. 4th ed. Washington, DC: American Psychiatric Publishing, Inc.; 2003:379–438.

Jarbin H, Ott Y, von Knorring A. Adult outcome of social function in adolescent-onset schizophrenia and affective psychosis. *J Am Acad Child Adolesc Psychiatry*. 2003;42:176–183.

Kelose JR. Arguments for the genetic basis of the bipolar spectrum. *J Affect Dis*. 2003;73:183–197.

Kilzieh N, Wood AE, Erdman J, Raskind M, Tapp A. Depression in Kraepelinian schizophrenia. *Comp Psychiatry*. 2003;44:1–6.

Lauriello J, Erickson BR, Keith SJ. Schizoaffective disorder, schizophreniform disorder, and brief psychotic disorder. In: Sadock BJ, Sadock VA, eds. *Kaplan & Sadock's Comprehensive Textbook of Psychiatry*. 7th ed. Vol. 1. Baltimore: Lippincott Williams & Wilkins; 2000:1232.

Marneros A. The schizoaffective phenomenon: The state of the art. *Acta Psychiatr Scand*. 2003;108:29–33.

Regnold WT, Thapar RK, Marano C, Gavirneri S, Kondapavuluru PV. Increased prevalence of type 2 diabetes mellitus among psychiatric inpatients with bipolar I affective and schizoaffective disorders independent of psychotropic drug use. *J Affect Disord*. 2003;70:19–26.

Soo Kwon J, Choi JS, Bahk WM, Yoon Kim C, Hyung Kim C, Chul Shin Y, Park BJ, Geun Oh C. Weight management program for treatment-emergent weight gain in olanzapine-treated patients with schizophrenia or schizoaffective disorder: A 12-week randomized controlled clinical trial. *J Clin Psychiatry*. 2006;67(4): 547–553.

▲ 14.3 Delusional Disorder and Shared Psychotic Disorder

Delusions are false fixed beliefs not in keeping with the culture. They are among the most interesting of psychiatric symptoms because of the great variety of false beliefs that can be held by so many people and because they are so difficult to treat. The diagnosis of delusional disorder is made when a person exhibits nonbizarre delusions of at least 1 month's duration that cannot be attributed to other psychiatric disorders. Definitions of the term delusion and types relevant to delusional disorders are presented in Table 14.3–1. *Nonbizarre* means that the delusions must be about situations that can occur in real life, such as being followed, infected, loved at a distance, and so on; that is, they usually have to do with phenomena that, although not real, are nonetheless possible. Several types of delusions may be present and the predominant type is specified when the diagnosis is made.

EPIDEMIOLOGY

An accurate assessment of the epidemiology of delusional disorder is hampered by the relative rareness of the disorder, as well as by its changing definitions in recent history. Moreover, delusional disorder may be underreported because delusional patients rarely seek psychiatric help unless forced to do so by their families or by the courts. Even with these limitations, however, the literature does support the contention that delusional disorder, although uncommon, has a relatively steady rate.

The prevalence of delusional disorder in the United States is currently estimated to be 0.025 to 0.03 percent. Thus, delusional disorder is much rarer than schizophrenia, which has a prevalence

Table 14.3–1
DSM-IV-TR Definition of Delusion and Certain Common Types Associated with Delusional Disorders

Delusion A false belief based on incorrect inference about external reality that is firmly sustained despite what almost everyone else believes and despite what constitutes incontrovertible and obvious proof of evidence to the contrary. The belief is not one ordinarily accepted by other members of the person's culture or subculture (e.g., it is not an article of religious faith). When a false belief involves a value judgment, it is regarded as a delusion only when the judgment is so extreme as to defy credibility. Delusional conviction occurs on a continuum and can sometimes be inferred from an individual's behavior. It is often difficult to distinguish between a delusion and an overvalued idea (in which case the individual has an unreasonable belief or idea but does not hold it as firmly as is the case with a delusion). Delusions are subdivided according to their content. Some of the more common types are listed below:

Bizarre—A delusion that involves a phenomenon that the person's culture would regard as totally implausible.

Delusional jealousy—The delusion that one's sexual partner is unfaithful.

Erotomanic—A delusion that another person, usually of higher status, is in love with the individual.

Grandiose—A delusion of inflated worth, power, knowledge, identity, or special relationship to a deity or famous person.

Mood-congruent—See mood-congruent psychotic features.

Mood-incongruent—See mood-incongruent psychotic features.

Of being controlled—A delusion in which feelings, impulses, thoughts, or actions are experienced as being under the control of some external force rather than being under one's own control.

Of reference—A delusion whose theme is that events, objects, or other persons in one's immediate environment have a particular and unusual significance. These delusions are usually of a negative or pejorative nature, but also may be grandiose in content. This differs from an idea of reference, in which the false belief is not as firmly held nor as fully organized into a true belief.

Persecutory—A delusion in which the central theme is that one (or someone to whom one is close) is being attacked, harassed, cheated, persecuted, or conspired against.

Somatic—A delusion whose main content pertains to the appearance or functioning of one's body.

Thought broadcasting—The delusion that one's thoughts are being broadcast out loud so that they can be perceived by others.

Thought insertion—The delusion that certain of one's thought are not one's own, but rather are inserted into one's mind.

Mood-congruent psychotic features—Delusions or hallucinations whose content is entirely consistent with the typical themes of a depressed or manic mood. If the mood is depressed, the content of the delusions or hallucinations would involve themes of personal inadequacy, guilt, disease, death, nihilism, or deserved punishment. The content of the delusion may include themes of persecution if these are based on self-derogatory concepts such as deserved punishment. If the mood is manic, the content of the delusions or hallucinations would involve themes of inflated worth, power, knowledge, or identity, or a special relationship to a deity or a famous person. The content of the delusion may include themes of persecution if these are based on concepts such as inflated worth or deserved punishment.

Mood-incongruent psychotic features—Delusions or hallucinations whose content is not consistent with the typical themes of a depressed or manic mood. In the case of depression, the delusions or hallucinations would not involve themes of personal inadequacy, guilt, disease, death, nihilism, or deserved punishment. In the case of mania, the delusions or hallucinations would not involve themes of inflated worth, power, knowledge, or identity, or a special relationship to a deity or a famous person. Examples of mood-incongruent psychotic features include persecutory delusions (without self-derogatory or grandiose content), thought insertion, thought broadcasting, and delusions of being controlled whose content has no apparent relationship to any of the themes listed above.

(From American Psychiatric Association. *Diagnostic and Statistical Manual of Mental Disorders.* 4th ed. Text rev. Washington, DC: American Psychiatric Association; copyright 2000, with permission.)

of about 1 percent, and the mood disorders, which have a prevalence of about 5 percent. The annual incidence of delusional disorder is 1 to 3 new cases per 100,000 persons. According to the text revision of the fourth edition of the *Diagnostic and Statistical Manual of Mental Disorders* (DSM-IV-TR), delusional disorders account for only 1 to 2 percent of all admissions to inpatient mental health facilities. The mean age of onset is about 40 years, but the range for age of onset runs from 18 years of age to the 90s. A slight preponderance of female patients exists. Men are more likely to develop paranoid delusions than women, who are more likely to develop delusions of erotomania. Many patients are married and employed, but some association is seen with recent immigration and low socioeconomic status.

ETIOLOGY

As with all major psychiatric disorders, the cause of delusional disorder is unknown. Moreover, patients currently classified as having delusional disorder probably have a heterogeneous group of conditions with delusions as the predominant symptom. The central concept about the cause of delusional disorder is its distinctness from schizophrenia and the mood disorders. Delusional disorder is much rarer than either schizophrenia or mood disorders, with a later onset than schizophrenia and a much less pronounced female predominance than the mood disorders. The most convincing data come from family studies that report an increased prevalence of delusional disorder and related personality traits (e.g., suspiciousness, jealousy, and secretiveness) in the relatives of delusional disorder probands. Family studies have reported neither an increased incidence of schizophrenia and mood disorders in the families of delusional disorder probands nor an increased incidence of delusional disorder in the families of probands with schizophrenia. Long-term follow-up of patients with delusional disorder indicates that the diagnosis of delusional disorder is relatively stable, with less than one fourth of the patients eventually being reclassified as having schizophrenia and less than 10 percent of patients eventually being reclassified as having a mood disorder. These data indicate that delusional disorder is not simply an early stage in the development of one or both of these two more common disorders.

Biological Factors

A wide range of nonpsychiatric medical conditions and substances, including clear-cut biological factors, can cause delusions, but not everyone with a brain tumor, for example, has delusions. Unique, and not yet understood, factors in a patient's brain and personality are likely to be relevant to the specific pathophysiology of delusional disorder.

The neurological conditions most commonly associated with delusions affect the limbic system and the basal ganglia. Patients whose delusions are caused by neurological diseases and who show no intellectual impairment tend to have complex delusions similar to those in patients with delusional disorder. Conversely, patients with neurological disorder with intellectual impairments often have simple delusions unlike those in patients with delusional disorder. Thus, delusional disorder may involve the limbic system or basal ganglia in patients who have intact cerebral cortical functioning.

Delusional disorder can arise as a normal response to abnormal experiences in the environment, the peripheral nervous system, or the central nervous system (CNS). Thus, if patients have erroneous sensory experiences of being followed (e.g., hearing footsteps), they may come to believe that they are actually being followed. This hypothesis hinges on the presence of hallucinatory-like experiences that need to be explained. The presence of such hallucinatory experiences in delusional disorder has not been proved.

Psychodynamic Factors

Practitioners have a strong clinical impression that many patients with delusional disorder are socially isolated and have attained less than expected levels of achievement. Specific psychodynamic theories about the cause and the evolution of delusional symptoms involve suppositions regarding hypersensitive persons and specific ego mechanisms: reaction formation, projection, and denial.

Freud's Contributions. Sigmund Freud believed that delusions, rather than being symptoms of the disorder, are part of a healing process. In 1896, he described projection as the main defense mechanism in paranoia. Later, Freud read *Memories of My Nervous Illness*, an autobiographical account by Daniel Paul Schreber. Although he never met Schreber, Freud theorized from his review of the autobiography that unconscious homosexual tendencies are defended against by denial and projection. According to classic psychodynamic theory, the dynamics underlying the formation of delusions for a female patient are the same as for a male patient. Careful studies of patients with delusions have been unable to corroborate Freud's theories, although they may be relevant in individual cases. Overall, no higher incidence of homosexual ideation or activity is found in patients with delusions than in other groups. Freud's major contribution, however, was to demonstrate the role of projection in the formation of delusional thought.

Paranoid Pseudocommunity. Norman Cameron described seven situations that favor the development of delusional disorders: an increased expectation of receiving sadistic treatment, situations that increase distrust and suspicion, social isolation, situations that increase envy and jealousy, situations that lower self-esteem, situations that cause persons to see their own defects in others, and situations that increase the potential for rumination over probable meanings and motivations. When frustration from any combination of these conditions exceeds the tolerable limit, persons become withdrawn and anxious; they realize that something is wrong, seek an explanation for the problem, and crystallize a delusional system as a solution. Elaboration of the delusion to include imagined persons and attribution of malevolent motivations to both real and imagined persons result in the organization of the *pseudocommunity*—a perceived community of plotters. This delusional entity hypothetically binds together projected fears and wishes to justify the patient's aggression and to provide a tangible target for the patient's hostilities.

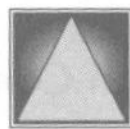

Table 14.3–2
Risk Factors Associated with Delusional Disorder

Advanced age
Sensory impairment or isolation
Family history
Social isolation
Personality features (e.g., unusual interpersonal sensitivity)
Recent immigration

Other Psychodynamic Factors. Clinical observations indicate that many, if not all, paranoid patients experience a lack of trust in relationships. A hypothesis relates this distrust to a consistently hostile family environment, often with an overcontrolling mother and a distant or sadistic father. Erik Erikson's concept of trust versus mistrust in early development is a useful model to explain the suspiciousness of the paranoid who never went through the healthy experience of having his or her needs satisfied by what Erikson termed the "outer-providers." Thus, they have a general distrust of their environment.

Defense Mechanisms. Patients with delusional disorder use primarily the defense mechanisms of reaction formation, denial, and projection. They use reaction formation as a defense against aggression, dependence needs, and feelings of affection and transform the need for dependence into staunch independence. Patients use denial to avoid awareness of painful reality. Consumed with anger and hostility and unable to face responsibility for the rage, they project their resentment and anger onto others and use projection to protect themselves from recognizing unacceptable impulses in themselves.

Other Relevant Factors. Delusions have been linked to a variety of additional factors such as social and sensory isolation, socioeconomic deprivation, and personality disturbance. The deaf, the visually impaired, and possibly immigrants with limited ability in a new language may be more vulnerable to delusion formation than the normal population. Vulnerability is heightened with advanced age. Delusional disturbance and other paranoid features are common in the elderly. In short, multiple factors are associated with the formation of delusions, and the source and pathogenesis of delusional disorders per se have yet to be specified (Table 14.3–2).

DIAGNOSIS AND CLINICAL FEATURES

The DSM-IV-TR diagnostic criteria for delusional disorder are listed in Table 14.3–3.

Mental Status

General Description. Patients are usually well groomed and well dressed, without evidence of gross disintegration of personality or of daily activities, yet they may seem eccentric, odd, suspicious, or hostile. They are sometimes litigious and may make this inclination clear to the examiner. The most remarkable feature of patients with delusional disorder is that the mental status examination shows them to be quite normal except for a markedly abnormal delusional system. Patients may attempt to engage clinicians as allies in their delusions, but a clinician should not pretend to accept the delusion; this collusion further

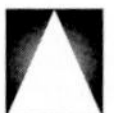

Table 14.3–3
DSM-IV-TR Diagnostic Criteria for Delusional Disorder

A. Nonbizarre delusions (i.e., involving situations that occur in real life, such as being followed, poisoned, infected, loved at a distance, or deceived by spouse or lover, or having a disease) of at least 1 month's duration.
B. Criterion A for schizophrenia has never been met. **Note:** Tactile and olfactory hallucinations may be present in delusional disorder if they are related to the delusional theme.
C. Apart from the impact of the delusion(s) or its ramifications, functioning is not markedly impaired and behavior is not obviously odd or bizarre.
D. If mood episodes have occurred concurrently with delusions, their total duration has been brief relative to the duration of the delusional periods.
E. The disturbance is not due to the direct physiological effects of a substance (e.g., a drug of abuse, a medication) or a general medical condition.

Specify type (the following types are assigned based on the predominant delusional theme):
Erotomanic type: delusions that another person, usually of higher status, is in love with the individual.
Grandiose type: delusions of inflated worth, power, knowledge, identity, or special relationship to a deity or famous person
Jealous type: delusions that the individual's sexual partner is unfaithful
Persecutory type: delusions that the person (or someone to whom the person is close) is being malevolently treated in some way
Somatic type: delusions that the person has some physical defect or general medical condition
Mixed type: delusions characteristic of more than one of the above types but no one theme predominates
Unspecified type

(From American Psychiatric Association. *Diagnostic and Statistical Manual of Mental Disorders.* 4th ed. Text rev. Washington, DC: American Psychiatric Association; copyright 2000, with permission.)

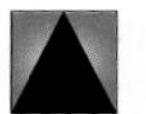

Table 14.3–4
ICD-10 Diagnostic Criteria for Delusional Disorders

Delusional disorder
A. A delusion or a set of related delusions, other than those listed as typically schizophrenic in Criterion G1(1)b or d for paranoid, hebephrenic, or catatonic schizophrenia (i.e., other than completely impossible or culturally inappropriate), must be present. The commonest examples are persecutory, grandiose, hypochondriacal, jealous (zelotypic), or erotic delusions.
B. The delusion(s) in Criterion A must be present for at least 3 months.
C. The general criteria for schizophrenia are not fulfilled.
D. There must be no persistent hallucinations in any modality (but there may be transitory or occasional auditory hallucinations that are not in the third person or giving a running commentary).
E. Depressive symptoms (or even a depressive episode) may be present intermittently, provided that the delusions persist at times when there is no disturbance of mood.
F. Most commonly used exclusion clause. There must be no evidence of primary or secondary organic mental disorder as listed under organic, including symptomatic, mental disorders, or of a psychotic disorder due to psychoactive substance use.

Specification for possible subtypes
The following types may be specified if desired: persecutory; litigious; self-referential; grandiose; hypochondriacal (somatic); jealous; erotomanic.

Other persistent delusional disorders
This is a residual category for persistent delusional disorders that do not meet the criteria for delusional disorder. Disorders in which delusions are accompanied by persistent hallucinatory voices or by schizophrenic symptoms that are insufficient to meet criteria for schizophrenia should be coded here. Delusional disorders that have lasted for less than 3 months should, however, be coded, at least temporarily, under acute and transient psychotic disorders.

Persistent delusional disorder, unspecified

(From World Health Organization. *The ICD-10 Classification of Mental and Behavioural Disorders: Diagnostic Criteria for Research.* Copyright, World Health Organization, Geneva, 1993, with permission.)

confounds reality and sets the stage for eventual distrust between the patient and the therapist.

Mood, Feelings, and Affect. Patients' moods are consistent with the content of their delusions. A patient with grandiose delusions is euphoric; one with persecutory delusions is suspicious. Whatever the nature of the delusional system, the examiner may sense some mild depressive qualities.

Perceptual Disturbances. By definition, patients with delusional disorder do not have prominent or sustained hallucinations. According to DSM-IV-TR, tactile or olfactory hallucinations may be present if they are consistent with the delusion (e.g., somatic delusion of body odor). A few delusional patients have other hallucinatory experiences—virtually always auditory rather than visual.

Thought. Disorder of thought content, in the form of delusions, is the key symptom of the disorder. The delusions are usually systematized and are characterized as being possible; for example, delusions of being persecuted, having an unfaithful spouse, being infected with a virus, or being loved by a famous person. These examples of delusional content contrast with the bizarre and impossible delusional content in some patients with schizophrenia. The delusional system itself can be complex or simple. Patients lack other signs of thought disorder, although some may be verbose, circumstantial, or idiosyncratic in their speech when they talk about their delusions. Clinicians should not assume that all unlikely scenarios are delusional; the veracity of a patient's beliefs should be checked before deeming their content to be delusional. Table 14.3–4 lists the tenth revision of *International Statistical Classification of Diseases and Related Health Problems* (ICD-10) diagnostic criteria for delusional disorder.

Sensorium and Cognition

ORIENTATION. Patients with delusional disorder usually have no abnormality in orientation unless they have a specific delusion about a person, place, or time.

MEMORY. Memory and other cognitive processes are intact in patients with delusional disorder.

Impulse Control. Clinicians must evaluate patients with delusional disorder for ideation or plans to act on their delusional material by suicide, homicide, or other violence. Although the incidence of these behaviors is not known, therapists should not hesitate to ask patients about their suicidal, homicidal, or other violent plans. Destructive aggression is most common in patients with a history of violence; if aggressive feelings existed in the past, therapists should ask patients how they managed those feelings. If patients cannot control their impulses, hospitalization is probably necessary. Therapists can sometimes help foster a therapeutic alliance by openly discussing how hospitalization can help patients gain additional control of their impulses.

Judgment and Insight. Patients with delusional disorder have virtually no insight into their condition and are almost always brought to the hospital by the police, family members, or employers. Judgment can best be assessed by evaluating the patient's past, present, and planned behavior.

Reliability. Patients with delusional disorder are usually reliable in their information, except when it impinges on their delusional system.

Types

Persecutory Type. The delusion of persecution is a classic symptom of delusional disorder; persecutory-type and jealousy-type delusions are probably the forms seen most frequently by psychiatrists. Patients with this subtype are convinced that they are being persecuted or harmed. The persecutory beliefs are often associated with querulousness, irritability, and anger, and the individual who acts out his or her anger may at times be assaultive or even homicidal. At other times, such individuals may become preoccupied with formal litigation against their perceived persecutors. In contrast to persecutory delusions in schizophrenia, the clarity, logic, and systematic elaboration of the persecutory theme in delusional disorder leave a remarkable stamp on this condition. The absence of other psychopathology, of deterioration in personality, or of deterioration in most areas of functioning also contrasts with the typical manifestations of schizophrenia.

Mrs. S, 62 years of age, was referred to a psychiatrist because of complaints of not being able to sleep. Before this episode, she worked full time taking care of children, played tennis almost every day, and managed her household chores. Her chief complaint was that her downstairs neighbor wanted to get her to move away and was doing a variety of things to harass her. At first, she based her belief on certain looks that he gave her and damage done to her mailbox, but later she believed he might be leaving empty bottles of cleaning solutions in the basement, so she would be overcome by fumes. As a result, the patient was fearful of falling asleep, convinced that she might be asphyxiated and not awaken in time to get help. She felt somewhat depressed and believed her appetite might be diminished from the stress of being harassed. She had not lost weight and still enjoyed playing tennis and going out with friends. At one point, she considered moving to another apartment but then decided to fight back. The episode had gone on for 8 months when her daughter persuaded her to have a psychiatric assessment. She was pleasant and cooperative in the interview. Except for the specific delusion and mild depressive symptoms, her mental status was normal.

Her history revealed that she was depressed 30 years before after the death of a close friend. She saw a counselor for several months, which she found helpful, but was not treated with medication. For the current episode, she agreed to take medications, although she believed her neighbor was more in need of treatment than she was. Her symptoms improved somewhat with oral risperidone (Risperdal), 2 mg every night, and oral clonazepam (Klonopin), 0.5 mg every morning and every night.

Jealous Type

Delusional disorder with delusions of infidelity has been called *conjugal paranoia* when it is limited to the delusion that a spouse has been unfaithful. The eponym *Othello syndrome* has been used to describe morbid jealousy that can arise from multiple concerns. The delusion usually afflicts men, often those with no prior psychiatric illness. It may appear suddenly and serve to explain a host of present and past events involving the spouse's behavior. The condition is difficult to treat and may diminish only on separation, divorce, or death of the spouse.

Marked jealousy (usually termed *pathological* or *morbid jealousy*) is thus a symptom of many disorders—including schizophrenia (in which female patients more commonly display this feature), epilepsy, mood disorders, drug abuse, and alcoholism—for which treatment is directed at the primary disorder. Jealousy is a powerful emotion; when it occurs in delusional disorder or as part of another condition, it can be potentially dangerous and has been associated with violence, notably both suicide and homicide (Fig. 14.3–1). The forensic aspects

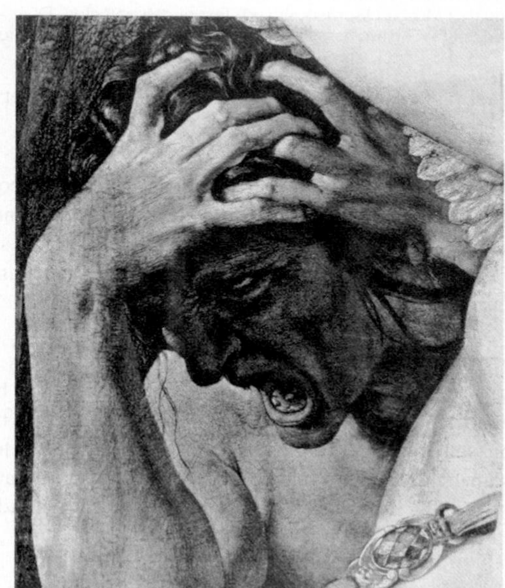

FIGURE 14.3–1

A detail from the painting *An Allegory with Venus and Cupid* by Bronzino depicting a jealous lover. There is a high risk of homicide when morbid jealousy becomes the dominant theme in a relationship in which one partner is jealous of the other. That rage is well-depicted in Bronzino's painting.

of the symptom have been noted repeatedly, especially its role as a motive for murder. Physical and verbal abuse occur more frequently, however, than do extreme actions among individuals with this symptom. Caution and care in deciding how to deal with such presentations are essential not only for diagnosis, but also from the point of view of safety.

F.M. was a 51-year-old married, white man who lived with his wife in their own home and worked full time driving a sanitation truck. He was admitted to the hospital reporting that he was depressed because his wife was having an affair. He began to follow her, kept notes on his observations, and badgered her constantly about this, often waking her up in the middle of the night to make accusations. Shortly before admission, these arguments led to physical violence, and he was brought to the hospital by police. He was treated with oral thioridazine (Mellaril), 50 mg every night, and noted that he was less worried about his wife's behavior. He was seen by a psychiatrist monthly, but on follow-up 10 years later, he continued to believe that his wife was unfaithful. His wife noted that he sometimes became agitated about the delusion but that he generally controlled the impulse to act on it.

Erotomanic Type

In erotomania, which has also been referred to as *de Clérambault syndrome* or *psychose passionelle*, the patient has the delusional conviction that another person, usually of higher status, is in love with him or her. Such patients also tend to be solitary, withdrawn, dependent, and sexually inhibited as well as to have poor levels of social or occupational functioning. The following operational criteria for the diagnosis of erotomania have been suggested: (1) a delusional conviction of amorous communication; (2) object of much higher rank; (3) object being the first to fall in love; (4) object being the first to make advances; (5) sudden onset (within a 7-day period); (6) object remains unchanged; (7) patient rationalizes paradoxical behavior of the object; (8) chronic course; and (9) absence of hallucinations. Besides being the key symptom in some cases of delusional disorder, it is known to occur in schizophrenia, mood disorder, and other organic disorders.

Patients with erotomania frequently show certain characteristics: They are generally unattractive women in low-level jobs who lead withdrawn, lonely lives; they are single and have few sexual contacts. They select secret lovers who differ substantially from them. They exhibit what has been called *paradoxical conduct*, the delusional phenomenon of interpreting all denials of love, no matter how clear, as secret affirmations of love. The course may be chronic, recurrent, or brief. Separation from the love object may be the only satisfactory intervention. Although men are less commonly afflicted by this condition than women, they may be more aggressive and possibly violent in their pursuit of love. Hence, in forensic populations, men with this condition predominate. The object of aggression may not be the loved individual but companions or protectors of the love object who are viewed as trying to come between the lovers. The tendency toward violence among men with erotomania may lead initially to police, rather than psychiatric, contact. In certain cases, resentment and rage in response to an absence of reaction from all forms of love communication may sufficiently escalate to put the love object in danger. So-called stalkers, who continually follow their perceived lovers, frequently have delusions. Although most stalkers are men, women also stalk and both groups have a high potential for violence.

Mrs. D was a 32-year-old nurse, married with two children, when she was referred to the clinic by her supervisor from a local hospital. She had assaulted one of the residents, claiming he was in love with her. She had worked in the hospital for 12 years and was considered a good nurse. She had previously fallen in love with another physician on the staff of the hospital. Her current delusion began when the young physician entered a room in which she was lying in bed after cosmetic surgery and pointed at her. She had not known him before, but at that moment, she became convinced that he was in love with her. She tried to approach him several times by letter and phone and, although he did not respond, she was sure he was trying to hide his love from her. She was convinced that he was trying to transmit his love through looks he gave her and through the tone of his voice. The resident met her and denied being in love with her, but she began stalking him. At that point, the head nurse forced her to go for a consultation. She was treated for several months during which she continued to work at the same unit and was able to avoid contact with the resident. She insisted that her husband did not know about this. She refused any medications. The therapist arranged a three-way meeting with himself, the patient, and the resident. As a result of this meeting, there was a small reduction in the intensity of her belief, but she continued to maintain it nonetheless. She subsequently agreed to take antipsychotic medications and was given perphenazine, 16 mg per day, but with no improvement. She continued to hold her belief, and the delusion subsided only after the resident moved to another hospital. (From *DSM-IV-TR Casebook*.)

Somatic Type

Delusional disorder with somatic delusions has been called *monosymptomatic hypochondriacal psychosis*. The condition differs from other conditions with hypochondriacal symptoms in the degree of reality impairment. In delusional disorder, the delusion is fixed, unarguable, and presented intensely, because the patient is totally convinced of the physical nature of the disorder. In contrast, persons with hypochondriasis often admit that their fear of illness is largely groundless. The content of the somatic delusion can vary widely from case to case. The three main types are (1) delusions of infestation (including parasitosis); (2) delusions of dysmorphophobia, such as of misshapenness, personal ugliness, or exaggerated size of body parts (this category seems closest to that of body dysmorphic disorder); and (3) delusions of foul body odors or halitosis. This third category, sometimes referred to as *olfactory reference syndrome*, appears somewhat different from the category of delusions of infestation in that patients with the former have an earlier age of onset (mean 25 years), male predominance, single status, and absence of past psychiatric treatment. Otherwise, the three groups, although individually low in prevalence, appear to overlap.

The onset of symptoms with the somatic type of delusional disorder may be gradual or sudden. In most patients, the illness is unremitting, although the delusion severity may fluctuate. Hyperalertness and high anxiety also characterize patients with this subtype. Some themes recur, such as concerns about infestation in delusional parasitosis, preoccupation with body features with the dysmorphic delusions, and delusional concerns about body odor, which are sometimes referred to as *bromosis*. In delusional parasitosis, tactile sensory phenomena are often linked to the delusional beliefs.

Patients with the somatic type of delusional disorder rarely present for psychiatric evaluation, and when they do, it is usually in the context of a psychiatric consultation or liaison service. Instead, patients generally present to a specific medical specialist for evaluation. Thus, these individuals are more often encountered by dermatologists, plastic surgeons, urologists, acquired immune deficiency syndrome (AIDS) specialists, and sometimes dentists or gastroenterologists.

Ms. G was a 56-year-old homemaker and mother of two who was hospitalized in the burn unit for wound care and skin grafting after sustaining chemical burns to her trunk and extremities. Six months before admission, Ms. G had become increasingly convinced that minute bugs had burrowed underneath her skin. She tried to rid herself of them by washing multiple times each day with medicated soap and lindane shampoo. She also visited several dermatologists and had shown them samples of "dead bugs" for them to examine under the microscope. All told her there was nothing wrong with her and suggested that her problems were psychiatric in nature. She became increasingly distressed by the infestation and worried that the bugs might invade her other organs if not eradicated. Consequently, she decided to asphyxiate the bugs by covering her body with gasoline and holding it against her skin with plastic wrap. She noted that her skin became red and felt as though it were burning, but she viewed this as a positive sign that the bugs were being killed and writhing around as they died. Several hours after she had applied the gasoline, her daughter came to the house, saw Ms. G's condition, and took her to the hospital. When evaluated in the burn unit, Ms. G spoke openly of her concerns about the bugs and was still unsure whether they were present or not. At the same time, she recognized that it had been a mistake to try to kill them with gasoline. She was oriented to person, place, and time and had no other delusional beliefs or auditory or visual hallucinations. She said her mood was "OK," although she was realistically concerned about the extensive treatment that she required and the difficult process of recovering from her injury. She reported no suicidal ideas or intent before admission and had no history of psychiatric treatment. She also did not report any use of substances except for drinking several beers socially approximately twice each month. During her stay in the hospital, she was treated with haloperidol in doses of up to 5 mg per day, with improvement in her concerns about the infestation. She continued to cooperate with treatment for her burns.

Grandiose Type

Delusions of grandeur (megalomania) have been noted for years. They were first described by Kraepelin.

A 51-year-old man was arrested for disturbing the peace. Police had been called to a local park to stop him from carving his initials and those of a recently formed religious cult into various trees surrounding a pond in the park. When confronted, he had scornfully argued that having been chosen to begin a new townwide religious revival, it was necessary for him to publicize his intent in a permanent fashion. The police were unsuccessful in preventing the man from cutting another tree and arrested him. Psychiatric examination was ordered at the state hospital, and the patient was observed there for several weeks. He denied any emotional difficulty and had never received psychiatric treatment. He had no history of euphoria or mood swings. The patient was angry about being hospitalized and only gradually permitted the doctor to interview him. In a few days, however, he was busy preaching to his fellow patients and letting them know that he had been given a special mandate from God to bring in new converts through his ability to heal. Eventually, his preoccupation with special powers diminished, and no other evidence of psychopathology was observed. The patient was discharged, having received no medication at all. Two months later he was arrested at a local theater, this time for disrupting the showing of a film that depicted subjects he believed to be satanic.

Mixed Type

The category mixed type applies to patients with two or more delusional themes. This diagnosis should be reserved for cases in which no single delusional type predominates.

Unspecified Type

The category unspecified type is reserved for cases in which the predominant delusion cannot be subtyped within the previous categories. A possible example is certain delusions of misidentification, for example, Capgras syndrome, named for the French psychiatrist who described the *illusion des sosies*, or the illusion of doubles. The delusion in Capgras syndrome is the belief that a familiar person has been replaced by an impostor. Others have described variants of the Capgras syndrome, namely, the delusion that persecutors or familiar persons can assume the guise of strangers (*Frégoli's phenomenon*) and the very rare delusion that familiar persons can change themselves into other persons at will (*intermetamorphosis*). Each disorder is not only rare but may be associated with schizophrenia, dementia, epilepsy, and other organic disorders. Reported cases have been predominantly in women, have had associated paranoid features, and have included feelings of depersonalization or derealization. The delusion may be short lived, recurrent, or persistent. It is unclear whether delusional disorder can appear with such a delusion. Certainly, the Frégoli and intermetamorphosis delusions have bizarre content and are unlikely, but the delusion in Capgras syndrome is a possible candidate for delusional disorder. The role of hallucination or perceptual disturbance in this condition needs to be explicated. Cases have appeared after sudden brain damage.

In the 19th century, the French psychiatrist Jules Cotard described several patients who suffered from a syndrome called *délire de négation*, sometimes referred to as *nihilistic delusional disorder* or *Cotard syndrome*. Patients with the syndrome complain of having lost not only possessions, status, and strength, but also their heart, blood, and intestines. The world beyond them is reduced to nothingness. This relatively rare syndrome is usually considered a precursor to a schizophrenic or depressive episode. With the common use today of antipsychotic drugs, the syndrome is seen even less frequently than in the past.

Shared Psychotic Disorder

Shared psychotic disorder (also referred to over the years as *shared paranoid disorder*, *induced psychotic disorder*, *folie á deux*, *folie impose*, and *double insanity*) was first described by

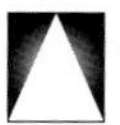

Table 14.3–5
DSM-IV-TR Diagnostic Criteria for Shared Psychotic Disorder

A. A delusion develops in an individual in the context of a close relationship with another person(s), who has an already-established delusion.
B. The delusion is similar in content to that of the person who already has the established delusion.
C. The disturbance is not better accounted for by another psychotic disorder (e.g., schizophrenia) or a mood disorder with psychotic features and is not due to the direct physiological effects of a substance (e.g., a drug of abuse, a medication) or a general medical condition.

(From American Psychiatric Association. *Diagnostic and Statistical Manual of Mental Disorders.* 4th ed. Text rev. Washington, DC: American Psychiatric Association; copyright 2000, with permission.)

two French psychiatrists, Lasegue and Falret in 1877. It is probably rare, but incidence and prevalence figures are lacking, and the literature consists almost entirely of case reports.

The disorder is characterized by the transfer of delusions from one person to another. Both persons are closely associated for a long time and typically live together in relative social isolation. In its most common form (which is covered by the DSM-IV-TR criteria in Table 14.3–5), the individual who first has the delusion (the primary case) is often chronically ill and typically is the influential member of a close relationship with a more suggestible person (the secondary case) who also develops the delusion. The person in the secondary case is frequently less intelligent, more gullible, more passive, or more lacking in self-esteem than the person in the primary case. If the pair separates, the secondary person may abandon the delusion, but this outcome is not seen uniformly. The occurrence of the delusion is attributed to the strong influence of the more dominant member. Old age, low intelligence, sensory impairment, cerebrovascular disease, and alcohol abuse are among the factors associated with this peculiar form of psychotic disorder. A genetic predisposition to idiopathic psychoses has also been suggested as a possible risk factor. The ICD-10 criteria for induced delusional disorder are given in Table 14.3–6.

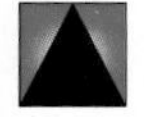

Table 14.3–6
ICD-10 Diagnostic Criteria for Induced Delusional Disorder

A. The individual(s) must develop a delusion or delusional system originally held by someone else with a disorder classified in schizophrenia, schizotypal disorder, persistent delusional disorder, or acute and transient psychotic disorders.
B. The people concerned must have an unusually close relationship with one another, and be relatively isolated from other people.
C. The individual(s) must not have held the belief in question before contact with the other person, and must not have suffered from any other disorder classified in schizophrenia, schizotypal disorder, persistent delusional disorder, or acute and transient psychotic disorders in the past.

(From World Health Organization. The *ICD-10 Classification of Mental and Behavioural Disorders: Diagnostic Criteria for Research.* Copyright, World Health Organization, Geneva, 1993, with permission.)

Other special forms have been reported, such as *folie simultanée*, in which two persons become psychotic simultaneously and share the same delusion. Occasionally, more than two individuals are involved (e.g., *folie á trois*, *quatre*, *cinq*; also *folie á famille*), but such cases are especially rare. The most common relationships in *folie á deux* are sister-sister, husband-wife, and mother-child, but other combinations have also been described. Almost all cases involve members of a single family.

Mrs. B, a 59-year-old woman, presented to the emergency department for evaluation of upper-thigh pain of 9 months' duration. She reported that, on a prior visit to another hospital, she had received an injection of an antiemetic medication in her left thigh while experiencing intense nausea and vomiting from a viral syndrome. Several weeks after that emergency department visit, she began to experience discomfort in her thigh that was typically a sharp pain, exacerbated by movement, but which was occasionally a dull pain that occurred even while motionless. She stated that she was convinced that the needle tip had broken off in her thigh and was continuing to cause her discomfort. She demanded that an X-ray of her leg be done and that a surgeon be called to remove the remaining portion of the needle. Physical examination showed no deformity or discoloration over the site of the reported discomfort and no tenderness on palpation. Neurological examination was nonfocal, and sensation was symmetrical and intact throughout. An X-ray of the left thigh disclosed no evidence of any object and showed no other abnormality. When this information was presented to the patient and her husband, they became outraged. Mr. B stated that he could not believe that five different hospitals had not been able to locate the retained piece of needle because he and his wife could feel it themselves. They both demanded to see a surgeon and refused to leave the emergency department until one was contacted. It was at this point that a psychiatric consultation was requested. Neither Mr. nor Mrs. B had any history of psychiatric disorder. They had been married for 40 years and had no children. Mr. B had worked as an accountant until his retirement 5 years previously, and Mrs. B was a homemaker. Neither described themselves as having many friends, and they generally spent their time together at home, reading, gardening, or watching television. Mr. B stated that at first he could not believe that a piece of the needle could have broken off in his wife's leg, but after the pain persisted for several months and his wife pointed out the irregular areas in her thigh, he became convinced that the needle was there and that something needed to be done about it. They both denied any plans to take legal action against the original facility and stated that their only goal was to have the problem addressed. They rejected all suggestions that psychiatric intervention might be of help, and Mrs. B signed herself out of the emergency department. (From *DSM-IV-TR Casebook.*)

DIFFERENTIAL DIAGNOSIS

Medical Conditions

In making a diagnosis of delusional disorder, the first step is to eliminate medical disorders as a potential cause of delusions. Many medical conditions can be associated with the development of delusions (Table 14.3–7), at times accompanying a delirious state.

Toxic-metabolic conditions and disorders affecting the limbic system and basal ganglia are most often associated with the emergence of delusional beliefs. Complex delusions occur more frequently in patients with subcortical pathology. In

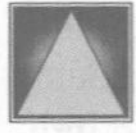

Table 14.3–7 Potential Medical Etiologies of Delusional Syndromes

Disease or Disorder Class	Examples
Neurodegenerative disorders	Alzheimer's disease, Pick's disease, Huntington's disease, basal ganglia calcification, multiple sclerosis, metachromatic leukodystrophy
Other central nervous system disorders	Brain tumors, especially temporal lobe and deep hemispheric tumors; epilepsy, especially complex partial seizure disorder; head trauma (subdural hematoma); anoxic brain injury; fat embolism
Vascular disease	Atherosclerotic vascular disease, especially when associated with diffuse, temporoparietal, or subcortical lesions; hypertensive encephalopathy; subarachnoid hemorrhage, temporal arteritis
Infectious disease	Human immunodeficiency virus or acquired immune deficiency syndrome, encephalitis lethargica, Creutzfeldt-Jakob disease, syphilis, malaria, acute viral encephalitis
Metabolic disorder	Hypercalcemia, hyponatremia, hypoglycemia, uremia, hepatic encephalopathy, porphyria
Endocrinopathies	Addison's disease, Cushing's syndrome, hyper- or hypothyroidism, panhypopituitarism
Vitamin deficiencies	Vitamin B_{12} deficiency, folate deficiency, thiamine deficiency, niacin deficiency
Medications	Adrenocorticotropic hormones, anabolic steroids, corticosteroids, cimetidine, antibiotics (cephalosporins, penicillin), disulfiram, anticholinergic agents
Substances	Amphetamines, cocaine, alcohol, cannabis, hallucinogens
Toxins	Mercury, arsenic, manganese, thallium

Huntington's disease and in individuals with idiopathic basal ganglia calcifications, for example, more than 50 percent of patients demonstrated delusions at some point in their illness. After right cerebral infarction, types of delusions that are more prevalent include anosognosia and reduplicative paramnesia (i.e., individuals believing they are in different places at the same time). Capgras syndrome has been observed in a number of medical disorders, including CNS lesions, vitamin B_{12} deficiency, hepatic encephalopathy, diabetes, and hypothyroidism. Focal syndromes have more often involved the right rather than the left hemisphere. Delusions of infestation, lycanthropy (i.e., the false belief that the patient is an animal, often a wolf or "werewolf"), heutoscopy (i.e., the false belief that one has a double), and erotomania have been reported in small numbers of patients with epilepsy, CNS lesions, or toxic-metabolic disorders.

Delirium, Dementia, and Substance-Related Disorders

Delirium and dementia should be considered in the differential diagnosis of a patient with delusions. Delirium can be differentiated by the presence of a fluctuating level of consciousness or impaired cognitive abilities. Delusions early in the course of a dementing illness, as in dementia of the Alzheimer's type, can give the appearance of a delusional disorder; however, neuropsychological testing usually detects cognitive impairment. Although alcohol abuse is an associated feature for patients with delusional disorder, delusional disorder should be distinguished from alcohol-induced psychotic disorder with hallucinations. Intoxication with sympathomimetics (including amphetamine), marijuana, or L-dopa is likely to result in delusional symptoms.

Other Disorders

The psychiatric differential diagnosis for delusional disorder includes malingering and factitious disorder with predominantly psychological signs and symptoms. The nonfactitious disorders in the differential diagnosis are schizophrenia, mood disorders, obsessive–compulsive disorder, somatoform disorders, and paranoid personality disorder. Delusional disorder is distinguished from schizophrenia by the absence of other schizophrenic symptoms and by the nonbizarre quality of the delusions; patients with delusional disorder also lack the impaired functioning seen in schizophrenia. The somatic type of delusional disorder may resemble a depressive disorder or a somatoform disorder. The somatic type of delusional disorder is differentiated from depressive disorders by the absence of other signs of depression and the lack of a pervasive quality to the depression. Delusional disorder can be differentiated from somatoform disorders by the degree to which the somatic belief is held by the patient. Patients with somatoform disorders allow for the possibility that their disorder does not exist, whereas patients with delusional disorder do not doubt its reality. Separating paranoid personality disorder from delusional disorder requires the sometimes difficult clinical distinction between extreme suspiciousness and frank delusion. In general, if clinicians doubt that a symptom is a delusion, the diagnosis of delusional disorder should not be made.

COURSE AND PROGNOSIS

Some clinicians and some research data indicate that an identifiable psychosocial stressor often accompanies the onset of delusional disorder. The nature of the stressor, in fact, may warrant some suspicion or concern. Examples of such stressors are recent immigration, social conflict with family members or friends, and social isolation. A sudden onset is generally thought to be more common than an insidious onset. Some clinicians believe that a person with delusional disorder is likely to have below-average intelligence and that the premorbid personality of such a person is likely to be extroverted, dominant, and hypersensitive. The person's initial suspicions or concerns gradually become elaborate, consume much of the person's attention, and finally become delusional. Persons may begin quarreling with coworkers, may seek protection from the Federal Bureau of Investigation (FBI) or the police, or may begin visiting many medical or surgical physicians to seek consultations, lawyers about suits, or police about delusional suspicions.

As mentioned, delusional disorder is considered a fairly stable diagnosis. About 50 percent of patients have recovered at long-term follow-up, 20 percent show decreased symptoms, and 30 percent exhibit no change. The following factors correlate with a good prognosis: high levels of occupational, social, and functional adjustments; female sex; onset before age 30; sudden onset; short duration of illness; and the presence of precipitating factors. Although reliable data are limited, patients with persecutory, somatic, and erotic delusions are thought to have a better prognosis than patients with grandiose and jealous delusions.

TREATMENT

Delusional disorder was generally regarded as resistant to treatment, and interventions often focused on managing the morbidity of the disorder by reducing the impact of the delusion on the patient's (and family's) life. In recent years, however, the outlook has become less pessimistic or restricted in planning effective treatment. The goals of treatment are to establish the diagnosis, to decide on appropriate interventions, and to manage complications (Table 14.3–8). The success of these goals depends on an effective and therapeutic doctor–patient relationship, which is far from easy to establish. The patients do not complain about psychiatric symptoms and often enter treatment against their will; even the psychiatrist may be drawn into their delusional nets.

In shared psychiatric disorder, the patients must be separated. If hospitalization is indicated, they should be placed on different units and have no contact. In general, the healthier of the two will give up the delusional belief (sometimes without any other therapeutic intervention). The sicker of the two will maintain the false fixed belief.

Psychotherapy

The essential element in effective psychotherapy is to establish a relationship in which patients begin to trust a therapist. Individual therapy seems to be more effective than group therapy; insight-oriented, supportive, cognitive, and behavioral therapies are often effective. Initially, a therapist should neither agree with nor challenge a patient's delusions. Although therapists must ask about a delusion to establish its extent, persistent questioning about it should probably be avoided. Physicians may stimulate the motivation to receive help by emphasizing a willingness to help patients with their anxiety or irritability, without suggesting that the delusions be treated, but therapists should not actively support the notion that the delusions are real.

Table 14.3–8
Diagnosis and Management of Delusional Disorder

Rule out other causes of paranoid features
Confirm the absence of other psychopathology
Assess consequences of delusion-related behavior
- Demoralization
- Despondency
- Anger, fear
- Depression
- Impact of search for "medical diagnosis," "legal solution," "proof of infidelity," etc. (i.e., financial, legal, personal, occupational, etc.)

Assess anxiety and agitation
Assess potential for violence, suicide
Assess need for hospitalization
Institute pharmacological and psychological therapies
Maintain connection through recovery

The unwavering reliability of therapists is essential in psychotherapy. Therapists should be on time and make appointments as regularly as possible, with the goal of developing a solid and trusting relationship with a patient. Overgratification may actually increase patients' hostility and suspiciousness because ultimately they must realize that not all demands can be met. Therapists can avoid overgratification by not extending the designated appointment period, by not giving extra appointments unless absolutely necessary, and by not being lenient about the fee.

Therapists should avoid making disparaging remarks about a patient's delusions or ideas but can sympathetically indicate to patients that their preoccupation with their delusions is both distressing to themselves and interferes with a constructive life. When patients begin to waver in their delusional beliefs, therapists may increase reality testing by asking the patients to clarify their concerns.

A useful approach in building a therapeutic alliance is to empathize with the patient's internal experience of being overwhelmed by persecution. It may be helpful to make such comments as, "You must be exhausted, considering what you have been through." Without agreeing with every delusional misperception, a therapist can acknowledge that from the patient's perspective, such perceptions create much distress. The ultimate goal is to help patients entertain the possibility of doubt about their perceptions. As they become less rigid, feelings of weakness and inferiority, associated with some depression, may surface. When a patient allows feelings of vulnerability to enter into the therapy, a positive therapeutic alliance has been established, and constructive therapy becomes possible.

When family members are available, clinicians may decide to involve them in the treatment plan. Without being delusionally seen as siding with the enemy, a clinician should attempt to enlist the family as allies in the treatment process. Consequently, both the patient and the family need to understand that the therapist maintains physician–patient confidentiality and that communications from relatives are discussed with the patient. The family may benefit from the therapist's support and, thus, may support the patient.

A good therapeutic outcome depends on a psychiatrist's ability to respond to the patient's mistrust of others and the resulting interpersonal conflicts, frustrations, and failures. The mark of successful treatment may be a satisfactory social adjustment rather than abatement of the patient's delusions.

Hospitalization

Patients with delusional disorder can generally be treated as outpatients, but clinicians should consider hospitalization for several reasons. First, patients may need a complete medical and neurological evaluation to determine whether a nonpsychiatric medical condition is causing the delusional symptoms. Second, patients need an assessment of their ability to control violent impulses (e.g., to commit suicide or homicide) that may be related to the delusional material. Third, patients' behavior about the delusions may have significantly affected their ability to function within their family or occupational settings; they may require professional intervention to stabilize social or occupational relationships.

If a physician is convinced that a patient would receive the best treatment in a hospital, then the physician should attempt to persuade the patient to accept hospitalization; failing that, legal commitment may be indicated. If a physician convinces a patient that hospitalization is inevitable, the patient often voluntarily enters a hospital to avoid legal commitment.

Pharmacotherapy

In an emergency, severely agitated patients should be given an antipsychotic drug intramuscularly. Although no adequately conducted clinical trials with large numbers of patients have been conducted, most clinicians consider antipsychotic drugs the treatment of choice for delusional disorder. Patients are likely to refuse medication because they can easily incorporate the administration of drugs into their delusional systems; physicians should not insist on medication immediately after hospitalization but, rather, should spend a few days establishing rapport with the patient. Physicians should explain potential adverse effects to patients, so that they do not later suspect that the physician lied.

A patient's history of medication response is the best guide to choosing a drug. A physician should often start with low doses (e.g., 2 mg of haloperidol [Haldol] or 2 mg of risperidone [Risperdal]) and increase the dose slowly. If a patient fails to respond to the drug at a reasonable dosage in a 6-week trial, antipsychotic drugs from other classes should be tried. Some investigators have indicated that pimozide may be particularly effective in delusional disorder, especially in patients with somatic delusions. A common cause of drug failure is noncompliance, which should also be evaluated. Concurrent psychotherapy facilitates compliance with drug treatment.

If the patient receives no benefit from antipsychotic medication, discontinue use of the drug. In patients who do respond to antipsychotic drugs, some data indicate that maintenance doses can be low. Although essentially no studies evaluate the use of antidepressants, lithium (Eskalith), or anticonvulsants (e.g., carbamazepine [Tegretol] and valproate [Depakene]) in the treatment of delusional disorder, trials with these drugs may be warranted in patients who do not respond to antipsychotic drugs. Trials of these drugs should also be considered when a patient has either the features of a mood disorder or a family history of mood disorders.

References

Caliyurt O, Vardar E, Tuglu C. Cotard's syndrome with schizophreniform disorder can be successfully treated with electroconvulsive therapy: Case report. *J Psychiatry Neurosci*. 2004;29:138–141.

Fennig S, Fochtmann LJ, Bromet EJ. Delusional disorder and shared psychotic disorder. In: Sadock BJ, Sadock VA, eds. *Kaplan & Sadock's Comprehensive Textbook of Psychiatry*. 8th ed. Vol. 1. Baltimore: Lippincott Williams & Wilkins; 2005:1525.

Goldstein RL, Laskin AM. De Clerambault's syndrome (erotomania) and claims of psychiatric malpractice. *J Forensic Sci*. 2002;47:852–855.

Mela M. *Folie à Trois* in a multilevel security forensic treatment center: Forensic and ethics-related implications. *J Am Acad Psychiatry Law*. 2005;33:3:310–316.

Noel-Jorand MC, Reinert M, Giudicelli S, Dassa D. Increased sense of identity in delusional disorders. *Psychol Rep*. 2004;94(3 Pt 1):926–930.

Pearn J, Gardner-Thorpe C. Jules Cotard (1840–1889): His life and the unique syndrome which bears his name. *Neurology*. 2002;58:1400–1403.

Reif A, Pfuhlmann B. Folie a deux versus genetically driven delusional disorder: Case reports and nosological considerations. *Compr Psychiatry*. 2004;45(2): 155–160.

Riecher-Rossler A, Hafner H, Hafner-Ranabauer W, Loffler W, Reinhard I. Late-onset schizophrenia versus paranoid psychoses: A valid diagnostic distinction? *Am J Geriatr Psychiatry*. 2003;11:595–604.

Rosenfeld B. Recidivism in stalking and obsessional harassment. *Law Hum Behav*. 2003;27:251–265.

Wehmeier PM, Barth N, Remschmidt H. Induced delusional disorder. A review of the concept and an unusual case of folie á famille. *Psychopathology*. 2003;36: 37–45.

▲ 14.4 Brief Psychotic Disorder, Psychotic Disorder Not Otherwise Specified, and Secondary Psychotic Disorders

BRIEF PSYCHOTIC DISORDER

Brief psychotic disorder is defined by the text revision of the fourth edition of *Diagnostic and Statistical Manual of Mental Disorders* (DSM-IV-TR) as a psychotic condition that involves the sudden onset of psychotic symptoms, which lasts 1 day or more but less than 1 month. Remission is full, and the individual returns to the premorbid level of functioning. Brief psychotic disorder is an acute and transient psychotic syndrome, thus, most individuals diagnosed with brief psychotic disorder under DSM-IV-TR are classified as having acute and transient psychotic disorders under the tenth revision of *International Statistical Classification of Diseases and Related Health Problems* (ICD-10).

History

Brief psychotic disorder has been poorly studied in psychiatry in the United States, partly because of the frequent changes in diagnostic criteria during the past 15 years. The diagnosis has been better appreciated and more completely studied in Scandinavia and other western European countries than in the United States. Patients with disorders similar to brief psychotic disorder were previously classified as having reactive, hysterical, stress, and psychogenic psychoses.

Reactive psychosis was often used as a synonym for good-prognosis schizophrenia, but the DSM-IV-TR diagnosis of brief psychotic disorder is not meant to imply a relation with schizophrenia. In 1913, Karl Jaspers described several essential features for the diagnosis of reactive psychosis, including an identifiable and extremely traumatic stressor, a close temporal relation between the stressor and the development of the psychosis, and a generally benign course for the psychotic episode. Jaspers also stated that the content of the psychosis often reflected the nature of the traumatic experience and that the development of the psychosis seemed to serve a purpose for the patient, often as an escape from a traumatic condition.

Epidemiology

The exact incidence and prevalence of brief psychotic disorder is not known, but it is generally considered uncommon. The disorder occurs more often among younger patients (20s and 30s) than among older patients. Reliable data on sex and sociocultural determinants are limited, although some findings suggest a higher incidence in women and persons in developing countries. Such epidemiological patterns are sharply distinct from those of schizophrenia. Some clinicians indicate that the disorder may be seen most frequently in patients from low socioeconomic classes and in those who have experienced disasters or major cultural changes (e.g., immigrants). The age of onset in industrialized settings may be higher than in developing countries. Persons who have gone through major psychosocial stressors may be at greater risk for subsequent brief psychotic disorder.

Comorbidity

The disorder is often seen in patients with personality disorders (most commonly, histrionic, narcissistic, paranoid, schizotypal, and borderline personality disorders).

Etiology

The cause of brief psychotic disorder is unknown. Patients who have a personality disorder may have a biological or psychological vulnerability for the development of psychotic symptoms, particularly those with borderline, schizoid, schizotypal, or paranoid qualities. Some patients with brief psychotic disorder have a history of schizophrenia or mood disorders in their families, but this finding is nonconclusive. Psychodynamic formulations have emphasized the presence of inadequate coping mechanisms and the possibility of secondary gain for patients with psychotic symptoms. Additional psychodynamic theories suggest that the psychotic symptoms are a defense against a prohibited fantasy, the fulfillment of an unattained wish, or an escape from a stressful psychosocial situation.

Diagnosis

The DSM-IV-TR describes a continuum of diagnoses for psychotic disorders, based primarily on the duration of the symptoms. For psychotic symptoms that last at least 1 day but less than 1 month and that are not associated with a mood disorder, a substance-related disorder, or a psychotic disorder caused by a general medical condition, a diagnosis of brief psychotic disorder is likely to be appropriate (Table 14.4–1).

By contrast, in the ICD-10, acute and transient psychotic disorders are diagnosed by setting up a "diagnostic sequence that reflects the order of priority given to selected key features," including sudden (within 48 hours) or abrupt (more than 48 hours but within 2 weeks) onset, typical syndromes, and associated acute distress. For psychotic symptoms that last more than 1 month, the appropriate diagnoses to consider are delusional disorder (if delusions are the primary psychotic symptoms), schizophreniform disorder (if the symptoms have lasted less than 6 months), and schizophrenia (if the symptoms have lasted more than 6 months). Table 14.4–2 lists the ICD-10 diagnostic criteria for acute and transient psychiatric disorder.

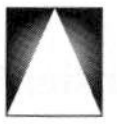

Table 14.4–1
DSM-IV-TR Diagnostic Criteria for Brief Psychotic Disorder

A. Presence of one (or more) of the following symptoms:
   (1) delusions
   (2) hallucinations
   (3) disorganized speech (e.g., frequent derailment or incoherence)
   (4) grossly disorganized or catatonic behavior
   Note: Do not include a symptom if it is a culturally sanctioned response pattern.
B. Duration of an episode of the disturbance is at least 1 day but less than 1 month, with eventual full return to premorbid level of functioning.
C. The disturbance is not better accounted for by a mood disorder with psychotic features, schizoaffective disorder, or schizophrenia and is not due to the direct physiological effects of a substance (e.g., a drug of abuse, a medication) or a general medical condition.

Specify if:
  With marked stressor(s) (brief reactive psychosis): if symptoms occur shortly after and apparently in response to events that, singly or together, would be markedly stressful to almost anyone in similar circumstances in the person's culture
  Without marked stressor(s): if psychotic symptoms do not occur shortly after, or are not apparently in response to events that, singly or together, would be markedly stressful to almost anyone in similar circumstances in the person's culture
  With postpartum onset: if onset within 4 weeks postpartum

(From American Psychiatric Association. *Diagnostic and Statistical Manual of Mental Disorders.* 4th ed. Text rev. Washington, DC: American Psychiatric Association; copyright 2000, with permission.)

The DSM-IV-TR describes three subtypes: (1) the presence of stressors, (2) the absence of stressors, and (3) a postpartum onset, each of which is discussed below.

As with other acutely ill psychiatric patients, the history necessary to make the diagnosis may not be obtainable solely from the patient. Although psychotic symptoms may be obvious, information about prodromal symptoms, previous episodes of a mood disorder, and a recent history of ingestion of a psychotomimetic substance may not be available from the clinical interview alone. In addition, clinicians may not be able to obtain accurate information about the presence or absence of precipitating stressors. Such information is usually best and most accurately obtained from a relative or a friend.

Clinical Features

The symptoms of brief psychotic disorder always include at least one major symptom of psychosis, usually with an abrupt onset, but do not always include the entire symptom pattern seen in schizophrenia. Some clinicians have observed that labile mood, confusion, and impaired attention may be more common at the onset of brief psychotic disorder than at the onset of eventually chronic psychotic disorders. Characteristic symptoms in brief psychotic disorder include emotional volatility, strange or bizarre behavior, screaming or muteness, and impaired memory for recent events. Some of the symptoms suggest a diagnosis of

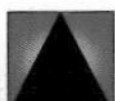

Table 14.4–2
ICD-10 Diagnostic Criteria for Acute and Transient Psychotic Disorders

G1. There is acute onset of delusions, hallucinations, incomprehensible or incoherent speech, or any combination of these. The time interval between the first appearance of any psychotic symptoms and the presentation of the fully developed disorder should not exceed 2 weeks.

G2. If transient states of perplexity, misidentification, or impairment of attention and concentration are present, they do not fulfill the criteria for organically caused clouding of consciousness as specified for delirium, not induced by alcohol and other psychoactive substances, criterion A.

G3. The disorder does not meet the symptomatic criteria for manic episode, depressive episode, or recurrent depressive disorder.

G4. There is insufficient evidence of recent psychoactive substance use to fulfill the criteria for intoxication, harmful use, dependence, or withdrawal states. The continued moderate and largely unchanged use of alcohol or drugs in amounts or with the frequency to which the individual is accustomed does not necessarily rule out the use of acute and transient psychotic disorders; this must be decided by clinical judgment and the requirements of the research project in question.

G5. *Most commonly used exclusion clause.* There must be no organic mental disorder or serious metabolic disturbances affecting the central nervous system (this does not include childbirth).

A fifth character should be used to specify whether the acute onset of the disorder is associated with acute stress (occurring 2 weeks or less before evidence of first psychotic symptoms):

Without associated acute stress
With associated acute stress

For research purposes, it is recommended that change of the disorder from a nonpsychotic to a clearly psychotic state is further specified as either abrupt (onset within 48 hours) or acute (onset in more than 48 hours but less than 2 weeks).

Acute polymorphic psychotic disorder without symptoms of schizophrenia

A. The general criteria for acute and transient psychotic disorders must be met.

B. Symptoms change rapidly in both type and intensity from day to day or within the same day.

C. Any type of either hallucinations or delusions occurs, for at least several hours, at any time from the onset of the disorder.

D. Symptoms from at least two of the following categories occur at the same time:
(1) emotional turmoil, characterized by intense feelings of happiness or ecstasy, or overwhelming anxiety or marked irritability;
(2) perplexity, or misidentification of people or places;
(3) increased or decreased motility, to a marked degree.

E. If any of the symptoms listed for schizophrenia, criterion G(1) and (2), are present, they are present only for a minority of the time from the onset; i.e., criterion B of acute polymorphic psychotic disorder with symptoms of schizophrenia is not fulfilled.

F. The total duration of the disorder does not exceed 3 months.

Acute polymorphic psychotic disorder with symptoms of schizophrenia

A. Criteria A, B, C, and D of acute polymorphic psychotic disorder must be met.

B. Some of the symptoms for schizophrenia must have been present for the majority of the time since the onset of the disorder, although the full criteria need not be met, i.e., at least one of the symptoms in criteria G1(1)a to G1(2)c.

C. The symptoms of schizophrenia in criterion B above do not persist for more than 1 month.

Acute schizophrenialike psychotic disorder

A. The general criteria for acute and transient psychotic disorders must be met.

B. The criteria for schizophrenia are met, with the exception of the criterion for duration.

C. The disorder does not meet criteria B, C, and D for acute polymorphic psychotic disorder.

D. The total duration of the disorder does not exceed 1 month.

Other acute predominantly delusional psychotic disorders

A. The general criteria for acute and transient psychotic disorders must be met.

B. Relatively stable delusions and/or hallucinations are present but do not fulfill the symptomatic criteria for schizophrenia.

C. The disorder does not meet the criteria for acute polymorphic psychotic disorder.

D. The total duration of the disorder does not exceed 3 months.

Other acute and transient psychotic disorders

Any other acute psychotic disorders that are not classifiable under any other category in acute and transient psychotic disorders (such as acute psychotic states in which definite delusions or hallucinations occur but persist for only small proportions of the time) should be coded here. States of undifferentiated excitement should also be coded here if more detailed information about the patient's mental state is not available, provided that there is no evidence of an organic cause.

Acute and transient psychotic disorder, unspecified

(From World Health Organization. *The ICD-10 Classification of Mental and Behavioural Disorders: Diagnostic Criteria for Research.* Copyright, World Health Organization, Geneva, 1993, with permission.)

delirium and warrant a medical workup, especially to rule out adverse reactions to drugs.

Scandinavian and other European literature describes several characteristic symptom patterns in brief psychotic disorder, although these may differ somewhat in Europe and America. The symptom patterns include acute paranoid reactions, and reactive confusion, excitation, and depression. Some data suggest that, in the United States, paranoia is often the predominant symptom in the disorder. In French psychiatry, bouffée délirante is similar to brief psychotic disorder.

H. is a 22-year-old student. She is in her first year of medical school in Egypt.

PROBLEM

Accompanied by her mother, H. came to see the physician at the psychiatric outpatient clinic. She was complaining about her nose. For the preceding week, from time to time she could smell a foul odor and was very afraid that it came from herself. She reported hearing voices talking about her behavior and telling her what to do. She had become extremely irritable and was unable to sleep. All these problems began 10 days after returning to her home in Alexandria on summer vacation from the medical school. She could find no obvious reason for the foul smell and the voices, but she thought the condition might be the result of witchcraft. She had developed a friendship with a young man, a fellow student at the medical school, and suddenly, just before the vacation, he had asked her to marry him. She was very surprised, became frightened, and had refused, which had upset him. She now suspected that her boyfriend had caused a spell to be cast on her because of her refusal. H.'s family said her condition was gradually getting worse. The foul smell and the voices seemed to affect her more each day.

HISTORY

H. was the first of two children born to a family of average income in Alexandria. Her father was a mechanic and seemed to be a rather shy and gentle person. The mother was ambitious and expressed great concern for her daughter's education. Her family reported that they had great hope that their first child would be a boy. The parents treated H. as if she were a boy for the first 3 years of her life until the birth of a second child, which was a son. There was no information about mental disorders in the family.

H. was introverted, thoughtful, and rather stubborn, with only a few friends. She had a high moral standard and had never dated or had sexual relations. She was doing very well at medical school and was determined to become a great physician in a culture where there is still some resistance to women physicians.

She had always been physically strong and had excellent health.

FINDINGS

On admission to the clinic, H. was found to be very self-conscious and tried to avoid being seen by other people. She appeared tense and sad and seemed close to tears. She was reluctant and mentioned with hesitation some "extraordinary experiences." These included the foul smell, which was like burned meat, and the voices that kept commenting on her behavior. She said the voices described what she was doing "here and now" and added comments. One example she gave of what the voices were saying was, "You are now speaking to the physician. You hope that he can help you, don't you? No hope. We shall overcome." She explained that she believed this was the result of the witchcraft to which she had been subjected. She seemed able to differentiate in her mind between normal and abnormal perceptual experiences. She stated that she was able to make this distinction but was unable to do anything about the voices.

She showed emotional response of normal modulation, and no abnormalities of speech were observed. She was fully oriented as to time, place, and person and showed no impairment of memory. Her attention seemed sharpened, but her concentration was slightly diminished.

Careful physical and neurological examinations revealed no abnormalities. An electroencephalogram with nasopharyngeal electrodes and a computed tomography scan also showed only normal results, and laboratory investigations, including thyroid parameters, were all normal.

COURSE

H. was prescribed haloperidol (3 mg per day) and a hypnotic. In the course of 4 days, the voices and the foul smell gradually disappeared. At the next visit to the clinic a week later, she complained of drowsiness and fatigue, aching and stiffness in the muscles, and difficulties with concentration. Her haloperidol was reduced to 1 mg per day, and the hypnotic was discontinued. After this she gradually improved, and after an additional 2 weeks she appeared well and was able to manage without medication. (Reprinted with permission from *ICD-10 Casebook.*)

Precipitating Stressors. The clearest examples of precipitating stressors are major life events that would cause any person significant emotional upset. Such events include the loss of a close family member or a severe automobile accident. Some clinicians argue that the severity of the event must be considered in relation to the patient's life. This view, although reasonable, may broaden the definition of precipitating stressor to include events unrelated to the psychotic episode. Others have argued that the stressor may be a series of modestly stressful events rather than a single markedly stressful event, but evaluating the amount of stress caused by a sequence of events calls for an almost impossibly high degree of clinical judgment.

A Norwegian lumberman was admitted to the psychiatric ward of a hospital shortly after starting his required military duty at 20 years of age. During the first week after his arrival at the military base, he believed the other recruits looked at him in a strange way. He watched the people around him to see whether they were out "to get" him. He heard voices calling his name several times. He became increasingly suspicious and after another week had to be admitted to the psychiatric department at the University of Oslo. There he was guarded, scowling, skeptical, and depressed. He gave the impression of being very shy and inhibited. His psychotic symptoms disappeared rapidly when he was treated with an antipsychotic drug. However, he had difficulties in adjusting to hospital life. Transfer to a long-term mental hospital was considered; but after 3 months, a decision was made to discharge him to his home in the forest. He was subsequently judged unfit to return to military services and was struck from the military lists.

The patient, the eldest of five siblings, was the son of a farm laborer in one of the valleys of Norway. His father was an intemperate drinker who became angry and brutal when drunk. The family was very poor, and there were constant quarrels between the parents. As a child, the patient was inhibited and fearful and often ran into the woods when troubled. He had academic difficulties and barely passed elementary school.

When the patient became older, he preferred to spend most of his time in the woods, where he worked as a lumberman from 15 years of age. He had his own horse, lived in a log cabin, and disliked being with people. He sometimes took part in the youth dances in the village. Although never a heavy drinker, he often got into fights in the village when he had a drink or two. At the age of 16 years, he began to keep company with a girl 1 year his junior who sometimes kept house for him in the woods. They eventually became engaged. (Courtesy of Ramin Mojtabai, M.D., Ph.D., M.P.H.)

Differential Diagnosis

Clinicians must not assume that the correct diagnosis for a patient who is briefly psychotic is brief psychotic disorder, even when a clear precipitating psychosocial factor is identified. Such a factor may be merely coincidental. If psychotic symptoms are present longer than 1 month, the diagnoses of schizophreniform disorder, schizoaffective disorder, schizophrenia, mood disorders with psychotic features, delusional disorder, and psychotic disorder not otherwise specified must be entertained. If psychotic symptoms of sudden onset are present for less than a month in response to an obvious stressor, however, the diagnosis of brief psychotic disorder is strongly suggested. Other diagnoses to consider in the differential diagnosis include factitious disorder with predominantly psychological signs and symptoms, malingering, psychotic disorder caused by a general medical condition, and substance-induced psychotic disorder. In factitious disorder, symptoms are intentionally produced; in malingering, a specific goal is involved in appearing psychotic (e.g., to gain admission to the hospital); and when associated with a medical condition or drugs, the cause becomes apparent with proper medical or drug workups. If the patient admits to using illicit substances, the clinician can make the assessment of substance intoxication or substance withdrawal without the use of laboratory testing. Patients with epilepsy or delirium can also show psychotic symptoms that resemble those seen in brief psychotic disorder. Additional psychiatric disorders to be considered in the differential diagnosis include dissociative identity disorder and psychotic episodes associated with borderline and schizotypal personality disorders.

Course and Prognosis

By definition, the course of brief psychotic disorder is less than 1 month. Nonetheless, the development of such a significant psychiatric disorder may signify a patient's mental vulnerability. Approximately half of patients who are first classified as having brief psychotic disorder later display chronic psychiatric syndromes such as schizophrenia and mood disorders. Patients with brief psychotic disorder, however, generally have good prognoses, and European studies have indicated that 50 to 80 percent of all patients have no further major psychiatric problems.

The length of the acute and residual symptoms is often just a few days. Occasionally, depressive symptoms follow the resolution of the psychotic symptoms. Suicide is a concern during both the psychotic phase and the postpsychotic depressive phase. Several indicators have been associated with a good prognosis (Table 14.4–3). Patients with the features listed in Table 14.4–3 are unlikely to have subsequent episodes, and schizophrenia or a mood disorder is unlikely to develop later.

Treatment

Hospitalization. A patient who is acutely psychotic may need brief hospitalization for both evaluation and protection. Evaluation requires close monitoring of symptoms and assessment of the patient's level of danger to self and others. In addition, the quiet, structured setting of a hospital may help patients regain their sense of reality. While clinicians wait for the setting or the drugs to have their effects, seclusion, physical restraints, or one-to-one monitoring of the patient may be necessary.

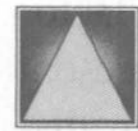

Table 14.4–3
Good Prognostic Features for Brief Psychotic Disorder

- Good premorbid adjustment
- Few premorbid schizoid traits
- Severe precipitating stressor
- Sudden onset of symptoms
- Affective symptoms
- Confusion and perplexity during psychosis
- Little affective blunting
- Short duration of symptoms
- Absence of schizophrenic relatives

Pharmacotherapy. The two major classes of drugs to be considered in the treatment of brief psychotic disorder are the antipsychotic drugs and the benzodiazepines. When an antipsychotic drug is chosen, a high-potency antipsychotic drug, such as haloperidol, may be used or a serotonin-dopamine agonist such as ziprasadone. In patients who are at high risk for the development of extrapyramidal adverse effects (e.g., young men), a serotonin-dopamine antagonist drug should be administered as prophylaxis against medication-induced movement disorder symptoms. Alternatively, benzodiazepines can be used in the short-term treatment of psychosis. Although benzodiazepines have limited or no usefulness in the long-term treatment of psychotic disorders, they can be effective for a short time and are associated with fewer adverse effects than the antipsychotic drugs. In rare cases, the benzodiazepines are associated with increased agitation and, more rarely still, with withdrawal seizures, which usually occur only with the sustained use of high dosages. The use of other drugs in the treatment of brief psychotic disorder, although reported in case studies, has not been supported in any large-scale studies. Anxiolytic medications, however, are often useful during the first 2 to 3 weeks after the resolution of the psychotic episode. Clinicians should avoid long-term use of any medication in the treatment of the disorder. If maintenance medication is necessary, a clinician may have to reconsider the diagnosis.

Psychotherapy. Although hospitalization and pharmacotherapy are likely to control short-term situations, the difficult part of treatment is the psychological integration of the experience (and possibly the precipitating trauma, if one was present) into the lives of the patients and their families. Psychotherapy is of use in providing an opportunity to discuss the stressors and the psychotic episode. Exploration and development of coping strategies are the major topics in psychotherapy. Associated issues include helping patients deal with the loss of self-esteem and to regain self-confidence. An individualized treatment strategy based on increasing problem-solving skills while strengthening the ego structure through psychotherapy appears to be the most efficacious. Family involvement in the treatment process may be crucial to a successful outcome.

PSYCHOTIC DISORDER NOT OTHERWISE SPECIFIED

Under the umbrella of psychosis not otherwise specified (NOS) is a variety of clinical presentations that do not fit within current diagnostic rubrics. In DSM-IV-TR, it includes "psychotic symptomatology (i.e., delusions, hallucinations, disorganized speech, grossly disorganized or catatonic behavior) about which there is inadequate information to make a specific diagnosis or about which there is contradictory information, or disorders with psychotic symptoms that do not meet the criteria for any specific Psychotic Disorder." DSM-IV-TR has listed some examples of the diagnosis to help guide clinicians (Table 14.4–4). ICD-10 criteria are listed in Table 14.4–5.

Autoscopic Psychosis

The characteristic symptom of autoscopic psychosis is a visual hallucination of all or part of the person's own body. The

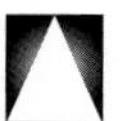

Table 14.4–4
DSM-IV-TR Diagnostic Criteria for Psychotic Disorder Not Otherwise Specified

This category includes psychotic symptomatology (i.e., delusions, hallucinations, disorganized speech, grossly disorganized or catatonic behavior) about which there is inadequate information to make a specific diagnosis or about which there is contradictory information, or disorders with psychotic symptoms that do not meet the criteria for any specific psychotic disorder.

Examples include

1. Postpartum psychosis that does not meet criteria for mood disorder with psychotic features, brief psychotic disorder, psychotic disorder due to a general medical condition, or substance-induced psychotic disorder
2. Psychotic symptoms that have lasted for less than 1 month but that have not yet remitted, so that the criteria for brief psychotic disorder are not met
3. Persistent auditory hallucinations in the absence of any other features
4. Persistent nonbizarre delusions with periods of overlapping mood episodes that have been present for a substantial portion of the delusional disturbance
5. Situations in which the clinician has concluded that a psychotic disorder is present, but is unable to determine whether it is primary, due to a general medical condition, or substance induced

(From American Psychiatric Association. *Diagnostic and Statistical Manual of Mental Disorders.* 4th ed. Text rev. Washington, DC: American Psychiatric Association; copyright 2000, with permission.)

hallucinatory perception, which is called a *phantom*, is usually colorless and transparent, and because the phantom imitates the person's movements, it is perceived as though appearing in a mirror. The phantom tends to appear suddenly and without warning.

Epidemiology. Autoscopy is a rare phenomenon. Some persons have an autoscopic experience only once or a few times; others have the experience more often. Although the data are limited, sex, age, heredity, and intelligence do not seem to be related to the occurrence of the syndrome.

Etiology. The cause of the autoscopic phenomenon is unknown. A biological hypothesis is that abnormal, episodic activity in areas of the temporoparietal lobes is involved with the sense of self, perhaps combined with abnormal activity in parts of the visual cortex. Psychological theories have associated the syndrome with personalities characterized by imagination, visual sensitivity, and, possibly, narcissistic personality disorder traits. Such persons may likely experience autoscopic phenomena during periods of stress.

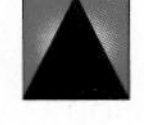

Table 14.4–5
ICD-10 Diagnostic Criteria for Other Nonorganic Psychotic Disorders

Psychotic disorders that do not meet the criteria for schizophrenia or for psychotic types of mood (affective) disorders, and psychotic disorders that do not meet the symptomatic criteria for persistent delusional disorder should be coded here (persistent hallucinatory disorder is an example). Combinations of symptoms not covered by the previous categories, such as delusions other than those listed as typically schizophrenic under criterion G1(1)b or d for schizophrenia (i.e., other than completely impossible or culturally inappropriate) plus catatonia, should also be included here.

(From World Health Organization. The *ICD-10 Classification of Mental and Behavioural Disorders: Diagnostic Criteria for Research.* Copyright, World Health Organization, Geneva, 1993, with permission.)

Course and Prognosis. The classic descriptions of the phenomenon indicate that, in most cases, the syndrome is neither progressive nor incapacitating. Affected persons usually maintain some emotional distance from the phenomenon, an observation that suggests a specific neuroanatomical lesion. Rarely do the symptoms reflect the onset of schizophrenia or other psychotic disorders.

Postpartum Psychosis

Postpartum psychosis (sometimes called *puerperal psychosis*) is an example of psychotic disorder not otherwise specified that occurs in women who have recently delivered a baby; the syndrome is most often characterized by the mother's depression, delusions, and thoughts of harming either her infant or herself. For a complete discussion on postpartum conditions and other disorders related to pregnancy see Chapter 30, *Psychiatry and Reproductive Medicine*.

PSYCHOTIC DISORDERS DUE TO A GENERAL MEDICAL CONDITION AND SUBSTANCE-INDUCED PSYCHOTIC DISORDER

The evaluation of a patient with psychotic disorders requires consideration of the possibility that the psychotic symptoms result from a general medical condition such as a brain tumor or the ingestion of a substance such as phencyclidine (PCP).

Epidemiology

Relevant epidemiological data about psychotic disorder caused by a general medical condition and substance-induced psychotic disorder are lacking. The disorders are most often encountered in patients who abuse alcohol or other substances on a long-term basis. The delusional syndrome that may accompany complex partial seizures is more common in women than in men.

Etiology

Physical conditions such as cerebral neoplasms, particularly of the occipital or temporal areas, can cause hallucinations. Sensory deprivation, as in people who are blind or deaf, can also result in hallucinatory or delusional experiences. Lesions involving the temporal lobe and other cerebral regions, especially the right hemisphere and the parietal lobe, are associated with delusions.

Psychoactive substances are common causes of psychotic syndromes. The most commonly involved substances are alcohol, indole hallucinogens, such as lysergic acid diethylamide (LSD), amphetamine, cocaine, mescaline, PCP, and ketamine. Many other substances, including steroids and thyroxine, can produce hallucinations. (*See* Table 13–9 for a list of general medical conditions and substances that can be associated with psychotic symptoms.)

Diagnosis

Psychotic Disorder Due to a General Medical Condition. The diagnosis of psychotic disorder due to a general medical condition (Table 14.4–6) is defined in DSM-IV-TR by specifying the predominant symptoms. When the diagnosis is used, the medical condition, along with the predominant symptoms pattern, should be included in the diagnosis; for example, psychotic disorder due to a brain tumor, with delusions. The DSM-IV-TR criteria further specify that the disorder does not occur exclusively while a patient is delirious or demented and that the symptoms are not better accounted for by another mental disorder.

Substance-Induced Psychotic Disorder

The diagnostic category of substance-induced psychotic disorder in DSM-IV-TR (Table 14.4–7) is reserved for those with substance-induced psychotic symptoms and impaired reality testing. People with substance-induced psychotic symptoms (e.g., hallucinations), but with intact reality testing, should be classified as having a substance-related disorder (e.g., PCP intoxication with perceptual disturbances). The diagnosis of substance-induced psychotic disorder is included with the other psychotic disorder diagnoses in DSM-IV-TR to prompt clinicians to consider the possibility that a substance is causally involved in the production of psychotic symptoms. The full diagnosis of substance-induced psychotic disorder should include the type of substance involved, the stage of substance use when the disorder began (e.g., during intoxication or withdrawal), and the clinical phenomena (e.g., hallucinations or delusions).

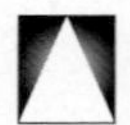

Table 14.4–6
DSM-IV-TR Diagnostic Criteria for Psychotic Disorder Due to a General Medical Condition

A. Prominent hallucinations or delusions
B. There is evidence from the history, physical examination, or laboratory findings that the disturbance is the direct physiological consequence of a general medical condition.
C. The disturbance is not better accounted for by another mental disorder.
D. The disturbance does not occur exclusively during the course of a delirium.

Code based on predominant symptom:
With delusions: if delusions are the predominant symptom
With hallucinations: if hallucinations are the predominant symptom

Coding note: Include the name of the general medical condition on Axis I, e.g., psychotic disorder due to malignant lung neoplasm, with delusions; also code the general medical condition on Axis III.

Coding note: If delusions are part of vascular dementia, indicate the delusions by coding the appropriate subtype, e.g., vascular dementia, with delusions.

(From American Psychiatric Association. *Diagnostic and Statistical Manual of Mental Disorders.* 4th ed. Text rev. Washington, DC: American Psychiatric Association; copyright 2000, with permission.)

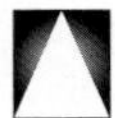

Table 14.4–7
DSM-IV-TR Diagnostic Criteria for Substance-Induced Psychotic Disorder

A. Prominent hallucinations or delusions. Note: Do not include hallucinations if the person has insight that they are substance induced.
B. There is evidence from the history, physical examination, or laboratory findings of either (1) or (2):
  (1) the symptoms in Criterion A developed during, or within a month of, substance intoxication or withdrawal
  (2) medication use is etiologically related to the disturbance
C. The disturbance is not better accounted for by a psychotic disorder that is not substance induced. Evidence that the symptoms are better accounted for by a psychotic disorder that is not substance induced might include the following: the symptoms precede the onset of the substance use (or medication use); the symptoms persist for a substantial period of time (e.g., about a month) after the cessation of acute withdrawal or severe intoxication, or are substantially in excess of what would be expected given the type or amount of the substance used or the duration of use; or there is other evidence that suggests the existence of an independent non–substance-induced psychotic disorder (e.g., a history of recurrent non–substance-related episodes).
D. The disturbance does not occur exclusively during the course of a delirium.

Note: This diagnosis should be made instead of a diagnosis of substance intoxication or substance withdrawal only when the symptoms are in excess of those usually associated with the intoxication or withdrawal syndrome and when the symptoms are sufficiently severe to warrant independent clinical attention.

Code [Specific substance]-induced psychotic disorder: (Alcohol, with delusions; alcohol, with hallucinations; amphetamine [or amphetaminelike substance], with delusions; amphetamine [or amphetaminelike substance], with hallucinations; cannabis, with delusions; cannabis, with hallucinations; cocaine, with delusions; cocaine, with hallucinations; hallucinogen, with delusions; hallucinogen, with hallucinations; inhalant, with delusions; inhalant, with hallucinations; opioid, with delusions; opioid, with hallucinations; phencyclidine [or phencyclidinelike substance], with delusions; phencyclidine [or phencyclidinelike substance], with hallucinations; sedative, hypnotic, or anxiolytic, with delusions; sedative, hypnotic, or anxiolytic, with hallucinations; other [or unknown] substance, with delusions; other [or unknown] substance, with hallucinations)

Specify if:
With onset during intoxication: if criteria are met for intoxication with the substance and the symptoms develop during the intoxication syndrome
With onset during withdrawal: if criteria are met for withdrawal from the substance and the symptoms develop during, or shortly after, a withdrawal syndrome

(From American Psychiatric Association. *Diagnostic and Statistical Manual of Mental Disorders.* 4th ed. Text rev. Washington, DC: American Psychiatric Association; copyright 2000, with permission.)

Clinical Features

Hallucinations. Hallucinations can occur in one or more sensory modalities. Tactile hallucinations (e.g., a sensation of bugs crawling on the skin) are characteristic of cocaine use. Auditory hallucinations are usually associated with psychoactive substance abuse; auditory hallucinations can also occur in persons who are deaf. Olfactory hallucinations can result from temporal lobe epilepsy; visual hallucinations can occur in persons who are blind because of cataracts. Hallucinations are either recurrent or persistent and are experienced in a state of full wakefulness and alertness; a hallucinating patient shows no significant changes in cognitive functions. Visual hallucinations often take the form of scenes involving diminutive (lilliputian) human figures or small animals. Rare musical hallucinations typically feature religious songs. Patients with psychotic disorder caused by a general medical condition and substance-induced psychotic disorder may act on their hallucinations. In alcohol-related hallucinations, threatening, critical, or insulting third-person voices speak about the patients and may tell them to harm either themselves or others. Such patients are dangerous and are at significant risk for suicide or homicide. Patients may or may not believe that the hallucinations are real.

Delusions. Secondary and substance-induced delusions are usually present in a state of full wakefulness. Patients experience no change in the level of consciousness, although mild cognitive impairment may be observed. Patients may appear confused, disheveled, or eccentric, with tangential or even incoherent speech. Hyperactivity and apathy may be present, and an associated dysphoric mood is thought to be common. The delusions can be systematized or fragmentary, with varying content, but persecutory delusions are the most common.

Differential Diagnosis

Psychotic disorder due to a general medical condition and substance-induced psychotic disorder must be distinguished from delirium (in which patients have a clouded sensorium), from dementia (in which patients have major intellectual deficits), and from schizophrenia (in which patients have other symptoms of thought disorder and impaired functioning). Psychotic disorder due to a general medical condition and substance-induced psychotic disorder must also be differentiated from psychotic mood disorders (in which other affective symptoms are pronounced).

Treatment

Treatment involves identifying the general medical condition or the particular substance involved. At this point, treatment is directed toward the underlying condition and the patient's immediate behavioral control. Hospitalization may be necessary to evaluate patients completely and to ensure their safety. Antipsychotic agents (e.g., olanzapine [Zyprexa] or haloperidol) may be necessary for immediate and short-term control of psychotic or aggressive behavior, although benzodiazepines may also be useful for controlling agitation and anxiety.

References

Caton CLM, Drake RE, Hasin DS, Dominguez B, Shrout PE, Samet S, Schanzer WB. Differences between early-phase primary psychotic disorders with concurrent substance use and substance-induced psychoses. *Arch Gen Psychiatry*. 2005;62(2):137–145.

Chabrol H. Chronic hallucinatory psychosis: Bouffe d'elirante, and the classification of psychosis in French psychiatry. *Curr Psychiatry Rep*. 2003;5:137–191.

Chaudron LH, Pies RW. The relationship between postpartum psychosis and bipolar disorder: A review. *J Clin Psychiatry*. 2003;64:1284–1292.

Crumlish N, Whitty P, Kamali M, Clarke M, Browne S, McTigue O, Lane A, Kinsella A, Larkin C, O'Callaghan E. Early insight predicts depression and attempted suicide after 4 years of first-episode schizophrenia and schizophreniform disorder. *Acta Psychiatr Scand*. 2005;112:449–455.

Degenhardt L, Hall W, Lynskey M. Testing hypotheses about the relationship between cannabis use and psychosis. *Drug Alcohol Depend*. 2003;71:37–48.

Fennig S, Fochtmann LJ. Psychosis not otherwise specified. In: Sadock BJ, Sadock VA, eds. *Kaplan & Sadock's Comprehensive Textbook of Psychiatry*. 8th ed. Vol. 1. Baltimore: Lippincott Williams & Wilkins; 2005:1542.

Jäger MDM, Hintermayr M, Bottlender R, Strauss A, Moller HJ. Course and outcome of first-admitted patients with acute and transient psychotic disorders (ICD-10:F23): Focus on relapses and social adjustment. *Eur Arch Psychiatry Clin Neurosci*. 2003;253:209.

Keri S, Kelemen O, Benedek G, Janka Z. Patients with schizophreniform disorder use verbal descriptions for the representation of visual categories. *Psychol Med*. 2004;34:247–253.

Malhotra S, Malhotra S. Acute and transient psychotic disorders: Comparison with schizophrenia. *Curr Psychiatry Rep*. 2003;5:178.

Mojtabai R. Acute and transient psychotic disorders and brief psychotic disorder. In: Sadock BJ, Sadock VA, eds. *Kaplan & Sadock's Comprehensive Textbook of Psychiatry*. 8th ed. Vol. 1. Baltimore: Lippincott Williams & Wilkins; 2005:1512.

Mojtabai R, Susser ES, Bromet EJ. Clinical characteristics, 4-year course, and DSM-IV classification of patients with nonaffective acute remitting psychosis. *Am J Psychiatry*. 2003;160:2108.

Naz B, Fochtmann LJ, Bromet EJ. In: Sadock BJ, Sadock VA, eds. *Kaplan & Sadock's Comprehensive Textbook of Psychiatry*. 8th ed. Vol. 1. Baltimore: Lippincott Williams & Wilkins; 2005:1536.

Pillmann F, Balzuweit S, Haring A, Bloink R, Marneros A. Suicidal behavior in acute and transient psychotic disorders. *Psychiatry Res*. 2003;117:199.

Sharma V. Pharmacotherapy of postpartum psychosis. *Exp Opin Pharmacother*. 2003;4:1651.

Sharma V, Mazmanian D. Sleep loss and postpartum psychosis. *Bipolar Disord*. 2003;5:98.

▲ 14.5 Culture-Bound Syndromes

The term *culture-bound syndrome* usually denotes specific arrays of behavioral and experiential phenomena that tend to present themselves preferentially in particular sociocultural contexts and that are readily recognized as illness behavior by most participants in that culture. The syndromes are commonly assigned culturally sanctioned explanations and interpretations that, in turn, generate a set of culturally congruent remedies, usually in the form of healing rituals performed by someone to whom the community assigns a therapeutic role.

Assessment of culture-bound syndromes must start with recognition that each human society has an indigenous body of beliefs and practices directed at explaining and treating disease and disorder and that patients internalize that worldview during the process of enculturation. They share their experiences and deal with distress through commonly understood symbols and meanings. In that light, the diagnostic encounter itself can be used as a point of entry into the patient's world. Although a person cannot become an anthropological expert about each and every possible cultural group, the clinician can try to learn by asking patients to share their cultural norms as they understand them.

EPIDEMIOLOGY

The last few decades have witnessed the production of significant research illuminating diverse aspects of cross-cultural practice. Of great interest for those responsible for the organization of psychiatric care are the ongoing findings of psychiatric epidemiology across cultures. Claims have repeatedly been made that African-Americans, Hispanics, Asians, and other minorities experience higher levels of psychological distress and disorder than the mainstream population. Lifetime rates for phobic disorder were significantly higher among African American respondents, with young Hispanics showing a higher prevalence of alcohol abuse. Other studies conducted by the Institute for Health Statistics demonstrated that, despite similar demographic characteristics, the prevalence of major depressive disorder for mainland Puerto Ricans was significantly higher than for island Puerto Ricans. Mexican-Americans with low acculturation status are reported to display low prevalence for most psychiatric disorders.

REPRESENTATIVE SYNDROMES

Table 14.5–1 lists representative culture-bound syndromes from around the world, with some of their clinical features. Two early descriptions of cases of cross-cultural syndromes are given below.

AMOK

The patient, a healthy young adult man, originally came from the hinterlands of Abau, in Papua, New Guinea. At the time of the act, he was working with a building gang on Ferguson Island. He was a foreigner to his work mates, one of whom called him an "Abau bush pig"—a grave insult. One night, at approximately 6:30 PM, the others were in their dormitory reading or lying down, when the patient came in with a 12-inch bush knife and suddenly attacked them, going from bed to bed hacking at them with the knife, mostly in the vicinity of the head and neck. Six died, then or later, some with terrible wounds, their heads being almost chopped off. Finally, another man in the vicinity heard the noise and came in with a rifle and one cartridge. The patient who has run amok attempted to attack him, was fired at, and still did not cease attacking. He was then put out of action by the butt of the rifle and died. (Courtesy of Manuel Trujillo, M.D.)

KORO

A Chinese patrol officer asked the physician A.H. Vorstman to accompany him to a village in the Singtan district to provide medical aid to a member of the native elite. The patient was found in bed, surrounded by a retinue and with an old man sitting at the foot of the bed. Having no information about the patient's symptoms during the preceding days, Vorstman's examination and questioning failed to yield much insight into the man's problem. Vorstman concluded that alcohol abuse, a common native habit, was the background for this case. The Chinese official who accompanied Vorstman related to him that, for the last 8 days, the patient's penis had withdrawn into his abdomen, and, as a preventive measure, the old man at the foot of the bed had been gripping his master's "obstinate limb." Vorstman was the first person to publish cases of Koro. (Courtesy of Manuel Trujillo, M.D.)

COURSE AND PROGNOSIS

Limited data on the longitudinal course of patients with culture-bound syndromes suggest that some of them eventually develop clinical features compatible with a diagnosis of schizophrenia, bipolar disorder, cognitive disorder, or other psychotic disorders. Thus, gathering information from all possible sources is crucial. Because clinical pictures evolve over time, thorough reevaluations should be conducted periodically to refine the diagnosis and improve clinical care.

TREATMENT

Treatment of a culture-bound syndrome poses several diagnostic challenges, the first of which is determining whether the symptomatology represents a culturally appropriate adaptive response to a situation. Clinicians are well advised to (1) know or search out the demographics of the local population or catchment area being served; (2) recognize that always a local pattern exists of conceptualization, naming, vocabulary, explanation, and treatment of patterns of distress that afflict a community, including mental disorders; and (3) talk with the family and learn about local customs or search out other modes of documentation. Persons within the culture will almost always recognize that one of their own is acting in a deviant manner, and their input can be extremely valuable in making an assessment of mental disorder.

When taking the history, ask the patients what they think could have caused the problem and how they explain it to themselves. Some useful questions: (1) What do you think has caused your problem? (2) Why do you think it started when it did? (3) What do you think your sickness does to you? How does it work? (4) How severe is your sickness? Will it have a short or long course? (5) What kind of treatment do you think you should receive?

Insight into the dynamics of the patient's world facilitates the clinician's efforts to adapt his or her techniques (e.g., general activity level, mode of verbal intervention, content of remarks, tone of voice) to the patient's cultural background. It implies acceptance of, and respect for, the patient's cultural frame of reference and opens the possibility of direct intervention in the lives of patients, who may be willing to cooperate when they feel understood.

Therapies. Much knowledge has accrued about the applications of standard, psychoanalytically based psychotherapy to populations and ethnic backgrounds, other than whites of Western origin. To the repeated observation that ethnic communities are accepted for psychotherapy treatment at lower rates and drop out earlier than their mainstream counterparts, researchers and clinicians have provided a bounty of adaptations ranging from preparations for psychotherapy to substantive framework modifications. The most daring step in this continuum is the development of culture-specific therapies empirically derived from culture-specific behavioral features. José Szapocznick, for example, has developed and proposed a model of family therapy for Miami's Cuban families guided by empirically derived values prevalent in that population, such as strong familial affiliation and a preference for hierarchical family structures.

While encouraging openness to such technologies, systems of care should establish standards and guidelines that aim to obtain clinical and functional outcomes equivalent to the mainstream state-of-the-art efficacy studies, equally avoiding, promoting, and discouraging particular approaches until unquestionable evidence of efficacy and effectiveness is developed.

Cognitive and cognitive behavior therapies may achieve some modicum of freedom from cultural bias to the degree that cognitive therapists work with the specific pathogenic beliefs of the patient, whatever the cultural origin of such beliefs. Its application to minority populations experiencing anxiety and depressive disorders may be an area of promising cross-cultural research.

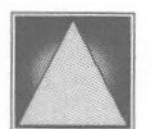

Table 14.5–1
Examples of Culture-Bound Syndromes

amok A dissociative episode characterized by a period of brooding followed by an outburst of violent, aggressive, or homicidal behavior directed at persons and objects. The episode tends to be precipitated by a perceived slight or insult and seems to be prevalent only among men. The episode is often accompanied by persecutory idea; automatism, amnesia, exhaustion, and a return to premorbid state following the episode. Some instances of amok may occur during a brief psychotic episode or constitute the onset or an exacerbation of a chronic psychotic process. The original reports that used this term were from Malaysia. A similar behavior pattern is found in Laos, Philippines, Polynesia (*cafard* or *cathard*), Papua New Guinea, and Puerto Rico (*mal de pelea*), and among the Navajo (*iich'aa*).

ataque de nervios An idiom of distress principally reported among Latinos from the Caribbean, but recognized among many Latin American and Latin Mediterranean groups. Commonly reported symptoms include uncontrollable shouting, attacks of crying, trembling, heat in the chest rising into the head, and verbal or physical aggression. Dissociative experiences, seizurelike or fainting episodes, and suicidal gestures are prominent in some attacks but absent in others. A general feature of an *ataque de nervios* is a sense of being out of control. *Ataques de nervios* frequently occur as a direct result of a stressful event relating to the family (e.g., death of a close relative, separation or divorce from a spouse, conflicts with a spouse or children, or witnessing an accident involving a family member). Persons may experience amnesia for what occurred during the *ataque de nervios*, but they otherwise return rapidly to their usual level of functioning. Although descriptions of some *ataques de nervios* most closely fit the DSM description of panic attacks, the association of most *ataques* with a precipitating event and the frequent absence of the hallmark symptoms of acute fear or apprehension distinguish them from panic disorder. *Ataques* span the range from normal expressions of distress not associated with a mental disorder to symptom presentations associated with anxiety, mood, dissociative, or somatoform disorders.

bilis and colera (also referred to as *muina*) The underlying cause is thought to be strongly experienced anger or rage. Anger is viewed among many Latino groups as a particularly powerful emotion that can have direct effects on the body and exacerbate existing symptoms. The major effect of anger is to disturb core body balances (which are understood as a balance between hot and cold valences in the body and between the material and spiritual aspects of the body). Symptoms can include acute nervous tension, headache, trembling, screaming, stomach disturbances, and, in more severe cases, loss of consciousness. Chronic fatigue may result from an acute episode.

bouff ée délirante A syndrome observed in West Africa and Haiti. The French term refers to a sudden outburst of agitated and aggressive behavior, marked confusion, and psychomotor excitement. It may sometimes be accompanied by visual and auditory hallucinations or paranoid ideation. The episodes may resemble an episode of brief psychotic disorder.

brain fag A term initially used in West Africa to refer to a condition experienced by high school or university students in response to the challenges of schooling. Symptoms include difficulties in concentrating, remembering, and thinking. Students often state that their brains are "fatigued." Additional somatic symptoms are usually centered around the head and neck and include pain, pressure or tightness, blurring of vision, heat, or burning. "Brain tiredness" or fatigue from "too much thinking" is an idiom of distress in many cultures, and resulting syndromes can resemble certain anxiety, depressive, and somatoform disorders.

dhat A folk diagnostic term used in India to refer to severe anxiety and hypochondriacal concerns associated with the discharge of semen, whitish discoloration of the urine, and feelings of weakness and exhaustion. Similar to *jiryan* (India), *sukra prameha* (Sri Lanka), and *shen-k'uei* (China).

falling-out or blackout Episodes that occur primarily in southern United States and Caribbean groups. They are characterized by a sudden collapse, which sometimes occurs without warming but is sometimes preceded by feelings of dizziness or "swimming" in the head. The person's eyes are usually open, but the person claims an inability to see. Those affected usually hear and understand what is occurring around them but feel powerless to move. This may correspond to a diagnosis of conversion disorder or a dissociative disorder.

ghost sickness A preoccupation with death and the deceased (sometimes associated with witchcraft), frequently observed among members of many American Indian tribes. Various symptoms can be attributed to ghost sickness, including bad dreams, weakness, feeling of danger, loss of appetite, fainting, dizziness, fear, anxiety, hallucinations, loss of consciousness, confusion, feelings of futility, and a sense of suffocation.

hwa-byung (also known as *wool-hwa-byung*) A Korean folk syndrome literally translated into English as "anger syndrome" and attributed to the suppression of anger. The symptoms include insomnia, fatigue, panic, fear of impending death, dysphoric affect, indigestion, anorexia, dyspnea, palpitations, generalized aches and pains, and a feeling of a mass in the epigastrium.

koro A term probably of Malaysian origin, that refers to an episode of sudden and intense anxiety that the penis (or, in women, the vulva and nipples) will recede into the body and possibly cause death. The syndrome is reported in South and East Asia, where it is known by a variety of local terms, such as *shuk yang, shook yong,* and *suo yang* (Chinese); *jinjinia bemar* (Assam); or *rok-joo* (Thailand). It is occasionally found in the West. *Koro* at times occurs in localized epidemic form in East Asian areas. The diagnosis is included in the second edition of *Chinese Classification of Mental Disorders* (*CCMD-2*).

latah Hypersensitivity to sudden fright, often with echopraxia, echolalia, command obedience, and dissociative or trancelike behavior. The term *latah* is of Malaysian or Indonesian origin, but the syndrome has been found in many parts of the world. Other terms for the condition are *amurakh, irkunil, ikota, olan, myriachit,* and *menkeiti* (Siberian groups); *bah tschi, bah-tsi, baah-ji* (Thailand); *imu* (Ainu, Sakhalin, Japan); and *mali-mali* and *silok* (Philippines). In Malaysia it is more frequent in middle-aged women.

locura A term used by Latinos in the United States and Latin America to refer to a severe form of chronic psychosis. The condition is attributed to an inherited vulnerability, to the effect of multiple life difficulties, or to a combination of both factors. Symptoms exhibited by persons with *locura* include incoherence, agitation, auditory and visual hallucinations, inability to follow rules of social interaction, unpredictability, and possibly violence.

mal de ojo A concept widely found in Mediterranean cultures and elsewhere in the world. *Mal de ojo* is a Spanish phrase translated into English as "evil eye." Children are especially at risk. Symptoms include fitful sleep, crying without apparent cause, diarrhea, vomiting and fever in a child or infant. Sometimes adults (especially women) have the condition.

nervios A common idiom of distress among Latinos in the United States and Latin America. A number of other ethnic groups have related, though often somewhat distinctive, ideas of nerves (such as *nerva* among Greeks in North America). *Nervios* refers both to a general state of vulnerability to stressful life experiences and to a syndrome brought on by difficult life circumstances. The term *nervios* includes a wide range of symptoms of emotional distress, somatic disturbance, and inability to function. Common symptoms include headaches and brain aches, irritability, stomach disturbances, sleep difficulties, nervousness, easy tearfulness, inability to concentrate, trembling, tingling sensations, and *mareos* (dizziness with occasional vertigolike exacerbations). *Nervios* tends to be an ongoing problem, although variable in the degree

(*continued*)

Table 14.5–1
(Continued)

of disability that is manifest. *Nervios* is a very broad syndrome that spans the range from patients free of a mental disorder to presentations resembling adjustment, anxiety, depressive, dissociative, somatoform, or psychotic disorders. Differential diagnosis depends on the constellation of symptoms experienced, the kinds of social events that are associated with the onset and progress of *nervios*, and the level of disability experienced.

piblokto An abrupt dissociative episode accompanied by extreme excitement of up to 30 minutes' duration and frequently followed by convulsive seizures and coma lasting up to 12 hours. It is observed primarily in Arctic and subarctic Eskimo communities, although regional variations in name exist. The person may be withdrawn or mildly irritable for a period of hours or days before the attack and typically reports complete amnesia for the attack. During the attack persons may tear off their clothing, break furniture, shout obscenities, eat feces, flee from protective shelters, or perform other irrational or dangerous acts.

***qi-gong* psychotic reactions** Acute, time-limited episodes characterized by dissociative, paranoid, or other psychotic or nonpsychotic symptoms that may occur after participation in the Chinese folk health-enhancing practice of *qi-gong* (exercise of vital energy). Especially vulnerable are persons who become overly involved in the practice. This diagnosis is included in CCMD-2.

rootwork A set of cultural interpretations that ascribe illness to hexing, witchcraft, sorcery, or evil influence of another person. Symptoms may include generalized anxiety and gastrointestinal complaints (e.g., nausea, vomiting, diarrhea), weakness, dizziness, the fear of being poisoned, and sometimes fear of being killed (voodoo death). Roots, spells, or hexes can be put or placed on other person, causing a variety of emotional and psychological problems. The hexed person may even fear death until the root has been taken off (eliminated), usually through the work of a root doctor (a healer in this tradition), who can also be called on to bewitched an enemy. Rootwork is found in the southern United States among both African-American and European-American populations and in Caribbean societies. It is also known as *mal puesto* or *brujeria* in Latino societies.

sangue dormido ("sleeping blood") A syndrome found among Portuguese Cape Verde Islanders (and immigrants from there to the United States). It includes pain, numbness, tremor, paralysis, convulsions, stroke, blindness, heart attack, infection, and miscarriages.

Shenjing shuariuo ("neurasthenia") In China a condition characterized by physical and mental fatigue, dizziness, headaches, other pains, concentration difficulties, sleep disturbance, and memory loss. Other symptoms include gastrointestinal problems, sexual dysfunction, irritability, excitability, and various signs suggesting disturbance of the autonomic nervous system. In many cases the symptoms would meet the criteria for a DSM mood or anxiety disorder. The diagnosis is included in CCMD-2.

shen-k'uei (Taiwan); *shenkui* (China) A Chinese folk label describing marked anxiety or panic symptoms with accompanying somatic complaints for which no physical cause can be demonstrated. Symptoms include dizziness, backache, fatigability, general weakness, insomnia, frequent dreams, and complaints of sexual dysfunction, such as premature ejaculation and impotence. Symptoms are attributed to excessive semen loss from frequent intercourse, masturbation, nocturnal emission, or passing of white turbid urine believed to contain semen. Excessive semen loss is feared because of the belief that it represents the loss of one's vital essence and can therefore be life threatening.

shin-byung A Korean folk label for a syndrome in which initial phases are characterized by anxiety and somatic complaints (general weakness, dizziness, fear, anorexia, insomnia, gastrointestinal problems), with subsequent dissociation and possession by ancestral spirits.

spell A trance state in which persons "communicate" with deceased relatives or spirits. At times the state is associated with brief periods of personality change. The culture-specific syndrome is seen among African-Americans and European-Americans from the southern United States. Spells are not considered to be medical events in the folk tradition but may be misconstrued as psychotic episodes in clinical settings.

susto (*frigh* or "soul loss") A folk illness prevalent among some Latinos in the United States and among people in Mexico, Central America, and South America. *Susto* is also referred to as *espanto, pasmo, tripa ida, perdida del alma,* or *chibih. Susto* is an illness attributed to a frightening event that causes the soul to leave the body and results in unhappiness and sickness. Persons with *susto* also experience significant strains in key social roles. Symptoms may appear any time from days to years after the fright is experienced. It is believed that in extreme cases, *susto* may result in death. Typical symptoms include appetite disturbances, inadequate or excessive sleep, troubled sleep or dreams, feelings of sadness, lack of motivation to do anything, and feelings of low self-worth or dirtiness. Somatic symptoms accompanying *susto* include muscle aches and pains, headache, stomachache, and diarrhea. Ritual healings are focused on calling the soul back to the body and cleansing the person to restore bodily and spiritual balance. Different experience of *susto* may be related to major depressive disorder, posttraumatic stress disorders, and somatoform disorders. Similar etiological beliefs and symptom configurations are found in many parts of the world.

taijin kyofu sho A culturally distinctive phobia in Japan, in some ways resembling social phobia in DSM. The syndrome refers to an intense fear that one's body, its parts or its functions, displease, embarrass, or are offensive to other people in appearance, odor, facial expressions, or movements. The syndrome is included in the official Japanese diagnostic system for mental disorders.

zar A general term applied in Ethiopia, Somalia, Egypt, Sudan, Iran, and other North African and Middle Eastern societies to the experience of spirits possessing a person. Persons possessed by a spirit may experience dissociative episodes that may include shouting, laughing, hitting the head against a wall, singing, or weeping. They may show apathy and withdrawal, refusing to eat or carry out daily tasks or may develop a long-term relationship with the possessing spirit. Such behavior is not considered pathological locally.

(From American Psychiatric Association. *Diagnostic and Statistical Manual of Mental Disorders.* 4th ed. Text rev. Washington, DC: American Psychiatric Association; copyright 2000, with permission.)

Indigenous Healers. One promising avenue is collaboration with indigenous healers. Several researchers have reported on their success in the use of indigenous and traditional healers in the treatment of psychiatric patients, especially those whose psychotic conditions are substantially connected to culture-specific beliefs (e.g., fear of voodoo death). Decisions about involving indigenous healers should be individualized and planned thoughtfully, taking into consideration the setting, the thoughtfulness and flexibility of the available healers, the type of psychopathology, and the patient's characteristics. The World Health Organization (WHO) has long advocated implementation at the local level of a policy of close collaboration between the conventional health system and traditional medicine, particularly between individual health professionals and traditional practitioners.

CULTURE AND PSYCHOPHARMACOLOGY

A rich lode of research findings must be codified by systems of psychiatric care that aim to improve the practice of ethnic psychopharmacology. Guidelines must include factual knowledge about differential pharmacogenetics and pharmacodynamics and relational knowledge regarding the impact of giving or withholding medications. Expectations about the use of medications, as well as the parallel use of traditional herbs, which is widespread in many cultures, are mediated by culture-specific beliefs about causation of illness and recovery and may need active inquiry by the clinician. The clinician and researcher must also consider additional factors, such as the patient's culturally based expectations of optimal psychiatric treatment (pharmacotherapy or psychotherapy), expected rate of recovery (fast or slow), target symptoms, and threshold and tolerance for adverse effects. If a Hispanic patient has the culturally shared expectation that psychological disorders are somatically based and best treated by an authoritative physician with medication, alternative treatment recommendations will be met with resistance and reduced compliance, unless extensive psychoeducational efforts are deployed. Alternatively, middle-class, educated, urban professionals may reject psychopharmacological prescriptions for their anxiety or depressive syndromes as simplistic, because they had expected psychotherapy or psychoanalysis.

Thus, the therapeutic relationship across the language or cultural barrier should be initiated by carefully eliciting the patient's explanatory framework of illness, anticipated path to recovery, and expectations for treatment. Clinicians must spend time and effort in an educational dialog with patients and their significant others and explain the reasons for an alternative to the patient's preferred course of treatment. Slow onset of action and the frequency of adverse effects interfere with the therapeutic cooperation of some Hispanic and Asian patients who expect rapid relief, fear toxicity, or are concerned with the addictive potential of medications to be taken long term. To obtain adequate compliance across the cultural barrier, the clinician must make tactful efforts to learn the patient's (and the immediate family's) latent, culturally shaped beliefs about the illness and its normative treatment, to provide therapeutic options compatible with the patient's culturally prescribed explanatory models, and to avoid having hidden miscommunication hinder the necessary compliance.

Pharmacogenetics

The field of pharmacogenetics grew out of observations of significant ethnic differences in response to drugs, in differential development, and in adverse-effect profiles, leading to the discovery of defects or deficiencies in the genetically controlled activity of enzyme systems responsible for the metabolism of psychotropic medications and toxins such as alcohol.

Acetylation Status. Observations of ethnic differences in the adverse-effects profile of the antituberculosis drug isoniazid (Nydrazid, Rifamate) led to the classification of persons as slow or rapid acetylators, which, among other biological effects, determines their metabolism of psychotropic medications such as clonazepam (Klonopin) and phenelzine (Nardil).

Alcohol Metabolism. P.H. Wolf, while studying racial differences in alcohol sensitivity, observed that about 80 percent of Asians and 50 percent of native Americans exhibited the flushing response to alcohol (compared with 10 percent of whites) and concluded that these differences had a genetic basis. They have been proved to be related to genetic polymorphism of isoenzymes of alcohol dehydrogenase (ADH) and aldehyde dehydrogenase (ALDH), enzymes critical for complete metabolism of alcohol and other neurotransmitters and which play a role in development of alcoholism or its avoidance. For example, Asians who are either homozygous or heterozygous for the atypical Asian-type *ALDH2* gene are alcohol sensitive and have a low risk for alcoholism and alcoholic liver disease.

Native Americans have a high frequency of both alcohol flushing and alcohol-related problems, and Akira Yoshida's research team reported in 1993 that they had practically no detectable Asian type *ADH2* and *ALDH2* genes, a major alcohol-rejecting genetic factor.

Cytochrome P450 Isoenzymes. The cytochrome P450 enzyme system is key in the metabolism of psychotropic and nonpsychotropic drugs as well as a great variety of environmental toxins that find their way into the diets of animals and humans. The genetic defects that render these enzymes less effective and make humans poor metabolizers are unequally distributed among ethnic populations. This is particularly the case for two cytochrome P450 (CYP) isoenzymes: CYP 2D6 (debrisoquin hydroxylase), and CYP 2Cmp (mephenytoin hydroxylase). The percentage of CYP 2D6-poor metabolizers is lower for Asians (0.5 to 2.4 percent), and higher for whites (2.9 to 10 percent). Similar interethnic variance exists in the frequency of poor metabolizers of CYP 2Cmp: low among whites (3 percent), intermediate for African-Americans (18 percent), and higher (up to 20 percent) in Asian and Japanese populations.

These interethnic differences in the P450 isoenzymes are of great importance in psychiatry and psychopharmacology because of their role in the metabolism of antipsychotics, antidepressants, sedatives such as barbiturates and benzodiazepines, and β-adrenergic receptor antagonists (beta-blockers) such as propranolol (Inderal).

Environmental Factors. In addition to being genetically regulated, enzymes that participate in the metabolism of psychotropic medications respond to environmental variables such as diet, alcohol, smoking status, and caffeine intake. All of these factors can accelerate or slow the metabolism of drugs through enzyme induction or inhibition.

Herbal Medicines. In parallel with available Western medicine-oriented psychiatric services, immigrants often retain their loyalty to ethnically based folk-medicine systems. Accounts by Vivian Garrison and Allan Hardwood document extensive use of folk healers by Puerto Ricans in New York City. Other investigators have reported that Mexican Americans are willing to accept prescribed medications from psychiatrists and herbs from a community healer, just as mainstream Americans use natural serotonin-enhancing herbs such as St. John's wort in addition to, or instead of, the more conventional psychotropics prescribed by their psychiatrists. Culturally competent psychopharmacologists need to inquire about their patients' use of the traditional herbal medicines of Asians, African-Americans, Hispanics, and other immigrants living in the United States. Many of these herbs possess high levels of psychoactive activity, such as anticholinergics (*Swertia japonica* used by Japanese patients or *Datura candida* used by Cubans), stimulants (the caffeine-loaded *Ibexguazusa* of Latin America), and sedatives (*Schumanniophyton problematicans* of the Nigerians). Others, such as ginseng and glycyrrhiza, may stimulate or inhibit cytochrome P450.

References

Ancis JR, Chen Y, Schultz D. Diagnostic challenges and the so-called culture-bound syndromes. In: Ancis JR, ed. *Culturally Responsive Interventions: Innovative Approaches to Working with Diverse Populations.* New York: Brunner-Routledge; 2004:197–209.

Belkin GS. Hard questions in court: Culture and psychiatry on trial. *Cult Med Psychiatry.* 2003;27:157–159.

Bhugra D, Mastrogianni A, Maharajh H, Harvey S. Prevalence of bulimic behaviours and eating attitudes in schoolgirls from Trinidad and Barbados. *Transcult Psychiatry.* 2003;40:408–428.

Castro-Blanco DR. Cultural sensitivity in conventional psychotherapy: A comment on Martinez-Taboas. *Psychotherapy: Theory, Research, Practice, Training*. 2005;42:14–16.

Chang DF, Myers HF, Yeung A, Zhang Y, Zhao J, Yu S. Shenjing Shuairuo and the DSM-IV: Diagnosis, distress, and disability in a Chinese primary care setting. *Transcult Psychiatry.* 2005;42(2):204–218.

Cohen S. Exotic deviance: Medicalizing cultural idioms from strangeness to illness. *Transcult Psychiatry.* 2005;42:151–154.

Faison WE, Armstrong D. Cultural aspects of psychosis in the elderly. *J Geriatr Psychiatry Neurol.* 2003;16:225–231.

Guarnaccia PJ, Martinez I, Ramirez R, Canino G. Are "Ataques de Nervios" in Puerto Rican children associated with psychiatric disorder? *J Am Acad Child Adolesc Psychiatry.* 2005;44(11):1184–1192.

Keel PK, Klump KL. Are eating disorders culture-bound syndromes? Implications for conceptualizing their etiology. *Psychological Bull.* 2003;129: 747–769.

Parzen MD. Towards a culture-bound syndrome-based insanity defense? *Cult Med Psychiatry.* 2003;27:131–155.

Trujillo M. Culture-bound syndromes. In: Sadock BJ, Sadock VA, eds. *Kaplan & Sadock's Comprehensive Textbook of Psychiatry*. 8th ed. Vol. 2. Baltimore: Lippincott Williams & Wilkins; 2005:2282.

15 Mood Disorders

▲ 15.1 Depression and Bipolar Disorder

Mood is a pervasive and sustained feeling tone that is experienced internally and that influences a person's behavior and perception of the world. Affect is the external expression of mood. Mood can be normal, elevated, or depressed. Healthy persons experience a wide range of moods and have an equally large repertoire of affective expressions; they feel in control of their moods and affects.

Mood disorders are a group of clinical conditions characterized by a loss of that sense of control and a subjective experience of great distress. Patients with elevated mood demonstrate expansiveness, flight of ideas, decreased sleep, and grandiose ideas. Patients with depressed mood experience a loss of energy and interest, feelings of guilt, difficulty in concentrating, loss of appetite, and thoughts of death or suicide. Other signs and symptoms of mood disorders include change in activity level, cognitive abilities, speech, and vegetative functions (e.g., sleep, appetite, sexual activity, and other biological rhythms). These disorders virtually always result in impaired interpersonal, social, and occupational functioning.

It is tempting to consider disorders of mood on a continuum with normal variations in mood. Patients with mood disorders, however, often report an ineffable, but distinct, quality to their pathological state. The concept of a continuum, therefore, may represent the clinician's overidentification with the pathology, thus possibly distorting his or her approach to patients with mood disorder.

Patients afflicted with only major depressive episodes are said to have *major depressive disorder* or *unipolar depression*. Patients with both manic and depressive episodes or patients with manic episodes alone are said to have *bipolar disorder*. The terms "unipolar mania" and "pure mania" are sometimes used for patients who are bipolar, but who do not have depressive episodes.

Three additional categories of mood disorders are hypomania, cyclothymia, and dysthymia. Hypomania is an episode of manic symptoms that does not meet the full text revision of the fourth edition of *Diagnostic and Statistical Manual of Mental Disorders* (DSM-IV-TR) criteria for manic episode. Cyclothymia and dysthymia are defined by DSM-IV-TR as disorders that represent less severe forms of bipolar disorder and major depression, respectively.

The field of psychiatry has considered major depression and bipolar disorder to be two separate disorders, particularly in the last 20 years. The possibility that bipolar disorder is actually a more severe expression of major depression has been reconsidered recently, however. Many patients given a diagnosis of a major depressive disorder reveal, on careful examination, past episodes of manic or hypomanic behavior that have gone undetected. Many authorities see considerable continuity between recurrent depressive and bipolar disorders. This has led to widespread discussion and debate about the bipolar spectrum, which incorporates classic bipolar disorder, bipolar II, and recurrent depressions.

HISTORY

The Old Testament story of King Saul describes a depressive syndrome, as does the story of Ajax's suicide in Homer's Iliad. About 400 BCE, Hippocrates used the terms *mania* and *melancholia* to describe mental disturbances. Around 30 AD, the Roman physician Celsus described melancholia (from Greek *melan* ["black"] and *chole* ["bile"]) in his work *De re medicina* as a depression caused by black bile.

In 1854, Jules Falret described a condition called *folie circulaire*, in which patients experience alternating moods of depression and mania. In 1882, the German psychiatrist Karl Kahlbaum, using the term *cyclothymia*, described mania and depression as stages of the same illness. In 1899, Emil Kraepelin, building on the knowledge of previous French and German psychiatrists, described manic-depressive psychosis using most of the criteria that psychiatrists now use to establish a diagnosis of bipolar I disorder. According to Kraepelin, the absence of a dementing and deteriorating course in manic-depressive psychosis differentiated it from dementia praecox (as schizophrenia was then called). Kraepelin also described a depression that came to be known as involutional melancholia, which has since come to be viewed as a form of mood disorder that begins in late adulthood (Fig. 15.1–1).

DSM-IV-TR CLASSIFICATION OF MOOD DISORDERS

Depression

According to DSM-IV-TR, a major depressive disorder occurs without a history of a manic, mixed, or hypomanic episode. A major depressive episode must last at least 2 weeks, and typically a person with a diagnosis of a major depressive episode also experiences at least four symptoms from a list that includes changes in appetite and weight, changes in sleep and activity,

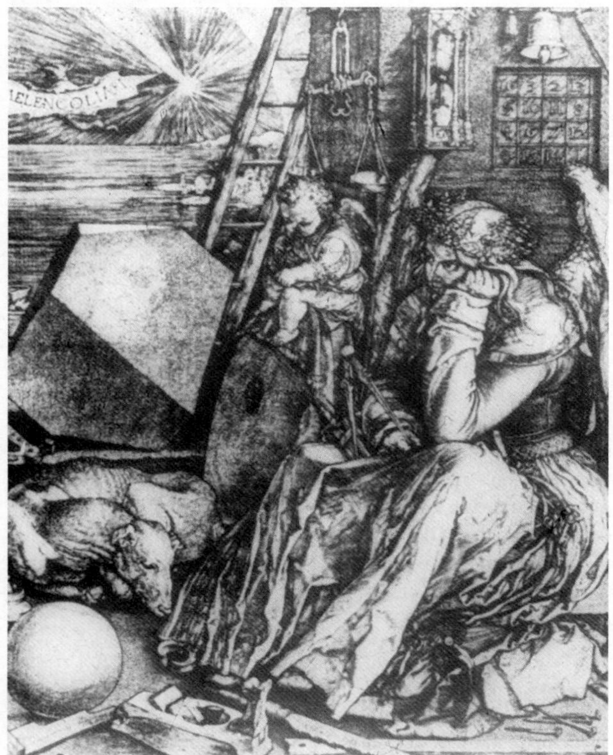

FIGURE 15.1–1
Melancholia (1514) by Albrecht Dürer.

lack of energy, feelings of guilt, problems thinking and making decisions, and recurring thoughts of death or suicide.

Mania

A manic episode is a distinct period of an abnormally and persistently elevated, expansive, or irritable mood lasting for at least 1 week, or less if a patient must be hospitalized. A hypomanic episode lasts at least 4 days and is similar to a manic episode except that it is not sufficiently severe to cause impairment in social or occupational functioning, and no psychotic features are present. Both mania and hypomania are associated with inflated self-esteem, decreased need for sleep, distractibility, great physical and mental activity, and overinvolvement in pleasurable behavior. According to DSM-IV-TR, bipolar I disorder is defined as having a clinical course of one or more manic episodes and, sometimes, major depressive episodes. A mixed episode is a period of at least 1 week in which both a manic episode and a major depressive episode occur almost daily. A variant of bipolar disorder characterized by episodes of major depression and hypomania rather than mania is known as *bipolar II disorder*.

Dysthymia and Cyclothymia

Two additional mood disorders, dysthymic disorder and cyclothymic disorder (discussed fully in Section 15.2), have also been appreciated clinically for some time. Dysthymic disorder and cyclothymic disorder are characterized by the presence of symptoms that are less severe than those of major depressive disorder and bipolar I disorder, respectively. DSM-IV-TR defines dysthymic disorder as characterized by at least 2 years of depressed mood that is not sufficiently severe to fit the diagnosis of major depressive episode. Cyclothymic disorder is characterized by at least 2 years of frequently occurring hypomanic symptoms that cannot fit the diagnosis of manic episode and of depressive symptoms that cannot fit the diagnosis of major depressive episode.

Other Categories

The DSM-IV-TR includes three mood disorder research categories (minor depressive disorder, recurrent brief depressive disorder, and premenstrual dysphoric disorder). Other DSM-IV-TR diagnoses are mood disorder due to a general medical condition and substance-induced mood disorder. These categories are designed to broaden the recognition of mood disorder diagnoses, to describe mood disorder symptoms more specifically than in the past, and to facilitate the differential diagnosis of mood disorders. Finally, DSM-IV-TR includes three residual disorders: bipolar disorder not otherwise specified, depressive disorder not otherwise specified, and mood disorder not otherwise specified (see Section 15.3).

EPIDEMIOLOGY

Incidence and Prevalence

Mood disorders are common. In the most recent surveys, major depressive disorder has the highest lifetime prevalence (almost 17 percent) of any psychiatric disorder. The lifetime prevalence rate of different forms of DSM-IV-TR unipolar depressive disorder, according to the eight major community surveys, are shown in Table 15.1–1. The yearly incidence of a major depression is 1.59 percent (women, 1.89 percent; men, 1.10 percent). The lifetime prevalence rates of different clinical forms of bipolar disorder are shown in Table 15.1–2. The annual incidence (number of new cases) of a major depressive episode is 1.59 percent (women, 1.89 percent; men, 1.10 percent). The annual incidence of bipolar illness is less than 1 percent, but it is difficult to estimate, because milder forms of bipolar disorder are often missed.

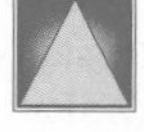

Table 15.1–1
Lifetime Prevalence Rates of Depressive Disorders

Type		Lifetime Prevalence (%)
Major depressive episode	Range	5–17
	Average	12
Dysthymic disorder	Range	3–6
	Average	5
Minor depressive disorder	Range	10
	Average	—
Recurrent brief depressive disorder	Range	16
	Average	—
Full unipolar spectrum		20–25

(Adapted from Rihmer Z, Angst A. Mood Disorders: Epidemiology. In: Sadock BJ, Sadock VA, eds. *Comprehensive Textbook of Psychiatry*. 8th ed. Baltimore: Lippincott Williams & Wilkins; 2004, with permission.)

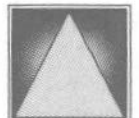

Table 15.1–2
Lifetime Prevalence Rates of Bipolar I, Bipolar II, Cyclothymic Disorder, and Hypomania

	Lifetime Prevalence (%)
Bipolar I disorder	0–2.4
Bipolar II disorder	0.3–4.8
Cyclothymia	0.5–6.3
Hypomania	2.6–7.8
Full bipolar spectrum	2.6–7.8

(Adapted from Rihmer Z, Angst A, Mood Disorders: Epidemiology. In: Sadock BJ, Sadock VA, eds. *Comprehensive Textbook of Psychiatry.* 8th ed. Baltimore: Lippincott Williams & Wilkins; 2004, with permission.)

Sex

An almost universal observation, independent of country or culture, is the twofold greater prevalence of major depressive disorder in women than in men. The reasons for the difference are hypothesized to involve hormonal differences, the effects of childbirth, differing psychosocial stressors for women and for men, and behavioral models of learned helplessness. In contrast to major depressive disorder, bipolar I disorder has an equal prevalence among men and women. Manic episodes are more common in men, and depressive episodes are more common in women. When manic episodes occur in women, they are more likely than men to present a mixed picture (e.g., mania and depression). Women also have a higher rate of being rapid cyclers, defined as having four or more manic episodes in a 1-year period.

Age

The onset of bipolar I disorder is earlier than that of major depressive disorder. The age of onset for bipolar I disorder ranges from childhood (as early as age 5 or 6) to 50 years or even older in rare cases, with a mean age of 30. The mean age of onset for major depressive disorder is about 40 years, with 50 percent of all patients having an onset between the ages of 20 and 50. Major depressive disorder can also begin in childhood or in old age. Recent epidemiological data suggest that the incidence of major depressive disorder may be increasing among people younger than 20 years of age. This may be related to the increased use of alcohol and drugs of abuse in this age group.

Marital Status

Major depressive disorder occurs most often in persons without close interpersonal relationships or in those who are divorced or separated. Bipolar I disorder is more common in divorced and single persons than among married persons, but this difference may reflect the early onset and the resulting marital discord characteristic of the disorder.

Socioeconomic and Cultural Factors

No correlation has been found between socioeconomic status and major depressive disorder. A higher than average incidence of bipolar I disorder is found among the upper socioeconomic groups. Bipolar I disorder is more common in persons who did not graduate from college than in college graduates, however, which may also reflect the relatively early age of onset for the disorder. Depression is more common in rural areas than in urban areas. The prevalence of mood disorder does not differ among races. A tendency exists, however, for examiners to underdiagnose mood disorder and overdiagnose schizophrenia in patients whose racial or cultural background differs from theirs.

COMORBIDITY

Individuals with major mood disorders are at an increased risk of having one or more additional comorbid Axis I disorders. The most frequent disorders are alcohol abuse or dependence, panic disorder, obsessive–compulsive disorder (OCD), and social anxiety disorder. Conversely, individuals with substance use disorders and anxiety disorders also have an elevated risk of lifetime or current comorbid mood disorder. In both unipolar and bipolar disorder, men more frequently present with substance use disorders, whereas women more frequently present with comorbid anxiety and eating disorders. In general, patients who are bipolar more frequently show comorbidity of substance use and anxiety disorders than do patients with unipolar major depression. In the Epidemiological Catchment Area (ECA) study, the lifetime history of substance use disorders, panic disorder, and OCD was approximately twice as high among patients with bipolar I disorder (61 percent, 21 percent, and 21 percent, respectively) than in patients with unipolar major depression (27 percent, 10 percent, and 12 percent, respectively). Comorbid substance use disorders and anxiety disorders worsen the prognosis of the illness and markedly increase the risk of suicide among patients who are unipolar major depressive and bipolar.

ETIOLOGY

Biological Factors

Many studies have reported biological abnormalities in patients with mood disorders. Until recently, the monoamine neurotransmitters—norepinephrine, dopamine, serotonin, and histamine—were the main focus of theories and research about the etiology of these disorders. A progressive shift has occurred from focusing on disturbances of single neurotransmitter systems in favor of studying neurobehavioral systems, neural circuits, and more intricate neuroregulatory mechanisms. The monoaminergic systems, thus, are now viewed as broader, neuromodulary systems, and disturbances are as likely to be secondary or epiphenomenal effects as they are directly or causally related to etiology and pathogenesis.

Biogenic Amines. Of the biogenic amines, norepinephrine and serotonin are the two neurotransmitters most implicated in the pathophysiology of mood disorders.

NOREPINEPHRINE. The correlation suggested by basic science studies between the downregulation or decreased sensitivity of β-adrenergic receptors and clinical antidepressant responses is probably the single most compelling piece of data indicating a direct role for the noradrenergic system in depression. Other evidence has also implicated the presynaptic β_2-receptors in depression, because activation of these receptors results in a decrease of the amount of norepinephrine released. Presynaptic β_2-receptors are also located on serotonergic neurons and regulate the amount of serotonin released. The clinical effectiveness of antidepressant drugs with noradrenergic effects—for example, venlafaxine (Effexor)—further supports a role for norepinephrine in the pathophysiology of at least some of the symptoms of depression.

SEROTONIN. With the huge effect that the selective serotonin reuptake inhibitors (SSRIs)—for example, fluoxetine (Prozac)—have made on the treatment of depression, serotonin has become the biogenic amine neurotransmitter most commonly associated with depression. The identification of multiple serotonin receptor subtypes has also increased the excitement within the research community about the development of even more specific treatments for depression. Besides that SSRIs and other serotonergic antidepressants are effective in the treatment of depression, other data indicate that serotonin is involved in the pathophysiology of depression. Depletion of serotonin may precipitate depression, and some patients with suicidal impulses have low cerebrospinal fluid (CSF) concentrations of serotonin metabolites and low concentrations of serotonin uptake sites on platelets.

DOPAMINE. Although norepinephrine and serotonin are the biogenic amines most often associated with the pathophysiology of depression, dopamine has also been theorized to play a role. The data suggest that dopamine activity may be reduced in depression and increased in mania. The discovery of new subtypes of the dopamine receptors and an increased understanding of the presynaptic and postsynaptic regulation of dopamine function have further enriched research into the relation between dopamine and mood disorders. Drugs that reduce dopamine concentrations—for example, reserpine (Serpasil)—and diseases that reduce dopamine concentrations (e.g., Parkinson's disease) are associated with depressive symptoms. In contrast, drugs that increase dopamine concentrations, such as tyrosine, amphetamine, and bupropion (Wellbutrin), reduce the symptoms of depression. Two recent theories about dopamine and depression are that the mesolimbic dopamine pathway may be dysfunctional in depression and that the dopamine D_1 receptor may be hypoactive in depression.

Other Neurotransmitter Disturbances. Acetylcholine (ACh) is found in neurons that are distributed diffusely throughout the cerebral cortex. Cholinergic neurons have reciprocal or interactive relationships with all three monoamine systems. Abnormal levels of choline, which is a precursor to ACh, have been found at autopsy in the brains of some depressed patients, perhaps reflecting abnormalities in cell phospholipid composition. Cholinergic agonist and antagonist drugs have differential clinical effects on depression and mania. Agonists can produce lethargy, anergia, and psychomotor retardation in healthy subjects, can exacerbate symptoms in depression, and can reduce symptoms in mania. These effects generally are not sufficiently robust to have clinical applications, and adverse effects are problematic. In an animal model of depression, strains of mice that are super- or subsensitive to cholinergic agonists have been found susceptible or more resistant to developing learned helplessness (discussed below). Cholinergic agonists can induce changes in hypothalamic-pituitary adrenal (HPA) activity and sleep that mimic those associated with severe depression. Some patients with mood disorders in remission, as well as their never-ill first-degree relatives, have a trait-like increase in sensitivity to cholinergic agonists.

γ-Aminobutyric acid (GABA) has an inhibitory effect on ascending monoamine pathways, particularly the mesocortical and mesolimbic systems. Reductions of GABA have been observed in plasma, CSF, and brain GABA levels in depression. Animal studies have also found that chronic stress can reduce and eventually can deplete GABA levels. By contrast, GABA receptors are upregulated by antidepressants, and some GABAergic medications have weak antidepressant effects.

The amino acids glutamate and glycine are the major excitatory and inhibitory neurotransmitters in the CNS. Glutamate and glycine bind to sites associated with the *N*-methyl-D-aspartate (NMDA) receptor, and an excess of glutamatergic stimulation can cause neurotoxic effects. Importantly, a high concentration of NMDA receptors exists in the hippocampus. Glutamate, thus, may work in conjunction with hypercortisolemia to mediate the deleterious neurocognitive effects of severe recurrent depression. Emerging evidence suggests that drugs that antagonize NMDA receptors have antidepressant effects.

Second Messengers and Intracellular Cascades. The binding of a neurotransmitter and a postsynaptic receptor triggers a cascade of membrane-bound and intracellular processes mediated by second messenger systems. Receptors on cell membranes interact with the intracellular environment via guanine nucleotide-binding proteins (G proteins). The G proteins, in turn, connect to various intracellular enzymes (e.g., adenylate cyclase, phospholipase C, and phosphodiesterase) that regulate utilization of energy and formation of second messengers, such as cyclic nucleotide (e.g., cyclic adenosine monophosphate [cAMP] and cyclic guanosine monophosphate [cGMP]), as well as phosphatidylinositols (e.g., inositol triphosphate and diacylglycerol) and calcium-calmodulin. Second messengers regulate the function of neuronal membrane ion channels. Increasing evidence also indicates that mood-stabilizing drugs act on G proteins or other second messengers.

Alterations of Hormonal Regulation. Lasting alterations in neuroendocrine and behavioral responses can result from severe early stress. Animal studies indicate that even transient periods of maternal deprivation can alter subsequent responses to stress. Activity of the gene coding for the neurokinin brain-derived neurotrophic growth factor (BDNF) is decreased after chronic stress, as is the process of neurogenesis. Protracted stress thus can induce changes in the functional status of neurons and, eventually, cell death. Recent studies in depressed humans indicate that a history of early trauma is associated with increased HPA activity accompanied by structural changes (i.e., atrophy or decreased volume) in the cerebral cortex.

Elevated HPA activity is a hallmark of mammalian stress responses and one of the clearest links between depression and the biology of chronic stress. Hypercortisolema in depression suggests one or more of the following central disturbances: decreased inhibitory serotonin tone; increased drive from norepinephrine (NE), ACh, or corticotropin releasing hormone (CRH); or decreased feedback inhibition from the hippocampus.

Evidence of increased HPA activity is apparent in 20 to 40 percent of depressed outpatients and 40 to 60 percent of depressed inpatients.

Elevated HPA activity in depression has been documented via excretion of urinary-free cortisol (UFC), 24-hour (or shorter time segments) intravenous (IV) collections of plasma cortisol levels, salivary cortisol levels, and tests of the integrity of feedback inhibition. A disturbance of feedback inhibition is tested by administration of dexamethasone (Decadron) (0.5 to 2.0 mg), a potent synthetic glucocorticoid, which normally suppresses HPA axis activity for 24 hours. Nonsuppression of cortisol secretion at 8:00 AM the following morning or subsequent escape from suppression at 4:00 PM or 11:00 PM is indicative of impaired feedback inhibition. Hypersecretion of cortisol and dexamethasone nonsuppression are imperfectly correlated (approximately 60 percent concordance). A more recent development to improve the sensitivity of the test involves infusion of a test dose of CRH after dexamethasone suppression.

These tests of feedback inhibition are not used as a diagnostic test because adrenocortical hyperactivity (albeit usually less prevalent) is observed in mania, schizophrenia, dementia, and other psychiatric disorders.

THYROID AXIS ACTIVITY. Approximately 5 to 10 percent of people evaluated for depression have previously undetected thyroid dysfunction, as reflected by an elevated basal thyroid-stimulating hormone (TSH) level or an increased TSH response to a 500-mg infusion of the hypothalamic neuropeptide thyroid-releasing hormone (TRH). Such abnormalities are often associated with elevated antithyroid antibody levels and, unless corrected with hormone replacement therapy, can compromise response to treatment. An even larger subgroup of depressed patients (e.g., 20 to 30 percent) shows a blunted TSH response to TRH challenge. To date, the major therapeutic implication of a blunted TSH response is evidence of an increased risk of relapse despite preventive antidepressant therapy. Of note, unlike the dexamethasone suppression test (DST), blunted TSH response to TRH does not usually normalize with effective treatment.

GROWTH HORMONE. Growth hormone (GH) is secreted from the anterior pituitary after stimulation by NE and Dopamine (DA). Secretion is inhibited by somatostatin, a hypothalamic neuropeptide, and CRH. Decreased CSF somatostatin levels have been reported in depression, and increased levels have been observed in mania.

PROLACTIN. Prolactin is released from the pituitary by serotonin stimulation and inhibited by DA. Most studies have not found significant abnormalities of basal or circadian prolactin secretion in depression, although a blunted prolactin response to various serotonin agonists has been described. This response is uncommon among premenopausal women, suggesting that estrogen has a moderating effect.

Alterations of Sleep Neurophysiology.

Depression is associated with a premature loss of deep (slow wave) sleep and an increase in nocturnal arousal. The latter is reflected by four types of disturbance: (1) an increase in nocturnal awakenings, (2) a reduction in total sleep time, (3) increased phasic rapid eye movement (REM) sleep, and (4) increased core body temperature. The combination of increased REM drive and decreased slow wave sleep results in a significant reduction in the first period of non-REM (NREM) sleep, a phenomenon referred to as *reduced REM latency*. Reduced REM latency and deficits of slow wave sleep typically persist after recovery of a depressive episode. Blunted secretion of GH after sleep onset is associated with decreased slow wave sleep and shows similar state-independent or trait-like behavior. The combination of reduced REM latency, increased REM density, and decreased sleep maintenance identifies approximately 40 percent of depressed outpatients and 80 percent of depressed inpatients. False–negative findings are commonly seen in younger, hypersomnolent patients, who may actually experience an increase in slow wave sleep during episodes of depression. Approximately 10 percent of otherwise healthy individuals have abnormal sleep profiles, and, as with dexamethasone nonsuppression, false–positive cases are not uncommonly seen in other psychiatric disorders.

Patients manifesting a characteristically abnormal sleep profile have been found to be less responsive to psychotherapy and to have a greater risk of relapse or recurrence and may benefit preferentially from pharmacotherapy.

Immunological Disturbance.

Depressive disorders are associated with several immunological abnormalities, including decreased lymphocyte proliferation in response to mitogens and other forms of impaired cellular immunity. These lymphocytes produce neuromodulators, such as corticotropin-releasing factor (CRF), and cytokines, peptides known as *interleukins*. There appears to be an association with clinical severity, hypercortisolism, and immune dysfunction, and the cytokine interleukin-1 may induce gene activity for glucocorticoid synthesis.

Structural and Functional Brain Imaging.

Computed axial tomography (CAT) and magnetic resonance imaging (MRI) scans have permitted sensitive, noninvasive methods to assess the living brain, including cortical and subcortical tracts, as well as white matter lesions. The most consistent abnormality observed in the depressive disorders is increased frequency of abnormal hyperintensities in subcortical regions, such as periventricular regions, the basal ganglia, and the thalamus. More common in bipolar I disorder and among the elderly, these hyperintensities appear to reflect the deleterious neurodegenerative effects of recurrent affective episodes. Ventricular enlargement, cortical atrophy, and sulcal widening also have been reported in some studies. Some depressed patients also may have reduced hippocampal or caudate nucleus volumes, or both, suggesting more focal defects in relevant neurobehavioral systems. Diffuse and focal areas of atrophy have been associated with increased illness severity, bipolarity, and increased cortisol levels.

The most widely replicated positron emission tomography (PET) finding in depression is decreased anterior brain metabolism, which is generally more pronounced on the left side. From a different vantage point, depression may be associated with a relative increase in nondominant hemispheric activity. Furthermore, a reversal of hypofrontality occurs after shifts from depression into hypomania, such that greater left hemisphere reductions are seen in depression compared with greater right hemisphere reductions in mania. Other studies have observed more specific reductions of reduced cerebral blood flow or metabolism, or both, in the dopaminergically innervated tracts of the mesocortical and mesolimbic systems in depression. Again, evidence suggests that antidepressants at least partially normalize these changes.

In addition to a global reduction of anterior cerebral metabolism, increased glucose metabolism has been observed in several limbic regions, particularly among patients with relatively severe recurrent depression and a family history of mood disorder. During episodes of depression, increased glucose metabolism is correlated with intrusive ruminations.

Neuroanatomical Considerations. Both the symptoms of mood disorders and biological research findings support the hypothesis that mood disorders involve pathology of the brain. Modern affective neuroscience focuses on the importance of four brain regions in the regulation of normal emotions: the prefrontal cortex (PFC), the anterior cingulate, the hippocampus, and the amygdala (*see* Color Plate 15.1–2 on page 493). The PFC is viewed as the structure that holds representations of goals and appropriate responses to obtain these goals. Such activities are particularly important when multiple, conflicting behavioral responses are possible or when it is necessary to override affective arousal. Evidence indicates some hemispherical specialization in PFC function. For example, left-sided activation of regions of the PFC is more involved in goal-directed or appetitive behaviors, whereas regions of the right PFC are implicated in avoidance behaviors and inhibition of appetitive pursuits. Subregions in the PFC appear to localize representations of behaviors related to reward and punishment.

The anterior cingulate cortex (ACC) is thought to serve as the point of integration of attentional and emotional inputs. Two subdivisions have been identified: an affective subdivision in the rostral and ventral regions of the ACC and a cognitive subdivision involving the dorsal ACC. The former subdivision shares extensive connections with other limbic regions, and the latter interacts more with the PFC and other cortical regions. It is proposed that activation of the ACC facilitates control of emotional arousal, particularly when goal attainment has been thwarted or when novel problems have been encountered.

The hippocampus is most clearly involved in various forms of learning and memory, including fear conditioning, as well as inhibitory regulation of the HPA axis activity. Emotional or contextual learning appears to involve a direct connection between the hippocampus and the amygdala.

The amygdala appears to be a crucial way station for processing novel stimuli of emotional significance and coordinating or organizing cortical responses. Located just above the hippocampi bilaterally, the amygdala has long been viewed as the heart of the limbic system. Although most research has focused on the role of the amygdala in responding to fearful or painful stimuli, it may be ambiguity or novelty, rather than the aversive nature of the stimulus per se, that brings the amygdala on line.

Genetic Factors

Numerous family, adoption, and twin studies have long documented the heritability of mood disorders. Recently, however, the primary focus of genetic studies has been to identify specific susceptibility genes using molecular genetic methods.

Family Studies. Family studies address the question of whether a disorder is familial. More specifically, is the rate of illness in the family members of someone with the disorder greater than that of the general population? Family data indicate that if one parent has a mood disorder, a child will have a risk of between 10 and 25 percent for mood disorder. If both parents are affected, this risk roughly doubles. The more members of the family who are affected, the greater the risk is to a child. The risk is greater if the affected family members are first-degree relatives rather than more distant relatives. A family history of bipolar disorder conveys a greater risk for mood disorders in general and, specifically, a much greater risk for bipolar disorder. Unipolar disorder is typically the most common form of mood disorder in families of bipolar probands. This familial overlap suggests some degree of common genetic underpinnings between these two forms of mood disorder. The presence of more severe illness in the family also conveys a greater risk.

Adoption Studies. Adoption studies provide an alternative approach to separating genetic and environmental factors in familial transmission. Only a limited number of such studies have been reported, and their results have been mixed. One large study found a threefold increase in the rate of bipolar disorder and a twofold increase in unipolar disorder in the biological relatives of bipolar probands. Similarly, in a Danish sample, a threefold increase in the rate of unipolar disorder and a sixfold increase in the rate of completed suicide in the biological relatives of affectively ill probands were reported. Other studies, however, have been less convincing and have found no difference in the rates of mood disorders.

Twin Studies. Twin studies provide the most powerful approach to separating genetic from environmental factors, or "nature" from "nurture." The twin data provide compelling evidence that genes explain only 50 to 70 percent of the etiology of mood disorders. Environment or other nonheritable factors must explain the remainder. Therefore, it is a predisposition or susceptibility to disease that is inherited. Considering unipolar and bipolar disorders together, these studies find a concordance rate for mood disorder in the monozygotic (MZ) twins of 70 to 90 percent compared with the same-sex dizygotic (DZ) twins of 16 to 35 percent. This is the most compelling data for the role of genetic factors in mood disorders.

Linkage Studies. DNA markers are segments of DNA of known chromosomal location, which are highly variable among individuals. They are used to track the segregation of specific chromosomal regions within families affected with a disorder. When a marker is identified with disease in families, the disease is said to be *genetically linked* (Table 15.1–3). Chromosomes 18q and 22q are the two regions with strongest evidence for linkage to bipolar disorder. Several linkage studies have found evidence for the involvement of specific genes in clinical subtypes. For example, the linkage evidence on 18q has been shown to be derived largely from bipolar II-bipolar II sibling pairs and from families in which the probands had panic symptoms.

Gene-mapping studies of unipolar depression have found very strong evidence of linkage to the locus for cAMP Response Element-Binding Protein (CREB1) on chromosome 2. Eighteen other genomic regions were found to be linked; some of these displayed interactions with the CREB1 locus. Another study has reported evidence for a gene–environment interaction in the development of major depression. Subjects who underwent adverse life events were shown, in general, to be at an increased risk for

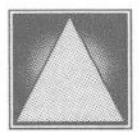

Table 15.1–3
Selected Chromosomal Regions with Evidence of Linkage to Bipolar Disorder

Chromosome 18	Data suggest the presence of as many as four different loci on this one chromosome. Studies have found linkage to 18q to preferentially occur in families in which affective illness was transmitted through the mother, suggesting a possible parent-of-origin effect
Chromosome 21q	Regions have shown linkage or association to both schizophrenia and bipolar disorder
Chromosome 22q	The breakpoint cluster region (BCR) gene is located on chromosome 22q11. The BCR gene encodes an activating protein, which is known to play important roles in neuron growth and axonal guidance

depression. Of such subjects, however, those with a variant in the serotonin transporter gene showed the greatest increase in risk. This is one of the first reports of a specific gene–environment interaction in a psychiatric disorder.

Psychosocial Factors

Life Events and Environmental Stress. A long-standing clinical observation is that stressful life events more often precede first, rather than subsequent, episodes of mood disorders. This association has been reported for both patients with major depressive disorder and patients with bipolar I disorder. One theory proposed to explain this observation is that the stress accompanying the first episode results in long-lasting changes in the brain's biology. These long-lasting changes may alter the functional states of various neurotransmitter and intraneuronal signaling systems, changes that may even include the loss of neurons and an excessive reduction in synaptic contacts. As a result, a person has a high risk of undergoing subsequent episodes of a mood disorder, even without an external stressor.

Some clinicians believe that life events play the primary or principal role in depression; others suggest that life events have only a limited role in the onset and timing of depression. The most compelling data indicate that the life event most often associated with development of depression is losing a parent before age 11. The environmental stressor most often associated with the onset of an episode of depression is the loss of a spouse. Another risk factor is unemployment; persons out of work are three times more likely to report symptoms of an episode of major depression than those who are employed.

Personality Factors. No single personality trait or type uniquely predisposes a person to depression; all humans, of whatever personality pattern, can and do become depressed under appropriate circumstances. Persons with certain personality disorders—OCD, histrionic, and borderline—may be at greater risk for depression than persons with antisocial or paranoid personality disorder. The latter can use projection and other externalizing defense mechanisms to protect themselves from their inner rage. No evidence indicates that any particular personality disorder is associated with later development of bipolar I disorder; however, patients with dysthymic disorder and cyclothymic disorder are at risk of later developing major depression or bipolar I disorder.

Recent stressful events are the most powerful predictors of the onset of a depressive episode. From a psychodynamic perspective, the clinician is always interested in the meaning of the stressor. Research has demonstrated that stressors that the patient experiences as reflecting negatively on his or her self-esteem are more likely to produce depression. Moreover, what may seem to be a relatively mild stressor to outsiders may be devastating to the patient because of particular idiosyncratic meanings attached to the event.

Psychodynamic Factors in Depression. The psychodynamic understanding of depression defined by Sigmund Freud and expanded by Karl Abraham is known as the classic view of depression. That theory involves four key points: (1) disturbances in the infant–mother relationship during the oral phase (the first 10 to 18 months of life) predispose to subsequent vulnerability to depression; (2) depression can be linked to real or imagined object loss; (3) introjection of the departed objects is a defense mechanism invoked to deal with the distress connected with the object's loss; and (4) because the lost object is regarded with a mixture of love and hate, feelings of anger are directed inward at the self.

Melanie Klein understood depression as involving the expression of aggression toward loved ones, much as Freud did. Edward Bibring regarded depression as a phenomenon that sets in when a person becomes aware of the discrepancy between extraordinarily high ideals and the inability to meet those goals. Edith Jacobson saw the state of depression as similar to a powerless, helpless child victimized by a tormenting parent. Silvano Arieti observed that many depressed people have lived their lives for someone else rather than for themselves. He referred to the person for whom depressed patients live as the dominant other, which may be a principle, an ideal, or an institution, as well as an individual. Depression sets in when patients realize that the person or ideal for which they have been living is never going to respond in a manner that will meet their expectations. Heinz Kohut's conceptualization of depression, derived from his self-psychological theory, rests on the assumption that the developing self has specific needs that must be met by parents to give the child a positive sense of self-esteem and self-cohesion. When others do not meet these needs, there is a massive loss of self-esteem that presents as depression. John Bowlby believed that damaged early attachments and traumatic separation in childhood predispose to depression. Adult losses are said to revive the traumatic childhood loss and so precipitate adult depressive episodes.

Psychodynamic Factors in Mania. Most theories of mania view manic episodes as a defense against underlying depression. Abraham, for example, believed that the manic episodes may reflect an inability to tolerate a developmental tragedy, such as the loss of a parent. The manic state may also result from a tyrannical superego, which produces intolerable self-criticism that is then replaced by euphoric self-satisfaction. Bertram Lewin regarded the manic patient's ego as overwhelmed by pleasurable impulses, such as sex, or by feared impulses, such as aggression. Klein also viewed mania as a defensive reaction to depression, using manic defenses such as omnipotence, in which the person develops delusions of grandeur.

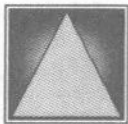

Table 15.1–4
Elements of Cognitive Theory

Element	Definition
Cognitive triad	Beliefs about oneself, the world, the future
Schemas	Ways of organizing and interpreting experiences
Cognitive distortions	
Arbitrary inference	Drawing a specific conclusion without sufficient evidence
Specific abstraction	Focus on a single detail while ignoring other, more important aspects of an experience
Overgeneralization	Forming conclusions based on too little and too narrow experience
Magnification and minimization	Over- or undervaluing the significance of a particular event
Personalization	Tendency to self-reference external events without basis
Absolutist, dichotomous thinking	Tendency to place experience into all-or-none categories

(Courtesy of Robert M.A. Hirschfeld, M.D., and M. Tracie Shea, Ph.D.)

Other Formulations of Depression

Cognitive Theory. According to cognitive theory, depression results from specific cognitive distortions present in persons susceptible to depression. Those distortions, referred to as *depressogenic schemata*, are cognitive templates that perceive both internal and external data in ways that are altered by early experiences. Aaron Beck postulated a cognitive triad of depression that consists of (1) views about the self—a negative self-precept; (2) about the environment—a tendency to experience the world as hostile and demanding, and (3) about the future—the expectation of suffering and failure. Therapy consists of modifying these distortions. The elements of cognitive theory are summarized in Table 15.1–4.

Learned Helplessness. The learned helplessness theory of depression connects depressive phenomena to the experience of uncontrollable events. For example, when dogs in a laboratory were exposed to electrical shocks from which they could not escape, they showed behaviors that differentiated them from dogs that had not been exposed to such uncontrollable events. The dogs exposed to the shocks would not cross a barrier to stop the flow of electric shock when put in a new learning situation. They remained passive and did not move. According to the learned helplessness theory, the shocked dogs learned that outcomes were independent of responses, so they had both cognitive motivational deficit (i.e., they would not attempt to escape the shock) and emotional deficit (indicating decreased reactivity to the shock). In the reformulated view of learned helplessness as applied to human depression, internal causal explanations are thought to produce a loss of self-esteem after adverse external events. Behaviorists who subscribe to the theory stress that improvement of depression is contingent on the patient's learning a sense of control and mastery of the environment.

DIAGNOSIS

In addition to the diagnostic criteria for major depressive disorder and bipolar disorders, DSM-IV-TR includes specific criteria for mood episodes (Tables 15.1–5 through 15.1–8) and criteria, such as severity (Tables 15.1–9 through 15.1–11) to qualify the most recent episode.

Major Depressive Disorder

The DSM-IV-TR lists the criteria for a major depressive episode separately from the diagnostic criteria for depression-related

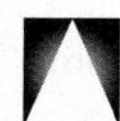

Table 15.1–5
DSM-IV-TR Criteria for Major Depressive Episode

A. Five (or more) of the following symptoms have been present during the same 2-week period and represent a change from previous functioning; at least one of the symptoms is either (1) depressed mood or (2) loss of interest or pleasure.
Note: Do not include symptoms that are clearly due to a general medical condition, or mood-incongruent delusions or hallucinations.
(1) depressed mood most of the day, nearly every day, as indicated by either subjective report (e.g., feels sad or empty) or observation made by others (e.g., appears tearful). **Note:** In children and adolescents, can be irritable mood
(2) markedly diminished interest or pleasure in all, or almost all, activities most of the day, nearly every day (as indicated by either subjective account or observation made by others)
(3) significant weight loss when not dieting or weight gain (e.g., a change of more than 5% of body weight in a month), or decrease or increase in appetite nearly every day. **Note:** In children, consider failure to make expected weight gains.
(4) insomnia or hypersomnia nearly every day
(5) psychomotor agitation or retardation nearly every day (observable by others, not merely subjective feelings of restlessness or being slowed down)
(6) fatigue or loss of energy nearly every day
(7) feelings of worthlessness or excessive or inappropriate guilt (which may be delusional) nearly every day (not merely self-reproach or guilt about being sick)
(8) diminished ability to think or concentrate, or indecisiveness, nearly every day (either by subjective account or as observed by others)
(9) recurrent thoughts of death (not just fear of dying), recurrent suicidal ideation without a specific plan, or a suicide attempt or a specific plan for committing suicide

B. The symptoms do not meet criteria for a mixed episode.

C. The symptoms cause clinically significant distress or impairment in social, occupational, or other important areas of functioning.

D. The symptoms are not due to the direct physiological effects of a substance (e.g., a drug of abuse, a medication) or a general medical condition (e.g., hypothyroidism).

E. The symptoms are not better accounted for by bereavement, i.e., after the loss of a loved one, the symptoms persist for longer than 2 months or are characterized by marked functional impairment, morbid preoccupation with worthlessness, suicidal ideation, psychotic symptoms, or psychomotor retardation.

(From American Psychiatric Association. *Diagnostic and Statistical Manual of Mental Disorders.* 4th ed. Text rev. Washington, DC: American Psychiatric Association; copyright 2000, with permission.)

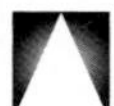

Table 15.1–6
DSM-IV-TR Criteria for Manic Episode

A. A distinct period of abnormally and persistently elevated, expansive, or irritable mood, lasting at least 1 week (or any duration if hospitalization is necessary).
B. During the period of mood disturbance, three (or more) of the following symptoms have persisted (four if the mood is only irritable) and have been present to a significant degree:
(1) inflated self-esteem or grandiosity
(2) decreased need for sleep (e.g., feels rested after only 3 hours of sleep)
(3) more talkative than usual or pressure to keep talking
(4) flight of ideas or subjective experience that thoughts are racing
(5) distractibility (i.e., attention too easily drawn to unimportant or irrelevant external stimuli)
(6) increase in goal-directed activity (either socially, at work or school, or sexually) or psychomotor agitation
(7) excessive involvement in pleasurable activities that have a high potential for painful consequences (e.g., engaging in unrestrained buying sprees, sexual indiscretions, or foolish business investments)
C. The symptoms do not meet criteria for a mixed episode.
D. The mood disturbance is sufficiently severe to cause marked impairment in occupational functioning or in usual social activities or relationships with others, or to necessitate hospitalization to prevent harm to self or others, or there are psychotic features.
E. The symptoms are not due to the direct physiological effects of a substance (e.g., a drug of abuse, a medication, or other treatment) or a general medical condition (e.g., hyperthyroidism).
Note: Manic-like episodes that are clearly caused by somatic antidepressant treatment (e.g., medication, electroconvulsive therapy, light therapy) should not count toward a diagnosis of bipolar I disorder.

(From American Psychiatric Association. *Diagnostic and Statistical Manual of Mental Disorders.* 4th ed. Text rev. Washington, DC: American Psychiatric Association; copyright 2000, with permission.)

diagnoses (Table 15.1–5) and also lists severity descriptors for a major depressive episode (Table 15.1–9).

Major Depressive Disorder, Single Episode. DSM-IV-TR specifies the diagnostic criteria for the first episode of major depressive disorder (Table 15.1–12). Differentiation between these patients and those who have two or more episodes of major depressive disorder is justified because of the uncertain course of the former patients' disorder. Several studies have reported data consistent with the notion that major depression covers a heterogeneous population of disorders. One type of study assessed the stability of a diagnosis of major depression in a patient over time. The study found that 25 to 50 percent of the patients were later reclassified as having a different psychiatric condition or a nonpsychiatric medical condition with psychiatric symptoms. A second type of study evaluated first-degree relatives of affectively ill patients to determine the presence and types of psychiatric diagnoses for these relatives over time. Both types of studies found that depressed patients with more depressive symptoms are more likely to have stable diagnoses over time and are more likely to have affectively ill relatives than are depressed patients with fewer depressive symptoms. Also, patients with bipolar I disorder and those with bipolar II disorder

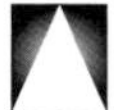

Table 15.1–7
DSM-IV-TR Criteria for Hypomanic Episode

A. A distinct period of persistently elevated, expansive, or irritable mood, lasting throughout at least 4 days, that is clearly different from the usual nondepressed mood.
B. During the period of mood disturbance, three (or more) of the following symptoms have persisted (four if the mood is only irritable) and have been present to a significant degree:
(1) inflated self-esteem or grandiosity
(2) decreased need for sleep (e.g., feels rested after only 3 hours of sleep)
(3) more talkative than usual or pressure to keep talking
(4) flight of ideas or subjective experience that thoughts are racing
(5) distractibility (i.e., attention too easily drawn to unimportant or irrelevant external stimuli)
(6) increase in goal-directed activity (either socially, at work or school, or sexually) or psychomotor agitation
(7) excessive involvement in pleasurable activities that have a high potential for painful consequences (e.g., the person engages in unrestrained buying sprees, sexual indiscretions, or foolish business investments)
C. The episode is associated with an unequivocal change in functioning that is uncharacteristic of the person when not symptomatic.
D. The disturbance in mood and the change in functioning are observable by others.
E. The episode is not severe enough to cause marked impairment in social or occupational functioning, or to necessitate hospitalization, and there are no psychotic features.
F. The symptoms are not due to the direct physiological effects of a substance (e.g., a drug of abuse, a medication, or other treatment) or a general medical condition (e.g., hyperthyroidism).
Note: Hypomanic-like episodes that are clearly caused by somatic antidepressant treatment (e.g., medication, electroconvulsive therapy, light therapy) should not count toward a diagnosis of bipolar II disorder.

(From American Psychiatric Association. *Diagnostic and Statistical Manual of Mental Disorders.* 4th ed. Text rev. Washington, DC: American Psychiatric Association; copyright 2000, with permission.)

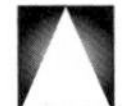

Table 15.1–8
DSM-IV-TR Criteria for Mixed Episode

A. The criteria are met both for a manic episode and for a major depressive episode (except for duration) nearly every day during at least a 1-week period.
B. The mood disturbance is sufficiently severe to cause marked impairment in occupational functioning or in usual social activities or relationships with others, or to necessitate hospitalization to prevent harm to self or others, or there are psychotic features.
C. The symptoms are not due to the direct physiological effects of a substance (e.g., a drug of abuse, a medication, or other treatment) or a general medical condition (e.g., hyperthyroidism).

Note: Mixed-like episodes that are clearly caused by somatic antidepressant treatment (e.g., medication, electroconvulsive therapy, light therapy) should not count toward a diagnosis of bipolar I disorder.

(From American Psychiatric Association. *Diagnostic and Statistical Manual of Mental Disorders.* 4th ed. Text rev. Washington, DC: American Psychiatric Association; copyright 2000, with permission.)

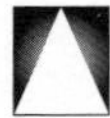

Table 15.1–9
DSM-IV-TR Criteria for Severity/Psychotic/Remission Specifiers for Current (or Most Recent) Major Depressive Episode

Note: Code in fifth digit. Mild, moderate, severe without psychotic features, and severe with psychotic features can be applied only if the criteria are currently met for a major depressive episode. In partial remission and in full remission can be applied to the most recent major depressive episode in major depressive disorder and to a major depressive episode in bipolar I or II disorder only if it is the most recent type of mood episode.

Mild: Few, if any, symptoms in excess of those required to make the diagnosis and symptoms result in only minor impairment in occupational functioning or in usual social activities or relationships with others.

Moderate: Symptoms or functional impairment between "mild" and "severe."

Severe without psychotic features: Several symptoms in excess of those required to make the diagnosis, and symptoms markedly interfere with occupational functioning or with usual social activities or relationships with others.

Severe with psychotic features: Delusions or hallucinations. If possible, specify whether the psychotic features are mood-congruent or mood-incongruent:

- **Mood-congruent psychotic features:** Delusions or hallucinations whose content is entirely consistent with the typical depressive themes of personal inadequacy, guilt, disease, death, nihilism, or deserved punishment.
- **Mood-incongruent psychotic features:** Delusions or hallucinations whose content does not involve typical depressive themes of personal inadequacy, guilt, disease, death, nihilism, or deserved punishment. Included are such symptoms as persecutory delusions (not directly related to depressive themes), thought insertion, thought broadcasting, and delusions of control.

In partial remission: Symptoms of a major depressive episode are present but full criteria are not met, or there is a period without any significant symptoms of a major depressive episode lasting less than 2 months following the end of the major depressive episode. (If the major depressive episode was superimposed on dysthymic disorder, the diagnosis of dysthymic disorder alone is given once the full criteria for a major depressive episode are no longer met.)

In full remission: During the past 2 months, no significant signs or symptoms of the disturbance were present.

Unspecified

(From American Psychiatric Association. *Diagnostic and Statistical Manual of Mental Disorders.* 4th ed. Text rev. Washington, DC: American Psychiatric Association; copyright 2000, with permission.)

(recurrent major depressive episodes with hypomania) are likely to have stable diagnoses over time.

Major Depressive Disorder, Recurrent. Patients who are experiencing at least a second episode of depression are classified in DSM-IV-TR as having major depressive disorder, recurrent (Table 15.1–13). The essential problem with diagnosing recurrent episodes of major depressive disorder is choosing the criteria to designate the resolution of each period. Two variables are the degree of resolution of the symptoms and the length of the resolution. DSM-IV-TR requires that distinct episodes of depression be separated by at least 2 months during which a patient has no significant symptoms of depression.

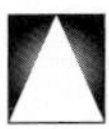

Table 15.1–10
DSM-IV-TR Criteria for Severity/Psychotic/Remission Specifiers for Current (or Most Recent) Manic Episode

Note: Code in fifth digit. Mild, moderate, severe without psychotic features, and severe with psychotic features can be applied only if the criteria are currently met for a manic episode. In partial remission and in full remission can be applied to a manic episode in bipolar I disorder only if it is the most recent type of mood episode.

Mild: Minimum symptom criteria are met for a manic episode.

Moderate: Extreme increase in activity or impairment in judgment.

Severe without psychotic features: Almost continual supervision required to prevent physical harm to self or others.

Severe with psychotic features: Delusions or hallucinations. If possible, specify whether the psychotic features are mood-congruent or mood-incongruent:

- **Mood-congruent psychotic features:** Delusions or hallucinations whose content is entirely consistent with the typical manic themes of inflated worth, power, knowledge, identity, or special relationship to a deity or famous person.
- **Mood-incongruent psychotic features:** Delusions or hallucinations whose content does not involve typical manic themes of inflated worth, power, knowledge, identity, or special relationship to a deity or famous person. Included are such symptoms as persecutory delusions (not directly related to grandiose ideas or themes), thought insertion, and delusions of being controlled.

In partial remission: Symptoms of a manic episode are present but full criteria are not met, or there is a period without any significant symptoms of a manic episode lasting less than 2 months following the end of the manic episode.

In full remission: During the past 2 months no significant signs or symptoms of the disturbance were present.

Unspecified

(From American Psychiatric Association. *Diagnostic and Statistical Manual of Mental Disorders.* 4th ed. Text rev. Washington, DC: American Psychiatric Association; copyright 2000, with permission.)

Bipolar I Disorder

The DSM-IV-TR criteria for a manic episode (Table 15.1–6) requires the presence of a distinct period of abnormal mood lasting at least 1 week and includes separate bipolar I disorder diagnoses for a single manic episode and a recurrent episode, based on the symptoms of the most recent episode as described below.

The designation bipolar I disorder is synonymous with what was formerly known as bipolar disorder—a syndrome in which a complete set of mania symptoms occurs during the course of the disorder. The diagnostic criteria for bipolar II disorder is characterized by depressive episodes and hypomanic episodes (Table 15.1–7) during the course of the disorder, but the episodes of manic-like symptoms do not quite meet the diagnostic criteria for a full manic syndrome.

Manic episodes clearly precipitated by antidepressant treatment (e.g., pharmacotherapy, electroconvulsive therapy [ECT]) do not indicate bipolar I disorder.

Bipolar I Disorder, Single Manic Episode. According to DSM-IV-TR, patients must be experiencing their first manic episode to meet the diagnostic criteria for bipolar I disorder,

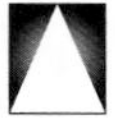

Table 15.1–11
DSM-IV-TR Criteria for Severity/Psychotic/Remission Specifiers for Current (or Most Recent) Mixed Episode

Note: Code in fifth digit. Mild, moderate, severe without psychotic features, and severe with psychotic features can be applied only if the criteria are currently met for a mixed episode. In partial remission and in full remission can be applied to a mixed episode in bipolar I disorder only if it is the most recent type of mood episode.

Mild: No more than minimum symptom criteria are met for both a manic episode and a major depressive episode.

Moderate: Symptoms or functional impairment between "mild" and "severe."

Severe without psychotic features: Almost continual supervision required to prevent physical harm to self or others.

Severe with psychotic features: Delusions or hallucinations. If possible, specify whether the psychotic features are mood-congruent or mood-incongruent:

- **Mood-congruent psychotic features:** Delusions or hallucinations whose content is entirely consistent with the typical manic or depressive themes.
- **Mood-incongruent psychotic features:** Delusions or hallucinations whose content does not involve typical manic or depressive themes. Included are such symptoms as persecutory delusions (not directly related to grandiose or depressive themes), thought insertion, and delusions of being controlled.

In partial remission: Symptoms of a mixed episode are present but full criteria are not met, or there is a period without any significant symptoms of a mixed episode lasting less than 2 months following the end of the mixed episode.

In full remission: During the past 2 months, no significant signs or symptoms of the disturbance were present.

Unspecified

(From American Psychiatric Association. *Diagnostic and Statistical Manual of Mental Disorders.* 4th ed. Text rev. Washington, DC: American Psychiatric Association; copyright 2000, with permission.)

single manic episode (Table 15.1–14). This requirement rests on the fact that patients who are having their first episode of bipolar I disorder depression cannot be distinguished from patients with major depressive disorder.

Bipolar I Disorder, Recurrent. The issues about defining the end of an episode of depression also apply to defining the end of an episode of mania. Manic episodes are considered distinct when they are separated by at least 2 months without significant symptoms of mania or hypomania. DSM-IV-TR specifies diagnostic criteria for recurrent bipolar I disorder on the basis of the symptoms of the most recent episode: bipolar I disorder, most recent episode manic (Table 15.1–15); bipolar I disorder, most recent episode hypomanic (Table 15.1–16); bipolar I disorder, most recent episode depressed (Table 15.1–17); bipolar I disorder, most recent episode mixed (Table 15.1–18); and bipolar I disorder, most recent episode unspecified (Table 15.1–19).

Bipolar II Disorder

The diagnostic criteria for bipolar II disorder specify the particular severity, frequency, and duration of the hypomanic symptoms. The diagnostic criteria for a hypomanic episode (Table 15.1–7) are listed separately from the criteria for bipolar II disorder

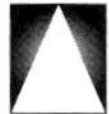

Table 15.1–12
DSM-IV-TR Diagnostic Criteria for Major Depressive Disorder, Single Episode

A. Presence of a single major depressive episode.
B. The major depressive episode is not better accounted for by schizoaffective disorder and is not superimposed on schizophrenia, schizophreniform disorder, delusional disorder, or psychotic disorder not otherwise specified.
C. There has never been a manic episode, a mixed episode, or a hypomanic episode. **Note:** This exclusion does not apply if all of the manic-like, mixed-like, or hypomanic-like episodes are substance or treatment induced or are due to the direct physiological effects of a general medical condition.

If the full criteria are currently met for a major depressive episode, specify its current clinical status and/or features:

Mild, moderate, severe without psychotic features/severe with psychotic features
Chronic
With catatonic features
With melancholic features
With atypical features
With postpartum onset

If the full criteria are not currently met for a major depressive episode, specify the current clinical status of the major depressive disorder or features of the most recent episode:

In partial remission, in full remission
Chronic
With catatonic features
With melancholic features
With atypical features
With postpartum onset

(From American Psychiatric Association. *Diagnostic and Statistical Manual of Mental Disorders.* 4th ed. Text rev. Washington, DC: American Psychiatric Association; copyright 2000, with permission.)

(Table 15.1–20). The criteria have been established to decrease overdiagnosis of hypomanic episodes and the incorrect classification of patients with major depressive disorder as patients with bipolar II disorder. Clinically, psychiatrists may find it difficult to distinguish euthymia from hypomania in a patient who has been chronically depressed for many months or years. As with bipolar I disorder, antidepressant-induced hypomanic episodes are not diagnostic of bipolar II disorder.

Specifiers Describing Most Recent Episode

In addition to the severity, psychotic, and remission specifiers (Tables 15.1–7 through 15.1–11), DSM-IV-TR defines additional symptom features that can be used to describe patients with various mood disorders. Two of the features (melancholic and atypical) are limited to describing depressive episodes. Two others (catatonic features and with postpartum onset) can be applied to depressive and manic episodes. These are described below.

With Psychotic Features. The presence of psychotic features (Table 15.1–7) in major depressive disorder reflects severe disease and is a poor prognostic indicator. A review of the literature comparing psychotic with nonpsychotic major depressive disorder indicates that the two conditions may be distinct in their pathogenesis. One difference is that bipolar I disorder is more common in the families of probands with psychotic depression than in the families of probands with nonpsychotic depression.

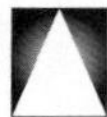

Table 15.1–13
DSM-IV-TR Diagnostic Criteria for Major Depressive Disorder, Recurrent

A. Presence of two or more major depressive episodes.
Note: To be considered separate episodes, there must be an interval of at least 2 consecutive months in which criteria are not met for a major depressive episode.
B. The major depressive episodes are not better accounted for by schizoaffective disorder and are not superimposed on schizophrenia, schizophreniform disorder, delusional disorder, or psychotic disorder not otherwise specified.
C. There has never been a manic episode, a mixed episode, or a hypomanic episode. **Note:** This exclusion does not apply if all of the manic-like, mixed-like, or hypomanic-like episodes are substance or treatment induced or are due to the direct physiological effects of a general medical condition.

If the full criteria are currently met for a major depressive episode, specify its current clinical status and/or features:
Mild, moderate, severe without psychotic features/severe with psychotic features
Chronic
With catatonic features
With melancholic features
With atypical features
With postpartum onset

If the full criteria are not currently met for a major depressive episode, specify the current clinical status of the major depressive disorder or features of the most recent episode:
In partial remission, in full remission
Chronic
With catatonic features
With melancholic features
With atypical features
With postpartum onset

Specify if:
Longitudinal course specifiers (with and without interepisode recovery)
With seasonal pattern

(From American Psychiatric Association. *Diagnostic and Statistical Manual of Mental Disorders.* 4th ed. Text rev. Washington, DC: American Psychiatric Association; copyright 2000, with permission.)

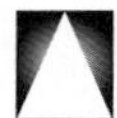

Table 15.1–14
DSM-IV-TR Diagnostic Criteria for Bipolar I Disorder, Single Manic Episode

A. Presence of only one manic episode and no past major depressive episodes.
Note: Recurrence is defined as either a change in polarity from depression or an interval of at least 2 months without manic symptoms.
B. The manic episode is not better accounted for by schizoaffective disorder and is not superimposed on schizophrenia, schizophreniform disorder, delusional disorder, or psychotic disorder not otherwise specified.

Specify if:
Mixed: if symptoms meet criteria for a mixed episode

If the full criteria are currently met for a manic, mixed, or major depressive episode, specify its current clinical status and/or features:
Mild, moderate, severe without psychotic features/severe with psychotic features
With catatonic features
With postpartum onset

If the full criteria are not currently met for a manic, mixed, or major depressive episode, specify the current clinical status of the bipolar I disorder or features of the most recent episode:
In partial remission, in full remission
With catatonic features
With postpartum onset

(From American Psychiatric Association. *Diagnostic and Statistical Manual of Mental Disorders.* 4th ed. Text rev. Washington, DC: American Psychiatric Association; copyright 2000, with permission.)

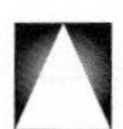

Table 15.1–15
DSM-IV-TR Diagnostic Criteria for Bipolar I Disorder, Most Recent Episode Manic

A. Currently (or most recently) in a manic episode.
B. There has previously been at least one major depressive episode, manic episode, or mixed episode.
C. The mood episodes in Criteria A and B are not better accounted for by schizoaffective disorder and are not superimposed on schizophrenia, schizophreniform disorder, delusional disorder, or psychotic disorder not otherwise specified.

If the full criteria are currently met for a manic episode, specify its current clinical status and/or features:
Mild, moderate, severe without psychotic features/severe with psychotic features
With catatonic features
With postpartum onset

If the full criteria are not currently met for a manic episode, specify the current clinical status of the bipolar I disorder and/or features of the most recent manic episode:
In partial remission, in full remission
With catatonic features
With postpartum onset

Specify if:
Longitudinal course specifiers (with and without interepisode recovery)
With seasonal pattern (applies only to the pattern of major depressive episodes)
With rapid cycling

(From American Psychiatric Association. *Diagnostic and Statistical Manual of Mental Disorders.* 4th ed. Text rev. Washington, DC: American Psychiatric Association; copyright 2000, with permission.)

The psychotic symptoms themselves are often categorized as either mood congruent, that is, in harmony with the mood disorder ("I deserve to be punished because I am so bad"), or mood incongruent, not in harmony with the mood disorder. Patients with mood disorder with mood-congruent psychoses have a psychotic type of mood disorder; however, patients with mood disorder with mood-incongruent psychotic symptoms may have schizoaffective disorder or schizophrenia.

The following factors have been associated with a poor prognosis for patients with mood disorders: long duration of episodes, temporal dissociation between the mood disorder and the psychotic symptoms, and a poor premorbid history of social adjustment. The presence of psychotic features also has significant treatment implications. These patients typically require antipsychotic drugs in addition to antidepressants or mood stabilizers and may need ECT to obtain clinical improvement.

With Melancholic Features. Melancholia is one of the oldest terms used in psychiatry, dating back to Hippocrates in the 4th century to describe the dark mood of depression. It is still used to refer to a depression characterized by severe anhedonia,

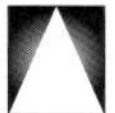

Table 15.1–16
DSM-IV-TR Diagnostic Criteria for Bipolar I Disorder, Most Recent Episode Hypomanic

A. Currently (or most recently) in a hypomanic episode.
B. There has previously been at least one manic episode or mixed episode.
C. The mood symptoms cause clinically significant distress or impairment in social, occupational, or other important areas of functioning.
D. The mood episodes in Criteria A and B are not better accounted for by schizoaffective disorder and are not superimposed on schizophrenia, schizophreniform disorder, delusional disorder, or psychotic disorder not otherwise specified.

Specify if:
Longitudinal course specifiers (with and without interepisode recovery)
With seasonal pattern (applies only to the pattern of major depressive episodes)
With rapid cycling

(From American Psychiatric Association. *Diagnostic and Statistical Manual of Mental Disorders.* 4th ed. Text rev. Washington, DC: American Psychiatric Association; copyright 2000, with permission.)

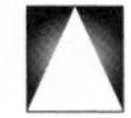

Table 15.1–17
DSM-IV-TR Diagnostic Criteria for Bipolar I Disorder, Most Recent Episode Depressed

A. Currently (or most recently) in a major depressive episode.
B. There has previously been at least one manic episode or mixed episode.
C. The mood episodes in Criteria A and B are not better accounted for by schizoaffective disorder and are not superimposed on schizophrenia, schizophreniform disorder, delusional disorder, or psychotic disorder not otherwise specified.

If the full criteria are currently met for a major depressive episode, specify its current clinical status and/or features:
Mild, moderate, severe without psychotic features/severe with psychotic features
Chronic
With catatonic features
With melancholic features
With atypical features
With postpartum onset

If the full criteria are not currently met for a major depressive episode, specify the current clinical status of the bipolar I disorder and/or features of the most recent major depressive episode:
In partial remission, in full remission
Chronic
With catatonic features
With melancholic features
With atypical features
With postpartum onset

Specify if:
Longitudinal course specifiers (with and without interepisode recovery)
With seasonal pattern (applies only to the pattern of major depressive episodes)
With rapid cycling

(From American Psychiatric Association. *Diagnostic and Statistical Manual of Mental Disorders.* 4th ed. Text rev. Washington, DC: American Psychiatric Association; copyright 2000, with permission.)

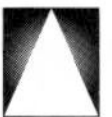

Table 15.1–18
DSM-IV-TR Diagnostic Criteria for Bipolar I Disorder, Most Recent Episode Mixed

A. Currently (or most recently) in a mixed episode.
B. There has previously been at least one major depressive episode, manic episode, or mixed episode.
C. The mood episodes in Criteria A and B are not better accounted for by schizoaffective disorder and are not superimposed on schizophrenia, schizophreniform disorder, delusional disorder, or psychotic disorder not otherwise specified.

If the full criteria are currently met for a mixed episode, specify its current clinical status and/or features:
Mild, moderate, severe without psychotic features/severe with psychotic features
With catatonic features
With postpartum onset

If the full criteria are not currently met for a mixed episode, specify the current clinical status of the bipolar I disorder and/or features of the most recent mixed episode:
In partial remission, in full remission
With catatonic features
With postpartum onset

Specify if:
Longitudinal course specifiers (with and without interepisode recovery)
With seasonal pattern (applies only to the pattern of major depressive episodes)
With rapid cycling

(From American Psychiatric Association. *Diagnostic and Statistical Manual of Mental Disorders.* 4th ed. Text rev. Washington, DC: American Psychiatric Association; copyright 2000, with permission.)

early morning awakening, weight loss, and profound feelings of guilt (often over trivial events). It is not uncommon for patients who are melancholic to have suicidal ideation. Melancholia is associated with changes in the autonomic nervous system and in endocrine functions. For that reason, melancholia is sometimes referred to as "endogenous depression" or depression that arises in the absence of external life stressors or precipitants. The DSM-IV-TR melancholic features can be applied to major depressive episodes in major depressive disorder, bipolar I disorder, or bipolar II disorder (Table 15.1–21).

With Atypical Features. The introduction of a formally defined depression with atypical features is a response to research and clinical data indicating that patients with atypical features have specific, predictable characteristics: overeating and oversleeping. These symptoms have sometimes been referred to as *reversed vegetative symptoms*, and the symptom pattern has sometimes been called *hysteroid dysphoria*. When patients with major depressive disorder with atypical features are compared with patients with typical depression features, the patients with atypical features are found to have a younger age of onset, more severe psychomotor slowing, and more frequent coexisting diagnoses of panic disorder, substance abuse or dependence, and somatization disorder. The high incidence and severity of anxiety symptoms in patients with atypical features have sometimes been correlated with the likelihood of their being misclassified as having an anxiety disorder rather than a mood disorder. Patients with atypical features may also have a long-term course, a diagnosis of bipolar I disorder, or a seasonal pattern to their disorder.

Table 15.1–19
DSM-IV-TR Diagnostic Criteria for Bipolar I Disorder, Most Recent Episode Unspecified

A. Criteria, except for duration, are currently (or most recently) met for a manic, a hypomanic, a mixed, or a major depressive episode.
B. There has previously been at least one manic episode or mixed episode.
C. The mood symptoms cause clinically significant distress or impairment in social, occupational, or other important areas of functioning.
D. The mood symptoms in Criteria A and B are not better accounted for by schizoaffective disorder and are not superimposed on schizophrenia, schizophreniform disorder, delusional disorder, or psychotic disorder not otherwise specified.
E. The mood symptoms in Criteria A and B are not due to the direct physiological effects of a substance (e.g., a drug of abuse, a medication, or other treatment) or a general medical condition (e.g., hyperthyroidism).

Specify if:
Longitudinal course specifiers (with and without interepisode recovery)
With seasonal pattern (applies only to the pattern of major depressive episodes)
With rapid cycling

(From American Psychiatric Association. *Diagnostic and Statistical Manual of Mental Disorders.* 4th ed. Text rev. Washington, DC: American Psychiatric Association; copyright 2000, with permission.)

The DSM-IV-TR atypical features can be applied to the most recent major depressive episode in major depressive disorder, bipolar I disorder, bipolar II disorder, or dysthymic disorder (Table 15.1–22).

Ms. G is a 17-year-old high school senior, referred for evaluation after she attempted suicide with an overdose of pills. Earlier on the night of the suicide attempt, she had a fight with her mother over a request to order pizza. Ms. G remembers her mother saying that she was a "spoiled brat" and asking whether she would be happier living elsewhere. Ms. G, feeling rejected and despondent, went to her room and wrote a note saying that she was having a mental breakdown and that she loved her parents but could not communicate with them. She added a request that her favorite glass animals be given to a particular friend. The parents, who had gone out to a movie, returned home later that evening to find their daughter comatose and immediately rushed her to the hospital emergency room.

During the last couple of months, Ms. G had been crying frequently and had lost interest in her friends, school, and social activities. She had been eating more and more and had recently begun to gain weight, which her mother is very unhappy about. Ms. G says that her mother is always harping about "taking care of herself," and in fact, the argument on the night of her suicide attempt was about Ms. G's desire to order a pizza that her mother did not think she needed. Ms. G's mother reports that all her daughter seems to want to do is sleep and that she never wants to go out with her friends or help around the house. When questioned about changes in her sleep habits, Ms. G admits that she has been feeling very tired lately and that she often feels as if there is nothing to make it worth getting out of bed. She does mention that she is excited about an upcoming visit from her boyfriend, who attends a college a considerable distance away and has not been home for several months.

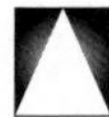

Table 15.1–20
DSM-IV-TR Diagnostic Criteria for Bipolar II Disorder

A. Presence (or history) of one or more major depressive episodes.
B. Presence (or history) of at least one hypomanic episode.
C. There has never been a manic episode or a mixed episode.
D. The mood symptoms in Criteria A and B are not better accounted for by schizoaffective disorder and are not superimposed on schizophrenia, schizophreniform disorder, delusional disorder, or psychotic disorder not otherwise specified.
E. The symptoms cause clinically significant distress or impairment in social, occupational, or other important areas of functioning.

Specify current or most recent episode:
Hypomanic: if currently (or most recently) in a hypomanic episode
Depressed: if currently (or most recently) in a major depressive episode

If the full criteria are currently met for a major depressive episode, specify its current clinical status and/or features:
Mild, moderate, severe without psychotic features/severe with psychotic features. Note: Fifth-digit codes cannot be used here because the code for bipolar II disorder already uses the fifth digit.
Chronic
With catatonic features
With melancholic features
With atypical features
With postpartum onset

If the full criteria are not currently met for a hypomanic or major depressive episode, specify the clinical status of the bipolar II disorder and/or features of the most recent major depressive episode (only if it is the most recent type of mood episode):
In partial remission, in full remission. Note: Fifth-digit codes cannot be used here because the code for bipolar II disorder already uses the fifth digit.
Chronic
With catatonic features
With melancholic features
With atypical features
With postpartum onset

Specify if:
Longitudinal course specifiers (with and without interepisode recovery)
With seasonal pattern (applies only to the pattern of major depressive episodes)
With rapid cycling

(From American Psychiatric Association. *Diagnostic and Statistical Manual of Mental Disorders.* 4th ed. Text rev. Washington, DC: American Psychiatric Association; copyright 2000, with permission.)

Upon evaluation, it is apparent that Ms. G, the third of three children of upper-middle-class and very intelligent parents, is struggling with a view of herself as less bright, clever, and attractive than her two siblings. She feels ignored and essentially rejected by her seemingly omnipresent mother. Ms. G is having difficulty developing a sense of separation from her mother and an individual sense of identity. She experiences her mother's directives as interference with her efforts to express autonomy and independence. (From *DSM-IV Case Studies.*)

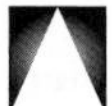

Table 15.1–21
DSM-IV-TR Criteria for Melancholic Features Specifier

Specify if:
With melancholic features (can be applied to the current or most recent major depressive episode in major depressive disorder and to a major depressive episode in bipolar I or bipolar II disorder only if it is the most recent type of mood episode)
A. Either of the following, occurring during the most severe period of the current episode:
(1) loss of pleasure in all, or almost all, activities
(2) lack of reactivity to usually pleasurable stimuli (does not feel much better, even temporarily, when something good happens)
B. Three (or more) of the following:
(1) distinct quality of depressed mood (i.e., the depressed mood is experienced as distinctly different from the kind of feeling experienced after the death of a loved one)
(2) depression regularly worse in the morning
(3) early morning awakening (at least 2 hours before usual time of awakening)
(4) marked psychomotor retardation or agitation
(5) significant anorexia or weight loss
(6) excessive or inappropriate guilt

(From American Psychiatric Association. *Diagnostic and Statistical Manual of Mental Disorders.* 4th ed. Text rev. Washington, DC: American Psychiatric Association; copyright 2000, with permission.)

With Catatonic Features. As a symptom, catatonia (Table 15.1–23) can be present in several mental disorders, most commonly, schizophrenia and the mood disorders. The presence of catatonic features in patients with mood disorders may have prognostic and treatment significance.

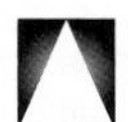

Table 15.1–22
DSM-IV-TR Criteria for Atypical Features Specifier

Specify if:
With atypical features (can be applied when these features predominate during the most recent 2 weeks of a current major depressive episode in major depressive disorder or in bipolar I or bipolar II disorder when a current major depressive episode is the most recent type of mood episode, or when these features predominate during the most recent 2 years of dysthymic disorder; if the major depressive episode is not current, it applies if the feature predominates during any 2-week period)
A. Mood reactivity (i.e., mood brightens in response to actual or potential positive events)
B. Two (or more) of the following features:
(1) significant weight gain or increase in appetite
(2) hypersomnia
(3) leaden paralysis (i.e., heavy, leaden feelings in arms or legs)
(4) long-standing pattern of interpersonal rejection sensitivity (not limited to episodes of mood disturbance) that results in significant social or occupational impairment
C. Criteria are not met for with melancholic features or with catatonic features during the same episode.

(From American Psychiatric Association. *Diagnostic and Statistical Manual of Mental Disorders.* 4th ed. Text rev. Washington, DC: American Psychiatric Association; copyright 2000, with permission.)

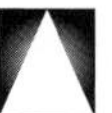

Table 15.1–23
DSM-IV-TR Criteria for Catatonic Features Specifier

Specify if:
With catatonic features (can be applied to the current or most recent major depressive episode, manic episode, or mixed episode in major depressive disorder, bipolar I disorder, or bipolar II disorder)
The clinical picture is dominated by at least two of the following:
(1) motoric immobility as evidenced by catalepsy (including waxy flexibility) or stupor
(2) excessive motor activity (that is apparently purposeless and not influenced by external stimuli)
(3) extreme negativism (an apparently motiveless resistance to all instructions or maintenance of a rigid posture against attempts to be moved) or mutism
(4) peculiarities of voluntary movement as evidenced by posturing (voluntary assumption of inappropriate or bizarre postures), stereotyped movements, prominent mannerisms, or prominent grimacing
(5) echolalia or echopraxia

(From American Psychiatric Association. *Diagnostic and Statistical Manual of Mental Disorders.* 4th ed. Text rev. Washington, DC: American Psychiatric Association; copyright 2000, with permission.)

The hallmark symptoms of catatonia—stuporousness, blunted affect, extreme withdrawal, negativism, and marked psychomotor retardation—can be seen in both catatonic and noncatatonic schizophrenia, major depressive disorder (often with psychotic features), and medical and neurological disorders. Clinicians often do not associate catatonic symptoms with bipolar I disorder because of the marked contrast between the symptoms of stuporous catatonia and the classic symptoms of mania. Because catatonic symptoms are a behavioral syndrome appearing in several medical and psychiatric conditions, catatonic symptoms do not imply a single diagnosis.

Postpartum Onset. DSM-IV-TR allows the specification of a postpartum mood disturbance if the onset of symptoms is within 4 weeks postpartum (Table 15.1–24). Postpartum mental disorders commonly include psychotic symptoms. (Postpartum psychosis is discussed in Section 14.4 and in Chapter 30 on reproductive psychiatry.)

Chronic. DSM-IV-TR allows the specification of chronic to describe major depressive episodes that occur as a part of major

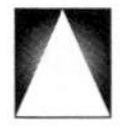

Table 15.1–24
DSM-IV-TR Criteria for Postpartum Onset Specifier

Specify if:
With postpartum onset (can be applied to the current or most recent major depressive, manic, or mixed episode in major depressive disorder, bipolar I disorder, or bipolar II disorder; or to brief psychotic disorder)
Onset of episode within 4 weeks postpartum

(From American Psychiatric Association. *Diagnostic and Statistical Manual of Mental Disorders.* 4th ed. Text rev. Washington, DC: American Psychiatric Association; copyright 2000, with permission.)

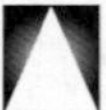

Table 15.1–25
DSM-IV-TR Criteria for Chronic Specifier

Specify if:

Chronic (can be applied to the current or most recent major depressive episode in major depressive disorder and to a major depressive episode in bipolar I or II disorder only if it is the most recent type of mood episode)

Full criteria for a major depressive episode have been met continuously for at least the past 2 years.

(From American Psychiatric Association. *Diagnostic and Statistical Manual of Mental Disorders.* 4th ed. Text rev. Washington, DC: American Psychiatric Association; copyright 2000, with permission.)

depressive disorder, bipolar I disorder, and bipolar II disorder (Table 15.1–25).

Describing Course of Recurrent Episodes

The DSM-IV-TR includes criteria for three distinct course specifiers for mood disorders. One of the course specifiers, with rapid cycling (Table 15.1–26), is restricted to bipolar I disorder and bipolar II disorder. Two other course specifiers, with seasonal pattern (Table 15.1–27) and with or without full interepisode recovery (Table 15.1–28), can be applied to bipolar I disorder, bipolar II disorder, and major depressive disorder, recurrent. The course specifier with postpartum onset can be applied to major depressive or manic episodes in bipolar I disorder, bipolar II disorder, major depressive disorder, and brief psychotic disorder.

Rapid Cycling. Patients with rapid cycling bipolar I disorder are likely to be female and to have had depressive and hypomanic episodes. No data indicate that rapid cycling has a familial pattern of inheritance and, thus, an external factor such as stress or drug treatment may be involved in the pathogenesis of rapid cycling. The DSM-IV-TR criteria specify that the patient must have at least four episodes within a 12-month period (Table 15.1–26).

When Mr. E's desperate wife finally got him to agree to a comprehensive inpatient evaluation, he was 37, unemployed, and had been essentially nonfunctional for several years. After a week during which he was partying all night and shopping all day, Mrs. E said that she would leave him if he did not check into a psychiatric hospital. The admitting psychiatrist found him to be a fast-talking, jovial, seductive man with no evidence of delusions or hallucinations.

Mr. E's troubles began 7 years before when he was working as an insurance adjuster and had a few months of mild, intermittent, depressive symptoms, anxiety, fatigue, insomnia, and loss of appetite. At the time, he attributed these symptoms to stress at work, and within a few months was back to his usual self.

A few years later an asymptomatic thyroid mass was noted during a routine physical examination. One month after removal of the mass, a papillary cyst, Mr. E noted dramatic mood changes. Twenty-five days of remarkable energy, hyperactivity, and euphoria were followed by 5 days of depression during which he slept a lot and felt that he could hardly move. This pattern of alternating periods of elation and depression, apparently with few "normal" days, repeated itself continuously over the following years.

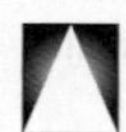

Table 15.1–26
DSM-IV-TR Criteria for Rapid-Cycling Specifier

Specify if:

With rapid cycling (can be applied to bipolar I disorder or bipolar II disorder)

At least four episodes of a mood disturbance in the previous 12 months that meet criteria for a major depressive, manic, mixed, or hypomanic episode.

Note: Episodes are demarcated either by partial or full remission for at least 2 months or a switch to an episode of opposite polarity (e.g., major depressive episode to manic episode).

(From American Psychiatric Association. *Diagnostic and Statistical Manual of Mental Disorders.* 4th ed. Text rev. Washington, DC: American Psychiatric Association; copyright 2000, with permission.)

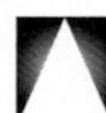

Table 15.1–27
DSM-IV-TR Criteria for Seasonal Pattern Specifier

Specify if:

With seasonal pattern (can be applied to the pattern of major depressive episodes in bipolar I disorder, bipolar II disorder, or major depressive disorder, recurrent)

A. There has been a regular temporal relationship between the onset of major depressive episodes in bipolar I or bipolar II disorder or major depressive disorder, recurrent, and a particular time of the year (e.g., regular appearance of the major depressive episode in the fall or winter).
Note: Do not include cases in which there is an obvious effect of seasonal-related psychosocial stressors (e.g., regularly being unemployed every winter).

B. Full remissions (or a change from depression to mania or hypomania) also occur at a characteristic time of the year (e.g., depression disappears in the spring).

C. In the last 2 years, two major depressive episodes have occurred that demonstrate the temporal seasonal relationships defined in Criteria A and B, and no nonseasonal major depressive episodes have occurred during that same period.

D. Seasonal major depressive episodes (as described above) substantially outnumber the nonseasonal major depressive episodes that may have occurred over the individual's lifetime.

(From American Psychiatric Association. *Diagnostic and Statistical Manual of Mental Disorders.* 4th ed. Text rev. Washington, DC: American Psychiatric Association; copyright 2000, with permission.)

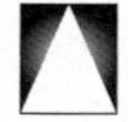

Table 15.1–28
DSM-IV-TR Criteria for Longitudinal Course Specifiers

Specify if (can be applied to recurrent major depressive disorder or bipolar I or II disorder):

With full interepisode recovery: if full remission is attained between the two most recent mood episodes

Without full interepisode recovery: if full remission is not attained between the two most recent mood episodes

(From American Psychiatric Association. *Diagnostic and Statistical Manual of Mental Disorders.* 4th ed. Text rev. Washington, DC: American Psychiatric Association; copyright 2000, with permission.)

During his energetic periods, Mr. E was optimistic and self-confident, but short tempered and easily irritated. His judgment at work was erratic. He spent large sums of money on unnecessary and, for him, uncharacteristic purchases, such as a high-priced stereo system and several Doberman pinschers. He also had several impulsive sexual flings.

During his depressed periods, he often stayed in bed all day because of fatigue, lack of motivation, and depressed mood. He felt guilty about the irresponsibility and excesses of the previous several weeks. He stopped eating, bathing, and shaving. After several days of this withdrawal, Mr. E would rise from bed one morning feeling better and, within 2 days, be back at work, often working feverishly, though ineffectively, to catch up on work he had let slide during his depressed periods.

Although both he and his wife denied any drug use, other than drinking binges during his hyperactive periods, Mr. E had been dismissed from his job 5 years previously because his supervisor was convinced that his overactivity must be due to drug use. His wife had supported him since then.

When he finally agreed to a psychiatric evaluation 2 years ago, Mr. E was minimally cooperative and noncompliant with several medications that were prescribed, including lithium, neuroleptics, and antidepressants. His mood swings had continued with few interruptions up to the current hospitalization.

In the hospital, results of his physical examination, blood chemistry, blood counts, computed tomography scan, and cognitive testing were unremarkable. Thyroid function testing revealed some laboratory evidence of thyroid hypofunction, but he was without clinical signs of thyroid disease. After a week he switched to his characteristic depressive state. (From *DSM-IV Casebook*.)

Seasonal Pattern. Patients with a seasonal pattern to their mood disorders tend to experience depressive episodes during a particular season, most commonly winter. The pattern has become known as seasonal affective disorder (SAD), although this term is not used in DSM-IV-TR (Table 15.1–27). Two types of evidence indicate that the seasonal pattern may represent a separate diagnostic entity. First, the patients are likely to respond to treatment with light therapy, although no studies with controls to evaluate light therapy in nonseasonally depressed patients have been conducted. Second, research has shown that patients evince decreased metabolic activity in the orbital frontal cortex and in the left inferior parietal lobe. Further studies are necessary to differentiate depressed persons with seasonal pattern from other depressed persons.

Longitudinal Course Specifiers. DSM-IV-TR includes specific descriptions of longitudinal courses for major depressive disorder, bipolar I disorder, and bipolar II disorder (Table 15.1–28). These longitudinal course specifiers help clinicians and researchers to identify appropriate treatment and prognosticate based on various longitudinal courses.

Non–DSM-IV-TR Types. Other systems that identify types of patients with mood disorders usually separate patients with good and poor prognoses or patients who may respond to one treatment or another. They also differentiate endogenous-reactive and primary-secondary schemes.

The endogenous-reactive continuum is a controversial division. It implies that endogenous depressions are biological and that reactive depressions are psychological, primarily on the basis of the presence or absence of an identifiable precipitating stress. Other symptoms of endogenous depression have been described as diurnal variation, delusions, psychomotor retardation, early morning awakening, and feelings of guilt; thus, endogenous depression is similar to the DSM-IV-TR diagnosis of major depressive disorder with psychotic features or melancholic features or both. Symptoms of reactive depression have included initial insomnia, anxiety, emotional lability, and multiple somatic complaints.

Primary depressions are what DSM-IV-TR refers to as mood disorders, except for the diagnoses of mood disorder caused by a general medical condition and substance-induced mood disorder, which are considered secondary depressions. Double depression is the condition in which major depressive disorder is superimposed on dysthymic disorder. A depressive equivalent is a symptom or syndrome that may be a *forme fruste* of a depressive episode. For example, a triad of truancy, alcohol abuse, and sexual promiscuity in a formerly well-behaved adolescent may constitute a depressive equivalent.

CLINICAL FEATURES

The two basic symptom patterns in mood disorders are depression and mania. Depressive episodes can occur in both major depressive disorder and bipolar I disorder. Researchers have attempted to find reliable differences between bipolar I disorder depressive episodes and episodes of major depressive disorder, but the differences are elusive. In a clinical situation, only the patient's history, family history, and future course can help differentiate the two conditions. Some patients with bipolar I disorder have mixed states with both manic and depressive features, and some seem to experience brief—minutes to a few hours—episodes of depression during manic episodes.

Depressive Episodes

A depressed mood and a loss of interest or pleasure are the key symptoms of depression. Patients may say that they feel blue, hopeless, in the dumps, or worthless. For a patient, the depressed mood often has a distinct quality that differentiates it from the normal emotion of sadness or grief. Patients often describe the symptom of depression as one of agonizing emotional pain and sometimes complain about being unable to cry, a symptom that resolves as they improve.

About two thirds of all depressed patients contemplate suicide, and 10 to 15 percent commit suicide. Those recently hospitalized with a suicide attempt or suicidal ideation have a higher lifetime risk of successful suicide than those never hospitalized for suicidal ideation. Some depressed patients sometimes seem unaware of their depression and do not complain of a mood disturbance, even though they exhibit withdrawal from family, friends, and activities that previously interested them. Almost all depressed patients (97 percent) complain about reduced energy; they have difficulty finishing tasks, are impaired at school and work, and have less motivation to undertake new projects. About 80 percent of patients complain of trouble sleeping, especially early morning awakening (i.e., terminal insomnia) and multiple awakenings at night, during which they ruminate about their problems. Many patients have decreased appetite and weight loss, but others experience increased appetite and weight gain and sleep longer than usual. These patients are classified in DSM-IV-TR as having atypical features.

Anxiety, a common symptom of depression, affects as many as 90 percent of all depressed patients. The various changes in food intake and rest can aggravate coexisting medical illnesses such as diabetes, hypertension, chronic obstructive lung disease, and heart disease. Other vegetative symptoms include abnormal menses and decreased interest and performance in sexual activities. Sexual problems can sometimes lead to inappropriate referrals, such as to marital counseling and sex therapy, when clinicians fail to recognize the underlying depressive disorder. Anxiety (including panic attacks), alcohol abuse, and somatic complaints (e.g., constipation and headaches) often complicate the treatment of depression. About 50 percent of all patients describe a diurnal variation in their symptoms, with increased severity in the morning and lessening of symptoms by evening. Cognitive symptoms include subjective reports of an inability to concentrate (84 percent of patients in one study) and impairments in thinking (67 percent of patients in another study).

Depression in Children and Adolescents. School phobia and excessive clinging to parents may be symptoms of depression in children. Poor academic performance, substance abuse, antisocial behavior, sexual promiscuity, truancy, and running away may be symptoms of depression in adolescents. (This subject is further discussed in Chapter 49.)

Depression in Older People. Depression is more common in older persons than it is in the general population. Various studies have reported prevalence rates ranging from 25 to almost 50 percent, although the percentage of these cases that are caused by major depressive disorder is uncertain. Several studies indicate that depression in older persons may be correlated with low socioeconomic status, the loss of a spouse, a concurrent physical illness, and social isolation. Other studies have indicated that depression in older persons is underdiagnosed and undertreated, perhaps particularly by general practitioners. The underrecognition of depression in older persons may occur because the disorder appears more often with somatic complaints in older, than in younger, age groups. Further, ageism may influence and cause clinicians to accept depressive symptoms as normal in older patients.

Manic Episodes

An elevated, expansive, or irritable mood is the hallmark of a manic episode. The elevated mood is euphoric and often infectious and can even cause a countertransferential denial of illness by an inexperienced clinician. Although uninvolved persons may not recognize the unusual nature of a patient's mood, those who know the patient recognize it as abnormal. Alternatively, the mood may be irritable, especially when a patient's overtly ambitious plans are thwarted. Patients often exhibit a change of predominant mood from euphoria early in the course of the illness to later irritability.

The treatment of manic patients in an inpatient ward can be complicated by their testing of the limits of ward rules, their tendency to shift responsibility for their acts onto others, their exploitation of the weaknesses of others, and their propensity to create conflicts among staff members. Outside the hospital, manic patients often drink alcohol excessively, perhaps in an attempt to self-medicate. Their disinhibited nature is reflected in excessive use of the telephone, especially in making long-distance calls during the early morning hours.

Pathological gambling, a tendency to disrobe in public places, wearing clothing and jewelry of bright colors in unusual or outlandish combinations, and inattention to small details (e.g., forgetting to hang up the telephone) are also symptomatic of the disorder. Patients act impulsively and at the same time with a sense of conviction and purpose. They are often preoccupied by religious, political, financial, sexual, or persecutory ideas that can evolve into complex delusional systems. Occasionally, manic patients become regressed and play with their urine and feces.

Mania in Adolescents. Mania in adolescents is often misdiagnosed as antisocial personality disorder or schizophrenia. Symptoms of mania in adolescents may include psychosis, alcohol or other substance abuse, suicide attempts, academic problems, philosophical brooding, OCD symptoms, multiple somatic complaints, marked irritability resulting in fights, and other antisocial behaviors. Although many of these symptoms are seen in normal adolescents, severe or persistent symptoms should cause clinicians to consider bipolar I disorder in the differential diagnosis.

Bipolar II Disorder

The clinical features of bipolar II disorder are those of major depressive disorder combined with those of a hypomanic episode. Although the data are limited, a few studies indicate that bipolar II disorder is associated with more marital disruption and with onset at an earlier age than bipolar I disorder. Evidence also indicates that patients with bipolar II disorder are at greater risk of both attempting and completing suicide than patients with bipolar I disorder and major depressive disorder.

Coexisting Disorders

Anxiety. In the anxiety disorders, DSM-IV-TR notes the existence of mixed anxiety–depressive disorder. Significant symptoms of anxiety can and often do coexist with significant symptoms of depression. Whether patients who exhibit significant symptoms of both anxiety and depression are affected by two distinct disease processes or by a single disease process that produces both sets of symptoms is not yet resolved. Patients of both types may constitute the group of patients with mixed anxiety–depressive disorder.

Alcohol Dependence. Alcohol dependence frequently coexists with mood disorders. Both patients with major depressive disorder and those with bipolar I disorder are likely to meet the diagnostic criteria for an alcohol use disorder. The available data indicate that alcohol dependence is more strongly associated with a coexisting diagnosis of depression in women than in men. In contrast, the genetic and family data about men who have both a mood disorder and alcohol dependence indicate that they are likely to have two genetically distinct disease processes.

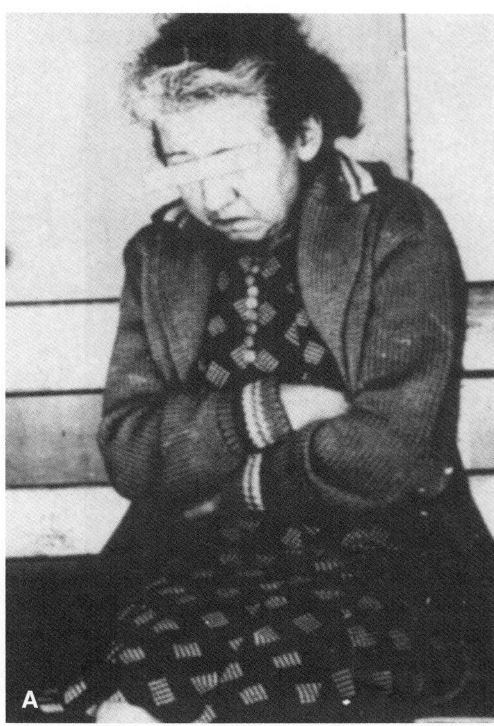

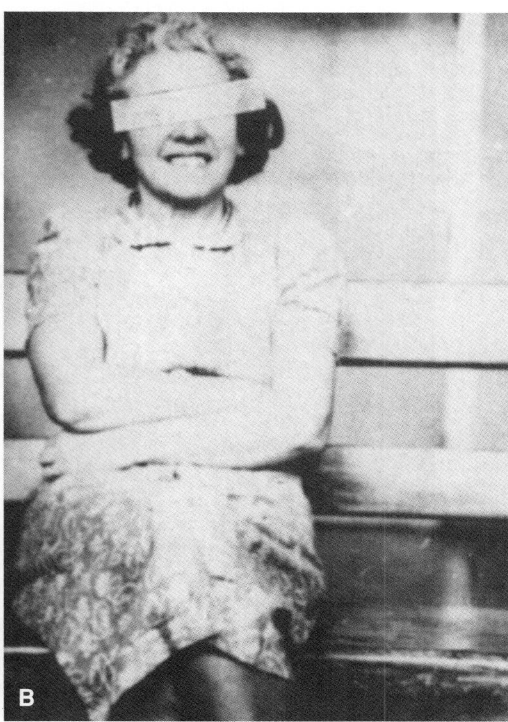

FIGURE 15.1–3
A 38-year-old woman during a state of deep retarded depression (**A**) and 2 months later, after recovery (**B**). The turned-down corners of her mouth, her stooped posture, her drab clothing, and her hairdo during the depressed episode are noteworthy. (Courtesy of Heinz E. Lehmann, M.D.)

Other Substance-Related Disorders. Substance-related disorders other than alcohol dependence are also commonly associated with mood disorders. The abuse of substances may be involved in precipitating an episode of illness or, conversely, may represent patients' attempts to treat their own illnesses. Although manic patients seldom use sedatives to dampen their euphoria, depressed patients often use stimulants, such as cocaine and amphetamines, to relieve their depression.

Medical Conditions. Depression commonly coexists with medical conditions, especially in older persons. When depression and medical conditions coexist, clinicians must try to determine whether the underlying medical condition is pathophysiologically related to the depression or whether any drugs that the patient is taking for the medical condition are causing the depression. Many studies indicate that treatment of a coexisting major depressive disorder can improve the course of the underlying medical disorder, including cancer.

MENTAL STATUS EXAMINATION

Depressive Episodes

General Description. Generalized psychomotor retardation is the most common symptom of depression, although psychomotor agitation is also seen, especially in older patients. Hand-wringing and hair-pulling are the most common symptoms of agitation. Classically, a depressed patient has a stooped posture, no spontaneous movements, and a downcast, averted gaze (Figs. 15.1–3 and 15.1–4). On clinical examination, depressed patients exhibiting gross symptoms of psychomotor retardation may appear identical to patients with catatonic schizophrenia. This fact is recognized in DSM-IV-TR by the inclusion of the symptom qualifier "with catatonic features" for some mood disorders.

Mood, Affect, and Feelings. Depression is the key symptom, although about 50 percent of patients deny depressive feelings and do not appear to be particularly depressed. Family members or employers often bring or send these patients for treatment because of social withdrawal and generally decreased activity.

Speech. Many depressed patients have decreased rate and volume of speech; they respond to questions with single words and exhibit delayed responses to questions. The examiner may literally have to wait 2 or 3 minutes for a response to a question.

Perceptual Disturbances. Depressed patients with delusions or hallucinations are said to have a major depressive episode with psychotic features. Even in the absence of delusions or hallucinations, some clinicians use the term *psychotic depression* for grossly regressed depressed patients—mute, not bathing, soiling. Such patients are probably better described as having catatonic features.

Delusions and hallucinations that are consistent with a depressed mood are said to be mood congruent. Mood-congruent delusions in a depressed person include those of guilt, sinfulness, worthlessness, poverty, failure, persecution, and terminal

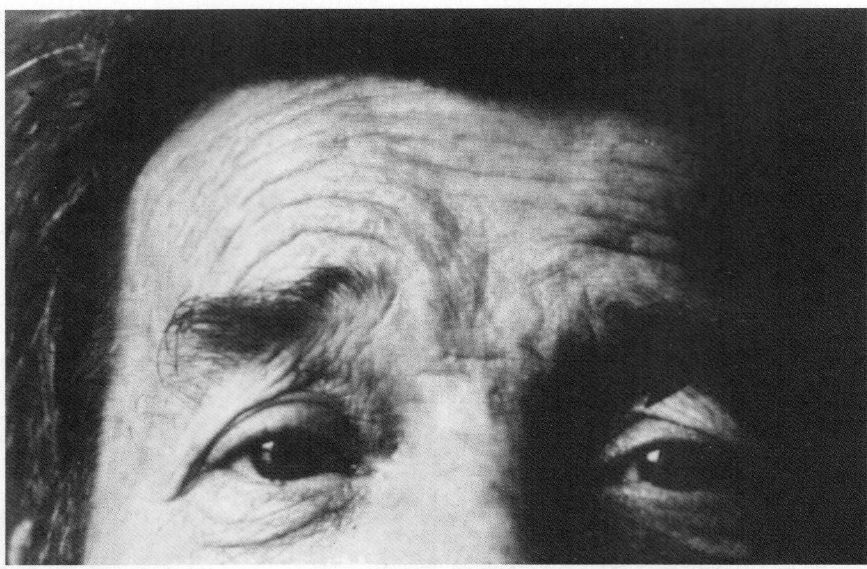

FIGURE 15.1–4
The Swiss neuropsychiatrist Otto Veraguth described a peculiar triangle-shaped fold in the nasal corner of the upper eyelid. The fold is often associated with depression and referred to as Veraguth's fold. The photograph illustrates this physiognomic feature in a 50-year-old man during a major depressive episode. Veraguth's fold may also be seen in persons who are not clinically depressed, usually while they are harboring a mild depressive affect. Distinct changes in the tone of the corrugator and zygomatic facial muscles accompany depression, as shown on electromyograms. (Courtesy of Heinz E. Lehmann, M.D.)

somatic illnesses (such as cancer and "rotting" brain). The content of mood-incongruent delusions or hallucinations is not consistent with a depressed mood. For example, a mood-incongruent delusion in a depressed person might involve grandiose themes of exaggerated power, knowledge, and worth. When that occurs, a schizophrenic disorder should be considered.

Thought. Depressed patients customarily have negative views of the world and of themselves. Their thought content often includes nondelusional ruminations about loss, guilt, suicide, and death. About 10 percent of all depressed patients have marked symptoms of a thought disorder, usually thought blocking and profound poverty of content.

Sensorium and Cognition

ORIENTATION. Most depressed patients are oriented to person, place, and time, although some may not have sufficient energy or interest to answer questions about these subjects during an interview.

MEMORY. About 50 to 75 percent of all depressed patients have a cognitive impairment, sometimes referred to as *depressive pseudodementia.* Such patients commonly complain of impaired concentration and forgetfulness.

Impulse Control. About 10 to 15 percent of all depressed patients commit suicide, and about two thirds have suicidal ideation. Depressed patients with psychotic features occasionally consider killing a person as a result of their delusional systems, but the most severely depressed patients often lack the motivation or the energy to act in an impulsive or violent way. Patients with depressive disorders are at increased risk of suicide as they begin to improve and regain the energy needed to plan and carry out a suicide (paradoxical suicide). It is usually clinically unwise to give a depressed patient a large prescription for a large number of antidepressants, especially tricyclic drugs, at the time of their discharge from the hospital. Similarly, drugs that may be activating, such as fluoxetine, may be prescribed in such a way that the energizing qualities are minimized (e.g., be given a benzodiazepine at the same time).

Judgment and Insight. Judgment is best assessed by reviewing patients' actions in the recent past and their behavior during the interview. Depressed patients' description of their disorder is often hyperbolic; they overemphasize their symptoms, their disorder, and their life problems. It is difficult to convince such patients that improvement is possible.

Reliability. In interviews and conversations, depressed patients overemphasize the bad and minimize the good. A common clinical mistake is to unquestioningly believe a depressed patient who states that a previous trial of antidepressant medications did not work. Such statements may be false, and they require confirmation from another source. Psychiatrists should not view patients' misinformation as an intentional fabrication; the admission of any hopeful information may be impossible for a person in a depressed state of mind.

Objective Rating Scales for Depression. Objective rating scales for depression can be useful in clinical practice for documenting the depressed patient's clinical state.

ZUNG. The Zung Self-Rating Depression Scale is a 20-item report scale. A normal score is 34 or less; a depressed score is 50 or more. The scale provides a global index of the intensity of a patient's depressive symptoms, including the affective expression of depression.

RASKIN. The Raskin Depression Scale is a clinician-rated scale that measures the severity of a patient's depression, as reported by the patient and as observed by the physician, on a five-point scale of three dimensions: verbal report, displayed behavior, and secondary symptoms. The scale has a range of 3 to 13; a normal score is 3, and a depressed score is 7 or more.

HAMILTON. The Hamilton Rating Scale for Depression (HAM-D) is a widely used depression scale with up to 24 items, each of which is rated 0 to 4 or 0 to 2, with a total score of 0 to 76. The clinician evaluates the patient's answers to questions about feelings of guilt, thoughts of suicide, sleep habits, and other symptoms of depression, and the ratings are derived from the clinical interview.

Manic Episodes

General Description. Manic patients are excited, talkative, sometimes amusing, and frequently hyperactive. At times, they are grossly psychotic and disorganized and require physical restraints and the intramuscular injection of sedating drugs.

Mood, Affect, and Feelings. Manic patients classically are euphoric, but they can also be irritable, especially when mania has been present for some time. They also have a low frustration tolerance, which can lead to feelings of anger and hostility. Manic patients may be emotionally labile, switching from laughter to irritability to depression in minutes or hours.

Speech. Manic patients cannot be interrupted while they are speaking, and they are often intrusive nuisances to those around them. Their speech is often disturbed. As the mania gets more intense, speech becomes louder, more rapid, and difficult to interpret. As the activated state increases, their speech is filled with puns, jokes, rhymes, plays on words, and irrelevancies. At a still greater activity level, associations become loosened, the ability to concentrate fades, and flight of ideas, clanging, and neologisms appear. In acute manic excitement, speech can be totally incoherent and indistinguishable from that of a person with schizophrenia.

Perceptual Disturbances. Delusions occur in 75 percent of all manic patients. Mood-congruent manic delusions are often concerned with great wealth, extraordinary abilities, or power. Bizarre and mood-incongruent delusions and hallucinations also appear in mania.

Thought. The manic patient's thought content includes themes of self-confidence and self-aggrandizement. Manic patients are often easily distracted, and their cognitive functioning in the manic state is characterized by an unrestrained and accelerated flow of ideas.

Sensorium and Cognition. Although the cognitive deficits of patients with schizophrenia have been much discussed, less has been written about similar deficits in patients with bipolar I disorder. These deficits can be interpreted as reflecting diffuse cortical dysfunction; subsequent work may localize the abnormal areas. Grossly, orientation and memory are intact, although some manic patients may be so euphoric that they answer questions testing orientation incorrectly. Emil Kraepelin called the symptom "delirious mania."

Impulse Control. About 75 percent of all manic patients are assaultive or threatening. Manic patients do attempt suicide and homicide, but the incidence of these behaviors is unknown.

Judgment and Insight. Impaired judgment is a hallmark of manic patients. They may break laws about credit cards, sexual activities, and finances and sometimes involve their families in financial ruin. Manic patients also have little insight into their disorder.

Reliability. Manic patients are notoriously unreliable in their information. Because lying and deceit are common in mania, inexperienced clinicians may treat manic patients with inappropriate disdain.

DIFFERENTIAL DIAGNOSIS

Major Depressive Disorder

Medical Disorders. The DSM-IV-TR diagnosis of mood disorder due to a general medical condition describes a mood disorder caused by a nonpsychiatric medical condition. The DSM-IV-TR diagnosis of substance-induced mood disorder describes a mood disorder caused by a substance. Both these diagnostic categories are discussed in Section 15.3.

Failure to obtain a good clinical history or to consider the context of a patient's current life situation can lead to diagnostic errors. Clinicians should have depressed adolescents tested for mononucleosis, and patients who are markedly overweight or underweight should be tested for adrenal and thyroid dysfunctions. Homosexuals, bisexual men, prostitutes, and persons who abuse a substance intravenously should be tested for acquired immune deficiency syndrome (AIDS). Older patients should be evaluated for viral pneumonia and other medical conditions.

Many neurological and medical disorders and pharmacological agents can produce symptoms of depression (*see* Table 15.3–9). Patients with depressive disorders often first visit their general practitioners with somatic complaints. Most medical causes of depressive disorders can be detected with a comprehensive medical history, a complete physical and neurological examination, and routine blood and urine tests. The workup should include tests for thyroid and adrenal functions, because disorders of both of these endocrine systems can appear as depressive disorders. In substance-induced mood disorder, a reasonable rule of thumb is that any drug a depressed patient is taking should be considered a potential factor in the mood disorder. Cardiac drugs, antihypertensives, sedatives, hypnotics, antipsychotics, antiepileptics, antiparkinsonian drugs, analgesics, antibacterials, and antineoplastics are all commonly associated with depressive symptoms.

NEUROLOGICAL CONDITIONS. The most common neurological problems that manifest depressive symptoms are Parkinson's disease, dementing illnesses (including dementia of the Alzheimer's type), epilepsy, cerebrovascular diseases, and tumors. About 50 to 75 percent of all patients with Parkinson's disease have marked symptoms of depressive disorder that do not correlate with the patient's physical disability, age, or duration of illness but do correlate with the presence of abnormalities found on neuropsychological tests. The symptoms of depressive disorder can be masked by the almost identical motor symptoms of Parkinson's disease. Depressive symptoms often respond to antidepressant drugs or ECT. The interictal changes associated with temporal lobe epilepsy can mimic a depressive disorder, especially if the epileptic focus is on the right side. Depression is a common complicating feature of cerebrovascular diseases, particularly in the 2 years after the episode. Depression is more common in anterior brain lesions than in posterior brain lesions and, in both cases, often responds to antidepressant medications. Tumors of the diencephalic and temporal regions are particularly likely to be associated with depressive disorder symptoms.

PSEUDODEMENTIA. Clinicians can usually differentiate the pseudodementia of major depressive disorder from the dementia of a disease, such as dementia of the Alzheimer's type, on clinical grounds. The cognitive symptoms in major depressive disorder have a sudden onset, and other symptoms of the disorder, such as self-reproach, are also present. A diurnal variation in the cognitive problems, which is not seen in primary dementias, may occur. Depressed patients with cognitive difficulties often do not try to answer questions ("I don't know"), whereas patients with dementia may confabulate. During an interview, depressed patients can sometimes be coached and encouraged into remembering, an ability that demented patients lack.

Mental Disorders. Depression can be a feature of virtually any mental disorder listed in DSM-IV-TR, but the mental disorders listed in Table 15.1–29 deserves particular consideration in the differential diagnosis.

Table 15.1–29
Mental Disorders That Commonly Have Depressive Features

- Adjustment disorder with depressed mood
- Alcohol use disorders
- Anxiety disorders
  - Generalized anxiety disorder
  - Mixed anxiety-depressive disorder
  - Panic disorder
  - Posttraumatic stress disorder
  - Obsessive–compulsive disorder
- Eating disorders
  - Anorexia nervosa
  - Bulimia nervosa
- Mood disorders
  - Bipolar I disorder
  - Bipolar II disorder
  - Cyclothymic disorder
  - Dysthymic disorder
  - Major depressive disorder
  - Minor depressive disorder
  - Mood disorder due to a general medical condition
  - Recurrent brief depressive disorder
  - Substance-induced mood disorder
- Schizophrenia
- Schizophreniform disorder
- Somatoform disorders (especially somatization disorder)

OTHER MOOD DISORDERS. Clinicians must consider a range of DSM-IV-TR diagnostic categories before arriving at a final diagnosis. Mood disorder caused by a general medical condition and substance-induced mood disorder must be ruled out. Clinicians must also determine whether a patient has had episodes of mania-like symptoms, indicating bipolar I disorder (complete manic and depressive syndromes), bipolar II disorder (recurrent major depressive episodes with hypomania), or cyclothymic disorder (incomplete depressive and manic syndromes). If a patient's symptoms are limited to those of depression, clinicians must assess the severity and duration of the symptoms to differentiate among major depressive disorder (complete depressive syndrome for 2 weeks), minor depressive disorder (incomplete but episodic depressive syndrome), recurrent brief depressive disorder (complete depressive syndrome but for less than 2 weeks per episode), and dysthymic disorder (incomplete depressive syndrome without clear episodes).

OTHER MENTAL DISORDERS. Substance-related disorders, psychotic disorders, eating disorders, adjustment disorders, somatoform disorders, and anxiety disorders are all commonly associated with depressive symptoms and should be considered in the differential diagnosis of a patient with depressive symptoms. Perhaps the most difficult differential is that between anxiety disorders with depression and depressive disorders with marked anxiety. The difficulty of distinguishing these is reflected in the inclusion of the diagnosis of mixed anxiety-depressive disorder in DSM-IV-TR. An abnormal result on the dexamethasone-suppression test, the presence of shortened REM latency on a sleep electroencephalogram (EEG), and a negative lactate infusion test result support a diagnosis of major depressive disorder in particularly ambiguous cases.

UNCOMPLICATED BEREAVEMENT. Uncomplicated bereavement is not considered a mental disorder, even though about one third of all bereaved spouses for a time meet the diagnostic criteria for major depressive disorder. Some patients with uncomplicated bereavement do develop major depressive disorder, but the diagnosis is not made unless no resolution of the grief occurs. The differentiation is based on the symptoms' severity and length. In major depressive disorder, common symptoms that evolve from unresolved bereavement are a morbid preoccupation with worthlessness, suicidal ideation, feelings that the person has committed an act (not just an omission) that caused the spouse's death, mummification (keeping the deceased's belongings exactly as they were), and a particularly severe anniversary reaction, which sometimes includes a suicide attempt.

In severe forms of bereavement depression, the patient simply pines away, unable to live without the departed person, usually a spouse. Such persons do have a serious medical condition. Their immune function is often depressed, and their cardiovascular status is precarious. Death can ensue within a few months of that of a spouse, especially among elderly men. Such considerations suggest that it would be clinically unwise to withhold antidepressants from many persons experiencing such an intense mourning.

A 75-year-old widow was brought to treatment by her daughter because of severe insomnia and total loss of interest in daily routines after her husband's death 1 year before. She had been agitated for the first 2 to 3 months and thereafter "sank into total inactivity—not wanting to get out of bed, not wanting to do anything, not wanting to go out." According to her daughter, she was married at 21 years of age, had four children, and had been a housewife until her husband's death from a heart attack. Past psychiatric history was negative; premorbid adjustment had been characterized by compulsive traits. During the interview, she was dressed in black, appeared moderately slowed, and sobbed intermittently, saying "I search everywhere for him. . . I don't find him." When asked about life, she said "everything I see is black." Although she expressed no interest in food, she did not seem to have lost an appreciable amount of weight. Her [dexamethasone suppression test] DST result was 18 mg/dL. The patient declined psychiatric care, stating that she "preferred to join her husband rather than get well." She was too religious to commit suicide, but, by refusing treatment, she felt that she would "pine away. . . find relief in death and reunion." (Courtesy of Hagop Akiskal, M.D.)

Schizophrenia. Much has been published about the clinical difficulty of distinguishing a manic episode from schizophrenia. Although difficult, a differential diagnosis is possible. Merriment, elation, and infectiousness of mood are much more common in manic episodes than in schizophrenia. The combination of a manic mood, rapid or pressured speech, and hyperactivity weighs heavily toward a diagnosis of a manic episode. The onset in a manic episode is often rapid and is perceived as a marked change from a patient's previous behavior. Half of all patients with bipolar I disorder have a family history of mood disorder. Catatonic features may be part of a depressive phase of bipolar I disorder. When evaluating patients with catatonia, clinicians should look carefully for a past history of manic or depressive episodes and for a family history of mood disorders. Manic symptoms in persons from minority groups (particularly blacks and Hispanics) are often misdiagnosed as schizophrenic symptoms.

Medical Conditions. In contrast to depressive symptoms, which are present in almost all psychiatric disorders, manic symptoms are more distinctive, although they can be caused by a wide range of medical and neurological conditions and substances. Antidepressant treatment can also be associated with the precipitation of mania in some patients.

Bipolar I Disorder

When a patient with bipolar I disorder has a depressive episode, the differential diagnosis is the same as that for a patient being considered for a diagnosis of major depressive disorder. When a patient is manic, however, the differential diagnosis includes bipolar I disorder, bipolar II disorder, cyclothymic disorder, mood disorder caused by a general medical condition, and substance-induced mood disorder. For manic symptoms, borderline, narcissistic, histrionic, and antisocial personality disorders need special consideration.

Bipolar II Disorder

The differential diagnosis of patients being evaluated for a mood disorder should include the other mood disorders, psychotic disorders, and borderline disorder. The differentiation between major depressive disorder and bipolar I disorder, on one hand, and bipolar II disorder, on the other hand, rests on the clinical evaluation of the mania-like episodes. Clinicians should not mistake euthymia in a chronically depressed patient for a hypomanic or manic episode. Patients with borderline personality disorder often have a severely disrupted life, similar to that of patients with bipolar II disorder, because of the multiple episodes of significant mood disorder symptoms.

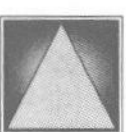

Table 15.1–30
Clinical Features Predictive of Bipolar Disorder

Early age at onset
Psychotic depression before 25 years of age
Postpartum depression, especially one with psychotic features
Rapid onset and offset of depressive episodes of short duration (<3 months)
Recurrent depression (more than five episodes)
Depression with marked psychomotor retardation
Atypical features (reverse vegetative signs)
Seasonality
Bipolar family history
High-density, three-generation pedigrees
Trait mood lability (cyclothymia)
Hyperthymic temperament
Hypomania associated with antidepressants
Repeated (at least three times) loss of efficacy of antidepressants after initial response
Depressive mixed state (with psychomotor excitement, irritable hostility, racing thoughts, and sexual arousal *during* major depression)

Major Depressive Disorder versus Bipolar Disorder

The question of whether a patient has major depressive disorder or bipolar disorder has emerged as a major challenge in clinical practice. Numerous studies have shown that bipolar disorder is not only confused with personality, substance use, and schizophrenic disorders, but also with depressive and anxiety disorders. Certain features—especially in combination—are predictive of bipolar disorder (Table 15.1–30).

More broad indicators of bipolarity include the following conditions, none of which, by themselves, confirm a bipolar diagnosis, but should raise clinical suspicion in that direction: agitated depression, cyclical depression, episodic sleep dysregulation, or a combination of these; refractory depression (failed antidepressants from three different classes); depression in someone with an extroverted profession, periodic impulsivity, such as gambling, sexual misconduct, and wanderlust, or periodic irritability, suicidal crises, or both; and depression with erratic personality disorders.

COURSE AND PROGNOSIS

Studies of the course and prognosis of mood disorders have generally concluded that mood disorders tend to have long courses and that patients tend to have relapses. Although mood disorders are often considered benign in contrast to schizophrenia, they exact a profound toll on affected patients.

Major Depressive Disorder

Course

ONSET. About 50 percent of patients having their first episode of major depressive disorder exhibited significant depressive symptoms before the first identified episode. Therefore, early identification and treatment of early symptoms may prevent the development of a full depressive episode. Although symptoms may have been present, patients with major depressive disorder usually have not had a premorbid personality disorder. The first depressive episode occurs before age 40 in about 50 percent of patients. A later onset is associated with the absence of a family history of mood disorders, antisocial personality disorder, and alcohol abuse.

DURATION. An untreated depressive episode lasts 6 to 13 months; most treated episodes last about 3 months. The withdrawal of antidepressants before 3 months has elapsed almost always results in the return of the symptoms. As the course of the disorder progresses, patients tend to have more frequent episodes that last longer. Over a 20-year period, the mean number of episodes is five or six.

DEVELOPMENT OF MANIC EPISODES. About 5 to 10 percent of patients with an initial diagnosis of major depressive disorder have a manic episode 6 to 10 years after the first depressive episode. The mean age for this switch is 32, and it often occurs after two to four depressive episodes. Although the data are inconsistent and controversial, some clinicians report that the depression of patients who are later classified as having bipolar I disorder is often characterized by hypersomnia, psychomotor retardation, psychotic symptoms, a history of postpartum episodes, a family history of bipolar I disorder, and a history of antidepressant-induced hypomania.

Prognosis. Major depressive disorder is not a benign disorder. It tends to be chronic, and patients tend to relapse. Patients who have been hospitalized for a first episode of major depressive disorder have about a 50 percent chance of recovering in the first year. The percentage of patients recovering after repeated hospitalization decreases with passing time. Many unrecovered patients remain affected with dysthymic disorder. About 25 percent of patients experience a recurrence of major depressive disorder in the first 6 months after release from a hospital, about 30 to 50 percent in the following 2 years, and about 50 to 75 percent in 5 years. The incidence of relapse is lower than these figures in patients who continue prophylactic psychopharmacological treatment and in patients who have had only one or two depressive episodes. Generally, as a patient experiences more and more depressive episodes, the time between the episodes decreases, and the severity of each episode increases.

PROGNOSTIC INDICATORS. Many studies have focused on identifying both good and bad prognostic indicators in the course of major depressive disorder. Mild episodes, the absence of psychotic symptoms, and a short hospital stay are good prognostic indicators. Psychosocial indicators of a good course include a history of solid friendships during adolescence, stable family functioning, and generally sound social functioning for the 5 years preceding the illness. Additional good prognostic signs are the absence of a comorbid psychiatric disorder and of a personality disorder, no more than one previous hospitalization for major depressive disorder, and an advanced age of onset. The possibility of a poor prognosis is increased by coexisting dysthymic disorder, abuse of alcohol and other substances, anxiety disorder symptoms, and a history of more than one previous depressive episode. Men are more likely than women to experience a chronically impaired course.

Bipolar I Disorder

Course. The natural history of bipolar I disorder is such that it is often useful to make a graph of a patient's disorder and to keep it up to date as treatment progresses (Fig. 15.1–5). Although cyclothymic disorder is sometimes diagnosed retrospectively in patients with bipolar I disorder, no identified personality traits are specifically associated with bipolar I disorder.

Bipolar I disorder most often starts with depression (75 percent of the time in women, 67 percent in men) and is a recurring disorder. Most patients experience both depressive and manic episodes, although 10 to 20 percent experience only manic episodes. The manic episodes typically have a rapid onset (hours or days), but may evolve over a few weeks. An untreated manic episode lasts about 3 months; therefore, clinicians should not discontinue giving drugs before that time. Of persons who have a single manic episode, 90 percent are likely to have another. As the disorder progresses, the time between episodes often decreases. After about five episodes, however, the interepisode interval often stabilizes at 6 to 9 months. Of persons with bipolar disorder, 5 to 15 percent have four or more episodes per year and can be classified as rapid cyclers.

BIPOLAR I DISORDER IN CHILDREN AND OLDER PERSONS. Bipolar I disorder can affect both the very young and older persons. The incidence of bipolar I disorder in children and adolescents is about 1 percent, and the onset can be as early as age 8. Common misdiagnoses are schizophrenia and oppositional defiant disorder.

Bipolar I disorder with such an early onset is associated with a poor prognosis. Manic symptoms are common in older persons, although the range of causes is broad and includes nonpsychiatric medical conditions, dementia, and delirium, as well as bipolar I disorder. The onset of true bipolar I disorder in older persons is relatively uncommon.

Prognosis. Patients with bipolar I disorder have a poorer prognosis than do patients with major depressive disorder. About 40 to 50 percent of patients with bipolar I disorder may have a second manic episode within 2 years of the first episode. Although lithium prophylaxis improves the course and prognosis of bipolar I disorder, probably only 50 to 60 percent of patients achieve significant control of their symptoms with lithium. One 4-year follow-up study of patients with bipolar I disorder found that a premorbid poor occupational status, alcohol dependence, psychotic features, depressive features, interepisode depressive features, and male gender were all factors that contributed a poor prognosis. Short duration of manic episodes, advanced age of onset, few suicidal thoughts, and few coexisting psychiatric or medical problems predict a better outcome.

About 7 percent of patients with bipolar I disorder do not have a recurrence of symptoms; 45 percent have more than one

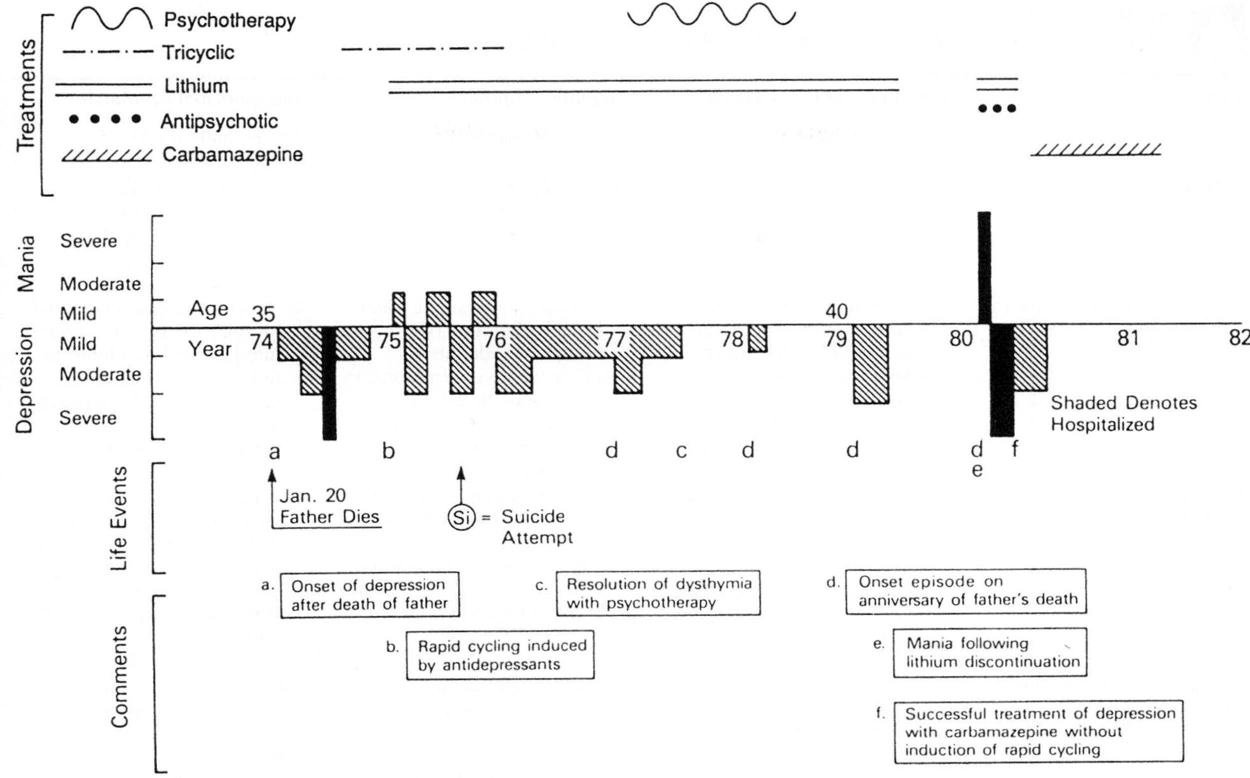

FIGURE 15.1–5
Graphing the course of a mood disorder. Prototype of a life chart. (Courtesy of Robert M. Post, M.D.)

episode, and 40 percent have a chronic disorder. Patients may have from 2 to 30 manic episodes, although the mean number is about 9. About 40 percent of all patients have more than ten episodes. On long-term follow-up, 15 percent of all patients with bipolar I disorder are well, 45 percent are well but have multiple relapses, 30 percent are in partial remission, and 10 percent are chronically ill. One third of all patients with bipolar I disorder have chronic symptoms and evidence of significant social decline.

Bipolar II Disorder

The course and prognosis of bipolar II disorder have just begun to be studied. Preliminary data indicate, however, that the diagnosis is stable, as shown by the high likelihood that patients with bipolar II disorder will have the same diagnosis up to 5 years later. Bipolar II disorder is a chronic disease that warrants long-term treatment strategies.

TREATMENT

Treatment of patients with mood disorders should be directed toward several goals. First, the patient's safety must be guaranteed. Second, a complete diagnostic evaluation of the patient is necessary. Third, a treatment plan that addresses not only the immediate symptoms but also the patient's prospective well-being should be initiated. Although current treatment emphasizes pharmacotherapy and psychotherapy addressed to the individual patient, stressful life events are also associated with increases in relapse rates. Thus, treatment should address the number and severity of stressors in patients' lives.

Overall, the treatment of mood disorders is rewarding for psychiatrists. Specific treatments are now available for both manic and depressive episodes, and data indicate that prophylactic treatment is also effective. Because the prognosis for each episode is good, optimism is always warranted and is welcomed by both the patient and the patient's family. Mood disorders are chronic, however, and the psychiatrist must educate the patient and the family about future treatment strategies.

Hospitalization

The first and most critical decision a physician must make is whether to hospitalize a patient or attempt outpatient treatment. Clear indications for hospitalization are the risk of suicide or homicide, a patient's grossly reduced ability to get food and shelter, and the need for diagnostic procedures. A history of rapidly progressing symptoms and the rupture of a patient's usual support systems are also indications for hospitalization.

A physician may safely treat mild depression or hypomania in the office if he or she evaluates the patient frequently. Clinical signs of impaired judgment, weight loss, or insomnia should be minimal. The patient's support system should be strong, neither overinvolved nor withdrawing from the patient. Any adverse changes in the patient's symptoms or behavior or the

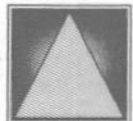

Table 15.1–31
Major Features of Three Psychotherapeutic Approaches to Depression

Feature	Psychodynamic Approach	Cognitive Approach	Interpersonal Approach
Major theorists	Freud, Abraham, Jacobson, Kohut	Plato, Adler, Beck, Rush	Meyer, Sullivan, Klerman, Weissman
Concepts of pathology and cause	Ego regression: damaged self-esteem and unresolved conflict due to childhood object loss and disappointment	Distorted thinking: dysphoria due to learned negative views of self, others, and the world	Impaired interpersonal relations: absent or unsatisfactory significant social bonds
Major goals and mechanisms of change	To promote personality change through understanding of past conflicts; to achieve insight into defenses, ego distortions, and superego defects; to provide a role model; to permit cathartic release of aggression	To provide symptomatic relief through alteration of target thoughts; to identify self-destructive cognitions; to modify specific erroneous assumptions; to promote self-control over thinking patterns	To provide symptomatic relief through solution of current interpersonal problems; to reduce stress involving family or work; to improve interpersonal communication skills
Primary techniques and practices	Expressive-empathic: fully or partially analyzing transference and resistance; confronting defenses; clarifying ego and superego distortions	Behavioral-cognitive: recording and monitoring cognitions; correcting distorted themes with logic and experimental testing; providing alternative thought content; homework	Communicative-environmental: clarifying and managing maladaptive relationships and learning new ones through communication and social skills training; providing information on illness
Therapist role-therapeutic relationship	Interpreter-reflector: establishment and exploration of transference; therapeutic alliance for benign dependence and empathic understanding	Educator-shaper: positive relationship instead of transference; collaborative empiricism as basis for joint scientific (logical) task	Explorer-prescriber: positive relationship-transference without interpretation; active therapist role for influence and advocacy
Marital-family role	Full individual confidentiality; exclusion of significant others except in life-threatening situations	Use of spouse as objective reporter; couples therapy for disturbed cognitions sustained in marital relationship	Integral role of spouse in treatment; examination of spouse's role in patient's predisposition to depression and effects of illness on marriage

(From Karasu TB. Toward a clinical model of psychotherapy for depression. I. Systematic comparison of three psychotherapies. *Am J Psychiatry.* 1990;147:141, with permission.)

attitude of the patient's support system may suffice to warrant hospitalization.

Patients with mood disorders are often unwilling to enter a hospital voluntarily, and may have to be involuntarily committed. These patients often cannot make decisions because of their slowed thinking, negative *Weltanschauung* (world view), and hopelessness. Patients who are manic often have such a complete lack of insight into their disorder that hospitalization seems absolutely absurd to them.

Psychosocial Therapy

Although most studies indicate—and most clinicians and researchers believe—that a combination of psychotherapy and pharmacotherapy is the most effective treatment for major depressive disorder, some data suggest another view: Either pharmacotherapy or psychotherapy alone is effective, at least in patients with mild major depressive episodes, and the regular use of combined therapy adds to the cost of treatment and exposes patients to unnecessary adverse effects.

Three types of short-term psychotherapies—cognitive therapy, interpersonal therapy, and behavior therapy—have been studied to determine their efficacy in the treatment of major depressive disorder. Although its efficacy in treating major depressive disorder is not as well researched as these three therapies, psychoanalytically oriented psychotherapy has long been used for depressive disorders, and many clinicians use the technique as their primary method. What differentiates the three short-term psychotherapy methods from the psychoanalytically oriented approach are the active and directive roles of the therapist, the directly recognizable goals, and the end points for short-term therapy.

Accumulating evidence is encouraging about the efficacy of dynamic therapy. In a randomized, controlled trial comparing psychodynamic therapy with cognitive behavior therapy, the outcome of the depressed patients was the same in the two treatments.

Table 15.1–31 summarizes the features of the psychodynamic, cognitive, and interpersonal approaches; Table 15.1–32 summarizes some nonselective and selective patient variables for psychotherapy; Table 15.1–33 summarizes the advantages and limitations of the three approaches; and Tables 15.1–34 and 15.1–35 summarize features that may affect the choice of pharmacotherapy or psychotherapy or combined therapy. The

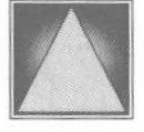

Table 15.1–32
Nonselective and Selective Patient Variables for Psychotherapy for Depression

	Selective Patient Variables		
Nonselective Patient Variables	**Psychodynamic Therapy**	**Cognitive Therapy**	**Interpersonal Therapy**
Feelings of hopelessness and helplessness Apathy, decreased enjoyment, diminished desire or gratification Too high ego ideals and expectations Oversleeping, morbid dreams or nightmares Feelings of restlessness or being slowed down Lack of motivation or will Low self-esteem, inappropriate or excessive guilt and self-reproach Distractibility, sluggish thinking or decision making Wish or intention to be dead Social withdrawal, fear of rejection or failure Psychosomatic complaints, hypochondriasis	Long-term sense of emptiness and underestimation of self-worth Loss or long separation in childhood Conflicts in past relationships (e.g., with parent, sexual partner) Capacity for insight Ability to modulate regression Access to dreams and fantasy Little need for direction and guidance Stable environment	Obvious distorted thoughts about self, world, and future Pragmatic (logical) thinking Real inadequacies (including poor response to other psychotherapies) Moderate to high need for direction and guidance Responsiveness to behavioral training and self-help (high degree of self-control)	Recent, focused dispute with spouse or significant other Social or communication problems Recent role transition or life change Abnormal grief reaction Modest to moderate need for direction and guidance Responsiveness to environmental manipulation (available support network)

(From Karasu TB. Toward a clinical model of psychotherapy for depression. II. An integrative and selective treatment approach. *Am J Psychiatry.* 1990;147:275, with permission.)

National Institute of Mental Health (NIMH) Treatment of Depression Collaborative Research Program found the following predictors of response to various treatments: low social dysfunction suggested a good response to interpersonal therapy; low cognitive dysfunction suggested a good response to cognitive-behavioral therapy and pharmacotherapy; high work dysfunction suggested a good response to pharmacotherapy; and high depression severity suggested a good response to interpersonal therapy and pharmacotherapy.

Cognitive Therapy. Cognitive therapy, originally developed by Aaron Beck, focuses on the cognitive distortions postulated to be present in major depressive disorder. Such distortions include selective attention to the negative aspects of circumstances and unrealistically morbid inferences about consequences. For example, apathy and low energy result from a patient's expectation of failure in all areas. The goal of cognitive therapy is to alleviate depressive episodes and prevent their recurrence by helping patients identify and test negative cognitions; develop alternative, flexible, and positive ways of thinking; and rehearse new cognitive and behavioral responses.

Studies have shown that cognitive therapy is effective in the treatment of major depressive disorder. Most studies found that cognitive therapy is equal in efficacy to pharmacotherapy and is associated with fewer adverse effects and better follow-up than pharmacotherapy. Some of the best controlled studies have indicated that the combination of cognitive therapy and pharmacotherapy is more efficacious than either therapy alone, although other studies have not found that additive effect. At least one study, the NIMH Treatment of Depression Collaborative Research Program, found that pharmacotherapy, either alone or with psychotherapy, may be the treatment of choice for patients with severe major depressive episodes.

Interpersonal Therapy. Interpersonal therapy, developed by Gerald Klerman, focuses on one or two of a patient's current interpersonal problems. This therapy is based on two assumptions. First, current interpersonal problems are likely to have their roots in early dysfunctional relationships. Second, current interpersonal problems are likely to be involved in precipitating or perpetuating the current depressive symptoms. Controlled trials have indicated that interpersonal therapy is effective in the treatment of major depressive disorder and, not surprisingly, may be specifically helpful in addressing interpersonal problems. Some studies indicate that interpersonal therapy may be the most effective method for severe major depressive episodes when the treatment choice is psychotherapy alone.

The interpersonal therapy program usually consists of 12 to 16 weekly sessions and is characterized by an active therapeutic approach. Intrapsychic phenomena, such as defense mechanisms and internal conflicts, are not addressed. Discrete behaviors—such as lack of assertiveness, impaired social skills, and distorted thinking—may be addressed but only in the context of their meaning in, or their effect on, interpersonal relationships.

Behavior Therapy. Behavior therapy is based on the hypothesis that maladaptive behavioral patterns result in a person's receiving little positive feedback and perhaps outright rejection from society. By addressing maladaptive behaviors in therapy, patients learn to function in the world in such a way that they receive positive reinforcement. Behavior therapy for major depressive disorder has not yet been the subject of many controlled studies. The limited data indicate that it is an effective treatment for major depressive disorder.

Psychoanalytically Oriented Therapy. The psychoanalytic approach to mood disorders is based on psychoanalytic theories about depression and mania. The goal of psychoanalytic

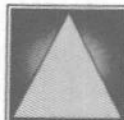

Table 15.1–33
Advantages and Limitations of Three Psychotherapeutic Approaches to Depression

Feature	Psychodynamic Approach	Cognitive Approach	Interpersonal Approach
Theory			
Advantages	Individual depth approach encourages patient to look inward for solutions, rather than depending on external sources	Cognitive-behavioral orientation is tangible and objective	Interpersonal orientation addresses broader (e.g., social, family) context, useful in focusing on man–woman relations
Limitations	Focus on intrapsychic phenomena may obscure other (e.g., interpersonal, environmental) factors; aggression-depression theory can be overgeneralized and lead to overreliance on catharsis	Cognitive-behavioral emphasis may neglect whole person, especially affective component; symptom-oriented perspective overlooks past history, complex problem areas, and hidden conflicts	Emphasis on four designated interpersonal problems can bias toward preconceived themes; interpersonal orientation may stress marital/family factors while underplaying intrapsychic forces
Goals			
Advantages	Enduring structural change transcends symptomatic relief; strengthened adaptive capacities can be useful beyond specific depressive pathology	Primary goal of symptom relief is expedient in itself and is first stage in changing cognitive style	Improvement of interpersonal relations is expedient in itself and may also result in relief of symptoms
Limitations	Personality alteration can be too ambitious and may be unnecessary or excessive for most depression diagnoses	Symptom reduction may be insufficient, superficial, or temporary; focus on current problems can preclude enduring modification of personality or prophylactic function of treatment	Symptom relief may be fragile and temporary if it is highly dependent on external factors
Structure			
Advantages	Indefinite duration allows long-term or flexible goals[a]	Brief or fixed duration is cost-effective and can foster results in short period, may heighten expectation of rapid change and encourage optimism	Predetermined duration is cost-effective; approach reengages family and may have preventive effect
Limitations	Long-term or open-ended treatment is uneconomical and difficult to evaluate[a]	Short or predetermined duration may be insufficient or inflexible	Time limitation predetermines the extent of personal growth and independence
Therapist role			
Advantages	Neutral, accepting stance ensures nonjudgmental attitude and objectivity; receptive listening encourages transference formation and ensuing analytic process	Active therapist can directly intervene to interrupt depressive schemata and suggest alternatives to faulty thinking	Therapist position between activity and reactivity can reassure patient and provide supportive person for patient to relate to
Limitations	Transference regression can produce overidealization of therapist and underestimation of patient self-worth; therapist silence may be misconstrued as rejection, which can perpetuate depression and cause premature termination	Active suggestion and direction can undermine patient responsibility and self-esteem by imposing therapist point of view or values	Supportive interpersonal role may encourage dependence and rage at withdrawal of therapist
Techniques			
Advantages	Free association provides verbal catharsis; interpretations provide new understanding of depressogenic conflicts and historical events	Specific approach is directly tailored to depressed population and aims at particular target symptoms; identification of depressogenic assumptions and homework to test new thinking foster cognitive modification	Specific approach is directly tailored to depressed population and can address particular current interpersonal maladaptions
Limitations	No specific techniques developed; focus on past events and spontaneous associations may encourage repetitive litany of depressive complaints at the expense of present therapeutic tasks	Emphasis on specific cognitive schemata may bias toward certain preconceived themes; overt simplicity of techniques may lead to underestimation of technical skill required	Identification of specific interpersonal problem areas may be overly restrictive, yet techniques are relatively nonspecific; legitimation of patient sick role may encourage passivity

(continued)

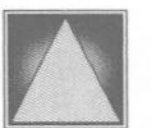

Table 15.1–33
(Continued)

Feature	Psychodynamic Approach	Cognitive Approach	Interpersonal Approach
Research status			
Advantages	Longitudinal case study approach useful for detailed examination and follow-up of individual patients	Operational manual allows for replication of treatment and training and empirical establishment of efficacy	Same as for cognitive approach
Limitations	Idiographic approach or anecdotal case history is not amenable to controlled or comparative research	Research-oriented operationalized approach may become oversimplified formula for complex clinical phenomena	Same as for cognitive approach
Relation to other modalities			
Advantages	Integrity of transference is maintained through elimination of outside influences	Competition with pharmacotherapy encourages research on relative efficacy, especially instances when cognitive therapy alone is most effective	Approach designed to be used alone or with drugs; it is especially amenable to combination with marital therapy
Limitations	Need for neutrality may limit use of other helpful treatment approaches (e.g., family therapy, drug treatment)	Competition with pharmacotherapy fosters polarization of approaches and partisan resistance to integration with drug treatment	Amenability to additive or eclectic modalities requires integrative theoretical model, clinical expertise in more than one modality, and ability to collaborate with other disciplines, which may lead to role diffusion and insufficient knowledge or training
Patient population			
Advantages	Special patient requisites (e.g., verbal orientation, psychological-mindedness) ensure maximal insight	Logical thinking ensures maximal potential to deal with and change depressogenic assumptions and thought patterns	Orientation toward interpersonal relations, especially marital interaction, can address gender issues in marriage, especially important given high prevalence of women among depressed patients
Limitations	Special patient requisites may limit usefulness to verbal, psychological-minded population	Cognitively impaired population may not benefit; sophisticated, introspective patients may find approach too simple-minded or superficial	Interpersonal orientation may overemphasize marriage; primarily female population may bias toward women; conjoint focus may bias against unmarried population

[a]Advantages and limitations of short-term psychodynamic therapy are similar to those for the cognitive and interpersonal approaches.
(From Karasu TB. Toward a clinical model of psychotherapy for depression. I. Systematic comparison of three psychotherapies. *Am J Psychiatry.* 1990;147:142, with permission.)

psychotherapy is to effect a change in a patient's personality structure or character, not simply to alleviate symptoms. Improvements in interpersonal trust, capacity for intimacy, coping mechanisms, the capacity to grieve, and the ability to experience a wide range of emotions are some of the aims of psychoanalytic therapy. Treatment often requires the patient to experience periods of heightened anxiety and distress during the course of therapy, which may continue for several years.

Family Therapy. Family therapy is not generally viewed as a primary therapy for the treatment of major depressive disorder, but increasing evidence indicates that helping a patient with a mood disorder to reduce and cope with stress can lessen the chance of a relapse. Family therapy is indicated if the disorder jeopardizes a patient's marriage or family functioning or if the mood disorder is promoted or maintained by the family situation. Family therapy examines the role of the mood-disordered member in the overall psychological well-being of the whole family; it also examines the role of the entire family in the maintenance of the patient's symptoms. Patients with mood disorders have a high rate of divorce, and about 50 percent of all spouses report that they would not have married or had children if they had known that the patient was going to develop a mood disorder.

Vagal Nerve Stimulation

Experimental stimulation of the vagus nerve in several studies designed for the treatment of epilepsy found that patients showed improved mood. This observation led to the use of left vagal nerve stimulation (VNS) using an electronic device implanted in the skin, similar to a cardiac pacemaker. Preliminary studies have shown that a number of patients with chronic,

Table 15.1–34
Indications for Psychotherapy and Pharmacotherapy in the Treatment of Depression

	Indication for Treatment [a]	
Variable	**Pharmacotherapy**	**Psychotherapy**
Symptom criteria for major depressive episode		
Depressed mood	Marked vegetative signs; extreme or uncontrolled mood	Mild to moderate situational or characterological depressed mood
Diminished interest or pleasure	Anhedonia; loss of libido; impaired sexual function or performance	Apathy, decreased enjoyment; diminished sexual desire or gratification
Weight loss or gain	Significant weight loss	Insignificant weight gain
Insomnia or hypersomnia	Early morning wakening	Oversleeping, morbid dreams or nightmares
Psychomotor agitation	Hyperactivity or motor retardation	Restlessness or feelings of being slowed down
Fatigue or loss of energy (anergia)	Depressive stupor	Lack of motivation or will
Feelings of worthlessness or excessive guilt	Nihilistic or self-deprecatory delusions, self-berating auditory hallucinations	Low self-esteem, inappropriate guilt feelings, self-reproach
Diminished ability to think or concentrate, indecisiveness	Loss of control over thinking, obsessive rumination, inability to focus or act	Distractibility, sluggish thinking or decision making; negative cognitions
Recurrent thoughts of death or suicide	Acute, episodic, and uncontrolled suicidal acts or plans[b]	Chronic feelings of hopelessness or helplessness[c]
Associated features	Panic (anxiety) attacks or phobias; persecutory delusions; pseudodementia; physical symptoms or somatic delusions	Social withdrawal or fears of rejection or failure; psychosomatic complaints or hypochondriasis
Family history	Genetic loading (bipolar disorder or depressive disorder)	No genetic loading (dysthymic disorder)
Predisposing factors	Other mental disorders, e.g., schizophrenia, alcohol dependence, anorexia nervosa	Psychosocial stressors, e.g., loss of significant other, change in status or role
Personality disorders	Borderline, histrionic, obsessive-compulsive	Dependent, inadequate, masochistic

[a]These are not mutually exclusive categories.
[b]Hospitalization may be required.
[c]Medication may also be useful.
(From Karasu TB. Toward a clinical model of psychotherapy for depression. II. An integrative and selective treatment approach. *Am J Psychiatry.* 1990;147:274, with permission.)

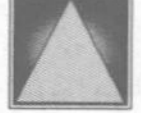

Table 15.1–35
Approach to Pharmacotherapy of Three Psychotherapies for Depression

Feature of Combined Treatment	Psychodynamic Therapy	Cognitive Therapy	Interpersonal Therapy
Basic stance	Medication is avoided except in life-threatening situation, used judiciously for severe vegetative signs	Pharmacotherapy and cognitive therapy alone are in ongoing competition, but drugs are used in case of poor response to cognitive therapy and for breaking psychotherapeutic impasses in severe depression when symptomatic relief is required	Interpersonal therapy and pharmacotherapy are considered having different effects and response timetables (early drug effects on vegetative symptoms, later psychotherapy effects on suicidal ideation, work, and interests)
Techniques	Personal (unconscious and conscious) meanings are explored and interpreted within therapy session	Information and rationale for use is provided; special tasks are assigned to increase adherence, e.g., postsession homework (lists of side effects); phone contact with therapist is encouraged	Information and rationale for use is provided, in line with medical model; time is set aside in each session to discuss pharmacological issues

(From Karasu TB. Toward a clinical model of psychotherapy for depression. II. An integrative and selective treatment approach. *Am J Psychiatry.* 1990;147:272, with permission.)

recurrent major depressive disorder went into remission when treated with VNS. The mechanism of action of VNS to account for improvement is unknown. The vagus nerve connects to the enteric nervous system and, when stimulated, may cause release of peptides that act as neurotransmitters. Extensive clinical trials are being conducted to determine the efficacy of VNS. Section 36.37 covers this and other brain stimulation methods.

Sleep Deprivation

Mood disorders are characterized by sleep disturbance. Mania tends to be characterized by a decreased need for sleep, whereas depression can be associated with either hypersomnia or insomnia. Sleep deprivation may precipitate mania in patients who are bipolar I and temporarily relieve depression in those who are unipolar. Approximately 60 percent of depressive disorder patients exhibit significant but transient benefit from total sleep deprivation. The positive results are typically reversed by the next night of sleep. Several strategies have been used in an attempt to achieve a more sustained response to sleep deprivation. One method used serial total sleep deprivation with a day or two of normal sleep in between. This method does not achieve a sustained antidepressant response because the depression tends to return with normal sleep cycles. Another approach used phase delay in the time patients go to sleep each night, or partial sleep deprivation. In this method, patients may stay awake from 2 AM to 10 PM daily. Up to 50 percent of patients get same-day antidepressant effects from partial sleep deprivation, but this benefit also tends to wear off in time. In some reports, however, serial partial sleep deprivation has been used successfully to treat insomnia associated with depression. The third, and probably most effective, strategy combines sleep deprivation with pharmacological treatment of depression. A number of studies have suggested that total and partial sleep deprivation followed by immediate treatment with an antidepressant or lithium (Eskalith) sustains the antidepressant effects of sleep deprivation. Likewise, several reports have suggested that sleep deprivation accelerates the response to antidepressants, including fluoxetine (Prozac) and nortriptyline (Aventyl, Pamelor). Sleep deprivation has also been noted to improve premenstrual dysphoria.

Phototherapy

Phototherapy (light therapy) was introduced in 1984 as a treatment for SAD (mood disorder with seasonal pattern). In this disorder, patients typically experience depression as the photoperiod of the day decreases with advancing winter. Women represent at least 75 percent of all patients with seasonal depression, and the mean age of presentation is 40. Patients rarely present over the age of 55 with seasonal affective disorder.

Phototherapy typically involves exposing the afflicted patient to bright light in the range of 1,500 to 10,000 lux or more, typically with a light box that sits on a table or desk. Patients sit in front of the box for approximately 1 to 2 hours before dawn each day, although some patients may also benefit from exposure after dusk. Alternatively, some manufacturers have developed light visors, with a light source built into the brim of the hat. These light visors allow mobility, but recent controlled studies have questioned the use of this type of light exposure. Trials have typically lasted 1 week, but longer treatment durations may be associated with greater response.

Phototherapy tends to be well tolerated. Newer light sources tend to use lower light intensities and come equipped with filters; patients are instructed not to look directly at the light source. As with any effective antidepressant, phototherapy, on rare occasions, has been implicated in switching some depressed patients into mania or hypomania.

In addition to seasonal depression, the other major indication for phototherapy may be in sleep disorders. Phototherapy has been used to decrease the irritability and diminished functioning associated with shift work. Sleep disorders in geriatric patients have reportedly improved with exposure to bright light during the day. Likewise, some evidence suggests that jet lag might respond to light therapy. Preliminary data indicate that phototherapy may benefit some patients with OCD that has a seasonal variation.

Pharmacotherapy

Once a diagnosis has been established, a pharmacological treatment strategy can be formulated. Accurate diagnosis is crucial, because unipolar and bipolar spectrum disorders require different treatment regimens.

The objective of pharmacologic treatment is symptom remission, not just symptom reduction. Patients with residual symptoms, as opposed to full remission, are more likely to experience a relapse or recurrence of mood episodes and to experience ongoing impairment of daily functioning.

Major Depressive Disorder. The use of specific pharmacotherapy approximately doubles the chances that a depressed patient will recover in 1 month. All currently available antidepressants may take up to 3 to 4 weeks to exert significant therapeutic effects, although they may begin to show their effects earlier. Choice of antidepressants is determined by the side effect profile least objectionable to a given patient's physical status, temperament, and lifestyle. That numerous classes of antidepressants (Table 15.1–36) are available, many with different mechanisms of action, represents indirect evidence for heterogeneity of putative biochemical lesions. Although the first antidepressant drugs, the monoamine oxidase inhibitors (MAOIs) and tricyclic antidepressants (TCAs), are still in use, newer compounds have made the treatment of depression more "clinician and patient friendly."

GENERAL CLINICAL GUIDELINES. The most common clinical mistake leading to an unsuccessful trial of an antidepressant drug is the use of too low a dosage for too short a time. Unless adverse events prevent it, the dosage of an antidepressant should be raised to the maximum recommended level and maintained at that level for at least 4 or 5 weeks before a drug trial is considered unsuccessful. Alternatively, if a patient is improving clinically on a low dosage of the drug, this dosage should not be raised unless clinical improvement stops before maximal benefit is obtained. When a patient does not begin to respond to appropriate dosages of a drug after 2 or 3 weeks, clinicians may decide to obtain a plasma concentration of the drug if the test is available for the particular drug being used. The test may indicate either noncompliance or particularly unusual pharmacokinetic disposition of the drug and may thereby suggest an alternative dosage.

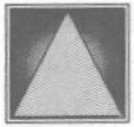

Table 15.1–36
Antidepressant Medications

Generic (Brand) Name	Usual Daily Dose (mg)	Common Side Effects	Clinical Caveats
NE Reuptake Inhibitors			
Desipramine (Norpramin, Pertofrane)	75–300	Drowsiness, insomnia, OSH, agitation, CA, weight ↑, anticholinergic[a]	Overdose may be fatal. Dose titration is needed.
Protriptyline (Vivactil)	20–60	Drowsiness, insomnia, OSH, agitation, CA, anticholinergic[a]	Overdose may be fatal. Dose titration is needed.
Nortriptyline (Aventyl, Pamelor)	40–200	Drowsiness, OSH, CA, weight ↑, anticholinergic[a]	Overdose may be fatal. Dose titration is needed.
Maprotiline (Ludiomil)	100–225	Drowsiness, CA, weight ↑, anticholinergic[a]	Overdose may be fatal. Dose titration is needed.
5-HT Reuptake Inhibitors			
Citalopram (Celexa)	20–60	All SSRIs may cause insomnia, agitation, sedation, GI distress, and sexual dysfunction	Many SSRIs inhibit various cytochrome P450 isoenzymes. They are better tolerated than tricyclics and have high safety in overdose. Shorter half-life SSRIs may be associated with discontinuation symptoms when abruptly stopped.
Escitalopram (Lexapro)	10–20		
Fluoxetine (Prozac)	10–40		
Fluvoxamine (Luvox)[b]	100–300		
Paroxetine (Paxil)	20–50		
Sertraline (Zoloft)	50–150		
NE and 5-HT Reuptake Inhibitors			
Amitriptyline (Elavil, Endep)	75–300	Drowsiness, OSH, CA, weight ↑, anticholinergic[a]	Overdose may be fatal. Dose titration is needed.
Doxepin (Triadapin, Sinequan)	75–300	Drowsiness, OSH, CA, weight ↑, anticholinergic[a]	Overdose may be fatal.
Imipramine (Tofranil)	75–300	Drowsiness, insomnia and agitation, OSH, CA, GI distress, weight ↑, anticholinergic[a]	Overdose may be fatal. Dose titration needed.
Trimipramine (Surmontil)	75–300	Drowsiness, OSH, CA, weight ↑, anticholinergic[a]	—
Venlafaxine (Effexor)	150–375	Sleep changes, GI distress, discontinuation syndrome	Higher doses may cause hypertension. Dose titration is needed. Abrupt discontinuation may result in discontinuation symptoms.
Duloxetine (Cymbalta)	30–60	GI distress, discontinuation syndrome	
Pre- and Postsynaptic Active Agents			
Nefazodone	300–600	Sedation	Dose titration is needed. No sexual dysfunction.
Mirtazapine (Remeron)	15–30	Sedation, weight ↑	No sexual dysfunction.
Dopamine Reuptake Inhibitor			
Bupropion (Wellbutrin)	200–400	Insomnia or agitation, GI distress	Twice-a-day dosing with sustained release. No sexual dysfunction or weight gain.
Mixed Action Agents			
Amoxapine (Asendin)	100–600	Drowsiness, insomnia/agitation, CA, weight ↑, OSH, anticholinergic[a]	Movement disorders may occur. Dose titration is needed.
Clomipramine (Anafranil)	75–300	Drowsiness, weight ↑	Dose titration is needed.
Trazodone (Desyrel)	150–600	Drowsiness, OSH, CA, GI distress, weight ↑	Priapism is possible.

Note: Dose ranges are for adults in good general medical health, taking no other medications, aged 18 to 60 years. Doses vary depending on the agent, concomitant medications, the presence of general medical or surgical conditions, age, genetic constitution, and other factors. Brand names are those used in the United States.
CA, cardiac arrhythmia; 5-HT, serotonin; GI, gastrointestinal; NE, norepinephrine; OSH, orthostatic hypotension; SSRI, selective serotonin reuptake inhibitor.
[a]Dry mouth, blurred vision, urinary hesitancy, and constipation.
[b]Not approved as an antidepressant in the United States by the US Food and Drug Administration.

DURATION AND PROPHYLAXIS. Antidepressant treatment should be maintained for at least 6 months or the length of a previous episode, whichever is greater. Prophylactic treatment with antidepressants is effective in reducing the number and severity of recurrences. One study concluded that when episodes are less than 2½ years apart, prophylactic treatment for 5 years is probably indicated. Another factor suggesting prophylactic treatment is the seriousness of previous depressive episodes. Episodes that have involved significant suicidal ideation or impairment of psychosocial functioning may indicate that clinicians should consider prophylactic treatment. When antidepressant treatment is stopped, the drug dose should be tapered gradually over 1 to 2 weeks, depending on the half-life of the particular compound. Several studies indicate that maintenance antidepressant medication appears to be safe and effective for the treatment of chronic depression.

Prevention of new mood episodes (i.e., recurrences) is the aim of the maintenance phase of treatment. Only those patients with recurrent or chronic depressions are candidates for maintenance treatment.

INITIAL MEDICATION SELECTION. The available antidepressants do not differ in overall efficacy, speed of response, or long-term effectiveness. Antidepressants, however, do differ in their pharmacology, drug–drug interactions, short- and long-term side effects, likelihood of discontinuation symptoms, and ease of dose adjustment. Failure to tolerate or to respond to one medication does not imply that other medications will also fail. Selection of the initial treatment depends on the chronicity of the condition, course of illness (a recurrent or chronic course is associated with increased likelihood of subsequent depressive symptoms without treatment), family history of illness and treatment response, symptom severity, concurrent general medical or other psychiatric conditions, prior treatment responses to other acute phase treatments, potential drug–drug interactions, and patient preference. In general, approximately 45 to 60 percent of all outpatients with uncomplicated (i.e., minimal psychiatric and general medical comorbidity), nonchronic, nonpsychotic major depressive disorder who begin treatment with medication respond (i.e., achieve at least a 50 percent reduction in baseline symptoms); however, only 35 to 50 percent achieve remission (i.e., the virtual absence of depressive symptoms).

TREATMENT OF DEPRESSIVE SUBTYPES. Clinical types of major depressive episodes may have varying responses to particular antidepressants, or to drugs other than antidepressants. Patients with major depressive disorder with atypical features (sometimes called *hysteriod dysphoria*) may preferentially respond to treatment with MAOIs or SSRIs. Antidepressants with dual action on both serotonergic and noradrenergic receptors demonstrate greater efficacy in melancholic depressions. Patients with seasonal winter depression can be treated with light therapy. Treatment of major depressive episodes with psychotic features may require a combination of an antidepressant and an atypical antipsychotic. Several studies have also shown that ECT is effective for this indication—perhaps more effective than pharmacotherapy. For those with atypical symptom features, strong evidence exists for the effectiveness of MAOIs. SSRIs and bupropion (Wellbutrin) are also of use in atypical depression.

COMORBID DISORDERS. The concurrent presence of another disorder can affect initial treatment selection. For example, the successful treatment of OCD associated with depressive symptoms usually results in remission of the depression. Similarly, when panic disorder occurs with major depression, medications with demonstrated efficacy in both conditions are preferred (e.g., tricyclics and SSRIs). In general, the nonmood disorder dictates the choice of treatment in comorbid states.

Concurrent substance abuse raises the possibility of a substance-induced mood disorder, which must be evaluated by history or by requiring abstinence for several weeks. Abstinence often results in remission of depressive symptoms in substance-induced mood disorders. For those with continuing significant depressive symptoms, even with abstinence, an independent mood disorder is diagnosed and treated.

General medical conditions are established risk factors in the development of depression. The presence of a major depressive episode is associated with increased morbidity or mortality of many general medical conditions (e.g., cardiovascular disease, diabetes, cerebrovascular disease, and cancer).

THERAPEUTIC USE OF SIDE EFFECTS. Choosing more sedating antidepressants (e.g., amitriptyline [Elavil, Endep]) for more anxious, depressed patients or more activating agents (e.g., desipramine) for more psychomotor-retarded patients is not generally helpful. For example, any short-term benefits with paroxetine, mirtazapine, or amitriptyline (more sedating drugs) on symptoms of anxiety or insomnia may become liabilities over time. These drugs often continue to be sedating in the longer run, which can lead to patients prematurely discontinuing medication and increase the risk of relapse or recurrence. Some practitioners use adjunctive medications (e.g., sleeping pills or anxiolytics) combined with antidepressants to provide more immediate symptom relief or to cover those side effects to which most patients ultimately adapt.

A patient's prior treatment history is important, because an earlier response typically predicts current response. A documented failure on a properly conducted trial of a particular antidepressant class (e.g., SSRIs, tricyclics, or MAOIs) suggests choosing an agent from an alternative class. The history of a first-degree relative responding to a particular drug is associated with a good response to the same class of agents in the patient.

ACUTE TREATMENT FAILURES. Patients may not respond to a medication, because (1) they cannot tolerate the side effects, even in the face of a good clinical response; (2) an idiosyncratic adverse event may occur; (3) the clinical response is not adequate; or (4) the wrong diagnosis has been made. Acute phase medication trials should last 4 to 6 weeks to determine if meaningful symptom reduction is attained. Most (but not all) patients who ultimately respond fully show at least a partial response (i.e., at least a 20 to 25 percent reduction in pretreatment depressive symptom severity) by week 4 if the dose is adequate during the initial weeks of treatment. Lack of a partial response by 4 to 6 weeks indicates that a treatment change is needed. Longer time periods—8 to 12 weeks or longer—are needed to define the ultimate degree of symptom reduction achievable with a medication. Approximately one half of patients require a second medication treatment trial because the initial treatment is poorly tolerated or ineffective.

SELECTING SECOND TREATMENT OPTIONS. When the initial treatment is unsuccessful, switching to an alternative treatment, or augmenting the current treatment is a common option. The choice between switching from the initial single treatment to a new single treatment (as opposed to adding a second treatment to the first one) rests on the patient's prior treatment history, the degree of benefit achieved with the initial treatment, and patient preference. As a rule, switching rather than augmenting is preferred after an initial medication failure. On the other hand, augmentation strategies are helpful with patients who have gained some benefit from the initial treatment but who have not achieved remission. The best-documented augmentation strategies involve lithium (Eskalith) or thyroid hormone. A combination of an SSRI and bupropion (Wellbutrin) is also widely employed. In fact, no combination strategy has been conclusively shown to be more effective than another. ECT is effective in psychotic and nonpsychotic forms of depression, but is recommended generally only for repeatedly nonresponsive cases or in patients with very severe disorders.

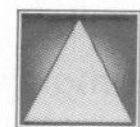

Table 15.1–37
US Food and Drug Administration (FDA)-Approved Medications for the Treatment of Bipolar Disorders

Agent	Mania	Maintenance
Aripiprazole (Abilify)	Yes (2004)	No
Carbamazepine XR (Equetro)	Yes (2004)	No
Divalproex (Depakote)	Yes (1996)	No
Lamotrigine (Lamictal)	No	Yes (2003)
Lithium (Lithobid)	Yes (1970)	Yes (1974)
Olanzapine (Zyprexa)	Yes (2000)	Yes (2004)
Risperidone (Risperdal)	Yes (2003)	No
Quetiapine (Seroquel)	Yes (2004)	No
Ziprasidone (Geodon)	Yes (2004)	No

COMBINED TREATMENT. Medication and formal psychotherapy are often combined in practice. If physicians view mood disorders as fundamentally evolving from psychodynamic issues, their ambivalence about the use of drugs may result in a poor response, noncompliance, and probably inadequate dosages for too short a treatment period. Alternatively, if physicians ignore the psychosocial needs of a patient, the outcome of pharmacotherapy may be compromised. Several trials of a combination of pharmacotherapy and psychotherapy for chronically depressed outpatients have shown a higher response and higher remission rates for the combination than for either treatment used alone.

Bipolar Disorders. The pharmacological treatment of bipolar disorders is divided into both acute and maintenance phases. Bipolar treatment, however, also involves the formulation of different strategies for the patient who is experiencing mania or hypomania or depression. Table 15.1–37 lists US Food and Drug Administration (FDA)-approved medications for the treatment of bipolar disorders. Each of these medications is associated with a unique side effect and safety profile, and no one drug is predictably effective for all patients. Often, it is necessary to try several so-called "mood stabilizers" before an optimal treatment is found.

TREATMENT OF ACUTE MANIA. The treatment of acute mania, or hypomania, usually is the easiest phases of bipolar disorders to treat. Agents can be used alone or in combination to bring the patient down from a high. Patients with severe mania are best treated in the hospital where aggressive dosing is possible and an adequate response can be achieved within days or weeks. Adherence to treatment, however, is often a problem, because patients with mania frequently lack insight into their illness, and refuse to take medication. Because impaired judgment, impulsivity, and aggressiveness combine to put the patient or others at risk, many patients in the manic phase are medicated to protect themselves and others from harm.

Lithium Carbonate. Lithium carbonate is considered the prototypical "mood stabilizer." Yet, because the onset of antimanic action with lithium can be slow, it usually is supplemented in the early phases of treatment by atypical antipsychotics, mood-stabilizing anticonvulsants, or high-potency benzodiazepines. Therapeutic lithium levels are between 0.6 and 1.2 mEq/L. The acute use of lithium has been limited in recent years by its unpredictable efficacy, problematic side effects, and the need for frequent laboratory tests. The introduction of newer drugs with more favorable side effects, lower toxicity, and less need for frequent laboratory testing has resulted in a decline in lithium use. For many patients, however, its clinical benefits can be remarkable.

Valproate. Valproate (valproic acid [Depakene] or divalproex sodium [Depakote]) has surpassed lithium in use for acute mania. Unlike lithium, Valproate is only indicated for acute mania, although most experts agree it also has prophylactic effects. Typical dose levels of valproic acid are 750 to 2,500 mg per day, achieving blood levels between 50 and 120 μg/mL. Rapid oral loading with 15 to 20 mg/kg of divalproex sodium from day 1 of treatment has been well tolerated and associated with a rapid onset of response. A number of laboratory tests are required during valproate treatment.

Carbamazepine and Oxcarbazepine. Carbamazepine has been used worldwide for decades as a first-line treatment for acute mania, but has only gained approval in the United States in 2004. Typical doses of carbamazepine to treat acute mania range between 600 and 1,800 mg per day associated with blood levels of between 4 and 12 μg/mL. The keto congener of carbamazepine, oxcarbazepine, may possess similar antimanic properties. Higher doses than those of carbamazepine are required, because 1,500 mg of oxcarbazepine approximates 1,000 mg of carbamazepine.

Clonazepam and Lorazepam. The high-potency benzodiazepine anticonvulsants used in acute mania include clonazepam (Klonopin) and lorazepam (Ativan). Both may be effective and are widely used for adjunctive treatment of acute manic agitation, insomnia, aggression, and dysphoria, as well as panic. The safety and the benign side effect profile of these agents render them ideal adjuncts to lithium, carbamazepine, or valproate.

Atypical and Typical Antipsychotics. All of the atypical antipsychotics—olanzapine, risperidone, quetiapine, ziprasidone, and aripiprazole—have demonstrated antimanic efficacy and are FDA approved for this indication. Compared with older agents, such as haloperidol (Haldol) and chlorpromazine (Thorazine), atypical antipsychotics have a lesser liability for excitatory postsynaptic potential and tardive dyskinesia; many do not increase prolactin. However, they have a wide range of substantial to no risk for weight gain with its associated problems of insulin resistance, diabetes, hyperlipidemia, hypercholesteremia, and cardiovascular impairment. Some patients, however, require maintenance treatment with an antipsychotic medication.

TREATMENT OF ACUTE BIPOLAR DEPRESSION. The relative usefulness of standard antidepressants in bipolar illness, in general, and in rapid cycling and mixed states, in particular, remains controversial because of their propensity to induce cycling, mania, or hypomania. Accordingly, antidepressant drugs are often enhanced by a mood stabilizer in the first-line treatment for a first or isolated episode of bipolar depression. A fixed combination of olanzapine and fluoxetine (Symbyax) has been shown to be effective in treating acute bipolar depression for an 8-week period without inducing a switch to mania or hypomania.

Paradoxically, many patients who are bipolar in the depressed phase do not respond to treatment with standard antidepressants. In these instances, lamotrigine or low dose ziprasidone (20 to 80 mg per day) may prove effective.

Electroconvulsive therapy may also be useful for bipolar depressed patients who do not respond to lithium or other mood stabilizers and their adjuncts, particularly in cases in which intense suicidal tendency presents as a medical emergency.

Other Agents. When standard treatments fail, other types of compounds may prove effective. The calcium channel antagonist verapamil (Calan, Isoptin) has acute antimanic efficacy. Gabapentin, topiramate, zonisamide, levetiracetam, and tiagabine have not been shown to have acute antimania effects, although some patients may benefit from a trial of these agents when standard therapies have failed. Lamotrigine does not possess acute antimanic properties, but does help prevent recurrence of manic episodes. Small studies suggest the potential acute antimanic and prophylactic efficacy of phenytoin. ECT is effective in acute mania. Bilateral treatments are required, as unilateral, nondominant treatments have been reported to be ineffective or even to exacerbate manic symptoms. ECT is reserved for the patient with rare refractory mania or for the patient with medical complications, as well as extreme exhaustion (malignant hyperthermia or lethal catatonia).

MAINTENANCE TREATMENT OF BIPOLAR DISORDER. Preventing recurrences of mood episodes is the greatest challenge facing the clinician. Not only must the chosen regimen achieve its primary goal—sustained euthymia—but the medications should not produce unwanted side effects that affect functioning. Sedation, cognitive impairment, tremor, weight gain, and rash are some side effects that lead to treatment discontinuation.

Lithium, carbamazepine, and valproic acid, alone or in combination, are the most widely used agents in the long-term treatment of patients who are bipolar. Lamotrigine has prophylactic antidepressant and, potentially, mood-stabilizing properties. Patients on lamotrigine with bipolar I disorder depression exhibit a rate of switch into mania that is the same as the rate with placebo. Lamotrigine appears to have superior acute and prophylactic antidepressant properties compared with antimanic properties. Given that breakthrough depressions are a difficult problem during prophylaxis, lamotrigine has a unique therapeutic role. Very slow increases of lamotrigine help avoid the rare side effect of lethal rash. A 200 mg per day dose appears to be the average in many studies. The incidence of severe rash (i.e., Stevens-Johnson syndrome, a toxic epidermal necrolysis) is now thought to be approximately 2 in 10,000 adults and 4 in 10,000 children.

Thyroid supplementation is frequently necessary during long-term treatment. Many patients treated with lithium develop hypothyroidism, and many patients with bipolar disorder have idiopathic thyroid dysfunction. T_3 (25 to 50 μg per day), because of its short half-life, is often recommended for acute augmentation strategies, whereas T_4 is frequently used for long-term maintenance. In some centers, hypermetabolic doses of thyroid

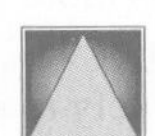

Table 15.1–38
Principles in the Treatment of Bipolar Disorders

- Maintain dual treatment focus: (1) acute short term and (2) prophylaxis.
- Chart illness retrospectively and prospectively.
- Mania as medical emergency: Treat first, chemistries later.
- Load valproate and lithium (Eskalith); titrate lamotrigine (Lamictal) slowly.
- Careful combination treatment can decrease adverse effects.
- Augment rather than substitute in treatment-resistant patient.
- Retain lithium in regimen for its antisuicide and neuroprotective effects.
- Taper lithium slowly, if at all.
- Educate patient and family about illness and risk-to-benefit ratios of acute and prophylactic treatments.
- Give statistics (i.e., 50 percent relapse in first 5 months off lithium).
- Assess compliance and suicidality regularly.
- Develop an early warning system for identification and treatment of emergent symptoms.
- Contract with patient as needed for suicide and substance use avoidance.
- Use regular visits; monitor course and adverse effects.
- Arrange for interval phone contact when needed.
- Develop fire drill for mania reemergence.
- Inquire about and address comorbid alcohol and substance abuse.
- Targeted psychotherapy; use medicalization of illness.
- Treat patient as a coinvestigator in the development of effective clinical approaches to the illness.
- If treatment is successful, be conservative in making changes, maintain the course, and continue full-dose pharmacoprophylaxis in absence of side effects.
- If treatment response is inadequate, be aggressive in searching for more effective alternatives.

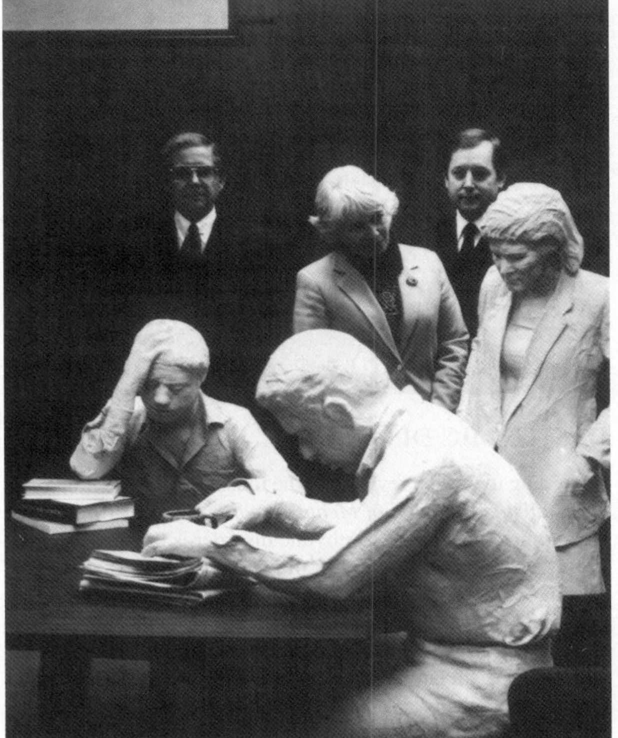

FIGURE 15.1–6
Statues from the Depression Awareness Recognition and Treatment (D/ART) campaign. (Courtesy of the National Library of Medicine.)

hormone are used. Data indicate improvement in both manic and depressive phases with hypermetabolic T_4 augmenting strategies. Table 15.1–38 summarizes the principles of treatment of bipolar disorders.

Depression Awareness, Recognition and Treatment

The Depression Awareness, Recognition and Treatment program (D/ART) is a multiphase information and education program designed to alert health professionals and the general public to the fact that depressive disorders are common, serious, and treatable. It was launched by the NIMH in 1988 to enhance the availability and quality of treatment for depression (Fig. 15.1–6).

References

Akiskal HS. Mood disorders: Historical introduction and conceptual overview. In: Sadock BJ, Sadock VA, eds. *Kaplan & Sadock's Comprehensive Textbook of Psychiatry*. 8th ed. Vol. 1. Baltimore: Lippincott Williams & Wilkins; 2005:1559.

Antonijevic IA. Depressive disorders—Is it time to endorse different pathophysiologies? *Psychoneuroendocrinology*. 2006;31:1–15.

Das AK, Olfson M, Gameroff MJ, Pilowsky DJ, Blanco C, Feder A, Gross R, Neria Y, Lantigua R, Shea S, Weissman MM. Screening for bipolar disorder in a primary care practice. *JAMA*. 2005;293:956–963.

Ginsberg DL. Anticonvulsants may reduce suicidality in bipolar disorder. *Primary Psychiatry*. 2003;10:19.

Hooley JM, Woodberry KA, Ferriter C. Family factors in schizophrenia and bipolar disorder. In: Hudson JL, Rapee RM, eds. *Psychopathology and the Family*. New York: Elsevier Science; 2005:205–223.

Keller J, Gomez RG, Kenna HA, Poesner J, DeBattista C, Flores B, Schatzberg AF. Detecting psychotic major depression using psychiatric rating scales. *J Psychiar Res*. 2006;40:22–29.

Krishnan KRR. Psychiatric and medical comorbidities of bipolar disorder. *Psycho Med*. 2005;67:1–8

Mitchell PB. Bipolar disorder 40 years ago: A critical period of transition. *Aust N Z J Psychiatry*. 2006;40:279–280.

Oquendo MA, Barrera A, Ellis SP, Li S, Burke AK, Grunebaum M, Endicott J, Mann JJ. Instability of symptoms in recurrent major depression: A prospective study. *Am J Psychiatry*. 2004;161:255–261.

Oquendo MA, Galfalvy H, Russo S, Ellis SP, Grunebaum MF, Burke A, Mann JJ. Prospective study of clinical predictors of suicidal acts after a major depressive episode in patients with major depressive disorder or bipolar disorder. *Am J Psychiatry*. 2004;161:1433–1441.

▲ 15.2 Dysthymia and Cyclothymia

DYSTHYMIC DISORDER

According to the text revision of the fourth edition of *Diagnostic and Statistical Manual of Mental Disorders* (DSM-IV-TR), the most typical features of dysthymic disorder is the presence of a depressed mood that lasts most of the day and is present almost continuously. There are associated feelings of inadequacy, guilt, irritability, and anger; withdrawal from society; loss of interest; and inactivity and lack of productivity. The term *dysthymia*, which means "ill humored," was introduced in 1980. Before that time, most patients now classified as having dysthymic disorder were classified as having depressive neurosis (also called neurotic depression).

Dysthymic disorder is distinguished from major depressive disorder by the fact that patients complain that they have always been depressed. Thus, most cases are of early onset, beginning in childhood or adolescence and certainly occurring by the time patients reach their 20s. A late-onset subtype, much less prevalent and not well characterized clinically, has been identified among middle-aged and geriatric populations, largely through epidemiological studies in the community.

Although dysthymia can occur as a secondary complication of other psychiatric disorders, the core concept of dysthymic disorder refers to a subaffective or subclinical depressive disorder with (1) low-grade chronicity for at least 2 years; (2) insidious onset, with origin often in childhood or adolescence; and (3) persistent or intermittent course. The family history of patients with dysthymia is typically replete with both depressive and bipolar disorders, which is one of the more robust findings supporting its link to primary mood disorder.

Epidemiology

Dysthymic disorder is common among the general population and affects 5 to 6 percent of all persons. It is seen among patients in general psychiatric clinics, where it affects between one half and one third of all patients. No gender differences are seen for incidence rates. The disorder is more common in women younger than 64 years of age than in men of any age and is more common among unmarried and young persons and in those with low incomes. Dysthymic disorder frequently coexists with other mental disorders, particularly major depressive disorder, and in persons with major depressive disorder there is less likelihood of full remission between episodes. The patients may also have coexisting anxiety disorders (especially panic disorder), substance abuse, and borderline personality disorder. The disorder is more common among those with first-degree relatives with major depressive disorder. Patients with dysthymic disorder are likely to be taking a wide range of psychiatric medications, including antidepressants, antimanic agents such as lithium (Eskalith) and carbamazepine (Tegretol), and sedative-hypnotics.

Etiology

Biological Factors. The biological basis for the symptoms of dysthymic disorder and major depressive disorder are similar, but the biological bases for the underlying pathophysiology in the two disorders differ.

SLEEP STUDIES. Decreased rapid eye movement (REM) latency and increased REM density are two state markers of depression in major depressive disorder that also occur in a significant proportion of patients with dysthymic disorder.

NEUROENDOCRINE STUDIES. The two most studied neuroendocrine axes in major depressive disorder and dysthymic disorder are the adrenal axis and the thyroid axis, which have been tested by using the dexamethasone-suppression test (DST) and the thyrotropin-releasing hormone (TRH)-stimulation test, respectively. Although the results of studies are not absolutely consistent, most indicate that patients with dysthymic disorder are less likely to have abnormal results on a DST than are patients with major depressive disorder.

Psychosocial Factors. Psychodynamic theories about the development of dysthymic disorder posit that the disorder results from personality and ego development and culminates in difficulty adapting to adolescence and young adulthood. Karl Abraham, for example, thought that the conflicts of depression center on oral- and anal-sadistic traits. Anal traits include excessive orderliness, guilt, and concern for others; they are postulated to be a defense against preoccupation with anal matter and with disorganization, hostility, and self-preoccupation. A major defense mechanism used is reaction formation. Low self-esteem, anhedonia, and introversion are often associated with the depressive character.

FREUD. In *Mourning and Melancholia*, Sigmund Freud asserted that an interpersonal disappointment early in life can cause a vulnerability to depression that leads to ambivalent love relationships as an adult; real or threatened losses in adult life then trigger depression. Persons susceptible to depression are orally dependent and require constant narcissistic gratification. When deprived of love, affection, and care, they become clinically depressed; when they experience a real loss, they internalize or introject the lost object and turn their anger on it and, thus, on themselves.

COGNITIVE THEORY. The cognitive theory of depression also applies to dysthymic disorder. It holds that a disparity between actual and fantasized situations leads to diminished self-esteem and a sense of helplessness. The success of cognitive therapy in the treatment of some patients with dysthymic disorder may provide some support for the theoretical model.

Diagnosis and Clinical Features

The DSM-IV-TR diagnosis criteria for dysthymic disorder (Table 15.2–1) stipulate the presence of a depressed mood most of the time for at least 2 years (or 1 year for children and adolescents). To meet the diagnostic criteria, a patient should not have symptoms that are better accounted for as major depressive disorder and should never have had a manic or hypomanic episode. DSM-IV-TR allows clinicians to specify whether the onset was early (before age 21) or late (age 21 or older). DSM-IV-TR also allows specification of atypical features in dysthymic disorder.

The profile of dysthymic disorder overlaps with that of major depressive disorder, but differs from it in that symptoms tend to outnumber signs (more subjective than objective depression). This means that disturbances in appetite and libido are uncharacteristic, and psychomotor agitation or retardation is not observed. This all translates into a depression with attenuated symptomatology. Subtle endogenous features are observed, however: inertia, lethargy, and anhedonia that are characteristically worse in the morning. Because patients presenting clinically often fluctuate in and out of a major depression, the core DSM-IV-TR criteria for dysthymic disorder tend to emphasize vegetative dysfunction, whereas the alternative Criterion B for dysthymic disorder (Table 15.2–2) in a DSM-IV-TR appendix lists cognitive symptoms.

Dysthymic disorder is quite heterogeneous. Anxiety is not a necessary part of its clinical picture, yet dysthymic disorder is often diagnosed in patients with anxiety and phobic disorders. That clinical situation is sometimes diagnosed as mixed anxiety depressive disorder. For greater operational clarity, it is best to restrict dysthymic disorder to a primary disorder, one that cannot be explained by another psychiatric disorder. The essential features of such primary dysthymic disorder include habitual gloom, brooding, lack of joy in life, and preoccupation with inadequacy. Dysthymic disorder then is best characterized as long-standing, fluctuating, low-grade depression, experienced as part of the habitual self and representing an accentuation of traits observed in the depressive temperament (Table 15.2–3). The clinical picture of dysthymic disorder is varied, with some patients proceeding to major depression, whereas others manifest the pathology largely at the personality level.

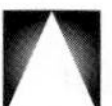

Table 15.2–1
DSM-IV-TR Diagnostic Criteria for Dysthymic Disorder

A. Depressed mood for most of the day, for more days than not, as indicated either by subjective account or observation by others, for at least 2 years. **Note:** In children and adolescents, mood can be irritable and duration must be at least 1 year.

B. Presence, while depressed, of two (or more) of the following:
   (1) poor appetite or overeating
   (2) insomnia or hypersomnia
   (3) low energy or fatigue
   (4) low self-esteem
   (5) poor concentration or difficulty making decisions
   (6) feelings of hopelessness

C. During the 2-year period (1 year for children or adolescents) of the disturbance, the person has never been without the symptoms in Criteria A and B for more than 2 months at a time.

D. No major depressive episode has been present during the first 2 years of the disturbance (1 year for children and adolescents); i.e., the disturbance is not better accounted for by chronic major depressive disorder, or major depressive disorder, in partial remission.

   Note: There may have been a previous major depressive episode provided there was a full remission (no significant signs or symptoms for 2 months) before development of the dysthymic disorder. In addition, after the initial 2 years (1 year in children or adolescents) of dysthymic disorder, there may be superimposed episodes of major depressive disorder, in which case both diagnoses may be given when the criteria are met for a major depressive episode.

E. There has never been a manic episode, a mixed episode, or a hypomanic episode, and criteria have never been met for cyclothymic disorder.

F. The disturbance does not occur exclusively during the course of a chronic psychotic disorder, such as schizophrenia or delusional disorder.

G. The symptoms are not due to the direct physiological effects of a substance (e.g., a drug of abuse, a medication) or a general medical condition (e.g., hypothyroidism).

H. The symptoms cause clinically significant distress or impairment in social, occupational, or other important areas of functioning.

Specify if:
   Early onset: if onset is before age 21 years
   Late onset: if onset is age 21 years or older

Specify (for most recent 2 years of dysthymic disorder) if
   With atypical features

(From American Psychiatric Association. *Diagnostic and Statistical Manual of Mental Disorders.* 4th ed. Text rev. Washington, DC: American Psychiatric Association; copyright 2000, with permission.)

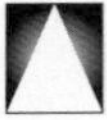

Table 15.2–2
DSM-IV-TR Alternative Research Criterion B for Dysthymic Disorder

B. Presence, while depressed, of three (or more) of the following:
(1) low self-esteem or self-confidence, or feelings of inadequacy
(2) feelings of pessimism, despair, or hopelessness
(3) generalized loss of interest or pleasure
(4) social withdrawal
(5) chronic fatigue or tiredness
(6) feelings of guilt, brooding about the past
(7) subjective feelings of irritability or excessive anger
(8) decreased activity, effectiveness, or productivity
(9) difficulty in thinking, reflected by poor concentration, poor memory, or indecisiveness

(From American Psychiatric Association. *Diagnostic and Statistical Manual of Mental Disorders.* 4th ed. Text rev. Washington, DC: American Psychiatric Association; copyright 2000, with permission.)

Leon is a 45-year-old postal employee who was evaluated at a clinic specializing in the treatment of depression. He claims to have felt constantly depressed since the first grade, without a period of "normal" mood for more than a few days at a time. His depression has been accompanied by lethargy, little or no interest or pleasure in anything, trouble concentrating, and feelings of inadequacy, pessimism, and resentfulness. His only periods of normal mood occur when he is home alone, listening to music or watching TV.

On further questioning, Leon reveals that he cannot ever remember feeling comfortable socially. Even before kindergarten, if he was asked to speak in front of a group of his parents' friends, his mind would "go blank." He felt overwhelming anxiety at children's social functions, such as birthday parties, which he either avoided or, if he went, attended in total silence. He could answer questions in class only if he wrote down the answers in advance; even then, he frequently mumbled and couldn't get the answer out. He met new children with his eyes lowered, fearing their scrutiny, expecting to feel humiliated and embarrassed. He was convinced that everyone around him thought he was "dumb" or "a jerk."

As he grew up, Leon had a couple of neighborhood playmates, but he never had a "best friend." His school grades were good, but suffered when oral classroom participation was expected. As a teenager he was terrified of girls, and to this day has never gone on a date or even asked a girl for a date. This bothers him, although he is so often depressed that he feels he has little energy or interest in dating.

Leon attended college and did well for a while, then dropped out as his grades slipped. He remained very self-conscious and "terrified" of meeting strangers. He had trouble finding a job because he was unable to answer questions in interviews. He worked at a few jobs for which only a written test was required. He passed a Civil Service exam at age 24, and was offered a job in the post office on the evening shift. He enjoyed this job as it involved little contact with others. He was offered, but refused, several promotions because he feared the social pressures. Although by now he supervises a number of employees, he still finds it difficult to give instructions, even to people he has known for years. He has no friends and avoids all invitations to socialize with co-workers. During the past several years, he has tried several therapies to help him get over his "shyness" and depression.

Leon has never experienced sudden anxiety or a panic attack in social situations or at other times. Rather, his anxiety gradually builds to a constant high level in anticipation of social situations. He has never experienced any psychotic symptoms. (Courtesy of *DSM-IV Casebook.*)

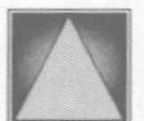

Table 15.2–3
Attributes, Assets, and Liabilities of Depressive and Hyperthymic Temperaments

Depressive	Hyperthymic
Gloomy, incapable of fun, complaining	Cheerful and exuberant
Humorless	Articulate and jocular
Pessimistic and given to brooding	Overoptimistic and carefree
Guilt-prone, low self-esteem, and preoccupied with inadequacy or failure	Overconfident, self-assured, boastful, and grandiose
Introverted with restricted social life	Extroverted and people seeking
Sluggish, living a life out of action	High energy level, full of plans
Few but constant interests	Versatile with broad interests
Passive	Overinvolved and meddlesome
Reliable, dependable, and devoted	Uninhibited and stimulus seeking

(Courtesy of Hagop S. Akiskal, M.D.)

Dysthymic Variants. Dysthymia is not uncommon in patients with chronically disabling physical disorders, particularly among elderly adults. Dysthymia-like, clinically significant, subthreshold depression lasting 6 or more months has also been described in neurological conditions, including stroke. According to a recent World Health Organization (WHO) conference, this condition aggravates the prognosis of the underlying neurological disease and, therefore, deserves pharmacotherapy.

Prospective studies on children have revealed an episodic course of dysthymia with remissions, exacerbations, and eventual complications by major depressive episodes, 15 to 20 percent of which might even progress to hypomanic, manic, or mixed episodes postpuberty. Persons with dysthymic disorder presenting clinically as adults tend to pursue a chronic unipolar course that may or may not be complicated by major depression. They rarely develop spontaneous hypomania or mania. When treated with antidepressants, however, some of them may develop brief hypomanic switches that typically disappear when the antidepressant dose is decreased.

Differential Diagnosis

The differential diagnosis for dysthymic disorder is essentially identical to that for major depressive disorder. Many substances and medical illnesses can cause chronic depressive symptoms. Two disorders are particularly important to consider in the differential diagnosis of dysthymic disorder—minor depressive disorder and recurrent brief depressive disorder.

Minor Depressive Disorder. Minor depressive disorder (discussed in Section 15.3) is characterized by episodes of depressive symptoms that are less severe than those seen in major depressive disorder. The difference between dysthymic disorder and minor depressive disorder is primarily the episodic nature of the symptoms in the latter. Between episodes, patients with minor depressive disorder have a euthymic mood, whereas patients with dysthymic disorder have virtually no euthymic periods.

Recurrent Brief Depressive Disorder. Recurrent brief depressive disorder (discussed in Section 15.3) is characterized by brief periods (less than 2 weeks) during which depressive episodes are present. Patients with the disorder would meet the diagnostic criteria for major depressive disorder if their episodes lasted longer. Patients with recurrent brief depressive disorder differ from patients with dysthymic disorder on two counts: They have an episodic disorder, and their symptoms are more severe.

Double Depression. An estimated 40 percent of patients with major depressive disorder also meet the criteria for dysthymic disorder, a combination often referred to as *double depression*. Available data support the conclusion that patients with double depression have a poorer prognosis than patients with only major depressive disorder. The treatment of patients with double depression should be directed toward both disorders, because the resolution of the symptoms of major depressive episode still leaves these patients with significant psychiatric impairment.

Alcohol and Substance Abuse. Patients with dysthymic disorder commonly meet the diagnostic criteria for a substance-related disorder. This comorbidity can be logical; patients with dysthymic disorder tend to develop coping methods for their chronically depressed state that involve substance abuse. Therefore, they are likely to use alcohol, stimulants such as cocaine, or marijuana, the choice perhaps depending primarily on a patient's social context. The presence of a comorbid diagnosis of substance abuse presents a diagnostic dilemma for clinicians; the long-term use of many substances can result in a symptom picture indistinguishable from that of dysthymic disorder.

Course and Prognosis

About 50 percent of patients with dysthymic disorder experience an insidious onset of symptoms before age 25. Despite the early onset, patients often suffer with the symptoms for a decade before seeking psychiatric help and may consider early-onset dysthymic disorder simply part of life. Patients with an early onset of symptoms are at risk for either major depressive disorder or bipolar I disorder in the course of their disorder. Studies of patients with the diagnosis of dysthymic disorder indicate that about 20 percent progressed to major depressive disorder, 15 percent to bipolar II disorder, and less than 5 percent to bipolar I disorder.

The prognosis for patients with dysthymic disorder varies. Antidepressive agents and specific types of psychotherapies (e.g., cognitive and behavior therapies) have positive effects on the course and prognosis of dysthymic disorder. The available data about previously available treatments indicate that only 10 to 15 percent of patients are in remission 1 year after the initial diagnosis. About 25 percent of all patients with dysthymic disorder never attain a complete recovery. Overall, however, the prognosis is good with treatment.

Treatment

Historically, patients with dysthymic disorder either received no treatment or were seen as candidates for long-term, insight-oriented psychotherapy. Contemporary data offer the most objective support for cognitive therapy, behavior therapy, and pharmacotherapy. The combination of pharmacotherapy and some form of psychotherapy may be the most effective treatment for the disorder.

Cognitive Therapy. Cognitive therapy is a technique in which patients are taught new ways of thinking and behaving to replace faulty negative attitudes about themselves, the world, and the future. It is a short-term therapy program oriented toward current problems and their resolution.

Behavior Therapy. Behavior therapy for depressive disorders is based on the theory that depression is caused by a loss of positive reinforcement as a result of separation, death, or sudden environmental change. The various treatment methods focus on specific goals to increase activity, to provide pleasant experiences, and to teach patients how to relax. Altering personal behavior in depressed patients is believed to be the most effective way to change the associated depressed thoughts and feelings. Behavior therapy is often used to treat the learned helplessness of some patients who seem to meet every life challenge with a sense of impotence.

Insight-Oriented (Psychoanalytic) Psychotherapy. Individual insight-oriented psychotherapy is the most common treatment method for dysthymic disorder, and many clinicians consider it the treatment of choice. The psychotherapeutic approach attempts to relate the development and maintenance of depressive symptoms and maladaptive personality features to unresolved conflicts from early childhood. Insight into depressive equivalents (e.g., substance abuse) or into childhood disappointments as antecedents to adult depression can be gained through treatment. Ambivalent current relationships with parents, friends, and others in the patient's current life are examined. Patients' understanding of how they try to gratify an excessive need for outside approval to counter low self-esteem and a harsh superego is an important goal in this therapy.

Interpersonal Therapy. In interpersonal therapy for depressive disorders, a patient's current interpersonal experiences and ways of coping with stress are examined to reduce depressive symptoms and to improve self-esteem. Interpersonal therapy lasts for about 12 to 16 weekly sessions and can be combined with antidepressant medication.

Family and Group Therapies. Family therapy may help both the patient and the patient's family deal with the symptoms of the disorder, especially when a biologically based subaffective syndrome seems to be present. Group therapy may help withdrawn patients learn new ways to overcome their interpersonal problems in social situations.

Pharmacotherapy. Because of long-standing and commonly held theoretical beliefs that dysthymic disorder is primarily a psychologically determined disorder, many clinicians avoid prescribing antidepressants for patients; however, many studies have shown therapeutic success with antidepressants. The data generally indicate that selective serotonin reuptake inhibitors (SSRIs) venlafaxine and bupropion are an effective treatment for patients with dysthymic disorder. Monoamine oxidase inhibitors (MAOIs) are effective in a subgroup of patients with dysthymic disorder, a group who may also respond to the judicious use of amphetamines.

Hospitalization. Hospitalization is usually not indicated for patients with dysthymic disorder, but particularly severe symptoms, marked social or professional incapacitation, the need for extensive diagnostic procedures, and suicidal ideation are all indications for hospitalization.

CYCLOTHYMIC DISORDER

Cyclothymic disorder is symptomatically a mild form of bipolar II disorder, characterized by episodes of hypomania and mild depression. In DSM-IV-TR, cyclothymic disorder is defined as a "chronic, fluctuating disturbance" with many periods of hypomania and of depression. The disorder is differentiated from bipolar II disorder, which is characterized by the presence of major (not minor) depressive and hypomanic episodes. As with dysthymic disorder, the inclusion of cyclothymic disorder with the mood disorders implies a relation, probably biological, to bipolar I disorder. Some psychiatrists, however, consider cyclothymic disorder to have no biological component and to result from chaotic object relations early in life.

Contemporary conceptualization of cyclothymic disorder is based to some extent on the observations of Emil Kraepelin and Kurt Schneider that one third to two thirds of patients with mood disorders exhibit personality disorders. Kraepelin described four types of personality disorders: depressive (gloomy), manic (cheerful and uninhibited), irritable (labile and explosive), and cyclothymic. He described the irritable personality as simultaneously depressive and manic and the cyclothymic personality as the alternation of the depressive and manic personalities.

Epidemiology

Patients with cyclothymic disorder may constitute from 3 to 5 percent of all psychiatric outpatients, perhaps particularly those with significant complaints about marital and interpersonal difficulties. In the general population, the lifetime prevalence of cyclothymic disorder is estimated to be about 1 percent. This figure is probably lower than the actual prevalence, because, as with patients with bipolar I disorder, the patients may not be aware that they have a psychiatric problem. Cyclothymic disorder, as with dysthymic disorder, frequently coexists with borderline personality disorder. An estimated 10 percent of outpatients and 20 percent of inpatients with borderline personality disorder have a coexisting diagnosis of cyclothymic disorder. The female-to-male ratio in cyclothymic disorder is about 3 to 2, and 50 to 75 percent of all patients have an onset between ages 15 and 25. Families of persons with cyclothymic disorder often contain members with substance-related disorder.

Etiology

As with dysthymic disorder, controversy exists about whether cyclothymic disorder is related to the mood disorders, either biologically or psychologically. Some researchers have postulated that cyclothymic disorder has a closer relation to borderline personality disorder than to the mood disorders. Despite these controversies, the preponderance of biological and genetic data favors the idea of cyclothymic disorder as a bona fide mood disorder.

Biological Factors. About 30 percent of all patients with cyclothymic disorder have positive family histories for bipolar I disorder; this rate is similar to the rate for patients with bipolar I disorder. Moreover, the pedigrees of families with bipolar I disorder often contain generations of patients with bipolar I disorder linked by a generation with cyclothymic disorder. Conversely, the prevalence of cyclothymic disorder in the relatives of patients with bipolar I disorder is much higher than the prevalence of cyclothymic disorder either in the relatives of patients with other mental disorders or in persons who are mentally healthy. The observations that about one third of patients with cyclothymic disorder subsequently have major mood disorders, that they are particularly sensitive to antidepressant-induced hypomania, and that about 60 percent respond to lithium, add further support to the idea of cyclothymic disorder as a mild or attenuated form of bipolar II disorder.

Psychosocial Factors. Most psychodynamic theories postulate that the development of cyclothymic disorder lies in traumas and fixations during the oral stage of infant development. Freud hypothesized that the cyclothymic state is the ego's attempt to overcome a harsh and punitive superego. Hypomania is explained psychodynamically as the lack of self-criticism and an absence of inhibitions occurring when a depressed person throws off the burden of an overly harsh superego. The major defense mechanism in hypomania is denial, by which the patient avoids external problems and internal feelings of depression.

Patients with cyclothymic disorder are characterized by periods of depression alternating with periods of hypomania. Psychoanalytic exploration reveals that such patients defend themselves against underlying depressive themes with their euphoric or hypomanic periods. Hypomania is frequently triggered by a profound interpersonal loss. The false euphoria generated in such instances is a patient's way to deny dependence on love objects and simultaneously disavowing any aggression or destructiveness that may have contributed to the loss of the loved person.

Diagnosis and Clinical Features

Although many patients seek psychiatric help for depression, their problems are often related to the chaos that their manic episodes have caused. Clinicians must consider a diagnosis of cyclothymic disorder when a patient appears with what may seem to be sociopathic behavioral problems. Marital difficulties and instability in relationships are common complaints because patients with cyclothymic disorder are often promiscuous and irritable while in manic and mixed states. Although there are anecdotal reports of increased productivity and creativity when patients are hypomanic, most clinicians report that their patients

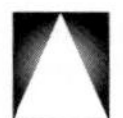

Table 15.2–4
DSM-IV-TR Diagnostic Criteria for Cyclothymic Disorder

A. For at least 2 years, the presence of numerous periods with hypomanic symptoms and numerous periods with depressive symptoms that do not meet criteria for a major depressive episode. **Note:** In children and adolescents, the duration must be at least 1 year.

B. During the above 2-year period (1 year in children and adolescents), the person has not been without the symptoms in Criterion A for more than 2 months at a time.

C. No major depressive episode, manic episode, or mixed episode has been present during the first 2 years of the disturbance.

Note: After the initial 2 years (1 year in children and adolescents) of cyclothymic disorder, there may be superimposed manic or mixed episodes (in which case both bipolar I disorder and cyclothymic disorder may be diagnosed) or major depressive episodes (in which case both bipolar II disorder and cyclothymic disorder may be diagnosed).

D. The symptoms in Criterion A are not better accounted for by schizoaffective disorder and are not superimposed on schizophrenia, schizophreniform disorder, delusional disorder, or psychotic disorder not otherwise specified.

E. The symptoms are not due to the direct physiological effects of a substance (e.g., a drug of abuse, a medication) or a general medical condition (e.g., hyperthyroidism).

F. The symptoms cause clinically significant distress or impairment in social, occupational, or other important areas of functioning.

(From American Psychiatric Association. *Diagnostic and Statistical Manual of Mental Disorders.* 4th ed. Text rev. Washington, DC: American Psychiatric Association; copyright 2000, with permission.)

become disorganized and ineffective in work and school during these periods.

The DSM-IV-TR diagnostic criteria for cyclothymic disorder (Table 15.2–4) stipulate that a patient has never met the criteria for a major depressive episode and did not meet the criteria for a manic episode during the first 2 years of the disturbance. The criteria also require the more or less constant presence of symptoms for 2 years (or 1 year for children and adolescents).

Signs and Symptoms. The symptoms of cyclothymic disorder are identical to the symptoms of bipolar II disorder, except that they are generally less severe. On occasion, however, the symptoms may be equally severe, but of shorter duration than those seen in bipolar II disorder. About half of all patients with cyclothymic disorder have depression as their major symptom, and these patients are most likely to seek psychiatric help while depressed. Some patients with cyclothymic disorder have primarily hypomanic symptoms and are less likely to consult a psychiatrist than are primarily depressed patients. Almost all patients with cyclothymic disorder have periods of mixed symptoms with marked irritability.

Most patients with cyclothymic disorder seen by psychiatrists have not succeeded in their professional and social lives as a result of their disorder, but a few have become high achievers who have worked especially long hours and have required little sleep. Some persons' ability to control the symptoms of the disorder successfully depends on multiple individual, social, and cultural attributes.

The lives of most patients with cyclothymic disorder are difficult. The cycles of the disorder tend to be much shorter than those in bipolar I disorder. In cyclothymic disorder, the changes in mood are irregular and abrupt and sometimes occur within hours. The unpredictable nature of the mood changes produces great stress. Patients often feel that their moods are out of control. In irritable, mixed periods, they may become involved in unprovoked disagreements with friends, family, and coworkers.

A 29-year-old car salesman was referred by his girlfriend, a psychiatric nurse, who suspected he had a mood disorder, even though the patient was reluctant to admit that he might be a "moody" person. According to him, since age 14 he has experienced repeated alternating cycles that he terms "good times and bad times." During a "bad" period, usually lasting 4 to 7 days, he oversleeps 10 to 14 hours daily, lacks energy, confidence, and motivation—"just vegetating," as he puts it. Often he abruptly shifts, characteristically upon waking up in the morning, to a 3-day to 4-day stretch of overconfidence, heightened social awareness, promiscuity, and sharpened thinking ("Things would flash in my mind"). At such times he indulges in alcohol to enhance the experience, but also to help him sleep. Occasionally the "good" periods last 7 to 10 days, but culminate in irritable and hostile outbursts, which often herald the transition back to another period of "bad" days. He admits to frequent use of marijuana, which he claims helps him "adjust" to daily routines.

In school, As and Bs alternated with Cs and Ds, with the result that the patient was considered a bright student whose performance was mediocre overall because of "unstable motivation." As a car salesman his performance has also been uneven, with "good days" canceling out the "bad days;" yet even during his "good days," he is sometimes argumentative with customers and loses sales that appeared sure. Although considered a charming man in many social circles, he alienates friends when he is hostile and irritable. He typically accumulates social obligations during the "bad" days and takes care of them all at once on the first day of a "good" period. (Courtesy of *DSM-IV Casebook.*)

Substance Abuse. Alcohol abuse and other substance abuse are common in patients with cyclothymic disorder, who use substances either to self-medicate (with alcohol, benzodiazepines, and marijuana) or to achieve even further stimulation (with cocaine, amphetamines, and hallucinogens) when they are manic. About 5 to 10 percent of all patients with cyclothymic disorder have substance dependence. Persons with this disorder often have a history of multiple geographical moves, involvements in religious cults, and dilettantism.

Differential Diagnosis

When a diagnosis of cyclothymic disorder is under consideration, all the possible medical and substance-related causes of depression and mania, such as seizures and particular substances (cocaine, amphetamine, and steroids), must be considered. Borderline, antisocial, histrionic, and narcissistic personality disorders should also be considered in the differential diagnosis. Attention-deficit/hyperactivity disorder (ADHD) can be difficult to differentiate from cyclothymic disorder in children and adolescents. A trial of stimulants helps most patients with ADHD and exacerbates the symptoms of most patients with cyclothymic disorder. The diagnostic category of bipolar II disorder (discussed in Section 15.1) is characterized by the combination of major depressive and hypomanic episodes.

Course and Prognosis

Some patients with cyclothymic disorder are characterized as having been sensitive, hyperactive, or moody as young children. The onset of frank symptoms of cyclothymic disorder often occurs insidiously in the teens or early 20s. The emergence of symptoms at that time hinders a person's performance in school and the ability to establish friendships with peers. The reactions of patients to such a disorder vary; patients with adaptive coping strategies or ego defenses have better outcomes than patients with poor coping strategies. About one third of all patients with cyclothymic disorder develop a major mood disorder, most often bipolar II disorder.

Treatment

Biological Therapy. The mood stabilizers and antimanic drugs are the first line of treatment for patients with cyclothymic disorder. Although the experimental data are limited to studies with lithium, other antimanic agents—for example, carbamazepine and valproate (Depakene)—are reported to be effective. Dosages and plasma concentrations of these agents should be the same as those in bipolar I disorder. Antidepressant treatment of depressed patients with cyclothymic disorder should be done with caution, because these patients have increased susceptibility to antidepressant-induced hypomanic or manic episodes. About 40 to 50 percent of all patients with cyclothymic disorder who are treated with antidepressants experience such episodes.

Psychosocial Therapy. Psychotherapy for patients with cyclothymic disorder is best directed toward increasing patients' awareness of their condition and helping them develop coping mechanisms for their mood swings. Therapists usually need to help patients repair any damage, both work and family related, done during episodes of hypomania. Because of the long-term nature of cyclothymic disorder, patients often require lifelong treatment. Family and group therapies may be supportive, educational, and therapeutic for patients and for those involved in their lives. The psychiatrist conducting psychotherapy is able to evaluate the degree of cyclothymia and so provide an early-warning system to prevent full-blown manic attacks before they occur.

References

Adler DA, Irish J, McLaughlin TJ, Perissinotto C, Chang H, Hood M, Lapitsky L, Rogers WH, Lerner D. The work impact of dysthymia in a primary care population. *Gen Hosp Psychiatry.* 2004;26(4):269–276.

Akiskal HS. Mood disorders: Clinical features. In: Sadock BJ, Sadock VA, eds. *Kaplan & Sadock's Comprehensive Textbook of Psychiatry.* 8th ed. Vol. 1. Baltimore: Lippincott Williams & Wilkins; 2005:1611.

Dougherty LR, Klein DN, Davila J. A growth curve analysis of the course of dysthymic disorder: The effects of chronic stress and moderation by adverse parent-child relationships and family history. *J Consult Clin Psychol.* 2004;72(6):1012–1021.

Dunner DL. Dysthymia and double depression. *Int Rev Psychiatry.* 2005;17(1):3–8.

Huprich SK, Porcerelli J, Binienda J, Karana D. Functional health status and its relationship to depressive personality disorder, dysthymia, and major depression: Preliminary findings. *Depress Anxiety.* 2005;22(4):168–176.

Klein DN, Shankman SA, Rose S. Ten-year prospective follow-up study of the naturalistic course of dysthymic disorder and double depression. *Am J Psychiatry.* 2006;163:872–880.

Markowitz JC, Kocsis JH, Bleiberg KL, Christos PJ, Sacks M. A comparative trial of psychotherapy and pharmacotherapy for "pure" dysthymic patients. *J Affect Disord.* 2005;89(1–3):167–175.

Markowitz JC, Skodol AE, Petkova E, Xie H, Cheng J, Hellerstein DJ, Gunderson JG, Sanislow CA, Grilo CM, McGlashan TH. Longitudinal comparison of depressive personality disorder and dysthymic disorder. *Compr Psychiatry.* 2005;46(4):239–245.

Ryder AG, Schuller DR, Bagby RM. Depressive personality and dysthymia: Evaluating symptom and syndrome overlap. *J Affect Disord.* 2006;91(2–3):217–227.

Schuyler D. Cognitive therapy for dysthymia. *Prim Care Companion J Clin Psychiatry.* 2004; 6(3):132–133.

▲ 15.3 Other Mood Disorders

DEPRESSIVE DISORDER NOT OTHERWISE SPECIFIED

The diagnostic category, depressive disorder not otherwise specified, is used for patients who exhibit depressive symptoms as the major feature, but who do not meet the diagnostic criteria for any other mood disorder (Table 15.3–1). Three disorders meet this criterion: (1) minor depressive disorder, (2) recurrent brief depressive disorder, and (3) premenstrual dysphoric disorder.

Minor Depressive Disorder

The literature in the United States on minor depressive disorder is limited, in part, because the term is used to describe a wide range of disorders, including dysthymic disorder, which is listed as a diagnosis in the text revision of the fourth revised edition of *Diagnostic and Statistical Manual of Mental Disorders* (DSM-IV-TR).

Epidemiology. Minor depressive disorder may be as common as major depressive disorder—that is, about 5 percent prevalence in the general population. The disorder is more common in women than in men and affects people of virtually any age, from childhood onward.

Etiology. The cause of minor depressive disorder is unknown. Both biological and psychological factors are implicated.

Diagnosis and Clinical Features. The criteria for minor depressive disorder include symptoms equal in duration to those of major depressive disorder, but less severe (Table 15.3–2). The central symptom of both disorders is the same—a depressed mood.

Differential Diagnosis. The differential diagnosis of minor depressive disorder includes dysthymic disorder and recurrent brief depressive disorder. Dysthymic disorder is characterized by the presence of chronic depressive symptoms, whereas recurrent brief depressive disorder is characterized by multiple brief episodes of severe depressive symptoms.

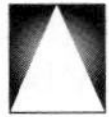

Table 15.3–1
DSM-IV-TR Diagnostic Criteria for Depressive Disorder Not Otherwise Specified

The depressive disorder not otherwise specified category includes disorders with depressive features that do not meet the criteria for major depressive disorder, dysthymic disorder, adjustment disorder with depressed mood, or adjustment disorder with mixed anxiety and depressed mood. Sometimes depressive symptoms can present as part of an anxiety disorder not otherwise specified. Examples of depressive disorder not otherwise specified include

1. Premenstrual dysphoric disorder: in most menstrual cycles during the past year, symptoms (e.g., markedly depressed mood, marked anxiety, marked affective lability, decreased interest in activities) regularly occurred during the last week of the luteal phase (and remitted within a few days of the onset of menses). These symptoms must be severe enough to markedly interfere with work, school, or usual activities and be entirely absent for at least 1 week postmenses.
2. Minor depressive disorder: episodes of at least 2 weeks of depressive symptoms but with fewer than the five items required for major depressive disorder.
3. Recurrent brief depressive disorder: depressive episodes lasting from 2 days up to 2 weeks, occurring at least once a month for 12 months (not associated with the menstrual cycle).
4. Postpsychotic depressive disorder of schizophrenia: a major depressive episode that occurs during the residual phase of schizophrenia.
5. A major depressive episode superimposed on delusional disorder, psychotic disorder not otherwise specified, or the active phase of schizophrenia.
6. Situations in which the clinician has concluded that a depressive disorder is present but is unable to determine whether it is primary, due to a general medical condition, or substance induced.

(From American Psychiatric Association. *Diagnostic and Statistical Manual of Mental Disorders.* 4th ed. Text rev. Washington, DC: American Psychiatric Association; copyright 2000, with permission.)

Course and Prognosis. No definitive data on the course and the prognosis of minor depressive disorder are available, but minor depressive disorder, as with major depressive disorder, has a long-term course that requires long-term treatment. Some cases remit spontaneously, however.

Treatment. The treatment of minor depressive disorder can include psychotherapy, pharmacotherapy, or both. Insight-oriented psychotherapy, cognitive therapy, interpersonal therapy, and behavior therapy are the psychotherapeutic treatments for major depressive disorder and, by implication, for minor depressive disorder. Patients with minor depressive disorder are probably responsive to pharmacotherapy, particularly selective serotonin reuptake inhibitors (SSRIs) and bupropion (Wellbutrin).

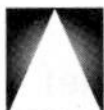

Table 15.3–2
DSM-IV-TR Research Criteria for Minor Depressive Disorder

A. A mood disturbance, defined as follows:
  (1) at least two (but less than five) of the following symptoms have been present during the same 2-week period and represent a change from previous functioning; at least one of the symptoms is either (a) or (b):
    (a) depressed mood most of the day, nearly every day, as indicated by either subjective report (e.g., feels sad or empty) or observation made by others (e.g., appears tearful). **Note**: In children and adolescents, can be irritable mood.
    (b) markedly diminished interest or pleasure in all, or almost all, activities most of the day, nearly every day (as indicated by either subjective account or observation made by others)
    (c) significant weight loss when not dieting or weight gain (e.g., a change of more than 5% of body weight in a month), or decrease or increase in appetite nearly every day. **Note**: In children, consider failure to make expected weight gains.
    (d) insomnia or hypersomnia nearly every day
    (e) psychomotor agitation or retardation nearly every day (observable by others, not merely subjective feelings of restlessness or being slowed down)
    (f) fatigue or loss of energy nearly every day
    (g) feelings of worthlessness or excessive or inappropriate guilt (which may be delusional) nearly every day (not merely self-reproach or guilt about being sick)
    (h) diminished ability to think or concentrate, or indecisiveness, nearly every day (either by subjective account or as observed by others)
    (i) recurrent thoughts of death (not just fear of dying), recurrent suicidal ideation without a specific plan, or a suicide attempt or a specific plan for committing suicide
  (2) the symptoms cause clinically significant distress or impairment in social, occupational, or other important areas of functioning
  (3) the symptoms are not due to the direct physiological effects of a substance (e.g., a drug of abuse, a medication) or a general medical condition (e.g., hypothyroidism)
  (4) the symptoms are not better accounted for by bereavement (i.e., a normal reaction to the death of a loved one)

B. There has never been a major depressive episode, and criteria are not met for dysthymic disorder.

C. There has never been a manic episode, a mixed episode, or a hypomanic episode, and criteria are not met for cyclothymic disorder. **Note**: This exclusion does not apply if all of the manic-, mixed-, or hypomanic-like episodes are substance or treatment induced.

D. The mood disturbance does not occur exclusively during schizophrenia, schizophreniform disorder, schizoaffective disorder, delusional disorder, or psychotic disorder not otherwise specified.

(From American Psychiatric Association. *Diagnostic and Statistical Manual of Mental Disorders.* 4th ed. Text rev. Washington, DC: American Psychiatric Association; copyright 2000, with permission.)

Recurrent Brief Depressive Disorder

Recurrent brief depressive disorder is characterized by multiple, relatively brief episodes (less than 2 weeks) of depressive symptoms that, except for their brief duration, meet the diagnostic criteria for major depressive disorder.

Epidemiology. The 10-year prevalence rate for the disorder is estimated to be 10 percent for people in their 20s; the 1-year prevalence rate for the general population is estimated to be 5 percent. These numbers indicate that recurrent brief depressive disorder is most common among young adults.

Etiology. Patients with recurrent brief depressive disorder may share several biological abnormalities with patients with

Table 15.3–3
DSM-IV-TR Research Criteria for Recurrent Brief Depressive Disorder

A. Criteria, except for duration, are met for a major depressive episode.
B. The depressive periods in Criterion A last at least 2 days but less than 2 weeks.
C. The depressive periods occur at least once a month for 12 consecutive months and are not associated with the menstrual cycle.
D. The periods of depressed mood cause clinically significant distress or impairment in social, occupational, or other important areas of functioning.
E. The symptoms are not due to the direct physiological effects of a substance (e.g., a drug of abuse, a medication) or a general medical condition (e.g., hypothyroidism).
F. There has never been a major depressive episode, and criteria are not met for dysthymic disorder.
G. There has never been a manic episode, a mixed episode, or a hypomanic episode, and criteria are not met for cyclothymic disorder. **Note:** This exclusion does not apply if all of the manic-, mixed-, or hypomanic-like episodes are substance or treatment induced.
H. The mood disturbance does not occur exclusively during schizophrenia, schizophreniform disorder, schizoaffective disorder, delusional disorder, or psychotic disorder not otherwise specified.

(From American Psychiatric Association. *Diagnostic and Statistical Manual of Mental Disorders.* 4th ed. Text rev. Washington, DC: American Psychiatric Association; copyright 2000, with permission.)

major depressive disorder. The variables include nonsuppression on the dexamethasone-suppression test (DST), a blunt response to thyrotropin-releasing hormone (TRH), and a shortening of rapid eye movement (REM) sleep latency. The data are consistent with the idea that recurrent brief depressive disorder is closely related to major depressive disorder in its cause and pathophysiology.

Diagnosis and Clinical Features. The criteria for recurrent brief depressive disorder specify that the symptom duration for each episode is less than 2 weeks (Table 15.3–3). Otherwise, the diagnostic criteria for recurrent brief depressive disorder and major depressive disorder are essentially identical. One subtle difference is that the frequent changes in their moods may make the lives of patients with recurrent brief depressive disorder seem more disrupted or chaotic than those of patients with major depressive disorder, whose depressive episodes occur at a measured pace.

Differential Diagnosis. Clinicians should consider bipolar disorder and major depressive disorder with seasonal pattern in the differential diagnosis. Recurrent brief depressive disorder can be associated with the rapid cycling type of bipolar disorder. Clinicians should also determine whether a seasonal pattern exists to the recurrence of depressive episodes.

Course and Prognosis. The course, including age of onset, and prognosis are similar to major depressive disorder.

Treatment. The treatment of patients with recurrent brief depressive disorder should be similar to the treatment of patients with major depressive disorder. Some of the treatments for bipolar I disorder—lithium (Eskalith) and anticonvulsants—may be of therapeutic value.

Premenstrual Dysphoric Disorder

Premenstrual dysphoric disorder is also called *late luteal phase dysphoric disorder*. The syndrome involves mood symptoms (e.g., lability), behavior symptoms (e.g., changes in eating patterns), and physical symptoms (e.g., breast tenderness, edema, and headaches). This pattern of symptoms occurs at a specific time during the menstrual cycle, and the symptoms resolve for some period of time between menstrual cycles. (Chapter 30 provides an extensive overview of this and other disorders related to the reproductive cycle.)

Postpsychotic Depressive Disorder of Schizophrenia

Postpsychotic depressive disorder in patients with schizophrenia is categorized in an appendix in DSM-IV-TR.

Epidemiology. The reported incidence of postpsychotic depression of schizophrenia varies widely, from less than 10 percent to more than 70 percent.

Etiology. The etiology is unknown. Psychologically, some patients became depressed after realizing their vulnerability to mental illness, which lowers their self-esteem.

Prognostic Significance. Patients with postpsychotic depressive disorder of schizophrenia are likely to have had poor premorbid adjustment, marked schizoid personality disorder traits, and an insidious onset of their psychotic symptoms. They are also likely to have first-degree relatives with mood disorders. Although the findings have not been consistent, postpsychotic depressive disorder of schizophrenia has been associated with a less-favorable prognosis, a higher likelihood of relapse, and a higher incidence of suicide than is seen in patients with schizophrenia without postpsychotic depressive disorder.

Diagnosis and Differential Diagnosis. The symptoms of postpsychotic depressive disorder of schizophrenia can closely resemble the symptoms of the residual phase of schizophrenia as well as the adverse effects of commonly used antipsychotic medications. Clinicians should not confuse the antipsychotic-induced adverse effects of akathisia and akinesia with symptoms of postpsychotic depressive disorder. Distinguishing the diagnosis from schizoaffective disorder, depressive type, is also difficult (Table 15.3–4).

Treatment. The use of antidepressants is indicated in the treatment of postpsychotic depressive disorder of schizophrenia, but response rates vary and are unpredictable.

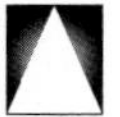

Table 15.3–4
DSM-IV-TR Research Criteria for Postpsychotic Depressive Disorder of Schizophrenia

A. Criteria are met for a major depressive episode.
Note: The major depressive episode must include Criterion A1: depressed mood. Do not include symptoms that are better accounted for as medication side effects or negative symptoms of schizophrenia.
B. The major depressive episode is superimposed on and occurs only during the residual phase of schizophrenia.
C. The major depressive episode is not due to the direct physiological effects of a substance or a general medical condition.

(From American Psychiatric Association. *Diagnostic and Statistical Manual of Mental Disorders.* 4th ed. Text rev. Washington, DC: American Psychiatric Association; copyright 2000, with permission.)

BIPOLAR DISORDER NOT OTHERWISE SPECIFIED

If patients exhibit depressive and manic symptoms as the major features of their disorder and do not meet the diagnostic criteria for any other mood disorder or other DSM-IV-TR mental disorder, the most appropriate diagnosis is bipolar disorder not otherwise specified (Table 15.3–5). This category should be used rarely.

Mixed Anxiety-Depressive Disorder

Mixed anxiety-depressive disorder is characterized by a persistent or recurrent depressed mood lasting at least 1 month and by symptoms of anxiety, such as sleep disturbance, fatigue or low energy, irritability, and worry (Table 15.3–6). The symptoms must cause clinically significant distress or impairment in social, occupational, or other important areas of functioning.

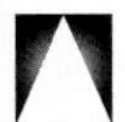

Table 15.3–5
DSM-IV-TR Diagnostic Criteria for Bipolar Disorder Not Otherwise Specified

The bipolar disorder not otherwise specified category includes disorders with bipolar features that do not meet criteria for any specific bipolar disorder. Examples include

1. Very rapid alternation (over days) between manic symptoms and depressive symptoms that meet symptom threshold criteria but not minimal duration criteria for manic, hypomanic, or major depressive episodes
2. Recurrent hypomanic episodes without intercurrent depressive symptoms
3. A manic or mixed episode superimposed on delusional disorder, residual schizophrenia, or psychotic disorder not otherwise specified
4. Hypomanic episodes, along with chronic depressive symptoms, that are too infrequent to qualify for a diagnosis of cyclothymic disorder
5. Situations in which the clinician has concluded that a bipolar disorder is present but is unable to determine whether it is primary, due to a general medical condition, or substance induced

(From American Psychiatric Association. *Diagnostic and Statistical Manual of Mental Disorders.* 4th ed. Text rev. Washington, DC: American Psychiatric Association; copyright 2000, with permission.)

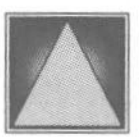

Table 15.3–6
Research Criteria for Mixed Anxiety-Depressive Disorder

A. Persistent or recurrent dysphoric mood lasting at least 1 month.
B. The dysphoric mood is accompanied by at least 1 month of four (or more) of the following symptoms:
(1) difficulty concentrating or mind going blank
(2) sleep disturbance (difficulty falling or staying asleep, or restless, unsatisfying sleep)
(3) fatigue or low energy
(4) irritability
(5) worry
(6) being easily moved to tears
(7) hypervigilance
(8) anticipating the worst
(9) hopelessness (pervasive pessimism about the future)
(10) low self-esteem or feelings of worthlessness
C. The symptoms cause clinically significant distress or impairment in social, occupational, or other important areas of functioning.
D. The symptoms are not due to the direct physiological effects of a substance (e.g., a drug of abuse, a medication) or a general medical condition.
E. All of the following:
(1) criteria have never been met for Major Depressive Disorder, Dysthymic Disorder, Panic Disorder, or Generalized Anxiety Disorder
(2) criteria are not currently met for any other Anxiety or Mood Disorder (including an Anxiety or Mood Disorder, In Partial Remission)
(3) the symptoms are not better accounted for by any other mental disorder

(From American Psychiatric Association. *Diagnostic and Statistical Manual of Mental Disorders.* 4th ed. Text rev. Washington DC: American Psychiatric Association; copyright 2000, with permission.)

Patients with mixed pictures are reportedly most prevalent in general medical settings because they have many somatic complaints about which they are anxious, one of the most prominent being chronic fatigue. In the 10th revision of *International Statistical Classification of Diseases and Related Health Problems* (ICD-10), these patients are diagnosed with neurasthenia. Some patients with chronic fatigue syndrome also have mixed anxiety and depressive symptomatology. This disorder is also discussed more fully in Chapter 18, which covers neurasthenia and chronic fatigue syndrome.

Atypical Depression

Atypical depression refers to fatigue superimposed on a history of somatic anxiety and phobias, together with reverse vegetative signs (mood worse in the evening, insomnia, tendency to oversleep and overeat), so that weight gain occurs rather than weight loss. Sleep is disturbed in the first half of the night in many persons with atypical depressive disorder, so irritability, hypersomnolence, and daytime fatigue would be expected. The temperaments of these patients are characterized by extreme sensitivity, especially to rejection. SSRIs and monoamine oxidase inhibitors (MAOIs) seem to show some specificity for such patients. Others are helped by psychostimulants, such as amphetamine.

OTHER DISORDERS NOT INCLUDED IN DSM-IV-TR

Several disorders with mood changes are not part of the official DSM nosological system. Some are included in the European diagnostic system and are found in the ICD-10.

Hysteroid Dysphoria

The category of non-DSM hysteroid dysphoria combines reverse vegetative signs with the following characteristics: (1) giddy responses to romantic opportunities and an avalanche of dysphoria (angry-depressive, even suicidal responses) on romantic disappointment; (2) impaired anticipatory pleasure, yet the capability to respond with pleasure when such is provided by others (i.e., preservation of consummatory reward); (3) craving for chocolate and sweets, which contain phenylethylamine compounds and sugars believed to facilitate cellular and neuronal intake of the amino acid L-tryptophan, hypothetically leading to synthesis of endogenous antidepressants in the brain. The word *hysteroid* was used to imply that the apparent character pathology was secondary to biological disturbances. Patients are treated symptomatically. Some respond to SSRIs, others to MAOIs and mood stabilizers, such as carbamazepine.

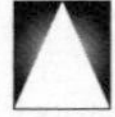

Table 15.3–7
DSM-IV-TR Diagnostic Criteria for Mood Disorder Due to a General Medical Condition

A. A prominent and persistent disturbance in mood predominates in the clinical picture and is characterized by either (or both) of the following:
   (1) depressed mood or markedly diminished interest or pleasure in all, or almost all, activities
   (2) elevated, expansive, or irritable mood

B. There is evidence from the history, physical examination, or laboratory findings that the disturbance is the direct physiological consequence of a general medical condition.

C. The disturbance is not better accounted for by another mental disorder (e.g., adjustment disorder with depressed mood in response to the stress of having a general medical condition).

D. The disturbance does not occur exclusively during the course of a delirium.

E. The symptoms cause clinically significant distress or impairment in social, occupational, or other important areas of functioning.

Specify type:

With depressive features: if the predominant mood is depressed but the full criteria are not met for a major depressive episode

With major depressive-like episode: if the full criteria are met (except Criterion D) for a major depressive episode

With manic features: if the predominant mood is elevated, euphoric, or irritable

With mixed features: if the symptoms of both mania and depression are present but neither predominates

Coding note: Include the name of the general medical condition on Axis I, e.g., mood disorder due to hypothyroidism, with depressive features; also code the general medical condition on Axis III.

Coding note: If depressive symptoms occur as part of a preexisting vascular dementia, indicate the depressive symptoms by coding the appropriate subtype, i.e., vascular dementia, with depressed mood.

(From American Psychiatric Association. *Diagnostic and Statistical Manual of Mental Disorders*. 4th ed. Text rev. Washington, DC: American Psychiatric Association; copyright 2000, with permission.)

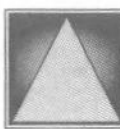

Table 15.3–8
Pharmacological Causes of Depression

1. Cardiac and antihypertensive drugs
2. Sedatives and hypnotics
3. Steroids and hormones
4. Stimulants and appetite suppressants
5. Psychotropic drugs
6. Neurological agents
7. Analgesics and anti-inflammatory drugs
8. Antibacterial and antifungal drugs
9. Antineoplastic drugs
10. Nonsteroidal anti-inflammatory drugs (NSAIDs)
11. Anticholinesterases

This is not an "official" DSM-IV-TR diagnosis; it can be considered an atypical variant of depression.

Motility Psychosis

The two forms of motility psychosis are akinetic and hyperkinetic. The akinetic form of motility psychosis has a clinical presentation similar to that of catatonic stupor. In contrast to the catatonic type of schizophrenia, however, akinetic motility psychosis has a rapidly resolving and favorable course that does not lead to personality deterioration. In its hyperkinetic form, motility psychosis can resemble manic or catatonic excitement. As with the akinetic form, the hyperkinetic form usually has a rapidly resolving and favorable course. Patients may switch from the akinetic to hyperkinetic form rapidly and may represent a danger to others during the excited phase. Mood is extremely labile in these patients. Motility psychosis is probably a variant of brief psychotic disorder.

Confusional Psychosis

As described originally, excited confusional psychosis is similar to mania, but was differentiated from mania by several characteristics: more anxiety, less distractibility, and a degree of speech incoherence out of proportion to the severity of the flight of ideas. Confusional psychosis

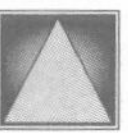

Table 15.3–9
Some Pharmacological Causes of Mania

Amphetamines
Baclofen
Bromide
Bromocriptine
Captopril
Cimetidine
Cocaine
Corticosteroids (including adrenocorticoid hormone [ACTH])
Cyclosporine
Disulfiram
Hallucinogens (intoxication and flashbacks)
Hydralazine
Isoniazid
Levodopa
Methylphenidate
Metrizamide (following myelography)
Opiates and opioids
Phencyclidine (PCP)
Procarbazine
Procyclidine
Yohimbine

(Adapted from Cummings JL. *Clinical Neuropsychiatry*. Orlando, FL: Grune & Stratton; 1985:187, with permission.)

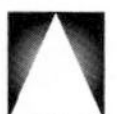

Table 15.3–10
DSM-IV-TR Diagnostic Criteria for Substance-Induced Mood Disorder

A. A prominent and persistent disturbance in mood predominates in the clinical picture and is characterized by either (or both) of the following:
   (1) depressed mood or markedly diminished interest or pleasure in all, or almost all, activities
   (2) elevated, expansive, or irritable mood

B. There is evidence from the history, physical examination, or laboratory findings of either (1) or (2):
   (1) the symptoms in Criterion A developed during, or within a month of, substance intoxication or withdrawal
   (2) medication use is etiologically related to the disturbance

C. The disturbance is not better accounted for by a mood disorder that is not substance induced. Evidence that the symptoms are better accounted for by a mood disorder that is not substance-induced might include the following: the symptoms precede the onset of the substance use (or medication use); the symptoms persist for a substantial period of time (e.g., about a month) after the cessation of acute withdrawal or severe intoxication or are substantially in excess of what would be expected given the type or amount of the substance used or the duration of use; or there is other evidence that suggests the existence of an independent non–substance-induced mood disorder (e.g., a history of recurrent major depressive episodes).

D. The disturbance does not occur exclusively during the course of a delirium.

E. The symptoms cause clinically significant distress or impairment in social, occupational, or other important areas of functioning.

Note: This diagnosis should be made instead of a diagnosis of substance intoxication or substance withdrawal only when the mood symptoms are in excess of those usually associated with the intoxication or withdrawal syndrome and when the symptoms are sufficiently severe to warrant independent clinical attention.

Code [Specific substance]-induced mood disorder:
Alcohol; amphetamine [or amphetamine-like substance]; cocaine; hallucinogen; inhalant; opioid; phencyclidine [or phencyclidine-like substance]; sedative, hypnotic, or anxiolytic; other [or unknown] substance

Specify type:
With depressive features: if the predominant mood is depressed
With manic features: if the predominant mood is elevated, euphoric, or irritable
With mixed features: if symptoms of both mania and depression are present and neither predominates

Specify if:
With onset during intoxication: if the criteria are met for intoxication with the substance and the symptoms develop during the intoxication syndrome
With onset during withdrawal: if criteria are met for withdrawal from the substance and the symptoms develop during, or shortly after, a withdrawal syndrome

(From American Psychiatric Association. *Diagnostic and Statistical Manual of Mental Disorders.* 4th ed. Text rev. Washington, DC: American Psychiatric Association; copyright 2000, with permission.)

is probably a clinical variation of the mania seen in bipolar I disorder. Patients may switch rapidly from the akinetic to the hyperkinetic form and may represent a danger to others during the excited phase.

Anxiety-Blissfulness Psychosis

Anxiety-blissfulness psychosis may resemble agitated depression but can also be characterized by so much inhibition that a patient can hardly move. Periodic states of overwhelming anxiety and paranoid ideas of reference are characteristic of the condition, but self-accusation, hypochondriacal preoccupation, other depressive symptoms, and hallucinations may also accompany it. The blissful phase manifests most frequently in expansive behavior and grandiose ideas, which are concerned less with self-aggrandizement than with the mission of making others happy and saving the world.

SECONDARY MOOD DISORDERS

Secondary mood disorders consist of two broad categories that must be considered in the differential diagnosis of any patient with mood disorder symptoms. They are (1) mood disorder caused by a general medical condition and (2) substance-induced mood disorder.

Mood Disorders Due to a General Medical Condition

When depressive or manic symptoms are present in a patient with a general medical condition, attributing the depressive symptoms either to the general medical condition or to a mood disorder can be difficult. Many general medical conditions present depressive symptoms, such as poor sleep, agitation, decreased appetite, increased appetite, and fatigue. Table 15.3–7 lists the DSM-IV-TR criteria for the disorder. This category is discussed extensively in Section 10.5.

Substance-Induced Mood Disorder

Substance-induced mood disorder must always be considered in the differential diagnosis of mood disorder symptoms. Clinicians should consider three possibilities: (1) a patient may be taking drugs for the treatment of nonpsychiatric medical problems; (2) a patient may have been accidentally, and perhaps unknowingly, exposed to neurotoxic chemicals; and (3) the patient may have taken a substance for recreational purposes or may be dependent on such a substance.

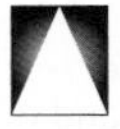

Table 15.3–11
DSM-IV-TR Diagnostic Criteria for Mood Disorder Not Otherwise Specified

This category includes disorders with mood symptoms that do not meet the criteria for any specific mood disorder and in which it is difficult to choose between depressive disorder not otherwise specified and bipolar disorder not otherwise specified (e.g., acute agitation).

(From American Psychiatric Association. *Diagnostic and Statistical Manual of Mental Disorders.* 4th ed. Text rev. Washington, DC: American Psychiatric Association; copyright 2000, with permission.)

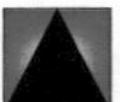

Table 15.3–12
ICD-10 Diagnostic Criteria for Mood [Affective] Disorders

Manic episode

Hypomania

A. The mood is elevated or irritable to a degree that is definitely abnormal for the individual concerned and sustained for at least 4 consecutive days.

B. At least three of the following signs must be present, leading to some interference with personal functioning in daily living:
 (1) increased activity or physical restlessness;
 (2) increased talkativeness;
 (3) distractibility or difficulty in concentration;
 (4) decreased need for sleep;
 (5) increased sexual energy;
 (6) mild overspending, or other types of reckless or irresponsible behavior;
 (7) increased sociability or overfamiliarity.

C. The episode does not meet the criteria for mania, bipolar affective disorder, depressive episode, cyclothymia, or anorexia nervosa.

D. *Most commonly used exclusion clause.* The episode is not attributable to psychoactive substance use or to any organic mental disorder.

Mania without psychotic symptoms

A. Mood must be predominantly elevated, expansive, or irritable, and definitely abnormal for the individual concerned. The mood change must be prominent and sustained for at least 1 week (unless it is severe enough to require hospital admission).

B. At least three of the following signs must be present (four if the mood is merely irritable), leading to severe interference with personal functioning in daily living:
 (1) increased activity or physical restlessness;
 (2) increased talkativeness ("pressure of speech");
 (3) flight of ideas or the subjective experience of thoughts racing;
 (4) loss of normal social inhibitions, resulting in behavior that is inappropriate to the circumstances;
 (5) decreased need for sleep;
 (6) inflated self-esteem or grandiosity;
 (7) distractibility or constant changes in activity or plans;
 (8) behavior that is foolhardy or reckless and whose risks the individual does not recognize, e.g., spending sprees, foolish enterprises, reckless driving;
 (9) marked sexual energy or sexual indiscretions.

C. There are no hallucinations or delusions, although perceptual disorders may occur (e.g., subjective hyperacusis, appreciation of colors as especially vivid).

D. *Most commonly used exclusion clause.* The episode is not attributable to psychoactive substance use or to any organic mental disorder.

Mania with psychotic symptoms

A. The episode meets the criteria for mania without psychotic symptoms with the exception of Criterion C.

B. The episode does not simultaneously meet the criteria for schizophrenia or schizoaffective disorder, manic type.

C. Delusions or hallucinations are present, other than those listed as typically schizophrenic in Criterion G1(1)b, c, and d for schizophrenia (i.e., delusions other than those that are completely impossible or culturally inappropriate, and hallucinations that are not in the third person or giving a running commentary). The commonest examples are those with grandiose, self-referential, erotic, or persecutory content.

D. *Most commonly used exclusion clause.* The episode is not attributable to psychoactive substance use or to any organic mental disorder.

Specify whether the hallucinations or delusions are congruent or incongruent with the mood:
 With mood-congruent psychotic symptoms (such as grandiose delusions or voices telling the individual that he or she has superhuman powers)
 With mood-incongruent psychotic symptoms (such as voices speaking to the individual about affectively neutral topics, or delusions of reference or persecution)

Other manic episodes

Manic episode, unspecified

Bipolar affective disorder

Note. Episodes are demarcated by a switch to an episode of opposite mixed polarity or by a remission.

Bipolar affective disorder, current episode hypomanic

A. The current episode meets the criteria for hypomania.

B. There has been at least one other affective episode in the past, meeting the criteria for hypomanic or manic episode, depressive episode, or mixed affective episode.

Bipolar affective disorder, current episode manic without psychotic symptoms

A. The current episode meets the criteria for mania without psychotic symptoms.

B. There has been at least one other affective episode in the past, meeting the criteria for hypomanic or manic episode, depressive episode, or mixed affective episode.

Bipolar affective disorder, current episode manic without psychotic symptoms

A. The current episode meets the criteria for mania without psychotic symptoms.

B. There has been at least one other affective episode in the past, meeting the criteria for hypomanic or manic episode, depressive episode, or mixed affective episode.

Specify whether the psychotic symptoms are congruent or incongruent with the mood:
 With mood-congruent psychotic symptoms
 With mood-incongruent psychotic symptoms

Bipolar affective disorder, current episode moderate or mild depression

A. The current episode meets the criteria for a depressive episode of either mild or moderate severity.

B. There has been at least one other affective episode in the past, meeting the criteria for hypomanic or manic episode, depressive episode, or mixed affective episode.

Specify the presence of the "somatic syndrome" in the current episode of depression:
 Without somatic syndrome
 With somatic syndrome

Bipolar affective disorder, current episode severe depression without psychotic symptoms

A. The current episode meets the criteria for a severe depressive episode without psychotic symptoms.

B. There has been at least one well-authenticated hypomanic or manic episode or mixed affective episode in the past.

Bipolar affective disorder, current episode severe depression with psychotic symptoms

A. The current episode meets the criteria for a severe depressive episode without psychotic symptoms.

B. There has been at least one well-authenticated hypomanic or manic episode or mixed affective episode in the past.

(*continued*)

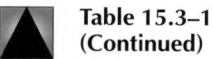

Table 15.3–12 (Continued)

Specify whether the psychotic symptoms are congruent or incongruent with the mood:

With mood-congruent psychotic symptoms
With mood-incongruent psychotic symptoms

Bipolar affective disorder, current episode mixed

A. The current episode is characterized by either a mixture or a rapid alternation (i.e., within a few hours) of hypomanic, manic, and depressive symptoms.
B. Both manic and depressive symptoms must be prominent most of the time during a period of at least 2 weeks.
C. There has been at least one well-authenticated hypomanic or manic episode, depressive episode, or mixed affective episode in the past.

Bipolar affective disorder, currently in remission

A. The current state does not meet the criteria for depressive or manic episode of any severity or for any other mood [affective] disorder (possibly because of treatment to reduce the risk of future episodes).
B. There has been at least one well-authenticated hypomanic or manic episode in the past and in addition at least one other affective episode (hypomanic or manic, depressive, or mixed).

Other bipolar affective disorders

Bipolar affective disorder, unspecified

Depressive episode

G1. The depressive episode should last for at least 2 weeks.
G2. There have been no hypomanic or manic symptoms sufficient to meet the criteria for hypomanic or manic episode at any time in the individual's life.
G3. *Most commonly used exclusion clause.* The episode is not attributable to psychoactive substance use or to any organic mental disorder.

Somatic syndrome

Some depressive symptoms are widely regarded as having special clinical significance and are here called "somatic." (Terms such as biological, vital, melancholic, or endogenomorphic are used for this syndrome in other classifications.)

A fifth character may be used to specify the presence or absence of the somatic syndrome. To qualify for the somatic syndrome, *four* of the following symptoms should be present:

(1) marked loss of interest or pleasure in activities that are normally pleasurable;
(2) lack of emotional reactions to events or activities that normally produce an emotional response;
(3) waking in the morning 2 hours or more before the usual time;
(4) depression worse in the morning;
(5) objective evidence of marked psychomotor retardation or agitation (remarked on or reported by other people);
(6) marked loss of appetite;
(7) weight loss (5% or more of body weight in the past month);
(8) marked loss of libido.

In *The ICD-10 Classification of Mental and Behavioural Disorders: Clinical Descriptions and Diagnostic Guidelines,* the presence or absence of the somatic syndrome is not specified for severe depressive episode, since it is presumed to be present in most cases. For research purposes, however, it may be advisable to allow for the coding of the absence of the somatic syndrome in severe depressive episode.

Mild depressive episode

A. The general criteria for depressive episode must be met.
B. At least two of the following three symptoms must be present:
   (1) depressed mood to a degree that is definitely abnormal for the individual, present for most of the day and almost every day, largely uninfluenced by circumstances, and sustained for at least 2 weeks;
   (2) loss of interest or pleasure in activities that are normally pleasurable;
   (3) decreased energy or increased fatigability.
C. An additional symptom or symptoms from the following list should be present, to give a total of at least *four*:
   (1) loss of confidence or self-esteem;
   (2) unreasonable feelings of self-reproach or excessive and inappropriate guilt;
   (3) recurrent thoughts of death or suicide, or any suicidal behavior;
   (4) complaints or evidence of diminished ability to think or concentrate, such as indecisiveness or vacillation;
   (5) change in psychomotor activity, with agitation or retardation (either subjective or objective);
   (6) sleep disturbance of any type;
   (7) change in appetite (decrease or increase) with corresponding weight change.

A fifth character may be used to specify the presence or absence of the "somatic syndrome":

Without somatic syndrome
With somatic syndrome

Moderate depressive episode

A. The general criteria for depressive episode must be met.
B. At least two of the three symptoms listed for Criterion B above must be present.
C. Additional symptoms from depressive episode, Criterion C, must be present, to give a total of at least *six*.

A fifth character may be used to specify the presence or absence of the "somatic syndrome":

Without somatic syndrome
With somatic syndrome

Severe depressive episode without psychotic symptoms

Note: If important symptoms such as agitation or retardation are marked, the patient may be unwilling or unable to describe many symptoms in detail. An overall grading of severe episode may still be justified in such a case.

A. The general criteria for depressive episode must be met.
B. All three of the symptoms in Criterion B, depressive episode, must be present.
C. Additional symptoms from depressive episode, Criterion C, must be present, to give a total of at least *eight*.
D. There must be no hallucinations, delusions, or depressive stupor.

Severe depressive episode with psychotic symptoms

A. The general criteria for depressive episode must be met.
B. The criteria for severe depressive episode without psychotic symptoms must be met with the exception of Criterion D.
C. The criteria for schizophrenia or schizoaffective disorder, depressive type, are not met.
D. Either of the following must be present:
   (1) delusions or hallucinations, other than those listed as typically schizophrenic in Criterion G1(1)b, c, and d for general criteria for paranoid, hebephrenic, catatonic, and undifferentiated schizophrenia (i.e., delusions other than those that are completely impossible or culturally inappropriate and hallucinations that are not in the third person or giving a running commentary), the commonest examples are those with depressive, guilty, hypochondriacal, nihilistic, self-referential, or persecutory content
   (2) depressive stupor

(*continued*)

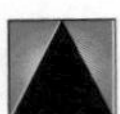

Table 15.3–12 (Continued)

A fifth character may be used to specify whether the psychotic symptoms are congruent or incongruent with mood:

With mood-congruent psychotic symptoms (i.e., delusions of guilt, worthlessness, bodily disease, or impending disaster, derisive or condemnatory auditory hallucinations)

With mood-incongruent psychotic symptoms (i.e., persecutory or self-referential delusions and hallucinations without an affective content)

Other depressive episodes

Episodes should be included here which do not fit the descriptions given for depressive episodes, but for which the overall diagnostic impression indicates that they are depressive in nature. Examples include fluctuating mixtures of depressive symptoms (particularly those of the somatic syndrome) with nondiagnostic symptoms such as tension, worry, and distress, and mixtures of somatic depressive symptoms with persistent pain or fatigue not due to organic causes (as sometimes seen in general hospital services).

Depressive episode, unspecified

Recurrent depressive disorder

G1. There has been at least one previous episode, mild, moderate, or severe, lasting a minimum of 2 weeks and separated from the current episode by at least 2 months free from any significant mood symptoms.

G2. At no time in the past has there been an episode meeting the criteria for hypomanic or manic episode.

G3. *Most commonly used exclusion clause.* The episode is not attributable to psychoactive substance use or to any organic mental disorder.

It is recommended that the predominant type of previous episodes is specified (mild, moderate, severe, uncertain).

Recurrent depressive disorder, current episode mild

A. The general criteria for recurrent depressive disorder are met.

B. The current episode meets the criteria for mild depressive episode.

A fifth character may be used to specify the presence or absence of the "somatic syndrome," in the current episode:

Without somatic syndrome
With somatic syndrome

Recurrent depressive disorder, current episode moderate

A. The general criteria for recurrent depressive disorder are met.

B. The current episode meets the criteria for moderate depressive episode.

A fifth character may be used to specify the presence or absence of the "somatic syndrome." in the current episode:

Without somatic syndrome
With somatic syndrome

Recurrent depressive disorder, current episode without psychotic symptoms

A. The general criteria for recurrent depressive disorder are met.

B. The current episode meets the criteria for severe depressive episode without psychotic symptoms.

Recurrent depressive disorder, current episode severe with psychotic symptoms

A. The general criteria for recurrent depressive disorder are met.

B. The current episode meets the criteria for severe depressive episode with psychotic symptoms.

A fifth character may be used to specify whether the psychotic symptoms are congruent or incongruent with the mood:

With mood-congruent psychotic symptoms
With mood-incongruent psychotic symptoms

Recurrent depressive disorder, currently in remission

A. The general criteria for recurrent depressive disorder have been met in the past.

B. The current state does not meet the criteria for a depressive episode of any severity or for any other disorder in mood [affective] disorders.

Comment

This category can still be used if the patient receives treatment to reduce the risk of further episodes.

Other recurrent depressive disorders

Recurrent depressive disorder, unspecified

Persistent mood [affective] disorders

Cyclothymia

A. There must have been a period of at least 2 years of instability of mood involving several periods of both depression and hypomania, with or without intervening periods of normal mood.

B. None of the manifestations of depression or hypomania during such a 2-year period should be sufficiently severe or long-lasting to meet criteria for manic episode or depressive episode (moderate or severe); however, manic or depressive episode(s) may have occurred before, or may develop after, such a period of persistent mood instability.

C. During at least some of the periods of depression at least three of the following should be present:

(1) reduced energy or activity;
(2) insomnia;
(3) loss of self-confidence or feelings of inadequacy;
(4) difficulty in concentrating;
(5) social withdrawal;
(6) loss of interest in or enjoyment of sex and other pleasurable activities;
(7) reduced talkativeness;
(8) pessimism about the future or brooding over the past.

D. During at least some of the periods of mood elevation at least three of the following should be present:

(1) increased energy or activity;
(2) decreased need for sleep;
(3) inflated self-esteem;
(4) sharpened or unusually creative thinking;
(5) increased gregariousness;
(6) increased talkativeness or wittiness;
(7) increased interest and involvement in sexual and other pleasurable activities;
(8) overoptimism or exaggeration of past achievements.

Note. If desired, time of onset may be specified as early (in late teenage or the 20s) or late (usually between age 30 and 50 years, following an affective episode).

Dysthymia

A. There must be a period of at least 2 years of constant or constantly recurring depressed mood. Intervening periods of normal mood rarely last for longer than a few weeks, and there are no episodes of hypomania.

B. None, or very few, of the individual episodes of depression within such a 2-year period should be sufficiently severe or long-lasting to meet the criteria for recurrent mild depressive disorder.

C. During at least some of the periods of depression at least three of the following should be present:

(1) reduced energy or activity;
(2) insomnia;
(3) loss of self-confidence or feelings of inadequacy;
(4) difficulty in concentrating;
(5) frequent tearfulness;

(*continued*)

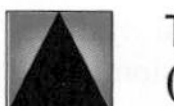

Table 15.3–12
(Continued)

(6) loss of interest in or enjoyment of sex and other pleasurable activities;
(7) feeling of hopelessness or despair;
(8) a perceived inability to cope with the routine responsibilities of everyday life;
(9) pessimism about the future or brooding over the past;
(10) social withdrawal;
(11) reduced talkativeness.

Note. If desired, time of onset may be specified as early (in late teenage or the 20s) or late (usually between age 30 and 50 years, following an affective episode).

Other persistent mood [affective] disorders

This is a residual category for persistent affective disorders that are not sufficiently severe or long-lasting to fulfill the criteria for cyclothymia or dysthymia but that are nevertheless clinically significant. Some types of depression previously called "neurotic" are included here, provided that they do not meet the criteria for either cyclothymia or dysthymia or for depressive episode of mild or moderate severity.

Persistent mood [affective] disorder, unspecified

Other mood [affective] disorders

There are so many possible disorders that could be listed that no attempt has been made to specify criteria, except for mixed affective episode and recurrent brief depressive disorder. Investigators requiring criteria more exact than those available in *Clinical Descriptions and Diagnostic Guidelines* should construct them according to the requirements of their studies.

Other single mood [affective] disorders

Mixed affective episode

A. The episode is characterized by either a mixture or a rapid alternation (i.e., within a few hours) of hypomanic, manic, and depressive symptoms.
B. Both manic and depressive symptoms must be prominent most of the time during a period of at least 2 weeks.
C. There is no history of previous hypomanic, depressive, or mixed episodes.

Other recurrent mood [affective] disorders

Recurrent brief depressive disorder

A. The disorder meets the symptomatic criteria for mild, moderate, or severe depressive episode.
B. The depressive episodes have occurred about once a month over the past year.
C. The individual episodes last less than 2 weeks (typically 2–3 days).
D. The episodes do not occur solely in relation to the menstrual cycle.

Other specified mood [affective] disorders

This is a residual category for affective disorders that do not meet the criteria for any other categories above.

(From World Health Organization. *The ICD-10 Classification of Mental and Behavioral Disorders: Diagnostic Criteria for Research.* Copyright, World Health Organization, Geneva, 1993, with permission.)

Epidemiology. The epidemiology of substance-induced mood disorder is unknown. The prevalence is probably high, given the widespread use of so-called recreational drugs, the many prescription drugs that can cause depression and mania, and the toxic chemicals that abound in the environment and the workplace.

Etiology. A wide range of drugs can produce depression (Table 15.3–8) and mania (Table 15.3–9).

Diagnosis and Clinical Features. When making the diagnosis of substance-induced mood disorder, the clinician should specify the substance involved, the time of onset (during intoxication or withdrawal), and the nature of the symptoms (e.g., manic or depressed) (Table 15.3–10). A maximum of 1 month between the use of the substance and the appearance of the symptoms is allowed in DSM-IV-TR, but the timeframe is usually much shorter.

Substance-induced manic and depressive features can be identical to those of bipolar I disorder and major depressive disorder. Substance-induced mood disorder, however, may show more waxing and waning of symptoms and a fluctuation in a patient's level of consciousness.

Differential Diagnosis. A history of mood disorders in the patient or the patient's family weighs toward the diagnosis of a primary mood disorder, although such a history does not rule out the possibility of substance-induced mood disorder. Substances can also trigger an underlying mood disorder in a patient who is biologically vulnerable to mood disorders.

Course and Prognosis. The course and prognosis of substance-induced mood disorder vary. Shortly after the substance has been cleared from the body, a normal mood usually returns. Sometimes, however, the substance exposure seems to precipitate a long-lasting mood disorder that may take weeks or months to resolve completely.

Treatment. The primary treatment of substance-induced mood disorder is the identification of the causally involved substance. Stopping the intake of the substance usually suffices to cause the mood disorder symptoms to abate. If the symptoms linger, treatment with appropriate psychiatric drugs may be necessary.

Mood Disorder Not Otherwise Specified

If patients exhibit mood symptoms that are difficult to distinguish between depression and mania and do not meet the diagnostic criteria for any other mood disorder or other DSM-IV-TR mental disorder, the most appropriate diagnosis is mood disorder not otherwise specified (Table 15.3–11). Clinicians are encouraged to try to make a more specific diagnosis, however.

ICD-10

The ICD-10 describes mood (affective) disorders as characterized by "a change in mood or affect, usually to depression (with or without associated anxiety) or to elation." A change in activity level accompanies the mood change, and "most other symptoms are either secondary to, or easily understood in the context of, such changes." These disorders are recurrent, and the onset of the episodes may be related to "stressful events or situations." The mood disorders also include those occurring in children. Table 15.3–12 lists the ICD-10 criteria for mood disorders.

References

Akiskal HS. Mood Disorders: Clinical features. In: Sadock BJ, Sadock VA, eds. *Kaplan & Sadock's Comprehensive Textbook of Psychiatry*. 8th ed. Vol. 1. Baltimore: Lippincott Williams & Wilkins; 2005:1611.

Albanese MJ, Pies R. The bipolar patient with comorbid substance use disorder: Recognition and management. *CNS Drugs*. 2004;18(9):585–596.

Grant BF, Stinson FS, Dawson DA, Chou SP, Dufour MC, Compton W, Pickering RP, Kaplan K. Prevalence and co-occurrence of substance use disorders and independent mood and anxiety disorders. *Arch Gen Psychiatry*. 2004;61:807–816.

Hill SK, Keshavan MS, Thase ME, Sweeney JA. Neuropsychological dysfunction in antipsychotic-naive first-episode unipolar psychotic depression. *Am J Psychiatry*. 2004;161:996–1003.

Iqbal Z, Birchwood M, Hemsley D, Jackson C, Morris E. Autobiographical memory and post-psychotic depression in first episode psychosis. *Br J Clin Psychol*. 2004;43(1):97–104.

Judd LL, Rapaport MH, Yonkers KA, Rush AJ, Frank E, Thase ME, Kupfer DJ, Plewes JM, Schettler PJ, Tollefson G. Randomized, placebo-controlled trial of fluoxetine for acute treatment of minor depressive disorder. *Am J Psychiatry*. 2004;161:1864–1871.

McGinn LK, Asnis GM, Suchday S, Kaplan M. Increased personality disorders and Axis I comorbidity in atypical depression. *Compr Psychiatry*. 2005;46(6):428–432.

Murray V, von Arbin M, Bartfai A, Berggren AL, Landtblom AM, Lundmark J, Nasman P, Olsson JE, Samuelsson M, Terent A, Varelius R, Asberg M, Martensson B. Double-blind comparison of sertraline and placebo in stroke patients with minor depression and less severe major depression. *J Clin Psychiatry*. 2005;66(6):708–716.

Spalletta G, Ripa A, Caltagirone C. Symptom profile of DSM-IV major and minor depressive disorders in first-ever stroke patients. *Am J Geriatr Psychiatry*. 2005;13:108–115.

Wilens TE, Biederman J, Kwon A, Ditterline J, Forkner P, Moore H, Swezey A, Snyder L, Henin A, Woznisk J, Faraone SV. Risk of substance use disorders in adolescents with bipolar disorder. *J Am Acad Child Adolesc Psychiatry*. 2004;43(11):1380–1386.

16 Anxiety Disorders

▲ 16.1 Overview

Anxiety disorders are among the most prevalent mental disorders in the general population. Nearly 30 million persons are affected in the United States, with women affected nearly twice as frequently as men. Anxiety disorders are associated with significant morbidity and often are chronic and resistant to treatment. Anxiety disorders can be viewed as a family of related but distinct mental disorders, which include the following as classified in the text revision of the fourth edition of *Diagnostic and Statistical Manual of Mental Disorders* (DSM-IV-TR): (1) panic disorder with or without agoraphobia; (2) agoraphobia with or without panic disorder; (3) specific phobia; (4) social phobia; (5) obsessive-compulsive disorder (OCD); (5) posttraumatic stress disorder (PTSD); (6) acute stress disorder; and (7) generalized anxiety disorder. Each of these disorders is discussed in detail in the sections that follow. For an overview of the features of all the anxiety disorders, see Table 16.1–1.

A fascinating aspect of anxiety disorders is the exquisite interplay of genetic and experiential factors. Little doubt exists that abnormal genes predispose to pathological anxiety states; however, evidence clearly indicates that traumatic life events and stress are also etiologically important. Thus, the study of anxiety disorders presents a unique opportunity to understand the relation between nature and nurture in the etiology of mental disorders.

NORMAL ANXIETY

Everyone experiences anxiety. It is characterized most commonly as a diffuse, unpleasant, vague sense of apprehension, often accompanied by autonomic symptoms such as headache, perspiration, palpitations, tightness in the chest, mild stomach discomfort, and restlessness, indicated by an inability to sit or stand still for long. The particular constellation of symptoms present during anxiety tends to vary among persons (Table 16.1–2).

Fear versus Anxiety

Anxiety is an alerting signal; it warns of impending danger and enables a person to take measures to deal with a threat. Fear is a similar alerting signal, but should be differentiated from anxiety. Fear is a response to a known, external, definite, or nonconflictual threat; anxiety is a response to a threat that is unknown, internal, vague, or conflictual.

This distinction between fear and anxiety arose accidentally. When Freud's early translator mistranslated *angst*, the German word for "fear," as anxiety, Freud himself generally ignored the distinction that associates anxiety with a repressed, unconscious object and fear with a known, external object. The distinction may be difficult to make because fear can also be caused by an unconscious, repressed, internal object displaced to another object in the external world. For example, a boy may fear barking dogs because he actually fears his father and unconsciously associates his father with barking dogs.

Nevertheless, according to postfreudian psychoanalytic formulations, the separation of fear and anxiety is psychologically justifiable. The emotion caused by a rapidly approaching car as a person crosses the street differs from the vague discomfort a person may experience when meeting new persons in a strange setting. The main psychological difference between the two emotional responses is the suddenness of fear and the insidiousness of anxiety.

In 1896, Charles Darwin gave the following psychophysiological description of acute fear merging into terror:

> Fear is often preceded by astonishment, and is so far akin to it, that both lead to the senses of sight and learning being instantly aroused. In both cases the eyes and mouth are widely opened, and the eyebrows raised. The frightened man at first stands like a statue motionless and breathless, or crouches down as if instinctively to escape observation. The heart beats quickly and violently, so that it palpitates or knocks against the ribs; but it is very doubtful whether it then works more efficiently than usual, so as to send a greater supply of blood to all parts of the body; for the skin instantly becomes pale, as during incipient faintness. This paleness of the surface, however, is probably in large part, or exclusively, due to the vasomotor center being affected in such a manner as to cause the contraction of the small arteries of the skin. That the skin is much affected under the sense of great fear, we see in the marvelous and inexplicable manner in which perspiration immediately exudes from it. This exudation is all the more remarkable, as the surface is then cold, and hence the term a cold sweat; whereas, the sudorific glands are properly excited into action when the surface is heated. The hairs also on the skin stand erect; and the superficial muscles shiver. In connection with the disturbed action of the heart, the breathing is hurried. The salivary glands act imperfectly; the mouth becomes dry, and is often opened and shut. I have also noticed that under slight fear there is a strong tendency to yawn. One of the best-marked symptoms is the trembling of all the muscles of the body; and this is often first seen in the lips. From this cause, and from the dryness of the mouth, the voice becomes husky or indistinct, or may altogether fail. . . .

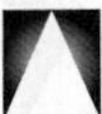

Table 16.1–1
Key Phenomenological Features of Major Anxiety Disorders As Defined by DSM-IV-TR

Panic disorder

- Recurrent unexpected panic attacks characterized by four or more of the following:
  - Palpitations
  - Sweating
  - Trembling or shaking
  - Shortness of breath
  - Feeling of choking (also known as *air hunger*)
  - Chest pain or discomfort
  - Nausea or abdominal distress
  - Feeling dizzy, lightheaded, or faint
  - Derealization or depersonalization
  - Fear of losing control or going crazy
  - Fear of dying
  - Numbness or tingling
  - Chills or hot flashes
- Persistent concern of future attacks
- Worry about the meaning of or consequences of the attacks (e.g., heart attack or stroke)
- Significant change in behavior related to the attacks (e.g., avoiding places at which panic attacks have occurred)
- ± Presence of agoraphobia

Agoraphobia

- Fear of being in places or situations from which escape might be difficult, embarrassing, or in which help may be unavailable in the event of having a panic attack
- Often results in avoidance of the feared places or situations, for example:
  - Crowds
  - Stores
  - Bridges
  - Tunnels
  - Traveling on a bus, train, or airplane
  - Theaters
  - Standing in a line
  - Small enclosed rooms

Social phobia

- Marked and persistent fear of one or more social or performance situations in which the person is concerned about negative evaluation or scrutiny by others, for example:
  - Public speaking
  - Writing, eating, or drinking in public
  - Initiating or maintaining conversations
- Fears humiliation or embarrassment, perhaps by manifesting anxiety symptoms (e.g., blushing or sweating)
- Feared social or performance situations are avoided or endured with intense anxiety or distress

Specific phobia

- Marked and persistent fear that is excessive, unreasonable, cued by the presence or anticipation of a specific object or situation, for example:
  - Flying
  - Enclosed spaces
  - Heights
  - Storms
  - Animals (e.g., snakes or spiders)
  - Receiving an injection
  - Blood
- Provokes an immediate anxiety response
- Recognition that the fear is excessive or unreasonable
- Avoidance, anticipatory anxiety, or distress is significantly impairing

Obsessive-compulsive disorder

- Has obsessions or compulsions
  - *Obsessions* are defined as recurrent and persistent thoughts, impulses, or images that are experienced as intrusive and inappropriate, for example:
    - Contamination
    - Repeated doubts
    - Order
    - Impulses
    - Sexual images
  - *Compulsions* are defined as repetitive behaviors or mental acts whose goal is to prevent or to reduce anxiety or distress, for example:
    - Hand washing
    - Ordering
    - Checking
    - Praying
    - Counting
    - Repeating words
- Recognition that the fear is excessive or unreasonable
- Obsessions cause marked distress, are time-consuming (more than 1 hour per day), or cause significant impairment in social, occupational or other daily functioning

Generalized anxiety disorder or overanxious disorder

- Excessive anxiety and worry about a number of events or activities (future oriented), occurring more days than not for at least 6 months
- Worry is difficult to control
- Worry is associated with at least three of the following symptoms:
  - Restlessness or feeling keyed up or on edge
  - Easily fatigued
  - Difficulty concentrating
  - Irritability
  - Muscle tension
  - Sleep disturbance
- Anxiety and worry cause significant distress and impairment in social, occupational, or other daily functioning

Separation anxiety disorder

- Developmentally inappropriate and excessive anxiety concerning separation from home or to an attachment figure. Characterized by three or more of the following:
  - Recurrent and excessive distress when separation from home or major attachment figure occurs or is anticipated
  - Persistent and excessive worry that major attachment figure will be lost or harmed
  - Persistent and excessive worry that an event will lead to separation from major attachment figure (e.g., getting kidnapped)
  - Persistent and recurring fear of being alone or without attachment figure at home
  - Reluctance or refusal to sleep away from home or without being near major attachment figure
  - Duration of at least 4 weeks
  - Age of onset before 18 years of age
  - Causes distress or impairment in functioning
  - Physical symptoms (e.g., headaches, stomachaches, nausea, and vomiting) when separation occurs or is anticipated

(From American Psychiatric Association. *Diagnostic and Statistical Manual of Mental Disorders*. 4th ed. Text rev. Washington, DC: American Psychiatric Association; copyright 2000, with permission.)

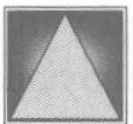

Table 16.1–2
Peripheral Manifestations of Anxiety

Diarrhea
Dizziness, light-headedness
Hyperhidrosis
Hyperreflexia
Hypertension
Palpitations
Pupillary mydriasis
Restlessness (e.g., pacing)
Syncope
Tachycardia
Tingling in the extremities
Tremors
Upset stomach ("butterflies")
Urinary frequency, hesitancy, urgency

As fear increases into an agony of terror, we behold, as under all violent emotions, diversified results. The heart beats wildly or may fail to act and faintness ensues; there is a deathlike pallor; the breathing is labored; the wings of the nostrils are widely dilated; there is a gasping and convulsive motion on the lips, a tremor on the hollow cheek, a gulping and catching of the throat; the uncovered and protruding eyeballs are fixed on the object of terror; or they may roll restlessly from side to side. The pupils are said to be enormously dilated. All the muscles of the body may become rigid, or may be thrown into convulsive movements. The hands are alternately clenched and opened, often with a twitching movement. The arms may be protruded, as if to avert some dreadful danger, or may be thrown wildly over the head. . . . In other cases there is a sudden and uncontrollable tendency to headlong flight; and so strong is this, that the boldest soldiers may be seized with a sudden panic.

Is Anxiety Adaptive?

Anxiety and fear both are alerting signals and act as a warning of an internal and external threat. Anxiety can be conceptualized as a normal and adaptive response that has lifesaving qualities, and warns of threats of bodily damage, pain, helplessness, possible punishment, or the frustration of social or bodily needs; of separation from loved ones; of a menace to one's success or status; and ultimately of threats to unity or wholeness. It prompts a person to take the necessary steps to prevent the threat or to lessen its consequences. This preparation is accompanied by increased somatic and autonomic activity controlled by the interaction of the sympathetic and parasympathetic nervous systems. Examples of a person warding off threats in daily life include getting down to the hard work of preparing for an examination, dodging a ball thrown at the head, sneaking into the dormitory after curfew to prevent punishment, and running to catch the last commuter train. Thus, anxiety prevents damage by alerting the person to carry out certain acts that forestall the danger.

Stress and Anxiety

Whether an event is perceived as stressful depends on the nature of the event and on the person's resources, psychological defenses, and coping mechanisms. All involve the ego, a collective abstraction for the process by which a person perceives, thinks, and acts on external events or internal drives. A person whose ego is functioning properly is in adaptive balance with both external and internal worlds; if the ego is not functioning properly and the resulting imbalance continues sufficiently long, the person experiences chronic anxiety.

Whether the imbalance is external, between the pressures of the outside world and the person's ego, or internal, between the person's impulses (e.g., aggressive, sexual, and dependent impulses) and conscience, the imbalance produces a conflict. Externally caused conflicts are usually interpersonal, whereas those that are internally caused are intrapsychic or intrapersonal. A combination of the two is possible, as in the case of employees whose excessively demanding and critical boss provokes impulses that they must control for fear of losing their jobs. Interpersonal and intrapsychic conflicts, in fact, are usually intertwined. Because human beings are social, their main conflicts are usually with other persons.

Symptoms of Anxiety

The experience of anxiety has two components: the awareness of the physiological sensations (e.g., palpitations and sweating) and the awareness of being nervous or frightened. A feeling of shame may increase anxiety—"Others will recognize that I am frightened." Many persons are astonished to find out that others are not aware of their anxiety or, if they are, do not appreciate its intensity.

In addition to motor and visceral effects (Table 16.1–2), anxiety affects thinking, perception, and learning. It tends to produce confusion and distortions of perception, not only of time and space but also of persons and the meanings of events. These distortions can interfere with learning by lowering concentration, reducing recall, and impairing the ability to relate one item to another—that is, to make associations.

An important aspect of emotions is their effect on the selectivity of attention. Anxious persons likely select certain things in their environment and overlook others in their effort to prove that they are justified in considering the situation frightening. If they falsely justify their fear, they augment their anxieties by the selective response and set up a vicious circle of anxiety, distorted perception, and increased anxiety. If, alternatively, they falsely reassure themselves by selective thinking, appropriate anxiety may be reduced, and they may fail to take necessary precautions.

PATHOLOGICAL ANXIETY

Epidemiology

The anxiety disorders make up one of the most common groups of psychiatric disorders. The National Comorbidity Study reported that one of four persons met the diagnostic criteria for at least one anxiety disorder and that there is a 12-month prevalence rate of 17.7 percent. Women (30.5 percent lifetime prevalence) are more likely to have an anxiety disorder than are men (19.2 percent lifetime prevalence). The prevalence of anxiety disorders decreases with higher socioeconomic status.

Contributions of Psychological Sciences

Three major schools of psychological theory—psychoanalytic, behavioral, and existential —have contributed theories about the causes of anxiety. Each theory has both conceptual and practical usefulness in treating anxiety disorders.

Psychoanalytic Theories. Although Freud originally believed that anxiety stemmed from a physiological buildup of libido, he ultimately redefined anxiety as a signal of the presence of danger in the unconscious. Anxiety was viewed as the result of psychic conflict between unconscious sexual or aggressive wishes and corresponding threats from the superego or external reality. In response to this signal, the ego mobilized defense mechanisms to prevent unacceptable thoughts and feelings from emerging into conscious awareness. In his classic paper "Inhibitions, Symptoms, and Anxiety," Freud states that "it was anxiety which produced repression and not, as I formerly believed, repression which produced anxiety." Today, many neurobiologists continue to substantiate many of Freud's original ideas and theories. One example is the role of the amygdala, which subserves the fear response without any reference to conscious memory and substantiates Freud's concept of an unconscious memory system for anxiety responses. One of the unfortunate consequences of regarding the symptom of anxiety as a disorder rather than a signal is that the underlying sources of the anxiety may be ignored. From a psychodynamic perspective, the goal of therapy is not necessary to eliminate all anxiety but to increase anxiety tolerance, that is, the capacity to experience anxiety and use it as a signal to investigate the underlying conflict that has created it. Anxiety appears in response to various situations during the life cycle and, although psychopharmacological agents may ameliorate symptoms, they may do nothing to address the life situation or its internal correlates that have induced the state of anxiety. In the following case a disturbing fantasy precipitated an anxiety attack.

> A married man 32 years of age was referred for therapy for severe and incapacitating anxiety, which was clinically manifested as repeated outbreaks of acute attacks of panic. Initially, he had absolutely no idea what had precipitated his attacks, nor were they associated with any conscious mental content. In the early weeks of treatment, he spent most of his time trying to impress the doctor with how hard he had worked and how effectively he had functioned before he was taken ill. At the same time, he described how fearful he was that he would fail at a new business venture he had embarked on. One day, with obvious acute anxiety that practically prevented him from talking, he revealed a fantasy that had suddenly popped into his mind a day or two before and had led to the outbreak of a severe anxiety attack. He had had the image of a large spike being driven through his penis. He also recalled that, as a child of 7, he was fascinated by his mother's clothing and that, on occasion, when she was out of the house, he dressed himself up in them. As an adult, he was fascinated by female lingerie and would sometimes find himself impelled by a desire to wear women's clothing. He had never yielded to the impulse, but on those occasions when the idea entered his consciousness, he became overwhelmed by acute anxiety and panic.

To understand fully a particular patient's anxiety from a psychodynamic view, it is often useful to relate the anxiety to developmental issues. At the earliest level, disintegration anxiety may be present. This anxiety derives from the fear that the self will fragment because others are not responding with needed affirmation and validation. Persecutory anxiety can be connected with the perception that the self is being invaded and annihilated by an outside malevolent force. Another source of anxiety involves the child who fears losing the love or approval of a parent or loved object. Freud's theory of castration anxiety is linked to the oedipal phase of development in boys, in which a powerful parental figure, usually the father, may damage the little boy's genitals or otherwise cause bodily harm. (See Section 6.1 for a discussion of Freud's theories.) At the most mature level, superego anxiety is related to guilt feelings about not living up to internalized standards of moral behavior derived from the parents. Often, a psychodynamic interview can elucidate the principal level of anxiety with which a patient is dealing. Some anxiety is obviously related to multiple conflicts at various developmental levels.

Behavioral Theories. The behavioral or learning theories of anxiety postulate that anxiety is a conditioned response to a specific environmental stimulus. In a model of classic conditioning, a girl raised by an abusive father, for example, may become anxious as soon as she sees the abusive father. Through generalization, she may come to distrust all men. In the social learning model, a child may develop an anxiety response by imitating the anxiety in the environment, such as in anxious parents.

Existential Theories. Existential theories of anxiety provide models for generalized anxiety, in which no specifically identifiable stimulus exists for a chronically anxious feeling. The central concept of existential theory is that persons experience feelings of living in a purposeless universe. Anxiety is their response to the perceived void in existence and meaning. Such existential concerns may have increased since the development of nuclear weapons and bioterrorism.

Contributions of Biological Sciences

Autonomic Nervous System. Stimulation of the autonomic nervous system causes certain symptoms—cardiovascular (e.g., tachycardia), muscular (e.g., headache), gastrointestinal (e.g., diarrhea), and respiratory (e.g., tachypnea). The autonomic nervous systems of some patients with anxiety disorder, especially those with panic disorder, exhibit increased sympathetic tone, adapt slowly to repeated stimuli, and respond excessively to moderate stimuli.

Neurotransmitters. The three major neurotransmitters associated with anxiety on the bases of animal studies and responses to drug treatment are norepinephrine (NE), serotonin, and γ-aminobutyric acid (GABA). Much of the basic neuroscience information about anxiety comes from animal experiments involving behavioral paradigms and psychoactive agents. One such experiment to study anxiety was the conflict test, in which the animal is simultaneously presented with stimuli that are positive (e.g., food) and negative (e.g., electric shock). Anxiolytic drugs (e.g., benzodiazepines) tend to facilitate the adaptation of the animal to this situation, whereas other drugs (e.g., amphetamines) further disrupt the animal's behavioral responses.

NOREPINEPHRINE. Chronic symptoms experienced by patients with anxiety disorder, such as panic attacks, insomnia, startle, and autonomic hyperarousal, are characteristic of increased noradrenergic function. The general theory about the role of norepinephrine in anxiety disorders is that affected patients may have a poorly regulated noradrenergic system with occasional bursts of activity. The cell bodies of the noradrenergic system are primarily localized to the locus ceruleus in the rostral pons, and they project their axons to the cerebral cortex, the limbic system, the brainstem, and the spinal cord. Experiments in primates have demonstrated that stimulation of the locus ceruleus produces a fear response in the animals and that ablation of the same area inhibits or completely blocks the ability of the animals to form a fear response.

Human studies have found that in patients with panic disorder, β-adrenergic receptor agonists (e.g., isoproterenol [Isuprel]) and α_2-adrenergic receptor antagonists (e.g., yohimbine [Yocon]) can provoke frequent and severe panic attacks. Conversely, clonidine (Catapres), an α_2-receptor agonist, reduces anxiety symptoms in some experimental and therapeutic situations. A less-consistent finding is that patients with anxiety disorders, particularly panic disorder, have elevated cerebrospinal fluid (CSF) or urinary levels of the noradrenergic metabolite 3-methoxy-4-hydroxyphenylglycol (MHPG).

HYPOTHALAMIC-PITUITARY-ADRENAL AXIS. Consistent evidence indicates that many forms of psychological stress increase the synthesis and release of cortisol. Cortisol serves to mobilize and to replenish energy stores and contributes to increased arousal, vigilance, focused attention, and memory formation; inhibition of the growth and reproductive system; and containment of the immune response. Excessive and sustained cortisol secretion can have serious adverse effects, including hypertension, osteoporosis, immunosuppression, insulin resistance, dyslipidemia, dyscoagulation, and, ultimately, atherosclerosis and cardiovascular disease. Alterations in hypothalamic-pituitary-adrenal (HPA) axis function have been demonstrated in PTSD. In patients with panic disorder, blunted adrenocorticoid hormone (ACTH) responses to corticotropin-releasing factor (CRF) have been reported in some studies and not in others.

CORTICOTROPIN-RELEASING HORMONE (CRH). One of the most important mediators of the stress response, CRH coordinates the adaptive behavioral and physiological changes that occur during stress. Hypothalamic levels of CRH are increased by stress, resulting in activation of the HPA axis and increased release of cortisol and dehydroepiandrosterone (DHEA). CRH also inhibits a variety of neurovegetative functions, such as food intake, sexual activity, and endocrine programs for growth and reproduction.

SEROTONIN. The identification of many serotonin receptor types has stimulated the search for the role of serotonin in the pathogenesis of anxiety disorders. Different types of acute stress result in increased 5-hydroxytryptamine (5-HT) turnover in the prefrontal cortex, nucleus accumbens, amygdala, and lateral hypothalamus. The interest in this relation was initially motivated by the observation that serotonergic antidepressants have therapeutic effects in some anxiety disorders—for example, clomipramine (Anafranil) in OCD. The effectiveness of buspirone (BuSpar), a serotonin 5-HT_{1A} receptor agonist, in the treatment of anxiety disorders also suggests the possibility of an association between serotonin and anxiety. The cell bodies of most serotonergic neurons are located in the raphe nuclei in the rostral brainstem and project to the cerebral cortex, the limbic system (especially, the amygdala and the hippocampus), and the hypothalamus. Several reports indicate that meta-chlorophenylpiperazine (mCPP), a drug with multiple serotonergic and nonserotonergic effects, and fenfluramine (Pondimin), which causes the release of serotonin, do cause increased anxiety in patients with anxiety disorders; and many anecdotal reports indicate that serotonergic hallucinogens and stimulants—for example, lysergic acid diethylamide (LSD) and 3,4-methylenedioxymethamphetamine (MDMA)—are associated with the development of both acute and chronic anxiety disorders in persons who use these drugs. Clinical studies of 5-HT function in anxiety disorders have had mixed results. One study found that patients with panic disorder had lower levels of circulating 5-HT compared with controls. Thus, no clear pattern of abnormality in 5-HT function in panic disorder has emerged from analysis of peripheral blood elements.

GABA. A role of GABA in anxiety disorders is most strongly supported by the undisputed efficacy of benzodiazepines, which enhance the activity of GABA at the GABA type A ($GABA_A$) receptor, in the treatment of some types of anxiety disorders. Although low-potency benzodiazepines are most effective for the symptoms of generalized anxiety disorder, high-potency benzodiazepines, such as alprazolam (Xanax), and clonazepam are effective in the treatment of panic disorder. Studies in primates have found that autonomic nervous system symptoms of anxiety disorders are induced when a benzodiazepine inverse agonist, β-carboline-3-carboxylic acid (BCCE), is administered. BCCE also causes anxiety in normal control volunteers. A benzodiazepine antagonist, flumazenil (Romazicon), causes frequent severe panic attacks in patients with panic disorder. These data have led researchers to hypothesize that some patients with anxiety disorders have abnormal functioning of their $GABA_A$ receptors, although this connection has not been shown directly.

APLYSIA. A neurotransmitter model for anxiety disorders is based on the study of *Aplysia Californica*, by Nobel Prize winner Eric Kandel, M.D. *Aplysia* is a sea snail that reacts to danger by moving away, withdrawing into its shell, and decreasing its feeding behavior. These behaviors can be classically conditioned, so that the snail responds to a neutral stimulus as if it were a dangerous stimulus. The snail can also be sensitized by random shocks, so that it exhibits a flight response in the absence of real danger. Parallels have previously been drawn between classic conditioning and human phobic anxiety. The classically conditioned *Aplysia* shows measurable changes in presynaptic facilitation, resulting in the release of increased amounts of neurotransmitter. Although the sea snail is a simple animal, this work shows an experimental approach to complex neurochemical processes potentially involved in anxiety disorders in humans.

NEUROPEPTIDE Y. Neuropeptide Y (NPY) is a highly conserved 36–amino acid peptide, which is among the most abundant peptides found in mammalian brain. Evidence suggesting the involvement of the amygdala in the anxiolytic effects of NPY is robust, and it probably occurs via the NPY-Y1 receptor. NPY has counter regulatory effects on CRH and LC-NE systems at brain sites that are important in the expression of anxiety, fear, and depression. Preliminary studies in special operations soldiers under extreme training stress indicate that high NPY levels are associated with better performance.

GALANIN. Galanin is a peptide that, in humans, contains 30 amino acids. It has been demonstrated to be involved in a number of physiological and behavioral functions, including learning and memory, pain control, food intake, neuroendocrine control, cardiovascular regulation, and, most recently, anxiety. A dense galanin immunoreactive fiber system originating in the LC innervates forebrain and midbrain structures, including the hippocampus, hypothalamus, amygdala, and prefrontal cortex. Studies in rats have shown that galanin administered centrally modulates anxiety-related behaviors. Galanin and NPY receptor agonists may be novel targets for antianxiety drug development.

Brain-Imaging Studies. A range of brain-imaging studies, almost always conducted with a specific anxiety disorder, has produced several possible leads in the understanding of anxiety disorders. Structural studies—for example, computed tomography (CT) and magnetic resonance imaging (MRI)—occasionally show some increase in the size of cerebral ventricles. In one study, the increase was correlated with the length of time patients had been taking benzodiazepines. In one MRI study, a specific defect in the right temporal lobe was noted in patients with panic disorder. Several other brain-imaging studies have reported

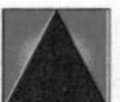

Table 16.1–3
ICD-10 Diagnostic Criteria for Phobic Anxiety Disorders

Agoraphobia

A. There is marked and consistently manifest fear in, or avoidance of, at least two of the following situations:
 (1) crowds;
 (2) public places;
 (3) traveling alone;
 (4) traveling away from home.

B. At least two symptoms of anxiety in the feared situation must have been present together, on at least one occasion since the onset of the disorder, and one of the symptoms must have been from items (1) to (4) listed below.

Autonomic arousal symptoms
 (1) palpitations or pounding heart, or accelerated heart rate;
 (2) sweating;
 (3) trembling or shaking;
 (4) dry mouth (not due to medication or dehydration);

Symptoms involving chest and abdomen
 (5) difficulty in breathing;
 (6) feeling of choking;
 (7) chest pain or discomfort;
 (8) nausea or abdominal distress (e.g., churning in stomach);

Symptoms involving mental state
 (9) feeling dizzy, unsteady, faint, or light-headed;
 (10) feelings that objects are unreal (derealization), or that the self is distant or "not really here" (depersonalization);
 (11) fear of losing control, "going crazy," or passing out;
 (12) fear of dying

General symptoms
 (13) hot flushes or cold chills;
 (14) numbness or tingling sensations.

C. Significant emotional distress is caused by the avoidance or by the anxiety symptoms, and the individual recognizes that these are excessive or unreasonable.

D. Symptoms are restricted to, or predominate in, the feared situations or contemplation of the feared situations.

E. *Most commonly used exclusion clause.* Fear or avoidance of situations (Criterion A) is not the result of delusions, hallucinations, or other disorders such as organic mental disorders, schizophrenia and related disorders, mood [affective] disorders, or obsessive-compulsive disorder, and is not secondary to cultural beliefs.

The presence or absence of panic disorder in a majority of agoraphobic situations may be specified by using a fifth character.

Without panic disorder

With panic disorder

Options for rating severity

Severity in agoraphobia may be rated by indicating the degree of avoidance, taking into account the specific cultural setting. Severity in social phobias may be rated by counting the number of panic attacks.

Social phobias

A. Either of the following must be present.
 (1) marked fear of being the focus of attention, or fear of behaving in a way that will be embarrassing or humiliating;
 (2) marked avoidance of being the focus of attention, or of situations in which there is fear of behaving in an embarrassing or humiliating way.

These fears are manifested in social situations, such as eating or speaking in public, encountering known individuals in public or entering or enduring small group situations (e.g., parties, meetings, classrooms).

B. At least two symptoms of anxiety in the feared situation as defined in agoraphobia, Criterion B, must have been manifest at some time since the onset of the disorder, together with at least one of the following symptoms:
 (1) blushing or shaking;
 (2) fear of vomiting;
 (3) urgency or fear of micturition or defecation.

C. Significant emotional distress is caused by the symptoms or by the avoidance, and the individual recognizes that these are excessive or unreasonable.

D. Symptoms are restricted to, or predominate in, the feared situations or contemplation of the feared situations.

E. *Most commonly used exclusion clause.* The symptoms listed in Criteria A and B are not the result of delusions, hallucinations, or other disorders such as organic mental disorders, schizophrenia and related disorders, mood [affective] disorders, or obsessive-compulsive disorder, and are not secondary to cultural beliefs.

Specific (isolated) phobias.

A. Either of the following must be present:
 (1) marked fear of a specific object or situation not included in agoraphobia or social phobia;
 (2) marked avoidance of a specific object or situation not included in agoraphobia or social phobia.

Among the most common objects and situations are animals, birds, insects, heights, thunder, flying, small enclosed spaces the sight of blood or injury, injections, dentists, and hospitals.

B. Symptoms of anxiety in the feared situation as defined in agoraphobia, Criterion B, must have been manifest at some time since the onset of the disorder.

C. Significant emotional distress is caused by the symptoms or by the avoidance, and the individual recognizes that these are excessive or unreasonable.

D. Symptoms are restricted to the feared situation or contemplation of the feared situation.

If desired, the specific phobias may be subdivided as follows.
—animal type (e.g., insects, dogs)
—nature-forces type (e.g., storms, water)
—blood, injection, and injury type.
—situation type (e.g., elevators, tunnels)
—other type

Other phobic anxiety disorders

Phobic anxiety disorder, unspecified

(From World Health Organization. *The ICD-10 Classification of Mental and Behavioural Disorders: Diagnostic Criteria for Research.* Copyright, World Health Organization, Geneva, 1993, with permission.)

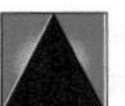

Table 16.1–4
ICD-10 Diagnostic Criteria for Other Anxiety Disorders

Panic disorder [episodic paroxysmal anxiety]

A. The individual experiences recurrent panic attacks that are not consistently associated with a specific situation or object and that often occur spontaneously (i.e., the episodes are unpredictable). The panic attacks are not associated with marked exertion or with exposure to dangerous or life-threatening situations.

B. A panic attack is characterized by all of the following:
  (1) it is a discrete episode of intense fear of discomfort;
  (2) it starts abruptly;
  (3) it reaches a maximum within a few minutes and lasts at least some minutes;
  (4) at least four of the symptoms listed below must be present, one of which must be from items (a) to (d):

Autonomic arousal symptoms
  (a) palpitations or pounding heart, or accelerated heart rate;
  (b) sweating;
  (c) trembling or shaking;
  (d) dry mouth (not due to medication or dehydration);

Symptoms involving chest and abdomen
  (e) difficulty in breathing;
  (f) feeling of choking;
  (g) chest pain or discomfort;
  (h) nausea or abdominal distress (e.g., churning in stomach);

Symptoms involving mental state
  (i) feeling dizzy, unsteady, faint, or light-headed;
  (j) feeling that objects are unreal (derealization), or that the self is distant or "not really here" (depersonalization);
  (k) fear of losing control, "going crazy," or passing out;
  (l) fear of dying;

General symptoms
  (m) hot flushes or cold chills;
  (n) numbness or tingling sensations.

C. *Most commonly used exclusion clause.* Panic attccks are not due to a physical disorder, organic mental disorder, or other mental disorders, such as schizophrenia and related disorders, mood [affective] disorders, or somatoform disorders.

The range of individual variation in both content and severity is so great that two grades, moderate and severe, may be specified, if desired, with a fifth character.

Panic disorder, moderate
At least four panic attacks in a 4-week period.

Panic disorder, severe
At least four panic attacks per week over a 4-week period.

Generalized anxiety disorder

Note. In children and adolescents the range of complaints by which the general anxiety is manifest is often more limited than in adults, and the specific symptoms of autonomic arousal are often less prominent. For these individuals, an alternative set of criteria is provided for use (in generalized anxiety disorder of childhood) if preferred.

A. There must have been a period of at least 6 months with prominent tension, worry, and feelings of apprehension about everyday events and problems.

B. At least four of the symptoms listed below must be present, at least one of which must be from items (1) to (4):

Autonomic arousal symptoms
  (1) palpitations or pounding heart, or accelerated heart rate;
  (2) sweating;
  (3) trembling or shaking;
  (4) dry mouth (not due to medication or dehydration);

Symptoms involving chest and abdomen
  (5) difficulty in breathing;
  (6) feeling of choking;
  (7) chest pain or discomfort;
  (8) nausea or abdominal distress (e.g., churning in stomach);

Symptoms involving mental state
  (9) feeling dizzy, unsteady, faint, or light-headed;
  (10) feelings that objects are unreal (derealization), or that the self is distant or "not really here" (depersonalization);
  (11) fear of losing control, "going crazy," or passing out;
  (12) fear of dying;

General symptoms
  (13) hot flushes or cold chills;
  (14) numbness or tingling sensations;

Symptoms of tension
  (15) muscle tension or aches and pains;
  (16) restlessness and inability to relax;
  (17) feeling keyed up, on edge, or mentally tense;
  (18) a sensation of a lump in the throat, or difficulty in swallowing;

Other nonspecific symptoms
  (19) exaggerated response to minor surprise or being startled;
  (20) difficulty in concentrating, or mind "going blank," because of worrying or anxiety;
  (21) persistent irritability;
  (22) difficulty in getting to sleep because of worrying.

C. The disorder does not meet the criteria for panic disorder, phobic anxiety disorders, obsessive-compulsive disorder, or hypochondriacal disorder.

D. *Most commonly used exclusion clause.* The anxiety disorder is not due to a physical disorder, such as hyperthyroidism, an organic mental disorder, or a psychoactive substance-related disorder, such as excess consumption of amphetaminelike substances or withdrawal from benzodiazepines.

Mixed anxiety and depressive disorder

There are so many possible combinations of comparatively mild symptoms for these disorders that specific criteria are not given other than those already in *Clinical Descriptions and Diagnostic Guidelines.* It is suggested that researchers wishing to study patients with these disorders should arrive at their own criteria within the guidelines, depending upon the setting and purpose of their studies.

Other mixed anxiety disorders

Other specified anxiety disorders

Anxiety disorder, unspecified

(From World Health Organization. *The ICD-10 Classification of Mental and Behavioural Disorders: Diagnostic Criteria for Research.* Copyright, World Health Organization, Geneva, 1993, with permission.)

abnormal findings in the right hemisphere but not the left hemisphere; this finding suggests that some types of cerebral asymmetries may be important in the development of anxiety disorder symptoms in specific patients. Functional brain-imaging (fMRI) studies—for example, positron emission tomography (PET), single photon emission computed tomography (SPECT), and electroencephalography (EEG)—of patients with anxiety disorder have variously reported abnormalities in the frontal cortex, the occipital and temporal areas, and, in a study of panic disorder, the parahippocampal gyrus. Several functional neuroimaging studies have implicated the caudate nucleus in the pathophysiology of OCD. In posttraumatic stress disorder, fMRI studies have found increased activity in the amygdala, a brain region associated with fear (*see* Color Plate Fig. 16.1–1 on p. 494). A conservative interpretation of these data is that some patients with anxiety disorders have a demonstrable functional cerebral pathological condition and that the condition may be causally relevant to their anxiety disorder symptoms.

Genetic Studies. Genetic studies have produced solid evidence that at least some genetic component contributes to the development of anxiety disorders. Heredity has been recognized as a predisposing factor in the development of anxiety disorders. Almost half of all patients with panic disorder have at least one affected relative. The figures for other anxiety disorders, although not as high, also indicate a higher frequency of the illness in first-degree relatives of affected patients than in the relatives of nonaffected persons. Although adoption studies with anxiety disorders have not been reported, data from twin registers also support the hypothesis that anxiety disorders are at least partially genetically determined. Clearly, a linkage exists between genetics and anxiety disorders, but no anxiety disorder is likely to result from a simple mendelian abnormality. One report has attributed about 4 percent of the intrinsic variability of anxiety within the general population to a polymorphic variant of the gene for the serotonin transporter, which is the site of action of many serotonergic drugs. Persons with the variant produce less transporter and have higher levels of anxiety.

In 2005, a scientific team, led by National Institute of Mental Health (NIMH) grantee and Noble Laureate Dr. Eric Kandel demonstrated that knocking out a gene in the brain's fear hub creates mice unperturbed by situations that would normally trigger instinctive or learned fear responses. The gene codes for *stathmin*, a protein that is critical for the amygdala to form fear memories. Stathmin knockout mice showed less anxiety when they heard a tone that had previously been associated with a shock, indicating less learned fear. The knockout mice also were more susceptible to explore novel open space and maze environments, a reflection of less innate fear. Kandel suggests that stathmin knockout mice can be used as a model of anxiety states of mental disorders with innate and learned fear components: these animals could be used to develop new antianxiety agents. Whether stathmin is similarly expressed and pivotal for anxiety in the human amygdala remains to be confirmed.

Neuroanatomical Considerations. The locus ceruleus and the raphe nuclei project primarily to the limbic system and the cerebral cortex. In combination with the data from brain-imaging studies, these areas have become the focus of much hypothesis-forming about the neuroanatomical substrates of anxiety disorders.

LIMBIC SYSTEM. In addition to receiving noradrenergic and serotonergic innervation, the limbic system also contains a high concentration of $GABA_A$ receptors. Ablation and stimulation studies in nonhuman primates have also implicated the limbic system in the generation of anxiety and fear responses. Two areas of the limbic system have received special attention in the literature: increased activity in the septohippocampal pathway, which may lead to anxiety, and the cingulate gyrus, which has been implicated particularly in the pathophysiology of OCD.

CEREBRAL CORTEX. The frontal cerebral cortex is connected with the parahippocampal region, the cingulate gyrus, and the hypothalamus and, thus, may be involved in the production of anxiety disorders. The temporal cortex has also been implicated as a pathophysiological site in anxiety disorders. This association is based in part on the similarity in clinical presentation and electrophysiology between some patients with temporal lobe epilepsy and patients with OCD.

ICD-10

In the 10th revision of *International Statistical Classification of Diseases and Related Health Problems* (ICD-10), neurotic (anxiety) disorders are grouped with stress-related and somatoform disorders because of "their historical association with the concept of neurosis and the association of a substantial (although uncertain) proportion of these disorders with psychological causation." In ICD-10, mixtures of symptoms are described

Table 16.1–5
ICD-10 Diagnostic Criteria for Obsessive-Compulsive Disorder

A. Either obsessions or compulsions (or both) are present on most days for a period of at least 2 weeks.
B. Obsessions (thoughts, ideas, or images) and compulsions (acts) share the following features, all of which must be present:
 (1) They are acknowledged as originating in the mind of the patient and are not imposed by outside persons or influences.
 (2) They are repetitive and unpleasant, and at least one obsession or compulsion that is acknowledged as excessive or unreasonable must be present.
 (3) The patient tries to resist them (but resistance to very long-standing obsessions or compulsions may be minimal). At least one obsession or compulsion that is unsuccessfully resisted must be present.
 (4) Experiencing the obsessive thought or carrying out the compulsive act is not in itself pleasurable. (This should be distinguished from the temporary relief of tension or anxiety.)
C. The obsessions or compulsions cause distress or interfere with the patient's social or individual functioning, usually by wasting time.
D. *Most commonly used exclusion clause.* The obsessions or compulsions are not the result of other mental disorders, such as schizophrenia and related disorders or mood [affective] disorders.

The diagnosis may be further specified by the following four-character codes:
 Predominantly obsessional thoughts and ruminations
 Predominantly compulsive acts [obsessional rituals]
 Mixed obsessional thoughts and acts
 Other obsessive-compulsive disorders
 Obsessive-compulsive disorder, unspecified

(From World Health Organization. *The ICD-10 Classification of Mental and Behavioural Disorders: Diagnostic Criteria for Research.* Copyright, World Health Organization, Geneva, 1993, with permission.)

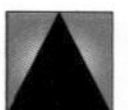

Table 16.1–6
ICD-10 Diagnostic Criteria for Reactions to Severe Stress

Acute stress reaction

A. The patient must have been exposed to an exceptional mental or physical stressor.

B. Exposure to the stressor is followed by an immediate onset of symptoms (within 1 hour).

C. Two groups of symptoms are given: the acute stress reaction is graded as:
Mild
Only Criterion (1) below is fulfilled.
Moderate
Criterion (1) is met, and there are any two symptoms from Criterion (2).
Severe
Either criterion (1) is met, and there are any four symptoms from criterion (2); *or* there is dissociative stupor.
(1) Criteria B, C, and D for generalized anxiety disorder are met.
(2) (a) Withdrawal from expected social interaction.
(b) Narrowing of attention
(c) Apparent disorientation
(d) Anger or verbal aggression
(e) Despair or hopelessness
(f) Inappropriate or purposeless overactivity
(g) Uncontrollable and excessive grief (judged by local cultural standards).

D. If the stressor is transient or can be relieved, the symptoms must begin to diminish after not more than 8 hours. If exposure to the stressor continues, the symptoms must begin to diminish after not more than 48 hours.

E. *Most commonly used exclusion clause.* The reaction must occur in the absence of any other concurrent mental or behavioral disorder in ICD-10 (except generalized anxiety disorder and personality disorders) and not within 3 months of the end of an episode of any other mental or behavioral disorder.

Posttraumatic stress disorder

A. The patient must have been exposed to a stressful event or situation (either short- or long-lasting) of an exceptionally threatening or catastrophic nature, which would be likely to cause pervasive distress in almost anyone.

B. There must be persistent remembering or "reliving" of the stressor in intrusive "flashbacks," vivid memories, or recurring dreams or in experiencing distress when exposed to circumstances resembling or associated with the stressor.

C. The patient must exhibit an actual or preferred avoidance of circumstances resembling or associated with the stressor, which was not present before exposure to the stressor.

D. Either of the following must be present:
(1) inability to recall, either partially or completely, some important aspects of the period of exposure to the stressor;
(2) persistent symptoms of increased psychological sensitivity and arousal (not present before exposure to the stressor), shown by any two of the following:
(a) difficulty in falling or staying asleep;
(b) irritability or outbursts of anger;
(c) difficulty in concentrating;
(d) hypervigilance;
(e) exaggerated startle response.

E. Criteria B, C, and D must all be met within 6 months of the stressful event or of the end of a period of stress. (For some purposes, onset delayed more than 6 months may be included, but this should be clearly specified.)

(From World Health Organization. *The ICD-10 Classification of Mental and Behavioural Disorders: Diagnostic Criteria for Research.* Copyright, World Health Organization, Geneva, 1993, with permission.)

as common, especially in less-severe varieties of these disorders, and a category for cases that cannot be based on a single main syndrome is provided. Although the idea of neurosis is no longer the organizing principle, "care has been taken to allow the easy identification of disorders that some users still might wish to regard as neurotic in their own usage of the term."

The main ICD-10 categories for "neurotic" anxiety disorders are phobic anxiety disorders (agoraphobia, social phobias, and specific phobias); other anxiety disorders (panic disorder, generalized anxiety disorder, and mixed anxiety and depressive disorder); and OCD (with predominantly obsessional thoughts, predominantly compulsive acts, or mixed obsessional thoughts and acts) (Tables 16.1–3 through 16.1–5).

In ICD-10, reaction to severe stress and adjustment disorders are grouped into one category, which is classed together with neurotic and somatoform disorders. The stress-related category differs from the other two categories, however, because it can be defined on the basis of both symptoms and one of two causative influences: a stressful life event causing an acute stress reaction or a significant life change producing an adjustment disorder. Stress-related disorders in all age groups, including children, fall into this category.

In this group, ICD-10 classifies reactions to severe stress (acute stress reaction, posttraumatic distress disorder) and adjustment disorders (see Chapter 26). ICD-10 also includes the dissociative (conversion) disorders in the category of stress-related disorders. (For a discussion of dissociative disorders, see Chapter 20.) The criteria for reactions to severe stress are given in Table 16.1–6.

References

Charney DS. Anxiety disorders: Introduction and overview. In: Sadock BJ, Sadock VA, eds. *Kaplan & Sadock's Comprehensive Textbook of Psychiatry*. 8th ed. Vol. 1. Baltimore: Lippincott Williams & Wilkins; 2005:1718.

Doyle AC, Pollack MH. Establishment of remission criteria for anxiety disorders. *J Clin Psychiatry*. 2003;64[Suppl 15]:40–45.

Hettema JM, Prescott CA, Myers JM, Neale MC, Kendler KS. The structure of genetic and environmental risk factors for anxiety disorders in men and women. *Arch Gen Psychiatry.* 2005;62:182–189.

Pigott TA. Anxiety disorders in women. *Psychiatr Clin North Am.* 2003;26: 621–672.

Schulz J, Gotto JG, Rapaport MH. The diagnosis and treatment of generalized anxiety disorder. *Primary Psychiatry.* 2005;12:58–67.

Schwartz CE, Wright CI, Shin LM, Kagan J, Rauch SL. Inhibited and uninhibited infants "grown up": Adult amygdala response to novelty. *Science.* 2003;300:1052–1053.

Stein MB. Attending to anxiety disorders in primary care. *J Clin Psychiatr.* 2003;64[Suppl 15]:35–39.

Sussman N. Anxiety disorders in the clinical setting. *Primary Psychiatry.* 2005;12:12.

Velting ON, Setzer NJ, Albano AM. Update on and advances in assessment and cognitive-behavioral treatment of anxiety disorders in children and adolescents. *Professional Psychology—Research & Practice.* 2004;35:42–54.

Wittchen HU, Beesdo K, Bittner A, Goodwin RD. Depressive episodes: Evidence for a causal role of primary anxiety disorders? *Eur Psychiatry.* 2003;18:384–393.

▲ 16.2 Panic Disorder and Agoraphobia

An acute intense attack of anxiety accompanied by feelings of impending doom is known as *panic disorder*. The anxiety is characterized by discrete periods of intense fear that can vary from several attacks during one day to only a few attacks during a year. Patients with panic disorder present with a number of comorbid conditions, most commonly agoraphobia, which refers to a fear of or anxiety regarding places from which escape might be difficult.

Agoraphobia can be the most disabling of the phobias, because it can significantly interfere with a person's ability to function in work and social situations outside the home. In the United States, most researchers of panic disorder believe that agoraphobia almost always develops as a complication in patients with panic disorder. That is, the fear of having a panic attack in a public place from which escape would be formidable is thought to cause the agoraphobia. Researchers in other countries as well as some researchers and clinicians in the United States disagree with this theory, but the text revision of the fourth edition of *Diagnostic and Statistical Manual of Mental Disorders* (DSM-IV-TR) establishes panic disorder as the predominant disorder in the dyad. DSM-IV-TR includes diagnoses for panic disorder with and without agoraphobia and also for agoraphobia without a history of panic disorder. Panic attacks can also occur in many mental disorders (e.g., depressive disorders) and medical conditions (e.g., substance withdrawal or intoxication), and the presence of a panic attack does not in itself necessitate a diagnosis of panic disorder.

HISTORY

The idea of panic disorder may have its roots in the concept of irritable heart syndrome, which the physician Jacob Mendes DaCosta (1833–1900) noted in soldiers in the American Civil War. DaCosta's syndrome included many psychological and somatic symptoms that have since been included among the diagnostic criteria for panic disorder. In 1895, Sigmund Freud introduced the concept of anxiety neurosis, consisting of acute and chronic psychological and somatic symptoms. Freud's acute anxiety neurosis was similar to panic disorder as defined in DSM-IV-TR, and Freud first noted the relation between panic attacks and agoraphobia. The term agoraphobia was coined in 1871 to describe the condition of patients who were afraid to venture alone into public places. The term is derived from the Greek words *agora* and *phobos*, meaning "fear of the marketplace."

EPIDEMIOLOGY

The lifetime prevalence of panic disorder is in the 1 to 4 percent range, with 6-month prevalence approximately 0.5 to 1.0 percent, and 3 to 5.6 percent for panic attacks. Women are two to three times more likely to be affected than men, although underdiagnosis of panic disorder in men may contribute to the skewed distribution. The differences among Hispanics, whites, and blacks are few. The only social factor identified as contributing to the development of panic disorder is a recent history of divorce or separation. Panic disorder most commonly develops in young adulthood—the mean age of presentation is about 25 years—but both panic disorder and agoraphobia can develop at any age. Panic disorder has been reported in children and adolescents, and it is probably underdiagnosed in these age groups.

The lifetime prevalence of agoraphobia is somewhat more controversial, varying between 2 to 6 percent across studies. The major factor leading to this wide range of estimates relates to disagreement about the conceptualization of agoraphobia's relationship to panic disorder. Although studies of agoraphobia in psychiatric settings have reported that at least three fourths of the affected patients have panic disorder as well, studies of agoraphobia in community samples have found that as many as half the patients have agoraphobia without panic disorder. The reasons for these divergent findings are unknown, but probably involve differences in ascertainment techniques. In many cases, the onset of agoraphobia follows a traumatic event.

COMORBIDITY

Of patients with panic disorder, 91 percent have at least one other psychiatric disorder as do 84 percent of those with agoraphobia. According to DSM-IV-TR, 10 to 15 percent of persons with panic disorder have comorbid major depressive disorder. About one third of persons with both disorders have major depressive disorder before the onset of panic disorder; about two thirds first experience panic disorder during or after the onset of major depression.

Anxiety disorders also commonly occur in persons with panic disorder and agoraphobia. Of persons with panic disorder, 15 to 30 percent also have social phobia, 2 to 20 percent have specific phobia, 15 to 30 percent have generalized anxiety disorder, 2 to 10 percent have posttraumatic stress disorder (PTSD), and up to 30 percent have obsessive-compulsive disorder (OCD). Other common comorbid conditions are hypochondriasis, personality disorders, and substance-related disorders.

ETIOLOGY

Biological Factors

Research on the biological basis of panic disorder has produced a range of findings; one interpretation is that the symptoms of panic disorder are related to a range of biological abnormalities in brain structure and function. Most work has used biological stimulants to induce panic attacks in patients with panic disorder. Considerable evidence indicates that abnormal regulation of brain noradrenergic systems is also involved in the pathophysiology of panic disorder. These and other studies have produced hypotheses implicating both peripheral and central nervous system (CNS) dysregulation in the pathophysiology of panic disorder. The autonomic nervous systems of some patients with panic disorder have been reported to exhibit increased sympathetic tone, to adapt slowly to repeated stimuli, and to respond excessively to moderate stimuli. Studies of the neuroendocrine status of these patients have shown several abnormalities, although the studies have been inconsistent in their findings.

The major neurotransmitter systems that have been implicated are those for norepinephrine, serotonin, and γ-aminobutyric acid (GABA). Serotonergic dysfunction is quite evident in panic disorder and various studies with mixed serotonin agonist-antagonist drugs have demonstrated increased rates of anxiety. Such responses may be caused by postsynaptic serotonin hypersensitivity in panic disorder. Preclinical evidence suggests that attenuation of local inhibitory GABAergic transmission in the basolateral amygdala, midbrain, and hypothalamus can elicit anxiety-like physiological responses. The biological data have led to a focus on the brainstem (particularly the noradrenergic neurons of the locus ceruleus and the serotonergic neurons of the median raphe nucleus), the limbic system (possibly responsible for the generation of anticipatory anxiety), and the prefrontal cortex (possibly responsible for the generation of phobic avoidance). Among the various neurotransmitters involved, the noradrenergic system has also attracted much attention, with the presynaptic α_2-adrenergic receptors, particularly, playing a significant role. Patients with panic disorder are sensitive to the anxiogenic effects of yohimbine in addition to having exaggerated plasma 3-methoxy-4-hydroxyphenylglycol (MHPG), cortisol, and cardiovascular responses. They have been identified by pharmacological challenges with the α_2-receptor agonist clonidine (Catapres) and the α_2-receptor antagonist yohimbine (Yocon), which stimulates firing of the locus ceruleus and elicits high rates of panic-like activity in those with panic disorder.

Panic-Inducing Substances. Panic-inducing substances (sometimes called *panicogens*) induce panic attacks in most patients with panic disorder and in a much smaller proportion of persons without panic disorder or a history of panic attacks. (The use of panic-inducing substances is strictly limited to research settings; no clinically indicated reasons exist to stimulate panic attacks in patients.) So-called respiratory panic-inducing substances cause respiratory stimulation and a shift in the acid-base balance. These substances include carbon dioxide (5 to 35 percent mixtures), sodium lactate, and bicarbonate. Neurochemical panic-inducing substances that act through specific neurotransmitter systems include yohimbine, an α_2-adrenergic receptor antagonist; m-chlorophenylpiperazine (mCPP), an agent with multiple serotonergic effects; m-Caroline drugs; $GABA_B$ receptor inverse agonists; flumazenil (Romazicon), a $GABA_B$ receptor antagonist; cholecystokinin; and caffeine. Isoproterenol (Isuprel) is also a panic-inducing substance, although its mechanism of action in inducing panic attacks is poorly understood. The respiratory panic-inducing substances may act initially at the peripheral cardiovascular baroreceptors and relay their signal by vagal afferents to the nucleus tractus solitarii and then on to the nucleus paragigantocellularis of the medulla. The hyperventilation in panic disorder patients may be caused by a hypersensitive suffocation alarm system whereby increasing P_{CO_2} and brain lactate concentrations prematurely activate a physiological asphyxia monitor. The neurochemical panic-inducing substances are presumed to primarily affect the noradrenergic, serotonergic, and GABA receptors of the CNS directly.

Brain Imaging. Structural brain-imaging studies, for example, magnetic resonance imaging (MRI), in patients with panic disorder have implicated pathological involvement in the temporal lobes, particularly the hippocampus and the amygdala. One MRI study reported abnormalities, especially cortical atrophy, in the right temporal lobe of these patients. Functional brain-imaging studies, for example, positron emission tomography (PET), have implicated dysregulation of cerebral blood flow (smaller increase or an actual decrease in cerebral blood flow). Specifically, anxiety disorders and panic attacks are associated with cerebral vasoconstriction, which may result in CNS symptoms, such as dizziness, and in peripheral nervous system symptoms that may be induced by hyperventilation and hypocapnia. Most functional brain-imaging studies have used a specific panic-inducing substance (e.g., lactate, caffeine, or yohimbine) in combination with PET or single photon emission computed tomography to assess the effects of the panic-inducing substance and the induced panic attack on cerebral blood flow.

Mitral Valve Prolapse. Although great interest was formerly expressed in an association between mitral valve prolapse and panic disorder, research has almost completely erased any clinical significance or relevance to the association. Mitral valve prolapse is a heterogeneous syndrome consisting of the prolapse of one of the mitral valve leaflets, resulting in a midsystolic click on cardiac auscultation. Studies have found that the prevalence of panic disorder in patients with mitral valve prolapse is the same as the prevalence of panic disorder in patients without mitral valve prolapse.

Genetic Factors

Although few well-controlled studies of the genetic basis of panic disorder and agoraphobia have been conducted, the data to date support the conclusion that the disorders have a distinct genetic component. In addition, some data indicate that panic disorder with agoraphobia is a severe form of panic disorder and, thus, is more likely to be inherited. Various studies have found that the first-degree relatives of patients with panic disorder have a fourfold to eightfold higher risk for panic disorder than first-degree relatives of other psychiatric patients. The twin studies conducted to date have generally reported that monozygotic twins are more likely to be concordant for panic disorder than are dizygotic twins. At this point, no data exist indicating an association between a specific chromosomal location or mode of transmission and this disorder.

Psychosocial Factors

Both cognitive-behavioral and psychoanalytic theories have been developed to explain the pathogenesis of panic disorder and agoraphobia. The success of cognitive-behavioral approaches in the treatment of these disorders may add credence to the cognitive-behavioral theories.

Cognitive-Behavioral Theories. Behavioral theories posit that anxiety is a response learned either from parental behavior or through the process of classic conditioning. In a classic conditioning approach to panic disorder and agoraphobia, a noxious stimulus (e.g., a panic attack) that occurs with a neutral stimulus (e.g., a bus ride) can result in the avoidance of the neutral stimulus. Other behavioral theories posit a linkage between the sensation of minor somatic symptoms (e.g., palpitations) and generation of a panic attack. Although cognitive-behavioral theories can help explain the development of agoraphobia or an increase in the number or severity of panic attacks, they do not explain the occurrence of the first unprovoked and unexpected panic attack that an affected patient experiences.

Psychoanalytic Theories. Psychoanalytic theories conceptualize panic attacks as arising from an unsuccessful defense against anxiety-provoking impulses. What was previously a mild signal anxiety becomes an overwhelming feeling of apprehension, complete with somatic symptoms. To explain agoraphobia, psychoanalytic theories emphasize the loss of a parent in childhood and a history of separation anxiety. Being alone in public places revives the childhood anxiety about being abandoned. The defense mechanisms used include repression, displacement, avoidance, and symbolization. Traumatic separations during childhood can affect children's developing nervous systems in such a manner that they become susceptible to anxieties in adulthood. A predisposing neurophysiological vulnerability may interact with certain kinds of environmental stressors to produce the resulting panic attack.

Many patients describe panic attacks as coming out of the blue, as though no psychological factors were involved, but psychodynamic exploration frequently reveals a clear psychological trigger for the panic attack. Although panic attacks are correlated neurophysiologically with the locus ceruleus, the onset of panic is generally related to environmental or psychological factors. Patients with panic disorder have a higher incidence of stressful life events (particularly loss) than control subjects in the months before the onset of panic disorder. Moreover, the patients typically experience greater distress about life events than control subjects do.

The hypothesis that stressful psychological events produce neurophysiological changes in panic disorder is supported by a study of female twins. The research findings revealed that panic disorder was strongly associated with both parental separation and parental death before children reached the age of 10. They were approximately seven- and fourfold times, respectively, more likely to be diagnosed with panic disorder with agoraphobia. Separation from the mother early in life was clearly more likely to result in panic disorder than was paternal separation in the cohort of 1,018 pairs of female twins. Another etiological factor in adult female patients appears to be childhood physical and sexual abuse. Approximately 60 percent of women with panic disorder have a history of childhood sexual abuse, compared with 31 percent of women with other anxiety disorders. Further support for psychological mechanisms in panic disorder can be inferred from a study of panic disorder in which patients received successful treatment with cognitive therapy. Before the therapy, the patients responded to panic attack induction with lactate. After successful cognitive therapy, lactate infusion no longer produced a panic attack.

The research indicates that the cause of panic attacks is likely to involve the unconscious meaning of stressful events and that the pathogenesis of the panic attacks may be related to neurophysiological factors triggered by the psychological reactions. Psychodynamic clinicians should always thoroughly investigate possible triggers whenever assessing a patient with panic disorder. The psychodynamics of panic disorder are summarized in Table 16.2–1.

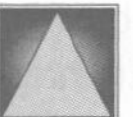

Table 16.2–1
Psychodynamic Themes in Panic Disorder

1. Difficulty tolerating anger
2. Physical or emotional separation from significant person both in childhood and in adult life
3. May be triggered by situations of increased work responsibilities
4. Perception of parents as controlling, frightening, critical, and demanding
5. Internal representations of relationships involving sexual or physical abuse
6. A chronic sense of feeling trapped
7. Vicious cycle of anger at parental rejecting behavior followed by anxiety that the fantasy will destroy the tie to parents
8. Failure of signal anxiety function in ego related to self-fragmentation and self-other boundary confusion
9. Typical defense mechanisms: reaction formation, undoing, somatization, and externalization.

DIAGNOSIS

Panic Attacks

The criteria for a panic attack are listed separately in the DSM-IV-TR (Table 16.2–2). Panic attacks can occur in mental disorders other than panic disorder, particularly in specific phobia, social phobia, and PTSD. Unexpected panic attacks occur at any time and are not associated with any identifiable situational stimulus, but panic attacks need not be unexpected. Attacks in patients with social and specific phobias are usually expected or cued to a recognized or specific stimulus. Some panic attacks do not fit easily into the distinction between unexpected and expected, and these attacks are referred to as *situationally predisposed panic attacks*. They may or may not occur when a patient is exposed to a specific trigger, or they may occur either immediately after exposure or after a considerable delay.

Panic Disorder

The DSM-IV-TR contains two diagnostic criteria for panic disorder, one without agoraphobia (Table 16.2–3) and the other with agoraphobia (Table 16.2–4), but both require the presence of panic attacks as described in Table 16.2–2. Some community surveys have indicated that panic attacks are common, and a major issue in developing diagnostic criteria for panic disorder was determining a threshold number or frequency of panic attacks required to meet the diagnosis. Setting the threshold too

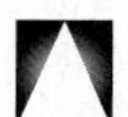

Table 16.2–2
DSM-IV-TR Criteria for Panic Attack

Note: A panic attack is not a codable disorder. Code the specific diagnosis in which the panic attack occurs (e.g., panic disorder with agoraphobia).

A discrete period of intense fear or discomfort, in which four (or more) of the following symptoms developed abruptly and reached a peak within 10 minutes:

(1) palpitations, pounding heart, or accelerated heart rate
(2) sweating
(3) trembling or shaking
(4) sensations of shortness of breath or smothering
(5) feeling of choking
(6) chest pain or discomfort
(7) nausea or abdominal distress
(8) feeling dizzy, unsteady, lightheaded, or faint
(9) derealization (feelings of unreality) or depersonalization (being detached from oneself)
(10) fear of losing control or going crazy
(11) fear of dying
(12) paresthesias (numbness or tingling sensations)
(13) chills or hot flushes

(From American Psychiatric Association. *Diagnostic and Statistical Manual of Mental Disorders.* 4th ed. Text rev. Washington, DC: American Psychiatric Association; copyright 2000, with permission.)

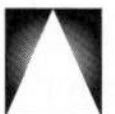

Table 16.2–3
DSM-IV-TR Diagnostic Criteria for Panic Disorder without Agoraphobia

A. Both (1) and (2):
  (1) recurrent unexpected panic attacks
  (2) at least one of the attacks has been followed by 1 month (or more) of one (or more) of the following:
    (a) persistent concern about having additional attacks
    (b) worry about the implications of the attack or its consequences (e.g., losing control, having a heart attack, "going crazy")
    (c) a significant change in behavior related to the attacks
B. Absence of agoraphobia
C. The panic attacks are not due to the direct physiological effects of a substance (e.g., a drug of abuse, a medication) or a general medical condition (e.g., hyperthyroidism).
D. The panic attacks are not better accounted for by another mental disorder, such as social phobia (e.g., occurring on exposure to feared social situations), specific phobia (e.g., on exposure to a specific phobic situation), obsessive-compulsive disorder (e.g., on exposure to dirt in someone with an obsession about contamination), posttraumatic stress disorder (e.g., in response to stimuli associated with a severe stressor), or separation anxiety disorder (e.g., in response to being away from home or close relatives).

(From American Psychiatric Association. *Diagnostic and Statistical Manual of Mental Disorders.* 4th ed. Text rev. Washington, DC: American Psychiatric Association; copyright 2000, with permission.)

low results in the diagnosis of panic disorder in patients who do not have an impairment from an occasional panic attack; setting the threshold too high results in a situation in which patients who are impaired by their panic attacks do not meet the diagnostic criteria. The vagaries of setting a threshold are evidenced by the range of thresholds set in various diagnostic criteria. The Research Diagnostic Criteria require six panic attacks during a 6-week period. The 10th revision of the *International Statistical Classification of Diseases and Related Health Problems* (ICD-10) requires three attacks in 3 weeks (for moderate disease) or four attacks in 4 weeks (for severe disease). DSM-IV-TR does not specify a minimal number of panic attacks or a time frame but does require that at least one attack be followed by at least a month-long period of concern about having another panic attack or about the implications of the attack or a significant change in behavior. DSM-IV-TR also requires that the panic attacks generally be unexpected, but allows for expected or situationally predisposed attacks.

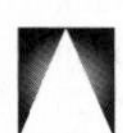

Table 16.2–4
DSM-IV-TR Diagnostic Criteria for Panic Disorder with Agoraphobia

A. Both (1) and (2):
  (1) recurrent unexpected panic attacks
  (2) at least one of the attacks has been followed by 1 month (or more) of one (or more) of the following:
    (a) persistent concern about having additional attacks
    (b) worry about the implications of the attack or its consequences (e.g., losing control, having a heart attack, "going crazy")
    (c) a significant change in behavior related to the attacks
B. The presence of agoraphobia
C. The panic attacks are not due to the direct physiological effects of a substance (e.g., a drug of abuse, a medication) or a general medical condition (e.g., hyperthyroidism).
D. The panic attacks are not better accounted for by another mental disorder, such as social phobia (e.g., occurring on exposure to feared social situations), specific phobia (e.g., on exposure to a specific phobic situation), obsessive-compulsive disorder (e.g., on exposure to dirt in someone with an obsession about contamination), posttraumatic stress disorder (e.g., in response to stimuli associated with a severe stressor), or separation anxiety disorder (e.g., in response to being away from home or close relatives).

(From American Psychiatric Association. *Diagnostic and Statistical Manual of Mental Disorders.* 4th ed. Text rev. Washington, DC: American Psychiatric Association; copyright 2000, with permission.)

Agoraphobia without History of Panic Disorder

Table 16.2–5 lists criteria for agoraphobia. The DSM-IV-TR diagnostic criteria for agoraphobia without history of panic disorder (Table 16.2–6) are based on the fear of a sudden incapacitating or embarrassing symptom. In contrast, the ICD-10 criteria require the presence of interrelated or overlapping phobias, but do not require fear of incapacitating or embarrassing symptoms.

The DSM-IV-TR criteria also address the avoidance of situations that are based on a concern related to a medical disorder (e.g., fear of a myocardial infarction in a patient with severe heart disease).

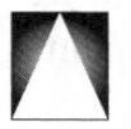

Table 16.2–5
DSM-IV-TR Criteria for Agoraphobia

Note: Agoraphobia is not a codable disorder. Code the specific disorder in which the agoraphobia occurs (e.g., panic disorder with agoraphobia or agoraphobia without history of panic disorder).

A. Anxiety about being in places or situations from which escape might be difficult (or embarrassing) or in which help may not be available in the event of having an unexpected or situationally predisposed panic attack or panic-like symptoms. Agoraphobic fears typically involve characteristic clusters of situations that include being outside the home alone; being in a crowd or standing in a line; being on a bridge; and traveling in a bus, train, or automobile.
   Note: Consider the diagnosis of specific phobia if the avoidance is limited to one or only a few specific situations, or social phobia if the avoidance is limited to social situations.
B. The situations are avoided (e.g., travel is restricted) or else are endured with marked distress or with anxiety about having a panic attack or panic-like symptoms, or require the presence of a companion.
C. The anxiety or phobic avoidance is not better accounted for by another mental disorder, such as social phobia (e.g., avoidance limited to social situations because of fear of embarrassment), specific phobia (e.g., avoidance limited to a single situation like elevators), obsessive-compulsive disorder (e.g., avoidance of dirt in someone with an obsession about contamination), posttraumatic stress disorder (e.g., avoidance of stimuli associated with a severe stressor), or separation anxiety disorder (e.g., avoidance of leaving home or relatives).

(From American Psychiatric Association. *Diagnostic and Statistical Manual of Mental Disorders.* 4th ed. Text rev. Washington, DC: American Psychiatric Association; copyright 2000, with permission.)

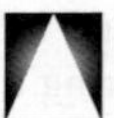

Table 16.2–6
DSM-IV-TR Diagnostic Criteria for Agoraphobia without History of Panic Disorder

A. The presence of agoraphobia related to fear of developing panic-like symptoms (e.g., dizziness or diarrhea).
B. Criteria have never been met for panic disorder.
C. The disturbance is not due to the direct physiological effects of a substance (e.g., a drug of abuse, a medication) or a general medical condition.
D. If an associated general medical condition is present, the fear described in Criterion A is clearly in excess of that usually associated with the condition.

(From American Psychiatric Association. *Diagnostic and Statistical Manual of Mental Disorders.* 4th ed. Text rev. Washington, DC: American Psychiatric Association; copyright 2000, with permission.)

CLINICAL FEATURES

Panic Disorder

The first panic attack is often completely spontaneous, although panic attacks occasionally follow excitement, physical exertion, sexual activity, or moderate emotional trauma. DSM-IV-TR emphasizes that at least the first attacks must be unexpected (uncued) to meet the diagnostic criteria for panic disorder. Clinicians should attempt to ascertain any habit or situation that commonly precedes a patient's panic attacks. Such activities may include the use of caffeine, alcohol, nicotine, or other substances; unusual patterns of sleeping or eating; and specific environmental settings, such as harsh lighting at work.

The attack often begins with a 10-minute period of rapidly increasing symptoms. The major mental symptoms are extreme fear and a sense of impending death and doom. Patients usually cannot name the source of their fear; they may feel confused and have trouble concentrating. The physical signs often include tachycardia, palpitations, dyspnea, and sweating. Patients often try to leave whatever situation they are in to seek help. The attack generally lasts 20 to 30 minutes and rarely more than an hour. A formal mental status examination during a panic attack may reveal rumination, difficulty speaking (e.g., stammering), and impaired memory. Patients may experience depression or depersonalization during an attack. The symptoms can disappear quickly or gradually. Between attacks, patients may have anticipatory anxiety about having another attack. The differentiation between anticipatory anxiety and generalized anxiety disorder can be difficult, although patients with pain disorder with anticipatory anxiety can name the focus of their anxiety.

Somatic concerns of death from a cardiac or respiratory problem may be the major focus of patients' attention during panic attacks. Patients may believe that the palpitations and chest pain indicate that they are about to die. As many as 20 percent of such patients actually have syncopal episodes during a panic attack. The patients may be seen in emergency rooms as young (20s), physically healthy persons who nevertheless insist that they are about to die from a heart attack. Rather than immediately diagnosing hypochondriasis, the emergency room physician should consider a diagnosis of panic disorder. Hyperventilation can produce respiratory alkalosis and other symptoms. The age-old treatment of breathing into a paper bag sometimes helps because it decreases alkalosis.

Ms. M is an attractive, stylishly dressed 25-year-old art director for a trade magazine who comes to an anxiety clinic after reading about the clinic program in the newspaper. She is seeking treatment for "panic attacks" that have occurred with increasing frequency over the past year, often two or three times a day. These attacks begin with a sudden intense wave of "horrible fear" that seems to come out of nowhere, sometimes during the day, sometimes waking her from sleep. She begins to tremble, is nauseated, sweats profusely, feels as though she is choking, and fears that she will lose control and do something crazy, like run screaming into the street.

Ms. M remembers first having attacks like this when she was in high school. She was dating a boy her parents disapproved of and had to do a lot of "sneaking around" to avoid confrontations with them. At the same time, she was under a lot of pressure as the principal designer of her high-school yearbook and was applying to Ivy League colleges. She remembers that her first panic attack occurred just after the yearbook went to press and she was accepted by Harvard, Yale, and Brown. The attacks lasted only a few minutes, and she would just "sit through them." She was otherwise perfectly healthy, and did not seek treatment.

Ms. M has had panic attacks intermittently over the 8 years since her first attack, sometimes not for many months, but sometimes, as now, several times a day. There have been extreme variations in the intensity of the attacks, some being so severe and debilitating that she has had to take a day off from work.

Ms. M has always functioned extremely well in school, at work, and in her social life, apart from her panic attacks and a brief period of depression at age 19 when she broke up with a boyfriend. She is a lively, friendly person who is respected by her friends and colleagues, both for her intelligence and creativity and for her ability to mediate disputes.

Ms. M has never limited her activities, even during the times that she was having frequent, severe attacks, although she might stay home from work for a day because she was exhausted from multiple attacks. She has never associated the attacks with particular places. She says, for example, that she is as likely to have an attack at home in her own bed as on the subway, so there is no point in avoiding the subway. Whether she has an attack on the subway, in a supermarket, or at home by herself, she says, "I just tough it out." (From *DSM-IV-TR Casebook.*)

Agoraphobia

Patients with agoraphobia rigidly avoid situations in which it would be difficult to obtain help. They prefer to be accompanied by a friend or a family member in busy streets, crowded stores, closed-in spaces (e.g., tunnels, bridges, and elevators), and closed-in vehicles (e.g., subways, buses, and airplanes). Patients may insist that they be accompanied every time they leave the house. The behavior can result in marital discord, which may be misdiagnosed as the primary problem. Severely affected patients may simply refuse to leave the house. Particularly before a correct diagnosis is made, patients may be terrified that they are going crazy.

Ms. A a 32-year-old medical secretary in Dublin, Ireland, is referred to a clinic for treatment of depression. She confides that the reason she is depressed is that for the last 5 months, she has been afraid that she will urinate in public. She has never actually done this; and in the safety of her own home, she considers the idea that it will actually happen to her to be nonsensical.

When Ms. A is away from home, the fear dominates her thinking, and she takes precautions to prevent its happening. She always wears sanitary napkins, never travels far from home, limits her intake of fluids, has stopped drinking alcohol, and has had her desk at work relocated near a toilet. For the 2 weeks before the consultation, she was unable to go to work because the fear had become so intense.

Ms. A vaguely recalls that her deceased father also had a fear of urinating in public. Before leaving for work each day, he urinated several times and avoided taking any fluids. Her younger sister had been successfully treated for a cleansing ritual.

Ms. A had psychiatric treatment 10 years ago when she began to fear that she had contracted syphilis, even though there was no clinical or laboratory evidence of infection. Up until 5 months ago, she had never feared that she would urinate in public. In addition to these specific fears, she has always been an anxious, insecure person, considered by her family to be overly cautious and perfectionistic. For the past year she has been upset about her boyfriend's impending return to his home country, after completing his medical studies in Ireland. She was divorced 5 years previously and is now living with her 7-year-old son and mother. Her mother disapproves of her boyfriend, and Ms. A has felt increased pressure to end the relationship. She believes that the onset of her current difficulties coincided with the stress of her relationship with her mother and the threat of her boyfriend's departure from the country.

When interviewed, Ms. A is visibly anxious. She remarks that she has been feeling despondent about her problems. She has trouble sleeping and has no energy during the day. Although her appetite is poor, she has not lost any weight. (From *DSM-IV-TR Casebook.*)

Associated Symptoms

Depressive symptoms are often present in panic disorder and agoraphobia, and in some patients, a depressive disorder coexists with the panic disorder. Some studies have found that the lifetime risk of suicide in persons with panic disorder is higher than it is in persons with no mental disorder. Clinicians should be alert to the risk of suicide. In addition to agoraphobia, other phobias and OCD can coexist with panic disorder. The psychosocial consequences of panic disorder and agoraphobia, in addition to marital discord, can include time lost from work, financial difficulties related to the loss of work, and alcohol and other substance abuse.

DIFFERENTIAL DIAGNOSIS

Panic Disorder

The differential diagnosis for a patient with panic disorder includes many medical disorders (Table 16.2–7), as well as many mental disorders.

Medical Disorders

Panic disorder, with or without agoraphobia, must be differentiated from a number of medical conditions that produce similar symptomatology. Panic attacks are associated with a variety of endocrinological disorders, including both hypo- and hyperthyroid states, hyperparathyroidism, and pheochromocytomas. Episodic hypoglycemia associated with insulinomas can also produce panic-like states, as can primary neuropathological processes. These include seizure disorders, vestibular dysfunction, neoplasms, or the effects of both prescribed and illicit substances on the CNS. Finally, disorders of the cardiac and pulmonary systems, including arrhythmias, chronic obstructive pulmonary disease, and asthma, can produce autonomic symptoms and accompanying crescendo anxiety that can be difficult to distinguish from panic disorder. Clues of an underlying medical etiology to panic-like symptoms include the presence of atypical features during panic attacks, such as ataxia, alterations in consciousness, or bladder dyscontrol; onset of panic disorder relatively late in life; and physical signs or symptoms indicative of a medical disorder.

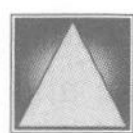

Table 16.2–7
Organic Differential Diagnosis for Panic Disorder

Cardiovascular Diseases	
Anemia	Hypertension
Angina	Mitral valve prolapse
Congestive heart failure	Myocardial infarction
Hyperactive β-adrenergic state	Paradoxical atrial tachycardia
Pulmonary Diseases	
Asthma	Pulmonary embolus
Hyperventilation	
Neurological Diseases	
Cerebrovascular disease	Migraine
Epilepsy	Multiple sclerosis
Huntington's disease	Transient ischemic attack
Infection	Tumor
Ménière's disease	Wilson's disease
Endocrine Diseases	
Addison's disease	Hypoglycemia
Carcinoid syndrome	Hypoparathyroidism
Cushing's syndrome	Menopausal disorders
Diabetes	Pheochromocytoma
Hyperthyroidism	Premenstrual syndrome
Drug Intoxications	
Amphetamine	Hallucinogens
Amyl nitrite	Marijuana
Anticholinergics	Nicotine
Cocaine	Theophylline
Drug Withdrawal	
Alcohol	Opiates and opioids
Antihypertensives	Sedative-hypnotics
Other Conditions	
Anaphylaxis	Systemic infections
B_{12} deficiency	Systemic lupus erythematosus
Electrolyte disturbances	Temporal arteritis
Heavy metal poisoning	Uremia

Mental Disorders

Panic disorder also must be differentiated from a number of psychiatric disorders, particularly other anxiety disorders. Panic attacks occur in many anxiety disorders, including social and specific phobia, PTSD, and even OCD. The key to correctly diagnosing panic disorder and differentiating the condition from other anxiety disorders involves the documentation of recurrent spontaneous panic attacks at some point in the illness. Differentiation from generalized anxiety disorder can also be difficult. Classically, panic attacks are characterized by their rapid onset (within minutes) and short duration (usually less than 10 to 15 minutes), in contrast to the anxiety associated with generalized anxiety disorder, which emerges and dissipates more slowly. Making this distinction can be difficult, however, because the anxiety surrounding panic attacks can be more diffuse and slower to dissipate than is typical. Because anxiety is a frequent concomitant of many other psychiatric disorders, including the psychoses and affective disorders, discrimination between panic disorder and a multitude of disorders can also be difficult.

Specific and Social Phobias.

DSM-IV-TR addresses the sometimes difficult diagnostic task of distinguishing between panic disorder with agoraphobia, on the one hand, and specific and social phobias, on the other hand. Some patients who experience a single panic attack in a specific setting (e.g., an elevator) may go on to have long-lasting avoidance of the specific setting, regardless of whether they ever have another panic attack. These patients meet the diagnostic criteria for a specific phobia, and clinicians must use their judgment about what is the most appropriate diagnosis. In another example, a person who experiences one or more panic attacks may then fear speaking in public. Although the clinical picture is almost identical to the clinical picture in social phobia, a diagnosis of social phobia is excluded because the avoidance of the public situation is based on fear of having a panic attack, rather than on fear of the public speaking itself. Because empirical data on the distinctions are limited, DSM-IV-TR advises clinicians to use their clinical judgment to diagnose difficult cases.

Agoraphobia without History of Panic Disorder

The differential diagnosis for agoraphobia without a history of panic disorder includes all the medical disorders that can cause anxiety or depression. The psychiatric differential diagnosis includes major depressive disorder, schizophrenia, paranoid personality disorder, avoidance personality disorder, and dependent personality disorder.

COURSE AND PROGNOSIS

Panic Disorder

Panic disorder usually has its onset in late adolescence or early adulthood, although onset during childhood, early adolescence, and midlife does occur. Some data implicate increased psychosocial stressors with the onset of panic disorder, although no psychosocial stressor can be definitely identified in most cases.

Panic disorder, in general, is a chronic disorder, although its course is variable, both among patients and within a single patient. The available long-term follow-up studies of panic disorder are difficult to interpret because they have not controlled for the effects of treatment. Nevertheless, about 30 to 40 percent of patients seem to be symptom free at long-term follow-up; about 50 percent have symptoms that are sufficiently mild not to affect their lives significantly; and about 10 to 20 percent continue to have significant symptoms.

After the first one or two panic attacks, patients may be relatively unconcerned about their condition; with repeated attacks, however, the symptoms may become a major concern. Patients may attempt to keep the panic attacks secret and thereby cause their families and friends concern about unexplained changes in behavior. The frequency and severity of the attacks can fluctuate. Panic attacks can occur several times in a day or less than once a month. Excessive intake of caffeine or nicotine can exacerbate the symptoms.

Depression can complicate the symptom picture in anywhere from 40 to 80 percent of all patients, as estimated by various studies. Although the patients do not tend to talk about suicidal ideation, they are at increased risk for committing suicide. Alcohol and other substance dependence occurs in about 20 to 40 percent of all patients, and OCD may also develop. Family interactions and performance in school and at work commonly suffer. Patients with good premorbid functioning and symptoms of brief duration tend to have good prognoses.

Agoraphobia

Most cases of agoraphobia are thought to be caused by panic disorder. When the panic disorder is treated, the agoraphobia often improves with time. For rapid and complete reduction of agoraphobia, behavior therapy is sometimes indicated. Agoraphobia without a history of panic disorder is often incapacitating and chronic, and depressive disorders and alcohol dependence often complicate its course.

TREATMENT

With treatment, most patients exhibit dramatic improvement in the symptoms of panic disorder and agoraphobia. The two most effective treatments are pharmacotherapy and cognitive-behavioral therapy. Family and group therapy may help affected patients and their families adjust to the patient's disorder and to the psychosocial difficulties that the disorder may have precipitated.

Pharmacotherapy

Overview. Alprazolam (Xanax) and paroxetine (Paxil) are the two drugs approved by the US Food and Drug Administration (FDA) for the treatment of panic disorder. In general, experience is showing superiority of the selective serotonin reuptake inhibitors (SSRIs) and clomipramine (Anafranil) over the benzodiazepines, monoamine oxidase inhibitors (MAOIs), and tricyclic and tetracyclic drugs in terms of effectiveness and tolerance of adverse effects. A few reports have suggested a role for venlafaxine (Effexor), and buspirone (BuSpar) has been suggested as an additive medication in some cases. Venlafaxine is approved by the FDA for treatment of generalized anxiety disorder and it may be useful in panic disorder combined with depression. β-adrenergic receptor antagonists have not been found to be particularly useful for panic disorder. A conservative approach is to begin treatment with paroxetine, sertraline (Zoloft), citalopram (Celexa), or fluvoxamine (Luvox) in isolated panic disorder. If rapid control of severe symptoms is desired, a brief course of alprazolam should be initiated concurrently with the SSRI, followed by slowly tapering use of the benzodiazepine. In long-term use, fluoxetine (Prozac) is an effective drug for panic with comorbid depression, although its initial activating properties may mimic panic symptoms for the first several weeks, and it may be poorly tolerated on this basis. Clonazepam (Klonopin) can be prescribed for patients who anticipate a situation in which

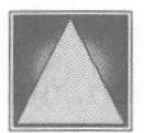

Table 16.2–8
Recommended Dosages for Antipanic Drugs (Daily Unless Indicated Otherwise)

Drug	Starting (mg)	Maintenance (mg)
SSRIs		
Paroxetine	5–10	20–60
Paroxetine CR	12.5–25	62.5
Fluoxetine	2–5	20–60
Sertraline	12.5–25	50–200
Fluvoxamine	12.5	100–150
Citalopram	10	20–40
Escitalopram	10	20
Tricyclic Antidepressants		
Clomipramine	5–12.5	50–125
Imipramine	10–25	150–500
Desipramine	10–25	150–200
Benzodiazepines		
Alprazolam	0.25–0.5 tid	0.5–2 tid
Clonazepam	0.25–0.5 bid	0.5–2 bid
Diazepam	2–5 bid	5–30 bid
Lorazepam	0.25–0.5 bid	0.5–2 bid
MAOIs		
Phenelzine	15 bid	15–45 bid
Tranylcypromine	10 bid	10–30 bid
RIMAs		
Moclobemide	50	300–600
Brofaromine	50	150–200
Atypical Antidepressants		
Venlafaxine	6.25–25	50–150
Venlafaxine XR	37.5	150–225
Other Agents		
Valproic acid	125 bid	500–750 bid
Inositol	6,000 bid	6,000 bid

SSRIs, selective serotonin reuptake inhibitors; MAOIs, monoamine oxidase inhibitors; RIMAs, reversible inhibitors of monamine oxidase type-A; bid, twice a day; tid, three times a day.

panic may occur (0.5 to 1 mg as required). Common dosages for antipanic drugs are listed in Table 16.2–8.

Selective Serotonin Reuptake Inhibitors. All SSRIs are effective for panic disorder. Paroxetine and paroxetine CR have sedative effects and tend to calm patients immediately, which leads to greater compliance and less discontinuation. Citalopram, escitalopram (Lexapro), fluvoxamine, and sertraline are the next best tolerated. Anecdotal reports suggest that patients with panic disorder are particularly sensitive to the activating effects of SSRIs, particularly fluoxetine, so they should be given initially at small dosages and titrated up slowly. Once at therapeutic dosages—for example, 20 mg a day of paroxetine—some patients may experience increased sedation. One approach for patients with panic disorder is to give 5 or 10 mg a day of paroxetine or 12.5 to 25 mg of paroxetine CR for 1 to 2 weeks, then increase the dosage by 10 mg of paroxetine or 12.5 mg of paroxetine CR a day every 1 to 2 weeks to a maximum of 60 mg of paroxetine or 62.5 mg of paroxetine CR. If sedation becomes intolerable, then taper the paroxetine dosage down to 10 mg a day of paroxetine or 12.5 mg of paroxetine CR and switch to fluoxetine at 10 mg a day and titrate upward slowly. Other strategies can be used, based on the experience of the clinician.

Benzodiazepines. Benzodiazepines have the most rapid onset of action against panic, often within the first week, and they can be used for long periods without the development of tolerance to the antipanic effects. Alprazolam has been the most widely used benzodiazepine for panic disorder, but controlled studies have demonstrated equal efficacy for lorazepam (Ativan), and case reports have also indicated that clonazepam may be effective. Some patients use benzodiazepines as needed when faced with a phobic stimulus. Benzodiazepines can reasonably be used as the first agent for treatment of panic disorder, while a serotonergic drug is being slowly titrated to a therapeutic dose. After 4 to 12 weeks, benzodiazepine use can be slowly tapered (over 4 to 10 weeks) while the serotonergic drug is continued. The major reservation among clinicians regarding the use of benzodiazepines for panic disorder is the potential for dependence, cognitive impairment, and abuse, especially after long-term use. Patients should be instructed not to drive, abstain from alcohol or other CNS depressant medications or operate dangerous equipment while taking benzodiazepines. Benzodiazepines elicit a sense of well-being, whereas discontinuation of benzodiazepines produces a well-documented and unpleasant withdrawal syndrome. Anecdotal reports and small case series have indicated that addiction to alprazolam is one of the most difficult to overcome, and it may require a comprehensive program of detoxification. Benzodiazepine dosage should be tapered slowly, and all anticipated withdrawal effects should be thoroughly explained to the patient.

Tricyclic and Tetracyclic Drugs. At the present time SSRIs are considered the first line agents for the treatment of panic disorder. Data, however, show that among tricyclic drugs, clomipramine and imipramine (Tofranil) are the most effective in the treatment of panic disorder. Clinical experience indicates that the dosages must be titrated slowly upward to avoid overstimulation and that the full clinical benefit requires full dosages and may not be achieved for 8 to 12 weeks. Some data support the efficacy of desipramine (Norpramin), and less evidence suggests a role for maprotiline (Ludiomil), trazodone (Desyrel), nortriptyline (Pamelor), amitriptyline (Elavil), and doxepin (Adapin). Tricyclic drugs are less widely used than SSRIs because the tricyclic drugs generally have more severe adverse effects at the higher dosages required for effective treatment of panic disorder.

Monoamine Oxidase Inhibitors. The most robust data support the effectiveness of phenelzine (Nardil), and some data also support the use of tranylcypromine (Parnate). MAOIs appear less likely to cause overstimulation than either SSRIs or tricyclic drugs, but they may require full dosages for at least 8 to 12 weeks to be effective. The need for dietary restrictions has limited the use of MAOIs, particularly since the appearance of the SSRIs.

Treatment Nonresponse. If patients fail to respond to one class of drugs, another should be tried. Recent data support the effectiveness of venlafaxine. The combination of an SSRI or a tricyclic drug and a benzodiazepine or of an SSRI and lithium or a tricyclic drug can be tried. Case reports have suggested the effectiveness of carbamazepine (Tegretol), valproate (Depakene), and calcium channel inhibitors. Buspirone may have a role in the augmentation of other medications but has little effectiveness by itself. Clinicians should reassess the patient, particularly to establish the presence of comorbid conditions such as depression, alcohol use, or other substance use.

Duration of Pharmacotherapy. Once it becomes effective, pharmacological treatment should generally continue for 8 to 12 months. Data indicate that panic disorder is a chronic, perhaps lifelong condition that recurs when treatment is discontinued. Studies have reported that 30 to 90 percent of patients with panic disorder who have had successful treatment have a relapse when their medication is discontinued. Patients may be likely to relapse if they have been given benzodiazepines and the benzodiazepine therapy is terminated in a way that causes withdrawal symptoms.

Cognitive and Behavior Therapies

Cognitive and behavior therapies are effective treatments for panic disorder. Various reports have concluded that cognitive and behavior therapies are superior to pharmacotherapy alone; other reports have concluded the opposite. Several studies and reports have found that the combination of cognitive or behavior therapy with pharmacotherapy is more effective than either approach alone. Several studies that included long-term follow-up of patients who received cognitive or behavior therapy indicate that the therapies are effective in producing long-lasting remission of symptoms.

Cognitive Therapy. The two major foci of cognitive therapy for panic disorder are instruction about a patient's false beliefs and information about panic attacks. The instruction about false beliefs centers on the patient's tendency to misinterpret mild bodily sensations as indicating impending panic attacks, doom, or death. The information about panic attacks includes explanations that when panic attacks occur, they are time limited and not life threatening.

Mr. J was a 27-year-old laboratory technician who began having full-blown panic attacks 8 months before seeking help. Although he was unable to identify specific situations that elicited attacks, he was particularly concerned about the possibility of their occurring while he was engaged in laboratory procedures with patients. His attacks typically involved a sudden explosion of autonomic arousal and included palpitations, sweating, dizziness, feelings of unreality, and tingling in his arms and legs. He dreaded the idea that the attacks might recur. In the beginning of his cognitive-behavioral program, he found an educational handout that described the myths of panic attacks (e.g., that they will lead to heart attacks, losing control, or going crazy) particularly reassuring. He began practicing diaphragmatic breathing each evening and, after several weeks, became effective in challenging his negative way of thinking about the consequences of panic attacks. In the latter few weeks of his 12-week program, he practiced exposing himself to physical sensations of panic by doing a variety of interoceptive exercises at home, including hyperventilating for 1 or 2 minutes at a time (designed to help Mr. J acclimate to the physical sensations associated with overbreathing), and spinning in a chair repeatedly (designed to help acclimate him to symptoms of dizziness and feelings of unreality). At the conclusion of the treatment program Mr. J's panic attacks had disappeared, and at 6-month follow-up he had maintained his treatment gains by attending "booster sessions" with his therapist once every 2 months.

Applied Relaxation. The goal of applied relaxation (e.g., Herbert Benson's relaxation training) is to instill in patients a sense of control over their levels of anxiety and relaxation. Through the use of standardized techniques for muscle relaxation and the imagining of relaxing situations, patients learn techniques that may help them through a panic attack.

Respiratory Training. Because the hyperventilation associated with panic attacks is probably related to some symptoms, such as dizziness and faintness, one direct approach to control panic attacks is to train patients to control the urge to hyperventilate. After such training, patients can use the technique to help control hyperventilation during a panic attack.

In Vivo Exposure. In vivo exposure used to be the primary behavior treatment for panic disorder. The technique involves sequentially greater exposure of a patient to the feared stimulus; over time, the patient becomes desensitized to the experience. Previously, the focus was on external stimuli; recently, the technique has included exposure of the patient to internal feared sensations (e.g., tachypnea and fear of having a panic attack).

Other Psychosocial Therapies

Family Therapy. Families of patients with panic disorder and agoraphobia may also have been affected by the family member's disorder. Family therapy directed toward education and support is often beneficial.

Insight-Oriented Psychotherapy. Insight-oriented psychotherapy can be of benefit in the treatment of panic disorder and agoraphobia. Treatment focuses on helping patients understand the hypothesized unconscious meaning of the anxiety, the symbolism of the avoided situation, the need to repress impulses, and the secondary gains of the symptoms. A resolution of early infantile and oedipal conflicts is hypothesized to correlate with the resolution of current stresses.

Combined Psychotherapy and Pharmacotherapy

Even when pharmacotherapy is effective in eliminating the primary symptoms of panic disorder, psychotherapy may be needed to treat secondary symptoms. Glen O. Gabbard wrote:

> Panic-disordered patients frequently require a combination of drug therapy and psychotherapy.... Even when patients with panic attacks and agoraphobia have their symptoms pharmacologically controlled, they are often reluctant to venture out into the world again and may require psychotherapeutic interventions to help overcome this fear.... Some patients will adamantly refuse any medication because they believe that it stigmatizes them as being mentally ill, so psychotherapeutic intervention is required to help them understand and eliminate their resistance to pharmacotherapy.... For a comprehensive and effective treatment plan, these patients require psychotherapeutic approaches in addition to appropriate medications. In all patients with symptoms of panic disorder or agoraphobia,

a careful psychodynamic evaluation will help weigh the contributions of biological and dynamic factors.

References

Bakker A, van Balkom AJLM, Stein DJ. Evidence-based pharmacotherapy of panic disorder. In: Stein DJ, Lerer B, Stahl S, eds. *Evidence-based Psychopharmacology*. New York: Cambridge University Press; 2005:105–120.

Bandelow B, Behnke K, Lenoir S, Hendriks GJ, Alkin T, Goebel C, Clary CM. Sertraline versus paroxetine in the treatment of panic disorder: An acute, double-blind noninferiority comparison. *J Clin Psychiatry*. 2004;65(3):405–413.

Grant BF, Hasin DS, Stinson FS, Dawson DA, Goldstein RB, Smith S, Huang B, Saha TD. The epidemiology of DSM-IV panic disorder and agoraphobia in the United States: Results from the National Epidemiologic Survey on Alcohol and Related Conditions. *J Clin Psychiatry*. 2006;67(3):363–374.

Kessler RC, Chiu WT, Jin R, Ruscio AM, Shear K, Walters EE. The epidemiology of panic attacks, panic disorder, and agoraphobia in the National Comorbidity Survey replication. *Arch Gen Psychiatry*. 2006;63:415–424.

Mitte K. A meta-analysis of the efficacy of psycho- and pharmacotherapy in panic disorder with and without agoraphobia. *J Affect Disord*. 2005;88:27–45.

Pilowsky DJ, Olfson M, Gameroff MJ, Wickramartane P, Blanco C, Feder A, Gross R, Neria Y, Weissman MM. Panic disorder and suicidal ideation in primary care. *Depress Anxiety*. 2006;23:11–16.

Sheehan DV, Burnham DB, Iyengar MK, Perera P. Efficacy and tolerability of controlled-release paroxetine in the treatment of panic disorder. *J Clin Psychiatry*. 2005;66(1):34–40.

Smits JAJ, O'Cleirigh CM, Otto MW. Panic and agoraphobia. In: Andrasik F, ed. *Comprehensive Handbook of Personality and Psychopathology: Vol 2: Adult Psychopathology*. Hoboken: John Wiley & Sons, Inc.; 2006:121–137.

Vanelli M. Improving treatment response in panic disorder. *Primary Psychiatry*. 2005;12:68–73.

Yonkers KA, Howell H. Panic and agoraphobia. *CNS Spectrums*. 2004;9:6–7.

▲ 16.3 Specific Phobia and Social Phobia

The term *phobia* refers to an excessive fear of a specific object, circumstance, or situation. A specific phobia is a strong, persisting fear of an object or situation, whereas a social phobia is a strong, persisting fear of situations in which embarrassment can occur. The diagnosis of both specific and social phobias requires the development of intense anxiety, even to the point of panic, when exposed to the feared object or situation. Persons with specific phobias may anticipate harm, such as being bitten by a dog, or may panic at the thought of losing control; for instance, if they fear being in an elevator, they may also worry about fainting after the door closes. Persons with social phobias (also called *social anxiety disorder*) have excessive fears of humiliation or embarrassment in various social settings, such as in speaking in public, urinating in a public rest room (also called shy bladder), and speaking to a date. A generalized social phobia, which is often a chronic and disabling condition characterized by a phobic avoidance of most social situations, can be difficult to distinguish from avoidant personality disorder.

EPIDEMIOLOGY

Phobias are one of the most common mental disorders in the United States, where approximately 5 to 10 percent of the population is estimated to be afflicted with these troubling and sometimes disabling disorders. Less-conservative estimates have ranged as high as 25 percent of the population. The distress associated with phobias, especially when they are not recognized or acknowledged as mental disorders, can lead to further psychiatric complications, including other anxiety disorders, major depressive disorder, and substance-related disorders, especially alcohol use disorders.

Although phobias are common mental disorders, many persons with phobias either do not seek help to overcome their phobias or their condition is misdiagnosed when they do seek psychiatric or medical attention. The lifetime prevalence of specific phobia is about 11 percent, and the lifetime prevalence of social phobia has been reported to be 3 to 13 percent.

Specific Phobia

Specific phobia is more common than social phobia. Specific phobia is the most common mental disorder among women and the second most common among men, second only to substance-related disorders. The 6-month prevalence of specific phobia is about 5 to 10 per 100 persons (Table 16.3–1). The rates of specific phobias in women (13.6 to 16.1 percent) were double those of men (5.2 to 6.7 percent), although the ratio is closer to 1 to 1 for the fear of blood, injection, or injury type. (Types of phobias are discussed below in this section.) The peak age of onset for the natural environment type and the blood-injection-injury type is in the range of 5 to 9 years, although onset also occurs at older ages. In contrast, the peak age of onset for the situational type (except fear of heights) is higher, in the mid-20s, which is closer to the age of onset for agoraphobia. The feared objects and situations in specific phobias (listed in descending frequency of appearance) are animals, storms, heights, illness, injury, and death.

Social Phobia

Various studies have reported a lifetime prevalence ranging from 3 to 13 percent for social phobia. The 6-month prevalence is about 2 to 3 per 100 persons (Table 16.3–2). In epidemiological studies, females are affected more often than males, but in clinical samples, the reverse is often true. The reasons for these varying observations are unknown. The peak age of onset for social phobia is in the teens, although onset is common as young as 5 years of age and as old as 35.

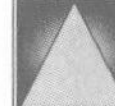

Table 16.3–1
Lifetime Prevalence Rates of Specific Phobia

Site	Men (%)	Women (%)	Total (%)
United States (National Comorbidity Survey)	6.7	15.7	11.3
United States (Epidemiological Catchment Area Study)	7.7	14.4	11.2
Puerto Rico	7.6	9.6	8.6
Edmonton, Canada	4.6	9.8	7.2
Korea	2.6	7.9	5.4
Zurich, Switzerland	5.2	16.1	10.7
The Netherlands	6.6	13.6	10.1

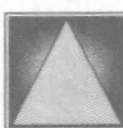

Table 16.3–2
Lifetime Prevalence Rates of Social Phobia

Site	Men (%)	Women (%)	Total (%)
United States (National Comorbidity Survey)	11.1	15.5	13.3
United States (Epidemiological Catchment Area Study)	2.1	3.1	2.6
Edmonton, Canada	1.3	2.1	1.7
Puerto Rico	0.8	1.1	1.0
Korea	0.1	1.0	0.5
Zurich, Switzerland	3.7	7.3	5.6
Taiwan	0.2	1.0	0.6
The Netherlands	5.9	9.7	7.8

COMORBIDITY

Persons with social phobia may have a history of other anxiety disorders, mood disorders, substance-related disorders, and bulimia nervosa. In addition, avoidant personality disorder frequently occurs in persons with generalized social phobia.

Reports of comorbidity in specific phobia range from 50 to 80 percent. Common comorbid disorders with specific phobia include anxiety, mood, and substance-related disorders.

ETIOLOGY

Both specific phobia and social phobia have types, and the precise causes of these types are likely to differ. Even within the types, as in all mental disorders, causative heterogeneity is found. The pathogenesis of the phobias, once it is understood, may prove to be a clear model for interactions between biological and genetic factors, on the one hand, and environmental events, on the other hand. In the blood-injection-injury type of specific phobia, affected persons may have inherited a particularly strong vasovagal reflex, which becomes associated with phobic emotions.

General Principles

Behavioral Factors. In 1920, John B. Watson wrote an article called "Conditioned Emotional Reactions," in which he recounted his experiences with Little Albert, an infant with a fear of rats and rabbits. Unlike Sigmund Freud's case of Little Hans, who had phobic symptoms (of horses) in the natural course of his maturation, Little Albert's difficulties were the direct result of the scientific experiments of two psychologists who used techniques that had successfully induced conditioned responses in laboratory animals.

Watson's hypothesis invoked the traditional pavlovian stimulus-response model of the conditioned reflex to account for the creation of the phobia: Anxiety is aroused by a naturally frightening stimulus that occurs in contiguity with a second inherently neutral stimulus. As a result of the contiguity, especially when the two stimuli are paired on several successive occasions, the originally neutral stimulus becomes capable of arousing anxiety by itself. The neutral stimulus, therefore, becomes a conditioned stimulus for anxiety production.

In the classic stimulus-response theory, the conditioned stimulus gradually loses its potency to arouse a response if it is not reinforced by periodic repetition of the unconditioned stimulus. In phobias, attenuation of the response to the stimulus does not occur; the symptom may last for years without any apparent external reinforcement. Operant conditioning theory provides a model to explain this phenomenon: Anxiety is a drive that motivates the organism to do whatever it can to obviate a painful affect. In the course of its random behavior, the organism learns that certain actions enable it to avoid the anxiety-provoking stimulus. These avoidance patterns remain stable for long periods as a result of the reinforcement they receive from their capacity to diminish anxiety. This model is readily applicable to phobias in that avoidance of the anxiety-provoking object or situation plays a central part. Such avoidance behavior becomes fixed as a stable symptom because of its effectiveness in protecting the person from the phobic anxiety.

Learning theory, which is particularly relevant to phobias, provides simple and intelligible explanations for many aspects of phobic symptoms. Critics contend, however, that learning theory deals mostly with surface mechanisms of symptom formation and is less useful than psychoanalytic theories in clarifying some of the complex underlying psychic processes involved.

Psychoanalytic Factors. Sigmund Freud's formulation of phobic neurosis is still the analytic explanation of specific phobia and social phobia. Freud hypothesized that the major function of anxiety is to signal the ego that a forbidden unconscious drive is pushing for conscious expression and to alert the ego to strengthen and marshall its defenses against the threatening instinctual force. Freud viewed the phobia—anxiety hysteria, as he continued to call it—as a result of conflicts centered on an unresolved childhood oedipal situation. Because sex drives continue to have a strong incestuous coloring in adults, sexual arousal can kindle an anxiety that is characteristically a fear of castration. When repression fails to be entirely successful, the ego must call on auxiliary defenses. In patients with phobias, the primary defense involved is displacement; that is, the sexual conflict is displaced from the person who evokes the conflict to a seemingly unimportant, irrelevant object or situation, which then has the power to arouse a constellation of affects, one of which is called *signal anxiety*. The phobic object or situation may have a direct associative connection with the primary source of the conflict and thus symbolizes it (the defense mechanism of symbolization).

Furthermore, the situation or the object is usually one that the person can avoid; with the additional defense mechanism of avoidance, the person can escape suffering serious anxiety. The end result is that the three combined defenses (repression, displacement, and symbolization) may eliminate the anxiety. The anxiety is controlled at the cost of creating a phobic neurosis, however. Freud first discussed the theoretical formulation of phobia formation in his famous case history of Little Hans, a 5-year-old boy who feared horses.

Although psychiatrists followed Freud's thought that phobias resulted from castration anxiety, recent psychoanalytic theorists have suggested that other types of anxiety may be involved. In agoraphobia, for example, separation anxiety clearly plays a leading role, and in erythrophobia (a fear of red that can be manifested as a fear of blushing), the element of shame implies the involvement of superego anxiety. Clinical observations have

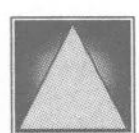

Table 16.3–3
Psychodynamic Themes in Phobias

- Principal defense mechanisms include displacement, projection, and avoidance.
- Environmental stressors, including humiliation and criticism from an older sibling, parental fights, or loss and separation from parents, interact with a genetic-constitutional diathesis.
- A characteristic pattern of internal object relations is externalized in social situations in the case of social phobia.
- Anticipation of humiliation, criticism, and ridicule is projected onto individuals in the environment.
- Shame and embarrassment are the principal affect states.
- Family members may encourage phobic behavior and serve as obstacles to any treatment plan.
- Self-exposure to the feared situation is a basic principle of all treatment.

led to the view that anxiety associated with phobias has a variety of sources and colorings.

Phobias illustrate the interaction between a genetic constitutional diathesis and environmental stressors. Longitudinal studies suggest that certain children are constitutionally predisposed to phobias because they are born with a specific temperament known as behavioral inhibition to the unfamiliar, but a chronic environmental stress must act on a child's temperamental disposition to create a full-blown phobia. Stressors, such as the death of a parent, separation from a parent, criticism or humiliation by an older sibling, and violence in the household, may activate the latent diathesis within the child, who then becomes symptomatic. An overview of psychodynamic aspects of phobias is summarized in Table 16.3–3.

COUNTERPHOBIC ATTITUDE. Otto Fenichel called attention to the fact that phobic anxiety can be hidden behind attitudes and behavior patterns that represent a denial, either that the dreaded object or situation is dangerous or that the person is afraid of it. Instead of being a passive victim of external circumstances, a person reverses the situation and actively attempts to confront and master whatever is feared. Persons with counterphobic attitudes seek out situations of danger and rush enthusiastically toward them. Devotees of potentially dangerous sports, such as parachute jumping and rock climbing, may be exhibiting counterphobic behavior. Such patterns may be secondary to phobic anxiety or may be normal means of dealing with a realistically dangerous situation. Children's play may exhibit counterphobic elements, as when children play doctor and give a doll the shot they received earlier that day in the pediatrician's office. This pattern of behavior may involve the related defense mechanism of identifying with the aggressor.

Specific Phobia

The development of specific phobia may result from the pairing of a specific object or situation with the emotions of fear and panic. Various mechanisms for the pairing have been postulated. In general, a nonspecific tendency to experience fear or anxiety forms the backdrop; when a specific event (e.g., driving) is paired with an emotional experience (e.g., an accident), the person is susceptible to a permanent emotional association between driving or cars and fear or anxiety. The emotional experience itself can be in response to an external incident, as a traffic accident, or to an internal incident, most commonly a panic attack. Although a person may never again experience a panic attack and may not meet the diagnostic criteria for panic disorder, he or she may have a generalized fear of driving, not an expressed fear of having a panic attack while driving. Other mechanisms of association between the phobic object and the phobic emotions include modeling, in which a person observes the reaction in another (e.g., a parent), and information transfer, in which a person is taught or warned about the dangers of specific objects (e.g., venomous snakes).

Genetic Factors. Specific phobia tends to run in families. The blood-injection-injury type has a particularly high familial tendency. Studies have reported that two thirds to three fourths of affected probands have at least one first-degree relative with specific phobia of the same type, but the necessary twin and adoption studies have not been conducted to rule out a significant contribution by nongenetic transmission of specific phobia.

Social Phobia

Several studies have reported that some children possibly have a trait characterized by a consistent pattern of behavioral inhibition. This trait may be particularly common in the children of parents who are affected with panic disorder, and it may develop into severe shyness as the children grow older. At least some persons with social phobia may have exhibited behavioral inhibition during childhood. Perhaps associated with this trait, which is thought to be biologically based, are the psychologically based data indicating that the parents of persons with social phobia, as a group, were less caring, more rejecting, and more overprotective of their children than were other parents. Some social phobia research has referred to the spectrum from dominance to submission observed in the animal kingdom. For example, dominant humans may tend to walk with their chins in the air and to make eye contact, whereas submissive humans may tend to walk with their chins down and to avoid eye contact.

Neurochemical Factors. The success of pharmacotherapies in treating social phobia has generated two specific neurochemical hypotheses about two types of social phobia. Specifically, the use of β-adrenergic receptor antagonists—for example, propranolol (Inderal)—for performance phobias (e.g., public speaking) has led to the development of an adrenergic theory for these phobias. Patients with performance phobias may release more norepinephrine or epinephrine, both centrally and peripherally, than do nonphobic persons, or such patients may be sensitive to a normal level of adrenergic stimulation. The observation that monoamine oxidase inhibitors (MAOIs) may be more effective than tricyclic drugs in the treatment of generalized social phobia, in combination with preclinical data, has led some investigators to hypothesize that dopaminergic activity is related to the pathogenesis of the disorder. One study has shown significantly lower homovanillic acid concentrations. Another study using single photon emission computed tomography (SPECT) demonstrated decreased striatal dopamine reuptake site density. Thus, some evidence suggests dopaminergic dysfunction in social phobia.

Genetic Factors. First-degree relatives of persons with social phobia are about three times more likely to be affected with social phobia than are first-degree relatives of those without mental disorders. And some preliminary data indicate that monozygotic twins are more often concordant than are dizygotic twins, although in social phobia it is particularly important to study twins reared apart to help control for environmental factors.

DIAGNOSIS

Specific Phobia

The text revision of the fourth edition of the *Diagnostic and Statistical Manual of Mental Disorders* (DSM-IV-TR) uses the term specific phobia to match the nomenclature in the 10th revision of the *International Statistical Classification of Diseases and Related Health Problems* (ICD-10). Table 16.3–4 lists the diagnostic criteria. Criteria A (excessive fear) and B (stimulus exposure) have been carefully worded in DSM-IV-TR to allow for the possibility that exposure to a phobic stimulus may result in a panic attack. In contrast to panic disorder, however, in specific phobia, the panic attack is situationally bound to the specific phobic stimulus. Criterion G (the anxiety attack) in DSM-IV-TR includes the words "not better accounted for" to emphasize the need for clinicians' judgment about diagnosing the symptoms. The specific content of the phobia and the strength of the relation (e.g., cued or noncued) between the stimulus and a panic attack also need to be considered.

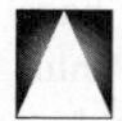

Table 16.3–4
DSM-IV-TR Diagnostic Criteria for Specific Phobia

A. Marked and persistent fear that is excessive or unreasonable, cued by the presence or anticipation of a specific object or situation (e.g., flying, heights, animals, receiving an injection, seeing blood).

B. Exposure to the phobic stimulus almost invariably provokes an immediate anxiety response, which may take the form of a situationally bound or situationally predisposed panic attack.
Note: In children, the anxiety may be expressed by crying, tantrums, freezing, or clinging.

C. The person recognizes that the fear is excessive or unreasonable.
Note: In children, this feature may be absent.

D. The phobic situation(s) is avoided or else is endured with intense anxiety or distress.

E. The avoidance, anxious anticipation, or distress in the feared situation(s) interferes significantly with the person's normal routine, occupational (or academic) functioning, or social activities or relationships, or there is marked distress about having the phobia.

F. In individuals under age 18 years, the duration is at least 6 months.

G. The anxiety, panic attacks, or phobic avoidance associated with the specific object or situation are not better accounted for by another mental disorder, such as obsessive-compulsive disorder (e.g., fear of dirt in someone with an obsession about contamination), posttraumatic stress disorder (e.g., avoidance of stimuli associated with a severe stressor), separation anxiety disorder (e.g., avoidance of school), social phobia (e.g., avoidance of social situations because of fear of embarrassment), panic disorder with agoraphobia, or agoraphobia without history of panic disorder.

Specify type:
Animal type
Natural environment type (e.g., heights, storms, water)
Blood-injection-injury type
Situational type (e.g., airplanes, elevators, enclosed places)
Other type (e.g., fear of choking, vomiting, or contracting an illness; in children, fear of loud sounds or costumed characters)

(From American Psychiatric Association. *Diagnostic and Statistical Manual of Mental Disorders*. 4th ed. Text rev. Washington, DC: American Psychiatric Association; copyright 2000, with permission.)

The DSM-IV-TR includes distinctive types of specific phobia: animal type, natural environment type (e.g., storms), blood-injection-injury type, situational type (e.g., cars), and other type (for specific phobias that do not fit into the previous four types). Preliminary data indicate that the natural environment type is most common in children younger than 10 years of age and the situational type most often occurs in persons in their early 20s. The blood-injection-injury type is differentiated from the others in that bradycardia and hypotension often follow the initial tachycardia that is common to all phobias. The blood-injection-injury type of specific phobia is particularly likely to affect many members and generations of a family. One type of recently reported specific phobia is space phobia, in which persons are afraid of falling when there is no nearby support like a wall or a chair. Some data indicate that affected persons may have abnormal right hemisphere function, possibly resulting in visual-spatial impairment. Balance disorders should also be ruled out in such patients.

Focus. Phobias have traditionally been classified according to the specific fear by means of Greek or Latin prefixes, as indicated in Table 16.3–5:

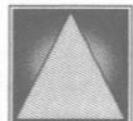

Table 16.3–5
Phobias

Acrophobia	fear of heights
Agoraphobia	fear of open places
Ailurophobia	fear of cats
Hydrophobia	fear of water
Claustrophobia	fear of closed spaces
Cynophobia	fear of dogs
Mysophobia	fear of dirt and germs
Pyrophobia	fear of fire
Xenophobia	fear of strangers
Zoophobia	fear of animals

Other phobias that are related to changes in the society are the fear of electromagnetic fields, of microwaves, and of society as a whole (amaxophobia).

Dr. B was a 32-year-old medical resident who was currently training in a large teaching hospital. He had a history of several years of extreme discomfort at the thought of doing a therapeutic removal of a fingernail or toenail for a patient. He first heard descriptions of this procedure while he was doing his undergraduate work in preparation for medical school. He recalled feeling nauseated, faint, and disgusted at the thought of doing this, although he had no similar squeamishness about the thought of performing other procedures. He stated that he would rather "take a cockroach out of a kid's ear" than take a fingernail off.

Dr. B was an active child who frequently had minor accidents requiring visits to his family doctor. He had a series of sprains and broken bones and recalled a finger getting smashed in a door when he was about 6 years old. He remembered the finger becoming swollen and bruised and the fingernail eventually coming off as the finger healed. Although he did not remember ever being extremely upset during his visits to the doctor, he did recall seeing his mother turn pale and look sick whenever he had to get a shot or stitches. He was always willing to try things with his buddies and described a self-induced fainting spell when he was 13 years old. He purposely hyperventilated and then stood up quickly and did a Valsalva maneuver. He passed out for about 10 seconds and remembered being very scared as he regained consciousness. He was aware that the voices of his friends seemed abnormal and their faces were distorted and blurry, and he had a sense of unreality and a brief feeling of terror.

During medical school, Dr. B successfully avoided doing a nail removal procedure but as a fourth-year student was forced to observe the procedure. He stood as far back as possible in the examination room and watched the physician remove a toenail. He began to feel sick, became sweaty, noticed his heart beginning to race, and then started to feel faint and weak. He had to sit down to avoid fainting. He explained that "nails are supposed to be there" and that he cannot stop thinking of the "excruciating pain" that might be experienced if the patient were not totally anesthetized.

During the first 2 years of his family medicine residency, Dr. B became known for his willingness to do surgical procedures. He often volunteered to help fellow residents and seemed to enjoy tasks such as setting bones, realigning joints, and even incision and drainage of cysts and boils and stitching acute lacerations. None of his colleagues were aware that he had never removed a nail—a procedure that was commonly done in this general practice. During an evening clinic when he was the only doctor available, a young girl was brought in and needed a nail removed. Unable to perform the procedure himself, he called a fellow resident at home and persuaded her to come in and help him. She agreed on the condition that he see a therapist to deal with the problem. (From DSM-IV-TR Case Studies.)

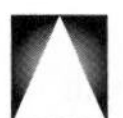

Table 16.3–6
DSM-IV-TR Diagnostic Criteria for Social Phobia

A. A marked and persistent fear of one or more social or performance situations in which the person is exposed to unfamiliar people or to possible scrutiny by others. The individual fears that he or she will act in a way (or show anxiety symptoms) that will be humiliating or embarrassing.
Note: In children, there must be evidence of the capacity for age-appropriate social relationships with familiar people and the anxiety must occur in peer settings, not just in interactions with adults.

B. Exposure to the feared social situation almost invariably provokes anxiety, which may take the form of a situationally bound or situationally predisposed panic attack.
Note: In children, the anxiety may be expressed by crying, tantrums, freezing, or shrinking from social situations with unfamiliar people.

C. The person recognizes that the fear is excessive or unreasonable.
Note: In children, this feature may be absent.

D. The feared social or performance situations are avoided or else are endured with intense anxiety or distress.

E. The avoidance, anxious anticipation, or distress in the feared social or performance situation(s) interferes significantly with the person's normal routine, occupational (academic) functioning, or social activities or relationships, or there is marked distress about having the phobia.

F. In individuals under age 18 years, the duration is at least 6 months.

G. The fear or avoidance is not due to the direct physiological effects of a substance (e.g., a drug of abuse, a medication) or a general medical condition and is not better accounted for by another mental disorder (e.g., panic disorder with or without agoraphobia, separation anxiety disorder, body dysmorphic disorder, a pervasive developmental disorder, or schizoid personality disorder).

H. If a general medical condition or another mental disorder is present, the fear in Criterion A is unrelated to it (e.g., the fear is not of stuttering, trembling in Parkinson's disease, or exhibiting abnormal eating behavior in anorexia nervosa or bulimia nervosa).

Specify if:
Generalized: if the fears include most social situations (also consider the additional diagnosis of avoidant personality disorder)

(From American Psychiatric Association. *Diagnostic and Statistical Manual of Mental Disorders.* 4th ed. Text rev. Washington, DC: American Psychiatric Association; copyright 2000, with permission.)

Social Phobia

The DSM-IV-TR diagnostic criteria for social phobia (Table 16.3–6) acknowledge that the disorder can be associated with panic attacks. DSM-IV-TR also includes a specifier for generalized type, which may be useful in predicting course, prognosis, and treatment response. DSM-IV-TR excludes a diagnosis of social phobia when the symptoms are a result of social avoidance stemming from embarrassment about another psychiatric or nonpsychiatric medical condition.

Andy, a 25-year-old single man, lives with his mother and brother. He works as a mail sorter at the post office, a job he has had since he dropped out of college after 2 years. He came to an anxiety disorders clinic after reading a newspaper advertisement of the availability of free treatment if he participated in a research study of anxiety disorders. His chief complaint is of "nervousness." He says that right now he is "just going through the motions" and wants "to lead a normal life and go back to college."

During his adolescence and young adulthood, Andy had no close friends and usually preferred to be by himself. When he entered college, he formed several close friendships but became "super self-conscious" when speaking to strangers, classmates, and sometimes even friends. He would feel nervous, and his face would become so "stiff" that he had difficulty speaking. He had a "buzzing" in his head, felt as if he were "outside [his] body," had hot flashes, and perspired. These "panic attacks" (his term) came on suddenly, within seconds, and only when he was with people. When a classmate spoke to him, he sometimes "couldn't hear" what the classmate was saying because of his nervousness.

Outside of class, Andy began to feel increasingly uncomfortable in social situations. "I think that I was afraid of saying or doing something stupid." He began to turn down invitations to parties and to withdraw from other social activities (e.g., a bowling league). Eventually, he dropped out of college entirely.

Andy explains that the reason he chose to work at the post office is that the job does not require him to deal with people. When asked about other things that make him nervous, he says he tries to avoid using public lavatories and feels more comfortable in a public bathroom when the lights are dim, when there are few people present, and when he can use a stall rather than a urinal.

Andy has two long-standing "best" friends with whom he socializes regularly and feels completely comfortable. However, he hasn't dated since college, and he totally avoids group settings, such as weddings and dances. He has no problem with authority figures, and even welcomes constructive criticism from his supervisor at the post office. "My problem is nervousness, not obstinacy." (From *DSM-IV-TR Casebook.*)

CLINICAL FEATURES

Phobias are characterized by the arousal of severe anxiety when patients are exposed to specific situations or objects or when patients even anticipate exposure to the situations or objects. DSM-IV-TR emphasizes the possibility that panic attacks can, and frequently do, occur in patients with specific and social phobias, but the panic attacks, except perhaps for the first few, are expected. Exposure to the phobic stimulus or anticipation of it almost invariably results in a panic attack in a person who is susceptible to them.

Persons with phobias, by definition, try to avoid the phobic stimulus; some go to great trouble to avoid anxiety-provoking situations. For example, a patient with a phobia may take a bus across the United States, rather than fly, to avoid contact with the object of the patient's phobia, an airplane. Perhaps as another way to avoid the stress of the phobic stimulus, many patients have substance-related disorders, particularly alcohol use disorders. Moreover, an estimated one third of patients with social phobia have major depressive disorder.

The major finding on the mental status examination is the presence of an irrational and ego-dystonic fear of a specific situation, activity, or object; patients are able to describe how they avoid contact with the phobia. Depression is commonly found on the mental status examination and may be present in as many as one third of all patients with phobia.

DIFFERENTIAL DIAGNOSIS

Specific phobia and social phobia need to be differentiated from appropriate fear and normal shyness, respectively. DSM-IV-TR aids in the differentiation by requiring that the symptoms impair the patient's ability to function appropriately. Nonpsychiatric medical conditions that can result in the development of a phobia include the use of substances (particularly hallucinogens and sympathomimetics), central nervous system tumors, and cerebrovascular diseases. Phobic symptoms in these instances are unlikely in the absence of additional suggestive findings on physical, neurological, and mental status examinations. Schizophrenia is also in the differential diagnosis of both specific phobia and social phobia, because patients with schizophrenia can have phobic symptoms as part of their psychoses. Unlike patients with schizophrenia, however, patients with phobia have insight into the irrationality of their fears and lack the bizarre quality and other psychotic symptoms that accompany schizophrenia.

In the differential diagnosis of both specific phobia and social phobia, clinicians must consider panic disorder, agoraphobia, and avoidant personality disorder. Differentiation among panic disorder, agoraphobia, social phobia, and specific phobia can be difficult in individual cases. In general, however, patients with specific phobia or nongeneralized social phobia tend to experience anxiety immediately when presented with the phobic stimulus. Furthermore, the anxiety or panic is limited to the identified situation; patients are not abnormally anxious when they are neither confronted with the phobic stimulus nor caused to anticipate the stimulus.

A patient with agoraphobia is often comforted by the presence of another person in an anxiety-provoking situation, whereas a patient with social phobia is made more anxious than before by the presence of other persons. Whereas breathlessness, dizziness, a sense of suffocation, and a fear of dying are common in panic disorder and agoraphobia, the symptoms associated with social phobia usually involve blushing, muscle twitching, and anxiety about scrutiny. Differentiation between social phobia and avoidant personality disorder can be difficult and can require extensive interviews and psychiatric histories.

Specific Phobia

Other diagnoses to consider in the differential diagnosis of specific phobia are hypochondriasis, obsessive-compulsive disorder (OCD), and paranoid personality disorder. Hypochondriasis is the fear of having a disease, whereas specific phobia of the illness type is the fear of contracting the disease. Some patients with OCD manifest behavior indistinguishable from that of a patient with specific phobia. For example, patients with OCD may avoid knives because they have compulsive thoughts about killing their children, whereas patients with specific phobia about knives may avoid them for fear of cutting themselves. Patients with paranoid personality disorder have generalized fear that distinguishes them from those with specific phobia.

Social Phobia

Two additional differential diagnostic considerations for social phobia are major depressive disorder and schizoid personality disorder. The avoidance of social situations can often be a symptom in depression, but a psychiatric interview with the patient is likely to elicit a broad constellation of depressive symptoms. In patients with schizoid personality disorder, the lack of interest in socializing, not the fear of socializing, leads to the avoidant social behavior.

COURSE AND PROGNOSIS

Specific phobia exhibits a bimodal age of onset, with a childhood peak for animal phobia, natural environment phobia, and blood-injection-injury phobia and an early adulthood peak for other phobias, such as situational phobia. As with other anxiety disorders, limited prospective epidemiological data exist on the natural course of specific phobia. Because patients with isolated specific phobias rarely present for treatment, research on the course of the disorder in the clinic is limited. The available information suggests that most specific phobias that begin in childhood and persist into adulthood continue to persist for many years. The severity of the condition is thought to remain relatively constant, without the waxing and waning course seen with other anxiety disorders.

> Mr. A was a successful businessman who presented for treatment following a change in his business schedule. While he had formerly worked largely from an office near his home, a promotion led to a schedule of frequent out-of-town meetings, requiring weekly flights. Mr. A reported being "deathly afraid" of flying. Even the thought of getting on an airplane led to thoughts of impending doom as he envisioned his airplane crashing to the ground. These thoughts were associated with intense fear, palpitations, sweating, clammy palms, and stomach upset. While the thought of flying was terrifying enough, Mr. A became nearly incapacitated when he went to the airport. Immediately before boarding, Mr. A often had to turn back from the plane and run to the bathroom to vomit. (Courtesy of Daniel S. Pine, M.D.)

Social phobia tends to have its onset in late childhood or early adolescence. Social phobia tends to be a chronic disorder, although as with the other anxiety disorders, prospective epidemiological data are limited. Both retrospective epidemiological studies and prospective clinical studies suggest that the disorder can profoundly disrupt the life of an individual over many years. This can include disruption in school or academic achievement and interference with job performance and social development.

TREATMENT

Behavior Therapy

The most studied and most effective treatment for phobias is probably behavior therapy. The key aspects of successful treatment are (1) the patient's commitment to treatment, (2) clearly identified problems and objectives, and (3) available, alternative strategies for coping with the feelings. A variety of behavioral treatment techniques have been used, the most common being systematic desensitization, a method pioneered by Joseph Wolpe. In this method, the patient is exposed serially to a predetermined list of anxiety-provoking stimuli graded in a hierarchy from the least to the most frightening. Through the use of antianxiety drugs, hypnosis, and instruction in muscle relaxation, patients are taught how to induce in themselves both mental and physical repose. Once they have mastered the techniques, patients are taught to use them to induce relaxation in the face of each anxiety-provoking stimulus. As they become desensitized to each stimulus in the scale, the patients move up to the next stimulus until, ultimately, what previously produced the most anxiety no longer elicits the painful affect.

Other behavioral techniques that have been used more recently involve intensive exposure to the phobic stimulus through either imagery or desensitization in vivo. In imaginal flooding, patients are exposed to the phobic stimulus for as long as they can tolerate the fear until they reach a point at which they can no longer feel it. Flooding (also known as implosion) in vivo requires patients to experience similar anxiety through exposure to the actual phobic stimulus.

Insight-Oriented Psychotherapy

Early in the development of psychoanalysis and the dynamically oriented psychotherapies, theorists believed that these methods were the treatments of choice for phobic neurosis, which was then thought to stem from oedipal-genital conflicts. Soon, however, therapists recognized that, despite progress in uncovering and analyzing unconscious conflicts, patients frequently failed to lose their phobic symptoms. Moreover, by continuing to avoid phobic situations, patients excluded a significant degree of anxiety and its related associations from the analytic process. Both Freud and his pupil Sandor Ferenczi recognized that if progress in analyzing these symptoms was to be made, therapists had to go beyond their analytic roles and actively urge patients with phobia to seek the phobic situation and experience the anxiety and resultant insight. Since then, psychiatrists have generally agreed that a measure of activity on the therapist's part is often required to treat phobic anxiety successfully. The decision to apply the techniques of psychodynamic insight-oriented therapy should be based not on the presence of phobic symptoms alone but on positive indications from the patient's ego structure and life patterns for the use of this method of treatment. Insight-oriented therapy enables patients to understand the origin of the phobia, the phenomenon of secondary gain, and the role of resistance and enables them to seek healthy ways of dealing with anxiety-provoking stimuli.

Other Therapeutic Modalities

Hypnosis, supportive therapy, and family therapy may be useful in the treatment of phobic disorders. Hypnosis is used to enhance the therapist's suggestion that the phobic object is not dangerous, and self-hypnosis can be taught to the patient as a method of relaxation when confronted with the phobic object. Supportive psychotherapy and family therapy are often useful in helping the patient actively confront the phobic object during treatment. Not only can family therapy enlist the aid of the family in treating the patient, but also it may help the family understand the nature of the patient's problem.

Specific Phobia

A common treatment for specific phobia is exposure therapy. In this method, therapists desensitize patients by using a series of gradual, self-paced exposures to the phobic stimuli, and they teach patients various techniques to deal with anxiety, including relaxation, breathing control, and cognitive approaches. The cognitive-behavioral approaches include reinforcing the realization that the phobic situation is, in fact, safe. The key aspects of successful behavior therapy are the patient's commitment to treatment, clearly identified problems and objectives, and alternative strategies for coping with the patient's feelings. In the special situation of blood-injection-injury phobia, some therapists recommend that patients tense their bodies and remain seated during the exposure to help avoid the possibility of fainting from a vasovagal reaction to the phobic stimulation. β-adrenergic receptor antagonists may be useful in the treatment of specific phobia, especially when the phobia is associated with panic attacks. Pharmacotherapy (e.g., benzodiazepines), psychotherapy, or combined therapy directed to the attacks may also be of benefit.

Social Phobia

Both psychotherapy and pharmacotherapy are useful in treating social phobias, and varying approaches are indicated for the generalized type and for performance situations. Some studies indicate that the use of both pharmacotherapy and psychotherapy produces better results than either therapy alone, although the finding may not be applicable to all situations and patients.

Effective drugs for the treatment of social phobia include (1) selective serotonin reuptake inhibitors (SSRIs), (2) the benzodiazepines, (3) venlafaxine (Effexor), and (4) buspirone (BuSpar). Most clinicians consider SSRIs the first-line treatment choice for patients with generalized social phobia. The benzodiazepines alprazolam (Xanax) and clonazepam (Klonopin) are also efficacious in both generalized and specific social phobia. Buspirone has shown additive effects when used to augment treatment with SSRIs.

In severe cases, successful treatment of social phobia with both irreversible MAOIs such as phenelzine (Nardil) and reversible inhibitors of monoamine oxidase such as moclobemide (Aurorix) and brofaromine (Consonar) (which are not available in the United States) has been reported. Therapeutic dosages of phenelzine range from 45 to 90 mg a day, with response rates ranging from 50 to 70 percent, and approximately 5 to 6 weeks are needed to assess the efficacy.

The treatment of social phobia associated with performance situations frequently involves the use of β-adrenergic receptor antagonists shortly before exposure to a phobic stimulus. The two compounds most widely used are atenolol (Tenormin), 50 to 100 mg every morning or 1 hour before the performance, and propranolol (20 to 40 mg). Another option to help with performance anxiety is a relatively short- or intermediate-acting benzodiazepine, such as lorazepam or alprazolam. Cognitive, behavioral, and exposure techniques are also useful in performance situations.

Psychotherapy for the generalized type of social phobia usually involves a combination of behavioral and cognitive methods, including cognitive retraining, desensitization, rehearsal during sessions, and a range of homework assignments.

References

Alfano CA, Beidel DC, Turner SM. Cognitive correlates of social phobia among children and adolescents. *J Abnorm Child Psychol*. 2006;34(2):182–194.

Belzer KD, McKee MB, Liebowitz MR. Social anxiety disorder: Current perspectives on diagnosis and treatment. *Primary Psychiatry*.2005;12:35–48.

Davidson JRT. Social phobia. Then, now, the future. In: Rothbaum BO, ed. *Pathological Anxiety: Emotional Processing in Etiology and Treatment*. New York: Guilford Press; 2006:115–131.

Dozois DJA, Frewen PA. Specificity of cognitive structure in depression and social phobia: A comparison of interpersonal and achievement content. *J Affect Disord*. 2006;90:101–109.

Gemignani A, Sebastiani L, Simoni A, Santarcangelo EL, Ghelarducci B. Hypnotic trait and specific phobia: EEG and autonomic output during phobic stimulation. *Brain Res Bull*. 2006;69(2):197–203.

Harvey AG, Ehlers A, Clark DM. Learning history in social phobia. *Behavioural and Cognitive Psychotherapy*. 2005;33:257–271.

Hofmann SG, Bogels SM. Recent advances in the treatment of social phobia: Introduction to the special issue. *Journal of Cognitive Psychotherapy*. 2006;20:3–5.

Rapee RM, Abbott MJ. Mental representation of observable attributes in people with social phobia. *J Behav Ther Exp Psychiatry*. 2006;37(2):113–126.

Stein DJ, Matsunaga H. Specific phobia: A disorder of fear conditioning and extinction. *CNS Spectrums*. 2006;11(4):248–251.

Van Ameringen M, Mancini C, Pipe B, Oakman J, Bennett M. An open trial of topiramate in the treatment of generalized social phobia. *J Clin Psychiatry*. 2004;65(12):1674–1678.

▲ 16.4 Obsessive-Compulsive Disorder

Obsessive-compulsive disorder (OCD) is represented by a diverse group of symptoms that include intrusive thoughts, rituals, preoccupations, and compulsions. These recurrent obsessions or compulsions cause severe distress to the person. The obsessions or compulsions are time-consuming and interfere significantly with the person's normal routine, occupational functioning, usual social activities, or relationships. A patient with OCD may have an obsession, a compulsion, or both.

An obsession is a recurrent and intrusive thought, feeling, idea, or sensation. In contrast to an obsession, which is a mental event, a compulsion is a behavior. Specifically, a compulsion is a conscious, standardized, recurrent behavior, such as counting, checking, or avoiding. A patient with OCD realizes the irrationality of the obsession and experiences both the obsession and the compulsion as ego-dystonic (i.e., unwanted behavior).

Although the compulsive act may be carried out in an attempt to reduce the anxiety associated with the obsession, it does not always succeed in doing so. The completion of the compulsive act may not affect the anxiety, and it may even increase the anxiety. Anxiety is also increased when a person resists carrying out a compulsion.

EPIDEMIOLOGY

The rates of OCD are fairly consistent, with a lifetime prevalence in the general population estimated at 2 to 3 percent. Some researchers have estimated that the disorder is found in as many as 10 percent of outpatients in psychiatric clinics. These figures make OCD the fourth most common psychiatric diagnosis after phobias, substance-related disorders, and major depressive disorder. Epidemiological studies in Europe, Asia, and Africa have confirmed these rates across cultural boundaries.

Among adults, men and women are equally likely to be affected, but among adolescents, boys are more commonly affected than girls. The mean age of onset is about 20 years, although men have a slightly earlier age of onset (mean about 19 years) than women (mean about 22 years). Overall, the symptoms of about two thirds of affected persons have an onset before age 25, and the symptoms of fewer than 15 percent have an onset after age 35. The onset of the disorder can occur in adolescence or childhood, in some cases as early as 2 years of age. Single persons are more frequently affected with OCD than are married persons, although this finding probably reflects the difficulty that persons with the disorder have maintaining a relationship. OCD occurs less often among blacks than among whites, although access to health care rather than differences in prevalence may explain the variation.

COMORBIDITY

Persons with OCD are commonly affected by other mental disorders. The lifetime prevalence for major depressive disorder in persons with OCD is about 67 percent and for social phobia, about 25 percent. Other common comorbid psychiatric diagnoses in patients with OCD include alcohol use disorders, generalized anxiety disorder, specific phobia, panic disorder, eating disorders, and personality disorders. OCD exhibits a superficial resemblance to obsessive-compulsive personality disorder, which is associated with an obsessive concern for details, perfectionism, and other similar personality traits. The incidence of Tourette's disorder in patients with OCD is 5 to 7 percent, and 20 to 30 percent of patients with OCD have a history of tics.

ETIOLOGY

Biological Factors

Neurotransmitters

SEROTONERGIC SYSTEM. The many clinical drug trials that have been conducted support the hypothesis that dysregulation of serotonin is involved in the symptom formation of obsessions and compulsions in the disorder. Data show that serotonergic drugs are more effective than drugs that affect other neurotransmitter systems, but whether serotonin is involved in the cause of OCD is not clear. Clinical studies have assayed cerebrospinal fluid (CSF) concentrations of serotonin metabolites (e.g., 5-hydroxyindoleacetic acid [5-HIAA]) and affinities and numbers of platelet-binding sites of tritiated imipramine (Tofranil), which binds to serotonin reuptake sites, and have reported variable findings of these measures in patients with OCD. In one study, the CSF concentration of 5-HIAA decreased after treatment with clomipramine (Anafranil), focusing attention on the serotonergic system.

NORADRENERGIC SYSTEM. Currently, less evidence exists for dysfunction in the noradrenergic system in OCD. Anecdotal reports show some improvement in OCD symptoms with use of oral clonidine (Catapres), a drug that lowers the amount of norepinephrine released from the presynaptic nerve terminals.

NEUROIMMUNOLOGY. Some interest exists in a positive link between streptococcal infection and OCD. Group A β-hemolytic streptococcal infection can cause rheumatic fever, and approximately 10 to 30 percent of the patients develop Sydenham's chorea and show obsessive-compulsive symptoms.

Brain-Imaging Studies. Neuroimaging in patients with OCD has produced converging data implicating altered function in the neurocircuitry between orbitofrontal cortex, caudate, and thalamus. Various functional brain-imaging studies—for example, positron emission tomography (PET)—have shown increased activity (e.g., metabolism and blood flow) in the frontal lobes, the basal ganglia (especially the caudate), and the cingulum of patients with OCD. The involvement of these areas in the pathology of OCD appears more associated with corticostriatal pathways than with the amygdala pathways that are the current focus of much anxiety disorder research. Pharmacological and behavioral treatments reportedly reverse these abnormalities (Fig. 16.4–1). Data from functional brain-imaging studies are consistent with data from structural brain-imaging studies. Both computed tomographic (CT) and magnetic resonance imaging (MRI) studies have found bilaterally smaller caudates in patients with OCD. Both functional and structural brain-imaging study results are also compatible with the observation that neurological procedures involving the cingulum are sometimes effective in the treatment of OCD. One recent MRI study reported increased T1 relaxation times in the frontal cortex, a finding consistent with the location of abnormalities discovered in PET studies.

Genetics. Available genetic data on OCD support the hypothesis that the disorder has a significant genetic component. Relatives of probands with OCD consistently have a three- to fivefold higher probability of having OCD or obsessive-compulsive features than families of control probands The data, however, do not yet distinguish the heritable factors from the influence of cultural and behavioral effects on the transmission of the disorder. Studies of concordance for the disorder in twins have consistently found a significantly higher concordance rate for monozygotic twins than for dizygotic twins. Some studies also demonstrate increased rates of a variety of conditions among relatives of OCD probands, including generalized anxiety disorder, tic disorders, body dysmorphic disorder, hypochondriasis, eating disorders, and habits such as nail-biting.

Other Biological Data. Electrophysiological studies, sleep electroencephalogram (EEG) studies, and neuroendocrine studies have contributed data that indicate some commonalities between depressive disorders and OCD. A higher than usual incidence of nonspecific EEG abnormalities occurs in patients with OCD. Sleep EEG studies have found abnormalities similar to those in depressive disorders, such as decreased rapid eye movement latency. Neuroendocrine studies have also produced some analogies to depressive disorders, such as nonsuppression on the dexamethasone-suppression test in about one third of patients and decreased growth hormone secretion with clonidine infusions.

As mentioned, studies have suggested a possible link between a subset of OCD cases and certain types of motor tic syndromes (i.e., Tourette's disorder and chronic motor tics). A higher rate of OCD, Tourette's disorder, and chronic motor tics are found in relatives of patients with Tourette's disorder than in relatives of controls, whether or not they had OCD. Most family studies of probands with OCD have found increased rates of Tourette's disorder and chronic motor tics only among the relatives of probands with OCD who also have some form of tic disorder. Evidence also suggests cotransmission of Tourette's syndrome, OCD, and chronic motor tics within families.

Behavioral Factors

According to learning theorists, obsessions are conditioned stimuli. A relatively neutral stimulus becomes associated with fear or anxiety through a process of respondent conditioning by being paired with events that are noxious or anxiety-producing. Thus, previously neutral objects and thoughts become conditioned stimuli capable of provoking anxiety or discomfort.

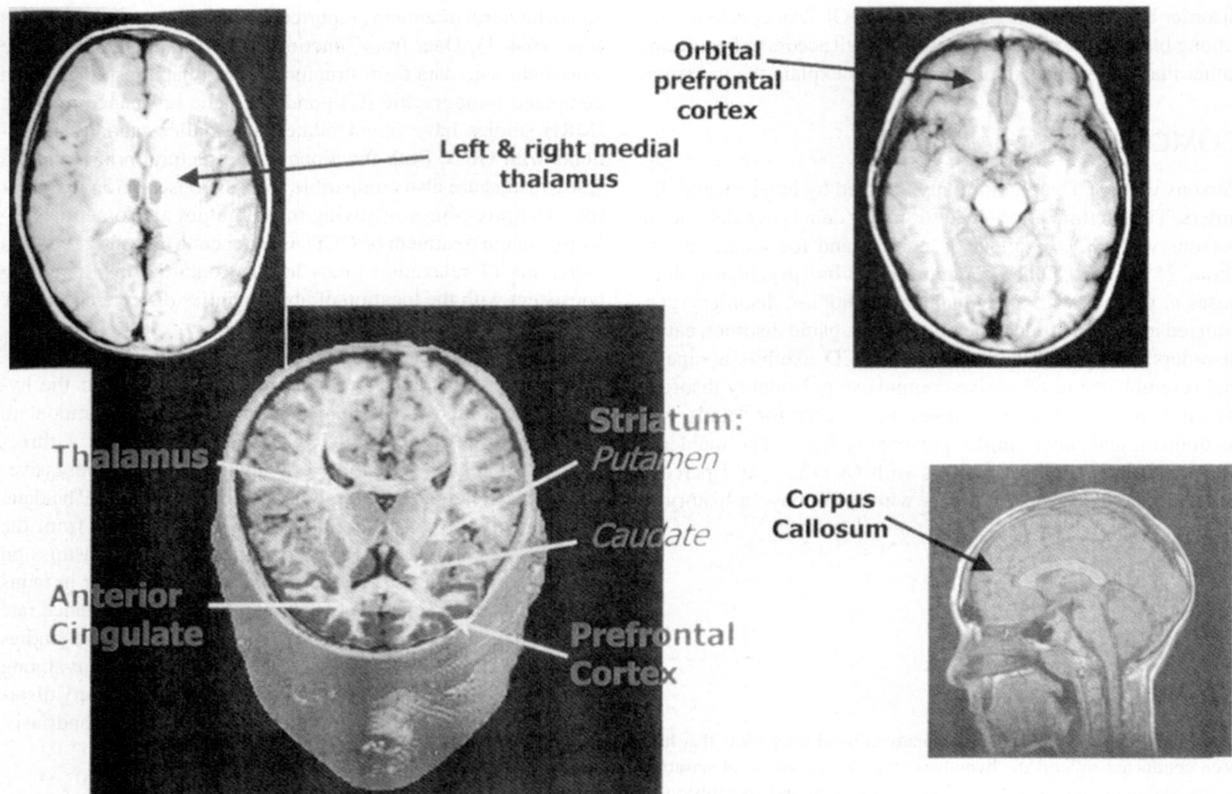

FIGURE 16.4–1
Brain regions implicated in the pathophysiology of obsessive-compulsive disorder. (From Rosenberg DR, MacMillan SN, Moore GJ. Brain anatomy and chemistry may predict treatment response in paediatric obsessive-compulsive disorder. *Int J Neuropsychopharmacol.* 2001;4:179, with permission.)

Compulsions are established in a different way. When a person discovers that a certain action reduces anxiety attached to an obsessional thought, he or she develops active avoidance strategies in the form of compulsions or ritualistic behaviors to control the anxiety. Gradually, because of their efficacy in reducing a painful secondary drive (anxiety), the avoidance strategies become fixed as learned patterns of compulsive behaviors. Learning theory provides useful concepts for explaining certain aspects of obsessive-compulsive phenomena—for example, the anxiety-provoking capacity of ideas not necessarily frightening in themselves and the establishment of compulsive patterns of behavior.

Psychosocial Factors

Personality Factors. OCD differs from obsessive-compulsive personality disorder, which is associated with an obsessive concern for details, perfectionism, and other similar personality traits. Most persons with OCD do not have premorbid compulsive symptoms, and such personality traits are neither necessary nor sufficient for the development of OCD. Only about 15 to 35 percent of patients with OCD have had premorbid obsessional traits.

Psychodynamic Factors. Psychodynamic insight may be of great help in understanding problems with treatment compliance, interpersonal difficulties, and personality problems accompanying the Axis I disorder. Many patients with OCD may refuse to cooperate with effective treatments such as selective serotonin reuptake inhibitors (SSRIs) and behavior therapy. Even though the symptoms of OCD may be biologically driven, psychodynamic meanings may be attached to them. Patients may become invested in maintaining the symptomatology because of secondary gains. For example, a male patient, whose mother stays home to take care of him, may unconsciously wish to hang on to his OCD symptoms because they keep the attention of his mother.

Another contribution of psychodynamic understanding involves the interpersonal dimensions. Studies have shown that relatives will accommodate the patient through active participation in rituals or significant modifications of their daily routines. This form of family accommodation is correlated with stress in the family, rejecting attitudes toward the patient, and poor family functioning. Often, the family members are involved in an effort to reduce the patient's anxiety or to control the patient's expressions of anger. This pattern of relatedness may become internalized and be recreated when the patient enters a treatment setting. By looking at recurring patterns of interpersonal relationships from a psychodynamic perspective, patients may learn how their illness affects others.

Finally, one other contribution of psychodynamic thinking is recognition of the precipitants that initiate or exacerbate symptoms. Often, interpersonal difficulties increase the patient's anxiety and, thus, increase the patient's symptomatology as well. Research suggests that OCD may be precipitated by a number of environmental stressors, especially those involving pregnancy, childbirth, or parental care of children. An understanding of the stressors may assist the clinician in an overall treatment plan that reduces the stressful events themselves or their meaning to the patient.

SIGMUND FREUD. In classic psychoanalytic theory, OCD was termed *obsessive-compulsive neurosis* and was considered a regression from the oedipal phase to the anal psychosexual phase of development. When patients with OCD feel threatened by anxiety about retaliation for unconscious impulses or by the loss of a significant object's love, they retreat from the oedipal position and regress to an intensely ambivalent emotional stage associated with the anal phase. The ambivalence is connected to the unraveling of the smooth fusion between sexual and aggressive drives characteristic of the oedipal phase. The coexistence of hatred and love toward the same person leaves patients paralyzed with doubt and indecision.

An example of how Freud viewed OCD symptoms is described by Otto Fenichel in the following case.

A patient, who was not analyzed, complained in the first interview that he suffered from the compulsion to look backward constantly, from fear that he might have overlooked something important behind him. These ideas were predominant; he might overlook a coin lying on the ground; he might have injured an insect by stepping on it; or an insect might have fallen on its back and need his help. The patient was also afraid of touching anything, and whenever he had touched an object he had to convince himself that he had not destroyed it. He had no vocation because the severe compulsions disturbed all his working activity; however, he had one passion: housecleaning. He liked to visit his neighbors and clean their houses, just for fun. Another symptom was described by the patient as his "clothes consciousness;" he was constantly preoccupied with the question whether or not his suit fitted. He, too, stated that sexuality did not play an important part in his life. He had sexual intercourse two or three times a year only, and exclusively with girls in whom he had no personal interest. Later on, he mentioned another symptom. As a child, he had felt his mother to be disgusting and had been terribly afraid of touching her. There was no real reason whatsoever for such a disgust, for the mother had been a nice person. (From Fenichel O. *The Psychoanalytic Theory of Neurosis*. New York: Norton; 1945:274, with permission.)

In this clinical picture, Freud believed the need to be clean and not to touch is related to anal sexuality, and the disgust for the mother is a reaction against incestuous fears.

One of the striking features of patients with OCD is the degree to which they are preoccupied with aggression or cleanliness, either overtly in the content of their symptoms or in the associations that lie behind them. The psychogenesis of OCD, therefore, may lie in disturbances in normal growth and development related to the anal-sadistic phase of development.

Ambivalence. Ambivalence is an important feature of normal children during the anal-sadistic developmental phase; children feel both love and murderous hate toward the same object, sometimes simultaneously. Patients with OCD often consciously experience both love and hate toward an object. This conflict of opposing emotions is evident in a patient's doing and undoing patterns of behavior and in paralyzing doubt in the face of choices.

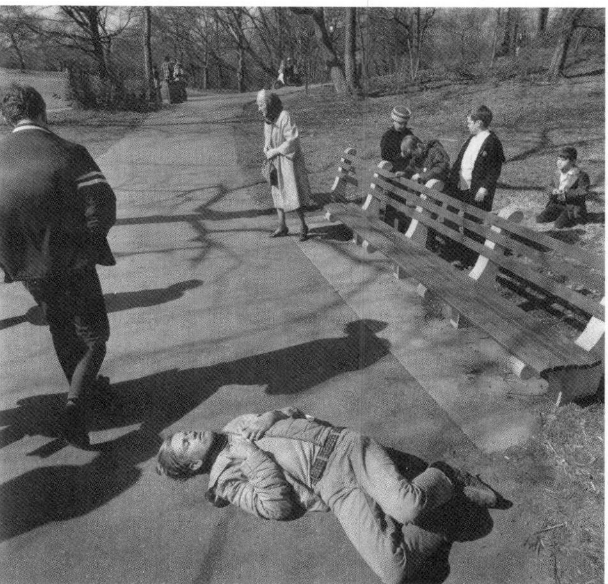

FIGURE 16.4–2
In magical thinking, one believes that the thought is equal to the deed, that wishing a person dead will make it happen as symbolized in this illustration. (Courtesy of Arthur Tress.)

Magical Thinking. In magical thinking, regression uncovers early modes of thought rather than impulses; that is, ego functions, as well as id functions, are affected by regression. Inherent in magical thinking is omnipotence of thought. Persons believe that merely by thinking about an event in the external world they can cause the event to occur without intermediate physical actions. This feeling causes them to fear having an aggressive thought (Fig. 16.4–2).

DIAGNOSIS

As part of the diagnostic criteria for OCD, the text revision of the fourth edition of *Diagnostic and Statistical Manual of Mental Disorders* (DSM-IV-TR) allows clinicians to specify that patients have the poor insight type of OCD if they generally do not recognize the excessiveness of their obsessions and compulsions (Table 16.4–1).

CLINICAL FEATURES

Patients with OCD often take their complaints to physicians other than psychiatrists (Table 16.4–2). Most patients with OCD have both obsessions and compulsions—up to 75 percent in some surveys. Some researchers and clinicians believe that the number may be much closer to 100 percent if patients are carefully assessed for the presence of mental compulsions in addition to behavioral compulsions. For example, an obsession about hurting a child may be followed by a mental compulsion to repeat a specific prayer a specific number of times. Other researchers and clinicians, however, believe that some patients do have only obsessive thoughts without compulsions. Such patients are likely to have repetitious thoughts of a sexual or aggressive act that

Table 16.4–1
DSM-IV-TR Diagnostic Criteria for Obsessive-Compulsive Disorder

A. Either obsessions or compulsions:
Obsessions as defined by (1), (2), (3), and (4):
(1) recurrent and persistent thoughts, impulses, or images that are experienced, at some time during the disturbance, as intrusive and inappropriate and that cause marked anxiety or distress
(2) the thoughts, impulses, or images are not simply excessive worries about real-life problems
(3) the person attempts to ignore or suppress such thoughts, impulses, or images, or to neutralize them with some other thought or action
(4) the person recognizes that the obsessional thoughts, impulses, or images are a product of his or her own mind (not imposed from without as in thought insertion)
Compulsions as defined by (1) and (2):
(1) repetitive behaviors (e.g., hand washing, ordering, checking) or mental acts (e.g., praying, counting, repeating words silently) that the person feels driven to perform in response to an obsession, or according to rules that must be applied rigidly
(2) the behaviors or mental acts are aimed at preventing or reducing distress or preventing some dreaded event or situation; however, these behaviors or mental acts either are not connected in a realistic way with what they are designed to neutralize or prevent or are clearly excessive

B. At some point during the course of the disorder, the person has recognized that the obsessions or compulsions are excessive or unreasonable.
Note: This does not apply to children.

C. The obsessions or compulsions cause marked distress, are time-consuming (take more than 1 hour a day), or significantly interfere with the person's normal routine, occupational (or academic) functioning, or usual social activities or relationships.

D. If another Axis I disorder is present, the content of the obsessions or compulsions is not restricted to it (e.g., preoccupation with food in the presence of an eating disorder; hair pulling in the presence of trichotillomania; concern with appearance in the presence of body dysmorphic disorder; preoccupation with drugs in the presence of a substance use disorder; preoccupation with having a serious illness in the presence of hypochondriasis; preoccupation with sexual urges or fantasies in the presence of a paraphilia; or guilty ruminations in the presence of major depressive disorder).

E. The disturbance is not due to the direct physiological effects of a substance (e.g., a drug of abuse, a medication) or a general medical condition.

Specify if:
With poor insight: if, for most of the time during the current episode, the person does not recognize that the obsessions and compulsions are excessive or unreasonable

(From American Psychiatric Association. *Diagnostic and Statistical Manual of Mental Disorders.* 4th ed. Text rev. Washington, DC: American Psychiatric Association; copyright 2000, with permission.)

is reprehensible to them. For clarity, it is best to conceptualize obsessions as thoughts and compulsions as behavior.

Obsessions and compulsions are the essential features of OCD. An idea or an impulse intrudes itself insistently and persistently into a person's conscious awareness. Typical obsessions associated with OCD include thoughts about contamination ("my hands are dirty") or doubts ("I forgot to turn off the stove").

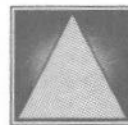

Table 16.4–2
Nonpsychiatric Clinical Specialists Likely to See Obsessive-Compulsive Disorder Patients

Specialist	Presenting Problem
Dermatologist	Chapped hands, eczematoid appearance
Family practitioner	Family member washing excessively, may mention counting or checking compulsions
Oncologist, infectious disease internist	Insistent belief that person has acquired immune deficiency syndrome
Neurologist	Obsessive-compulsive disorder associated with Tourette's disorder, head injury, epilepsy, choreas, other basal ganglia lesions or disorders
Neurosurgeon	Severe, intractable obsessive-compulsive disorder
Obstetrician	Postpartum obsessive-compulsive disorder
Pediatrician	Parent's concern about child's behavior, usually excessive washing
Pediatric cardiologist	Obsessive-compulsive disorder secondary to Sydenham's chorea
Plastic surgeon	Repeated consultations for "abnormal" features
Dentist	Gum lesions from excessive teeth cleaning

(From Rapoport JL. The neurobiology of obsessive-compulsive disorder. *JAMA.* 1988;260:2889, with permission.)

A feeling of anxious dread accompanies the central manifestation and the key characteristic of a compulsion is that it reduces the anxiety associated with the obsession. The obsession or the compulsion is ego-alien; that is, it is experienced as foreign to the person's experience of himself or herself as a psychological being. No matter how vivid and compelling the obsession or compulsion, the person usually recognizes it as absurd and irrational. The person suffering from obsessions and compulsions usually feels a strong desire to resist them. Nevertheless, about half of all patients offer little resistance to compulsions, although about 80 percent of all patients believe that the compulsion is irrational. Sometimes, patients overvalue obsessions and compulsions—for example, they may insist that compulsive cleanliness is morally correct, even though they have lost their jobs because of time spent cleaning.

Symptom Patterns

The presentation of obsessions and compulsions is heterogeneous in adults (Table 16.4–3) and in children and adolescents (Table 16.4–4). The symptoms of an individual patient can overlap and change with time, but OCD has four major symptom patterns.

Contamination. The most common pattern is an obsession of contamination, followed by washing or accompanied by compulsive avoidance of the presumably contaminated object. The feared object is often hard to avoid (e.g., feces, urine, dust, or germs). Patients may literally rub the skin off their hands by excessive hand washing or may be unable to leave their homes because of fear of germs. Although anxiety is the most common emotional response to the feared object, obsessive shame and disgust are also common. Patients with contamination

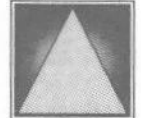

Table 16.4–3
Obsessive-Compulsive Symptoms in Adults

Variable	%
Obsessions (*N* = 200)	
Contamination	45
Pathological doubt	42
Somatic	36
Need for symmetry	31
Aggressive	28
Sexual	26
Other	13
Multiple obsessions	60
Compulsions (*N* = 200)	
Checking	63
Washing	50
Counting	36
Need to ask or confess	31
Symmetry and precision	28
Hoarding	18
Multiple comparisons	48
Course of illness (*N* = 100)[a]	
Type	
Continuous	85
Deteriorative	10
Episodic	2
Not present	71
Present	29

[a]Age at onset: men, 17.5 ± 6.8 years; women, 20.8 ± 8.5 years.
(From Rasmussen SA, Eiser JL. The epidemiology and differential diagnosis of obsessive compulsive disorder. *J Clin Psychiatry*. 1992;53[4 Suppl]: 6, with permission.)

obsessions usually believe that the contamination is spread from object to object or person to person by the slightest contact.

Pathological Doubt. The second most common pattern is an obsession of doubt, followed by a compulsion of checking. The obsession often implies some danger of violence (e.g., forgetting to turn off the stove or not locking a door). The checking may involve multiple trips back into the house to check the stove, for example. The patients have an obsessional self-doubt and always feel guilty about having forgotten or committed something.

Intrusive Thoughts. In the third most common pattern, there are intrusive obsessional thoughts without a compulsion. Such obsessions are usually repetitious thoughts of a sexual or aggressive act that is reprehensible to the patient. Patients obsessed with thoughts of aggressive or sexual acts may report themselves to police or confess to a priest.

Symmetry. The fourth most common pattern is the need for symmetry or precision, which can lead to a compulsion of slowness. Patients can literally take hours to eat a meal or shave their faces.

Other Symptom Patterns. Religious obsessions and compulsive hoarding are common in patients with OCD. Trichotillomania (compulsive hair pulling) and nail biting may be compulsions related to OCD. Masturbation may also be compulsive.

Mental Status Examination

On mental status examinations, patients with OCD may show symptoms of depressive disorders. Such symptoms are present in about 50 percent of all patients. Some patients with OCD have character traits suggesting obsessive-compulsive personality disorder (e.g., excessive need for preciseness and neatness), but most do not. Patients with OCD, especially men, have a higher than average celibacy rate. Married patients have a greater than usual amount of marital discord.

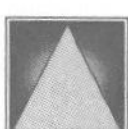

Table 16.4–4
Reported Obsessions and Compulsions for 70 Consecutive Child and Adolescent Patients

Major Presenting Symptom	No. (%) Reporting Symptom at Initial Interview[a]
Obsession	
Concern or disgust with bodily wastes or secretions (urine, stool, saliva), dirt, germs, environmental toxins	30 (43)
Fear something terrible may happen (fire, death or illness of loved one, self, or others)	18 (24)
Concern or need for symmetry, order, or exactness	12 (17)
Scrupulosity (excessive praying or religious concerns out of keeping with patient's background)	9 (13)
Lucky and unlucky numbers	6 (8)
Forbidden or perverse sexual thoughts, images, or impulses	3 (4)
Intrusive nonsense sounds, words, or music	1 (1)
Compulsion	
Excessive or ritualized hand washing, showering, bathing, toothbrushing, or grooming	60 (85)
Repeating rituals (e.g., going in and out of door, up and down from chair)	36 (51)
Checking doors, locks, stove, appliances, car brakes	32 (46)
Cleaning and other rituals to remove contact with contaminants	16 (23)
Touching	14 (20)
Ordering and arranging	12 (17)
Measures to prevent harm to self or others (e.g., hanging clothes a certain way)	11 (16)
Counting	13 (18)
Hoarding and collecting	8 (11)
Miscellaneous rituals (e.g., licking, spitting, special dress pattern)	18 (26)

[a]Multiple symptoms recorded, so total exceeds 70.
(From Rapoport JL. The neurobiology of obsessive-compulsive disorder. *JAMA*. 1988;260:2889, with permission.)

Ms. A is a 30-year-old elementary schoolteacher with a 5-year history of repetitively checking report card grades; retracing her driving route; and having persistent thoughts about harm coming to her parents, excessive concern about her health, and difficulty grocery shopping alone.

Ms. A first developed checking behaviors during high school, when she would repeatedly check that the stove and her curling iron were turned off before going out of the house. She reports that her checking rituals grew progressively worse during college and, at that time, she began rereading pages in books over and over before exams.

During the past 5 years, Ms. A has experienced further escalation of her symptoms. She often spends 3 to 4 hours a day engaged in checking behaviors. She spends at least an hour going back and forth between her curling iron, the stove, and the front door. After she is finally convinced that everything is as it should be, the thought comes to her that she should check it all again because, if she doesn't, the house may burn down or a burglar may get in. She often retraces her driving path for fear that she has run over someone or something. Report card time is a nightmare for Ms. A because she repetitively checks and rechecks for hours the grades she has recorded. She reports an association between obsessional thoughts about harm coming to her parents and her behaviors. For instance, she feels that she must call her mother every day, both in the morning and evening, no matter how inconvenient this may be. She says that she is obsessed with the thought that if she misses a phone call to check on her, her mother may have a stroke and die and it will be her fault for failing to call.

In the context of discussing this in the clinician's office, Ms. A can admit that this fear is unrealistic; however, she says that it is almost impossible for her not to make these daily calls without becoming excessively anxious and scared.

Over the past 5 years, Ms. A has become increasingly isolated because of her checking behaviors and obsessional thoughts. She will not go grocery shopping alone because she is terrified that she will do something to "embarrass" herself if she is out alone. Therefore, she will go to shopping malls or grocery stores only when she is with her husband or a friend. Her social isolation and need to be with her husband when she goes out have resulted in increased marital tension. In addition to her tendency to keep herself isolated, the patient is beginning to have doubts about whether she wants a child. Her ambivalence about a possible pregnancy is also contributing to the martial conflict.

Her medical history is unremarkable, with the exception of mild mood swings before the onset of menses. She denies any history of head trauma or central nervous system (CNS) infection. Her family history is notable for superstitions, hoarding behaviors, and extreme meticulousness in her mother and maternal grandmother. There is also a positive family history of motor tics in the patient's father and two paternal uncles. Ms. A has no history of alcohol or other substance abuse.

On initial evaluation, the patient's mental status examination is notable for increased motor movements, a dysthymic/anxious effect, and intermittent tearfulness. There is no abnormality of thought process or thought content. (From *DSM-IV-TR Case Studies*.)

The DSM-IV-TR diagnostic requirement of personal distress and functional impairment differentiates OCD from ordinary or mildly excessive thoughts and habits.

DIFFERENTIAL DIAGNOSIS

Medical Conditions

A number of primary medical disorders can produce syndromes bearing a striking resemblance to OCD. The current conceptualization of OCD as a disorder of the basal ganglia derives from the phenomenological similarity between idiopathic OCD and OCD-like disorders that are associated with basal ganglia diseases, such as Sydenham's chorea and Huntington's disease. Neurological signs of such basal ganglia pathology must be assessed when considering the diagnosis of OCD in a patient presenting for psychiatric treatment. It should also be noted that OCD frequently develops before age 30 years, and new-onset OCD in an older individual should raise questions about potential neurological contributions to the disorder.

Tourette's Disorder

Obsessive-compulsive disorder is closely related to Tourette's syndrome, as the two conditions frequently co-occur, both in individuals over time and within families. About 90 percent of persons with Tourette's disorder have compulsive symptoms, and as many as two thirds meet the diagnostic criteria for OCD.

In its classic form, Tourette's syndrome is associated with a pattern of recurrent vocal and motor tics that bears only a slight resemblance to OCD. The premonitory urges that precede tics often strikingly resemble obsessions, however, and many of the more complicated motor tics are very similar to compulsions.

Other Psychiatric Conditions

Obsessive-compulsive behavior is found in a host of other psychiatric disorders, and the clinician must also rule out these conditions when diagnosing OCD. OCD exhibits a superficial resemblance to obsessive-compulsive personality disorder, which is associated with an obsessive concern for details, perfectionism, and other similar personality traits. The conditions are easily distinguished in that only OCD is associated with a true syndrome of obsessions and compulsions.

Psychotic symptoms often lead to obsessive thoughts and compulsive behaviors that can be difficult to distinguish from OCD with poor insight, in which obsessions border on psychosis. The keys to distinguishing OCD from psychosis are (1) patients with OCD can almost always acknowledge the unreasonable nature of their symptoms, and (2) psychotic illnesses are typically associated with a host of other features that are not characteristic of OCD. Similarly, OCD can be difficult to differentiate from depression, because the two disorders often occur comorbidly, and major depression is often associated with obsessive thoughts that, at times, border on true obsessions such as those that characterize OCD. The two conditions are best distinguished by their courses. Obsessive symptoms associated with depression are only found in the presence of a depressive episode, whereas true OCD persists despite remission of depression.

COURSE AND PROGNOSIS

More than half of patients with OCD have a sudden onset of symptoms. The onset of symptoms for about 50 to 70 percent of patients occurs after a stressful event, such as a pregnancy, a sexual problem, or the death of a relative. Because many persons manage to keep their symptoms secret, they often delay 5 to 10 years before coming to psychiatric attention, although the delay is probably shortening with increased awareness of the disorder. The course is usually long but variable; some patients experience a fluctuating course, and others experience a constant one.

About 20 to 30 percent of patients have significant improvement in their symptoms, and 40 to 50 percent have moderate improvement. The remaining 20 to 40 percent of patients either remain ill or their symptoms worsen.

About one third of patients with OCD have major depressive disorder, and suicide is a risk for all patients with OCD. A poor prognosis is indicated by yielding to (rather than resisting) compulsions, childhood onset, bizarre compulsions, the need for hospitalization, a coexisting major depressive disorder, delusional beliefs, the presence of overvalued ideas (i.e., some acceptance of obsessions and compulsions), and the presence of a personality disorder (especially schizotypal personality disorder). A good prognosis is indicated by good social and occupational adjustment, the presence of a precipitating event, and an episodic nature of the symptoms. The obsessional content does not seem to be related to the prognosis.

TREATMENT

With mounting evidence that OCD is largely determined by biological factors, classic psychoanalytic theory has fallen out of favor. Moreover, because OCD symptoms appear to be largely refractory to psychodynamic psychotherapy and psychoanalysis, pharmacological and behavioral treatments have become common. But psychodynamic factors may be of considerable benefit in understanding what precipitates exacerbations of the disorder and in treating various forms of resistance to treatment, such as noncompliance with medication.

Many patients with OCD tenaciously resist treatment efforts. They may refuse to take medication and may resist carrying out therapeutic homework assignments and other activities prescribed by behavior therapists. The obsessive-compulsive symptoms themselves, no matter how biologically based, may have important psychological meanings that make patients reluctant to give them up. Psychodynamic exploration of a patient's resistance to treatment may improve compliance.

Well-controlled studies have found that pharmacotherapy, behavior therapy, or a combination of both is effective in significantly reducing the symptoms of patients with OCD. The decision about which therapy to use is based on the clinician's judgment and experience and the patient's acceptance of the various modalities.

Pharmacotherapy

The efficacy of pharmacotherapy in OCD has been proved in many clinical trials and is enhanced by the observation that the studies find a placebo response rate of only about 5 percent.

The drugs, some of which are used to treat depressive disorders or other mental disorders, can be given in their usual dosage ranges. Initial effects are generally seen after 4 to 6 weeks of treatment, although 8 to 16 weeks are usually needed to obtain maximal therapeutic benefit. Treatment with antidepressant drugs is still controversial, and a significant proportion of patients with OCD who respond to treatment with antidepressant drugs seem to relapse if the drug therapy is discontinued.

The standard approach is to start treatment with an SSRI or clomipramine and then move to other pharmacological strategies if the serotonin-specific drugs are not effective. The serotonergic drugs have increased the percentage of patients with OCD who are likely to respond to treatment to the range of 50 to 70 percent.

Serotonin-Specific Reuptake Inhibitors. Each of the SSRIs available in the United States—fluoxetine (Prozac), fluvoxamine (Luvox), paroxetine (Paxil), sertraline (Zoloft), citalopram (Celexa)—has been approved by the US Food and Drug Administration (FDA) for the treatment of OCD. Higher dosages have often been necessary for a beneficial effect, such as 80 mg a day of fluoxetine. Although the SSRIs can cause sleep disturbance, nausea and diarrhea, headache, anxiety, and restlessness, these adverse effects are often transient and are generally less troubling than the adverse effects associated with tricyclic drugs, such as clomipramine. The best clinical outcomes occur when SSRIs are used in combination with behavioral therapy.

Clomipramine. Of all the tricyclic and tetracyclic drugs, clomipramine is the most selective for serotonin reuptake versus norepinephrine reuptake and is exceeded in this respect only by the SSRIs. The potency of serotonin reuptake of clomipramine is exceeded only by sertraline and paroxetine. Clomipramine was the first drug to be FDA approved for the treatment of OCD. Its dosing must be titrated upward over 2 to 3 weeks to avoid gastrointestinal adverse effects and orthostatic hypotension, and as with other tricyclic drugs, it causes significant sedation and anticholinergic effects, including dry mouth and constipation. As with SSRIs, the best outcomes result from a combination of drug and behavioral therapy.

Other Drugs. If treatment with clomipramine or an SSRI is unsuccessful, many therapists augment the first drug by the addition of valproate (Depakene), lithium (Eskalith), or carbamazepine (Tegretol). Other drugs that can be tried in the treatment of OCD are venlafaxine (Effexor), pindolol (Visken), and the monoamine oxidase inhibitors (MAOIs), especially phenelzine (Nardil). Other pharmacological agents for the treatment of unresponsive patients include buspirone (BuSpar), 5-hydroxytryptamine (5-HT), l-tryptophan, and clonazepam (Klonopin). Adding an atypical antipsychotic such as risperidol has helped in some cases.

Behavior Therapy

Although few head-to-head comparisons have been made, behavior therapy is as effective as pharmacotherapies in OCD, and some data indicate that the beneficial effects are longer lasting with behavior therapy. Many clinicians, therefore, consider behavior therapy the treatment of choice for OCD. Behavior therapy can be conducted in both outpatient and inpatient settings. The principal behavioral approaches in OCD are exposure and response prevention. Desensitization, thought stopping, flooding, implosion therapy, and aversive conditioning have also been used in patients with OCD. In behavior therapy, patients must be truly committed to improvement.

Psychotherapy

In the absence of adequate studies of insight-oriented psychotherapy for OCD, any valid generalizations about its effectiveness are hard to make, although there are anecdotal reports of successes. Individual analysts have seen striking and lasting changes for the better in patients with obsessive-compulsive personality disorder, especially when they are able to come to terms with the aggressive impulses underlying their character traits. Likewise, analysts and dynamically oriented psychiatrists have observed marked symptomatic improvement in patients with OCD in the course of analysis or prolonged insight psychotherapy.

Supportive psychotherapy undoubtedly has its place, especially for those patients with OCD who, despite symptoms of varying degrees of severity, are able to work and make social adjustments. With continuous and regular contact with an interested, sympathetic, and encouraging professional person, patients may be able to function by virtue of this help, without which their symptoms would incapacitate them. Occasionally, when obsessional rituals and anxiety reach an intolerable intensity, it is necessary to hospitalize patients until the shelter of an institution and the removal from external environmental stresses diminish symptoms to a tolerable level.

A patient's family members are often driven to the verge of despair by the patient's behavior. Any psychotherapeutic endeavors must include attention to the family members through provision of emotional support, reassurance, explanation, and advice on how to manage and respond to the patient.

Other Therapies

Family therapy is often useful in supporting the family, helping reduce marital discord resulting from the disorder, and building a treatment alliance with the family members for the good of the patient. Group therapy is useful as a support system for some patients.

For extreme cases that are treatment resistant and chronically debilitating, electroconvulsive therapy (ECT) and psychosurgery are considerations. ECT is not as effective as psychosurgery, but it should be tried before surgery. A common psychosurgical procedure for OCD is cingulotomy, which is successful in treating 25 to 30 percent of otherwise treatment-unresponsive patients. Other surgical procedures (e.g., subcaudate tractotomy, also known as *capsulotomy*) have also been used for this purpose. Nonablative surgical techniques involving indwelling electrodes in various basal ganglia nuclei (deep brain stimulation) are under investigation to treat both OCD and Tourette's disorder. All of these are all increasingly being performed using MRI-guided stereotactic techniques. The most common complication of psychosurgery is the development of seizures, which are almost always controlled by treatment with phenytoin (Dilantin). Some patients who do not respond to psychosurgery alone and who do not respond to pharmacotherapy or behavior therapy before the operation do respond to pharmacotherapy or behavior therapy after psychosurgery.

References

Besiroglu L, Agargun MY, Ozbebit O, Aydin A. A discrimination based on autogenous versus reactive obsessions in obsessive-compulsive disorder and related clinical manifestations. *CNS Spectrum*. 2006;11(3):179–186.

Burgy M. Psychopathology of obsessive-compulsive disorder: A phenomenological approach. *Psychopathology*. 2005;38:291–300.

Crino R, Slade T, Andrews G. The changing prevalence and severity of obsessive-compulsive disorder criteria from DSM-III to DSM-IV. *Am J Psychiatry*. 2005;162:876–882.

De Silva P, Rachman S. *Obsessive-Compulsive Disorder: The Facts*. New York: Oxford University Press; 2006.

Roth RM, Milovan D, Baribeau J, O'Connor K. Neuropsychological functioning in early- and late-onset obsessive-compulsive disorder. *J Neuropsychiatry Clin Neurosci*. 2005;17:208–213.

Simpson HB, Huppert JD, Petkova E, Foa EB, Liebowitz MR. Response versus remission in obsessive-compulsive disorder. *J Clin Psychiatry*. 2006;67(2): 269–276.

Stewart SE, Jenike MA, Keuthen NJ. Severe obsessive-compulsive disorder with and without comorbid hair pulling: Comparisons and clinical implications. *J Clin Psychiatry*. 2005;66(7):864–869.

Taylor S, Abramowitz JS, McKay D, Calamari JE, Sookman D, Kyrios M, Wilhelm S, Carmin C. Do dysfunctional beliefs play a role in all types of obsessive-compulsive disorder? *J Anxiety Disord*. 2006;20(1):85–97.

Vulink NC, Denys D, Westenberg HG. Bupropion for patients with obsessive-compulsive disorder: An open-label, fixed-dose study. *J Clin Psychiatry*. 2005;66(2):228–230.

Yaryura-Tobias JA. An overview on delusions, obsessions and overvalued ideas: An intimate cluster of thought pathology. *Clinical Neuropsychiatry: Journal of Treatment Evaluation*. 2004;1:5–12.

▲ 16.5 Posttraumatic Stress Disorder and Acute Stress Disorder

Posttraumatic stress disorder (PTSD) is a condition marked by the development of symptoms after exposure to traumatic life events. The person reacts to this experience with fear and helplessness, persistently relives the event, and tries to avoid being reminded of it. Kagan has suggested that children who are behaviorally inhibited may be especially susceptible to anxiety or PTSD after threatening events.

To make the diagnosis, the symptoms must last for more than a month after the event and must significantly affect important areas of life, such as family and work. The text revision of the fourth edition of *Diagnostic and Statistical Manual of Mental Disorders* (DSM-IV-TR) defines a disorder that is similar to PTSD called *acute stress disorder*, which occurs earlier than PTSD (within 4 weeks of the event) and remits within 2 days to 4 weeks. If symptoms persist after that time, a diagnosis of PTSD is warranted.

The stressors causing both acute stress disorder and PTSD are sufficiently overwhelming to affect almost anyone. They can arise from experiences in war, torture, natural catastrophes, assault, rape, and serious accidents, for example, in cars and in burning buildings. Persons reexperience the traumatic event in their dreams and their daily thoughts; they are determined to evade anything that would bring the event to mind and they undergo a numbing of responsiveness along with a state of hyperarousal. Other symptoms are depression, anxiety, and cognitive difficulties, such as poor concentration.

HISTORY

Because of the presence of autonomic cardiac symptoms, "soldier's heart" was the name given during the US Civil War to a syndrome similar to PTSD. Jacob DaCosta's 1871 paper, "On Irritable Heart," described soldiers with the syndrome. In the 1900s, the influence of psychoanalysis was strong, particularly in the United States, and clinicians applied the diagnosis of traumatic neurosis to the condition. In World War I, the syndrome was called *shell shock* and was hypothesized to result from brain trauma caused by exploding shells. In 1941, the survivors of a fire in a crowded Boston nightclub, the Coconut Grove, showed increased nervousness, fatigue, and nightmares. World War II veterans, survivors of Nazi concentration camps, and survivors of the atomic bombings in Japan had similar symptoms, sometimes

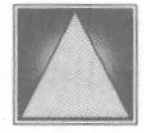

Table 16.5–1
Eponyms and Symptoms of Posttraumatic Stress Disorders in Various US Wars

War	Disorder
Civil War	"Irritable heart": fatigue, shortness of breath, palpitations, headache, excessive sweating, dizziness, disturbed sleep, fainting
World War I	"Effort syndrome": fatigue, shortness of breath, palpitations, headache, excessive sweating, dizziness, disturbed sleep, fainting, difficulty concentrating
World War II	"Combat stress reaction": fatigue, shortness of breath, palpitations, headache, excessive sweating, dizziness, disturbed sleep, fainting, difficulty concentrating, forgetfulness
Vietnam War	"Posttraumatic stress disorder": fatigue, shortness of breath, palpitations, headache, muscle and joint pain, dizziness, disturbed sleep, difficulty concentrating, forgetfulness
Gulf War	"Gulf War syndrome": fatigue, shortness of breath, headache, muscle and joint pain, disturbed sleep, difficulty concentrating, forgetfulness

(Adapted from Hymans KC, Wignall FS, Roswell P. War, syndromes and their evaluation: from the US Civil War to the Persian Gulf War. *Ann Intern Med.* 1996;125:398, with permission.)

called *combat neurosis* or *operational fatigue* (Table 16.5–1). The psychiatric morbidity associated with Vietnam War veterans finally brought the concept of PTSD, as it is currently known, to fruition and was first introduced as a psychiatric diagnosis in the late 1980s. In all these traumatic situations, the appearance of the disorder roughly correlated with the severity of the stressor; the most severe stresses (e.g., incarceration in concentration camps) resulted in the occurrence of the syndrome in more than 75 percent of the victims.

EPIDEMIOLOGY

The lifetime incidence of PTSD is estimated to be 9 to 15 percent and the lifetime prevalence of PTSD is estimated to be about 8 percent of the general population, although an additional 5 to 15 percent may experience subclinical forms of the disorder. Among high-risk groups whose members experienced traumatic events, the lifetime prevalence rates range from 5 to 75 percent. About 30 percent of Vietnam veterans experienced PTSD, and an additional 25 percent experienced subclinical forms of the disorder. The lifetime prevalence ranges from about 10 to 12 percent among women and 5 to 6 percent among men. Although PTSD can appear at any age, it is most prevalent in young adults, because they tend be more exposed to precipitating situations. Children can also have the disorder (discussed below). Men and women differ in the types of traumas to which they are exposed and their liability to develop PTSD. The lifetime prevalence is significantly higher in women, and a higher proportion of women go on to develop the disorder. Historically, men's trauma was usually combat experience, and women's trauma was most commonly assault or rape. The disorder is most likely to occur in those who are single, divorced, widowed, socially withdrawn, or of low socioeconomic level. The most important risk factors, however, for this disorder are the severity, duration, and proximity of a person's exposure to the actual trauma. A familial pattern seems to exist for this disorder, and first-degree biological relatives of persons with a history of depression have an increased risk for developing PTSD following a traumatic event.

COMORBIDITY

Comorbidity rates are high among patients with PTSD, with about two thirds having at least two other disorders. Common comorbid conditions include depressive disorders, substance-related disorders, other anxiety disorders, and bipolar disorders. Comorbid disorders make persons more vulnerable to developing PTSD.

ETIOLOGY

Stressor

By definition, a stressor is the prime causative factor in the development of PTSD. Not everyone experiences the disorder after a traumatic event, however. The stressor alone does not suffice to cause the disorder. The response to the traumatic event must involve intense fear or horror. Clinicians must also consider individual preexisting biological and psychosocial factors and events that happened before and after the trauma. For example, a member of a group who lived through a disaster can sometimes deal with trauma because others shared the experience. The stressor's subjective meaning to a person is also important. For example, survivors of a catastrophe may experience guilt feelings (survivor guilt) that can predispose to, or exacerbate, PTSD.

Risk Factors

As mentioned, even when faced with overwhelming trauma, most persons do not experience PTSD symptoms. The National Comorbidity Study found that 60 percent of males and 50 percent of females had experienced some significant trauma, whereas the reported lifetime prevalence of PTSD was only 6.7 percent. Similarly, events that may appear mundane or less than catastrophic to most persons can produce PTSD in some. Evidence indicates of a dose–response relationship between the degree of trauma and the likelihood of symptoms. Table 16.5–2 summarizes vulnerability factors that appear to play etiological roles in the disorder.

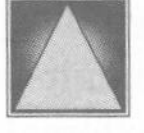

Table 16.5–2
Predisposing Vulnerability Factors in Posttraumatic Stress Disorder

Presence of childhood trauma
Borderline, paranoid, dependent, or antisocial personality disorder traits
Inadequate family or peer support system
Being female
Genetic vulnerability to psychiatric illness
Recent stressful life changes
Perception of an external locus of control (natural cause) rather than an internal one (human cause)
Recent excessive alcohol intake

Table 16.5–3
Psychodynamic Themes in Posttraumatic Stress Disorder

- The subjective meaning of a stressor may determine its traumatogenicity.
- Traumatic events can resonate with childhood traumas.
- Inability to regulate affect can result from trauma.
- Somatization and alexithymia may be among the aftereffects of trauma.
- Common defenses used include denial, minimization, splitting, projective disavowal, dissociation, and guilt (as a defense against underlying helplessness).
- Mode of object relatedness involves projection and introjection of the following roles: omnipotent rescuer, abuser, and victim.

Psychodynamic Factors

The psychoanalytic model of the PTSD hypothesizes that the trauma has reactivated a previously quiescent, yet unresolved psychological conflict. The revival of the childhood trauma results in regression and the use of the defense mechanisms of repression, denial, reaction formation, and undoing. According to Freud, a splitting of consciousness occurs in patients who reported a history of childhood sexual trauma. A preexisting conflict might be symbolically reawakened by the new traumatic event. The ego relives and thereby tries to master and reduce the anxiety. Psychodynamic themes in PTSD are summarized in Table 16.5–3. Persons who suffer from alexithymia, the inability to identify or verbalize feeling states, are incapable of soothing themselves when under stress.

Cognitive-Behavioral Factors

The cognitive model of PTSD posits that affected persons cannot process or rationalize the trauma that precipitated the disorder. They continue to experience the stress and attempt to avoid experiencing it by avoidance techniques. Consistent with their partial ability to cope cognitively with the event, persons experience alternating periods of acknowledging and blocking the event. The attempt of the brain to process the massive amount of information provoked by the trauma is thought to produce these alternating periods. The behavioral model of PTSD emphasizes two phases in its development. First, the trauma (the unconditioned stimulus) that produces a fear response is paired, through classic conditioning, with a conditioned stimulus (physical or mental reminders of the trauma, such as sights, smells, or sounds). Second, through instrumental learning, the conditioned stimuli elicit the fear response independent of the original unconditioned stimulus, and persons develop a pattern of avoiding both the conditioned stimulus and the unconditioned stimulus. Some persons also receive secondary gains from the external world, commonly monetary compensation, increased attention or sympathy, and the satisfaction of dependency needs. These gains reinforce the disorder and its persistence.

Biological Factors

The biological theories of PTSD have developed both from preclinical studies of animal models of stress and from measures of biological variables in clinical populations with the disorder. Many neurotransmitter systems have been implicated by both sets of data. Preclinical models of learned helplessness, kindling, and sensitization in animals have led to theories about norepinephrine, dopamine, endogenous opioids, and benzodiazepine receptors and the hypothalamic-pituitary-adrenal (HPA) axis. In clinical populations, data have supported hypotheses that the noradrenergic and endogenous opiate systems, as well as the HPA axis, are hyperactive in at least some patients with PTSD. Other major biological findings are increased activity and responsiveness of the autonomic nervous system, as evidenced by elevated heart rates and blood pressure readings and by abnormal sleep architecture (e.g., sleep fragmentation and increased sleep latency). Some researchers have suggested a similarity between PTSD and two other psychiatric disorders, major depressive disorder and panic disorder.

Noradrenergic System. Soldiers with PTSD-like symptoms exhibit nervousness, increased blood pressure and heart rate, palpitations, sweating, flushing, and tremors—symptoms associated with adrenergic drugs. Studies found increased 24-hour urine epinephrine concentrations in veterans with PTSD and increased urine catecholamine concentrations in sexually abused girls. Further, platelet α_2- and lymphocyte β-adrenergic receptors are downregulated in PTSD, possibly in response to chronically elevated catecholamine concentrations. About 30 to 40 percent of patients with PTSD report flashbacks after yohimbine (Yocon) administration. Such findings are strong evidence for altered function in the noradrenergic system in PTSD.

Opioid System. Abnormality in the opioid system is suggested by low plasma β-endorphin concentrations in PTSD. Combat veterans with PTSD demonstrate a naloxone (Narcan)-reversible analgesic response to combat-related stimuli, raising the possibility of opioid system hyperregulation similar to that in the HPA axis. One study showed that nalmefene (Revex), an opioid receptor antagonist, was of use in reducing symptoms of PTSD in combat veterans.

Corticotropin-Releasing Factor and the HPA Axis. Several factors point to dysfunction of the HPA axis. Studies have demonstrated low plasma and urinary free cortisol concentrations in PTSD. More glucocorticoid receptors are found on lymphocytes, and challenge with exogenous corticotropin-releasing factor (CRF) yields a blunted ACTH response. Further, suppression of cortisol by challenge with low-dose dexamethasone (Decadron) is enhanced in PTSD. This indicates hyperregulation of the HPA axis in PTSD. Also, some studies have revealed cortisol hypersuppression in trauma-exposed patients who develop PTSD, compared with patients exposed to trauma who do not develop PTSD, indicating that it might be specifically associated with PTSD and not just trauma. Overall, this hyperregulation of the HPA axis differs from the neuroendocrine activity usually seen during stress and in other disorders such as depression. Recently, the role of the hippocampus in PTSD has received increased attention, although the issue remains controversial. Animal studies have shown that stress is associated with structural changes in the hippocampus, and studies of combat veterans with PTSD have revealed a lower average volume in the hippocampal region of the brain. Structural changes in the amygdala, an area of the brain associated with fear, have also been demonstrated.

DIAGNOSIS

The DSM-IV-TR diagnostic criteria for PTSD (Table 16.5–4) specify that the symptoms of experiencing, avoidance, and hyperarousal must have lasted more than 1 month. For patients whose symptoms have been present less than 1 month, the appropriate diagnosis may be acute stress disorder (Table 16.5–5). The DSM-IV-TR diagnostic criteria for PTSD allow clinicians to specify whether the disorder is acute (if the symptoms have lasted less than 3 months) or chronic (if the symptoms have lasted 3 months or more). DSM-IV-TR also allows clinicians to specify that the disorder was with delayed onset if the onset of the symptoms was 6 months or more after the stressful event. An example of an acute stress disorder not progressing to PTSD as a result of timely therapy is given in the following vignette.

A 40-year-old man saw the September 11, 2001, terrorist attack on the World Trade Center (discussed below) on television. Immediately thereafter he developed feelings of panic associated with thoughts that he was going to die. The panic disappeared within a few hours; however, for the next few nights he had nightmares with obsessive thoughts about dying. He sought consultation and reported to the psychiatrist that his wife had been killed in a plane crash 10 years earlier. He described having adapted to the loss "normally" and was aware that his current symptoms were probably related to that traumatic event. On further exploration in brief psychotherapy, he realized that his reactions to his wife's death were muted and that his relationship with her was ambivalent. At the time of her death he was contemplating divorce and frequently had wished her dead. He had never fully worked through the mourning process for his wife, and his catastrophic reaction to the terrorist attack was related, in part, to those suppressed feelings. He was able to recognize his feelings of guilt related to his wife and his need for punishment manifested by thinking he was going to die.

CLINICAL FEATURES

The principal clinical features of PTSD are painful reexperiencing of the event, a pattern of avoidance and emotional numbing, and fairly constant hyperarousal. The disorder may not develop until months or even years after the event. The mental status examination often reveals feelings of guilt, rejection, and humiliation. Patients may also describe dissociative states and panic attacks, and illusions and hallucinations may be present. Associated symptoms can include aggression, violence, poor impulse control, depression, and substance-related disorders. Cognitive testing may reveal that patients have impaired memory and attention. Patients have elevated Sc, D, F, and Ps scores on the Minnesota Multiphasic Personality Inventory, and the Rorschach test findings often include aggressive and violent material.

Mr. R, a burly, full-bearded, 37-year-old Irish fireman, was hospitalized for second- and third-degree burns over a third of his body. During the month he spent on the burn unit, he was the model stoic patient, but a week after discharge, during his first appointment in

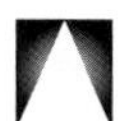

Table 16.5–4
DSM-IV-TR Diagnostic Criteria for Posttraumatic Stress Disorder

A. The person has been exposed to a traumatic event in which both of the following were present:
   (1) the person experienced, witnessed, or was confronted with an event or events that involved actual or threatened death or serious injury, or a threat to the physical integrity of self or others
   (2) the person's response involved intense fear, helplessness, or horror. **Note**: In children, this may be expressed instead by disorganized or agitated behavior.

B. The traumatic event is persistently reexperienced in one (or more) of the following ways:
   (1) recurrent and intrusive distressing recollections of the event, including images, thoughts, or perceptions. **Note**: In young children, repetitive play may occur in which themes or aspects of the trauma are expressed.
   (2) recurrent distressing dreams of the event. **Note**: In children, there may be frightening dreams without recognizable content.
   (3) acting or feeling as if the traumatic event were recurring (includes a sense of reliving the experience, illusions, hallucinations, and dissociative flashback episodes, including those that occur on awakening or when intoxicated). **Note**: In young children, trauma-specific reenactment may occur.
   (4) intense psychological distress at exposure to internal or external cues that symbolize or resemble an aspect of the traumatic event
   (5) physiological reactivity on exposure to internal or external cues that symbolize or resemble an aspect of the traumatic event

C. Persistent avoidance of stimuli associated with the trauma and numbing of general responsiveness (not present before the trauma), as indicated by three (or more) of the following:
   (1) efforts to avoid thoughts, feelings, or conversations associated with the trauma
   (2) efforts to avoid activities, places, or people that arouse recollections of the trauma
   (3) inability to recall an important aspect of the trauma
   (4) markedly diminished interest or participation in significant activities
   (5) feeling of detachment or estrangement from others
   (6) restricted range of affect (e.g., unable to have loving feelings)
   (7) sense of a foreshortened future (e.g., does not expect to have a career, marriage, children, or a normal life span)

D. Persistent symptoms of increased arousal (not present before the trauma), as indicated by two (or more) of the following:
   (1) difficulty falling or staying asleep
   (2) irritability or outbursts of anger
   (3) difficulty concentrating
   (4) hypervigilance
   (5) exaggerated startle response

E. Duration of the disturbance (symptoms in Criteria B, C, and D) is more than 1 month.

F. The disturbance causes clinically significant distress or impairment in social, occupational, or other important areas of functioning.

Specify if:
   Acute: if duration of symptoms is less than 3 months
   Chronic: if duration of symptoms is 3 months or more

Specify if:
   With delayed onset: if onset of symptoms is at least 6 months after the stressor

(From American Psychiatric Association. *Diagnostic and Statistical Manual of Mental Disorders*. 4th ed. Text rev. Washington, DC: American Psychiatric Association; copyright 2000, with permission.)

Table 16.5–5
DSM-IV-TR Diagnostic Criteria for Acute Stress Disorder

A. The person has been exposed to a traumatic event in which both of the following were present:
   (1) the person experienced, witnessed, or was confronted with an event or events that involved actual or threatened death or serious injury, or a threat to the physical integrity of self or others
   (2) the person's response involved intense fear, helplessness, or horror
B. Either while experiencing or after experiencing the distressing event, the individual has three (or more) of the following dissociative symptoms:
   (1) a subjective sense of numbing, detachment, or absence of emotional responsiveness
   (2) a reduction in awareness of his or her surroundings (e.g., "being in a daze")
   (3) derealization
   (4) depersonalization
   (5) dissociative amnesia (i.e., inability to recall an important aspect of the trauma)
C. The traumatic event is persistently reexperienced in at least one of the following ways: recurrent images, thoughts, dreams, illusions, flashback episodes, or a sense of reliving the experience; or distress on exposure to reminders of the traumatic event.
D. Marked avoidance of stimuli that arouse recollections of the trauma (e.g., thoughts, feelings, conversations, activities, places, people).
E. Marked symptoms of anxiety or increased arousal (e.g., difficulty sleeping, irritability, poor concentration, hypervigilance, exaggerated startle response, motor restlessness).
F. The disturbance causes clinically significant distress or impairment in social, occupational, or other important areas of functioning or impairs the individual's ability to pursue some necessary task, such as obtaining necessary assistance or mobilizing personal resources by telling family members about the traumatic experience.
G. The disturbance lasts for a minimum of 2 days and a maximum of 4 weeks and occurs within 4 weeks of the traumatic event.
H. The disturbance is not due to the direct physiological effects of a substance (e.g., a drug of abuse, a medication) or a general medical condition, is not better accounted for by brief psychotic disorder, and is not merely an exacerbation of a preexisting Axis I or Axis II disorder.

(From American Psychiatric Association. *Diagnostic and Statistical Manual of Mental Disorders.* 4th ed. Text rev. Washington, DC: American Psychiatric Association; copyright 2000, with permission.)

the surgical clinic, he is tremulous, stammering, and unresponsive to the surgeon's assurances. Deeply concerned, the surgeon pages the burn unit's consultant-liaison psychiatrist and introduces him to Mr. R, who shakes hands and mumbles, "I sort of expected you'd be calling in the shrinks."

Although Mr. R tries to appear confident, he chain-smokes, glances around furtively, squirms in his chair, and at times bursts into tears. When he is able to calm down somewhat, he explains that he cannot stop thinking about how, for the first time in his distinguished career, he entered a burning building alone, in a manner contrary to the safety procedures he was responsible for teaching, and sustained near-fatal burns. He tells the interviewer, "You see before you the wreck of what once was a pretty good man."

His hospitalization was bearable because the staff on the burn unit was very supportive, but he admits now that during that month he was troubled by frequent terrible nightmares about the fire. He did not say anything about them because he thought they would pass. Now that he is home, he admits he is constantly jumpy and nervous and drinks to calm his nerves and to sleep. He feels humiliated about his mistake at the fire and cannot stop replaying it in his mind. His recurrent nightmares, in which he reexperiences the fire over and over again, have worsened since he has been home, and he is having great difficulty going to sleep—perchance to dream. At the invitation of his co-workers, Mr. R. recently visited the fire station with great reluctance. When a fire alarm sounded, he "nearly leapt out of what was left of my skin" and began to tremble and sweat. He left hurriedly, pleading illness. He is very ashamed about having to face his co-workers in his present condition—shaky, sweating, and frightened—instead of his usual brash and fearless self. He is scheduled to return to his duties on a part-time basis in 2 weeks but doesn't think he ever will be able to stand going back to the firehouse or going out to fight a fire again. He feels that he is cracking up. He paces the floor; is afraid to leave the house on his own; and frequently feels dizzy, numb, and detached. He says he doesn't feel like himself anymore and does not want to talk to anyone. He also expresses a sense of total helplessness and horror about how he looks. For the first time, he has begun to wonder whether life is worth living. (From *DSM-IV-TR Case Studies.*)

PTSDs in Children and Adolescents

PTSD occurs in children and adolescents, but most studies of the disorder have focused on adults. DSM-IV-TR has little to say about PTSD as it affects young children except to describe symptoms such as repetitive dreams of the event, nightmares of monsters, and the development of physical symptoms such as stomachaches and headaches.

High rates of PTSD have been documented in children exposed to such life-threatening events as combat and other war-related trauma, kidnapping, severe illness or burns, bone marrow transplantation, and a number of natural and man-made disasters. Studies on young victims or witneses to criminal assault, domestic violence, and community violence have revealed high psychiatric morbidity following exposure to violence. As might be expected, the prevalence of PTSD is higher in children than in adults exposed to the same stressor. In certain situations, up to 90 percent of children will develop the disorder. In general, PTSD has been underestimated in children and adolescents.

Child risk factors include demographic factors (e.g., age, sex, socioeconomic status), other life events (positive and negative), social and cultural cognitions, psychiatric comorbidity, and inherent coping strategies. Family factors (e.g., parental psychopathology and functioning, marital status, and education) play key roles in determining symptoms of a child. Parents' responses to traumatic events particularly influence young children who may not completely understand the nature of the trauma or its inherent danger.

Stressor. Stressors in children may be sudden, single-incident trauma or ongoing or chronic trauma, such as physical or sexual abuse. Children also suffer as the result of "indirect" exposure—that is, the unwitnessed death or injury of a loved one, as in situations of disaster, war, or community violence.

Reenactment and Reexperiencing. Children, as with adults, reexperience the traumatic event in the form of distressing, intrusive thoughts or memories, flashbacks, and dreams. Children's nightmares may be linked specifically to a trauma theme or may generalize to other fears. Flashbacks occur in children as well as in their adolescent or adult victim counterparts. "Traumatic play," a specific form of reexperiencing seen in young children, consists of repetitive acting out of the trauma or trauma-related themes in play. Older children may incorporate aspects of the trauma into their lives in a process termed *reenactment*. Fantasized actions of intervention or revenge are common; adolescents should be considered at increased risk for impulsive acting out secondary to anger and revenge fantasies. Related behaviors in child and adolescent victims of trauma include sexual acting out, substance use, and delinquency. Children often withdraw and show reduced interest in previously enjoyable activities. Regressive behaviors, such as enuresis or fear of sleeping alone, may also occur. (See Section 51.2 for further discussion.)

Gulf War Syndrome

In the Persian Gulf War against Iraq, which began in 1990 and ended in 1991, approximately 700,000 American soldiers served in the coalition forces. On their return, more than 100,000 US veterans reported a vast array of health problems, including irritability, chronic fatigue, shortness of breath, muscle and joint pain, migraine headaches, digestive disturbances, rash, hair loss, forgetfulness, and difficulty concentrating. Collectively, these symptoms were called the *Gulf War syndrome*. The US Department of Defense acknowledges that up to 20,000 troops serving in the combat area may have been exposed to chemical weapons and the best evidence indicates that the condition is a disorder that in some cases may have been precipitated by exposure to an unidentified toxin (Table 16.5–6). One study of loss of memory found structural change in the right parietal lobe and damage to the basal ganglia with associated neurotransmitter dysfunction. A significant number of veterans have developed amyotrophic lateral sclerosis (ALS), thought to be the result of genetic mutations.

In a 1997 editorial in the *Journal of the American Medical Association*, the relationship of the Persian Gulf War syndrome and stress was stated as follows:

> Physicians need to acknowledge that many Gulf War veterans are experiencing stress-related disorders and the physical consequences of stress. These conditions should not be hidden or denied, but rather are well-recognized entities that have been studied extensively in survivors of past wars, most notably the Vietnam conflict. As physicians, we should not accept a diagnosis of stress-related disorder in veterans prior to excluding treatable physical factors, but at the same time, we need to recognize the pervasive presence of stress-related illness such as hypertension, fibromyalgia, and chronic fatigue among Persian Gulf War veterans and manage these illnesses appropriately. As a nation, we need to get beyond the fallacious idea that diseases of the mind either are not real or are shameful and to better recognize that the mind and the body are inextricably linked.

In addition, thousands of Gulf War veterans developed PTSD and the differentiation between the two disorders has proved difficult. PTSD is caused by psychological stress and the Gulf War syndrome is presumed to be caused by environmental biological stressors. Signs and symptoms often overlap and both conditions may exist at the same time.

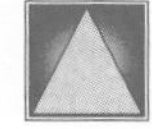

Table 16.5–6
Syndromes Associated with Toxic Exposure[a]

Syndrome	Characteristics	Possible Toxins
1	Impaired cognition	Insect repellant containing N,N′-diethyl-m-toluamide (DEET[b]) absorbed through skin
2	Confusion-ataxia	Exposure to chemical weapons, e.g., sarin
3	Arthromyoneuropathy	Insect repellant containing DEET[b] in combination with oral pyridostigmine[c]

[a]The three syndromes involve a relatively small group ($N = 249$) of veterans and are based on self-reported descriptions and selection. Data are from R. W. Haley and T. L. Kurt.
[b]DEET is a carbonate compound used as an insect repellant. Concentrations above 30 percent DEET are neurotoxic in children. The military repellant contained 75 percent. (DEET is available in 100 percent concentrations as an unregulated over-the-counter preparation usually sold in sports stores.)
[c]Most US troops took low-dose pyridostigmine (Mestinon, 30 mg every 8 hours) for about 5 days in 1991 to protect against exposure to the nerve agent soman.

9/11/01

On September 11, 2001, terrorist activity destroyed the World Trade Center (Fig. 16.5–1) in New York City and damaged the Pentagon in Washington. It resulted in more than 3,500 deaths and injuries and left many citizens in need of therapeutic intervention. One survey found a prevalence rate of 11.4 percent for PTSD and 9.7 percent for depression in US citizens 1 month after 9/11. As of 2004, it is estimated that more than 25,000 people continue to suffer symptoms of PTSD related to the 9/11 attacks beyond the 1 year mark.

Iraq and Afghanistan

In October 2001, the United States, along with Australia, Canada, and the United Kingdom, began the invasion of Afghanistan in the wake of the September 11, 2001 attacks. On March 20, 2003, US forces, along with allies, invaded Iraq, marking the beginning of the Iraq War.

Both wars are ongoing and PTSD is a rising problem with an estimated 17 percent of returning soldiers having PTSD. The rate of PTSD is higher in women soldiers. Women account for 11 percent of those who served in Iraq and Afghanistan and for 14 percent of patients at Veterans Affairs (VA) hospitals and clinics. Women soldiers are more likely to seek help than men soldiers.

Natural Disasters

Tsunami. On December 26, 2004, a massive tsunami struck the shores of Indonesia, Sri Lanka, South India, and Thailand and caused serious damage and deaths as far west as the coast of Africa and South Africa (Fig. 16.5–2). The tsunami caused nearly 300,000 deaths and left more than 1 million people without homes. Many survivors continue to

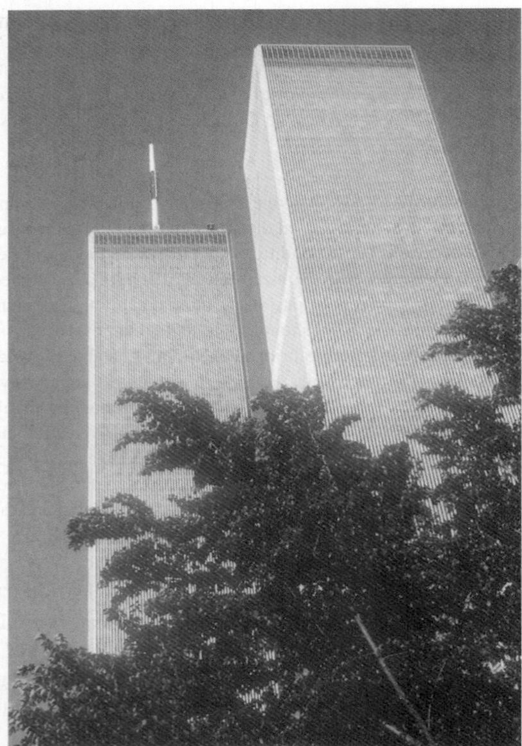

FIGURE 16.5–1
The World Trade Center, New York City, prior to 9/11/01. (Courtesy of Kimsamoon, Inc.)

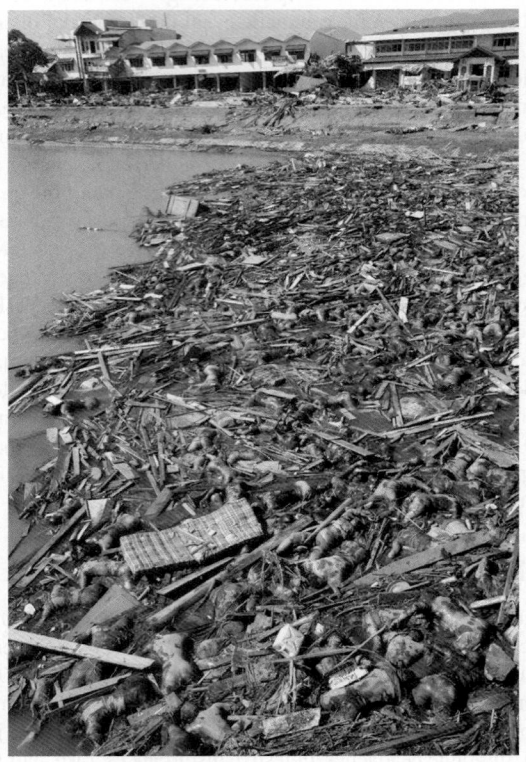

FIGURE 16.5–2
In December 2004, an undersea earthquake in the Indian Ocean caused a tsunami that killed more than 283,000 people. Inhabitants of the countries devastated by the tsunami were unaware of its approach because no tsunami warning systems were in place. Note the dead bodies through the debris. (Courtesy of the US Navy.)

live in fear and show signs of PTSD; fishermen fear venturing out to sea, children fear playing at beaches they once enjoyed, and many families have trouble sleeping in fear of another tsunami.

Hurricane. In August 2005, a category 5 hurricane, Hurricane Katrina, ravaged the Gulf of Mexico, the Bahamas, South Florida, Louisiana, Mississippi, and Alabama (Fig. 16.5–3). Its high winds and torrential rainfall breached the levee system that protected New Orleans, Louisiana causing major flooding. More than 1,300 people were killed and tens of thousands were left stranded.

Earthquake. On October 8, 2005, a 7.6 magnitude earthquake hit South Asia, affecting Pakistan, Afghanistan and Northern India. The area of Kashmir in South Asia was the worse hit. More than 85,000 casualties have occurred (Fig. 16.5–4). Up to 3 million people were left homeless. Many cases of PTSD developed among those who experienced these disasters.

Torture

The intentional physical and psychological torture of one human by another can have emotionally damaging effects comparable to, and possibly worse than, those seen with combat and other types of trauma. As defined by the United Nations, torture is any deliberate infliction of severe mental pain or suffering, usually through cruel, inhuman, or degrading treatment or punishment. This broad definition includes various forms of interpersonal violence, from chronic domestic abuse to broad-scale genocide. According to Amnesty International, torture is common and widespread in most of the 150 countries worldwide where human rights violations have been documented. Recent figures estimate that between 5 and 35 percent of the world's 14 million refugees have had at least one torture experience, and these numbers do not even account for the consequences of the current political, regional, and religious disputes in Eastern Europe, the former Yugoslavia, and the Middle East.

Torture is distinct from most other types of trauma because it is human inflicted and intentional. One individual working for himself or for a higher authority may abuse another to punish, exact retribution, or obtain information from the victim. Methods can be physical (e.g., beatings, burning of the skin, electric shock, or asphyxiation) or psychological, through threats, humiliation, or being forced to watch others, often loved ones, being tortured. One distinct method of torture that may combine physical and psychological aspects is brainwashing (see Chapter 20, Dissociative disorders and Chapter 30, additional conditions that may be a focus of clinical attention). Although many forms of torture can leave lasting physical scars, which themselves serve as constant reminders of the trauma, it seems that the true purpose is the psychological effect—the torturer invokes fear, helplessness, and, ultimately, physical and mental weakness in the victim. Reported prevalence rates of PTSD among survivors of torture are about 36 percent, much higher than the average lifetime prevalence, and researchers concur that the severity and duration of PTSD may be greater when the stressors are of human design. Studies have also revealed substantial comorbidity with depression and other anxiety disorders in victims of torture.

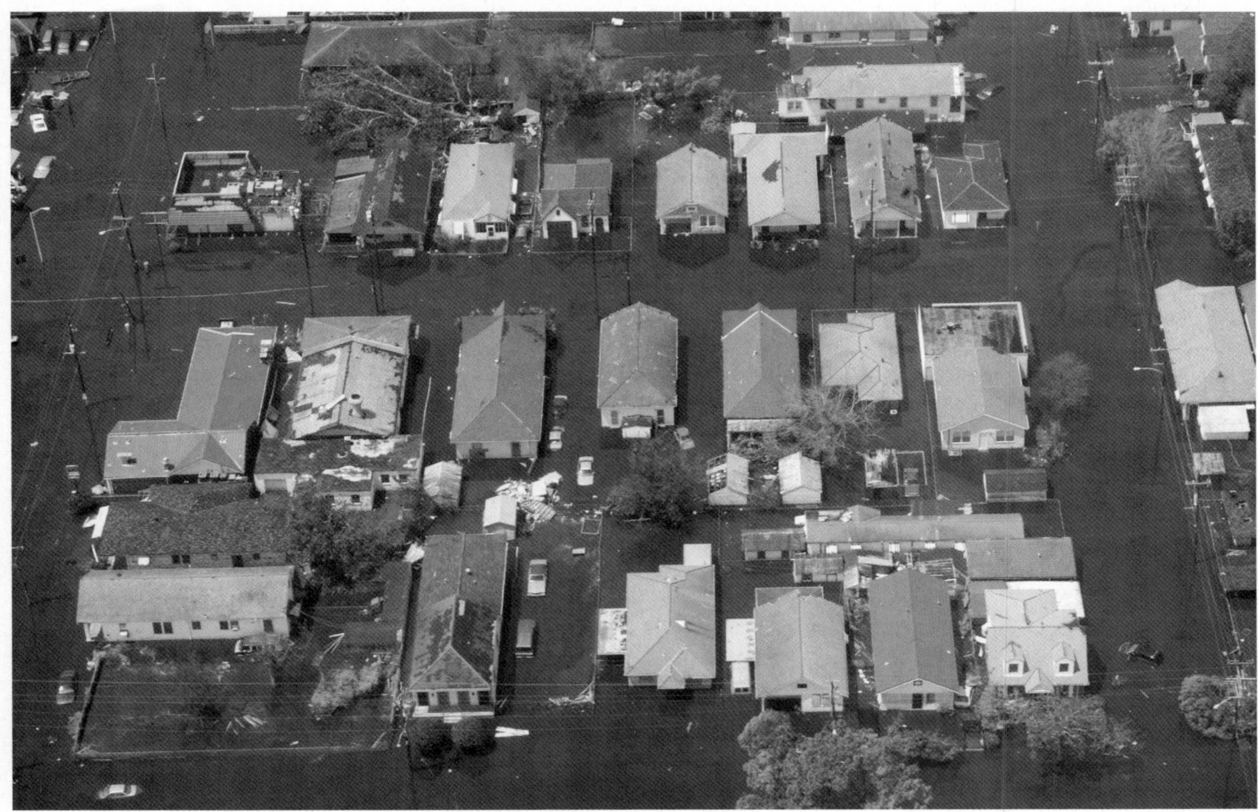

FIGURE 16.5–3
In August 2005, Hurricane Katrina, a category 5 hurricane hit land in Florida before crossing over the Gulf of Mexico and making a second landfall in Louisiana. The hurricane devastated the southern states, leaving millions without power. Thousands of homes were destroyed by the 175-mph winds and by the hurricane's storm surge, which ultimately left about 80% of New Orleans underwater. Hurricane Katrina caused the deaths of at least 1,380 people; others are still missing or unaccounted for. (Courtesy of www.fema.gov.)

Other common psychological complaints include somatization, obsessive-compulsive symptoms, anger-hostility, phobias, paranoid ideation, and psychotic episodes.

Treatment methods for survivors of torture are the same as those for other posttraumatic symptoms and disorders, but clinicians must be especially sensitive to the array of stressful life events that victims of torture have experienced. Many survivors who present for treatment are refugees who face new posttrauma stressors over and above the effects of torture, such as separation from family, difficulty finding work, difficulty obtaining health services, language barriers, loneliness, poverty, and racial discrimination. Religious faith, political education and commitment, strong social support, and mental preparedness for the possibility of torture seem to serve as protective factors against developing PTSD and other psychological consequences after torture. Moreover, cultural and religious factors that influence coping styles may also affect treatment response in survivors of torture.

DIFFERENTIAL DIAGNOSIS

Because patients often exhibit complex reactions to trauma, the clinician must be careful to exclude other syndromes as well when evaluating patients presenting in the wake of trauma. It is particularly important to recognize potentially treatable medical contributors to posttraumatic symptomatology, especially head injury during the trauma. Medical contributors can usually be detected through a careful history and physical examination. Other organic considerations that can both cause and exacerbate the symptoms are epilepsy, alcohol-use disorders, and other substance-related disorders. Acute intoxication or withdrawal from some substances may also present a clinical picture that is difficult to distinguish from the disorder until the effects of the substance have worn off.

Symptoms of PTSD can be difficult to distinguish from both panic disorder and generalized anxiety disorder, because all three syndromes are associated with prominent anxiety and autonomic arousal. Keys to correctly diagnosing PTSD involve a careful review of the time course relating the symptoms to a traumatic event. PTSD is also associated with reexperiencing and avoidance of a trauma, features typically not present in panic or generalized anxiety disorder. Major depression is also a frequent concomitant of PTSD. Although the two syndromes are not usually difficult to distinguish phenomenologically, it is important to note the presence of comorbid depression, because this can influence treatment of PTSD. PTSD must be differentiated from a series of related disorders that can exhibit phenomenological similarities, including borderline personality disorder, dissociative disorders, and factitious disorders. Borderline personality disorder can be difficult to distinguish from PTSD. The two

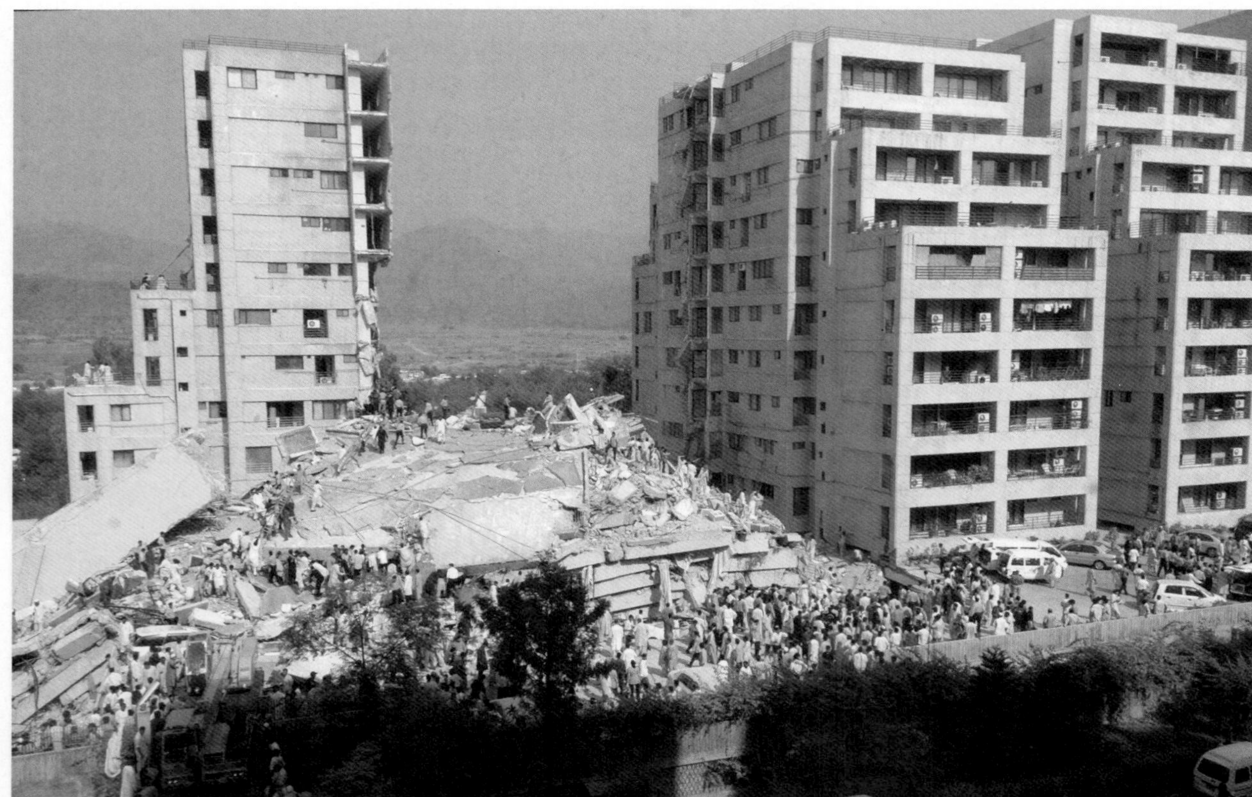

FIGURE 16.5–4
On October 8, 2005, a 7.6 magnitude earthquake hit South Asia leaving millions homeless and more than 87,000 people dead. The disputed area of Kashmir, shown in this figure, was hit worst. (Courtesy of Samoon Ahmad, M.D.)

disorders can coexist or even be causally related. Patients with dissociative disorders do not usually have the degree of avoidance behavior, the autonomic hyperarousal, or the history of trauma that patients with PTSD report.

COURSE AND PROGNOSIS

PTSD usually develops some time after the trauma. The delay can be as short as 1 week or as long as 30 years. Symptoms can fluctuate over time and may be most intense during periods of stress. Untreated, about 30 percent of patients recover completely, 40 percent continue to have mild symptoms, 20 percent continue to have moderate symptoms, and 10 percent remain unchanged or become worse. After 1 year, about 50 percent of patients will recover. A good prognosis is predicted by rapid onset of the symptoms, short duration of the symptoms (less than 6 months), good premorbid functioning, strong social supports, and the absence of other psychiatric, medical, or substance-related disorders or other risk factors.

In general, the very young and the very old have more difficulty with traumatic events than do those in midlife. For example, about 80 percent of young children who sustain a burn injury show symptoms of PTSD 1 or 2 years after the initial injury; only 30 percent of adults who suffer such an injury have a PTSD after 1 year. Presumably, young children do not yet have adequate coping mechanisms to deal with the physical and emotional insults of the trauma. Likewise, older persons are likely to have more rigid coping mechanisms than younger adults and to be less able to muster a flexible approach to dealing with the effects of trauma. Furthermore, the traumatic effects can be exacerbated by physical disabilities characteristic of late life, particularly disabilities of the nervous system and the cardiovascular system, such as reduced cerebral blood flow, failing vision, palpitations, and arrhythmias. Preexisting psychiatric disability, whether a personality disorder or a more serious condition, also increases the effects of particular stressors. PTSD that is comorbid with other disorders is often more severe and perhaps more chronic and may be difficult to treat. The availability of social supports may also influence the development, severity, and duration of PTSD. In general, patients who have a good network of social support are less likely to have the disorder and to experience it in its severe forms, and are more likely to recover faster.

TREATMENT

When a clinician is faced with a patient who has experienced a significant trauma, the major approaches are support, encouragement to discuss the event, and education about a variety of coping mechanisms (e.g., relaxation). The use of sedatives and hypnotics can also be helpful. When a patient experienced a traumatic event in the past and now has PTSD, the emphasis should be on education about the disorder and its treatment, both pharmacological and psychotherapeutic. The clinician should also work to destigmatize the notion of mental illness and PTSD. Additional support for the patient and the family can be obtained through local and national support groups for patients with PTSD.

Pharmacotherapy

Selective serotonin reuptake inhibitors (SSRIs), such as sertraline (Zoloft) and paroxetine (Paxil), are considered first-line treatments for PTSD, owing to their efficacy, tolerability, and safety ratings. SSRIs reduce symptoms from all PTSD symptom clusters and are effective in improving symptoms unique to PTSD, not just symptoms similar to those of depression or other anxiety disorders. Buspirone (BuSpar) is serotonergic and may also be of use.

The efficacy of imipramine (Tofranil) and amitriptyline (Elavil), two tricyclic drugs, in the treatment of PTSD is supported by a number of well-controlled clinical trials. Although some trials of the two drugs have had negative findings, most of these trials had serious design flaws, including too short a duration. Dosages of imipramine and amitriptyline should be the same as those used to treat depressive disorders, and an adequate trial should last at least 8 weeks. Patients who respond well should probably continue the pharmacotherapy for at least 1 year before an attempt is made to withdraw the drug. Some studies indicate that pharmacotherapy is more effective in treating the depression, anxiety, and hyperarousal than in treating the avoidance, denial, and emotional numbing.

Other drugs that may be useful in the treatment of PTSD include the monoamine oxidase inhibitors (MAOIs) (e.g., phenelzine [Nardil]), trazodone (Desyrel), and the anticonvulsants (e.g., carbamazepine [Tegretol], valproate [Depakene]). Some studies have also revealed improvement in PTSD in patients treated with reversible monoamine oxidase inhibitors (RIMAs). Use of clonidine (Catapres) and propranolol (Inderal), which are antiadrenergic agents, is suggested by the theories about noradrenergic hyperactivity in the disorder. Almost no positive data concern the use of antipsychotic drugs in the disorder, so the use of drugs such as haloperidol (Haldol) should be reserved for the short-term control of severe aggression and agitation.

Psychotherapy

Psychodynamic psychotherapy may be useful in the treatment of many patients with PTSD. In some cases, reconstruction of the traumatic events with associated abreaction and catharsis may be therapeutic, but psychotherapy must be individualized because reexperiencing the trauma overwhelms some patients.

Psychotherapeutic interventions for PTSD include behavior therapy, cognitive therapy, and hypnosis. Many clinicians advocate time-limited psychotherapy for the victims of trauma. Such therapy usually takes a cognitive approach and also provides support and security. The short-term nature of the psychotherapy minimizes the risk of dependence and chronicity, but issues of suspicion, paranoia, and trust often adversely affect compliance. Therapists should overcome patients' denial of the traumatic event, encourage them to relax, and remove them from the source of the stress. Patients should be encouraged to sleep, using medication if necessary. Support from persons in their environment (e.g., friends and relatives) should be provided. Patients should be encouraged to review and abreact emotional feelings associated with the traumatic event and to plan for future recovery. Abreaction—experiencing the emotions associated with the event—may be helpful for some patients. The amobarbital (Amytal) interview has been used to facilitate this process.

Psychotherapy after a traumatic event should follow a model of crisis intervention with support, education, and the development of coping mechanisms and acceptance of the event. When PTSD has developed, two major psychotherapeutic approaches can be taken. The first is exposure therapy, in which the patient reexperiences the traumatic event through imaging techniques or in vivo exposure. The exposures can be intense, as in implosive therapy, or graded, as in systematic desensitization. The second approach is to teach the patient methods of stress management, including relaxation techniques and cognitive approaches to coping with stress. Some preliminary data indicate that, although stress management techniques are effective more rapidly than exposure techniques, the results of exposure techniques last longer.

Another psychotherapeutic technique that is relatively novel and somewhat controversial is eye movement desensitization and reprocessing (EMDR), in which the patient focuses on the lateral movement of the clinician's finger while maintaining a mental image of the trauma experience. The general belief is that symptoms can be relieved as patients work through the traumatic event while in a state of deep relaxation. Proponents of this treatment state it is as effective, and possibly more effective, than other treatments for PTSD and that it is preferred by both clinicians and patients who have tried it.

In addition to individual therapy techniques, group therapy and family therapy have been reported to be effective in cases of PTSD. The advantages of group therapy include sharing of traumatic experiences and support from other group members. Group therapy has been particularly successful with Vietnam veterans and survivors of catastrophic disasters such as earthquakes. Family therapy often helps sustain a marriage through periods of exacerbated symptoms. Hospitalization may be necessary when symptoms are particularly severe or when a risk of suicide or other violence exists.

References

Cary J, O'Donnell ML, Creamer M. Delayed-onset PTSD: A prospective study of injury survivors. *J Affect Disord.* 2006;90:257–261.

Cavanagh SR, Shin LM, Rauch SL. Brain imaging in posttraumatic stress disorder. *Directions in Psychiatry.* 2006;26:33–48.

Classen CC, Pain C, Field NP, Woods P. Posttraumatic personality disorder: A reformulation of complex posttraumatic stress disorder and borderline personality disorder. *Psychiatr Clin North Am.* 2006;29:87–112.

Gurvits TV, Metzger LJ, Lasko NB, Cannistraro PA, Tarhan AS, Gilbertson MW, Orr SP, Charbonneau AM, Wedig MM, Pitman RK. Subtle neurologic compromise as a vulnerability factor for combat-related posttraumatic stress disorder. *Arch Gen Psychiatry.* 2006;63:571–576.

Hoge CW, Castro CA, Messer SC, McGurk D, Cotting DI, Koffman RL. Combat duty in Iraq and Afghanistan, Mental Health Problem, and Barriers to Care. *N Engl J Med.* 2004;351:13.

McFarland BH. Introduction: Disaster dangers and decisions. *Community Ment Health J.* 2005;41:631–632.

Nemeroff CB, Bremner JD, Foa EB, Mayberg HS, North CS, Stein MB. Posttraumatic stress disorder: A state-of-the-science review. *J Psychiatr Res.* 2006;40: 1–21.

Oquendo M, Brent DA, Birmaher B, Greenhill L, Kolko D, Stanley B, Zelazny J, Burke AK, Firinciogullari S, Ellis SP, Mann JJ. Posttraumatic stress disorder

comorbid with major depression: Factors mediating the association with suicidal behavior. *Am J Psychiatry*. 2005;162:560–566.
Palyo SA, Beck JG. Post-traumatic stress disorder symptoms, pain, and perceived life control: Associations with psychosocial and physical functioning. *Pain*. 2005;117:121–127.
Wilson JP, Drozdek B, Turkovic S. Posttraumatic Shame and Guilt. *Trauma, Violence & Abuse*. 2006;7:122–141.

▲ 16.6 Generalized Anxiety Disorder

Anxiety can be conceptualized as a normal and adaptive response to threat that prepares the organism for flight or fight. Persons who seem to be anxious about almost everything, however, are likely to be classified as having generalized anxiety disorder. The text revision of the fourth edition of the *Diagnostic and Statistical Manual of Mental Disorders* (DSM-IV-TR) defines generalized anxiety disorder as excessive anxiety and worry about several events or activities for most days during at least a 6-month period. The worry is difficult to control and is associated with somatic symptoms, such as muscle tension, irritability, difficulty sleeping, and restlessness. The anxiety is not focused on features of another Axis I disorder, is not caused by substance use or a general medical condition, and does not occur only during a mood or psychiatric disorder. The anxiety is difficult to control, is subjectively distressing, and produces impairment in important areas of a person's life.

EPIDEMIOLOGY

Generalized anxiety disorder is a common condition; reasonable estimates for its 1-year prevalence range from 3 to 8 percent. The ratio of women to men with the disorder is about 2 to 1, but the ratio of women to men who are receiving inpatient treatment for the disorder is about 1 to 1. A lifetime prevalence is close to 5 percent with the Epidemiological Catchment Area (ECA) study suggesting a lifetime prevalence as high as 8 percent. In anxiety disorder clinics about 25 percent of patients have generalized anxiety disorder. The disorder usually has its onset in late adolescence or early adulthood, although cases are commonly seen in older adults. Also, some evidence suggests that the prevalence of generalized anxiety disorder is particularly high in primary care settings.

COMORBIDITY

Generalized anxiety disorder is probably the disorder that most often coexists with another mental disorder, usually social phobia, specific phobia, panic disorder, or a depressive disorder. Perhaps 50 to 90 percent of patients with generalized anxiety disorder have another mental disorder. As many as 25 percent of patients eventually experience panic disorder. Generalized anxiety disorder is differentiated from panic disorder by the absence of spontaneous panic attacks. An additional high percentage of patients are likely to have major depressive disorder. Other common disorders associated with generalized anxiety disorder are dysthymic disorder and substance-related disorders.

ETIOLOGY

The cause of generalized anxiety disorder is not known. As currently defined, generalized anxiety disorder probably affects a heterogeneous group of persons. Perhaps because a certain degree of anxiety is normal and adaptive, differentiating normal anxiety from pathological anxiety and differentiating biological causative factors from psychosocial factors are difficult. Biological and psychological factors probably work together.

Biological Factors

The therapeutic efficacies of benzodiazepines and the azaspirones (e.g., buspirone [BuSpar]) have focused biological research efforts on the γ-aminobutyric acid and serotonin neurotransmitter systems. Benzodiazepines (which are benzodiazepine receptor agonists) are known to reduce anxiety, whereas flumazenil (Romazicon) (a benzodiazepine receptor antagonist) and the β-carbolines (benzodiazepine receptor reverse agonists) are known to induce anxiety. Although no convincing data indicate that the benzodiazepine receptors are abnormal in patients with generalized anxiety disorder, some researchers have focused on the occipital lobe, which has the highest concentrations of benzodiazepine receptors in the brain. Other brain areas hypothesized to be involved in generalized anxiety disorder are the basal ganglia, the limbic system, and the frontal cortex. Because buspirone is an agonist at the serotonin 5-HT_{1A} receptor, there is the hypothesis that the regulation of the serotonergic system in generalized anxiety disorder is abnormal. Other neurotransmitter systems that have been the subject of research in generalized anxiety disorder include the norepinephrine, glutamate, and cholecystokinin systems. Some evidence indicates that patients with generalized anxiety disorder may have subsensitivity of their α_2-adrenergic receptors, as indicated by a blunted release of growth hormone after clonidine (Catapres) infusion.

Brain-imaging studies of patients with generalized anxiety disorder have revealed significant findings. One positron emission tomography study reported a lower metabolic rate in basal ganglia and white matter in patients with generalized anxiety disorder than in normal control subjects (Fig. 16.6–1). A few genetic studies have also been conducted in the field. One study found that a genetic relation might exist between generalized anxiety disorder and major depressive disorder in women. Another study showed a distinct, but difficult-to-quantitate, genetic component in generalized anxiety disorder. About 25 percent of first-degree relatives of patients with generalized anxiety disorder are also affected. Male relatives are likely to have an alcohol use disorder. Some twin studies report a concordance rate of 50 percent in monozygotic twins and 15 percent in dizygotic twins. Table 16.6–1 lists relative genetic risks in selected anxiety disorders.

A variety of electroencephalogram (EEG) abnormalities has been noted in alpha rhythm and evoked potentials. Sleep EEG studies have reported increased sleep discontinuity, decreased delta sleep, decreased stage 1 sleep, and reduced rapid eye movement sleep. These changes in sleep architecture differ from the changes seen in depressive disorders.

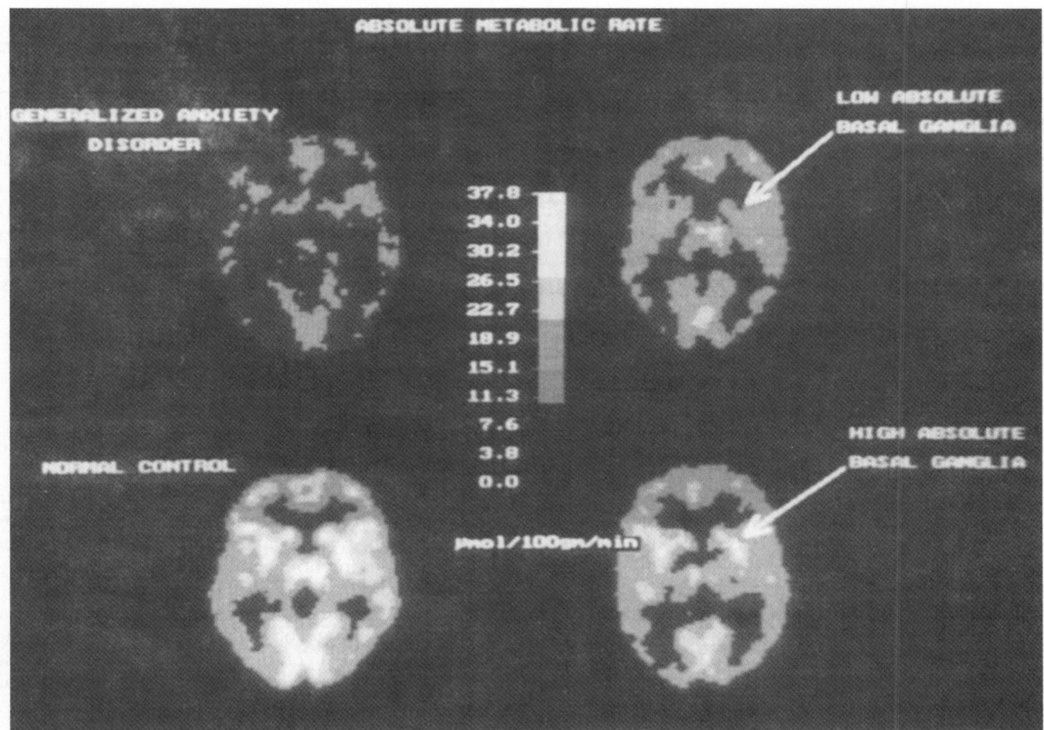

FIGURE 16.6–1
Basal ganglia metabolism. A common glucose scale shows the decrease in absolute glucose metabolic rate in the basal ganglia of two typical subjects with generalized anxiety disorder **(top row)** compared with two normal control subjects **(bottom row)**. (From Wu JC, Buchsbaum MS, Hershey TG, Hazlett E, Sicotte N, Johnson JC. PET in generalized anxiety disorder. *Biol Psychiatry* 1991;29:1188, with permission.)

Psychosocial Factors

The two major schools of thought about psychosocial factors leading to the development of generalized anxiety disorder are the cognitive-behavioral school and the psychoanalytic school. According to the cognitive-behavioral school, patients with generalized anxiety disorder respond to incorrectly and inaccurately perceived dangers. The inaccuracy is generated by selective attention to negative details in the environment, by distortions in information processing, and by an overly negative view of the person's own ability to cope. The psychoanalytic school hypothesizes that anxiety is a symptom of unresolved, unconscious conflicts. Sigmund Freud first presented this psychological theory in 1909 with his description of Little Hans; before then, Freud had conceptualized anxiety as having a physiological basis. An example of Freudian theory as applied to general anxiety can be seen in the following case:

Mrs. B, a 26-year-old married woman, was admitted to the hospital for the evaluation of persistent anxiety that had begun 8 months earlier and was becoming increasingly disabling. Especially disturbing to the patient was the spontaneous intrusion of intermittent images in her mind's eye of her father and herself locked in a naked sexual embrace. The images were not only frightening, but they puzzled her greatly, for she had always disliked her father intensely. Not only was he "poison" to her, but she tried to avoid any contact with him and found it difficult to talk to him if she was forced to be in his company.

As the patient described the difficulty of her relationship with her father, she suddenly recalled that her anxiety had begun at a time when her father was seemingly being more intrusive than ever as he tried to help her and her husband over a period of financial difficulty.

As the patient continued to revile her father, she suddenly commented that her mother had told her that her father "had been good to me when I was little and he used to sing songs to me and take me on his lap, but I don't remember. I only remember when he was mean to me. I just am glad when he keeps on talking mean to me the way he always has. I just wouldn't know what to do if he was nice to me." When asked by the interviewer if there might have been a time when she had wanted him to be nice to her, the patient replied, "When I was little, I just wanted to know that he did love me a little. I guess I always wanted him to be nice to me. But when I stop to think about it, I guess I didn't want him to be nice to me." The doctor then

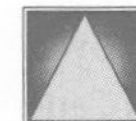

Table 16.6–1
Familial Relative Risks in Selected Anxiety Disorders

Disorder	Population Prevalence (%)	Familial Relative Risk[a]
Panic disorder	1–3	2–20
Generalized anxiety disorder	3–5	6
Obsessive-compulsive disorder	1–3	3–5

[a]Ratio of risk to relatives of cases versus risk to relatives of controls.

commented, "It sounds as if a part of you wants to be close to your father." In response, the patient burst into agitated sobs and blurted out, "I don't know how to be close to my father! I am too old to care about my father now!"

When the patient regained her composure, she recalled the memory of an event she had not thought of since it had occurred 15 years earlier. When she was 11, she reported, while in the living room with her father, she had suddenly had the mental image of being in a sexual embrace with him. Terrified, she had run into the kitchen to find her mother. There had been no recurrence of that image until the onset of the current illness, and the incident had remained forgotten until its recall during the interview. Its emergence into consciousness amplified the history of the patient's illness and disclosed an earlier transient outbreak of the same symptoms she had experienced as an adult. After the patient had recovered her composure, she recalled further hitherto forgotten memories. She had slept in her parents' bedroom until she was 6, during which period her father, on one occasion, had taken her into bed and told her stories and, on another, had yelled at her very angrily as she lay in her crib.

During a clinical interview the next day, the patient revealed a fact that she had forgotten in her earlier account of her illness: At the end of the period during which her father had been making the friendly overtures that had so deeply troubled her, and the night before the sudden onset of her symptoms, she had had a nightmare. She was, she dreamed, at a zoo. It was night, and she heard strange noises in the darkness. She asked an attendant standing next to her what the noises were. "Oh," the attendant replied casually, "that's only the animals mating." She then noticed a large, gray elephant lying on its right side in the grass in front of her. As she watched, she noticed the creature moving its left hind leg up and down as if it were trying to get to its feet. At that point she awoke from the dream with a feeling of terror and, afterward, during the morning, experienced the first episode of the frightening imagery of sexual activity with her father.

In direct association to the dream, the patient recalled a long-forgotten childhood memory of an incident that had occurred during her fourth or fifth year. She had awoken one night while in her crib in her parents' bedroom to observe her parents having sexual intercourse. They suddenly became aware of her watching them and sprang apart. The patient remembered seeing her mother hastily pulling up the bedclothes around her to cover her nakedness. Her father, meanwhile, rolled over half on his back, half on his left side. The patient noticed his erection and then saw him lift up his left leg as he sat up and yelled at her angrily to go to sleep.

It was not easy for the patient to communicate these memories. She spoke haltingly, in a low voice and was visibly ashamed and anxious throughout the whole recital of the dream and its associations. She discharged a great quantity of affect, but after doing so, appeared considerably relaxed, relieved, and composed. On her return to the psychiatric ward, she was observed to be cheerful and outgoing with the ward personnel and other patients. Of particular note was that she no longer experienced any anxiety and had no recurrence of the sexual images involving her father that had previously been so deeply distressing. The patient was discharged a short while later after a further series of psychotherapeutic interviews, and when seen for a follow-up visit 2 months later, she reported continued emotional calm and comfort, without recurrence of psychiatric symptoms.

DIAGNOSIS

Generalized anxiety disorder, according to DSM-IV-TR, is characterized by a pattern of frequent, persistent worry and anxiety that is out of proportion to the impact of the event or circumstance that is the focus of the worry (Table 16.6–2). The distinction between generalized anxiety disorder and normal anxiety is emphasized by the use of the words "excessive" and "difficult to control" in the criteria and by the specification that the symptoms cause significant impairment or distress.

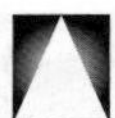

Table 16.6–2
DSM-IV-TR Diagnostic Criteria for Generalized Anxiety Disorder

A. Excessive anxiety and worry (apprehensive expectation), occurring more days than not for at least 6 months, about a number of events or activities (such as work or school performance).
B. The person finds it difficult to control the worry.
C. The anxiety and worry are associated with three (or more) of the following six symptoms (with at least some symptoms present for more days than not for the past 6 months).
Note: Only one item is required in children.
(1) restlessness or feeling keyed up or on edge
(2) being easily fatigued
(3) difficulty concentrating or mind going blank
(4) irritability
(5) muscle tension
(6) sleep disturbance (difficulty falling or staying asleep, or restless unsatisfying sleep)
D. The focus of the anxiety and worry is not confined to features of an Axis I disorder, e.g., the anxiety or worry is not about having a panic attack (as in panic disorder), being embarrassed in public (as in social phobia), being contaminated (as in obsessive-compulsive disorder), being away from home or close relatives (as in separation anxiety disorder), gaining weight (as in anorexia nervosa), having multiple physical complaints (as in somatization disorder), or having a serious illness (as in hypochondriasis), and the anxiety and worry do not occur exclusively during posttraumatic stress disorder.
E. The anxiety, worry, or physical symptoms cause clinically significant distress or impairment in social, occupational, or other important areas of functioning.
F. The disturbance is not due to the direct physiological effects of a substance (e.g., a drug of abuse, a medication) or a general medical condition (e.g., hyperthyroidism) and does not occur exclusively during a mood disorder, a psychotic disorder, or a pervasive developmental disorder.

(From American Psychiatric Association. *Diagnostic and Statistical Manual of Mental Disorders.* 4th ed. Text rev. Washington, DC: American Psychiatric Association; copyright 2000, with permission.)

CLINICAL FEATURES

The essential characteristics of generalized anxiety disorder are sustained and excessive anxiety and worry accompanied by a number of physiological symptoms, including motor tension, autonomic hyperactivity, and cognitive vigilance (Table 16.6–3). The anxiety is excessive and interferes with other aspects of a person's life. This pattern must occur more days than not for at least 6 months. The motor tension is most commonly manifested as shakiness, restlessness, and headaches. The autonomic hyperactivity is commonly manifested by shortness of breath, excessive sweating, palpitations, and various gastrointestinal symptoms. The cognitive vigilance is evidenced by irritability and the ease with which patients are startled.

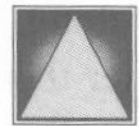

Table 16.6–3
Physiological Symptoms of Anxiety Disorders Explicitly Mentioned in DSM-IV-TR

Panic disorder
- Palpitations, pounding heart, or accelerated heart rate
- Sweating
- Trembling or shaking
- Sensation of shortness of breath or smothering
- Feeling of choking
- Chest pain or discomfort
- Nausea or abdominal distress
- Feeling dizzy, unsteady, lightheaded, or faint
- Chills or hot flushes

Posttraumatic stress disorder
- Physiological reactivity on exposure to trauma-related cues
- Difficulties falling asleep or staying asleep
- Exaggerated startle response

Generalized anxiety disorder
- Muscle tension
- Sleep disturbance

Acute stress disorder
- Marked symptoms of arousal

Patients with generalized anxiety disorder usually seek out a general practitioner or internist for help with a somatic symptom. Alternatively, the patients go to a specialist for a specific symptom (e.g., chronic diarrhea). A specific nonpsychiatric medical disorder is rarely found, and patients vary in their doctor-seeking behavior. Some patients accept a diagnosis of generalized anxiety disorder and the appropriate treatment; others seek additional medical consultations for their problems. Generalized anxiety disorders can be disabling as in the following case.

A 27-year-old married electrician complained of dizziness, sweating palms, heart palpitations, and ringing of the ears of more than 18 months' duration. He also experienced dry mouth and throat, periods of extreme muscle tension, and a constant "edgy" and watchful feeling that had often interfered with his ability to concentrate. These feelings had been present most of the time over the previous 2 years; they had not been limited to discrete periods. Although these symptoms made him feel "discouraged," he denied feeling depressed and continued to enjoy activities with his family.

Because of these symptoms the patient had seen a family practitioner, a neurologist, a neurosurgeon, a chiropractor, and an ear-nose-throat specialist. He had been placed on a hypoglycemic diet, received physiotherapy for a pinched nerve, and been told he might have "an inner ear problem."

He also had many worries. He constantly worried about the health of his parents. His father, in fact, had a myocardial infarction 2 years previously, but is now feeling well. He also worried about whether he is "a good father," whether his wife will ever leave him (there is no indication that she is dissatisfied with the marriage), and whether he is liked by co-workers on the job. Although he recognizes that his worries are often unfounded, he can't stop worrying.

For the past 2 years the patient has had few social contacts because of his nervous symptoms. Although he sometimes had to leave work when the symptoms became intolerable, he continues to work for the same company he joined for his apprenticeship following high-school graduation. He tends to hide his symptoms from his wife and children, to whom he wants to appear "perfect." (Adapted from *DSM-IV-TR Casebook.*)

DIFFERENTIAL DIAGNOSIS

As with other anxiety disorders, generalized anxiety disorder must be differentiated from both medical and psychiatric disorders. Neurological, endocrinological, metabolic, and medication-related disorders similar to those considered in the differential diagnosis of panic disorder must be considered in the differential diagnosis of generalized anxiety disorder. Common co-occurring anxiety disorders also must be considered, including panic disorder, phobias, obsessive-compulsive disorder (OCD), and posttraumatic stress disorder (PTSD). To meet criteria for generalized anxiety disorder, patients must both exhibit the full syndrome and their symptoms also cannot be explained by the presence of a comorbid anxiety disorder. To diagnose generalized anxiety disorder in the context of other anxiety disorders, it is most important to document anxiety or worry related to circumstances or topics that are either unrelated, or only minimally related, to other disorders. Proper diagnosis involves both definitively establishing the presence of generalized anxiety disorder and properly diagnosing other anxiety disorders. Patients with generalized anxiety disorder frequently develop major depressive disorder. As a result, this condition must also be recognized and distinguished. The key to making a correct diagnosis is documenting anxiety or worry that is unrelated to the depressive disorder.

COURSE AND PROGNOSIS

The age of onset is difficult to specify; most patients with the disorder report that they have been anxious for as long as they can remember. Patients usually come to a clinician's attention in their 20s, although the first contact with a clinician can occur at virtually any age. Only one third of patients who have generalized anxiety disorder seek psychiatric treatment. Many go to general practitioners, internists, cardiologists, pulmonary specialists, or gastroenterologists, seeking treatment for the somatic component of the disorder. Because of the high incidence of comorbid mental disorders in patients with generalized anxiety disorder, the clinical course and prognosis of the disorder are difficult to predict. Nonetheless, some data indicate that life events are associated with the onset of generalized anxiety disorder: The occurrence of several negative life events greatly increases the likelihood that the disorder will develop. By definition, generalized anxiety disorder is a chronic condition that may well be lifelong.

TREATMENT

The most effective treatment of generalized anxiety disorder is probably one that combines psychotherapeutic, pharmacotherapeutic, and supportive approaches. The treatment may take a significant amount of time for the involved clinician, whether the clinician is a psychiatrist, a family practitioner, or another specialist.

Psychotherapy

The major psychotherapeutic approaches to generalized anxiety disorder are cognitive-behavioral, supportive, and insight oriented. Data are still limited on the relative merits of those approaches, although the most sophisticated studies have examined cognitive-behavioral techniques, which seem to have both short-term and long-term efficacy. Cognitive approaches address patients' hypothesized cognitive distortions directly, and behavioral approaches address somatic symptoms directly. The major techniques used in behavioral approaches are relaxation and biofeedback. Some preliminary data indicate that the combination of cognitive and behavioral approaches is more effective than either technique used alone. Supportive therapy offers patients reassurance and comfort, although its long-term efficacy is doubtful. Insight-oriented psychotherapy focuses on uncovering unconscious conflicts and identifying ego strengths. The efficacy of insight-oriented psychotherapy for generalized anxiety disorder is found in many anecdotal case reports, but large controlled studies are lacking.

Most patients experience a marked lessening of anxiety when given the opportunity to discuss their difficulties with a concerned and sympathetic physician. If clinicians discover external situations that are anxiety provoking, they may be able—alone or with the help of the patients or their families—to change the environment and, thus, reduce the stressful pressures. A reduction in symptoms often allows patients to function effectively in their daily work and relationships and, thus, gain new rewards and gratification that are themselves therapeutic.

In the psychoanalytic perspective, anxiety sometimes signals unconscious turmoil that deserves investigation. The anxiety can be normal, adaptive, maladaptive, too intense, or too mild, depending on the circumstances. Anxiety appears in numerous situations over the course of the life cycle; in many cases, symptom relief is not the most appropriate course of action.

For patients who are psychologically minded and motivated to understand the sources of their anxiety, psychotherapy may be the treatment of choice. Psychodynamic therapy proceeds with the assumption that anxiety can increase with effective treatment. The goal of the dynamic approach may be to increase the patient's anxiety tolerance (a capacity to experience anxiety without having to discharge it), rather than to eliminate anxiety. Empirical research indicates that many patients who have successful psychotherapeutic treatment may continue to experience anxiety after termination of the psychotherapy, but their increased ego mastery allows them to use the anxiety symptoms as a signal to reflect on internal struggles and to expand their insight and understanding. A psychodynamic approach to patients with generalized anxiety disorder involves a search for the patient's underlying fears.

Pharmacotherapy

The decision to prescribe an anxiolytic to patients with generalized anxiety disorder should rarely be made on the first visit. Because of the long-term nature of the disorder, a treatment plan must be carefully thought out. The three major drugs to be considered for the treatment of generalized anxiety disorder are benzodiazepines, the serotonin-specific reuptake inhibitors (SSRIs), buspirone (BuSpar), and venlafaxine (Effexor). Other drugs that may be useful are the tricyclic drugs (e.g., imipramine [Tofranil]), antihistamines, and the β-adrenergic antagonists (e.g., propranolol [Inderal]).

Although drug treatment of generalized anxiety disorder is sometimes seen as a 6- to 12-month treatment, some evidence indicates that treatment should be long term, perhaps lifelong. About 25 percent of patients relapse in the first month after the discontinuation of therapy, and 60 to 80 percent relapse over the course of the next year. Although some patients become dependent on the benzodiazepines, tolerance rarely develops to the therapeutic effects of the benzodiazepines, buspirone, venlafaxine, or the SSRIs.

Benzodiazepines. Benzodiazepines have been the drugs of choice for generalized anxiety disorder. They can be prescribed on an as-needed basis, so that patients take a rapidly acting benzodiazepine when they feel particularly anxious. The alternative approach is to prescribe benzodiazepines for a limited period, during which psychosocial therapeutic approaches are implemented.

Several problems are associated with the use of benzodiazepines in generalized anxiety disorder. About 25 to 30 percent of all patients fail to respond, and tolerance and dependence can occur. Some patients also experience impaired alertness while taking the drugs and, therefore, are at risk for accidents involving automobiles and machinery.

The clinical decision to initiate treatment with a benzodiazepine should be considered and specific. The patient's diagnosis, the specific target symptoms, and the duration of treatment should all be defined, and the information should be shared with the patient. Treatment for most anxiety conditions lasts for 2 to 6 weeks, followed by 1 or 2 weeks of tapering drug use before it is discontinued. The most common clinical mistake with benzodiazepine treatment is routinely to continue treatment indefinitely.

For the treatment of anxiety, it is usual to begin giving a drug at the low end of its therapeutic range and to increase the dosage to achieve a therapeutic response. The use of a benzodiazepine with an intermediate half-life (8 to 15 hours) will likely avoid some of the adverse effects associated with the use of benzodiazepines with long half-lives, and the use of divided doses prevents the development of adverse effects associated with high peak plasma levels. The improvement produced by benzodiazepines may go beyond a simple antianxiety effect. For example, the drugs may cause patients to regard various occurrences in a positive light. The drugs can also have a mild disinhibiting action, similar to that observed after ingesting modest amounts of alcohol.

Buspirone. Buspirone is a 5-HT_{1A} receptor partial agonist and is most likely effective in 60 to 80 percent of patients with generalized anxiety disorder. Data indicate that buspirone is more effective in reducing the cognitive symptoms of generalized anxiety disorder than in reducing the somatic symptoms. Evidence also indicates that patients who have previously had treatment with benzodiazepines are not likely to respond to treatment with buspirone. The lack of response may be caused by the absence, with buspirone treatment, of some of the nonanxiolytic effects of benzodiazepines (e.g., muscle relaxation and the additional sense of well-being). The major disadvantage of buspirone is that its effects take 2 to 3 weeks to become evident, in contrast to the almost immediate anxiolytic effects of the benzodiazepines. One approach is to initiate benzodiazepine and buspirone use simultaneously, then taper off the benzodiazepine use after 2 to 3 weeks, at which point the buspirone should have reached its maximal effects. Some studies have also reported that long-term combined treatment with benzodiazepine and buspirone may be more effective than either drug alone. Buspirone is not an effective treatment for benzodiazepine withdrawal.

Venlafaxine. Venlafaxine is effective in treating the insomnia, poor concentration, restlessness, irritability, and excessive muscle tension associated with generalized anxiety disorder. Venlafaxine is a nonselective inhibitor of the reuptake of three biogenic amines—serotonin, norepinephrine, and, to a lesser extent, dopamine.

Selective Serotonin Reuptake Inhibitors. SSRIs may be effective, especially for patients with comorbid depression. The prominent disadvantage of SSRIs, especially fluoxetine (Prozac), is that they can transiently increase anxiety and cause agitated states. For this reason, the SSRIs sertraline (Zoloft), citalopram (Celexa), or paroxetine (Paxil) are better choices in patients with high anxiety disorder. It is reasonable to begin treatment with sertraline, citalopram, or paroxetine plus a benzodiazepine, then to taper benzodiazepine use after 2 to 3 weeks. Further studies are needed to determine whether SSRIs are as effective for generalized anxiety disorder as they are for panic disorder and OCD.

Other Drugs. If conventional pharmacological treatment (e.g., with buspirone or a benzodiazepine) is ineffective or not completely effective, then a clinical reassessment is indicated to rule out comorbid conditions, such as depression, or to better understand the patient's environmental stresses. Other drugs that have proved useful for generalized anxiety disorder include the tricyclic and tetracyclic drugs. The β-adrenergic receptor antagonists may reduce the somatic manifestations of anxiety, but not the underlying condition, and their use is usually limited to situational anxieties, such as performance anxiety.

References

Ball SG, Kuhn A, Wall D, Shekhar A, Goddard AW. Selective serotonin reuptake inhibitor treatment for generalized anxiety disorder: A double-blind, prospective comparison between paroxetine and sertraline. *J Clin Psychiatry.* 2005;66(1):94–99.

Brawman-Mintzer O, Monnier J, Wolitzky KB, Falsetti SA. Patients with generalized anxiety disorder and a history of trauma: Somatic symptom endorsement. *Journal of Psychiatric Practice.* 2005;11(3):212–215.

Ginsberg DL, ed. Women and anxiety disorders: Implications for diagnosis and treatment. *CNS Spectrums.* 2004;9:1–16.

Heimberg RG, Turk CL, Mennin DS, eds. *Generalized Anxiety Disorder: Advances in Research and Practice.* New York: Guilford Press; 2004.

Le Roux H, Gatz M, Wetherell JL. Age at onset of generalized anxiety disorder in older adults. *Am J Geriatr Psychiatry.* 2005;13:23–30.

Rickels K, Rynn M, Iyengar M, Duff D. Remission of generalized anxiety disorder: A review of the paroxetine clinical trials database. *J Clin Psychiatry.* 2006;67(1):41–47.

Rodriguez BF, Bruce SE, Pagano ME, Keller MB. Relationships among psychosocial functioning, diagnostic comorbidity, and the recurrence of generalized anxiety disorder, panic disorder, and major depression. *J Anxiety Disord.* 2005;19(7):752–766.

Rollman BL, Belnap BH, Mazumdar S, Zhu F, Kroenke K, Schulberg HC, Shear MK. Symptomatic severity on Prime-MD diagnosed episodes of panic and generalized anxiety disorder in primary care. *J Gen Intern Med.* 2005;20: 623–628.

Shear K, Belnap BH, Mazumdar S, Houck P, Rollman BL. Generalized anxiety disorder severity scale (GADSS): A preliminary validation study. *Depress Anxiety.* 2006;23(2):77–82.

Steffens DC, McQuoid DR. Impact of symptoms of generalized anxiety disorder on the course of late-life depression. *Am J Geriatr Psychiatry.* 2005;13:40–47.

▲ 16.7 Other Anxiety Disorders

ANXIETY DISORDER DUE TO A GENERAL MEDICAL CONDITION

Many medical disorders are associated with anxiety. Symptoms can include panic attacks, generalized anxiety, obsessions and compulsions, and other signs of distress. In all cases, the signs and symptoms will be due to the direct physiological effects of the medical condition.

Epidemiology

The occurrence of anxiety symptoms related to general medical conditions is common, although the incidence of the disorder varies for each specific general medical condition.

Etiology

A wide range of medical conditions can cause symptoms similar to those of anxiety disorders (Table 16.7–1). Hyperthyroidism (*see* Color Plate 16.7–1 on page 494), hypothyroidism, hypoparathyroidism, and vitamin B_{12} deficiency are frequently associated with anxiety symptoms. A pheochromocytoma produces epinephrine, which can cause paroxysmal episodes of anxiety symptoms. Certain lesions of the brain and postencephalitic states reportedly produce symptoms identical to those seen in obsessive-compulsive disorder (OCD). Other medical conditions, such as cardiac arrhythmia, can produce physiological symptoms of panic disorder. Hypoglycemia can also mimic the symptoms of an anxiety disorder. The diverse medical conditions that can cause symptoms of anxiety disorder may do so through a common mechanism, the noradrenergic system, although the effects on the serotonergic system are also under study. Each of these conditions is characterized by prominent anxiety that arises as the direct result of some underlying physiological perturbation.

Diagnosis

The text revision of the fourth edition of *Diagnostic and Statistical Manual of Mental Disorders* (DSM-IV-TR) diagnosis of anxiety disorder due to a general medical condition (Table 16.7–2) requires the presence of symptoms of an anxiety disorder. DSM-IV-TR allows clinicians to specify whether the disorder is characterized by symptoms of generalized anxiety, panic attacks, or obsessive-compulsive symptoms.

Clinicians should have an increased level of suspicion for the diagnosis when chronic or paroxysmal anxiety is associated with a physical disease known to cause such symptoms in some patients. Paroxysmal bouts of hypertension in an anxious patient may indicate that a workup for a pheochromocytoma is appropriate. A general medical workup may reveal diabetes, an adrenal tumor, thyroid disease, or a neurological condition. For example, some patients with complex partial epilepsy have extreme

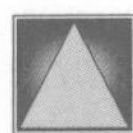

Table 16.7–1
Disorders Associated with Anxiety

Neurological disorders	Miscellaneous conditions
Cerebral neoplasms	Hypoglycemia
Cerebral trauma and postconcussive syndromes	Carcinoid syndrome
Cerebrovascular disease	Systemic malignancies
Subarachnoid hemorrhage	Premenstrual syndrome
Migraine	Febrile illnesses and chronic infections
Encephalitis	Porphyria
Cerebral syphilis	Infectious mononucleosis
Multiple sclerosis	Posthepatitis syndrome
Wilson's disease	Uremia
Huntington's disease	Toxic conditions
Epilepsy	Alcohol and drug withdrawal
Systemic conditions	Amphetamines
Hypoxia	Sympathomimetic agents
Cardiovascular disease	Vasopressor agents
Cardiac arrhythmias	Caffeine and caffeine withdrawal
Pulmonary insufficiency	Penicillin
Anemia	Sulfonamides
Endocrine disturbances	Cannabis
Pituitary dysfunction	Mercury
Thyroid dysfunction	Arsenic
Parathyroid dysfunction	Phosphorus
Adrenal dysfunction	Organophosphates
Pheochromocytoma	Carbon disulfide
Virilization disorders of females	Benzene
Inflammatory disorders	Aspirin intolerance
Lupus erythematosus	Idiopathic psychiatric disorders
Rheumatoid arthritis	Depression
Polyarteritis nodosa	Mania
Temporal arteritis	Schizophrenia
Deficiency states	Anxiety disorders
Vitamin B_{12} deficiency	Generalized anxiety
Pellagra	Panic attacks
	Phobic disorders
	Posttraumatic stress disorder

(From Cumming JL. *Clinical Neuropsychiatry.* Orlando, FL: Grune & Stratton; 1985:214, with permission.)

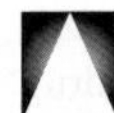

Table 16.7–2
DSM-IV-TR Diagnostic Criteria for Anxiety Disorder Due to a General Medical Condition

A. Prominent anxiety, panic attacks, or obsessions or compulsions predominate in the clinical picture.

B. There is evidence from the history, physical examination, or laboratory findings that the disturbance is the direct physiological consequence of a general medical condition.

C. The disturbance is not better accounted for by another mental disorder (e.g., adjustment disorder with anxiety in which the stressor is a serious general medical condition).

D. The disturbance does not occur exclusively during the course of a delirium.

E. The disturbance causes clinically significant distress or impairment in social, occupational, or other important areas of functioning.

Specify if:

With generalized anxiety: if excessive anxiety or worry about a number of events or activities predominates in the clinical presentation

With panic attacks: if panic attacks predominate in the clinical presentation

With obsessive-compulsive symptoms: if obsessions or compulsions predominate in the clinical presentation

Coding note: Include the name of the general medical condition on Axis I, e.g., anxiety disorder due to pheochromocytoma, with generalized anxiety; also code the general medical condition on Axis III.

(From American Psychiatric Association. *Diagnostic and Statistical Manual of Mental Disorders.* 4th ed. Text rev. Washington, DC: American Psychiatric Association; copyright 2000, with permission.)

episodes of anxiety or fear as their only manifestation of the epileptic activity.

Clinical Features

The symptoms of anxiety disorder due to a general medical condition can be identical to those of the primary anxiety disorders. A syndrome similar to panic disorder is the most common clinical picture, and a syndrome similar to a phobia is the least common.

Panic Attacks. Patients who have cardiomyopathy may have the highest incidence of panic disorder secondary to a general medical condition. One study reported that 83 percent of patients with cardiomyopathy awaiting cardiac transplantation had panic disorder symptoms. Increased noradrenergic tone in these patients may be the provoking stimulus for the panic attacks. In some studies, about 25 percent of patients with Parkinson's disease and chronic obstructive pulmonary disease have symptoms of panic disorder. Other medical disorders associated with panic disorder include chronic pain, primary biliary cirrhosis, and epilepsy, particularly when the focus is in the right parahippocampal gyrus.

A 78-year-old, retired lumber-company president sought help for the onset of a series of attacks in which he experienced marked apprehension, restlessness, and the need to be outdoors to relieve his sense of discomfort. He described the most recent event as having occurred at 3 AM a week earlier: he awoke from sleep and felt "the walls were caving in" on him. He denied that this was related to dreaming and said that he was fully awake at the time. He arose, dressed, and went outside in subzero weather; once outside, he noted gradual improvement (but not full resolution) of his symptoms. Complete resolution took a full day.

In response to pointed questioning, the patient denied dyspnea, palpitations, choking sensations, paresthesias, or nausea. He reported trembling and some sweating, together with intermittent dizziness. He imagined that he would die (or lose consciousness) if he could not "escape" from his house. He spoke of a need "to be active."

On questioning, the patient recalled a similar series of attacks almost 30 years earlier following eye surgery for an injury. He described bilateral patching of his eyes and being confined to bed for days, with his head sandbagged to preclude movement. Once ambulatory, he had experienced these attacks for more than a year.

The patient denied recent sleep dysfunction, change in appetite or weight, crying spells, or decreased energy. He had been taking diazepam for approximately 2 months for feelings of increased nervousness and tension. He had noted mild memory problems of late.

Further inquiry established a problem with balance and intermittent pain in the right arm, and a complaint of indigestion and intermittent diarrhea. The patient had stopped gardening the past summer because of his balance problem. On examination he was found to have a "beefy" red tongue (which he said was painful), difficulty with tandem gait and rapid alternating motion, and a mild intention tremor. He denied urinary incontinence.

Laboratory studies revealed a macrocytic anemia and vitamin B_{12} deficiency. The patient was given B_{12} replacement, and his attacks did not recur. (From *DSM-IV-TR Casebook*.)

Generalized Anxiety. A high prevalence of generalized anxiety disorder symptoms has been reported in patients with Sjögren's syndrome, and this rate may be related to the effects of Sjögren's syndrome on cortical and subcortical functions and thyroid function. The highest prevalence of generalized anxiety disorder symptoms in a medical disorder seems to be in Graves' disease (hyperthyroidism), in which as many as two thirds of all patients meet the criteria for generalized anxiety disorder.

Obsessive-Compulsive Symptoms. Reports have associated the development of OCD symptoms with Sydenham's chorea.

A 12-year-old girl had a sudden onset of high fever, lethargy, and sore throat with purulent tonsillar exudate. Streptococci were found in the infected site, and she was treated successfully with penicillin. Following recovery, mild athetoid movements of the upper torso and facial tics were noted and diagnosed as sequelae of the infection. She was kept on antibiotics (to prevent reinfection) until the neurological complication subsided spontaneously after 1 year.

Phobias. Symptoms of phobias appear to be uncommon, although one study reported a 17 percent prevalence of symptoms of social phobia in patients with Parkinson's disease. Older persons with balance difficulties often complain of a fear of falling, which may express itself by their being unwilling or fearful of walking.

Differential Diagnosis

Anxiety, as a symptom, can be associated with many psychiatric disorders in addition to the anxiety disorders themselves. A mental status examination is necessary to determine the presence of mood symptoms or psychotic symptoms that may suggest another psychiatric diagnosis. For a clinician to conclude that a patient has an anxiety disorder caused by a general medical condition, the patient should clearly have anxiety as the predominant symptom and should have a specific causative nonpsychiatric medical disorder. To ascertain the degree to which a general medical condition is causative for the anxiety, the clinician should know whether the medical condition and the anxiety symptoms have been related closely in the literature, the age of onset (primary anxiety disorders usually have their onset before age 35), and the patient's family history of both anxiety disorders and relevant general medical conditions (e.g., hyperthyroidism). A diagnosis of adjustment disorder with anxiety must also be considered in the differential diagnosis.

Course and Prognosis

The unremitting experience of anxiety can be disabling and can interfere with every aspect of life, including social, occupational, and psychological functioning. A sudden increase in anxiety level may prompt an affected person to seek medical or psychiatric help more quickly than when the onset is insidious. The treatment or the removal of the primary medical cause of the anxiety usually initiates a clear course of improvement in the anxiety disorder symptoms. In some cases, however, the anxiety disorder symptoms continue even after the primary medical condition is treated (e.g., after an episode of encephalitis). Some symptoms, particularly OCD symptoms, linger for a longer time than other anxiety disorder symptoms. When anxiety disorder symptoms are present for a significant period after the medical disorder has been treated, the remaining symptoms should probably be treated as if they were primary—that is, with psychotherapy, pharmacotherapy, or both.

Treatment

The primary treatment for anxiety disorder due to a general medical condition is to treat the underlying medical condition. If a patient also has an alcohol or other substance use disorder, this disorder must also be addressed therapeutically to gain control of the anxiety disorder symptoms. If the removal of the primary medical condition does not reverse the anxiety disorder symptoms, treatment of these symptoms should follow the treatment guidelines for the specific mental disorder. In general, behavioral modification techniques, anxiolytic agents, and serotonergic antidepressants have been the most effective treatment modalities.

SUBSTANCE-INDUCED ANXIETY DISORDER

Substance-induced disorder is the direct result of a toxic substance, including drugs of abuse, medication, poison, and alcohol, among others.

Epidemiology

Substance-induced anxiety disorder is common, both as the result of the ingestion of so-called recreational drugs and as the result of prescription drug use.

Etiology

A wide range of substances can cause symptoms of anxiety that can mimic any of the DSM-IV-TR anxiety disorders. Although sympathomimetics, such as amphetamine, cocaine, and caffeine, have been most associated with the production of anxiety disorder symptoms, many serotonergic drugs (e.g., lysergic acid diethylamide [LSD] and methylenedioxymethamphetamine [MDMA]) can also cause both acute and chronic anxiety syndromes in users. A wide range of prescription medications is also associated with the production of anxiety disorder symptoms in susceptible persons.

Diagnosis

The DSM-IV-TR diagnostic criteria for substance-induced anxiety disorder require the presence of prominent anxiety, panic attacks, obsessions, or compulsions (Table 16.7–3). The DSM-IV-TR guidelines state that the symptoms should have developed during the use of the substance or within a month of the cessation of substance use, but DSM-IV-TR encourages clinicians to use appropriate clinical judgment to assess the relation between substance exposure and anxiety symptoms. The structure of the diagnosis includes specification of (1) the substance (e.g., cocaine), (2) the appropriate state during the onset (e.g., intoxication), and (3) the specific symptom pattern (e.g., panic attacks).

Table 16.7–3
DSM-IV-TR Diagnostic Criteria for Substance-Induced Anxiety Disorder

A. Prominent anxiety, panic attacks, or obsessions or compulsions predominate in the clinical picture.
B. There is evidence from the history, physical examination, or laboratory findings of either (1) or (2):
(1) the symptoms in Criterion A developed during, or within 1 month of, substance intoxication or withdrawal
(2) medication use is etiologically related to the disturbance
C. The disturbance is not better accounted for by an anxiety disorder that is not substance induced. Evidence that the symptoms are better accounted for by an anxiety disorder that is not substance induced might include the following: the symptoms precede the onset of the substance use (or medication use); the symptoms persist for a substantial period of time (e.g., about a month) after the cessation of acute withdrawal or severe intoxication or are substantially in excess of what would be expected given the type or amount of the substance used or the duration of use; or there is other evidence suggesting the existence of an independent non–substance-induced anxiety disorder (e.g., a history of recurrent non–substance-related episodes).
D. The disturbance does not occur exclusively during the course of a delirium.
E. The disturbance causes clinically significant distress or impairment in social, occupational, or other important areas of functioning.

Note: This diagnosis should be made instead of a diagnosis of substance intoxication or substance withdrawal only when the anxiety symptoms are in excess of those usually associated with the intoxication or withdrawal syndrome and when the anxiety symptoms are sufficiently severe to warrant independent clinical attention.

Code [Specific substance]-induced anxiety disorder
Alcohol; amphetamine (or amphetaminelike substance); caffeine; cannabis; cocaine; hallucinogen; inhalant; phencyclidine (or phencyclidinelike substance); sedative, hypnotic, or anxiolytic; other [or unknown] substance

Specify if:
With generalized anxiety: if excessive anxiety or worry about a number of events or activities predominates in the clinical presentation
With panic attacks: if panic attacks predominate in the clinical presentation
With obsessive-compulsive symptoms: if obsessions or compulsions predominate in the clinical presentation
With phobic symptoms: if phobic symptoms predominate in the clinical presentation

Specify if:
With onset during intoxication: if the criteria are met for intoxication with the substance and the symptoms develop during the intoxication syndrome
With onset during withdrawal: if criteria are met for withdrawal from the substance and the symptoms develop during, or shortly after, a withdrawal syndrome

(From American Psychiatric Association. *Diagnostic and Statistical Manual of Mental Disorders*. 4th ed. Text rev. Washington, DC: American Psychiatric Association; copyright 2000, with permission.)

Clinical Features

The associated clinical features of substance-induced anxiety disorder vary with the particular substance involved. Even infrequent use of psychostimulants can result in anxiety disorder symptoms in some persons. Cognitive impairments in comprehension, calculation, and memory can be associated with anxiety disorder symptoms. These cognitive deficits are usually reversible when the substance use is stopped.

Virtually everyone who drinks alcohol, on at least a few occasions, has used it to reduce anxiety, most often social anxiety. In contrast, carefully controlled studies have found that the effects of alcohol on anxiety are variable and can be significantly affected by gender, the amount of alcohol ingested, and cultural attitudes. Nevertheless, alcohol use disorders and other substance-related disorders are commonly associated with anxiety disorders. Alcohol use disorders are about four times more common among patients with panic disorder than among the general population, about three and a half times more common among patients with OCD, and about two and a half times more common among patients with phobias. Several studies have reported data indicating that genetic diatheses for both anxiety disorders and alcohol use disorders can exist in some families.

Differential Diagnosis

The differential diagnosis for substance-induced anxiety disorder includes the primary anxiety disorders, anxiety disorder due to a general medical condition (for which the patient may be receiving an implicated drug), and mood disorders, which are frequently accompanied by symptoms of anxiety disorders. Personality disorders and malingering must be considered in the differential diagnosis, particularly in some urban emergency rooms.

Course and Prognosis

The course and prognosis generally depend on removal of the causally involved substance and the long-term ability of the affected person to limit use of the substance. The anxiogenic effects of most drugs are reversible. When the anxiety does not reverse with cessation of the drug, clinicians should reconsider the diagnosis of substance-induced anxiety disorder or consider the possibility that the substance caused irreversible brain damage.

Treatment

The primary treatment for substance-induced anxiety disorder is the removal of the causally involved substance. Treatment then must focus on finding an alternative treatment if the substance was a medically indicated drug, on limiting the patient's exposure if the substance was introduced through environmental exposure, or on treating the underlying substance-related disorder.

If anxiety disorder symptoms continue even after stopping substance use, treatment of the anxiety disorder symptoms with appropriate psychotherapeutic or pharmacotherapeutic modalities may be appropriate.

ANXIETY DISORDER NOT OTHERWISE SPECIFIED

Some patients have symptoms of anxiety disorders that do not meet the criteria for any specific DSM-IV-TR anxiety disorder or adjustment disorder with anxiety or mixed anxiety and depressed mood. Such patients are most appropriately classified as having anxiety disorder not otherwise specified. DSM-IV-TR includes four examples of conditions that are appropriate for the diagnosis (Table 16.7–4). One of the examples is mixed anxiety-depressive disorder.

Mr. W came into the emergency room of a New York hospital complaining of malaise, fever, and a cough. An upper respiratory infection was diagnosed. As the doctor was writing out a prescription, Mr. W tearfully revealed that he had no home to go to, was depressed, and felt that life was not worth living. A psychiatric resident was called to see the patient and obtained the following additional information.

For the past month Mr. W had been living in the basement of his apartment building, eating in restaurants, and using a health club for showers. He was eating and sleeping poorly. His own apartment was so full of newspapers, magazines, and books that he could no longer get in the door, but he could not bring himself to get rid of any of his "stuff."

When he was 12, Mr. W began collecting baseball cards and then books and magazines. His parents were poor immigrants from Eastern Europe, and the idea of holding on to things that might someday be valuable was not strange to them. Eventually, however, the apartment became so cluttered that they threw out much of his collection. He retrieved it from the garbage, and from that point on his "collecting" became a focus of conflict with family and employers.

Mr. W does not go out of his way to obtain things, but once he has a newspaper, book, or magazine, he cannot throw it away because "there might be something of value written in it." The thought of throwing things out makes him extremely anxious, and, in the end, he simply cannot do it.

For many years he worked as a doorman in elegant apartment buildings, but invariably was fired because he brought his "stuff" to store in his workplace, and sometimes got into fistfights with the building maintenance people who tried to throw it out. He was married for 10 years, and has a 25-year-old son. His wife finally left him, unable to tolerate his behavior. He rarely sees his son.

Mr. W first entered treatment not because of his collecting, but because at age 20, "my mood took a turn for the worse. I had a breakdown." He stopped doing virtually everything—working, eating, sleeping. "It was an effort even to lift my leg." He began seeing a psychiatrist as an outpatient, and over the years has been in therapy much of the time, treated with a variety of antidepressants and anxiolytics.

After his divorce, 10 years ago, he moved some of his collection into his own apartment and rented storage space for the rest. Gradually his new apartment filled up with newspapers, magazines, and books, and it became a struggle just to get in the front door and make his way to his bed. Finally, last month, he injured his shoulder trying to push things aside, and then abandoned the apartment for a cot in the basement of the building He understands that his inability to throw things out is irrational, but the thought of starting to do it makes him intolerably anxious. (From *DSM-IV-TR Casebook.*)

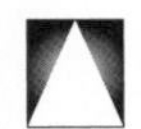

Table 16.7–4
DSM-IV-TR Diagnostic Criteria for Anxiety Disorder Not Otherwise Specified

This category includes disorders with prominent anxiety or phobic avoidance that do not meet criteria for any specific anxiety disorder, adjustment disorder with anxiety, or adjustment disorder with mixed anxiety and depressed mood. Examples include

1. Mixed anxiety-depressive disorder: clinically significant symptoms of anxiety and depression, but the criteria are not met for either a specific mood disorder or a specific anxiety disorder
2. Clinically significant social phobic symptoms that are related to the social impact of having a general medical condition or mental disorder (e.g., Parkinson's disease, dermatological conditions, stuttering, anorexia nervosa, body dysmorphic disorder)
3. Situations in which the disturbance is severe enough to warrant a diagnosis of an anxiety disorder but the individual fails to report enough symptoms for the full criteria for any specific anxiety disorder to have been met; for example, an individual who reports all of the features of panic disorder without agoraphobia except that the panic attacks are all limited-symptom attacks
4. Situations in which the clinician has concluded that an anxiety disorder is present but is unable to determine whether it is primary, due to a general medical condition, or substance induced

(From American Psychiatric Association. *Diagnostic and Statistical Manual of Mental Disorders.* 4th ed. Text rev. Washington, DC: American Psychiatric Association; copyright 2000, with permission.)

MIXED ANXIETY-DEPRESSIVE DISORDER

Mixed anxiety-depressive disorder describes patients with both anxiety and depressive symptoms who do not meet the diagnostic criteria for either an anxiety disorder or a mood disorder. The combination of depressive and anxiety symptoms results in significant functional impairment for the affected person. The condition may be particularly prevalent in primary care practices and outpatient mental health clinics. Opponents have argued that the availability of the diagnosis may discourage clinicians from taking the necessary time to obtain a complete psychiatric history to differentiate true depressive disorders from true anxiety disorders. In Europe, and especially, in China, many of these patients are given a diagnosis of neurasthenia (see Chapter 18).

Epidemiology

The coexistence of major depressive disorder and panic disorder is common. As many as two thirds of all patients with depressive symptoms have prominent anxiety symptoms, and one third may meet the diagnostic criteria for panic disorder. Researchers have reported that 20 to 90 percent of all patients with panic disorder have episodes of major depressive disorder. These data suggest that the coexistence of depressive and anxiety symptoms, neither of which meets the diagnostic criteria for other depressive or anxiety disorders, may be common. Presently, however, formal epidemiological data on mixed anxiety-depressive disorder are not available. Nevertheless, some clinicians and researchers have estimated that the prevalence of the disorder in the general population is as high as 10 percent and in primary care clinics, as high as 50 percent, although conservative estimates suggest a prevalence of about 1 percent in the general population.

Etiology

Four principal lines of evidence suggest that anxiety symptoms and depressive symptoms are causally linked in some affected patients. First, several investigators have reported similar neuroendocrine findings in depressive disorders and anxiety disorders, particularly panic disorder, including blunted cortisol response to adrenocorticotropic hormone, blunted growth hormone response to clonidine (Catapres), and blunted thyroid-stimulating hormone and prolactin responses to thyrotropin-releasing hormone. Second, several investigators have reported data indicating that hyperactivity of the noradrenergic system is causally relevant to some patients with depressive disorders and with panic disorder. Specifically, these studies have found elevated concentrations of the norepinephrine metabolite 3-methoxy-4-hydroxyphenyglycol (MHPG) in the urine, the plasma, or the cerebrospinal fluid (CSF) of depressed patients and patients with panic disorder who were actively experiencing a panic attack. As with other anxiety and depressive disorders, serotonin and γ-aminobutyric acid (GABA) may also be causally involved in mixed anxiety-depressive disorder. Third, many studies have found that serotonergic drugs, such as fluoxetine (Prozac) and clomipramine (Anafranil), are useful in treating both depressive and anxiety disorders. Fourth, a number of family studies have reported data indicating that anxiety and depressive symptoms are genetically linked in at least some families.

Diagnosis

The DSM-IV-TR criteria (Table 16.7–5) require the presence of subsyndromal symptoms of both anxiety and depression and the presence of some autonomic symptoms, such as tremor, palpitations, dry mouth, and the sensation of a churning stomach. Some preliminary studies have indicated that the sensitivity of general practitioners to a syndrome of mixed anxiety-depressive disorder is low, although this lack of recognition may reflect the lack of an appropriate diagnostic label for the patients.

Clinical Features

The clinical features of mixed anxiety-depressive disorder combine symptoms of anxiety disorders and some symptoms of depressive disorders. In addition, symptoms of autonomic nervous system hyperactivity, such as gastrointestinal complaints, are common and contribute to the high frequency with which the patients are seen in outpatient medical clinics.

Table 16.7–5
DSM-IV-TR Research Criteria for Mixed Anxiety-Depressive Disorder

A. Persistent or recurrent dysphoric mood lasting at least 1 month.

B. The dysphoric mood is accompanied by at least 1 month of four (or more) of the following symptoms:
   (1) difficulty concentrating or mind going blank
   (2) sleep disturbance (difficulty falling or staying asleep, or restless, unsatisfying sleep)
   (3) fatigue or low energy
   (4) irritability
   (5) worry
   (6) being easily moved to tears
   (7) hypervigilance
   (8) anticipating the worst
   (9) hopelessness (pervasive pessimism about the future)
   (10) low self-esteem or feelings of worthlessness

C. The symptoms cause clinically significant distress or impairment in social, occupational, or other important areas of functioning.

D. The symptoms are not due to the direct physiological effects of a substance (e.g., a drug of abuse, a medication) or a general medical condition.

E. All of the following:
   (1) criteria have never been met for major depressive disorder, dysthymic disorder, panic disorder, or generalized anxiety disorder
   (2) criteria are not currently met for any other anxiety or mood disorder (including an anxiety or mood disorder, in partial remission)
   (3) the symptoms are not better accounted for by any other mental disorder

(From American Psychiatric Association. *Diagnostic and Statistical Manual of Mental Disorders.* 4th ed. Text rev. Washington, DC: American Psychiatric Association; copyright 2000, with permission.)

Differential Diagnosis

The differential diagnosis includes other anxiety and depressive disorders and personality disorders. Among the anxiety disorders, generalized anxiety disorder is most likely to overlap with mixed anxiety-depressive disorder. Among the mood disorders, dysthymic disorder and minor depressive disorder are most likely to overlap with mixed anxiety-depressive disorder. Among the personality disorders, avoidant, dependent, and obsessive-compulsive personality disorders may have symptoms that resemble those of mixed anxiety-depressive disorder. A diagnosis of a somatoform disorder should also be considered. Only a psychiatric history, a mental status examination, and a working knowledge of the specific DSM-IV-TR criteria can help clinicians differentiate among these conditions. The prodromal signs of schizophrenia may show itself as a mixed picture of mounting anxiety and depression with eventual onset of psychotic symptoms.

Course and Prognosis

On the basis of clinical data to date, patients seem to be equally likely to have prominent anxiety symptoms, prominent depressive symptoms, or an equal mixture of the two symptoms at onset. During the course of the illness, anxiety or depressive symptoms may alternate in their predominance. The prognosis is not known.

Treatment

Because adequate studies comparing treatment modalities for mixed anxiety-depressive disorder are not available, clinicians are probably most likely to provide treatment based on the symptoms present, their severity, and the clinician's own level of experience with various treatment modalities. Psychotherapeutic approaches may involve time-limited approaches, such as cognitive therapy or behavior modification, although some clinicians use a less-structured psychotherapeutic approach, such as insight-oriented psychotherapy. Pharmacotherapy for mixed anxiety-depressive disorder can include antianxiety drugs, antidepressant drugs, or both. Among the anxiolytic drugs, some data indicate that the use of triazolobenzodiazepines (e.g., alprazolam [Xanax]) may be indicated because of their effectiveness in treating depression associated with anxiety. A drug that affects the serotonin 5-HT_{1A} receptor, such as buspirone (BuSpar), may also be indicated. Among the antidepressants, despite the noradrenergic theories linking anxiety disorders and depressive disorders, the serotonergic antidepressants may be most effective in treating mixed anxiety-depressive disorder. Venlafaxine (Effexor) is an effective antidepressant that has been approved by the US Food and Drug Administration (FDA) for the treatment of depression as well as generalized anxiety disorder and is a drug of choice in the combined disorder.

References

Cassidy EL, Lauderdale S, Sheikh JI. Mixed anxiety and depression in older adults: clinical characteristics and management. *J Geriatr Psychiatry Neurol.* 2005;18(2):83–88.

Coryell W, Pine D, Fyer A, Klein D. Anxiety responses to CO2 inhalation in subjects at high-risk for panic disorder. *J Affect Disord.* 2006;92(1):63–70.

Grant BF, Stinson FS, Dawson DA, Chou SP, Dufour MC, Compton W, Pickering RP, Kaplan K. Prevalence and co-occurrence of substance use disorders and independent mood and anxiety disorders: Results from the National Epidemiologic Survey on Alcohol and Related Conditions. *Arch Gen Psychiatry.* 2004;61(8):807–816.

Malyszczak K, Pawlowski T. Distress and functioning in mixed anxiety and depressive disorder. *Psychiatry Clin Neurosci.* 2006;60(2):168–173.

McCabe RE, Chudzik SM, Antony MM, Young L, Swinson RP, Zolvensky MJ. Smoking behaviors across anxiety disorders. *J Anxiety Disord.* 2004;18(1):7–18.

Nandi A, Galea S, Ahern J, Vlahov D. Probable cigarette dependence, PTSD, and depression after an urban disaster: Results from a population survey of New York City residents 4 months after September 11, 2001. *Psychiatry.* 2005;68(4): 299–310.

Schoevers RA, Deeg DJ, van Tilburg W, Beekman AT. Depression and generalized anxiety disorder: Co-occurrence and longitudinal patterns in elderly patients. *Am J Geriatr Psychiatry.* 2005;13(1):31–39.

Weisberg RB, Maki KM, Culpepper L, Keller MB. Is anyone really M.A.D.?: The occurrence and course of mixed anxiety-depressive disorder in a sample of primary care patients. *J Nerv Ment Dis.* 2005;193(4):223–230.

Welkowitz J, Welkowitz LA, Struening E, Hellman F, Guardino M. Panic and comorbid anxiety symptoms in a national anxiety screening sample: Implications for clinical interventions. *Psychotherapy: Theory, Research, Practice Training.* 2004;41:69–75.

Woodward SH, Kaloupek DG, Streeter CC, Kimble MO, Reiss AL, Eliez S, Wald LL, Renshaw PF, Frederick BB, Lane B, Sheikh JI, Stegman WK, Kutter CJ, Stewart LP, Prestel RS, Arsenault NJ. Hippocampal volume, PTSD, and alcoholism in combat veterans. *Am J Psychiatry.* 2006;163(4):674–681.

17 Somatoform Disorders

Seven somatoform disorders are listed in the revised fourth edition of the *Diagnostic and Statistical Manual of Mental Disorders* (DSM-IV-TR): (1) somatization disorder, characterized by many physical complaints affecting many organ systems; (2) conversion disorder, characterized by one or two neurological complaints; (3) hypochondriasis, characterized less by a focus on symptoms than by patients' beliefs that they have a specific disease; (4) body dysmorphic disorder, characterized by a false belief or exaggerated perception that a body part is defective; (5) pain disorder, characterized by symptoms of pain that are either solely related to, or significantly exacerbated by, psychological factors; (6) undifferentiated somatoform disorder, which includes somatoform disorders not otherwise described that have been present for 6 months or longer; and (7) somatoform disorder not otherwise specified, which is the category for somatoform symptoms that do not meet any of the somatoform disorder diagnoses mentioned above (Table 17–1).

The term *somatoform* derives from the Greek *soma* for body, and the somatoform disorders are a broad group of illnesses that have bodily signs and symptoms as a major component. These disorders encompass mind–body interactions in which the brain, in ways still not well understood, sends various signals that impinge on the patient's awareness, indicating a serious problem in the body. Additionally, minor or as yet undetectable changes in neurochemistry, neurophysiology, and neuroimmunology may result from unknown mental or brain mechanisms that cause illness.

From a nosological perspective, somatoform disorders were grouped together for the first time in 1980 in the third edition of DSM (DSM-III) as those disorders in which bodily sensations or functions, as the patient's predominant focus, are influenced by a disorder of the mind. This clustering was not based on theoretical construct or laboratory findings. In fact, physical and laboratory examinations persistently fail to show significant substantiating data about the patient's complaints, which, nevertheless, are vigorous and sincere. Patients with somatoform disorders are convinced that their suffering comes from some type of presumably undetected and untreated bodily derangement. As Charles Beard stated about neurasthenia in 1881: "The complaints are not imaginary." The modern physician who dismisses his or her patient with the statement that the complaint is imaginary does a disservice to both the patient and the profession.

SOMATIZATION DISORDER

Somatization disorder is an illness of multiple somatic complaints in multiple organ systems that occurs over a period of several years and results in significant impairment or treatment seeking, or both. Somatization disorder is the prototypic somatoform disorder and has the best evidence of any of the somatoform disorders for being a stable and reliably measured entity over many years in individuals with the disorder. Somatization disorder differs from other somatoform disorders because of the multiplicity of the complaints and the multiple organ systems (e.g., gastrointestinal and neurological) that are affected. The disorder is chronic and is associated with significant psychological distress, impaired social and occupational functioning, and excessive medical-help-seeking behavior.

Somatization disorder has been recognized since the time of ancient Egypt. An early name for somatization disorder was *hysteria*, a condition incorrectly thought to affect only women. (The word hysteria is derived from the Greek word for uterus, *hystera*.) In the 17th century, Thomas Sydenham recognized that psychological factors, which he called "antecedent sorrows," were involved in the pathogenesis of the symptoms. In 1859, Paul Briquet, a French physician, observed the multiplicity of symptoms and affected organ systems and commented on the usually chronic course of the disorder. Because of these clinical observations, the disorder was called "Briquet's syndrome" until the term *somatization disorder* became the standard in the United States.

Epidemiology

The lifetime prevalence of somatization disorder in the general population is estimated to be 0.2 percent to 2 percent in women and 0.2 percent in men. Women with somatization disorder outnumber men 5 to 20 times, but the highest estimates may be because of the early tendency not to diagnose somatization disorder in male patients. Nevertheless, it is not an uncommon disorder. With a 5-to-1 female-to-male ratio, the lifetime prevalence of somatization disorder among women in the general population may be 1 or 2 percent. Among patients in the offices of general practitioners and family practitioners, 5 to 10 percent may meet the diagnostic criteria for somatization disorder. The disorder is inversely related to social position and occurs most often among patients who have little education and low incomes. Somatization disorder is defined as beginning before age 30; it usually begins during a person's teenage years.

Several studies have noted that somatization disorder commonly coexists with other mental disorders. About two thirds of all patients with somatization disorder have identifiable psychiatric symptoms, and up to half have other mental disorders. Commonly associated personality traits or personality disorders are those characterized by avoidant, paranoid, self-defeating, and obsessive-compulsive features. Two disorders not seen more commonly in patients with somatization disorder than in the general population are bipolar I disorder and substance abuse.

Table 17–1
Clinical Features of Somatoform Disorders

Diagnosis	Clinical Presentation	Demographic and Epidemiological Features	Diagnostic Features	Management Strategy	Prognosis	Associated Disturbances	Primary Differential Presentation	Psychological Processes Contributing to Symptoms	Motivation for Symptom Production
Somatization disorder	Polysymptomatic Recurrent and chronic Sickly by history	Young age Female predominance 20 to 1 Familial pattern 5%–10% incidence in primary care populations	Review of systems profusely positive Multiple clinical contacts Polysurgical	Therapeutic alliance Regular appointments Crisis intervention	Poor to fair	Histrionic personality disorder Antisocial personality disorder Alcohol and other substance abuse Many life problems Conversion disorder	Physical disease Depression	Unconscious Cultural and developmental	Unconscious psychological factors
Conversion disorder	Monosymptomatic Mostly acute Simulates disease	Highly prevalent Female predominance Young age Rural and low social class Little-educated and psychologically unsophisticated	Simulation incompatible with known physiological mechanisms or anatomy	Suggestion and persuasion Multiple techniques	Excellent except in chronic conversion disorder	Alcohol and other substance dependence Antisocial personality disorder Somatization disorder Histrionic personality disorder	Depression Schizophrenia Neurological disease	Unconscious Psychological stress or conflict may be present	Unconscious psychological factors
Hypochondriasis	Disease concern *or* preoccupation	Previous physical disease Middle or old age Male-female ratio equal	Disease conviction amplifies symptoms Obsessional	Document symptoms Psychosocial review Psychotherapeutic	Fair to good Waxes and wanes	Obsessive-compulsive personality disorder Depressive and anxiety disorders	Depression Physical disease Personality disorder Delusional disorder	Unconscious Stress–bereavement Developmental factors	Unconscious psychological factors
Body dysmorphic disorder	Subjective feelings of ugliness or concern with body defect	Adolescence or young adult Female predominance	Pervasive bodily concerns	Therapeutic alliance Stress management Psychotherapies Antidepressant medications	Guarded	Anorexia nervosa Psychosocial distress Plastic surgery addiction	Delusional disorder Depressive disorders Somatization disorder	Unconscious Self-esteem factors	Unconscious psychological factors
Pain disorder	Pain syndrome simulated	Female predominance 2 to 1 Older: 4th or 5th decade Familial pattern Up to 40% of pain populations	Simulation or intensity incompatible with known physiological mechanisms or anatomy	Therapeutic alliance Redefine goals of treatment Antidepressant medications	Guarded, variable	Depressive disorders Alcohol and other substance abuse Dependent or histrionic personality disorder	Depression Psychophysio-logical Physical disease Malingering and disability syndrome	Unconscious Acute stressor and developmental Physical trauma may predispose	Unconscious psychological factors

(Adapted from Folks DG, Ford CV, Houck CA. Somatoform disorders, factitious disorders, and malingering. In: Stoudemire A, ed. *Clinical Psychiatry for Medical Students.* Philadelphia: JB Lippincott; 1990:233, with permission.)

Etiology

Psychosocial Factors. The cause of somatization disorder is unknown. Psychosocial formulations of the cause involve interpretations of the symptoms as social communication whose result is to avoid obligations (e.g., going to a job a person does not like), to express emotions (e.g., anger at a spouse), or to symbolize a feeling or a belief (e.g., a pain in the gut). Strict psychoanalytic interpretations of symptoms rest on the hypothesis that the symptoms substitute for repressed instinctual impulses.

A behavioral perspective on somatization disorder emphasizes that parental teaching, parental example, and ethnic mores may teach some children to somatize more than others. In addition, some patients with somatization disorder come from unstable homes and have been physically abused. Social, cultural, and ethnic factors may also be involved in the development of symptoms.

Biological Factors. Some studies point to a neuropsychological basis for somatization disorder. These studies propose that the patients have characteristic attention and cognitive impairments that result in the faulty perception and assessment of somatosensory inputs. The reported impairments include excessive distractibility, inability to habituate to repetitive stimuli, grouping of cognitive constructs on an impressionistic basis, partial and circumstantial associations, and lack of selectivity, as indicated in some studies of evoked potentials. A limited number of brain-imaging studies have reported decreased metabolism in the frontal lobes and the nondominant hemisphere.

GENETICS. Genetic data indicate that, in at least some families, the transmission of somatization disorder has genetic components. Somatization disorder tends to run in families and occurs in 10 to 20 percent of the first-degree female relatives of probands of patients with somatization disorder. Within these families, first-degree male relatives are susceptible to substance abuse and antisocial personality disorder. One study also reported a concordance rate of 29 percent in monozygotic twins and 10 percent in dizygotic twins, an indication of a genetic effect. The male relatives of women with somatization disorder show an increased risk of antisocial personality disorder and substance-related disorders. Having a biological or adoptive parent with any of these three disorders increases the risk of developing antisocial personality disorder, a substance-related disorder, or somatization disorder.

CYTOKINES. Cytokines are messenger molecules that the immune system uses to communicate within itself and with the nervous system, including the brain. Examples of cytokines are interleukins, tumor necrosis factor, and interferons. Some preliminary experiments indicate that cytokines contribute to some of the nonspecific symptoms of disease, such as hypersomnia, anorexia, fatigue, and depression. The hypothesis that abnormal regulation of the cytokine system may result in some of the symptoms seen in somatoform disorders is under investigation.

Diagnosis

For the diagnosis of somatization disorder, DSM-IV-TR requires onset of symptoms before age 30 (Table 17–2). During the course of the disorder, patients must have complained of at least four pain symptoms, two gastrointestinal symptoms, one sexual symptom, and one pseudoneurological symptom, none of which is completely explained by physical or laboratory examinations.

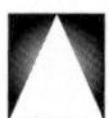

Table 17–2
DSM-IV-TR Diagnostic Criteria for Somatization Disorder

A. A history of many physical complaints beginning before age 30 years that occur over a period of several years and result in treatment being sought or significant impairment in social, occupational, or other important areas of functioning.

B. Each of the following criteria must have been met, with individual symptoms occurring at any time during the course of the disturbance:
  (1) four pain symptoms: a history of pain related to at least four different sites or functions (e.g., head, abdomen, back, joints, extremities, chest, rectum, during menstruation, during sexual intercourse, or during urination)
  (2) two gastrointestinal symptoms: a history of at least two gastrointestinal symptoms other than pain (e.g., nausea, bloating, vomiting other than during pregnancy, diarrhea, or intolerance of several different foods)
  (3) one sexual symptom: a history of at least one sexual or reproductive symptom other than pain (e.g., sexual indifference, erectile or ejaculatory dysfunction, irregular menses, excessive menstrual bleeding, vomiting throughout pregnancy)
  (4) one pseudoneurological symptom: a history of at least one symptom or deficit suggesting a neurological condition not limited to pain (conversion symptoms such as impaired coordination or balance, paralysis or localized weakness, difficulty swallowing or lump in throat, aphonia, urinary retention, hallucinations, loss of touch or pain sensation, double vision, blindness, deafness, seizures; dissociative symptoms such as amnesia; or loss of consciousness other than fainting)

C. Either (1) or (2):
  (1) after appropriate investigation, each of the symptoms in Criterion B cannot be fully explained by a known general medical condition or the direct effects of a substance (e.g., a drug of abuse, a medication)
  (2) when there is a related general medical condition, the physical complaints or resulting social or occupational impairment are in excess of what would be expected from the history, physical examination, or laboratory findings

D. The symptoms are not intentionally produced or feigned (as in factitious disorder or malingering).

Clinical Features

Patients with somatization disorder have many somatic complaints and long, complicated medical histories. Nausea and vomiting (other than during pregnancy), difficulty swallowing, pain in the arms and legs, shortness of breath unrelated to exertion, amnesia, and complications of pregnancy and menstruation are among the most common symptoms. Patients frequently believe that they have been sickly most of their lives. Pseudoneurological symptoms suggest, but are not pathognomonic of, a neurological disorder. According to DSM-IV-TR, they include impaired coordination or balance, paralysis or localized weakness, difficulty swallowing or lump in throat, aphonia, urinary retention, hallucinations, loss of touch or pain sensation, double vision, blindness, deafness, seizures, or loss of consciousness other than fainting.

Psychological distress and interpersonal problems are prominent; anxiety and depression are the most prevalent psychiatric conditions. Suicide threats are common, but actual suicide is rare. If suicide does occur, it is often associated with substance abuse. Patients' medical histories are often circumstantial, vague, imprecise, inconsistent, and disorganized. Patients classically (but not always) describe their complaints in a dramatic, emotional, and exaggerated fashion, with vivid and colorful language; they may confuse temporal sequences and cannot clearly distinguish current from past symptoms. Female patients with somatization disorder may dress in an exhibitionistic manner. Patients may be perceived as dependent, self-centered, hungry for admiration or praise, and manipulative.

Somatization disorder is commonly associated with other mental disorders, including major depressive disorder, personality disorders, substance-related disorders, generalized anxiety disorder, and phobias. The combination of these disorders and the chronic symptoms results in an increased incidence of marital, occupational, and social problems.

A 34-year-old female temporary clerk presented with chronic and intermittent dizziness, paresthesias, pain in multiple areas of her body, and intermittent nausea and diarrhea. On further history, the patient said that the symptoms had been present most of the time, although they had been undulating since she was approximately 24 years of age. In addition to the symptoms previously mentioned, she had mild depression, was disinterested in many things in life, including sexual activity, and had been to many doctors to try to find out what was wrong with her. Even though she had seen many doctors and had many tests, she stated that "no one can find out what's wrong" with her. She wanted another opinion. She commented that she had been "sick a lot" since childhood and had been on various medications on and off. Physical examination revealed a normotensive, slightly overweight female in no acute distress. She had diffuse and mild abdominal tenderness, without true guarding or rebound tenderness. Her neurological examination was normal. She winced when physical examination was conducted on various parts of her body, although this wincing went away when the physician was speaking with her while conducting the examination. (Courtesy of Michael A. Hollifield, M.D.)

Differential Diagnosis

Table 17–3 shows the vast differential diagnosis for somatization phenomena. The three features that most suggest a diagnosis of somatization disorder instead of another medical disorder are (1) the involvement of multiple organ systems, (2) early onset and chronic course without development of physical signs or structural abnormalities, and (3) absence of laboratory abnormalities that are characteristic of the suggested medical condition. In the process of diagnosis, the astute clinician considers other medical disorders that are characterized by vague, multiple, and confusing somatic symptoms, such as thyroid disease, hyperparathyroidism, intermittent porphyria, multiple sclerosis (MS), and systemic lupus erythematosus.

Table 17–3
Differential Diagnosis of the Somatizing Patient

Psychophysiological symptoms
- Psychological factors affecting physical illness
- Nonpathological, transient psychogenic somatic symptoms (all are acute but may become chronic)
- Grief and bereavement, with physical symptoms
- Fear, with physical symptoms
- Exaggeration or elaboration of physical symptoms (e.g., postaccident, when litigation or compensation is involved)
- Sleep deprivation, with physical symptoms
- Sensory overload or deprivation, with physical symptoms

Psychiatric syndromes (other than somatoform disorders)
- Mood disorders (e.g., major depression and dysthymia)
- Anxiety disorders (e.g., panic disorders)
- Substance use, abuse, and withdrawal
- Psychotic disorders (e.g., schizophrenia, psychotic depression, and monosymptomatic hypochondriasis)
- Adjustment disorders with anxiety or depression, or both
- Personality disorders
- Dementias

Somatoform disorders
- Somatization disorder
- Hypochondriasis
- Body dysmorphic disorder
- Somatoform pain disorder
- Conversion disorder
- Somatoform disorder, not otherwise specified

Voluntary psychogenic symptoms or syndromes
- Factitious, with physical symptoms (e.g., Munchausen syndrome)
- Malingering, with physical symptoms

(Adapted from Rubin RH, Voss C, Derksen DJ, et al., eds. *Medicine: A Primary Care Approach.* Philadelphia: WB Saunders; 1996:390, with permission.)

Mood and anxiety disorders often, but not always, have prominent somatic symptoms, which do not exist separately from the mood or anxiety disorder. Somatization disorder may be diagnosed, however, as a comorbid condition with mood and anxiety disorders. Schizophrenia and other psychotic disorders with multiple somatic delusions need to be differentiated from the nondelusional somatic complaints of individuals with somatization disorder. Hallucinations can occur as pseudoneurological symptoms and must be distinguished from the typical hallucinations seen in schizophrenia. Somatization disorder symptoms are usually easier to distinguish from psychotic disorders than is the case for hypochondriasis, the disease fears of which can reach delusional quality.

Course and Prognosis

Somatization disorder is a chronic, undulating, and relapsing disorder that rarely remits completely. It is unusual for the individual with somatization disorder to be free of symptoms for greater than 1 year, during which time they may see a doctor several times. Research has indicated that a person diagnosed with somatization disorder has approximately an 80 percent chance of being diagnosed with this disorder 5 years later. Although patients with this disorder consider themselves to be medically ill, good evidence is that they are no more likely to develop another medical illness in the next 20 years than people without somatization disorder.

Treatment

Somatization disorder is best treated when the patient has a single identified physician as primary caretaker. When more than one clinician is involved, patients have increased opportunities to express somatic complaints. Primary physicians should see patients during regularly scheduled visits, usually at monthly intervals. The visits should be relatively brief, although a partial physical examination should be conducted to respond to each new somatic complaint. Additional laboratory and diagnostic procedures should generally be avoided. Once somatization disorder has been diagnosed, the treating physician should listen to the somatic complaints as emotional expressions rather than as medical complaints. Nevertheless, patients with somatization disorder can also have bona fide physical illnesses; therefore, physicians must always use their judgment about what symptoms to work up and to what extent. A reasonable long-range strategy for a primary care physician who is treating a patient with somatization disorder is to increase the patient's awareness of the possibility that psychological factors are involved in the symptoms until the patient is willing to see a mental health clinician. In complex cases with many medical presentations, a psychiatrist is better able to judge whether or not to seek a medical or surgical consultation because of his or her medical training; however, a nonmedical mental health professional can explore the psychological antecedents of the disorder as well, especially if consulting closely with a physician.

Psychotherapy, both individual and group, decreases these patients' personal health care expenditures by 50 percent, largely by decreasing their rates of hospitalization. In psychotherapy settings, patients are helped to cope with their symptoms, to express underlying emotions, and to develop alternative strategies for expressing their feelings.

Giving psychotropic medications whenever somatization disorder coexists with a mood or anxiety disorder is always a risk, but psychopharmacological treatment, as well as psychotherapeutic treatment, of the coexisting disorder is indicated. Medication must be monitored, because patients with somatization disorder tend to use drugs erratically and unreliably. Few available data indicate that pharmacological treatment is effective in patients without coexisting mental disorders.

CONVERSION DISORDER

Conversion disorder is an illness of symptoms or deficits that affect voluntary motor or sensory functions, which suggest another medical condition, but that is judged to be caused by psychological factors because the illness is preceded by conflicts or other stressors. The symptoms or deficits of conversion disorder are not intentionally produced, are not caused by substance use, are not limited to pain or sexual symptoms, and the gain is primarily psychological and not social, monetary, or legal (Table 17–4).

The syndrome currently known as *conversion disorder* was originally combined with the syndrome known as *somatization disorder* and was referred to as hysteria, conversion reaction, or dissociative reaction. Paul Briquet and Jean-Martin Charcot contributed to the development of the concept of conversion disorder by noting the influence of heredity on the symptom and the common association with a traumatic event. The term conversion was introduced by Sigmund Freud, who, based on his work with Anna O, hypothesized that the symptoms of conversion disorder reflect unconscious conflicts.

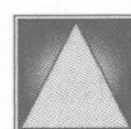

Table 17–4
Common Symptoms of Conversion Disorder

Motor Symptoms	Sensory Deficits
Involuntary movements	Anesthesia, especially of extremities
Tics	Midline anesthesia
Blepharospasm	Blindness
Torticollis	Tunnel vision
Opisthotonos	Deafness
Seizures	**Visceral Symptoms**
Abnormal gait	Psychogenic vomiting
Falling	Pseudocyesis
Astasia-abasia	Globus hystericus
Paralysis	Swooning or syncope
Weakness	Urinary retention
Aphonia	Diarrhea

(Courtesy of Frederick G. Guggenheim, M.D.)

Epidemiology

Some symptoms of conversion disorder that are not sufficiently severe to warrant the diagnosis may occur in up to one third of the general population sometime during their lives. Reported rates of conversion disorder vary from 11 of 100,000 to 300 of 100,000 in general population samples. Among specific populations, the occurrence of conversion disorder may be even higher than that, perhaps making conversion disorder the most common somatoform disorder in some populations. Several studies have reported that 5 to 15 percent of psychiatric consultations in a general hospital and 25 to 30 percent of admissions to a Veterans Administration hospital involve patients with conversion disorder diagnoses.

The ratio of women to men among adult patients is at least 2 to 1 and as much as 10 to 1; among children, an even higher predominance is seen in girls. Symptoms are more common on the left than on the right side of the body in women. Women who present with conversion symptoms are more likely subsequently to develop somatization disorder than women who have not had conversion symptoms. An association exists between conversion disorder and antisocial personality disorder in men. Men with conversion disorder have often been involved in occupational or military accidents. The onset of conversion disorder is generally from late childhood to early adulthood and is rare before 10 years of age or after 35 years of age, but onset as late as the ninth decade of life has been reported. When symptoms suggest a conversion disorder onset in middle or old age, the probability of an occult neurological or other medical condition is high. Conversion symptoms in children younger than 10 years of age are usually limited to gait problems or seizures.

Data indicate that conversion disorder is most common among rural populations, persons with little education, those with low intelligence quotients, those in low socioeconomic groups, and military personnel who have been exposed to combat situations. Conversion disorder is commonly associated with comorbid diagnoses of major depressive disorder, anxiety disorders, and schizophrenia and shows an increased frequency in relatives of probands with conversion disorder. Limited data suggest that conversion symptoms are more frequent in relatives of people with conversion disorder. An increased risk of conversion disorder in monozygotic, but not dizygotic, twin pairs has been reported.

Comorbidity

Medical and, especially, neurological disorders occur frequently among patients with conversion disorders. What is typically seen in these comorbid neurological or medical conditions is an elaboration of symptoms stemming from the original organic lesion.

Among the Axis I psychiatric conditions, depressive disorders, anxiety disorders, and somatization disorders are especially noted for their association with conversion disorder. Conversion in schizophrenia is reported, but it is uncommon. Studies of patients admitted to a psychiatric hospital for conversion disorder reveal, on further study, that one quarter to one half have a clinically significant mood disorder or schizophrenia.

Personality disorders also frequently accompany conversion disorder, especially the histrionic type (in 5 to 21 percent of cases) and the passive-dependent type (9 to 40 percent of cases). Conversion disorders can occur, however, in persons with no predisposing medical, neurological, or psychiatric disorder.

Etiology

Psychoanalytic Factors. According to psychoanalytic theory, conversion disorder is caused by repression of unconscious intrapsychic conflict and conversion of anxiety into a physical symptom. The conflict is between an instinctual impulse (e.g., aggression or sexuality) and the prohibitions against its expression. The symptoms allow partial expression of the forbidden wish or urge but disguise it, so that patients can avoid consciously confronting their unacceptable impulses; that is, the conversion disorder symptom has a symbolic relation to the unconscious conflict—for example, vaginismus protects the patient from expressing unacceptable sexual wishes. Conversion disorder symptoms also allow patients to communicate that they need special consideration and special treatment. Such symptoms may function as a nonverbal means of controlling or manipulating others.

Learning Theory. In terms of conditioned learning theory, a conversion symptom can be seen as a piece of classically conditioned learned behavior; symptoms of illness, learned in childhood, are called forth as a means of coping with an otherwise impossible situation.

Biological Factors. Increasing data implicate biological and neuropsychological factors in the development of conversion disorder symptoms. Preliminary brain-imaging studies have found hypometabolism of the dominant hemisphere and hypermetabolism of the nondominant hemisphere and have implicated impaired hemispheric communication in the cause of conversion disorder. The symptoms may be caused by an excessive cortical arousal that sets off negative feedback loops between the cerebral cortex and the brainstem reticular formation. Elevated levels of corticofugal output, in turn, inhibit the patient's awareness of bodily sensation, which may explain the observed sensory deficits in some patients with conversion disorder. Neuropsychological tests sometimes reveal subtle cerebral impairments in verbal communication, memory, vigilance, affective incongruity, and attention in these patients.

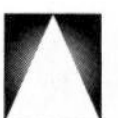

Table 17–5
DSM-IV-TR Diagnostic Criteria for Conversion Disorder

A. One or more symptoms or deficits affecting voluntary motor or sensory function that suggest a neurological or other general medical condition.

B. Psychological factors are judged to be associated with the symptom or deficit because the initiation or exacerbation of the symptom or deficit is preceded by conflicts or other stressors.

C. The symptom or deficit is not intentionally produced or feigned (as in factitious disorder or malingering).

D. The symptom or deficit cannot, after appropriate investigation, be fully explained by a general medical condition, or by the direct effects of a substance, or as a culturally sanctioned behavior or experience.

E. The symptom or deficit causes clinically significant distress or impairment in social, occupational, or other important areas of functioning or warrants medical evaluation.

F. The symptom or deficit is not limited to pain or sexual dysfunction, does not occur exclusively during the course of somatization disorder, and is not better accounted for by another mental disorder.

Specify type of symptom or deficit:

With motor symptom or deficit
With sensory symptom or deficit
With seizures or convulsions
With mixed presentation

(From American Psychiatric Association. *Diagnostic and Statistical Manual of Mental Disorders.* 4th ed. Text rev. Washington, DC: American Psychiatric Association; copyright 2000, with permission.)

Diagnosis

The DSM-IV-TR limits the diagnosis of conversion disorder to those symptoms that affect a voluntary motor or sensory function, that is, neurological symptoms (Table 17–5). Physicians cannot explain the neurological symptoms solely on the basis of any known neurological condition.

The diagnosis of conversion disorder requires that clinicians find a necessary and critical association between the cause of the neurological symptoms and psychological factors, although the symptoms cannot result from malingering or factitious disorder. The diagnosis of conversion disorder also excludes symptoms of pain and sexual dysfunction and symptoms that occur only in somatization disorder. DSM-IV-TR allows specification of the type of symptom or deficit seen in conversion disorder (Table 17–5).

Clinical Features

Paralysis, blindness, and mutism are the most common conversion disorder symptoms. Conversion disorder may be most commonly associated with passive-aggressive, dependent, antisocial, and histrionic personality disorders. Depressive and anxiety disorder symptoms often accompany the symptoms of conversion disorder, and affected patients are at risk for suicide.

Mr. J is a 28-year-old single man who is employed in a factory. He was brought to an emergency department by his father, complaining that he had lost his vision while sitting in the back seat on the way home from a family gathering. He had been playing volleyball at the gathering but had sustained no significant injury except for the volleyball hitting him in the head a few times. As was usual for this man, he had been reluctant to play volleyball because of the lack of his athletic skills, and was placed on a team at the last moment. He recalls having some problems with seeing during the game, but his vision did not become ablated until he was in the car on the way home. By the time he got to the emergency department, his vision was improving, although he still complained of blurriness and mild diplopia. The double vision could be attenuated by having him focus on items at different distances.

On examination, Mr. J was fully cooperative, somewhat uncertain about why this would have occurred, and rather nonchalant. Pupillary, oculomotor, and general sensorimotor examinations were normal. After being cleared medically, the patient was sent to a mental health center for further evaluation.

At the mental health center, the patient recounts the same story as he did in the emergency department, and he was still accompanied by his father. He began to recount how his vision started to return to normal when his father pulled over on the side of the road and began to talk to him about the events of the day. He spoke with his father about how he had felt embarrassed and somewhat conflicted about playing volleyball and how he had felt that he really should play because of external pressures. Further history from the patient and his father revealed that this young man had been shy as an adolescent, particularly around athletic participation. He had never had another episode of visual loss. He did recount feeling anxious and sometimes not feeling well in his body during athletic activities.

Discussion with the patient at the mental health center focused on the potential role of psychological and social factors in acute vision loss. The patient was somewhat perplexed by this but was also amenable to discussion. He stated that he clearly recognized that he began seeing and feeling better when his father pulled off to the side of the road and discussed things with him. Doctors admitted that they did not know the cause of the vision loss and that it would likely not return. The patient and his father were satisfied with the medical and psychiatric evaluation and agreed to return for care if there were any further symptoms. The patient was appointed a follow-up time at the outpatient psychiatric clinic. (Courtesy of Michael A. Hollifield, M.D.)

Sensory Symptoms. In conversion disorder, anesthesia and paresthesia are common, especially of the extremities. All sensory modalities can be involved, and the distribution of the disturbance is usually inconsistent with either central or peripheral neurological disease. Thus, clinicians may see the characteristic stocking-and-glove anesthesia of the hands or feet or the hemianesthesia of the body beginning precisely along the midline.

Conversion disorder symptoms may involve the organs of special sense and can produce deafness, blindness, and tunnel vision. These symptoms can be unilateral or bilateral, but neurological evaluation reveals intact sensory pathways. In conversion disorder blindness, for example, patients walk around without collisions or self-injury, their pupils react to light, and their cortical evoked potentials are normal.

Motor Symptoms. The motor symptoms of conversion disorder include abnormal movements, gait disturbance, weakness, and paralysis. Gross rhythmical tremors, choreiform movements, tics, and jerks may be present. The movements generally worsen when attention is called to them. One gait disturbance seen in conversion disorder is *astasia-abasia*, which is a wildly ataxic, staggering gait accompanied by gross, irregular, jerky truncal movements and thrashing and waving arm movements. Patients with the symptoms rarely fall; if they do, they are generally not injured.

Other common motor disturbances are paralysis and paresis involving one, two, or all four limbs, although the distribution of the involved muscles does not conform to the neural pathways. Reflexes remain normal; the patients have no fasciculations or muscle atrophy (except after long-standing conversion paralysis); electromyography findings are normal.

Seizure Symptoms. Pseudoseizures are another symptom in conversion disorder. Clinicians may find it difficult to differentiate a pseudoseizure from an actual seizure by clinical observation alone. Moreover, about one third of the patient's pseudoseizures also have a coexisting epileptic disorder. Tongue-biting, urinary incontinence, and injuries after falling can occur in pseudoseizures, although these symptoms are generally not present. Pupillary and gag reflexes are retained after pseudoseizure, and patients have no postseizure increase in prolactin concentrations.

Other Associated Features. Several psychological symptoms have also been associated with conversion disorder.

PRIMARY GAIN. Patients achieve primary gain by keeping internal conflicts outside their awareness. Symptoms have symbolic value; they represent an unconscious psychological conflict.

SECONDARY GAIN. Patients accrue tangible advantages and benefits as a result of being sick; for example, being excused from obligations and difficult life situations, receiving support and assistance that might not otherwise be forthcoming, and controlling other persons' behavior.

LA BELLE INDIFFÉRENCE. La belle indifférence is a patient's inappropriately cavalier attitude toward serious symptoms; that is, the patient seems to be unconcerned about what appears to be a major impairment. That bland indifference is also seen in some seriously ill medical patients who develop a stoic attitude. The presence or absence of la belle indifférence is not pathnognomonic of conversion disorder, but it is often associated with the condition.

IDENTIFICATION. Patients with conversion disorder may unconsciously model their symptoms on those of someone important to them. For example, a parent or a person who has recently died may serve as a model for conversion disorder. During pathological grief reaction, bereaved persons commonly have symptoms of the deceased.

Differential Diagnosis

One of the major problems in diagnosing conversion disorder is the difficulty of definitively ruling out a medical disorder. Concomitant nonpsychiatric medical disorders are common in hospitalized patients with conversion disorder, and evidence of a current or previous neurological disorder or a systemic disease affecting the brain has been reported in 18 to 64 percent of such patients. An estimated 25 to 50 percent of patients classified as having conversion disorder eventually receive diagnoses of neurological or nonpsychiatric medical disorders that could have caused their earlier symptoms. Thus, a thorough medical and neurological workup is essential in all cases. If the symptoms can be resolved by suggestion, hypnosis, or parenteral amobarbital (Amytal) or lorazepam (Ativan), they are probably the result of conversion disorder.

Neurological disorders (e.g., dementia and other degenerative diseases), brain tumors, and basal ganglia disease must be considered in the differential diagnosis. For example, weakness may be confused with myasthenia gravis, polymyositis, acquired myopathies, or MS. Optic neuritis may be misdiagnosed as conversion disorder blindness. Other diseases that can cause confusing symptoms are Guillain-Barré syndrome, Creutzfeldt-Jakob disease, periodic paralysis, and early neurological manifestations of acquired immunodeficiency syndrome (AIDS). Conversion disorder symptoms occur in schizophrenia, depressive disorders, and anxiety disorders, but these other disorders are associated with their own distinct symptoms that eventually make differential diagnosis possible.

Sensorimotor symptoms also occur in somatization disorder. But somatization disorder is a chronic illness that begins early in life and includes symptoms in many other organ systems. In hypochondriasis, patients have no actual loss or distortion of function; the somatic complaints are chronic and are not limited to neurological symptoms, and the characteristic hypochondriacal attitudes and beliefs are present. If the patient's symptoms are limited to pain, pain disorder can be diagnosed. Patients whose complaints are limited to sexual function are classified as having a sexual dysfunction, rather than conversion disorder.

In both malingering and factitious disorder, the symptoms are under conscious, voluntary control. A malingerer's history is usually more inconsistent and contradictory than that of a patient with conversion disorder, and a malingerer's fraudulent behavior is clearly goal directed.

Table 17–6 lists examples of important tests that are relevant to conversion disorder symptoms.

Course and Prognosis

The onset of conversion disorder is usually acute, but a crescendo of symptomatology may also occur. Symptoms or deficits are usually of short duration, and approximately 95 percent of acute cases remit spontaneously, usually within 2 weeks in hospitalized patients. If symptoms have been present for 6 months or longer, the prognosis for symptom resolution is less than 50 percent and diminishes further the longer that conversion is present. Recurrence occurs in one fifth to one fourth of people within 1 year of the first episode. Thus, one episode is a predictor for future episodes. A good prognosis is heralded by acute onset, presence of clearly identifiable stressors at the time of onset, a short interval between onset and the institution of treatment, and above average intelligence. Paralysis, aphonia, and blindness are associated with a good prognosis, whereas tremor and seizures are poor prognostic factors.

Treatment

Resolution of the conversion disorder symptom is usually spontaneous, although it is probably facilitated by insight-oriented supportive or behavior therapy. The most important feature of the therapy is a relationship with a caring and confident therapist. With patients who are resistant to the idea of psychotherapy, physicians can suggest that the psychotherapy will focus on issues of stress and coping. Telling such patients that their symptoms are imaginary often makes them worse. Hypnosis, anxiolytics, and behavioral relaxation exercises are effective in some cases. Parenteral amobarbital or lorazepam may be helpful

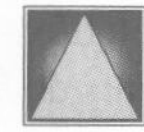

Table 17–6
Distinctive Physical Examination Findings in Conversion Disorder

Condition	Test	Conversion Findings
Anesthesia	Map dermatomes	Sensory loss does not conform to recognized pattern of distribution
Hemianesthesia	Check midline	Strict half-body split
Astasia-abasia	Walking, dancing	With suggestion, those who cannot walk may still be able to dance; alteration of sensory and motor findings with suggestion
Paralysis, paresis	Drop paralyzed hand onto face	Hand falls next to face, not on it
	Hoover test	Pressure noted in examiner's hand under paralyzed leg when attempting straight leg raising
	Check motor strength	Give-away weakness
Coma	Examiner attempts to open eyes	Resists opening; gaze preference is away from doctor
	Ocular cephalic maneuver	Eyes stare straight ahead, do not move from side to side
Aphonia	Request a cough	Essentially normal coughing sound indicates cords are closing
Intractable sneezing	Observe	Short nasal grunts with little or no sneezing on inspiratory phase; little or no aerosolization of secretions: minimal facial expression; eyes open; stops when asleep; abates when alone
Syncope	Head-up tilt test	Magnitude of changes in vital signs and venous pooling do not explain continuing symptoms
Tunnel vision	Visual fields	Changing pattern on multiple examinations
Profound monocular blindness	Swinging flashlight sign (Marcus Gunn)	Absence of relative afferent pupillary defect
	Binocular visual fields	Sufficient vision in "bad eye" precludes plotting normal physiological blind spot in good eye
Severe bilateral blindness	"Wiggle your fingers, I'm just testing coordination"	Patient may begin to mimic new movements before realizing the slip
	Sudden flash of bright light	Patient flinches
	"Look at your hand"	Patient does not look there
	"Touch your index fingers"	Even blind patients can do this by proprioception

(Courtesy of Frederick G. Guggenheim, M.D.)

in obtaining additional historic information, especially when a patient has recently experienced a traumatic event. Psychodynamic approaches include psychoanalysis and insight-oriented psychotherapy, in which patients explore intrapsychic conflicts and the symbolism of the conversion disorder symptoms. Brief and direct forms of short-term psychotherapy have also been used to treat conversion disorder. The longer the duration of these patients' sick role and the more they have regressed, the more difficult the treatment.

HYPOCHONDRIASIS

Hypochondriasis is characterized by 6 months or more of a general and nondelusional preoccupation with fears of having, or the idea that one has, a serious disease based on the person's misinterpretation of bodily symptoms. This preoccupation causes significant distress and impairment in one's life; it is not accounted for by another psychiatric or medical disorder; and a subset of individuals with hypochondriasis has poor insight about the presence of this disorder. The term *hypochondriasis* is derived from the old medical term hypochondrium, ("below the ribs") and reflects the common abdominal complaints of many patients with the disorder, but they may occur in any part of the body.

Epidemiology

One recent study reported a 6-month prevalence of hypochondriasis of 4 to 6 percent in a general medical clinic population, but it may be as high as 15 percent. Men and women are equally affected by hypochondriasis. Although the onset of symptoms can occur at any age, the disorder most commonly appears in persons 20 to 30 years of age. Some evidence indicates that the diagnosis is more common among blacks than among whites, but social position, education level, and marital status do not appear to affect the diagnosis. Hypochondriacal complaints reportedly occur in about 3 percent of medical students, usually in the first 2 years, but they are generally transient.

Etiology

In the diagnostic criteria for hypochondriasis, DSM-IV-TR indicates that the symptoms reflect a misinterpretation of bodily symptoms. Much data indicate that persons with hypochondriasis augment and amplify their somatic sensations; they have low thresholds for, and low tolerance of, physical discomfort. For example, what persons normally perceive as abdominal pressure, persons with hypochondriasis experience as abdominal pain. They may focus on bodily sensations, misinterpret them, and become alarmed by them because of a faulty cognitive scheme.

A second theory is that hypochondriasis is understandable in terms of a social learning model. The symptoms of hypochondriasis are viewed as a request for admission to the sick role made by a person facing seemingly insurmountable and insolvable problems. The sick role offers an escape that allows a patient to avoid noxious obligations, to postpone unwelcome challenges, and to be excused from usual duties and obligations.

A third theory suggests that hypochondriasis is a variant form of other mental disorders, among which depressive disorders and anxiety disorders are most frequently included. An estimated 80 percent of patients with hypochondriasis may have coexisting depressive or anxiety disorders. Patients who meet the diagnostic criteria for hypochondriasis may be somatizing subtypes of these other disorders.

The psychodynamic school of thought has produced a fourth theory of hypochondriasis. According to this theory, aggressive and hostile wishes toward others are transferred (through repression and displacement) into physical complaints. The anger of patients with hypochondriasis originates in past disappointments, rejections, and losses, but the patients express their anger in the present by soliciting the help and concern of other persons and then rejecting them as ineffective. Hypochondriasis is also viewed as a defense against guilt, a sense of innate badness, an expression of low self-esteem, and a sign of excessive self-concern. Pain and somatic suffering, thus, become means of atonement and expiation (undoing) and can be experienced as deserved punishment for past wrongdoing (either real or imaginary) and for a person's sense of wickedness and sinfulness.

Diagnosis

The DSM-IV-TR diagnostic criteria for hypochondriasis require that patients be preoccupied with the false belief that they have a serious disease, based on their misinterpretation of physical signs or sensations (Table 17–7). The belief must last at least 6 months, despite the absence of pathological findings on medical and neurological examinations. The diagnostic criteria also stipulate that the belief cannot have the intensity of a delusion (more appropriately diagnosed as delusional disorder) and cannot be restricted to distress about appearance (more appropriately diagnosed as body dysmorphic disorder). The symptoms of hypochondriasis must be sufficiently intense to cause emotional distress or impair the patient's ability to function in important areas of life. Clinicians may specify the presence of poor insight; patients do

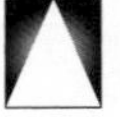

Table 17–7
DSM-IV-TR Diagnostic Criteria for Hypochondriasis

A. Preoccupation with fears of having, or the idea that one has, a serious disease based on the person's misinterpretation of bodily symptoms.
B. The preoccupation persists despite appropriate medical evaluation and reassurance.
C. The belief in Criterion A is not of delusional intensity (as in delusional disorder, somatic type) and is not restricted to a circumscribed concern about appearance (as in body dysmorphic disorder).
D. The preoccupation causes clinically significant distress or impairment in social, occupational, or other important areas of functioning.
E. The duration of the disturbance is at least 6 months.
F. The preoccupation is not better accounted for by generalized anxiety disorder, obsessive-compulsive disorder, panic disorder, a major depressive episode, separation anxiety, or another somatoform disorder.

Specify if:
With poor insight: if, for most of the time during the current episode, the person does not recognize that the concern about having a serious illness is excessive or unreasonable

(From American Psychiatric Association. *Diagnostic and Statistical Manual of Mental Disorders.* 4th ed. Text rev. Washington, DC: American Psychiatric Association; copyright 2000, with permission.)

not consistently recognize that their concerns about disease are excessive.

Clinical Features

Patients with hypochondriasis believe that they have a serious disease that has not yet been detected, and they cannot be persuaded to the contrary. They may maintain a belief that they have a particular disease or, as time progresses, they may transfer their belief to another disease. Their convictions persist despite negative laboratory results, the benign course of the alleged disease over time, and appropriate reassurances from physicians. Yet, their beliefs are not sufficiently fixed to be delusions. Hypochondriasis is often accompanied by symptoms of depression and anxiety and commonly coexists with a depressive or anxiety disorder.

Although DSM-IV-TR specifies that the symptoms must be present for at least 6 months, transient hypochondriacal states can occur after major stresses, most commonly the death or serious illness of someone important to the patient, or a serious (perhaps life-threatening) illness that has been resolved but that leaves the patient temporarily hypochondriacal in its wake. Such states that last fewer than 6 months should be diagnosed as somatoform disorder not otherwise specified. Transient hypochondriacal responses to external stress generally remit when the stress is resolved, but they can become chronic if reinforced by persons in the patient's social system or by health professionals.

Differential Diagnosis

Hypochondriasis must be differentiated from nonpsychiatric medical conditions, especially disorders that show symptoms that are not necessarily easily diagnosed. Such diseases include AIDS, endocrinopathies, myasthenia gravis, MS, degenerative diseases of the nervous system, systemic lupus erythematosus, and occult neoplastic disorders.

Hypochondriasis is differentiated from somatization disorder by the emphasis in hypochondriasis on fear of having a disease and emphasis in somatization disorder on concern about many symptoms. Patients with hypochondriasis usually complain about fewer symptoms than patients with somatization disorder. Somatization disorder usually has an onset before age 30, whereas hypochondriasis has a less specific age of onset. Patients with somatization disorder are more likely to be women; hypochondriasis is equally distributed among men and women.

Hypochondriasis must also be differentiated from the other somatoform disorders. Conversion disorder is acute and generally transient and usually involves a symptom rather than a particular disease. The presence or absence of la belle indifférence is an unreliable feature with which to differentiate the two conditions. Pain disorder is chronic, as is hypochondriasis, but the symptoms are limited to complaints of pain. Patients with body dysmorphic disorder wish to appear normal, but believe that others notice that they are not, whereas those with hypochondriasis seek out attention for their presumed diseases.

Hypochondriacal symptoms can also occur in patients with depressive disorders and anxiety disorders. If a patient meets the full diagnostic criteria for both hypochondriasis and another major mental disorder, such as major depressive disorder or generalized anxiety disorder, the patient should receive both diagnoses, unless the hypochondriacal symptoms occur only during episodes of the other mental disorder. Patients with panic disorder may initially complain that they are affected by a disease (e.g., heart trouble), but careful questioning during the medical history usually uncovers the classic symptoms of a panic attack. Delusional hypochondriacal beliefs occur in schizophrenia and other psychotic disorders, but can be differentiated from hypochondriasis by their delusional intensity and by the presence of other psychotic symptoms. In addition, schizophrenic patients' somatic delusions tend to be bizarre, idiosyncratic, and out of keeping with their cultural milieus.

Hypochondriasis is distinguished from factitious disorder with physical symptoms and from malingering in that patients with hypochondriasis actually experience and do not simulate the symptoms they report.

Course and Prognosis

The course of hypochondriasis is usually episodic; the episodes last from months to years and are separated by equally long quiescent periods. There may be an obvious association between exacerbations of hypochondriacal symptoms and psychosocial stressors. Although no well-conducted large outcome studies have been reported, an estimated one third to one half of all patients with hypochondriasis eventually improve significantly. A good prognosis is associated with high socioeconomic status, treatment-responsive anxiety or depression, sudden onset of symptoms, the absence of a personality disorder, and the absence of a related nonpsychiatric medical condition. Most children with hypochondriasis recover by late adolescence or early adulthood.

Treatment

Patients with hypochondriasis usually resist psychiatric treatment, although some accept this treatment if it takes place in a medical setting and focuses on stress reduction and education in coping with chronic illness. Group psychotherapy often benefits such patients, in part because it provides the social support and social interaction that seem to reduce their anxiety. Other forms of psychotherapy, such as individual insight-oriented psychotherapy, behavior therapy, cognitive therapy, and hypnosis may be useful.

Frequent, regularly scheduled physical examinations help to reassure patients that their physicians are not abandoning them and that their complaints are being taken seriously. Invasive diagnostic and therapeutic procedures should only be undertaken, however, when objective evidence calls for them. When possible, the clinician should refrain from treating equivocal or incidental physical examination findings.

Pharmacotherapy alleviates hypochondriacal symptoms only when a patient has an underlying drug-responsive condition, such as an anxiety disorder or major depressive disorder. When hypochondriasis is secondary to another primary mental disorder, that disorder must be treated in its own right. When hypochondriasis is a transient situational reaction, clinicians must help patients cope with the stress without reinforcing their illness behavior and their use of the sick role as a solution to their problems.

BODY DYSMORPHIC DISORDER

Body dysmorphic disorder is characterized by a preoccupation with an imagined defect in appearance that causes clinically significant distress or impairment in important areas of functioning. If a slight physical anomaly is actually present, the person's concern with the anomaly is excessive and bothersome.

The disorder was recognized and named *dysmorphophobia* more than 100 years ago by Emil Kraepelin, who considered it a compulsive neurosis; Pierre Janet called it *obsession de la honte du corps* (obsession with shame of the body). Freud wrote about the condition in his description of the Wolf-Man, who was excessively concerned about his nose. Although dysmorphophobia was widely recognized and studied in Europe, it was not until the publication of DSM-III in 1980 that dysmorphophobia, as an example of a typical somatoform disorder, was specifically mentioned in the US diagnostic criteria. In DSM-IV-TR, the condition is known as body dysmorphic disorder, because the DSM editors believed that the term *dysmorphophobia* inaccurately implied the presence of a behavioral pattern of phobic avoidance.

Epidemiology

Body dysmorphic disorder is a poorly studied condition, partly because patients are more likely to go to dermatologists, internists, or plastic surgeons than to psychiatrists. One study of a group of college students found that more than 50 percent had at least some preoccupation with a particular aspect of their appearance, and in about 25 percent of the students, the concern had at least some significant effect on their feelings and functioning.

Available data indicate that the most common age of onset is between 15 and 30 years and that women are affected somewhat more often than men. Affected patients are also likely to be unmarried. Body dysmorphic disorder commonly coexists with other mental disorders. One study found that more than 90 percent of patients with body dysmorphic disorder had experienced a major depressive episode in their lifetimes; about 70 percent had experienced an anxiety disorder; and about 30 percent had experienced a psychotic disorder.

Etiology

The cause of body dysmorphic disorder is unknown. The high comorbidity with depressive disorders, a higher-than-expected family history of mood disorders and obsessive-compulsive disorder (OCD), and the reported responsiveness of the condition to serotonin-specific drugs indicate that, in at least some patients, the pathophysiology of the disorder may involve serotonin and may be related to other mental disorders. Stereotyped concepts of beauty emphasized in certain families and within the culture at large may significantly affect patients with body dysmorphic disorder. In psychodynamic models, body dysmorphic disorder is seen as reflecting the displacement of a sexual or emotional conflict onto a nonrelated body part. Such an association occurs through the defense mechanisms of repression, dissociation, distortion, symbolization, and projection.

Diagnosis

The DSM-IV-TR diagnostic criteria for body dysmorphic disorder stipulate preoccupation with an imagined defect in appearance or overemphasis of a slight defect (Table 17–8). The preoccupation causes patients significant emotional distress or markedly impairs their ability to function in important areas.

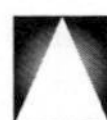

Table 17–8
DSM-IV-TR Diagnostic Criteria for Body Dysmorphic Disorder

A. Preoccupation with an imagined defect in appearance. If a slight physical anomaly is present, the person's concern is markedly excessive.
B. The preoccupation causes clinically significant distress or impairment in social, occupational, or other important areas of functioning.
C. The preoccupation is not better accounted for by another mental disorder (e.g., dissatisfaction with body shape and size in anorexia nervosa).

(From American Psychiatric Association. *Diagnostic and Statistical Manual of Mental Disorders.* 4th ed. Text rev. Washington, DC: American Psychiatric Association; copyright 2000, with permission.)

Clinical Features

The most common concerns (Table 17–9) involve facial flaws, particularly those involving specific parts (e.g., the nose). Sometimes the concern is vague and difficult to understand, such as extreme concern over a "scrunchy" chin. One study found that, on average, patients had concerns about four body regions during

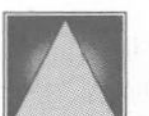

Table 17–9
Location of Imagined Defects in 30 Patients with Body Dysmorphic Disorder[a]

Location	*N*	%
Hair[b]	19	63
Nose	15	50
Skin[c]	15	50
Eyes	8	27
Head, face[d]	6	20
Overall body build, bone structure	6	20
Lips	5	17
Chin	5	17
Stomach, waist	5	17
Teeth	4	13
Legs, knees	4	13
Breasts, pectoral muscles	3	10
Ugly face (general)	3	10
Ears	2	7
Cheeks	2	7
Buttocks	2	7
Penis	2	7
Arms, wrists	2	7
Neck	1	3
Forehead	1	3
Facial muscles	1	3
Shoulders	1	3
Hips	1	3

[a]Total is greater than 100% because most patients had "defects" in more than one location.
[b]Involved head hair in 15 cases, beard growth in 2 cases, and other body hair in 3 cases.
[c]Involved acne in 7 cases, facial lines in 3 cases, and other skin concerns in 7 cases.
[d]Involved concerns with shape in 5 cases and size in 1 case.
(From Phillips KA, McElroy SL, Keck PE Jr, Pope HG, Hudson JL. Body dysmorphic disorder: 30 cases of imagined ugliness. *Am J Psychiatry.* 1993;150:303, with permission.)

the course of the disorder. Other body parts of concern are hair, breasts, and genitalia. A proposed variant of dysmorphic disorder among men is the desire to "bulk up" and develop large muscle mass, which can interfere with ordinary living, holding a job, or staying healthy. The specific body part may change during the time a patient is affected with the disorder. Common associated symptoms include ideas or frank delusions of reference (usually about persons' noticing the alleged body flaw), either excessive mirror checking or avoidance of reflective surfaces, and attempts to hide the presumed deformity (with makeup or clothing). The effects on a person's life can be significant; almost all affected patients avoid social and occupational exposure. As many as one third of the patients may be housebound because of worry about being ridiculed for the alleged deformities, and approximately one fifth attempt suicide. As discussed, comorbid diagnoses of depressive disorders and anxiety disorders are common, and patients may also have traits of OCD, schizoid, and narcissistic personality disorders.

Ms. J, a 30-year-old single unemployed woman, presents to a psychiatrist with this chief complaint: "My biggest wish is to be invisible so that no one can see how ugly I am. My biggest fear is that people are laughing at me thinking I'm ugly." In reality, Ms. J is an attractive woman who has been preoccupied with her supposed ugliness since 12 years of age. At that time, she became "obsessed" with her nose, which she thought was too "big and shiny." Before the onset of this concern, Ms. J had been confident, a good student, and socially active. However, as a result of her fixation on her nose, she became socially withdrawn and was unable to concentrate in school; her grades plummeted from As to Ds and Fs.

When she was 18 years old, Ms. J dropped out of school because of her concern about her nose. Shortly after this, she took a job she disliked and, at that time, also became excessively focused on her minimal acne. She frequently picked at her few "blemishes"—sometimes all night long—with tweezers and needles, a behavior she found difficult to resist. Over the following years, Ms. J developed additional excessive preoccupations with the appearance of her hair, which "wasn't smooth and neat enough;" her breasts, which she thought were too small; her supposedly thin lips; and her supposedly large buttocks. Ms. J thinks about her "defects" nearly all day long and states that "I always have two tapes playing—one saying not to worry and the other saying I'm ugly."

Ms. J frequently checks her supposed defects in mirrors and other reflecting surfaces, such as windows, car bumpers, and spoons. Before she can leave her house, she asks her family members "at least 30 times" whether she looks OK, but she cannot be reassured by their responses. She also combs her hair excessively and attempts to camouflage her supposed defects with clothing, posture, and elaborate makeup that takes several hours a day to apply. Despite her efforts to hide her "ugliness," Ms. J thinks that others are probably taking special notice of her, staring at her. or laughing at her behind her back. She sometimes drives through red lights, because she is "unable to tolerate people looking at me." On one occasion, when she was stuck in a traffic jam, Ms. J became so anxious over her belief that other drivers were staring at her nose, skin, and hair that she fled her car and left it in the middle of the highway.

Ms. J thinks that her view of her appearance and her belief that others are ridiculing her are probably accurate. However, she is able to acknowledge that she has "a small amount of doubt" about her beliefs, noting that it is possible—although unlikely—that she has a distorted view of her defects. Nonetheless, Ms. J occasionally briefly feels "100 percent" convinced that she is hideously ugly and is "completely certain" that others are taking special notice of her, as happened when she abandoned her car. At these times, she firmly believes that the neighbors are staring at her through binoculars, and she hides where she thinks they cannot see her.

As a result of her preoccupation with her appearance, Ms. J has been able to work only briefly and intermittently. She became increasingly socially isolated and avoided dating and other social interactions. As her concern intensified, Ms. J began to go out only at night when she could not be seen. Finally, after more than a decade of symptoms, Ms. J stopped working altogether and went on disability. She also became completely housebound, even hiding when relatives came to visit. As she explains, "I didn't leave my house because I didn't want people to see how ugly I was." Although Ms. J relies on her family members to buy her clothes, food, and other necessities, she is unable to tell them about her concerns about her appearance, because she is too embarrassed. She has become increasingly depressed, with poor sleep, appetite, and energy, and has suicidal ideation. As a result of her social isolation and her feelings of hopelessness about her appearance, Ms. J has made two suicide attempts and has been hospitalized on several occasions.

Before she became housebound, Ms. J received antibiotics from several dermatologists, but this did not alleviate her concerns about her appearance. She was refused a rhinoplasty by a plastic surgeon she consulted. Ms. J also sought outpatient psychiatric treatment but was never able to discuss her preoccupations with her therapist, because she was too embarrassed to do so. (Courtesy of Michael A. Hollifield, M.D.)

Differential Diagnosis

The diagnosis of body dysmorphic disorder should not be made if the excessive bodily preoccupation is better accounted for by another psychiatric disorder. Excessive bodily preoccupation is generally restricted to concerns about being fat in anorexia nervosa, to discomfort with, or a sense of wrongness about, his or her primary and secondary sex characteristics occurring in gender identity disorder, and to mood-congruent cognitions involving appearance that occur exclusively during a major depressive episode. Individuals with avoidant personality disorder or social phobia may worry about being embarrassed by imagined or real defects in appearance, but this concern is usually not prominent, persistent, distressing, or impairing. Taijin kyofu-sho, a diagnosis in Japan, is similar to social phobia but has some features that are more consistent with body dysmorphic disorder, such as the belief that the person has an offensive odor or body parts that are offensive to others. Although individuals with body dysmorphic disorder have obsessional preoccupations about their appearance and may have associated compulsive behaviors (e.g., mirror checking), a separate or additional diagnosis of OCD is made only when the obsessions or compulsions are not restricted to concerns about appearance and are ego-dystonic. An additional diagnosis of delusional disorder, somatic type, can be made in people with body dysmorphic disorder only if their preoccupation with the imagined defect in appearance is held with a delusional intensity. Unlike normal concerns about appearance, the preoccupation with appearance and specific imagined defects in body dysmorphic disorder and the changed behavior because of the preoccupation are excessively time-consuming and are associated with significant distress or impairment.

Course and Prognosis

Body dysmorphic disorder usually begins during adolescence, although it may begin later after a protracted dissatisfaction with the body. Age of onset is not well understood because variably a long delay occurs between symptom onset and treatment seeking. The onset can be gradual or abrupt. The disorder usually has a long and undulating course with few symptom-free intervals. The part of the body on which concern is focused may remain the same or may change over time.

Treatment

Treatment of patients with body dysmorphic disorder with surgical, dermatological, dental, and other medical procedures to address the alleged defects is almost invariably unsuccessful. Although tricyclic drugs, monoamine oxidase inhibitors (MAOIs), and pimozide (Orap) have reportedly been useful in individual cases, other data indicate that serotonin-specific drugs—for example, clomipramine (Anafranil) and fluoxetine (Prozac)—reduce symptoms in at least 50 percent of patients. In any patient with a coexisting mental disorder, such as a depressive disorder or an anxiety disorder, the coexisting disorder should be treated with the appropriate pharmacotherapy and psychotherapy. How long treatment should be continued after the symptoms of body dysmorphic disorder have remitted is unknown. Augmentation of the selective serotonin reuptake inhibitor (SSRI) with clomipramine (Anafranil), buspirone (BuSpar), lithium (Eskalith), methylphenidate (Ritalin), or antipsychotics may improve the response rate.

Relation to Plastic Surgery

Few data exist about the number of patients seeking plastic surgery who have body dysmorphic disorder. One study found that only 2 percent of the patients in a plastic surgery clinic had the diagnosis. The overall percentage may be much higher, however. Surgical requests are varied: removal of facial sags, jowls, wrinkles, or puffiness; rhinoplasty; breast reduction or enhancement; and penile enlargement. Men who request penile enlargements and women who request cosmetic surgery of the labia of the vagina or the lips of the mouth often are suffering from this disorder. Commonly associated with the belief about appearance is an unrealistic expectation of how much surgery will correct the defect. As reality sets in, the person realizes that life's problems are not solved by altering the perceived cosmetic defect. Ideally, such patients will seek out psychotherapy to understand the true nature of their neurotic feelings of inadequacy. Absent that, patients may take out their anger by suing their plastic surgeons—who have one of highest malpractice-suit rates of any specialty—or by developing a clinical depression.

PAIN DISORDER

A pain disorder is characterized by the presence of, and focus on, pain in one or more body sites and is sufficiently severe to come to clinical attention. Psychological factors are necessary in the genesis, severity, or maintenance of the pain, which causes significant distress or impairment, or both. The physician does not have to judge the pain to be "inappropriate" or "in excess of what would be expected." Rather, the phenomenological and diagnostic focus is on the importance of psychological factors and the degree of impairment caused by the pain. The disorder has been called somatoform pain disorder, psychogenic pain disorder, idiopathic pain disorder, and atypical pain disorder.

Epidemiology

The prevalence of pain disorder appears to be common. Recent work indicates that the 6-month and lifetime prevalence is approximately 5 percent and 12 percent, respectively. It has been estimated that 10 to 15 percent of adults in the United States have some form of work disability because of back pain alone in any year. Approximately 3 percent of people in a general practice have persistent pain, with at least 1 day per month of activity restriction because of the pain.

Pain disorder can begin at any age. The gender ratio is unknown. Pain disorder is associated with other psychiatric disorders, especially affective and anxiety disorders. Chronic pain appears to be most frequently associated with depressive disorders, and acute pain appears to be more commonly associated with anxiety disorders. The associated psychiatric disorders may precede the pain disorder, may co-occur with it, or may result from it. Depressive disorders, alcohol dependence, and chronic pain may be more common in relatives of individuals with chronic pain disorder. Individuals whose pain is associated with severe depression and those whose pain is related to a terminal illness, such as cancer, are at increased risk for suicide. Differences may exist in how various ethnic and cultural groups respond to pain, but the usefulness of cultural factors for the clinician remains obscure to the treatment of individuals with pain disorder because of a lack of good data and because of high individual variability.

Etiology

Psychodynamic Factors. Patients who experience bodily aches and pains without identifiable and adequate physical causes may be symbolically expressing an intrapsychic conflict through the body. Patients suffering from alexithymia, who are unable to articulate their internal feeling states in words, express their feelings with their bodies. Other patients may unconsciously regard emotional pain as weak and somehow lacking legitimacy. By displacing the problem to the body, they may feel that they have a legitimate claim to the fulfillment of their dependency needs. The symbolic meaning of body disturbances may also relate to atonement for perceived sin, to expiation of guilt, or to suppressed aggression. Many patients have intractable and unresponsive pain because they are convinced that they deserve to suffer.

Pain can function as a method of obtaining love, a punishment for wrongdoing, and a way of expiating guilt and atoning for an innate sense of badness. Among the defense mechanisms used by patients with pain disorder are displacement, substitution, and repression. Identification plays a part when a patient takes on the role of an ambivalent love object who also has pain, such as a parent.

Behavioral Factors. Pain behaviors are reinforced when rewarded and are inhibited when ignored or punished. For example, moderate pain symptoms may become intense when followed by the solicitous and attentive behavior of others, by monetary gain, or by the successful avoidance of distasteful activities.

Interpersonal Factors. Intractable pain has been conceptualized as a means for manipulation and gaining advantage in interpersonal relationships, for example, to ensure the devotion of a family member or to stabilize a fragile marriage. Such secondary gain is most important to patients with pain disorder.

Biological Factors. The cerebral cortex can inhibit the firing of afferent pain fibers. Serotonin is probably the main neurotransmitter in the descending inhibitory pathways, and endorphins also play a role in the central nervous system modulation of pain. Endorphin deficiency seems to correlate with augmentation of incoming sensory stimuli. Some patients may have pain disorder, rather than another mental disorder, because of sensory and limbic structural or chemical abnormalities that predispose them to experience pain.

Diagnosis

The DSM-IV-TR diagnostic criteria for pain disorder require the presence of clinically significant complaints of pain (Table 17–10). The complaints of pain must be judged to be significantly affected by psychological factors, and the symptoms must result in a patient's significant emotional distress or functional impairment (e.g., social or occupational). DSM-IV-TR requires that the pain disorder be associated primarily with psychological factors or with both psychological factors and a general medical condition. DSM-IV-TR further specifies that pain disorder associated solely with a general medical condition be diagnosed as an Axis III condition; it also allows clinicians to specify whether the pain disorder is acute or chronic, depending on whether the duration of symptoms has been 6 months or more.

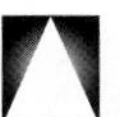

Table 17–10
DSM-IV-TR Diagnostic Criteria for Pain Disorder

A. Pain in one or more anatomical sites is the predominant focus of the clinical presentation and is of sufficient severity to warrant clinical attention.
B. The pain causes clinically significant distress or impairment in social, occupational, or other important areas of functioning.
C. Psychological factors are judged to have an important role in the onset, severity, exacerbation, or maintenance of the pain.
D. The symptom or deficit is not intentionally produced or feigned (as in factitious disorder or malingering).
E. The pain is not better accounted for by a mood, anxiety, or psychotic disorder and does not meet criteria for dyspareunia.

Code as follows:

Pain disorder associated with psychological factors: psychological factors are judged to have the major role in the onset, severity, exacerbation, or maintenance of the pain. (If a general medical condition is present, it does not have a major role in the onset, severity, exacerbation, or maintenance of the pain.) This type of pain disorder is not diagnosed if criteria are also met for somatization disorder.

Specify if:
Acute: duration of less than 6 months
Chronic: duration of 6 months or longer

Pain disorder associated with both psychological factors and a general medical condition: both psychological factors and a general medical condition are judged to have important roles in the onset, severity, exacerbation, or maintenance of the pain. The associated general medical condition or anatomical site of the pain (see below) is coded on Axis III.

Specify if:
Acute: duration of less than 6 months
Chronic: duration of 6 months or longer

Note: The following is not considered to be a mental disorder and is included here to facilitate differential diagnosis.

Pain disorder associated with a general medical condition: a general medical condition has a major role in the onset, severity, exacerbation, or maintenance of the pain. (If psychological factors are present, they are not judged to have a major role in the onset, severity, exacerbation, or maintenance of the pain.) The diagnostic code for the pain is selected based on the associated general medical condition if one has been established or on the anatomical location of the pain if the underlying general medical condition is not yet clearly established—for example, low back, sciatic, pelvic, headache, facial, chest, joint, bone, abdominal, breast, renal, ear, eye, throat, tooth, and urinary.

(From American Psychiatric Association. *Diagnostic and Statistical Manual of Mental Disorders.* 4th ed. Text rev. Washington, DC: American Psychiatric Association; copyright 2000, with permission.)

Clinical Features

Patients with pain disorder are not a uniform group, but a heterogeneous collection of persons with low back pain, headache, atypical facial pain, chronic pelvic pain, and other kinds of pain. A patient's pain may be posttraumatic, neuropathic, neurological, iatrogenic, or musculoskeletal; to meet a diagnosis of pain disorder, however, the disorder must have a psychological factor judged to be significantly involved in the pain symptoms and their ramifications.

Patients with pain disorder often have long histories of medical and surgical care. They visit many physicians, request many medications, and may be especially insistent in their desire for surgery. Indeed, they can be completely preoccupied with their pain and cite it as the source of all their misery. Such patients often deny any other sources of emotional dysphoria and insist that their lives are blissful except for their pain. Their clinical picture can be complicated by substance-related disorders, because these patients attempt to reduce the pain through the use of alcohol and other substances.

At least one study has correlated the number of pain symptoms to the likelihood and severity of symptoms of somatization disorder, depressive disorders, and anxiety disorders. Major depressive disorder is present in about 25 to 50 percent of patients with pain disorder, and dysthymic disorder or depressive disorder symptoms are reported in 60 to 100 percent of the patients. Some investigators believe that chronic pain is almost always a variant of a depressive disorder, a masked or somatized form ofdepression. The most prominent depressive symptoms in patients with pain disorder are anergia, anhedonia, decreased libido, insomnia, and irritability; diurnal variation, weight loss, and psychomotor retardation appear to be less common.

A 36-year-old London meter maid was referred for psychiatric examination by her solicitor. Six months previously, moments after she had written a ticket and placed it on the windshield of an illegally parked car, a man came dashing out of a barbershop, ran up to her, swearing and shaking his fist, swung, and hit her in the jaw with enough force to knock her down. A fellow worker came to her aid and summoned the police, who caught the man a few blocks away and placed him under arrest.

The patient was taken to the hospital, where a hairline fracture of the jaw was diagnosed by X-ray. The fracture did not require that her jaw be wired, but the patient was placed on a soft diet for 4 weeks. Several different physicians, including her own, found her physically fit to return to work after 1 month. The patient, however, complained of severe pain and muscle tension in her neck and back that virtually immobilized her. She spent most of her days sitting in a chair or lying on a bedboard on her bed. She enlisted the services of a solicitor as the Workman's Compensation Board was cutting off her payments and her employer was threatening her with suspension if she did not return to work.

The patient shuffled slowly and laboriously into the psychiatrist's office and lowered herself with great care into a chair. She was attractively dressed and well made up and wore a neck brace. She related the story with vivid detail and considerable anger directed at her assailant (whom she repeatedly referred to as "that bloody foreigner"), her employer, and the compensation board. It was as if the incident had occurred yesterday. Regarding her ability to work, she said that she wanted to return to the job and would soon be severely strapped financially, but was physically not up to even the lightest office work.

She denied any previous psychological problems and initially described her childhood and family life as storybook perfect. In subsequent interviews, however, she admitted that as a child, she had frequently been beaten by her alcoholic father and had once had a broken arm as a result, and that she had often been locked in a closet for hours at a time as punishment for misbehavior. (Courtesy of *DSM-IV-TR Casebook.*)

Differential Diagnosis

Purely physical pain can be difficult to distinguish from purely psychogenic pain, especially because the two are not mutually exclusive. Physical pain fluctuates in intensity and is highly sensitive to emotional, cognitive, attentional, and situational influences. Pain that does not vary and is insensitive to any of these factors is likely to be psychogenic. When pain does not wax and wane and is not even temporarily relieved by distraction or analgesics, clinicians can suspect an important psychogenic component.

Pain disorder must be distinguished from other somatoform disorders, although some somatoform disorders can coexist. Patients with hypochondriacal preoccupations may complain of pain, and aspects of the clinical presentation of hypochondriasis, such as bodily preoccupation and disease conviction, can also be present in patients with pain disorder. Patients with hypochondriasis tend to have many more symptoms than patients with pain disorder, and their symptoms tend to fluctuate more than those of patients with pain disorder. Conversion disorder is generally short-lived, whereas pain disorder is chronic. In addition, pain is, by definition, not a symptom in conversion disorder. Malingering patients consciously provide false reports, and their complaints are usually connected to clearly recognizable goals.

The differential diagnosis can be difficult because patients with pain disorder often receive disability compensation or a litigation award. Muscle contraction (tension) headaches, for example, have a pathophysiological mechanism to account for the pain and so are not diagnosed as pain disorder. Patients with pain disorder are not pretending to be in pain, however. As in all of the somatoform disorders, symptoms are not imaginary.

Course and Prognosis

The pain in pain disorder generally begins abruptly and increases in severity for a few weeks or months. The prognosis varies, although pain disorder can often be chronic, distressful, and completely disabling. Acute pain disorders have a more favorable prognosis than chronic pain disorders. A wide range of variability is seen in the onset and course of chronic pain disorder. In many cases, the pain has been present for many years by the time the individual comes to psychiatric care, owing to the reluctance of patient and physician to see pain as a psychiatric disorder. People with pain disorder who resume participation in regularly scheduled activities, despite the pain, have a more favorable prognosis than people who allow the pain to become the determining factor in their lifestyle.

Treatment

Because it may not be possible to reduce the pain, the treatment approach must address rehabilitation. Clinicians should discuss the issue of psychological factors early in treatment and should frankly tell patients that such factors are important in the cause and consequences of both physical and psychogenic pain. Therapists should also explain how various brain circuits that are involved with emotions (e.g., the limbic system) can influence the sensory pain pathways. For example, persons who hit their head while happy at a party can seem to experience less pain than when they hit their head while angry and at work. Nevertheless, therapists must fully understand that the patient's experiences of pain are real.

Pharmacotherapy. Analgesic medications do not generally benefit most patients with pain disorder. In addition, substance abuse and dependence are often major problems for such patients who receive long-term analgesic treatment. Sedatives and antianxiety agents are not especially beneficial and are also subject to abuse, misuse, and adverse effects.

Antidepressants, such as tricyclics and SSRIs, are the most effective pharmacological agents. Whether antidepressants reduce pain through their antidepressant action or exert an independent, direct analgesic effect (possibly by stimulating efferent inhibitory pain pathways) remains controversial. The success of SSRIs supports the hypothesis that serotonin is important in the pathophysiology of the disorder. Amphetamine, which has analgesic effects, may benefit some patients, especially when used as an adjunct to SSRIs, but dosages must be monitored carefully.

Psychotherapy. Some outcome data indicate that psychodynamic psychotherapy benefits patients with pain disorder. The first step in psychotherapy is to develop a solid therapeutic alliance by empathizing with the patient's suffering. Clinicians should not confront somatizing patients with comments such as "This is all in your head." For the patient, the pain is real, and clinicians must acknowledge the reality of the pain, even as they understand that it is largely intrapsychic in origin. A useful entry point into the emotional aspects of the pain is to examine its interpersonal ramifications in the patient's life. In marital therapy, for example, the psychotherapist may soon get to the source of the patient's psychological pain and the function of the physical complaints in significant relationships. Cognitive therapy has been used to alter negative thoughts and to foster a positive attitude.

Other Therapies. Biofeedback can be helpful in the treatment of pain disorder, particularly with migraine pain, myofacial pain, and muscle tension states, such as tension headaches. Hypnosis, transcutaneous nerve stimulation, and dorsal column stimulation also have been used. Nerve blocks and surgical ablative procedures are effective for some patients with pain disorder; but these procedures must be repeated, because the pain returns after 6 to 18 months.

Pain Control Programs. Sometimes it may be necessary to remove patients from their usual settings and place them in a comprehensive inpatient or outpatient pain control program or clinic. Multidisciplinary pain units use many modalities, such as cognitive, behavior, and group therapies. They provide extensive physical conditioning through physical therapy and exercise and offer vocational evaluation and rehabilitation. Concurrent mental disorders are diagnosed and treated, and patients who are dependent on analgesics and hypnotics are detoxified. Inpatient multimodal treatment programs generally report encouraging results.

UNDIFFERENTIATED SOMATOFORM DISORDER

Undifferentiated somatoform disorder is characterized by one or more unexplained physical symptoms of at least 6 months' duration, which are below the threshold for a diagnosis of somatization disorder (Table 17–11). These symptoms are not caused, or fully explained, by another medical, psychiatric, or substance abuse disorder, and they cause clinically significant distress or impairment.

Two types of symptom patterns may be seen in patients with undifferentiated somatoform disorder: those involving the autonomic nervous system and those involving sensations of fatigue or weakness. In what is sometimes referred to as *autonomic arousal disorder*, some patients are affected with somatoform disorder symptoms that are limited to bodily functions innervated by the autonomic nervous system. Such patients have complaints involving the cardiovascular, respiratory, gastrointestinal, urogenital, and dermatological systems. Other patients complain of mental and physical fatigue, physical weakness and exhaustion, and inability to perform many everyday activities because of their symptoms. Some clinicians believe this syndrome is neurasthenia, a diagnosis used primarily in Europe and Asia. The syndrome may overlap chronic fatigue syndrome, which various research reports have hypothesized to involve psychiatric, virological, and immunological factors. (See Chapter 18, which discusses chronic fatigue syndrome and neurasthenia in depth.)

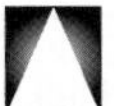

Table 17–11
DSM-IV-TR Diagnostic Criteria for Undifferentiated Somatoform Disorder

A. One or more physical complaints (e.g., fatigue, loss of appetite, gastrointestinal or urinary complaints).
B. Either (1) or (2):
   (1) after appropriate investigation, the symptoms cannot be fully explained by a known general medical condition or the direct effects of a substance (e.g., a drug of abuse, a medication)
   (2) when there is a related general medical condition, the physical complaints or resulting social or occupational impairment is in excess of what would be expected from the history, physical examination, or laboratory findings
C. The symptoms cause clinically significant distress or impairment in social, occupational, or other important areas of functioning.
D. The duration of the disturbance is at least 6 months.
E. The disturbance is not better accounted for by another mental disorder (e.g., another somatoform disorder, sexual dysfunction, mood disorder, anxiety disorder, sleep disorder, or psychotic disorder).
F. The symptom is not intentionally produced or feigned (as in factitious disorder or malingering).

(From American Psychiatric Association. *Diagnostic and Statistical Manual of Mental Disorders.* 4th ed. Text rev. Washington, DC: American Psychiatric Association; copyright 2000, with permission.)

Somatoform Disorder Not Otherwise Specified

The DSM-IV-TR diagnostic category of somatoform disorder not otherwise specified (Table 17–12) is a residual category for patients who have symptoms suggesting a somatoform disorder, but do not meet the specific diagnostic criteria for other somatoform disorders. Such patients may have a symptom not covered in the other somatoform disorders (e.g., pseudocyesis) or

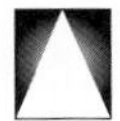

Table 17–12
DSM-IV-TR Diagnostic Criteria for Somatoform Disorder Not Otherwise Specified

This category includes disorders with somatoform symptoms that do not meet the criteria for any specific somatoform disorder. Examples include

1. Pseudocyesis: a false belief of being pregnant that is associated with objective signs of pregnancy, which may include abdominal enlargement (although the umbilicus does not become everted), reduced menstrual flow, amenorrhea, subjective sensation of fetal movement, nausea, breast engorgement and secretions, and labor pains at the expected date of delivery. Endocrine changes may be present, but the syndrome cannot be explained by a general medical condition that causes endocrine changes (e.g., a hormone-secreting tumor).
2. A disorder involving nonpsychotic hypochondriacal symptoms of less than 6 months' duration.
3. A disorder involving unexplained physical complaints (e.g., fatigue or body weakness) of less than 6 months' duration that are not due to another mental disorder.

(From American Psychiatric Association. *Diagnostic and Statistical Manual of Mental Disorders.* 4th ed. Text rev. Washington, DC: American Psychiatric Association; copyright 2000, with permission.)

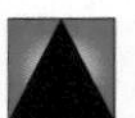

Table 17–13
ICD-10 Diagnostic Criteria for Somatoform Disorders

Somatization disorder

A. There must be a history of at least 2 years' complaints of multiple and variable physical symptoms that cannot be explained by any detectable physical disorders. (Any physical disorders that are known to be present do not explain the severity, extent, variety, and persistence of the physical complaints, or the associated social disability.) If some symptoms clearly due to autonomic arousal are present, they are not a major feature of the disorder in that they are not particularly persistent or distressing.

B. Preoccupation with the symptoms causes persistent distress and leads the patient to seek repeated (three or more) consultations or sets of investigations with either primary care or specialist doctors. In the absence of medical services within either the financial or physical reach of the patient, there must be persistent self-medication or multiple consultations with local healers.

C. There is persistent refusal to accept medical reassurance that there is no adequate physical cause for the physical symptoms. (Short-term acceptance of such reassurance, i.e., for a few weeks during or immediately after investigations, does not exclude this diagnosis.)

D. There must be a total of six or more symptoms from the following list, with symptoms occurring in at least two separate groups:

Gastrointestinal symptoms
(1) abdominal pain;
(2) nausea;
(3) feeling bloated or full of gas;
(4) bad taste in mouth, or excessively coated tongue;
(5) complaints of vomiting or regurgitation of food;
(6) complaints of frequent and loose bowel motions or discharge of fluids from anus;

Cardiovascular symptoms
(7) breathlessness without exertion;
(8) chest pains;

Genitourinary symptoms
(9) dysuria or complaints of frequency of micturition;
(10) unpleasant sensations in or around the genitals;
(11) complaints of unusual or copious vaginal discharge;

Skin and pain symptoms
(12) blotchiness or discoloration of the skin;
(13) pain in the limbs, extremities, or joints;
(14) unpleasant numbness or tingling sensations.

E. *Most commonly used exclusion clause.* Symptoms do not occur only during any of the schizophrenic or related disorders, any of the mood [affective] disorders, or panic disorder.

Undifferentiated somatoform disorder

A. Criteria A, C, and E for somatization disorder are met, except that the duration of the disorder is at least 6 months.

B. One or both of Criteria B and D for somatization disorder are incompletely fulfilled.

Hypochondriacal disorder

A. Either of the following must be present:
(1) a persistent belief, of at least 5 months' duration, of the presence of a maximum of two serious physical diseases (of which at least one must be specifically named by the patient);
(2) a persistent preoccupation with a presumed deformity or disfigurement (body dysmorphic disorder).

B. Preoccupation with the belief and the symptoms cause persistent distress or interference with personal functioning in daily living and leads the patient to seek medical treatment or investigations (or equivalent help from local healers).

C. There is persistent refusal to accept medical reassurance that there is no physical cause for the symptoms or physical abnormality. (Short-term acceptance of such reassurance, i.e., for a few weeks during or immediately after investigations, does not exclude this diagnosis.)

D. *Most commonly used exclusion clause.* The symptoms do not occur only during any of the schizophrenic and related disorders or any of the mood [affective] disorders.

Somatoform autonomic dysfunction

A. There must be symptoms of autonomic arousal that are attributed by the patient to a physical disorder of one or more of the following systems or organs:
(1) heart and cardiovascular system;
(2) upper gastrointestinal tract (esophagus and stomach);
(3) lower gastrointestinal tract;
(4) respiratory system;
(5) genitourinary system.

B. Two or more of the following autonomic symptoms must be present:
(1) palpitations;
(2) sweating (hot or cold);
(3) dry mouth;
(4) flushing or blushing;
(5) epigastric discomfort, "butterflies," or churning in the stomach.

C. One or more of the following symptoms must be present:
(1) chest pains or discomfort in and around the precordium;
(2) dyspnea or hyperventilation;
(3) excessive tiredness on mild exertion;
(4) aerophagy, hiccough, or burning sensations in chest or epigastrium;
(5) reported frequent bowel movements;
(6) increased frequency of micturition or dysuria;
(7) feeling of being bloated, distended, or heavy.

D. There is no evidence of a disturbance of structure or function in the organs or systems about which the patient is concerned.

E. *Most commonly used exclusion clause.* These symptoms do not occur only in the presence of phobic disorders or panic disorder.

A fifth character is to be used to classify the individual disorders in this group, indicating the organ or system regarded by the patient as the origin of the symptoms:

Heart and cardiovascular system
Includes: cardiac neurosis, neurocirculatory asthenia, da Costa's syndrome.

Upper gastrointestinal tract
Includes: psychogenic aerophagy, hiccough, gastric neurosis.

Lower gastrointestinal tract
Includes: psychogenic irritable bowel syndrome, psychogenic diarrhea, gas syndrome.

Respiratory system
Includes: hyperventilation.

Genitourinary system
Includes: psychogenic increase of frequency of micturition and dysuria.

Other organ or system

Persistent somatoform pain disorder

A. There is persistent severe and distressing pain (for at least 6 months, and continuously on most days), in any part of the body, which cannot be explained adequately by evidence of a physiological process or a physical disorder and which is consistently the main focus of the patient's attention.

B. *Most commonly used exclusion clause.* This disorder does not occur in the presence of schizophrenia or related disorders, or only during any of the mood [affective] disorders, somatization disorder, undifferentiated somatoform disorder, or hypochondriacal disorder.

Other somatoform disorders

In these disorders the presenting complaints are not mediated through the autonomic nervous system, and are limited to specific systems or parts of the body, such as the skin. This is in contrast to the multiple and often changing complaints of the origin of symptoms and distress found in somatization disorder and undifferentiated somatoform disorder. Tissue damage is not involved. Any other disorder of sensation not due to physical disorder, which are closely associated in time with stressful events or problems, or which result in significantly increased attention for the patient, either personal or medical, should also be classified here.

Somatoform disorder, unspecified

(From World Health Organization. *The ICD 10 Classification of Mental and Behavioural Disorders: Diagnostic Criteria for Research*. Copyright, World Health Organization, Geneva, 1993, with permission.)

may not have met the 6-month criterion of the other somatoform disorders.

ICD-10

In the 10th revision of *International Statistical Classification of Diseases and Related Health Problems* (ICD-10), somatoform disorders are described as a "repeated presentation of physical symptoms, together with persistent requests for medical investigation," although patients have been reassured by their physicians that the symptoms have no physical basis. If physical disorders are present, they cannot account for patients' symptoms or for their distress (Table 17–13).

This nosology overlaps with DSM-IV-TR classification, yet important differences are apparent from the criteria. The DSM-IV-TR has conversion disorder and body dysmorphic disorder in its classification, whereas the ICD-10 does not, but instead specifies somatoform autonomic dysfunction and other somatoform disorders. In the ICD-10, conversion is classified as a dissociative disorder, and somatoform autonomic dysfunction is similar to the symptoms associated with anxiety and depressive disorders in the DSM-IV-TR. In the ICD-10, body dysmorphic disorder is subsumed under hypochondriacal disorder.

References

Brown RJ, Schrag A, Trimble MR. Dissociation, childhood interpersonal trauma, and family functioning in patients with somatization disorder. *Am J Psychiatry*. 2005;162:899–905.

Grabe HJ, Meyer C, Hapke U, Rumpf HJ, Freyberger HJ, Dilling H, John U. Specific somatoform disorder in the general population. *Psychosomatics*. 2003;44:304.

Guggenheim FG. Somatoform disorders. In: Sadock BJ, Sadock VA, eds. *Kaplan & Sadock's Comprehensive Textbook of Psychiatry*. 7th ed. Vol. 1. Baltimore: Lippincott William & Wilkins; 2000:1504.

Guz H, Doganay Z, Ozkan A, Colak E, Tomac A, Sarisoy G. Conversion and somatization disorders: Dissociative symptoms and other characteristics. *J Psychosom Res*. 2004;56:287–291.

Hollifield MA. Somatoform disorders. In: Sadock BJ, Sadock VA, eds. *Kaplan & Sadock's Comprehensive Textbook of Psychiatry*. 8th ed. Vol. 1. Baltimore: Lippincott William & Wilkins; 2005:1800.

Mayou R, Kirmayer LJ, Simon G, Kroenke K, Sharpe M. Somatoform disorders: Time for a new approach in DSM-V. *Am J Psychiatry*. 2005;162(5):847–855.

Noyes R Jr, Stuart SP, Langbehn DR, Happel RL, Longley SL, Muller BA, Yagla SJ. Test of an interpersonal model of hypochondriasis. *Psychosom Med*. 2003;65:292.

Sansone RA, Pole M, Dakroub H, Butler M. Childhood trauma, borderline personality symptomatology, and psychophysiological and pain disorders in adulthood. *Psychosomatics: Journal of Consultation Liaison Psychiatry*. 2006;47: 158–162.

Stone J, Smyth R, Carson A, Lewis S, Prescott R, Warlow C, Sharpe M. Systematic review of misdiagnosis of conversion symptoms and "hysteria". *BMJ*. 2005; 331(7523):989.

Tezcan E, Atmaca M, Kuloglu M, Gecici O, Buyukbayram A, Tutkun H. Dissociative disorders in Turkish inpatients with conversion disorder. *Comp Psychiatry*. 2003;44:324.

18 Chronic Fatigue Syndrome

CHRONIC FATIGUE SYNDROME

Chronic fatigue syndrome (CFS) (referred to as *myalgic encephalomyelitis* in the United Kingdom and Canada) is characterized by 6 months or more of severe, debilitating fatigue, often accompanied by myalgia, headaches, pharyngitis, low-grade fever, cognitive complaints, gastrointestinal symptoms, and tender lymph nodes. The search continues for an infectious cause of chronic fatigue because of the high percentage of patients who report abrupt onset after a severe flu-like illness.

In 1988, the US Centers for Disease Control and Prevention (CDC) defined specific diagnostic criteria for chronic fatigue syndrome. Since then, the disorder has captured the attention of both the medical profession and the general public. The disorder is classified in the 10th revision of *International Statistical Classification of Diseases and Related Health Problems* (ICD-10) as an ill-defined condition of unknown etiology under the heading "Malaise and Fatigue" and is subdivided into asthenia and unspecified disability.

Epidemiology

The exact incidence and prevalence of chronic fatigue syndrome are unknown, but the incidence ranges from 0.007 percent to 2.8 percent in the general adult population. The illness is observed primarily in young adults (ages 20 to 40). Chronic fatigue syndrome also occurs in children and adolescents but at a lower rate. Women are at least twice as likely as men to be affected.

In the United States, studies show that about 25 percent of the general adult population experiences fatigue lasting 2 weeks or longer. When the fatigue persists beyond 6 months, it is defined as chronic fatigue. The symptoms of chronic fatigue often coexist with other illnesses, such as fibromyalgia, irritable bowel syndrome, and temporomandibular joint disorder.

Etiology

The cause of the disorder is unknown. The diagnosis can be made only after all other medical and psychiatric causes of chronic fatiguing illness have been excluded. Scientific studies have validated no pathognomonic signs or diagnostic tests for this condition.

Investigators have tried to implicate the Epstein-Barr virus (EBV) as the etiological agent in chronic fatigue syndrome. EBV infection, however, is associated with specific antibodies and atypical lymphocytosis, which are absent in chronic fatigue syndrome. Results of tests for other viral agents, such as enteroviruses, herpesvirus, and retroviruses, have been negative. Some investigators have found nonspecific markers of immune abnormalities in patients with chronic fatigue syndrome; for example, reduced proliferation responses of peripheral blood lymphocytes, but these responses are similar to those detected in some patients with major depression.

Several reports have shown of disruption in the hypothalamic-pituitary-axis (HPA) in patients with chronic fatigue syndrome, with mild hypocortisolism. Because of this, exogenous cortisol has been used to reduce fatigue but with equivocal results.

Chronic fatigue syndrome may be familial. In one study, the correlation within twin pairs for monozygotic twins was more than 2.5 times greater than the correlation for dizygotic twins. Further studies are needed, however.

Diagnosis and Clinical Features

Because chronic fatigue syndrome has no pathognomonic features, diagnosis is difficult. Physicians should attempt to delineate as many signs and symptoms as possible to facilitate the process. Although chronic fatigue is the most common complaint, most patients have many other symptoms (Table 18–1). As a patient's history unfolds, clinicians are likely to think of a variety of disease states that fall within the range of neurological, metabolic, or psychiatric disorders to account for the patient's distress. In most cases, however, no picture of any disorder clearly emerges from history taking alone.

The physical examination is also an unreliable source of diagnostic certainty. In addition to chronic fatigue, for example, patients may complain of feeling warm or having chills with normal body temperature, and others may complain of lymph node tenderness in the absence of node enlargement. These and other equivocal findings neither confirm nor rule out the disorder.

The CDC diagnostic criteria for chronic fatigue syndrome, which are listed in Table 18–2, include fatigue for at least 6 months, impaired memory or concentration, sore throat, tender or enlarged lymph nodes, muscle pain, arthralgias, headache, sleep disturbance, and postexertional malaise. Fatigue, the most obvious symptom, is characterized by severe mental and physical exhaustion, sufficient to cause a 50 percent reduction in patients' activities. The onset is usually gradual, but some patients have an acute onset that resembles a flu-like illness.

In some cases, a noticeable correlation exists between CFS and neuearlly mediated hypotension, an autonomic nervous system dysfunction. It has been suggested that patients presenting with CFS symptoms undergo a tilt-table test to delineate

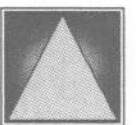

Table 18–1
Signs and Symptoms Reported by Patients with Chronic Fatigue Syndrome

Fatigue or exhaustion	Double vision
Headache	Sensitivity to bright lights
Malaise	Numbness and/or tingling in extremities
Short-term memory loss	
Muscle pain	Fainting spells
Difficulty concentrating	Light-headedness
Joint pain	Dizziness
Depression	Clumsiness
Abdominal pain	Insomnia
Lymph node pain	Fever or sensation of fever
Sore throat	Chills
Lack of restful sleep	Night sweats
Muscle weakness	Weight gain
Bitter or metallic taste	Allergies
Balance disturbance	Chemical sensitivities
Diarrhea	Palpitations
Constipation	Shortness of breath
Bloating	Flushing rash of the face and cheeks
Panic attacks	Swelling of the extremities or eyelids
Eye pain	Burning on urination
Scratchiness in eyes	Sexual dysfunction
Blurring of vision	Hair loss

(Adapted from Bell DS. *The Doctor's Guide to Chronic Fatigue Syndrome: Understanding, Treating, and Living with CFIDS*. Reading: Addison-Wesley; 1995:10, with permission.)

symptoms attributable to hypotension so that they may be placed on appropriate pharmacotherapy.

The following case illustrates many of the uncertainties and difficulties involved in diagnosis and treatment.

Ms. J was a 35-year-old single white librarian with a benign medical past and no psychiatric symptoms prior to developing a flu-like illness. After 10 days, the acute episode passed, but she continued to feel lethargic and fatigued readily. Two weeks after the onset of this illness, she returned to work but was unable to complete her usual 8-hour days because of increasing exhaustion and newly developed, gradually evolving, diffuse muscle and joint pain.

Her primary care physician suggested naproxen (Naprosyn) and encouraged her while counseling patience. The physician noted nothing unusual about her mood, and prescribed hypnotic agents to improve her sleep. There was no improvement, however, from 10 mg of zolpidem (Ambien). She then started having squeezing bi-temporal headaches. After 3 months, she was referred to a rheumatologist who tried to give her amitriptyline (Elavil) 50 mg at night. She protested vehemently, saying that she was not depressed, just in pain.

Previously, she had been a conscientious employee and had rarely taken leave or missed work because of illness. After 3 months of this illness, however, she was forced to take a leave of absence, returning to live with her mother, because she no longer had any income. She continued to "hurt all over," was lethargic and irritable, and slept poorly because of pain. When she slept, she reported that she no longer awoke refreshed.

Six months after the onset of her original symptoms, she self-referred to an academic health center's rheumatology clinic, where she presented as an afebrile and otherwise healthy woman who was angry about her protracted illness and her living situation. She admitted to difficulty with concentration. Joint examination revealed full range of motion with no red, hot, or swollen joints; tender points were present at all 18 sites.

Her rheumatologist prescribed amitriptyline 25 mg at night for 4 days and then told her to increase the dose by one tablet until she achieved better sleep or reached a dosage of 150 mg. Still protesting that she was not depressed, she took the antidepressant medication because she was desperate for relief. A month later she returned to the rheumatology clinic, still hostile and impatient, with little change, and she was then prescribed 20 mg of fluoxetine (Prozac) in the morning in addition to the amitriptyline at night.

Within a month of this regimen, she was somewhat improved in her mood, sleep, and joint symptoms. However, she still continues to have episodes of fatigue, usually related to stressful life events. She had not yet returned to the work force. (Courtesy of Brian Anthony Fallan, M.D.)

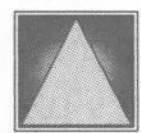

Table 18–2
Centers for Disease Control and Prevention (CDC) Criteria for Chronic Fatigue Syndrome

A. Severe unexplained fatigue for over 6 months that is:
 (1) of a new or definite onset
 (2) not due to continuing exertion
 (3) not resolved by rest
 (4) functionally impairing

B. The presence of four or more of the following new symptoms:
 (1) impaired memory or concentration
 (2) sore throat
 (3) tender lymph nodes
 (4) muscle pain
 (5) pain in several joints
 (6) new pattern of headaches
 (7) unrefreshing sleep
 (8) postexertional malaise lasting more than 24 hours

Differential Diagnosis

Chronic fatigue must be differentiated from endocrine disorders (e.g., hypothyroidism), neurological disorders (e.g., multiple sclerosis [MS]), infectious disorders (e.g., acquired immune deficiency syndrome [AIDS], infectious mononucleosis), and psychiatric disorders (e.g., depressive disorders). The evaluation process is complex, and a diagnostic scheme is listed in Table 18–3.

Up to 80 percent of patients with chronic fatigue syndrome meet the diagnostic criteria for major depression. The correlation is so high that many psychiatrists believe that all cases of this syndrome are depressive disorders, yet patients with chronic fatigue syndrome rarely report feelings of guilt, suicidal ideation, or anhedonia and show little or no weight loss. Also, usually no family history of depression or other genetic loading for psychiatric disorder is found and few, if any, stressful events have occurred in patients' lives that might precipitate or account for a depressive illness. In addition, although some patients respond to antidepressant medication, many eventually become refractory to all psychopharmacological agents. Regardless of diagnostic labeling, however, depressive comorbidity requires treatment with either antidepressants, cognitive-behavioral therapy, or a combination of both.

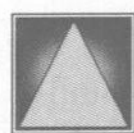

Table 18–3
Approach to the Assessment of Persistent Fatigue

History

- Record the medical and psychosocial circumstances at onset of symptoms.
- Assess previous physical and psychological health.
- Seek clues to underlying medical disorder (e.g., fevers, weight loss, dyspnea).
- Assess the impact of the symptoms on the patient's lifestyle.

Characteristic symptoms of chronic fatigue syndrome (CFS) include fatigue, myalgia, arthralgia, impaired memory and concentration, and unrefreshing sleep.

↓

Physical examination

- Seek abnormalities to suggest an underlying medical disorder:
  - Hypothyroidism
  - Chronic hepatitis
  - Chronic anemia
  - Neuromuscular disease
  - Sleep apnea syndrome
  - Occult malignancy, etc.

The physical examination in patients with CFS characteristically shows no abnormalities.

↓

Mental state examination

- Past or family history of psychiatric disorder, notably depression, anxiety
- Past history of frequent episodes of medically unexplained symptoms
- Past history of alcohol or substance abuse
- Current symptoms: depression, anxiety, self-destructive thoughts, and use of over-the-counter medications
- Current signs of psychomotor retardation
- Evaluate psychosocial support system

CFS patients have depressive symptoms, but not guilt, suicidal ideation, or observable psychomotor slowing.

↓

Laboratory investigation

- Screening tests:
  - Urinalysis
  - Blood count and differential
  - Erythrocyte sedimentation rate
  - Renal function tests
  - Liver function tests
  - Calcium, phosphate
  - Random blood glucose
  - Thyroid function tests (including thyroid stimulating hormone level)
- Additional investigations as clinically indicated (e.g., sleep study)

The diagnosis of CFS is primarily one of exclusion of alternative conditions.

↓

Chronic fatigue syndrome

- *Unexplained, persistent, or relapsing chronic fatigue lasting 6 or more consecutive months* that is of new or definite onset; is not the result of ongoing exertion; in not substantially relieved by rest; and results in substantial reduction in previous levels of occupational, educational, social, or personal activities; and

Four more of the following symptoms occurring concurrently: (1) impairment of short-term memory or concentration; (2) sore throat; (3) tender cervical or axillary lymph nodes; (4) muscle pain, or multijoint pain; (5) headaches; (6) unrefreshing sleep; and (7) postexertional malaise.

(From Hickie JB, Lloyd AR, Wakefield D. Chronic fatigue syndrome: Current perspectives on evaluation and management. *Med J Aust.* 1995;163:315, with permission.)

Course and Prognosis

Spontaneous recovery is rare in patients with chronic fatigue syndrome, but improvement does occur. At present, most reports on course and prognosis are based on small samples. In one study, 63 percent of patients with the syndrome, followed for up to 4 years, reported improvement. Patients with the best prognosis have had no previous or concurrent psychiatric illness, are able to maintain social contacts, and continue to work, even at reduced levels.

Treatment

Treatment of chronic fatigue syndrome is mainly supportive. Physicians must first establish rapport and not dismiss patients' complaints as being without foundation. The complaints are not imaginary. A careful medical examination is necessary, and a psychiatric evaluation is indicated, both of which are geared to rule out other causes for the symptoms.

No effective medical treatment is known. Antiviral agents and corticosteroids are not useful, although a few patients have shown a lessening of fatigue with the antiviral drug amantadine (Symmetrel). Symptomatic treatment (e.g., analgesics for arthralgias and muscular pain) is the usual approach, but nonsteroidal anti-inflammatory drugs (NSAIDs) are not effective. Patients must be encouraged to continue their daily activities and to resist their fatigue as much as possible. A reduced workload is far better than absence from work. Several studies have reported a positive effect from graded exercise therapy (GET).

Psychiatric treatment is desirable, especially when depression is present. In many cases, symptoms improve markedly when patients are in psychotherapy. Cognitive-behavioral therapy is especially useful. Therapy is geared to helping patients overcome and correct mistaken beliefs, such as fear that any activity causing fatigue worsens the disorder. Pharmacological agents, especially antidepressants with nonsedating qualities, such as bupropion (Wellbutrin), may be helpful. Nefazodone (Serzone) was reported to decrease pain and improve sleep and

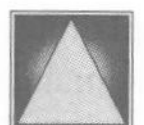

Table 18–4
Recommendations for a Logical Pharmacotherapy of Chronic Fatigue

- Establish a collaborative patient/physician treatment framework.
- Avoid premature diagnostic closure.
- Determine what self-administered, over-the-counter medications the patient is already taking and assess closely for interaction with the proposed medication.
- Discuss the role of medication and identify clear treatment goals:
  Psychiatric syndromes
  Domains of symptomatic distress (e.g., musculoskeletal pain, poor sleep quality, fatigue, subjective cognitive changes, and mood or anxiety symptoms)
- Choice of agent should be based on:
  The predicted side-effect profile
  The patient's preference
  Medical contraindications to the use of a particular medication
- Begin therapy at the lowest possible dose, and increase the dose gradually; observe and discuss side effects during treatment, clarifying issues of significant medical concern.
- Attempt thorough trial to known optimal target dose of drug or until maximum clinical effect is evident.
- Ongoing discussion of the patient's specific response pattern should occur, clarifying the patient's expectations about the treatment.
- Do not continue treatment indefinitely without evidence of clear clinical response; if necessary, discontinue treatment and reassess during medication-free state.
- Avoid polypharmacy; assess treatment response to one agent at a time.
- Frame pharmacotherapy with respect to other aspects of the treatment plan; use medication as setting a context for a multidimensional treatment framework.

(From Demitrack MA. Psychopharmacological principles in the treatment of chronic MA, Abbey SE, eds. *Chronic Fatigue Syndrome.* New York: Guilford; 1996:281, with permission.)

memory in some patients. Analeptics (e.g., amphetamine or methylphenidate [Ritalin]) may help reduce fatigue. Table 18–4 contains recommendations for a general approach to pharmacotherapy.

Self-help groups have helped patients with chronic fatigue syndrome. They derive benefit from the group dynamic of instilling hope, offering identification, sharing experiences, and imparting information. The cohesion of members in such groups also raises self-esteem, which is usually impaired in these patients, who often feel that their physicians are not taking them seriously. For this reason, many persons with the syndrome rely on vitamins, minerals, and miscellaneous herbal products or treatment methods that fall under the rubric of alternative medicine. Neither these nor other unidentified general tonics have been peer reviewed in the medical literature, and they are of little or no benefit.

NEURASTHENIA

The term neurasthenia ("nervous exhaustion") was introduced in the 1860s by the American neuropsychiatrist George Miller Beard, who applied it to a condition characterized by chronic fatigue and disability. This term is not used frequently now, but it does appear in the psychiatric literature, and it remains a diagnostic entity in ICD-10, where it is classified as one of the neurotic disorders. According to current nosology in the United States, the disorder is not considered a distinct diagnosis. The text revision of the fourth edition of *Diagnostic and Statistical Manual of Mental Disorders* (DSM-IV-TR) categorizes neurasthenia as undifferentiated somatoform disorder.

This disorder is a prime example of cultural differences influencing the classification and manifestations of diseases. Neurasthenia is an accepted condition in Europe and Asia, where it is characterized by fatigue, headache, insomnia, and other vague somatic complaints and is thought to result from chronic stress rather than from unconscious psychological conflicts. In many cultures (especially China), in which persons resist being categorized as having a mental disorder, neurasthenia is a preferred diagnosis. Thus, the disorder is most commonly diagnosed in Eastern Asia.

Epidemiology

Difficulties investigating the epidemiology of neurasthenia stem from its occurring in connection with other conditions, such as anxiety, depression, and somatoform disorders, and it has not been studied sufficiently as an independent disorder. Beard considered neurasthenia one of the most frequently observed conditions in 19th century United States, although no statistics were available to support his observation. A 1994 study in Switzerland (using ICD-10 criteria) found a prevalence rate of 12 percent. A World Health Organization (WHO) study found an incidence of about 2 percent, which increased to 6 percent when depressive symptoms were present.

Etiology

According to Beard, the cause of neurasthenia was "nervous exhaustion," which referred to depletion of the "stored nutrient" in the nerve cell (neuron). This depletion resulted from stress, such as overwork. Beard considered the disorder to have a physiological cause in which (as described by Arthur Noyes) "the nervous system is drained of its energy in the manner of a partially discharged battery of low voltage." Beard postulated a "nervous diathesis" theory, in which a person has a specific vulnerability that, when acted on by a stressful environmental influence (either biological or psychological), allowed the symptoms of neurasthenia to develop.

Sigmund Freud was acquainted with the disorder. He agreed with Beard that stress was involved, but Freud thought that neurasthenia was produced by a disturbance in sexual functioning (one of the neuroses), specifically the inadequate discharge of sexual energy that occurred when masturbation replaced normal intercourse. Psychoanalysts after Freud considered neurasthenia a reaction to unconscious factors, such as feelings of rejection, low self-esteem, a sense of worthlessness, and repressed anger.

Depletion Hypothesis. The present-day depletion hypothesis, which holds that prolonged stress lowers the levels of neurotransmitters in neurons, bears a striking resemblance to Beard's concept of nervous exhaustion. Depletion of brain amines causes symptoms of anxiety or depression. Low neuronal dopamine activity occurs in depression; the noradrenergic and adrenergic systems are affected in anxiety disorder and depression; and serotonin levels are low in depressive disorder.

A variety of neuroendocrine dysregulations have been reported in patients with mood and anxiety disorders, with the major ones affecting the adrenal, thyroid, and growth hormone axes. Other neuroendocrine abnormalities include decreased nocturnal secretion of melatonin, decreased basal levels of follicle-stimulating hormone (FSH) and luteinizing hormone (LH), and decreased testosterone levels. These hormones are also altered in prolonged stress states and, presumably, in neurasthenia as well.

Table 18–5
ICD-10 Diagnostic Criteria for Neurasthenia

A. Either of the following must be present:
(1) persistent and distressing complaints of feelings of exhaustion after a minor mental effort (such as performing or attempting to perform everyday tasks that do not require unusual mental effort);
(2) persistent and distressing complaints of feelings of fatigue and bodily weakness after minor physical effort;
At least one of the following symptoms must be present:
(1) feelings of muscular aches and pains;
(2) dizziness;
(3) tension headaches;
(4) sleep disturbances;
(5) inability to relax;
(6) irritability
The patient is unable to recover from the symptoms in Criterion A (1) or (2) by means of rest, relaxation, or entertainment.
The duration of the disorder is at least 3 months.
Most commonly used exclusion clause. The disorder does not occur in the presence of organic emotionally labile disorder, postencephalitic syndrome, postconcussional syndrome, mood disorders, panic disorder, or generalized anxiety disorder.

(From World Health Organization. *The ICD-10 Classification of Mental and Behavioural Disorders: Diagnostic Criteria for Research.* Copyright, World Health Organization, Geneva, 1993, with permission.)

Diagnosis and Clinical Features

According to ICD-10, neurasthenia is not used as a diagnostic category in all countries. In the United States, for example, many of the cases so diagnosed would meet the criteria for depressive disorder, somatoform disorder, or anxiety disorder. Some patients, however, have such varied symptoms that neurasthenia is the preferred diagnosis. These patients' conditions may be diagnosed using the ICD-10 diagnostic criteria (Table 18–5), or they may receive a diagnosis of undifferentiated somatoform disorder according to the DSM-IV-TR criteria (*see* Table 17–11).

The ICD-10 describes two types of the disorder, with substantial overlap between them. In the first type, the main feature is increased fatigue after mental effort, often associated with some decrease in occupational performance or coping efficiency in daily tasks. The mental fatigability is typically described as an unpleasant intrusion of distracting association or recollections, difficulty concentrating, and generally inefficient thinking. The second type emphasizes feelings of bodily or physical weakness and exhaustion after only minimal effort, accompanied by muscular aches and pains and an inability to relax. In both types, other unpleasant physical feelings, such as dizziness, tension headaches, and a sense of general instability, are common. Worry about decreasing mental and physical well-being, irritability, anhedonia, and varying degrees of both depression and anxiety may be present. Sleep is frequently disturbed in its initial and middle phases, but hypersomnia may also be prominent.

If the DSM-IV-TR criteria are used, neurasthenia would be associated with one of the two forms of undifferentiated somatoform disorders, that is, with the group of physical complaints including chronic fatigue and loss of appetite.

Differential Diagnosis

Neurasthenia must be distinguished from anxiety disorders, depressive disorder, and the somatoform disorders. Because so many signs and symptoms of neurasthenia overlap with, and appear in, each of these disorders, differential diagnosis can be exceedingly difficult. For example, patients with anxiety disorder uncommonly do not have depressive symptomatology; patients with hypochondriasis often complain of anxiety; and patients with body dysmorphic disorder can have somatic complaints.

Clinicians must rigorously apply the diagnostic criteria for anxiety, depressive, and somatoform disorders before making a diagnosis of neurasthenia. Hallmarks of neurasthenia are a patient's emphasis on fatigability and weakness and concern about lowered mental and physical efficiency (in contrast to the somatoform disorders, in which bodily complaints and preoccupation with physical disease dominate the picture). If the neurasthenic syndrome develops in the aftermath of a physical illness (particularly, influenza, viral hepatitis, or infectious mononucleosis), the diagnosis of the illness should also be recorded. Chronic fatigue syndrome must also be considered, and differentiating the two disorders is difficult.

Course and Prognosis

Neurasthenia most often occurs during adolescence or middle age. Untreated, the disorder is usually chronic, and patients may become incapacitated by one or more symptoms so that all areas of functioning become impaired. In childhood, difficulties in school functioning, including poor grades and truancy, are likely. In adulthood, work performance deteriorates, or patients may become so disabled that work is impossible. Similarly, social, marital, and interpersonal relationships suffer.

The range of therapeutic options now available is broad, and with treatment, the prognosis should be favorable; but the long-term prognosis is unknown. For patients first having this diagnosis in childhood, the prognosis without treatment is guarded, with chronic symptoms being the most likely outcome. Sometimes, it is difficult to distinguish the prodromal signs of schizophrenia or bipolar disorder from neurasthenia.

Treatment

The key concept in the current treatment of neurasthenia is clinicians' understanding that a patient's symptoms are not imaginary. The symptoms are objective and are produced by emotions that influence the autonomic nervous system, which in turn affects bodily functions. Stress can cause structural change in an organ system, and the result can be life threatening. Therapy, therefore, must begin with a careful medical workup to determine whether the somatic symptoms are amenable to therapy, and if so, what treatment is likely to produce the best results. Patients should be reassured that the administration of medication (analgesics, laxatives, and so on) to relieve medical symptoms will be useful, but only when combined with concurrent psychotherapeutic intervention. Patients must be helped to recognize the stresses in their lives and the coping mechanisms they use to deal with these stresses, to gain insight into the interaction between mind and body. Without such insight-oriented psychotherapy, the neurasthenic condition is likely to continue unabated.

The availability of psychopharmacological agents has markedly improved therapeutic options. Serotonergic agents (e.g., fluoxetine), which have both antidepressant and antianxiety effects, are the most useful class of drugs. Other antidepressants, such as nefazodone and mirtazapine (Remeron), are also effective. Physicians should take care in prescribing drugs with abuse potential, such as benzodiazepines, because of these patients' predilection for self-medication and drug misuse. Such drugs may be useful, for brief periods and under careful supervision, to deal with overwhelming anxiety, phobias, or insomnia. Similarly, small doses of analeptics, such as amphetamine or methylphenidate, may help to treat chronic fatigue and anhedonia. In some cases, it may be necessary to prescribe these medications for long periods of time. In these situations, patients generally stabilize the dose of drugs taken (e.g., 15 mg of amphetamine per day in divided doses). Tolerance does not usually develop, and the clinician should rarely increase the dose lest drug dependence develop. Testosterone replacement can be tried in men with demonstrated low or borderline testosterone levels, but long-term treatment with testosterone may be associated with serious adverse effects, such as prostatic cancer.

References

Blacker CV, Greenwood DT, Wesnes KA, Wilson R, Woodward C, Howe I, Ali T. Effect of galantamine hydrobromide in chronic fatigue syndrome: A randomized controlled trial. *JAMA*. 2004;292(10):1195–1204.

Blockmans D, Persoons P, Van Houdenhove B, Bobbaers H. Does methylphenidate reduce the symptoms of chronic fatigue syndrome? *Am J Med*. 2006;119(2):167.

Carruthers BM, Jain AK, de Meirleir KL, Peterson DL, Klimas NG, Lerner AM, Bested AC, Flor-Henry P, Joshi P, Powles ACP, Sherkey JA, van de Sande MI. Myalgic encephalomyelitis/chronic fatigue syndrome: Clinical working case definition, diagnostic treatment protocols. *Journal of Chronic Fatigue Syndrome*. 2003;11:7–115.

Elena Garralda M, Chalder T. Practitioner review: Chronic fatigue syndrome in childhood. *J Child Psychol Psychiatry*. 2005;46(11):1143–1151.

Gullickson T. Chronic fatigue syndrome: An integrative approach to evaluation and treatment. *PsycCRITIQUES*. 2004.

Hampton T. Researchers find genetic clues to chronic fatigue syndrome. *JAMA*. 2006;295(21):2466–2467.

Jones JF, Nicholson A, Nisenbaum R, Papanicolaou DA, Solomon L, Boneva R, Heim C, Reeves WC. Orthostatic instability in a population-based study of chronic fatigue syndrome. *Am J Med*. 2005;118(12):1415.

Luthra A, Wessely S. Unloading the trunk: Neurasthenia, CFS and race. *Soc Sci Med*. 2004;58:2363–2369.

Rollin H. 'Neurasthenia'. *Br J Psych*. 2004;184:545.

Solomon L, Reeves WC. Factors influencing the diagnosis of chronic fatigue syndrome. *Arch Intern Med*. 2004;164(20):2241–2245.

19 Factitious Disorders

Persons with factitious disorder fake illness. They simulate, induce, or aggravate illness, often inflicting painful, deforming, or even life-threatening injury on themselves or those under their care. Unlike malingerers who have material goals, such as monetary gain or avoidance of duties, patients with factitious disorder undertake these tribulations primarily to gain the emotional care and attention that comes with playing the role of the patient. In doing so, they practice artifice and art, creating hospital drama that often causes frustration and dismay. The disorders have a compulsive quality, but the behaviors are considered voluntary in that they are deliberate and purposeful, even if they cannot be controlled. Clinicians can assess whether a symptom is intentional both by direct evidence and by excluding other causes.

In a 1951 article in *Lancet*, Richard Asher coined the term "Munchausen syndrome" to refer to a syndrome in which patients embellish their personal history, chronically fabricate symptoms to gain hospital admission, and move from hospital to hospital. The syndrome was named after Baron Hieronymus Friedrich Freiherr von Munchausen (1720–1791), a German cavalry officer (Fig. 19–1).

EPIDEMIOLOGY

No comprehensive epidemiological data on factitious disorder exist. Limited studies indicate that patients with factitious disorder may comprise approximately 0.8 to 1.0 percent of psychiatry consultation patients. According to the text revision of the fourth edition of *Diagnostic and Statistical Manual of Mental Disorders* (DSM-IV-TR), factitious disorder is diagnosed in about 1 percent of patients who are seen in psychiatric consultation in general hospitals. The prevalence appears to be greater in highly specialized treatment settings. Cases of feigned psychological signs and symptoms are reported much less commonly than those of physical signs and symptoms. A data bank of persons who feign illness has been established to alert hospitals about such patients, many of whom travel from place to place, seek admission under different names, or simulate different illnesses.

Approximately two thirds of patients with Munchausen syndrome are male. They tend to be white, middle-aged, unemployed, unmarried, and without significant social or family attachments. Patients diagnosed with factitious disorders with physical signs and symptoms are mostly women who outnumber men 3 to 1. They are usually 20 to 40 years of age with a history of employment or education in nursing or a health care occupation. Factitious physical disorders usually begin for patients in their 20s or 30s, although the literature contains cases ranging from 4 to 79 years of age.

Factitious disorder by proxy (discussed separately below) is most commonly perpetrated by mothers against infants or young children. Rare or underrecognized, it accounts for less than 0.04 percent, or 1,000 of 3 million cases of child abuse reported in the United States each year. Good epidemiological data are lacking, however.

COMORBIDITY

Many persons diagnosed with factitious disorder have comorbid psychiatric diagnoses (e.g., mood disorders, personality disorders, or substance-related disorders).

ETIOLOGY

Psychosocial Factors

The psychodynamic underpinnings of factitious disorders are poorly understood because the patients are difficult to engage in an exploratory psychotherapy process. They may insist that their symptoms are physical and that psychologically oriented treatment is therefore useless. Anecdotal case reports indicate that many of the patients suffered childhood abuse or deprivation, resulting in frequent hospitalizations during early development. In such circumstances, an inpatient stay may have been regarded as an escape from a traumatic home situation, and the patient may have found a series of caretakers (e.g., doctors, nurses, and hospital workers) to be loving and caring. In contrast, the patients' families of origin included a rejecting mother or an absent father. The usual history reveals that the patient perceives one or both parents as rejecting figures who are unable to form close relationships. The facsimile of genuine illness, therefore, is used to recreate the desired positive parent–child bond. The disorders are a form of repetitional compulsion, repeating the basic conflict of needing and seeking acceptance and love while expecting that they will not be forthcoming. Hence, the patient transforms the physicians and staff members into rejecting parents.

Patients who seek out painful procedures, such as surgical operations and invasive diagnostic tests, may have a masochistic personality makeup in which pain serves as punishment for past sins, imagined or real. Some patients may attempt to master the past and the early trauma of serious medical illness or hospitalization by assuming the role of the patient and reliving the painful and frightening experience over and over again through multiple hospitalizations. Patients who feign psychiatric illness may have had a relative who was hospitalized with the illness they are simulating. Through identification, patients hope to reunite with the relative in a magical way.

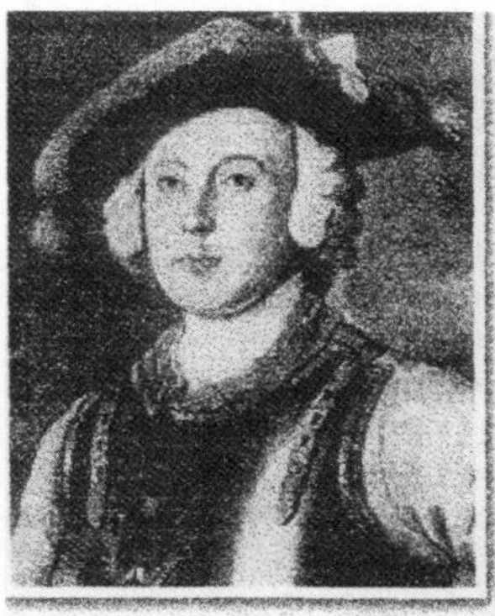
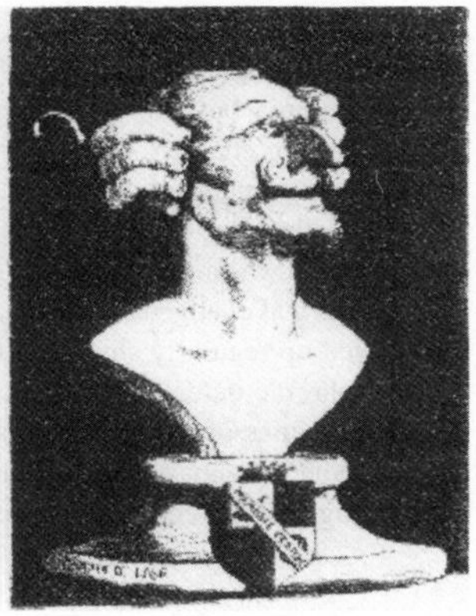

FIGURE 19–1

The Baron Karl Friedrich Hieronymus Freiherr von Munchhausen (1720–1797). **Left:** The Baron wears military armor in this 1750 portrait by G. Bruckner. An honorable nobleman who served in the Russian army in the war against the Turks, the Baron entertained friends in his retirement with embellished stories of his war adventures. His tales gained fame when published by Rudolph E. Raspe. **Right:** The Baron appears as a caricature in this drawing by 19th-century artist Gustave Dore. As was the case with the Baron, patients with factitious disorders are persons deserving of respect, even though they often present themselves as caricatures. (Portrait courtesy of Bernhard Wiebel, *http://www.muenchhausen.ch.* The actual portrait was lost in World War II. Caricature from *The Adventures of Baron Munchausen: One Hundred and Sixty Illustrations by Gustave Dore.* New York: Pantheon Books, Inc.; 1944, with permission.)

Many patients have the poor identity formation and disturbed self-image that is characteristic of someone with borderline personality disorder. Some patients are *as-if personalities* who have assumed the identities of those around them. If these patients are health professionals, they are often unable to differentiate themselves from the patients with whom they come in contact. The cooperation or encouragement of other persons in simulating a factitious illness occurs in a rare variant of the disorder. Although most patients act alone, friends or relatives participate in fabricating the illness in some instances.

Significant defense mechanisms are repression, identification with the aggressor, regression, and symbolization.

Biological Factors

Some researchers have proposed that brain dysfunction may be a factor in factitious disorders. It has been hypothesized that impaired information processing contributes to the *pseudologia fantastica* and aberrant behavior of patients with Munchausen disorder; however, no genetic patterns have been established, and electroencephalographic (EEG) studies noted no specific abnormalities in patients with factitious disorders.

DIAGNOSIS AND CLINICAL FEATURES

The diagnostic criteria for factitious disorder in DSM-IV-TR are given in Table 19–1. The psychiatric examination should emphasize securing information from any available friends, relatives, or other informants, because interviews with reliable outside sources often reveal the false nature of the patient's illness. Although time-consuming and tedious, verifying all the facts presented by the patient about previous hospitalizations and medical care is essential.

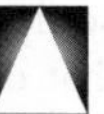

Table 19–1
DSM-IV-TR Diagnostic Criteria for Factitious Disorder

A. Intentional production or feigning of physical or psychological signs or symptoms.
B. The motivation for the behavior is to assume the sick role.
C. External incentives for the behavior (such as economic gain, avoiding legal responsibility, or improving physical well-being, as in malingering) are absent.

Code based on type:

With predominantly psychological signs and symptoms: if psychological signs and symptoms predominate in the clinical presentation

With predominantly physical signs and symptoms: if physical signs and symptoms predominate in the clinical presentation

With combined psychological and physical signs and symptoms: if both psychological and physical signs and symptoms are present but neither predominates in the clinical presentation

(From American Psychiatric Association. *Diagnostic and Statistical Manual of Mental Disorders.* 4th ed. Text rev. Washington, DC: American Psychiatric Association; copyright 2000, with permission.)

Psychiatric evaluation is requested on a consultation basis in about 50 percent of cases, usually after a simulated illness is suspected. The psychiatrist is often asked to confirm the diagnosis of factitious disorder. Under these circumstances, it is necessary to avoid pointed or accusatory questioning that may provoke truculence, evasion, or flight from the hospital. A danger may exist of provoking frank psychosis if vigorous confrontation is used; in some instances, the feigned illness serves an adaptive function and is a desperate attempt to ward off further disintegration.

Factitious Disorder with Predominantly Psychological Signs and Symptoms

Some patients show psychiatric symptoms judged to be feigned. This determination can be difficult and is often made only after a prolonged investigation (Table 19–1). The feigned symptoms frequently include depression, hallucinations, dissociative and conversion symptoms, and bizarre behavior. Because the patient's condition does not improve after routine therapeutic measures are administered, he or she may receive large doses of psychoactive drugs and may undergo electroconvulsive therapy.

Factitious psychological symptoms resemble the phenomenon of pseudomalingering, conceptualized as satisfying the need to maintain an intact self-image, which would be marred by admitting psychological problems that are beyond the person's capacity to master through conscious effort. In this case, deception is a transient ego-supporting device.

Recent findings indicate that factitious psychotic symptoms are more common than had previously been suspected. The presence of simulated psychosis as a feature of other disorders, such as mood disorders, indicates a poor overall prognosis.

Inpatients who are psychotic and found to have factitious disorder with predominantly psychological signs and symptoms—that is, exclusively simulated psychotic symptoms—generally have a concurrent diagnosis of borderline personality disorder. In these cases, the outcome appears to be worse than that of bipolar I disorder or schizoaffective disorder.

Patients may appear depressed and may explain their depression by offering a false history of the recent death of a significant friend or relative. Elements of the history that may suggest factitious bereavement include a violent or bloody death, a death under dramatic circumstances, and the dead person's being a child or a young adult. Other patients may describe either recent and remote memory loss or both auditory and visual hallucinations. According to DSM-IV-TR:

> The individual may surreptitiously use psychoactive substances for the purpose of producing symptoms that suggest a mental disorder (e.g., stimulants to produce restlessness or insomnia, hallucinogens to induce altered perceptual states, analgesics to induce euphoria, and hypnotics to induce lethargy). Combinations of psychoactive substances can produce very unusual presentations.

Other symptoms, which also appear in the physical type of factitious disorder, include pseudologia fantastica and impostorship. In pseudologia fantastica, limited factual material is mixed with extensive and colorful fantasies. The listener's interest pleases the patient and, thus, reinforces the symptom. The history or the symptoms are not the only distortions of truth. Patients often give false and conflicting accounts about other areas of their lives (e.g., they may claim the death of a parent, to play on the sympathy of others). Imposture is commonly related to lying in these cases. Many patients assume the identity of a prestigious person. Men, for example, report being war heroes and attribute their surgical scars to wounds received during battle or in other dramatic and dangerous exploits. Similarly, they may say that they have ties to accomplished or renowned figures.

Table 19–2 lists various syndromes feigned by patients who want to be seen as having a mental illness.

Ms. MA was 24 years of age when she first presented in 1973 after an overdose. She gave a history of recurrent overdoses and wrist-slashing attempts since 1969, and, on admission, she stated that she was controlled by her dead sister who kept telling her to take her own life. Her family history was negative.

She was found to be carrying a list of schneiderian first-rank symptoms in her handbag; she behaved bizarrely, picking imaginary objects out of the wastepaper basket and opening imaginary doors in the waiting room. She admitted to visual hallucinations and offered four of the first-rank symptoms on her list, but her mental state reverted to normal after 2 days. When she was presented at a case conference, the consensus view was that she had been simulating schizophrenia but had a gross personality disorder; however, the consultant in charge dissented from that general view, feeling that she was genuinely psychotic.

On follow-up, this turned out to be the case. She was readmitted in 1975 and was mute, catatonic, grossly thought disordered, and the diagnosis was changed to that of a schizophrenic illness. She has been followed up regularly since and now presents the picture of a mild schizophrenic defect state; she takes regular depot medication but still complains of auditory hallucinations, hearing her dead sister's voice. She is a day patient. (Courtesy of Dora Wang, M.D., Deepa N. Nadiga, M.D., and James J. Jenson, M.D.)

Table 19–2
Presentations in Factitious Disorder with Predominantly Psychological Signs and Symptoms

Bereavement	Eating disorder
Depression	Amnesia
Posttraumatic stress disorder	Substance-related disorder
Pain disorder	Paraphillias
Psychosis	Hypersomnia
Bipolar I disorder	Transsexualism
Dissociative identity disorder	

(Adapted from Feldman MD, Eisendrath SJ. *The Spectrum of Factitious Disorders.* Washington, DC: American Psychiatric Press; 1996, with permission.)

Chronic Factitious Disorder with Predominantly Physical Signs and Symptoms (Munchausen Syndrome)

Factitious disorder with predominantly physical signs and symptoms is the best known type of Munchausen syndrome. The disorder has also been called hospital addiction, polysurgical addiction—producing the so-called washboard abdomen, and professional patient syndrome, among other names.

The essential feature of patients with the disorder is their ability to present physical symptoms so well that they can gain admission to, and stay in, a hospital (Table 19–1). To support their history, these patients may feign symptoms suggesting a disorder involving any organ system (*see* Color Plate 19–2 on page 494). They are familiar with the diagnoses of most disorders that usually require hospital admission or medication and can give excellent histories capable of deceiving even experienced clinicians. Clinical presentations are myriad and include hematoma, hemoptysis, abdominal pain, fever, hypoglycemia, lupus-like syndromes, nausea, vomiting, dizziness, and seizures. Urine is contaminated with blood or feces; anticoagulants are taken to simulate bleeding disorders; insulin is used to produce hypoglycemia; and so on. Such patients often insist on surgery and claim adhesions from previous surgical procedures. They may acquire a "gridiron" or washboard-like abdomen from multiple procedures. Complaints of pain, especially that simulating renal colic, are common, with the patients wanting narcotics. In about half the reported cases, these patients demand treatment with specific medications, usually analgesics. Once in the hospital, they continue to be demanding and difficult. As each test is returned with a negative result, they may accuse doctors of incompetence, threaten litigation, and become generally abusive. Some may sign out abruptly shortly before they believe they are going to be confronted with their factitious behavior. They then go to another hospital in the same or another city and begin the cycle again. Specific predisposing factors are true physical disorders during childhood leading to extensive medical treatment, a grudge against the medical profession, employment as a medical paraprofessional, and an important relationship with a physician in the past.

Factitious Disorder with Combined Psychological and Physical Signs and Symptoms

In combined forms of factitious disorder, both psychological and physical signs and symptoms are present. If neither type predominates in the clinical presentation, a diagnosis of factitious disorder with combined psychological and physical signs and symptoms should be made (Table 19–1). In one representative report, a patient alternated between feigned dementia, bereavement, rape, and seizures.

Mr. MT was a man who appeared to be middle-aged but who arrived at a children's psychiatric hospital claiming to be 17 years of age and suicidal. As he held a gun to his head, staff called security officers who promptly recognized him as the patient with Munchausen syndrome who arrived in early May each year. He was denied admission.

Late that evening, he presented to the emergency room (ER) of the main hospital claiming that he was diabetic, dizzy, and weak. Intern physicians found his blood glucose to be low and immediately admitted him. Hospital staff on the wards recognized him as "that Munchausen syndrome patient," and a psychiatric consultation was requested. The patient continued to insist that he was 17 years of age and that he was the son of famous golfer Lee Trevino. Hospital legal counsel revealed that he used at least two other pseudonyms and social security numbers and was wanted for health insurance fraud in at least two other states.

When the psychiatry consultants greeted him with familiarity, the patient immediately claimed suicidal tendency, but, when denied psychiatric admission, he left the hospital against medical advice. An inquisitive medical student called local pharmacies, which informed him that, if a customer claimed to be diabetic, traveling, and without insulin, they would give the customer insulin even without a prescription to avoid liability. In this manner, Mr. MT could have procured insulin to induce hypoglycemia.

At a care conference, a psychiatry consultant expressed that, in the past, common practice was to call ERs in town to alert them to patients with Munchausen syndrome, giving all possibly helpful descriptions and information. However, because of heightened attention to confidentiality rights, she now instead advocated calling ERs and simply warning them about the possible appearance of a patient with factitious hypoglycemia. An ER physician, however, stated that he would go ahead and give a detailed description of the patient to friends in each ER in town. The May of the following year, the patient failed to appear for the first time in several years. (Courtesy of Dora Wang, M.D., Deepa N. Nadiga, M.D., and James J. Jenson, M.D.)

Factitious Disorder Not Otherwise Specified

Some patients with factitious signs and symptoms do not meet the DSM-IV-TR criteria for a specific factitious disorder and should be classified as having factitious disorder not otherwise specified (Table 19–3). The most notable example of the diagnosis is factitious disorder by proxy, which is also included in a DSM-IV-TR appendix (Table 19–4). In this diagnosis, a person intentionally produces physical signs or symptoms in another person who is under the first person's care. One apparent purpose of the behavior is for the caretaker to indirectly assume the sick role; another is to be relieved of the caretaking role by having the child hospitalized (Table 19–5). The most common case of factitious disorder by proxy involves a mother who deceives medical personnel into believing that her child is ill. The deception may involve a false medical history, contamination of

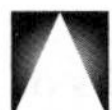

Table 19–3
DSM-IV-TR Diagnostic Criteria for Factitious Disorder Not Otherwise Specified

This category includes disorders with factitious symptoms that do not meet the criteria for factitious disorder. An example is factitious disorder by proxy: the intentional production or feigning of physical or psychological signs or symptoms in another person who is under the individual's care for the purpose of indirectly assuming the sick role (see Table 19-4 for suggested research criteria).

(From American Psychiatric Association. *Diagnostic and Statistical Manual of Mental Disorders.* 4th ed. Text rev. Washington, DC: American Psychiatric Association; copyright 2000, with permission.)

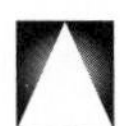

Table 19–4
DSM-IV-TR Research Criteria for Factitious Disorder by Proxy

A. Intentional production or feigning of physical or psychological signs or symptoms in another person who is under the individual's care.
B. The motivation for the perpetrator's behavior is to assume the sick role by proxy.
C. External incentives for the behavior (such as economic gain) are absent.
D. The behavior is not better accounted for by another mental disorder.

(From American Psychiatric Association. *Diagnostic and Statistical Manual of Mental Disorders.* 4th ed. Text rev. Washington, DC: American Psychiatric Association; copyright 2000, with permission.)

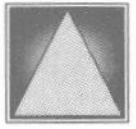

Table 19–5
Clinical Indicators That May Suggest Factitious Disorder by Proxy

The symptoms and pattern of illness are extremely unusual, or inexplicable physiologically.
Repeated hospitalizations and workups by numerous caregivers fail to reveal a conclusive diagnosis or cause.
Physiological parameters are consistent with induced illness; e.g., apnea monitor tracings disclose massive muscle artifact prior to respiratory arrest, suggesting that the child has been struggling against an obstruction to the airways.
The patient fails to respond to appropriate treatments.
The vitality of the patient is inconsistent with the laboratory findings.
The signs and symptoms abate when the mother has not had access to the child.
The mother is the only witness to the onset of signs and symptoms.
Unexplained illnesses have occurred in the mother or her other children.
The mother has had medical or nursing education, or exposure to models of the illnesses afflicting the child (e.g., a parent with sleep apnea).
The mother welcomes even invasive and painful tests.
The mother grows anxious if the child improves.
Maternal lying is proved.
Medical observations yield information that is inconsistent with parental reports.

(Adapted from Feldman MD, Eisendrath SJ. *The Spectrum of Factitious Disorders.* Washington, DC: American Psychiatric Press; 1996, with permission.)

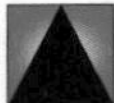

Table 19–6
ICD-10 Diagnostic Criteria for Other Disorders of Adult Personality and Behavior Elaboration of Physical Symptoms for Psychological Reasons

A. Physical symptoms originally due to a confirmed physical disorder, disease, or disability become exaggerated or prolonged in excess of what can be explained by the physical disorder itself.
B. There is evidence for a psychological causation for the excess symptoms (such as evident fear of disability or death, possible financial compensation, disappointment at the standard of care experienced).

Intentional production or feigning of symptoms or disabilities, either physical or psychological [factitious disorder]

A. The individual exhibits a persistent pattern of intentional production or feigning of symptoms and/or self-infliction of wounds in order to produce symptoms.
B. No evidence can be found for an external motivation such as financial compensation, escape from danger, or more medical care. (If such evidence can be found, the category, malingering, should be used.)
C. *Most commonly* used exclusion clause. There is no confirmed physical or mental disorder that could explain the symptoms.

Other specified disorders of adult personality and behavior

This category should be used for coding any specified disorder of adult personality and behavior that cannot be classified under any one of the preceding headings.

(From World Health Organization. *The ICD-10 Classification of Mental and Behavioural Disorders: Diagnostic Criteria for Research.* Copyright, World Health Organization, Geneva, 1993, with permission.)

laboratory samples, alteration of records, or induction of injury and illness in the child.

ICD-10

The 10th revision of *International Statistical Classification of Diseases and Related Health Problems* (ICD-10) notes that "the condition is best interpreted as a disorder of illness behavior and the sick role. Individuals with this pattern of behavior usually show signs of... other marked abnormalities of personality and relationships." ICD-10 also includes a category called *elaboration of physical symptoms for psychological reasons*. The ICD-10 criteria for both conditions are presented in Table 19–6. In ICD-10, these conditions exclude factitious dermatitis, and "Munchausen by proxy" is classified under child abuse, not factitious disorders.

PATHOLOGY AND LABORATORY EXAMINATION

Psychological testing may reveal specific underlying pathology in individual patients. Features that are overrepresented in patients with factitious disorder include normal or above-average intelligence quotient (IQ); absence of a formal thought disorder; poor sense of identity, including confusion over sexual identity; poor sexual adjustment; poor frustration tolerance; strong dependence needs; and narcissism. An invalid test profile and elevations of all clinical scales on the Minnesota Multiphasic Personality Inventory-2 (MMPI-2) indicate an attempt to appear more disturbed than is the case ("fake bad").

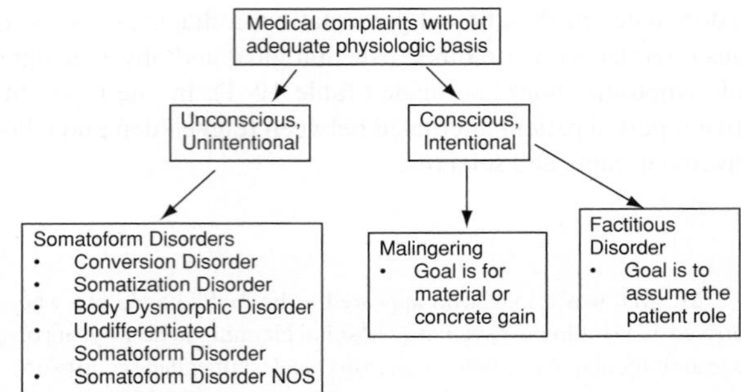

FIGURE 19–3
Differential diagnosis of factitious disorder with predominantly physical signs and symptoms. NOS, not otherwise specified.

No specific laboratory tests are available for factitious disorders. Certain tests (e.g., drug screening), however, may help confirm or rule out specific mental or medical disorders.

DIFFERENTIAL DIAGNOSIS

Any disorder in which physical signs and symptoms are prominent should be considered in the differential diagnosis, and the possibility of authentic or concomitant physical illness must always be explored. Additionally, a history of many surgeries in patients with factous disorder may predispose such patients to complications or actual diseases, necessitating even further surgery. Factitious disorder is on a continuum between somatoform disorders and malingering, the goal being to assume the sick role. On one hand it is unconscious and nonvolitional (somatoform) and on the other hand it is conscious and willful (malingering) (Fig. 19–3).

Somatoform Disorders

A factitious disorder is differentiated from somatization disorder (Briquet's syndrome) by the voluntary production of factitious symptoms, the extreme course of multiple hospitalizations, and the seeming willingness of patients with a factitious disorder to undergo an extraordinary number of mutilating procedures. Patients with conversion disorder are not usually conversant with medical terminology and hospital routines, and their symptoms have a direct temporal relation or symbolic reference to specific emotional conflicts.

Hypochondriasis differs from factitious disorder in that the hypochondriacal patient does not voluntarily initiate the production of symptoms, and hypochondriasis typically has a later age of onset. As with somatization disorder, patients with hypochondriasis do not usually submit to potentially mutilating procedures. (Somatoform disorders are discussed in Chapter 17.)

Personality Disorders

Because of their pathological lying, lack of close relationships with others, hostile and manipulative manner, and associated substance abuse and criminal history, patients with factitious disorder are often classified as having antisocial personality disorder. Antisocial persons, however, do not usually volunteer for invasive procedures or resort to a way of life marked by repeated or long-term hospitalization.

Because of attention seeking and an occasional flair for the dramatic, patients with factitious disorder may be classified as having histrionic personality disorder. But not all such patients have a dramatic flair; many are withdrawn and bland.

Consideration of the patient's chaotic lifestyle, history of disturbed interpersonal relationships, identity crisis, substance abuse, self-damaging acts, and manipulative tactics may lead to the diagnosis of borderline personality disorder. Persons with factitious disorder usually do not have the eccentricities of dress, thought, or communication that characterize schizotypal personality disorder patients. (Personality disorders are discussed in Chapter 27.)

Schizophrenia

The diagnosis of schizophrenia is often based on patients' admittedly bizarre lifestyles, but patients with factitious disorder do not usually meet the diagnostic criteria for schizophrenia unless they have the fixed delusion that they are actually ill and act on this belief by seeking hospitalization. Such a practice seems to be the exception; few patients with factitious disorder show evidence of a severe thought disorder or bizarre delusions.

Malingering

Factitious disorders must be distinguished from malingering. Malingerers have an obvious, recognizable environmental goal in producing signs and symptoms. They may seek hospitalization to secure financial compensation, evade the police, avoid work, or merely obtain free bed and board for the night, but they always have some apparent end for their behavior. Moreover, these patients can usually stop producing their signs and symptoms when they are no longer considered profitable or when the risk becomes too great. (Malingering is discussed in Chapter 33.)

Substance Abuse

Although patients with factitious disorders may have a complicating history of substance abuse, they should be considered not merely as substance abusers but as having coexisting diagnoses.

Ganser's Syndrome

Ganser's syndrome, a controversial condition most typically associated with prison inmates, is characterized by the use of approximate answers. Persons with the syndrome respond to simple questions with astonishingly incorrect answers. For example, when asked about the color of a blue car, the person answers "red" or answers "2 plus 2 equals 5." Ganser's syndrome may be a variant of malingering, in that the patients avoid punishment or responsibility for their actions. Ganser's syndrome is classified in DSM-IV-TR as a dissociative disorder not otherwise specified and in ICD-10 under other dissociative or conversion disorders. Patients with factitious disorder with predominantly psychological signs and symptoms may intentionally give approximate answers, however. (See Chapter 20: Dissociative Disorders for a further discussion.)

COURSE AND PROGNOSIS

Factitious disorders typically begin in early adulthood, although they can appear during childhood or adolescence. The onset of the disorder or of discrete episodes of seeking treatment may follow real illness, loss, rejection, or abandonment. Usually, the patient or a close relative had a hospitalization in childhood or early adolescence for a genuine physical illness. Thereafter, a long pattern of successive hospitalizations begins insidiously and evolves. As the disorder progresses, the patient becomes knowledgeable about medicine and hospitals. The onset of the disorder in patients who had early hospitalizations for actual illness is earlier than generally reported.

Factitious disorders are incapacitating to the patient and often produce severe trauma or untoward reactions related to treatment. A course of repeated or long-term hospitalization is obviously incompatible with meaningful vocational work and sustained interpersonal relationships. The prognosis in most cases is poor. A few patients occasionally spend time in jail, usually for minor crimes, such as burglary, vagrancy, and disorderly conduct. Patients may also have a history of intermittent psychiatric hospitalization.

Although no adequate data are available about the ultimate outcome for the patients, a few of them probably die as a result of needless medication, instrumentation, or surgery. In view of the patients' often expert simulation and the risks that they take, some may die without the disorder being suspected. Possible features that indicate a favorable prognosis are (1) the presence of a depressive-masochistic personality; (2) functioning at a borderline, not a continuously psychotic, level; and (3) the attributes of an antisocial personality disorder with minimal symptoms.

TREATMENT

No specific psychiatric therapy has been effective in treating factitious disorders. It is a clinical paradox that patients with the disorders simulate serious illness and seek and submit to unnecessary treatment while they deny to themselves and others their true illness and thus avoid possible treatment for it. Ultimately, the patients elude meaningful therapy by abruptly leaving the hospital or failing to keep follow-up appointments.

Treatment, thus, is best focused on management rather than on cure. Guidelines for the treatment and management of factitious disorder are given in Table 19-7. The three major goals in the treatment and management of factitious disorders are (1) to reduce the risk of morbidity and mortality, (2) to address the underlying emotional needs or psychiatric diagnosis underlying factitious illness behavior, and (3) to be mindful of legal and ethical issues. Perhaps the single most important factor in successful management is a physician's early recognition of the disorder. In this way, physicians can forestall a multitude of painful and potentially dangerous diagnostic procedures for these patients. Good liaison between psychiatrists and the medical or surgical staff is strongly advised. Although a few cases of individual psychotherapy have been reported in the literature, no consensus exists about the best approach. In general, working in concert with the patient's primary care physician is more effective than working with the patient in isolation.

The personal reactions of physicians and staff members are of great significance in treating and establishing a working alliance

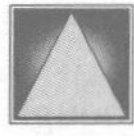

Table 19–7
Guidelines for Management and Treatment of Factitious Disorder

Active pursuit of a prompt diagnosis can minimize the risk of morbidity and mortality.
Minimize harm. Avoid unnecessary tests and procedures, especially if invasive. Treat according to clinical judgment, keeping in mind that subjective complaints may be deceptive.
Regular interdisciplinary meetings to reduce conflict and splitting among staff. Manage staff countertransference.
Consider facilitating healing by using the double-bind technique or face-saving behavioral strategies, such as self-hypnosis or biofeedback.
Steer the patient toward psychiatric treatment in an empathic, nonconfrontational, face-saving manner. Avoid aggressive direct confrontation.
Treat underlying psychiatric disturbances, such as Axis I disorders and Axis II disorders. In psychotherapy, address coping strategies and emotional conflicts.
Appoint a primary care provider as a gatekeeper for all medical and psychiatric treatment.
Consider involving risk management professionals and bioethicists from an early point.
Consider appointing a guardian for medical and psychiatric decisions.
Consider prosecution for fraud, as a behavioral disincentive.

with the patients, who invariably evoke feelings of futility, bewilderment, betrayal, hostility, and even contempt. In essence, staff members are forced to abandon a basic element of their relationship with patients—accepting the truthfulness of the patients' statements. One appropriate psychiatric intervention is to suggest to the staff ways of remaining aware that even though the patient's illness is factitious, the patient is ill.

Physicians should try not to feel resentment when patients humiliate their diagnostic prowess, and they should avoid any unmasking ceremony that sets up the patients as adversaries and precipitates their flight from the hospital. The staff should not perform unnecessary procedures or discharge patients abruptly, both of which are manifestations of anger.

Clinicians who find themselves involved with patients with factitious disorders may become angry at the patients for lying and deceiving them. Hence, therapists must be mindful of countertransference whenever they suspect factitious disorder. Often, the diagnosis is unclear because a definitive physical cause cannot be entirely ruled out. Although the use of confrontation is controversial, at some point in the treatment, patients must be made to face reality. Most patients simply leave treatment when their methods of gaining attention are identified and exposed. In some cases, clinicians should reframe the factitious disorder as a cry for help, so that patients do not view the clinicians' responses as punitive. A major role for psychiatrists working with patients with factitious disorder is to help other staff members in the hospital deal with their own sense of outrage at having been duped. Education about the disorder and some attempt to understand the patient's motivations may help staff members maintain their professional conduct in the face of extreme frustration.

In cases of factitious disorder by proxy, legal intervention has been obtained in several instances, particularly with children. The senselessness of the disorder and the denial of false action by parents are obstacles to successful court action and often make conclusive proof unobtainable. In such cases, the child welfare services should be notified, and arrangements made for ongoing monitoring of the children's health.

Pharmacotherapy of factitious disorders is of limited use. Comorbid Axis I disorder (e.g., schizophrenia) will respond to antipsychotic medication; however, in all cases, medication should be administered carefully because of the potential for abuse. Selective serotonin reuptake inhibitors (SSRIs) may be useful in decreasing impulsive behavior when that is a major component in acting-out factitious behavior.

References

Awadalla N, Vaughan A, Franco K, Munir F, Sharaby N, Goldfarb J. Muchausen by proxy: A case, chart series, and literature review of older victims. *Child Abuse Negl.* 2005;29:931–941.

Eisendrath SJ, McNeil DE. Factitious disorders in civil litigation: Twenty cases illustrating the spectrum of abnormal illness-affirming behavior. *J Am Acad Psychiatry Law.* 2002;30:391.

Eisendrath SJ, McNiel DE. Factitious physical disorders, litigation, and morality. *Psychosomatics: Journal of Consultation Liaison Psychiatry.* 2004;45:350–353.

Feldman MD, Ford VF. Factitious disorders. In: Sadock BJ, Sadock VA, eds. *Kaplan & Sadock's Comprehensive Textbook of Psychiatry*. 7th ed. Vol. 1. Baltimore: Lippincott Williams & Wilkins; 2000:1533.

Krahn LE, Li H, O'Connor MK. Patients who strive to be ill: Factitious disorder with physical symptoms. *Am J Psychiatry.* 2003;160:1163.

Peebles R, Sabella C, Franco K, Goldfarb J. Factitious disorder and malingering in adolescent girls: Case series and literature review. *Clin Pediatr (Phil).* 2005;44:237–243.

Rogers R, Jackson RL, Kaminski PL. Factitious psychological disorders: The overlooked response style in forensic evaluations. *Journal of Forensic Psychology Practice.* 2005;5:21–41.

Schrier H. Munchausen by proxy defined. *Pediatrics.* 2003;110:958.

Turner MA. Factitious disorder: Reformulating the DSM-IV criteria. *Psychosomatics: Journal of Consultation Liaison Psychiatry.* 2006;47:23–32.

Wang D, Nadiga DN, Jenson JJ. Factitious disorders. In: Sadock BJ, Sadock VA, eds. *Kaplan & Sadock's Comprehensive Textbook of Psychiatry*. 8th ed. Vol. 1. Baltimore: Lippincott Williams & Wilkins; 2005:1829.

20 Dissociative Disorders

According to the text revision of the fourth edition of the *Diagnostic and Statistical Manual of Mental Disorders* (DSM-IV-TR), "the essential feature of the dissociative disorders is a disruption in the usually integrated functions of consciousness, memory, identity, or perception of the environment. The disturbance may be sudden or gradual, transient or chronic." The DSM-IV-TR dissociative disorders are dissociative identity disorder, depersonalization disorder, dissociative amnesia, dissociative fugue, and dissociative disorder not otherwise specified (NOS).

DISSOCIATIVE AMNESIA

According to DSM-IV-TR (Table 20–1), the essential feature of dissociative amnesia is an inability to recall important personal information, usually of a traumatic or stressful nature, that is too extensive to be explained by normal forgetfulness. The disturbance does not occur exclusively during the course of dissociative identity disorder, dissociative fugue, posttraumatic stress disorder (PTSD), acute stress disorder, or somatization disorder and does not result from the direct physiological effects of a substance or a neurological or other general medical condition. This disturbance can be based on neurobiological changes in the brain caused by traumatic stress. The different patterns of dissociative amnesia are listed in Table 20–2.

A 45-year-old, divorced, left-handed, male bus dispatcher was seen in psychiatric consultation on a medical unit. He had been admitted with an episode of chest discomfort, light headedness, and left-arm weakness. He had a history of hypertension and had a medical admission in the past year for ischemic chest pain, although he had not suffered a myocardial infarction. Psychiatric consultation was called, because the patient complained of memory loss for the previous 12 years, behaving and responding to the environment as if it were 12 years previously (e.g., he didn't recognize his 8-year-old son, insisted that he was unmarried, and denied recollection of current events, such as the current president). Physical and laboratory findings were unchanged from the patient's usual baseline. Brain computed tomography (CT) scan was normal.

On mental status examination, the patient displayed intact intellectual function but insisted that the date was 12 years earlier, denying recall of his entire subsequent personal history and of current events for the last 12 years. He was perplexed by the contradiction between his memory and current circumstances. The patient described a family history of brutal beatings and physical discipline. He was a decorated combat veteran, although he described amnestic episodes for some of his combat experiences. In the military, he had been a champion golden glove boxer noted for his powerful left hand.

He was educated about his disorder and given the suggestion that his memory could return as he could tolerate it, perhaps overnight during sleep or perhaps over a longer time. If this strategy was unsuccessful, hypnosis or an amobarbital interview was proposed. (Adapted from case of Richard J. Loewenstein, M.D., and Frank W. Putnam, M.D.)

Epidemiology

Dissociative amnesia, as defined by DSM-IV-TR, has been reported in approximately 6 percent of the general population. No known difference is seen in incidence between men and women. Cases generally begin to be reported in late adolescence and adulthood. Dissociative amnesia can be especially difficult to assess in preadolescent children because of their more limited ability to describe subjective experience.

Etiology

Amnesia and Extreme Intrapsychic Conflict. In many cases of acute dissociative amnesia, the psychosocial environment out of which the amnesia develops is massively conflictual, with the patient experiencing intolerable emotions of shame, guilt, despair, rage, and desperation. These usually result from conflicts over unacceptable urges or impulses, such as intense sexual, suicidal, or violent compulsions.

Betrayal Trauma. *Betrayal trauma* attempts to explain amnesia by the intensity of trauma and by the extent that a negative event represents a betrayal by a trusted, needed other. This betrayal is thought to influence the way in which the event is processed and remembered. Information about the abuse is not linked to mental mechanisms that control attachment and attachment behavior.

Diagnosis and Clinical Features

Classic Presentation. The classic disorder is an overt, florid, dramatic clinical disturbance that frequently results in the patient being brought quickly to medical attention, specifically for symptoms related to the dissociative disorder. It is frequently found in those who have experienced extreme acute trauma. It also commonly develops, however, in the context of profound intrapsychic conflict or emotional stress. Patients may present with intercurrent somatoform or conversion symptoms, alterations

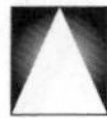

Table 20–1
DSM-IV-TR Diagnostic Criteria for Dissociative Amnesia

A. The predominant disturbance is one or more episodes of inability to recall important personal information, usually of a traumatic or stressful nature, that is too extensive to be explained by ordinary forgetfulness.
B. The disturbance does not occur exclusively during the course of dissociative identity disorder, dissociative fugue, posttraumatic stress disorder, acute stress disorder, or somatization disorder and is not due to the direct physiological effects of a substance (e.g., a drug of abuse, a medication) or a neurological or other general medical condition (e.g., amnestic disorder due to head trauma).
C. The symptoms cause clinically significant distress or impairment in social, occupational, or other important areas of functioning.

(From American Psychiatric Association. *Diagnostic and Statistical Manual of Mental Disorders.* 4th ed. Text rev. Washington, DC: American Psychiatric Association; 2000, with permission.)

in consciousness, depersonalization, derealization, trance states, spontaneous age regression, and even ongoing anterograde dissociative amnesia. Depression and suicidal ideation are reported in many cases. No single personality profile or antecedent history is consistently reported in these patients, although a prior personal or family history of somatoform or dissociative symptoms has been shown to predispose individuals to develop acute amnesia during traumatic circumstances. Many of these patients have histories of prior adult or childhood abuse or trauma. In wartime cases, as in other forms of combat-related posttraumatic disorders, the most important variable in the development of dissociative symptoms, however, appears to be the intensity of combat.

Nonclassic Presentation. These patients frequently come to treatment for a variety of symptoms, such as depression or mood swings, substance abuse, sleep disturbances, somatoform symptoms, anxiety and panic, suicidal or self-mutilating impulses and acts, violent outbursts, eating problems, and interpersonal problems. Self-mutilation and violent behavior in these patients may also be accompanied by amnesia. Amnesia may also occur for flashbacks or behavioral reexperiencing episodes related to trauma.

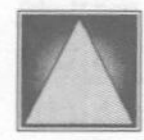

Table 20–2
Types of Dissociative Amnesia

Localized amnesia
Inability to recall events related to a circumscribed period of time
Selective amnesia
Ability to remember some, but not all, of the events occurring during a circumscribed period of time
Generalized amnesia
Failure to recall one's entire life
Continuous amnesia
Failure to recall successive events as they occur
Systematized amnesia
Amnesia for certain categories of memory, such as all memories relating to one's family or to a particular person

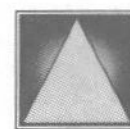

Table 20–3
Differential Diagnosis of Dissociative Amnesia

Ordinary forgetfulness
- Age-related cognitive decline

Nonpathological forms of amnesia
- Infantile and childhood amnesia
- Amnesia for sleep and dreaming
- Hypnotic amnesia

Dementia
Delirium
Amnestic disorders
Neurological disorders with discrete memory loss episodes
- Posttraumatic amnesia
- Transient global amnesia
- Amnesia related to seizure disorders

Substance-related amnesia
- Alcohol
- Sedative-hypnotics
- Anticholinergic agents
- Steroids
- Marijuana
- Narcotic analgesics
- Psychedelics
- Phencyclidine
- Methyldopa (Aldomet)
- Pentazocine (Talwin)
- Hypoglycemic agents
- β-blockers
- Lithium carbonate
- Many others

Other dissociative disorders
- Dissociative fugue
- Dissociative identity disorder
- Dissociative disorder not otherwise specified

Acute stress disorder
Posttraumatic stress disorder
Somatization disorder
Psychotic episode
- Lack of memory for psychotic episode when returns to nonpsychotic state

Mood disorder episode
- Lack of memory for aspects of episode of mania when depressed and vice versa or when euthymic

Factitious disorder
Malingering

Differential Diagnosis

The differential diagnosis of dissociative amnesia is listed in Table 20-3.

Ordinary Forgetfulness and Nonpathological Amnesia. The DSM-IV-TR diagnostic criteria for dissociative amnesia specify that the disturbance must be "too extensive to be explained by normal forgetfulness." Furthermore, nonpathological forms of amnesia have been described, such as infantile and childhood amnesia, amnesia for sleep and dreaming, and hypnotic amnesia.

Dementia, Delirium, and Organic Amnestic Disorders. In patients with dementia, organic amnestic disorders, and delirium, the memory loss for personal information is embedded in a far more extensive set of cognitive, language, attentional, behavioral, and memory problems. Loss of memory for personal identity is usually not found without evidence of a marked disturbance in many domains of cognitive function. Causes of organic amnestic disorders include Korsakoff's psychosis, cerebral vascular accident (CVA), postoperative amnesia, postinfectious amnesia, anoxic amnesia, and transient global amnesia. Electroconvulsive therapy (ECT) may also cause a marked temporary amnesia, as well as persistent memory problems in some cases. Here, however, memory loss for autobiographical experience is unrelated to traumatic or overwhelming experiences and seems to involve many different types of personal experience, most commonly that occurring just before or during the ECT treatments.

Posttraumatic Amnesia. In posttraumatic amnesia caused by brain injury is usually seen a history of a clear-cut physical trauma, a period of unconsciousness or amnesia, or both, and objective clinical evidence of brain injury.

Seizure Disorders. In most seizure cases, the clinical presentation differs significantly from that of dissociative amnesia, with clear-cut ictal events and sequelae. Patients with pseudoepileptic seizures may also have dissociative symptoms, such as amnesia and an antecedent history of psychological trauma. Rarely, patients with recurrent, complex partial seizures present with ongoing bizarre behavior, memory problems, irritability, or violence, leading to a differential diagnostic puzzle. In some of these cases, the diagnosis can be clarified only by telemetry or ambulatory electroencephalographic (EEG) monitoring.

Substance-Related Amnesia. A variety of substances and intoxicants have been implicated in the production of amnesia. Common offending agents are listed in Table 20–3.

Transient Global Amnesia. Transient global amnesia can be mistaken for a dissociative amnesia, especially because stressful life events may precede either disorder. In transient global amnesia, however, there is the sudden onset of complete anterograde amnesia and learning abilities; pronounced retrograde amnesia; preservation of memory for personal identity; anxious awareness of memory loss with repeated, often perseverative, questioning; overall normal behavior; lack of gross neurological abnormalities in most cases; and rapid return of baseline cognitive function, with a persistent short retrograde amnesia. The patient usually is older than 50 years of age and shows risk factors for cerebrovascular disease, although epilepsy and migraine have been etiologically implicated in some cases.

Dissociative Disorders. Patients with dissociative identity disorder can present with acute forms of amnesia and fugue episodes. These patients, however, are characterized by a plethora of symptoms, only some of which are usually found in patients with dissociative amnesia. With respect to amnesia, most patients with dissociative identity disorder and those with dissociative disorder NOS with dissociative identity disorder features report multiple forms of complex amnesia, including recurrent blackouts, fugues, unexplained possessions, and fluctuations in skills, habits, and knowledge.

Acute Stress Disorder, Posttraumatic Stress Disorder, and Somatoform Disorders. Most forms of dissociative amnesia are best conceptualized as part of a group of trauma spectrum disorders that includes acute stress disorder, PTSD, and somatization disorder. Many patients with dissociative amnesia meet full or partial diagnostic criteria for acute stress disorder, PTSD, or somatization disorder, or a combination of these. Amnesia is a criterion symptom of each of the latter disorders. DSM-IV-TR stipulates that, to be diagnosed, the dissociative amnesia must be distinct from the course of acute stress disorder, PTSD, or somatization disorder. In practice, clinical judgment usually determines whether the extent of the amnesia warrants a separate dissociative diagnosis.

Malingering and Factitious Amnesia. No absolute way exists to differentiate dissociative amnesia from factitious or malingered amnesia. Malingerers have been noted to continue their deception even during hypnotically or barbiturate-facilitated interviews. A patient who presents to psychiatric attention asking to recover repressed memories as a chief complaint most likely has a factitious disorder or has been subject to suggestive influences. Most of these individuals actually do not describe bona fide amnesia when carefully questioned, but are often insistent that they must have been abused in childhood to explain their unhappiness or life dysfunction.

Course and Prognosis

Little is known about the clinical course of dissociative amnesia. Acute dissociative amnesia frequently spontaneously resolves once the person is removed to safety from traumatic or overwhelming circumstances. At the other extreme, some patients do develop chronic forms of generalized, continuous, or severe localized amnesia and are profoundly disabled and require high levels of social support, such as nursing home placement or intensive family caretaking. Clinicians should try to restore patients' lost memories to consciousness as soon as possible; otherwise, the repressed memory may form a nucleus in the unconscious mind around which future amnestic episodes may develop.

Treatment

Cognitive Therapy. Cognitive therapy may have specific benefits for individuals with trauma disorders. Identifying the specific cognitive distortions that are based in the trauma may provide an entrée into autobiographical memory for which the patient experiences amnesia. As the patient is becomes able to correct cognitive distortions, particularly about the meaning of prior trauma, more detailed recall of traumatic events may occur.

Hypnosis. Hypnosis can be used in a number of different ways in the treatment of dissociative amnesia. In particular, hypnotic interventions can be used to contain, modulate, and titrate the intensity of symptoms; to facilitate controlled recall of dissociated memories; to provide support and ego strengthening for the patient; and, finally, to promote working through and integration of dissociated material.

In addition, the patient can be taught self-hypnosis to apply containment and calming techniques in his or her everyday life. Successful use of containment techniques, whether hypnotically facilitated or not, also increases the patient's sense that he or she can more effectively be in control of alternations between intrusive symptoms and amnesia.

Somatic Therapies. No known pharmacotherapy exists for dissociative amnesia other than pharmacologically facilitated interviews. A variety of agents have been used for this purpose, including sodium amobarbital, thiopental (Pentothal), oral benzodiazepines, and amphetamines.

Pharmacologically facilitated interviews using intravenous amobarbital or diazepam are used primarily in working with acute amnesias and conversion reactions, among other indications, in general hospital medical and psychiatric services. This procedure is also occasionally useful in refractory cases of chronic dissociative amnesia when patients are unresponsive to other interventions. The material uncovered in a pharmacologically facilitated interview needs to be processed by the patient in his or her usual conscious state.

Group Psychotherapy. Time-limited and longer-term group psychotherapies have been reported to be helpful for combat veterans with PTSD and for survivors of childhood abuse. During group sessions, patients may recover memories for which they have had amnesia. Supportive interventions by the group members or the group therapist, or both, may facilitate integration and mastery of the dissociated material.

DEPERSONALIZATION DISORDER

The DSM-IV-TR identifies the essential feature of depersonalization as the persistent or recurrent feeling of detachment or estrangement from one's self. The individual may report feeling like an automaton or as if in a dream or watching himself or herself in a movie (Fig. 20–1). According to DSM-IV-TR, "there may be a sensation of being an outside observer of one's mental processes, one's body, or parts of one's body." Often, the patient has a sense of an absence of control over his or her actions. The current DSM-IV-TR definition of depersonalization disorder is found in Table 20–4.

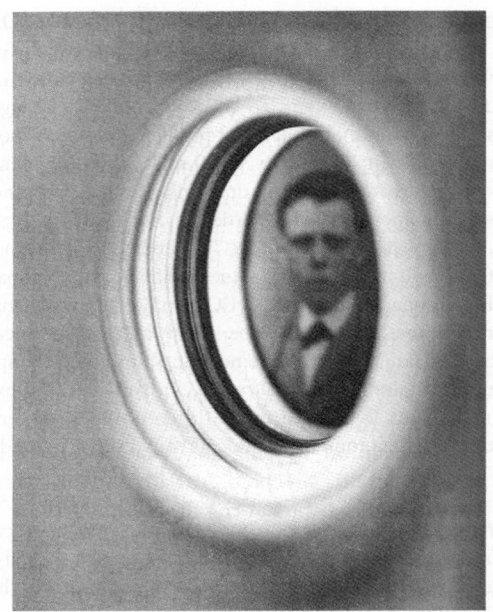

FIGURE 20–1
Dissociative states are characterized by feelings of unreality, as evoked in this photograph. (Courtesy of Arthur Tress for Magnum Photos, Inc.)

Epidemiology

Transient experiences of depersonalization and derealization are extremely common in normal and clinical populations. They are the third most commonly reported psychiatric symptoms, after depression and anxiety. One survey found a 1-year prevalence of 19 percent in the general population. It is common in seizure patients and migraine sufferers; they can also occur with use of psychedelic drugs, especially marijuana, lysergic acid diethylamide (LSD), and mescaline; and less frequently as a side effect of some medications, such as anticholinergic agents. They have been described after certain types of meditation, deep hypnosis, extended mirror or crystal gazing, and sensory deprivation experiences. They are also common after mild to moderate head injury, wherein little or no loss of consciousness occurs, but they are significantly less likely if unconsciousness lasts for more than 30 minutes. They are also common after life-threatening experiences, with or without serious bodily injury. Depersonalization is found two to four times more in women than in men.

Etiology

Psychodynamic. Traditional psychodynamic formulations have emphasized the disintegration of the ego or have viewed depersonalization as an affective response in defense of the ego.

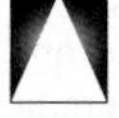

Table 20–4
DSM-IV-TR Diagnostic Criteria for Depersonalization Disorder

A. Persistent or recurrent experiences of feeling detached from, and as if one is an outside observer of, one's mental processes or body (e.g., feeling like one is in a dream).
B. During the depersonalization experience, reality testing remains intact.
C. The depersonalization causes clinically significant distress or impairment in social, occupational, or other important areas of functioning.
D. The depersonalization experience does not occur exclusively during the course of another mental disorder, such as schizophrenia, panic disorder, acute stress disorder, or another dissociative disorder, and is not due to the direct physiological effects of a substance (e.g., a drug of abuse, a medication) or a general medical condition (e.g., temporal lobe epilepsy).

(From American Psychiatric Association. *Diagnostic and Statistical Manual of Mental Disorders.* 4th ed. Text rev. Washington, DC: American Psychiatric Association; 2000, with permission.)

These explanations stress the role of overwhelming painful experiences or conflictual impulses as triggering events.

Traumatic Stress. A substantial proportion, typically one third to one half, of patients in clinical depersonalization case series report histories of significant trauma. Several studies of accident victims find as much as 60 percent of those with a life-threatening experience report at least transient depersonalization during the event or immediately thereafter. Military training studies find that symptoms of depersonalization and derealization are commonly evoked by stress and fatigue and are inversely related to performance.

Neurobiological Theories. The association of depersonalization with migraines and marijuana, its generally favorable response to selective serotonin reuptake inhibitor (SSRI) drugs, and the increase in depersonalization symptoms seen with the depletion of L-tryptophan, a serotonin precursor, point to serotoninergic involvement. Depersonalization is the primary dissociative symptom elicited by the drug-challenge studies described in the section on neurobiological theories of dissociation. These studies strongly implicate the *N*-Methyl-D-aspartate (NMDA) subtype of the glutamate receptor as central to the genesis of depersonalization symptoms.

Diagnosis and Clinical Features

A number of distinct components comprise the experience of depersonalization, including a sense of (1) bodily changes, (2) duality of self as observer and actor, (3) being cut off from others, and (4) being cut off from one's own emotions. Patients experiencing depersonalization often have great difficulty expressing what they are feeling. Trying to express their subjective suffering with banal phrases, such as "I feel dead," "nothing seems real," or "I'm standing outside of myself," depersonalized patients may not adequately convey to the examiner the distress they experience. While complaining bitterly about how this is ruining their life, they may nonetheless appear remarkably undistressed.

Ms. R was a 27-year-old, unmarried, graduate student with a master's degree in Biology. She complained about intermittent episodes of "standing back," usually associated with anxiety-provoking social situations. When asked about a recent episode, she described presenting in a seminar course. "All of a sudden, I was talking, but it didn't feel like it was me talking. It was very disconcerting. I had this feeling, 'who's doing the talking?' I felt like I was just watching someone else talk. Listening to words come out of my mouth, but I wasn't saying them. It wasn't me. It went on for a while. I was calm, even sort of peaceful. It was as if I was very far away. In the back of the room somewhere—just watching myself. But the person talking didn't even seem like me really. It was like I was watching someone else." The feeling lasted the rest of that day and persisted into the next, during which time it gradually dissipated. She thought that she remembered having similar experiences during high school, but was certain that they occurred at least once a year during college and graduate school.

As a child, Ms. R reported frequent intense anxiety from overhearing or witnessing the frequent violent arguments and periodic physical fights between her parents. In addition, the family was subject to many unpredictable dislocations and moves owing to the patient's father's intermittent difficulties with finances and employment. The patient's anxieties did not abate when the parents divorced when she was a late adolescent. Her father moved away and had little further contact with her. Her relationship with her mother became increasingly angry, critical, and contentious. She was unsure if she experienced depersonalization during childhood while listening to her parents' fights. (Adapted from case of Richard J. Loewenstein, M.D., and Frank W. Putnam, M.D.)

Differential Diagnosis

The variety of conditions associated with depersonalization complicate the differential diagnosis of depersonalization disorder. Depersonalization can result from a medical condition or neurological condition, intoxication or withdrawal from illicit drugs; as a side effect of medications; or can be associated with panic attacks, phobias, PTSD, or acute stress disorder, schizophrenia, or another dissociative disorder. A thorough medical and neurological evaluation is essential, including standard laboratory studies, an EEG, and any indicated drug screens. Drug-related depersonalization is typically transient, but persistent depersonalization can follow an episode of intoxication with a variety of substances, including marijuana, cocaine, and other psychostimulants. A range of neurological conditions, including seizure disorders, brain tumors, postconcussive syndrome, metabolic abnormalities, migraine, vertigo, and Ménière's disease, have been reported as causes. Depersonalization caused by organic conditions tends to be primarily sensory without the elaborated descriptions and personalized meanings common to psychiatric etiologies.

Course and Prognosis

Depersonalization after traumatic experiences or intoxications commonly remits spontaneously after removal from the traumatic circumstances or ending of the episode of intoxication. Depersonalization accompanying mood, psychotic, or other anxiety disorders commonly remits with definitive treatment of these conditions.

Depersonalization disorder itself may have an episodic, relapsing and remitting, or chronic course. Many patients with chronic depersonalization may have a course characterized by severe impairment in occupational, social, and personal functioning. Mean age of onset is thought to be in late adolescence or early adulthood in most cases.

Treatment

Clinicians working with patients with depersonalization disorder often find them to be a singularly clinically refractory group. Some systematic evidence indicates that SSRI antidepressants, such as fluoxetine (Prozac), may be helpful to patients with depersonalization disorder. Two recent, double-blind, placebo-controlled studies, however, found no efficacy for fluvoxetine (Luvox) and lamotrigine, respectively, for depersonalization disorder. Some patients with depersonalization disorder respond at best sporadically and partially to the usual groups of psychiatric medications, singly or in combination: antidepressants, mood stabilizers, typical and atypical neuroleptics, anticonvulsants, and so forth.

Many different types of psychotherapy have been used to treat depersonalization disorder: psychodynamic, cognitive, cognitive-behavioral, hypnotherapeutic, and supportive. Many such patients do not have a robust response to these specific types of standard psychotherapy. Stress management strategies, distraction techniques, reduction of sensory stimulation, relaxation training, and physical exercise may be somewhat helpful in some patients.

DISSOCIATIVE FUGUE

The essential feature of dissociative fugue (Table 20-5) is described as sudden, unexpected travel away from home or one's customary place of daily activities, with inability to recall some or all of one's past. This is accompanied by confusion about personal identity or even the assumption of a new identity. The disturbance does not occur exclusively during the course of dissociative identity disorder and is not due to the direct physiological effects of a substance or a general medical condition. The symptoms must cause clinically significant distress or impairment in social, occupational, or other important areas of functioning.

Etiology

Traumatic circumstances (i.e., combat, rape, recurrent childhood sexual abuse, massive social dislocations, natural disasters), leading to an altered state of consciousness dominated by a wish to flee, are the underlying cause of most fugue episodes. In some cases is seen a similar antecedent history, although a psychological trauma is not present at the onset of the fugue episode. In these cases, instead of, or in addition to, external dangers or traumas, the patients are usually struggling with extreme emotions or impulses (i.e., overwhelming fear, guilt, shame, or intense incestuous, sexual, suicidal, or violent urges) that are in conflict with the patient's conscience or ego ideals.

Table 20–5
DSM-IV-TR Diagnostic Criteria for Dissociative Fugue

A. The predominant disturbance is sudden, unexpected travel away from home or one's customary place of work, with inability to recall one's past.

B. Confusion about personal identity or assumption of a new identity (partial or complete).

C. The disturbance does not occur exclusively during the course of dissociative identity disorder and is not due to the direct physiological effects of a substance (e.g., a drug of abuse, a medication) or a general medical condition (e.g., temporal lobe epilepsy).

D. The symptoms cause clinically significant distress or impairment in social, occupational, or other important areas of functioning.

(From American Psychiatric Association. *Diagnostic and Statistical Manual of Mental Disorders.* 4th ed. Text rev. Washington, DC: American Psychiatric Association; 2000, with permission.)

Epidemiology

The disorder is thought to be more common during natural disasters, wartime, or times of major social dislocation and violence, although no systematic data exist on this point. No adequate data exist to demonstrate a gender bias to this disorder; however, most cases describe men, primarily in the military. Dissociative fugue is usually described in adults.

Diagnosis and Clinical Features

Dissociative fugues have been described to last from minutes to months. Some patients report multiple fugues. In most cases in which this was described, a more chronic dissociative disorder, such as dissociative identity disorder, was not ruled out.

In some extremely severe cases of PTSD, nightmares may be terminated by a waking fugue in which the patient runs to another part of the house or runs outside. Children or adolescents may be more limited than adults in their ability to travel. Thus, fugues in this population may be brief and involve only short distances.

A teenage girl was continually sexually abused by her alcoholic father and another family friend. She was threatened with perpetration of sexual abuse on her younger siblings if she told anyone about the abuse. The girl became suicidal but felt that she had to stay alive to protect her siblings. She precipitously ran away from home after being raped by her father and several of his friends as a "birthday present" for one of them. She traveled to a part of the city where she had lived previously with the idea that she would find her grandmother with whom she had lived before the abuse began. She traveled by public transportation and walked the streets, apparently without attracting attention. After approximately 8 hours, she was stopped by the police in a curfew check. When questioned, she could not recall recent events or give her current address, insisting that she lived with her grandmother. On initial psychiatric examination, she was aware of her identity, but she believed that it was 2 years earlier, giving her age as 2 years younger and insisting that none of the events of recent years had occurred. (Courtesy of Richard J. Loewenstein, M.D., and Frank W. Putnam, M.D.)

After the termination of a fugue, the patient may experience perplexity, confusion, trance-like behaviors, depersonalization, derealization, and conversion symptoms, in addition to amnesia. Some patients may terminate a fugue with an episode of generalized dissociative amnesia.

As the patient with dissociative fugue begins to become less dissociated, he or she may display mood disorder symptoms, intense suicidal ideation, and PTSD or other anxiety disorder symptoms. In the classic cases, an alter identity is created under whose auspices the patient lives for a period of time. Many of these latter cases are better classified as dissociative identity disorder or dissociative disorder NOS with features of dissociative identity disorder.

Differential Diagnosis

Individuals with dissociative amnesia may engage in confused wandering during an amnesia episode. In dissociative fugue, however, there is *purposeful* travel away from the individual's home or customary place of daily activities, usually with the individual preoccupied by a single idea that is accompanied by a wish to run away.

Patients with dissociative identity disorder may have symptoms of dissociative fugue, usually recurrently throughout their lives. Patients with dissociative identity disorder have multiple forms of complex amnesias and, usually, multiple alter identities that develop, starting in childhood.

In complex partial seizures, patients have been noted to exhibit wandering or semipurposeful behavior, or both, during seizures or in postictal states, for which subsequent amnesia occurs. Seizure patients in an epileptic fugue often exhibit abnormal behavior, however, including confusion, perseveration, and abnormal or repetitive movements. Other features of seizures are typically reported in the clinical history, such as an aura, motor abnormalities, stereotyped behavior, perceptual alterations, incontinence, and a postictal state. Serial or telemetric EEGs, or both, usually show abnormalities associated with behavioral pathology.

Wandering behavior during a variety of general medical conditions, toxic and substance-related disorders, delirium, dementia, and organic amnestic syndromes could theoretically be confused with dissociative fugue. In most cases, however, the somatic, toxic, neurological, or substance-related disorder can be ruled in by the history, physical examination, laboratory tests, or toxicological and drug screening. Use of alcohol or substances may be involved in precipitating an episode of dissociative fugue.

Wandering and purposeful travel can occur during the manic phase of bipolar disorder or schizoaffective disorder. Patients who are manic may not recall behavior that occurred in the euthymic or depressed state and vice versa. In purposeful travel owing to mania, however, the patient is usually preoccupied with grandiose ideas and often calls attention to himself or herself because of inappropriate behavior. Assumption of an alternate identity does not occur.

Similarly, peripatetic behavior can occur in some patients with schizophrenia. Memory for events during wandering episodes in such patients may be difficult to ascertain owing to the patient's thought disorder. Patients with dissociative fugue, however, do not demonstrate a psychotic thought disorder or other symptoms of psychosis.

Malingering of dissociative fugue can occur in individuals who are attempting to flee a situation involving legal, financial, or personal difficulties, as well as in soldiers who are attempting to avoid combat or unpleasant military duties. No test, battery of tests, or set of procedures exist that invariably distinguish true dissociative symptoms from those that are malingered. Malingering of dissociative symptoms, such as reports of amnesia for purposeful travel during an episode of antisocial behavior, can be maintained even during hypnotic or pharmacologically facilitated interviews. Many malingerers confess spontaneously or when confronted. In the forensic context, the examiner should always carefully consider the diagnosis of malingering when fugue is claimed.

Course and Prognosis

Most fugues are relatively brief, lasting from hours to days. Most individuals appear to recover, although refractory dissociative amnesia may persist in rare cases. Some studies have described recurrent fugues in most individuals presenting with an episode of dissociative fugue. No systematic modern data exist that attempt to differentiate dissociative fugue from dissociative identity disorder with recurrent fugues.

Treatment

Dissociative fugue is usually treated with an eclectic, psychodynamically oriented psychotherapy that focuses on helping the patient recover memory for identity and recent experience. Hypnotherapy and pharmacologically facilitated interviews are frequently necessary adjunctive techniques to assist with memory recovery. Patients may need medical treatment for injuries sustained during the fugue, food, and sleep.

Clinicians should be prepared for the emergence of suicidal ideation or self-destructive ideas and impulses as the traumatic or stressful prefugue circumstances are revealed. Psychiatric hospitalization may be indicated if the patient is an outpatient.

Family, sexual, occupational, or legal problems that were part of the original matrix that generated the fugue episode may be substantially exacerbated by the time the patient's original identity and life situation are detected. Thus, family treatment and social service interventions may be necessary to help resolve such complex difficulties.

When dissociative fugue involves assumption of a new identity, it is useful to conceptualize this entity as psychologically vital to protecting the person. Traumatic experiences, memories, cognitions, identifications, emotions, strivings, or self-perceptions, or a combination of these, have become so conflicting and, yet, so peremptory that the person can resolve them only by embodying them in an alter identity. The therapeutic goal in such cases is neither suppression of the new identity nor fascinated explication of all its attributes. As in dissociative identity disorder, the clinician should appreciate the importance of the psychodynamic information contained within the alter personality state and the intensity of the psychological forces that necessitated its creation. In these cases, the most desirable therapeutic outcome is fusion of the identities, with the person working through and integrating the memories of the experiences that precipitated the fugue.

DISSOCIATIVE IDENTITY DISORDER

According to DSM-IV-TR, dissociative identity disorder, previously called *multiple personality disorder*, "is characterized by the presence of two or more distinct identities or personality states that recurrently take control of the individual's behavior accompanied by an inability to recall important personal information that is too extensive to be explained by ordinary forgetfulness." The identities or personality states, sometimes called *alters*, *self-states*, *alter identities*, or *parts*, among other terms, differ from one another in that each presents as having "its own relatively enduring pattern of perceiving, relating to, and thinking about the environment and self".

Epidemiology

Few systematic epidemiological data exist for dissociative identity disorder. Clinical studies report female to male ratios between 5 to 1 and 9 to 1 for diagnosed cases.

Etiology

Dissociative identity disorder is strongly linked to severe experiences of early childhood trauma, usually maltreatment. The rates of reported severe childhood trauma for child and adult patients with dissociative identity disorder range from 85 to 97 percent of cases. Physical and sexual abuse are the most frequently reported sources of childhood trauma. The contribution of genetic factors is only now being systematically assessed, but preliminary studies have not found evidence of a significant genetic contribution.

Diagnosis and Clinical Features

Table 20-6 lists the DSM-IV-TR criteria for dissociative identity disorder.

Dimensions of Trauma. A number of common dimensions underlie traumatic sequelae. Affect modulation is frequently disturbed, giving rise to mood swings, depression, suicidal tendency, and generalized irritability. Impulse control is often impaired, leading to risk-taking, substance abuse, and inappropriate or self-destructive behaviors. High levels of anxiety and panic are common. A variety of disturbances in sense of self, from the identity diffusion seen in patients who are borderline to the alter identities of dissociative identity disorder, reflects disruptions in the psychological integration of traumatic and nontraumatic aspects of self. Eating disorders are common in a subgroup of trauma patients and may also relate to disorders of body image and identity. Frequent somatization, conversion, and psychophysiological disorders may represent disruptions in the integration of psychic and somatic representations of overwhelming recollections, intolerable affects, posttraumatic cognitive schema, and intrapsychic conflicts. Childhood sexual abuse survivors with psychophysiological disorders are more likely to have a lower threshold for experiencing physiological phenomena as noxious or painful.

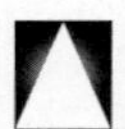

Table 20–6
DSM-IV-TR Diagnostic Criteria for Dissociative Identity Disorder

A. The presence of two or more distinct identities or personality states (each with its own relatively enduring pattern of perceiving, relating to, and thinking about the environment and self).

B. At least two of these identities or personality states recurrently take control of the person's behavior.

C. Inability to recall important personal information that is too extensive to be explained by ordinary forgetfulness.

D. The disturbance is not due to the direct physiological effects of a substance (e.g., blackouts or chaotic behavior during alcohol intoxication) or a general medical condition (e.g., complex partial seizures). **Note:** In children, the symptoms are not attributable to imaginary playmates or other fantasy play.

(From American Psychiatric Association. *Diagnostic and Statistical Manual of Mental Disorders.* 4th ed. Text rev. Washington, DC: American Psychiatric Association; 2000, with permission.)

Memory and Amnesia Symptoms. Dissociative disturbances of memory are manifest in several basic ways and are frequently observable in clinical settings (Table 20–7). As part of the general mental status examination, clinicians should routinely inquire about experiences of losing time, black-out spells, and major gaps in the continuity of recall for personal information. Dissociative time loss experiences are too extensive to be explained by normal forgetting and typically have sharply demarcated onsets and offsets.

Patients with dissociative disorder often report significant gaps in autobiographical memory, especially for childhood events. Dissociative gaps in autobiographical recall are usually sharply demarcated and do not fit the normal decline in autobiographical recall for younger ages.

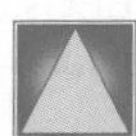

Table 20–7
Amnesia and Memory Symptoms

Blackouts or time loss
Disremembered behavior
Fugues
Unexplained possessions
Inexplicable changes in relationships
Fluctuations in skills, habits, and knowledge
Fragmentary recall of entire life history
Chronic mistaken identity experiences
Microdissociations

Mental status examination questions for dissociative amnesia

If answers are positive, ask the patient to describe the event. Make sure to specify that the symptom does not occur during an episode of intoxication.

(1) Do you ever have blackouts? Blank spells? Memory lapses?
(2) Do you lose time? Have gaps in your experience of time?
(3) Have you ever traveled a considerable distance without recollection of how you did this or where you went exactly?
(4) Do people tell you of things you have said and done that you do not recall?
(5) Do you find objects in your possession (such as clothes, personal items, groceries in your grocery cart, books, tools, equipment, jewelry, vehicles, weapons, and so on) that you do not remember acquiring? Out-of-character items? Items that a child might have? Toys? Stuffed animals?
(6) Have you ever been told or found evidence that you have talents and abilities that you did not know that you had? For example, musical, artistic, mechanical, literary, athletic, or other talents? Do your tastes seem to fluctuate a lot? For example, food preference, personal habits, taste in music or clothes, and so forth.
(7) Do you have gaps in your memory of your life? Are you missing parts of your memory for your life history? Are you missing memories of some important events in your life? For example, weddings, birthdays, graduations, pregnancies, birth of children, and so on.
(8) Do you lose track of or tune out conversations or therapy sessions as they are occurring? Do you find that, while you are listening to someone talk, you did not hear all or part of what was just said?
(9) What is the longest period of time that you have lost? Minutes? Hours? Days? Weeks? Months? Years? Describe.

(Adapted from Loewenstein RJ. An office mental status examination for chronic complex dissociative symptoms and multiple personality disorder. *Psychiatr Clin North Am.* 1991;14:567–604, with permission.)

Ms. A, a 33-year-old married woman employed as a librarian in a school for disturbed children, presented to psychiatric attention after discovering her 5-year-old daughter "playing doctor" with several neighborhood children. Although this event was of little consequence, the patient began to become fearful that her daughter would be molested. The patient was seen by her internist and was treated with antianxiety agents and antidepressants, but with little improvement. She sought psychiatric consultation from several clinicians, but repeated, good trials of antidepressants, antianxiety agents, and supportive psychotherapy resulted in limited improvement. After the death of her father from complications of alcoholism, the patient became more symptomatic. He had been estranged from the family since the patient was approximately 12 years of age, owing to his drinking and associated antisocial behavior.

Psychiatric hospitalization was precipitated by the patient's arrest for disorderly conduct in a nearby city. She was found in a hotel, in revealing clothing, engaged in an altercation with a man. She denied knowledge of how she had come to the hotel, although the man insisted that she had come there under a different name for a voluntary sexual encounter.

On psychiatric examination, the patient described dense amnesia for the first 12 years of her life, with the feeling that her "life started at 12 years old." She reported that, for as long as she could remember, she had an imaginary companion, an elderly black woman, who advised her and kept her company. She reported hearing other voices in her head: several women and children, as well as her father's voice repeatedly speaking to her in a derogatory way. She reported that much of her life since 12 years of age was also punctuated by episodes of amnesia: for work, for her marriage, for the birth of her children, and for her sex life with her husband. She reported perplexing changes in skills; for example, she was often told that she played the piano well but had no conscious awareness that she could do so. Her husband reported that she had always been "forgetful" of conversations and family activities. He also noted that, at times, she would speak like a child; at times, she would adopt a southern accent; and, at other times, she would be angry and provocative. She frequently had little recall of these episodes.

Questioned more closely about her early life, the patient appeared to enter a trance and stated, "I just don't want to be locked in the closet" in a child-like voice. Inquiry about this produced rapid shifts in state between alter identities who differed in manifested age, facial expression, voice tone, and knowledge of the patient's history. One spoke in an angry, expletive-filled manner and appeared irritable and preoccupied with sexuality. She discussed the episode with the man in the hotel and stated that it was she who had arranged it. Gradually, the alters described a history of family chaos, brutality, and neglect during the first 12 years of the patient's life, until her mother, also alcoholic, achieved sobriety and fled her husband, taking her children with her. The patient, in the alter identities, described episodes of physical abuse, sexual abuse, and emotional torment by the father, her siblings, and her mother.

After assessment of family members, the patient's mother also met diagnostic criteria for dissociative identity disorder, as did her older sister, who also had been molested. A brother met diagnostic criteria for PTSD, major depression, and alcohol dependence. (Adapted from case of Richard J. Loewenstein, M.D., and Frank W. Putnam, M.D.)

Dissociative Alterations in Identity. Clinically, dissociative alterations in identity may first be manifested by odd first-person plural or third-person singular or plural self-references. In addition, patients may refer to themselves using their own first names or make depersonalized self-references, such as "the body," when describing themselves and others. Patients often describe a profound sense of concretized internal division or personified internal conflicts between parts of themselves. In some instances, these parts may have proper names or may be designated by their predominate affect or function, for example, "the angry one" or "the wife." Patients may suddenly change the way in which they refer to others, for example, "the son" instead of "my son."

Other Associated Symptoms. Because dissociative identity disorder is conceptualized as a trauma spectrum disorder, most of these patients also meet diagnostic criteria for PTSD (Table 20–8). Approximately 70 percent of patients with dissociative identity disorder have been shown to meet diagnostic criteria for PTSD by DSM-IV-TR criteria.

Patients with dissociative identity disorder commonly exhibit multiple types of psychophysiological, somatoform, and conversion symptoms. Of patients with dissociative identity disorder, 40 to 60 percent also meet diagnostic criteria for somatization disorder, and many others meet diagnostic criteria for undifferentiated somatoform disorder, somatoform pain disorder, or conversion disorder, or a combination of these.

Most patients with dissociative identity disorder meet criteria for a mood disorder, usually one of the depression spectrum disorders. Frequent, rapid mood swings are common, but these are usually caused by posttraumatic and dissociative phenomena, not a true cyclic mood disorder. Considerable overlap may

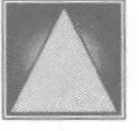

Table 20–8
Dissociative Identity Disorder–Associated Symptoms Commonly Found in Dissociative Identity Disorder

Posttraumatic stress disorder symptoms
- Intrusive symptoms
- Hyperarousal
- Avoidance and numbing symptoms

Somatoform symptoms
- Conversion and pseudoneurological symptoms
- Seizure-like episodes
- Somatization disorder or Briquet's syndrome
- Somatoform pain symptoms
- Headache, abdominal, musculoskeletal, pelvic pain
- Undifferentiated somatoform disorder
- Psychophysiological symptoms or disorders
- Asthma and breathing problems
- Perimenstrual disorders
- Irritable bowel syndrome
- Gastroesophageal reflux disease
- Somatic memory

Affective symptoms
- Depressed mood, dysphoria, or anhedonia
- Brief mood swings or mood lability
- Suicidal thoughts and attempts or self-mutilation
- Guilt and survivor guilt
- Helpless and hopeless feelings

Obsessive-compulsive symptoms
- Ruminations about trauma
- Obsessive counting, singing
- Arranging
- Washing
- Checking

exist between PTSD symptoms of anxiety, disturbed sleep, and dysphoria and mood disorder symptoms.

Obsessive-compulsive personality traits are common in dissociative identity disorder, and intercurrent obsessive-compulsive disorder (OCD) symptoms are regularly found in patients with dissociative identity disorder, with a subgroup manifesting severe OCD symptoms. OCD symptoms commonly have a posttraumatic quality: checking repeatedly to be sure that no one can enter the house or the bedroom, compulsive washing to relieve a feeling of being dirty because of abuse, and repetitive counting or singing in the mind to distract from anxiety over being abused, for example.

Child and Adolescent Presentations. Children and adolescents manifest the same core dissociative symptoms and secondary clinical phenomena as adults. Age-related differences in autonomy and lifestyle, however, may significantly influence the clinical expression of dissociative symptoms in youth. Younger children, in particular, have a less linear and less continuous sense of time and often are not able to self-identify dissociative discontinuities in their behavior. Often additional informants, such as teachers and relatives, are available to help document dissociative behaviors.

A number of normal childhood phenomena, such as imaginary companionship and elaborated daydreams, must be carefully differentiated from pathological dissociation in younger children. The clinical presentation may be that of an elaborated or autonomous imaginary companionship, with the imaginary companions taking control of the child's behavior, often experienced through passive influence experiences or auditory pseudohallucinations, or both, that command the child to behave in certain ways.

Differential Diagnosis

Table 20–9 lists the most common disorders that must be differentiated from dissociative identity disorder.

Factitious, Imitative, and Malingered Dissociative Identity Disorder. Indicators of falsified or *imitative dissociative identity disorder* are reported to include those typical of other factitious or malingering presentations. These include symptom exaggeration, lies, use of symptoms to excuse antisocial behavior (e.g., amnesia only for bad behavior), amplification of symptoms when under observation, refusal to allow collateral contacts, legal problems, and pseudologia fantastica. Patients with genuine dissociative identity disorder are usually confused, conflicted, ashamed, and distressed by their symptoms and trauma history. Those with nongenuine disorder frequently show little dysphoria about their disorder.

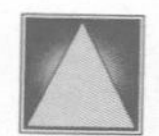

Table 20–9
Differential Diagnosis of Dissociative Identity Disorder

Comorbidity versus differential diagnosis
Affective disorders
Psychotic disorders
Anxiety disorders
Posttraumatic stress disorder
Personality disorders
Cognitive disorders
Neurological and seizure disorders
Somatoform disorders
Factitious disorders
Malingering
Other dissociative disorders
Deep-trance phenomena, such as the hidden observer or ego states

Course and Prognosis

Little is known about the natural history of untreated dissociative identity disorder. Some individuals with untreated dissociative identity disorder are thought to continue involvement in abusive relationships or violent subcultures, or both, that may result in the traumatization of their children, with the potential for additional family transmission of the disorder. Many authorities believe that some percentage of patients with undiagnosed or untreated dissociative identity disorder die by suicide or as a result of their risk-taking behaviors.

Prognosis is poorer in patients with comorbid organic mental disorders, psychotic disorders (*not* dissociative identity disorder pseudopsychosis), and severe medical illnesses. Refractory substance abuse and eating disorders also suggest a poorer prognosis. Other factors that usually indicate a poorer outcome include significant antisocial personality features, current criminal activity, ongoing perpetration of abuse, and current victimization, with refusal to leave abusive relationships. Repeated adult traumas with recurrent episodes of acute stress disorder may severely complicate the clinical course.

Treatment

Psychotherapy. Successful psychotherapy for the patient with dissociative identity disorder requires the clinician to be comfortable with a range of psychotherapeutic interventions and be willing to actively work to structure the treatment. These modalities include psychoanalytic psychotherapy, cognitive therapy, behavioral therapy, hypnotherapy, and a familiarity with the psychotherapy and psychopharmacological management of the traumatized patient. Comfort with family treatment and systems theory is helpful in working with a patient who subjectively experiences himself or herself as a complex system of selves with alliances, family-like relationships, and intragroup conflict. A grounding in work with patients with somatoform disorders may also be helpful in sorting through the plethora of somatic symptoms with which these patients commonly present.

Cognitive Therapy. Many cognitive distortions associated with dissociative identity disorder are only slowly responsive to cognitive therapy techniques, and successful cognitive interventions may lead to additional dysphoria. A subgroup of patients with dissociative identity disorder does not progress beyond a long-term supportive treatment entirely directed toward stabilization of their multiple multiaxial difficulties. To the extent that they can be engaged in treatment at all, these patients require a long-term treatment focus on symptom containment and management of their overall life dysfunction, as would be the case with any other severely and persistently ill psychiatric patient.

Hypnosis. Hypnotherapeutic interventions can often alleviate self-destructive impulses or reduce symptoms, such as flashbacks, dissociative hallucinations, and passive-influence experiences. Teaching the patient self-hypnosis may help with crises outside of sessions. Hypnosis can be useful for accessing specific alter personality states and their sequestered affects and memories. Hypnosis is also used to create relaxed mental states in which negative life events can be examined without overwhelming anxiety. Clinicians using hypnosis should be trained in its use in general and in trauma populations. Clinicians should be aware of current controversies over the impact of hypnosis on accurate reporting of recollections and should use appropriate informed consent for its use.

Psychopharmacological Interventions. Antidepressant medications are often important in the reduction of depression and stabilization of mood. A variety of PTSD symptoms, especially intrusive and hyperarousal symptoms, are partially medication responsive. Clinicians report some success with SSRI, tricyclic, and monamine oxidase (MAO) antidepressants, β-blockers, clonidine (Catapres), anticonvulsants, and benzodiazepines in reducing intrusive symptoms, hyperarousal, and anxiety in patients with dissociative identity disorder. Recent research suggests that the α_1-adrenergic antagonist, prazosin (Minipress), may be helpful for PTSD nightmares. Case reports suggest that aggression may respond to carbamazepine in some individuals if EEG abnormalities are present. Patients with obsessive-compulsive symptoms may respond to antidepressants with antiobsessive efficacy. Open-label studies suggest that naltrexone (ReVia) may be helpful for amelioration of recurrent self-injurious behaviors in a subset of traumatized patients.

The atypical neuroleptics, such as risperidone (Risperdal), quetiapine (Seroquel), ziprasidone (Geodon), and olanzapine (Zyprexa), may be more effective and better tolerated than typical neuroleptics for overwhelming anxiety and intrusive PTSD symptoms in patients with dissociative identity disorder. Occasionally, an extremely disorganized, overwhelmed, chronically ill patient with dissociative identity disorder, who has not responded to trials of other neuroleptics, responds favorably to a trial of clozapine (Clozaril).

Electroconvulsive Therapy. For some patients, ECT is helpful in ameliorating refractory mood disorders and does not worsen dissociative memory problems. Clinical experience in tertiary care settings for severely ill patients with dissociative identity disorder suggests that a clinical picture of major depression with persistent, refractory melancholic features across all alter states may predict a positive response to ECT. This response is usually only partial, however, as is typical for most successful somatic treatments in the dissociative identity disorder population.

Target symptoms and somatic treatments for dissociative identity disorder are listed in Table 20–10.

Adjunctive Treatments

GROUP THERAPY. In therapy groups including general psychiatric patients, the emergence of alter personalities can be disruptive to the group process by eliciting excess fascination or by frightening other patients. Therapy groups composed only of patients with dissociative identity disorder are reported to be more successful, although the groups must be carefully structured, must provide firm limits, and should generally focus only on here-and-now issues of coping and adaptation.

FAMILY THERAPY. Family or couples therapy is often important for long-term stabilization and to address pathological family and marital processes that are common in patients with dissociative identity disorder and their family members. Education of family and concerned others about dissociative identity disorder and dissociative identity disorder treatment may help family members cope more effectively with dissociative identity disorder and PTSD symptoms in their loved ones. Group interventions for education and support of family members have also been found helpful. Sex therapy may be an important part of couple's

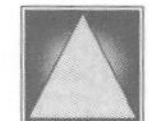

Table 20–10
Medications for Associated Symptoms in Dissociative Identity Disorder

Medications and somatic treatments for PTSD, affective disorders, anxiety disorders, and OCD
- Selective serotonin reuptake inhibitors (no preferred agent, except for OCD symptoms)
- Fluvoxamine (Luvox) (for OCD presentations)
- Clomipramine (Anafranil) (for OCD presentations)
- Tricyclic antidepressants
- Monoamine oxidase inhibitors (if patient can reliably maintain diet safely)
- Electroconvulsive therapy (for refractory depression with persistent melancholic features across all dissociative identity disorder alters)
- Mood stabilizers (more useful for PTSD and anxiety than mood swings)
- Divalproex (Depakote)
- Lamotrigine (Lamictal)
- Gabapentin (Neurontin)
- Topiramate (Topamax)
- Carbamazepine (Tegretol)
- Benzodiazepines
- Clonazepam (Klonopin) and lorazepam (Ativan) have best track records
- Atypical neuroleptics
- Typical neuroleptics (if patient fails trials of atypicals)
- β-blockers (for PTSD hyperarousal symptoms)
- Clonidine (Catapres) (for PTSD hyperarousal symptoms)
- Prazosin (Minipress) (for PTSD nightmares)

Medications for thought disorder
- Atypical neuroleptics preferred

Medications for acute dyscontrol
- Oral or intramuscular neuroleptics
- Oral or intramuscular benzodiazepines

Medications for sleep problems
- Low-dose trazodone (Desyrel)
- Low-dose mirtazapine (Remeron)
- Low-dose tricyclic antidepressants
- Low-dose neuroleptics
- Benzodiazepines (often less helpful for sleep problems in this population)
- Zolpidem (Ambien)
- Anticholinergic agents (diphenhydramine [Benadryl], hydroxyzine [Vistaril])
- Chloral hydrate (primarily for inpatient use)

Medications for self-injury, addictions
- Naltrexone (ReVia)

OCD, obsessive-compulsive disorder; PTSD, posttraumatic stress disorder.

treatment, because the patient with dissociative identity disorder may become intensely phobic of intimate contact for periods of time, and spouses may have little idea how to deal with this in a helpful way.

SELF-HELP GROUPS. Patients with dissociative identity disorder usually have a negative outcome to self-help groups or 12-step groups for incest survivors. A variety of problematic issues occur in these settings, including intensification of PTSD symptoms because of discussion of trauma material without clinical safeguards, exploitation of the patient with dissociative identity disorder by predatory group members, contamination of that patient's recall by group discussions of trauma, and a feeling of alienation even from these other reputed sufferers of trauma and dissociation.

EXPRESSIVE AND OCCUPATIONAL THERAPIES. Expressive and occupational therapies, such as art and movement therapy, have proved particularly helpful in treatment of patients with dissociative identity disorder. Art therapy may be used to help with containment and structuring of severe dissociative identity disorder and PTSD symptoms, as well as to permit these patients safer expression of thoughts, feelings, mental images, and conflicts that they have difficulty verbalizing. Movement therapy may facilitate normalization of body sense and body image for these severely traumatized patients. Occupational therapy may help the patient with focused, structured activities that can be completed successfully and may help with grounding and symptom management.

DISSOCIATIVE DISORDER NOT OTHERWISE SPECIFIED

The category of dissociative disorder NOS covers all of the conditions characterized by a primary dissociative response that do not meet diagnostic criteria for one of the other DSM-IV-TR dissociative disorders. Dissociative disorder NOS cases must also fail to exclusively meet diagnostic criteria for acute stress disorder, PTSD, or somatization disorder, which all include dissociative symptoms among their criteria (Table 20–11).

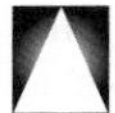

Table 20–11
DSM-IV-TR Diagnostic Criteria for Dissociative Disorder Not Otherwise Specified

This category is included for disorders in which the predominant feature is a dissociative symptom (i.e., a disruption in the usually integrated functions of consciousness, memory, identity, or perception of the environment) that does not meet the criteria for any specific dissociative disorder. Examples include the following:

(1) Clinical presentations similar to dissociative identity disorder that fail to meet full criteria for this disorder. Examples include presentations in which (a) there are not two or more distinct personality states or (b) amnesia for important personal information does not occur.
(2) Derealization unaccompanied by depersonalization in adults.
(3) States of dissociation that occur in individuals who have been subjected to periods of prolonged and intense coercive persuasion (e.g., brainwashing, thought reform, or indoctrination while captive).
(4) Dissociative trance disorder: single or episodic disturbances in the state of consciousness, identity, or memory that are indigenous to particular locations and cultures. Dissociative trance involves narrowing of awareness of immediate surroundings or stereotyped behaviors or movements that are experienced as being beyond one's control. Possession trance involves replacement of the customary sense of personal identity by a new identity, attributed to the influence of a spirit, power, deity, or other person and associated with stereotyped involuntary movements or amnesia, and is perhaps the most common dissociative disorder in Asia. Examples include *amok* (Indonesia), *bebainan* (Indonesia), *latah* (Malaysia), *pibloktoq* (Arctic), *ataque de nervios* (Latin America), and possession (India). The dissociative or trance disorder is not a normal part of a broadly accepted collective cultural or religious practice.
(5) Loss of consciousness, stupor, or coma not attributable to a general medical condition.
(6) Ganser syndrome: the giving of approximate answers to questions (e.g., 2 + 2 = 5) when not associated with dissociative amnesia or dissociative fugue.

(From American Psychiatric Association. *Diagnostic and Statistical Manual of Mental Disorders.* 4th ed. Text rev. Washington, DC: American Psychiatric Association; 2000, with permission.)

Dissociative Trance Disorder

Dissociative trance disorder is manifest by a temporary, marked alteration in the state of consciousness or by loss of the customary sense of personal identity without the replacement by an alternate sense of identity (Table 20–12). A variant of this, possession trance, involves single or episodic alternations in the state of consciousness, characterized by the exchange of the person's customary identity by a new identity usually attributed to a spirit, divine power, deity, or another person. In this possessed state, the individual exhibits stereotypical and culturally determined behaviors or experiences being controlled by the possessing entity. There must be partial or full amnesia for the event. The trance or possession state must not be a normally accepted part of a cultural or religious practice and must cause significant distress or functional impairment in one or more of the usual domains. Finally, the dissociative trance state must not occur exclusively during the course of a psychotic disorder and is not the result of any substance use or general medical condition.

Brainwashing

DSM-IV-TR describes this dissociative disorder as "states of dissociation that occur in individuals who have been subjected to periods of prolonged and intense coercive persuasion (e.g., brainwashing, thought reform, or indoctrination while captive)." Brainwashing occurs largely in the setting of political reform, as has been described at length with the Cultural Revolution in communist China, war imprisonment, torture of political dissidents, terrorist hostages, and, more familiarly in Western culture: totalitarian cult indoctrination. It implies that under conditions of adequate stress and duress, individuals can be made to comply with the demands of those in power, thereby undergoing major changes in their personality, beliefs, and behaviors. Persons submitted to such conditions can undergo considerable harm,

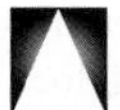

Table 20–12
DSM-IV-TR Research Criteria for Dissociative Trance Disorder

A. Either (1) or (2):
 (1) Trance, that is, temporary marked alteration in the state of consciousness or loss of customary sense of personal identity without replacement by an alternate identity, associated with at least one of the following:
  (a) Narrowing of awareness of immediate surroundings or unusually narrow and selective focusing on environmental stimuli
  (b) Stereotyped behaviors or movements that are experienced as being beyond one's control
 (2) Possession trance, a single or episodic alteration in the state of consciousness characterized by the replacement of customary sense of personal identity by a new identity. This is attributed to the influence of a spirit, power, deity, or other person, as evidenced by one or more of the following:
  (a) Stereotyped and culturally determined behaviors or movements that are experienced as being controlled by the possessing agent
  (b) Full or partial amnesia for the event

B. The trance or possession trance state is not accepted as a normal part of a collective cultural or religious practice.

C. The trance or possession trance state causes clinically significant distress or impairment in social, occupational, or other important areas of functioning.

D. The trance or possession trance state does not occur exclusively during the course of a psychotic disorder (including mood disorder with psychotic features and brief psychotic disorder) or dissociative identity disorder and is not due to the direct physiological effects of a substance or a general medical condition.

(From American Psychiatric Association. *Diagnostic and Statistical Manual of Mental Disorders*. 4th ed. Text rev. Washington, DC: American Psychiatric Association; 2000, with permission.)

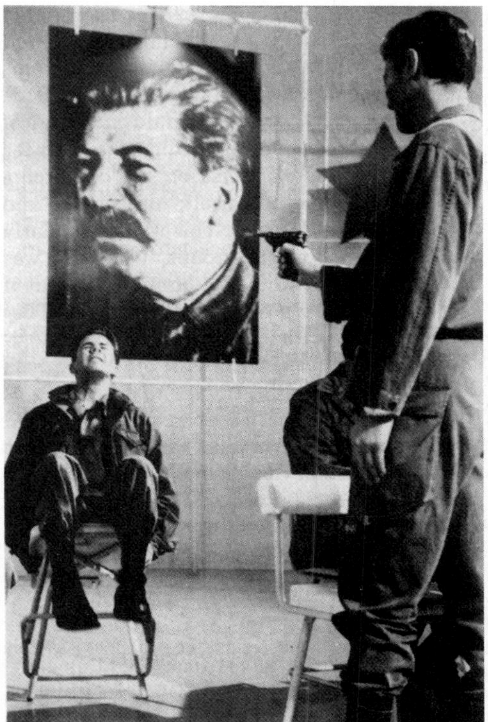

FIGURE 20–2
In the motion picture, *The Manchurian Candidate*, from which this still photograph is taken, US prisoners of war were brainwashed by their communist captors. The actor holding the gun is being programmed to shoot a fellow prisoner and, after his planned release from captivity, to assassinate the American presidential candidate. (Courtesy of Culver Pictures, Inc.)

including loss of health and life, and they typically manifest a variety of posttraumatic and dissociative symptoms.

The first stage in coercive processes has been likened to the artificial creation of an identity crisis, with the emergence of a new pseudoidentity that manifests characteristics of a dissociative state. Under circumstances of extreme and malignant dependency, overwhelming vulnerability, and danger to one's existence, individuals develop a state characterized by extreme idealization of their captors, with ensuing identification with the aggressor and externalization of their superego, regressive adaptation known as *traumatic infantilism*, paralysis of will, and a state of frozen fright. The coercive techniques that are typically used to induce such a state in the victim have been amply described and include isolation of the subject, degradation, control over all communications and basic daily functions, induction of fear and confusion, peer pressure, assignment of repetitive and monotonous routines, unpredictability of environmental supplies, renunciation of past relationships and values, and various deprivations. Even though physical or sexual abuse, torture, and extreme sensory deprivation and physical neglect can be parts of this process, they are not required to define a coercive process. As a result, victims manifest extensive posttraumatic and dissociative symptomatology, including drastic alteration of their identity, values, and beliefs; reduction of cognitive flexibility with regression to simplistic perceptions of good-evil and dominance-submission; numbing of experience and blunting of affect; trance-like states and diminished environmental responsiveness; and, in some cases, more severe dissociative symptoms such as amnesia, depersonalization, and shifts in identity (Fig. 20–2).

The treatment of the victims of coercion can vary considerably, depending on their particular background, the circumstances involved, and the setting in which help is sought. Although no systematic studies exist in this domain, basic principles involve validation of the traumatic experience and coercive techniques used, cognitive reframing of the events that transpired, exploration of preexisting psychopathology and vulnerabilities (when applicable), and general techniques used in treating posttraumatic and dissociative states. In addition, family interventions and therapy may be required, at least in cases of cult indoctrination, because significant family duress and disruption commonly occur.

Recovered Memory Syndrome

Under hypnosis or during psychotherapy, a patient may recover a memory of a painful experience or conflict—particularly of sexual or physical abuse—that is etiologically significant. When the repressed material is brought back to consciousness, the person not only may recall the experience but may relive it, accompanied by the appropriate affective response (a process called *abreaction*). If the event recalled never really happened but the person believes it to be true and reacts accordingly, it is known as *false memory syndrome*.

The syndrome has led to lawsuits involving accusations of child abuse. However, Thomas E. Gutheil describes memory as a "slender reed—insufficiently strong to bear the weight of a court case." Even if the memory of abuse is real, the perpetrator is not the present person, but the person of the past. Gutheil does not believe that litigation usually serves the patient's psychological goals. Clinical attention should probably be directed toward helping patients cast aside the limiting restrictive role of victim and transcend their past traumas, work through them, and try to get on with their lives.

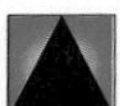

Table 20–13
ICD-10 Diagnostic Criteria for Dissociative (Conversion) Disorders

G1. There must be no evidence of a physical disorder that can explain the characteristic symptoms of this disorder (although physical disorders may be present that give rise to other symptoms).
G2. There are convincing associations in time between the onset of symptoms of the disorder and stressful events, problems, or needs.

Dissociative amnesia
A. The general criteria for dissociative disorder must be met.
B. There must be amnesia, partial or complete, for recent events or problems that were or still are traumatic or stressful.
C. The amnesia is too extensive and persistent to be explained by ordinary forgetfulness (although its depth and extent may vary from one assessment to the next) or by intentional simulation.

Dissociative fugue
A. The general criteria for dissociative disorder must be met.
B. The individual undertakes an unexpected yet organized journey away from home or from the ordinary places of work and social activities, during which self-care is largely maintained.
C. There is amnesia, partial or complete, for the journey, which also meets Criterion C for dissociative amnesia.

Dissociative stupor
A. The general criteria for dissociative disorder must be met.
B. There is profound diminution or absence of voluntary movements and speech and of normal responsiveness to light, noise, and touch.
C. Normal muscle tone, static posture, and breathing (and often limited coordinated eye movements) are maintained.

Trance and possession disorders
A. The general criteria for dissociative disorder must be met.
B. Either of the following must be present:
(1) *Trance.* There is temporary alteration of the state of consciousness, shown by any two of the following:
(a) Loss of the usual sense of personal identity
(b) Narrowing of awareness of immediate surroundings or unusually narrow and selective focusing on environmental stimuli
(c) Limitation of movements, postures, and speech to repetition of a small repertoire
(2) *Possession disorder.* The individual is convinced that he or she has been taken over by a spirit, power, deity, or other person.
C. (1) and (2) of Criterion B must be unwanted and troublesome, occurring outside, or being a prolongation of, similar states in religious or other culturally accepted situations.
D. *Most commonly used exclusion clause.* The disorder does not occur at the same time as schizophrenia or related disorders, or mood (affective) disorders with hallucinations or delusions.

Dissociative motor disorders
A. The general criteria for dissociative disorder must be met.
B. Either of the following must be present:
(1) Complete or partial loss of the ability to perform movements that are normally under voluntary control (including speech)
(2) Various or variable degrees of incoordination or ataxia, or inability to stand unaided

Dissociative convulsions
A. The general criteria for dissociative disorder must be met.
B. The individual exhibits sudden and unexpected spasmodic movements, closely resembling any of the varieties of epileptic seizure but not followed by loss of consciousness.
C. The symptoms in Criterion B are not accompanied by tongue biting, serious bruising or laceration due to falling, or urinary incontinence.

Dissociative anesthesia and sensory loss
A. The general criteria for dissociative disorder must be met.
B. Either of the following must be present:
(1) Partial or complete loss of any or all of the normal cutaneous sensations over part or all of the body (specify: touch, pin prick, vibration, heat, cold)
(2) Partial or complete loss of vision, hearing, or smell (specify)

Mixed dissociative (conversion) disorders
Other dissociative (conversion) disorders
This residual code may be used to indicate other dissociative and conversion states that meet Criteria G1 and G2 for dissociative (conversion) disorders but do not meet the criteria for the dissociative disorders listed previously.
Ganser syndrome (approximate answers)
Multiple personality disorder
A. Two or more distinct personalities exist within the individual, only one being evident at a time.
B. Each personality has its own memories, preferences, and behavior patterns and, at some time (and recurrently), takes full control of the individual's behavior.
C. There is inability to recall important personal information, which is too extensive to be explained by ordinary forgetfulness.
D. The symptoms are not due to organic mental disorders (e.g., in epileptic disorders) or psychoactive substance-related disorders (e.g., intoxication or withdrawal).

Transient dissociative (conversion) disorders occurring in childhood and adolescence
Other specified dissociative (conversion) disorders
Specific research criteria are not given for all disorders mentioned previously, because these other dissociative states are rare and not well described. Research workers studying these conditions in detail should specify their own criteria according to the purpose of their studies.

Dissociative (conversion) disorder, unspecified

(From World Health Organization. *The ICD-10 Classification of Mental and Behavioural Disorders: Diagnostic Criteria for Research.* Geneva: World Health Organization; 1993, with permission.)

Ganser Syndrome

Ganser syndrome is a poorly understood condition characterized by the giving of approximate answers (paralogia) together with a clouding of consciousness, and frequently accompanied by hallucinations and other dissociative, somatoform, or conversion symptoms.

Epidemiology. Cases have been reported in a variety of cultures, but the overall frequency of such reports has declined with time. Men outnumber women by approximately 2 to 1. Three of Ganser's first four cases were convicts, leading some authors to consider it to be a disorder of penal populations and, thus, an indicator of potential malingering.

Etiology. Some case reports identify precipitating stressors, such as personal conflicts and financial reverses, whereas others note organic brain syndromes, head injuries, seizures, and medical or psychiatric illness. Psychodynamic explanations are common in the older literature, but organic etiologies are stressed in more recent case studies. It is speculated that the organic insults may act as acute stressors, precipitating the syndrome in vulnerable individuals. Some patients have reported significant histories of childhood maltreatment and adversity.

Diagnosis and Clinical Features. The symptom of *passing over* (*vorbeigehen*) the correct answer for a related, but incorrect one, is the hallmark of Ganser syndrome. The approximate answers often just miss the mark but bear an obvious relation to the question, indicating that it has been understood. When asked how old she was, a 25-year-old woman answered, "I'm not five." If asked to do simple calculations (e.g., 2 + 2 = 5); for general information (the capital of the United States is New York); to identify simple objects (a pencil is a key); or to name colors (green is gray), the patient with Ganser syndrome gives erroneous but comprehensible answers.

A clouding of consciousness also occurs, usually manifest by disorientation, amnesias, loss of personal information, and some impairment of reality testing. Visual and auditory hallucinations occur in roughly one half of the cases. Neurological examination may reveal what Ganser called *hysterical stigmata*, for example, a nonneurological analgesia or shifting hyperalgesia. It must be accompanied by other dissociative symptoms, such as amnesias, conversion symptoms, or trance-like behaviors.

Differential Diagnosis. Given the reported frequent history of organic brain syndromes, seizures, head trauma, and psychosis in Ganser syndrome, a thorough neurological and medical evaluation is warranted. Differential diagnoses include organic dementia, depressive pseudodementia, the confabulation of Korsakoff's syndrome, organic dysphasias, and reactive psychoses. Patients with dissociative identity disorder occasionally may also exhibit Ganser-like symptoms.

Treatment. No systematic treatment studies have been conducted, given the rarity of this condition. In most case reports, the patient has been hospitalized and has been provided with a protective and supportive environment. In some instances, low doses of antipsychotic medications have been reported to be beneficial. Confrontation or interpretations of the patient's approximate answers are not productive, but exploration of possible stressors may be helpful. Hypnosis and amobarbital narcosynthesis have also been used successfully to help patients reveal the underlying stressors that preceded the development of the syndrome, with concomitant cessation of the Ganser symptoms. Usually, a relatively rapid return to normal function occurs within days, although some cases may take a month or more to resolve. The individual is typically amnesic for the period of the syndrome.

ICD-10

The tenth edition of the *International Statistical Classification of Diseases and Related Health Problems* (ICD-10) classifies the dissociative disorders among the *neurotic*, *stress-related*, and *somatoform disorders*. The ICD-10 explicitly states that the term *hysteria* should be avoided because of its lack of precision. The ICD-10 dissociative [conversion] disorders include dissociative amnesia, dissociative fugue, dissociative stupor, trance and possession disorder, and dissociative disorders of movement and sensation (roughly equivalent to the DSM-IV-TR conversion disorder diagnosis). The latter includes dissociative motor disorders, dissociative convulsions, and dissociative anesthesia and sensory loss. Ganser syndrome and multiplex personality disorder are classified under *other* dissociative disorders. Depersonalization disorder is classified separately. The ICD-10 diagnostic criteria for these disorders are found in Table 20–13.

References

Anderson MC, Ochsner KN, Kuhl B, Cooper J, Robertson E, Gabrieli SW, Glover GH, Gabrieli JDE. Neural systems underlying the suppression of unwanted memories. *Science*. 2004;303:232–235.

Foote B, Smolin Y, Kaplan M, Legatt ME, Lipschitz D. Prevalence of dissociative disorders in psychiatric outpatients. *Am J Psychiatry*. 2006;163(4): 623–629.

Hunter ECM, Baker D, Phillips ML, Sierra M, David AS. Cognitive-behaviour therapy for depersonalization disorder: An open study. *Behaviour Research and Therapy*. 2005;43:1121–1130.

Isaac M, Chand PK. Dissociative and conversion disorder: Defining boundaries. *Current Opinion in Psychiatry*. 2006;19:61–66.

Lanius RA, Williamson PC, Densmore M, Boksman K, Neufeld RWJ, Gati JS, Menon R. The nature of traumatic memories: A 4-T fMRI functional connectivity analysis. *Am J Psychiatry*. 2004;161:36–44.

Loewenstein RJ, Putnam FW. Dissociative disorders. In: Sadock BJ, Sadock VA, eds. *Kaplan & Sadock's Comprehensive Textbook of Psychiatry*. 8th ed. Vol. 1. Baltimore: Lippincott Williams & Wilkins; 2005;1844.

Maaranen P, Tanskanen A, Honkalampi K, Haatainen K, Hintikka J, Viinamaki H. Factors associated with pathological dissociation in the general population. *Aust N Z J Psychiatry*. 2005;39:387–394.

Markowitsch HJ. Psychogenic amnesia. *Neuroimage*. 2003;20:S132–S138.

Middleton W. Owning the past, claiming the present: Perspectives on the treatment of dissociative patients. *Australasian Psychiatry*. 2005;13: 40–49.

Reinders AA, Nijenhuis ERS, Paans AMJ, Korf J, Willemsen ATM, den Boer JA. One brain, two selves. *Neuroimage*. 2003;20:2119–2125.

Simeon D, Knutelska M, Nelson D, Guralnik O. Feeling unreal: A depersonalization disorder update of 117 cases. *J Clin Psychiatry*. 2003;64:990–997.

21 Human Sexuality

▲ 21.1 Normal Sexuality

Sexuality has been a consistent focus of curiosity, interest, and analysis to humankind. Depictions of sexual behavior have existed from the time of prehistoric cave drawings through da Vinci's anatomical illustrations of intercourse to current pornographic sites available on the Internet.

Sexuality is determined by anatomy, physiology, the culture in which a person lives, relationships with others, and developmental experiences throughout the life cycle. It includes the perception of being male or female and private thoughts and fantasies as well as behavior. To the average normal person, sexual attraction to another person and the passion and love that follow are deeply associated with feelings of intimate happiness.

Normal sexual behavior brings pleasure to oneself and one's partner, involves stimulation of the primary sex organs including coitus; it is devoid of inappropriate feelings of guilt or anxiety and is not compulsive. Recreational, as opposed to relational sex, that is sex outside a committed relationship, masturbation, and various forms of stimulation involving other than the primary sex organs, constitutes normal behavior in some contexts.

TERMS

Sexuality and total personality are so entwined that to speak of sexuality as a separate entity is virtually impossible. The term *psychosexual*, therefore, is used to describe personality development and functioning as these are affected by sexuality. The term *psychosexual* applies to more than sexual feelings and behavior, and it is not synonymous with *libido* in the broad freudian sense.

Sigmund Freud's generalization that all pleasurable impulses and activities are originally sexual has given laypersons a somewhat distorted view of sexual concepts and has presented psychiatrists a confused picture of motivation. For example, some oral activities are directed toward obtaining food, and others are directed toward achieving sexual gratification. Both activities are pleasure seeking and use the same organ, but they are not, as Freud contended, both necessarily sexual. Labeling all pleasure-seeking behaviors sexual makes it impossible to specify precise motivations. Persons may also use sexual activities for gratification of nonsexual needs, such as dependency, aggression, power, and status. Although sexual and nonsexual impulses can jointly motivate behavior, the analysis of behavior depends on understanding the underlying individual motivations and their interactions.

CHILDHOOD SEXUALITY

Before Freud described the effects of childhood experiences on adults' personalities, the universality of sexual activity and sexual learning in children was unrecognized. Most sexual learning experiences in childhood occur without the parents' knowledge, but awareness of a child's sex does influence parental behavior. Male infants, for instance, tend to be handled more vigorously and female infants tend to be cuddled more. Fathers spend more time with their infant sons than with their daughters, and they also tend to be more aware of their sons' adolescent concerns than of their daughters' anxieties. Boys are more likely than girls to be physically disciplined. A child's sex affects parental tolerance for aggression and reinforcement or extinction of activity and of intellectual, aesthetic, and athletic interests.

Observation of children reveals that genital play in infants is part of normal development. According to Harry Harlow, interaction with mothers and peers is necessary for the development of effective adult sexual behavior in monkeys, a finding that has relevance to the normal socialization of children. During a critical period in development, infants are especially susceptible to certain stimuli; later, they may be immune to these stimuli. The detailed relation of critical periods to psychosexual development has yet to be established; Freud's stages of psychosexual development—oral, anal, phallic, latent, and genital—presumably provide a broad framework.

PSYCHOSEXUAL FACTORS

Sexuality depends on four interrelated psychosexual factors: sexual identity, gender identity, sexual orientation, and sexual behavior. These factors affect personality, growth, development, and functioning. Sexuality is something more than physical sex, coital or noncoital, and something less than all behaviors directed toward attaining pleasure.

Sexual Identity and Gender Identity

Sexual identity is the pattern of a person's biological sexual characteristics: chromosomes, external genitalia, internal genitalia, hormonal composition, gonads, and secondary sex characteristics. In normal development, these characteristics form a cohesive pattern that leaves a person in no doubt about his or her sex. Gender identity is a person's sense of maleness or femaleness. Sexual identity and gender identity are interactive. Genetic influences and hormones affect behavior and the environment affects hormonal production and gene expression.

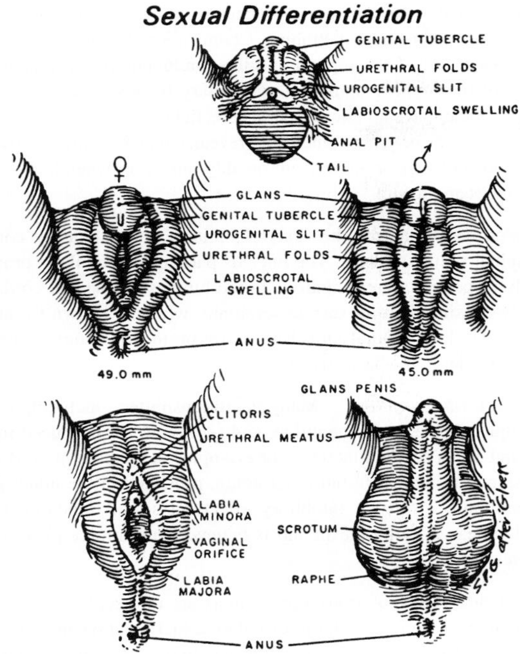

FIGURE 21.1–1

Differentiation of male and female external genitalia from indifferent primordia. Male differentiation occurs only in the presence of androgenic stimulation during the first 12 weeks of fetal life. (Redrawn from Van Wyk and Grumbach, 1968; from Brobeck JR, ed. *Best & Taylor's Physiological Basis of Medical Practice*, 9th ed. Baltimore: Williams & Wilkins; 1973, with permission.)

Sexual Identity. Modern embryological studies have shown that all mammalian embryos, whether genetically male (XY genotype) or genetically female (XX genotype) are anatomically female during the early stages of fetal life. Differentiation of the male from the female results from the action of fetal androgens; the action begins about the sixth week of embryonic life and is completed by the end of the third month (Fig. 21.1–1). Recent research has focused on the possible roles of key genes in fetal sexual development. A testis develops as a result of SRY and SOX9 action and an ovary in the absence of such action. DAX1 plays a part in the fetal development of both sexes and WNT4 action is needed for the development of the mullerian ducts in the female. Other studies have explained the effects of fetal hormones on the masculinization or feminization of the brain. In animals, prenatal hormonal stimulation of the brain is necessary for male and female reproductive and copulatory behavior. The fetus is also vulnerable to exogenously administered androgens during that period. For instance, if a pregnant woman receives sufficient exogenous androgens, her female fetus possessing ovaries can develop external genitalia resembling those of a male (Table 21.1–1).

Gender Identity. By 2 to 3 years of age, almost everyone has a firm conviction that "I am male" or "I am female." Yet, even if maleness and femaleness develop normally, persons must still develop a sense of masculinity or femininity.

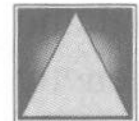

Table 21.1–1
Classification of Intersexual Disorders[a]

Syndrome	Description
Virilizing adrenal hyperplasia (adrenogenital syndrome)	Results from excess androgens in fetus with XX genotype; most common female intersex disorder; associated with enlarged clitoris, fused labia, hirsutism in adolescence
Turner's syndrome	Results from absence of second female sex chromosome (XO); associated with web neck, dwarfism, cubitus valgus; no sex hormones produced; infertile
Klinefelter's syndrome	Genotype is XXY; male habitus present with small penis and rudimentary testes because of low androgen production; weak libido; usually assigned as male
Androgen insensitivity syndrome (testicular-feminizing syndrome)	Congenital X-linked recessive disorder that results in inability of tissues to respond to androgens; external genitals look female and cryptorchid testes present; in extreme form patient has breasts, normal external genitals, short blind vagina, and absence of pubic and axillary hair
Enzymatic defects in XY genotype (e.g., 5-α-reductase deficiency, 17-hydroxy-steroid deficiency)	Congenital interruption in production of testosterone that produces ambiguous genitals and female habitus
Hermaphroditism	True hermaphrodite is rare and characterized by both testes and ovaries in same person (may be 46 XX or 46 XY)
Pseudohermaphroditism	Usually the result of endocrine or enzymatic defect (e.g., adrenal hyperplasia) in persons with normal chromosomes; female pseudohermaphrodites have masculine-looking genitals but are XX; male pseudohermaphrodites have rudimentary testes and external genitals and are XY

[a] Intersexual disorders include a variety of syndromes that produce persons with gross anatomical or physiological aspects of the opposite sex.

Gender identity, according to Robert Stoller, "connotes psychological aspects of behavior related to masculinity and femininity." He considers gender social and sex biological: "Most often the two are relatively congruent, that is, males tend to be manly and females womanly." But sex and gender can develop in conflicting or even opposite ways. Gender identity results from an almost infinite series of cues derived from experiences with family members, teachers, friends, and coworkers and from cultural phenomena. Physical characteristics derived from a person's biological sex—such as physique, body shape, and physical dimensions—interrelate with an intricate system of stimuli, including rewards and punishment and parental gender labels, to establish gender identity.

Thus, formation of gender identity arises from parental and cultural attitudes, the infant's external genitalia, and a genetic influence, which is physiologically active by the sixth week of fetal life. Although family, cultural, and biological influences may complicate establishment of a sense of masculinity or femininity, persons usually develop a relatively secure sense of identification with their biological sex—a stable gender identity.

GENDER ROLE. Related to, and in part derived from, gender identity is gender role behavior. John Money and Anke Ehrhardt described gender role behavior as all those things that a person says or does to disclose himself or herself as having the status of boy or man, girl or woman, respectively. A gender role is not established at birth but is built up cumulatively through (1) experiences encountered and transacted through casual and unplanned learning, (2) explicit instruction and inculcation, and (3) spontaneously putting two and two together to make sometimes four and sometimes five. The usual outcome is a congruence of gender identity and gender role. Although biological attributes are significant, the major factor in achieving the role appropriate to a person's sex is learning.

Research on sex differences in children's behavior reveals more psychological similarities than differences. Girls, however, are found to be less susceptible to tantrums after the age of 18 months than are boys, and boys generally are more physically and verbally aggressive than are girls from age 2 onward. Little girls and little boys are similarly active, but boys are more easily stimulated to sudden bursts of activity when they are in groups. Some researchers speculate that, although aggression is a learned behavior, male hormones may have sensitized boys' neural organizations to absorb these lessons more easily than do girls.

Persons' gender roles can seem to be opposed to their gender identities. Persons may identify with their own sex and yet adopt the dress, hairstyle, or other characteristics of the opposite sex. Or, they may identify with the opposite sex and yet for expediency adopt many behavioral characteristics of their own sex. A further discussion of gender issues appears in Chapter 22.

Sexual Orientation

Sexual orientation describes the object of a person's sexual impulses: heterosexual (opposite sex), homosexual (same sex), or bisexual (both sexes). A group of people have defined themselves as "asexual" and assert this as a positive identity. Some researchers believe this lack of attraction to any object is a manifestation of a desire disorder.

Sexual Behavior

The Central Nervous System and Sexual Behavior

THE BRAIN

Cortex. The cortex is involved both in controlling sexual impulses and in processing sexual stimuli that may lead to sexual activity. In studies of young men, some areas of the brain have been found to be more active during sexual stimulation than others. These include the orbitofrontal cortex, which is involved in emotions; the left anterior cingulate cortex, which is involved in hormone control and sexual arousal; and the right caudate nucleus, whose activity is a factor in whether sexual activity follows arousal.

Limbic System. In all mammals, the limbic system is directly involved with elements of sexual functioning. Chemical or electrical stimulation of the lower part of the septum and the contiguous preoptic area, the fimbria of the hippocampus, the mammilary bodies, and the anterior thalamic nuclei have all elicited penile erections.

Studies of the brain in women have revealed that those areas activated by emotions of fear or anxiety are notably quiescent when the woman experiences an orgasm.

Brainstem. Brainstem sites exert inhibitory and excitatory control over spinal sexual reflexes. The nucleus paragigantocellularis projects directly to pelvic efferent neurons in the lumbosacral spinal cord, apparently causing them to secrete serotonin, which is known to inhibit orgasms. The lumbosacral cord also receives projections from other serotonergic nuclei in the brainstem.

Brain Neurotransmitters. Many neurotransmitters, including dopamine, epinephrine, norepinephrine, and serotonin, are produced in the brain and affect sexual function. For example, an increase in dopamine is presumed to increase libido. Serotonin, produced in the upper pons and midbrain, exerts an inhibitory effect on sexual function. Oxytocin is released with orgasm and is believed to reinforce pleasurable activities.

Spinal Cord. Sexual arousal and climax are ultimately organized at the spinal level. Sensory stimuli related to sexual function are conveyed via afferents from the pudendal, pelvic, and hypogastric nerves. Several separate experiments suggest that sexual reflexes are mediated by spinal neurons in the central gray region of the lumbosacral segments.

Physiological Responses.

Sexual response is a true psychophysiological experience. Arousal is triggered by both psychological and physical stimuli; levels of tension are experienced both physiologically and emotionally; and, with orgasm, normally a subjective perception of a peak of physical reaction and release occurs. Psychosexual development, psychological attitudes toward sexuality, and attitudes toward one's sexual partner are directly involved with, and affect, the physiology of human sexual response.

Normally, men and women experience a sequence of physiological responses to sexual stimulation. In the first detailed description of these responses, William Masters and Virginia Johnson observed that the physiological process involves increasing levels of vasocongestion and myotonia (tumescence) and the subsequent release of the vascular activity and muscle tone as a result of orgasm (detumescence). Tables 21.1–2 and 21.1–3 describe the male and female sexual response cycles. The text revision of the fourth edition of *Diagnostic and Statistical Manual of Mental Disorders* (DSM-IV-TR) defines a four-phase response cycle: phase 1, desire; phase 2, excitement; phase 3, orgasm; phase 4, resolution. It is important to remember that the sequence of responses can overlap and fluctuate. Additionally, a person's subjective experiences are as important to sexual satisfaction as the objective physiologic response.

PHASE 1: DESIRE. The classification of the desire (or appetitive) phase, which is distinct from any phase identified solely through physiology, reflects the psychiatric concern with motivations, drives, and personality. The phase is characterized by sexual fantasies and the desire to have sexual activity.

PHASE 2: EXCITEMENT. The excitement and arousal phase, brought on by psychological stimulation (fantasy or the presence of a love object) or physiological stimulation (stroking or kissing) or a combination of the two, consists of a subjective sense of pleasure. During this phase, penile

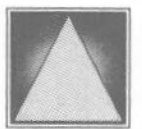

Table 21.1–2
Male Sexual Response Cycle[a]

Organ	Excitement Phase	Orgasmic Phase	Resolution Phase
	Lasts several minutes to several hours; heightened excitement before orgasm, 30 seconds to 3 minutes	3 to 15 seconds	10 to 15 minutes; if no orgasm, 1/2 to 1 day
Skin	Just before orgasm: sexual flush inconsistently appears; maculopapular rash originates on abdomen and spreads to anterior chest wall, face, and neck and can include shoulders and forearms	Well-developed flush	Flush disappears in reverse order of appearance; inconsistently appearing film of perspiration on soles of feet and palms of hands
Penis	Erection in 10 to 30 seconds caused by vasocongestion of erectile bodies of corpus cavernosa of shaft; loss of erection may occur with introduction of asexual stimulus, loud noise; with heightened excitement, size of glands and diameter of penile shaft increase further	Ejaculation; emission phase marked by three to four 0.8-second contractions of vas, seminal vesicles, prostate; ejaculation proper marked by 0.8-second contractions of urethra and ejaculatory spurt of 12 to 20 inches at age 18, decreasing with age to seepage at 70	Erection: partial involution in 5 to 10 seconds with variable refractory period; full detumescence in 5 to 30 minutes
Scrotum and testes	Tightening and lifting of scrotal sac and elevation of testes; with heightened excitement, 50% increase in size of testes over unstimulated state and flattening against perineum, signaling impending ejaculation	No change	Decrease to baseline size because of loss of vasocongestion; testicular and scrotal descent within 5 to 30 minutes after orgasm; involution may take several hours if no orgasmic release takes place
Cowper's glands	2 to 3 drops of mucoid fluid that contain viable sperm are secreted during heightened excitement	No change	No change
Other	Breasts: inconsistent nipple erection with heightened excitement before orgasm Myotonia: semispastic contractions of facial, abdominal, and intercostal muscles Tachycardia: up to 175 beats a minute Blood pressure: rise in systolic 20 to 80 mm; in diastolic 10 to 40 mm Respiration: increased	Loss of voluntary muscular control Rectum: rhythmical contractions of sphincter Heart rate: up to 180 beats a minute Blood pressure: up to 40 to 100 mm systolic; 20 to 50 mm diastolic Respiration: up to 40 respirations a minute	Return to baseline state in 5 to 10 minutes

[a]A desire phase consisting of sex fantasies and desire to have sex precedes excitement phase.
(Table by Virginia Sadock, M.D.)

tumescence leads to erection in men and vaginal lubrication occurs in women. The nipples of both sexes become erect, although nipple erection is more common in women than in men. A woman's clitoris becomes hard and turgid, and her labia minora become thicker as a result of venous engorgement. Initial excitement may last from several minutes to several hours. With continued stimulation, a man's testes increase 50 percent in size and elevate. A woman's vaginal barrel shows a characteristic constriction along the outer third, known as the orgasmic platform. The clitoris elevates and retracts behind the symphysis pubis, and as a result is not easily accessible. Stimulation of the area, however, causes traction on the labia minora and the prepuce and intrapreputial movement of the clitoral shaft. Women's breast size increases 25 percent. Continued engorgement of the penis and the vagina produces color changes, particularly in the labia minora, which become bright or deep red. Voluntary contractions of large muscle groups occur, heartbeat and respiration rates increase, and blood pressure rises. Heightened excitement lasts from 30 seconds to several minutes.

PHASE 3: ORGASM. The orgasm phase consists of a peaking of sexual pleasure, with the release of sexual tension and the rhythmic contraction of the perineal muscles and the pelvic reproductive organs. A subjective sense of ejaculatory inevitability triggers men's orgasms. The forceful emission of semen follows. The male orgasm is also associated with four to five rhythmic spasms of the prostate, seminal vesicles, vas, and urethra. In women, orgasm is characterized by 3 to 15 involuntary contractions of the lower third of the vagina and by strong sustained contractions of the uterus, flowing from the fundus downward to the cervix. Both men and women have involuntary contractions of the internal and external anal sphincters. These and the other contractions during orgasm occur at 0.8-second intervals. Other manifestations include voluntary and involuntary movements of the large muscle groups, including facial grimacing and carpopedal spasm. Blood pressure rises 20 to 40 mm (both systolic and diastolic), and the heart rate increases up to 160 beats per minute. Orgasm lasts from 3 to 25 seconds and is associated with a slight clouding of consciousness (Figs. 21.1–2 and 21.1–3).

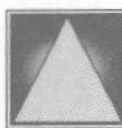

Table 21.1–3
Female Sexual Response Cycle[a]

Organ	Excitement Phase	Orgasmic Phase	Resolution Phase
	Lasts several minutes to several hours; heightened excitement before orgasm, 30 seconds to 3 minutes	3 to 15 seconds	10 to 15 minutes; if no orgasm, 1/2 to 1 day
Skin	Just before orgasm: sexual flush inconsistently appears; maculopapular rash originates on abdomen and spreads to anterior chest wall, face, and neck; can include shoulders and forearms	Well-developed flush	Flush disappears in reverse order of appearance; inconsistently appearing film of perspiration on soles of feet and palms of hands
Breasts	Nipple erection in two thirds of women, venous congestion and areolar enlargement; size increases to one fourth over normal	Breasts may become tremulous	Return to normal in about 30 minutes
Clitoris	Enlargement in diameter of glands and shaft; just before orgasm, shaft retracts into prepuce	No change	Shaft returns to normal position in 5 to 10 seconds; detumescence in 5 to 30 minutes; if no orgasm, detumescence takes several hours
Labia majora	Nullipara: elevate and flatten against perineum Multipara: congestion and edema	No change	Nullipara: decrease to normal size in 1 to 2 minutes Multipara: decrease to normal size in 10 to 15 minutes
Labia minora	Size increased two to three times over normal; change to pink, red, deep red before orgasm	Contractions of proximal labia minora	Return to normal within 5 minutes
Vagina	Color change to dark purple; vaginal transudate appears 10 to 30 seconds after arousal; elongation and ballooning of vagina; lower third of vagina constricts before orgasm	3 to 15 contractions of lower third of vagina at intervals of 0.8 second	Ejaculate forms seminal pool in upper two thirds of vagina; congestion disappears in seconds or, if no orgasm, in 20 to 30 minutes
Uterus	Ascends into false pelvis; labor-like contractions begin in heightened excitement just before orgasm	Contractions throughout orgasm	Contractions cease, and uterus descends to normal position
Other	Myotonia A few drops of mucoid secretion from Bartholin's glands during heightened excitement Cervix swells slightly and is passively elevated with uterus	Loss of voluntary muscular control Rectum: rhythmical contractions of sphincter Hyperventilation and tachycardia	Return to baseline status in seconds to minutes Cervix color and size return to normal, and cervix descends into seminal pool

[a]A desire phase consisting of sex fantasies and desire to have sex precedes excitement phase.
(Table by Virginia Sadock, M.D.)

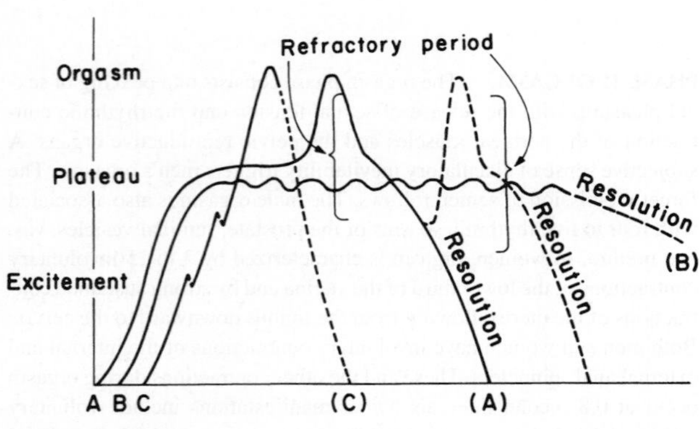

FIGURE 21.1–2
Male sexual response. An individual man may experience any of these three patterns (**A, B,** or **C**) during a particular sexual experience. (From Walker JI, ed. *Essentials of Clinical Psychiatry*. Philadelphia: JB Lippincott; 1985:276, with permission.)

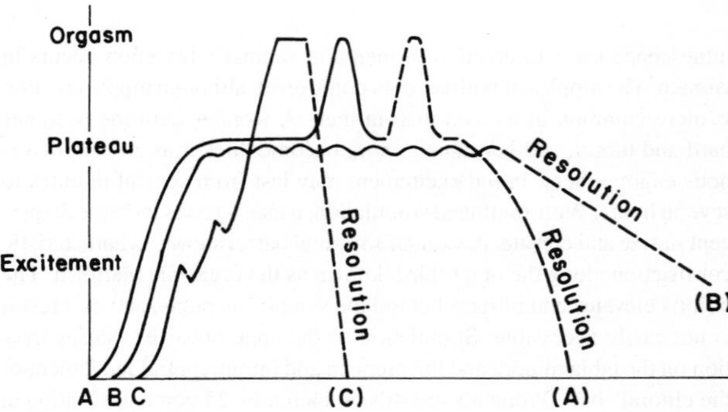

FIGURE 21.1–3
Female sexual response. An individual woman may experience any of these three patterns (**A, B,** or **C**) during a particular sexual experience. (From Walker JI, ed. *Essentials of Clinical Psychiatry*, Philadelphia: JB Lippincott; 1985:276. with permission.)

PHASE 4: RESOLUTION. Resolution consists of the disgorgement of blood from the genitalia (detumescence), which brings the body back to its resting state. If orgasm occurs, resolution is rapid and is characterized by a subjective sense of well-being, general relaxation, and muscular relaxation. If orgasm does not occur, resolution may take from 2 to 6 hours and may be associated with irritability and discomfort. After orgasm, men have a refractory period that may last from several minutes to many hours; in that period they cannot be stimulated to further orgasm. Women do not have a refractory period and are capable of multiple and successive orgasms.

HORMONES AND SEXUAL BEHAVIOR

In general, substances that increase dopamine levels in the brain increase desire, whereas substances that augment serotonin decrease desire. Testosterone increases libido in both men and women, although estrogen is a key factor in the lubrication involved in female arousal and may increase sensitivity in the woman to stimulation. Progesterone mildly depresses desire in men and women as do excessive prolactin and cortisol. Oxytocin is involved in pleasurable sensations during sex and is found in higher levels in men and women following orgasm.

Gender Differences in Desire and Erotic Stimuli

Sexual impulses and desire exist in men and women. If measuring desire by the frequency of spontaneous sexual thoughts, interest in participating in sexual activity, and alertness to sexual cues, males generally possess a higher baseline level of desire than do women, which may be biologically determined.

Although explicit sexual fantasies are common to both sexes, the external stimuli for the fantasies frequently differ for men and women. Many men respond sexually to visual stimuli of nude or barely dressed women. Women report responding sexually to romantic stories with a tender, demonstrative hero whose passion for the heroine impels him toward a lifetime commitment to her. A complicating factor is that a woman's subjective sense of arousal is not always congruent with her physiological state of arousal. Specifically, her sense of excitement may reflect a readiness to be aroused rather than physiological lubrication. Conversely, she may experience the physical signs of arousal without being aware of them. This situation rarely occurs in men.

Masturbation

Masturbation is usually a normal precursor of object-related sexual behavior. No other form of sexual activity has been more frequently discussed, more roundly condemned, and more universally practiced than masturbation. Research by Alfred Kinsey into the prevalence of masturbation indicated that nearly all men and three fourths of all women masturbate sometime during their lives.

Longitudinal studies of development show that sexual self-stimulation is common in infancy and childhood. Just as infants learn to explore the functions of their fingers and mouths, they learn to do the same with their genitalia. At about 15 to 19 months of age, both sexes begin genital self-stimulation. Pleasurable sensations result from any gentle touch to the genital region. Those sensations, coupled with the ordinary desire for exploration of the body, produce a normal interest in masturbatory pleasure at that time. Children also develop an increased interest in the genitalia of others—parents, children, and even animals. As youngsters acquire playmates, the curiosity about their own and others' genitalia motivates episodes of exhibitionism or genital exploration. Such experiences, unless blocked by guilty fear, contribute to continued pleasure from sexual stimulation.

With the approach of puberty, the upsurge of sex hormones, and the development of secondary sex characteristics, sexual curiosity intensifies, and masturbation increases. Adolescents are physically capable of coitus and orgasm, but are usually inhibited by social restraints. The dual and often conflicting pressures of establishing their sexual identities and controlling their sexual impulses produce a strong physiological sexual tension in teenagers that demands release, and masturbation is a normal way to reduce sexual tensions. In general, males learn to masturbate to orgasm earlier than females and masturbate more frequently. An important emotional difference between the adolescent and the youngster of earlier years is the presence of coital fantasies during masturbation in the adolescent. These fantasies are an important adjunct to the development of sexual identity; in the comparative safety of the imagination, the adolescent learns to perform the adult sex role. This autoerotic activity is usually maintained into the young adult years, when it is normally replaced by coitus.

Couples in a sexual relationship do not abandon masturbation entirely. When coitus is unsatisfactory or is unavailable because of illness or the absence of the partner, self-stimulation often serves an adaptive purpose, combining sensual pleasure and tension release. Kinsey reported that when women masturbate, most prefer clitoral stimulation. Masters and Johnson stated that women prefer the shaft of the clitoris to the glans because the glans is hypersensitive to intense stimulation. Most men masturbate by vigorously stroking the penile shaft and glans.

Moral taboos against masturbation have generated myths that masturbation causes mental illness or decreased sexual potency. No scientific evidence supports such claims. Masturbation is a psychopathological symptom only when it becomes a compulsion beyond a person's willful control. Then, it is a symptom of emotional disturbance, not because it is sexual but because it is compulsive. Masturbation is probably a universal aspect of psychosexual development and, in most cases, it is adaptive.

Several studies found that in men, orgasm from masturbation raised the serum prostate-specific antigen (PSA) significantly. Male patients scheduled for PSA tests should be advised not to masturbate (or have coitus) for at least 7 days prior to the examination.

HOMOSEXUALITY

In 1973 homosexuality was eliminated as a diagnostic category by the American Psychiatric Association, and in 1980, it was removed from DSM. The 10th revision of the *International Statistical Classification of Diseases and Related Health Problems* (ICD-10) states: "Sexual orientation alone is not to be regarded as a disorder." This change reflects a change in the understanding of homosexuality, which is now considered to occur with some regularity as a variant of human sexuality, not as a pathological disorder. As David Hawkins wrote, "The presence of homosexuality does not appear to be a matter of choice; the expression of it is a matter of choice."

Definition

The term *homosexuality* often describes a person's overt behavior, sexual orientation, and sense of personal or social identity. Many persons prefer to identify sexual orientation by using terms such as *lesbians* and *gay men*, rather than *homosexual*, which may imply pathology and etiology based on its origin as a medical term, and refer to sexual behavior with terms such as *same sex* and *male–female*. Hawkins wrote that the terms *gay* and *lesbian* refer to a combination of self-perceived identity and social identity; they reflect a person's sense of belonging to a social group that is similarly labeled. Homophobia is a negative attitude toward, or fear of, homosexuality or homosexuals. Heterosexism is the belief that a heterosexual relationship is preferable to all others; it implies discrimination against those practicing other forms of sexuality.

Prevalence

Recent research reports rates of homosexuality in 2 to 4 percent of the population. A 1994 survey by the US Bureau of the Census concluded that the male prevalence rate for homosexuality is 2 to 3 percent. A 1989 University of Chicago study showed that less than 1 percent of both sexes are exclusively homosexual. The Alan Guttmacher Institute found in 1993 that 1 percent of men reported exclusively same-sex activity in the previous year and that 2 percent reported a lifetime history of homosexual experiences.

Some lesbians and gay men, particularly the latter, report being aware of same-sex romantic attractions before puberty. According to Kinsey's data, about half of all prepubertal boys have had some genital experience with a male partner. These experiences are often exploratory, particularly when shared with a peer, not an adult, and typically lack a strong affective component. Most gay men recall the onset of romantic and erotic attractions to same-sex partners during early adolescence. For women, the onset of romantic feelings toward same-sex partners may also be in preadolescence, but the clear recognition of a same-sex partner preference typically occurs in middle to late adolescence or in young adulthood. More lesbians than gay men appear to have engaged in heterosexual experiences. In one study, 56 percent of lesbians had experienced heterosexual intercourse before their first genital homosexual experience, compared with 19 percent of gay men who had sampled heterosexual intercourse first. Nearly 40 percent of the lesbians had had heterosexual intercourse during the year preceding the survey.

Theoretical Issues

Psychological Factors. The determinants of homosexual behavior are enigmatic. Freud viewed homosexuality as an arrest of psychosexual development and mentioned castration fears and fears of maternal engulfment in the preoedipal phase of psychosexual development. According to psychodynamic theory, early-life situations that can result in male homosexual behavior include a strong fixation on the mother; lack of effective fathering; inhibition of masculine development by the parents; fixation at, or regression to, the narcissistic stage of development; and losses when competing with brothers and sisters. Freud's views on the causes of female homosexuality included a lack of resolution of penis envy in association with unresolved oedipal conflicts.

Freud did not consider homosexuality a mental illness. In "Three Essays on the Theory of Sexuality," he wrote that homosexuality "is found in persons who exhibit no other serious deviations from normal whose efficiency is unimpaired and who are indeed distinguished by especially high intellectual development and ethical culture." In "Letter to an American Mother," Freud wrote, "Homosexuality is assuredly no advantage, but it is nothing to be ashamed of, no vice, no degradation, it cannot be classified as an illness; we consider it to be a variation of the sexual functions produced by a certain arrest of sexual development."

New Concepts of Psychoanalytic Factors. Some psychoanalysts have advanced new psychodynamic formulations that contrast with classic psychoanalytic theory. According to Richard Isay, gay men have described same-sex fantasies that occurred when they were 3 to 5 years of age, at about the same age that heterosexuals have male-female fantasies. Isay wrote that same-sex erotic fantasies in gay men center on the father or the father surrogate.

The child's perception of, and exposure to, these erotic feelings may account for such "atypical" behavior as greater secretiveness than other boys, self-isolation, and excessive emotionality. Some "feminine" traits may also be caused by identification with the mother or a mother surrogate. Such characteristics usually develop as a way of attracting the father's love and attention in a manner similar to the way the heterosexual boy may pattern himself after his father to gain his mother's attention.

The psychodynamics of homosexuality in women may be similar. The little girl does not give up her original fixation on the mother as a love object and continues to seek it in adulthood.

Biological Factors. Recent studies indicate that genetic and biological components may contribute to sexual orientation. Gay men reportedly exhibit lower levels of circulatory androgens than do heterosexual men. Prenatal hormones appear to play a role in the organization of the central nervous system: The effective presence of androgens in prenatal life is purported to contribute to a sexual orientation toward females, and a deficiency of prenatal androgens (or tissue insensitivity to them) may lead to a sexual orientation toward males. Preadolescent girls exposed to large amounts of androgens before birth are uncharacteristically aggressive, and boys exposed to excessive female hormones in utero are less athletic, less assertive, and less aggressive than other boys. Women with hyperadrenocorticalism are lesbian and bisexual in greater proportion than women in the general population.

Genetic studies have shown a higher incidence of homosexual concordance among monozygotic twins than among dizygotic twins; these results suggest a genetic predisposition, but chromosome studies have been unable to differentiate homosexuals from heterosexuals. Gay men show a familial distribution; they have more brothers who are gay than do heterosexual men. One study found that 33 of 40 pairs of gay brothers shared a genetic marker on the bottom half of the X chromosome. Another study found that a group of cells in the hypothalamus was smaller in women and in gay men than in heterosexual men. Neither of these studies has been replicated.

Sexual Behavior Patterns. The behavioral features of gay men and lesbian women are as varied as those of heterosexuals. Gay men and lesbians engage in the same sexual practices as heterosexuals, with the obvious differences imposed by anatomy.

Many ongoing relationship patterns occur among gay men and lesbians. Some same-sex pairs live in a common household in either a

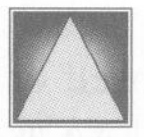

Table 21.1–4
Taking a Sex History

I. Identifying data
   A. Age
   B. Sex
   C. Occupation
   D. Relationship status—single, married, number of times previously married, separated, divorced, cohabiting, serious involvement, casual dating (difficulty forming or keeping relationships should be assessed throughout the interview)
   E. Sexual orientation—heterosexual, homosexual, or bisexual (this may also be ascertained later in the interview)
II. Current functioning
   A. Unsatisfactory to highly satisfactory
   B. If unsatisfactory, why?
   C. Feeling about partner satisfaction
   D. Dysfunctions?—e.g., lack of desire, erectile disorder, inhibited female arousal, anorgasmia, premature ejaculation, retarded ejaculation, pain associated with intercourse (dysfunction discussed below)
      1. Onset—lifelong or acquired
         a. If acquired, when?
         b. Did onset coincide with drug use (medications or illegal recreational drugs), life stresses (e.g., loss of job, birth of child), interpersonal difficulties
      2. Generalized—occurs in most situations or with most partners
      3. Situational
         a. Only with current partner
         b. In any committed relationship
         c. Only with masturbation
         d. In socially proscribed circumstance (e.g., affair)
         e. In definable circumstance (e.g., very late at night, in parental home, when partner initiated sex play)
   E. Frequency—partnered sex (coital and noncoital sex play)
   F. Desire/libido—how often are sexual feelings, thoughts, fantasies, dreams, experienced? (per day, week, etc.)
   G. Description of typical sexual interaction
      1. Manner of initiation or invitation (e.g., verbal or physical? Does same person always initiate?)
      2. Presence, type, and extent of foreplay (e.g., kissing, caressing, manual or oral genital stimulation)
      3. Coitus? positions used?
      4. Verbalization during sex? if so, what kind?
      5. Afterplay? (whether sex act is completed or disrupted by dysfunction); typical activities (e.g., holding, talking, return to daily activities, sleeping)
      6. Feeling after sex: relaxed, tense, angry, loving
   H. Sexual compulsivity?—intrusion of sexual thoughts or participation in sexual activities to a degree that interferes with relationships or work, requires deception and may endanger the patient
III. Past sexual history
   A. Childhood sexuality
      1. Parental attitudes about sex—degree of openness of reserve (assess unusual prudery or seductiveness)
      2. Parents' attitudes about nudity and modesty
      3. Learning about sex
         a. From parents? (initiated by child's questions or parent volunteering information? which parent? what was child's age?) subjects covered (e.g., pregnancy, birth, intercourse, menstruation, nocturnal emission, masturbation)
         b. From books, magazines, or friends at school or through religious group?
         c. Significant misinformation
         d. Feeling about information
      4. Viewing or hearing primal scene—reaction?
      5. Viewing sex play or intercourse of person other than parent
      6. Viewing sex between pets or other animals
   B. Childhood sex activities
      1. Genital self-stimulation before adolescence; age? reaction if apprehended?
      2. Awareness of self as boy or girl; bathroom sensual activities? (regarding urine, feces, odor, enemas)
      3. Sexual play or exploration with another child (playing doctor)—type of activity (e.g., looking, manual touching, genital touching); reactions or consequences if apprehended (by whom?)
IV. Adolescence
   A. Age of onset of puberty—development of secondary sex characteristics, age of menarche for girl, wet dreams or first ejaculation for boy (preparation for and reaction to)
   B. Sense of self as feminine or masculine—body image, acceptance by peers (opposite sex and same sex), sense of sexual desirability, onset of coital fantasies
   C. Sex activities
      1. Masturbation—age begun; ever punished or prohibited? method used, accompanying fantasies, frequency (questions about masturbation and fantasies are among the most sensitive for patients to answer)
      2. Homosexual activities—ongoing or rare and experimental episodes, approached by others? If homosexual, has there been any heterosexual experimentation?
      3. Dating—casual or steady, description of first crush, infatuation, or first love
      4. Experiences of kissing, necking, petting ("making out" or "fooling around"), age begun, frequency, number of partners, circumstances, type(s) of activity
      5. Orgasm—when first experienced? (may not be experienced during adolescence), with masturbation, during sleep, or with partner? with intercourse or other sex play? frequency?
      6. First coitus—age, circumstances, partner, reactions (may not be experienced during adolescence); contraception and/or safe sex precautions used
V. Adult sexual activities (may be experienced by some adolescents)
   A. Premarital sex
      1. Types of sex play experiences—frequency of sexual interactions, types and number of partners
      2. Contraception and/or safe sex precautions used
      3. First coitus (if not experienced in adolescence) age, circumstances, partner
      4. Cohabitation—age begun, duration, description of partner, sexual fidelity, types of sexual activity, frequency, satisfaction, number of cohabiting relationships, reasons for breakup(s)
      5. Engagement—age, activity during engagement period with fiancé(e), with others; length of engagement
   B. Marriage (if multiple marriages have occurred, explore sexual activity, reasons for marriage, and reasons for divorce in each marriage)
      1. Types and frequency of sexual interaction—describe typical sexual interaction (see above), satisfaction with sex life? view of partner's feeling
      2. First sexual experience with spouse—when? what were the circumstances? was it satisfying? disappointing?
      3. Honeymoon—setting, duration, pleasant or unpleasant, sexually active, frequency? problems? compatibility?
      4. Effect of pregnancies and children on marital sex
      5. Extramarital sex—number of incidents, partner; emotional attachment to extramarital partners? feelings about extramarital sex
      6. Postmarital masturbation—frequency? effect on marital sex?
      7. Extramarital sex by partner—effect on interviewee
      8. Ménage à trois or multiple sex (swinging)
      9. Areas of conflict in marriage (e.g., parenting, finances, division of responsibilities, priorities)
VI. Sex after widowhood, separation, divorce—celibacy, orgasms in sleep, masturbation, noncoital sex play, intercourse (number of and relationship to partners), other
VII. Special issues
   A. History of rape, incest, sexual or physical abuse
   B. Spousal abuse (current)
   C. Chronic illness (physical or psychiatric)
   D. History or presence of sexually transmitted diseases
   E. Fertility problems
   F. Abortions, miscarriages, or unwanted or illegitimate pregnancies
   G. Gender identity conflict—(e.g., transsexualism, wearing clothes of opposite sex)
   H. Paraphilias—(e.g., fetishes, voyeurism, sadomasochism)

monogamous or a primary relationship for decades; other gay men and lesbians typically have only fleeting sexual contacts. Although many gay men form stable relationships, male–male relationships appear to be less stable and more fleeting than female–female relationships. Gay-male couples are subjected to civil and social discrimination and do not have the legal social support system of marriage or the biological capacity for childbearing that bonds some otherwise incompatible heterosexual couples. Lesbian couples appear to experience less social stigmatization and to have more enduring monogamous or primary relationships.

Psychopathology. The range of psychopathology that may be found among distressed lesbians and gay men parallels that found among heterosexuals; some studies have reported a high suicide rate, however. Distress resulting only from conflict between gay men and lesbians and the societal value structure is not classifiable as a disorder. If the distress is sufficiently severe to warrant a diagnosis, adjustment disorder or a depressive disorder should be considered. Some gay men and lesbians with major depressive disorder may experience guilt and self-hatred that become directed toward their sexual orientation; then the desire for sexual reorientation is only a symptom of the depressive disorder. According to ICD-10 ego-dystonic sexual orientation occurs when

> The gender identity or sexual preference is not in doubt but the individual wishes it were different because of associated psychological and behavioural disorders and may seek treatment in order to change it.

Coming Out. According to Rochelle Klinger and Robert Cabaj, coming out is a "process by which an individual acknowledges his or her sexual orientation in the face of societal stigma and with successful resolution accepts himself or herself." The authors wrote:

> Successful coming out involves the individual accepting his or her sexual orientation and integrating it into all spheres (e.g., social, vocational, and familial). Another milestone that individuals and couples must eventually confront is the degree of disclosure of sexual orientation to the external world. Some degree of disclosure is probably necessary for successful coming out.

Difficulty negotiating coming out and disclosure is a common cause of relationship difficulties. For each person, problems resolving the coming out process can contribute to poor self-esteem caused by internalized homophobia and lead to deleterious effects on the person's ability to function in the relationship. Conflict can also arise within a relationship when partners disagree on the degree of disclosure.

LOVE AND INTIMACY

Freud postulated that psychological health could be determined by a person's ability to function well in two spheres, work and love. A person able to give and receive love with a minimum of fear and conflict has the capacity to develop genuinely intimate relationships with others. A desire to maintain closeness to the love object typifies being in love. Mature love is marked by the intimacy that is a special attribute of the relationship between two persons. When involved in an intimate relationship, the person actively strives for the growth and happiness of the loved person. Sex frequently acts as a catalyst in forming and maintaining intimate relationships. The quality of intimacy in a mature sexual relationship is what Rollo May called "active receiving," in which a person, while loving, permits himself or herself to be loved. May describes the value of sexual love as an expansion of self-awareness, the experience of tenderness, an increase of self-affirmation and pride, and sometimes, at the moment of orgasm, loss of feeling of separateness. In that setting, sex and love are reciprocally enhancing and healthily fused.

Some persons suffer from conflicts that prevent them from fusing tender and passionate impulses. This can inhibit the expression of sexuality in a relationship, interfere with feelings of closeness to another person, and diminish a person's sense of adequacy and self-esteem. When these problems are severe, they may prevent the formation of, or commitment to, an intimate relationship.

SEX AND THE LAW

Medicine and the law both assess the impact of sexuality on the individual and society and determine what is healthy or legal behavior. Appropriateness or legality of sexual behavior, however, is not always viewed the same way by both professions. The issues at the interface of sexual science and the law often are emotionally charged and reflect cultural divisions about acceptable sexual mores. They include abortion, pornography, prostitution, sex education, the treatment of sex offenders, and the right to sexual privacy, among other issues. Laws regarding these issues (e.g., criminalization of oral or anal sex by consenting adults, or the need for parental permission by minors requesting an abortion) vary from state to state.

TAKING A SEX HISTORY

A sex history provides important information about patients, regardless of the presence of a sexual disorder or whether that is the patient's chief complaint. The information can be obtained gradually, through open-ended questions. The outline in Table 21.1–4 provides a guide to the topics to be covered and a structure that can be used when time is limited.

REFERENCES

Arnold P, Agate RJ, Carruth LL. Hormonal and nonhormonal mechanisms of sexual differentiation of the brain. In: Legato M, ed. *Principles of Gender Specific Medicine*. San Diego: Elsevier Science; 2004:84.

Bancroft J. Alfred C. Kinsey and the politics of sex research. *Ann Rev Sex Res.* 2004;15:1–39.

Drescher J, Stein TS, Byne WM. Homosexuality, gay and lesbian identities and homosexual behavior. In: Sadock BJ, Sadock VA, eds. *Kaplan & Sadock's Comprehensive Textbook of Psychiatry*. 8th ed. Vol. 1. Baltimore: Lippincott Williams & Wilkins; 2005:1936.

Federman DD. Current concepts: The biology of human sex differences. *N Engl J Med.* 2006;354(14):1507.

Federman DD. Perspective: Three facets of sexual differentiation. *N Engl J Med.* 2004; 350:323–324.

Freud S. Letter to an American mother. *Am J Psychiatry*. 1951;102:786.

Freud S. Three essays on the theory of sexuality. In: *Standard Edition of the Complete Psychological Works of Sigmund Freud*. Vol. 16. London: Hogarth Press; 1966:135.

Freud S. General theory of the neuroses. In: *Standard Edition of the Complete Psychological Works of Sigmund Freud*. Vol. 16. London: Hogarth Press; 1966:241.

Gutmann P. About confusions of the mind due to abnormal conditions to the sexual organs. *History of Psychiatry*. 2006;17:107–111.

Hawkins DM. Group psychotherapy with gay men and lesbians. In: Kaplan HI, Sadock BJ, ed. *Comprehensive Group Psychotherapy*. 3rd ed. Baltimore: Williams & Wilkins; 1993:506.

Hines M. *Brain Gender*. New York: Oxford University Press; 2004.

MacLaughlin DT, Donahoe PK. Mechanisms of disease: Sex determination and differentiation. *N Engl J Med.* 2004;350:369.

Melby T. Asexuality: Is it a sexual orientation? *Contemporary Sexuality*. 2005;39(11):1.
Person ES. As the wheel turns: A centennial reflection on Freud's three essays on the theory of sexuality. *J Am Psychoanal Assoc*. 2005;53:1257–1282.
Sadock VA. Normal human sexuality and sexual dysfunctions. In: Sadock BJ, Sadock VA, eds. *Kaplan & Sadock's Comprehensive Textbook of Psychiatry*. 8th ed. Vol. 1. Baltimore: Lippincott Williams & Wilkins; 2005:1902.

▲ 21.2 Abnormal Sexuality and Sexual Dysfunctions

In the text revision of the 4th edition of the *Diagnostic and Statistical Manual of Mental Disorders* (DSM-IV-TR), sexual dysfunctions are categorized as Axis I disorders. The syndromes listed are correlated with the sexual physiological response, which is divided into the four phases (Table 21.2–1). The essential feature of the sexual dysfunctions is inhibition in one or more of the phases, including disturbance in the subjective sense of pleasure or desire or in the objective performance. Either type of disturbance can occur alone or in combination. Sexual dysfunctions are diagnoses only when they are a major part of the clinical picture. They can be lifelong or acquired, generalized or situational, and result from psychological factors, physiological factors, or combined factors. If they are attributable entirely to a general medical condition, substance use, or adverse effects of medication, then sexual dysfunction due to a general medical condition or substance-induced sexual dysfunction is diagnosed. Sexual dysfunctions not associated with the sexual response cycle are listed in Table 21.2–2.

With the possible exception of premature ejaculation and anorgasmia, sexual dysfunctions are rarely found separate from other psychiatric syndromes. Sexual disorders can lead to or result from relational problems, and patients invariably develop an increasing fear of failure and

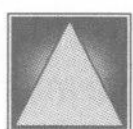

Table 21.2–2
Sexual Dysfunction Not Correlated with Phases of the Sexual Response Cycle

Category	Dysfunctions
Sexual pain disorders	Vaginismus (female) Dyspareunia (female and male)
Other	Sexual dysfunctions not otherwise specified. Examples: 1. No erotic sensation despite normal physiological response to sexual stimulation (e.g., orgasmic anhedonia) 2. Female analogue of premature ejaculation 3. Genital pain occurring during masturbation

self-consciousness about their sexual performance. Sexual dysfunctions are frequently associated with other mental disorders, such as depressive disorders, anxiety disorders, personality disorders, and schizophrenia. In many instances, a sexual dysfunction may be diagnosed in conjunction with another psychiatric disorder; in other cases, however, it is only one of many signs or symptoms of the psychiatric disorder.

In DSM-IV-TR, a sexual dysfunction is defined as a disturbance in the sexual response cycle or as pain with sexual intercourse. Seven major categories of sexual dysfunction are listed in DSM-IV-TR: sexual desire disorders, sexual arousal disorders, orgasm disorders, sexual pain disorders, sexual dysfunction caused by a general medical condition, substance-induced sexual dysfunction, and sexual dysfunction not otherwise specified.

Sexual dysfunctions can be symptomatic of biological (biogenic) problems or intrapsychic or interpersonal (psychogenic) conflicts or a combination of these factors. Sexual function can be adversely affected by stress of any kind, by emotional disorders, or by ignorance of sexual function and physiology. The dysfunction may be lifelong or acquired—that is, it can develop after a period of normal functioning. The dysfunction may be generalized or limited to a specific partner or a certain situation.

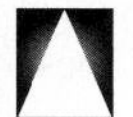

Table 21.2–1
DSM-IV-TR Phases of the Sexual Response Cycle and Associated Sexual Dysfunctions[a]

Phases	Characteristics	Dysfunction
1. Desire	Distinct from any identified solely through physiology and reflects the patient's motivations, drives, and personality; characterized by sexual fantasies and the desire to have sex	Hypoactive sexual desire disorder; sexual aversion disorder; hypoactive sexual desire disorder due to a general medical condition (male or female); substance-induced sexual dysfunction with impaired desire
2. Excitement	Subjective sense of sexual pleasure and accompanying physiological changes; all physiological responses noted in Masters and Johnson's excitement and plateau phases are combined in this phase	Female sexual arousal disorder; male erectile disorder (may also occur in stages 3 and 4); male erectile disorder due to a general medical condition; dyspareunia due to a general medical condition (male or female); substance-induced sexual dysfunction with impaired arousal
3. Orgasm	Peaking of sexual pleasure, with release of sexual tension and rhythmic contraction of the perineal muscles and pelvic reproductive organs	Female orgasmic disorder; male orgasmic disorder; premature ejaculation; other sexual dysfunction due to a general medical condition (male or female); substance-induced sexual dysfunction with impaired orgasm
4. Resolution	A sense of general relaxation, well-being, and muscle relaxation; men are refractory to orgasm for a period of time that increases with age, whereas women can have multiple orgasms without a refractory period	Postcoital dysphoria; postcoital headache

[a]DSM-IV-TR consolidates the Masters and Johnson excitement and plateau phases into a single excitement phase, which is preceded by the desire (appetitive) phase. The orgasm and resolution phases remain the same as originally described by Masters and Johnson.

In considering each of the disorders, clinicians need to rule out an acquired medical condition and the use of a pharmacological substance that could account for, or contribute to, the dysfunction. If the disorder is biogenic, it is coded on Axis III unless substantial evidence indicates dysfunctional episodes apart from the onset of physiological or pharmacological influences. In some cases, a patient has more than one dysfunction—for example, premature ejaculation and male erectile disorder.

SEXUAL DESIRE DISORDERS

Sexual desire disorders are divided into two classes: hypoactive sexual desire disorder, characterized by a deficiency or absence of sexual fantasies and desire for sexual activity (Table 21.2–3); and sexual aversion disorder, characterized by an aversion to, and avoidance of, genital sexual contact with a sexual partner or by masturbation (Table 21.2–4). The former condition is more common than the latter and more common among women than among men. Minimal spontaneous sexual thinking or minimal desire for sex ahead of sexual experiences does not necessarily constitute a desire disorder in women, particularly if desire is triggered during the sexual encounter. Low desire has been reported by 10 to 15 percent of women in various countries. In the United States, an estimated 20 percent of persons have hypoactive sexual desire disorder.

A variety of causative factors are associated with sexual desire disorders. Patients with desire problems often use inhibition of desire defensively, to protect against unconscious fears about sex. Sigmund Freud conceptualized low sexual desire as the result of inhibition during the phallic psychosexual phase of development and of unresolved oedipal conflicts. Some men, fixated at the phallic state of development, are fearful of the vagina and believe that they will be castrated if they approach it. Freud called this concept *vagina dentata*; because men unconsciously believe that the vagina has teeth, they avoid contact with the female genitalia. Equally, women may suffer from unresolved developmental conflicts that inhibit desire. Lack of desire can also result from chronic stress, anxiety, or depression.

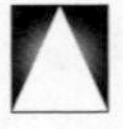

Table 21.2–3
DSM-IV-TR Diagnostic Criteria for Hypoactive Sexual Desire Disorder

A. Persistently or recurrently deficient (or absent) sexual fantasies and desire for sexual activity. The judgment of deficiency or absence is made by the clinician, taking into account factors that affect sexual functioning, such as age and the context of the person's life.
B. The disturbance causes marked distress or interpersonal difficulty.
C. The sexual dysfunction is not better accounted for by another Axis I disorder (except another sexual dysfunction) and is not due exclusively to the direct physiological effects of a substance (e.g., a drug of abuse, a medication) or a general medical condition.

Specify type:
Lifelong type
Acquired type

Specify type:
Generalized type
Situational type

Specify:
Due to psychological factors
Due to combined factors

(From American Psychiatric Association. *Diagnostic and Statistical Manual of Mental Disorders.* 4th ed. Text rev. Washington, DC: American Psychiatric Association; copyright 2000, with permission.)

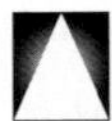

Table 21.2–4
DSM-IV-TR Diagnostic Criteria for Sexual Aversion Disorder

A. Persistent or recurrent extreme aversion to, and avoidance of, all (or almost all) genital sexual contact with a sexual partner.
B. The disturbance causes marked distress or interpersonal difficulty.
C. The sexual dysfunction is not better accounted for by another Axis I disorder (except another sexual dysfunction).

Specify type:
Lifelong type
Acquired type

Specify type:
Situational type
Generalized type

Specify:
Due to psychological factors
Due to combined factors

(From American Psychiatric Association. *Diagnostic and Statistical Manual of Mental Disorders.* 4th ed. Text rev. Washington, DC: American Psychiatric Association; copyright 2000, with permission.)

Abstinence from sex for a prolonged period sometimes results in suppression of sexual impulses. Loss of desire may also be an expression of hostility to a partner or the sign of a deteriorating relationship. In one study of young married couples who ceased having sexual relations for 2 months, marital discord was the reason most frequently given for the cessation or inhibition of sexual activity.

The presence of desire depends on several factors: biological drive, adequate self-esteem, the ability to accept oneself as a sexual person, previous good experiences with sex, the availability of an appropriate partner, and a good relationship in nonsexual areas with a partner. Damage to, or absence of, any of these factors can diminish desire.

In making the diagnosis, clinicians must evaluate a patient's age, general health, and life stresses and must attempt to establish a baseline of sexual interest before the disorder began. The need for sexual contact and satisfaction varies among persons and over time in any given person. In a group of 100 couples with stable marriages, 8 percent reported having intercourse less than once a month. In another group of couples, one third reported episodic lack of sexual relations for periods averaging 8 weeks. Married couples have coitus three times a month, on average. The diagnosis should not be made unless the lack of desire is a source of distress to a patient.

SEXUAL AROUSAL DISORDERS

The sexual arousal disorders are divided by DSM-IV-TR into female sexual arousal disorder, characterized by the persistent or recurrent partial or complete failure to attain or maintain the lubrication-swelling response of sexual excitement until the completion of the sexual act (Table 21.2–5), and male erectile disorder, characterized by the recurrent and persistent partial or complete failure to attain or maintain an erection to perform the sex act (Table 21.2–6). The diagnosis takes into account the

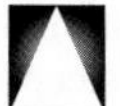

Table 21.2–5
DSM-IV-TR Diagnostic Criteria for Female Sexual Arousal Disorder

A. Persistent or recurrent inability to attain, or to maintain until completion of the sexual activity, an adequate lubrication-swelling response of sexual excitement.
B. The disturbance causes marked distress or interpersonal difficulty.
C. The sexual dysfunction is not better accounted for by another Axis I disorder (except another sexual dysfunction) and is not due exclusively to the direct physiological effects of a substance (e.g., a drug of abuse, a medication) or a general medical condition.

Specify type:
Lifelong type
Acquired type

Specify type:
Generalized type
Situational type

Specify:
Due to psychological factors
Due to combined factors

(From American Psychiatric Association. *Diagnostic and Statistical Manual of Mental Disorders.* 4th ed. Text rev. Washington, DC: American Psychiatric Association; copyright 2000, with permission.)

focus, intensity, and duration of the sexual activity in which patients engage. If sexual stimulation is inadequate in focus, intensity, or duration, the diagnosis should not be made.

Female Sexual Arousal Disorder

The DSM-III-R defines female sexual arousal disorder in terms of the physiological arousal response. A subjective sense of arousal is often poorly correlated, however, with genital lubrication in both dysfunctional and normal women. A woman complaining of lack of arousal may lubricate vaginally, but may not experience a subjective sense of excitement. Some studies using functional magnetic resonance imaging (fMRI) have revealed a low correlation between brain activation in areas controlling genital response and simultaneous ratings of subjective arousal.

Physiological studies of sexual dysfunctions indicate that a hormonal pattern may contribute to responsiveness in women who have excitement-phase dysfunction. William Masters and Virginia Johnson found women particularly desirous of sex before the onset of the menses. Other women report feeling the greatest sexual excitement immediately after the menses or at the time of ovulation. Alterations in testosterone, estrogen, prolactin, and thyroxin levels have been implicated in female sexual arousal disorder. Also, medications with antihistaminic or anticholinergic properties cause a decrease in vaginal lubrication.

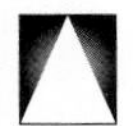

Table 21.2–6
DSM-IV-TR Diagnostic Criteria for Male Erectile Disorder

A. Persistent or recurrent inability to attain, or to maintain until completion of the sexual activity, an adequate erection.
B. The disturbance causes marked distress or interpersonal difficulty.
C. The erectile dysfunction is not better accounted for by another Axis I disorder (other than a sexual dysfunction) and is not due exclusively to the direct physiological effects of a substance (e.g., a drug of abuse, a medication) or a general medical condition.

Specify type:
Lifelong type
Acquired type

Specify type:
Generalized type
Situational type

Specify:
Due to psychological factors
Due to combined factors

(From American Psychiatric Association. *Diagnostic and Statistical Manual of Mental Disorders.* 4th ed. Text rev. Washington, DC: American Psychiatric Association; copyright 2000, with permission.)

Male Erectile Disorder

Male erectile disorder is also called *erectile dysfunction* and *impotence*. A man with lifelong male erectile disorder has never been able to obtain an erection sufficient for vaginal insertion. In acquired male erectile disorder, a man has successfully achieved vaginal penetration at some time in his sexual life but is later unable to do so. In situational male erectile disorder, a man is able to have coitus in certain circumstances but not in others; for example, he may function effectively with a prostitute but be impotent with his wife.

Acquired male erectile disorder has been reported in 10 to 20 percent of all men. Freud declared it common among his patients. Impotence is the chief complaint of more than 50 percent of all men treated for sexual disorders. Lifelong male erectile disorder is rare; it occurs in about 1 percent of men under age 35, but the incidence increases with age. It has been reported in about 8 percent of the young adult population. Alfred Kinsey reported that 75 percent of all men were impotent at age 80. All men over 40, Masters and Johnson reported, have a fear of impotence, which the researchers believed reflects the masculine fear of loss of virility with advancing age. Male erectile disorder, however, is not universal in aging men; having an available sex partner is related to continuing potency, as is a history of consistent sexual activity and the absence of vascular disease.

Male erectile disorder can be organic or psychological or a combination of both, but in young and middle-aged men the cause is usually psychological. A good history is of primary importance in determining the cause of the dysfunction. If a man reports having spontaneous erections at times when he does not plan to have intercourse, having morning erections, or having good erections with masturbation or with partners other than his usual one, the organic causes of his impotence can be considered negligible, and costly diagnostic procedures can be avoided. Male erectile disorder caused by a general medical condition or a pharmacological substance is discussed below in this section.

Freud ascribed one type of impotence to an inability to reconcile feelings of affection toward a woman with feelings of desire for her. Men with such conflicting feelings can function only with women whom they see as degraded (Madonna–Putana complex). Other factors that have been cited as contributing to impotence include a punitive superego, an inability to trust, and feelings of inadequacy or a sense of being undesirable as a partner. A man may be unable to express a sexual impulse because of fear, anxiety, anger, or moral prohibition. In an ongoing relationship, impotence may reflect difficulties between the partners, particularly when a man cannot communicate his needs or his anger in a direct and constructive way. In addition, episodes of impotence are reinforcing, with the man becoming increasingly anxious before each sexual encounter.

ORGASM DISORDERS

Female Orgasmic Disorder

Female orgasmic disorder, sometimes called *inhibited female orgasm* or *anorgasmia*, is defined as the recurrent or persistent inhibition of female orgasm, as manifested by the recurrent delay in, or absence of, orgasm after a normal sexual excitement phase that a clinician judges to be adequate in focus, intensity, and duration—in short, a woman's inability to achieve orgasm by masturbation or coitus (Table 21.2–7). Women who can achieve orgasm by one of these methods are not necessarily categorized as anorgasmic, although some sexual inhibition may be postulated.

Research on the physiology of the female sexual response has shown that orgasms caused by clitoral stimulation and those caused by vaginal stimulation are physiologically identical. Freud's theory that women must give up clitoral sensitivity for vaginal sensitivity to achieve sexual maturity is now considered misleading, but some women report that they gain a special sense of satisfaction from an orgasm precipitated by coitus. Some researchers attribute this satisfaction to the psychological feeling of closeness engendered by the act of coitus, but others maintain that the coital orgasm is a physiologically different experience. Many women achieve orgasm during coitus by a combination of manual clitoral stimulation and penile vaginal stimulation.

A woman with lifelong female orgasmic disorder has never experienced orgasm by any kind of stimulation. A woman with acquired orgasmic disorder has previously experienced at least one orgasm, regardless of the circumstances or means of stimulation, whether by masturbation or while dreaming during sleep. Kinsey found that only 5 percent of married women over 35 years of age had never achieved orgasm by any means. The incidence of orgasm increases with age. According to Kinsey, the first orgasm occurs during adolescence in about 50 percent of women as a result of masturbation or genital caressing with a partner; the rest usually experience orgasm as they get older. Lifelong female orgasmic disorder is more common among unmarried women than married women. Increased orgasmic potential in women over 35 years of age has been explained on the basis of less psychological inhibition, greater sexual experience, or both.

Table 21.2–7
DSM-IV-TR Diagnostic Criteria for Female Orgasmic Disorder

A. Persistent or recurrent delay in, or absence of, orgasm following a normal sexual excitement phase. Women exhibit wide variability in the type or intensity of stimulation that triggers orgasm. The diagnosis of female orgasmic disorder should be based on the clinician's judgment that the woman's orgasmic capacity is less than would be reasonable for her age, sexual experience, and the adequacy of sexual stimulation she receives.
B. The disturbance causes marked distress or interpersonal difficulty.
C. The orgasmic dysfunction is not better accounted for by another Axis I disorder (except another sexual dysfunction) and is not due exclusively to the direct physiological effects of a substance (e.g., a drug of abuse, a medication) or a general medical condition.

Specify type:
Lifelong type
Acquired type

Specify type:
Generalized type
Situational type

Specify:
Due to psychological factors
Due to combined factors

(From American Psychiatric Association. *Diagnostic and Statistical Manual of Mental Disorders.* 4th ed. Text rev. Washington, DC: American Psychiatric Association; copyright 2000, with permission.)

Acquired female orgasmic disorder is a common complaint in clinical populations. One clinical treatment facility reported having about four times as many nonorgasmic women in its practice as patients with all other sexual disorders. In another study, 46 percent of women complained of difficulty reaching orgasm. The true prevalence of problems maintaining excitement is not known, but inhibition of excitement and orgasmic problems often occur together. The overall prevalence of female orgasmic disorder from all causes is estimated to be 30 percent. A recent twin study suggests that orgasmic dysfunction in some females has a genetic basis and cannot be attributed solely to cultural differences. That study demonstrated an estimated heritability for difficulty reaching orgasm with intercourse of 34 percent and an estimated heritability in women who could not climax with masturbation of 45 percent.

Numerous psychological factors are associated with female orgasmic disorder. They include fears of impregnation, rejection by a sex partner, and damage to the vagina; hostility toward men; and feelings of guilt about sexual impulses. Some women equate orgasm with loss of control or with aggressive, destructive, or violent impulses; their fear of these impulses may be expressed through inhibition of excitement or orgasm. Cultural expectations and social restrictions on women are also relevant. Many women have grown up to believe that sexual pleasure is not a natural entitlement for so-called decent women. Nonorgasmic women may be otherwise symptom free or may experience frustration in a variety of ways; they may have such pelvic complaints as lower abdominal pain, itching, and vaginal discharge, as well as increased tension, irritability, and fatigue.

Male Orgasmic Disorder

In male orgasmic disorder, sometimes called *inhibited orgasm* or *retarded ejaculation*, a man achieves ejaculation during coitus with great difficulty, if at all (Table 21.2–8). A man with lifelong orgasmic disorder has never been able to ejaculate during coitus. The disorder is diagnosed as acquired if it develops after previously normal functioning. Some researchers think that orgasm and ejaculation should be differentiated, especially in the case of men who ejaculate but complain of a decreased or absent subjective sense of pleasure during the orgasmic experience (orgasmic anhedonia).

The incidence of male orgasmic disorder is much lower than the incidence of premature ejaculation or impotence. Masters and Johnson reported an incidence of male orgasmic disorder of only 3.8 percent in one group of 447 men with sexual dysfunctions. A general prevalence of 5 percent has been reported.

Lifelong male orgasmic disorder indicates severe psychopathology. A man may come from a rigid, puritanical background; he may perceive sex as sinful and the genitals as dirty; and he may have conscious or unconscious incest wishes and guilt. He usually has difficulty with closeness in areas beyond those of sexual relations. In a few cases, the

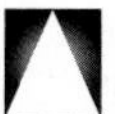

Table 21.2–8
DSM-IV-TR Diagnostic Criteria for Male Orgasmic Disorder

A. Persistent or recurrent delay in, or absence of, orgasm following a normal sexual excitement phase during sexual activity that the clinician, taking into account the person's age, judges to be adequate in focus, intensity, and duration.
B. The disturbance causes marked distress or interpersonal difficulty.
C. The orgasmic dysfunction is not better accounted for by another Axis I disorder (except another sexual dysfunction) and is not due exclusively to the direct physiological effects of a substance (e.g., a drug of abuse, a medication) or a general medical condition.

Specify type:
 Lifelong type
 Acquired type

Specify type:
 Generalized type
 Situational type

Specify:
 Due to psychological factors
 Due to combined factors

(From American Psychiatric Association. *Diagnostic and Statistical Manual of Mental Disorders*. 4th ed. Text rev. Washington, DC: American Psychiatric Association; copyright 2000, with permission.)

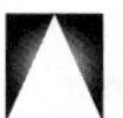

Table 21.2–9
DSM-IV-TR Diagnostic Criteria for Premature Ejaculation

A. Persistent or recurrent ejaculation with minimal sexual stimulation before, on, or shortly after penetration and before the person wishes it. The clinician must take into account factors that affect duration of the excitement phase, such as age, novelty of the sexual partner or situation, and recent frequency of sexual activity.
B. The disturbance causes marked distress or interpersonal difficulty.
C. The premature ejaculation is not due exclusively to the direct effects of a substance (e.g., withdrawal from opioids).

Specify type:
 Lifelong type
 Acquired type

Specify type:
 Generalized type
 Situational type

Specify:
 Due to psychological factors
 Due to combined factors

(From American Psychiatric Association. *Diagnostic and Statistical Manual of Mental Disorders*. 4th ed. Text rev. Washington, DC: American Psychiatric Association; copyright 2000, with permission.)

condition is aggravated by an attention-deficit disorder. A man's distractibility prevents sufficient arousal for climax to occur.

In an ongoing relationship, acquired male orgasmic disorder frequently reflects interpersonal difficulties. The disorder may be a man's way of coping with real or fantasized changes in a relationship, such as plans for pregnancy about which the man is ambivalent, the loss of sexual attraction to the partner, or demands by the partner for greater commitment as expressed by sexual performance. In some men, the inability to ejaculate reflects unexpressed hostility toward a woman. The problem is more common among men with obsessive-compulsive disorder (OCD) than among others.

Premature Ejaculation

In premature ejaculation, men persistently or recurrently achieve orgasm and ejaculation before they wish to. No definite timeframe exists within which to define the dysfunction; the diagnosis is made when a man regularly ejaculates before or immediately after entering the vagina. Clinicians need to consider factors that affect the duration of the excitement phase, such as age, the novelty of the sex partner, and the frequency and duration of coitus (Table 21.2–9). Masters and Johnson conceptualized the disorder in terms of the couple and considered a man a premature ejaculator if he could not control ejaculation sufficiently long enough during intravaginal containment to satisfy his partner in at least half their episodes of coitus. This definition assumes that the female partner is capable of an orgasmic response. As with the other sexual dysfunctions, premature ejaculation is not diagnosed when it is caused exclusively by organic factors or when it is not symptomatic of any other clinical psychiatric syndrome.

Premature ejaculation is more commonly reported among college-educated men than among men with less education. The complaint is thought to be related to their concern for partner satisfaction, but the true cause of this increased frequency has not been determined. Premature ejaculation is the chief complaint of about 35 to 40 percent of men treated for sexual disorders. Some researchers divide men who experience premature ejaculation into two groups: those who are physiologically predisposed to climax quickly because of shorter nerve latency time and those with a psychogenic or behaviorally conditioned cause. Difficulty in ejaculatory control can be associated with anxiety regarding the sex act, with unconscious fears about the vagina, or with negative cultural conditioning. Men whose early sexual contacts occurred largely with prostitutes who demanded that the sex act proceed quickly or whose sexual contacts took place in situations in which discovery would be embarrassing (e.g., in the back seat of a car or in the parental home) might have been conditioned to achieve orgasm rapidly. With young, inexperienced men, who are more likely to have the problem, it may resolve in time. In ongoing relationships, the partner has a great influence on a premature ejaculator, and a stressful marriage exacerbates the disorder. The developmental background and the psychodynamics found in premature ejaculation and in impotence are similar.

SEXUAL PAIN DISORDERS

Dyspareunia

Dyspareunia is recurrent or persistent genital pain occurring in either men or women before, during, or after intercourse. Much more common in women than in men, dyspareunia is related to, and often coincides with, vaginismus. Repeated episodes of vaginismus can lead to dyspareunia and vice versa; in either case, somatic causes must be ruled out. Dyspareunia should not be diagnosed when an organic basis for the pain is found or when, in a woman, it is caused exclusively by vaginismus or by a lack of lubrication (Table 21.2–10). The incidence of dyspareunia is unknown.

In most cases, dynamic factors are considered causative. Chronic pelvic pain is a common complaint in women with a history of rape or childhood sexual abuse. Painful coitus can result from tension and anxiety about the sex act that cause women to involuntarily contract their vaginal muscles. The pain is real and makes intercourse unpleasant or unbearable. Anticipation of further pain may cause women to avoid coitus altogether. If a partner proceeds with intercourse regardless of a woman's state of readiness, the condition is aggravated. Dyspareunia can also

Table 21.2–10
DSM-IV-TR Diagnostic Criteria for Dyspareunia

A. Recurrent or persistent genital pain associated with sexual intercourse in either a male or a female.
B. The disturbance causes marked distress or interpersonal difficulty.
C. The disturbance is not caused exclusively by vaginismus or lack of lubrication, is not better accounted for by another Axis I disorder (except another sexual dysfunction), and is not due exclusively to the direct physiological effects of a substance (e.g., a drug of abuse, a medication) or a general medical condition.

Specify type:
Lifelong type
Acquired type

Specify type:
Generalized type
Situational type

Specify:
Due to psychological factors
Due to combined factors

(From American Psychiatric Association. *Diagnostic and Statistical Manual of Mental Disorders.* 4th ed. Text rev. Washington, DC: American Psychiatric Association; copyright 2000, with permission.)

occur in men, but it is uncommon and is usually associated with an organic condition, such as herpes, prostatitis, or Peyronie's disease, which consists of sclerotic plaques on the penis that cause penile curvature.

Vaginismus

Vaginismus is an involuntary muscle constriction of the outer third of the vagina that interferes with penile insertion and intercourse. This response may occur during a gynecological examination when involuntary vaginal constriction prevents the introduction of the speculum into the vagina. The diagnosis is not made when the dysfunction is caused exclusively by organic factors or when it is symptomatic of another Axis I mental disorder (Table 21.2–11).

Vaginismus is less prevalent than female orgasmic disorder. It most often afflicts highly educated women and those in high socioeconomic groups. Women with vaginismus may consciously wish to have coitus, but unconsciously wish to keep a penis from entering their bodies. A sexual trauma, such as rape, may cause vaginismus; women with psychosexual conflicts may perceive the penis as a weapon. In some cases, pain or the anticipation of pain at the first coital experience causes vaginismus. Clinicians have noted that a strict religious upbringing in which sex is associated with sin is frequent in these patients. Other women have problems in dyadic relationships; if women feel emotionally abused by their partners, they may protest in this nonverbal fashion.

SEXUAL DYSFUNCTION DUE TO A GENERAL MEDICAL CONDITION

The category sexual dysfunction due to a general medical condition covers sexual dysfunction that results in marked distress and interpersonal difficulty; the history, physical examination, or laboratory findings must provide evidence of a general medical condition judged to be causally related to the sexual dysfunction (Table 21.2–12).

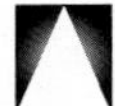

Table 21.2–11
DSM-IV-TR Diagnostic Criteria for Vaginismus

A. Recurrent or persistent involuntary spasm of the musculature of the outer third of the vagina that interferes with sexual intercourse.
B. The disturbance causes marked distress or interpersonal difficulty.
C. The disturbance is not better accounted for by another Axis I disorder (e.g., somatization disorder) and is not due exclusively to the direct physiological effects of a general medical condition.

Specify type:
Lifelong type
Acquired type

Specify type:
Generalized type
Situational type

Specify:
Due to psychological factors
Due to combined factors

(From American Psychiatric Association. *Diagnostic and Statistical Manual of Mental Disorders.* 4th ed. Text rev. Washington, DC: American Psychiatric Association; copyright 2000, with permission.)

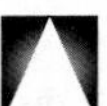

Table 21.2–12
DSM-IV-TR Diagnostic Criteria for Sexual Dysfunction Due to a General Medical

A. Clinically significant sexual dysfunction that results in marked distress or interpersonal difficulty predominates in the clinical picture.
B. There is evidence from the history, physical examination, or laboratory findings that the sexual dysfunction is fully explained by the direct physiological effects of a general medical condition.
C. The disturbance is not better accounted for by another mental disorder (e.g., major depressive disorder).

Select code and term based on the predominant sexual dysfunction:

Female hypoactive sexual desire disorder due to . . . [indicate the general medical condition]: if deficient or absent sexual desire is the predominant feature
Male hypoactive sexual desire disorder due to . . . [indicate the general medical condition]: if deficient or absent sexual desire is the predominant feature
Male erectile disorder due to . . . [indicate the general medical condition]: if male erectile dysfunction is the predominant feature
Female dyspareunia due to . . . [indicate the general medical condition]: if pain associated with intercourse is the predominant feature
Male dyspareunia due to . . . [indicate the general medical condition]: if pain associated with intercourse is the predominant feature
Other female sexual dysfunction due to . . . [indicate the general medical condition]: if some other feature is predominant (e.g., orgasmic disorder) or no feature predominates
Other male sexual dysfunction due to . . . [indicate the general medical condition]: if some other feature is predominant (e.g., orgasmic disorder) or no feature predominates

Coding note: Include the name of the general medical condition on Axis I, e.g., male erectile disorder due to diabetes mellitus; also code the general medical condition on Axis III.

(From American Psychiatric Association. *Diagnostic and Statistical Manual of Mental Disorders.* 4th ed. Text rev. Washington, DC: American Psychiatric Association; copyright 2000, with permission.)

Male Erectile Disorder Due to a General Medical Condition

The incidence of psychological, as opposed to organic, male erectile disorder has been the focus of many studies. Statistics indicate that 20 to 50 percent of men with erectile disorder have an organic basis for the disorder. The organic causes of male erectile disorder are listed in Table 21.2–13. Side effects of medication can impair male sexual functioning in a variety of ways (Table 21.2–14). Castration (removal of the testes) does not always lead to sexual dysfunction, because erection may still occur. A reflex arc, fired when the inner thigh is stimulated, passes through the sacral cord erectile center to account for the phenomenon.

A number of procedures, benign and invasive, are used to help differentiate organically caused impotence from functional impotence. The procedures include monitoring nocturnal penile tumescence (erections that occur during sleep), normally associated with rapid eye movement; monitoring tumescence with a strain gauge; measuring blood pressure in the penis with a penile plethysmograph or an ultrasound (Doppler) flowmeter, both of which assess blood flow in the internal pudendal artery; and measuring pudendal nerve latency time. Other diagnostic tests that delineate organic bases for impotence include glucose tolerance tests, plasma hormone assays, liver and thyroid function tests, prolactin and follicle-stimulating hormone (FHS) determinations, and cystometric examinations. Invasive diagnostic studies include penile arteriography, infusion cavernosonography, and radioactive xenon penography. Invasive procedures require expert interpretation and are used only for patients who are candidates for vascular reconstructive procedures.

Dyspareunia Due to a General Medical Condition

An estimated 30 percent of all surgical procedures on the female genital area result in temporary dyspareunia. In addition, 30 to 40 percent of women with the complaint who are seen in sex therapy clinics have pelvic pathology. Organic abnormalities leading to dyspareunia and vaginismus include irritated or infected hymenal remnants, episiotomy scars, Bartholin's gland infection, various forms of vaginitis and cervicitis, and endometriosis. Postcoital pain has been reported by women with myomata and endometriosis and is attributed to the uterine contractions during orgasm. Postmenopausal women may have dyspareunia resulting from thinning of the vaginal mucosa and reduced lubrication.

Two conditions not readily apparent on physical examination that produce dyspareunia are vulvar vestibulitis and interstitial cystitis. The former may present with chronic vulvar pain and the latter produces pain most intensely following orgasm. Dyspareunia can also occur in men, but it is uncommon and is usually associated with an organic condition, such as Peyronie's disease, which consists of sclerotic plaques on the penis that cause penile curvature.

Hypoactive Sexual Desire Disorder Due to a General Medical Condition

Sexual desire commonly decreases after major illness or surgery, particularly when the body image is affected after such procedures as mastectomy, ileostomy, hysterectomy, and

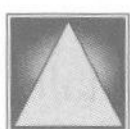

Table 21.2–13
Diseases and Other Medical Conditions Implicated in Male Erectile Disorder

Infectious and parasitic diseases
- Elephantiasis
- Mumps

Cardiovascular disease[a]
- Atherosclerotic disease
- Aortic aneurysm
- Leriche's syndrome
- Cardiac failure

Renal and urological disorders
- Peyronie's disease
- Chronic renal failure
- Hydrocele and varicocele

Hepatic disorders
- Cirrhosis (usually associated with alcohol dependence)

Pulmonary disorders
- Respiratory failure

Genetics
- Klinefelter's syndrome
- Congenital penile vascular and structural abnormalities

Nutritional disorders
- Malnutrition
- Vitamin deficiencies
- Obesity

Endocrine disorders[a]
- Diabetes mellitus
- Dysfunction of the pituitary-adrenal-testis axis
- Acromegaly
- Addison's disease
- Chromophobe adenoma
- Adrenal neoplasia
- Myxedema
- Hyperthyroidism

Neurological disorders
- Multiple sclerosis
- Transverse myelitis
- Parkinson's disease
- Temporal lobe epilepsy
- Traumatic and neoplastic spinal cord diseases[a]
- Central nervous system tumor
- Amyotrophic lateral sclerosis
- Peripheral neuropathy
- General paresis
- Tabes dorsalis

Pharmacological factors
- Alcohol and other dependence-inducing substances (heroin, methadone, morphine, cocaine, amphetamines, and barbiturates)
- Prescribed drugs (psychotropic drugs, antihypertensive drugs, estrogens, and antiandrogens)

Poisoning
- Lead (plumbism)
- Herbicides

Surgical procedures[a]
- Perineal prostatectomy
- Abdominal-perineal colon resection
- Sympathectomy (frequently interferes with ejaculation)
- Aortoiliac surgery
- Radical cystectomy
- Retroperitoneal lymphadenectomy

Miscellaneous
- Radiation therapy
- Pelvic fracture
- Any severe systemic disease or debilitating condition

[a]In the United States an estimated 2 million men are impotent because they suffer from diabetes mellitus; an additional 300,000 are impotent because of other endocrine diseases; 1.5 million are impotent as a result of vascular disease; 180,000 because of multiple sclerosis; 400,000 because of traumas and fractures leading to pelvic fractures or spinal cord injuries; and another 650,000 are impotent as a result of radical surgery, including prostatectomies, colostomies, and cystectomies.

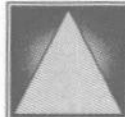

Table 21.2–14
Some Pharmacological Agents Implicated in Male Sexual Dysfunctions

Drug	Impairs Erection	Impairs Ejaculation
Psychiatric drugs		
Cyclic drugs[a]		
Imipramine (Tofranil)	+	+
Protriptyline (Vivactil)	+	+
Desipramine (Pertofrane)	+	+
Clomipramine (Anafranil)	+	+
Amitriptyline (Elavil)	+	+
Trazodone (Desyrel)[b]	−	−
Monoamine oxidase inhibitors		
Tranylcypromine (Parnate)	+	
Phenelzine (Nardil)	+	+
Pargyline (Eutonyl)	−	+
Isocarboxazid (Marplan)	−	+
Other mood-active drugs		
Lithium (Eskalith)	+	
Amphetamines	+	+
Fluoxetine (Prozac)[e]	−	+
Antipsychotics[c]		
Fluphenazine (Prolixin)	+	
Thioridazine (Mellaril)	+	+
Chlorprothixene (Taractan)	−	+
Mesoridazine (Serentil)	−	+
Perphenazine (Trilafon)	−	+
Trifluoperazine (Stelazine)	−	+
Reserpine (Serpasil)	+	+
Haloperidol (Haldol)	−	+
Antianxiety agent[d]		
Chlordiazepoxide (Librium)	−	+
Antihypertensive drugs		
Clonidine (Catapres)	+	
Methyldopa (Aldomet)	+	+
Spironolactone (Aldactone)	+	−
Hydrochlorothiazide	+	−
Guanethidine (Ismelin)	+	+
Commonly abused substances		
Alcohol	+	+
Barbiturates	+	+
Cannabis	+	−
Cocaine	+	+
Heroin	+	+
Methadone	+	−
Morphine	+	+
Miscellaneous drugs		
Antiparkinsonian agents	+	+
Clofibrate (Atromid-S)	+	−
Digoxin (Lanoxin)	+	−
Glutethimide (Doriden)	+	+
Indomethacin (Indocin)	+	−
Phentolamine (Regitine)	−	+
Propranodol (Inderal)	+	−

[a]The incidence of male erectile disorder associated with the use of tricyclic drugs is low.
[b]Trazodone has been causative in some cases of priapism.
[c]Impairment of sexual function is not a common complication of the use of antipsychotics. Priapism has occasionally occurred in association with the use of antipsychotics.
[d]Benzodiazepines have been reported to decrease libido, but in some patients the diminution of anxiety caused by those drugs enhances sexual function.
[e]All selective serotonergic reuptake inhibitors can produce sexual dysfunction, more commonly, in men.

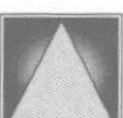

Table 21.2–15
Neurophysiology of Sexual Dysfunction

	DA	5-HT	NE	ACh	Clinical Correlation
Erection	↑	○	α, β ↓↑	M	Antipsychotics may lead to erectile dysfunction (DA block): DA agonists may lead to enhanced erection and libido; priapism with trazodone (α_1, block); β-blockers may lead to impotence
Ejaculation and orgasm	○	± ↓	α_1 ↑	M	α_1-Blockers (tricyclic drugs, MAOIs, thioridazine) may lead to impaired ejaculation; 5-HT agents may inhibit orgasm

↑, facilities; ↓, inhibits or decreases; ±, some; ACh, acetylcholine; DA dopamine; 5-HT serotonin; M, modulates; NE, norepinephrine; ○, minimal.
(Reprinted with permission from Segraves R. *Psychiatric Times*, 1990.)

prostatectomy. Illnesses that deplete a person's energy, chronic conditions that require physical and psychological adaptation, and serious illnesses that can cause a person to become depressed can all markedly lessen sexual desire in both men and women.

In some cases, biochemical correlates are associated with hypoactive sexual desire disorder (Table 21.2–15). A recent study found markedly lower levels of serum testosterone in men complaining of low desire than in normal controls in a sleep-laboratory situation. Drugs that depress the central nervous system (CNS) or decrease testosterone production can decrease desire.

Other Male Sexual Dysfunction Due to a General Medical Condition

When another dysfunctional feature is predominant (e.g., orgasmic disorder) or when no feature predominates, the category other male sexual dysfunction due to a general medical condition is used.

Male orgasmic disorder can have physiological causes and can occur after surgery on the genitourinary tract, such as prostatectomy. It may also be associated with Parkinson's disease and other neurological disorders involving the lumbar or sacral sections of the spinal cord. The antihypertensive drug guanethidine monosulfate (Ismelin), methyldopa (Aldomet), the phenothiazines, the tricyclic drugs, and the selective serotonin reuptake inhibitors (SSRIs), among others, have been implicated in retarded ejaculation. Male orgasmic disorder must also be differentiated from retrograde ejaculation, in which ejaculation occurs but the seminal fluid passes backward into the bladder. Retrograde ejaculation always has an organic cause. It can develop after genitourinary surgery and is also associated with

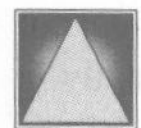

Table 21.2–16
Some Antipsychotic Drugs Implemented in Inhibited Female Orgasm[a]

Tricyclic antidepressants
- Imipramine (Tofranil)
- Clomipramine (Anafranil)
- Nortriptyline (Aventyl)

Monoamine oxidase inhibitors
- Tranylcypromine (Parnate)
- Phenelzine (Nardil)
- Isocarboxazid (Marplan)

Dopamine receptor antagonists
- Thioridazine (Mellaril)
- Trifluoperazine (Stelazine)

Selective serotonergic receptor inhibitors
- Fluoxetine (Prozac)
- Paroxetine (Paxil)
- Sertraline (Zoloft)
- Fluvoxamine (Luvox)
- Citalopram (Celexa)

[a]The interrelation between female sexual dysfunction and pharmacological agents has been less extensively evaluated than male reactions. Oral contraceptives are reported to decrease libido in some women, and some drugs with anticholinergic side effects may impair arousal as well as orgasm. Benzodiazepines have been reported to decrease libido, but in some patients the diminution of anxiety caused by those drugs enhances sexual function. Both increase and decrease in libido have been reported with psychoactive agents. It is difficult to separate those effects from the underlying condition or from improvement of the condition. Sexual dysfunction associated with the use of a drug disappears when use of the drug is discontinued.

medications that have anticholinergic adverse effects, such as the phenothiazines, especially thioridazine (Mellaril).

Other Female Sexual Dysfunction Due to a General Medical Condition

Some medical conditions—specifically, endocrine diseases such as hypothyroidism, diabetes mellitus, and primary hyperprolactinemia—can affect a woman's ability to have orgasms. Several drugs also affect some women's capacity to have orgasms (Table 21.2–16). Antihypertensive medications, CNS stimulants, tricyclic drugs, SSRIs, and, frequently, monoamine oxidase inhibitors (MAOIs) have interfered with female orgasmic capacity. One study of women taking MAOIs, however, found that after 16 to 18 weeks of pharmacotherapy, the adverse effect of the medication disappeared and the women were able to reexperience orgasms, although they continued taking an undiminished dosage of the drug.

SUBSTANCE-INDUCED SEXUAL DYSFUNCTION

The diagnosis of substance-induced sexual dysfunction is used when evidence of substance intoxication or withdrawal is apparent from the history, physical examination, or laboratory findings. Distressing sexual dysfunction occurs within a month of significant substance intoxication or withdrawal (Table 21.2–17). Specified substances include alcohol, amphetamines or related substances, cocaine, opioids, sedatives, hypnotics, or anxiolytics, and other or unknown substances.

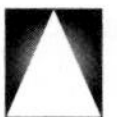

Table 21.2–17
DSM-IV-TR Diagnostic Criteria for Substance-Induced Sexual Dysfunction

A. Clinically significant sexual dysfunction that results in marked distress or interpersonal difficulty predominates in the clinical picture.
B. There is evidence from the history, physical examination, or laboratory findings that the sexual dysfunction is fully explained by substance use as manifested by either (1) or (2):
   (1) the symptoms in Criterion A developed during, or within a month of, substance intoxication
   (2) medication use is etiologically related to the disturbance
C. The disturbance is not better accounted for by a sexual dysfunction that is not substance induced. Evidence that the symptoms are better accounted for by a sexual dysfunction that is not substance induced might include the following: the symptoms precede the onset of the substance use or dependence (or medication use); the symptoms persist for a substantial period of time (e.g., about a month) after the cessation of intoxication, or are substantially in excess of what would be expected given the type or amount of the substance used or the duration of use; or there is other evidence that suggests the existence of an independent non–substance-induced sexual dysfunction (e.g., a history of recurrent non–substance-related episodes).

Note: This diagnosis should be made instead of a diagnosis of substance intoxication only when the sexual dysfunction is in excess of that usually associated with the intoxication syndrome and when the dysfunction is sufficiently severe to warrant independent clinical attention.

Code [Specific substance]-induced sexual dysfunction: Alcohol; amphetamine [or amphetamine-like substance]; cocaine; opioid; sedative, hypnotic, or anxiolytic; other [or unknown] substance

Specify if:
With impaired desire
With impaired arousal
With impaired orgasm
With sexual pain

Specify if:
With onset during intoxication: if the criteria are met for intoxication with the substance and the symptoms develop during the intoxication syndrome

(From American Psychiatric Association. *Diagnostic and Statistical Manual of Mental Disorders*. 4th ed. Text rev. Washington, DC: American Psychiatric Association; copyright 2000, with permission.)

Abused recreational substances affect sexual function in various ways. In small doses, many substances enhance sexual performance by decreasing inhibition or anxiety or by causing a temporary elation of mood. With continued use, however, erectile engorgement and orgasmic and ejaculatory capacities become impaired. The abuse of sedatives, anxiolytics, hypnotics, and particularly opiates and opioids nearly always depresses desire. Alcohol may foster the initiation of sexual activity by removing inhibition, but it also impairs performance. Cocaine and amphetamines produce similar effects. Although no direct evidence indicates that sexual drive is enhanced, users initially have feelings of increased energy and may become sexually active. Ultimately, dysfunction occurs. Men usually go through two stages: an experience of prolonged erection without ejaculation, then a gradual loss of erectile capability.

Patients recovering from substance dependency may need therapy to regain sexual function, partly because of psychological readjustment to a nondependent state. Many substance abusers have always had difficulty with intimate interactions. Others who spent their crucial developmental years under the influence of a substance have missed the experiences that would have enabled them to learn social and sexual skills.

PHARMACOLOGICAL AGENTS IMPLICATED IN SEX DYSFUNCTION

Almost every pharmacological agent, particularly those used in psychiatry, has been associated with an effect on sexuality. In men, these effects include decreased sex drive, erectile failure (impotence), decreased volume of ejaculate, and delayed or retrograde ejaculation. In women, decreased sex drive, decreased vaginal lubrication, inhibited or delayed orgasm, and decreased or absent vaginal contractions may occur. Drugs may also enhance the sexual responses and increase the sex drive, but this is less common than adverse effects (Table 21.2–18).

Psychoactive Drugs

Antipsychotic Drugs. Most antipsychotic drugs are dopamine receptor antagonists that also block adrenergic and cholinergic receptors, thus accounting for adverse sexual effects. Chlorpromazine (Thorazine), thioridazine, and trifluoperazine (Stelazine) are potent anticholinergics and they impair erection and ejaculation, in which the seminal fluid backs up into the bladder rather than being propelled through the penile urethra. Patients still have a pleasurable sensation, but the orgasm is dry. When urinating after orgasm, the urine may be milky white because it contains the ejaculate. The condition is startling but harmless and may occur in up to 50 percent of patients taking the drug. Paradoxically, some rare cases of priapism have been reported with antipsychotics.

Antidepressant Drugs. The tricyclic and tetracyclic antidepressants have anticholinergic effects that interfere with erection and delay ejaculation. Because the anticholinergic effects vary among the cyclic antidepressants, those with the fewest effects (e.g., desipramine [Norpramin]) produce the fewest sexual adverse effects. The effects of the tricyclics and tetracyclics have not been documented sufficiently in women; however, few women seem to complain of any effects.

Some men report increased sensitivity of the glans that is pleasurable and that does not interfere with erection, although it delays ejaculation. In some cases, however, the tricyclic causes painful ejaculation, perhaps as the result of interference with seminal propulsion caused by interference with, in turn, urethral, prostatic, vas, and epididymal smooth muscle contractions. Clomipramine (Anafranil) has been reported to increase sex drive in some persons. Selegiline (Deprenyl), a selective MAO type B (MAO_B) inhibitor, and bupropion (Wellbutrin) have also been reported to increase sex drive, possibly by dopaminergic activity and increased production of norepinephrine.

Venlafaxine (Effexor) and the SSRIs most often have adverse effects because of the rise in serotonin levels. A lowering of the sex drive and difficulty reaching orgasm occur in both sexes. Reversal of those negative effects has been achieved with cyproheptadine (Periactin), an antihistamine with antiserotonergic effects, and with methylphenidate (Ritalin), which has adrenergic effects. Trazodone (Desyrel) is associated with the rare occurrence of priapism, the symptom of prolonged erection in the absence of sexual stimuli. That symptom appears to result from the α_2-adrenergic antagonism of trazodone.

The MAOIs affect biogenic amines broadly. Accordingly, they produce impaired erection, delayed or retrograde ejaculation, vaginal dryness, and inhibited orgasm. Tranylcypromine (Parnate) has a paradoxical sexually stimulating effect in some persons, possibly as a result of its amphetamine-like properties.

GENERAL EFFECTS. Because depression is associated with a decreased libido, varying levels of sexual dysfunction and anhedonia are part of the disease process. Some patients report improved sexual functioning as their depression improves as a result of antidepressant medication. The phenomenon makes the evaluation of sexual side effects difficult; also, the side effects may disappear with time, perhaps because a biogenic amine homeostatic mechanism comes into play.

Lithium. Lithium (Eskalith) regulates mood and, in the manic state, may reduce hypersexuality, possibly by a dopamine antagonist activity. In some patients, impaired erection has been reported.

Sympathomimetics. Psychostimulants, which are sometimes used in the treatment of depression, include amphetamines, methylphenidate, and pemoline (Cylert), which raise the plasma levels of norepinephrine and dopamine. Libido is increased; however, with prolonged use, men may experience a loss of desire and erections.

α-Adrenergic and β-Adrenergic Receptor Antagonists. α-Adrenergic and β-adrenergic receptor antagonists are used in the treatment of hypertension, angina, and certain cardiac arrhythmias. They diminish tonic sympathetic nerve outflow from vasomotor centers in the brain. As a result, they can cause impotence, decrease the volume of ejaculate, and produce retrograde ejaculation. Changes in libido have been reported in both sexes.

Suggestions have been made to use the side effects of drugs therapeutically. Thus, a drug that delays or interferes with ejaculation (e.g., fluoxetine [Prozac]) might be used to treat premature ejaculation.

Anticholinergics. The anticholinergics block cholinergic receptors and include such drugs as amantadine (Symmetrel) and benztropine (Cogentin). They produce dryness of the mucous membranes (including those of the vagina) and impotence. However, amantadine may reverse SSRI-induced orgasmic dysfunction through its dopaminergic effect.

Antihistamines. Drugs such as diphenhydramine (Benadryl) have anticholinergic activity and are mildly hypnotic. They may inhibit

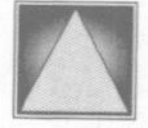

Table 21.2–18
Diagnostic Issues with Sex and Some Antipsychotic Drugs

Differential diagnosis of drug-induced sexual dysfunction	Problem after drug therapy started or drug overdose Problem not situation or partner specific Not a lifelong or recurrent problem No obvious nonpharmacological precipitant Dissipates with drug discontinuation
Antipsychotic drugs and ejaculatory problems	Perphenazine Chlorpromazine Trifluoperazine Haloperidol Mesoridazine Thioridazine Chlorprothixene
Antipsychotic drugs and priapism	Perphenazine Mesoridazine Chlorpromazine Thioridazine Fluphenazine Molindone Risperidone Clozapine

(Table by R. T. Seagraves, M.D.)

sexual function as a result. Cyproheptadine, although an antihistamine, also has potent activity as a serotonin antagonist. It is used to block the serotonergic sexual adverse effects produced by SSRIs, such as delayed orgasm and impotence.

Antianxiety Agents. The major class of anxiolytics is the benzodiazepines (e.g., diazepam [Valium]). They act on the γ-aminobutyric acid (GABA) receptors, which are believed to be involved in cognition, memory, and motor control. Because they decrease plasma epinephrine concentrations, they diminish anxiety, and as a result they improve sexual function in persons inhibited by anxiety.

Alcohol. Alcohol suppresses CNS activity generally and can produce erectile disorders in men as a result. Alcohol has a direct gonadal effect that decreases testosterone levels in men; paradoxically, it can produce a slight rise in testosterone levels in women. The latter finding may account for women reporting increased libido after drinking small amounts of alcohol. The long-term use of alcohol reduces the ability of the liver to metabolize estrogenic compounds. In men, that produces signs of feminization (such as gynecomastia as a result of testicular atrophy).

Opioids. Opioids, such as heroin, have adverse sexual effects, such as erectile failure and decreased libido. The alteration of consciousness may enhance the sexual experience in occasional users.

Hallucinogens. The hallucinogens include lysergic acid diethylamide (LSD), phencyclidine (PCP), psilocybin (from some mushrooms), and mescaline (from peyote cactus). In addition to inducing hallucinations, the drugs cause loss of contact with reality and an expanding and heightening of consciousness. Some users report that the sexual experience is similarly enhanced, but others experience anxiety, delirium, or psychosis, which clearly interferes with sexual function.

Cannabis. The altered state of consciousness produced by cannabis may enhance sexual pleasure for some persons. Its prolonged use depresses testosterone levels.

Barbiturates and Similarly Acting Drugs. Barbiturates and similarly acting sedative-hypnotic drugs may enhance sexual responsiveness in persons who are sexually unresponsive as a result of anxiety. They have no direct effect on the sex organs; however, they do produce an alteration in consciousness that some persons find pleasurable. They are subject to abuse and can be fatal when combined with alcohol or other CNS depressants.

Methaqualone (Quaalude) acquired a reputation as a sexual enhancer, which had no biological basis in fact. It is no longer marketed in the United States.

SEXUAL DYSFUNCTION NOT OTHERWISE SPECIFIED

The category sexual dysfunction not otherwise specified covers sexual dysfunctions that cannot be classified under the categories described above (Table 21.2–19). Examples include persons who experience the physiological components of sexual excitement and orgasm, but report no erotic sensation or even anesthesia (orgasmic anhedonia). Women with conditions analogous to premature ejaculation in men are classified here. Orgasmic women who desire, but have not experienced, multiple orgasms can be classified under this heading as well. Also, disorders of excessive, rather than inhibited, dysfunction, such as compulsive masturbation or coitus (sex addiction), or those with genital pain occurring during masturbation may be classified here. Other unspecified disorders are found in persons who have one or more sexual fantasies about which they feel guilty or otherwise dysphoric, but the range of common sexual fantasies is broad.

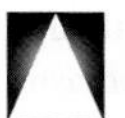

Table 21.2–19
DSM-IV-TR Diagnostic Criteria for Sexual Dysfunction Not Otherwise Specified

This category includes sexual dysfunctions that do not meet criteria for any specific sexual dysfunction. Examples include:

1. No (or substantially diminished) subjective erotic feelings despite otherwise normal arousal and orgasm
2. Situations in which the clinician has concluded that a sexual dysfunction is present but is unable to determine whether it is primary, due to a general medical condition, or substance induced

(From American Psychiatric Association. *Diagnostic and Statistical Manual of Mental Disorders.* 4th ed. Text rev. Washington, DC: American Psychiatric Association; copyright 2000, with permission.)

Female Premature Orgasm

Data on female premature orgasm are lacking; no separate category of premature orgasm for women is included in DSM-IV-TR. A case of multiple spontaneous orgasms without sexual stimulation was seen in a woman; the cause was an epileptogenic focus in the temporal lobe. Instances have been reported of women taking antidepressants (e.g., fluoxetine and clomipramine) who experience spontaneous orgasm associated with yawning.

Postcoital Headache

Postcoital headache, characterized by headache immediately after coitus, may last for several hours. It is usually described as throbbing and is localized in the occipital or frontal area. The cause is unknown. There may be vascular, muscle-contraction (tension), or psychogenic causes. Coitus may precipitate migraine or cluster headaches in predisposed persons.

Orgasmic Anhedonia

Orgasmic anhedonia is a condition in which a person has no physical sensation of orgasm, even though the physiological component (e.g., ejaculation) remains intact. Organic causes, such as sacral and cephalic lesions that interfere with afferent pathways from the genitalia to the cortex, must be ruled out. Psychiatric causes usually relate to extreme guilt about experiencing sexual pleasure. These feelings produce a dissociative response that isolates the affective component of the orgasmic experience from consciousness.

Masturbatory Pain

Persons may experience pain during masturbation. Organic causes should always be ruled out; a small vaginal tear or early Peyronie's disease can produce a painful sensation. The condition should be differentiated from compulsive masturbation. Persons may masturbate to the extent that they do physical damage to their genitals and eventually experience pain during subsequent masturbatory acts. Such cases constitute a separate sexual disorder and should be so classified.

Certain masturbatory practices have resulted in what has been called autoerotic asphyxiation. The practices involve persons masturbating while hanging by the neck to heighten the erotic sensations and the orgasm's intensity through the mechanism of mild hypoxia. Although the persons intend to release themselves from the noose after orgasm, an estimated 500 to 1,000 persons a year accidentally kill themselves by hanging. Most who indulge in the practice are male; transvestism is often associated with the habit, and most deaths occur among adolescents. Such masochistic practices are usually associated with severe mental disorders, such as schizophrenia and major mood disorders.

TREATMENT

Before 1970, the most common treatment of sexual dysfunctions was individual psychotherapy. Classic psychodynamic theory holds that sexual inadequacy has its roots in early developmental conflicts, and the sexual disorder is treated as part of a pervasive emotional disturbance. Treatment focuses on the exploration of unconscious conflicts, motivation, fantasy, and various interpersonal difficulties. One of the assumptions of therapy is that removal of the conflicts allows the sexual impulse to become structurally acceptable to the ego, and thereby the patient finds appropriate means of satisfaction in the environment. The symptoms of sexual dysfunctions, however, frequently become secondarily autonomous and continue to persist, even when other problems evolving from the patients' pathology have been resolved. The addition of behavioral techniques is often necessary to cure the sexual problem.

Dual-Sex Therapy

The theoretical basis of dual-sex therapy is the concept of the marital unit or dyad as the object of therapy; the approach represents the major advance in the diagnosis and treatment of sexual disorders in the 20th century. The methodology was originated and developed by Masters and Johnson. In dual-sex therapy, treatment is based on a concept that the couple must be treated when a dysfunctional person is in a relationship. Because both are involved in a sexually distressing situation, both must participate in the therapy program. The sexual problem often reflects other areas of disharmony or misunderstanding in the marriage so that the entire marital relationship is treated, with emphasis on sexual functioning as a part of the relationship.

The keystone of the program is the roundtable session in which a male and female therapy team clarifies, discusses, and works through problems with the couple. The four-way sessions require active participation by the patients. Therapists and patients discuss the psychological and physiological aspects of sexual functioning, and therapists have an educative attitude. Therapists suggest specific sexual activities, which the couple follow in the privacy of their home. The aim of the therapy is to establish or reestablish communication within the marital unit. Sex is emphasized as a natural function that flourishes in the appropriate domestic climate, and improved communication is encouraged toward that end. In a variation of this therapy that has proved effective, one therapist may treat the couple. Treatment is short-term and behaviorally oriented. The therapists attempt to reflect the situation as they see it, rather than interpret underlying dynamics. An undistorted picture of the relationship presented by the therapists often corrects the myopic, narrow view held by each marriage partner. This new perspective can interrupt the couple's distructive pattern of relating and can encourage improved, more effective communication. Specific exercises are prescribed for the couple to treat their particular problems. Sexual inadequacy often involves lack of information, misinformation, and performance fear. Therefore, the couple are specifically prohibited from any sexual play other than that prescribed by the therapists. Beginning exercises usually focus on heightening sensory awareness to touch, sight, sound, and smell. Initially, intercourse is interdicted, and the couple learn to give and receive bodily pleasure without the pressure of performance or penetration. At the same time, they learn how to communicate nonverbally in a mutually satisfactory way, and they learn that sexual foreplay is an enjoyable alternative to intercourse and orgasm.

During the sensate focus exercises, the couple receive much reinforcement to reduce their anxiety. They are urged to use fantasies to distract them from obsessive concerns about performance (spectatoring). The needs of both the dysfunctional partner and the nondysfunctional partner are considered. If either partner becomes sexually excited by the exercises, the other is encouraged to bring him or her to orgasm by manual or oral means. Open communication between the partners is urged, and the expression of mutual needs is encouraged. Resistances, such as claims of fatigue or not enough time to complete the exercises, are common and must be dealt with by the therapists. Issues of body image, fear of being touched, and difficulty touching oneself arise frequently. Genital stimulation is eventually added to general body stimulation. The couple is instructed sequentially to try various positions for intercourse, without necessarily completing the act, and to use varieties of stimulating techniques before they are instructed to proceed with intercourse.

Psychotherapy sessions follow each new exercise period, and problems and satisfactions, both sexual and in other areas of the couple's lives, are discussed. Specific instructions and the introduction of new exercises geared to the individual couple's progress are reviewed in each session. Gradually, the couple gains confidence and learns to communicate, verbally and sexually. Dual-sex therapy is most effective when the sexual dysfunction exists apart from other psychopathology.

Specific Techniques and Exercises

Various techniques are used to treat the various sexual dysfunctions. In cases of vaginismus, a woman is advised to dilate her vaginal opening with her fingers or with size graduated dilators. Dilators are also used to treat cases of dyspareunia. Sometimes, treatment is coordinated with specially trained physiotherapists who work with the patients to help them relax the perineal muscles.

In cases of premature ejaculation, an exercise known as the squeeze technique is used to raise the threshold of penile excitability. In this exercise, the man or the woman stimulates the erect penis until the earliest sensations of impending ejaculation are felt. At this point, the woman forcefully squeezes the coronal ridge of the glans, the erection is diminished, and ejaculation is inhibited. The exercise program eventually raises the threshold of the sensation of ejaculatory inevitability and allows the man to focus on sensations of arousal without anxiety and develop confidence in his sexual performance. A variant of the exercise is the stop-start technique developed by James H. Semans, in which the woman stops all stimulation of the penis when the man first senses an impending ejaculation. No squeeze is used. Research has shown that the presence or absence of circumcision has no bearing on a man's ejaculatory control; the glans is equally sensitive in the two states. Sex therapy has been most successful in the treatment of premature ejaculation.

A man with a sexual desire disorder or male erectile disorder is sometimes told to masturbate to prove that full erection and ejaculation are possible. Male orgasmic disorder is managed initially by extravaginal ejaculation and then by gradual vaginal entry after stimulation to a point near ejaculation. Most importantly, the early exercises forbid ejaculation to remove the pressure to climax and allow the man to immerse himself in sexual pleasuring.

In cases of lifelong female orgasmic disorder, the woman is directed to masturbate, sometimes using a vibrator. The shaft of the clitoris is the masturbatory site most preferred by women, and orgasm depends on adequate clitoral stimulation. An area on the anterior wall of the vagina has been identified in some women as a site of sexual excitation, known as the *G-spot*; but reports of an ejaculatory phenomenon at orgasm in women following the stimulation of the G-spot have not been satisfactorily verified.

Hypnotherapy

Hypnotherapists focus specifically on the anxiety-producing situation—that is, the sexual interaction that results in dysfunction. The successful use of hypnosis enables patients to gain control over the symptom that has been lowering self-esteem and disrupting psychological homeostasis. The patient's cooperation is first obtained and encouraged during a series of nonhypnotic sessions with the therapist. Those discussions permit the development of a secure doctor–patient relationship, a sense of physical and psychological comfort on the part of the patient, and the establishment of mutually desired treatment goals. During this time, the therapist assesses the patient's capacity for the trance experience. The nonhypnotic sessions also permit the clinician to take a psychiatric history and perform a mental status examination before beginning hypnotherapy. The focus of treatment is on symptom removal and attitude alteration. The patient is instructed in developing alternative means of dealing with the anxiety-provoking situation, the sexual encounter.

Patients are also taught relaxation techniques to use on themselves before sexual relations. With these methods to alleviate anxiety, the physiological responses to sexual stimulation can readily result in pleasurable excitation and discharge. Psychological impediments to vaginal lubrication, erection, and orgasms are removed, and normal sexual functioning ensues. Hypnosis may be added to a basic individual psychotherapy program to accelerate the effects of psychotherapeutic intervention.

Behavior Therapy

Behavioral approaches were initially designed for the treatment of phobias but are now used to treat other problems as well. Behavior therapists assume that sexual dysfunction is learned maladaptive behavior, which causes patients to be fearful of sexual interaction. Using traditional techniques, therapists set up a hierarchy of anxiety-provoking situations, ranging from least threatening (e.g., the thought of kissing) to most threatening (the thought of penile penetration). The behavior therapist enables the patient to master the anxiety through a standard program of systematic desensitization, which is designed to inhibit the learned anxious response by encouraging behaviors antithetical to anxiety. The patient first deals with the least anxiety-producing situation in fantasy and progresses by steps to the most anxiety-producing situation. Medication, hypnosis, and special training in deep muscle relaxation are sometimes used to help with the initial mastery of anxiety.

Assertiveness training is helpful in teaching patients to express sexual needs openly and without fear. Exercises in assertiveness are given in conjunction with sex therapy; patients are encouraged to make sexual requests and to refuse to comply with requests perceived as unreasonable. Sexual exercises may be prescribed for patients to perform at home, and a hierarchy may be established, starting with those activities that have proved most pleasurable and successful in the past.

One treatment variation involves the participation of the patient's sexual partner in the desensitization program. The partner, rather than the therapist, presents items of increasing stimulation value to the patient. A cooperative partner is necessary to help the patient carry gains made during treatment sessions to sexual activity at home.

Group Therapy

Group therapy has been used to examine both intrapsychic and interpersonal problems in patients with sexual disorders. A therapy group provides a strong support system for a patient who feels ashamed, anxious, or guilty about a particular sexual problem. It is a useful forum in which to counteract sexual myths, correct misconceptions, and provide accurate information about sexual anatomy, physiology, and varieties of behavior.

Groups for the treatment of sexual disorders can be organized in several ways. Members may all share the same problem, such as premature ejaculation; members may all be of the same sex with different sexual problems; or groups may be composed of both men and women who are experiencing a variety of sexual problems. Group therapy can be an adjunct to other forms of therapy or the prime mode of treatment. Groups organized to treat a particular dysfunction are usually behavioral in approach.

Groups composed of married couples with sexual dysfunctions have also been effective. A group provides the opportunity to gather accurate information, offers consensual validation of individual preferences, and enhances self-esteem and self-acceptance. Techniques, such as role playing and psychodrama, may be used in treatment. Such groups are not indicated for couples when one partner is uncooperative, when a patient has a severe depressive disorder or psychosis, when a patient finds explicit sexual audiovisual material repugnant, or when a patient fears or dislikes groups.

Analytically Oriented Sex Therapy

One of the most effective treatment modalities is the use of sex therapy integrated with psychodynamic and psychoanalytically oriented psychotherapy. The sex therapy is conducted over a longer period than usual, which allows learning or relearning of sexual satisfaction under the realities of patients' day-to-day lives. The addition of psychodynamic conceptualizations to behavioral techniques used to treat sexual dysfunctions allows the treatment of patients with sexual disorders associated with other psychopathology.

The material and dynamics that emerge in patients in analytically oriented sex therapy are the same as those in psychoanalytic therapy, such as dreams, fear of punishment, aggressive feelings, difficulty trusting a partner, fear of intimacy, oedipal feelings, and fear of genital mutilation. The combined approach of analytically oriented sex therapy is used by the general psychiatrist who carefully judges the optimal timing of sex therapy and the ability of patients to tolerate the directive approach that focuses on their sexual difficulties.

Biological Treatments

Biological treatments, including pharmacotherapy, surgery, and mechanical devices, are used to treat specific cases of sexual disorder. Most of the recent advances involve male sexual dysfunction. Current studies are under way to test biological treatment of sexual dysfunction in women.

Pharmacotherapy. The major new medications to treat sexual dysfunction are sildenafil (Viagra) and its congeners (Table 21.2–20); oral phentolamine (Vasomax); alprostadil (Caverject), an injectable prostaglandin; and a transurethral alprostadil (MUSE), all used to treat erectile disorder.

Sildenafil is a nitric oxide enhancer that facilitates the inflow of blood to the penis necessary for an erection. The drug takes effect about 1 hour after ingestion, and its effect can last up to 4 hours. Sildenafil is not effective in the absence of sexual stimulation. The most common adverse events associated with its use are headaches, flushing, and dyspepsia. The use of sildenafil is contraindicated for persons taking organic nitrates. The concomitant action of the two drugs can result in large, sudden, and sometimes fatal drops in systemic blood pressure. Sildenafil is not effective in all cases of erectile dysfunction. It fails to produce an erection rigid enough for penetration in about 50 percent of men who have had radical prostate surgery or in those with long-standing insulin-dependent diabetes. It is also ineffective in certain cases of nerve damage.

A small number of patients developed Nonarteritic Ischemic Optic Neuropathy (NAION) soon after use of sildenafil. Six patients had vision loss within 24 hours after use of the agent. Both eyes were affected in one individual. All affected individuals had pre-existing hypertension, diabetes, elevated cholesterol, or hyperlipidemia. Although very rare, sildenafil may provoke NAION in individuals with an arteriosclerotic risk profile.

Sildenafil use in women results in vaginal lubrication, but not in increased desire. Anecdotal reports, however, describe individual women who have experienced intensified excitement with sildenafil.

Oral phentolamine and apomorphine are not US Food and Drug Administration (FDA) approved at present, but have proved effective as potency enhancers in men with minimal erectile dysfunction. Phentolamine reduces sympathetic tone and relaxes corporeal smooth muscle. Adverse events include hypotension, tachycardia, and dizziness. Apomorphine effects are mediated

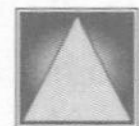

Table 21.2–20
Pharmacokinetics of the PDE-5 Inhibitors

	Sildenafil 100 mg	Vardenafil 20 mg	Tadalafil 20 mg
Maximum concentration	450 ng/mL	20.9 ng/mL	378 ng/mL
Time to maximum concentration	1.0 hours	0.7 hours	2.0 hours
Half-life	4 hours	3.9 hours	17.5 hours

(From Arnold LM. Vardenafil & Tadalafil: Options for erectile dysfunction. *Current Psychiatry.* 2004;3(2):46, with permission.)

by the autonomic nervous system and result in vasodilatation that facilitates the inflow of blood to the penis. Adverse events include nausea and sweating.

In contrast to the oral medications, injectable and transurethral alprostadil act locally on the penis and can produce erections in the absence of sexual stimulation. Alprostadil contains a naturally occurring form of prostaglandin E, a vasodilating agent. Alprostadil may be administered by direct injection into the corpora cavernosa or by intraurethral insertion of a pellet through a canula. The firm erection produced within 2 to 3 minutes after administration of the drug may last as long as 1 hour. Infrequent and reversible adverse effects of injections include penile bruising and changes in liver function test results. Possible hazardous sequelae exist, including priapism and sclerosis of the small veins of the penis. Users of transurethral alprostadil sometimes complain of burning sensations in the penis.

Two small trials found different topical agents effective in alleviating erectile dysfunction. One cream consists of three vasoactive substances known to be absorbed through the skin: aminophylline, isosorbide dinitrate, and co-dergocrine mesylate, which is a mixture of ergot alkaloids. The other is a gel containing alprostadil and an additional ingredient, which temporarily makes the outer layer of the skin more permeable.

A cream incorporating alprostadil also has been developed to treat female sexual arousal disorder. The initial results are promising. Also, vaginally applied phentolamine mesylate, an α-receptor antagonist, significantly increased vasocongestion and a subjective sense of arousal in a trial of postmenopausal women with arousal problems who were already on hormonal therapy. A nasal inhalant, bremekinotide, set to enter phase 3 of clinical trials, affects the brain and has been shown to activate the same neural circuitry that is activated when a person feels desire. If approved, it will be offered as a stimulant of desire to both men and women.

The pharmacological treatments described above are useful in the treatment of arousal dysfunction of various causes: neurogenic, arterial insufficiency, venous leakage, psychogenic, and mixed. When coupled with insight-oriented or behavioral sex therapy, the use of medications can reverse psychogenic arousal disorder resistant to psychotherapy alone, the ultimate goal being pharmacologically unassisted sexual functioning.

Other Pharmacological Agents

Numerous other pharmacological agents have been used to heal the various sexual disorders. Intravenous methohexital sodium (Brevital) has been used in desensitization therapy. Antianxiety agents may have some application in tense patients, although these drugs can also interfere with the sexual response. The side effects of antidepressants, in particular the SSRIs and tricyclic drugs, have been used to prolong the sexual response in patients with premature ejaculation. This approach is particularly useful in patients refractory to behavioral techniques who may fall into the category of physiologically disposed premature ejaculators. The use of antidepressants has also been advocated in treatment for patients who are phobic of sex and in those with a posttraumatic stress disorder following rape. Trazodone is an antidepressant that improves nocturnal erections. The risks of taking such medications must be carefully weighed against their possible benefits. Bromocriptine (Parlodel) is used in the treatment of hyperprolactinemia, which is frequently associated with hypogonadism. In such patients, it is necessary to rule out pituitary tumors. Bromocriptine, a dopamine agonist, may improve sexual function impaired by hyperprolactinemia.

A number of substances have popular standing as aphrodisiacs; for example, ginseng root and yohimbine (Yocon). Studies, however, have not confirmed any aphrodisiac properties. Yohimbine, an α-receptor antagonist, may cause dilation of the penile artery; however the American Urologic Association does not recommend its use to treat organic erectile dysfunction. Many recreational drugs, including cocaine, amphetamines, alcohol, and cannabis, are considered enhancers of sexual performance. Although they may provide the user with an initial benefit because of their tranquilizing, disinhibiting, or mood-elevating effects, consistent or prolonged use of any of these substances impairs sexual functioning.

Dopaminergic agents have been reported to increase libido and improve sex function. Those drugs include L-dopa, a dopamine precursor, and bromocriptine, a dopamine agonist. The antidepressant bupropion has dopaminergic effects and has increased sex drive in some patients. Selegiline, an MAOI, is selective for MAO_B and is dopaminergic. It improves sexual functioning in older persons.

Hormone Therapy. Androgens increase the sex drive in women and in men with low testosterone concentrations. Women may experience virilizing effects, some of which are irreversible (e.g., deepening of the voice). In men, prolonged use of androgens produces hypertension and prostatic enlargement. Testosterone is most effective when given parenterally; however, effective oral and transdermal preparations are available.

Women who use estrogens for replacement therapy or for contraception may report decreased libido; in such cases, a combined preparation of estrogen and testosterone has been used effectively. Estrogen itself prevents thinning of the vaginal mucous membrane and facilitates lubrication. Two new forms of estrogen, vaginal rings and vaginal tablets, provide alternate administration routes to treat women with arousal problems or genital atrophy. Because tablets and rings do not significantly increase circulating estrogen levels, these devices may be considered for patients with breast cancer with arousal problems.

Antiandrogens and Antiestrogens. Estrogens and progesterone are antiandrogens that have been used to treat compulsive sexual behavior in men, usually in sex offenders. Clomiphene (Clomid) and tamoxifen (Nolvadex) are both antiestrogens, and both stimulate gonadotropin-releasing hormone (GnRH) secretion and increase testosterone concentrations, thereby increasing libido. Women being treated for breast cancer with tamoxifen report an increased libido. However, tamoxifen may cause uterine cancer.

Mechanical Treatment Approaches

In male patients with arteriosclerosis (especially of the distal aorta, known as Leriche's syndrome), the erection may be lost during active pelvic thrusting. The need for increased blood in the gluteal muscles and others served by the ilial or hypogastric arteries takes blood away (steals) from the pudendal artery and, thus, interferes with penile blood flow. Relief may be obtained by decreasing pelvic thrusting, which is also aided by the woman's superior coital position.

Vacuum Pump. Vacuum pumps are mechanical devices that patients without vascular disease can use to obtain erections. The blood drawn into the penis following the creation of the vacuum is kept there by a ring placed around the base of the penis. This device has no adverse effects, but it is cumbersome, and partners must be willing to accept its use. Some women complain that the penis is redder and cooler than when erection is produced by natural circumstances, and they find the process and the result objectionable.

A similar device, called EROS, has been developed to create clitoral erections in women. EROS is a small suction cup that fits over the clitoral region and draws blood into the clitoris. Studies have reported its success in treating female sexual arousal disorder. Vibrators used to stimulate the clitoral area have been successful in treating anorgasmic women.

Surgical Treatment

Male Prostheses. Surgical treatment is infrequently advocated, but penile prosthetic devices are available for men with inadequate erectile responses who are resistant to other treatment methods or who have medically caused deficiencies. The two main types of prostheses are (1) a semirigid rod prosthesis that produces a permanent erection that can be positioned close to the body for concealment and (2) an inflatable type that is implanted with its own reservoir and pump for inflation and deflation. The latter type is designed to mimic normal physiological functioning.

Vascular Surgery. When vascular insufficiency is present due to atherosclerosis or other blockage, bypass surgery of penile arteries has been attempted in selected cases with some success.

Outcome

Demonstrating the effectiveness of traditional outpatient psychotherapy is just as difficult when therapy is oriented to sexual problems as it is in general. The more severe the psychopathology associated with a problem of long duration, the more adverse the outcome is likely to be. The results of different treatment methods have varied considerably since Masters and Johnson first reported positive results for their treatment approach in 1970. Masters and Johnson studied the failure rates of their patients (defined as the failure to initiate reversal of the basic symptom of the presenting dysfunction). They compared initial failure rates with 5-year follow-up findings for the same couples. Although some have criticized their definition of the percentage of presumed successes, other studies have confirmed the effectiveness of their approach.

The more difficult treatment cases involve couples with severe marital discord. Desire disorders are particularly difficult to treat. They require longer, more intensive therapy than some other disorders, and their outcomes vary greatly.

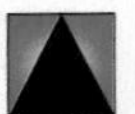

Table 21.2–21
ICD-10 Diagnostic Criteria for Sexual Dysfunction, Not Caused by Organic Disorder or Disease

G1. The subject is unable to participate in a sexual relationship as he or she would wish.
G2. The dysfunction occurs frequently, but may be absent on some occasions.
G3. The dysfunction has been present for at least 6 months.
G4. The dysfunction is not entirely attributable to any of the other mental and behavioral disorders in ICD-10, physical disorders (such as endocrine disorder), or drug treatment.

Comments

Measurement of each form of dysfunction can be based on rating scales that assess severity as well as frequency of the problem. More than one type of dysfunction can coexist.

Lack or loss of sexual desire

A. The general criteria for sexual dysfunction must be met.
B. There is a lack or loss of sexual desire, manifest by diminution of seeking out sexual cues, or thinking about sex with associated feelings of desire or appetite, or of sexual fantasies.
C. There is a lack of interest in initiating sexual activity either with a partner or as solitary masturbation, resulting in a frequency of activity clearly lower than expected, taking into account age and context, or in a frequency very clearly reduced from previous much higher levels.

Sexual aversion and lack of sexual enjoyment

Sexual aversion

A. The general criteria for sexual dysfunction must be met.
B. The prospect of sexual interaction with a partner produces sufficient aversion, fear, or anxiety that sexual activity is avoided, or, if it occurs, is associated with strong negative feelings and an inability to experience any pleasure.
C. The aversion is not the result of performance anxiety (reaction to previous failure of sexual response).

Lack of sexual enjoyment

A. The general criteria for sexual dysfunction must be met.
B. Genital response (orgasm and/or ejaculation) occurs during sexual stimulation, but is not accompanied by pleasurable sensations or feelings of pleasant excitement.
C. There is no manifest and persistent fear or anxiety during sexual activity (see sexual aversion).

Failure of genital response

A. The general criteria for sexual dysfunction must be met. In addition, for men:
B. Erection sufficient for intercourse fails to occur when intercourse is attempted. The dysfunction takes one of the following forms:
  (1) full erection occurs during the early stages of lovemaking but disappears or declines when intercourse is attempted (before ejaculation if it occurs);
  (2) erection does occur, but only at times when intercourse is not being considered;
  (3) partial erection, insufficient for intercourse, occurs, but not full erection;
  (4) no penile tumescence occurs at all.

In addition, for women:

B. There is failure of genital response, experienced as failure of vaginal lubrication, together with inadequate tumescence of the labia. The dysfunction takes one of the following forms.
  (1) general lubrication fails in all relevant circumstances;
  (2) lubrication may occur initially but fails to persist for long enough to allow comfortable penile entry;
  (3) Situational: lubrication occurs only in some situations (e.g., with one partner but not another, or during masturbation, or when vaginal intercourse is not being contemplated).

Orgasmic dysfunction

A. The general criteria for sexual dysfunction must be met.
B. There is orgasmic dysfunction (either absence or marked delay of orgasm), which takes one of the following forms:
  (1) orgasm has never been experienced in any situation;
  (2) orgasmic dysfunction has developed after a period of relatively normal response:
    (a) general: orgasmic dysfunction occurs in all situations and with any partner;
    (b) situational:

    For *women*: orgasm does occur in certain situations (e.g., when masturbating or with certain partners); For *men*, one of the following can be applied:

      i) orgasm occurs only during sleep, never during the waking state;
      ii) orgasm never occurs in the presence of the partner;
      iii) orgasm occurs in the presence of the partner but not during intercourse.

Premature ejaculation

A. The general criteria for sexual dysfunction must be met.
B. There is an inability to delay ejaculation sufficiently to enjoy lovemaking, manifest as either of the following:
  (1) occurrence of ejaculation before or very soon after the beginning of intercourse (if a time limit is required: before or within 15 seconds of the beginning of intercourse);
  (2) ejaculation occurs in the absence of sufficient erection to make intercourse possible.
C. The problem is not the result of prolonged abstinence from sexual activity.

Nonorganic vaginismus

A. The general criteria for sexual dysfunction must be met.
B. There is spasm of the perivaginal muscles, sufficient to prevent penile entry or make it uncomfortable. The dysfunction takes one of the following forms:
  (1) normal response has never been experienced;
  (2) vaginismus has developed after a period of relatively normal response;
    (a) when vaginal entry is not attempted, a normal sexual response may occur;
    (b) any attempt at sexual contact leads to generalized fear and efforts to avoid vaginal entry (e.g., spasm of the adductor muscles of the thighs).

Nonorganic dyspareunia

A. The general criteria for sexual dysfunction must be met.

In addition, for women:

B. Pain is experienced at the entry of the vagina, either throughout sexual intercourse or only when deep thrusting of the penis occurs.
C. The disorder is not attributable to vaginismus or failure of lubrication, dyspareunia of organic origin should be classified according to the underlying disorder.

In addition, for men:

B. Pain or discomfort is experienced during sexual response. (The timing of the pain and the exact localization should be carefully recorded.)
C. The discomfort is not the result of local physical factors. If physical factors are found, the dysfunction should be classified elsewhere.

Excessive sexual drive

No research criteria are attempted for this category. Researchers studying this category are recommended to design their own criteria.

Other sexual dysfunction, not caused by organic disorder or disease

Unspecified sexual dysfunction, not caused by organic disorder or disease

(From World Health Organization. *The ICD-10 Classification of Mental and Behavioural Disorders: Diagnostic Criteria for Research*. Copyright, World Health Organization, Geneva, 1993, with permission.)

When behavioral approaches are used, empirical criteria that predict outcome are more easily isolated. Using these criteria, for instance, couples who regularly practice assigned exercises appear to have a much greater likelihood of success than do more resistant couples or those whose interaction involves sadomasochistic or depressive features or mechanisms of blame and projection. Attitude flexibility is also a positive prognostic factor. Overall, younger couples tend to complete sex therapy more often than older couples. Couples whose interactional difficulties center on their sex problems, such as inhibition, frustration, or fear of performance failure, are also likely to respond well to therapy.

Although most therapists prefer to treat a couple for sexual dysfunction, treatment of individual persons has also been successful. In general, methods that have proved effective singly or in combination include training in behavioral sexual skills, systematic desensitization, directive marital counseling, traditional psychodynamic approaches, group therapy, and pharmacotherapy.

ICD-10

According to the 10th revision of *International Statistical Classification of Diseases and Related Health Problems* (ICD-10), sexual dysfunction refers to a person's inability to "participate in a sexual relationship as he or she would wish." This dysfunction is expressed in various ways: a lack of desire or of pleasure or a physiological inability to begin, maintain, or complete sexual interaction. Because sexual response is psychosomatic, it may be difficult to determine "the relative importance of psychological and/or organic factors."

Sexual dysfunction, such as lack of desire, can occur in both men and women, but women complain more often of the "subjective quality" of the experience than of the "failure of a specific response." ICD-10 advises looking "beyond the presenting complaint to find the most appropriate diagnostic category." Table 21.2–21 presents the ICD-10 diagnostic criteria.

References

Arnold LM. Vardenafil and tadalafil: Options for erectile dysfunction. *Current Psychiatry.* 2004;13(2):51.

Basson R. Sexual desire and arousal disorders in women. *N Engl J Med.* 2006;354(15):1497.

Fava M, Rankin M. Sexual functioning and SSRIs. *J Clin Psychiatry.* 2002;63[Suppl 5]:13.

Fisher WA, Rosen RC, Mollen M, Brock G, Karlin G, Pommerville P, Goldstein I, Bangerter K, Bandel TJ, Derogatis LR, Sand M. Improving the sexual quality of life of couples affected by erectile dysfunction: A double-blind, randomized, placebo-controlled trial of vardenafil. *Journal of Sexual Medicine.*2005;2(5):699.

Freud S. Three essays on the theory of sexuality. In: *Standard Edition of the Complete Psychological Works of Sigmund Freud.* Vol. 7. London: Hogarth Press; 1953:125.

Frohman EM. Sexual dysfunction in neurological disease. *Clin Neuropharmacol.* 2002;25:126.

Fugl-Meyer KS, Oberg K, Lundberg PO, Lewin B, Fugl-Meyer A. On orgasm, sexual techniques, and erotic perceptions in 18- to 74-year-old Swedish women. *Journal of Sexual Medicine.* 2006;3:56–68.

Gopalakrishnan R, Jacob KS , Kuruvilla A, Vasantharaj B, John JK. Sildenafil in the treatment of antipsychotic-induced erectile dysfunction: A randomized, double-blind, placebo-controlled, flexible-dose, two-way crossover trial. *Am J Psych.* 2006;163:494–499.

Gross G, Blundo R. Viagra: Medical technology constructing aging masculinity. *Journal of Sociology & Social Welfare.* 2005;32:85–97.

Pauls RN,Kleeman SD, Karram MM. Female sexual dysfunction: Principles of diagnosis and therapy. *Obstet Gynecol Surv.* 2005;60(3):196–205.

Rhoden EL, Morgentaler A. Risks of testosterone-replacement therapy and recommendations deficiency. *N Engl J Med.* 2004;350:482.

Rosen R, Shabsigh R, Berber M, Assalian P, Menza M, Rodriguez-Vela L, Porto R, Bangerter K, Seger M, Montorsi F, The Vardenafil Study Site Investigators. Efficacy and tolerability of vardenafil in men with mild depression and erectile dysfunction: The depression-related improvement with vardenafil for erectile response study. *Am J Psychiatry.* 2006;163:79–87.

Sadock BJ, Kaplan HI, Freedman AM, eds. *The Sexual Experience.* Baltimore: Williams & Wilkins; 1976.

Sadock VA. Normal human sexuality and sexual dysfunction. In: Sadock BJ, Sadock VA, eds. *Kaplan & Sadock's Comprehensive Textbook of Psychiatry.* 8th ed. Vol. 1. Baltimore: Lippincott Williams & Wilkins; 2005:1902.

Thompson IM, Tangen CM, Goodman PJ. Erectile dysfunction and subsequent cardiovascular disease. *JAMA.* 2005;294(23):2996.

▲ 21.3 Paraphilias and Sexual Disorder Not Otherwise Specified

PARAPHILIAS

Paraphilias or perversions are sexual stimuli or acts that are deviations from normal sexual behaviors, but are necessary for some persons to experience arousal and orgasm. These individuals can experience sexual pleasure, but are inhibited from responding to stimuli that are normally considered erotic. The paraphiliac's sexuality is restricted to specific deviant stimuli or acts. Persons that occasionally experiment with paraphiliac behavior (e.g., infrequent episode of bondage or dressing in costumes), but are capable of responding to more typical erotic stimuli, are not diagnosed as suffering from paraphilias.

Paraphilias can range from nearly normal behavior to behavior that is destructive or hurtful only to a person's self or to a person's self and partner, and finally to behavior that is deemed destructive or threatening to the community at large. The text revision of the 4th edition of *Diagnostic and Statistical Manual of Mental Disorders* (DSM-IV-TR) addresses these differences by designating impulses toward pedophilia, frotteurism, voyeurism, exhibitionism, and sexual sadism clinically significant if the person has acted on these fantasies or if these fantasies cause marked distress or interpersonal difficulty. The remaining paraphilias, such as transvestic fetishism, sexual masochism, or those not otherwise specified (e.g., as zoophilia), meet the criteria for clinical significance only if they cause marked distress or impairment in social, occupational, or other important areas of functioning, even if the urges have been expressed behaviorally.

A special fantasy with its unconscious and conscious components is the pathognomonic element of the paraphilia, with sexual arousal and orgasm being associated phenomena that *reinforce the fantasy or impulse*. The influence of these fantasies and their behavioral manifestations often extend beyond the sexual sphere to pervade people's lives.

The major functions of human sexual behavior are to assist in bonding, to create mutual pleasure in cooperation with a partner, to express and enhance love between two persons, and to procreate. Paraphilias are divergent behaviors in that those acts involve aggression, victimization, and extreme one-sidedness. The behaviors exclude or harm others and disrupt the potential for bonding between persons. Moreover, paraphiliac sexual scripts often serve other vital psychic functions. They may assuage anxiety, bind aggression, or stabilize identity.

Epidemiology

Paraphilias are practiced by only a small percentage of the population, but the insistent, repetitive nature of the disorders results in a high frequency of such acts. Thus, a large proportion of the population has been victimized by persons with paraphilias. DSM-IV-TR suggests that the prevalence of paraphilias is significantly higher than the number of cases diagnosed in general clinical facilities, based on the large commercial market in paraphilic pornography and paraphernalia.

Among legally identified cases of paraphilias, pedophilia is most common. Of all children, 10 to 20 percent have been molested by age 18. Because a child is the object, the act is taken more seriously, and greater effort is spent tracking down the culprit than in other paraphilias. Persons with exhibitionism who publicly display themselves to young children are also commonly apprehended. Those with voyeurism may be apprehended, but their risk is not great. Of adult females, 20 percent have been the targets of persons with exhibitionism and voyeurism. Sexual masochism and sexual sadism are underrepresented in any prevalence estimates. Sexual sadism usually comes to attention only in sensational cases of rape, brutality, and lust murder. The excretory paraphilias are scarcely reported, because activity usually takes place between consenting adults or between prostitute and client. Persons with fetishism rarely become entangled in the legal system. Those with transvestic fetishism may be arrested occasionally for disturbing the peace or on other misdemeanor charges if they are obviously men dressed in women's clothes, but arrest is more common among those with gender identity disorders. Zoophilia as a true paraphilia is rare.

As usually defined, the paraphilias seem to be largely male conditions. Fetishism almost always occurs in men. More than 50 percent of all paraphilias have their onset before age 18. Patients with paraphilia frequently have three to five paraphilias, either concurrently or at different times in their lives. This pattern of occurrence is especially the case with exhibitionism, fetishism, sexual masochism, sexual sadism, transvestic fetishism, voyeurism, and zoophilia (Table 21.3–1). The occurrence of paraphiliac behavior peaks between ages 15 and 25 and gradually declines; in men of 50, criminal paraphiliac acts are rare. Those that occur are practiced in isolation or with a cooperative partner.

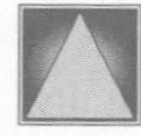

Table 21.3–1
Frequency of Paraphiliac Acts Committed by Patients with Paraphilia Seeking Outpatient Treatment

Diagnostic Category	Patients with Paraphilia Seeking Outpatient Treatment (%)	Paraphiliac Acts per Patient with Paraphilia[a]
Pedophilia	45	5
Exhibitionism	25	50
Voyeurism	12	17
Frotteurism	6	30
Sexual masochism	3	36
Transvestic fetishism	3	25
Sexual sadism	3	3
Fetishism	2	3
Zoophilia	1	2

[a]Median number.
(Courtesy of Gene G. Abel, M.D.)

Etiology

Psychosocial Factors. In the classic psychoanalytic model, persons with a paraphilia have failed to complete the normal developmental process toward heterosexual adjustment, but the model has been modified by new psychoanalytic approaches. What distinguishes one paraphilia from another is the method chosen by a person (usually male) to cope with the anxiety caused by the threat of castration by the father and separation from the mother. However bizarre its manifestation, the resulting behavior provides an outlet for the sexual and aggressive drives that would otherwise have been channeled into normal sexual behavior.

Failure to resolve the oedipal crisis by identifying with the father-aggressor (for boys) or mother-aggressor (for girls) results either in improper identification with the opposite-sex parent or in an improper choice of object for libido cathexis. Classic psychoanalytic theory holds that transsexualism and transvestic fetishism are disorders because each involves identification with the opposite-sex parent instead of the same-sex parent; for instance, a man dressing in women's clothes is believed to identify with his mother. Exhibitionism and voyeurism may be attempts to calm anxiety about castration because the reaction of the victim or the arousal of the voyeur reassures the paraphiliac that the penis is intact. Fetishism is an attempt to avoid anxiety by displacing libidinal impulses to inappropriate objects. A person with a shoe fetish unconsciously denies that women have lost their penises through castration by attaching libido to a phallic object, the shoe, which symbolizes the female penis. Persons with pedophilia and sexual sadism have a need to dominate and control their victims to compensate for their feelings of powerlessness during the oedipal crisis. Some theorists believe that choosing a child as a love object is a narcissistic act. Persons with sexual masochism overcome their fear of injury and their sense of powerlessness by showing that they are impervious to harm. Another theory proposes that the masochist directs the aggression inherent in all paraphilias toward herself or himself. Although recent developments in psychoanalysis place more emphasis on treating defense mechanisms than on oedipal traumas, psychoanalytic therapy for patients with a paraphilia remains consistent with Sigmund Freud's theory.

Other theories attribute the development of a paraphilia to early experiences that condition or socialize children into committing a paraphiliac act. The first shared sexual experience can be important in that regard. Molestation as a child can predispose a person to accept continued abuse as an adult or, conversely, to become an abuser of others. Also, early experiences of abuse that is not specifically sexual, such as spanking, enemas, or verbal humiliation, can be sexualized by a child and can form the basis for a paraphilia. Such experiences can result in the development of an *eroticized child*. The onset of paraphiliac acts can result from persons' modeling their behavior on the behavior of others who have carried out paraphiliac acts, mimicking sexual behavior depicted in the media, or recalling emotionally laden events from the past, such as their own molestation. Learning theory indicates that because the fantasizing of paraphiliac interests begins at an early age and because personal fantasies and thoughts are not shared with others (who could block or discourage them), the use and misuse of paraphiliac fantasies and urges continue uninhibited until late in life. Only then do persons begin to realize that such paraphiliac interests and urges are inconsistent with societal norms. By that time, however, the repetitive use of such fantasies has become ingrained, and the sexual thoughts and behaviors have become associated with, or conditioned to, paraphiliac fantasies.

Biological Factors. Several studies have identified abnormal organic findings in persons with paraphilias. None has used random samples of such persons; instead, they have extensively investigated patients with paraphilia who were referred to large medical centers. Among these patients, those with positive organic findings included 74 percent with abnormal hormone levels, 27 percent with hard or soft neurological signs, 24 percent with chromosomal abnormalities, 9 percent with seizures, 9 percent with dyslexia, 4 percent with abnormal electroencephalograms (EEGs), 4 percent with major mental disorders, and 4 percent with mental handicaps. The question is whether these abnormalities are causally related to paraphiliac interests or are incidental findings that bear no relevance to the development of paraphilia.

Psychophysiological tests have been developed to measure penile volumetric size in response to paraphiliac and nonparaphiliac stimuli. The procedures may be of use in diagnosis and treatment, but are of questionable diagnostic validity because some men are able to suppress their erectile responses.

Diagnosis and Clinical Features

In DSM-IV-TR, the diagnostic criteria for paraphilias include the presence of a pathognomonic fantasy and an intense urge to act out the fantasy or its behavior elaboration. The fantasy, which may distress a patient, contains unusual sexual material that is relatively fixed and shows only minor variations. Arousal and orgasm depend on the mental elaboration or the behavioral playing out of the fantasy. Sexual activity is ritualized or stereotyped and makes use of degraded, reduced, or dehumanized objects.

Exhibitionism. Exhibitionism is the recurrent urge to expose the genitals to a stranger or to an unsuspecting person (Table 21.3–2). Sexual excitement occurs in anticipation of the exposure, and orgasm is brought about by masturbation during or after the event. In almost 100 percent of cases, those with exhibitionism are men exposing themselves to women. The dynamic of men with exhibitionism is to assert their masculinity by showing their penises and by watching the victims' reactions—fright, surprise, and disgust. In this situation, men unconsciously feel castrated and impotent. Wives of men with exhibitionism often substitute for the mothers to whom the men were excessively attached during childhood. In other related paraphilias, the central themes involve derivatives of looking or showing.

Table 21.3–2
DSM-IV-TR Diagnostic Criteria for Exhibitionism

A. Over a period of at least 6 months, recurrent, intense sexually arousing fantasies, sexual urges, or behaviors involving the exposure of one's genitals to an unsuspecting stranger.
B. The person has acted on these sexual urges, or the sexual urges or fantasies cause marked distress or interpersonal difficulty.

(From American Psychiatric Association. *Diagnostic and Statistical Manual of Mental Disorders.* 4th ed. Text rev. Washington, DC: American Psychiatric Association; copyright 2000, with permission.)

Fetishism. In fetishism the sexual focus is on objects (e.g., shoes, gloves, pantyhose, and stockings) that are intimately associated with the human body (Table 21.3–3). The particular fetish is linked to someone closely involved with a patient during childhood and has a quality associated with this loved, needed, or even traumatizing person. Usually, the disorder begins by adolescence, although the fetish may have been established in childhood. Once established, the disorder tends to be chronic.

Sexual activity may be directed toward the fetish itself (e.g., masturbation with or into a shoe), or the fetish may be incorporated into sexual intercourse (e.g., the demand that high-heeled shoes be worn). The disorder is almost exclusively found in men. According to Freud, the fetish serves as a symbol of the phallus to persons with unconscious castration fears. Learning theorists believe that the object was associated with sexual stimulation at an early age.

A single, 32-year-old male freelance photographer presented with the chief complaint of "abnormal sex drive." The patient related that although he was somewhat sexually attracted by women, he was far more attracted by "their panties."

To the best of the patient's memory, sexual excitement began at about age 7, when he came upon a pornographic magazine and felt stimulated by pictures of partially nude women wearing "panties." His first ejaculation occurred at age 13 via masturbation to fantasies of women wearing panties. He masturbated into his older sister's panties, which he had stolen without her knowledge. Subsequently he stole panties from her friends and from other women he met socially. He found pretexts to "wander" into the bedrooms of women during social occasions, and would quickly rummage through their possessions until he found a pair of panties to his satisfaction. He later used these to masturbate into and then "saved them" in a "private cache." The pattern of masturbating into women's underwear had been his preferred method of achieving sexual excitement and orgasm from adolescence until the present consultation.

The patient first had sexual intercourse at age 18. Since then he had had intercourse on many occasions, and his preferred partner was a prostitute paid to wear panties, with the crotch area cut away,

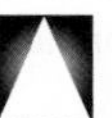

Table 21.3–3
DSM-IV-TR Diagnostic Criteria for Fetishism

A. Over a period of at least 6 months, recurrent, intense sexually arousing fantasies, sexual urges, or behaviors involving the use of nonliving objects (e.g., female undergarments).
B. The fantasies, sexual urges, or behaviors cause clinically significant distress or impairment in social, occupational, or other important areas of functioning.
C. The fetish objects are not limited to articles of female clothing used in cross-dressing (as in transvestic fetishism) or devices designed for the purpose of tactile genital stimulation (e.g., a vibrator).

(From American Psychiatric Association. *Diagnostic and Statistical Manual of Mental Disorders.* 4th ed. Text rev. Washington, DC: American Psychiatric Association; copyright 2000, with permission.)

during the act. On less common occasions when sexual activity was attempted with a partner who did not wear panties, his sexual excitement was sometimes weak.

The patient felt uncomfortable dating "nice women" as he felt that friendliness might lead to sexual intimacy and that they would not understand his sexual needs. He avoided socializing with friends who might introduce him to such women. He recognized that his appearance, social style, and profession all resulted in his being perceived as a highly desirable bachelor. He felt anxious and depressed because his social life was limited by his sexual preference.

The patient sought consultation shortly after his mother's sudden and unexpected death. Despite the fact that he complained of loneliness, he admitted that the pleasure he experienced from his unusual sexual activity made him unsure about whether or not he wished to give it up. (Courtesy of *DSM-IV-TR Casebook.*)

Frotteurism. Frotteurism is usually characterized by a man's rubbing his penis against the buttocks or other body parts of a fully clothed woman to achieve orgasm (Table 21.3–4). At other times, he may use his hands to rub an unsuspecting victim. The acts usually occur in crowded places, particularly in subways and buses. Those with frotteurism are extremely passive and isolated, and frottage is often their only source of sexual gratification. The expression of aggression in this paraphilia is readily apparent.

Pedophilia. Pedophilia involves recurrent intense sexual urges toward, or arousal by, children 13 years of age or younger, over a period of at least 6 months. Persons with pedophilia are at least 16 years of age and at least 5 years older than the victims (Table 21.3–5). When a perpetrator is a late adolescent involved in an ongoing sexual relationship with a 12- or 13-year-old, the diagnosis is not warranted.

Most child molestations involve genital fondling or oral sex. Vaginal or anal penetration of children occurs infrequently, except in cases of incest. Although most child victims coming to public attention are girls, this finding appears to be a product of the referral process. Offenders report that when they touch a child, most (60 percent) of the victims are boys. This figure is in sharp contrast to the figure for nontouching victimization of children, such as window peeping and exhibitionism; 99 percent of all such cases are perpetrated against girls. Of those with pedophilia, 95 percent are heterosexual, and 50 percent have consumed alcohol to excess at the time of the incident. In addition to their pedophilia, a significant number of the perpetrators are concomitantly or have previously been involved in exhibitionism, voyeurism, or rape.

Incest is related to pedophilia by the frequent selection of an immature child as a sex object, the subtle or overt element of coercion, and occasionally the preferential nature of the adult–child liaison.

Table 21.3–4
DSM-IV-TR Diagnostic Criteria for Frotteurism

A. Over a period of at least 6 months, recurrent, intense sexually arousing fantasies, sexual urges, or behaviors involving touching and rubbing against a nonconsenting person.
B. The person has acted on these sexual urges, or the sexual urges or fantasies cause marked distress or interpersonal difficulty.

(From American Psychiatric Association. *Diagnostic and Statistical Manual of Mental Disorders.* 4th ed. Text rev. Washington, DC: American Psychiatric Association; copyright 2000, with permission.)

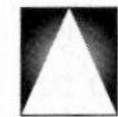

Table 21.3–5
DSM-IV-TR Diagnostic Criteria for Pedophilia

A. Over a period of at least 6 months, recurrent, intense sexually arousing fantasies, sexual urges, or behaviors involving sexual activity with a prepubescent child or children (generally age 13 years or younger).
B. The person has acted on these sexual urges, or the sexual urges or fantasies cause marked distress or interpersonal difficulty.
C. The person is at least age 16 years and at least 5 years older than the child or children in Criterion A.

Note: Do not include an individual in late adolescence involved in an ongoing sexual relationship with a 12- or 13-year-old.

Specify if:
Sexually attracted to males
Sexually attracted to females
Sexually attracted to both

Specify if:
Limited to incest

Specify type:
Exclusive type (attracted only to children)
Nonexclusive type

(From American Psychiatric Association. *Diagnostic and Statistical Manual of Mental Disorders.* 4th ed. Text rev. Washington, DC: American Psychiatric Association; copyright 2000, with permission.)

Dr. C, a single, 35-year-old child psychiatrist, had been arrested and convicted of fondling several neighborhood boys, ages 6 to 12. Friends and colleagues were shocked and dismayed, as he had been considered by all to be particularly caring and supportive of children. Not only had he chosen a profession involving their care, but he had been a Cub Scout leader for many years and also a member of the local Big Brothers.

Dr. C was from a stable family. His father, who had also been a physician, was described as a workaholic, spending little time with his three children. Dr. C never married and, when interviewed by a psychiatrist as part of his presentence investigation, admitted that he experienced little, if any, sexual attraction toward females, either adults or children. He also denied sexual attraction toward adult men. In presenting the history of his psychosexual development, he reported that he had become somewhat dismayed as a child when his boyfriends began expressing rudimentary awareness of an attraction toward girls. His "secret" at the time was that he was attracted more to other boys, eventually progressing to mutual masturbation with some of his boyfriends.

His first sexual experience was at age 6, when a 15-year-old male camp counselor performed fellatio on him several times over the course of the summer—an experience that he had always kept to himself. As he reached his teenage years, he began to suspect that he was homosexual. As he grew older, he was surprised to notice that the age range of males who attracted him sexually did not change, and he continued to have recurrent erotic urges and fantasies about boys between the ages of 6 and 12. Whenever he masturbated, he would fantasize about a boy in that age range, and on a couple of occasions over the years had felt himself to be in love with such a youngster.

Intellectually, Dr. C knew that others would disapprove of his many sexual involvements with young boys. He never believed, however, that he had caused any of these youngsters harm, feeling instead that they were simply sharing pleasurable feelings together. He yearned to be able to experience the same sort of feelings toward women, but he never was able to do so. He frequently prayed for help and that his actions would go undetected. He kept promising himself that he would stop, but he could not. He was so fearful of destroying his reputation, his friendships, and his career that he had never been able to bring himself to tell anyone about his problem. (Courtesy of *DSM-IV-TR Casebook.*)

Sexual Masochism. Masochism takes its name from the activities of Leopold von Sacher-Masoch, a 19th century Austrian novelist whose characters derived sexual pleasure from being abused and dominated by women. According to DSM-IV-TR, persons with sexual masochism have a recurrent preoccupation with sexual urges and fantasies involving the act of being humiliated, beaten, bound, or otherwise made to suffer (Table 21.3–6). Sexual masochistic practices are more common among men than among women. Freud believed masochism resulted from destructive fantasies turned against the self. In some cases, persons can allow themselves to experience sexual feelings only when punishment for the feelings follows. Persons with sexual masochism may have had childhood experiences that convinced them that pain is a prerequisite for sexual pleasure. About 30 percent of those with sexual masochism also have sadistic fantasies. Moral masochism involves a need to suffer, but is not accompanied by sexual fantasies.

A 25-year-old female graduate student asked for a consultation because of depression and martial discord. The patient had been married for 5 years, during which time both she and her husband were in school. For the past 3 years, her academic performance had been consistently better than his, and she attributed their frequent, intense arguments to this. She noted that she experienced a feeling of sexual excitement when her husband screamed at her or hit her in rage. Sometimes she would taunt him until he had sexual intercourse with her in a brutal fashion, as if she were being raped. She experienced the brutality and sense of being punished as sexually exciting.

One year before the consultation, the patient had found herself often ending arguments by storming out of the house. On one such occasion she went to a "singles bar," picked up a man, and got him to slap her as part of their sexual activity. She found the "punishment" sexually exciting and subsequently fantasized about being beaten during masturbation to orgasm. The patient then discovered that she enjoyed receiving physical punishment at the hands of strange men more than any other type of sexual stimulus. In a setting in which she could be whipped or beaten, all aspects of sexual activity, including the quality of orgasms, were far in excess of anything she had previously experienced.

This sexual preference was not the reason for the consultation, however. She complained that she could not live without her husband, yet could not live with him. She had suicidal fantasies stemming from the fear that he would leave her.

She recognized that her sexual behavior was dangerous to herself and felt mildly ashamed of it. She was unaware of any possible reasons for its emergence and was not sure she wished treatment for "it," because it gave her so much pleasure. (Courtesy of *DSM-IV-TR Casebook.*)

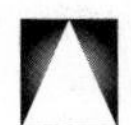

Table 21.3–6
DSM-IV-TR Diagnostic Criteria for Sexual Masochism

A. Over a period of at least 6 months, recurrent, intense sexually arousing fantasies, sexual urges, or behaviors involving the act (real, not simulated) of being humiliated, beaten, bound, or otherwise made to suffer.
B. The fantasies, sexual urges, or behaviors cause clinically significant distress or impairment in social, occupational, or other important areas of functioning.

(From American Psychiatric Association. *Diagnostic and Statistical Manual of Mental Disorders.* 4th ed. Text rev. Washington, DC: American Psychiatric Association; copyright 2000, with permission.)

Sexual Sadism. The DSM-IV-TR diagnostic criteria for sexual sadism are presented in Table 21.3–7. The onset of the disorder is usually before the age of 18 years, and most persons with sexual sadism are male. According to psychoanalytic theory, sadism is a defense against fears of castration; persons with sexual sadism do to others what they fear will happen to them and derive pleasure from expressing their aggressive instincts. The disorder was named after the Marquis de Sade, an 18th century French author and military officer who was repeatedly imprisoned for his violent sexual acts against women. Sexual sadism is related to rape, although rape is more aptly considered an expression of power. Some sadistic rapists, however, kill their victims after having sex (so-called lust murders). In many cases, these persons have underlying schizophrenia. John Money believes that lust murderers have dissociative identity disorder and perhaps a history of head trauma. He lists five contributory causes of sexual sadism: hereditary predisposition, hormonal malfunctioning, pathological relationships, a history of sexual abuse, and the presence of other mental disorders.

A controlling, narcissistic physician, raised alone by his widowed mother since age 2, has been preoccupied with spanking's erotic charge for him since age 6. Socially awkward during adolescence

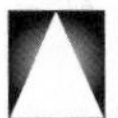

Table 21.3–7
DSM-IV-TR Diagnostic Criteria for Sexual Sadism

A. Over a period of at least 6 months, recurrent, intense sexually arousing fantasies, sexual urges, or behaviors involving acts (real, not simulated) in which the psychological or physical suffering (including humiliation) of the victim is sexually exciting to the person.
B. The person has acted on these sexual urges with a nonconsenting person, or the sexual urges or fantasies cause marked distress or interpersonal difficulty.

(From American Psychiatric Association. *Diagnostic and Statistical Manual of Mental Disorders.* 4th ed. Text rev. Washington, DC: American Psychiatric Association; copyright 2000, with permission.)

and his 20s, he married the first woman he dated and gradually introduced her to his secret arousal pattern of imagining himself spanking women. Although horrified, she episodically agreed to indulge him on an infrequent schedule to supplement their frequent ordinary sexual behavior. He ejaculated only when imagining spanking. Following her sixth episode of anxious, sullen depression in 20 years of marriage, her psychologist instructed her to tell him "No more." He fell into despair, was diagnosed with a major depressive disorder, and wrote a long letter to her about why he was entitled to spank her. He claimed to have had little idea that her participation in this humiliation was negatively affecting her mental health ("She even had orgasms sometimes after I spanked her!"). He became suicidal as a solution to the dilemma of choosing between his or her happiness and becoming conscious that what he was asking was abusive. He was shocked to discover that she had long considered suicide as a solution to her marital trap of loving an otherwise good husband and father who had an unexplained sick sexual need.

Voyeurism. Voyeurism, also known as *scopophilia*, is the recurrent preoccupation with fantasies and acts that involve observing persons who are naked or engaged in grooming or sexual activity (Table 21.3–8). Masturbation to orgasm usually accompanies or follows the event. The first voyeuristic act usually occurs during childhood and the paraphilia is most common in men. When persons with voyeurism are apprehended, the charge is usually loitering.

One man, best described as polymorphous perverse, spent the early years of his marriage avoiding sex with his wife while sneaking glances of a woman across the courtyard dressing and undressing. This man, as with many other voyeurs, had a number of coexisting paraphilias; he preferred watching his spouse insert the tube of an enema bag into her vagina, so as to masturbate rather than having intercourse with her. He associated this preference to having once seen his mother naked in her bathroom, holding a douche bag or an enema bag. In his therapy sessions, he frequently closed his eyes. He eventually disclosed that, during such moments, he had flash fantasies in which he visualized women in a number of erotic poses. (Courtesy of Ethel Spector Person, M.D.)

Transvestic Fetishism. Transvestic fetishism is described as fantasies and sexual urges to dress in opposite gender clothing as a means of arousal and as an adjunct to masturbation or coitus (Table 21.3–9). Transvestic fetishism typically begins in childhood or early adolescence. As years pass, some men with transvestic fetishism want to dress and live permanently as women. More rarely, women want to dress and live as men. These persons are classified in DSM-IV-TR as persons with transvestic fetishism and gender dysphoria. Usually, a person wears more than one article of opposite sex clothing; frequently, an entire wardrobe is involved. When a man with transvestic fetishism is cross-dressed, the appearance of femininity may be striking, although not usually to the degree found in transsexualism. When not dressed in women's clothes, men with transvestic fetishism may be hypermasculine in appearance and occupation. Cross-dressing can be graded from solitary, depressed, guilt-ridden dressing to ego-syntonic, social membership in a transvestite subculture.

The overt clinical syndrome of transvestic fetishism may begin in latency, but is more often seen around pubescence or in adolescence. Frank dressing in opposite sex clothing usually does not begin until mobility and relative independence from parents are well established.

Table 21.3–8
DSM-IV-TR Diagnostic Criteria for Voyeurism

A. Over a period of at least 6 months, recurrent, intense sexually arousing fantasies, sexual urges, or behaviors involving the act of observing an unsuspecting person who is naked, in the process of disrobing, or engaging in sexual activity.
B. The person has acted on these sexual urges, or the sexual urges or fantasies cause marked distress or interpersonal difficulty.

(From American Psychiatric Association. *Diagnostic and Statistical Manual of Mental Disorders.* 4th ed. Text rev. Washington, DC: American Psychiatric Association; copyright 2000, with permission.)

Table 21.3–9
DSM-IV-TR Diagnostic Criteria for Transvestic Fetishism

A. Over a period of at least 6 months, in a heterosexual male, recurrent, intense sexually arousing fantasies, sexual urges, or behaviors involving cross-dressing.
B. The fantasies, sexual urges, or behaviors cause clinically significant distress or impairment in social, occupational, or other important areas of functioning.

Specify if:
With gender dysphoria: if the person has persistent discomfort with gender role or identity

(From American Psychiatric Association. *Diagnostic and Statistical Manual of Mental Disorders.* 4th ed. Text rev. Washington, DC: American Psychiatric Association; copyright 2000, with permission.)

Mr. H is a 46-year-old married transvestic fetishist, a successful lawyer who loves his work. He and his wife have two grown children, who no longer live at home. Ambitious and competitive, he masks his aggression behind a gentle facade. He views himself as helpful to other people and is proud of his ability to assert himself when necessary.

Mr. H was the youngest of two siblings with a sister who was 3 years older. His parents had a tempestuous marriage and, after multiple separations, ultimately divorced when Mr. H was 7 years of age. During the separations, and after the divorce, he and his sister stayed with their maternal grandparents. Mr. H was living with them on a consistent basis even before his parents finally divorced. He saw his mother only irregularly. He has obliterated all memory of his father. His mother was outgoing and loving to Mr. H when she saw him, but, with each separation, he feared he might never see her again and was overwhelmed with sadness. As he grew older, his grandparents left him on his own. He would disappear and stay with friends for several days, and no one questioned why. Although he sometimes recounts this as a positive experience, the fact is that he felt abandoned throughout childhood, commenting that he largely raised himself. He was never effeminate, and he never played with girls. He was a good student, and, after college, he went to law school.

His grandmother's ministrations were tender and, at times, seductive. She fondled him, combed his hair, and rubbed him down with oil. He remembers an early attachment to her mohair blankets but denies that she ever cross-dressed him. He began to cross-dress in his grandmother's clothes at 8 years of age. It was always in secret, and he was never discovered. Cross-dressing was initially nonerotic and produced a safe form of relaxation—like alcohol. Only in adolescence did he begin to eroticize female clothing and to have spontaneous ejaculations while cross-dressed. In his late teens, he had sexual intercourse for the first time with an older female neighbor whom he married while he was still in his early 20s.

His cross-dressing escalated after the birth of his first child. At the same time, his sexual drive toward his wife began to diminish. He continues to have an increasing urge to cross-dress under stress. He entered treatment, because the cross-dressing preoccupied him more and more, and his wife was threatening divorce in response to his loss of sexual interest in her. As with many other transvestic fetishists, he continues to have a pronounced interest in masculine activities. (Courtesy of Ethel Spector Person, M.D.)

Paraphilia Not Otherwise Specified. The classification of paraphilia not otherwise specified includes various paraphilias that do not meet the criteria for any of the aforementioned categories (Table 21.3–10).

TELEPHONE AND COMPUTER SCATOLOGIA. Telephone scatologia is characterized by obscene phone calling and involves an unsuspecting partner. Tension and arousal begin in anticipation of phoning; the recipient of the call listens while the telephoner (usually male) verbally exposes his preoccupations or induces her to talk about her sexual activity. The conversation is accompanied by masturbation, which is often completed after the contact is interrupted.

Persons also use interactive computer networks, sometimes compulsively, to send obscene messages by electronic mail and to transmit sexually explicit messages and video images. Because of the anonymity of the users in chat rooms who use aliases, on-line or computer sex (cybersex) allows some persons to play the role of the opposite sex ("genderbending"), which represents an alternative method of expressing transvestic or transsexual fantasies. A danger of on-line cybersex is that pedophiles often make contact with children or adolescents who are lured into meeting them and are then molested. Many on-line contacts develop into off-line liaisons. Although some persons report that the off-line encounters develop into meaningful relationships, most such meetings are filled with disappointment and disillusionment, as the fantasized person fails to meet unconscious expectations of perfection. In other situations, when adults meet, rape or even homicide may occur.

NECROPHILIA. Necrophilia is an obsession with obtaining sexual gratification from cadavers. Most persons with this disorder find corpses in morgues, but some have been known to rob graves or even to murder to satisfy their sexual urges. In the few cases studied, those with necrophilia believed that they were inflicting the greatest conceivable humiliation on their lifeless victims. According to Richard von Krafft-Ebing, the diagnosis of psychosis is, under all circumstances, justified.

PARTIALISM. Persons with the disorder of partialism concentrate their sexual activity on one part of the body to the exclusion of all others. Mouth–genital contact—such as cunnilingus (oral contact with a woman's external genitals), fellatio (oral contact with the penis), and anilingus (oral contact with the anus)—is normally associated with foreplay; Freud recognized the mucosal surfaces of the body as erotogenic and capable of producing pleasurable sensation. But when a person uses these activities as the sole source of sexual gratification and cannot have or refuses to have coitus, a paraphilia exists. It is also known as *oralism*.

ZOOPHILIA. In zoophilia, animals—which may be trained to participate—are preferentially incorporated into arousal fantasies or sexual activities, including intercourse, masturbation, and oral–genital contact. Zoophilia as an organized paraphilia is rare. For many persons, animals are the major source of relatedness, so it is not surprising that a broad variety of domestic animals are used sensually or sexually.

Sexual relations with animals may occasionally be an outgrowth of availability or convenience, especially in parts of the world where rigid convention precludes premarital sexuality and in situations of enforced isolation. Because masturbation is also available in such situations, however, a predilection for animal contact is probably present in opportunistic zoophilia.

COPROPHILIA AND KLISMAPHILIA. Coprophilia is sexual pleasure associated with the desire to defecate on a partner, to be defecated on, or to eat feces (coprophagia). A variant is the compulsive utterance of obscene words (coprolalia). These paraphilias are associated with fixation at the anal stage of psychosexual development. Similarly, klismaphilia, the use of enemas as part of sexual stimulation, is related to anal fixation.

UROPHILIA. Urophilia, a form of urethral eroticism, is interest in sexual pleasure associated with the desire to urinate on a partner or to be urinated on. In both men and women, the disorder may be associated with masturbatory techniques involving the insertion of foreign objects into the urethra for sexual stimulation.

MASTURBATION. Masturbation is a normal activity that is common in all stages of life from infancy to old age, but this viewpoint was not always accepted. Freud believed that neurasthenia was caused by excessive masturbation. In the early 1900s, masturbatory insanity was a common diagnosis in hospitals for the criminally insane in the United States. Masturbation can be defined as a person's achieving sexual pleasure—which usually results in orgasm—by himself or herself (autoeroticism). Alfred Kinsey found it to be more prevalent in males than in females, but this difference may no longer exist. The frequency of masturbation varies from three to four times a week in adolescence to one to two times a week in adulthood. It is common among married persons; Kinsey reported that it occurred on the average of once a month among married couples.

The techniques of masturbation vary in both sexes and among persons. The most common technique is direct stimulation of the clitoris or penis with the hand or the fingers. Indirect stimulation can also be used, such as rubbing against a pillow or squeezing

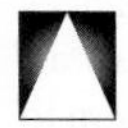

Table 21.3–10
DSM-IV-TR Diagnostic Criteria for Paraphilia Not Otherwise Specified

This category is included for coding paraphilias that do not meet the criteria for any of the specific categories. Examples include, but are not limited to, telephone scatologia (obscene phone calls), necrophilia (corpses), partialism (exclusive focus on part of body), zoophilia (animals), coprophilia (feces), klismaphilia (enemas), and urophilia (urine).

(From American Psychiatric Association. *Diagnostic and Statistical Manual of Mental Disorders.* 4th ed. Text rev. Washington, DC: American Psychiatric Association; copyright 2000, with permission.)

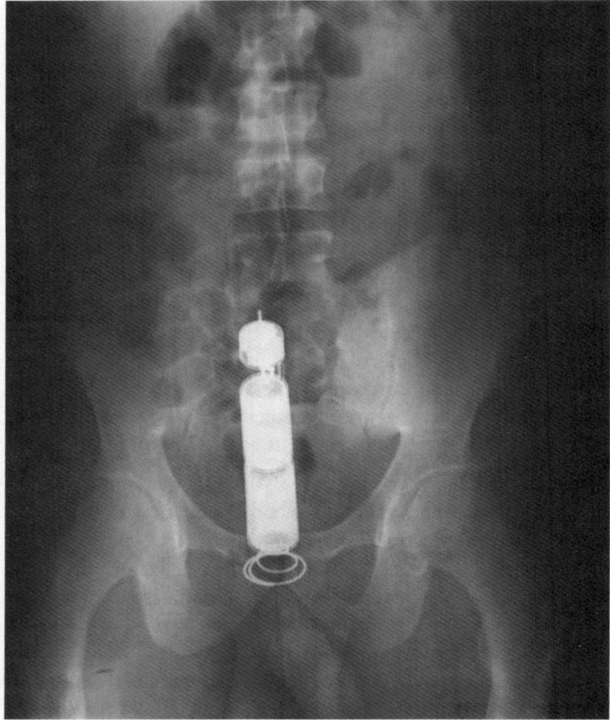

FIGURE 21.3–1

A man who masturbated compulsively with a large electrically powered vibrator by inserting the head of the instrument into his anus was unable to retrieve it when it was inserted too far into the anal canal. (Courtesy of Stephen Baker, M.D.)

the thighs. Kinsey found that 2 percent of women are capable of achieving orgasm through fantasy alone. Men and women have been known to insert objects in the urethra to achieve orgasm. The hand vibrator is now used as a masturbatory device by both sexes.

Masturbation is abnormal when it is the only type of sexual activity performed in adulthood, when its frequency indicates a compulsion or sexual dysfunction, or when it is consistently preferred to sex with a partner (Fig. 21.3–1).

HYPOXYPHILIA. Hypoxyphilia is the desire to achieve an altered state of consciousness secondary to hypoxia while experiencing orgasm. Persons may use a drug (e.g., a volatile nitrite or nitrous oxide) to produce hypoxia. Autoerotic asphyxiation is also associated with hypoxic states, but it should be classified as a form of sexual masochism. (A discussion of autoerotic asphyxiation appears in Section 21.2 of this chapter.)

Differential Diagnosis

Clinicians must differentiate a paraphilia from an experimental act that is not recurrent or compulsive and that is done for its novelty. Paraphiliac activity most likely begins during adolescence. Some paraphilias (especially the bizarre types) are associated with other mental disorders, such as schizophrenia. Brain diseases can also release perverse impulses.

Course and Prognosis

The difficulty in controlling or curing paraphilias rests in the fact that it is hard for people to give up sexual pleasure with no assurance that new routes to sexual gratification will be secured. A poor prognosis for paraphilias is associated with an early age of onset, a high frequency of acts, no guilt or shame about the act, and substance abuse. The course and the prognosis are better when patients have a history of coitus in addition to the paraphilia and when they are self-referred rather than referred by a legal agency.

Treatment

Five types of psychiatric interventions are used to treat persons with paraphilias: external control, reduction of sexual drives, treatment of comorbid conditions (e.g., depression or anxiety), cognitive-behavioral therapy, and dynamic psychotherapy.

Prison is an external control mechanism for sexual crimes that usually does not contain a treatment element. When victimization occurs in a family or work setting, the external control comes from informing supervisors, peers, or other adult family members of the problem and advising them about eliminating opportunities for the perpetrator to act on urges.

Drug therapy, including antipsychotic or antidepressant medication, is indicated for the treatment of schizophrenia or depressive disorders if the paraphilia is associated with these disorders. Antiandrogens, such as cyproterone acetate in Europe and medroxyprogesterone acetate (depo-Provera) in the United States, may reduce the drive to behave sexually by decreasing serum testosterone levels to subnormal concentrations. Serotonergic agents, such as fluoxetine (Prozac), have been used with limited success in some patients with paraphilia.

Cognitive-behavioral therapy is used to disrupt learned paraphiliac patterns and modify behavior to make it socially acceptable. The interventions include social skills training, sex education, cognitive restructuring (confronting and destroying the rationalizations used to support victimization of others), and development of victim empathy. Imaginal desensitization, relaxation technique, and learning what triggers the paraphiliac impulse so that such stimuli can be avoided are also taught. In modified aversive behavior rehearsal, perpetrators are videotaped acting out their paraphilia with a mannequin. Then the patient with paraphilia is confronted by a therapist and a group of other offenders who ask questions about feelings, thoughts, motives associated with the act and repeatedly try to correct cognitive distortions and point out lack of victim empathy to the patient.

Insight-oriented psychotherapy is a long-standing treatment approach. Patients have the opportunity to understand their dynamics and the events that caused the paraphilia to develop. In particular, they become aware of the daily events that cause them to act on their impulses (e.g., a real or fantasized rejection). Treatment helps them deal with life stresses better and enhances their capacity to relate to a life partner. Psychotherapy also allows patients to regain self-esteem, which in turn allows them to approach a partner in a more normal sexual manner. Sex therapy is an appropriate adjunct to the treatment of patients who suffer from specific sexual dysfunctions when they attempt nondeviant sexual activities.

Good prognostic indicators include the presence of only one paraphilia, normal intelligence, the absence of substance abuse, the absence of nonsexual antisocial personality traits, and the presence of a successful adult attachment. Paraphilias, however, remain significant treatment challenges even under these circumstances.

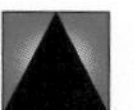

Table 21.3–11
ICD-10 Diagnostic Criteria for Disorders of Sexual Preference

G1. The individual experiences recurrent intense sexual urges and fantasies involving unusual objects of activities.
G2. The individual either acts on the urges or is markedly distressed by them.
G3. The preference has been present for at least 6 months.

Fetishism

A. The general criteria for disorders of sexual preference must be met.
B. The fetish (some nonliving object) is the most important source of sexual stimulation or is essential for satisfactory sexual response.

Fetishistic transvestism

A. The general criteria for disorders of sexual preference must be met.
B. The individual wears articles of clothing of the opposite sex in order to create the appearance and feeling of being a member of the opposite sex.
C. The cross dressing is closely associated with sexual arousal. Once orgasm occurs and sexual arousal declines, there is a strong desire to remove the clothing.

Exhibitionism

A. The general criteria for disorders of sexual preference must be met.
B. There is either a recurrent or a persistent tendency to expose the genitalia to unsuspecting strangers (usually of the opposite sex) which is almost invariably associated with sexual arousal and masturbation.
C. There is no intention or invitation to have sexual intercourse with the "witness(es)."

Voyeurism

A. The general criteria for disorders of sexual preference must be met.
B. There is either a recurrent or a persistent tendency to look at people engaging in sexual or intimate behaviour such as undressing, which is associated with sexual excitement and masturbation.
C. There is no intention to reveal one's presence.
D. There is no intention of sexual involvement with the person(s) observed.

Pedophilia

A. The general criteria for disorders of sexual preference must be met.
B. There is a persistent or predominant preference for sexual activity with a prepubescent child or children.
C. The individual is at least 16 years old and at least 5 years older than the child or children in Criterion B.

Sadomasochism

A. The general criteria for disorders of sexual preference must be met.
B. There is preference for sexual activity, as recipient (masochism) or provider (sadism), or both, which involves at least one of the following:
(1) pain;
(2) humiliation;
(3) bondage.
C. The sadomasochistic activity is the most important source of stimulation or is necessary for sexual gratification.

Multiple disorders of sexual preference

The likelihood of more than one abnormal sexual preference occurring in one individual is greater than would be expected by chance. For research purposes the different types of preference, and their relative importance to the individual, should be listed. The most common combination is fetishism, transvestism, and sadomasochism.

Other disorders of sexual preference

A variety of other patterns of sexual preference and activity may occur, each being relatively uncommon. These include such activities as making obscene telephone calls, rubbing up against people for sexual stimulation in crowded public places (frotteurism), sexual activity with animals, use of strangulation or anoxia for intensifying sexual excitement, and a preference for partners with some particular anatomical abnormality such as an amputated limb.

Erotic practices are too diverse and many too rare or idiosyncratic to justify a separate term for each. Swallowing urine, smearing feces, or piercing foreskin or nipples may be part of the behavioral repertiore in sadomasochism. Masturbatory rituals of various kinds are common, but the more extreme practices, such as the insertion of objects into the rectum or penile urethra, or partial self-strangulation, when they take the place of ordinary sexual contacts, amount to abnormalities. Necrophilia should also be coded here.

Disorder of sexual preference, unspecified

(From World Health Organization. *The ICD-10 Classification of Mental and Behavioural Disorders: Diagnostic Criteria for Research.* Copyright, World Health Organization, Geneva, 1993, with permission.)

ICD-10

In the 10th revision of *International Statistical Classification of Diseases and Related Health Problems* (ICD-10), the paraphilias are classified as disorders of sexual preference. In ICD-10, six specific disorders—fetishism, fetishistic transvestism, exhibitionism, voyeurism, pedophilia, and sadomasochism—and three residual categories are listed (Table 21.3–11).

SEXUAL DISORDER NOT OTHERWISE SPECIFIED

Many sexual disorders are not classifiable as sexual dysfunctions or as paraphilias. These unclassified disorders are rare, poorly documented, not easily classified, or not specifically described in DSM-IV-TR (Table 21.3–12). ICD-10 has a similar residual category for problems related to sexual development or preference (Table 21.3–13).

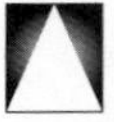

Table 21.3–12
DSM-IV-TR Diagnostic Criteria for Sexual Disorder Not Otherwise Specified

This category is included for coding a sexual disturbance that does not meet the criteria for any specific sexual disorder and is neither a sexual dysfunction nor a paraphilia. Examples include

1. Marked feelings of inadequacy concerning sexual performance or other traits related to self-imposed standards of masculinity or femininity
2. Distress about a pattern of repeated sexual relationships involving a succession of lovers who are experienced by the individual only as things to be used
3. Persistent and marked distress about sexual orientation

(From American Psychiatric Association. *Diagnostic and Statistical Manual of Mental Disorders.* 4th ed. Text rev. Washington, DC: American Psychiatric Association; copyright 2000, with permission.)

Postcoital Dysphoria

Not listed in DSM-IV-TR, postcoital dysphoria occurs during the resolution phase of sexual activity, when persons normally experience a sense of general well-being and muscular and psychological relaxation. Some persons, however, undergo postcoital dysphoria at this time and, after an otherwise satisfactory sexual experience, become depressed, tense, anxious, and irritable and show psychomotor agitation. They often want to get away from their partners and may become verbally or even physically abusive. The incidence of the disorder is unknown, but it is more common in men than in women. The causes relate to the person's attitude toward sex in general and toward the partner in particular. The disorder may occur in adulterous sex and in contacts with prostitutes. The fear of acquired immune deficiency syndrome (AIDS) causes some persons to experience postcoital dysphoria. Treatment requires insight-oriented psychotherapy to help patients understand the unconscious antecedents to their behavior and attitudes.

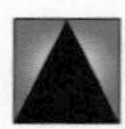

Table 21.3–13
ICD-10 Diagnostic Criteria for Psychological and Behavioral Disorders Associated with Sexual Development and Orientation

This section is intended to cover those types of problems that derive from variations of sexual development or orientation, when the sexual preference per se is not necessarily problematic or abnormal.

Sexual maturation disorder
The patient suffers from uncertainty about his or her gender identity or sexual orientation, which causes anxiety or depression.

Ego-dystonic sexual orientation
The gender identity or sexual preference is not in doubt, but the individual wishes it were different.

Sexual relationship disorder
The abnormality of gender identity or sexual preference is responsible for difficulties in forming or maintaining a relationship with a sexual partner.

Other psychosexual development disorders
Psychosexual development disorder, unspecified

(Reprinted with permission from World Health Organization. *The ICD-10 Classification of Mental and Behavioural Disorders: Diagnostic Criteria for Research.* Copyright, World Health Organization, Geneva, 1993.)

Couple Problems

At times, a complaint arises from the spousal unit or the couple, rather than from an individual dysfunction. For example, one partner may prefer morning sex, but the other functions more readily at night, or the partners have unequal frequencies of desire.

Unconsummated Marriage

A couple involved in an unconsummated marriage have never had coitus and are typically uninformed and inhibited about sexuality. Their feelings of guilt, shame, or inadequacy are increased by their problem, and they experience conflict between their need to seek help and their need to conceal their difficulty. Couples may seek help for the problem after having been married several months or several years. William Masters and Virginia Johnson reported one unconsummated marriage of 17 years' duration.

Frequently, the couple does not seek help directly; the woman may reveal the problem to her gynecologist on a visit ostensibly concerned with vague vaginal or other somatic complaints. On examining her, the gynecologist may find an intact hymen. In some cases, however, the wife may have undergone a hymenectomy to resolve the problem, but the surgery may aggravate the situation without solving the basic problem. The surgical procedure is another stress and often increases the couple's feelings of inadequacy. The wife may feel put upon, abused, or mutilated, and the husband's concern about his manliness may increase. An inquiry by a physician who is comfortable dealing with sexual problems may be the first opening to a frank discussion of the couple's distress. Often, the pretext of the medical visit is a discussion of contraceptive methods or—even more ironically—a request for an infertility workup. Once presented, the complaint can often be treated successfully. The duration of the problem does not significantly affect the prognosis or the outcome of the case.

The causes of unconsummated marriage are varied: lack of sex education, sexual prohibitions overly stressed by parents or society, problems of an oedipal nature, immaturity in both partners, overdependence on primary families, and problems in sexual identification. Religious orthodoxy, with severe control of sexual and social development, and the equation of sexuality with sin or uncleanliness has also been cited as a dominant cause. Many women involved in an unconsummated marriage have distorted concepts about their vaginas. They may fear that it is too small or too soft, or they may confuse the vagina with the rectum and thus feel unclean. Men may share these distortions about the vagina and perceive it as dangerous to themselves. Similarly, both partners may have distortions about the man's penis and perceive it as a weapon, as too large, or as too small. Many patients can be helped by simple education about genital anatomy and physiology, by suggestions for self-exploration, and by correct information from a physician. The problem of unconsummated marriage is best treated by seeing both members of the couple. Dual-sex therapy involving a male-female cotherapist team has been markedly effective. Other forms of conjoint therapy, marital counseling, traditional psychotherapy on a one-to-one basis, and counseling from a sensitive family physician, gynecologist, or urologist are also helpful.

Body Image Problems

Some persons are ashamed of their bodies and experience feelings of inadequacy related to self-imposed standards of masculinity or femininity. They may insist on sex only during total darkness, not allow certain body parts to be seen or touched, or seek unnecessary operative procedures to deal with their imagined inadequacies. Body dysmorphic disorder should be ruled out.

Sex Addiction and Compulsivity

The concept of sex addiction developed over the past two decades to refer to persons who compulsively seek out sexual experiences and whose behavior becomes impaired if they are unable to gratify their sexual impulses. The concept of sex addiction derived from the model of addiction to such drugs as heroin or addiction to behavioral patterns, such as gambling. Addiction implies psychological dependence, physical dependence, and the presence of a withdrawal syndrome if the substance (e.g., the drug) is unavailable or the behavior (e.g., gambling) is frustrated.

In DSM-IV-TR the term *sex addiction* is not used, nor is it a disorder that is universally recognized or accepted. Nevertheless, the phenomenon of a person whose entire life revolves around sex-seeking behavior and activities, who spends an excessive amount of time in such behavior, and who often tries to stop such behavior but is unable to do so is well known to clinicians. Such persons show repeated and increasingly frequent attempts to have a sexual experience, deprivation of which gives rise to symptoms of distress. Sex addiction is a useful concept heuristically, in that it can alert the clinician to seek an underlying cause for the manifest behavior. There is interest in making it a new official diagnostic category, which the authors support.

Diagnosis. Sex addicts are unable to control their sexual impulses, which can involve the entire spectrum of sexual fantasy or behavior. Eventually, the need for sexual activity increases, and the person's behavior is motivated solely by the persistent desire to experience the sex act. The history usually reveals a long-standing pattern of such behavior, which the person repeatedly has tried to stop, but without success. Although a patient may have feelings of guilt and remorse after the act, these feelings do not suffice to prevent its recurrence. The patient may report that the need to act out is most severe during stressful periods or when angry, depressed, anxious, or otherwise dysphoric. Most acts culminate in a sexual orgasm. Eventually, the sexual activity interferes with the person's social, vocational, or marital life, which begins to deteriorate. The signs of sexual addiction are listed in Table 21.3–14.

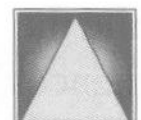

Table 21.3–14
Signs of Sexual Addiction

1. Out-of-control behavior
2. Severe adverse consequences (medical, legal, interpersonal) due to sexual behavior
3. Persistent pursuit of self-destructive or high-risk sexual behavior
4. Repeated attempts to limit or stop sexual behavior
5. Sexual obsession and fantasy as a primary coping mechanism
6. The need for increasing amounts of sexual activity
7. Severe mood changes related to sexual activity (e.g., depression, euphoria)
8. Inordinate amount of time spent in obtaining sex, being sexual, or recovering from sexual experience
9. Interference of sexual behavior in social, occupational, or recreational activities

(Data from Carnes P. *Don't Call It Love.* New York: Bantam Books; 1991.)

Types of Behavioral Patterns. The paraphilias constitute the behavioral patterns most often found in the sex addict. As defined in DSM-IV-TR, the essential features of a paraphilia are recurrent, intense sexual urges or behaviors, including exhibitionism, fetishism, frotteurism, sadomasochism, cross-dressing, voyeurism, and pedophilia. Paraphilias are associated with clinically significant distress and almost invariably interfere with interpersonal relationships, and they often lead to legal complications. In addition to the paraphilias, however, sex addiction can also include behavior that is considered normal, such as coitus and masturbation, except that it is promiscuous and uncontrolled.

In the 19th century, Krafft-Ebing reported on several cases of abnormally increased sexual desire. One involved a 36-year-old married teacher, the father of seven children, who masturbated repeatedly while sitting at his desk in front of his pupils, after which he was "penitent and filled with shame." He indulged in coitus three or four times a day in addition to his repeated masturbatory act. In another case, a young woman masturbated almost incessantly and was unable to control her impulses. She had frequent coitus with many men, but neither coitus nor masturbation sufficed, and she eventually was placed in an institution. Krafft-Ebing referred to the condition as "sexual hyperaesthesia," which he believed could occur in otherwise normal persons.

In many cases, sex addiction is the final common pathway of a variety of other disorders. In addition to the paraphilias that are often present, the patient may have an associated major mood disorder or schizophrenia. Antisocial personality disorder and borderline personality disorder are common.

DON JUANISM. Some men who appear to be hypersexual, as manifested by their need to have many sexual encounters or conquests, use their sexual activities to mask deep feelings of inferiority. Some have unconscious homosexual impulses, which they deny by compulsive sexual contacts with women. After having sex, most Don Juans are no longer interested in the woman. The condition is sometimes referred to as *satyriasis* or *sex addiction.*

NYMPHOMANIA. Nymphomania signifies a woman's excessive or pathological desire for coitus. Of the few scientific studies of the condition, those patients who were studied usually have had one or more sexual disorders, often including female orgasmic disorder. The woman often has an intense fear of losing love and, through her actions, attempts to satisfy her dependence needs rather than gratify her sexual impulses. This disorder is a form of sex addiction.

Comorbidity. Comorbidity (dual diagnosis) refers to the presence of an addiction that coexists with another psychiatric disorder. For example, about 50 percent of patients with substance-use disorder also have an additional psychiatric disorder. Similarly, many sex addicts have an associated psychiatric disorder. Dual diagnosis implies that the psychiatric illness and the addiction are separate disorders; one does not cause the other. The diagnosis of comorbidity is often difficult to make because addictive behavior (of all types) can produce extreme anxiety and severe disturbances in mood and affect, especially while the addictive behavior is treated. If, after a period of abstinence, symptoms of a psychiatric disorder remain, the comorbid condition is more easily recognized and diagnosed than during the addictive period. Finally, a high correlation is found between sex addiction and substance-use disorders (up to 80 percent in some studies), which not only complicates the task of diagnosis, but also complicates treatment.

Treatment. Self-help groups based on the 12-step concept used in Alcoholics Anonymous (AA) have been used successfully with many sex addicts. They include such groups as Sexaholics Anonymous (SA), Sex and Love Addicts Anonymous (SLAA), and Sex Addicts Anonymous (SAA). The groups differ in that some are for men or women, or for married persons or couples. All advocate some abstinence from either the addictive behavior or sex in general. Should a substance-use disorder also be present, the patient often requires referral to AA or Narcotics Anonymous (NA) as well. Patients may enter an inpatient treatment unit when they lack sufficient motivation to control their behavior on an outpatient basis or may be a danger to themselves or others. Additionally, severe medical or psychiatric symptoms may require careful supervision and treatment best carried out in a hospital.

A 42-year-old married businessman with two children was considered a model of virtue in his community. He was active in his church and on the boards of several charitable organizations. He was living a secret life, however, and would lie to his wife, telling her that he was at a board meeting when he was actually visiting massage parlors for paid sex. He eventually was engaging in the behavior four to five times a day, and although he tried to quit many times, he was unable to do so. He knew that he was harming himself by putting his reputation and marriage at risk.

The patient presented himself to the psychiatric emergency room, stating that he would prefer to be dead rather than continue the behavior described. He was admitted with a diagnosis of major depressive disorder and started on a daily dose of 20 mg of fluoxetine. In addition, he received 100 mg of medroxyprogesterone intramuscularly once a day. His need to masturbate diminished markedly and ceased entirely on the third hospital day, as did his mental preoccupation with sex. The medroxyprogesterone was discontinued on the sixth day, when he was discharged. He continued to take fluoxetine, enrolled in a local SA group, and entered individual and couples psychotherapy. His addictive behavior eventually stopped, he was having satisfactory sexual relations with his wife, and he was no longer suicidal or depressed.

Psychotherapy. Insight-oriented psychotherapy may help patients understand the dynamics of their behavioral patterns. Supportive psychotherapy can help repair the interpersonal, social, or occupational damage that occurs. Cognitive behavioral therapy helps the patient recognize dysphoric states that precipitate sexual acting out. Marital therapy or couples therapy can help the patient regain self-esteem, which is severely impaired by the time a treatment program is begun. Finally, psychotherapy may be of help in the treatment of any associated psychiatric disorder.

Pharmacotherapy. Most specialists in general addiction avoid the use of psychotropic agents, especially in the early stages of treatment. Substance-dependent persons have a tendency to abuse those agents, especially agents with a high abuse potential, such as the benzodiazepines. Pharmacotherapy is of use in the treatment of associated psychiatric disorders, such as major depressive disorders and schizophrenia.

Certain medications may be of use in treating sex addiction, however, because of their specific effects on reducing the sex drive. Serotonin-specific reuptake inhibitors (SSRIs) reduce libido in some persons, a side effect that is used therapeutically. Compulsive masturbation is an example of a behavioral pattern that may benefit from such medication. Medroxyprogesterone acetate diminishes libido in men and, thus, makes it easier to control sexually addictive behavior.

The use of antiandrogens in women to control hypersexuality has not been tested sufficiently, but because androgenic compounds contribute to the sex drive in women, antiandrogens could be of benefit. Antiandrogenic agents (cyproterone acetate) are not available in the United States but are used in Europe with varying success.

Persistent and Marked Distress about Sexual Orientation

Distress about sexual orientation is characterized by dissatisfaction with sexual arousal patterns and it is usually applied to dissatisfaction with homosexual arousal patterns, a desire to increase heterosexual arousal, and strong negative feelings about being homosexual. Occasional statements to the effect that life would be easier if the speaker were not homosexual do not constitute persistent and marked distress about sexual orientation.

Treatment of sexual orientation distress is controversial. One study reported that with a minimum of 350 hours of psychoanalytic therapy, about a third of 100 bisexual and gay men achieved a heterosexual reorientation at a 5-year follow-up; this study has been challenged, however. Behavior therapy and avoidance conditioning techniques have also been used, but these techniques may change behavior only in the laboratory setting. Prognostic factors weighing in favor of heterosexual reorientation for men include being under 35 years of age, having some experience of heterosexual arousal, and feeling highly motivated to reorient.

Another and more prevalent style of intervention is directed at enabling persons with persistent and marked distress about sexual orientation to live comfortably with homosexuality without shame, guilt, anxiety, or depression. Gay counseling centers are engaged with patients in such treatment programs. At present, outcome studies of such centers have not been reported in detail.

Few data are available about the treatment of women with persistent and marked distress about sexual orientation, and these are primarily from single-case studies with variable outcomes. (Section 21.1 of this chapter presents a further discussion of sexual orientation, homosexuality, and coming out.)

References

Carnes PJ, Murray R, Charpantier L. Addiction interaction disorder. In: Combs RH, ed. *Handbook of Addictive Disorders: A Practical Guide to Diagnosis and Treatment.* Hoboken, NJ: John Wiley & Sons, Inc.; 2004:31.

Carnes PJ. Sexual addiction. In: Sadock BJ, Sadock VA, eds. *Kaplan & Sadock's Comprehensive Textbook of Psychiatry*. 8th ed. Vol. 1. Baltimore: Lippincott Williams & Wilkins; 2005:1991.

Ceccarelli P. Perversion on the other side of the couch. *International Forum of Psychoanalysis*. 2005;14:176–182.

Chirban JT. Integrative strategies for treating internet sexuality: A case study of paraphillias. *Clinical Case Studies*. 2006;5:126–141.

Coleman E, Raymond N, McBean A. Assessment and treatment of compulsive sexual behavior. *Minn Med.* 2003;86:42.

Dimen M. Perversion is us? Eight notes. In: *Sexuality, Intimacy, Power*. Hillsdale, NJ: The Analytic Press; 2003:257–291.

Jacobson L. On the use of "sexual addiction": The case for "perversion." *Contemp Psychoanal.* 2003;39:107–113.

Kafka MP. The monoamine hypothesis for the pathophysiology of paraphilic disorders: An update. *Ann N Y Acad Sci.* 2003;989:86.

Kafka MP. Sex offending and sexual appetite: The clinical and theoretical relevance of hypersexual desire. *Int J Offender Ther Comp Criminol.* 2003;47: 439.

Kafka MP, Hennen J. Hypersexual desire in males: Are males with paraphilias different from males with paraphilia-related disorders? *Sex Abuse.* 2003;15: 307.

Nestler EJ, Malenka RC. The addicted brain. *Sci Am.* 2004;290:78.

Person ES. Paraphilias. In: Sadock BJ, Sadock VA, eds. *Kaplan & Sadock's Comprehensive Textbook of Psychiatry*. 8th ed. Vol. 1. Baltimore: Lippincott Williams & Wilkins; 2005:1965.

Raymond NC, Coleman E, Miner MH. Psychiatric comorbidity and compulsive/impulsive traits in compulsive sexual behavior. *Compr Psychiatry.* 2003;44:370.

Richards AK. A fresh look at perversion. *J Am Psychoanal Assoc.* 2003;51:1199–1218.

22 Gender Identity Disorders

Gender identity refers to the sense one has of being male or being female which corresponds, normally, to the person's anatomical sex. The revised 4th edition of the *Diagnostic and Statistical Manual of Mental Disorders* (DSM-IV-TR) defines *gender identity disorders* as a group whose common feature is a strong, persistent preference for living as a person of the other sex. The affective component of gender identity disorders is gender dysphoria, discontent with one's designated birth sex and a desire to have the body of the other sex, and to be regarded socially as a person of the other sex. Gender identity disorder in adults was referred to in early versions of the DSM as *transsexualism*.

In DSM-IV-TR, no distinction is made for the overriding diagnostic term *gender identity disorder* as a function of age. In children, it can manifest as statements of wanting to be the other sex and as a broad range of sex-typed behaviors conventionally shown by children of the other sex. Gender identity crystallizes in most persons by age 2 or 3 years.

EPIDEMIOLOGY

Children

Most children with gender identity disorder are referred for clinical evaluation in early grade school years. Parents, however, typically report that the cross-gender behaviors were apparent before 3 years of age. Among a sample of boys under age 12 referred for a range of clinical problems, the reported desire to be the opposite sex was 10 percent. For clinically referred girls under age 12, the reported desire to be the opposite sex was 5 percent.

The sex ratio of referred children is 4 to 5 boys for each girl.

Adults

The best estimate of gender identity disorder or transsexualism in adults emanates from Europe with a prevalence of 1 in 30,000 men and 1 in 100,000 women. Most clinical centers report a sex ratio of three to five male patients for each female patient. Most adults with gender identity disorder report having felt different from other children of their same sex, although, in retrospect, many could not identify the source of that difference. Many report feeling extensively cross-gender identified from the earliest years, with the cross-gender identification becoming more profound in adolescence and young adulthood. Many adults with gender identity disorder may well have qualified for gender identity disorder in childhood.

ETIOLOGY

Biological Factors

For mammals, the resting state of tissue is initially female; as the fetus develops, a male is produced only if androgen (set off by the Y chromosome, which is responsible for testicular development) is introduced. Without testes and androgen, female external genitalia develop. Thus, maleness and masculinity depend on fetal and perinatal androgens. Lower animals' sexual behavior is governed by sex steroids, but this effect diminishes as the evolutionary tree is scaled. Sex steroids influence the expression of sexual behavior in mature men or women; that is, testosterone can increase libido and aggressiveness in women, and estrogen can decrease libido and aggressiveness in men. But masculinity, femininity, and gender identity result more from postnatal life events than from prenatal hormonal organization.

The same principle of masculinization or feminization has been applied to the brain. Testosterone affects brain neurons that contribute to the masculinization of the brain in such areas as the hypothalamus. Whether testosterone contributes to so-called masculine or feminine behavioral patterns in gender identity disorders remains a controversial issue.

Psychosocial Factors

Children usually develop a gender identity consonant with their sex of rearing (also known as *assigned sex*). The formation of gender identity is influenced by the interaction of children's temperament and parents' qualities and attitudes. Culturally acceptable gender roles exist: Boys are not expected to be effeminate, and girls are not expected to be masculine. There are boys' games (e.g., cops and robbers) and girls' toys (e.g., dolls and dollhouses). These roles are learned, although some investigators believe that some boys are temperamentally delicate and sensitive and that some girls are aggressive and energized—traits that are stereotypically known in today's culture as feminine and masculine, respectively. However, greater tolerance for mild cross-gender activity in children has developed in the past few decades.

Sigmund Freud believed that gender identity problems resulted from conflicts experienced by children within the oedipal triangle. These conflicts are fueled by both real family events and children's fantasies. Whatever interferes with a child's loving the opposite-sex parent and identifying with the same-sex parent interferes with normal gender identity.

The quality of the mother–child relationship in the first years of life is paramount in establishing gender identity. During this period, mothers normally facilitate their children's awareness of, and pride in, their gender: Children are valued as little boys and girls, but devaluing, hostile mothering can result in gender problems. At the same time, the separation-individuation process is unfolding. When gender problems become associated with separation-individuation problems, the result can be the use of sexuality to remain in relationships characterized by shifts between a desperate infantile closeness and a hostile, devaluing distance.

Some children are given the message that they would be more valued if they adopted the gender identity of the opposite sex. Rejected or abused children may act on such a belief. Gender identity problems can also be triggered by a mother's death, extended absence, or depression, to which a young boy may react by totally identifying with her—that is, by becoming a mother to replace her.

The father's role is also important in the early years, and his presence normally helps the separation-individuation process. Without a father, mother and child may remain overly close. For a girl, the father is normally the prototype of future love objects; for a boy, the father is a model for male identification.

DIAGNOSIS AND CLINICAL FEATURES

Current diagnostic criteria for children and adults are organized under two main groupings: *cross-gender identification* and *discomfort with assigned gender role*. For children, this includes the intense desire to participate in the games and pastimes of the other sex and may include rejection of gender-conventional toys and games. The essential features, for all ages, are a persistent and intense distress about his or her assigned sex and a desire to be of the other sex. Table 22–1 lists the DSM-IV-TR criteria for the disorder.

Children

At the extreme of gender identity disorder in children are boys who, by the standards of their cultures, are as feminine as the most feminine of girls and girls who are as masculine as the most masculine of boys. No sharp line can be drawn on the continuum of gender identity disorder between children who should receive a formal diagnosis and those who should not. Girls with the disorder regularly have male companions and an avid interest in sports and rough-and-tumble play; they show no interest in dolls or playing house (unless they play the father or another male role). They may refuse to urinate in a sitting position, claim that they have or will grow a penis and not want to grow breasts or to menstruate, and assert that they will grow up to become a man (not merely to play a man's role).

Boys with the disorder are usually preoccupied with stereotypically female activities. They may have a preference for dressing in girls' or women's clothes or may improvise such items from available material when the genuine articles are not available. (The cross-dressing typically does not cause sexual excitement, as in transvestic fetishism.) They often have a compelling desire to participate in the games and pastimes of girls. Female dolls are often their favorite toys, and girls are regularly their preferred playmates. When playing house, they take a girl's role. Their gestures and actions are often judged to be feminine, and they are usually subjected to male peer group teasing and rejection, a phenomenon that rarely occurs with boyish girls until adolescence. Boys with the disorder may assert that they will grow up to become a woman (not merely in role). They may claim that their penis or testes are disgusting or will disappear or that it would be better not to have a penis or testes. Some children refuse to attend school because of teasing or the

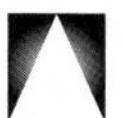

Table 22–1
DSM-IV-TR Diagnostic Criteria for Gender Identity Disorder

A. A strong and persistent cross-gender identification (not merely a desire for any perceived cultural advantages of being the other sex).

In children, the disturbance is manifested by four (or more) of the following:
(1) repeatedly stated desire to be, or insistence that he or she is, the other sex
(2) in boys, preference for cross-dressing or simulating female attire; in girls, insistence on wearing only stereotypical masculine clothing
(3) strong and persistent preferences for cross-sex roles in make-believe play or persistent fantasies of being the other sex
(4) intense desire to participate in the stereotypical games and pastimes of the other sex
(5) strong preference for playmates of the other sex

In adolescents and adults, the disturbance is manifested by symptoms such as a stated desire to be the other sex, frequent passing as the other sex, desire to live or be treated as the other sex, or the conviction that he or she has the typical feelings and reactions of the other sex.

B. Persistent discomfort with his or her sex or sense of inappropriateness in the gender role of that sex.

In children, the disturbance is manifested by any of the following: in boys, assertion that his penis or testes are disgusting or will disappear or assertion that it would be better not to have a penis, or aversion toward rough-and-tumble play and rejection of male stereotypical toys, games, and activities; in girls, rejection of urinating in a sitting position, assertion that she has or will grow a penis, or assertion that she does not want to grow breasts or menstruate, or marked aversion toward normative feminine clothing.

In adolescents and adults, the disturbance is manifested by symptoms such as preoccupation with getting rid of primary and secondary sex characteristics (e.g., request for hormones, surgery, or other procedures to physically alter sexual characteristics to simulate the other sex) or belief that he or she was born the wrong sex.

C. The disturbance is not concurrent with a physical intersex condition.

D. The disturbance causes clinically significant distress or impairment in social, occupational, or other important areas of functioning.

Code based on current age:
Gender identity disorder in children
Gender identity disorder in adolescents or adults

Specify if (for sexually mature individuals):
Sexually attracted to males
Sexually attracted to females
Sexually attracted to both
Sexually attracted to neither

(From American Psychiatric Association. *Diagnostic and Statistical Manual of Mental Disorders.* 4th ed. Text rev. Washington, DC: American Psychiatric Association; copyright 2000, with permission.)

pressure to dress in attire stereotypical of their assigned sex. Most children deny being disturbed by the disorder, except that it brings them into conflict with the expectations of their families or peers.

The parents of a 7-year-old boy came for consultation because the boy had told his parents on several occasions that he would like to be a girl. From 2 to 3 years of age, he showed interest in dressing in his older sister's clothing. Initially, both parents thought that their son's interest in his sister's and, occasionally, his mother's clothes was cute. They were reassured of its transient nature by their family doctor. Preschool teachers told them that many boys dress up and that it was normal. When his parents kept the clothes from him, he would improvise with a towel for long hair and a large t-shirt for a dress. When playing mother–father games, he would be mother, and he imitated female characters from children's stories. Most of his playmates were girls. He played often with his sister's discarded dolls and did not like sports. At school, he was teased by age-mates, notably boys, for cross-gender activities. At consultation, the father was concerned that his son would grow up to be gay. Mother was less concerned with this potential but was more worried that he was becoming a loner and unhappy at school in consequence of peer stigma. (Adapted from case of Richard Green, M.D.)

Differential Diagnosis of Children. Children with a gender identity disorder must be distinguished from other gender-atypical children. For girls, tomboys without gender identity disorder prefer functional and gender-neutral clothing. By contrast, gender identity-disordered girls adamantly refuse to wear girls' clothes and reject gender-neutral clothes. They make repeated statements of being or wanting to be a boy and wanting to grow up to be a man, along with repeated cross-sex fantasy play, so that, in mother–father games or other games imitating characters from mass media, they are male. This accompanies a marked aversion to traditionally feminine activities.

For boys, the differential diagnosis must distinguish those who do not conform to traditional masculine sex-typed expectations, but do not show extensive cross-gender identification and are not discontent with being male. It is not uncommon for boys to reject rough-and-tumble play or sports and to prefer nonathletic activities or occasionally to role play as a girl, to play with a doll, or to dress up in girl's or women's costumes. Such boys do not necessarily have a gender identity disorder. Boys who do have a gender identity disorder state a preference for being a girl and for growing up to become a woman, along with repeated cross-sex fantasy play, as in mother–father games, a strong preference for traditionally female-typed activities, cross-dressing, and a female peer group.

Because the diagnosis of gender identity disorder excludes children with anatomical intersex, a medical history needs to be taken with the focus on any suggestion of hermaphrodism in the child. With doubt, referral to a pediatric endocrinologist is indicated.

Adolescents and Adults

Similar signs and symptoms are seen in adolescents and adults. Adolescents and adults with the disorder manifest a stated desire to be the other sex; they frequently try to pass as a member of the other sex and they desire to live or to be treated as the other sex. In addition, they desire to acquire the sex characteristics of the opposite sex. They may believe that they were born the wrong sex and may make such characteristic statements as, "I feel that I'm a woman trapped in a male body" or vice versa.

Adolescents and adults frequently request medical or surgical procedures to alter their physical appearance. Although the term transsexual is not used in DSM-IV-TR, many clinicians find the term useful and will probably continue to use it. In addition, transsexualism appears in the 10th revision of *International Statistical Classification of Diseases and Related Health Problems* (ICD-10), and persons refer to themselves as transsexuals. Transsexual persons have a persistent preoccupation with getting rid of their primary and secondary sex characteristics and acquiring the sex characteristics of the other sex. The wish to dress and live as a member of the other sex is always present.

Most retrospective studies of transsexuals report gender identity problems during childhood, but prospective studies of children with gender identity disorders indicate that few become transsexuals and want to change their sex. The disorder is much more common in men (1 per 30,000) than in women (1 per 100,000). Adult transsexuals usually complain that they are uncomfortable wearing the clothes of their assigned sex; therefore, they dress the way the other sex dresses and engage in activities associated with the other sex. They find their genitals repugnant, a feeling that can lead to persistent requests for surgery. This desire may override all other wishes.

Men take estrogen to create breasts and other feminine contours, have electrolysis to remove their male hair, and have surgery to remove the testes and the penis and to create an artificial vagina. Women bind their breasts or have a double mastectomy, a hysterectomy, and an oophorectomy; they take testosterone to build up muscle mass and deepen the voice and have surgery in which an artificial phallus is created. These procedures may make a person indistinguishable from members of the other sex. Some investigators describe behavior in sex-reassigned persons as almost a caricature of the newly assumed male or female role.

A 27-year-old anatomical woman referred to a gender identity clinic reported having felt different as a child from other girls, although unable then to identify its source. As a young girl, she enjoyed playing sports with girls and boys, but generally preferred the companionship of boys. She preferred wearing unisex or boyish clothes and resisted wearing a skirt or dress. Everyone referred to her as a tomboy. She tried to hide her breast development by wearing loose fitting tops and stooping forward. Menses were embarrassing and poignantly reminded her of her femaleness, which was becoming increasingly alienating. As sexual attractions evolved, they were exclusively directed to female partners. In her late teens, she had one sexual experience with a man, and it was aversive. She began socializing in lesbian circles, but did not feel comfortable there and did not consider herself lesbian but more a man. For sexual partners, she wanted heterosexual women and wanted to be considered by the partner as a man. As gender dysphoric feelings became increasingly pronounced, she consulted transsexual sites on the Internet and contacted a female-to-male transsexual community support group. She then set into motion the process of clinical referral. She transitioned to living as a man, had a name change, and was administered androgen injections. Voice deepened, facial and body hair grew, menses stopped, and sex drive increased, along with clitoral hypertrophy. After 2 years, the patient underwent bilateral mastectomy and is on the wait list for phalloplasty and hysterectomy-ovariectomy. Employment as a man continues, as does a 3-year relationship with a female partner. The partner has a child from a previous marriage. (Adapted from case of Richard Green, M.D.)

Gender identity disorders can be associated with other diagnoses. Although some patients with gender identity disorder have a history of major psychosis, including schizophrenia or major affective disorder, most do not. When a diagnosis of gender identity disorder is made, as well as another DSM Axis I diagnosis, it is necessary to consider whether the diagnoses are distinct. A variety of Axis II personality disorders may be found in patients with gender identity disorder, particularly borderline personality, but none is specific. A proportion of nonhomosexual men with gender identity disorder report a history of erotic arousal in association with cross-dressing, and some would still qualify for a concurrent diagnosis of fetishistic transvestism. Some are more sexually aroused by imagining themselves with a female body or by seeing themselves cross-dressed in a mirror (autogynephilia) than by items of women's clothing per se.

COURSE AND PROGNOSIS

Children

Boys begin to have the disorder before the age of 4 years, and peer conflict develops during the early school years, at about the age of 7 or 8 years. Grossly feminine mannerisms may lessen as boys grow older, especially if attempts are made to discourage such behavior. Cross-dressing may be part of the disorder, and 75 percent of boys who cross-dress begin to do so before age 4. The age of onset is also early for girls, but most give up masculine behavior by adolescence.

In both sexes, homosexuality is likely to develop in one third to two thirds of all cases, although, for reasons that are unclear, fewer girls than boys have a homosexual orientation. Steven Levine reported that follow-up studies of gender-disturbed boys consistently indicated that homosexual orientation was the usual adolescent outcome.

Adults

Adult male patients who are gender dysphoric and sexually attracted to male partners may have a continuous development of gender dysphoria from childhood. Some manifestations of their gender dysphoria may be driven underground, however, in an effort, during their teens and, perhaps, early 20s, to merge with the larger community. They may also hope or think that their gender dysphoria will disappear. Sexual interest in male partners begins in early puberty, and some may consider themselves to be homosexual. They find, however, that they do not integrate effectively into the gay community. Approximately two thirds of adult men with gender identity disorder are sexually attracted to men only.

Gender identity disorders in men sexually attracted to female partners may be characterized as more progressive disorders with insidious onset. The course is fairly continuous in some cases; in others, the intensity of symptoms fluctuates. Some experience a lifelong struggle with feminine identification that changes in intensity from time to time and may temporarily recede in the face of conflicting desires, such as marriage and family. In most cases, the first outward manifestation is cross-dressing in childhood, dressing in mother's or sister's clothing, and many patients report that they first began wishing to be female during that period. The extent of their cross-gender behavior in childhood does not usually warrant diagnosis of gender identity disorder, however.

Female patients may experience adolescence in which they initially consider themselves lesbian because of sexual attraction to female partners. They come to define themselves as distinct from lesbians, however, because they consider themselves to be men in their relationships with women. They insist that their partners treat them as men and that the partners are heterosexual women. Female patients are often, more often than male patients, in a romantic or sexual relationship at the time of initial clinical assessment.

In earlier clinical experience, it was the rare female-to-male transsexual who reported sexual attractions to male partners. This has changed. Some gender identity clinics report approximately one tenth of patients born female have a sexual partner orientation to men and consider themselves to be gay men.

TREATMENT

Children

At present, no convincing evidence indicates that psychiatric or psychological intervention for children with gender identity disorder affects the direction of subsequent sexual orientation. Transsexualism, however, can be affected. Transsexuals or adults with gender identity disorder are unable to cope socially as persons of their anatomical birth sex. The treatment of gender identity disorder in children is directed largely at developing social skills and comfort in the sex role expected by birth anatomy. To the extent that treatment is successful, transsexual development may be interrupted. The low prevalence of transsexualism in the general population, however, even in the special population of cross-gender children, thwarts the testing of this assumption.

No hormonal or psychopharmacological treatments for gender identity disorder in childhood have been identified.

Adolescents

Adolescents whose gender identity disorder has persisted beyond puberty present unique treatment problems. One is how to manage the rapid emergence of unwanted secondary sex characteristics. Thus, a new area of treatment management has evolved with respect to slowing down or stopping pubertal changes expected by anatomical birth sex and then implementing cross-sex body changes with cross-sex hormones.

Young persons whose previous gender identity disorder has remitted may experience new conflicts should homosexual feelings emerge. This may be a source of anxiety in the adolescent and may cause conflict within the family. Teenagers should be reassured about the prevalence and nonpathological aspects of a same-sex partner preference. Parents must also be informed of the nonpathological nature of same-sex orientation. The goal of family intervention is to keep the family stable and to provide a supportive environment for the teenager.

Adults

Adult patients coming to a gender identity clinic usually present with straightforward requests for hormonal and surgical sex reassignment. No drug treatment has been shown to be effective in reducing cross-gender desires per se. When patient gender dysphoria is severe and intractable, sex reassignment may be the best solution.

Sex-Reassignment Surgery. Sex reassignment surgery for a person born anatomically male consists principally of removal of the penis, scrotum, and testes, construction of labia, and vaginoplasty. Some clinicians attempt to construct a neoclitoris from the former frenulum of the penis. The neoclitoris may have erotic sensation. Postoperative complications include urethral strictures, rectovaginal fistulas, vaginal stenosis, and inadequate width or depth.

Some male patients who do not have adequate breast development from years of hormone treatment may elect augmentation mammaplasty. Some also have thyroid cartilage shaved to reduce the male-appearing thyroid cartilage. Patients need to undergo vocal retraining, and those who do not have a fully effective response may undergo a cricothyroid approximation procedure, which can raise vocal pitch. The results of these operations are variable.

Female-to-male patients typically may undergo bilateral mastectomy and construct a neophallus. Because of increased technical skills in phalloplasty, more female-to-male patients are now electing these procedures.

Uncertainty and controversy exist with respect to the capacity for sexual arousal by the patient postsurgery. Some patients maintain that they are orgasmic. They describe the sensation of orgasm as more gradual and attenuated than their orgasms preoperatively. On the other hand, some patients report little sexual responsivity postsurgery. To date, no adequate assessments have been made of the physiological functioning of postoperative male-to-female transsexuals with respect to the human sexual response cycle. Many patients, however, report satisfaction with being able to have vaginal intercourse with a male partner.

Hormonal Treatment

Persons born male are typically treated with daily doses of oral estrogen. This may be conjugated equine estrogens or ethinylestradiol or estrogen patches. These hormones produce breast enlargement, the amount being largely determined by genetic predisposition, which continues for approximately 2 years. Other major effects of estrogen treatment are testicular atrophy, decreased libido, and diminished erectile capacity. Also, a decrease occurs in the density of body hair and, perhaps, an arrest of male pattern baldness. Side effects of endocrine treatment can be elevated levels of prolactin, blood lipids, fasting blood sugar, and hepatic enzymes. Patients should be monitored with appropriate blood tests. Smoking is a contraindication of endocrine treatment, because it increases the risk of deep vein thrombosis and pulmonary embolism. There is no effect on voice. Facial hair removal is required by laser treatment or electrolysis.

Biological women are treated with monthly or three weekly injections of testosterone. Because the effects of exogenous testosterone are more profound than those of estrogen, clinicians should be more cautious about commencing female patients on hormone treatment. The pitch of the voice drops permanently into the male range as the vocal cords thicken. The clitoris enlarges to two or three times its pretreatment length and is often accompanied by increased libido. Hair growth changes to the male pattern, and a full complement of facial hair may grow. Menses cease. Male pattern baldness may develop, and acne may be a complication.

Ethinylestradiol in male-to-female transsexuals increases regional fat depots and thigh muscle mass. Conversely, female-to-male transsexuals receiving testosterone may have increased thigh muscle and reduced subcutaneous fat deposition. Thus, cross-sex steroid hormones affect general body fat and muscle distribution, as well as promote breast development in patients born male.

GENDER IDENTITY DISORDER NOT OTHERWISE SPECIFIED

The diagnosis of gender identity disorder not otherwise specified is reserved for persons who cannot be classified as having a gender identity disorder with the characteristics described above (Table 22–2). Three examples are listed in DSM-IV-TR: persons with intersex conditions and gender dysphoria; adults with transient, stress-related cross-dressing behavior; and persons who have a persistent preoccupation with castration or penectomy without a desire to acquire the sex characteristics of the other sex.

Intersex Conditions

Intersex conditions include a variety of syndromes in which persons have gross anatomical or physiological aspects of the opposite sex.

Congenital Virilizing Adrenal Hyperplasia. Congenital virilizing adrenal hyperplasia was formerly called *the adrenogenital syndrome*. An enzymatic defect in the production of adrenal cortisol, beginning prenatally, leads to overproduction of adrenal androgens and virilization of the female fetus.

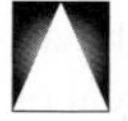

Table 22–2
DSM-IV-TR Diagnostic Criteria for Gender Identity Disorder Not Otherwise Specified

This category is included for coding disorders in gender identity that are not classifiable as a specific gender identity disorder. Examples include

1. Intersex conditions (e.g., partial androgen insensitivity syndrome or congenital adrenal hyperplasia) and accompanying gender dysphoria
2. Transient, stress-related cross-dressing behavior
3. Persistent preoccupation with castration or penectomy without a desire to acquire the sex characteristics of the other sex

(From American Psychiatric Association. *Diagnostic and Statistical Manual of Mental Disorders.* 4th ed. Text rev. Washington, DC: American Psychiatric Association; copyright 2000, with permission.)

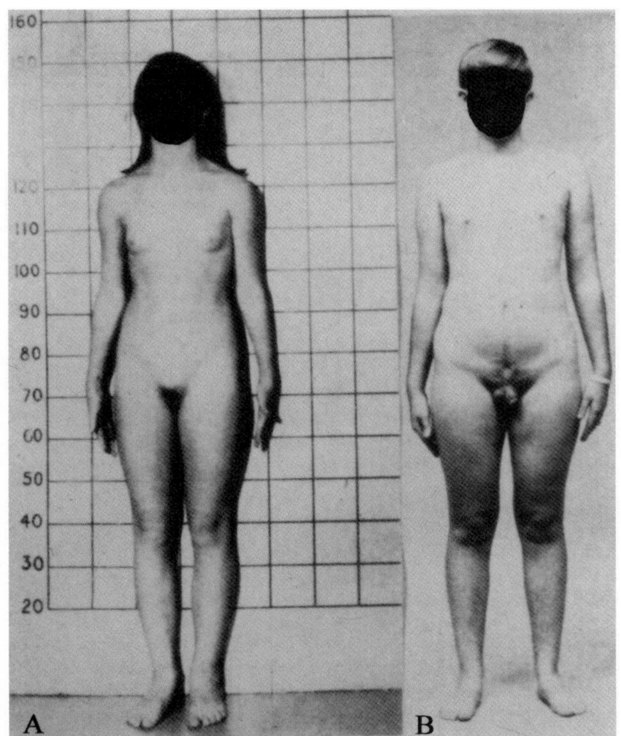

FIGURE 22–1
Two patients with adrenogenital syndrome. The patient in **A** was raised as a female and the patient in **B** was raised as a male.

Postnatally, excessive adrenal androgen can be controlled by steroid administration.

The androgenization can range from mild clitoral enlargement to external genitals that look like a normal scrotal sac, testes, and a penis, but hidden behind these external genitals are a vagina and a uterus (Fig. 22–1). The patients are otherwise normally female. At birth, if the genitals look male, children are assigned to the male sex and so reared; the result is usually a clear sense of maleness and unremarkable masculinity. If the children are assigned to the female sex and so reared, a sense of femaleness and femininity usually results. If the parents are uncertain about the sex of their child, a hermaphroditic identity results. The resultant gender identity usually reflects the rearing practices, but androgens may help determine behavior. Children raised unequivocally as girls have a more intense tomboy quality than that found in a control group. The girls most often have a heterosexual orientation. Some of these children experience gender identity conflicts and do not feel comfortable in the sex of assignment. Higher rates of bisexual or homosexual behavior in adulthood have been reported.

Androgen Insensitivity Syndrome. Androgen insensitivity syndrome was formerly called *testicular feminization*. In these persons with the XY karyotype, tissue cells are unable to use testosterone or other androgens. Therefore, the person appears to be a normal female at birth and is raised as a girl. She is later found to have cryptorchid testes, which produce the testosterone to which the tissues do not respond, and minimal or absent internal sexual organs. Secondary sex characteristics at puberty are female because of the small, but sufficient, amount of estrogens, which results from the conversion of testosterone into estradiol. The patients usually sense themselves as females and are feminine. However, some experience gender conflicts and distress.

TURNER'S SYNDROME. In Turner's syndrome, one sex chromosome is missing, such that the sex karyotype is simply X. Children have female genitalia, are short, and, possibly, anomalies such as a shield-shaped chest and a webbed neck. As a consequence of dysfunctional ovaries, they require exogenous estrogen to develop female secondary sex characteristics. Gender identity is female (Fig. 22–2).

KLINEFELTER'S SYNDROME. An extra X chromosome is present in Klinefelter's syndrome, such that the karyotype is XXY. At birth, patients appear to be normal males. Excessive gynecomastia may occur in adolescence. Testes are small, usually without sperm production. They are tall, and body habitus is eunuchoid. Reports suggest a higher rate of gender identity disorder.

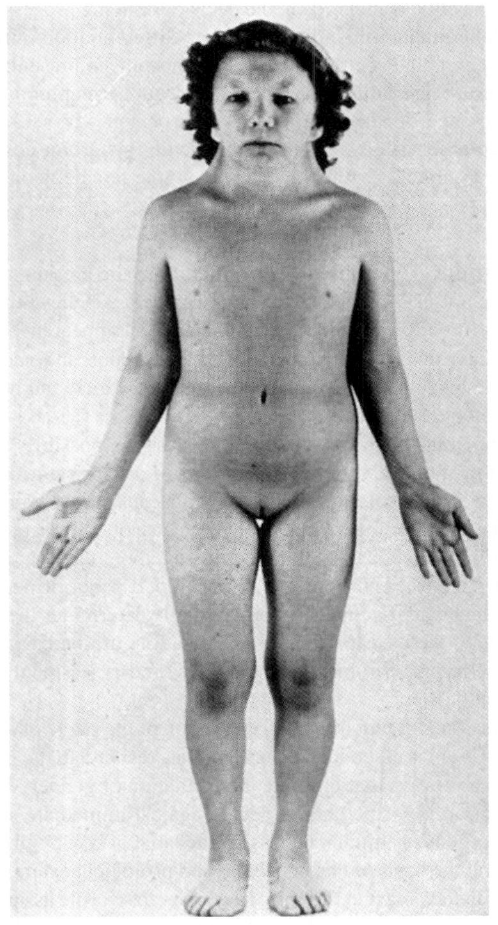

FIGURE 22–2
Turner's syndrome in a patient aged 23. Note webbed neck, increased carrying angle, failure of breast development, and lack of pubic hair. (From Douthwaite AH, ed. *French's Index of Differential Diagnosis*. 7th ed. Baltimore: Williams & Wilkins; 234.)

5-α-Reductase Deficiency. In 5-α-reductase deficiency, an enzymatic defect prevents the conversion of testosterone to dihydrotestosterone, which is required for prenatal virilization of the genitalia. At birth, the affected person appears to be female, although some anomaly is visible. In earlier generations, before childhood identification of the disorder was common, these persons, raised as girls, virilized at puberty and changed their gender identity to male. Later generations were expected to virilize and, thus, may have been raised with ambiguous gender. Recently, there are reports of a small number of patients for whom early removal of the testes and socialization as girls have resulted in a female gender identity.

Pseudohermaphroditism. Infants born with ambiguous genitals are pseudohermaphrodites. True hermaphroditism is characterized by the presence of both testes and ovaries in the same person. It is a rare condition. Sex assignment, based on the genitals' appearance at birth, determines gender identity, which is male, female, or hermaphroditic, depending on the family's conviction about the child's sex. Recently, treatment has changed, postponing sex assignment at birth based on the appearance of the genitalia to delay sex assignment until adolescence when the child is included in the decision-making process. Male pseudohermaphroditism is incomplete differentiation of the external genitalia even though a Y chromosome is present; testes are present but rudimentary. Female pseudohermaphroditism is the presence of virilized genitals in a person who is XX, the most common cause being the adrenogenital syndrome described above. Figure 22–3 illustrates a phenotypic female with an XY karyotype.

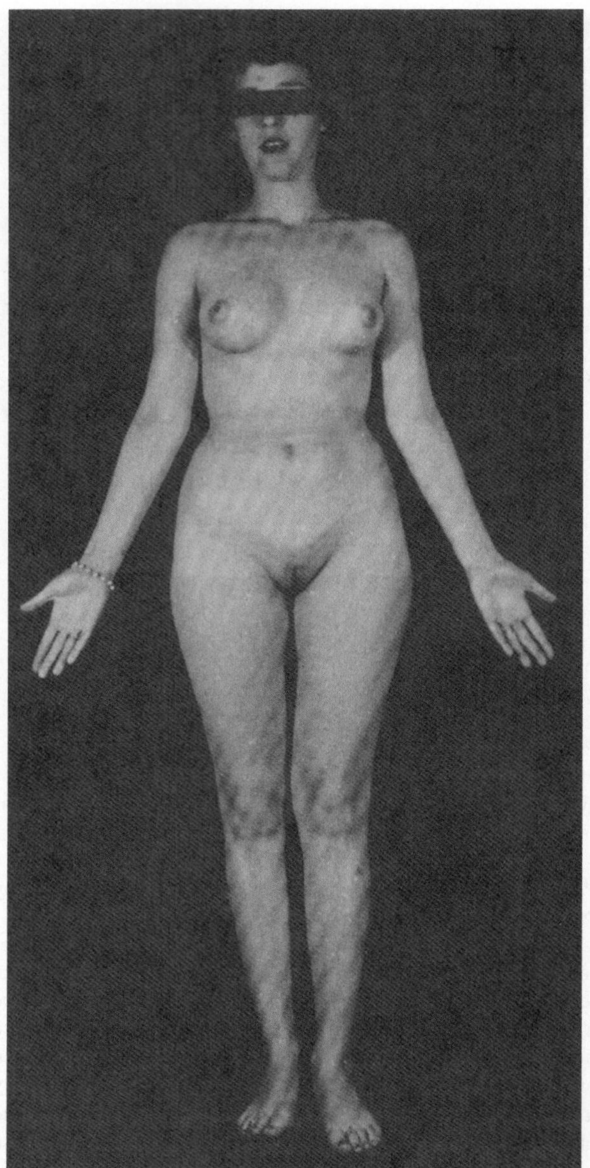

FIGURE 22–3
A phenotypic female with abdominal testes and an XY chromosomal karyotype. Note the excellent breast development and the absence of pubic hair. A normal blind vagina was present without clitoral enlargement.

Treatment. Because intersex conditions are present at birth, treatment must be timely, and some physicians believe the conditions to be true medical emergencies. The appearance of the genitalia in diverse conditions is often ambiguous, and a decision must be made about the assigned sex (boy or girl) and how the child should be reared.

Problems should be addressed as early as possible, so that the entire family can regard the child in a consistent, relaxed manner. This is particularly important because intersex patients may have gender identity problems because of complicated biological influences and familial confusion about their actual sex. When intersex conditions are discovered, a panel of pediatric, urological, and psychiatric experts usually determines the sex of rearing on the basis of clinical examination, urological studies, buccal smears, chromosomal analyses, and assessment of the parental wishes.

Education of parents and presentation of the range of options open to them is essential, because parents respond to the infant's genitalia in ways that promote the formation of gender identity. One option is for parents to decide against immediate surgery for ambiguous genitalia, but assign the label of boy or girl to the infant on the basis of chromosomal and urological examination. They can then react to the child according to sex role assignment with leeway to adjust the sex assignment should the child act definitively as a member of the sex opposite to the one designated.

If the parents decide on surgery to normalize genital appearance, it is generally undertaken before the age of 3 years. It is easier to assign a child to be female than to assign one to be male, because male-to-female genital surgical procedures are far more advanced than female-to-male procedures. That is an insufficient reason, however, to assign a chromosomal male to be female.

Some groups oppose surgical interventions on principle. The Intersex Society of North America, one such group, proposes that change is cosmetic at best and at worst may interfere with later sexual functioning. Some advocate that the US Congress pass laws prohibiting doctors from performing such surgery, especially because the infant cannot consent. The goal of treatment however, is to have genitals concordant with chromosomal, biological, physiological, and other genetic antecedents, thus allowing the development of a person with healthy gender identity. If this cannot be determined with certainty, then treatment can and should wait.

Cross-Dressing

The DSM-IV-TR lists cross-dressing—dressing in clothes of the opposite sex—as a gender identity disorder if it is transient and related to stress. If the disorder is not stress related, persons who cross-dress are classified as having transvestic fetishism, which is described as a paraphilia in DSM-IV-TR. An essential feature of transvestic fetishism is that it produces sexual excitement. Stress-related cross-dressing may sometimes produce sexual excitement, but it also reduces a patient's tension and anxiety. Patients may harbor fantasies of cross-dressing, but act them out only under stress. Male adult cross-dressers may have the fantasy that they are female, in whole or in part.

Cross-dressing is commonly known as *transvestism*, and the cross-dresser as a *transvestite*. Although these terms are no longer used in DSM-IV-TR, they remain in common parlance. Cross-dressing phenomena range from the occasional solitary wearing of clothes of the other sex to extensive feminine identification in men and masculine identification in women, with involvement in a transvestic subculture. More than one article of clothing of the other sex is involved, and a person may dress entirely as a member of the opposite sex. The degree to which a cross-dressed person appears as a member of the other sex varies, depending on mannerisms, body habitus, and cross-dressing skill. When not cross-dressed, these persons usually appear as unremarkable members of their assigned sex. Cross-dressing can coexist with paraphilias, such as sexual sadism, sexual masochism, and pedophilia.

Cross-dressing differs from transsexualism in that the patients have no persistent preoccupation with getting rid of their primary and secondary sex characteristics and acquiring the sex characteristics of the other sex. Some persons with the disorder once had transvestic fetishism, but no longer become sexually aroused by cross-dressing. Other persons with the disorder are homosexual men and women who cross-dress. The disorder is most common among female impersonators (Fig. 22–4).

Treatment. A combined approach, using psychotherapy and pharmacotherapy, is often useful in the treatment of cross-dressing. The stress factors that precipitate the behavior are identified in therapy. The goal is to help patients cope with the stressors appropriately and, if possible, eliminate them. Intrapsychic dynamics about attitudes toward men and women are examined, and unconscious conflicts are identified. Medication, such as antianxiety and antidepressant agents, is used to treat the symptoms. Because cross-dressing can occur impulsively, medications that reinforce impulse control may be helpful, such as fluoxetine (Prozac). Behavior therapy, aversive conditioning, and hypnosis are alternative methods that may be of use in selected patients.

Preoccupation with Castration

The category of preoccupation with castration is reserved for men and women who have a persistent preoccupation with castration

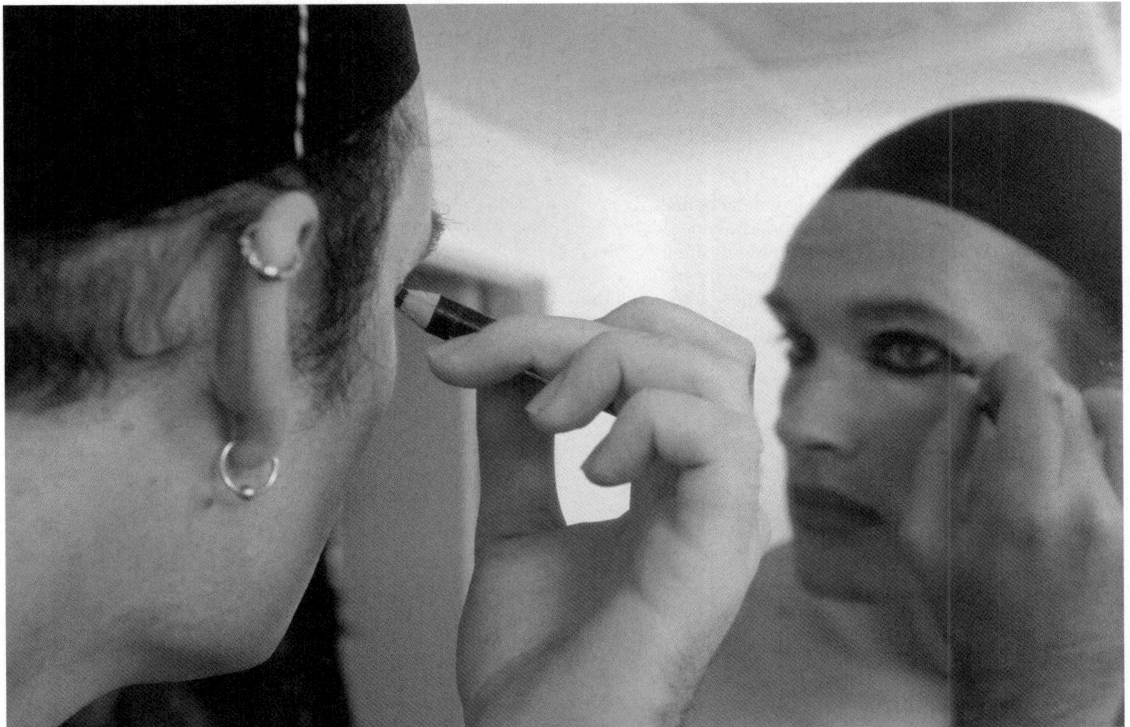

FIGURE 22–4
Female impersonator making up, reflected image. (Courtesy of Corbis.)

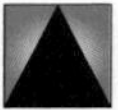

Table 22–3
ICD-10 Diagnostic Criteria for Gender Identity Disorders

Transsexualism

A. The individual desires to live and be accepted as a member of the opposite sex, usually accompanied by the wish to make his or her body as congruent as possible with the preferred sex through surgery and hormonal treatment.
B. The transsexual identity has been present persistently for at least 2 years.
C. The disorder is not a symptom of another mental disorder, such as schizophrenia, nor is it associated with chromosome abnormality.

Dual-role transvestism

A. The individual wears clothes of the opposite sex in order to experience temporarily membership of the opposite sex.
B. There is no sexual motivation for the cross-dressing.
C. The individual has no desire for a permanent change to the opposite sex.

Gender identity disorder of childhood

For girls:

A. The individual shows persistent and intense distress about being a girl, and has a stated desire to be a boy (not merely a desire for any perceived cultural advantages to being a boy), or insists that she is a boy.
B. Either of the following must be present:
  (1) persistent marked aversion to normative feminine clothing and insistence on wearing stereotypical masculine clothing, e.g., boy's underwear and other accessories;
  (2) persistent repudiation of female anatomical structures, as evidenced by at least one of the following:
    (a) an assertion that she has, or will grow, a penis;
    (b) rejection of urinating in a sitting position;
    (c) assertion that she does not want to grow breasts or menstruate.
C. The girl has not yet reached puberty.
D. The disorder must have been present for at least 6 months.

For boys:

A. The individual shows persistent and intense distress about being a boy, and has an intense desire to be a girl or, more rarely, insists that he is a girl.
B. Either of the following must be present:
  (1) preoccupation with stereotypical female activities, as shown by a preference for either cross-dressing or simulating female attire, or by an intense desire to participate in the games and pastimes of girls and rejection of stereotypical male toys, games, and activities;
  (2) persistent repudiation of male anatomical structures, as indicated by at least one of the following repeated assertions:
    (a) that he will grow up to become a woman (not merely in role);
    (b) that his penis or testes are disgusting or will disappear;
    (c) that it would be better not to have a penis or testes;
C. The boy has not yet reached puberty.
D. The disorder must have been present for at least 6 months.

Other gender identity disorders
Gender identity disorder, unspecified

(Reprinted with permission from World Health Organization. *The ICD-10 Classification of Mental and Behavioural Disorders: Diagnostic Criteria for Research*. Copyright, World Health Organization, Geneva, 1993.)

or penectomy without a desire to acquire the sex characteristics of the opposite sex. They are clearly uncomfortable with their assigned sex and their lives are driven by the fantasy of what it would be like to be a different gender. They may be asexual and lack sexual interest in either men or women.

A 45-year-old married male was admitted to the hospital after amputating the glans of his penis with a carving knife. He claimed that he heard voices telling him to carry out the act. He had been diagnosed with schizophrenia at age 25 after an episode of paranoid ideation in which he felt that persons were going to harm him. Although married, he had had repeated homosexual encounters since adolescence. He was able to function in the community when taking antipsychotic medications, but at the time of the event, he had not taken medication for more than 1 year.

ICD-10

The tenth edition of the ICD (ICD-10) includes, under the category gender identity disorders, *transsexualism*, *dual-role transvestism*, and *gender identity disorder of childhood*. *Gender identity disorders* are placed in the section on disorders of adult personality and behavior, although including gender identity disorder of childhood (Table 22–3).

References

Garofalo R, Deleon J, Osmer E, Doll M, Harper GW. Overlooked, misunderstood and at-risk: Exploring the lives and HIV risk of ethnic minority male-to-female transgender youth. *J Adolesc Health*. 2006;38:230–236.

Green R. Gender identity disorder. In: Sadock BJ, Sadock VA, eds. *Kaplan & Sadock's Comprehensive Textbook of Psychiatry*. 8th ed. Vol. 1. Baltimore: Lippincott Williams & Wilkins; 2005:1979.

Haraldsen IR, Egeland T, Haug F, Finset A, Stein O. Cross-sex hormone treatment does not change sex-sensitive cognitive performance in gender identity disorder patients. *Psychiatry Res*. 2005;137:161–174.

Hepp U, Kraemer B, Schnyder U, Miller N, Delsignore A. Psychiatric comorbidity in gender identity disorder. *J Psychosom Res*. 2005;58(3):259–261.

Hill DB, Rozanski C, Caragnini J. Gender identity disorders in childhood and adolescence: A critical inquiry. *Journal of Psychology and Human Sexuality*. 2005;17(3–4):7.

Maguen S, Shipherd JC, Harris HN. Providing culturally sensitive care for transgender patients. *Cognitive and Behavioral Practice*. 2005;12:479–490.

McFalls JA Jr., Gallagher BJ III, Halluska M. Surgery vs. therapy: Attitudes of psychiatrists concerning the treatment of transsexualism. *Psychology and Education: An Interdisciplinary Journal*. 2005;42:14–19.

Meyer-Bahlburg HFL. Introduction: Gender dysphoria and gender change in persons with intersexuality. *Arch Sex Behav*. 2005;34:371–373.

Schaefer LC, Wheeler CC. Guilt in cross-gender identity conditions: Presentations and treatment. In: Leli U, Drescher J, eds. *Transgender Subjectivities: A Clinician's Guide*. New York: Hawthorn Press; 2004:117–127.

Selvaggi G, Ceulemans P, de Cuypere G, van Landuyt K, Blondeel P, Handi M, Bowman C, Monstrey S. Gender identity disorder: General overview and surgical treatment for vaginoplasty in male-to-female transsexuals. *Plast Reconstr Surg*. 2005;116(16):135e–145e.

Smith YLS, van Goozen SHM, Kuiper AJ, Cohen-Kettenis PT. Transexual subtypes: Clinical and theoretical significance. *Psychiatry Res*. 2005;137:151–160.

Wilson I, Griffin C, Wren B. The interaction between young people with atypical gender identity organization and their peers. *Journal of Health Psychology*. 2005;10(3):307–315.

Winters K. Gender dissonance: Diagnostic reform of gender identity disorder for adults. *Journal of Psychology and Human Sexuality*. 2005;17(3–4):71.

Zamboni BD. Therapeutic considerations in working with the family, friends, and partners of transgendered individuals. *Family Journal: Counseling and Therapy for Couples and Families*. 2006;14:174–179.

23 Eating Disorders

▲ 23.1 Anorexia Nervosa

The term *anorexia nervosa* is derived from the Greek term for "loss of appetite" and a Latin word implying nervous origin. Anorexia nervosa is a syndrome characterized by three essential criteria. The first is a self-induced starvation to a significant degree; the second is a relentless drive for thinness or a morbid fear of fatness; and the third is the presence of medical signs and symptoms resulting from starvation. Anorexia nervosa is often associated with disturbances of body image, the perception that one is distressingly large despite obvious thinness. In the text revision of the fourth edition of *Diagnostic and Statistical Manual of Mental Disorders* (DSM-IV-TR), anorexia nervosa is characterized as a disorder in which persons refuse to maintain a minimally normal weight, intensely fear gaining weight, and significantly misinterpret their body and its shape. DSM-IV-TR also notes that the term anorexia ("lack of appetite") is misleading because loss of appetite rarely occurs in the early stage of the disorder.

Approximately half of anorexic persons will lose weight by drastically reducing their total food intake. The other half of these patients will not only diet but will regularly engage in binge eating followed by purging behaviors. Some patients routinely purge after eating small amounts of food. Anorexia nervosa is much more prevalent in females than in males and usually has its onset in adolescence. Hypotheses of an underlying psychological disturbance in young women with the disorder include conflicts surrounding the transition from girlhood to womanhood. Psychological issues related to feelings of helplessness and difficulty establishing autonomy have also been suggested as contributing to the development of the disorder. Bulimic symptoms can occur as a separate disorder (bulimia nervosa, which is discussed in Section 23.2) or as part of anorexia nervosa. Persons with either disorder are excessively preoccupied with weight, food, and body shape. The outcome of anorexia nervosa varies from spontaneous recovery to a waxing and waning course to death.

EPIDEMIOLOGY

Eating disorders of various kinds have been reported in up to 4 percent of adolescent and young adult students. Anorexia nervosa has been reported more frequently over the past several decades, with increasing reports of the disorder in prepubertal girls and in boys. The most common ages of onset of anorexia nervosa are the midteens, but up to 5 percent of anorectic patients have the onset of the disorder in their early 20s. According to DSM-IV-TR, the most common age of onset is between 14 and 18 years. Anorexia nervosa is estimated to occur in about 0.5 to 1 percent of adolescent girls. It occurs 10 to 20 times more often in females than in males. The prevalence of young women with some symptoms of anorexia nervosa who do not meet the diagnostic criteria is estimated to be close to 5 percent. Although the disorder was initially reported most often among the upper classes, recent epidemiological surveys do not show that distribution. It seems to be most frequent in developed countries, and it may be seen with greatest frequency among young women in professions that require thinness, such as modeling and ballet.

COMORBIDITY

Anorexia nervosa is associated with depression in 65 percent of cases, social phobia in 34 percent of cases, and obsessive-compulsive disorder in 26 percent of cases.

ETIOLOGY

Biological, social, and psychological factors are implicated in the causes of anorexia nervosa. Some evidence points to higher concordance rates in monozygotic twins than in dizygotic twins. Sisters of patients with anorexia nervosa are likely to be afflicted, but this association may reflect social influences more than genetic factors. Major mood disorders are more common in family members than in the general population. Neurochemically, diminished norepinephrine turnover and activity are suggested by reduced 3-methoxy-4-hydroxyphenylglycol (MHPG) levels in the urine and the cerebrospinal fluid (CSF) of some patients with anorexia nervosa. An inverse relation is seen between MHPG and depression in these patients; an increase in MHPG is associated with a decrease in depression.

Biological Factors

Endogenous opioids may contribute to the denial of hunger in patients with anorexia nervosa. Preliminary studies show dramatic weight gains in some patients given opiate antagonists. Starvation results in many biochemical changes, some of which are also present in depression, such as hypercortisolemia and nonsuppression by dexamethasone. Thyroid function is suppressed as well. These abnormalities are corrected by realimentation. Starvation produces amenorrhea, which reflects lowered hormonal levels (luteinizing, follicle-stimulating, and gonadotropin-releasing hormones). Some patients with anorexia nervosa, however, become amenorrheic before significant weight

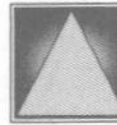

Table 23.1–1
Neuroendocrine Changes in Anorexia Nervosa and Experimental Starvation

Hormone	Anorexia Nervosa	Weight Loss
Corticotropin-releasing hormone (CRH)	Increased	Increased
Plasma cortisol levels	Mildly increased	Mildly increased
Diurnal cortisol difference	Blunted	Blunted
Luteinizing hormone (LH)	Decreased, prepubertal pattern	Decreased
Follicle-stimulating hormone (FSH)	Decreased, prepubertal pattern	Decreased
Growth hormone (GH)	Impaired regulation Increased basal levels and limited response to pharmacological probes	Same
Somatomedin C	Decreased	Decreased
Thyroxine (T_4)	Normal or slightly decreased	Normal or slightly decreased
Triiodothyronine (T_3)	Mildly decreased	Mildly decreased
Reverse T3	Mildly increased	Mildly increased
Thyrotropin-stimulating hormone (TSH)	Normal	Normal
TSH response to thyrotropin-releasing hormone (TRH)	Delayed or blunted	Delayed or blunted
Insulin	Delayed release	–
C-peptide	Decreased	–
Vasopressin	Secretion uncoupled from osmotic challenge	–
Serotonin	Increased function with weight restoration	
Norepinephrine	Reduced turnover	Reduced turnover
Dopamine	Blunted response to pharmacological probes	–

loss. Several computed tomographic (CT) studies reveal enlarged CSF spaces (enlarged sulci and ventricles) in anorectic patients during starvation, a finding that is reversed by weight gain. In one positron emission tomographic (PET) scan study, caudate nucleus metabolism was higher in the anorectic state than after realimentation.

Some authors have proposed a hypothalamic-pituitary axis (neuroendocrine) dysfunction. Some studies have shown evidence for dysfunction in serotonin, dopamine, and norepinephrine, three neurotransmitters involved in regulating eating behavior in the paraventricular nucleus of the hypothalamus. Other humoral factors that may be involved include corticotropin-releasing factor (CRF), neuropeptide Y, gonadotropin-releasing hormone, and thyroid-stimulating hormone. Table 23.1–1 lists neuroendocrine changes associated with anorexia nervosa.

Social Factors

Patients with anorexia nervosa find support for their practices in society's emphasis on thinness and exercise. No family constellations are specific to anorexia nervosa, but some evidence indicates that these patients have close, but troubled, relationships with their parents. Families of children who present with eating disorders, especially binge eating or purging subtypes, may exhibit high levels of hostility, chaos, and isolation and low levels of nurturance and empathy. An adolescent with a severe eating disorder may tend to draw attention away from strained marital relationships.

Vocational and avocational interests interact with other vulnerability factors to increase the probability of developing eating disorders. In young women, participation in strict ballet schools increases the probability of developing anorexia nervosa at least sevenfold. In high school boys, wrestling is associated with a prevalence of full or partial eating-disordered syndromes during wrestling season of approximately 17 percent, with a minority developing an eating disorder and not improving spontaneously at the end of training. Although these athletic activities probably select for perfectionistic and persevering youth in the first place, pressures regarding weight and shape generated in these social milieus reinforce the likelihood that these predisposing factors will be channeled toward eating disorders.

A gay orientation in men is a proved predisposing factor, not because of sexual orientation or sexual behavior per se, but because norms for slimness, albeit muscular slimness, are very strong in the gay community, only slightly lower than for heterosexual women. In contrast, a lesbian orientation may be slightly protective, because lesbian communities may be more tolerant of higher weights and a more normative natural distribution of body shapes than their heterosexual female counterparts.

Psychological and Psychodynamic Factors

Anorexia nervosa appears to be a reaction to the demand that adolescents behave more independently and increase their social and sexual functioning. Patients with the disorder substitute their preoccupations, which are similar to obsessions, with eating and weight gain for other, normal adolescent pursuits. These patients typically lack a sense of autonomy and selfhood. Many experience their bodies as somehow under the control of their parents, so that self-starvation may be an effort to gain validation as a unique and special person. Only through acts of extraordinary self-discipline can an anorectic patient develop a sense of autonomy and selfhood.

Psychoanalytic clinicians who treat patients with anorexia nervosa generally agree that these young patients have been unable to separate psychologically from their mothers. The body may be perceived as though it were inhabited by the introject of an intrusive and unempathic mother. Starvation may unconsciously mean arresting the growth of this intrusive internal object and thereby destroying it. Often, a projective identification process is involved in the interactions between the patient and

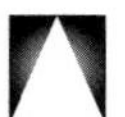

Table 23.1–2
DSM-IV-TR Diagnostic Criteria for Anorexia Nervosa

A. Refusal to maintain body weight at or above a minimally normal weight for age and height (e.g., weight loss leading to maintenance of body weight less than 85% of that expected; or failure to make expected weight gain during period of growth, leading to body weight less than 85% of that expected).
B. Intense fear of gaining weight or becoming fat, even though underweight.
C. Disturbance in the way in which one's body weight or shape is experienced, undue influence of body weight or shape on self-evaluation, or denial of the seriousness of the current low body weight.
D. In postmenarcheal females, amenorrhea, i.e., the absence of at least three consecutive menstrual cycles. (A woman is considered to have amenorrhea if her periods occur only following hormone, e.g., estrogen, administration.)

Specify type:
Restricting type: during the current episode of anorexia nervosa, the person has not regularly engaged in binge-eating or purging behavior (i.e., self-induced vomiting or the misuse of laxatives, diuretics, or enemas)
Binge-eating/purging type: during the current episode of anorexia nervosa, the person has regularly engaged in binge-eating or purging behavior (i.e., self-induced vomiting or the misuse of laxatives, diuretics, or enemas)

(From American Psychiatric Association. *Diagnostic and Statistical Manual of Mental Disorders.* 4th ed. Text rev. Washington, DC: American Psychiatric Association; copyright 2000, with permission.)

the patient's family. Many anorectic patients feel that oral desires are greedy and unacceptable; therefore, these desires are projectively disavowed. Other theories have focused on fantasies of oral impregnation. Parents respond to the refusal to eat by becoming frantic about whether the patient is actually eating. The patient can then view the parents as the ones who have unacceptable desires and can projectively disavow them; that is, others may be voracious and ruled by desire but not the patient.

DIAGNOSIS AND CLINICAL FEATURES

The onset of anorexia nervosa usually occurs between the ages of 10 and 30 years. It is present when (1) an individual voluntarily reduces and maintains an unhealthy degree of weight loss or fails to gain weight proportional to growth; (2) an individual experiences an intense fear of becoming fat, has a relentless drive for thinness despite obvious medical starvation, or both; (3) an individual experiences significant starvation-related medical symptomatology, often, but not exclusively, abnormal reproductive hormone functioning, but also hypothermia, bradycardia, orthostasis, and severely reduced body fat stores; and (4) the behaviors and psychopathology are present for at least 3 months. The DSM-IV-TR diagnostic criteria for anorexia nervosa are given in Table 23.1–2.

An intense fear of gaining weight and becoming obese is present in all patients with the disorder and undoubtedly contributes to their lack of interest in, and even resistance to, therapy. Most aberrant behavior directed toward losing weight occurs in secret. Patients with anorexia nervosa usually refuse to eat with their families or in public places. They lose weight by drastically reducing their total food intake, with a disproportionate decrease in high-carbohydrate and fatty foods.

As mentioned, the term *anorexia* is a misnomer, because loss of appetite is usually rare until late in the disorder. Evidence that patients are constantly thinking about food is their passion for collecting recipes and for preparing elaborate meals for others. Some patients cannot continuously control their voluntary restriction of food intake and so have eating binges. These binges usually occur secretly and often at night and are frequently followed by self-induced vomiting. Patients abuse laxatives and even diuretics to lose weight, and ritualistic exercising, extensive cycling, walking, jogging, and running are common activities.

Patients with the disorder exhibit peculiar behavior about food. They hide food all over the house and frequently carry large quantities of candies in their pockets and purses. While eating meals, they try to dispose of food in their napkins or hide it in their pockets. They cut their meat into very small pieces and spend a great deal of time rearranging the pieces on their plates. If the patients are confronted with their peculiar behavior, they often deny that their behavior is unusual or flatly refuse to discuss it.

Obsessive-compulsive behavior, depression, and anxiety are other psychiatric symptoms of anorexia nervosa most frequently noted in the literature. Patients tend to be rigid and perfectionist, and somatic complaints, especially epigastric discomfort, are usual. Compulsive stealing, usually of candies and laxatives but occasionally of clothes and other items, is common.

Poor sexual adjustment is frequently described in patients with the disorder. Many adolescent patients with anorexia nervosa have delayed psychosocial sexual development; in adults, a markedly decreased interest in sex often accompanies onset of the disorder. An unusual minority of anorectic patients have a premorbid history of promiscuity, substance abuse, or both and during the disorder do not show a decreased interest in sex.

Patients usually come to medical attention when their weight loss becomes apparent. As the weight loss grows profound, physical signs such as hypothermia (as low as 35°C), dependent edema, bradycardia, hypotension, and lanugo (the appearance of neonatal-like hair) appear, and patients show a variety of metabolic changes (Fig. 23.1–1). Some female patients with anorexia nervosa come to medical attention because of amenorrhea, which often appears before their weight loss is noticeable. Some patients induce vomiting or abuse purgatives and diuretics; such behavior causes concern about hypokalemic alkalosis. Impaired water diuresis may be noted.

Electrocardiographic (ECG) changes, such as T wave flattening or inversion, ST segment depression, and lengthening of the QT interval, have been noted in the emaciated stage of anorexia nervosa. ECG changes may also result from potassium loss, which can lead to death. Gastric dilation is a rare complication of anorexia nervosa. In some patients, aortography has

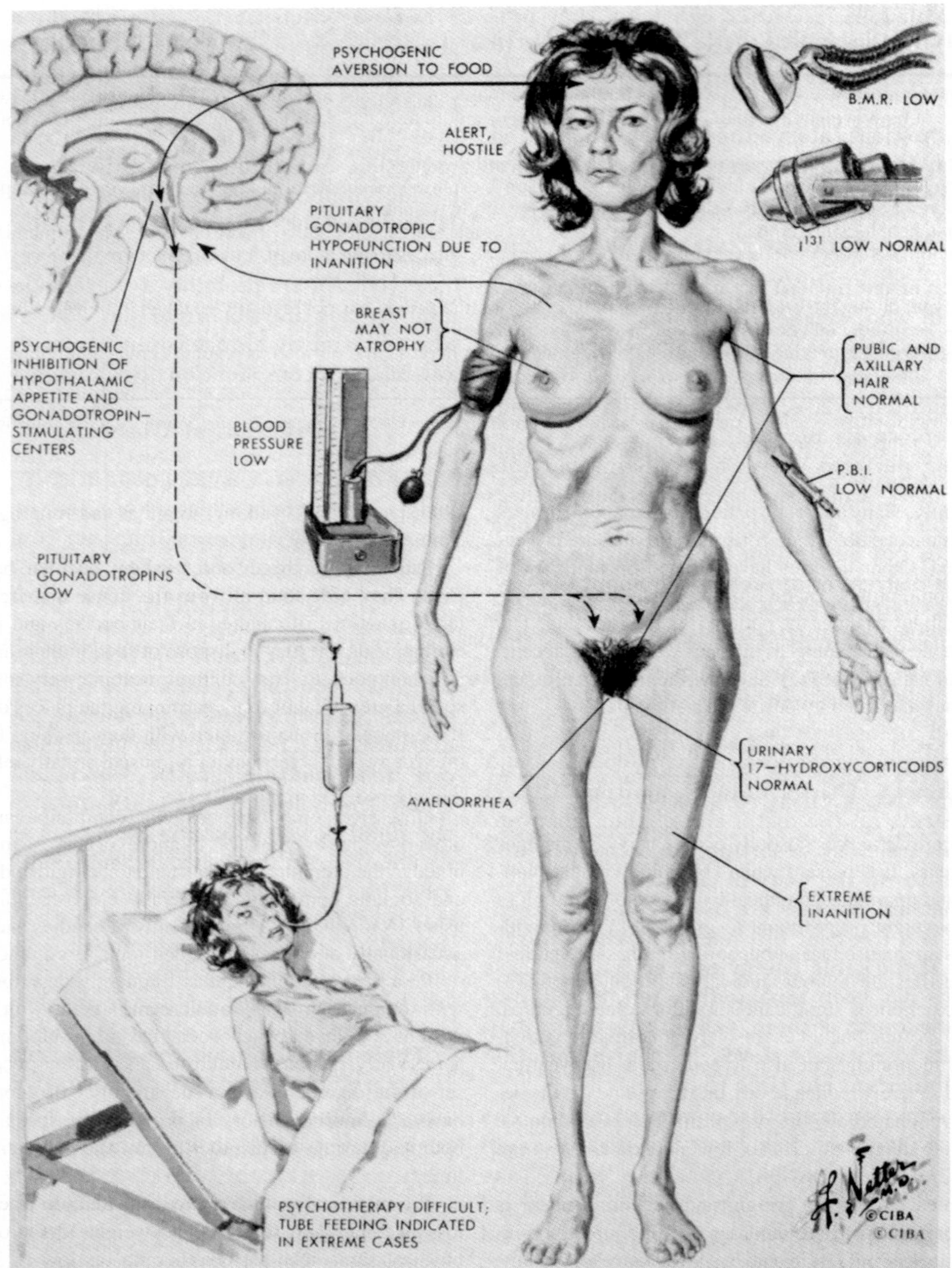

FIGURE 23.1–1

Anorexia nervosa. (Copyright 1959 CIBA Pharmaceutical Company, Division of CIBA-GEIGY Corporation. Reproduced with permission from *The CIBA Collection of Medical Illustrations* by Frank H. Netter, M.D. All rights reserved.)

shown a superior mesenteric artery syndrome. Other medical complications of eating disorders are listed in Table 23.1–3.

Subtypes

Anorexia nervosa has been divided into two subtypes—the food-restricting category and the binge-eating or purging category. In the food-restricting category, present in approximately 50 percent of cases, food intake is highly restricted (usually with attempts to consume fewer than 300 to 500 calories per day and no fat grams), and the patient may be relentlessly and compulsively overactive, with overuse athletic injuries. In the binge-eating or purging subtype, patients alternate attempts at rigorous dieting with intermittent binge or purge episodes, with the binges, if present, being either subjective (more than the patient intended, or because of social pressure, but not enormous) or objective. Purging represents a secondary compensation for the unwanted calories, most often accomplished by self-induced vomiting, frequently by laxative abuse, less frequently by diuretics, and occasionally with emetics. Sometimes, repetitive purging occurs

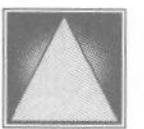

Table 23.1–3
Medical Complications of Eating Disorders

Related to weight loss
Cachexia: Loss of fat, muscle mass, reduced thyroid metabolism (low T3 syndrome), cold intolerance, and difficulty in maintaining core body temperature
Cardiac: Loss of cardiac muscle; small heart; cardiac arrhythmias, including atrial and ventricular premature contractions, prolonged His bundle transmission (prolonged QT interval), bradycardia, ventricular tachycardia; sudden death
Digestive-gastrointestinal: Delayed gastric emptying, bloating, constipation, abdominal pain
Reproductive: Amenorrhea, low levels of luteinizing hormone (LH) and follicle-stimulating hormone (FSH)
Dermatological: Lanugo (fine baby-like hair over body), edema
Hematological: Leukopenia
Neuropsychiatric: Abnormal taste sensation (?zinc deficiency), apathetic depression, mild cognitive disorder
Skeletal: Osteoporosis

Related to purging (vomiting and laxative abuse)
Metabolic: Electrolyte abnormalities, particularly hypokalemic, hypochloremic alkalosis; hypomagnesemia
Digestive-gastrointestinal: Salivary gland and pancreatic inflammation and enlargement with increase in serum amylase, esophageal and gastric erosion, dysfunctional bowel with haustral dilation
Dental: Erosion of dental enamel, particularly of front teeth, with corresponding decay
Neuropsychiatric: Seizures (related to large fluid shifts and electrolyte disturbances), mild neuropathies, fatigue and weakness, mild cognitive disorder

(From Yager I. Eating disorders. In: Stoudemire A, ed. *Clinical Psychiatry for Medical Students.* Philadelphia: JB Lippincott; 1990:324, with permission.)

without prior binge eating, after ingesting only relatively few calories. Both may be socially isolated and have depressive disorder symptoms and diminished sexual interest. Overexercising and perfectionistic traits are common in both types.

Those who practice binge eating and purging share many features with persons who have bulimia nervosa without anorexia nervosa. Those who binge eat and purge tend to have families in which some members are obese, and they themselves have histories of heavier body weights before the disorder than do persons with the restricting type. Binge eating–purging persons are likely to be associated with substance abuse, impulse control disorders, and personality disorders. Persons with restricting anorexia nervosa often have obsessive-compulsive traits with respect to food and other matters. Some persons with anorexia nervosa may purge but not binge.

Persons with anorexia nervosa have high rates of comorbid major depressive disorders; major depressive disorder or dysthymic disorder has been reported in up to 50 percent of patients with anorexia nervosa. The suicide rate is higher in persons with the binge eating–purging type of anorexia nervosa than in those with the restricting type.

Patients with anorexia nervosa are often secretive, deny their symptoms, and resist treatment. In almost all cases, relatives or intimate acquaintances must confirm a patient's history. The mental status examination usually shows a patient who is alert and knowledgeable on the subject of nutrition and who is preoccupied with food and weight.

A patient must have a thorough general physical and neurological examination. If the patient is vomiting, a hypokalemic alkalosis may be present. Because most patients are dehydrated, serum electrolyte levels must be determined initially and periodically during hospitalization.

When Peggy was first evaluated for admission to an inpatient eating disorder program, she was a 20-year-old woman who had difficulty supporting her 5'3" body with a weight of only 67 pounds. She had begun to lose weight 4 years earlier, initially dieting to lose an unwanted 6 pounds. Encouraged by compliments on her new body, she proceeded to lose 8 more pounds. Over the next 2 years she continued to lose weight, increased her physical activity until her weight reached a low of 64 pounds, and stopped menstruating. She was admitted to a medical unit, treated for peptic ulcer disease, and discharged, only to be admitted 3 months thereafter to the psychiatric unit of a general hospital. During that 8-week hospitalization, she went from 84 pounds to 100 pounds. She did well until she went off to college, where, with increased academic and social demands, she again began to diet until she weighed only 67 pounds. Her eating habits were ritualized: she cut food into very small pieces, moved them around on the plate, and ate very slowly. She resisted eating foods with high fat and carbohydrate content. She was troubled by the changes in her body, and became increasingly anxious as her figure developed. She was forced to drop out of school and to accept another hospitalization.

Peggy was motivated to comply with treatment, but her fears of gaining weight and becoming obese affected her progress. She was expected to gain a minimum of 2 pounds every week, and she was restricted to bed rest if she failed to gain sufficient weight. In psychotherapy Peggy was gradually guided to discuss her feelings and to actually look at herself in the mirror. She was initially instructed to look at one part of her body for a minimum of 10 seconds, and the time was progressively increased until she could look at her whole body without any anxiety. Her menses returned at a weight of 93 pounds. After 7 months of individual and family treatment, she was discharged at a weight of 100 pounds. Peggy returned to college, worked part time, and lived with her parents. (Courtesy of the *DSM-IV Casebook.*)

PATHOLOGY AND LABORATORY EXAMINATION

A complete blood count often reveals leukopenia with a relative lymphocytosis in emaciated patients with anorexia nervosa. If binge eating and purging are present, serum electrolyte determination reveals hypokalemic alkalosis. Fasting serum glucose concentrations are often low during the emaciated phase, and serum salivary amylase concentrations are often elevated if the patient is vomiting. The ECG may show ST segment and T-wave changes, which are usually secondary to electrolyte disturbances; emaciated patients have hypotension and bradycardia. Young girls may have a high serum cholesterol level. All these values revert to normal with nutritional rehabilitation and cessation of purging behaviors. Endocrine changes that occur, such as amenorrhea, mild hypothyroidism, and hypersecretion of corticotrophin-releasing hormone are caused by the underweight condition and revert to normal with weight gain.

DIFFERENTIAL DIAGNOSIS

The differential diagnosis of anorexia nervosa is complicated by patients' denial of the symptoms, the secrecy surrounding their bizarre eating rituals, and their resistance to seeking treatment. Thus, it may be difficult to identify the mechanism of weight loss and the patient's associated ruminative thoughts about distortions of body image.

Clinicians must ascertain that a patient does not have a medical illness that can account for the weight loss (e.g., a brain tumor or cancer). Weight loss, peculiar eating behaviors, and vomiting can occur in several mental disorders. Depressive disorders and anorexia nervosa have several features in common, such as depressed feelings, crying spells, sleep disturbance, obsessive ruminations, and occasional suicidal thoughts. The two disorders, however, have several distinguishing features. Generally, a patient with a depressive disorder has decreased appetite, whereas a patient with anorexia nervosa claims to have normal appetite and to feel hungry; only in the severe stages of anorexia nervosa do patients actually have decreased appetite. In contrast to depressive agitation, the hyperactivity seen in anorexia nervosa is planned and ritualistic. The preoccupation with recipes, the caloric content of foods, and the preparation of gourmet feasts is typical of patients with anorexia nervosa, but is absent in patients with a depressive disorder. In depressive disorders, patients have no intense fear of obesity or disturbance of body image.

Weight fluctuations, vomiting, and peculiar food handling may occur in somatization disorder. On rare occasions, a patient fulfills the diagnostic criteria for both somatization disorder and anorexia nervosa; in such a case, both diagnoses should be made. Generally, the weight loss in somatization disorder is not as severe as that in anorexia nervosa, nor does a patient with somatization disorder express a morbid fear of becoming overweight, as is common in those with anorexia nervosa. Amenorrhea for 3 months or longer is unusual in somatization disorder.

In patients with schizophrenia, delusions about food are seldom concerned with caloric content. More likely, they believe the food to be poisoned. Patients with schizophrenia are rarely preoccupied with a fear of becoming obese and do not have the hyperactivity that is seen in patients with anorexia nervosa. Patients with schizophrenia have bizarre eating habits but not the entire syndrome of anorexia nervosa.

Anorexia nervosa must be differentiated from bulimia nervosa, a disorder in which episodic binge eating, followed by depressive moods, self-deprecating thoughts, and often self-induced vomiting, occurs while patients maintain their weight within a normal range. Patients with bulimia nervosa seldom lose 15 percent of their weight, but the two conditions frequently coexist.

Rare conditions of unknown etiology are seen in which hyperactivity of the vagus nerve causes changes in eating patterns that are associated with weight loss, sometimes of severe degree. In such cases are seen bradycardia, hypotension and other parasympathomimetic signs and symptoms. Because the vagus nerve relates to the enteric nervous system, eating may be associated with gastric distress such as nausea or bloating. Patients do not generally lose their appetite. Treatment is symptomatic and anticholinergic drugs can reverse hypotension and bradycardia, which may be life threatening.

COURSE AND PROGNOSIS

The course of anorexia nervosa varies greatly—spontaneous recovery without treatment, recovery after a variety of treatments, a fluctuating course of weight gains followed by relapses, and a gradually deteriorating course resulting in death caused by complications of starvation. A recent study reviewing subtypes of anorectic patients found that restricting-type anorectic patients seemed less likely to recover than those of the binge eating-purging type. The short-term response of patients to almost all hospital treatment programs is good. Those who have regained sufficient weight, however, often continue their preoccupation with food and body weight, have poor social relationships, and exhibit depression. In general, the prognosis is not good. Studies have shown a range of mortality rates from 5 to 18 percent.

Indicators of a favorable outcome are admission of hunger, lessening of denial and immaturity, and improved self-esteem. Such factors as childhood neuroticism, parental conflict, bulimia nervosa, vomiting, laxative abuse, and various behavioral manifestations (e.g., obsessive-compulsive, hysterical, depressive, psychosomatic, neurotic, and denial symptoms) have been related to poor outcome in some studies, but not in others.

Ten-year outcome studies in the United States have shown that about one fourth of patients recover completely and another one half are markedly improved and functioning fairly well. The other one fourth includes an overall 7 percent mortality rate and those who are functioning poorly with a chronic underweight condition. Swedish and English studies over a 20- and 30-year period show a mortality rate of 18 percent. About half of patients with anorexia nervosa eventually will have the symptoms of bulimia, usually within the first year after the onset of anorexia nervosa.

TREATMENT

In view of the complicated psychological and medical implications of anorexia nervosa, a comprehensive treatment plan, including hospitalization when necessary and both individual and family therapy, is recommended. Behavioral, interpersonal, and cognitive approaches and, in some cases, medication should be considered.

Hospitalization

The first consideration in the treatment of anorexia nervosa is to restore patients' nutritional state; dehydration, starvation, and electrolyte imbalances can seriously compromise health and, in some cases, lead to death. The decision to hospitalize a patient is based on the patient's medical condition and the amount of structure needed to ensure patient cooperation. In general, patients with anorexia nervosa who are 20 percent below the expected weight for their height are recommended for inpatient programs, and patients who are 30 percent below their expected weight require psychiatric hospitalization for 2 to 6 months.

Inpatient psychiatric programs for patients with anorexia nervosa generally use a combination of a behavioral management approach, individual psychotherapy, family education and therapy, and, in some cases, psychotropic medications. Successful treatment is promoted by the ability of staff members to maintain a firm yet supportive approach to patients, often through a combination of positive reinforcers (praise) and negative reinforcers (restriction of exercise and purging behavior). The program must have some flexibility for individualizing treatment to meet patients' needs and cognitive abilities. Patients must become willing participants for treatment to succeed in the long run.

Most patients are uninterested in psychiatric treatment and even resist it; they are brought to a doctor's office unwillingly by agonizing relatives or friends. The patients rarely accept the recommendation of hospitalization without arguing and criticizing the proposed program. Emphasizing the benefits, such as relief of insomnia and depressive signs and symptoms, may help persuade the patients to admit themselves willingly to the hospital. Relatives' support and confidence in the physicians and treatment team are essential when firm recommendations must be carried out. Patients' families should be warned that the patients will resist admission and, for the several weeks of treatment, will make many dramatic pleas for the family's support to obtain release from the hospital program. Compulsory admission or commitment should be obtained only when the risk of death from the complications of malnutrition is likely. On rare occasions, patients prove that doctor's statements about the probable failure of outpatient treatment are wrong. Some patients may gain a specified amount of weight by the time of each outpatient visit, but such behavior is uncommon, and a period of inpatient care is usually necessary.

The following considerations apply to the general management of patients with anorexia nervosa during a hospitalized treatment program. Patients should be weighed daily, early in the morning after emptying the bladder. The daily fluid intake and urine output should be recorded. If vomiting is occurring, hospital staff members must monitor serum electrolyte levels regularly and watch for the development of hypokalemia. Because food is often regurgitated after meals, the staff may be able to control vomiting by making the bathroom inaccessible for at least 2 hours after meals or by having an attendant in the bathroom to prevent vomiting. Constipation in these patients is relieved when they begin to eat normally. Stool softeners may occasionally be given, but never laxatives. If diarrhea occurs, it usually means that patients are surreptitiously taking laxatives. Because of the rare complication of stomach dilation and the possibility of circulatory overload when patients immediately start eating an enormous number of calories, the hospital staff should give patients about 500 calories over the amount required to maintain their present weight (usually 1,500 to 2,000 calories a day). It is wise to give these calories in six equal feedings throughout the day, so that patients need not eat a large amount of food at one sitting. Giving patients a liquid food supplement such as Sustagen may be advisable, because they may be less apprehensive about gaining weight slowly with the formula than by eating food. After patients are discharged from the hospital, clinicians usually find it necessary to continue outpatient supervision of the problems identified in the patients and their families.

Psychotherapy

Cognitive-Behavioral Therapy. Cognitive and behavioral therapy principles can be applied in both inpatient and outpatient settings. Behavior therapy has been found effective for inducing weight gain; no large, controlled studies of cognitive therapy with behavior therapy in patients with anorexia nervosa have been reported. Monitoring is an essential component of cognitive-behavioral therapy. Patients are taught to monitor their food intake, their feelings and emotions, their binging and purging behaviors, and their problems in interpersonal relationships. Patients are taught cognitive restructuring to identify automatic thoughts and to challenge their core beliefs. Problem-solving is a specific method whereby patients learn how to think through and devise strategies to cope with their food-related and interpersonal problems. Patients' vulnerability to rely on anorectic behavior as a means of coping can be addressed if they can learn to use these techniques effectively.

Dynamic Psychotherapy. Dynamic expressive-supportive psychotherapy is sometimes used in the treatment of patients with anorexia nervosa, but their resistance may make the process difficult and painstaking. Because patients view their symptoms as constituting the core of their specialness, therapists must avoid excessive investment in trying to change their eating behavior. The opening phase of the psychotherapy process must be geared to building a therapeutic alliance. Patients may experience early interpretations as though someone else were telling them what they really feel and thereby minimizing and invalidating their own experiences. Therapists who empathize with patients' points of view and take an active interest in what their patients think and feel, however, convey to patients that their autonomy is respected. Above all, psychotherapists must be flexible, persistent, and durable in the face of patients' tendencies to defeat any efforts to help them.

Family Therapy. A family analysis should be done for all patients with anorexia nervosa who are living with their families, as a basis for a clinical judgment on what type of family therapy or counseling is advisable. In some cases, family therapy is not possible; however, issues of family relationships can then be addressed in individual therapy. Sometimes, brief counseling sessions with immediate family members is the extent of family therapy required. In one controlled family therapy study in London, anorectic patients under the age of 18 benefited from family therapy, whereas patients over the age of 18 did worse in family therapy than with the control therapy. No controlled studies have been reported on the combination of individual and family therapy; however, in actual practice, most clinicians provide individual therapy and some form of family counseling in managing patients with anorexia nervosa.

Pharmacotherapy

Pharmacological studies have not yet identified any medication that yields definitive improvement of the core symptoms of

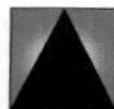

Table 23.1–4
ICD-10 Diagnostic Criteria for Eating Disorders

Anorexia nervosa

A. There is weight loss or, in children, a lack of weight gain, leading to a body weight at least 15% below the normal or expected weight for age and height.
B. The weight loss is self-induced by avoidance of "fattening foods."
C. There is self-perception of being too fat, with an intrusive dread of fatness, which leads to a self-imposed low weight threshold.
D. A widespread endocrine disorder involving the hypothalamic-pituitary-gonadal axis is manifest in women as amenorrhea and in men as a loss of sexual interest and potency. (An apparent exception is the persistence of vaginal bleeding in anorexic women who are on replacement hormonal therapy, most commonly taken as a contraceptive pill.)
E. The disorder does not meet Criteria A and B for bulimia nervosa.

Comments

The following features support the diagnosis but are not essential elements: self-induced vomiting, self-induced purging, excessive exercise, and use of appetite suppressants and/or diuretics.

If onset is prepubertal, the sequence of pubertal events is delayed or even arrested (growth ceases; in girls the breasts do not develop, and there is a primary amenorrhea; in boys the genitals remain juvenile). With recovery, puberty is often completed normally, but the menarche is late.

Atypical anorexia nervosa

Researchers studying atypical forms of anorexia nervosa are recommended to make their own decisions about the number and type of criteria to be fulfilled.

Bulimia nervosa

A. There are recurrent episodes of overeating (at least twice a week over a period of 3 months) in which large amounts of food are consumed in short periods.
B. There is persistent preoccupation with eating and a strong desire or a sense of compulsion to eat (craving).
C. The patient attempts to counteract the "fattening" effects of food by one or more of the following:
  (1) self-induced vomiting;
  (2) self-induced purging;
  (3) alternating periods of starvation;
  (4) use of drugs such as appetite suppressants, thyroid preparations, or diuretics; when bulimia occurs in diabetic patients, they may choose to neglect their insulin treatment.
D. There is self-perception of being too fat, with an intrusive dread of fatness (usually leading to underweight).

Atypical bulimia nervosa

Researchers studying atypical forms of bulimia nervosa, such as those involving normal or excessive body weight, are recommended to make their own decisions about the number and type of criteria to be fulfilled.

Overeating associated with other psychological disturbances

Researchers wishing to use this category are recommended to design their own criteria.

Vomiting associated with other psychological disturbances

Researchers wishing to use this category are recommended to design their own criteria.

Other eating disorders

Eating disorder, unspecified

(Adapted from World Health Organization. *The ICD-10 Classification of Mental and Behavioural Disorders: Diagnostic Criteria for Research*. Copyright, World Health Organization, Geneva, 1993, with permission.)

anorexia nervosa. Some reports support the use of cyproheptadine (Periactin), a drug with antihistaminic and antiserotonergic properties, for patients with the restricting type of anorexia nervosa. Amitriptyline (Elavil) has also been reported to have some benefit. Other medications that have been tried by patients with anorexia nervosa with variable results include clomipramine, pimozide (Orap), and chlorpromazine (Thorazine). Trials of fluoxetine have resulted in some reports of weight gain, and serotonergic agents may yield positive responses in the future. In patients with anorexia nervosa and coexisting depressive disorders, the depressive condition should be treated. Concern exists about the use of tricyclic drugs in low-weight, depressed patients with anorexia nervosa, who may be vulnerable to hypotension, cardiac arrhythmia, and dehydration. Once an adequate nutritional status has been attained, the risk of serious adverse effects from the tricyclic drugs may decrease; in some patients, the depression improves with weight gain and normalized nutritional status.

ICD-10

The 10th revision of the *International Statistical Classification of Diseases and Related Health Disorders* (ICD-10) describes anorexia nervosa as a deliberate, severe weight loss caused by the patient. According to ICD-10, its causes remain unknown, but a combination of sociocultural and biological factors apparently contributes to the disorder, along with a vulnerable personality and other psychological processes. Undernutrition produces endocrine and metabolic changes and disturbs bodily functions. Whether the endocrine disorder is completely caused by the eating disorder or whether other factors are also at work is uncertain. The ICD-10 criteria for eating disorders are presented in Table 23.1–4.

References

Andersen AE, Yager J. Eating Disorders. In: Sadock BJ, Sadock VA, eds. *Kaplan & Sadock's Comprehensive Textbook of Psychiatry*. 8th ed. Vol. 1. Baltimore: Lippincott Williams & Wilkins; 2005:2002.

Bulik CM, Reba L, Siega-Riz AM, Reichborn-Kjennerud T. Anorexia nervosa: Definition, epidemiology, and cycle of risk. *Int J Eat Disord.* 2005;37[Suppl 1]:S2–S9.
Bulik CM, Sullivan PF, Tozzi F, Furberg H, Lichtenstein P, Pedersen NL. Prevalence, heritability, and prospective risk factors for anorexia nervosa. *Arch Gen Psychiatry.* 2006;63:305–312.
de Zwaan M, Roerig J. Pharmacological treatment, in evidence and experience in psychiatry. In: Halmi KA, Maj M, eds. *Eating Disorders.* Vol. 6. World Psychiatric Association, England: John Wiley; 2003.
Keel PK, Dorer DJ, Franko DL, Jackson SC, Herzog DB. Postremission predictors of relapse in women with eating disorder. *Am J Psychiatry.* 2005;162:2263–2268.
Lock J, le Grange D, Agras WS, Dare C. *Treatment Manual for Anorexia Nervosa.* New York: Guilford Press; 2002.
McIntosh VV, Jordan J, Carter FA, Luty SE, McKenzie JM, Bulik CM, Frampton CM, Joyce PR. Three psychotherapies for anorexia nervosa: a randomized, controlled trial. *Am J Psychiatry.* 2005;162(4):741–747.
O'Reardon JP, Peshek A, Allison KC. Night eating syndrome: Diagnosis, epidemiology and management. *CNS Drugs.* 2005;19:997–1008.
Robb AS, Silber TJ, Orrell-Valente JK, Valadez-Meltzer A, Ellis N, Dadson MJ, Chatoor I. Supplemental nocturnal nasogastric refeeding for better short-term outcome in hospitalized adolescent girls with anorexia nervosa. *Am J Psychiatry.* 2002;159(8):1347–1353.
Sysko R, Walsh BT, Schebendach J, Wilson GT. Eating behavior among women with anorexia nervosa. *Am J Clin Nutr.* 2005;82(2):296–301.
Treasure J, Schmidt U. *Anorexia Nervosa. Clinical Evidence 7.* London: BMJ Publishing Group; 2002:161–162.

▲ 23.2 Bulimia Nervosa and Eating Disorder Not Otherwise Specified

BULIMIA NERVOSA

Bulimia nervosa, in many ways, represents a failed attempt at anorexia nervosa, sharing the goal of becoming very thin, but occurring in an individual less able to sustain prolonged semistarvation or severe hunger as consistently as classic restricting anorexia nervosa patients. These eating binges provoke panic as individuals feel that their eating has been out of control. The unwanted binges lead to secondary attempts to avoid the feared weight gain by a variety of compensatory behaviors, such as purging or excessive exercise (Fig. 23.2–1).

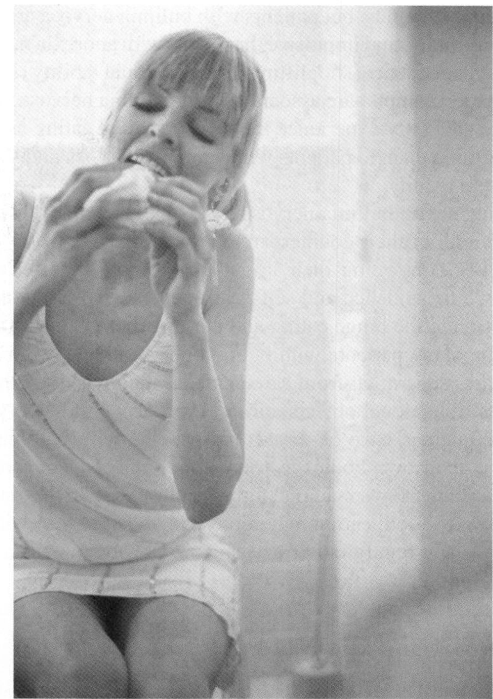

FIGURE 23.2–1
Young woman eating a hamburger in a bathroom. These patients will often vomit immediately after gorging themselves, use laxatives, or enemas in an effort not to gain weight. (Courtesy of Corbis.)

In the text revision of the 4th edition of *Diagnostic and Statistical Manual of Mental Disorders* (DSM-IV-TR), bulimia nervosa is defined as binge eating combined with inappropriate ways of stopping weight gain. Social interruption or physical discomfort—that is, abdominal pain or nausea—terminates the binge eating, which is often followed by feelings of guilt, depression, or self-disgust. Unlike patients with anorexia nervosa, those with bulimia nervosa may maintain a normal body weight.

Epidemiology

Bulimia nervosa is more prevalent than anorexia nervosa. Estimates of bulimia nervosa range from 2 to 4 percent of young women. As with anorexia nervosa, bulimia nervosa is significantly more common in women than in men, but its onset is often later in adolescence than that of anorexia nervosa. According to DSM-IV-TR, the rate of occurrence in males is one tenth of that in females. The onset may even occur in early adulthood. Approximately 20 percent of college women experience transient bulimic symptoms at some point during their college years. Although bulimia nervosa is often present in normal-weight young women, they sometimes have a history of obesity. In industrialized countries, the prevalence is about 1 percent of the general population.

Etiology

Biological Factors. Some investigators have attempted to associate cycles of binging and purging with various neurotransmitters. Because antidepressants often benefit patients with bulimia nervosa and because serotonin has been linked to satiety, serotonin and norepinephrine have been implicated. Because plasma endorphin levels are raised in some bulimia nervosa patients who vomit, the feeling of well-being after vomiting that some of these patients experience may be mediated by raised endorphin levels. According to DSM-IV-TR, increased frequency of bulimia nervosa is found in first-degree relatives of persons with the disorder.

Social Factors. Patients with bulimia nervosa, as with those with anorexia nervosa, tend to be high achievers and to respond to societal pressures to be slender. As with anorexia nervosa patients, many patients with bulimia nervosa are depressed and have increased familial depression, but the families of patients with bulimia nervosa are generally less close and more conflictual than the families of those with anorexia nervosa. Patients with bulimia nervosa describe their parents as neglectful and rejecting.

Psychological Factors. Patients with bulimia nervosa, as with those with anorexia nervosa, have difficulties with adolescent demands, but patients with bulimia nervosa are more outgoing, angry, and impulsive than those with anorexia nervosa. Alcohol dependence, shoplifting, and emotional lability (including suicide attempts) are associated with bulimia nervosa. These patients generally experience their uncontrolled eating as more ego-dystonic than do patients with anorexia nervosa and so seek help more readily.

Patients with bulimia nervosa lack superego control and the ego strength of their counterparts with anorexia nervosa. Their difficulties controlling their impulses are often manifested by substance dependence and self-destructive sexual relationships in addition to the binge eating and purging that characterize the disorder. Many patients with bulimia nervosa have histories of difficulties separating from caretakers, as manifested by the absence of transitional objects during their early childhood years. Some clinicians have observed that patients with bulimia nervosa use their own bodies as transitional objects. The struggle for separation from a maternal figure is played out in the ambivalence toward food; eating may represent a wish to fuse with the caretaker, and regurgitating may unconsciously express a wish for separation.

Diagnosis and Clinical Features

According to DSM-IV-TR, bulimia nervosa is present when (1) episodes of binge eating occur relatively frequently (twice a week or more) for at least 3 months; (2) compensatory behaviors are practiced after binge eating to prevent weight gain, primarily self-induced vomiting, laxative abuse, diuretics, or abuse of emetics (80 percent of cases), and, less commonly, severe dieting and strenuous exercise (20 percent of cases); (3) weight is not severely lowered as in anorexia nervosa; and (4) the patient has a morbid fear of fatness, a relentless drive for thinness, or both and a disproportionate amount of self-evaluation depends on body weight and shape (Table 23.2–1). When making a diagnosis of bulimia nervosa, clinicians should explore the possibility that the patient has experienced a brief or prolonged prior bout of anorexia nervosa, present in approximately half of those with bulimia nervosa. Binging usually precedes vomiting by about 1 year.

Vomiting is common and is usually induced by sticking a finger down the throat, although some patients are able to vomit at will. Vomiting decreases the abdominal pain and the feeling of being bloated and allows patients to continue eating without fear of gaining weight. Depression, sometimes called *postbinge anguish*, often follows the episode. During binges, patients eat food that is sweet, high in calories, and generally soft or smooth textured, such as cakes and pastry. Some patients prefer bulky foods without regard to taste. The food is eaten secretly and rapidly and is sometimes not even chewed.

Most patients with bulimia nervosa are within their normal weight range, but some may be underweight or overweight. These patients are concerned about their body image and their appearance, worry about how others see them, and are concerned about their sexual attractiveness. Most are sexually active, compared with anorexia nervosa patients, who are not interested in sex. Pica and struggles during meals are sometimes revealed in the histories of patients with bulimia nervosa.

Bulimia nervosa occurs in persons with high rates of mood disorders and impulse control disorders. Bulimia nervosa is also reported to occur in those at risk for substance-related disorders and a variety of personality disorders. Patients with bulimia nervosa also have increased rates of anxiety disorders, bipolar I disorder, and dissociative disorders, and histories of sexual abuse.

Subtypes. Evidence indicates that bulimic persons who purge differ from binge eaters who do not purge in that the latter tend to have less body-image disturbance and less anxiety concerning eating. Those with bulimia nervosa who do not purge tend to be obese. Distinct physiological differences also exist between patients with bulimia who purge and those who do not. Because of all these differences, the diagnosis of bulimia nervosa is subtyped into a purging type, for those who regularly engage in self-induced vomiting or the use of laxatives or diuretics; and a nonpurging type, for those who use strict dieting, fasting, or vigorous exercise but do not regularly engage in purging.

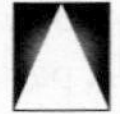

Table 23.2–1
DSM-IV-TR Diagnostic Criteria for Bulimia Nervosa

A. Recurrent episodes of binge eating. An episode of binge eating is characterized by both of the following:
   (1) eating, in a discrete period of time (e.g., within any 2-hour period), an amount of food that is definitely larger than most people would eat during a similar period of time and under similar circumstances
   (2) a sense of lack of control over eating during the episode (e.g., a feeling that one cannot stop eating or control what or how much one is eating)

B. Recurrent inappropriate compensatory behavior in order to prevent weight gain, such as self-induced vomiting; misuse of laxatives, diuretics, enemas, or other medications; fasting; or excessive exercise.

C. The binge eating and inappropriate compensatory behaviors both occur, on average, at least twice a week for 3 months.

D. Self-evaluation is unduly influenced by body shape and weight.

E. The disturbance does not occur exclusively during episodes of anorexia nervosa.

Specify type:

Purging type: during the current episode of bulimia nervosa, the person has regularly engaged in self-induced vomiting or the misuse of laxatives, diuretics, or enemas

Nonpurging type: during the current episode of bulimia nervosa, the person has used other inappropriate compensatory behaviors, such as fasting or excessive exercise, but has not regularly engaged in self-induced vomiting or the misuse of laxatives, diuretics, or enemas

(From American Psychiatric Association. *Diagnostic and Statistical Manual of Mental Disorders.* 4th ed. Text rev. Washington, DC: American Psychiatric Association; copyright 2000, with permission.)

Patients with the purging type of bulimia nervosa may be at risk for certain medical complications, such as hypokalemia from vomiting or laxative abuse and hypochloremic alkalosis. Those who vomit repeatedly are at risk for gastric and esophageal tears, although these complications are rare. Patients who purge may have a different course from that of patients who binge and then diet or exercise.

Abby Thurmond, age 42, had not had a food binge for over 2 years when she flew from Miami to Chicago to attend the wedding of her friend's daughter. Single, independent, and devoted to her work, Abby had just sold her first screenplay. She was pleased, but she was also experiencing the "postpartum" letdown that always occurred when she finished a major project. Despite knowing, from 2 years in Overeaters Anonymous (OA), that she needed to keep a safe distance from food, especially in emotionally hard times, Abby spent the entire day of the wedding rehearsal party in the company of food. She stood in her friend's kitchen for hours—cutting, chopping, sorting, arranging, and, eventually, picking at the food.

When night and the guests came, the flurry of activity made it easy for Abby to disappear—physically and emotionally—into a binge. She started with a plate of what would have been an "abstinent" meal (an OA concept for whatever is included on one's meal plan): pasta salad, green salad, cold cuts, and a roll. Although the portions were generous, Abby wanted more. She spent the next 5 hours eating, at first trying to graze among the guests, but then, when shame set in, retreating to dark corners of the room to take frantic, stolen bites. Abby stuffed herself with crackers, cheeses, breads, chicken, turkey, pasta, and salads, but all that was a prelude to what she really wanted—sugar. She'd been waiting for the guests to leave the dining room, where the desserts were. When they finally did, she cut herself two pieces of cake, then two more, then ate directly from the serving tray, shoveling the food into her mouth. She reached for cookies, more cake, and cookies again. Heart racing, terrified of being discovered, Abby finally tore herself away and slipped out onto the terrace.

By now, in what she thought of as a "food trance," Abby piled her plate with bread, onto which she smeared some unidentifiable spread. Though the food tasted like mud, Abby kept eating. Soon, other guests came out to the terrace, leaving Abby feeling she had to move again, which she did, stepping into the kitchen—and the light. When Abby glanced down at her plate, she was horrified; ants were crawling all over it. Instead of reflexively spitting out the food, Abby, overcome by shame, could only swallow. Then her eyes began to search the debris on her plate for uncontaminated morsels. Witnessing her own madness, Abby began to cry. She flung the plate into the trash and ran to her room.

That event marked the beginning of a 6-month relapse into binge eating—Abby's worst experience with bingeing since the problem began 15 years earlier. During the relapse, she binged on sugar foods and refined carbohydrates, returned to cigarette smoking to control the bingeing, and once again was driven to "get rid" of the calories by incessant exercise after each binge, walking 4 or 5 hours at a time, dragging her bicycle up and down six flights of stairs, and biking for miles after dark in a dangerous city park. (Courtesy of *DSM-IV-TR Casebook*.)

Pathology and Laboratory Examinations

Bulimia nervosa can result in electrolyte abnormalities and various degrees of starvation, although it may not be as obvious as in low-weight patients with anorexia nervosa. Thus, even normal-weight patients with bulimia nervosa should have laboratory studies of electrolytes and metabolism. In general, thyroid function remains intact in bulimia nervosa, but patients may show nonsuppression on the dexamethasone-suppression test. Dehydration and electrolyte disturbances are likely to occur in patients with bulimia nervosa who purge regularly. These patients commonly exhibit hypomagnesemia and hyperamylasemia. Although not a core diagnostic feature, many patients with bulimia nervosa have menstrual disturbances. Hypotension and bradycardia occur in some patients.

Differential Diagnosis

The diagnosis of bulimia nervosa cannot be made if the binge-eating and purging behaviors occur exclusively during episodes of anorexia nervosa. In such cases, the diagnosis is anorexia nervosa, binge eating-purging type.

Clinicians must ascertain that patients have no neurological disease, such as epileptic-equivalent seizures, central nervous system tumors, Klüver-Bucy syndrome, or Kleine-Levin syndrome. The pathological features manifested by Klüver-Bucy syndrome are visual agnosia, compulsive licking and biting, examination of objects by the mouth, inability to ignore any stimulus, placidity, altered sexual behavior (hypersexuality), and altered dietary habits, especially hyperphagia. The syndrome is exceedingly rare and is unlikely to cause a problem in differential diagnosis. Kleine-Levin syndrome consists of periodic hypersomnia lasting for 2 to 3 weeks and hyperphagia. As in bulimia nervosa, the onset is usually during adolescence, but the syndrome is more common in men than in women.

Patients with bulimia nervosa who have concurrent seasonal affective disorder and patterns of atypical depression (with overeating and oversleeping in low-light months) may manifest seasonal worsening of both bulimia nervosa and depressive features. In these cases, binges are typically much more severe during winter months. Bright light therapy (10,000 lux for 30 minutes, in early morning, at 18 to 22 inches from the eyes) may be a useful component of comprehensive treatment of an eating disorder with seasonal affective disorder.

Some patients with bulimia nervosa—perhaps 15 percent—have multiple comorbid impulsive behaviors, including substance abuse, and lack of ability to control themselves in such diverse areas as money management (resulting in impulse buying and compulsive shopping) and sexual relationships (often resulting in brief, passionate attachments and promiscuity). They exhibit self-mutilation, chaotic emotions, and chaotic sleeping patterns. They often meet criteria for borderline personality disorder and other mixed personality disorders and, not infrequently, bipolar II disorder.

Course and Prognosis

Bulimia nervosa is characterized by higher rates of partial and full recovery compared with anorexia nervosa. As noted in the treatment section, those treated fare much better than those untreated. Patients untreated tend to remain chronic or may show small, but generally unimpressive degrees of improvement with time. In a 10-year follow-up study of patients who had previously participated in treatment programs, the number of women who continued to meet full criteria for bulimia nervosa declined as the duration of follow-up increased. Approximately 30 percent continued to engage in recurrent binge-eating or purging behaviors. A history of substance use problems and a longer duration of the disorder at presentation predicted worse outcome. Depending on definitions, 38 to 47 percent of women were fully recovered at follow-up.

Treatment

Most patients with uncomplicated bulimia nervosa do not require hospitalization. In general, patients with bulimia nervosa are not as secretive about their symptoms as patients with anorexia nervosa. Therefore, outpatient treatment is usually not difficult, but psychotherapy is frequently stormy and may be prolonged. Some obese patients with bulimia nervosa who have had prolonged psychotherapy do surprisingly well. In some cases—when eating binges are out of control, outpatient treatment does not work, or a patient exhibits such additional psychiatric symptoms as suicidality and substance abuse—hospitalization may become necessary. In addition, electrolyte and metabolic disturbances resulting from severe purging may necessitate hospitalization.

Psychotherapy

COGNITIVE-BEHAVIORAL THERAPY. Cognitive-behavioral therapy (CBT) should be considered the benchmark, first-line treatment for bulimia nervosa. The data supporting the efficacy of CBT are based on strict adherence to rigorously implemented, highly detailed, manual-guided treatments that include about 18 to 20 sessions over 5 to 6 months. CBT implements a number of cognitive and behavioral procedures to (1) interrupt the self-maintaining behavioral cycle of bingeing and dieting and (2) alter the individual's dysfunctional cognitions; beliefs about food, weight, body image; and overall self-concept.

DYNAMIC PSYCHOTHERAPY. Psychodynamic treatment of patients with bulimia nervosa has revealed a tendency to concretize introjective and projective defense mechanisms. In a manner analogous to splitting, patients divide food into two categories: items that are nutritious and those that are unhealthy. Food that is designated nutritious may be ingested and retained because it unconsciously symbolizes good introjects. But junk food is unconsciously associated with bad introjects and, therefore, is expelled by vomiting, with the unconscious fantasy that all destructiveness, hate, and badness are being evacuated. Patients can temporarily feel good after vomiting because of the fantasized evacuation, but the associated feeling of "being all good" is short-lived because it is based on an unstable combination of splitting and projection.

Pharmacotherapy. Antidepressant medications have been shown to be helpful in treating bulimia. This includes the selective serotonin reuptake inhibitors (SSRIs), such as fluoxetine. This may be based on elevating central 5-hydroxytryptamine levels. Antidepressant medications can reduce binge eating and purging independent of the presence of a mood disorder. Thus, antidepressants have been used successfully for particularly difficult binge-purge cycles that do not respond to psychotherapy alone. Imipramine (Tofranil), desipramine (Norpramin), trazodone (Desyrel), and monoamine oxidase inhibitors (MAOIs) have been helpful. In general, most of the antidepressants have been effective at dosages usually given in the treatment of depressive disorders. Dosages of fluoxetine that are effective in decreasing binge eating, however, may be higher (60 to 80 mg a day) than those used for depressive disorders. Medication is helpful in patients with comorbid depressive disorders and bulimia nervosa. Carbamazepine (Tegretol) and lithium (Eskalith) have not shown impressive results as treatments for binge eating, but they have been used in the treatment of patients with bulimia nervosa with comorbid mood disorders, such as bipolar I disorder. Evidence indicates that the use of antidepressants alone results in a 22 percent rate of abstinence from bingeing and purging; other studies show that CBT and medications are the most effective combination.

EATING DISORDER NOT OTHERWISE SPECIFIED

The DSM-IV-TR diagnostic classification eating disorder not otherwise specified is a residual category used for eating disorders that do not meet the criteria for a specific eating disorder (Table 23.2–2). Binge-eating disorder—that is, recurrent episodes of binge eating in the absence of the inappropriate compensatory behaviors characteristic of bulimia nervosa (Table 23.2–3)—falls into this category. Such patients are not fixated on body shape and weight.

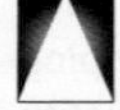

Table 23.2–2
DSM-IV-TR Diagnostic Criteria for Eating Disorder Not Otherwise Specified

The eating disorder not otherwise specified category is for disorders of eating that do not meet the criteria for any specific eating disorder. Examples include

1. For females, all of the criteria for anorexia nervosa are met except that the individual has regular menses.
2. All of the criteria for anorexia nervosa are met except that, despite significant weight loss, the individual's current weight is in the normal range.
3. All of the criteria for bulimia nervosa are met except that the binge eating and inappropriate compensatory mechanisms occur at a frequency of less than twice a week or for a duration of less than 3 months.
4. The regular use of inappropriate compensatory behavior by an individual of normal body weight after eating small amounts of food (e.g., self-induced vomiting after the consumption of two cookies).
5. Repeatedly chewing and spitting out, but not swallowing, large amounts of food.
6. Binge-eating disorder: recurrent episodes of binge eating in the absence of the regular use of inappropriate compensatory behaviors characteristic of bulimia nervosa.

(From American Psychiatric Association. *Diagnostic and Statistical Manual of Mental Disorders.* 4th ed. Text rev. Washington, DC: American Psychiatric Association; copyright 2000, with permission.)

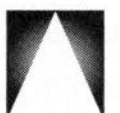

Table 23.2–3
DSM-IV-TR Research Criteria for Binge-Eating Disorder

A. Recurrent episodes of binge eating. An episode of binge eating is characterized by both of the following:
 (1) eating, in a discrete period of time (e.g., within any 2-hour period), an amount of food that is definitely larger than what most people would eat in a similar period of time under similar circumstances
 (2) a sense of lack of control over eating during the episode (e.g., a feeling that one cannot stop eating or control what or how much one is eating)
B. The binge-eating episodes are associated with three (or more) of the following:
 (1) eating much more rapidly than normal
 (2) eating until feeling uncomfortably full
 (3) eating large amounts of food when not feeling physically hungry
 (4) eating alone because of being embarrassed by how much one is eating
 (5) feeling disgusted with oneself, depressed, or very guilty after overeating
C. Marked distress regarding binge eating is present.
D. The binge eating occurs, on average, at least 2 days a week for 6 months.
 Note: The method of determining frequency differs from that used for bulimia nervosa; future research should address whether the preferred method of setting a frequency threshold is counting the number of days on which binges occur or counting the number of episodes of binge eating.
E. The binge eating is not associated with the regular use of inappropriate compensatory behaviors (e.g., purging, fasting, excessive exercise) and does not occur exclusively during the course of anorexia nervosa or bulimia nervosa.

(From American Psychiatric Association. *Diagnostic and Statistical Manual of Mental Disorders.* 4th ed. Text rev. Washington, DC: American Psychiatric Association; copyright 2000, with permission.)

ICD-10

The 10th revision of *International Statistical Classification of Diseases and Related Health Problems* (ICD-10) describes bulimia nervosa as repeated bouts of overeating and a preoccupation about controlling weight that lead to self-induced vomiting; in turn, vomiting produces physical complications, electrolyte disturbances, and severe weight loss (*see* Table 23.1–4).

In the category of eating disorders, ICD-10 also includes atypical anorexia, atypical bulimia nervosa, overeating associated with other psychological disturbances, vomiting associated with other psychological disturbances, other eating disorders, and eating disorders, unspecified.

References

Andersen AE, Yager J. Eating Disorders. In: Sadock BJ, Sadock VA, eds. *Kaplan & Sadock's Comprehensive Textbook of Psychiatry*. 8th ed. Vol. 1. Baltimore: Lippincott Williams & Wilkins; 2005:2002.

Chamay-Weber C, Narring F, Michaud PA. Partial eating disorders among adolescents: A review. *J Adolesc Health*. 2005;37:416–426.

Constantino MJ, Arnow BA, Blasey C, Agras WS. The association between patient characteristics and the therapeutic alliance in cognitive-behavioral and interpersonal therapy for bulimia nervosa. *J Consult Clin Psychol*. 2005;73(2):203–211.

Cummins LH, Simmons AM, Zane NW. Eating disorders in Asian populations: A critique of current approaches to the study of culture, ethnicity, and eating disorders. *Am J Orthopsychiatry*. 2005;75:553–574.

de Zwaan M, Roerig J. Pharmacological treatment, in evidence and experience in psychiatry. In: Halmi KA, Maj M, eds. *Eating Disorders*. Vol. 6. World Psychiatric Association. England: John Wiley; 2003.

Engelberg MJ, Gauvin L, Steiger H. A naturalistic evaluation of the relation between dietary restraint, the urge to binge, and actual binge eating: A clarification. *Int J Eat Disord*. 2005;38:355–360.

Favaro A, Tenconi E, Santonastaso P. Perinatal factors and the risk of developing anorexia nervosa and bulimia nervosa. *Arch Gen Psychiatry*. 2006;63:82–88.

Johnson JG, Cohen P, Kasen S, Brook JS. Eating disorders during adolescence and the risk for physical and mental disorders during early adulthood. *Arch Gen Psychiatry*. 2002;59(6):545–552.

Morgan JF, Lacey JH, Chung E. Risk of postnatal depression, miscarriage, and preterm birth in bulimia nervosa: Retrospective controlled study. *Psychosom Med*. 2006;68(3):487–492.

Palmer RL, Birchall H, McGrain L, Sullivan V. Self-help for bulimic disorders: a randomised controlled trial comparing minimal guidance with face-to-face or telephone guidance. *Br J Psychiatry*. 2002;181:230–235.

▲ 23.3 Obesity

Obesity is a complex disease resulting from a combination of genetic susceptibility, increased availability of high-energy foods, and decreased requirement for physical activity in modern society. The prevalence of obesity has reached epidemic proportions in industrialized countries and is now considered the leading cause of preventable death in the United States. Because it is associated with significant increases in morbidity and mortality, the health care costs directly attributable to obesity also have dramatically increased over the past few decades.

Obesity refers to an excess of body fat (Fig. 23.3–1). In healthy individuals, body fat accounts for approximately 25 percent of body weight in women and 18 percent in men. Overweight refers to weight above some reference norm, typically standards derived from actuarial or epidemiological data. In most cases, increasing weight reflects increasing obesity, but not always. Muscular individuals might be overweight (weight might be high for height) but not be obese, and a person might have normal weight but have high body fat.

Indexes have been developed using height and weight to estimate level of obesity. The most common of these is the body mass index (BMI). BMI is calculated by dividing weight in kilograms by height in meters squared. Although there is debate about the ideal BMI, it is generally thought that a BMI of 20 to 25 kg/m^2 represents healthy weight, a BMI of 25 to 27 kg/m^2 is associated with somewhat elevated risk, a BMI above 27 kg/m^2 represents clearly increased risk, and a BMI above 30 kg/m^2 carries greatly increased risk. Figure 23.3–2 presents a chart for determining BMI from height and weight.

EPIDEMIOLOGY

Obesity rates continue to grow at epidemic proportions in the United States and other industrialized nations, representing a serious public health threat to millions of people. In the United States, 34 percent of the population is overweight (defined as a

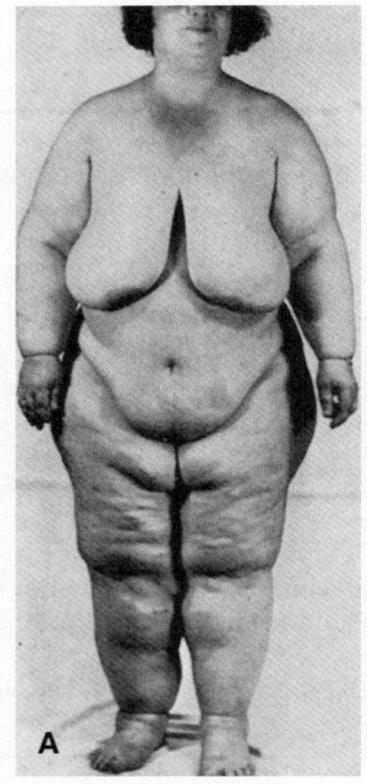

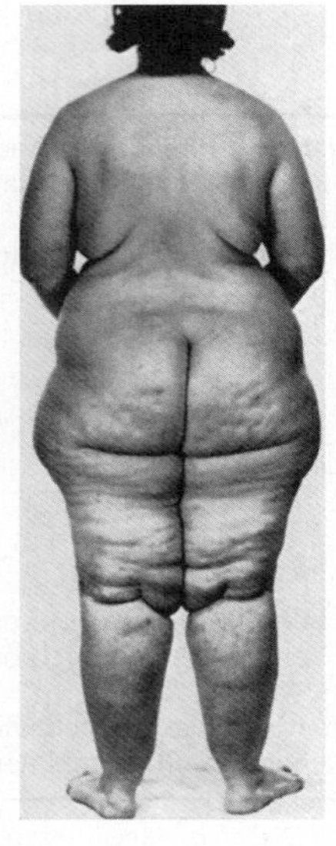

FIGURE 23.3–1

A. Gross obesity, frontal view. **B.** Same patient, rear view. (From Douthwait AH, ed. *French's Index of Differential Diagnosis*, 7th ed. Baltimore: Williams & Wilkins.)

BMI of 25.0 to 29.9 kg/m^2), whereas 30 percent is obese (defined as a BMI >30 kg/m^2). Obesity (BMI >30 kg/m^2) among adults increased from 30 percent in 2000 to 32.2 percent in 2004. Extreme obesity (BMI $\geq$40 kg/m^2) also increased significantly during the same time period now standing at 2.8 percent in men and 6.9 percent in women.

The prevalence of obesity is highest in minority populations, particularly among non-Hispanic black women. More than one-half of these individuals, 40 years of age or older, are obese, and more than 80 percent are overweight. The prevalence of overweight and obesity in children and adolescents in the United States has also increased substantially from about 15 percent in 2000 to about 18 percent in 2004. About 10 percent of 2- to 5-year-olds are overweight.

ETIOLOGY

Persons accumulate fat by eating more calories than are expended as energy; thus intake of energy exceeds its dissipation. If fat is to be removed from the body, fewer calories must be put in or more calories must be taken out than are put in. An error of no more than 10 percent in either intake or output would lead to a 30-pound change in body weight in 1 year.

	Height (ft,in)																	
Weight (lb)	4'10"	4'11"	5'0"	5'1"	5'2"	5'3"	5'4"	5'5"	5'6"	5'7"	5'8"	5'9"	5'10"	5'11"	6'0"	6'1"	6'2"	
125	26	25	24	24	23	22	22	21	20	20	19	18	18	17	17	17	16	
130	27	26	25	25	24	23	22	22	21	20	20	19	19	18	18	17	17	Underweight
135	28	27	26	26	25	24	23	23	22	21	21	20	19	19	18	18	17	
140	29	28	27	27	26	25	24	23	23	22	21	21	20	20	19	19	18	
145	30	29	28	27	27	26	25	24	23	23	22	21	21	20	20	19	19	
150	31	30	29	28	27	27	26	25	24	24	23	22	22	21	20	20	19	
155	32	31	30	29	28	28	27	26	25	24	24	23	22	22	21	20	20	
160	33	32	31	30	29	28	28	27	26	25	24	24	23	22	22	21	21	
165	34	33	32	31	30	29	28	28	27	26	25	24	24	23	22	22	21	
170	35	34	33	32	31	30	29	28	28	27	26	25	24	24	23	22	22	Normal Weight
175	36	35	34	33	32	31	30	29	28	27	27	26	25	24	24	23	23	
180	37	36	35	34	33	32	31	30	29	28	27	27	26	25	25	24	23	
185	38	37	36	35	34	33	32	31	30	29	28	27	27	26	25	24	24	
190	39	38	37	36	35	34	33	32	31	30	29	28	27	27	26	25	24	
195	40	39	38	37	36	35	34	33	32	31	30	29	28	27	27	26	25	
200	41	40	39	38	37	36	34	33	32	31	30	30	29	28	27	26	26	
205	42	41	40	39	38	36	35	34	33	32	31	30	29	29	28	27	26	
210	43	43	41	40	38	37	36	35	34	33	32	31	30	29	29	28	27	Overweight
215	44	44	42	41	39	38	37	36	35	34	33	32	31	30	29	28	28	
220	45	45	43	42	40	39	38	37	36	35	34	33	32	31	30	29	28	
225	46	46	44	43	41	40	39	38	36	35	34	33	32	31	31	30	29	
230	47	47	45	44	42	41	40	38	37	36	35	34	33	32	31	30	30	
235	48	48	46	44	43	42	40	39	38	37	36	35	34	33	32	31	30	
240	49	49	47	45	44	43	41	40	39	38	37	36	35	34	33	32	31	
245	50	50	48	46	45	43	42	41	40	38	37	36	35	34	33	32	32	
250	51	51	49	47	46	44	43	42	40	39	38	37	36	35	34	33	32	
255	52	52	50	48	47	45	44	43	41	40	39	38	37	36	35	34	33	Obese
260	54	53	51	49	48	46	45	43	42	41	40	38	37	36	36	34	33	
265	56	54	52	50	49	47	46	44	43	42	40	39	38	37	36	35	34	
270	57	55	53	51	49	48	46	45	44	42	41	40	39	38	37	36	35	
275	58	56	54	52	50	49	47	46	44	43	42	41	40	38	37	36	35	

FIGURE 23.3–2

Body mass index (BMI) chart. To determine BMI, find the patient's weight on the left of the graph and their height on the top of the graph. Follow the two categories toward the middle of the graph until they intersect. This point represents the patient's BMI.

Satiety

Satiety is the feeling that results when hunger is satisfied. Persons stop eating at the end of a meal because they have replenished nutrients that had been depleted. Persons become hungry again when nutrients restored by earlier meals are once again depleted. It seems reasonable that a metabolic signal, derived from food that has been absorbed, is carried by the blood to the brain, where the signal activates receptor cells, probably in the hypothalamus, to produce satiety. Some studies have shown evidence for dysfunction in serotonin, dopamine, and norepinephrine involvement in regulating eating behavior through the hypothalamus. Other hormonal factors that may be involved include corticotrophin releasing factor (CRF), neuropeptide Y, gonadotropin-releasing hormone, and thyroid-stimulating hormone. A new substance obestatin, made in the stomach, is a hormone that in animal experiments produces satiety and may have potential use as a weight loss agent in humans. Hunger results from a decrease in the strength of metabolic signals, secondary to the depletion of critical nutrients.

Cannabinoid receptors are related to appetite and are stimulated with cannabis (marijuana). A cannabinoid inverse antagonist has been developed that blocks appetite.

Satiety occurs soon after the beginning of a meal and before the total caloric content of the meal has been absorbed; therefore satiety is only one regulatory mechanism controlling food intake. Appetite, defined as the desire for food, is also involved. A hungry person may eat to full satisfaction when food is available, but appetite can also induce a person to overeat past the point of satiety. Appetite may be increased by psychological factors such as thoughts or feelings, and an abnormal appetite may result in an abnormal increase in food intake. Eating is also affected by cannabinoid receptors which when stimulated increases appetite. Marijuana acts on that receptor which accounts for the "munchies" associated with marijuana use. A drug called rimonabaut is an inverse agonist to the cannabidiol receptor, meaning that it blocks appetite. It may have clinical use.

The olfactory system may play a role in satiety. Experiments have shown that strong stimulation of the olfactory bulbs in the nose with food odors by use of an inhaler saturated with a particular smell produces satiety for that food. This may have implications for therapy of obesity.

Genetic Factors

The existence of numerous forms of inherited obesity in animals and the ease with which adiposity can be produced by selective breeding make it clear that genetic factors can play a role in obesity. These factors must also be presumed to be important in human obesity.

About 80 percent of patients who are obese have a family history of obesity. This fact can be accounted for not only by genetic factors but also in part by identification with fat parents and by learned oral methods for coping with anxiety. Nonetheless, studies show that identical twins raised apart can both be obese, an observation that suggests a hereditary role. To date, no specific genetic marker of obesity has been found. Table 23.3–1 lists the genetic factors affecting body weight.

Developmental Factors

Early in life, adipose tissue grows by increases in both cell number and cell size. Once the number of adipocytes has been established, it does not seem to be susceptible to change. Obesity that begins early in life is characterized by adipose tissue with an increased number of adipocytes of increased size. Obesity that begins in adult life, on the other hand, results solely from an increase in the size of the adipocytes. In both instances, weight reduction produces a decrease in cell size. The greater number and size of adipocytes in patients with juvenile-onset diabetes may be a factor in their widely recognized difficulties with weight reduction and the persistence of their obesity.

The distribution and amount of fat vary in individuals, and fat in different body areas has different characteristics. Fat cells around the waist, flanks, and abdomen (the so-called potbelly) are more active metabolically than those in the thighs and buttocks. The former pattern is more common in men and has a

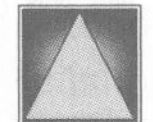

Table 23.3–1
Genetic Factors Affecting Body Weight

	Genetic Factor Description
Leptin	Highly expressed in areas of the hypothalamus that control feeding behavior, hunger, body temperature, and energy expenditure. The mechanisms by which leptin suppresses feeding and exerts its effects on metabolism are largely unknown.
Neuropeptide Y	Synthesized in many areas of the brain; it is a potent stimulator of feeding. Leptin appears to suppress feeding in part by inhibiting expression of neuropeptide Y.
Ghrelin	An acylated, 28–amino acid peptide secreted primarily by the stomach. Ghrelin circulates in the blood and activates neuropeptide Y neurons in the hypothalamic arcuate nucleus, thereby stimulating food intake.
Melanocortins	Acts on certain hypothalamic neurons that inhibit feeding. Targeted disruptions of the melanocortin-4 receptor in mice are associated with development of obesity.
Carboxypeptidase E	The enzyme necessary for processing proinsulin and perhaps other hormones, such as neuropeptide Y. Mice with mutations in this gene gradually become obese as they age and develop hyperglycemia that can be suppressed by treatment with insulin.
Mitochondrial uncoupling proteins	First discovered in brown fat and subsequently identified in white fat and muscle cells. May play an important role in energy expenditure and body weight regulation.
Tubby protein	Highly expressed in the paraventricular nucleus of the hypothalamus and other regions of the brain. Mice with naturally occurring or engineered mutations in the tubby gene show adult onset of obesity, but the mechanisms involved are not known.

(Adapted from Comuzzie AG, Williams JT, Martin LJ, Blanger J. Searching for genes underlying normal variation in human adiposity. *J Mol Med.* 2001;79:57.)

higher correlation with cardiovascular disease than does the latter pattern. Women, whose fat distribution is in the thighs and buttocks, may become obsessed with nostrums that are advertised to reduce fat in these areas (so-called cellulite, which is not a medical term); but no externally applied preparation to reduce this fat pattern exists. Men with abdominal fat may attempt to reduce their girth with machines that exercise the abdominal muscles, but exercise has no effect on fat loss.

A hormone called leptin, made by fat cells, acts as a fat thermostat. When the blood level of leptin is low, more fat is consumed; when high, less fat is consumed. Further research is needed to determine whether this might lead to new ways of managing obesity.

Physical Activity Factors

The marked decrease in physical activity in affluent societies seems to be the major factor in the rise of obesity as a public health problem. Physical inactivity restricts energy expenditure and may contribute to increased food intake. Although food intake increases with increasing energy expenditure over a wide range of energy demands, intake does not decrease proportionately when physical activity falls below a certain minimum level.

Brain-Damage Factors

Destruction of the ventromedial hypothalamus can produce obesity in animals, but this is probably a very rare cause of obesity in humans. There is evidence that the central nervous system, particularly in the lateral and ventromedial hypothalamic areas, adjusts to food intake in response to changing energy requirements so as to maintain fat stores at a baseline determined by a specific set point. This set point varies from one person to another and depends on height and body build.

Health Factors

In only a small number of cases is obesity the consequence of identifiable illness. Such cases include a variety of rare genetic disorders, such as Prader-Willi syndrome, as well as neuroendocrine abnormalities (Table 23.3–2). Hypothalamic obesity results from damage to the ventromedial region of the hypothalamus (VMH), which has been studied extensively in laboratory animals and is a known center of appetite and weight regulation. In humans, damage to the VMH may result from trauma, surgery, malignancy, or inflammatory disease.

Some forms of depression, particularly seasonal affective disorder, are associated with weight gain. Most persons who live in seasonal climates report increases in appetite and weight during the fall and winter months, with decreases in the spring and summer. Depressed patients usually lose weight; but some will gain weight.

Other Clinical Factors

A variety of clinical disorders are associated with obesity. Cushing's disease is associated with a characteristic fat distribution and moon-like face (Fig. 23.3-3). Myxedema is associated with weight gain, although not invariably. Other neuroendocrine disorders include adiposogenital dystrophy (Fröhlich's syndrome), which is characterized by obesity and sexual and skeletal abnormalities.

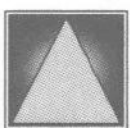

Table 23.3–2
Illnesses That Can Explain Some Cases of Obesity

Genetic (dysmorphic) obesities
- Autosomal recessive
- X-linked
- Chromosomal (e.g., Prader-Willi syndrome)

Neuroendocrine obesities
- Hypothalamic syndromes
- Cushing's syndrome
- Hypothyroidism
- Polycystic ovarian syndrome (Stein-Leventhal syndrome)
- Pseudohypoparathyroidism
- Hypogonadism
- Growth hormone deficiency
- Insulinoma and hyperinsulinism

Iatrogenic obesities
- Drugs (psychiatric)
- Hypothalamic surgery (neuroendocrine)

(Adapted from Bray GA. An approach to the classification and evaluation of obesity. In: Bjorntorp P, Brodoff BN, eds. *Obesity.* Philadelphia: Lippincott Williams & Wilkins; 1992.)

Psychotropic Drugs

Long-term use of steroid medications is associated with significant weight gain, as is the use of several psychotropic agents. Patients treated for major depression, psychotic disturbances, and bipolar disorder typically gain 3 to 10 kg, with even larger gains with chronic use. This can produce the so-called metabolic syndrome discussed below.

Psychological Factors

Although psychological factors are evidently crucial to the development of obesity, how such psychological factors result in obesity is not known. The food-regulating mechanism is susceptible to environmental influence, and cultural, family, and psychodynamic factors have all been shown to contribute to the development of obesity. Although many investigators have proposed that specific family histories, precipitating factors, personality structures, or unconscious conflicts cause obesity, overweight persons may suffer from every conceivable psychiatric disorder and come from a variety of disturbed backgrounds. Many obese patients are emotionally disturbed persons who, because of the availability of the overeating mechanism in their environments, have learned to use hyperphagia as a means of coping with psychological problems. Some patients may show signs of serious mental disorder when they attain normal weight because they no longer have that coping mechanism.

DIAGNOSIS AND CLINICAL FEATURES

The diagnosis of obesity, if done in a sophisticated way, involves the assessment of body fat. As this is rarely practical, the use of height and weight to calculate BMI is recommended (Fig. 23.3–2).

In most cases of obesity, it is not possible to identify the precise etiology, given the multitude of possible causes and their

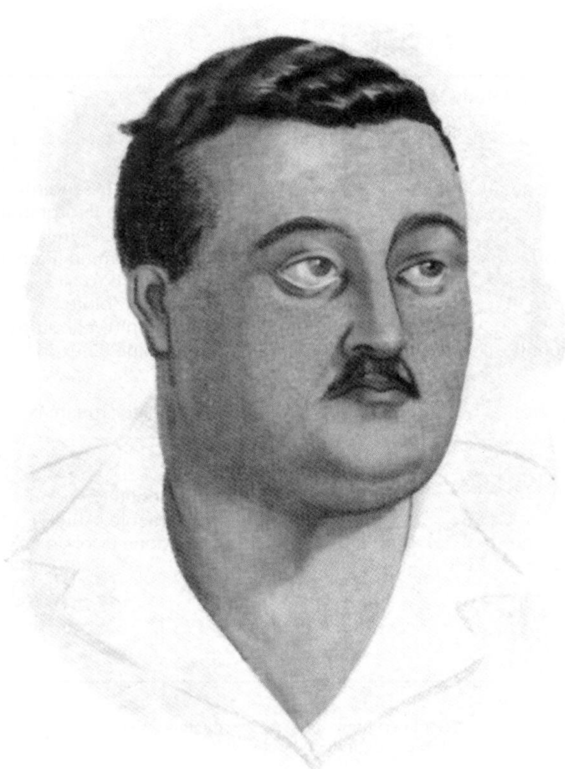

FIGURE 23.3–3
Cushing's syndrome. Plethoric, 'moon-faced' with 'sun-fish' mouth. (From Douthwait AH, ed. *French's Index of Differential Diagnosis,* 7th ed. Baltimore: Williams & Wilkins; 513.)

interactions. Instances of secondary obesity (described in Table 23.3–3) are rare but should not be overlooked.

The habitual eating patterns of many obese persons often seem similar to patterns found in experimental obesity. Impaired satiety is a particularly important problem. Obese persons seem inordinately susceptible to food cues in their environment, to the palatability of foods, and to the inability to stop eating if food is available. Obese persons are usually susceptible to all kinds of external stimuli to eating, but they remain relatively unresponsive to the usual internal signals of hunger. Some are unable to distinguish between hunger and other kinds of dysphoria.

DIFFERENTIAL DIAGNOSIS

Other Syndromes

The night-eating syndrome, in which persons eat excessively after they have had their evening meal, seems to be precipitated by stressful life circumstances and, once present, tends to recur daily until the stress is alleviated. Night-eating may also occur as a result of using sedatives to sleep which may produce sleep-walking and eating. This has been reported with the use of Zolpidem (Ambien) in patients.

The binge-eating syndrome (bulimia) is characterized by sudden, compulsive ingestion of very large amounts of food in a short time, usually with great subsequent agitation and self-condemnation. Binge eating also appears to represent a reaction to stress. In contrast to the night-eating syndrome, however, these bouts of overeating are not periodic, and they are far more often linked to specific precipitating circumstances. (See Chapter 23, Section 23.2, for a complete discussion of bulimia.) The Pickwickian syndrome is said to exist when a person is 100 percent over desirable weight and has associated respiratory and cardiovascular pathology.

Body Dysmorphic Disorder (Dysmorphophobia)

Some obese persons feel that their bodies are grotesque and loathsome and that others view them with hostility and contempt. This feeling is closely associated with self-consciousness and impaired social functioning. Emotionally healthy obese persons have no body image disturbances, and only a minority of neurotic obese persons has such disturbances. The disorder is confined mainly to persons who have been obese since childhood; even among them, less than half suffer from it. (Body dysmorphic disorder is discussed further in Chapter 18 on somatoform disorders.)

Metabolic Syndrome

The metabolic syndrome consists of a cluster of metabolic abnormalities associated with obesity and that contribute to an increased risk of cardiovascular disease and type II diabetes. The syndrome is diagnosed when a patient has three or more of the following five risk factors: (1) abdominal obesity, (2) high triglyceride level, (3) low HDL cholesterol level, (4) hypertension, and (5) an elevated fasting blood glucose level. Table 23.3–4 lists the criteria as set forth by the World Health Organization (WHO). The syndrome is believed to occur in about 30 percent of the American population, but is also well known in other industrialized countries around the world.

The cause of the syndrome is unknown but obesity, insulin resistance and a genetic vulnerability are involved. Treatment involves weight loss, exercise and the use of statins and antihypertensives as needed to lower lipid levels and blood pressure. Because of the increased risk of mortality it is important that the syndrome be recognized early and treated.

Second generation (atypical) antipsychotic medication has been implicated as a cause of metabolic syndrome. In patients with schizophrenia, treatment with these medications can cause a rapid increase in body weight in the first few months of therapy that may continue on for more than a year. In addition, insulin resistance leading to Type II diabetes has been associated with an artherogenic lipid profile.

Clozapine and olanzapine (Zyprexa) are the two drugs most implicated but other atypical antipsychotics may also be involved.

Patients prescribed second generation antipsychotic medication should be monitored periodically with fasting blood glucose levels at the beginning of treatment and during its course. Lipid profiles should also be obtained. Table 23.3–5 lists screening procedures for patients taking these medications.

Psychological reactions to the metabolic syndrome depend on the signs and symptoms experienced by the patient. Those who suffer primarily from obesity must deal with self-esteem issues from being overweight as well as the stress of participating in weight loss programs. In many cases of obesity, eating is a way of satisfying deep seated dependency needs. As weight is lost, some patients become depressed or anxious. Cases of psychosis have been reported in a few markedly obese patients during or after the process of losing a vast amount of weight. Other metabolic discrepancies, particularly variations in blood sugar, may be accompanied by irritability or other mood changes. Finally, fatigue is a common occurrence in patients with this syndrome. As the condition

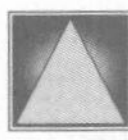

Table 23.3–3
Psychiatric Medications and Changes in Body Weight

Tendency to Increase Appetite and Body Weight		
Greatest	**Intermediate**	**Least**
Antidepressant drugs		
Amitriptyline (Elavil)	Doxepin (Adapin, Sinequan)	Amoxapine (Asendin)
	Imipramine (Tofranil)	Desipramine (Norpramin)
	Mirtazapine (Remeron)	Trazodone (Desyrel)
	Nortriptyline (Pamelor)	Tranylcypromine (Parnate)
		Fluoxetine (Prozac)[a]
	Phenelzine (Nardil)	Sertraline (Zoloft)[a]
		Bupropion (Wellbutrin)[a]
	Trimipramine (Surmontil)	Venlafaxine (Effexor)[a]
Mood stabilizers		
Lithium (Eskalith)	Carbamazepine (Tegretol)	Topiramate (Topamax)
Valproic acid (Depakene)		
Antipsychotic drugs		
Chlorpromazine (Thorazine)	Haloperidol (Haldol)	Ziprasidone (Geodon)
		Aripiprazole (Abilify)
Clozapine (Clozaril)	Trifluoperazine (Stelazine)	Molindone (Moban)[a]
Thioridazine (Mellaril)	Perphenazine (Trilafon)	
Mesoridazine (Serentil)	Thiothixene (Navane)	
Olanzapine (Zyprexa)	Fluphenazine (Permitil, Prolixin)	
Sertindole (Serdolect)		
Risperidone (Risperdal)		

[a]May decrease appetite and facilitate weight loss.
(Adapted from Allison DB, Mentore JL, Heo M, Chandler LP, Capeller JC, Infante MC, Weiden PJ. Antipsychotic-induced weight gain: A comprehensive research synthesis. *Am J Psychiatry.* 1999;156:1686; and Bernstein JG. Management of psychotropic drug-induced obesity. In: Bjorntorp P, Brodoff BN, eds. *Obesity.* Philadelphia: Lippincott Williams & Wilkins; 1992.)

improves, especially if exercise is part of the regimen, fatigue eventually diminishes; but patients may be misdiagnosed as having a dysthymic disorder or chronic fatigue syndrome if metabolic causes of fatigue are not considered.

COURSE AND PROGNOSIS

Effects on Health

Obesity has adverse effects on health and is associated with a broad range of illnesses (Table 23.3–6). There is a strong correlation between obesity and cardiovascular disorders. Hypertension (blood pressure higher than 160/95) is three times higher for persons who are overweight, and hypercholesterolemia (blood cholesterol over 250 mg/dL) is twice as common. Studies show that blood pressure and cholesterol levels can be reduced by weight reduction. Diabetes, which has clear genetic determinations, can often be reversed with weight reduction, especially type II diabetes (mature-onset or non-insulin-dependent diabetes mellitus).

According to National Institutes of Health data, obese men, regardless of smoking habits, have a higher mortality from colon, rectal, and prostate cancer than men of normal weight. Obese women have a higher mortality from cancer of the gallbladder, biliary passages, breast (postmenopause), uterus (including cervix and endometrium), and ovaries than women of normal weight.

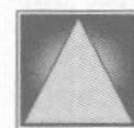

Table 23.3–4
WHO Clinical Criteria for Metabolic Syndrome

Insulin resistance, identified by 1 of the following:
- Type II diabetes
- Impaired fasting glucose
- Impaired glucose tolerance
- Or for those with normal fasting glucose levels (<110 mg/dL), glucose uptake below the lowest quartile for background population under investigation under hyperinsulinemic, euglycemic conditions

Plus any 2 of the following:
- Antihypertensive medication and/or high blood pressure ($\geq$140 mm Hg systolic or $\geq$90 mm Hg diastolic)
- Plasma triglycerides $\geq$150 mg/dL ($\geq$1.7 mmol/L)
- BMI >30 kg/m^2 and/or waist:hip ratio >0.9 in men, >0.85 in women
- Urinary albumin excretion rate $\geq$20 μg/min or albumin:creatinine ratio $\geq$30 mg/g

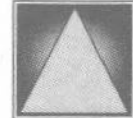

Table 23.3–5
Screen Patients Before Prescribing Antipsychotics

- Personal history of obesity
- Family history of obesity
- Diabetes
- Dyslipidemias
- Hypertension
- Cardiovascular disease
- Body mass index
- Waist circumference at level of umbilicus
- Blood pressure
- Fasting plasma glucose
- Fasting lipid profile

(Data from American Diabetes Association; 2004.)

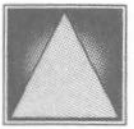

Table 23.3–6
Health Disorders Thought to Be Caused or Exacerbated by Obesity

Heart
- Premature coronary heart disease
- Left ventricular hypertrophy
- Angina pectoris
- Sudden death (ventricular arrhythmia)
- Congestive heart failure

Vascular system
- Hypertension
- Cerebrovascular disorder (cerebral infarction or hemorrhage)
- Venous stasis (with lower-extremity edema, varicose veins)

Respiratory system
- Obstructive sleep apnea
- Pickwickian syndrome (alveolar hypoventilation)
- Secondary polycythemia
- Right ventricular hypertrophy (sometimes leading to failure)

Hepatobiliary system
- Cholelithiasis and cholecystitis
- Hepatic steatosis

Hormonal and metabolic functions
- Diabetes mellitus (insulin independent)
- Gout (hyperuricemia)
- Hyperlipidemias (hypertriglyceridemia and hypercholesterolemia)

Kidney
- Proteinuria and, in very severe obesity, nephrosis
- Renal vein thrombosis

Joints, muscles, and connective tissue
- Osteoarthritis of knees
- Bone spurs of the heel
- Osteoarthrosis of spine (in women)
- Aggravation of preexisting postural faults

Neoplasia
- In women: increased risk of cancer of endometrium, breast, cervix, ovary, gallbladder, and biliary passages
- In men: increased risk of cancer of colon, rectum, and prostate

(Reprinted with permission from Vanitallie TB. Obesity: adverse effects on health and longevity. *Am J Clin Nutr.* 1979;32:2723.)

Longevity

Reliable studies indicate that the more overweight a person is, the higher is that person's risk for death. A person who reduces weight to acceptable levels has a mortality decline to normal rates. Weight reduction may be lifesaving for patients with extreme obesity, defined as weight that is twice the desirable weight. Such patients may have cardiorespiratory failure, especially when asleep (sleep apnea).

A number of studies have demonstrated that decreasing caloric intake by 30 percent or more in young or middle-aged laboratory animals prevents or retards age-related chronic diseases and significantly prolongs maximal life span. The mechanisms through which this effect is mediated are not known, but may include reductions in metabolic rate, oxidative stress and inflammation, improved insulin sensitivity, and changes in neuroendocrine and sympathetic nervous system function. Whether long-term calorie restriction with adequate nutrition slows aging in humans is not yet known.

Prognosis

The prognosis for weight reduction is poor, and the course of obesity tends toward inexorable progression. Of patients who lose significant amounts of weight, 90 percent regain it eventually. The prognosis is particularly poor for those who become obese in childhood. Juvenile-onset obesity tends to be more severe, more resistant to treatment, and more likely to be associated with emotional disturbance than is adult obesity.

Discrimination Toward the Obese. Overweight and obese individuals are subject to significant prejudice and discrimination in the United States and other industrialized nations. In a culture in which beauty ideals are thin and highly unrealistic, overweight people are blamed for their condition and are the subject of teasing, bias, and discrimination (sometimes called "fatism"). Income and earning power are suppressed in overweight people, and untoward social conditions, such as absence of romantic relationships, are more common. Furthermore, obese individuals face limited access to health care and may receive biased diagnoses and treatment from medical and mental health providers.

TREATMENT

As mentioned above many patients routinely treated for obesity may develop anxiety or depression. A high incidence of emotional disturbances has been reported among obese persons undergoing long-term, in-hospital treatment by fasting or severe calorie restriction. Obese persons with extensive psychopathology, those with a history of emotional disturbance during dieting, and those in the midst of a life crisis should attempt weight reduction, if at all, cautiously and under careful supervision.

Diet

The basis of weight reduction is simple—establish a caloric deficit by bringing intake below output. The simplest way to reduce caloric intake is by means of a low-calorie diet. The best long-term effects are achieved with a balanced diet that contains readily available foods. For most persons, the most satisfactory reducing diet consists of their usual foods in amounts determined with the aid of tables of food values that are available in standard books on dieting. Such a diet gives the best chance of long-term maintenance of weight loss. Total unmodified fasts are used for short-term weight loss, but they have associated morbidity including orthostatic hypotension, sodium diuresis, and impaired nitrogen balance.

Ketogenic diets are high-protein, high-fat diets used to promote weight loss. They have high cholesterol content and produce ketosis, which is associated with nausea, hypotension, and lethargy. Many obese persons find it tempting to use a novel or even bizarre diet. Whatever effectiveness these diets may have in large part results from their monotony. When a dieter stops the diet and returns to the usual fare, the incentives to overeat are multiplied.

In general, the best method of weight loss is a balanced diet of 1,100 to 1,200 calories. Such a diet can be followed for long periods but should be supplemented with vitamins, particularly iron, folic acid, zinc, and vitamin B6.

Exercise

Increased physical activity is an important part of a weight-reduction regimen. Because caloric expenditure in most forms of physical activity is directly proportional to body weight, obese persons expend more calories than persons of normal weight with the same amount of activity. Furthermore, increased physical activity may actually decrease food intake by formerly sedentary persons. This combination of increased caloric expenditure and decreased food intake makes an increase in physical activity a highly desirable feature of any weight-reduction program. Exercise also helps maintain weight loss. It is essential in the treatment of the metabolic syndrome.

Pharmacotherapy

Various drugs, some more effective than others, are used to treat obesity. Table 23.3–7 lists the drugs currently available. Drug treatment is effective because it suppresses appetite, but tolerance to this effect may develop after several weeks of use. An initial trial period of 4 weeks with a specific drug can be used; then, if the patient responds with weight loss, the drug can be continued to see whether tolerance develops. If a drug remains effective, it can be dispensed for a longer time until the desired weight is achieved.

The other weight-loss medication approved by the Food and Drug Administration (FDA) for long-term use (in 1999) is orlistat (Xenical), which is a selective gastric and pancreatic lipase inhibitor that reduces the absorption of dietary fat (which is then excreted in stool). In clinical trials orlistat (120 mg, three times a day), in combination with a low-calorie diet, induced losses of approximately 10 percent of initial weight in the first 6 months, which were generally well maintained for periods up to 24 months. Because of its peripheral mechanism of action, orlistat is generally free of the central nervous system effects (i.e., increased pulse, dry mouth, insomnia, etc.) that are associated with most weight-loss medications. The principal adverse effects of orlistat are gastrointestinal; patients must consume 30 percent or fewer calories from fat to prevent adverse events that include oily stool, flatulence with discharge, and fecal urgency. Sibutramine (Meridia) is a β-phenylethylamine that inhibits the reuptake of serotonin and norepinephrine (and dopamine to a limited extent). It was approved by the FDA in 1997 for weight loss and the maintenance of weight loss (i.e., long-term use).

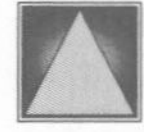

Table 23.3–7
Drugs for the Treatment of Obesity

Generic Name	Trade Name(s)	Usual Dosage Range (mg/day)
Amphetamine and dextroamphetamine	Biphetamine	12.5–20
Methamphetamine	Desoxyn	10–15
Benzphetamine	Didrex	75–150
Phendimetrazine	Bontril, Plegine, Prelu-2, X-Trozine	105
Phentermine		
Hydrochloride	Adipex-P, Fastin, Oby-trim	18.75–37.5
Resin	Ionamin	15–30
Diethylpropion hydrochloride	Tenuate	75
Mazindol	Sanorex, Mazanor	3–9
Sibutramine	Meridia	10–15
Orlistat	Xenical	360

Rimonabant. Dopamine receptor agonists, or sympathomimetics, are among the most widely used appetite suppressants. An alternative to psychostimulants, rimonabant, has a unique mechanism of action: It is a selective cannabinoid-1 receptor (CB1) blocker. Rimonabant has been shown to reduce body weight and improve cardiovascular risk factors in obese patients. The effects of rimonabant on metabolic risk factors have been studied in clinical trials of high-risk patients who are overweight or obese and have dyslipidemia. At a dose of 20 mg rimonabant causes significant weight loss, reduction in waist circumference, increase in HDL cholesterol, and reduction in triglycerides. At that dose it also increases in plasma adiponectin levels. Adiponectin is a protein hormone that modulates glucose regulation and fatty acid catabolism. Adiponectin is exclusively secreted from adipose tissue and its plasma levels are inversely correlated with body mass index (BMI). It appears to help suppress metabolic abnormalities that lead to type 2 diabetes, obesity, and atherosclerosis. Rimonabant has not been studied in patients with psychiatric disorders. It should thus be used with caution in that population since the most frequent adverse events resulting in discontinuation of the drug in clinical trials were nausea, depression, and anxiety. However, since weight gain is such a common side effect of many psychiatric drugs, and the use of rimonabant to mitigate drug-induced metabolic disturbances may be justified in some patients.

Surgery

Surgical methods that cause malabsorption of food or reduce gastric volume have been used in persons who are markedly obese. *Gastric bypass* is a procedure in which the stomach is made smaller by transecting or stapling one of the stomach curvatures. In *gastroplasty* the size of the stomach stoma is reduced so that the passage of food slows. Results are successful, although vomiting, electrolyte imbalance, and obstruction may occur. A syndrome called dumping, which consists of palpitations, weakness, and sweating may follow surgical procedures in some patients if they ingest large amounts of carbohydrates in a single meal. The surgical removal of fat (lipectomy) has no effect on weight loss in the long run nor does liposuction (Fig. 23.3–4) which has value only for cosmetic reasons. Bariatric surgery is now recommended in individuals who have serious obesity-related health complications and a BMI of greater than 35 kg/m^2 (or a BMI >40 kg/m^2 in the absence of major health complications). Before surgery, candidates should have tried to lose weight using the safer, more traditional options of diet, exercise, and weight loss medication.

Psychotherapy

The psychological problems of obese persons vary, and there is no particular personality type that is obese. Some patients may respond to insight-oriented psychodynamic therapy with weight loss, but this treatment has not had much success. Uncovering the unconscious causes of overeating may not alter the behavior of persons who overeat in response to stress although it may

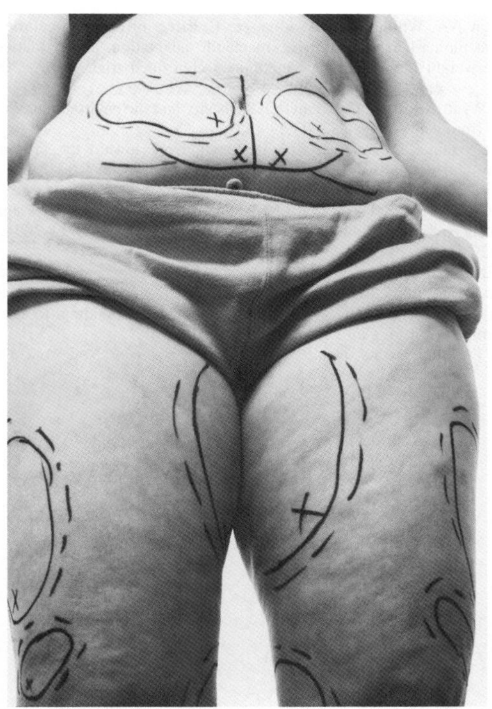

FIGURE 23.3–4
Woman with liposuction markings prior to surgery. (Courtesy of Corbis.)

serve to augment other treatment methods. Years after successful psychotherapy many persons who overeat under stress continue to do so. Obese persons seem particularly vulnerable to overdependency on a therapist and the inordinate regression that may occur during the uncovering psychotherapies should be carefully monitored.

Behavior modification has been the most successful of the therapeutic approaches for obesity and is considered the method of choice. Patients are taught to recognize external cues that are associated with eating and to keep diaries of foods consumed in particular circumstances, such as at the movies or while watching television, or during certain emotional states, such as anxiety or depression. Patients are also taught to develop new eating patterns, such as eating slowly, chewing food well, not reading while eating, and not eating between meals or when not seated. Operant conditioning therapies that use rewards such as praise or new clothes to reinforce weight loss have also been successful. Group therapy helps to maintain motivation, to promote identification among members who have lost weight, and to provide education about nutrition.

Comprehensive Approach

The National Heart, Lung, and Blood Institute formulated key recommendations for patients and the public regarding weight loss. These are listed in Table 23.3–8.

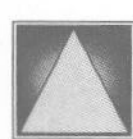

Table 23.3–8
Key Recommendations for Healthy Weight (formulated from the Obesity Education Institute, National Institute of Health)

- Weight loss to lower elevated blood pressure in overweight and obese persons with high blood pressure.
- Weight loss to lower elevated levels of total cholesterol, LDL-cholesterol, and triglycerides, and to raise low levels of HDL-cholesterol in overweight and obese persons with dyslipidemia.
- Weight loss to lower elevated blood glucose levels in overweight and obese persons with type 2 diabetes.
- Use the BMI to classify overweight and obesity and to estimate relative risk of disease compared to normal weight.
- The waist circumference should be used to assess abdominal fat content.
- The initial goal of weight loss therapy should be to reduce body weight by about 10 percent from baseline. With success, and if warranted, further weight loss can be attempted.
- Weight loss should be about 1 to 2 pounds per week for a period of 6 months, with the subsequent strategy based on the amount of weight lost.
- Low calorie diets (LCD) for weight loss in overweight and obese persons. Reducing fat as part of an LCD is a practical way to reduce calories.
- Reducing dietary fat alone without reducing calories is not sufficient for weight loss. However, reducing dietary fat, along with reducing dietary carbohydrates, can help reduce calories.
- A diet that is individually planned to help create a deficit of 500 to 1,000 kcal/day should be an integral part of any program aimed at achieving a weight loss of 1 to 2 pounds per week.
- Physical activity should be part of a comprehensive weight loss therapy and weight control program because it: (1) modestly contributes to weight loss in overweight and obese adults, (2) may decrease abdominal fat, (3) increases cardiorespiratory fitness, and (4) may help with maintenance of weight loss.
- Physical activity should be an integral part of weight loss therapy and weight maintenance. Initially, moderate levels of physical activity for 30 to 45 minutes, 3 to 5 days a week, should be encouraged. All adults should set a long-term goal of accumulate at least 30 minutes or more of moderate-intensity physical activity on most, and preferably all, days of the week.
- The combination of a reduced calorie diet and increased physical activity is recommended since it produces weight loss that may also result in decreases in abdominal fat and increases in cardiorespiratory fitness.
- Behavior therapy is a useful adjunct when incorporated into treatment for weight loss and weight maintenance.
- Weight loss and weight maintenance therapy should employ the combination of LCD's, increased physical activity, and behavior therapy.
- After successful weight loss, the likelihood of weight loss maintenance is enhanced by a program consisting of dietary therapy, physical activity, and behavior therapy, which should be continued indefinitely. Drug therapy can also be used. However, drug safety and efficacy beyond 1 year of total treatment have not been established.
- A weight maintenance program should be a priority after the initial 6 months of weight loss therapy.

References

Brownell KD, Battle Horgen K. *Food Fight: The Inside Story of the Food Industry, America's Obesity Crisis, and What We Can Do About It.* New York: McGraw-Hill; 2004.

Brownell KD, Wadden TA, Phelan S. Obesity. In: Sadock BJ, Sadock VA, eds. *The Comprehensive Textbook of Psychiatry*. 8th ed. Baltimore: Lippincott Williams & Wilkins; 2004.

Cummings DE, Shannon MH. Roles for ghrelin in the regulation of appetite and body weight. *Arch Surg*. 2003;138:389.

Fairburn CG, Brownell KD. *Eating Disorders and Obesity: A Comprehensive Handbook*. New York: Guilford; 2002.

Flegal KM, Graubard BI, Williamson DF, Gail MH. Excess deaths associated with underweight, overweight, and obesity. *JAMA*. 2005;293:1861–1867.

Foster GD, Wyatt HR, Hill JO, McGuckin BG, Brill C, Mohammed BS, Szapary PO, Rader DJ, Edman JS, Klein S. A randomized trial of a low-carbohydrate diet for obesity. *N Engl J Med*. 2003;348:2082.

Heilbronn LK, De Jonge L, Frisard MI, Delany JP, Larson-Meyer DE, Rood J, Nguyen T, Martin CK, Volavfova J, Most MK, Greenway FL, Smith SR, Deutsch WA, Williamson DA, Ravussin E. Effect of 6-month calorie restriction on biomarkers of longevity, metabolic adaptation, and oxidative stress in overweight individuals: A randomized controlled trial. *JAMA*. 2006;295: 1539.

Hill JO, Wyatt HR, Reed GW, Peters JC. Obesity and the environment: Where do we go from here? *Science*. 2003;299:853.

Neumark-Sztainer D. Can we simultaneously work toward the prevention of obesity and eating disorders in children and adolescents? *Int J Eat Disord*. 2005;38:220–227.

Ogden CL, Carroll MD, Curtin LR, McDowell MA, Tabak CJ, Flegal KM. Prevalence of overweight and obesity in the United States, 1999–2004. *JAMA*. 2006;295:1549.

Taylor EN, Stampfer MJ, Curhan GC. Obesity, weight gain, and the risk of kidney stones. *JAMA*. 2005;293(4):455–462.

Wadden TA, Brownell KD, Foster GD. Obesity: Responding to the global epidemic. *J Consult Clin Psychol*. 2002;70:510.

Wadden TA, Stunkard AJ. *Handbook of Obesity Treatment*. New York: Guilford; 2002.

24 Normal Sleep and Sleep Disorders

▲ 24.1 Normal Sleep

Sleep is a universal behavior that has been demonstrated in every animal species studied, from insects to mammals. It is one of the most significant of human behaviors, occupying roughly one third of human life. Although the exact functions of sleep are still unknown, it is clearly necessary for survival, because prolonged sleep deprivation leads to severe physical and cognitive impairment and, finally, death. Sleep is particularly relevant to psychiatry, because sleep disturbances occur in virtually all psychiatric illnesses and are frequently part of the diagnostic criteria for specific disorders.

The ancient Greeks ascribed the need for sleep to the god Hypnos (sleep) and his son Morpheus, also a creature of the night, who brought dreams in human forms. The dreams have played an important role in psychoanalysis. Freud believed the dreams to be the "royal road to the unconscious." They have figured prominently in art and literature from ancient times to the present (Fig. 24.1–1).

ELECTROPHYSIOLOGY OF SLEEP

Sleep is made up of two physiological states: non-rapid eye movement (NREM) sleep and rapid eye movement (REM) sleep. In NREM sleep, which is composed of stages 1 through 4, most physiological functions are markedly lower than in wakefulness. REM sleep is a qualitatively different kind of sleep, characterized by a high level of brain activity and physiological activity levels similar to those in wakefulness. About 90 minutes after sleep onset, NREM yields to the first REM episode of the night. This REM latency of 90 minutes is a consistent finding in normal adults; shortening of REM latency frequently occurs with such disorders as depressive disorders and narcolepsy.

For clinical and research applications, sleep is typically scored in epochs of 30 seconds, with stages of sleep defined by the visual scoring of three parameters: electroencephalogram (EEG), electrooculogram (EOG), and electromyogram (EMG) recorded beneath the chin. The EEG records the rapid conjugate eye movements that are the identifying feature of the sleep state (no or few rapid eye movements occur in NREM sleep); the EEG pattern consists of low-voltage, random, fast activity with sawtooth waves; the EMG shows a marked reduction in muscle tone (Fig. 24.1–2). The criteria defined by Allan Rechtschaffen and Anthony Kales in 1968 are accepted in clinical practice and for research around the world (Table 24.1–1).

In normal persons, NREM sleep is a peaceful state relative to waking. The pulse rate is typically slowed five to ten beats a minute below the level of restful waking and is very regular. Respiration is similarly affected, and blood pressure also tends to be low, with few minute-to-minute variations. The body musculature resting muscle potential is lower in REM sleep than in a waking state. Episodic, involuntary body movements are present in NREM sleep. There are few, if any, REMs and seldom do any penile erections occur in men. Blood flow through most tissues, including cerebral blood flow, is slightly reduced.

The deepest portions of NREM sleep—stages 3 and 4—are sometimes associated with unusual arousal characteristics. When persons are aroused 30 minutes to 1 hour after sleep onset—usually in slow-wave sleep—they are disoriented, and their thinking is disorganized. Brief arousals from slow-wave sleep are also associated with amnesia for events that occur during the arousal. The disorganization during arousal from stage 3 or stage 4 may result in specific problems, including enuresis, somnambulism, and stage 4 nightmares or night terrors.

Polygraphic measures during REM sleep show irregular patterns, sometimes close to aroused waking patterns. Otherwise, if researchers were unaware of the behavioral stage and happened to be recording a variety of physiological measures (aside from muscle tone) during REM periods, they undoubtedly would conclude that the person or animal they were studying was in an active waking state. Because of this observation, REM sleep has also been termed *paradoxical sleep*. Pulse, respiration, and blood pressure in humans are all high during REM sleep—much higher than during NREM sleep and often higher than during waking. Even more striking than the level or rate is the variability from minute to minute. Brain oxygen use increases during REM sleep. The ventilatory response to increased levels of carbon dioxide (CO_2) is depressed during REM sleep, so that no increase in tidal volume occurs as the partial pressure of carbon dioxide (PCO_2) increases. Thermoregulation is altered during REM sleep. In contrast to the homoeothermic condition of temperature regulation during wakefulness or NREM sleep, a poikilothermic condition (a state in which animal temperature varies with the changes in the temperature of the surrounding medium) prevails during REM sleep. Poikilothermia, which is characteristic of reptiles, results in a failure to respond to changes in ambient temperature with shivering or sweating, whichever is appropriate to maintaining body temperature. Almost every REM period in men is accompanied by a partial or full penile erection. This finding is clinically significant in evaluating the cause of impotence; the nocturnal penile tumescence study is one of the most commonly requested sleep laboratory tests. Another physiological change that occurs during REM sleep is the near-total paralysis of the skeletal (postural) muscles. Because of this motor inhibition,

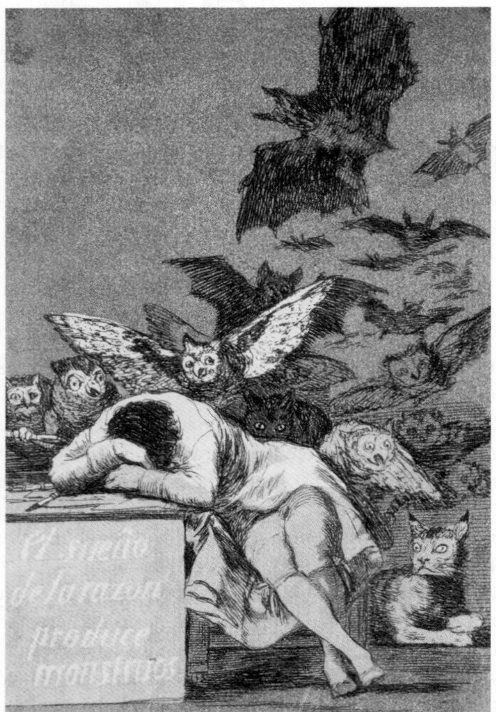

FIGURE 24.1–1
The Sleep of Reason Produces Monsters by Francisco de Goya (1746–1828). This print is number 43 from the series *Los Caprichos* by Francisco de Goya. Goya understood that unconscious mental processes were released during sleep. (Courtesy of Corbis.)

body movement is absent during REM sleep. Probably the most distinctive feature of REM sleep is dreaming. Persons awakened during REM sleep frequently (60 to 90 percent of the time) report that they had been dreaming. Dreams during REM sleep are typically abstract and surreal. Dreaming does occur during NREM sleep, but it is typically lucid and purposeful.

The cyclical nature of sleep is regular and reliable; a REM period occurs about every 90 to 100 minutes during the night (Fig. 24.1–3). The first REM period tends to be the shortest, usually lasting less than 10 minutes; later REM periods may last 15 to 40 minutes each. Most REM periods occur in the last third of the night, whereas most stage 4 sleep occurs in the first third of the night.

These sleep patterns change over a person's life span. In the neonatal period, REM sleep represents more than 50 percent of total sleep time, and the EEG pattern moves from the alert state directly to the REM state without going through stages 1 through 4. Newborns sleep about 16 hours a day, with brief periods of wakefulness. By 4 months of age, the pattern shifts so that the total percentage of REM sleep drops to less than 40 percent, and entry into sleep occurs with an initial period of NREM sleep. By young adulthood, the distribution of sleep stages is as follows:

NREM (75 percent)
Stage 1: 5 percent
Stage 2: 45 percent
Stage 3: 12 percent
Stage 4: 13 percent
REM (25 percent)

This distribution remains relatively constant into old age, although a reduction occurs in both slow-wave sleep and REM sleep in older persons.

SLEEP REGULATION

Most researchers think that there is not one simple sleep control center but a small number of interconnecting systems or centers that are located chiefly in the brainstem and that mutually activate and inhibit one another. Many studies also support the role of serotonin in sleep regulation. Prevention of serotonin synthesis or destruction of the dorsal raphe nucleus of the brainstem, which contains nearly all the brain's serotonergic cell bodies, reduces sleep for a considerable time. Synthesis and release of serotonin by serotonergic neurons are influenced by the availability of amino acid precursors of this neurotransmitter, such as L-tryptophan. Ingestion of large amounts of L-tryptophan (1 to 15 g) reduces sleep latency and nocturnal awakenings. Conversely, L-tryptophan deficiency is associated with less time spent in REM sleep. Norepinephrine-containing neurons with cell bodies located in the locus ceruleus play an important role in controlling normal sleep patterns. Drugs and manipulations that increase the firing of these noradrenergic neurons markedly reduce REM sleep (REM-off neurons) and increase wakefulness. In humans with implanted electrodes (for the control of spasticity), electrical stimulation of the locus ceruleus profoundly disrupts all sleep parameters. Brain acetylcholine is also involved in sleep, particularly in the production of REM sleep. In animal studies, the injection of cholinergic-muscarinic agonists into pontine reticular formation neurons (REM-on neurons) results in a shift from wakefulness to REM sleep. Disturbances in central cholinergic activity are associated with the sleep changes observed in major depressive disorder. Compared with healthy persons and nondepressed psychiatric controls, patients who are depressed have marked disruptions of REM sleep patterns. These disruptions include shortened REM latency (60 minutes or less), an increased percentage of REM sleep, and a shift in REM distribution from the last half to the first half of the night. Administration of a muscarinic agonist, such as arecoline, to depressed patients during the first or second NREM period results in a rapid onset of REM sleep. Depression can be associated with an underlying supersensitivity to acetylcholine. Drugs that reduce REM sleep, such as antidepressants, produce beneficial effects in depression. Indeed, about half the patients with major depressive disorder experience temporary improvement when they are deprived of sleep or when sleep is restricted. Conversely, reserpine (Serpasil), one of the few drugs that increase REM sleep, also produces depression. Patients with dementia of the Alzheimer's type have sleep disturbances characterized by reduced REM and slow-wave sleep. The loss of cholinergic neurons in the basal forebrain has been implicated as the cause of these changes. Melatonin secretion from the pineal gland is inhibited by bright light, so the lowest serum melatonin concentrations occur during the day. The suprachiasmatic nucleus of the hypothalamus may act as the anatomical site of a circadian pacemaker that regulates melatonin secretion and the entrainment of the brain to a 24-hour sleep-wake cycle. Evidence shows that dopamine has an alerting effect. Drugs that increase dopamine concentrations in the brain tend to produce arousal and wakefulness. In contrast, dopamine blockers, such as pimozide (Orap) and the phenothiazines, tend

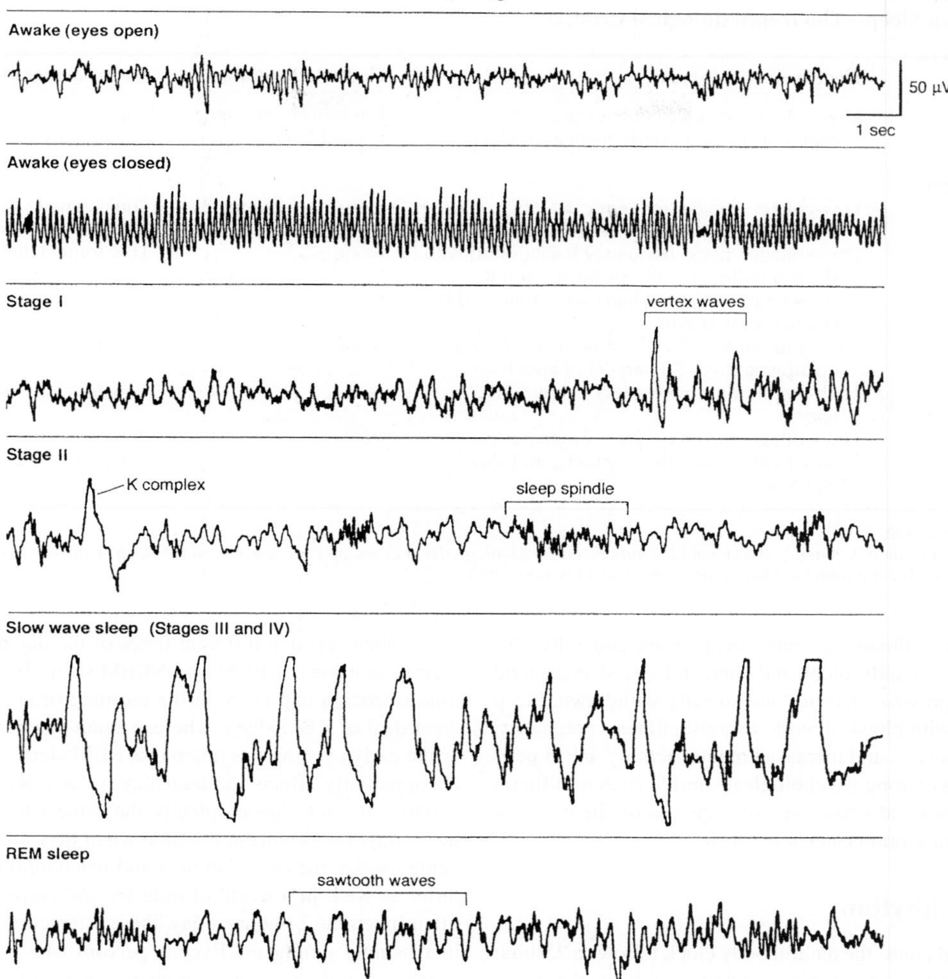

FIGURE 24.1–2
Electroencephalogram patterns for stages of human sleep and wakefulness. REM, rapid eye movement. (From Butkov N. *Atlas of Clinical Polysomnography.* Medford, OR: Synapse Media; 1996, with permission.)

to increase sleep time. A hypothesized homeostatic drive to sleep, perhaps in the form of an endogenous substance—process S—may accumulate during wakefulness and act to induce sleep. Another compound—process C—may act as a regulator of body temperature and sleep duration.

FUNCTIONS OF SLEEP

The functions of sleep have been examined in a variety of ways. Most investigators conclude that sleep serves a restorative, homeostatic function and appears to be crucial for normal thermoregulation and energy conservation. As NREM sleep increases after exercise and starvation, this stage may be associated with satisfying metabolic needs.

Sleep Deprivation

Prolonged periods of sleep deprivation sometimes lead to ego disorganization, hallucinations, and delusions. Depriving persons of REM sleep by awakening them at the beginning of REM cycles increases the number of REM periods and the amount of REM sleep (rebound increase) when they are allowed to sleep without interruption. REM-deprived patients may exhibit irritability and lethargy. In studies with rats, sleep deprivation produces a syndrome that includes a debilitated appearance, skin lesions, increased food intake, weight loss, increased energy expenditure, decreased body temperature, and death. The neuroendocrine changes include increased plasma norepinephrine and decreased plasma thyroxine levels.

Sleep Requirements

Some persons are normally short sleepers who require fewer than 6 hours of sleep each night to function adequately. Long sleepers are those who sleep more than 9 hours each night to function adequately. Long sleepers have more REM periods and more rapid eye movements within each period (known as *REM density*) than short sleepers. These movements are sometimes considered a measure of the intensity of REM sleep and are related

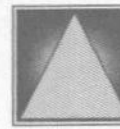

Table 24.1–1
Stages of Sleep—Electrophysiological Criteria

	Electroencephalogram	Electrooculogram	Electromyogram
Wakefulness	Low-voltage, mixed frequency activity Alpha (8–13 cps) activity with eyes closed	Eye movements and eye blinks	High tonic activity and voluntary movements
Nonrapid eye movement sleep			
Stage I	Low-voltage, mixed frequency activity Theta (3–7 cps) activity, vertex sharp waves	Slow eye movements	Tonic activity slightly decreased from wakefulness
Stage II	Low-voltage, mixed frequency background with sleep spindles (12–14 cps bursts) and K complexes (negative sharp wave followed by positive slow wave)	None	Low tonic activity
Stage III	High-amplitude (≥75 μV) slow waves (≤2 cps) occupying 20 to 50 percent of epoch	None	Low tonic activity
Stage IV	High-amplitude slow waves occupy >50% of epoch	None	Low tonic activity
REM sleep	Low-voltage, mixed frequency activity Saw-tooth waves, theta activity, and slow alpha activity	REMs	Tonic atonia with phasic twitches

REM, rapid eye movement.
Criteria from Rechtchaffen A, Kales A. *A Manual of Standardized Terminology, Techniques, and Scoring System for Sleep Stages of Human Subjects.* UCLA, Los Angeles: Brain Information Service/Brain Research Institute; 1968.

to the vividness of dreaming. Short sleepers are generally efficient, ambitious, socially adept, and content. Long sleepers tend to be mildly depressed, anxious, and socially withdrawn. Sleep needs increase with physical work, exercise, illness, pregnancy, general mental stress, and increased mental activity. REM periods increase after strong psychological stimuli, such as difficult learning situations and stress, and after the use of chemicals or drugs that decrease brain catecholamines.

Sleep-Wake Rhythm

Without external clues, the natural body clock follows a 25-hour cycle. The influence of external factors—such as the light-dark cycle, daily routines, meal periods, and other external synchronizers—entrain persons to the 24-hour clock. Sleep is also influenced by biological rhythms. Within a 24-hour period, adults sleep once, sometimes twice. This rhythm is not present at birth but develops over the first 2 years of life. Some women exhibit sleep pattern changes during the phases of the menstrual cycle. Naps taken at different times of the day differ greatly in their proportions of REM and NREM sleep. In a normal nighttime sleeper, a nap taken in the morning or at noon includes a great deal of REM sleep, whereas a nap taken in the afternoon or the early evening has much less REM sleep. A circadian cycle apparently affects the tendency to have REM sleep. Sleep patterns are not physiologically the same when persons sleep in the daytime or during the time when they are accustomed to being awake; the psychological and behavioral effects of sleep differ as well. In a world of industry and communications that often functions 24 hours a day, these interactions are becoming increasingly significant. Even in persons who work at night, interference with the various rhythms can produce problems. The best-known example is jet lag, in which, after flying east to west, persons try to convince their bodies to go to sleep at a time that is out of phase with some body cycles. Most persons adapt within a few days, but some require more time. Conditions in these persons' bodies apparently involve long-term cycle disruption and interference.

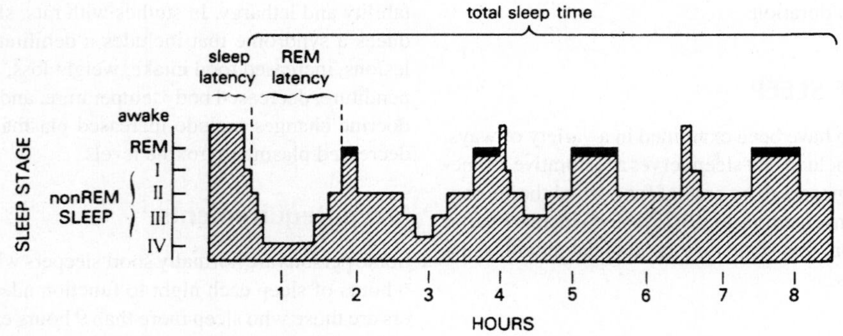

FIGURE 24.1–3
Sleep pattern in a young, healthy subject. REM, rapid eye movement. (From Gillian JC, Seifritz E, Zoltoltoski RK, Salin-Pascual RJ. Basic science of sleep. In: Sadock BJ, Sadock VA, eds. *Kaplan & Sadock's Comprehensive Textbook of Psychiatry.* 7th ed. Vol. 1. Baltimore: Lippincott Williams & Wilkins; 2000:199, with permission.)

REFERENCES

Benca RM, Cirelli C, Rattenborg NC, Tononi G. Basic science of sleep. In: Sadock BJ, Sadock VA, eds. *Kaplan & Sadock's Comprehensive Textbook of Psychiatry.* 8th ed. Vol. 1. Baltimore: Lippincott Williams & Wilkins; 2005:280.

Feldman JB. Epidemiology of sleep: Age, gender, and ethnicity. *Am J Clin Hypns.* 2005;48:58–60.

Ferri R, Bruni O, Miano S, Plazzi G, Spruyt K, Gozal D, Terzano MG. The time structure of the cyclic alternating pattern during sleep. *Sleep.* 2006;29(5):693–699.

Gillin JC, Seifritz E, Zoltoski RK, Salin-Pascual R. Basic science of sleep. In: Sadock BJ, Sadock VA, eds. *Kaplan & Sadock's Comprehensive Textbook of Psychiatry.* 7th ed. Vol. 1. Baltimore: Lippincott Williams & Wilkins; 2000:199.

Hirshkowitz M, Sharafkhaneh A. Clinical and technologic approaches to sleep evaluation. *Neurol Clin.* 2005;23:991–1005.

Richardson GS. The human circadian system in normal and disordered sleep. *J Clin Psychiatry.* 2005;66[Suppl 9]:3–9.

Roth T, Drake CL. Understanding the effects of age on "normal" human sleep. *Sleep: Journal of Sleep and Sleep Disorder Research.* 2004;27:1238–1239.

Roth T. Characteristics and determinants of normal sleep. *J Clin Psychol.* 2004;65[Suppl 16]:8–11.

Tononi G, Cirelli C. Sleep and synaptic homeostasis: A hypothesis. *Brain Res Bull.* 2003;62:2:143.

Van Dongen HP, Maislin G, Mullington JM, Dinges DF. The cumulative cost of additional wakefulness: Dose-response effects on neurobehavioral functions and sleep physiology from chronic sleep restriction and total sleep deprivation. *Sleep.* 2003;26:117.

▲ 24.2 Sleep Disorders

The text revision of the 4th edition of *Diagnostic and Statistical Manual of Mental Disorders* (DSM-IV-TR) divides primary sleep disorders into *dyssomnias* and *parasomnias*. The dyssomnias, disorders of quantity or timing of sleep, are divided into *insomnia* and *hypersomnia.* Insomnia is a perceived disturbance in the quantity or quality of sleep, which, depending on the specific condition, may be associated with disturbances in objectively measured sleep. Forms of insomnia include the primary insomnias and circadian rhythm sleep disturbances. Hypersomnias represent conditions that are clinically expressed as excessive sleepiness. Parasomnias are abnormal behaviors during sleep or the transition between sleep and wakefulness. Often, they reflect the appearance of normal sleep processes at inappropriate times. The symptoms often overlap and are described below. Table 24.2–1 lists the terms used in this section to diagnose and describe sleep disorders.

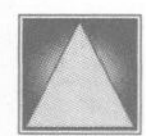

Table 24.2–1
Common Polysomnographic Measures

Sleep latency: Period of time from turning out the lights until the appearance of stage II sleep

Early morning awakening: Time of being continuously awake from the last stage of the sleep until the end of the sleep record (usually at 7 AM)

Sleep efficiency: Total sleep time or total time of the sleep record × 100

Apnea index: Number of apneas longer than 10 seconds per hour of sleep

Nocturnal myoclonus index: Number of periodic leg movements per hour

Rapid eye movement (REM) latency: Period of time from the onset of sleep until the first REM period of the night

Sleep-onset REM period: REM sleep within the first 10 minutes of sleep.

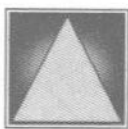

Table 24.2–2
Common Causes of Insomnia

Symptom	Insomnia Secondary to Medical Conditions	Insomnia Secondary to Psychiatric or Environmental Conditions
Difficulty falling asleep	Any painful or uncomfortable condition Central nervous system (CNS) lesions Conditions listed below, at times	Anxiety Tension anxiety, muscular Environmental changes Circadian rhythm sleep disorder
Difficulty remaining asleep	Sleep apnea syndromes Nocturnal myoclonus and restless legs syndrome Dietary factors (probably) Episodic events (parasomnias) Direct substance effects (including alcohol) Substance withdrawal effects (including alcohol) Substance interactions Endocrine or metabolic diseases Infectious, neoplastic, or other diseases Painful or uncomfortable conditions Brainstem or hypothalamic lesions or diseases Aging	Depression, especially primary depression Environmental changes Circadian rhythm sleep disorder Posttraumatic stress disorder Schizophrenia

(Courtesy of Ernest L. Hartmann, M.D.)

Insomnia

Insomnia is difficulty initiating or maintaining sleep. It is the most common sleep complaint and may be transient or persistent. Population surveys show a 1-year prevalence rate of 30 to 45 percent in adults. Common causes of insomnia are given in Table 24.2-2.

A brief period of insomnia is most often associated with anxiety, either as a sequela to an anxious experience or in anticipation of an anxiety-provoking experience (e.g., an examination or an impending job interview). In some persons, transient insomnia of this kind may be related to grief, loss, or almost any life change or stress. The condition is not likely to be serious, although a psychotic episode or a severe depression sometimes begins with acute insomnia. Specific treatment for the condition is usually not required. When treatment with hypnotic medication is indicated, both the physician and the patient should be clear that the treatment is of short duration and that some symptoms, including a brief recurrence of the insomnia, may be expected when the medication is discontinued.

Persistent insomnia is composed of a fairly common group of conditions in which the problem is most often difficulty falling asleep rather than remaining asleep. This insomnia involves two sometimes separable, but often intertwined, problems: somatized tension and anxiety, and a conditioned associative response. Patients often have no clear complaint other than insomnia. They

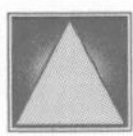

Table 24.2–3
Common Causes of Hypersomnia

Symptom	Chiefly Medical	Chiefly Psychiatric or Environmental
Excessive sleep (hypersomnia)	Kleine-Levin syndrome Menstrual-associated somnolence Metabolic or toxic conditions Encephalitic conditions Alcohol and depressant medications Withdrawal from stimulants	Depression (some) Avoidance reactions
Excessive daytime sleepiness	Narcolepsy and narcolepsy-like syndromes Sleep apneas Hypoventilation syndrome Hyperthyroidism and other metabolic and toxic conditions Alcohol and depressant medications Withdrawal from stimulants Sleep deprivation or insufficient sleep Any condition producing serious insomnia	Depression (some) Avoidance reactions Circadian rhythm sleep disorder

(Courtesy of Ernest L. Hartmann, M.D.)

may not experience anxiety per se but discharge the anxiety through physiological channels; they may complain chiefly of apprehensive feeling or ruminative thoughts that appear to keep them from falling asleep. Sometimes (but not always) a patient describes the condition's exacerbation at times of stress at work or at home and its remission during vacations.

Hypersomnia

Hypersomnia manifests as excessive amounts of sleep, excessive daytime sleepiness (somnolence), or sometimes both. The term *somnolence* should be reserved for patients who complain of sleepiness and have a clearly demonstrable tendency to fall asleep suddenly in the waking state, who have sleep attacks, and who cannot remain awake; it should not be used for persons who are simply physically tired or weary. The distinction, however, is not always clear. Complaints of hypersomnia are much less frequent (5 percent of adults) than complaints of insomnia, but they are by no means rare if clinicians are alert to them. More than 100,000 persons with narcolepsy are estimated to live in the United States, and narcolepsy is just one well-known condition that clearly produces hypersomnia. If substance-related conditions are included, hypersomnia is a common symptom.

Table 24.2–3 lists some common causes of hypersomnia. As with insomnia, hypersomnia is associated with conditions that are hard to classify and idiopathic cases. According to a recent survey, the most common conditions responsible for hypersomnia sufficiently severe to be evaluated by all-night recordings at a sleep disorders center were sleep apnea and narcolepsy.

Transient and situational hypersomnia is a disruption of the normal sleep-wake pattern; it is marked by excessive difficulty in remaining awake and a tendency to remain in bed for unusually long periods or to return to bed to nap frequently during the day. The pattern is experienced suddenly in response to an identifiable recent life change, conflict, or loss and is much less common than insomnia. It is seldom marked by definite sleep attacks or unavoidable sleep but, rather, is characterized by tiredness or by falling asleep sooner than usual and by difficulty arising in the morning.

Parasomnia

Parasomnia is an unusual or undesirable phenomenon that appears suddenly during sleep or that occurs at the threshold between waking and sleeping. Parasomnia usually occurs in stages III and IV and, thus, is associated with poor recall of the disturbance.

Sleep-Wake Schedule Disturbance. Sleep-wake schedule disturbance involves the displacement of sleep from its desired circadian period. Patients commonly cannot sleep when they wish to sleep, although they are able to sleep at other times. Correspondingly, they cannot be fully awake when they want to be fully awake, but they are able to be awake at other times. The disturbance does not precisely produce insomnia or somnolence, although the initial complaint is often either insomnia or somnolence; the inabilities to sleep and be awake are elicited only on careful questioning. Sleep-wake schedule disturbance can be considered a misalignment between sleep and wake behaviors. A sleep history questionnaire is helpful in diagnosing a patient's sleep disorder (Table 24.2–4).

CLASSIFICATION

DSM-IV-TR

The DSM-IV-TR classifies sleep disorders on the basis of clinical diagnostic criteria and presumed etiology. The three major categories of sleep disorders in DSM-IV-TR are primary sleep disorders, sleep disorders related to another mental disorder, and other sleep disorders (due to a general medical condition or are substance induced). The disorders described in DSM-IV-TR are only a fraction of the known sleep disorders; they provide a framework for clinical assessment.

ICSD

The most detailed classification of sleep disorders appears in the American Sleep Disorders Association's *International Classification of Sleep Disorders: Diagnostic and Coding Manual* (ICSD). ICSD divides sleep disorders into four categories: dyssomnias, parasomnias, sleep disorders associated with medical-psychiatric disorders, and proposed sleep disorders. Table 24.2–5 presents an outline of this classification.

ICD-10

In the 10th revision of *International Statistical Classification of Diseases and Related Health Problems* (ICD-10), the subject of sleep disorders covers only those of nonorganic type. These disorders are classified as dyssomnias, psychogenic conditions "in which the predominant

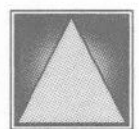

Table 24.2–4
Sleep History Questionnaire

Patient name ______________________
Date ______________________
Please check the appropriate box or give short answers for the following:

	Yes	No
1. Do you feel sleepy or have sleep attacks during the day?	☐	☐
2. Do you nap during the day?	☐	☐
3. Do you have trouble concentrating during the day?	☐	☐
4. Do you have trouble falling asleep when you first go to bed?	☐	☐
5. Do you awaken during the night?	☐	☐
6. Do you awaken more than once?	☐	☐
7. Do you awaken too early in the morning?	☐	☐
8. How long have you had trouble sleeping? What do you think precipitated the problem? ______________________		
9. How would you describe your usual night's sleep (hours of sleep, quality of sleep, etc.)? ______________________		
10. Does your schedule for sleep and rising on the weekend differ from what it is during the week?	☐	☐
11. Do others live at home who interrupt your sleep?	☐	☐
12. Are you regularly awakened at night by pain or the need to use the bathroom?	☐	☐
13. Does your job require shift changes or travel?	☐	☐
14. Do you drink caffeinated beverages (coffee, tea, or soft drinks)?	☐	☐
15. Apart from difficulty in sleeping, what, if any, other medical problems do you have? ______________________		
16. What sleep medications, prescription or nonprescription, do you take? (Please include the dosage, how often you take it, and for how many months or years you have taken it.) ______________________		
17. What other prescription and over-the-counter medications do you regularly use? (Again, please include the dosage, the frequency, and the duration.) ______________________		
18. Have you ever suffered from depression, anxiety, or similar problems?	☐	☐
19. Do you snore?	☐	☐
Questions for the sleep partner		
1. Does your sleep partner snore?	☐	☐
2. Does your sleep partner seem to stop breathing repeatedly during the night?	☐	☐
3. Does your sleep partner jerk his or her legs or kick you while he or she is sleeping?	☐	☐
4. Have you ever experienced trouble sleeping? Please explain. ______________________	☐	☐

disturbances . . . [are] in the amount, quality, or timing of sleep" because of emotional causes, and parasomnias, "abnormal episodic events occurring during sleep." The dyssomnias include insomnia, hypersomnia, and disorder of the sleep-wake schedule. The parasomnias in childhood are related to development; those in adulthood are psychogenic and include sleepwalking, sleep terrors, and nightmares. Sleep disorders of organic origin, nonpsychogenic disorders such as narcolepsy and cataplexy, and sleep apnea and episodic movement disorders are discussed under other categories.

The ICD-10 notes that sleep disorders are often symptoms of other disorders, but even when they are not, the specific sleep disorder should be diagnosed along with as many other relevant diagnoses as necessary to describe the "psychopathology and/or pathophysiology involved in a given case." Table 24.2–6 presents the ICD-10 criteria for nonorganic sleep disorders.

PRIMARY SLEEP DISORDERS

The DSM-IV-TR defines primary sleep disorders as those not caused by another mental disorder, a physical condition, or a substance but, rather, are caused by an abnormal sleep-wake mechanism and often by conditioning. The two main primary sleep disorders are dyssomnias and parasomnias. Dyssomnias are a heterogeneous group of sleep disorders that includes primary insomnia, primary hypersomnia, narcolepsy, breathing-related sleep disorder, circadian rhythm sleep disorder (sleep-wake schedule disorder), and dyssomnia not otherwise specified. Parasomnias include nightmare disorder (dream anxiety disorder), sleep terror disorder, sleepwalking disorder, and parasomnia not otherwise specified.

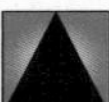

Table 24.2–5
International Classification of Sleep Disorders (ICSD)

1. Dyssomnias
   - A. Intrinsic sleep disorders
     1. Psychophysiological insomnia
     2. Sleep state misperception
     3. Idiopathic insomnia
     4. Narcolepsy
     5. Recurrent hypersomnia
     6. Idiopathic hypersomnia
     7. Posttraumatic hypersomnia
     8. Obstructive sleep apnea syndrome
     9. Central sleep apnea syndrome
     10. Central alveolar hypoventilation syndrome
     11. Periodic limb movement disorder
     12. Restless legs syndrome
     13. Intrinsic sleep disorder NOS
   - B. Extrinsic sleep disorder
     1. Inadequate sleep hygiene
     2. Environmental sleep disorder
     3. Altitude insomnia
     4. Adjustment sleep disorder
     5. Insufficient sleep syndrome
     6. Limit-setting sleep disorder
     7. Sleep-onset association disorder
     8. Food allergy insomnia
     9. Nocturnal eating (drinking) syndrome
     10. Hypnotic-dependent sleep disorder
     11. Stimulant-dependent sleep disorder
     12. Alcohol-dependent sleep disorder
     13. Toxin-induced sleep disorder
     14. Extrinsic sleep disorder NOS
   - C. Circadian rhythm sleep disorders
     1. Time zone change (jet lag) syndrome
     2. Shift work sleep disorder
     3. Irregular sleep–wake pattern
     4. Delayed sleep phase syndrome
     5. Advanced sleep phase syndrome
     6. Non-24-hour sleep–wake disorder
     7. Circadian rhythm sleep disorder NOS
2. Parasomnias
   - A. Arousal disorders
     1. Confusional arousals
     2. Sleepwalking
     3. Sleep terrors
   - B. Sleep–wake transition disorders
     1. Rhythmic movement disorder
     2. Sleep starts
     3. Sleep talking
     4. Nocturnal leg cramps
   - C. Parasomnias usually associated with REM sleep
     1. Nightmares
     2. Sleep paralysis
     3. Impaired-sleep-related penile erections
     4. Sleep-related painful erections
     5. REM-sleep-related sinus arrest
     6. REM sleep behavior disorder
   - D. Other parasomnias
     1. Sleep bruxism
     2. Sleep enuresis
     3. Sleep-related abnormal swallowing syndrome
     4. Nocturnal paroxysmal dystonia
     5. Sudden unexplained nocturnal death syndrome
     6. Primary snoring
     7. Infant sleep apnea
     8. Congenital central hypoventilation syndrome
     9. Sudden infant death syndrome
     10. Benign neonatal sleep myoclonus
     11. Other parasomnia NOS
3. Sleep disorders associated with medical-psychiatric disorders
   - A. Associated with mental disorders
     1. Psychoses
     2. Mood disorders
     3. Anxiety disorders
     4. Panic disorders
     5. Alcoholism
   - B. Associated with neurological disorders
     1. Cerebral degenerative disorders
     2. Dementia
     3. Parkinsonism
     4. Fatal familial insomnia
     5. Sleep-related epilepsy
     6. Electrical status epilepticus of sleep
     7. Sleep-related headaches
   - C. Associated with other medical disorders
     1. Sleeping sickness
     2. Nocturnal cardiac ischemia
     3. Chronic obstructive pulmonary disease
     4. Sleep-related asthma
     5. Sleep-related gastroesophageal reflux
     6. Peptic ulcer disease
     7. Fibrositis syndrome
4. Proposed sleep disorders
   1. Short sleeper
   2. Long sleeper
   3. Subwakefulness syndrome
   4. Fragmentary myoclonus
   5. Sleep hyperhidrosis
   6. Menstrual-associated sleep disorder
   7. Pregnancy-associated sleep disorder
   8. Terrifying hypnagogic hallucinations
   9. Sleep-related neurogenic tachypnea
   10. Sleep-related laryngospasm
   11. Sleep choking syndrome

NOS, not otherwise specified.

Dyssomnias

Primary Insomnia. Primary insomnia is diagnosed when the chief complaint is nonrestorative sleep or difficulty in initiating or maintaining sleep, and the complaint continues for at least a month (Table 24.2–7). (According to ICD-10, the disturbance must occur at least three times a week for a month.) The term *primary* indicates that the insomnia is independent of any known physical or mental condition. Primary insomnia is often characterized both by difficulty falling asleep and by repeated awakening. Increased nighttime physiological or psychological arousal and negative conditioning for sleep are frequently evident. Patients with primary insomnia are generally preoccupied with getting enough sleep. The more they try to sleep, the greater the sense of frustration and distress and the more elusive sleep becomes.

TREATMENT. Treatment of primary insomnia is among the most difficult problems in sleep disorders. When the conditioned component is prominent, a deconditioning technique may be useful. Patients are asked to use their beds for sleeping and for nothing else; if they are not asleep after 5 minutes in bed, they are

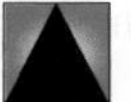

Table 24.2–6
ICD-10 Diagnostic Criteria for Nonorganic Sleep Disorders

Note: A more comprehensive classification of sleep disorders is available (*International Classification of Sleep Disorders*[a]), but it should be noted that this is organized differently from ICD-10.
For some research purposes, where particularly homogeneous groups of sleep disorders are required, four or more events occurring within a 1-year period may be considered as a criterion for use of categories sleepwalking (somnambulism), sleep terrors (night terrors), and nightmares.

Nonorganic insomnia

A. The individual complains of difficulty falling asleep, difficulty maintaining sleep, or nonrefreshing sleep.
B. The sleep disturbance occurs at least 3 times a week for at least 1 month.
C. The sleep disturbance results in marked personal distress or interference with personal functioning in daily living.
D. There is no known causative organic factor, such as a neurological or other medical condition, psychoactive substance use disorder, or a medication.

Nonorganic hypersomnia

A. The individual complains of excessive daytime sleepiness or sleep attacks or of prolonged transition to the fully aroused state upon awakening (sleep drunkenness), which is not accounted for by an inadequate amount of sleep.
B. This sleep disturbance occurs nearly every day for at least 1 month or recurrently for shorter periods of time and causes either marked distress or interference with personal functioning in daily living.
C. There are no auxiliary symptoms of narcolepsy (cataplexy, sleep paralysis, hypnagogic hallucinations) and no clinical evidence for sleep apnea (nocturnal breath cessation, typical intermittent snorting sounds, etc.).
D. There is no known causative organic factor, such as a neurological or other medical condition, psychoactive substance use disorder, or a medication.

Nonorganic disorder of the sleep–wake schedule

A. The individual's sleep–wake pattern is out of synchrony with the desired sleep–wake schedule, as imposed by societal demands and shared by most people in the individual's environment.
B. As a result of disturbance of the sleep–wake schedule, the individual experiences insomnia during the major sleep period or hypersomnia during the waking period, nearly every day for at least 1 month or recurrently for shorter periods of time.
C. The unsatisfactory quantity, quality, and timing of sleep causes either marked personal distress or interference with personal functioning in daily living.
D. There is no known causative organic factor such as a neurological or other medical condition, psychoactive substance use disorder, or a medication.

Sleepwalking (somnambulism)

A. The predominant symptom is repeated (two or more) episodes of rising from bed, usually during the first third of nocturnal sleep, and walking about for between several minutes and half an hour.
B. During an episode, the individual has a blank, staring face, is relatively unresponsive to the efforts of others to influence the event or to communicate with him or her, and can be awakened only with considerable difficulty.
C. Upon awakening (either from an episode or the next morning), the individual has amnesia for the episode.
D. Within several minutes of awakening from the episode, there is no impairment of mental activity or behavior, although there may initially be a short period of some confusion and disorientation.
E. There is no evidence of an organic mental disorder, such as dementia, or a physical disorder, such as epilepsy.

Sleep terrors (night terrors)

A. Repeated (two or more) episodes in which the individual gets up from sleep with a panicky scream and intense anxiety, body motility, and autonomic hyperactivity (such as tachycardia, heart pounding, rapid breathing, and sweating).
B. The episodes occur mainly during the first third of sleep.
C. The duration of the episode is less than 10 minutes.
D. If others try to comfort the individual during the episode, there is a lack of response followed by disorientation and preservative movements.
E. The individual has limited recall of the event.
F. There is no known causative organic factor, such as neurological or other medical condition, psychoactive substance use disorder, or a medication.

Nightmares

A. The individual wakes from nocturnal sleep or naps with detailed and vivid recall or intensely frightening dreams, usually involving threats to survival, security, or self-esteem. The awakening may occur during any part of the sleep period, but typically during the second half.
B. Upon awakening from the frightening dreams, the individual rapidly becomes oriented and alert.
C. The dream experience itself and the disturbance of sleep resulting from the awakenings associated with the episodes cause marked distress to the individual.
D. There is no known causative organic factor, such as neurological or other medical condition, psychoactive substance use disorder, or a medication.

Other nonorganic sleep disorders
Nonorganic sleep disorder, unspecified

[a]Diagnostic Classification Steering Committee: *International Classification of Sleep Disorders: Diagnostic and Coding Manual.* Rochester, MN: American Sleep Disorders Association; 1990.
(From World Health Organization. *The ICD-10 Classification of Mental and Behavioural Disorders: Diagnostic Criteria for Research.* Copyright, World Health Organization, Geneva, 1993, with permissions).

instructed simply to get up and do something else. Sometimes, changing to another bed or to another room is useful. When somatized tension or muscle tension is prominent, relaxation tapes, transcendental meditation, and practicing the relaxation response and biofeedback are occasionally helpful. Psychotherapy has not been very useful in the treatment of primary insomnia. Satisfying sexual experiences promote sleep, more so in men than in women.

THERAPY. Primary insomnia is commonly treated with benzodiazepines, zolpidem, zaleplon (Sonata), and other hypnotics. Hypnotic drugs should be used with care. Over-the-counter sleep aids have limited effectiveness. Long-acting sleep medications (e.g., flurazepam [Dalmane], quazepam [Doral]) are best for middle-of-the-night insomnia; short-acting drugs (e.g., zolpidem, triazolam [Halcion]) are useful for persons who have difficulty falling asleep. In general, sleep medications should not be

Table 24.2–7
DSM-IV-TR Diagnostic Criteria for Primary Insomnia

A. The predominant complaint is difficulty initiating or maintaining sleep, or nonrestorative sleep, for at least 1 month.
B. The sleep disturbance (or associated daytime fatigue) causes clinically significant distress or impairment in social, occupational, or other important areas of functioning.
C. The sleep disturbance does not occur exclusively during the course of narcolepsy, breathing-related sleep disorder, circadian rhythm sleep disorder, or a parasomnia.
D. The disturbance does not exclusively occur during the course of another mental disorder (e.g., major depressive disorder, generalized anxiety disorder, a delirium).
E. The disturbance is not due to the direct physiological effects of a substance (e.g., a drug of abuse, a medication) or a general medical condition.

(From American Psychiatric Association. *Diagnostic and Statistical Manual of Mental Disorders*. 4th ed. Text rev. Washington, DC: American Psychiatric Association; copyright 2000, with permission.)

prescribed for more than 2 weeks because tolerance and withdrawal may result.

Some dietary supplements used for insomnia include melatonin and L-tryptophan. Melatonin is an endogenous hormone produced by the pineal gland, which is linked to the regulation of sleep. Administration of exogenous melatonin has yielded mixed results, however, in clinical research. Melatonin's precursor L-tryptophan was used previously with the same rationale; however, in addition to having uncertain efficacy, it was found to be contaminated with a substance causing eosinophilic myalgia, a possibly deadly dyscrasia. These substances are available worldwide, however, and may be obtained by patients in the United States. Other concerns with L-tryptophan include serotonin syndrome if used in conjunction with a selective serotonin reuptake inhibitor (SSRI). Dietary supplement use has increased during the past decade.

Various nonspecific measures—so-called sleep hygiene—can help improve sleep (Table 24.2–8). Physicians must reassure

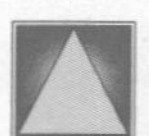

Table 24.2–8
Nonspecific Measures to Induce Sleep (Sleep Hygiene)

1. Arise at the same time daily.
2. Limit daily in-bed time to the usual amount present before the sleep disturbance.
3. Discontinue central nervous system (CNS)-acting drugs (caffeine, nicotine, alcohol, stimulants).
4. Avoid daytime naps (except when sleep chart shows they induce better night sleep).
5. Establish physical fitness by means of a graded program of vigorous exercise early in the day.
6. Avoid evening stimulation; substitute radio or relaxed reading for television.
7. Try very hot, 20-minute, body-temperature-raising bath soaks near bedtime.
8. Eat at regular times daily; avoid large meals near bedtime.
9. Practice evening relaxation routines, such as progressive muscle relaxation or meditation.
10. Maintain comfortable sleeping conditions.

patients with insomnia that their health is not at risk if they do not get 6 to 8 hours of sleep. Light therapy is also used.

INADEQUATE SLEEP HYGIENE. A common finding is that a patient's lifestyle leads to sleep disturbance. This is usually phrased as *inadequate sleep hygiene*, referring to a problem in following generally accepted practices to aid sleep. These include, for instance, keeping regular hours of bedtime and arousal, avoiding excessive caffeine, not eating heavy meals before bedtime, and getting adequate exercise. DSM-IV-TR indicates that inadequate sleep hygiene sometimes falls within the primary insomnia classification, depending on the specific sleep hygiene factor involved. Many behaviors can interfere with sleep and may do so by increasing nervous system arousal near bedtime or by altering circadian rhythms. Treatment should focus on only two or three problem areas at a time. Overwhelming the patient with too many lifestyle changes or a complex regimen seldom succeeds. Some general "dos and don'ts" are instructive.

PSYCHOPHYSIOLOGICAL INSOMNIA. Psychophysiological insomnia typically presents as a primary complaint of difficulty in going to sleep. A patient may describe this as having gone on for years and usually denies that it is associated with stressful periods in his or her life. Objects associated with sleep (e.g., the bed, the bedroom) likewise become conditioned stimuli that evoke insomnia. Thus, psychophysiological insomnia is sometimes called *conditioned insomnia*. Psychophysiological insomnia often occurs in combination with other causes of insomnia, including episodes of stress and anxiety disorders, delayed sleep phase syndrome, and hypnotic drug use and withdrawal. In contrast to the insomnia in patients with psychiatric disorders, daytime adaptation is generally good. Work and relationships are satisfying; however, extreme tiredness can exist. Other features include (1) excessive worry about not being able to sleep; (2) trying too hard to sleep; (3) rumination, inability to clear one's mind while trying to sleep; (4) increased muscle tension when attempting to sleep; (5) other somatic manifestations of anxiety; (6) being able to sleep better away from one's own bedroom; and (7) being able to fall asleep when not trying (e.g., watching TV). The sleep complaint becomes fixed over time. Interestingly, many patients with psychophysiological insomnia sleep well in the laboratory.

Treatment can be difficult. Sleeping pills should be used sparingly and at the lowest effective dose. Sleeplessness during withdrawal from long-term sleeping pill use typically exacerbates the problem. Stimulus control therapy is recommended to break the conditioning and improve the association between going to bed and being able to fall asleep. Because many patients with psychophysiological insomnia have developed poor sleep habits, improving sleep hygiene is usually beneficial if muscle tension and rumination at bedtime are prominent features; relaxation therapy is a useful ancillary treatment.

SLEEP STATE MISPERCEPTION. Sleep state misperception (also known as *subjective insomnia*) is characterized by a dissociation between the patient's experience of sleeping and the objective polygraphic measures of sleep. The ultimate cause of this dissociation is not yet understood, although it appears to be a specific case of a general phenomenon seen in many areas of medicine. Sleep state misperception is diagnosed when a patient complains of difficulty initiating or maintaining sleep and no objective evidence of sleep disruption is found. For example, a patient sleeping in the laboratory reports taking more than an hour to fall asleep, awakening more than 30 times, and sleeping less than 2 hours the entire night. By contrast, the polysomnogram shows sleep onset occurring within 15 minutes, few awakenings, a 90 percent sleep efficiency, and total sleep time exceeding 7 hours. Sleep state misperception can occur in individuals who are apparently free from psychopathology or it can represent a somatic delusion or hypochondriasis. Some patients with sleep state misperception have obsessional features concerning somatic functions. Short-term sleep state misperception can occur during periods of stress, and some clinicians believe it can result from latent or ineffectively treated anxiety or depressive disorders. Cognitive relabeling, diffusing the worry about being unable to sleep, or both can help. Interestingly, anxiolytics can profoundly reduce the perception of sleeplessness without markedly changing sleep physiologically.

IDIOPATHIC INSOMNIA. Idiopathic insomnia typically starts early in life, sometimes at birth, and continues throughout life. As the name implies, its cause is unknown; suspected causes include neurochemical imbalance in brainstem reticular formation, impaired regulation of brainstem sleep generators (e.g., raphe nuclei, locus ceruleus), or basal forebrain dysfunction. Treatment is difficult, but improved sleep hygiene, relaxation therapy, and judicious use of hypnotic medicines are reportedly helpful.

Primary Hypersomnia.

Primary hypersomnia is diagnosed when no other cause can be found for excessive somnolence occurring for at least 1 month. Some persons are long sleepers who, as with short sleepers, show a normal variation. Their sleep, although long, is normal in architecture and physiology. Sleep efficiency and the sleep-wake schedule are normal. This pattern is without complaints about the quality of sleep, daytime sleepiness, or difficulties with the awake mood, motivation, and performance. Long sleep may be a lifetime pattern, and it appears to have a familial incidence. Many persons are variable sleepers and may become long sleepers at certain times in their lives.

Some persons have subjective complaints of feeling sleepy without objective findings. They do not have a tendency to fall asleep more often than is normal and do not have any objective signs. Clinicians should try to rule out clear-cut causes of excessive somnolence. According to DSM-IV-TR, the disorder should be coded as recurrent if patients have periods of excessive sleepiness lasting at least 3 days and occurring several times a year for at least 2 years (Table 24.2–9).

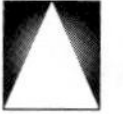

Table 24.2–9
DSM-IV-TR Diagnostic Criteria for Primary Hypersomnia

A. The predominant complaint is excessive sleepiness for at least 1 month (or less if recurrent) as evidenced by either prolonged sleep episodes or daytime sleep episodes that occur almost daily.
B. The excessive sleepiness causes clinically significant distress or impairment in social, occupational, or other important areas of functioning.
C. The excessive sleepiness is not better accounted for by insomnia and does not occur exclusively during the course of another sleep disorder (e.g., narcolepsy, breathing-related sleep disorder, circadian rhythm sleep disorder, or a parasomnia) and cannot be accounted for by an inadequate amount of sleep.
D. The disturbance does not occur exclusively during the course of another mental disorder.
E. The disturbance is not due to the direct physiological effects of a substance (e.g., a drug of abuse, a medication) or a general medical condition.

Specify if:
Recurrent: if there are periods of excessive sleepiness that last at least 3 days occurring several times a year for at least 2 years

(From American Psychiatric Association. *Diagnostic and Statistical Manual of Mental Disorders.* 4th ed. Text rev. Washington, DC: American Psychiatric Association; copyright 2000, with permission.)

A 55-year-old businessman had had excessive sleepiness since age 21, which he had described to his new family physician, who then referred him to a sleep specialist. Typically, he slept regularly from 10:15 A.M., and 1:30 P.M. and 2:00 P.M. and 8:30 P.M. When napping at work, on his office floor, he deferred all calls. He awoke temporarily refreshed. Delay of his naps caused overwhelming fatigue. He had no sudden loss of muscle tone (as in cataplexy) or other symptoms suggesting narcolepsy and neither snored nor had any other symptoms suggesting a Breathing-Related Sleep Disorder.

The patient owned a television station in Birmingham, Alabama. He was spared obligatory hard work as his staff could run the operation. Nevertheless, he was an organized, motivated person. He was in good health and jogged 4-5 miles daily. He lived with his wife and youngest son. He enjoyed socializing with his married children and their families and dabbling in local politics. He would take a longer afternoon nap in anticipation of any evening activity, which he always left early in favor of his regular bedtime.

His father had taken a nap daily after lunch, and his paternal grandfather had been excessively sleepy. During childhood the patient had had some nightmares, but no other sleep problem. He had been athletic and spontaneously ran along his paper route.

The patient drank about two beers a week, but avoided additional alcohol, caffeine, and other drugs. Previous physical exams had revealed good health, with a resting heart rate maintained in the 50s, blood pressures that ran around 110/70 to 105/70 mm Hg, normal thyroid function, and normal fasting blood sugar.

When interviewed, the patient was friendly, informative, and self-assured. He denied depressed mood or loss of interest or pleasure. He regarded his sleepiness as a difficulty with which he had come to terms, but would be grateful for further relief.

Test of daytime vigilance indicated impaired arousal. He had an average interval to sleep onset of 11 minutes during five polygraphically recorded naps, which is within the normal range. During a nighttime polygraphic recording, he had normal-appearing sleep that continued uninterrupted for $9^1/_2$ hours until he had to be awakened. (Courtesy of *DSM-IV-TR Casebook.*)

TREATMENT. Treatment of primary hypersomnia consists mainly of stimulant drugs, such as amphetamines, given in the morning or evening. Nonsedating antidepressant drugs, such as SSRIs, may be of value in some patients.

Narcolepsy.

Narcolepsy is a condition characterized by excessive sleepiness, as well as auxiliary symptoms that represent the intrusion of aspects of REM sleep into the waking

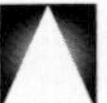

Table 24.2–10
DSM-IV-TR Diagnostic Criteria for Narcolepsy

A. Irresistible attacks of refreshing sleep that occur daily over at least 3 months.
B. The presence of one or both of the following:
  (1) cataplexy (i.e., brief episodes of sudden bilateral loss of muscle tone, most often in association with intense emotion)
  (2) recurrent intrusions of elements of rapid eye movement (REM) sleep into the transition between sleep and wakefulness, as manifested by either hypnopompic or hypnagogic hallucinations or sleep paralysis at the beginning or end of sleep episodes
C. The disturbance is not due to the direct physiological effects of a substance (e.g., a drug of abuse, a medication) or another general medical condition.

(From American Psychiatric Association. *Diagnostic and Statistical Manual of Mental Disorders.* 4th ed. Text rev. Washington, DC: American Psychiatric Association; copyright 2000, with permission.)

state (Table 24.2–10). The sleep attacks of narcolepsy represent episodes of irresistible sleepiness, leading to perhaps 10 to 20 minutes of sleep, after which the patient feels refreshed, at least briefly. They can occur at inappropriate times (e.g., while eating, talking, or driving and during sex). The REM sleep includes hypnagogic and hypnopompic hallucinations, cataplexy, and sleep paralysis. The appearance of REM sleep within 10 minutes of sleep onset (sleep-onset REM periods) is also considered evidence of narcolepsy. The disorder can be dangerous because it can lead to automobile and industrial accidents.

Narcolepsy is not as rare as was once thought. It is estimated to occur in 0.02 to 0.16 percent of adults and shows some familial incidence. Narcolepsy is neither a type of epilepsy nor a psychogenic disturbance. It is an abnormality of the sleep mechanisms—specifically, REM-inhibiting mechanisms—and it has been studied in dogs, sheep, and humans. Narcolepsy can occur at any age, but it most frequently begins in adolescence or young adulthood, generally before the age of 30. The disorder either progresses slowly or reaches a plateau that is maintained throughout life.

The most common symptom is sleep attacks: Patients cannot avoid falling asleep. Often associated with the problem (close to 50 percent of long-standing cases) is cataplexy, a sudden loss of muscle tone, such as jaw drop, head drop, weakness of the knees, or paralysis of all skeletal muscles with collapse. Patients often remain awake during brief cataplectic episodes; the long episodes usually merge with sleep and show the electroencephalographic (EEG) signs of REM sleep.

Other symptoms include hypnagogic or hypnopompic hallucinations, which are vivid perceptual experiences, either auditory or visual, occurring at sleep onset or on awakening. Patients are often momentarily frightened, but within a minute or two they return to an entirely normal frame of mind and are aware that nothing was actually there.

Another uncommon symptom is sleep paralysis, most often occurring on awakening in the morning; during the episode, patients are apparently awake and conscious but unable to move a muscle. If the symptom persists for more than a few seconds, as it often does in narcolepsy, it can become extremely uncomfortable. (Isolated brief episodes of sleep paralysis occur in many

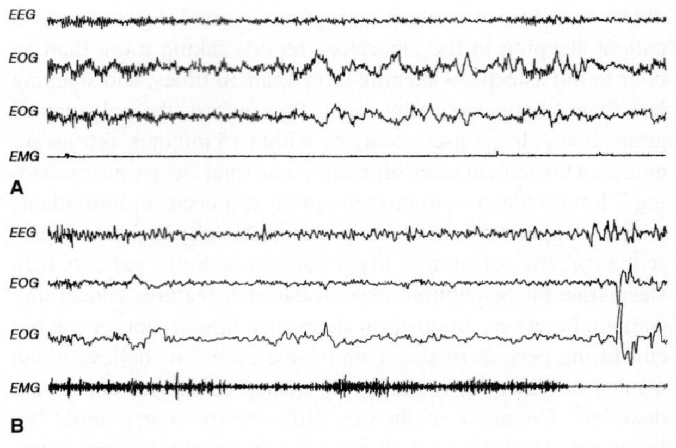

FIGURE 24.2–1
Polygraphic tracing comparing normal sleep onset with that of a patient with narcolepsy. Each panel illustrates approximately 30 seconds of polysomnographic recording beginning with relaxed wakefulness. **A:** (Normal sleep progression) shows reduced encephalographic (EEG) alpha activity and development of slow rolling eye movements. **B:** Shows the normally expected abatement of EEG alpha activity associated with increased theta activity and the appearance of a few slow eye movements. However, within 25 seconds (*far right of figure*) a swift loss of muscle tone occurs accompanied by rapid eye movements (REM). This appearance of sleep-onset REM sleep characterizes narcolepsy and is part of the diagnostic criteria. (Courtesy of Constance A. Moore, M.D., Robert W. Williams, M.D. and Max Hirshkowitz, Ph.D.)

nonnarcoleptic persons.) Patients with narcolepsy report falling asleep quickly at night but often experience broken sleep.

When the diagnosis is not clinically clear, a nighttime polysomnographic recording reveals a characteristic sleep-onset REM period (Fig. 24.2–1). A test of daytime multiple sleep latency (several recorded naps at 2-hour intervals) shows rapid sleep onset and usually one or more sleep-onset REM periods. A type of human leukocyte antigen called HLA-DR2 is found in 90 to 100 percent of patients with narcolepsy and only 10 to 35 percent of unaffected persons. One recent study showed that patients with narcolepsy are deficient in the neurotransmitter hypocretin, which stimulates appetite and alertness. Another study found that the number of hypocretin neurons (Hrct cells) in narcoleptics is 85 to 95 percent lower than in nonnarcoleptic brains.

TREATMENT. No cure exists for narcolepsy, but symptom management is possible. A regimen of forced naps at a regular time of day occasionally helps patients with narcolepsy and, in some cases, the regimen alone, without medication, can almost cure the condition. When medication is required, stimulants are most commonly used.

Modafinil (Provigil), an α_1-adrenergic receptor agonist, has been approved by the US Food and Drug Administration (FDA) to reduce the number of sleep attacks and to improve psychomotor performance in narcolepsy. This observation suggests the involvement of noradrenergic mechanisms in the disorder. Modafinil lacks some of the adverse effects of traditional psychostimulants. Nonetheless, the clinician must monitor its use and be sensitive to developing tolerance.

Sleep specialists often prescribe tricyclic drugs or SSRIs to reduce cataplexy. This approach capitalizes on the REM sleep-suppressant

Table 24.2–11
DSM-IV-TR Diagnostic Criteria for Breathing-Related Sleep Disorder

A. Sleep disruption, leading to excessive sleepiness or insomnia, that is judged to be due to a sleep-related breathing condition (e.g., obstructive or central sleep apnea syndrome or central alveolar hypoventilation syndrome).
B. The disturbance is not better accounted for by another mental disorder and is not due to the direct physiological effects of a substance (e.g., a drug of abuse, a medication) or another general medical condition (other than a breathing-related disorder).

Coding note: Also code sleep-related breathing disorder on Axis III.

(From American Psychiatric Association. *Diagnostic and Statistical Manual of Mental Disorders.* 4th ed. Text rev. Washington, DC: American Psychiatric Association; copyright 2000, with permission.)

properties of these drugs. Because cataplexy is presumably an intrusion of REM sleep phenomena into the awake state, the rationale is clear. Many reports indicate that imipramine (Tofranil), modafinil (Provigil), and fluoxetine are effective in reducing or eliminating cataplexy. Although drug therapy is the treatment of choice, the overall therapeutic approach should include scheduled naps, lifestyle adjustment, psychological counseling, drug holidays to reduce tolerance, and careful monitoring of drug refills, general health, and cardiac status.

Breathing-Related Sleep Disorder. Breathing-related sleep disorder is characterized by sleep disruption leading to excessive sleepiness or insomnia caused by a sleep-related breathing disturbance (Table 24.2–11). Breathing disturbances that can occur during sleep include apneas, hypopneas, and oxygen desaturations. These disturbances invariably cause hypersomnia. Two disorders of the respiratory system that can produce hypersomnia are sleep apnea and central alveolar hypoventilation. Both disorders can also cause insomnia, but more commonly produce hypersomnia.

Obstructive Sleep Apnea Syndrome. Obstructive sleep apnea (OSA) is characterized by periods of functional obstruction of the upper airway during sleep, resulting in decreases in arterial oxygen saturation and a transient arousal, after which respiration (at least briefly) resumes normally. It tends to occur in patients who snore, although most snorers do not have sleep apnea, and results in a sensation that sleep has not been refreshing. Many, although by far not all, patients are overweight, and it appears more frequently in patients with smaller jaws or true micrognathia, acromegaly, and hypothyroidism. Studies of the upper airway suggest that, as a group, these patients have smaller airways than normal sleepers, but there is a great deal of overlap. Medical consequences include cardiac arrhythmias, systemic and pulmonary hypertension, and decreased sexual drive or function. The exact relationship of obesity, OSA, and hypertension is a matter under investigation, some arguing that hypertension is a consequence of OSA, whereas others believe that OSA and hypertension can best be viewed as difficulties arising from a common etiology, including obesity. It tends to be an illness of middle age, primarily in men, but can occur at any age, including children.

On the polysomnograrm, episodes of OSA in adults are characterized by multiple periods of at least 10 seconds in duration in which nasal and oral airflow ceases completely (an apnea) or partially (a hypopnea), while the abdominal and chest expansion leads indicate continuing efforts of the diaphragm and accessory muscles of respiration to move air through the obstruction (Fig. 24.2–2). The arterial oxygen saturation drops and, often is seen a bradycardia that may be accompanied by other arrhythmias, such as premature ventricular contractions. At the end, an arousal reflex takes place, seen as a waking signal and possibly, as a motor artifact on the EEG channels. At this moment, sometimes called the *breakthrough*, the patient can be observed making brief restless movements in bed. The patient then returns to sleep, with normal respirations. These events can occur in NREM or REM sleep, the former usually more frequently, the latter usually more severely.

Central sleep apnea (CSA), which tends to occur in the elderly, results from periodic failure of central nervous system (CNS) mechanisms that stimulate breathing. The original teaching was that OSA results in a complaint of excessive sleepiness, whereas CSA is manifest as insomnia, but later case series have emphasized that either symptom may appear in either disorder. The polysomnogramic features of CSA are similar to those of OSA, except that, during the periods of apnea, a cessation of respiratory effort is seen in the abdominal and chest expansion leads.

Several features of OSA and CSA are significant in psychiatric practice. These include decreased ability to concentrate, decreased libido, memory complaints, and deficits in neuropsychological testing. Many or even most patients have dysthymic features and, although many patients manifest OSA and major depression, it is not certain that they occur more often than would be seen by chance. One study has indicated that, among patients with OSA, those with a history of treatment for affective disorder show greater decrements in ventilatory measurements. Although systematic data are minimal, many clinicians believe that if OSA is found and treated in cases of refractory depression, the depressive symptoms may improve. Neuropsychological testing indicates that most, but not all, deficits can be relieved by treatment.

Patients sometimes awaken from apneas with a sensation of being unable to breathe, and these episodes need to be distinguished from nocturnal panic attacks. In taking a history, it should be noted that perhaps one third of patients with daytime panic attacks also have these episodes during sleep, but it is rare to have panic attacks purely at night. Similar awakenings can occur in cases of paradoxical vocal cord movement: in this situation, however, there is usually a history of trauma or surgery of the neck. Sleep apnea episodes also need to be distinguished from nocturnal laryngospasm, in which patients report that they are unable to speak or can only whisper for a few minutes after awakening.

Nasal continuous positive airway pressure (nCPAP) is the treatment of choice for OSA (Fig. 24.2–3). Other procedures include weight loss, nasal surgery, tracheostomy, and uvulopalatoplasty. Some medications may normalize sleep in patients with apnea. SSRIs and heterocyclic antidepressant drugs sometimes help treat sleep apnea by decreasing the amount of time spent in REM sleep, the stage of sleep in which apneic episodes occur most often. In addition, theophylline has been shown to decrease the number of episodes of apnea; however, it may interfere with the overall quality of sleep, limiting its general utility. When

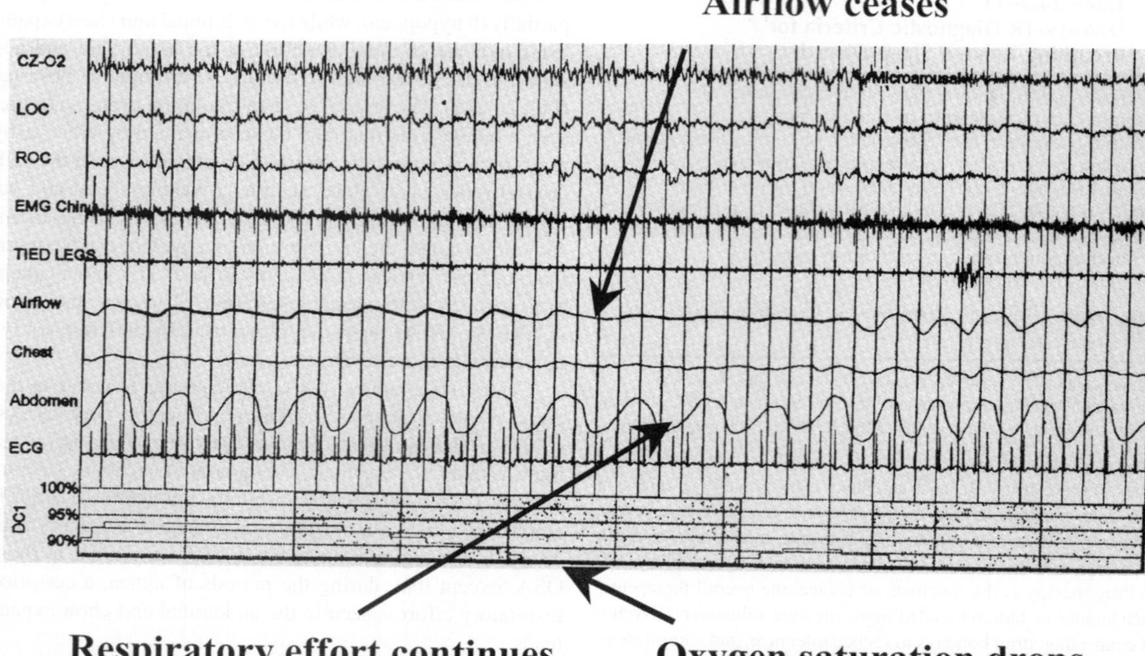

FIGURE 24.2–2
Example of an obstructive sleep apnea event on polysomnogram. CZ-O2, electroencephalogram channel; ECG, electrocardiogram; EMG, electromyogram; LOC, left electroculogram; ROC, right electroculogram.

sleep apnea is established or suspected, patients must avoid the use of sedative medication, including alcohol, because it can considerably exacerbate the condition, which may then become life threatening.

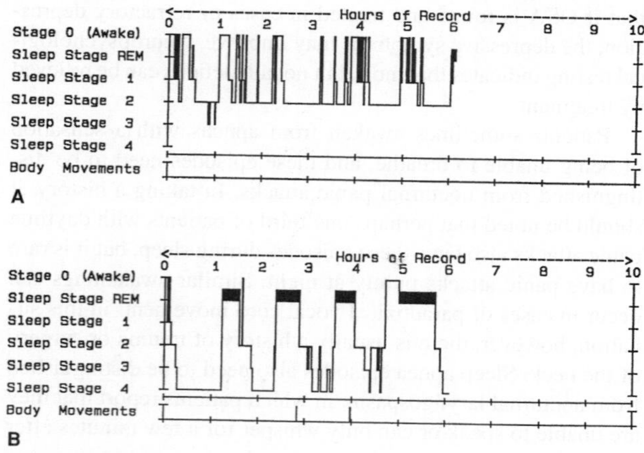

FIGURE 24.2–3
Sleep stage histogram illustrating the immediate, dramatic improvement in sleep architecture produced be treating obstructive sleep apnea with continuous positive airway pressure (CPAP) therapy. **A:** Illustrates the abnormal sleep pattern on a night when the patient had more than 200 episodes of obstructive sleep apnea. Sleep is disturbed by frequent awakenings while rapid eye movement (REM) and slow-wave (stages III and IV) sleep are nearly absent. **B:** Data from the same patient being treated with CPAP on the next night. Normalization of sleep continuity with a massive rebound in REM and slow-wave sleep is evident. (Courtesy of Constance A. Moore, M.D., Robert L. Williams, M.D., and Max Hirshkowitz, Ph. D.)

Central Alveolar Hypoventilation. Central alveolar hypoventilation refers to several conditions marked by impaired ventilation in which the respiratory abnormality appears or greatly worsens only during sleep and in which no significant apneic episodes are present. The ventilatory dysfunction is characterized by inadequate tidal volume or respiratory rate during sleep. Death may occur during sleep (Ondine's curse). Central alveolar hypoventilation is treated with some form of mechanical ventilation (e.g., nasal ventilation).

Circadian Rhythm Sleep Disorder. Circadian rhythm sleep disorder includes a wide range of conditions involving a misalignment between desired and actual sleep periods. DSM-IV-TR lists four types of circadian rhythm sleep disorders: delayed sleep phase type, jet lag type, shift work type, and unspecified (Table 24.2–12).

DELAYED SLEEP PHASE TYPE. In delayed sleep-phase syndrome, the circadian system is operating in a delayed, but stable, relationship to the day-night cues of the external world. It is marked by sleep and wake times that are intractably later than desired, actual sleep times at virtually the same daily clock hour, no reported difficulty in maintaining sleep once begun, and an inability to advance the sleep phase by enforcing conventional sleep and wake times. The patients' major complaint is often the difficulty of falling asleep at a desired conventional time, and their disorder may appear to be similar to sleep onset insomnia. Daytime sleepiness often occurs secondary to sleep loss.

The first major therapy for delayed sleep-phase syndrome is chronotherapy, in which the patient is instructed to shift his or her hours of sleep and waking progressively later each night,

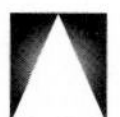

Table 24.2–12
DSM-IV-TR Diagnostic Criteria for Circadian Rhythm Sleep Disorder

A. A persistent or recurrent pattern of sleep disruption leading to excessive sleepiness or insomnia that is due to a mismatch between the sleep-wake schedule required by a person's environment and his or her circadian sleep-wake pattern.
B. The sleep disturbance causes clinically significant distress or impairment in social, occupational, or other important areas of functioning.
C. The disturbance does not occur exclusively during the course of another sleep disorder or other mental disorder.
D. The disturbance is not due to the direct physiological effects of a substance (e.g., a drug of abuse, a medication) or a general medical condition.

Specify type:

Delayed sleep phase type: a persistent pattern of late sleep onset and late awakening times, with an inability to fall asleep and awaken at a desired earlier time
Jet lag type: sleepiness and alertness that occur at an inappropriate time of day relative to local time, occurring after repeated travel across more than one time zone
Shift work type: insomnia during the major sleep period or excessive sleepiness during the major awake period associated with night shift work or frequently changing shift work
Unspecified type

(From American Psychiatric Association. *Diagnostic and Statistical Manual of Mental Disorders.* 4th ed. Text rev. Washington, DC: American Psychiatric Association; copyright 2000, with permission.)

until he or she has moved around the clock to a point at which he or she has a more traditional bedtime. An alternative approach is bright-light therapy in which the patient is exposed to bright artificial light in the early morning.

JET LAG TYPE. Depending on the length of the east-to-west trip and individual sensitivity, jet lag sleep disorder usually disappears spontaneously in 2 to 7 days; no specific treatment is required. Some persons find that they can prevent the symptoms by altering their mealtimes and sleep times in an appropriate direction before traveling. Others find that what appear to be symptoms of jet lag (fatigue and so on) are actually associated with sleep deprivation and that simply obtaining enough sleep helps. Melatonin taken orally at prescribed times is useful for some persons. Maximizing light exposure during the new daytime and minimizing light during the new nighttime are also helpful.

SHIFT WORK TYPE. Shift work can induce sleep disturbances, as well as other difficulties, including accidents because of sleepiness during nighttime working hours and, in more extreme cases, a *shift-work syndrome* characterized by gastrointestinal (GI) and cardiovascular disorders. A common experience among night shift workers is to come home in the early morning, to go to bed feeling exhausted, to sleep only 2 to 3 hours, and to awaken feeling unrefreshed but unable to continue sleeping. The treatments for shift work are complex and vary with the type of work schedule. Various strategies, including napping before going into work in the evening or taking a scheduled nap during nighttime work hours, may be helpful. Using bright light at night and avoiding light during the day have been proposed. It may be helpful, for instance, for a night-shift worker driving home in the morning to wear sunglasses, so as not to get a large light exposure immediately before going to bed. It has been demonstrated that using circadian principles to design industrial work schedules can reduce absenteeism and medical difficulties. Treatment with melatonin has been found to be less successful than timed bright light exposure in aiding adjustment to shift work.

A particular problem occurs in the training of physicians, who are often required to work 36 to 48 hours without sleeping. This condition is dangerous to both doctors and their patients. It behooves medical educators to develop more shifts for doctors in training.

UNSPECIFIED

Advanced Sleep Phase Syndrome. The advanced sleep phase syndrome is characterized by sleep onsets and wake times that are intractably earlier than desired, actual sleep times at virtually the same daily clock hour, no reported difficulty in maintaining sleep once begun, and an inability to delay the sleep phase by enforcing conventional sleep and wake times. Unlike delayed sleep phase type, the condition does not interfere with the work or school day. The major presenting complaint is the inability to stay awake in the evening and to sleep in the morning until desired conventional times. It is particularly common in the elderly, who have a phase advance of approximately 1 hour in terms of their temperature and melatonin rhythms. This condition can be treated by administering bright light in the early evening, resulting in a phase delay of the pacemaker, such that the sleep-wake signal is in closer concert with traditional hours for bedtime and arising.

Disorganized Sleep-Wake Pattern. Disorganized sleep-wake pattern is defined as irregular, variable sleep and waking behavior that disrupts the regular sleep-wake pattern. The condition is associated with frequent daytime naps at irregular times and excessive bed rest. Sleep at night is not adequately long, and the condition may seem to be insomnia, although the total amount of sleep in 24 hours is normal for the patient's age.

Dyssomnia Not Otherwise Specified.

According to DSM-IV-TR, dyssomnia not otherwise specified includes insomnias, hypersomnias, and circadian rhythm disturbances that do not meet the criteria for any specific dyssomnia (Table 24.2–13).

PERIODIC LIMB MOVEMENT SYNDROME. Periodic limb movement syndrome (PLMS) (also known as *nocturnal myoclonus*) consists of highly stereotyped abrupt contractions of certain leg muscles during sleep. These movements include extension of the toes, as well as flexion of the ankle and knee. The patient is usually unaware that these movements occur, although the bed partner may be only too aware. The result of these events is usually insomnia, although hypersomnia may also appear. The condition is associated with renal disease, as well as iron and vitamin B_{12} anemia; some investigators believe that it is exacerbated by tricyclic antidepressants, although there are differing views regarding this issue. The disorder tends to be a problem of middle age in both sexes, with increasing frequency with advancing age.

On the polysomnogram, periodic limb movements are 0.5 to 5.0 seconds in duration and occur every 20 to 40 seconds (Fig. 24.2–4) during periods of NREM sleep. Often, they are accompanied by a K-complex or brief arousal signal in the EEG

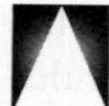

Table 24.2–13
DSM-IV-TR Diagnostic Criteria for Dyssomnia Not Otherwise Specified

The dyssomnia not otherwise specified category is for insomnias, hypersomnias, or circadian rhythm disturbances that do not meet criteria for any specific dyssomnia. Examples include

1. Complaints of clinically significant insomnia or hypersomnia that are attributable to environmental factors (e.g., noise, light, frequent interruptions).
2. Excessive sleepiness that is attributable to ongoing sleep deprivation.
3. "Restless legs syndrome": This syndrome is characterized by a desire to move the legs or arms, associated with uncomfortable sensations typically described as creeping, crawling, tingling, burning, or itching. Frequent movements of the limbs occur in an effort to relieve the uncomfortable sensations. Symptoms are worse when the individual is at rest and in the evening or night, and they are relieved temporarily by movement. The uncomfortable sensations and limb movements can delay sleep onset, awaken the individual from sleep, and lead to daytime sleepiness or fatigue. Sleep studies demonstrate involuntary periodic limb movements during sleep in a majority of individuals with restless legs syndrome. A minority of individuals have evidence of anemia or reduced serum iron stores. Peripheral nerve electrophysiological studies and gross brain morphology are usually normal. Restless legs syndrome can occur in an idiopathic form, or it can be associated with general medical or neurological conditions, including normal pregnancy, renal failure, rheumatoid arthritis, peripheral vascular disease, or peripheral nerve dysfunction. Phenomenologically, the two forms are indistinguishable. The onset of restless legs syndrome is typically in the second or third decade, although up to 20% of individuals with this syndrome may have symptoms before age 10. The prevalence of restless legs syndrome is between 2% and 10% in the general population and as high as 30% in general medical populations. Prevalence increases with age and is equal in males and females. Course is marked by stability or worsening of symptoms with age. There is a positive family history in 50%–90% of individuals. The major differential diagnoses include medication-induced akathisia, peripheral neuropathy, and nocturnal leg cramps. Worsening at night and periodic limb movements are more common in restless legs syndrome than in medication-induced akathisia or peripheral neuropathy. Unlike restless legs syndrome, nocturnal leg cramps do not present with the desire to move the limbs nor are there frequent limb movements.
4. Periodic limb movements: Periodic limb movements are repeated low-amplitude brief limb jerks, particularly in the lower extremities. These movements begin near sleep onset and decrease during stage 3 or 4 non-rapid eye movement (NREM) and rapid eye movement (REM) sleep. Movements usually occur rhythmically every 20–60 seconds and are associated with repeated, brief arousals. Individuals are often unaware of the actual movements, but may complain of insomnia, frequent awakenings, or daytime sleepiness if the number of movements is very large. Individuals may have considerable variability in the number of periodic limb movements from night to night. Periodic limb movements occur in the majority of individuals with restless legs syndrome, but they may also occur without the other symptoms of restless legs syndrome. Individuals with normal pregnancy or with conditions such as renal failure, congestive heart failure, and posttraumatic stress disorder may also develop periodic limb movements. Although typical age at onset and prevalence in the general population are unknown, periodic limb movements increase with age and may occur in more than one-third of individuals over age 65. Men are more commonly affected than women.
5. Situations in which the clinician has concluded that a dyssomnia is present but is unable to determine whether it is primary, due to a general medical condition, or substance induced.

(From American Psychiatric Association. *Diagnostic and Statistical Manual of Mental Disorders.* 4th ed. Text rev. Washington, DC: American Psychiatric Association; copyright 2000, with permission.)

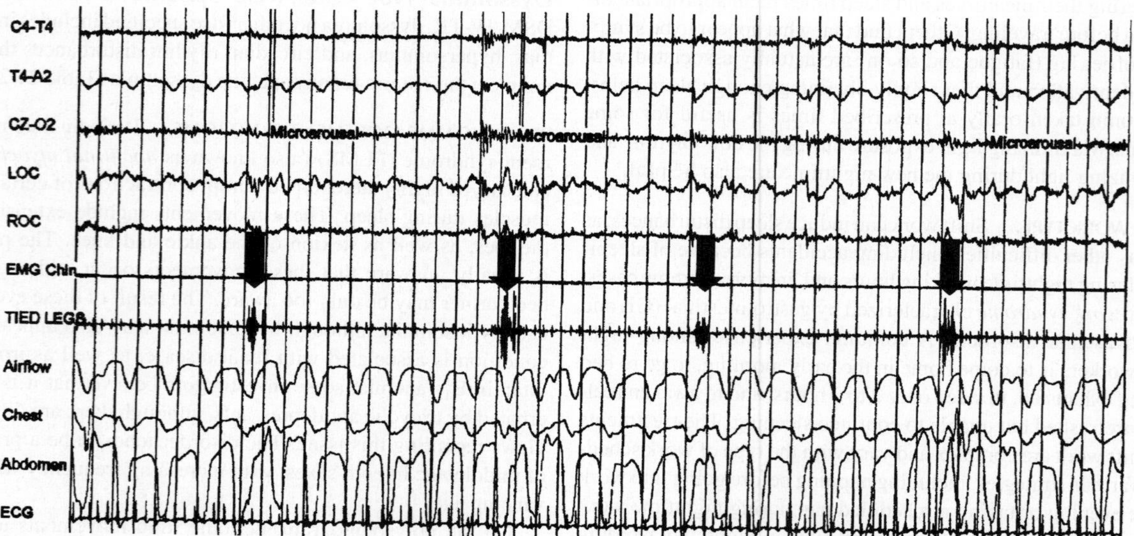

FIGURE 24.2–4

Example of periodic leg movements (*arrows*) seen on the polysomnogram. CZ-O2, electroencephalogram channel; ECG, electrocardiogram; EMG, electromyogram; LOC, left electroculogram; ROC, right electroculogram.

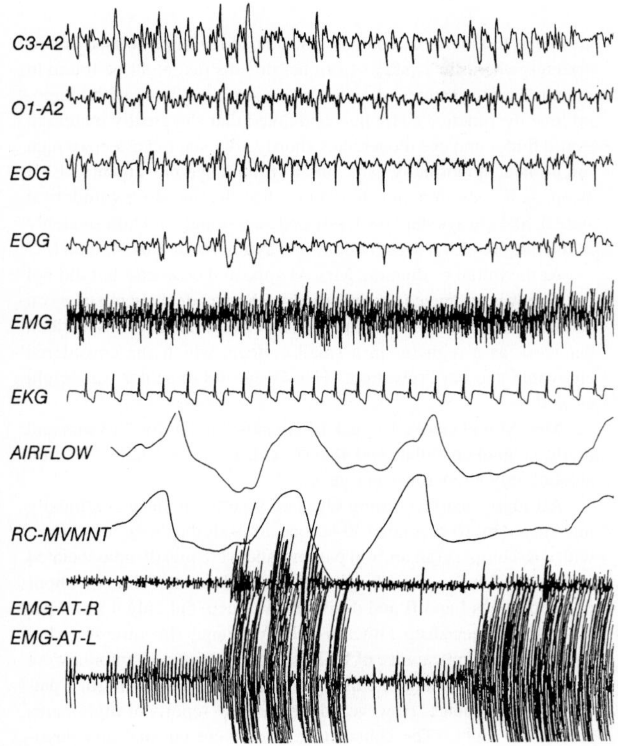

FIGURE 24.2–5

Restless legs syndrome. This patient presented with complaints of uncomfortable, crawling sensations in the legs when trying to fall asleep. Patients commonly report an urge to move the leg to dispel the sensation. This figure shows a bilateral pattern of leg electromyogram (EMG) activity; however, the discharge is more pronounced in the left anterior tibialis (*EMG-AT-L*) than the right (*EMG-AT-R*). This pattern continued for more than an hour as the patient attempted to fall asleep; note that the sharp activity in central and occipital encephalogram (EEG) (*C3 – A2* and *O1 – A2*, respectively) and electroculogram (EOG) is an electrocardiographic (ECG) artifact and not an EEG abnormality. (Courtesy of Constance A. Moore, M.D., Robert L. Williams, M.D., and Max Hirshkowitz, Ph. D.)

channels of a polysomnogram. Clinicians differ to whether to count only those that are accompanied by EEG evidence of arousal or to count all PLMs regardless of EEG consequences. A diagnosis of PLMS requires a PLM index of at least five per hour. No treatment for nocturnal myoclonus is universally effective. Treatments that may be useful include benzodiazepines, levodopa (Larodopa), quinine, and, in rare cases, opioids.

RESTLESS LEGS SYNDROME. Restless limbs syndrome (RLS) (also known as *Ekbom syndrome*) is an uncomfortable, subjective sensation of the limbs, usually the legs, sometimes described as a "creepy crawly" feeling or as the sensation of ants walking on the skin. It tends to be worse at night, and is relieved by walking or moving about (Fig. 24.2–5). It appears as a cause of sleep initiation insomnia, because the patient may find it difficult to lie still in bed, needing to get up to relieve the discomfort. The ultimate cause is unknown, but it appears often in pregnancy, iron or vitamin B_{12} deficiency anemia, and renal disease.

The first step in treatment is looking for anemia and treating it, if found. Benzodiazepines are relatively ineffective. The off-label use of L-dopa and carbidopa (Sinemet), bromocriptine (Parlodel), and pergolide (Permax) is often helpful. In rare patients who are severely affected, the off-label use of narcotic analgesics can help when other treatments have been tried and have failed. Ropinirole (Requip), a dopamine agonist already available for treatment of Parkinson's disease, is now the first drug approved by the FDA for treatment of moderate to severe RLS.

KLEINE-LEVIN SYNDROME. Kleine-Levin syndrome is a relatively rare condition consisting of recurrent periods of prolonged sleep (from which patients may be aroused) with intervening periods of normal sleep and alert waking. During the hypersomniac episodes, wakeful periods are usually marked by withdrawal from social contacts and return to bed at the first opportunity; patients may also display apathy, irritability, confusion, voracious eating, loss of sexual inhibitions, delusions, hallucinations, frank disorientation, memory impairment, incoherent speech, excitation or depression, and truculence. Unexplained fevers have occurred in a few such patients.

Kleine-Levin syndrome is uncommon. About 100 cases with features suggesting the diagnosis have been reported. In most cases, several periods of hypersomnia, each lasting for one or several weeks, are experienced by patients over a year. With few exceptions, the first attack occurs between the ages of 10 and 21 years. Rare instances of onset in the fourth and fifth decades of life have been reported. The syndrome appears to be almost invariably self-limited, and enduring remission occurs spontaneously before age 40 in early-onset cases.

MENSTRUAL-ASSOCIATED SYNDROME. Some women experience intermittent marked hypersomnia, altered behavioral patterns, and voracious eating at, or shortly before, the onset of their menses. Nonspecific EEG abnormalities similar to those associated with Kleine-Levin syndrome have been documented in several instances. Endocrine factors are probably involved, but no specific abnormalities in laboratory endocrine measures have been reported. Increased cerebrospinal fluid (CSF) serotonin levels were found in one patient.

SLEEP DISTURBANCE IN PREGNANCY. Sleep disturbance is common in pregnant women. Several hormonal factors contribute to this disturbance, including changes in levels of estrogen, progesterone, cortisol, and melatonin from baseline. In addition, changes in maternal respiratory physiology, body habitus, and, in the third trimester, movements of the fetus can all act to diminish the quantity and quality of sleep.

INSUFFICIENT SLEEP. Insufficient sleep is defined as an earnest complaint of daytime sleepiness and associated waking symptoms by a person who persistently fails to obtain sufficient daily sleep to support alert wakefulness. The person is voluntarily, but often unwittingly, chronically sleep deprived. The diagnosis can usually be made on the basis of the history, including a sleep log. Some persons, especially students and shift workers, who want to maintain an active daytime life and perform their nighttime jobs, may seriously deprive themselves of sleep and, thus, produce somnolence during waking hours.

SLEEP DRUNKENNESS. Sleep drunkenness is an abnormal form of awakening in which the lack of a clear sensorium in the transition from sleep to full wakefulness is prolonged and exaggerated. A confusional state develops that often leads to individual or social inconvenience and sometimes to criminal acts. The diagnosis requires the absence of sleep deprivation. It is a rare condition, and there may be a familial tendency. Before making the diagnosis, clinicians should examine patients' sleep and rule out such conditions as apnea, nocturnal myoclonus, narcolepsy, and excessive use of alcohol and other substances.

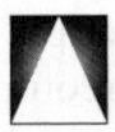

Table 24.2–14
DSM-IV-TR Diagnostic Criteria for Nightmare Disorder

A. Repeated awakenings from the major sleep period or naps with detailed recall of extended and extremely frightening dreams, usually involving threats to survival, security, or self-esteem. The awakenings generally occur during the second half of the sleep period.
B. On awakening from the frightening dreams, the person rapidly becomes oriented and alert (in contrast to the confusion and disorientation seen in sleep terror disorder and some forms of epilepsy).
C. The dream experience, or the sleep disturbance resulting from the awakening, causes clinically significant distress or impairment in social, occupational, or other important areas of functioning.
D. The nightmares do not occur exclusively during the course of another mental disorder (e.g., a delirium, posttraumatic stress disorder) and are not due to the direct physiological effects of a substance (e.g., a drug of abuse, a medication) or a general medical condition.

(From American Psychiatric Association. *Diagnostic and Statistical Manual of Mental Disorders.* 4th ed. Text rev. Washington, DC: American Psychiatric Association; copyright 2000, with permission.)

Parasomnias

Nightmare Disorder. Nightmares are vivid dreams that become progressively more anxiety producing, ultimately resulting in an awakening (Table 24.2–14). As with other dreams, nightmares almost always occur during REM sleep and usually after a long REM period late in the night. Some persons have frequent nightmares as a lifelong condition; others experience them predominantly at times of stress and illness. About 50 percent of the adult population may report occasional nightmares. No specific treatment is usually required for nightmare disorder. Agents that suppress REM sleep, such as tricyclic drugs, may reduce the frequency of nightmares, and benzodiazepines have also been used. Contrary to popular belief, no harm results from awakening a person who is having a nightmare.

Mrs. M, a 35-year-old woman, had nightmares every night, beginning in her early teenage years. She came to a sleep specialist at the insistence of her husband, who was fed up with her behavior both while sleeping and while awake. One to four times a night, she awoke out of a dream, the content of which was always disturbing. Often she dreamt of yelling at other people or of menacing confrontations. In the dreams she felt angry and frustrated. Typically, she awoke from the dreams feeling extremely tense.

During the day Mrs. M often had uncontrollable outbursts of temper. These could be precipitated by minor frustrations, such as a delay in finding her eyeglasses. In the midst of an outburst she sometimes felt that it was wrong to behave thus, that her outburst was unwarranted, but she was powerless to stop it. After the outburst she apologized for it.

Mrs. M slept excessively, sometimes 12–13 hours consecutively on weekends, and often took 3-hour to 4-hour naps. She was sleepy while driving on the turnpike, but managed to stay awake by having the temperature cold and the radio "blasting."

She denied having sudden, irresistible attacks of sleepiness, cataplexy (sudden loss of motor power), hypogogic hallucinations (hallucinations while awakening), or sleep paralysis (motor weakness and brief inability to move upon sudden awakening), all of which are characteristic of narcolepsy. She denied feeling confused or disoriented when she awakens from her dreams (as might be found in impaired arousal states, such as in episodes associated with temporal lobe dysfunction). Her husband noted that she greatly increased eyelid flutter and eye movements shortly after she fell asleep (which might mean abnormally early onset of rapid eye movement [REM] sleep, as is seen in major depressive disorder and drug withdrawal states). She always slept restlessly and occasionally hit him suddenly in the middle of the night (a common symptom of Parasomnias).

At the initial evaluation, Mrs. M appeared downcast but did not cry. She was organized and informative. She made three mistakes on serial sevens, but her sensorium was otherwise intact. She described her work as a registrar in a small college, which she considered enjoyable and her "salvation." Her 4-year-old daughter was bright as well.

Mrs. M had smoked a pack of cigarettes a day for 25 years and drank a cup of chocolate and 48 oz of cola beverages daily. She took alcohol only a few times per year.

All-night sleep recording revealed 9 hours of sleep continually interrupted by 10-second to 30-second arousals that frequently began with a K-complex (an arousal pattern) and were mostly unassociated with prior body movements. These happened about 35 times per hour in sleep stages I and II and during REM sleep, but only 4 times per hour during deep sleep. Otherwise, REM latency (the time spent before the initial appearance of REM sleep), density, and amount were normal, and other stages, although interrupted, were of normal pattern and percentage. However, there were no reports of nightmares during the night. (The constant arousals were unusual and possibly related to the abnormalities noted in the electroencephalogram.) (Courtesy of *DSM-IV-TR Casebook.*)

Sleep Terror Disorder. Sleep terror disorder is an arousal in the first third of the night during deep NREM (stages III and IV) sleep. It is almost invariably inaugurated by a piercing scream or cry and accompanied by behavioral manifestations of intense anxiety bordering on panic (Table 24.2–15).

Typically, patients sit up in bed with a frightened expression, scream loudly, and sometimes awaken immediately with a sense of intense terror. Patients may remain awake in a disoriented state, but more often fall asleep, and as with sleepwalking,

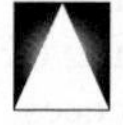

Table 24.2–15
DSM-IV-TR Diagnostic Criteria for Sleep Terror Disorder

A. Recurrent episodes of abrupt awakening from sleep, usually occurring during the first third of the major sleep episode and beginning with a panicky scream.
B. Intense fear and signs of autonomic arousal, such as tachycardia, rapid breathing, and sweating, during each episode.
C. Relative unresponsiveness to efforts of others to comfort the person during the episode.
D. No detailed dream is recalled and there is amnesia for the episode.
E. The episodes cause clinically significant distress or impairment in social, occupational, or other important areas of functioning.
F. The disturbance is not due to the direct physiological effects of a substance (e.g., a drug of abuse, a medication) or a general medical condition.

(From American Psychiatric Association. *Diagnostic and Statistical Manual of Mental Disorders.* 4th ed. Text rev. Washington, DC: American Psychiatric Association; copyright 2000, with permission.)

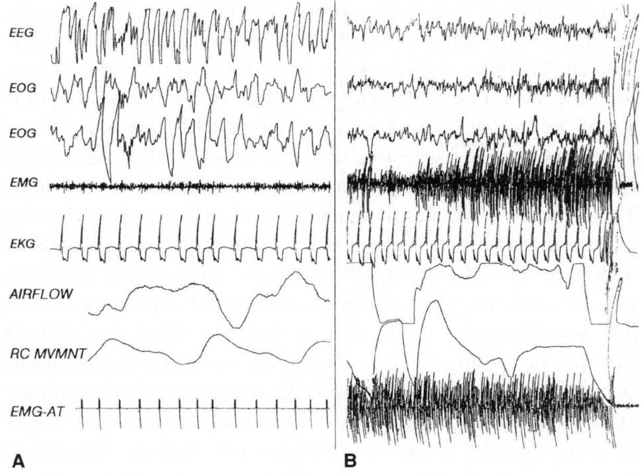

FIGURE 24.2–6

Polysomnogram of a sleep terror. **A:** Approximately 14 seconds of tracing occurring immediately before the sleep terror. Prominent encephalographic (EEG) slow-wave activity and other characteristics of stage IV sleep are seen. **B:** The awakening, accompanied by tachycardia and movement. EEG activity is ambiguous, and the patient eventually disconnected his electrodes as he thrashed about in bed (visible at *far right of figure*). Although the patient was screaming and greatly agitated, no dreaming was reported. In the morning, he had little recollection of anything having occurred during the night. (Courtesy of Constance A. Moore, M.D., Robert L. Williams, M.D., and Max Hirshkowitz, Ph. D.)

they forget the episodes. A night terror episode after the original scream frequently develops into a sleepwalking episode. Polygraphic recordings of night terrors are somewhat like those of sleepwalking; in fact, the two conditions appear to be closely related. Night terrors, as isolated episodes, are especially frequent in children. About 1 to 6 percent of children have the disorder, which is more common in boys than in girls and which tends to run in families.

Night terrors may reflect a minor neurological abnormality, perhaps in the temporal lobe or underlying structures, because when night terrors begin in adolescence and young adulthood, they turn out to be the first symptom of temporal lobe epilepsy. In a typical case of night terrors, however, no signs of temporal lobe epilepsy or other seizure disorders are seen, either clinically or on EEG recordings (Fig. 24.2–6).

Although night terrors are closely related to sleepwalking and are occasionally related to enuresis, they differ from nightmares. Night terrors are associated with simply awakening in terror. Patients generally have no dream recall but may occasionally recall a single frightening image.

Specific treatment for night terror disorder is seldom required. Investigation of stressful family situations may be important, and individual or family therapy is sometimes useful. In the rare cases when medication is required, diazepam (Valium) in small doses at bedtime improves the condition and sometimes completely eliminates the attacks.

Sleepwalking Disorder. Sleepwalking, also known as *somnambulism*, consists of a sequence of complex behaviors that are initiated in the first third of the night during deep NREM (stage III and IV) sleep and frequently, although not always, progress—without full consciousness or later memory of the episode—to leaving bed and walking about (Table 24.2–16).

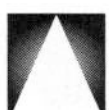

Table 24.2–16
DSM-IV-TR Diagnostic Criteria for Sleepwalking Disorder

A. Repeated episodes of rising from bed during sleep and walking about, usually occurring during the first third of the major sleep episode.
B. While sleepwalking, the person has a blank, staring face, is relatively unresponsive to the efforts of others to communicate with him or her, and can be awakened only with great difficulty.
C. On awakening (either from the sleepwalking episode or the next morning), the person has amnesia for the episode.
D. Within several minutes after awakening from the sleepwalking episode, there is no impairment of mental activity or behavior (although there may initially be a short period of confusion or disorientation).
E. The sleepwalking causes clinically significant distress or impairment in social, occupational, or other important areas of functioning.
F. The disturbance is not due to the direct physiological effects of a substance (e.g., a drug of abuse, a medication) or a general medical condition.

(From American Psychiatric Association. *Diagnostic and Statistical Manual of Mental Disorders.* 4th ed. Text rev. Washington, DC: American Psychiatric Association; copyright 2000, with permission.)

Patients sit up and sometimes perform preservative motor acts, such as walking, dressing, going to the bathroom, talking, screaming, and even driving. The behavior occasionally terminates in awakening, with several minutes of confusion; more frequently, the person returns to sleep without any recollection of the sleepwalking event. An artificially induced arousal from stage IV sleep can sometimes produce the condition. For instance, in children, especially those with a history of sleepwalking, an attack can sometimes be provoked by standing them on their feet and thus producing a partial arousal during stage IV sleep.

Sleepwalking usually begins between ages 4 and 8 and tends to dissipate in adolescence. Peak prevalence is at about 12 years of age. The disorder is more common in boys than in girls, and about 15 percent of children have an occasional episode. It tends to run in families. A minor neurological abnormality probably underlies the condition; the episodes should not be considered purely psychogenic, although stressful periods are associated with increased sleepwalking in affected persons. Extreme tiredness or previous sleep deprivation exacerbates attacks. The disorder is occasionally dangerous because of the possibility of accidental injury. Treatment consists primarily of educating and reassuring the parents. Although it can be exacerbated by periods of stress or sleep deprivation, in childhood, it is not associated with psychiatric illness. Some cases of sleepwalking can be induced by medication. Medical intervention is rarely needed for typical night terrors or sleepwalking. In difficult cases, some clinicians try the off-label use of benzodiazepines, which decrease slow-wave sleep. Recent reports of sleepwalking associated with the use of the sedative Zolpidem (Ambien) require further study.

An 11-year-old girl asked her mother to take her to a psychiatrist because she feared she might be "going crazy." Several times during the last 2 months she had awakened confused about where she was until she realized she was on the living room couch or in her little sister's bed, even though she went to bed in her own room. When she recently woke up in her older brother's bedroom, she became very concerned and felt quite guilty about it. Her younger sister said that she had seen the patient walking during the night, looking like a "zombie," that she didn't answer when she called her, and that the patient had done that several times, but usually went back to her bed. The patient feared she might have "amnesia" because she had no memory of anything happening during the night.

There is no history of seizures or of similar episodes during the day. An EEG and physical examination proved normal. The patient's mental status was unremarkable except for some anxiety about her symptoms and the usual early adolescent concerns. School and family functioning were excellent. (From *DSM-IV Casebook.*)

Parasomnia Not Otherwise Specified. The diagnostic criteria for parasomnia not otherwise specified are given in Table 24.2–17.

SLEEP-RELATED BRUXISM. Bruxism, tooth grinding, occurs throughout the night, most prominently in stage II sleep. According to dentists, 5 to 10 percent of the population has sufficient bruxism to produce noticeable damage to teeth. The condition often goes unnoticed by the sleepers, except for an occasional jaw ache in the morning, but bed partners and roommates are consistently awakened by the sound. Treatment consists of a dental bite plate and corrective orthodontic procedures.

REM SLEEP BEHAVIOR DISORDER. REM behavior disorder is characterized by episodes of complex, often violent, behavior and is thought to represent a patient acting out his or her dreams. It is more common in older men, and often a history exists of a small stroke or other CNS insult in the last months or year. It can also appear as an early event in the evolution of Parkinson's disease. If an episode is captured on the polygraph, it shows motor artifact appearing out of REM sleep. If a patient with REM behavior disorder does not have an episode while in the laboratory, the sleep study may show a failure of the normal hypotonia of the weight-bearing muscles during REM sleep. In cats, a syndrome that is suggestive of REM behavior disorder can be induced by lesions of the areas surrounding the locus ceruleus, a brainstem noradrenergic center. The initial view was that the clinical disorder represents a malfunction of the descending pathway to the spinal cord, which produces atonia during REM; its prevalence in the elderly and in patients with Parkinson's disease has suggested a more complex etiology involving alteration of function in pontine areas, including the nucleus pedunculopontine, where integration of sleep-wake regulation with locomotor systems takes place. The most widely used treatment for REM behavior disorder is the off-label administration of clonazepam (Klonopin), 0.5 to 2.0 mg a day. Carbamazepine, 100 mg three times a day, is also effective in controlling the disorder.

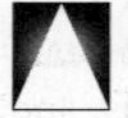

Table 24.2–17
DSM-IV-TR Diagnostic Criteria for Parasomnia Not Otherwise Specified

The parasomnia not otherwise specified category is for disturbances that are characterized by abnormal behavioral or physiological events during sleep or sleep-wake transitions, but that do not meet criteria for a more specific parasomnia. Examples include

1. REM sleep behavior disorder: motor activity, often of a violent nature, that arises during rapid eye movement (REM) sleep. Unlike sleepwalking, these episodes tend to occur later in the night and are associated with vivid dream recall.
2. Sleep paralysis: an inability to perform voluntary movement during the transition between wakefulness and sleep. The episodes may occur at sleep onset (hypnagogic) or with awakening (hypnopompic). The episodes are usually associated with extreme anxiety and, in some cases, fear of impending death. Sleep paralysis occurs commonly as an ancillary symptom of narcolepsy and, in such cases, should not be coded separately.
3. Situations in which the clinician has concluded that a parasomnia is present but is unable to determine whether it is primary, due to a general medical condition, or substance induced.

(From American Psychiatric Association. *Diagnostic and Statistical Manual of Mental Disorders.* 4th ed. Text rev. Washington, DC: American Psychiatric Association; copyright 2000, with permission.)

SLEEPTALKING (SOMNILOQUY). Sleeptalking is common in children and adults. It has been studied extensively in the sleep laboratory and is found in all stages of sleep. The talking usually involves a few words that are difficult to distinguish. Long episodes of talking involve the sleeper's life and concerns, but sleeptalkers do not relate their dreams during sleep, nor do they often reveal deep secrets. Episodes of sleeptalking sometimes accompany night terrors and sleepwalking. Sleeptalking alone requires no treatment.

SLEEP-RELATED HEAD BANGING (JACTATIO CAPITIS NOCTURNA). Sleep-related head banging is the term for a sleep behavior consisting chiefly of rhythmic to-and-fro head rocking (less commonly, total body rocking) occurring just before or during sleep. Usually, it is observed in the immediate presleep period and is sustained into light sleep. It uncommonly persists into, or occurs in, deep NREM sleep. Treatment consists of measures to prevent injury.

SLEEP PARALYSIS. Familial sleep paralysis is characterized by a sudden inability to execute voluntary movements, either just at the onset of sleep or on awakening during the night or in the morning.

SLEEP DISORDERS RELATED TO ANOTHER MENTAL DISORDER. DSM-IV-TR defines a sleep disorder related to another mental disorder as a complaint of sleep disturbance caused by a diagnosable mental disorder, but sufficiently severe to merit clinical attention on its own.

Insomnia Related to Axis I or Axis II Disorder

Insomnia that occurs for at least 1 month and is clearly related to the psychological and behavioral symptoms of the clinically well-known mental disorders is classified here (Table 24.2–18). The category consists of a heterogeneous group of conditions. The sleep problem is usually, but not always, difficulty falling asleep secondary to anxiety that is part of any of the various mental disorders listed. The insomnia is more common in women than in men. In clear-cut cases in which the anxiety has psychological roots, psychiatric treatment of the anxiety (e.g.,

Table 24.2–18
DSM-IV-TR Diagnostic Criteria for Insomnia Related to Another Mental Disorder

A. The predominant complaint is difficulty initiating or maintaining sleep, or nonrestorative sleep, for at least 1 month that is associated with daytime fatigue or impaired daytime functioning.
B. The sleep disturbance (or daytime sequelae) causes clinically significant distress or impairment in social, occupational, or other important areas of functioning.
C. The insomnia is judged to be related to another Axis I or Axis II disorder (e.g., major depressive disorder, generalized anxiety disorder, adjustment disorder with anxiety) but is sufficiently severe to warrant independent clinical attention.
D. The disturbance is not better accounted for by another sleep disorder (e.g., narcolepsy, breathing-related sleep disorder, a parasomnia).
E. The disturbance is not due to the direct physiological effects of a substance (e.g., a drug of abuse, a medication) or a general medical condition.

individual psychotherapy, group psychotherapy, or family therapy) often relieves the insomnia.

The insomnia associated with major depressive disorder involves relatively normal sleep onset, but repeated awakenings during the second half of the night and premature morning awakening (Fig. 24.2–7), usually with an uncomfortable mood in the morning. (Morning is the worst time of day for many patients with major depressive disorder.) Polysomnography shows reduced stage III and IV sleep, often a short REM latency, and a long first REM period. The use of partial or total sleep deprivation can accelerate the response to antidepressant medication.

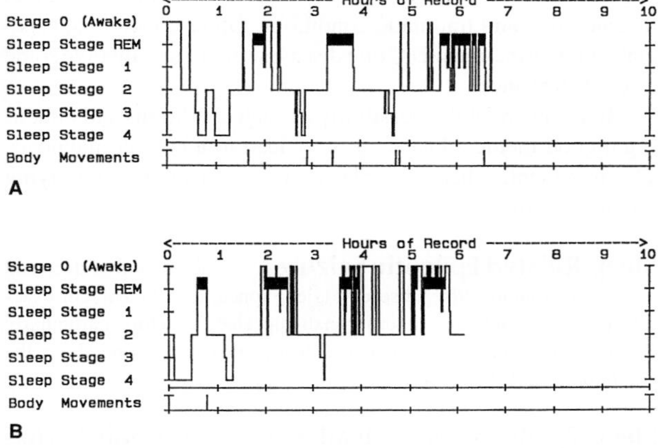

FIGURE 24.2–7
Sleep stage histograms comparing normal sleep **(A)** with that found in a patient with major depressive disorders **(B).** Difficulty maintaining sleep and early morning awakenings are common complaints in patients with depression. **B:** The electrophysiological correlates of these complaints beginning after approximately 2 hours of sleep. Sleep continuity becomes disrupted as morning approaches. Also present is a markedly reduced latency to rapid eye movement (REM) sleep, a feature characteristic of this patient population and thought by some to reflect cholinergic-aminergic imbalance. (Courtesy of Constance A. Moore, M.D., Robert L. Williams, M.D., and Max Hirshkowitz, Ph. D.)

B.A. awoke in the middle of the night gasping for breath, sweating, shaking, and experiencing palpitations. He felt his pulse; it was 120. He thought, "I could be dying." It was his third attack of the week and at least his tenth that month that had awakened him from sleep. The problem, which had begun 2 years previously when he turned 50, was getting much worse: not only was he having trouble staying asleep because of similar attacks, but after such nights he felt tired all day. He decided to take a friend's advice and seek help from the psychiatrist who specialized in sleep problems.

The psychiatrist elicited this additional history. Attacks of panic occurring during the day had begun at age 12 and had recurred every few months since that time. They did not begin to occur during sleep until the patient turned 50, 2 years earlier. A few months ago the attacks had become much rarer, after the patient had discontinued drinking the 8 to 10 beers he had drunk every weekend for most of his adult life. His weight had fallen from 227 pounds to a mildly overweight 181 pounds, and the mild hypertension he had had for several years disappeared.

In addition to the recurrent attacks, for most of his life the patient had also felt anxious in anticipation of particular situations, including being shut inside airplanes or elevators or traveling in the middle lane of a road. On a turnpike he counted the exits until he could leave, fearing that he would have a panic attack.

He described a fear of falling apart if he ever got too far from his "support system," his term for a beer cooler, which he carried with him always, although he rarely drank the beer. In anticipation of an airplane flight, however, he would drink six to eight beers. He almost always had a company employee, his son, or a friend accompany him, and particularly disliked plane flights when he was not with a familiar person. The night after he drank, the anxiety almost always occurred, awakening him from sleep.

Mr. A ran a successful auto parts business and consulted for several others. Recently, however, anxiety had prevented his accepting a huge government contract to set up an international distribution system for retail stores on military bases. He felt he would be too exposed to scrutiny and would therefore fail. He also worried that some long plane rides would be unavoidable.

During the interview Mr. A was highly verbal, informative, cheerful, friendly, and engaging. He talked about uncomfortable subjects frankly and productively. He had two sisters and two daughters who had "agoraphobia"; one of the daughters was housebound.

Initially, the patient was thought to have sleep apnea (recurrent periods of not breathing during sleep), on the basis of the loud snoring that he reported and the awakening provoked by drinking alcohol, relieved by weight loss, and the presence of mild hypertension. (From *DSM-IV-TR Casebook.*)

Panic disorder may be associated with paroxysmal awakenings or with entering stage III and IV sleep. The emotional and cognitive symptoms of a panic attack are present, along with tachycardia and increased respiratory rate. Patients with manic episodes and bipolar II disorder appear to be extreme cases of short sleepers. They sometimes appear to have difficulty falling asleep, but most often do not complain of sleep problems. They awaken refreshed after 2 to 4 hours of sleep and appear to have a true reduction in their need for sleep during the course of the manic or hypomanic episode. In schizophrenia, total sleep time and slow-wave sleep are reduced. REM sleep is often reduced early during an exacerbation. Other conditions associated with insomnia include posttraumatic stress disorder (nightmares), obsessive-compulsive disorder (rituals), and eating disorders. Attention-deficit/hyperactivity disorder (ADHD) has been linked to higher than normal rates of sleep disturbance (usually difficulty falling asleep). At times, this can be exacerbated by the patient's schedule of stimulant administration; special care should be taken when designing a medication regimen.

Hypersomnia Related to Axis I or Axis II Disorder

Hypersomnia that occurs for at least 1 month and is associated with a mental disorder is found in a variety of conditions, including mood disorders. Excessive daytime sleepiness may be reported in the initial stages of many mild depressive disorders and characteristically in the depressed phase of bipolar I disorder. For a few weeks, hypersomnia sometimes is associated with uncomplicated grief. Other mental disorders—such as personality disorders, dissociative disorders, somatoform disorders, dissociative fugue, and amnestic disorders—can produce hypersomnia (Table 24.2–19). Treatment of the primary disorder should resolve the hypersomnia.

OTHER SLEEP DISORDERS

The DSM-IV-TR defines a sleep disorder caused by a medical condition as a complaint of sleep disturbance produced by a physiological effect of the medical condition on the sleep-wake system. A substance-induced sleep disorder arises from the use, or the recently discontinued use, of a substance.

Sleep Disorder Due to a General Medical Condition

Any sleep disturbance (e.g., insomnia, hypersomnia, parasomnia, or a combination) can be caused by a general medical condition (Table 24.2–20). Almost any medical condition associated with pain and discomfort (e.g., arthritis or angina) can produce insomnia. Some conditions are associated with insomnia even when pain and discomfort are not specifically present. These conditions include neoplasms, vascular lesions, infections, and degenerative and traumatic conditions. Other conditions, especially endocrine and metabolic diseases, frequently involve some sleep disturbance.

Being aware of the possibility of such conditions and obtaining a good medical history usually lead to a correct diagnosis. The treatment, when possible, is treatment of the underlying medical condition.

Table 24.2–19
DSM-IV-TR Diagnostic Criteria for Hypersomnia Related to Another Mental Disorder

A. The predominant complaint is excessive sleepiness for at least 1 month as evidenced by either prolonged sleep episodes or daytime sleep episodes that occur almost daily.
B. The excessive sleepiness causes clinically significant distress or impairment in social, occupational, or other important areas of functioning.
C. The hypersomnia is judged to be related to another Axis I or Axis II disorder (e.g., major depressive disorder, dysthymic disorder) but is sufficiently severe to warrant independent clinical attention.
D. The disturbance is not better accounted for by another sleep disorder (e.g., narcolepsy, breathing-related sleep disorder, a parasomnia) or by an inadequate amount of sleep.
E. The disturbance is not due to the direct physiological effects of a substance (e.g., a drug of abuse, a medication) or a general medical condition.

(From American Psychiatric Association. *Diagnostic and Statistical Manual of Mental Disorders.* 4th ed. Text rev. Washington, DC: American Psychiatric Association; copyright 2000, with permission.)

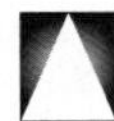

Table 24.2–20
DSM-IV-TR Diagnostic Criteria for Sleep Disorder Due to a General Medical Condition

A. A prominent disturbance in sleep that is sufficiently severe to warrant independent clinical attention.
B. There is evidence from the history, physical examination, or laboratory findings that the sleep disturbance is the direct physiological consequence of a general medical condition.
C. The disturbance is not better accounted for by another mental disorder (e.g., an adjustment disorder in which the stressor is a serious medical illness).
D. The disturbance does not occur exclusively during the course of a delirium.
E. The disturbance does not meet the criteria for breathing-related sleep disorder or narcolepsy.
F. The sleep disturbance causes clinically significant distress or impairment in social, occupational, or other important areas of functioning.

Specify type:
Insomnia type: if the predominant sleep disturbance is insomnia
Hypersomnia type: if the predominant sleep disturbance is hypersomnia
Parasomnia type: if the predominant sleep disturbance is a parasomnia
Mixed type: if more than one sleep disturbance is present and none predominates

Coding note: Include the name of the general medical condition on Axis I, e.g., sleep disorder due to chronic obstructive pulmonary disease, insomnia type; also code the general medical condition on Axis III.

(From American Psychiatric Association. *Diagnostic and Statistical Manual of Mental Disorders.* 4th ed. Text rev. Washington, DC: American Psychiatric Association; copyright 2000, with permission.)

Sleep-Related Epileptic Seizures. The relation of sleep and epilepsy is complex. Sleep disorders (sleep apnea, in particular) can exacerbate seizures. Seizures, in turn, can disrupt sleep structure, particularly REM sleep. When seizures occur almost exclusively during sleep, the condition is called *sleep epilepsy*.

Sleep-Related Cluster Headaches and Chronic Paroxysmal Hemicrania. Sleep-related cluster headaches are agonizingly severe unilateral headaches that often appear during sleep and are marked by an on-off pattern of attacks. Chronic paroxysmal hemicrania is a similar unilateral headache that occurs every day with more frequent, but short-lived, onsets that are without a preponderant sleep distribution. Both types of vascular headaches are examples of sleep-exacerbated conditions and appear in association with REM sleep periods; paroxysmal hemicrania is virtually REM sleep locked.

Sleep-Related Abnormal Swallowing Syndrome. Abnormal swallowing syndrome is a condition during sleep in which inadequate swallowing results in aspiration of saliva, coughing, and choking. It is intermittently associated with brief arousals or awakenings.

Sleep-Related Asthma. Asthma that is exacerbated by sleep in some persons can result in significant sleep disturbances.

Sleep-Related Cardiovascular Symptoms. Sleep-related cardiovascular symptoms derive from disorders of cardiac rhythm, myocardial incompetence, coronary artery insufficiency, and blood pressure variability, which may be induced or exacerbated by sleep-altered or sleep-state-modified cardiovascular physiology.

Sleep-Related Gastroesophageal Reflux. Sleep-related gastroesophageal reflux is a disorder in which patients awaken from sleep with burning, substernal pain or a feeling of general pain or tightness in the chest or a sour taste in the mouth. Coughing, choking, and vague respiratory discomfort may also occur repeatedly.

Sleep-Related Hemolysis (Paroxysmal Nocturnal Hemoglobinuria). Paroxysmal nocturnal hemoglobinuria is a rare, acquired, chronic hemolytic anemia in which intravascular hemolysis results in hemoglobinemia and hemoglobinuria. The hemolysis and consequent hemoglobinuria are accelerated during sleep, and the morning urine is brownish red. Hemolysis is linked to the sleep period, even when the period is shifted.

Substance-Induced Sleep Disorder

Any sleep disturbance (e.g., insomnia, hypersomnia, parasomnia, or a combination) can be caused by a substance (Table 24.2–21). According to DSM-IV-TR, clinicians should also specify whether the onset of the disorder occurred during intoxication or withdrawal.

Somnolence related to tolerance or withdrawal from a CNS stimulant is common in persons withdrawing from amphetamines, cocaine, caffeine, and related substances. The somnolence may be associated with severe depression, which occasionally reaches suicidal proportions. Sustained use of a CNS depressant, such as alcohol, can cause somnolence. Heavy alcohol use in the evening produces sleepiness and difficulty arising the next day. This reaction may present a diagnostic problem when patients do not admit alcohol abuse.

Insomnia is associated with tolerance to, or withdrawal from, sedative-hypnotic drugs, such as benzodiazepines, barbiturates, and chloral hydrate. With the sustained use of such agents—usually undertaken to treat insomnia arising from a different source—tolerance increases, and the drugs lose their sleep-inducing effects; patients then often increase the dosage. On sudden discontinuation of the drug, severe sleeplessness supervenes, often accompanied by the general features of substance withdrawal. Typically, patients experience a temporary increase in the severity of the insomnia.

Long-term use (more than 30 days) of a hypnotic agent is well tolerated by some patients, but others begin to complain of sleep disturbance, most often multiple brief awakenings during the night. Recordings show a disruption of sleep architecture, reduced stage III and IV sleep, increased stage I and II sleep, and fragmentation of sleep throughout the night.

Clinicians should be aware of CNS stimulants as a possible cause of insomnia and should remember that various medications for weight reduction, beverages containing caffeine, and, occasionally, adrenergic drugs taken by asthmatic patients may all produce this insomnia. Alcohol may help induce sleep, but frequently results in nocturnal awakening. Alcohol use during the cocktail hour can produce difficulty falling asleep later in the evening.

For reasons that are not always clear, a wide variety of drugs occasionally produce sleep problems as a side effect. These drugs include antimetabolites and other cancer chemotherapeutic

Table 24.2–21
DSM-IV-TR Diagnostic Criteria for Substance-Induced Sleep Disorder

A. A prominent disturbance in sleep that is sufficiently severe to warrant independent clinical attention.
B. There is evidence from the history, physical examination, or laboratory findings of either (1) or (2):
   (1) the symptoms in Criterion A developed during, or within a month of, substance intoxication or withdrawal
   (2) medication use is etiologically related to the sleep disturbance
C. The disturbance is not better accounted for by a sleep disorder that is not substance induced. Evidence that the symptoms are better accounted for by a sleep disorder that is not substance induced might include the following: the symptoms precede the onset of the substance use (or medication use); the symptoms persist for a substantial period of time (e.g., about a month) after the cessation of acute withdrawal or severe intoxication or are substantially in excess of what would be expected given the type or amount of the substance used or the duration of use; or there is other evidence that suggests the existence of an independent non–substance-induced sleep disorder (e.g., a history of recurrent non–substance-related episodes).
D. The disturbance does not occur exclusively during the course of a delirium.
E. The sleep disturbance causes clinically significant distress or impairment in social, occupational, or other important areas of functioning.

Note: This diagnosis should be made instead of a diagnosis of substance intoxication or substance withdrawal only when the sleep symptoms are in excess of those usually associated with the intoxication or withdrawal syndrome and when the symptoms are sufficiently severe to warrant independent clinical attention.

Code [Specific substance]-induced sleep disorder:
Alcohol; amphetamine; caffeine; cocaine; opioid; sedative, hypnotic, or anxiolytic; other [or unknown] substance

Specify type:
- **Insomnia type:** if the predominant sleep disturbance is insomnia
- **Hypersomnia type:** if the predominant sleep disturbance is hypersomnia
- **Parasomnia type:** if the predominant sleep disturbance is a parasomnia
- **Mixed type:** if more than one sleep disturbance is present and none predominates

Specify if:
- **With onset during intoxication:** if the criteria are met for intoxication with the substance and the symptoms develop during the intoxication syndrome
- **With onset during withdrawal:** if criteria are met for withdrawal from the substance and the symptoms develop during, or shortly after, a withdrawal syndrome

(From American Psychiatric Association. *Diagnostic and Statistical Manual of Mental Disorders.* 4th ed. Text rev. Washington, DC: American Psychiatric Association; copyright 2000, with permission) agents, thyroid preparations, anticonvulsant agents, antidepressant drugs, adrenocorticotropic hormone (ACTH)-like drugs, oral contraceptives, α-methyldopa, and β-adrenergic receptor antagonists.

Other agents do not produce sleep disturbance while being used, but may have this effect after withdrawal. Almost any sedating or tranquilizing agents, including at times the benzodiazepines, the phenothiazines, the sedating tricyclic drugs, and various street drugs, including marijuana and opioids, can have this effect.

Alcohol is a CNS depressant and produces the serious problems of other CNS depressants, both during administration—perhaps related to the development of tolerance—and after withdrawal. The insomnia after long-term alcohol consumption is sometimes severe and lasts for weeks or longer. Clinicians should not give potentially addicting medications to patients who have just recovered from an addiction; if possible, sleeping medications should be avoided.

Among cigarette smokers, the combination of a relaxing ritual and the tendency of low doses of nicotine to cause sedation may actually help sleep, but high doses of nicotine can interfere with sleep, particularly sleep onset. Cigarette smokers typically sleep less than nonsmokers. Nicotine withdrawal can cause drowsiness or arousal.

Ms. M, a 28-year-old lawyer, described her problems to a psychiatrist. She frequently felt anxious and upset around bedtime. On these nights it would take her an hour or more to fall asleep. She dreaded going to bed and would engross herself in reading murder mysteries until late hours. Her bedtime varied from 7:00 PM to 2:00 AM. On awakening in the morning, she felt groggy and incapacitated, hardly able to crawl out of bed. Some mornings she missed work completely. She slept until noon on weekends. Worry about her tardiness getting to work motivated her to seek a consultation.

Ms. M had had bronchial asthma since age 18 months. Her mother had constantly worried that Ms. M would die during the night. As a teenager Ms. M used epinephrine inhalers to remain awake until 1:00 AM to 3:00 AM, reading. She remembered her father screaming at her to turn out the lights. She always considered the late night hours, when everyone else was asleep, a "safe time," free from interference by others.

Ms. M was particularly prone to nocturnal asthma attacks, which typically occurred around 4:00 AM. Wheezing at night led to feelings of terror and fear of dying ("I feel out of control"). The current treatment for her asthma was aminophylline 400 mg/day plus 2 puffs on a beclomethasone inhaler twice daily. She also used an albuterol inhaler irregularly, sometimes at bedtime. About once a year, an exacerbation of asthma would require a short course of systemic steroids.

Ms. M drank five to eight cups of coffee daily. Alcoholic beverages precipitated wheezing and aggravated the delay in onset of sleep. Short-acting sedatives at bedtime caused a noticeable decrease in her ability to concentrate on work the following day. Evening relaxation exercises precipitated fears of being alone with a breathing problem and made her feel like "a skeleton with a pair of lungs."

During the consultation, Ms. M was articulate, smiling and cheerful and had a full range of affect. She seemed to enjoy her own idiosyncrasies. She was quite talkative, organized, and informative and easily able to discuss her feelings. She noted that it was ironic that she feared death so much yet loved to read about murders in fiction. "I guess it's been my way of feeling some sense of control." (From *DSM-IV-TR Casebook*.)

References

Anders TF. Sleep disorders in infancy through adolescence. In: Wiener JM, Dulcan MK, eds. *The American Psychiatric Publishing Textbook of Child and Adolescent Psychiatry*. 3rd ed. Washington, DC: American Psychiatric Publishing, Inc.; 2004:727–742.

Baillargeon L, Landreville P, Verreault R, Beauchemin JP, Gregoire JP, Morin CM. Discontinuation of benzodiazepines among older insomniac adults treated with cognitive-behavioural therapy combined with gradual tapering: A randomized trial. *CMAJ*. 2003;169:1015–1020.

Kamel NS, Gammack JK. Insomnia in the elderly: Cause, approach, and treatment. *Am J Med*. 2006;119(6):463–469.

Krystal A, Walsh J, Roth T, Amato DA. The sustained efficacy and safety of eszopiclone over six months of nightly treatment: A placebo-controlled study in patients with chronic insomnia. *Sleep*. 2003;26[Suppl]:A310.

Mendelson W. Sleep disorders. In: Sadock BJ, Sadock VA, eds. *Kaplan & Sadock's Comprehensive Textbook of Psychiatry*. 8th ed. Vol. 1. Baltimore: Lippincott Williams & Wilkins; 2005:2022.

Morin CM, Rodriguez S, Ivers H. Role of stress, arousal, and coping skills in primary insomnia. *Psychosom Med*. 2003;65:259–267.

Ng AT, Qian J, Cistulli PA. Oropharyngeal collapse predicts treatment response with oral appliance therapy in obstructive sleep apnea. *Sleep*. 2006;29(5):666–671.

Schmidt LE, Johnson KP, Martin A, eds. A clinical guide to pediatric sleep: Diagnosis and management of sleep problems. *J Am Acad Child Adolesc Psychiatry*. 2005;44:720–721.

Silber MH. Chronic insomnia. *N Engl J Med*. 2005;353:803–810.

Zadra A, Pilon M, Donderi DC. Variety and intensity of emotions in nightmares and bad dreams. *J Nerv Ment Dis*. 2006;194(4):249–254.

25 Impulse-Control Disorders Not Elsewhere Classified

Six conditions comprise the category of *impulse-control disorders, not elsewhere specified.* They include (1) intermittent explosive disorder, (2) kleptomania, (3) pyromania, (4) pathological gambling, (5) trichotillomania, and (6) impulse-control disorder not otherwise specified (NOS). Each disorder is characterized by the inability to resist an intense impulse, drive, or temptation to perform a particular act that is obviously harmful to self or others, or both. Before the event, the individual usually experiences mounting tension and arousal, sometimes—but not consistently—mingled with conscious anticipatory pleasure. Completing the action brings immediate gratification and relief. Within a variable time afterward, the individual experiences a conflation of remorse, guilt, self-reproach, and dread. These feelings may stem from obscure unconscious conflicts or awareness of the deed's impact on others (including the possibility of serious legal consequences in syndromes such as kleptomania). Shameful secretiveness about the repeated impulsive activity frequently expands to pervade the individual's entire life, often significantly delaying treatment.

Etiology

Psychodynamic, psychosocial, and biological factors all play an important role in impulse-control disorders; however, the primary causal factor remains unknown. Some impulse-control disorders may have common underlying neurobiological mechanisms. Fatigue, incessant stimulation, and psychic trauma can lower a person's resistance to control impulses.

Psychodynamic Factors

An impulse is a disposition to act to decrease heightened tension caused by the buildup of instinctual drives or by diminished ego defenses against the drives. The impulse disorders have in common an attempt to bypass the experience of disabling symptoms or painful affects by acting on the environment. In his work with adolescents who were delinquent, August Aichhorn described impulsive behavior as related to a weak superego and weak ego structures associated with psychic trauma produced by childhood deprivation.

Otto Fenichel linked impulsive behavior to attempts to master anxiety, guilt, depression, and other painful affects by means of action. He thought that such actions defend against internal danger and that they produce a distorted aggressive or sexual gratification. To observers, impulsive behaviors may appear irrational and motivated by greed, but they may actually be endeavors to find relief from pain.

Heinz Kohut considered many forms of impulse-control problems, including gambling, kleptomania, and some paraphiliac behaviors, to be related to an incomplete sense of self. He observed that when patients do not receive the validating and affirming responses that they seek from persons in significant relationships with them, the self might fragment. As a way of dealing with this fragmentation and regaining a sense of wholeness or cohesion in the self, persons may engage in impulsive behaviors that to others appear self-destructive. Kohut's formulation has some similarities to Donald Winnicott's view that impulsive or deviant behavior in children is a way for them to try to recapture a primitive maternal relationship. Winnicott saw such behavior as hopeful in that the child searches for affirmation and love from the mother rather than abandoning any attempt to win her affection.

Patients attempt to master anxiety, guilt, depression, and other painful affects by means of actions, but such actions aimed at obtaining relief seldom succeed even temporarily.

Psychosocial Factors

Psychosocial factors implicated causally in impulse-control disorders are related to early-life events. The growing child may have had improper models for identification, such as parents who had difficulty controlling impulses. Other psychosocial factors associated with the disorders include exposure to violence in the home, alcohol abuse, promiscuity, and antisocial behavior.

Biological Factors

Many investigators have focused on possible organic factors in the impulse-control disorders, especially for patients with overtly violent behavior. Experiments have shown that impulsive and violent activity is associated with specific brain regions, such as the limbic system, and that the inhibition of such behaviors is associated with other brain regions. A relation has been found between low cerebrospinal fluid (CSF) levels of 5-hydroxyindoleacetic acid (5-HIAA) and impulsive aggression. Certain hormones, especially testosterone, have also been associated with violent and aggressive behavior. Some reports have described a relation between temporal lobe epilepsy and certain impulsive violent behaviors, as well as an association of aggressive behavior in patients who have histories of head trauma with increased numbers of emergency room visits and other potential organic antecedents. A high incidence of mixed cerebral dominance may be found in some violent populations.

Considerable evidence indicates that the serotonin neurotransmitter system mediates symptoms evident in impulse-control disorders. Brainstem and CSF levels of 5-HIAA are decreased, and serotonin-binding sites are increased in persons who have committed suicide. The dopaminergic and noradrenergic systems have also been implicated in impulsivity.

Impulse-control disorder symptoms can continue into adulthood in persons whose disorder has been diagnosed as childhood attention-deficit/hyperactivity disorder (ADHD). Lifelong or acquired mental deficiency, epilepsy, and even reversible brain syndromes have long been implicated in lapses in impulse control.

INTERMITTENT EXPLOSIVE DISORDER

Intermittent explosive disorder manifests as discrete episodes of losing control of aggressive impulses; these episodes can result in serious assault or the destruction of property. The aggressiveness expressed is grossly out of proportion to any stressors that may have helped elicit the episodes. The symptoms, which patients may describe as spells or attacks, appear within minutes or hours and, regardless of duration, remit spontaneously and quickly. After each episode, patients usually show genuine regret or self-reproach, and signs of generalized impulsivity or aggressiveness are absent between episodes. The diagnosis of intermittent explosive disorder should not be made if the loss of control can be accounted for by schizophrenia, antisocial or borderline personality disorder, ADHD, conduct disorder, or substance intoxication.

The term *epileptoid personality* has been used to convey the seizure-like quality of the characteristic outbursts, which are not typical of the patient's usual behavior, and to convey the suspicion of an organic disease process, for example, damage to the central nervous system. Several associated features suggest the possibility of an epileptoid state: the presence of auras; postictal-like changes in the sensorium, including partial or spotty amnesia; and hypersensitivity to photic, aural, or auditory stimuli.

Epidemiology

Intermittent explosive disorder is underreported. The disorder appears to be more common in men than in women. The men are likely to be found in correctional institutions and the women in psychiatric facilities. In one study, about 2 percent of all persons admitted to a university hospital psychiatric service had disorders that were diagnosed as intermittent explosive disorder; 80 percent were men.

Evidence indicates that intermittent explosive disorder is more common in first-degree biological relatives of persons with the disorder than in the general population. Many factors other than a simple genetic explanation may be responsible.

Comorbidity

High rates of fire setting in patients with intermittent explosive disorder have been reported. Other disorders of impulse control and substance use and mood, anxiety, and eating disorders have also been associated with intermittent explosive disorder.

Etiology

Psychodynamic Factors. Psychoanalysts have suggested that explosive outbursts occur as a defense against narcissistic injurious events. Rage outbursts serve as interpersonal distance and protect against any further narcissistic injury.

Psychosocial Factors. Typical patients have been described as physically large, but dependent, men whose sense of masculine identity is poor. A sense of being useless and impotent or of being unable to change the environment often precedes an episode of physical violence, and a high level of anxiety, guilt, and depression usually follows an episode.

An unfavorable childhood environment often filled with alcohol dependence, beatings, and threats to life is usual in these patients. Predisposing factors in infancy and childhood include perinatal trauma, infantile seizures, head trauma, encephalitis, minimal brain dysfunction, and hyperactivity. Workers who have concentrated on psychogenesis as causing episodic explosiveness have stressed identification with assaultive parental figures as symbols of the target for violence. Early frustration, oppression, and hostility have been noted as predisposing factors. Situations that are directly or symbolically reminiscent of early deprivations (e.g., persons who directly or indirectly evoke the image of the frustrating parent) become targets for destructive hostility.

Biological Factors. Some investigators suggest that disordered brain physiology, particularly in the limbic system, is involved in most cases of episodic violence. Compelling evidence indicates that serotonergic neurons mediate behavioral inhibition. Decreased serotonergic transmission, which can be induced by inhibiting serotonin synthesis or by antagonizing its effects, decreases the effect of punishment as a deterrent to behavior. The restoration of serotonin activity, by administering serotonin precursors such as L-tryptophan or drugs that increase synaptic serotonin levels, restores the behavioral effect of punishment. Restoring serotonergic activity by administration of L-tryptophan or drugs that increase synaptic serotonergic levels appears to restore control of episodic violent tendencies. Low levels of CSF 5-HIAA have been correlated with impulsive aggression. High CSF testosterone concentrations are correlated with aggressiveness and interpersonal violence in men. Antiandrogenic agents have been shown to decrease aggression.

Familial and Genetic Factors. First-degree relatives of patients with intermittent explosive disorder have higher rates of impulse-control disorders, depressive disorders, and substance use disorders. Biological relatives of patients with the disorder were more likely to have histories of temper or explosive outbursts than the general population.

Diagnosis and Clinical Features

The diagnosis of intermittent explosive disorder should be the result of history-taking that reveals several episodes of loss of control associated with aggressive outbursts (Table 25–1). One

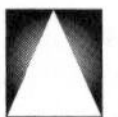

Table 25–1
DSM-IV-TR Diagnostic Criteria for Intermittent Explosive Disorder

A. Several discrete episodes of failure to resist aggressive impulses that result in serious assaultive acts or destruction of property.
B. The degree of aggressiveness expressed during the episodes is grossly out of proportion to any precipitating psychosocial stressors.
C. The aggressive episodes are not better accounted for by another mental disorder (e.g., antisocial personality disorder, borderline personality disorder, a psychotic disorder, a manic episode, conduct disorder, or attention-deficit/hyperactivity disorder) and are not due to the direct physiological effects of a substance (e.g., a drug of abuse, a medication) or a general medical condition (e.g., head trauma, Alzheimer's disease).

(From American Psychiatric Association. *Diagnostic and Statistical Manual of Mental Disorders.* 4th ed. Text rev. Washington, DC: American Psychiatric Association; copyright 2000, with permission.)

discrete episode does not justify the diagnosis. The histories typically describe a childhood in an atmosphere of alcohol dependence, violence, and emotional instability. Patients' work histories are poor; they report job losses, marital difficulties, and trouble with the law. Most patients have sought psychiatric help in the past but to no avail. Anxiety, guilt, and depression usually follow an outburst, but this is not a constant finding. Neurological examination sometimes reveals soft neurological signs, such as left-right ambivalence and perceptual reversal. Electroencephalographic (EEG) findings are frequently normal or show nonspecific changes.

A 36-year-old real estate agent sought assistance for difficulty with his anger. He was quite competent at his job, although he frequently lost clients when he became enraged over their indecisiveness. On a number of occasions, he became verbally abusive, leading clients to find ways out of escrow closings. The impulsive aggression also led to termination of multiple relationships because sudden angry outbursts contained demeaning accusations toward his girlfriends. This occurred frequently in the absence of any clear conflict. On multiple occasions, the patient became so uncontrollably enraged that he threw things across the room, including books, his desk, and the contents of the refrigerator. Between episodes, he was a kind and likable individual with many friends. He enjoyed drinking on the weekends and had a history of two arrests for driving while intoxicated. On one of these occasions, he became involved in a verbal altercation with a police officer. He had a history of drug experimentation in college that included cocaine and marijuana.

Mental status examination revealed a generally cooperative patient. However, he became quite defensive when questioned about his anger and easily felt accused and blamed by the interviewer for his past behaviors. He had no significant medical history and no signs of neurological problems. He had never been in psychiatric treatment prior to this evaluation. He was on no medications. He denied any symptoms of a mood disorder or any other antisocial activity.

Treatment included the use of carbamazepine (Tegretol) and a combination of supportive and cognitive-behavioral psychotherapy. The patient's angry outbursts improved as he became aware of early signs that he was about to lose control. He learned techniques to avoid confrontation when he was faced with these warning signs. (Courtesy of Vivien K. Burt, M.D., Ph.D., and Jeffrey William Katzman, M.D.)

Physical Findings and Laboratory Examination

Persons with the disorder have a high incidence of soft neurological signs (e.g., reflex asymmetries), nonspecific EEG findings, abnormal neuropsychological testing results (e.g., letter reversal difficulties), and accident susceptibility. Blood chemistry (liver and thyroid function tests, fasting blood glucose, electrolytes), urinalysis (including drug toxicology), and syphilis serology may help rule out other causes of aggression. Magnetic resonance imagery (MRI) may reveal changes in the prefrontal cortex, which is associated with loss of impulse control.

Differential Diagnosis

The diagnosis of intermittent explosive disorder can be made only after disorders associated with the occasional loss of control of aggressive impulses have been ruled out as the primary cause. These other disorders include psychotic disorders, personality change because of a general medical condition, antisocial or borderline personality disorder, and substance intoxication (e.g., alcohol, barbiturates, hallucinogens, and amphetamines), epilepsy, brain tumors, degenerative diseases, and endocrine disorders.

Conduct disorder is distinguished from intermittent explosive disorder by its repetitive and resistant pattern of behavior, as opposed to an episodic pattern. Intermittent explosive disorder differs from the antisocial and borderline personality disorders because, in the personality disorders, aggressiveness and impulsivity are part of patients' characters and, thus, are present between outbursts. In paranoid and catatonic schizophrenia, patients may display violent behavior in response to delusions and hallucinations, and they show gross impairments in reality testing. Hostile patients with mania may be impulsively aggressive, but the underlying diagnosis is generally apparent from their mental status examinations and clinical presentations.

Amok is an episode of acute violent behavior for which the person claims amnesia. Amok is usually seen in southeastern Asia, but it has been reported in North America. Amok is distinguished from intermittent explosive disorder by a single episode and prominent dissociative features.

Course and Prognosis

Intermittent explosive disorder may begin at any stage of life, but usually appears between late adolescence and early adulthood. The onset can be sudden or insidious, and the course can be episodic or chronic. In most cases, the disorder decreases in severity with the onset of middle age, but heightened organic impairment can lead to frequent and severe episodes.

Treatment

A combined pharmacological and psychotherapeutic approach has the best chance of success. Psychotherapy with patients who have intermittent explosive disorder is difficult, however, because of their angry outbursts. Therapists may have problems with countertransference and limit-setting. Group psychotherapy may be helpful, and family therapy is useful, particularly when the explosive patient is an adolescent or a young adult. A goal of therapy is to have the patient recognize and verbalize the thoughts or feelings that precede the explosive outbursts instead of acting them out.

Anticonvulsants have long been used, with mixed results, in treating explosive patients. Lithium (Eskalith) has been reported useful in generally lessening aggressive behavior, and carbamazepine, valproate (Depakene) or divalproex (Depakote), and phenytoin (Dilantin) have been reported helpful. Some clinicians have also used other anticonvulsants (e.g., gabapentin [Neurontin]). Benzodiazepines are sometimes used but have been reported to produce a paradoxical reaction of dyscontrol in some cases.

Antipsychotics (e.g., phenothiazines and serotonin-dopamine antagonists) and tricyclic drugs have been effective in some cases, but clinicians must then question whether schizophrenia or a mood disorder is the true diagnosis. With a likelihood of subcortical seizure-like activity, medications that lower the seizure threshold can aggravate the situation. Selective serotonin reuptake inhibitors (SSRIs), trazodone (Desyrel), and buspirone (BuSpar) are useful in reducing impulsivity and aggression.

Propranolol (Inderal) and other β-adrenergic receptor antagonists and calcium channel inhibitors have also been effective in some cases. Some neurosurgeons have performed operative treatments for intractable violence and aggression. No evidence indicates that such treatment is effective.

KLEPTOMANIA

The essential feature of kleptomania is a recurrent failure to resist impulses to steal objects not needed for personal use or for monetary value. The objects taken are often given away, returned surreptitiously, or kept and hidden. Persons with kleptomania usually have the money to pay for the objects they impulsively steal.

As with other impulse-control disorders, kleptomania is characterized by mounting tension before the act, followed by gratification and lessening of tension with or without guilt, remorse, or depression after the act. The stealing is not planned and does not involve others. Although the thefts do not occur when immediate arrest is probable, persons with kleptomania do not always consider their chances of being apprehended, although repeated arrests lead to pain and humiliation. These persons may feel guilt and anxiety after the theft, but they do not feel anger or vengeance. Furthermore, when the object stolen is the goal, the diagnosis is not kleptomania; in kleptomania, the act of stealing is itself the goal.

Epidemiology

The prevalence of kleptomania is not known, but it is estimated to be about 0.6 percent. The range varies from 3.8 to 24 percent of those arrested for shoplifting. DSM-IV-TR reports that it occurs in fewer than 5 percent of identified shoplifters. The male-to-female ratio is 1:3 in clinical samples.

Comorbidity

Patients with kleptomania are said to have a high lifetime comorbidity of major affective illness (usually, but not exclusively, depressive) and various anxiety disorders. Associated conditions also include other impulse-control disorders (notably, pathological gambling and compulsive shopping), eating disorders, and substance abuse disorders, alcoholism in particular.

Etiology

Psychosocial Factors. The symptoms of kleptomania tend to appear in times of significant stress, for example, losses, separations, and endings of important relationships. Some psychoanalytic writers have stressed the expression of aggressive impulses in kleptomania; others have discerned a libidinal aspect. Those who focus on symbolism see meaning in the act itself, the object stolen, and the victim of the theft.

Analytic writers have focused on stealing by children and adolescents. Anna Freud pointed out that the first thefts from mother's purse indicate the degree to which all stealing is rooted in the oneness between mother and child. Karl Abraham wrote of the central feeling of being neglected, injured, or unwanted. One theoretician established seven categories of stealing in chronically acting-out children:

1. As a means of restoring the lost mother–child relationship
2. As an aggressive act
3. As a defense against fears of being damaged (perhaps a search by girls for a penis or a protection against castration anxiety in boys)
4. As a means of seeking punishment
5. As a means of restoring or adding to self-esteem
6. In connection with, and as a reaction to, a family secret
7. As excitement (*lust angst*) and a substitute for a sexual act

One or more of these categories can also apply to adult kleptomania.

Biological Factors. Brain diseases and mental retardation have been associated with kleptomania, as they have with other disorders of impulse control. Focal neurological signs, cortical atrophy, and enlarged lateral ventricles have been found in some patients. Disturbances in monoamine metabolism, particularly of serotonin, have been postulated.

Family and Genetic Factors. In one study, 7 percent of first-degree relatives had obsessive-compulsive disorder (OCD). In addition, a higher rate of mood disorders has been reported in family members.

Diagnosis and Clinical Features

The essential feature of kleptomania is recurrent, intrusive, and irresistible urges or impulses to steal unneeded objects (Table 25–2). Patients with kleptomania may also be distressed about the possibility or actuality of being apprehended and may manifest signs of depression and anxiety. Patients feel guilty, ashamed, and embarrassed about their behavior. They often have serious problems with interpersonal relationships and often show signs of personality disturbance. In one study of patients with kleptomania, the frequency of stealing ranged from less than 1 to 120 episodes a month. Most patients with kleptomania steal

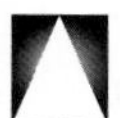

Table 25–2
DSM-IV-TR Diagnostic Criteria for Kleptomania

A. Recurrent failure to resist impulses to steal objects that are not needed for personal use or for their monetary value.
B. Increasing sense of tension immediately before committing the theft.
C. Pleasure, gratification, or relief at the time of committing the theft.
D. The stealing is not committed to express anger or vengeance and is not in response to a delusion or a hallucination.
E. The stealing is not better accounted for by conduct disorder, a manic episode, or antisocial personality disorder.

(From American Psychiatric Association. *Diagnostic and Statistical Manual of Mental Disorders.* 4th ed. Text rev. Washington, DC: American Psychiatric Association; copyright 2000, with permission.)

from retail stores, but they may also steal from family members in their own households.

Jane was a 42-year-old, highly successful, single executive from a wealthy background. She called herself a "shop-'til-you-drop type" and had always been able to afford the expensive designer clothing that she loved. Since college, her "legit" shopping had been paralleled by "boosting" cheap panties and brassieres from discount stores. She did not wear the stolen items; indeed, she considered them "sleazy." She could never bring herself to get rid of them either and kept boxes filled with pilfered lingerie in a storage facility.

Jane talked or bought her way out of trouble until her 30s, when she was arrested while stealing pantyhose from the same K-Mart for the third time in as many months. As a condition of probation, she was ordered to see a psychiatrist. Her attendance was sporadic, and several more thefts occurred over the next 2 years. She also experienced substantial depression, which she tried to alleviate by heavy drinking.

Jane finally began taking her problem seriously after yet another arrest precipitated a suicidal gesture. She began keeping appointments regularly and consented to taking citalopram (Celexa) and naltrexone (ReVia). She believes that her participation in an AA group for high-pressured executives has been at least as effective—if not more so—in controlling her stealing. (Courtesy of Harvey Roy Greenberg, M.D.)

Differential Diagnosis

Episodes of theft occasionally occur during psychotic illness, for example, acute mania, major depression with psychotic features, or schizophrenia. Psychotic stealing is obviously a product of pathological elevation or depression of mood or command hallucinations or delusions. Theft in individuals with antisocial personality disorder is deliberately undertaken for personal gain, with some degree of premeditation and planning, often executed with others. Antisocial stealing regularly involves the threat of harm or actual violence, particularly to elude capture. Guilt and remorse are distinctively lacking, or patients are patently insincere. Shoplifting has become a national epidemic. Few shoplifters have true kleptomania; most are teenagers and young adults who "boost" in pairs or small groups for "kicks," as well as goods, and do not have a major psychiatric disorder. Acute intoxication with drugs or alcohol may precipitate theft in an individual with another psychiatric disorder or without significant psychopathology. Patients with Alzheimer's disease or other dementing organic illness may leave a store without paying, owing to forgetfulness, rather than larcenous intent. Malingering kleptomania is common in apprehended antisocial types, as well as nonantisocial youthful shoplifters. Given a sufficiently intelligent perpetrator, the fictive version can be difficult to distinguish from the genuine disorder.

Course and Prognosis

Kleptomania may begin in childhood, although most children and adolescents who steal do not become kleptomaniac adults. The onset of the disorder generally is late adolescence. Women are more likely to present for psychiatric evaluation or treatment than are men. Men are more likely to be sent to prison. Men tend to present with the disorder at about 50 years of age and women, at about 35 years of age. In quiescent cases, new bouts of the disorder may be precipitated by loss or disappointment.

The course of the disorder waxes and wanes, but tends to be chronic. Persons sometimes have bouts of being unable to resist the impulse to steal, followed by free periods that last for weeks or months. Its spontaneous recovery rate is unknown.

Serious impairment and complications are usually secondary to being caught, particularly to being arrested. Many persons seem never to have consciously considered the possibility of facing the consequences of their acts, a feature that agrees with some descriptions of patients with kleptomania (sometimes, as persons who feel wronged and therefore entitled to steal). Often, the disorder in no way impairs a person's social or work functioning.

The prognosis with treatment can be good, but few patients come for help of their own accord.

Treatment

Because true kleptomania is rare, reports of treatment tend to be individual case descriptions or a short series of cases. Insight-oriented psychotherapy and psychoanalysis have been successful, but depend on patients' motivations. Those who feel guilt and shame may be helped by insight-oriented psychotherapy because of their increased motivation to change their behavior.

Behavior therapy, including systematic desensitization, aversive conditioning, and a combination of aversive conditioning and altered social contingencies, has been reported successful, even when motivation was lacking. The reports cite follow-up studies of up to 2 years. SSRIs, such as fluoxetine (Prozac) and fluvoxamine (Luvox), appear to be effective in some patients with kleptomania. Case reports indicated successful treatment with tricyclic drugs, trazodone, lithium, valproate, naltrexone and electroconvulsive therapy.

PYROMANIA

Pyromania is the recurrent, deliberate, and purposeful setting of fires. Associated features include tension or affective arousal before setting the fires; fascination with, interest in, curiosity about, or attraction to fire and the activities and equipment associated with firefighting; and pleasure, gratification, or relief when setting fires or when witnessing or participating in their aftermath. Patients may make considerable advance preparations before starting a fire. Pyromania differs from arson in that the latter is done for financial gain, revenge, or other reasons and is planned beforehand.

Epidemiology

No information is available on the prevalence of pyromania, but only a small percentage of adults who set fires can be classified as having pyromania. The disorder is found far more often in men than in women with a male to female ratio of approximately 8 to 1. More than 40 percent of arrested arsonists are younger than 18 years of age.

Comorbidity

Pyromania is significantly associated with substance abuse disorder (especially alcoholism); affective disorders, depressive or bipolar; other impulse control disorders, such as kleptomania in female fire setters; and various personality disturbances, such as inadequate and borderline personality disorders. Attention-deficit disorder and learning disabilities may be conspicuously associated with childhood pyromania; this constellation frequently persists into adulthood. Persons who set fires are more likely to be mildly retarded than are those in the general population. Some studies have noted an increased incidence of alcohol use disorders in persons who set fires. Fire setters also tend to have a history of antisocial traits, such as truancy, running away from home, and delinquency. Enuresis has been considered a common finding in the history of fire setters, although controlled studies have failed to confirm this. Studies, however, have found an association between cruelty to animals and fire setting. Childhood and adolescent fire setting is often associated with ADHD or adjustment disorders.

Etiology

Psychosocial. Freud saw fire as a symbol of sexuality. He believed the warmth radiated by fire evokes the same sensation that accompanies a state of sexual excitation, and a flame's shape and movements suggest a phallus in activity. Other psychoanalysts have associated pyromania with an abnormal craving for power and social prestige. Some patients with pyromania are volunteer firefighters who set fires to prove themselves brave, to force other firefighters into action, or to demonstrate their power to extinguish a blaze. The incendiary act is a way to vent accumulated rage over frustration caused by a sense of social, physical, or sexual inferiority. Several studies have noted that the fathers of patients with pyromania were absent from the home. Thus, one explanation of fire setting is that it represents a wish for the absent father to return home as a rescuer, to put out the fire, and to save the child from a difficult existence.

Female fire setters, in addition to being much fewer in number than male fire setters, do not start fires to put firefighters into action as men frequently do. Frequently noted delinquent trends in female fire setters include promiscuity without pleasure and petty stealing, often approaching kleptomania.

Table 25–3
DSM-IV-TR Diagnostic Criteria for Pyromania

A. Deliberate and purposeful fire setting on more than one occasion.
B. Tension or affective arousal before the act.
C. Fascination with, interest in, curiosity about, or attraction to fire and its situational contexts (e.g., paraphernalia, uses, consequences).
D. Pleasure, gratification, or relief when setting fires, or when witnessing or participating in their aftermath.
E. The fire setting is not done for monetary gain, as an expression of sociopolitical ideology, to conceal criminal activity, to express anger or vengeance, to improve one's living circumstances, in response to a delusion or hallucination, or as a result of impaired judgment (e.g., in dementia, mental retardation, substance intoxication).
F. The fire setting is not better accounted for by conduct disorder, a manic episode, or antisocial personality disorder.

Biological Factors. Significantly low CSF levels of 5-HIAA and 3-methoxy-4-hydroxyphenylglycol (MHPG) have been found in fire setters, which suggests possible serotonergic or adrenergic involvement. The presence of reactive hypoglycemia, based on blood glucose concentrations on glucose tolerance tests, has been put forward as a cause of pyromania. Further studies are needed, however.

Diagnosis and Clinical Features

Persons with pyromania often regularly watch fires in their neighborhoods, frequently set off false alarms, and show interest in firefighting paraphernalia (Table 25–3). Their curiosity is evident, but they show no remorse and may be indifferent to the consequences for life or property. Fire setters may gain satisfaction from the resulting destruction; frequently, they leave obvious clues. Commonly associated features include alcohol intoxication, sexual dysfunctions, below-average intelligence quotient (IQ), chronic personal frustration, and resentment toward authority figures. Some fire setters become sexually aroused by the fire.

Differential Diagnosis

Clinicians should have little trouble distinguishing between pyromania and the fascination of many young children with matches, lighters, and fire as part of the normal investigation of their environments. Pyromania must also be separated from incendiary acts of sabotage carried out by dissident political extremists or by paid torches, termed arsonists in the legal system.

When fire setting occurs in conduct disorder and antisocial personality disorder, it is a deliberate act, not a failure to resist an impulse. Fires may be set for profit, sabotage, or retaliation. Patients with schizophrenia or mania may set fires in response to delusions or hallucinations. Patients with brain dysfunction (e.g., dementia), mental retardation, or substance intoxication may set fires because of a failure to appreciate the consequences of the act.

Course and Prognosis

Although fire setting often begins in childhood, the typical age of onset of pyromania is unknown. When the onset is in adolescence or adulthood, the fire setting tends to be deliberately destructive. Fire setting in pyromania is episodic and may wax and wane in frequency. The prognosis for treated children is good, and complete remission is a realistic goal. The prognosis for adults is guarded, because they frequently deny their actions, refuse to take responsibility, are dependent on alcohol, and lack insight.

Treatment

Little has been written about the treatment of pyromania, and treating fire setters has been difficult because of their lack of motivation. No single treatment has been proved effective; thus a number of modalities, including behavioral approaches, should be tried. Because of the recurrent nature of pyromania, any treatment program should include supervision of patients to prevent a repeated episode of fire setting. Incarceration may be the only method of preventing a recurrence. Behavior therapy can then be administered in the institution.

Fire setting by children must be treated with the utmost seriousness. Intensive interventions should be undertaken when possible, but as therapeutic and preventive measures, not as punishment. In the case of children and adolescents, treatment of pyromania or fire setting should include family therapy.

PATHOLOGICAL GAMBLING

Pathological gambling is characterized by persistent and recurrent maladaptive gambling that causes economic problems and significant disturbances in personal, social, or occupational functioning. Aspects of the maladaptive behavior include (1) a preoccupation with gambling; (2) the need to gamble with increasing amounts of money to achieve the desired excitement; (3) repeated unsuccessful efforts to control, cut back, or stop gambling; (4) gambling as a way to escape from problems; (5) gambling to recoup losses; (6) lying to conceal the extent of the involvement with gambling; (7) the commission of illegal acts to finance gambling; (8) jeopardizing or losing personal and vocational relationships because of gambling; and (9) a reliance on others for money to pay off debts.

Epidemiology

Although comprehensive worldwide statistics have yet to be compiled, excellent local studies all point to a 3 to 5 percent rate of problem gamblers in the general population and an approximate 1 percent rate of individuals meeting the requirements for pathological gambling.

The typical patient in treatment studies is a white man from a comfortable economic background, 35 to 50 years of age. Surveys of more extensive nontreatment populations indicate, however, that pathological gambling cuts across every ethnic, class, age, and occupational divide (according to anonymous casino personnel, physicians are among their most consistent heavy players and losers).

As every type of gambling has become increasingly accessible over the past few decades, the rate of normal and pathological gambling has risen spectacularly, especially in locales with legalized gaming. Escalation has been noted in the poor, notably poor minorities; adolescents; elderly retirees; and women. One of three pathological gamblers is now female: It has been suggested that women are gambling more because an increased presence in the workplace gives them more cash. These groups are all still greatly underserved with regard to research and treatment.

Family histories of pathological gamblers show an increased rate of substance abuse (particularly alcoholism) and depressive disorders. A parent or influential relative of the patient often has been a problem or pathological gambler. The family circle is likely to be competitively and materialistically oriented, evincing intense admiration for money and associated symbols of success. In this respect, compulsive gambling has been called the dark side of the American dream.

Comorbidity

Significant comorbidity occurs between pathological gambling and mood disorders (especially, major depression and bipolarity) and substance abuse disorders (notably, alcohol and cocaine abuse and caffeine and nicotine dependence). Comorbidity also exists with ADHD (particularly in childhood), various personality disorders (notably, narcissistic, antisocial, and borderline personality disorders), and other impulse-control disorders. Although many pathological gamblers have obsessive personality traits, full-blown OCD is uncommon.

Etiology

Psychosocial Factors. Several factors may predispose persons to develop the disorder: loss of a parent by death, separation, divorce, or desertion before a child is 15 years of age; inappropriate parental discipline (absence, inconsistency, or harshness); exposure to, and availability of, gambling activities for adolescents; a family emphasis on material and financial symbols; and a lack of family emphasis on saving, planning, and budgeting.

Psychoanalytic theory has focused on a number of core character difficulties. Freud suggested that compulsive gamblers have an unconscious desire to lose, and gamble to relieve unconscious feelings of guilt. Another suggestion is that the gamblers are narcissists whose grandiose and omnipotent fantasies lead them to believe they can control events and even predict their outcome. Learning theorists view uncontrolled gambling as resulting from erroneous perceptions regarding control of impulses.

Biological Factors. Several studies have suggested that gamblers' risk-taking behavior may have an underlying neurobiological cause. These theories have centered on both serotonergic and noradrenergic receptor systems. Male pathological gamblers may have subnormal MHPG concentrations in plasma, increased MHPG concentrations in the CSF, and increased urinary output of norepinephrine. Evidence also implicates serotonergic regulatory dysfunction in the pathological gambler. Chronic gamblers have low platelet monoamine oxidase (MAO) activity, a marker of serotonin activity, also linked to difficulties with inhibition. Further studies are needed to confirm these findings.

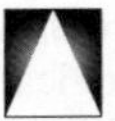

Table 25–4
DSM-IV-TR Diagnostic Criteria for Pathological Gambling

A. Persistent and recurrent maladaptive gambling behavior as indicated by five (or more) of the following:
(1) is preoccupied with gambling (e.g., preoccupied with reliving past gambling experiences, handicapping or planning the next venture, or thinking of ways to get money with which to gamble)
(2) needs to gamble with increasing amounts of money in order to achieve the desired excitement
(3) has repeated unsuccessful efforts to control, cut back, or stop gambling
(4) is restless or irritable when attempting to cut down or stop gambling
(5) gambles as a way of escaping from problems or of relieving a dysphoric mood (e.g., feelings of helplessness, guilt, anxiety, depression)
(6) after losing money gambling, often returns another day to get even ("chasing" one's losses)
(7) lies to family members, therapist, or others to conceal the extent of involvement with gambling
(8) has committed illegal acts such as forgery, fraud, theft, or embezzlement to finance gambling
(9) has jeopardized or lost a significant relationship, job, or educational or career opportunity because of gambling
(10) relies on others to provide money to relieve a desperate financial situation caused by gambling

B. The gambling behavior is not better accounted for by a manic episode.

(From American Psychiatric Association. *Diagnostic and Statistical Manual of Mental Disorders.* 4th ed. Text rev. Washington, DC: American Psychiatric Association; copyright 2000, with permission.)

Diagnosis and Clinical Features

In addition to the features already described, pathological gamblers often appear overconfident, somewhat abrasive, energetic, and free-spending. They often show obvious signs of personal stress, anxiety, and depression (Table 25–4). They commonly have the attitude that money is both the cause of, and the solution to, all their problems. As their gambling increases, they are usually forced to lie to obtain money and to continue gambling while hiding the extent of their gambling. They make no serious attempt to budget or save money. When their borrowing resources are strained, they are likely to engage in antisocial behavior to obtain money for gambling. Their criminal behavior is typically nonviolent, such as forgery, embezzlement, or fraud, and they consciously intend to return or repay the money. Complications include alienation from family members and acquaintances, the loss of life accomplishments, suicide attempts, and association with fringe and illegal groups. Arrest for nonviolent crimes may lead to imprisonment.

Frank was a 32-year-old businessman whose uncle was a compulsive horse player. His maternal grandmother committed suicide with sleeping pills. He was an avid card player and sports bettor since his early teens, taking pride in being a small but steady winner. Frank found formal education boring and dropped out of college in his freshman year to take over his father's appliance store. He expanded the business to a chain of electronic equipment outlets. Over the next decade, he prospered, married happily, had three children, and lived in substantial luxury.

During the same time, Frank's inveterate gambling slowly increased. Besides his weekly poker game and weekend sports betting, he enjoyed occasional Saturday outings with his poker buddies to a casino that had opened at a nearby Indian reservation. He mostly broke even or sustained small losses, but he was immensely exhilarated by several big scores at blackjack and craps, games that he had not played much before.

After his father's sudden death from a stroke, Frank began traveling more often to the casino and started playing at higher stakes. Soon, he found himself betting hundreds, then thousands, of dollars on the turn of a card or the throw of the dice. The size of sports betting similarly increased. He visited the casino most weekends and many weekday nights, lying about his whereabouts to colleagues and family.

Within 2 years, Frank accumulated several million dollars in gambling debts. Now, he gambled not to win but to catch up—still fervently believing that "one streak would put me straight." He invaded business and personal finances, juggled accounts, charged his credit cards beyond the maximal limit, and borrowed money from loan sharks at exorbitant rates. He had always shielded his wife and family from his problem. Profoundly depressed, he considered killing himself in a car accident, so that "everyone would be taken care of." He used cocaine to alleviate his despair.

The grim reality of Frank's indebtedness and its cause was unmasked when his wife discovered that he had plundered the children's college funds to pay off a loan shark who had threatened to have his family killed. At first, she wanted to divorce him, but then her wealthy father intervened and bailed Frank out. He swore that he would never gamble again, entered Gamblers Anonymous (GA), and, within a few months, was back at the casino.

Several more episodes of recovery and relapse did lead to divorce and left Frank penniless. He finally entered a pilot program for pathological gamblers, where he was diagnosed as also having atypical bipolar disorder. Treatment has included individual and group counseling, medication with an antidepressant and mood regulator, family therapy (his wife is now willing to see him, but not to live with him), and a program of restitution. He works as a delicatessen clerk, has been abstinent for 6 months, and says that "not a day goes by that I don't miss the action." (Courtesy of Harvey Roy Greenberg, M.D.)

Psychological Testing and Laboratory Examination

Males with the disorders have shown abnormalities in platelet MAO activity. Patients with pathological gambling often display high levels of impulsivity on neuropsychological tests. German studies have demonstrated increased cortisol levels in the saliva of gamblers while they gamble, which can account for the euphoria that occurs during the experience and its addictive potential.

Differential Diagnosis

Social gambling is distinguished from pathological gambling in that the former occurs with friends, on special occasions, and with predetermined acceptable and tolerable losses. Gambling that is symptomatic of a manic episode can usually be distinguished from pathological gambling by the history of a marked mood change and the loss of judgment preceding the gambling.

Manic-like mood changes are common in pathological gambling, but they always follow winning and are usually succeeded by depressive episodes because of subsequent losses. Persons with antisocial personality disorder may have problems with gambling. When both disorders are present, both should be diagnosed.

Course and Prognosis

Pathological gambling usually begins in adolescence for men and late in life for women. The disorder waxes and wanes and tends to be chronic. Four phases are seen in pathological gambling:

1. The winning phase, ending with a big win, equal to about a year's salary, which hooks patients. Women usually do not have a big win, but use gambling as an escape from problems.
2. The progressive-loss phase, in which patients structure their lives around gambling and then move from being excellent gamblers to being stupid ones who take considerable risks, cash in securities, borrow money, miss work, and lose jobs.
3. The desperate phase, with patients frenziedly gambling with large amounts of money, not paying debts, becoming involved with loan sharks, writing bad checks, and possibly embezzling.
4. The hopeless stage of accepting that losses can never be made up, but the gambling continues because of the associated arousal or excitement. The disorder may take up to 15 years to reach the last phase, but then, within a year or two, patients have deteriorated totally.

Treatment

Gamblers seldom come forward voluntarily to be treated. Legal difficulties, family pressures, or other psychiatric complaints bring gamblers to treatment. GA was founded in Los Angeles in 1957 and modeled on Alcoholics Anonymous (AA); it is accessible, at least in large cities, and is an effective treatment for gambling in some patients. GA is a method of inspirational group therapy that involves public confession, peer pressure, and the presence of reformed gamblers (as with sponsors in AA) available to help members resist the impulse to gamble. The dropout rate from GA is high, however. In some cases, hospitalization may help by removing patients from their environments. Insight-oriented psychotherapy should not be sought until patients have been away from gambling for 3 months. At this point, patients who are pathological gamblers may become excellent candidates for this form of psychotherapy. Family therapy is often valuable. Cognitive-behavioral therapy (e.g., relaxation techniques combined with visualization of gambling avoidance) has had some success.

Little is known about the efficacy of pharmacotherapy for treating patients with pathological gambling. One study reported that 7 of 10 patients remained completely abstinent over 8 weeks after taking fluvoxamine. Also, case reports indicate successful treatment with lithium and clomipramine (Anafranil). If gambling is associated with depressive disorders, mania, anxiety, or other mental disorders, pharmacotherapy with antidepressants, lithium, or antianxiety agents is useful.

TRICHOTILLOMANIA

Trichotillomania is a chronic disorder characterized by repetitive hair pulling, driven by escalating tension and causing variable hair loss that is usually—but not always—visible to others. The disorder was known at least as far back as the 12th century. Formation of *trichobezoars*—hairballs accumulating in the alimentary tract from hair pulling and swallowing—was described in the late 18th century. The term *trichotillomania* was coined by a French dermatologist, Francois Hallopeau, in 1889.

Trichotillomania was once deemed rare, and little about it was described beyond phenomenology. The condition is now regarded as more common. With a substantial increase in research, treatment has greatly improved since the 1980s.

Epidemiology

The prevalence of trichotillomania may be underestimated because of accompanying shame and secretiveness. The diagnosis encompasses at least two categories of hair pullers differing in incidence, severity, age of presentation, and gender ratio. Other subsets may exist.

The potentially most serious, chronic form of the disorder usually begins in early to mid-adolescence, with a lifetime prevalence ranging from 0.6 percent to as high as 3.4 percent in general populations and with a female to male ratio as high as 9 to 1. The number of men may actually be higher, because men are even more likely than women to conceal hair pulling. A patient with chronic trichotillomania is likely to be the only or oldest child in the family.

A childhood type of trichotillomania occurs approximately equally in girls and boys. It is said to be more common than the adolescent or young adult syndrome and is generally far less serious dermatologically and psychologically.

An estimated 33 to 40 percent of patients with trichotillomania chew or swallow the hair that they pull out at one time or another. Of this group, approximately 37.5 percent develop potentially hazardous bezoars.

Comorbidity

Significant comorbidity is found between trichotillomania and OCD (as well as other anxiety disorders); Tourette's syndrome; affective illness, especially depressive conditions; eating disorders; and various personality disorders—particularly obsessive-compulsive, borderline, and narcissistic personality disorders. Comorbid substance abuse disorder is not encountered as frequently as it is in pathological gambling, kleptomania, and other disorders.

Etiology

Although trichotillomania is regarded as multidetermined, its onset has been linked to stressful situations in more than one fourth of all cases. Disturbances in mother-child relationships, fear of being left alone, and recent object loss are often cited as critical factors contributing to the condition. Substance abuse may encourage development of the disorder. Depressive dynamics are often cited as predisposing factors, but no particular personality

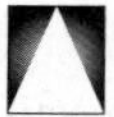

Table 25–5
DSM-IV-TR Diagnostic Criteria for Trichotillomania

A. Recurrent pulling out of one's hair resulting in noticeable hair loss.
B. An increasing sense of tension immediately before pulling out the hair or when attempting to resist the behavior.
C. Pleasure, gratification, or relief when pulling out the hair.
D. The disturbance is not better accounted for by another mental disorder and is not due to a general medical condition (e.g., a dermatological condition).
E. The disturbance causes clinically significant distress or impairment in social, occupational, or other important areas of functioning.

(From American Psychiatric Association. *Diagnostic and Statistical Manual of Mental Disorders*. 4th ed. Text rev. Washington, DC: American Psychiatric Association; copyright 2000, with permission.)

trait or disorder characterizes patients. Some see self-stimulation as the primary goal of hair pulling.

Trichotillomania is increasingly being viewed as having a biologically determined substrate that may reflect inappropriately released motor activity or excessive grooming behaviors. Biological theories have also pointed to metabolic differences in the serotonin and opioid systems. Family members of trichotillomania patients often have a history of tics, impulse-control disorders, and obsessive-compulsive symptoms, further supporting a possible genetic predisposition.

Diagnosis and Clinical Features

Before engaging in the behavior, patients with trichotillomania experience an increasing sense of tension and achieve a sense of release or gratification from pulling out their hair (Table 25–5). All areas of the body may be affected, most commonly the scalp (Fig. 25–1). Other areas involved are eyebrows, eyelashes, and beard; trunk, armpits, and pubic area are less commonly involved (Fig. 25–2). Hair loss is often characterized by short, broken strands appearing together with long, normal hairs in the affected areas. No abnormalities of the skin or scalp are present. Hair pulling is not reported to be painful, although pruritus and tingling may occur in the involved area. Trichophagy, mouthing of the hair, may follow the hair plucking. Complications of trichophagy include trichobezoars, malnutrition, and intestinal obstruction. Patients usually deny the behavior and often try to hide the resultant alopecia. Head banging, nail biting, scratching, gnawing, excoriation, and other acts of self-mutilation may be present.

Kathy was a 24-year-old editor who had suffered from trichotillomania since 17 years of age. Typical hair-pulling behavior began during junior year at a highly competitive private high school in the setting of increasing torment by ruminations about not getting into the "right" college. She plucked, chewed, and swallowed hair from the top and sides of her scalp, as well as her eyebrows. She concealed hair pulling from her family and friends, because she thought "I was going nuts." She finally blurted out her symptoms to a trusted pediatrician during a routine office visit.

Kathy's parents were professionals who made intense academic demands on all of their children; family life was otherwise not notably problematic. As a child, she was extremely critical of herself and afraid of failure. Her father experienced mild periodic depression since college. One brother developed obsessions and compulsions during his late teens. Both responded well to fluoxetine (Prozac).

Kathy had received analytic psychotherapy, behavioral therapy, and medication (recently fluoxetine and clomipramine) elsewhere. Although she made reasonably good progress psychologically, she was never able to stop pulling her hair long enough for it to grow back. She had a wide circle of friends but still kept romance at arm's length, fearing that a potential lover would be frightened off if he found out her "secret." She could not bring herself to replace the "ratty" wig that she had been wearing since her late teens. "It makes me look dowdy," she said, "but buying a new one would be like telling myself I'll never get better."

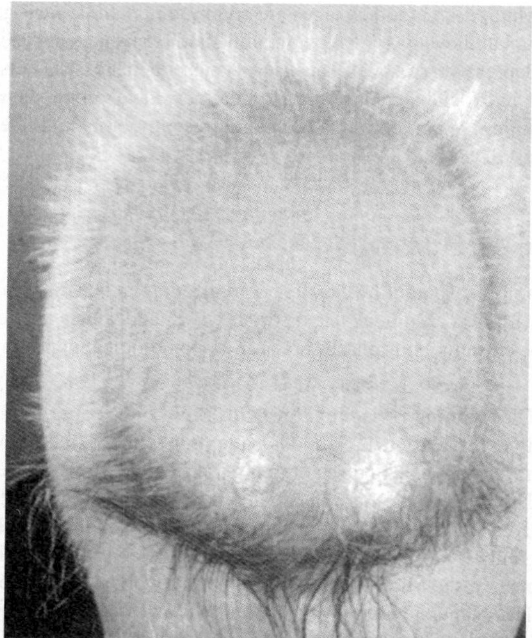

FIGURE 25–1
Example of plucking of the hair of the scalp because of trichotillomania.

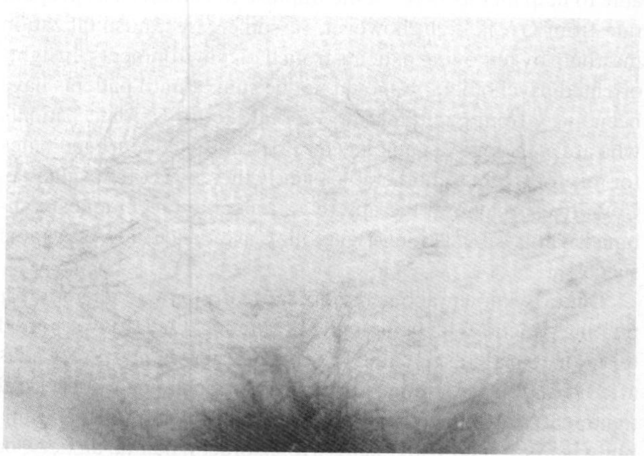

FIGURE 25–2
Example of plucking of the pubic hair because of trichotillomania.

Kathy sought treatment chiefly for regulation of her medication but quickly proved amenable to weekly psychotherapy sessions. Her clomipramine was increased, while she explored the sense of damage and "freakiness" that made her fend off men who liked her. She was much helped by weekly meetings at a trichotillomania support group. After 6 months, her self-esteem had improved, she had fewer bouts of hair pulling and had begun dating hesitantly. She arrived at her last session displaying an attractive new wig, stating ironically: "It isn't my real hair yet, but at least it's better than my old rug." (Courtesy of Harvey Roy Greenberg, M.D.)

Pathology and Laboratory Examination

If necessary, the clinical diagnosis of trichotillomania can be confirmed by punch biopsy of the scalp. In patients with a trichobezoar, blood count may reveal a mild leukocytosis and hypochromic anemia due to blood loss. Appropriate chemistries and radiological studies should also be performed, depending on the bezoar's suspected location and impact on the gastrointestinal (GI) tract.

Differential Diagnosis

Hair pulling may be a wholly benign condition or it may occur in the context of several mental disorders. The phenomenology of trichotillomania and OCD overlap. As with OCD, trichotillomania is often chronic and recognized by patients as undesirable. Unlike those with OCD, patients with trichotillomania do not experience obsessive thoughts, and the compulsive activity is limited to one act, hair pulling. Patients with factitious disorder with predominantly physical signs and symptoms actively seek medical attention and the patient role and deliberately simulate illness toward these ends. Patients who malinger or who have factitious disorder may mutilate themselves to get medical attention, but they do not acknowledge the self-inflicted nature of the lesions. Patients with stereotypic movement disorder have stereotypical and rhythmic movements, and they usually do not seem distressed by their behavior. A biopsy may be necessary to distinguish trichotillomania from alopecia areata and tinea capitis.

Course and Prognosis

The mean age at onset of trichotillomania is in the early teens, most frequently before age 17, but onsets have been reported much later in life. The course of the disorder is not well known; both chronic and remitting forms occur. An early onset (before age 6) tends to remit more readily and responds to suggestion, support, and behavioral strategies. Late onset (after age 13) is associated with an increased likelihood of chronicity and poorer prognosis than the early-onset form. About a third of persons presenting for treatment report a duration of 1 year or less, whereas in some cases, the disorder has persisted for more than two decades.

Treatment

No consensus exists on the best treatment modality for trichotillomania. Treatment usually involves psychiatrists and dermatologists in a joint endeavor. Psychopharmacological methods that have been used to treat psychodermatological disorders include topical steroids and hydroxyzine hydrochloride (Vistaril), an anxiolytic with antihistamine properties; antidepressants; serotonergic agents; and antipsychotics. Whether depression is present or not, antidepressant agents can lead to dermatological improvement. Current evidence strongly points to the efficacy of drugs that alter central serotonin turnover. Patients who respond poorly to SSRIs may improve with augmentation with pimozide (Orap), a dopamine receptor antagonist. A report of successful lithium treatment for trichotillomania cited the possible effect of the drug on aggression, impulsivity, and mood instability as an explanation. Lithium also possesses serotonergic activity. Case reports indicate successful treatment with buspirone, clonazepam (Klonopin), and trazodone. In one placebo-controlled study, patients taking naltrexone had a reduction in symptom severity.

Successful behavioral treatments, such as biofeedback, self-monitoring, covert desensitization, and habit reversal, have been reported, but most studies have been based on individual cases or a small series of cases with relatively short follow-up periods. Further controlled study of the treatments is warranted. Chronic trichotillomania has been treated successfully with insight-oriented psychotherapy. Hypnotherapy and behavior therapy have been mentioned as potentially effective in the treatment of dermatological disorders in which psychological factors may be involved; the skin has been shown to be susceptible to hypnotic suggestion. Most of the work has been research oriented, with little effect on clinical management.

IMPULSE-CONTROL DISORDER NOT OTHERWISE SPECIFIED

The DSM-IV-TR diagnostic category of impulse-control disorder not otherwise specified (Table 25–6) is a residual category for disorders of impulse control that do not meet the criteria for a specific impulse-control disorder. Some of the impulse disorders are listed below as compulsive disorders. Important, although subtle, distinctions exist between the two terms. An *impulse* is a tension state that can exist without an action; a *compulsion* is a tension state that always has an action component. The disorders are classified here as compulsions because the patients feel "compelled" to act out their pathological behavior; they cannot resist the impulse to do so. Impulses are acted on with the expectation of receiving pleasure; compulsions are usually

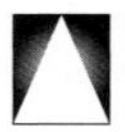

Table 25–6
DSM-IV-TR Diagnostic Criteria for Impulse-Control Disorder Not Otherwise Specified

This category is for disorders of impulse control (e.g., skin picking) that do not meet the criteria for any specific impulse-control disorder or for another mental disorder having features involving impulse control described elsewhere in the manual (e.g., substance dependence, a paraphilia).

(From American Psychiatric Association. *Diagnostic and Statistical Manual of Mental Disorders*. 4th ed. Text rev. Washington, DC: American Psychiatric Association; copyright 2000, with permission.)

ego-dystonic; for example, the patient does not like having to perform the act even though compelled to do so. An exception to the rule that impulses are associated with pleasure involves those cases in which feelings of guilt follow the act and disturb the sense of pleasure. Similarly, not all compulsions are ego-dystonic; for example, certain compulsive video game playing may have a pleasurable component. Both impulsive and compulsive behaviors are characterized by their repetitive nature; however, the repeated acting out of impulses leads to psychosocial impairment, whereas compulsive behavior does not always carry that risk. Because of the repetitive and pleasurable nature of many of the behavioral patterns in this group of disorders, they are often referred to as addictions.

Compulsive Buying

Originally referred to as *oniomania* and recognized by Emil Kraeplin and Eugen Bleuler, compulsive buying is not listed as a separate diagnostic category in DSM-IV-TR and ICD-10. Proposed diagnostic criteria are listed in Table 25–7. Compulsive buying is estimated to affect 1.1 to 5.9 percent of the general population. It is more common in women than in men.

The cause of the disorder is unknown. Psychodynamic theories have implicated low self-esteem, anxiety, and the need to reduce stress. Comorbid conditions include other disorders of impulse control (e.g., kleptomania), mood disorders, and OCD. A diagnosis of compulsive buying should not be made if the behavior occurs as part of a hypomanic or manic episode.

The onset of the disorder is usually about 18 years of age; however, patients do not seek treatment until their 20s or 30s, usually because they have developed serious financial problems. Compulsive buyers usually buy with credit and have many credit cards. Serious financial problems are usual, and some persons must declare bankruptcy. One study reported an average debt in compulsive shoppers of $23,000. The disorder may be chronic with urges to buy occurring hourly or as infrequently as once a month. Patients often try to limit their behavior but are unsuccessful.

Treatment of compulsive buying is difficult. Some patients are helped with supportive therapy, insight-oriented therapy, and self-help groups, such as Debtors Anonymous. Pharmacological therapies include antidepressants, antimanic drugs, anxiolytics, and antipsychotics to treat any comorbid conditions. The SSRIs have been used to limit compulsive behavior and may be of use in this condition, which has compulsive aspects.

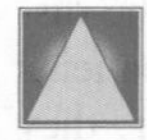

Table 25–7
Diagnostic Criteria for Compulsive Buying

A. Maladaptive preoccupation with buying or shopping, or maladaptive buying or shopping impulses or behavior, as indicated by at least one of the following:
   1. Frequent preoccupation with buying or impulses to buy that are experienced as irresistible, intrusive, and/or senseless.
   2. Frequent buying of more than can be afforded, frequent buying of items that are not needed, or shopping for longer periods of time than intended.

B. The buying preoccupations, impulses, or behaviors cause marked distress, are time consuming, significantly interfere with social or occupational functioning, or result in financial problems (e.g., indebtedness or bankruptcy).

C. The excessive buying or shopping behavior does not occur exclusively during periods of hypomania or mania.

(From McElroy SL, Keck PE Jr, Pope HG Jr, Smith JM, Strakowski SM. Compulsive buying: A report of 20 cases. *J Clin Psychiatry*. 1994;55:242, with permission.)

Internet Compulsion

Also called *Internet Addiction*, such persons spend almost all their waking hours at the computer terminal. Their patterns of use are repetitive and constant, and they are unable to resist strong urges to use the computer or to "surf the Web." Internet addicts may gravitate to certain sites that meet specific needs (e.g., shopping, sex, and interactive games, among others). Video game compulsive behavior is a variant behavioral pattern.

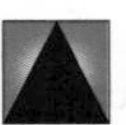

Table 25–8
ICD-10 Diagnostic Criteria for Habit and Impulse Disorders

Pathological gambling

A. Two or more episodes of gambling occur over a period of at least 1 year.
B. These episodes do not have a profitable outcome for the individual but are continued despite personal distress and interference with personal functioning in daily living.
C. The individual describes an intense urge to gamble which is difficult to control and reports that he or she is unable to stop gambling by an effort of will.
D. The individual is preoccupied with thoughts or mental images of the act of gambling or the circumstances surrounding the act.

Pathological fire setting (pyromania)

A. There are two or more acts of fire setting without apparent motive.
B. The individual describes an intense urge to set fire to objects, with a feeling of tension before the act and relief afterward.
C. The individual is preoccupied with thoughts or mental images of fire setting or of the circumstances surrounding the act (e.g., abnormal interest in fire engines or in calling out the fire service).

Pathological stealing (kleptomania)

A. There are two or more thefts in which the individual steals without any apparent motive of personal gain or gain for another person.
B. The individual describes an intense urge to steal, with a feeling of tension before the act and relief afterward.

Trichotillomania

A. Noticeable hair loss is caused by the individual's persistent and recurrent failure to resist impulses to pull out hairs.
B. The individual describes an intense urge to pull out hairs, with mounting tension before the act and a sense of relief afterward.
C. There is no preexisting inflammation of the skin, and the hair pulling is not in response to a delusion or hallucination.

Other habit and impulse disorders

This category should be used for other kinds of persistently repeated maladaptive behaviors that are not secondary to a recognized psychiatric syndrome and in which it appears that there is repeated failure to resist impulses to carry out the behavior. There is a prodromal period of tension with a feeling of release at the time of the act.

Habit and impulse disorder, unspecified

(From World Health Organization. The *ICD-10 Classification of Mental and Behavioural Disorders: Diagnostic Criteria for Research.* Copyright World Health Organization, Geneva, 1993, with permission.)

Cellular or Mobile Phone Compulsion

Some persons compulsively use mobile phones to call others—friends, acquaintances, or business associates. They justify their need to contact others by giving plausible reasons for calling; but underlying conflicts may be expressed in the behavior, such as fear of being alone, the need to satisfy unconscious dependency needs, or undoing a hostile wish toward a loved one, among others (e.g., "I just want to make sure you are OK.").

Repetitive Self-Mutilation

Persons who repeatedly cut themselves or do damage to their bodies may do so in a compulsive manner. In all cases, another disorder will be found. Parasuicidal behavior is common in borderline personality disorder. Compulsive body piercing or tattooing may be a symptom of a paraphilia or a depressive equivalent.

Compulsive Sexual Behavior

Some persons repeatedly seek out sexual gratification, often in perverse ways (e.g., exhibitionism). They are unable to control their behavior and may not experience feelings of guilt after an episode of acting-out behavior. Sometimes called *sexual addiction*, this condition is discussed extensively in Chapter 21, "Human Sexuality."

ICD-10

The category of *habit and impulse disorder* in the tenth edition of the *International Statistical Classification of Diseases and Related Health Problems* (ICD-10) (Table 25–8) is analogous to the DSM-IV-TR's *impulse-control disorders, not elsewhere specified*. Intermittent explosive disorder is not mentioned per se in the ICD-10 schema. Habitual use of alcohol or drugs, as well as addictive or otherwise pathological sexual and eating disorders, is specifically excluded.

In the ICD-10, habit and impulse disorders are characterized by repeated acts with no clear rational motive that cannot be controlled by the patient and are usually harmful to the interests of self and others. ICD-10 states the causes of these conditions are unknown, further asserting that they are only grouped together because of broad descriptive similarities, "not because they are known to share any other important features."

References

Chambers RO, Potenza MN. Neurodevelopment, impulsivity, and adolescent gambling. *J Gambl Stud.* 2003;19:53.

Dannon PN. Topiramate for the treatment of kleptomania: A case series and review of the literature. *Clin Neuropharmacol.* 2003;26:1.

Grant JE, Kim SW, Potenza MN. Advances in the pharmacological treatment of pathological gambling. *J Gambl Stud.* 2003;19:85.

Grant JE, Potenza MN. Impulse control disorders: Clinical characteristics and pharmacological management. *Ann Clin Psychiatry.* 2004;16:27–34.

Greenberg HR. Impulse-control disorders not elsewhere classified. In: Sadock BJ, Sadock VA, eds. *Kaplan & Sadock's Comprehensive Textbook of Psychiatry.* 8th ed. Vol. 1. Baltimore: Lippincott Williams & Wilkins; 2005:2035.

Hollander E, Baker BR, Kahn J, Stein DJ. Conceptualizing and assessing impulse-control disorders. In: In: Hollander E, Stein DJ, eds. *Clinical Manual of Impulse-Control Disorders.* Washington, DC: American Psychiatric Publishing, Inc.; 2006:1–18.

Kuzma JM, Black DW. Disorders characterized by poor impulse control. *Ann Clin Psychiatry.* 2005;17:219–226.

Lyke J. A psychiatric perspective on the variety of impulsive behaviors. *PsychCRITIQUES.* 2006;51.

Reist C, Nakamura K, Sagart E, Sokolski KN, Fujimoto KA. Impulsive aggressive behavior: Open-label treatment with citalopram. *J Clin Psychiatry.* 2003;64:81.

Stein DJ, Harvey B, Seedat S, Hollander E. Treatment of impulse-control disorders. In: Hollander E, Stein DJ, eds. *Clinical Manual of Impulse-Control Disorders.* Washington, DC: American Psychiatric Publishing, Inc.; 2006:309–325.

Tavares H, Zilberman ML, el-Guebaly N. Are there cognitive and behavioural approaches specific to the treatment of pathological gambling? *Can J Psychiatry.* 2003;48:22.

26 Adjustment Disorders

The adjustment disorders are a diagnostic category characterized by an emotional response to a stressful event. Typically, the stressor involves financial issues, a medical illness, or a relationship problem. The symptom complex that develops may involve anxious or depressive affect or may present with a disturbance of conduct. By definition, the symptoms must begin within 3 months of the stressor and must remit within 6 months of removal of the stressor. A variety of subtypes of adjustment disorder are identified in the text revision of the fourth edition of *Diagnostic and Statistical Manual of Mental Disorders* (DSM-IV-TR), varying on the particular predominant affective presentation. These include adjustment disorder with depressed mood, anxious mood, mixed anxiety and depressed mood, disturbance of conduct, mixed disturbance of emotions and conduct, and unspecified type.

EPIDEMIOLOGY

According to DSM-IV-TR, the prevalence of the disorder is estimated to be from 2 to 8 percent of the general population. Women are diagnosed with the disorder twice as often as men, and single women are generally overly represented as most at risk. In children and adolescents, boys and girls are equally diagnosed with adjustment disorders. The disorders can occur at any age, but are most frequently diagnosed in adolescents. Among adolescents of either sex, common precipitating stresses are school problems, parental rejection and divorce, and substance abuse. Among adults, common precipitating stresses are marital problems, divorce, moving to a new environment, and financial problems.

Adjustment disorders are one of the most common psychiatric diagnoses for disorders of patients hospitalized for medical and surgical problems. In one study, 5 percent of persons admitted to a hospital over a 3-year period were classified as having an adjustment disorder. Up to 50 percent of persons with specific medical problems or stressors have been diagnosed with adjustment disorders. Furthermore, 10 to 30 percent of mental health outpatients and up to 12 percent of general hospital inpatients referred for mental health consultations have been diagnosed with adjustment disorders.

ETIOLOGY

By definition, an adjustment disorder is precipitated by one or more stressors. The severity of the stressor or stressors does not always predict the severity of the disorder; the stressor severity is a complex function of degree, quantity, duration, reversibility, environment, and personal context. For example, the loss of a parent is different for a child 10 years of age than for a person 40 years of age. Personality organization and cultural or group norms and values also contribute to the disproportionate responses to stressors.

Stressors may be single, such as a divorce or the loss of a job, or multiple, such as the death of a person important to a patient, which coincides with the patient's own physical illness and loss of a job. Stressors may be recurrent, such as seasonal business difficulties, or continuous, such as chronic illness or poverty. A discordant intrafamilial relationship can produce an adjustment disorder that affects the entire family system, or the disorder may be limited to a patient who was perhaps the victim of a crime or who has a physical illness. Sometimes, adjustment disorders occur in a group or community setting, and the stressors affect several persons, as in a natural disaster or in racial, social, or religious persecution. Specific developmental stages, such as beginning school, leaving home, getting married, becoming a parent, failing to achieve occupational goals, having the last child leave home, and retiring, are often associated with adjustment disorders.

Psychodynamic Factors

Pivotal to understanding adjustment disorders is an understanding of three factors: the nature of the stressor, the conscious and unconscious meanings of the stressor, and the patient's preexisting vulnerability. A concurrent personality disorder or organic impairment may make a person vulnerable to adjustment disorders. Vulnerability is also associated with the loss of a parent during infancy or being reared in a dysfunctional family. Actual or perceived support from key relationships can affect behavioral and emotional responses to stressors.

Several psychoanalytic researchers have pointed out that the same stress can produce a range of responses in various persons. Throughout his life, Sigmund Freud remained interested in why the stresses of ordinary life produce illness in some and not in others, why an illness takes a particular form, and why some experiences and not others predispose a person to psychopathology. He gave considerable weight to constitutional factors and viewed them as interacting with a person's life experiences to produce fixation.

Psychoanalytic research has emphasized the role of the mother and the rearing environment in a person's later capacity to respond to stress. Particularly important was Donald Winnicott's concept of the good-enough mother, a person who adapts to the infant's needs and provides sufficient support to enable the growing child to tolerate the frustrations in life.

Clinicians must undertake a detailed exploration of a patient's experience of the stressor. Certain patients commonly place all the blame on a particular event when a less obvious event may have had more significant psychological meaning for the patient. Current events may reawaken past traumas or disappointments from childhood, so patients should be encouraged to think about how the current situation relates to similar past events.

Throughout early development, each child develops a unique set of defense mechanisms to deal with stressful events. Because of greater amounts of trauma or greater constitutional vulnerability, some children have less mature defensive constellations than other children. This disadvantage may cause them as adults to react with substantially impaired functioning when they are faced with a loss, a divorce, or a financial setback; those who have developed mature defense mechanisms are less vulnerable and bounce back more quickly from the stressor. Resilience is also crucially determined by the nature of children's early relationships with their parents. Studies of trauma repeatedly indicate that supportive, nurturant relationships prevent traumatic incidents from causing permanent psychological damage.

Psychodynamic clinicians must consider the relation between a stressor and the human developmental life cycle. When adolescents leave home for college, for example, they are at high developmental risk for reacting with a temporary symptomatic picture. Similarly, if the young person who leaves home is the last child in the family, the parents may be particularly vulnerable to a reaction of adjustment disorder. Moreover, middle-aged persons who are confronting their own mortality may be especially sensitive to the effects of loss or death.

Family and Genetic Factors

Some studies suggest that certain persons appear to be at increased risk both for the occurrence of these adverse life events and for the development of pathology once they occur. Findings from a study of more than 2,000 twin pairs indicate that life events and stressors are modestly correlated in twin pairs, with monozygotic twins showing greater concordance than dizygotic twins. Family environmental and genetic factors each accounted for approximately 20 percent of the variance in that study. Another twin study that examined genetic contributions to the development of posttraumatic stress disorder (PTSD) symptoms (not necessarily at the level of full disorder and, therefore, relevant to adjustment disorders) also concluded that the likelihood of developing symptoms in response to traumatic life events is partially under genetic control.

DIAGNOSIS AND CLINICAL FEATURES

Although by definition adjustment disorders follow a stressor, the symptoms do not necessarily begin immediately. Up to 3 months may elapse between a stressor and the development of symptoms. Symptoms do not always subside as soon as the stressor ceases; if the stressor continues, the disorder may be chronic. The disorder can occur at any age, and its symptoms vary considerably, with depressive, anxious, and mixed features most common in adults. Physical symptoms, which are most common in children and the elderly, can occur in any age group. Manifestations may also include assaultive behavior and reckless driving, excessive drinking, defaulting on legal responsibilities, withdrawal, vegetative signs, insomnia, and suicidal behavior.

The clinical presentations of adjustment disorder can vary widely. DSM-IV-TR lists six adjustment disorders, including an unspecified category (Table 26–1).

Adjustment Disorder with Depressed Mood

In adjustment disorder with depressed mood, the predominant manifestations are depressed mood, tearfulness, and hopelessness. This type must be distinguished from major depressive

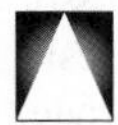

Table 26–1
DSM-IV-TR Diagnostic Criteria for Adjustment Disorders

A. The development of emotional or behavioral symptoms in response to an identifiable stressor(s) occurring within 3 months of the onset of the stressor(s).
B. These symptoms or behaviors are clinically significant as evidenced by either of the following:
 (1) marked distress that is in excess of what would be expected from exposure to the stressor
 (2) significant impairment in social or occupational (academic) functioning
C. The stress-related disturbance does not meet the criteria for another specific Axis I disorder and is not merely an exacerbation of a preexisting Axis I or Axis II disorder.
D. The symptoms do not represent bereavement.
E. Once the stressor (or its consequences) has terminated, the symptoms do not persist for more than an additional 6 months.

Specify if:

Acute: if the disturbance lasts less than 6 months
Chronic: if the disturbance lasts for 6 months or longer

Adjustment disorders are coded based on the subtype, which is selected according to the predominant symptoms. The specific stressor(s) can be specified on Axis IV.

With depressed mood
With anxiety
With mixed anxiety and depressed mood
With disturbance of conduct
With mixed disturbance of emotions and conduct
Unspecified

(From American Psychiatric Association. *Diagnostic and Statistical Manual of Mental Disorders.* 4th ed. Text rev. Washington, DC: American Psychiatric Association; copyright 2000.)

disorder and uncomplicated bereavement. Adolescents with this type of adjustment disorder are at increased risk for major depressive disorder in young adulthood.

Adjustment Disorder with Anxiety

Symptoms of anxiety, such as palpitations, jitteriness, and agitation, are present in adjustment disorder with anxiety, which must be differentiated from anxiety disorders.

Adjustment Disorder with Mixed Anxiety and Depressed Mood

In adjustment disorder with mixed anxiety and depressed mood, patients exhibit features of both anxiety and depression that do not meet the criteria for an already established anxiety disorder or depressive disorder.

A 48-year-old married woman, in good health, with no previous psychiatric difficulties, presented to the emergency room reporting that she had overdosed on a handful of antihistamines shortly before she arrived. She described her problems as having started 2 months earlier, soon after her husband unexpectedly requested a divorce. She felt betrayed after having devoted much of her 20-year marriage to being a wife, mother, and homemaker. She was sad and tearful at times, and she occasionally had difficulty sleeping. Otherwise, she had no vegetative symptoms and enjoyed time with family and friends. She felt desperate and suicidal after she realized that "he no longer loved me." After crisis intervention in the emergency setting, she responded well to individual psychotherapy over a 3-month period. She occasionally required benzodiazepines for anxiety during the period of treatment. By the time of discharge, she had returned to her baseline function. She came to terms with the possibility of life after divorce and was exploring her best options under the circumstances. (Courtesy of Jeffrey William Katz, M.D., and Oladapo Tomori, M.D.)

Adjustment Disorder with Disturbance of Conduct

In adjustment disorder with disturbance of conduct, the predominant manifestation involves conduct in which the rights of others are violated or age-appropriate societal norms and rules are disregarded. Examples of behavior in this category are truancy, vandalism, reckless driving, and fighting. The category must be differentiated from conduct disorder and antisocial personality disorder.

Adjustment Disorder with Mixed Disturbance of Emotions and Conduct

A combination of disturbances of emotions and of conduct sometimes occurs. Clinicians are encouraged to try to make one or the other diagnosis in the interest of clarity.

Adjustment Disorder Unspecified

Adjustment disorder unspecified is a residual category for atypical maladaptive reactions to stress. Examples include inappropriate responses to the diagnosis of physical illness, such as massive denial, severe noncompliance with treatment, and social withdrawal, without significant depressed or anxious mood.

DIFFERENTIAL DIAGNOSIS

Although uncomplicated bereavement often produces temporarily impaired social and occupational functioning, the person's dysfunction remains within the expectable bounds of a reaction to the loss of a loved one and, thus, is not considered adjustment disorder. Other disorders from which adjustment disorder must be differentiated include major depressive disorder, brief psychotic disorder, generalized anxiety disorder, somatization disorder, substance-related disorder, conduct disorder, academic problem, occupational problem, identity problem, and PTSD. These diagnoses should be given precedence in all cases that meet their criteria, even in the presence of a stressor or group of stressors that served as a precipitant. Patients with an adjustment disorder are impaired in social or occupational functioning and show symptoms beyond the normal and expectable reaction to the stressor. Because no absolute criteria help to distinguish an adjustment disorder from another condition, clinical judgment is necessary. Some patients may meet the criteria for both an adjustment disorder and a personality disorder. If the adjustment disorder follows a physical illness, the clinician must make sure that the symptoms are not a continuation or another manifestation of the illness or its treatment.

Acute and Posttraumatic Stress Disorders

The presence of a stressor is a requirement in the diagnosis of adjustment disorder, PTSD, and acute stress disorder. PTSD and acute stress disorder have the nature of the stressor better characterized and are accompanied by a defined constellation of affective and autonomic symptoms. In contrast, the stressor in adjustment disorder can be of any severity, with a wide range of possible symptoms. When the response to an extreme stressor does not meet the acute stress or posttraumatic disorder threshold, the adjustment disorder diagnosis would be appropriate. PTSD is discussed fully in Chapter 16.5.

COURSE AND PROGNOSIS

With appropriate treatment, the overall prognosis of an adjustment disorder is generally favorable. Most patients return to their previous level of functioning within 3 months. Some persons (particularly adolescents) who receive a diagnosis of an adjustment disorder later have mood disorders or substance-related disorders. Adolescents usually require a longer time to recover than adults.

TREATMENT

Psychotherapy

Psychotherapy remains the treatment of choice for adjustment disorders. Group therapy can be particularly useful for patients who have had similar stresses—for example, a group of retired persons or patients having renal dialysis. Individual psychotherapy offers the opportunity to explore the meaning of the stressor to the patient so that earlier traumas can be worked through. After successful therapy, patients sometimes emerge from an adjustment disorder stronger than in the premorbid period, although no pathology was evident during that period. Because a stressor can be clearly delineated in adjustment disorders, it is often believed that psychotherapy is not indicated and that the disorder will remit spontaneously. This viewpoint, however, ignores the fact that many persons exposed to the same stressor experience different symptoms, and in adjustment disorders, the response is pathological. Psychotherapy can help persons adapt to stressors that are not reversible or time limited and can serve as a preventive intervention if the stressor does remit. Psychiatrists treating adjustment disorders must be particularly aware of problems of secondary gain. The illness role may be rewarding to some normally healthy persons who have had little experience with illness's capacity to free them from responsibility. Thus, patients can find therapists' attention, empathy, and understanding, which are necessary for success, rewarding in their own right, and therapists may thereby reinforce patients' symptoms. Such considerations must be weighed before intensive psychotherapy is begun; when a secondary gain has already been established, therapy is difficult. Patients with an adjustment disorder that includes a conduct disturbance may have difficulties with the law, authorities, or school. Psychiatrists should not attempt to rescue such patients from the consequences of their actions. Too often, such kindness only reinforces socially unacceptable means of tension reduction and hinders the acquisition of insight and subsequent emotional growth. In these cases, family therapy can help.

Crisis Intervention. Crisis intervention and case management are short-term treatments aimed at helping persons with adjustment disorders resolve their situations quickly by supportive techniques, suggestion, reassurance, environmental modification, and even hospitalization, if necessary. The frequency and length of visits for crisis support vary according to patients' needs; daily sessions may be necessary, sometimes two or three times each day. Flexibility is essential in this approach.

Pharmacotherapy

No studies have assessed the efficacy of pharmacological interventions in individuals with adjustment disorder, but it may be reasonable to use medication to treat specific symptoms for a brief time. The judicious use of medications can help patients with adjustment disorders, but they should be prescribed for brief periods. Depending on the type of adjustment disorder, a patient may respond to an antianxiety agent or to an antidepressant. Patients with severe anxiety bordering on panic can benefit from anxiolytics such as diazepam (Valium), and those in withdrawn or inhibited states may be helped by a short course of psychostimulant medication. Antipsychotic drugs may be used if there are signs of decompensation or impending psychosis. Selective serotonin reuptake inhibitors have been found useful in treating symptoms of traumatic grief. Recently, there has been an increase in antidepressant use to augment psychotherapy in patients with adjustment disorders. Pharmacological intervention in this population is most often used, however, to augment psychosocial strategies rather than serving as the primary modality.

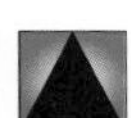

Table 26–2
ICD-10 Diagnostic Criteria for Adjustment Disorders

A. Onset of symptoms must occur within 1 month of exposure to an identifiable psychosocial stressor, not of an unusual or catastrophic type.

B. The individual manifests symptoms or behavior disturbance of the types found in any of the affective disorders (except for delusions and hallucinations), any disorder in neurotic, stress-related, and somatoform disorders, and conduct disorders, but the criteria for an individual disorder are not fulfilled. Symptoms may be variable in both form and severity.

The predominant feature of the symptoms may be further specified.

Brief depressive reaction
A transient mild depressive state of a duration not exceeding 1 month.

Prolonged depressive reaction
A mild depressive state occurring in response to a prolonged exposure to a stressful situation but of a duration not exceeding 2 years.

Mixed anxiety and depressive reaction
Both anxiety and depressive symptoms are prominent, but at levels no greater than those specified for mixed anxiety and depressive disorder or other mixed anxiety disorders.

With predominant disturbance of other emotions
The symptoms are usually of several types of emotions, such as anxiety, depression, worry, tensions, and anger. Symptoms of anxiety and depression may meet the criteria for mixed anxiety and depressive disorder or for other mixed anxiety disorders, but they are not so predominant that other more specific depressive or anxiety disorders can be diagnosed. This category should also be used for reactions in children in whom regressive behavior such as bed-wetting or thumb-sucking is also present.

With predominant disturbance of conduct
The main disturbance is one involving conduct, e.g., an adolescent grief reaction resulting in aggressive or dissocial behavior.

With mixed disturbance of emotions and conduct
Both emotional symptoms and disturbances of conduct are prominent features.

With other specified predominant symptoms

C. Except in prolonged depressive reaction, the symptoms do not persist for more than 6 months after the cessation of the stress or its consequences. However, this should not prevent a provisional diagnosis being made if this criterion is not yet fulfilled.

(Reprinted with permission from World Health Organization. The *ICD-10 Classification of Mental and Behavioural Disorders: Diagnostic Criteria for Research.* Copyright, World Health Organization, Geneva, 1993.)

ICD-10

The 10th revision of the *International Statistical Classification of Diseases and Related Health Problems* (ICD-10) also contains a category of adjustment disorders. The diagnosis is similar to the DSM-IV-TR entity in outlining the development of psychological symptoms following a stressor. In ICD-10, however, the symptoms must appear within 1 month of the stressor, instead of the 3-month temporal course of DSM-IV-TR (Table 26–2). The ICD-10 criteria share with DSM-IV-TR the requirement that symptoms must not persist for longer than 6 months after the removal of the stressor. The ICD-10 and DSM-IV-TR differ in their consideration of chronicity. Whereas the DSM-IV-TR requires the specification of *acute* or *chronic* for all subtypes of adjustment disorder, the ICD-10 only refers to *chronicity* if the primary experience involved is a depressed state. In this case, the diagnosis of prolonged depressive reaction is used to describe symptoms lasting for as long as 2 years.

References

Akizuki N, Akechi T, Nakanishi T, Yoshikawa E, Okamura M, Nakano T, Murakami Y, Uchitomi Y. Development of a brief screening interview for adjustment disorders and major depression in patients with cancer. *Cancer.* 2003;97:2605.

Gonzalez-Jaimes EI, Turbull-Plaza B. Selection of psychotherapeutic treatment for adjustment disorder with depressive mood due to acute myocardial infarction. *Arch Med Res.* 2003;34:298.

Judy DH. Seasons change: Adjustment disorder as summons to new life structure. In: Mijares SG, Khalsa GS, eds. *The Psychospiritual Clinician's Handbook: Alternative Methods for Understanding and Treating Mental Disorders.* New York: Haworth Press, Inc.; 2005:33–50.

Katz JW, Tomori O. Adjustment disorders. In: Sadock BJ, Sadock VA, eds. *Kaplan & Sadock's Comprehensive Textbook of Psychiatry.* 8th ed. Vol. 2. Baltimore: Lippincott Williams & Wilkins; 2005:2055.

Kim KJ, Conger RD, Elder GH Jr, Lorenz FO. Reciprocal influences between stressful life events and adolescent internalizing and externalizing problems. *Child Dev.* 2003;74:127.

Levitas AS, Hurley AD. Diagnosis and treatment of adjustment disorders in people with intellectual disability. *Mental Health Aspects of Developmental Disabilities.* 2005;8:52–60.

Linden M. Posttraumatic embitterment disorder. *Psychother Psychosom.* 2003;72:195.

Newcorn JH, Strain JJ, Mezzich JE. Adjustment disorders. In: Sadock BJ, Sadock VA, eds. *Kaplan & Sadock's Comprehensive Textbook of Psychiatry.* 7th ed. Vol. 2. Baltimore: Lippincott Williams & Wilkins; 2000:1714.

Portzky G, Audenaert K, van Heeringen K. Adjustment disorder and the course of the suicidal process in adolescents. *J Affect Disord.* 2005;87:265–270.

Powell S, McCone D. Treatment of adjustment disorder with anxiety: A September 11, 2001, case study with a 1-year follow-up. *Cognitive and Behavioral Practice.* 2004;11:331–336.

Van der Klink JJ, van Dijk FJ. Dutch practice guidelines for managing adjustment disorders in occupational and primary health care. *Scand J Work Environ Health.* 2003;29:478.

27 Personality Disorders

Personality disorder is a common and chronic disorder. Its prevalence is estimated between 10 and 20 percent in the general population, and its duration is expressed in decades. Persons with personality disorder are frequently labeled as *aggravating*, *demanding*, or *parasitic* and are generally considered to have poor prognosis. Approximately one half of all psychiatric patients have personality disorder, which is frequently comorbid with Axis I conditions. Personality disorder is also a predisposing factor for other psychiatric disorders (e.g., substance use, suicide, affective disorders, impulse-control disorders, eating disorders, and anxiety disorders) in which it interferes with treatment outcomes of Axis I syndromes and increases personal incapacitation, morbidity, and mortality of these patients.

Persons with personality disorders are far more likely to refuse psychiatric help and to deny their problems than persons with anxiety disorders, depressive disorders, or obsessive-compulsive disorder. Personality disorder symptoms are alloplastic (i.e., able to adapt to, and alter, the external environment) and ego-syntonic (i.e., acceptable to the ego). Persons with personality disorders do not feel anxiety about their maladaptive behavior. Because they do not routinely acknowledge pain from what others perceive as their symptoms, they often seem disinterested in treatment and impervious to recovery.

CLASSIFICATION

The text revision of the fourth edition of the *Diagnostic and Statistical Manual of Mental Disorders* (DSM-IV-TR) defines personality disorders as enduring subjective experiences and behavior that deviate from cultural standards, are rigidly pervasive, have an onset in adolescence or early adulthood, are stable through time, and lead to unhappiness and impairment. When personality traits are rigid and maladaptive and produce functional impairment or subjective distress, a personality disorder may be diagnosed (Table 27–1).

Personality disorder subtypes classified in DSM-IV-TR are: *schizotypal*, *schizoid*, and *paranoid* (Cluster A); *narcissistic*, *borderline*, *antisocial*, and *histrionic* (Cluster B); and *obsessive-compulsive*, *dependent*, and *avoidant* (Cluster C). Cluster A includes three disorders with odd, aloof features, such as paranoid, schizoid, and schizotypal. Cluster B includes four disorders with dramatic, impulsive, and erratic features, such as borderline, antisocial, narcissistic, and histrionic. Cluster C includes three disorders sharing anxious and fearful features, such as avoidant, dependent, and obsessive-compulsive. Many persons exhibit traits that are not limited to a single personality disorder. When a patient meets the criteria for more than one personality disorder, clinicians should diagnose each. Personality disorders are coded on Axis II of DSM-IV-TR.

ETIOLOGY

Genetic Factors

The best evidence that genetic factors contribute to personality disorders comes from investigations of 15,000 pairs of twins in the United States. Among monozygotic twins, the concordance for personality disorders was several times that among dizygotic twins. Moreover, according to one study, monozygotic twins reared apart are about as similar as monozygotic twins reared together. Similarities include multiple measures of personality and temperament, occupational and leisure-time interests, and social attitudes.

Cluster A personality disorders are more common in the biological relatives of patients with schizophrenia than in control groups. More relatives with schizotypal personality disorder occur in the family histories of persons with schizophrenia than in control groups. Less correlation exists between paranoid or schizoid personality disorder and schizophrenia.

Cluster B personality disorders apparently have a genetic base. Antisocial personality disorder is associated with alcohol use disorders. Depression is common in the family backgrounds of patients with borderline personality disorder. These patients have more relatives with mood disorders than do control groups, and persons with borderline personality disorder often have a mood disorder as well. A strong association is found between histrionic personality disorder and somatization disorder (Briquet's syndrome); patients with each disorder show an overlap of symptoms.

Cluster C personality disorders may also have a genetic base. Patients with avoidant personality disorder often have high anxiety levels. Obsessive-compulsive traits are more common in monozygotic twins than in dizygotic twins, and patients with obsessive-compulsive personality disorder show some signs associated with depression—for example, shortened rapid eye movement (REM) latency period and abnormal dexamethasone-suppression test (DST) results.

Biological Factors

Hormones. Persons who exhibit impulsive traits also often show high levels of testosterone, 17-estradiol, and estrone. In

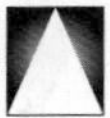

Table 27–1
DSM-IV-TR General Diagnostic Criteria for a Personality Disorder

A. An enduring pattern of inner experience and behavior that deviates markedly from the expectations of the individual's culture. This pattern is manifested in two (or more) of the following areas:
   (1) cognition (i.e., ways of perceiving and interpreting self, other people, and events)
   (2) affectivity (i.e., the range, intensity, lability, and appropriateness of emotional response)
   (3) interpersonal functioning
   (4) impulse control
B. The enduring pattern is inflexible and pervasive across a broad range of personal and social situations.
C. The enduring pattern leads to clinically significant distress or impairment in social, occupational, or other important areas of functioning.
D. The pattern is stable and of long duration, and its onset can be traced back at least to adolescence or early adulthood.
E. The enduring pattern is not better accounted for as a manifestation or consequence of another mental disorder.
F. The enduring pattern is not due to the direct physiological effects of a substance (e.g., a drug of abuse, a medication) or a general medical condition (e.g., head trauma).

(From American Psychiatric Association. *Diagnostic and Statistical Manual of Mental Disorders.* 4th ed. Text rev. Washington, DC: American Psychiatric Association; copyright 2000, with permission.)

nonhuman primates, androgens increase the likelihood of aggression and sexual behavior, but the role of testosterone in human aggression is unclear. DST results are abnormal in some patients with borderline personality disorder who also have depressive symptoms.

Platelet Monoamine Oxidase. Low platelet monoamine oxidase (MAO) levels have been associated with activity and sociability in monkeys. College students with low platelet MAO levels report spending more time in social activities than students with high platelet MAO levels. Low platelet MAO levels have also been noted in some patients with schizotypal disorders.

Smooth Pursuit Eye Movements. Smooth pursuit eye movements are saccadic (i.e., jumpy) in persons who are introverted, who have low self-esteem and tend to withdraw, and who have schizotypal personality disorder. These findings have no clinical application, but they do indicate the role of inheritance.

Neurotransmitters. Endorphins have effects similar to those of exogenous morphine, such as analgesia and the suppression of arousal. High endogenous endorphin levels may be associated with persons who are phlegmatic. Studies of personality traits and the dopaminergic and serotonergic systems indicate an arousal-activating function for these neurotransmitters. Levels of 5-hydroxyindoleacetic acid (5-HIAA), a metabolite of serotonin, are low in persons who attempt suicide and in patients who are impulsive and aggressive.

Raising serotonin levels with serotonergic agents such as fluoxetine (Prozac) can produce dramatic changes in some character traits of personality. In many persons, serotonin reduces depression, impulsiveness, and rumination, and can produce a sense of general well-being. Increased dopamine concentrations in the central nervous system, produced by certain psychostimulants (e.g., amphetamines) can induce euphoria. The effects of neurotransmitters on personality traits have generated much interest and controversy about whether personality traits are inborn or acquired.

Electrophysiology. Changes in electrical conductance on the electroencephalogram (EEG) occur in some patients with personality disorders, most commonly antisocial and borderline types; these changes appear as slow-wave activity on EEGs.

Psychoanalytic Factors

Sigmund Freud suggested that personality traits are related to a fixation at one psychosexual stage of development. For example, those with an oral character are passive and dependent because they are fixated at the oral stage, when the dependence on others for food is prominent. Those with an anal character are stubborn, parsimonious, and highly conscientious because of struggles over toilet training during the anal period.

Wilhelm Reich subsequently coined the term *character armor* to describe persons' characteristic defensive styles for protecting themselves from internal impulses and from interpersonal anxiety in significant relationships. Reich's theory has had a broad influence on contemporary concepts of personality and personality disorders. For example, each human being's unique stamp of personality is considered largely determined by his or her characteristic defense mechanisms. Each personality disorder in Axis II has a cluster of defenses that help psychodynamic clinicians recognize the type of character pathology present. Persons with paranoid personality disorder, for instance, use projection, whereas schizoid personality disorder is associated with withdrawal.

When defenses work effectively, persons with personality disorders master feelings of anxiety, depression, anger, shame, guilt, and other affects. They often view their behavior as ego-syntonic; that is, it creates no distress for them, even though it may adversely affect others. They may also be reluctant to engage in a treatment process; because their defenses are important in controlling unpleasant affects, they are not interested in surrendering them.

In addition to characteristic defenses in personality disorders, another central feature is internal object relations. During development, particular patterns of self in relation to others are internalized. Through introjection, children internalize a parent or another significant person as an internal presence that continues to feel like an object rather than a self. Through identification, children internalize parents and others in such a way that the traits of the external object are incorporated into the self and the child "owns" the traits. These internal self-representations and object representations are crucial in developing the personality and, through externalization and projective identification, are played out in interpersonal scenarios in which others are coerced into playing a role in the person's internal life. Hence, persons with personality disorders are also identified by particular patterns of interpersonal relatedness that stem from these internal object relations patterns.

Defense Mechanisms. To help those with personality disorders, psychiatrists must appreciate patients' underlying defenses, the unconscious mental processes that the ego uses to resolve conflicts among the four lodestars of the inner life: instinct (wish or need), reality, important persons, and conscience. When defenses are most effective, especially in those with personality disorders, they can abolish anxiety and depression. Thus, abandoning a defense increases conscious anxiety and depression—a major reason that those with personality disorders are reluctant to alter their behavior.

Although patients with personality disorders may be characterized by their most dominant or rigid mechanism, each patient uses several defenses. Therefore, the management of defense mechanisms used by patients with personality disorders is discussed here as a general topic and not as an aspect of the specific disorders. Many formulations presented here in the language of psychoanalytic psychiatry can be translated into principles consistent with cognitive and behavioral approaches.

FANTASY. Many persons who are often labeled schizoid—those who are eccentric, lonely, or frightened—seek solace and satisfaction within themselves by creating imaginary lives, especially imaginary friends. In their extensive dependence on fantasy, these persons often seem to be strikingly aloof. Therapists must understand that the unsociableness of these patients rests on a fear of intimacy. Rather than criticizing them or feeling rebuffed by their rejection, therapists should maintain a quiet, reassuring, and considerate interest without insisting on reciprocal responses. Recognition of patients' fear of closeness and respect for their eccentric ways are both therapeutic and useful.

DISSOCIATION. Dissociation or denial is a Pollyanna-like replacement of unpleasant affects with pleasant ones. Persons who frequently dissociate are often seen as dramatizing and emotionally shallow; they may be labeled histrionic personalities. They behave like anxious adolescents who, to erase anxiety, carelessly expose themselves to exciting dangers. Accepting such patients as exuberant and seductive is to overlook their anxiety, but confronting them with their vulnerabilities and defects makes them still more defensive. Because these patients seek appreciation of their courage and attractiveness, therapists should not behave with inordinate reserve. While remaining calm and firm, clinicians should realize that these patients are often inadvertent liars, but they benefit from ventilating their own anxieties and may in the process "remember" what they "forgot." Often therapists deal best with dissociation and denial by using displacement. Thus, clinicians may talk with patients about an issue of denial in an unthreatening circumstance. Empathizing with the denied affect without directly confronting patients with the facts may allow them to raise the original topic themselves.

ISOLATION. Isolation is characteristic of the orderly, controlled persons who are often labeled obsessive-compulsive personalities. Unlike those with histrionic personality, persons with obsessive-compulsive personality remember the truth in fine detail but without affect. In a crisis, patients may show intensified self-restraint, overly formal social behavior, and obstinacy. Patients' quests for control may annoy clinicians or make them anxious. Often, such patients respond well to precise, systematic, and rational explanations and value efficiency, cleanliness, and punctuality as much as they do clinicians' effective responsiveness. Whenever possible, therapists should allow such patients to control their own care and should not engage in a battle of wills.

PROJECTION. In projection, patients attribute their own unacknowledged feelings to others. Patients' excessive faultfinding and sensitivity to criticism may appear to therapists as prejudiced, hypervigilant injustice collecting, but should not be met by defensiveness and argument. Instead, clinicians should frankly acknowledge even minor mistakes on their part and should discuss the possibility of future difficulties. Strict honesty, concern for patients' rights, and maintaining the same formal, concerned distance as used with patients who use fantasy defenses are all helpful. Confrontation guarantees a lasting enemy and early termination of the interview. Therapists need not agree with patients' injustice collecting, but they should ask whether both can agree to disagree.

The technique of counterprojection is especially helpful. Clinicians acknowledge and give paranoid patients full credit for their feelings and perceptions; they neither dispute patients' complaints nor reinforce them, but agree that the world described by patients is conceivable. Interviewers can then talk about real motives and feelings, misattributed to someone else, and begin to cement an alliance with patients.

SPLITTING. In splitting, persons toward whom patients' feelings are, or have been, ambivalent are divided into good and bad. For example, in an inpatient setting, a patient may idealize some staff members and uniformly disparage others. This defense behavior can be highly disruptive on a hospital ward and can ultimately provoke the staff to turn against the patient. When staff members anticipate the process, discuss it at staff meetings, and gently confront the patient with the fact that no one is all good or all bad, the phenomenon of splitting can be dealt with effectively.

PASSIVE AGGRESSION. Persons with passive-aggressive defense turn their anger against themselves. In psychoanalytic terms this phenomenon is called *masochism* and includes failure, procrastination, silly or provocative behavior, self-demeaning clowning, and frankly self-destructive acts. The hostility in such behavior is never entirely concealed. Indeed, in a mechanism such as wrist cutting, others feel as much anger as if they themselves had been assaulted and view the patient as a sadist, not a masochist. Therapists can best deal with passive aggression by helping patients to ventilate their anger.

ACTING OUT. In acting out, patients directly express unconscious wishes or conflicts through action to avoid being conscious of either the accompanying idea or the affect. Tantrums, apparently motiveless assaults, child abuse, and pleasureless promiscuity are common examples. Because the behavior occurs outside reflective awareness, acting out often appears to observers to be unaccompanied by guilt, but when acting out is impossible, the conflict behind the defense may be accessible. The clinician faced with acting out, either aggressive or sexual, in an interview situation, must recognize that the patient has lost control, that anything the interviewer says will probably be misheard, and that getting the patient's attention is of paramount importance. Depending on the circumstances, a clinician's response may be, "How can I help you if you keep screaming?" Or, if the patient's loss of control seems to be escalating, say, "If you continue screaming, I'll leave." An interviewer who feels genuinely frightened of the patient can simply leave and, if necessary, ask for help from ward attendants or the police.

PROJECTIVE IDENTIFICATION. The defense mechanism of projective identification appears mainly in borderline personality disorder and consists of three steps. First, an aspect of the self is projected onto someone else. The projector then tries to coerce the other person into identifying with what has been projected. Finally, the recipient of the projection and the projector feel a sense of oneness or union.

PARANOID PERSONALITY DISORDER

Persons with paranoid personality disorder are characterized by long-standing suspiciousness and mistrust of persons in general. They refuse responsibility for their own feelings and assign responsibility to others. They are often hostile, irritable, and angry. Bigots, injustice collectors, pathologically jealous spouses, and litigious cranks often have paranoid personality disorder.

Epidemiology

The prevalence of paranoid personality disorder is 0.5 to 2.5 percent of the general population. Those with the disorder rarely seek treatment themselves; when referred to treatment by a spouse or an employer, they can often pull themselves together and appear undistressed. Relatives of patients with schizophrenia show a higher incidence of paranoid personality disorder than controls. The disorder is more common in men than in women and does not appear to have a familial pattern. The prevalence among persons who are homosexual is no higher than usual, as was once thought, but it is believed to be higher among minority groups, immigrants, and persons who are deaf than it is in the general population.

Diagnosis

On psychiatric examination, patients with paranoid personality disorder may be formal in manner and act baffled about having to seek psychiatric help. Muscular tension, an inability to relax, and a need to scan the environment for clues may be evident, and the patient's manner is often humorless and serious. Although some premises of their arguments may be false, their speech is goal directed and logical. Their thought content shows evidence of projection, prejudice, and occasional ideas of reference. The DSM-IV-TR diagnostic criteria are listed in Table 27–2.

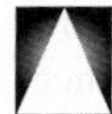

Table 27–2
DSM-IV-TR Diagnostic Criteria for Paranoid Personality Disorder

A. A pervasive distrust and suspiciousness of others such that their motives are interpreted as malevolent, beginning by early adulthood and present in a variety of contexts, as indicated by four (or more) of the following:
  (1) suspects, without sufficient basis, that others are exploiting, harming, or deceiving him or her
  (2) is preoccupied with unjustified doubts about the loyalty or trustworthiness of friends or associates
  (3) is reluctant to confide in others because of unwarranted fear that the information will be used maliciously against him or her
  (4) reads hidden demeaning or threatening meanings into benign remarks or events
  (5) persistently bears grudges, i.e., is unforgiving of insults, injuries, or slights
  (6) perceives attacks on his or her character or reputation that are not apparent to others and is quick to react angrily or to counterattack
  (7) has recurrent suspicions, without justification, regarding fidelity of spouse or sexual partner

B. Does not occur exclusively during the course of schizophrenia, a mood disorder with psychotic features, or another psychotic disorder and is not due to the direct physiological effects of a general medical condition.
Note: If criteria are met prior to the onset of schizophrenia, add "premorbid," e.g., "paranoid personality disorder (premorbid)."

(From American Psychiatric Association. *Diagnostic and Statistical Manual of Mental Disorders.* 4th ed. Text rev. Washington, DC: American Psychiatric Association; copyright 2000, with permission.)

Clinical Features

The hallmarks of paranoid personality disorder are excessive suspiciousness and distrust of others expressed as a pervasive tendency to interpret actions of others as deliberately demeaning, malevolent, threatening, exploiting, or deceiving. This tendency begins by early adulthood and appears in a variety of contexts. Almost invariably, those with the disorder expect to be exploited or harmed by others in some way. They frequently dispute, without any justification, friends' or associates' loyalty or trustworthiness. Such persons are often pathologically jealous and, for no reason, question the fidelity of their spouses or sexual partners. Persons with this disorder externalize their own emotions and use the defense of projection; they attribute to others the impulses and thoughts that they cannot accept in themselves. Ideas of reference and logically defended illusions are common.

Persons with paranoid personality disorder are affectively restricted and appear to be unemotional. They pride themselves on being rational and objective, but such is not the case. They lack warmth and are impressed with, and pay close attention to, power and rank. They express disdain for those they see as weak, sickly, impaired, or in some way defective. In social situations, persons with paranoid personality disorder may appear business-like and efficient, but they often generate fear or conflict in others.

Differential Diagnosis

Paranoid personality disorder can usually be differentiated from delusional disorder by the absence of fixed delusions. Unlike persons with paranoid schizophrenia, those with personality disorders have no hallucinations or formal thought disorder. Paranoid personality disorder can be distinguished from borderline personality disorder because patients who are paranoid are rarely capable of overly involved, tumultuous relationships with others. Patients with paranoia lack the long history of antisocial behavior of persons with antisocial character. Persons with schizoid personality disorder are withdrawn and aloof and do not have paranoid ideation.

Course and Prognosis

No adequate, systematic long-term studies of paranoid personality disorder have been conducted. In some, paranoid personality disorder is lifelong; in others, it is a harbinger of schizophrenia.

In still others, paranoid traits give way to reaction formation, appropriate concern with morality, and altruistic concerns as they mature or as stress diminishes. In general, however, those with paranoid personality disorder have lifelong problems working and living with others. Occupational and marital problems are common.

Treatment

Psychotherapy. Psychotherapy is the treatment of choice for paranoid personality disorder. Therapists should be straightforward in all their dealings with these patients. If a therapist is accused of inconsistency or a fault, such as lateness for an appointment, honesty and an apology are preferable to a defensive explanation. Therapists must remember that trust and toleration of intimacy are troubled areas for patients with this disorder. Individual psychotherapy, thus, requires a professional and not overly warm style from therapists. Clinicians' overzealous use of interpretation—especially interpretation about deep feelings of dependence, sexual concerns, and wishes for intimacy—increase patients' mistrust significantly. Patients who are paranoid usually do not do well in group psychotherapy, although it can be useful for improving social skills and diminishing suspiciousness through role playing. Many cannot tolerate the intrusiveness of behavior therapy, also used for social skills training.

At times, patients with paranoid personality disorder behave so threateningly that therapists must control or set limits on their actions. Delusional accusations must be dealt with realistically but gently and without humiliating patients. Patients who are paranoid are profoundly frightened when they feel that those trying to help them are weak and helpless; therefore, therapists should never offer to take control unless they are willing and able to do so.

Pharmacotherapy. Pharmacotherapy is useful in dealing with agitation and anxiety. In most cases, an antianxiety agent such as diazepam (Valium) suffices. It may be necessary, however, to use an antipsychotic such as haloperidol (Haldol) in small dosages and for brief periods to manage severe agitation or quasi-delusional thinking. The antipsychotic drug pimozide (Orap) has successfully reduced paranoid ideation in some patients.

SCHIZOID PERSONALITY DISORDER

Schizoid personality disorder is diagnosed in patients who display a lifelong pattern of social withdrawal. Their discomfort with human interaction, their introversion, and their bland, constricted affect are noteworthy. Persons with schizoid personality disorder are often seen by others as eccentric, isolated, or lonely.

Epidemiology

The prevalence of schizoid personality disorder is not clearly established, but the disorder may affect 7.5 percent of the general population. The sex ratio of the disorder is unknown; some studies report a 2-to-1 male-to-female ratio. Persons with the disorder tend to gravitate toward solitary jobs that involve little or no contact with others. Many prefer night work to day work, so that they need not deal with many persons.

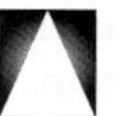

Table 27–3
DSM-IV-TR Diagnostic Criteria for Schizoid Personality Disorder

A. A pervasive pattern of detachment from social relationships and a restricted range of expression of emotions in interpersonal settings, beginning by early adulthood and present in a variety of contexts, as indicated by four (or more) of the following:
   (1) neither desires nor enjoys close relationships, including being part of a family
   (2) almost always chooses solitary activities
   (3) has little, if any, interest in having sexual experiences with another person
   (4) takes pleasure in few, if any, activities
   (5) lacks close friends or confidants other than first-degree relatives
   (6) appears indifferent to the praise or criticism of others
   (7) shows emotional coldness, detachment, or flattened affectivity

B. Does not occur exclusively during the course of schizophrenia, a mood disorder with psychotic features, another psychotic disorder, or a pervasive developmental disorder and is not due to the direct physiological effects of a general medical condition.
   Note: If criteria are met prior to the onset of schizophrenia, add "premorbid," e.g., "schizoid personality disorder (premorbid)."

(From American Psychiatric Association. *Diagnostic and Statistical Manual of Mental Disorders.* 4th ed. Text rev. Washington, DC: American Psychiatric Association; copyright 2000, with permission.)

Diagnosis

On an initial psychiatric examination, patients with schizoid personality disorder may appear ill at ease. They rarely tolerate eye contact, and interviewers may surmise that such patients are eager for the interview to end. Their affect may be constricted, aloof, or inappropriately serious, but underneath the aloofness, sensitive clinicians can recognize fear. These patients find it difficult to be lighthearted: Their efforts at humor may seem adolescent and off the mark. Their speech is goal-directed, but they are likely to give short answers to questions and to avoid spontaneous conversation. They may occasionally use unusual figures of speech, such as an odd metaphor, and may be fascinated with inanimate objects or metaphysical constructs. Their mental content may reveal an unwarranted sense of intimacy with persons they do not know well or whom they have not seen for a long time. Their sensorium is intact, their memory functions well, and their proverb interpretations are abstract. The DSM-IV-TR diagnostic criteria are listed in Table 27–3.

Clinical Features

Persons with schizoid personality disorder seem to be cold and aloof; they display a remote reserve and show no involvement with everyday events and the concerns of others. They appear quiet, distant, seclusive, and unsociable. They may pursue their own lives with remarkably little need or longing for emotional ties, and they are the last to be aware of changes in popular fashion.

The life histories of such persons reflect solitary interests and success at noncompetitive, lonely jobs that others find difficult to tolerate. Their sexual lives may exist exclusively in fantasy, and they may postpone mature sexuality indefinitely. Men may not marry because they are unable to achieve intimacy; women may passively agree to marry an aggressive man who wants the marriage. Persons with schizoid personality disorder usually reveal a lifelong inability to express anger directly. They can invest enormous affective energy in nonhuman interests, such as mathematics and astronomy, and they may be very attached to animals. Dietary and health fads, philosophical movements, and social improvement schemes, especially those that require no personal involvement, often engross them.

Although persons with schizoid personality disorder appear self-absorbed and lost in daydreams, they have a normal capacity to recognize reality. Because aggressive acts are rarely included in their repertoire of usual responses, most threats, real or imagined, are dealt with by fantasized omnipotence or resignation. They are often seen as aloof, yet such persons can sometimes conceive, develop, and give to the world genuinely original, creative ideas.

Differential Diagnosis

Schizoid personality disorder is distinguished from schizophrenia, delusional disorder, and affective disorder with psychotic features based on periods with positive psychotic symptoms, such as delusions and hallucinations in the latter. Although patients with paranoid personality disorder share many traits with those with schizoid personality disorder, the former exhibit more social engagement, a history of aggressive verbal behavior, and a greater tendency to project their feelings onto others. If just as emotionally constricted, patients with obsessive-compulsive and avoidant personality disorders experience loneliness as dysphoric, possess a richer history of past object relations, and do not engage as much in autistic reverie. Theoretically, the chief distinction between a patient with schizotypal personality disorder and one with schizoid personality disorder is that the patient who is schizotypal is more similar to a patient with schizophrenia in oddities of perception, thought, behavior, and communication. Patients with avoidant personality disorder are isolated but strongly wish to participate in activities, a characteristic absent in those with schizoid personality disorder. Schizoid personality disorder is distinguished from autistic disorder and Asperger's syndrome by more severely impaired social interactions and stereotypical behaviors and interests than in those two disorders.

Course and Prognosis

The onset of schizoid personality disorder usually occurs in early childhood. As with all personality disorders, schizoid personality disorder is long lasting, but not necessarily lifelong. The proportion of patients who incur schizophrenia is unknown.

Treatment

Psychotherapy. The treatment of patients with schizoid personality disorder is similar to that of those with paranoid personality disorder. Patients who are schizoid tend toward introspection, however, these tendencies are consistent with psychotherapists' expectations, and such patients may become devoted, if distant, patients. As trust develops, patients who are schizoid may, with great trepidation, reveal a plethora of fantasies, imaginary friends, and fears of unbearable dependence—even of merging with the therapist.

In group therapy settings, patients with schizoid personality disorder may be silent for long periods; nonetheless, they do become involved. The patients should be protected against aggressive attack by group members for their proclivity to be silent. With time, the group members become important to patients who are schizoid and may provide the only social contact in their otherwise isolated existence.

Pharmacotherapy. Pharmacotherapy with small dosages of antipsychotics, antidepressants, and psychostimulants has benefitted some patients. Serotonergic agents may make patients less sensitive to rejection. Benzodiazepines may help diminish interpersonal anxiety.

SCHIZOTYPAL PERSONALITY DISORDER

Persons with schizotypal personality disorder are strikingly odd or strange, even to laypersons. Magical thinking, peculiar notions, ideas of reference, illusions, and derealization are part of a schizotypal person's everyday world.

Epidemiology

Schizotypal personality disorder occurs in about 3 percent of the population. The sex ratio is unknown. A greater association of cases exists among the biological relatives of patients with schizophrenia than among controls, and a higher incidence among monozygotic twins than among dizygotic twins (33 percent versus 4 percent in one study).

Diagnosis

Schizotypal personality disorder is diagnosed on the basis of the patients' peculiarities of thinking, behavior, and appearance. Taking a history may be difficult because of the patients' unusual way of communicating. The DSM-IV-TR diagnostic criteria for schizotypal personality disorder are given in Table 27–4.

Clinical Features

Patients with schizotypal personality disorder exhibit disturbed thinking and communicating. Although frank thought disorder is absent, their speech may be distinctive or peculiar, may have meaning only to them, and often needs interpretation. As with patients with schizophrenia, those with schizotypal personality disorder may not know their own feelings and yet are exquisitely sensitive to, and aware of, the feelings of others, especially negative affects such as anger. These patients may be superstitious or claim powers of clairvoyance and may believe that they have other special powers of thought and insight. Their inner world may be filled with vivid imaginary relationships and child-like fears and fantasies. They may admit to perceptual illusions or macropsia and confess that other persons seem wooden and all the same.

Because persons with schizotypal personality disorder have poor interpersonal relationships and may act inappropriately,

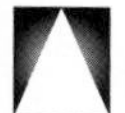

Table 27–4
DSM-IV-TR Diagnostic Criteria for Schizotypal Personality Disorder

A. A pervasive pattern of social and interpersonal deficits marked by acute discomfort with, and reduced capacity for, close relationships as well as by cognitive or perceptual distortions and eccentricities of behavior, beginning by early adulthood and present in a variety of contexts, as indicated by five (or more) of the following:
(1) ideas of reference (excluding delusions of reference)
(2) odd beliefs or magical thinking that influences behavior and is inconsistent with subcultural norms (e.g., superstitiousness, belief in clairvoyance, telepathy, or "sixth sense"; in children and adolescents, bizarre fantasies or preoccupations)
(3) unusual perceptual experiences, including bodily illusions
(4) odd thinking and speech (e.g., vague, circumstantial, metaphorical, overelaborate, or stereotyped)
(5) suspiciousness or paranoid ideation
(6) inappropriate or constricted affect
(7) behavior or appearance that is odd, eccentric, or peculiar
(8) lack of close friends or confidants other than first-degree relatives
(9) excessive social anxiety that does not diminish with familiarity and tends to be associated with paranoid fears rather than negative judgments about self

B. Does not occur exclusively during the course of schizophrenia, a mood disorder with psychotic features, another psychotic disorder, or a pervasive developmental disorder.

Note: If criteria are met prior to the onset of schizophrenia, add "premorbid," e.g., "schizotypal personality disorder (premorbid)."

(From American Psychiatric Association. *Diagnostic and Statistical Manual of Mental Disorders.* 4th ed. Text rev. Washington, DC: American Psychiatric Association; copyright 2000, with permission.)

they are isolated and have few, if any, friends. Patients may show features of borderline personality disorder, and indeed, both diagnoses can be made. Under stress, patients with schizotypal personality disorder may decompensate and have psychotic symptoms, but these are usually brief. Patients with severe cases of the disorder may exhibit anhedonia and severe depression.

A 41-year-old man was referred to a community mental health center's activities program for help in improving his social skills. He had a lifelong pattern of social isolation, with no real friends, and spent long hours worrying that his angry thoughts about his older brother would cause his brother harm. He had previously worked as a clerk in civil service, but had lost his job because of poor attendance and low productivity.

On interview, the patient was distant and somewhat distrustful. He described in elaborate and often irrelevant detail his rather uneventful and routine daily life. He told the interviewer that he had spent an hour and a half in a pet store deciding which of two brands of fish food to buy and explained their relative merits. For 2 days he had studied the washing instructions on a new pair of jeans—Did "Wash before wearing" mean that the jeans were to be washed before wearing the first time, or did they need, for some reason, to be washed each time before they were worn? He did not regard concerns such as these as senseless, though he acknowledged that the amount of time spent thinking about them might be excessive. He described how he often would buy several different brands of the same item, such as different kinds of can openers, and then would keep them in their original bags in his closet, expecting that at some future time he would find them useful. He was, however, usually very reluctant to spend money on things that he actually needed, although he had a substantial bank account. He could recite from memory his most recent monthly bank statement, including the amount of every check and the running balance as each check was written. He knew his balance on any particular day, but sometimes got anxious if he considered whether a certain check or deposit had actually cleared.

He asked the interviewer whether, if he joined the program, he would be required to participate in groups. He said that groups made him very nervous because he felt that if he revealed too much personal information, such as the amount of money that he had in the bank, people would take advantage of him or manipulate him for their own benefit. (From *DSM-IV-TR Casebook.*)

Differential Diagnosis

Theoretically, persons with schizotypal personality disorder can be distinguished from those with schizoid and avoidant personality disorders by the presence of oddities in their behavior, thinking, perception, and communication and perhaps by a clear family history of schizophrenia. Patients with schizotypal personality disorder can be distinguished from those with schizophrenia by their absence of psychosis. If psychotic symptoms do appear, they are brief and fragmentary. Some patients meet the criteria for both schizotypal personality disorder and borderline personality disorder. Patients with paranoid personality disorder are characterized by suspiciousness, but lack the odd behavior of patients with schizotypal personality disorder.

Course and Prognosis

A long-term study by Thomas McGlashan reported that 10 percent of those with schizotypal personality disorder eventually committed suicide. Retrospective studies have shown that many patients thought to have had schizophrenia actually had schizotypal personality disorder and, according to current clinical thinking, the schizotype is the premorbid personality of the patient with schizophrenia. Some, however, maintain a stable schizotypal personality throughout their lives and marry and work, despite their oddities.

Treatment

Psychotherapy. The principles of treatment of schizotypal personality disorder do not differ from those of schizoid personality disorder, but clinicians must deal sensitively with the former. These patients have peculiar patterns of thinking, and some are involved in cults, strange religious practices, and the occult. Therapists must not ridicule such activities or be judgmental about these beliefs or activities.

Pharmacotherapy. Antipsychotic medication may be useful in dealing with ideas of reference, illusions, and other symptoms of the disorder and can be used in conjunction with psychotherapy. Antidepressants are useful when a depressive component of the personality is present.

ANTISOCIAL PERSONALITY DISORDER

Antisocial personality disorder is an inability to conform to the social norms that ordinarily govern many aspects of a person's adolescent and adult behavior. Although characterized by continual antisocial or criminal acts, the disorder is not synonymous with criminality (the 10th revision of *International Statistical Classification of Diseases and Related Health Problems* [ICD-10] uses the name *dissocial personality disorder*).

Epidemiology

The prevalence of antisocial personality disorder is 3 percent in men and 1 percent in women. It is most common in poor urban areas and among mobile residents of these areas. Boys with the disorder come from larger families than girls with the disorder. The onset of the disorder is before the age of 15. Girls usually have symptoms before puberty, and boys even earlier. In prison populations, the prevalence of antisocial personality disorder may be as high as 75 percent. A familial pattern is present; the disorder is five times more common among first-degree relatives of men with the disorder than among controls.

Diagnosis

Patients with antisocial personality disorder can fool even the most experienced clinicians. In an interview, patients can appear composed and credible, but beneath the veneer (or, to use Hervey Cleckley's term, *the mask of sanity*) lurks tension, hostility, irritability, and rage. A stress interview, in which patients are vigorously confronted with inconsistencies in their histories, may be necessary to reveal the pathology.

A diagnostic workup should include a thorough neurological examination. Because patients often show abnormal EEG results and soft neurological signs suggesting minimal brain damage in childhood, these findings can be used to confirm the clinical impression. The DSM-IV-TR diagnostic criteria are listed in Table 27–5.

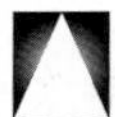

Table 27–5
DSM-IV-TR Diagnostic Criteria for Antisocial Personality Disorder

A. There is a pervasive pattern of disregard for and violation of the rights of others occurring since age 15 years, as indicated by three (or more) of the following:
   (1) failure to conform to social norms with respect to lawful behaviors as indicated by repeatedly performing acts that are grounds for arrest
   (2) deceitfulness, as indicated by repeated lying, use of aliases, or conning others for personal profit or pleasure
   (3) impulsivity or failure to plan ahead
   (4) irritability and aggressiveness, as indicated by repeated physical fights or assaults
   (5) reckless disregard for safety of self or others
   (6) consistent irresponsibility, as indicated by repeated failure to sustain consistent work behavior or honor financial obligations
   (7) lack of remorse, as indicated by being indifferent to or rationalizing having hurt, mistreated, or stolen from another

B. The individual is at least age 18 years.

C. There is evidence of conduct disorder with onset before age 15 years.

D. The occurrence of antisocial behavior is not exclusively during the course of schizophrenia or a manic episode.

(From American Psychiatric Association. *Diagnostic and Statistical Manual of Mental Disorders*. 4th ed. Text rev. Washington, DC: American Psychiatric Association; copyright 2000, with permission.)

Clinical Features

Patients with antisocial personality disorder can often seem to be normal and even charming and ingratiating. Their histories, however, reveal many areas of disordered life functioning. Lying, truancy, running away from home, thefts, fights, substance abuse, and illegal activities are typical experiences that patients report as beginning in childhood. These patients often impress opposite-sex clinicians with the colorful, seductive aspects of their personalities, but same-sex clinicians may regard them as manipulative and demanding. Patients with antisocial personality disorder exhibit no anxiety or depression, a lack that may seem grossly incongruous with their situations, although suicide threats and somatic preoccupations may be common. Their own explanations of their antisocial behavior make it seem mindless, but their mental content reveals the complete absence of delusions and other signs of irrational thinking. In fact, they frequently have a heightened sense of reality testing and often impress observers as having good verbal intelligence.

Persons with antisocial personality disorder are highly representative of so-called con men. They are extremely manipulative and can frequently talk others into participating in schemes for easy ways to make money or to achieve fame or notoriety. These schemes may eventually lead the unwary to financial ruin or social embarrassment or both. Those with this disorder do not tell the truth and cannot be trusted to carry out any task or adhere to any conventional standard of morality. Promiscuity, spousal abuse, child abuse, and drunk driving are common events in their lives. A notable finding is a lack of remorse for these actions; that is, they appear to lack a conscience.

A 19-year-old youth sporting a punk-style haircut and T-shirt with "Twisted Sister" written across the front was brought, by ambulance, at midnight to a hospital emergency room. He was accompanied by a 23-year-old male friend who called the ambulance because he was afraid his companion "was going to die like that basketball player" (a reference to a famous basketball player who died from a cocaine overdose).

The patient was agitated and argumentative, his breathing was irregular and rapid, his pulse was rapid, and his pupils were dilated. Reluctantly, the patient's friend admitted they used a lot of cocaine that evening.

By the time the patient's mother arrived, his condition had improved somewhat, although he created a commotion in the emergency room with his loud singing and gesticulations. The mother, looking disheveled and smelling of alcohol, was distraught and tearful. She told a disorganized story about her son's problems at home: he was disobedient and resentful of authority, unwilling to take part in family activities, and violently argumentative when confronted about his carrying on and partying at all hours of the night. She reported that he had been arrested twice for shoplifting and once for driving while intoxicated and that he spent almost all of his time with an older crowd. "They drag race a lot and hang out in the streets," she said.

Divorced for almost 15 years, the mother admitted that not having a stable father figure in the household made disciplining quite difficult. She suspected that her son used drugs because she had heard him talk to his friends about drugs, but she did not have any direct evidence. She claimed that her son was not all bad, that he was a fairly good student and even a star member of the basketball team. (In fact, the son was quite successful in deceiving his nonvigilant mother into believing that. Actually, the patient never completed high school, had poor or failing grades, and never played on the school's basketball team.) When asked about her own drinking habits, the mother became defensive and claimed she drank only occasionally and in small amounts.

Within 24 hours the patient was physically well and quite willing to talk. He stated, almost boastfully, that he had been using alcohol and other drugs regularly since age 13. He told of repeated instances in which he and his friends had each consumed an entire case of beer in a day ("I can drink a lot before I feel anything. We call ourselves the 'Andre the Giant Club'.") in addition to using other drugs. These drug orgies had often included a dangerous game called "hurricane drag racing," in which intoxicated contestants engaged in drag racing on side roads until somebody "chickens out" to avoid an oncoming car. During this heavy drug use, it was common for him to skip school because of the drug activity; when he had to be in school, he typically was intoxicated. To help support his drug involvement, he had devised various schemes for acquiring money, such as "borrowing" money from friends that would never be repaid or stealing car radios from the student parking lot, plus blatant stealing of money from his mother. This behavior was justified by a "Robin Hood" attitude: "I take from people who have a lot of money anyway."

Despite the patient's admission of heavy drug involvement, he stopped short of admitting that he had a real problem. In response to a question about his ability to control drug use, he replied in a hostile manner, "Of course I could. No problem. I just don't see any damn good reason to stop."

Somewhat fidgety and restless, the patient said he was finished with the interview. Before the interviewer had an opportunity to press him further about seeking treatment, the patient began to roam around the hospital unit, looking for someone who had an extra cigarette. (From *DSM-IV-TR Casebook*.)

Differential Diagnosis

Antisocial personality disorder can be distinguished from illegal behavior in that antisocial personality disorder involves many areas of a person's life. When antisocial behavior is the only manifestation, patients are classified in the DSM-IV-TR category of additional conditions that may be a focus of clinical attention—specifically, adult antisocial behavior. Dorothy Lewis found that many of these persons have a neurological or mental disorder that has been either overlooked or undiagnosed. More difficult is the differentiation of antisocial personality disorder from substance abuse. When both substance abuse and antisocial behavior begin in childhood and continue into adult life, both disorders should be diagnosed. When, however, the antisocial behavior is clearly secondary to premorbid alcohol abuse or other substance abuse, the diagnosis of antisocial personality disorder is not warranted.

In diagnosing antisocial personality disorder, clinicians must adjust for the distorting effects of socioeconomic status, cultural background, and sex. Furthermore, the diagnosis of antisocial personality disorder is not warranted when mental retardation, schizophrenia, or mania can explain the symptoms.

Course and Prognosis

Once an antisocial personality disorder develops, it runs an unremitting course, with the height of antisocial behavior usually occurring in late adolescence. The prognosis varies. Some reports indicate that symptoms decrease as persons grow older. Many patients have somatization disorder and multiple physical complaints. Depressive disorders, alcohol use disorders, and other substance abuse are common.

Treatment

Psychotherapy. If patients with antisocial personality disorder are immobilized (e.g., placed in hospitals), they often become amenable to psychotherapy. When patients feel that they are among peers, their lack of motivation for change disappears. Perhaps for this reason, self-help groups have been more useful than jails in alleviating the disorder.

Before treatment can begin, firm limits are essential. Therapists must find ways of dealing with patients' self-destructive behavior. And to overcome patients' fear of intimacy, therapists must frustrate patients' desire to run from honest human encounters. In doing so, a therapist faces the challenge of separating control from punishment and of separating help and confrontation from social isolation and retribution.

Pharmacotherapy. Pharmacotherapy is used to deal with incapacitating symptoms such as anxiety, rage, and depression, but because patients are often substance abusers, drugs must be used judiciously. If a patient shows evidence of attention-deficit/hyperactivity disorder, psychostimulants such as methylphenidate (Ritalin) may be useful. Attempts have been made to alter catecholamine metabolism with drugs and to control impulsive behavior with antiepileptic drugs, for example, carbamazepine (Tegretol) or valproate (Depakote), especially if abnormal waveforms are noted on an EEG. β-Adrenergic receptor antagonists have been used to reduce aggression.

BORDERLINE PERSONALITY DISORDER

Patients with borderline personality disorder stand on the border between neurosis and psychosis and they are characterized by extraordinarily unstable affect, mood, behavior, object relations, and self-image. The disorder has also been called *ambulatory schizophrenia*, *as-if personality* (a term coined by Helene Deutsch), *pseudoneurotic schizophrenia* (described by Paul Hoch and Phillip Politan), and *psychotic character disorder* (described by John Frosch). ICD-10 uses the term *emotionally unstable personality disorder*.

Epidemiology

No definitive prevalence studies are available, but borderline personality disorder is thought to be present in about 1 to 2 percent of the population and is twice as common in women as in men. An increased prevalence of major depressive disorder, alcohol use disorders, and substance abuse is found in first-degree relatives of persons with borderline personality disorder.

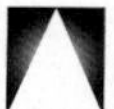

Table 27–6
DSM-IV-TR Diagnostic Criteria for Borderline Personality Disorder

A pervasive pattern of instability of interpersonal relationships, self-image, and affects, and marked impulsivity beginning by early adulthood and present in a variety of contexts, as indicated by five (or more) of the following:
(1) frantic efforts to avoid real or imagined abandonment. **Note**: Do not include suicidal or self-mutilating behavior covered in Criterion 5.
(2) a pattern of unstable and intense interpersonal relationships characterized by alternating between extremes of idealization and devaluation
(3) identity disturbance: markedly and persistently unstable self-image or sense of self
(4) impulsivity in at least two areas that are potentially self-damaging (e.g., spending, sex, substance abuse, reckless driving, binge eating). **Note**: Do not include suicidal or self-mutilating behavior covered in Criterion 5.
(5) recurrent suicidal behavior, gestures, or threats, or self-mutilating behavior
(6) affective instability due to a marked reactivity of mood (e.g., intense episodic dysphoria, irritability, or anxiety usually lasting a few hours and only hours and only rarely more than a few days)
(7) chronic feelings of emptiness
(8) inappropriate, intense anger or difficulty controlling anger (e.g., frequent displays of temper, constant anger, recurrent physical fights)
(9) transient, stress-related paranoid ideation or severe dissociative symptoms

(From American Psychiatric Association. *Diagnostic and Statistical Manual of Mental Disorders.* 4th ed. Text rev. Washington, DC: American Psychiatric Association; copyright 2000, with permission.)

Diagnosis

According to DSM-IV-TR, the diagnosis of borderline personality disorder can made by early adulthood when patients show at least five of the criteria listed in Table 27–6. Biological studies may aid in the diagnosis; some patients with borderline personality disorder show shortened REM latency and sleep continuity disturbances, abnormal DST results, and abnormal thyrotropin-releasing hormone test results. Those changes, however, are also seen in some patients with depressive disorders.

Clinical Features

Persons with borderline personality disorder almost always appear to be in a state of crisis. Mood swings are common. Patients can be argumentative at one moment, depressed the next, and later complain of having no feelings. Patients can have short-lived psychotic episodes (so-called *micropsychotic episodes*) rather than full-blown psychotic breaks, and the psychotic symptoms of these patients are almost always circumscribed, fleeting, or doubtful. The behavior of patients with borderline personality disorder is highly unpredictable, and their achievements are rarely at the level of their abilities. The painful nature of their lives is reflected in repetitive self-destructive acts. Such patients may slash their wrists and perform other self-mutilations to elicit help from others, to express anger, or to numb themselves to overwhelming affect.

Because they feel both dependent and hostile, persons with this disorder have tumultuous interpersonal relationships. They can be dependent on those with whom they are close and, when frustrated, can express enormous anger toward their intimate friends. Patients with borderline personality disorder cannot tolerate being alone, and they prefer a frantic search for companionship, no matter how unsatisfactory, to their own company. To assuage loneliness, if only for brief periods, they accept a stranger as a friend or behave promiscuously. They often complain about chronic feelings of emptiness and boredom and the lack of a consistent sense of identity (identity diffusion); when pressed, they often complain about how depressed they usually feel, despite the flurry of other affects.

Otto Kernberg described the defense mechanism of projective identification that occurs in patients with borderline personality disorder. In this primitive defense mechanism, intolerable aspects of the self are projected onto another; the other person is induced to play the projected role, and the two persons act in unison. Therapists must be aware of this process so that they can act neutrally toward such patients.

Most therapists agree that these patients show ordinary reasoning abilities on structured tests, such as the Wechsler Adult Intelligence Scale, and show deviant processes only on unstructured projective tests, such as the Rorschach test.

Functionally, patients with borderline personality disorder distort their relationships by considering each person to be either all good or all bad. They see persons as either nurturing attachment figures or as hateful, sadistic figures who deprive them of security needs and threaten them with abandonment whenever they feel dependent. As a result of this splitting, the good person is idealized, and the bad person devalued. Shifts of allegiance from one person or group to another are frequent. Some clinicians use the concepts of panphobia, pananxiety, panambivalence, and chaotic sexuality to delineate these patients' characteristics.

Differential Diagnosis

The disorder is differentiated from schizophrenia on the basis that the patient with borderline personality lacks prolonged psychotic episodes, thought disorder, and other classic schizophrenic signs. Patients with schizotypal personality disorder show marked peculiarities of thinking, strange ideation, and recurrent ideas of reference. Those with paranoid personality disorder are marked by extreme suspiciousness. Patients with borderline personality disorder generally have chronic feelings of emptiness and short-lived psychotic episodes; they act impulsively and demand extraordinary relationships; they may mutilate themselves and make manipulative suicide attempts.

Course and Prognosis

Borderline personality disorder is fairly stable; patients change little over time. Longitudinal studies show no progression toward schizophrenia, but patients have a high incidence of major depressive disorder episodes. The diagnosis is usually made before the age of 40, when patients are attempting to make occupational, marital, and other choices and are unable to deal with the normal stages of the life cycle.

Treatment

Table 27–7 summarizes the American Psychiatric Association guidelines for treating this disorder.

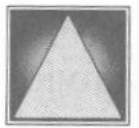

Table 27–7
Common Features of Recommended Psychotherapy for Borderline Personality Disorder

Therapy is not expected to be brief.
A strong helping relationship develops between patient and therapist.
Clear roles and responsibilities of patient and therapist are established.
Therapist is active and directive, not a passive listener.
Patient and therapist mutually develop a hierarchy of priorities.
Therapist conveys empathic validation plus the need for patient to control his/her behavior.
Flexibility is needed as new circumstances, including stresses, develop.
Limit setting, preferably mutually agreed upon, is used.
Concomitant individual and group approaches are used.

(From Oldham JM. A 44-year-old woman with borderline personality disorder. *JAMA*. 2002;287:1034, with permission.)

Psychotherapy. Psychotherapy for patients with borderline personality disorder is an area of intensive investigation and has been the treatment of choice. For best results, pharmacotherapy has been added to the treatment regimen.

Psychotherapy is difficult for patient and therapist alike. Patients regress easily, act out their impulses, and show labile or fixed negative or positive transferences, which are difficult to analyze. Projective identification may also cause countertransference problems when therapists are unaware that patients are unconsciously trying to coerce them to act out a particular behavior. The splitting defense mechanism causes patients to alternately love and hate therapists and others in the environment. A reality-oriented approach is more effective than in-depth interpretations of the unconscious.

Therapists have used behavior therapy to control patients' impulses and angry outbursts and to reduce their sensitivity to criticism and rejection. Social skills training, especially with videotape playback, helps enable patients to see how their actions affect others and thereby improve their interpersonal behavior.

Patients with borderline personality disorder often do well in a hospital setting in which they receive intensive psychotherapy on both an individual and a group basis. In a hospital, they can also interact with trained staff members from a variety of disciplines and can be provided with occupational, recreational, and vocational therapy. Such programs are especially helpful when the home environment is detrimental to a patient's rehabilitation because of intrafamilial conflicts or other stresses, such as parental abuse. Within the protected environment of the hospital, patients who are excessively impulsive, self-destructive, or self-mutilating can be given limits, and their actions can be observed. Under ideal circumstances, patients remain in the hospital until they show marked improvement, up to 1 year in some cases. Patients can then be discharged to special support systems, such as day hospitals, night hospitals, and halfway houses.

A particular form of psychotherapy called dialectical behavior therapy (DBT) has been used for patients with borderline personality disorder, especially those with parasuicidal behavior, such as frequent cutting. (For further discussion of DBT see Section 35.5 in Chapter 35.)

Pharmacotherapy. Pharmacotherapy is useful to deal with specific personality features that interfere with patients' overall functioning. Antipsychotics have been used to control anger, hostility, and brief psychotic episodes. Antidepressants improve the depressed mood common in patients with borderline personality disorder. The MAO inhibitors (MAOIs) have successfully modulated impulsive behavior in some patients. Benzodiazepines, particularly alprazolam (Xanax), help anxiety and depression, but some patients show a disinhibition with this class of drugs. Anticonvulsants, such as carbamazepine, may improve global functioning for some patients. Serotonergic agents such as selective serotonin reuptake inhibitors (SSRIs) have been helpful in some cases.

HISTRIONIC PERSONALITY DISORDER

Persons with histrionic personality disorder are excitable and emotional and behave in a colorful, dramatic, extroverted fashion. Accompanying their flamboyant aspects, however, is often an inability to maintain deep, long-lasting attachments.

Epidemiology

According to DSM-IV-TR, limited data from general population studies suggest a prevalence of histrionic personality disorder of about 2 to 3 percent. Rates of about 10 to 15 percent have been reported in inpatient and outpatient mental health settings when structured assessment is used. The disorder is diagnosed more frequently in women than in men. Some studies have found an association with somatization disorder and alcohol use disorders.

Diagnosis

In interviews, patients with histrionic personality disorder are generally cooperative and eager to give a detailed history. Gestures and dramatic punctuation in their conversations are common; they may make frequent slips of the tongue, and their language is colorful. Affective display is common, but, when pressed to acknowledge certain feelings (e.g., anger, sadness, and sexual wishes), they may respond with surprise, indignation, or denial. The results of the cognitive examination are usually normal, although a lack of perseverance may be shown on arithmetic or concentration tasks, and the patients' forgetfulness of affect-laden material may be astonishing. The DSM-IV-TR diagnostic criteria are listed in Table 27–8.

Clinical Features

Persons with histrionic personality disorder show a high degree of attention-seeking behavior. They tend to exaggerate their thoughts and feelings and make everything sound more important than it really is. They display temper tantrums, tears, and accusations when they are not the center of attention or are not receiving praise or approval.

Seductive behavior is common in both sexes. Sexual fantasies about persons with whom patients are involved are common, but patients are inconsistent about verbalizing these fantasies and may be coy or flirtatious rather than sexually aggressive. In fact, histrionic patients may have a psychosexual dysfunction; women may be anorgasmic, and men may be impotent. Their need for

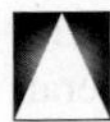

Table 27–8
DSM-IV-TR Diagnostic Criteria for Histrionic Personality Disorder

A pervasive pattern of excessive emotionality and attention seeking, beginning by early adulthood and present in a variety of contexts, as indicated by five (or more) of the following:
(1) is uncomfortable in situations in which he or she is not the center of attention
(2) interaction with others is often characterized by inappropriate sexually seductive or provocative behavior
(3) displays rapidly shifting and shallow expression of emotions
(4) consistently uses physical appearance to draw attention to self
(5) has a style of speech that is excessively impressionistic and lacking in detail
(6) shows self-dramatization, theatricality, and exaggerated expression of emotion
(7) is suggestible, i.e., easily influenced by others or circumstances
(8) considers relationships to be more intimate than they actually are

(From American Psychiatric Association. *Diagnostic and Statistical Manual of Mental Disorders.* 4th ed. Text rev. Washington, DC: American Psychiatric Association; copyright 2000, with permission.)

reassurance is endless. They may act on their sexual impulses to reassure themselves that they are attractive to the other sex. Their relationships tend to be superficial, however, and they can be vain, self-absorbed, and fickle. Their strong dependence needs make them overly trusting and gullible.

The major defenses of patients with histrionic personality disorder are repression and dissociation. Accordingly, such patients are unaware of their true feelings and cannot explain their motivations. Under stress, reality testing easily becomes impaired.

Differential Diagnosis

Distinguishing between histrionic personality disorder and borderline personality disorder is difficult, but in borderline personality disorder, suicide attempts, identity diffusion, and brief psychotic episodes are more likely. Although both conditions may be diagnosed in the same patient, clinicians should separate the two. Somatization disorder (Briquet's syndrome) may occur in conjunction with histrionic personality disorder. Patients with brief psychotic disorder and dissociative disorders may warrant a coexisting diagnosis of histrionic personality disorder.

Course and Prognosis

With age, persons with histrionic personality disorder show fewer symptoms, but because they lack the energy of earlier years, the difference in number of symptoms may be more apparent than real. Persons with this disorder are sensation seekers, and they may get into trouble with the law, abuse substances, and act promiscuously.

Treatment

Psychotherapy. Patients with histrionic personality disorder are often unaware of their own real feelings; clarification of their inner feelings is an important therapeutic process. Psychoanalytically oriented psychotherapy, whether group or individual, is probably the treatment of choice for histrionic personality disorder.

Pharmacotherapy. Pharmacotherapy can be adjunctive when symptoms are targeted (e.g., the use of antidepressants for depression and somatic complaints, antianxiety agents for anxiety, and antipsychotics for derealization and illusions).

NARCISSISTIC PERSONALITY DISORDER

Persons with narcissistic personality disorder are characterized by a heightened sense of self-importance and grandiose feelings of uniqueness.

Epidemiology

According to DSM-IV-TR, estimates of the prevalence of narcissistic personality disorder range from 2 to 16 percent in the clinical population and less than 1 percent in the general population. Persons with the disorder may impart an unrealistic sense of omnipotence, grandiosity, beauty, and talent to their children; thus, offspring of such parents may have a higher than usual risk for developing the disorder themselves. The number of cases of narcissistic personality disorder reported is increasing steadily.

Diagnosis

Table 27–9 gives the DSM-IV-TR diagnostic criteria for narcissistic personality disorder.

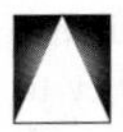

Table 27–9
DSM-IV-TR Diagnostic Criteria for Narcissistic Personality Disorder

A pervasive pattern of grandiosity (in fantasy or behavior), need for admiration, and lack of empathy, beginning by early adulthood and present in a variety of contexts, as indicated by five (or more) of the following:
(1) has a grandiose sense of self-importance (e.g., exaggerates achievements and talents, expects to be recognized as superior without commensurate achievements)
(2) is preoccupied with fantasies of unlimited success, power, brilliance, beauty, or ideal love
(3) believes that he or she is "special" and unique and can only be understood by, or should associate with, other special or high-status people (or institutions)
(4) requires excessive admiration
(5) has a sense of entitlement, i.e., unreasonable expectations of especially favorable treatment or automatic compliance with his or her expectations
(6) is interpersonally exploitative, i.e., takes advantage of others to achieve his or her own ends
(7) lacks empathy: is unwilling to recognize or identify with the feelings and needs of others
(8) is often envious of others or believes that others are envious of him or her
(9) shows arrogant, haughty behaviors or attitudes

(From American Psychiatric Association. *Diagnostic and Statistical Manual of Mental Disorders.* 4th ed. Text rev. Washington, DC: American Psychiatric Association; copyright 2000, with permission.)

Clinical Features

Persons with narcissistic personality disorder have a grandiose sense of self-importance; they consider themselves special and expect special treatment. Their sense of entitlement is striking. They handle criticism poorly and may become enraged when someone dares to criticize them, or they may appear completely indifferent to criticism. Persons with this disorder want their own way and are frequently ambitious to achieve fame and fortune. Their relationships are fragile, and they can make others furious by their refusal to obey conventional rules of behavior. Interpersonal exploitiveness is commonplace. They cannot show empathy, and they feign sympathy only to achieve their own selfish ends. Because of their fragile self-esteem, they are susceptible to depression. Interpersonal difficulties, occupational problems, rejection, and loss are among the stresses that narcissists commonly produce by their behavior—stresses they are least able to handle.

Differential Diagnosis

Borderline, histrionic, and antisocial personality disorders often accompany narcissistic personality disorder, so a differential diagnosis is difficult. Patients with narcissistic personality disorder have less anxiety than those with borderline personality disorder; their lives tend to be less chaotic, and they are less likely to attempt suicide. Patients with antisocial personality disorder have a history of impulsive behavior, often associated with alcohol or other substance abuse, which frequently gets them into trouble with the law. Patients with histrionic personality disorder show features of exhibitionism and interpersonal manipulativeness that resemble those of patients with narcissistic personality disorder.

Course and Prognosis

Narcissistic personality disorder is chronic and difficult to treat. Patients with the disorder must constantly deal with blows to their narcissism resulting from their own behavior or from life experience. Aging is handled poorly; patients value beauty, strength, and youthful attributes, to which they cling inappropriately. They may be more vulnerable, therefore, to midlife crises than are other groups.

Treatment

Psychotherapy. Because patients must renounce their narcissism to make progress, the treatment of narcissistic personality disorder is difficult. Psychiatrists such as Kernberg and Heinz Kohut have advocated using psychoanalytic approaches to effect change, but much research is required to validate the diagnosis and to determine the best treatment. Some clinicians advocate group therapy for their patients so they can learn how to share with others and, under ideal circumstances, can develop an empathic response to others.

Pharmacotherapy. Lithium (Eskalith) has been used with patients whose clinical picture includes mood swings. Because patients with narcissistic personality disorder tolerate rejection poorly and are susceptible to depression, antidepressants, especially serotonergic drugs, may also be of use.

AVOIDANT PERSONALITY DISORDER

Persons with avoidant personality disorder show extreme sensitivity to rejection and may lead a socially withdrawn life. Although shy, they are not asocial and show a great desire for companionship, but they need unusually strong guarantees of uncritical acceptance. Such persons are commonly described as having an inferiority complex. (ICD-10 uses the term *anxious personality disorder*.)

Epidemiology

Avoidant personality disorder is common. The prevalence of the disorder is 1 to 10 percent of the general population. No information is available on sex ratio or familial pattern. Infants classified as having a timid temperament may be more susceptible to the disorder than those who score high on activity-approach scales.

Diagnosis

In clinical interviews, patients' most striking aspect is anxiety about talking with an interviewer. Their nervous and tense manner appears to wax and wane with their perception of whether an interviewer likes them. They seem vulnerable to the interviewer's comments and suggestions and may regard a clarification or interpretation as criticism. The DSM-IV-TR diagnostic criteria for avoidant personality disorder are listed in Table 27–10.

Clinical Features

Hypersensitivity to rejection by others is the central clinical feature of avoidant personality disorder, and patients' main personality trait is timidity. These persons desire the warmth and

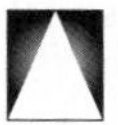

Table 27–10
DSM-IV-TR Diagnostic Criteria for Avoidant Personality Disorder

A pervasive pattern of social inhibition, feelings of inadequacy, and hypersensitivity to negative evaluation, beginning by early adulthood and present in a variety of contexts, as indicated by four (or more) of the following:

(1) avoids occupational activities that involve significant interpersonal contact, because of fears of criticism, disapproval, or rejection
(2) is unwilling to get involved with people unless certain of being liked
(3) shows restraint within intimate relationships because of the fear of being shamed or ridiculed
(4) is preoccupied with being criticized or rejected in social situations
(5) is inhibited in new interpersonal situations because of feelings of inadequacy
(6) views self as socially inept, personally unappealing, or inferior to others
(7) is unusually reluctant to take personal risks or to engage in any new activities because they may prove embarrassing

(From American Psychiatric Association. *Diagnostic and Statistical Manual of Mental Disorders.* 4th ed. Text rev. Washington, DC: American Psychiatric Association; copyright 2000, with permission.)

security of human companionship, but justify their avoidance of relationships by their alleged fear of rejection. When talking with someone, they express uncertainty, show a lack of self-confidence, and may speak in a self-effacing manner. Because they are hypervigilant about rejection, they are afraid to speak up in public or to make requests of others. They are apt to misinterpret other persons' comments as derogatory or ridiculing. The refusal of any request leads them to withdraw from others and to feel hurt.

In the vocational sphere, patients with avoidant personality disorder often take jobs on the sidelines. They rarely attain much personal advancement or exercise much authority, but seem shy and eager to please. These persons are generally unwilling to enter relationships unless they are given an unusually strong guarantee of uncritical acceptance. Consequently, they often have no close friends or confidants.

Differential Diagnosis

Patients with avoidant personality disorder desire social interaction, unlike patients with schizoid personality disorder, who want to be alone. Patients with avoidant personality disorder are not as demanding, irritable, or unpredictable as those with borderline and histrionic personality disorders. Avoidant personality disorder and dependent personality disorder are similar. Patients with dependent personality disorder are presumed to have a greater fear of being abandoned or unloved than those with avoidant personality disorder, but the clinical picture may be indistinguishable.

Course and Prognosis

Many persons with avoidant personality disorder are able to function in a protected environment. Some marry, have children, and live their lives surrounded only by family members. Should their support system fail, however, they are subject to depression, anxiety, and anger. Phobic avoidance is common, and patients with the disorder may give histories of social phobia or incur social phobia in the course of their illness.

Treatment

Psychotherapy. Psychotherapeutic treatment depends on solidifying an alliance with patients. As trust develops, a therapist must convey an accepting attitude toward the patient's fears, especially the fear of rejection. The therapist eventually encourages a patient to move out into the world to take what are perceived as great risks of humiliation, rejection, and failure. But therapists should be cautious when giving assignments to exercise new social skills outside therapy; failure can reinforce a patient's already poor self-esteem. Group therapy may help patients understand how their sensitivity to rejection affects them and others. Assertiveness training is a form of behavior therapy that may teach patients to express their needs openly and to enlarge their self-esteem.

Pharmacotherapy. Pharmacotherapy has been used to manage anxiety and depression when they are associated with the disorder. Some patients are helped by β-adrenergic receptor antagonists, such as atenolol (Tenormin), to manage autonomic nervous system hyperactivity, which tends to be high in patients with avoidant personality disorder, especially when they approach feared situations. Serotonergic agents may help rejection sensitivity. Theoretically, dopaminergic drugs might engender novelty-seeking behavior in these patients; however, the patient must be psychologically prepared for any new experience that might result.

DEPENDENT PERSONALITY DISORDER

Persons with dependent personality disorder subordinate their own needs to those of others, get others to assume responsibility for major areas of their lives, lack self-confidence, and may experience intense discomfort when alone for more than a brief period. The disorder has been called *passive-dependent personality*. Freud described an oral-dependent personality dimension characterized by dependence, pessimism, fear of sexuality, self-doubt, passivity, suggestibility, and lack of perseverance; his description is similar to the DSM-IV-TR categorization of dependent personality disorder.

Epidemiology

Dependent personality disorder is more common in women than in men. One study diagnosed 2.5 percent of all personality disorders as falling into this category. It is more common in young children than in older ones. Persons with chronic physical illness in childhood may be most susceptible to the disorder.

Diagnosis

In interviews, patients appear compliant. They try to cooperate, welcome specific questions, and look for guidance. The DSM-IV-TR diagnostic criteria for dependent personality disorder are listed in Table 27–11.

Clinical Features

Dependent personality disorder is characterized by a pervasive pattern of dependent and submissive behavior. Persons with the disorder cannot make decisions without an excessive amount of advice and reassurance from others. They avoid positions of responsibility and become anxious if asked to assume a leadership role. They prefer to be submissive. When on their own, they find it difficult to persevere at tasks, but may find it easy to perform these tasks for someone else.

Because persons with the disorder do not like to be alone, they seek out others on whom they can depend; their relationships, thus, are distorted by their need to be attached to another person. In folie à deux (shared psychotic disorder), one member of the pair usually has dependent personality disorder; the submissive partner takes on the delusional system of the more aggressive, assertive partner on whom he or she depends.

Pessimism, self-doubt, passivity, and fears of expressing sexual and aggressive feelings all typify the behavior of persons with dependent personality disorder. An abusive, unfaithful, or alcoholic spouse may be tolerated for long periods to avoid disturbing the sense of attachment.

Table 27–11
DSM-IV-TR Diagnostic Criteria for Dependent Personality Disorder

A pervasive and excessive need to be taken care of that leads to submissive and clinging behavior and fears of separation, beginning by early adulthood and present in a variety of contexts, as indicated by five (or more) of the following:

(1) has difficulty making everyday decisions without an excessive amount of advice and reassurance from others
(2) needs others to assume responsibility for most major areas of his or her life
(3) has difficulty expressing disagreement with others because of fear of loss of support or approval. **Note:** Do not include realistic fears of retribution
(4) has difficulty initiating projects or doing things on his or her own (because of a lack of self-confidence in judgment or abilities rather than a lack of motivation or energy)
(5) goes to excessive lengths to obtain nurturance and support from others, to the point of volunteering to do things that are unpleasant
(6) feels uncomfortable or helpless when alone because of exaggerated fears of being unable to care for himself or herself
(7) urgently seeks another relationship as a source of care and support when a close relationship ends
(8) is unrealistically preoccupied with fears of being left to take care of himself or herself

(From American Psychiatric Association. *Diagnostic and Statistical Manual of Mental Disorders.* 4th ed. Text rev. Washington, DC: American Psychiatric Association; copyright 2000, with permission.)

Differential Diagnosis

The traits of dependence are found in many psychiatric disorders, so differential diagnosis is difficult. Dependence is a prominent factor in patients with histrionic and borderline personality disorders, but those with dependent personality disorder usually have a long-term relationship with one person, rather than a series of persons on whom they are dependent, and they do not tend to be overtly manipulative. Patients with schizoid and schizotypal personality disorders may be indistinguishable from those with avoidant personality disorder. Dependent behavior can occur in patients with agoraphobia, but these patients tend to have a high level of overt anxiety or even panic.

Course and Prognosis

Little is known about the course of dependent personality disorder. Occupational functioning tends to be impaired, because persons with the disorder cannot act independently and without close supervision. Social relationships are limited to those on whom they can depend, and many suffer physical or mental abuse because they cannot assert themselves. They risk major depressive disorder if they lose the person on whom they depend, but with treatment, the prognosis is favorable.

Treatment

Psychotherapy. The treatment of dependent personality disorder is often successful. Insight-oriented therapies enable patients to understand the antecedents of their behavior, and with the support of a therapist, patients can become more independent, assertive, and self-reliant. Behavioral therapy, assertiveness training, family therapy, and group therapy have all been used, with successful outcomes in many cases.

A pitfall may arise in treatment when a therapist encourages a patient to change the dynamics of a pathological relationship (e.g., supports a physically abused wife in seeking help from the police). At this point, patients may become anxious and unable to cooperate in therapy; they may feel torn between complying with the therapist and losing a pathological external relationship. Therapists must show great respect for these patients' feelings of attachment, no matter how pathological these feelings may seem.

Pharmacotherapy. Pharmacotherapy has been used to deal with specific symptoms, such as anxiety and depression, which are common associated features of dependent personality disorder. Patients who experience panic attacks or who have high levels of separation anxiety may be helped by imipramine (Tofranil). Benzodiazepines and serotonergic agents have also been useful. If a patient's depression or withdrawal symptoms respond to psychostimulants, they may be used.

OBSESSIVE-COMPULSIVE PERSONALITY DISORDER

Obsessive-compulsive personality disorder is characterized by emotional constriction, orderliness, perseverance, stubbornness, and indecisiveness. The essential feature of the disorder is a pervasive pattern of perfectionism and inflexibility. (ICD-10 uses the name *anancastic personality disorder.*)

Epidemiology

The prevalence of obsessive-compulsive personality disorder is unknown. It is more common in men than in women and is diagnosed most often in oldest children. The disorder also occurs more frequently in first-degree biological relatives of persons with the disorder than in the general population. Patients often have backgrounds characterized by harsh discipline. Freud hypothesized that the disorder is associated with difficulties in the anal stage of psychosexual development, generally around the age of 2, but various studies have failed to validate this theory.

Diagnosis

In interviews, patients with obsessive-compulsive personality disorder may have a stiff, formal, and rigid demeanor. Their affect is not blunted or flat, but can be described as constricted. They lack spontaneity, and their mood is usually serious. Such patients may be anxious about not being in control of the interview. Their answers to questions are unusually detailed. The defense mechanisms they use are rationalization, isolation, intellectualization, reaction formation, and undoing. The DSM-IV-TR diagnostic criteria for obsessive-compulsive personality disorder are listed in Table 27–12.

Clinical Features

Persons with obsessive-compulsive personality disorder are preoccupied with rules, regulations, orderliness, neatness, details,

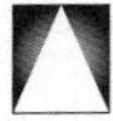

Table 27–12
DSM-IV-TR Diagnostic Criteria for Obsessive-Compulsive Personality Disorder

A pervasive pattern of preoccupation with orderliness, perfectionism, and mental and interpersonal control, at the expense of flexibility, openness, and efficiency, beginning by early adulthood and present in a variety of contexts, as indicated by four (or more) of the following:

(1) is preoccupied with details, rules, lists, order, organization, or schedules to the extent that the major point of the activity is lost
(2) shows perfectionism that interferes with task completion (e.g., is unable to complete a project because his or her own overly strict standards are not met)
(3) is excessively devoted to work and productivity to the exclusion of leisure activities and friendships (not accounted for by obvious economic necessity)
(4) is overconscientious, scrupulous, and inflexible about matters of morality, ethics, or values (not accounted for by cultural or religious identification)
(5) is unable to discard worn-out or worthless objects even when they have no sentimental value
(6) is reluctant to delegate tasks or to work with others unless they submit to exactly his or her way of doing things
(7) adopts a miserly spending style toward both self and others; money is viewed as something to be hoarded for future catastrophes
(8) shows rigidity and stubbornness

and the achievement of perfection. These traits account for the general constriction of the entire personality. They insist that rules be followed rigidly and cannot tolerate what they consider infractions. Accordingly, they lack flexibility and are intolerant. They are capable of prolonged work, provided it is routinized and does not require changes to which they cannot adapt.

Persons with obsessive-compulsive personality disorder have limited interpersonal skills. They are formal and serious and often lack a sense of humor. They alienate persons, are unable to compromise, and insist that others submit to their needs. They are eager to please those whom they see as more powerful than they are, however, and they carry out these persons' wishes in an authoritarian manner. Because they fear making mistakes, they are indecisive and ruminate about making decisions. Although a stable marriage and occupational adequacy are common, persons with obsessive-compulsive personality disorder have few friends. Anything that threatens to upset their perceived stability or the routine of their lives can precipitate much anxiety otherwise bound up in the rituals that they impose on their lives and try to impose on others.

The patient was a 45-year-old lawyer who sought treatment at his wife's insistence. She was fed up with their marriage; she could no longer tolerate his emotional coldness, rigid demands, bullying behavior, sexual disinterest, long work hours, and frequent business trips. The patient felt no particular distress in his marriage and had agreed to the consultation only to humor his wife.

It soon developed, however, that the patient was troubled by problems at work. He was known as that hardest-driving member of a hard-driving law firm. He was the youngest full partner in the firm's history and is famous for being able to handle many cases at the same time. Lately, he found himself increasingly unable to keep up. He was too proud to turn down a new case and too much of a perfectionist to be satisfied with the quality of work performed by his assistants. Displeased by their writing style and sentence structure, he found himself constantly correcting their briefs and, therefore, unable to stay abreast of his schedule. People at work complained that his attention to detail and inability to delegate responsibility were reducing his efficiency. He has had two or three secretaries a year for 15 years. No one could tolerate working for him for very long because he was so critical of any mistakes made by others. When assignments got backed up, he could not decide which to address first, started making schedules for himself and his staff, but then was unable to meet them and worked 15 hours a day. He found it difficult to be decisive now that his work had expanded beyond his own direct control.

The patient discussed his children as if they were mechanical dolls, but also with a clear underlying affection. He described his wife as a "suitable mate" and had trouble understanding why she was dissatisfied. He was punctilious in his manners and dress and slow and ponderous in his speech, dry and humorless, with a stubborn determination to get his point across.

The patient was the son of two upwardly mobile, extremely hard-working parents. He grew up feeling that he was never working hard enough, that he had much to achieve and very little time. He was a superior student, a "bookworm," awkward and unpopular in adolescent social pursuits. He had always been competitive and a high achiever. He had trouble relaxing on vacations, developed elaborate activity schedules for every family member, and became impatient and furious if they refused to follow his plans. He liked sports but had little time for them and refused to play if he couldn't be at the top of his form. He was a ferocious competitor on the tennis courts and a poor loser. (From the *DSM-IV-TR Casebook*.)

Differential Diagnosis

When recurrent obsessions or compulsions are present, obsessive-compulsive disorder should be noted on Axis I. Perhaps the most difficult distinction is between outpatients with some obsessive-compulsive traits and those with obsessive-compulsive personality disorder. The diagnosis of personality disorder is reserved for those with significant impairments in their occupational or social effectiveness. In some cases, delusional disorder coexists with personality disorders and should be noted.

Course and Prognosis

The course of obsessive-compulsive personality disorder is variable and unpredictable. From time to time, persons may develop obsessions or compulsions in the course of their disorder. Some adolescents with obsessive-compulsive personality disorder evolve into warm, open, and loving adults; in others, the disorder can be either the harbinger of schizophrenia or—decades later and exacerbated by the aging process—major depressive disorder.

Persons with obsessive-compulsive personality disorder may flourish in positions demanding methodical, deductive, or detailed work, but they are vulnerable to unexpected changes, and their personal lives may remain barren. Depressive disorders, especially those of late onset, are common.

Treatment

Psychotherapy. Unlike patients with the other personality disorders, those with obsessive-compulsive personality disorder are often aware of their suffering, and they seek treatment on their own. Overtrained and oversocialized, these patients value free association and no-directive therapy highly. Treatment, however, is often long and complex, and countertransference problems are common.

Group therapy and behavior therapy occasionally offer certain advantages. In both contexts, it is easy to interrupt the patients in the midst of their maladaptive interactions or explanations. Preventing the completion of their habitual behavior raises patients' anxiety and leaves them susceptible to learning new coping strategies. Patients can also receive direct rewards for change in group therapy, something less often possible in individual psychotherapies.

Pharmacotherapy. Clonazepam (Klonopin), a benzodiazepine with anticonvulsant use, has reduced symptoms in patients with severe obsessive-compulsive disorder. Whether it is of use in the personality disorder is unknown. Clomipramine (Anafranil) and such serotonergic agents as fluoxetine, usually at dosages of 60 to 80 mg a day, may be useful if obsessive-compulsive signs and symptoms break through. Nefazodone (Serzone) may benefit some patients.

PERSONALITY DISORDER NOT OTHERWISE SPECIFIED

In DSM-IV-TR, the category personality disorder not otherwise specified is reserved for disorders that do not fit into any of the personality disorder categories described above. Passive-aggressive personality disorder and depressive personality disorder are now listed as examples of personality disorder not otherwise specified. A narrow spectrum of behavior or a particular trait—such as oppositionalism, sadism, or masochism—can also be classified in this category. A patient with features of more than one personality disorder but without the complete criteria of any one disorder can be assigned this classification. The DSM-IV-TR criteria for personality disorder not otherwise specified are presented in Table 27–13.

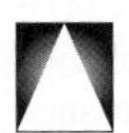

Table 27–13
DSM-IV-TR Diagnostic Criteria for Personality Disorder Not Otherwise Specified

This category is for disorders of personality functioning that do not meet criteria for any specific personality disorder. An example is the presence of features of more than one specific personality disorder that do not meet the full criteria for any one personality disorder ("mixed personality"), but that together cause clinically significant distress or impairment in one or more important areas of functioning (e.g., social or occupational). This category can also be used when the clinician judges that a specific personality disorder that is not included in the classification is appropriate. Examples include depressive personality disorder and passive-aggressive personality disorder.

(From American Psychiatric Association. *Diagnostic and Statistical Manual of Mental Disorders.* 4th ed. Text rev. Washington, DC: American Psychiatric Association; copyright 2000, with permission.)

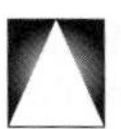

Table 27–14
DSM-IV-TR Research Criteria for Passive-Aggressive Personality Disorder

A. A pervasive pattern of negativistic attitudes and passive resistance to demands for adequate performance, beginning by early adulthood and present in a variety of contexts, as indicated by four (or more) of the following:
   (1) passively resists fulfilling routine social and occupational tasks
   (2) complains of being misunderstood and unappreciated by others
   (3) is sullen and argumentative
   (4) unreasonably criticizes and scorns authority
   (5) expresses envy and resentment toward those apparently more fortunate
   (6) voices exaggerated and persistent complaints of personal misfortune
   (7) alternates between hostile defiance and contrition
B. Does not occur exclusively during major depressive episodes and is not better accounted for by dysthymic disorder.

(From American Psychiatric Association. *Diagnostic and Statistical Manual of Mental Disorders.* 4th ed. Text rev. Washington, DC: American Psychiatric Association; copyright 2000, with permission.)

Passive-Aggressive Personality Disorder

Persons with passive-aggressive personality disorder are characterized by covert obstructionism, procrastination, stubbornness, and inefficiency. Such behavior is a manifestation of passively expressed underlying aggression. In DSM-IV-TR, the disorder is also called *negativistic personality disorder*.

Epidemiology. No data are available about the epidemiology of the disorder. Sex ratio, familial patterns, and prevalence have not been adequately studied.

Diagnosis. The criteria for passive-aggressive personality disorder are presented in Table 27–14.

Clinical Features. Patients with passive-aggressive personality disorder characteristically procrastinate, resist demands for adequate performance, find excuses for delays, and find fault with those on whom they depend; yet they refuse to extricate themselves from the dependent relationships. They usually lack assertiveness and are not direct about their own needs and wishes. They fail to ask needed questions about what is expected of them and may become anxious when forced to succeed or when their usual defense of turning anger against themselves is removed.

In interpersonal relationships, these persons attempt to manipulate themselves into a position of dependence, but others often experience this passive, self-detrimental behavior as punitive and manipulative. Persons with this disorder expect others to do their errands and to carry out their routine responsibilities. Friends and clinicians may become enmeshed in trying to assuage the patients' many claims of unjust treatment. The close relationships of persons with passive-aggressive personality disorder, however, are rarely tranquil or happy. Because they are bound to their resentment more closely than to their satisfaction, they may never even formulate goals for finding enjoyment in life. Persons with the disorder lack self-confidence and are typically pessimistic about the future.

Differential Diagnosis. Passive-aggressive personality disorders must be differentiated from histrionic and borderline personality disorders. Patients with passive-aggressive personality disorder, however, are less flamboyant, dramatic, affective, and openly aggressive than those with histrionic and borderline personality disorders.

Course and Prognosis. In a follow-up study averaging 11 years of 100 inpatients with passive-aggressive disorder, Ivor Small found that the primary diagnosis in 54 was passive-aggressive personality disorder; 18 were also alcohol abusers, and 30 could be clinically labeled as depressed. Of the 73 former patients located, 58 (79 percent) had persistent psychiatric difficulties, and 9 (12 percent) were considered symptom free. Most seemed irritable, anxious, and depressed; somatic complaints were numerous. Only 32 (44 percent) were employed full time as workers or homemakers. Although neglect of responsibility and suicide attempts were common, only one patient had committed suicide in the interim. Twenty-eight (38 percent) had been readmitted to a hospital, but only three had been diagnosed as having schizophrenia.

Treatment. Patients with passive-aggressive personality disorder who receive supportive psychotherapy have good outcomes, but psychotherapy for these patients has many pitfalls. Fulfilling their demands often supports their pathology, but refusing their demands rejects them. Therapy sessions, thus, can become a battleground on which a patient expresses feelings of resentment against a therapist on whom the patient wishes to become dependent. With these patients, clinicians must treat suicide gestures as any covert expression of anger, and not as object loss in major depressive disorder. Therapists must point out the probable consequences of passive-aggressive behaviors as they occur. Such confrontations may be more helpful than a correct interpretation in changing patients' behavior.

Antidepressants should be prescribed only when clinical indications of depression and the possibility of suicide exist. Depending on the clinical features, some patients have responded to benzodiazepines and psychostimulants.

Depressive Personality Disorder

Persons with depressive personality disorder are characterized by lifelong traits that fall along the depressive spectrum. They are pessimistic, anhedonic, duty bound, self-doubting, and chronically unhappy. The disorder is newly classified in DSM-IV-TR, but melancholic personality was described by early 20th century European psychiatrists such as Ernst Kretschmer.

Epidemiology. Because depressive personality disorder is a new category, no epidemiological data are available. On the basis of the prevalence of depressive disorders in the overall population, however, depressive personality disorder seems to be common, to occur equally in men and women, and to occur in families in which depressive disorders are found.

Etiology. The cause of depressive personality disorder is unknown, but the same factors involved in dysthymic disorder and major depressive disorder may be at work. Psychological theories involve early loss, poor parenting, punitive superegos, and extreme feelings of guilt. Biological theories involve the hypothalamic-pituitary-adrenal-thyroid axis, including the noradrenergic and serotonergic amine systems. Genetic predisposition, as indicated by Stella Chess's studies of temperament, may also play a role.

Diagnosis and Clinical Features. A classic description of depressive personality was provided in 1963 by Arthur Noyes and Laurence Kolb:

> They feel but little of the normal joy of living and are inclined to be lonely and solemn, to be gloomy, submissive, pessimistic, and self-deprecatory. They are prone to express regrets and feelings of inadequacy and hopelessness. They are often meticulous, perfectionistic, overconscientious, preoccupied with work, feel responsibility keenly, and are easily discouraged under new conditions. They are fearful of disapproval, tend to suffer in silence and perhaps to cry easily, although usually not in the presence of others. A tendency to hesitation, indecision, and caution betrays an inherent feeling of insecurity.

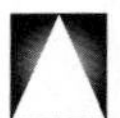

Table 27–15
DSM-IV-TR Research Criteria for Depressive Personality Disorder

A. A pervasive pattern of depressive cognitions and behaviors beginning by early adulthood and present in a variety of contexts, as indicated by five (or more) of the following:
   (1) usual mood is dominated by dejection, gloominess, cheerlessness, joylessness, unhappiness
   (2) self-concept centers around beliefs of inadequacy, worthlessness, and low self-esteem
   (3) is critical, blaming, and derogatory toward self
   (4) is brooding and given to worry
   (5) is negativistic, critical, and judgmental toward others
   (6) is pessimistic
   (7) is prone to feeling guilty or remorseful

B. Does not occur exclusively during major depressive episodes and is not better accounted for by dysthymic disorder.

(From American Psychiatric Association. *Diagnostic and Statistical Manual of Mental Disorders.* 4th ed. Text rev. Washington, DC: American Psychiatric Association; copyright 2000, with permission.)

More recently, Hagop Akiskal described seven groups of depressive traits: quiet, introverted, passive, and nonassertive; gloomy, pessimistic, serious, and incapable of fun; self-critical, self-reproachful, and self-derogatory; skeptical, critical of others, and hard to please; conscientious, responsible, and self-disciplined; brooding and given to worry; and preoccupied with negative events, feelings of inadequacy, and personal shortcomings.

Patients with depressive personality disorder complain of chronic feelings of unhappiness. They admit to low self-esteem and difficulty finding anything in their lives about which they are joyful, hopeful, or optimistic. They are self-critical and derogatory and are likely to denigrate their work, themselves, and their relationships with others. Their physiognomy often reflects their mood—poor posture, depressed facies, hoarse voice, and psychomotor retardation. The DSM-IV-TR criteria are listed in Table 27–15.

Differential Diagnosis. Dysthymic disorder is a mood disorder characterized by greater fluctuation in mood than occurs in depressive personality disorder. The personality disorder is chronic and lifelong, whereas dysthymic disorder is episodic, can occur at any time, and usually has a precipitating stressor. The depressive personality can be conceptualized as part of a spectrum of affective conditions in which dysthymic disorder and major depressive disorder are more severe variants. Patients with avoidant personality disorder are introverted and dependent, but they tend to be more anxious than depressed, compared with persons with depressive personality disorder.

Course and Prognosis. Persons with depressive personality disorder may be at great risk for dysthymic disorder and major depressive disorder. In a recent study by Donald Klein and Gregory Mills, subjects with depressive personality exhibited significantly higher rates of current mood disorder, lifetime mood disorder, major depression, and dysthymia than subjects without depressive personality.

Treatment. Psychotherapy is the treatment of choice for depressive personality disorder. Patients respond to insight-oriented psychotherapy, and because their reality testing is good, they can gain insight into the psychodynamics of their illness and appreciate its effects on their interpersonal relationships. Treatment is likely to be long term. Cognitive therapy helps patients understand the cognitive manifestations of their low self-esteem and pessimism. Group psychotherapy and interpersonal therapy are also useful. Some persons respond to self-help measures.

Psychopharmacological approaches include the use of antidepressant medications, especially such serotonergic agents as sertraline (Zoloft), 50 mg a day. Some patients respond to small dosages of psychostimulants, such as amphetamine, 5 to 15 mg a day. In all cases, psychopharmacological agents should be combined with psychotherapy to achieve maximum effects.

Sadomasochistic Personality Disorder

Some personality types are characterized by elements of sadism or masochism or a combination of both. Sadomasochistic personality disorder is listed here because it is of major clinical and historical interest in psychiatry. It is not an official diagnostic category in DSM-IV-TR or its appendix, but it can be diagnosed as personality disorder not otherwise classified.

Sadism is the desire to cause others pain by being either sexually abusive or generally physically or psychologically abusive. It is named for the Marquis de Sade, a late 18th century writer of erotica describing persons who experienced sexual pleasure while inflicting pain on others. Freud believed that sadists ward off castration anxiety and are able to achieve sexual pleasure only when they can do to others what they fear will be done to them.

Masochism, named for Leopold von Sacher-Masoch, a 19th century German novelist, is the achievement of sexual gratification by inflicting pain on the self. So-called moral masochists generally seek humiliation and failure rather than physical pain. Freud believed that masochists' ability to achieve orgasm is disturbed by anxiety and guilt feelings about sex, which are alleviated by suffering and punishment.

Clinical observations indicate that elements of both sadistic and masochistic behavior are usually present in the same person. Treatment with insight-oriented psychotherapy, including psychoanalysis, has been effective in some cases. As a result of therapy, patients become aware of the need for self-punishment secondary to excessive unconscious guilt and also come to recognize their repressed aggressive impulses, which originate in early childhood.

Sadistic Personality Disorder

Sadistic personality disorder is not included in DSM-IV-TR, but it still appears in the literature and may be of descriptive use. Beginning in early adulthood, persons with sadistic personality disorder show a pervasive pattern of cruel, demeaning, and aggressive behavior that is directed toward others. Physical cruelty or violence is used to inflict pain on others, not to achieve another goal, such as mugging a person to steal. Persons with the disorder like to humiliate or demean persons in front of others and have usually treated or disciplined persons uncommonly harshly, especially children. In general, persons with sadistic personality disorder are fascinated by violence, weapons, injury, or torture. To be included in this category, such persons cannot be motivated solely by the desire to derive sexual arousal from their behavior; if they are so motivated, the paraphilia of sexual sadism should be diagnosed.

PERSONALITY CHANGE DUE TO A GENERAL MEDICAL CONDITION

Personality change due to a general medical condition (*see* Table 10.5–13) deserves some discussion here. ICD-10 includes the category personality and behavioral disorders due to brain disease, damage, and dysfunction, which includes organic personality disorder (*see* Table 10.5–18), postencephalitic syndrome, and postconcussional syndrome. Personality change due to a general medical condition is characterized by a marked change in personality style and traits from a previous level of functioning. Patients must show evidence of a causative organic factor antedating the onset of the personality change.

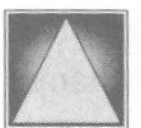

Table 27–16
Medical Conditions Associated with Personality Change

Head trauma
Cerebrovascular diseases
Cerebral tumors
Epilepsy (particularly, complex partial epilepsy)
Huntington's disease
Multiple sclerosis
Endocrine disorders
Heavy metal poisoning (manganese, mercury)
Neurosyphilis
Acquired immune deficiency syndrome (AIDS)

Etiology

Structural damage to the brain is usually the cause of the personality change, and head trauma is probably the most common cause. Cerebral neoplasms and vascular accidents, particularly of the temporal and frontal lobes, are also common causes. The conditions most often associated with personality change are listed in Table 27–16.

Diagnosis and Clinical Features

A change in personality from previous patterns of behavior or an exacerbation of previous personality characteristics is notable. Impaired control of the expression of emotions and impulses is a cardinal feature. Emotions are characteristically labile and shallow, although euphoria or apathy may be prominent. The euphoria may mimic hypomania, but true elation is absent, and patients may admit to not really feeling happy. There is a hollow and silly ring to their excitement and facile jocularity, particularly when the frontal lobes are involved. Also associated with damage to the frontal lobes, the so-called frontal lobe syndrome, is prominent indifference and apathy, characterized by a lack of concern for events in the immediate environment. Temper outbursts, which can occur with little or no provocation, especially after alcohol ingestion, can result in violent behavior. The expression of impulses may be manifested by inappropriate jokes, a coarse manner, improper sexual advances, and antisocial conduct resulting in conflicts with the law, such as assaults on others, sexual misdemeanors, and shoplifting. Foresight and the ability to anticipate the social or legal consequences of actions are typically diminished. Persons with temporal lobe epilepsy characteristically show humorlessness, hypergraphia, hyperreligiosity, and marked aggressiveness during seizures.

Persons with personality change due to a general medical condition have a clear sensorium. Mild disorders of cognitive function often coexist, but do not amount to intellectual deterioration. Patients may be inattentive, which may account for disorders of recent memory. With some prodding, however, patients are likely to recall what they claim to have forgotten. The diagnosis should be suspected in patients who show marked changes in behavior or personality involving emotional lability and impaired impulse control, who have no history of mental disorder, and whose personality changes occur abruptly or over a relatively brief time. The DSM-IV-TR diagnostic criteria appear in Table 10.5–13.

Anabolic Steroids. An increasing number of high school and college athletes and bodybuilders are using anabolic steroids as a shortcut to maximize physical development. Anabolic steroids include oxymetholone (Anadrol), somatropin (Humatrope), stanozolol (Winstrol), and testosterone.

DSM-IV-TR does not include a diagnostic category for substance-induced personality disorder, so it is unclear whether a personality change caused by steroid abuse is better diagnosed as personality change due to a general medical condition or as one of the other (or unknown) substance use disorders. It is mentioned here because anabolic steroids can cause persistent alterations of personality and behavior. Anabolic steroid abuse is discussed in Section 12.13.

Differential Diagnosis

Dementia involves global deterioration in intellectual and behavioral capacities, of which personality change is just one category. A personality change may herald a cognitive disorder that eventually will evolve into dementia. In these cases, as deterioration begins to encompass significant memory and cognitive deficits, the diagnosis of the disorder changes from personality change caused by a general medical condition to dementia. In differentiating the specific syndrome from other disorders in which personality change may occur—such as schizophrenia, delusional disorder, mood disorders, and impulse control disorders—physicians must consider the most important factor, the presence in personality change disorder of a specific organic causative factor.

Course and Prognosis

Both the course and the prognosis of personality change due to a general medical condition depend on its cause. If the disorder results from structural damage to the brain, the disorder tends to persist. The disorder may follow a period of coma and delirium in cases of head trauma or vascular accident and may be permanent. The personality change can evolve into dementia in cases of brain tumor, multiple sclerosis, and Huntington's disease. Personality changes produced by chronic intoxication, medical illness, or drug therapy (such as levodopa [Larodopa] for parkinsonism) may be reversed if the underlying cause is treated. Some patients require custodial care or at least close supervision to meet their basic needs, avoid repeated conflicts with the law, and protect themselves and their families from the hostility of others and from destitution resulting from impulsive and ill-considered actions.

Treatment

Management of personality change disorder involves treatment of the underlying organic condition when possible. Psychopharmacological treatment of specific symptoms may be indicated in some cases, such as imipramine or fluoxetine for depression.

Patients with severe cognitive impairment or weakened behavioral controls may need counseling to help avoid difficulties at work or to prevent social embarrassment. As a rule, patients' families need emotional support and concrete advice on how to help minimize patients' undesirable conduct. Alcohol should be avoided, and social engagements should be curtailed when patients tend to act in a grossly offensive manner.

PSYCHOBIOLOGICAL MODEL OF TREATMENT

The psychobiological model of treatment combines psychotherapy and pharmacotherapy and is based on the established structural, clinical, and postulated neurochemical characteristics of temperament and character. Pharmacotherapy and psychotherapy can be systematically matched to the personality structure and stage of character development of each patient—clearly a unique advantage over other available approaches.

The newest development is treating personality disorders pharmacologically. Target symptoms are identified, and particular drugs with known effects on personality traits (e.g., harm avoidance) are used. Table 27–17 summarizes drug choices for various target symptoms of personality disorders.

In his book, *Listening to Prozac*, Peter Kramer described dramatic personality changes when serotonin levels are raised by fluoxetine administration, such as decreased sensitivity to rejection, increased assertiveness, improved self-esteem, and the ability to tolerate stress. These changes in personality traits occur in patients with a wide range of psychiatric conditions as well as in persons without diagnosable mental disorders. Using medications to treat specific traits in a person who is otherwise normal (i.e., does not meet the criteria for a full-blown personality disorder) is controversial. It has been called "cosmetic psychopharmacology" by its critics.

Biological Character Traits

Four character traits have been described (Table 27–18), each with certain neurochemical and neurophysiological substrates. Some workers postulate specific genes for some traits, e.g., novelty seeking gene.

Harm Avoidance. Harm avoidance involves a heritable bias in the inhibition of behavior in response to signals of punishment and nonreward. High harm avoidance is observed as fear of uncertainty, social inhibition, shyness with strangers, rapid fatigability, and pessimistic worry in anticipation of problems, even in situations that do not worry other persons. Persons low in harm avoidance are carefree, courageous, energetic, outgoing, and optimistic, even in situations that worry most persons.

The psychobiology of harm avoidance is complex. Benzodiazepines disinhibit avoidance by γ-aminobutyric acid (GABA)-ergic inhibition of serotonergic neurons originating in the dorsal raphe nuclei.

Positron emission tomography (PET) at the National Institute of Mental Health (NIMH) with [^{18}F]-deoxyglucose (FDG) in 31 healthy adult volunteers during a simple, continuous, performance task showed that harm avoidance was associated with increased activity in the anterior paralimbic circuit, specifically the right amygdala and insula, the right orbitofrontal cortex, and the left medial prefrontal cortex.

High GABA concentrations in plasma have also been correlated with low harm avoidance. Plasma GABA concentration has also been correlated with other measures of anxiety susceptibility, and it correlates highly with GABA concentration in the brain. Finally, a gene on chromosome 17q12 that regulates the expression of the serotonin transporter accounts for 4 to 9 percent of the total variance in harm avoidance. These findings support a role for both GABA and serotonergic projections from the dorsal raphe underlying individual differences in behavioral inhibition as measured by harm avoidance. Persons given serotonin drugs show decreased harm avoidance behavior.

Novelty Seeking. Novelty seeking reflects a heritable bias in the initiation or activation of appetitive approach in response to novelty, approach to signals of reward, active avoidance of conditioned signals of punishment, and escape from unconditioned punishment (all of which are hypothesized to covary as part of one heritable system of learning). Novelty seeking is observed as exploratory activity in response to novelty, impulsiveness, extravagance in approach to cues of reward, and active avoidance of frustration. Individuals high in novelty seeking are

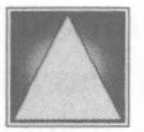

Table 27–17
Pharmacotherapy of Target Symptom Domains of Personality Disorders

Target Symptom	Drug of Choice	Contraindication[a]
I. Behavior dyscontrol		
Aggression/impulsivity		
Affective aggression (hot temper with normal EEG)	Lithium[a] Serotonergic drugs[a] Anticonvulsants[a] Low-dosage antipsychotics	? Benzodiazepines Stimulants
Predatory aggression (hostility/cruelty)	Antipsychotics[a] Lithium β-Adrenergic receptor antagonists	Benzodiazepines Stimulants
Organic-like aggression	Imipramine[a] Cholinergic agonists (donepezil)	
Ictal aggression (abnormal EEG)	Carbamazepine[a] Diphenylhydantoin[a] Benzodiazepines	Antipsychotics Stimulants
II. Mood dysregulation		
Emotional lability	Lithium[a] Antipsychotics	? Tricyclic drugs
Depression		
Atypical depression, dysphoria	MAOIs[a] Serotonergic drugs[a] Antipsychotics	
Emotional detachment	Serotonin-dopamine antagonists[a] Atypical antipsychotics	? Tricyclic drugs
III. Anxiety		
Chronic cognitive	Serotonergic drugs[a] MAOIs[a] Benzodiazepines	Stimulants
Chronic somatic	MAOIs[a] β-Adrenergic receptor antagonists	
Severe anxiety	Low-dose antipsychotics MAOIs	
IV. Psychotic symptoms		
Acute and psychosis	Antipsychotics[a]	Stimulants
Chronic and low-level psychotic-like symptoms	Low-dose antipsychotics[a]	

[a]Drug of choice or major contraindication.
EEG, electroencephalogram; MAOIs, monamine oxidase inhibitors.

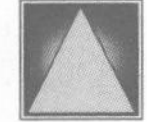

Table 27–18
Descriptors of Individuals Who Score High and Low on the Four Temperament Dimensions

	Descriptors of Extreme Variants	
Temperament Dimension	High	Low
Harm avoidance	Pessimistic Fearful Shy Fatigable	Optimistic Daring Outgoing Energetic
Novelty seeking	Exploratory Impulsive Extravagant Irritable	Reserved Deliberate Thrifty Stoical
Reward dependence	Sentimental Open Warm Affectionate	Detached Aloof Cold Independent
Persistence	Industrious Determined Enthusiastic Perfectionist	Lazy Spoiled Underachieving Pragmatic

quick-tempered, curious, easily bored, impulsive, extravagant, and disorderly. Persons low in novelty seeking are slow tempered, uninquiring, stoical, reflective, frugal, reserved, tolerant of monotony, and orderly.

Dopaminergic projections have a crucial role in novelty seeking. Novelty seeking involves increased reuptake of dopamine at presynaptic terminals, thereby requiring frequent stimulation to maintain optimal levels of postsynaptic dopaminergic stimulation. Novelty seeking leads to various pleasure-seeking behaviors, including cigarette smoking, which may explain the frequent observation of low platelet MAO type B (MAO_B) activity, because cigarette smoking inhibits MAO_B activity in platelets and brain.

Studies of genes involved in dopamine neurotransmission, such as the dopamine transporter gene (*DAT1*) and the type 4 dopamine receptor gene (*DRD4*) have provided evidence of association with novelty seeking or risk-taking behavior.

Reward Dependence. Reward dependence reflects maintenance of behavior in response to cues of social reward. Individuals high in reward dependence are tender hearted, sensitive, socially dependent, and sociable. Individuals low in reward dependence are practical, tough minded, cold, socially insensitive, irresolute, and indifferent if alone.

Noradrenergic projections from the locus ceruleus and serotonergic projections from the median raphe are thought to influence such reward conditioning. High reward dependence is associated with increased activity in the thalamus. The 3-methoxy-4-hydroxyphenylglycol (MHPG) concentration is low in persons with high reward dependence.

Persistence. Persistence reflects maintenance of behavior, despite frustration, fatigue, and intermittent reinforcement. Highly persistent persons are hard-working, perseverant, and ambitious overachievers who tend to intensify their effort in response to anticipated reward and view frustration and fatigue as a personal challenge. Individuals low in persistence are indolent, inactive, unstable, and erratic; they tend to give up easily when faced with frustration, rarely strive for higher accomplishments, and manifest little perseverance even in response to intermittent reward.

Recent work in rodents related the integrity of the partial reinforcement extinction effect to hippocampal connections and glutamate metabolism. Persistence may be enhanced by psychostimulants.

ICD-10

In ICD-10, personality disorders are described as severe disturbances of personality and behavior that are pronounced deviations from normal cultural patterns. ICD-10's diagnostic guidelines include disturbances of long-standing duration in several areas of functioning; pervasive and maladaptive behavior; onset in childhood or adolescence; continuation into adulthood; considerable personality distress (although sometimes apparent only late in the disorder's course); and usually, but not always, significant problems in work and in social behavior. ICD-10 also allows for the possibility of criteria developed to describe personality disorders in different cultures. The diagnostic criteria for specific personality disorders appear in Table 27–1.

References

Cloninger CR. *Feeling Good: The Science of Well Being*. New York: Oxford University Press; 2004.

Crawford TN, Cohen P, Johnson JG, Sneed Joel R, Brook JS. The course and psychosocial correlates of personality disorder symptoms in adolescence: Erikson's developmental theory revisited. *J Youth Adolesc*. 2004;33:373–387.

Helgeland MI, Kjelsberg E, Torgersen S. Continuities between emotional and disruptive behavior disorders in adolescence and personality disorders in adulthood. *Am J Psych*. 2005;162:1941–1947.

Johnson JG, First MB, Cohen P, Skodol AE, Kasen S, Brook JS. Adverse outcomes associated with personality disorder not otherwise specified in a community sample. *Am J Psych*. 2005;162:1926–1932.

Nickel MK, Muehlbacher M, Nickel C, Kettler C, Pedrosa Gil F, Bachler E, Buschmann W, Rother N, Fartacek R, Egger C, Anvar J, Rother WK, Loew TH, Kaplan P. Aripiprazole in the treatment of patients with borderline personality disorder: A double-blind, placebo-controlled study. *Am J Psychiatry*. 2006;163(5):833–838.

Ozkan M, Altindag A. Comorbid personality disorders in subjects with panic disorder: Do personality disorders increase clinical severity? *Compr Psychiatry*. 2005;46:20–26.

Pagan JL, Oltmanns TF, Whitmore MJ, Turkheimer E. Personality disorder not otherwise specified: Searching for an empirically based diagnostic threshold. *J Personal Disord*. 2005;19:674–689.

Sussman N. Borderline personality and bipolar disorders: Is there a connection? *Primary Psychiatry*. 2004;11:13.

Svrakic DM, Cloninger CR. Personality disorders. In: Sadock BJ, Sadock VA, eds. *Kaplan & Sadock's Comprehensive Textbook of Psychiatry*. 8th ed. Vol. 2. Baltimore: Lippincott Williams & Wilkins; 2005:2063.

Zimmerman M, Rothschild L, Chelminski I. The prevalence of DSM-IV personality disorders in psychiatric outpatients. *Am J Psychiatry*. 2005;162:1911–1918.

28 Psychosomatic Medicine

▲ 28.1 Psychological Factors Affecting Physical Conditions

Psychosomatic (psychophysiological) medicine has been a specific area of study within the field of psychiatry for more than 75 years. It is informed by two basic assumptions: There is a unity of mind and body (reflected in the term mind-body medicine); and psychological factors must be taken into account when considering all disease states.

Concepts derived from the field of psychosomatic medicine influenced both the emergence of complementary and alternative medicine (CAM), which relies heavily on examining psychological factors in the maintenance of health, and the field of holistic medicine with its emphasis on examining and treating the whole patient, not just his or her disease or disorder. The concepts of psychosomatic medicine also influenced the field of behavioral medicine, which integrates the behavioral sciences and the biomedical approach to the prevention, diagnosis, and treatment of disease. Psychosomatic concepts have contributed greatly to those approaches to medical care.

No classification for psychosomatic disease is listed in the revised fourth edition of *Diagnostic and Statistical Manual of Mental Disorders* (DSM-IV-TR). The concepts of psychosomatic medicine are subsumed in the diagnostic entity called *Psychological Factors Affecting Medical Conditions*. This category covers physical disorders caused by emotional or psychological factors. It also applies to mental or emotional disorders caused or aggravated by physical illness.

In 2005, the American Board of Medical Specialties and the American Board of Psychiatry and Neurology approved a separate board to be called the American Board of Psychosomatic Medicine. That decision recognizes the importance of the field and also brings the term *psychosomatic* back into common use.

CLASSIFICATION

The DSM-IV-TR diagnostic criteria for psychological factors affecting medical condition are presented in Table 28.1–1. Excluded are (1) classic mental disorders that have physical symptoms as part of the disorder (e.g., conversion disorder, in which a physical symptom is produced by psychological conflict); (2) somatization disorder, in which the physical symptoms are not based on organic pathology; (3) hypochondriasis, in which patients have an exaggerated concern with their health; (4) physical complaints that are frequently associated with mental disorders (e.g., dysthymic disorder, which usually has such somatic accompaniments as muscle weakness, asthenia, fatigue, and exhaustion); and (5) physical complaints associated with substance-related disorders (e.g., coughing associated with nicotine dependence). Criteria in the 10th revision of the *International Statistical Classification of Diseases and Related Health Problems* (ICD-10) are more general than the DSM-IV-TR criteria and are listed in Table 28.1–2.

STRESS THEORY

Stress can be described as a circumstance that disturbs, or is likely to disturb, the normal physiological or psychological functioning of a person. In the 1920s, Walter Cannon (1875–1945) conducted the first systematic study of the relation of stress to disease. He demonstrated that stimulation of the autonomic nervous system, particularly the sympathetic system, readied the organism for the "fight or flight" response characterized by hypertension, tachycardia, and increased cardiac output. This was useful in the animal who could fight or flee; but in the person who could do neither by virtue of being civilized, the ensuing stress resulted in disease (e.g., produced a cardiovascular disorder).

In the 1950s, Harold Wolff (1898–1962) observed that the physiology of the gastrointestinal (GI) tract appeared to correlate with specific emotional states. Hyperfunction was associated with hostility, and hypofunction with sadness. Wolff regarded such reactions as nonspecific, believing that the patient's reaction is determined by the general life situation and perceptual appraisal of the stressful event. Earlier, William Beaumont (1785–1853), an American military surgeon, had a patient named Alexis St. Martin, who became famous because of a gunshot wound that resulted in a permanent gastric fistula. Beaumont noted that during highly charged emotional states the mucosa could become either hyperemic or blanch, indicating that blood flow to the stomach was influenced by emotions.

Hans Selye (1907–1982) developed a model of stress that he called the *general adaptation syndrome*. It consisted of three phases: (1) the alarm reaction; (2) the stage of resistance, in which adaptation is ideally achieved; and (3) the stage of exhaustion, in which acquired adaptation or resistance may be lost. He considered stress a nonspecific bodily response to any demand caused by either pleasant or unpleasant conditions. Selye believed that stress, by definition, need not always be unpleasant. He called unpleasant stress distress. Accepting both types of stress requires adaptation.

The body reacts to stress—in this sense defined as anything (real, symbolic, or imagined) that threatens an individual's

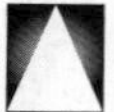

Table 28.1–1
DSM-IV-TR Diagnostic Criteria for Psychological Factors Affecting General Medical Condition

A. A general medical condition (coded on Axis III) is present.
B. Psychological factors adversely affect the general medical condition in one of the following ways:
(1) the factors have influenced the course of the general medical condition as shown by a close temporal association between the psychological factors and the development or exacerbation of, or delayed recovery from, the general medical condition
(2) the factors interfere with the treatment of the general medical condition
(3) the factors constitute additional health risks for the individual
(4) stress-related physiological responses precipitate or exacerbate symptoms of the general medical condition

Choose name based on the nature of the psychological factors (if more than one factor is present, indicate the most prominent):
Mental disorder affecting... [indicate the general medical condition] (e.g., an Axis I disorder such as major depressive disorder delaying recovery from a myocardial infarction)
Psychological symptoms affecting... [indicate the general medical condition] (e.g., depressive symptoms delaying recovery from surgery; anxiety exacerbating asthma)
Personality traits or coping style affecting... [indicate the general medical condition] (e.g., pathological denial of the need for surgery in a patient with cancer; hostile, pressured behavior contributing to cardiovascular disease)
Maladaptive health behaviors affecting... [indicate the general medical condition] (e.g., overeating; lack of exercise; unsafe sex)
Stress-related physiological response affecting... [indicate the general medical condition] (e.g., stress-related exacerbations of ulcer, hypertension, arrhythmia, or tension headache)
Other or unspecified psychological factors affecting... [indicate the general medical condition] (e.g., interpersonal, cultural, or religious factors)

(From American Psychiatric Association. *Diagnostic and Statistical Manual of Mental Disorders.* 4th ed. Text rev. Washington, DC: American Psychiatric Association; copyright 2000, with permission.)

survival—by putting into motion a set of responses that seeks to diminish the impact of the stressor and restore homeostasis. Much is known about the physiological response to acute stress, but considerably less is known about the response to chronic stress. Many stressors occur over a prolonged period of time or have long-lasting repercussions. For example, the loss of a spouse may be followed by months or years of loneliness and a violent sexual assault may be followed by years of apprehension and worry. Neuroendocrine and immune responses to such events help explain why and how stress can have deleterious effects.

Neurotransmitter Responses to Stress

Stressors activate noradrenergic systems in the brain (most notably in the locus ceruleus) and cause release of catecholamines from the autonomic nervous system. Stressors also activate serotonergic systems in the brain, as evidenced by increased serotonin turnover. Recent evidence suggests that, although glucocorticoids tend to enhance overall serotonin functioning, differences may exist in glucocorticoid regulation of serotonin-receptor subtypes, which can have implications for serotonergic functioning in depression and related illnesses. For example, glucocorticoids can increase serotonin 5-hydroxytryptamine (5-HT_2)-mediated actions, thus contributing to the intensification of actions of these receptor types, which have been implicated in the pathophysiology of major depressive disorder. Stress also increases dopaminergic neurotransmission in mesoprefrontal pathways.

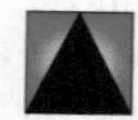

Table 28.1–2
ICD-10 Diagnostic Criteria for Psychological and Behavioral Factors Associated with Disorders or Diseases Classified Elsewhere

This category should be used to record the presence of psychological or behavioral factors thought to have influenced the manifestation, or affected the course, of physical disorders that can be classified using other chapters of ICD-10. Any resulting mental disturbances are usually mild and often prolonged (such as worry, emotional conflict, apprehension) and do not of themselves justify the use of any of the categories described in the rest of this book. An additional code should be used to identify the physical disorder. (In the rare instances in which an overt psychiatric disorder is thought to have caused a physical disorder, a second additional code should be used to record the psychiatric disorder.)

(Reprinted with permission from World Health Organization. *International Classification of Mental and Behavioural Disorders: Diagnostic Criteria for Research.* Copyright, World Health Organization, Geneva, 1993.)

Amino acid and peptidergic neurotransmitters are also intricately involved in the stress response. Studies have shown that corticotropin-releasing factor (CRF) (as a neurotransmitter, not just as a hormonal regulator of hypothalamic-pituitary-adrenal [HPA] axis functioning), glutamate (through *N*-methyl-D-aspartate [NMDA] receptors), and γ-aminobutyric acid (GABA) all play important roles in generating the stress response or in modulating other stress-responsive systems, such as dopaminergic and noradrenergic brain circuitry.

Endocrine Responses to Stress

In response to stress, CRF is secreted from the hypothalamus into the hypophysial-pituitary-portal system. CRF acts at the anterior pituitary to trigger release of adrenocorticotropic hormone (ACTH). Once ACTH is released, it acts at the adrenal cortex to stimulate the synthesis and release of glucocorticoids. Glucocorticoids themselves have myriad effects within the body, but their actions can be summarized in the short term as promoting energy use, increasing cardiovascular activity (in the service of the "flight or fight" response), and inhibiting functions such as growth, reproduction, and immunity.

This HPA axis is subject to tight negative feedback control by its own end products (i.e., ACTH and cortisol) at multiple levels, including the anterior pituitary, the hypothalamus, and such suprahypothalamic brain regions as the hippocampus. In addition to CRF, numerous secretagogues (i.e., substances that elicit ACTH release) exist that can bypass CRF release and act directly to initiate the glucocorticoid cascade. Examples of such secretagogues include catecholamines, vasopressin, and oxytocin. Interestingly, different stressors (e.g., cold stress versus hypotension) trigger different patterns of secretagogue release, again demonstrating that the notion of a uniform stress response to a generic stressor is an oversimplification.

Immune Response to Stress

Part of the stress response consists of the inhibition of immune functioning by glucocorticoids. This inhibition may reflect a compensatory action of the HPA axis to mitigate other physiological effects of stress. Conversely, stress can also cause immune activation through a variety of pathways. CRF itself can stimulate norepinephrine release via CRF receptors located on the locus ceruleus, which activates the sympathetic nervous system, both centrally and peripherally, and increases epinephrine release from the adrenal medulla. In addition, direct links of norepinephrine neurons synapse on immune target cells. Thus, in the face of stressors, profound immune activation also occurs, including the release of humoral immune factors (cytokines) such as interleukin-1 (IL-1) and IL-6. These cytokines can themselves cause further release of CRF, which in theory serves to increase glucocorticoid effects and thereby self-limit the immune activation. An extensive discussion of the immune response can be found in Section 3.5.

Life Events

A life event or situation, favorable or unfavorable (Selye's distress), often occurring by chance, generates challenges to which the person must adequately respond. Thomas Holmes and Richard Rahe constructed a social readjustment rating scale after asking hundreds of persons from varying backgrounds to rank the relative degree of adjustment required by changing life events. Holmes and Rahe listed 43 life events associated with varying amounts of disruption and stress in average persons' lives and assigned each of them a certain number of units: for example, the death of a spouse, 100 life-change units; divorce, 73 units; marital separations, 65 units; and the death of a close family member, 63 units. Accumulation of 200 or more life-change units in a single year increases the risk of developing a psychosomatic disorder in that year. Of interest, persons who face general stresses optimistically, rather than pessimistically, are less apt to experience psychosomatic disorders; if they do, they are more apt to recover easily. Table 28.1–3 lists the top 15 stressors and their units in the social readjustment scale.

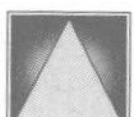

Table 28.1–3
Social Readjustment Rating Scale

Life Event	Mean Value
1. Death of spouse	100
2. Divorce	73
3. Marital separation from mate	65
4. Detention in jail or other institution	63
5. Death of a close family member	63
6. Major personal injury or illness	53
7. Marriage	50
8. Being fired at work	47
9. Marital reconciliation with mate	45
10. Retirement from work	45
11. Major change in the health or behavior of a family member	44
12. Pregnancy	40
13. Sexual difficulties	39
14. Gaining a new family member (through birth, adoption, oldster moving in, etc.)	39
15. Major business readjustment (merger, reorganization, bankruptcy, etc.)	39

(From Holmes T. Life situations, emotions, and disease. *Psychosom Med.* 1978;9:747, with permission.)

Specific versus Nonspecific Stress Factors

In addition to life stresses such as a divorce or the death of a spouse, some investigators have suggested that specific personalities and conflicts are associated with certain psychosomatic diseases. A specific personality or a specific unconscious conflict may contribute to the development of a specific psychosomatic disorder. Researchers first identified specific personality types in connection with coronary disease. An individual with a coronary personality is a hard-driving, competitive, aggressive person who is predisposed to coronary artery disease. Meyer Friedman and Ray Rosenman first defined two types: (1) type A—similar to the coronary personality—and (2) type B personalities—calm, relaxed, and not susceptible to coronary disease (See discussion below).

Franz Alexander was a major proponent of the theory that specific unconscious conflicts are associated with specific psychosomatic disorders. For example, persons susceptible to having a peptic ulcer were believed to have strong ungratified dependency needs. Persons with essential hypertension were considered to have hostile impulses about which they felt guilty. Patients with bronchial asthma had issues with separation anxiety. The specific psychic stress theory is no longer considered a reliable indicator of who will develop which disorder; the nonspecific stress theory is more acceptable to most workers in the field today. Nevertheless, chronic stress, usually with the intervening variable of anxiety, predisposes certain persons to psychosomatic disorders. The vulnerable organ may be anywhere in the body. Some persons are "stomach reactors," others are "cardiovascular reactors," "skin reactors," and so on. The diathesis or susceptibility of an organ system to react to stress is probably of genetic origin; but it may also result from acquired vulnerability (e.g., lungs weakened by smoking). According to psychoanalytic theory, the choice of the afflicted region is determined by unconscious factors, a concept known as *somatic compliance*. For example, Freud reported on a male patient with fears of homosexual impulses who developed *pruritis ani* and a woman with guilt over masturbation who developed vulvodynia.

Another nonspecific factor is the concept of alexithymia, developed by Peter Sifneos and John Nemiah, in which persons cannot express feelings because they are unaware of their mood. Such patients develop tension states that leave them susceptible to develop somatic diseases.

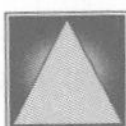

Table 28.1–4
Functional Gastrointestinal Disorders

Functional esophageal disorders	
Globus	Lump in throat, common transient response to emotional distress
Rumination	Repetitive regurgitation of gastric contents
Noncardiac chest pain	Angina-like chest pain thought to be esophageal in origin; motor abnormalities include nonspecific high-amplitude esophageal contractions, especially in the distal esophagus (*nutcracker esophagus*) and diffuse esophageal motor spasms; symptoms particularly sensitive to emotional distress
Functional heartburn	Acid reflux without anatomical abnormality or esophagitis
Functional dysphagia	Difficulty swallowing solids or liquids in the absence of anatomical abnormality; intermittent esophageal motor disorder can be present
Unspecified functional esophageal disorder	Other nonspecific esophageal symptoms
Functional gastroduodenal disorder	
Functional dyspepsia	Symptoms localized to epigastrium include pain, bloating, early satiety, nausea, or vomiting, often associated with heartburn
Aerophagia	Repetitive air swallowing and belching
Functional bowel disorder	
Irritable bowel syndrome	See discussion in text.
Burbulence	Bloating, fullness, borborygmi, and flatulence
Functional constipation	A wide range of patterns that are difficult to categorize; generally fewer than three bowel movements a week with hardened stools, causing discomfort in defecation; abdominal pain is variably present; diarrhea suggests diagnosis of irritable bowel syndrome
Functional diarrhea	Loose or watery stools more than 75% of time, often with urgency or incontinence, which may or may not have pain, but lack other aspects of irritable bowel syndrome
Unspecified functional bowel disorder	Catch-all category for symptoms that are not sufficient to allow clear diagnosis of another functional disorder; includes isolated symptomatic abdominal pain with or without change in stool habits, mucus, urgency, runny or loose stools, distention, heartburn, or borborygmi
Functional abdominal pain	
Functional abdominal pain	Diffuse abdominal pain without symptoms that are diagnostic of irritable bowel syndrome
Functional biliary pain	Right upper quadrant pain; sphincter of Oddi dyskinesia, fibrosis, or other anatomical abnormalities commonly identified
Functional anorectal disorder	
Functional incontinence	Commonly associated with fecal impaction; must differentiate from anatomical (scarring) or neurological disorders of rectum
Functional anorectal pain	Chronic, severe, persistent rectal pain (levator syndrome) or intermittent sharp pain lasting seconds to minutes and disappearing completely (proctalgia fugax)
Obstructed defecation	Caused by spastic pelvic floor (pelvic floor dyssynergia; most common in young and middle-aged women)
Dyschezia	Difficulty with evacuation

(Adapted from Drossman DA, Thomspson WG, Talley NJ, et al. Identification of sub-groups of functional gastrointestinal disorders. *Gastroenterol Int.* 1990;3:159, with permission.)

SPECIFIC ORGAN SYSTEMS

Gastrointestinal System

Gastrointestinal disorders rank high in medical illnesses associated with psychiatric consultation. This ranking reflects the high prevalence of GI disorders and the link between psychiatric disorders and GI somatic symptoms. A significant proportion of GI disorders are functional disorders. Psychological and psychiatric factors commonly influence onset, severity, and outcome in the functional GI disorders.

Functional Gastrointestinal Disorders. Table 28.1–4 outlines the spectrum of functional GI disorders, which can include symptoms identified throughout the GI tract.

The following case history is presented to illustrate the relationship between psychiatric illness, GI disease, and GI disorders.

A freshman, male, college cross-country athlete was referred for psychiatric consultation with complaints of frequent belching and anxiety. The patient had been a successful high school runner, but had struggled in his early adjustment to college athletics. His performance was below that of his high school level. Consultation with a gastroenterologist failed to find a physical cause for his complaints.

On psychiatric consultation, the patient noted anxiety about his ability to compete at the college level. Many more talented runners were in practice and meets than he had previously experienced. He reported an urge to belch frequently and feelings of abdominal fullness. When he tried to run, he reported difficulty breathing, and feeling excess gas in his stomach prohibited him from taking a full breath. He reported significant worry with insomnia and feeling "edgy" during the day. There was no history of alcohol or drug use and no previous psychiatric history.

Further interview information was consistent with aerophagia and adjustment disorder with anxious mood. He was referred for relaxation training and brief psychotherapy to address his target anxiety symptoms. The therapy focused on reducing his fear of failing as a college athlete and reducing dysfunctional cognitions about his performance. The therapist advised the coaching staff that performance anxiety significantly contributed to the patient's symptoms. Suggestions to reduce performance anxiety in this athlete were made to the coaching staff. Citalopram (Celexa), 20 mg, was prescribed.

Over the next 6 weeks, the patient reported significant improvement in his breathing, feelings of fullness, anxiety, and sleep disturbance. His running began to improve, but had not yet returned to the expected level of performance. His coaches, however, were happy with his improvement and optimistic about his probability of eventually making a contribution to the team. (Courtesy of William R. Yates, M.D.)

Extensive reports in the literature attest to the link between stress, anxiety, and physiological responsivity of the GI system. Anxiety can produce disturbances in GI function through a central control mechanism or via humoral effects, such as the release of catecholamines. Electrical stimulation studies suggest that sympathetic autonomic responses can be generated in the lateral hypothalamus, a region with neural interactions within the limbic forebrain. Parasympathetic autonomic responses also influence GI function. Parasympathetic impulses originate in the periventricular and lateral hypothalamus and travel to the dorsal motor nucleus of the vagus, the main parasympathetic output pathway. The vagus is modulated by the limbic system linking an emotions-gut pathway of response.

Acute stress can induce physiological responses in several GI target organs. In the esophagus, acute stress increases resting tone of the upper esophageal sphincter and increases contraction amplitude in the distal esophagus. Such physiological responses may result in symptoms that are consistent with globus or esophageal spasm syndrome. In the stomach, acute stress induces decreased antral motor activity, potentially producing functional nausea and vomiting. In the small intestine, reduced migrating motor function can occur, whereas in the large intestine, myoelectrical and motility activity can be increased under acute stress. These effects in the small and large intestine may be responsible for bowel symptoms associated with irritable bowel syndrome (IBS).

Patients with contraction abnormalities and functional esophageal syndromes demonstrate high rates of psychiatric comorbidity. Functional esophageal symptoms include globus, dysphagia, chest pain, and regurgitation. Such symptoms can occur in conjunction with esophageal smooth muscle contraction abnormalities in the esophagus. Not all patients with functional esophageal symptoms display contraction abnormalities. Anxiety disorders ranked highest in a study of psychiatric comorbidity in functional esophageal spasm, being present in 67 percent of subjects referred to a GI motility laboratory for testing. Generalized anxiety disorder topped the list of anxiety disorder diagnoses in this series. Many patients in this study had anxiety disorder symptoms before the onset of esophageal symptoms. This suggests that anxiety disorder may induce physiological changes in the esophagus that can produce functional esophageal symptoms.

Peptic Ulcer Disease. *Peptic ulcer* refers to mucosal ulceration involving the distal stomach or proximal duodenum. Symptoms of peptic ulcer disease include a gnawing or burning epigastric pain that occurs 1 to 3 hours after meals and is relieved by food or antacids. Accompanying symptoms can include nausea, vomiting, dyspepsia, or signs of GI bleeding, such as hematemesis or melena. Lesions generally are small, 1 cm or less in diameter.

Early theories identified excess gastric acid secretion as the most important etiological factor. Infection with the bacteria *Helicobacter pylori* has been associated with 95 to 99 percent of duodenal ulcers and 70 to 90 percent of gastric ulcers. Antibiotic therapy that targets *H. pylori* results in much higher healing and cure rates than antacid and histamine blocker therapy.

Early studies of peptic ulcer disease suggested a role of psychological factors in the production of ulcer vulnerability. This effect was believed to be mediated through the increased gastric acid excretion associated with psychological stress. Studies of prisoners of war during World War II documented rates of peptic ulcer formation twice as high as controls. Recent evidence for a primary role of *H. pylori* in peptic ulcer initiation suggests that psychosocial factors may play primarily a role in the clinical expression of symptoms. Stressful life events may also reduce immune responses, resulting in a higher vulnerability to infection with *H. pylori*. No consensus exists on specific psychiatric disorders being related to peptic ulcer disease.

Ulcerative Colitis. Ulcerative colitis is an inflammatory bowel disease affecting primarily the large intestine. The cause of ulcerative colitis is unknown. The predominant symptom of ulcerative colitis is bloody diarrhea. Extracolonic manifestations can include uveitis, iritis, skin diseases, and primary sclerosing cholangitis. Diagnosis is made mainly by colonoscopy or proctoscopy. Surgical resection of portions of the large bowel or entire bowel can result in cure for some patients.

For individual patients, psychiatric factors may play a key role in the presentation and complexity of the disorders such as ulcerative colitis. Some workers have reported an increased prevalence of dependent personalities in these patients. No generalizations about psychological mechanisms for ulcerative colitis can be made, however.

Crohn's Disease. Crohn's disease is an inflammatory bowel disease affecting primarily the small intestine and colon. Common symptoms in Crohn's disease include diarrhea, abdominal pain, and weight loss.

Because Crohn's disease is a chronic illness, most studies of psychiatric comorbidity focus on psychiatric disorders occurring after the onset of the disorder. A study of psychiatric symptoms in patients with Crohn's disease before the onset of symptoms found high rates (23 percent) of preexisting panic disorder compared with control subjects and subjects with ulcerative colitis. No statistically significant preexisting psychiatric comorbidity in ulcerative colitis occurred in this study. Longitudinal studies and careful retrospective studies in chronic GI disorders can be helpful in sorting out psychiatric disorder as a risk factor, consequence, or chance association with specific GI disorder.

Psychotropic Drug Side Effects on Gastrointestinal Function. Psychotropic drugs can produce significant changes in GI function, resulting in adverse effects. These GI adverse effects can produce several clinical challenges. First, patients may elect to discontinue necessary treatment because of the GI side effects. Second, prescribers may need to consider the possibility of serious GI illness or exacerbation of functional GI disturbances when drug-induced symptoms develop. Clinicians may need to carefully consider the side effect profile of specific psychotropic drugs when treating patients with GI disorders.

Serotonin is found in the gut and the selective serotonin reuptake inhibitors (SSRIs) can produce significant GI symptoms. These GI adverse effects tend to be noted at the initiation of therapy and to be dose related, with higher doses producing higher rates of adverse effects. Nausea and diarrhea are significant adverse effects in the profile of the SSRI compounds.

Standard tricyclic antidepressants (TCAs) also can produce GI effects, specifically, dry mouth and constipation. These effects appear to be primarily related to the anticholinergic effect of tricyclic compounds.

Treatment

PSYCHOTROPIC TREATMENT. Psychotropic drug use is common in the treatment of a variety of GI disorders. Psychotropic drug treatment in patients with GI disease is complicated by disturbances in gastric motility and absorption, and metabolism is related to the underlying GI disorder. Many GI effects of psychotropic drugs can be used for therapeutic effects with functional GI disorders. An example of a beneficial side effect would be using a TCA to reduce gastric motility in IBS with diarrhea. Psychotropic GI side effects, however, can exacerbate a GI disorder. An example of a potential adverse side effect would be prescribing a TCA to treat a depressed patient with gastroesophageal reflux.

Psychotropic drug treatment is complicated by acute and chronic liver disease. Most of the psychotropic agents are metabolized by the liver. Many of these agents can be associated with hepatotoxicity. When acute changes in liver function tests occur with TCAs, carbamazepine, or the antipsychotics, it may be necessary to discontinue the drugs. During periods of discontinuation, lorazepam or lithium can be used, because they are excreted by the kidney. Electroconvulsive therapy (ECT) could also be used in the patient with liver disease, although the anesthesiologist needs to carefully choose anesthetic agents with minimal risk for hepatotoxicity.

PSYCHOTHERAPY. Psychotherapy can be a key component in the stepped-care approach to the treatment of IBS and other functional GI disorders. Multiple different models of psychotherapy have been used. These include short-term, dynamically oriented, individual psychotherapy; supportive psychotherapy; hypnotherapy; relaxation techniques; and cognitive therapy.

COMBINED PHARMACOTHERAPY AND PSYCHOTHERAPY MANAGEMENT. The combination of pharmacotherapy and psychotherapy is receiving increasing attention in effectiveness studies for a variety of disorders. Many GI disorders present opportunities for clinicians to consider combined therapy options. Because GI tolerability may be limited in these populations, psychotherapy augmentation strategies increase in importance.

Cardiovascular Disorders

Cardiovascular disorders are the leading cause of death in the United States and the industrialized world. Depression, anxiety, type A behavior, hostility, anger, and acute mental stress have been evaluated as risk factors for the development and expression of coronary disease. Negative affect in general, low socioeconomic status, and low social support have been shown to have significant relationships with each of these individual psychological factors, and some investigators have proposed these latter characteristics as more promising indices of psychological risk. Data from the Normative Aging Study on 498 men with mean age of 60 years demonstrate a dose-response relationship between negative emotions, a combination of anxiety and depression symptoms, and the incidence of coronary disease. At present, however, the strongest evidence available pertains to depression.

Studies of patients with preexisting coronary artery disease (CAD) also demonstrate a near doubling of risk for adverse coronary disease-related outcomes, including myocardial infarction (MI), revascularization procedures for unstable angina, and death, in association with depression. Severe depression 6 months after coronary artery bypass graft (CABG) surgery, or persistence of even moderate depression symptoms beginning before surgery at 6-month postoperative follow-up, predicts increased risk of death over 5-year follow-up.

Type A Behavior Pattern, Anger, and Hostility.

The relationship between a behavior pattern characterized by easily aroused anger, impatience, aggression, competitive striving, and time urgency (type A) and CAD found the type A pattern to be associated with a nearly twofold increased risk of incident MI and CAD-related mortality. Group therapy to modify a type A behavior pattern was associated with reduced reinfarction and mortality in a 4.5-year study of patients with prior MI. Type A behavior modification therapy has also been demonstrated to reduce episodes of silent ischemia seen on ambulatory electrocardiographic (ECG) monitoring.

Hostility is a core component of the type A concept. Low hostility is associated with low CAD risk in studies of workplace populations. High hostility is associated with increased risk of death in 16-year follow-up of survivors of a previous MI. In addition, hostility is associated with several physiological processes that, in turn, are associated with CAD, such as reduced parasympathetic modulation of heart rate, increased circulating catecholamines, increased coronary calcification, and increased lipid levels during interpersonal conflict. Conversely, submissiveness has been found to be protective against CAD risk in women. Adrenergic receptor function is downregulated in hostile men, presumably an adaptive response to heightened sympathetic drive and chronic overproduction of catecholamines caused by chronic and frequent anger.

Stress Management.

A recent meta-analysis of 23 randomized, controlled trials evaluated the additional impact of psychosocial treatment on rehabilitation from documented CAD. Relaxation training, stress management, and group social support were the predominant modalities of psychosocial intervention. Anxiety, depression, biological risk factors, mortality, and recurrent cardiac events were the clinical endpoints studied. These studies included a total of 2,024 patients in intervention groups and 1,156 control subjects. Patients having psychosocial treatment had greater reductions in emotional distress, systolic blood pressure, heart rate, and blood cholesterol level than comparison subjects. Patients who did not receive psychosocial intervention had 70 percent greater mortality and 84 percent higher cardiac recurrent event rates during 2 years of follow-up. Cardiac rehabilitation itself may reduce high levels of hostility, as well as anxiety and depression symptoms, in patients after MI. A meta-analytical review of psychoeducational programs for patients with CAD concluded that they led to a substantial improvement in blood pressure, cholesterol, body weight, smoking behavior, physical exercise, and eating habits and to a 29 percent reduction in MI and 34 percent reduction in mortality, without achieving significant effects on mood and anxiety. These programs included health education and stress management components.

Cardiac Arrhythmias and Sudden Cardiac Death.

A comprehensive overview of cardiac arrhythmias is beyond the scope of this chapter. Among the many subtypes of cardiac arrhythmia, of greatest importance to psychiatrists are sinus node dysfunction and atrioventricular (AV) conduction disturbances resulting in bradyarrhythmias and tachyarrhythmias that may be lethal or symptomatic yet benign.

Because autonomic cardiac modulation is profoundly sensitive to acute emotional stress, such as intense anger, fear, or sadness, it is not surprising that acute emotions can stimulate arrhythmias. Indeed, instances of sudden cardiac death related to sudden emotional distress have been noted throughout history in all cultures. Two studies have demonstrated that, in addition to depression, a high level of anxiety symptoms raises the risk of further coronary events in patients after MI by two to five times that for nonanxious comparison patients. High anxiety symptom levels are associated with a tripling of risk of sudden cardiac death.

Heart Transplantation. Heart transplantation is available to approximately 2,500 patients annually in the United States. It provides approximately 75 percent 5-year survival for patients with severe heart failure, who would otherwise have a less than 50 percent 2-year survival. Candidates for heart transplantation typically experience a series of adaptive challenges as they proceed through the process of evaluation, waiting, perioperative management, postoperative recuperation, and long-term adaptation to life with a transplant. These stages of adaptation typically elicit anxiety, depression, elation, and working through of grief. Mood disorders are common in transplant recipients, in part because of chronic prednisone therapy.

Hypertension. Hypertension is a disease characterized by an elevated blood pressure of 160/95 mm Hg or above. It is primary (essential hypertension of unknown etiology) or secondary to a known medical illness. Some patients have labile blood pressure (e.g., "white coat" hypertension, in which elevations occur only in a physician's office and are related to anxiety). Personality profiles associated with essential hypertension include persons who have a general readiness to be aggressive, which they try to control, albeit unsuccessfully. The psychoanalyst Otto Fenichel observed that the increase in essential hypertension is probably connected to the mental situation of persons who have learned that aggressiveness is bad and must live in a world for which an enormous amount of aggressiveness is required.

Vasovagal Syncope. Vasovagal syncope is characterized by a sudden loss of consciousness (fainting) caused by a vasodepressor response decreasing cerebral perfusion. Sympathetic autonomic activity is inhibited, and parasympathetic vagal nerve activity is augmented; the result is decreased cardiac output, decreased vascular peripheral resistance, vasodilation, and bradycardia. This reaction decreases ventricular filling, lowers the blood supply to the brain, and leads to brain hypoxia and loss of consciousness. Because patients with vasomotor syncope normally put themselves, or fall into, a prone position, the decreased cardiac output is corrected. Raising the patient's legs also helps correct the physiological imbalance. When syncope is related to orthostatic hypotension, as an adverse effect of psychotropic medication, patients should be advised to shift slowly from a sitting to a standing position. The specific physiological triggers of vasovagal syncope have not been identified, but acutely stressful situations are known etiological factors.

Respiratory System

Psychological distress may become manifest in disrupted breathing, as in the tachypnea seen in anxiety disorders or sighing respirations in the depressed or anxious patient. Disturbances of breathing can likewise perturb any sense of psychic calm, as in the terror of any asthma patient with severe airway obstruction or marked hypoxemia.

Asthma. Asthma is a chronic, episodic illness characterized by extensive narrowing of the tracheobronchial tree. Symptoms include coughing, wheezing, chest tightness, and dyspnea. Nocturnal symptoms and exacerbations are common. Although patients with asthma are characterized as having excessive dependency needs, no specific personality type has been identified; however, up to 30 percent of persons with asthma meet the criteria for panic disorder or agoraphobia. The fear of dyspnea can directly trigger asthma attacks, and high levels of anxiety are associated with increased rates of hospitalization and asthma-associated mortality. Certain personality traits in patients with asthma are associated with greater use of corticosteroids and bronchodilators and longer hospitalizations than would be predicted from pulmonary function alone. These traits include intense fear, emotional lability, sensitivity to rejection, and lack of persistence in difficult situations.

Family members of patients with severe asthma tend to have higher than predicted prevalence rates of mood disorders, posttraumatic stress disorder, substance use, and antisocial personality disorder. How these conditions contribute to the genesis or maintenance of asthma in an individual patient is unknown. The familial and current social environment may interact with a genetic predisposition for asthma to influence the timing and severity of the clinical picture. This interaction may be especially insidious in adolescents whose need for, and fear of, emotional separation from the family often becomes entangled in battles over medication adherence as well as other modes of diligent self-care.

Hyperventilation Syndrome. Patients with hyperventilation syndrome breathe rapidly and deeply for several minutes, often unaware that they are doing so. They soon complain of feelings of suffocation, anxiety, giddiness, and lightheadedness. Tetany, palpitations, chronic pain, and paresthesias about the mouth and in the fingers and toes are associated symptoms. Finally, syncope may occur. The symptoms are caused by an excessive loss of CO_2 resulting in respiratory alkalosis. Cerebral vasoconstriction results from low cerebral tissue Pco_2.

The attack can be aborted by having patients breathe into a paper (not plastic) bag or hold their breath for as long as possible, which raises the plasma Pco_2. Another useful treatment technique is to have patients deliberately hyperventilate for 1 or 2 minutes and then describe the syndrome to them. This can also be reassuring to patients who fear they have a progressive, if not fatal, disease.

Chronic Obstructive Pulmonary Disease (COPD). *COPD* refers to a spectrum of disorders that are characterized by three pathophysiological aspects: (1) chronic cough and sputum production; (2) emphysema usually associated with smoking or α_1-antitrypsin deficiency; and (3) inflammation, which produces fibrosis and narrowing of the airways. As for asthma, prevalence rates for panic disorder and anxiety disorders are increased among patients with COPD. Anxiety disorders occur at rates of 16 to 34 percent, which are greater than the rate of 15 percent for the general population. Panic disorder prevalence rates among patients with COPD range from 8 to 24 percent, higher than the general prevalence of 1.5 percent.

Patients with COPD can benefit from the use of inhaled sympathomimetic agents, but two points deserve emphasis. First, use of high doses can produce hypokalemia. Second, refractory symptoms can lead to the excessive use of oral α_2-agonists, which have a high incidence of side effects, including tremor, anxiety, and interference with sleep.

> A 59-year-old female smoker with known COPD presented to the emergency room with chronic fatigue and dyspnea and an acute syndrome of depressed mood, suicidal ideation, and confusion. She lived alone and had exhausted her tank of supplemental oxygen that she only occasionally used at a low flow rate. One week earlier, to more aggressively treat the patient's worsened sputum production, her pulmonary physician had changed the oral corticosteroid to 10 mg dexamethasone (Decadron) per day from 10 mg prednisone per day. Arterial blood gases revealed moderate hypoxemia and hypercapnia and a chronic compensated respiratory acidosis—all essentially unchanged from previous studies. On examination, the patient appeared agitated and could not specify the date, the weekday, or her physician's name. The consulting psychiatrist considered delirium likely and ordered serum electrolytes, which yielded a blood glucose of 580 mg%. The psychiatrist made a diagnosis of organic mental disorder and secondary mood disturbance due to severe hyperglycemia. The change to a high-potency corticosteroid with intense glucocorticoid activity had provoked the massive rise in blood sugar and, in this elderly patient with poor oxygenation, resulted in delirium and a severe mood disturbance. The patient was admitted and treated for the hyperglycemia with intravenous (IV) saline and small doses of insulin. By the next day, her mental status had returned to normal, and the suicidal ideation and depressed mood had disappeared. (Courtesy of Michael G. Moran, M.D.)

Endocrine System

An understanding of endocrine disorders is important, not only because they are widespread, but also because they can produce symptoms that are indistinguishable from psychiatric illnesses. Physical manifestations of endocrine disease provide clues to the diagnosis but are not always present. The effect of endocrinopathies on psychiatric symptomatology has been studied, particularly for disorders of the thyroid and adrenal glands. Less is known about psychiatric sequelae of other endocrine disorders, such as reproductive disturbances, acromegaly, prolactin (PRL)-secreting tumors, and hyperparathyroidism.

Hyperthyroidism. Hyperthyroidism, or thyrotoxicosis, results from overproduction of thyroid hormone by the thyroid gland. The most common cause is exophthalmic goiter, also called Graves' disease (Fig. 28.1–1). Toxic nodular goiter causes another 10 percent of cases among middle-aged and elderly patients. Physical signs of hyperthyroidism include increased pulse, arrhythmias, elevated blood pressure, fine tremor, heat intolerance, excessive sweating, weight loss, tachycardia, menstrual irregularities, muscle weakness, and exophthalmos. Psychiatric features include nervousness, fatigue, insomnia, mood lability, and dysphoria. Speech may be pressured, and patients may exhibit a heightened activity level. Cognitive symptoms include a short attention span, impaired recent memory, and an exaggerated startle response. Patients with severe hyperthyroidism may exhibit visual hallucinations, paranoid ideation, and delirium. Although some symptoms of hyperthyroidism resemble those of a manic episode, an association between hyperthyroidism and mania has rarely been observed; however, both disorders may exist in the same patient.

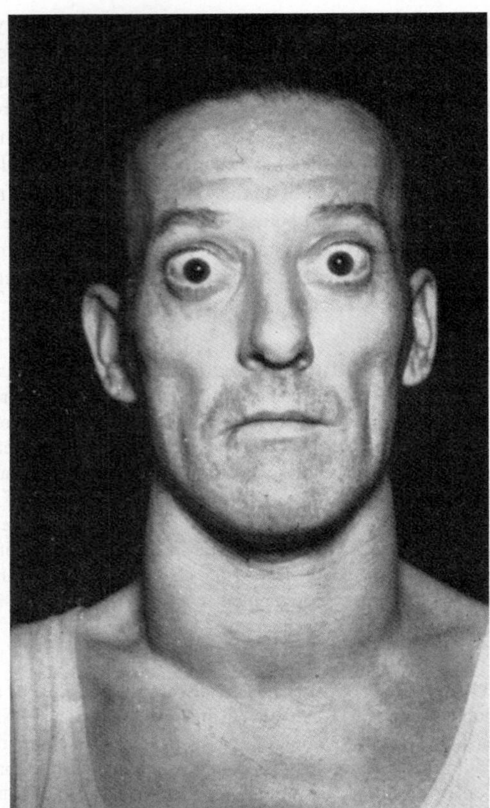

FIGURE 28.1–1
Exophthalmic goiter. Note lid retraction and enlarged thyroid. (From Douthwaite AH, ed. *French's Index of Differential Diagnosis.* 7th ed. Baltimore: Williams & Wilkins; 1954, with permission.)

Treatments for Graves' disease are (1) propylthiouracil (PTU) and antithyroid drugs, (2) radioactive iodine (RAI), and (3) surgical thyroidectomy. β-Adrenergic receptor antagonists (e.g., propranolol [Inderal]) can provide symptomatic relief.

Treatment of thyroid nodular goiter consists of β-adrenergic receptor antagonists and RAI. Treatment of thyroiditis consists of a brief course (a few weeks) of β-adrenergic receptor antagonists, because this condition is short-lived. For patients with psychotic symptoms, medium-potency antipsychotics are preferable to low-potency drugs, because the latter can worsen tachycardia. Tricyclic drugs should be used with caution, if at all, for the same reason. Depressed patients often respond to SSRIs. In general, the psychiatric symptoms resolve with successful treatment of the hyperthyroidism.

Hypothyroidism. Hypothyroidism results from inadequate synthesis of thyroid hormone and is categorized as either overt or subclinical. In overt hypothyroidism, thyroid hormone concentrations are abnormally low, thyroid-stimulating hormone (TSH) levels are elevated, and patients are symptomatic; in subclinical hypothyroidism, patients have normal thyroid hormone concentrations but elevated TSH levels.

Psychiatric symptoms of hypothyroidism include depressed mood, apathy, impaired memory, and other cognitive defects. Also, hypothyroidism can contribute to treatment-refractory depression. A psychotic syndrome of auditory hallucinations and paranoia, named "myxedema madness," has been described in some patients. Urgent psychiatric treatment is necessary for patients presenting with severe psychiatric symptoms (e.g., psychosis or suicidal depression). Psychotropic agents should be given at low doses initially, because the reduced metabolic rate of patients with hypothyroidism may reduce breakdown and result in higher concentrations of medications in blood, as in the following case.

Mr. DS was a 52-year-old white man who was admitted for melancholia after a suicide attempt. On admission, he acknowledged having a negative mood and poor memory for 1 year. These symptoms worsened after he was fired from his job. Mental status examination revealed time disorientation, poor memory of recent events, and inability to perform simple calculations. Laboratory tests were as follows: computed axial tomography (CAT) scan was negative, electroencephalogram (EEG) showed diffuse slowing, lumbar puncture was normal, TSH and other thyroid indices were within normal limits. Medical history was remarkable for a thyroid ablation for Graves' disease 4 years earlier, after which Mr. DS had not received thyroid replacement. He began doxepin 300 mg per day and T_4 250 μg per day and, within 4 weeks, experienced marked improvement in mood, sleep, energy, and cognition. Six weeks after initiation of thyroid hormone, his TSH level was normal at 4.5 mIU/L. (Courtesy of Natalie L. Rasgon, M.D., Ph.D., Victoria C. Hendrick, M.D., and Thomas R. Garrick, M.D.)

SUBCLINICAL HYPOTHYROIDISM. Subclinical hypothyroidism can produce depressive symptoms and cognitive deficits, although they are less severe than those produced by overt hypothyroidism. The lifetime prevalence of depression in patients with subclinical hypothyroidism is approximately double that in the general population. These patients display a lower response rate to antidepressants and a greater likelihood of responding to liothyronine (Cytomel) augmentation than euthyroid patients with depression.

Diabetes Mellitus.

Diabetes mellitus is a disorder of metabolism and the vascular system, manifested by disturbances in the body's handling of glucose, lipid, and protein. It results from impaired insulin secretion or action. It is also a serious long term side effect of serotonin-dopamine antagonist drugs (SDAs) used to treat psychosis. Heredity and family history are important in the onset of diabetes; however, sudden onset is often associated with emotional stress, which disturbs the homeostatic balance in persons who are predisposed to the disorder. Psychological factors that seem significant are those provoking feelings of frustration, loneliness, and dejection. Patients with diabetes must usually maintain some dietary control over their diabetes. When they are depressed and dejected, they often overeat or overdrink self-destructively and cause their diabetes to get out of control. This reaction is especially common in patients with juvenile, or type I, diabetes. Terms such as oral, dependent, seeking maternal attention, and excessively passive have been applied to persons with this condition.

Supportive psychotherapy helps achieve cooperation in the medical management of this complex disease. Therapists should encourage patients to lead as normal a life as possible, recognizing that they have a chronic but manageable disease. In patients with known diabetes, ketoacidosis can produce some violence and confusion. More commonly, hypoglycemia (often occurring when a patient with diabetes drinks alcohol) can produce severe anxiety states, confusion, and disturbed behavior. Inappropriate behavior caused by hypoglycemia must be distinguished from that caused by simple drunkenness.

Adrenal Disorders

Cushing's Syndrome.

Spontaneous Cushing's syndrome results from adrenocortical hyperfunction and can develop from either excessive secretion of ACTH (which stimulates the adrenal gland to produce cortisol) or from adrenal pathology (e.g., a cortisol-producing adrenal tumor). Cushing's disease, the most common form of spontaneous Cushing's syndrome, results from excessive pituitary secretion of ACTH, usually from a pituitary adenoma.

The clinical features of Cushing's disease include a characteristic "moon facies," or rounded face, from accumulation of adipose tissue around the zygomatic arch (Fig. 28.1–2). Truncal obesity, a "buffalo hump" appearance, results from cervicodorsal adipose tissue deposition. The catabolic effects of cortisol on protein produce muscle wasting, slow wound healing, easy bruising, and thinning of the skin leading to abdominal striae. Bones become osteoporotic, sometimes resulting in pathological fractures and loss of height. Psychiatric symptoms are common and vary from severe depression to elation with or without evidence of psychotic features.

The treatment of pituitary ACTH-producing tumors involves surgical resection or pituitary irradiation. Medications that antagonize cortisol production (e.g., metyrapone) or suppress ACTH (e.g., serotonin antagonists such as cyproheptadine [Periactin]) are sometimes used but have met with limited success.

Hypercortisolism.

Psychiatric symptoms are myriad. Most patients experience fatigue and approximately 75 percent report depressed mood. Of these, approximately 60 percent

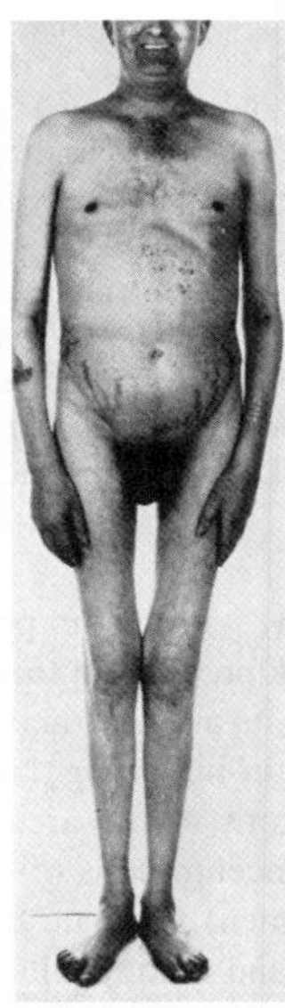

FIGURE 28.1–2

Cushing's syndrome. Legs thin owing to atrophy of thigh muscles. Some abdominal obesity with marked striae. (From Douithwaite AH, ed. *French's Index of Differential Diagnosis.* 7th ed. Baltimore: Williams & Wilkins; 1954, with permission.)

experience moderate or severe depression. Depression severity does not appear to be influenced by the etiology underlying the Cushing's syndrome. Depressive symptoms occur more commonly in female patients than in male patients with Cushing's syndrome.

Emotional lability, irritability, decreased libido, anxiety, and hypersensitivity to stimuli are common. Somatic symptoms and elevated neuroticism scores on the Eysenck Personality Inventory have also been reported, with significant improvements after normalization of cortisol levels. Social withdrawal may develop as a result of shame regarding one's physical appearance. Paranoia, hallucinations, and depersonalization are estimated to occur in 5 to 15 percent of cases. Cognitive changes are common, with approximately 83 percent of patients experiencing deficits in concentration and memory. The severity of these deficits correlates with plasma cortisol and ACTH levels.

Manic and psychotic symptoms occur much less frequently than depression, at a rate of approximately 3 to 8 percent of patients, but rising to as high as 40 percent in patients with adrenal carcinomas. In cases of iatrogenic hypercortisolism and adrenal carcinomas, however, mania and psychosis may predominate. The psychiatric disturbances in prednisone-treated patients tend to appear within the first 2 weeks of treatment and occur more commonly in women than in men.

The withdrawal of steroids can also produce psychiatric disturbances, particularly depression, weakness, anorexia, and arthralgia. Other steroid-induced withdrawal symptoms include emotional lability, memory impairment, and delirium. Withdrawal symptoms have been noted to persist for as long as 8 weeks after corticosteroid withdrawal.

Patients presenting with mood lability or depression in association with muscle weakness, obesity, diabetes, easy bruising, cutaneous striae, acne, hypertension, and, in women, hirsutism and oligomenorrhea or amenorrhea benefit from an endocrinological evaluation.

> Ms. TS was a 40-year-old white woman who was diagnosed with membranoproliferative glomerulonephritis and began treatment with prednisone, 20 mg per day. Within 10 days of beginning the steroid treatment, her mood became elevated, her speech was pressured, her sleep diminished from 8 to 6 hours a night, and her activity level was heightened. She reported that her house "has never been so clean!" Within 2 weeks of discontinuing the prednisone, her mental state returned to baseline. (Courtesy of Natalie L. Rasgon, M.D., Ph.D., Victoria C. Hendrick, M.D., and Thomas R. Garrick, M.D.)

Hyperprolactinemia. Prolactin, produced by the anterior pituitary, stimulates milk production from the breast and modulates maternal behavior. Its production is inhibited by dopamine (also known as prolactin-inhibiting factor) produced by the tuberoinfundibular neurons of the arcuate nucleus of the hypothalamus. Normal concentrations (5 to 25 ng/mL in women and 5 to 15 ng/mL in men) fluctuate during the day, peaking during sleep. Exercise and emotional stress can increase prolactin concentration. Medications that block dopamine action (e.g., antipsychotics) raise prolactin concentrations up to 20 times. All antipsychotics appear equally likely to raise prolactin concentrations, with the exception of clozapine (Clozaril) and olanzapine (Zyprexa). Other medications that may increase prolactin concentrations include oral contraceptives, estrogens, tricyclic drugs, serotonergic antidepressants, and propranolol. Hypothyroidism raises prolactin concentration because thyrotropin-releasing hormone (TRH) stimulates prolactin release. Physiological hyperprolactinemia occurs in pregnant and breast-feeding women; nipple stimulation also increases prolactin concentrations.

Traumatic childhood experiences, such as separation from parents or living with an alcoholic father, have been reported to predispose to hyperprolactinemia. Stressful life events are also associated with galactorrhea, even in the absence of increased prolactin concentrations. Low prolactin levels are associated with decreased libido. Hyperprolactinemia can cause sexual dysfunction, such as erectile disorder and anorgasmia.

Skin Disorders

Psychocutaneous disorders encompass a wide variety of dermatological diseases that may be affected by the presence of psychiatric symptoms or stress and psychiatric illnesses in which the skin is the target of disordered thinking, behavior, or perception. Although the link between stress and several dermatological disorders has been suspected for years, few well-controlled studies of treatments of dermatological disorders have assessed whether stress reduction or treatment of psychiatric comorbidity improves their outcome. Although evidence of interactions between the nervous, immune, and endocrine systems has improved the understanding of psychocutaneous disorders, more study of these often disabling disorders and their treatment is needed.

Atopic Dermatitis. Atopic dermatitis (also called *atopic eczema* or *neurodermatitis*) is a chronic skin disorder characterized by pruritus and inflammation (eczema), which often begins as an erythematous, pruritic, maculopapular eruption. Patients with atopic dermatitis tend to be more anxious and depressed than clinical and disease-free control groups. Anxiety or depression exacerbates atopic dermatitis by eliciting scratching behavior, and depressive symptoms appear to amplify the itch perception. Studies of children with atopic dermatitis found that those with behavior problems had more severe illness. In families that encouraged independence, children had less severe symptoms, whereas parental overprotectiveness reinforced scratching.

Psoriasis. Psoriasis is a chronic, relapsing disease of the skin, with lesions characterized by silvery scales with a glossy, homogeneous erythema under the scales (Fig. 28.1–3). It is difficult to control the adverse effect of psoriasis on quality of life. It can lead to stress that, in turn, can trigger more psoriasis. Patients who report that stress triggered psoriasis often describe disease-related stress resulting from the cosmetic disfigurement and social stigma of psoriasis, rather than stressful major life events. Psoriasis-related stress may have more to do with psychosocial difficulties inherent in the interpersonal relationships of patients with psoriasis than with the severity or chronicity of psoriasis activity.

Controlled studies have found that patients with psoriasis have high levels of anxiety and depression and significant comorbidity with a wide array of personality disorders including schizoid, avoidant, passive-aggressive, and obsessive-compulsive personality disorders. Patients' self-report of

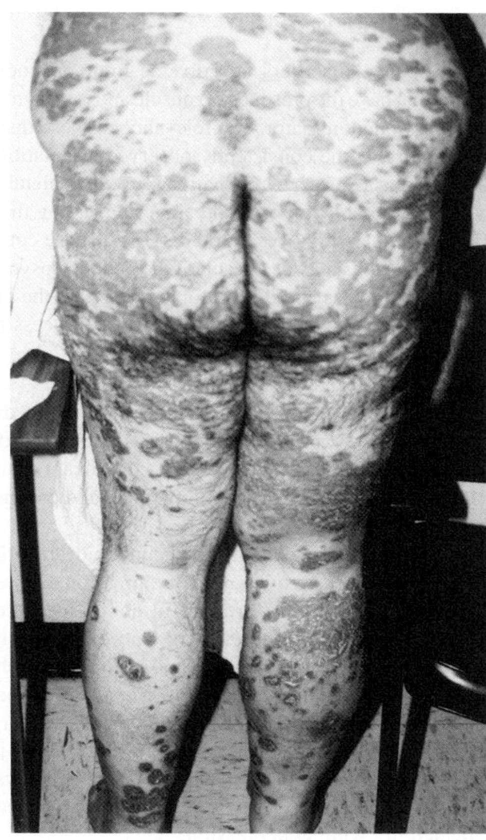

FIGURE 28.1–3
Psoriasis. The characteristic lesions have clear-cut borders and silvery scales. (Courtesy of D.F. Mutasim.)

psoriasis severity correlated directly with depression and suicidal ideation, and comorbid depression reduced the threshold for pruritus in patients with psoriasis. Heavy alcohol consumption (more than 80 grams of ethanol daily) by male patients with psoriasis may predict a poor treatment outcome.

Psychogenic Excoriation. Psychogenic excoriations (also called *psychogenic pruritus*) are lesions caused by scratching or picking in response to an itch or other skin sensation or because of an urge to remove an irregularity on the skin from preexisting dermatoses, such as acne. Lesions are typically found in areas that the patient can easily reach (e.g., the face, upper back, and the upper and lower extremities) and are a few millimeters in diameter and weeping, crusted, or scarred, with occasional postinflammatory hypopigmentation or hyperpigmentation (Fig. 28.1–4). The behavior in psychogenic excoriation sometimes resembles obsessive-compulsive disorder in that it is repetitive, ritualistic, and tension reducing, and patients attempt (often unsuccessfully) to resist excoriating. The skin is an important erogenous zone, and Freud believed it susceptible to unconscious sexual impulses.

A 55-year-old woman with a history of recurrent major depressive disorder presented with a 1-year history of excoriation blemishes on her face, scalp, and upper back. She was obsessed with removing any infection from her skin and reported "constantly messing" with her skin in an attempt to rid herself of blemishes. When a blemish formed, she worried constantly about infection and would repeatedly wash the blemish, put ointment on it, and pick at it to remove any pus and reduce the swelling. She worked at the blemishes for hours at a time, becoming completely focused on the behavior. At other times, she found herself picking the lesions automatically while watching television. She tried to resist the urge to excoriate the blemishes but felt she had little control over the behavior. She reported feeling tension build with the urge to pick her face and feeling some relief of tension and anxiety on acting. She developed a deep skin ulcer on her chin because of repeated picking of her skin. (Courtesy of Lesley M. Arnold, M.D.)

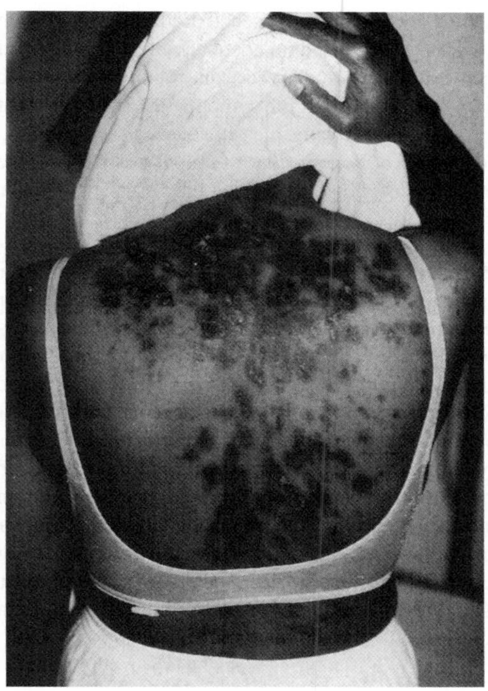

FIGURE 28.1–4
Psychogenic excoriation. The self-induced nature of the condition is suggested by the relative sparing of the lateral upper back, where the patient cannot easily reach.

Localized Pruritus.

PRURITUS ANI. The investigation of pruritus ani commonly yields a history of local irritation (e.g., threadworms, irritant discharge, fungal infection) or general systemic factors (e.g., nutritional deficiencies, drug intoxication). After running a conventional course, however, pruritus ani often fails to respond to therapeutic measures and acquires a life of its own, apparently perpetuated by scratching and superimposed inflammation. It is a distressing complaint that often interferes with work and social activity. Investigation of many patients with the disorder has revealed that personality deviations often precede the condition and that emotional disturbances often precipitate and maintain it.

PRURITUS VULVAE. As with pruritus ani, specific physical causes, either localized or generalized, may be demonstrable in pruritus vulvae, and the presence of glaring psychopathology in no way lessens the need for adequate medical investigation. In some patients, pleasure derived from rubbing and scratching is conscious—they realize it is a symbolic form of masturbation—but more often than not, the pleasure element is repressed. Some patients may give a long history of sexual frustration, which was frequently intensified at the time of the onset of the pruritus.

Hyperhidrosis. States of fear, rage, and tension can induce increased sweat secretion that appears primarily on the palms, the soles, and the axillae. The sensitivity of sweating in response to emotion serves as the basis for measurement of sweat by the galvanic skin response (an important tool of psychosomatic research), biofeedback, and the polygraph (lie detector test). Under conditions of prolonged emotional stress, excessive sweating (hyperhidrosis) can lead to secondary skin changes, rashes, blisters, and infections; therefore, hyperhidrosis may underlie several other dermatological conditions that are not primarily related to emotions. Basically, hyperhidrosis can be viewed as an anxiety phenomenon mediated by the autonomic nervous system, and it must be differentiated from drug-induced states of hyperhidrosis.

Urticaria. Psychiatric factors have been implicated in the development of some types of urticaria. Most psychiatric studies have focused on chronic idiopathic urticaria. Early psychodynamic theories about urticaria have been abandoned because no association between a specific personality conflict and urticaria could be proved. Patients with chronic idiopathic urticaria are frequently depressed and anxious, however, and women are more likely to experience significant psychiatric symptoms. Whether the psychiatric symptoms resulted from urticaria or were a contributing causal factor in its development or exacerbation is unclear, however. Controlled studies found an association between stressful life events and the onset of urticaria. Stress can lead to the secretion of such neuropeptides as vasoactive intestinal peptide and substance P, which can cause vasodilation and contribute to the development of urticarial wheals (Fig. 28.1–5).

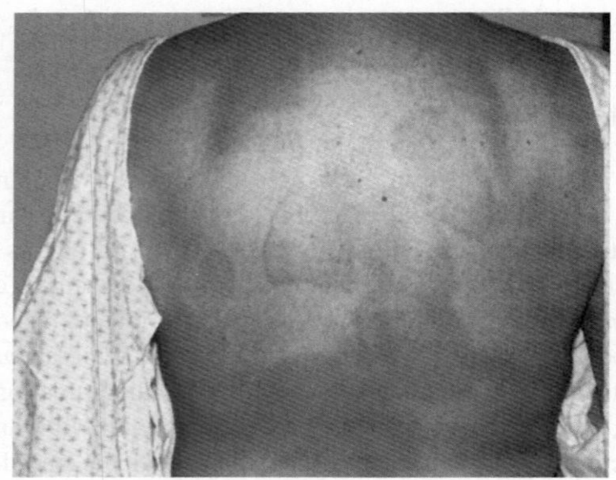

FIGURE 28.1–5
Urticaria. Dermal vasodilatation occurs, with no epidermal change (scale). (From Goodheart HP. *Goodheart's Photoguide of Common Skin Disorders.* 2nd ed. Philadelphia: Lippincott Williams & Wilkins; 2003:165, with permission.)

Musculoskeletal System

The musculoskeletal disorders are a diverse group of syndromes and diseases that have the presence of muscle and joint symptoms as their common denominator. The relevance of these disorders to the psychiatrist is the consistently observed correlation with psychiatric illness. Many patients with a musculoskeletal disorder exhibit additional symptoms and signs suggesting the presence of an accompanying psychiatric disorder. These comorbid psychiatric conditions may be a result of the patient's psychological response to the loss and discomfort imposed by the disease or may be produced by the effect of the disease process on the central nervous system (CNS).

Rheumatoid Arthritis. Rheumatoid arthritis is a disease characterized by chronic musculoskeletal pain arising from inflammation of the joints. The disorder's significant causative factors are hereditary, allergic, immunological, and psychological.

Stress can predispose patients to rheumatoid arthritis and other autoimmune diseases by immune suppression. Depression is comorbid with rheumatoid arthritis in about 20 percent of individuals. Those who get depressed are more likely to be unmarried, have a longer duration of illness, and have a higher occurrence of medical comorbidity. Individuals with rheumatoid arthritis and depression commonly demonstrate poorer functional status, and they report more of the following: painful joints, pronounced experience of pain, health care use, bed days, and inability to work than do patients with similar objective measures of arthritic activity without depression.

Psychotropic agents may be of use in some patients. Sleep, which is often disrupted by pain, can be assisted by the combination of a nonsteroidal anti-inflammatory drug (NSAID) and trazodone (Desyrel) or mirtazapine (Remeron), with appropriate cautionary advice regarding orthostatic hypotension. Tricyclic drugs exert mild anti-inflammatory effects independent of their mood-altering benefit; however, anticholinergic effects (prominent among the tricyclic drugs and also present with some serotonergic agents) can aggravate dry oral and ocular membranes in some patients with the disorder.

Systemic Lupus Erythematosus. Systemic lupus erythematosus is a connective tissue disease of unclear etiology, characterized by recurrent episodes of destructive inflammation of several organs, including the skin, joints, kidneys, blood vessels, and CNS (Fig 28.1–6). This disorder is highly unpredictable, often incapacitating, and potentially disfiguring, and its treatment requires administration of potentially toxic drugs. The psychiatrist can assist in promoting positive interactions between patients and the program staff and ensuring a tolerant attitude on the part of these staff members. Supportive psychotherapy can help patients acquire the knowledge and maturity necessary to deal with the disorder as effectively as possible.

Low Back Pain. Low back pain affects almost 15 million Americans and is one of the major reasons for days lost from work and for disability claims paid to workers by insurance companies. Signs and symptoms vary from patient to patient, most often consisting of excruciating pain, restricted movement, paresthesias, and weakness or numbness, all of which may be

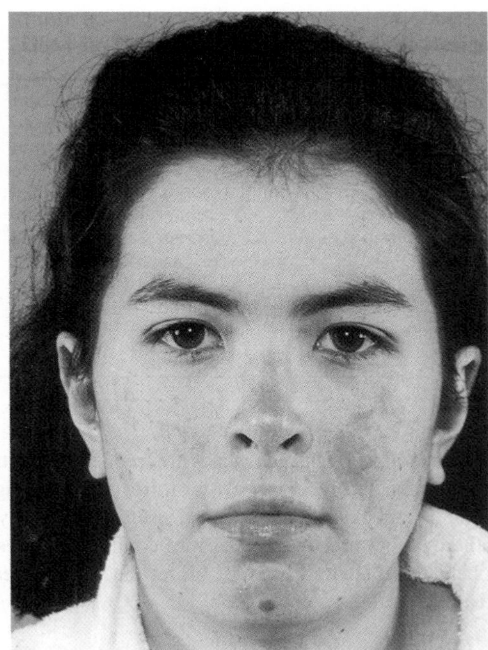

FIGURE 28.1–6
Woman with lupus erythematosus malar rash. (Courtesy of M. Kevin O'Connor, M.D.)

accompanied by anxiety, fear, or even panic. The areas most affected are the lower lumbar, lumbosacral, and sacroiliac regions. It is often accompanied by sciatica, with pain radiating down one or both buttocks or following the distribution of the sciatic nerve. Although low back pain can be caused by a ruptured intervertebral disk, a fracture of the back, congenital defects of the lower spine, or a ligamentous muscle strain, many instances are psychosomatic. Examining physicians should be particularly alert to patients who give a history of minor back trauma followed by severe disabling pain. Patients with low back pain often report that the pain began at a time of psychological trauma or stress, but others (perhaps 50 percent) develop pain gradually over a period of months. Patients' reaction to the pain is disproportionately emotional, with excessive anxiety and depression. Furthermore, the pain distribution rarely follows a normal neuroanatomical distribution and may vary in location and intensity.

There are two approaches to treatment. In the first or conventional method, treatment is symptomatic. Analgesics, such as aspirin (up to 4 g a day) can be used for pain. Muscle relaxants, such as diazepam (Valium, 2.5 to 5 mg every 4 to 6 hours for 2 or 3 days) are used to reduce muscle spasms and anxiety. Physical therapy is prescribed for the person in severe pain with restricted movement. Some patients respond to relaxation therapy and biofeedback. Many techniques have been proposed to treat low back pain, most of which are untested and unproved in overall effectiveness. These include various forms of massage, acupressure, acupuncture, injections of anesthetics or steroids, traction, bed rest, electrical stimulation, ultrasound, and hot packs and cold packs.

The second approach, developed by John Sarno, is psychoeducational. This treatment is based on the premise that the back is structurally sound without any abnormality to account for symptoms. To assure both patient and doctor, a careful physical examination is recommended, including a neurological examination and magnetic resonance imaging (MRI), if necessary. An MRI study that shows some abnormality does not automatically implicate it as the cause of the pain. To the contrary, normal changes in spinal morphology occur with age, and most such patients are asymptomatic. Additionally, many patients who have MRI studies show spinal abnormalities as an incidental finding and have never complained of back pain. These include bulging or herniated intervertebral disks, osteophytes, spinal stenosis, and other osteoarthritic changes, but they are not responsible for pain or any neurological symptom.

According to Sarno, the pathophysiology involved is vasospasm of blood vessels that supply the involved muscle, nerve, or tendon. Vasospasm is mediated by the autonomic nervous system, which is extraordinarily sensitive to changes in emotional tone, chronic emotional stress, and unconscious affects. The ischemia and oxygen deprivation cause pain in the areas involved. An analogy can be drawn to the vasospasm of coronary arteries that cause angina.

Treatment includes educating patients about the physiological component (vasospasm) and helping them understand the working of the unconscious mind and conflicts that arise from unconscious affects, especially that of rage. The patient understands that the mind is substituting physical pain for emotional pain so that the conscious mind does not have to deal with conflict. Physical activity should be resumed as quickly as possible, and treatments such as spinal manipulation and mandatory physical therapy sessions used minimally if it all.

Fibromyalgia. Fibromyalgia is characterized by pain and stiffness of the soft tissues, such as muscles, ligaments, and tendons. Local areas of tenderness are referred to as "trigger points." The cervical and thoracic areas are affected most often, but the pain may be located in the arms, shoulders, low back, or legs. It is more common in women than in men. The etiology is unknown; however, it is often precipitated by stress that causes localized arterial spasm that interferes with perfusion of oxygen in the affected areas. Pain results, with associated symptoms of anxiety, fatigue, and inability to sleep because of the pain. There are no pathognomonic laboratory findings. The diagnosis is made after excluding rheumatic disease or hypothyroidism (Table 28.1–5). Fibromyalgia is often present in chronic fatigue syndrome and depressive disorders.

Analgesics, such as aspirin and acetaminophen, are useful for pain. Narcotics should be avoided. Some patients may respond to NSAIDs. Patients with more severe cases may respond to injections of an anesthetic (e.g., procaine) into the affected area; steroid injections are usually unwarranted. The relation between stress, spasms, and pain should be explained. Relaxation exercises and massage of the trigger points may also be of use. Antidepressants, especially sertraline (Zoloft), have shown encouraging results. Psychotherapy may be warranted for patients

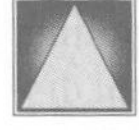

Table 28.1–5
The 1990 American College of Rheumatology Criteria for the Classification of Fibromyalgia

I. Widespread pain
Pain must be present for 3 months, widespread and not localized to one area. Involvement includes left and right side of the body, above and below the waist, and axial-skeletal pain.

II. Presence of 11 of 18 tender-point sites
Digital palpation must elicit pain in at least 11 of possible 18 tender-point sites. These bilateral sites include occiput, lower cervical, trapezius, supraspinatus, second rib, lateral epicondyle, gluteal, greater trochanter, and knees.

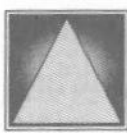

Table 28.1–6
Clinical Features of Episodic and Chronic Tension-Type Headache Compared with Migraine without Aura

Feature	Episodic Tension-Type Headache	Chronic Tension-Type Headache	Migraine/No Aura
Duration	30 min to 7 days	>15 days/mo	4 to 72 hr
Nausea/vomiting	Rare nausea	Occasional nausea	Nausea/vomiting
Pain	Bilateral/pressing, tightening/mild to moderate	Bilateral/pressing, tightening/moderate	Unilateral/pulsates/moderate to severe
Worse on activity	No	Occasionally	Yes
Age at onset	Usually over 18 yr	Usually over 18 yr	25% before 10 yr
Onset on wakening	Uncommon	Common	Common
Medication overuse	No	Occasional opiate/barbiturate	No
Prevalence	Up to 80%	2% to 4%	11%

(From Welch KM. A 47-year-old woman with tension-type headaches. *JAMA*, with permission. 2001;286:960.)

who are able to gain insight into the nature of the disorder and also to help them identify and deal with psychosocial stressors.

Headaches

Headaches are the most common neurological symptom and one of the most common medical complaints. Every year about 80 percent of the population has at least one headache, and 10 to 20 percent go to physicians with headache as their primary complaint. Headaches are also a major cause of absenteeism from work and avoidance of social and personal activities.

Most headaches are not associated with significant organic disease; many persons are susceptible to headaches at times of emotional stress. Moreover, in many psychiatric disorders, including anxiety and depressive disorders, headache is frequently a prominent symptom. Patients with headaches are often referred to psychiatrists by primary care physicians and neurologists after extensive biomedical workups, which often include MRI of the head. Most workups for common headache complaints have negative findings, and such results may be frustrating for both patient and physician. Physicians not well versed in psychological medicine may attempt to reassure such patients by telling them that they have no disease. But this reassurance may have the opposite effect—it may increase patients' anxiety and even escalate into a disagreement about whether the pain is real or imagined. Psychological stress usually exacerbates headaches, whether their primary underlying cause is physical or psychological.

Migraine (Vascular) and Cluster Headaches. Migraine (vascular) headache is a paroxysmal disorder characterized by recurrent unilateral headaches, with or without related visual and gastrointestinal disturbances (e.g., nausea, vomiting, and photophobia). They are probably caused by a functional disturbance in the cranial circulation. Migraines can be precipitated by cycling estrogen, which may account for their higher prevalence in women. Stress is also a precipitant, and many persons with migraine are overly controlled, perfectionists, and unable to suppress anger. Cluster headaches are related to migraines. They are unilateral, occur up to eight times a day, and are associated with miosis, ptosis, and diaphoresis.

Migraines and cluster headaches are best treated during the prodromal period with ergotamine tartrate (Cafergot) and analgesics. Prophylactic administration of propranolol or verapamil (Isoptin) is useful when the headaches are frequent. Sumatriptan (Imitrex) is indicated for the short-term treatment of migraine and can abort attacks. SSRIs are also useful for prophylaxis. Psychotherapy to diminish the effects of conflict and stress and certain behavioral techniques (e.g., biofeedback) have been reported to be useful.

Tension (Muscle Contraction) Headaches. Emotional stress is often associated with prolonged contraction of head and neck muscles, which over several hours may constrict the blood vessels and result in ischemia. A dull, aching pain, sometimes feeling like a tightening band, often begins suboccipitally and may spread over the head. The scalp may be tender to the touch and, in contrast to a migraine, the headache is usually bilateral and not associated with prodromata, nausea, or vomiting. Tension headaches may be episodic or chronic and need to be differentiated from migraine headaches, especially with and without aura (Table 28.1–6).

Tension headaches are frequently associated with anxiety and depression and occur to some degree in about 80 percent of persons during periods of emotional stress. Tense, high-strung, competitive personalities are especially susceptible to the disorder. In the initial stage, persons may be treated with antianxiety agents, muscle relaxants, and massage or heat application to the head and neck; antidepressants may be prescribed when an underlying depression is present. Psychotherapy is an effective treatment for persons chronically afflicted by tension headaches. Learning to avoid or cope better with tension is the most effective long-term management approach. Biofeedback using electromyogram (EMG) feedback from the frontal or temporal muscles may help some patients. Relaxation exercises and meditation also benefit some patients.

TREATMENT OF PSYCHOSOMATIC DISORDERS

A major role of psychiatrists and other physicians working with patients with psychosomatic disorders is mobilizing the patient to change behavior in ways that optimize the process of healing. This may require a general change in lifestyle (e.g., taking vacations) or a more specific behavioral change (e.g., giving up smoking). Whether or not this occurs depends in large measure on the quality of the relationship between doctor and patient.

Failure of the physician to establish good rapport accounts for much of the ineffectiveness in getting patients to change.

Ideally, both physician and patient collaborate and decide on a course of action. At times this may resemble a negotiation in which doctor and patient discuss various options and reach a compromise about an agreed-on goal. Aaron Lazare described specific negotiating strategies to achieve behavioral changes:

1. Direct education. Explain the problem, goals, and methods to achieve goals. Education must be geared to the patient's socioeconomic level and cultural traditions. If the patient has questions, they should be answered frankly. Explanations in keeping with the patient's capacity to understand should be given. Such factors as intelligence, sophistication in regard to personality reactions, and degree and type of illness should influence the vocabulary and content of the physician's response. Every effort should be made to convey to belligerent patients both understanding and tolerance for their feelings.
2. Third-party intervention. Family members, friends, and other clinicians can provide support and encourage the patient to follow a course of action. This may occur in a group setting, which is especially effective in motivating patients who have substance abuse problems to obtain treatment (called an intervention).
3. Exploration of options. There may be alternative methods for achieving a desired goal. For example, quitting smoking can be done with support groups, nicotine patches or gum, psychotropic drugs, or "cold turkey," among others.
4. Provision of sample treatment. If a patient fears a particular course of action or considers change impossible, a treatment trial can be implemented. The patient always may opt out of the prescribed program.
5. Control sharing. Some patients resent any approach that appears to be authoritarian. They may wish to set the pace of a withdrawal program or titrate their medication depending on adverse effects.
6. Concession making. The clinician may grant the patient something that he or she wants (e.g., medication) as a bargaining chip to get the patient to comply with advice.
7. Empathic confrontation. Patients who resist change may do so because of fear or other uncomfortable emotions of which they are unaware. The doctor can try to "step into the patients' shoes" in an effort to raise their level of awareness. Doctors should be prepared to answer the patient's question: "What would you do if you were in my place?"
8. Standard setting. Guidelines or standards (sometimes called milestones) should be set to evaluate the progress of an agreed-upon program (e.g., the loss of 1 pound of weight every 2 weeks to achieve a weight loss of 10 pounds in 20 weeks).

In rare cases in which negotiations break down and an impasse is reached it may be necessary to threaten to terminate the relationship.

Stress Management and Relaxation Therapy

Cognitive-behavioral therapy methods are increasingly used to help individuals better manage their responses to stressful life events. These treatment methods are based on the notion that cognitive appraisals about stressful events and the coping efforts related to these appraisals play a major role in determining stress responding. Cognitive-behavioral therapy approaches to stress management have three major aims: (1) to help individuals become more aware of their own cognitive appraisals of stressful events, (2) to educate individuals about how their appraisals of stressful events can influence negative emotional and behavioral responses and to help them reconceptualize their abilities to alter these appraisals, and (3) to teach individuals how to develop and maintain the use of a variety of effective cognitive and behavioral stress management skills.

Stress-Management Training. Five skills form the core of almost all stress-management programs: self-observation, cognitive restructuring, relaxation training, time management, and problem-solving.

SELF-OBSERVATION. A daily diary format is used, with patients being asked to keep a record of how they responded to challenging or stressful events that occurred each day. A particular stress (e.g., argument with spouse) may precipitate a sign or symptom (e.g., pain in the neck).

COGNITIVE RESTRUCTURING. Helping participants become aware of, and change, their maladaptive thoughts, beliefs, and expectations. Patients are taught to substitute negative assumptions with positive assumptions.

RELAXATION EXERCISES

Relaxation Techniques. Edmund Jacobson in 1938 developed a method called *progressive muscle relaxation* to teach relaxation without using instrumentation as is used in biofeedback. Patients were taught to relax muscle groups, such as those involved in "tension headaches." When they encountered, and were aware of, situations that caused tension in their muscles, the patients were trained to relax. This method is a type of systematic desensitization—a type of behavior therapy.

Herbert Benson in 1975 used concepts developed from transcendental meditation in which a patient maintained a more passive attitude, allowing relaxation to occur on its own. Benson derived his techniques from various Eastern religions and practices, such as yoga. All of these techniques have in common a position of comfort, a peaceful environment, a passive approach, and a pleasant mental image on which to concentrate.

HYPNOSIS. Hypnosis is effective in smoking cessation and dietary change augmentation. It is used in combination with aversive imagery (e.g., cigarettes taste obnoxious). Some patients exhibit a moderately high relapse rate and may require repeated programs of hypnotic therapy (usually three to four sessions).

BIOFEEDBACK. Neal Miller in 1969 published his pioneering paper "Learning of Visceral and Glandular Responses," in which he reported that, in animals, various visceral responses regulated by the involuntary autonomic nervous system could be modified by learning accomplished through operant conditioning carried out in the laboratory. This led to humans being able to learn to control certain involuntary physiological responses (called *biofeedback*) such as blood vessel vasoconstriction, cardiac rhythm, and heart rate. These physiological changes seem to play a significant role in the development and treatment or cure of certain psychosomatic disorders. Such studies, in fact, confirmed that conscious learning could control heart rate and systolic pressure in humans.

Biofeedback and related techniques have been useful in tension headaches, migraine headaches, and Raynaud's disease. Although biofeedback techniques initially produced encouraging results in treating essential hypertension, relaxation therapy has produced more significant long-term effects than biofeedback.

TIME MANAGEMENT. Time-management methods are designed to help individuals restore a sense of balance to their lives. The first step in training in time-management skills is designed to enhance awareness of current patterns of time use. To accomplish this goal, individuals might be asked to keep a record of how they spend their time each day, noting the amount of time spent in important categories, such as work, family, exercise, or leisure activities. Alternatively, they may be asked to list the important areas in their lives and, then, asked to provide two time estimates: (1) the amount of time they currently spend engaging in these activities and (2) the amount of time they would like to spend engaging in these activities. Frequently, a substantial difference is seen in the time individuals would like to spend on important activities and the amount of time they actually spend on such activities. With awareness of this difference comes increased motivation to make changes.

Problem-Solving. The final step is problem-solving in which patients basically try to apply the best solution to the problem situation and then review their progress with the therapist.

In the following case, a traumatic event and its effect on the patient was treated with several modalities.

> A 55-year-old married man was seen in psychiatric consultation because of symptoms of profound anxiety and depression after the destruction of his home in an earthquake. Although he and his family survived intact, his home was a total loss. He developed chest pains and a myocardial infarction while trying to argue with insurance adjusters regarding the loss. In the coronary care unit, he was apprehensive, tremulous, and tearful.
>
> In the coronary care unit, he was treated with low-dose benzodiazepines to alleviate some of his anxiety symptoms. He made an uneventful recovery. During the next 6 months, frequent aftershocks occurred, and he became fearful, complained of difficulty sleeping, and felt guilty for not having taken better earthquake precautions to preserve his former house. Symptoms progressed to frank depression, and his chest pain symptoms worsened. The depression responded to treatment with an SSRI; however, he continued to be preoccupied about his losses and the unpredictability of the future.
>
> In cognitive-behavioral therapy, he began to chart the occurrence of his worries about future earthquakes and noted that the worries were more evident when he was paying bills for house renovation. He began to attend to some of the negative thoughts associated with the bills ("I'll never receive enough insurance reimbursement." "My credit rating will be destroyed unless I pay the bill immediately."). In addition, he began a program of cardiac rehabilitation with exercise training, which reassured him that he was recovering well. He also began regular meditation twice daily, which he found helpful for his anxiety symptoms. After 10 weeks of treatment, he reported considerable improvement in his symptoms. (Courtesy of Joel E. Dimsdale, M.D., Michael Irwin, M.D., Francis J. Keefe, Ph.D., and Murray B. Stein, M.D.)

REFERENCES

Desan P. Psychosomatic medicine revisited. *Primary Psychiatry*. 2005;12:35.

Drossman DA, Toner BB, Whitehead WE, Diamant NE, Dalton CB, Duncan S, Emmott S, Proffitt V, Akman D, Frusciante K, Le T, Meyer K, Bradshaw B, Mikula K, Morris CB, Blackman CJ, Hu Y, Jia H, Li JZ, Koch GG, Bangdiwala SI. Cognitive-behavioral therapy versus education and desipramine versus placebo for moderate to severe functional bowel disorders. *Gastroenterology.* 2003;125:19.

Fava GA, Sonino N. The clinical domains of psychosomatic medicine. *J Clin Psychiatry*. 2005;66:849–858.

Goodwin RD, Olfson M, Shea S, Lantigua RA, Carrasquilo O, Gameroff MJ, Weissman MM. Asthma and mental disorders in primary care. *Gen Hosp Psychiatry.* 2004;25:479–483.

Halder SL, Locke GR 3rd, Talley NJ, Fett SL, Zinsmeister AR, Melton LJ 3rd. Impact of functional gastrointestinal disorders on health-related quality of life: A population-based case-control study. *Aliment Pharmacol Ther.* 2004;19: 233.

Keefe FJ, Abernethy AP, Campbell LC. Psychological approaches to understanding and treating disease-related pain. *Annu Rev Psychol*. 2005;56:601–630.

Lesperance F, Frasure-Smith N, Theroux P, Irwin M. The association between major depression and levels of soluble intercellular adhesion molecule 1, interleukin-6, and C-reactive protein in patients with recent acute coronary syndromes. *Am J Psychiatry*. 2004;161:271–277.

Matthews KA, Gump BB, Harris KF, Haney TL, Barefoot JC. Hostile behaviors predict cardiovascular mortality among men enrolled in the multiple risk factor intervention trial. *Circulation*. 2004;109:66–70.

McLean DE, Bowen S, Drezner K, Rowe A, Sherman P, Schroeder S, Redlener K. Asthma among homeless children: Undercounting and undertreating the underserved. *Arch Pediatr Adolesc Med.* 2004;158:244–249.

Moran MG. Respiratory disorders. In: Sadock BJ, Sadock VA, eds. *Kaplan & Sadock's Comprehensive Textbook of Psychiatry*. 8th ed. Vol. 2. Baltimore: Lippincott Williams & Wilkins; 2005:2148.

Poricelli P, Affatati V, Bellomo A, De Carne M, Todarello O, Taylor GJ. Alexithymia and psychopathology in patients with psychiatric and functional gastrointestinal disorders. *Psychother Psychosom*. 2004;73:84.

Rietveld S, Creer TL. Psychiatric factors in asthma: Implications for diagnosis and therapy. *Am J Respir Med.* 2004;2:1–10.

Shapiro PA. Cardiovascular disorders. In: Sadock BJ, Sadock VA, eds. *Kaplan & Sadock's Comprehensive Textbook of Psychiatry*. 8th ed. Vol. 2. Baltimore: Lippincott Williams & Wilkins; 2005: 2136.

Smith TW. Hostility and health: Current status of psychosomatic hypothesis. In: Salovey P, Rothman AJ, eds. *Social Psychology of Health*. New York: Psychology Press; 2003:325–341.

Yates WR. Gastrointestinal disorders. In: Sadock BJ, Sadock VA, eds. *Kaplan & Sadock's Comprehensive Textbook of Psychiatry*. 8th ed. Vol. 2. Baltimore: Lippincott Williams & Wilkins; 2005:2112.

▲ 28.2 Consultation-Liaison Psychiatry

Consultation-liaison (C-L) psychiatry is the study, practice, and teaching of the relation between medical and psychiatric disorders. In C-L psychiatry, psychiatrists serve as consultants to medical colleagues (either another psychiatrist or, more commonly, a nonpsychiatric physician) or to other mental health professionals (psychologist, social worker, or psychiatric nurse). In addition, C-L psychiatrists consult regarding patients in medical or surgical settings and provide follow-up psychiatric treatment as needed. C-L psychiatry is associated with all the diagnostic, therapeutic, research, and teaching services that psychiatrists perform in the general hospital and serves as a bridge between psychiatry and other specialties.

In the medical wards of the hospital, C-L psychiatrists must play many roles: skillful and brief interviewer, good psychiatrist and psychotherapist, teacher, and knowledgeable physician who understands the medical aspects of the case. The C-L is part of the medical team, who makes a unique contribution to the patient's total medical treatment. The scope of C-L psychiatry is outlined in Table 28.2–1.

DIAGNOSIS

Knowledge of psychiatric diagnosis is essential to C-L psychiatrists. Both dementia and delirium frequently complicate medical illness, especially among hospital patients. Delirium occurs in 15

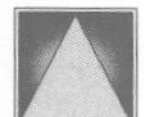

Table 28.2–1
Scope of Consultation-Liaison Psychiatry

1. Understand the impact of medical illness and the system in which it is treated and how this affects the presentation, experience, and impact of psychiatric and psychosocial morbidity.
2. Conduct a biopsychosociocultural assessment, create a formulation, and implement appropriate treatment in the context of the general hospital including effective communication with the rest of the treatment team.
3. Assess reactions to illness, and differentiate the presentation of depression and anxiety in the medical setting.
4. Understand the combined trajectories of illness and the developmental issues of the person with mental health problems and mental illness.
5. Ability to assess and treat somatization and somatoform disorders.
6. Ability to assess and manage common neuropsychiatric disorders, with a particular emphasis on delirium.
7. Understand the particular needs of special populations with psychiatric and psychosocial morbidity in the medical settings, including the young, the old, the indigenous, and those with intellectual disabilities.
8. Assess and manage acute and emergency presentations of psychiatric morbidity in the general medical setting.

(From the Royal Australian and New Zealand College of Psychiatry.)

to 30 percent of hospitalized patients. Psychoses and other mental disorders often complicate the treatment of medical illness, and deviant illness behavior, such as suicide, is a common problem in patients who are organically ill. C-L psychiatrists must be aware of the many medical illnesses that can have psychiatric symptoms. Lifetime prevalence of mental illness in chronically physically ill patients is more than 40 percent, particularly substance abuse and mood and anxiety disorders. Interviews and serial clinical observations are the C-L psychiatrist's tools for diagnosis. The purposes of the diagnosis are to identify (1) mental disorders and psychological responses to physical illness, (2) patients' personality features, and (3) patients' characteristic coping techniques to recommend the most appropriate therapeutic intervention for patients' needs. Table 28.8–2 provides a comprehensive survey of the broad range of medical conditions that can present with psychiatric symptoms.

TREATMENT

The C-L psychiatrists' principal contribution to medical treatment is a comprehensive analysis of a patient's response to illness, psychological and social resources, coping style, and psychiatric illness, if any. This assessment is the basis of the patient treatment plan. In discussing the plan, C-L psychiatrists provide their patient assessment to nonpsychiatric health professionals. Psychiatrists' recommendations should be clear, concrete guidelines for action. A C-L psychiatrist may recommend a specific therapy, suggest areas for further medical inquiry, inform doctors and nurses of their roles in the patient's psychosocial care, recommend a transfer to a psychiatric facility for long-term psychiatric treatment, or suggest or undertake brief psychotherapy with the patient on the medical ward.

The C-L psychiatrists must deal with a broad range of psychiatric disorders, the most common symptoms being anxiety, depression, and disorientation. Treatment problems account for 50 percent of the consultation requests made of psychiatrists.

Common Consultation-Liaison Problems

Suicide Attempt or Threat. Suicide rates are higher in persons with medical illness than in those without medical or surgical problems. High-risk factors for suicide are men over 45 years of age, no social support, alcohol dependence, previous attempt, and incapacitating or catastrophic medical illness, especially if accompanied by severe pain. If suicide risk is present, the patient should be transferred to a psychiatric unit or started on 24-hour nursing care.

Depression. As mentioned, suicidal risk must be assessed in every depressed patient. Depression without suicidal ideation is not uncommon in hospitalized patients and treatment with antidepressant medication can be started if necessary. A careful assessment of drug-drug interactions must be made before prescribing, which should be undertaken in collaboration with the patient's primary physician. Antidepressants should be used cautiously in cardiac patients because of conduction side effects and orthostatic hypotension.

Agitation. Agitation is often related to the presence of a cognitive disorder, or associated with withdrawal from drugs (e.g., opioids, alcohol, sedative-hypnotics). Antipsychotic medications (e.g., haloperidol [Haldol]) are very useful drugs for excessive agitation. Physical restraints should be used with great caution and only as a last resort. The patient should be examined for command hallucinations or paranoid ideation to which he or she is responding to in an agitated manner. Toxic reactions to medications that cause agitation should always be ruled out. Table 28.2–3 compares different agitated states, their cause and treatment.

Hallucinations. The most common cause of hallucinations is delirium tremens, which usually begins 3 to 4 days after hospitalization. Patients in intensive care units who experience sensory isolation may respond with hallucinatory activity. Conditions such as brief psychotic disorder, schizophrenia, and cognitive disorders are associated with hallucinations, and they respond rapidly to antipsychotic medication. Fornication in which the patient believes that bugs are crawling over the skin is often associated with cocainism.

Sleep Disorder. A common cause of insomnia in hospitalized patients is pain, which when treated, solves the sleep problem. Early morning awakening is associated with depression and difficulty falling asleep is associated with anxiety. Depending on the cause, antianxiety or antidepressant agents may be prescribed. Early substance withdrawal as a cause of insomnia should be considered in the differential diagnosis.

Confusion. Delirium is the most common cause of confusion or disorientation among hospitalized patients in general hospitals. The causes are myriad and relate to metabolic status, neurological findings, substance abuse, and mental illness, among many others. Small doses of antipsychotics may be used when major agitation occurs in conjunction with the confused state; however, sedatives, such as benzodiazepines, can worsen the condition and cause sundowner syndrome (ataxia, disorientation). If sensory deprivation is a contributing factor, the environment can be modified so that the patient has sensory cues (e.g., radio, clock, no curtains around the bed) Table 28.2–4 lists probable causes of confusional states that require urgent attention.

Noncompliance or Refusal to Consent to Procedure. Issues such as noncompliance and refusal to consent to a procedure can sometimes be traced to the relationship of the patient and his or her treating doctor, which should be explored. A negative transference

(Text continues on page 834)

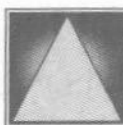

Table 28.2–2
Medical Conditions That Present with Psychiatric Symptoms

Disease	Common Medical Symptoms	Psychiatric Symptoms and Complaints	Impaired Performance and Behavior	Laboratory Tests and Findings	Diagnostic Problems
Hyperthyroidism (thyrotoxicosis)	Heat intolerance Excessive sweating Diarrhea Weight loss Tachycardia Palpitations Vomiting	Nervousness Excitability Irritability Pressured speech Insomnia May express fear of impending death Psychosis	Fine tremor Impaired cognition Decreased concentration Hyperactivity Intrusiveness	Free T_4 increased T_3 increased TSH decreased T_3 uptake decreased ECG: Tachycardia, atrial fibrillation, P and T wave changes	Full range of symptoms may not be present Hyperthyroidism and anxiety states may coexist Rule out occult malignancy, cardiovascular disease, amphetamine intoxication, cocaine intoxication, anxiety states, mania
Hypothyroidism (myxedema)	Cold intolerance Dry skin Constipation Weight gain Brittle hair Goiter	Lethargy Depressed affect Personality change Maniclike psychosis Paranoia Hallucinations	Muscle weakness Decreased concentration Psychomotor slowing Apathy Unusual sensitivity to barbiturates	TSH increased TSH low if pituitary disease Free T_4 decreased ECG: Bradycardia	More common in women Associated with lithium carbonate therapy Rule out pituitary disease, hypothalamic disease, major depressive disorder, bipolar I disorder
Hypoglycemia	Sweating Drowsiness Stupor Coma Tachycardia	Anxiety Confusion Agitation	Tremor Restlessness Seizures	Hypoglycemia Tachycardia	Excess insulin often complicated by exercise, alcohol, decreased food intake Rule out insulinoma, postictal states, agitated depression, paranoid psychosis
Hyperglycemia	Polyuria Anorexia Nausea Vomiting Dehydration Abdominal complaints	Anxiety Agitation Delirium	Acetone breath Seizures	Hyperglycemia Serum ketones Urine ketones Anion gap acidosis	Almost always associated with brittle diabetes in young juvenile diabetics and elderly non—insulin-dependent diabetics Rule out depressive disorders, anxiety disorders
Brain neoplasms	Headache Vomiting Papilledema Focal findings on neurology examination	Personality changes		Lumbar puncture: increased CSF pressure, skull X-ray, CT scan, EEG, MRI	40%–50% gliomas most common in 40–50-year-olds Cerebellar tumors most common in children
Frontal lobe tumor		Mood changes Irritability Facetiousness Impaired judgment Impaired memory Delirium	Seizures Loss of speech Loss of smell	Angiogram: space-occupying lesion	Rule out intracranial abscess, aneurysm, subdural hematoma, seizure disorder, cerebrovascular disease, reactive depression, mania, schizophreniform disorder, dementia
Parietal lobe tumor	Hyperreflexia Babinski's sign Astereognosis		Sensory and motor abnormalities Contralateral hemiparesis Focal seizures		
Occipital lobe tumor	Headache Papilledema Homonymous hemianopsia	Aura Visual hallucinations	Visual problems Seizures		

(*continued*)

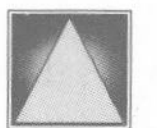

Table 28.2–2 (Continued)

Disease	Common Medical Symptoms	Psychiatric Symptoms and Complaints	Impaired Performance and Behavior	Laboratory Tests and Findings	Diagnostic Problems
Temporal lobe tumor	Contralateral homonymous field cut		Psychomotor seizures Aphasia, olfactory hallucinations		
Cerebellar tumor	Early evidence of increased intracranial pressure		Disturbed equilibrium Disturbed coordination		
Head trauma	History or evidence of head trauma Headache Dizziness Bleeding from ear Altered level of consciousness Loss of consciousness Focal neurological findings	Confusion Personality changes Memory impairment	Seizures Paralysis	Lumbar puncture, skull X-rays, CT scan shows, evidence of bleeding or increased intracranial pressure Cerebral angiogram EEG	History of blow to head or bleeding confirms cause of ALS Rule out cerebrovascular disease, seizure disorder, alcohol dependence, diabetes mellitus, hepatic encephalopathy, depression, dementia
Acquired immuno-deficiency syndrome (AIDS)	Fever Weight loss Ataxia Incontinence Focal findings on neurological examination	Progressive dementia Personality changes Depression Loss of libido Psychosis Mutism	Impaired memory Decreased concentration Seizures	HIV testing CT, MRI, lumbar puncture, CSF, and blood cultures	>60% of patients have neuropsychiatric symptoms; always consider in high-risk populations and young patients with signs of dementia Rule out other infections, brain neoplasms, dementia, depression, schizophreniform disorder
Injuries requiring ambulatory surgical evaluation and treatment (for example, wrist slashing)	Alcohol abuse and other substance abuse Recent surgery Chronic pain Chronic illness Terminal illness	>90% have major psychiatric disease History of prior suicide attempts Depressed mood Postpartum psychosis in women	Frequent accidents Repeated emergency room visits Eager to leave emergency room before full evaluation		Suicidal behavior is a symptom of underlying psychiatric illness Knowledge of risk factors is helpful but not a substitute for good clinical judgment Prediction is best done through assessment of current risk projected into the immediate future
Hyponatremia	Excessive thirst Polydipsia Stupor Coma	Confusion Lethargy Personality changes	Seizures Speech abnormalities	Decreased serum Na^+ Serum Na^+ and osmolalities to document syndrome of inappropriate secretion of antidiuretic hormone (SIADH)	Caused by excessive free water for level of total body Na^+ Often abnormal SIADH May be psychogenic Rule out nephrotic syndrome, liver disease, congestive heart failure, schizophreniform disorder, schizotypal personality disorder
Pancreatic carcinoma	Weight loss Abdominal pain	Depression Lethargy Anhedonia	Apathy Decreased energy	Elevated amylase	Always consider in depressed middle-aged patients Rule out other GI illness, major depressive disorder

(continued)

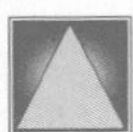

Table 28.2–2 (Continued)

Disease	Common Medical Symptoms	Psychiatric Symptoms and Complaints	Impaired Performance and Behavior	Laboratory Tests and Findings	Diagnostic Problems
Cushing's syndrome	Central obesity Purple striae Easy bruising Osteoporosis Proximal muscle weakness Hirsutism	Depression Insomnia Emotional lability Suicidality Euphoria Mania Psychosis Delirium	Disturbed sleep Decreased energy Agitation Difficulty concentrating	Elevated blood pressure Poor glucose tolerance Dexamethasone-suppression test (may be falsely positive)	Must distinguish other causes—e.g., cancer from exogenous steroid excess Suicide rate in untreated cases is about 10% Rule out major depressive disorder, bipolar I disorder
Adrenocortical insufficiency (Addison's disease)	Nausea Vomiting Anorexia Stupor Coma Hyperpigmentation	Lethargy Depression Psychosis Delirium	Fatigue	Decreased blood pressure Decreased Na^+ Increased K^+ Eosinophilia	May be primary (Addison's disease) or secondary Rule out eating disorders, mood disorders
Seizure disorder	Sensory distortions Aura	Confusion Psychosis Dissociative states Catatoniclike state	Violence Motor automatisms Belligerence Bizarre behavior	EEG, including NP leads	Consider complex partial seizures in all dissociative states Rule out postictal states, catatonic schizophrenia
Hyperparathyroidism	Constipation Polydipsia Nausea	Depression Paranoia Confusion		Increased Ca^{2-} PTH variable ECG; shortened QT interval	Causes hypercalcemia Rule out major depressive disorder, schizoaffective disorder
Hypoparathyroidism	Headache Paresthesias Tetany Carpopedal spasm Laryngeal spasm Abdominal pain	Anxiety Agitation Depression Confusion	Impaired memory	Low Ca^{2+}, normal albumin Low blood pressure ECG; QT prolongation, ventricular arrhythmias	Causes hypocalcemia Rule out anxiety disorders, mood disorders
Systemic lupus erythematosus	Fever Photosensitivity Butterfly rash Joint pains Headache	Depression Mood disturbances Psychosis Delusions Hallucinations	Fatigue	Positive ANA Positive lupus erythematosus test Anemia Thrombocytopenia Chest X-ray: pleural effusion, pericarditis	Multisystemic autoimmune disease most frequent in women Psychiatric symptoms are present in 50% of patients Steroid treatment can cause psychiatric symptoms Rule out depressive disorders, paranoid psychosis psychotic mood disorder
Multiple sclerosis	Sudden transient motor and sensory disturbances Impaired vision Diffuse neurological signs with remissions and exacerbations	Anxiety Euphoria Mania	Slurred speech Incontinence	Cerebrospinal fluid (CSF) may show increased gamma globulin CT: degenerative patches in brain and spinal cord	Onset usually in young adults Rule out tertiary syphilis, other degenerative diseases, hysteria, mania (late)

(*continued*)

Table 28.2–2 (Continued)

Disease	Common Medical Symptoms	Psychiatric Symptoms and Complaints	Impaired Performance and Behavior	Laboratory Tests and Findings	Diagnostic Problems
Acute intermittent porphyria	Abdominal pain Fever Nausea Vomiting Constipation Peripheral neuropathy Paralysis	Acute depression Agitation Paranoia Visual hallucinations	Restlessness Diaphoresis Weakness	Leukocytosis Elevated δ-aminolevulinic acid Elevated porphobilinogen Tachycardia	Autosomal dominant More common in women ages 20–40 May be precipitated by a variety of drugs Rule out acute abdominal disease, acute psychiatric episode, schizophreniform disorder, major depressive disorder
Hepatic encephalopathy	Asterixis Hyperreflexia Spider angiomata Palmar erythema Ecchymoses Liver enlargement and atrophy	Euphoria Disinhibition Psychosis Depression	Restlessness Decreased activities of daily living (ADL) Impaired cognition Impaired concentration Ataxia Dysarthria	Abnormal liver function test results Abnormal albumin EEG: diffuse slowing	May be acute or chronic depending on cause Rule out substance intoxication, mania, depressive disorder, dementia
Injuries requiring inpatient surgical evaluation and treatment (e.g., suicide attempts, self-mutilation)	Alcohol abuse and other substance abuse Serious injury Major blood loss Damage to genitals, eyes, face, etc.	99% have severe psychiatric disease associated with psychosis, psychotic depression Impaired mental status secondary to substance intoxication Bizarre, inappropriate affect	Remain at great risk for suicide		Must assess and treat the underlying psychiatric condition on a priority basis Maintain a high index of suspicion for suicide risk
Pheochromocytoma	Paroxysmal hypertension Headache	Anxiety Apprehension Feeling of impending doom	Panic Diaphoresis Tremor	Hypertension Elevated VMA in 24-h urine Tachycardia	Adrenal medulla secreting catecholamines Rule out anxiety disorders
Wilson's disease	Kayser-Fleischer corneal ring Hepatitislike picture	Mood disturbances Delusions Hallucinations	Choreoathetoid movements Gait disturbance Clumsiness Rigidity	Decreased serum ceruloplasmin Increased copper in urine	Hepatolenticular degeneration Autosomal recessive disorder of copper metabolism Often presents in adolescence, early adulthood Rule out extrapyramidal reactions, schizophreniform disorder, mood disorders
Huntington's disease	Family history	Depression Euphoria	Rigidity Choreoathetoid movements		Autosomal dominant Rule out mood disorders, mania, schizophrenia
Vitamin deficiencies					
Thiamine	Neuropathy Cardiomyopathy Wernicke-Korsakoff syndrome	Confusion Confabulation	General malaise Inability to sustain a conversation Poor concentration	Low thiamine level	Most common in alcoholic persons Rule out hypomania, depressive disorder, dementia

(*continued*)

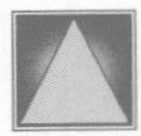

Table 28.2–2 (Continued)

Disease	Common Medical Symptoms	Psychiatric Symptoms and Complaints	Impaired Performance and Behavior	Laboratory Tests and Findings	Diagnostic Problems
	Nystagmus Headache Amnesia				
Nicotinamide	Diarrhea Stocking-glove dermatitis	Confusion Irritability Insomnia Depression Psychosis Dementia	Memory disturbances		Rule out mood disorders, mania, schizophreniform disorder, dementia
Pyridoxine		Apathy Irritability	Memory disturbance Muscle weakness Seizures		Often caused by medication: isoniazid Rule out mood disorders, dementia
Vitamin B_{12}	Pallor Dizziness Peripheral neuropathy Dorsal column signs	Irritability Inattentiveness Psychosis Dementia	Fatigue Ataxia	Low B_{12} level Schilling test Megaloblastic anemia	Often due to pernicious anemia Rule out dementia, mania, mood disorders
Tertiary syphilis	Skin lesions Leukoplakia Periostitis Arthritis Respiratory distress Progressive cardiovascular distress	Personality changes Irritability Confusion Psychosis	Irresponsible behavior Decreased attention to activities of daily living (ADLs)	VDRL, treponema antibody test CSF abnormal	General paresis Rule out neoplasias, meningitis, dementia, psychotic mood disorder, schizophrenia

CT, computed tomography; EEG, electroencephalogram; MRI, magnetic resonance imaging; HIV, human immunodeficiency virus; PTH, Parathyroid hormone; ECG, electrocardiogram; ANA, antinuclear antibodies; VMA, vanillyl mandelic acid.

toward the physician is a common cause of noncompliance. Patients who fear medication or who fear a procedure often respond well to education and reassurance. Patients whose refusal to give consent is related to impaired judgment can be declared incompetent, but only by a judge. Cognitive disorder is the main cause of impaired judgment in hospitalized patients.

No Organic Basis for Symptoms. The C-L psychiatrist is often called in when the physician cannot find evidence of medical or surgical disease to account for the patient's symptoms. In these instances, several psychiatric conditions must be considered, including conversion disorder, somatization disorder, factitious disorders, and malingering. Glove and stocking anesthesia with autonomic nervous system symptoms is seen in conversion disorder; multiple bodily complaints are present in somatization disorder; the wish to be in the hospital occurs in factitious disorder; and obvious secondary gain is observed in patients who are malingering (e.g., compensation cases).

C-L Psychiatry in Special Situations

Intensive Care Units (ICUs). All ICUs deal with patients who experience anxiety, depression, and delirium. ICUs also impose extraordinarily high stress on staff and patients, which is related to the intensity of the problems. Patients and staff members alike frequently observe cardiac arrests, deaths, and medical disasters, which leave them all autonomically aroused and psychologically defensive. ICU nurses and their patients experience particularly high levels of anxiety and depression. As a result, nurse burnout and high turnover rates are common.

The problem of stress among ICU staff receives much attention, especially in the nursing literature. Much less attention is given to the house staff, especially those on the surgical services. All persons in ICUs must to be able to deal directly with their feelings about their extraordinary experiences and difficult emotional and physical circumstances. Regular support groups in which persons can discuss their feelings are important to the ICU staff and the house staff. Such support groups protect staff members from the otherwise predictable psychiatric morbidity that some may experience and also protect their patients from the loss of concentration, decreased energy, and psychomotor-retarded communications that some staff members otherwise exhibit.

Hemodialysis Units. Hemodialysis units present a paradigm of complex modern medical treatment settings. Patients are coping with lifelong, debilitating, and limiting disease; they are totally dependent on a multiplex group of caretakers for access to a machine controlling their well-being. Dialysis is scheduled three times a week and takes 4 to 6 hours; thus, it disrupts patient's previous living routines.

In this context, patients first and foremost fight the disease. Invariably, however, they also must come to terms with a level of dependence on others probably not experienced since childhood. Predictably, patients entering dialysis struggle for their independence; regress to childhood states; show denial by acting out against doctor's orders, by breaking their diet, or by missing

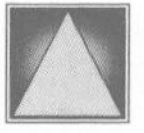

Table 28.2–3
Substance-Induced Organic Mental Disorders versus Functional Disorders in Patients Presenting with Agitated Behavior[1]

	Physical Examination	Probable Cause	Treatment
Agitation with blank stare,[2] anxiety, stupor, aggression, panic, bizarre behavior	Elevated blood pressure and heart rate, vertical and horizontal nystagmus, analgesia to pinprick, muscular rigidity, salivation, vomiting	Phencyclidine (PCP)	Minimal intervention (no talking down) Sensory deprivation with observation at a distance Diazepam for intoxication Haloperidol for psychosis No phenothiazines Diazepam for seizures α-Blockers or diazoxide for severe hypertension
Agitation with persecutory delusions or euphoria with irritability	Sympathetic signs: blood pressure elevation, tachycardia, tachypnea, mydriasis, diaphoresis, motor restlessness, tremor	Amphetamine or cocaine or other sympathomimetics	Controlled environment Acidify urine Control hyperpyrexia, seizures (diazepam), behavior (haloperidol) No sedatives
	No sympathetic signs	Consider schizophrenia, schizophreniform disorder, paranoid disorder, bipolar disorder, brief reactive psychosis, atypical psychosis	
Sensory distortion, hypersensitivity of all senses, euphoria, hallucinations, pseudohallucinations	Sympathetic excess Minimal changes	Epinephrine-type hallucinogens; STP, mescaline, nutmeg Indole-type hallucinogens; LSD, psilocybin	Controlled environment, support and reassurance (talking down); haloperidol for behavior control
Undistinguishable acute delirium	Muscarinic blockade: dilated and sluggishly reactive pupils, blurred vision, flushed face, paralytic ileus, constipation, urinary retention, fever, and hyperreflexia	Pilocarpine or methacholine	Physostigmine
	Muscarinic blockade not present	Reclassify patient by physical examination; if the findings are not clear, consider mixed or unusual presentation; consider polydrug ingestion when psychological and physical presentations are contradictory or confusing	Conservative, with observation and protection as needed

(From E. L. Bassuk, A. E. Skodol. The first few minutes: Identifying and managing life-threatening emergencies. In: Bassuk, E L, Birk A W, eds. *Emergency Psychiatry: Concepts, Methods, and Practices.* Plenum: New York, 1984: 26, with permission.)
[1]Adapted from A DiSclafani, R C Hall, E R Gardner. Drug-induced psychosis: Emergency diagnosis and management. *Psychosomatics.* 22:1981.
[2]The patient with moderate-dose or high-dose PCP ingestion may present with stupor or coma and later exhibit low-dose signs and symptoms.
LSD, lysergic acid diethylamide; STP, 2,5 Dimethoxy-4-methylamphetamine.

sessions; show anger directed against staff members; bargain and plead or become infantilized and obsequious; however, most often they are accepting and courageous. The determinants of patients' responses to entering dialysis include personality styles and previous experiences with this or another chronic illness. Patients who have had time to react and adapt to their chronic renal failure face less new psychological work of adaptation than those with recent renal failure and machine dependence.

Although little has been written about social factors, the effects of culture in reaction to dialysis and the management of the dialysis unit are known to be important. Units run with a firm hand, which is consistent in dealing with patients; clear contingencies are in place for behavioral failures; and adequate psychological support available for staff members tend to produce the best results.

Complications of dialysis treatment can include psychiatric problems, such as depression, and suicide is not rare. Sexual problems can be neurogenic, psychogenic, or related to gonadal dysfunction and testicular atrophy. Dialysis dementia is a rare condition that evidences loss of memory, disorientation, dystonias, and seizures. The disorder occurs in patients who have been receiving dialysis treatment for many years. The cause is unknown.

The psychological treatment of dialysis patients falls into two areas. First, careful preparation before dialysis, including the work of adaptation to chronic illness, is important, especially in dealing with denial and unrealistic expectations. Predialysis, all patients should have a psychosocial evaluation. Second, once in a dialysis program, patients need periodic specific inquiries about adaptation that do not encourage dependence or the sick role.

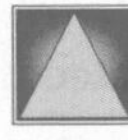

Table 28.2–4
Some Clues to Causes of Acute Confusional States Demanding Urgent Attention

Metabolic disorders

1. Hypoglycemia: history of diabetes or alcoholism; reduced level of consciousness, shaky, sweaty, perhaps combative
2. Hyperglycemia: history of diabetes; complaints of increased thirst, urination, or flulike symptoms
3. Hyponatremia: underlying illness like lung cancer, recent stroke, chronic pulmonary infections, heart failure, cirrhosis, diuretic use
4. Hypernatremia: dehydration from inadequate fluid intake or excessive fluid loss without replacement
5. Hypercalcemia: underlying disorder such as cancer metastatic to bone, sarcoidosis, lung and renal cell cancer, multiple myeloma, and/or prolonged immobilization
6. Hypoxia: inadequate oxygen supplied to the brain because of poor pulmonary or cardiac function or carbon monoxide poisoning
7. Hypercarbia: history of chronic lung disease characterized by carbon dioxide retention; may use oxygen at home
8. Hepatic encephalopathy: history of chronic liver disease or alcoholism; probably jaundiced; ascites
9. Uremia: history of kidney disease, enlarged prostate, recent inability to pass urine
10. Thiamine deficiency (Wernicke's encephalopathy): variable degrees of ophthalmoplegia, ataxia, and mental disturbance; history of nutritional deficiency secondary to alcoholism, particularly of thiamine; since remaining thiamine in the body is rapidly used when the patient is given intravenous glucose, any patient with alcoholism should immediately receive intramuscular thiamine before glucose infusion to prevent precipitating this encephalopathy; untreated, the disorder rapidly progresses to a permanent memory disorder (Korsakoff's syndrome) and, in some advanced cases, death
11. Hypothyroidism: history of progressive fatigue, constipation, sensitivity to cold, weight gain, coarsening of hair and skin, mental slowing; examination shows abnormally low temperature and enlarged heart and slow pulse; may be precipitated by the effects of lithium on thyroid function
12. Hyperthyroidism: patient may be either hyperactive or apathetic; history may reveal rapid weight loss, diarrhea, heat intolerance, and emotional instability; examination shows goiter, silky fine hair, warm moist skin, proptosis and wide-eyed stare, fine tremor, rapid or irregular pulse; in elderly patients muscle weakness and heart failure may be most apparent

Systemic illness

1. Decreased cardiac output from various causes, such as congestive heart failure, arrhythmia, pulmonary embolus, and myocardial infarction; acute myocardial infarction presents with confusion as the major symptom in 13% of elderly patients; aged patients do not complain of typical pain; often they complain of indigestion; vital signs may be abnormal, and patient may look ill (ashen coloring, weak, nauseated, sweaty) and be confused
2. Pneumonia: recent history of a cold, becoming bedridden and aspirating; fever may not be apparent, but tachycardia or hypotension are evident on vital signs
3. Urinary tract infection: especially in patients with indwelling urinary catheters, prostatic hypertrophy, diabetes, neurogenic bladder
4. Anemia: especially with acute blood loss (injury, intestinal bleeding), chronic illness, occult gastrointestinal malignancy
5. Acute surgical emergencies: infarction of the bowel, appendicitis, and volvulus are common and often present only with confusion and no other complaints
6. Hypertension: sustained or rapid increase in blood pressure may cause encephalopathy; often has history of elevated blood pressure; may occur in patient on MAO inhibitor antidepressants who has eaten food containing tyramine
7. Vasculitides: e.g., systemic lupus erythematosus; confusion arises from cerebral involvement or treatment with steroids
8. Any febrile illness and infection can cause confusion in the aged

Central nervous system disorders

1. Subdural or epidural hematoma: may or may not have history of head trauma; fluctuating mental status often present; may have no focal neurological signs
2. Seizure: unwitnessed seizure may be suggested if patient was found on floor with evidence of incontinence or vomiting; history of seizure disorder or alcoholism
3. Stroke: history of transient ischemic attacks or strokes; may have no signs except confusion
4. Infection: meningitis (bacterial, fungal, or tuberculous), viral encephalitis
5. Tumor, primary or metastatic: with a growing mass, raised intracranial pressure may cause local compression of vital structures or herniation of the brain; in the elderly, brain atrophy allows for greater space inside the skull so that symptoms may not appear until the mass is quite large
6. Normal pressure hydrocephalus: presents with triad of gait disturbance, incontinence, dementia; surgery may be curative

Drugs and medication

1. Almost all drugs are capable of causing confusion in the elderly; the most commonly implicated drugs include those with strong anticholinergic effects (antidepressants, antipsychotics, and antiparkinsonian drugs, and many over-the-counter preparations), sedative-hypnotics (barbiturates, benzodiazepines), cardiac medications (digoxin, propranolol, lidocaine, quinidine), antihypertensives, anticonvulsants, cimetidene, nonnarcotic and narcotic analgesics, and corticosteroids
2. Alcohol: intoxication and withdrawal syndromes occur as in young patients, but poor health in the elderly may put geriatric patients at greater risk
3. Drug abuse: far less common in elderly persons, but chronic intoxication with bromides, minor tranquilizers (especially meprobamate, barbiturates) occurs

(From S L Minden. Elderly psychiatric emergency patients. In: E L Bassuk; A W Birk, ed. *Emergency Psychiatry.* New York: Plenum, 1984: 360, with permission.)

Staff members should be sensitive to the likelihood of depression and sexual problems. Group sessions function well for support, and patient self-help groups restore a useful social network, self-esteem, and self-mastery. When needed, tricyclic drugs or phenothiazines can be used for dialysis patients. Psychiatric care is most effective when brief and problem oriented.

The use of home dialysis units has improved treatment attitude. Patients treated at home can integrate the treatment into their daily lives more easily, and they feel more autonomous and less dependent on others for their care than do those who are treated in the hospital.

Surgical Units. Some surgeons believe that patients who expect to die during surgery will. This belief now seems less superstitious than it once did. Chase Patterson Kimball and others have studied the premorbid psychological adjustment of patients scheduled for surgery and have shown that those who show evident depression or anxiety and deny it have a higher risk for morbidity and mortality than those who, given similar depression or anxiety, can express it. Even better results occur in those with a positive attitude toward impending surgery. The factors that contribute to an improved outcome for surgery are informed consent and education so that patients know what they can expect to feel, where they will be (e.g., it is useful to show patients the recovery room), what loss of function to expect, what tubes and gadgets will be in place, and how to cope with the anticipated pain. If patients will not be able to talk or see after surgery, it is helpful to explain before surgery what they can do to compensate for these losses. If postoperative states such as confusion, delirium, and pain can be predicted, they should be discussed with patients in advance so they do not experience them as unwarranted or as signs of danger. Constructive family support members can help both before and after surgery.

Transplantation Issues. Transplantation programs have expanded over the past decade, and C-L psychiatrists play an important role in helping patients and their families deal with the many psychosocial issues involved: (1) which and when patients on a waiting list will receive organs, (2) anxiety about the procedure, (3) fear of death, (4) organ rejection, and (5) adaptation to life after successful transplantation. After transplant, patients require complex aftercare, and achieving compliance with medication may be difficult without supportive psychotherapy. This is particularly relevant to patients who have received liver transplants as a result of hepatitis C brought on by promiscuous sexual behavior and to drug addicts who use contaminated needles.

Group therapy with patients who have had similar transplantation procedures benefits members who can support one another and share information and feelings about particular stressors related to their disease. Groups may be conducted or supervised by the psychiatrist. Psychiatrists must be especially concerned about psychiatric complication. Within 1 year of transplant, almost 20 percent of patients experience a major depression or an adjustment disorder with depressed mood. In such cases, evaluation for suicidal ideation and risk is important. In addition to depression, another 10 percent of patients experience signs of posttraumatic stress disorder, with nightmares and anxiety attacks related to the procedure. Other issues concern whether or not the transplanted organ came from a cadaver or from a living donor who may or may not be related to the patient. Pretransplant consulting sessions with potential organ donors helps to deal with fears about surgery and concerns about who will receive the donated organ. Sometimes, both the recipient and donor may be counseled together, as in cases where one sibling is donating a kidney to another. Peer support groups with both donors and recipients have also been used to facilitate coping with transplantation issues.

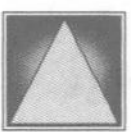

Table 28.2–5
Medical Conditions Associated with Delirium in Cancer Patients

Metabolic encephalopathy
Vital organ failure
Electrolyte imbalance (such as hypercalcemia in patients with bony metastases or those receiving tamoxifen, diethylstilbestrol, or chlorotrianisene)
Hypoxia, especially in patients with pulmonary involvement or severe anemia
Nutritional deficiencies, such as thiamine, folic acid, and vitamin B_{12}
Infections, especially in immunosuppressed hosts
Vascular disorders, especially in patients with coagulopathies
Endocrine and hormonal abnormalities

(Courtesy of Marguerite S. Lederberg, M.D., and Jimmie C. Holland, M.D.)

PSYCHO-ONCOLOGY

Psycho-oncology seeks to study both the impact of cancer on psychological functioning and the role that psychological and behavioral variables may play in cancer risk and survival. A hallmark of psycho-oncology research has been intervention studies that attempt to influence the course of illness in patients with cancer. A landmark study by David Spiegel found that women with metastatic breast cancer who received weekly group psychotherapy survived an average of 18 months longer than control patients randomly assigned to routine care. In another study, patients with malignant melanoma who received structured group intervention exhibited a statistically significant lower recurrence of cancer and a lower mortality rate than patients who did not receive such therapy. Patients with malignant melanoma who received the group intervention also exhibited significantly more large

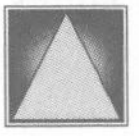

Table 28.2–6
Causes of Mood Disorders Common in Cancer Patients

Drugs
- Chemotherapeutic agents such as prednisone, dexamethasone, procarbazine, vincristine, vinblastine, L-asparaginase, tamoxifen, interferon
- Additive effect of narcotics and many other drugs known to cause depression, such as antihypertensives, benzodiazepines, antiparkinson agents, and β-adrenergic receptor antagonists

Tumor effects
- Hormone-secreting tumors
- Central nervous system tumors

Associated medical conditions
- Uremia
- Viral encephalopathies
- Electrolyte imbalances

(Courtesy of Marguerite S. Lederberg, M.D., and Jimmie C. Holland, M.D.)

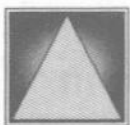

Table 28.2–7
Suicide Vulnerability Factors in Cancer Patients

Depression and hopelessness
Poorly controlled pain
Mild delirium (disinhibition)
Feeling of loss of control
Exhaustion
Anxiety
Preexisting psychopathology (substance abuse, character pathology, major psychiatric disorder)
Family problems
Threats and history of prior attempts of suicide
Positive family history of suicide
Other usually described risk factors in psychiatric patients

(Adapted from Breitbart W. Suicide in cancer patients. *Oncology.* 1987;1:49, with permission.)

granular lymphocytes and natural killer (NK) cells as well as indications of increased NK cell activity, suggesting an increased immune response. Another study used a group behavioral intervention (relaxation, guided imagery, and biofeedback training) for patients with breast cancer, who demonstrated higher NK cell activity and lymphocyte mitogen responses than the controls.

Because new treatment protocols, in many cases, have transformed cancer from an incurable to frequently chronic and often curable disease, the psychiatric aspects of cancer—the reactions to both the diagnosis and the treatment—are increasingly important. At least half of the persons who contract cancer in the United States each year are alive 5 years later. Currently, an estimated 3 million cancer survivors have no evidence of the disease.

About half of all cancer patients have mental disorders. The largest groups are those with adjustment disorder (68 percent), and major depressive disorder (13 percent) and delirium (8 percent) are the next most common diagnoses. Most of these disorders are thought to be reactive to the knowledge of having cancer. Some of the most common causes of delirium are listed in Table 28.2–5, and some conditions associated with mood disorders in cancer patients are listed in Table 28.2–6.

When persons learn that they have cancer, their psychological reactions include fear of death, disfigurement, and disability; fear of abandonment and loss of independence; fear of disruption in relationships, role functioning, and financial standings; and denial, anxiety, anger, and guilt. Although suicidal thoughts and wishes are frequent in persons with cancer, the actual incidence of suicide is only slightly higher than that in the general population. Factors that signal vulnerability to suicide in persons with cancer are listed in Table 28.2–7.

Psychiatrists should make a careful assessment of psychiatric and medical issues in every patient. Special attention should be given to family factors, in particular, preexisting intrafamily conflicts, family abandonment, and family exhaustion.

REFERENCES

Aladjem AD. Consultation-liaison psychiatry. In: Sadock BJ, Sadock VA, eds. *Kaplan & Sadock's Comprehensive Textbook of Psychiatry*. 8th ed. Vol. 2. Baltimore: Lippincott Williams & Wilkins; 2005:2225.

Huffman JC, Popkin MK, Stern TA. Psychiatric considerations in the patient receiving organ transplantation: A clinical case conference. *Gen Hosp Psychiatry.* 2003;25:484–491.

Jenkins V, Shilling V, Fallowfield L, Howell A, Hutton S. Does hormone therapy for the treatment of breast cancer have a detrimental effect on memory and cognition? A pilot study. *Psychooncology.* 2004;13:61–66.

Jorsh MS. Somatoform disorders: The role of consultation liaison psychiatry. *International Review of Psychiatry*. 2006;18:61–65.

Karvonen JT, Veijola J, Jokelainen J, Laksy K, Jarvelin M-R, Joukamaa M. Somatization disorder in the young adult population. *Gen Hosp Psychiatry.* 2004;26:9–12.

Lederberg MS. Psycho-oncology. In: Sadock BJ, Sadock VA, eds. *Kaplan & Sadock's Comprehensive Textbook of Psychiatry*. 8th ed. Vol. 2. Baltimore: Lippincott Williams & Wilkins; 2005:2196.

Matthews SC, Camacho A, Mills PJ, Dimsdale JE. The internet for medical information about cancer: Help or hindrance? *Psychosomatics.* 2003;44:100–103.

Miller AH, ed.. Mechanisms of psychosocial effects on disease: Implications for cancer control. *Brain Behav Immun.* 2003;17[Suppl 1]:1–135.

Musselman DL, Betan E, Larsen H, Phillips LS. Relationship of depression to diabetes types 1 and 2: Epidemiology, biology, and treatment. *Biol Psychiatry.* 2003;54:317–329.

Potter VT, Wiseman CE, Dunn SM, Boyle FM. Patient barriers to optimal cancer pain control. *Psychooncology.* 2003;12:153–160.

Sollner W, Diefenbacher A, Creed F. Future developments in consultation-liaison psychiatry and psychosomatics. *J Psychosom Res.* 2005;58:111–112.

Stark D, Kiely M, Smith A, Velikova G, House A, Selby P. Anxiety disorders in cancer patients: Their nature, associations, and relation to quality of life. *J Clin Oncol.* 2002;20:3137–3148.

Strain JJ, Strain JJ, Mustafa S, Sultana K, Cartagena-Rochas A, Guillermo Flores LR, Smith G, Mayou R, Carvalho S, Chiu NM, Zimmerman P, Fraguas R Jr., Lyons J, Tsopolis N, Malt U. Consultation-liaison psychiatry literature database: 2003 update and national lists. *Gen Hosp Psychiatry.* 2003;25:377–378.

Turkel SB, Braslow K, Tavare CJ, Trzepacz PT. The delirium rating scale in children and adolescents. *Psychosomatics.* 2003;44:126–129.

Wagner EH. Chronic disease care [Editorial]. *BMJ.* 2004;328:177–178.

Wise MG, Rundell JR. *Clinical Manual of Psychosomatic Medicine: A Guide to Consultation-Liaison Psychiatry*. Washington DC: American Psychiatric Publishing, Inc.; 2005.

29 Complementary and Alternative Medicine in Psychiatry

Complementary and alternative medicine (CAM) practices are being used by an increasing number of persons in the United States and abroad. Patients who present to psychiatrists or other physicians may be treating their conditions by taking herbal supplements, practicing meditative breathing, consulting a specialist in botanical essences, or using any of the other methods discussed in this chapter. These practices may or may not be efficacious and, more importantly, may pose a safety risk, especially when combined with certain conventional treatments.

The term *complementary and alternative medicine* refers to the various disease-treating or disease-preventing practices whose methods and efficacy differ from traditional or conventional biomedical treatment. The term *practice* is preferred to *therapy* by some authors, because many of the clinical benefits and safety profiles of these approaches have not been proved effective. In complementary medicine, some approaches can be and are used in conjunction with traditional therapeutic methods. Other terms used to describe these therapeutic approaches are *integrative medicine* and *holistic medicine*. This is not a new concept in psychiatry. The idea of emphasizing the whole patient and the need to evaluate psychosocial, environmental, and lifestyle factors in health and disease is subsumed under the heading of psychosomatic or mind-body medicine. The work of physician George Engel, who pioneered the biopsychosocial approach to treating the patient, is entirely consistent with the approach that focuses on the whole person and not simply the disease.

Traditional medicine, as practiced in the United States and elsewhere in the Western world, is based on the scientific method—the use of experiments to validate a hypothesis or determine the probability of a theory being correct. Traditional medicine presumes that the body is a biological and physiological system and that disorders have a cause that can be treated with medications, surgery, and complex technological methods to produce a cure. Traditional medicine is thus also referred to as *biomedicine* or *technomedicine*.

Traditional medicine is also known as *allopathic medicine*. The term allopathy, derived from the Greek word *allos* ("other"), refers to the use of outside agents or medications to counteract the signs and symptoms of disease; for example, antipyretics to treat fever. *Allopathy* is the type of medicine taught in medical schools in the United States. Samuel Hahnemann (1755–1843), a German physician, coined the term to distinguish this form of medicine from *homeopathy* (derived from the Greek word *homos* ["same"]), in which specially formulated medicinal remedies, different from allopathic medicine, are used. Allopathy is the most prevalent form of medicine practiced in the Western world. (Homeopathy is discussed more fully later in this chapter.)

NATIONAL CENTER FOR COMPLEMENTARY MEDICINE AND ALTERNATIVE MEDICINE

The widespread adoption of CAM practices led the US government to establish the National Center for Complementary Medicine and Alternative Medicine (NCCAM) within the National Institute of Health (NIH). NCCAM's mission is to evaluate the usefulness and safety of a broad range of unrelated, nonorthodox healing practices and provide scientific explanations for their possible effectiveness, train CAM researchers, and disseminate information to the public.

An NCCAM study in 2002 revealed that more than one third of Americans used some form of CAM in a 12-month period. When prayer was included, the percentage rose to more than 60 percent. Prayer for one's own health was most prominent (43 percent), followed by prayer by others for one's own health (24 percent), natural products (19 percent), deep-breathing exercises (12 percent), group prayer (10 percent), meditation (8 percent), chiropractic care (8 percent), yoga (5 percent), massage (5 percent), and diet-based therapies (4 percent). Echinacea, ginseng, Gingko biloba, garlic supplements, glucosamine, and St. John's wort were the most common natural products used. Back, head, and neck pain were the most common conditions treated. The CAM practices were most likely to be embraced by those with more education, women, former smokers, and those recently hospitalized. Most users of CAM practices believed the greatest benefits were achieved in combination with conventional treatment.

At present, NCCAM is coordinating more than 300 clinical trials at the NIH and academic research institutions to investigate the benefits of various CAM practices on a spectrum of diseases and disorders, ranging from psychiatric conditions to cancer, osteoporosis, and multiple sclerosis. Completed studies have validated the following: acupuncture is beneficial to treat functional impairment and osteoarthritic pain of the knee; no prophylactic benefit was found for low dose *Echinacea augustifoli* in the prevention of cold symptoms; combined glucosamine and chondroitin sulfate supplements do not provide significant relief for osteoarthritic pain in most cases, but does benefit a smaller subset with more severe pain; and St. John's wort *(Hypericum perforatum)* is no more effective for treating major depression of moderate severity than placebo. St. John's wort is being further investigated as a treatment for posttraumatic stress disorder (PTSD), anxiety, and minor depression (see *Herbal Medicine* below).

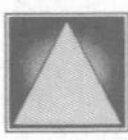

Table 29–1
Complementary and Alternative Medicine Practices

Whole Medical Systems	Biologically Based Practices	Manipulative and Body-Based Practice
Anthroposophically extended medicine	Cell treatment	Acupressure or acupuncture
Ayurveda	Chelation therapy	Alexander technique
Environmental medicine	Diet	Aromatherapy
Homeopathy	Atkins diet	Biofield therapeutics
Kampo medicine	Macrobiotic diet	Chiropractic medicine
Native American medicine	Ornish diet	Feldenkrais method
Naturopathic medicine	Pritikin diet	Massage therapy
Tibetan medicine	Vegetarian diet	Osteopathic medicine
Mind-Body Interventions	Zone diet	Reflexology
Art therapy	Dietary supplements	Rolfing
Biofeedback	Gerson therapy	Therapeutic touch
Dance therapy	Herbal products	Trager method
Guided imagery	Echinacea	**Energy Medicine**
Humor therapy	St. John's wort	Blue light treatment and artificial treatment
Meditation	Gingko biloba extract	Electroacupuncture
Mental healing	Ginseng root	Electromagnetic field therapy
Past life therapy	Garlic supplements	Electrostimulation and Neuromagnetic stimulation
Prayer and counseling	Peppermint	Magnetoresonance therapy
Psychotherapy	Metabolic therapy	Qi Gong
Sound, music therapy	Megavitamin	Reiki
Yoga exercise	Nutritional supplements	Therapeutic touch
Traditional Chinese medicine	Oxidizing agents (ozone, hydrogen peroxide)	Zone therapy

The NCCAM has compiled a classification of alternative medical practices designed to support research (Table 29–1). Including a practice in the classification does not imply an endorsement of the method. Indeed, many complementary and alternative health practices are based on no known scientific principles and are considered quackery.

Some health maintenance organizations (HMOs) have approved alternative medical therapies for reimbursement. Chiropractic treatment is covered by many large HMOs and an increasing number offer acupuncture coverage. The HMOs claim to be responding to public pressure, but many health experts believe that these HMOs are motivated solely by financial considerations. Persons who visit alternative practitioners are reimbursed at lower rates than those who visit traditional practitioners. Some HMOs allow their members to self-refer to these practitioners. In contrast, referral to a traditional medical specialist may only be initiated by the patient's primary care physician. The practice of self-referral may endanger the health of the general public by encouraging persons to seek alternative treatment that may not help them.

Many systems of treatment discussed in this chapter are centuries old, and it would be presumptuous for traditional biomedical practitioners to dismiss them lightly as worthless. Nevertheless, without rigorous scientific evidence to the contrary, physicians must approach many of these treatments with skepticism. The influence of the mind on the body and the effect of psychological factors in health and disease are well known to physicians, especially to psychiatrists. Suggestion is a potent remedy, and the well-established placebo effect, in which an inert substance is effective in curing a disorder, serves to confirm the importance of mind–body interaction in health and disease.

Currently, more than half the medical schools in the United States offer some form of complementary and alternative medicine education. Several have developed centers for alternative medicine research, with professors of mind–body or integrative medicine drawn largely from the ranks of such traditional specialties as internal medicine and psychiatry. This trend is likely to continue, with the goal of determining which of the many existing alternative medical systems have scientific merit. Only when and if they can withstand rigorous clinical trials can certain of these techniques be integrated into traditional medicine.

Listed below in alphabetical order are some of the most visible complementary and alternative health practices that have been used in the treatment of (broadly defined) psychiatric conditions. The discussion of therapies should not be considered definitive; new therapies continue to emerge. The number of alternative healing practices available in the United States is unknown and probably soars into the hundreds.

ACUPRESSURE AND ACUPUNCTURE

Acupressure and acupuncture are Chinese healing techniques that are mentioned in ancient medical texts dating back to 5000 BC, and continue to be an important medical intervention in the East. A basic tenet of Chinese medicine is the belief that vital energy (*qi* or *chi*) flows along specific pathways (meridians) that have about 350 major points (acupoints) whose manipulation corrects imbalances by stimulating or removing blockages to energy flow. Another fundamental concept is the idea of two opposing energy fields (*yin* and *yang*) that must be in balance for health to be sustained. In acupressure, the acupoints are manipulated by the fingers; in acupuncture, sterilized silver or gold needles (some the diameter of a human hair) are inserted into the skin to varying depths (0.5 mm to 1.5 cm) and are rotated or left in place for varying periods to correct any imbalance of *qi*.

In the West, acupressure and acupuncture are explained on the basis of nerve stimulation that releases endogenous neurotransmitters, endorphins and enkephalins to help cure illness. The benefits of acupuncture have been validated in a variety of conditions, most notably pain management, postoperative nausea and vomiting, osteoarthritis of the knee, fibromyalgia, and headaches. Other conditions treated with these techniques are asthma, dysmenorrhea, cervical pain, insomnia, anxiety, depression, and substance abuse, including smoking cessation (see the description of moxibustion below). Most pain management clinics in the United Kingdom use acupuncture treatment. A variation of acupuncture, which uses mild electric current to augment therapeutic effects (electroacupuncture), is most often used for analgesia or during surgery. Acupuncture applied to the ear (auricolocupuncture) is also common.

ALEXANDER TECHNIQUE

The Alexander technique was developed by F. M. Alexander (1869–1955), who was born in Tasmania and eventually became a well-known stage actor. After developing aphonia, he experimented on himself by changing his body posture and eventually regained his voice. Alexander developed a theory of the proper use of body musculature to help alleviate somatic and mental illness. Techniques involve corrective manipulation of the muscles involving the head and neck, torso, pelvis, and extremities to improve posture. Treatment improves cardiovascular, respiratory, and gastrointestinal functioning as well as mood. A small, devoted group of

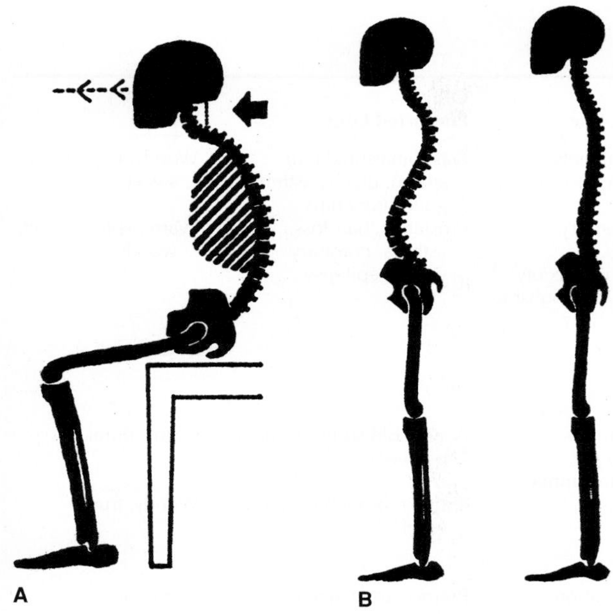

FIGURE 29–1

A. Position of pelvis, back, neck, and head in slumped position. **B.** Standing in hunched position (*left*) and well balanced (*right*). (From Barlow W. *The Alexander Principle*. London: Gollancz; 1973, with permission.)

Alexander practitioners is found in the United States and throughout the world. The Alexander technique may deserve consideration, if for no other reason than that so many persons in the United States have poor posture (Fig. 29–1).

ANTHROPOSOPHICALLY EXTENDED MEDICINE

Anthroposophically extended medicine is a form of healing developed by the Austrian philosopher Rudolf Steiner (1861–1925). The healing process involves the use of conscious understanding, which Steiner called anthroposophy, or the "wisdom of life." Anthroposophy focuses on mental exercises that enable persons to find a balance between mind and body to ensure health maintenance. Steiner founded a school of thought represented in this country by the Rudolf Steiner School, which teaches children these concepts as they apply to civilization, besides a standard educational curriculum.

AROMATHERAPY

Aromatherapy is the therapeutic use of plant oils. Named by the French chemist Maurice René-Maurice Gattefosse in 1928, aromatherapy is one of the fastest growing alternative therapies in the United States and Europe. The essential oils of plants are organic compounds that are benzene derivatives. Aromatic substances were used in ancient civilization as both medicines and perfumes. Today, plant oils are inhaled using atomizers or are absorbed through the skin using massage (aromatherapy massage). Plant oils have many therapeutic effects—analgesic, psychological, antimicrobial—some of which have been demonstrated scientifically. Aromatherapy is used to reduce stress and anxiety and to alleviate gastrointestinal and musculoskeletal disorders. In psychiatry, olfactory stimulation has been used to elicit feeling tones, memories, and emotions during psychotherapy. Aromatherapy can cause skin irritation or allergic reactions in some people. Table 29–2 lists essential oils and their effects.

Pheromones are chemical substances secreted and smelled by humans, which affects their physiological and behavioral responses, usually related to sex. Women who are exposed to the smell of androstenol, which occurs in male underarm sweat, show increased social exchanges with men, hightened sexual arousal and improved mood. Androstenol also affects the length and timing of the menstrual cycle as a result of changes in the level and release of gonadotrophic releasing hormone (GnRH) and luteinizing hormone (LH). Female pheromones, known as copulins are present in female underarm sweat and in vaginal secretions. Males perceive the odor of copulines as most pleasant during the woman's ovulatory cycle when such odors are most volatile. The synchronization of the menstrual cycle of women living together (a well-documented phenomenon) is also related to the effect of copulins. Olfactory sexual signaling is being investigated extensively and whether or not these studies have therapeutic potential remains to be seen.

AYURVEDA

Ayurveda means "knowledge of life." The technique originated in India about 3000 BC and is believed to be one of the oldest and most comprehensive medical systems in the world. Ayurveda is similar to Chinese medicine in its beliefs about energy points on the body and a vital force (*prana*) that must be in balance to maintain health. Ayurveda practitioners diagnose illness by examining the pulse, the urine, and the heat or coldness of the body. Treatment relies on diet, medicines, purification, enemas, and bloodletting. (See also *Tibetan Medicine*.)

BATES METHOD

The Bates method, designed to treat vision problems, was devised by William H. Bates. It is aimed at naturally strengthening the eye muscles and includes the following basic exercises: splashing closed eyes 20 times with warm water, then 20 times with cold water; alternately focusing on near and distant objects; focusing on an object while gently swaying the body; remembering objects in the mind's eye to facilitate the actual perception of these objects in reality; and closing the eyes, cupping them with the palms of both hands (without touching the eyes), and focusing on pleasant thoughts. Bates practitioners claim that persons who need glasses to correct refraction errors will not need them if these methods are followed rigorously.

BIOENERGETICS

Bioenergetics, based on the belief that dammed-up energy produces maladaptive behavioral patterns, evolved from the work of the Austrian psychoanalyst Wilhelm Reich (1897–1957), who studied with Sigmund Freud. Reich believed that energy fields were propelled by sexual impulses called ergs and that satisfactory orgasms indicated healthy bodily functioning. Modern-day practitioners look for areas of muscular tension in the body that are thought to be associated with repressed memories and emotions. Therapists try to bring these repressions to consciousness through a variety of relaxation techniques, including massage.

CHELATION

Chelation therapy is a traditional medical procedure used to treat accidental poisoning with heavy metals, such as lead, arsenic, and mercury. A chelating agent (ethylenediaminetetraacetic acid [EDTA]) is infused into the bloodstream and binds to the metal, which is then excreted from the body. As an alternative medical practice, chelation therapy is used as a form of preventive medicine to remove lead, cadmium, and aluminum from the body. These substances are presumed by some to be associated with premature aging, memory loss, and the symptoms of Alzheimer's disease. Chelation therapy has also been used to treat atherosclerosis and coronary artery disease.

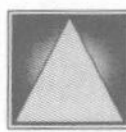

Table 29–2
Common Aromatherapies

Compound	Possible Properties	Purported Psychiatric Use	Other Purported Uses	Aroma
Angelica	Sedative, muscle relaxant, antibiotic, antifungal	Anorexia, anxiety, insomnia	Gastrointestinal (GI) spasm, ulcers, asthma, gout, bronchitis	Woody, pepper, sweet
Basil	Antispasmotic, active on sympathetic nervous system, narcotic, antiviral, insect repellant, aphrodisiac, antiinflammative, stimulant for the adrenal cortex, GI and urogenital tracts, cerebral or memory stimulator, hepatostimulative	Fatigue, memory problems, depression, anxiety, delirium, alcoholism	Prostatitis, hair loss, asthma, coronary spasm, epilepsy	Warm, spicy, sweet, woody
Bergamot	Antidepressant, sedative, antiseptic, antiinflammatory	Depression, hyperactivity, anxiety, insomnia	Acne, cold sores, eczema, psoriasis	Citrus, floral
Frankincense or oil of olibanum	Antitumor, antidepressant, expectorant, immunostimulant, antiinflammatory	Depression	Asthma, bronchitis, pain relief	Woody, fruity
Geranium (*P.g* or *P.x a*) pelargonium	Pancreatic stimulant, antiinflammatory, antibiotic, relaxant, hemostatic	Anxiety, agitation, fatigue	Premenstrual syndrome (PMS), menopause	Floral, dry
Jasmine	Antidepressant, stimulant, analgesic	Depression, stress, fatigue	Menstrual problems, headaches	Floral, musky
Lavender	Sedative, muscular relaxant, antiinflammatory	Depression, jet lag, insomnia, restlessness	Acne, burns, hiccups, ulcers	Powder, floral
Mandarin	Antispasmodic, sedative, hypnotic	Hyperactivity, anxiety, insomnia	Cardiovascular spasm, pain, dyspnea	Sweet, fruity
Marjoram	Diuretic, analgesic, spasmolytic, parasympathotonic	Anxiety, excessive sexual desire, psychosis, insomnia	Hyperthyroid, cardiovascular disease, vertigo, epilepsy	Nutty, woody, warm
Melissa	Sedative, antiinflammatory, antispasmodic	Anger, agitation, insomnia	Herpes, hypertension, asthma	Citrus, herb
Myrrh	Antiinflammatory, analgesic, antifungal	Sexual overexcitation	Dysentery, hemorrhoids	Fruity, clean
Neroli	Antidepressant, stimulant	Depression, fatigue, insomnia, anxiety, postpartum depression	Hemorrhoids, tuberculosis	Floral, powder, spicy
Spikenard	Sedative, antifungal, antiseptic, insect repellent	Insomnia, depression, anxiety	Psoriasis, epilepsy	Earthy, woody
Tuberose	Anxiety, sedative, analgesic	Agitation	Pain	Earthy, tropical

(Table by Marissa Kaminsky, M.D.)

References: Herbweb. Natural Resources Industries, Pure and Natural Essential Oils from Nepal. http://www.msinp.com/herbs/index.html; Ontario Ministry of Agriculture, Food and Rural Affairs. http://www.omafra.gov.on.ca/english/index.html; Rose, Jeanne. *375 Essential Oils and Hydrosols.* Berkeley, CA: Frog, Ltd. North Atlantic Books, 1999; Schnaubelt Kurt. *Medical Aromatherapy.* Berkeley, CA: Frog, Ltd. North Atlantic Books, 1999.

CHIROPRACTIC

Chiropractic is concerned with the diagnosis and treatment of disorders of the musculoskeletal system, especially those of the spine. It was developed by a Canadian, Daniel David Palmer (1845–1913) (Fig. 29–2), who moved to the United States in 1895. Palmer believed that disease could be attributed to spinal misalignment leading to abnormal nerve transmission.

Chiropractors diagnose illness by clinical examination and X-ray. Treatment involves manual manipulation of bones, joints, and musculature to restore biomechanical function. Chiropractic is the largest independent alternative health profession in the Western world, with more than 50,000 chiropractors in the United States. They are recognized by government and insurance agencies and treat more than 20 million persons in the United States annually.

COLONIC IRRIGATION

Colonic irrigation is a technique known since antiquity that consists of flushing the intestinal colon with large quantities of water, sometimes with minerals or other substances (e.g., coffee) added. It is a method used to eliminate autointoxication, a concept originating from the Pasteur Institute in France in 1908 that holds that retained fecal matter and undigested food ferment in the bowel producing toxins that cause disease. Special colon hydrotherapy machines force fluids via the rectum to clean the colon of this matter thus eliminating such toxins. Colon cleansing using powerful laxatives and enemas is an alternative way of achieving the same result. Anecdotal reports of improved general health as a result of such practices are common; however there are risks of electrolyte imbalance and intestinal perforation. The practice is poorly regulated although some states attempts to monitor therapists and equipment.

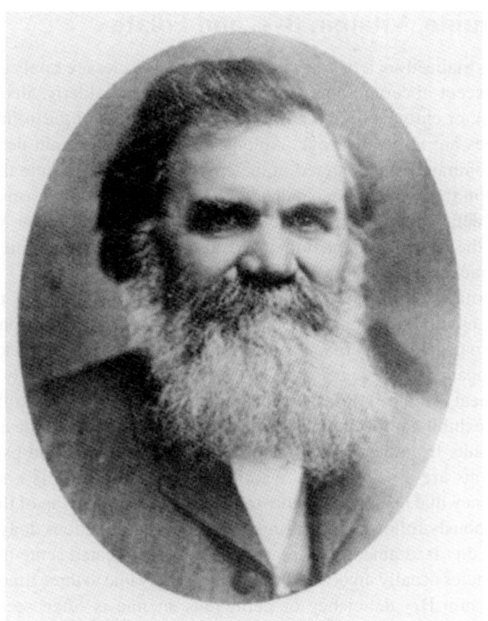

FIGURE 29–2
Daniel David Palmer (1845–1913), the founder of chiropractic. (Reprinted with permission from Shealy CN, ed. *The Complete Family Guide to Alternative Medicine: An Illustrated Encyclopedia of Natural Healing.* New York: Barnes & Noble Books; 1996:39.)

COLOR THERAPY

In color therapy, different colors are thought to affect mood, and this has been used to address specific health problems. For example, blue is believed to be sedating, and red, excitatory. A Swiss psychologist, Max Lüscher, devised a color test in which a subject's mood at a particular time is determined by exposing the subject to various colors. Lüscher also experimented with the effect of color on the autonomic nervous system and found that pure red is sympathomimetic and can cause an increase in blood pressure, heart rate, and respiration. Blue is parasympathomimetic and produces opposite effects.

DANCE THERAPY

Dance therapy was formally recognized in 1942, with the hiring of pioneer dance therapist Marian Chace (1896–1990) at St. Elisabeth's Hospital in Washington, DC. The terms *dance* and *movement* are used synonymously; however, each actually describes a point of view. *Movement* encompasses the world of physical motion, whereas *dance* is a specific creative act within that world. The American Dance Therapy Association defines dance therapy as "the psychotherapeutic use of movement which furthers the emotional and physical integration of the individual." Dance therapy sessions have four basic goals: the development of body awareness; the expression of feelings; the fostering of interaction and communication; and the integration of the physical, emotional, and social experiences that result in a sense of increased self-confidence and contentment.

DIET AND NUTRITION

Nutritional methods to prevent or cure disease have an important place in modern medicine, and their efficacy has been proved by scientific evidence. The federal government has established recommended daily allowances (RDAs) to meet the nutritional needs of average persons in the United States. Table 29–3 depicts the recommendations for a 40-year-old sedentary man. Whole grain, lean meat, and green vegetable consumption are encouraged, and excess intake of unrefined sugar products is discouraged. Critics have faulted the federal guidelines for being unduly influenced by the meat and dairy industries. Nutritional experts and dieticians have developed alternate recommendations, especially for children, adolescents, diabetics, and pregnant women.

Many alternative diets exist, and specific vitamin and mineral supplementation programs have been developed to deal with specific diseases or bodily processes. Diets low in fat have been recommended for the treatment of cardiovascular disease and diabetes. The Pritikin diet developed

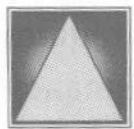

Table 29–3
United States Department of Agriculture Food Guide for a 40-Year-Old Sedentary Male

Grains 8 Ounces	Vegetables 3 Cups	Fruits 2 Cups	Milk 3 Cups	Meat and beans 6 1/2 Ounces
Make half your grains whole	**Vary your veggies** Aim for these amounts **each week:**	**Focus on fruits**	**Get your calcium-rich foods**	**Go lean with protein**
Aim for at least **4 ounces** of whole grains a day	**Dark green veggies** = 3 cups **Orange veggies** = 2 cups **Dry beans & peas** = 3 cups **Starchy veggies** = 6 cups **Other veggies** = 7 cups	Eat a variety of fruit Go easy on fruit juices	Go low-fat or fat-free when you choose milk, yogurt, or cheese	Choose low-fat or lean meats and poultry Vary your protein routine—choose more fish, beans, peas, nuts, and seeds

Find your balance between food and physical activity.

Be physically active for at least **30 minutes** most days of the week.
Your results are based on a 2,400 calorie pattern.

Know your limits on fats, sugars, and sodium.
Your allowance for oils is **7 teaspoons a day.**
Limit extras—solid fats and sugars—to **360 calories a day.**
Name: ________________

Referenced from USDA site: http://www.mypyramid.gov

by Nathan Pritikin is extremely low in fat (less than 10 percent of daily calories), high in complex carbohydrates, and high in fiber. The Ornish diet, developed by physician Dean Ornish, is vegetarian: No meat, poultry, or fish is allowed, and only 10 percent of calories are obtained from fat. The low carbohydrate, high protein diet developed by Robert Atkins, M.D. (1930–2003) has proved effective in short-term weight loss, most likely because of increased compliance. Concern exists around the risk of ketoacidosis and the lack of long-term studies on health. This diet has also been used to treat refractory childhood epilepsy. All of these diets include an exercise program, a component proved to increase cardiac performance. Studies have shown that weight loss alone can reduce cholesterol, decrease blood pressure, and eliminate the need for drugs in newly diagnosed cases of adult-onset diabetes.

Diets from other cultures may have certain health benefits. In Asia, diets are low in fat, and there is a low incidence of cardiac disease; diets in Mediterranean countries are high in olive oil, garlic, and grains and are associated with a low incidence of colon cancer and cardiac disease. Food allergies have been implicated in many conditions: arthritis, asthma, hyperactivity, and ulcerative colitis, among others.

DIETARY SUPPLEMENTS

In addition to herbs (discussed below) a variety of dietary supplements are used to promote health. Dietary supplements are products that contain vitamins, minerals, or amino acids. In many cases, the supplement is actually an extract, metabolite, or combination of those. They are intended to *supplement* a healthy diet; they do not comprise a diet or meal. Nutritional supplements have long been familiar to Americans in the form of multivitamins, but they are now available in a vast array of other compounds that can be purchased in grocery stores, pharmacies, health food stores, and over the Internet. As of 2005, annual sales of dietary supplements in the US totaled \$20.3 billion. Of Americans, 75 percent currently use some form of nutritional supplement on a regular basis. Although medicinal benefits are well documented in some supplements, especially vitamins, others vary greatly in safety and consistency. As a general rule, supplements should not be taken by pregnant or lactating women. In psychiatry, nutritional supplements are being used to treat a wide spectrum of illness including cognitive, mood, psychotic, sleep, and conduct disorders; however, little scientific evidence currently supports their efficacy. Table 29–4 lists some of the more common supplements being used to treat psychiatric illness.

Nutritional status has long been deemed important in mental health, and vitamin deficiencies can produce psychiatric symptoms. Severe niacin deficiency results in pellagra with its characteristic triad of skin lesions, gastrointestinal disorder, and psychiatric symptoms. The psychiatric symptoms include irritability and emotional instability progressing to severe depression and then to disorientation, memory impairment, hallucinations, and paranoia. Folic acid deficiency is associated with depression and dementia, whereas vitamin B_{12} deficiency is associated with cognitive impairment, depression, and other affective symptoms. Severe malnutrition can result in apathy and emotional instability.

In 1968, the eminent chemist and Nobel Prize winner Linus Pauling coined the term *orthomolecular* to refer to the connection between the mind and nutrition. In his book *Orthomolecular Psychiatry*, research articles were compiled supporting the notion that taking many times the recommended minimal daily dose of vitamins is useful in the treatment of schizophrenia and other psychiatric disorders. As mentioned, some severe vitamin deficiencies can result in syndromes with a psychiatric component; however, empirical data and an American Psychiatric Association (APA) task force failed to find evidence supporting the notion that schizophrenia and other disorders respond to vitamin therapies.

Evidence indicates that severe vitamin deficiencies can result in psychiatric symptoms and that amino acid supplements may be pharmacologically useful in the treatment of some disorders. These are briefly reviewed below.

Thiamine, Vitamin B_{12}, and Folate

In industrialized societies, severe vitamin deficiencies are rarely encountered except in certain populations. Those who are elderly, alcohol dependent, or chronically ill or who have certain types of gastrointestinal surgeries are at greatest risk. Among the forms of vitamin deficiency most commonly encountered in the emergency room is acute thiamine depletion from alcohol dependence. Whereas the chronic forms of thiamine deficiency that lead to beriberi are rarely seen in the Western world, the fulminant depletion of already low stores of thiamine results in Wernicke's encephalopathy and Korsakoff's syndrome.

Wernicke's encephalopathy classically presents with the triad of ataxia, ophthalmoplegia, and mental confusion, but confusion and a staggering gait are perhaps most common. Although Wernicke's encephalopathy is an acute process, Korsakoff's syndrome may be the permanent residue of this encephalopathy. Patients with Korsakoff's syndrome exhibit a well-circumscribed retrograde and anterograde amnesia that results from destruction of the mammillary bodies, and psychotic symptoms are also reported. Wernicke's encephalopathy is a medical emergency that responds to short-term treatment with 50 mg of thiamine intravenously followed by 250-mg intramuscular injections daily until a normal diet is attained. The treatment of uncomplicated acute thiamine deficiencies usually involves 100 mg given orally one to three times a day.

Vitamin B_{12} deficiency or pernicious anemia is often seen in elderly adults, patients with gastric surgery, and malnourished depressed patients. The most typical psychiatric presentations include apathy, malaise, depressed mood, confusion, and memory deficits. Vitamin B_{12} concentrations of 150 mg/mL of serum are sometimes associated with these symptoms. Vitamin B_{12} deficiency is a more common cause of reversible dementia and is typically assessed in dementia evaluations. The treatment of pernicious anemia usually involves daily intramuscular injections of 1,000 mg of vitamin B_{12} for approximately 1 week, followed by maintenance doses of 1,000 mg every 1 to 2 months.

Folate deficiency has been associated with depression, paranoia, psychosis, agitation, and dementia. Folate deficiency can result from anorexia in depressed patients and can also contribute to depression by interfering with the synthesis of norepinephrine and serotonin. Folate deficiency has been associated with anticonvulsant use, particularly phenytoin (Dilantin), primidone (Mysoline), and phenobarbital (Solfoton), and the sex steroids, including oral contraceptives and estrogen replacement. The most common cause of folate deficiency is the malnourishment associated with alcoholism. Many folate deficiencies respond to 1 mg of folate orally per day; however, some more severe forms may require dosages of 5 mg up to three times a day. Folate deficiency in pregnancy is associated with neural tube defects (e.g., spina bifida, anecephaly).

ENVIRONMENTAL MEDICINE

The field of environmental medicine began to emerge in the 1950s when physicians such as Theron Randolf, professor of allergy and immunology at Northwestern University School of Medicine, began to examine some persons' allergic reactions to various foods. Other workers studied the effects on the body of pollutants in water and air, and eventually the field expanded to include the total environment in which humans exist. As a result, environmental medicine now concerns itself with issues such as food additives; electromagnetic fields from electric utility wires; fertilizers and hormones used in food production; microwaves from appliances such as microwave ovens, television sets, and cellular telephones; and nuclear radiation. Practitioners of environmental medicine believe that many persons are extraordinarily sensitive to environmental contaminants that can trigger a disease process. Some issues are highly controversial. For instance, despite claims to the contrary, studies fail to demonstrate a higher incidence of cancer in persons exposed to electromagnetic fields; however, a correlation exists between higher cancer rates and living near oil refineries

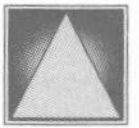

Table 29–4
Dietary Supplements used in Psychiatry

Name	Ingredients/ What Is It?	Uses	Adverse Effects	Interactions	Dosage	Comments
Docosahexaenoic acid (DHA)	Omega-3 polyunsaturated fatty acid	ADD, dyslexia, cognitive impairment, dementia	Anticoagulant properties, mild GI distress	Warfarin	Varies with indication	Stop using prior to surgery
Choline	Choline	Fetal brain development, manic conditions, cognitive disorders, tardive dyskinesia, cancers	Restrict in patients with primary genetic trimethyluria, sweating, hypotension, depression	Methotrexate, works with B_6, B_{12}, and folic acid in metabolism of homocysteine	300–1,200 mg doses >3 g associated with fishy body odor	Needed for structure and function of all cells
L-α-Glycerylphosphorylcholine (α-GPC)	Derived from soy lecithin	To increase growth hormone secretion, cognitive disorders	None known	None known	500 mg–1 g daily	Remains poorly understood
Phosphatidylcholine	Phospholipid that is part of cell membranes	Manic conditions, Alzheimer's disease and cognitive disorders, tardive dyskinesia	Diarrhea, steatorrhea in those with malabsorption, avoid with antiphospholipid antibody syndrome	None known	3–9 g per day in divided doses	Soybeans, sunflower, rapeseed are major sources
Phosphatidylserine	Phospholipid isolated from soya and egg yolks	Cognitive impairment including Alzheimer's disease, may reverse memory problems	Avoid with antiphospholipid antibody syndrome, GI side effects	None known	For soya-derived variety, 100 mg tid	Type derived from bovine brain carries hypothetical risk of bovine spongiform encephalopathy
Zinc	Metallic element	Immune impairment, wound healing, cognitive disorders, prevention of neural tube defects	GI distress, high doses can cause copper deficiency, immunosuppression	Bisphosphonates, quinolones, tetracycline, penicillamine, copper, cysteine-containing foods, caffeine, iron	Typical dose 15 mg per day, adverse effects >30 mg	Claims that zinc can prevent and treat the common cold are supported in some studies but not in others; more research needed
Acetyl-L-carnitine	Acetyl ester of L-carnitine	Neuroprotection, Alzheimer's disease, Down's syndrome, strokes, antiaging, depression in geriatric patients	Mild GI distress, seizures, increased agitation in some with Alzheimer's disease	Nucleoside analogs, valproic acid and pivalic acid–containing antibiotics	500 mg–2 g daily in divided doses	Found in small amounts in milk and meat
Huperzine A	Plant alkaloid derived from Chinese club moss	Alzheimer's disease, age-related memory loss, inflammatory disorders	Seizures, arrhythmias, asthma, irritable bowel disease	Acetylcholinesterase inhibitors and cholinergic drugs	60 μg–200 μg per day	*Huperzia serrata* has been used in Chinese folk medicine for the treatment of fevers and inflammation
NADH (nicotinamide adenine dinucleotide)	Dinucleotide located in mitochondria and cytosol of cells	Parkinson's disease, Alzheimer's disease, chronic fatigue, CV disease	GI distress	None known	5 mg per day or 5 mg bid	Precursor of NADH is nicotinic acid
S-Adenosyl-L-methionine (SAMe)	Metabolite of essential amino acid L-methionine	Mood elevation, osteoarthritis	Hypomania, hyperactive muscle movement, caution in patients with cancer	None known	200–1,600 mg daily in divided doses	Several trials demonstrate some efficacy in the treatment of depression
5-Hydroxytryptophan (5-HTP)	Immediate precursor of serotonin	Depression, obesity, insomnia, fibromyalgia, headaches	Possible risk of serotonin syndrome in those with carcinoid tumors or taking MAOIs	SSRIs, MAOIs, methyldopa, St. John's wort, phenoxybenzamine, 5-HT antagonists, 5-HT receptor agonists	100 mg–2 g daily, safer with carbidopa	5-HTP along with carbidopa is used in Europe for the treatment of depression

(*continued*)

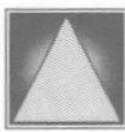

Table 29–4 (Continued)

Name	Ingredients/ What Is It?	Uses	Adverse Effects	Interactions	Dosage	Comments
Phenylalanine	Essential amino acid	Depression, analgesia, vitiligo	Contraindicated in patients with PKU, may exacerbate tardive dyskinesia or hypertension	MAOIs and neuroleptic drugs	Comes in 2 forms: 500 mg–1.5 g daily for DL-phenylalanine, 375 mg–2.25 g for DL-phenylalanine	Found in vegetables, juices, yogurt, and miso
Myoinositol	Major nutritionally active form of inositol	Depression, panic attacks, OCD	Caution in patients with bipolar disorder, GI distress	Possible additive effects with SSRIs and 5-HT receptor agonists (sumatriptan)	12 g in divided doses for depression and panic attacks	Studies have *not* shown effectiveness in treating Alzheimer's disease, autism, or schizophrenia
Vinpocetine	Semisynthetic derivative of vincamine (plant derivative)	Cerebral ischemic stroke, dementias	GI distress, dizziness, insomnia, dry mouth, tachycardia, hypotension, flushing	Warfarin	5–10 mg daily with food, no more than 20 mg per day	Used in Europe, Mexico, and Japan as pharmaceutical agent for treatment of cerebrovascular and cognitive disorders
Vitamin E family	Essential fat-soluble vitamin, family made of tocopherols and tocotrienols	Immune-enhancing, antioxidant, some cancers, protection in CV disease, neurologic disorders, diabetes, premenstrual syndrome	May increase bleeding in those with propensity to bleed, possible increased risk of hemorrhagic stroke, thrombophlebitis	Warfarin, antiplatelet drugs, neomycin, may be additive with statins	Depends on form: tocotrienols, 200–300 mg daily with food; tocopherols, 200 mg per day	Stop members of vitamin E family 1 month prior to surgical procedures
Glycine	Amino acid	Schizophrenia, alleviating spasticity and seizures	Avoid in those who are anuric or have hepatic failure	Additive with antispasmodics	1 g per day in divided doses for supplement; 40–90 g per day for schizophrenia	
Melatonin	Hormone of pineal gland	Insomnia, sleep disturbances, jet lag, cancer	May inhibit ovulation in 1 g doses, seizures, grogginess, depression, headache, amnesia	Aspirin, NSAIDs, β-blockers, INH, sedating drugs, corticosteroids, valerian, kava kava, 5-HTP, alcohol	0.3–3 mg hs for short periods of time	Melatonin sets the timing of circadian rhythms and regulates seasonal responses
Fish oil	Lipids found in fish	Bipolar disorder, lowering triglycerides, hypertension, decrease blood clotting	Caution in hemophiliacs, mild GI upset, "fishy"-smelling excretions	Coumadin, aspirin, NSAIDs, garlic, ginkgo	Varies depending on form and indication—usually about 3–5 g daily	Stop prior to any surgical procedure

Table by Mercedes Blackstone, M.D.

ADD, attention-deficit disorder; CV, cardiovascular; OCD obsessive-compulsive disorder; GI, gastrointestinal; MAOIs; monamine oxidase inhibitors; PKU, phenylketonuria; SSRIs, serotonin reuptake inhibitors; NSAIDs, nonsteroidal anti-inflammatory drugs; INH, isoniazid; 5-HTP, 5-hydroxytryptophan.

and chemical plants. Environmental medicine is a form of preventative medicine that focuses on increased individual awareness of environmental hazards and the control or elimination of these hazards. (See also *Naturopathy*.)

EXERCISE

Exercise improves quality of life through better physical function, reduced morbidities, and improved mental health. The positive effects of exercise on cardiovascular, musculoskeletal, and immune system functions are well documented. These benefits extend to the cognitive and emotional realms and, thus, validate the mind–body connection that is central to many CAM physical practices—yoga, tai-chi, qi-gong. Exercise has been shown to ameliorate depression, anxiety, and PTSD; improve cognitive function and self-esteem; and reduce psychotic symptoms in schizophrenic populations. These effects can be accounted for neurochemically, because exercise promotes secretion of neurotransmitters, such serotonin, adrenaline, and endogenous opiates. Studies have also associated weight loss with increased social interaction, distraction from stress, recreational enjoyment, and mastery of challenge.

Exercise offers many benefits to people with serious mental illness because they more likely suffer from serious medical conditions, such as obesity, diabetes, and hypertension; live sedentary lifestyles; and smoke. Studies of adults with schizophrenia have shown a moderate exercise program reduces body mass index, improves aerobic fitness, raises self-esteem, and results in fewer psychiatric symptoms. Exercise may prove useful in remediating the weight gain from antipsychotic medications and improve compliance.

Although presently underused, exercise holds significant potential benefit as a therapeutic intervention in the mental health care setting.

A structured aerobic exercise program consisting of 45-minute sessions three times per week showed significant gains in cardiovascular fitness, self-esteem, and quality of life, and in altering mood and depression. Unstructured programs benefited those who have adhered to the exercise regimen. No drawbacks are found to moderate exercise, and the health gains are significant.

FELDENKRAIS METHOD

The Feldenkrais method was developed by Moshe Feldenkrais (1904–1982), a Russian-born physicist who developed a theory evolved from Freud's work. Feldenkrais thought that the body should be emphasized as much as the mind and that proprioception (somatic sensations from muscles and other organs) can influence behavior. He believed that posture and the positions of the body reflected conflict; therefore, retraining the body was part of his treatment program. Practitioners of the Feldenkrais method are active throughout the world. Those learning the Feldenkrais method are referred to as students rather than patients, to reinforce the view that the work is primarily an educational process. Lessons generally last from 30 to 60 minutes and consist of structured movement that involves thinking, sensing, moving, and imagining. The method has been used in central nervous system disorders, such as multiple sclerosis, cerebral palsy, and stroke. Older persons who use the method claim that they retain or regain their ability to move without strain or discomfort.

HERBAL MEDICINE

Herbal medicine (Table 29–5) relies on plants to cure illnesses and to maintain health. Probably the oldest known system of medicine, it originated in China about 4000 BC. Ancient texts of Chinese medicine are still in use, and modern Chinese medicine relies on herbs in addition to other methods, such as acupuncture, massage, diet, and exercise, to correct imbalances in the body. A Greco-Roman medical text by Pedanius Dioscorides, *De Materia Medica*, describes the use of more than 500 plants and herbs to cure disease.

The decline of herbal medicine in the late 20th century was related to scientific and technological advances that led to the use of synthetic pharmaceuticals; nevertheless, according to some estimates, at least 25 percent of current medicines are derived from the active ingredients of plants. The examples are many: digitalis from foxglove; ephedrine from ephedra; morphine from the opium poppy; paclitaxel (Taxol) from the yew tree; and quinine from the bark of the cinchona tree.

Herbal medicine is becoming more and more popular. As of 2005, approximately $4.3 billion a year was spent in the United States on herbal medicines, which are classified as dietary supplements. Western herbalists use plants to treat various disorders related to the respiratory, gastrointestinal, cardiovascular, and nervous systems; as with most prescription medicines, these plants contain active compounds that produce physiological effects. As a result, they must be used in appropriate doses if toxic results are to be prevented. They are not subject to US Food and Drug Administration (FDA) approval, and no uniform standards exist for quality control or potency in herbal preparations. Indeed, some preparations have no active ingredients or are adulterated. Herbal supplement producers need only prove safety and truth in labeling, not efficacy to be sold. The herbal industry attempts to regulate itself through organizations such as the Council for Responsible Nutrition and the American Herbal Association, but according to the Federal Trade Commission, fraudulent practices and false advertising still exist. In 2003, the FDA

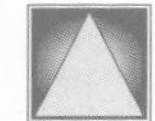

Table 29–5
Herbal Medicine and Other Dietary Supplement-Related Sites on the World Wide Web*

Organization	Web Address	Site Information
Center for Food Safety and Applied Nutrition, Food and Drug Administration	http://vm.cfsan.fda.gov	Clinicians should use this site to report adverse events associated with herbal medicines and other dietary supplements. Sections also contain safety, industry, and regulatory information.
National Center for Complementary and Alternative Medicine, National Institutes of Health	http://nccam.nih.gov	This site contains information about alternative therapies, research studies, consensus reports, and databases.
Agricultural Research Service, United States Department of Agriculture	http://www.ars-grin.gov/npgs/index.html	The site contains an extensive phytochemical database with search capabilities.
Quackwatch	http://www.quackwatch.com	Although this site addresses all aspects of health care, a considerable amount of information covers complementary and herbal therapies.
National Council Against Health Fraud	http://www.ncahf.org	This site focuses on health fraud with a position paper on over-the-counter herbal remedies.
HerbMed	http://www.herbmed.org	This site contains information on almost 200 herbal medications, with evidence for activity, warnings, preparations, mixtures, and mechanisms of action. There are short summaries of important research publications with MEDLINE links.
ConsumerLab	http://www.consumerlab.com	This site is maintained by a corporation that conducts independent laboratory investigations of dietary supplements and other health products.

*Sites updated to 2007.
(From Ang-Lee MK, Moss J, Yuan CS. Herbal Medicines and Perioperative Care. *JAMA.* 2001;286:213.)

banned ephedra (ma huang)-based diet products because of significant risk to cardiovascular health. There is now a *Physicians Desk Reference* for both herbal products and nutritional supplements.

One herb that has caught the attention of Western psychiatry is St. John's wort (*Hypericum*) for the treatment of major depressive disorders. St. John's wort has been used in folk medicine for hundreds of years and is still commonly used in Europe. In Germany, several million prescriptions for hypericum are obtained annually and covered by insurance for the treatment of depression, anxiety, and sleep problems. Studies have compared St. John's wort with placebo, tricyclic drugs, and selective serotonin reuptake inhibitors (SSRIs) and found that *Hypericum* extracts were more effective than placebo in the treatment of mild to moderate depression. Many of these studies lacked of rigor in the diagnosis of depression, sample size, and the assessment of efficacy. NCCAM sponsored studies and other researchers are working to determine the active ingredients, effective dosing, and toxicities associated this plant and other biologically derived supplements using spectrographic and other scientific analyses.

Mrs. J, a 68-year-old retired school teacher in good health was experiencing ahedonia after the death of her spouse and was started on a low dose SSRI by her psychiatrist. After several weeks, her symptoms began to improve. One morning while at the local health food store, she inquired if there were any natural products that improved mood. The store manager informed her that St. John's wort "works just like an SSRI." The patient proceeded to take the recommended daily dose of three capsules that day, each containing 300 mg of 0.3 percent *Hypericin*. Later that evening, she began to feel anxious and could not fall asleep. After several hours of doing needlework to pass the time, she began to sweat profusely. She became concerned for her health when she felt her heart racing. She drove herself to the emergency room of a local hospital. On examination, she was observed to be extremely anxious and hyperactive, tachycardic, and mildly hypertensive. She was given a short-acting, fast-onset benzodiazepine. After 4 hours, the patient reported feeling calm and her vital signs had returned to baseline. The emergency room physician informed Mrs. J that although she had only taken a single daily dose of St. John's wort, she had most likely experienced the side effects of an interaction between the plant extract and the SSRI. Known interactions include a manic reaction and serotonin syndrome. The patient agreed to discontinue the St. John's wort. She was discharged and a follow-up appointment was scheduled with her psychiatrist to discuss treatment options.

PSYCHOACTIVE HERBS

Many phytomedicinals (from the Greek *phyto*, meaning "plant") have psychoactive properties that are used, or have been used, to treat a variety of psychiatric conditions. Adverse effects are possible, and toxic interactions with other drugs can occur with all phytomedicinals. Clinicians should always attempt to obtain a history of herbal use during the psychiatric evaluation. Adulteration is common, and no consistent standard preparations are available for most herbs. Safety profiles and knowledge of adverse effects of most of these substances are lacking; many, if not all, of these herbs are secreted in breast milk and are contraindicated during lactation and should be avoided during pregnancy.

Many cultures have used hallucinogens, including mescaline, psilocybin, and ergots, for thousands of years to gain spiritual and personal insight. Lysergic acid diethylamide (LSD), synthesized in the 1930s, was marketed to psychiatrists and other practitioners in the late 1940s under the trade name Delysid as a tool for understanding psychosis and for facilitating psychotherapy. Using LSD reportedly helped patients capture repressed memories and deal with anxiety, and it allowed patients to gain insight through an analysis of the primary process induced by the hallucinogen. Oral doses of 150 to 250 mg were administered occasionally by psychiatrists throughout the 1950s and early 1960s to facilitate psychotherapy with some patients. In the 1960s, Timothy Leary advocated the widespread use of hallucinogens, but the drugs were outlawed as class I controlled substances in 1965.

Although no longer used for therapeutic purposes in the United States, LSD has fulfilled part of its early promise as a probe for psychosis. More recent understanding of the pharmacology of LSD and its affinity to serotonin (5-hydroxytryptamine [5-HT]) type 2 (5-HT2) receptors has supported the interest in developing serotonin-dopamine antagonists (atypical antipsychotics) with the 5-HT2-receptor blocking properties. Recently, studies using methylenedioxymethamphetamine (MDMA, "ecstasy") have been approved by the NIH to determine whether psychotherapy is facilitated when the patient is under the influence of the drug, which can affect interpersonal relationships positively by promoting feelings of empathy.

It is important not to be judgmental in dealing with patients who use phytomedicinals. They are used for various reasons: (1) as part of their cultural tradition, (2) because they mistrust physicians or are dissatisfied with conventional medicine, or (3) because they experience relief of symptoms. If psychotropic agents are prescribed, the clinician must be extraordinarily alert to the possibility of adverse effects as a result of drug–drug interactions, because many phytomedicinals have ingredients that produce physiological changes in the body. More than 200 herbal drugs are in use; only those with psychoactive properties are listed in Table 29–6.

HOMEOPATHY

Homeopathic healing was developed in the early 1800s by Samuel Hahnemann, a German physician (Fig. 29–3). It is based on the concept that self-healing is a basic characteristic of human life and that special medications can aid this inherent process. The homeopathic pharmacopoeia is unique in several ways. First, it contains more than 2,000 medications, including those from plants, such as aconite, ergot, and hellebore; minerals, such as silver, copper, gold, and iodine; and animals, such as snake and jellyfish venom and tissue extracts. Second, medications are prepared as tinctures (i.e., mixed with 95 percent grain alcohol) or as pills with lactose fillers. Finally, medications are dispersed in infinitesimally dilute solutions, such as 1:1,020,000, which prevents the medication from being detected by conventional chemical methods. Homeopaths claim that the therapeutic effect is based on "molecular medicine."

Hahnemann based his drug treatment on the following assumptions: medical substances elicit a standard array of signs and symptoms in healthy people and the medicine whose effect in normal persons most closely resembles the illness being treated is the one most likely to initiate a curative response. Thus, a medication that produces nausea would be used to treat nausea, except that it would be given in dilute amounts. This law of similars—*Similia similibus curantur* ("Let like be cured by like")—led to coining of the word homeopathy ("similar experiences"). In traditional medicine, such highly dilute substances are considered to have no effect, and no pharmacological research studies demonstrate otherwise.

No longer are any homeopathic medical schools found in the United States (the last one was Hahnemann University Medical School, which closed in 1994); nevertheless, the practice of homeopathy is increasing in the United States and around the world. In Europe, homeopathy is extraordinarily popular. Homeopathic medicines are sold over the counter in the United States. Homeopathic remedies sold in the United States must meet the standards of monographs in the Homeopathic

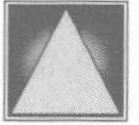

Table 29–6
Phytomedicinals with Psychoactive Effect

Name	Ingredients	Use	Adverse Effects[a]	Interactions	Dosage[a]	Comments
Areca, areca nut, betel nut, *L. Areca catechu*	Arecoline, guvacoline	For alteration of consciousness to reduce pain and elevate mood	Parasympathomimetic overload; increased salivation, tremors, bradycardia, spasms, gastrointestinal disturbances, ulcers of the mouth	Avoid with parasympathomimetic drugs; atropinelike compounds reduce effect	Undetermined; 8–10 g is toxic dose for humans	Used by chewing the nut; used in the past as a chewing balm for gum disease and as a vermifuge; long-term use may result in malignant tumors of the oral cavity
Belladonna, *L. Atropa belladonna,* deadly nightshade	Atropine, scopolamine, flavonoids[b]	Anxiolytic	Tachycardia, arrhythmias, xerostomia, mydriasis, difficulties with micturition and constipation	Synergistic with anticholinergic drugs; avoid with tricyclic antidepressants, amantadine, and quinidine	0.05–0.10 mg a day; maximum single dose is 0.20 mg	Has a strong smell, tastes sharp and bitter, and is poisonous
Bitter orange flower, *Citrus aurantium*	Flavonoids, limonene	Sedative, anxiolytic, hypnotic	Photosensitization	Undetermined	Tincture 2–3 g per day, drug 4–6 g per day, extract 1–2 g per day	Contradictory evidence; some refer to it as a gastric stimulant
Black cohosh, *L. Cimicifuga racemosa*	Triterpenes, isoferulic acid	For premenstrual syndrome, menopausal symptoms, dysmenorrhea	Weight gain, gastrointestinal disturbances	Possible adverse interaction with male or female hormones	1–2 g per day; over 5 g can cause vomiting, headache, dizziness, cardiovascular collapse	Estrogenlike effects questionable because root may act as estrogen-receptor blocker
Black haw, cramp bark, *L. Viburnum prunifolium*	Scopoletin, flavonoids, caffeic acids, triterpenes	Sedative, antispasmodic action on uterus; for dysmenorrhea	Undetermined	Anticoagulant-enhanced effects	1–3 g per day	
California poppy, *L. Eschscholtzia californica*	Isoquinoline alkaloids, cyanogenic glycosides	Sedative, hypnotic, anxiolytic; for depression	Lethargy	Combination of California poppy, valerian, St. John's wort, and passion flowers can result in agitation	2 g per day	Clinical or experimental documentation of effects is unavailable
Catnip, *L. Nepeta cataria*	Valeric acid	Sedative, antispasmodic; for migraine	Headache, malaise, nausea, hallucinogenic effects	Undetermined	Undetermined	Delirium produced in children
Chamomile, *L. Matricaria chamomilla*	Flavonoids	Sedative, anxiolytic	Allergic reaction	Undetermined	2–4 g per day	May be GABAergic
Corydalis, *L. Corydalis cava*	Isoquinoline alkaloids	Sedative, antidepressant; for mild depression	Hallucination, lethargy	Undetermined	Undetermined	Clonic spasms and muscular tremor with overdose
Cyclamen, *L. Cyclamen europaeum*	Triterpene	Anxiolytic; for menstrual complaints	Small doses (e.g., 300 mg) can lead to nausea, vomiting, and diarrhea	Undetermined	Undetermined	High doses can lead to respiratory collapse
Echinacea, *L. Echinacea purpurea*	Flavonoids, polysaccharides, caffeic acid derivatives, alkamides	Stimulates immune system; for lethargy, malaise, respiratory and lower urinary tract infections	Allergic reaction, fever, nausea, vomiting	Undetermined	1–3 g per day	Use in HIV and AIDS patients is controversial; potential for immunosuppression with long-term use. NCCAM studied.
Ephedra, ma-huang *L. Ephedra sinica*	Ephedrine, pseudoephedrine	Stimulant; for lethargy, malaise, diseases of respiratory tract	Sympathomimetic overload; arrhythmias, increased blood pressure, headache, irritability, nausea, vomiting	Synergistic with sympathomimetics, serotonergic agents; avoid with MAOIs	1–2 g per day	Administer for short periods as tachyphylaxis and dependence can occur; risk of myocardial ischemia and stroke. Banned in US diet supplement.

(continued)

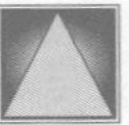

Table 29–6 (Continued)

Name	Ingredients	Use	Adverse Effects[a]	Interactions	Dosage[a]	Comments
Ginkgo, *L. Ginkgo biloba*	Flavonoids, ginkgolide A, B	Symptomatic relief of delirium, dementia; improves concentration and memory deficits; possible antidote to SSRI-induced sexual dysfunction	Allergic skin reactions, gastrointestinal upset, muscle spasms, headache	Anticoagulant: use with caution because of its inhibitory effect on platelet-activating factor (PAF); increased bleeding possible	120–240 mg per day	Studies indicate improved cognition in Alzheimer's patients after 4–5 weeks of use, possibly because of increased blood flow
Ginseng, *L. Panax ginseng*	Triterpenes, ginsenosides	Stimulant; for fatigue, elevation of mood, immune system	Insomnia, hypertonia, and edema (called ginseng abuse syndrome)	Not to be used with sedatives, hypnotic agents, MAOIs, antidiabetic agents, or steroids; has anticoagulant action (discontinue 7 days before surgery)	1–2 g per day	Several varieties exist: Korean (most highly valued), Chinese, Japanese, American (*Panax quinquefolius*)
Heather, *L. Calluna vulgaris*	Flavonoids, catechin, triterpenes, β-sitosterol	Anxiolytic, hypnotic	Undetermined	Undetermined	Undetermined	Efficacy for claimed uses is not documented
Hops, *L. Humulus lupulus*	Humulone, lupulone, flavonoids	Sedative, anxiolytic, hypnotic; for mood disturbances, restlessness	Contraindicated in patients with estrogen-dependent tumors (breast, uterine, cervical)	Hyperthermia effects with phenothiazine antipsychotics and with CNS depressants	0.5 g per day	May decrease plasma levels of drugs metabolized by CPY450 system
Horehound, *L. Ballota nigra*	Diterpenes, tannins	Sedative	Arrhythmias, diarrhea, hypoglycemia, possible spontaneous abortions	May enhance serotonergic drug effects, may augmen-thypoglycemic effects of drugs	1–4 g per day	May cause abortion
Jambolan, *L. Syzygium cumini*	Oleic acid, myristic acid, palmitic and linoleic acid, tannins	Anxiolytic, antidepressant	Undetermined	Undetermined	1–2 g per day	In folk medicine, a single dose is 30 seeds (1.9 g) of powder
Kava kava, *L. Piperis methysticum*	Kava lactones, kava pyrone	Sedative, hypnotic antispasmodic	Lethargy, impaired cognition, dermatitis with long-term unreported usage	Synergistic with anxiolytics, alcohol; avoid with levodopa and dopaminergic agents	600–800 mg per day	May be GABAergic; contraindicated in patients with endogenous depression; may increase the danger of suicide
Lavender, *L. Lavandula angustifolia*	Hydroxycoumarin, tannins, caffeic acid	Sedative, hypnotic	Headache, nausea, confusion	Synergistic with other sedatives	3–5 g per day	May cause death in overdose
Lemon balm, sweet Mary, *L. Melissa officinalis*	Flavonoids, caffeic acid, triterpenes	Hypnotic, anxiolytic, sedative	Undetermined	Potentiates CNS depressant; adverse reaction with thyroid hormone	8–10g per day	
Mistletoe, *L. Viscum album*	Flavonoids, triterpenes, lectins, polypeptides	Anxiolytic; for mental and physical exhaustion	Berries said to have emetic and laxative effects	Contraindicated in patients with chronic infections, e.g., tuberculosis	10 per day	Berries have caused death in children
Mugwort, *L. Artemisia vulgaris*	Sesquitemene lactones, flavonoids	Sedative, antidepressant, anxiolytic	Anaphylaxis, contact dermatitis	Potentiates anticoagulants	5–15 g per day	May stimulate uterine contractions
Nux vomica, *L. strychnos nux vomica*, poison nut	Indole alkaloids: strychnine and brucine, polysaccharides	Antidepressant; for migraine, menopausal symptoms	Convulsions, liver damage, death; severely toxic because of strychnine	Undetermined	0.02–0.05 g per day	Symptoms of poisoning can occur after ingestion of one bean; lethal dose is 1–2 g

(*continued*)

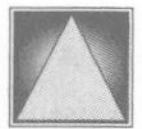

Table 29–6 (Continued)

Name	Ingredients	Use	Adverse Effects[a]	Interactions	Dosage[a]	Comments
Oats, *L. Avena sativa*	Flavonoids, oligo-and polysac-charides	Anxiolytic, hypnotic; for stress, insomnia, opium and tobacco withdrawal	Bowel obstruction or other bowel dysmotility syndromes, flatulence	Undetermined	3 g per day	Oats have sometimes been contaminated with aflatoxin, a fungal toxin linked with some cancers
Passion flower, *L. Passiflora incarnata*	Flavonoids, cyanogenic glycosides	Anxiolytic, sedative, hypnotic	Cognitive impairment	Undetermined	4–8 g per day	Overdose causes depression
St. John's wort, *L. Hypericum perforatum*	Hypericin, flavonoids, xanthones	Antidepressant, sedative, anxiolytic	Headaches, photosensitivity (may be severe), constipation	Report of manic reaction when used with sertraline (Zoloft); do not combine with SSRIs or MAOIs: possible serotonin syndrome; do not use with alcohol, opioids; discontinue 5 days before surgery	100–950 mg per day	Under investigation by the National Institutes of Health (NIH); may act as MAOI or SSRI; 4- to 6-week trial for mild depressive moods if no apparent improvement, another therapy should be tried
Scarlet pimpernel, *L. Anagallis arvensis*	Flavonoids, triterpenes, cucurbitacins, caffeic acids	Antidepressant	Overdose or long-term doses may lead to gastroenteritis and nephritis	Undetermined	1.8 g of powder 4 times a day	Flowers are poisonous
Skullcap, *L. Scutellaria laterflora*	Flavonoid, monoterpenes	Anxiolytic, sedative, hypnotic	Cognitive impairment, hepatotoxicity	Disulfiramlike reaction may occur if used with alcohol	1–2 g per day	Little information exists to support the use of this herb in humans
Strawberry leaf, *L. Fragaria vesca*	Flavonoids, tannins	Anxiolytic	Contraindicated with strawberry allergy	Undetermined	1 g per day	Little information exists to support the use of this herb in humans
Tarragon, *L. Artemisia dracunculus*	Flavonoids, hydroxycou-marins	Hypnotic, appetite stimulant	Undetermined	Undetermined	Undetermined	Little information exists to support the use of this herb in humans
Valerian, *L. Valeriana officinalis*	Valepotriates, valerenic acid, caffeic acid	Sedative, muscle relaxant, hypnotic	Cognitive and motor impairment, gastrointestinal upset, hepatotoxicity; long-term use: contact allergy, headache, restlessness, insomnia, mydriasis, cardiac dysfunction	Avoid concomitant use with alcohol or CNS depressants	1–2 g per day	May be chemically unstable

[a]No reliable, consistent, or valid data exist on dosages or adverse affects of most phytomedicinals.
[b]Flavonoids are common to many herbs. They are plant by-products that act as antioxidants, i.e., agents that prevent the deterioration of material such as DNA via oxidation.
MAOIs, monamine oxidase inhibitors; CNS, central nervous system; SSRIs, serotonin reuptake inhibitors; NCCAM, National Center for Complementary Medicine and Alternative Medicine.

Pharmacopoeia of the United States (HPUS), which was recognized in the Food, Drug and Cosmetic Act with authority equivalent to that of the United States Pharmacopeia (USP).

LIGHT AND MELATONIN THERAPY

Light therapy is based on the concept that humans are subject to circadian rhythms (from the Latin words *circa* ["around"] and *dies* ["day"]) that affect physiological processes in predictable ways. There are 24-hour cycles of rest and activity that include changing levels of corticosteroids, electrolyte excretion, and physiological processes; for instance, blood pressure is higher during the day than at night. By varying light exposure, circadian rhythms can be altered. The concentration of the hormone melatonin, produced by the pineal gland, is highest in the bloodstream at night and is low or absent during the daylight. Melatonin is believed to regulate sleep, and exogenous melatonin (available over the counter) produces drowsiness in normal people. Artificial bright-light therapy (over 2,500 lux) is a proved method used to treat depressive disorder with seasonal pattern (see Section 15.2 in Chapter 15), which is seen during the winter months when daylight hours are reduced.

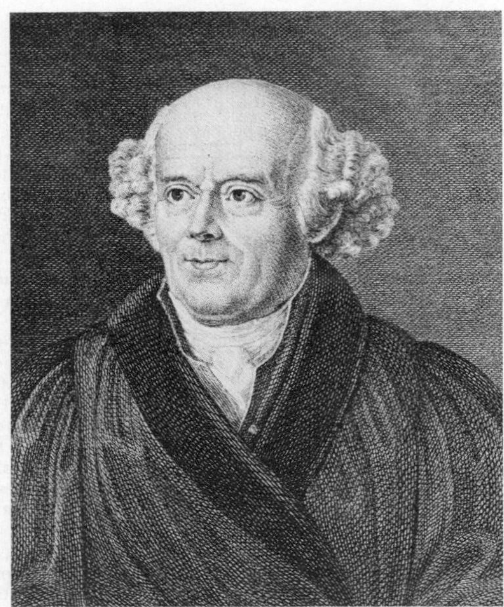

FIGURE 29–3
Samuel Hahnemann. (From the New York Academy of Medicine, New York, NY, with permission.)

MACROBIOTICS

Macrobiotics (from the Greek words *makros* ["long"] and *bios* ["life"]) is a health practice that focuses on living in harmony with nature, using mainly a balanced diet. Macrobiotics became associated with the biblical patriarchs, the Chinese sages, and the Ethiopians of Africa, who were said to live 120 years or more. In 1797, a German physician and philosopher, Christoph W. Hufeland wrote an influential book on diet and health, *Macrobiotics or the Art of Prolonging Life*.

Macrobiotic foods are classified as yin (cold and wet) and yang (hot and dry); the goal is to keep yin and yang in balance. The diet consists of 50 percent grain products, 25 percent cooked or raw vegetables, 10 percent protein, 10 percent vegetable or fish soup, and 5 percent teas and fruits. Prolonged use of the diet can result in vitamin and mineral deficiencies.

MASSAGE

Massage is a treatment that involves manipulation of the soft tissues and the surfaces of the body. It was prescribed for the treatment of diseases more than 5,000 years ago by Chinese physicians, and Hippocrates considered it to be a method of maintaining health.

Massage is believed to affect the body in several ways: it increases blood circulation, improves the flow of lymph through the lymphatic vessels, improves the tone of the musculoskeletal system, and has a tranquilizing effect on the mind. Massage techniques have been described in various ways: stroking, kneading, pinching, rubbing, knuckling, tapping, or applying friction. Massage is most often done with the hands and fingers, but vibrating machines and electrical stimulation are also used. The different types of massage therapies that have evolved over the years are more similar than different. These include Swedish, Oriental, Shiatsu, and Esalen massages. Studies have proved massage useful to reduce anxiety and pain perception. Most persons who experience massage find it physically and mentally restorative.

MEDITATION

Meditation is a technique that involves entering a trance state by focusing thought on a word or sound (a mantra), an object (e.g., a burning candle), or a movement (e.g., an oscillating disk). During the trance, the person experiences a state of calm. A meditative trance has physiological effects, all associated with decreased anxiety: heart and respiratory rates slow, blood pressure decreases, and alpha brain waves increase.

Transcendental meditation (TM), developed by the Indian mystic Maharishi Majesh Yogi, was introduced into the United States in the 1950s. TM uses mantras based on personal characteristics to induce a trance state. In the 1960s, a physician, Herbert Benson, developed the relaxation response, which used mantras and breath control as a treatment for stress and stress-related disorders.

MOXIBUSTION

Moxibustion is based on theories of Oriental medicine in which energy forces are balanced by applying heat to stimulate specific acupoints. The heat is generated by burning dry mugwort leaves (*Artemisia vulgaris*, known as *moxa*). Heat is applied either directly or indirectly. In the direct method, dried moxa is rolled into small cones and placed on the skin. The tops of the cones are lit, but they are extinguished as soon as heat is felt. In the indirect method, a burning cigar-like moxa is held near the skin at acupoints.

Moxibustion is used in musculoskeletal disorder, arthritis, asthma, and eczema. As with many other alternative therapies, however, no scientific clinical trials are available to show its effectiveness.

NATUROPATHY

Naturopathy is a health care system intended to ensure a healthy mind and body based on maintaining healthy nutrition, pollution-free air and water supplies, and exercising regularly. The treatment is based on the belief that the body has the power to heal itself; it requires the patient's active participation in the health maintenance program.

Naturopathy developed in Germany in the later 19th century under the guidance of Benedict Lusz, who prescribed hydrotherapy (alternating hot and cold water) as a form of natural healing. Lusz came to the United States, became an osteopathic physician, and founded the American School of Naturopathy in 1902. Since then, naturopathic medicine has grown into a major form of health care, which uses an eclectic group of methods in addition to hydrotherapy. These methods include eating specialized diets, homeopathy, breathing ionized air, using fomentations (the application of hot and cold compresses), taking colonic irrigations and enemas, drinking pollution-free water, eating foods grown organically, and using massage therapy, herbs, and rest therapy. Naturopathic physicians are licensed in several states (Alaska, Connecticut, New Hampshire, among others), but because no standard regulation of the field exists, persons with minimal or no educational background set up practices.

ORIENTAL MEDICINE

Oriental medicine is a broad term covering the traditional medicines of China, Korea, Japan, Vietnam, Tibet, and other Asian countries. In general, the techniques of Oriental medicine were first developed in China and include acupuncture, moxibustion, herbology, massage, cupping, *gwa sha* (scraping away toxins), breath work, *qi gong* (see below), and exercise (*tai chi*). Chinese medicine is a coherent and independent system of thought and practice based on ancient texts. It is the result of a continuous process of critical thinking, extensive clinical observation, and testing, and it represents a thorough exposition of material by respected clinicians and theoreticians. It is rooted in philosophy, logic, sensibility, and habits of civilization foreign to Western civilization and, therefore, is difficult for Western physicians to understand. The basic theory is that a life force, called chi energy, flows in us in a harmonious, balanced way. This harmony and balance signify health. When the life force does not flow properly, disharmony and imbalance, or illness, result.

OSTEOPATHIC MEDICINE

The scope of osteopathic medicine is similar to allopathic medicine and is best indicated by the fact that doctors of osteopathy (D.O.s) are licensed to practice in every state and are accepted into medical, surgical, and psychiatric residency programs and the military on the same basis as M.D.s; they are qualified to practice in every branch of clinical medicine and take the same licensure examinations as M.D.s. Their medical education is identical to that of medical doctors, except that they have additional training in disorders of the musculoskeletal system, in which D.O.s consider themselves more knowledgeable than M.D.s.

Nineteen osteopathic medical schools exist in the United States. Approximately 35,000 osteopaths treat about 20 million patients each year. Osteopathy was developed by Andrew Taylor Still, M.D. (1828–1917), who founded the American School of Osteopathy in Kirksville, Missouri (now Kirksville College of Osteopathic Medicine), in 1892. Disease is viewed in the same way as in allopathic medicine; however, special emphasis is placed on proper musculoskeletal alignment as a prerequisite for health maintenance. Osteopaths may rely on the manipulation of body parts, particularly the craniosacral spinal axis, as part of a treatment plan. Osteopathic manipulation therapy is perceived as an adjunct, not a substitute, to traditional medical, surgical, and pharmacological intervention.

OZONE THERAPY

Ozone, which acts as an antioxidant and disinfectant, is used conventionally for water purification, odor control, and air purification. Ozone therapy is based on the assumption that most illness is caused by viral and bacterial infection; ozone is used to treat medical conditions that range from influenza to cancer and acquired immunodeficiency syndrome (AIDS). The first ozone generators were developed by Werner von Siemens in Germany in 1857, and ozone was used therapeutically to purify blood shortly thereafter in Germany and other European countries.

Ozone therapy introduces ozone into the body in various ways. These include drinking ozonated water; ozone limb bagging, in which ozone is pumped into an airtight bag that covers an arm or leg; breathing ozone bubbled through olive oil or topically applying ozonated olive oil; insufflations, in which a catheter is inserted into the rectum or vagina with ozone administered at a slow flow rate; and autohemotherapy, in which a person's own ozonized blood is reintroduced into the body.

PAST LIFE MEDICINE

In past life medicine, the healing process is aided by contact with spiritual beings who are believed to have the ability to reverse illness and maintain health. The spirits are approached through the use of altered states of consciousness, so-called *channeling*, higher states of awareness, and transmissions from spiritually evolved beings. Past life regression using hypnosis allows a person to experience past life events (via imagery).

A 40-year-old man, in good health, with an obsessive fear of death was referred to an integrative psychiatrist to deal with his preoccupations about dying. The patient was placed in a trance state under hypnosis and asked to imagine and describe a past life. He described himself as an itinerant silk merchant living in 16th century France. He was married, had eight children, and was content with his life. He was asked to describe his death and proceeded to do so. He was 90 years old when he died, surrounded by his family who were at his bedside. He knew he was dying and described the process as a "peaceful falling away." Following the session, his fears about dying diminished; when he became anxious about death, he remembered the past life narrative and was able to relax.

PRAYER

The pervasive interest in faith healing, the curative anecdotes of television evangelists, and the millions of hopeful individuals visiting religious shrines in search of relief give witness to the continuing interest in, and prevalence of, prayer and spirituality in the process of healing. Some religious groups specifically recommend against standard psychiatric therapies and offer their own approach as the only valid alternative for mental and spiritual health. Others view prayer as a form of distant healing defined by the psychic Elizabeth Targ as any purely mental effort undertaken by one person with the intention of improving the physical or emotional well-being of another.

Some advocate the use of shared prayer, silent prayer, and distant or "intercessory" prayer (praying on behalf of someone else for a specific purpose) to benefit patients. Studies to date are inconclusive, however, on the impact of prayer on medical outcomes. Surveys indicate that 92 percent of a sample of inner city homeless women reported one or more spiritual or religious practice. Some 48 percent reported that prayer was significantly related to less use of alcohol or street drugs or both and fewer perceived worries and depression. Recent epidemiological research indicates that religious beliefs and practices are negatively correlated with substance abuse and positively correlated with health status. Also 12-step programs have a long history of successfully incorporating prayer and spirituality in the treatment of addictive behavior. Personal belief in religion and active attendance at worship has been correlated with a moderately decreased incidence of depression and hypertension.

QI GONG

Chinese *Qi gong* has been practiced for more than 2,000 years. Translated directly, *Qi Gong* means the skill or work (*Gong*) of cultivating energy (*Qi*). It is a Chinese exercise system that attracts and directs the vital life energy (see *Oriental Medicine*), enabling practitioners to build up their health, prevent illness, and increase vitality. 'Still' Qi Gong is practiced as a motionless meditation with the emphasis on breath and intentional thoughts. 'Moving' Qi Gong involves external movements under the conscious direction of the mind. Electroencephalogram studies have detected measurable differences in the brain patterns of practitioners. Purported benefits include increased autoimmune cell production, reduced hypertension, and decreased incidence of falls in the elderly.

REFLEXOLOGY

Reflexology is the gentle massaging of the feet, hands, and ears to stimulate the body's natural healing power. It is used to alleviate tension by clearing crystalline deposits under the skin that may interfere with the natural flow of the body's energy. Reflexologists believe that all body parts can be mapped out on the soles or sides of the feet; for instance, the tip of the second toe represents the eye. Applying pressure to a particular area of the foot can relieve disorders related to the represented body parts.

REIKI

Reiki is a Japanese word with the general meaning of "healing." (*Rei* means "universal" or "spiritual," and *Ki* is "life force energy.") The two degrees of Reiki healing are as follows. First-degree Reiki practitioners use light, nonmanipulative touch to precipitate a flow of healing energy, called *Reiki*, drawn through the practitioner and into the patient according to the recipient's needs. Second-degree healing enables practitioners to access this energy for distant healing when touch is impossible. Reiki treatment typically creates an almost immediate feeling of relaxation, which may reduce the biochemical effects of prolonged stress. First-degree Reiki is easily learned and is a method that patients use to decrease anxiety, insomnia, and pain. Recipients may experience the energy as heat or cold, or as a sense of flow throughout the body, not limited to where the practitioner's hands are placed. Reiki is also used in hospices for pain management, to support a peaceful death, and to provide emotional support for family members.

ROLFING

Rolfing is a type of massage that was developed by an American biochemist, Ida Rolf (1896–1979), to relieve tension in muscle, connective tissue, and fascia, which she believed caused musculoskeletal diseases, such as arthritis and fibromyalgia. Therapy consists of deep, sometimes painful, massage to produce flexible planes between muscle groups throughout the body. Rolf discovered that she could achieve remarkable changes in posture and structure by manipulating the body's myofascial system; as various parts of the body are massaged, past memories and emotional states are often released. In this sense, rolfing is a psychophysiological experience.

SHAMANISM

A shaman (Fig. 29–4) is an individual who is believed to have the power to heal the sick and communicate with the spirit world. Individuals having this designation can be found in many parts of the world, including American aboriginal groups (Native Americans and Alaskan natives). Qualifications of a medicine man (or woman) are determined by a series of initiatory trials and teaching and "certification" by qualified, recognized elders. Shamanistic practices often include cleansing ceremonies, such as fasting or sweating, and so-called vision quests, which are accompanied by hallucinations. The ceremony is sometimes facilitated by rhythmic sounds, dancing, physical pain or privation, and the use of "spiritual herbs." Through this process, the shaman escorts the soul of the dying to the afterlife. Shamanistic practices are also used to provide solutions to insolvable personal or social problems.

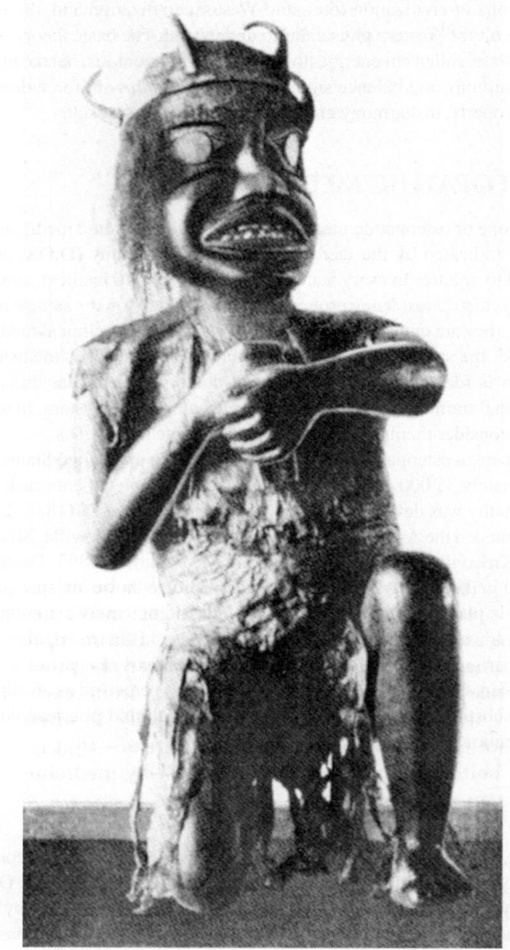

FIGURE 29–4
Wooden statue of shaman. North Pacific coast.

SOUND AND MUSIC THERAPY

Sound therapy is an ancient technique in which sounds (e.g., chants, bell rings, or drum beats) are used to create vibrations in the body and believed to have healing powers. Practitioners claim that a sense of relaxation can also be achieved. Sound therapy is used in Ayurveda to promote health, with claims of reducing tumor growth by using certain sounds known as *Sama Veda*. Music therapy uses the sound of musical instruments, such as the flute, to achieve similar results. In the Bible, David attempted to treat King Saul's depression by playing the harp. The effect of music and sound on psychophysiological processes is under investigation at various academic centers.

TAI CHI CHUAN

Tai chi chuan, or tai chi, is one of the most popular Asian movement arts used in the West. This ancient Chinese technique is designed to increase the life force in the body through a series of slow circular movements. It is a moving form of meditation and is based, as are other Chinese methods, on the search for perfect balance between yin and yang energies.

The practitioner performs sequences of movements that last from 5 to 30 minutes. A session may last a couple of hours and is typically performed in early morning. The practitioner is expected to focus on breathing and its precise synchronization with the movements. Tai chi chuan is believed to help mainly stress-related problems and conditions and so is primarily used to treat anxiety, depression, muscular tension, high blood pressure, and other cardiovascular conditions.

THERAPEUTIC TOUCH

Therapeutic touch is the technique of healing with hands. It was developed by a nurse, Dolores Krieger, in the 1970s. Energy is believed to be transferred by laying the hands over specific parts of the body to aid in the process of healing. Therapeutic touch has gained popularity in the nursing profession, as well as among some physicians.

TIBETAN MEDICINE

The Tibetan health system dates to about the 7th century AD. The Tibetan king Songsten Gampo is credited with its creation from the synthesis of various, more ancient sources. It has elements of Arabic, Indian, and

Chinese health systems. In Tibet, its practice is closely related to religion and magic. Disease is believed to be the result of imbalance between the three components or humors of the living organism: wind (breathing and movement in general), bile (related to digestion and temperament), and phlegm (related to sleep, joint mobility, and skin elasticity). Imbalance can be caused by ignorance of health principles, environmental assaults, or improper diet. Treatment consists of restoring the balance between the different humors through the use of herbal medicine and accessory therapies, such as massage, moxibustion, acupuncture, appropriate diet, religious rituals, and purification techniques.

TRAGER METHOD

The Trager method, developed by Milton Trager, a Chicago physician, is a technique of movement reduction to aid individuals suffering from polio and other neuromuscular disorders. The client, typically in 60- to 90-minute sessions, is instructed to relax all conscious muscles and to allow the unconscious to choose natural, less restrictive body movements, as guided by the practitioner. This method is particularly suitable to individuals with back pain and severely restricted movement.

YOGA

Yoga ("yoking" or "union" in Sanskrit) is a comprehensive philosophical system with the goal of preparing an individual to unite with the supreme being. The technique of early yoga seeks to bring into balance all the disparate aspects of body, mind, and personality. Early evidence of yoga practice dates back to 5,000 years ago in India, and it has been practiced as a religion and health system ever since. The West grew familiar with yoga through the practice of Hatha Yoga and an emphasis on the physical collection of *asanas* (postures). The other aspects of the system, *pranayama* (breathing exercises) and *dhyana* (meditation), and other forms of yoga are gaining adoption. Yoga is used to reduce stress and to treat anxiety, high blood pressure, and musculoskeletal conditions. Studies have proved its benefits for depression.

INTEGRATIVE PSYCHIATRY

A new type of psychiatry, called *integrative psychiatry*, selectively incorporates elements of complementary and alternative medicine into practice methods. It emphasizes treatment rather than diagnosis and views the patient holistically, taking into account not only mind–body issues and interactions but spiritual values as well. Integrative psychiatry also is concerned with prevention of illness, emphasized by having the patient pay attention to lifestyle factors such as diet and exercise. Stress reduction involves use of yoga, meditation, or other relaxation exercises. Attention is paid to stress factors related to work and interpersonal relationships.

History

At one time, hypnosis and biofeedback were considered alternative therapies out of the mainstream of traditional psychiatric practice. These modalities are now incorporated into standard psychiatric practice. Hypnosis, for example, is used by psychiatrists for a variety of disorders, and dynamically oriented psychiatrists use hypnotherapy in their work to enable a patient to recover feelings and memories that are repressed and not otherwise available for analysis. In the middle of the 20th century, workers such as Paul Schilder, in his book *The Image and Appearance of the Human Body*, described how one's physiology and physiognomy could be influenced by psychological experiences during various developmental stages. More recently, mainstream psychiatrists, such as Brian Weiss, have described their use of past life regression as a therapeutic method and a means of accessing unconscious material.

Methods

Any of the complementary methods described in this section can be integrated into standard psychotherapeutic practice, although some lend themselves better than others. For example, during a Reiki treatment, a patient tends to be in a relaxed state and may have feeling tones, images, or thoughts that would not ordinarily be discussed. In an integrative therapy session, those mental and physical phenomena would be verbalized and subject to analysis and interpretation. Similarly, a patient having past life regression may have an elaborate narrative about his or her past life that would be carefully examined by the integrative psychiatrist for its relevance to current life experiences. Most integrative psychiatrists view past-life narratives as dynamic representations of the patient's unconscious wishes and fears; some view them as representations of actual past lives. In either case, the material is used to help patients gain greater insight and understanding of themselves in their current life.

Complementary and alternative techniques that involve body manipulation (e.g., craniosacral manipulation, massage, or the Alexander technique) lend themselves to integrative psychiatric therapy. As mentioned, the image persons have of their body and the way in which the body is held (e.g., stooped posture) are heavily influenced both by genetics and by life experiences. Depressive facies, Veraguth's folds, and other physiologic correlates of mood have long been recognized in the psychiatric literature. The integrative psychiatrist uses this and other bodily markers as a way to gain access to previously unrecognized neurotic conflict. Patients with somatoform disorders, such as dysmorphophobia, are often helped by such approaches, as are patients with eating disorders who have major body image distortions.

Any technique that involves manipulation of a body part can potentially elicit an image, thought, or feeling related to the experience. A patient experiencing a back rub may have myriad associations to the experience that are examined in the session. Some patients cannot tolerate being touched, a trait that is almost always related to some past traumatic experience. Body manipulation can be geared to correcting abnormalities. In the Alexander technique, careful attention is paid to posture and body alignment. As the corrective procedures unfold, patients may gain understanding and insight into what caused the defective or inefficient postural attitude in the first place.

Finally, spiritual beliefs derived from Judeo-Christian, Native American, and Eastern religious thought can be integrated into traditional psychotherapy. Workers such as Alan Watts incorporated Zen Buddhism into Western psychotherapy more than 50 years ago. Psychiatrists are working with Native American healers to help patients diminish anxiety, especially regarding death and dying.

Other Issues

Ideally, the psychiatrist practicing integrative therapy should be schooled in one or more of the complementary methods he or she plans to employ. In some cases, a complementary practitioner may work in conjunction with the psychiatrist, especially if the psychiatrist is not schooled in a particular method. At times, patients may be expert in a field (e.g., yoga) and seek out the integrative psychiatrist to enlarge on their experience. Integrative psychiatrists may use psychoactive herbs and homeopathic medicinals alone or in conjunction with traditional psychopharmacologic agents, mindful of the possibility of adverse drug–drug interactions.

Ethical Issues

The same standards that apply to traditional psychiatric practice and psychotherapy apply to integrative psychiatry. Because some of the techniques involve a laying on of hands or place the patient in a more dependent and vulnerable state than traditional psychotherapy techniques, boundary issues must be carefully evaluated. Currently, no standards of practice exist for this method other than those to which physicians have always been held, including to do no harm. As in complementary and alternative medicine generally, careful outcome studies are needed if this new amalgam is to prove its worth.

References

Astrup A. Atkins and other low-carbohydrate diets: hoax or effective tool for weight loss? The *Lancet*. 2004;364(9437):897–899.

Barnes P. *Complementary and Alternative Medicine Use among Adults: United States, 2002*. Washington, DC: US Department of Health and Human Services. Advance Data 304; May, 2004.

Beebe L, Tian L, Morris N, Goodwin A, Allen S, Kuldau J. Effects of exercise on mental and physical health parameter of persons with schizophrenia. *Issues Ment Health Nurs*. 2005;26(6):661–676.

Callahan P. Exercise: A neglected intervention in mental health care? *J Psychiatr Ment Health Nurs*. 2004;11(4):476–483.

Block K. Challenges of complementary and alternative medicine research. *Integr Cancer Ther*. 2005;4(3):207–209.

Frisch MJ, Franko DL, Herzog DB. Arts-based therapies in the treatment of eating disorders. *Eat Disord*. 2006;14(2):131–142.

Fogarty M, Happell B. Exploring the benefits of an exercise program for people with schizophrenia: A qualitative study. *Issues Ment Health Nurs*. 2005;26(3):341–351.

Fowler NA. Aromatherapy, used as an integrative tool for crisis management by adolescents in a residential treatment center. *J Child Adolesc Psychiatr Nurs*. 2006;19(2):69.

Kiresuk TJ, Trachtenberg A. Alternative and complementary health practices. In: Sadock BJ, Sadock VA, eds. *Kaplan & Sadock's Comprehensive Textbook of Psychiatry*. 8th ed. Vol. 2. Baltimore: Lippincott Williams & Wilkins; 2005:2406.

Knüppel L. Adverse effects of St. John's wort: A systematic review. *J Clin Psychiatry*. 2004; 65(11):1470–1480.

Larson EB, Wang L, Bowen JD, McCormick WC, Teri L, Crane P, Kukull W. Exercise is associated with reduced risk for incident dementia among persons 65 years of age and older. *Ann Intern Med*. 2006;114(2):73–81.

Moyer CA, Rounds J, Hannum JW. A meta-analysis of massage therapy research. *Psychol Bull*. 2004;130:3.

Overstreet DH, Keung WM, Rezvani AH, Massi M, Lee DY. Herbal remedies for alcoholism: Promises and possible pitfalls. *Alcohol Clin Exp Res*. 2003;27:177.

Shaw K, Turner J, Del Mar C. *Tryptophan and 5-hydroxytryptophan for depression*. Cochrane Collection: Cochrane Library, Vol. 1, 2003.

Townsend M, Kladder V, Ayele H, Mulligan T. Systematic review of clinical trials examining the effects of religion on health. *South Med J*. 2002;95(12):1429–1434.

30 Psychiatry and Reproductive Medicine

Reproductive events and processes have profound psychological effects, some of which can progress to overt psychopathological states. This section addresses such events, including pregnancy, infertility, abortion, menopause, and sterilization, among others.

REPRODUCTIVE PHYSIOLOGY

The physiological processes associated with menarche, menstrual cycling, pregnancy, postpartum, and menopause occur within the context of a woman's physiological and interpersonal life, interfacing with psychosocial functioning throughout adolescence, young adulthood, midlife, and late life. The fields of psychiatry and reproductive medicine are just beginning to elaborate the multiple mechanisms by which psyche and soma interact to determine a woman's gynecological and psychological function. This chapter illustrates how reproductive processes interact with psychosocial events and aims ultimately to improve the approach to both gynecologic and psychiatric treatments.

Menstrual Physiology

Menstrual cyclicity results directly from ovarian cyclicity. Each ovarian cycle starts with the development of a group or cohort of follicles, one of which becomes dominant. The follicles are composed of an oocyte surrounded by granulosa cells, which, in turn, are surrounded by theca cells.

As shown at the top of Figure 30–1, follicular development is initiated by the hypothalamic release of gonadotropin-releasing hormones (GnRH) at a pulse frequency of approximately one pulse every 90 minutes. GnRH stimulates the release of the pituitary gonadotropins, luteinizing hormone (LH), and follicle-stimulating hormone (FSH). In turn, LH stimulates ovarian theca cells to synthesize and secrete androgens; FSH induces granulosa cell development, including the enzyme aromatase, which converts the thecally produced androgens to estrogens. In the presence of a constant GnRH pulse frequency of one pulse each 90 minutes, the secretion of LH and FSH in the follicular phase will be regulated primarily by estradiol feedback at the level of the pituitary. Rising estradiol concentrations suppress FSH, thereby limiting the number of follicles that become mature oocytes capable of ovulating.

As illustrated in the middle panel of Figure 30–1, when estradiol concentrations rise exponentially to exceed a critical threshold and remain elevated for at least 36 hours, which is the pattern one fully mature follicle produces, an LH surge is triggered and ovulation (release of the ovum from the follicle sac) ensues approximately 36 hours later. Thereafter, granulosa cells transform into progesterone-secreting luteal cells, and the ovulated follicle is then referred to as the *corpus luteum*, which secretes progesterone.

Figure 30–1 displays the levels of LH, FSH, estradiol, and progesterone throughout the menstrual cycle and corresponding follicular events. The target tissues for ovarian steroids include the endometrium, whose developmental sequence is illustrated along the bottom panel, and the hypothalamic GnRH pulse generator, whose frequency, as indicated in the top right panel, is slowed dramatically by the combination of estrogen and progesterone secreted during the postovulatory or luteal phase of the menstrual cycle. This inhibition of GnRH is followed by decreased secretion of LH and FSH so that new follicular development is prevented until the corpus luteum regresses. As progesterone concentrations decline, GnRH pulsatility increases, and gonadotropin, especially FSH, secretion rises. The phases of the menstrual cycle can be termed *follicular* and *luteal* in reference to ovarian events or *proliferative* and *secretory* in reference to endometrial events.

Premenstrual Syndrome (PMS) and Premenstrual Dysphoric Disorder (PDD) occur during the late luteal phase of the menstrual cycle and are usually relieved by the onset of menses or shortly thereafter. Both disorders are discussed in detail below.

PREGNANCY

Biology of Pregnancy

The first presumptive sign of pregnancy is the absence of menses for 1 week. Other presumptive signs are breast engorgement and tenderness, changes in breast size and shape, nausea with or without vomiting (morning sickness), frequent urination, and fatigue. A diagnosis can be made 10 to 15 days after fertilization by testing for human chorionic gonadotropin (hCG), which is produced by the placenta. The definitive diagnosis requires a doubling of hCG levels and the presence of fetal heart sounds. Transvaginal ultrasound scanning can reveal a pregnant uterus as early as 4 weeks after fertilization, by visualization of a gestational sac.

Stages of Pregnancy

Pregnancy is commonly divided into three trimesters, starting from the first day of the last menstrual cycle and ending with the delivery of a

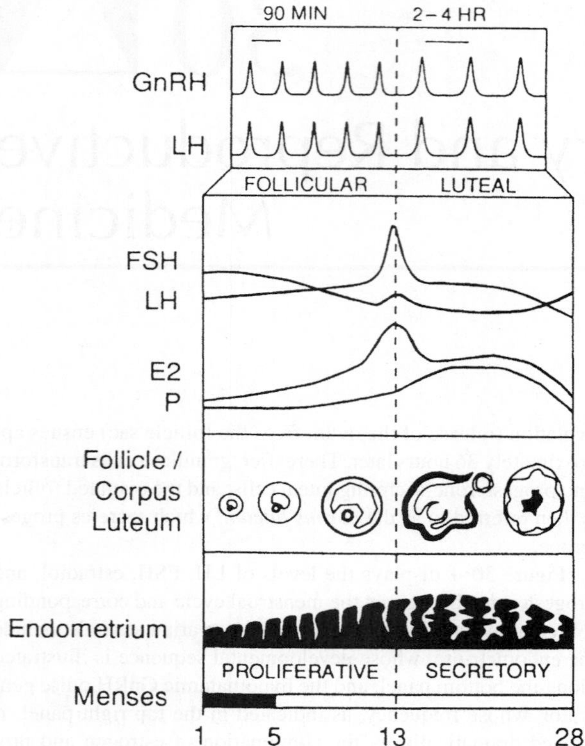

FIGURE 30–1
Schematization of the human menstrual cycle. Es, estradiol; FSH, follicule-stimulating hormone; GnRH, gonadotropin-releasing hormone; LH, luteinizing hormone; P, progesterone.

baby. During the first trimester, the woman must adapt to changes in her body, such as fatigue, nausea and vomiting, breast tenderness and mood lability. The second trimester is often the most rewarding for women. A return of energy and the end of nausea and vomiting allow women to feel better and experience the excitement of starting to look pregnant. The third trimester is associated with physical discomfort for many women. All systems—cardiovascular, renal, pulmonary, gastrointestinal, and endocrine—have undergone profound changes that can produce a heart murmur, weight gain, exertional dyspnea, and heartburn. Some women require reassurance that those changes are not evidence of disease and that they will return to normal shortly after delivery—generally in 4 to 6 weeks.

Psychology of Pregnancy

Pregnant women undergo marked psychological changes. Their attitudes toward pregnancy reflect deeply felt beliefs about all aspects of reproduction, including whether the pregnancy was planned and whether the baby is wanted. The relationship with the infant's father, the age of the mother, and her sense of identity also affect a woman's reaction to prospective motherhood. Prospective fathers also face psychological challenges.

Psychologically healthy women often find pregnancy a means of self-realization. Many women report that being pregnant is a creative act gratifying a fundamental need. Other women use pregnancy to diminish self-doubts about femininity or to reassure themselves that they can function as women in the most basic sense. Still others view pregnancy negatively; they may fear childbirth or feel inadequate about mothering.

During early stages of their own development, women must undergo the experience of separating from their mothers and of establishing an independent identity; this experience later affects their own success at mothering. If a woman's mother was a poor role model, a woman's sense of maternal competence may be impaired, and she may lack confidence before and after her baby's birth. Women's unconscious fears and fantasies during early pregnancy often center on the idea of fusion with their own mothers.

Psychological attachment to the fetus begins in utero and, by the beginning of the second trimester, most women have a mental picture of the infant. Even before being born, the fetus is viewed as a separate being, endowed with a prenatal personality. Many mothers talk to their unborn children. Recent evidence suggests that emotional talk with the fetus is related not only to early mother–infant bonding but also to the mother's efforts to have a healthy pregnancy, for example, by giving up cigarettes and caffeine. According to psychoanalytic theorists, the child-to-be is a blank screen on which a mother projects her hopes and fears. In rare instances, these projections account for postpartum pathological states, such as a mother's desire to harm her infant, whom she views as a hated part of herself. Normally, however, giving birth to a child fulfills a woman's need to create and nurture life.

Fathers are also profoundly affected by pregnancy. Impending parenthood demands a synthesis of such developmental issues as gender role and identity, separation-individuation from a man's own father, sexuality, and, as Erik Erikson proposed, generativity. Pregnancy fantasies in men and wishes to give birth in boys reflect early identification with their mothers as well as the wish to be as powerful and creative as they perceive mothers to be. For some men, getting a woman pregnant is proof of their potency, a dynamic that plays a large part in adolescent fatherhood.

Marriage and Pregnancy

The prospective mother–wife and father–husband must redefine their roles as a couple and as individuals. They face readjustments in their relationships with friends and relatives and must deal with new responsibilities as caretakers of the newborn and each other. Both parents may experience anxiety about their adequacy as parents; one or both partners may be consciously or unconsciously ambivalent about the addition of the child to the family and about the effects on the dyadic (two-person) relationship. A husband may feel guilty about his wife's discomfort during pregnancy and parturition, and some men experience jealousy or envy of the experience of pregnancy. Accustomed to gratifying each other's dependency needs, the couple must attend to the unremitting needs of a new infant and a developing child. Although most couples respond positively to these demands, some do not. Under ideal conditions, the decision to become a parent and have a child should be agreed on by both partners, but sometimes parenthood is rationalized as a way to achieve intimacy in a conflicted marriage or to avoid having to deal with other life circumstance problems.

Attitudes toward the Pregnant Woman. In general, others' attitudes toward a pregnant woman reflect a variety of factors: intelligence, temperament, cultural practices, and myths of the society and the subculture into which the person was born. Married men's responses to pregnancy are generally positive. For some men, however, reactions vary from a misplaced sense of pride that they are able to impregnate the woman to fear of increased responsibility and subsequent termination of the relationship. A woman's risk of abuse by her husband or boyfriend increases during pregnancy, particularly during the first trimester. One study found that 6 percent of pregnant women are abused. Domestic abuse adds significantly to the cost of health care during pregnancy, and abused women are more likely than nonabused controls to have histories of miscarriage, abortion, and neonatal death. The reasons for abuse vary. Some men fear being neglected and not having excessive dependency needs gratified; others may see the fetus as a rival. In most cases, however, one finds a history of abuse before the woman was pregnant.

Alternative Lifestyle Pregnancy

Some lesbian couples decide that one partner should become pregnant through artificial insemination. Societal attitudes may put stress on this arrangement, but if the two women have a secure relationship, they tend to bond strongly together as a family unit. Men in committed gay relationships are fathering children through artificial insemination with surrogate mothers. Recent studies show that children raised in same sex couple households are not measurably different from children raised by heterosexual parents with respect to personality development, psychological development, and gender identity. These children are also not more likely to be gay or lesbian themselves.

Some single, never-married women who do not wish to marry but do want to become pregnant may do so through artificial or natural insemination. Such women constitute a group who believe that motherhood is the fulfillment of female identity, without which they view their lives to be incomplete. Most of these women have considered the consequence of single parenthood and feel able to rise to the challenges.

Sexual Behavior

The effects of pregnancy on sexual behavior vary. Some women experience an increased sex drive as pelvic vasocongestion produces a more sexually responsive state. Others are more responsive than before the pregnancy, because they no longer fear becoming pregnant. Some have diminished desire or lose interest in sexual activity altogether. Libido may be decreased because of higher estrogen levels or feelings of unattractiveness. Avoidance of sex may also result from physical discomfort or an association of motherhood with asexuality. Men with a Madonna complex view pregnant women as sacred and not to be defiled by the sexual act. Either a man or a woman may erroneously consider intercourse potentially harmful to the developing fetus and, thus, something to be avoided. Men who have extramarital affairs during their wives' pregnancies usually do so during the last trimester.

Coitus. Most obstetricians place no prohibitions on coitus during pregnancy. Some suggest that sexual intercourse cease 4 to 5 weeks antepartum. If bleeding occurs early in pregnancy, an obstetrician may prohibit coitus temporarily as a therapeutic measure. Bleeding in the first 20 days of pregnancy occurs in 20 to 25 percent of women and approximately half of that group experience spontaneous abortion. Maternal death resulting from forcibly blowing air into the vagina during cunnilingus has been reported; the deaths presumably result from air emboli in the placental–maternal circulation.

Parturition

Fears regarding pain and bodily harm during delivery are universal and, to some extent, warranted. Preparation for childbirth affords a sense of familiarity and can ease anxieties, which facilitates delivery. Continuous emotional support during labor reduces the rate of cesarean section and forceps deliveries, the need for anesthesia, the use of oxytocin, and the duration of labor. A technically difficult or even painful delivery, however, does not appear to influence the decision to bear additional children.

Men's responses to pregnancy and labor have not been well studied, but the recent trend toward inclusion of fathers in the birth process eases their anxieties and elicits a fuller sense of participation. Fathers do not parent the same way as mothers, and new mothers often need to be encouraged to respect these differences and view them positively.

Lamaze Method. Also known as natural childbirth, the Lamaze method originated with the French obstetrician Fernand Lamaze. In this method, women are fully conscious during labor and delivery, and no analgesic or anesthetic is used. The expectant mother and father attend special classes, during which they are taught relaxation and breathing exercises designed to facilitate the birth process. Women who have such training often report minimal pain during labor and delivery. Participating in the birth process may help a fearful or ambivalent father bond to his newborn infant.

Prenatal Screening

Prenatal screening for potential or actual fetal malformation is conducted in most pregnant women. Sonograms are noninvasive and can detect structural fetal abnormalities. Maternal α-fetoprotein (AFP) is measured between 15 and 20 weeks, screening for neural tube defects and Down syndrome. The sensitivity of Down syndrome testing is increased when a triple screen is done (AFP, hCG, and estriol). Amniocentesis is indicated for women over 35 years, those with a sibling or parent with a known chromosome anomaly, and those with abnormal AFP or any other risk for severe genetic disorder. Amniocentesis is usually done between 16 and 18 weeks and carries a risk that 1 in 300 women will miscarry after the procedure. In the first trimester, chorionic villus sampling (CVS) can be done, which reveals the same information concerning chromosomal status, enzyme levels, and DNA patterns. With CVS, there is a risk that 1 in 100 women will have a spontaneous abortion after the procedure.

Screening in the first trimester allows women to choose early termination, which may be physically and emotionally easier on the woman. Profound ethical questions are involved in whether or not to abort a fetus with a known defect. Some women choose not to terminate and report a strong loving bond that lasts throughout the life of the child, who usually predeceases the parent.

Lactation

Lactation occurs because of a complex psychoneuroendocrine cascade that is triggered by the abrupt decline in estrogen and progesterone concentrations at parturition. In general, babies should be fed as needed, rather than by schedule. Breast-feeding has many benefits. The composition of breast milk supports timely neuronal development, confers passive immunity, and reduces food allergies in the child. In subsistence-level cultures in which children are allowed to nurse as long as they want (a practice supported by La Leche League, a breast-feeding advocacy group), most babies will wean themselves between ages 3 and 5 if not encouraged by the mother to do so earlier. Women who decide to breast-feed need good teaching and social support, which if lacking may lead to frustration and feelings of inadequacy. Women must not feel pressured or coerced into breast-feeding if they are opposed or ambivalent. In the long term, no discernible difference exists between bottle-fed and breast-fed children as adults.

An incidental finding about lactation is that some women experience sexual sensations during lactation, which in rare cases can lead to orgasm. In the early 1990s a woman who called a help line about such feelings was put in jail and had her infant taken from her on allegations of sexual abuse. Common sense ultimately prevailed, however, and mother and infant were reunited.

Perinatal Death

Perinatal death, defined as death sometime between the 20th week of gestation and the first month of life, includes spontaneous abortion (miscarriage), fetal demise, stillbirth, and neonatal death. In previous years, the intense bond between the expectant or new parent and the fetus or neonate was underestimated, but perinatal loss is now recognized as a significant trauma for both parents. Parents who experience such a loss go through a period of mourning much as that experienced when any loved one is lost.

Intrauterine fetal death, which can occur at any time during the pregnancy, is an emotionally traumatic experience. In the early months of pregnancy, a woman is usually unaware of fetal death and learns of it only from her doctor. Later in pregnancy, after fetal movements and heart tones have been experienced, a woman may be able to detect fetal demise. When given the diagnosis of fetal death, most women want the dead fetus removed; depending on the trimester, labor may be induced, or the woman may have to wait for spontaneous expulsion of the uterine contents. Many couples consider sexual relations during the period of waiting not only undesirable but psychologically unacceptable as well.

A sense of loss also accompanies the birth of a stillborn child and induced abortion of an abnormal fetus detected by antenatal diagnosis. As mentioned, attachment to an unborn child begins before birth, and grief and mourning occur after a loss at any time. The grief experienced after a third-trimester loss, however, is generally greater than that experienced after a first-trimester loss. Some parents do not wish to view a stillborn child, and their wishes should be respected. Others wish to hold the stillborn, and this act can assist the mourning process. A subsequent pregnancy may diminish overt feelings of grief, but it does not eliminate the need to mourn. So-called replacement children are at risk for overprotection and future emotional problems.

CONCEPTION

Infertility

Infertility is the inability of a couple to conceive after 1 year of coitus without the use of a contraceptive. In the United States, about 15 percent of married couples are unable to have children. Until recently, women were blamed when couples did not have children, and feelings of guilt, depression, and inadequacy frequently accompanied the perception of being barren. Today, causes of infertility are attributed to disorders in women in 40 percent of cases, disorders in men in 40 percent, and disorders of both in 20 percent. Tests in an infertility workup (Table 30–1) usually reveal the specific cause; however, 10 to 20 percent of couples have no identifiable cause.

The inability to have a child can produce severe psychological stress on one or both partners in a marriage. Self-blame increases the likelihood of psychological problems. Women—but not men—are at increased risk for psychological distress if they are older and do not already have biological children. If one or both partners are unwilling to take advantage of assisted reproductive techniques, the marriage may falter. A psychiatric evaluation of the couple may be advisable. Marital disharmony or emotional conflicts about intimacy, sexual relations, or parenting roles can directly affect endocrine function and such physiological processes as erection, ejaculation, and ovulation. No evidence exists, however, for any simple, causal relation between stress and infertility.

When preexisting conflict gives rise to problems of identity, self-esteem, and guilt, the disturbance may be severe and may manifest through regression; extreme dependence on a physician, mate, or parent; diffuse anger; impulsive behavior; or depression. The problem is further complicated when hormone therapy is used to treat the infertility, because the therapy may temporarily increase depression in some patients. Mood and cognition can be altered by pharmacological agents used to treat disorders of ovulation or to hyperstimulate the ovaries.

Persons who have difficulty conceiving may experience shock, disbelief, and a general sense of helplessness, and they develop an understandable preoccupation with the problem. Involvement in the infertility workup and the development of expertise about infertility can be a constructive defense against feelings of inadequacy and the humiliating, sometimes painful aspects of the workup itself. Worries about attractiveness and sexual desirability are common. Partners may feel ugly or impotent, and episodes of sexual dysfunction and loss of desire are reported. These problems are aggravated when a couple is scheduling sexual relations according to temperature charts or ovulatory cycles. Treatments for infertility (Table 30–2) are expensive and consume much time and energy. Both men and women can be overwhelmed by complexity, cost, invasiveness, and uncertainty associated with medical intervention.

Single persons who are aware of their own infertility may shy away from relationships for fear of being rejected once their "defect" is known. Persons who are infertile may have particular difficulty in their adult relationships with their own parents. The identification and equality that come from sharing the experience

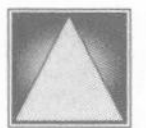

Table 30–1
Focused History for Infertility Workup

Medical History	Female Partner	Male Partner
Medical history and review of systems	Current medical problems and medication, allergies, hirsutism, thyroid dysfunction, weight gain, diabetes mellitus	Current medical problems and medication, allergies, erectile function, exposure to high temperatures
Surgical history	Fallopian tube surgery, ectopic pregnancy, appendectomy, pelvic surgery	Hernia repair, testicular or varicocele surgery
Sexual history	Frequency of intercourse, timing of intercourse with ovulation kit, dyspareunia	History of contraception use, excessive use of lubricants
Infertility history	Prior fertility, history of infertility treatments, duration of infertility	Prior fertility or infertility
Social history	Use of tobacco, caffeine, tetrahydrocannabinol (THC), recreational drugs, exposure to chemotherapy or radiation, psychosocial stressors	Use of tobacco, caffeine, THC, recreational drugs, exposure to chemotherapy or radiation
Developmental history	Menarche, breast development, dysmenorrhea, history of sexually transmitted diseases, use of prior contraception, diethylstibestrol (DES) exposure, history of abnormal Papanicolaou smear and subsequent treatment	Degree of virilization, testicular infections, genital trauma, undescended testes, pubertal development, history of sexually transmitted diseases

(Adapted from Frey KA, Patel KS. Initial evaluation and management of infertility. *Mayo Clin Proc.* 2004;79(11):1439–1443, with permission.)

of parenthood must be replaced by internal reserves and other generative aspects of their lives.

Professional intervention may be necessary to help infertile couples ventilate their feelings and go through the process of mourning for their lost biological functions and the children they cannot have. Couples who remain infertile must cope with an actual loss. Couples who decide not to pursue parenthood may develop a renewed sense of love, dedication, and identity as a pair. Others may need help in exploring the options of husband or donor insemination, laboratory implantation, and adoption.

FAMILY PLANNING AND CONTRACEPTION

Family planning is the process of choosing when, and if, to bear children. One form of family planning is contraception, the prevention of fecundation, or fertilization of the ovum. The choice of a contraceptive method (Table 30–3) is a complex decision

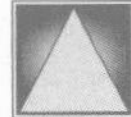

Table 30–2
Assisted Reproduction Techniques

Method	Indication	Procedure
Intrauterine insemination (IUI)	Mild male factor Minimal endometriosis Unexplained infertility	Concentrated sperm is injected into the cervix at ovulation
Therapeutic donor insemination (TDI)	Severe male factor Women without partners Lesbian couples	Timed insemination from anonymous donor. Frozen donor from commercial sperm bank
Ovulation induction or augmentation	Ovulatory dysfunction Polycystic Ovarian Disease (PCOD) Hyperprolactinemia Hypothalamic amenorrhea Premature ovarian failure	Stimulates multifollicular development and ovulation. May produce multiple births
In vitro fertilization and embryo transfer (IVF-ET)	Tubal factor Severe endometriosis Unexplained infertility Male factor Premature ovarian failure Perimenopause	Ovarian hyperstimulation followed by human chorionic gonadotropin (hCG) administration. Retrieved oocytes then combined with sperm in Petri dish for fertilization. Embryos incubated in growth media and transferred back into uterus. May be performed with cryoembryo transfer or donor oocytes.
Intracytoplasmic sperm injection (ICSI)	Congenital absence of vas deferens Azoospermia Previous vasectomy	Injection in vitro of sperm head or sperm DNA directly to cytoplasm of oocyte to cause fertilization and production of embryos
Gestational carrier	Women without a uterus Women with medical conditions precluding carrying term pregnancy Gay male couples	IVF with transfer of embryos to a woman with a uterus to carry pregnancy to term. A highly controversial technique with unclear legal ramifications.

(Adapted from Brigham and Women's Hospital. *Infertility: A Guide to Evaluation, Treatment, and Counseling.* Boston, MA: Brigham and Women's Hospital; 2003:11, with permission.)

Table 30–3
Current Methods of Contraception

Type	Efficacy	Advantages	Disadvantages	Potential Complications
Barrier (Chemical or Mechanical)				
Spermicidal agents	Moderate	Readily available and easy to use	Messy; loss of spontaneity	Allergic reactions Does not prevent sexually transmitted diseases (STDs)
Diaphragm Cervical cap	Moderate	Inexpensive Does not interfere with menstrual cycle or hormones	Requires prescription and professional fitting User familiarity required	Recurrent urinary tract infections Requires refit with >10 lb. change in weight Allergic reactions Does not prevent STDs
Male condom	Moderate	Readily available and easy to use Protects against STDs	Loss of spontaneity	Allergy to latex is rare
Female condom	Moderate	Readily available and easy to use Protects against STDs	Loss of spontaneity Expensive	Allergy to latex is rare
Hormonal (suppresses ovulation and/or impairs endometrial development)				
Oral contraceptives (estrogen/progesterone concentrations vary)	High	Inexpensive; potential absolute efficiency; not coitally connected	Pharmacological side effects Daily or weekly ingestion Requires professional visit and prescription	Increased risk of thromboembolism, migraine headaches, and hypertension depression Nausea May be contraindicated in some medical conditions and smokers
Progestin implants (Norplant rods)	High	Effective for 5 years Effective for dysfunctional uterine bleeding	Irregular bleeding Requires minor surgery to implant and remove	Amenorrhea Minimal risk of infections For use only with patients with a low risk of STDs
Injectable steroids	High	Injections every three months Useful for compliance or if OCPs not an option	Slow return of ovarian function after last use Significant bone loss	Amenorrhea Irritability and depression Irregular bleeding Acne Hair loss Weight gain
Estrogen-progestin patch	High	Transdermal patch applied weekly for 1 month	Back-up method required if patch falls off	Increased exposure to estrogen over OCPs, which increases risk of clotting, myocardial infarction, and stroke
Vaginal ring	High	Use for 3 weeks for continual absorption of hormones	Back-up method required if ring is removed for >3 hours	Rare vaginal irritation and discharge
Intrauterine Device (IUD)				
Copper T IUD or Levonorgesterel IUD	High	Reversible Effective emergency contraception May be used up to 10 years	Requires professional insertion Annual checkup required	No protection against STDs May increase menstrual bleeding
Sterilization				
Male sterilization (vasectomy)	High	Failure very rare; 20-minute office procedure	Morbidity in 1% to 2% of patients includes infections, clots	Can be reversed in only 80% of cases; rare neurotic impotence reaction
Female sterilization	High	Almost 100% protection; no impairment of sexual function or pleasure	More complex procedure than vasectomy; reversal is complicated and difficult	Surgical morbidity Risk of ectopic pregnancy in those who do become pregnant
Emergency				
Oral steroid	Moderate	Accessible and easy to administer Levonorgesterel (Plan B) or OCP combination dosages	75% efficacy	Nausea Abdominal pain Menstrual irregularity Headache

(continued)

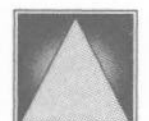

Table 30–3 (Continued)

Type	Efficacy	Advantages	Disadvantages	Potential Complications
Copper T IUD	High	Insertion within 5 days of intercourse 99% efficacy	Requires physician insertion	For use when efficacy is most important and for continued use of IUD
Mifepristone	Moderate	Single dose of 10 mg within 5 days of intercourse 99% efficacy	Emergency dose not available in the United States	Dose of 600 mg is an abortifactant dose
Other				
Rhythm Withdrawal Coitus interruptus	Low	No cost or health risks No professional help required	Imposed coital timing	Essentially none
Natural family planning	Moderate	Readily available	Must monitor cervical mucus and basal body temperature Imposed coital timing	Essentially none

(Adapted and modified from Brigham and Women's Hospital by Seeba Anam, M.D. *Contraception and Family Planning: A Guide to Counseling and Management.* Boston, MA: Brigham and Women's Hospital; 2005, with permission.)

involving both women and their partners. Factors influencing the decision include a woman's age and medical condition, her access to medical care, the couple's religious beliefs, and the need for coital spontaneity. The woman and her partner can weigh the risks and benefits of the various forms of contraception and make their decision on the basis of their current lifestyle and other factors. The success of contraceptive technology has enabled career-minded couples to delay child-bearing into their 30s and 40s. Such a delay, however, may increase infertility problems. Consequently, many women with careers feel their biological clocks ticking and plan to have children while in their early 30s to avoid the risk of not being able to have them at all.

Sterilization

Sterilization is a procedure that prevents a man or a woman from producing offspring. In a woman, the procedure is usually salpingectomy, ligation of the fallopian tubes, a procedure with low morbidity and low mortality. A man is usually sterilized by vasectomy, excision of part of the vas deferens, which is a simpler procedure than salpingectomy, and can be performed in a physician's office. Voluntary sterilization, especially vasectomy, has become the most popular form of birth control in couples married for more than 10 years.

A small proportion of patients who elect sterilization may suffer a neurotic poststerilization syndrome, which can manifest through hypochondriasis, pain, loss of libido, sexual unresponsiveness, depression, and concerns about masculinity or femininity. One study of a group of women who regretted sterilization reported they had chosen the procedure while in poor relationships, frequently with abusive partners. Regret is most prevalent when a woman forms a new relationship and wishes to have a child with a new partner. Psychiatric consultation may be necessary to separate persons seeking sterilization for irrational or psychotic reasons from those who have made the decision after some time and thought.

In the United States, involuntary sterilization procedures have been performed to prevent the reproduction of traits considered genetically undesirable, and various statutes allowed sterilization of hereditary criminals, sex offenders, syphilitic patients, mentally retarded persons, and persons with epilepsy. Some of these statutes have been declared unconstitutional, and human rights and civil liberties groups have challenged the legality and ethical standing of such sterilization procedures with increasing vigor.

The operative procedures for sterilization, namely vasectomy and tubal ligation, have assumed less importance than in the past because of the advent of contraceptives and the relative ease of obtaining abortions. Nonetheless, sterilization procedures are still chosen by men and women who, for a variety of reasons, want to permanently end their ability to produce children.

Abortion

Induced abortion is the planned termination of a pregnancy. About 1.3 million abortions are performed in the United States each year—246 abortions for every 1,000 live births. Over the last decade, the number of abortions has declined by about 15 percent. Family planning experts believe that more sex education and greater availability of contraceptive devices keep the number of abortions down. In Western countries, most women who obtain abortions are young, unmarried, and primiparous; in emerging countries, abortion is most common among married women with two or more children.

Of abortions, 60 percent are performed before 8 weeks of gestation, 88 percent are performed before 13 weeks, and 4.1 percent between 16 and 20 weeks, with 1.4 percent occurring after 21 weeks. Table 30–4 summarizes the most common abortion techniques. Table 30–5 compares medical and surgical abortion techniques.

Abortion has become a political and philosophical issue in the United States. The country is sharply divided between prochoice (pro-abortion) and pro-life (anti-abortion) factions. In recent years, anti-abortion demonstrators have picketed abortion clinics and have provoked angry confrontations with patients. The atmosphere of moral condemnation and intimidation may make the decision to terminate a pregnancy difficult.

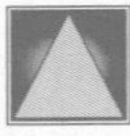

Table 30–4
Pregnancy Termination

Method	Description	Comments
Surgical		
Suction curettage	First trimester. Cervical dilatation is performed using rods, then a cannula is inserted into the uterus and uterine contents are aspirated.	May be performed as soon as intrauterine pregnancy is confirmed, 5 to 13 weeks. Can be performed under local anesthesia in an outpatient setting. Cervical laceration and uterine perforations are rare complications. Most common risks are infection, bleeding, or need for repeat procedure for blood clots.
Dilatation and extraction	Second trimester. On the first day, the cervix is dilated with *laminaria. Misoprostol or second day of laminaria is sometimes necessary for further dilatation. Extraction is performed on the second or third day.	Morbidity is lower than with induction of labor. Hemorrhage from uterine perforation, cervical laceration, uterine atony, or retained products of conception. Complication rates increase with advancing gestational age and are greatest over 20 weeks gestation.
Induction of labor with misoprostol, oxytocin, or prostaglandin gel	Second trimester. *Laminaria are placed for cervical dilatation, then labor is induced with misoprostol.	Risk of hemorrhage, infection, uterine rupture. Risk of failure or retained placenta requiring dilatation and extraction or curettage.
Medical		
Mifepristone	First trimester, within 9 weeks of pregnancy.	92%–98% rate of complete termination when given with Misoprostol. Associated with gastrointestinal discomfort, vaginal bleeding. Requires access to ultrasonography and surgical back-up, as well as transfusion resources in case of serious bleeding or incomplete abortion. Reliable follow-up required.

*Laminaria: a sterile rod made of kelp (*genus Laminaria*), which is hydrophilic, and, when placed in the cervical canal, absorbs moisture, swells, and gradually dilates the cervix.

(Adapted from Brigham and Women's Hospital. *Contraception and Family Planning: A Guide to Counseling and Management.* Boston, MA: Brigham and Women's Hospital; 2005:15, with permission.)

Psychological Reactions to Abortion. Recent studies demonstrate that most women who have an abortion for an unwanted pregnancy (i.e., induced abortion) were satisfied with their decision with few, if any, negative psychological sequelae. Women who had miscarriages however, (i.e., spontaneous abortion) reported a high rate of dysphoric reactions. The difference can be explained, in part, by the fact that most women who induced abortion did so because they did not want the child. Women who spontaneously miscarried presumably wanted their babies. In the long term, however, women who had induced abortion were more likely to be upset about the procedure than women who had a miscarriage.

Second-trimester abortions are more psychologically traumatic than first-trimester abortions. The most common reason for late abortions is the discovery (via amniocentesis or ultrasound) of an abnormal karyotype or fetal anomaly. Thus, late abortions usually involve the loss of a wanted child with whom the mother has already formed a bond.

Before the legalization of abortion in the United States in 1973, many women sought illegal abortions, often performed by untrained practitioners under nonsterile conditions. Considerable morbidity and mortality were associated with these abortions, and women who were denied abortion sometimes chose suicide over continuation of an unwanted pregnancy. When a woman is forced to carry a fetus to term, the risk increases of infanticide, abandonment, and neglect of the unwanted newborn.

Abortion can also be a significant experience for men. If a man has a close relationship with the woman, he may wish to play an active role in the abortion by accompanying her to the hospital or abortion clinic and providing emotional support. Fathers may experience considerable grief over the termination of a wanted pregnancy.

Table 30–5
Comparison of Medical and Surgical Pregnancy Termination

Termination	Medical	Surgical
Timing	Up to 9 weeks gestation	As soon as intrauterine pregnancy confirmed, as early as 5 weeks
Anesthesia	None	Required
Side Effects	Pain, bleeding expected	Usually minimal side effects
Efficacy	92% to 98% effective	98% to 99% effective
Privacy	Termination likely to occur at home	Procedure in surgical suite or office

(Adapted from Brigham and Women's Hospital. *Contraception and Family Planning: A Guide to Counseling and Management.* Boston, MA: Brigham and Women's Hospital; 2005:15, with permission.)

Reproductive Senescence

Both men and women age and experience an age-related decline in reproductive capacity, but only women experience complete gonadal cessation. Loss of reproductive capacity may present a psychological challenge to those who are not reconciled to the loss of fertility. Even with gonadal failure, however, the availability of donor oocytes and sperm means that pregnancy can be initiated in a menopausal woman with an intact uterus who elects to pursue that option. Studies have shown that older men may develop a genetic sperm mutation giving rise to a higher incidence of autistic or schirophienic offspring.

Menopause

Menopause, the cessation of ovulation, generally occurs between 47 and 53 years of age. The hypoestrogenism that follows can lead to hot flashes, sleep disturbances, vaginal atrophy and dryness, and cognitive and affective disturbances. Women are at increased risk for osteoporosis, dementia, and cardiovascular disease. Depression at menopause has been attributed to the "empty nest syndrome." Many women, however, report an enhanced sense of well-being and enjoy opportunities to pursue goals postponed because of child rearing.

PSYCHIATRIC ASPECTS OF PREGNANCY

Postpartum Depression

Many women experience some affective symptoms during the postpartum period, 4 to 6 weeks following delivery. Most of these women report symptoms consistent with "baby blues," a transient mood disturbance characterized by mood lability, sadness, dysphoria, subjective confusion, and tearfulness. These feelings, which may last several days, have been ascribed to rapid changes in women's hormonal levels, the stress of childbirth, and the awareness of the increased responsibility that motherhood brings. No professional treatment is required other than education and support for the new mother. If the symptoms persist longer than 2 weeks, evaluation is indicated for postpartum depression.

Postpartum depression is characterized by a depressed mood, excessive anxiety, insomnia, and change in weight. The onset is generally within 12 weeks after delivery. No conclusive evidence indicates that "baby blues" will lead to a subsequent episode of depression. Several studies do indicate that an episode of postpartum depression increases the risk of lifetime episodes of major depression. Treatment of postpartum depression is not well studied because of the risk of transmitting antidepressants to newborns during lactation. Table 30–6 differentiates postpartum "baby blues" from postpartum depression.

A syndrome described in fathers is characterized by mood changes during their wives' pregnancies or after the babies are born. These fathers are affected by several factors: added responsibility, diminished sexual outlet, decreased attention from his wife, and the belief that the child is a binding force in an unsatisfactory marriage.

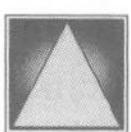

Table 30–6
Comparison of "Baby Blues" and Postpartum Depression

Characteristic	"Baby Blues"	Postpartum Depression
Incidence	30% to 75% of women who give birth	10% to 15% of women who give birth
Time of onset	3 to 5 days after delivery	Within 3 to 6 months after delivery
Duration	Days to weeks	Months to years, if untreated
Associated stressors	No	Yes, especially lack of support
Sociocultural influence	No; present in all cultures and socioeconomic classes	Strong association
History of mood disorder	No association	Strong association
Family history of mood disorder	No association	Some association
Tearfulness	Yes	Yes
Mood lability	Yes	Often present, but sometimes mood is uniformly depressed
Anhedonia	No	Often
Sleep disturbance	Sometimes	Nearly always
Suicidal thoughts	No	Sometimes
Thoughts of harming the baby	Rarely	Often
Feelings of guilt, inadequacy	Absent or mild	Often present and excessive

(From Miller LJ. How "baby blues" and postpartum depression differ. *Women's Psychiatric Health.* 1995:13, with permission. Copyright 1995, The KSF Group.)

Postpartum Psychosis

Postpartum psychosis (sometimes called *puerperal psychosis*) is an example of psychotic disorder not otherwise specified that occurs in women who have recently delivered a baby. The syndrome is often characterized by the mother's depression, delusions, and thoughts of harming either herself or her infant. Such ideation of suicide or infanticide must be carefully monitored; although rare, some mothers have acted on these ideas. Most available data suggest a close relation between postpartum psychosis and mood disorders, particularly bipolar disorder and major depressive disorder.

The incidence of postpartum psychosis is about 1 to 2 per 1,000 childbirths. About 50 to 60 percent of affected women have just had their first child, and about 50 percent of cases involve deliveries associated with nonpsychiatric perinatal complications. About 50 percent of the affected women have a family history of mood disorders. The most robust data indicate that an episode of postpartum psychosis is essentially an episode of a mood disorder, usually a bipolar disorder but possibly a depressive disorder. Relatives of those with postpartum psychosis have an incidence of mood disorders that is similar to the incidence in relatives of persons with mood disorders. As many as two thirds of the patients have a second episode of an underlying affective disorder during the year after baby's birth. The delivery process may best be seen as a nonspecific stress that causes the development of an episode of a major mood disorder, perhaps through a major hormonal mechanism.

The symptoms of postpartum psychosis can often begin within days of the delivery, although the mean time to onset is within 2 to 3 weeks and almost always within 8 weeks of delivery. Characteristically, patients begin to complain of fatigue, insomnia, and restlessness, and they may have episodes of tearfulness and emotional lability. Later, suspiciousness, confusion, incoherence, irrational statements, and obsessive concerns about the baby's health and welfare may be present. Delusional material may involve the idea that the baby is dead or defective.

Patients may deny the birth and express thoughts of being unmarried, virginal, persecuted, influenced, or perverse. Hallucinations with similar content may involve voices telling the patient to kill the baby or herself. Complaints regarding the inability to move, stand, or walk are also common.

The onset of florid psychotic symptoms is usually preceded by prodromal signs such as insomnia, restlessness, agitation, lability of mood, and mild cognitive deficits. Once the psychosis occurs, the patient may be a danger to herself or to her newborn, depending on the content of her delusional system and her degree of agitation. In one study, 5 percent of patients committed suicide and 4 percent committed infanticide. A favorable outcome is associated with a good premorbid adjustment and a supportive family network. Subsequent pregnancies are associated with an increased risk of another episode, sometimes as high as 50 percent.

As with any psychotic disorder, clinicians should consider the possibility of either a psychotic disorder caused by a general medical condition or a substance-induced psychotic disorder. Potential general medical conditions include hypothyroidism and Cushing's syndrome. Substance-induced psychotic disorder can be associated with the use of pain medications such as pentazocine (Talwin) or of antihypertensive drugs during pregnancy. Other potential medical causes include infections, toxemia, and neoplasms.

Postpartum psychosis is a psychiatric emergency. Antipsychotic medications and lithium (Eskalith), often in combination with an antidepressant, are the treatments of choice. No pharmacological agents should be prescribed to a woman who is breastfeeding. Suicidal patients may require transfer to a psychiatric unit to help prevent a suicide attempt.

The mother is usually helped by contact with her baby if she so desires, but the visits must be closely supervised, especially if the mother is preoccupied with harming the infant. Psychotherapy is indicated after the period of acute psychosis, and therapy is usually directed at helping the patient accept and be at ease with the mothering role. Changes in environmental factors may also be indicated, such as increased support from the husband and others in the environment. Most studies report high rates of recovery from the acute illness.

Mrs. Z is a 30-year-old high school teacher living in Lagos, Nigeria. She is married and has five children. The birth of her last child was complicated by hemorrhage and sepsis, and she was still hospitalized on the gynecology service for 13 days after delivery when her gynecologist requested a psychiatric consultation. Mrs. Z was agitated and seemed to be in a daze. She said to the psychiatrist: "I am a sinner. I have to die. My time is past. I cannot be a good Christian again. I need to be reborn. Jesus Christ should help me. He is not helping me." A diagnosis of postpartum psychosis was made. An antipsychotic drug, chlorpromazine (Thorazine), was prescribed, and Mrs. Z was soon well enough to go home. Three weeks later, she was readmitted, this time to the psychiatric ward, claiming she "had had a vision of the spirits" and was "wrestling with the spirits." Her relatives reported that at home she had been fasting and "keeping a vigil" through the nights and was not sleeping. She had complained to the neighbors that there was a witch in her house. The witch turned out to be her mother. Mrs. Z's husband, who was studying engineering in Europe, hurriedly returned and took over the running of the household, sending his mother-in-law away and supervising Mrs. Z's treatment himself. She improved rapidly on an antidepressant medication and was discharged in 2 weeks. Her improvement, however, was short-lived. She threw away her medications and began to attend mass whenever one was given, pursuing the priests to ask questions about scriptures. Within 1 week, she was readmitted. On the ward, she accused the psychiatrist of shining powerful torchlights on her and taking pictures of her, opening her chest, using her as a guinea pig, poisoning her food, and planning to bury her alive. She claimed to receive messages from Mars and Jupiter and announced that there was a riot in town. She clutched her Bible to her breast and accused all the doctors of being "idol worshippers," calling down the wrath of her god on all of them. After considerable resistance, Mrs. Z was finally convinced to accept electroconvulsive treatment, and she became symptom free after six treatments. At this point, she attributed her illness to a difficult childbirth, the absence of her husband, and her unreasonable mother. She saw no further role for doctors, called for her priest, and began to speak of her illness as a religious experience that was similar to the experience of religious leaders throughout history. However, her symptoms did not return, and she was discharged after 6 weeks of hospitalization. (Courtesy of Bushra Naz, M.D., Laura J. Fochtmann, M.D., and Evelyn J. Bromet, Ph.D.)

Psychotropic Medications in Pregnancy

No definitive answers exist to the questions of which psychotropic medications are safest during pregnancy and lactation. In patients with worsening psychiatric illness during pregnancy, outpatient psychotherapy, hospitalization, and milieu therapy should be attempted before routine use of psychotropic medication. The risks and benefits of treatment with psychotropics versus maternal psychiatric illness must be carefully evaluated on an individual basis. If the patient, her psychiatrist, and her obstetrician decide to continue psychiatric medications throughout pregnancy, the dosage should be calibrated to the physiological changes each trimester. Although no antidepressant medications have been associated with intrauterine death or major birth defects, both selective serotonin reuptake inhibitors (SSRIs) and tricyclic antidepressants (TCAs) are associated with a transient perinatal syndrome. Studies demonstrate that fluoxetine (Prozac) has been found in amniotic fluid. Mood stabilizers are associated with more consequential teratogenic risks, namely cardiac anomalies and neural tube defects, but women with bipolar disorder are at a significant risk of relapse without medication maintenance. Lithium has been associated with an increased risk of Ebstein's anomaly, a congenital downward displacement of the tricuspid valve into the right ventricle.

The US Food and Drug Administration (FDA) rates drugs in five categories of safety for use in pregnancy (Table 30–7). In general, all medications that are not absolutely essential should be avoided during pregnancy.

Teratogens

Teratogens are drugs or other agents that cause abnormal fetal development. Infections such as varicella, toxoplasmosis, and herpes simplex, among others, can interfere with normal development. Pregnant women who smoke are subject to premature births, and congenital defects are more common in smokers than in nonsmokers. Alcohol abuse is associated with fetal alcohol syndrome (see Section 12.2). Other drugs of abuse, such

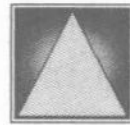

Table 30–7
FDA Rating of Drug Safety in Pregnancy

Category	Definition	Drug Examples
A	No fetal risks in controlled human studies	Iron
B	No fetal risk in animal studies, but no controlled human studies or fetal risk in animals, but no risk in well-controlled human studies	Acetaminophen
C	Adverse fetal effects in animals and no human data available	Aspirin, haloperidol, chlorpromazine
D	Human fetal risk seen (may be used in life-threatening situation)	Lithium, tetracycline, ethanol
X	Proved fetal risk in humans (no indication for use, even in life-threatening situations)	Valproic acid, thalidomide

as cocaine and heroin, produce drug-dependent newborns. In general, pregnant women should not use prescription and over-the-counter drugs and phytomedicinals. Drugs given in the third trimester are rarely teratogenic. Retinoids (used to treat acne) taken early in pregnancy have been associated with fetal abnormalities.

Premenstrual Dysphoric Disorder (PMDD)

Premenstrual dysphoric disorder is a somatopsychic illness triggered by changing levels of sex steroids that accompany an ovulatory menstrual cycle. It occurs about 1 week before the onset of menses and is characterized by irritability, emotional lability, headache, anxiety, and depression. Somatic symptoms include edema, weight gain, breast pain, syncope, and paresthesias. Approximately 5 percent of women have the disorder. Treatment is symptomatic and includes analgesics for pain and sedatives for anxiety and insomnia. Some patients respond to short courses of SSRIs. Fluid retention is relieved with diuretics.

An appendix in the 4th edition revised of the *Diagnostic and Statistical Manual of Mental Disorders* (DSM-IV-TR) includes suggested diagnostic criteria for PMDD to help researchers and clinicians evaluate the validity of the diagnosis (Table 30–8). Nevertheless, the generally recognized syndrome involves mood symptoms (e.g., lability), behavior symptoms (e.g., changes in eating patterns), and physical symptoms (e.g., breast tenderness, edema, and headaches). This pattern of symptoms occurs at a specific time during the menstrual cycle, and the symptoms resolve for some period of time between menstrual cycles. The hormonal changes occurring during the menstrual cycle are probably involved in producing symptoms, although the exact etiology is unknown.

Because of the absence of generally agreed-on diagnostic criteria, the epidemiology of premenstrual dysphoria is not known with certainty. Up to 80 percent of all women experience some alteration in mood, sleep, or somatic symptoms during the premenstrual period, and about 40 percent of these women have at least mild to moderate premenstrual symptoms prompting them to seek medical advise. Only 3 to 7 percent of women have symptoms that meet the full diagnostic criteria for PMDD.

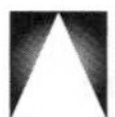

Table 30–8
DSM-IV-TR Research Criteria for Premenstrual Dysphoric Disorder

A. In most menstrual cycles during the past year, five (or more) of the following symptoms were present for most of the time during the last week of the luteal phase, began to remit within a few days after the onset of the follicular phase, and were absent in the week postmenses, with at least one of the symptoms being either (1), (2), (3), or (4):
  (1) markedly depressed mood, feelings of hopelessness, or self-deprecating thoughts
  (2) marked anxiety, tension, feelings of being "keyed up," or "on edge"
  (3) marked affective lability (e.g., feeling suddenly sad or tearful or increased sensitivity to rejection)
  (4) persistent and marked anger or irritability or increased interpersonal conflicts
  (5) decreased interest in usual activities (e.g., work, school, friends, hobbies)
  (6) subjective sense of difficulty in concentrating
  (7) lethargy, easy fatigability, or marked lack of energy
  (8) marked change in appetite, overeating, or specific food cravings
  (9) hypersomnia or insomnia
  (10) a subjective sense of being overwhelmed or out of control
  (11) other physical symptoms, such as breast tenderness or swelling, headaches, joint or muscle pain, a sensation of "bloating," weight gain

  Note: In menstruating females, the luteal phase corresponds to the period between ovulation and the onset of menses, and the follicular phase begins with menses. In nonmenstruating females (e.g., those who have had a hysterectomy), the timing of luteal and follicular phases may require measurement of circulating reproductive hormones.

B. The disturbance markedly interferes with work or school or with usual social activities and relationships with others (e.g., avoidance of social activities, decreased productivity and efficiency at work or school).

C. The disturbance is not merely an exacerbation of the symptoms of another disorder, such as major depressive disorder, panic disorder, dysthymic disorder, or a personality disorder (although it may be superimposed on any of these disorders).

D. Criteria A, B, and C must be confirmed by prospective daily ratings during at least two consecutive symptomatic cycles. (The diagnosis may be made provisionally prior to this confirmation.)

(From American Psychiatric Association. *Diagnostic and Statistical Manual of Mental Disorders.* 4th ed. Text rev. Washington, DC: American Psychiatric Association; copyright 2000, with permission.)

Given that most women who experience changes in affect or somatic symptoms during the premenstrual period are not severely functionally impaired, it is important to distinguish these women from those who are diagnosed with PMDD. Premenstrual syndrome is distinguished from PMDD by the severity and number of symptoms, as well as the degree to which function is impaired. Table 30–9 lists the diagnostic criteria for PMS in which the patient reports at least one of the affective or somatic symptoms during the 5 days before menses in each of the three prior menstrual cycles.

The course and the prognosis of PMDD have not been studied sufficiently to reach any reasonable conclusions. Anecdotally, the symptoms tend to be chronic unless effective treatment is initiated. Treatment of PMDD includes support for the patient

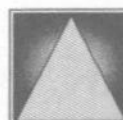

Table 30–9
Diagnostic Criteria for Premenstrual Syndrome

Affective Symptoms	Somatic Symptoms
Depression	Breast tenderness
Irritability	Abdominal bloating
Anxiety	Headache
Confusion	Swelling of extremities
Social withdrawal	

(Adapted from American College of Obstetricians and Gynecologists [ACOG] Practice Bulletin #15, April 2000, with permission.)

about the presence and recognition of the symptoms. SSRIs, for example, fluoxetine and alprazolam (Xanax), have all been reported to be effective, although no treatment has been conclusively demonstrated to be effective in multiple, well-controlled trials. If symptoms are present throughout the menstrual cycle, with no intercycle symptom relief, clinicians should consider one of the nonmenstrual cycle-related mood disorders and anxiety disorders. The presence of especially severe symptoms, even if cyclical, should prompt clinicians to consider other mood disorders and anxiety disorder. A thorough medical workup is necessary to rule out medical or surgical conditions to account for symptoms (e.g., endometriosis).

OTHER ISSUES

Sexually Transmitted Diseases

A sexually transmitted disease (STD) is a contagious disease acquired as a result of a physical sexual interaction. From the 1950s through 1970s, the infections were considered treatable and not life threatening. Acquired immune deficiency syndrome (AIDS), which is caused by infection with human immunodeficiency virus (HIV), is currently incurable, life threatening, and transmissible from mother to fetus. The specter of AIDS has captured the popular imagination. Although it was initially found in male homosexuals and intravenous drug abusers, HIV knows no boundaries.

A sequela of STDs, such as gonorrhea and chlamydia, is pelvic inflammatory disease (PID). Untreated, PID can develop into bilateral tuboovarian abscesses and necessitate hysterectomy and bilateral salpingo-oophorectomy. Early antibiotic treatment is advocated to prevent development of the abscesses and to reduce the likelihood of infertility, chronic pelvic pain, and ectopic pregnancy from tubal damage. These infections also can lead to obstruction of the vas deferens and chronic prostatitis and subsequent male infertility.

Another STD that can have serious consequences is venereal warts, or human papillomavirus (HPV). Genital infections with certain subtypes of HPV can lead to premalignant changes of the penis, vulva, vagina, and cervix and are thought to cause cervical cancer. Venereal warts can be removed chemically or surgically, but are difficult to eradicate completely. Women who contract HPV are encouraged to have regular gynecological examinations and Papanicolaou smears to detect premalignant lesions. An HPV vaccine exists which is recommended for all girls 11 to 12 years of age to decrease the incidence of certain strains of HPV virus. This vaccine would then decrease the incidence of genital warts and cervical cancer.

Sexual monogamy and abstinence, which will prevent most STDs, are advocated as public health measures. Libidinal impulses, however, can be difficult to control and restrict. Therefore, measures such as condom use are strongly recommended as an alternative public health measure. Adolescents, in particular, need to know the potential consequences of sexual activity with regard to STDs and pregnancy. Admonishing teens to remain chaste is unlikely to be completely effective and may be counterproductive. The risks of sexual intercourse may be forgotten or seem minimal in comparison to the need for affection or escape. Persons with low self-esteem or under stress may view sex as a means of bolstering their self-image or escaping their stresses. The reinforcing properties of sex ensure that the problem of STDs will endure. Studies in Europe, especially Holland, have shown that easy availability of condoms (e.g., in schools) reduces both STDs and unwanted pregnancies.

Pelvic Pain

Pelvic pain can have many causes, including endometriosis, pelvic adhesions, ovarian or adnexal masses, hernias, and bowel or rectal disease. Pelvic pain can also be secondary to psychogenic causes such as guilt, fertility, or fears of infertility, and the emotional disturbances associated with ongoing or past incest or sexual abuse. Pelvic pain should not be attributed to psychogenic causes unless a thorough evaluation has excluded organic causes. In most instances, the evaluation should include a diagnostic laparoscopy. Likewise, dyspareunia or pain with intercourse should not be assumed to have a psychogenic origin unless all anatomical causes have been excluded.

Pseudocyesis

Pseudocyesis (false pregnancy) is the development of the classic symptoms of pregnancy—amenorrhea, nausea, breast enlargement and pigmentation, abdominal distention (Fig. 30–2), and labor pains—in a nonpregnant woman. Pseudocyesis demonstrates the ability of the psyche to dominate the soma, probably via central input at the level of the hypothalamus. Predisposing psychological processes are thought to include a pathological wish for, and fear of, pregnancy; ambivalence or conflict regarding gender, sexuality, or childbearing; and a grief reaction to loss following a miscarriage, tubal ligation, or hysterectomy. The patient may have a true somatic delusion that is not subject to reality testing, but often a negative pregnancy test result or pelvic ultrasound scan leads to resolution. Psychotherapy is recommended during or after a presentation of pseudocyesis to evaluate and treat the underlying psychological dysfunction. A related event, couvade, occurs in some cultures in which the father of the child undergoes simulated labor, as though he were giving birth. In those societies couvade is a normal phenomenon.

Miss S, aged 16, thought she had become pregnant after her first coital experience, which occurred without contraception. Shortly after she read about the signs and symptoms of pregnancy, her menses stopped. She related that she felt tingling in her breasts, which she believed were enlarged. She also reported nausea and vomiting in the morning, which was observed by her mother. On examination, the uterus was enlarged, breasts were developed with dark areola and

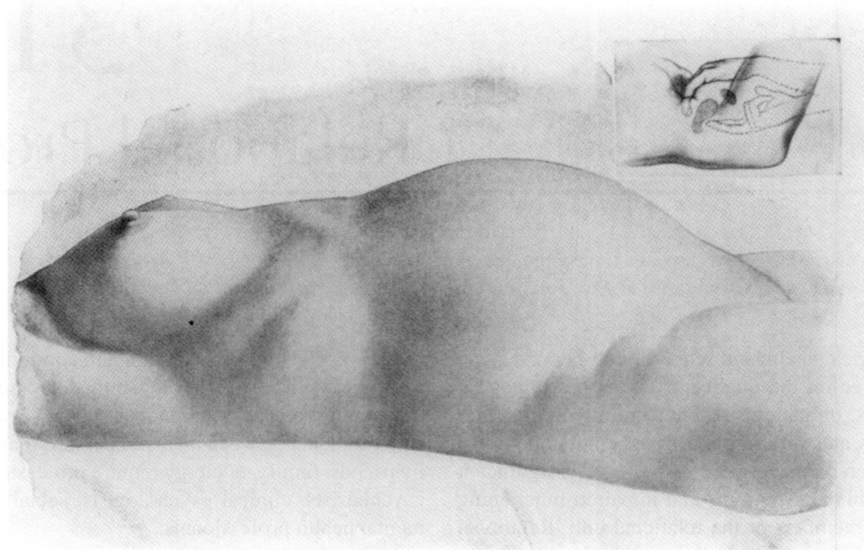

FIGURE 30–2
Patient at 36th (?) week. Bimanual examination revealed uterus normal in size and position.

contained milk, and a pigmented line was observed from the umbilicus to the pubis. The abdomen was not enlarged, but she believed she felt fetal movement. A pregnancy test had negative results and the patient was so informed; however, she could not be dissuaded of her belief that she was pregnant. She entered psychotherapy, and within 2 months her menses returned and she accepted the fact that she was not pregnant.

Hyperemesis Gravidarum

Hyperemesis gravidarum is differentiated from morning sickness in that vomiting is chronic, persistent, and frequent, leading to ketosis, acidosis, weight loss, and dehydration. The prognosis is excellent for both mother and fetus with prompt treatment. Most women can be treated as outpatients, with changing to smaller meals, discontinuing iron supplements, and avoiding certain foods. In severe cases, hospitalization may be necessary. Although the cause is unknown, a psychological component may exist. Women with histories of anorexia nervosa or bulimia nervosa may be at risk.

Pica

Pica is the repeated ingestion of nonnutritive substances, such as dirt, clay, starch, sand, and feces. This eating disorder is most often seen in young children, but is common in pregnant women in some subcultures, most notably among African American women in the rural South, who may eat clay or starch (e.g., Argo). The cause of pica is unknown, but it may be related to nutritional deficiencies in the mother.

References

Berga SL, Marcus MD, Loucks TL, Hlastala S, Ringham R, Krohn MA. Recovery of ovarian activity in women with functional hypothalamic amenorrhea who were treated with cognitive behavior therapy. *Fertil Steril*. 2003;80:976–981.

Berga SL, Parry PL, Cyranowski JM. Psychiatry and reproductive medicine. In: Sadock BJ, Sadock VA, eds. *Kaplan & Sadock's Comprehensive Textbook of Psychiatry*. 8th ed. Vol. 2. Baltimore: Lippincott Williams & Wilkins; 2005: 2293.

Bloch M, Rotenberg N, Koren D, Klein E. Risk factors for early postpartum depressive symptoms. *Gen Hosp Psychiatry*. 2006;28(1):3–8.

Dell DL. Premenstrual syndrome, premenstrual dysphoric disorder, and the premenstrual exacerbation of another disorder. *Clin Obstet Gynec*. 2004;47: 571.

Kroll R, Rapkin AJ. Treatment of premenstrual disorders. *J Reprod Med*. 2006;51[4 Suppl]:359 –370.

Lamberg L. Risks and benefits key to psychotropic use during pregnancy and postpartum period. *JAMA*. 2005;294:1604–1608.

Nelson HD, Humphrey LL, Nygen P. Postmenopausal hormone replacement therapy: Scientific review. *JAMA*. 2002;288:882.

Rosenberg R, Greening D, Windell J. *Conquering Postpartum Depression: A Proven Plan for Recovery*. Cambridge, MA: Perseus Pub.; 2003.

Seyfried LS, Marcus SM. Postpartum mood disorders. *International Review of Psychiatry*. 2003;15:231–242.

Yonkers KA, Wisner KL, Stowe Z, Leibenluft E, Cohen L, Miller L, Manber R, Viguera A, Suppes T, Altshuler L. Management of bipolar disorder during pregnancy and the postpartum period. *Am J Psychiatry*. 2004;161:608–620.

31 Relational Problems

An adult's psychological health and sense of well-being depend to a significant degree on the quality of his or her important relationships—that is, on patterns of interaction with a partner and children, parents and siblings, and friends and colleagues. Problems in the interaction between any of these significant others can lead to clinical symptoms and impaired functioning among one or more members of the relational unit. Relational problems may be a focus of clinical attention (1) when a relational unit is distressed and dysfunctional or threatened with dissolution and (2) when the relational problems precede, accompany, or follow other psychiatric or medical disorders. Indeed, other medical or psychiatric symptoms can be influenced by the relational context of the patient. Conversely, the functioning of a relational unit is affected by a member's general and other medical or psychiatric illness. Relational disorders require a different clinical approach than other disorders. Instead of focusing primarily on the link between symptoms, signs, and the workings of the individual mind, the clinician must also focus on interactions between the individuals involved and how these interactions are related to the general and other medical or psychiatric symptoms in a meaningful way.

DEFINITION

According to the text revision of the fourth edition of *Diagnostic and Statistical Manual of Mental Disorders* (DSM-IV-TR), relational problems are patterns of interaction between members of a relational unit that are associated with symptoms or significantly impaired functioning in one or more individual members or with significantly impaired functioning of the relational unit itself. DSM-IV-TR distinguishes five categories of relational problems: (1) relational problem related to a mental or general medical condition; (2) parent–child relational problem; (3) partner relational problem; (4) sibling relational problem; and (5) relational problem not otherwise specified.

EPIDEMIOLOGY

No reliable figures are available on the prevalence of relational problems. They can be assumed to be ubiquitous; however, most relational problems resolve without professional intervention. The nature, frequency, and effects of the problem on those involved are elements that must be considered before a diagnosis of relational problem is made. For example, divorce, which occurs in just under 50 percent of marriages, is a problem between partners that is resolved through the legal remedy of divorce and need not be diagnosed as a relational problem. If the persons cannot resolve their disputation and continue to live together in a sadomasochistic or pathologically depressed relationship with unhappiness and abuse, then they should be so labeled. Relationship problems between involved persons that cannot be resolved by friends, family, or clergy require professional intervention by psychiatrists, clinical psychologists, social workers, and other mental health professionals.

RELATIONAL PROBLEM RELATED TO A MENTAL DISORDER OR GENERAL MEDICAL CONDITION

According to DSM-IV-TR, the category of relational problem related to a mental disorder or general medical condition "should be used when the focus of clinical attention is a pattern of impaired interaction associated with a psychiatric disorder or a general medical condition in a family member."

Studies indicate that satisfying relationships may have a health-protective influence, whereas relationship distress tends to be associated with an increased incidence of illness. The influence of relational systems on health has been explained through psychophysiological mechanisms that link the intense emotions generated in human attachment systems to vascular reactivity and immune processes. Thus, stress-related psychological or physical symptoms can be an expression of family dysfunction.

Adults must often assume responsibility for caring for aging parents while they are still caring for their own children, and this dual obligation can create stress. When adults take care of their parents, both parties must adapt to a reversal of their former roles, and the caretakers not only face the potential loss of their parents, but also must cope with evidence of their own mortality.

Some caretakers abuse their aging parents—a problem that is now receiving attention. Abuse is most likely to occur when the caretaking offspring have substance abuse problems, are under economic stress, and have no relief from their caretaking duties, or when the parent is bedridden or has a chronic illness requiring constant nursing attention. More women are abused than men, and most abuse occurs in persons over age 75.

The development of a chronic illness in a family member stresses the family system and requires adaptation by both the sick person and the other family members. The person who has become sick must frequently face a loss of autonomy, an increased sense of vulnerability, and sometimes a taxing medical regimen. The other family members must experience the loss of the person as he or she was before the illness, and they usually have substantial caretaking responsibility—for example, in debilitating neurological diseases, including dementia of the Alzheimer's type, and in diseases such as acquired immunodeficiency syndrome (AIDS) and cancer. In these cases, the whole family must deal with the stress of prospective death as well as the current illness. Some families use the anger engendered by such situations to create support organizations, increase public awareness of the disease, and rally around the sick member. But chronic illness frequently produces depression in family members and can cause them to withdraw from, or attack, one another. The burden of caring for ill family members falls disproportionately on the women in a family—mothers, daughters, and daughters-in-law.

Chronic emotional illness also requires major adaptations by families. For instance, family members may react with chaos or fear to the psychotic productions of a family member with schizophrenia. The regression, exaggerated emotions, frequent hospitalizations, and economic and social dependence of a person with schizophrenia can stress the family system. Family members may react with hostile feelings (referred to as expressed emotion) that are associated with a poor prognosis for the person who is sick. Similarly, a family member with bipolar I disorder can disrupt a family, particularly during manic episodes.

Family devastation can occur when illness (1) suddenly strikes a previously healthy person, (2) occurs earlier than expected in the life cycle (some impairment of physical capacities is expected in old age, although many older persons are healthy), (3) affects the economic stability of the family, and (4) when little can be done to improve or ease the condition of the sick family member.

PARENT–CHILD RELATIONAL PROBLEM

Parents differ widely in sensing the needs of their infants. Some quickly note their child's moods and needs; others are slow to respond. Parental responsiveness interacts with the child's temperament to affect the quality of the attachment between child and parent. According to DSM-IV-TR, the diagnosis of parent–child relational problem applies when the focus of clinical attention is a pattern of interaction between parent and child that is associated with clinically significant impairment in individual or family functioning or with clinically significant symptoms. Examples include impaired communication, overprotection, and inadequate discipline.

Research on parenting skills has isolated two major dimensions: (1) a permissive-restrictive dimension and (2) a warm-and-accepting versus cold-and-hostile dimension. A typology that separates parents on these dimensions distinguishes between *authoritarian* (restrictive and cold), *permissive* (minimally restrictive and accepting), and *authoritative* (restrictive as needed, but also warm and accepting) parenting styles. Children of authoritarian parents tend to be withdrawn or conflicted; those of permissive parents are likely to be more aggressive, impulsive, and low achievers; and children of authoritative parents seem to function at the highest level, socially and cognitively. Yet, switching from an authoritarian to a permissive mode may create a negative reinforcement pattern.

Difficulties in many situations stress the usual parent–child interaction. Substantial evidence indicates that marital discord leads to problems in children, from depression and withdrawal to conduct disorder and poor performance at school. This negative effect may be partly mediated through *triangulation* of the parent–child relationships, which is a process in which conflicted parents attempt to win the sympathy and support of their child, who is recruited by one parent as an ally in the struggle with the partner. Divorces and remarriages stress the parent–child relationship and may create painful loyalty conflicts. Stepparents often find it difficult to assume a parental role and may resent the special relationship that exists between their new marital partner and the children from that partner's previous marriages. The resentment of a stepparent by a stepchild and the favoring of a natural child are usual reactions in a new family's initial phases of adjustment. When a second child is born, both familial stress and happiness may result, although happiness is the dominant emotion in most families. The birth of a child can also be troublesome when parents had adopted a child in the belief that they were infertile. Single-parent families usually consist of a mother and children, and their relationship is often affected by financial and emotional problems.

Other situations that can produce a parent–child problem are the development of fatal, crippling, or chronic illness, such as leukemia, epilepsy, sickle-cell anemia, or spinal cord injury, in either parent or child. The birth of a child with congenital defects, such as cerebral palsy, blindness, and deafness, may also produce parent–child problems. These situations, which are not rare, challenge the emotional resources of those involved. Parents and child must face present and potential loss and must adjust their day-to-day lives physically, economically, and emotionally. These situations can strain the healthiest families and produce parent–child problems not only with the sick person but also with the unaffected family members. In a family with a severely sick child, parents may resent, prefer, or neglect the other children because the ill child requires so much time and attention.

Parents with children who have emotional disorders face particular problems, depending on the child's illness. In families with a child with schizophrenia, family treatment is beneficial and improves the social adjustment of the patient. Similarly, family therapy is useful when a child has a mood disorder. In families with a substance-abusing child or adolescent, family involvement is crucial to help control the drug-seeking behavior and to allow family members to verbalize the feelings of frustration and anger that are invariably present.

Normal developmental crises can also be related to parent–child problems. For instance, adolescence is a time of frequent conflict, as the adolescent resists rules and demands increasing autonomy, and, at the same time, elicits protective control by displaying immature and dangerous behavior.

> The parents of sons aged 18, 15, and 11 years presented with distress about the behavior of their middle child. The family had been cohesive with satisfactory relationships among all members until 6 months before this consultation. At that time, the 15-year-old began seeing a girl from a comparatively unsupervised household. Frequent arguments had developed between parents and son regarding going out on school nights, curfews, and neglect of schoolwork. The son's combativeness and lowered academic achievement upset his parents a great deal. They had not experienced similar conflicts with their oldest child. The adolescent, however, maintained a good relationship with his siblings and friends, was not a behavior problem at school, continued to participate on the school basketball team, and was not a substance user.

Day Care Centers

Quality of care during the first 3 years of life is crucial to neuropsychological development. A 1997 study from the National Institute of Child Health and Human Development indicated that day care was not harmful to children, when the caregivers and day care teachers provided consistent, empathetic, nurturing care. Not all day care centers can meet that level of care, however, especially those located in poor urban areas. Children receiving less than optimal caring exhibit decreased intellectual and verbal skills that indicate delayed neurocognitive development. They may also become irritable, anxious, or depressed, which interferes with the parent–child bonding experience, and they are less assertive and less effectively toilet trained by the age of 5.

Currently, more than 55 percent of women are in the work force, many of whom have no choice but to place their children in day care centers. Approximately 40 percent of entering medical students are women; few medical centers, however, make adequate provisions for on-site day care centers for their students or staff. Similarly, corporations need to provide on-site, high-quality care for the children of their employees. Not only will that approach benefit the children, but also corporate economic benefits will accrue as a result of reduced absenteeism, increased productivity, and happier working mothers. Such programs have the added benefit of decreasing stresses on marriages.

PARTNER RELATIONAL PROBLEM

According to DSM-IV-TR, clinicians should use the category partner relational problem when the focus of clinical attention is a pattern of interaction between the spouses or partners. These patterns are characterized by negative communication (e.g., criticisms), distorted communication (e.g., unrealistic expectations), or noncommunication (e.g., withdrawal), associated with clinically significant impairment in individual or family functioning or symptoms in one or both partners.

When persons have partner relational problems, psychiatrists must assess whether a patient's distress arises from the relationship or from a mental disorder. Mental disorders are more common in single persons—those who never married or who are widowed, separated, or divorced—than among married persons. Clinicians should evaluate developmental, sexual, and occupational and relationship histories, for purposes of diagnosis. (Divorce is discussed in Chapter 2, Section 2.4, and couples therapy is discussed in Chapter 35, Section 35.4.)

Marriage demands a sustained level of adaptation from both partners. In a troubled marriage, a therapist can encourage the partners to explore areas such as the extent of communication between the partners, their ways of solving disputes, their attitudes toward child-bearing and child-rearing, their relationships with their in-laws, their attitudes toward social life, their handling of finances, and their sexual interaction. The birth of a child, an abortion or miscarriage, economic stresses, moves to new areas, episodes of illness, major career changes, and any situations that involve a significant change in marital roles can precipitate stressful periods in a relationship. Illness in a child exerts the greatest strain on a marriage, and marriages in which a child has died through illness or accident more often than not end in divorce. Complaints of lifelong anorgasmia or impotence by marital partners usually indicate intrapsychic problems, although sexual dissatisfaction is involved in many cases of marital maladjustment.

Adjustment to marital roles can be a problem when partners are from different backgrounds and have grown up with different value systems. For example, members of low socioeconomic status groups perceive a wife as making most of the decisions in the family, and they accept physical punishment as a way to discipline children. Middle-class persons perceive family decision-making processes as shared, with the husband often being the final arbiter, and they prefer to discipline children verbally. Problems involving conflicts in values, adjustment to new roles, and poor communication are handled most effectively when therapist and partners examine the couple's relationship, as in marital therapy.

Epidemiological surveys show that unhappy marriages are a risk factor for major depressive disorder. Marital discord also affects physical health. For example, in a study of women aged 30 to 65 years with coronary artery disease, marital stress worsened the prognosis 2.9 times for recurrent coronary events. Marital conflict was also associated with a 46 percent higher relative death risk among female patients having hemodialysis, and with elevations in serum epinephrine, norepinephrine, and corticotrophin levels in both men and women. In one study, high levels of hostile marital behavior were associated with slower healing of wounds, lower production of proinflammatory cytokines, and higher cytokine production in peripheral blood. Overall, women show greater psychological and physiological responsiveness to conflict than men.

Physician Marriages

Physicians have a higher risk of divorce than other occupational groups. The incidence of divorce among physicians is about 25 to 30 percent. Specialty choice influenced divorce. The highest rate of divorce occurred in psychiatrists (50 percent), followed by surgeons (33 percent) and internists, pediatricians, and pathologists (31 percent). The average age at first marriage was 26 years among all groups.

It is not clear why physicians are at high risk for divorce. Factors implicated include the stresses of dealing with dying patients, making life-and-death decisions, working long hours, and the constant risk of malpractice litigation. Such stressors may predispose physicians to a variety of emotional ills, with the most common being depression and substance abuse, including alcoholism. Such persons generally cannot deal with the complex interactions required to maintain successful long-term relationships of any kind, and marriage requires the most interpersonal skills of all.

SIBLING RELATIONAL PROBLEM

According to DSM-IV-TR, the category of sibling relational problem "should be used when the focus of clinical attention is a pattern of interaction between siblings, associated with clinically significant impairment of family functioning, or symptoms in one or more of the siblings."

Sibling relationships tend to be characterized by competition, comparison, and cooperation. Intense sibling rivalry can occur with the birth of a child and can persist as the children grow up, compete for parental approval, and measure their accomplishments against one another. Alliances between siblings are equally common. Siblings may learn to protect one another against parental control or aggression. In households with three children, one pair tends to become closely involved with one another, leaving the extra child in the position of outsider.

Relational problems can arise when siblings are not treated equally; for instance, when one child is being idealized, while another is cast in the role of the family scapegoat. Differences in gender roles and expectations expressed by the parents can underlie sibling rivalry. Parent–child relationships also are dependent on personality interactions. A child's resentment directed at a parental figure or a child's own disavowed dark emotions can be projected onto a sibling and can fuel an intense hate relationship.

A child's general, other medical or psychiatric condition always stresses the sibling relationships. Parental concern and attention to the sick child can elicit envy in the siblings. In addition, chronic disability can leave the sick child feeling devalued and rejected by siblings, and the latter may develop a sense of superiority and may feel embarrassed about having a disabled sister or brother.

RELATIONAL PROBLEM NOT OTHERWISE SPECIFIED

According to DSM-IV-TR, the category of relational problem not otherwise specified "should be used when the focus of clinical attention is on relational problems not classifiable by any of the specific problems above (e.g., difficulties with superiors and coworkers)."

People, across the life cycle, may become involved in relational problems with leaders and others in their community at large. In such relationships, conflicts are common and can bring about stress-related symptoms. Many relational problems of children occur in the school setting and involve peers. Impaired peer relationships can be the chief complaint in attention-deficit or conduct disorders, as well as in depressive and other psychiatric disorders of childhood, adolescence, and adulthood.

Racial, ethnic, and religious prejudices and ignorance cause problems in interpersonal relationships. In the workplace and in communities at large, sexual harassment is often a combination of inappropriate sexual interactions, inappropriate displays of abuse of power and dominance, and expressions of negative gender stereotypes, primarily toward women and gay men, although also toward children and adolescents of both sexes.

REFERENCES

Bernstein AC. Gender in stepfamilies: Daughters and fathers. In: Silverstein LB, Goodrich TJ, eds. *Feminist Family Therapy: Empowerment in Social Context.* Washington, DC: American Psychological Association; 2003.

Dickstein LJ. Relational problems. In: Sadock BJ, Sadock VA, eds. *Kaplan & Sadock's Comprehensive Textbook of Psychiatry.* 8th ed. Vol. 2. Baltimore: Lippincott Williams & Wilkins; 2005:2241.

Drescher J, D'Ercole A, Schoenberg E, eds. *Psychotherapy with Gay Men and Lesbians: Contemporary Dynamic Approaches.* Binghampton, NY: The Harrington Park Press/The Haworth Press, Inc.; 2003.

Edward J. The loving side of the sibling bond: A force for growth or conflict. *Issues in Psychoanalysis and Psychology.* 2003;25:27–43.

Kirkpatrick DC, Duck S, Foley MK, eds. *Relating Difficulty: The Processes of Constructing and Managing Difficult Interaction.* Mahwah, NJ: Lawrence Erlbaum Associates Publishers; 2006.

Lasenza S. Sexuality: Psychoanalytic perspectives. *J Sex Marital Ther.* 2004;30:53–56.

Looy HA. Gender and sexuality: Constancy and change. In: Vander Stoep SW, ed. *Science and the Soul: Christian Faith and Psychological Research.* Lantham, MD: University Press of America, Inc.; 2003.

Morrongiello BA, Hogg K. Mothers' reactions to children misbehaving in ways that can lead to injury: Implications for gender differences in children's risk taking and injuries. *Sex Roles.* 2004;50:103–118.

Nemeroff CB. Neurobiological consequences of childhood trauma. *J Clin Psychiatry.* 2004;65[Suppl 1]:18–28.

Riley S. Art therapy with couples. In: Malchiodi CA, ed. *Handbook of Art Therapy.* New York: Guilford Press; 2003.

Sanford K. Expectancies and communication behavior in marriage: Distinguishing proximal level effects from distal level effects. *Journal of Social and Personal Relationships.* 2003;20:391–402.

Sholerane G, Pirooz MD, eds with LD Schwoer. *Textbook of Family and Couples Therapy: Clinical Applications.* Washington, DC: American Psychiatric Press, Inc.; 2003.

Stern DN. The motherhood constellation: Therapeutic approaches to early relational problems. In: Sameroff AJ, McDonough SC, Rosenalum KL, eds. *Treating Parent–Infant Relationship Problems: Strategies for Intervention.* New York: Guilford Press; 2004:29-42.

Vandervoort D, Rokach A. Posttraumatic relationship syndrome: The conscious processing of the world of trauma. *Social Behavior and Personality.* 2003;31:675–686.

Walzer S, Oles TP. Managing conflict after marriages end: A qualitative study of narratives of ex-spouses. *Families in Society.* 2003;84:192–200.

32 Problems Related to Abuse or Neglect

The text revision of the fourth edition of *Diagnostic and Statistical Manual of Mental Disorders* (DSM-IV-TR) specifies five problems related to abuse or neglect: (1) physical abuse of child, (2) sexual abuse of child, (3) neglect of child, (4) physical abuse of adult, and (5) sexual abuse of adult (Table 32–1). Physical abuse of an adult includes spouse or partner abuse and abuse of elderly persons. Sexual abuse of an adult includes rape, sexual coercion, and sexual harassment.

CHILD ABUSE AND NEGLECT

Physical and sexual abuse occurs in girls and boys of all ages, in all ethnic groups, and at all socioeconomic levels. The abuses vary widely with respect to severity and duration, but any form of continued abuse constitutes an emergency situation for the child. Fear, guilt, anxiety, depression, and ambivalence regarding disclosure commonly surround the child who has been abused.

In child neglect, a child's physical, mental, or emotional condition has been impaired because of a parent's or caretaker's inability to provide adequate food, shelter, education, or supervision. In its extreme form, neglect can contribute to failure to thrive. Failure to thrive typically occurs under circumstances in which adequate nourishment is available yet a disturbance within the relationship between the caretaker and the child results in a child who does not eat enough to grow and develop. For a further discussion of failure to thrive, see Section 34.3, Psychiatric Emergencies in Children.

Epidemiology

Each year, the Children's Bureau, an agency within the Department of Health and Human Services, collects data on child maltreatment. The results are published in an annual document called *Child Maltreatment*. The agency estimated that, in 2004, approximately 3 million alleged victims were reported to child protective services. Of those reports, more than 870,000 were substantiated; this represents 2.03 of every 1,000 children. The substantiated cases were distributed as follows: neglect, 62 percent; physical abuse, 18 percent; sexual abuse, 10 percent; and emotional abuse, 7 percent. The Children's Bureau estimated that 1,400 children died as the result of abuse or neglect in 2004: 36 percent from neglect and 28 percent from physical abuse. Approximately 81 percent of these deaths were children younger than 4 years of age.

The data were analyzed for patterns of maltreatment by the sex and age of victims. Rates of many types of maltreatment were similar for boys and girls, but the sexual abuse rate for girls was higher than the sexual abuse rate for boys. Examining the age distribution of victims, the age group from 0 to 3 years of age had the highest victimization rate, and the rate of victimization declined as the age of the victims increased. For example, the rate for infants (0 to 3 years of age) was 16 per 1,000, whereas the rate for adolescents (16 to 17 years of age) was 6 per 1,000. Regarding the perpetrators of abuse, it was reported that, overall, 58 percent were female, and 42 percent were male.

Etiology

Many factors contribute to child abuse and neglect. Abusive parents have themselves often been victims of physical and sexual abuse and of long-term exposure to violent home lives of pain and physical torment, which are powerful promoters of aggression. Thus, parents brought up with harsh corporal punishment and cruel treatment by their own families may continue the abuse tradition with their children. In some cases, adults believe that their methods are acceptable ways of teaching discipline. In other cases, parents are ambivalent about their methods of abusive parenting, but find themselves without coping mechanisms and so fall into behaviors similar to those of their own parents.

Stressful living conditions, such as overcrowding and poverty, can contribute to aggressive behavior and may contribute to physical abuse toward children. Social isolation, the lack of a support system, and parental substance abuse increase the potential for abusive and neglectful treatment of children. When such environmental crises as unemployment, housing problems, and financial need heighten stress levels in vulnerable families, neglect or abuse may ensue. Mental disorders can play a role in child abuse and neglect insofar as a parent's judgment and thought processes may be impaired. Parents who are depressed or psychotic or who have severe personality disorders may view their children as bad or as trying to drive them crazy.

Certain characteristics can increase a child's vulnerability to neglect and physical and sexual abuse. Children who are premature, mentally retarded, or physically disabled and those who cry excessively or are unusually demanding—the so-called difficult child—may be at high risk for abuse or neglect. Many abused children are perceived by their parents as different, slow in development, bad, selfish, or hard to discipline. Children who are

Table 32–1
DSM-IV-TR Problems Related to Abuse or Neglect

Physical abuse of child
This category should be used when the focus of clinical attention is physical abuse of a child.
Sexual abuse of child
This category should be used when the focus of clinical attention is sexual abuse of a child.
Neglect of child
This category should be used when the focus of clinical attention is child neglect.
Physical abuse of adult
This category should be used when the focus of clinical attention is physical abuse of an adult (e.g., spouse beating, abuse of elderly parent).
Sexual abuse of adult
This category should be used when the focus of clinical attention is sexual abuse of an adult (e.g., sexual coercion, rape).

(Reprinted with permission from American Psychiatric Association. *Diagnostic and Statistical Manual of Mental Disorders.* 4th ed. Copyright, Washington, DC: American Psychiatric Association; 1994.)

hyperactive are particularly vulnerable to abuse, especially when they are born to parents with limited capacities for nurturing behavior. A child who is the object of physical abuse is also known as a *battered child.*

The perpetrator of physical abuse is more often the mother than the father. One parent is usually the active batterer, and the other passively accepts the battering. Of a group of perpetrators studied, 80 percent were regularly living in the homes of the children they abused. More than 80 percent of the children studied were living with married parents, and about 20 percent were living with a single parent. The average age of a mother who abuses her children is reportedly about 26 years; the father's average age is 30 years. Many abused children come from poor homes, and the families tend to be socially isolated.

Abusive parents have inappropriate expectations of their children, with a reversal of dependence needs. Parents treat an abused child as if the child were older than the parents. A parent often turns to the child for reassurance, nurturing, comfort, and protection and expects a loving response. Of such parents, 90 percent were severely physically abused by their own mothers or fathers.

Men usually perpetrate sexual abuse, although women acting in concert with men or alone are also involved, especially in child pornography. Men are the perpetrators in about 95 percent of cases of sexual abuse of girls and about 80 percent of cases of sexual abuse of boys. Perpetrators of sexual abuse are usually known to the child and, in many cases, have been victims of physical or sexual abuse. In some circumstances, pedophilia is a factor; the adult perpetrator is more aroused by children than by adult partners. Many times, however, the perpetrator has no preference for child sexual partners. In some cases, sexual abuse is mixed with physical abuse.

Diagnosis and Clinical Features

Physical Abuse of Child. Clinicians must always consider physical abuse when a child shows bruises or injuries that cannot be adequately explained or that are incompatible with the history that the parent gives. Suspicious physical indicators are bruises and marks that form symmetrical patterns, such as injuries to both sides of the face and regular patterns on the back, buttocks, and thighs; accidental injuries are unlikely to result in symmetrical patterns. Bruises may have the shape of the instrument used to make them, such as a belt buckle or a cord. Burns by cigarettes result in symmetrical, round scars, and immersions in boiling water produce burns that look like socks or gloves or that are doughnut-shaped. Physical aggression can cause multiple and spiral fractures, especially in a young baby; retinal hemorrhages in an infant may result from shaking.

Children repeatedly brought to hospitals for treatment of peculiar or puzzling problems by overly cooperative parents may be victims of Munchausen syndrome by proxy, that is, factitious disorder. In this abuse scenario, a parent repeatedly inflicts illness on, or causes injury to, a child—by injecting toxins or by inducing the child to ingest drugs or toxins to cause diarrhea, dehydration, or other symptoms—and then eagerly seeks medical attention. Because the pathological parents are stealthy and superficially compliant, this is a difficult diagnosis to make.

In hospital emergency rooms, severely abused children show external evidence of body trauma, bruises, abrasions, cuts, lacerations, burns, soft tissue swellings, and hematomas (Fig. 32-1). Hypernatremic dehydration, after periodic water deprivation of children by mothers who are usually psychotic, is another form of child abuse. Inability to move certain extremities because of dislocations and fractures associated with neurological signs of intracranial damage can also indicate inflicted trauma. Other clinical signs and symptoms attributed to inflicted abuse may include injury to the viscera. Abdominal trauma can result in unexplained ruptures of the stomach, the bowel, the liver, or the pancreas, with manifestations of an injured abdomen. Children with the most severe maltreatment injuries arrive at the hospital or physician's office in a coma or in convulsions; some arrive dead.

Behaviorally, abused children may appear withdrawn and frightened or may show aggressive behavior and labile mood. They often exhibit depression, poor self-esteem, and anxiety. They may try to physically cover up injuries and are usually reticent to disclose the abuse for fear of retaliation. Abused children often show some delay in developmental milestones; they may have difficulties with peer relationships and may engage in self-destructive or suicidal behaviors.

Carol, 4 years of age, had a change in her behavior at preschool approximately 3 months after the birth of her sister. Her teacher saw Carol push other children and hit a classmate with a wooden block, causing a laceration of the child's lip. When Carol's teacher took her aside to talk about her behavior, she noticed what seemed to be belt marks on Carol's abdomen and forehead. The teacher reported possible child abuse to protective services. Also, the family was referred for psychiatric evaluation.

Carol's baby sister was colicky and slept only for short periods of time throughout the day and night. She stopped crying only when her mother held her. Her mother, therefore, had little time for Carol, and Carol's father took over her care on evenings after day care and on weekends. He began to drink more than usual and became increasingly irritable. The parents argued over the mother's attention to the infant and the requirement that the father take care of Carol. Carol, who was a bright, curious, and talkative child, constantly asked questions and often asked to carry the baby. When refused,

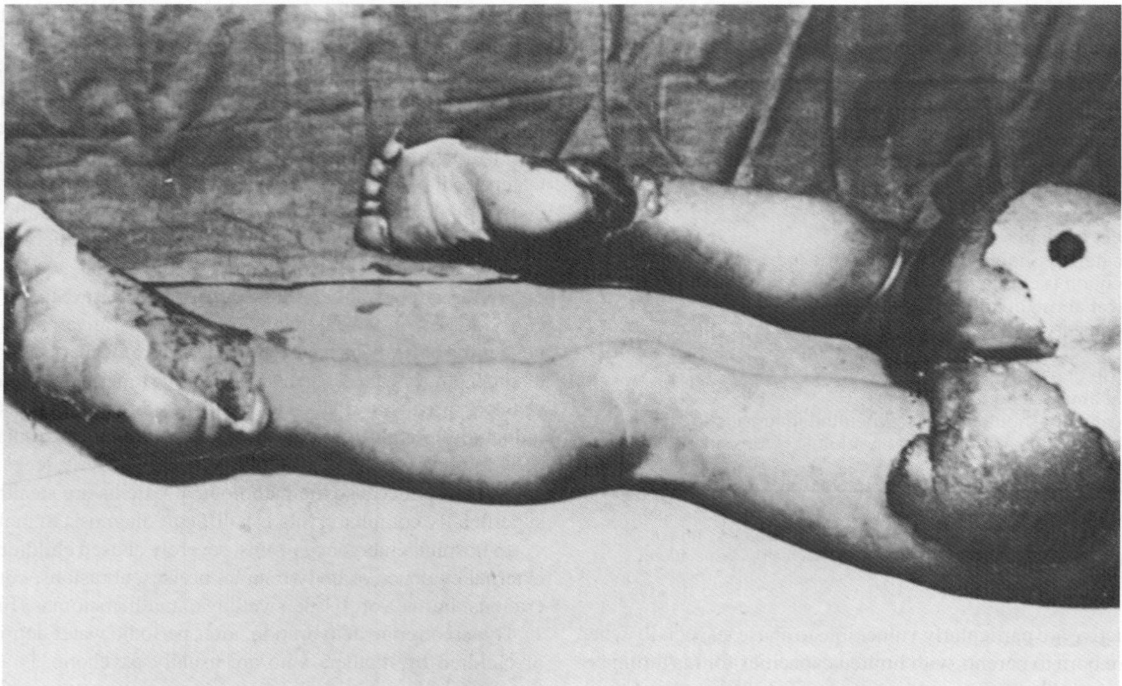

FIGURE 32–1
A $3^1/_2$-year-old boy, brought into an emergency room by his mother, had second-degree burns of his buttocks, perineum, hands, and feet. His mother related that the child accidentally fell into a tub of hot water while preparing to take a bath. Physical examination revealed no evidence of burns along the body area. The location of the burns led physicians to suspect that the child's buttocks were forced into boiling water, and, in an attempt to keep himself from being submerged, he extended his feet and hands into the water. Scalding injury to his feet, perineum, and buttocks caused burn areas corresponding to the child's posture on dunking. His mother later admitted that a boyfriend had placed the child into a tub of hot water while she was out shopping. (Courtesy of Vincent J. Fontana, M.D.)

she would lie on the floor and have a tantrum. She also began to have difficulty falling asleep and awoke repeatedly during the night. Carol's father was unable to cope with her requests for attention and often told her to shut up and slapped her when she continued her demands. On many occasions, he responded to her tantrums or repeated questions by hitting her with his belt.

While protective services monitored the situation, Carol and her parents began a family therapy program that included parenting training and behavioral therapy for Carol, which was coordinated with the preschool. Carol's father attended Alcoholics Anonymous (AA) meetings and stopped drinking. He was able to control his anger at his daughter. Six months later, Carol's aggressive behavior ceased. She was doing well with peers, was sleeping through the night, and stopped having temper tantrums. (Courtesy of William Bernet, M.D.)

Sexual Abuse of Child. Adults within the immediate or extended family of a child perpetrate most child sexual abuse. Thus, children commonly know the sexual abuser, who is often a highly trusted family member with a position of authority and with wide access to the child (Table 32–2). Most cases of sexual abuse involving children are never revealed because of the victim's feelings of guilt, shame, ignorance, and tolerance, compounded by some physicians' reluctance to recognize and report sexual abuse, the court's insistence on strict rules of evidence, and families' fears of dissolution if the sexual abuse is discovered. Despite their familial roles, sexual abusers often threaten to hurt, kill, or abandon the children if the events are disclosed.

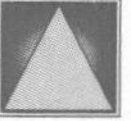

Table 32–2
Sexual Abuse of Children

Reported cases in the United States, 1985[a]	123,000
Prevalence of male abuse	3% to 31%
Prevalence of female abuse	6% to 62%
Perpetrators	
Father or stepfather	7% to 8%
Uncles or older siblings	16% to 42%
Friends	32% to 60%
Strangers	1%
Sexual activity	
Coitus	16% to 29%
Oral sex and intercourse	3% to 11%
Touching genitals	13% to 33%
Age	Peak between ages 9 and 12 25% below age 8
High-risk factors	Child living in single-parent home Marital conflict History of physical abuse Increase in sexual abuse
Reported motivation of abuser	Pedophilic impulses No other sexual object Inability to delay gratification

[a]Current estimates are 150,000 to 200,000 new cases each year.
Data are from Finklehor D. The sexual abuse of children: current research reviewed. *Psychiatr Ann.* 1987;7:4. Percentages may total more than 100% because of overlapping studies.

The incidence of sexual abuse and of child pornography, which is a form of sexual abuse, is much higher than had been previously assumed. Children may be sexually abused as early as infancy and as late as adolescence. Sexual abuse has been reported in schools, day care centers, and group homes, where adult caretakers are the major offenders.

The overwhelming fear, shame, and guilt that contribute to a child's reticence to disclose sexual abuse also complicate identifying the abuse. Most often, no definitive physical evidence can prove the occurrence of sexual abuse. Physical indicators of sexual abuse include bruises, pain, and itching in the genital region. Genital or rectal bleeding may be a sign of sexual molestation. Recurrent urinary tract infections and vaginal discharges may be related to abuse. Sexually transmitted diseases and difficulty walking and sitting raise suspicions of sexual abuse.

No specific behavioral manifestations prove that sexual abuse has taken place, but children may exhibit many possible significant behaviors. Young children who have a detailed knowledge of sexual acts have usually witnessed or participated in sexual behavior. Young sexually abused children often exhibit their sexual knowledge through play and may initiate sexual behaviors with their peers. Aggressive behavior is common among abused children. Children who are extremely fearful of adults, particularly men, may have been subjected to sexual abuse. Clinicians should listen carefully to children who report sexual assaults even when parts of their stories are not consistent. When a child begins to disclose information about sexual assaults, retractions and contradictions are typical, and anxiety may prevent full disclosure.

The diagnosis of sexual abuse in children is full of pitfalls. An estimated 2 to 8 percent of allegations of sexual abuse are false. A much higher percentage of reports cannot be substantiated. Many investigations are done hastily or are carried out by inexperienced evaluators. In custody cases, an allegation of sexual abuse can be a maneuver to limit a parent's visitation rights. Alleged sexual abuse of a preschool-aged child is particularly difficult to evaluate because of the child's immature cognitive and language development. The use of anatomically correct dolls has grown in popularity, but is controversial. Patient and careful evaluations by experienced, objective professionals are necessary, and leading questions must be avoided. Children under the age of 3 years are unlikely to produce a verbal memory of past trauma or abuses, but their experience may be reflected in play or fantasies. Some abused children meet the DSM-IV-TR diagnostic criteria for posttraumatic stress disorder (PTSD).

No specific psychiatric symptom results universally from sexual abuse. Vulnerability to the sequelae of sexual abuse depends on the type of abuse, its chronicity, the age of the child, and the overall relationship of the victim and the abuser. The psychological and physical effects of sexual abuse can be devastating and long lasting. Children who are sexually stimulated by an adult feel anxiety and overexcitement, lose confidence in themselves, and become mistrustful of adults. Seduction, incest, and rape are important predisposing factors to later symptom formations, such as phobias, anxiety, and depression. Abused children tend to be hyperalert to external aggression as shown by an inability to deal with their own aggressive impulses toward others or with others' hostility directed toward them.

Depressive feelings, usually combined with shame, guilt, and a sense of permanent damage, are commonly reported among children who have been sexually abused. Adolescents who have undergone sexual abuse are said to show high rates of poor impulse control and self-destructive and suicidal behaviors. PTSD and dissociative disorders are common in adults who have been sexually abused as children. Sexual abuse is a common preexisting factor in the development of dissociative identity disorder (also known as *multiple personality disorder*). Signs of dissociation include periods in which the children are amnestic, do not feel the pain, or feel that they are somewhere else. Borderline personality disorder has been reported in some patients with histories of sexual abuse. Substance abuse has also been reported with high frequency among adolescents and adults who were sexually abused as children.

INCEST. *Incest* is defined as the occurrence of sexual relations between close blood relatives. A broader definition describes incest as sexual intercourse between participants who are related to each other by a formal or informal kinship bond that is culturally regarded as a bar to sexual relations. For example, sexual relations between stepparents and stepchildren or among stepsiblings are usually considered incestuous, even though no blood relationships exist.

Sociologists have underlined the role of incest prohibitions as socialization factors, and biological factors also support the taboo. Inbreeding groups risk unmasking lethal or detrimental recessive genes and the progeny of inbred groups are generally less fit than less closely related offspring. Anthropologists have observed that different cultures have different types of incest taboos. In *Totem and Taboo*, Sigmund Freud developed the concept of the primal horde, in which young men collectively murdered the group's patriarch, who had kept all the women to himself. According to Freud, the incest taboo arose both from guilt about the murder and from a group's desire to prevent a repetition of the act, further rivalry after the murder, and subsequent disintegration of the horde.

Fathers, stepfathers, uncles, and older siblings most commonly abuse children. A passive, sick, absent, or somehow incapacitated mother, a daughter who takes on a maternal role in the family, a father who abuses alcohol, and overcrowding are features of father–daughter incest common in many homes. Mother–son incest is the strongest and most nearly universal taboo and is the rarest form of incest. Such behavior usually indicates more severe psychopathology in the participants than is the case in father–daughter and sibling incest.

Accurate figures on the incidence of incest are difficult to obtain because of families' shame and embarrassment. Girls are victims more often than are boys; in the United States, about 15 million women have been the objects of incestuous attention, and one third of all sexually abused persons were molested before the age of 9.

Incestuous behavior is reported much more frequently among families of low socioeconomic status than among other families. This difference may be caused by greater contact with reporting officials, such as welfare workers, public health personnel, and law enforcement agents, and does not truly reflect a higher incidence in these families. Incest is more easily hidden by economically stable families than by those of low socioeconomic status.

Social, cultural, physiological, and psychological factors all contribute to the breakdown of the incest taboo. Incestuous behavior has been associated with alcohol abuse, overcrowding, increased physical proximity, and rural isolation that prevents adequate extrafamilial contacts. Some communities are more tolerant of incestuous behavior than is the whole of society. Major mental disorders and intellectual deficiencies can contribute to clinical incest. Some family therapists view incest as a defense designed to maintain a dysfunctional family unit. The older and stronger participant in incestuous behavior is usually male. Thus, incest may be viewed as a form of child abuse, a pedophilia, or a variant of rape.

About 75 percent of reported cases involve father–daughter incest, but parents often deny the occurrence of sibling incest. Other instances of sibling incest involve nearly normal interaction of prepubertal sexual play and exploration. In many cases of father–daughter incest, the daughter has had a close relationship with her father throughout her childhood and may appear to be pleased when he approaches her sexually. The incestuous behavior usually begins when the daughter is 10 years of age. As the behavior continues, however, the abused daughter becomes bewildered, confused, and frightened, and when she nears adolescence, she undergoes physiological changes that add to her confusion. She never knows whether her father is a parent or sexual partner. Her mother may be alternately caring and competitive and may often refuse to believe her daughter's reports or to confront her husband with her suspicion. The daughter's relationships with her siblings are also affected; they sense her special position with her father and treat her as an outsider. The father, fearing that his daughter may expose their relationship and often jealously possessive of her, interferes with her development of normal peer relationships.

Physicians must be aware that intrafamilial sexual abuse can cause a wide variety of emotional and physical symptoms, including abdominal pain, genital irritations, separation anxiety disorder, phobias, nightmares, and school problems. When incest is suspected, clinicians must interview the child apart from the rest of the family.

Homosexual Incest. Father–son and mother–daughter incest are rarely reported, but a family in which same-sex incest occurs is usually highly disturbed, with a violent, alcohol-dependent, or antisocial father; a dependent or disabled mother who is unable to protect her children; and an absence of the usual family roles and individual identities. A son involved in father–son incest is frequently the eldest child, and, if there is a daughter, the father often sexually abuses her as well. Fathers in this situation do not necessarily have any other history of homosexual behavior. Sons may experience homicidal or suicidal ideation and may first consult or be sent to a psychiatrist because of self-destructive behavior.

STATUTORY RAPE. Intercourse is unlawful between a man over 16 years of age and a woman under the age of consent, which varies from 14 to 21 years, depending on the jurisdiction. Thus, a man of 18 and a girl of 15 may have consensual intercourse, yet the man may be held for statutory rape. Statutory rape can vary dramatically from other types of rape in being nonassaultive and nonviolent, and it is not a deviant act unless the age discrepancy is sufficiently large for the man to be defined as a pedophile—that is, when the girl is less than 13 years of age. Parents of a consenting girl, rather than the girl herself, usually press charges of statutory rape.

Neglect of Child.

A maltreated child often shows no obvious signs of being battered, but has multiple minor physical evidences of emotional and, at times, nutritional deprivation, neglect, and abuse. A maltreated child, often brought to a hospital or to a private physician, has a history of failure to thrive, malnutrition, poor skin hygiene, irritability, withdrawal, and other signs of psychological and physical neglect.

Children who have been neglected may show overt failure to thrive at less than 1 year of age. Their physical and emotional development is drastically impaired; they may be physically small and unable to display appropriate social interaction. Hunger, chronic infections, poor hygiene, inappropriate dress, and eventual malnutrition may all be evident. Behaviorally, children who are chronically neglected can be indiscriminately affectionate, even with strangers, or socially unresponsive, even in familiar situations. Neglected children may be runaways or exhibit conduct disorder.

An extreme form of failure to thrive in children 5 years or older is psychosocial dwarfism, in which a chronically deprived child does not grow and develop, even when offered adequate amounts of food. Such children have normal proportions, but are exceedingly small for their age. They often have reversible endocrinological changes resulting in decreased growth hormone, and they cease to grow for a time. Children with this disorder exhibit bizarre eating behaviors and disturbed social relationships. Binge eating, ingestion of garbage or inedible substances, drinking of toilet water, and induced vomiting have been reported.

Parents who neglect their children are often overwhelmed, depressed, isolated, and impoverished. Unemployment, the absence of a two-parent family, and substance abuse can exacerbate the situation. There are several possible prototypes of neglectful mothers. Some young, inexperienced, socially isolated, and ignorant mothers may temporarily be unable to care for their children. Other neglectful mothers are chronically passive and withdrawn women who may have been raised in chaotic, abusive, and neglectful homes. In these cases, once the situation comes to the attention of a child protective agency, the mother often accepts help. Mothers with major mental disorders who view their children as evil or as purposely driving them crazy are difficult to help.

Female Genital Mutilation.

Commonly called "female circumcision," female genital mutilation is performed on an estimated 2 million girls worldwide each year. It is practiced across diverse socioeconomic classes and different ethnic, cultural, and religious groups. Commonly, girls are circumcised between 4 and 10 years of age, but the procedure may be performed on infants, postponed until just before marriage, or done after the birth of the first child. Some cultures consider it part of a ceremonial induction into adult society. Female circumcision, in the mildest form, consists of clitoridectomy, the anatomical equivalent of penile amputation. In its most severe form, total infibulation involves removal of the clitoris and labia minora plus incision of the labia major to create raw surfaces that are then stitched together. This practice has been widely criticized, including opposition by the World Health Organization and other major health care groups. In the United States, female circumcision is generally considered child abuse. Efforts have been made to educate immigrant communities about the health risks and legal liabilities of the practice. Compromise may be possible by finding a way to satisfy the cultural requirements without using mutilation; for example, adopting a nonmutilative ritual incision that results in only small scars on the labia.

Male genital mutilation (circumcision) is not usually considered child abuse, but it does have its critics. Although this simple procedure is one of the most common operations performed worldwide, serious complications may result. These complications include hemorrhage, infection, and penile amputation. In 1999, the American Academy of Pediatrics recommended it not be done as a routine procedure on newborns.

Pathology and Laboratory Examination. Although no definitive laboratory tests are available to help clinicians diagnose child physical or sexual abuse or neglect, a physical examination to detect physical stigmata is indicated when abuse is suspected. In cases of failure to thrive, endocrinological screening is indicated. An external genital examination is indicated in cases of suspected child sexual abuse to detect scars, tears, and genital infections. X-ray evidence of fractures may be present in various stages of reparative changes, but when no fractures or dislocations are apparent on examination, bone repair may become evident within weeks after the specific bone trauma.

Roentgenological examinations of unrecognized traumatic fractures reveal several unusual bone changes (Fig. 32-2). Metaphyseal fragmentation is caused by twisting or pulling of the afflicted extremity. Squaring of the long bones secondary to the new bone formation may be seen on the metaphyseal fragments. Periosteal hemorrhages are frequently noted because the periosteum of infants is not securely attached to the underlying bone. Periosteal calcification follows this hemorrhaging and begins to become apparent 5 to 7 days after the inflicted trauma. A layer of calcification around the shaft of the bone should cause suspicion of inflicted abuse. Epiphyseal separations and periosteal shearing usually result from traction and torsion of the affected extremity. X-ray findings of reparative changes involving excessive new bone formation or previously healed fractures with periosteal reactions may be diagnostic when correlated with other manifestations of child abuse.

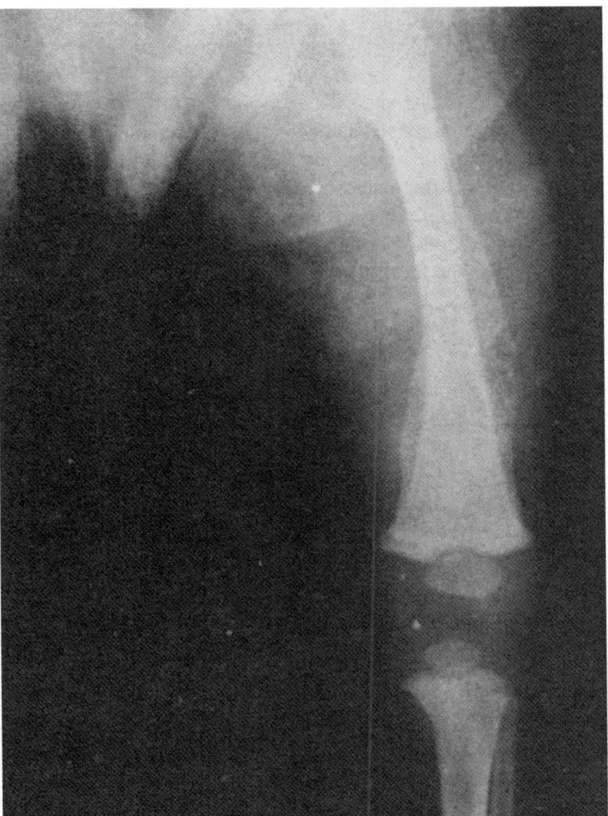

FIGURE 32–2
Follow-up X-ray of a maltreated 6-month-old infant taken 4 weeks after inflicted trauma to the upper thigh. Extensive reparative changes are noted in association with new bone formation, external cortical thickening, and squaring of the metaphysis—diagnostic evidence of bone changes after trauma. The layer of calcification around the shaft of the bone and the presence of bone fragments at the ends of the bone should be evidence for suspicion of inflicted trauma and should prompt further investigations into the causes of the X-ray findings. The X-ray changes may be diagnostic when correlated with other manifestations of physical abuse of child. (Courtesy of Vincent J. Fontana, M.D.)

Differential Diagnosis

Parental feuding and custody disputes are among the factors that complicate identifying and substantiating abuse and neglect situations. When marital discord is severe, children are often caught in the line of fire. A mother who is overwhelmingly hostile toward a separated father may be convinced and may convince a child that the father is abusive. In some cases, parents have gone so far as to fabricate entire abuse scenarios and coach children to repeat them. In other instances, parents may refuse to accept the possibility that a spouse or close relative is the perpetrator of abuse, and they may repeatedly insist that a child stop telling lies, and coerce a child into retracting the disclosures. In either scenario, the child suffers profoundly, and the alleged abuse situation is never disentangled.

When a child speaks in a manner consistent with his or her language development stage, does not sound rehearsed, and does not use adult-like phrasing, the abuse allegations may be true. Distress, the display of precocious sexual behavior, and a knowledge of, or preoccupation with, sexual material also support the possibility of sexual abuse. A child who has not been abused but who is coached to report sexual or physical abuse is also placed under unbearable duress. Therefore, clinicians must recognize that severe chronic parental conflict in which a child is caught can be as destructive as physical and sexual abuse.

Controversies are now arising in the courts because children are accusing caretakers and teachers of sexual abuse, and the children's veracity is being challenged. See Chapter 20 for a discussion of the recovered or false memory syndrome.

Course and Prognosis

The outcome of child physical and sexual abuse and neglect is multifactorial, depending on the severity, duration, and nature of the abuse, and on the child's vulnerabilities. Children who already suffer from mental retardation, pervasive developmental disorders, physical disabilities, disruptive behavior, and attention-deficit disorders are likely to have a poorer outcome than children who are unhampered by mental or physical disorders. Children who are abused for long periods, from the time they are babies or toddlers into adolescence, are likely to be more profoundly damaged than those who have experienced only brief episodes of abuse. The development of mental disorders—such as major depressive disorder, suicidal behavior, PTSD, dissociative identity disorder, and substance abuse—further complicates the long-term prognosis, as does the nature of the relationship between victim and abuser and the adult support figures available to children after disclosure. The best outcomes occur when children are cognitively intact, the abuse is recognized and interrupted in an early phase, and the entire family is capable of participating in treatment.

Treatment

Child. The first part of treating child abuse and neglect is to ensure the child's safety and well-being. Children may need to be removed from abusive or neglectful families to ensure their protection; yet, on an emotional level, a child may feel additionally vulnerable in an unfamiliar setting. Because of the high risk for psychiatric symptoms in abused and neglected children, a comprehensive psychiatric evaluation is in order. Next, along with providing specific treatments for any mental disorders present, a therapist may have to deal with the immediate situation and the long-term implications of the abuse or neglect. Therapists must address several psychotherapeutic issues: dealing with the child's fears, anxieties, and self-esteem; building a trusting adult relationship in which the child is not exploited or betrayed; and ultimately gaining a helpful perspective of the factors contributing to the child's victimization at home.

Ideally, each abused and neglected child should receive an intervention plan based on the assessment of the factors responsible for the parental psychopathology. The plan should include an overall prognosis for parents' achieving adequate parenting skills; the time estimated to achieve meaningful change in their ability to parent; an estimate of whether the parental dysfunction is confined to this child or involves other children, whether the parents' overall malfunctioning, if that is the case, is short term or long term, and whether a mother's malfunctioning is confined to infants as opposed to older children (i.e., when the incidence of abuse is inversely related to a child's age); willingness of those involved to participate in the intervention plan; the availability of personnel and physical resources to implement the various intervention strategies; and the risk of the child sustaining additional physical or sexual abuse by remaining in the home.

Parents. On the basis of the information obtained, several options can be selected to improve parental functioning: (1) eliminate or diminish the social or environmental stresses; (2) lessen the adverse psychological effects of social factors on the parents; (3) reduce the demands on the mother to a level within her capacity through day care placement of the child or provision of a housekeeper or baby-sitter; (4) provide emotional support, encouragement, sympathy, stimulation, instruction in maternal care, and aid in learning to plan for, assess, and meet the needs of the infant (supportive casework); and (5) resolve or diminish the parents' inner psychic conflicts (psychotherapy). Some clinics provide group counseling for nonoffending parents.

INCESTUOUS BEHAVIOR. The first step in the treatment of incestuous behavior is its disclosure. Once a breakthrough of family members' denial, collusion, and fear has been achieved, incest is unlikely to recur. When the participants have severe psychopathology, treatment must be directed toward the underlying illness. Family therapy is useful to reestablish the group as a functioning unit and to develop healthier role definitions for each member. While the participants are learning to develop internal restraints and appropriate ways to gratify their needs, the external control provided by therapy helps prevent further incestuous behavior. At times, legal agencies must help enforce external controls.

Reporting. In cases of suspected child abuse and neglect, physicians should diagnose the suspected maltreatment; secure the child's safety by admitting the child to a hospital or arranging out-of-home placement; report the case to the appropriate social service department, child protection unit, or central registry; make an assessment with the help of a history, a physical examination, a skeletal survey, and photographs; request a social worker's report and appropriate surgical and medical consultations; confer with members of a child abuse committee within 72 hours; arrange a program of care for the child and the parents; and arrange for social service follow-up. Among those generally included as mandated child-abuse reporters are physicians, psychologists, school officials, police officers, hospital personnel engaged in the treatment of patients, district attorneys, and providers of child day care and foster care.

Prevention. To prevent child abuse and neglect, clinicians must identify those families at high risk and intervene before a child becomes a victim. Once high-risk families have been identified, a comprehensive program should include psychiatric monitoring of the families, including the identified high-risk child. Families can be educated to recognize when they are being neglectful or abusive, and alternative coping strategies can be suggested.

In general, child abuse and neglect prevention and treatment programs should try to prevent the separation of parents and children if possible, prevent the placement of children in institutions, encourage parental attainment of self-care status, and encourage the family's attainment of self-sufficiency. As a last resort and to prevent further abuse and neglect, children may have to be removed from families who are unwilling or unable to profit from the treatment program. In cases of sexual abuse, the licensing of day care centers and the psychological screening of persons who work in them should be mandatory to prevent further abuses. Education of the medical profession, members of allied health fields, and all who come in contact with children aid in early detection. Providing support services to stressed families helps to prevent the problem in the first place.

On January 11, 2006, 7-year-old Nixzmary Brown was found dead in what the family called "the dirty room" in an apartment in Brooklyn, New York. She was allegedly bound to a chair, tortured, sexually molested, and starved for weeks. She died from a blow to the head while being dunked in a tub of cold water repeatedly by stepfather, 27-year-old Cesar Rodriguez, over a missing cup of yogurt and a broken printer. Nixzmary weighed only 36 pounds at the time of death.

Two reports were made to the Administration for Children's Services (ACS) in New York City before Nixzmary's death. The first was filed in May, 2004 by school employees after Nixzmary was absent from school for weeks. After speaking with her mother, 27-year-old Nixzaliz Santiago, and Cesar Rodriguez, the case worker found no evidence of neglect or abuse. The second was filed on December 1, 2005 from a person who saw Nixzmary with a swollen eye. The doctor who examined her found her condition to be consistent with the explanation that she fell. ACS kept the case open and continued to communicate with her family to no avail.

Cesar Rodriguez was charged with second-degree murder, sex abuse, and child endangerment. Nixzaliz Santiago was charged with second-degree manslaughter and child endangerment. The five other children living in the household, ages 6 months to 9 years, were removed from the home and placed in the care of the child welfare agency. Three ACS workers who were charged with mishandling the case were terminated.

PHYSICAL ABUSE OF ADULT

Spouse Abuse

Spouse abuse (also known as *domestic violence*) is defined as physical assault within the home in which one spouse is repeatedly assaulted by the other (Fig. 32-3). Spouse abuse is estimated to occur in 2 to 12 million families in the United States. This aspect of domestic violence has been recognized as a severe problem, largely because of recent cultural emphasis on civil rights and the work of feminist groups, but the problem itself is long-standing.

The major problem in spouse abuse is wife abuse. One study estimated that 1.8 million wives are battered in the United States, excluding divorced women and women battered on dates. Wife beating occurs in families of every racial and religious background and in all socioeconomic strata. It is most frequent in families with problems of substance abuse, particularly alcohol and crack abuse. Behavioral, cultural, intrapsychic, and interpersonal factors all contribute to the problem. Abusive men are likely to have come from violent homes where they witnessed wife beating or were abused themselves as children. The act itself is reinforcing; once a man has beaten his wife, he is likely to do so again. Abusive husbands tend to be immature, dependent, and nonassertive and to suffer from strong feelings of inadequacy.

The husbands' aggression is bullying behavior designed to humiliate their wives and to build up their own low self-esteem. Impatient, impulsive, abusive husbands physically displace aggression provoked by others onto their wives. The abuse most likely occurs when a man feels threatened or frustrated at home, at work, or with his peers. The dynamics include identification with an aggressor (father, boss), testing behavior (Will she stay with me, no matter how I treat her?), distorted desires to express manhood, and dehumanization of women. As in rape, aggression is deemed permissible when a woman is perceived as property. About 50 percent of battered wives grew up in violent homes, and their most common trait is dependence.

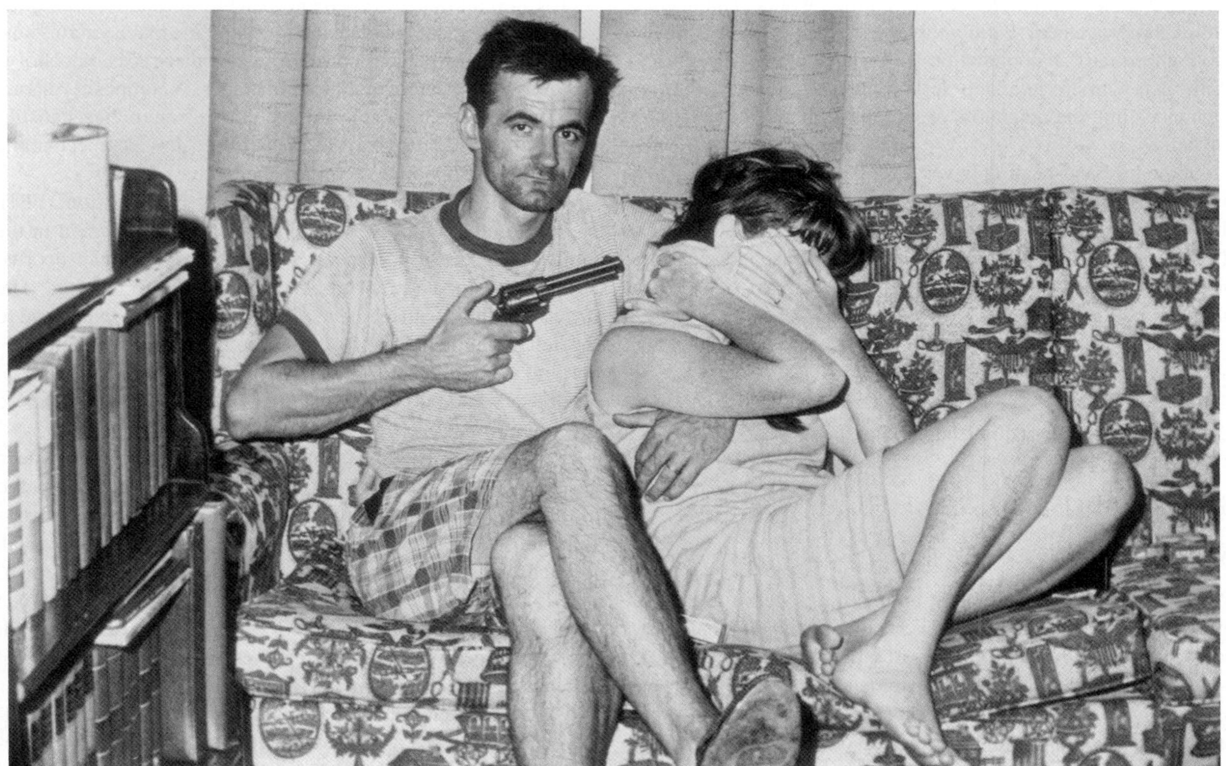

FIGURE 32–3
Photo of a husband holding a pistol aimed at his wife. Shortly after this dramatic photo was taken he agreed to be interviewed by a television reporter. As he stepped from the house using his wife as a shield, he apparently tripped, causing the gun to discharge with a bullet striking his wife in the neck. After the shot, police fired at the husband who was killed. The wife survived her wounds. (Courtesy of Corbis.)

The Surgeon General's office has identified pregnancy as a high-risk period for battering; 15 to 25 percent of pregnant women are physically abused while pregnant, and the abuse often results in birth defects. Hot lines, emergency shelters for women, and other organizations (e.g., the National Coalition Against Domestic Violence) have been established to aid battered wives and to educate the public. One major problem of abused women is finding a place to go when they leave home, frequently in fear of their lives.

Battering is often severe, involving broken limbs, broken ribs, internal bleeding, and brain damage. When an abused wife tries to leave her husband, he often becomes doubly intimidating and threatens to "get" her. If the woman has small children to care for, her problem is compounded. The abusive husband wages a conscious campaign to isolate his wife and make her feel worthless. Women face risks when they leave an abusive husband; they have a 75 percent greater chance of being killed by their batterers than women who stay. New York State prepared a physician reference card to alert and guide doctors about domestic violence (Table 32–3).

Some men feel remorse and guilt after an episode of violent behavior and so become particularly loving. If this behavior gives the wife hope, she remains until the next, inevitable cycle of violence.

When a man is convinced that a woman will no longer tolerate the situation and when she begins to exert control over his behavior, change is initiated. By leaving for a prolonged period, if she is physically and economically able to do so, and by making therapy for the man a condition of return, a woman can begin a cycle of improvement. Family therapy is effective in treating the problem, usually in conjunction with social and legal agencies. With men who are relatively less impulsive, external controls, such as calling the neighbors or the police, may suffice to stop the behavior.

Some husband-beating wives have been also reported. Husbands complain of fear of ridicule if they expose the problem; they fear charges of counterassault and often feel unable to leave the situation because of financial difficulties. Husband abuse has also been reported when a frail, elderly man is married to a much younger woman.

Elder Abuse

Elder abuse is discussed in Chapter 56.

SEXUAL ABUSE OF ADULT

Rape

Rape is the forceful coercion of an unwilling victim to engage in a sexual act, usually sexual intercourse, although anal intercourse and fellatio can also be acts of rape. Using this definition, one survey found that one of six women and 1 of 33 men have experienced an attempted or completed rape as a child or as an adult in the United States. Rape can occur between married partners and between persons of the same sex. The crime of rape requires only slight penile penetration of the victim's outer vulva; full erection and ejaculation are unnecessary for defining the crime. Forced acts of fellatio and anal penetration, although they frequently accompany rape, are legally considered sodomy.

The problem of rape is most appropriately discussed under the heading of aggression. Rape is an act of violence and humiliation that happens to be expressed through sexual means. Rape expresses power or anger; sex is rarely the dominant issue because sexuality is used in the service of nonsexual needs.

Rape of Women. Between 680,000 and 1.5 million women are raped annually in the United States. One of every eight adult women, or at least 12.1 million American women, is estimated to become the victim of forcible rape sometime in her lifetime. The male rapist can be categorized into separate groups: sexual sadists, who are aroused by the pain of their victims; exploitive predators, who use their victims as objects for their gratification in an impulsive way; inadequate men, who believe that no woman would voluntarily sleep with them and who are obsessed with fantasies about sex; and men for whom rape is a displaced expression of anger and rage. Some believe that the anger was originally directed toward a wife or mother, but feminist theory proposes that a woman serves as an object for the displacement of aggression that a rapist cannot express directly toward other men. Women are considered men's property or vulnerable possessions, a rapist's instrument for revenge against other men.

Rape often accompanies another crime. Rapists always threaten their victims, with fists, a knife, or a gun, and frequently harm them in nonsexual ways as well. Victims can be beaten, wounded, and killed.

Statistics show that most men who commit rapes are between 25 and 44 years of age; 51 percent are white and tend to rape white victims, 47 percent are black and tend to rape black victims, and the remaining 2 percent come from all other races. Alcohol is involved in 34 percent of all forcible rapes. A composite characterization of the archetypical rapist drawn from police statistics portrays a single 19-year-old man from a low socioeconomic group who has a police record of acquisitive offenses.

According to the Federal Bureau of Investigation (FBI), 97,464 forcible rapes were reported to law enforcement in the United States in 1995. Rape, however, is a highly underreported crime: An estimated four to five of ten rapes are reported. The underreporting is attributed to victims' feelings of shame and to the belief that there is no recourse through the legal system. According to the FBI Uniform Crime Reporting program, in 1995, 72 of every 100,000 females in the United States were reported rape victims.

Persons who are raped can be of any age. Cases have been reported in which the victims were as young as 15 months and as old as 82 years, but women ages 16 to 24 are at highest risk. Rape most commonly occurs in a woman's own neighborhood, frequently inside or near her own home. Most rapes are premeditated; about half are committed by strangers and half by men known, to varying degrees, by the victims. Seven percent of all rapes are perpetrated by close relatives of the victim; 10 percent of rapes involve more than one attacker.

A woman being raped is frequently in a life-threatening situation. During the rape, she experiences shock and fright approaching panic; her prime motivation is to stay alive. In most cases, rapists choose victims slightly smaller than themselves. Rapists may urinate or defecate on their victims, ejaculate into their faces and hair, force anal intercourse, and insert foreign objects into their vaginas and rectums.

Table 32–3
Physician Reference Card

PHYSICIAN REFERENCE CARD
RECOGNIZING AND TREATING VICTIMS OF DOMESTIC VIOLENCE BASED ON THE AMERICAN MEDICAL ASSOCIATION'S DIAGNOSTIC AND TREATMENT GUIDELINES ON DOMESTIC VIOLENCE

If you treat women, whether in private practice or a hospital setting, you are almost certainly treating some patients who are victims of domestic violence.

The following decision tree is designed to help you assess a patient's risk of domestic violence and offer appropriate help to those in need of it.

Identifying Victims of Domestic Violence

Although many women who are victims of abuse will not volunteer any information, they will discuss it if asked simple, direct questions in a nonjudgmental way and in a confidential setting. *The patient should be interviewed alone, without her partner present.*

You may want to offer a statement such as: "Because violence is so common in many women's lives, I've begun to ask about it routinely." Then you can ask a direct question, such as: "At any time, has your partner hit, kicked, or otherwise hurt or frightened you?"

IF PATIENT ANSWERS YES, THE FOLLOWING STEPS ARE SUGGESTED:

1. *Encourage her to talk about it:*
   "Would you like to talk about what has happened to you?"
   "How do you feel about it?"
   "What would you like to do about this?"
2. *Listen nonjudgmentally.*
   This serves both to begin the healing process for the woman and to give you an idea of what kind of referrals she needs.
3. *Validate:*
   Victims of domestic violence are frequently not believed, and the fear they report is minimized. The physician can express support through simple statements such as
   - You are not alone.
   - You don't deserve to be treated this way.
   - You are not to blame.
   - You are not crazy.
   - What happened to you is a crime.
   - Help is available for you.
4. *Document:*
   - The patient's complaints and symptoms as well as the results of the observation and assessment. (Complaints should be described in the patient's own words whenever possible.)
   - The patient's complete medical and trauma history and relevant social history.
   - A detailed description of the injuries, including type, number, size, location, resolution, possible causes, and explanations given.
   - An opinion on whether the injuries were inconsistent with the patient's explanation.
   - Results of all pertinent laboratory and other diagnostic procedures.
   - Color photographs and imaging studies, if applicable.
   - If the police are called, the name of the investigating officer and any action taken (the police should be called only if patient requests this or exhibits a reportable injury).
   - Child abuse and neglect is a reportable offense. If you suspect that children in the patient's home are also being abused, you are mandated to report the situation to the NYS Department of Social Services at 1-800-342-3720.
5. *Assess the danger to your patient:*
   Assess your patient's safety *before she leaves the medical setting.* The most important determinants of risk are the woman's level of fear and her appraisal of her immediate and future safety. Discussing the following indicators with the patient can help you determine if she is in escalating danger:
   - an increase in the frequency or severity of the assaults
   - increasing or new threats of homicide or suicide by the partner
   - threats to her children
   - the presence or availability of a firearm
6. *Provide appropriate treatment referral and support:*
   - Treat the patient's injuries as indicated. In prescribing medication, keep in mind that medications which hinder the patient's ability to protect herself or to flee from a violent partner may endanger her life.
   - If your patient is in imminent danger, determine if she has friends or family with whom she can stay. If this is not an option, ask if she wants immediate access to a shelter for battered women. If none is available, can she be admitted to the hospital?
   - If she doesn't need immediate access to a shelter, offer written information about shelters and other community resources. Remember that it may be dangerous for the woman to have these in her possession. Don't insist that she take them if she is reluctant to do so.

   Give your patient the telephone number of the local domestic violence hotline or the toll-free NYS Domestic Violence hotline (1-800-942-6906; 1-800-942-6908 for Spanish-speaking callers). It may be safest for your patient if you write the number on a prescription blank or an appointment card. You may wish to give her the opportunity to call from a private phone in your office.

IF THE PATIENT ANSWERS NO, OR WILL NOT DISCUSS THE TOPIC:

1. *Be aware of clinical findings that may indicate abuse:*
   - injury to the head, neck, torso, breasts, abdomen, or genitals
   - bilateral or multiple injuries
   - delay between onset of injury and seeking treatment
   - explanation by the patient which is inconsistent with the type of injury
   - any injury during pregnancy, especially to the abdomen or breasts
   - prior history of trauma
   - chronic pain symptoms for which no etiology is apparent
   - psychological distress, such as depression, suicidal ideation, anxiety, and/or sleep disorders
   - a partner who seems overly protective or who will not leave the woman's side
2. *If any of the above clinical signs is present, it is appropriate to ask more specific questions. Be sure that the patient's partner is not present.* Some examples of questions that may elicit more information about the patient's situation are:
   - It looks as though someone may have hurt you. Could you tell me how it happened?
   - Sometimes when people come for health care with physical symptoms like yours, we find that there may be trouble at home. We are concerned that someone is hurting or abusing you. Is this happening?
   - Sometimes when people feel the way you do, it's because they may have been hurt or abused at home. Is this happening to you?
3. *If patient answers YES:*
   See the suggestions for assessment and treatment that begin on the other side of this card.

   If patient answers NO:
   If the patient denies abuse, but you strongly suspect that it is taking place, you can let her know that your office can provide referrals to local programs, should she choose to pursue such options in the future.
   - You may want to write the Domestic Violence hotline number (1-800-942-6906 English; 1-800-942-6908 Spanish) on a prescription blank or on an appointment card.

   Don't judge the success of the intervention by the patient's action. A woman is most at risk of serious injury or even homicide when she attempts to leave an abusive partner, and it may take her a long time before she can finally do so. It is frustrating for the physician when a patient stays in an abusive situation. Be reassured that if you have acknowledged and validated her situation and offered appropriate referrals, you have done what you can to help her.

(From Office for Prevention of Domestic Violence, Medical Society of the State of New York, New York State Department of Health, with permission.)

After a rape, a woman often experiences shame, humiliation, confusion, fear, and rage. The type and duration of the reactions vary, but women report that the effects last for a year or longer. Many women experience the symptoms of PTSD. Some women, particularly those who have always felt sexually adequate, are able to resume sexual relations with men, but others become phobic about sexual interaction or exhibit such symptoms as vaginismus. Few women emerge from the assault completely unscathed. The manifestations and the degree of damage depend on the violence of the attack itself, the vulnerability of the woman, and the support system available to her immediately after the attack.

A rape victim fares best when she receives immediate support and can ventilate her fear and rage to loving family members, sympathetic physicians, and law enforcement officials. Knowing that she has socially acceptable means of recourse, such as the arrest and conviction of the rapist, can help a rape victim.

Unless a woman has a severe underlying disorder, therapy usually has a supportive approach and focuses on restoring a victim's sense of adequacy and control over her life; it also aims to relieve feelings of helplessness, dependence, and obsession with the assault, which frequently follow the rape. Group therapy with homogeneous groups of persons who have been raped is a particularly effective form of treatment.

In addition to the physical and psychological trauma experienced when they are assaulted, until recently rape victims also faced skepticism from those to whom they reported the crime (if they had sufficient strength to do so) or accusations of having provoked or desired the assault. In reality, the National Commission on the Causes and Prevention of Violence found discernible victim participation in rape in only 4.4 percent of all cases. This statistic is lower than that of any other crime of violence. Educating police officers and assigning policewomen to deal with rape victims have helped increase reporting of the crime. Rape crisis centers and telephone hot lines are available for immediate aid and information for victims. Volunteer groups work in emergency rooms in hospitals and with physician education programs to assist in the treatment of victims.

Legally, women no longer must prove in court that they actively struggled against a rapist, and testimony about a victim's previous sexual history has been declared inadmissible as evidence in several states. Because penalties for first-time rapists have been reduced, juries are likely to consider a conviction. In some states, wives can now prosecute husbands for rape.

In her book, *Against Our Will: Men, Women, and Rape*, feminist writer and historian Susan Brownmiller (Fig. 32-4) theorized that rape is a conscious process of intimidation to keep a group of people in fear. She suggested that the crime can be eliminated "when men cease aggression and when women cease to identify their femininity with submission and passivity."

DATE RAPE. *Date rape* and *acquaintance rape* are terms applied to rapes in which the rapist is known to the victim. The assault can occur on a first date or after the man and woman have known

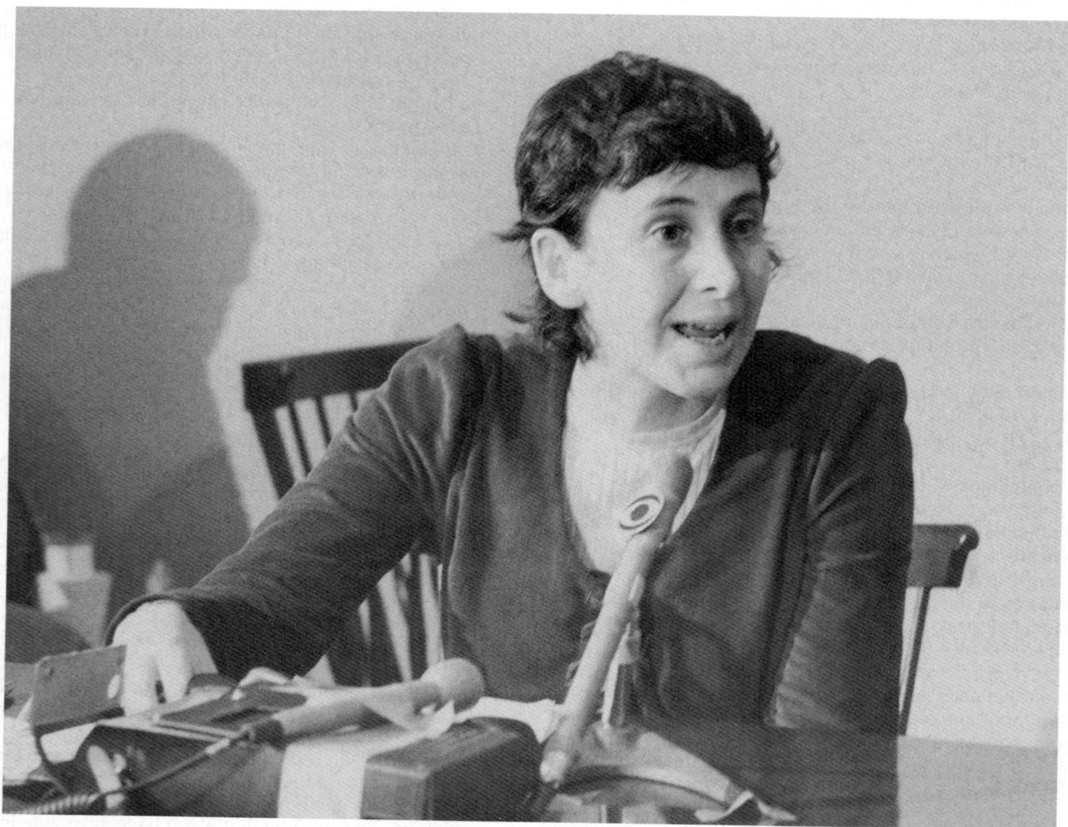

FIGURE 32–4
Susan Brownmiller speaking at a conference. (Courtesy of Corbis.)

each other for many months. Considerable data on date rape have been gathered from college populations. In one study, 38 percent of male students said that they would commit rape if they thought they could get away with it, and 11 percent stated that they had committed rape; 16 percent of female students said that they had been raped by men they knew or were dating. In addition to suffering the symptoms of all rape survivors, victims of date rape berate themselves for exercising poor judgment in their choice of male friends and are more likely to blame themselves for provoking the rapist than are other victims. Many colleges and universities have set up programs for rape prevention and for counseling those who have been assaulted.

Rape of Men. In some states the definition of rape is being changed to substitute the word *person* for *female*. In most states, male rape is legally defined as sodomy. Homosexual rape is much more frequent among men than among women and occurs frequently in closed institutions such as prisons and maximum-security hospitals.

The dynamics are identical to those of heterosexual rape. The crime enables the rapist to discharge aggression and to aggrandize himself. The victim is usually smaller than the rapist, is always perceived as passive and unmanly (weaker), and is used as an object. A rapist selecting a male victim may be heterosexual, bisexual, or homosexual. The most common act is anal penetration of the victim; the second most common is fellatio.

Homosexual-rape victims often feel (as raped women do) that they have been ruined. Some also fear that they will become homosexual because of the attack.

Sexual Coercion

Sexual coercion is a term used in DSM-IV-TR for incidents in which one person dominates another by force or compels the other person to perform a sexual act.

Stalking. Stalking is defined as a pattern of harassing or menacing behavior coupled with a threat to do harm. In 1990, California passed the first antistalking law, and most states now prohibit stalking, although some will not intervene unless an act of violence has occurred. In states with stalking laws, the person can be arrested on the basis of a pattern of harassment and can be charged with either a misdemeanor or felony. Some stalkers continue the activity for years; others, for only a few months. The court may mandate that stalkers undergo counseling sessions. The best means of deterrent is to report all stalkers to law enforcement agencies. Most stalkers are men, but women who stalk are just as likely as men to attack their victims violently.

Sexual Harassment. Sexual harassment refers to sexual advances, requests for sexual favors, or verbal or physical conduct of a sexual nature—all of which are unwelcomed by the victim. In more than 95 percent of cases the perpetrator is a man and the victim, a woman. If a man is being harassed, it is almost always by another man. A woman sexually harassing a man is an extremely rare event. The victim of harassment reacts to the experience in various ways. Some blame themselves and become depressed; others become anxious or angry. In general, harassment most commonly occurs in the workplace, and many organizations have developed procedures to deal with the problem. All too often, however, the victim is unwilling to step forward and lodge a complaint because of fear of retribution, of being humiliated, of being accused of lying (which is exceedingly rare), or ultimately of being fired from the job.

The types of behaviors that make up sexual harassment are broad. They include abusive language, requests for sexual favors, sexual jokes, staring, ogling, and giving massages, among others.

To reduce harassment, organizations may distribute educational material (Table 32–4). Employers are obligated to investigate every complaint, which most often are addressed to the Equal Employment Opportunity Commission. Appropriate organizational responses range from a written reprimand to firing the offender.

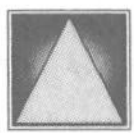

Table 32–4
Educational Material to Reduce Sexual Harassment

WHAT YOU SHOULD KNOW ABOUT SEXUAL HARASSMENT
WHAT IS SEXUAL HARASSMENT?
WHAT IS PROHIBITED?
The 1980 Equal Opportunity Employment Commission Guidelines for Sexual Harassment encompass:
1. Unwelcomed sexual advances.
2. Requests for sexual favors.
3. Verbal conduct of a sexual nature.
4. Physical conduct of a sexual nature.

UNDER WHAT CONDITIONS?
When such conduct has the purpose or effect of:
1. Unreasonably interfering with an individual's work performance.
2. Creating an intimidating, hostile or offensive working environment. (This can be interpreted to include the "terms, conditions or privileges of unemployment" such as the psychological and emotional work environment and subjecting female employees to anxiety and debilitation.)
3. When submission to or rejection of the conduct is made either explicitly or implicitly a term or condition of an individual's employment or
4. Is the basis for employment decisions affecting the individual.

WHO IS RESPONSIBLE?
1. The employer who is committing the act.
2. The employer, even if its agents and supervisors committed the act regardless of whether the acts were authorized or even forbidden.
3. The employer for acts committed by an employee's co-worker.
4. The employer for conduct by a non-employee (such as a customer or supplier) if the employer "knows or should have known of the conduct and fails to take an immediate and appropriate action."
5. The employer, if timely corrective actions are not taken.

(From Tulin DiversiTeam Associates, Philadelphia, with permission.)

References

Bernet W. Child maltreatment. In: Sadock BJ, Sadock VA, eds. *Kaplan & Sadock's Comprehensive Textbook of Psychiatry*. 8th ed. Vol. 2. Baltimore: Lippincott Williams & Wilkins; 2005:3412.

Borrego J Jr, Terao SY. The consideration of cultural factors in the context of child maltreatment. In: Talley PF, ed. *Handbook for the Treatment of Abused and Neglected Children*. Binghamton, NY: Haworth Social Work Practice Press; 2005:341–357.

Cohen JA, Deblinger E, Mannarino AP, Steer R. A multi-site randomized controlled trial for children with sexual abuse-related PTSD symptoms. *J Am Acad Child Adolesc Psychiatry.* 2004;43:393.

English DJ, Bangdiwala SI, Runyan DK. The dimensions of maltreatment: Introduction. *Child Abuse Negl.* 2005;29(5):441–460.

Harder J. Research implications for the prevention of child abuse and neglect. *Families in Society.* 2005;86(4):491–501.

Jones LM, Finkelhor D, Halter S. Child maltreatment trends in the 1990s: Why does neglect differ from sexual and physical abuse? *Child Maltreatment: Journal of the American Professional Society of the Abuse of Children.* 2006;11(2):107–120.

Manly JT. Advances in research definitions of child maltreatment. *Child Abuse Negl.* 2005;29(5):425–439.

Portwood SG. What we know—and don't know—about preventing child maltreatment. *Journal of Aggression, Maltreatment & Trauma.* 2006;12(3–4):5–80.

Runyon MK, Deblinger E, Ryan EE, Thakkar-Kolar R. An overview of child physical abuse: Developing an integrated parent-child cognitive-behavioral treatment system. *Trauma Violence Abuse.* 2004;5:65.

Schneider MW, Ross A, Graham JC, Zielinski A. Do allegations of emotional maltreatment predict developmental outcomes beyond that of other forms of maltreatment? *Child Abuse Negl.* 2005;29(5):513–532.

Swenson CC, Chaffin M. Beyond psychotherapy: Treating abused children by changing their social ecology. *Aggression and Violent Behavior.* 2006;11(2):120–137.

Trocme N, Bala N. False allegations of abuse and neglect when parents separate. *Child Abuse Negl.* 2005;29(12):1333–1345.

US Department of Health and Human Services, Administration for Children and Families. *Child Maltreatment 2002*. Washington, DC: US Government Printing Office; 2004.

van der Kolk BA. Physical and sexual abuse of adults. In: Sadock BJ, Sadock VA, eds. *Kaplan & Sadock's Comprehensive Textbook of Psychiatry*. 8th ed. Vol. 2. Baltimore: Lippincott Williams & Wilkins; 2005:2393.

Zielinski DS, Bradshaw CP. Ecological influences on the sequelae of child maltreatment: A review of the literature. *Child Maltreatment: Journal of the American Professional Society on the Abuse of Children.* 2006;11:49–62.

33 Additional Conditions That May Be a Focus of Clinical Attention

As defined in the text revision of the fourth edition of *Diagnostic and Statistical Manual of Mental Disorders* (DSM-IV-TR), conditions that may be a focus of clinical attention have led to contact with the mental health care system, but without sufficient evidence to justify a diagnosis of a mental disorder. In some instances, one of these conditions will be noted during the course of a psychiatric evaluation, although no mental disorder has been found. In other instances, the diagnostic evaluation reveals no mental disorder, but a need is seen to note the primary reason for contact with the mental health care system.

In some cases, a mental disorder may eventually be found, but the focus of attention or treatment is on a condition that is not caused by a mental disorder. For example, a patient with an anxiety disorder may receive treatment for a marital problem that is unrelated to the anxiety disorder itself.

Thirteen conditions make up the diagnostic category of additional disorders that may be a focus of clinical attention. Nine of these conditions are discussed in this chapter: malingering, bereavement, occupational problems, adult antisocial behavior, religious or spiritual problem, acculturation problem, phase of life problem, noncompliance with treatment for a mental disorder, and age-associated memory decline. (Four other conditions included in the DSM-IV-TR are discussed in Chapter 53: borderline intellectual functioning, academic problem, childhood or adolescent antisocial behavior, and identity problem.)

MALINGERING

According to the DSM-IV-TR:

> The essential feature of Malingering is the intentional production of false or grossly exaggerated physical or psychological symptoms, motivated by external incentives such as avoiding military duty, avoiding work, obtaining financial compensation, evading criminal prosecution, or obtaining drugs. Under some circumstances, malingering may represent adaptive behavior—for example, feigning illness while a captive of the enemy during wartime.

Malingering should be strongly suspected if any combination of the following is noted: (1) medicolegal context of presentation (e.g., the person is referred by an attorney to the clinician for examination or is incarcerated), (2) evident discrepancy between the individual's claimed stress or disability and the objective findings, (3) lack of cooperation during the diagnostic evaluation and in complying with the prescribed treatment regimen, and (4) the presence of antisocial personality disorder.

Epidemiology

A 1 percent prevalence of malingering has been estimated among mental health patients in civilian clinical practice, with the estimate rising to 5 percent in the military. In a litigious context, during interviews of criminal defendants, the estimated prevalence of malingering is much higher—between 10 and 20 percent. Approximately 50 percent of children presenting with conduct disorders are described as having serious lying-related issues.

Although no familial or genetic patterns have been reported and no clear sex bias or age at onset has been delineated, malingering does appear to be highly prevalent in certain military, prison, and litigious populations and, in Western society, in men from youth through middle age. Associated disorders include conduct disorder and anxiety disorders in children and antisocial, borderline, and narcissistic personality disorders in adults.

Etiology

Although no biological factors have been found to be causally related to malingering, its frequent association with antisocial personality disorder raises the possibility that hypoarousability may be an underlying metabolic factor. Still, no predisposing genetic, neurophysiological, neurochemical, or neuroendocrinological forces are presently known.

Diagnosis and Clinical Features

Avoidance of Criminal Responsibility, Trial, and Punishment. Criminals may pretend to be incompetent to avoid standing trial; they may feign insanity at the time of perpetration of the crime, malinger symptoms to receive a less harsh penalty, or attempt to act too incapacitated (incompetent) to be executed.

Avoidance of Military Service or of Particularly Hazardous Duties. Persons may malinger to avoid conscription into the armed forces and, once conscripted, they may feign illness to escape from particularly onerous or hazardous duties.

Financial Gain. Modern malingerers may seek financial gain in the form of undeserved disability insurance, veterans' benefits, workers' compensation, or tort damages for purported psychological injury.

Avoidance of Work, Social Responsibility, and Social Consequences. Individuals may malinger to escape from unpleasant vocational or social circumstances or to avoid the social and litigation-related consequences of vocational or social improprieties.

An owner of a previously successful photographic equipment supplier declared bankruptcy in a way that the government maintained was illegal. Subsequently, the government indicted the defendant on various counts of fraud. The defendant's counsel maintained that the defendant was too depressed to cooperate with him and that, because of that depression, he experienced memory loss that made it impossible to understand what had occurred and, therefore, impossible to provide a meaningful defense. The government's forensic psychiatrist evaluated the defendant to ascertain the nature of his depression and to determine whether it was causing cognitive problems.

When asked early in his evaluation when his birthday was, he responded, "Oh, what does it matter, it was in the 40s or 50s." Similarly, when queried about where he was born, he said, "Some place in Hungary." Even when pressed for more specifics, he refused to elaborate. Yet, at many points later in his evaluation, he responded with complete, often detailed, information about transactions not related to those for which he had been indicted. It was the impression of the evaluator that the defendant was malingering in a gross and inconsistent fashion, incompatible with the kinds of decreases in cognitive skills that occasionally attend major depression. (Adapted from case of Mark J. Mills, J.D., M.D., and Mark S. Lipian, M.D., Ph.D.)

Facilitation of Transfer from Prison to Hospital. Prisoners may malinger (fake bad) with the goal of obtaining a transfer to a psychiatric hospital from which they may hope to escape or in which they expect to do "easier time." The prison context may also give rise to dissimulation (faking good), however; the prospect of an indeterminate number of days on a mental health ward may prompt an inmate with true psychiatric symptoms to make every effort to conceal them.

Admission to a Hospital. In this era of deinstitutionalization and homelessness, individuals may malinger in an effort to gain admission to a psychiatric hospital. Such institutions may be seen as providing free room and board, a safe haven from the police, or refuge from rival gang members or disgruntled drug cronies who have made street life even more unbearable and hazardous than it usually is.

A robust, neatly attired man presented to the psychiatric emergency department in the early-morning hours. He stated that "the voices" were worse and that he wished to be readmitted to the hospital. When the psychiatrist challenged him, observing that he had just been discharged that afternoon, that he routinely left the hospital in the morning and demanded rehospitalization at night, and that, despite multiple hospitalizations, his reported history of hallucinations had been increasingly doubted, the man became belligerent. When the psychiatrist still refused to admit him, the patient grabbed the psychiatrist's clothes, threatening him but inflicting no harm. The psychiatrist asked the hospital police to escort him off the grounds. The patient was told he could seek readmission to his regular ward during the day. Subsequent contact with the patient's ward revealed that their diagnoses were substance abuse and homelessness; his apparent schizophrenia appeared never to have been an actual issue in his treatment. (Courtesy of Mark J. Mills, J.D., M.D., and Mark S. Lipian, M.D., Ph.D.)

Drug-Seeking. Malingerers may feign illness in an effort to obtain favored medications, either for personal use or, in a prison setting, as currency to barter for cigarettes, protection, or other inmate-provided favors.

The plaintiff, a woman in her late 20s, was injured while dancing at a club. Although her claim initially appeared bona fide, subsequent investigation cast doubt on the mechanism of injury that she claimed—namely, that a misplaced electrical cord under a carpet caused her to slip. This was true, she claimed, despite that she had to be dancing in a particularly jerky manner that could have easily caused problems without tripping.

Subsequently, she sought medical and surgical treatment for torn cartilage in her injured knee. Despite that the initial surgery went well, she kept reinjuring the knee with various "slips." As a result, she requested narcotic analgesics. A careful medical record review revealed that she was obtaining such medications from multiple practitioners and that she had apparently forged at least one prescription.

In reviewing the case before binding arbitration, it was the opinion of the orthopedic and psychiatric consultants that, although the initial injury and reported pain were real, the plaintiff consciously elaborated her injuries to obtain the desired narcotic analgesics. (Courtesy of Mark J. Mills, J.D., M.D., and Mark S. Lipian, M.D., Ph.D.)

Child Custody. Minimizing difficulties or faking good for the sake of obtaining child custody can occur when one party accurately accuses the other of being an unfit parent because of psychological conditions. The accused party may feel compelled to minimize symptoms or to portray him- or herself in a positive light to reduce chances of being deemed unfit and losing custody.

Differential Diagnosis

Malingering must be differentiated from the actual physical or psychiatric illness suspected of being feigned. Furthermore, the possibility of partial malingering, which is an exaggeration of existing symptoms, must be entertained. Also the possibility exists of unintentional, dynamically driven misattribution of genuine symptoms (e.g., of depression) to an incorrect environmental cause (e.g., to sexual harassment rather than to narcissistic injury).

It should also be remembered that a real psychiatric disorder and malingering are not mutually exclusive.

Factitious disorder is distinguished from malingering by motivation (sick role versus tangible pain), whereas the somatoform disorders involve no conscious volition. In conversion disorder,

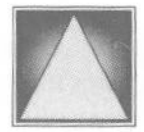

Table 33–1
Factors Aiding in the Differentiation between Malingering and Conversion Disorder

1. Malingerers are more likely to be suspicious, uncooperative, aloof, and unfriendly; patients with conversion disorder are likely friendly, cooperative, appealing, dependent, and clinging.
2. Malingerers may try to avoid diagnostic evaluations and refuse recommended treatment; patients with conversion disorder likely welcome evaluation and treatment, "searching for an answer."
3. Malingerers likely refuse employment opportunities designed to circumvent their disability; patients with conversion disorder likely accept such opportunities.
4. Malingerers are more likely to provide extremely detailed and exacting descriptions of events precipitating their "illness;" patients with conversion disorder are more likely to report historical gaps, inaccuracies, and vagaries.

as in malingering, objective signs cannot account for subjective experience, and differentiation between the two disorders can be difficult. Table 33-1 lists some variables that may aid in distinguishing between these two conditions.

Course and Prognosis

Malingering persists as long as the malingerer believes it will likely produce the desired rewards. In the absence of concurrent diagnoses, once the rewards have been attained, the feigned symptoms disappear. In some structured settings, such as the military or prison units, ignoring the malingered behavior may result in its disappearance, particularly if an expectation of continued productive performance, despite complaints, is made clear. In children, malingering is most likely associated with a predisposing anxiety or conduct disorder; proper attention to this developing problem may alleviate the child's propensity to malinger.

Treatment

The appropriate stance for the psychiatrist is clinical neutrality. If malingering is suspected, a careful differential investigation should ensue. If, at the conclusion of the diagnostic evaluation, malingering seems most likely, the patient should be tactfully, but firmly confronted with the apparent outcome. The reasons underlying the ruse need to be elicited, however, and alternative pathways to the desired outcome explored. Coexisting psychiatric disorders should be thoroughly assessed. Only if the patient is utterly unwilling to interact with the physician under any terms other than manipulation should the therapeutic (or evaluative) interaction be abandoned.

BEREAVEMENT

Normal bereavement begins immediately after, or within a few months of, the loss of a loved one. Typical signs and symptoms include feelings of sadness, preoccupation with thoughts about the deceased, tearfulness, irritability, insomnia, and difficulties concentrating and carrying out daily activities. On the basis of the cultural group, bereavement is limited to a varying time, usually 6 months, but it can be longer. Normal bereavement, however, can lead to a full depressive disorder that requires treatment.

The DSM-IV-TR includes the following description of bereavement:

> This category can be used when the focus of clinical attention is a reaction to the death of a loved one. As part of their reaction to the loss, some grieving individuals present with symptoms characteristic of a Major Depressive Episode (e.g., feelings of sadness and associated symptoms such as insomnia, poor appetite, and weight loss). The bereaved individual typically regards the depressed mood as "normal," although the person may seek professional help for relief of associated symptoms such as insomnia or anorexia. The duration and expression of "normal" bereavement vary considerably among different cultural groups. The diagnosis of Major Depressive Disorder is generally not given unless the symptoms are still present 2 months after the loss. However, the presence of certain symptoms that are not characteristic of a "normal" grief reaction may be helpful in differentiating bereavement from a Major Depressive Episode. These include (1) guilt about things other than actions taken or not taken by the survivor at the time of the death; (2) thoughts of death other than the survivor feeling that he or she would be better off dead or should have died with the deceased person; (3) morbid preoccupation with worthlessness; (4) marked psychomotor retardation; (5) prolonged and marked functional impairment; and (6) hallucinatory experiences other than thinking that he or she hears the voice of, or transiently sees the image of, the deceased person. (Chapter 2.6 presents a further discussion of bereavement.)

OCCUPATIONAL PROBLEM

The DSM-IV-TR includes the following statement about occupational problem:

> This category can be used when the focus of clinical attention is an occupational problem that is not due to a mental disorder or, if it is due to a mental disorder, is sufficiently severe to warrant independent clinical attention. Examples include job dissatisfaction and uncertainty about career choices.

Occupational problems often arise during stressful changes in work, namely, at initial entry into the workforce or when making job changes within the same organization to a higher position because of good performance or to a parallel position because of corporate need. Distress occurs particularly if these changes are not sought and no preparatory training has taken place, as well as during layoffs and at retirement, especially if retirement is mandatory and the person is unprepared for this event. Work distress can result if initially agreed-to-conditions change to work overload or lack of challenge and opportunity to experience work satisfaction; if an individual feels unable to fulfill conflicting expectations or feels that work conditions prevent accomplishing assignments because of lack of legitimate power; or if an individual believes he or she works in a hierarchy with harsh and unreasonable superiors.

Work Choices and Changes

Young adults without role models or guidance from families, mentors, or others in their communities too often underestimate their lifetime potential abilities to learn a trade or earn a college or postgraduate degree. In addition, women and members of minority groups often feel less prepared to accept work challenges, fear rejection, and do not apply for jobs for which they are qualified. On the other hand, men, in fields in which they are underrepresented, often and confidently move up the career ladder faster (glass elevator). As part of initial interviews for evaluation of occupational problems, patients should be encouraged to consider their heretofore unrecognized, unadmitted talents; long-held, yet unexpressed, dreams and goals regarding work; actual successes in work and school; and motivation to risk learning what they would find satisfying.

Minorities and those in low-paying and low-skilled jobs too often have less job security. Business and institutional reorganization and consequent downsizing, factory closings, and moves affect many, often leaving these workers feeling hopeless and helpless about future employment, on welfare, angry, and depressed.

With ongoing and often sudden downsizing of corporations and businesses, men and women continue to struggle with unexpected job loss and premature retirement, even when finances are not an issue. In addition, men, in particular, define themselves by their work roles, and, thus, experience more occupational distress from these changes. Women may adjust faster to retirement, but they often have less financial security than men do (white women earn approximately 80 cents on the dollar, and African American and Hispanic women earn even less for comparable work); women have generally been in lower-status work positions, find themselves widowed more often than men, and are more likely to be caring for children, grandchildren, and elderly relatives. Women represent more of the single working parent group and the working poor.

Stress and the Workplace

More than 30 percent of workers report that they are under stress at work. Workplace distress is implicated in at least 15 percent of occupational disability claims. Expected distress follows recognized and uncontrollable work changes—downsizing, mergers and acquisitions, work overload, and chronic physical strains, including work noise, temperature, bodily injuries, and strain from performing computer work. According to one study, the top ten most stressful jobs in 1998 were (1) President of the United States, (2) firefighter, (3) senior corporate executive, (4) race car driver, (5) taxi driver, (6) surgeon, (7) astronaut, (8) police officer, (9) football player, and (10) air traffic controller. People who work under deadlines, such as bus drivers, are subject to hypertension.

Work frustration can also arise from an individual worker's unrecognized (and therefore unresolved) psychodynamic issues, such as working appropriately with superiors and not relating to one's supervisor as a parent figure. Other developmental issues include unresolved problems with competition, assertiveness, envy, fear of success, and inability to communicate verbally in a constructive manner.

After the September 11, 2001, World Trade Center tragedy, a 32-year-old, married, male firefighter, who had been away on vacation that day with his wife and children, began to exhibit changed behaviors at home and at work. At home, he appeared not to listen to his two latency-aged children and, instead, focused his attention on television sporting events. At work, he also appeared to be more focused on cooking the same dinners for his peers and watching television than on interacting verbally with his remaining peers and the new chief. In the course of several months, a chaplain visited the station several times and talked to the firefighters about survivor guilt and the 9/11 tragedy, and the firefighter began to return somewhat to his former healthier behaviors. (Courtesy of Leah J. Dickstein, M.D.)

Often, work conflicts reflect similar conflicts in the worker's personal life, and referral for treatment, unless there is insight, is in order. Some studies have found that massage therapy, meditation, and yoga at intervals during the work day relieve stress when used on a regular basis. Approaches using cognitive therapy have also helped people reduce work pressure.

Suicide Risk

Some occupations—health professionals, financial service workers, and police, the first and latter groups because of easier access to lethal drugs and weapons—both attract persons with a high suicide risk and involve increased chronic distress that may lead to higher suicide rates.

Career and Job Problems of Women

Most women work outside the home out of necessity to support themselves or their dependents (whether children or adults) or as part of a working couple. With the divorce rate remaining at the 50 percent level, many women find themselves economically poorer after a divorce than when married, although divorced men usually find their economic status improved. Despite more than four decades of increasing knowledge about, and concern for, women's status in the workplace, unique gender issues, bias, and lack of accommodation to their unique needs at certain life stages (i.e., pregnancy and postpartum, major responsibility for young healthy and ill children) continue. Yet, women were the largest group establishing new small businesses in the 1990s. Many have left large corporations where they were not valued for their efforts because of their gender, termed *contra culture*. Women experience problems when they are the sole woman in a man's field. Despite increasing recognition of the need for men in relationships with women to assume home and family responsibilities, less than 25 percent of men do so equitably.

Women of childbearing and child-rearing ages continue to find themselves in conflict with job expectations, opportunities, and personal responsibilities. High-quality, on-site, dependent-care facilities with extended hours are rare and often out of range financially. Major unresolved work issues that are unique to women at certain life stages include flextime and paid and unpaid dependent leave options. Beyond dependent care issues, women in the workforce continue to experience distress after chronic and repeated sexual harassment, despite its illegality and media attention. Increasingly, more women have travel responsibilities, work long hours, work shifts beyond daylight hours, and experience personal workplace violence.

Among dual-career families and partners, the woman is more likely to move when the man chooses to move for a work opportunity than vice versa. Consequently, a woman's career is interrupted more often. Less reluctance is seen, however, to have the two members of a relationship work for the same organization than previously, albeit usually in different departments. Work distress may also stem from continuous miscommunication, especially that based on gender.

Working Teenagers

With unemployment increasing, many teenagers work part-time while attending high school. Consequently, stress can arise because of less parent–teenager interaction and constructive parental control issues about teens' use of earnings, time spent away from home, and consequent behaviors both in and outside the home. When both parents or a single parent, as well as the teenager, work outside the home, often on different schedules, parent–teen verbal communication must be proactive, clear, and ongoing.

Working within the Home

Although most women with children of all ages must work outside the home, at times they may be home full time or part time or may work at home. When their husbands or significant others work full time outside the home, problems may develop from each one's perceived expectations of the other. Women who care for children and their home exclusively may be seen by their partners as not only economically dependent and inferior, but also not as competent and not understanding of the man's stressors and needs. Ongoing respectful listening and verbal communication must be encouraged.

People in organizations are increasingly taking work home as their work expectations increase. This work-at-home experience can and does interfere with personal lives and satisfaction, which can then have further repercussions at work.

Chronic Illness

As general and other medical and psychiatric treatments for chronic diseases improve, employers have been increasingly concerned about accommodating patients with acquired immunodeficiency syndrome (AIDS), diabetes mellitus, and other disorders. The issue of mandatory testing for AIDS and substance abuse (alcohol and other illegal substances) continues to be of concern. Employee assistance programs offering education about general and mental health topics have proved timely and cost-effective.

Domestic Violence

Although occurring in the home, signs and symptoms that interfere with work often trigger identification of those who experience domestic violence. Trained professionals must question all employees experiencing work distress about domestic violence and, when indicated, refer individuals for assistance, which includes safety in the workplace.

Job Loss

Regardless of the reason for job loss, most people experience distress, at least temporarily, including symptoms of normal grief, loss of self-esteem, anger, reactive depressive and anxiety symptoms, as well as somatic symptoms, and, possibly, the onset of, or increase in, substance abuse or domestic violence. Timely education, support programs, and vocational guidance should be instituted and access to treatment made available, if indicated.

Vocational Rehabilitation

Rehabilitation is often necessary for those traumatized by stresses in the workplace, those who had to take a leave of absence because of medical or psychiatric reasons, or those who have been fired. Individual or group counseling enables persons to improve personal relationships, raise self-esteem, or learn new work skills. Patients with schizophrenia may benefit from sheltered workshops in which they perform work that is geared to their level of function. Some patients with schizophrenia or autism do well in tasks that are repetitive or require obsessive concern with details.

ADULT ANTISOCIAL BEHAVIOR

Characterized by activities that are illegal, immoral, or both, antisocial behavior usually begins in childhood and often persists throughout life. DSM-IV-TR includes the following statements about adult antisocial behavior:

> This category can be used when the focus of clinical attention is adult antisocial behavior that is not due to a mental disorder (e.g., Conduct Disorder, Antisocial Personality Disorder, or an Impulse-Control Disorder). Examples include the behavior of some professional thieves, racketeers, or dealers in illegal substances.

The term *antisocial behavior* somewhat confusingly applies both to persons' actions that are not due to a mental disorder and to actions by those who never received a neuropsychiatric workup to determine the presence or absence of a mental disorder. As Dorothy Lewis noted, the term can apply to behavior by normal persons who "struggle to make a dishonest living."

Epidemiology

Depending on the criteria and the sampling, estimates of the prevalence of adult antisocial behavior range from 5 to 15 percent of the population. Within prison populations, investigators report prevalence figures between 20 and 80 percent. Men account for more adult antisocial behavior than do women.

Etiology

Antisocial behaviors in adulthood are characteristic of a variety of persons, ranging from those with no demonstrable psychopathology to those who are severely impaired and have psychotic disorders, cognitive disorders, and retardation, among other conditions. A comprehensive neuropsychiatric assessment of antisocial adults is indicated and may reveal potentially treatable psychiatric and neurological impairments that can easily be overlooked. Only in the absence of mental disorders can patients be categorized as displaying adult antisocial behavior. Adult antisocial behavior may be influenced by genetic and social factors.

Genetic Factors. Data supporting the genetic transmission of antisocial behavior are based on studies that found a 60 percent concordance rate in monozygotic twins and about a 30 percent concordance rate in dizygotic twins. Adoption studies show a high rate of antisocial behavior in the biological relatives of adoptees identified with antisocial behavior and a high incidence of antisocial behavior in the adopted-away offspring of those with antisocial behavior. The prenatal and perinatal periods of those who subsequently display antisocial behavior often are associated with low birthweight, mental retardation, and prenatal exposure to alcohol and other drugs of abuse.

Social Factors. Studies have shown that in neighborhoods in which families with low socioeconomic status (SES) predominate, the sons of unskilled workers are more likely to commit more offenses and more serious criminal offenses than do the sons of middle-class and skilled workers, at least during adolescence and early adulthood. These data are not as clear for women, but the findings are generally similar in studies from many countries. Areas of family training differ by SES group. Middle-SES parents use love-oriented techniques in discipline. They withdraw affection rather than impose physical punishment as is done in low-SES groups. Negative parental attitudes toward aggressive behavior, attempts to curb aggressive behavior, and the ability to communicate parental values are more characteristic of middle- and high-SES groups than of low ones. Adult antisocial behavior is associated with the use and abuse of alcohol and other substances and with the easy availability of handguns.

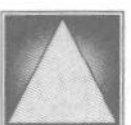

Table 33–2
Symptoms of Adult Antisocial Behavior

Life Area	Antisocial Patients with Significant Problems in Area (%)
Work problems	85
Marital problems	81
Financial dependence	79
Arrests	75
Alcohol abuse	72
School problems	71
Impulsiveness	67
Sexual behavior	64
Wild adolescence	62
Vagrancy	60
Belligerence	58
Social isolation	56
Military record (of those serving)	53
Lack of guilt	40
Somatic complaints	31
Use of aliases	29
Pathological lying	16
Drug abuse	15
Suicide attempts	11

Data are from Robins L. *Deviant Children Grown Up: A Sociological and Psychiatric Study of Sociopathic Personality.* Baltimore: Williams & Wilkins; 1966.

Diagnosis and Clinical Features

The diagnosis of adult antisocial behavior is one of exclusion. Substance dependence in such behavior often makes it difficult to separate the antisocial behavior related primarily to substance dependence from disordered behaviors that occurred either before substance use or during episodes unrelated to substance dependence.

During the manic phases of bipolar I disorder, certain aspects of behavior, such as wanderlust, sexual promiscuity, and financial difficulties, can be similar to adult antisocial behavior. Patients with schizophrenia may have episodes of adult antisocial behavior, but the symptom picture is usually clear, especially regarding thought disorder, delusions, and hallucinations on the mental status examination.

Neurological conditions can be associated with adult antisocial behavior, and electroencephalograms (EEGs), computed tomography (CT) scans, magnetic resonance imaging (MRI), and complete neurological examinations are indicated. Temporal lobe epilepsy should be considered in the differential diagnosis. When a clear-cut diagnosis of temporal lobe epilepsy or encephalitis can be made, the disorder may be considered to contribute to the adult antisocial behavior. Abnormal EEG findings are prevalent among violent offenders: An estimated 50 percent of aggressive criminals have abnormal EEG findings.

Persons with adult antisocial behavior have difficulties in work, marriage, and money matters and conflicts with various authorities. The symptoms of adult antisocial behavior are summarized in Table 33-2. (Antisocial personality disorder is discussed in Chapter 27.)

Treatment

In general, therapists are pessimistic about treating adult antisocial behavior. They have little hope of changing a pattern that has been present almost continuously throughout a person's life. Psychotherapy has not been effective, and no major breakthroughs with biological treatments, including medications, have occurred.

Therapists show more enthusiasm for the use of therapeutic communities and other forms of group treatment, although the data provide little basis for optimism. Many adult criminals who are incarcerated in institutional settings have shown some response to group therapy approaches. The history of violence, criminality, and antisocial behavior has shown that such behaviors seem to decrease after age 40. Recidivism in criminals, which can reach 90 percent in some studies, also decreases in middle age.

Prevention. Because antisocial behavior often begins during childhood, the major focus must be on delinquency prevention. Any measures that improve the physical and mental health of socioeconomically disadvantaged children and their families are likely to reduce delinquency and violent crime. Often, recurrently violent persons have sustained many insults to the central nervous system (CNS), prenatally and throughout childhood and adolescence. Consequently, programs must be developed to educate parents about the dangers to their children of CNS injury from maltreatment, including the effects of psychoactive substances on the brain of the growing fetus. Public education about the releasing effect of alcohol on violent behaviors (not to mention its contribution to vehicular homicide) may also reduce crime.

In a Surgeon General's Report on Violence and Public Health issued more than 15 years ago, the Committee on the Prevention of Assault and Homicide emphasized the importance of discouraging corporal punishment in the home, forbidding it in the schools, and even abolishing capital punishment by the state, saying that all are models and sanctions for violence. Since that time, capital punishment has been instituted in states that did not have it, such as New York. No evidence indicates that capital punishment reduces crime in states that have it. Opponents of capital punishment see it as "vengeance," not punishment.

Although persons disagree about the contribution of violence in the media to violent crime, the propaganda potential of the media is universally recognized. The extent to which the media, such as television, can be used to transmit positive social values has not yet been realized. The guidelines issued by the television industry to indicate the amount of sex and violence in programs is an attempt to deal with the issue; however, program content that espouses traditional societal values would be beneficial.

The most successful preventive measures within the field of medicine have come from community-wide public health programs (e.g., campaigns against smoking) and from programs that detect individual vulnerabilities (e.g., individual monitoring of blood pressure). Studies of adult antisocial behavior reveal the contribution of broad cultural factors and constellations of individual biopsychosocial vulnerabilities. Prevention programs must recognize and address both kinds of factors.

RELIGIOUS OR SPIRITUAL PROBLEM

According to DSM-IV-TR,

> This category can be used when the focus of clinical attention is a religious or spiritual problem. Examples include distressing experiences that involve loss or questioning of faith, problems associated with conversion to a new faith, or questioning other spiritual values which may not necessarily be related to an organized church or religious institution.

Psychiatrists must enable and assist patients to distinguish religious thought or experience from psychopathology and, if this is a problem, encourage patients to work through the issues independently or with assistance. Religious imagery may be recognized in mental illness when persons state they believe they have been commanded by God to take a dangerous or grandiose action.

A midcareer male surgeon who was very successful but long overcommitted to his private practice and his academic responsibilities revealed to his often-neglected wife that, at age 9, he was approached by his religious leader to get close physically. Believing it was his fault, he never told anyone and decided, then, never to have children. In the weeks after this disclosure, he and his wife began to spend more private time together and even discussed the possibility of starting a family.

Cults

Recently, cults have appeared to be less popular and less attractive to naïve late adolescents and young adults seeking assistance in discovering who they are as they struggle to develop more mature relationships with their parents. Cults are led by charismatic leaders, often out of control themselves, with inappropriate and often unethical values, but purporting to offer acceptance and guidance to troubled followers. Cult members are strongly controlled and forced to dissolve allegiance to family and others to serve the cult leader's directives and personal needs. These young members often come from educated families who then seek professional help in persuading their children to leave the cult and enter deprogramming therapy to restore personal psychological stability to the former cult members. Deprogramming and adjustment back into family, society, and an independent life are time-intensive and long-term with resultant posttraumatic stress disorder (PTSD), which must be recognized and treated.

ACCULTURATION PROBLEM

The DSM-IV-TR includes the following statement about acculturation problem:

> This category can be used when the focus of clinical attention is a problem involving adjustment to a different culture (e.g., following migration).

Culture Shock

Major cultural change can evoke severe distress, termed *culture shock.* This condition arises when individuals suddenly find themselves in a new culture in which they feel completely alien. They may also feel conflict over which lifestyles to maintain, change, or adopt. Children and young adult immigrants often adapt more easily than do middle-aged and elderly immigrants. Younger immigrants often learn the new language more easily and continue to mature in the new culture, whereas those who are more senior, having had more stability and unchanging routines in their former culture, struggle more to adapt. Culture shock from immigration clearly differs from the restless and continuous moving of psychiatric patients secondary to their illness.

Culture shock can occur within a person's own country with geographic, school, and work changes, such as joining the military, experiencing school busing, moving across country, or moving to a vastly different neighborhood or from a rural area to a metropolis. Reactive symptoms, which are understandable, include anxiety, depression, isolation, fear, and a sense of loss of identity as the person adjusts. If the person is part of a family or group making this transition and the move is positive and planned, stress can be lower. Furthermore, if selected cultural mores can be safely maintained as persons integrate into the new culture, stress is also minimized.

Constant geographic moves because of chosen work opportunities or necessity involve a large proportion of workers in the United States. Joining activities in the new community and actively trying to meet neighbors and coworkers can lessen the culture shock.

An 18-year-old, first-year female college student offered an academic scholarship by a small southern college with a major in her field of interest realized on her return home to the Midwest for winter break that she felt like a misfit among her dorm peers. They were friendly, yet generally kept their distance from her after class. At home, she discussed her experiences with high school friends, who replied that they had heard about such cultural dissonance from peers at their midwestern colleges. The student returned to college feeling that it was not her fault or imagination and slowly began to reach out more assertively to her peers so they could get to know her beyond stereotypical beliefs and so she could do the same.

Brainwashing. First practiced by the Chinese Communists on American prisoners during the Korean War, *brainwashing* is the deliberate creation of culture shock. Individuals are isolated, intimidated, and made to feel different and out of place to break their spirits and destroy their coping skills. Once a person appears mentally weak and helpless, the aggressors impose new ideas on them that they would never have accepted in their normal state. As with those involved in cults, on release and return to their homes, brainwashed individuals with PTSD require deprogramming treatment, including reeducation and ongoing supportive psychotherapy, both on an individual and group basis. Treatment is usually long term to rebuild healthy self-esteem and coping skills. (See also Chapter 20: *Dissociative Disorders*.)

Prisoners of War and Torture Victims. Prisoners who survive war or torture experiences do so because of personal inner strengths developed in their earlier lives, beginning within their emotionally strong and caring families; if they come from troubled families, they are more likely to commit suicide during imprisonment and torture. Prisoners must constantly cope with ongoing anxiety, fear, isolation from known lives, and complete loss of all control over their lives. Those who appear to cope best believe they must survive for a reason (e.g., to tell others what they experienced or to find and return to loved ones). Prisoners who cope best describe living simultaneously on two levels—coping in the here and now to survive the situation while maintaining constant mental connections to their past values and experiences and those important to them (Fig. 33-1).

Beyond the surviving prisoner's personal difficulties, including PTSD disorder, if and when his or her survival behavior continues, his or her family may be affected by the surviving prisoner's inordinate fear of police and strangers, overprotection and overburdening of children to replace those significant others lost, lack of sharing of the past, continued isolation from current communities, or inappropriate expressed anger. Thus, another generation (i.e., children of survivors) can be affected in their personal development and psychological functioning and may require psychiatric evaluation and treatment. (See also Chapter 16.5: *Posttraumatic Stress Disorder and Acute Stress Disorder*.)

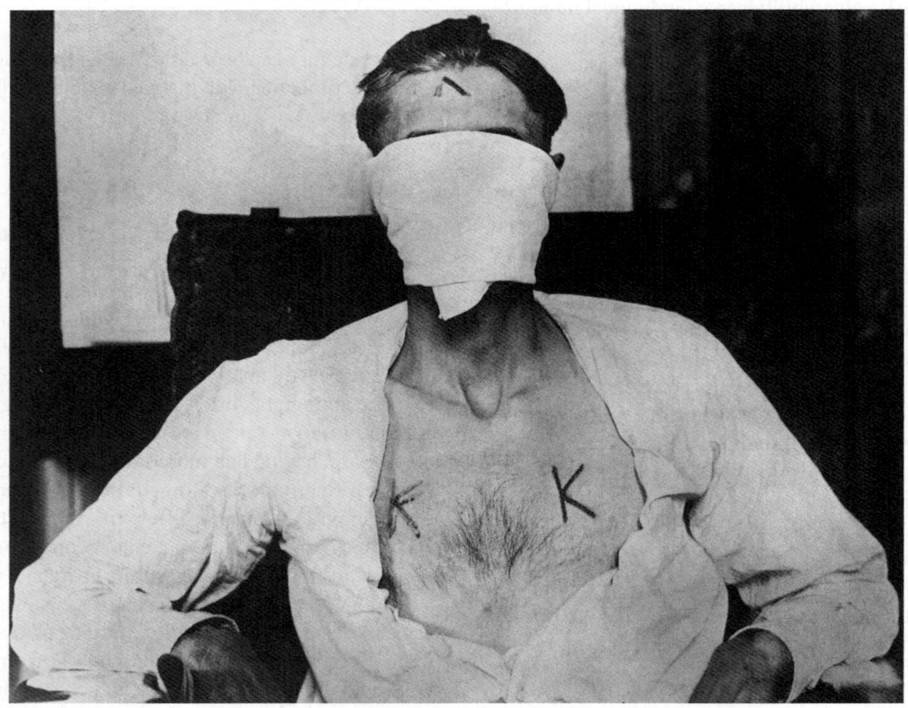

FIGURE 33–1

Nelson Burroughs displays the initials "KK" which were branded onto his chest and forehead by the Ku Klux Klan with a hot iron during his 17 days of captivity after his kidnapping near Haverhill, Massachusetts in 1925. The kidnappers were attempting to force Burroughs to renounce the Catholic Church. (Courtesy of Corbis.)

A 75-year-old, Catholic, female survivor of the Pawiak prison in Warsaw, Poland, and then of a concentration camp after her capture as a member of the underground in World War II stated that she had wanted to become a painter. In camp, she carved the Madonna and Child on her toothbrush and sent it home to her mother. She made other clandestine carvings for several women in her barracks to send home to their families, which pleased everyone. After the war, she became a well-known sculptress with exhibits throughout Europe. Many of her art pieces taught people about suffering and respect for others who are of different religions and cultures.

PHASE OF LIFE PROBLEM

The DSM-IV-TR description of phase of life problem includes the following:

> This category can be used when the focus of clinical attention is a problem associated with a particular developmental phase or some other life circumstance that is not due to a mental disorder or, if it is due to a mental disorder, is sufficiently severe to warrant independent clinical attention. Examples include: problems associated with entering school, leaving parental control, starting a new job or career, and changes involved in marriage, divorce, relationship loss, illness, and retirement.

Although, on some level, adults recognize that life events will intrude on expected plans in the course of a lifetime, unexpected, multiple, major negative occurrences, especially if they are chronic, overwhelm a person's ability to recover and function constructively. Common phase of life problems include relationship changes, such as a changed significant personal relationship or its loss, job crises, and parenthood.

Because of sex role socialization and consequent cultural expectations, men appear externally better able to handle these phases of life problems, whereas women, the poor, and minority group members appear more vulnerable to negative experiences, perhaps because they feel less empowered psychologically. Major life changes precipitate distress in the form of anxiety and depressive symptoms, inability to express reactive emotions directly, and, often, difficulties in coping with ongoing or changed life responsibilities.

Individuals with positive attitudes, strong family and personal relationships, and mature defense mechanisms and coping styles, including basic trust in self and others, good verbal communication skills, a capacity for creative and positive thinking, and the ability to be flexible, reliable, and energetic, appear to be best able to cope with phase of life problems. Furthermore, a capacity for sublimation, adequate financial and work status, solid values, and healthy feasible goals can enable people to face, accept, and deal realistically with expected and unexpected life problems and changes.

NONCOMPLIANCE WITH TREATMENT

The DSM-IV-TR contains the following statement regarding noncompliance with treatment:

> This category can be used when the focus of clinical attention is noncompliance with an important aspect of the treatment for a mental disorder or a general medical condition. The reasons for noncompliance may include discomfort resulting from treatment (e.g., medication side effects), expense of treatment, decisions based on personal value judgments, religious or cultural beliefs about the advantages and disadvantages of the proposed treatment, maladaptive personality traits or coping styles (e.g., denial of illness), or the presence of a mental disorder (e.g., Schizophrenia, Avoidant Personality Disorder). This category should be used only when the problem is sufficiently severe to warrant independent clinical attention.

Compliance is closely connected to the doctor–patient relationship, and a thorough discussion of noncompliance and compliance appears in Chapter 1: *The Patient–Doctor Relationship*.

AGE-RELATED COGNITIVE DECLINE

The DSM-IV-TR includes the following comment regarding age-related cognitive decline:

> This category can be used when the focus of clinical attention is an objectively identified decline in cognitive functioning consequent to the aging process that is within normal limits given the person's age. Individuals with this condition may report problems remembering names or appointments or may experience difficulty in solving complex problems. This category should be considered only after it has been determined that the cognitive impairment is not attributable to a specific mental disorder or neurological condition.

Attempts to delay age-related cognitive decline are myriad. They include daily intake of vitamin E (200 to 600 mg), daily intake of nonsteroidal anti-inflammatory drugs (NSAIDs), use of the herb ginkgo biloba, and use of male and female sex steroids. Cognitive decline is lower in persons who exercise, do not smoke, drink little or no alcohol, and who challenge their intellect at work or play (e.g., crossword puzzles). The ability to learn new material is maintained through old age; however, it takes longer and requires more practice than in young persons.

REFERENCES

Barzilai-Pesach V, Sheiner EK, Sheiner E, Potashnik G, Shoham-Vardi I. The effect of women's occupational psychologic stress on outcome of fertility treatments. *J Occup Environ Med.* 2006;48(1):56–62.

Bhugra D. Migration and depression. *Acta Psychiatr Scand Suppl.* 2003;418:67–72.

Bogduk N. Diagnostic blocks: A truth serum for malingering. *Clin J Pain.* 2004;20(6):409–414.

Bosco SM, Harvey D. Effects of terror attacks on employment plans and anxiety levels of college students. *College Student Journal.* 2003;37:438–446.

Campagna AF. Sexual abuse of males: The SAM model of theory and practice. *J Am Acad Child Adolesc Psychiatry.* 2005;44(10):1064–1065.

Caruso KA, Benedek DM, Auble PM, Bernet W. Concealment of psychopathology in forensic evaluations: A pilot study of intentional and uninsightful dissimulators. *J Am Acad Psychiatry Law.* 2003;31(4):444–450.

Costigan CL, Cox MJ, Cauce AM. Work–parenting linkage among dual earner couples at the transition to parenthood. *J Fam Psychol.* 2003;17:397–408.

Dagan E, Gil S. BRCA1/2 mutation carriers: Psychological distress and ways of coping. *Journal of Psychosocial Oncology*. 2004;22(3):93–106.

Dickstein LJ. Other additional conditions that may be a focus of clinical attention. In: Sadock BJ, Sadock VA, eds. *Kaplan & Sadock's Comprehensive Textbook of Psychiatry*. 8th ed. Vol. 2. Baltimore: Lippincott Williams & Wilkins; 2005:2277.

Feldman MD. *Playing Sick? Untangling the Web of Munchausen Syndrome, Munchausen by Proxy, Malingering, and Factitious Disorder*. New York: Brunner-Routledge; 2004.

Guriel J, Fremouw W. Assessing malingered posttraumatic disorder: A critical review. *Clin Psychol Rev*. 2003;23(7):881–904.

Larrabee GJ. Detection of malingering using atypical performance patterns on standard neuropsychological tests. *Clin Neuropsychol*. 2003;17(3):410–425.

Mills MJ, Lipian MS. Malingering. In: Sadock BJ, Sadock VA, eds. *Kaplan & Sadock's Comprehensive Textbook of Psychiatry*. 8th ed. Vol. 2. Baltimore: Lippincott Williams & Wilkins. 2005: 2247.

O'Bryant SE, Hilsabeck RC, Fisher JM, McCaffrey RJ. Utility of the trail making test in the assessment of malingering in a sample of mild traumatic brain injury litigants. *Clin Neuropsychol*. 2003;17(1):69–74.

Zierold KM, Anderson H. The relationship between work permits, injury, and safety training among working teenagers. *Am J Ind Med*. 2006;49(5):360–366.

34 Emergency Psychiatric Medicine

▲ 34.1 Suicide

Suicide is the primary emergency for the mental health professional, with homicide and failure to diagnose an underlying potentially fatal medical illness representing other, but less common, emergencies. Suicide is also a major public health problem: More than 30,000 persons commit suicide each year in the United States with more than 600,000 suicide attempts. Although suicide is impossible to predict precisely, numerous clues can be seen, which are enumerated in this section to help the practitioner reduce the risk for his or her patients. Also, some generally accepted standards of care exist that facilitate risk reduction, as well as lessen the likelihood of successful litigation, should a patient death occur and a lawsuit be filed. Suicide also needs to be considered in terms of the devastating legacy that it leaves for those who have survived a loved one's suicide, as well as the ramifications for the clinicians who cared for the decedents. Perhaps the most important concept regarding suicide is that it is almost always the result of a mental illness, usually depression, and is amenable to psychological and pharmacological treatment.

Suicide is derived from the Latin word for "self-murder." It is a fatal act that represents the person's wish to die. There is a range, however, between thinking about suicide and acting it out. Some persons have ideas of suicide that they will never act on; some plan for days, weeks, or even years before acting; and others take their lives seemingly on impulse, without premeditation. Lost in the definition are intentional misclassifications of the cause of death, accidents of undetermined cause, and so-called chronic suicides—for example, death through alcohol and other substance abuse and consciously poor adherence to medical regimens for addiction, obesity, and hypertension.

EPIDEMIOLOGY

As mentioned approximately 30,000 deaths are attributed to suicide each year in the United States. This is in contrast to approximately 20,000 deaths annually from homicide. Although significant shifts were seen in the suicide death rates for certain subpopulations during the last century (e.g., increased adolescent and decreased elderly rates), the rate has remained fairly constant, averaging about 12.5 per 100,000 through the 20th century and into the 21st. Whereas the overall suicide rate remained relatively stable, however, the rate for those 15 to 24 years of age has increased two- to threefold. Suicide is currently ranked the 8th overall cause of death in the United States, after heart disease, cancer, cerebrovascular disease, chronic obstructive pulmonary disease, accidents, pneumonia and influenza, and diabetes mellitus.

Suicide rates in the United States are at the midpoint of the rates for industrialized countries as reported to the United Nations. Internationally, suicide rates range from highs of more than 25 per 100,000 persons in Scandinavia, Switzerland, Germany, Austria, the eastern European countries (the so-called suicide belt), and Japan, to fewer than 10 per 100,000 in Spain, Italy, Ireland, Egypt, and the Netherlands.

A state-by-state analysis of suicides in the last decade among persons between the ages of 15 and 44 revealed that New Jersey had the nation's lowest suicide rates for both sexes. Nevada and New Mexico had the highest rates for men, and Nevada and Wyoming had the highest rates for women. Women in Nevada killed themselves at a higher frequency than did men in New Jersey. The prime suicide site of the world is the Golden Gate Bridge in San Francisco, with more than 800 suicides committed there since the bridge opened in 1937.

Risk Factors

Gender Differences. Men commit suicide more than four times as often as women, a rate that is stable over all ages. Women, however, are four times more likely to attempt suicide than men. Men's higher rate of completed suicide is related to the methods they use: firearms, hanging, or jumping from high places. Women more commonly take an overdose of psychoactive substances or a poison, but their use of firearms is increasing. In states with gun control laws, the use of firearms has decreased as a method of suicide. Globally, the most common method of suicide is hanging (Fig 34.1-1).

Age. Suicide rates increase with age and underscore the significance of the midlife crisis. Among men, suicides peak after age 45; among women, the greatest number of completed suicides occurs after age 55. Rates of 40 per 100,000 population occur in men age 65 and older. Older persons attempt suicide less often than younger persons, but are more often successful. Although they are only 10 percent of the total population, older persons account for 25 percent of suicides. The rate for those 75 or older is more than three times the rate among young persons.

The suicide rate, however, is rising most rapidly among young persons, particularly males 15 to 24 years of age, and the rate is still rising. The suicide rate for females in the same age group is increasing more slowly than that for males. Among men 25 to 34 years of age, the suicide rate increased almost 30 percent over the past decade. Suicide is the third leading cause of death in those 15 to 24 years of age, after accidents and homicides, and attempted suicides in this age group number between 1 million and 2 million annually. Most suicides now occur among those aged 15 to 44. Suicide is rare before puberty. (See Chapter 49: *Mood*

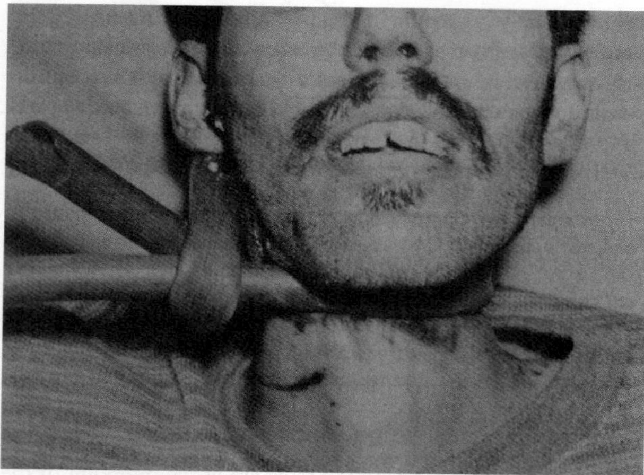

FIGURE 34.1–1
A suicidal hanging by means of a rubber hose. (Courtesy of New York University School of Medicine.)

Disorders and Suicide in Children and Adolescents for a thorough discussion of this topic.)

Race. Two of every three suicides are white males. White male and female rates are approximately two to three times as high as African American male and female rates across the life cycle. Among young persons who live in inner cities and certain Native American and Inuit groups, suicide rates have greatly exceeded the national rate. Suicide rates among immigrants are higher than those in the native-born population.

Religion. Historically, suicide rates among Roman Catholic populations have been lower than rates among Protestants and Jews. The degree of orthodoxy and integration may be a more accurate measure of risk in this category than simple institutional religious affiliation.

Marital Status. Marriage lessens the risk of suicide significantly, especially if there are children in the home. Single, never-married persons register an overall rate nearly double that of married persons. Divorce increases suicide risk, with divorced men three times more likely to kill themselves as divorced women. Widows and widowers also have high rates. Suicide occurs more frequently than usual in persons who are socially isolated and have a family history of suicide (attempted or real). Persons who commit so-called anniversary suicides take their lives on the day a member of their family did.

Occupation. The higher a person's social status, the greater the risk of suicide, but a fall in social status also increases the risk. Work, in general, protects against suicide. Among occupational rankings, professionals, particularly physicians, have traditionally been considered to be at greatest risk. Other high risk occupations include law enforcement, dentists, artists, mechanics, lawyers, and insurance agents. Suicide is higher among the unemployed than among employed persons. The suicide rate increases during economic recessions and depressions and decreases during times of high unemployment and during wars.

PHYSICIAN SUICIDES. The weight of current evidence supports the conclusion that both male and female physicians in the United States have elevated rates of suicide, with females at particularly high risk. Recent United Kingdom and Scandinavian data show that the suicide rate for male physicians is two to three times that found in the general male population of the same age. Female physicians have a higher risk of suicide than other women. In the United States, the annual suicide rate for female physicians is about 41 per 100,000, compared with 12 per 100,000 among all white women over 25 years of age. Studies show that physicians who commit suicide have a mental disorder, most often depressive disorder, substance dependence, or both. Both male and female physicians commit suicide significantly more often by substance overdoses and less often by firearms than persons in the general population; drug availability and knowledge about toxicity are important factors in physician suicides. Among physicians, psychiatrists are considered to be at greatest risk, followed by ophthalmologists and anesthesiologists, but all specialties are vulnerable.

Climate. No significant seasonal correlation with suicide has been found. Suicides increase slightly in spring and fall but, contrary to popular belief, not during December and holiday periods.

Physical Health. The relation of physical health and illness to suicide is significant. Previous medical care appears to be a positively correlated risk indicator of suicide: About one third of all persons who commit suicide have had medical attention within 6 months of death and a physical illness is estimated to be an important contributing factor in about half of suicides.

Factors associated with illness and contributing to both suicides and suicide attempts are loss of mobility, especially when physical activity is important to occupation or recreation; disfigurement, particularly among women; and chronic, intractable pain. Patients on hemodialysis are at high risk. In addition to the direct effects of illness, the secondary effects—for example, disruption of relationships and loss of occupational status—are prognostic factors.

Certain drugs can produce depression, which may lead to suicide in some cases. Among these drugs are reserpine (Serpasil), corticosteroids, antihypertensives, and some anticancer agents. Alcohol-related illnesses, such as cirrhosis, are associated with higher suicide rates.

Mental Illness. Almost 95 percent of all persons who commit or attempt suicide have a diagnosed mental disorder. Depressive disorders account for 80 percent of this figure, schizophrenia accounts for 10 percent, and dementia or delirium for 5 percent. Among all persons with mental disorders, 25 percent are also alcohol dependent and have dual diagnoses. Persons with delusional depression are at highest risk of suicide. A history of impulsive behavior or violent acts increases the risk of suicide as does previous psychiatric hospitalization for any reason. Among adults who commit suicide, significant differences between young and old exist for both psychiatric diagnoses and antecedent stressors. Diagnoses of substance abuse and antisocial personality disorder occurred most often among suicides in persons less than 30 years of age, and diagnoses of mood disorders and cognitive disorders most often among suicides in those age 30 and above. Stressors associated with suicide in those under 30 were separation, rejection, unemployment, and legal troubles; illness stressors most often occurred among suicide victims over 30.

Psychiatric Patients. Psychiatric patients' risk for suicide is 3 to 12 times that of nonpatients. The degree of risk varies, depending on age, sex, diagnosis, and inpatient or outpatient status. Male and female psychiatric patients who have at some time been inpatients have five and ten times higher suicide risks, respectively, than their counterparts in the general population. For male and female outpatients who have never been admitted to a hospital for psychiatric treatment, the suicide risks are three and four times greater, respectively, than those of their counterparts in the general population. The higher suicide risk for psychiatric patients who have been inpatients reflects that patients with severe mental disorders tend to be hospitalized—for example, patients with depressive disorder who require electroconvulsive therapy (ECT). The psychiatric diagnosis with greatest risk of suicide in both sexes is a mood disorder.

Those in the general population who commit suicide tend to be middle-aged or older, but studies increasingly report that psychiatric patients who commit suicide tend to be relatively young. In one study, the mean age of male suicides was 29.5 years and that of women 38.4 years. The relative youthfulness of these suicide cases was partly because that two early-onset, chronic mental disorders—schizophrenia and recurrent major depressive disorder—accounted for just over half of these suicides and so reflected an age and diagnostic pattern found in most studies of psychiatric patient suicides.

A small, but significant, percentage of psychiatric patients who commit suicide do so while they are inpatients. Most of these do not kill themselves in the psychiatric ward itself, but on the hospital grounds, while on a pass or weekend leave, or when absent without leave. For both sexes, the suicide risk is highest in the first week of the psychiatric admission; after 3 to 5 weeks, inpatients have the same risk as the general population. Times of staff rotation, particularly of the psychiatric residents, are periods associated with inpatient suicides. Epidemics of inpatient suicides tend to be associated with periods of ideological change on the ward, staff disorganization, and staff demoralization.

The period after discharge from the hospital is a time of increased suicide risk. A follow-up study of 5,000 patients discharged from an Iowa psychiatric hospital showed that in the first 3 months after discharge, the rate of suicide for female patients was 275 times that of all Iowa women; the rate of suicide for male patients was 70 times that of all Iowa men. Studies show that one third or more of depressed patients who commit suicide do so within 6 months of leaving a hospital; presumably they have relapsed.

The main risk groups are patients with depressive disorders, schizophrenia, and substance abuse, and patients who make repeated visits to the emergency room. Patients, especially those with panic disorder, who frequent emergency services, also have an increased suicide risk. Thus, mental health professionals working in emergency services must be well trained in assessing suicidal risk and making appropriate dispositions. They must also be aware of the need to contact patients at risk who fail to keep follow-up appointments.

DEPRESSIVE DISORDERS. Mood disorders are the diagnoses most commonly associated with suicide. The psychopharmacological advances of the past 25 years may have reduced the suicide risk among patients with depressive disorder. Nevertheless, the age-adjusted suicide rates for patients with mood disorders have been estimated to be 400 per 100,000 for male patients and 180 per 100,000 for female patients.

More patients with depressive disorders commit suicide early in the illness than later; more depressed men than women commit suicide; and the chance of depressed persons' killing themselves increases if they are single, separated, divorced, widowed, or recently bereaved. Patients with depressive disorder in the community who commit suicide tend to be middle-aged or older.

Social isolation enhances suicidal tendencies among depressed patients. This finding is in accord with the data from epidemiological studies showing that persons who commit suicide may be poorly integrated into society. Suicide among depressed patients is likely at the onset or the end of a depressive episode. As with other psychiatric patients, the months after discharge from a hospital are a time of high risk.

Regarding outpatient treatment, most depressed suicidal patients had a history of therapy; however, less than half were receiving psychiatric treatment at the time of suicide. Of those who were in treatment, studies have shown that treatment was less than adequate. For example, most patients who received antidepressants were prescribed subtherapeutic doses of the medication.

SCHIZOPHRENIA. The suicide risk is high among patients with schizophrenia: Up to 10 percent die by committing suicide. In the United States, an estimated 4,000 patients with schizophrenia commit suicide each year. The onset of schizophrenia is typically in adolescence or early adulthood, and most of these patients who commit suicide do so during the first few years of their illness; therefore, those patients with schizophrenia who commit suicide are young.

Thus, the risk factors for suicide among patients with schizophrenia are young age, male gender, single marital status, a previous suicide attempt, a vulnerability to depressive symptoms, and a recent discharge from a hospital. Having three or four hospitalizations during their 20s probably undermines the social, occupational, and sexual adjustment of possibly suicidal patients with schizophrenia. Consequently, potential suicide victims are likely to be male, unmarried, unemployed, socially isolated, and living alone—perhaps in a single room. After discharge from their last hospitalization, they may experience a new adversity or return to ongoing difficulties. As a result, they become dejected, experience feelings of helplessness and hopelessness, reach a depressed state, and have, and eventually act on, suicidal ideas. Only a small percentage committed suicide because of hallucinated instructions or a need to escape persecutory delusions. Up to 50 percent of suicides among patients with schizophrenia occur during the first few weeks and months after discharge from a hospital; only a minority commit suicide while inpatients.

ALCOHOL DEPENDENCE. Up to 15 percent of all alcohol-dependent persons commit suicide. The suicide rate for those who are alcoholic is estimated to be about 270 per 100,000 annually; in the United States, between 7,000 and 13,000 alcohol-dependent persons commit suicide each year.

About 80 percent of all alcohol-dependent suicide victims are male, a percentage that largely reflects the sex ratio for alcohol dependence. Alcohol-dependent suicide victims tend to be white, middle-aged, unmarried, friendless, socially isolated, and currently drinking. Up to 40 percent have made a previous suicide attempt. Up to 40 percent of all suicides by persons who are alcohol dependent occur within a year of the patient's last hospitalization; older alcohol-dependent patients are at particular risk during the postdischarge period.

Studies show that many alcohol-dependent patients who eventually commit suicide are rated depressed during hospitalization and that up to two thirds are assessed as having mood disorder symptoms during the period in which they commit suicide. As many as 50 percent of all alcohol-dependent suicide victims have experienced the loss of a close, affectionate relationship during the previous year. Such interpersonal losses and other types of undesirable life events are probably brought about by the alcohol dependence and contribute to the development of the mood disorder symptoms, which are often present in the weeks and months before the suicide.

The largest group of male alcohol-dependent patients is composed of those with an associated antisocial personality disorder. Studies show that such patients are particularly likely to attempt suicide; to abuse other substances; to exhibit impulsive, aggressive, and criminal behaviors; and to be found among alcohol-dependent suicide victims.

OTHER SUBSTANCE DEPENDENCE. Studies in various countries have found an increased suicide risk among those who abuse substances. The suicide rate for persons who are heroin dependent is about 20 times the rate for the general population. Adolescent girls who use intravenous substances also have a high suicide rate. The availability of a lethal amount of substances, intravenous use, associated antisocial personality disorder, a chaotic lifestyle, and impulsivity are some of the factors that predispose substance-dependent persons to suicidal behavior, particularly when they are dysphoric, depressed, or intoxicated.

PERSONALITY DISORDERS. A high proportion of those who commit suicide have various associated personality difficulties or disorders. Having a personality disorder may be a determinant of suicidal behavior in several ways: by predisposing to major mental disorders such as depressive disorders or alcohol dependence; by leading to difficulties in relationships and social adjustment; by precipitating undesirable life events; by impairing the ability to cope with a mental or physical disorder;

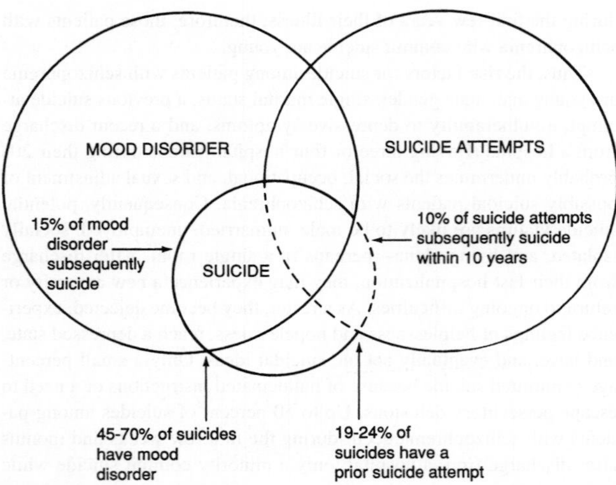

FIGURE 34.1–2

Venn diagram summarizing suicide data and its relation to mood disorder and suicide attempts. (Courtesy of Alec Roy, M.D.)

and by drawing persons into conflicts with those around them, including family members, physicians, and hospital staff members.

An estimated 5 percent of patients with antisocial personality disorder commit suicide. Suicide is three times more common among prisoners than among the general population. More than one third of prisoner suicides have had past psychiatric treatment, and half have made a previous suicide threat or attempt, often in the previous 6 months.

ANXIETY DISORDER. Uncompleted suicide attempts are made by almost 20 percent of patients with a panic disorder and social phobia. If depression is an associated feature, however, the risk of completed suicide rises.

Previous Suicidal Behavior.

A past suicide attempt is perhaps the best indicator that a patient is at increased risk of suicide. Studies show that about 40 percent of depressed patients who commit suicide have made a previous attempt. The risk of a second suicide attempt is highest within 3 months of the first attempt. The relation between a mood disorder, completed suicide, and attempts at suicide is shown in Figure 34.1-2.

Depression is associated with both completed suicide and serious attempts at suicide. The clinical feature most often associated with the seriousness of the intent to die is a diagnosis of a depressive disorder. This is shown by studies that relate the clinical characteristics of suicidal patients with various measures of the medical seriousness of the attempt or of the intent to die. Also, intent-to-die scores correlate significantly with both suicide risk scores and the number and severity of depressive symptoms. Patients having high suicide intent are more often male, older, single or separated, and living alone than those with low intent. In other words, depressed patients who seriously attempt suicide more closely resemble suicide victims than they do suicide attempters.

ETIOLOGY

Sociological Factors

Durkheim's Theory.

The first major contribution to the study of the social and cultural influences on suicide was made at the end of the 19th century by the French sociologist Emile Durkheim. In an attempt to explain statistical patterns, Durkheim divided suicides into three social categories: egoistic, altruistic, and anomic. Egoistic suicide applies to those who are not strongly integrated into any social group. The lack of family integration explains why unmarried persons are more vulnerable to suicide than married ones and why couples with children are the best protected group. Rural communities have more social integration than urban areas and, thus, fewer suicides. Protestantism is a less cohesive religion than Roman Catholicism, and so Protestants have a higher suicide rate than Catholics.

Altruistic suicide applies to those susceptible to suicide stemming from their excessive integration into a group, with suicide being the outgrowth of the integration—for example, a Japanese soldier who sacrifices his life in battle. Anomic suicide applies to persons whose integration into society is disturbed so that they cannot follow customary norms of behavior. Anomie explains why a drastic change in economic situation makes persons more vulnerable than they were before their change in fortune. In Durkheim's theory, anomie also refers to social instability, and a general breakdown of society's standards and values.

Psychological Factors

Freud's Theory.

Sigmund Freud offered the first important psychological insight into suicide. He described only one patient who made a suicide attempt, but he saw many depressed patients. In his paper "Mourning and Melancholia," Freud stated his belief that suicide represents aggression turned inward against an introjected, ambivalently cathected love object. Freud doubted that there would be a suicide without an earlier repressed desire to kill someone else.

Menninger's Theory.

Building on Freud's ideas, Karl Menninger, in *Man against Himself*, conceived of suicide as inverted homicide because of a patient's anger toward another person. This retroflexed murder is either turned inward or used as an excuse for punishment. He also described a self-directed death instinct (Freud's concept of Thanatos) plus three components of hostility in suicide: the wish to kill, the wish to be killed, and the wish to die.

Recent Theories.

Contemporary suicidologists are not persuaded that a specific psychodynamic or personality structure is associated with suicide. They believe that much can be learned about the psychodynamics of suicidal patients from their fantasies about what would happen and what the consequences would be if they commit suicide. Such fantasies often include wishes for revenge, power, control, or punishment; atonement, sacrifice, or restitution; escape or sleep; rescue, rebirth, reunion with the dead; or a new life. The suicidal patients most likely to act out suicidal fantasies may have lost a love object or received a narcissistic injury, may experience overwhelming affects like rage and guilt, or may identify with a suicide victim. Group dynamics underlie mass suicides such as those at Masada, at Jonestown, and by the Heaven's Gate cult.

Depressed persons may attempt suicide just as they appear to be recovering from their depression. A suicide attempt can cause a long-standing depression to disappear, especially if it fulfills a patient's need for punishment. Of equal relevance, many suicidal patients use a preoccupation with suicide as a way of fighting off intolerable depression and a sense of hopelessness. A study by Aaron Beck showed that hopelessness was one of the most accurate indicators of long-term suicidal risk.

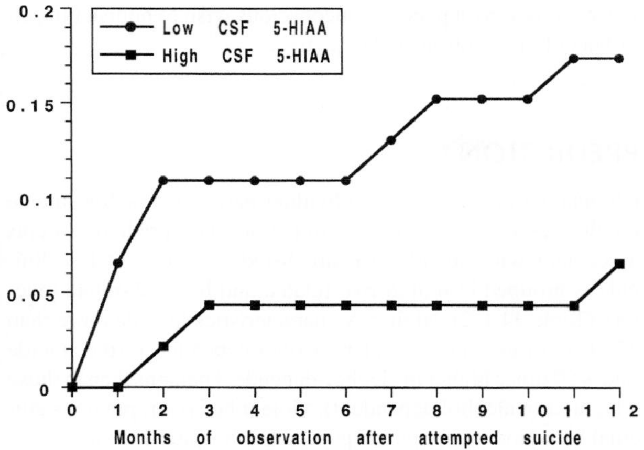

FIGURE 34.1–3

Cumulative suicide risk during first year after attempted suicide in patients with low versus high CSF concentrations of 5-HIAA. *Filled circles* indicate CSF 5-HIAA concentrations below the sample median and *filled squares* indicate concentrations above the sample median (87 nM). (From Nordstrom P, Samuelsson M, Asberg M, et al. CSF concentrations 5-HIAA predicts suicide risk after attempted suicide. *Suicide Life Threat Behav.* 1994;24:1, with permission.)

Biological Factors. Diminished central serotonin plays a role in suicidal behavior. A group at the Karolinska Institute in Sweden first noted that low concentrations of the serotonin metabolite 5-hydroxyindoleacetic acid (5-HIAA) in the lumbar cerebrospinal fluid (CSF) were associated with suicidal behavior. This finding has been replicated many times and in different diagnostic groups. Postmortem neurochemical studies have reported modest decreases in serotonin itself or 5-HIAA in either the brainstem or the frontal cortex of suicide victims. Postmortem receptor studies have reported significant changes in presynaptic and postsynaptic serotonin binding sites in suicide victims. Together, these CSF, neurochemical, and receptor studies support the hypothesis that reduced central serotonin is associated with suicide. Recent studies also report some changes in the noradrenergic system of suicide victims.

Low concentrations of 5-HIAA in CSF also predict future suicidal behavior. For example, the Karolinska group examined completed suicide in a sample of 92 depressed patients who had attempted suicide. They found that 8 of the 11 patients who committed suicide within 1 year belonged to the subgroup with below-median concentrations of 5-HIAA in CSF. The suicide risk in that subgroup was 17 percent, compared with 7 percent among those with above-median concentrations of 5-HIAA in CSF (Fig. 34.1-3). Also, the cumulative number of patient-months survived during the first year after attempted suicide was significantly lower in the subgroup with low 5-HIAA concentrations. The Karolinska group concluded that low 5-HIAA concentrations in CSF predict short-range suicide risk in the high-risk group of depressed patients who have attempted suicide. Low 5-HIAA concentrations in CSF have also been demonstrated in adolescents who kill themselves.

Genetic Factors. Suicidal behavior, as with other psychiatric disorders, tends to run in families. For example, Margaux Hemingway's 1997 suicide was the fifth suicide among four generations of Ernest Hemingway's family. In psychiatric patients, a family history of suicide increases the risk of attempted suicide and that of completed suicide in most diagnostic groups. In medicine, the strongest evidence for involvement of genetic factors comes from twin and adoption studies and from molecular genetics. Such studies in suicide are reviewed below.

Twin Studies. A landmark study in 1991 investigated 176 twin pairs in which one twin had committed suicide. In nine of these twin pairs, both twins had committed suicide. Seven of these nine pairs concordant for suicide were found among the 62 monozygotic pairs, whereas two pairs concordant for suicide were found among the 114 dizygotic twin pairs. This twin group difference for concordance for suicide (11.3 versus 1.8 percent) is statistically significant ($P < .01$).

Another study collected a group of 35 twin pairs in which one twin had committed suicide, and the living co-twin was interviewed. Ten of the 26 living monozygotic co-twins had themselves attempted suicide, compared with 0 of the 9 living dizygotic co-twins ($P < .04$). Although monozygotic and dizygotic twins may have some differing developmental experiences, these results show that monozygotic twin pairs have significantly higher concordance for both suicide and attempted suicide, which suggests that genetic factors may play a role in suicidal behavior.

Danish-American Adoption Studies. The strongest evidence suggesting the presence of genetic factors in suicide comes from adoption studies carried out in Denmark. A screening of the registers of causes of death revealed that 57 of 5,483 adoptees in Copenhagen eventually committed suicide. They were matched with adopted controls. Searches of the causes of death revealed that 12 of the 269 biological relatives of these 57 adopted suicide victims had themselves committed suicide, compared with only 2 of the 269 biological relatives of the 57 adopted controls. This is a highly significant difference for suicide between the two groups of relatives. None of the adopting relatives of either the suicide or control group had committed suicide.

In a further study of 71 adoptees with mood disorder, adoptee suicide victims with a situational crisis or impulsive suicide attempt or both (particularly) had more biological relatives who had committed suicide than controls had. This led to the suggestion that a genetic factor lowering the threshold for suicidal behavior may lead to an inability to control impulsive behavior. Psychiatric disorder or environmental stress may serve "as potentiating mechanisms which foster or trigger the impulsive behavior, directing it toward a suicidal outcome."

Molecular Genetic Studies. Tryptophan hydroxylase (TPH) is an enzyme involved in the biosynthesis of serotonin. A polymorphism in the human TPH gene has been identified, with two alleles—U and L. Because low concentrations of 5-HIAA in CSF are associated with suicidal behavior, it was hypothesized that such individuals may have alterations in genes controlling serotonin synthesis and metabolism. It was found that impulsive alcoholics, who had low CSF 5-HIAA concentrations, had more LL and UL genotypes. Furthermore, a history of suicide attempts was significantly associated with TPH genotype in all the violent alcoholics; 34 of the 36 violent subjects who attempted suicide had either the UL or LL genotype. Thus, it was concluded that the presence of the L allele was associated with an increased risk of suicide attempts.

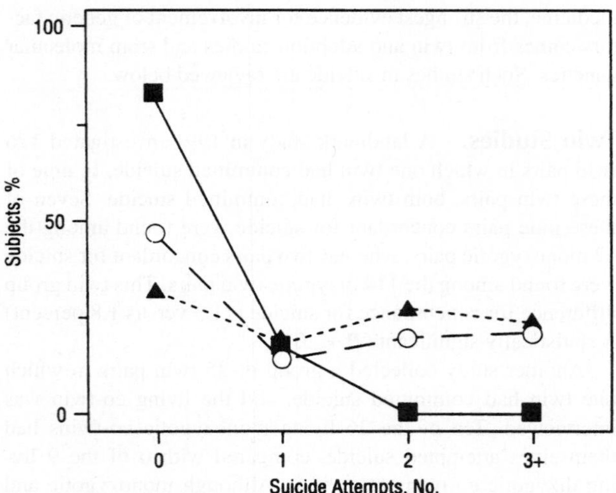

FIGURE 34.1–4
Relation between tryptophan hydroxylase (TPH) genotype and lifetime history of multiple suicide attempts. For each genotype, the fraction of subjects having each genotype (UU, *squares*; UL, *circles*; LL, *triangles*) is plotted against the number of suicide attempts they have made in their lives. (From Nielsen D, Goldman D, Virkkunen M, et al. Suicidality and 5-hydroxyindoleacetic acid concentration associated with a tryptophan hydroxylase polymorphism. *Arch Gen Psychiatry*. 1994;51:34, with permission.)

Also, a history of multiple suicide attempts was found most often in subjects with the LL genotype and to a lesser extent among those with the UL genotype (Fig. 34.1-4). This led to the suggestion that the L allele was associated with repetitive suicidal behavior. The presence of one TPH*L allele may indicate a reduced capacity to hydroxylate tryptophan to 5-hydroxytryptophan in the synthesis of serotonin, producing low central serotonin turnover and, thus, a low concentration of 5-HIAA in CSF.

Parasuicidal Behavior. *Parasuicide* is a term introduced to describe patients who injure themselves by self-mutilation (e.g., cutting the skin), but who usually do not wish to die. Studies show that about 4 percent of all patients in psychiatric hospitals have cut themselves; the female-to-male ratio is almost 3 to 1. The incidence of self-injury in psychiatric patients is estimated to be more than 50 times that in the general population. Psychiatrists note that so-called cutters have cut themselves over several years. Self-injury is found in about 30 percent of all abusers of oral substances and 10 percent of all intravenous users admitted to substance-treatment units.

These patients are usually in their 20s and may be single or married. Most cut delicately, not coarsely, usually in private with a razor blade, knife, broken glass, or mirror. The wrists, arms, thighs, and legs are most commonly cut; the face, breasts, and abdomen are cut infrequently. Most persons who cut themselves claim to experience no pain and give reasons, such as anger at themselves or others, relief of tension, and the wish to die. Most are classified as having personality disorders and are significantly more introverted, neurotic, and hostile than controls. Alcohol abuse and other substance abuse are common, and most cutters have attempted suicide. Self-mutilation has been viewed as localized self-destruction, with mishandling of aggressive impulses caused by a person's unconscious wish to punish himself or herself or an introjected object.

PREDICTION

Clinicians must assess an individual patient's risk for suicide on the basis of a clinical examination. The predictive items associated with suicide risk are listed in Table 34.1-1. Suicide is grouped into high-risk-related and low-risk-related factors (Table 34.1-2). High-risk characteristics include more than 45 years of age, male gender, alcohol dependence (the suicide rate is 50 times higher in alcohol-dependent persons than in those who are not alcohol dependent), violent behavior, previous suicidal behavior, and previous psychiatric hospitalization.

It is important that questions about suicidal feelings and behaviors be asked, often directly. Asking depressed patients whether or not they have had thoughts of wanting to kill themselves does not plant the seed of suicide. To the contrary, it may be the first opportunity a patient has had to talk about suicidal ideation that may have been present for some time.

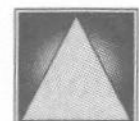

Table 34.1–1
Variables Enhancing Risk of Suicide among Vulnerable Groups

Adolescence and late life
Bisexual or homosexual gender identity
Criminal behavior
Cultural sanctions for suicide
Delusions
Disposition of personal property
Divorced, separated, or single marital status
Early loss or separation from parents
Family history of suicide
Hallucinations
Homicide
Hopelessness
Hypochondriasis
Impulsivity
Increasing agitation
Increasing stress
Insomnia
Lack of future plans
Lack of sleep
Lethality of previous attempt
Living alone
Low self-esteem
Male sex
Physical illness or impairment
Previous attempts that could have resulted in death
Protestant or nonreligious status
Recent childbirth
Recent loss
Repression as a defense
Secondary gain
Severe family pathology
Severe psychiatric illness
Sexual abuse
Signals of intent to die
Suicide epidemics
Unemployment
White race

(From Slaby AE. Outpatient management of suicidal patients in the era of managed care. *Prim Psychiatry*. 1995;Apr:43, with permission.)

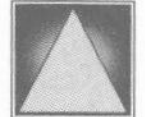

Table 34.1–2
Evaluation of Suicide Risk

Variable	High Risk	Low Risk
Demographic and Social Profile		
Age	Over 45 years	Below 45 years
Sex	Male	Female
Marital status	Divorced or widowed	Married
Employment	Unemployed	Employed
Interpersonal relationship	Conflictual	Stable
Family background	Chaotic or conflictual	Stable
Health		
Physical	Chronic illness	Good health
	Hypochondriac	Feels healthy
	Excessive substance intake	Low substance use
Mental	Severe depression	Mild depression
	Psychosis	Neurosis
	Severe personality disorder	Normal personality
	Substance abuse	Social drinker
	Hopelessness	Optimism
Suicidal activity		
Suicidal ideation	Frequent, intense, prolonged	Infrequent, low intensity, transient
Suicide attempt	Multiple attempts	First attempt
	Planned	Impulsive
	Rescue unlikely	Rescue inevitable
	Unambiguous wish to die	Primary wish for change
	Communication internalized (self-blame)	Communication externalized (anger)
	Method lethal and available	Method of low lethality or not readily available
Resources		
Personal	Poor achievement	Good achievement
	Poor insight	Insightful
	Affect unavailable or poorly controlled	Affect available and appropriately controlled
Social	Poor rapport	Good rapport
	Socially isolated	Socially integrated
	Unresponsive family	Concerned family

(From Adam K. Attempted suicide. *Psychiatr Clin North Am.* 1985;8:183, with permission.)

The American Psychiatric Association (APA) developed practice guidelines for treating patients with suicidal behaviors and Table 34.1-3 lists a host of questions that can help the clinician assess suicide risk.

TREATMENT

Most suicides among psychiatric patients are preventable, because evidence indicates that inadequate assessment or treatment is often associated with suicide. Some patients experience suffering so great and intense, or so chronic and unresponsive to treatment, that their eventual suicides may be perceived as inevitable. Such patients are relatively uncommon, however. Other patients have severe personality disorders, are highly impulsive, and commit suicide spontaneously, often when dysphoric or intoxicated or both.

The evaluation for suicide potential involves a complete psychiatric history; a thorough examination of the patient's mental state; and an inquiry about depressive symptoms, suicidal thoughts, intents, plans, and attempts. A lack of future plans, giving away personal property, making a will, and having recently experienced a loss all imply increased risk of suicide. The decision to hospitalize a patient depends on diagnosis, depression severity and suicidal ideation, the patient's and the family's coping abilities, the patient's living situation, availability of social support, and the absence or presence of risk factors for suicide.

Inpatient versus Outpatient Treatment

Whether to hospitalize patients with suicidal ideation is the most important clinical decision to be made. Not all such patients require hospitalization; some can be treated on an outpatient basis. But the absence of a strong social support system, a history of impulsive behavior, and a suicidal plan of action are indications for hospitalization. To decide whether outpatient treatment is feasible, clinicians should use a straightforward clinical approach: Ask patients who are considered suicidal to agree to call when they become uncertain about their ability to control their suicidal impulses. Patients who can make such an agreement with a doctor with whom they have a relationship reaffirm the belief that they have sufficient strength to control such impulses and to seek help.

In return for a patient's commitment, clinicians should be available to the patient 24 hours a day. If a patient who is considered seriously suicidal cannot make the commitment, immediate emergency hospitalization is indicated; both the patient and the patient's family should be so advised. If, however, the patient is to be treated on an outpatient basis, the therapist should note the patient's home and work telephone numbers for emergency reference; occasionally, a patient hangs up unexpectedly during a late night call or gives only a name to the answering service. If the patient refuses hospitalization, the family must take the responsibility to be with the patient 24 hours a day.

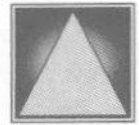

Table 34.1–3
Questions about Suicidal Feelings and Behaviors*

Begin with questions that address the patient's feeling about living

Have you ever felt that life was not worth living?
Did you ever wish you could go to sleep and just not wake up?

Follow on with specific questions that ask about thoughts of death, self-harm, or suicide

Is death something you have thought about recently?
Have things ever reached the point that you have thought of harming yourself?

For individuals who have thoughts of self-harm or suicide

When did you first notice such thoughts?
What led up to the thoughts (e.g., interpersonal and psychosocial precipitants, including real or imagined losses; specific symptoms such as mood changes, anhedonia, hopelessness, anxiety, agitation, psychosis)?
How often have those thoughts occurred, including frequency, obsessional quality, controllability?
How close have you come to acting on those thoughts?
How likely do you think it is that you will act on them in the future?
Have you ever started to harm (or kill) yourself but stopped before doing something (e.g., holding knife or gun to your body but stopping before acting, going to edge of bridge but not jumping)?
What do you envision happening if you actually killed yourself (e.g., escape, reunion with significant other, rebirth, reactions of others)?
Have you made a specific plan to harm or kill yourself? (If so, what does the plan include?)
Do you have guns or other weapons available to you?
Have you made any particular preparations (e.g., purchasing specific items, writing a note or a will, making financial arrangements, taking steps to avoid discovery, rehearsing the plan)?
Have you spoken to anyone about your plans?
How does the future look to you?
What things would lead you to feel more (or less) hopeful about the future (e.g., treatment, reconciliation of relationship, resolution of stressors)?
What things would make it more (or less) likely that you would try to kill yourself?
What things in your life would lead you to want to escape from life or be dead?
What things in your life make you want to go on living?
If you began to have thoughts of harming or killing yourself again, what would you do?

For individuals who have attempted suicide or engaged in self-damaging action(s), parallel questions to those in the previous section can address the prior attempt(s). Additional questions can be asked in general terms or can refer to the specific method used and may include:

Can you describe what happened (e.g., circumstances, precipitants, view of future, use of alcohol or other substances, method, intent, seriousness of injury)?
What thoughts were you having beforehand that led up to the attempt?
What did you think would happen (e.g., going to sleep versus injury versus dying, getting a reaction out of a particular person)?
Were other people present at the time?
Did you seek help afterward yourself, or did someone get help for you?
Had you planned to be discovered, or were you found accidentally?
How did you feel afterward (e.g., relief versus regret at being alive)?
Did you receive treatment afterward (e.g., medical versus psychiatric, emergency department versus inpatient versus outpatient)?
Has your view of things changed, or is anything different for you since the attempt?
Are there other times in the past when you have tried to harm (or kill) yourself?

For individuals with repeated suicidal thoughts or attempts

About how often have you tried to harm (or kill) yourself?
When was the most recent time?
Can you describe your thoughts at the time that you were thinking most seriously about suicide?
When was your most serious attempt at harming or killing yourself?
What led up to it, and what happened afterward?

For individuals with psychosis, ask specifically about hallucinations and delusions

Can you describe the voices (e.g., single versus multiple, male versus female, internal versus external, recognizable versus nonrecognizable)?
What do the voices say (e.g., positive remarks versus negative remarks versus threats)? (If the remarks are commands, determine if they are for harmless versus harmful acts; ask for examples.)
How do you cope with (or respond to) the voices?
Have you ever done what the voices ask you to do? (What led you to obey the voices? If you tried to resist them, what made it difficult?)
Have there been times when the voices told you to hurt or kill yourself? (How often? What happened?)
Are you worried about having a serious illness or that your body is rotting?
Are you concerned about your financial situation even when others tell you there's nothing to worry about?
Are there things that you've been feeling guilty about or blaming yourself for?

Consider assessing the patient's potential to harm others in addition to him- or herself

Are there others who you think may be responsible for what you are experiencing (e.g., persecutory ideas, passivity experiences)?
Are you having any thoughts of harming them?
Are there other people you would want to die with you?
Are there others who you think would be unable to go on without you?

*Direct and specific questions about suicide are essential in suicide assessment. The psychiatrist should ask about suicidal thoughts, plans, and behaviors. Accepting a negative response to an initial question about suicidal ideation may not be enough to determine actual suicide risk. A denial of suicidal ideation that is inconsistent with the patient's presentation or current depressive symptomatology may indicate a need for additional questioning or collateral sources of information. These questions may be helpful when asking about specific aspects of a patient's suicidal thoughts, plans and behaviors.

(From the *Practice Guidelines for Assessment and Treatment of the Suicidal Patient*, 2nd ed. *American Psychiatric Association Practice Guidelines for the Treatment of Psychiatric Disorders Compendium*, [Copyright 2004], with permission.)

According to ES Shneidman, a clinician has several practical preventive measures for dealing with a suicidal person: reducing the psychological pain by modifying the patient's stressful environment, enlisting the aid of the spouse, the employer, or a friend; building realistic support by recognizing that the patient may have a legitimate complaint; and offering alternatives to suicide.

Many psychiatrists believe that any patient who has attempted suicide, despite its lethality, should be hospitalized. Although most of these patients voluntarily enter a hospital, the danger to self is one of the few clear-cut indications currently acceptable in all states for involuntary hospitalization. In a hospital, patients can receive antidepressant or antipsychotic medications as indicated; individual therapy, group therapy, and family therapy are available, and patients receive the hospital's social support and sense of security. Other therapeutic measures depend on patients' underlying diagnoses. For example, if alcohol dependence is an associated problem, treatment must be directed toward alleviating that condition.

Although patients classified as acutely suicidal may have favorable prognoses, chronically suicidal patients are difficult to treat, and they exhaust the caretakers. Constant observation by special nurses, seclusion, and restraints cannot prevent suicide when a patient is resolute. ECT may be necessary for some severely depressed patients, who may require several treatment courses.

Useful measures for the treatment of depressed suicidal inpatients include searching patients and their belongings on arrival in the ward for objects that could be used for suicide and repeating the search at times of exacerbation of the suicidal ideation. Ideally, suicidally depressed inpatients should be treated on a locked ward where the windows are shatterproof, and the patient's room should be located near the nursing station to maximize observation by the nursing staff. The treatment team must assess how much to restrict the patient and whether to make regular checks or use continuous direct observation.

Vigorous treatment with antidepressant or antipsychotic medication should be initiated, depending on the underlying disorder. Some medications (e.g., risperidone [Risperdal]) have both antipsychotic and antidepressant effects and are useful when the patient has signs and symptoms of both psychosis and depression.

Supportive psychotherapy by a psychiatrist shows concern and may alleviate some of a patient's intense suffering. Some patients may be able to accept the idea that they are suffering from a recognized illness and that they will probably make a complete recovery. Patients should be dissuaded from making major life decisions while they are suicidally depressed, because such decisions are often morbidly determined and may be irrevocable. The consequences of such bad decisions can cause further anguish and misery when the patient has recovered.

Patients recovering from a suicidal depression are at particular risk. As the depression lifts, patients become energized and, thus, are able to put their suicidal plans into action (paradoxical suicide). A further complication is the activating effect of serotonergic drugs, such as fluoxetine, which are effective antidepressants, especially with suicidally depressed patients. Such agents may improve psychomotor withdrawal, thus permitting the patient to act on preexisting suicidal impulses because they have more energy. Sometimes, depressed patients, with or without treatment, suddenly appear to be at peace with themselves because they have reached a secret decision to commit suicide. Clinicians should be especially suspicious of such a dramatic clinical change, which may portend a suicide attempt. Although rare, some patients lie to the psychiatrist about their suicidal intent, thus subverting the most careful clinical assessment.

A patient may commit suicide even when in the hospital. According to one survey, about 1 percent of all suicides were committed by patients who were being treated in general medical-surgical or psychiatric hospitals, but the annual suicide rate in psychiatric hospitals is only 0.003 percent.

Table 34.1-4 lists guidelines for selecting a treatment setting for suicidal patients.

Legal and Ethical Factors. Liability issues stemming from suicides in psychiatric hospitals frequently involve questions about a patient's rate of deterioration, the presence during hospitalization of clinical signs indicating risk, and psychiatrists' and staff members' awareness of, and response to, these clinical signs.

In about half of cases in which suicides occur while patients are on a psychiatric unit, a lawsuit results. Courts do not require zero suicide rates, but do require periodic patient evaluation for suicidal risk, formulation of a treatment plan with a high level of security, and having staff members follow the treatment plan.

Currently, suicide and attempted suicide are variously viewed as a felony and a misdemeanor, respectively; in some states, the acts are considered not crimes but unlawful under common law and statutes. Aiding and abetting a suicide adds another dimension to the legal morass; some court decisions have held that, although neither suicide nor attempted suicide is punishable, anyone who assists in the act may be punished. (Doctor-assisted suicide is discussed in Chapter 57: *End of Life and Palliative Care*.)

National Strategy for Suicide Prevention

In 2001, Surgeon General David Satcher organized the National Strategy for Suicide Prevention, under the auspices of the National Institutes of Health (NIH). The National Strategy of Suicide Prevention of NIH has set specific goals and objectives to reduce suicide (Table 34.1-5).

The National Strategy for Suicide Prevention creates a framework for suicide prevention for the nation. It is designed to encourage and empower groups and individuals to work together. The stronger and broader the support and collaboration on suicide prevention, the greater the chance of success for this public health initiative. Suicide and suicidal behaviors can be reduced as the general public gains more understanding about (1) the extent to which suicide is a problem, (2) the ways in which it can be prevented, and (3) the roles individuals and groups can play in prevention efforts.

SUICIDES INVOLVING OTHER DEATHS

Victim-Precipitated Homicide

The phenomenon of using others, usually police, to kill oneself is well known to law enforcement personnel. Described by Marvin Wolfgang, the classic situation is exemplified by a person holding

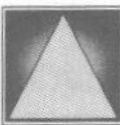

Table 34.1–4
Guidelines for Selecting a Treatment Setting for Patients at Risk for Suicide or Suicidal Behaviors*

Admission generally indicated: high risk of suicide	
After a suicide attempt or aborted suicide attempt if:	
Patient is psychotic Attempt was violent, near-lethal, or premediated Precautions were taken to avoid rescue or discovery Persistent plan and/or intent is present Distress is increased or patient regrets surviving Patient is male, >45 years of age, especially with new onset of psychiatric illness or suicidal thinking	Patient has limited family and/or social support, including lack of stable living situation Current impulsive behavior, severe agitation, poor judgment, or refusal of help is evident Patient has change in mental status with a metabolic, toxic, infectious, or other etiology requiring further workup in a structured setting
In the presence of suicidal ideation with:	
Specific plan with high lethality	High suicidal intent
Admission may be necessary: moderate risk of suicide	
After a suicide attempt or aborted suicide attempt, except in circumstances for which admission is generally indicated in the presence of suicidal ideation with:	
Psychosis Major psychiatric disorder Past attempts, particularly if medically serious Possibly contributing medical condition (e.g., acute neurological disorder, cancer, infection) Lack of response to or inability to cooperate with partial hospital or outpatient treatment Need for supervised setting for medication trial or electroconvulsive therapy	Need for skilled observation, clinical tests, or diagnostic assessments that require a structured setting Limited family and/or social support, including lack of stable living situation Lack of an ongoing clinician-patient relationship or lack of access to timely outpatient follow-up In the absence of suicide attempts or reported suicidal ideation/plan/intent but evidence from the psychiatric evaluation and/or history from others suggests a high level of suicide risk and a recent acute increase in risk
Release from emergency department with follow-up recommendations may be possible: lesser risk	
After a suicide attempt or in the presence of suicidal ideation/plan when:	
Suicidality is a reaction to precipitating events (e.g., exam failure, relationship difficulties), particularly if the patient's view of situation has changed since coming to emergency department Plan/method and intent have low lethality	Patient has stable and supportive living situation Patient is able to cooperate with recommendations for follow-up, with treater contacted, if possible, if patient is currently in treatment
Outpatient treatment may be more beneficial than hospitalization: lesser risk of suicide	
Patient has chronic suicidal ideation and/or self-injury without prior medically serious attempts, if a safe and supportive living situation is available and outpatient psychiatric care is ongoing	

*Suicide occurs infrequently, even in high-risk populations. This statistical rarity makes suicide prediction, based on risk factors, either alone or in combination, impossible. Psychiatrists, however, can use knowledge of suicide risk factors to help determine appropriate treatment settings and individual treatment plans. The objective of suicide risk assessment is to clarify the presence or absence of risk and protective factors, and then estimate the patient's individual risk for suicide. The primary and ongoing goal of this assessment is to reduce the patient's suicide risk.

(From the *Practice Guidelines for Assessment and Treatment of the Suicidal Patient,* 2nd ed. *The American Psychiatric Association Practice Guidelines for the Treatment of Psychiatric Disorders Compendium,* [Copyright 2004], with permission.)

up a gas station or all-night store and brandishing a gun, which he threatens to use on the police when they arrive. They then shoot him, thinking that it is in self-defense. The psychology of such victims is not clear, except that they apparently believe that this is the only way that they can die.

A 25-year-old, white, divorced father of twin 3-year-old boys had been threatening to his wife, and, consequently, she had an order of restraint placed on him. Nonetheless, one evening, he went to her home, carrying a realistic-looking toy pistol in his pocket "to give her a scare." She refused to admit him, and, when he began to create a scene, she called the police. When three police officers arrived, he refused to leave, pointed the toy pistol at them and taunted them to shoot him. They drew their revolvers, ordered him to drop his "weapon" (which he did), and restrained him. They took him to a local emergency department, where the nurse's admission note read: "divorced and angry man threatened others with a toy pistol." The on-call psychiatrist saw him briefly; the patient denied suicidal or homicidal intent; and the psychiatrist concluded that it was safe to discharge him (as a "situational problem–marital issues"). The following day, he killed himself by using carbon monoxide. Although this was not a case of "completed" victim-precipitated homicide, hospital staff failed to perceive that this represented "attempted," victim-precipitated homicide and was an act of high risk. Noting that he "threatened others with a toy pistol," trivialized the gravity of pointing what appears to be a genuine gun at armed police and telling them to shoot. In effect, he had given up control over this life-threatening situation to the police, and only their self-restraint protected him from being killed that evening.

Murder-Suicides

Murder-suicides receive a disproportionate amount of attention, because they are dramatic and tragic. Unless it is a pact between two truly consenting adults, such events testify to the enormous amount of aggression inherent in many suicides—in addition to the depression. Furthermore, what appears to be a pact is often, in fact, more of a coercion (or flat-out murder) than a true pact among equals. Pacts tend to be made more often by females or elderly couples.

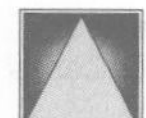

Table 34.1–5
Goals to Reduce Suicide

1. Promote awareness that suicide is a public health problem that is preventable
2. Develop broad-based support for suicide prevention
3. Develop and implement strategies to reduce the stigma associated with being a consumer of mental health, substance abuse, and suicide prevention services
4. Develop and implement suicide prevention programs
5. Promote efforts to reduce access to lethal means and methods of self-harm
6. Implement training for recognition of at-risk behavior and delivery of effective treatment
7. Develop and promote effective clinical and professional practices
8. Improve access to, and community linkages with, mental health and substance abuse services
9. Improve reporting and portrayals of suicidal behavior, mental illness, and substance abuse in the entertainment and news media
10. Promote and support research on suicide and suicide prevention
11. Improve and expand surveillance systems

SURVIVING SUICIDE

To be a *suicide survivor* refers to those who have lost a loved one to suicide, not to someone who has attempted suicide but lived. The toll on suicide survivors appears greater than that by other deaths, mainly because the opportunities for guilt are so great. Survivors feel that the loved one intentionally and willfully took his or her life and that if only the survivor had done something differently, the decedent would still be here. Because the decedent cannot tell them otherwise, survivors are at the mercy of their often merciless consciences. What is generally more accurate is that the decedents were not entirely willful but were themselves victims of their own genetic or lifetime experience predispositions to depression and suicide. For children, in particular, the loss of a parent to suicide feels like a shameful abandonment for which the child may blame himself or herself. For parents of children who have killed themselves, their grief is compounded not only by having lost a part of themselves, but also by having failed in what they perceive as their responsibility for the total feelings of their child. To provide mutual support, survivors of suicide groups have appeared throughout the United States, generally led by nonprofessional survivors themselves. Therapists who have lost patients to suicide comprise another survivor group—one too often ignored and unsupported, despite their own considerable suffering and sense of guilt, and compounded by the specter of litigation potentially being brought to bear.

References

APA practice guidelines for the assessment and treatment of suicidal behaviors. *Am J Psychiatry.* 2003;160:3.

Bauer MS, Mitchener L. What is a mood stabilizer? An evidence-based response. *Am J Psychiatry.* 2004;161:3.

Brown GK, Ten Have T, Henriques GR, Xie SX, Hollander JE, Beck AT. Cognitive therapy for the prevention of suicide attempts: A randomized controlled trial. *JAMA.* 2005;294(5):563–570.

Geddes JR, Burgess S, Hawton K, Jamison K, Goodwin GM. Long-term lithium therapy for bipolar disorder: Systematic review and meta-analysis of randomized controlled trials. *Am J Psychiatry.* 2004;161:217.

Gibbons RD, Hur K, Bhaumik DK, Mann JJ. The relationship between antidepressant medication use and rate of suicide. *Arch Gen Psychiatry.* 2005;62:165–172.

Goodwin F, Fireman B, Simon GE, Honkeler EM, Lee J, Revicki D. Suicide risk in bipolar disorder during treatment with lithium and divalproex. *JAMA.* 2003;290:1467.

Kessler RC, Berglund P, Borges G, Nock M, Wang PS. Trends in suicide ideation, plans, gestures, and attempts in the United States, 1990–1992 to 2001–2003. *JAMA.* 2005;293:2487–2495.

Shneidman ES. *The Suicidal Mind.* New York: Oxford University Press; 1996.

Simon GE, Savarino J, Operskalski B, Wang PS. Suicide risk during antidepressant treatment. *Am J Psych.* 2006;163:41–47.

Sudack HS. Suicide. In: Sadock BJ, Sadock VA, eds. *Kaplan & Sadock's Comprehensive Textbook of Psychiatry.* 8th ed. Vol. 2. Baltimore: Lippincott Williams & Wilkins; 2005:2442.

▲ 34.2 Psychiatric Emergencies in Adults

A psychiatric emergency is any disturbance in thoughts, feelings, or actions for which immediate therapeutic intervention is necessary. For a variety of reasons—such as the growing incidence of violence, the increased appreciation of the role of medical disease in altered mental status, and the epidemic of alcoholism and other substance use disorders—the number of emergency patients is on the rise. The widening scope of emergency psychiatry goes beyond general psychiatric practice to include such specialized problems as the abuse of substances, children, and spouses; violence in the form of suicide, homicide, and rape; and such social issues as homelessness, aging, competence, and acquired immune deficiency syndrome (AIDS). The emergency psychiatrist must be up to date on medicolegal issues and managed care. This section provides an overview of psychiatric emergencies in general and in adults in particular. The next section covers psychiatric emergencies in children.

TREATMENT SETTINGS

Most emergency psychiatric evaluations are done by nonpsychiatrists in a general medical emergency room setting, but specialized psychiatric services are increasingly favored. Regardless of the type of setting, an atmosphere of safety and security must prevail. An adequate number of staff members—including psychiatrists, nurses, aides, and social workers—must be present at all times. Additional personnel to help out in times of overcrowding should be available. Specific responsibilities, such as the use of restraints, should be clearly defined and practiced by the entire emergency team. Clear communication and lines of authority are essential. The organization of the staff into multidisciplinary teams is desirable.

Children and young adolescents are best served in a pediatric setting (see Section 34.3). Unless there is a risk of behavioral problems or of their leaving the hospital against advice, they need not be sent to the adult psychiatric emergency service.

Immediate access to the medical emergency room and to appropriate diagnostic services is necessary because one third of medical conditions present with psychiatric manifestations. The full spectrum of psychopharmacological options should be available to the psychiatrist.

Violence in the emergency service cannot be condoned or tolerated. The code of conduct expected of staff members and patients must be posted and understood from the time of the patient's arrival in the emergency room. Security is best managed as a clinical issue by the clinical staff, not by law enforcement personnel. Whenever possible, agitated and threatening patients should be sequestered from the nonagitated. Seclusion and restraint rooms should be located close to the nursing station for close observation.

The entire staff must understand that patients in physical and emotional distress are fragile and that various expectations and fantasies, often unrealistic, influence their responses to treatment. For example, a man with impaired reality testing who is brought in by the police against his will may not understand that the clinician is interested in helping him. Other patients, influenced by previous unsatisfactory treatment experiences, may be hostile. A high percentage of patients believe that psychiatrists can read minds or are only interested in admitting patients to lock them away. Such people see little point in openly discussing their problems. Many people have an inaccurate understanding of their rights as patients. All clinical interventions must take those expectations and attitudes into account to minimize the possibility of misunderstanding and consequent problems.

EPIDEMIOLOGY

Psychiatric emergency rooms are used equally by men and women and more by single than by married persons. About 20 percent of these patients are suicidal, and about 10 percent are violent. The most common diagnoses are mood disorders (including depressive disorders and manic episodes), schizophrenia, and alcohol dependence. About 40 percent of all patients seen in psychiatric emergency rooms require hospitalization. Most visits occur during the night hours, but usage difference is not based on the day of the week or the month of the year. Contrary to popular belief, studies have not found that use of psychiatric emergency rooms increases during the full moon or the Christmas season.

EVALUATION

The primary goal of an emergency psychiatric evaluation is the timely assessment of the patient in crisis. To that end, the physician must make an initial diagnosis, identify the precipitating factors and immediate needs, and begin treatment or refer the patient to the most appropriate treatment setting. In view of the unpredictable nature of emergency room work, with many patients presenting both physical and emotional complaints, and in view of the limited space and the competition for ancillary services, a pragmatic approach to the patient is required. Sometimes, moving the patient out of the emergency room into the most appropriate diagnostic or treatment setting is best for the patient. Medical emergencies are generally better managed elsewhere in the system. Keeping the number of emergency patients in one place to a minimum reduces the chance of agitation and violence.

The standard psychiatric interview—consisting of a history, a mental status examination, and, when appropriate and depending on the rules of the emergency room, a full physical examination and ancillary tests—is the cornerstone of the emergency room evaluation. The emergency room psychiatrist, however, must be ready to introduce modifications as needed. For example, the emergency psychiatrist may have to structure the interview with a rambling manic patient, medicate or restrain an agitated patient, or forgo the usual rules of confidentiality to assess an adolescent's risk of suicide. In general, any strategy introduced in the emergency room to accomplish the goal of assessing the patient is considered consistent with good clinical practice as long as the rationale for the strategy is documented in the medical record.

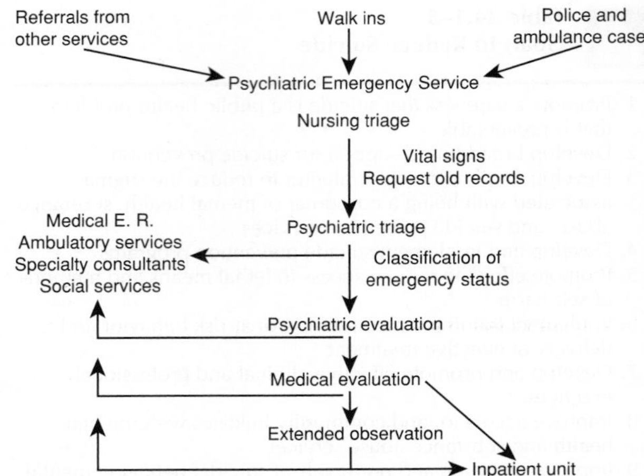

FIGURE 34.2–1
Evaluation and treatment of psychiatric emergencies.

What constitutes a psychiatric emergency is highly subjective. The emergency room has increasingly come to serve as an admitting area, a holding room, a detoxification center, and a private office. Such medical conditions as head traumas, acute intoxications, withdrawal states, and AIDS encephalopathies may present with acute psychiatric manifestations. The emergency psychiatrists must rapidly assess and distinguish the truly emergency psychiatric patients from those who are less acutely ill and from nonpsychiatric emergencies. A triage system using psychiatrists, nurses, and psychiatric social workers is an efficient and effective way to identify emergency, urgent, and nonurgent patients, who can then be prioritized for care (Fig. 34.2-1).

In one model, every patient who comes to the emergency room is assessed by a triage nurse on arrival to ascertain the patient's chief complaint, clinical condition, and vital signs. The psychiatrist then briefly meets with the patient and other significant people involved in the case—family members, emergency medical service technicians, and police—to assign the patient to one of the three categories—emergency, urgent, and nonurgent—or to refer the patient to an appropriate treatment setting, such as the medical emergency room. Having a senior clinician perform that task ensures a rapid identification of the most urgent and troublesome cases, an appropriate allocation of resources, and an answer to the most common question heard in the emergency room: "When am I going to see a doctor?"

The psychiatrist then assigns clinical responsibility for each patient to the appropriate personnel. As the evaluation often stretches over more than one shift, a careful procedure to transfer responsibility and to pass along information from tour to tour must be built into the system by using visual, oral, and written communications. A request for old records should be made automatically for every patient who is assigned to the emergency room. Each emergency should be judged on its own merits, but information from previous records and from workers in the field and family members can be of crucial importance is assessing patients, especially patients who are psychotic, frightened, or otherwise unable or unwilling to cooperate in giving a good history.

A multilingual staff and a hospital language bank that lists bilingual staff members and other translation services should be readily available to the psychiatrist. The use of the patient's friends or family members

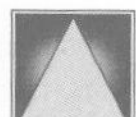

Table 34.2–1
General Strategy in Evaluating the Patient

I. Self-protection
- A. Know as much as possible about the patients before meeting them.
- B. Leave physical restraint procedures to those who are trained.
- C. Be alert to risks of impending violence.
- D. Attend to the safety of the physical surroundings (e.g., door access, room objects).
- E. Have others present during the assessment if needed.
- F. Have others in the vicinity.
- G. Attend to developing an alliance with the patient (e.g., do not confront or threaten patients with paranoid psychoses).

II. Prevent harm
- A. Prevent self-injury and suicide. Use whatever methods are necessary to prevent patients from hurting themselves during the evaluation.
- B. Prevent violence toward others. During the evaluation, briefly assess the patient for the risk of violence. If the risk is deemed significant, consider the following options:
  1. Inform the patient that violence is not acceptable.
  2. Approach the patient in a nonthreatening manner.
  3. Reassure, calm, or assist the patient's reality testing.
  4. Offer medication.
  5. Inform the patient that restraint or seclusion will be used if necessary.
  6. Have teams ready to restrain the patient.
  7. When patients are restrained, always closely observe them, and frequently check their vital signs. Isolate restrained patients from surrounding agitating stimuli. Immediately plan a further approach—medication, reassurance, medical evaluation.

III. Rule out organic mental disorders.

IV. Rule out impending psychosis.

as translators is not desirable because of the possibility of unconscious or deliberate denial or distortion of the clinical picture stemming from their involvement with the patient.

An initial assessment of the patient's total biopsychosocial needs is optimal, but the patient's emergency status, other patients waiting to be seen, and the constraints of the emergency room setting often make such a full assessment a moot point. At a minimum, the emergency evaluation should address the following five questions before any disposition is decided on: (1) Is it safe for the patient to be in the emergency room? (2) Is the problem organic or functional or a combination? (3) Is the patient psychotic? (4) Is the patient suicidal or homicidal? (5) To what degree is the patient capable of self-care? Table 34.2-1 provides a general strategy in evaluating patients.

Patient Safety

Physicians should consider the question of the patient's safety before evaluating every patient. The answer must address the issues of the emergency room's physical layout, staffing patterns and communication, and patient population. Psychiatrists must then take stock of themselves: Are they in the proper frame of mind to conduct an evaluation? Do any issues in the case spark countertransference reactions? The self-assessment should go on throughout the evaluation. The physical and emotional safety of the patient takes priority over all other considerations. If verbal interventions fail or are contraindicated, the use of medication or restraints must be considered and, if necessary, ordered. Careful attention to the possible outbreak of agitation or disruptive behavior beyond acceptable limits is often the best insurance against untoward occurrences.

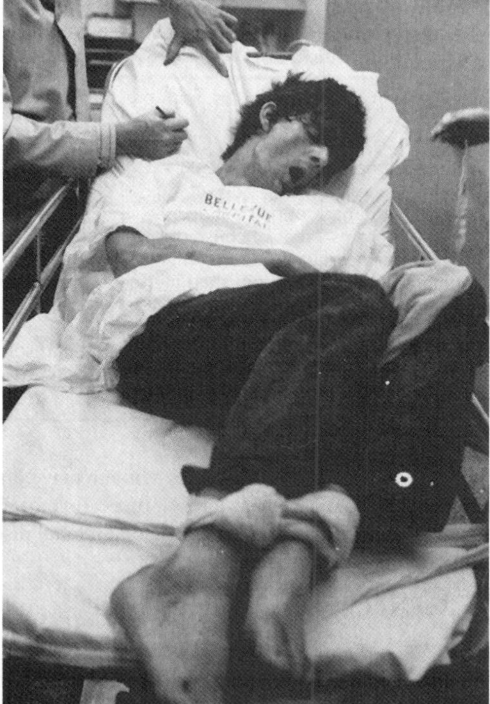

FIGURE 34.2–2
Bellevue Hospital emergency ward: a drug addict brought in after having taken an overdose. (Courtesy of Leonard Freed for Magnum Photos, Inc.)

Medical or Psychiatric?

The most important question for the emergency psychiatrist to address is whether the problem is medical or psychiatric or both. Medical conditions—such as diabetes mellitus, thyroid disease, acute intoxications, withdrawal states, AIDS, and head traumas—can present with prominent mental status changes that mimic common psychiatric illnesses (Fig. 34.2-2). Such conditions may be life-threatening if not treated promptly. Generally, the treatment of a medical illness is more definitive and the prognosis is better than for a functional psychiatric disorder. The psychiatrist must consider all casual possibilities.

Once patients are labeled psychiatric, their complaints may not be taken seriously by nonmental health professionals, however, and such patients' conditions may deteriorate, especially if they have a major Axis I syndrome. Because of such factors as deinstitutionalization, homelessness, and chronic alcoholism, the mentally ill are at great risk of tuberculosis, vitamin deficiencies, and other easily overlooked, but easily treated conditions. Symptoms such as paranoia, internal preoccupation, and acute psychosis can make a routine medical diagnosis exceedingly difficult. Each patient must be assessed for the possibility that an organic illness is combined with an underlying psychiatric illness. A young man who comes to the emergency room intoxicated or

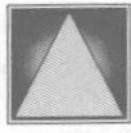

Table 34.2–2
Features That Point to a Medical Cause of a Mental Disorder

Acute onset (within hours or minutes, with prevailing symptoms)
First episode
Geriatric age
Current medical illness or injury
Significant substance abuse
Nonauditory disturbances of perception
Neurological symptoms—loss of consciousness, seizures, head injury, change in headache pattern, change in vision
Classic mental status signs—diminished alertness, disorientation, memory impairment, impairment in concentration and attention, dyscalculia, concreteness
Other mental status signs—speech, movement, or gait disorders
Constructional apraxia—difficulties in drawing clock, cube, intersecting pentagons, Bender gestalt design

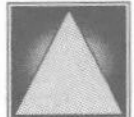

Table 34.2–3
History, Signs, and Symptoms of Suicidal Risk

1. Previous attempt or fantasized suicide
2. Anxiety, depression, exhaustion
3. Availability of means of suicide
4. Concern for effect of suicide on family members
5. Verbalized suicidal ideation
6. Preparation of a will, resignation after agitated depression
7. Proximal life crisis, such as mourning or impending surgery
8. Family history of suicide
9. Pervasive pessimism or hopelessness

in alcohol withdrawal two or three times a month may come one day with a subdural hematoma as a result of a fall. Table 34.2-2 lists features that point to a medical cause of a mental disorder.

SPECIFIC INTERVIEW SITUATIONS

Psychosis

Whether the patient is psychotic refers not so much to the diagnosis as to the severity of the patient's symptoms and the degree of life disruption. The patient's degree of withdrawal from objective reality, level of affectivity, intellectual functioning, and degree of regression are other important parameters. Impairment in any of those areas may lead to difficulties in conducting an evaluation. Agitated, assaultive behavior or failure to comply with treatment recommendations may also result. A paranoid, hypervigilent patient may misperceive a staff member's offer of help as an attack and may lash out in self-defense. Command auditory hallucinations may cause a patient to deny symptoms and to throw prescriptions in the garbage immediately after leaving the emergency room. The psychiatrist should be alert to the complications that can arise with patients whose reality testing is impaired and should modify the approach accordingly.

All communication with patients must be straightforward. All clinical interventions should be briefly explained in language the patient can understand. Psychiatrists should not assume that the patient trusts or believes them or even wants their help. Clinicians must be prepared to structure or to terminate an interview to limit the potential for agitation and regression.

Depression and Potentially Suicidal Patients

The clinician should always ask about suicidal ideas as part of every mental status examination, especially if the patient is depressed. The patient may not realize that such symptoms as waking during the night and increased somatic complaints are related to depressive disorders. The patient should be asked directly, "Are you or have you ever been suicidal?" "Do you want to die?" "Do you feel so bad that you might hurt yourself?" Eight of 10 persons who eventually kill themselves give warnings of their intent. If the patient admits to a plan of action, that is a particularly dangerous sign. If a patient who has been threatening suicide becomes quiet and less agitated than before, that may be an ominous sign. The clinician should be especially concerned with the factors listed in Table 34.2-3.

A suicide note, a family history of suicide, or previous suicidal behavior on the part of the patient increases the risk of suicide. Evidence of impulsivity or of pervasive pessimism about the future also places the patient at risk. If the physician decides that the patient is in imminent risk for suicidal behavior, the patient must be hospitalized or otherwise protected. A difficult situation arises when the risk does not seem to be immediate but the potential for suicide is present as long as the patient remains depressed. If the psychiatrist decides not to hospitalize the patient immediately, the doctor should insist that the patient promise to call whenever the suicidal pressure mounts.

Violent Patients

Patients may be violent for many reasons, and the interview with a violent patient must attempt to ascertain the underlying cause of the violent behavior, because cause determines intervention. The differential diagnosis of violent behavior includes psychoactive substance-induced organic mental disorder, antisocial personality disorder, catatonic schizophrenia, medical infections, cerebral neoplasms, decompensating obsessive-compulsive personality disorder, dissociative disorders, impulse control disorders, sexual disorders, alcohol idiosyncratic intoxication, delusional disorder, paranoid personality disorder, schizophrenia, temporal lobe epilepsy, bipolar disorder, and uncontrollable violence secondary to interpersonal stress.

The psychiatric interview must include questions that attempt to sort out the differential for violent behavior and questions directed toward the prediction of violence.

The best predictors of violent behavior are (1) excessive alcohol intake; (2) a history of violent acts, with arrests or criminal activity; and (3) a history of childhood abuse. Table 34.2-4 lists some of the most significant factors in assessing and predicting violence.

Rape and Sexual Abuse

Rape is the forceful coercion of an unwilling victim to engage in a sexual act, usually sexual intercourse, although anal intercourse and fellatio can also be acts of rape. As with other acts of violence, rape is a psychiatric emergency that requires immediate, appropriate intervention. Rape victims may suffer sequelae that persist for a lifetime. Rape is a life-threatening experience in which the victim has almost always been threatened with physical harm, often with a weapon. In addition to rape, other forms of sexual abuse include genital manipulation with foreign objects, infliction of pain, and forced sexual activity.

Most rapists are male, and most victims are female. Male rape does occur, however, often in institutions where men are detained (e.g., prisons). Women between the ages of 16 and 24 years are in the highest risk category, but female victims as young as 15 months and as old as 82 years have been raped. More than a third of all rapes are committed by rapists known to the victim, 7 percent by close relatives. A fifth of all rapes involve more than one rapist (gang rape).

Typical reactions in both rape and sexual abuse victims include shame, humiliation, anxiety, confusion, and outrage. Many victims wonder whether they are partly responsible and somehow invited the assault. In fact, victim behavior is less important in precipitating a rape than it

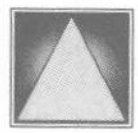

Table 34.2–4
Assessing and Predicting Violent Behavior

1. Signs of impending violence
   a. Very recent acts of violence, including property violence
   b. Verbal or physical threats (menacing)
   c. Carrying weapons or other objects that may be used as weapons (e.g., forks, ashtrays)
   d. Progressive psychomotor agitation
   e. Alcohol or drug intoxication
   f. Paranoid features in a psychotic patient
   g. Command violent auditory hallucinations—some but not all patients are at high risk
   h. Organic mental disorders, global or with frontal lobe findings; less commonly with temporal lobe findings (controversial)
   i. Patients with catatonic excitement
   j. Certain patients with mania
   k. Certain patients with agitated depression
   l. Personality disorder patients prone to rage, violence, or impulse dyscontrol
2. Assess the risk of violence
   a. Consider violent ideation, wish, intention, plan, availability of means, implementation of plan, wish for help.
   b. Consider demographics—sex (male), age (15–24), socioeconomic status (low), social supports (few).
   c. Consider past history: violence, nonviolent antisocial acts, impulse dyscontrol (e.g., gambling, substance abuse, suicide or self-injury, psychosis).
   d. Consider overt stressors (e.g., marital conflict, real or symbolic loss).

is in precipitating a homicide or a robbery. Rape and sexual abuse victims are often confused after the assault. Clinicians should be reassuring, supportive, and nonjudgmental. Inform the patient about the availability of medical and legal services and about rape crisis centers that provide multidisciplinary services.

If possible, a female clinician should evaluate the patient, because the victim may find it easier to talk with a woman than with a man. The evaluation should take place in private. When rape or sexual abuse has not been acknowledged openly, it is usually because many victims hesitate to discuss the assault and thus avoid the topic. If the patient appears to be anxious when questioned about sexual history and avoids the discussion, it is important to validate the patient's avoidance. Recognize that the rape victim has undergone an unanticipated, life-threatening stress. It is legally and therapeutically important to take a detailed and complete history of the attack.

With the patient's written consent, collect evidence, such as semen and pubic hair, that may be used to identify the rapist. Take photographs of the evidence, if possible. The medical record may be used as evidence in criminal proceedings; therefore, meticulous objective documentation of all aspects of the evaluation is essential.

TREATMENT OF EMERGENCIES

Psychotherapy

In an emergency psychiatric intervention, all attempts are made to help patients' self-esteem. Empathy is critical to healing in a psychiatric emergency. The acquired knowledge of how biogenetic, situational, developmental, and existential forces converge at one point in history to create a psychiatric emergency is tantamount to the maturation of skill in emergency psychiatry. Adjustment disorder in all age groups may result in tantrum-like outbursts of rage. These outbursts are particularly common in marital quarrels, and police are often summoned by neighbors distressed by the sounds of a violent altercation. Such family quarrels should be approached with caution, because they may be complicated by alcohol use and the presence of dangerous weapons. The warring couple frequently turn their combined fury on an unwary outsider. Wounded self-esteem is a major issue, and clinicians must avoid patronizing or contemptuous attitudes and try to communicate an attitude of respect and an authentic peacemaking concern.

In family violence, psychiatrists should note the special vulnerability of selected close relatives. A wife or husband may have a curious masochistic attachment to the spouse and can provoke violence by taunting and otherwise undermining a partner's self-esteem. Such relationships often end in the murder of the provoking partner and sometimes in the suicide of the other partner—the dynamics behind most so-called suicide pacts. As with many suicidal patients, many violent patients require hospitalization and usually accept the offer of inpatient care with a sense of relief.

More than one psychotherapist or type of psychotherapy is frequently used in emergency therapy. For example, a 28-year-old man, depressed and suicidal after a colostomy for intractable colitis, whose wife was threatening to leave him because of his irritability and their constant altercations, may be referred to a psychiatrist for supportive psychotherapy and antidepressant medication, to a marital therapist with his wife to improve their marital functioning, and to a colostomy support group to learn ways of coping with a colostomy. Emergency psychiatric clinicians are pragmatic; they use every necessary mode of therapeutic intervention available to resolve the crisis and facilitate value exploration and growth, with less concern than usual about diluting a therapeutic relationship. Emergency therapy emphasizes how various psychiatric modalities act synergistically to enhance recovery.

No single approach is appropriate for all persons in similar situations. What does a doctor say to a patient and a family experiencing a psychiatric emergency, such as a suicide attempt or a schizophrenic break? For some, a genetic rationale helps; the information that an illness has a strong biological component relieves some persons. For others, however, this approach underlines a lack of control and increases depression and anxiety. All feel helpless because neither the family nor the patient can alter the behavior to minimize the likelihood of recurrence. Some persons may benefit from an explanation of family or individual dynamics. Others only want someone to listen to them; in time, they reach their own understanding.

In an emergency situation as in any other psychiatric situation, when a clinician does not know what to say, the best approach is to listen. Persons in crisis reveal how much they need support, denial, ventilation, and words to conceptualize the meaning of their crisis and to discover paths to resolution.

Pharmacotherapy

The major indications for the use of psychotropic medication in an emergency room include violent or assaultive behavior, massive anxiety or panic, and extrapyramidal reactions, such as dystonia and akathisia as adverse effects of psychiatric drugs. Laryngospasm is a rare form of dystonia, and psychiatrists should be prepared to maintain an open airway with intubation if necessary.

Persons who are paranoid or in a state of catatonic excitement require tranquilization. Episodic outbursts of violence respond to haloperidol (Haldol), β-adrenergic receptor antagonists (beta-blockers), carbamazepine (Tegretol), and lithium. If a history suggests a seizure disorder, use clinical studies to confirm the diagnosis and an evaluation to ascertain the cause. If the findings are positive, anticonvulsant therapy is initiated or appropriate surgery is provided (e.g., in the case of a cerebral mass). Conservative measures may suffice for intoxication from drugs of abuse. Sometimes, drugs such as haloperidol (5 to 10 mg every half-hour to an hour) are needed until a patient is stabilized. Benzodiazepines may be used instead of, or in addition to, antipsychotics (to reduce the antipsychotic dosage). When a recreational drug has strong anticholinergic properties, benzodiazepines are more appropriate than antipsychotics. Persons with allergic or aberrant responses to antipsychotics and benzodiazepines are treated with amobarbital (Amytal), 130 mg orally or intramuscularly (IM), paraldehyde, or diphenhydramine (Benadryl), 50 to 100 mg orally or IM.

Violent, struggling patients are subdued most effectively with an appropriate sedative or antipsychotic. Diazepam (Valium), 5 to 10 mg, or lorazepam (Ativan), 2 to 4 mg, may be given slowly intravenously (IV) over 2 minutes. Clinicians must give IV medication with great care to avoid respiratory arrest. Patients who require IM medication can be sedated with haloperidol, 5 to 10 mg IM. If the furor is caused by alcohol or is part of a postseizure psychomotor disturbance, the sleep produced by a relatively small amount of an IV medication may go on for hours. On awakening, patients are often entirely alert and rational and typically have complete amnesia about the violent episode.

If the disturbance is part of an ongoing psychotic process and returns as soon as the IV medication wears off, continuous medication may be given. It is sometimes better to use small IM or oral doses at half-hour to 1-hour intervals (e.g., haloperidol, 2 to 5 mg, or diazepam, 20 mg) until the patient is controlled than to use large dosages initially, which can result in an overmedicated patient. As the disturbed behavior is brought under control, successively smaller and less frequent doses should be used. During the preliminary treatment, a patient's blood pressure and other vital signs should be monitored.

Restraints

Restraints are used when patients are so dangerous to themselves or others that they pose a severe threat that cannot be controlled in any other way. Patients may be restrained temporarily to receive medication or for long periods if medication cannot be used. Usually, patients in restraints quiet down after a time. On a psychodynamic level, such patients may even welcome the control of their impulses provided by restraints. See Table 34.2-5 for a summary of the use of restraints.

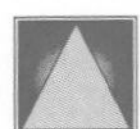

Table 34.2–5
Use of Restraints

Preferably five or a minimum of four persons should be used to restrain the patient. Leather restraints are the safest and surest type of restraint.

Explain to the patient why he or she is going into restraints.

A staff member should always be visible and reassuring the patient who is being restrained. Reassurance helps alleviate the patient's fear of helplessness, impotence, and loss of control.

Patients should be restrained with legs spread-eagled and one arm restrained to one side and the other arm restrained over the patient's head.

Restraints should be placed so that intravenous fluids can be given, if necessary.

The patient's head is raised slightly to decrease the patient's feelings of vulnerability and to reduce the possibility of aspiration.

The restraints should be checked periodically for safety and comfort.

After the patient is in restraints, the clinician begins treatment, using verbal intervention.

Even in restraints, most patients still take antipsychotic medication in concentrated form.

After the patient is under control, one restraint at a time should be removed at 5-minute intervals until the patient has only two restraints on. Both of the remaining restraints should be removed at the same time, because it is inadvisable to keep a patient in only one restraint.

Always thoroughly document the reason for the restraints, the course of treatment, and the patient's response to treatment while in restraints.

Data from Dubin WR, Weiss KJ. Emergency psychiatry. In: Michaels R, Cooper A, Guze SB, et al., eds. *Psychiatry*. Vol. 2. Philadelphia: JB Lippincott; 1991.

Disposition

In some cases, the usual option of admitting or discharging the patient is not considered optimal. Suspected toxic psychoses, brief decompensations in a patient with a personality disorder, and adjustment reactions to traumatic events, for example, may be best managed in an extended-observation setting. Allowing the patient additional time in a secure environment can result in sufficient improvement or clarification of the issues to make traditional inpatient treatment unnecessary. It can also spare the patient the trauma and stigma of a psychiatric admission and can free up bed space for needier patients. Crisis intervention for victims of rape and other traumas can also be done in an extended-observation setting.

When the decision is to admit the patient to the hospital, it is preferable to do so on a voluntary basis. Allowing patients that option gives them a sense of control over their lives and of participation in the treatment decisions. Patients who clearly meet involuntary admission criteria on the basis of dangerousness to themselves or to others cannot leave the hospital without further review and can always be converted to involuntary status if warranted.

Because the initial evaluation is often inconclusive, definitive treatment is best deferred until the patient can be further assessed on the inpatient unit or in the outpatient department. When the diagnosis is clear, however, and the patient's response to previous treatment is known, nothing is gained by delay. For example, a patient with chronic schizophrenia that has decompensated after discontinuing the usual regimen of antipsychotic medication is best served by prompt resumption of treatment.

Even if patients feel comfortable coming to the emergency room in times of need, the emergency psychiatrist should always direct or redirect them to the most appropriate treatment setting. Patients in the psychopharmacology clinic who have missed their regular appointments should be given only enough medication

(Text continues on page 918.)

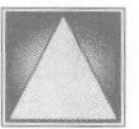

Table 34.2–6
Common Psychiatric Emergencies

Syndrome	Emergency Manifestations	Treatment Issues
Abuse of child or adult	Signs of physical trauma	Management of medical problems; psychiatric evaluation; report to authorities
Acquired immune deficiency syndrome (AIDS)	Changes in behavior secondary to organic causes; changes in behavior secondary to fear and anxiety; suicidal behavior	Management of neurological illness; management of psychological concomitants; reinforcement of social support
Adolescent crises	Suicidal attempts and ideation; substance abuse, truancy, trouble with law, pregnancy, running away; eating disorders; psychosis	Evaluation of suicidal potential, extent of substance abuse, family dynamics; crisis-oriented family and individual therapy; hospitalization if necessary; consultation with appropriate extrafamilial authorities
Agoraphobia	Panic; depression	Alprazolam (Xanax), 0.25 mg to 2 mg; propranolol (Inderal); antidepressant medication
Agranulocytosis (clozapine [Clozaril]-induced)	High fever, pharyngitis, oral and perianal ulcerations	Discontinue medication immediately; administer granulocyte colony-stimulating factor
Akathisia	Agitation, restlessness, muscle discomfort; dysphoria	Reduce antipsychotic dosage; propranolol (30 to 120 mg a day); benzodiazepines; diphenhydramine (Benadryl) orally or IV; benztropine (Cogentin) IM
Alcohol-related emergencies		
Alcohol delirium	Confusion, disorientation, fluctuating consciousness and perception, autonomic hyperactivity; may be fatal	Chlordiazepoxide (Librium); haloperidol (Haldol) for psychotic symptoms may be added if necessary
Alcohol intoxication	Disinhibited behavior, sedation at high doses	With time and protective environment, symptoms abate
Alcohol persisting amnestic disorder	Confusion, loss of memory even for all personal identification data	Hospitalization; hypnosis; amobarbital (Amytal) interview; rule out organic cause
Alcohol persisting dementia	Confusion, agitation, impulsivity	Rule out other causes for dementia; no effective treatment; hospitalization if necessary
Alcohol psychotic disorder with hallucinations	Vivid auditory (fat times visual) hallucinations with affect appropriate to content (often fearful); clear sensorium	Haloperidol for psychotic symptoms
Alcohol seizures	Grand mal seizures; rarely status epilepticus	Diazepam (Valium), phenytoin (Dilantin); prevent by using chlordiazepoxide (Librium) during detoxification
Alcohol withdrawal	Irritability, nausea, vomiting, insomnia, malaise, autonomic hyperactivity, shakiness	Fluid and electrolytes maintained; sedation with benzodiazepines; restraints; monitoring of vital signs; 100 mg thiamine IM
Idiosyncratic alcohol intoxication	Marked aggressive or assaultive behavior	Generally no treatment required other than protective environment
Korsakoff's syndrome	Alcohol stigmata, amnesia, confabulation	No effective treatment; institutionalization often needed
Wernicke's encephalopathy	Oculomotor disturbances, cerebellar ataxia; mental confusion	Thiamine, 100 mg IV or IM, with $MgSO_4$ given before glucose loading
Amphetamine (or related substance) intoxication	Delusions, paranoia; violence; depression (from withdrawal); anxiety, delirium	Antipsychotics; restraints; hospitalization if necessary; no need for gradual withdrawal; antidepressants may be necessary
Anorexia nervosa	Loss of 25% of body weight of the norm for age and sex	Hospitalization; electrocardiogram (ECG), fluid and electrolytes; neuroendocrine evaluation
Anticholinergic intoxication	Psychotic symptoms, dry skin and mouth, hyperpyrexia, mydriasis, tachycardia, restlessness, visual hallucinations	Discontinue drug, IV physostigmine (Antilirium), 0.5 to 2 mg, for severe agitation or fever, benzodiazepines; antipsychotics contraindicated
Anticonvulsant intoxication	Psychosis; delirium	Dosage of anticonvulsant is reduced
Benzodiazepine intoxication	Sedation, somnolence, and ataxia	Supportive measures; flumazenil (Romazicon), 7.5 to 45 mg a day, titrated as needed, should be used only by skilled personnel with resuscitative equipment available
Bereavement	Guilt feelings, irritability; insomnia; somatic complaints	Must be differentiated from major depressive disorder; antidepressants not indicated; benzodiazepines for sleep; encouragement of ventilation

(*continued*)

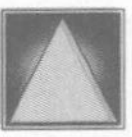

Table 34.2–6 (Continued)

Syndrome	Emergency Manifestations	Treatment Issues
Borderline personality disorder	Suicidal ideation and gestures; homicidal ideations and gestures; substance abuse; micropsychotic episodes; burns, cut marks on body	Suicidal and homicidal evaluation (if great, hospitalization); small dosages of antipsychotics; clear follow-up plan
Brief psychotic disorder	Emotional turmoil, extreme lability; acutely impaired reality testing after obvious psychosocial stress	Hospitalization often necessary; low dosage of antipsychotics may be necessary but often resolves spontaneously
Bromide intoxication	Delirium; mania; depression; psychosis	Serum levels obtained (>50 mg a day); bromide intake discontinued; large quantities of sodium chloride IV or orally; if agitation, paraldehyde or antipsychotic is used
Caffeine intoxication	Severe anxiety, resembling panic disorder; mania; delirium; agitated depression; sleep disturbance	Cessation of caffeine-containing substances; benzodiazepines
Cannabis intoxication	Delusions; panic; dysphoria; cognitive impairment	Benzodiazepines and antipsychotics as needed; evaluation of suicidal or homicidal risk; symptoms usually abate with time and reassurance
Catatonic schizophrenia	Marked psychomotor disturbance (either excitement or stupor); exhaustion; can be fatal	Rapid tranquilization with antipsychotics; monitor vital signs; amobarbital may release patient from catatonic mutism or stupor but can precipitate violent behavior
Cimetidine psychotic disorder	Delirium; delusions	Reduce dosage or discontinue drug
Clonidine withdrawal	Irritability; psychosis; violence; seizures	Symptoms abate with time, but antipsychotics may be necessary; gradual lowering of dosage
Cocaine intoxication and withdrawal	Paranoia and violence; severe anxiety; manic state; delirium: schizophreniform psychosis; tachycardia, hypertension, myocardial infarction, cerebrovascular disease; depression and suicidal ideation	Antipsychotics and benzodiazepines; antidepressants or ECT for withdrawal depression if persistent; hospitalization
Delirium	Fluctuating sensorium; suicidal and homicidal risk; cognitive clouding; visual, tactile, and auditory hallucinations; paranoia	Evaluate all potential contributing factors and treat each accordingly; reassurance, structure, clues to orientation; benzodiazepines and low-dosage, high-potency antipsychotics must be used with extreme care because of their potential to act paradoxically and increase agitation
Delusional disorder	Most often brought in to emergency room involuntarily; threats directed toward others	Antipsychotics if patient will comply (IM if necessary); intensive family intervention; hospitalization if necessary
Dementia	Unable to care for self; violent outbursts; psychosis; depression and suicidal ideation; confusion	Small dosages of high-potency antipsychotics; clues to orientation; organic evaluation, including medication use; family intervention
Depressive disorders	Suicidal ideation and attempts; self-neglect; substance abuse	Assessment of danger to self; hospitalization if necessary, nonpsychiatric causes of depression must be evaluated
L-Dopa intoxication	Mania; depression; schizophreniform disorder, may induce rapid cycling in patients with bipolar I disorder	Lower dosage or discontinue drug
Dystonia, acute	Intense involuntary spasm of muscles of neck, tongue, face, jaw, eyes, or trunk	Decrease dosage of antipsychotic; benztropine or diphenhydramine IM
Group hysteria	Groups of people exhibit extremes of grief or other disruptive behavior	Group is dispersed with help of other health care workers; ventilation, crisis-oriented therapy; if necessary, small dosages of benzodiazepines
Hallucinogen-induced psychotic disorder with hallucinations	Symptom picture is result of interaction of type of substance, dose taken, duration of action, user's premorbid personality, setting; panic; agitation; atropine psychosis	Serum and urine screens; rule out underlying medical or mental disorder; benzodiazepines (2 to 20 mg) orally; reassurance and orientation; rapid tranquilization; often responds spontaneously
Homicidal and assaultive behavior	Marked agitation with verbal threats	Seclusion, restraints, medication

(continued)

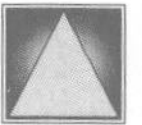

Table 34.2–6 (Continued)

Syndrome	Emergency Manifestations	Treatment Issues
Homosexual panic	Not seen with men or women who are comfortable with their sexual orientation; occurs in those who adamantly deny having any homoerotic impulses; impulses are aroused by talk, a physical overture, or play among same-sex friends, such as wrestling, sleeping together, or touching each other in a shower or hot tub; panicked person sees others as sexually interested in him or her and defends against them	Ventilation, environmental structuring, and, in some instances, medication for acute panic (e.g., alprazolam, 0.25 to 2 mg) or antipsychotics may be required; opposite-sex clinician should evaluate the patient whenever possible, and the patient should not be touched save for the routine examination; patients have attached physicians who were examining an abdomen or performing a rectal examination (e.g., on a man who harbors thinly veiled unintegrated homosexual impulses)
Hypertensive crisis	Life-threatening hypertensive reaction secondary to ingestion of tyramine-containing foods in combination with MAOIs; headache, stiff neck, sweating, nausea, vomiting	α-Adrenergic blockers (e.g., phentolamine [Regitinel]); nifedipine (Procardia) 10 mg orally; chlorpromazine (Thorazine); make sure symptoms are not secondary to hypotension (side effect of monoamine oxidase inhibitors [MAOIs] alone)
Hyperthermia	Extreme excitement or catatonic stupor or both; extremely elevated temperature; violent hyperagitation	Hydrate and cool; may be drug reaction, so discontinue any drug; rule out infection
Hyperventilation	Anxiety, terror, clouded consciousness; giddiness, faintness; blurring vision	Shift alkalosis by having patient breathe into paper bag; patient education; antianxiety agents
Hypothermia	Confusion; lethargy; combativeness; low body temperature and shivering; paradoxical feeling of warmth	IV fluids and rewarming, cardiac status must be carefully monitored; avoidance of alcohol
Incest and sexual abuse of child	Suicidal behavior; adolescent crises; substance abuse	Corroboration of charge, protection of victim; contact social services; medical and psychiatric evaluation; crisis intervention
Insomnia	Depression and irritability; early morning agitation; frightening dreams; fatigue	Hypnotics only in short term; e.g., triazolam (Halcion), 0.25 to 0.5 mg, at bedtime; treat any underlying mental disorder; rules of sleep hygiene
Intermittent explosive disorder	Brief outbursts of violence; periodic episodes of suicide attempts	Benzodiazepines or antipsychotics for short term; long-term evaluation with computed tomography (CT) scan, sleep-deprived electroencephalogram (EEG), glucose tolerance curve
Jaundice	Uncommon complication of low-potency phenothiazine use (e.g., chlorpromazine)	Change drug to low dosage of a low-potency agent in a different class
Leukopenia and agranulocytosis	Side effects within the first 2 months of treatment with antipsychotics	Patient should call immediately for sore throat, fever, etc., and obtain immediate blood count; discontinue drug; hospitalize if necessary
Lithium toxicity	Vomiting; abdominal pain; profuse diarrhea; severe tremor, ataxia; coma; seizures; confusion; dysarthria; focal neurological signs	Lavage with wide-bore tube; osmotic diuresis; medical consultation; may require ICU treatment
Major depressive episode with psychotic features	Major depressive episode symptoms with delusions; agitation, severe guilt; ideas of reference; suicide and homicide risk	Antipsychotics plus antidepressants; evaluation of suicide and homicide risk; hospitalization and ECT if necessary
Manic episode	Violent, impulsive behavior; indiscriminate sexual or spending behavior; psychosis; substance abuse	Hospitalization; restraints if necessary; rapid tranquilization with antipsychotics; restoration of lithium levels
Marital crises	Precipitant may be discovery of an extramarital affair, onset of serious illness, announcement of intent to divorce, or problems with children or work; one or both members of the couple may be in therapy or may be psychiatrically ill; one spouse may be seeking hospitalization for the other	Each should be questioned alone regarding extramarital affairs, consultations with lawyers regarding divorce, and willingness to work in crisis-oriented or long-term therapy to resolve the problem; sexual, financial, and psychiatric treatment histories from both, psychiatric evaluation at the time of presentation; may be precipitated by onset of untreated mood disorder or affective symptoms caused by medical illness or insidious-onset dementia; referral for management of the illness reduces

(*continued*)

Table 34.2–6
(Continued)

Syndrome	Emergency Manifestations	Treatment Issues
		immediate stress and enhances the healthier spouse's coping capacity; children may give insights available only to someone intimately involved in the social system
Migraine	Throbbing, unilateral headache	Sumatriptan (Imitrex) 6 mg IM
Mitral valve prolapse	Associated with panic disorder; dyspnea and palpitations; fear and anxiety	Echocardiogram; alprazolam or propranolol
Neuroleptic malignant syndrome	Hyperthermia; muscle rigidity; autonomic instability; parkinsonian symptoms; catatonic stupor; neurological signs; 10% to 30% fatality; elevated creatine phosphokinase	Discontinue antipsychotic; IV dantrolene (Dantrium); bromocriptine (Parlodel) orally; hydration and cooling; monitor CPK levels
Nitrous oxide toxicity	Euphoria and light-headedness	Symptoms abate without treatment within hours of use
Nutmeg intoxication	Agitation; hallucinations; severe headaches; numbness in extremities	Symptoms abate within hours of use without treatment
Opioid intoxication and withdrawal	Intoxication can lead to coma and death; withdrawal is not life-threatening	IV naloxone, narcotic antagonist; urine and serum screens; psychiatric and medical illnesses (e.g., AIDS) may complicate picture
Panic disorder	Panic, terror; acute onset	Must differentiate from other anxiety-producing disorders, both medical and psychiatric; ECG to rule out mitral valve prolapse; propranolol (10 to 30 mg); alprazolam (0.25 to 2.0 mg); long-term management may include an antidepressant
Paranoid schizophrenia	Command hallucinations; threat to others or themselves	Rapid tranquilization; hospitalization; long-acting depot medication; threatened persons must be notified and protected
Parkinsonism	Stiffness, tremor, bradykinesia, flattened affect, shuffling gait, salivation, secondary to antipsychotic medication	Oral antiparkinsonian drug for 4 weeks to 3 months; decrease dosage of the antipsychotic
Perioral (rabbit) tremor	Perioral tumor (rabbitlike facial grimacing) usually appearing after long-term therapy with antipsychotics	Decrease dosage or change to a medication in another class
Phencyclidine (or phencyclidine-like intoxication)	Paranoid psychosis; can lead to death; acute danger to self and others	Serum and urine assay; benzodiazepines may interfere with excretion; antipsychotics may worsen symptoms because of anticholinergic side effects; medical monitoring and hospitalization for severe intoxication
Phenelzine-induced psychotic disorder	Psychosis and mania in predisposed people	Reduce dosage or discontinue drug
Phenylpropanolamine toxicity	Psychosis; paranoia; insomnia; restlessness; nervousness; headache	Symptoms abate with dosage reduction or discontinuation (found in over-the-counter diet aids and oral and nasal decongestants)
Phobias	Panic, anxiety; fear	Treatment same as for panic disorder
Photosensitivity	Easy sunburning secondary to use of antipsychotic medication	Patient should avoid strong sunlight and use high-level sunscreens
Pigmentary retinopathy	Reported with dosages of thioridazine (Mellaril) of 800 mg a day or above	Remain below 800 mg a day of thioridazine
Postpartum psychosis	Childbirth can precipitate schizophrenia, depression, reactive psychoses, mania, and depression; affective symptoms are most common; suicide risk is reduced during pregnancy but increased in the postpartum period	Danger to self and others (including infant) must be evaluated and proper precautions taken; medical illness presenting with behavioral aberrations is included in the differential diagnosis and must be sought and treated; care must be paid to the effects on father, infant, grandparents, and other children
Posttraumatic stress disorder	Panic, terror; suicidal ideation; flashbacks	Reassurance; encouragement of return to responsibilities; avoid hospitalization if possible to prevent chronic invalidism; monitor suicidal ideation
Priapism (trazodone [Desyrel]-induced)	Persistent penile erection accompanied by severe pain	Intracorporeal epinephrine; mechanical or surgical drainage
Propranolol toxicity	Profound depression; confusional states	Reduce dosage or discontinue drug; monitor suicidality

(*continued*)

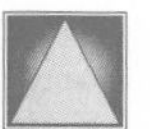

Table 34.2–6 (Continued)

Syndrome	Emergency Manifestations	Treatment Issues
Rape	Not all sexual violations are reported; silent rape reaction is characterized by loss of appetite, sleep disturbance, anxiety, and, sometimes, agoraphobia; long periods of silence, mounting anxiety, stuttering, blocking, and physical symptoms during the interview when the sexual history is taken; fear of violence and death and of contracting a sexually transmitted disease or being pregnant	Rape is a major psychiatric emergency; victim may have enduring patterns of sexual dysfunction; crisis-oriented therapy, social support, ventilation, reinforcement of healthy traits, and encouragement to return to the previous level of functioning as rapidly as possible; legal counsel; thorough medical examination and tests to identify the assailant (e.g., obtaining samples of pubic hairs with a pubic hair comb, vaginal smear to identify blood antigens in semen); if a woman, methoxyprogesterone or diethylstilbestrol orally for 5 days to prevent pregnancy; if menstruation does not commence within one week of cessation of the estrogen, all alternatives to pregnancy, including abortion, should be offered; if the victim has contracted a venereal disease, appropriate antibiotics; witnessed written permission is required for the physician to examine, photograph, collect specimens, and release information to the authorities; obtain consent, record the history in the patient's own words, obtain required tests, record the results of the examination, save all clothing, defer diagnosis, and provide protection against disease, psychic trauma, and pregnancy; men's and women's responses to rape affectively are reported similarly, although men are more hesitant to talk about homosexual assault for fear they will be assumed to have consented
Reserpine intoxication	Major depressive episodes; suicidal ideation; nightmares	Evaluation of suicidal ideation; lower dosage or change drug; antidepressants of ECT may be indicated
Schizoaffective disorder	Severe depression; manic symptoms; paranoia	Evaluation of dangerousness to self or others; rapid tranquilization if necessary; treatment of depression (antidepressants alone can enhance schizophrenic symptoms); use of antimanic agents
Schizophrenia	Extreme self-neglect; severe paranoia; suicidal ideation or assaultiveness; extreme psychotic symptoms	Evaluation of suicidal and homicidal potential; identification of any illness other than schizophrenia; rapid tranquilization
Schizophrenia in exacerbation	Withdrawn; agitation; suicidal and homicidal risk	Suicide and homicide evaluation; screen for medical illness; restraints and rapid tranquilization if necessary; hospitalization if necessary; reevaluation of medication regimen
Sedative, hypnotic, or anxiolytic intoxication and withdrawal	Alterations in mood, behavior, thought—delirium; derealization and depersonalization; untreated, can be fatal; seizures	Naloxone (Narcan) to differentiate from opioid intoxication; slow withdrawal with phenobarbital (Luminal) or sodium thiopental or benzodiazepine; hospitalization
Seizure disorder	Confusion; anxiety; derealization and depersonalization; feelings of impending doom; gustatory or olfactory hallucinations; fuguelike state	Immediate EEG; admission and sleep-deprived and 24-hour EEG; rule out pseudoseizures; anticonvulsants
Substance withdrawal	Abdominal pain; insomnia, drowsiness; delirium; seizures; symptoms of tardive dyskinesia may emerge; eruption of manic or schizophrenic symptoms	Symptoms of psychotropic drug withdrawal disappear with time or disappear with reinstitution of the substance; symptoms of antidepressant withdrawal can be successfully treated with anticholinergic agents, such as atropine; gradual withdrawal of psychotropic substances over two to four weeks generally obviates development of symptoms
Sudden death associated with antipsychotic medication	Seizures; asphyxiation; cardiovascular causes; postural hypotension; laryngeal-pharyngeal dystonia; suppression of gag reflex	Specific medical treatments

(*continued*)

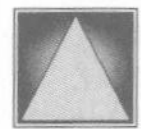

Table 34.2–6 (Continued)

Syndrome	Emergency Manifestations	Treatment Issues
Sudden death of psychogenic origin	Myocardial infarction after sudden psychic stress; voodoo and hexes; hopelessness, especially associated with serious physical illness	Specific medical treatments; folk healers
Suicide	Suicidal ideation; hopelessness	Hospitalization, antidepressants
Sympathomimetic withdrawal	Paranoia; confusional states; depression	Most symptoms abate without treatment; antipsychotics; antidepressants if necessary
Tardive dyskinesia	Dyskinesia of mouth, tongue, face, neck, and trunk; choreoathetoid movements of extremities; usually but not always appearing after long-term treatment with antipsychotics, especially after a reduction in dosage; incidence highest in the elderly and brain-damaged; symptoms are intensified by antiparkinsonian drugs and masked but not cured by increased dosages of antipsychotic	No effective treatment reported; may be prevented by prescribing the least amount of drug possible for as little time as is clinically feasible and using drug-free holidays for patients who need to continue taking the drug; decrease or discontinue drug at first sign of dyskinetic movements
Thyrotoxicosis	Tachycardia; gastrointestinal dysfunction; hyperthermia; panic, anxiety, agitation; mania; dementia; psychosis	Thyroid function test (T_3, T_4, thyroid-stimulating hormone [TSH]); medical consultation
Toluene abuse	Anxiety; confusion; cognitive impairment	Neurological damage is nonprogressive and reversible if toluene use in discontinued early
Vitamin B_{12} deficiency	Confusion; mood and behavior changes; ataxia	Treatment with vitamin B_{12}
Volatile nitrates	Alternations of mood and behavior; light-headedness; pulsating headache	Symptoms abate with cessation of use

to sustain them until they can be seen in the clinic. Feedback to others treating them should be a matter of course.

The emergency room is often the gateway to the department of psychiatry or the general hospital. First impressions carry a great deal of weight. The kind of attention and concern shown to patients on arrival in the emergency room strongly affects how they will respond to staff members and treatment recommendations and even their treatment compliance long after they have left the emergency room.

Documentation

In the interests of good care, respect for patients' rights, cost control, and medicolegal concerns, documentation has become a central focus for the emergency physician. The medical record should convey a concise picture of the patient, highlighting all pertinent positive and negative findings. Gaps in information and their reason should be mentioned. The names and the telephone numbers of interested parties should be noted. A provisional diagnosis or differential diagnosis must be made. An initial treatment plan or recommendations should clearly follow from the findings of the patient's history, mental status examination and other diagnostic tests, and the medical evaluation. The writing must be legible. The emergency physician has unusual latitude under the law to perform an adequate initial assessment; however, all interventions and decisions must be thought out, discussed, and documented in the patient's record.

Specific Psychiatric Emergencies

Table 34.2-6 outlines common psychiatric emergencies in alphabetical order. Readers are referred to the index and to specific chapters of this textbook for a thorough discussion of each disorder.

References

Albanese MJ, Shaffer HJ. Treatment considerations in patients with addictions. *Prim Psychiatry.* 2003;10:55.

Correll CU, Leucht S, Kane JM. Lower risk for tardive dyskinesia associated with second-generation antipsychotics: A systematic review of 1-year studies. *Am J Psychiatry.* 2004;161:414.

Ganesan S, Levy M, Bilsker D, Khanbhai I. Effectiveness of quetiapine for the management of aggressive psychosis in the emergency psychiatric setting: A naturalistic uncontrolled trial. *International Journal of Psychiatry in Clinical Practice.* 2005;9(3):199–203.

Kessing LV. Severity of depressive episodes according to ICD-10 predictions of risk of relapse and suicide. *Br J Psychiatry.* 2004;184:153.

Lukens TW, Wolf SJ, Edlow JA, Shahabuddin S, Allen MH, Currier GW, Jagoda AS. Clinical policy: Critical issues in the diagnosis and management of the adult psychiatric patient in the emergency department. *Ann Emerg Med.* 2006;47(1):79–99.

Mann JJ. Searching for triggers of suicidal behavior. *Am J Psychiatry.* 2004;161:395.

Marco CA, Vaughan J. Emergency management of agitation in schizophrenia. *Am J Emerg Med.* 2005;23(6):767–776.

Matthews M, Matthews M, Matthews S. Recognition and treatment of depression in the elderly. *Prim Psychiatry.* 2004;11:33.

Sailas E, Wahlbeck K. Restraint and seclusion in psychiatric inpatient wards. *Current Opinion in Psychiatry.* 2005;18(5):555–559.

Slaby AE, Dubin WR, Baron DA. Other psychiatric emergencies. In: Sadock BJ, Sadock VA, eds. *Kaplan & Sadock's Comprehensive Textbook of Psychiatry.* 8th ed. Vol. 2. Baltimore: Lippincott Williams & Wilkins; 2005:2442.

▲ 34.3 Psychiatric Emergencies in Children

Few children or adolescents seek psychiatric intervention on their own, even during crisis; thus, most of their emergency evaluations are initiated by parents, relatives, teachers, therapists,

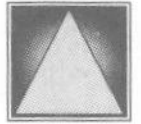

Table 34.3–1
Familial Risk Factors

Physical and sexual abuse
Recent family crisis: loss of a parent, divorce, loss of job, family move
Severe family dysfunction, including parental mental illness

physicians, and child protective service workers. Some referrals are for the evaluation of life-threatening situations for the child or for others, such as suicidal behavior, physical abuse, and violent or homicidal behavior. Other urgent but non–life-threatening referrals pertain to children and adolescents with exacerbations of clear-cut serious psychiatric disorders, such as mania, depression, florid psychosis, and school referral. Less diagnostically obvious situations occur when children and adolescents present with a history of a wide range of disruptive, aberrant behaviors, and are accompanied by an overwhelmed, anxious, and distraught adult who perceive the child's actions as an emergency, despite the absence of life-threatening behavior of an obvious psychiatric disorder. In those cases, the spectrum of contributing factors is not immediately clear, and the emergency psychiatrist must assess the entire family or system involved with the child. Familial stressors and parental discord can contribute to the evolution of a crisis for a child. For example, immediate evaluations are sometimes legitimately indicated for a child caught in the crossfire of feuding parents or in a seemingly irreconcilable conflict between a set of parents and a school, therapist, or protective service worker regarding the needs of the child (Table 34.3-1).

An emergency setting is often the site of an initial evaluation of a chronic problem behavior. For example, an identified problem—such as severe tantrums, violence, and destructive behavior in a child—may have been present for months or even years. Yet, the initial contact with the mental health system in the emergency room or private office may be the first opportunity for the child or adolescent to disclose underlying stressors, such as physical or sexual abuse.

In view of the integral relation of severe family dysfunction to childhood behavioral disturbance, the emergency psychiatrist must assess familial discord and psychiatric disorder in family members during an urgent evaluation. One way to make the assessment is to interview the child and the individual family members, both alone and together, and to obtain a history from informants outside the family whenever possible. Noncustodial parents, therapists, and teachers may add valuable information regarding the child's daily functioning. Many families, especially those with mental illness and severe dysfunction, may have little or no inclination to seek psychiatric help on a nonurgent basis; therefore, the emergency evaluation becomes the only way to engage them in an extensive psychiatric treatment program.

LIFE-THREATENING EMERGENCIES

Suicidal Behavior

Assessment. Suicidal behavior is the most common reason for an emergency evaluation in adolescents. Despite the minimal risk for a complete suicide in a child less than 12 years of age, suicidal ideation or behavior in a child of any age must be carefully evaluated, with particular attention to the psychiatric status of the child and the ability of the family or the guardians to provide the appropriate supervision. The assessment must determine the circumstances of the suicidal ideation or behavior, its lethality, and the persistence of the suicidal intention. An evaluation of the family's sensitivity, supportiveness, and competence must be done to assess their ability to monitor the child's suicidal potential. Ultimately, during the course of an emergency evaluation, the psychiatrist must decide whether the child may return home to a safe environment and receive outpatient follow-up care or whether hospitalization is necessary. A psychiatric history, a mental status examination, and an assessment of family functioning help establish the general level of risk.

Management. When self-injurious behavior has occurred, the adolescent likely requires hospitalization on a pediatric unit for treatment of the injury or for the observation of medical sequelae after a toxic ingestion. If the adolescent is medically clear, the psychiatrist must decide whether the adolescent needs psychiatric admission. If the patient persists in suicidal ideation and shows signs of psychosis, severe depression (including hopelessness), or marked ambivalence about suicide, psychiatric admission is indicated. An adolescent who is taking drugs or alcohol should not be released until an assessment can be done when the patient is in a nonintoxicated state. Patients with high-risk profiles—such as late-adolescent males, especially those with substance abuse and aggressive behavior disorders, and those who have severe depression or who have made prior suicide attempts, particularly with lethal weapons—warrant hospitalization. Young children who have made suicide attempts, even when the attempt had a low lethality, need psychiatric admission if the family is so chaotic, dysfunctional, and incompetent that follow-up treatment is unlikely. (See Chapter 49: *Mood Disorders and Suicide in Children and Adolescents* for further discussion of suicide in children.)

Violent Behavior and Tantrums

Assessment. The first task in an emergency evaluation of a violent child or adolescent is to make sure that both the child and the staff members are physically protected so that nobody gets hurt. If the child appears to be calming down in the emergency area, the clinician may indicate to the child that it would be helpful if the child recounted what happened and may ask whether the child feels in sufficient control to do so. If the child agrees and the clinician judges the child to be in good control, the clinician may approach the child with the appropriate backup close at hand. If not, the clinician may either give the child several minutes to calm down before reassessing the situation or, with an adolescent, suggest that a medication may help the adolescent relax.

If the adolescent is clearly combative, physical restraint may be necessary before anything else is attempted. Some rageful children and adolescents brought to an emergency setting by overwhelmed families are able to regain control of themselves without the use of physical or pharmacological restraint. Children and adolescents are most likely to calm down if approached calmly in a nonthreatening manner and given a chance to tell their side of the story to a nonjudgmental adult. At this time, the psychiatrist should look for any underlying psychiatric disorder that may be mediating the aggression. The psychiatrist should speak to family members and others who have been witnessing the episode to understand the context in which it occurred and the extent to which the child has been out of control.

Management. Prepubertal children, in the absence of major psychiatric illness, rarely require medication to keep them safe, because they are generally small enough to be physically restrained if they begin to hurt themselves or others. It is not immediately necessary to administer medication to a child or an adolescent who was in a rage but is in a calm state when examined. Adolescents and older children who are assaultive, extremely agitated, or overtly self-injurious and who may be difficult to subdue physically may require medication before a dialogue can take place.

Children who have a history of repeated, self-limited, severe tantrums may not require admission to a hospital if they are able to calm down during the course of the evaluation. Yet the pattern, no doubt, will reoccur unless ongoing outpatient treatment for the child and the family is arranged. For adolescents who continue to pose a danger to themselves or others during the evaluation period, admission to a hospital is necessary.

Fire Setting

Assessment. A sense of emergency and panic often surrounds the parents of a child who has set a fire. Parents or teachers often request an emergency evaluation, even for a very young child who has accidentally lit a fire. Many children, during the course of normal development, become interested in fire, but in most cases, a school-age child who has set a fire has done so accidentally while playing with matches and seeks help to put it out. When a child has a strong interest in playing with matches, the level of supervision by family members must be clarified, so that no further accidental fires occur. The clinician must distinguish between a child who accidentally or even impulsively sets a single fire and a child who engages in repeated fire setting with premeditation and subsequently leaves the fire without making any attempt to extinguish it. In repeated fire setting, the risk is obviously greater than in a single occurrence, and the psychiatrist must determine whether underlying psychopathology exists in the child or in the family members. The psychiatrist should also evaluate family interactions, because any factors that interfere with effective supervision and communication—such as high levels of marital discord and harsh, punitive parenting styles—can impede appropriate intervention.

Fire setting is one of a triad of symptoms—enuresis, cruelty to animals, and fire setting—that were believed, some years ago, to be typical of children with conduct disorders; however, no evidence indicates that the three symptoms are truly linked, although conduct disorder is the most frequent psychiatric disorder that occurs with pathological fire setting.

Management. The critical component of management and treatment for fire setters is to prevent further incidents while treating any underlying psychopathology. In general, fire setting alone is not an indication for hospitalization, unless a continued direct threat exists that the patient will set another fire. The parents of children with a pattern of fire setting must be emphatically counseled that the child must not be left alone at home and should never be left to take care of younger siblings without direct adult supervision. Children who exhibit a pattern of concurrent aggressive behaviors and other forms of destructive behavior are likely to have a poor outcome. Outpatient treatment should be arranged for children who repeatedly set fires. Behavioral techniques that involve both the child and the family are helpful in decreasing the risk for further fire setting, as is positive reinforcement for alternate behaviors.

Child Abuse: Physical and Sexual

Assessment. Physical and sexual abuse occurs in girls and boys of all ages, in all ethnic groups, and at all socioeconomic levels. The abuses vary widely with respect to severity and duration, but any form of continued abuse constitutes an emergency situation for a child (Fig. 34.3-1). No single psychiatric syndrome is a *sine qua non* of physical or sexual abuse, but fear, guilt, anxiety, depression, and ambivalence regarding disclosure commonly surrounds the child who has been abused.

Young children who are being sexually abused may exhibit precocious sexual behavior with peers and present a detailed sexual knowledge that reflects exposure beyond their developmental level. Children who endure sexual or physical abuse often display sadistic and aggressive behaviors themselves. Children who are abused in any manner are likely to have been threatened with severe and frightening consequences by the perpetrator if they reveal the situation to anyone. Frequently, an abused child who is victimized by a family member is placed in the irreconcilable position of having either to endure continued abuse silently or to defy the abuser by disclosing the experiences and be responsible for destroying the family and risk being disbelieved or abandoned by the family.

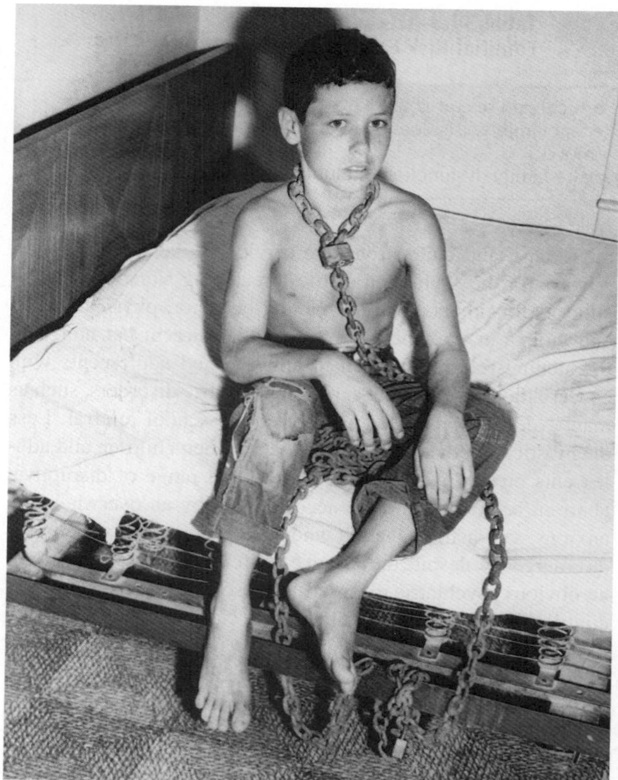

FIGURE 34.3–1
Boy chained by neck to his bed. This 11-year-old boy was found chained to the bed in his home. The boy said that he had spent the night before sleeping in the doghouse in his backyard rather than going into the house to be mistreated. His parents were charged with abusing a minor before a domestic relations court. (Courtesy of Corbis.)

In cases of suspected abuse, the child and other family members must be interviewed individually to give each member a chance to speak privately. If possible, the clinician should observe the child with each parent individually to get a sense of the spontaneity, warmth, fear, anxiety, or other prominent features of the relationships. One observation is generally not sufficient to make a final judgment about the family relationship, however; abused children almost always have mixed emotions toward abusive parents.

Physical indicators of sexual abuse in children include sexually transmitted diseases (e.g., gonorrhea); pain, irritation, and itching of the genitalia and the urinary tract; and discomfort while sitting and walking. In many instances of suspected sexual abuse, however, physical evidence is not present. Thus, a careful history is essential. The physician should speak directly about the issues without leading the child in any direction, because already frightened children may be easily influenced to endorse what they think the examiner wants to hear. Furthermore, children who have been abused often retract all or part of what has been disclosed during the course of an interview.

The use of anatomically correct dolls in the assessment of sexual abuse can help the child identify body parts and show what has happened, but no conclusive evidence supports sexual play with dolls as a means of validating abuse. (See Chapter 32: *Problems Related to Abuse or Neglect* for a full discussion of child abuse.)

Neglect: Failure to Thrive

Assessment. In child neglect, a child's physical, mental, or emotional condition has been impaired because of the inability of a parent or caretaker to provide adequate food, shelter, education, or supervision. Similar to abuse, any form of continued neglect is an emergency situation for the child. Parents who neglect their children range widely and may include parents who are very young and ignorant about the emotional and concrete needs of a child, parents with depression and significant passivity, substance-abusing parents, and parents with a variety of incapacitating mental illnesses.

In its extreme form, neglect can contribute to failure to thrive—that is, an infant, usually under 1 year of age, becomes malnourished in the absence of an organic cause (Figs. 34.3-2 and 34.3-3). Failure to thrive typically occurs under circumstances in which adequate nourishment is available yet a disturbance within the relationship between the caretaker and the child results in a child who does not eat sufficiently to grow and develop. A negative pattern may exist between the mother and the child in which the child refuses feedings and the mother feels rejected and eventually withdraws. She may then avoid offering food as frequently as the infant needs it. Observation of the mother and the child together may reveal a nonspontaneous, tense interaction, with withdrawal on both sides, resulting in a seeming apathy in the mother. Both the mother and the child may seem depressed.

A rare form of failure to thrive in children who are at least several years old and are not necessarily malnourished is the syndrome of psychosocial dwarfism. In that syndrome, marked growth retardation and delayed epiphyseal malnutrition accompany a disturbed relationship between the parent and the child, along with bizarre social and eating behaviors in the child. Those behaviors sometimes include eating from garbage cans, drinking toilet water, binging and vomiting, and diminished outward response to pain. Half of the children with the syndrome have decreased growth hormone. Once the children are removed from the troubled environment and placed in another setting, such as a psychiatric hospital with appropriate supervision and guidance regarding meals, the endocrine abnormalities normalize, and the children begin to grow at a more rapid rate.

Management. In cases of child neglect, as with physical and sexual abuse, the most important decision to be made during the initial evaluation is whether the child is safe in the home environment. Whenever neglect is suspected, it must be reported to the local child protective service agency. In mild cases, the decision to refer the family for outpatient services, as opposed to hospitalizing the child, depends on the clinician's conviction that the family is cooperative and willing to be educated and to enter into treatment and that the child is not in danger. Before a neglected child is released from an emergency setting, a follow-up appointment must be made.

Education for the family must begin during the evaluation; the family must be told, in a nonthreatening manner, that failure to thrive can become life-threatening, that the entire family needs to monitor the child's progress, and that they will receive some help in overcoming the many possible obstacles interfering with the child's emotional and physical well-being.

Anorexia Nervosa

Anorexia nervosa occurs in females about ten times as often as in males. It is characterized by the refusal to maintain body weight, leading to a weight at least 15 percent below the expected, by a distorted body image, by a persistent fear of becoming fat, and by the absence of at least three menstrual cycles. The disorder usually begins after puberty, but it has occurred in children of 9 to 10 years of age, in whom expected weight gain does not occur, rather than a loss of 15 percent of body weight. The disorder reaches medical emergency proportions when the weight loss approaches 30 percent of body weight or when metabolic disturbances become severe. Hospitalization then becomes necessary to control the

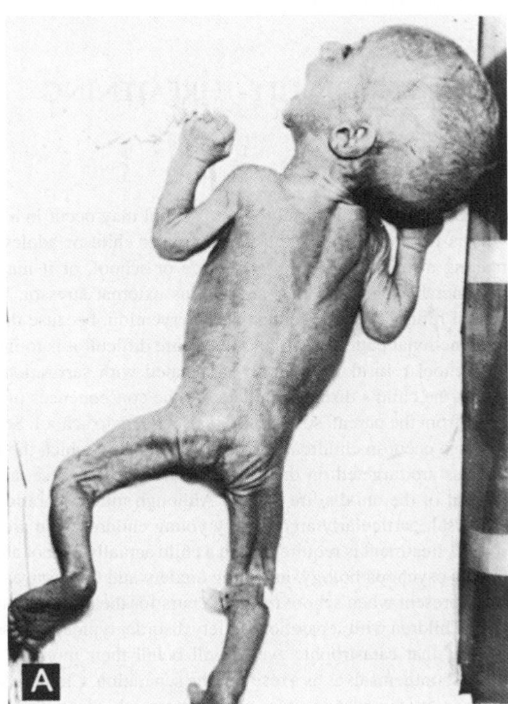

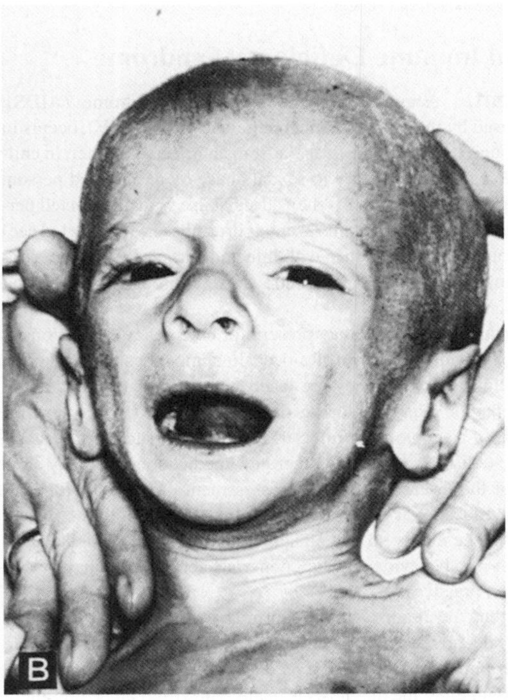

FIGURE 34.3–2
A 3-month-old baby suffering from failure to thrive secondary to caloric deprivation. Weight is only 1 ounce over birthweight. (Courtesy of Barbon Schmitt, M.D., Children's Hospital, Denver, CO.)

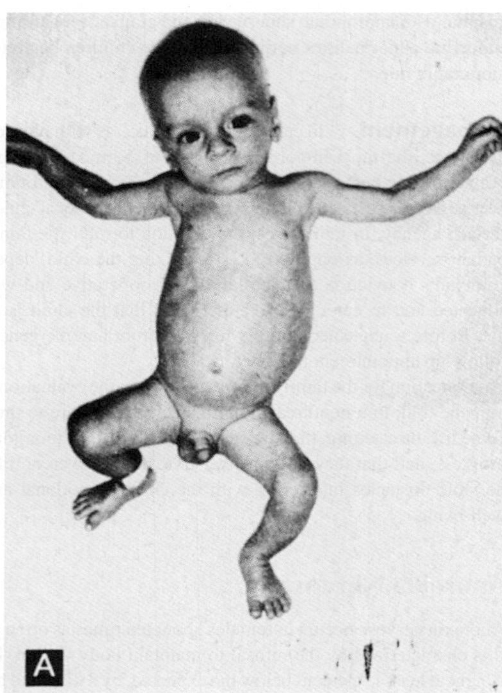

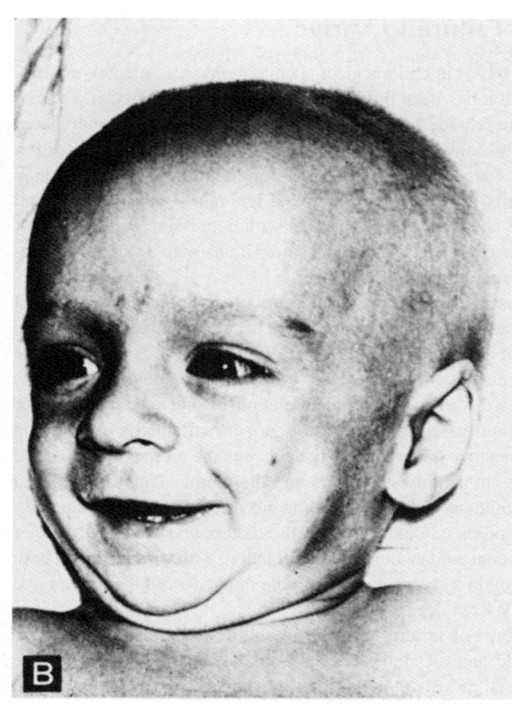

FIGURE 34.3–3
The same infant as in Figure 34.3-2, 3 weeks later, after hospitalization. (Courtesy of Barbon Schmitt, M.D., Children's Hospital, Denver, CO.)

ongoing process of starvation, potential dehydration, and the medical complications of starvation, including electrolyte imbalances, cardiac arrhythmias, and hormonal changes. (See Chapter 23: *Eating Disorders* for a further discussion of anorexia nervosa and other eating disorders.)

Acquired Immune Deficiency Syndrome

Assessment. Acquired immune deficiency syndrome (AIDS), which is caused by the human immunodeficiency virus (HIV), occurs in neonate through perinatal transmission from an infected mother, in children and adolescents secondary to sexual abuse by an infected person, and in adolescents through intravenous drug abuse with an infected person, and in adolescents through intravenous drug abuse with infected needles and through sexual activities with infected partners. Child and adolescent hemophiliac patients may contract AIDS through tainted blood transfusions.

Children and adolescents may present for emergency evaluations at the urging of a family member of a peer; in some cases, they take the initiative themselves when they are faced with anxiety or panic about high-risk behavior. Early screening of high-risk persons may lead to the treatment of asymptomatic infected patients with such drugs as azidothymidine (AZT) and possibly other new medications that may slow the course of the disease. During the assessment of the risks for HIV infection, an educational process can be initiated with both the patient and the rest of the family so that an adolescent who is not infected, but exhibits high-risk behavior, can be counseled about that behavior and about safe-sex practices.

In children, the brain is often a primary site for HIV infection; encephalitis, decreased brain development, and such neuropsychiatric symptoms as impairment in memory, concentration, and attention span may be present before the diagnosis is made. The virus can be present in the cerebrospinal fluid before it shows up in the bloodstream. Changes in cognitive function, frontal lobe disinhibition, social withdrawal, slowed information processing, and apathy constitute some common symptoms of the AIDS dementia complex. Organic mood disorders, organic personality disorder, and frank psychosis can also occur in patients infected with HIV. (HIV is discussed in Chapter 11: *Neuropsychiatric Aspects of HIV Infection and AIDS*.)

URGENT NON-LIFE-THREATENING SITUATIONS

School Refusal

Assessment. Refusal to go to school may occur in a young child who is first entering school or in an older child or adolescent who is making a transition into a new grade or school, or it may emerge in a vulnerable child without an obvious external stressor. In any case, school refusal requires immediate intervention, because the longer the dysfunctional pattern continues, the more difficult it is to interrupt.

School refusal is generally associated with separation anxiety, in which the child's distress is related to the consequences of being separated from the parent, so the child resists going to school. School refusal can also occur in children with school phobia, in which the fear and the distress are targeted on the school itself. In either case, a serious disruption of the child's life occurs. Although mild separation anxiety is universal, particularly among very young children who are first facing school, treatment is required when a child actually cannot attend school. Severe psychopathology, including anxiety and depressive disorders, is often present when school refusal occurs for the first time in an adolescent. Children with separation anxiety disorder typically present extreme worries that catastrophic events will befall their mothers, attachment figures, or themselves as a result of the separation. Children with separation anxiety disorder may also exhibit many other fears and symptoms of depression, including such somatic complaints such as headaches, stomachaches, and nausea. Severe tantrums and desperate pleas may ensue when preoccupation that a parent will be harmed during the separation is frequently verbalized; in adolescents, the stated reasons for refusing to go to school are often physical complaints.

As part of an urgent assessment, the psychiatrist must ascertain the duration of the patient's absence from school and must assess the parents' ability to participate in a treatment plan that will undoubtedly involve firm parental guidelines to ensure the child's return to school. The parents of a child with separation anxiety disorder often exhibit excessive separation anxiety or other anxiety disorders themselves, thereby compounding the child's problem. When the parents are unable to participate in a treatment program from home, hospitalization should be considered.

Management. When school refusal caused by separation anxiety is identified during an emergency evaluation, the underlying disorder can be explained to the family, and an intervention can be started immediately. In severe cases, however, a multidimensional, long-term family-oriented treatment plan is necessary. Whenever possible, a separation-anxious child should be brought back to school the next school day, despite the distress, and a contact person within the school (counselor, guidance counselor, or teacher) should be involved to help the child stay in school while praising the child for tolerating the school situation.

When school refusal has been going on for months or years or when the family members are unable to cooperate, a treatment program to move the child back to school from the hospital should be considered. When the child's anxiety is not diminished by behavioral methods alone, tricyclic antidepressants, such as imipramine (Tofranil), are helpful. Medication is generally prescribed not at the initial evaluation but after a behavioral intervention has been tried.

Munchausen Syndrome by Proxy

Assessment. Munchausen syndrome by proxy, essentially, is a form of child abuse in which a parent, usually the mother, or a caretaker repeatedly fabricates or actually inflicts injury or illness in a child for whom medical intervention is then sought, often in an emergency setting. Although it is a rare scenario, mothers who inflict injury often have some prior knowledge of medicine, leading to sophisticated symptoms; the mothers sometimes engage in inappropriate camaraderie with the medical staff regarding the treatment of the child. Careful observation may reveal that the mothers often do not exhibit appropriate signs of distress on hearing the details of the child's medical symptoms. Prototypically, such mothers tend to present themselves as highly accomplished professionals in ways that seem inflated or blatantly untrue.

The illnesses appearing in the child can involve any organ system, but certain symptoms are commonly presented: bleeding from one or may sites, including the gastrointestinal (GI) tract, the genitourinary system, and the respiratory system; seizures; and central nervous system (CNS) depression. At times, the illness is simulated, rather than actually inflicted. This syndrome is covered in Chapter 19.

OTHER CHILDHOOD DISTURBANCES

Posttraumatic Stress Disorder

Children who have been subjected to a severe catastrophic or traumatic event may present for a prompt evaluation because they have extreme fears of the specific trauma occurring again or sudden discomfort with familiar places, people, or situations that previously did not evoke anxiety. Within weeks of a traumatic event, a child may re-create the event in play, in stories, and in dreams that directly replay the terrifying situation. A sense of reliving the experience may occur, including hallucinations and flashback (dissociative) experiences, and intrusive memories of the event come and go. Many traumatized children, over time, go on to reproduce parts of the event through their own victimization behaviors toward others, without being aware that those behaviors reflect their own traumatic experiences. (See Section 50.2: *Posttraumatic Stress Disorder of Infancy, Childhood, and Adolescence* for further discussion of this topic.)

Dissociative Disorders

Dissociative states—including the extreme form, multiple personality disorder—are believed most likely to occur in children who have been subjected to severe and repetitive physical, sexual, or emotional abuse. Children with dissociative symptoms may be referred for evaluation because family members or teachers observe that the children sometimes seem to be spaced out or distracted or act like different persons. Dissociative states are occasionally identified during the evaluation of violent and aggressive behavior, particularly in patients who truly do not remember chunks of their own behavior.

When a child who dissociates is violent or self-destructive or endangers others, hospitalization is necessary. A variety of psychotherapy methods have been used in the complex treatment of children with dissociative disorders, including play techniques and, in some cases, hypnosis. (See Chapter 20: *Dissociative Disorders* for a complete discussion of this condition.)

References

Arnow BA. Relationships between childhood maltreatment, adult health and psychiatric outcomes, and medical utilization. *J Clin Psychiatry.* 2004;65[Suppl 12]:10–15.

Donaldson D, Spirito A, Esposito-Smythers C. Treatment for adolescents following a suicide attempt: Results of a pilot trial. *J Am Acad Child Adolesc Psychiatry.* 2005;44(2):113–120.

Dorfman DH, Mehta S. Restraint use for psychiatric patients in the pediatric emergency department. *Pediatr Emerg Care.* 2006;22(1):7–12.

Goldstein AB, Silverman MAC, Phillips S, Lichenstein R. Mental health visits in a pediatric emergency department and their relationship to the school calendar. *Pediatr Emerg Care.* 2005;21(10):653–657.

Huey SJ Jr, Henggeler SW, Rowland MD, Halliday-Boykins CA, Cunningham PB, Pickrel SG. Predictors of treatment response for suicidal youth referred for emergency psychiatric hospitalization. *J Clin Child Adolesc Psychol.* 2005;34(3):582–589.

Katz LY, Cox BJ, Gunasekara S, Miller AL. Feasibility of dialectical behavior therapy for suicidal adolescent inpatients. *J Am Acad Child Adolesc Psychiatry.* 2004;43(3):276–282.

Londino DL, Mabe PA, Josephson AM. Child and adolescent psychiatric emergencies: Family psychodynamic issues. *Child and Adolescent Psychiatric Clinics of North America.* 2003;12(4):629–647.

Sharp DL, Blaakman SW, Cole EC, Cole RE. Evidence-based multidisciplinary strategies for working with children who set fires. *Journal of the American Psychiatric Nurses Association.* 2005;11(6):329–337.

Sorrentino A. Chemical restraints for the agitated, violent, or psychotic pediatric patient in the emergency department: Controversies and recommendations. *Curr Opin Pediatr.* 2004;16(2):201–205.

Tardif M, Auclair N, Jacob M, Carpentier J. Sexual abuse by adult and juvenile females: An ultimate attempt to resolve a conflict associated with maternal identity. *Child Abuse Negl.* 2005;29(2):153–167.

35 Psychotherapies

▲ 35.1 Psychoanalysis and Psychoanalytic Psychotherapy

Psychoanalysis is virtually synonymous with the renowned name of its founding father, Sigmund Freud (Freud and his theories are discussed in Section 6.1). It is also referred to as "classic" or "orthodox" psychoanalysis to distinguish it from more recent variations known as *psychoanalytic psychotherapy* (discussed below).

Psychoanalysis is based on the theory of sexual repression and traces the unfulfilled infantile libidinal wishes in the individual's unconscious memories. It remains unsurpassed as a method to discover the meaning and motivation of behavior, especially the unconscious elements informing thoughts and feelings.

As broadly practiced today, psychoanalytic treatment encompasses a wide range of uncovering strategies used in varied degrees and blends. Despite the inevitable blurring of boundaries in actual application, the original modality of classic psychoanalysis and major modes of psychoanalytic psychotherapy (expressive and supportive) are delineated separately here (Table 35.1-1). Analytical practice in all its complexity resides on a continuum. Individual technique is always a matter of emphasis, as the therapist titrates the treatment according to the needs and capacities of the patient at every moment.

PSYCHOANALYSIS

Psychoanalytic Process

The psychoanalytic process involves bringing to the surface repressed memories and feelings by means of a scrupulous unraveling of hidden meanings of verbalized material and of the unwitting ways in which the patient wards off underlying conflicts through defensive forgetting and repetition of the past.

The overall process of analysis is one in which unconscious neurotic conflicts are recovered from memory and verbally expressed, reexperienced in the transference, reconstructed by the analyst, and, ultimately, resolved through understanding. Freud referred to these processes as *recollection*, *repetition*, and *working through*, which make up the totality of remembering, reliving, and gaining insight. *Recollection* entails the extension of memory back to early childhood events, a time in the distant past when the core of neurosis was formed. The actual reconstruction of these events comes through reminiscence, associations, and autobiographical linking of developmental events. *Repetition* involves more than mere mental recall; it is an emotional replay of former interactions with significant individuals in the patient's life. The replay occurs within the special context of the analyst as projected parent, a fantasized object from the patient's past with whom the latter unwittingly reproduces forgotten, unresolved feelings and experiences from childhood. Finally, *working through* is both an affective and cognitive integration of previously repressed memories that have been brought into consciousness and through which the patient is gradually set free (cured of neurosis). The analytical course can be subdivided into three major stages (Table 35.1-2).

Indications and Contraindications

In general, all of the so-called *psychoneuroses* are suitable for psychoanalysis. These include anxiety disorders, obsessional thinking, compulsive behavior, conversion disorder, sexual dysfunction, depressive states, and many other nonpsychotic conditions, such as personality disorders. Significant suffering must be present so that patients are motivated to make the sacrifices of time and financial resources required for psychoanalysis. Patients who enter analysis must have a genuine wish to understand themselves, not a desperate hunger for symptomatic relief. They must be able to withstand frustration, anxiety, and other strong affects that emerge in analysis without fleeing or acting out their feelings in a self-destructive manner. They must also have a reasonable, mature superego that allows them to be honest with the analyst. Intelligence must be at least average, and above all, they must be psychologically minded in the sense that they can think abstractly and symbolically about the unconscious meanings of their behavior.

Many contraindications for psychoanalysis are the flip side of the indications. The absence of suffering, poor impulse control, inability to tolerate frustration and anxiety, and low motivation to understand are all contraindications. The presence of extreme dishonesty or antisocial personality disorder contraindicates analytic treatment. Concrete thinking or the absence of psychological mindedness is another contraindication. Some patients who might ordinarily be psychologically minded are not suitable for analysis because they are in the midst of a major upheaval or life crisis, such as a job loss or a divorce. Serious physical illness can also interfere with a person's ability to invest in a long-term treatment process. Patients of low intelligence generally do not understand the procedure or cooperate in the process. An age older than 40 years was once considered a contraindication, but today

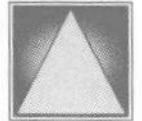

Table 35.1–1
Scope of Psychoanalytic Practice: A Clinical Continuum[a]

		Psychoanalytic Psychotherapy	
Feature	**Psychoanalysis**	**Expressive Mode**	**Supportive Mode**
Frequency	Regular four to five times/wk; "50-minute hour"	Regular one to three times/wk; $^1/_2$ to full hr	Flexible one time/wk or less; or as needed $^1/_2$ to full hr
Duration	Long-term; usually 3 to 5+ yrs	Short- or long-term; several sessions to months or years	Short- or intermittent long-term; single session to lifetime
Setting	Patient primarily on couch with analyst out of view	Patient and therapist face-to-face; occasional use of couch	Patient and therapist face-to-face; couch contraindicated
Modus operandi	Systematic analysis of all positive and negative transference and resistance; primary focus on analyst and intrasession events; transference neurosis facilitated; regression encouraged	Partial analysis of dynamics and defenses; focus on current interpersonal events and transference to others outside of sessions; analysis of negative transference; positive transference left unexplored unless impedes progress; limited regression encouraged	Formation of therapeutic alliance and real object relationship; analysis of transference contraindicated with rare exceptions; focus on conscious external events; regression discouraged
Analyst/therapist role	Absolute neutrality; frustration of patient; reflector/mirror role	Modified neutrality; implicit gratification of patient and greater activity	Neutrality suspended; limited explicit gratification, direction, and disclosure
Mutative change agents	Insight predominates within relatively deprived environment	Insight within more empathic environment; identification with benevolent object	Auxiliary or surrogate ego as temporary substitute; holding environment; insight to degree possible
Patient population	Neuroses; mild character psychopathology	Neuroses; mild to moderate character psychopathology, especially narcissistic and borderline disorders	Severe character disorders, latent or manifest psychoses, acute crises, physical illness
Patient requisites	High motivation, psychological-mindedness; good previous object relationships; ability to maintain transference neurosis; good frustration tolerance	High to moderate motivation and psychological-mindedness; ability to form therapeutic alliance; some frustration tolerance	Some degree of motivation and ability to form therapeutic alliance
Basic goals	Structural reorganization of personality; resolution of unconscious conflicts; insight into intrapsychic events; symptom relief an indirect result	Partial reorganization of personality and defenses; resolution of preconscious and conscious derivatives of conflicts; insight into current interpersonal events; improved object relations; symptom relief a goal or prelude to further exploration	Reintegration of self and ability to cope; stabilization or restoration of preexisting equilibrium; strengthening of defenses; better adjustment or acceptance of pathology; symptom relief and environmental restructuring as primary goals
Major techniques	Free association method predominates; full dynamic interpretation (including confrontation, clarification, and working through), with emphasis on genetic reconstruction	Limited free association; confrontation, clarification, and partial interpretation predominate, with emphasis on here-and-now interpretation and limited genetic interpretation	Free association method contraindicated; suggestion (advise) predominates; abreaction useful; confrontation, clarification, and interpretation in the here-and-now secondary; genetic interpretation contraindicated
Adjunct treatment	Primarily avoided; if applied, all negative and positive meanings and implications are thoroughly analyzed	May be necessary—e.g., psychotropic drugs as temporary measure; if applied, its negative implications explored and diffused	Often necessary— e.g., psychotropic drugs, family rehabilitative therapy, or hospitalization; if applied, its positive implications are emphasized

[a]This division is not categorical; all practice resides on a clinical continuum.

analysts recognize that patients are malleable and analyzable in their 60s or 70s. One final contraindication is a close relationship with the analyst. Analysts should avoid analyzing friends, relatives, or persons with whom they have other involvements.

Patient Requisites

The most important patient requisites for psychoanalysis are listed in Table 35.1-3.

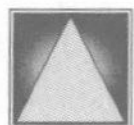

Table 35.1–2
Stages of Psychoanalysis

Stage one: Patient becomes familiar with the methods, routines, and requirements of analysis, and a realistic therapeutic alliance is formed between patient and analyst. Basic rules are established; the patient describes his or her problems; there is some review of history, and the patient gains initial relief through catharsis and a sense of security before delving more deeply into the source of the illness. The patient is primarily motivated by the wish to get well.

Stage two: Transference neurosis emerges that substitutes for the actual neurosis of the patient and in which the wish for health comes into direct conflict with the simultaneous wish to receive emotional gratification from the analyst. There is a gradual surfacing of unconscious conflicts; an increased irrational attachment to the analyst, with regressive and dependent concomitants of that bond; a developmental return to earlier forms of relating (sometimes compared to that of mother and infant); and a repetition of childhood patterns and recall of traumatic memories through transfer to the analyst of unresolved libidinal wishes.

Stage three: The termination phase is marked by the dissolution of the analytical bond as the patient prepares for leave-taking. The irrational attachment to the analyst in the transference neurosis has subsided because it has been worked through, and more rational aspects of the psyche preside, providing greater mastery and more mature adaptation to the patient's problems. Termination is not a hard-and-fast event, and the patient invariably has to continue to work through any problems outside of the therapy situation without the analyst or may need intermittent assistance after analysis has technically terminated.

Courtesy of T. Byram Karasu, M.D.

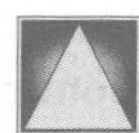

Table 35.1–3
Patient Prerequisites for Psychoanalysis

1. *High motivation.* The patient needs a strong motivation to persevere, in light of the rigors of intense and lengthy treatment. The desire for health and self-understanding must surpass the neurotic need for unhappiness. The patient must be willing to face issues of time and money and to endure the pain and frustration associated with sacrificing rapid relief in favor of future cure and with foregoing the secondary gains of illness.
2. *Ability to form a relationship.* The capacity to form and maintain, as well as to detach from, a trusting object relationship is essential. The patient also has to withstand a frustrating and regressive transference without decompensating or becoming excessively attached. Patients with a history of impaired or transient interpersonal relations who cannot establish a viable connection to another human make poor candidates for psychoanalysis.
3. *Psychological-mindedness and capacity for insight.* As an introspective process, psychoanalysis requires curiosity about oneself and the capacity for self-scrutiny. Those who are unable to articulate and comprehend their inner thoughts and feelings cannot negotiate with the fundamental analytical coin-words and their meanings. The inability to examine one's own motivations and behaviors precludes benefits from the analytical method.
4. *Ego strength.* Ego strength is the integrative capacity to oscillate appropriately between two antithetical types of ego functioning: On the one hand, the patient must be able to reflect temporarily, to relinquish reality for fantasy, and to be dependent and passive. On the other hand, the patient has to be able to accept analytical rules, to integrate interpretations, to defer important decisions, to shift perspectives to become an observer of his or her intrapsychic processes, and to function in a sustained interpersonal relationship as a responsible adult.

Courtesy of T. Byram Karasu, M.D.

Goals

Stated in developmental terms, psychoanalysis aims at the gradual removal of amnesias rooted in early childhood based on the assumption that when all gaps in memory have been filled, the morbid condition will cease because the patient no longer needs to repeat or remain fixated to the past. The patient should be better able to relinquish former regressive patterns and to develop new, more adaptive ones, particularly as he or she learns the reasons for his or her behavior. A related goal of psychoanalysis is for the patient to achieve some measure of self-understanding or insight.

Psychoanalytic goals are often considered formidable (e.g., a total personality change), involving the radical reorganization of old developmental patterns based on earlier affects and the entrenched defenses built up against them. Goals may also be elusive, framed as they are in theoretical intrapsychic terms (e.g., greater ego strength) or conceptually ambiguous ones (resolution of the transference neurosis). Criteria for successful psychoanalysis may be largely intangible and subjective and they are best regarded as conceptual endpoints of treatment that must be translated into more realistic and practical terms.

In practice, the goals of psychoanalysis for any patient naturally vary, as do the many manifestations of neuroses. The form that the neurosis takes—unsatisfactory sexual or object relationships, inability to enjoy life, underachievement, and fear of work or academic success, or excessive anxiety, guilt, or depressive ideation—determines the focus of attention and the general direction of treatment, as well as the specific goals. Such goals may change at any time during the course of analysis, especially as many years of treatment may be involved.

Major Approach and Techniques

Structurally, *psychoanalysis* usually refers to individual (dyadic) treatment that is frequent (four or five times per week) and long-term (several years). All three features take their precedent from Freud himself.

The dyadic arrangement is a direct function of the freudian theory of neurosis as an intrapsychic phenomenon, which takes place within the person as instinctual impulses continually seek discharge. Because dynamic conflicts must be internally resolved if structural personality reorganization is to take place, the individual's memory and perceptions of the repressed past are pivotal.

Freud initially saw patients 6 days a week for 1 hour each day, a routine now reduced to four or five sessions of the classic 50-minute hour, which leaves time for the analyst to take notes and organize relevant thoughts before the next patient. Long intervals between sessions are avoided so that the momentum gained in uncovering conflictual material is not lost and confronted defenses do not have time to restrengthen.

Freud's belief that successful psychoanalysis always takes a long time because profound changes in the mind occur slowly still holds. The process can be likened to the fluid sense of time that is characteristic of our unconscious processes. Moreover, because psychoanalysis involves a detailed recapitulation of present and past events, any compromise in time presents the risk of losing pace with the patient's mental life.

Psychoanalytic Setting. As with other forms of psychotherapy, psychoanalysis takes place in a professional setting, apart from the realities of everyday life, in which the patient is offered a temporary sanctuary in which to ease psychic pain and reveal intimate thoughts to an accepting expert. The psychoanalytic environment is designed to promote relaxation and regression. The setting is usually spartan and sensorially neutral, and external stimuli are minimized.

USE OF THE COUCH. The couch has several clinical advantages that are both real and symbolic: (1) the reclining position is relaxing because it is associated with sleep and so eases the patient's conscious control of thoughts; (2) it minimizes the intrusive influence of the analyst, thus curbing unnecessary cues; (3) it permits the analyst to make observations of the patient without interruption; and (4) it holds symbolic value for both parties, a tangible reminder of the freudian legacy that gives credibility to the analyst's professional identity, allegiance, and expertise. The reclining position of the patient with analyst nearby can also generate threat and discomfort, however, as it recalls anxieties derived from the earlier parent–child configuration that it physically resembles. It may also have personal meanings—for some, a portent of dangerous impulses or of submission to an authority figure; for others, a relief from confrontation by the analyst (e.g., fear of use of the couch and overeagerness to lie down may reflect resistance and, thus, need to be analyzed). Although the use of the couch is requisite to analytical technique, it is not applied automatically; it is introduced gradually and can be suspended whenever additional regression is unnecessary or countertherapeutic.

FUNDAMENTAL RULE. The fundamental rule of free association requires patients to tell the analyst everything that comes into their heads—however disagreeable, unimportant, or nonsensical—and to let themselves go as they would in a conversation that leads you from "cabbages to kings." It differs decidedly from ordinary conversation—instead of connecting personal remarks with a rational thread, the patient is asked to reveal those very thoughts and events that are objectionable precisely because of being averse to doing so.

This directive represents an ideal because free association does not arise freely but is guided and inhibited by a variety of conscious and unconscious forces. The analyst must not only encourage free association through the physical setting and a nonjudgmental attitude toward the patient's verbalizations, but also examine those very instances when the flow of associations is diminished or comes to a halt— they are as important analytically as the content of the associations. The analyst should also be alert to how individual patients use or misuse the fundamental rule.

Aside from its primary purpose of eliciting recall of deeply hidden early memories, the fundamental rule reflects the analytical priority placed on verbalization, which translates the patient's thoughts into words so that they are not channeled physically or behaviorally. As a direct concomitant of the fundamental rule, which prohibits action in favor of verbal expression, patients are expected to postpone making major alterations in their lives, such as marrying or changing careers, until they discuss and analyze them within the context of treatment.

PRINCIPLE OF EVENLY SUSPENDED ATTENTION. As a reciprocal corollary to the rule that patients communicate everything that occurs to them without criticism or selection, the principle of evenly suspended attention requires the analyst to suspend judgment and to give impartial attention to every detail equally. The method consists simply of making no effort to concentrate on anything specific, while maintaining a neutral, quiet attentiveness to all that is said.

ANALYST AS MIRROR. A second principle is the recommendation that the analyst be impenetrable to the patient and, as a mirror, reflect only what is shown. Analysts are advised to be neutral blank screens and not to bring their own personalities into treatment. This means that they are not to bring their own values or attitudes into the discussion or to share personal reactions or mutual conflicts with their patients, although they may sometimes be tempted to do so. The bringing in of reality and external influences can interrupt or bias the patient's unconscious projections. Neutrality also allows the analyst to accept without censure all forbidden or objectionable responses.

RULE OF ABSTINENCE. The fundamental rule of abstinence does not mean corporal or sexual abstinence, but refers to the frustration of emotional needs and wishes that the patient may have toward the analyst or part of the transference. It allows the patient's longings to persist and serve as driving forces for analytical work and motivation to change. Freud advised that the analyst carry through the analytical treatment in a state of renunciation. The analyst must deny the patient who is longing for love the satisfaction he or she craves.

Limitations. At present, the predominant treatment constraints are often economic, relating to the high cost in time and money, both for patients and in the training of future practitioners. In addition, because clinical requirements emphasize such requisites as psychological-mindedness, verbal and cognitive ability, and stable life situation, psychoanalysis may be unduly restricted to a diagnostically, socioeconomically, or intellectually advantaged patient population. Other intrinsic issues pertain to the use and misuse of its stringent rules, whereby overemphasis on technique may interfere with an authentic human encounter between analyst and patient, and to the major long-term risk of interminability, in which protracted treatment may become a substitute for life. Reification of the classic analytical tradition may interfere with a more open and flexible application of its tenets to meet changing needs. It may also obstruct a comprehensive view of patient care that includes a greater appreciation of other treatment modalities in conjunction with, or as an alternative to, psychoanalysis.

Ms. A, a 25-year-old articulate and introspective medical student, began analysis complaining of mild, chronic anxiety, dysphoria, and a sense of inadequacy, despite above-average intelligence and performance. She also expressed difficulty in long-term relationships with her male peers.

Ms. A began the initial phase of analysis with enthusiastic self-disclosure, frequent reports of dreams and fantasies, and overidealization of the analyst; she tried to please him by being a compliant, good patient, just as she had been a good daughter to her father (a professor of medicine) by going to medical school.

Over the next several months, Ms. A gradually developed a strong attachment to the analyst and settled into a phase of excessive preoccupation with him. Simultaneously, however, she began dating an older psychiatrist and proceeded to complain about the analyst's coldness and unresponsiveness, even considering dropping out of analysis because he did not meet her demands.

In the course of analysis, through dreams and associations, Ms. A recalled early memories of her ongoing competition with her mother for her father's attention and realized that, failing to obtain his exclusive love, she had tried to become like him. She was also able to see how her increasing interest in becoming a psychiatrist (rather than following her original plan to be a pediatrician), as well as her recent choice of a man to date, were recapitulations of the past vis-à-vis the analyst. As this repeated pattern was recognized, the patient began to relinquish her intense erotic and dependent tie to the analyst, viewing him more realistically and beginning to appreciate the ways in which his quiet presence reminded her of her mother. She also became less disturbed by the similarities she shared with her mother and was able to disengage from her father more comfortably. By the fifth year of analysis, she was happily married to a classmate, was pregnant, and was a pediatric chief resident. Her anxiety was now attenuated and situation-specific (that is, she was concerned about motherhood and the termination of analysis). (Courtesy of T. Byram Karasu, M.D.)

PSYCHOANALYTIC PSYCHOTHERAPY

Psychoanalytic psychotherapy, which is based on fundamental dynamic formulations and techniques that derive from psychoanalysis, is designed to broaden its scope. Psychoanalytic psychotherapy, in its narrowest sense, is the use of insight-oriented methods only. As generically applied today to an ever-larger clinical spectrum, it incorporates a blend of uncovering and suppressive measures.

The strategies of psychoanalytic psychotherapy currently range from expressive (insight-oriented, uncovering, evocative, or interpretive) techniques to supportive (relationship-oriented, suggestive, suppressive, or repressive) techniques. Although those two types of methods are sometimes regarded as antithetical, their precise definitions and the distinctions between them are by no means absolute.

The duration of psychoanalytic psychotherapy is generally shorter and more variable than in psychoanalysis. Treatment may be brief, even with an initially agreed-on or fixed time limit, or may extend to a less-definite number of months or years. Brief treatment is chiefly used for selected problems or highly focused conflict, whereas longer treatment may be applied in more chronic conditions or for intermittent episodes that require ongoing attention to deal with pervasive conflict or recurrent decompensation. Unlike psychoanalysis, psychoanalytic psychotherapy rarely uses the couch; instead, patient and therapist sit face to face. This posture helps to prevent regression because it encourages the patient to look on the therapist as a real person from whom to receive direct cues, even though transference and fantasy will continue. The couch is considered unnecessary because the free-association method is rarely used, except when the therapist wishes to gain access to fantasy material or dreams to enlighten a particular issue.

Expressive Psychotherapy

Indications and Contraindications. Diagnostically, psychoanalytic psychotherapy in its expressive mode is suited to a range of psychopathology with mild to moderate ego weakening, including neurotic conflicts, symptom complexes, reactive conditions, and the whole realm of nonpsychotic character disorders, including those disorders of the self that are among the more transient and less profound on the severity-of-illness spectrum, such as narcissistic behavior disorders and narcissistic personality disorders. It is also one of the treatments recommended for patients with borderline personality disorders, although special variations may be required to deal with the associated turbulent personality characteristics, primitive defense mechanisms, tendencies toward regressive episodes, and irrational attachments to the analyst.

The persons best suited for the expressive psychotherapy approach have fairly well integrated egos and the capacity to both sustain and detach from a bond of dependency and trust. They are, to some degree, psychologically minded and self-motivated, and they are generally able, at least temporarily, to tolerate doses of frustration without decompensating. They must also have the ability to manage the rearousal of painful feelings outside the therapy hour without additional contact. Patients must have some capacity for introspection and impulse control, and they should be able to recognize the cognitive distinction between fantasy and reality.

Goals. The overall goals of expressive psychotherapy are to increase the patient's self-awareness and to improve object relations through exploration of current interpersonal events and perceptions. In contrast to psychoanalysis, major structural changes in ego function and defenses are modified in light of patient limitations. The aim is to achieve a more limited and, thus, select and focused understanding of one's problems. Rather than uncovering deeply hidden and past motives and tracing them back to their origins in infancy, the major thrust is to deal with preconscious or conscious derivatives of conflicts as they became manifest in present interactions. Although insight is sought, it is less extensive; instead of delving to a genetic level, greater emphasis is on clarifying recent dynamic patterns and maladaptive behaviors in the present.

Major Approach and Techniques. The major modus operandi involves establishment of a therapeutic alliance and early recognition and interpretation of negative transference. Only limited or controlled regression is encouraged, and positive transference manifestations are generally left unexplored, unless they are impeding therapeutic progress; even here, the emphasis is on shedding light on current dynamic patterns and defenses.

Limitations. A general limitation of expressive psychotherapy, as of psychoanalysis, is the problem of emotional integration of cognitive awareness. The major danger for patients who are at the more disorganized end of the diagnostic spectrum, however, may have less to do with the overintellectualization that is sometimes seen in neurotic patients than with the threat of decompensation from, or acting out of, deep or frequent interpretations that the patient is unable to integrate properly.

Some therapists fail to accept the limitations of a modified insight-oriented approach and so apply it inappropriately to modulate the techniques and goals of psychoanalysis. Overemphasis on dreams and fantasies, zealous efforts to use the couch, indiscriminate deep interpretations, and continual focus on the analysis of transference may have less to do with the patient's needs than with those of a therapist who is unwilling or unable to be flexible.

Ms. B, an intelligent and verbal 34-year-old divorced woman, presented with complaints of being unappreciated at work. Always angry and irritable, she considered quitting her job and even leaving the city. Her social life was also being negatively affected; her boyfriend had threatened to leave her because of her extremely hostile, clinging behavior (the same reason her ex-husband had given when he left her 9 years earlier after only 16 months of marriage).

Her past included promiscuity and experimentation with various drugs, and, currently, she indulged in heavy drinking on weekends and occasionally smoked marijuana. She had held many jobs and had lived in various cities. The eldest of three children of a middle-class family, she came from an unhappy and unstable home: her brother had been in and out of psychiatric hospitals; her sister had left home at the age of 16 after becoming pregnant and being forced to marry; and her overly controlling parents had subjected their children to psychological (and occasionally physical) abuse, alternating between heated arguments and passionate reconciliations.

Initially, Ms. B attempted to contain her rage in treatment, but it frequently surfaced and alternated with child-like helplessness; she interrogated the psychiatrist regarding his credentials, ridiculed psychodynamic concepts, constantly challenged statements, and would demand practical advice but then denigrate or fail to follow the guidance given. The psychiatrist remained unprovoked by her aggression and explored with her the need to engage him negatively. Her response was to question and test his continued concern.

When her boyfriend finally left her, she attempted suicide (she cut her wrists superficially), was briefly hospitalized, and, on discharge, was placed on selective serotonin reuptake inhibitors (SSRIs) for 6 months for her minor, but protracted depression. The psychiatrist maintained their regular frequency of sessions despite her greater demands. Although she was puzzled by the steadiness of his interest, she gradually felt safe enough to express her vulnerabilities. As they explored her lack of full commitment to work, friends, and therapy, she began to understand the meaning of her anger in terms of the early abusive relationship with her parents and her tendency to bring it into contemporary relationships. With the psychiatrist's encouragement, she also began to seek work and make small strides in relationship-oriented efforts. By the end of her second year of treatment, she had decided to remain in the city, to stay at her place of employment, and to continue therapy. She needed to experience and practice her somewhat fragile new self, which included greater intimacy in relationships, additional mastery of work skills, and a more cohesive sense of self. (Courtesy of T. Byram Karasu, M.D.)

Supportive Psychotherapy

Supportive psychotherapy aims at the creation of a therapeutic relationship as a temporary buttress or bridge for the deficient patient. It has roots in virtually every therapy that recognizes the ameliorative effects of emotional support and a stable, caring atmosphere in the management of patients. As a nonspecific attitude toward mental illness, it predates scientific psychiatry, with foundations in 18th-century moral treatment, whereby for the first time patients were treated with understanding and kindness in a humane interpersonal environment free from mechanical restraints.

Supportive psychotherapy has been the chief form used in the general practice of medicine and rehabilitation, frequently to augment extratherapeutic measures, such as prescriptions of medication to suppress symptoms, rest to remove the patient from excessive stimulation, or hospitalization to provide a structured therapeutic environment, protection, and control of the patient. It can be applied as primary or ancillary treatment. The global perspective of supportive psychotherapy (often part of a combined treatment approach) places major etiological emphasis on external rather than intrapsychic events, particularly on stressful environmental and interpersonal influences on a severely damaged self. Table 35.1-4 outlines supportive psychotherapy.

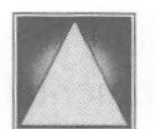

Table 35.1–4
Supportive Psychotherapy

Goal	Support reality testing Provide ego support Maintain or reestablish usual level of functioning
Selection criteria	Very healthy patient faced with overwhelming crises Patient with ego deficits
Duration	Days, months, or years—as needed
Technique	Therapist predictably available Interpretation used to strengthen defenses Therapist maintains working, reality-based relationship based on support, concern, and problem solving Suggestion, reinforcement, advice, reality testing, cognitive restructuring, and reassurance Psychodynamic life narrative Medication

(From Ursano RJ, Silberman EK. Individual psychotherapies. In: Talbott JA, Hales RE, Yudofsky SC, eds. *The American Psychiatric Press Textbook of Psychiatry*. Washington, DC: American Psychiatric Press; 1988:878, with permission.)

Indications and Contraindications. Supportive psychotherapy is generally indicated for those patients for whom classic psychoanalysis or insight-oriented psychoanalytic psychotherapy is typically contraindicated—those who have poor ego strength and whose potential for decompensation is high. Amenable patients fall into the following major areas: (1) individuals in acute crisis or a temporary state of disorganization and inability to cope (including those who might otherwise be well functioning) whose intolerable life circumstances have produced extreme anxiety or sudden turmoil (e.g., individuals going through grief reactions, illness, divorce, job loss, or who were victims of crime, abuse, natural disaster, or accident); (2) patients with chronic severe pathology with fragile or deficient ego functioning (e.g., those with latent psychosis, impulse disorder, or severe character disturbance); (3) patients whose cognitive deficits and physical symptoms make them particularly vulnerable and, thus, unsuitable for an insight-oriented approach (e.g., certain psychosomatic or medically ill persons); (4) individuals who are psychologically unmotivated, although not necessarily characterologically resistant to a depth approach (e.g., patients who come to treatment in response to family or agency pressure and are interested only in immediate relief or those who need assistance in very specific problem areas of social adjustment as a possible prelude to more exploratory work).

Because support forms a tacit part of every therapeutic modality, it is rarely contraindicated as such. The typical attitude regards better-functioning patients as unsuitable not because they will be harmed by a supportive approach, but because they will not be sufficiently benefited by it. In aiming to maximize the patient's potential for further growth and change, supportive therapy tends to be regarded as relatively restricted and superficial and, thus, is not recommended as the treatment of choice if the patient is available for, and capable of, a more in-depth approach.

Goals. The general aim of supportive treatment is the amelioration or relief of symptoms through behavioral or environmental restructuring within the existing psychic framework. This often means helping the patient to adapt better to problems and to live more comfortably with his or her psychopathology. To restore the disorganized, fragile, or decompensated patient to a state of relative equilibrium, the major goal is to suppress or control symptomatology and to stabilize the patient in a protective and reassuring benign atmosphere that militates against overwhelming external and internal pressures. The ultimate goal is to maximize the integrative or adaptive capacities so that the patient increases the ability to cope, while decreasing vulnerability by reinforcing assets and strengthening defenses.

Major Approach and Techniques. Supportive therapy uses several methods, either singly or in combination, including warm, friendly, strong leadership; partial gratification of dependency needs; support in the ultimate development of legitimate independence; help in developing pleasurable activities (e.g., hobbies); adequate rest and diversion; removal of excessive strain, when possible; hospitalization, when indicated; medication to alleviate symptoms; and guidance and advice in dealing with current issues. This therapy uses techniques to help patients feel secure, accepted, protected, encouraged, safe, and not anxious.

Limitations. To the extent that much supportive therapy is spent on practical, everyday realities and on dealing with the external environment of the patient, it may be viewed as more mundane and superficial than depth approaches. Because those patients are seen intermittently and less frequently, the interpersonal commitment may not be as compelling on the part of either the patient or the therapist. Greater severity of illness (and possible psychoses) also makes such treatment potentially more erratic, demanding, and frustrating. The need for the therapist to deal with other family members, caretakers, or agencies (auxiliary treatment, hospitalization) can become an additional complication, because the therapist comes to serve as an ombudsman to negotiate with the outside world of the patient and with other professional peers. Finally, the supportive therapist must be able to accept personal limitations and the patient's limited psychological resources and to tolerate the often unrewarded efforts until small gains are made.

Mr. C, a 50-year-old married man with two sons, the owner of a small construction company, was referred by his internist after recovery from bypass surgery because of frequent, unfounded physical complaints. He was taking minor tranquilizers in increasing doses, not complying with his daily regimen, avoiding sexual contact with his wife, and he had dropped out of group therapy for postsurgical patients after one session.

He came to his first appointment 20 minutes late, after having "forgotten" two previous appointments. He was extremely anxious, often lost in his train of thought, and was semidelusional about his wife and sons, suggesting that they might want to have him locked up. He briefly told his life history, which included his coming from a strict and hard-working but caring middle-class family and the death of his mother when he was only 11 years old. He had joined his father's business (taking over after his father's death 2 years earlier), with both of his sons as associates. Describing himself as successful in work and marriage, he claimed that "the only test I ever failed was the stress test."

Mr. C explained his lack of compliance with diet restrictions as a lack of will and his constant contact with the internist as his having real physical problems not yet diagnosed; he rejected the idea of addiction to tranquilizers, insisting that he could quit any time. He had no fantasy life, remembered no dreams, made it clear that he had entered treatment on his internist's instruction only, and started each session by stating that he had nothing to talk about.

After suggesting that Mr. C was coming to sessions just to pass the "sanity test" and that there was no reason to have him locked up, the psychiatrist encouraged the patient to join him in figuring out the real reasons for his anxiety. Initial sessions were devoted to discussing the patient's medical condition and providing factual information about heart and bypass surgery. The therapist likened the patient's condition to that of an older house getting new plumbing, trying to allay his unrealistic fears of impending death. As Mr. C's anxiety declined, he became less defensive and more psychologically accessible. As the therapist began to explore his difficulty in accepting help, Mr. C was able to talk about his inability to admit problems (i.e., weaknesses). The therapist's explicit recognition of the patient's strength in admitting his weaknesses encouraged the patient to reveal more about himself—how he had welcomed his father's death and his belief that perhaps his illness was punishment. The psychiatrist also encouraged him to speak about his unrealistic guilt and, at the same time, helped him recognize his suspicion of his sons as the reflection of his own wishes concerning his father and his lack of commitment to his medical regimen as a wish to die so as to expiate guilt. After steady urging by the therapist, Mr. C returned to work. He agreed to meet monthly with the psychiatrist and to taper off his use of tranquilizers. He even agreed that he might see the psychiatrist for "deep analysis" in the future because his wife now jokingly complained of his obsessive dieting, his uncompromising exercise regimens, and his regularly scheduled sexual activities. (Courtesy of T. Byram Karasu, M.D.)

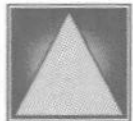

Table 35.1–5
Indications for Expressive or Supportive Emphasis in Psychotherapy

Insight-Oriented (Expressive)	Supportive
Strong motivation to understand	Significant ego defects of a long-term nature
Significant suffering	Severe life crisis
Ability to regress in the service of the ego	
Tolerance for frustration	Poor frustration tolerance
Capacity for insight (psychological-mindedness)	Lack of psychological-mindedness
Intact reality testing	Poor reality testing
Meaningful object relations	Severely impaired object relations
Good impulse control	Poor impulse control
Ability to sustain work	Low intelligence
Capacity to think in terms of analogy and metaphor	Little capacity for self-observation
Reflective responses to trial interpretations	Organically based cognitive dysfunction
	Tenuous ability to form a therapeutic alliance

(From Gabbard GO. *Psychodynamic Psychotherapy in Clinical Practice.* 3rd ed. Washington, DC: American Psychiatric Press; 2000:108, with permission.)

CORRECTIVE EMOTIONAL EXPERIENCE. The relationship between therapist and patient gives a therapist an opportunity to display behavior different from the destructive or unproductive behavior of a patient's parent. At times, such experiences seem to neutralize or reverse some effects of the parents' mistakes. If the patient had overly authoritarian parents, the therapist's friendly, flexible, nonjudgmental, nonauthoritarian—but at times firm and limit setting—attitude gives the patient an opportunity to adjust to, be led by, and identify with, a new parent figure. Franz Alexander described this process as a corrective emotional experience. It draws on elements of both psychoanalysis and psychoanalytic psychotherapy.

Table 35.1-5 summarizes indications for insight-oriented (expressive) therapy versus supportive therapy.

References

Buckley P. Revolution and evolution: A brief intellectual history of American psychoanalysis during the past two decades. *Am J Psychother*. 2003;57:1–17.

Canestri J. Some reflections on the use and meaning of conflict in contemporary psychoanalysis. *Psychoanal Q*. 2005;74(1):295–326.

Dasgupta C. The lure of the norm and the challenge of children. In: King L, Randall R, eds. *The Future of Psychoanalytic Psychotherapy*. Philadelphia: Whurr Publishers, Ltd., 2003:130–142.

Furlong A. Confidentiality with respect to third parties: A psychoanalytic view. *Int J Psychoanal*. 2005;86(2):375–394.

Joannidis C. Psychoanalysis and psychoanalytic psychotherapy. *Psychoanalytic Psychotherapy*. 2006;20(1):30–39.

Kandel ER. *Psychiatry, Psychoanalysis, and the New Biology of Mind*. Washington, DC: American Psychiatric Publishing; 2005.

Karasu TB. Psychoanalysis and psychoanalytic psychotherapy. In: Sadock BJ, Sadock VA, eds. *Kaplan & Sadock's Comprehensive Textbook of Psychiatry*. 8th ed. Vol. 2. Baltimore: Lippincott Williams & Wilkins; 2005: 2472.

Karasu TB. *The Art of Serenity*. New York: Simon and Schuster; 2003.

McWilliams N. *Psychoanalytic Psychotherapy: A Practitioner's Guide*. New York: Guilford Press; 2004.

Person ES, Cooper AM, Gabbard GO, eds. *The American Psychiatric Publishing Textbook of Psychoanalysis*. Washington, DC: American Psychiatric Publishing; 2005.

Shulman DG. The analyst's equilibrium, countertransferential management, and the action of psychoanalysis. *Psychoanal Rev*. 2005;92(3):469–478.

Siegel E. Psychoanalysis as a traditional form of knowledge: An inquiry into the methods of psychoanalysis. *International Journal of Applied Psychoanalytic Studies*. 2006;2(2):146–163.

Strenger C. *The Designed Self: Psychoanalysis and Contemporary Identities*. Hillsdale, NJ: The Analytic Press Inc.; 2005.

Varvin S. Which patients should avoid psychoanalysis, and which professionals should avoid psychoanalytic training? A critical evaluation. *Scandinavian Psychoanalytic Review*. 2003;26:109–122.

▲ 35.2 Brief Psychodynamic Psychotherapy

Brief psychodynamic psychotherapy is a time-limited treatment (10 to 12 sessions) that is based on psychoanalysis and psychodynamic theory. It is used to help persons with depression, anxiety, and posttraumatic stress disorder, among others. There are several methods, each having its own treatment technique and specific criteria for selecting patients; however, they are more similar than different. Brief psychodynamic psychotherapy has gained widespread popularity, partly because of the great pressure on health care professionals to contain treatment costs. It is also easier to evaluate treatment efficacy by comparing groups of persons who have had short-term therapy for mental illness with control groups than it is to measure the results of long-term psychotherapy. Thus, short-term therapies have been the subject of much research, especially on outcome measures, which have found them to be effective. Other short-term methods include interpersonal therapy discussed in Section 35.11 and cognitive behavioral therapy discussed in Section 35.9.

In 1946, Franz Alexander and Thomas French identified the basic characteristics of brief psychodynamic psychotherapy. They described a therapeutic experience designed to put patients at ease, to manipulate the transference, and to use trial interpretations flexibly. Alexander and French conceived psychotherapy as a corrective emotional experience capable of repairing traumatic events of the past and convincing patients that new ways of thinking, feeling, and behaving are possible. At about the same time, Eric Lindemann established a consultation service at the Massachusetts General Hospital in Boston for persons experiencing a crisis. He developed new treatment methods to deal with these situations and eventually applied these techniques to persons who were not in crisis, but who were experiencing various kinds of emotional distress. Since then, the field has been influenced by many workers such as David Malan in England, Peter Sifneos in the United States, and Habib Davanloo in Canada.

TYPES

Brief Focal Psychotherapy (Tavistock–Malan)

Brief focal psychotherapy was originally developed in the 1950s by the Balint team at the Tavistock Clinic in London. Malan, a member of the team, reported the results of the therapy. Malan's selection criteria for treatment included eliminating absolute contraindications, rejecting patients for whom certain dangers seemed inevitable, clearly assessing patients' psychopathology, and determining patients' capacities to consider problems in emotional terms, face disturbing material, respond to interpretations, and endure the stress of the treatment. Malan found that high motivation invariably correlated with a successful outcome. Contraindications to treatment were serious suicide attempts, substance dependence, chronic alcohol abuse, incapacitating chronic obsessional symptoms, incapacitating chronic phobic symptoms, and gross destructive or self-destructive acting out.

Requirements and Techniques. In Malan's routine, therapists should identify the transference early and interpret it and the negative transference. They should then link the transferences to patients' relationships to their parents. Both patients and therapists should be willing to become deeply involved and to bear the ensuing tension. Therapists should formulate a circumscribed focus and set a termination date in advance, and patients should work through grief and anger about termination. An experienced therapist should allow about 20 sessions as an average length for the therapy; a trainee should allow about 30 sessions. Malan himself did not exceed 40 interviews with his patients. Tables 35.2-1 and 35.2-2 summarize Malan's techniques and exclusion criteria.

Time-Limited Psychotherapy (Boston University–Mann)

A psychotherapeutic model of exactly 12 interviews focusing on a specified central issue was developed at Boston University by James Mann and his colleagues in the early 1970s. In

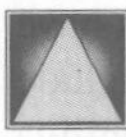

Table 35.2–1
Malan and the Tavistock Group: Brief Focal Psychotherapy

Goal	Clarify the nature of the defense, the anxiety, and the impulse
	Link the present, the past, and the transference
Selection criteria	Patient able to think in feeling terms
	High motivation
	Good response to trial interpretation
Duration	Up to one year
	Mean, 20 sessions
Focus	Internal conflict present since childhood
Termination	Set definite date at beginning of treatment

(From Ursano RJ, Silberman EK. Individual psychotherapies. In: Talbott JA, Hales RE, Yudofsky SC, eds. *The American Psychiatric Press Textbook of Psychiatry.* Washington, DC: American Psychiatric Press; 1988:861, with permission.)

contrast with Malan's emphasis on clear-cut selection and rejection criteria, Mann has not been as explicit about the appropriate candidates for time-limited psychotherapy. Mann considered the major emphases of his theory to be determining a patient's central conflict reasonably correctly and exploring young persons' maturational crises with many psychological and somatic complaints. Mann's exceptions, similar to his rejection criteria, include persons with major depressive disorder that interferes with the treatment agreement, those with acute psychotic states, and desperate patients who need, but cannot tolerate, object relations.

Requirements and Techniques. Mann's technical requirements included strict limitation to 12 sessions, positive transference predominating early, specification and strict adherence to a central issue involving transference, positive identification, making separation a maturational event for patients, absolute prospect of termination to avoid development of dependence, clarification of present and past experiences and resistances, active therapists who support and encourage patients, and education of patients through direct information, reeducation, and manipulation. The conflicts likely to be encountered included independence versus dependence, activity versus passivity, unresolved or delayed grief, and adequate versus inadequate self-esteem. Table 35.2-3 summarizes the features of Mann's time-limited psychotherapy.

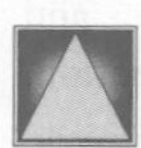

Table 35.2–2
Malan and the Tavistock Group's Exclusion Criteria for Brief Focal Psychotherapy

1. Patient is unavailable to therapeutic contact.
2. Therapist anticipates that prolonged work will be needed to
   - generate motivation
   - penetrate rigid defenses
   - deal with complex or deep-seated issues
   - resolve unfavorable, intense transference, dependent or other, that may develop
3. Depressive or psychotic disturbance may intensify

(From Ursano RJ, Silberman EK. Individual psychotherapies. In: Talbott JA, Hales RE, Yudofsky SC, eds. *The American Psychiatric Press Textbook of Psychiatry.* Washington, DC: American Psychiatric Press; 1988:861, with permission.)

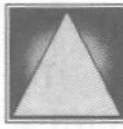

Table 35.2–3
Mann: Time-Limited Psychotherapy

Goal	Resolution of the present and chronically endured pain and the patient's negative self-image
Selection criteria	High ego strength
	Able to engage and disengage
	Therapist quickly able to identify a central issue
	Excludes major depressive disorder, acute psychosis, and borderline personality disorder
Duration	12 treatment hours
Focus	Present and chronically endured pain
	Particular image of the self
Termination	Specific last session set at beginning of treatment
	Termination a major focus of the therapy work

(From Ursano RJ, Silberman EK. Individual psychotherapies. In: Talbott JA, Hales RE, Yudofsky SC, eds. *The American Psychiatric Press Textbook of Psychiatry.* Washington, DC: American Psychiatric Press; 1988:864, with permission.)

Short-Term Dynamic Psychotherapy (McGill University–Davanloo)

As conducted by Davanloo at McGill University, short-term dynamic psychotherapy encompasses nearly all varieties of brief psychotherapy and crisis intervention. Patients treated in Davanloo's series are classified as those whose psychological conflicts are predominantly oedipal, those whose conflicts are not oedipal, and those whose conflicts have more than one focus. Davanloo also devised a specific psychotherapeutic technique for patients with severe, long-standing neurotic problems, specifically those with incapacitating obsessive-compulsive disorders and phobias.

Davanloo's selection criteria emphasize evaluating those ego functions of primary importance to psychotherapeutic work: the establishment of a psychotherapeutic focus; the psychodynamic formulation of the patient's psychological problems; the ability to interact emotionally with evaluators; a history of give-and-take relationships with a significant person in the patient's lives; the patient's ability to experience and tolerate anxiety, guilt, and depression; the patient's motivations for change, psychological-mindness, and ability to respond to interpretation and to link evaluators with persons in the present and past. Both Malan and Davanloo emphasized a patient's responses to interpretation as an important selection and prognostic criterion.

Requirements and Techniques. The highlights of Davanloo's psychotherapeutic approach are flexibility (therapists should adapt the technique to the patient's needs), control, the patient's regressive tendencies, active intervention to avoid having the patient develop overdependence on a therapist, and the patient's intellectual insight and emotional experiences in the transference. These emotional experiences become corrective as a result of the interpretation. Table 35.2-4 summarizes the features of Davanloo's short-term dynamic psychotherapy.

Short–Term Anxiety-Provoking Psychotherapy (Harvard University–Sifneos)

Sifneos developed short-term anxiety-provoking psychotherapy at the Massachusetts General Hospital in Boston during the

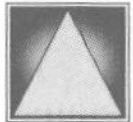

Table 35.2–4
Davanloo: Short-Term Dynamic Psychotherapy

Goal	Resolution of oedipal conflict, loss focus, or multiple foci
Selection criteria	Psychological-mindedness
	At least one past meaningful relationship
	Able to tolerate affect
	Good response to trial transference interpretation
	High motivation
	Flexible defenses
	Lack of projection, splitting, and denial
Duration	5–40 sessions, usually 5–25
	Longer durations for seriously ill
Termination	No specific termination date
	Patient is told that treatment will be short

(From Ursano RJ, Silberman EK. Individual psychotherapies. In: Talbott JA, Hales RE, Yudofsky SC, eds. *The American Psychiatric Press Textbook of Psychiatry.* Washington, DC: American Psychiatric Press; 1988:865, with permission.)

1950s. He used the following criteria for selection: a circumscribed chief complaint (implying a patient's ability to select one of a variety of problems to be given top priority and the patient's desire to resolve the problem in treatment), one meaningful or give-and-take relationship during early childhood, the ability to interact flexibly with an evaluator and to express feelings appropriately, above-average psychological sophistication (implying not only above-average intelligence but also an ability to respond to interpretations), a specific psychodynamic formulation (usually a set of psychological conflicts underlying a patient's difficulties and centering on an oedipal focus), a contract between therapist and patient to work on the specified focus and the formulation of minimal expectations of outcome, and good to excellent motivation for change, not just for symptom relief.

Requirements and Techniques. Treatment can be divided into four major phases: patient–therapist encounter, early therapy, height of treatment, and evidence of change and termination. Therapists use the following techniques during the four phases.

PATIENT–THERAPIST ENCOUNTER. A therapist establishes a working alliance by using the patient's quick rapport with, and positive feelings for, the therapist that appear in this phase. Judicious use of open-ended and forced-choice questions enables the therapist to outline and concentrate on a therapeutic focus. The therapist specifies the minimal expectations of outcome to be achieved by the therapy.

EARLY THERAPY. In transference, feelings for the therapist are clarified as soon as they appear, a technique that leads to the establishment of a true therapeutic alliance.

HEIGHT OF THE TREATMENT. Height of treatment emphasizes active concentration on the oedipal conflicts that have been chosen as the therapeutic focus; repeated use of anxiety-provoking questions and confrontations; avoidance of pregenital characterological issues, which the patient uses defensively to avoid dealing with the therapist's anxiety-provoking techniques; avoidance at all costs of a transference neurosis; repetitive demonstration of the patient's neurotic ways or maladaptive patterns of behavior; concentration on the anxiety-laden material, even before the defense mechanisms have been clarified; repeated demonstrations of parent-transference links by the use of properly timed interpretations based on material given by the patient; establishment of a corrective emotional experience; encouragement and support of the patient, who becomes anxious while struggling to understand the conflicts; new learning and problem-solving patterns; and repeated presentations and recapitulations of the patient's psychodynamics until the defense mechanisms used in dealing with oedipal conflicts are understood.

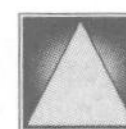

Table 35.2–5
Short-Term Anxiety-Provoking Psychotherapy

Goal	Resolution of oedipal conflict
Selection criteria	Above-average intelligence
	At least one past meaningful relationship
	High motivation
	Specific chief complaint
	Able to interact with evaluator
	Able to express feelings
	Flexible
Duration	A few months
Focus	Oedipal (triangular) conflict
Termination	No specific date given

(From Ursano RJ, Silberman EK. Individual psychotherapies. In: Talbott JA, Hales RE, Yudofsky SC, eds. *The American Psychiatric Press Textbook of Psychiatry.* Washington, DC: American Psychiatric Press; 1988:863, with permission.)

EVIDENCE OF CHANGE AND TERMINATION OF PSYCHOTHERAPY. The final phase of therapy emphasizes the tangible demonstration of change in the patient's behavior outside therapy, evidence that adaptive patterns of behavior are being used, and initiation of talk about terminating the treatment. Table 35.2-5 summarizes features of the Sifneos short-term anxiety-provoking psychotherapy.

Overview and Results

The shared techniques of all the brief psychotherapies described above outdistance their differences. They share the therapeutic alliance or dynamic interaction between therapist and patient, the use of transference, the active interpretation of a therapeutic focus or central issue, the repetitive links between parental and transference issues, and the early termination of therapy.

The outcomes of these brief treatments have been investigated extensively. Contrary to prevailing ideas that the therapeutic factors in psychotherapy are nonspecific, controlled studies and other assessment methods (e.g., interviews with unbiased evaluators, patients' self-evaluations) point to the importance of the specific techniques used. The capacity for genuine recovery in certain patients is far greater than was thought. A certain type of patient receiving brief psychotherapy can benefit greatly from a practical working through of his or her nuclear conflict in the transference. Such patients can be recognized in advance through a process of dynamic interaction, because they are responsive, motivated, and able to face disturbing feelings and because a circumscribed focus can be formulated for them. The more radical the technique in terms of transference, depth of interpretation, and the link to childhood, the more radical the therapeutic effects will be. For some disturbed patients, a carefully chosen partial focus can be therapeutically effective.

References

Abbass A. Five cards to play for major depression: Brief psychotherapy options. *The Canadian Journal for Continuing Medical Education.* 2005.

Beutel ME, Höflich A, Kurth RA, Reimer CH. Who benefits from inpatient short-term psychotherapy in the long run? Patients' evaluations, outpatient after-care and determinants of outcome. *Psychology and Psychotherapy: Theory, Research and Practice*. 2005;78(2):219–234.

Bianchi-DeMicheli F, Zutter AM. Intensive short-term dynamic sex therapy: A proposal. *Journal of Sex & Marital Therapy*. 2005;31(1):57–72.

Book HE. *How to practice Brief Psychodynamic Psychotherapy*. Washington, DC: American Psychological Association; 2003.

Davanloo H. *Basic Principles and Technique of Short Term Dynamic Psychotherapy*. New York: Spectrum; 1978.

Davanloo H. Intensive short-term dynamic psychotherapy. In: Sadock BJ, Sadock VA, eds. *Kaplan & Sadock's Comprehensive Textbook of Psychiatry*. 8th ed. Vol. 2. Baltimore: Lippincott Williams & Wilkins; 2005:2628.

Fonagy P, Roth A, Higgitt A. Psychodynamic psychotherapies: Evidence-based practice and clinical wisdom. *Bull Menninger Clin*. 2005;69(1): 1–58.

Hersoug AG. Assessment of therapists' and patients' personality: Relationship to therapeutic technique and outcome in brief dynamic psychotherapy. *J Pers Assess*. 2004;83(3):191–200.

Leichsenring F, Rabung S, Leibing E. The efficacy of short-term psychodynamic psychotherapy in specific psychiatric disorders: A meta-analysis. *Arch Gen Psychiatry*. 2004;61(12):1208–1216.

McCullough L, Osborn KA. Short term dynamic psychotherapy goes to Hollywood: The treatment of performance anxiety in cinema. *J Clin Psychol*. 2004;60(8):841–852.

Peretz J. Treating affect phobia: A manual for short-term dynamic psychotherapy. *Psychotherapy Research*. 2004;14(2):261–263.

Powers TA, Alonso A. Dynamic psychotherapy and the problem of time. *Journal of Contemporary Psychotherapy*. 2004;34(2):125–139.

Price JL, Hilsenroth MJ, Callahan KL, Petretic-Jackson PA, Bonge D. A pilot study of psychodynamic psychotherapy for adult survivors of childhood sexual abuse. *Clinical Psychology & Psychotherapy*. 2004;11(6):378–391.

Svartberg M, Stiles TC, Seltzer MH. Randomized, controlled trial of the effectiveness of short-term dynamic psychotherapy and cognitive therapy for cluster C personality disorders. *Am J Psychiatry*. 2004;161:810–817.

▲ 35.3 Group Psychotherapy, Combined Individual and Group Psychotherapy, and Psychodrama

A widely accepted psychiatric treatment modality, group psychotherapy uses therapeutic forces within the group, constructive interactions between members, and interventions of a trained leader to change the maladaptive behavior, thoughts, and feelings of emotionally distressed individuals. In an era of increasingly stringent financial constraints, decreasing emphasis on individual psychotherapies, and expanding use of psychopharmacological approaches, more patients have been treated with group psychotherapy than with any other form of verbal therapy. Group therapy is applicable to inpatient and outpatient settings, institutional work, partial hospitalization units, halfway houses, community settings, and private practice. Group psychotherapy is also widely used by those who are not mental health professionals in the adjuvant treatment of physical disorders. The principles of group psychotherapy have also been applied with success in the fields of business and education in the form of training, sensitivity, and role-playing.

Group psychotherapy is a treatment in which carefully selected persons who are emotionally ill meet in a group guided by a trained therapist and help one another effect personality change. By using a variety of technical maneuvers and theoretical constructs, the leader directs group members' interactions to bring about changes.

CLASSIFICATION

Group therapy at present has many approaches. Some clinicians work within a psychoanalytic frame of reference. Others use therapy techniques, such as transactional group therapy, which was devised by Eric Berne and emphasizes the here-and-now interactions among group members; behavioral group therapy, which relies on conditioning techniques based on learning theory; Gestalt group therapy, which was created from the theories of Frederick Perls, enables patients to abreact and express themselves fully; and client-centered group psychotherapy, which was developed by Carl Rogers and is based on the nonjudgmental expression of feelings among group members. Table 35.3-1 outlines the major group psychotherapy approaches.

PATIENT SELECTION

To determine a patient's suitability for group psychotherapy, a therapist needs a great deal of information, which is gathered in a screening interview. The psychiatrist should take a psychiatric history and perform a mental status examination to obtain certain dynamic, behavioral, and diagnostic information. Table 35.3-2 outlines the general criteria for the selection of patients for group therapy.

Authority Anxiety

Those patients whose primary problem is their relationship to authority and who are extremely anxious in the presence of authority figures may do well in group therapy because they are more comfortable in a group and more likely will do better in a group than in a dyadic (one-to-one) setting. Patients with a great deal of authority anxiety may be blocked, anxious, resistant, and unwilling to verbalize thoughts and feelings in an individual setting, generally for fear of the therapist's censure or disapproval. Thus, they may welcome the suggestion of group psychotherapy to avoid the scrutiny of the dyadic situation. Conversely, if a patient reacts negatively to the suggestion of group psychotherapy or openly resists the idea, the therapist should consider the possibility that the patient has high peer anxiety.

Peer Anxiety

Patients with conditions such as borderline and schizoid personality disorders who have destructive relationships with their peer groups or who have been extremely isolated from peer group contact generally react negatively or anxiously when placed in a group setting. When such patients can work through their anxiety, however, group therapy can be beneficial.

Robert entered therapy seeking to understand why he was unable to maintain close or lasting relationships. A handsome and successful businessman, he had made a painful and courageous transition away from self-centered, dysfunctional parents early in his life. Although he made good initial impressions in his jobs, he was always puzzled and disappointed when his superiors gradually lost interest in him and his colleagues avoided him. In one-on-one therapy, he was charming and entertaining, but was easily injured

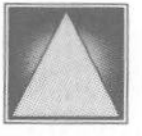

Table 35.3–1
Comparison of Types of Group Psychotherapy

Parameters	Supportive Group Therapy	Analytically Oriented Group Therapy	Psychoanalysis of Groups	Transactional Group Therapy	Behavioral Group Therapy
Frequency	Once a week	One to three times a week	One to five times a week	One to three times a week	One to three times a week
Duration	Up to 6 months	1 to 3+ years	1 to 3+ years	1 to 3 years	Up to 6 months
Primary indications	Psychotic and anxiety disorders	Anxiety disorders, borderline states, personality disorders	Anxiety disorders, personality disorders	Anxiety and psychotic disorders	Phobias, passivity, sexual problems
Individual screening interview	Usually	Always	Always	Usually	Usually
Communication content	Primarily environmental factors	Present and past life situations, intragroup and extragroup relationships	Primarily past life experiences, intragroup relationships	Primarily intragroup relationships; rarely, history; here and now stressed	Specific symptoms without focus on causality
Transference	Positive transference encouraged to promote improved functioning	Positive and negative transference evoked and analyzed	Transference neurosis evoked and analyzed	Positive relationships fostered, negative feelings analyzed	Positive relationships fostered, no examination of transference
Dreams	Not analyzed	Analyzed frequently	Always analyzed and encouraged	Analyzed rarely	Not used
Dependence	Intragroup dependence encouraged; members rely on leader to great extent	Intragroup dependence encouraged; dependence on leader variable	Intragroup dependence not encouraged; dependence on leader variable	Intragroup dependence encouraged; dependence on leader not encouraged	Intragroup dependence not encouraged; reliance on leader is high
Therapist activity	Strengthen existing defenses, active, give advice	Challenge defenses, active, give advice or personal response	Challenge defense, passive, give no advice or personal response	Challenge defenses, active, give personal response, rather than advice	Create new defenses, active and directive
Interpretation	No interpretation of unconcious conflict	Interpretation of unconscious conflict	Interpretation of unconscious conflict extensive	Interpretation of current behavioral patterns in the here and now	Not used
Major group processes	Universalization, reality testing	Cohesion, transference, reality testing	Transference, ventilation, catharsis, reality testing	Abreaction, reality testing	Cohesion, reinforcement, conditioning
Socialization outside of group	Encouraged	Generally discouraged	Discouraged	Variable	Discouraged
Goals	Improved adaptation to environment	Moderate reconstruction of personality dynamics	Extensive reconstruction of personality dynamics	Alteration of behavior through mechanism of conscious control	Relief of specific psychiatric symptoms

by perceived narcissistic slights and would become angry and attacking. Group psychotherapy was suggested when his transference feelings remained intense and therapy was at a seeming impasse. Initially, Robert charmed the group and strove to be the center of attention. Visibly annoyed whenever he felt the group leader was paying more attention to other members, Robert was especially critical and hostile toward older people in the group and displayed little empathy for others. After repeated and forceful confrontations from the group about his antagonistic behavior, he gradually realized that he was repeating childhood patterns in his family of desperately seeking the attention of unloving parents and then entering violent rages when they lost interest. (Courtesy of Normund Wong, M.D.)

Diagnosis

The diagnosis of patients' disorders is important in determining the best therapeutic approach and in evaluating patients' motivations for treatment, capacities for change, and personality structure strengths and weaknesses. Few contraindications exist to group therapy. Antisocial patients generally do poorly in a heterogeneous group setting because they cannot adhere to group standards; but if the group is composed of other antisocial patients, they may respond better to peers than to perceived authority figures. Depressed patients profit from group therapy after they have established a trusting relationship with the therapist. Patients who are actively suicidal or severely depressed should not be treated solely in a group setting. Patients who are

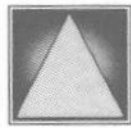

Table 35.3–2
Therapist's Basic Tasks in Group Therapy

1. Decision to establish a therapy group:
   Determine setting and size of the group
   Choose frequency and length of group sessions
   Decide on open versus closed group
   Select a cotherapist for the group
   Formulate policy on group therapy with other therapeutic modalities
2. Act of creating a therapy group:
   Formulate appropriate goals
   Select patients who can perform the group task
   Prepare patients for group therapy
3. Construction and maintenance of a therapeutic environment:
   Build the culture of the group explicitly and implicitly identify and resolve common problems (membership turnover, subgrouping, conflict)

(From Vinogradov S, Yalom ID. Group therapy. In: Talbott JA, Hales RE, Yudofsky SC, eds. *The American Psychiatric Press Textbook of Psychiatry.* Washington, DC: American Psychiatric Press; 1988:964, with permission.)

manic are disruptive but, once under pharmacological control, do well in the group setting. Patients who are delusional and who may incorporate the group into their delusional system should be excluded, as should patients who pose a physical threat to other members because of uncontrollable aggressive outbursts.

PREPARATION

Patients prepared by a therapist for a group experience tend to continue in treatment longer and report less initial anxiety than those who are not prepared. The preparation consists of having a therapist explain the procedure in as much detail as possible and answer the patient's questions before the first session.

STRUCTURAL ORGANIZATION

Table 35.3-2 summarizes some of the critical tasks that a group therapist must face when organizing a group.

Size

Group therapy has been successful with as few as 3 members and as many as 15, but most therapists consider 8 to 10 members the optimal size. Interaction may be insufficient with fewer members unless they are especially verbal, and with more than 10 members, the interaction may be too great for the members or the therapist to follow.

Frequency and Length of Sessions

Most group psychotherapists conduct group sessions once a week. Maintaining continuity in sessions is important. When there are alternate sessions, the group meets twice a week, once with and once without the therapist. Group sessions generally last anywhere from 1 to 2 hours, but the time limit should be constant.

Marathon groups were most popular in the 1970s, but are much less common today. In time-extended therapy (marathon group therapy), the group meets continuously for 12 to 72 hours. Enforced interactional proximity and, during the longest time-extended sessions, sleep deprivation break down certain ego defenses, release affective processes, and theoretically promote open communication. Time-extended sessions, however, can be dangerous for patients with weak ego structures, such as persons with schizophrenia or borderline personality disorder.

Homogeneous versus Heterogeneous Groups

Most therapists believe that groups should be as heterogeneous as possible to ensure maximal interaction. Members with different diagnostic categories and varied behavioral patterns; from all races, social levels, and educational backgrounds; and of varying ages and both sexes should be brought together. Patients between the ages of 20 and 65 years can be included effectively in the same group. Age differences help in developing parent–child and brother–sister models, and patients have the opportunity to relive and rectify interpersonal difficulties that may have appeared insurmountable.

Both children and adolescents are best treated in groups composed mostly of persons in their own age groups. Some adolescent patients are capable of assimilating the material of an adult group, regardless of content, but they should not be deprived of a constructive peer experience that they might otherwise not have.

Open versus Closed Groups

Closed groups have a set number and composition of patients. If members leave, no new members are accepted. In open groups, membership is more fluid, and new members are taken on whenever old members leave.

MECHANISMS

Group Formation

Each patient approaches group therapy differently and, in this sense, groups are microcosms. Patients use typical adaptive abilities, defense mechanisms, and ways of relating, and when these tactics are ultimately reflected back to them by the group, they learn to be introspective about their personality functioning. A process inherent in group formation requires that patients suspend their previous ways of coping. In entering the group, they allow their executive ego functions—reality testing, adaptation to and mastery of the environment, and perception—to be assumed, to some degree, by the collective assessment provided by the total membership, including the leader.

Therapeutic Factors

Table 35.3-3 outlines 20 significant therapeutic factors that account for change in group psychotherapy. Table 35.3-4 summarizes the forces that shape learning and change secondary to the nature of the group as a social microcosm.

ROLE OF THE THERAPIST

Although opinions differ about how active or passive a group therapist should be, the consensus is that the therapist's role

Table 35.3–3
Twenty Therapeutic Factors in Group Psychotherapy

Factor	Definition
Abreaction	A process by which repressed material, particularly a painful experience or conflict, is brought back to consciousness. In the process, the person not only recalls but relives the material, which is accompanied by the appropriate emotional response; insight usually results from the experience.
Acceptance	The feeling of being accepted by other members of the group; differences of opinion are tolerated, and there is an absence of censure.
Altruism	The act of one member helping another; putting another person's need before one's own and learning that there is value in giving to others. The term was originated by Auguste Comte (1798–1857), and Sigmund Freud believed it was a major factor in establishing group cohesion and community feeling.
Catharsis	The expression of ideas, thoughts, and suppressed material that is accompanied by an emotional response that produces a state of relief in the patient.
Cohesion	The sense that the group is working together toward a common goal; also referred to as a sense of "we-ness"; believed to be the most important factor related to positive therapeutic effects.
Consensual validation	Confirmation of reality by comparing one's own conceptualizations with those of other group members; interpersonal distortions are thereby corrected. The term was introduced by Harry Stack Sullivan; Trigant Burrow had used the phrase "consensual observation" to refer to the same phenomenon.
Contagion	The process in which the expression of emotion by one member stimulates the awareness of a similar emotion in another member.
Corrective familial experience	The group re-creates the family of origin for some members who can work through original conflicts psychologically through group interaction (e.g., sibling rivalry, anger toward parents).
Empathy	The capacity of a group member to put himself or herself into the psychological frame of reference of another group member and thereby understand his or her thinking, feeling, or behavior.
Identification	An unconscious defense mechanism in which the person incorporates the characteristics and the qualities of another person or object into his or her ego system.
Imitation	The conscious emulation or modeling of one's behavior after that of another (also called *role modeling*); also known as spectator therapy, as one patient learns from another.
Insight	Conscious awareness and understanding of one's own psychodynamics and symptoms of maladaptive behavior. Most therapists distinguish two types: (1) intellectual insight—knowledge and awareness without any changes in maladaptive behavior; (2) emotional insight—awareness and understanding leading to positive changes in personality and behavior.
Inspiration	The process of imparting a sense of optimism to group members; the ability to recognize that one has the capacity to overcome problem; also known as instillation of hope.
Interaction	The free and open exchange of ideas and feelings among group members; effective interaction is emotionally charged.
Interpretation	The process during which the group leader formulates the meaning or significance of a patient's resistance, defenses, and symbols; the result is that the patient has a cognitive framework within which to understand his or her behavior.
Learning	Patients acquire knowledge about new areas, such as social skills and sexual behavior; they receive advice, obtain guidance, and attempt to influence and are influenced by other group members.
Reality testing	Ability of the person to evaluate objectively the world outside the self; includes the capacity to perceive oneself and other group members accurately. *See also* Consensual validation.
Transference	Projection of feelings, thoughts, and wishes onto the therapist, who has come to represent an object from the patient's past. Such reactions, while perhaps appropriate for the condition prevaling in the patient's earlier life, are inappropriate and anachronistic when applied to the therapist in the present. Patients in the group may also direct such feelings toward one another, a process called *multiple transferences*.
Universalization	The awareness of the patient that he or she is not alone in having problems; others share similar complaints or difficulties in learning; the patient is not unique.
Ventilation	The expression of suppressed feelings, ideas, or events to other group members; the sharing of personal secrets that ameliorate a sense of sin or guilt (also referred to as *self-disclosure*).

is primarily facilitative. Ideally, the group members themselves are the primary source of cure and change. The climate produced by the therapist's personality is a potent agent of change. The therapist is more than an expert applying techniques; he or she exerts a personal influence that taps such variables as empathy, warmth, and respect.

INPATIENT GROUP PSYCHOTHERAPY

Group therapy is an important part of hospitalized patients' therapeutic experiences. Groups can be organized in many ways on a ward. In a community meeting, an entire inpatient unit meets with all the staff members (e.g., psychiatrists, psychologists, and nurses). In team meetings, 15 to 20 patients and staff members meet; a regular or small group composed of 8 to 10 patients may meet with 1 or 2 therapists, as in traditional group therapy. Although the goals of each group vary, they all have common purposes: to increase patients' awareness of themselves through their interactions with the other group members, who provide feedback about their behavior; to provide patients with improved interpersonal and social skills; to help the members adapt to an inpatient setting; and to improve communication between patients and staff. In addition, one type of group meeting is attended only by inpatient hospital staff and is meant to improve communication among the staff members and to provide mutual support and encouragement in their day-to-day work with patients. Community meetings and team meetings are more helpful for dealing with patient treatment problems than they are for

Table 35.3–4
Learning from Behavioral Patterns in the Social Microcosm of the Therapy Group

Display of interpersonal pathology
↓
Feedback and self-observation
↓
Sharing reactions
↓
Examining the results of sharing reactions
↓
Understanding one's opinion of self
↓
Developing a sense of responsibility
↓
Realizing one's power to effect change
↓
High affect potentiates change

(From Vinogradov S, Yalom ID. Group therapy. In: Talbott JA, Hales RE, Yudofsky SC, eds. *The American Psychiatric Press Textbook of Psychiatry*. Washington, DC: American Psychiatric Press; 1988:982, with permission.)

providing insight-oriented therapy, which is the province of the small-group therapy meeting.

Group Composition

Two key factors of inpatient groups common to all short-term therapies are the heterogeneity of the members and the rapid turnover of patients. Outside the hospital, therapists have large caseloads from which to select patients for group therapy. On the ward, therapists have a limited number of patients to choose from and are further restricted to those patients who are both willing to participate and suitable for a small-group experience. In certain settings, group participation may be mandatory (e.g., in substance abuse and alcohol dependence units), but mandatory attendance does not usually apply in a general psychiatry unit. In fact, most group experiences are more productive when the patients themselves choose to enter them.

More sessions are preferable to fewer. During patients' hospital stays, groups may meet daily to allow interactional continuity and the carryover of themes from one session to the next. A new member of a group can be brought up to date quickly, either by the therapist in an orientation meeting or by one of the members. A newly admitted patient has often learned many details about the small-group program from another patient before actually attending the first session. The less frequently the group sessions are held, the greater the need for a therapist to structure the group and be active in it.

Inpatient versus Outpatient Groups

Although the therapeutic factors that account for change in small inpatient groups are similar to those in the outpatient settings, there are qualitative differences. For example, the relatively high turnover of patients in inpatient groups complicates the process of cohesion. But the fact that all the group members are together in the hospital aids cohesion, as do the therapists' efforts to foster the process. Sharing of information, universalization, and catharsis are the main therapeutic factors at work in inpatient groups. Although insight more likely occurs in outpatient groups because of their long-term nature, some patients can obtain a new understanding of their psychological makeup within the confines of a single group session. A unique quality of inpatient groups is the patients' extragroup contacts, which are extensive because they live together on the same ward. Verbalizing their thoughts and feelings about such contacts in the therapy sessions encourages interpersonal learning. In addition, conflicts between patients or between patients and staff members can be anticipated and resolved.

Twelve former psychiatric inpatients who attended the monthly medication clinic would meet for 1 hour before their individual appointments with the psychiatrist to review their current social situation and medications. All had been treated by the same ward doctor and had known one another while on the inpatient service. The psychiatrist who performed the medication reviews also served as the group leader. Periodically, he was assisted by a staff member who was also familiar with the patients. Coffee was available, and the patients often brought pastries from home. The patients socialized with each other during the hour and frequently exchanged helpful ideas and tips about job opportunities. Those without cars shared rides with other members. The group was open ended and well attended. Most of the patients were single and had a long history of psychotic illness. For most, this meeting was their only opportunity to socialize and be among peers. Frequently, on learning that a member had been rehospitalized, many in the group would visit their colleague on the ward. (Courtesy of Normund Wong, M.D.)

SELF-HELP GROUPS

Self-help groups are composed of persons who are trying to cope with a specific problem or life crisis and are usually organized with a particular task in mind. Such groups do not attempt to explore individual psychodynamics in great depth or to change personality functioning significantly, but self-help groups have improved the emotional health and well-being of many persons.

A distinguishing characteristic of the self-help groups is their homogeneity. The members have the same disorders and share their experiences—good and bad, successful and unsuccessful—with one another. By so doing, they educate each other, provide mutual support, and alleviate the sense of alienation usually felt by persons drawn to this kind of group.

Self-help groups emphasize cohesion, which is exceptionally strong in these groups. Because the group members have similar problems and symptoms, they develop a strong emotional bond. Each group may have its unique characteristics, to which the members can attribute magical qualities of healing. Examples of self-help groups are Alcoholics Anonymous (AA), Gamblers Anonymous (GA), and Overeaters Anonymous (OA).

The self-help group movement is presently in ascendancy. These groups meet their members' needs by providing acceptance, mutual support, and help in overcoming maladaptive patterns of behavior or states of feeling that traditional mental health and medical professionals have not generally dealt with successfully. Self-help groups and therapy groups have begun to converge. Self-help groups have enabled their members to give up patterns of unwanted behavior; therapy groups have helped their members understand why and how they got to be the way they were or are.

COMBINED INDIVIDUAL AND GROUP PSYCHOTHERAPY

In combined individual and group psychotherapy, patients see a therapist individually and also take part in group sessions. The therapist for the group and individual sessions is usually the same person. Groups can vary in size from 3 to 15 members, but the most helpful size is 8 to 10. Patients must attend all group sessions. Attendance at individual sessions is also important, and failure to attend either group or individual sessions should be examined as part of the therapeutic process.

Combined therapy is a particular treatment modality, not a system by which individual therapy is augmented by an occasional group session or a group therapy in which a participant meets alone with a therapist from time to time. Rather, it is an ongoing plan in which meaningful integration of the group experience with the individual sessions yields reciprocal feedback to help form an integrated therapeutic experience. Although the one-to-one doctor–patient relationship makes a deep examination of the transference reaction possible for some patients, it may not provide other patients with the corrective emotional experiences necessary for therapeutic change. The group gives patients a variety of persons with whom they can have transferential reactions. In the microcosm of the group, patients can relive and work through familial and other important influences.

Techniques

Differing techniques based on varying theoretical frameworks have been used in the combined therapy format. Some clinicians increase the frequency of individual sessions to encourage the emergence of the transference neurosis. In the behavioral model, individual sessions are scheduled regularly, but they tend to be less frequent than in other approaches. Whether patients use a couch or a chair during individual sessions depends on a therapist's orientation. Techniques such as alternate meetings or "after-sessions" without the therapist present may be used. A combined therapy approach called *structured interactional group psychotherapy* has a different group member as the focus of each weekly group session who is discussed in depth by the other members.

Results

Most workers in the field believe that combined therapy has the advantages of both dyadic and group settings, without sacrificing the qualities of either. Generally, the dropout rate in combined therapy is lower than that in group therapy alone. In many cases, combined therapy appears to bring problems to the surface and to resolve them more quickly than might be possible with either method alone.

PSYCHODRAMA

Psychodrama is a method of group psychotherapy originated by the Viennese-born psychiatrist Jacob Moreno in which personality makeup, interpersonal relationships, conflicts, and emotional problems are explored by means of special dramatic methods. Therapeutic dramatization of emotional problems includes the protagonist or patient, the person who acts out problems with the help of auxiliary egos, persons who enact varying aspects of the patient, and the director, psychodramatist, or therapist, the person who guides those in the drama toward the acquisition of insight.

Roles

Director. The director is the leader or therapist and so must be an active participant. He or she has a catalytic function by encouraging the members of the group to be spontaneous. The director must also be available to meet the group's needs without superimposing his or her values. Of all the group psychotherapies, psychodrama requires the most participation from the therapist.

Protagonist. The protagonist is the patient in conflict. The patient chooses the situation to portray in the dramatic scene, or the therapist chooses it if the patient so desires.

Auxiliary Ego. An auxiliary ego is another group member who represents something or someone in the protagonist's experience. The auxiliary egos help account for the great range of therapeutic effects available in psychodrama.

Group. The members of the psychodrama and the audience make up the group. Some are participants, and others are observers, but all benefit from the experience to the extent that they can identify with the ongoing events. The concept of spontaneity in psychodrama refers to the ability of each member of the group, especially the protagonist, to experience the thoughts and feelings of the moment and to communicate emotion as authentically as possible.

Techniques

The psychodrama can focus on any special area of functioning (a dream, a family, or a community situation), a symbolic role, an unconscious attitude, or an imagined future situation. Such symptoms as delusions and hallucinations can also be acted out in the group. Techniques to advance the therapeutic process and to increase productivity and creativity include the soliloquy (a recital of overt and hidden thoughts and feelings), role reversal (the exchange of the patient's role for the role of a significant person), the double (an auxiliary ego acting as the patient), the multiple double (several egos acting as the patient did on varying occasions), and the mirror technique (an ego imitating the patient and speaking for him or her). Other techniques include the use of hypnosis and psychoactive drugs to modify the acting behavior in various ways.

ETHICAL AND LEGAL ISSUES

Confidentiality

Except where disclosure is required by law, the group therapist legally and ethically gives information about the group members to others only after obtaining appropriate patient consent. The therapist is obligated to take appropriate steps to be responsible to society, as well as to patients, when patients pose a danger to themselves or to others. The guidelines for ethics of the American Group Psychotherapy Association state that therapists must obtain specific permission to confer with the referring therapist or with the individual therapist when the patient is in conjoint therapy.

Although the group members, as well as the therapist, should protect the identity of the members and maintain confidentiality, the group members are not legally bound to do so. During the preparation of patients for group psychotherapy, therapists should routinely instruct the prospective members to keep all material discussed in the group confidential. Theoretically, in a legal case, one member of a group can be asked to testify against another, but such a situation has not yet occurred.

A therapist must exercise clinical judgment and caution in placing a patient in a group if he or she thinks that the burdens of maintaining secrets will be too great for some potential members or if a prospective group patient harbors a secret of such magnitude or notoriety that membership in a group would not be wise.

Violence and Aggression

Although reports of violence and aggression are rare, the potential exists that a group member may physically attack another patient or a therapist. The attack may occur within the group or outside the group. The likelihood of such an event can be diminished through the careful selection of group members. Patients with a demonstrated history of assaultive behavior and psychotic patients who pose a potential for violence should not be placed in a group. In institutional settings, in which group therapy is commonly practiced, sufficient safeguards must be in place to discourage any physical danger to others—for example, guards or attendants can act as observers.

Sexual Behavior

For therapists, sexual intercourse with a patient or a former patient is unethical; in many states, such behavior is considered a criminal act. The issue is complicated in group psychotherapy, however, because members may engage in sexual activities with one another. The issues of pregnancy, rape, and the transmission of acquired immunodeficiency syndrome (AIDS) by group members are open questions. If a patient is injured as a result of sexual activity by group members, the therapist could be held accountable for not preventing such behavior. The therapist should advise prospective group members that each patient is responsible for reporting any sexual contact between members. The therapist cannot anticipate every group sexual encounter or prevent sexual relationships from developing, but he or she is obligated to provide patients with guidelines of acceptable behavior. The therapist should identify sexual, vulnerable, or exploitive patients in the selection and preparation of patients for the group. Sociopathic patients who sexually exploit others should be informed that such behavior is explicitly not acceptable in the group and that such behavior should be verbalized rather than acted out. The group must be conducted in such a way that the therapist does not encourage or tacitly allow sexual activity. Patients with AIDS are encouraged to reveal that they harbor the virus. To protect members if sexual relationships occur, some therapists do not accept patients with AIDS into a group unless they agree to reveal their condition. In those situations, the therapist discusses the issue of AIDS with the patient and the group into which the patient is to be placed.

References

Billow RM. Bonding in group: The therapist's contribution. *Int J Group Psychother*. 2003;53:83.

Burlingame GM, Fuhriman A, Mosier J. The differential effectiveness of group psychotherapy: A meta-analytic perspective. *Group Dynamics*. 2003;7:3.

Higaki Y, Ueda S, Hatton H, Arikawa J, Kawamoto K, Kamo T, Kawasima M. The effects of group psychotherapy in the quality of life of adult patients with atopic dermatitis. *J Psychosom Res*. 2003;55:162.

Ogrodniczuk JS, Piper WE, Joyce AS. Treatment compliance in different types of group psychotherapy: Exploring the effect of age. *J Nerv Ment Dis*. 2006;194(4):287–293.

Paparella LR. Group psychotherapy and Parkinson's disease: When members and therapist share the diagnosis. *Int J Group Psychother*. 2004;54(3):401–409.

Segalla R. Selfish and unselfish behavior: Scene stealing and scene sharing in group psychotherapy. *Int J Group Psychother*. 2006;56(1):33–46.

Scheidlinger S. Group psychotherapy and related helping groups today: An overview. *Am J Psychother*. 2004;58(3):265–280.

Tyminski R. Long-term group psychotherapy for children with pervasive developmental disorders: Evidence for group development. *Int J Group Psychother*. 2005;55(2):189–210.

Wong N. Group psychotherapy and combined individual and group psychotherapy. In: Sadock BJ, Sadock VA, eds. *Kaplan & Sadock's Comprehensive Textbook of Psychiatry*. 8th ed. Vol. 2. Baltimore: Lippincott Williams & Wilkins; 2005:2568.

Zoger S, Suedland J, Holgers K. Benefits from group psychotherapy in treatment of severe refractory tinnitus. *J Psychosom Res*. 2003;55:134.

▲ 35.4 Family Therapy and Couples Therapy

FAMILY THERAPY

Family therapy can be defined as any psychotherapeutic endeavor that explicitly focuses on altering the interactions between or among family members and seeks to improve the functioning of the family as a unit, or its subsystems, and/or the functioning of individual members of the family. Both family and couple therapy aim at some change in relational functioning. In most cases, they also aim at some other change, typically in the functioning of specific individuals in the family. Family therapy meant to heal a rift between parents and their adult children is an example of the use of family therapy centered on relationship goals. Family therapy aimed at increasing the family's coping with schizophrenia and at reducing the family's expressed emotion is an example of family therapy aimed at individual goals (in this case, the functioning of the person with schizophrenia), as well as family goals. In the early years of family therapy, change in the family system was seen as being sufficient to produce individual change. More recent treatments aimed at change in individuals, as well as in the family system, tend to supplement the interventions that focus on interpersonal relationships with specific strategies that focus on individual behavior.

Indications

The presence of a relational difficulty is a clear indication for family and couple therapy. Couple and family therapies are the only treatments that have been shown to be efficacious for such problems as marital maladjustment, and other methods, such as individual therapy, have been shown to often have deleterious effects in these situations. Couple and family therapy has also been demonstrated to have a clear and important role in the treatment of numerous specific psychiatric disorders, often as a component within a multimethod treatment.

Of course, as with any therapy, the indications for family and couple therapy are broad and vary from case to case. Family therapy is a therapeutic collage of ideas regarding the underpinnings of family and individual stability and change, psychopathology, and problems in living, as well as relational ethics. Family therapy might better be called *systemically sensitive therapy* and, in this sense, reflects a basic worldview as much as a clinical treatment methodology. For therapists thus inclined, then, all clinical problems involve salient interactional components; thus, some kind of family (or other functionally significant others') involvement in therapy is always called for, even in treatment that emphasizes individual problems.

An impressive array now exists of common clinical disorders and problems, including child, adolescent, and adult disorders, for which research has demonstrated family or couple treatment methods to be effective. In a few instances, couple and family interventions are probably even the treatment of choice, and for several disorders, the research argues for family intervention to be an essential part of treatment.

Techniques

Initial Consultation. Family therapy is familiar enough to the general public for families with a high level of conflict to request it specifically. When the initial complaint is about an individual family member, however, pretreatment work may be needed. Underlying resistance to a family approach typically includes fears by parents that they will be blamed for their child's difficulties, that the entire family will be pronounced sick, that a spouse will object, and that open discussion of one child's misbehavior will have a negative influence on siblings. Refusal by an adolescent or young adult patient to participate in family therapy is frequently a disguised collusion with the fears of one or both parents.

Interview Technique. The special quality of a family interview springs from two important facts. A family comes to treatment with its history and dynamics firmly in place. To a family therapist, the established nature of the group, more than the symptoms, constitutes the clinical problem. Family members usually live together and, at some level, depend on one another for their physical and emotional well-being. Whatever transpires in the therapy session is known to all. Central principles of technique also derive from these facts. For example, the therapist must carefully channel the catharsis of anger by one family member toward another. The person who is the object of the anger will react to the attack, and the anger may escalate into violence and fracture relationships, with one or more member withdrawing from therapy. For another example, free association is inappropriate in family therapy because it can encourage one person to dominate a session. Thus, therapists must always control and direct the family interview.

Table 35.4-1, "Rationale for Family-Life Chronology," summarizes the principles in which the history of the family is examined in an effort to understand how that history informs the current familial interactions.

Frequency and Length of Treatment. Unless an emergency arises, sessions are usually held no more than once a week. Each session, however, may require as much as 2 hours. Long sessions can include an intermission to give the therapist time to organize the material and plan a response. A flexible schedule is necessary when geography or personal circumstances make it physically difficult for the family to get together. The length of treatment depends both on the nature of the problem and on the therapeutic model. Therapists who use problem-solving models exclusively may accomplish their goals in a few sessions, whereas therapists using growth-oriented models may work with a family for years and may schedule sessions at long intervals. Table 35.4-2 summarizes one model for treatment termination.

Models of Intervention

Many models of family therapy exist, none of which is superior to the others. The particular model used depends on the training received, the context in which therapy occurs, and the personality of the therapist.

Psychodynamic-Experiential Models. Psychodynamic-experiential models emphasize individual maturation in the context of the family system and are free from unconscious patterns of anxiety and projection rooted in the past. Therapists seek to establish an intimate bond with each family member, and sessions alternate between the therapist's exchanges with the members and the members' exchanges with one another. Clarity of communication and honestly admitted feelings are given high priority. Toward this end, family members may be encouraged to change their seats, to touch each other, and to make direct eye contact. Their use of metaphor, body language, and parapraxes helps reveal the unconscious pattern of family relationships. The therapist may also use family sculpting, in which family members physically arrange one another in tableaus depicting their personal view of relationships, past or present. The therapist both interprets the living sculpture and modifies it in a way to suggest new relationships. In addition, the therapist's subjective responses to the family are given great importance. At appropriate moments, the therapist expresses these responses to the family to form yet another feedback loop of self-observation and change.

Bowen Model. Murray Bowen called his model *family systems*, but in the family therapy field it rightfully carries the name of its originator. The hallmark of the Bowen model is persons' differentiation from their family of origin, their ability to be their true selves in the face of familial or other pressures that threaten the loss of love or social position. Problem families are assessed on two levels: the degree of their enmeshment versus the degree of their ability to differentiate and the analysis of emotional triangles in the problem for which they seek help.

An emotional triangle is defined as a three-party system (and many of these can exist within a family) arranged so that the closeness of two members expressed as either love or repetitive conflict tends to exclude a third. When the excluded third person attempts to join with one of the other two or when one of the involved parties shifts in the direction of the excluded one, emotional cross-currents are activated. The therapist's role is, first, to stabilize or shift the "hot" triangle—the one producing the presenting symptoms—and, second, to work with the most psychologically available family members, individually if necessary, to achieve sufficient personal differentiation so that the hot triangle does not recur. To preserve his or her neutrality in the family's triangles, the therapist minimizes emotional contact with family members.

Bowen also originated the genogram, a theoretical tool that is a historical survey of the family, going back several generations.

Structural Model. In a structural model, families are viewed as single, interrelated systems assessed in terms of significant alliances and

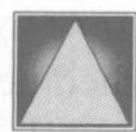

Table 35.4–1
Rationale for Family-Life Chronology

The family therapist enters a session knowing little or nothing about the family.
- The therapist may know who the identified patient is and what symptoms the patient manifests, but that is usually all. So the therapist must get clues about the meaning of the symptom.
- The therapist may know that pain exists in the marital relationship, but needs to get clues about how the pain shows itself.
- The therapist needs to know how the mates have tried to cope with their problems.
- The therapist may know that the mates both operate from models (from what they saw going on between their own parents), but needs to find out how those models have influenced each mate's expectations about how to be a mate and how to be a parent.

The family therapist enters a session knowing that the family, in fact, has had a history, but that is usually all.
- Every family, as a group, has gone through or jointly experienced many events. Certain events (e.g., deaths, childbirth, sickness, geographical moves, and job changes) occur in almost all families.
- Certain events primarily affect the mates and only indirectly the children. (Maybe the children were not born yet or were too young to fully comprehend the nature of an event as it affected their parents. They may have only sensed periods of parental remoteness, distraction, anxiety, or annoyance.)
- The therapist can profit from answers to just about every question asked.

Family members enter therapy with a great deal of fear.
- Therapist structuring helps decrease the threats. It says, "I am in charge of what will happen here. I will see to it that nothing catastrophic happens here."
- All members are covertly feeling to blame that nothing seems to have turned out right (even though they may overtly blame the identified patient or the other mate).
- Parents, especially, need to feel that they did the best they could as parents. They need to tell the therapist, "This is why I did what I did. This is what happened to me."
- A family-life chronology that deals with such facts as names, dates, labeled relationships, and moves, seems to appeal to the family. It asks questions that members can answer, questions that are relatively nonthreatening. It deals with life as the family understands it.

Family members enter therapy with a great deal of despair.

Therapist structuring helps stimulate hope.
- As far as family members are concerned, past events are part of them. They now can tell the therapist, "I existed." And they can also say, "I am not just a big blob of pathology. I succeeded in overcoming many handicaps."
- If the family knew what questions needed asking, they would not need to be in therapy. So the therapist does not say, "Tell me what you want to tell me." Family members will simply tell the therapist what they have been telling themselves for years. The therapist's questions say, "I know what to ask. I take responsibility for understanding you. We are going to go somewhere."

The family therapist also knows that, to some degree, the family has focused on the identified patient to relieve marital pain. The therapist also knows that, to some degree, the family will resist any effort to change that focus. A family-life chronology is an effective, nonthreatening way to change from an emphasis on the "sick" or "bad" family member to an emphasis on the marital relationship.

The family-life chronology serves other useful therapy purposes, such as providing the framework within which a reeducation process can take place. The therapist serves as a model in checking out information or correcting communication techniques and placing questions and eliciting answers to begin the process. In addition, when taking the chronology, the therapist can introduce in a relatively nonfrightening way some of the crucial concepts to induce change.

(Adapted from Satir V. *Conjoint Family Therapy*. Palo Alto, CA: Science and Behavior; 1967:57, with permission.)

splits among family members, hierarchy of power (parents in charge of children), clarity and firmness of boundaries between the generations, and family tolerance for each other. The structural model uses concurrent individual and family therapy.

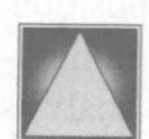

Table 35.4–2
Criteria for Treatment Termination

Treatment is completed:
- When family members can complete transactions, check, ask
- When they can interpret hostility
- When they can see how others see them
- When they can see how they see themselves
- When one member can tell others how they manifest themselves
- When one member can tell others what is hoped, feared, and expected from them
- When they can disagree
- When they can make choices
- When they can learn through practice
- When they can free themselves from the harmful effects of past models
- When they can give clear message—that is, be congruent in their behavior—with a minimum of difference between feelings and communication and with a minimum of hidden messages.

(Adapted from Satir V. *Conjoint Family Therapy*. Palo Alto, CA: Science and Behavior; 1967:133, with permission.)

General Systems Model. Based on general systems theory, a general systems model holds that families are systems and that every action in a family produces a reaction in one or more of its members. Families have external boundaries and internal rules. Every member is presumed to play a role (e.g., spokesperson, persecutor, victim, rescuer, symptom bearer, nurturer), which is relatively stable, but which member fills each role may change. Some families try to scapegoat one member by blaming him or her for the family's problems (the identified patient). If the identified patient improves, another family member may become the scapegoat. The general systems model overlaps with some of the other models presented, particularly the Bowen and structural models.

Modifications of Techniques

Family Group Therapy. Family group therapy combines several families into a single group. Families share mutual problems and compare their interactions with those of the other families in the group. Treatment of schizophrenia has been effective in multiple family groups. Parents of disturbed children may also meet together to share their situations.

Social Network Therapy. In social network therapy, the social community or network of a disturbed patient meets in group sessions with the patient. The network includes those with whom the patient comes into contact in daily life, not only the immediate family but also relatives, friends, tradespersons, teachers, and coworkers.

Paradoxical Therapy. With the paradoxical therapy approach, which evolved from the work of Gregory Bateson, a therapist suggests that the patient intentionally engage in the unwanted behavior (called the paradoxical injunction) and, for example, avoid a phobic object or perform a compulsive ritual. Although paradoxical therapy and the use of paradoxical injunctions seem to be counterintuitive, the therapy can create new insights for some patients. It is used in individual therapy as well as in family therapy.

Reframing. Reframing, also known as *positive connotation*, is a relabeling of all negatively expressed feelings or behavior as positive. When the therapist attempts to get family members to view behavior from a new frame of reference, "This child is impossible" becomes "This child is desperately trying to distract and protect you from what he or she perceives as an unhappy marriage." Reframing is an important process that allows family members to view themselves in new ways that can produce change.

Goals

Family therapy has several goals: to resolve or reduce pathogenic conflict and anxiety within the matrix of interpersonal relationships; to enhance the perception and fulfillment by family members of one another's emotional needs; to promote appropriate role relationships between the sexes and generations; to strengthen the capacity of individual members and the family as a whole to cope with destructive forces inside and outside the surrounding environment; and to influence family identity and values so that members are oriented toward health and growth. The therapy ultimately aims to integrate families into the large systems of society, extended family, and community groups and social systems, such as schools, medical facilities, and social, recreational, and welfare agencies.

COUPLES (MARITAL) THERAPY

Couples or marital therapy is a form of psychotherapy designed to psychologically modify the interaction of two persons who are in conflict with each other over one parameter or a variety of parameters—social, emotional, sexual, or economic. In couples therapy, a trained person establishes a therapeutic contract with a patient-couple and, through definite types of communication, attempts to alleviate the disturbance, to reverse or change maladaptive patterns of behavior, and to encourage personality growth and development.

Marriage counseling may be considered more limited in scope than marriage therapy: Only a particular familial conflict is discussed, and the counseling is primarily task oriented, geared to solving a specific problem, such as child rearing. Marriage therapy, by contrast, emphasizes restructuring a couple's interaction and sometimes explores the psychodynamics of each partner. Both therapy and counseling stress helping marital partners cope effectively with their problems. Most important is the definition of appropriate and realistic goals, which may involve extensive reconstruction of the union or problem-solving approaches or a combination of both.

Types of Therapies

Individual Therapy. In individual therapy, the partners may consult different therapists, who do not necessarily communicate with each other and indeed may not even know each other. The goal of treatment is to strengthen each partner's adaptive capacities. At times, only one of the partners is in treatment; and, in such cases, it is often helpful for the person who is not in treatment to visit the therapist. The visiting partner may give the therapist data about the patient that may otherwise be overlooked; overt or covert anxiety in the visiting partner as a result of change in the patient can be identified and dealt with; irrational beliefs about treatment events can be corrected; and conscious or unconscious attempts by the partner to sabotage the patient's treatment can be examined.

Individual Couples Therapy. In individual couples therapy, each partner is in therapy, which is either concurrent, with the same therapist, or collaborative, with each partner seeing a different therapist.

Conjoint Therapy. In conjoint therapy, the most common treatment method in couples therapy, either one or two therapists treat the partners in joint sessions. Cotherapy with therapists of both sexes prevents a particular patient from feeling ganged up on when confronted by two members of the opposite sex.

Four-Way Session. In a four-way session, each partner is seen by a different therapist, with regular joint sessions in which all four persons participate. A variation of the four-way session is the roundtable interview, developed by William Masters and Virginia Johnson for the rapid treatment of sexually dysfunctional couples. Two patients and two opposite-sex therapists meet regularly.

Group Psychotherapy. Group therapy for couples allows a variety of group dynamics to affect the participants. Groups usually consist of three to four couples and one or two therapists. The couples identify with one another and recognize that others have similar problems; each gains support and empathy from fellow group members of the same or opposite sex. They explore sexual attitudes and have an opportunity to gain new information from their peer groups, and each receives specific feedback about his or her behavior, either negative or positive, which may have more meaning and be better assimilated coming from a neutral, nonspouse member, for example, than from the spouse or the therapist.

Combined Therapy. *Combined therapy* refers to all or any of the preceding techniques used concurrently or in combination. Thus, a particular patient-couple may begin treatment with one or both partners in individual psychotherapy, continue in conjoint therapy with the partner, and terminate therapy after a course of treatment in a married couples group. The rationale for combined therapy is that no single approach to marital problems has been shown to be superior to another. A familiarity with a variety of approaches thus allows therapists a flexibility that provides maximal benefit for couples in distress.

Indications

Whatever the specific therapeutic technique, initiation of couples therapy is indicated when individual therapy has failed to resolve the relationship difficulties, when the onset of distress in one or both partners is clearly a relational problem, and when couples therapy is requested by a couple in conflict. Problems in communication between partners are a prime indication for couples therapy. In such instances, one spouse may be intimidated by the other, may become anxious when attempting to tell the other about thoughts or feelings, or may project unconscious expectations onto the other. The therapy is geared toward enabling each partner to see the other realistically.

Conflicts in one or several areas, such as the partners' sexual life, are also indications for treatment. Similarly, difficulty in establishing satisfactory social, economic, parental, or emotional roles implies that a couple needs help. Clinicians should evaluate all aspects of the marital relationship before attempting to treat only one problem, which could be a symptom of a pervasive marital disorder.

Contraindications

Contraindications for couples therapy include patients with severe forms of psychosis, particularly patients with paranoid elements and those in whom the marriage's homeostatic mechanism is a protection against psychosis, marriages in which one or both partners really want to divorce, and marriages in which one spouse refuses to participate because of anxiety or fear.

Goals

Nathan Ackerman defined the aims of couples therapy as follows: The goals of therapy for partner relational problems are to alleviate emotional distress and disability and to promote the levels of well-being of both partners together and of each as an individual. Ideally, therapists move toward these goals by strengthening the shared resources for problem solving, by encouraging the substitution of adequate controls and defenses for pathogenic ones, by enhancing both the immunity against the disintegrative effects of emotional upset and the complementarity of the relationship, and by promoting the growth of the relationship and of each partner.

Part of a therapist's task is to persuade each partner in the relationship to take responsibility in understanding the psychodynamic makeup of personality. Each person's accountability for the effects of behavior on his or her own life, the life of the partner, and the lives of others in the environment is emphasized, and the result is often a deep understanding of the problems that created the marital discord.

Couples therapy does not ensure the maintenance of any marriage or relationship. Indeed, in certain instances, it may show the partners that they are in a nonviable union that should be dissolved. In these cases, couples may continue to meet with therapists to work through the difficulties of separating and obtaining a divorce, a process that has been called *divorce therapy*.

References

Goldenberg I, Goldenberg H. *Family Therapy: An Overview*. 6th ed. Pacific Grove, CA: Brooks/Cole; 2004.

Gurman AS. Brief integrative marital therapy. In: Gurman AS, Jacobson NS, eds. *Clinical Handbook of Couple Therapy*. 3rd ed. New York: Guilford Press; 2003:180.

Gurman AS, Jacobson NS, eds. *Clinical Handbook of Couple Therapy*. 3rd ed. New York: Guilford Press; 2003.

Gurman AS, Lebow JL. Family therapy and couple's therapy. In: Sadock BJ, Sadock VA, eds. *Kaplan & Sadock's Comprehensive Textbook of Psychiatry*. 8th ed. Vol. 2. Baltimore: Lippincott Williams & Wilkins; 2005:2584.

Johnson SM, Greenman PS. The path to a secure bond: Emotionally focused couple therapy. *J Clin Psychol*. 2006; 62(5):597—609.

Johnson SM, Whiffen VE, eds. *Attachment Processes in Couple and Family Therapy*. New York: Guilford Press; 2003.

McGoldrick M, Giordano J, Garcia-Preto N, eds. *Ethnicity and Family Therapy*. 3rd ed. New York: Guilford Press; 2005.

Nichols MP, Schwartz RC. *Family Therapy: Concepts and Methods*. 6th ed. Boston: Allyn & Bacon; 2004.

Scholevar GP, Schwoeri LW, eds. *Family and Couples Therapy: Clinical Applications*. Washington, DC: American Psychiatric Publishing; 2003.

Snyder DK, Whisman MA, eds. *Treating Difficult Couples*. New York: Guilford Press; 2003.

▲ 35.5 Dialectical Behavior Therapy

Dialectical behavior therapy (DBT) is a type of psychotherapy that was originally developed for chronically self-injurious patients with borderline personality disorder and parasuicidal behavior. In recent years, its use has extended to other forms of mental illness. The method is eclectic, drawing on concepts derived from supportive, cognitive, and behavioral therapies. Some elements can be traced to Franz Alexander's view of therapy as a corrective emotional experience, and other elements from certain Eastern philosophical schools (e.g., Zen).

Patients are seen weekly, with the goal of improving interpersonal skills and decreasing self-destructive behavior using techniques involving advice, metaphor, storytelling, and confrontation, among others. Patients with borderline personality disorder especially are helped to deal with the ambivalent feelings that are characteristic of the disorder. Marsha Linehan, Ph.D., developed the treatment method, based on her theory that such patients cannot identify emotional experiences and cannot tolerate frustration or rejection. As with other behavioral approaches, DBT assumes all behavior (including thoughts and feelings) is learned and that patients with borderline personality disorder behave in ways that reinforce or even reward their behavior, regardless of how maladaptive it is.

FUNCTIONS OF DIALECTICAL BEHAVIOR THERAPY

As described by its originator, there are five essential "functions" in treatment: (1) to enhance and expand the patient's repertoire of skillful behavioral patterns; (2) to improve patient motivation to change by reducing reinforcement of maladaptive behavior, including dysfunctional cognition and emotion; (3) to ensure that new behavioral patterns generalize from the therapeutic to the natural environment; (4) to structure the environment so that

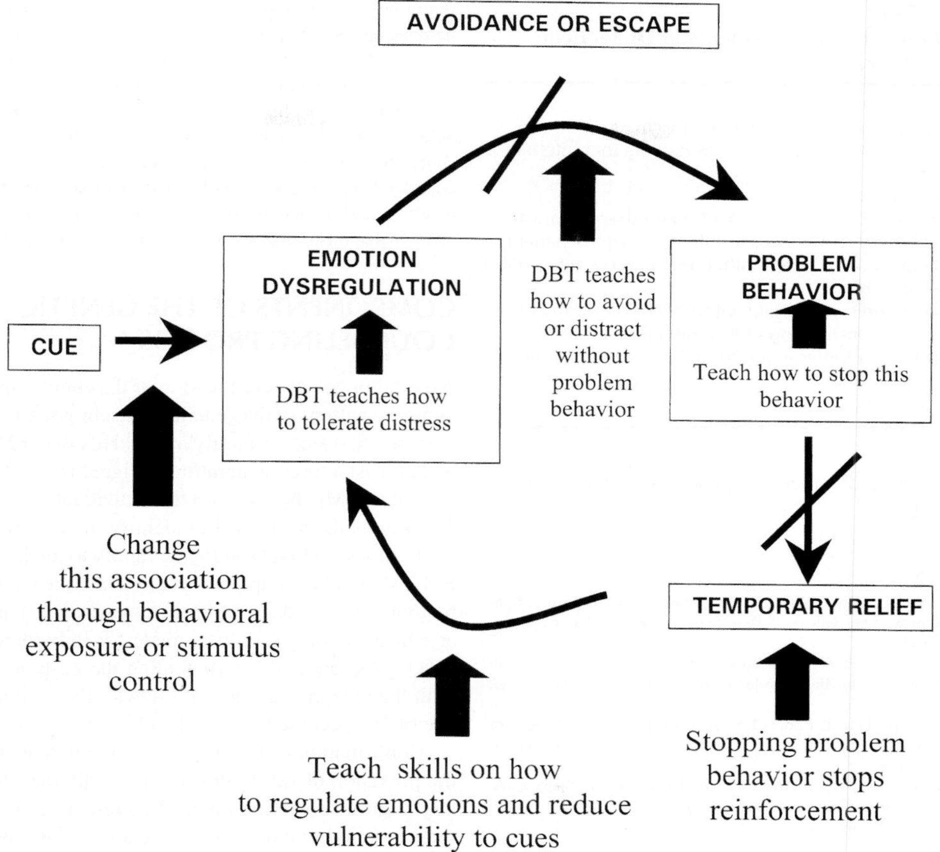

FIGURE 35.5–1
How dialectical behavior therapy (DBT) works.

effective behaviors, rather than dysfunctional behaviors, are reinforced; and (5) to enhance the motivation and capabilities of the therapist so that effective treatment is rendered. Figure 35.5-1 illustrates how DBT breaks the cycle of problem behavior being used to avoid emotional distress.

The four modes of treatment in DBT are as follows: (1) group skills training, (2) individual therapy, (3) phone consultations, and (4) consultation team. Other ancillary treatments used are pharmacotherapy and hospitalization, when needed. These are described below.

Group Skills Training

In group format, patients learn specific behavioral, emotional, cognitive, and interpersonal skills. Unlike traditional group therapy, observations about others in the group are discouraged. Rather, a didactic approach, using specific exercises taken from a skills training manual, is used, many of which are geared to control emotional dysregulation and impulsive behavior.

Individual Therapy

Sessions in DBT are held weekly, generally for 50 to 60 minutes, in which skills learned during group training are reviewed and life events in the previous week examined. Particular attention is paid to episodes of pathological behavioral patterns that could have been corrected if learned skills had been put into effect. Patients are encouraged to record their thoughts, feelings, and behavior on diary cards which are analyzed in the session.

Telephone Consultation

Therapists are available for phone consultation 24 hours per day. Patients are encouraged to call when they feel themselves heading toward some crisis that might lead to injurious behavior to themselves or others. Calls are intended to be brief and usually last about 10 minutes.

Consultation Team

Therapists meet in weekly meetings to review their work with their patients. By doing so, they provide support for one another and maintain motivation in their work. The meetings enable them to compare techniques used and to validate those that are most effective (Table 35.5-1).

RESULTS

A study evaluating the effect of DBT for patients with borderline personality disorder found that such therapy was positive. Patients had a low dropout rate from treatment; the incidence of parasuicidal behaviors declined; self-report of angry affect decreased; and social adjustment and work performance improved. The method is now being applied to other disorders, including

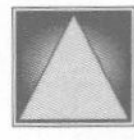

Table 35.5–1
Consultation Team Agreements in Dialectical Behavior Therapy

Meet weekly for 1 to 2 hr
Discuss cases according to the treatment hierarchy (i.e., self-injurious/life-threatening behavior, behaviors that interfere with treatment or quality of life).
Accept a dialectical philosophy.
Consult with the patient on how to interact with other therapists, but do not tell other therapists how to interact with the patient.
Consistency of therapists with one another (even across the same patient) is not expected.
All therapists observe their own limits without fear of judgmental reactions from other consultation group members.
Search for nonpejorative empathic interpretation of the patient's behavior.
All therapists are fallible.

substance abuse, eating disorders, schizophrenia, and posttraumatic stress disorder.

References

Brown MZ, Comtois KA, Linehan MM. Reasons for suicide attempts and nonsuicidal self-injury in women with borderline personality disorder. *J Abnorm Psychol*. 2002;111:198.

Krause ED, Mendelson T, Lynch TR. Childhood emotion invalidation and adult psychological distress: The mediating role of inhibition. *Child Abuse Negl*. 2003;27:199–213.

Lynch TL, Morse JQ, Mendelson T, Robins CJ. Dialectical behavior therapy for depressed older adults: A randomized pilot study. *Am J Geriatr Psychiatry*. 2003;11:33–45.

Rosenthal MZ, Lynch TR. Dialectical behavior therapy. In: Sadock BJ, Sadock VA, eds. *Kaplan & Sadock's Comprehensive Textbook of Psychiatry*. 8th ed. Vol. 2. Baltimore: Lippincott Williams & Wilkins; 2005:2619.

35.6 Genetic Counseling

Genetic counseling is a process that provides information (medical, technical, and probabilistic) to the patient (and family) at risk for developing a specific disorder. The provision of information occurs in conjunction with helping them adapt emotionally and psychologically to the diagnosis (or threat of it), thus facilitating informed decision making. The process aims to minimize distress, to increase one's feeling of personal control, and to facilitate informed decision making.

GENETICS AND MENTAL HEALTH

Disorders can recur in families for many reasons, including the functioning of genes (single genes versus polygenic), shared environmental exposures, a combination of genetic and environmental factors (multifactorial), and cultural transmission. *Single gene disorders* are caused by defects in one particular gene, and they often have simple and predictable inheritance patterns. By contrast, most psychiatric disorders are *multifactorial* in etiology, influenced by multiple genes as well as environmental factors, making them more difficult to predict.

Two phenomena that further complicate genetic counseling include penetrance and expressivity. *Penetrance* refers to the portion of individuals with a specific genotype who also manifest that genotype at the phenotype level. If all individuals who carry the dominant gene show any phenotype of the gene, the gene is said to be *completely penetrant*. Currently, only rare examples exist of known genes for mental disorders that demonstrate complete penetrance of symptoms in the presence of a single gene. One such example is early-onset familial Alzheimer's disease resulting from mutations in the amyloid precursor protein (APP) located on the long arm of chromosome 21. In contrast, *expressivity* refers to the extent to which a genotype is expressed. In the case of variable expressivity, the trait can vary in expression from mild to severe, but is never completely unexpressed in individuals who have the gene. The genes that result in most mental disorders are believed to regulate a wide spectrum of traits demonstrating variability of expression (spectrum disorders).

COMPONENTS OF THE GENETIC COUNSELING PROCESS

Ascertainment and clarification of the client's specific questions and expectations of the genetic counseling session are a basic and essential first step. A family medical history (FMH) is collected, and at least a three-generation pedigree is constructed. The collection of FMH begins with the individual seeking information. *Proband* is the term used to identify the affected person within the family who first brought the family to medical attention. The FMH should be comprehensive and include the following information: ages (or dates of birth) of each family member, the age at which the diagnosis was made for individuals with the disorder, pregnancy losses (including the gestational length along with the recognized cause, if known), the recognized cause and age of any deceased family members, and ethnic backgrounds.

Confirmation or clarification of the diagnosis is essential to the provision of valid information within the session. This usually requires obtaining medical records to clarify or to confirm the suspected diagnosis in the relatives. Depending on the situation, genetic testing may be available for at-risk members in families with single-gene disorders; but because DNA testing for most mental disorders is not yet an option, risk assessment is based solely on analysis of the pedigree.

The topics that are most often included in counseling sessions are a definition of the disorder and its natural history; explanation of the possible modes of inheritance and their associated recurrence risks; options for medical management, prevention or treatment; and the availability of genetic testing and the associated risks, benefits, and limitations. The provision of understandable and meaningful information, coupled with empathy, compassion, and sensitivity, moves a simple educational effort to a multifaceted genetic counseling encounter.

The collection and review of the FMH with the patient might elicit or recall intense feelings of sadness, guilt, anxiety, or anger. Furthermore, the graphic presentation of the family history may bring to light a more concrete realization of an individual's risks; therefore, attention to the patient's affect is important throughout the process. The following case study brings this potential to light (Fig. 35.6-1):

A couple in their mid 30s contacts a local psychiatrist regarding the woman's diagnosis of bipolar disorder and her use of lithium carbonate during her recently recognized first pregnancy. She has not been able to function well without the medication during her 5-year history with the disorder. They are concerned about the use of medication during the pregnancy. In addition, the husband expressed concern about his partner's family history of other psychiatric disorders, such as schizophrenia. As the family history unfolded, the

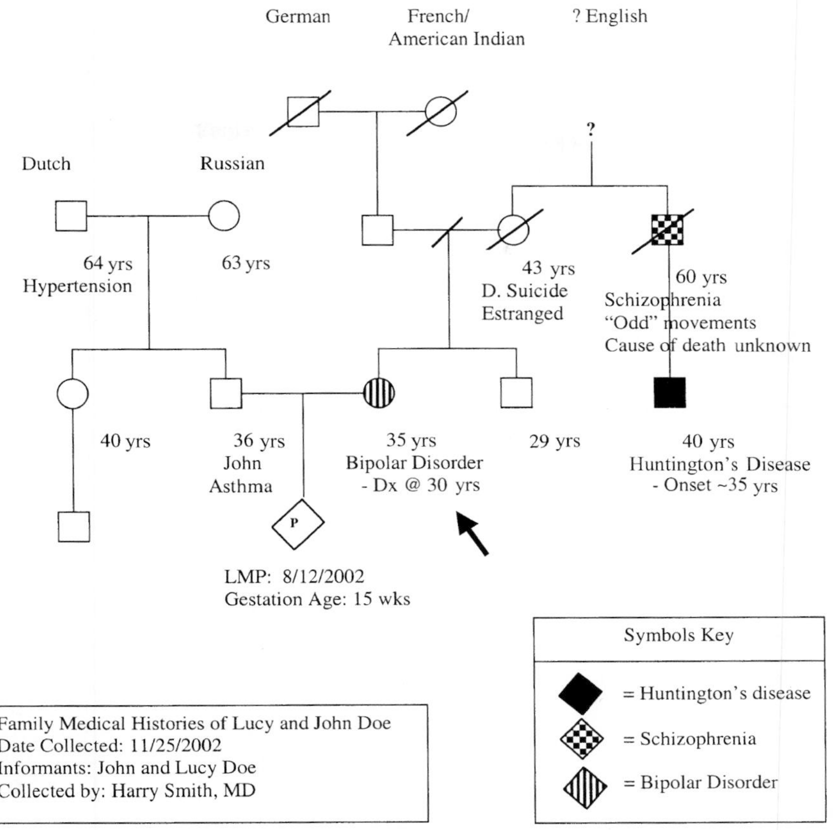

FIGURE 35.6–1
Family medical histories of Lucy and John Doe. Dx, diagnosis; LMP, last menstrual period.

husband learned of the diagnosis of Huntington's disease in his wife's first cousin.

Patients with Huntington's disease develop significant personality changes (72 percent), affective psychosis (20 to 90 percent), or schizophrenic psychosis (4 to 12 percent). After a description of clinical features associated with Huntington's disease, the couple realized that the woman's symptoms might be presenting signs of Huntington's disease. In this particular case, the woman developed significant anxiety that worsened in response to her husband's anger regarding the discovery.

Issues recognized by the psychiatrist and needing attention in this case include the teratogenic effects of the lithium carbonate, increased risk for chromosomal anomalies because of maternal age, and an assessment of recurrence risks for mental illness and Huntington's disease. Anticipation of a wide variety of emotions may prepare the psychiatrist to assist the couple in their initial adaptation to the various identified risks.

Communication of Risk and Decision Making

Individuals vary in their level of understanding risks. The provision of risk information is best approached in a balanced and accurate manner that is tailored to the patient as much as possible. There is the temptation to use nonnumeric phrases of probability (e.g., often, rarely, most likely); however, the meaning of these nonnumeric phrases is highly subjective and their use in the genetic counseling session introduces the potential for bias.

Ideally, risks should be presented in several different ways, taking clues from interactions with the client that inform the approach. Some examples of approaches to assist the client's understanding of risks include stating numeric risks as percentages (25 percent) and as fractional risks (one-in-four chance). It is important to frame risks from the perspective of a negative and a positive outcome; for example, there is a 1 percent chance that the test will result in a complication and a 99 percent chance that there will be no complication.

Owing to the high rate of co-occurring disorders and the wide phenotypic range of psychiatric disorders, patients should be informed of potential risks for disorders other than those that brought them to genetic counseling. An example of this is the risk to first-degree relatives of an individual diagnosed with bipolar disorder. In this situation, the risk for bipolar disorder is increased for first-degree relatives, as are the risks for unipolar disorder, schizoaffective disorder, and cyclothymia.

It should be made clear that the risks are determined from populations and not derived from individuals and, therefore, are estimates at best. Table 35.6-1 provides a compilation of recurrence risks from various referenced sources in the literature.

CHALLENGES POSED BY PRESYMPTOMATIC AND SUSCEPTIBILITY GENETIC TESTING

Psychiatrists will be on the front line for receiving requests for genetic counseling and testing because of their established

Table 35.6–1
Empiric Risks for Selected Mental Disorders

	Schizophrenia (%)	Bipolar Disorder (%)	Major Depressive Disorder		Schizo-affective Disorder (%)	Obsessive-Compulsive Disorder (%)	Panic Disorder (%)	Generalized Anxiety Disorder (%)	Alcohol Dependence		Phobia (%)	Anorexia Nervosa (%)	ADHD (%)
			Men (%)	Women (%)					Men (%)	Women (%)			
Affected relative													
General population	1[a]	0.8–1.6[b,c,d,e]	1–15[b,c]	2–23[b,c]	0.5–<1[b,c,d]	1.5–3[a,p]	1.5–3.5[a,n]	3.5[a]	14[a]	3[a]	4–11[a]	0.1[a]	3–5[f]
First degree (pooled)	9[a]	5–20[b,c,e]	9[a]	18[a]	1–10[b,c,d]	17–25[a,p]	15–25[a,n]	20[a]	27[a]	5[a]	12–31[a]	5–10[a]	?
Siblings	9–16[d,i,j,k]	5–20[b,c,e,h,i]	5–30[b,c,h,i]	5–30[b,c,h,i]	—	25–35[l]	—	—	—	—	—	—	17–25[g]
Parent	5–13[g,i,j,k,o]	15[c,d,e,h,m]	7–19[h,i]	7–19[h,i]	—	25–35[l]	—	—	—	—	—	—	—
Sibling and one parent	15[h]	20[h]	—	—	—	—	—	—	—	—	—	—	—
Both parents	45[h,i]	50–75 for affective disorder[b,d,h,i]	—	—	—	—	—	—	—	—	—	—	—
Second degree (pooled)	2–6[h,j]	5[h]	—	—	—	—	—	—	—	—	—	—	—
Uncle/aunt	1–4[i,j]	—	—	—	—	—	—	—	—	—	—	—	—
Nephew/niece	2–4[i,j,o]	—	—	—	—	—	—	—	—	—	—	—	—
Grandparent	2–8[i,j]	—	—	—	—	—	—	—	—	—	—	—	—
Half-sibling	4[i,j]	—	—	—	—	—	—	—	—	—	—	—	—
Third degree	—	—	—	—	—	—	—	—	—	—	—	—	—
First cousin	2–6[i,j]	—	—	—	—	—	—	—	—	—	—	—	—
Risks for additional mental disorders	Spectrum disorders Schizoaffective disorder Unipolar and major depression	Unipolar disorder Alcohol dependence Schizoaffective disorder Cyclothymia	Anxiety disorders Alcohol dependence Dysthymia ADHD	Schizophrenia Other psychoses Bipolar disorder Unipolar disorder	—	—	—	—	—	—	—	—	—
Notes	Early onset and severe phenotype may increase recurrence risks	Early onset may increase risks; female relatives at greatest risk for any affective disorder	Early onset and recurrent episodes may increase risk to first-degree relatives; female to male ratio is 2–3:1	Recurrence risks highest for unipolar disorder (5–27)	—	—	—	—	—	—	—	—	—

ADHD, attention-deficit/hyperactivity disorder.
[a]Moldin SO. Psychiatric genetic counseling, In: Guze SB, ed. *Washington University Adult Psychiatry.* Mosby-Year Book; 1997.
[b]Duffy A, Grof P. The implications of genetic studies of major mood disorders for clinical practice. *J Clin Psychiatry.* 2000;61:630–637.
[c]Gershon ES. A family study of schizoaffective, bipolar I, bipolar II, unipolar and normal control probands. *Arch Gen Psychiatry.* 1982;39:1157–1167.
[d]Gershon ES. A controlled family study of chronic psychosis. *Arch Gen Psychiatry.* 1988;45:328–336.
[e]Potash JB. Searching high and low: A review of the genetics of bipolar disorder. *Bipolar Disord.* 2000;2:8–26.
[f]Barkley RA: Attention deficit hyperactivity disorder. *Sci Am.* 1998;9:66–71.
[g]Biederman J. *Arch Gen Psychiatry.* 1992;49:728–738.
[h]Harper PS. *Practical Genetic Counseling.* 4th ed. Oxford, UK: Butterworth-Heinemann; 1994:348.
[i]Nurnberger J Jr, Berretini W. *Psychiatric Genetics.* 1st ed. London: Chapman and Hall; 1998:164.
[j]Hodgkinson KA. Genetic counseling for schizophrenia in the era of molecular genetics. *Can J Psychiatry.* 2001;46:123–130.
[k]Kendler KS, McGuire M. An epidemiologic, clinical and family study of simple schizophrenia in county Roscommon, Ireland. *Am J Psychiatry.* 1994;151:27–34.
[l]Rasmussen SA, Tsuang MT. The epidemiology of obsessive compulsive disorder. *J Clin Psychiatry.* 1984;45:450–457.
[m]Goodwin FK, Jamison KR. *Manic Depressive Illness,* New York: Oxford University Press; 1990:938.
[n]Crowe RR, Noyes R, Pauls DL. A family study of panic disorder. *Arch Gen Psychiatry.* 1983;40:1065.
[o]Gottesman II, Shields J. *Schizophrenia: The Epigenetic Puzzle.* New York: Cambridge University Press: 1982.
[p]Swedo SE, Rapoport IL, Leonard H. Obsessive-compulsive disorder in children and adolescence. *Arch Gen Psychiatry.* 1989;46:335–341.

relationship between patients and families with mental disorders. The identification of these risks will most likely occur before the discovery or availability of preventative options. The option of knowing risks without preventative options raises concerns regarding the impact of such knowledge on the individual's mood, anxiety, distress, self-image, reproductive decisions, career decisions, family relationships, insurability, employment, and, potentially, other areas.

A model for the provision of presymptomatic genetic testing is provided through the protocol developed for Huntington's disease (see the Hereditary Disease Foundation Web site at http://www.hdfoundation.org). This model recommends conducting education, counseling, and evaluative sessions over an extended period of time (3 to 4 months), during which time information is provided, questions are addressed, and counseling is initiated, thus maximizing informed decision making. The process is most appropriately undertaken in the absence of other stressful events (e.g., death of a family member, diagnosis of the disease in another family member, job loss, and divorce).

Studies suggest that most individuals receiving information of their increased risk for the disease in their family experience significantly more anxiety, depression, and psychological distress and have poorer perception of their health over the short term (within 1 month after receiving test results) compared with their baseline levels, but no difference over the long term (as long as 1 year after the receipt of results) compared with pretest levels. Consideration should also be given to the impact of such information on the spouse, because initial studies have suggested that the spouse may experience higher levels of depression related to the presymptomatic diagnosis than the client. Furthermore, partners of gene-positive individuals may experience increased levels of intrusive thoughts, avoidance, and hopelessness over the short and long term compared with baseline levels.

ETHICAL, LEGAL, AND SOCIAL CONSIDERATIONS

Certain individuals and families may experience significant levels of stigma associated with the identification of a genetic disorder, a situation already familiar to individuals and families with mental illness. The added knowledge of a hereditary component may heighten stigmatization. Conversely, having an identified, biological basis may supplant current public perceptions that mental illness is somehow a personal or family failure in moral, spiritual, or attitudinal perspectives.

Questions frequently arise about the privacy of an individual's genetic information, the ability of employers or insurers to access such information, and the potential of using the information against them by denying insurance, raising rates to unreasonable levels, or denying jobs, and a host of other possible concerns. Currently, no overarching federal laws comprehensively protect citizens of the United States from the potential of these abuses, although significant efforts are continuing in this regard. The status of existing and proposed state and federal laws can be reviewed through the Web site of the National Human Genome Research Institute (http://www.genome.gov).

References

Erblich J, Lerman C, Self DW, Diaz GA, Bovbjerg DH. Stress-induced cigarette craving: Effects of the DRD2 TaqI RFLP and SLC6A3 VNTR polymorphisms. *Pharmacogenomics J.* 2004;4:102–109.

Howes OD, McDonald C, Cannon M, Arseneault L, Boydell J, Murray RM. Pathways to schizophrenia: The impact of environmental factors. *Int J Neuropsychopharmacol.* 2004;7[Suppl 1]:S7–S13.

Noble EP. D2 dopamine receptor gene in psychiatric and neurologic disorders and its phenotypes. *Am J Med Genet.* 2003;116B:103–125.

Nussbaum RL, McInnes RR, Willard HF. *Thompson & Thompson: Genetics in Medicine.* Philadelphia: WB Saunders; 2001.

Pilnick A, Dingwall R. Research directions in genetic counseling: A review of the literature. *Patient Education and Counseling.* 2001;44:95–105.

Resta RG. *Psyche and Helix: Psychological Aspects of Genetic Counseling.* New York: Wiley-Liss; 2000.

Roberts JS, LaRusse SA, Katzen H, Whitehouse PJ, Barber M, Post SG, Relkin N, Quaid K, Pietrzak RH, Cupples LA, Farrer LA, Brown T, Green RC. Reasons for seeking genetic susceptibility testing among first-degree relatives of people with Alzheimer's disease. *Alzheimer Dis Assoc Disord.* 2003;17:86–93.

Xu Q, Jia YB, Zhang BY, Zou K, Tao YB, Wang YP, Qiang BQ, Wu GY, Shen Y, Ji HK, Huang Y, Sun XQ, Ji L, Li YD, Yuan YB, Shu L, Yu X, Shen YC, Yu YQ, Ju GZ. Association study of an SNP combination pattern in the dopaminergic pathway in paranoid schizophrenia: A novel strategy for complex disorders. *Mol Psychiatry.* 2004:1–12.

▲ 35.7 Biofeedback

Biofeedback involves the recording and display of small changes in the physiological levels of the feedback parameter. The display can be visual, such as a big meter or a bar of lights, or auditory. Patients are instructed to change the levels of the parameter, using the feedback from the display as a guide. Biofeedback is based on the idea that the autonomic nervous system can come under voluntary control through operant conditioning. Biofeedback can be used by itself or in combination with relaxation. For example, patients with urinary incontinence use biofeedback alone to regain control over the pelvic musculature. Biofeedback is also used in the rehabilitation of neurological disorders. The benefits of biofeedback may be augmented by the relaxation that patients are trained to facilitate.

THEORY

Neal Miller demonstrated the medical potential of biofeedback by showing that the normally involuntary autonomic nervous system can be operantly conditioned by use of appropriate feedback. By means of instruments, patients acquire information about the status of involuntary biological functions, such as skin temperature and electrical conductivity, muscle tension, blood pressure, heart rate, and brain wave activity. Patients then learn to regulate one or more of these biological states that affect symptoms. For example, a person can learn to raise the temperature of his or her hands to reduce the frequency of migraines, palpitations, or angina pectoris. Presumably, patients lower the sympathetic activation and voluntarily self-regulate arterial smooth muscle vasoconstrictive tendencies.

METHODS

Instrumentation

The feedback instrument used depends on the patient and the specific problem. The most effective instruments are the electromyogram (EMG), which measures the electrical potentials of muscle fibers; the electroencephalogram (EEG), which measures alpha waves that occur in relaxed states; the galvanic skin response (GSR) gauge, which shows decreased skin conductivity during a relaxed state; and the thermistor, which measures skin temperature (which drops during tension because of peripheral vasoconstriction). Patients are attached to one of the instruments that measures a physiological function and translates the measurement into an audible or visual signal that patients use to gauge their responses. For example, in the treatment of bruxism, an EMG is attached to the masseter muscle. The EMG emits a high tone when the muscle is contracted and a low tone when at rest. Patients can learn to alter the tone to indicate relaxation. Patients receive feedback about the masseter muscle, the tone reinforces the learning, and the condition ameliorates—all of these events interacting synergistically.

Many less-specific clinical applications (e.g., treating insomnia, dysmenorrhea, and speech problems; improving athletic performance; treating volitional disorders; achieving altered states of consciousness; managing stress; and supplementing psychotherapy for anxiety associated with somatoform disorders) use a model in which frontalis muscle EMG biofeedback is combined with thermal biofeedback and verbal instructions in progressive relaxation. Table 35.7-1 outlines some important clinical applications of biofeedback and shows that a wide variety of biofeedback modalities have been used to treat numerous conditions.

Table 35.7–1
Biofeedback Applications

Condition	Effects
Asthma	Both frontal electromyogram (EMG) and airway resistance biofeedback have been reported as producing relaxation from the panic associated with asthma, as well as improving air flow rate.
Cardiac arrhythmias	Specific biofeedback of the electrocardiogram has permitted patients to lower the frequency of premature ventricular contractions.
Fecal incontinence and enuresis	The timing sequence of internal and external anal sphincters has been measured, using triple lumen rectal catheters providing feedback to incontinent patients to allow them to reestablish normal bowel habits in a relatively small number of biofeedback sessions. An actual precursor of biofeedback dating to 1938 was a buzzer sounding for sleeping enuretic children at the first sign of moisture (the pad and bell).
Grand mal epilepsy	A number of electroencephalogram (EEG) biofeedback procedures have been used experimentally to suppress seizure activity prophylactically in patients not responsive to anticonvulsant medication. The procedures permit patients to enhance the sensorimotor brain wave rhythm or to normalize brain activity as computed in real-time power spectrum displays.
Hyperactivity	EEG biofeedback procedures have been used with children with attention-deficit/hyperactivity disorder to train them to reduce their motor restlessness.
Idiopathic hypertension and orthostatic hypotension	A variety of specific (direct) and nonspecific biofeedback procedures—including blood pressure feedback, galvanic skin response, and foot-hand thermal feedback combined with relaxation procedures—have been used to teach patients to increase or decrease their blood pressure. Some follow-up data indicate that the changes may persist for years and often permit the reduction or elimination of antihypertensive medications.
Migraine	The most common biofeedback strategy with classic or common vascular headaches has been thermal biofeedback from a digit accompanied by autogenic self-suggestive phrases encouraging hand warming and head cooling. The mechanism is thought to help prevent excessive cerebral artery vasoconstriction, often accompanied by an ischemic prodromal symptom, such as scintillating scotomata, followed by rebound engorgement of arteries and stretching of vessel wall pain receptors.
Myofacial and temporomandibular joint (TMJ) pain	High levels of EMG activity over the powerful muscles associated with bilateral TMJs have been decreased, using biofeedback in patients who are jaw clenchers or have bruxism.
Neuromuscular rehabilitation	Mechanical devices or an EMG measurement of muscle activity displayed to a patient increases the effectiveness of traditional therapies, as documented by relatively long clinical histories in peripheral nerve–muscle damage, spasmodic torticollis, selected cases of tardive dyskinesia, cerebral palsy, and upper motor neuron hemiplegias.
Raynaud's syndrome	Cold hands and cold feet are frequent concomitants of anxiety and also occur in Raynaud's syndrome, caused by vasospasm of arterial smooth muscle. A number of studies report that thermal feedback from the hand, an inexpensive and benign procedure compared with surgical sympathectomy, is effective in about 70 percent of cases of Raynaud's syndrome.
Tension headaches	Muscle contraction headaches are most frequently treated with two large active electrodes spaced on the forehead to provide visual or auditory information about the levels of muscle tension. The frontal electrode placement is sensitive to EMG activity regarding the frontalis and occipital muscles, which the patient learns to relax.

Relaxation Therapy

Muscle relaxation is used as a component of treatment programs (e.g., systematic desensitization) or as treatment in its own right (relaxation therapy). Relaxation is characterized by (1) immobility of the body, (2) control over the focus of attention, (3) low muscle tone, and (4) cultivation of a specific frame of mind, described as contemplative, nonjudgmental, detached, or mindful.

Progressive relaxation was developed by Edmund Jacobson in 1929. Jacobson observed that

> When an individual lies "relaxed," in the ordinary sense, the following clinical signs reveal the presence of residual tension: respiration is slightly irregular in time or force; the pulse-rate, although often normal, is in some instances moderately increased as compared with later tests; voluntary or local reflex activities are revealed in such slight marks as wrinkling of the forehead, frowning, movements of the eye balls, frequent or rapid winking, restless shifting of the head, a limb or even a finger; finally, the mind

continues to be active, and once started, worry or oppressive emotion will persist. It is amazing that a faint degree of tension can be responsible for all this.

Learning relaxation, therefore, involves cultivating a muscle sense. To develop the muscle sense further, patients are taught to isolate and contract specific muscles or muscle groups, one at a time. For example, patients flex the forearm while the therapist holds it back to observe tenseness in the biceps muscle. (Jacobson used the word "tenseness" rather than "tension" to emphasize the patient's role in tensing the muscles.) Once this sensation is reported, Jacobson would say, "This is your doing! What we wish is the reverse of this—simply not doing." Patients are repeatedly reminded that relaxation involves no effort. In fact "making an effort is being tense and therefore is not to relax." As the session progresses, patients are instructed to let go further and further, even past the point when the body part seems perfectly relaxed.

Patients would work in this fashion with different muscle groups, often over more than 50 sessions. For example, an entire session might be devoted to relaxing the biceps muscle. Another feature of Jacobson's method was that instructions were given tersely so they would not interfere with a patient's focus on muscle sensations; suggestions commonly used today (e.g., "your arm is becoming limp") were avoided. Patients were also frequently left alone, while the therapist attended to other patients.

In psychiatry, relaxation therapy is mainly used as a component of multifaceted broad-spectrum programs. Its use in desensitization was mentioned previously. Relaxing breathing exercises are often helpful for patients with panic disorder, especially that considered to be related to hyperventilation. In the treatment of patients with anxiety disorders, relaxation can serve as an occasion-setting stimulus (i.e., as a context of safety in which other specific intervention can be confidently tried).

Later Adaptation of Progressive Muscular Relaxation

Joseph Wolpe chose progressive relaxation as a response incompatible with anxiety when designing his systematic desensitization treatment (discussed below). For this purpose, Jacobson's original method was too lengthy to be practical. Wolpe abbreviated the program to 20 minutes during the first six sessions (devoting the remainder of these sessions to other things, such as behavioral analysis). In a later modification of progressive relaxation, patients completed work with all the principal muscle groups in one session. The specific muscle groups and instructions for this type of progressive relaxation are listed in Table 35.7-2. Once the patients have mastered this procedure (typically after three sessions), these groups are combined into larger groups. Finally, patients practice relaxation by recall (i.e., without tensing the muscles).

Autogenic Training

Autogenic training is a method of self-suggestion that originated in Germany. It involves the patients directing their attention to specific bodily areas and hearing themselves think certain phrases reflecting a relaxed state. In the original German version, patients progressed through six themes over many sessions. The six areas are listed in Table 35.7-3 along with representative autogenic phrases. Autogenic relaxation is an American modification of autogenic training, in which all six areas are covered in one session.

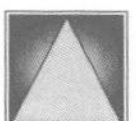

Table 35.7–2
Outline of Initial Progressive Relaxation Session, All Muscle Groups

Muscle Group	Instruction
Dominant hand and forearm	Make a tight fist, now
Dominant biceps, triceps	Make your upper arm tense by counterposing muscles
Nondominant arm, forearm	Make a tight fist, now
Nondominant biceps	Make your upper arm tense by counterposing muscles
Forehead	Lift eyebrows
Orbital and nose muscles	Squint and wrinkle your nose
Lower cheeks and jaws	Bite your teeth together and pull the corners of your mouth back
Neck and throat	Pull your chin toward your chest, but prevent it from happening by counterposing muscles in front and back
Chest, shoulders, upper back	Take a deep breath, hold it, and pull the shoulder blades upward (if sitting) or backward (if supine)
Abdominal or stomach region	Make your stomach hard, as if you were going to hit yourself
Dominant thigh	Counterpose extensors and flexors
Dominant lower leg	Dorsiflex foot
Dominant foot	Curl toes upward (not down to avoid cramps)
Nondominant thigh	Counterpose extensors and flexors
Nondominant calf	Dorsiflex foot
Nondominant foot	Curl toes upward (not down, to avoid cramps)

(Adapted from Bernstein DA, Borkovec TD. *Progressive Relaxation Training: A Manual for the Helping Professions.* Champaign, IL: Research Press; 1973, with permission.)

Applied Tension

Applied tension is a technique that is the opposite of relaxation; applied tension can be used to counteract the fainting response. The treatment extends over four sessions. In the first session, patients learn to tense the muscles of the arms, legs, and torso for 10 to 15 seconds (as if they were bodybuilders). The tension is maintained long enough for a sensation of warmth to develop in the face. The patients then release the tension, but do not

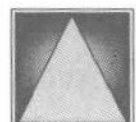

Table 35.7–3
Sample Autogenic Phrases

Theme	Examples of Self-Statements
Heaviness	"My left arm is heavy."
Warmth	"My left arm is warm."
Cardiac regulation	"My heartbeat is calm and regular."
Breathing adjustment	"It breathes me."
Solar plexus	"My solar plexus is warm."
Forehead	"My forehead is cool."

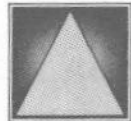

Table 35.7–4
Steps in Applied Relaxation

Technique	Instructions
Progressive relaxation	Session 1: hands, arms, face, neck, and shoulders Session 2: back, chest, stomach, breathing, hips, legs, and feet
Release-only relaxation	As with progressive relaxation, except that the tension phase is omitted; when release-only relaxation is mastered, the patient can relax within 5 to 7 mins
Cue-controlled relaxation	A stimulus—the word *relax*—is presented just before exhalation; patients focus on their breathing while already in a relaxed state; the therapist says the word *inhale* just before each inhalation and the word *relax* just before each exhalation; after approximately five cycles, the patient mentally says these words (optionally dropping the *inhale*)
Differential relaxation	Patients can remain relaxed and move at the same time by differentially keeping muscles unrelated to the movement in a relaxed state; after achieving a relaxed state, patients lift an arm or a leg or look around in the room, while keeping movements and tension in other body parts at a minimum; patients also perform differential relaxation in other settings, including sitting in different chairs, sitting at a desk while writing, talking on the phone, and walking.
Rapid relaxation	Patients relax by taking one to three breaths with slow exhalations, thinking the word *relax* before each exhalation and scanning their bodies for areas of tension; with this practice, relaxation is shortened to 20 to 30 secs; patients are instructed to relax in this manner 15 to 20 times per day at certain predetermined events in their natural environment (e.g., when they look at the watch or make a telephone call. As a reminder, colored dots might be taped on the watch or phone. After some time, the dots are changed to a different color to keep their reminding power fresh).
Application training	Patients relax just before entering the target situation; they stay in the situation for 10 to 15 mins, using their relaxation skills as a coping technique; patients may initially be accompanied by the therapist; alternatively, if the patient's problem is panic attacks or generalized anxiety, imagery or physical exercise is used to induce fearful sensations, which then are used for application training.

progress to a state of relaxation. The maneuver is repeated five times at half-minute intervals. This method can be augmented with feedback of the patient's blood pressure during the muscle contraction; increased blood pressure suggests that appropriate muscle tension was achieved. The patients continue to practice the technique five times a day. An adverse effect of treatment that sometimes develops is headache. In this case, the intensity of the muscle contraction and the frequency of treatment are reduced.

Patients with blood and injury phobia show a unique, biphasic response when exposed to a phobic stimulus. The first phase is associated with increased heart rate and blood pressure. In the second phase, however, blood pressure suddenly falls and the patient faints. To treat the problem, patients are shown a series of slides that are provocative (e.g., mutilated bodies). They are coached in identifying early warning signs of fainting, such as queasiness, cold sweats, or dizziness, and in applying the learned muscle tension response quickly, contingent on these warning signs. Patients can also perform applied tension while donating blood or watching a surgical operation. The technique of isometric tension raises blood pressure, which prevents fainting.

Applied Relaxation

Applied relaxation involves eliciting a relaxation response in the stressful situation itself. The previous discussion showed that this is not advisable right away because of the possible ironic effects of relaxation. Therefore, patients should first practice relaxation in nonstressful circumstances. The method developed by Lars-Göran Öst and coworkers in Sweden has been proved efficacious for panic disorder and generalized anxiety disorder. Establishing the relaxation response in the patient's natural environment consists of seven phases of one to two sessions each: progressive relaxation, release-only relaxation, cue-controlled relaxation, differential relaxation, rapid relaxation, application training, and maintenance. Details are provided in Table 35.7-4.

RESULTS

Biofeedback, progressive relaxation, and applied tension have been shown to be effective treatment methods for a broad range of disorders. They form one basis of behavioral medicine in which the patient changes (or learns how to change) behavior that contributes to illness. They form a basis on which many complementary and alternative medical procedures are effective (e.g., yoga and Reiki) in which relaxation is an important component. Relaxation also informs more mainstream treatments, such as hypnosis.

References

Enger T, Gruzelier JH. EEG Biofeedback of low beta band components: Frequency-specific effects on variables of attention and event-related brain potentials. *Clin Neurophysiol*. 2004;115;131–139.

Jacob RG, Pelham WE. Behavior therapy. In: Sadock BJ, Sadock VA, eds. *Kaplan & Sadock's Comprehensive Textbook of Psychiatry*. 8th ed. Baltimore: Lippincott Williams & Wilkins; 2005:2498.

Mitani S, Fujita M, Sakamoto S, Shirakawa T. Effect of autogenic training on cardiac autonomic nervous activity in high-risk fire service workers for post-traumatic stress disorder. *J Psychosom Res*. 2006;60(5):439–444.

Nanke A, Rief W. Biofeedback in somatoform disorders and related syndromes. *Current Opinion in Psychiatry*. 2004;17(2):133–138.

Othmer S, Pollock V, Miller N. The subjective response to neurofeedback. In: Earleywine M, ed. *Mind-Altering Drugs: The Science of Subjective Experience*. New York: Oxford University Press; 2005:345–365.

Ritz T, Dahme B, Roth WT. Behavioral interventions in asthma: Biofeedback techniques. *J Psychosom Res*. 2004;56(6):711–720.

Schwartz MS, Andrasik F, eds. *Biofeedback: A Practitioner's Guide*. 3rd ed. New York: Guilford Press; 2003.

Scott WC, Kaiser D, Othmer S, Sideroff SI. Effects of an EEG biofeedback protocol on a mixed substance abusing population. *Am J Drug Alcohol Abuse*. 2005;31(3):455–469.

Seo JT, Choe JH, Lee WS, Kim KH. Efficacy of functional electrical stimulation-biofeedback with sexual cognitive-behavioral therapy as treatment of vaginismus. *Urology*. 2005;66(1):77–81.

Thornton KE, Carmody DP. Electroencephalogram biofeedback for reading disability and traumatic brain injury. *Child Adolesc Psychiatric Clin N Am*. 2005;14:137–162.

Yucha C, Gilbert C. *Evidence-Based Practice in Biofeedback and Neurofeedback*. Wheat Ridge, CO: Association for Applied Psychophysiology and Biofeedback; 2004.

▲ 35.8 Behavior Therapy

The term *behavior* in *behavior therapy* refers to a person's observable actions and responses. Behavior therapy involves changing the behavior of patients to reduce dysfunction and to improve quality of life. Behavior therapy includes a methodology, referred to as *behavior analysis*, for the strategic selection of behaviors to change, and a technology to bring about behavior change, such as modifying antecedents or consequences or giving instructions. Behavior therapy has not only influenced mental health care, but, under the rubric of behavioral medicine, it has also made inroads into other medical specialties.

Behavior therapy represents clinical applications of the principles developed in learning theory. Behavioral psychology, or behaviorism, arose in the early 20th century in reaction to the method of introspection that dominated psychology at the time. John B. Watson, the father of behaviorism, had initially studied animal psychology. This background made it a small conceptual leap to argue that psychology should concern itself only with publicly observable phenomena (i.e., overt behavior). According to behavioristic thinking, because mental content is not publicly observable, it cannot be subjected to rigorous scientific inquiry. Consequently, behaviorists developed a focus on overt behaviors and their environmental influences.

Today, different behavioral schools continue to share a focus on verifiable behavior. Behavioral views differ from cognitive views in holding that physical, rather than mental, events control behavior. According to behaviorism, mental phenomena or speculations about them are of little or no scientific interest.

HISTORY

As early as the 1920s, scattered reports about the application of learning principles to the treatment of behavioral disorders began to appear, but they had little effect on the mainstream of psychiatry and clinical psychology. Not until the 1960s did behavior therapy emerge as a systematic and comprehensive approach to psychiatric (behavioral) disorders; at that time, it arose independently on three continents. Joseph Wolpe and his colleagues in Johannesburg, South Africa, used pavlovian techniques to produce and eliminate experimental neuroses in cats. From this research, Wolpe developed systematic desensitization, the prototype of many current behavioral procedures for the treatment of maladaptive anxiety produced by identifiable stimuli in the environment. At about the same time, a group at the Institute of Psychiatry of the University of London, particularly Hans Jurgen Eysenck and M. B. Shapiro, stressed the importance of an empirical, experimental approach to understanding and treating individual patients, using controlled, single-case experimental paradigms and modern learning theory. The third origin of behavior therapy was work inspired by the research of Harvard psychologist B. F. Skinner. Skinner's students began to apply his operant-conditioning technology, developed in animal-conditioning laboratories, to human beings in clinical settings.

SYSTEMATIC DESENSITIZATION

Developed by Wolpe, systematic desensitization is based on the behavioral principle of counterconditioning, whereby a person overcomes maladaptive anxiety elicited by a situation or an object by approaching the feared situation gradually, in a psychophysiological state that inhibits anxiety. In systematic desensitization, patients attain a state of complete relaxation and are then exposed to the stimulus that elicits the anxiety response. The negative reaction of anxiety is inhibited by the relaxed state, a process called *reciprocal inhibition*. Rather than using actual situations or objects that elicit fear, patients and therapists prepare a graded list or hierarchy of anxiety-provoking scenes associated with a patient's fears. The learned relaxation state and the anxiety-provoking scenes are systematically paired in treatment. Thus, systematic desensitization consists of three steps: relaxation training, hierarchy construction, and desensitization of the stimulus.

Relaxation Training

As described in Section 35.7, relaxation produces physiological effects opposite to those of anxiety: slow heart rate, increased peripheral blood flow, and neuromuscular stability. A variety of relaxation methods have been developed. Some, such as yoga and Zen, have been known for centuries. Most methods use so-called progressive relaxation, developed by the psychiatrist Edmund Jacobson. Patients relax major muscle groups in a fixed order, beginning with the small muscle groups of the feet and working cephalad or vice versa. Some clinicians use hypnosis to facilitate relaxation or use tape-recorded exercise to allow patients to practice relaxation on their own. Mental imagery is a relaxation method in which patients are instructed to imagine themselves in a place associated with pleasant relaxed memories. Such images allow patients to enter a relaxed state or experience (as Herbert Benson termed it) the *relaxation response*.

The physiological changes that take place during relaxation are the opposite of those induced by the adrenergic stress responses that are part of many emotions. Muscle tension, respiration rate, heart rate, blood pressure, and skin conductance decrease. Finger temperature and blood flow to the finger usually increase. Relaxation increases respiratory heart rate variability, an index of parasympathetic tone.

Hierarchy Construction

When constructing a hierarchy, clinicians determine all the conditions that elicit anxiety, and then patients create a hierarchy list of 10 to 12 scenes in order of increasing anxiety. For example, an acrophobic hierarchy may begin with a patient's imagining standing near a window on the second floor and end with being on the roof of a 20-story building, leaning on a guard rail and looking straight down. Table 35.8-1 provides an example of a hierarchy construction for fear of water and heights.

Desensitization of the Stimulus

In the final step, called *desensitization*, patients proceed systematically through the list from the least, to the most, anxiety-provoking scene while in a deeply relaxed state. The rate at

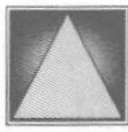

Table 35.8–1
Hierarchy Construction (Least Anxious to Most Anxious): Fear of Water and Heights

1. Taking a bath at home.
2. Taking a shower at home.
3. Going into the shallow end of the swimming pool.
4. Starting to swim at the shallow end of the swimming pool, breaststroke only.
5. Swimming at the shallow end, doing the crawl.
6. Jumping into the swimming pool at the shallow end.
7. Jumping into the pool and then doing the crawl.
8. Swimming at the shallow end, first breaststroke, then the crawl.
9. Pushing away from the bars and causing a splash.
10. Swimming in the middle of the pool at a depth of 5 feet 3 inches.
11. Swimming at the shallow end and then at the deep end (10 feet 3 inches).
12. Going into the deep end of the swimming pool.
13. Watching people jump from the diving boards.
14. Standing on a step at the deep end of the pool and making a little jump into the water.
15. Backstroke at the shallow end of the pool.
16. Jumping into the water at the shallow end of the pool (belly-flop dive).
17. Belly-flop dive at the deep end of the pool.
18. Racing dive at the shallow end of the pool.
19. Racing dive at the deep end of the pool.
20. Swimming three times across the deep end of the pool without stopping:
    (a) breaststroke
    (b) crawl
    (c) backstroke
21. Jumping into the pool at a depth of:
    (a) 5 feet 3 inches
    (b) 6 feet
    (c) 7 feet
22. Several jumps at 6 feet and 7 feet, alternating them, and then remaining at the 7-foot depth.
23. Going onto the first diving board and jumping into the water.
24. Jumping off the first diving board, then diving from the first board.
25. Diving off the first board.
26. Jumping from the first diving board, jumping from the second diving board, then diving from the first diving board.
27. Jumping off the first, second, and third diving boards, then diving from the first diving board.
28. Jumping off the first, second, and third diving boards, then diving from the first and then the second diving board.
29. Jumping off the fourth diving board, then diving off the second diving board.
30. Jumping off the fifth diving board, then diving off the third diving board.
31. Jumping off the fifth diving board, then diving off the fourth diving board.
32. Jumping off the top board, then diving off the fourth diving board.
33. Jumping off the top board, then diving off the fifth diving board.
34. Diving off the top diving board.
35. Random stimuli.
36. Looking around before jumping off the third diving board.
37. Looking around before jumping off the fourth diving board.
38. Looking around before jumping off the fifth diving board.
39. Diving from the fifth diving board and looking around before diving.
40. Diving from the top board and looking around before diving.

(From Kraft T. The use of behavior therapy in a psychotherapeutic context. In: Lazarus AA, ed. *Clinical Behavior Therapy*. New York: Brunner/Mazel; 1972:222, with permission.)

which patients progress through the list is determined by their responses to the stimuli. When patients can vividly imagine the most anxiety-provoking scene of the hierarchy with equanimity, they experience little anxiety in the corresponding real-life situation.

Adjunctive Use of Drugs

Clinicians have used various drugs to hasten relaxation, but drugs should be used cautiously and only by clinicians trained and experienced in potential adverse effects. Either the ultrarapidly acting barbiturate sodium methohexital (Brevital) or diazepam (Valium) is given intravenously in subanesthetic doses. If the procedural details are followed carefully, almost all patients find the procedure pleasant, with few unpleasant side effects. The advantages of pharmacological desensitization are that preliminary training in relaxation can be shortened, almost all patients can relax adequately, and the treatment itself seems to proceed more rapidly than without the drugs.

Indications

Systematic desensitization works best in cases of a clearly identifiable anxiety-provoking stimulus. Phobias, obsessions, compulsions, and certain sexual disorders have been treated successfully with this technique.

THERAPEUTIC-GRADED EXPOSURE

Therapeutic-graded exposure is similar to systematic desensitization, except that relaxation training is not involved and treatment is usually carried out in a real-life context. This means that the individual must be brought in contact with (i.e., be exposed to) the warning stimulus to learn firsthand that no dangerous consequences will ensue. Exposure is graded according to a hierarchy. Patients afraid of cats, for example, might progress from looking at a picture of a cat to holding one.

FLOODING

Flooding (sometimes called *implosion*) is similar to graded exposure in that it involves exposing the patient to the feared object in vivo; however, there is no hierarchy. Flooding is based on the premise that escaping from an anxiety-provoking experience reinforces the anxiety through conditioning. Thus, clinicians can extinguish the anxiety and prevent the conditioned avoidance behavior by not allowing patients to escape the situation. Clinicians encourage patients to confront feared situations directly, without a gradual buildup, as in systematic desensitization or graded exposure. No relaxation exercises are used, as in systematic desensitization. Patients experience fear, which gradually subsides after a time. The success of the procedure depends on having patients remain in the fear-generating situation until they are calm and feel a sense of mastery. Prematurely withdrawing from the situation or prematurely terminating the fantasized scene is equivalent to an escape, which then reinforces both the conditioned anxiety and the avoidance behavior and produces the opposite of the desired effect. In a variant, called *imaginal flooding*, the feared object or situation is confronted only in the imagination, not in real life. Many patients refuse flooding because of the psychological discomfort involved. It is also contraindicated when intense anxiety would be hazardous to a patient (e.g., those with heart disease or fragile psychological adaptation). The technique works best with specific phobias. An example of in vivo flooding follows.

The patient was a 33-year-old woman with social fears of eating in public. In particular, she was afraid of being observed by others when chewing and swallowing, particularly at dinner parties. A contrived situation was arranged in which the patient came to the session with a prepared meal and drink. She entered a conference room in which five persons in professional attire were already seated along a table. The patient was instructed to eat her meal in front of these individuals. Between bites, she was instructed to look at them often, and they had been instructed to avoid staring contests. She was not to distract herself from her anxiety symptoms. She was to eat her meal slowly, paying attention to the behavior of the observers and to her anxiety symptoms (e.g., dry mouth or difficulty swallowing). No conversation between the patient and observers was permitted. The observers would look at her and observe her chewing and swallowing behaviors, at times writing comments in a notebook. Occasionally, observers would communicate by whispering to each other, exchanging written notes, or giving knowing glances and smiles.

The only other communication occurred between the patient and therapist, and this was limited to the patient providing her subjective units of distress rating. The session lasted 90 minutes. **Note**: this situation may seem quite traumatizing. Because the exposure session is long and continues until ratings decline, the patient becomes desensitized. (Courtesy of Rolf G. Jacob, M.D., and William H. Pelham, M.D.)

PARTICIPANT MODELING

In participant modeling, patients learn a new behavior by imitation, primarily by observation, without having to perform the behavior until they feel ready. Just as irrational fears can be acquired by learning, they can be unlearned by observing a fearless model confront the feared object. The technique has been useful with phobic children who are placed with other children of their own age and sex who approach the feared object or situation. With adults, a therapist may describe the feared activity in a calm manner that a patient can identify. Or, the therapist may act out the process of mastering the feared activity with a patient. Sometimes, a hierarchy of activities is established, with the least anxiety-provoking activity being dealt with first. The participant-modeling technique has been used successfully with agoraphobia by having a therapist accompany a patient into the feared situation. In a variant of the procedure, called *behavior rehearsal*, real-life problems are acted out under a therapist's observation or direction.

The following is a self-report by a patient with a contamination phobia, who is afraid to touch objects for fear of being infected or contaminated. She describes her reactions.

[The therapist] started touching everything very slowly. I was told to follow behind and touch everything she touched. It was like we were spreading the contamination. She touched doorknobs, light switches, walls, pictures, and woodwork. She opened drawers in each bedroom and touched the contents. She opened closets and touched clothes hanging on the rods. She touched the towels and sheets in the linen closet. She went through the children's rooms, touching dolls, stuffed animals, models, Star Wars figures, Transformers, and books.

[The therapist] kept talking to me quietly and calmly all the time we went along. I had been anxious when we started, but as we continued, my anxiety level decreased. At one point, when I had begun to think the worst was over, she pointed to the attic door and said we were going inside. I said, "No, that's where the mice were." She told me I didn't want to have a place in my home that was off limits. I agreed but became very anxious. It was very hard for me to go inside. I began touching the boxes too, but I was very upset. Then, she put her hands down on the floor and wanted me to do the same. I said, "I can't. I just can't." Julie said, "Yes you can."

[The therapist] spent several hours with me that day. Before she left, she made a list of things for me to do by myself. Twice a day I was to go through the house touching everything the way she had done with me. I was to invite a friend of mine who had a pet to come and visit and also friends of my children who had pets. (Courtesy of Rolf G. Jacobs, M.D., and William H. Pelham, M.D.)

EXPOSURE TO STIMULI PRESENTED IN VIRTUAL REALITY

Advances in computer technology have made it possible to present environmental cues in virtual reality for exposure treatment. Beneficial effects have been reported with virtual reality exposure of patients with height phobia, fear of flying, spider phobia, and claustrophobia. Much experimental work is being done in the field. One model uses an avatar of the patient walking through a crowded supermarket filled with other avatars (including one of the therapists) as a way of conquering agoraphobia.

ASSERTIVENESS TRAINING

Assertiveness is defined as follows: Assertive behavior enables a person to act in his or her own best interest, to stand up for herself or himself without undue anxiety, to express honest feelings comfortably, and to exercise personal rights without denying the rights of others.

Two types of situations frequently call for assertive behaviors: (1) setting limits on pushy friends or relatives and (2) commercial situations, such as countering a sales pitch or being persistent when returning defective merchandise. Early assertiveness training programs tended to define specific behaviors as assertive or nonassertive. For example, individuals were encouraged to assert themselves if somebody got in front of them in a supermarket checkout line. Increasing attention is now given to context, that is, what would be assertive behavior in this situation depends on circumstances.

SOCIAL SKILLS TRAINING

The negative symptoms in patients with schizophrenia constitute behavioral deficits that go beyond difficulties with assertiveness.

These patients have inadequate expressive behaviors and inappropriate stimulus control of their social behaviors (i.e., they do not pick up social cues). Similarly, patients with depression often experience a lack of social reinforcement because of a lack of social skills, and social skills training has been found to be efficacious for depression. Patients with social phobia similarly often have not acquired adolescents' social skills. In fact, their social defensive behaviors (e.g., avoiding eye contact, making brief statements, and minimizing self-disclosure) increase the probability of the rejection that they fear.

Social skills training programs for patients with schizophrenia cover skills in the following areas: conversation, conflict management, assertiveness, community living, friendship and dating, work and vocation, and medication management. Each of these skills has several components. For example, assertiveness skills include making requests, refusing requests, making complaints, responding to complaints, expressing unpleasant feelings, asking for information, making apologies, expressing fear, and refusing alcohol and street drugs. Each component involves specific steps. For example, conflict management includes skills in negotiating, compromising, tactful disagreeing, responding to untrue accusations, and leaving overly stressful situations. A situation in which conflict management skills might be used is when the patient and a friend decide to go to a movie and their choice of movie differs.

Negotiating and compromising, for example, involves the following steps:

1. Explain one's viewpoint briefly.
2. Listen to the other person's viewpoint.
3. Repeat the other person's viewpoint.
4. Suggest a compromise.

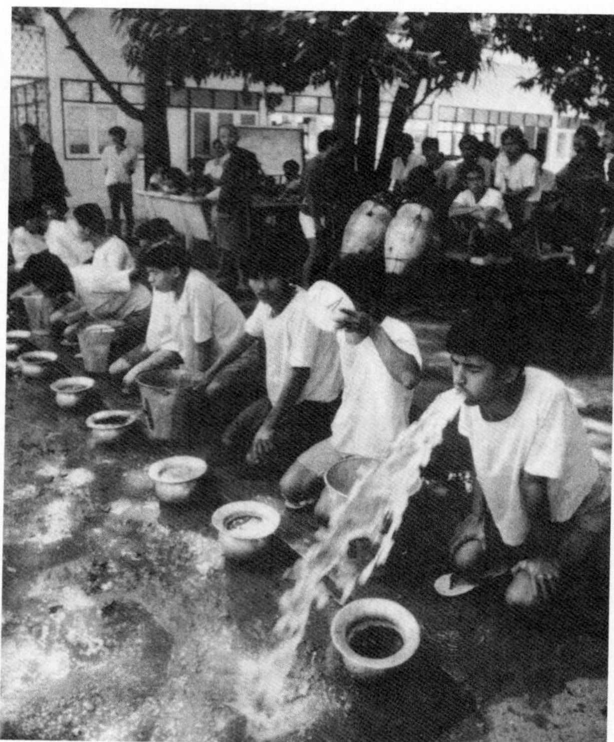

FIGURE 35.8–1

Treatment of addicts at Tham Krabok Monastery in Thailand results in a 70 percent success rate, according to its records. The 10-day free treatment begins with a vow to Buddha never to use narcotics again. Then, patients are given an herbal medicine that makes them vomit immediately. (From White PT, Raymer S. The poppy—for good and evil. *National Geographic.* 1985;167:187, with permission.)

AVERSION THERAPY

When a noxious stimulus (punishment) is presented immediately after a specific behavioral response, theoretically, the response is eventually inhibited and extinguished. Many types of noxious stimuli are used: electric shocks, substances that induce vomiting, corporal punishment, and social disapproval. The negative stimulus is paired with the behavior, which is thereby suppressed. The unwanted behavior may disappear after a series of such sequences. Aversion therapy has been used for alcohol abuse, paraphilias, and other behaviors with impulsive or compulsive qualities, but this therapy is controversial for many reasons. For example, punishment does not always lead to the expected decreased response and can sometimes be positively reinforcing. Aversion therapy has been used with good effect in some cultures in the treatment of opioid addicts (Fig. 35.8-1).

EYE MOVEMENT DESENSITIZATION AND REPROCESSING

Saccadic eye movements are rapid oscillations of the eyes that occur when a person tracks an object that is moved back and forth across the line of vision. A few studies have demonstrated that inducing saccades while a person is imagining or thinking about an anxiety-producing event can yield a positive thought or image that results in decreased anxiety. Eye movement desensitization and reprocessing has been used in posttraumatic stress disorders and phobias.

POSITIVE REINFORCEMENT

When a behavioral response is followed by a generally rewarding event, such as food, avoidance of pain, or praise, it tends to be strengthened and to occur more frequently than before the reward. This principle has been applied in a variety of situations. On inpatient hospital wards, patients with mental disorder receive a reward for performing a desired behavior, such as tokens that they can use to purchase luxury items or certain privileges. The process, known as token economy, has successfully altered behavior. Table 35.8-2 gives a summary of some clinical applications of behavior therapy.

RESULTS

Behavior therapy has been used successfully for a variety of disorders (Table 35.8-2) and can be easily taught (Table 35.8-3). It requires less time than other therapies and is less expensive to administer. Although useful for circumscribed behavioral symptoms, the method cannot be used to treat global areas of dysfunction (e.g., neurotic conflicts, personality disorders). Controversy

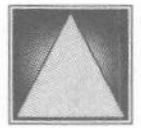

Table 35.8–2
Some Common Clinical Applications of Behavior Therapy

Disorder	Comments
Agoraphobia	Graded exposure and flooding can reduce the fear of being in crowded places. About 60% of patients so treated improve. In some cases, the spouse can serve as the model while accompanying the patient into the fear situation; however, the patient cannot get a secondary gain by keeping the spouse nearby and displaying symptoms.
Alcohol dependence	Aversion therapy in which the alcohol-dependent patient is made to vomit (by adding an emetic to the alcohol) every time a drink is ingested is effective in treating alcohol dependence. Disulfiram (Antabuse) can be given to alcohol-dependent patients when they are alcohol free. Such patients are warned of the severe physiological consequences of drinking (e.g., nausea, vomiting, hypotension, collapse) with disulfiram in the system.
Anorexia nervosa	Observe eating behavior; contingency management; record weight
Bulimia nervosa	Record bulimic episodes; log moods
Hyperventilation	Hyperventilation test; controlled breathing; direct observation
Other phobias	Systematic desensitization has been effective in treating phobias, such as fears of heights, animals, and flying. Social skills training has also been used for shyness and fear of other people.
Paraphilias	Electric shocks or other noxious stimuli can be applied at the time of a paraphilic impulse, and eventually the impulse subsides. Shocks can be administered by either the therapist or the patient. The results are satisfactory but must be reinforced at regular intervals.
Schizophrenia	The token economy procedure, in which tokens are awarded for desirable behavior and can be used to buy ward privileges, has been useful in treating inpatients with schizophrenia. Social skills training teaches patients with schizophrenia how to interact with others in a socially acceptable way so that negative feedback is eliminated. In addition, the aggressive behavior of some patients with schizophrenia can be diminished through those methods.
Sexual dysfunctions	Sex therapy, developed by William Masters and Virginia Johnson, is a behavior therapy technique used for various sexual dysfunctions, especially male erectile disorder, orgasm disorders, and premature ejaculation. It uses relaxation, desensitization, and graded exposure as the primary techniques.
Shy bladder	Inability to void in a public bathroom; relaxation exercises
Type A behavior	Physiological assessment, muscle relaxation, biofeedback (on electromyogram [EMG]

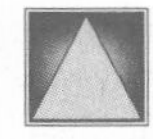

Table 35.8–3
Social Skills Competence Checklist of Therapist-Trainer Behaviors

1. Actively helps the patient set and elicit specific interpersonal goals.
2. Promotes favorable expectations, a therapeutic orientation, and motivation before role playing begins.
3. Assists the patient in building possible scenes in terms of "What emotion or communication?" "Who is the interpersonal target?" "Where and when?"
4. Structures the role playing by setting the scene and assigning roles to the patient and surrogates.
5. Engages the patient in behavioral rehearsal—getting the patient to role-play with others.
6. Uses self or other group members in modeling appropriate alternatives for the patient.
7. Prompts and cues the patient during the role playing.
8. Uses an active style of training through coaching, shadowing, being physically out of a seat, and closely monitoring and supporting the patient.
9. Gives the patient positive feedback for specific verbal and nonverbal behavioral skills.
10. Identifies the patient's specific verbal and nonverbal behavioral deficits or excesses and suggests constructive alternatives.
11. Ignores or suppresses inappropriate and interfering behavior.
12. Shapes behavioral improvements in small, attainable increments.
13. Solicits from the patient or suggests an alternative behavior for a problem situation that can be used and practiced during the behavioral rehearsal or role playing.
14. Evaluates deficits in social perception and problem solving and remedies them.
15. Gives specific attainable and functional homework assignments.

(Courtesy of Robert Paul Liberman, M.D., and Jeffrey Bedell, Ph.D.)

continues between behaviorists and psychoanalysts, which is epitomized by Eysenck's statement: "Learning theory regards neurotic symptoms as simply learned habits; there is no neurosis underlying the symptoms, but merely the symptom itself. Get rid of the symptom and you have eliminated the neurosis." Analytically-oriented theorists have criticized behavior therapy by noting that simple symptom removal can lead to symptom substitution: When symptoms are not viewed as consequences of inner conflicts and the core cause of the symptoms is not addressed or altered, the result is the production of new symptoms. Whether this occurs remains open to question, however.

BEHAVIORAL MEDICINE

Behavioral medicine uses the concepts and methods described above to treat a variety of physical diseases. Emphasis is placed on the role of stress and its influence on the body, particularly on the endocrine system. Attempts to relieve stress are made with the expectation that either the disease state will lessen or the patient's ability to tolerate the disease state will strengthen.

One study measured the effects of a behavioral medicine program on symptoms of acquired immunodeficiency syndrome (AIDS). The treatment group received training in biofeedback, guided imagery, and hypnosis. Results included significant decreases in fever, fatigue, pain, headache, nausea, and insomnia; and increased vigor and hardiness.

Another study of immunological and psychological outcomes of a stress reduction program was conducted with patients with malignant melanoma. Results included significant increases in large granular lymphocytes (defined as CD 57 with Leu-7) and natural killer (NK) cells (defined as CD16 with Leu-II and CD56 with NKHI), along with indications of increased NK cytotoxic activity. Also noted were significantly lower levels of psychological distress, and higher levels of positive coping methods in comparison with patients who were not part of the group.

Many other applications of behavior therapy are used in medical care. In general, most patients feel they benefit from such interventions, especially in their ability to cope with chronic illness. For a further discussion of behavioral medicine see Chapter 28: *Psychosomatic Medicine*.

References

Abramowitz JS, Whiteside S, Kalsy SA, Tolin DF. Thought control strategies in obsessive-compulsive disorder: A replication and extension. *Behav Res Ther.* 2003;41:529.

Bear RA. Mindfulness training as a clinical intervention. *Clin Psychol Sci Pract.* 2003;10:125.

Bisson JI. Single-session early psychological interventions following traumatic events. *Clin Psychol Rev.* 2003;23:481.

Emmons RA, Paloutzian RF. The psychology of religion. *Annu Rev Psychol.* 2003;54:377.

Gilbert C. Clinical applications of breathing regulation—Beyond anxiety management. *Behav Modif.* 2003;27:692.

Hanley GP, Iwata BA, McCord BE. Functional analysis of problem behavior, a review. *J Appl Behav Anal.* 2003;36:147.

Harmon-Jones E. Anger and the behavioral approach system. *Personality and Individual Differences.* 2003;995.

Harvey AG, Bryant RA, Tarrier N. Cognitive behaviour therapy for posttraumatic stress disorder. *Clin Psychol Rev.* 2003;23:501.

Haug TT, Blomhoff S, Hellstrom K, Holme I, Humble M, Madsbu HP, Wold JE. Exposure therapy and sertraline in social phobia: 1-year follow-up of a randomised controlled trial. *Br J Psychiatry.* 2003;182:312.

Havermans RC, Jansen ATM. Increasing the efficacy of cue exposure treatment in preventing relapse of addictive behavior. *Addict Behav.* 2003;28:989.

Hayes SC, Strosahl KD, Wilson KG. *Acceptance and Commitment Therapy: An Experiential Approach to Behavior Change.* New York: Guilford Press; 2003.

Jacob RG, Pelham WH. Behavior therapy. In: Sadock BJ, Sadock VA, eds. *Kaplan & Sadock's Comprehensive Textbook of Psychiatry.* 8th ed. Vol. 2. Baltimore: Lippincott Williams & Wilkins; 2005:2498.

Moulds ML, Nixon RD. In vivo flooding for anxiety disorders: Proposing its utility in the treatment of posttraumatic stress disorder. *J Anxiety Disord.* 2006;20(4): 498–509.

▲ 35.9 Cognitive Therapy

Cognitive therapy is a short-term, structured therapy that uses active collaboration between patient and therapist to achieve its therapeutic goals, which are oriented toward current problems and their resolution. Cognitive therapy is used with depression, panic disorder, obsessive-compulsive disorder, personality disorders, and somatoform disorders. Therapy is usually conducted on an individual basis, although group methods are sometimes helpful. A therapist may also prescribe drugs in conjunction with therapy.

The treatment of depression can serve as a paradigm of the cognitive approach.

Cognitive therapy assumes that perception and experiencing, in general, are active processes that involve both inspective and introspective data. The patient's cognitions represent a synthesis of internal and external stimuli. The way persons appraise a situation is generally evident in their cognitions (thoughts and visual images).

Those cognitions constitute their stream of consciousness or phenomenal field, which reflects their configuration of themselves, their world, their past, and their future.

Alterations in the content of their underlying cognitive structures affect their affective state and behavioral pattern. Through psychological therapy, patients can become aware of their cognitive distortions. Correction of faulty dysfunctional constructs can lead to clinical improvement.

COGNITIVE THEORY OF DEPRESSION

According to the cognitive theory of depression, cognitive dysfunctions are the core of depression, and affective and physical changes and other associated features of depression are consequences of cognitive dysfunctions. For example, apathy and low energy result from a person's expectation of failure in all areas. Similarly, paralysis of will stems from a person's pessimism and feelings of hopelessness. From a cognitive perspective, depression can be explained by the cognitive triad, which explains that negative thoughts are about the self, the world, and the future.

The goal of therapy is to alleviate depression and to prevent its recurrence by helping patients to identify and test negative cognitions, to develop alternative and more flexible schemas, and to rehearse both new cognitive and behavioral responses. Changing the way a person thinks can alleviate the psychiatric disorder.

STRATEGIES AND TECHNIQUES

Therapy is relatively short and lasts about 25 weeks. If a patient does not improve in this time, the diagnosis should be reevaluated. Maintenance therapy can be carried out over years. As with other psychotherapies, therapists' attributes are important to successful therapy. Therapists must exude warmth, understand the life experience of each patient, and be genuine and honest with themselves and with their patients. They must be able to relate skillfully and interactively with their patients. Cognitive therapists set the agenda at the beginning of each session, assign homework to be performed between sessions, and teach new skills. Therapist and patient collaborate actively (Table 35.9-1). The three components of cognitive therapy are didactic aspects, cognitive techniques, and behavioral techniques.

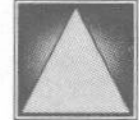

Table 35.9–1
Cognitive Psychotherapy

Goal	Identify and alter cognitive distortions that maintain symptoms
Selection criteria	Primarily used in dysthymic disorder Nonendogenous depressive disorders Symptoms not sustained by pathological family
Duration	Time-limited, usually 15 to 25 weeks, once-weekly meetings
Techniques	Collaborative empiricism Structured and directive Assigned readings Homework and behavioral techniques Identification of irrational beliefs and automatic thoughts Identification of attitudes and assumptions underlying negatively biased thoughts

Reprinted from Ursano RJ, Silberman EK. Individual psychotherapies. In: Talbott JA, Hales RE, Yudofsky SC, eds. *The American Psychiatric Press Textbook of Psychiatry.* Washington, DC: American Psychiatric Press; 1988:872, with permission.

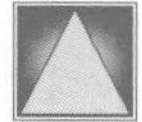

Table 35.9–2
Cognitive Profile of Psychiatric Disorders

Disorder	Core Belief
Depressive disorder	Negative view of self, experience, and future
Hypomanic episode	Inflated view of self, experience, and future
Anxiety disorders	Fear of physical or psychological danger
Panic disorder	Catastrophic misinterpretation of bodily and mental experiences
Phobias	Danger in specific, avoidable situations
Paranoid personality disorder	Negative bias, interference, and so forth by others
Conversion disorder	Concept of motor or sensory abnormality
Obsessive-compulsive disorder	Repeated warning or doubting about safety and repetitive acts to ward off threat
Suicidal behavior	Hopelessness and deficit in problem solving
Anorexia nervosa	Fear of being fat or unshapely
Hypochondriasis	Attribution of serious medical disorder

Courtesy of Aaron Beck, M.D., and A. John Rush, M.D.

Didactic Aspects

The therapy's didactic aspects include explaining to patients the cognitive triad, schemas, and faulty logic. Therapists must tell patients that they will formulate hypotheses together and test them over the course of the treatment. Cognitive therapy requires a full explanation of the relationship between depression and thinking, affect, and behavior, as well as the rationale for all aspects of treatment. This explanation contrasts with psychoanalytically oriented therapies, which require little explanation.

Cognitive Techniques

The therapy's cognitive approach includes four processes: eliciting automatic thoughts, testing automatic thoughts, identifying maladaptive underlying assumptions, and testing the validity of maladaptive assumptions.

Eliciting Automatic Thoughts. Automatic thoughts, also called cognitive distortions, are cognitions that intervene between external events and a person's emotional reaction to the event. For example, the belief that "people will laugh at me when they see how badly I bowl" is an automatic thought that occurs to someone who has been asked to go bowling and responds negatively. Another example is the thought, "She doesn't like me," when someone passes in the hall without saying, "Hello." Every psychopathological disorder has its own specific cognitive profile of distorted thought, which, if known, provides a framework for specific cognitive interventions (Table 35.9-2).

Testing Automatic Thoughts. Acting as a teacher, a therapist helps a patient test the validity of automatic thoughts. The goal is to encourage the patient to reject inaccurate or exaggerated automatic thoughts after careful examination. Patients often blame themselves when things that are outside their control go awry. The therapist reviews the entire situation with the patient and helps reassign the blame or cause of the unpleasant events. Generating alternative explanations for events is another way of undermining inaccurate and distorted automatic thoughts.

Identifying Maladaptive Assumptions. As the patient and therapist continue to identify automatic thoughts, patterns usually become apparent. The patterns represent rules or maladaptive general assumptions that guide a patient's life. Samples of such rules are "In order to be happy, I must be perfect" and "If anyone doesn't like me, I'm not lovable." Such rules inevitably lead to disappointments and failure and, ultimately, to depression (Fig. 35.9-1).

Testing the Validity of Maladaptive Assumptions. Testing the accuracy of maladaptive assumptions is similar to testing the validity of automatic thoughts. In a particularly effective test, therapists ask patients to defend the validity of their assumptions. For example, patients may state that they should always work up to their potential, and a therapist may ask, "Why is that so important to you?" Table 35.9-3 gives examples of some interventions designed to elicit, identify, test, and correct the cognitive distortions that lead to depressive and other painful affects.

BEHAVIORAL TECHNIQUES

Behavioral and cognitive techniques go hand in hand; behavioral techniques test and change maladaptive and inaccurate cognitions. The overall purposes of such techniques are to help patients understand the inaccuracy of their cognitive assumptions and learn new strategies and ways of dealing with issues.

Among the behavioral techniques in cognitive therapy are scheduling activities, mastery and pleasure, graded task assignments, cognitive rehearsal, self-reliance training, role-playing, and diversion techniques. One of the first things done in therapy is scheduling activities on an hourly basis. Patients keep records of the activities and review them with the therapist. In addition to scheduling activities, patients are asked to rate the amount of mastery and pleasure their activities bring them. Patients are often surprised to learn that they have much more mastery of activities and enjoy them more than they had thought.

To simplify the situation and allow mini accomplishments, therapists often break tasks into subtasks, as in graded task assignments, to show patients that they can succeed. In cognitive rehearsal, patients imagine and rehearse the various steps in meeting and mastering a challenge.

Patients (especially inpatients) are encouraged to become self-reliant by doing such simple things as making their own beds, doing their own shopping, and preparing their own meals. This process is called self-reliance training. Role-playing is a particularly powerful and useful technique to elicit automatic thoughts and to learn new behaviors. Diversion techniques are useful in helping patients get through difficult times and include physical activity, social contact, work, play, and visual imagery.

Imagery or thought stoppage can treat impulsive or obsessive behavior. For instance, patients imagine a stop sign with

AUTOMATIC THOUGHT RECORD

Directions: When you notice your mood getting worse, ask yourself, **"What's going through my mind right now?"** and as soon as possible jot down the thought or mental image in the Automatic Thoughts column.

DATE/ TIME	SITUATION	AUTOMATIC THOUGHT(S)	EMOTION(S)	ALTERNATIVE RESPONSE	OUTCOME
	1. What event, daydream, or recollection led to the unpleasant emotion? 2. What (if any) distressing physical sensations did you have?	1. What thought(s) and/or image(s) went through your mind? 2. How much did you believe each one at the time?	1. What emotion(s) (sad, anxious, angry, etc.) did you feel at the time? 2. How intense (0-100%) was the emotion?	1. (optional) What cognitive distortion did you make? (e.g., all-or-nothing thinking, mind-reading, catastrophizing) 2. Use questions at bottom to compose a response to the automatic thought(s). 3. How much do you believe each response?	1. How much do you now believe each automatic thought? 2. What emotion(s) do you feel now? How intense (0-100%) is the emotion? 3. What will or did you do?
Friday 7:30 PM	I called Sally to go out, as we talked about. I got her answering machine. Felt a sinking sensation.	1) They have all gone out and forgotten about me, because I'm not important to them anymore. (90% believable) 2) I'm left out again. (90% believable) 3) I'm going to have to spend another Friday night alone. (100% believable) 4) I just don't fit in anywhere in this world. (70% believable)	1) Angry (60% intensity) 2) Lonely (95% intensity) 3) Depressed (95% intensity)	I'm engaging in arbitrary inference, overgeneralization, personalization, and catastrophization. 1) It could all be an innocent misunderstanding. (40% believable) 2) I have spent a lot of time with Sally and the others and I know they like me. (60% believable) 3) Being at home alone is not the end of the world. (50% believable)	1) 30% 2) 10% 3) 50% 4) 0% Angry (5%) Lonely (40%) Depressed (20%) Calm (70%) I will call back in an hour if I don't hear from Sally.

Questions to help compose an alternative response: (1) What is the evidence that the automatic thought is true? Not true? (2) Is there an alternative explanation? (3) What's the worst that could happen? Could I live through it? What's the best that could happen? What's the most realistic outcome? (4) What's the effect of my believing the automatic thought? What could be the effect of changing my thinking? (5) What should I do about it? (6) If ___________ (friend's name) was in the situation and had this thought, what would I tell him/her?

FIGURE 35.9–1
Sample automatic thought record.

a police officer nearby or another image that evokes inhibition at the same time that they recognize an impulse or obsession that is alien to the ego. Similarly, obesity can be treated by having patients visualize themselves as thin, athletic, trim, and well muscled, and then training them to evoke this image whenever they have an urge to eat. Hypnosis or autogenic training can enhance such imagery. In a technique called guided imagery, therapists encourage patients to have fantasies that can be interpreted as wish fulfillments or attempts to master disturbing affects or impulses.

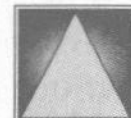

Table 35.9–3
Cognitive Errors Derived from Assumptions

Cognitive Error	Assumption	Intervention
Overgeneralizing	If it's true in one case, it applies to any case that is even slightly similar.	Exposure of faulty logic. Establish criteria of which cases are similar to what degree.
Selective abstraction	The only events that matter are failures, deprivation, etc. Should measure self by errors, weaknesses, etc.	Use log to identify successes patient forgot.
Excessive responsibility (assuming personal causality)	I am responsible for all bad things, failures, etc.	Disattribution technique.
Assuming temporal causality (predicting without sufficient evidence)	If it has been true in the past, it's always going to be true.	Expose faulty logic. Specify factors that could influence outcome other than past events.
Self-references	I am the center of everyone's attention—especially my bad performances. I am the cause of misfortunes.	Establish criteria to determine when patient is the focus of attention and also the probable facts that cause bad experiences.
Catastrophizing	Always think of the worst. It's almost likely to happen to you.	Calculate real probabilities. Focus on evidence that the worst did not happen.
Dichotomous thinking	Everything is either one extreme or another (black or white, good or bad).	Demonstrate that events may be evaluated on a continuum.

From Beck AT, Rush AJ, Shaw BF, Emery G. *Cognitive Therapy of Depression*. New York: Guilford Press; 1979:48, with permission.

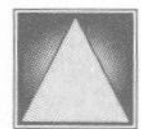

Table 35.9–4
Indications for Cognitive Therapy

Criteria that justify the administration of cognitive therapy alone:
- Failure to respond to adequate trials of two antidepressants
- Partial response to adequate dosages of antidepressants
- Failure to respond or only a partial response to other psychotherapies
- Diagnosis of dysthymic disorder
- Variable mood reactive to environmental events
- Variable mood that correlates with negative cognitions
- Mild somatoform disorders (sleep, appetite, weight, libidinal)
- Adequate reality testing (i.e., no hallucinations or delusions), span of concentration, and memory function
- Inability to tolerate medication effects or evidence that excessive risk is associated with pharmacotherapy

Features that suggest cognitive therapy alone is not indicated:
- Evidence of coexisting schizophrenia, dementia, substance-related disorders, mental retardation
- Patient has medical illness or is taking medication that is likely to cause depression
- Obvious memory impairment or poor reality testing (hallucinations, delusions)
- History of manic episode (bipolar I disorder)
- History of family member who responded to antidepressant
- History of family member with bipolar I disorder
- Absence of precipitating or exacerbating environmental stresses
- Little evidence of cognitive distortions
- Presence of severe somatoform disorders (e.g., pain disorder)

Indications for combined therapies (medication plus cognitive therapy):
- Partial or no response to trial of cognitive therapy alone
- Partial but incomplete response to adequate pharmacotherapy alone
- Poor compliance with medication regimen
- Historical evidence of chronic maladaptive functioning with depressive syndrome on intermittent basis
- Presence of severe somatoform disorders and marked cognitive distortions (e.g., hopelessness)
- Impaired memory and concentration and marked psychomotor difficulty
- Major depressive disorder with suicidal danger
- History of first-degree relative who responded to antidepressants
- History of manic episode in relative or patient

Adapted from Beck AT, Rush AJ, Shaw BF, Emery G. *Cognitive Therapy of Depression.* New York: Guilford Press; 1979:42.

EFFICACY

Cognitive therapy can be used alone in the treatment of mild to moderate depressive disorders or in conjunction with antidepressant medication for major depressive disorder. Studies have clearly shown that cognitive therapy is effective and in some cases is superior or equal to medication alone. It is one of the most useful psychotherapeutic interventions currently available for depressive disorders, and it shows promise in the treatment of other disorders.

Cognitive therapy has also been studied as a way of increasing compliance with lithium (Eskalith) prescription by patients with bipolar I disorder and as an adjunct in treating withdrawal from heroin. Table 35.9-4 outlines Beck's criteria for determining when cognitive therapy is indicated.

References

Beck AT, Freeman A, Davis DD. *Cognitive Therapy of Personality Disorders.* 2nd ed. New York: Guilford; 2003.

Beck AT, Newman CF. Cognitive therapy. In: Sadock BJ, Sadock VA, eds. *Kaplan & Sadock's Comprehensive Textbook of Psychiatry.* 8th ed. Vol 2. Baltimore: Lippincott Williams & Wilkins; 2005:2595.

Hollon SD. Does cognitive therapy have an enduring effect? *Cognit Ther Res.* 2003;27:71–75.

Lam DH, Watkins ER, Hayward P, Bright J, Wright K, Kerr N, Parr-Davis G, Pak S. A randomized controlled study of cognitive therapy for relapse prevention for bipolar affective disorder: Outcome of the first year. *Arch Gen Psychiatry.* 2003;60:145–152.

Leahy RL, ed. *Contemporary Cognitive Therapy: Theory, Research, and Practice.* New York: Guilford Press, 2004.

Rector NA, Seeman MV, Segal ZV. Cognitive therapy for schizophrenia: A preliminary randomized controlled trial. *Schiz Res.* 2003;63:1–11.

Reinecke MA, Clark DA. *Cognitive Therapy Across the Lifespan: Evidence and Practice.* Cambridge, UK: Cambridge University Press; 2003.

Sturmey P. On some recent claims for the efficacy of cognitive therapy for people with intellectual disabilities. *J of Applied Research in Intellectual Disabilities.* 2006;19:109-117.

▲ 35.10 Hypnosis

Hypnosis, in contemporary lay thought, is often steeped in mystery and its powers believed to border on magic. In reality, hypnosis is a powerful means of directing innate capabilities of imagination, imagery, and attention. During the hypnotic trace, focal attention and imagination are enhanced and simultaneously peripheral awareness is decreased. This trance may be induced by a hypnotist through formalized induction procedures, but it can also occur spontaneously. The capacity to be hypnotized and, relatedly, the occurrence of spontaneous trance states is a trait that varies between individuals, but is relatively stable throughout a person's life cycle.

HISTORY

Descriptions of trance states, ecstatic states, and spontaneous dissociative states abound in the Eastern and Western religious, literary, and philosophical traditions. Anton Franz Anton Mesmer (1734–1815) first formally described hypnosis as a therapeutic modality in the 18th century and believed it to be the result of a magnetic energy or an invisible fluid that the therapist channels into the patient to correct imbalances, restoring health. James Braid (1795–1860), an English physician and surgeon, used eye fixation and closure to induce trance states. Later, Dr. Jean Martin Charcot (1825–1893) theorized the hypnotic state to be a neurophysiologic phenomenon that was a sign of mental illness. Contemporaneously, Dr. Hippolyte Bernheim (1837–1919) believed it to be a function of the normal brain.

Early in his career, Dr. Sigmund Freud (1856–1939) used hypnosis as part of his psychoanalysis and noticed that patients in a trance could relive traumatic events, a process called *abreaction.* Later, Freud switched from hypnosis to free association because he wanted to minimize the transference that sometimes accompanies the trance state. Importantly, the switch did not eliminate the occurrence of spontaneous trance during the analysis.

World War I produced many shell-shocked soldiers and Dr. Ernst Simmel (1882–1947), a German psychoanalyst, developed a technique for accessing repressed material that he named *hypnoanalysis.* During World War II, hypnosis played a prominent role in the treatment of pain, combat fatigue, and neurosis. Formal recognition of hypnosis as a therapeutic modality did not occur, however, until the 1950s. The British Medical Society recommended its teaching in medical schools in 1955 and the American Medical Association and American Psychiatric Association officially stated its safety and efficacy in 1958.

DEFINITION

Hypnosis is currently understood as a normal activity of a normal mind through which attention is more focused, critical judgment is partially suspended, and peripheral awareness is diminished. The trance state, being a function of the subject's mind, cannot be forcibly projected by an outside person. The hypnotist, however, may aid in the achievement of the state and use its uncritical, intense focus to facilitate the acceptance of new thoughts and feelings, thereby accelerating therapeutic change. For the subject, hypnosis is typified by a feeling of involuntariness and movements seem automatic.

TRAIT OF HYPNOTIZABILITY

A person's degree of hypnotizability is a trait that is relatively stable throughout the life cycle and is measurable. The process of hypnosis takes the hypnotizability trait and transforms it into the hypnotized state. Experiencing the hypnotic concentration state requires a convergence of three essential components: absorption, dissociation, and suggestibility.

Absorption is an ability to reduce peripheral awareness that results in a greater focal attention. It can be metaphorically described as a psychological zoom lens that increases attention to the given thought or emotion to the increasing exclusion of all context, even including orientation to time and space.

Dissociation is the separating out from consciousness elements of the patient's identity, perception, memory, or motor response as the hypnotic experience deepens. The result is that components of self-awareness, time, perception, and physical activity can occur without being known to the patient's consciousness and so may seem involuntary.

Suggestibility is the tendency of the hypnotized patient to accept signals and information with a relative suspension of normal critical judgment; it is controversial whether critical judgment can be completely suspended. This trait will vary from an almost compulsive response to input in the highly hypnotizable to a sense of automaticity in the less hypnotizable individual. Table 35.10-1 lists the indicators of trance development.

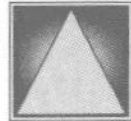

Table 35.10–1
Indicators of Trance Development

Autonomous ideation
Balanced tonicity (catalepsy)
Changed voice quality
Comfort, relaxation
Economy of movement
Eye changes/closure
Facial features ironed out
Feeling distant
Feeling good after trance
Lack of body movement
Lack of startle response
Literalism
Objective and impersonal ideation
Pupillary changes
Response attentiveness
Retardation of reflexes:
Swallowing
Blinking
Sensory, muscular, and body changes
Slowing pulse
Slowing and loss of blink reflex
Slowing respiration
Spontaneous hypnotic phenomena:
Amnesia
Anesthesia
Catalepsy
Regression
Time distortion
Time lag in motor and conceptual behavior

(From Erickson M, Rossi EL, Rossi SI. *Hypnotic Realities: The Induction of Clinical Hypnosis and Forms of Indirect Suggestion.* New York: Irvington; 1976:98, with permission.)

QUANTIFICATION OF HYPNOTIZABILITY

Quantifying a patient's degree of hypnotizability is useful in a clinical setting because it predicts the effectiveness of hypnosis as a therapeutic modality. Quantification also provides useful information about the way patients relate to themselves and the social environment. Highly hypnotizable patients have an increased incidence of spontaneous trance-like states and so may be unduly influenced by ideas and emotions that are not being appropriately self-critiqued.

NEUROPHYSIOLOGICAL CORRELATES OF HYPNOSIS

Neurological testing of individuals in the hypnotized state and those with a high degree of hypnotizability has led to some interesting findings, but no set of changes has been shown to be sensitive or specific for the trance state or hypnotizability trait.

Electroencephalographic (EEG) studies have shown that hypnotized persons exhibit electrical patterns that are similar to those of fully awake and attentive persons and not like those found during sleep. Increased alpha activity and theta power in the left frontal region has been reported in highly hypnotizable patients as compared with those who are less hypnotizable; these differences exist in the trance and nontrance states.

Positron emission tomography (PET) studies that compare regional blood flow in the brain in both hypnotized and nonhypnotized subjects lend further evidence to the hypothesis that hypnosis exerts some of its effects at lower level modalities of the brain. Hypnotic suggestions to add color to a visual image result in increased blood flow to the lingual and fusiform gyri, the color vision processing centers of the brain; suggestions to remove color have the opposite effect. Similarly, the intensity and noxiousness of pain are believed to be processed by different regions of the brain, because different areas of reduced blood flow result when each is minimized through hypnosis.

The role of the anterior brain regions, such as the frontal lobes, in hypnosis has been shown physiologically by the positive correlation between homovanillic acid concentrations in the cerebrospinal fluid and degree of hypnotizability. The frontal cortex and basal ganglia have a large number of neurons that use dopamine, of which the metabolite is homovanillic acid. This may explain why pharmacological enhancement of hypnotizability, although difficult, is primarily accomplished with dopaminergic agents, such as amphetamine. The increased activation of the basal ganglia may relate to the increased automaticity of hypnotic motor behavior.

CLINICAL ASSESSMENT OF HYPNOTIC CAPACITY

Two major procedures exist to clinically evaluate hypnotic capacity, the *Stanford Hypnotic Susceptibility Scale* and the *Hypnotic Induction Profile* (HIP) (Table 35.10-2). The *Stanford Hypnotic Susceptibility Scale* is a long laboratory-based test that has been modified for clinical evaluation and requires approximately 20 minutes to perform. It primarily measures behavioral compliance and suggestibility. The HIP is a shorter test that uses the eye roll sign as a biological indicator and measures cognitive flow, which differentiates those with no hypnotic capacity because of mental pathology from those mentally normal patients with any inherent hypnotic capacity (Fig. 35.10-1).

INDUCTION

Many different induction protocols follow the same basic principles and pattern, but may be better suited to the patients with different levels of hypnotizability.

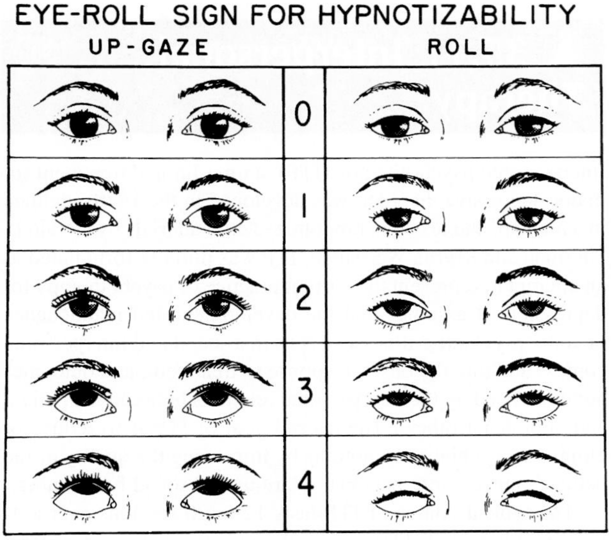

EYE-ROLL SIGN FOR HYPNOTIZABILITY

UP-GAZE | ROLL

0

1

2

3

4

FIGURE 35.10–1

Administration of the *Hypnotic Induction Profile* can be a routine part of the initial visit and evaluation. The test begins with the eye-roll sign, a presumptive measure of biological ability to experience dissociation. In the test procedure for eye-roll sign measurement, the patient is told "Hold your head looking straight forward; while holding your head in that position, look upward, toward your eyebrows—now toward the top of your head [up-gaze]. While continuing to look upward, close your eyelids slowly [roll]."

The up-gaze and roll are scored on a 0 to 4 scale by observing the amount of sclera visible between the lower eyelid and the lower edge of the cornea. If an internal squint occurs, the degree is scored on a 1 to 3 scale. The squint score is added to the roll score. This procedure takes about 5 seconds. The eye-roll is a part of the hypnotic induction, which is also scored as an initial indicator of the potential for hypnotic experience. (Courtesy of Herbert Spiegel, M.D., Marcia Greenleaf, Ph.D., and Davig Spiegel, M.D.).

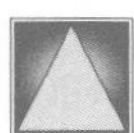

Table 35.10–2
HIP-derived Method of Self-Hypnosis

One, look up toward your eyebrows, all the way up; two, close your eyelids slowly and take a deep breath; count to three, exhale, let your eyes relax, and let your body float.

As you feel yourself floating, you permit one hand or the other to feel like a buoyant balloon and allow it to float upward. As it does, your elbow bends, and your forearm floats into an upright position. When your hand reaches this upright position, it becomes a signal for you to enter a state of meditation and to increase your receptivity to new thoughts and feelings.

In this state of meditation, you concentrate on this feeling of imaginary floating and, at the same time, concentrate on the following critical points (e.g., the three critical points to stop smoking in the following discussion).

Reflect on the implications of these critical points, and then bring yourself out of this state of concentration called self-hypnosis by counting backward in this manner: Three, get ready; two, with your eyelids closed, roll up your eyes (do it now); and, one, let your eyelids open slowly. Then, when your eyes are back in focus, slowly make a fist with the hand that is up; and, as you open your fist slowly, your usual sensation and control returns. Let your hand float down. That is the end of the exercise, but you can retain a general overall feeling of floating.

By doing this exercise ten different times each day, you can float into this state of buoyant repose. Give yourself this island of time, 20 seconds, ten times a day, in which to use this extra receptivity to reimprint these critical points. Reflect on them, then float back to your usual state of awareness, and then continue with what you ordinarily do.

HIP, Hypnotic Induction Profile.
(Herbert Spiegel M.D., Marcia Greenleaf Ph.D., David Spiegel M.D.)

Doctor: Take a long, deep, breath—inhale and exhale; now close your eyes and relax. Pay particular attention to the muscles in and about your eyes—relax them to the point that they just won't work. Are you trying to do that? Good. If you really have them relaxed, right at this very moment, no matter how hard you try, they just won't open. Test them. The harder you try, the faster they stick together, just as if they were glued together. That's fine!

Now you can open your eyes; that's good. When I tell you to and not before, open and close your eyes once more, and, when you close them this time, you will be ten times as relaxed as you are right now. Go ahead, open and close, and feel that surge of relaxation go through your whole body, from the top of your head to the tip of your toes. Very good!

Now once again, open and close your eyes, and this time, when you close them, you will double the relaxation that you now have. Fine.

If you have followed my suggestions, right at this very moment, when I lift your hand and let it drop into your lap, it will drop like a wet cloth, heavy and limp. That's very, very good.

You now have good physical relaxation, but medical relaxation consists of two phases: physical, which you now have, and mental, which I will now show you how to achieve.

When I ask you to and not before, I want you to start counting backward from 100. I know you can count; that is not what we're after. I just want you to relax mentally. As you say each number, pause momentarily until you feel a wave of relaxation cover your whole body, from the top of your head to the tip of your toes. When you feel this wave of relaxation, then say the next number, and each time you say a number, you will double the relaxation you had before you said the number. If you do this properly, an interesting thing will happen—as you say the numbers and relax, the succeeding numbers will start to disappear and vanish from your mind. Command your mind to dispel these numbers. Now, aloud and slowly, start counting backward from 100.

Patient: One hundred.

Doctor: Very good.

Patient: Ninety-nine.

Doctor: Make them start to disappear now.

Patient: Ninety-eight.

Doctor: Now they're fading away, and after the next number they'll all be gone. Make them disappear. Let the numbers go.

Patient: Ninety-seven.

Doctor: And now they're all gone. Are they gone? Fine. If there are any numbers still lurking in your mind, when I lift your hand and drop it, they will all disappear. (Courtesy of William Holt, M.D.)

INDICATIONS

A patient's degree of hypnotizability and the technique of hypnosis are clinically useful in diagnosis and in treatment, respectively.

The existence of spontaneous, trance-like states in everyday life and the potential of individuals to uncritically accept emotions and information in these states make a person's degree of hypnotizability a factor in the way the world is viewed and processed. A relationship is seen between various Axis I and Axis II conditions and hypnotizability. For example, patients with paranoid personality disorder are low and patients who are histrionic higher on the hypnotizability spectrum. Patients with dissociative identity disorder are highly hypnotizable. Patients with eating disorders are difficult to hypnotize.

Therapeutically, hypnosis' effectiveness in facilitating acceptance of new thoughts and feelings makes it useful in treating habitual problems and also with symptom management. Smoking, overeating, phobias, anxiety, conversion symptoms, and chronic pain are all indications for hypnosis. They can often be treated in a single session, in which a patient is taught to perform self-hypnosis. Hypnosis can also aid in psychotherapy, notably for posttraumatic stress disorder, and it has been used for memory retrieval.

CONTRAINDICATIONS

No intrinsic dangers to the hypnotic process exist. Because of the increased dependence that the hypnotized patient has towards the therapist, a strong transference may occur, however, in which the patient exhibits feelings for the therapist that are inappropriate in regards to their relationship. Strong attachments may occur and it is important that these are respected and properly interpreted. Negative emotions may also be brought out in the patient, especially those who are emotionally fragile or who have poor reality testing. To minimize the likelihood of this negative transference, caution should be taken when choosing patients who have problems with basic trust, such as those who are paranoid or who require high levels of control The hypnotized patient also has a reduced ability to critically evaluate hypnotic suggestions and, thus, the hypnotist must have a strong ethical value system. Controversy exists about whether patients can perform acts during a trance state that they would otherwise find repugnant or that run contrary to their moral system.

References

Faymonville ME, Roediger L, Del Fiore G, Delgueldre C, Phillips C, Lamy M, Luxen A, Maquet P, Laureys S. Increased cerebral functional connectivity underlying the antinociceptive effects of hypnosis. *Brain Res Cogn Brain Res.* 2003;17:255.

Finkelstein S. Rapid hypnotic inductions and therapeutic strategies in the dental setting. *Int J Clin Exp Hypn.* 2003;51:77.

Ginandes C, Brooks P, Sando W, Jones C, Aker J. Can medical hypnosis accelerate post-surgical wound healing? Results of a clinical trial. *Am J Clin Hypn.* 2003;45:333.

Gullickson T. Hypnosis and hypnotherapy with children. *PsycCRITIQUES.* 2004.

Liossi C, Hatira P. Clinical hypnosis in the alleviation of procedure-related pain in pediatric oncology patients. *Int J Clin Exp Hypn.* 2003;51:4.

Patterson DR, Jensen MP. Hypnosis and clinical pain. *Psychol Bull.* 2003;129:495.

Ploghaus A, Becerra L, Borras C, Borsook D. Neural circuitry underlying pain modulation: Expectation, hypnosis, placebo. *Trends in Cognitive Science.* 2003;7:197.

Raz A, Landzberg KS, Schweizer HR, Zephrani ZR, Shapiro T, Fan J, Posner MI. Posthypnotic suggestion and the modulation of Stroop interference under cycloplegia. *Conscious Cogn.* 2003;12:332.

Santarcangelo EL, Busse K, Carli G. Frequency of occurrence of the F wave in distal flexor muscles as a function of hypnotic susceptibility and hypnosis. *Brain Res Cogn Brain Res.* 2003;16:99.

Spiegel D. Negative and positive visual hypnotic hallucinations: Attending inside and out. *Int J Clin Exp Hypn.* 2003;51:130.

Spiegel H, Greenleaf M, Spiegel D. Hypnosis. In: Sadock BJ, Sadock VA, eds. *Kaplan & Sadock's Comprehensive Textbook of Psychiatry.* 8th ed. Vol. 2. Baltimore: Lippincott Williams & Wilkins; 2005:2548.

Spiegel H, Spiegel D. *Trance and Treatment: Clinical Uses of Hypnosis*, 2nd ed. Washington, DC: American Psychiatric Press; 2004.

▲ 35.11 Interpersonal Therapy

Interpersonal psychotherapy (ITP), a time-limited treatment for major depressive disorder, was developed in the 1970s, defined in a manual, and tested in randomized clinical trials by Gerald L. Klerman and Myrna Weissman. ITP was initially formulated as an attempt to represent the current practice of psychotherapy for depression. It assumes that the development and maintenance of some psychiatric illnesses occur in a social and interpersonal context and that the onset, response to treatment, and outcomes are influenced by the interpersonal relations between the patient and significant others. The overall goal of ITP is to reduce or eliminate psychiatric symptoms by improving the quality of the patient's current interpersonal relations and social functioning.

The typical course of ITP lasts 12 to 20 sessions over a 4- to 5-month period. ITP moves through three defined phases: (1) The initial phase is dedicated to identifying the problem area that will be the target for treatment; (2) the intermediate phase is devoted to working on the target problem area(s); and (3) the termination phase is focused on consolidating gains made during treatment and preparing the patients for future work on their own (Table 35.11-1).

TECHNIQUES

Individual Interpersonal Psychotherapy

Initial Phase. Sessions 1 through 5 typically constitute the initial phase of ITP. After assessing the patient's current psychiatric symptoms and obtaining a history of these symptoms,

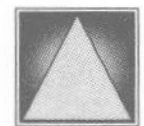

Table 35.11–1
Phases of Interpersonal Psychotherapy

Initial phase: sessions 1–5
- Give the syndrome a name; provide information about prevalence and characteristics of the disorder
- Describe the rationale and nature of interpersonal psychotherapy
- Conduct the interpersonal inventory to identify the current interpersonal problem area(s) associated with the onset or maintenance of the psychiatric symptoms
- Review significant relationships, past and present
- Identify interpersonal precipitants of episodes of psychiatric symptoms
- Select and reach consensus about the interpersonal psychotherapy problem area(s) and treatment plan with patient

Intermediate phase: sessions 6–15
- Implement strategies specific to the identified problem area(s)
- Encourage and review work on goals specific to the problem area
- Illuminate connections between symptoms and interpersonal events during the week
- Work with the patient to identify and manage negative or painful affects associated with his or her interpersonal problem area
- Relate issues about psychiatric symptoms to the interpersonal problem area

Termination phase: sessions 16–20
- Discuss termination explicitly
- Educate patient about the end of treatment as a potential time of grieving; encourage patient to identify associated emotions
- Review progress to foster feelings of accomplishment and competence
- Outline goals for remaining work; identify areas and warning signs of anticipated future difficulty
- Formulate specific plans for continued work after termination of treatment

the therapist gives the patient a formal diagnosis from the revised fourth edition of the *Diagnostic and Statistical Manual of Mental Disorders* (DSM-IV-TR). Therapist and patient then discuss the diagnosis, as well as what might be expected from treatment. Assignment of the sick role during this phase serves the dual function of granting the patient both the permission to recover and the responsibility to recover. The therapist explains the rationale of ITP, underscoring that therapy will focus on identifying and altering dysfunctional interpersonal patterns related to psychiatric symptomatology. To determine the precise focus of treatment, the therapist conducts an interpersonal inventory with the patient and develops an interpersonal formulation based on this. In the interpersonal formulation, the therapist links the patient's psychiatric symptomatology to one of the four interpersonal problem areas—grief, interpersonal deficits, interpersonal role disputes, or role transitions. The patient's concurrence with the therapist's identification of the problem area and agreement to work on this area are essential before beginning the intermediate treatment phase.

Intermediate Phase. The intermediate phase—typically sessions 8 to 10—constitutes the "work" of the therapy. An essential task throughout the intermediate phase is to strengthen the connections the patient makes between the changes he or she is making in his or her interpersonal life and the changes in his or her psychiatric symptoms. During the intermediate phase, the therapist implements the treatment strategies specific to the identified problem area as specified in Table 35.11-2.

Termination Phase. In the termination phase (usually, sessions 16 through 20), the therapist discusses termination explicitly with the patient and assists him or her in understanding that the end of treatment is a potential time of grief. During this phase, patients are encouraged to describe specific changes in their psychiatric symptoms, especially as they relate to improvements in the identified problem area(s). The therapist also assists the patient in evaluating and consolidating gains, detailing plans for maintaining improvements in the identified interpersonal problem area(s), and outlining remaining work for the patient to continue on his or her own. Patients are also encouraged to identify early warning signs of symptom recurrence and to identify plans of action.

Ms. G is a 51-year-old woman who presented for treatment of binge-eating disorder. She is college educated, has her own business, and is a divorced mother of one adult son in his early 20s. Before treatment, she had a body mass index (BMI) of 42 and had been binge eating approximately 10 to 15 days per month for the last 8 years. Along with her current diagnosis of binge-eating disorder, Ms. G struggled with recurrent major depression.

During the initial phase, Ms. G and her therapist began to review her history and the interpersonal events that were associated with her binge eating. Ms. G shared that she began overeating and gaining weight at age 14. When she was 18 years of age, she moved to a foreign country with her parents. Soon after the move, Ms. G's father left her and her mother to return to the United States. Ms. G was enraged at her father for leaving them and still gets very tearful and angry when discussing the separation. She and her mother decided to stay abroad, because she had started university and her mother was working. Both had developed strong social ties and felt comfortable in their new home. During this time, Ms. G continued to gain weight and started dieting. Shortly after graduating from university, Ms. G met and married a foreign national and, at the age of 28, delivered their only son. Two years later, she and her husband went through a very bitter divorce. Although Ms. G described this as a terrible time in her life, she maintained close ties with her friends and her mother. During this time, she began to diet and reached her lowest adult weight. At the age of 35, when her mother died of a heart condition, Ms. G had her first episode of major depression, which was treated and resolved with antidepressants and a brief course of psychotherapy. Although she had previous cycles of weight loss and weight regain, she did not evidence any sign of eating disturbance at this point. She continued to maintain close social ties and enjoyed her close relationship with her son. When Ms. G was in her early 40s, an economic downturn in her adopted country forced her to return to the United States. Having lost all of her savings, she struggled financially while she looked for work. During this time, she started binge eating and gaining weight. Within 1 year of this move, Ms. G's son decided to return to live with his father (who was very wealthy). Ms. G felt angry and betrayed. Yet, when her son would visit, she would assume a subservient role with him, because she was afraid of losing his affection. He, in turn, became quite demanding and critical of her. Before seeking treatment, her heightened feelings of isolation and loneliness were leading to increased binge eating, depression, and weight gain.

By session 3 of the initial phase, Ms. G's therapist began to consider which problem area would be the focus of the remainder of treatment. Ms. G had a history of important relationship losses and

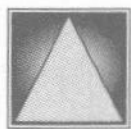

Table 35.11–2
Interpersonal Problem Areas: Description, Goals, and Strategies

Interpersonal Problem Area	Description	Goals	Strategies
Grief	Complicated bereavement after the death of a loved one	Facilitate the mourning process Help patient reestablish interest in new activities and relationships to substitute for what has been lost	Reconstruct the patient's relationship with the deceased Explore associated feelings (negative and positive) Consider ways of becoming reinvolved with others
Interpersonal deficits	A history of social impoverishment, inadequate or unsustaining interpersonal relationships	Reduce patient's social isolation Enhance quality of any existing relationships Encourage the formation of new relationships	Review past significant relationships, including negative and positive aspects Explore repetitive patterns in relationships Note problematic interpersonal patterns in the session and relate them to similar patterns in the patient's life
Interpersonal role disputes	Conflicts with a significant other—a partner, other family member, coworker, or close friend	Identify the nature of the dispute Explore options to resolve the dispute Modify expectations and faulty communication to bring about a satisfactory resolution If modification is unworkable, encourage patient to reassess the expectations for the relationship and to generate options to either resolve it or dissolve it and mourn its loss	Determine the stage of the dispute: renegotiation (calm down participants to facilitate resolution); impasse (increase disharmony to reopen negotiation); dissolution (assist mourning and adaptation) Understand how nonreciprocal role expectations relate to the dispute Identify available resources to bring about change in the relationship
Role transitions	Economic or family change—the beginning or end of a relationship or career, a move, promotion, retirement, graduation, diagnosis of a medical illness	Mourn and accept the loss of the old role Recognize the positive and negative aspects of the new role and assets and liabilities of the old role Restore self-esteem by developing a sense of mastery regarding the demands of the new role	Review positive and negative aspects of old and new roles Explore feelings about what is lost Encourage development of social support system and new skills called for in new role

(From Treasure J, Schmidt U, van Furth E. *Handbook of Eating Disorders.* 2nd ed. Hoboken, NJ: John Wiley & Sons; 2003:258, with permission.)

subsequent grief—the loss of her father, her husband, her mother, and, most recently, her son. However, none of these losses was associated with the development of binge-eating problems (although her dieting was clearly linked to her feelings of anger after the divorce from her husband and her depression was intimately linked with her mother's death). Ms. G's anger at her son for returning to live with the enemy was clearly a role dispute, yet her binge eating had begun 2 years before his departure (although it clearly worsened after he left). Because neither of these problem areas was directly linked to the onset of the eating disorder, Ms. G's therapist decided that the focus of treatment would be to assist her in managing her role transition. Her move back to the United States, with the subsequent loss of her support and friendship networks, was clearly associated with the onset and continued maintenance of her binge eating. During the fourth session of the initial phase, Ms. G's therapist shared her formulation of the problem area with her: From what you have described, your binge eating really began after you returned to the United States. After that transition, you were more isolated and alone than you have ever been. It seems that binge eating was a way for you to manage that transition and the subsequent feelings of isolation and loneliness. Your transition has also had a negative impact on your relationship with your son. Even though you are a very social person and enjoy the company of others, you have yet to develop the kind of support that you had before you moved. Although you have struggled with some very significant issues over the course of your life—your father leaving, the pain of the divorce, and the death of your mother—your friends and support systems sustained you. If we work together to help you find and develop more intimate and supportive relationships here, I believe you will be much less likely to turn to food and binge eating as a source of support or comfort.

Ms. G agreed with the formulation and worked with her therapist to establish some treatment goals to help her resolve the problem area. First, she was encouraged to become more aware of her feelings (especially isolation and loneliness) when she was binge eating and of how binge eating seemed to be the way she managed those feelings. A second goal was for her to take steps to increase her social contacts and develop more friendships. The third goal, which was identified as a secondary problem area, centered on helping Ms. G resolve the role dispute with her son. Specifically, the therapist developed a goal with her to help her establish a clearer parental role with her son.

During the intermediate phase, the therapist helped Ms. G grieve the loss of her previous role and the extensive support that she once had. Ms. G and her therapist worked to identify several sources of support and friendships of which she had not been aware. Soon after, Ms. G reported significant progress in initiating and establishing relationships with others. This change appeared to help give her confidence in her new roles. In fact, she had begun to receive a few social invitations. She was more attuned to the ways that she would rely on food, especially when she felt lonely or felt that she was not receiving enough time from others. The connection between the lack of supportive contacts and binge eating was becoming very clear to her in these intermediate sessions. During this phase, the therapist also assisted her in setting appropriate limits in her relationship with her adult son and in recognizing his adult-like responses in return. By the termination phase, Ms. G reported that she no longer felt so lonely and isolated and that her binge eating had all but disappeared. She remarked how the quality of her relationship with her son had changed dramatically. He was more supportive and respectful, visited more frequently, and stayed with her for longer periods of time. In the final sessions, she talked about her need to let go of the past and move on with her life as it is now, assuming her new roles more fully. She worked closely with her therapist to develop a plan to maintain the gains that she had made in treatment and used the final session to review the important work that she had accomplished. (Courtesy of Denise E. Wilfley, Ph.D.)

Interpersonal Psychotherapy Delivered in a Group Format

A recent approach in the ongoing development of ITP has been its use in a group format. ITP delivered in a group format has many potential benefits in comparison with individual treatment. For example, a group format in which membership is based on diagnostic similarity (e.g., depression, social phobia, eating disorders) can help alleviate patients' concerns that they are the only one with a particular psychiatric disorder, while offering a social environment for patients who have become isolated, withdrawn, or disconnected from others. Given the number and different types of interpersonal interactions in a group setting, the interpersonal skills that are developed may be more readily transferable to the patient's outside social life than are the relationship patterns that are addressed in a one-on-one setting. Moreover, a group modality has therapeutic features not present in individual psychotherapy (e.g., interpersonal learning). The group format also facilitates the identification of problems common to many patients and provides a cost-effective alternative to individual treatment. Table 35.11-3 links the phases of ITP to the stages of group development.

Timeline and Structure of Treatment. The typical course of group ITP lasts 20 sessions over a 5-month period. It is recommended that group size range from six to nine members, with one or two group leaders, depending on resources and training needs. The three individual meetings (pre-, mid-, and postgroup), sequenced to correspond with critical time points in the three phases of ITP, in combination with other techniques, were designed to maintain the exclusive and strategic focus on individual patients' interpersonal problem areas—the hallmark of ITP.

Pregroup Meeting. The pretreatment meeting is crucial for facilitating a patient's individualized work in the first phase of group ITP. The focus of the 2-hour pretreatment meeting is to identify interpersonal problem areas, establish an explicit treatment contract to work on problem areas, and prepare patients for group treatment. After identifying a patient's interpersonal problem(s) (i.e., interpersonal deficits, role disputes, role transitions, or grief), the therapist works collaboratively with the patient to formulate concrete prescriptions for change, in addition to the specific steps the patient will take to improve social relationships and patterns of relating. These goals of treatment are expressed in language that is as specific and personally meaningful to the patient as possible. Before the start of the group, each group

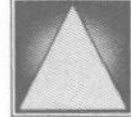

Table 35.11–3
Linking the Phases of Interpersonal Psychotherapy to the Stages of Group Development

Interpersonal Psychotherapy Phases/Tasks	Group Stages	Members' Work	Therapist Interventions
Initial: sessions 1–5; identify problem areas	Engagement: sessions 1–2	Members look for structure as they grapple with the anxiety of being in a group and sharing their problems.	Establish a structure that encourages appropriate self-disclosure. Facilitate norms for effective communication.
	Differentiation: sessions 3–5	Members work to manage negative feelings over interpersonal differences as they emerge in the group.	Help members understand their reactions in the context of interpersonal differences in their outside social lives.
Middle: sessions 6–15; work on goals	Work: sessions 6–15	Members work out differences and strive toward common goals.	Facilitate connections among members as they share their work with each other. Encourage practice of newly acquired interpersonal skills in and outside of the group.
Final: sessions 16–20; consolidate treatment	Termination: sessions 16–20	Members struggle with how to manage the impending loss of connection with other group members.	Help members to consolidate their work and to plan continued work. Assist members in grieving the loss of the group.

(From Wilfley DE, MacKenzie KR, Welch RR, et al. *Interpersonal Psychotherapy for Group.* New York: Basic Books; 2000:20, with permission.)

member is given a written summary of his or her goals and told that these goals will guide his or her work in the group.

Another important element of the pregroup meeting involves adequately preparing patients for group treatment. That is, patients are encouraged to think of the group as an "interpersonal laboratory" in which they can experiment with new approaches to handling challenging interpersonal situations. In this regard, patients are informed about the important interpersonal skills that are learned while participating in a group (e.g., interpersonal confrontation, honest communication, expression of feelings) and are encouraged to learn from others as they see changes occur. The therapist stresses to patients the importance of keeping their work in the group focused on changing their current interpersonal situations or intensifying important existing relationships and not using the group as a substitute social network.

Initial Phase. The first five sessions of the group treatment comprise the initial phase in group ITP. During this phase, the therapist works to cultivate positive group norms and group cohesion, while emphasizing the commonality of symptoms among members and how they will be addressed in the group context. During this phase, group members are encouraged to review their goals with the group and begin to make some initial changes in their respective interpersonal problem areas. As members begin to experiment with the changes outlined in their goals, the therapist works collaboratively with each group member to refine and make any alterations in the target areas before the beginning of the intermediate phase.

Intermediate Phase. During the intermediate "work" phase of group ITP (sessions 6 through 15), the therapist works to facilitate connections among members as they share the work on their goals with one another. In contrast to other interactive group approaches, the group interpersonal psychotherapist is much less likely to focus on intragroup processes and relationships unless they are specific to the work on a member's interpersonal problem area (e.g., interpersonal deficits). The therapist, however, consistently and continuously encourages group members to practice newly acquired interpersonal skills both inside and, most importantly, outside of the group. As is the case with individual ITP, an essential task throughout the intermediate phase is to strengthen the connections the group members make between difficulties in their interpersonal lives and their psychiatric problems.

MIDTREATMENT MEETING. The midtreatment meeting is held midway (usually between sessions 10 and 11) through the intermediate phase. This meeting provides an opportunity to conduct a detailed review of each group member's progress on his or her individual problems and to refine interpersonal goals. The therapist(s) recontract with group members during this meeting as a means of outlining and emphasizing the work that remains, both inside and outside of the group, before the conclusion of treatment.

Termination Phase. In the termination phase (sessions 16 through 20), the therapist discusses termination explicitly with the group members and begins to help them recognize that the end of treatment is a time of possible grief and loss. The therapist helps members recognize their own progress and the progress made by other group members. During this phase, group members are encouraged to describe the specific changes in their psychiatric symptoms, especially as they relate to improvements in the identified problem area(s) and relationships. Although it is common for group members to want to keep meeting on their own or to have frequent reunions, group members are encouraged to use this phase of the group to formally say goodbye to one another and to the therapist(s). The therapist(s) also uses this time to encourage members to detail their plans for maintaining improvements in their identified interpersonal problem area(s) and to outline their remaining work.

POSTTREATMENT MEETING. The posttreatment meeting is scheduled within 1 week after the final group session. The therapist(s) use this final individual meeting to develop an individualized plan for each group member's continued work on his or her interpersonal goals. The therapist(s) reviews the group experience and the changes the patient has made in his or her interpersonal problem area and significant relationships.

REFERENCES

Bolton P, Bass J, Neugebauer R, Verdeli H, Clougherty KF, Wickramaratne P, Speelman L, Ndogoni L, Weissman M. Group interpersonal psychotherapy for depression in rural Uganda: A randomized controlled trial. *JAMA*. 2003;289:3117.

Markowitz JC. Interpersonal psychotherapy for chronic depression. *J Clin Psychol*. 2003;59:847.

Miller MD, Frank E, Cornes C, Houck PR, Reynolds CF 3rd. The value of maintenance interpersonal psychotherapy (IPT) in older adults with different IPT foci. *Am J Geriatr Psychiatry*. 2003;11:97.

Spinelli MG, Endicott J. Controlled clinical trial of interpersonal psychotherapy versus parenting education program for depressed pregnant women. *Am J Psychiatry*. 2003;160:555.

Swartz HA, Frank E, Shear MK, Thase ME, Fleming MA, Scott J. A pilot study of brief interpersonal psychotherapy for depression among women. *Psychiatr Serv*. 2004;55:448.

Wilfley DE. Interpersonal psychotherapy. In: Sadock BJ, Sadock VA, eds. *Kaplan & Sadock's Comprehensive Textbook of Psychiatry*. 8th ed. Vol. 2. Baltimore: Lippincott Williams & Wilkins; 2005:2610.

▲ 35.12 Psychiatric Rehabilitation

Psychiatric rehabilitation denotes a wide range of interventions designed to help people with disabilities caused by mental illness improve their functioning and quality of life by enabling them to acquire the skills and supports needed to be successful in usual adult roles and in the environments of their choice. Normative adult roles include living independently, attending school, working in competitive jobs, relating to family, having friends, and having intimate relationships. Psychiatric rehabilitation emphasizes independence rather than reliance on professionals, community integration rather than isolation in segregated settings for persons with disabilities, and patient preferences rather than professional goals.

VOCATIONAL REHABILITATION

Impairment of vocational role performance is a common complication related to schizophrenia. Studies across the United States show that less than 15 percent of patients with severe mental illnesses, such as schizophrenia, are employed. Nevertheless, studies also show that competitive employment is a primary goal for 50 to 75 percent of patients with schizophrenia. Because of patient interests and historical factors, vocational rehabilitation has always been a centerpiece of psychiatric rehabilitation.

Antonio is a 45-year-old man who has been a client of a mental health agency for more than 10 years. He attended the rehabilitative day treatment program until it was converted to a supported employment program. His case manager encouraged him to think about the possibility of working part-time. Antonio told his case manager that he could not work because of his schizophrenia and because he was helping to raise his two kids and needed to be home at 3 PM, when they returned from school every day. The case manager explained to Antonio that getting a job does not necessarily mean working 40 hours a week and that lots of people in the agency's supported employment program were working in part-time jobs, even jobs that only require a few hours a week.

Antonio agreed to meet one of the employment specialists to discuss the possibility of work. Over the next couple of weeks, the employment specialist met with Antonio several times, read his clinical record, and talked with his case manager and psychiatrist. The employment specialist learned that Antonio loved to drive his car. He also learned that Antonio had attendance problems in past jobs because he felt unappreciated. The employment specialist found Antonio to be a sociable and likable person.

Antonio told the employment specialist that he was willing to do any job. He did not have one specific job in mind. After discussing options with Antonio and with the team, the employment specialist suggested a job at Meals on Wheels as a driver for the lunch delivery. Antonio was hired and loved it right from the start. Absenteeism was never a problem, because he liked driving around and knew that people were counting on him for their meals. The hours were perfect (10 AM to 2 PM), so he could be at home when his kids returned from school. He became good friends with the other workers. He told his case manager that it was wonderful to be bringing home a paycheck again. And best of all, he said, was that his kids saw him going to work just like their friends' dads. (Courtesy of Robert E. Drake, M.D., Ph.D., and Alan S. Bellack, Ph.D.)

SOCIAL SKILLS REHABILITATION

Social dysfunction is a defining characteristic of schizophrenia. People with the illness have difficulty fulfilling social roles, such as worker, spouse, and friend, and have difficulty meeting their needs when social interaction is required (e.g., negotiating with merchants, requesting assistance to solve problems). Social dysfunction is semi-independent of symptomatology and plays an important role in the course and outcome of the illness. As shown in Table 35.12-1, social competence is based on three component skills: (1) social perception, or receiving skills; (2) social cognition, or processing skills; and (3) behavioral response, or expressive skills. Social perception is the ability to read or decode social inputs accurately. This includes accurate detection of affect cues, such as facial expressions and nuances of voice, gesture, and body posture, as well as verbal content and contextual information. Social cognition involves effective analysis of the social stimulus, integration of current information with historical information, and planning of an effective response. This domain is also referred to as *social problem solving*.

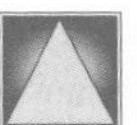

Table 35.12–1
Components of Social Skill

Expressive behaviors
Speech content
Paralinguistic features
Voice volume
Speech rate
Pitch
Intonation
Nonverbal behaviors
Eye contact (gaze)
Posture
Facial expression
Proxemics
Kinesics
Receptive skills (social perception)
Attention to and interpretation of relevant cues
Emotion recognition
Processing skills
Analysis of the situation demands
Incorporation of relevant contextual information
Social problem solving
Interactive behaviors
Response timing
Use of social reinforcers
Turn taking
Situational factors
Social "intelligence" (knowledge of social mores and the demands of the specific situation)

Methods

The primary modality of social skills training is role play of simulated conversations. The trainer first provides instructions on how to perform the skill and then models the behavior to demonstrate how it is performed. After identifying a relevant social situation in which the skill might be used, the patient engages in role play with the trainer. The trainer next provides feedback and positive reinforcement, which are followed by suggestions for how the response can be improved. The sequence of role play followed by feedback and reinforcement is repeated until the patient can perform the response adequately. Training is typically conducted in small groups (six to eight patients), in which case patients each practice role playing for three to four trials and provide feedback and reinforcement to one another. Teaching is tailored to the individual—for example, a highly impaired group member might simply practice saying "no" to a simple request, whereas a less cognitively impaired peer might learn to negotiate and compromise.

Richard was a single, white man first diagnosed with schizophrenia at age 22, when he was a freshman at college. He was hospitalized briefly but was unable to return to school and moved back home with his parents. He attended a day treatment program intermittently over the next 6 years, before he was referred for help with getting a job and dating.

Richard had missed out on a critical period of adult development and had never learned dating skills or the social skills needed to get or maintain a job. He was appropriately groomed and did not present himself as a patient, but he seemed quite uncomfortable in social interactions. He scarcely made eye contact, staring at the floor when he spoke, and did not initiate conversation, responding to questions with brief answers.

Richard was invited to participate in a social skills training group for 3 months with six other patients. The focus of the group was employment skills. Patients were taught critical social skills for getting and maintaining a job, such as how to participate in job interviews; how to approach a supervisor to understand how to do a job or for help with work-related problems; how and when to make requests or explain problems, such as getting to work late because of traffic or needing to leave early to go to a doctor's appointment; and socializing with coworkers. Simultaneously, Richard was enrolled in a supported employment program and worked with a case manager to find a job as a computer support person. He found a 24-hours-per-week job at a small company and continued to attend the skills group, using the sessions to work on interpersonal issues at work, including engaging in casual conversation with coworkers and dealing with unreasonable requests from people.

When the vocational skills group ended, Richard was scheduled for a dating group with seven other male and female patients who had similar interests. This group focused on finding someone to date, dating etiquette, asking someone out (or being asked out), appropriate conversation for dates, sexual interactions, and safe sex practices. In addition to role play and discussion, the group shared ideas on how to meet people and what to do on dates.

Richard responded well to treatment. He had maintained the computer job at follow-up, 6 months after he concluded the dating skills group. His case manger also reported that he had a girlfriend, a woman that he had met at his church group. He had also expressed an interest in enrolling in college classes at night. He was still living at home with his parents, but, for the first time, was seriously considering what he would need to do to move out. (Courtesy of Robert E. Drake, M.D., Ph.D., and Alan S. Bellack, Ph.D.)

Goals

In a treatment setting, there are four major goals of social skills training: (1) improved social skills in specific situations, (2) moderate generalization of acquired skills to similar situations, (3) acquisition or relearning of social and conversational skills, and (4) decreased social anxiety. Learning, however, is tedious or almost nonexistent when patients are floridly ill with positive symptoms and high levels of distractibility.

Some findings limit the applicability of social skills training. It is more difficult to teach complex conversational skills than to teach briefer, more discrete verbal and nonverbal responses in social situations. Because complex behaviors are more critical for generating social support in the community, methods have been developed to improve the learning and durability of conversational skills. These training methods, focusing on training in social skills and information-processing skills, are discussed below.

Training in Social Perception Skills. Recently, efforts have been made to develop strategies for training patients in affect and social cue recognition. Patients with chronic psychotic disorders, such as schizophrenia, often have difficulty perceiving and interpreting the subtle affective and cognitive cues that are critical elements of communication. Social perception abilities are considered the first step in effective interpersonal problem solving; difficulties in this area are likely to lead to a cascade of deficits in social behavior. Training skills in social perception address these deficits and help provide a foundation for developing more specific social and coping skills.

Despite attending several social gatherings, Matt felt apart from the rest of the group. He reported that these events seemed like "a jumble of sights and sounds." His therapist, recognizing Matt's difficulty with social perception, gave him a series of questions designed to help him organize and give meaning to the social stimuli he encountered. For example, when Matt was confused about a conversation someone was having with him, he would ask himself, "What is this person's short-term goal? At what level of disclosure should I be? Should I be talking now or listening?" Identifying the rules and goals of a particular social interaction provided a template for Matt to recognize, and react to, a greater variety of social cues, thus enhancing his behavioral repertoire. (Courtesy of Robert Paul Liberman, M.D., Alex Kopelowicz, M.D., and Thomas E. Smith, M.D.)

Information-Processing Model of Training. Methods of training that follow a cognitive perspective teach patients to use a set of generative rules that can be adapted for use in various situations. For example, a six-step problem-solving strategy has developed as an outline for helping patients overcome interpersonal dilemmas: (1) adopt a problem-solving attitude, (2) identify the problem, (3) brainstorm alternative solutions, (4) evaluate solutions and pick one to implement, (5) plan the implementation and carry it out, and (6) evaluate the efficacy of the effort and, if ineffective, choose another alternative. Although the step-wise, structured, linear process of problem solving occurs intuitively, without conscious awareness in normal persons, it can be a useful interpersonal crutch to help cognitively impaired mental patients cope with the information needed to fill their social and personal needs.

MILIEU THERAPY

The locus of milieu is a living, learning, or working environment. The defining characteristics of treatment are the use of a team to provide treatment and the time the patient spends in the environment. Recent adaptations of milieu therapy include 24-hour-a-day programs situated in community locales frequented by patients, which provide in vivo support, case management, and training in living skills.

Most milieu therapy programs emphasize group and social interaction; rules and expectations are mediated by peer pressure for normalization of adaptation. When patients are viewed as responsible human beings, the patient role becomes blurred. Milieu therapy stresses a patient's rights to goals and to have freedom of movement and informal relationship with staff; it also emphasizes interdisciplinary participation and goal-oriented, clear communication.

Token Economy

The use of tokens, points, or credits as secondary or generalized reinforcers can be seen as normalizing a mental hospital or day hospital environment with a program mimicking society's use of money to meet instrumental needs. Token economies establish the rules and culture of a hospital inpatient unit or partial hospitalization program, offering coherence and consistency to the interdisciplinary team as it struggles to promote therapeutic progress in difficult patients. These programs are challenging to establish, however, and their widespread dissemination has suffered because of the organizational prerequisites and the

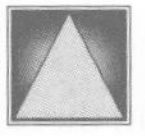

Table 35.12–2
Contingencies of Reinforcement in the Token Economy Used at the Camarillo–UCLA Clinical Research Unit[a]

Token earnings	
Morning rising from bed and getting dressed on time	3
Satisfactory completion of morning activities of daily living	3
Satisfactory participation in a social skills training group or recreational therapy activity	10
Satisfactory participation in individual behavioral therapy session	10
Satisfactory participation in leisure time activities (per activity)	5
Meets criteria for dress and grooming checks during day (per check)	3
Showers satisfactorily	3
Completes assigned jobs or tasks on unit (per job or task)	4
Participates in off-unit vocational rehabilitation or adult education activity (per half-day)	10
Token fines	
Smoking rule violation	5
Lying on floor	5
Stealing	10
Forgery of token credit card	10
Assault or property destruction	20
Late return from grounds privileges	20
Reinforcers available for tokens	
Cigarettes	4
Drinks (coffee, tea, sodas, hot chocolate)	10
Snacks (potato chips, pretzels, ice cream, candy)	10
Grounds privileges (per half-hour)	4
Music time (per half-hour)	4
Private room time (per half-hour)	4
Nintendo, Walkman stereo, private TV (per half-hour)	4

[a]This token economy uses a card that can be punched with holes to document token earnings and purchases. The token economy has three levels, which differ in the immediacy and type of reinforcement and privileges. At the highest level of performance, the patient carries a "credit card" and has full access to all unit privileges and rewards without having to pay with tokens.
(Courtesy of Robert Paul Liberman, M.D.)

additional resources and rewards needed to create a truly positively reinforcing environment. Table 35.12-2 lists behaviors that can be reinforced by tokens.

COGNITIVE REHABILITATION

Increased recognition of the prevalence and importance of neurocognitive deficits over the last decade has stimulated increasing interest in remediation strategies. Much of the work in this area has focused on psychopharmacological approaches, especially on the new-generation antipsychotics. New-generation medications appear to have a positive effect on neurocognitive test performance, but the effect size for any of the medications is small to medium, and little evidence indicates that these medications have a clinically meaningful impact on neurocognitive functioning in the community. As a result, a parallel interest has arisen in the potential for *rehabilitation* or *cognitive remediation*. This body of work is distinguished from cognitive-behavioral therapy and cognitive therapy, which focus on reducing psychotic symptoms.

A study at the National Institutes of Health (NIH) found that patients with schizophrenia were unable to benefit from explicit instructions and practice on the Wisconsin Card Sorting Test (WCST), a widely used test of executive functioning. The study was linked to data demonstrating that patients had diminished prefrontal blood flow in dorsolateral prefrontal cortex while responding to the WCST, implying that schizophrenia was marked by an unmodifiable abnormality of the dorsolateral prefrontal cortex. The NIH work stimulated a series of mostly successful laboratory demonstrations that WCST performance deficits, albeit widespread, are neither endemic to the illness nor immutable. For example, one study demonstrated that WCST performance could be enhanced by financial reinforcement and specific instructions. Other laboratories have since produced comparable and enduring effects using similar training strategies and extended practice alone.

ETHICAL ISSUES

The ethics of conducting rehabilitation strategies are generally the same as for conducting other psychotherapies. Two issues come up regularly, however: avoiding infantilization and maintaining confidentiality. The first concerns the risk of viewing the patient as unable to make adult choices, such as whether to participate in rehabilitation, where to live, whether or not to work, and whether or not to use drugs and alcohol. Although it may be more of a value than an ethical standard, psychiatric rehabilitation is based on the assumption that the practitioner and the patient are in a partnership to facilitate recovery and improve quality of life. The basic model involves collaboration and shared decision making and does not portray the practitioner as an authority or parental figure. When patients make what appear to be bad choices, the practitioner must consider the patient's right to choose and whether the choice is dangerous versus simply not the choice the practitioner would make. If the choice, in fact, is potentially harmful, a collaborative process of considering alternatives is more likely to produce good choices than an authoritative, admonitory approach.

Failure to consider the patient as a partner also leads to violations of confidentiality. Practitioners sometimes assume that they are the primary arbiters of what information to share with parents, other clinicians, and other agencies. In fact, in most circumstances that do not involve the safety of patients or others, the patient should be the arbiter of what information is shared with whom. For example, in supported employment, the patients always determine whether to disclose information about their illnesses to employers.

REFERENCES

Becker DR, Drake RE. *A Working Life for People with Severe Mental Illness*. New York: Oxford University Press; 2003.

Drake RE, Bellack AS. Psychiatric rehabilitation. In: Sadock BJ, Sadock VA, eds. *Kaplan & Sadock's Comprehensive Textbook of Psychiatry.* 8th ed. Vol. 1. Baltimore: Lippincott Williams & Wilkins; 2005:1476.

Ganju V. Implementation of evidence-based practices in state mental health systems: Implications for research and effectiveness studies. *Schizophr Bull.* 2003;29:125–131.

Mueser KT, Noordsy DL, Drake RE, Fox L. *Integrated Treatment for Dual Disorders: Effective Intervention for Severe Mental Illness and Substance Abuse.* New York: Guilford Press; 2003.

Twamley EW, Jeste DV, Bellack AS. A review of cognitive training in schizophrenia. *Schizophr Bull.* 2003;29(2):359–382.

▲ 35.13 Combined Psychotherapy and Pharmacology

The use of psychotropic drugs in combination with psychotherapy has become widespread. In fact, it has become the standard of care for many patients seen by psychiatrists. In this therapeutic approach, psychotherapy is augmented by the use of pharmacological agents. It should not be a system in which the therapist meets with the patient on an occasional or irregular basis to monitor the effects of medication or to make notations on a rating scale to assess progress or side effects; rather, it should be a system in which both therapies are integrated and synergistic. In many cases, it has been demonstrated that the results of combined therapy are superior to either type of therapy used alone. The term *pharmacotherapy-oriented psychotherapy* is used by some practitioners to refer to the combined approach. The methods of psychotherapy used can vary immensely and all can be combined with pharmacotherapy.

INDICATIONS FOR COMBINED THERAPY

A major indication for using medication when conducting psychotherapy, particularly for those patients with major mental disorders such as schizophrenia or bipolar disorder is that psychotropics reduce anxiety and hostility. This improves the patient's capacity to communicate and to participate in the psychotherapeutic process. Another indication for combined therapy is to relieve distress when the signs and the symptoms of the patient's disorder are so prominent that they require more rapid amelioration than psychotherapy alone may be able to offer. In addition, each technique may facilitate the other; psychotherapy may enable the patient to accept a much needed pharmacological agent, and the psychoactive drug may enable the patient to overcome resistance to entering or continuing psychotherapy (Table 35.13-1).

The reduction of symptoms, especially anxiety, does not decrease the patient's motivation for psychoanalysis or other insight-oriented psychotherapy. In practice, drug-induced symptom reduction improves communication and motivation. All therapies have a cognitive base, and anxiety generally interferes with the patient's ability to gain cognitive understanding of the illness. Drugs that decrease anxiety facilitate cognitive understanding. They improve attention, concentration, memory, and learning.

NUMBER OF TREATING CLINICIANS

Any number of clinicians can be involved in treatment of a psychiatric disorder. In *one-person therapy*, the psychiatrist provides individual psychotherapy and medication treatment. Multiperson therapy is a form of treatment in which one therapist (who may be a psychiatrist, psychologist, or a social worker) conducts psychotherapy while the other therapist (always a psychiatrist) prescribes medications. Other therapists may oversee marriage or family therapy or group therapy. The terms *cotherapy* or *triangular therapy* are sometimes used to describe permutations of multiperson therapy.

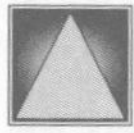

Table 35.13–1
Benefits of Combined Therapy

Improved medication compliance
Better monitoring of clinical status
Decreased number and length of hospitalizations
Decreased risk of relapse
Improved social and occupational functioning

Communication Among Therapists

Whenever more than one clinician is involved in treatment, there should be regular exchanges of information. Some patients split the transference between the two; one therapist may be seen as giving and nurturing, and the other may be seen as withholding and aloof. Similarly, countertransference issues, such as one therapist's identifying with the patient's idealized or devalued image of the other therapist, can interfere with therapy. Those issues must be worked out, and the cotherapists must be compatible and respectful of each other's orientation, so that the therapy program can succeed.

A therapist may have some concerns about the quality of the psychopharmacology or that the existing regimen needs to be reconsidered. For example, a patient may not be doing well on medication, experiencing significant side effects, or showing lack of sufficient improvement. Some patients may also be taking many different medications. When and if it is deemed in the patient's interest to question the medication regimen or the prescriber's skill, these misgivings should not be shared with the patient without first conferring with the prescribing physician.

If the therapist or pharmacologist, after a good-faith effort to understand the methods and course of treatment, still has misgivings about treatment, he or she should inform his or her counterpart that a second opinion would be useful. This should then be suggested to the patient without necessarily raising undue alarm. Communication between treating clinicians should take place as frequently as needed. No standard exists for how frequent that should be.

ORIENTATIONS OF TREATING CLINICIANS

The orientation of the treating psychiatrist or other clinician can influence the therapeutic process during combination treatment. Clinicians invariably bring a theoretical bias to the treatment setting. Some, for example, are oriented, by preference and training, to practice a specific form of psychotherapy, such as psychoanalysis, cognitive-behavioral therapy (CBT), or group therapy. To these clinicians, psychotherapy is seen as the primary treatment modality, with pharmacological agents being used as an adjunct. Conversely, to a psychopharmacologically oriented psychiatrist, psychotherapy is seen as augmenting the use of medication. Although disagreement may arise on which approach represents the most active ingredient in clinical response, the optimal use of both modalities should complement one another.

In addition to having extensive training in one or more psychoanalytic or psychotherapeutic techniques, the psychiatrist who practices pharmacotherapy-oriented psychotherapy must have a comprehensive knowledge of psychopharmacology. That knowledge must include a thorough understanding of the indications for the use of each drug, the contraindications, the pharmacokinetics and pharmacodynamics, the drug–drug interactions (with all pharmacological agents, not only the psychoactive agents), and the adverse effects of medications. The psychiatrist must be able both to identify adverse effects and to treat them.

Nonpsychiatric physicians often use psychoactive agents inaccurately (too small or too large a dose for too short or too long a course), because they lack the requisite psychopharmacological knowledge, training, and experience. Psychotherapists who work with primary care physicians instead of psychiatrists should understand the limitations in depth of knowledge that these practitioners have and should seek a consultation with a psychiatrist if a patient is not responding to, or tolerating, medication. In some

Table 35.13–2
Clinical Situations in Which It Is Advantageous for One Psychiatrist to Provide Medication and Psychotherapy

Patients with schizophrenia and other psychotic disorders who are not compliant with prescribed medication
Patients with bipolar I disorder who deny illness and do not cooperate with the treatment plan
Patients with serious or unstable medical conditions
Patients with severe borderline personality disorders
Impulsive and severely suicidal patients who are likely to require hospitalization
Patients with eating disorders who present complicated management problems
Patients who present a clinical picture in which the need for medication is unclear, thus requiring ongoing assessment

situations, it is preferable for psychotherapy and pharmacotherapy to be carried out by the same clinician; however, this is often not possible for a variety of reasons, including therapist availability, time limitations, and economic restraints, among others (Table 35.13-2).

Therapist Attitudes

Psychiatrists trained primarily as psychotherapists may prescribe medication more reluctantly than those who are more oriented to biological psychiatry. Conversely, those who view medication as the preferred intervention for most psychiatric disorders may be reluctant to refer patients for psychotherapy. Therapists who are pessimistic about the value of psychotherapy or who misjudge the patient's motivation may prescribe medications because of their own beliefs; others may withhold medication if they overvalue psychotherapy or undervalue pharmacological treatments. When a patient is in psychotherapy with someone other than the clinician prescribing medication, it is important to recognize treatment bias and to avoid contentious turf battles that put the patient in the middle of such conflict.

Linkage Phenomenon

At some point, patients may view the improvement being made in therapy as the result of a conscious or unconscious linkage between the psychopharmacological agent and the therapist. In fact, after being weaned from medication, patients often carry a pill with them for reassurance. In that sense, the pill acts as a transitional object between the patient and the therapist. Some patients with anxiety disorders, for example, may carry a single benzodiazepine tablet, which they take when they think that they are about to have an anxiety attack. Then, the patient may report that the attack was aborted—before the medication could even have been absorbed into the bloodstream. In other cases, the pill is never taken, because the patient knows that the pill is available and gains reassurance from that fact. The linkage phenomenon is usually not seen unless the patient is in a positive transference to the therapist. Indeed, the therapist may use this phenomenon to his or her advantage by suggesting that the patient carry medication to use as needed. Eventually, the behavior has to be analyzed, and often findings are that the patient has attributed magical properties to the therapist that are then transferred to the medication. Some clinicians believe the effect to be the result of conditioning. After repeated trials, the sight of the medicine can decrease anxiety. The positive transference may also cause *transference cure* or *flight into health*, in which the patient feels better in an unconscious attempt to meet the presumed expectations of the prescribing physician. Therapists should consider this phenomenon if the patient reports rapid improvement well before a particular medication may reach its therapeutic level.

COMPLIANCE AND PATIENT EDUCATION

Compliance

Compliance is the degree to which a patient carries out the recommendations of the treating physician. Compliance is fostered when the doctor–patient relationship is a positive one, and the patient's refusal to take medication may provide insight into a negative transferential situation. In some cases, the patient acts out hostilities by noncompliance, rather than by becoming aware of, and ventilating, such negative feelings toward the doctor. Medication noncompliance may provide the psychiatrist with the first clue that a negative transference is present in an otherwise compliant patient who had appeared to be agreeable and cooperative.

Education

Patients should know the target signs and symptoms that the drug is supposed to reduce, the length of time that they will be taking the drug, the expected and unexpected adverse effects, and the treatment plan to be followed if the current drug is unsuccessful. Although some psychiatric disorders interfere with patients' abilities to comprehend that information, the psychiatrist should relay as much of the information as possible. The clear presentation of such material is often less frightening than are patients' fantasies about drug treatment. The psychiatrist should tell patients when they may expect to begin to receive benefits from the drug. That information is most critical when the patient has a mood disorder and may not observe any therapeutic effects for 3 to 4 weeks.

Some patients' ambivalent attitudes toward drugs often reflect the confusion about drug treatment that exists in the field of psychiatry. Patients often believe that taking a psychotherapeutic drug means that they are not in control of their lives or that they may become addicted to the drug and have to take it forever. Psychiatrists should explain the difference between drugs of abuse that affect the normal brain and psychiatric drugs that are used to treat emotional disorders. They should also point out to patients that antipsychotics, antidepressants, and antimanic drugs are not addictive in the way in which, for example, heroin is addictive. The psychiatrist's clear and honest explanation of how long the patient should take the drug helps the patient adjust to the idea of chronic maintenance medication if that is the treatment plan. In some cases, the psychiatrist may appropriately give the patient increasing responsibility for adjusting the medications as the treatment progresses. Doing so often helps the patient feel less controlled by the drug and supports a collaborative role with the therapist.

ATTRIBUTION THEORY

Attribution theory is concerned with how persons perceive the causes of behavior. According to attribution theory, persons are likely to attribute changes in their own behavior to external events, but are likely to attribute another's behavior to internal dispositions, such as that person's personality traits. Research on drug effects by attribution theorists has shown that, when patients take medication and their behaviors change, they attribute it to the drug and not to any changes that occur within themselves. Accordingly, it may be unwise to describe a drug as extremely strong or effective, because, if it does have the desired effect, the patient may believe that is the only reason that he or she got better; if the drug does not work, he or she may assume his or her condition is incurable. Therapists do best by presenting the use of drugs and psychotherapy as complementary or adjunctive, as neither standing alone, and as both being needed for improvements or cure to occur.

MENTAL DISORDERS

Depressive Disorders

Some patients and clinicians fear that medication covers over the depression and that psychotherapy is impeded. Instead, medication should be viewed as a facilitator in overcoming the anergia that can inhibit a communication process between doctor and patient. The psychiatrist should explain to the patient that depression interferes with interpersonal activity in a variety of ways. For instance, depression produces withdrawal and irritability, which alienate significant others who may otherwise gratify the strong dependency needs that make up much of depressive psychodynamics.

If medication is stopped, the psychiatrist should be alert for signs and symptoms of a recurrent major depressive episode. Medication may have to be reinstituted. Before doing so, however, carefully review any stress, especially rejections, that could have precipitated recurrent major depressive disorder. A new episode of depression may occur because the patient is in a stage of negative transference, and the psychiatrist must try to elicit negative feelings. In many cases, the ventilation of angry feelings toward the therapist without an angry response can serve as a corrective emotional experience, and a major depressive episode necessitating medication can thereby be forestalled. Depressed patients are generally maintained on their medication for 6 months or longer after clinical improvement. The cessation of pharmacotherapy before that time is likely to result in a relapse.

Combined treatment has been shown to be superior to either therapy used alone in the treatment of major depression. It is associated with improved social and occupational functioning and improved quality of life compared with either therapy alone.

Bipolar I Disorder

Patients taking lithium or other treatments for bipolar I disorder are usually medicated for an indefinite period of time to prevent episodes of mania or depression. Most psychotherapists insist that patients with bipolar I disorder be medicated before starting any insight-oriented therapy. Without such premedication, most patients with bipolar I disorder are unable to make the necessary therapeutic alliance. When those patients are depressed, their abulia seriously disrupts their flow of thoughts, and the sessions are nonproductive. When they are manic, their flow of associations can be rapid, and their speech can be so pressured that the therapist may be flooded with material and may be unable to make appropriate interpretations or to assimilate the material into the patient's disrupted cognitive framework.

The practice guideline of the American Psychiatric Association (APA) for bipolar disorder recommend combined therapy as the best approach. It increases compliance, decreases relapse, and reduces the need for hospitalization.

Substance Abuse

Patients who abuse alcohol or drugs present the most difficult challenge in combined therapy. They are often impulsive, and, although they may promise not to abuse a substance, they may do so repeatedly. In addition, they frequently withhold information from the psychiatrist about episodes of abuse. For that reason, some psychiatrists do not prescribe any medication to such patients, especially not those substances with a high abuse potential, such as benzodiazepines, barbiturates, and amphetamines. Drugs with no abuse potential, such as amitriptyline (Elavil) and fluoxetine, have an important role in treating the anxiety or depression that almost always accompanies substance-related disorders. The psychiatrist conducting psychotherapy with such patients should have no reservations about sending the patient to a laboratory for random urine toxicological tests.

Anxiety Disorders

Anxiety disorders encompass obsessive-compulsive disorder (OCD), posttraumatic stress disorder (PTSD), generalized anxiety disorder, phobic disorders, and panic disorder with or without agoraphobia. Many drugs are effective in managing distressing signs and symptoms. As the symptoms are controlled by medication, patients are reassured and develop confidence that they will not be incapacitated by the disorder. That effect is particularly strong in panic disorder, which is often associated with anticipatory anxiety about the attack. Depression can also complicate the symptom picture in patients with anxiety disorders and has to be addressed pharmacologically and psychotherapeutically. Studies have shown that patients with anxiety disorders who receive ongoing psychotherapy are less likely to experience relapse compared with patients who receive medication alone.

Schizophrenia and Other Psychotic Disorders

Included in the group of schizophrenia and other disorders are schizophrenia, delusional disorder, schizoaffective disorder, schizophreniform disorder, and brief psychotic disorder. Drug treatment for those disorders is always indicated, and hospitalization is often necessary for diagnostic purposes, to stabilize medication, to prevent danger to self or others, and to establish a psychosocial treatment program that may include individual psychotherapy. In attempting individual psychotherapy, the therapist must establish a treatment relationship and a therapeutic alliance with the patient. The patient with schizophrenia defends against closeness and trust and often becomes suspicious, anxious, hostile, or regressed in therapy. Before the advent of psychotropics, many psychiatrists were fearful for their own safety when working with such patients. Indeed, many assaults occurred.

Individual psychotherapy for schizophrenia is labor intensive, expensive, and not often attempted. The recognition that combined psychotherapy and pharmacotherapy have a greater chance of success than does either type of therapy alone may reverse that situation. The psychiatrist who conducts such combined therapy must be especially empathic and must be able to tolerate the bizarre manifestations of the illness. The patient with schizophrenia is exquisitely sensitive to rejection, and individual psychotherapy should never be started unless the therapist is willing to make a total commitment to the process.

OTHER ISSUES

Evidence suggests that therapy can induce physical changes in the nervous system. Eric Kandel has provided elegant proof, winning the Nobel Prize for demonstrating that environmental stimuli produce lasting changes in the synaptic architecture of living organisms. Imaging studies have begun to show that patients who show clinical improvement from psychotherapy show changes in brain metabolism that are similar to that seen in patients successfully treated with medications.

Still, some patients do well on only one form of treatment. Even with identical diagnoses, not all patients respond to the same treatment regimens. Success may be as dependent on the knowledge and quality of the clinician as on the potential benefit of a particular drug.

A real dilemma when combining treatment is the additional direct costs of two treatments. Although successful treatment results in reduced costs to society, the cost of treatment is usually narrowly defined by the patient as out-of-pocket expenses and by insurance and managed care companies as payments to the physician or hospital. Restrictions placed on the frequency and cost of visits to mental health professionals by managed care organizations, however, encourage the use of medication rather than psychotherapy.

References

Arean PA, Cook BL. Psychotherapy and combined psychotherapy/pharmacotherapy for late life depression. *Biol Psychiatry.* 2002;52:293–303.

Anton RF, O'Malley SS, Ciraulo DA, Cisler RA, Couper D, Donovan DM, Gastfriend DR, Hosking JD, Johnson BA, LoCastro JS, Longabaugh R, Mason BJ, Mattson ME, Miller WR, Pettinati HM, Randall CL, Swift R, Weiss RD, Williams LD, Zweben A. Combined pharmacotherapies and behavioral interventions for alcohol dependence: The COMBINE study: A randomized controlled trial. *JAMA.* 2006;295:2003.

Beitman BD, Blinder BJ, Thase ME, Riba M, Safer DL. *Integrating Psychotherapy and Pharmacotherapy: Dissolving the Mind-Brain Barrier.* New York: WW Norton & Co.; 2003.

Brent DA, Birmhaher B. Adolescent depression. *N Engl J Med.* 2002;347:667–671.

Burnand Y, Andreoli A, Kolatte E, Venturini A, Rosset N. Psychodynamic psychotherapy and clomipramine in the treatment of major depression. *Psychiatr Serv.* 2002;53:585–590.

Friedman MA, Detweiler-Bedell JB, Leventhal HE, Horne R, Keitner GI, Miller IW. Combination psychotherapy and pharmacotherapy for the treatment of major depressive disorder. *Clinical Psychology: Science and Practice.* 2004;11:47–68.

Karon BP. *Effective Psychoanalytic Therapy of Schizophrenia and Other Severe Disorders.* Washington, DC: American Psychological Association; 2002.

Otto MW, Smits JAJ, Reese HE. Combination psychotherapy and pharmacotherapy for mood and anxiety disorders in adults: Review and analysis. *Clinical Psychology: Science and Practice.* 2005;12:72–86.

Overholser JC. Where has all the psyche gone? Searching for treatments that focus on psychological issues. *J Contemp Psychother.* 2003;33:49–61.

Preskorn SH. Psychopharmacology and psychotherapy: What's the connection? *J Psychiatr Pract.* 2006;12(1):41.

Ray WA, Daugherty JR, Meador KG. Effect of a mental health "carve-out" program on the continuity of antipsychotic therapy. *N Engl J Med.* 2003;348:1885–1894.

Sadock BJ, Sussman N. Combined psychotherapy and pharmacology. In: Sadock BJ, Sadock VA, eds. *Kaplan & Sadock's Comprehensive Textbook of Psychiatry.* 8th ed. Vol. 2. Baltimore: Lippincott Williams & Wilkins; 2005:2669.

Schmidt NB. Combining psychotherapy and pharmacological service provision for anxiety pathology. *Journal of Cognitive Psychotherapy.* 2005;19(4):307.

Ver Eecke W. In understanding and treating schizophrenia: A rejoinder to the PORT report's condemnation of psychoanalysis. *J Am Acad Psychanal.* 2003;31:11–29.

36 Biological Therapies

36.1 General Principles of Psychopharmacology

Psychopharmacologic advances continue dramatically to expand the parameters of psychiatric treatments. Greater understanding of how the brain functions has led to more effective, less toxic, better-tolerated, and more specifically targeted therapeutic agents. With the ever-increasing sophistication and array of treatment options, clinicians, however, must remain aware of potential adverse effects, drug–drug (and drug–food or drug–supplement) interactions, and how to manage the emergence of unwanted or unintended consequences. Newer drugs may lead ultimately to side effects that are not recognized initially. Keeping up with the latest research findings is increasingly important as these findings proliferate. A thorough understanding of the management of medication-induced side effects (either through treating the effect with another agent or substituting another primary agent) is necessary.

GUIDE TO USE

An alphabetical list of generic drug names is presented in Table 36.1–1, with cross-references to the sections in which they or their class is discussed.

CLASSIFICATION

Medications used to treat psychiatric disorders are referred to as *psychotropic drugs*. These drugs are commonly described by their major clinical application, for example, *antidepressants*, *antipsychotics*, *mood stabilizers*, *anxiolytics*, *hypnotics*, *cognitive enhancers*, and *stimulants*. A problem with this approach is that, in many instances, drugs have multiple indications. For example, drugs such as the selective serotonin reuptake inhibitors (SSRIs) are both antidepressants and anxiolytics, and the serotonin-dopamine antagonists (SDAs) are both antipsychotics and mood stabilizers.

Psychotropic drugs have also been organized according to structure (e.g., tricyclic), mechanism (e.g., monoamine oxidase inhibitor [MAOI]), history (e.g., first generation, traditional), uniqueness (e.g., atypical), or indication (e.g., antidepressant). A further problem is that many drugs used to treat medical and neurological conditions are routinely used to treat psychiatric disorders.

In addition, psychotropic drug terminology can be confusing. The first pharmaceutical agents used to treat schizophrenia were termed *tranquilizers*. When newer drugs emerged as therapies for anxiety, a distinction was drawn between *major* and *minor tranquilizers*. At first, antidepressants were tricyclic antidepressants (TCAs) or MAOIs. In the 1970s and 1980s, as newer antidepressant drugs emerged, they were labeled as *second-* or *third-generation antidepressants*. More recently, older agents used as treatments for psychosis became known as *typical*, *conventional*, or *traditional* neuroleptics. Newer ones became *atypical neuroleptics*. In order to eliminate much of this confusion, in this chapter, drugs are presented according to shared mechanism of action or by similarity of structure to provide consistency, ease of reference, and comprehensiveness.

PHARMACOLOGICAL ACTIONS

Both genetic and environmental factors influence individual response to, and tolerability of, psychotropic agents. Thus, a drug that may not prove effective in many patients with a disorder can dramatically improve symptoms in others. In these cases, identification of characteristics that might predict potential candidates for that drug becomes important, but often remains elusive.

Drugs, even within the same class, are distinguished from one another by often subtle differences in molecular structure, types of interactions with neurotransmitter systems, differences in pharmacokinetics, the presence or absence of active metabolites, and protein binding. These differences, combined with the biochemistry of the patient, account for the profile of efficacy, tolerability, and safety and the risk-to-benefit ratio for the individual. These multiple variables, some poorly understood, make it difficult to predict a drug's effect with certainty. Nevertheless, knowledge of the nature of each property increases the likelihood of successful treatment. The clinical effects of drugs are best understood in terms of pharmacokinetics, which describes *what the body does to a drug*, and pharmacodynamics, which describes *what the drug does to the body*.

Pharmacokinetics and pharmacodynamics need to be seen in the context of the underlying variability among patients with respect to how drug effects are expressed clinically. Patients differ in their therapeutic response to a drug and the experience of side effects. It is increasingly clear that these differences have a strong genetic basis. Pharmacogenetics research is attempting to identify the role of genetics in drug response.

DRUG SELECTION

Although all US Food and Drug Administration (FDA)-approved psychotropics are similar in overall effectiveness for their indicated disorder, they differ considerably in their pharmacology and in their efficacy and adverse effects on individual patients.

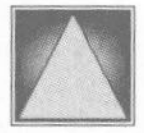

Table 36.1–1
Cross-References by Generic Name of Drug

Generic Name	Brand Name	Section Title	Section Number
Acamprosate	Campral	Disulfiram and Acamprosate	36.16
Acebutolol	Sectral	β-Adrenergic Receptor Antagonists	36.4
Acetophenazine	Tindal	Dopamine Receptor Antagonists (Typical Antipsychotics)	36.18
Alprazolam	Xanax	Benzodiazepines and Drugs Acting at Benzodiazepine Receptors	36.9
Amantadine	Symmetrel	Anticholinergics and Amantadine	36.5
Amitriptyline	Elavil, Endep	Tricyclics and Tetracyclics	36.34
Amlodipine	Lotrel, Norvasc	Calcium Channel Inhibitors	36.12
Amobarbital	Amytal	Barbiturates and Similarly Acting Drugs	36.8
Amoxapine	Asendin	Tricyclics and Tetracyclics	36.34
Amphetamine	—	Sympathomimetics and Related Drugs	36.31
Apomorphine	Apokyn	Dopamine Receptor Agonists and Precursors: Bromocriptine, Levodopa, Pergolide, Pramipexole, and Ropirinole	36.17
Aprobarbital	Alurate	Barbiturates and Similarly Acting Drugs	36.8
Aripiprazole	Abilify	Serotonin-Dopamine Antagonists (Atypical Antipsychotics)	36.30
Atenolol	Tenormin	β-Adrenergic Receptor Antagonists	36.4
Atomoxetine	Strattera	Sympathomimetics and Related Drugs	36.31
Benzphetamine	Didrex	Sympathomimetics and Related Drugs	36.31
Benztropine	Cogentin	Anticholinergics and Amantadine	36.5
Biperiden	Akineton	Anticholinergics and Amantadine	36.5
Brofaromine	Consonar	Monoamine Oxidase Inhibitors	36.23
Bromocriptine	Parlodel	Dopamine Receptor Agonists and Precursors: Bromocriptine, Levodopa, Pergolide, Pramipexole, and Ropirinole	36.17
Buprenorphine	Subutex	Opioid Receptor Agonists: Methadone, Levomethadyl, and Buprenorphine	36.25
Bupropion	Wellbutrin, Zyban	Bupropion	36.10
Buspirone	BuSpar	Buspirone	36.11
Butabarbital	Butisol	Barbiturates and Similarly Acting Drugs	36.8
Butalbital	—	Barbiturates and Similarly Acting Drugs	36.8
Butaperazine	Repoise	Dopamine Receptor Antagonists (Typical Antipsychotics)	36.18
Carbamazepine	Tegretol (Equetro)	Carbamazepine and Oxcarbazepine	36.13
Carbidopa	Lodosyn	Dopamine Receptor Agonists and Precursors: Bromocriptine, Levodopa, Pergolide, Pramipexole, and Ropirinole	36.17
Carisprodol	Soma	Barbiturates and Similarly Acting Drugs	36.8
Carphenazine	Proketazine	Dopamine Receptor Antagonists (Typical Antipsychotics)	36.18
Certirizine	Zyrtec	Antihistamines	36.7
Chloral hydrate	Noctec	Barbiturates and Similarly Acting Drugs	36.8
Chlorpromazine	Thorazine	Dopamine Receptor Antagonists (Typical Antipsychotics)	36.18
Chlorprothixene	Taractan	Dopamine Receptor Antagonists (Typical Antipsychotics)	36.18
Citalopram	Celexa	Selective Serotonin Reuptake Inhibitors	36.29
Clomipramine	Anafranil	Tricyclics and Tetracyclics	36.34
Clonazepam	Klonopin	Benzodiazepines and Drugs Acting at Benzodiazepine Receptors	36.9
Clonidine	Catapres	α_2-Adrenergic Receptor Agonists: Clonidine and Guanfacine	36.3
Clorgyline	—	Monoamine Oxidase Inhibitors	36.23
Clozapine	Clozaril	Serotonin-Dopamine Antagonists (Atypical Antipsychotics)	36.30
Cycrimine	Pagitane	Anticholinergics and Amantadine	36.5
Cyproheptadine	Periactin	Antihistamines	36.7
Dantrolene	Dantrium	Dantrolene	36.15
Desipramine	Norpramin, Pertofrane	Tricyclics and Tetracyclics	36.34
Desvenlafaxine	Pristiq	Selective Serotonin-Norepinephrine Reuptake Inhibitors	36.28
Dexfenfluramine	—	Sympathomimetics and Related Drugs	36.31
Dextroamphetamine	Dexedrine	Sympathomimetics and Related Drugs	36.31
Diazepam	Valium	Benzodiazepines and Drugs Acting at Benzodiazepine Receptors	36.9
Diethylpropion	Tenuate	Sympathomimetics and Related Drugs	36.31
Diltiazem	Cardizem	Calcium Channel Inhibitors	36.12
Diphenhydramine	Benadryl	Antihistamines	36.7
Disulfiram	Antabuse	Disulfiram and Acamprosate	36.16
Divalproex	Depakote	Valproate	36.35
Donepezil	Aricept	Cholinesterase Inhibitors	36.14
Doxepin	Adapin, Sinequan	Tricyclics and Tetracyclics	36.34
Droperidol	Inapsine	Dopamine Receptor Antagonists (Typical Antipsychotics)	36.18
Duloxetine	Cymbalta	Selective Serotonin–Norepinephrine Reuptake Inhibitors	36.28
Escitalopram	Lexapro	Selective Serotonin Reuptake Inhibitors	36.29
Estazolam	ProSom	Benzodiazepines and Drugs Acting at Benzodiazepine Receptors	36.9
Eszopiclone	Lunesta	Benzodiazepines and Drugs Acting at Benzodiazepine Receptors	36.9
Ethopropazine	Parsidol	Anticholinergics and Amantadine	36.5
Ethchlorvynol	Placidyl	Barbiturates and Similarly Acting Drugs	36.8
Ethinamate	Valmid	Barbiturates and Similarly Acting Drugs	36.8
Ethopropazine	Parsidol	Anticholinergics and Amantadine	36.5

(continued)

Table 36.1–1 (Continued)

Generic Name	Brand Name	Section Title	Section Number
Fenfluramine	Pondimin	Sympathomimetics and Related Drugs	36.31
Fexofenadine	Allegra	Antihistamines	36.7
Flumazenil	Romazicon	Benzodiazepines and Drugs Acting at Benzodiazepine Receptors	36.9
Fluoxetine	Prozac	Selective Serotonin Reuptake Inhibitors	36.29
Fluphenazine	Prolixin, Permitil	Dopamine Receptor Antagonists (Typical Antipsychotics)	36.18
Flurazepam	Dalmane	Benzodiazepines and Drugs Acting at Benzodiazepine Receptors	36.9
Fluvoxamine	Luvox	Selective Serotonin Reuptake Inhibitors	36.29
Gabapentin	Neurontin	Anticonvulsants: Gabapentin, Pregabalin, Tiagabine, Levetiracetam, Topiramate, and Zonisamide	36.6
Galanthamine	Reminyl	Cholinsterase Inhibitors	36.14
Glutethimide	Doriden	Barbiturates and Similarly Acting Drugs	36.8
Halazepam	Paxipam	Benzodiazepines and Drugs Acting at Benzodiazepine Receptors	36.9
Haloperidol	Haldol	Dopamine Receptor Antagonists (Typical Antipsychotics)	36.18
Hydroxyzine	Atarax, Vistaril	Antihistamines	36.7
Imipramine	Tofranil	Tricyclics and Tetracyclics	36.34
Indipon	—	Benzodiazepines and Drugs Acting at Benzodiazepine Receptor	36.9
Isocarboxazid	Marplan	Monoamine Oxidase Inhibitors	36.23
Isradipine	DynaCirc	Calcium Channel Inhibitors	36.12
Labetalol	Normodyne, Trandate	β-Adrenergic Receptor Antagonists	36.4
Lamotrigine	Lamictal	Lamotrigine	36.19
Levetiracetam	Keppra	Anticonvulsants: Gabapentin, Pregabalin, Tiagabine, Levetiracetam, Topiramate, and Zonisamide	36.6
Levodopa	Larodopa	Dopamine Receptor Agonists and Precursors: Bromocriptine, Levodopa, Pergolide, Pramipexole, and Ropirinole	36.17
Levomethadyl acetate	ORLAAM	Opioid Receptor Agonists: Methadone, Levomethadyl, and Buprenorphine	36.25
Levothyroxine	Levoxine, Levothroid, Synthroid	Thyroid Hormones	36.32
Liothyronine	Cytomel	Thyroid Hormones	36.32
Lithium	Eskalith, Lithobid, Lithonate	Lithium	36.20
Loratadine	Claritin	Antihistamines	36.7
Lorazepam	Ativan	Benzodiazepines and Drugs Acting at Benzodiazepine Receptors	36.9
Loxapine	Loxitane	Dopamine Receptor Antagonists (Typical Antipsychotics)	36.18
Maprotiline	Ludiomil	Tricyclics and Tetracyclics	36.34
Mazindol	Mazanor, Sanorex	Sympathomimetics and Related Drugs	36.31
Memantine	Namenda	Cholinesterase Inhibitors	36.14
Mephobarbital	Mebaral	Barbiturates and Similarly Acting Drugs	36.8
Meprobamate	Miltown	Barbiturates and Similarly Acting Drugs	36.8
Mesoridazine	Serentil	Dopamine Receptor Antagonists (Typical Antipsychotics)	36.18
Metformin	Glucophage	General Principles of Psychopharmacology	36.1
Methadone	Dolophine, Methadone	Opioid Receptor Agonists: Methadone, Levomethadyl, and Buprenorphine	36.25
Methamphetamine	Desoxyn	Sympathomimetics and Related Drugs	36.31
Metharbital	Gemonil	Barbiturates and Similarly Acting Drugs	36.8
Methohexital	Brevital	Barbiturates and Similarly Acting Drugs	36.8
Methylphenidate	Ritalin	Sympathomimetics and Related Drugs	36.31
Methyprylon	Noludar	Barbiturates and Similarly Acting Drugs	36.8
Metoprolol	Lopressor, Toprol	β-Adrenergic Receptor Antagonists	36.4
Midazolam	Versed	Benzodiazepines and Drugs Acting at Benzodiazepine Receptors	36.9
Milnacipran	—	Selective Serotonin-Norepinephrine Reuptake Inhibitors	36.28
Mirtazapine	Remeron	Mirtazapine	36.22
Moclobemide	Manerix	Monoamine Oxidase Inhibitors	36.23
Modafinil	Provigil	Sympathomimetics and Related Drugs	36.31
Molindone	Moban	Dopamine Receptor Antagonists (Typical Antipsychotics)	36.18
Nadolol	Corgard	β-Adrenergic Receptor Antagonists	36.4
Nalmefene	Revex	Opioid Receptor Antagonists: Naltrexone and Nalmefene	36.26
Naloxone	Narcan	Opioid Receptor Antagonists: Naltrexone and Nalmefene	36.26
Naltrexone	ReVia	Opioid Receptor Antagonists: Naltrexone and Nalmefene	36.26
Nefazodone	Serzone	Nefazodone	36.24
Nifedipine	Adalat, Procardia	Calcium Channel Inhibitors	36.12
Nimodipine	Nimotop	Calcium Channel Inhibitors	36.12
Nortriptyline	Pamelor, Aventyl	Tricyclics and Tetracyclics	36.34
Olanzapine	Zyprexa	Serotonin-Dopamine Antagonists (Atypical Antipsychotics)	36.30
Orphenadrine	Norflex, Dispal	Anticholinergics and Amantadine	36.5
Oxazepam	Serax	Benzodiazepines and Drugs Acting at Benzodiazepine Receptors	36.9
Oxcarbazepine	Trileptal	Carbamazepine and Oxcarbazepine	36.13
Oxybutyin	Ditropan	General Principles of Psychopharmacology	36.1
Paliperidone	Invega	Serotonin-Dopamine Antagonists (Atypical Antipsychotics)	36.30
Paraldehyde	PARAL	Barbiturates and Similarly Acting Drugs	36.8

(continued)

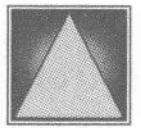

Table 36.1–1 (Continued)

Generic Name	Brand Name	Section Title	Section Number
Paroxetine	Paxil	Selective Serotonin Reuptake Inhibitors	36.29
Pemoline	Cylert	Sympathomimetics and Related Drugs	36.31
Pentobarbital	Nembutal	Barbiturates and Similarly Acting Drugs	36.8
Pergolide	Permax	Dopamine Receptor Agonists and Precursors: Bromocriptine, Levodopa, Pergolide, Pramipexole, and Ropirinole	36.17
Perphenazine	Trilafon	Dopamine Receptor Antagonists (Typical Antipsychotics)	36.18
Phendimetrazine	Adipost, Bontril	Sympathomimetics and Related Drugs	36.31
Phenelzine	Nardil	Monoamine Oxidase Inhibitors	36.23
Phenmetrazine	Prelude	Sympathomimetics and Related Drugs	36.31
Phenobarbital	Solfoton, Luminal	Barbiturates and Similarly Acting Drugs	36.8
Phentermine	Adipex-P, Fastin, Ionamine	Sympathomimetics and Related Drugs	36.31
Pimozide	Orap	Dopamine Receptor Antagonists (Typical Antipsychotics)	36.18
Pindolol	Visken	β-Adrenergic Receptor Antagonists	36.4
Piperacetazine	Quide	Dopamine Receptor Antagonists (Typical Antipsychotics)	36.18
Prazepam	Centrax	Benzodiazepines and Drugs Acting at Benzodiazepine Receptors	36.9
Pregabalin	Lyrica	Anticonvulsants: Gabapentin, Pregabalin, Tiagabine, Levetiracetam, Topiramate, and Zonisamide	36.6
Prochlorperazine	Compazine	Dopamine Receptor Antagonists (Typical Antipsychotics)	36.18
Procyclidine	Kemadrin	Anticholinergics and Amantadine	36.5
Promazine	Sparine	Dopamine Receptor Antagonists (Typical Antipsychotics)	36.18
Promethazine	Phenergan	Antihistamines	36.7
Propranolol	Inderal	β-Adrenergic Receptor Antagonists	36.4
Protriptyline	Vivactil	Benzodiazepines and Drugs Acting at Benzodiazepine Receptors	36.9
Quazepam	Doral	Benzodiazepines and Drugs Acting at Benzodiazepine Receptors	36.9
Quetiapine	Seroquel	Serotonin-Dopamine Antagonists (Atypical Antipsychotics)	36.30
Ramelteon	Rozerem	Melatonin Agonists: Ramelteon and Melatonin	36.21
Reboxetine	Edronax, Norebox	Selective Serotonin Reuptake Inhibitors	36.29
Reserpine	Diupres	Dopamine Receptor Antagonists (Typical Antipsychotics)	36.18
Risperidone	Risperdal	Serotonin-Dopamine Antagonists (Atypical Antipsychotics)	36.30
Rivastigmine	Exelon	Cholinsterase Inhibitors	36.14
Ropinirole	Requip	Dopamine Receptor Agonists and Precursors: Bromocriptine, Levodopa, Pergolide, Pramipexole, and Ropirinole	36.17
Secobarbital	Seconal	Barbiturates and Similarly Acting Drugs	36.8
Selegiline	Eldepryl	Monoamine Oxidase Inhibitors	36.23
Selegiline Patch	EmSam	Monoamine Oxidase Inhibitors	36.23
Sertraline	Zoloft	Selective Serotonin Reuptake Inhibitors	36.29
Sildenafil	Viagra	Phosphodiesterase-5 Inhibitors	36.27
Sulpiride	Dogmatil, Sesif	Dopamine Receptor Antagonists (Typical Antipsychotics)	36.18
Tacrine	Cognex	Cholinesterase Inhibitors	36.14
Temazepam	Restoril	Benzodiazepines and Drugs Acting at Benzodiazepine Receptor	36.9
Thiopental	Pentothal	Barbiturates and Similarly Acting Drugs	36.8
Thioridazine	Mellaril	Dopamine Receptor Antagonists (Typical Antipsychotics)	36.18
Thiothixene	Navane	Dopamine Receptor Antagonists (Typical Antipsychotics)	36.18
Tiagabine	Gabitril	Anticonvulsants: Gabapentin, Pregabalin, Tiagabine, Levetiracetam, Topiramate, and Zonisamide	36.6
Topiramate	Topamax	Anticonvulsants: Gabapentin, Pregabalin, Tiagabine, Levetiracetam, Topiramate, and Zonisamide	36.6
Tranylcypromine	Parnate	Monoamine Oxidase Inhibitors	36.23
Trazodone	Desyrel	Trazodone	31.28
Triazolam	Halcion	Benzodiazepines and Drugs Acting at Benzodiazepine Receptor	36.9
Trifluoperazine	Stelazine	Dopamine Receptor Antagonists (Typical Antipsychotics)	36.18
Triflupromazine	Vesprin	Dopamine Receptor Antagonists (Typical Antipsychotics)	36.18
Trihexyphenidyl	Artane	Anticholinergics and Amantadine	36.5
Trimipramine	Surmontil	Tricyclics and Tetracyclics	36.34
Valproic acid	Depakene	Valproate	36.35
Vardenafil	Levitra	Phosphodiesterase-5 Inhibitors	36.27
Venlafaxine	Effexor	Selective Serotonin–Norepinephrine Reuptake Inhibitors	36.28
Verapamil	Calan, Isoptin	Calcium Channel Inhibitors	36.12
Vigabatrin	Sabril	Anticonvulsants: Gabapentin, Pregabalin, Tiagabine, Levetiracetam, Topiramate, and Zonisamide	36.6
Yohimbine	Yocon	Yohimbine	36.36
Zaleplon	Sonata	Benzodiazepines and Drugs Acting at Benzodiazepine Receptors	36.9
Ziprasidone	Geodon	Serotonin-Dopamine Antagonists (Atypical Antipsychotics)	36.30
Zolpidem	Ambien	Benzodiazepines and Drugs Acting at Benzodiazepine Receptors	36.9
Zonisamide	Zonegran	Anticonvulsants: Gabapentin, Pregabalin, Tiagabine, Levetiracetam, Topiramate, and Zonisamide	36.6

The clinician should always consult *Physicians' Desk Reference* (PDR) or contact the manufacturer of the drug for the latest information on toxicity and lethality.

The ability of a drug to prove effective, thus, is only partially predictable and is dependent on poorly understood patient variables. Nevertheless, it is possible that some drugs have a niche in which they can be uniquely helpful for a subgroup of patients, without demonstrating any overall superiority in efficacy. No drug is universally effective, and no evidence indicates the unambiguous superiority of any single agent as a treatment for any major psychiatric disorders. The only exception, clozapine, has been approved by the FDA as a treatment for cases of treatment-refractory schizophrenia.

Decisions about drug selection and use are made on a case-by-case basis, relying on the individual judgment by the physician. Other factors in drug selection are the characteristics of the drug and the nature of the patients illness. Each of these components affects the probability of a successful outcome.

DRUG FACTORS

Pharmacodynamics

The time course and intensity of a drug's effects are referred to as its *pharmacodynamics*. Major pharmacodynamic considerations include receptor mechanisms, the dose-response curve, the therapeutic index, and the development of tolerance, dependence, and withdrawal phenomena. Drug mechanism of action is subsumed under pharmacodynamics. The clinical response to a drug, including adverse reactions, results from an interaction between that drug and a patient's susceptibility to those actions. Pharmacogenetic studies are beginning to identify genetic polymorphisms linked to individual differences in treatment response and sensitivity to side effects.

Mechanisms

The mechanisms through which most psychotropic drugs produce their therapeutic effects remain poorly understood. Standard explanations focus on ways that drugs alter synaptic concentrations of dopamine, serotonin, norepinephrine, histamine, γ-aminobutyric acid (GABA), or acetylcholine. These changes are said to result from receptor antagonists or agonists, interference with neurotransmitter reuptake, enhancement of neurotransmitter release, or inhibition of enzymes. Specific drugs are associated with permutations or combinations of these actions. For example, a drug can be an agonist for a receptor, thus stimulating the specific biological activity of the receptor, or an antagonist, thus inhibiting the biological activity. Some drugs are partial agonists, because they are not capable of fully activating a specific receptor. Some psychotropic drugs also produce clinical effects through mechanisms other than receptor interactions. For example, lithium can act by directly inhibiting the enzyme inositol-1-phosphatase. Some effects are closely linked to a specific synaptic effect. For example, most medications that treat psychosis share the ability to block the dopamine type 2 (D_2) receptor. Similarly, benzodiazepine agonists bind a receptor complex that contains benzodiazepine and GABA receptors.

Accounts of so-called mechanisms of action should nevertheless be kept in perspective. Explanations of how psychotropic drugs actually work that focus on synaptic elements represent an oversimplification of a complex series of events. If merely raising or lowering levels of neurotransmitter activity is associated with the clinical effects of a drug, then all drugs that cause these changes should produce equivalent benefits. This is not the case. Multiple obscure actions, several steps removed from events at neuronal receptor sites, are probably responsible for the therapeutic effects of psychotropic drugs. These *downstream* elements are postulated to represent the actual reasons that these drugs produce clinical improvement. A glossary of terms related to receptor drug interactions is given in Table 36.1–2.

SIDE EFFECTS

Side effects are an unavoidable risk of medication treatment. Although it is impossible to have an encyclopedic knowledge of all possible adverse drug effects, prescribing clinicians should be familiar with the more common adverse effects, as well as those with serious medical consequences. No single text or document, including the product information, contains a complete list of possible treatment-emergent events.

Side effect considerations include the probability of its occurrence, its impact on a patient's quality of life, its time course, and its cause. Just as no one drug is certain to produce clinical improvement in all patients, no side effect, no matter how common, occurs in every patient. When concurrent medical disorders or a history of a similar adverse reaction puts a patient at increased risk for a side effect, it is logical to consider prescribing a compound not typically associated with that adverse reaction.

Side effects can result from the same pharmacological action that is responsible for a drug's therapeutic activity or from an unrelated property. In examples of the latter, some of the most common adverse effects of the TCAs are caused by blockade of muscarinic acetylcholine receptors or histamine 2 receptors. If a patient is sensitive to these effects, alternative agents without these properties should be prescribed. When side effects are manifestations of the drug's presumed mechanism of action, side effects may be unavoidable. Thus, blockade of serotonin reuptake by SSRIs can cause nausea and sexual dysfunction. The D_2 blockade of drugs used to treat psychosis can cause extrapyramidal side effects. Agonist action of benzodiazepine receptors can cause ataxia and daytime sleepiness. In these cases, additional medications are frequently used to make the primary agent better tolerated.

Time Course

Adverse effects differ in terms of their onset and duration. Some side effects appear at the outset of treatment and then rapidly diminish. Nausea occurring with SSRIs or venlafaxine (Effexor) and sedation occurring with mirtazapine (Remeron) are good examples of early, time-limited side effects. Early-onset, but persistent, side effects include dry mouth that is associated with noradrenergic reuptake inhibition or antimuscarinic activity. Some side effects appear later in treatment (*late-appearing side effects*) and, sometimes, may be just the opposite of adverse events early in treatment. For example, patients may typically lose weight during early treatment with SSRIs, only to find, over time, a reversal occurs, so that they gain weight. Similarly, early activation or agitation may be followed by constant fatigue or apathy. Because most data about new drugs come from short-term studies, generally 8 weeks in duration, early-onset side effects are overrepresented in product information and descriptions of newly marketed information. It is essential that clinicians follow the letters to the editor sections of journals and other sources of

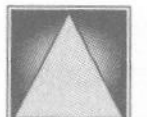

Table 36.1–2
Glossary of Receptor Drug Interactions

Receptor Interaction	Definition	Examples and Comments
Agonist (Full Agonist)	A drug or medication that binds to a specific receptor producing an effect identical to that usually produced by the neurotransmitter affecting that receptor. Drugs are often designed as receptor agonists to treat a variety of diseases and disorders in which the original neurotransmitter is missing or diminished.	Full agonists include opioids such as morphine, methadone, oxycodone, hydrocodone, heroin, codeine, meperidine, propoxyphene, and fentanyl. Benzodiazepines act as agonists at the GABA receptor complex.
Antagonist	A compound that binds to a receptor that blocks or reduces the action of another substance (agonist) at the receptor site involved. Antagonists that compete with an agonist for a receptor are *competitive antagonists.* Those that antagonize by other means are *non-competitive antagonists.*	Flumazenil is a competitive benzodiazepine receptor antagonist. It competitively inhibits the activity at the benzodiazepine recognition site on the GABA/benzodiazepine receptor complex. It is the purest antagonist synthesized. Drugs used in the treatment of schizophrenia block dopamine D_2 receptors. Examples of opioid antagonists include naltrexone and naloxone.
Partial Agonist (Mixed Agonist)	A compound which (even when fully occupying a receptor) possesses affinity for a receptor, but elicits a partial pharmacological response at the receptor involved. Partial agonists are often structural analogs of agonist molecules. If neurotransmitter concentrations are low, partial agonists may behave as an agonist. This is why these medications are sometimes called mixed agonists.	Buprenorphine is a partial agonist that produces typical opioid agonist effects and side effects, such as euphoria and respiratory depression, but its maximal effects are less than those of full agonists like heroin and methadone. When used at low doses buprenorphine produces sufficient agonist effect to enable opioid-addicted individuals to discontinue the drugs with fewer withdrawal symptoms.
Inverse Agonist	An inverse agonist is an agent that binds to the same receptor as an agonist for that receptor but produces the opposite pharmacological effect.	Several inverse agonists are currently in clinical development. One particular example is R015-4513 which the inverse agonist of the benzodiazepine class of drugs R015-4513 and the benzodiazepines both utilize the same GABA binding site on neurons, yet R015-4513 has the opposite effect, producing severe anxiety rather than the sedative and anxiolytic effects associated with benzodiazepines. Cannabinoid inverse agonists have been found to reduce appetite, the opposite of the craving effect associated with cannibus.

(Table by Norman Sussman, M.D.)
GABA, γ-aminobutyric acid.

information to update their understanding of the true side effect profile of a drug.

Adverse effects differ in their impact on compliance and potential to cause harm. Depending on a patient's threshold of tolerance for a side effect and the impact on quality of life, side effects can lead to drug discontinuation. Examples of serious side effects include agranulocytosis (clozapine [Clozaril]), Stevens-Johnson syndrome (lamotrigine [Lamictal]), hepatic failure (nefazodone [Serzone]), stroke (phenelzine [Nardil]), and heart block (thioridazine [Mellaril]). Overall, the risk of life-threatening side effects with psychotropics is low. Drugs that carry such a risk should be monitored more closely, and the prescribing physician should take into account whether the potential clinical benefits justify the additional risk. Any drug with a serious risk, as reflected in a black box warning, is generally used less extensively than would otherwise be the case.

In the case of haloperidol (Haldol) and other dopamine receptor antagonists, long-term complications, such as tardive dyskinesia, have been well documented. Emerging evidence also suggests that the use of dopamine antagonists is associated with a small increase in the risk of breast cancer and that this is related to larger cumulative doses. In cases in which serious risk is associated with a drug, closer medical monitoring of medication treatment is warranted. Because the most widely used psychotropics, such as the SSRIs and serotonin-dopamine antagonists, have only been in use since the 1980s or 1990s, there is less certainty about long-term effects, but no evidence indicates that side effects are not merely extensions of those already evident during initial therapy. It should also be kept in mind that most drugs used in the treatment of chronic medical disorders have not been in use sufficiently long to provide assurances about unintended long-term adverse effects.

Suicidal Ideation and Antidepressant Treatment

The issue of antidepressant-associated suicide has become front-page news, the result of an analysis suggesting a link between medication use and suicidal ideation among children, adolescents, and adults up to age 24 in short-term (4 to 16 weeks), placebo-controlled trials of nine newer antidepressant drugs. The data from trials involving more than 4,400 patients suggested that the average risk of suicidal thinking or behavior (suicidality) during the first few months of treatment in those receiving antidepressants was 4 percent, twice the placebo risk of 2 percent. No suicides occurred in these trials. The analysis also showed no increase in suicide risk among the 25 to 65 age group. Antidepressants reduced suicidality among those over age 65.

Following public hearings on the subject, in October 2004, the FDA requested the addition of "black box" warnings—the most serious warning placed on the labeling of a prescription medication—to all antidepressant drugs, old and new. This action raised alarm bells among parents and physicians and prompted an explosion of advertisements by malpractice attorneys. Most importantly, antidepressant prescriptions written for adolescents declined, whereas those for adults flattened, after years of growth.

A large study of real world patients published in the January 2006 issue of the *American Journal of Psychiatry* raises serious doubt about true antidepressants and suicidality, and about the wisdom of the FDA's decision to change the labeling. The study examined suicides and hospitalizations for suicide attempts in the medical records of 65,103 members of a nonprofit insurer in the Pacific Northwest that covers about 500,000 people who received antidepressants from 1992 to 2003. It found that (1) newer antidepressants were associated with a more rapid and greater reduction in risk than older types of antidepressants and (2) patients were significantly more likely to attempt or commit suicide in the month before they began drug therapy than in the 6 months after starting it.

This is not the first time credible evidence has contradicted a significant link between antidepressant use and increased risk of suicide. At the hearings that led to the black box warning, John Mann, M.D., of Columbia University presented population data showing that since 1987, the year before fluoxetine (Prozac) became the first marketed SSRI, suicide rates in the United States began dropping, and that area in the United States with the highest SSRI prescription rates had the biggest decline in suicides. For every 10 percent increase in prescription rates, the US suicide rate declined 3 percent.

Another study, a review of 588 case files of patients aged 10 to 19 (October 2003 *Archives of General Psychiatry*) found that a 1 percent increase in antidepressant use was associated with a decrease of 0.23 suicides per 100,000 adolescents per year.

For now, the question of whether antidepressants pose an increased risk of suicide remains unsettled. A more important question, given how slight the risk may be, if indeed it exists, is whether as a result of the FDA's ill-considered actions, some depressed patients are not getting potentially life-saving treatment.

Side Effects Associated with Newer Medications

All medications are associated with side effects. The clinician should be aware of these, be able to recognize them, and take appropriate measures to treat them.

Somnolence. Sedation is often an intended effect of many psychotropic drugs, especially when used to treat insomnia, anxiety, or agitation. Daytime sleepiness, or somnolence, is also an unwanted adverse event, however. It is important for the clinician to alert patients to the possibility of sedation and to document that the person was advised to exercise caution when operating any type of vehicle or mechanical equipment. Some somnolence results from a carryover of nighttime use of drugs as hypnotics. Even with drugs, such as the SSRIs, which are activating to many patients, somnolence can be problematic. In some instances, it results from impairment of sleep quality. Chronic use of SSRIs can cause some patients to experience a subjective sense of fatigue, exhaustion, or yawning, even with adequate amounts of sleep. Management of unwanted somnolence includes adjustment of dose or timing of administration, switching to alternative medications, addition of small doses of stimulants, or the addition of modafanil (Provigil).

Gastrointestinal Disturbances. The major gastrointestinal (GI) side effects of the older antidepressant and antipsychotic drugs consisted primarily of constipation and dry mouth, a consequence of their antimuscarinic activity. Most of the newer drugs have little antimuscarinic activity, but do have effects on the serotonin system. Most of the body's serotonin is in the GI tract, and serotonergic drugs often cause varying degrees of stomach pain, nausea, flatulence, and diarrhea. In most cases, these side effects are transient, but some persons never accommodate and must switch to another class of drugs. Initial use of lower doses or use of delayed release preparations are the most effective strategies for minimizing GI side effects.

Movement Disorders. The introduction of serotonin-dopamine antagonists has greatly reduced the incidence of medication-induced movement disorders, but varying degrees of dose-related parkinsonism, akathisia, and dystonia still occur. Risperidone (Risperdal) most closely resembles the older agents in terms of these side effects. Olanzapine (Zyprexa) also causes more extrapyramidal effects than clinical trials suggested. There have been rare reports of SSRI-induced movement disorders, ranging from akathisia to tardive dyskinesia.

Sexual Dysfunction. The use of psychiatric drugs can be associated with sexual dysfunction—decreased libido, impaired ejaculation and erection, and inhibition of female orgasm. In clinical trials with the SSRIs, the extent of sexual side effects was grossly underestimated, because data were based on spontaneous reports by patients. The rate of sexual dysfunction in the original fluoxetine product information, for example, was less than 5 percent. In subsequent studies in which information about sexual side effects was elicited by specific questions, the rate of SSRI-associated sexual dysfunction was found to be between 35 and 75 percent. In clinical practice, patients are not likely to report sexual dysfunction spontaneously to the physician, so it is important to ask about this side effect. Also, some sexual dysfunctions may be related to the primary psychiatric disorder. Nevertheless, if sexual dysfunction emerges after pharmacotherapy has begun, and the primary response to treatment has been positive, it may be worthwhile to attempt to treat the symptoms. Long lists of possible antidotes to these side effects have evolved, but few interventions are consistently effective, and few have more than anecdotal evidence to support their use. The clinician and patient should consider the possibility of sexual side effects with a patient when selecting a drug and switching treatment to another drug that is less or not at all associated with sexual dysfunction if this adverse effect is not acceptable to the patient.

Weight Gain. Weight gain accompanies the use of many psychotropic drugs as a result of retained fluid, increased caloric intake, decreased exercise, or altered metabolism. Weight gain can also occur as a symptom of disorder, as in bulimia or atypical depression, or as a sign of recovery from an episode of illness. Treatment-emergent increase in body weight is a common reason for noncompliance with a drug regimen. No specific mechanisms have been identified as causing weight gain, and it appears that the histamine and serotonin systems mediate changes in weight associated with many drugs used to treat depression and psychosis. Metformin (Glucophage) has been reported to facilitate weight loss among patients whose weight gain is attributed to use of serotonin-dopamine reuptake inhibitors and valproic acid (Depakene). Valproate, as well as olanzapine, has been linked to the development of insulin resistance, which could induce appetite increase, with subsequent weight increase. Weight gain is a noteworthy side effect of clozapine (Clozaril) and olanzapine. Genetic factors that regulate body weight, as well as the related problem of diabetes mellitus, seem to involve the 5-HT_{2C} receptor. There is a genetic polymorphism of the promoter region of this receptor, with significantly less weight gain in patients with the variant allele than in those without this allele. Drugs with a strong 5-HT_{2C} affinity would be expected to have a greater impact on body weight of patients with a polymorphism of the 5-HT_{2C} receptor promoter region.

Weight Loss. Initial weight loss is associated with SSRI treatment but is usually transient, with most weight being regained within the first few months. Bupropion (Wellbutrin) has been shown to cause modest weight loss that is sustained. When combined with diet and lifestyle changes, bupropion can facilitate more significant weight loss. Topiramate (Topamax) and zonisamide (Zonegran), marketed as treatments for epilepsy, sometimes produce substantial, sustained loss of weight.

Glucose Changes. Increased risk of glucose abnormalities, including diabetes mellitus, is associated with weight increase during psychotropic drug therapy. Clozapine and olanzapine are associated with a greater risk than other serotonin-dopamine antagonists of abnormalities in fasting glucose levels, as well as hyperosmolar diabetes and ketoacidosis.

Hyponatremia. Hyponatremia is associated with oxcarbazepine (Trileptal) and SSRI treatment, especially in elderly patients. Confusion, agitation, and lethargy are common symptoms.

Cognitive Impairment. Cognitive impairment means a disturbance in the capacity to think. Some agents, such as the benzodiazepine agonists, are recognized as causes of cognitive impairment. Other widely used psychotropics, such as the SSRIs, lamotrigine (Lamictal), gabapentin (Neurontin), lithium (Eskalith), TCAs, and bupropion, however, are also associated with varying degrees of memory impairment and word-finding difficulties. In contrast to the benzodiazepine-induced anterograde amnesia, these agents cause a more subtle type of absentmindedness. Drugs with anticholinergic properties are likely to worsen memory performance.

Sweating. Severe perspiration unrelated to ambient temperature is associated with TCAs, SSRIs, and venlafaxine. This side effect is often socially disabling. Attempts can be made to treat this side effect with alpha agents, such as terazosin (Hytrin) and oxybutynin (Ditropan).

Cardiovascular Disturbances. Newer agents are less likely to have direct cardiac effects. Many older agents, such as TCAs and phenothiazines, affected blood pressure and cardiac conduction. The drug thioridazine (Mellaril), which has been in use for decades, has been shown to prolong the QTc interval in a dose-related manner and may increase the risk of sudden death by delaying ventricular repolarization and causing torsades de pointes. Newer drugs are now routinely scrutinized for evidence of cardiac effects. A promising treatment for psychosis, sertindole (Serlect), was not marketed because the FDA would have required a black box warning. Slight QTc effects noted with ziprasidone (Geodon) delayed the marketing of that drug. Clozapine [Clozaril] can cause myocarditis in rare cases of which the clinician should be aware.

Rash. Any medication is a potential source of a drug rash. Some psychotropics, such as carbamazepine (Equetro, Tegretol) and lamotrigine (Lamictal), have been linked to an increased risk of serious exfoliative dermatitis. Commonly referred to as Stevens-Johnson syndrome, this condition is a systemic, immune-mediated reaction that can prove fatal or result in permanent scarring or blindness. All patients should be informed about the potential seriousness of lesions that are widespread, that occur above the neck, that involve the mucous membranes, and that may be associated with fever and lymphadenopathy. If such symptoms manifest, a patient should be instructed at the time that the medication is prescribed to go immediately to an emergency department.

Idiosyncratic and Paradoxical Drug Responses

Idiosyncratic reactions occur in a very small percentage of patients taking a drug. The reactions are not related to the known pharmacologic properties, and most likely represent a genetically based abnormal sensitivity to a drug. A paradoxical response represents the manifestation of a clinical effect the opposite of what is expected. In March 2007, the FDA reported dissociative-like states associated with certain sedative-hypnotics. These included behaviors such as sleepwalking, binge-eating, aggressive outbursts and night driving of which the patient was unaware. Table 36.1–3 lists the drugs required to have warning labels for that effect.

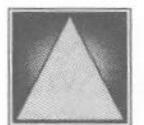

Table 36.1–3
Sedative Hypnotics Cited by the FDA

Drug	Manufacturer
Zolpidem (Ambien/Ambien CR)	Sanofi Aventis
Butabarbital (Butisol Sodium)	MedPointe Pharmaceuticals
Pentubabital and carbromal (Carbrital)	Parke-Davis
Flurazepam (Dalmane)	Valeant Pharmaceuticals
Quazepam (Doral)	Questcor Pharmaceuticals
Triazolam (Halcion)	Pfizer
Eszopiclone (Lunesta)	Sepracor
Ethylchloravynol (Placidyl)	Abbott
Estazolam (Prosom)	Abbott
Temazepam (Restoril)	Tyco Healthcare
Ramelteon (Rozerem)	Takeda
Secobarbital (Seconal)	Lilly
Zalepzon (Sonata)	King Pharmaceuticals

Therapeutic Index

Therapeutic index is a relative measure of the toxicity or safety of a drug and is defined as the ratio of the median toxic dose to the median effective dose. The median toxic dose is the dose at which 50 percent of patients experience a specific toxic effect, and the median effective dose is the dose at which 50 percent of patients have a specified therapeutic effect. When the therapeutic index is high, as it is for haloperidol, it is reflected by the wide range of dosages in which that drug is prescribed. Conversely, the therapeutic index for lithium is quite low, thus requiring careful monitoring of serum lithium levels in patients for whom the drug is prescribed.

Overdose

Safety in overdose is always a consideration in drug selection. Almost all of the newer agents, however, have a wide margin of safety when taken in overdose. By contrast, a 1-month supply of TCAs could be fatal. The depressed patients they were used to treat were the group most at risk to attempt suicide. Because even the safest drugs can sometimes produce severe medical complications, especially when combined with other agents, clinicians must recognize that the prescribed medication can be used in an attempt to commit suicide. Although it is prudent to write nonrefillable prescriptions for small quantities, this practice passes along increased copay costs to the patient. In fact, many pharmacy benefit management programs encourage the prescribing of a 3-month supply of medication.

In cases in which suicide is a major concern, an attempt should be made to verify that the medication is not being hoarded for a later overdose attempt. Random pill counts or asking a family member to dispense daily doses may be helpful. Some patients attempt suicide just as they are beginning to recover. Large quantities of medications with a low therapeutic index should be prescribed judiciously. Another reason to limit the number of pills prescribed is the possibility of accidental ingestion of medications by children in the household. Psychotherapeutic medications should be kept in a safe place.

Physicians who work in emergency rooms should know which drugs can be hemodialyzed. The issues involved are complex and are not based on any single chemical property of the drug. For example, it is generally presumed that drugs with low protein-binding are good candidates for dialysis. Venlafaxine, however, is only 27 percent protein bound and is too large as a molecule dialyzed. Hemodialysis is effective for treating overdose of valproic acid (Depakene).

Pharmacokinetics

Pharmacokinetic drug interactions are the effects of drugs on the plasma concentrations of each other, and pharmacodynamic drug interactions are the effects of drugs on the biological activities of each other. Pharmacokinetic concepts are used to describe and to predict the time course of drug concentrations in different parts of the body, such as plasma, adipose tissue, and the central nervous system (CNS). From a clinical perspective, pharmacokinetic methods help explain or predict the onset and duration of drug activity and interactions between drugs that alter their metabolism or excretion.

Pharmacogenetic research focuses on finding variant alleles that alter drug pharmacokinetics and pharmacodynamics. Researchers are attempting to identify genetic differences in how enzymes metabolize psychotropics, as well as CNS proteins directly involved in drug action. Likely, identification of patient genotypes will facilitate prediction of clinical response to different types of drugs.

Most clinicians need to consult charts or computer programs to determine when potential interactions may occur and, if so, how clinically relevant they may be. Whenever possible, it is preferable to use a medication that produces minimal risk of drug interactions. Also, it is recommended that prescribers know the interaction profiles of the drugs that they most commonly prescribe.

Examples of pharmacokinetic interactions include one drug increasing or decreasing the concentrations of a coadministered compound. These types of interactions can also lead to altered concentrations of metabolites. In some cases, there may also be interference with the conversion of a drug to its active metabolite. Enormous variability exists among patients with respect to pharmacokinetic parameters, such as drug absorption and metabolism. Another type of interaction is represented by interactions involving the kidney. Commonly used medications, such as angiotensin-converting enzyme (ACE) inhibitors, nonsteroidal anti-inflammatory drugs (NSAIDs), and thiazides, decrease renal clearance of lithium, increasing the likelihood of severe elevations of lithium. Drug interactions can occur pharmacokinetically or pharmacodynamically.

Pharmacogenetics is being used to study why patients differ in the way that they metabolize drugs. In patients who are ultrarapid or extensive metabolizers, the concentrations of a drug may be lower than expected.

PATIENT-RELATED FACTORS

Response to medication and sensitivity to side effects are influenced by factors related to the patient. This is why there is no one-size-fits-all approach to pharmacological treatment. Patient-related variables include diagnosis, genetic factors, lifestyle, overall medical status, concurrent disorders, and history of drug response. A patient's attitude toward medication in general, aversion to certain types of side effects, and preference for a specific agent also need to be considered.

Diagnosis

Failure to correctly diagnose a disorder diminishes the likelihood of optimal drug selection. Misdiagnosis not only can result in a missed opportunity, but also can, at times, produce worsening of symptoms. Inadvertently diagnosing a patient in the depressed phase of bipolar disorder as having unipolar depression can induce mania or rapid cycling. Treatment failure or exacerbation of symptoms should prompt a reassessment of the working diagnosis.

Past Treatment Response

A specific drug should be selected according to the patient's history of drug response (compliance, therapeutic response, adverse effects), the patient's family history of drug response, the profile of adverse effects for that drug with regard to the particular patient, and the prescribing clinician's usual practice. If a drug has previously been effective in treating a patient or a family member, the same drug should be used again. For reasons that are not understood, however, some patients fail to respond to a previously effective agent when challenged again. A history of severe adverse effects from a specific drug is a strong indicator that the patient would not be compliant with that particular drug.

It is helpful if patients can recall the details of past psychotropic drug treatment: the drugs prescribed, in what dosages, for how long, and in what combinations. Because of their mental disorders, many patients, however, are poor historians. If possible, patients' medical records should be obtained to confirm their reports. Family members are a good source of collateral information.

Response in Family Members

It is widely held that drug responses cluster in families. Thus, response to a drug in a relative is an indicator of whether a patient might also benefit from that medication. Although no conclusive evidence supports this as a consideration in drug selection, existing studies do confirm that a history of positive response to treatment with a drug should be considered in making treatment decisions.

Concurrent Medical or Psychiatric Disorders

Initial assessment should elicit information about coexisting medical disorders. In some cases, a medical disorder may be responsible for the symptoms. Patients with thyroid disease who are not adequately treated may appear depressed. Sleep apnea produces depression and cognitive impairment. Rare conditions, such as Kleine-Levin syndrome, can mimic bipolar disorder. A drug should be selected that minimally exacerbates any preexisting medical problems that a particular patient may have.

Recreational drug use, excessive consumption of alcohol, and frequent ingestion of caffeine-containing beverages can complicate and even undermine psychotropic drug treatment. These compounds possess significant psychoactive properties and, in some cases, may represent the source of the patient's symptoms.

It is reasonable to ask patients to abstain from use of these substances, at least until the benefits of psychotropic drug treatment have been unequivocally established. Gradual reintroduction of moderate amounts of alcohol, tea, and coffee can then take place. Patients can then observe for themselves whether there are any untoward effects on their clinical status.

INFORMED CONSENT AND PATIENT EDUCATION

Establishing trust and providing motivation to comply with the medication regimen are essential components of successful treatment. Patients should be informed about treatment options and the probable side effects and unique benefits of each treatment. Patient preference should be respected, unless a compelling advantage exists involving efficacy, tolerability, or safety with an alternative agent. If a particular medication is being recommended, the reasons for this recommendation should be explained. Patients are more likely to continue taking their medication if they fully understand the reasons why it is being prescribed.

A strong therapeutic alliance between a clinician and a patient is always helpful. Given the unpredictability of medication response, the frequent occurrence of side effects, and underlying ambivalence about, or fear of taking, medication, a positive, trusting relationship serves to improve patient compliance. Repeated failed trials may be needed before a response is seen. A patient's confidence in the physician's knowledge and judgment enables medication trials and more complex regimens, such as the use of multiple medications.

Discussions about drug selection should be documented in notes, but a signed informed consent is not needed. Surprisingly, patients who are informed of potential adverse effects report a higher incidence of side effects, but do not have higher rates of premature discontinuation.

How the patient and family are engaged in the treatment plan can determine the success of treatment. The psychodynamic meaning of pharmacotherapy to the patient and family and environmental influences, psychosocial stressors, and support should be explored. Some patients may view drug treatment as a panacea, and others may view it as the enemy. With the patient's consent, relatives and other clinicians should be instructed about the reasons for the drug treatment, as well as the expected benefits and potential risks.

DOSING, DURATION, AND MONITORING

Dosing

The clinically effective dose for treatment depends on the characteristics of the drug and patient factors, such as inherited sensitivity and ability to metabolize a drug, concurrent medical disorders, use of concurrent medications, and history of exposure to previous medications.

Plasma concentrations of many psychotropics can vary up to tenfold. Thus, to some extent, the optimal dose for an individual is ultimately determined by trial and error, guided by the empirical evidence of the usual dose range for that drug. Some drugs demonstrate a clear relationship between increases in dose and clinical response. This dose-response curve plots the drug concentration against the effects of the drug.

The *potency* of a drug refers to the relative dose required to achieve certain effects, not to its efficacy. Haloperidol, for example, is more potent than chlorpromazine, because approximately 5 mg of haloperidol is required to achieve the same therapeutic effect as 100 mg of chlorpromazine. These drugs, however, are equal in their clinical efficacy—that is, the maximal clinical response achievable by administration of a drug.

Drugs must be used in effective dosages for sufficient periods. Although drug tolerability and safety are always a consideration, subtherapeutic doses and incomplete therapeutic trials should be avoided. The use of inadequate doses merely exposes the patient to the risk of side effects, without providing the probability of therapeutic benefit. In view of the wide margin of safety associated with most currently prescribed medications, more risk exists in underdosing than in overshooting the recommended dose range.

Time of dosing is usually based on the plasma half-life of a drug and its side effect profile. Sedating drugs are given all at night or with disproportionate daily doses at night. The opposite is true with activating drugs. The frequency of dosing is less clear cut. Most dosing regimens of psychotropic drugs, such as once-a-day versus divided doses, are based on measurements of plasma concentrations rather than receptor occupancy in the brain. Evidence suggests a significant dissociation exists between brain and plasma kinetics. Reliance on plasma kinetics as the basis for dosing regimens leads to misunderstanding of necessary schedules.

As a rule, psychotropic drugs should be used continuously. Exceptions are the use of drugs for insomnia, acute agitation, and severe situational anxiety. A common mistake is the use of high-potency benzodiazepines, such as alprazolam (Xanax) and clonazepam (Klonopin), only after an attack has begun. These drugs should be used as part of a regular schedule to prevent attacks.

Some patients who experience sexual dysfunction while being treated with SSRIs take a drug holiday, that is, they skip a daily dose from time to time to facilitate sexual performance.

Intermittent dosing regimens of SSRIs have been found to be effective as a treatment for premenstrual dysphoric disorder. The drugs are taken daily during the 2-week luteal phase of the menstrual cycle.

Duration of Treatment

A common question from a patient: "How long do I need to take the medication?" The answer depends on multiple variables, including the nature of the disorder, the duration of symptoms, the family history, and the extent to which the patient tolerates and benefits from the medication. Patients can be given a reasonable explanation of the probabilities but should be told that it is first best to see if the medication works for him or her and whether the side effects are acceptable. Any more definitive discussion of treatment duration can be held once the degree of success is clear. Even patients with a philosophical aversion to the use of psychotropic drugs may elect to stay on medication indefinitely if the magnitude of improvement is great. Most psychiatric disorders have high rates of chronicity and relapse. Because of this, long-term treatment is often needed to prevent recurrence. Nevertheless, the fact remains that psychotropic drugs are not said to cure the disorders they treat, but rather to help control the symptoms.

Treatment is conceptually broken down into three phases: the initial therapeutic trial, the continuation, and the maintenance phase. The initial period of treatment should last at least several weeks because of the delay in therapeutic effects that characterizes most classes of psychotropic drugs. The required duration of a *therapeutic trial* of a drug should be discussed at the outset of treatment, so that the patient does not have unrealistic expectations of an immediate improvement in symptoms. Patients are more likely to experience side effects early in the course of pharmacotherapy than any relief from their disorder. In some cases, medication may even exacerbate some symptoms. Patients should be counseled that a poor initial reaction to medication is not an indicator of the ultimate outcome of treatment. For instance, many patients with panic disorder develop jitteriness or an increase in panic attacks after starting on tricyclic or SSRI treatment. Benzodiazepine agonists are an exception to the rule that clinical onset is delayed. In most cases, their hypnotic and antianxiety effects are evident immediately.

Ongoing use of medication, however, does not provide absolute protection against relapse. Continuation therapy provides clinically and statistically significant protective effects against relapse. The optimal duration of continuation or maintenance therapy is variable and dependent on the clinical history of the patient. Early-onset chronic major depression, for example, has a more severe course and greater comorbidity than late-onset chronic major depression. In addition to early onset, a history of multiple past episodes, and severity and length of current episode would make longer, even indefinite, treatment appropriate.

Frequency of Visits

Until an unequivocal response to treatment occurs, patients should be seen as frequently as circumstances warrant. The frequency of follow-up or monitoring visits is determined by clinical judgment. In severely ill patients, this might mean several times a week. Patients on maintenance therapy, even when stable, need monitoring, but no consensus exists on the frequency of follow-up therapy. Three months is a reasonable interval between visits, but 6 months may be adequate after long-standing treatment.

LABORATORY TESTS AND THERAPEUTIC BLOOD MONITORING

Laboratory testing and therapeutic blood monitoring should be based on clinical circumstances and the drugs being used. For most commonly used psychotropic drugs, routine testing is not required. No currently available laboratory test can confirm the diagnosis of a mental disorder.

Pretreatment tests are routine as part of a workup to establish baseline values and to rule out underlying medical problems that may be causing the psychiatric symptoms or that might complicate treatment with drugs. Results of recently performed tests should be obtained. With agents known to cause cardiac conduction changes, a pretreatment electrocardiogram (ECG) should be obtained before initiating treatment. With lithium and clozapine, the possibility of serious changes in thyroid, renal, hepatic, or hematological functions requires pretreatment and ongoing monitoring with appropriate laboratory tests.

As a result of both anecdotal and research findings of sometimes severe glucose dysregulation during treatment primarily with SDA's, the FDA has suggested that patients being treated with any atypical antipsychotic be monitored for the emergence of diabetes.

Certain circumstances present in which it is necessary or useful to use plasma concentrations to monitor a patient's condition. These include the monitoring of drugs with narrow therapeutic indexes, such as lithium; drugs with a therapeutic window, the optimal dose range for a therapeutic response; drug combinations that can lead to interactions that raise drug concentrations of medications or their metabolites, which can cause toxicity; unexplained toxicity at normal therapeutic doses; and failure to respond in a patient who may be noncompliant. A clinician should have no reservations about requesting random urine toxicological tests in a patient who abuses substances.

TREATMENT OUTCOMES

The goal of psychotropic treatment is to eliminate all manifestations of disorder, thus enabling the patient to regain the ability to function as well and to enjoy life as fully as before he or she became ill. This degree of improvement to below the syndromal threshold is defined as *remission*.

Response and Remission

Remission is the preferred outcome of treatment, not only because of the immediate impact on functioning and state of mind, but also because emerging evidence suggests that patients in remission are less likely to experience relapse and recurrence of their disorder.

Patients who improve but do not experience a full resolution are considered to be responders. They may exhibit significant improvement, but continue to experience symptoms. In depression studies, *response* is usually defined as a 50 percent or greater decrease from baseline on a standard rating scale, such as the Hamilton Depression (HAM-D) Scale or the Montgomery-Asberg Depression Rating Scale (MADRS). *Remission* is defined as an absolute score of seven or less on the HAM-D or ten or less on the MADRS. Expectations about the likely degree of improvement should be based on what is known about the responsiveness of specific disorders to medication therapy. Obsessive-compulsive disorder (OCD) and schizophrenia, for example, are more likely to be associated with residual manifestations of illness than major depression or panic disorder. The probability of full remission from OCD with SSRI treatment alone over a 2-year period is less than 12 percent, and the probability of partial remission is approximately 47 percent.

Treatment Failure

The initial treatment plan should anticipate the possibility that the medication may be ineffective. A next-step strategy should be in place at the initiation of treatment. Repeated drug failures should prompt reassessment of the patient. First, was the original diagnosis correct? In answering this question, the clinician should include the possibility of an undiagnosed medical condition or recreational drug use as the cause of the psychiatric symptoms. Second, are the observed symptoms related to the original disorder, or are they actually adverse effects of the drug treatment? Some antipsychotic drugs, for example, can produce akinesia, which resembles psychotic withdrawal, or akathisia and neuroleptic malignant syndrome, which resemble increased psychotic agitation. Long-term use of SSRIs can produce emotional blunting, which can mimic depression.

Intolerance of side effects may be the most common reason for treatment failure. Third, was the drug administered at an appropriate dosage for a sufficient length of time? Because absorption and metabolism of drugs can vary greatly in patients, the clinician may need to measure plasma levels of a drug to ensure a sufficient dose of the drug. Fourth, did a pharmacokinetic or pharmacodynamic interaction with another drug that the patient was taking reduce the efficacy of the newly prescribed drug? Fifth, did the patient take the drug as directed? Drug noncompliance is a common clinical problem that arises as a result of complicated drug regimens (more than one drug in more than one daily dosage), adverse effects (especially if unnoticed by the clinician), and poor patient education about the drug treatment plan. Patients may discontinue medication when they recover, thinking that they are cured and no longer benefiting from the medication.

Treatment Resistance

Some patients fail to respond to repeated trials of medication. No single factor can explain the ineffectiveness of the various interventions in these cases. Strategies in these cases include the use of drug combinations, high-dose therapy, and use of unconventional drugs. Limited evidence is available on the comparative success rates associated with any given strategy.

Tolerance

The development of tolerance is marked by a need, over time, to use increased doses of a drug for it to maintain a clinical effect. This decreased responsiveness to a drug occurs after repeated doses. Tolerance also describes decreased sensitivity to adverse effects of the drug, such as nausea. This phenomenon is used as the basis for starting some drugs at subtherapeutic doses, with the plan to adjust the schedule once the patient can tolerate higher doses. Clinical tolerance appears to represent changes in the CNS, such as altered receptor configuration or density. Drugs with similar pharmacological actions often exhibit cross-tolerance.

Sensitization

Clinically manifested as the reverse of tolerance, sensitization is said to occur when sensitivity to a drug effect increases over time. In these cases, the same dose typically produces more pronounced effects as treatment progresses.

Withdrawal

The development of physiological adaptation to a drug, with a subsequent risk of withdrawal symptoms, has been reported for many classes of psychotropic drugs. Technically, withdrawal should be considered a side effect. The probability and severity of these reactions are remote with most drugs and more common with others. As a general rule, the more abruptly a drug is stopped and the shorter its elimination half-life, the more likely it is that clinically significant withdrawal symptoms will occur. When using some short-acting drugs, withdrawal reactions can result from missed doses and during daily intervals between doses. Gradual tapering of medications after prolonged use is recommended, when possible. Although this reduces the risk of withdrawal reactions, it does not ensure that they will not occur. So-called sedative hypnotics and opiates are the agents most often associated with mentally and physically distressing discontinuation reactions. In some cases, such as barbiturate use, withdrawal can be fatal.

Marked differences are found among agents, even within a given class, with respect to the probability and severity of discontinuation effects. For example, among the benzodiazepines, alprazolam and triazolam (Halcion) commonly produce more immediate and intense withdrawal symptoms than other compounds. Among the SSRIs, there is a well-described withdrawal syndrome that appears to be more frequent and severe with paroxetine (Paxil). It can, however, occur with any SSRI. Even fluoxetine can be associated with discontinuation symptoms, but the symptoms may be delayed and attenuated because of the long elimination half-life of its active metabolite. These manifestations are subtle and are delayed for weeks after the last dose. Venlafaxine also produces a severe SSRI-like withdrawal syndrome.

In addition to half-life, many variables can influence the likelihood and degree of discontinuation symptoms. Changes in the rate of drug metabolism, as an example, can play a role. Paroxetine is primarily metabolized by the cytochrome P450 (CYP) 2D6 isoenzyme. Paroxetine, however, is also a potent inhibitor of CYP 2D6. This results in *autoinhibition*, a dose-dependent inhibition of its own metabolism, with a subsequent increase in plasma concentrations of paroxetine. If the dose of paroxetine is decreased or the drug is stopped, the decline in its plasma concentrations can be steep, causing withdrawal to occur. Withdrawal can occur in rare cases in which the dosage of a drug is not decreased, but a second agent, which had been inhibiting its metabolism, was stopped. For example, alprazolam is metabolized via the CYP 3A3/4 enzyme system. Nefazodone inhibits that enzyme. If a patient taking both agents for several weeks discontinues the nefazodone, it could result in a rapid increase in the rate of alprazolam metabolism and a consequent drop in plasma concentrations.

The development of sustained-release versions of drugs, such as alprazolam, paroxetine, and venlafaxine, has not reduced the severity of their withdrawal reactions. The prolonged half-life of those agents results from delayed absorption rather than prolongation of the elimination phase. The frequency of drug dosing is reduced but not the rate of fall-off in plasma concentrations.

Poor bioavailability with a generic agent may account for unexpected loss of clinical effect in emergence of withdrawal symptoms. The occurrence of these events soon after refilling a prescription should prompt examination of the new medication. It should be confirmed whether the dispensed medication and dose are both correct. It is difficult to ascertain whether generic medications are truly equivalent, so the possibility exists that differences in potency may underlie adverse changes in clinical status.

Withdrawal symptoms invariably occur hours or days after dose reduction or discontinuation. Symptoms resolve within a few weeks, so the persistence of symptoms argues against withdrawal. Although depletion studies have been shown to provoke rapid return of symptoms, in clinical practice, psychotic and mood symptoms do not usually reappear abruptly after long-term treatment.

COMBINATION OF DRUGS

According to the American Psychiatric Association Practice Guidelines for the Treatment of Psychiatric Disorders, "the use of multiple agents should be avoided if possible" in the treatment of psychiatric disorders. Although *monotherapy* represents the ideal, *polypharmacy*, the simultaneous use of psychotropic medications, has been commonplace since chlorpromazine (Thorazine) was combined with reserpine (Diupres) in the early 1950s. The practice of combining drugs and the merits of various *augmentation* or *combination* strategies are routinely discussed in the literature and at scientific meetings. The mean number of simultaneously prescribed medications has increased in recent decades. Among psychiatric inpatients, the mean number of psychotropics prescribed is approximately three. Fixed combinations—drugs that contain more than one active ingredient—have been successfully marketed in the past, and research on new combinations is ongoing. A fluoxetine-olanzapine fixed combination has been approved as a treatment for bipolar disorder. The use of such drugs may increase the patients' compliance by simplifying the drug regimen. A problem with combination drugs, however, is that the clinician has less flexibility in adjusting the dosage of one of the components; that is, the use of combination drugs can cause two drugs to be administered when only one drug continues to be necessary for therapeutic efficacy (Table 36.1–4).

Sometimes distinctions are made between augmentation and combination therapy. When two psychotropics with the same approved indications are used concurrently, this is termed *combination therapy*. Adding a drug with another indication is termed *augmentation*. Augmentation often entails use of a drug that is not primarily considered a psychotropic. For example, in treating depression, it is not common to add thyroid hormone to an approved antidepressant.

Almost all patients with bipolar disorder are taking more than one psychotropic agent. Combination treatment with drugs that treat depression and dopamine receptor antagonist or serotonin-dopamine antagonist has long been held as preferable in patients with psychotic depression. Similarly, SSRIs typically produce partial improvement in patients with OCD, so that the addition of a serotonin-dopamine antagonist may be helpful.

Medications also can be combined to counteract side effects, to treat specific symptoms, and as a temporary measure to transition from one drug to another. It is common practice to add a new medication without the discontinuation of a prior drug, particularly when the first drug has provided partial benefit. This can be done as part of a plan to transition from an agent that is not producing a satisfactory response or as an attempt to maintain the patient on combined therapy.

Advantages of combining drugs include building on existing response, which may be less demoralizing, and the possibility that combinations produce new mechanisms that no single agent

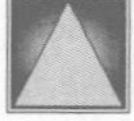

Table 36.1–4
Combination Drugs Used in Psychiatry

Ingredients	Preparation	Amount of Each	Recommended Dosage	Indications
Perphenazine and amitriptyline	—	Tablet—2:25, 4:25, 4:50, 2:10, 4:10	Initial therapy: tablet of 2:25 or 4:25 q.i.d. Maintenance therapy: tablet 2:25 or 4:25 b.i.d. or q.i.d.	Depression and associated anxiety
Dextroamphetamine and amphetamine	Adderal	Tablet: 5, 7.5, 10.0, 12.5, 15.0, 20.0, 30.0 mg	3 to 5 yrs: 2.5 mg/day; 6 yrs and older: 5 mg/day	Attention Deficit/ Hyperactivity Disorder
	Adderal XR	Capsule: 5, 10, 15, 20, 25, 30 mg	—	—
Chlordiazepoxide and clidinium bromide	—	Capsule—5:25	One or two capsules t.i.d. or q.i.d. before meals and at bedtime	Peptic ulcer, gastritis, duodenitis, irritable bowel syndrome, spastic colitis, and mild ulcerative colitis
Chlordiazepoxide and amitriptyline	—	Tablet—5.0:12.5, 10:25	Tablet of 5:12.5 t.i.d. or q.i.d.; tablet of 10:25 t.i.d. or q.i.d., initially, then may increase to six tablets daily as required	Depression and associated anxiety
Olanzapine and fluoxetine	Symbyax	6:25, 6:50, 12:25, 12:50	Once daily in the evening in a dose range of olanzapine 6 to 12 mg and fluoxetine 25 to 50 mg	Depressive episodes associated with bipolar I disorder

DEA, Drug Enforcement Administration; q.i.d., four times daily; b.i.d., twice daily; t.i.d., three times daily.

can provide. One limitation is that noncompliance and adverse effects increase and that the clinician may not be able to determine whether it was the second drug alone or the combination of drugs that resulted in a therapeutic success or a particular adverse effect. Combining drugs can create a broad spectrum effect and also changes the ratio of metabolites.

COMBINED PSYCHOTHERAPY AND PHARMACOTHERAPY

Many psychiatrists believe that patients are best treated with a combination of medication and psychotherapy. Studies have demonstrated that the results of combined therapy are superior to those of either type of therapy alone. When pharmacotherapy and psychotherapy are used together, the approach should be coordinated, integrated, and synergistic. If the psychotherapy and the pharmacotherapy are directed by two separate clinicians, the clinicians must communicate with each other clearly and often.

SPECIAL POPULATIONS

Although every patient brings a unique combination of demographic and clinical variables to the clinical setting, certain patient populations require special consideration. When treating the young, the elderly, those with medical disorders, and women who want to conceive, are pregnant, or are nursing, awareness of risks associated with medication assumes increased importance. Data derived from clinical trials are of limited value in guiding many decisions, because populations in these studies consisted of healthy young adults and, until recently, excluded many women of child-bearing age. Studies of children and adolescents have become more common, so that understanding of treatment effects in this population has grown.

Children

Understanding of the safety and efficacy of most psychotropic drugs when used to treat children is based more on clinical experience than on evidence from large clinical trial data. Other than attention-deficit/hyperactivity disorder (ADHD) and OCD, commonly used psychotropic drugs have no labeling for pediatric use, so results from adult studies are extrapolated to children. This is not necessarily appropriate because of developmental differences in pharmacokinetics and pharmacodynamics. Dosing is another special consideration in drug use with children. Although the small volume of distribution suggests the use of lower doses than those used in adults, a child's higher rate of metabolism suggests that a higher ratio of milligrams of drug to kilograms of body weight should be used. In practice, it is best to begin with a small dose and to increase it until clinical effects are observed. The clinician should not hesitate, however, to use adult dosages in children if these dosages are effective, and the adverse effects are acceptable.

The paucity of research data is a legacy of many years in which manufacturers avoided conducting trials in children because of liability concerns, small market share, and, hence, limited profit potential represented by this population. To correct this problem, the FDA Modernization Act (FDAMA) of 1997 provided for special encouragement and incentives to study drugs for pediatric use.

Pregnant and Nursing Women

No definitive assurances exist that any drug is completely without risk during pregnancy and lactation. No psychotropic medication is absolutely contraindicated during pregnancy, although drugs with known risks of birth defects, premature birth, or neonatal complications should be avoided if acceptable alternatives are available.

Women who are pregnant or lactating are excluded from clinical trials and it is only recently that women of child-bearing age have been able to participate in these studies. As a result, there are large gaps in knowledge of the effects of psychotropic agents on the developing fetus and on the neonate. Most of what is known is the result of anecdotal reports or data from registries. The basic rule is to avoid administering any drug to a woman who is pregnant (particularly during the first trimester) or who is breast-feeding a child, unless the mother's psychiatric disorder is severe, and it is determined that the therapeutic value of the drug outweighs the theoretical adverse effects on the fetus or newborn. A woman may elect to continue on medication, because she does not want to chance a possible recurrence of painful or disabling symptoms.

Among the newer antidepressants, paroxetine is the only one to carry a warning from the FDA, the result of an increase risk of cardiac malformation. The agents with the most well-documented risk of specific birth defects are lithium, carbamazepine, and valproate. Lithium administration during pregnancy is associated with Ebstein's anomaly, a serious abnormality in cardiac development, although recent evidence suggests that the risk is not as great as previously believed. Carbamazepine and valproic acid are associated with neural tube defects, which can be prevented by use of folate during pregnancy. Lamotrigine can cause oral-clefts when used during the first trimester. Some experts advise that all women of child-bearing age who are treated with psychotropics take supplemental folate.

The administration of psychotherapeutic drugs at or near delivery can cause the baby to be overly sedated at delivery, thus requiring a respirator, or to be physically dependent on the drug, requiring detoxification and the treatment of a withdrawal syndrome. Reports exist of a neonatal withdrawal syndrome associated with third trimester use of SSRIs in pregnant women. They have also been implicated in producing pulmonary hypertension in newborns.

Virtually all psychiatric drugs are secreted in the milk of a nursing mother; therefore, mothers on those agents should be advised not to breast-feed their infants.

Elderly Patients

The two major concerns when treating geriatric patients with psychotherapeutic drugs are that elderly persons may be more susceptible to adverse effects (particularly, cardiac effects) and may metabolize and excrete drugs more slowly, thus requiring lower dosages of medication. In practice, clinicians should begin treating geriatric patients with a small dose, usually approximately one half of the usual starting dose. The dosage should be raised in small increments, more slowly than for middle-aged adults, until a clinical benefit is achieved or unacceptable adverse effects appear. Although many geriatric patients require a small dosage of medication, many others require a full therapeutic dosage.

Elderly patients account for approximately one third of all prescription drug use and a substantial percentage of over-the-counter preparations, as well. Even more significant is the incidence of polypharmacy. Recent surveys have found that elderly patients in the community are taking between three and five medications and that hospitalized elderly patients are treated with an average of ten drugs. Nearly one half of all patients in long-term care facilities are prescribed one or more psychotropic agents. In view of these statistics, clinicians need to consider potential types and likelihood of drug interactions when selecting medications.

Psychotropic drugs have been shown to be causally related to falls in the elderly. Discontinuation of psychotropic drugs results in an estimated 40 percent risk reduction for falls. This association between psychotropics and falls and hip fractures may weaken as newer agents become widely used. As a rule, new-generation compounds produce less unwanted sedation, dizziness, parkinsonism, and postural hypotension.

Age-related changes in renal clearance and hepatic metabolism make it more important to be conservative with the starting doses of medication, as well as the rate of dose titration. Within any class of psychotropic agents, those with potentially serious consequences, such as hypotension, cardiac conduction abnormalities, anticholinergic activity, and respiratory depression, are not suitable choices. Drugs that cause cognitive impairment, such as benzodiazepines and anticholinergics, can mimic or exacerbate symptoms of dementia. Similarly, dopamine receptor antagonists can worsen or induce Parkinson's disease, another age-related disorder. Some side effects, such as SSRI-associated syndrome of inappropriate secretion of antidiuretic hormone (SIADH) and oxcarbazepine-associated hyponatremia, occur more commonly in older patients.

A common ethical dilemma with the medically ill elderly or those with dementia is the question of their capacity to give informed consent before treatment with psychotropic drugs or electroconvulsive therapy (ECT).

Medically Ill Patients

There are special considerations, diagnostic and therapeutic, when administering psychiatric drugs to medically ill patients. The medical disorder should be ruled out as a cause of the psychiatric symptoms. For example, patients with neurological or endocrine disorders or those infected with human immunodeficiency virus (HIV) may experience disturbances of mood and cognition. Common medications, such as corticosteroids and L-dopa, are associated with induction of mania.

A patient with diabetes mellitus is better treated with an agent without the risk of weight gain or glucose dysregulation. Depending on the diagnosis, drugs that might treat the primary psychiatric disorder and also cause weight loss, drugs such as bupropion, topiramate (Topamax), and zonisamide (Zonegran), should be prescribed for these patients. Patients with obstructive pulmonary disease should not be given sedating drugs, which raise the arousal threshold and suppress respiration. Patients with medical disorders are also taking other medications, which can result in pharmacodynamic and pharmacokinetic interactions. Combined treatment with an inducer of multiple CYP enzymes and a drug that is a substrate for those enzymes could result in subtherapeutic levels, leading to inadequate symptom control. Use of the tuberculosis treatment rifampicin (Rifadin) with carbamazepine is an example of this. Use of drugs that inhibit CYP 2D6, agents such as paroxetine and fluoxetine, can prevent the conversion of hydrocodone (Robidone) and other opiates into an active analgesic form. NSAIDs are also a rare cause of perceptual disturbances and psychotic symptoms.

Other issues include a potentially increased sensitivity to adverse effects, including increased or decreased metabolism and excretion of the drug, and interactions with other medications. Drug interactions are an obvious concern when drugs with a narrow therapeutic range are being used. Any change in the rate of metabolism or interference with the formation and elimination of metabolites can profoundly influence the activity of that drug. Similarly, interactions that interfere with drug metabolism can produce an increase in side effects and toxicity.

As with children and geriatric patients, the most reasonable clinical practice is to begin with a small dosage, to increase it slowly, and to watch for clinical benefit and adverse effects. Determining the plasma drug concentrations may be helpful for such patients, but therapeutic blood concentrations for most psychotropic drugs are neither necessary nor routinely available.

Substance Abuse

Many patients who seek or need treatment for a psychiatric disorder engage in chronic use of illicit substances or drink excessive amounts of alcohol. Marijuana is the most commonly used illicit drug in the United States.

Discontinuation of chronic drug or alcohol use can result not only in craving, but also in clinically significant psychiatric and physiological withdrawal symptoms. For many patients, successful treatment of their underlying psychiatric disorder may not be possible in the presence of ongoing marijuana, cocaine, and alcohol use. If several trials of medications fail, hospitalization for detoxification may be necessary. Little research and no consensus exist about how to use psychotropic agents in patients who are regular users of cocaine, marijuana, or other recreational drugs.

Table 36.1–4 lists combination drugs used in psychiatry.

REGULATORY ISSUES

The FDA has the authority to approve a drug for clinical use, and to ensure that product labeling is truthful and contains all information pertinent to the safe and effective use of that drug.

Product information that is FDA approved for marketed drugs appears as a package insert that lists potential side effects, drug interactions, the need for special monitoring, and restrictions for use. In some cases, these adverse reactions and potential safety hazards warrant a special warning label called a "black box." The FDA typically negotiates final labeling language with the company; however, in cases where a company refuses to satisfy the FDA, the agency may initiate proceedings to remove the drug from clinical use. In recent years, warning labels have been applied to entire classes of psychotropic drugs, including the serotonin dopamine antagonists and antidepressants such as the SSRIs.

The product information may also contain a "Contraindications" heading. This section describes instances in which the drug should not be used because the risk of using it clearly outweighs the benefit. If no contraindications are known, this section of the labeling will state "None known."

A precautions section may contain precautions for most individuals taking the drug, as well as for specific groups, such as pregnant women, nursing mothers, or children. In this section, one will find recommendations for patients to ensure safe and effective use of the drug. For example, there may be precautions about driving when taking the medication or using substances such as other drugs, food, or alcohol that may have harmful effects if taken while using the medication. The Precautions Section also provides information about laboratory tests needed to track responses or to identify adverse reactions to the drug or about known interactions with other drugs, foods, or ingredients.

Every product label has an Adverse Reaction section that lists the frequency of undesirable effects that may be associated with use of a drug. Causes of adverse reactions can include medication errors, such as overdosage, or interactions between different drugs or between drugs and certain foods.

NONAPPROVED DOSAGES AND USES

It is now common practice to treat psychiatric disorders with drugs that are approved for nonpsychiatric conditions. Some examples include propranolol (Inderal) for social anxiety and treatment of lithium-induced tremor; verapamil (Calan, Isoptin) for mania and treatment of MAOI-induced hypertensive crisis; levothyroxine (Levoxyl) for antidepressant augmentation; clonidine (Catapres) and guanfacine (Tenex) for ADHD and posttraumatic stress disorder (PTSD); dextroamphetamine (Dexedrine) for antidepressant augmentation; and riluzole (Rilutek) for self-injurious behavior. Off-label use of a drug is not a violation of law or a departure from good medical practice. The FDA does not limit the manner in which a physician may use an approved drug. Medications can be prescribed for any reason shown to be medically indicated for the welfare of the patient. Once a drug is approved for commercial use, a physician can, as part of the practice of medicine, lawfully prescribe a different dosage for a patient or may otherwise vary the conditions of use from what is approved in the package labeling without notifying the FDA or obtaining its approval.

Failure to follow the information on the drug label does not in itself impose liability and should not preclude a physician from using good clinical judgment in the service of the patient. Physicians are permitted to use a drug for indications not included on the drug's official labeling without violating the FDA rules. This fact, however, does not absolve the physician of responsibility for an untoward result from treatment. Patients can still sue for possible medical malpractice with the reasoning that the failure to follow the FDA-approved label can be interpreted as deviating from the prevailing standard of care.

When using a drug for an unapproved indication or in a dose outside the usual range, good clinical practice is to explain to the patient and to document in the chart why a drug is being used instead of an approved agent. In cases if doubt about a plan to use a drug off-label, a consultation with a colleague should be obtained.

In some cases, a drug has obtained a limited approval for an indication. Divalproex (Depakote), quetiapine (Seroquel), and risperidone, for example, are approved by the FDA for the acute, but not long-term, treatment of mania. Nevertheless, these drugs are routinely used for long-term prevention of recurrences of mania and bipolar disorder. In the case of lamotrigine, it was accepted as a first-choice agent for the treatment of bipolar disorder long before the FDA granted approval for that indication.

PLACEBOS

Pharmacologically inactive substances have long been known to sometimes produce significant clinical benefits. A patient who believes that a compound is helpful may often derive considerable benefit from taking that substance, whether it is known to be pharmacologically active or not. For many psychiatric disorders, including mild to moderate depression and some anxiety disorders, well over 30 percent of patients can exhibit significant improvement or remission of symptoms on a placebo. For other conditions, such as schizophrenia, manic episodes, and psychotic depression, the placebo response rate is very low. Whereas suggestion is undoubtedly important in the efficacy of placebos (and active drugs), placebos can produce biological effects. For example, placebo-induced analgesia may sometimes be blocked by naloxone (Narcan), which suggests that endorphins may mediate the analgesia derived from taking a placebo. It is conceivable that placebos may also stimulate endogenous anxiolytic and antidepressant factors, resulting in clinical improvement in patients with depression and anxiety disorders.

Just as placebos can produce benefit, they can also have adverse effects. In many studies, some adverse effects are likely to be more common with placebos than with the active drug. Some patients will not tolerate placebos despite the fact that they are supposedly inert, and they exhibit adverse effects (called the *nocebo phenomenon*). It is easy to discount such patients as overly suggestible; however, if beneficial endogenous factors can be stimulated by placebos, perhaps toxic endogenous factors can also be produced.

Prudence is needed in contemplating the use of a placebo in clinical practice. Treating a patient with a placebo without consent can seriously undermine a patient's confidence in the physician if, and when, it is discovered.

REFERENCES

Chuang DM. The antiapoptotic actions of mood stabilizers: Molecular mechanisms and therapeutic potentials. *Ann NY Acad Sci*. 2005;1053:195–204.

DeVeaugh-Geiss J, March J, Shapiro M, Andreason PJ, Emslie G, Ford LM, Greenhill L, Murphy D, Prentice E, Roberts R, Silva S, Swanson JM, van Zwieten-Boot B, Vitiello B, Wagner KD, Mangum B. Child and adolescent psychopharmacology in the new millennium: A workshop for academia, industry, and government. *J Am Acad Child Adolesc Psychiatry*. 2006;45(3):261–270.

Ginsberg DL. Psychopharmacology reviews: Diazepam-associated gynecomastia. *Primary Psychiatry*. 2005;12(7):27.

Grippo AJ, Francis J, Weiss RM, Felder RB, Johnson AK. Cytokine mediation of experimental heart failure-induced anhedonia. *Am J Physiol Regul Integr Comp Physiol*. 2003;284:R666–R673.

Heisler LK, Cowley MA, Tecott LH, Fan W, Low MJ, Smart JL, Rubinstein M, Tatro JB, Marcus JN, Holstege H, Lee CE, Cone RD, Elmquist JK. Activation of central melanocortin pathways by fenfluramine. *Science*. 2002;297:609–611.

Khan A, Khan SR, Leventhal RM, Krishnan RR, Gorman JM. An application of the revised CONSORT standards to FDA summary reports of recently approved antidepressants and antipsychotics. *Biol Psychiatry*. 2002;52:62–67.

King C, Voruganti LN. What's in a name? The evolution of nomenclature of antipsychotic drugs. *J Psychiatry Neurosci*. 2002;27:168–175.

Kosky N. A possible association between high normal and high dose olanzapine and prolongation of the PR interval. *J Psychopharmacol*. 2002;16:181–182.

Malizia AL. The role of emission tomography in pharmacokinetic and pharmacodynamic studies in clinical psychopharmacology. *J Psychopharmacol*. 2006;20[Suppl 4]:100–107.

Preskorn SH. Pharmacogenomics, informatics, and individual drug therapy in psychiatry: past, present and future. *J Psychopharmacol*. 2006;20[Suppl 4]: 85–94.

Ray WA, Daugherty JR, Meador KG. Effect of a mental health "carve-out" program on the continuity of antipsychotic therapy. *N Engl J Med*. 2003;348:1885–1894.

Sussman N. General principles of psychopharmacology. In: Sadock BJ, Sadock VS, eds. *Kaplan & Sadock's Comprehensive Textbook of Psychiatry*. 8th ed. Vol. 2. Baltimore: Lippincott Williams & Wilkins; 2005:2676.

Wadsworth EJK, Moss SC, Simpson SA, Smith AP. Psychotropic medication use and accidents, injuries, and cognitive failures. *Human Psychopharmaocology: Clinical and Experimental*. 2005;20(6):391–400.

Wang PS, Walker AM, Tsuang MT, Orav EJ, Glynn RJ, Levin R, Avorn J. Dopamine antagonists and the development of breast cancer. *Arch Gen Psychiatry*. 2002;59:1147–1154.

Zajecka J, Goldstein C. Combining and augmenting: Choosing the right therapies for treatment-resistant depression. *Psychiatric Annals*. 2005;35(12):994–1000.

▲ 36.2 Medication-Induced Movement Disorders

The text revision of the fourth edition of the *Diagnostic and Statistical Manual of Mental Disorders* (DSM-IV-TR) includes in the category of "medication-induced movement disorders" both such disorders and any medication-induced adverse effect that becomes a focus of clinical attention. The most common neuroleptic-related movement disorders are parkinsonism, acute dystonia, and acute akathisia. Neuroleptic malignant syndrome is a life-threatening and often misdiagnosed condition. Neuroleptic-induced tardive dyskinesia is a late-appearing adverse effect of neuroleptic drugs and can be irreversible; recent data, however, indicate that the syndrome, although still serious and potentially disabling, is less pernicious than was previously thought in patients taking dopamine receptor antagonists (DRAs). The newer antipsychotics, the serotonin-dopamine antagonists (SDAs), block binding to dopamine receptors to a much lesser degree and thereby are less likely to produce such movement disorders. Table 36.2–1 lists the selected medications associated with movement disorders and their impact on relevant neuroreceptors.

NEUROLEPTIC-INDUCED PARKINSONISM

Diagnosis, Signs, and Symptoms

Symptoms include muscle stiffness (lead pipe rigidity), cogwheel rigidity, shuffling gait, stooped posture, and drooling. The pill-rolling tremor of idiopathic parkinsonism is rare, but a regular, coarse tremor similar to essential tremor may be present. The so-called *rabbit syndrome,* a tremor affecting the lips and perioral muscles, is another parkinsonian effect seen with antipsychotics, although perioral tremor is more likely than other tremors to occur late in the course of treatment.

Epidemiology

Parkinsonian adverse effects occur in about 15 percent of patients who are treated with antipsychotics, usually within 5 to 90 days of the initiation of treatment. Patients who are elderly and female are at the highest risk for neuroleptic-induced parkinsonism, although the disorder can occur at all ages.

Etiology

Neuroleptic-induced parkinsonism is caused by the blockade of dopamine type 2 (D_2) receptors in the caudate at the termination of the nigrostriatal dopamine neurons. All antipsychotics can cause the symptoms, especially high-potency drugs with low levels of anticholinergic activity (e.g., trifluoperazine [Stelazine]). Chlorpromazine (Thorazine) and thioridazine (Mellaril) are not likely to be involved. The newer, atypical antipsychotics (e.g., aripiprazole [Abilify], olanzapine [Zyprexa], and quetiapine [Seroquel]) are less likely to cause parkinsonism.

Differential Diagnosis

Included in the differential diagnosis are idiopathic parkinsonism, other organic causes of parkinsonism, and depression, which can also be associated with parkinsonian symptoms.

Treatment

Parkinsonism can be treated with anticholinergic agents, benztropine (Cogentin), amantadine (Symmetrel), or diphenhydramine (Benadryl) (Table 36.2–2). Anticholinergics should be withdrawn after 4 to 6 weeks to assess whether tolerance to the parkinsonian effects has developed; about half of patients with neuroleptic-induced parkinsonism require continued treatment. Even after the antipsychotics are withdrawn, parkinsonian symptoms can last up to 2 weeks and even up to 3 months in elderly patients. With such patients, the clinician may continue the anticholinergic drug after the antipsychotic has been stopped until the parkinsonian symptoms resolve completely.

NEUROLEPTIC-INDUCED ACUTE DYSTONIA

Diagnosis, Signs, and Symptoms

Dystonias are brief or prolonged contractions of muscles that result in obviously abnormal movements or postures, including oculogyric crises, tongue protrusion, trismus, torticollis, laryngeal–pharyngeal dystonias, and dystonic postures of the limbs and trunk. Other dystonias include blepharospasm and glossopharyngeal dystonia; the latter results in dysarthria, dysphagia, and even difficulty in breathing, which can cause cyanosis. Children are particularly likely to evidence opisthotonos, scoliosis, lordosis, and writhing movements. Dystonia can be painful and frightening and often results in noncompliance with future drug treatment regimens.

Epidemiology

The development of dystonic symptoms is characterized by their early onset during the course of treatment with neuroleptics and their high incidence in men, in patients younger than age 30 years, and in patients given high dosages of high-potency medications.

Etiology

Although it is most common with intramuscular doses of high-potency antipsychotics, dystonia can occur with any antipsychotic. The mechanism of action is thought to be dopaminergic hyperactivity in the basal ganglia that occurs when central nervous system (CNS) levels of the antipsychotic drug begin to fall between doses.

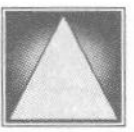

Table 36.2–1
Selected Medications Associated with Movement Disorders: Impact on Relevant Neuroreceptors

Type (Subtype)	Name (Brand)	D_2 Blockade	5-HT_2 Blockade	mACh Blockade
Antipsychotics				
Phenothiazine (Aliphatic)	Chlorpromazine (Thorazine)	Low	High	High
Phenothiazine (Piperidines)	Thioridazine (Mellaril)	Low	Med	High
	Mesoridazine (Serentil)	Low	Med	High
Phenothiazine (Piperazines)	Trifluoperazine (Stelazine)	Med	Med	Med
	Fluphenazine (Prolixin)	High	Low	Low
	Perphenazine (Trilafon)	High	Med	Low
Thioxanthenes	Thiothixene (Navane)	High	Med	Low
	Chlorprothivene (Taractan)	Med	High	Med
Dibenzoxazepines	Loxapine (Lovitane)	Med	High	Low
Butyrophenones	Haloperidol (Haldol)	High	Low	Low
	Droperidol (Inapsine)	High	Med	—
Diphenyl-butylpiperidines	Pimozide (Orap)	High	Med	Low
Dihydroindolones	Molindone (Moban)	Med	Low	Low
Dibenzodiazepines	Clozapine (Clozaril)	Low	High	High
Benzisoyazole	Risperidone (Risperdal)	High	High	Low
Thienobenzodiazepines	Olanzapine (Zvprexa)	Low	High	High
Dibenzothiazepines	Quetiapine (Seroquel)	Low/med	Low/med	Low
Benzisothiazolvils	Ziprasidone (Geodon)	Med	High	Low
Quinolones	Aripiprazole (Abilify)	High (as partial agonist)	High	Low
Nonantipsychotic psychotropics	Lithium (Eskalith)	N/A	N/A	N/A
Anticonvulsants		Low	Low	Low
Antidepressants		Low (except amoxapine)	(Varies)	(Varies)
Nonpsychotropics	Prochlorperazine (Compazine)	High	Med	Low
	Metoclopramide (Reglan)	High	High	—

D_2, dopamine type 2; 5-HT_2, 5-hydroxytryptomine type 2; mACh, mustarinic acetylcholine; N/A, not applicable.
(Adapted from Jantcak PG, David JM, Preshorn SH, et al. *Principles and Practice of Psychopharmacotherapy.* 3rd ed. Philadelphia: Lippincott Williams & Wilkins; 2001, with permission.)

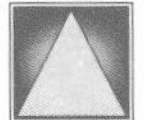

Table 36.2–2
Drug Treatment of Extrapyramidal Disorders

Generic Name	Trade Name	Usual Daily Dosage	Indications
Anticholinergics			
Benztropine	Cogentin	PO 0.5 to 2 mg tid; IM or IV 1 to 2 mg	Acute dystonia, parkinsonism, akinesia, akathisia
Biperiden	Akineton	PO 2 to 6 mg tid; IM or IV 2 mg	
Procyclidine	Kemadrin	PO 2.5 to 5 mg bid-qid	
Trihexyphenidyl	Artane, Tremin	PO 2 to 5 mg tid	
Orphenodrine	Norflex, Dispal	PO 50 to 100 mg bid-qid; IV 60 mg	Rabbit syndrome
Antihistamine			
Diphenhydramine	Benadryl	PO 25 mg qid; IM or IV 25 mg	Acute dystonia, parkinsonism, akinesia, rabbit syndrome
Amantadine	Symmetrel	PO 100 to 200 mg bid	Parkinsonism, akinesia rabbit syndrome
β-Adrenergic antagonist			
Propranolol	Inderal	PO 20 to 40 mg tid	Akathisia, tremor
α-Adrenergic antagonist			
Clonidine	Catapres	PO 0.1 mg tid	Akathisia
Benzodiazepines			
Clonazepam	Klonopin	PO 1 mg bid	Akathisia, acute dystonia
Lorazepam	Ativan	PO 1 mg tid	
Buspirone	BuSpar	PO 20 to 40 mg qid	Tardive dyskinesia
Vitamin E	—	PO 1200 to 1600 IU/day	Tardive dyskinesia

PO, oral; IM, intramuscular; IV, intravenous; qd, per day; bid, twice a day; tid, three times a day; qid; four times a day.

Differential Diagnosis

The differential diagnosis includes seizures and tardive dyskinesia.

Course and Prognosis

Dystonia can fluctuate spontaneously and respond to reassurance, so that the clinician acquires the false impression that the movement is hysterical or completely under conscious control.

Treatment

Prophylaxis with anticholinergics or related drugs (Table 36.2–2) usually prevents dystonia, although the risks of prophylactic treatment weigh against that benefit. Treatment with intramuscular anticholinergics or intravenous or intramuscular diphenhydramine (50 mg) almost always relieves the symptoms. Diazepam (Valium) (10 mg intravenously), amobarbital (Amytal), caffeine sodium benzoate, and hypnosis have also been reported to be effective. Although tolerance for the adverse effects usually develops, it is sometimes prudent to change the antipsychotic if the patient is particularly concerned that the reaction may recur.

NEUROLEPTIC-INDUCED ACUTE AKATHISIA

Diagnosis, Signs, and Symptoms

Akathisia is subjective feelings of restlessness, objective signs of restlessness, or both. Examples include a sense of anxiety, inability to relax, jitteriness, pacing, rocking motions while sitting, and rapid alternation of sitting and standing. Akathisia has been associated with the use of a wide range of psychiatric drugs, including antipsychotics, antidepressants, and sympathomimetics. Once akathisia is recognized and diagnosed, the antipsychotic dose should be reduced to the minimal effective level. Akathisia may be associated with a poor treatment outcome.

Epidemiology

Middle-aged women are at increased risk of akathisia, and the time course is similar to that for neuroleptic-induced parkinsonism.

Treatment

Three basic steps in the treatment of akathisia are reducing medication dosage, attempting treatment with appropriate drugs, and considering changing the neuroleptic. The most efficacious drugs are β-adrenergic receptor antagonists, although anticholinergic drugs, benzodiazepines, and cyproheptadine (Periactin) may benefit some patients. In some cases of akathisia, no treatment seems to be effective.

NEUROLEPTIC-INDUCED TARDIVE DYSKINESIA

Diagnosis, Signs, and Symptoms

Tardive dyskinesia is a delayed effect of antipsychotics; it rarely occurs until after 6 months of treatment. The disorder consists of abnormal, involuntary, irregular choreoathetoid movements of the muscles of the head, limbs, and trunk. The severity of the movements ranges from minimal—often missed by patients and their families—to grossly incapacitating. Perioral movements are the most common and include darting, twisting, and protruding movements of the tongue; chewing and lateral jaw movements; lip puckering; and facial grimacing. Finger movements and hand clenching are also common. Torticollis, retrocollis, trunk twisting, and pelvic thrusting occur in severe cases. In the most serious cases, patients may have breathing and swallowing irregularities that result in aerophagia, belching, and grunting. Respiratory dyskinesia has also been reported. Dyskinesia is exacerbated by stress and disappears during sleep.

Epidemiology

Tardive dyskinesia develops in about 10 percent to 20 percent of patients who are treated for more than a year. About 20 percent to 40 percent of patients having long-term hospitalization have tardive dyskinesia. Women are more likely to be affected than men. Children, patients who are more than 50 years of age, and patients with brain damage or mood disorders are also at high risk.

Course and Prognosis

Between 5 percent and 40 percent of all cases of tardive dyskinesia eventually remit, and between 50 percent and 90 percent of all mild cases remit. Tardive dyskinesia is less likely to remit in elderly patients than in young patients, however.

Treatment

The three basic approaches to tardive dyskinesia are prevention, diagnosis, and management. Prevention is best achieved by using antipsychotic medications only when clearly indicated and in the lowest effective doses. The atypical antipsychotics are associated with less tardive dyskinesia than the older antipsychotics. Clozapine is the only antipsychotic to have minimal risk of tardive dyskinesia, and can even help improve preexisting symptoms of tardive dyskinesia. This has been attributed to its low affinity for D_2 receptors and high affinity for 5-hydroxytryptamine (5HT) receptor antagonism. Patients who are receiving antipsychotics should be examined regularly for the appearance of abnormal movements, preferably with the use of a standardized rating scale (Table 36.2–3). Patients frequently experience an exacerbation of their symptoms when the DRA is withheld, whereas substitution of an SDA may limit the abnormal movements without worsening the progression of the dyskinesia.

Once tardive dyskinesia is recognized, the clinician should consider reducing the dose of the antipsychotic or even stopping the medication altogether. Alternatively, the clinician may switch the patient to clozapine or to one of the new SDAs. In patients who cannot continue taking any antipsychotic medication, lithium, carbamazepine (Tegretol), or benzodiazepines may effectively reduce the symptoms of both the movement disorder and the psychosis.

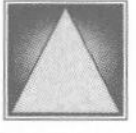

Table 36.2–3
Abnormal Involuntary Movement Scale (AIMS) Examination Procedure

Patient Identification **Date**

Rated by

Either before or after completing the examination procedure, observe the patient unobtrusively at rest (e.g., in waiting room).
The chair to be used in this examination should be a hard, firm one without arms.
After observing the patient, rate him or her on a scale of 0 (none), 1 (minimal), 2 (mild), 3 (moderate), and 4 (severe), according to the severity of the symptoms.
Ask patient whether there is anything in his or her mouth (e.g., gum, candy) and, if so, to remove it.
Ask patient about the current condition of his or her teeth. Ask patient if he or she wears dentures. Do teeth or dentures bother patient now?
Ask patient whether he or she notices movement in mouth, face, hands, or feet. If yes, ask patient to describe and indicate to what extent movements currently bother patient or interfere with his or her activities.
0 1 2 3 4 Have patient sit in chair with hands on knees, legs slightly apart, and feet flat on floor. (Look at entire body for movement while in this position.)
0 1 2 3 4 Ask patient to sit with hands hanging unsupported. If male, between legs; if female and wearing a dress, hanging over knees. (Observe hands and other body areas.)
0 1 2 3 4 Ask patient to open mouth. (Observe tongue at rest within mouth.) Do this twice.
0 1 2 3 4 Ask patient to protrude tongue. (Observe abnormalities of tongue movement.) Do this twice.
0 1 2 3 4 Ask patient to tap thumb, with each finger, as rapidly as possible for 10 to 15 seconds; separately with right hand, then with left hand. (Observe focial and leg movements.)
0 1 2 3 4 Flex and extend patient's left and right arms. (One at a time.)
0 1 2 3 4 Ask patient to stand up. (Observe in profile. Observe all body areas again, hips included.)
0 1 2 3 4 [a]Ask patient to extend both arms outstretched in front with palms down. (Observe trunk, legs, and mouth.)
0 1 2 3 4 [a]Have patient walk a few paces, turn, and walk back to chair. (Observe hands and gait.)
Do this twice.

[a] Activated movements.

NEUROLEPTIC MALIGNANT SYNDROME

Diagnosis, Signs, and Symptoms

Neuroleptic malignant syndrome is a life-threatening complication that can occur anytime during the course of antipsychotic treatment. The motor and behavioral symptoms include muscular rigidity and dystonia, akinesia, mutism, obtundation, and agitation. The autonomic symptoms include high fever, sweating, and increased pulse and blood pressure. Laboratory findings include an increased white blood cell count and increased levels of creatinine phosphokinase, liver enzymes, plasma myoglobin, and myoglobinuria, occasionally associated with renal failure.

Epidemiology

Men are affected more frequently than women, and young patients are affected more commonly than elderly patients. The mortality rate can reach 10 percent to 20 percent or even higher when depot antipsychotic medications are involved. The prevalence of the syndrome is estimated to be 0.02 percent to 2.4 percent of patients exposed to DRAs.

Course and Prognosis

The symptoms usually evolve over 24 to 72 hours, and the untreated syndrome lasts 10 to 14 days. The diagnosis is often

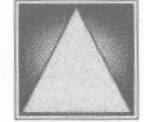

Table 36.2–4
Treatment of Neuroleptic Malignant Syndrome

Intervention	Dosing	Effectiveness
Amantadine	200 to 400 mg PO/day in divided doses	Beneficial as monotherapy or in combination; decrease in death rate
Bromocriptine	2.5 mg PO bid or tid, may increase to a total of 45 mg/day	Mortality reduced as a single or combined agent
Levodopa/carbidopa	Levodopa 50 to 100 mg/day IV as continuous infusion	Case reports of dramatic improvement
Electroconvulsive therapy	Reports of good outcome with both unilateral and bilateral treatments; response may occur in as few as three treatments	Effective when medications have failed; also may treat underlying psychiatric disorder
Dantrolene	1 mg/kg/day for 8 days, then continue as PO for 7 additional days	Benefits may occur in minutes or hours as a single agent or in combination
Benzodiazepines	1 to 2 mg IM as test dose; if effective, switch to PO; consider use if underlying disorder has catatonic symptoms	Has been reported effective when other agents have failed
Supportive measures	IV hydration, cooling blankets, ice packs, ice-water enema, oxygenation, antipyretics	Often effective as initial approach early in the episode

PO, oral; bid, twice a day; tid, three times a day; IV, intravenously; IM, intramuscularly.
Adapted from Davis JM. Caroif SN, Mann SC. Treatment of neuroleptic malignant syndrome. *Psychiatr Ann.* 2000;30:325–331, with permission.)

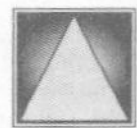

Table 36.2–5
Drug-Induced Central Hyperthermic Syndromes[a]

Condition (and Mechanism)	Common Drug Causes	Frequent Symptoms	Possible Treatment[b]	Clinical Course
Hyperthermia (↓ heat dissipation) (↑ heat production)	Atropine, lidocaine, meperidine NSAID toxicity, pheochromocytoma, thyrotoxicosis	Hyperthermia, diaphoresis, malaise	Acetaminophen per rectum (325 mg every 4 hrs), diazepam oral or per rectum (5 mg every 8 hrs) for febrile seizures	Benign, febrile seizures in children
Malignant hyperthemia (↑ heat production)	NMJ blockers (succinylcholine), halathone	Hyperthermia muscle rigidity, arrthythmias, ischemia,[c] hypotension, rhabdomyolysis; disseminated intravascular coagulation	Dantrolene sodium (1–2 mg/kg/min IV infusion)[d]	Familial, 10% mortality if untreated
Tricyclic overdose (↑ heat production)	Tricyclic antidepressants, cocaine	Hyperthermia, confusion, visual hallucinations, agitation, hyperreflexia, muscle relaxation, anticholinergic effects (dry skin, pupil dilation), arrhythmias	Sodium bicarbonate (1 mEq/kg IV bolus) if arrhythmia is present, physostigmine (1–3 mg IV) with cardiac monitoring	Fatalities have occurred if untreated
Autonomic hyperreflexia (↑ heat production)	CNS stimulants (amphetamines)	Hyperthermia excitement, hyperreflexia	Trimethaphan (0.3–7 mg/min IV infusion)	Reversible
Lethal catatonia (↓ heat dissipation)	Lead poisoning	Hyperthermia, intense anxiety, destructive behavior, psychosis	Lorazepam (1–2 mg IV every 4 hrs), antipsychotics may be contraindicated	High mortality if untreated
Neuroleptic malignant syndrome (mixed; hypothalamic, ↓ heat dissipation, ↑ heat production)	Antipsychotics (neuroleptics), methyldopa, reserpine	Hyperthermia, muscle rigidity, diaphoresis (60%), leukocytosis, delirium, rhabdomyolysis, elevated CPK, autonomic deregulation, extrapyramidal symptoms	Bromocriptine (2–10 mg every 8 hrs orally or nsagastric tube), lisuride (0.02–0.1 mg/hr IV infusion), carbidopa-levodopa (Sinemet) (25/100 PO every 8 hrs), dantrolene sodium (0.3–1 mg/kg IV every 6 hrs)	Rapid onset, 20% mortality if untreated

[a]Boldface indicates features that may be used to distinguish one syndrome from another. NSAID, nonsteroidal anti-inflammatory drug; MAOI, monoamine oxidase inhibitor; NMJ, neuromuscular junction; CNS, central nervous system; CPK, creatine phosphokinase; IV, intravenously.
[b]Gastric lavage and supportive measures, including cooling, are required in most cases.
[c]Oxygen consumption increases by 7% for every 1°F up in body temperature.
[d]Has been associated with idiosyncratic hepatocellular injury, as well as severe hypotension in one case.
(From Theoharides TC, Harris RS, Weckstein D. Neuroleptic malignant-like syndrome due to cyclobenzaprine? [letter]. *J Clin Psychopharmacol* 1995;15:80, with permission.)

missed in the early stages, and the withdrawal or agitation may mistakenly be considered to reflect an exacerbation of the psychosis.

Treatment

In addition to supportive medical treatment, the most commonly used medications for the condition are dantrolene (Dantrium) and bromocriptine (Parlodel), although amantadine (Symmetrel) is sometimes used. Bromocriptine and amantadine pose direct DRA effects and may serve to overcome the antipsychotic-induced dopamine receptor blockade. The lowest effective dosage of the antipsychotic drug should be used to reduce the chance of neuroleptic malignant syndrome. Antipsychotic drugs with anticholinergic effects seem less likely to cause neuroleptic malignant syndrome (Table 36.2–4). Electroconvulsive therapy (ECT) has been used successfully and is preferred by some clinicians.

MEDICATION-INDUCED POSTURAL TREMOR

Diagnosis, Signs, and Symptoms

Tremor is a rhythmic alteration in movement that is usually faster than one beat per second.

Epidemiology

Typically, tremors decrease during periods of relaxation and sleep and increase with stress or anxiety.

Etiology

Whereas all the above diagnoses specifically include an association with a neuroleptic, a range of psychiatric medications can produce tremor—most notably, lithium, antidepressants, and valproate (Depakene).

Treatment

The treatment involves four principles:

1. The lowest possible dose of the psychiatric drug should be taken.
2. Patients should minimize caffeine consumption.
3. The psychiatric drug should be taken at bedtime to minimize the amount of daytime tremor.
4. β-adrenergic receptor antagonists (e.g., propranolol [Inderal]) can be given to treat drug-induced tremors.

OTHER MOVEMENT DISORDERS

Nocturnal Myoclonus

Nocturnal myoclonus consists of highly stereotyped, abrupt contractions of certain leg muscles during sleep. Patients lack any subjective awareness of the leg jerks. The condition may be present in about 40 percent of persons over 65 years of age. The cause is unknown, but it is a rare side effect of selective serotonin reuptake inhibitors (SSRIs).

The repetitive leg movements occur every 20 to 60 seconds, with extensions of the large toe and flexion of the ankle, the knee, and the hips. Frequent awakenings, unrefreshing sleep, and daytime sleepiness are major symptoms. No treatment for nocturnal myoclonus is universally effective. Treatments that may be useful include benzodiazepines, levodopa (Larodopa), quinine, and, in rare cases, opioids.

Restless Leg Syndrome

In restless leg syndrome, persons feel deep sensations of creeping inside the calves whenever sitting or lying down. The dysesthesias are rarely painful, but are agonizingly relentless and cause an almost irresistible urge to move the legs; thus, this syndrome interferes with sleep and with falling asleep. It peaks in middle age and occurs in 5 percent of the population. The cause is unknown, but it is a rare side effect of SSRIs.

Symptoms are relieved by movement and by leg massage. The dopamine receptor agonist ropinirole (Requip) is effective in treating this syndrome. Other treatments include the benzodiazepines, levodopa, quinine, opioids, propranolol (Inderal), valproate (Depakene), and carbamazepine (Tegretol).

HYPERTHERMIC SYNDROMES

All the medication-induced movement disorders may be associated with hyperthermia. Table 36.2–5 lists the various conditions associated with hyperthermia.

References

Caroff SN, Mann SC, Campbell EC, Sullivan KA. Movement disorders associated with atypical antipsychotic drugs. *J Clin Psychiatry*. 2002;63[Suppl 4]:12–19.

Earley CJ. Restless legs syndrome. *N Engl J Med*. 2003;348(21):2103.

Factor SA, Lang AE, Weiner WJ, eds. *Drug Induced Movement Disorders*. 2nd ed. Malden, MA: Blackwell Futura; 2005.

Janicak PG, Beedle D. Medication-induced movement disorders. In: Sadock BJ, Sadock VA, eds. *Kaplan & Sadock's Comprehensive Textbook of Psychiatry*. 8th ed. Vol. 2. Baltimore: Lippincott Williams & Wilkins; 2005:2712.

Janno S, Holi M, Tuisku K, Wahlbeck K. Prevalence of neuroleptic-induced movement disorders in chronic schizophrenic inpatients. *Am J Psychiatry*. 2004;161:160–163.

Lee PE, Sykora K, Gill SS, Mamdani M, Marras C, Anderson G, Shulman KI, Stukel T, Normand SL, Rochon PA. Antipsychotic medications and drug-induced movement disorders other than parkinsonism: A population-based cohort study in older adults. *J Am Geriatr Soc*. 2005;53(8):1374–1379.

Lyons KE, Pahwa R. Efficacy and tolerability of levetiracetam in Parkinson disease patients with levodopa-induced dyskinesia. *Clin Neuropharmacol*. 2006;29(3):148–153.

Papapetropoulos S, Wheeler S, Singer C. Tardive dystonia associated with ziprasidone. *Am J Psychiatry*. 2005;162(11):2191.

Saint-Cyr JA. Neuropsychology for movement disorders neurosurgery. *Can J Neurol Sci*. 2003;30[Suppl 1]:S83093.

Thomas M, Jankovic J. Psychogenic movement disorders: Diagnosis and management. *CNS Drugs*. 2004;18(7):437.

Watts RL, Koller WC. *Movement Disorders Neurologic Principles and Practice*. 2nd ed. New York: McGraw Hill; 2004.

▲ 36.3 α_2-Adrenergic Receptor Agonists: Clonidine and Guanfacine

Clonidine (Catapres) and guanfacine (Tenex) are presynaptic α_2-adrenergic receptor agonists approved for use as antihypertensive agents. Stimulation of α_2-adrenergic receptors reduces the firing rate of noradrenergic neurons and of plasma concentrations of norepinephrine. Because of the widespread actions of the noradrenergic system, clonidine has also been adopted for use as a psychopharmacologic agent. The most important clinical applications in psychiatry are as therapy for attention-deficit/hyperactivity disorder (ADHD), opioid withdrawal, Tourette's disorder, and suppression of agitation in posttraumatic stress disorder (PTSD). Their role as a treatment for selected mental disorders is generally limited to instances in which other interventions have failed to ameliorate symptoms adequately.

CHEMISTRY

The molecular structures of clonidine and guanfacine are shown in Figure 36.3–1.

PHARMACOLOGIC ACTIONS

Clonidine and guanfacine are well absorbed from the gastrointestinal (GI) tract and reach peak plasma levels 1 to 3 hours after oral administration. The half-life of clonidine is 6 to 20 hours and that of guanfacine is 10 to 30 hours.

The agonist effects of clonidine and guanfacine on presynaptic α_2-adrenergic receptors in the sympathetic nuclei of the brain result in a decrease in the amount of norepinephrine released from the presynaptic nerve terminals. This serves generally to reset the body's sympathetic tone at a lower level and decrease arousal.

Clonidine

Guanfacine

FIGURE 36.3–1
Molecular structures of clonidine and guanfacine.

THERAPEUTIC INDICATIONS

Clinical psychiatry has considerably more experience with clonidine than with guanfacine. Recent interest in the use of guanfacine for the same indications that respond to clonidine centers on guanfacine's longer half-life and relative lack of sedative effects.

Withdrawal from Opioids, Alcohol, Benzodiazepines, or Nicotine

Clonidine and guanfacine are effective in reducing the autonomic symptoms of rapid opioid withdrawal (e.g., hypertension, tachycardia, dilated pupils, sweating, lacrimation, and rhinorrhea), but not the associated subjective sensations. Clonidine administration (0.1 to 0.2 mg two to four times a day) is initiated before detoxification and is then tapered off over 1 to 2 weeks (Table 36.3–1).

Clonidine and guanfacine can reduce symptoms of alcohol and benzodiazepine withdrawal, including anxiety, diarrhea, and tachycardia. Clonidine and guanfacine can reduce craving, anxiety, and irritability symptoms of nicotine withdrawal. The transdermal patch formulation of clonidine is associated with better long-term compliance for purposes of detoxification than is the tablet formulation.

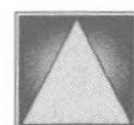

Table 36.3–1
Oral Clonidine Protocols for Opioid Detoxification

Clonidine 0.1 to 0.2 mg PO qid; hold for systolic BP <90 mm Hg or bradycardia; stabilize for 2 to 3 days, then taper over 5 to 10 days

OR

Clonidine 0.1 to 0.2 mg PO q4h to q6h as needed for withdrawal signs or symptoms; stabilize for 2 to 3 days, then taper over 5 to 10 days

OR

Test dose with clonidine 0.1 to 0.2 mg PO or sublingually (for patients weighing over 200 lb); check BP after 1 hr. If diastolic BP >70 mm Hg and no symptoms of hypotension, begin treatment as follows:

Weight (lb)	Number of clonidine patches
<110	1
110–160	2
160–200	2
>200	2

OR

Test dose of oral clonidine 0.1 mg; check BP after 1 h (if systolic BP <90, do not give patch)
Place two TTS-2 clonidine patches (or three patches if patient weighs >150 lb) on hairless area of upper body; then
For first 23 hrs after patch application, give oral clonidine 0.2 mg q6h; then
For next 24 hrs, give oral clonidine 0.1 mg q6h
Change patches weekly
After 2 weeks of two patches, switch to one patch (or two patches if patient weighs >150 lb)
After 1 week of one patch, discontinue patches

PO, oral; BP, blood pressure; hr, hour; TTS, through the skin; q4h, every four hours; q6h, every six hours; qid, four times a day.
(From American Society of Addiction Medicine. Detoxification: Principle and Protocols. In: *The Principles Update Series: Topics in Addiction Medicine,* section 11. American Society of Addiction, 1997, with permission.)

Tourette's Disorder

Clonidine and guanfacine are effective drugs for the treatment of Tourette's disorder. Most clinicians begin treatment for Tourette's disorder with the standard dopamine receptor antagonists (DRAs), haloperidol (Haldol) and pimozide (Orap), and the serotonin-dopamine antagonists, risperidone (Risperdal) and olanzapine (Zyprexa). If concerned about the adverse effects of these drugs, the clinician, however, may begin treatment with clonidine or guanfacine. The starting child dosage of clonidine is 0.05 mg a day; it can be raised to 0.3 mg a day in divided doses. Three months are needed before the beneficial effects of clonidine can be seen in Tourette's disorder. The response rate has been reported to be up to 70 percent.

Other Tic Disorders

Clonidine and guanfacine reduce the frequency and severity of tics in persons with tic disorder with or without comorbid ADHD symptoms.

Hyperactivity and Aggression in Children

Clonidine and guanfacine can be useful alternatives for the treatment of ADHD. They are used in place of sympathomimetics and antidepressants, which can produce paradoxical worsening of hyperactivity in some children with mental retardation, aggression, or features on the spectrum of autism. Clonidine and guanfacine can improve mood, reduce activity level, and improve social adaptation. Some multiply impaired children may respond favorably to clonidine, whereas others may simply become sedated. The starting dosage is 0.05 mg a day; it can be raised to 0.3 mg a day in divided doses. The efficacy of clonidine and guanfacine for control of hyperactivity and aggression often diminishes over several months of use.

Clonidine or guanfacine can be combined with methylphenidate (Ritalin) or amphetamine to treat hyperactivity and inattentiveness, respectively. A few cases have been reported of sudden death of children taking clonidine together with methylphenidate; however, it has not been conclusively demonstrated that these medications contributed to these deaths. The clinician should explain to the family that the efficacy and safety of this combination have not been investigated in controlled trials. Periodic cardiovascular assessments, including vital signs and electrocardiograms, are warranted if this combination is used.

Posttraumatic Stress Disorder

Acute exacerbations of PTSD may be associated with hyperadrenergic symptoms, such as hyperarousal, exaggerated startle response, insomnia, vivid nightmares, tachycardia, agitation, hypertension, and perspiration. These symptoms may respond to the use of clonidine or, especially for overnight benefit, to the use of guanfacine.

Other Disorders

Other potential indications for clonidine include other anxiety disorders (panic disorder, phobias, obsessive-compulsive disorder, and generalized anxiety disorder) and mania, in which it may be synergistic with lithium (Eskalith) or carbamazepine (Tegretol). Anecdotal reports have noted the efficacy of clonidine in schizophrenia and tardive dyskinesia. A clonidine patch can reduce the hypersalivation and dysphagia caused by clozapine (Clozaril).

PRECAUTIONS AND ADVERSE REACTIONS

The most common adverse effects associated with clonidine are dry mouth and eyes, fatigue, sedation, dizziness, nausea, hypotension, and constipation, which result in discontinuation of therapy by about 10 percent of all persons taking the drug. Some persons also experience sexual dysfunction. Tolerance may develop to these adverse effects. A similar but milder adverse effect profile is seen with guanfacine, especially at doses of 3 mg or more per day. Clonidine and guanfacine should not be taken by adults with blood pressure (BP) below 90/60 or with cardiac arrhythmias, especially bradycardia. Development of bradycardia warrants gradual, tapered discontinuation of the drug. Clonidine, in particular, is associated with sedation, and tolerance does not usually develop to this adverse effect. Uncommon central nervous system (CNS) adverse effects of clonidine include insomnia, anxiety, and depression; rare CNS adverse effects include vivid dreams, nightmares, and hallucinations. Fluid retention associated with clonidine use can be treated with diuretics.

The transdermal patch formulation of clonidine can cause local skin irritation, which can be minimized by rotating the application sites.

Overdose

Persons who take an overdose of clonidine can present with coma and constricted pupils, symptoms similar to those of an opioid overdose. Other symptoms of overdose are decreased BP, pulse, and respiratory rates. Guanfacine overdose produces a milder version of these symptoms. Clonidine and guanfacine should be used with caution in persons with heart disease, any type of vascular disease, renal disease, Raynaud's syndrome, or a history of depression. Clonidine and guanfacine should be avoided during pregnancy and by nursing mothers. Elderly persons are more sensitive to the drug than are younger adults. Children are susceptible to the same adverse effects as are adults.

Withdrawal

Abrupt discontinuation of clonidine can cause anxiety, restlessness, perspiration, tremor, abdominal pain, palpitations, headache, and a dramatic rise in BP. These symptoms may appear about 20 hours after the last dose of clonidine and, thus, may be seen if one or two doses are skipped. A similar set of symptoms occasionally occurs 2 to 4 days after discontinuation of guanfacine, but the usual course is a gradual return to baseline BP over 2 to 4 days. Because of the possibility of discontinuation symptoms, dosages of clonidine and guanfacine should be tapered slowly.

DRUG INTERACTIONS

Coadministration of clonidine and tricyclic drugs can reduce the hypotensive effects of clonidine. Clonidine and guanfacine may enhance the CNS depressive effects of barbiturates, alcohol, other sedative-hypnotics, and trazodone (Desyrel). Clonidine and guanfacine can have an unwanted synergistic hypotensive effect if coadministered with other antihypertensive drugs. The α_2-adrenergic receptor antagonist yohimbine (Yocon) blocks the effects of clonidine and guanfacine. The concomitant use of β-adrenergic receptor antagonists can increase the severity of rebound phenomena when clonidine and guanfacine are discontinued.

LABORATORY INTERFERENCES

No known laboratory interferences are associated with the use of clonidine or guanfacine.

DOSAGE AND CLINICAL GUIDELINES

Clonidine is available in 0.1-, 0.2-, and 0.3-mg tablets. The usual starting dosage is 0.1 mg orally twice a day; the dosage can be raised by 0.1 mg a day to an appropriate level (up to 1.2 mg per day). Clonidine must always be tapered when it is discontinued to avoid rebound hypertension, which may occur about 20 hours after the last clonidine dose. A weekly transdermal formulation of clonidine is available at doses of 0.1, 0.2, and 0.3 mg per day. The usual starting dosage is the 0.1-mg-a-day patch, which is changed each week for adults and every 5 days for children; the dose can be increased, as needed, every 1 to 2 weeks. Transition from the oral to the transdermal formulations should be accomplished gradually by overlapping them for 3 to 4 days.

Guanfacine is available in 1- and 2-mg tablets. The usual starting dose is 1 mg before sleep, and this can be increased to 2 mg before sleep after 3 to 4 weeks, if necessary. Regardless of the indication for which clonidine or guanfacine is being used, the drug should be withheld if a person becomes hypotensive (BP below 90/60).

Table 36.3–2 provides a summary of the α_2-adrenergic receptor agonists used in psychiatry.

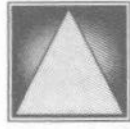

Table 36.3–2
α2-Adrenergic Receptor Agonists Used in Psychiatry[a]

Drug	Preparations	Usual Child Starting Dosage	Usual Child Dosage Range	Usual Starting Adult Dosage	Usual Adult Dosage
Clonidine tablets (Catapres)	0.1, 0.2, 0.3 mg	0.05 mg a day	Up to 0.3 mg a day tablets in divided doses	0.1 to 0.2 mg two to four times a day (0.2 to 0.8 mg a day)	0.3 to 1.2 mg a day, two to three times a day (1.2 mg a day maximal dosage)
Clonidine transdermal system (Catapres-TTS)	0.1, 0.2, 0.3 mg a day	0.05 mg a day	Up to 0.3 mg a day patch every 5 days (0.5 mg a day every 5 days maximal dosage)	0.1 mg a day every 7 days	0.1 mg a day patch per week 0.6 mg a day every 7 days
Guanfacine (Tenex)	1–2-mg tablets	1 mg a day at bedtime	1 to 2 mg a day at bedtime (3 mg a day maximal dosage)	1 mg a day at bedtime	1 to 2 mg at bedtime (3 mg a day maximal dosage)

[a]Dosages for medical indications, such as hypertension, vary.

References

Hazell PL, Stuart J. A randomized controlled trial of clonidine added to psychostimulant medication for hyperactive and aggressive children. *J Am Acad Child Adolesc Psychiatry*. 2003;42(8):886–894.

Ishiyama T, Kashimoto S, Oguchi T, Furuya A, Fukushima H, Kumazawa T. Clonidine-ephedrine combination reduces pain on injection of propofol and blunts hemodynamic stress responses during the induction sequence. *J Clin Anesth*. 2006;18(3):211–215.

Johnston JA, Ye W, Van Brunt DL, Pohl G, Sumner CR. Decreased use of clonidine following treatment with atomoxetine in children with ADHD. *J Clin Psychopharmacol*. 2006;26(4):389–395.

King D, Etzel JP, Chopra S, Smith J, Cadman PE, Rao F, Funk SD, Rana BK, Schork NJ, Insel PA, O'Connor DT. Human response to alpha$_2$-adrenergic agonist stimulation studied in an isolated vascular bed in vivo: Biphasic influence of dose, age, gender, and receptor genotype. *Clin Pharmacol Ther*. 2005;77(5):388–403.

Nemeroff CB, Putnam JS. α_2-adrenergic receptor agonists: Clonidine and guanfacine. In: Sadock BJ, Sadock VA, eds. *Kaplan & Sadock's Comprehensive Textbook of Psychiatry*. 8th ed. Vol. 2. Baltimore: Lippincott Williams & Wilkins; 2005:2718.

Park L, Nigg JT, Waldman ID, Nummy KA, Huang-Pollock C, Rappley M, Friderici KH. Association and linkage of α_{2A} adrenergic receptor gene polymorphisms with childhood ADHD. *Mol Psychiatry*. 2005;10:572.

Posey DJ, Puntney JI, Sasher TM, Kem DL, McDougle CJ. Guanfacine treatment of hyperactivity and inattention in pervasive developmental disorders: A retrospective analysis of 80 cases. *J Child Adolesc Psychopharmacol*. 2004;14(2):233–241.

Schnoes CJ, Kuhn BR, Workman EF, Ellis CR. Pediatric prescribing practices for clonidine and other pharmacologic agents for children with sleep disturbance. *Clin Pediatr (Phila)*. 2006;45(3):229–238.

Szot P, Lester M, Laughlin ML, Palmiter RD, Liles LC, Weinshenker D. The anticonvulsant and proconvulsant effects of α_2-adrenoreceptor agonists are mediated by distinct populations of α_{2A}-adrenoreceptors. *Neuroscience*. 2004;126(3):795.

Webber MA, Szwast SJ, Steadman TM, Frazer A, Malloy FW, Lightfoot JD, Shekhar A. Guanfacine treatment of clozapine-induced sialorrhea. *J Clin Psychopharmacol*. 2004;24(6):675–676.

▲ 36.4 β-Adrenergic Receptor Antagonists

The β-adrenergic receptor antagonists, which are variously referred to as *β-blockers* and *β-antagonists,* are commonly used in medical practice for their peripheral effects in the treatment of hypertension, angina, certain cardiac arrhythmias, and migraine. Their effectiveness as peripherally and centrally acting agents has been well demonstrated for social phobia (e.g., performance anxiety), lithium-induced postural tremor, control of aggressive behavior, and neuroleptic-induced akathisia (Table 36.4–1). Figure 36.4–1 depicts the structure of the human β_2-adrenergic receptor.

CHEMISTRY

The β-receptor antagonists most commonly used in psychiatry are propranolol (Inderal), nadolol (Corgard), pindolol (Visken), labetalol (Normodyne, Trandate), atenolol (Tenormin), metoprolol (Lopressor, Toprol), and acebutolol (Sectral). The molecular structures of these drugs are shown in Figure 36.4–2.

PHARMACOLOGIC ACTIONS

The β-receptor antagonists differ with regard to lipophilicities, metabolic routes, β-receptor selectivity, and half-lives (Table 36.4–2). The absorption of the β-receptor antagonists from the gastrointestinal (GI) tract is variable. The agents that are most soluble in lipids (i.e., are lipophilic) are likely to cross the blood–brain barrier and enter the brain; those agents that are least lipophilic are less likely to enter the brain. When central nervous system (CNS) effects are desired, a lipophilic drug may be

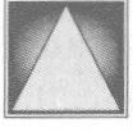

Table 36.4–1
Psychiatric Uses for β-Adrenergic Receptor Antagonists

Definitely effective
- Performance anxiety
- Lithium-induced tremor
- Neuroleptic-induced akathisia

Probably effective
- Adjunctive therapy for alcohol withdrawal and other substance-related disorders
- Adjunctive therapy for aggressive or violent behavior

Possibly effective
- Antipsychotic augmentation
- Antidepressant augmentation

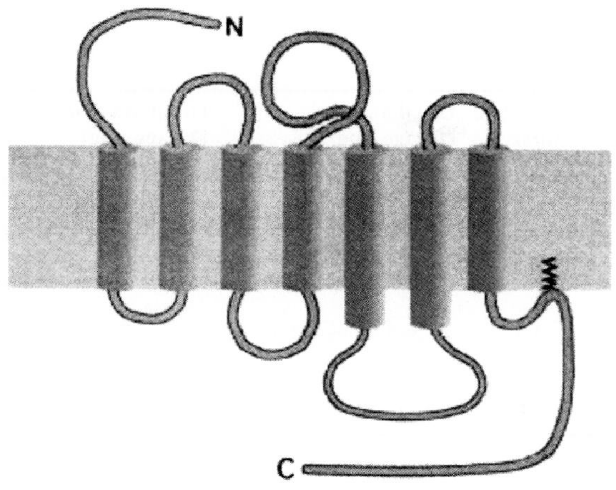

FIGURE 36.4–1
Snake diagram of the human β_2-adrenergic receptor. (Adapted from Gerthur U. Uncovering molecular mechanisms involved in activation of G protein coupled receptors. *Endocr Rev.* 2002;21(1): 90–113, with permission.)

preferred; when only peripheral effects are desired, a less lipophilic drug may be indicated.

Propranolol, nadolol, pindolol, and labetalol have essentially equal potency at both the β_1- and β_2-receptors, whereas metoprolol, atenolol, and acebutolol have greater affinity for the β_1-receptor than for the β_2-receptor. Relative β_1-selectivity confers few pulmonary and vascular effects on these drugs, although they must be used with caution in asthmatic persons, because the drugs retain some activity at the β_2-receptors.

Pindolol has sympathomimetic effects in addition to its β-antagonist effects, which has permitted its use for augmentation of antidepressant drugs. Pindolol, propranolol, and nadolol possess some antagonist activity at the serotonin 5-HT_{1A} receptors.

THERAPEUTIC INDICATIONS

Anxiety Disorders

Propranolol is useful for the treatment of social phobia, primarily of the performance type (e.g., disabling anxiety before a musical performance). Data are also available for its use in treatment of panic disorder, posttraumatic stress disorder (PTSD), and generalized anxiety disorder. In social phobia, the common

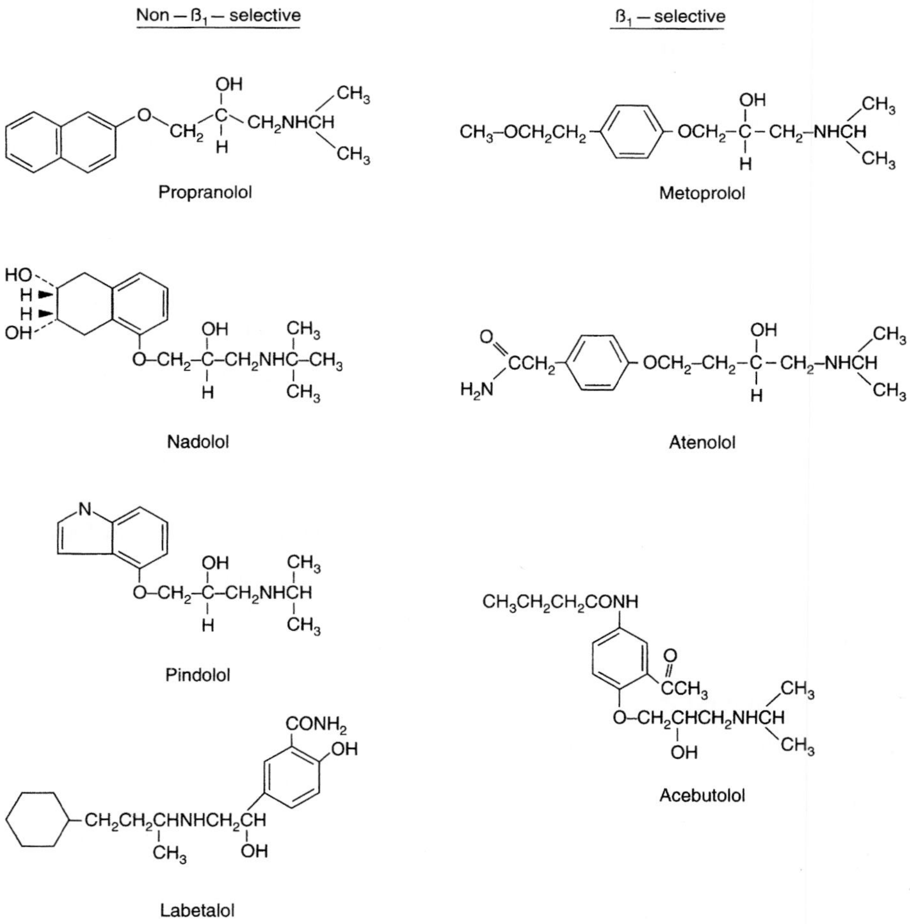

Non – β_1 – selective

Propranolol

Nadolol

Pindolol

Labetalol

β_1 – selective

Metoprolol

Atenolol

Acebutolol

FIGURE 36.4–2
Molecular structure of β_2-adrenergic receptor antagonists.

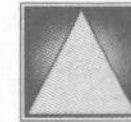

Table 36.4–2
β-Adrenergic Drugs Used in Psychiatry

Generic Name	Trade Name	Lipophilic	Metabolism	Receptor Selectivity	Half-Life (hrs)	Usual Starting Dosage (mg)	Usual Maximum Dosage (mg)
Propranolol	Inderal	Yes	Hepatic	$\beta_1 = \beta_2$	3 to 6	10 to 20 two or three times a day	30 to 40 three times a day
Nadolol	Corgard	No	Renal	$\beta_1 = \beta_2$	14 to 24	40 once daily	30 to 240 once daily
Pindolol	Visken	Intermediate	Hepatic	$\beta_1 = \beta_2$	3 to 4	5 two times a day	30 two times a day
Labetalol	Normodyne, Trandate	Intermediate	Hepatic	$\beta_1 = \beta_2$	4 to 6	100 two times a day	400 to 800 three times a day
Metoprolol	Lopressor	Yes	Hepatic	$\beta_1 > \beta_2$	3 to 4	50 two times a day	75 to 150 two times a day
Atenolol	Tenormin	No	Renal	$\beta_1 > \beta_2$	5 to 8	50 once daily	50 to 100 once daily
Acebutolol	Sectral	No	Hepatic	$\beta_1 > \beta_2$	3 to 4	400 once daily	600 two times a day

treatment approach is to take 10 to 40 mg of propranolol 20 to 30 minutes before the anxiety-provoking situation. A test run of the β-receptor antagonist can be tried before using it before an anxiety-provoking situation to be sure that the patient does not experience any adverse effects from the drug or the dosage. β-receptor antagonists may blunt cognition in some people. The β-receptor antagonists are less effective for the treatment of panic disorder than are benzodiazepines or selective serotonin reuptake inhibitors (SSRIs).

Lithium-Induced Postural Tremor

The β-receptor antagonists are beneficial for lithium-induced postural tremor and other medication-induced postural tremors—for example, those induced by tricyclic drugs and valproate (Depakene). The initial approach to this movement disorder includes lowering the dose of lithium, eliminating aggravating factors, such as caffeine, and administering lithium at bedtime. If these interventions are inadequate, however, propranolol in the range of 20 to 160 mg a day, given two or three times daily, is generally effective for the treatment of lithium-induced postural tremor.

Neuroleptic-Induced Acute Akathisia

Many studies have shown that β-receptor antagonists can be effective in the treatment of neuroleptic-induced acute akathisia. Most clinicians believe that β-receptor antagonists are more effective for this indication than are anticholinergics and benzodiazepines. The β-receptor antagonists are not effective in the treatment of such neuroleptic-induced movement disorders as acute dystonia and parkinsonism.

Aggression and Violent Behavior

The β-receptor antagonists may be effective in reducing the number of aggressive and violent outbursts in persons with impulse disorders, schizophrenia, and aggression associated with brain injuries, such as trauma, tumors, anoxic injury, encephalitis, alcohol dependence, and degenerative disorders (e.g., Huntington's disease). Many studies have added a β-receptor antagonist to the ongoing therapy (e.g., antipsychotics, anticonvulsants, lithium); therefore, it is difficult to distinguish additive effects from independent effects.

Alcohol Withdrawal

Propranolol is reported to be useful as an adjuvant to benzodiazepines, but not as a sole agent in the treatment of alcohol withdrawal. The following dose schedule is suggested: no propranolol for a pulse rate below 50; 50 mg propranolol for a pulse rate between 50 and 79; and 100 mg propranolol for a pulse rate of 80 or above.

Antidepressant Augmentation

Pindolol has been used to augment and hasten the antidepressant effects of SSRIs, tricyclic drugs, and electroconvulsive therapy. Small studies have shown that pindolol administered at the onset of antidepressant therapy may shorten the usual 2- to 4-week latency of antidepressant response by several days. Because the β-receptor antagonists may possibly induce depression in some persons, augmentation strategies with these drugs need to be further clarified in controlled trials.

Other Disorders

A number of case reports and controlled studies have reported data indicating that β-receptor antagonists may be of modest benefit for persons with schizophrenia and with manic symptoms. They have also been used in some cases of stuttering.

PRECAUTIONS AND ADVERSE REACTIONS

The β-receptor antagonists are contraindicated for use in people with asthma, insulin-dependent diabetes, congestive heart failure, significant vascular disease, persistent angina, and hyperthyroidism. The contraindication in diabetic persons is because of the drugs' antagonizing the normal physiologic response to hypoglycemia. The β-receptor antagonists can worsen atrioventricular (AV) conduction defects and lead to complete AV heart block and death. If the clinician decides that the risk-to-benefit ratio warrants a trial of a β-receptor antagonist in a person with one of these coexisting medical conditions, a β_1-selective agent should be the first choice. All currently available β-receptor antagonists are excreted in breast milk and should be administered with caution to nursing women.

The most common adverse effects of β-receptor antagonists are hypotension and bradycardia. In persons at risk for these

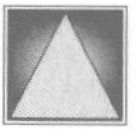

Table 36.4–3
Adverse Effects and Toxicity of β-Adrenergic Receptor Antagonists

Cardiovascular
- Hypotension
- Bradycardia
- Dizziness
- Congestive heart failure (in patients with compromised myocardial function)

Respiratory
- Asthma (less risk with β_1-selective drugs)

Metabolic
- Worsened hypoglycemia in diabetic patients on insulin or oral agents

Gastrointestinal (GI)
- Nausea
- Diarrhea
- Abdominal pain

Sexual function
- Impotence

Neuropsychiatric
- Lassitude
- Fatigue
- Dysphoria
- Insomnia
- Vivid nightmares
- Depression (rare)
- Psychosis (rare)

Other (rare)
- Raynaud's phenomenon
- Peyronie's disease

Withdrawal syndrome
- Rebound worsening of preexisting angina pectoris when β-adrenergic receptor antagonists are discontinued

adverse effects, a test dosage of 20 mg a day of propranolol can be given to assess reaction to the drug. Depression has been associated with lipophilic β-receptor antagonists, such as propranolol, but it is probably rare. Nausea, vomiting, diarrhea, and constipation can also be caused by treatment with these agents. Serious CNS adverse effects (e.g., agitation, confusion, and hallucinations) are rare. Table 36.4–3 lists the possible adverse affects of β-receptor antagonists.

DRUG INTERACTIONS

Concomitant administration of propranolol results in increases in plasma concentrations of antipsychotics, anticonvulsants, theophylline (Theo-Dur, Slo-bid), and levothyroxine (Synthroid). Other β-receptor antagonists possibly have similar effects. The β-receptor antagonists that are eliminated by the kidneys may have similar effects on drugs that are also eliminated by the renal route. Barbiturates, phenytoin (Dilantin), and cigarette smoking increase the elimination of β-receptor antagonists that are metabolized by the liver. Several reports have associated hypertensive crises and bradycardia with the coadministration of β-receptor antagonists and monoamine oxidase inhibitors. Depressed myocardial contractility and AV nodal conduction can occur from concomitant administration of a β-receptor antagonist and calcium channel inhibitors.

LABORATORY INTERFERENCES

The β-receptor antagonists do not interfere with standard laboratory tests.

DOSAGE AND CLINICAL GUIDELINES

Propranolol is available in 10-, 20-, 40-, 60-, 80-, and 90-mg tablets; 4-, 8-, and 80-mg/mL solutions; and 60-, 80-, 120-, and 160-mg sustained-release capsules. Nadolol is available in 20-, 40-, 80-, 120-, and 160-mg tablets. Pindolol is available in 5- and 10-mg tablets. Labetalol is available in 100-, 200-, and 300-mg tablets. Metoprolol is available in 50- and 100-mg tablets; and 50-, 100-, and 200-mg sustained-release tablets. Atenolol is available in 25-, 50-, and 100-mg tablets. Acebutolol is available in 200- and 400-mg capsules.

For the treatment of chronic disorders, propranolol administration is usually initiated at 10 mg by mouth three times a day or 20 mg by mouth twice daily. The dosage can be raised by 20 to 30 mg a day until a therapeutic effect begins to emerge. The dosage should be leveled off at the appropriate range for the disorder under treatment. The treatment of aggressive behavior sometimes requires dosages up to 800 mg a day, and therapeutic effects may not be seen until the person has been receiving the maximal dosage for 4 to 8 weeks. For the treatment of social phobia, primarily the performance type, the patient should take 10 to 40 mg of propranolol 20 to 30 minutes before the performance.

Pulse and BP readings should be taken regularly, and the drug should be withheld if the pulse rate is below 50 or the systolic BP is below 90. The drug should be temporarily discontinued if it produces severe dizziness, ataxia, or wheezing. Treatment with β-receptor antagonists should never be discontinued abruptly. Propranolol should be tapered by 60 mg a day until a dosage of 60 mg a day is reached, after which the drug should be tapered by 10 to 20 mg a day every 3 or 4 days.

References

Butler J, Young JB, Abraham WT, Bourge RC, Adams KF Jr, Clare R, O'Connor C. Beta-blocker use and outcomes among hospitalized heart failure patients. *J Am Coll Cardiol.* 2006;47(12):2462–2469.

Connolly SJ, Dorian P, Roberts RS, Gent M, Bailin S, Fain ES, Thorpe K, Champagne J, Talajic M, Coutu B, Gronefeld GC, Hohnloser SH. Comparison of β-blockers, amiodarone plus β-blockers, or sotalol for prevention of shocks from implantable cardioverter defibrillators. *JAMA.* 2006;295:165–171.

Go AS, Iribarren C, Chandra M, Lathon PV, Fortmann SP, Quertermous T, Hlatky MA. Statin and β-blocker therapy and the initial presentation of coronary heart disease. *Ann Intern Med.* 2006;144(4):229.

Kang EH, Yu BH. Anxiety and β-adrenergic receptor function in a normal population. *Prog Neuropsychopharmacol Biol Psychiatry.* 2005;29(5):733–737.

Kim YR, Min SK, Yu BH. Difference in β-adrenergic receptor sensitivity between women and men with panic disorder. *Eur Neuropsychopharmacol.* 2004;14(6):515–520.

Lanfear DE, Jones PG, Marsh S, Cresci S, McLeod HL, Spertus JA. β-2-adrenergic receptor genotype and survival among patients receiving β-blocker therapy after an acute coronary syndrome. *JAMA.* 2005;294:1526–1533.

Lindenauer PK, Fitzgerald J, Hoople N, Benjamin EM. The potential preventability of postoperative myocardial infarction: Underuse of perioperative beta-adrenergic blockade. *Arch Intern Med.* 2004;164(7):762–766.

Nemeroff CB, Putnam JS. β-adrenergic receptor antagonists. In: Sadock BJ, Sadock VA, eds. *Kaplan & Sadock's Comprehensive Textbook of Psychiatry.* 8th ed. Vol. 2. Baltimore: Lippincott Williams & Wilkins; 2005:2722.

Schlienger RG, Kraenzlin ME, Jick SS, Meier CR. Use of beta-blockers and risk of fractures. *JAMA.* 2004;292(11):1326–1332.

Siddiqui AK, Ahmed S, Delbeau H, Conner D, Mattana J. Lack of physician concordance with guidelines on the perioperative use of β-blockers. *Arch Intern Med.* 2004;164:664–667.

▲ 36.5 Anticholinergics and Amantadine

In the clinical practice of psychiatry, the anticholinergic drugs are primarily used to treat medication-induced movement disorders, particularly neuroleptic-induced parkinsonism, neuroleptic-induced acute dystonia, and medication-induced postural tremor. Amantadine (Symmetrel) is used primarily for the treatment of medication-induced movement disorders, such as neuroleptic-induced parkinsonism. It is also used as an antiviral agent for the prophylaxis and treatment of influenza A infection.

ANTICHOLINERGICS

Chemistry

The molecular structures of representative anticholinergic drugs are shown in Figure 36.5–1.

Pharmacologic Actions

All anticholinergic drugs are well absorbed from the gastrointestinal (GI) tract after oral administration, and all are sufficiently lipophilic to enter the central nervous system (CNS). Trihexyphenidyl (Artane) and benztropine (Cogentin) reach peak plasma concentrations in 2 to 3 hours after oral administration and their duration of action is 1 to 12 hours. Benztropine is absorbed equally rapidly by intramuscular (IM) and intravenous (IV) administration; IM administration is preferred because of its low risk for adverse effects.

All five anticholinergic drugs listed in this section block muscarinic acetylcholine receptors, and benztropine also has some antihistaminergic effects. None of the available anticholinergic drugs has any effects on the nicotinic acetylcholine receptors. Of the five drugs, trihexyphenidyl is the most stimulating agent, perhaps acting through dopaminergic neurons, and benztropine is the least stimulating and, thus, is least associated with abuse potential.

Therapeutic Indications

The primary indication for the use of anticholinergics in psychiatric practice is for the treatment of *neuroleptic-induced parkinsonism*, characterized by tremor, rigidity, cogwheeling, bradykinesia, sialorrhea, stooped posture, and festination. All the available anticholinergics are equally effective in the treatment of parkinsonian symptoms. Neuroleptic-induced parkinsonism is most common in the elderly and is most frequently seen with high-potency dopamine receptor antagonists (DRAs), for example, haloperidol (Haldol). The onset of symptoms usually occurs after 2 or 3 weeks of treatment. The incidence of neuroleptic-induced parkinsonism is lower with the newer antipsychotic drugs of the serotonin-dopamine antagonist (SDA) class.

Another indication is for the treatment of *neuroleptic-induced acute dystonia,* which is most common in young men. The syndrome often occurs early in the course of treatment, is commonly associated with high-potency DRAs (e.g., haloperidol),

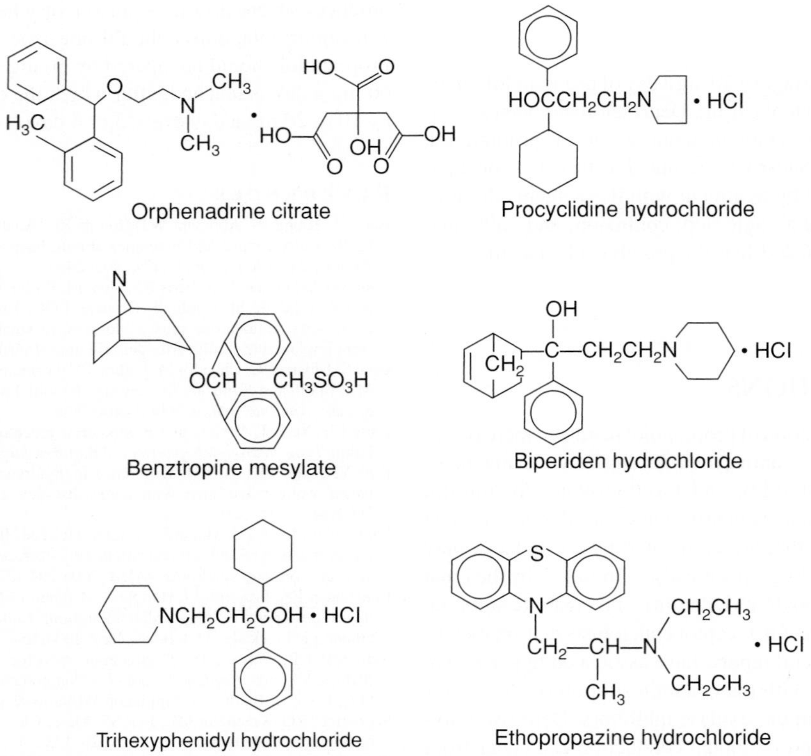

Orphenadrine citrate

Procyclidine hydrochloride

Benztropine mesylate

Biperiden hydrochloride

Trihexyphenidyl hydrochloride

Ethopropazine hydrochloride

FIGURE 36.5–1
Molecular structures of selected anticholinergic drugs.

and most commonly affects the muscles of the neck, the tongue, the face, and the back. Anticholinergic drugs are effective both in the short-term treatment of dystonias and in prophylaxis against neuroleptic-induced acute dystonias.

Akathisia is characterized by a subjective and objective sense of restlessness, anxiety, and agitation. Although a trial of anticholinergics for the treatment of neuroleptic-induced acute akathisia is reasonable, these drugs are not generally considered as effective as the β-adrenergic receptor antagonists, the benzodiazepines, and clonidine (Catapres).

Precautions and Adverse Reactions

The adverse effects of the anticholinergic drugs result from blockade of muscarinic acetylcholine receptors. Anticholinergic drugs should be used cautiously, if at all, by persons with prostatic hypertrophy, urinary retention, and narrow-angle glaucoma. The anticholinergics are occasionally used as drugs of abuse because of their mild mood-elevating properties, most notably, trihexyphenidyl.

The most serious adverse effect associated with anticholinergic toxicity is anticholinergic intoxication, which can be characterized by delirium, coma, seizures, agitation, hallucinations, severe hypotension, supraventricular tachycardia, and peripheral manifestations—flushing, mydriasis, dry skin, hyperthermia, and decreased bowel sounds. Treatment should begin with the immediate discontinuation of all anticholinergic drugs. The syndrome of anticholinergic intoxication can be diagnosed and treated with physostigmine (Antilirium, Eserine), an inhibitor of anticholinesterase, 1 to 2 mg IV (1 mg every 2 minutes) or IM every 30 or 60 minutes. Treatment with physostigmine should be used only in severe cases and only when emergency cardiac monitoring and life-support services are available, because physostigmine can lead to severe hypotension and bronchial constriction. Table 36.5–1 lists the major adverse effects of antichoinergics.

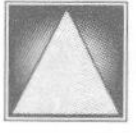

Table 36.5–1
Adverse Effects of Anticholinergics

Anticholinergics
Cardiovascular system
Tachycardia
Digestive system
Constipation
Dry mouth
Nausea
Nervous system
Confusion
Disorientation
Memory impairment
Visual system
Blurred vision
Dilated pupils
Worsening of narrow-angle glaucoma
Urogenital system
Urinary retention
Amantadine
Cardiovascular system
Arrhythmia
Tachycardia
Nervous system
Delirium
Paranoia
Paresthesias

Drug Interactions

The most common drug–drug interactions with the anticholinergics occur when they are coadministered with psychotropics that also have high anticholinergic activity, such as DRAs, tricyclic and tetracyclic drugs, and monoamine oxidase inhibitors (MAOIs). Many other prescription drugs and over-the-counter cold preparations also induce significant anticholinergic activity. The coadministration of those drugs can result in a life-threatening anticholinergic intoxication syndrome. Anticholinergic drugs can also delay gastric emptying, thereby decreasing the absorption of drugs that are broken down in the stomach and usually absorbed in the duodenum (e.g., levodopa [Larodopa] and DRAs).

Laboratory Interferences

No known laboratory interferences have been associated with anticholinergics.

Dosage and Clinical Guidelines

The five anticholinergic drugs discussed in this chapter are available in a range of preparations (Table 36.5–2).

Neuroleptic-Induced Parkinsonism. For the treatment of neuroleptic-induced parkinsonism, the equivalent of 1 to 3 mg of benztropine should be given one to two times daily. The anticholinergic drug should be administered for 4 to 8 weeks, and then it should be discontinued to assess whether the person still requires the drug. Anticholinergic drugs should be tapered over a period of 1 to 2 weeks.

Treatment with anticholinergics as prophylaxis against the development of neuroleptic-induced parkinsonism is usually not indicated, because onset of its symptoms are usually sufficiently mild and gradual to allow the clinician to initiate treatment only after it is clearly indicated. In young men, prophylaxis may be indicated, however, especially if a high-potency DRA is being used. The clinician should attempt to discontinue the antiparkinsonian agent in 4 to 6 weeks to assess whether its continued use is necessary.

Neuroleptic-Induced Acute Dystonia. For the short-term treatment and prophylaxis of neuroleptic-induced acute dystonia, 1 to 2 mg of benztropine or its equivalent in another drug should be given IM. The dose can be repeated in 20 to 30 minutes, as needed. If the person still does not improve in another 20 to 30 minutes, a benzodiazepine (e.g., 1 mg IM or IV lorazepam [Ativan]) should be given. Laryngeal dystonia is a medical emergency and should be treated with benztropine, up to 4 mg in a 10-minute period, followed by 1 to 2 mg of lorazepam, administered slowly by the IV route.

Prophylaxis against dystonias is indicated in persons who have had one episode or in persons at high risk (young men taking high-potency DRAs). Prophylactic treatment is given for 4 to 8 weeks and then gradually tapered over 1 to 2 weeks to allow assessment of its continued need. The prophylactic use of anticholinergics in persons requiring antipsychotic drugs has

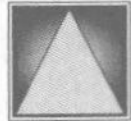

Table 36.5–2
Anticholinergic Drugs

Generic Name	Brand Name	Tablet Size	Injectable	Usual Daily Oral Dosage	Short-term Intramuscular or Intravenous Dosage
Benztropine	Cogentin	0.5, 1, 2 mg	1 mg/mL	1–4 mg one to three times	1–2 mg
Biperiden	Akineton	2 mg	5 mg/mL	2 mg one to three times	2 mg
Ethopropazine	Parsidol	10, 50 mg	—	50–100 mg one to three times	—
Orphenadrine	Norflex, Dispal	100 mg	30 mg/mL	50–100 mg three times	60 mg IV given over 5 min
Procyclidine	Kemadrin	5 mg	—	2, 5–5 mg three times	—
Trihexyphenidyl	Artane, Trihexane, Trihexy-5	2, 5 mg elixir 2 mg/5 mL	—	2–5 mg two to four times	—

IV, intravenous.

largely become a moot issue because of the availability of SDAs, which are relatively free of parkinsonian effects.

Akathisia. As mentioned, anticholinergics are not the drugs of choice for this syndrome. The β-adrenergic receptor antagonists (Section 36.4) and perhaps the benzodiazepines (Section 36.9) and clonidine (Section 36.3) are preferable drugs to try initially.

AMANTADINE

Chemistry

Amantadine's molecular structure is given in Figure 36.5–2.

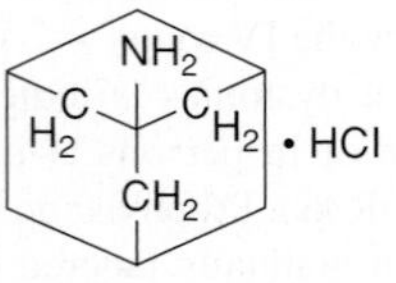

FIGURE 36.5–2
Molecular structure of amantadine.

Pharmacologic Actions

Amantadine is well absorbed from the GI tract after oral administration, reaches peak plasma concentrations in approximately 2 to 3 hours, has a half-life of about 12 to 18 hours, and attains steady-state concentrations after approximately 4 to 5 days of therapy. Amantadine is excreted unmetabolized in the urine. Amantadine plasma concentrations can be twice as high in elderly persons as in younger adults. Patients with renal failure accumulate amantadine in their bodies.

Amantadine augments dopaminergic neurotransmission in the CNS; however, the precise mechanism for the effect is unknown. The mechanism may involve dopamine release from presynaptic vesicles, blocking reuptake of dopamine into presynaptic nerve terminals, or an agonist effect on postsynaptic dopamine receptors.

Therapeutic Indications

The primary indication for amantadine use in psychiatry is to treat extrapyramidal signs and symptoms, such as parkinsonism, akinesia, and so-called rabbit syndrome (focal perioral tremor of the choreoathetoid type) caused by the administration of DRA or SDA drugs. Amantadine is as effective as the anticholinergics (e.g., benztropine [Cogentin]) for these indications and results in improvement in approximately one half of all persons who take it. Amantadine, however, is not generally considered as effective as the anticholinergics for the treatment of acute dystonic reactions and is not effective in treating tardive dyskinesia and akathisia.

Amantadine is a reasonable compromise for persons with extrapyramidal symptoms who would be sensitive to additional anticholinergic effects, particularly those taking a low-potency DRA or the elderly. Elderly persons are susceptible to anticholinergic adverse effects, both in the CNS, such as anticholinergic delirium, and in the peripheral nervous system, such as urinary retention. Amantadine is associated with less memory impairment than are the anticholinergics.

Amantadine has been reported to be of benefit in treating some selective serotonin reuptake inhibitor (SSRI)-associated side effects, such as lethargy, fatigue, anorgasmia, and ejaculatory inhibition.

Amantadine is used in general medical practice for the treatment of parkinsonism of all causes, including idiopathic parkinsonism.

Precautions and Adverse Effects

The most common CNS effects of amantadine are mild dizziness, insomnia, and impaired concentration (dosage related), which occur in 5 percent to 10 percent of all persons. Irritability, depression, anxiety, dysarthria, and ataxia occur in 1 percent to 5 percent of persons. More severe CNS adverse effects, including seizures and psychotic symptoms, have been reported. Nausea is the most common peripheral adverse effect of amantadine. Headache, loss of appetite, and blotchy spots on the skin have also been reported.

Livedo reticularis of the legs (a purple discoloration of the skin, caused by dilation of blood vessels) has been reported in up to 5 percent of persons who take the drug for over a month. It usually diminishes with elevation of the legs and resolves in almost all cases when drug use is terminated.

Amantadine is relatively contraindicated in persons with renal disease or a seizure disorder. Amantadine should be used with caution in persons with edema or cardiovascular disease. Some evidence indicates that amantadine is teratogenic and, therefore, should not be taken by pregnant women. Because amantadine is excreted in milk, women who are breast-feeding should not take the drug.

Suicide attempts with amantadine overdosages are life threatening. Symptoms can include toxic psychoses (confusion, hallucinations, aggressiveness) and cardiopulmonary arrest. Emergency treatment beginning with gastric lavage is indicated.

Drug Interactions

Coadministration of amantadine with phenelzine (Nardil) or other MAOIs can result in a significant increase in resting blood pressure (BP). The coadministration of amantadine with CNS stimulants can result in insomnia, irritability, nervousness, and possibly seizures or irregular heartbeat. Amantadine should not be coadministered with anticholinergics because unwanted side effects—such as confusion, hallucinations, nightmares, dry mouth, and blurred vision—may be exacerbated.

Dosage and Clinical Guidelines

Amantadine is available in 100-mg capsules and as a 50-mg/5 mL syrup. The usual starting dosage of amantadine is 100 mg given orally twice a day, although the dosage can be cautiously increased up to 200 mg given orally twice a day if indicated. Amantadine should be used in persons with renal impairment *only* in consultation with the physician treating the renal condition. If amantadine is successful in the treatment of the drug-induced extrapyramidal symptoms, it should be continued for 4 to 6 weeks and then discontinued to see whether the person has become tolerant to the neurologic adverse effects of the antipsychotic medication. Amantadine should be tapered over 1 to 2 weeks once a decision has been made to discontinue the drug. Persons taking amantadine should not drink alcoholic beverages.

References

Bright RA, Shay DK, Shu B, Cox NJ, Klimov AI. Adamantane resistance among influenza A viruses isolated early during the 2005–2006 influenza season in the United States. *JAMA*. 2006;295(8):891.

Carroll BT, Thomas C, Jayanti K. Amantadine and memantine in catatonic schizophrenia. *Ann Clin Psychiatry*. 2006;18(2):133.

Friedman JH. Anticholinergics in dementia and other confounding problems. *Am J Geriatr Psychiatry*. 2006;14(4):384.

Gironell A, Kulisevsky J, Pascual-Sedano B, Flamarich D. Effect of amantadine in essential tremor: A randomized, placebo-controlled trial. *Mov Disord*. 2006;21(4):441.

Graham KA, Gu H, Lieberman JA, Harp JB, Perkins DO. Double-blind, placebo-controlled investigation of amantadine for weight loss in subjects who gained weight with olanzapine. *Am J Psychiatry*. 2005;162:1744.

Minzenberg MJ, Poole JH, Benton C, Vinogradov S. Association of anticholinergic load with impairment of complex attention and memory in schizophrenia. *Am J Psychiatry*. 2004;161:116.

Nemeroff CB, Putnam JS. Anticholinergics and amantadine. In: Sadock BJ, Sadock VA, eds. *Kaplan & Sadock's Comprehensive Textbook of Psychiatry*. 8th ed. Vol. 2. Baltimore: Lippincott Williams & Wilkins; 2005:2727.

Ness J, Hoth A, Barnett MJ, Shorr RI, Kaboli PJ. Anticholinergic medications in community-dwelling older veterans: Prevalence of anticholinergic symptoms, symptom burden, and adverse drug events. *American Journal of Geriatric Pharmacotherapy*. 2006;4(1):42–51.

Van Arendonk KJ, Austin JC, Boyt MA, Cooper CS. Frequency of wetting is predictive of response to anticholinergic treatment in children with overactive bladder. *Urology*. 2006;67(5):1049–1053.

Wenning GK. Placebo-controlled trial of amantadine in multiple-system atrophy. *Clin Neuropharmacol*. 2005;28(5):225–227.

▲ 36.6 Anticonvulsants: Gabapentin, Pregabalin, Tiagabine, Levetiracetam, Topiramate, and Zonisamide

Despite the absence of large placebo-controlled trials proving their efficacy as psychotropics, six anticonvulsant drugs—gabapentin (Neurontin), pregabalin (Lyrica), tiagabine (Gabitril), levetiracetam (Keppra), topiramate (Topamax), and zonisamide (Zonegran)—are occasionally used in psychiatry. Anecdotal evidence suggests that some patients benefit from treatment with each of these drugs in certain clinical circumstances; however, their routine use in place of proved treatments is not recommended. These drugs differ in chemical structure (Fig. 36.6–1). The pharmacokinetics and dosing of these agents, which also vary, are summarized in Table 36.6–1.

GABAPENTIN

Gabapentin indirectly increases brain γ-aminobutyric acid (GABA) levels. It is well absorbed, but its bioavailability decreases as doses are increased, because of saturation of the neutral amino acid membrane transporter system in the gut. Because higher amounts are not absorbed, doses should not exceed 1,800 mg per single dose or 5,400 mg a day. Gabapentin absorption is unaffected by food. Steady-state half-life of 5 to 9 hours is reached in 2 days when taken three times a day. Gabapentin does not bind to plasma proteins and is not metabolized. It is excreted unchanged in the urine.

Therapeutic Indications

Gabapentin is used as a hypnotic agent, because of its sedating effects. It also has anxiolytic properties, providing benefit to patients with panic attacks and social anxiety disorder. Gabapentin decreases craving for alcohol, helping patients to remain abstinent, and facilitates detoxification. In some cases, patients can be switched to gabapentin following benzodiazepine-facilitated alcohol detoxification. Because gabapentin is renally excreted, it is well suited for use among patients with liver disease. To the extent that gabapentin reduces alcohol use among patients with bipolar disorder, it may prove useful as an adjunct to standard mood stabilizer regimens. Gabapentin is approved by the US Food and Drug Administration (FDA) for the treatment of postherpetic neuralgia. Other pain conditions responsive to gabapentin include trigeminal neuralgia; central pain syndromes; and compression neuropathies, such as carpal tunnel syndrome, radiculopathies, and meralgia paresthetica. Pregabalin, an analog of gabapentin, has been approved for the management of neuropathic pain associated with diabetic peripheral neuropathy and postherpetic neuralgia.

Clinical Guidelines

Gabapentin dosage can be escalated to the maintenance range within 2 to 3 days, with sedation being the only dose-related side

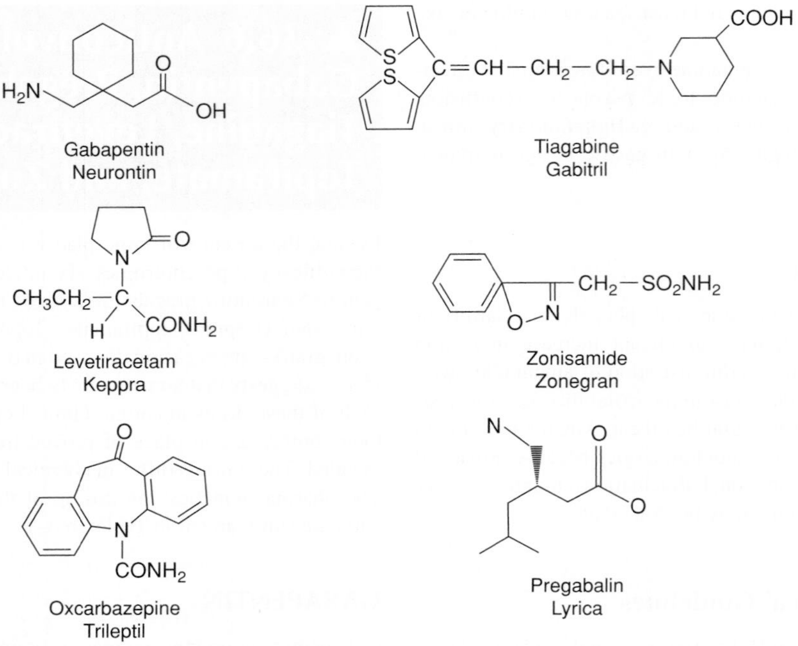

Gabapentin
Neurontin

Tiagabine
Gabitril

Levetiracetam
Keppra

Zonisamide
Zonegran

Oxcarbazepine
Trileptil

Pregabalin
Lyrica

FIGURE 36.6–1
Molecular structures of anticonvulsants.

effect. Other frequent adverse effects of gabapentin are dizziness, ataxia, fatigue, and nystagmus, which are usually transient. Some patients experience peripheral edema, memory impairment, weight gain, and orgasmic dysfunction. Gabapentin has no significant hepatic cytochrome P450 or pharmacodynamic interactions. Antacids containing aluminum hydroxide and magnesium hydroxide (Maalox) decrease gabapentin absorption by 20 percent if administered concurrently, but negligibly if administered 2 hours before taking the dose of gabapentin. Gabapentin can cause false-positive readings with the Ames N-Multistix SG dipstick test for urinary protein. The drug should be used cautiously in patients with renal disease or on dialysis.

Gabapentin is available as 100-, 300-, and 400-mg capsules and as 600- and 800-mg tablets. The starting dosage of gabapentin is 300 mg three times a day, and the dosage can be rapidly titrated up to a maximum of 1,800 mg three times a day over a period of a few days. Most people achieve satisfactory benefit within the range of 600 to 900 mg three times a day. Although abrupt discontinuation of gabapentin does not cause withdrawal effects, use of all anticonvulsant drugs should be gradually tapered.

PREGABALIN

Pregabalin is pharmacologically similar to gabapentin. It is believed to work by inhibiting the release of excess excitatory neurotransmitters, presumably by binding to the α-2-Δ subunit protein of voltage-dependent calcium channels in the brain and spinal cord. It also increases neurnal γ-aminobutyric acid (GABA) levels. The binding affinity of pregabalin for the α-2-Δ subunit is six times more potent than gabapentin and has a longer half-life.

Therapeutic Indications

Pregabalin is approved for the management of diabetic peripheral neuropathy and postherpetic neuralgia and for adjunctive treatment of partial onset seizures.

Pregabalin has been found to be of benefit to some patients with generalized anxiety disorder. In studies, no consistent dose response relationship was found, although 300-mg pregabalin per day was more effective than 150 mg or 450 mg.

Although rejected for that indication by the FDA, the Committee for Medicinal Products for Human Use (CHMP) of the European Medicines Agency issued a positive opinion recommending marketing authorization of pregabalin. Some patients with panic disorder or social anxiety disorder may benefit from pregabalin, but little evidence supports its routine use in treating those disorders.

Clinical Guidelines

Pregabalin exhibits linear pharmacokinetics. It is extremely and rapidly absorbed in proportion to its dose. The time to maximal plasma concentration is about 1 hour and to steady state within 24 to 48 hours. Pregabalin demonstrates high bioavailability, and has a mean elimination half-life of about 6.5 hours. Food does not affect absorption. Pregabalin does not bind to plasma proteins and is excreted virtually unchanged (less than 2 percent metabolism) by the kidneys. It is not subject to hepatic metabolism and does not induce or inhibit liver enzymes such as the cytochrome P450 system. Dose adjustment may be necessary in patients with creatinine clearance (CLcr) less than 60 mL per minute. A 50 percent reduction in pregabalin daily dose is recommended for patients with CLcr between 30 and 60 mL per

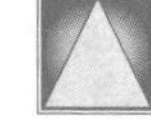

Table 36.6–1
Anticonvulsants: Doses, Levels, Kinetics, and Metabolism

Drug	Starting Dose	Usual Dose Range[a] (mg/day) (Typical)	Steady-State Blood Levels (μg/mL)	Nonliniear Kinetics	Percent Protein Bound	Enzyme	Metabolism	Half-Life (hrs)		↑ Metabolism and Clearance of Oral Contraceptives[b]
								Acute (Chronic)	With Induces[c]	
Zonisamide (Zonegran)	25 to 100	100 to 600	15 to 40	[d]	60	—	CYP 3A4, glucuronldation, renal acetylation	57 to 68	27 to 37	—
Topiramate (Topamax)	25	200 to 1,000 (100 to 200)	3 to 5?	—	15	Inducer CYP 3A4	Oxidation, renal excretion	19 to 25	9 to 12	↑
Gabapentin (Neurontin)	100	400 to 4,800 (1,200)	6 to 21	[e]	0	—	Renal excretion (no interactions)	5 to 9	?	—
Pregabalin (Lyrica)	50	100 to 300	24 to 48	—	0	—	Renal excretion (no interactions)	6 to 7	—	—
Tiagabine (Gabitril)	1	4 to 32 (12)	—	—	98	—	CYP 3A4, oxidation, glucuronidation	4 to 13	2 to 5	—
Levetiracetam (Keppra)	250	500–3,000 (1,500–2,000)	–40?	—	0	—	Nonhepatic hydrolysis, renal excretion (no interactions)	6 to 8	?	—

[a]In epilepsy.
[b]Increases in metabolism and clearance of oral contraceptive should propel use of higher estrogen formulations or use of other types of contraceptives.
[c]Elimination of half-life when administered in conjunction with a liver cytochrome P450 enzyme inducer.
[d]Due to saturation of metabolism.
[e]Due to saturation of gastrointestinal absorption.

minute compared with those with CLcr greater than 60 mL per minute. Daily doses should be further reduced by approximately 50 percent for each additional 50 percent decrease in CLcr. Pregabalin is highly cleared by hemodialysis, so additional doses may be needed for patients on chronic hemodialysis treatment after each hemodialysis treatment.

The most common adverse events associated with pregabalin use are dizziness, somnolence, blurred vision, peripheral edema, amnesia or loss of memory, and tremors. Pregabalin potentiates sedating effects of alcohol, antihistamines, benzodiazepines, and other central nervous system (CNS) depressants. It remains to be seen if pregabalin is associated with benzodiazepine-type withdrawal symptoms.

The recommended dosage for postherpetic neuralgia is 50 or 100 mg orally three times a day. The recommended dosage for diabetic peripheral neuropathy is 100 to 200 mg orally three times a day. Pregabalin is available as 25, 50, 75, 100, 150, 200, 225, and 300 mg capsules.

TOPIRAMATE

Topiramate is a selective inhibitor of Glu AMPA receptors, blocks Na^+ receptors, and has indirect GABAergic activity. It potentiates the action of GABA at a non–benzodiazepine-, non–barbiturate-sensitive $GABA_A$ receptor, is rapidly and completely absorbed, and has a steady-state half-life of 21 hours. Food does not affect its absorption. It is 15 percent protein bound in the plasma and 70 percent of an oral dose of topiramate is excreted unchanged in the urine, together with small amounts of several inactive metabolites. Topiramate is an inhibitor of state-dependent sodium channels.

Therapeutic Indications

Despite initial reports of mood-stabilizing properties, a series of large, placebo-controlled studies failed to find any evidence of antimanic activity. The fact that some patients lose a substantial amount of weight while taking topiramate is exploited in psychiatry, mainly to counteract the weight gain caused by many psychotropic drugs. Topiramate has been shown to benefit patients with primary alcoholism and posttraumatic stress disorder. Topiramate may reduce the frequency of cutting and other forms of self-mutilating behavior in patients with borderline personality disorder. It is effective in treating neuropathic pain and migraine and is also highly effective in treating binge-eating disorder.

The most common non–dose-related adverse effects of topiramate used in combination with other antiepileptic drugs include psychomotor slowing; speech and language problems, especially word-finding difficulties; somnolence; dizziness; ataxia; nystagmus; and paresthesias. The most common dose-related adverse effects are fatigue, nervousness, poor concentration, confusion, taste perversion, depression, anorexia, anxiety, mood problems, weight loss, and tremor. Some 1.5 percent of persons taking topiramate develop renal calculi, a rate ten times that associated with placebo. Patients at risk for calculi should be encouraged to drink plenty of fluids.

Clinical Guidelines

Topiramate has a few well-characterized drug interactions with other anticonvulsant drugs. Topiramate can increase phenytoin concentrations up to 25 percent and valproic acid concentrations 11 percent; it does not affect the concentrations of carbamazepine or its epoxide, phenobarbital (Luminal), or primidone. Topiramate concentrations are decreased by 40 percent to 48 percent with concomitant administration of carbamazepine or phenytoin and by 14 percent with concurrent administration of valproic acid. Topiramate also slightly decreases digoxin (Lanoxin) bioavailability and the efficacy of estrogenic oral contraceptives. Addition of topiramate, a weak inhibitor of carbonic anhydrase, to other inhibitors of carbonic anhydrase, such as acetazolamide (Diamox) or dichlorphenamide (Daranide), may promote development of renal calculi and is to be avoided. Topiramate does not interfere with any laboratory tests.

Topiramate is available as unscored 25-, 100-, and 200-mg tablets. To reduce the risk of adverse cognitive and sedative effects, topiramate dosage is titrated gradually over 8 weeks to a maximum of 200 mg twice a day. Higher doses are not associated with increased efficacy. Persons with renal insufficiency should reduce doses by half.

TIAGABINE

Tiagabine is a potent and selective reuptake inhibitor of GABA. It also has mild blocking effects of H_1, serotonin I_B, benzodiazepine, and chloride channel receptors. More than 95 percent of tiagabine is rapidly absorbed. The rate of absorption is slowed by food. Absolute bioavailability of tiagabine is 95 percent, and it is 96 percent protein bound. It has a half-life of 7 to 9 hours and is metabolized by the hepatic CYP450 3A system. Tiagabine concentrations are about 40 percent lower in the evening than in the morning.

Tiagabine is occasionally used as an anxiolytic or hypnotic agent in patients who have not responded to, or tolerated, standard treatments. It has not been found to be useful in treating manic symptoms, whether used alone or as adjunctive therapy.

Animal studies have found teratogenic effects in rats. Ophthalmic changes can occur with chronic use. CNS side effects include sedation, cognitive impairment, ataxia, dizziness, tremor, paresthesias, confusion, and depression. Other side effects include ecchymosis, nausea, abdominal pain, muscle weakness, and flushing. Cases of serious rash can occur, including Stevens-Johnson syndrome. Lower doses of tiagabine should be used in patients with hepatic impairment. Patients being treated with tiagabine for bipolar disorder have experienced new-onset seizures. Reports of seizures in patients without epilepsy being treated with tiagabine have prompted an FDA warning about its use. Consequently, this drug should not be considered for off-label psychiatric use.

ZONISAMIDE

Zonisamide is sometimes used as an alternative treatment for acute mania and as a weight loss agent for drug-induced weight gain.

Zonisamide blocks sodium channels and may weakly potentiate dopamine and serotonin activity. It also inhibits carbonic anhydrase. Some evidence suggests that it might block calcium channels. Zonisamide is metabolized by the hepatic CYP450 3A system, so enzyme-inducing agents, such as carbamazepine, alcohol, and phenobarbital, increase the clearance and reduce the availability of the drug. Zonisamide does not affect the metabolism of other drugs.

Zonisamide can elevate hepatic alkaline phosphatase and increase blood urea nitrogen and creatinine. Zonisamide is a sulfonamide and, thus, may cause fatal rash and blood dyscrasias, although these events are rare. About 4 percent of patients develop kidney stones. The most common side effects are drowsiness, cognitive impairment, insomnia, ataxia, nystagmus, paresthesia, speech abnormalities, constipation, diarrhea, nausea, and dry mouth. Weight loss is also a common side effect, which has been exploited as a therapy for patients who have gained weight during treatment with psychotropics or who have ongoing difficulty controlling their eating.

Zonisamide is available in 100- and 200-mg capsules. In epilepsy, the dose range is 100 to 400 mg per day, with side effects becoming more pronounced at doses above 300 mg. Because of its long half-life, zonisamide can be given once a day.

LEVETIRACETAM

Levetiracetam has been used to treat acute mania, as add-on therapy to antidepressants to prevent the emergence of mania or cycling, and as an anxiolytic.

The CNS effects of levetiracetam are poorly understood, but it appears to indirectly enhance GABA inhibition. It is rapidly and completely absorbed. Peak concentrations are reached in 1 hour. Food delays the rate of absorption and decreases the amount of absorption. Levetiracetam is not significantly plasma protein bound and is not metabolized through the hepatic CYP system. Its metabolism involves hydrolysis of its acetamide group. No significant drug interactions have been noted. Serum concentrations are not correlated with any therapeutic effect.

The most common side effects of levetiracetam are drowsiness, dizziness, ataxia, diplopia, memory impairment, apathy, and paresthesia. More notably, some patients develop behavioral disturbances during treatment, and hallucinations can occur. Suicidality was noted in a few patients during clinical trials.

Levetiracetam is available as 250-, 500-, and 750-mg tablets. In epilepsy, it is given twice a day, with daily dosage ranging from 500 mg to 3,000 mg. The typical daily dose in epilepsy is 1,000 mg.

References

Barbosa L, Berk M, Vorster M. A double-blind, randomized, placebo-controlled trial of augmentation with lamotrigine or placebo in patients concomitantly treated with fluoxetine for resistant major depressive episodes. *J Clin Psychiatry*. 2003;64:403–407.

Brandes JL, Saper JR, Diamond M, Couch JR, Lewis DW, Schmitt J, Neto W, Schwabe S, Jacobs D. Topiramate for migraine prevention: A randomized controlled trial. *JAMA*. 2004;291:965–973.

Cookson J, Elliott B. The use of anticonvulsants in the aftermath of mania. *J Psychopharmacol*. 2006;20(2):23.

Ginsberg DL. Psychopharmacology reviews: Gabapentin-induced dystonia. *Primary Psychiatry*. 2005;12(7):27–28.

Ginsberg DL. Sudden pregabalin discontinuation associated with focal brain edema. *Primary Psychiatry*. 2005;12(9):26–27.

Ketter TA. Lamotrigine. In: Sadock BJ, Sadock VA, eds. *Kaplan & Sadock's Comprehensive Textbook of Psychiatry*. 8th ed. Vol. 2. Baltimore: Lippincott Williams & Wilkins; 2005:2749.

Ketter TA. Gabapentin. In: Sadock BJ, Sadock VA, eds. *Kaplan & Sadock's Comprehensive Textbook of Psychiatry*. 8th ed. Vol. 2. Baltimore: Lippincott Williams & Wilkins; 2005:2746.

Ketter TA. Topiramate. In: Sadock BJ, Sadock VA, eds. *Kaplan & Sadock's Comprehensive Textbook of Psychiatry*. 8th ed. Vol. 2. Baltimore: Lippincott Williams & Wilkins; 2005:2753.

Montgomery SA, Tobias K, Zornberg GL, Kasper S, Pande AC. Efficacy and safety of pregabalin in the treatment of generalized anxiety disorder: A 6-week, multicenter, randomized, double-blind, placebo-controlled comparison of pregabalin and venlafaxine. *J Clin Psychiatry*. 2006;67(5):771.

Penland HR, Ostroff RB. Combined use of lamotrigine and electroconvulsive therapy in bipolar depression: a case series. *J ECT*. 2006;22(2):142.

Post RM, Altshuler LL, Frye MA, Suppes T, McElroy SL, Keck PE Jr, Leverich GS, Kupka R, Nolen WA, Luckenbaugh DA, Walden J, Grunze H. Preliminary observations on the effectiveness of levetiracetam in the open adjunctive treatment of refractory bipolar disorder. *J Clin Psychiatry*. 2005;66(3):370–374.

Sierra M, Phillips ML, Ivin G, Krystal J, David AS. A placebo-controlled, crossover trial of lamotrigine in depersonalization disorder. *J Psychopharmacol*. 2003;17:103–105.

Zito JM, Safer DJ, Gardner JF, Soeken K, Ryu J. Anticonvulsant treatment for psychiatric and seizure indications among youths. *Psychiatr Serv*. 2006;57(5):681.

▲ 36.7 Antihistamines

In clinical psychiatry, certain antihistamines (antagonists of histamine H_1 receptors) are used to treat neuroleptic-induced parkinsonism and neuroleptic-induced acute dystonia and also as hypnotics and anxiolytics. Diphenhydramine (Benadryl) is used to treat neuroleptic-induced parkinsonism and neuroleptic-induced acute dystonia and sometimes as a hypnotic. Hydroxyzine hydrochloride (Atarax) and hydroxyzine pamoate (Vistaril) are used as anxiolytics. Promethazine (Phenergan) is used for its sedative and anxiolytic effects. Cyproheptadine (Periactin) has been used for the treatment of anorexia nervosa and inhibited male and female orgasm caused by serotonergic agents. The antihistamines most commonly used in psychiatry are listed in Table 36.7–1. Fexofenadine (Allegra), loratadine (Claritin), and cetirizine (Zyrtec) are less commonly used in psychiatric practice. Terfenadine (Seldane) and astemizole (Hismanal) were withdrawn from commercial availability because they were associated with serious cardiac arrhythmias when coadministered with some drugs (e.g., nefazodone [Serzone], selective serotonin reuptake inhibitors [SSRIs]).

Table 36.7–2 lists antihistaminic drugs not used in psychiatry, but which may have psychiatric adverse effects or drug-drug interactions.

CHEMISTRY

The molecular structures of representative first-generation antihistamines used in psychiatry are shown in Figure 36.7–1.

PHARMACOLOGIC ACTIONS

The H_1 antagonists used in psychiatry are well absorbed from the gastrointestinal (GI) tract. The antiparkinsonian effects of

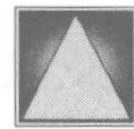

Table 36.7–1
Histamine Antagonists Commonly Used in Psychiatry

Generic Name	Trade Name	Duration of Action (hrs)
Diphenhydramine	Benadryl	4 to 6
Hydroxyzine	Atarax, Vistaril	6 to 24
Promethazine	Phenergan	4 to 6
Cyproheptadine	Periactin	4 to 6

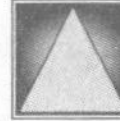

Table 36.7–2
Other Histamine Antagonists Often Prescribed

Class	Generic Name	Trade Name
Second-generation histamine 1 receptor antagonists	Cetirizine	Zyrtec
	Loratadine	Claritin
	Fexofenadine	Allegra
Histamine 2 receptor antagonists	Nizatidine	Axid
	Famotidine	Pepcid
	Ranitidine	Zantac
	Cimetidine	Tagamet

intramuscular (IM) diphenhydramine have their onset in 15 to 30 minutes, and the sedative effects of diphenhydramine peak in 1 to 3 hours. The sedative effects of hydroxyzine and promethazine begin after 20 to 60 minutes and last for 4 to 6 hours. Because all three drugs are metabolized in the liver, persons with hepatic disease, such as cirrhosis, may attain high plasma concentrations with long-term administration. Cyproheptadine is well absorbed after oral administration, and its metabolites are excreted in the urine.

Activation of H_1 receptors stimulates wakefulness; therefore, receptor antagonism causes sedation. All four agents also possess some antimuscarinic cholinergic activity. Cyproheptadine is unique among the drugs, because it has both potent antihistamine and serotonin 5-HT_2 receptor antagonist properties.

THERAPEUTIC INDICATIONS

Antihistamines are useful as a treatment for neuroleptic-induced parkinsonism, neuroleptic-induced acute dystonia, and neuroleptic-induced akathisia. They are an alternative to anticholinergics and amantadine for these purposes. The antihistamines are relatively safe hypnotics, but they are not superior to the benzodiazepines, which have been much better studied in terms of efficacy and safety. The antihistamines have not been proved effective for long-term anxiolytic therapy; therefore, either the benzodiazepines, buspirone (BuSpar), or SSRIs are preferable for such treatment. Cyproheptadine is sometimes used to treat impaired orgasms, especially delayed orgasm resulting from treatment with serotonergic drugs.

Because it promotes weight gain, cyproheptadine may be of some use in the treatment of eating disorders, such as anorexia nervosa. Cyproheptadine can reduce recurrent nightmares with posttraumatic themes. The antiserotonergic activity of cyproheptadine may counteract the serotonin syndrome caused by concomitant use of multiple serotonin-activating drugs, such as SSRIs and monoamine oxidase inhibitors (MAOIs).

PRECAUTIONS AND ADVERSE REACTIONS

Antihistamines are commonly associated with sedation, dizziness, and hypotension, all of which can be severe in elderly persons, who are also likely to be affected by the anticholinergic effects of those drugs. Paradoxical excitement and agitation are adverse effects seen in a small number of persons. Poor motor coordination can result in accidents; therefore, persons should be warned about driving and operating dangerous machinery. Other common adverse effects include epigastric distress, nausea, vomiting, diarrhea, and constipation. Because of mild anticholinergic activity, some people experience dry mouth, urinary retention, blurred vision, and constipation. For this reason also, antihistamines should be used only at very low doses, if at all, by persons with narrow-angle glaucoma or obstructive GI, prostate, or bladder conditions. A central anticholinergic syndrome with psychosis may be induced by either cyproheptadine or diphenhydramine.

In addition to the above adverse effects, antihistamines have some potential for abuse. The coadministration of antihistamines and opioids can increase the euphoria experienced by persons with substance dependence. Overdoses of antihistamines can be fatal. Antihistamines are excreted in breast milk, so their

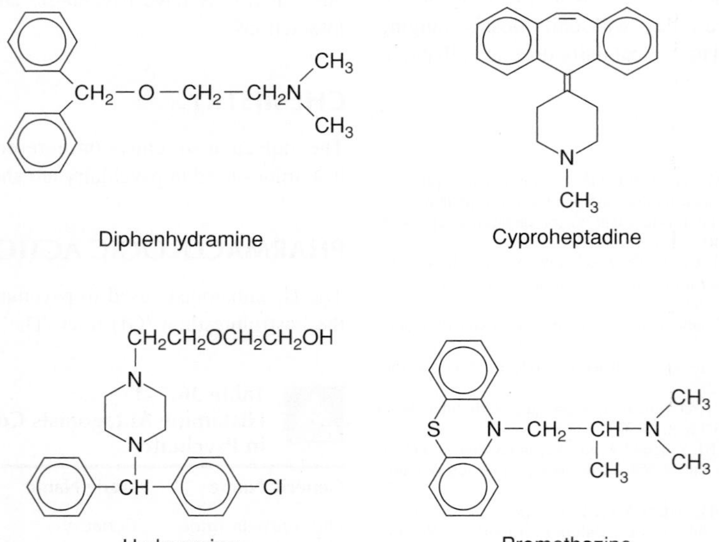

Diphenhydramine

Cyproheptadine

Hydroxyzine

Promethazine

FIGURE 36.7–1
Molecular structures of antihistamines used in psychiatry.

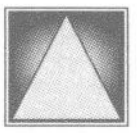

Table 36.7–3
Dosage and Administration of Common Histamine Antagonists

Medication	Route	Preparation	Common Dosage
Diphenhydramine (Benadryl)	PO	Capsules and tablets: 25 mg, 50 mg Liquid: 12.5 mg/5.0 mL	Adults: 25 to 50 mg three to four times per day Children: 5 mg/kg three to four times per day, not to exceed 300 mg/day
	Deep IM or IV	Solution: 10 or 50 mg/mL	Same as oral
Hydroxyzine Hydrochloride (Atarax)	PO	Tablets: 10, 25, 50, and 100 mg Syrup: 10 mg/5 mL	Adults: 50 to 100 mg three to four times daily Children younger than 6 yrs of age: 2 mg/kg/day in divided doses Children older than 6 yrs of age: 12.5 to 25.0 mg, three to four times daily
	IM	Solution: 25 or 50 mg/mL	Same as oral
Pamoate (Vistaril)	PO	Suspension: 25 mg/mL Capsules: 25, 50, and 100 mg	Same as dosages for hydrochloride
Promethazine (Phenergan)	PO	Tablets: 15.2, 25.0, and 50.0 mg Syrup: 3.25 mg/5 mL	Adults: 50 to 100 mg three to four times daily for sedation Children: 12.5 to 25.0 mg at night for sedation
	Rectal	Suppositories: 12.5, 25.0, and 50.0 mg	
	IM	Solution: 25 and 50 mg/mL	
Cyproheptadine (Periactin)	PO	Tablets: 4 mg Syrup: 2 mg/5 mL	Adults: 4 to 20 mg/day Children 2 to 7 yrs of age: 2 mg two to three times daily (maximum of 12 mg/day) Children 7 to 14 yrs of age: 4 mg two to three times daily (maximum of 16 mg/day)

PO, oral; IM, intramuscular; IV, intravenous.

use should be avoided by nursing mothers. Because of some potential for teratogenicity, the use of antihistamines should also be avoided by pregnant women.

Drug Interactions

The sedative property of antihistamines can be additive with other central nervous system (CNS) depressants, such as alcohol, other sedative-hypnotic drugs, and many psychotropic drugs, including tricyclic drugs and dopamine receptor antagonists (DRAs). The anticholinergic activity can also be additive with that of other anticholinergic drugs and can sometimes result in severe anticholinergic symptoms or intoxication. The beneficial effects of SSRIs can be antagonized by cyproheptadine.

LABORATORY INTERFERENCES

H_1 antagonists may eliminate the wheal and induration that form the basis of allergy skin tests. Promethazine can interfere with pregnancy tests and can increase blood glucose concentrations. Diphenhydramine may yield a false-positive urine test result for phencyclidine (PCP). Hydroxyzine use can falsely elevate the results of certain tests for urinary 17-hydroxycorticosteroids.

DOSAGE AND CLINICAL GUIDELINES

The antihistamines are available in a variety of preparations (Table 36.7–3). Intramuscular injections should be deep, because superficial administration can cause local irritation.

Intravenous (IV) administration of 25 to 50 mg of diphenhydramine is an effective treatment for neuroleptic-induced acute dystonia, which may immediately disappear. Treatment with 25 mg three times a day—up to 50 mg four times a day, if necessary—can be used to treat neuroleptic-induced parkinsonism, akinesia, and buccal movements. Diphenhydramine can be used as a hypnotic at a 50-mg dose for mild transient insomnia. Doses of 100 mg have not been shown to be superior to doses of 50 mg, but they produce more anticholinergic effects than doses of 50 mg.

Hydroxyzine is most commonly used as a short-term anxiolytic. Hydroxyzine should not be given IV, because it is irritating to the blood vessels. Dosages of 50 to 100 mg given orally four times a day for long-term treatment or 50 to 100 mg IM every 4 to 6 hours for short-term treatment are usually effective.

Anorgasmia induced by SSRIs may sometimes be reversed with 4 to 16 mg a day of cyproheptadine taken by mouth 1 or 2 hours before anticipated sexual activity. A number of case reports and small studies have also reported that cyproheptadine may be of some use in the treatment of eating disorders, such as anorexia nervosa. Cyproheptadine is available in 4-mg tablets and a 2-mg/5 mL solution. Children and elderly patients are more sensitive to the effects of antihistamines than are young adults.

REFERENCE

Nemeroff CB, Putnam JS. Antihistamines. In: Sadock BJ, Sadock VA, eds. *Kaplan & Sadock's Comprehensive Textbook of Psychiatry*. 8th ed. Vol. 2. Baltimore: Lippincott Williams & Wilkins; 2005:2772.

▲ 36.8 Barbiturates and Similarly Acting Drugs

Barbiturates were widely used as sedative-hypnotic agents in the first half of the 20th century. Many problems are associated with these drugs, including high abuse and addiction potential, a narrow therapeutic range with low therapeutic index, and unfavorable side effects. The use of barbiturates and similar compounds such as meprobamate (Miltown) has been practically eliminated by the benzodiazepines, other anxiolytics such as buspirone (BuSpar), and hypnotics such as zolpidem (Ambien) and zaleplon (Sonata), which have a lower abuse potential and a higher therapeutic index than the barbiturates. Nevertheless, the barbiturates and similarly acting drugs still have a role in the treatment of certain mental disorders.

CHEMISTRY

The various clinically available barbiturates are derived from the same barbituric acid substrate, differing primarily in their substitutions at the C_5 position of the parent molecule. The molecular structures of the various barbiturates are shown in Figure 36.8–1.

PHARMACOLOGIC ACTIONS

The barbiturates are well absorbed after oral administration. The binding of barbiturates to plasma proteins is high, but lipid solubility varies. The individual barbiturates are metabolized by the liver and excreted by the kidneys. The half-lives of specific barbiturates range from 1 to 120 hours (Table 36.8–1). Barbiturates may also induce hepatic enzymes (cytochrome P450), thereby reducing the levels of both the barbiturate and any other concurrently administered drugs metabolized by the liver. The mechanism of action of barbiturates involves the γ-aminobutyric acid (GABA) receptor–benzodiazepine receptor–chloride ion channel complex.

General Formula:

R_3, N 3, (or S=)[b] O=C 2, 5 C, R_{5a}, R_{5b}, H, O, O

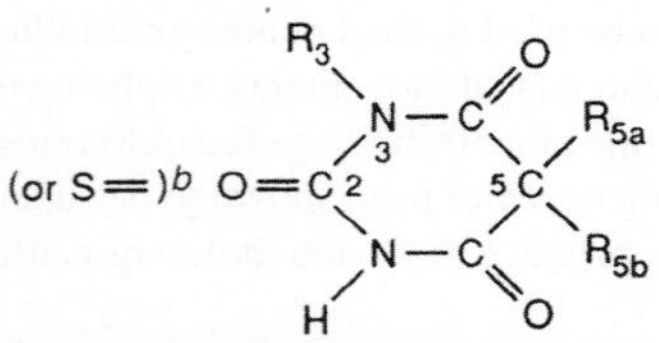

Barbiturate	R_{5a}	R_{5b}
Amobarbital	Ethyl	Isopentyl
Aprobarbital	Allyl	Isopropyl
Butabarbital	Ethyl	*Sec*-Butyl
Butalbital	Allyl	Isobutyl
Mephobarbital[a]	Ethyl	Phenyl
Methohexital[a]	Allyl	1-Methyl-2-Pentynyl
Pentobarbital	Ethyl	1-Methylbutyl
Phenobarbital	Ethyl	Phenyl
Secobarbital	Allyl	1-Methylbutyl
Thiamylal[b]	Allyl	1-Methylbutyl
Thiopental[b]	Ethyl	1-Methylbutyl

[a] R_3 = H_1 except in mephobarbital and methohexital, where it is replaced by CH_3.
[b] O, except in thiamylal and thiopental, where it is replaced by S.

FIGURE 36.8–1

Molecular structures and names of barbiturates available in the United States. (From Rall TW. Hypnotics and sedatives: Ethanol. In: Goodman A, Gilman AG, Rall TW, et al., eds. *Goodman and Gilman's The Pharmacological Basis of Therapeutics,* 8th ed. New York: McGraw-Hill, 1990, with permission.)

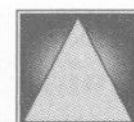

Table 36.8–1
Half-Life, Onset, and Duration of Action of Selected Barbiturates

Barbiturate	Half-Life (hrs)	Onset (mins)	Duration (hrs)
Amobarbital (Amytal)	10 to 40	60	10 to 12
Aprobarbital (Alurate)	14 to 34	45 to 60	6 to 8
Butabarbital (Butisol)	35 to 50	45 to 60	6 to 8
Mephobarbital (Mebaral)	10 to 70	60+	10 to 12
Pentobarbital (Nembutal)	15 to 50	10 to 15	3 to 4
Phenobarbital (Luminal)	80 to 120	60+	10 to 12
Secobarbital (Seconal)	15 to 40	10 to 15	3 to 4

THERAPEUTIC INDICATIONS

Electroconvulsive Therapy

Methohexital (Brevital) is commonly used as an anesthetic agent for electroconvulsive therapy (ECT). It has lower cardiac risks than other barbiturate anesthetics. Used intravenously, methohexital produces rapid unconsciousness and, because of rapid redistribution, it has a brief duration of action (5 to 7 minutes). Typical dosing for ECT is 0.7 to 1.2 mg/kg. Methohexital can also be used to abort prolonged seizures in ECT or to limit postictal agitation.

Seizures

Phenobarbital (Solfoton, Luminal), the most commonly used barbiturate for treatment of seizures, has indications for the treatment of generalized tonic-clonic and simple partial seizures. Parenteral barbiturates are used in the emergency management of seizures independent of cause. Intravenous (IV) phenobarbital should be administered slowly, 10 to 20 mg/kg for status epilepticus.

Narcoanalysis

Amobarbital (Amytal) has been used historically as a diagnostic aid in a number of clinical conditions, including conversion reactions, catatonia, hysterical stupor, and unexplained muteness, and to differentiate stupor of depression, schizophrenia, and structural brain lesions.

The *Amytal interview* is performed by placing the patient in a reclining position and administering amobarbital intravenously, 50 mg a minute. Infusion is continued until lateral nystagmus is sustained or drowsiness is noted, usually at 75 to 150 mg. Following this, 25 to 50 mg can be administered every 5 minutes to maintain narcosis. The patient should be allowed to rest for 15 to 30 minutes after the interview before attempting to walk.

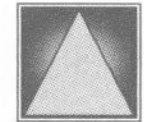

Table 36.8–2
Pentobarbital Challenge Test

1. Give pentobarbital 200 mg p.o.
2. Observe for intoxication after 1 hr (e.g., sleepiness, slurred speech, or nystagmus).
3. If patient is not intoxicated, give another 100 mg of pentobarbital every 2 hr (maximum 500 mg over 6 hrs).
4. Total dose given to produce mild intoxication is equivalent to daily abuse level of barbiturates.
5. Substitute phenobarbital 30 mg (longer half-life) for each 100 mg of pentobarbital.
6. Dosage by about 10% a day.
7. Adjust rate if signs of intoxication or withdrawal are present.

p.o., oral.

Sleep

The barbiturates reduce sleep latency and the number of awakenings during sleep, although tolerance to these effects generally develops within 2 weeks. Discontinuation of barbiturates often leads to rebound increases on electroencephalogram (EEG) measures of sleep and a worsening of the insomnia.

Withdrawal from Sedative-Hypnotics

Barbiturates are sometimes used to determine the extent of tolerance to barbiturates or other hypnotics to guide detoxification. Once intoxication has resolved, a test dose of pentobarbital (200 mg) is given orally. An hour later the patient is examined. Tolerance and dose requirements are determined by the degree to which the patient is affected. If the patient is not sedated, another 100 mg of pentobarbital can be administered every 2 hours, up to three times (maximum, 500 mg over 6 hours). The amount needed for mild intoxication corresponds to the approximate daily dose of barbiturate used. Phenobarbital (30 mg) may then be substituted for each 100 mg of pentobarbital. This daily dose requirement can be administered in divided doses and gradually tapered by 10 percent a day, with adjustments made according to withdrawal signs (Table 36.8–2).

PRECAUTIONS AND ADVERSE REACTIONS

Some adverse effects of barbiturates are similar to those of benzodiazepines, including paradoxical dysphoria, hyperactivity, and cognitive disorganization. Rare adverse effects associated with barbiturate use include the development of Stevens-Johnson syndrome, megaloblastic anemia, and neutropenia.

A major difference between the barbiturates and the benzodiazepines is the low therapeutic index of the barbiturates. An overdose of barbiturates can easily prove fatal. In addition to narrow therapeutic indexes, the barbiturates are associated with a significant risk of abuse potential and the development of tolerance and dependence. Barbiturate intoxication is manifested by confusion, drowsiness, irritability, hyporeflexia or areflexia, ataxia, and nystagmus. The symptoms of barbiturate withdrawal are similar to, but more marked than, those of benzodiazepine withdrawal.

Because of some evidence of teratogenicity, barbiturates should not be used by pregnant women or women who are breast-feeding. Barbiturates should be used with caution by patients with a history of substance abuse, depression, diabetes, hepatic impairment, renal disease, severe anemia, pain, hyperthyroidism, or hypoadrenalism. Barbiturates are also contraindicated in patients with acute intermittent porphyria, impaired respiratory drive, or limited respiratory reserve.

DRUG INTERACTIONS

The primary area for concern about drug interactions is the potentially additive effects of respiratory depression. Barbiturates should be used with great caution with other prescribed central nervous system (CNS) drugs (including antipsychotic and antidepressant drugs) and nonprescribed CNS agents (e.g., alcohol). Caution must also be exercised when prescribing barbiturates to patients who are taking other drugs that are metabolized in the liver, especially cardiac drugs and anticonvulsants. Because individual patients have a wide range of sensitivities to barbiturate-induced enzyme induction, it is not possible to predict the degree to which the metabolism of concurrently administered medications is affected. Drugs that may have their metabolism enhanced by barbiturate administration include opioids, antiarrhythmic agents, antibiotics, anticoagulants, anticonvulsants, antidepressants, β-adrenergic receptor antagonists, dopamine receptor antagonists (DRAs), contraceptives, and immunosuppressants (Table 36.8–3).

LABORATORY INTERFERENCES

No known laboratory interferences are associated with the administration of barbiturates.

DOSAGE AND CLINICAL GUIDELINES

Barbiturates and other drugs described below begin to act within 1 to 2 hours of administration. The dosages of barbiturates vary (Table 36.8–4), and treatment should begin with low dosages that are increased to achieve a clinical effect. Children and older

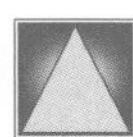

Table 36.8–3
Drug Interactions

The metabolism of the following drugs has been reported to be increased with long-term use of barbiturates. Others unlisted may also be affected.
Analgesics—acetaminophen, fenoprofen
Antiarrhythmics—digitalis, lidocaine, mexiletine
Antibiotics—chloramphenicol, metronidazole, rifampin, tetracycline, griseofulvin
Anticoagulants—warfarin
Anticonvulsants—carbamazepine, phenytoin
Antidepressants—amitriptyline, desipramine, paroxetine, protriptyline
Antihypertensives—methyldopa
Antipsychotics—haloperidol, thioridazine, loxapine
β-adrenergic receptor antagonists—labetalol, propranolol, metoprolol
Benzodiazepines—clonazepam, diazepam
Contraceptives—all containing estrogens
Immunosuppressant—corticosteroids, cyclophosphamide, cyclosporine, decarbazine
Xanthines—aminophylline, caffeine, theophylline

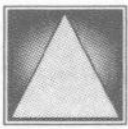

Table 36.8–4
Barbiturate Dosages (Adult)

Drug	Trade Name	Available Preparations	Hypnotic Dose Range	Anticonvulsant Dose Range
Amobarbital	Amytal	200 mg	50 to 300 mg	65 to 500 mg IV
Aprobarbital	Alurate	40-mg/5-mL elixir	40 to 120 mg	Not established
Butabarbital	Butisol	15-, 30-, and 50-mg tablets 30-mg/5-mL elixir	45 to 120 mg	Not established
Mephobarbital	Mebaral	32-, 50-, and 100-mg tablets	100 to 200 mg	200 to 600 mg
Methohexital	Brevital	500 mg/50 cc	1 mg/kg for electroconvulsive therapy	Not established
Pentobarbital	Nembutal	50- and 100-mg capsules 50-mg/mL injection or elixir 30-, 60-, 120-, and 200-mg suppository	100 to 200 mg	100 mg IV, each minute up to 500 mg
Phenobarbital	Luminal	Tablets range from 15–100 mg 20-mg/5-mL elixir 30- to 130-mg/mL injection	30 to 150 mg	100 to 300 mg IV, up to 600 mg/day
Secobarbital	Seconal	100-mg capsule, 50-mg/mL injection	100 mg	5.5 mg/kg IV

IV, intravenous.

people are more sensitive to the effects of the barbiturates than are young adults. The most commonly used barbiturates are available in a variety of dose forms. Barbiturates with half-lives in the 15- to 40-hour range are preferable, because long-acting drugs tend to accumulate in the body. Clinicians should instruct patients clearly about the adverse effects and the potential for dependence associated with barbiturates.

Although determining plasma concentrations of barbiturates is rarely necessary in psychiatry, monitoring of phenobarbital concentrations is standard practice when the drug is used as an anticonvulsant. The therapeutic blood concentrations for phenobarbital in this indication range from 15 to 40 mg/L, although some patients may experience significant adverse effects in that range.

Barbiturates are contained in combination products with which the clinician should be familiar (Table 36.8–5).

OTHER SIMILARLY ACTING DRUGS

A number of agents that act similarly to the barbiturates are used in the treatment of anxiety and insomnia. Three such available drugs are paraldehyde (Paral), meprobamate, and chloral hydrate. These drugs are rarely used because of their abuse potential and potential toxic effects.

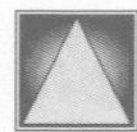

Table 36.8–5
Barbiturate-Containing Medications

Brand-Name Product	Barbiturate	Other Contents
Fiorinal with codeine	Butalbital (Butisol), 50 mg	Aspirin (Bayer), 325 mg; caffeine, 40 mg; codeine, 30 mg
Fioricet with codeine	Butalbital, 50 mg	Acetaminophen (Tylenol), 325 mg; caffeine, 40 mg; codeine, 30 mg
Esgic	Butalbital, 50 mg	Caffeine, 40 mg; acetaminophen, 325 mg
Donnatal	Phenobarbital (Luminal), 16.2 mg	Atropine, 0.02 mg; hyoscyamine (Anaspaz), 0.1 mg; scopolamine (Transderm-Scop), 6.5 μg

Paraldehyde

Paraldehyde is a cyclic ether, first used in 1882 as a hypnotic. It has also been used to treat epilepsy, alcohol withdrawal symptoms, and delirium tremens. Because of its low therapeutic index, it has been supplanted by the benzodiazepines and other anticonvulsants.

Chemistry. The molecular structure of paraldehyde is shown in Figure 36.8–2.

Pharmacologic Actions. Paraldehyde is rapidly absorbed from the gastrointestinal (GI) tract and from intramuscular (IM) injections. It is primarily metabolized to acetaldehyde by the liver, and unmetabolized drug is expired by the lungs. Reported half-lives range from 3.4 to 9.8 hours. Onset of action is 15 to 30 minutes.

Therapeutic Indications. Paraldehyde is not indicated as an anxiolytic or a hypnotic and has little place in current psychopharmacology.

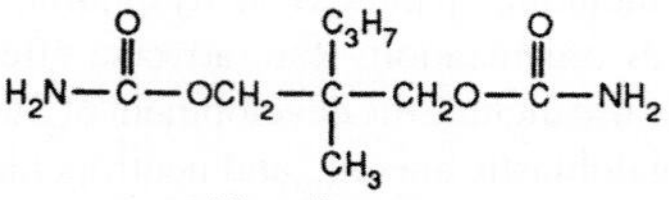

Meprobamate

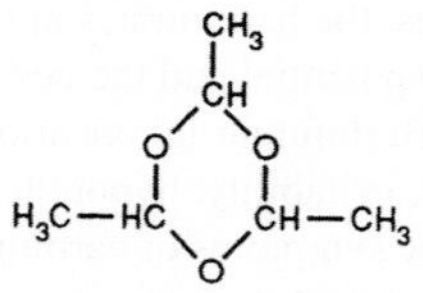

Paraldehyde

FIGURE 36.8–2
Molecular structures of similarly acting drugs.

Precautions and Adverse Reactions. Paraldehyde frequently causes foul breath because of expired unmetabolized drug. It can inflame pulmonary capillaries and cause coughing. It can also cause local thrombophlebitis with IV use. Patients may experience nausea and vomiting with oral use. Overdose leads to metabolic acidosis and decreased renal output. There is risk of abuse among drug addicts.

Drug Interactions. Disulfiram (Antabuse) inhibits acetaldehyde dehydrogenase and reduces metabolism of paraldehyde, leading to possible toxic concentration of paraldehyde. Paraldehyde has addictive sedating effects in combination with other CNS depressants such as alcohol or benzodiazepines.

Laboratory Interferences. Paraldehyde can interfere with the metyrapone, phentolamine, or urinary 17-hydroxycorticosteroid tests.

Dosage and Clinical Guidelines. Paraldehyde is available in 30-mL vials for oral, IV, or rectal use. For seizures in adults, up to 12 mL (diluted to a 10 percent solution) can be administered by gastric tube every 4 hours. For children the oral dose is 0.3 mg/kg.

Meprobamate

Meprobamate, a carbamate, was introduced shortly before the benzodiazepines, specifically to treat anxiety. It is also used for muscle relaxant effects.

Chemistry. The molecular structure of meprobamate is shown in Figure 36.8–2.

Pharmacologic Actions. Meprobamate is rapidly absorbed from the GI tract and from IM injections. It is primarily metabolized by the liver, and a small portion is excreted unchanged in urine. The plasma half-life is approximately 10 hours.

Therapeutic Indications. Meprobamate is indicated for short-term treatment of anxiety disorders. It has also been used as a hypnotic and is prescribed as a muscle relaxant.

Precautions and Adverse Reactions. Meprobamate can cause CNS depression and death in overdose and carries the risk of abuse by patients with drug or alcohol dependence. Abrupt cessation following long-term use can lead to withdrawal syndrome, including seizures and hallucinations. Meprobamate can exacerbate acute intermittent porphyria. Other rare side effects include hypersensitivity reactions, wheezing, hives, paradoxical excitement, and leukopenia. It should not be used in patients with hepatic compromise.

Drug Interactions. Meprobamate has additive sedating effects in combination with other CNS depressants such as alcohol, barbiturates, or benzodiazepines.

Laboratory Interferences. Meprobamate can interfere with the metyrapone, phentolamine, or urinary 17-hydroxycorticosteroid tests.

Dosage and Clinical Guidelines. Meprobamate is available in 200-, 400-, and 600-mg tablets; 200- and 400-mg extended-release capsules; and various combinations, for example, aspirin, 325 mg and 200 mg of meprobamate (Equagesic) for oral use. For adults, the usual dosage is 400 to 800 mg twice daily. Elderly patients and children ages 6 to 12 years require half the adult dose.

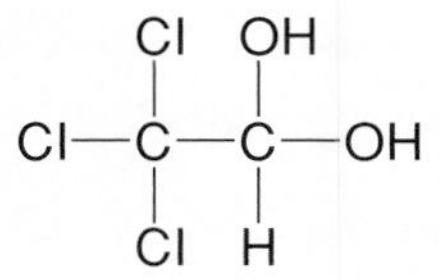

```
   Cl OH
   |  |
Cl—C——C—OH
   |  |
   Cl H
```

FIGURE 36.8–3
Molecular structure of chloral hydrate.

Chloral Hydrate

Chloral hydrate is a hypnotic agent rarely used in psychiatry because numerous safer options, such as benzodiazepines, are available.

Chemistry. The molecular structure of chloral hydrate is shown in Figure 36.8–3.

Pharmacologic Actions. Chloral hydrate is well absorbed from the GI tract. The parent compound is metabolized within minutes by the liver to the active metabolite trichloroethanol, which has a half-life of 8 to 11 hours. A dose of chloral hydrate induces sleep in about 30 to 60 minutes and maintains sleep for 4 to 8 hours. It probably potentiates GABAergic neurotransmission, which suppresses neuronal excitability.

Therapeutic Indications. The major indication for chloral hydrate is to induce sleep. It should be used for no more than 2 or 3 days, because longer-term treatment is associated with an increased incidence and severity of adverse effects. Tolerance develops to the hypnotic effects of chloral hydrate after 2 weeks of treatment. The benzodiazepines are superior to chloral hydrate for all psychiatric uses.

Precautions and Adverse Reactions. Chloral hydrate has adverse effects on the CNS, GI system, and skin. High doses (over 4 g) may be associated with stupor, confusion, ataxia, falls, or coma. The GI effects include nonspecific irritation, nausea, vomiting, flatulence, and an unpleasant taste. With long-term use and overdose, gastritis and gastric ulceration can develop. In addition to the development of tolerance, dependence on chloral hydrate can occur, with symptoms similar to those of alcohol dependence. The lethal dose of chloral hydrate is between 5,000 and 10,000 mg, thus making it a particularly poor choice for potentially suicidal persons.

Drug Interactions. It is because of metabolic interference that chloral hydrate should be strictly avoided with alcohol, a notorious concoction known as a *Mickey Finn*. Chloral hydrate may displace warfarin (Coumadin) from plasma proteins and enhance anticoagulant activity; this combination should be avoided.

Laboratory Interferences. Chloral hydrate administration can lead to false-positive results for urine glucose determinations that use cupric sulfate (e.g., Clinitest), but not in tests that use glucose oxidase (e.g., Clinistix and Tes-Tape). Chloral hydrate can also interfere with the determination of urinary catecholamines in 17-hydroxycorticosteroids.

Dosage and Clinical Guidelines. Chloral hydrate is available in 500-mg capsules, 500-mg/5 mL solution, and 324-, 500-, and 648-mg rectal suppositories. The standard dose of chloral hydrate is 500 to 2,000 mg at bedtime. Because the drug is a GI irritant, it should be administered with excess water, milk, other liquids, or antacids to decrease gastric irritation.

Reference

Nemeroff CB, Putnam JS. Barbiturates and similarly acting substances. In: Sadock BJ, Sadock VA, eds. *Kaplan & Sadock's Comprehensive Textbook of Psychiatry*. 8th ed. Vol. 2. Baltimore: Lippincott Williams & Wilkins; 2005:2775.

▲ 36.9 Benzodiazepines and Drugs Acting on Benzodiazepine Receptors

The benzodiazepines derive their name from their molecular structure. They share a common effect on receptors that have been termed *benzodiazepine receptors*, which in turn modulate γ-aminobutyric acid (GABA) activity. Nonbenzodiazepine agonists, such zolpidem (Ambien), zaleplon (Sonata), and eszopiclone (Lunesta)—the so-called “Z drugs”—are discussed in this chapter because their clinical effects result from interactions with GABA-receptor complexes at binding domains located close to or coupled to benzodiazepine receptors. Flumazenil (Romazicon), a benzodiazepine receptor antagonist used to reverse benzodiazepine-induced sedation and in emergency care of benzodiazepine overdosage, is also covered here.

Because benzodiazepines have a rapid anxiolytic sedative effect, they are most commonly used for immediate treatment of insomnia, acute anxiety, and agitation or anxiety associated with any psychiatric disorder. In addition, the benzodiazepines are used as anesthetics, anticonvulsants, and muscle relaxants. Because of the risk of psychological and physical dependence, long-term use of benzodiazepines should be in conjunction with psychotherapy and in cases where alternative agents have been tried and proved ineffective or poorly tolerated.

CHEMISTRY

The structural formulas of the benzodiazepines are shown in Figure 36.9–1; zolpidem, zaleplon, and eszopiclone in Figure 36.9–2; and flumazenil in Figure 36.9–3.

PHARMACOLOGIC ACTIONS

With the exception of clorazepate (Tranxene), all the benzodiazepines are completely absorbed unchanged from the gastrointestinal (GI) tract. The absorption, the attainment of peak concentrations, and the onset of action are quickest for diazepam (Valium), lorazepam (Ativan), alprazolam (Xanax), triazolam (Halcion), and estazolam (ProSom). The rapid onset of effects is important to persons who take a single dose of a benzodiazepine to calm an episodic burst of anxiety or to fall asleep rapidly. Several benzodiazepines are effective following intravenous (IV) injection, whereas only lorazepam and midazolam (Versed) have rapid and reliable absorption following intramuscular (IM) administration.

Diazepam, chlordiazepoxide, clonazepam (Klonopin), clorazepate, flurazepam (Dalmane), prazepam (Centrax), quazepam (Doral), and halazepam (Paxipam) have plasma half-lives of 30 to more than 100 hours and, therefore, are the longest-acting benzodiazepines. The plasma half-lives of these compounds can be as high as 200 hours in persons whose metabolism is genetically slow. Because the attainment of steady-state plasma concentrations of the drugs can take up to 2 weeks, persons may experience symptoms and signs of toxicity after only 7 to 10 days of treatment with a dosage that seemed initially to be in the therapeutic range.

The half-lives of lorazepam, oxazepam (Serax), temazepam (Restoril), and estazolam are between 8 and 30 hours. Alprazolam has a half-life of 10 to 15 hours and triazolam has the shortest half-life (2 to 3 hours) of all the orally administered benzodiazepines.

The advantages of long half-life drugs over short half-life drugs include less-frequent dosing, less variation in plasma concentration, and less-severe withdrawal phenomena. The disadvantages include drug accumulation, increased risk of daytime psychomotor impairment, and increased daytime sedation. The advantages of the short half-life drugs over the long half-life drugs include no drug accumulation and less daytime sedation. The disadvantages include more-frequent dosing and earlier and more-severe withdrawal syndromes. Rebound insomnia and anterograde amnesia are thought to be more of a problem with the short half-life drugs than with the long half-life drugs.

Zaleplon, zolpidem, and eszopiclone are structurally distinct and vary in their binding to the GABA receptor subunits. Benzodiazepines activate all three specific GABA–benzodiazepine (GABA–BZ) binding sites of the GABA type a ($GABA_A$)-receptor, which opens chloride channels and reduces the rate of neuronal and muscle firing. Zolpidem, zaleplon, and eszopiclone have selectivity for certain subunits of the GABA receptor. This may account for their selective sedative effects and relative lack of muscle relaxant and anticonvulsant effects.

Zolpidem, zaleplon, and eszopiclone are rapidly and well absorbed after oral administration, although absorption can be delayed by as much as 1 hour if they are taken with food. Zolpidem reaches peak plasma concentrations in 1.6 hours and has a half-life of 2.6 hours. Zaleplon reaches peak plasma concentrations in 1 hour and has a half-life of 1 hour. If taken immediately after a high-fat/heavy meal, the peak is delayed by approximately

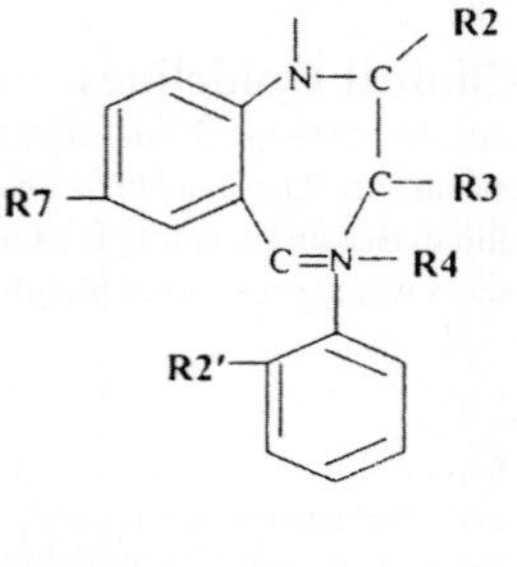

Benzodiazepine	R1	R2	R3	R7	R2′
Alprazolam	Fused triazolo ring		-H	-Cl	-H
Chlordiazepoxide	-	$-NHCH_3$	-H	-Cl	-H
Clonazepam	-H	=O	-H	NO_2	-Cl
Diazepam	$-CH_3$	=O	-H	-Cl	-H

FIGURE 36.9–1
Basic benzodiazepine structure.

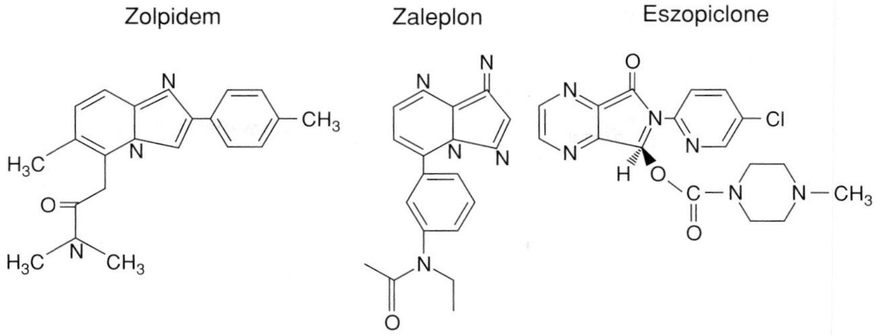

FIGURE 36.9–2
Molecular structures of zolpidem, zaleplon, and eszopiclone.

1 hour, reducing the effects of eszopiclone on sleep onset. The terminal-phase elimination half-life is approximately 6 hours in healthy adults. Eszopiclone is weakly bound to plasma protein (52 to 59 percent).

The rapid metabolism and lack of active metabolites of zolpidem, zaleplon, and eszopiclone avoid the accumulation of plasma concentrations with long-term use of benzodiazepines.

Gaboxatal. This is a new hypnotic agent which works on the α-4 GABA receptor subtype rather than on the α-1 GABA subtype which the other benzodiazepines effect. α-4 GABA is expressed at high levels in the thalmus.

THERAPEUTIC INDICATIONS

Insomnia

Because insomnia can be a symptom of a physical or psychiatric disorder, hypnotics should not be used for more than 7 to 10 consecutive days without a thorough investigation of the cause of the insomnia. In fact, however, many patients have longstanding sleep difficulties and benefit greatly from chronic use of hypnotic agents. Temazepam, flurazepam, and triazolam are benzodiazepines with a sole indication for insomnia. Zolpidem, zaleplon, and eszopiclone are also indicated only for insomnia. Whereas these "Z-drugs" are not usually associated with rebound insomnia after the discontinuation of their use for short periods, some patients experience increased sleep difficulties the first few nights after discontinuing their use. Use of zolpidem, zaleplon, and eszopiclone for periods longer than 1 month is not associated with the delayed emergence of adverse effects. No development of tolerance to any parameter of sleep measurement was observed over 6 months in clinical trials of eszopiclone.

Flurazepam, temazepam, quazepam, estazolam, and triazolam are the benzodiazepines approved for use as hypnotics. The benzodiazepine hypnotics differ principally in their half-lives; flurazepam has the longest half-life, and triazolam has the shortest. Flurazepam may be associated with minor cognitive impairment on the day after its administration, and triazolam may be associated with mild rebound anxiety and anterograde amnesia. Quazepam may be associated with daytime impairment when used for a long time. Temazepam or estazolam may be a reasonable compromise for most adults. Estazolam produces rapid onset of sleep and a hypnotic effect for 6 to 8 hours.

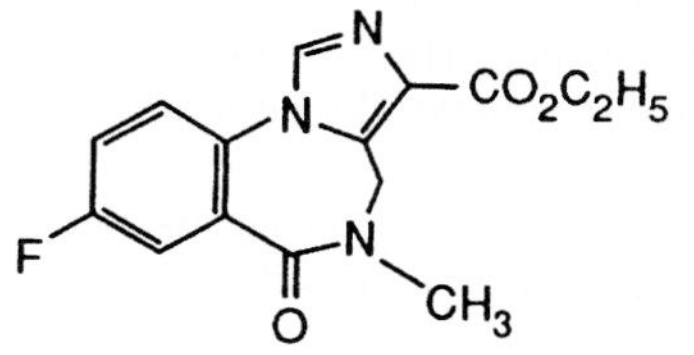

FIGURE 36.9–3
Molecular structure of flumazenil.

Anxiety Disorders

Generalized Anxiety Disorder. Benzodiazepines are highly effective for the relief of anxiety associated with generalized anxiety disorder. Most persons should be treated for a predetermined, specific, and relatively brief period. Because generalized anxiety disorder is a chronic disorder with a high rate of recurrence, some persons with generalized anxiety disorder may warrant long-term maintenance treatment with benzodiazepines.

Panic Disorder. Alprazolam and clonazepam, both high-potency benzodiazepines, are commonly used medications for panic disorder, with or without agoraphobia. Although the selective serotonin reuptake inhibitors (SSRIs) are also indicated for treatment of panic disorder, benzodiazepines have the advantage of working quickly and of not causing significant sexual dysfunction and weight gain. SSRIs are still often preferred, however, because they target common comorbid conditions, such as depression or obsessive-compulsive disorder (OCD). Benzodiazepines and SSRIs can be initiated together to treat acute panic symptoms; use of the benzodiazepine can be tapered after 3 to 4 weeks once the therapeutic benefits of the SSRI have emerged.

Social Phobia. Clonazepam has been shown to be an effective treatment for social phobia. In addition, several other benzodiazepines (e.g., diazepam) have been used as adjunctive medications for treatment of social phobia.

Other Anxiety Disorders. Benzodiazepines are used adjunctively for treatment of adjustment disorder with anxiety, pathological anxiety associated with life events (e.g., after an accident), OCD, and posttraumatic stress disorder.

Mixed Anxiety–Depressive Disorder

Alprazolam is indicated for the treatment of anxiety associated with depression. The availability of several antidepressant drugs with more favorable safety profiles makes alprazolam a second-line drug for this indication; however, some patients respond to this medication when other drugs have had minimal effect.

Bipolar I Disorder

Clonazepam, lorazepam, and alprazolam are effective in the management of acute manic episodes and as an adjuvant to maintenance therapy in lieu of antipsychotics. As an adjuvant to lithium (Eskalith) or lamotrigine (Lamictal), clonazepam may result in an increased time between cycles and fewer depressive episodes.

Akathisia

The first-line drug for akathisia is most commonly a β-adrenergic receptor antagonist. Benzodiazepines are also effective in treating some patients with akathisia, however.

Parkinson's Disease

A few persons with idiopathic Parkinson's disease will respond to long-term use of zolpidem with reduced bradykinesia and rigidity. Zolpidem dosages of 10 mg four times daily may be tolerated without sedation for several years.

Other Psychiatric Indications

Chlordiazepoxide (Librium) is used to manage the symptoms of alcohol withdrawal. The benzodiazepines (especially IM lorazepam) are used to manage agitation, both substance-induced (except amphetamine) and psychotic, in the emergency room. Benzodiazepines have been used instead of amobarbital (Amytal) for drug-assisted interviewing. Benzodiazepines have also been used in the treatment of catatonia. Some patients with delusional disorders with associated anxiety or panic have benefited from the use of benzodiazepines.

Flumazenil for Benzodiazepine Overdosage

Flumazenil is used to reverse the adverse psychomotor, amnesic, and sedative effects of benzodiazepine receptor agonists, including benzodiazepines, zolpidem, and zaleplon. Flumazenil is administered IV and has a half-life of 7 to 15 minutes. The most common adverse effects of flumazenil are nausea, vomiting, dizziness, agitation, emotional lability, cutaneous vasodilation, injection-site pain, fatigue, impaired vision, and headache. The most common serious adverse effect associated with use of flumazenil is the precipitation of seizures, which is especially likely to occur in persons with seizure disorders, those who are physically dependent on benzodiazepines, or those who have ingested large quantities of benzodiazepines. Flumazenil alone may impair memory retrieval.

In mixed-drug overdosage, the toxic effects (e.g., seizures and cardiac arrhythmias) of other drugs (e.g., tricyclic drugs) may emerge with the reversal of the benzodiazepine effects of flumazenil. For example, seizures caused by an overdosage of tricyclic drugs may have been partially treated in a person who had also taken an overdosage of benzodiazepines. With flumazenil treatment, the tricyclic-induced seizures or cardiac arrhythmias may appear and result in a fatal outcome. Flumazenil does not reverse the effects of ethanol, barbiturates, or opioids.

For the initial management of a known or suspected benzodiazepine overdosage, the recommended initial dosage of flumazenil is 0.2 mg (2 mL) administered IV over 30 seconds. If the desired consciousness is not obtained after 30 seconds, a further dose of 0.3 mg (3 mL) can be administered over 30 seconds. Further doses of 0.5 mg (5 mL) can be administered over 30 seconds at 1-minute intervals up to a cumulative dose of 3.0 mg. The clinician should not rush the administration of flumazenil. A secure airway and IV access should be established before the administration of the drug. Persons should be awakened gradually.

Most persons with a benzodiazepine overdosage respond to a cumulative dose of 1 to 3 mg of flumazenil; doses above 3 mg of flumazenil do not reliably produce additional effects. If a person has not responded 5 minutes after receiving a cumulative dose of 5 mg of flumazenil, the major cause of sedation is probably not benzodiazepine receptor agonists, and additional flumazenil is unlikely to have an effect.

Sedation can return in 1 to 3 percent of persons treated with flumazenil. It can be prevented or treated by giving repeated dosages of flumazenil at 20-minute intervals. For repeat treatment, no more than 1 mg (given as 0.5 mg a minute) should be given at any one time, and no more than 3 mg should be given in any 1 hour.

PRECAUTIONS AND ADVERSE REACTIONS

The most common adverse effect of benzodiazepines is drowsiness, which occurs in about 10 percent of all persons. Because of this adverse effect, persons should be advised to be careful while driving or using dangerous machinery when taking the drugs. Drowsiness can be present during the day after the use of a benzodiazepine for insomnia the previous night, so-called *residual daytime sedation*. Some persons also experience ataxia (less than 2 percent) and dizziness (less than 1 percent). These symptoms can result in falls and hip fractures, especially in elderly persons. The most serious adverse effects of benzodiazepines occur when other sedative substances, such as alcohol, are taken concurrently. These combinations can result in marked drowsiness, disinhibition, or even respiratory depression. Infrequently, benzodiazepine receptor agonists cause mild cognitive deficits.

High-potency benzodiazepines, especially triazolam, and zolpidem can cause anterograde amnesia. An unusual, paradoxical increase in aggression has been reported in persons given benzodiazepines, although this effect may be most common in persons with preexisting brain damage. Allergic reactions to the drugs are rare, but a few studies report maculopapular rashes and generalized itching. The symptoms of benzodiazepine intoxication include confusion, slurred speech, ataxia, drowsiness, dyspnea, and hyporeflexia.

Triazolam has received significant attention in the media because of an alleged association with serious aggressive behavioral manifestations. The manufacturer, therefore, recommends that the drug be used for no more than 10 days for treatment of insomnia and that physicians carefully evaluate the emergence of any abnormal thinking or behavioral changes in persons treated with triazolam, giving appropriate consideration to all potential causes. Triazolam was banned in Great Britain in 1991.

Persons with hepatic disease and elderly persons are particularly likely to have adverse effects and toxicity from the benzodiazepines, including hepatic coma, especially when the drugs are administered repeatedly or in high dosages. Benzodiazepines can produce clinically significant impairment of respiration in persons with chronic obstructive pulmonary disease and sleep apnea. Alprazolam can exert a direct appetite stimulant effect and may cause weight gain. Benzodiazepines should be used with caution by persons with a history of substance abuse, cognitive disorders, renal disease, hepatic disease, porphyria, central nervous system (CNS) depression, or myasthenia gravis.

Some data indicate that benzodiazepines are teratogenic; therefore, their use during pregnancy is not advised. Moreover, the use of benzodiazepines in the third trimester can precipitate a withdrawal syndrome in the newborn. The drugs are secreted in breast milk in sufficient concentrations to affect the newborn. Benzodiazepines can cause dyspnea, bradycardia, and drowsiness in nursing babies.

Zolpidem and zaleplon are generally well tolerated. At zolpidem dosages of 10 mg per day and zaleplon dosages above 10 mg per day, a small number of persons will experience dizziness, drowsiness, dyspepsia, or diarrhea. Zolpidem and zaleplon are secreted in breast milk and, therefore, are contraindicated for use by nursing mothers. The dosage of zolpidem and zaleplon should be reduced in the elderly and in persons with hepatic impairment.

In rare cases, zolpidem can cause hallucinations and behavioral changes. The coadministration of zolpidem and SSRIs can extend the duration of hallucinations in susceptible patients.

Eszopiclone exhibits a dose-response relationship in elderly adults for the side effects of pain, dry mouth, and unpleasant taste, with this relationship clearest for unpleasant taste.

Tolerance, Dependence, and Withdrawal

When benzodiazepines are used for short periods (1 to 2 weeks) in moderate dosages, they usually cause no significant tolerance, dependence, or withdrawal effects. The short-acting benzodiazepines (e.g., triazolam) may be an exception to this rule, because some persons have reported increased anxiety the day after taking a single dosage of the drug. Some persons also report a tolerance for the anxiolytic effects of benzodiazepines and require increased dosages to maintain the clinical remission of symptoms.

The appearance of a withdrawal syndrome, also called a *discontinuation syndrome*, depends on the length of time the person has been taking a benzodiazepine, the dosage the person has been taking, the rate at which the drug is tapered, and the half-life of the compound. Benzodiazepine withdrawal syndrome consists of anxiety, nervousness, diaphoresis, restlessness, irritability, fatigue, light-headedness, tremor, insomnia, and weakness (Table 36.9–1). Abrupt discontinuation of benzodiazepines, particularly those with short half-lives, is associated with severe withdrawal symptoms, which can include depression, paranoia, delirium, and seizures. These severe symptoms are more likely to occur if flumazenil is used for rapid reversal of the benzodiazepine receptor agonist effects. Some features of the syndrome

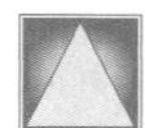

Table 36.9–1
Signs and Symptoms of Benzodiazepine Withdrawal

Anxiety	Tremor
Irritability	Depersonalization
Insomnia	Hyperesthesia
Hyperacusis	Myoclonus
Nausea	Delirium
Difficulty concentrating	Seizures

can occur in as many as 90 percent of the persons treated with the drugs. The development of a severe withdrawal syndrome is seen only in persons who have taken high dosages for long periods. The appearance of the syndrome can be delayed for 1 or 2 weeks in persons who had been taking benzodiazepines with long half-lives. Alprazolam seems to be particularly associated with an immediate and severe withdrawal syndrome and should be tapered gradually.

When the medication is to be discontinued, the drug must be tapered slowly (25 percent a week); otherwise, recurrence or rebound of symptoms is likely. Monitoring of any withdrawal symptoms (possibly with a standardized rating scale) and psychological support of the person are helpful in the successful accomplishment of benzodiazepine discontinuation. Concurrent use of carbamazepine (Tegretol) during benzodiazepine discontinuation has been reported to permit a more rapid and better-tolerated withdrawal than does a gradual taper alone. The dosage range of carbamazepine used to facilitate withdrawal is 400 to 500 mg a day. Some clinicians report particular difficulty in tapering and discontinuing alprazolam, especially in persons who have been receiving high dosages for long periods. There have been reports of successful discontinuation of alprazolam by switching to clonazepam, which is then gradually withdrawn.

Zolpidem and zaleplon can produce a mild withdrawal syndrome lasting 1 day after prolonged use at higher therapeutic dosages. Rarely, a person taking zolpidem has self-titrated up the daily dosage to 300 to 400 mg a day. Abrupt discontinuation of such a high dosage of zolpidem can cause withdrawal symptoms for 4 or more days. Tolerance does not appear to develop to the sedative effects of zolpidem and zaleplon.

DRUG INTERACTIONS

The most common and potentially serious benzodiazepine receptor agonist interaction results in excessive sedation and respiratory depression occurring when benzodiazepines, zolpidem, or zaleplon are administered concomitantly with other CNS depressants, such as alcohol, barbiturates, tricyclic and tetracyclic drugs, dopamine receptor antagonists (DRAs), opioids, and antihistamines. Ataxia and dysarthria may likely occur when lithium, antipsychotics, and clonazepam are combined. The combination of benzodiazepines and clozapine (Clozaril) has been reported to cause delirium and should be avoided. Cimetidine (Tagamet), disulfiram (Antabuse), isoniazid, estrogen, and oral contraceptives increase the plasma concentrations of diazepam, chlordiazepoxide, clorazepate, flurazepam, prazepam, and halazepam. Cimetidine increases the plasma concentrations of zaleplon. The plasma concentrations of triazolam and alprazolam are increased to potentially toxic concentrations by nefazodone

(Serzone) and fluvoxamine (Luvox). The manufacturer of nefazodone recommends that the dosage of triazolam be lowered by 75 percent and the dosage of alprazolam lowered by 50 percent when given concomitantly with nefazodone. Over-the-counter preparations of kava plant, advertised as a "natural tranquilizer," can potentiate the action of benzodiazepine receptor agonists through synergistic overactivation of GABA receptors. Carbamazepine can lower the plasma concentration of alprazolam. Antacids and food can decrease the plasma concentrations of benzodiazepines, and smoking can increase the metabolism of benzodiazepines. Rifampin (Rifadin), phenytoin (Dilantin), carbamazepine, and phenobarbital (Solfoton, Luminal) significantly increase the metabolism of zaleplon. The benzodiazepines can increase the plasma concentrations of phenytoin and digoxin (Lanoxin). SSRIs may prolong and exacerbate the severity of zolpidem-induced hallucinations.

LABORATORY INTERFERENCES

No known laboratory interferences are associated with the use of benzodiazepines, zolpidem, and zaleplon.

DOSAGE AND CLINICAL GUIDELINES

The clinical decision to treat an anxious person with a benzodiazepine should be carefully considered. Medical causes of anxiety (e.g., thyroid dysfunction, caffeinism, and prescription medications) should be ruled out. Benzodiazepine use should be started at a low dosage, and the person should be instructed regarding the drug's sedative properties and abuse potential. An estimated length of therapy should be decided at the beginning of treatment, and the need for continued therapy should be reevaluated at least monthly because of the problems associated with long-term use. Certain persons with anxiety disorders, however, are unresponsive to treatments other than benzodiazepines in long term use.

Benzodiazepines are available in a wide range of formulations. Clonazepam is available in a wafer formulation that facilitates its use in patients who have trouble swallowing pills. Alprazolam is available in an extended-release form, which reduces the frequency of dosing. Some benzodiazepines are more potent than others in that one compound requires a relatively smaller dosage than another compound to achieve the same effect. For example, clonazepam requires 0.25 mg to achieve the same effect as 5 mg of diazepam; thus, clonazepam is considered a high-potency benzodiazepine. Conversely, oxazepam has an approximate dosage equivalence of 15 mg and is a low-potency drug.

Zaleplon is available in 5- and 10-mg capsules. A single 10-mg dose is the usual adult dose. The dose can be increased to a maximum of 20 mg as tolerated. A single dose of zaleplon can be expected to provide 4 hours of sleep with minimal residual impairment. For persons over age 65 or persons with hepatic impairment, an initial dose of 5 mg is advised.

Eszopiclone is available in 1-, 2-, and 3-mg tablets. The starting dose should not exceed 1 mg in patients with severe hepatic impairment or those taking potent CYP 3A4 inhibitors. The recommended dosing to improve sleep onset or maintenance is 2 or 3 mg for adult patients (ages 18 to 64) and 2 mg for older adult patients (ages 65 and older). The 1-mg dose is for sleep onset in older adult patients whose primary complaint is difficulty falling asleep.

Table 36.9–2 lists preparations and doses of medications discussed in this chapter.

RAMELTEON (See also chapter 36.21)

Ramelteon (Rozerem), a new treatment for insomnia, was approved by the US Food and Drug Administration (FDA) in 2005.

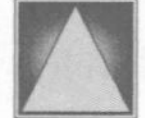

Table 36.9–2
Preparations and Doses of Medications Acting on the Benzodiazepine Receptor

Medication	Brand Name	Dose Equivalent	Usual Adult Dose (mg)	How Supplied
Diazepam	Valium	5	2.5 to 40.0	2-, 5-, and 10-mg tablets 15-mg slow release
Clonazepam	Klonopin	0.5	0.5 to 4.0	0.5-, 1.0-, and 2.0-mg tablets
Alprazolam	Xanax	0.25	0.5 to 6.0	0.125-, 0.25-, 0.5-, 1.0-, and 2.0-mg orally and disintegrating tablets 1.5-mg sustained-release tablet
Lorazepam	Ativan	1	0.5 to 6.0	0.5-, 1.0-, and 2.0-mg tablets 4 mg/mL parenteral
Oxazepam	Serax	10	15 to 120	7.5-, 10.0-, 15.0-, and 30.0-mg capsules 15-mg tablet
Chlordiazepoxide	Librium	15	10 to 100	5-, 10-, and 25-mg capsules and tablets
Clorazepate	Tranxene	7.5	15 to 60	3.75-, 7.50-, and 15.00-mg tablets 11.25- and 22.50-mg slow-release tablets
Halazepam	Paxipam	20	60 to 160	20- and 40-mg tablets
Midazolam	Versed	0.25	1 to 50	5 mg/mL parental 1-, 2-, 5-, and 10-mL vials
Flurazepam	Dalmane	5	15 to 30	15- and 30-mg capsules
Temazepam	Restoril	5	7.5 to 30.0	7.5-, 15.0-, and 30.0-mg capsules
Triazolam	Halcion	0.125	0.125 to 0.250	0.125- and 0.250-mg tablets
Estazolam	ProSom	0.33	1 to 2	1- and 2-mg tablets
Quazepam	Doral	5	7.5 to 15.0	7.5- and 15.0-mg tablets
Zolpidem	Ambien	2.5	5 to 10	5- and 10-mg tablets
Zaleplon	Sonata	2	5 to 20	5- and 10-mg capsules
Flumazenil	Romazicon	0.05	0.2 to 0.5/min	0.1 mg/mL 5- and 10-mL vials

Pharmacologic Actions

Unlike the other hypnotic agents discussed in this section, ramelteon does not act on the benzodiazepine or GABA system. It specifically targets the melatonin MT1 and MT2 receptors in the brain's suprachiasmatic nucleus (SCN). The SCN regulates 24-hour, or circadian, rhythms including the sleep–wake cycle.

Ramelteon is absorbed rapidly, with peak concentrations occurring 30 to 90 minutes after fasting oral administration. The elimination half-life of ramelteon is 1 to 2.6 hours, and that of its active metabolite is 2 to 5 hours.

Therapeutic Indications

Ramelteon is indicated for the treatment of insomnia characterized by difficulty with sleep onset.

Precautions and Adverse Events

The most common adverse events seen with ramelteon were somnolence, dizziness, and fatigue. Ramelteon has been associated with decreased testosterone levels and increased prolactin levels. No evidence suggests abuse or dependence, and the drug is not designated as a controlled substance.

Drug Interactions

CYP1A2 is the major isozyme involved in the hepatic metabolism of ramelteon.

Laboratory Intereferences

Ramelteon is not known to interfere with laboratory tests. Prolactin and testosterone levels should be monitored if patients develop signs and symptoms affecting lactation, menses, libido, or fertility during treatment.

Dosage and Clinical Guidelines

The recommended dose for long-term use in adults is 8 mg taken within 30 minutes before going to bed. Ramelteon should not be combined with fluvoxamine and should not be used by patients with severe hepatic impairment.

References

Ashton H. Calming the brain: Benzodiazepines and related drugs from laboratory to clinic. *J Psychopharmacology*. 2005;19(6):680–681.

Casellas P, Galiegue S, Basile AS. Peripheral benzodiazepine receptors and mitochondrial function. *Neurochem Int*. 2002;40:475–486.

Decaudin D, Castedo M, Nemati F, Beurdeley-Thomas A, de Pinieux G, Caron A, Pouillart P, Wijdenes J, Rouillard D, Groemer G, Poupon M-F. Peripheral benzodiazepine receptor ligands reverse apoptosis resistance of cancer cells in vitro and in vivo. *Cancer Res*. 2002;62:1388–1393.

Dubovsky S. Benzodiazepine receptor agonists and antagonists. In: Sadock BJ, Sadock VA, eds. *Kaplan & Sadock's Comprehensive Textbook of Psychiatry*. 8th ed. Vol. 2. Baltimore: Lippincott Williams & Wilkins; 2005:2781.

Lane SD, Tcheremissine OV, Lieving LM, Nouvion S, Cherek DR. Acute effects of alprazolam on risky decision making in humans. *Psychopharmacology*. 2005;181(2):364–373.

Mol AJJ, Oude VRC, Gorgels WJMJ, Breteler MHM, van Balkom AJLM, van de Lisdonk EH, Kan CC, Mulder J, Zitman FG. The absence of benzodiazepine craving in a general practice benzodiazepine trial. *Addict Behav*. 2006;31(2):211–222.

Strohmmeir R, Roller M, Sanger N, Knecht R, Kuhl H. Modulation of tamoxifen-induced apoptosis by peripheral benzodiazepine receptor ligands in breast cancer. *Biochem Pharmacol*. 2002;64:99–107.

Witek MW, Rojas V, Alonso C, Minami H, Silva RR. Review of benzodiazepine use in children and adolescents. *Psychiatr Q*. 2005;76(3):283–296.

▲ 36.10 Bupropion

Unlike other currently used antidepressants, bupropion (Wellbutrin, Wellbutrin SR, Wellbutrin XL) does not act on the serotonin system. It is a norepinephrine and dopamine reuptake inhibitor. This results in a side-effect profile characterized by little risk of sexual dysfunction or sedation, and with modest weight loss during acute and long-term treatment. No withdrawal syndrome has been linked to discontinuation of bupropion. Bupropion is the only medication approved by the US Food and Drug Administration (FDA) for the prevention of seasonal depressive episodes of patients with seasonal affective disorder (SAD). Although increasingly used as first-line monotherapy, a significant percentage of bupropion use occurs as add-on therapy to other antidepressants, most commonly selective serotonin reuptake inhibitors (SSRIs). This practice has not been systematically studied and is essentially based on the premise that combining agents with differing mechanisms of action may increase efficacy or mitigate side effects. Bupropion has also been marketed under the name Zyban for use in smoking cessation regimens.

CHEMISTRY

Bupropion is a monocyclic aminoketone that resembles amphetamine and the diet drug diethylpropion (Tenuate) in its molecular structure (Fig. 36.10–1).

PHARMACOLOGIC ACTIONS

Three formulations of bupropion are available: immediate release (taken three times daily); sustained release (taken twice daily); and extended release (taken once daily). The different versions of the drug contain the same active ingredient, but differ in their pharmacokinetics and dosing.

Immediate-release bupropion is well absorbed from the gastrointestinal (GI) tract. Peak plasma concentrations of bupropion are usually reached within 2 hours of oral administration, and peak levels of the sustained-release version are seen after 3 hours. The mean half-life of the compound is 12 hours, ranging from 8 to 40 hours. Peak levels of extended-release bupropion occur 5 hours after ingestion. This provides a longer time to maximal plasma concentration (t_{max}) but comparable

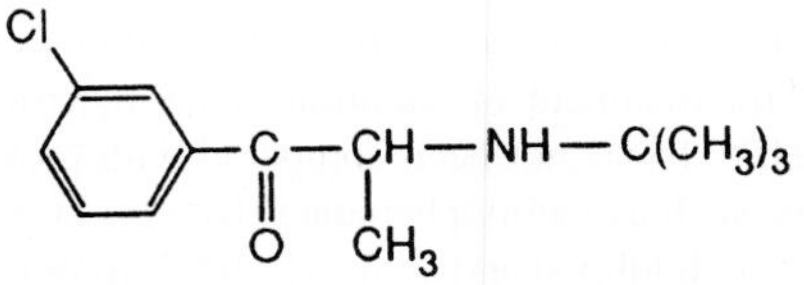

Cl

C—CH—NH—C(CH$_3$)$_3$

O CH$_3$

FIGURE 36.10–1
Molecular structure of bupropion (Wellbutrin).

peak and trough plasma concentrations. The 24-hour exposure occurring after administration of the extended-release version of 300 mg once daily is equivalent to that provided by sustained release of 150 mg twice daily. Clinically, this permits the drug to be taken once a day in the morning. Plasma levels are also reduced in the evening, making it less likely for some patients to experience treatment-related insomnia.

The mechanism of action for the antidepressant effects of bupropion is poorly understood, although it presumably involves inhibition of dopamine and norepinephrine reuptake. Bupropion binds to the dopamine transporter in the brain. The effects of bupropion on smoking cessation may be related to its effects on dopamine reward pathways or to inhibition of nicotinic acetylcholine receptors.

THERAPEUTIC INDICATIONS

Depression

Although overshadowed by the SSRIs as first-line treatment for major depression, the therapeutic efficacy of bupropion in depression is well established in both outpatient and inpatient settings. Observed rates of response and remission are comparable to those seen with SSRIs.

Seasonal Affective Disorder

Seasonal affective disorder is characterized by recurring fall/winter onset of depressive symptoms that include weight gain, lethargy, and increased sleep. Bupropion has been found to prevent seasonal major depressive episodes in patients with a history of SAD.

Smoking Cessation

As the brand name Zyban, bupropion is indicated for use in combination with behavioral modification programs for smoking cessation. It is intended to be used in patients who are highly motivated and who receive some form of structured behavioral support. Bupropion is most effective when combined with nicotine substitutes (NicoDerm, Nicotrol).

Bipolar Disorders

Bupropion is less likely than tricyclics to precipitate mania in persons with bipolar I disorder and less likely than other antidepressants to exacerbate or induce rapid-cycling bipolar II disorder; however, the evidence about use of bupropion in the treatment of patients who are bipolar is limited.

Attention-Deficit/Hyperactivity Disorder

Bupropion is used as a second-line agent, after the sympathomimetics, for treatment of attention-deficit/hyperactivity disorder (ADHD). It has not been compared with proved ADHD medications, such as methylphenidate (Ritalin) or atomoxetine (Strattera), for childhood and adult ADHD. Bupropion is an appropriate choice for persons with comorbid ADHD and depression or persons with comorbid ADHD, conduct disorder, or substance abuse. It may also be considered for use in patients who develop tics when treated with psychostimulants.

Cocaine Detoxification

Bupropion may be associated with a euphoric feeling; thus, it may be contraindicated in persons with histories of substance abuse. Because of its dopaminergic effects, bupropion, however, has been explored as a treatment to reduce the cravings for cocaine in persons who have withdrawn from the substance. Results have been inconclusive, with some patients showing a reduction in drug craving and others finding their cravings increased.

Hypoactive Sexual Desire Disorder

Bupropion is often added to drugs, such as SSRIs, to counteract sexual side effects and may be helpful as a treatment for nondepressed individuals with hypoactive sexual desire disorder. Bupropion may improve sexual arousal, orgasm completion, and sexual satisfaction.

PRECAUTIONS AND ADVERSE REACTIONS

Headache, insomnia, dry mouth, tremor, and nausea are the most common side effects of bupropion use. Restlessness, agitation, and irritability may also occur. Patients with severe anxiety or panic disorder should not be started on bupropion. Most likely because of its potentiating effects on dopaminergic neurotransmission, bupropion can cause psychotic symptoms, including hallucinations, delusions, and catatonia, as well as delirium. Some bupropion-treated patients experience word-finding difficulties and memory impairment. Most notable about bupropion is the absence of significant drug-induced orthostatic hypotension, weight gain, daytime drowsiness, and anticholinergic effects. Some persons, however, may experience dry mouth or constipation and weight loss. Hypertension can occur in some patients, but bupropion causes no other significant cardiovascular or clinical laboratory changes. Bupropion exerts indirect sympathomimetic activity, producing positive inotropic effects in human myocardium, an effect that may reflect catecholamine release.

Concern about seizure has deterred some physicians from prescribing bupropion. Studies show that at dosages of 300 mg a day or less of sustained-release bupropion, the incidence of seizures is 0.05 percent, which is no worse than the incidence of seizures with other antidepressants. The risk of seizures increases to about 0.1 percent with dosages of 400 mg a day. Risk factors for seizures include a history of seizures, use of alcohol, recent benzodiazepine withdrawal, organic brain disease, head trauma, or epileptiform discharges on electroencephalogram (EEG).

The use of bupropion by pregnant women is not associated with specific risk of increased rate of birth defects. Bupropion is secreted in breast milk, so the use of bupropion in nursing women should be based on the clinical circumstances of the patient and the judgment of the clinician.

Few deaths have been reported following overdoses of bupropion. Poor outcomes are associated with cases of huge doses and mixed-drug overdoses. Seizures occur in about one third of all overdoses and are dose-dependent, with those having seizures ingesting a significantly higher median dose. Fatalities can involve uncontrollable seizures, sinus bradycardia, and cardiac arrest. Symptoms of poisoning most often involve seizures, sinus tachycardia, hypertension, GI symptoms, hallucinations, and agitation. All seizures are typically brief and self-limited. In general, however, bupropion is safer in overdose cases than are other antidepressants, except perhaps SSRIs.

DRUG INTERACTIONS

Given that bupropion is frequently combined with SSRIs or venlafaxine (Effexor), potential interactions are significant. Bupropion has been found to have an effect on the pharmacokinetics of venlafaxine. One study noted a significant increase in venlafaxine levels, and a consequent decrease in its main metabolite O-desmethylvenlafaxine, during combined treatment with sustained-release bupropion. Bupropion hydroxylation is weakly inhibited by venlafaxine. No significant changes in plasma levels of the SSRIs paroxetine and fluoxetine have been reported. A few case reports, however, indicate that the combination of bupropion and fluoxetine (Prozac) may be associated with panic, delirium, or seizures. Bupropion in combination with lithium (Eskalith) may rarely cause CNS toxicity, including seizures.

Because of the possibility of inducing a hypertensive crisis, bupropion should not be used concurrently with monoamine oxidase inhibitors (MAOIs). At least 14 days should pass after the discontinuation of an MAOI before initiating treatment with bupropion. In some cases, the addition of bupropion may permit persons taking antiparkinsonian medications to lower the doses of their dopaminergic drugs. Delirium, psychotic symptoms, and dyskinetic movements may, however, be associated with the coadministration of bupropion and dopaminergic agents such as levodopa (Larodopa), pergolide (Permax), ropinirole (Requip), pramipexole (Mirapex), amantadine (Symmetrel), and bromocriptine (Parlodel). Sinus bradycardia may occur when bupropion is combined with metoprolol.

Carbamazepine (Tegretol) may decrease plasma concentrations of bupropion, and bupropion may increase plasma concentrations of valproic acid (Depakene).

In vitro biotransformation studies of bupropion have found that formation of a major active metabolite, hydroxybupropion, is mediated by CYP 2B6. Bupropion has some inhibitory effect on CYP 2D6.

LABORATORY INTERFERENCES

Bupropion may give a false-positive result on urinary amphetamine screens. No other reports have appeared of laboratory interferences clearly associated with bupropion treatment. Clinically nonsignificant changes in the electrocardiogram (premature beats and nonspecific ST-T changes) and decreases in the white blood cell (WBC) count (by about 10 percent) have been reported in a small number of persons.

DOSAGE AND CLINICAL GUIDELINES

Immediate-release bupropion is available in 75-, 100-, and 150-mg tablets. Sustained-release bupropion is available in 100-, 150- , 200-, and 300-mg tablets. Extended-release bupropion comes in 150- and 300-mg strengths, and a 450-mg strength is in development.

Initiation of immediate-release bupropion in the average adult person should be 75 mg orally twice a day. On the fourth day of treatment, the dosage can be raised to 100 mg three times a day. Because 300 mg is the recommended dosage, the person should be maintained on this dosage for several weeks before increasing it further. The maximal dosage, 450 mg a day, should be given as 150 mg three times a day. Because of the risk of seizures, increases in dosage should never exceed 100 mg in a 3-day period; a single dose of immediate-release bupropion should never exceed 150 mg, and the total daily dosage should not exceed 450 mg. The maximum of 400 mg of the sustained-release version should be used as a twice-a-day regimen of either 200 mg twice daily or 300 mg in the morning and 100 mg in the afternoon. A starting dose of the sustained-release version, 100 mg once a day, can be increased to 100 mg twice a day after 4 days. Then, 150 mg twice a day may be used. A single dose of sustained-release bupropion should never exceed 300 mg. The maximal dose is 200 mg twice a day of the immediate-release or extended-release formulations. An advantage of the extended-release preparation is that, after appropriate titration, a total of 450 mg can be given all at once in the morning.

For smoking cessation, the patient should start taking 150 mg a day of sustained-release bupropion 10 to 14 days before quitting smoking. On the fourth day, the dosage should be increased to 150 mg twice daily. Treatment generally lasts 7 to 12 weeks.

References

Ahluwalia IS, Harris KJ, Catley D, Okuyemi KS, Mayo MS. Sustained-release bupropion for smoking cessation in African Americans: A randomized controlled trial. *JAMA*. 2002;288:497.

Clayton AH, Warnock JK, Kornstein SG, Pinkerton R, Sheldon-Keller A, McGarvey EL. A placebo-controlled trial of bupropion SR as an antidote for selective serotonin reuptake inhibitor-induced sexual dysfunction. *J Clin Psychiatry*. 2004;65(1):62.

Fava M, Rush AJ, Thase ME, Clayton A, Stahl SM, Pradko JF, Johnston JA. 15 years of clinical experience with bupropion HCl: From bupropion to bupropion SR to bupropion XL. *Prim Care Companion J Clin Psychiatry*. 2005; 7(3):106.

Gadde KM, Zhang W, Foust MS. Bupropion treatment of olanzapine-associated weight gain: An open-label, prospective trial. *J Clin Psychopharmacol*. 2006;26(4):409.

Jefferson JW, Rush AJ, Nelson JC, Vanmeter SA, Krishen A, Hampton KD, Wightman DS, Modell JG. Extended-release bupropion for patients with major depressive disorder presenting with symptoms of reduced energy, pleasure, and interest: Findings from a randomized, double-blind, placebo-controlled study. *J Clin Psychiatry*. 2006;67(6):865.

Killen JD, Fortmann SP, Murphy GM Jr., Hayward C, Arredondo C, Cromp D, Celio M, Abe L, Wang Y, Schatzburg AF. Extended treatment with bupropion SR for cigarette smoking cessation. *J Consult Clin Psychol*. 2006; 74(2):286.

Papakostas GI, Worthington JJ 3rd, Iosifescu DV, Kinrys G, Burns AM, Fisher LB, Homberger CH, Mischoulon D, Fava M. The combination of duloxetine and bupropion for treatment-resistant major depressive disorder. *Depress Anxiety*. 2006;23(3):178.

Rush JA, Hudziak J, Rettew DC. Bupropion. In: Sadock BJ, Sadock VA, eds. *Kaplan & Sadock's Comprehensive Textbook of Psychiatry*. 8th ed. Vol. 2. Baltimore: Lippincott Williams & Wilkins. 2005:2791.

Rush AJ, Trivedi MH, Wisniewski SR, Stewart JW, Nierenberg AA, Thase ME, Ritz L, Biggs MM, Warden D, Luther JF, Shores-Wilson K, Niederehe G, Fava M. Bupropion-SR, sertraline, or venlafaxine-XR after failure of SSRIs for depression. *N Engl J Med*. 2006;354(12):1231.

Weihs KL, Houser TL, Batey SR, Ascher JA, Bolden-Watson C, Donahue RM, Metz A. Continuation phase treatment with bupropion SR effectively decreases the risk for relapse of depression. *Biol Psychiatry*. 2002;51:753.

Wilens TE, Haight BR, Horrigan JP, Hudziak JJ, Rosenthal NE, Connor DF, Hampton KD, Richard NE, Modell JG. Bupropion XL in adults with attention-deficit/hyperactivity disorder: A randomized, placebo-controlled study. *Biol Psychiatry*. 2005;57(7):793.

▲ 36.11 Buspirone

Buspirone (BuSpar) was introduced in 1986 as the first nonsedating drug specifically indicated for the treatment of generalized anxiety disorder. At that time, it was considered highly novel because, in contrast to existing antianxiety drugs such as the benzodiazepines and barbiturates, it did not cause sedation and was devoid of dependence risk, abuse potential, or a withdrawal syndrome. It also was distinct from those drugs in not having hypnotic, muscle-relaxant, or anticonvulsant properties. Despite these seeming advantages, buspirone has never achieved widespread use. This has been attributed to unrealistic expectations that patients on benzodiazepines could be easily switched to buspirone, and the introduction in 1988 of the first selective serotonin reuptake inhibitor (SSRI), fluoxetine. The SSRIs were subsequently found to treat a wider spectrum of mood and anxiety disorders than buspirone and, thus, became anxiolytics of choice.

CHEMISTRY

Buspirone is classified as an azaperone and is chemically distinct from other psychotropic agents (Fig. 36.11–1).

PHARMACOLOGIC ACTIONS

Buspirone is well absorbed from the gastrointestinal (GI) tract, but absorption is delayed by food ingestion. Peak plasma levels are achieved 40 to 90 minutes after oral administration. At doses of 10 to 40 mg, single-dose linear pharmacokinetics are observed. Nonlinear pharmacokinetics are observed after multiple doses. Because of a short half-life (2 to 11 hours), buspirone is dosed three times daily. An active metabolite of buspirone, 1-pyrimidinylpiperazine (1-PP), is about 20 percent less potent than buspirone, but up to 30 percent more concentrated in the brain than the parent compound. The elimination half-life of 1-PP is 6 hours.

Buspirone acts as an agonist, partial agonist, or antagonist on serotonin 5-HT_{1A} receptors. Its most pronounced action, as a presynaptic agonist at these receptors, inhibits release of serotonin, with consequent antianxiety effects. Action as an agonist at postsynaptic receptors appears to account for antidepressant activity.

Buspirone has no effect on the γ-aminobutyric acid (GABA)-associated chloride ion channel on that receptor mechanism or the serotonin reuptake transporter, targets of other drugs that are effective in generalized anxiety disorder. Buspirone also has activity at 5-HT_2 and dopamine type 2 (D_2) receptors, although the significance of the effects at these receptors is unknown. At D_2 receptors, it has properties of both an agonist and an antagonist.

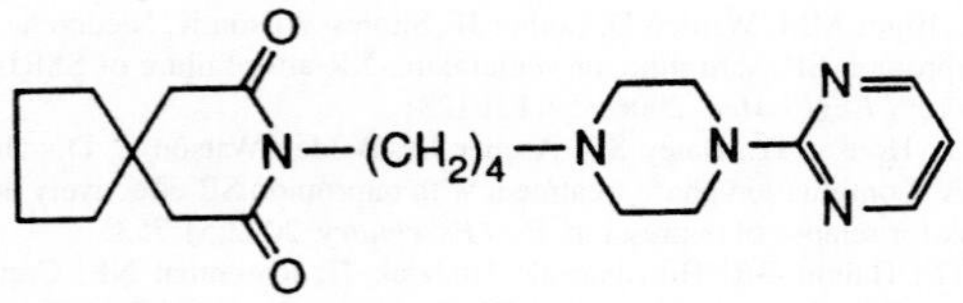

N—$(CH_2)_4$—N N—

FIGURE 36.11–1
Molecular structure of buspirone.

That buspirone takes 2 to 3 weeks to exert its therapeutic effects implies that, whatever its initial effects, they involve the modulation of several neurotransmitters and intraneuronal mechanisms.

THERAPEUTIC INDICATIONS

Generalized Anxiety Disorder

Buspirone is a narrow-spectrum antianxiety agent, with demonstrated efficacy only in the treatment of generalized anxiety disorder. In contrast to the SSRIs or venlafaxine (Effexor), buspirone is not effective in the treatment of panic disorder, obsessive-compulsive disorder (OCD), or social phobia. Buspirone, however, has an advantage over these agents in that it does not typically cause sexual dysfunction or weight gain.

Some evidence suggests that, compared with benzodiazepines, buspirone is generally more effective for symptoms of anger and hostility, equally effective for psychic symptoms of anxiety, and less effective for somatic symptoms of anxiety. The full benefit of buspirone is evident only at dosages above 30 mg a day. Compared with the benzodiazepines, buspirone has a delayed onset of action and lacks any euphoric effect. Unlike benzodiazepines, buspirone has no immediate effects, and the patient should be told that a full clinical response may take 2 to 4 weeks. If an immediate response is needed, the patient can be started on a benzodiazepine and then withdrawn from the drug after buspirone's effects begin. Sometimes the sedative effects of benzodiazepines, which are not found with buspirone, are desirable; however, these sedative effects can cause impaired motor performance and cognitive deficits.

Other Disorders

Many other clinical uses of buspirone have been reported, but most have not been confirmed in controlled trials. Evidence of the efficacy of high-dosage buspirone (30 to 90 mg a day) for depressive disorders is mixed. Buspirone appears to have weak antidepressant activity, which has led to its use as an augmenting agent in patients who have failed standard antidepressant therapy. Buspirone is sometimes used to augment SSRIs in the treatment of OCD. Some reports indicate that buspirone may be beneficial against the increased arousal and flashbacks associated with posttraumatic stress disorder.

Because buspirone does not act on the GABA–chloride ion channel complex, the drug is not recommended for the treatment of withdrawal from benzodiazepines, alcohol, or sedative-hypnotic drugs, except as treatment of comorbid anxiety symptoms.

Scattered trials suggests that buspirone reduces aggression and anxiety in persons with organic brain disease or traumatic brain injury, SSRI-induced bruxism and sexual dysfunction, and nicotine craving, and in attention-deficit/hyperactivity disorder (ADHD).

PRECAUTIONS AND ADVERSE REACTIONS

Buspirone does not cause weight gain, sexual dysfunction, discontinuation symptoms, or significant sleep disturbance. It does not produce sedation or cognitive and psychomotor impairment. The most common adverse effects of buspirone are headache, nausea, dizziness, and, rarely, insomnia. No sedation is associated with buspirone. Some persons may report a minor feeling of restlessness, although that symptom may reflect an incompletely treated anxiety disorder. No deaths have been reported from overdoses of buspirone, and the median lethal dose (LD_{50}) is estimated to be 160 to 550 times the recommended daily dose. Buspirone should be used with caution by persons with hepatic and renal impairment, pregnant women, and nursing mothers. Buspirone can be used safely by the elderly.

DRUG INTERACTIONS

The coadministration of buspirone and haloperidol (Haldol) results in increased blood concentrations of haloperidol. Buspirone should not be used with monoamine oxidase inhibitors (MAOIs) to avoid hypertensive episodes, and a 2-week washout period should pass between the discontinuation of MAOI use and the initiation of treatment with buspirone. Drugs or foods that inhibit CYP450 3A4, for example, erythromycin (E-mycin), itraconazole (Sporanox), nefazodone (Serzone), and grapefruit juice, increase buspirone plasma concentrations.

LABORATORY INTERFERENCES

Single doses of buspirone can cause transient elevations in growth hormone, prolactin, and cortisol concentrations, although the effects are not clinically significant.

DOSAGE AND CLINICAL GUIDELINES

Buspirone is available in single-scored 5- and 10-mg tablets and triple-scored 15- and 30-mg tablets; treatment is usually initiated with either 5 mg orally three times daily or 7.5 mg orally twice daily. The dosage can be raised 5 mg every 2 to 4 days to the usual dosage range of 15 to 60 mg a day.

Switching from a Benzodiazepine to Buspirone

Buspirone is not cross-tolerant with benzodiazepines, barbiturates, or alcohol. A common clinical problem, therefore, is how to initiate buspirone therapy in a person who is currently taking benzodiazepines. The two alternatives are as follows: First, the clinician can start buspirone treatment gradually while the benzodiazepine is being withdrawn. Second, the clinician can start buspirone treatment and bring the person up to a therapeutic dosage for 2 to 3 weeks, while the person is still receiving the regular dosage of the benzodiazepine, and then slowly taper the benzodiazepine dosage. Patients who have received benzodiazepines in the past, especially in recent months, may find that buspirone is not as effective as the benzodiazepines in treating their anxiety. This might be explained by the absence of the immediate mildly euphoric and sedative effects of the benzodiazepines. The coadministration of buspirone and benzodiazepines may be effective in the treatment of anxiety disorders that have not responded to treatment with either drug alone.

REFERENCES

Birudaraj R, Berner B, Shen S, Li X. Buccal permeation of buspirone: Mechanistic studies on transport pathways. *J Pharm Sci*. 2005;94(1):70.

Buydens-Branchey L, Branchey M, Reel-Brander C. Efficacy of buspirone in the treatment of opioid withdrawal. *J Clin Psychopharmacol*. 2005;25(3):230.

Commissaris RL, Fomum EA, Leavell BJ. Effects of buspirone and alprazolam treatment on the startle-potentiated startle response. *Depress Anxiety*. 2004;19(3):146.

Cooper JP. Buspirone for anxiety and agitation in dementia. *J Psychiatry Neurosci*. 2003;28(6):469.

Edwards DJ, Chugani DC, Chugani HT, Chehab J, Malian M, Aranda JV. Pharmacokinetics of buspirone in autistic children. *J Clin Pharmacol*. 2006;46(5):508.

Helvink B, Holroyd S. Buspirone for stereotypic movements in elderly with cognitive impairment. *J Neuropsychiatry Clin Neurosci*. 2006;18(2):242.

Hudziak J, Waterman GS. Buspirone. In: Sadock BJ, Sadock VA, eds. *Kaplan & Sadock's Comprehensive Textbook of Psychiatry*. 8th ed. Vol. 2. Baltimore: Lippincott Williams & Wilkins; 2005:2797.

McRae AL, Sonne SC, Brady KT, Durkalski V, Palesch Y. A randomized, placebo-controlled trial of buspirone for the treatment of anxiety in opioid-dependent individuals. *Am J Addict*. 2004;13:53.

Pavlovic ZM. Buspirone to improve compliance in venlafaxine-induced movement disorder. *Int J Neuropsychopharmacol*. 2004;7(4):523.

Shim JC, Kim YH, Kelly DL, Lee JG, Conley RR. Tardive dyskinesia predicts prolactin response to buspirone challenge in people with schizophrenia. *J Neuropsychiatry Clin Neurosci*. 2005;17(2):221.

▲ 36.12 Calcium Channel Inhibitors

Calcium channel inhibitors are used in psychiatry as antimanic agents for persons who are refractory to, or cannot tolerate, treatment with first-line mood-stabilizing agents. Calcium channel inhibitors include nifedipine (Procardia, Adalat), nimodipine (Nimotop), isradipine (DynaCirc), amlodipine (Norvasc, Lotrel), nicardipine (Cardene), nisoldipine (Sular), nitrendipine, and verapamil (Calan). They are used to control mania and ultradian bipolar disorder (mood cycling in less than 24 hours).

CHEMISTRY

Different classes of calcium channel blockers have significantly different molecular structures. The structures of the calcium channel inhibitors that are most relevant to psychiatry are shown in Figure 36.12–1.

PHARMACOLOGIC ACTIONS

The calcium channel inhibitors are nearly completely absorbed after oral use, with significant first-pass hepatic metabolism. Considerable intraindividual and interindividual variations are seen in the plasma concentrations of the drugs after a single dose. Peak plasma levels of most of these agents are achieved within 30 minutes. Amlodipine does not reach peak plasma levels for about 6 hours. The half-life of verapamil after the first dose is 2 to 8 hours; the half-life increases to 5 to 12 hours after the first few days of therapy. The half-lives of the other calcium channel blockers range from 1 to 2 hours for nimodipine and isradipine to 30 to 50 hours for amlodipine (Table 36.12–1).

The primary mechanism of action of calcium channel blockers in bipolar illness is not known. The calcium channel inhibitors discussed in this section inhibit the influx of calcium into neurons through L-type (long-acting) voltage-dependent calcium channels.

THERAPEUTIC INDICATIONS

Bipolar Disorder

Nimodipine and verapamil have been demonstrated to be effective as maintenance therapy in bipolar illness. Patients who

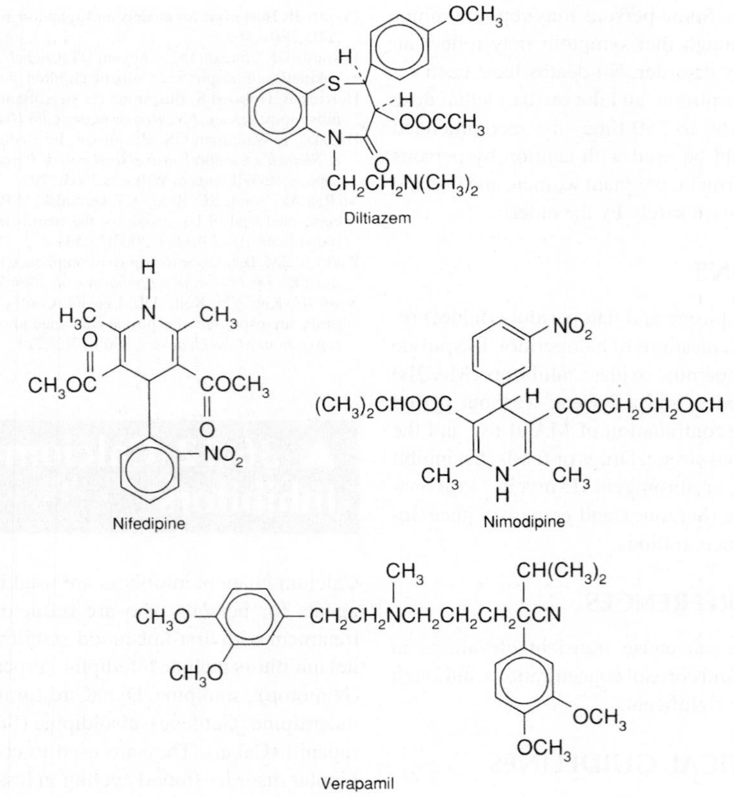

FIGURE 36.12–1
Molecular structures of calcium channel inhibitors.

respond to lithium appear to also respond to treatment with verapamil. Nimodipine may be useful for ultradian cycling and recurrent brief depression. The clinician should begin treatment with a short-acting drug, such as nimodipine or isradipine, beginning with a low dosage and increasing the dosage every 4 to 5 days until a clinical response is seen or adverse effects appear. Once symptoms are controlled, a longer-acting drug, such as amlodipine, can be substituted as maintenance therapy. Failure to respond to verapamil does not exclude a favorable response to one of the other drugs. Verapamil has been shown to prevent antidepressant-induced mania. Calcium channel blockers can be combined with other agents, such as carbamazepine, in patients who are partial responders to monotherapy.

Depression

None of the calcium channel blockers is effective as treatment for depression and, in fact, may prevent response to antidepressants.

Other Psychiatric Indications

Nifedipine is used to treat hypertensive crises associated with use of monoamine oxidase inhibitors. Isradipine may reduce the

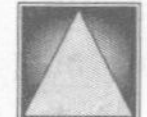

Table 36.12–1
Half-Lives, Dosages, and Effectiveness of Selected Calcium Channel Inhibitors in Psychiatric Disorders

	Verapamil (Calan, Isoftin)	Nimodipine (Nimotop)	Isradipine (DynaCirc)	Amlodipine (Norvasc)
Half-Life	Short (5 to 12 hrs)	Short (1 to 2 hrs)	Short (1 to 2 hrs)	Long (30 to 50 hrs)
Starting dosage	30 mg tid	30 mg tid	2.5 mg bid	5 mg hs
Peak daily dosage	480 mg	240 to 450 mg	15 mg	10 to 15 mg
Antimanic	++	++	++	[a]
Antidepressant	±	+	+	[a]
Antiultradian[b]	±	++	(++)	[a]

bid, twice a day; tid, three times a day; hs, half strength.
[a]No systematic studies, only case reports.
[b]Rapid-cycling bipolar disorder.
(Table adapted from Robert M. Post, M.D.)

subjective response to methamphetamine. Calcium channel inhibitors may be beneficial in Tourette's disorder, Huntington's disease, panic disorder, intermittent explosive disorder, and tardive dyskinesia.

PRECAUTIONS AND ADVERSE REACTIONS

The most common adverse effects associated with calcium channel inhibitors are those caused by vasodilation: dizziness, headache, tachycardia, nausea, dysesthesias, and peripheral edema. Verapamil and diltiazem (Cardizem), in particular, can cause hypotension, bradycardia, and atrioventricular (AV) heart block, all of which necessitate close monitoring and sometimes discontinuation of the drugs. In all patients with cardiovascular disease, the drugs should be used with caution. Other common adverse effects include constipation, fatigue, rash, coughing, and wheezing. Adverse effects noted with diltiazem include hyperactivity, akathisia, and parkinsonism; with verapamil, delirium, hyperprolactinemia, and galactorrhea; with nimodipine, a subjective sense of chest tightness and skin flushing; and with nifedipine, depression. The drugs have not been evaluated for safety in pregnant women and are best avoided. Because the drugs are secreted in breast milk, nursing mothers should also avoid the drugs.

DRUG INTERACTIONS

Verapamil raises serum levels of carbamazepine, digoxin, and other CYP 34A substrates. Verapamil and diltiazem, but not nifedipine, have been reported to precipitate carbamazepine-induced neurotoxicity. Calcium channel inhibitors should not be used by persons taking β-adrenergic receptor antagonists, hypotensives (e.g., diuretics, vasodilators, and angiotensin-converting enzyme inhibitors), or antiarrhythmic drugs (e.g., quinidine and digoxin) without consultation with an internist or cardiologist. Cimetidine (Tagamet) has been reported to increase plasma concentrations of nifedipine and diltiazem. Some patients who are treated with lithium and calcium channel inhibitors concurrently may be at increased risk for the signs and symptoms of neurotoxicity, and deaths have occurred.

LABORATORY INTERFERENCES

No known laboratory interferences are associated with the use of calcium channel inhibitors.

DOSAGE AND CLINICAL GUIDELINES

Verapamil is available in 40-, 80-, and 120-mg tablets; 120-, 180- and 240-mg sustained-release tablets; and 100-, 120-, 180-, 200-, 240-, 300-, and 360-mg sustained-release capsules. The starting dosage is 40 mg orally three times a day and can be raised in increments every 4 to 5 days up to 80 to 120 mg three times a day. The patient's blood pressure (BP), pulse, and electrocardiogram (ECG) (in patients more than 40 years of age or with a history of cardiac illness) should be routinely monitored.

Nifedipine is available in 10- and 20-mg capsules and 30-, 60-, and 90-mg extended-release tablets. Administration should be started at 10 mg orally three or four times a day and can be increased up to a maximal dosage of 120 mg a day.

Nimodipine is available in 30-mg capsules. It has been used at 60 mg every 4 hours for ultrarapid-cycling bipolar disorder and sometimes briefly at up to 630 mg per day.

Isradipine is available in 2.5- and 5-mg capsules and 5- or 10-mg controlled-release tablets. Administration should be started at 2.5 mg a day and can be increased up to a maximum of 15 mg a day in divided doses.

Amlodipine is available in 2.5-, 5-, and 10-mg tablets. Administration should start at 5 mg once at night and can be increased to a maximal dosage of 10 to 15 mg a day.

Diltiazem is available in 30-, 60-, 90-, and 120-mg tablets; 60-, 90-, 120-, 180-, 240-, 300-, and 360-mg extended-release capsules; and 60-, 90-, 120-, 180-, 240-, 300-, and 360-mg extended-release tablets. Administration should start with 30 mg orally four times a day and can be increased up to a maximum of 360 mg a day.

Elderly persons are more sensitive to the calcium channel inhibitors than are younger adults. No specific information is available regarding the use of these agents for children.

REFERENCES

Dubovsky S. Calcium channel inhibitors. In: Sadock BJ, Sadock VA, eds. *Kaplan & Sadock's Comprehensive Textbook of Psychiatry*. 8th ed. Vol. 2. Baltimore: Lippincott Williams & Wilkins; 2005:2801.

Post RM, Gavin CS. Calcium channel blockers in bipolar disorder. *Directions in Psychiatry*. 2005;25:71.

Wisner KL, Peindl KS, Perel JM, Hanusa BH, Piontek CM, Baab S. Verapamil treatment for women with bipolar disorder. *Biol Psychiatry*. 2002;51:745–752.

▲ 36.13 Carbamazepine and Oxcarbazepine

Carbamazepine (Equetro, Carbatrol, Tegretol) was first used to treat partial- and generalized-onset epilepsy and trigeminal neuralgia. Outside the United States, carbamazepine has been used for decades as a first-line agent for acute and maintenance treatment for bipolar I disorder. Despite its proved efficacy, carbamazepine was not approved as a treatment for bipolar disorder by the US Food and Drug Administration (FDA) until 2004 and only in the extended release form. An analog of carbamazepine, oxcarbazepine (Trileptal), was marketed in the United States in 2000, after being used as a treatment for pediatric epilepsy in Europe since 1990. Very small studies and anecdotal reports suggest that oxcarbazepine may possess mood-stabilizing properties, which, however, has not been confirmed in large, placebo-controlled trials.

CHEMISTRY

Both carbamazepine and oxcarbazepine are iminostilbenes. As seen in Figure 36.13–1, both drugs are almost structurally identical and are similar to the tricyclic antidepressants. Oxcarbazepine differs structurally from carbamazepine as a result of the replacement of a carbohydrate (CH) group with a carboxy (CO) moiety. The resulting change in metabolism leads to products that are both safer and better tolerated than carbamazepine. The therapeutic effects of carbamazepine have been linked to blockade of type 2 or batrachotoxin-sensitive sodium channels, action on mitochondrial receptors, and activity at adenosine A_1

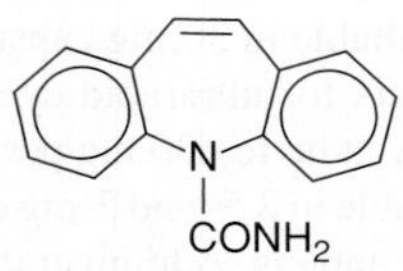

FIGURE 36.13–1
Molecular structure of carbamazepine and oxcarbazepine.

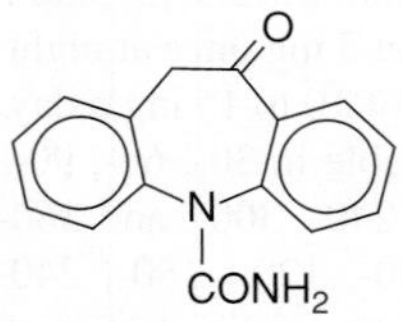

receptors. Numerous other receptor effects of carbamazepine have also been described. The primary biochemical effect of oxcarbazepine is potent blockade of sodium channels.

CARBAMAZEPINE

Pharmacologic Actions

Absorption of carbamazepine is slow and unpredictable. Food enhances absorption. Peak plasma concentrations are reached 2 to 8 hours after a single dose, and steady-state levels are reached after 2 to 4 days on a steady dosage. It is 70 percent to 80 percent protein bound. The half-life of carbamazepine ranges from 18 to 54 hours, with an average of 26 hours. With chronic administration, however, the half-life of carbamazepine decreases to an average of 12 hours. This results from induction of hepatic CYP450 enzymes by carbamazepine, and specifically autoinduction of carbamazepine metabolism. The induction of hepatic enzymes reaches its maximal level after about 3 to 5 weeks of therapy.

The pharmacokinetics of carbamazepine are different for two long-acting preparations of carbamazepine, each of which uses slightly different technology. One formulation, Tegretol XR, requires food to ensure normal gastrointestinal (GI) transit time. The other preparation, Carbatrol, relies on a combination of intermediate, extended-release, and very slow-release beads, making it suitable for bedtime administration.

Carbamazepine is metabolized in the liver, and the 10, 11-epoxide metabolite is active as an anticonvulsant. Its activity in the treatment of bipolar disorders is unknown. Long-term use of carbamazepine is associated with an increased ratio of the epoxide-to-the-parent molecule.

The anticonvulsant effects of carbamazepine are thought to be mediated mainly by binding to voltage-dependent sodium channels in the inactive state and prolonging their inactivation. This secondarily reduces voltage-dependent calcium channel activation and, therefore, synaptic transmission. Additional effects include reduction of currents through *N*-methyl-D-aspartate (NMDA) glutamate-receptor channels, competitive antagonism of adenosine A_1 receptors, and potentiation of central nervous system (CNS) catecholamine neurotransmission. Whether any or all of these mechanisms also result in mood stabilization is not known.

Therapeutic Indications

Bipolar Disorder

ACUTE MANIA. The acute antimanic effects of carbamazepine are typically evident within the first several days of treatment. A 50 percent to 70 percent response is seen within 2 to 3 weeks of initiation. Studies suggest that carbamazepine may be especially effective in persons who are not responsive to lithium, such as persons with dysphoric mania, rapid cycling, or a negative family history of mood disorders. The antimanic effects of carbamazepine can be, and often are, augmented by concomitant administration of lithium, valproic acid, thyroid hormones, dopamine receptor antagonists, or serotonin-dopamine antagonists. Some persons may respond to carbamazepine but not lithium or valproic acid, and vice versa. Comparative data with more recently approved serotonin-dopamine antagonists, also known as the atypical neuroleptics, all of which are also indicated for acute mania, are not available.

PROPHYLAXIS. Carbamazepine is effective in preventing relapses, particularly among patients with bipolar II illness, schizoaffective disorder, and dysphoric mania.

ACUTE DEPRESSION. A subgroup of treatment-refractory patients with acute depression responds well to carbamazepine. Patients with more severe episodic and less chronic depressions seem to be better responders to carbamazepine. Nevertheless, carbamazepine remains an alternative drug for depressed persons who have not responded to conventional treatments, including electroconvulsive therapy (ECT).

Other Disorders. Carbamazepine helps to control symptoms associated with acute alcohol withdrawal. Although lacking the abuse potential of benzodiazepines in this population, the lack of any advantage of carbamazepine over the benzodiazepines for alcohol withdrawal and the potential risk of adverse effects with carbamazepine limit use in this role. Carbamazepine has been suggested as a treatment for the paroxysmal recurrent component of posttraumatic stress disorder. Uncontrolled studies suggest that carbamazepine is effective in controlling impulsive, aggressive behavior in persons of all ages who are not psychotic, including children and the elderly. Carbamazepine is also effective in controlling nonacute agitation and aggressive behavior in patients with schizophrenia and schizoaffective disorder. Persons with prominent positive symptoms (e.g., hallucinations) may likely respond, as are persons who display impulsive aggressive outbursts.

Precautions and Adverse Reactions

Carbamazepine is relatively well tolerated. Mild GI (nausea, vomiting, gastric distress, constipation, diarrhea, and anorexia) and CNS (ataxia, drowsiness) are the most common side effects. The severity of these adverse effects is reduced if the dosage of carbamazepine is increased slowly and kept at the minimal effective plasma concentration. In contrast to lithium and valproate, other drugs used to manage bipolar disorder, carbamazepine does not appear to cause weight gain. Because of the phenomenon of autoinduction, with consequent reductions in carbamazepine concentrations, side-effect tolerability may improve over time.

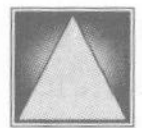

Table 36.13–1
Adverse Events Associated with Carbamazepine

Dosage-Related Adverse Effects	Idiosyncratic Adverse Effects
Double or blurred vision	Agranulocytosis
Vertigo	Stevens-Johnson syndrome
Gastrointestinal (GI) disturbances	Aplastic anemia
Task performance impairment	Hepatic failure
Hematologic effects	Rash
	Pancreatitis

Most of the adverse effects of carbamazepine are correlated with plasma concentrations above 9 μg/mL. The rarest but most serious adverse effects of carbamazepine are blood dyscrasias, hepatitis, and serious skin reactions (Table 36.13–1).

Blood Dyscrasias. The drug's hematologic effects are not dose related. Severe blood dyscrasias (aplastic anemia, agranulocytosis) occur in about 1 in 125,000 persons treated with carbamazepine. A correlation does not appear to exist between the degree of benign white blood cell suppression (leukopenia), which is seen in 1 percent to 2 percent of persons, and the emergence of life-threatening blood dyscrasias. Persons should be warned that the emergence of such symptoms as fever, sore throat, rash, petechiae, bruising, and easy bleeding can potentially herald a serious dyscrasia and the person should seek medical evaluation immediately. Routine hematologic monitoring in carbamazepine-treated persons is recommended at 3, 6, 9, and 12 months. With no significant evidence of bone marrow suppression by that time, many experts would reduce the interval of monitoring. Even assiduous monitoring, however, may fail to detect severe blood dyscrasias before they cause symptoms.

Hepatitis

Within the first few weeks of therapy, carbamazepine can cause both a hepatitis associated with increases in liver enzymes, particularly transaminases, and a cholestasis associated with elevated bilirubin and alkaline phosphatase. Mild transaminase elevations warrant observation only, but persistent elevations more than three times the upper limit of normal indicate the need to discontinue the drug. Hepatitis can recur if the drug is reintroduced to the person and can result in death.

Dermatologic Effects. About 10 percent to 15 percent of persons treated with carbamazepine develop a benign maculopapular rash within the first 3 weeks of treatment. Stopping the medication usually leads to resolution of the rash. Some patients may experience life-threatening dermatologic syndromes, including exfoliative dermatitis, erythema multiforme, Stevens-Johnson syndrome, and toxic epidermal necrolysis. The possible emergence of these serious dermatologic problems causes most clinicians to discontinue carbamazepine use in a person who develops any type of rash. The risk of drug rash is about equal between valproic acid and carbamazepine in the first 2 months of use, but is subsequently much higher for carbamazepine. If carbamazepine seems to be the only effective drug for a person who has a benign rash with carbamazepine treatment, a retrial of the drug can be undertaken. Many patients can be rechallenged without re-emergence of the rash. Pretreatment with prednisone (40 mg a day) may suppress the rash, although other symptoms of an allergic reaction (e.g., fever and pneumonitis) may develop, even with steroid pretreatment.

Renal Effects. Carbamazepine is occasionally used to treat diabetes insipidus not associated with lithium use. This activity results from direct or indirect effects at the vasopressin receptor. It also can lead to the development of hyponatremia and water intoxication in some patients, particularly the elderly or when used in high doses.

Other Adverse Effects. Carbamazepine decreases cardiac conduction (although less than the tricyclic drugs do) and, thus, can exacerbate preexisting cardiac disease. Carbamazepine should be used with caution in persons with glaucoma, prostatic hypertrophy, diabetes, or a history of alcohol abuse. Carbamazepine occasionally activates vasopressin receptor function, which results in a condition resembling the syndrome of secretion of inappropriate antidiuretic hormone (SIADH), characterized by hyponatremia and, rarely, water intoxication. This is the opposite of the renal effects of lithium (i.e., nephrogenic diabetes insipidus). Augmentation of lithium with carbamazepine does not reverse the lithium effect, however. Emergence of confusion, severe weakness, or headache in a person taking carbamazepine should prompt measurement of serum electrolytes.

Carbamazepine use rarely elicits an immune hypersensitivity response consisting of fever, rash, eosinophilia, and possibly fatal myocarditis.

Minor cranial facial abnormalities, fingernail hypoplasia, and spina bifida in infants may be associated with the maternal use of carbamazepine during pregnancy. Pregnant women should not use carbamazepine unless absolutely necessary. All women with childbearing potential should take 1 to 4 mg of folic acid daily, even if they are not trying to conceive. Carbamazepine is secreted in breast milk.

Drug Interactions

Carbamazepine decreases serum concentrations of numerous drugs as a result of prominent induction of hepatic CYP 3A4 (Table 36.13–2). Monitoring for a decrease in clinical effects is frequently indicated. Carbamazepine can decrease the blood concentrations of oral contraceptives, resulting in breakthrough bleeding and uncertain prophylaxis against pregnancy. Carbamazepine should not be administered with monoamine oxidase inhibitors (MAOIs), which should be discontinued at least 2 weeks before initiating treatment with carbamazepine. Grapefruit juice inhibits the hepatic metabolism of carbamazepine. When carbamazepine and valproate are used in combination, the dosage of carbamazepine should be decreased, because valproate displaces carbamazepine binding on proteins, and the dosage of valproate may need to be increased.

Laboratory Interferences

Circulating increased levels of thyroxine (T_4) and triiodothyronine (T_3) without an associated increase in thyroid-stimulating hormone (TSH) may be associated with carbamazepine

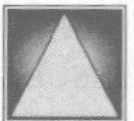

Table 36.13–2
Carbamazepine-Drug Interactions

Effect of Carbamazepine on Plasma Concentrations of Concomitant Agents	Agents That May Affect Carbamazepine Plasma Concentrations
Carbamazepine may decrease drug plasma concentration of	*Agents that may increase carbamazepine plasma concentration*
Acetaminophen	Aliopurinol
Alprazolam	Climetidine
Amitriptyline	Clorithromycin
Bupropion	Danazol
Clomipramine	Dilthiazem
Clonazepam	Erythromycin
Clozapine	Fluoxetine
Cyclosporine	Fluvoxamine
Desipramine	Gemfibrozil
Dicumarol	Itraconazole
Doxepin	Ketoconazole
Doxycycline	Isoniazid[a]
Ethosuximide	Itraconazole
Felbamate	Lomotrigine
Fentanyl	Loratadine
Fluphenazine	Macrolides
Haloperidol	Nefazodone
Hormonal contraceptives	Nicotinamide
Imipramine	Propoxyphene
Lamotrigine	Terfenadine
Methadone	Troleandomycin
Methsuximide	Valproate[a]
Methylprednisolone	Verapamil
Nimodipine	Viloxazine
Pancuronium	*Drugs that may decrease carbamazepine plasma concentrations*
Phensuximide	Carbamazepine (autoinduction)
Phenytoin	Cisplatin
Primidone	Doxorubicin HCl
Theophylline	Felbamate
Valproate	Phenobarbital
Warfarin	Phenytoin
Carbamazepine may increase drug plasma concentrations of	Primidone
Clomipramine	Rifampin[b]
Phenytoin	Theophylline
Primidone	Valproate

[a]Increased concentrations of the active 10, 11-epoxide.
[b]Decreased concentrations of carbamazepine and increased concentrations of the 10, 11-epoxide.
(Table courtesy of Carlos A. Zarate, Jr., M.D., and Mauricio Tohen, M.D.)

treatment. Carbamazepine is also associated with an increase in total serum cholesterol, primarily by increasing high-density lipoproteins. The thyroid and cholesterol effects are not clinically significant. Carbamazepine can interfere with the dexamethasone suppression test and may also cause false-positive pregnancy test results.

Dosing and Administration

The target dose for antimanic activity is 1,200 mg a day, although this varies considerably. Immediate-release carbamazepine needs to be taken three or four times a day, which leads to lapses in compliance. Extended-release formulations are thus preferred, because they can be taken just once or twice a day. One form of extended-release carbamazepine, Carbatrol, comes as 100-, 200-, and 300-mg capsules. Another form called Equatro is identical to Carbetrol and marketed as a treatment for bipolar disorder. These capsules contain tiny beads with three different types of coatings so that they dissolve at different times. Capsules should not be crushed or chewed. The contents can be sprinkled over food, however, without affecting the extended-release qualities. This formulation can be taken either with or without meals. The entire daily dose can be given at bedtime. The rate of absorption is faster when it is given with a high-fat meal. Another extended-release form of carbamazepine, Tegretol XR, uses a different drug-delivery system than Carbatrol. It is available in 100-, 200-, and 300-mg tablets.

Preexisting hematologic, hepatic, and cardiac diseases can be relative contraindications for carbamazepine treatment. Persons with hepatic disease require only one third to one half the usual dosage; the clinician should be cautious about raising the dosage in such persons and should do so only slowly and gradually. The laboratory examination should include a complete blood count with platelet count, liver function tests, serum electrolytes, and an electrocardiogram in persons more than 40 years of age or those with a preexisting cardiac disease. An electroencephalogram (EEG) is not necessary before the initiation of treatment, but it may be helpful in some cases for the documentation of objective changes correlated with clinical improvement.

Routine Laboratory Monitoring. Serum levels for antimanic efficacy have not been established. The anticonvulsant blood concentration range for carbamazepine is 4 to 12 μg/mL and this range should be reached before determining that carbamazepine is not effective in the treatment of a mood disorder. A clinically insignificant suppression of the white blood count commonly occurs during carbamazepine treatment. This benign decrease can be reversed by adding lithium, which enhances colony-stimulating factor. Potential serious hematologic effects of carbamazepine, such as pancytopenia, agranulocytosis, and aplastic anemia, occur in about 1 of 125,000 patients. Complete laboratory blood assessments may be performed every 2 weeks for the first 2 months of treatment and quarterly thereafter, but the FDA has revised the package insert for carbamazepine to suggest that blood monitoring be performed at the discretion of the physician. Patients should be informed that fever, sore throat, rash, petechiae, bruising, or unusual bleeding may indicate a hematologic problem and should prompt immediate notification of a physician. This approach is probably more effective than is frequent blood monitoring during long-term treatment. It has also been suggested that liver and renal function tests be conducted quarterly, although the benefit of conducting tests this frequently has been questioned. It seems reasonable, however, to assess hematologic status, along with liver and renal functions, whenever a routine examination of the person is being conducted. A monitoring protocol is listed in Table 36.13–3.

Carbamazepine treatment should be discontinued, and a consult with a hematologist be obtained, if the following laboratory values are found: total white blood cell count below 3,000/mm^3, erythrocytes below 4.0 × 10^6/mm^3, neutrophils below 1,500/mm^3, hematocrit less than 32 percent, hemoglobin less than 11 g/100 mL, platelet count below 100,000/mm^3,

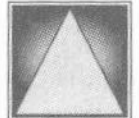

Table 36.13–3
Laboratory Monitoring of Carbamazepine for Adult Psychiatric Disorders

	Baseline	Weekly to Stability	Monthly for 6 Months	6 to 12 Months
CBC	+	+	+	+
Bilirubin	+		+	+
Alanine aminotransferase	+		+	+
Aspartate aminotransferase	+		+	+
Alkaline phosphatase	+		+	+
Carbamazepine level	+	+		+

CBC, Complete blood count.

reticulocyte count below 0.3 percent, and a serum iron concentration below 150 mg/100 mL.

OXCARBAZEPINE

Although structurally related to carbamazepine, the usefulness of oxcarbazepine as a treatment for mania or other psychiatric disorders has not been established in controlled trials.

Pharmacokinetics

Absorption is rapid and unaffected by food. Peak concentrations occur after about 45 minutes. The elimination half-life of the parent compound is 2 hours, which remains stable over long-term treatment. The monohydroxide has a half-life of 9 hours. Most of the drug's anticonvulsant activity is presumed to result from this monohydroxy derivative.

Side Effects

The most common side effects are sedation and nausea. Less frequent side effects are cognitive impairment, ataxia, diplopia, nystagmus, dizziness, and tremor. In contrast to carbamazepine, oxcarbazepine does not have an increased risk of serious blood dyscrasias, so hematologic monitoring is not necessary. The frequency of benign rash is lower than observed with carbamazepine, and serious rashes are extremely rare. About 25 percent to 30 percent of patients who develop an allergic rash on carbamazepine also, however, develop a rash with oxcarbazepine. Oxcarbazepine is more likely to cause hyponatremia than carbamazepine. Approximately 3 percent to 5 percent of patients taking oxcarbazepine develop this side effect. It is advisable to obtain serum sodium concentrations early in the course of treatment, because hyponatremia may be clinically silent. In severe cases, confusion and seizure may occur.

Dosing and Administration

Oxcarbazepine dosing for psychiatric disorders has not been established. It is available in 150-, 300-, and 600-mg tablets. The dose range may vary from 150 to 2,400 mg per day, given in divided doses twice a day. In clinical trials for mania, the doses typically used were from 900 to 1,200 mg per day, with a starting dose of 150 or 300 mg at night.

Drug Interactions

Drugs such as phenobarbital and alcohol, which induce CYP 3A4, increase the clearance and reduce oxcarbazepine concentrations. Oxcarbazepine induces CYP 3A4/5 and inhibits CYP 2C19, which may affect the metabolism of drugs that utilize that pathway. Women taking oral contraceptives should be told to consult with their gynecologist because oxcarbazepine may reduce concentrations of their contraceptive and, thus, decrease its efficacy.

References

Elias A, Madhusoodanan S, Pudukkadan D, Antony JT. Angioedema and maculopapular eruptions associated with carbamazepine administration. *CNS Spectrums*. 2006;11(5):352.

Garnett WR, Gilbert TD, O'Connor P. Patterns of care, outcomes, and direct health plan costs of antiepileptic therapy: A pharmacoeconomic analysis of the available carbamazepine formulations. *Clinical Therapeutics: The International Peer-Reviewed J of Drug Therapy*. 2005;27(7):1092.

Ketter TA, Ginsberg DL, Akiskal HS, Keck PE Jr., Fuller MA, Weisler RH, Hirschfeld RMA, Hollander E. Reassessing carbamazepine in the treatment of bipolar disorder clinical implications of new data. *CNS Spectrum*. 2005;10(6).

▲ 36.14 Cholinesterase Inhibitors and Memantine

Donepezil (Aricept), rivastigmine (Exelon), galantamine (Reminyl), and tacrine (Cognex) are cholinesterase inhibitors used to treat mild to moderate cognitive impairment in dementia of the Alzheimer's type. They reduce the inactivation of the neurotransmitter acetylcholine and, thus, potentiate cholinergic neurotransmission, which in turn produces a modest improvement in memory and goal-directed thought. Memantine (Namenda) is not a cholinesterase inhibitor, producing its effects through blockade of *N*-methyl-D-aspartate (NMDA) receptors. Unlike the cholinesterase inhibitors, which are indicated for the mild to moderate stages of Alzheimer's disease, memantine is indicated for the moderate to severe stages of the disease. Tacrine, the first cholinesterase inhibitor to be introduced, is rarely used because of its multiple daily dosing regimens, its potential for hepatotoxicity, and the consequent need for frequent laboratory monitoring.

CHEMISTRY

The molecular structures of donepezil, rivastigmine, tacrine, and galantamine are shown in Figure 36.14–1.

PHARMACOLOGIC ACTIONS

Donepezil is absorbed completely from the gastrointestinal (GI) tract. Peak plasma concentrations are reached about 3 to 4 hours after oral dosing. The half-life of donepezil is 70 hours in the elderly, and it is taken only once daily. Steady-state levels are achieved within about 2 weeks. Presence of stable alcoholic cirrhosis reduces clearance of donepezil by 20 percent. Rivastigmine is rapidly and completely absorbed from the GI tract and reaches peak plasma concentrations in 1 hour, but this is

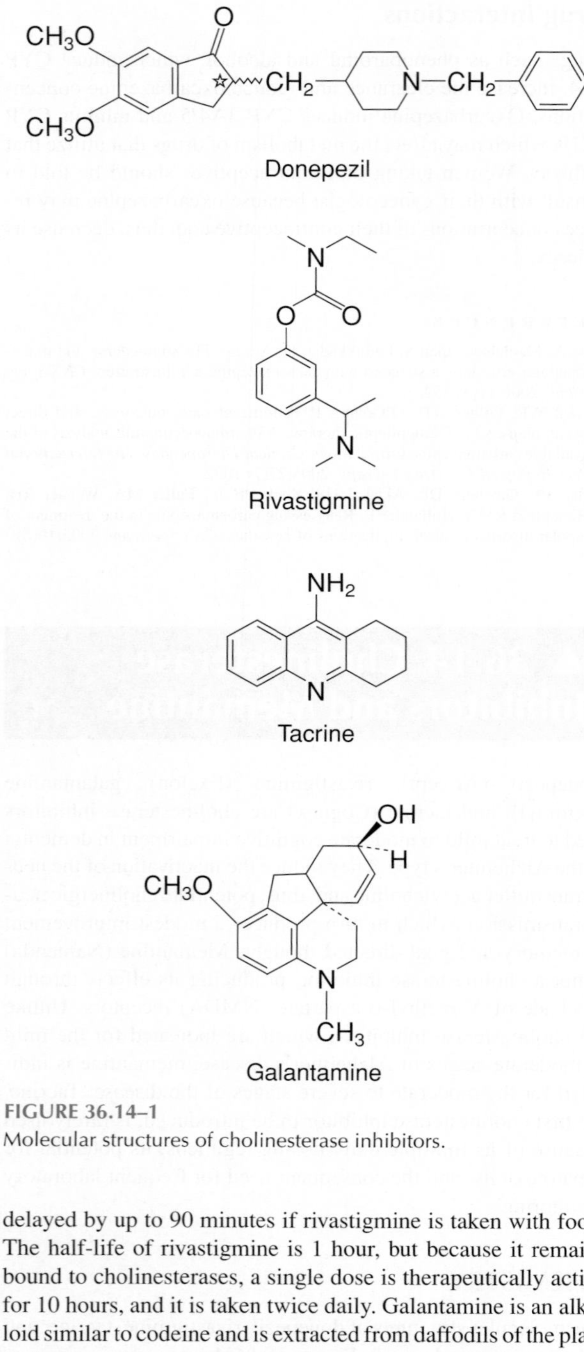

FIGURE 36.14–1
Molecular structures of cholinesterase inhibitors.

delayed by up to 90 minutes if rivastigmine is taken with food. The half-life of rivastigmine is 1 hour, but because it remains bound to cholinesterases, a single dose is therapeutically active for 10 hours, and it is taken twice daily. Galantamine is an alkaloid similar to codeine and is extracted from daffodils of the plant *Galanthus nivalis*. It is readily absorbed, with maximal concentrations reached after 30 minutes to 2 hours. Food decreases the maximal concentration by 25 percent. The elimination half-life of galantamine is approximately 6 hours.

Tacrine is absorbed rapidly from the GI tract. Peak plasma concentrations are reached about 90 minutes after oral dosing. The half-life of tacrine is about 2 to 4 hours, thereby necessitating four-times-daily dosing.

The primary mechanism of action of cholinesterase inhibitors is reversible, nonacylating inhibition of acetylcholinesterase and butyrylcholinesterase, the enzymes that catabolize acetylcholine in the central nervous system (CNS). The enzyme inhibition increases synaptic concentrations of acetylcholine, especially in the hippocampus and cerebral cortex. Unlike tacrine, which is nonselective for all forms of acetylcholinesterase, donepezil appears to be selectively active within the CNS and to have little activity in the periphery. Donepezil's favorable side-effect profile appears to correlate with its lack of inhibition of cholinesterases in the GI tract. Rivastigmine appears to have somewhat more peripheral activity than donepezil and, thus, is more likely to cause GI adverse effects than is donepezil.

THERAPEUTIC INDICATIONS

Cholinesterase inhibitors are effective for the treatment of mild to moderate cognitive impairment in dementia of the Alzheimer's type. In long-term use, they slow the progression of memory loss and diminish apathy, depression, hallucinations, anxiety, euphoria, and purposeless motor behaviors. Functional autonomy is less well preserved. Some persons note immediate improvement in memory, mood, psychotic symptoms, and interpersonal skills. Others note little initial benefit, but are able to retain their cognitive and adaptive faculties at a relatively stable level for many months. A practical benefit of cholinesterase inhibitor use is a delay or reduction of the need for nursing home placement.

Donepezil and rivastigmine may be beneficial for patients with Parkinson's disease and Lewy body disease and for the treatment of cognitive deficits caused by traumatic brain injury. Donepezil is under study for treatment of mild cognitive impairment less severe than that caused by Alzheimer's disease. People with vascular dementia may respond to acetylcholinesterase inhibitors. Occasionally, cholinesterase inhibitors elicit an idiosyncratic catastrophic reaction, with signs of grief and agitation, which is self-limited once the drug is discontinued. Use of cholinesterase inhibitors to improve cognition by nondemented individuals should be discouraged.

PRECAUTIONS AND ADVERSE REACTIONS

Donepezil

Donepezil is generally well tolerated at recommended dosages. Less than 3 percent of persons taking donepezil experience nausea, diarrhea, and vomiting. These mild symptoms are more common with a 10-mg dose than with a 5-mg dose and, when present, they tend to resolve after 3 weeks of continued use. Donepezil can cause weight loss. Donepezil treatment has been infrequently associated with bradyarrhythmias, especially in persons with underlying cardiac disease. A few persons experience syncope.

Rivastigmine

Rivastigmine is generally well tolerated, but recommended dosages may need to be scaled back in the initial period of treatment to limit GI and CNS adverse effects. These mild symptoms are more common at dosages above 6 mg a day and, when present, they tend to resolve once the dosage is lowered. The most common adverse effects associated with rivastigmine are nausea, vomiting, dizziness, headache, diarrhea, abdominal pain, anorexia, fatigue, and somnolence. Rivastigmine can cause weight loss, but it does not appear to cause hepatic, renal, hematologic, or electrolyte abnormalities.

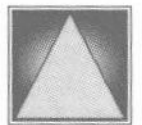

Table 36.14–1
Incidence (%) of Major Adverse Side Effects with Cholinesterase Inhibitors

Drug	Dose (mg/day)	Nausea	Vomiting	Diarrhea	Dizziness	Muscle Cramps	Insomnia
Donepezil	5	4	3	9	15	9	7
Donepezil	10	17	10	17	13	12	8
Rivastigmine	1 to 4	14	7	10	15	NR	NR
Rivastigmine	6 to 12	48	27	17	24	NR	NR
Galantamine	8	5.7	3.6	5	NR	NR	NR
Galantamine	16	13.3	6.1	12.2	NR	NR	NR
Galantamine	24	16.5	9.9	5.5	NR	NR	NR

NR, not reported from clinical trial data; incidence <5.0%.

Galantamine

The most common side effects of galantamine are dizziness, headache, nausea, vomiting, diarrhea, and anorexia. These side effects tend to be mild and transient.

Tacrine

Tacrine is the least used of the cholinesterase inhibitors, but its use requires more discussion with the patient than the others because it is cumbersome to titrate and use, and it poses the risk of potentially significant elevations in hepatic transaminase levels. These increases occur in 25 percent to 30 percent of persons. Aside from elevated transaminase levels, the most common specific adverse effects associated with tacrine treatment are nausea, vomiting, myalgia, anorexia, and rash, but only nausea, vomiting, and anorexia have been found to have a clear relation to the dosage. Transaminase elevations characteristically develop during the first 6 to 12 weeks of treatment and cholinergically mediated events are dosage related.

Hepatotoxicity. Tacrine is associated with increases in the plasma activities of alanine aminotransferase (ALT) and aspartate aminotransferase (AST). The ALT measurement is the more sensitive indicator of the hepatic effects of tacrine. About 95 percent of patients who develop elevated ALT serum levels do so in the first 18 weeks of treatment. Four weeks is the average length of time for elevated ALT concentrations to return to normal after stopping tacrine treatment.

For routine monitoring of hepatic enzymes, AST and ALT activities should be measured weekly for the first 18 weeks, every month for the second 4 months, and every 3 months thereafter. Weekly assessments of AST and ALT should be performed for at least 6 weeks after any increase in dosage. Patients with mildly elevated ALT activity should be monitored weekly and not be rechallenged with tacrine until the ALT activity returns to the normal range. For any patient with elevated ALT activity and jaundice, tacrine treatment should be stopped, and the patient should not be given the drug again.

Table 36.14–1 summarizes the incidence of major adverse side effects associated with each of the cholinesterase inhibitors.

DRUG INTERACTIONS

All cholinesterase inhibitors should be used cautiously with drugs that also possess cholinomimetic activity, such as succinylcholine (Anectine) or bethanechol (Urecholine). The coadministration of cholinesterase inhibitors and drugs that have cholinergic antagonist activity (e.g., tricyclic drugs) is probably counterproductive. Paroxetine has the most marked anticholinergic effects of any of the newer antidepressant and anxiolytic drugs and should be avoided for that reason, as well as for its inhibiting effect on the metabolism of some of the cholinesterase inhibitors.

Donepezil undergoes extensive metabolism via both CYP 2D6 and 3A4 isozymes. The metabolism of donepezil may be increased by phenytoin (Dilantin), carbamazepine (Tegretol), dexamethasone (Decadron), rifampin (Rifadin), or phenobarbital (Solfoton). Commonly used agents, such as paroxetine, ketoconazole, and erythromycin, can significantly increase donepezil concentrations. Donepezil is highly protein bound, but it does not displace other protein-bound drugs, such as furosemide (Lasix), digoxin (Lanoxin), or warfarin (Coumadin). Rivastigmine circulates mostly unbound to serum proteins and has no significant drug interactions.

As with donepezil, galantamine is metabolized by both CYP 2D6 and 3A4 isozymes and, thus, may interact with drugs that inhibit these pathways. Paroxetine and ketoconazole should be used with great caution.

LABORATORY INTERFERENCES

No laboratory interferences have been associated with use of cholinesterase inhibitors.

DOSAGE AND CLINICAL GUIDELINES

Before initiating cholinesterase inhibitor therapy, potentially treatable causes of dementia should be ruled out and the diagnosis of dementia of the Alzheimer's type established.

Donepezil is available in 5- and 10-mg tablets. Treatment should be initiated at 5 mg each night. If well tolerated and of some discernible benefit after 4 weeks, the dosage should be increased to a maintenance dosage of 10-mg each night. Donepezil absorption is unaffected by meals.

Rivastigmine is available in 1.5-, 3-, 4.5-, and 6-mg capsules. The recommended initial dosage is 1.5 mg twice daily for a minimum of 2 weeks, after which increases of 1.5 mg a day can be made at intervals of at least 2 weeks to a target dosage of 6 mg a day, taken in two equal dosages. If tolerated, the dosage can be further titrated upward to a maximum of 6 mg twice daily. The risk of adverse GI events can be reduced by administration of rivastigmine with food.

Galantamine is available in 4-, 8-, and 16-mg tablets. The suggested dose range is 16 to 32 mg per day given twice a day. The higher dose is actually better tolerated than the lower dose. The initial dosage is 8 mg per day and, after a minimum of 4 weeks, the dose can be raised. All subsequent dosage increases should occur at 4-week intervals and should be based on tolerability.

Tacrine is available in 10-, 20-, 30-, and 40-mg capsules. Before the initiation of tacrine treatment, a complete physical and laboratory examination should be conducted, with special attention to liver function tests and baseline hematologic indexes. Treatment should be initiated at 10 mg four times a day and then raised by increments of 10 mg a dose every 6 weeks up to 160 mg a day; the person's tolerance of each dosage is indicated by the absence of unacceptable side effects and lack of elevation of ALT activity. Tacrine should be given four times daily—ideally 1 hour before meals, because tacrine absorption is reduced by about 25 percent when it is taken during the first 2 hours after meals. If tacrine is used, the specific guidelines for tacrine-induced ALT listed above should be followed.

MEMANTINE

Chemistry

The molecular structure of memantine is shown in Figure 36.14–2.

Pharmacologic Actions

Memantine is well absorbed after oral administration with peak concentrations reached in about 3 to 7 hours. Food has no effect on the absorption of memantine. Memantine has linear pharmacokinetics over the therapeutic dose range and has a terminal elimination half-life of about 60 to 80 hours. Plasma protein binding is 45 percent.

Memantine undergoes little metabolism, with most (57 percent to 82 percent) of an administered dose excreted unchanged in urine; the remainder is converted primarily to three polar metabolites: the N-gludantan conjugate, 6-hydroxy memantine, and 1-nitroso-deaminated memantine. These metabolites possess minimal NMDA receptor antagonist activity. Memantine is a low to moderate affinity NMDA receptor antagonist. It is thought that overexcitation of NMDA receptors by the neurotransmitter glutamate may play a role in Alzheimer's disease, because glutamate plays an integral role in the neural pathways associated with learning and memory. Excess glutamate overstimulates NMDA receptors to allow too much calcium into nerve cells, leading to the eventual cell death observed in Alzheimer's disease. Memantine may protect cells against excess glutamate by partially blocking NMDA receptors associated with abnormal transmission of glutamate, while allowing for physiologic transmission associated with normal cell functioning.

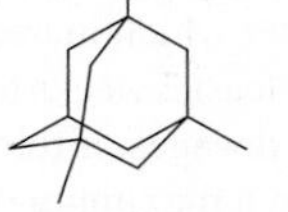

$NH_2 \cdot HCl$

FIGURE 36.14–2
Molecular structure of memantine.

Therapeutic Indications

Memantine is the only approved therapy in the United States for moderate to severe Alzheimer's disease.

Precautions and Adverse Reactions

Memantine is safe and well tolerated. The most common adverse effects are dizziness, headache, constipation, and confusion. The use of memantine in patients with severe renal impairment is not recommended. In a documented case of an overdose with up to 400 mg of memantine, the patient experienced restlessness, psychosis, visual hallucinations, somnolence, stupor, and loss of consciousness. The patient recovered without permanent sequelae.

Drug Interactions

In vitro studies conducted with marker substrates of CYP450 enzymes (CYP 1A2, 2A6, 2C9, 2D6, 2E1, and 3A4) showed minimal inhibition of these enzymes by memantine. No pharmacokinetic interactions with drugs metabolized by these enzymes are expected.

Because memantine is eliminated in part by tubular secretion, coadministration of drugs that use the same renal cationic system, including hydrochlorothiazide triamterene, cimetidine, ranitidine, quinidine, and nicotine, could potentially result in altered plasma levels of both agents. Coadministration of memantine and a combination of hydrochlorothiazide and triamterene did not affect the bioavailability of either memantine or triamterene, and the bioavailability of hydrochlorothiazide decreased by 20 percent.

Urine pH is altered by diet, drugs (e.g., carbonic anhydrase inhibitors, topiramate, sodium bicarbonate), and the clinical state of the patient (e.g., renal tubular acidosis or severe infections of the urinary tract). Memantine clearance is reduced by about 80 percent under alkaline urine conditions at pH 8. Therefore, alterations of urine pH toward the alkaline condition may lead to an accumulation of the drug with a possible increase in adverse effects. Hence, memantine should be used with caution under these conditions.

Laboratory Interferences

No laboratory interferences have been associated with use of memantine.

Dosage and Clinical Guidelines

Memantine is supplied as 5- and 10-mg tablets. It should be given twice per day for doses above 5 mg. The recommended dosage is 5 mg twice daily following a 4-week titration. There should be a minimal interval of 1 week between dose increases.

Patients with mild to moderate disease receiving memantine in combination with a cholinesterase inhibitor have not been found to experience significantly greater benefit in cognition or overall function than those who receive a cholinesterase inhibitor alone.

REFERENCES

Jann MW, Small GW. Cholinesterase inhibitors and similarly acting compounds. In: Sadock BJ, Sadock VA, eds. *Kaplan & Sadock's Comprehensive Textbook of Psychiatry*. 8th ed. Vol 2. Baltimore: Lippincott Williams & Wilkins; 2005:2808.

Mori E, Hashimoto M, Krishnan KR, Doraiswamy PM. What constitutes clinical evidence for neuroprotection in Alzheimer's disease: Support for the cholinesterase inhibitors? *Alzheimer's Dis Assoc Disord.* 2006;20[2, Suppl 1]:S19.
Nordberg A. Mechanisms behind the neuroprotective action of cholinesterase inhibitors in Alzheimer's disease. *Alzheimer's Dis Assoc Disord.* 2006;20[2, Suppl 1]:S12.
Reisberg B, Doody R, Stoffer A, Schmidt F, Ferris S, Mobius HJ for the Memantine Study Group. Memantine in moderate-to-severe Alzheimer's disease. *N Engl J Med.* 2003;348:1333–1341.
Rogawski MA, Wenk GL. The neuropharmacological basis for the use of memantine in the treatment of Alzheimer's disease. *CNS Drug Reviews.* 2003;9:275–308.
Tariot PN, Farlow MR, Grossberg GT, Graham SM, McDonald S, Gergel I for the Memantine Study Group. Memantine treatment in patients with moderate to severe Alzheimer's disease already receiving donepezil. *JAMA.* 2004;291:317–324.
Wimo A, Winblad B, Stoffer A, Wirth Y, Mobius HJ. Resource utilization and cost analysis of memantine in patients with moderate to severe Alzheimer's disease. *Pharmacoeconomics.* 2003;21:327–340.

▲ 36.15 Dantrolene

Dantrolene (Dantrium) is a direct-acting skeletal muscle relaxant, which is used to treat neuroleptic malignant syndrome.

CHEMISTRY

The molecular structure of dantrolene is shown in Figure 36.15–1.

PHARMACOLOGIC ACTIONS

About one third of orally administered dantrolene is slowly absorbed from the gastrointestinal (GI) tract. Peak plasma concentrations are seen about 5 hours after oral administration, and the elimination half-life of dantrolene is about 9 hours. Dantrolene is metabolized by the liver and excreted in the urine.

Dantrolene produces skeletal muscle relaxation by directly affecting the contractile response of the muscles at a site inside the skeletal muscle cell. The skeletal muscle relaxant effect is the basis of its efficacy in reducing the muscle destruction and hyperthermia associated with neuroleptic malignant syndrome.

THERAPEUTIC INDICATIONS

Intravenous (IV) dantrolene reduces muscle spasm in about 80 percent of persons with neuroleptic malignant syndrome. Dantrolene is almost always used in conjunction with appropriate supportive measures and a dopamine receptor antagonist (DRA). Muscle relaxation and a general and dramatic improvement in symptoms can appear within minutes of administration, although in most cases, the beneficial effects can take several hours to appear. Some evidence indicates that dantrolene treatment must be continued for some time, perhaps days to a week or more, to minimize the risk of the recurrence of symptoms. Dantrolene has been used in efforts to treat other psychiatric conditions characterized by life-threatening muscle rigidity, such as catatonia and serotonin syndrome.

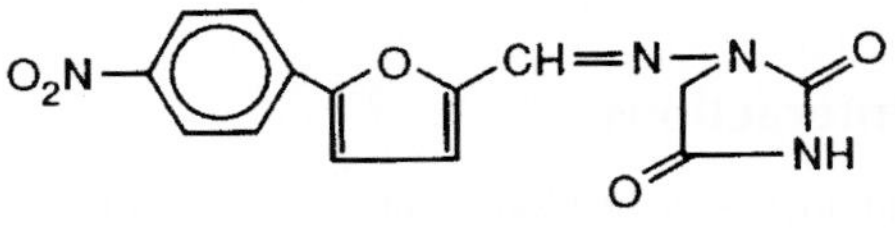

O_2N — CH=N—N — O — NH — O

FIGURE 36.15–1
Molecular structure of dantrolene.

PRECAUTIONS AND ADVERSE REACTIONS

The most common adverse effects of dantrolene include muscle weakness, drowsiness, dizziness, light-headedness, nausea, diarrhea, malaise, and fatigue. These effects are generally transient. The central nervous system (CNS) effects of dantrolene include slurred speech, headache, visual disturbances, alteration of taste, depression, confusion, hallucinations, nervousness, and insomnia. More serious adverse effects, which appear only with long-term use, include hepatitis, seizures, and pleural effusion with pericarditis. Dantrolene should be used with caution by patients with hepatic, renal, or chronic lung disease.

Dantrolene can cross the placenta and, thus, is contraindicated for pregnant women and should not be used by nursing mothers except in emergency situations, such as neuroleptic malignant syndrome. No data are available regarding the use of dantrolene by the elderly, and no unique problems have been associated with its use by children.

DRUG INTERACTIONS

The risk of liver toxicity may be increased in patients who are also taking estrogens. Dantrolene should be used with caution by patients who are using other drugs that produce drowsiness, most notably the benzodiazepines. In the case of neuroleptic malignant syndrome, however, the general guidelines regarding dantrolene must be weighed against the severity of the syndrome. Dantrolene should not be given by IV in combination with calcium channel blockers.

LABORATORY INTERFERENCES

No known laboratory interferences are associated with dantrolene, although experience with its use in patients with neuroleptic malignant syndrome is still limited.

DOSAGE AND CLINICAL GUIDELINES

In addition to the immediate discontinuation of antipsychotic drugs, medical support to cool the patient, and the monitoring of vital signs and renal output, dantrolene in doses of 1 mg/kg can be given orally four times daily, or 1 to 5 mg/kg can be given by IV to reduce muscle spasms in patients with neuroleptic malignant syndrome. Although some clinicians have recommended low dosages (2.5 mg/kg per day) because of the adverse effects, other clinicians indicate that daily dosages of 10 mg/kg are most likely to be effective. Dantrolene is supplied as 25-, 50-, and 100-mg capsules and in a 20-mg parenteral preparation for reconstitution with 60 mL of sterile water.

REFERENCES

Andre N, Boyer M, Coze C, Delorme J, Rome A, Gentet JC, Bernard JL. Can dantrolene contribute to methotrexate toxicity? *Ann Pharmacother.* 2006;40(9): 1695–6.

Inada H, Jinno S, Kohase H, Fukayama H, Umino M. Postoperative hyperthermia of unknown origin treated with dantrolene sodium. *Anesth Prog*. 2005;52(1):21–3.
Kang M, Lisk G, Hollingworth S, Baylor SM, Desai SA. Malaria parasites are rapidly killed by dantrolene derivatives specific for the plasmodial surface anion channel. *Mol Pharmacol*. 2005;68(1):34–40.
Kobayashi S, Bannister ML, Gangopadhyay JP, Hamada T, Parness J, Ikemoto N. Dantrolene stabilizes domain interactions within the ryanodine receptor. *J Biol Chem*. 2005;280(8):6580–7.
Lin CM, Neeru S, Doufas AG, Liem E, Muneer Shah Y, Wadhwa A, Lenhardt R, Bjorksten A, Taguchi A, Kabon B, Sessler DI, Kurz A. Dantrolene reduces the threshold and gain for shivering. *Anesth Analg*. 2004;98(5):1318–24.
Paul-Pletzer K, Yamamoto T, Ikemoto N, Jimenez LS, Morimoto H, Williams PG, Ma J, Parness J. Probing a putative dantrolene-binding site on the cardiac ryanodine receptor. *Biochem J*. 2005;387(Pt 3):905–9.
Pierobon N, Renard-Rooney DC, Gaspers LD, Thomas AP. Ryanodine receptors in liver. *J Biol Chem*. 2006;281(45):34086–95.
Strawn JR, Keck PE Jr. Early bicarbonate loading and dantroline for ziprasidone/haloperidol-induced neuroleptic malignant syndrome. *J Clin Psychiatry*. 2006;67(4):677.
Voermans NC, Poels PJ, Kluijtmans LA, van Engelen BG. The effect of dantrolene sodium in Very Long Chain Acyl-CoA Dehydrogenase Deficiency. *Neuromuscul Disord*. 2005;15(12):844–6.
Wray CJ, Sun X, Gang GI, Hasselgren PO. Dantrolene downregulates the gene expression and activity of the ubiquitin-proteasome proteolytic pathway in septic skeletal muscle. *J Surg Res*. 2002;104(2):82–7.

▲ 36.16 Disulfiram and Acamprosate

Disulfiram (Antabuse) and acamprosate (Campral) are used to treat alcohol dependence. Disulfiram is an alcohol-sensitizing agent—it deters use of alcohol by producing a rapid and violently unpleasant reaction in a person who ingests even a small amount of alcohol. Many clinicians have stopped prescribing disulfiram because of the risk of severe and even fatal disulfiram–alcohol reactions. Unlike disulfiram, acamprosate does not produce aversive side effects when combined with alcohol, but it reduces the craving that is experienced by alcohol-dependent patients.

Other drugs useful in reducing alcohol consumption include naltrexone (ReVia, Trexan), nalmefene (Revex), topiramate (Topamax), and gabapentin (Neurontin). These agents are discussed in their respective chapters.

DISULFIRAM

Chemistry

The structural formula of disulfiram is shown in Figure 36.16–1.

Pharmacologic Actions

Disulfiram is almost completely absorbed from the gastrointestinal (GI) tract after oral administration. Its half-life is estimated to be 60 to 120 hours. Therefore, 1 or 2 weeks may be needed before disulfiram is totally eliminated from the body after the last dose has been taken.

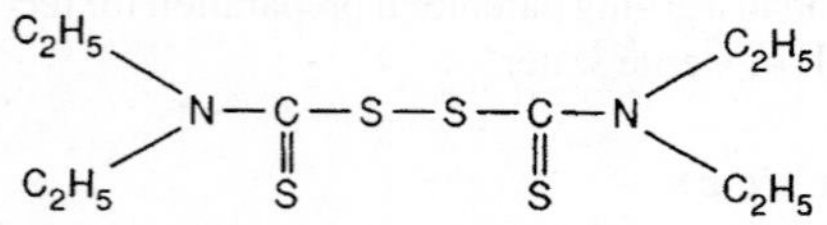

$$(C_2H_5)_2N-\underset{\underset{S}{\|}}{C}-S-S-\underset{\underset{S}{\|}}{C}-N(C_2H_5)_2$$

FIGURE 36.16–1
Molecular formula of disulfiram.

The metabolism of ethanol proceeds through oxidation via alcohol dehydrogenase to the formation of acetaldehyde, which is further metabolized to acetyl-coenzyme A (acetyl-CoA) by aldehyde dehydrogenase. Disulfiram is an aldehyde dehydrogenase inhibitor that interferes with the metabolism of alcohol by producing a marked increase in blood acetaldehyde concentration. The accumulation of acetaldehyde (to a level up to ten times higher than occurs in the normal metabolism of alcohol) produces a wide array of unpleasant reactions, called the *disulfiram–alcohol reaction*, characterized by nausea, throbbing headache, vomiting, hypertension, flushing, sweating, thirst, dyspnea, tachycardia, chest pain, vertigo, and blurred vision. The reaction occurs almost immediately after the ingestion of one alcoholic drink and can last from 30 minutes to 2 hours.

Therapeutic Indications

The primary indication for disulfiram use is as an aversive conditioning treatment for alcohol dependence. Either the fear of having a disulfiram–alcohol reaction or the memory of having had one is meant to condition the person not to use alcohol. Usually, describing the severity and the unpleasantness of the disulfiram–alcohol reaction sufficiently graphically discourages the person from imbibing alcohol. Disulfiram treatment should be combined with such treatments as psychotherapy, group therapy, and support groups such as Alcoholics Anonymous (AA). Treatment with disulfiram requires careful monitoring, because a person can simply decide not to take the medication.

Precautions and Adverse Reactions

With Alcohol Consumption. The intensity of the disulfiram–alcohol reaction varies with each person. In extreme cases it is marked by respiratory depression, cardiovascular collapse, myocardial infarction, convulsions, and death. Therefore, disulfiram is contraindicated for a person with significant pulmonary or cardiovascular disease. In addition, disulfiram should be used with caution, if at all, by a person with nephritis, brain damage, hypothyroidism, diabetes, hepatic disease, seizures, polydrug dependence, or an abnormal electroencephalogram (EEG). Most fatal reactions occur in persons who are taking more than 500 mg a day of disulfiram and who consume more than 3 ounces of alcohol. The treatment of a severe disulfiram–alcohol reaction is primarily supportive to prevent shock.

Without Alcohol Consumption. The adverse effects of disulfiram in the absence of alcohol consumption include fatigue, dermatitis, impotence, optic neuritis, a variety of mental changes, and hepatic damage. A metabolite of disulfiram inhibits dopamine-β-hydroxylase, the enzyme that metabolizes dopamine into norepinephrine and epinephrine and, thus, may exacerbate psychosis in persons with psychotic disorders. Catatonic reactions can also occur.

Drug Interactions

Disulfiram increases the blood concentration of diazepam (Valium), paraldehyde, phenytoin (Dilantin), caffeine, tetrahydrocannabinol (the active ingredient in marijuana), barbiturates, anticoagulants, isoniazid (Nydrazid), and tricyclic drugs. Disulfiram should not be administered concomitantly with paraldehyde, because paraldehyde is metabolized to acetaldehyde in the liver.

Laboratory Interferences

In rare instances, disulfiram has been reported to interfere with the incorporation of iodine-131 into protein-bound iodine. Disulfiram can reduce urinary concentrations of homovanillic acid, the major metabolite of dopamine, because of its inhibition of dopamine hydroxylase.

Dosage and Clinical Guidelines

Disulfiram is supplied in 250- and 500-mg tablets. The usual initial dosage is 500 mg a day taken by mouth for the first 1 or 2 weeks, followed by a maintenance dosage of 250 mg a day. The dosage should not exceed 500 mg a day. The maintenance dosage range is 125 to 500 mg a day.

The person taking disulfiram must be instructed that the ingestion of even the smallest amount of alcohol will bring on a disulfiram–alcohol reaction, with all its unpleasant effects. In addition, the person should be warned against ingesting any alcohol-containing preparations, such as cough drops, tonics of any kind, and alcohol-containing foods and sauces. Some reactions have occurred in patients who used alcohol-based aftershave lotions, toilet water, colognes, or perfumes and inhaled the fumes; therefore, precautions must be explicit and should include any topically applied preparations containing alcohol, such as perfume.

Disulfiram should not be administered until the person has abstained from alcohol for at least 12 hours. Persons should be warned that the disulfiram–alcohol reaction can occur as long as 1 or 2 weeks after the last dose of disulfiram. Persons taking disulfiram should carry identification cards describing the disulfiram–alcohol reaction and listing the name and the telephone number of the physician to be called.

ACAMPROSATE

Chemistry

Acamprosate has a chemical structure similar to that of the amino acid taurine and is structurally similar to γ-aminobutyric acid (GABA). Its molecular structure is shown in Figure 36.16–2.

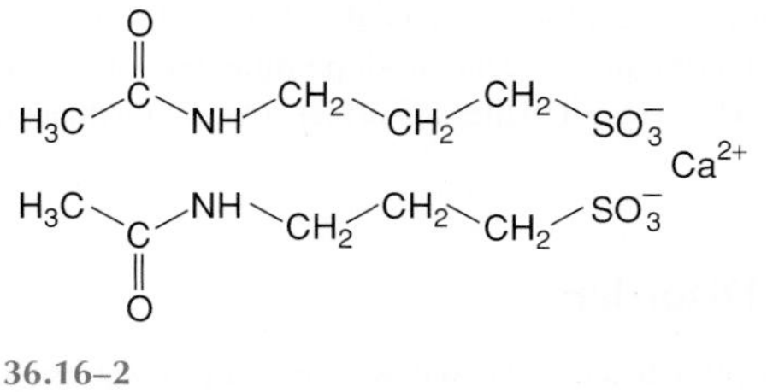

$$H_3C-C(=O)-NH-CH_2-CH_2-CH_2-SO_3^-$$
$$Ca^{2+}$$
$$H_3C-C(=O)-NH-CH_2-CH_2-CH_2-SO_3^-$$

FIGURE 36.16–2
Molecular formula of acamprosate.

Pharmacologic Actions

Acamprosate's mechanism of action is not fully understood, but it is thought to antagonize neuronal overactivity related to the actions of the excitatory neurotransmitter glutamate. In part, this may result from antagonism of *N*-methyl- D-aspartate (NMDA) receptors.

Indications

Acamprosate is used for treating alcohol-dependent individuals seeking to continue to remain alcohol-free after they have stopped drinking. Its efficacy in promoting abstinence has not been demonstrated in persons who have not undergone detoxification and who have not achieved alcohol abstinence before beginning treatment.

Precautions and Adverse Effects

Side effects, which are mostly seen early in treatment, are usually mild and transient in nature. The most common side effects are headache, diarrhea, flatulence, abdominal pain, paresthesias, and various skin reactions. No adverse events occur following abrupt withdrawal of acamprosate, even after long-term use. No evidence indicates addiction to the drug. Patients with severe renal impairment (creatinine clearance of <30 mL/min) should not be given acamprosate.

Drug Interactions

The concomitant intake of alcohol and acamprosate does not affect the pharmacokinetics of either alcohol or acamprosate. Administration of disulfiram or diazepam does not affect the pharmacokinetics of acamprosate. Coadministration of naltrexone with acamprosate produces an increase in concentrations of acamprosate. No adjustment of dosage is recommended in such patients. The pharmacokinetics of naltrexone and its major metabolite 6-β-naltrexol were unaffected following coadministration with acamprosate. During clinical trials, patients taking acamprosate concomitantly with antidepressants more commonly reported both weight gain and weight loss, compared with patients taking either medication alone.

Laboratory Interferences

Acamprosate has not been shown to interfere with commonly done laboratory tests.

Dosage and Clinical Guidelines

It is important to remember that acamprosate should not be used to treat alcohol withdrawal symptoms. It should only be started after the individual has been successfully weaned off the alcohol. Patients should show a commitment to remaining abstinent, and treatment should be part of a comprehensive management program that includes counseling or support group attendance.

Each tablet contains acamprosate calcium 333 mg, which is equivalent to 300 mg of acamprosate. The dose of acamprosate is different for different patients. The recommended dosage is two 333-mg tablets (each dose should total 666 mg) taken three times daily. Although dosing may be done without regard to meals, dosing with meals was used during clinical trials and is suggested as an aid to compliance in those patients who regularly eat three meals daily. A lower dose may be effective in some patients. A missed dose should be taken as soon as possible. If it is almost time for the next dose, however, the missed dose should be skipped, and then the regular dosing schedule should be resumed. Doses should not be doubled up. For patients with moderate renal impairment (creatinine clearance of 30 to 50 mL/min), a starting dosage of one 333-mg tablet taken three times daily is recommended.

References

Kulig CC, Beresford TP. Hepatitis C in alcohol dependence: Drinking versus disulfiram. *J Addict Dis*. 2005;24(2):77.

Suh JJ, Pettinati HM, Kampman KM, O'Brien CP. The status of disulfiram: A half of a century later. *J Clin Psychopharmacol*. 2006;26(3):290.

▲ 36.17 Dopamine Receptor Agonists and Precursors: Apomorphine, Bromocriptine, Levodopa, Pergolide, Pramipexole, and Ropinirole

Dopamine receptor agonists and precursors were developed to treat idiopathic Parkinson's disease. On occasion, they are used by psychiatrists to treat such adverse effects of antipsychotic drugs as (1) parkinsonism, (2) extrapyramidal symptoms, (3) akinesia, (4) focal perioral tremors, (5) hyperprolactinemia, (6) galactorrhea, and (7) neuroleptic malignant syndrome. The drugs in this class most commonly prescribed are bromocriptine (Parlodel), levodopa also called L-Dopa, (Larodopa), and carbidopa-levodopa (Sinemet). New dopamine receptor agonists include ropinirole (Requip), pramipexole (Mirapex), pergolide (Permax), and apomorphine (Apokyn).

CHEMISTRY

Levodopa is the natural precursor of dopamine. The formulation of levodopa combined with carbidopa reduces the incidence of noncentral nervous system (non-CNS) adverse effects experienced with use of levodopa alone. Bromocriptine and pergolide are ergotamine derivatives. Pramipexole is a nonergot dopamine agonist. Apomorphine, also a nonergot dopamine agonist, has been used in medicine for more than a century. It has been available since the 1970s in Europe and Canada, but was only approved for use in the United States in 2004. It is indicated for the treatment of motor symptoms associated with late-stage Parkinson's disease. Apomorphine is structurally related to morphine and other opioids. The molecular structures of dopamine receptor agonists and carbidopa (Lodosyn) are shown in Figure 36.17–1.

PHARMACOLOGIC ACTIONS

L-Dopa is rapidly absorbed after oral administration, and peak plasma levels are reached after 30 to 120 minutes. The half-life of L-Dopa is 90 minutes. Absorption of L-Dopa can be significantly reduced by changes in gastric pH and by ingestion with meals. Bromocriptine, pergolide, and ropinirole are rapidly absorbed, but undergo first-pass metabolism such that only about 30 percent to 55 percent of the dose is bioavailable. Peak concentrations are achieved 1.5 to 3 hours after oral administration. Pergolide has a half-life of about 27 hours, and a single dose has 5 to 6 hours of clinical activity. The half-life of ropinirole is 6 hours. Pramipexole is rapidly absorbed with little first-pass metabolism and reaches peak concentrations in 2 hours. Its half-life is 8 hours. Oral forms of apomorphine have been studied, although they are not available in the United States. Subcutaneous apomorphine injection results in rapid and controlled systemic delivery, with linear pharmacokinetics over a dose ranging from 2 to 8 mg.

Once L-Dopa enters the dopaminergic neurons of the CNS, it is converted into the neurotransmitter dopamine. Apomorphine, bromocriptine, pergolide, ropinirole, and pramipexole act directly on dopamine receptors. Dopamine, pramipexole, and ropinirole bind about 20 times more selectively to dopamine D_3 than D_2 receptors; the corresponding ratio for pergolide is 5:1 and for bromocriptine is less than 2:1. Apomorphine binds selectively to D_1 and D_2 receptors, with little affinity for D_3 and D_4 receptors. L-Dopa, pramipexole, and ropinirole have no significant activity at nondopaminergic receptors, but pergolide and bromocriptine bind to serotonin 5-HT_1 and 5-HT_2, and α_1-, α_2-, and β-adrenergic receptors.

THERAPEUTIC INDICATIONS

Medication-induced Movement Disorders

In present-day clinical psychiatry, dopamine receptor agonists are used to treat medication-induced parkinsonism, extrapyramidal symptoms, akinesia, and focal perioral tremors. Their use has diminished, however, because the incidence of medication-induced movement disorders is much lower with the use of the newer, atypical antipsychotics (serotonin–dopamine antagonists [SDAs]). Dopamine receptor agonists are effective in treating idiopathic restless leg syndrome and may also be helpful when this is a medication side effect.

For the treatment of medication-induced movement disorders, most clinicians rely on anticholinergics, amantadine (Symmetrel), and antihistamines because they are equally effective and have few adverse effects. Bromocriptine remains in use in the treatment of neuroleptic malignant syndrome; however, the incidence of this disorder is diminishing with the decreasing use of dopamine receptor antagonists.

Dopamine receptor agonists are also used to counteract the hyperprolactinemic effects of dopamine receptor antagonists (DRAs), which result in the side effects of amenorrhea and galactorrhea.

Mood Disorders

Bromocriptine has long been used to enhance response to antidepressant drugs in refractory patients. Ropinirole and pergolide

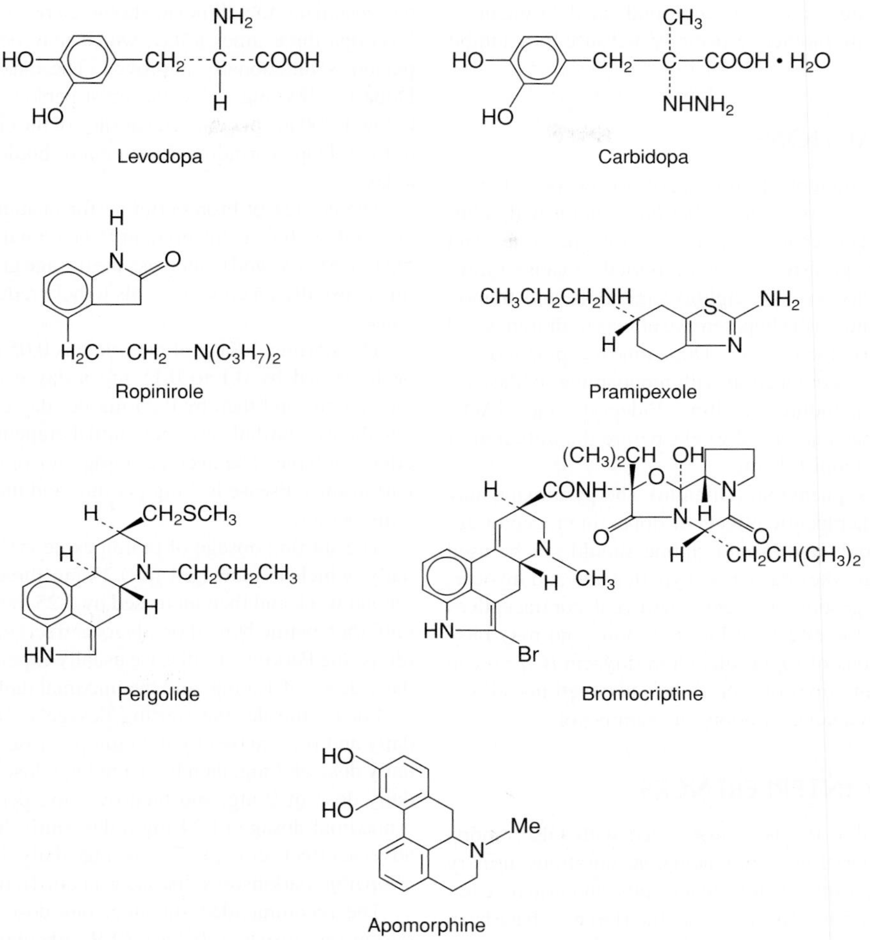

FIGURE 36.17–1
Molecular structures of dopamine receptors and carbidopa.

have been reported to be useful as augmentation to antidepressant therapy and to treat medication-resistant bipolar II depression. Ropinirole may also be helpful in the treatment of antidepressant-induced sexual dysfunction.

Sexual Dysfunction

All dopamine receptor agonists can improve erectile dysfunction. They are rarely used, however, because, at therapeutic dosages, they frequently cause adverse effects. Recently introduced phosphodiesterase-5 inhibitors (PDE-5) agents are better tolerated and more effective.

PRECAUTIONS AND ADVERSE REACTIONS

Adverse effects are common with dopamine receptor agonists, thus limiting the usefulness of these drugs. Adverse effects, which are dosage dependent, include nausea, vomiting, orthostatic hypotension, headache, dizziness, and cardiac arrhythmias. To reduce the risk of orthostatic hypotension, the initial dosage of all dopamine receptor agonists should be quite low, with incremental increases in dose at intervals of at least 1 week. These drugs should be used with caution in persons with hypertension, cardiovascular disease, and hepatic disease. After long-term use, persons, particularly elderly persons, may experience choreiform and dystonic movements and psychiatric disturbances—including hallucinations, delusions, confusion, depression, and mania—and other behavioral changes.

Long-term use of bromocriptine and pergolide can produce retroperitoneal and pulmonary fibrosis, pleural effusions, and pleural thickening.

In general, ropinirole and pramipexole have a similar but much milder adverse effect profile than L-Dopa, bromocriptine, and pergolide. Pramipexole and ropinirole can cause irresistible sleep attacks that occur suddenly without warning and have caused motor vehicle accidents.

The most common adverse effects of apomorphine are yawning, dizziness, nausea, vomiting, drowsiness, bradycardia, syncope, and perspiration. Hallucinations have also been reported. Apomorphine's sedative effects are exacerbated with concurrent use of alcohol or other CNS depressants.

Dopamine receptor agonists are contraindicated during pregnancy and for nursing mothers especially, because they inhibit lactation.

DRUG INTERACTIONS

Dopamine receptor antagonists are capable of reversing the effects of dopamine receptor agonists, but this is not usually clinically significant. The concurrent use of tricyclic drugs and dopamine receptor agonists has been reported to cause symptoms of neurotoxicity, such as rigidity, agitation, and tremor. They may also potentiate the hypotensive effects of diuretics and other antihypertensive medications. Dopamine receptor agonists should not be used in conjunction with monoamine oxidase inhibitors (MAOIs), including selegiline (Eldepryl), and MAOIs should be discontinued at least 2 weeks before the initiation of dopamine receptor agonist therapy.

Benzodiazepines, phenytoin (Dilantin), and pyridoxine may interfere with the therapeutic effects of dopamine receptor agonists. Ergot alkaloids and bromocriptine should not be used concurrently, because they can cause hypertension and myocardial infarction. Progestins, estrogens, and oral contraceptives may interfere with the effects of bromocriptine and may raise plasma concentrations of ropinirole. Ciprofloxacin (Cipro) can raise plasma concentrations of ropinirole, and cimetidine (Tagamet) can raise plasma concentrations of pramipexole.

LABORATORY INTERFERENCES

L-Dopa administration has been associated with false reports of elevated serum and urinary uric acid concentrations, urinary glucose test results, urinary ketone test results, and urinary catecholamine concentrations. No laboratory interferences have been associated with the administration of the other dopamine receptor agonists.

DOSAGE AND CLINICAL GUIDELINES

Table 36.17–1 lists the various dopamine receptor agonists and their formulations. For the treatment of antipsychotic-induced parkinsonism, the clinician should start with a 100-mg dose of levodopa three times a day, which may be increased until the person is functionally improved. The maximum dosage of L-Dopa is 2,000 mg a day, but most persons respond to dosages below 1,000 mg per day. The dosage of the carbidopa component of the L-Dopa-carbidopa formulation should total at least 75 mg a day.

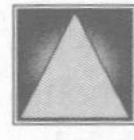

Table 36.17–1
Available Preparations of Dopamine Receptor Agonists and Carbidopa

Generic Name	Trade Name	Preparations
Bromocriptine	Parlodel	2.5-mg, 5-mg tablets
Carbidopa	Lodosyn	25 mg[a]
Levodopa (L-Dopa)	Larodopa	100-, 250-, 500-mg tablets
Levodopa-carbidopa (cocareldopa)	Sinemet, Atamet	100/10-mg, 100/25-mg, 250/25-mg tablets; 100/25-, 200/50-extended-release tablets
Pergolide	Permax	0.05-, 0.25-, 1-mg tablets
Pramipexole	Mirapex	0.125-, 0.25-, 0.5-, 1-, 1.5-mg tablets
Ropinirole	Requip	0.25-, 0.5-, 1-, 2-, 5-mg tablets

[a] Drug only available directly through the manufacturer.

The dosage of bromocriptine for mental disorders is uncertain, although it seems prudent to begin with low dosages (1.25 mg twice daily) and to increase the dosage gradually. Bromocriptine is usually taken with meals to help reduce the likelihood of nausea.

The starting dosage of pergolide is 0.05 mg daily, which can be increased by 0.1 to 0.15 mg a day every 3 days for four increments, and then by 0.25 mg per day every 3 days divided into three equal daily dosages, until therapeutic benefit or adverse effects emerge. The average dosage for treatment of idiopathic Parkinson's disease is 3 mg per day, and the maximal dosage is 5 mg per day.

The starting dosage of pramipexole is 0.125 mg three times daily, which is increased to 0.25 mg three times daily in the second week and then increased by 0.25 mg per dose each week until therapeutic benefit or adverse effects emerge. Persons with idiopathic Parkinson's disease usually experience benefit at total daily doses of 1.5 mg, and the maximal daily dose is 4.5 mg.

For ropinirole, the starting dosage is 0.25 mg three times daily and is increased by 0.25 mg per dose each week to a total daily dose of 3 mg, then by 0.5 mg per dose each week to a total daily dose of 9 mg, and then by 1 mg per dose each week to a maximal dosage of 24 mg a day, until therapeutic benefit or adverse effects emerge. The average daily dose for persons with idiopathic Parkinson's disease is about 16 mg.

The recommended subcutaneous dose of apomorphine in Parkinson's disease is 0.2 to 0.6 mL subcutaneously during acute hypomobility episodes, delivered via metered injector pen. Apomorphine can be administered three times daily, with a maximal dose of 0.6 mL five times daily.

REFERENCES

Arnold G, Gasser T, Storch A, Lipp A, Kupsch A, Hundemer JP, Schwartz J. High doses of pergolide improve clinical global impression in advance Parkinson's disease—A preliminary open label study. *Arch Gerontol Geriatr*. 2005;41(3):239.

Gibbs SEB, D'Esposito M. A functional MRI study of the effects of bromocriptine, a dopamine receptor agonist, on component processes of working memory. *Psychopharmacology*. 2005;180(4):644.

Gorelick DA, Wilkins JN. Bromocriptine treatment for cocaine addiction: Association with plasma prolactin levels. *Drug Alcohol Depend*. 2006;81(2):189.

Guptsa S, Vincent JL, Frank B. Pramipexole. Augmentation in the treatment of depressive symptoms. *CNS Spectrums*. 2006;11(3):172.

Lieberman JA. Dopamine partial agonists: A new class of antipsychotic. *CNS Drugs*. 2004;18(4):251.

Perea E, Robbins BV, Hutto B. Psychosis related to ropinirole. *Am J Psychiatry*. 2006;163(3):346.

Pellecchia MT, Vitale C, Sabatini M, Longo K, Amboni M, Bonavita V, Barone P. Ropinirole as a treatment of restless leg syndrome in patients on chronic hemodialysis: An open randomized crossover trial versus levodopa sustained release. *Clin Neuropharmacol*. 2004;27(4):178.

Pomerantz JM. Pramipexole as a psychiatric medication. *Drug Benefit Trends*. 2003;15(4):25.

Roach ES. Initial Parkinson disease therapy: Levodopa, dopamine agonists, or both? *Arch Neurol*. 2004;61(12):1972.

Smail DB, Samuel C, Rouy-Thenaisy K, Regnault J, Azouvi P. Bromocriptine in traumatic brain injury. *Brain Injury*. 2006;20(1):111.

▲ 36.18 Dopamine Receptor Antagonists: Typical Antipsychotics

Chlorpromazine (Thorazine), which was introduced in the mid-1950s, was the first drug that significantly and consistently reduced symptoms of psychosis. Other drugs with similar clinical effects were introduced over the next two decades. Antipsychotic activity was related to high-affinity antagonism of dopamine D_2 receptors. Accordingly, these agents are called dopamine receptor antagonists (DRAs). Other terms used to refer to these drugs are *first-generation, typical, traditional,* or *conventional* antipsychotics.

The DRAs are no longer the mainstay of the treatment of schizophrenia or other conditions associated with psychotic symptoms. Newer antipsychotic agents, the serotonin–dopamine antagonists (SDAs) and partial dopamine agonists (PDAs), also called *second-generation, novel,* or *atypical* antipsychotics, have largely replaced the DRAs as first-line treatments for the same spectrum of disorders. Not only do the newer agents cause fewer extrapyramidal side effects, but they may have greater effects against negative symptoms of schizophrenia, cognitive defects and depression that may coexist with psychosis. These drugs are covered in Section 36.30.

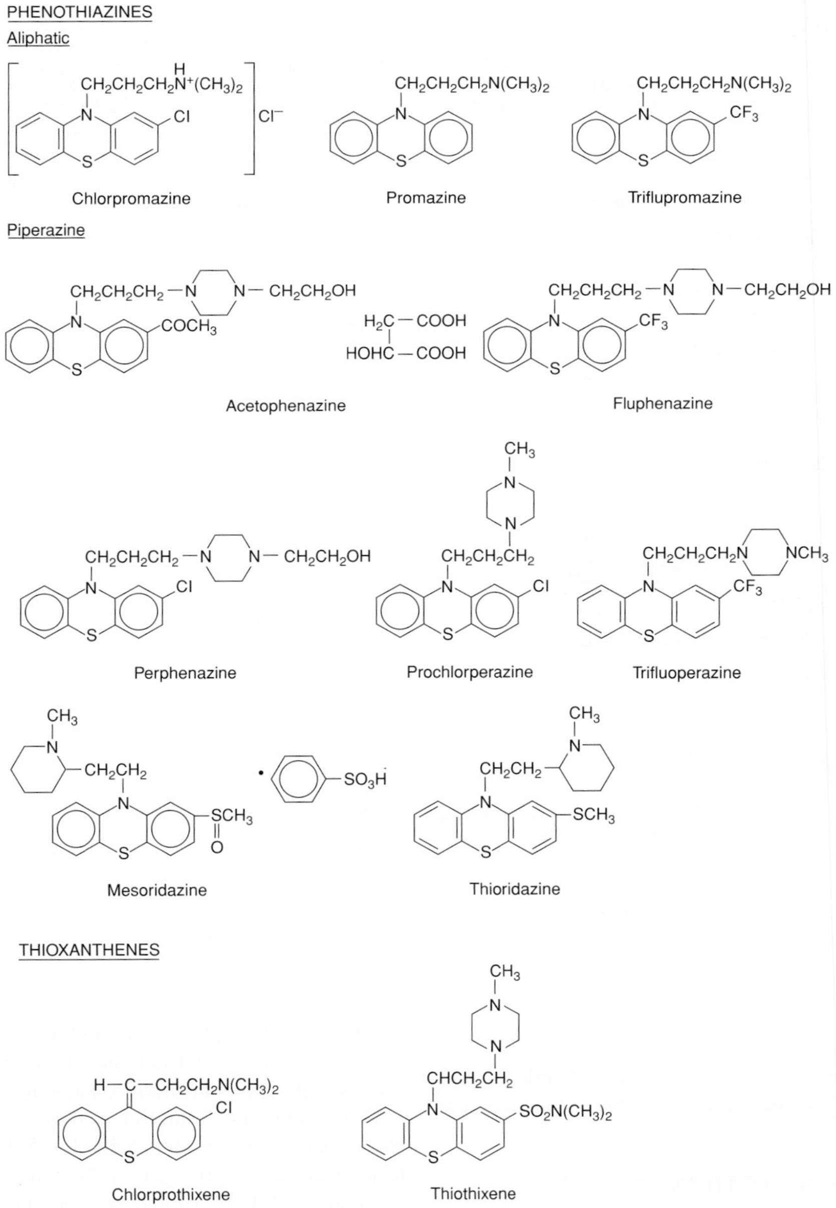

PHENOTHIAZINES

Aliphatic

Chlorpromazine

Promazine

Triflupromazine

Piperazine

Acetophenazine

Fluphenazine

Perphenazine

Prochlorperazine

Trifluoperazine

Mesoridazine

Thioridazine

THIOXANTHENES

Chlorprothixene

Thiothixene

FIGURE 36.18–1

Molecular structure of dopamine receptor antagonists and reserpine. (*continued*)

Dibenzoxazepine

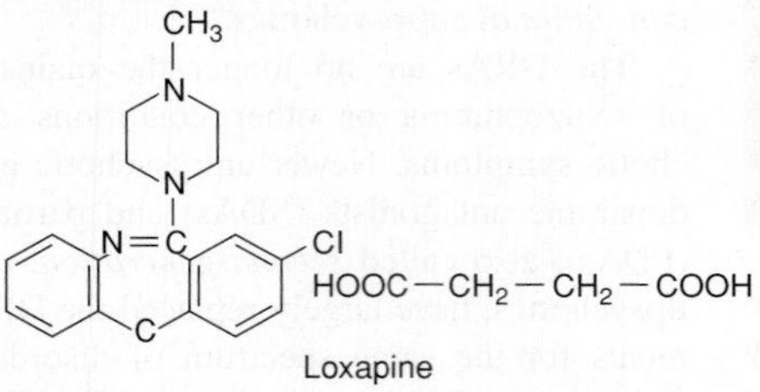

Loxapine

Dihydroindole

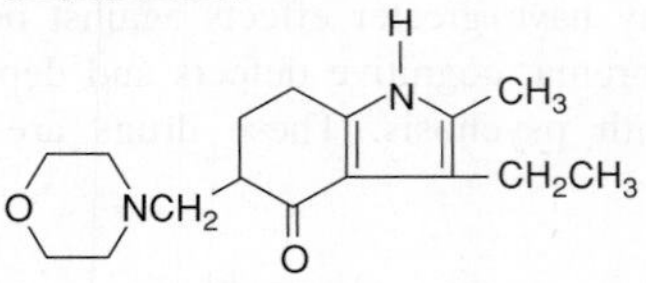

Molindone

Butyrophenones

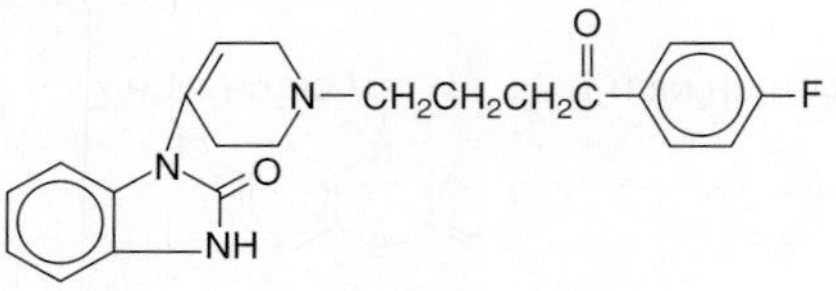

Droperidol

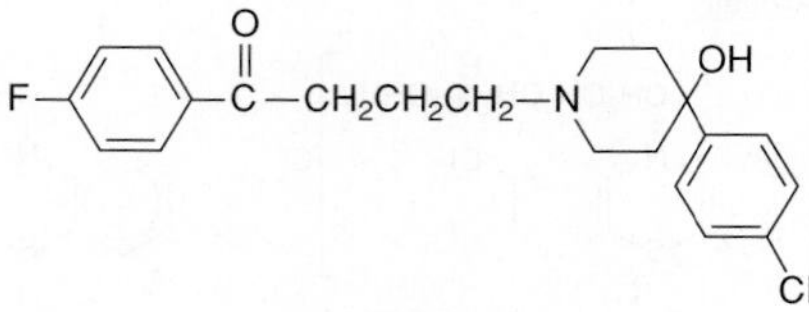

Haloperidol

Diphenylbutylpiperidine

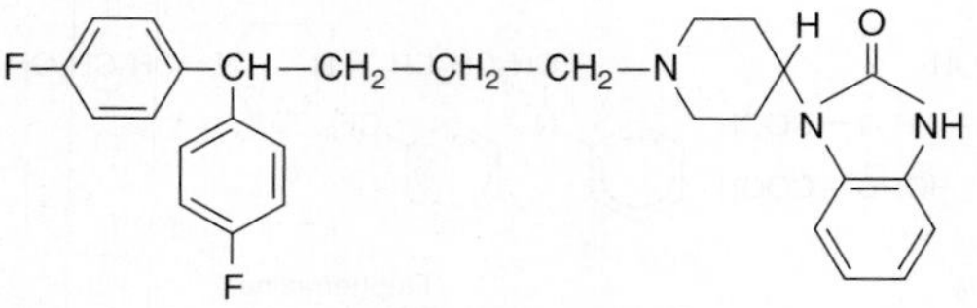

Pimozide

Benzamide

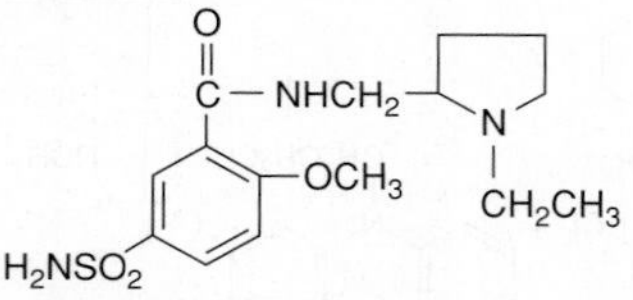

Sulpiride (not available in U.S.)

Rauwolfia Alkaloid

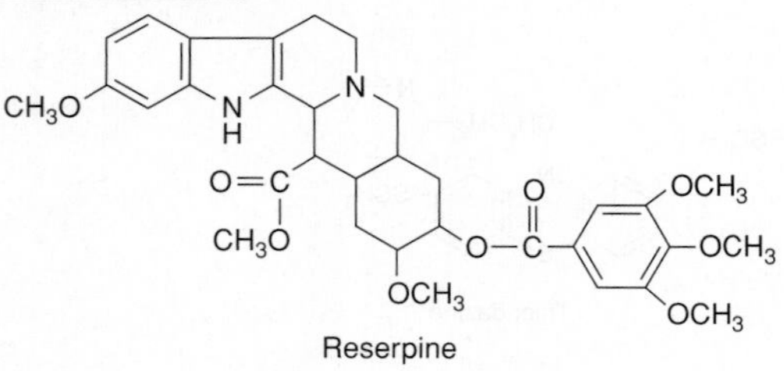

Reserpine

FIGURE 36.18–1
(Continued)

CHEMISTRY

The DRAs are subclassified according to their chemical structures. The molecular structures of the DRAs are shown in Figure 36.18–1.

PHARMACOLOGIC ACTIONS

All the DRAs are well absorbed after oral administration, with liquid preparations being absorbed more efficiently than tablets or capsules. Peak plasma concentrations are usually reached 1 to 4 hours after oral administration and 30 to 60 minutes after parenteral administration. Smoking, coffee, antacids, and food interfere with absorption of these drugs. Steady-state levels are reached in approximately 3 to 5 days. The half-lives of these drugs are approximately 24 hours. All can be given in one daily oral dose, if tolerated, once the person is in a stable condition. Most DRAs are highly protein bound. Parenteral formulation of DRAs results in more rapid and more reliable onset

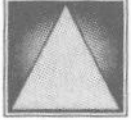

Table 36.18–1
Factors Influencing the Pharmacokinetics of Antipsychotics

Age	Elderly patients may demonstrate reduced clearance rates.
Medical condition	Decreased hepatic blood flow can reduce clearance.
	Hepatic disease can decrease clearance.
Enzyme inducers	Carbamazepine, phenytoin, ethambutol, barbiturates
Clearance inhibitors	Include selective serotonin reuptake inhibitors, tricyclic antidepressants, cimetidine, β-blockers, isoniazid, methylphenidate, erythromycin, triazolobenzodiazepines, ciprofloxacin, ketoconazole.
Changes in binding protein	Hypoalbuminemia can occur with malnutrition or hepatic failure.

(Adapted from Ereshefsky L. Pharmacokinetics and drug interactions: Update for new antipsychotics. *J Clin Psychiatry,* 1996;57[Suppl 1]1:12–25, with permission.)

of action. Bioavailability is also up to tenfold higher with parenteral administration. Most DRAs are metabolized by CYP 2D6 and 3A isozymes; however, differences exist among the specific agents.

Long-acting depot parenteral formulations of haloperidol (Haldol) and fluphenazine (Prolixin) are available in the United States. They are usually administered once every 1 to 4 weeks, depending on the dose and the person. It can take up to 6 months of treatment with depot formulations to reach steady-state plasma levels, indicating that oral therapy should be continued during the first month or so of depot antipsychotic treatment.

Antipsychotic activity derives from inhibition of dopaminergic neurotransmission. The DRAs are effective when approximately 60 percent of D_2 receptors in the brain are occupied. At 80 percent one sees the beginning of extrapyramidial signs. The DRAs also block noradrenergic, cholinergic, and histaminergic receptors, with different drugs having different effects on these receptor systems.

Some generalizations can be made about the DRAs based on their potency. Potency refers to the amount of drug that is required to achieve therapeutic effects. Low-potency drugs, such as chlorpromazine and thioridazine, given in doses of several hundred milligrams per day, typically produce more weight gain and sedation than high-potency agents, such as haloperidol and fluphenazine, usually given in doses of less than 10 mg per day. High-potency agents are also more likely to cause extrapyramidal side effects. Some factors influencing the pharmacologic actions of DRAs are listed in Table 36.18–1.

THERAPEUTIC INDICATIONS

Many types of psychiatric and neurologic disorders may benefit from treatment with DRAs. Some of these indications are shown in Table 36.18–2.

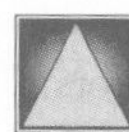

Table 36.18–2
Indications for Dopamine Receptor Antagonists

Acute psychotic episodes in schizophrenia and schizoaffective disorder
Maintenance treatment in schizophrenia and schizoaffective disorders
Mania
Depression with psychotic symptoms
Delusional disorder
Borderline personality disorder
Substance-induced psychotic disorder
Delirium and dementia
Mental disorders due to a medical condition
Childhood schizophrenia
Pervasive developmental disorder
Tourette's syndrome
Huntington's disease

Schizophrenia and Schizoaffective Disorder

Dopamine receptor antagonists are effective in both the short-term and the long-term management of schizophrenia and schizoaffective disorder. They reduce both acute symptoms and prevent future exacerbations. The DRAs produce their most dramatic effects against the positive symptoms of schizophrenia (e.g., hallucinations, delusions, and agitation). Negative symptoms (e.g., emotional withdrawal and ambivalence) are less likely to improve significantly, and they may appear to worsen because these drugs produce constriction of facial expression and akinesia, side effects that mimic negative symptoms.

Schizophrenia and schizoaffective disorder are characterized by remission and relapse. DRAs decrease the risk of reemergence of psychosis in patients who have recovered while on medication. Following a first episode of psychosis, patients should be maintained on medication for 1 to 2 years; after multiple episodes, for 2 to 5 years. Some clinicians recommend lifelong treatment.

Mania

The DRAs are effective to treat psychotic symptoms of acute mania. Because antimanic agents (e.g., lithium) generally have a slower onset of action than do antipsychotics in the treatment of acute symptoms, it is standard practice initially to combine either a DRA or an SDA with lithium (Eskalith), lamotrigine (Lamictal), or carbamazepine (Tegretol) and then gradually withdraw the antipsychotic.

Depression with Psychotic Symptoms

Combination treatment with an antipsychotic and an antidepressant is one of the treatments of choice for major depressive disorder with psychotic features; the other is electroconvulsive therapy (ECT).

Delusional Disorder

Patients with delusional disorder often respond favorably to treatment with these drugs.

Severe Agitation and Violent Behavior

Severely agitated and violent patients, regardless of diagnosis, can be treated with DRAs. Symptoms, such as extreme irritability, lack of impulse control, severe hostility, gross hyperactivity, and agitation, respond to short-term treatment with these drugs. Mentally handicapped children, especially those with profound mental retardation and autistic disorder, often have associated episodes of violence, aggression, and agitation that respond to treatment with antipsychotic drugs; however, the repeated administration of antipsychotics to control disruptive behavior in children is controversial.

Tourette's Syndrome

Dopamine receptor antagonists are used to treat Tourette's disorder, a neurobehavioral disorder marked by motor and vocal tics. Haloperidol and pimozide (Orap) are the drugs most frequently used, but other DRAs are also effective. Some clinicians prefer to use clonidine (Catapres) for this disorder because of its lower risk of neurologic side effects. Pimozide is used less frequently because of adverse cardiac effects.

Borderline Personality Disorder

Patients with borderline personality disorder who experience transient psychotic symptoms, such as perceptual disturbances, suspiciousness, ideas of reference, and aggression, may need to be treated with a DRA. This disorder is also associated with mood instability, so patients should be evaluated for possible treatment with mood-stabilizing agents.

Dementia and Delirium

About two thirds of agitated, elderly patients with various forms of dementia improve when given a DRA. Low doses of high-potency drugs (e.g., 0.5 to 1 mg a day of haloperidol) are used. DRAs are also used to treat psychotic symptoms and agitation associated with delirium. The cause of the delirium needs to be determined, because toxic deliriums caused by anticholinergic agents can be exacerbated by low-potency DRAs, which often have significant antimuscarinic activity.

Substance-Induced Psychotic Disorder

Intoxication with cocaine, amphetamines, alcohol, phencyclidine, or other drugs can cause psychotic symptoms. Because these symptoms tend to be time limited, it is preferable to avoid use of a DRA unless the patient is severely agitated and aggressive. Usually, benzodiazepines can be used to calm the patient. Benzodiazepines should be used instead of DRAs in cases of phencyclidine intoxication because of the anticholinergic effects of the DRAs. In cases where patients are experiencing hallucinations or delusions as a result of alcohol withdrawal, DRAs may increase the risk of seizure.

Childhood Schizophrenia

Children with schizophrenia benefit from treatment with antipsychotic medication, although considerably less research has been devoted to this population. Studies are currently under way to determine if intervention with medication at the very earliest signs of disturbance in children genetically at risk for schizophrenia can prevent the emergence of more florid symptoms. Careful consideration needs to be given to side effects, especially those involving cognition and alertness.

Other Psychiatric and Nonpsychiatric Indications

The DRAs reduce the chorea in the early stages of Huntington's disease. Patients with this disease may develop hallucinations, delusions, mania, or hypomania. These and other psychiatric symptoms respond to DRAs. High-potency DRAs should be used. Clinicians should be aware, however, that patients with the rigid form of this disorder may experience acute extrapyramidal symptoms. The use of DRAs to treat impulse-control disorders should be reserved for patients where other interventions have failed. Patients with pervasive developmental disorder may exhibit hyperactivity, screaming, and agitation with combativeness. Some of these symptoms respond to high-potency DRAs, but little research evidence supports their benefits in these patients.

The rare neurologic disorders ballismus and hemiballismus (which affects only one side of the body), characterized by propulsive movements of the limbs away from the body, also respond to treatment with antipsychotic agents. Other miscellaneous indications for the use of DRAs include the treatment of nausea, emesis, intractable hiccups, and pruritus. Endocrine disorders and temporal lobe epilepsy may be associated with psychosis that responds to antipsychotic treatment.

The most common side effects of DRAs are neurologic. Medication-induced movement disorders, such as parkinsonism, dystonia, akathisia, and tardive dyskinesia, are discussed in Section 36.2. As a rule, low-potency drugs cause most nonneurologic adverse effects, while the high-potency drugs cause most neurologic adverse effects.

PRECAUTIONS AND ADVERSE REACTIONS

Table 36.18–3 summarizes the most common adverse events associated with the use of DRAs. Table 36.18–4 summarizes the neurological side effects of DRAs.

Neuroleptic Malignant Syndrome

A potentially fatal side effect of DRA treatment, neuroleptic malignant syndrome, can occur at any time during the course of DRA treatment. Symptoms include extreme hyperthermia, severe muscular rigidity and dystonia, akinesia, mutism, confusion, agitation, and increased pulse rate and blood pressure (BP) leading to cardiovascular collapse. Laboratory findings include increased white blood cell (WBC) count, creatinine phosphokinase, liver enzymes, plasma myoglobin, and myoglobinuria, occasionally associated with renal failure. The symptoms usually evolve over 24 to 72 hours, and the untreated syndrome lasts 10 to 14 days. The diagnosis is often missed in the early stages, and the withdrawal or agitation may mistakenly be considered to reflect increased psychosis. Men are affected more frequently than are women, and young persons are affected more commonly than are elderly persons. The mortality rate can reach 20 percent to 30 percent or even higher when depot medications are involved. Rates are also increased when high doses of high-potency agents are used.

If neuroleptic malignant syndrome is suspected, the DRA should be stopped immediately and the following done: medical support to cool the person; monitoring of vital signs, electrolytes, fluid balance, and renal output; and symptomatic treatment

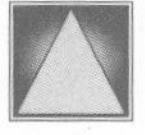

Table 36.18–3
Dopamine Receptor Antagonists: Potency and Adverse Effects

Drug Name	Chemical Classification	Therapeutically Equivalent Oral Dose (mg)	Side Effects: Sedation	Autonomic[a]	Extrapyramidal Reactions[b]
Pimozide[c] Orap	Diphenylbutylpiperidine	1.5	+	+	+++
Fluphenazine Permitil Prolixin	Phenothiazine: piperazine compound	2	+	+	+++
Haloperidol Haldol	Butyrophenone	2	+	+	+++
Thiothixene Navane	Thioxanthene	4	+	+	+++
Trifluoperazine Stelazine	Phenothiazine: piperazine compound	5	++	+	+++
Perphenazine Trilafon	Phenothiazine: piperazine compound	8	++	+	++/+++
Molindone Moban	Dihydroindolone	10	++	+	+
Loxapine Loxitane	Dibenzoxazepine	10	++	+/++	++/+++
Prochlorperazine[c] Compazine	Phenothiazine: piperazine compound	15	++	+	+++
Acetophenazine Tindal	Phenothiazine: piperazine compound	20	++	+	++/+++
Triflupromazine Vesprin	Phenothiazine: aliphatic compound	25	+++	++/+++	++
Mesoridazine Serentil	Phenothiazine: piperidine compound	50	+++	++	+
Chlorpromazine Thorazine	Phenothiazine: aliphatic compound	100	+++	+++	++
Chlorprothixene Taractan	Thioxanthene	100	+++	+++	+/++
Thioridazine Mellaril	Phenothiazine: piperidine compound	100	+++	+++	+

[a] Anti–α-adrenergic and anticholinergic effects.
[b] Excluding tardive dyskinesia, which appears to be produced to the same degree and frequency by all agents with equieffective antipsychotic dosages.
[c] Pimozide is used principally in the treatment of Tourette's syndrome; prochlorperazine is used rarely, if ever, as an antipsychotic agent.
(Adapted from American Medical Association. *AMA Drug Evaluations: Annual 1992.* Chicago: American Medical Association; 1992, with permission.)

of fever. Antiparkinsonian medications may reduce some of the muscle rigidity. Dantrolene (Dantrium), a skeletal muscle relaxant (0.8 to 2.5 mg/kg every 6 hours, up to a total dosage of 10 mg a day) may be useful in the treatment of this disorder. Once the person can take oral medications, dantrolene can be given in doses of 100 to 200 mg a day. Bromocriptine (20 to 30 mg a day in four divided doses) or amantadine can be added to the regimen. Treatment should usually be continued for 5 to 10 days. When drug treatment is restarted, the clinician should consider switching to a low-potency drug or an SDA, although these agents—including clozapine—can also cause neuroleptic malignant syndrome.

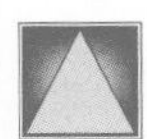

Table 36.18–4
Neurological Side Effects of Dopamine Receptor Antagonists

Acute extrapyramidal syndromes
Akathisia
Acute dystonia
Drug-induced parkinsonism
Neuroleptic malignant syndrome
Chronic extrapyramidal syndromes
Tardive dyskinesia and dystonia
Perioral tremor

Seizure Threshold

The DRAs may lower the seizure threshold. Chlorpromazine, thioridazine, and other low-potency drugs are thought to be more epileptogenic than are high-potency drugs. Molindone may be the least epileptogenic of the DRA drugs. The risk of inducing a seizure by drug administration warrants consideration when the person already has a seizure disorder or brain lesion.

Sedation

Blockade of histamine H_1 receptors is the usual cause of sedation associated with DRAs. Chlorpromazine is the most sedating typical antipsychotic. The relative sedative properties of the drugs are summarized in Table 36.18–3. Giving the entire daily dose at bedtime usually eliminates any problems from sedation, and tolerance for this adverse effect often develops.

Central Anticholinergic Effects

The symptoms of central anticholinergic activity include severe agitation; disorientation to time, person, and place; hallucinations; seizures; high fever; and dilated pupils. Stupor and coma may ensue. The treatment of anticholinergic toxicity consists of discontinuing the causal agent or agents, close medical supervision, and physostigmine (Antilirium, Eserine), 2 mg by slow intravenous (IV) infusion, repeated within 1 hour as necessary. Too much physostigmine is dangerous, and symptoms of physostigmine toxicity include hypersalivation and sweating. Atropine sulfate (0.5 mg) can reverse the effects of physostigmine toxicity.

Cardiac Effects

The DRAs decrease cardiac contractility, disrupt enzyme contractility in cardiac cells, increase circulating levels of catecholamines, and prolong atrial and ventricular conduction time and refractory periods. Low-potency DRAs are more cardiotoxic than are high-potency drugs. Chlorpromazine causes prolongation of the QT and PR intervals, blunting of the T waves, and depression of the ST segment. Thioridazine and mesoridazine, in particular, are associated with substantial QT prolongation and risk of torsade de pointes. These drugs, thus, are indicated only when other agents have been ineffective.

Sudden Death

Occasional reports of sudden cardiac death during treatment with DRAs may be the result of cardiac arrhythmias. Other causes may include seizure, asphyxiation, malignant hyperthermia, heat stroke, and neuroleptic malignant syndrome. An overall increase in the incidence of sudden death linked to the use of antipsychotics does not appear to exist, however.

Orthostatic (Postural) Hypotension

Orthostatic (postural) hypotension is most common with low-potency drugs, particularly chlorpromazine, thioridazine, and chlorprothixene. When using intramuscular (IM) low-potency DRAs, the clinician should measure the person's BP (lying and standing) before and after the first dose and during the first few days of treatment.

Orthostatic hypotension is mediated by adrenergic blockade and occurs most frequently during the first few days of treatment. Tolerance often develops for this side effect, which is why initial dosing of these drugs is lower than the usual therapeutic dose. Fainting or falls, although uncommon, can lead to injury. Patients should be warned of this side effect and instructed to rise slowly after sitting or reclining. Patients should avoid all caffeine and alcohol; they should drink at least 2 L of fluid a day and, if not under treatment for hypertension, should add liberal amounts of salt to their diet. Support hose may help some persons.

Hypotension can usually be managed by having patients lie down with their feet higher than their heads, and pump their legs as if bicycling. Volume expansion or vasopressor agents, such as norepinephrine (Levophed), may be indicated in severe cases. Because hypotension is produced by α-adrenergic blockade, the drugs also block the α-adrenergic stimulating properties of epinephrine, leaving the β-adrenergic stimulating effects untouched. Therefore, the administration of epinephrine results in a paradoxical worsening of hypotension and is contraindicated in cases of antipsychotic-induced hypotension. Pure α-adrenergic pressor agents, such as metaraminol (Aramine) and norepinephrine, are the drugs of choice in the treatment of the disorder.

Hematologic Effects

A temporary leukopenia with a WBC count of about 3,500 is a common, but not serious problem. Agranulocytosis, a life-threatening hematologic problem, occurs in about 1 of 10,000 persons treated with DRAs. Thrombocytopenic or nonthrombocytopenic purpura, hemolytic anemias, and pancytopenia may occur rarely in persons treated with DRAs. Although routine complete blood counts (CBCs) are not indicated, if a person reports a sore throat and fever, a CBC should be done immediately to check for the possibility. If the blood indexes are low, administration of DRAs should be stopped, and the person should be transferred to a medical facility. The mortality rate for the complication may be as high as 30 percent.

Peripheral Anticholinergic Effects

Peripheral anticholinergic effects, consisting of dry mouth and nose, blurred vision, constipation, urinary retention, and mydriasis, are common, especially with low-potency DRAs, for example, chlorpromazine, thioridazine, mesoridazine (Serentil). Some persons also have nausea and vomiting.

Constipation should be treated with the usual laxative preparations, but severe constipation can progress to paralytic ileus. A decrease in the DRA dosage or a change to a less anticholinergic drug is warranted in such cases. Pilocarpine (Salagen) can be used to treat paralytic ileus, although the relief is only transitory. Bethanechol (Urecholine) (20 to 40 mg a day) may be useful in some persons with urinary retention.

Weight gain is associated with increased mortality and morbidity and with medication noncompliance. Low-potency DRAs can cause significant weight gain but not as much as is seen with the SDAs olanzapine (Zyprexa) and clozapine (Clozaril). Molindone (Moban) and, perhaps, loxapine (Loxitane) appear to be least likely to cause weight gain.

Endocrine Effects

Blockade of the dopamine receptors in the tuberoinfundibular tract results in the increased secretion of prolactin, which can result in breast enlargement, galactorrhea, amenorrhea, and inhibited orgasm in women and impotence in men. The SDAs, with the exception of risperidone, are not particularly associated with an increase in prolactin levels and may be the drugs of choice for persons experiencing disturbing side effects from increased prolactin release.

Sexual Adverse Effects

Both men and women taking DRAs can experience anorgasmia and decreased libido. As many as 50 percent of men taking antipsychotics report ejaculatory and erectile disturbances. Sildenafil (Viagra), vardenafil (Levitra), or tadalafil (Cialis) are often used to treat psychotropic-induced orgasmic dysfunction, but they have not been studied in combination with DRAs. Thioridazine is particularly associated with decreased libido and retrograde ejaculation in men. Priapism and reports of painful orgasms have also been described, both possibly resulting from α_1-adrenergic antagonist activity.

Skin and Eye Effects

Allergic dermatitis and photosensitivity can occur, especially with low-potency agents. Urticarial, maculopapular, petechial, and edematous eruptions can occur early in treatment, generally in the first few weeks, and remit spontaneously. A photosensitivity reaction that resembles a severe sunburn also occurs in some persons taking chlorpromazine. Persons should be warned of this adverse effect, spend no more than 30 to 60 minutes in the sun, and use sunscreens. Long-term chlorpromazine use is associated with blue-gray discoloration of skin areas exposed to sunlight. The skin changes often begin with a tan or golden brown color and progress to such colors as slate gray, metallic blue, and purple. These discolorations resolve when the patient is switched to another medication.

Irreversible retinal pigmentation is associated with use of thioridazine at dosages above 1,000 mg a day. An early symptom of the side effect can sometimes be nocturnal confusion related to difficulty with night vision. The pigmentation can progress even after thioridazine administration is stopped, finally resulting in blindness. It is for this reason that the maximal recommended dosage of thioridazine is 800 mg per day.

Patients taking chlorpromazine can develop a relatively benign pigmentation of the eyes, characterized by whitish brown granular deposits concentrated in the anterior lens and posterior cornea and visible only by slit-lens examination. The deposits can progress to opaque white and yellow-brown granules, often stellate. Occasionally, the conjunctiva is discolored by a brown pigment. No retinal damage is seen, and vision is almost never impaired. This condition gradually resolves when the chlorpromazine is discontinued.

Jaundice

Elevations of liver enzymes during treatment with a DRA tend to be transient and not clinically significant. When chlorpromazine first came into use, cases of obstructive or cholestatic jaundice were reported. It usually occurred in the first month of treatment and was heralded by symptoms of upper abdominal pain, nausea, and vomiting. This was followed by fever, rash, eosinophilia, bilirubin in the urine, and increases in serum bilirubin, alkaline phosphatase, and hepatic transaminases. Reported cases are now extremely rare, but if jaundice occurs, the medication should be discontinued.

Overdoses

Overdoses typically consist of exaggerated DRA side effects. Symptoms and signs include central nervous system (CNS) depression, extrapyramidal symptoms, mydriasis, rigidity, restlessness, decreased deep tendon reflexes, tachycardia, and hypotension. The severe symptoms of overdose include delirium, coma, respiratory depression, and seizures. Haloperidol may be among the safest typical antipsychotics in overdose. After an overdose, the electroencephalogram (EEG) shows diffuse slowing and low voltage. Extreme overdose can lead to delirium and coma, with respiratory depression and hypotension. Life-threatening overdose usually involves ingestion of other CNS depressants, such as alcohol or benzodiazepines.

Activated charcoal, if possible, and gastric lavage should be administered if the overdose is recent. Emetics are not indicated, because the antiemetic actions of DRAs inhibit their efficacy. Seizures can be treated with IV diazepam (Valium) or phenytoin (Dilantin). Hypotension can be treated with either norepinephrine or dopamine, but not epinephrine.

Pregnancy and Lactation

A low correlation exists between the use of antipsychotics during pregnancy and congenital malformations. Nevertheless, antipsychotics should be avoided during pregnancy, particularly in the first trimester, unless the benefit outweighs the risk. High-potency drugs, particularly fluphenazine (Prolixon), are preferable to low-potency drugs, because the low-potency drugs are associated with hypotension.

The DRAs are secreted in the breast milk, although concentrations are low. Women taking these agents should be advised against breast-feeding.

DRUG INTERACTIONS

Many pharmacokinetic and pharmacodynamic drug interactions are associated with these drugs (Table 36.18–5). CYP 2D6 is the most common hepatic isozyme involved in DRA pharmacokinetic interactions. Other common drug interactions affect the absorption of the DRAs.

Antacids, activated charcoal, cholestyramine, kaolin, pectin, and cimetidine (Tagamet) taken within 2 hours of antipsychotic administration can reduce the absorption of these drugs. Anticholinergics can decrease the absorption of DRAs. The additive anticholinergic activity of DRAs, anticholinergics, and tricyclic drugs can result in anticholinergic toxicity. Digoxin and steroids, both of which decrease gastric motility, can increase DRA absorption.

Phenothiazines, especially thioridazine, can decrease the metabolism of, and cause toxic concentrations of, phenytoin. Barbiturates can increase the metabolism of DRAs, and these drugs may lower the person's seizure threshold.

Tricyclic drugs and selective serotonin reuptake inhibitors (SSRIs) that inhibit CYP 2D6—paroxetine, fluoxetine, and fluvoxamine—interact with DRAs, resulting in increased plasma concentrations of both drugs. The anticholinergic, sedative, and hypotensive effects of the drugs may also be additive.

Typical antipsychotics may inhibit the hypotensive effects of α-methyldopa (Aldomet). Conversely, typical antipsychotics may have an additive effect on some hypotensive drugs. Antipsychotic drugs have a variable effect on the hypotensive effects of clonidine. Propranolol coadministration increases the blood concentrations of both drugs.

The DRAs potentiate the CNS-depressant effects of sedatives, antihistamines, opiates, opioids, and alcohol, particularly in persons with impaired respiratory status. When these agents are taken with alcohol, the risk for heat stroke may be increased.

Cigarette smoking may decrease the plasma levels of typical antipsychotic drugs. Epinephrine has a paradoxical hypotensive effect in persons taking typical antipsychotics. These drugs may decrease the blood concentration of warfarin (Coumadin), resulting in decreased bleeding time. Phenothiazines, thioridazine, and

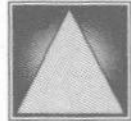

Table 36.18–5
Antipsychotic Drug Interactions

Interacting Medication	Mechanism	Clinical Effect
Drug interactions assessed to have major severity		
β-adrenergic receptor antagonists	Synergistic pharmacologic effect; antipsychotic inhibits metabolism of propranolol; antipsychotic increases plasma concentrations	Severe hypotension
Anticholinergics	Pharmacodynamic effects Additive anticholinergic effect	Decreased antipsychotic effect Anticholinergic toxicity
Barbiturates	Phenobarbital induces antipsychotic metabolism	Decreased antipsychotic concentrations
Carbamazepine	Induces antipsychotic metabolism	Up to 50% reduction in antipsychotic concentrations
Charcoal	Reduces GI absorption of antipsychotic and adsorbs drug during enterohepatic circulation	May reduce antipsychotic effect or cause toxicity when during overdose or for GI disturbances
Cigarette smoking	Induction of microsomal enzymes	Reduced plasma concentrations of antipsychotic agents
Epinephrine, norepinephrine	Antipsychotic antagonizes pressor effect	Hypotension
Ethanol	Additive CNS depression	Impaired psychomotor status
Fluvoxamine	Fluvoxamine inhibits metabolism of haloperidol and clozapine	Increased concentrations of haloperidol and clozapine
Guanethidine	Antipsychotic antagonizes guanethidine reuptake	Impaired antihypertensive effect
Lithium	Unknown	Rare reports of neurotoxicity
Meperidine	Additive CNS depression	Hypotension and sedation
Drug interactions assessed to have minor or moderate severity		
Amphetamines anorexiants	Decreased pharmacologic effect of amphetamine	Diminished weight loss effect; amphetamines may exacerbate psychosis; treatment-refractory schizophrenics may improve
Angiotensin-converting enzyme inhibitors	Additive hypotensive crisis	Hypotension, postural intolerance
Antacids containing aluminum	Insoluble complex formed in GI tract	Possible reduced antipsychotic effect
AD nonspecific	Decreased metabolism of AD through competitive inhibition	Increased AD concentration
Benzodiazepines	Increased pharmacologic effect of the benzodiazepine	Respiratory depression, stupor, hypotension
Bromocriptine	Antipsychotic antagonizes dopamine receptor stimulation	Increased prolactin
Caffeinated beverages	Form precipitate with antipsychotic solutions	Possible diminished antipsychotic effect
Cimetidine	Reduced antipsychotic absorption and clearance	Decreased antipsychotic effect
Clonidine	Antipsychotic potentiates α-adrenergic hypotensive effect	Hypotension or hypertension
Disulfiram	Impairs antipsychotic metabolism	Increased antipsychotic concentrations
Methyldopa	Unknown	BP elevations
Phenytoin	Induction of antipsychotic metabolism; decreased phenytoin metabolism	Decreased antipsychotic concentrations; increased phenytoin levels
Selective-serotonin reuptake inhibitors	Impair antipsychotic metabolism; pharmacodynamic interaction	Sudden onset of extrapyramidal symptoms
Valproic acid	Antipsychotic inhibits valproic acid metabolism	Increased valproic acid half-life and levels

GI, gastrointestinal; CNS, central nervous system; AD, antidepressant; BP, blood pressure.
(From Ereshosky L, Overman GP, Karp JK. Current psychotropic dosing and monitoring guidelines. *Prim Psychiatry* 1996;3:21, with permission.)

pimozide should not be coadministered with other agents that prolong the QT interval. Thioridazine is contraindicated in patients taking drugs that inhibit the cytochrome P450 (CYP) 2D6 isoenzyme or in patients with reduced levels of CYP 2D6.

LABORATORY INTERFERENCES

Chlorpromazine and perphenazine (Trilafon) may cause both false-positive and false-negative results in immunologic pregnancy tests and falsely elevated bilirubin (with reagent test strips) and urobilinogen (with Ehrlich's reagent test) values. These drugs have also been associated with an abnormal shift in results of the glucose tolerance test, although that shift may reflect the effects of the drugs on the glucose-regulating system. Phenothiazines have been reported to interfere with the measurement of 17-ketosteroids and 17-hydroxycorticosteroids and produce false-positive results in tests for phenylketonuria.

DOSAGE AND CLINICAL GUIDELINES

Contraindications to the use of DRAs include (1) a history of a serious allergic response, (2) the possible ingestion of a substance that will interact with the antipsychotic to induce CNS depression (e.g., alcohol, opioids, barbiturates, and benzodiazepines) or anticholinergic delirium (e.g., scopolamine and possibly phencyclidine [PCP]), (3) the presence of a severe cardiac abnormality,

(4) a high risk for seizures, (5) the presence of narrow-angle glaucoma or prostatic hypertrophy if a drug with high anticholinergic activity is to be used, and (6) the presence or a history of tardive dyskinesia. Antipsychotics should be administered with caution in persons with hepatic disease, because impaired hepatic metabolism can result in high plasma concentrations. The usual assessment should include a CBC with WBC indexes, liver function tests, and an electrocardiogram, especially in women over 40 years of age and men over 30 years of age. The elderly and children are more sensitive to side effects than are young adults, so the dosage of the drug should be adjusted accordingly.

Various patients may respond to widely different dosages of antipsychotics; therefore, no set dosage exists for any given antipsychotic drug. Because tolerance develops to many side effects, it is reasonable clinical practice to begin at a low dosage and increase it as necessary. It is important to remember that the maximal effects of a particular dosage may not be evident for 4 to 6 weeks. Available preparations and dosages of dopamine receptor antagonists are given in Table 36.18–6.

Short-term Treatment

The equivalent of 5 to 20 mg of haloperidol is a reasonable dose for an adult person in an acute state. A geriatric person may benefit from as little as 1 mg of haloperidol. The administration of more than 25 mg of chlorpromazine in one injection can result in serious hypotension. Administration of the antipsychotic IM results in peak plasma levels in about 30 minutes, versus 90 minutes using the oral route. Doses of drugs for IM administration are about half those given by the oral route. In a short-term treatment setting, the person should be observed for 1 hour after the first dose of medication. After that time, most clinicians administer a second dose or a sedative agent (e.g., a benzodiazepine) to achieve effective behavioral control. Possible sedatives include lorazepam (Ativan) (2 mg IM) and amobarbital (Amytal) (50 to 250 mg IM).

Rapid Neuroleptization

Rapid neuroleptization (also called *psychotolysis*) is the practice of administering hourly IM doses of antipsychotic medications until marked sedation of the person is achieved. Several research studies have shown, however, that merely waiting several more hours after one dose yields the same clinical improvement as is seen with repeated doses. Nevertheless, clinicians must be careful to keep persons from becoming violent while they are psychotic. Clinicians can help prevent violent episodes by using adjuvant sedatives or by temporarily using physical restraints until the persons can control their behavior.

Early Treatment

A full 6 weeks may be necessary to evaluate the extent of the improvement in psychotic symptoms. Agitation and excitement usually improve quickly with antipsychotic treatment, however. About 75 percent of persons with a short history of illness show significant improvement in their psychosis. Psychotic symptoms, both positive and negative, usually continue to improve 3 to 12 months after the initiation of treatment.

About 5 mg of haloperidol or 300 mg of chlorpromazine is the usual effective daily dose. In the past, much higher doses were used, but evidence suggests that this resulted in more side effects without additional benefits. A single daily dose is usually given at bedtime to help induce sleep and to reduce the incidence of adverse effects. Bedtime dosing for elderly persons may increase their risk of falling, however, if they get out of bed during the night. The sedative effects of typical antipsychotics last only a few hours, in contrast to the antipsychotic effects, which last for 1 to 3 days.

Intermittent Medications

It is common clinical practice to order medications to be given intermittently as needed (p.r.n.). Although this practice may be reasonable during the first few days that a person is hospitalized, the amount of time the person takes antipsychotic drugs, rather than an increase in dosage, is what produces therapeutic improvement. Clinicians on in-patient services may feel pressured by staff members to write p.r.n. antipsychotic orders; such orders should include specific symptoms, how often the drugs should be given, and how many doses can be given each day. Clinicians may choose to use small doses for the p.r.n. doses (e.g., 2 mg of haloperidol) or use a benzodiazepine instead (e.g., 2 mg of lorazepam IM). If p.r.n. doses of an antipsychotic are necessary after the first week of treatment, the clinician may want to consider increasing the standing daily dosage of the drug.

Maintenance Treatment

The first 3 to 6 months after a psychotic episode is usually considered a period of stabilization. After that time, the dosage of the antipsychotic can be decreased about 20 percent every 6 months until the minimal effective dosage is found. A person is usually maintained on antipsychotic medications for 1 to 2 years after the first psychotic episode. Antipsychotic treatment is often continued for 5 years after a second psychotic episode, and lifetime maintenance is considered after the third psychotic episode, although attempts to reduce the daily dosage can be made every 6 to 12 months.

Antipsychotic drugs are effective in controlling psychotic symptoms, but persons may report that they prefer being off the drugs because they feel better without them. This problem is less common with the newer antipsychotic SDAs. The clinician must discuss maintenance medication with patients and take into account their wishes, the severity of their illnesses, and the quality of their support systems. It is essential for the clinician to know enough about the patient's life to try to predict upcoming stressors that might require increasing the dosage or closely monitoring compliance.

Long-acting Depot Medications

Long-acting depot preparations may be needed to overcome problems with compliance. IM preparations are typically given once every 1 to 4 weeks.

Two depot preparations, a decanoate and an enanthate, of fluphenazine and a decanoate preparation of haloperidol are available in the United States. The preparations are injected IM into an area of large muscle tissue, from which they are absorbed

Table 36.18–6
Dopamine Receptor Antagonists

Name							Adult Dose Range (mg/day)	
Generic or Chemical	Trade	Tablets (mg)	Capsules (mg)	Solution	Parenteral	Rectal Suppositories (mg)	Acute	Maintenance
Chlorpromazine	Thorazine	10, 25, 50, 100, 200	30, 75, 150, 200, 300	10 mg/5 mL, 30 mg/mL, 100 mg/mL	25 mg/mL	25, 100	100 to 1,600 p.o. 25 to 400 IM	50 to 400 p.o.
Prochlorperazine	Compazine	5, 10, 25	10, 15, 30	5 mg/5 mL	5 mg/mL	2.5, 5, 25	15 to 200 p.o. 40 to 80 IM	15 to 60 p.o.
Perphenazine	Trilafon	2, 4, 8, 16	—	16 mg/5 mL	5 mg/mL	—	12 to 64 p.o. 15 to 30 IM	8 to 24 p.o.
Trifluoperazine	Stelazine	1, 2, 5, 10	—	10 mg/mL	2 mg/mL	—	4 to 40 p.o. 4 to 10 IM	5 to 20 p.o.
Fluphenazine	Prolixin	1, 2.5, 5, 10	—	2.5 mg/5 mL, 5 mg/mL	2.5 mg/mL (IM only)	—	2.5 to 40.0 p.o. 5 to 20 IM	1.0 to 15.0 p.o. 12.5 to 50.0 IM (decanoate or enanthate, weekly or biweekly)
Fluphenazine decanoate		—	—	—	2.5 mg/mL	—		
Fluphenazine enanthate	—	—	—	2.5 mg/mL	—			
Thioridazine	Mellaril	10, 15, 25, 50, 100, 150, 200	—	25 mg/5 mL, 100 mg/5 mL, 30 mg/mL, 100 mg/mL	—	—	200 to 800 p.o.	100 to 300 p.o.
Mesoridazine	Serentil	10, 25, 50, 100	—	25 mg/mL	25 mg/mL	—	100 to 400 p.o. 25 to 200 IM	30 to 150 p.o.
Haloperidol	Haldol	0.5, 1, 2, 5, 10, 20	—	2 mg/5 mL	5 mg/mL (IM only)	—	5 to 20 p.o.	1 to 10 p.o.
Haloperidol decanoate		—	—	—	50 mg/mL, 100 mg/mL (IM only)	—	12.5 to 25 IM	25 to 200 IM (decanoate, monthly)
Chlorprothixene	Taractan	10, 25, 50, 100	—	100 mg/5 mL (suspension)	12.5 mg/mL	—	75 to 600 p.o. 75 to 200 IM	50 to 400
Thiothixene	Navane	—	1, 2, 5, 10, 20	5 mg/mL	5 mg/mL (IM only), 20 mg/mL (IM only)	—	6 to 100 p.o. 8 to 30 IM	6 to 30
Loxapine	Loxitane	—	5, 10, 25, 50	25 mg/5 mL	50 mg/mL	—	20 to 250, 20 to 75 IM	20 to 100
Molindone	Moban	5, 10, 25, 50, 100	—	20 mg/mL	—	—	50 to 225	5 to 150
Pimozide	Orap	2	—	—	—	—	0.5 to 20	0.5 to 5.0

p.o., oral; IM, intramuscular.

slowly into the blood. Decanoate preparations can be given less frequently than enanthate preparations because they are absorbed more slowly. Although stabilizing a person on the oral preparation of the specific drugs is not necessary before initiating the depot form, it is good practice to give at least one oral dose of the drug to assess the possibility of an adverse effect, such as severe extrapyramidal symptoms or an allergic reaction.

It is reasonable to begin with either 12.5 mg (0.5 mL) of fluphenazine preparation or 25 mg (0.5 mL) of haloperidol decanoate. If symptoms emerge in the next 2 to 4 weeks, the person can be treated temporarily with additional oral medications or with additional small depot injections. After 3 to 4 weeks, the depot injection can be increased to a single dose equal to the total of the doses given during the initial period.

A good reason to initiate depot treatment with low doses is that the absorption of the preparations may be faster than usual at the onset of treatment, resulting in frightening episodes of dystonia that eventually discourage compliance with the medication. Some clinicians keep persons drug free for 3 to 7 days before initiating depot treatment and give small doses of the depot preparations (3.125 mg of fluphenazine or 6.25 mg of haloperidol) every few days to avoid those initial problems.

Plasma Concentrations

Genetic differences among persons and pharmacokinetic interactions with other drugs influence the metabolism of the antipsychotics. If a person has not improved after 4 to 6 weeks of treatment, the plasma concentration of the drug should be determined, if feasible. After a patient has been on a particular dosage for at least five times the half-life of the drug and, thus, approaches steady-state concentrations, blood levels may be helpful. It is standard practice to obtain plasma samples at trough levels—just before the daily dose is given, usually at least 12 hours after the previous dose and most commonly 20 to 24 hours after the previous dose. In fact, most antipsychotics have no well-defined dose–response curve. The best-studied drug is haloperidol, which may have a therapeutic window ranging from 2 to 15 ng/mL. Other therapeutic ranges that have been reasonably well documented are 30 to 100 ng/mL for chlorpromazine and 0.8 to 2.4 ng/mL for perphenazine.

Treatment-resistant Persons

Approximately 10 percent to 35 percent of persons with schizophrenia, however, do not obtain significant benefit from the antipsychotic drugs. Treatment resistance is failure on at least two adequate trials of antipsychotics from two pharmacologic classes. It is useful to determine plasma concentrations for such persons, because they may be slow or rapid metabolizers or may not be taking their medication. Clozapine has been conclusively shown to be effective when given to patients who have failed multiple trials of DRAs.

Adjunctive Medications

It is common practice to use DRAs in conjunction with other psychotropic agents, either to treat side effects or further improve symptoms. Most commonly, this involves the use of lithium or other mood stabilizing agents, SSRIs, or benzodiazepines. It was once held that antidepressant drugs exacerbated psychosis in patients with schizophrenia. In all likelihood, this observation involved patients with bipolar disorder who were misdiagnosed as being schizophrenic. Abundant evidence suggests that antidepressants, in fact, lessen symptoms of depression in patients with schizophrenia. In some cases, amphetamines can be added to DRAs if patients remain withdrawn and apathetic.

Choice of Drug

Given their proved efficacy in managing acute psychotic symptoms and that prophylactic administration of antiparkinsonian medication prevents or minimizes acute motor abnormalities, DRAs are still valuable—especially for short-term therapy. Considerable cost advantage exists to a DRA antiparkinsonian regimen as compared with monotherapy with a newer antipsychotic agent. Concern about the development of DRA-induced tardive dyskinesia is the major deterrent to long-term use of these drugs, yet it is not clear that SDAs are completely risk free of this complication. Side effects, such as extreme weight gain are more common with SDAs than with DRAs which can contribute to the risk of diabetes mellitus. Thus, DRAs still occupy an important role in psychiatric treatment. DRAs are not predictably interchangeable. For reasons that cannot be explained, some patients do better on one drug than another. Choice of a particular DRA should be based on the known adverse-effect profile of the drugs. Other than a significant advantage in terms of medication cost, the choice currently would be an SDA. If a DRA is felt to be preferable, a high-potency antipsychotic is favored even though it may be associated with more neurologic adverse effects, mainly because a higher incidence exists of other adverse effects (e.g., cardiac, hypotensive, epileptogenic, sexual, and allergic) with the low-potency drugs. If sedation is a desired goal, either a low-potency antipsychotic can be given in divided doses or a benzodiazepine can be coadministered.

An unpleasant or dysphoric reaction (a subjective sense of restlessness, oversedation, and acute dystonia) to the first dose of an antipsychotic predicts future poor response and noncompliance. Prophylactic use of antiparkinsonian medications may prevent this reaction.

References

Aruna AS, Murungi JH. Fluphenazine-induced neuroleptic malignant syndrome in a schizophrenic patient. *Ann Pharmacother*. 2005 Jun;39(6):1131–5.

Conley RR, Kelly DL, Nelson MW, Richardson CM, Feldman S, Benham R, Steiner P, Yu Y, Khan I, McMullen R, Gale E, Mackowick M, Love RC. Risperidone, quetiapine, and fluphenazine in the treatment of patients with therapy-refractory schizophrenia. *Clin Neuropharmacol*. 2005 Jul–Aug;285(4):163–8.

Duncan E, Dunlop WB, Boshoven W, Woolson SL, Hamer RM, Phillips LS. Relative risk of glucose elevation during antipsychotic exposure in a Veterans Administration population. *Int Clin Psychopharmacol*. 2007;22(1):1–11.

Kelly DL, Conley RR. Thyroid function in treatment-resistant schizophrenia patients treated with quetiapine, risperidone, or fluphenazine. *J Clin Psychiatry*. 2005;66(1):80–4.

Kinon BJ, Liu-Seifert H, Adams DH, Citrome L. Differential rates of treatment discontinuation in clinical trials as a measure of treatment effectiveness for olanzapine and comparator atypical antipsychotics for schizophrenia. *J Clin Psychopharmacol*. 2006 Dec;26(6):632–7.

Khorram B, Lang DJ, Kopala LC, Vandorpe RA, Rui Q, Goghari VM, Smith GN, Honer WG. Reduced thalamic volume in patients with chronic schizophrenia after switching from typical antipsychotic medications to olanzapine. *Am J Psychiatry*. 2006;163(11):2005–7.

Lo Y, Chia YY, Liu K, Ko NH. Morphine sparing with droperidol in patient-controlled analgesia. *J Clin Anesth*. 2005;17(4):271–5.

Marder SR, van Kammen DP. Dopamine receptor antagonists (typical antipsychotics). In: Sadock BJ, Sadock VA, eds. *Kaplan & Sadock's Comprehensive*

Textbook of Psychiatry. 8th ed. Vol. 2. Baltimore: Lippincott Williams & Wilkins; 2005:2817.

Murray M. Role of CYP pharmacogenetics and drug-drug interactions in the efficacy and safety of atypical and other antipsychotic agents. *J Pharm Pharmacol*. 2006;58(7):871–85.

Zirnheld PJ, Carroll CA, Kieffaber PD, O'Donnell BF, Shekhar A, Hetrick WP. Haloperidol impairs learning and error-related negativity in humans. *J Cogn Neurosci*. 2004;16(6):1098–1112.

▲ 36.19 Lamotrigine

Lamotrigine (Lamictal) was originally developed as an antiepileptic drug used as adjunctive therapy for general and partial seizures in adults and pediatric patients. It was approved by the US Food and Drug Administration (FDA) for maintenance treatment of bipolar I disorder in 2003. In clinical trials, it was shown to keep patients euthymic longer and was particularly effective in preventing depressive episodes. As a maintenance treatment, lamotrigine can be used in situations where lithium has traditionally been prescribed.

Although comparatively new when compared with lithium, the gold standard of bipolar maintenance therapy, lamotrigine has very real advantages compared with that agent in terms of tolerability, safety, and convenience. For example, lamotrigine treatment is associated with no significant metabolic or neurologic effects, and does not require laboratory testing of plasma concentrations. In contrast to lithium however, lamotrigine does not have any acute antimanic effects.

CHEMISTRY

Lamotrigine is a novel three-ringed (phenyltriazine) compound. Its structural formula is shown in Figure 36.19–1. It has antiglutamatergic and sodium channel blocking effects, as well as other properties.

PHARMACOLOGIC ACTIONS

Lamotrigine is completely absorbed, has bioavailability of 98 percent, and has a steady-state plasma half-life of 25 hours. The rate of lamotrigine's metabolism varies, however, over a sixfold range, depending on which other drugs are administered concomitantly. Dosing is escalated slowly to twice-a-day maintenance dosing. Food does not affect its absorption, and it is 55 percent protein bound in the plasma; 94 percent of lamotrigine and its inactive metabolites are excreted in the urine. Among the better-delineated biochemical actions of lamotrigine are blockade of voltage-sensitive sodium channels, which in turn modulate release of glutamate and aspartate, and a slight effect on calcium channels. Lamotrigine modestly increases plasma serotonin concentrations, possibly through inhibition of serotonin reuptake, and is a weak inhibitor of serotonin 5-HT_3 receptors.

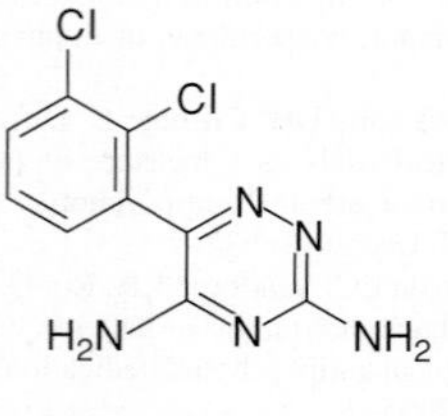

Cl
Cl
N
N
H_2N
N
NH_2
Lamotrigine

FIGURE 36.19–1
Molecular structure of lamotrigine.

THERAPEUTIC INDICATIONS

Bipolar Disorder

Lamotrigine is indicated in the maintenance treatment of bipolar disorder and may prolong the time between episodes of depression and mania. It is more effective in lengthening the intervals between depressive episodes than manic episodes. It is also effective as treatment for rapid-cycling bipolar disorder.

Other Indications

Therapeutic benefit has been reported in the treatment of borderline personality disorder and in the treatment for various pain syndromes.

PRECAUTIONS AND ADVERSE REACTIONS

Lamotrigine is remarkably well tolerated. The absence of sedation, weight gain, or other metabolic effects is noteworthy. The most common adverse effects—dizziness, ataxia, somnolence, headache, diplopia, blurred vision, and nausea—are typically mild. Cognitive impairment and joint or back pain may occur.

The appearance of a rash, which is common and occasionally very severe, is a source of concern. About 8 percent of patients started on lamotrigine develop a benign maculopapular rash during the first 4 months of treatment, and the drug should be discontinued if a rash develops. Although these rashes are benign, concern is that in some cases, they may represent early manifestations of a Stevens-Johnson syndrome or toxic epidermal necrolysis. Nevertheless, even if lamotrigine is discontinued immediately on development of rash or other signs of hypersensitivity reaction, such as fever and lymphadenopathy, this may not prevent subsequent development of a life-threatening rash or permanent disfiguration.

Estimates of the rate of serious rash vary, depending on the source of the data. In some studies, the incidence of serious rashes was 0.08 percent in adult patients receiving lamotrigine as initial monotherapy and 0.13 percent in adult patients receiving lamotrigine as adjunctive therapy. German registry data, based on clinical practice, suggest that the risk of rash may be as low as 1 of 5,000 patients. The appearance of any type of rash necessitates immediate discontinuation of drug administration (*see* Color Plate 36.19–2 on page 494).

It is known that the likelihood of a rash increases if the recommended starting dose and speed of dose increase exceed what is recommended. Concomitant administration of valproic acid also increases risk, and should be avoided if possible. If valproate is used, a more conservative dosing regimen is followed. Children and adolescents under 16 years of age appear to be more susceptible to rash with lamotrigine. If patients miss more than four consecutive days of lamotrigine treatment, they need to restart

Table 36.19–1
Gradual Introduction of Lamotrigine in Adults with Bipolar Disorder

	Lamotrigine with Valproate (mg/day)	Lamotrigine with Carbamazepine (mg/day)	Lamotrigine with Neither (mg/day)
Weeks 1 and 2 dose	12.5	50	25
Weeks 3 and 4 dose	25	100	50
Week 5 dose	50	200	100
Subsequent weekly dose increments	25 to 50	100	50 to 100
FDA target dose	100	400	200
Typical final dose range	100 to 200	400 to 800	200 to 400

FDA, US Food and Drug Administration.

therapy at the initial starting dose and titrate upward as if they had not already been on the medication.

Pregnancy registry data suggest a possible association between lamotrigine and an increased risk of nonsyndromic oral clefts in infants exposed to lamotrigine during the first trimester of pregnancy.

LABORATORY TESTING

No proven correlation exists between lamotrigine blood concentrations and either antiseizure effects or efficacy in bipolar disorders. Laboratory tests are not useful in predicting the occurrence of adverse events.

DRUG INTERACTIONS

Lamotrigine has significant, well-characterized drug interactions involving other anticonvulsants. The most potentially serious lamotrigine drug interaction involves concurrent use of valproic acid, which doubles serum lamotrigine concentrations conversely. Lamotrigine decreases the plasma concentration of valproic acid by 25 percent. Sertraline (Zoloft) also increases plasma lamotrigine concentrations, but to a lesser extent than does valproic acid. Lamotrigine concentrations are decreased by 40 percent to 50 percent with concomitant administration of carbamazepine, phenytoin, or phenobarbital. Combinations of lamotrigine and other anticonvulsants have complex effects on the time of peak plasma concentration and the plasma half-life of lamotrigine.

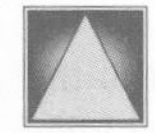

Table 36.19–2
Lamotrigine Dosing (mg/day)

Treatment	Weeks 1–2	Weeks 3–4	Weeks 4–5
Lamotrigine monotherapy	25	50	100 to 200 mg (500 maximum)*
Lamotrigine plus carbamazepine	50	100	200 to 500 mg (700 maximum)
Lamotrigine plus valproate	25 every other day	25	50 to 200 mg (200 maximum)

*For bipolar disorder efficacy above 200 mg not established.

LABORATORY INTERFERENCES

Lamotrigine and topiramate do not interfere with any laboratory tests.

DOSAGE AND ADMINISTRATION

In the clinical trials leading to the approval of lamotrigine as a treatment for bipolar disorder, no consistent increase in efficacy was associated with doses above 200 mg per day (Table 36.19–1). Most patients should take between 100 and 200 mg a day. In epilepsy, the drug is administered twice daily: in bipolar disorder, however, the total dose can be taken once a day, either in the morning or at night, depending on whether the patient finds the drug activating or sedating.

Lamotrigine is available as unscored 25-, 100-, 150-, and 200-mg tablets. The major determinant of lamotrigine dosing is minimization of the risk of rash. Lamotrigine should not be taken by anyone under the age of 16 years. Because valproic acid markedly slows the elimination of lamotrigine, concomitant administration of these two drugs necessitates a much slower titration (Table 36.19–2). People with renal insufficiency should aim for a lower maintenance dosage. Appearance of any type of rash necessitates immediate discontinuation of lamotrigine administration. Lamotrigine should usually be discontinued gradually over 2 weeks unless a rash emerges, in which case it should be discontinued over 1 to 2 days.

Chewable dispersible tablets of 2, 5, and 25 mg are also available.

References

Barbosa L, Berk M, Vorster M. A double-blind, randomized, placebo-controlled trial of augmentation with lamotrigine or placebo in patients concomitantly treated with fluoxetine for resistant major depressive episodes. *J Clin Psychiatry.* 2003;64:403–407.

Bowden CL, Calabrese JR, Sachs G, Yatham LN, Asghar SA, Hompland M, Montgomery P, Earl N, Smoot TM, DeVeaugh-Geiss J. A placebo-controlled 18-month trial of lamotrigine and lithium maintenance treatment in recently manic or hypomanic patients with bipolar I disorder. *Arch Gen Psychiatry.* 2003;60:392–400.

Calabrese JR, Bowden CL, Sachs G, Yatham LN, Behnke K, Mehtonen OP, Montgomery P, Ascher J, Paska W, Earl N, DeVeaugh-Geiss J. A placebo-controlled 18-month trial of lamotrigine and lithium maintenance treatment in recently depressed patients with bipolar I disorder. *J Clin Psychiatry.* 2003;64:1013–1024.

Goldsmith DR, Wagstaff AJ, Ibbotson T, Perry CM. Lamotrigine: A review of its use in bipolar disorder. *Drugs.* 2003;63:2029–2050.

Ketter TA. Lamotrigine. In: Sadock BJ, Sadock VA, eds. *Kaplan & Sadock's Comprehensive Textbook of Psychiatry.* 8th ed. Vol. 2. Baltimore: Lippincott Williams & Wilkins; 2005:2749.

Ketter TA, Manji HK, Post RM. Potential mechanisms of action of lamotrigine in the treatment of bipolar disorders. *J Clin Psychopharmacol*. 2003;23:484–495.
Ketter TA, Wang PW. The emerging differential roles of GABAergic and antiglutamatergic agents in bipolar disorders. *J Clin Psychiatry*. 2003;64[Suppl 3]:15–20.
Ketter TA, Wang PW, Becker OV, Nowakowska C, Yang YS. The diverse roles of anticonvulsants in bipolar disorders. *Ann Clin Psychiatry*. 2003;15:95–108.

▲ 36.20 Lithium

Lithium (Eskalith, Lithobid, Lithonate) was approved by the US Food and Drug Administration (FDA) for the treatment of mania in 1970, more than 20 years after the first favorable reports by John F. J. Cade, an Australian psychiatrist. It is used for short-term, long-term, and prophylactic treatment of bipolar I disorder. Until recently, it was the only drug approved for both acute and maintenance treatment. It is also used as an adjunctive medication in the treatment of major depressive disorder.

CHEMISTRY

Lithium (Li), a monovalent ion, is a member of the group IA alkaline metals on the periodic table, a group that also includes sodium, potassium, rubidium, cesium, and francium. Lithium exists in nature as both ^{6}Li (7.42 percent) and ^{7}Li (92.58 percent). The latter isotope allows the imaging of lithium by magnetic resonance spectroscopy. Some 300 mg of lithium is contained in 1,597 mg of lithium carbonate (Li_2CO_3). Most lithium used in the United States is obtained from dry lake mining in Chile and Argentina.

PHARMACOLOGIC ACTIONS

Lithium is rapidly and completely absorbed after oral administration, with peak serum concentrations occurring in 1 to 1.5 hours with standard preparations and in 4 to 4.5 hours with slow- and controlled-released preparations. Lithium does not bind to plasma proteins, is not metabolized, and is excreted through the kidneys. The plasma half-life is initially 1.3 days and is 2.4 days after administration for more than 1 year. The blood–brain barrier permits only slow passage of lithium, which is why a single overdose does not necessarily cause toxicity and why long-term lithium intoxication is slow to resolve. The elimination half-life of lithium is 18 to 24 hours in young adults, but is shorter in children and longer in the elderly. Renal clearance of lithium is decreased with renal insufficiency. Equilibrium is reached after 5 to 7 days of regular intake. Obesity is associated with higher rates of lithium clearance. The excretion of lithium is complex during pregnancy; excretion increases during pregnancy, but decreases after delivery. Lithium is excreted in breast milk and in insignificant amounts in the feces and sweat. Thyroid and renal concentrations of lithium are higher than serum levels.

An explanation for the mood-stabilizing effects of lithium remains elusive. Theories include alterations of ion transport and effects on neurotransmitters and neuropeptides, signal transduction pathways, and second messenger systems.

THERAPEUTIC INDICATIONS

Bipolar I Disorder

Manic Episodes. Lithium controls acute mania and prevents relapse in about 80 percent of persons with bipolar I disorder and in a somewhat smaller percentage of persons with mixed (mania and depression) episodes, rapid-cycling bipolar disorder, or mood changes in encephalopathy. Lithium has a relatively slow onset of action when used and exerts its antimanic effects over 1 to 3 weeks. Thus, a benzodiazepine, dopamine receptor antagonist, serotonin–dopamine antagonist, or valproic acid is usually administered for the first few weeks. Patients with mixed or dysphoric mania, rapid cycling, comorbid substance abuse, or organicity respond less well to lithium than those with classic mania.

Bipolar Depression. Lithium has been shown to be effective in the treatment of depression associated with bipolar I disorder, as well as in add-on therapy for patients with severe major depressive disorder. Augmentation of lithium therapy with valproate (Depakene) or carbamazepine (Tegretol) is usually well tolerated, with little risk of mania precipitation.

When a depressive episode occurs in a person taking maintenance lithium, the differential diagnosis should include lithium-induced hypothyroidism, substance abuse, and lack of compliance with the lithium therapy. Possible treatment approaches include increasing the lithium concentration (up to 1 to 1.2 mEq/L), adding supplemental thyroid hormone (e.g., 25 μg a day of liothyronine [Cytomel]) even in the presence of normal findings on thyroid function tests, augmentation with valproate or carbamazepine, the judicious use of antidepressants, or electroconvulsive therapy (ECT). Once the acute depressive episode resolves, other therapies should be tapered off in favor of lithium monotherapy, if clinically tolerated.

Maintenance. Maintenance treatment with lithium markedly decreases the frequency, the severity, and the duration of manic and depressive episodes in persons with bipolar I disorder. Lithium provides relatively more effective prophylaxis for mania than for depression, and supplemental antidepressant strategies may be necessary, either intermittently or continuously. Lithium maintenance is almost always indicated after the second episode of bipolar I disorder depression or mania and should be considered after the first episode for adolescents or for persons who have a family history of bipolar I disorder. Others who benefit from lithium maintenance are those who have poor support systems, had no precipitating factors for the first episode, have a high suicide risk, had a sudden onset of the first episode, or had a first episode of mania. Clinical studies have shown that lithium reduces the incidence of suicide in patients with bipolar I disorder sixfold or sevenfold. Lithium is also effective treatment for persons with severe cyclothymic disorder.

Initiating maintenance therapy after the first manic episode is considered a wise approach based on several observations. First, each episode of mania increases the risk of subsequent episodes. Second, among people responsive to lithium, relapses are 28 times more likely after lithium use is discontinued. Third, case reports describe persons who initially responded to lithium, discontinued taking it, and then had a relapse but no longer responded to lithium in subsequent episodes. Continued maintenance treatment with lithium is often associated with increasing efficacy and reduced mortality. An episode of depression or mania that occurs after a relatively short time of lithium maintenance, therefore, does not necessarily represent treatment failure. Lithium treatment alone may begin, however, to lose its effectiveness after several years of successful use. If this occurs, then supplemental treatment with carbamazepine or valproate may be useful.

Maintenance lithium dosages often can be adjusted to achieve plasma concentration somewhat lower than that needed for treatment of acute mania. If lithium use is to be discontinued, then the dosage should be slowly tapered. Abrupt discontinuation of lithium therapy is associated with increased risk of recurrence of manic and depressive episodes.

A patient had two manic episodes in 2 years, one resolving spontaneously and one with ECT, followed by 18 euthymic years without any treatment before the next episode occurred. Had she been treated with lithium after the second manic episode, the subsequent 18 years would have been considered a testimonial to the therapeutic effectiveness of lithium. (Courtesy of James W. Jefferson, M.D., and John H. Greist, M.D.)

Major Depressive Disorder

Lithium is effective in the long-term treatment of major depression, but is not more effective than antidepressant drugs. The most common role for lithium in major depressive disorder is as an adjuvant to antidepressant use in persons who have failed to respond to the antidepressants alone. About 50 percent to 60 percent of antidepressant nonresponders do respond when lithium, 300 mg three times daily, is added to the antidepressant regimen. In some cases, a response may be seen within days, but most often, several weeks are required to see the efficacy of the regimen. Lithium alone may effectively treat depressed persons who have bipolar I disorder but have not yet had their first manic episode. Lithium has been reported to be effective in persons with major depressive disorder whose disorder has a particularly marked cyclicity.

Schizoaffective Disorder and Schizophrenia

Persons with prominent mood symptoms—either bipolar type or depressive type—with schizoaffective disorder are more likely to respond to lithium than are those with predominant psychotic symptoms. Whereas serotonin–dopamine antagonists (SDAs) and dopamine receptor antagonists (DRAs) are the treatments of choice for persons with schizoaffective disorder, lithium is a useful augmentation agent. This is particularly true for persons whose symptoms are resistant to treatment with SDAs and DRAs. Lithium augmentation of an SDA or DRA treatment may be effective for persons with schizoaffective disorder even in the absence of a prominent mood disorder component. Some persons with schizophrenia who cannot take antipsychotic drugs may benefit from lithium treatment alone.

Other Indications

Over the years, reports have appeared about the use of lithium to treat a wide range of other psychiatric and nonpsychiatric conditions (Tables 36.20–1 and 36.20–2). The effectiveness and safety of lithium for most of these disorders has not been confirmed. Lithium has antiaggressive activity that is separate from its effects on mood. Aggressive outbursts in persons with schizophrenia, violent prison inmates, and children with conduct disorder, and aggression or self-mutilation in persons with mental retardation can sometimes be controlled with lithium.

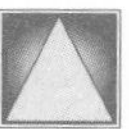

Table 36.20–1
Psychiatric Uses of Lithium

Historical
- Gouty mania

Well established (FDA-approved)
- Manic episode
- Maintenance therapy

Reasonably well established
- Bipolar I disorder
  - Depressive episode
  - Bipolar II disorder
  - Rapid-cycling bipolar I disorder
  - Cyclothymic disorder
- Major depressive disorder
  - Acute depression (as an augmenting agent)
  - Maintenance therapy
- Schizoaffective disorder

Evidence of benefit in particular groups
- Schizophrenia
- Aggression (episodic), explosive behavior, and self-mutilation
- Conduct disorder in children and adolescents
- Mental retardation
- Cognitive disorders
- Prisoners

Anecdotal, controversial, unresolved, or doubtful
- Alcohol and other substance-related disorders
  - Cocaine abuse
  - Substance-induced mood disorder with manic features
- Anxiety disorders
  - Obsessive-compulsive disorder
  - Phobias
  - Posttraumatic stress disorder
- Attention-deficit/hyperactivity disorder (ADHD)
- Eating disorders
  - Anorexia nervosa
  - Bulimia nervosa
- Impulse-control disorders
- Kleine-Levin syndrome
- Mental disorders due to a general medical condition (e.g., mood disorder due to a general medical condition with manic features)
- Periodic catatonia
- Periodic hypersomnia
- Personality disorders (e.g., antisocial, borderline, emotionally unstable, schizotypal)
- Premenstrual dysphoric disorder
- Sexual disorders
  - Transvestic fetishism
  - Exhibitionism

Pathological hypersexuality

FDA, Food and Drug Administration; ADHD, attention-deficit/hyperactivity disorder.

PRECAUTIONS AND ADVERSE EFFECTS

More than 80 percent of patients taking lithium experience side effects. It is important to minimize the risk of adverse events through monitoring of lithium blood levels and to use appropriate

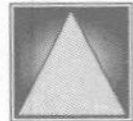

Table 36.20–2
Nonpsychiatric Uses of Lithium[a]

Historical
- Gout and other uric acid diatheses
- Lithium bromide as anticonvulsant

Neurologic
- Epilepsy
- Headache (chronic cluster, hypnic, migraine, particularly cyclic)
- Ménière's disease (not supported by controlled studies)
- Movement disorders
- Huntington's disease
- L-Dopa-induced hyperkinesias
- On–off phenomenon in Parkinson's disease (controlled study found decreased akinesia, but development of dyskinesia in a few cases)
- Spasmodic torticollis
- Tardive dyskinesia (not supported by controlled studies, and pseudoparkinsonism has been reported)
- Tourette's disorder
- Pain (facial pain syndrome, painful shoulder syndrome, fibromyalgia)
- Periodic paralysis (hypokalemic and hypermagnesic but not hyperkalemic)

Hematologic
- Aplastic anemia
- Cancer—chemotherapy-induced and radiotherapy-induced
- Neutropenia (one study found increased risk of sudden death in patients with preexisting cardiovascular disorder)
- Drug-induced neutropenia (e.g., from carbamazepine, antipsychotics, immunosuppressives, and zidovudine)
- Felty's syndrome
- Leukemia

Endocrine
- Thyroid cancer, as adjunct to radioactive iodine
- Thyrotoxicosis
- Syndrome of inappropriate antidiuretic hormone secretion

Cardiovascular
- Antiarrhythmic agent (animal data only)

Dermatologic
- Genital herpes (controlled studies support topical and oral use)
- Eczematoid dermatitis
- Seborrheic dermatitis (controlled study supports)

Gastrointestinal
- Cyclic vomiting
- Gastric ulcers
- Pancreatic cholera
- Ulcerative colitis

Respiratory
- Asthma (controlled study did not support)
- Cystic fibrosis

Other
- Bovine spastic paresis

[a] All the uses listed here are experimental and do not have FDA approved labeling. There are conflicting reports about many of these uses—some have negative findings in controlled studies, and a few involve reports of possible adverse effects.

L-Dopa, levodopa; FDA, Food and Drug Administration.

pharmacologic interventions to counteract unwanted effects when they occur. The most common adverse effects are summarized in Table 36.20–3. Patient education can play an important role in reducing the incidence and severity of side effects. Patients taking lithium should be advised that changes in the body's water and salt content can affect the amount of lithium excreted, resulting in either increases or decreases in lithium concentrations.

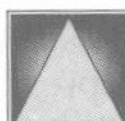

Table 36.20–3
Adverse Effects of Lithium

Neurologic
- Benign, nontoxic: dysphoria, lack of spontaneity, slowed reaction time, memory difficulties
- Tremor: postural, occasional extrapyramidal
- Toxic: coarse tremor, dysarthria, ataxia, neuromuscular irritability, seizures, coma, death
- Miscellaneous: peripheral neuropathy, benign intracranial hypertension, myasthenia gravis-like syndrome, altered creativity, lowered seizure threshold

Endocrine
- Thyroid: goiter, hypothyroidism, exophthalmos, hyperthyroidism (rare)
- Parathyroid: hyperparathyroidism, adenoma

Cardiovascular
- Benign T-wave changes, sinus node dysfunction

Renal
- Concentrating defect, morphologic changes, polyuria (nephrogenic diabetes insipidus), reduced GFR, nephrotic syndrome, renal tubular acidosis

Dermatologic
- Acne, hair loss, psoriasis, rash

Gastrointestinal
- Appetite loss, nausea, vomiting, diarrhea

Miscellaneous
- Altered carbohydrate metabolism, weight gain, fluid retention

GFR, glomerular filtration rate.

Excessive sodium intake (e.g., a dramatic dietary change) lowers lithium concentrations. Conversely, too little sodium (e.g., fad diets) can lead to potentially toxic concentrations of lithium. Decreases in body fluid (e.g., excessive perspiration) can lead to dehydration and lithium intoxication. Patients should report whenever medications are prescribed by another clinician, because many commonly used agents can affect lithium concentrations.

Gastrointestinal Effects

Gastrointestinal (GI) symptoms—which include nausea, decreased appetite, vomiting, and diarrhea—can be diminished by dividing the dosage, administering the lithium with food, or switching to another lithium preparation. The lithium preparation least likely to cause diarrhea is lithium citrate. Some lithium preparations contain lactose, which can cause diarrhea in lactose-intolerant persons. Persons taking slow-release formulations of lithium who experience diarrhea because of unabsorbed medication in the lower part of the GI tract may experience less diarrhea than with standard-release preparations. Diarrhea may also respond to antidiarrheal preparations such as loperamide (Imodium, Kaopectate), bismuth subsalicylate (Pepto-Bismol), or diphenoxylate with atropine (Lomotil).

Weight Gain

Weight gain results from a poorly understood effect of lithium on carbohydrate metabolism. Weight gain can also result from lithium-induced hypothyroidism, lithium-induced edema, or excessive consumption of soft drinks and juices to quench lithium-induced thirst.

Neurologic Effects

Tremor. A lithium-induced postural tremor can occur that is usually 8 to 12 Hz and is most notable in outstretched hands, especially in the fingers, and during tasks involving fine manipulations. The tremor can be reduced by dividing the daily dosage, using a sustained-release formulation, reducing caffeine intake, reassessing the concomitant use of other medicines, and treating comorbid anxiety. β-adrenergic receptor antagonists, such as propranolol, 30 to 120 mg a day in divided doses, and primidone (Mysoline), 50 to 250 mg a day, are usually effective in reducing the tremor. In persons with hypokalemia, potassium supplementation may improve the tremor. When a person taking lithium has a severe tremor, the possibility of lithium toxicity should be suspected and evaluated.

Cognitive Effects. Lithium use has been associated with dysphoria, lack of spontaneity, slowed reaction times, and impaired memory. The presence of these symptoms should be noted carefully, because they are a frequent cause of noncompliance. The differential diagnosis for such symptoms should include depressive disorders, hypothyroidism, hypercalcemia, other illnesses, and other drugs. Some, but not all, persons have reported that fatigue and mild cognitive impairment decrease with time.

Other Neurologic Effects. Uncommon neurologic adverse effects include symptoms of mild parkinsonism, ataxia, and dysarthria, although the latter two symptoms may also be caused by lithium intoxication. Lithium is rarely associated with development of peripheral neuropathy, benign intracranial hypertension (pseudotumor cerebri), findings resembling myasthenia gravis, and increased risk of seizures.

Renal Effects

The most common adverse renal effect of lithium is polyuria with secondary polydipsia. The symptom is particularly a problem in 25 percent to 35 percent of persons taking lithium who may have a urine output of more than 3 L a day (normal, 1 to 2 L a day). The polyuria primarily results from lithium antagonism to the effects of antidiuretic hormone, which thus causes diuresis. When polyuria is a significant problem, the person's renal function should be evaluated and followed up with 24-hour urine collections for creatinine clearance determinations. Treatment consists of fluid replacement, the use of the lowest effective dosage of lithium, and single daily dosing of lithium. Treatment can also involve the use of a thiazide or potassium-sparing diuretic—for example, amiloride (Midamor), spironolactone (Aldactone), triamterene (Dyrenium), or amiloride-hydrochlorothiazide (Moduretic). If treatment with a diuretic is initiated, the lithium dosage should be halved, and the diuretic should not be started for 5 days because the diuretic is likely to increase lithium retention.

The most serious renal adverse effects, which are rare and associated with continuous lithium administration for 10 years or more, involve appearance of nonspecific interstitial fibrosis, associated with gradual decreases in glomerular filtration rate and increases in serum creatinine concentrations, and rarely with renal failure. Lithium occasionally is associated with nephrotic syndrome and features of distal renal tubular acidosis. It is prudent for persons taking lithium to check their serum creatinine concentration, urine chemistries, and 24-hour urine volume at 6-month intervals.

A 62-year-old man, successfully stabilized on lithium for 27 years, experienced a gradual increase in serum creatinine to 3.6 mg/dL (range of normal, 0.6 to 1.3 mg/dL). A thorough evaluation by a nephrologist produced no other explanation, and lithium was felt to be the most likely cause. (Courtesy of James W. Jefferson, M.D., and John H. Greist, M.D.)

Thyroid Effects

Lithium causes a generally benign and often transient diminution in the concentrations of circulating thyroid hormones. Reports have attributed goiter (5 percent of persons), benign reversible exophthalmos, hyperthyroidism, and hypothyroidism (7 percent to 10 percent of persons) to lithium treatment. Lithium-induced hypothyroidism is more common in women (14 percent) than in men (4.5 percent). Women are at highest risk during the first 2 years of treatment. Persons taking lithium to treat bipolar disorder are twice as likely to develop hypothyroidism if they develop rapid cycling. About 50 percent of persons receiving long-term lithium treatment have laboratory abnormalities, such as an abnormal thyrotropin-releasing hormone (TRH) response, and about 30 percent have elevated concentrations of thyroid-stimulating hormone (TSH). If symptoms of hypothyroidism are present, replacement with levothyroxine (Synthroid) is indicated. Even in the absence of hypothyroid symptoms, some clinicians treat persons with significantly elevated TSH concentrations with levothyroxine. In lithium-treated persons, TSH concentrations should be measured every 6 to 12 months. Lithium-induced hypothyroidism should be considered when evaluating depressive episodes that emerge during lithium therapy.

Cardiac Effects

The cardiac effects of lithium resemble those of hypokalemia on the electrocardiogram (ECG). They are caused by the displacement of intracellular potassium by the lithium ion. The most common changes on the ECG are T-wave flattening or inversion. The changes are benign and disappear after the lithium is excreted from the body.

Lithium depresses the pacemaking activity of the sinus node, sometimes resulting in sinus dysrhythmias, heart block, and episodes of syncope. Lithium treatment, therefore, is contraindicated in persons with sick sinus syndrome. In rare cases, ventricular arrhythmias and congestive heart failure have been associated with lithium therapy. Lithium cardiotoxicity is more prevalent in persons on a low-salt diet, those taking certain diuretics or angiotensin-converting enzyme (ACE) inhibitors, and those with fluid-electrolyte imbalances or any renal insufficiency.

Dermatologic Effects

Dermatologic effects may be dose dependent. They include acneiform, follicular and maculopapular eruptions; pretibial ulcerations; and worsening of psoriasis. Occasionally, aggravated psoriasis or acneiform eruptions may force the discontinuation of lithium treatment. Alopecia has also been reported. Many of those conditions respond favorably to changing to another lithium preparation and the usual dermatologic measures. Lithium concentrations should be monitored if tetracycline is used for the treatment of acne, because it can increase lithium retention.

Lithium Toxicity and Overdoses

The early signs and symptoms of lithium toxicity include neurologic symptoms, such as coarse tremor, dysarthria, and ataxia; GI symptoms; cardiovascular changes; and renal dysfunction. The later signs and symptoms include impaired consciousness, muscular fasciculations, myoclonus, seizures, and coma. Signs and symptoms of lithium toxicity are outlined in Table 36.20–4. Risk factors include exceeding the recommended dosage, renal impairment, low-sodium diet, drug interaction, and dehydration. Elderly persons are more vulnerable to the effects of increased serum lithium concentrations. The greater the degree and duration of elevated lithium concentrations are, the worse are the symptoms of lithium toxicity.

Lithium toxicity is a medical emergency, potentially causing permanent neuronal damage and death. In cases of toxicity (Table 36.20–5), lithium should be stopped and dehydration treated. Unabsorbed lithium can be removed from the GI tract by ingestion of polystyrene sulfonate (Kayexalate) or polyethylene glycol solution (GoLYTELY) but not activated charcoal. Ingestion of a single large dose may create clumps of medication in the stomach, which can be removed by gastric lavage with a wide-bore tube. The value of forced diuresis is still debated. In severe cases, hemodialysis rapidly removes excessive amounts of serum lithium. Postdialysis serum lithium concentrations may rise as lithium is redistributed from tissues to blood, so repeat dialysis may be needed. Neurologic improvement may lag behind clearance of serum lithium by several days, because lithium crosses the blood–brain barrier slowly.

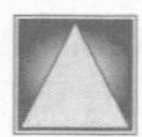

Table 36.20–4
Signs and Symptoms of Lithium Toxicity

Mild to moderate intoxication (lithium level = 1.5 to 2.0 mEq/L)	
GI	Vomiting
	Abdominal pain
	Dryness of mouth
Neurologic	Ataxia
	Dizziness
	Slurred speech
	Nystagmus
	Lethargy or excitement
	Muscle weakness
Moderate to severe intoxication (lithium level = 2.0 to 2.5 mEq/L)	
GI	Anorexia
	Persistent nausea and vomiting
Neurologic	Blurred vision
	Muscle fasciculations
	Clonic limb movements
	Hyperactive deep tendon reflexes
	Choreoathetoid movements
	Convulsions
	Delirium
	Syncope
	Electroencephalographic changes
	Stupor
	Coma
	Circulatory failure (lowered BP, cardiac arrhythmias, and conduction abnormalities)
Severe lithium intoxication (lithium level >2.5 mEq/L)	
Generalized convulsions	
Oliguria and renal failure	
Death	

GI, gastrointestinal; BP, blood pressure.
(From Marangell LB, Silver JM, Yudofsky SC. Psychopharmacology and electroconvulsive therapy. In: *The American Psychiatric Press Textbook of Psychiatry.* 3rd ed. Washington, DC: American Psychiatric Press, 1999, with permission.)

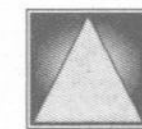

Table 36.20–5
Management of Lithium Toxicity

1. The patient should immediately contact his or her personal physician or go to a hospital emergency room.
2. Lithium should be discontinued and the patient instructed to ingest fluids, if possible.
3. Physical examination should be completed, including vital signs and a neurologic examination with complete formal mental status examination.
4. Lithium level, serum electrolytes, renal function tests, and ECG should be obtained as soon as possible.
5. For significant acute ingestion, residual gastric contents should be removed by induction of emesis, gastric lavage, and absorption with activated charcoal.
6. Vigorous hydration and maintenance of electrolyte balance are essential.
7. For any patient with a serum lithium level greater than 4.0 mEq/L or with serious manifestations of lithium toxicity, hemodialysis should be initiated.
8. Repeat dialysis may be required every 6 to 10 hours, until the lithium level is within nontoxic range and the patient has no signs or symptoms of lithium toxicity.

ECG, electrocardiogram.
(From Marangell LB, Silver JM, Yudofsky SC. Psychopharmacology and electroconvulsive therapy. In: *The American Psychiatric Press Textbook of Psychiatry.* 3rd ed. Washington, DC: American Psychiatric Press, 1999, with permission.)

Adolescents

The serum lithium concentrations for adolescents are similar to that for adults. Weight gain and acne associated with lithium use can be particularly troublesome to an adolescent.

Elderly Persons

Lithium is a safe and effective drug for the elderly. Treatment of elderly persons taking lithium may be complicated, however, by the presence of other medical illnesses, decreased renal function, special diets that affect lithium clearance, and generally increased sensitivity to lithium. Elderly persons should initially be given low dosages, their dosages should be switched less frequently than are those of younger persons, and a longer time must be allowed for renal excretion to equilibrate with absorption before lithium can be assumed to have reached its steady-state concentrations.

A 60-year-old man was treated with 900 mg a day of lithium carbonate. The dosage was continued unchanged for 10 years, despite laboratory evidence of gradually increasing serum lithium and creatinine concentrations. Even as the clinical symptoms of toxicity were being reported, a thiazide diuretic was added to treat hypertension. Three weeks later, the patient was hospitalized with a serum lithium concentration of 4.2 mEq/L and marked neurological impairment that never fully resolved. (Courtesy of James W. Jefferson, M.D., and John H. Greist, M.D.)

Pregnant Women

Lithium should not be administered to pregnant women in the first trimester because of the risk of birth defects. The most common malformations involve the cardiovascular system, most commonly Ebstein's anomaly of the tricuspid valves. The risk of Ebstein's malformation in lithium-exposed fetuses is 1 of 1,000, which is 20 times the risk in the general population. The possibility of fetal cardiac anomalies can be evaluated with fetal echocardiography. The teratogenic risk of lithium (4 percent to 12 percent) is higher than that for the general population (2 percent to 3 percent), but appears to be lower than that associated with use of valproate or carbamazepine. A woman who continues to take lithium during pregnancy should use the lowest effective dosage. The maternal lithium concentration must be monitored closely during pregnancy and especially after pregnancy, because of the significant decrease in renal lithium excretion as renal function returns to normal in the first few days after delivery. Adequate hydration can reduce the risk of lithium toxicity during labor. Lithium prophylaxis is recommended for all women with bipolar disorder as they enter the postpartum period. Lithium is excreted into breast milk and should be taken by a nursing mother only after careful evaluation of potential risks and benefits. Signs of lithium toxicity in infants include lethargy, cyanosis, abnormal reflexes, and sometimes hepatomegaly.

Miscellaneous Effects

Lithium should be used with caution in diabetic persons, who should monitor their blood glucose concentrations carefully to avoid diabetic ketoacidosis. Benign, reversible leukocytosis is commonly associated with lithium treatment. Dehydrated, debilitated, and medically ill persons are most susceptible to adverse effects and toxicity.

DRUG INTERACTIONS

Lithium drug interactions are summarized in Table 36.20–6.

Lithium is commonly used in conjunction with DRAs. This combination is typically effective and safe. Coadministration of higher dosages of a DRA and lithium may, however, result in a synergistic increase in the symptoms of lithium-induced neurologic side effects and neuroleptic extrapyramidal symptoms. In rare instances, encephalopathy has been reported with this combination.

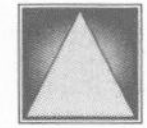

Table 36.20–6
Drug Interactions with Lithium

Drug Class	Reaction
Antipsychotics	Case reports of encephalopathy, worsening of extrapyramidal adverse effects, and neuroleptic malignant syndrome; inconsistent reports of altered red blood cell and plasma concentrations of lithium, antipsychotic drug, or both
Antidepressants	Occasional reports of a serotonin-like syndrome with potent serotonin reuptake inhibitors
Anticonvulsants	No significant pharmacokinetic interactions with carbamazepine or valproate; reports of neurotoxicity with carbamazepine; combinations helpful for treatment resistance
NSAIDs	May reduce renal lithium clearance and increase serum concentration; toxicity reported (exception is aspirin)
Diuretics	
Thiazides	Well-documented reduced renal lithium clearance and increased serum concentration; toxicity reported
Potassium sparing	Limited data, may increase lithium concentration
Loop	Lithium clearance unchanged (some case reports of increased lithium concentration)
Osmotic (mannitol, urea)	Increase renal lithium clearance and decrease lithium concentration
Xanthine (aminophylline, caffeine, theophylline)	Increase renal lithium clearance and decrease lithium concentration
Carbonic anhydrase inhibitors (acetazolamide)	Increase renal lithium clearance
ACE inhibitors	Reports of reduced lithium clearance, increased concentrations, and toxicity
Calcium channel inhibitors	Case reports of neurotoxicity; no consistent pharmacokinetic interactions
Miscellaneous	
Succinylcholine, pancuronium	Reports of prolonged neuromuscular blockade
Metronidazole	Increased lithium concentration
Methyldopa	Few reports of neurotoxicity
Sodium bicarbonate	Increased renal lithium clearance
Iodides	Additive antithyroid effects
Propranolol	Used for lithium tremor; possible slight increase in lithium concentration

NSAID, nonsteroidal anti-inflammatory drug; ACE, angiotensin-converting enzyme.

The coadministration of lithium and carbamazepine, lamotrigine, valproate, and clonazepam may increase lithium concentrations and aggravate lithium-induced neurologic adverse effects. Treatment with the combination should be initiated at slightly lower dosages than usual, and the dosages should be increased gradually. Changes from one to another treatment for mania should be made carefully, with as little temporal overlap between the drugs as possible.

Most diuretics (e.g., thiazide and potassium sparing) can increase lithium concentrations; when treatment with such a diuretic is stopped, the clinician may need to increase the person's daily lithium dosage. Osmotic and loop diuretics, carbonic anhydrase inhibitors, and xanthines (including caffeine) can reduce lithium concentrations to below therapeutic concentrations. ACE inhibitors can cause an increase in lithium concentrations, whereas the AT_1 angiotensin II receptor inhibitors losartan (Cozaar) and irbesartan (Avapro) do not alter lithium concentrations. A wide range of nonsteroidal anti-inflammatory drugs (NSAIDs) can decrease lithium clearance, thereby increasing lithium concentrations. These drugs include indomethacin (Indocin), phenylbutazone (Azolid), diclofenac (Voltaren), ketoprofen (Orudis), oxyphenbutazone (Oxalid), ibuprofen (Motrin, Advil), piroxicam (Feldene), and naproxen (Naprosyn). Aspirin and sulindac (Clinoril) do not affect lithium concentrations.

The coadministration of lithium and quetiapine (Seroquel) can cause somnolence, but is otherwise well tolerated. The coadministration of lithium and ziprasidone (Geodon) may modestly increase the incidence of tremor. The coadministration of lithium and calcium channel inhibitors should be avoided because of potentially fatal neurotoxicity.

A person taking lithium who is about to undergo ECT should discontinue taking lithium 2 days before beginning ECT to reduce the risk of delirium.

LABORATORY INTERFERENCES

Lithium does not interfere with any laboratory tests, but lithium-induced alterations include increased white blood cell (WBC) count, decreased serum thyroxine, and increased serum calcium. Blood collected in a lithium–heparin anticoagulant tube will produce falsely elevated lithium concentrations.

DOSAGE AND CLINICAL GUIDELINES

Initial Medical Workup

All patients should have a routine laboratory workup and physical examination before being started on lithium. The laboratory tests should include serum creatinine concentration (or a 24-hour urine creatinine if the clinician has any reason to be concerned about renal function), electrolytes, thyroid function (TSH, T_3, and T_4), a complete blood count (CBC), ECG, and a pregnancy test in women of child-bearing age.

Dosage Recommendations

Table 36.20–7 lists the lithium preparations available in the United States. Lithium formulations include immediate-release 150-, 300-, and 600-mg lithium carbonate capsules (Eskalith and generic), 300-mg lithium carbonate tablets (Lithotabs), 450-mg controlled-release lithium carbonate capsules (Eskalith CR and Lithonate), and 8 mEq/5 mL of lithium citrate syrup.

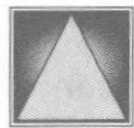

Table 36.20–7
Lithium Preparations Available in the United States

Lithium carbonate capsules	150, 300, 600 mg
Lithium carbonate tablets	300 mg
Lithium carbonate controlled-release tablets	450 mg
Lithium carbonate slow-release tablets	300 mg
Lithium citrate syrup	8 mEq/5 mL

The starting dosage for most adults is 300 mg of the regular-release formulation three times daily. The starting dosage for elderly persons or persons with renal impairment should be 300 mg once or twice daily. After stabilization, dosages between 900 and 1,200 mg a day usually produce a therapeutic plasma concentration of 0.6 to 1 mEq/L, and a daily dose of 1,200 to 1,800 mg usually produces a therapeutic concentration of 0.8 to 1.2 mEq/L. Maintenance dosing can be given either in two or three divided doses of the regular-release formulation or in a single dosage of the sustained-release formulation equivalent to the combined daily dosage of the regular-release formulation. The use of divided doses reduces gastric upset and avoids single high-peak lithium concentrations. Discontinuation of lithium should be gradual to minimize the risk of early recurrence of mania and also to permit recognition of early signs of recurrence.

Laboratory Monitoring

Regular monitoring of serum lithium concentrations is essential. Lithium levels should be obtained every 2 to 6 months, except when signs of toxicity are seen, during dosage adjustments, and in persons suspected to be noncompliant with the prescribed dosages. Baseline ECGs are essential and should be repeated annually.

When obtaining blood for lithium levels, patients should be at steady-state lithium dosing (usually after 5 days of constant dosing), preferably using a twice- or three-times daily dosing regimen, and the blood sample must be drawn 12 hours (±30 minutes) after a given dose. Lithium concentrations 12 hours postdose in persons treated with sustained-release preparations are generally about 30 percent higher than the corresponding concentrations obtained from those taking the regular-release preparations. Because available data are based on a sample population following a multiple-dosage regimen, regular-release formulations given at least twice daily should be used for initial determination of the appropriate dosages. Factors that can cause fluctuations in lithium measurements include dietary sodium intake, mood state, activity level, body position, and use of an improper blood sample tube.

Laboratory values that do not seem to correspond to clinical status may result from the collection of blood in a tube with a lithium–heparin anticoagulant (which can give results falsely elevated by as much as 1 mEq/L) or aging of the lithium ion-selective electrode (which can cause inaccuracies of up to 0.5 mEq/L). Once the daily dose has been set, it is reasonable to change to the sustained-release formulation given once daily.

Effective serum concentrations for mania are 1.0 to 1.5 mEq/L, a level associated with 1,800 mg a day. The recommended range for maintenance treatment is 0.4 to 0.8 mEq/L,

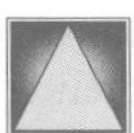

Table 36.20–8
Instructions to Patients Taking Lithium

Lithium can be remarkably effective in treating your disorder. If not used appropriately and not monitored closely, it can be ineffective and potentially harmful. It is important to keep the following instructions in mind.

Dosing

Take lithium exactly as directed by your doctor—never take more or less than the prescribed dose.

Do not stop taking without speaking to your doctor.

If you miss a dose, take it as soon as is possible. If it is within 4 hours of the next dose, skip the missed dose (about 6 hours in the case of extended- or slow-release preparations). Never double up doses.

Blood Tests

Comply with the schedule of recommended regular blood tests.

Despite their inconvenience and discomfort, your lithium blood levels, thyroid function, and kidney status need to be monitored as long as you take lithium.

When going to have lithium levels checked, you should have taken your last lithium dose 12 hours earlier.

Use of Other Medications

Do not start any prescription or over-the-counter medications without telling your doctor.

Even drugs such as ibuprofen (Advil, Motrin) or naproxen (Aleve) can significantly raise lithium levels.

Diet and Fluid Intake

Avoid sudden changes in your diet or fluid intake. If you do go on a diet, your doctor may need to increase the frequency of blood tests.

Caffeine and alcohol act as diuretics and can lower your lithium concentrations.

During treatment with lithium, it is recommended that you drink about 2 or 3 quarts of fluid daily, and use normal amounts of salt.

Inform your doctor if you start or stop a low-salt diet.

Recognizing Potential Problems

If you engage in vigorous exercise or have an illness that causes sweating, vomiting, or diarrhea, consult your doctor, because these might affect lithium levels.

Nausea, constipation, shakiness, increased thirst, frequency of urination, weight gain, or swelling of the extremities should be reported to your doctor.

Blurred vision, confusion, loss of appetite, diarrhea, vomiting, muscle weakness, lethargy, shakiness, slurred speech, dizziness, loss of balance, inability to urinate, or seizures could indicate severe toxicity, and should prompt immediate medical attention.

which is usually achieved with a daily dose of 900 to 1,200 mg. A few persons will not achieve therapeutic benefit with a lithium concentration of 1.5 mEq/L yet will have no signs of toxicity. For such persons, titration of the lithium dosage to achieve a concentration above 1.5 mEq/L may be warranted. Some patients can be maintained at concentrations below 0.4 mEq/L. Considerable variation is seen from patient to patient, so it is best to follow the maxim "treat the patient, not the laboratory results." The only way to establish an optimal dose for a patient may be through trial and error.

If no response occurs after 2 weeks at a concentration that is beginning to cause adverse effects, then the person should taper off lithium use over 1 to 2 weeks and should try other mood-stabilizing drugs.

Patient Education

Lithium has a narrow therapeutic index and many factor
upset the balance between lithium concentrations that are
tolerated and produce therapeutic benefit and those that pro
side effects or toxicity. Thus, it is imperative that persons
ing lithium be educated about signs and symptoms of toxi
factors that affect lithium levels, how and when to obtain lab
tory testing, and the importance of regular communication w
the prescribing physician. Common factors, such as excess
sweating caused by ambient heat or exercise or use of wid
prescribed agents, such as ACE inhibitors or NSAIDs, can s
riously disrupt lithium concentrations. Patients may stop takin
their lithium because they are feeling well, or because they a
experiencing side effects. They should be advised against dis
continuing or modifying their lithium regimen. Table 36.20–
lists some important instructions for patients.

References

Bratti IM, Baldessarini RJ, Baethge C, Tondo L. Pretreatment episode count and response to lithium treatment in manic-depressive illness. *Harv Rev Psychiatry*. 2003;11:245.

Brunello N, Tascedda F. Cellular mechanisms and second messengers: relevance to the psychopharmacology of bipolar disorders. *Int J Neuropsychopharmacol*. 2003;6:181.

Geddes JR, Burgess S, Hawton K, Jamison K, Goodwin GM. Long-term lithium therapy for bipolar disorder: Systematic review and metaanalysis of randomized controlled trials. *Am J Psychiatry*. 2004;161:217.

Goodwin FK, Fireman B, Simon GE, Hunkeler EM, Lee J, Revicki D. Suicide risk in bipolar disorder during treatment with lithium and divalproex. *JAMA*. 2003;290:1467.

Jefferson JW, Greist JH. Lithium. In: Sadock BJ, Sadock VA, eds. *Kaplan & Sadock's Comprehensive Textbook of Psychiatry*. 8th ed. Vol. 2. Baltimore: Lippincott Williams & Wilkins; 2005:2839.

▲ 36.21 Melatonin Agonists: Ramelteon and Melatonin

RAMELTEON (See also chapter 36.9)

Ramelteon (Rozerem) is a melatonin receptor agonist used to treat sleep onset insomnia. Unlike benzodiazepines, ramelteon has no appreciable affinity for the γ-aminobutyric acid (GABA) receptor complex.

Pharmacologic Actions

Ramelteon essentially mimics melatonin's sleep-promoting properties. It has high affinity for melatonin MT1 and MT2 receptors in the brain. These receptors are believed to be critical in the regulation of the body's sleep-wake cycle. Melatonin (N-acetyl-5 methoxytryptamine) is a hormone mainly produced at night in the pineal gland. Its secretion is stimulated by the dark and inhibited by light. It is naturally synthesized from the amino acid tryptophan. Tryptophan is converted to serotonin and finally converted to melatonin. The suprachiasmatic nuclei (SCN) of the hypothalamus have melatonin receptors and melatonin may have a direct action on SCN to influence "circadian" rhythms. These include jet lag and sleep disturbances. Melatonin is also produced in the retina and gastrointestinal (GI) tract.

ɔccurs between 30 and 90 minutes after in-
e of ramelteon is between 1 and 2.6 hours.

ndications

y shortens latency to sleep onset and, to a lesser total duration of sleep.

ls and animal studies failed to find evidence of nia or withdrawal effects.

ns and Adverse Events

s the most common side effect. Other adverse ef- nelteon may include somnolence, fatigue, dizziness, insomnia, depression, nausea, and diarrhea. This drug ɩt be used in patients with severe hepatic impairment. not recommended in patients with severe sleep apnea e chronic obstructive pulmonary disease (COPD).

ɩelteon has been found to sometimes decrease blood cor- nd testosterone and to raise prolactin. Female patients d be monitored for cessation of menses or galactorrhea, ased libido, or fertility problems. Safety and effectiveness melteon in children has not been established. Its use is not ɔmmended during lactation.

rug Interactions

CYP1A2 is the major isozyme involved in the hepatic metabolism of ramelteon. Accordingly, fluvoxamine (Luvox) and other CYP1A2 inhibitors may increase side effects of ramelteon.

Efficacy of ramelteon may be reduced when it is used in combination with potent CYP enzyme inducers, such as rifampin.

Rozerem should be administered with caution in patients taking other CYP1A2 inhibitors, strong CYP3A4 inhibitors such as, ketoconazole, and strong CYP2C9 inhibitors, such as fluconazole (Diflucan). No clinically meaningful interactions were found when ramelteon was coadministered with omeprazole, theophylline, dextromethorphan, midazolam, digoxin, and warfarin.

Dosage and Clinical Guidelines

The usual dose of ramelteon is 8 mg within 30 minutes of going to bed. It should not be taken with or immediately after high fat meals.

MELATONIN

Ingested melatonin has been shown to be capable of reaching and binding to melatonin binding sites in the brains of mammals, and to produce somnolence when used at higher doses. Accordingly, melatonin has become available as a dietary supplement. It is not a medication, however, and few well-controlled clinical trials have been conducted to determine its effectiveness in treating such conditions as insomnia, jet lag, and sleep disturbances related to shift work.

Melatonin can cause severe headaches, mental impairment, and mood changes. Melatonin concentrations are increased when taken in combination with monoamine oxidase inhibitors (MAOIs) because MAOIs inhibit the breakdown of melatonin by the body. Melatonin can suppress libido by inhibiting secretion of luteinizing hormone (LH) and follicle-stimulating hormone (FSH) from the anterior pituitary gland. Beta blockers may decrease nocturnal melatonin release. The elimination half life of melatonin is 32 to 40 minutes.

Over-the-counter melatonin is available in the following formulations: 1 mg, 2.5 mg, 3 mg, and 5 mg capsules; 1 mg/mL or 1 mg/4mL liquid; 0.5 mg and 3 mg lozenges; 2.5 mg sublingual tablets; 1 mg, 2 mg, and 3 mg timed-release tablets.

AGOMELATINE (VALDOXAN)

Agomelatine (Valdoxan) is structurally related to melatonin and is being investigated as a treatment of major depressive disorder. It acts as an agonist at melatonin (MT_1 and MT_2) receptors. It is also an antagonist at serotonin-2C ($5\text{-}HT_{2C}$) receptors. It is hypothesized that the antidepressant-like activity agomelatine most probably involves a combination of both its melatonin agonist and $5\text{-}HT_{2C}$ receptor antagonist properties. The effective dose in clinical trials is 25 mg/day. If found to be effective and safe, this compound could be very useful because sleep complaints are a feature of depression.

References

Bellon A. Searching for new options for treating insomnia: Are melatonin and ramelteon beneficial? *J Psychiatr Pract*. 2006 Jul;12(4):229–43.

Borja NL, Daniel KL. Ramelteon for the treatment of insomnia. *Clin Ther*. 2006;28(10):1540–55.

Cagnacci A, Cannoletta M, Renzi A, Baldassari F, Arangino S, Volpe A. Prolonged melatonin administration decreases nocturnal blood pressure in women. *Am J Hypertens*. 2005;18(12 Pt 1):1614–8.

Grossman E, Laudon M, Yalcin R, Zengil H, Peleg E, Sharabi Y, kamari Y, Shen-Orr Z, Zisapel N. Melatonin reduces night blood pressure in patients with nocturnal hypertension. *Am J Med*. 2006;119(10):898–902.

Johnson MW, Suess PE, Griffiths RR. Ramelteon: a novel hypnotic lacking abuse liability and sedative adverse effects. *Arch Gen Psychiatry*. 2006;63(10):1149–57.

Jung B, Ahmad N. Melatonin in cancer management: progress and promise. *Cancer Res*. 2006;66(20):9789–93.

Karim A, Tolbert D, Cao C. Disposition kinetics and tolerance of escalating single doses of ramelteon, a high-affinity MT1 and MT2 melatonin receptor agonist indicated for treatment of insomnia. *J Clin Pharmacol*. 2006;46(2):140–8.

Laustsen G, Andersen M. Ramelteon (rozerem) a novel approach for insomnia treatment. *Nurse Pract*. 2006;31(4):52–5.

Saha L, Malhotra S, Rana S, Bhasin D, Pandhi P. A preliminary study of melatonin in irritable bowel syndrome. *J Clin Gastroenterol*. 2007;41(1):29–32.

Thomas KA, Burr RL. Melatonin level and pattern in postpartum versus nonpregnant nulliparous women. *J Obstet Gynecol Neonatal Nurs*. 2006;35(5):608–15.

▲ 36.22 Mirtazapine

Mirtazapine (Remeron) is unique among drugs used to treat major depression in that it increases both norepinephrine and serotonin through a mechanism other than reuptake blockade (as in the case of tricyclic agents or selective serotonin reuptake inhibitors [SSRIs]) or monoamine oxidase inhibition (as in the case of phenelzine or tranylcypromine). Mirtazapine is also more likely to reduce rather than cause nausea and diarrhea, the result of its effects on serotonin $5\text{-}HT_3$ receptors. Characteristic side effects include increased appetite and sedation.

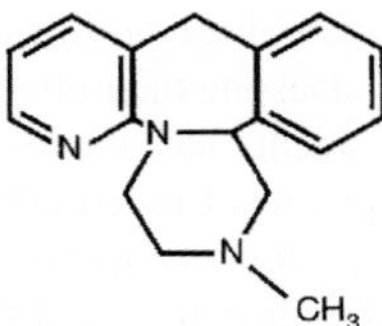

FIGURE 36.22–1
The molecular structure of mirtazapine.

CHEMISTRY

The molecular structure of mirtazapine is shown in Figure 36.22-1.

PHARMACOLOGIC ACTIONS

Mirtazapine is administered orally and is rapidly and completely absorbed. It has a half-life of about 30 hours. Peak concentration is achieved within 2 hours of ingestion and steady-state is reached after 6 days. Plasma clearance may be slowed up to 30 percent in persons with impaired hepatic function, up to 50 percent in those with impaired renal function, up to 40 percent slower in elderly males, and up to 10 percent slower in elderly females.

The mechanism of action of mirtazapine is antagonism of central presynaptic α_2-adrenergic receptors and blockade of postsynaptic serotonin 5-HT_2 and 5-HT_3 receptors. The α_2-adrenergic receptor antagonism causes increased firing of norepinephrine and serotonin neurons. The potent antagonist of serotonin 5-HT_2 and 5-HT_3 receptors serves to decrease anxiety, relieve insomnia, and stimulate appetite. Mirtazapine is a potent antagonist of histamine H_1 receptors and is a moderately potent antagonist at α_1-adrenergic and muscarinic-cholinergic receptors.

THERAPEUTIC INDICATIONS

Mirtazapine is effective for the treatment of depression. It is highly sedating, making it a reasonable choice for use in depressed patients with severe or long-standing insomnia. Some patients find the residual daytime sedation associated with initiation of treatment to be quite pronounced. The more extreme sedating properties of the drug generally lessen over the first week of treatment. Combined with the tendency to cause a sometimes ravenous appetite, mirtazapine is well suited for depressed patients with melancholic features such as insomnia, weight loss, and agitation. Elderly depressed patients, in particular, are good candidates for mirtazapine, whereas young adults are more likely to object to this side-effect profile.

Mirtazapine's blockade of 5-HT_3 receptors, a mechanism associated with medications used to combat the severe gastrointestinal (GI) side effects of cancer chemotherapy agents, has led to use of the drug in a similar role. In this population, sedation and stimulation of appetite clearly could be seen as being beneficial, instead of unwelcome side effects.

Mirtazapine is often combined with SSRIs or venlafaxine (Effexor) to augment antidepressant response or counteract serotonergic side effects of those drugs, particularly nausea, agitation, and insomnia. Mirtazapine has no significant pharmacokinetic interactions with other antidepressants.

PRECAUTIONS AND ADVERSE REACTIO

Somnolence, the most common adverse effect of mirtaz
occurs in over 50 percent of persons (Table 36.22–1). Pe
starting mirtazapine, thus, should exercise caution when dr
or operating dangerous machinery, or even when getting o
bed at night. This adverse effect is why mirtazapine is al
always given before sleep. Mirtazapine potentiates the seda
effects of other central nervous system (CNS) depressants
potentially sedating prescription or over-the-counter drugs
alcohol should be avoided during use of mirtazapine. Mirta
pine also causes dizziness in 7 percent of persons. It does n
appear to increase the risk for seizures. Mania or hypoman
occurred in clinical trials at a rate similar to that of other antid
pressant drugs.

Mirtazapine increases appetite in about one third of patients
Mirtazapine may also increase serum cholesterol concentratio
to 20 percent or more above the upper limit of normal in 15
percent of persons and increase triglycerides to 500 mg/dL or more in 6 percent of persons. Elevations of alanine transaminase (ALT) levels to more than three times the upper limit of normal were seen in 2 percent of mirtazapine-treated persons, as opposed to 0.3 percent of placebo controls.

In limited premarketing experience, the absolute neutrophil count dropped to 500/mm^3 or less within 2 months of onset of use in 0.3 percent of persons, some of whom developed symptomatic infections. This hematologic condition, which was reversible in all cases, was more likely to occur when other risk factors for neutropenia were present. Increases in the frequency of neutropenia, however, have not been reported during the extensive postmarketing period. Persons who develop fever, chills, sore throat, mucous membrane ulceration, or other signs of infection should nevertheless be evaluated medically. If a low white blood cell (WBC) count is found, mirtazapine should be immediately discontinued, and the infectious disease status should be followed closely.

A few persons experience orthostatic hypotension while taking mirtazapine. Although no data exist regarding effects on fetal development, mirtazapine should be used with caution during pregnancy.

Mirtazapine use by pregnant women has not been studied; because the drug may be excreted in breast milk, it should not be taken by nursing mothers. Because of the risk of agranulocytosis associated with mirtazapine use, persons should be attuned to signs of infection, as discussed above. Because of the sedating effects of mirtazapine, persons should determine the degree

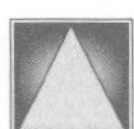

Table 36.22–1
Adverse Reactions Reported with Mirtazapine

Event	Percentage (%)
Somnolence	54
Dry mouth	25
Increased appetite	17
Constipation	13
Weight gain	12
Dizziness	7
Myalgias	5
Disturbing dreams	4

:ted before engaging in driving or other activities.

CTIONS

tentiate the sedation of alcohol and benzodi- ›ine should not be used within 14 days of use ›xidase inhibitor.

RY INTERFERENCES

nterferences have yet been described for mirtaza-

AND ADMINISTRATION

e is available in 15-, 30-, and 45-mg scored tablets. ıe is also available in 15-, 30- and 45-mg orally dis- g tablets for persons who have difficulty swallowing ›ersons fail to respond to the initial dose of 15 mg of ›ine before sleep, the dosage may be increased in 15-mg ents every 5 days to a maximum of 45 mg before sleep. dosages may be necessary in elderly persons or persons ·enal or hepatic insufficiency.

FERENCES

bek N, Kargili A, Akcay A, Kaya A. Recurrent hyponatremia associated with :italopram and mirtazapine. *Am J Kidney Dis.* 2006;48(4):e61–2.

ıvidson JR, Weisler RH, Butterfield MI, Casat CD, Connor KM, Barnett S, van Meter S. Mirtazapine vs. placebo in posttraumatic stress disorder: A pilot trial. *Biol Psychiatry.* 2003;53:188.

Djulus J, Koren G, Einarson TR, Wilton L, Shakir S, Diav-Citrin O, Kennedy D, Voyer Lavigne S, De Santis M, Einarson A. Exposure to mirtazapine during pregnancy: a prospective, comparative study of birth outcomes. *J Clin Psychiatry.* 2006;67(8):1280–4.

Kirkton C, McIntyre IM. Therapeutic and toxic concentrations of mirtazapine. *J Anal Toxicol.* 2006;30(9):687–91.

Kim SW, Shin IS, Kim JM, Kang HC, Mun JU, Yang SJ, Yoon JS. Mirtazapine for severe gastroparesis unresponsive to conventional prokinetic treatment. *Psychosomatics.* 2006;47(5):440–2.

Kim SW, Shin IS, Kim JM, Lim SY, Yang SJ, Yoon JS. Mirtazapine treatment for pathological laughing and crying after stroke. *Clin Neuropharmacol.* 2005;28(5):249–51.

Laimer M, Kramer-Reinstadler K, Rauchenzauner M, Lechner-Schoner T, Strauss R, Engl J, Deisenhammer EA, Hinterhuber H, Patsch JR, Ebenbichler CF. Effect of mirtazapine treatment on body composition and metabolism. *J Clin Psychiatry.* 2006;67(3):421–4.

Norman TR. Mechanism of action of mirtazapine: Dual action or dual effect? *Aust N Z J Psychiatry.* 2004;38(4):267–269.

Prospero-Garcia KA, Torres-Ruiz A, Ramirez-Bermudez J, Velazquez-Moctezuma J, Arana-Lechuga Y, Teran-Perez G. Fluoxetine-mirtazapine interaction may induce restless legs syndrome: report of 3 cases from a clinical trial. *J Clin Psychiatry.* 2006;67(11):1820.

Thase ME. Mirtazapine. In: Sadock BJ, Sadock VA, eds. *Kaplan & Sadock's Comprehensive Textbook of Psychiatry.* 8th ed. Vol 2. Philadelphia: Lippincott Williams & Wilkins; 2005:2851.

▲ 36.23 Monoamine Oxidase Inhibitors

The monoamine oxidase inhibitors (MAOIs), which were introduced as antidepressants in 1957, are effective in treating both depression and panic disorder. The first of these drugs were hydrazine derivatives developed as treatments for tuberculosis. Their antidepressant properties were discovered by chance, when some of the patients were observed to experience elevation of mood during treatment. Despite their effectiveness, prescription of MAOIs as first-line agents has always been limited by concern about the development of potentially lethal hypertension and the consequent need for a restrictive diet. Use of MAOIs declined further after the introduction of the selective serotonin reuptake inhibitors (SSRIs) and other new agents. They are now mainly relegated to use in treatment-resistant cases. Thus, the second-line status of MAOIs has less to do with considerations of efficacy than with concerns for safety. The currently available MAOIs include phenelzine (Nardil), isocarboxazid (Marplan), tranylcypromine (Parnate), and selegiline (Eldepryl). Oral Selegiline is a selective inhibitor of MAO_B used for the treatment of parkinsonism. A transdermal delivery system to administer selegiline has been developed for use as an antidepressant. Reversible inhibitors of MAO_A (RIMAs), which are not available in the United States (e.g., moclobemide [Manerix] and befloxatone), require few dietary restrictions.

CHEMISTRY

Isocarboxazid and phenelzine are derivatives of hydrazine, whereas tranylcypromine is structurally similar to amphetamine. The molecular structures of phenelzine, isocarboxazid, tranylcypromine, and moclobemide are shown in Figure 36.23–1.

PHARMACOLOGIC ACTIONS

Phenelzine, tranylcypromine, and isocarboxazid are readily absorbed after oral administration and reach peak plasma concentrations within 2 hours. Their plasma half-lives are in the range of 2 to 3 hours, whereas their tissue half-lives are considerably longer. Because they irreversibly inactivate MAOs, the

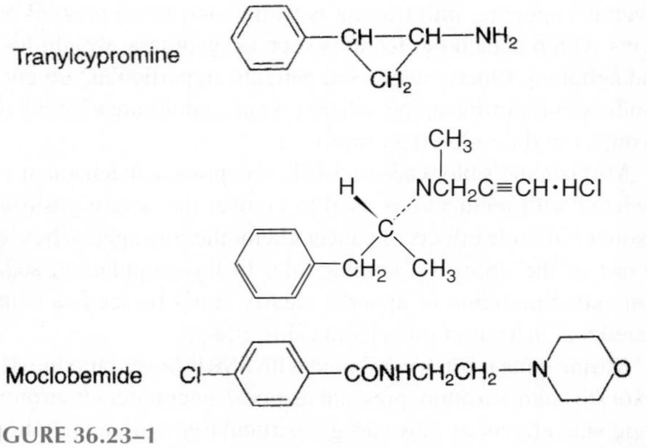

FIGURE 36.23–1
Molecular structure of monoamine oxidase inhibitors (MAOIs) used in psychiatry.

therapeutic effect of a single dose of irreversible MAOIs may persist for as long as 2 weeks. The RIMA moclobemide is rapidly absorbed and has a half-life of 0.5 to 3.5 hours. Because it is a reversible inhibitor, moclobemide has a much briefer clinical effect following a single dose than do irreversible MAOIs.

The MAO enzymes are found on the outer membranes of mitochondria where they degrade cytoplasmic and extraneuronal monoamine neurotransmitters, such as norepinephrine, serotonin, dopamine, epinephrine, and tyramine. MAOIs act in the central nervous system (CNS), the sympathetic nervous system, the liver, and the gastrointestinal (GI) tract. The two types of MAOs are MAO_A and MAO_B. MAO_A primarily metabolizes norepinephrine, serotonin, and epinephrine; dopamine and tyramine are metabolized by both MAO_A and MAO_B.

THERAPEUTIC INDICATIONS

The MAOIs are used to treat depression. Some research indicates that phenelzine is more effective than tricyclic antidepressants (TCAs) in depressed patients with mood reactivity, extreme sensitivity to interpersonal loss or rejection, prominent anergia, hyperphagia, and hypersomnia—a constellation of symptoms conceptualized as atypical depression. Evidence also indicates that MAOIs are more effective than TCAs as a treatment for bipolar depression.

A 38-year-old divorced mother of two teenage daughters presented at the Mood Disorders Clinic with a history of failed antidepressant treatment trials. Two years earlier, she had become increasingly irritable, exhausted, and tearful after the breakup of her marriage. She could not tolerate fluoxetine (Prozac) or sertraline (Zoloft) and discontinued each of these SSRIs after only a few days because of GI symptoms. Although she could tolerate desipramine (Norpramin) up to 300 mg daily, she felt no benefit after 4 months and was reluctant to continue this tricyclic antidepressant medication because of adverse effects (weight gain and sweating, in particular). Because of her increasing fatigue and sleep needs, and generally atypical profile, she was offered a trial of phenelzine. After 4 weeks, at a dosage of 60 mg daily, she reported significant improvement in her energy level, mood, and sleep pattern. Two years later, she continues to take 45 mg of phenelzine daily with some adverse effects (occasional insomnia and anorgasmia). (Courtesy of Sidney H. Kennedy, M.D., Andrew Holt, Ph.D., and Glen B. Baker, Ph.D., D.Sc.)

Patients with panic disorder and social phobia respond well to MAOIs. MAOIs have also been used to treat bulimia nervosa, posttraumatic stress disorder, anginal pain, atypical facial pain, migraine, attention deficit disorder, idiopathic orthostatic hypotension, and depression associated with traumatic brain injury.

PRECAUTIONS AND ADVERSE REACTIONS

The most frequent adverse effects of MAOIs are orthostatic hypotension, insomnia, weight gain, edema, and sexual dysfunction. Orthostatic hypotension can lead to dizziness and falls. Thus, cautious upward tapering of the dosage should be used to determine the maximal tolerable dosage. Treatment for orthostatic hypotension includes avoidance of caffeine, intake of 2 L of fluid per day, addition of dietary salt or adjustment of pertensive drugs (if applicable), support stockings, and, in cases, treatment with fludrocortisone (Florinef), a minera ticoid, 0.1 to 0.2 mg a day. Orthostatic hypotension asso with tranylcypromine use can usually be relieved by dividi daily dosage.

Insomnia can be treated by dividing the dose, not givin medication after dinner, and using trazodone (Desyrel) or a zodiazepine hypnotic, if necessary. Weight gain, edema, and ual dysfunction often do not respond to any treatment and warrant switching to another agent. When switching from MAOI to another, the clinician should taper and stop use of first drug for 10 to 14 days before beginning use of the seco drug.

Paresthesias, myoclonus, and muscle pains are occasional seen in persons treated with MAOIs. Paresthesias may be sec ondary to MAOI-induced pyridoxine deficiency, which may re spond to supplementation with pyridoxine, 50 to 150 mg orally each day. Occasionally, persons complain of feeling drunk or confused, perhaps indicating that the dosage should be reduced and then increased gradually. Reports that the hydrazine MAOIs are associated with hepatotoxic effects are relatively uncommon. MAOIs are less cardiotoxic and less epileptogenic than are the tricyclic and tetracyclic drugs.

The most common adverse effects of the RIMA moclobemide are dizziness, nausea, and insomnia or sleep disturbance. RIMAs cause fewer GI adverse effects than do SSRIs. Moclobemide does not have adverse anticholinergic or cardiovascular effects, and it has not been reported to interfere with sexual function.

Persons with renal disease, cardiovascular disease, or hyperthyroidism should use the MAOIs with caution. MAOIs may alter the dosage of a hypoglycemic agent required by diabetic persons. MAOIs have been particularly associated with induction of mania in persons in the depressed phase of bipolar I disorder and triggering of a psychotic decompensation in persons with schizophrenia. MAOIs are contraindicated during pregnancy, although data on their teratogenic risk are minimal. MAOIs should not be taken by nursing women because the drugs can pass into the breast milk.

Tyramine-induced Hypertensive Crisis

The most worrisome side effect of MAOIs is the tyramine-induced hypertensive crisis. The amino acid tyramine is normally transformed via GI metabolism. MAOIs, however, inactivate GI metabolism of dietary tyramine, thus allowing intact tyramine to enter the circulation. A hypertensive crisis may subsequently occur as a result of a powerful pressor effect of the amino acid. It is to allow resynthesis of adequate concentrations of MAOs that tyramine-containing foods be avoided until 2 weeks after the last dose of an irreversible MAOI.

Accordingly, foods rich in tyramine (Table 36.23–1) or other sympathomimetic amines, such as ephedrine, pseudoephedrine (Sudafed), or dextromethorphan (Trocal), should be avoided by persons who are taking irreversible MAOIs. Patients should be advised to continue the dietary restrictions for 2 weeks after they stop MAOI treatment to allow the body to resynthesize the enzyme. Bee stings may cause a hypertensive crisis. In addition to severe hypertension, other symptoms may

Foods to be Avoided in Planning

[a] (≥2 mg of tyramine a serving)
ton; blue cheese; white (3 years old); extra
; Danish blue; mozzarella; cheese snack

, sausage; pâtés and organs: salami:
-dried sausage
ages[b]: liqueurs and concentrated after-dinner

entrated yeast extract)

ine content[a] (0.5 to 1.99 mg of tyramine a

iss Gruyere; muenster; feta; parmesan; gorgonzola:
ese dressing: Black Diamond
d meats, sausage, pâtés and organs: chicken liver (5
d): bologna; aged sausage smoked meat; salmon
e
ic beverages: Beer and ale (12 oz per bottle)—Amstel,
rt Draft, Blue Light, Guinness Extra Stout, Old Vienna,
adian, Miller Light, Export, Heineken, Blue Wines (per 4
glass)—Rioja (red wine)

amine content[a] (0.01 to >0.49 mg of tyramine a serving)
ese: Brie, Camembert, Cambozola with or without rind
, cured meat, sausage, organs, and pâtés pickled herring;
moked fish: kielbasa sausage; chicken livers, liverwurst
(<2 days old)
lcoholic beverages: red wines; sherry; scotch[c]
Others: banana or avocado (ripe or not); banana peel

AOI, monoamine oxidase inhibitor.
Any food left out to age or spoil can spontaneously develop tyramine through fermentation.
[b]Alcohol can produce profound orthostasis interacting with MAOIs, but cannot produce direct hypotensive reactions.
[c]White wines, gin, and vodka have no tyramine content.
(Table by Jonathan M. Himmelhoch, M.D.)

include headache, stiff neck, diaphoresis, nausea, and vomiting. A patient with these symptoms should seek immediate medical treatment.

An MAOI-induced hypertensive crisis should be treated with α-adrenergic antagonists—for example, phentolamine (Regitine) or chlorpromazine (Thorazine). These drugs lower blood pressure (BP) within 5 minutes. Intravenous (IV) furosemide (Lasix) can be used to reduce fluid load and a β-adrenergic receptor antagonist can control tachycardia. A sublingual 10-mg dose of nifedipine (Procardia) can be given and repeated after 20 minutes. MAOIs should not be used by persons with thyrotoxicosis or pheochromocytoma.

The risk of tyramine-induced hypertensive crises is relatively low for persons who are taking RIMAs, such as moclobemide and befloxatone. These drugs have relatively little inhibitory activity for MAO_B and, because they are reversible, normal activity of existing MAO_A returns within 16 to 48 hours of the last dose of a RIMA. Therefore, the dietary restrictions are less stringent for RIMAs, applying only to foods containing high concentrations of tyramine, which need be avoided for only 3 days after the last dose of a RIMA. A reasonable dietary recommendation for persons taking RIMAs is not to eat tyramine-containing foods for a period from 1 hour before to 2 hours after taking a RIMA.

Spontaneous, non–tyramine-induced hypertensive crisis is a rare occurrence, usually shortly after the first exposure an MAOI. Persons experiencing such a crisis should avoid MAOIs altogether.

> A 57-year-old man had been successfully treated with tranylcypromine for 10 years after failing to respond to previous antidepressants. At his follow-up appointments, he admitted to being somewhat complacent about following a low-tyramine diet, because there appeared to be no hazardous sequelae. A confirmed hypertensive crisis occurred some time later and was successfully treated with sublingual nifedipine (Procardia; 10 mg). The cause of this reaction was ultimately traced to a change in his beer-drinking habit. For years, he had consumed one or two standard domestic beers every week. Just before the reaction, he sampled a microbrewery bottled draft beer that, on subsequent analysis, turned out to have a high tyramine content. (Courtesy of Sidney H. Kennedy, M.D., Andrew Holt, Ph.D., and Glen B. Baker, Ph.D., D.Sc.)

Withdrawal

Abrupt cessation of regular doses of MAOIs can cause a self-limited discontinuation syndrome consisting of arousal, mood disturbances, and somatic symptoms. To avoid these symptoms when discontinuing use of an MAOI, dosages should be gradually tapered over several weeks.

Overdose

Often, an asymptomatic period of 1 to 6 hours occurs after an MAOI overdose before the occurrence of the symptoms of toxicity. MAOI overdose is characterized by agitation that progresses to coma with hyperthermia, hypertension, tachypnea, tachycardia, dilated pupils, and hyperactive deep tendon reflexes. Involuntary movements may be present, particularly in the face and the jaw. Acidification of the urine markedly hastens the excretion of MAOIs, and dialysis can be of some use. Phentolamine or chlorpromazine may be useful if hypertension is a problem. Moclobemide alone in overdosage causes relatively mild and reversible symptoms.

DRUG INTERACTIONS

The major drug–drug and food–drug interactions involving MAOIs are listed in Table 36.23–2. Most antidepressants, as well as precursor agents, should be avoided. Persons should be instructed to tell any other physicians or dentists who are treating them that they are taking an MAOI. MAOIs may potentiate the action of CNS depressants, including alcohol and barbiturates. MAOIs should not be coadministered with serotonergic drugs, such as SSRIs and clomipramine (Anafranil), because this combination can trigger a serotonin syndrome. Use of lithium or tryptophan with an irreversible MAOI may also induce a serotonin syndrome. Initial symptoms of a serotonin syndrome can include tremor, hypertonicity, myoclonus, and autonomic signs, which can then progress to hallucinosis, hyperthermia, and even death. Fatal reactions have occurred when MAOIs were combined with meperidine (Demerol) or fentanyl (Sublimaze).

When switching from an irreversible MAOI to any other type of antidepressant drug, persons should wait at least 14 days after the last dose of the MAOI before beginning use of the next drug to allow replenishment of the body's MAOs. When switching

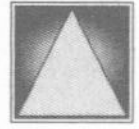

Table 36.23–2
Drugs to be Avoided During MAOI Treatment (Part of Listing)

Never use
- Antiasthmatics
- Antihypertensives (methyldopa, guanethidine, reserpine)
- Buspirone
- Levodopa
- Opioids (especially meperidine, dextromethorphan, propoxyphene, tramadol; morphine or codeine may be less dangerous)
- Cold, allergy, or sinus medications containing dextromethorphan or sympathomimetics
- SSRIs, clomipromine, venlafaxine, sibutramine
- Sympathomimetics (amphetamines, cocaine, methylphenidate, dopamine, epinephrine, norepinephrine, isoproterenol, ephedrine, pseudoephedrine, phenylpropanolamine)
- L-tryptophan

Use carefully
- Anticholinergics
- Antihistamines
- Disulfiram
- Bromocriptine
- Hydralazine
- Sedative-hypnotics
- Terpin hydrate with codeine
- Tricyclics and tetracyclics (avoid clomipramine)

MAOI, monoamine oxidase inhibitor; SSRIs, selective serotonin reuptake inhibitors.

from an antidepressant to an irreversible MAOI, persons should wait 10 to 14 days (or 5 weeks for fluoxetine [Prozac]) before starting use of the MAOI to avoid drug–drug interactions. In contrast, MAO activity recovers completely 24 to 48 hours after the last dose of a RIMA.

The effects of the MAOIs on hepatic enzymes are poorly studied. Tranylcypromine inhibits CYP 2C19. Moclobemide inhibits CYP 2D6, CYP 2C19, and CYP 1A2, and is a substrate for 2C19.

Cimetidine (Tagamet) and fluoxetine significantly reduce the elimination of moclobemide. Modest doses of fluoxetine and moclobemide administered concurrently may be well tolerated, with no significant pharmacodynamic or pharmacokinetic interactions.

LABORATORY INTERFERENCES

The MAOIs may lower blood glucose concentrations. MAOIs artificially raise urinary metanephrine concentrations and may cause a false-positive test result for pheochromocytoma or neuroblastoma. MAOIs have been reported to be associated with a minimal false elevation in thyroid function test results.

DOSAGE AND CLINICAL GUIDELINES

No definitive rationale exists for choosing one irreversible MAOI over another. Table 36.23–3 lists MAOI preparations and typical dosages. Phenelzine use should begin with a test dose of 15 mg on the first day. The dosage can be increased to 15 mg three times daily during the first week and increased by 15 mg a day each week thereafter until the dosage of 90 mg a day, in divided doses, is reached by the end of the fourth week. Tranylcypromine and isocarboxazid use should begin with a test dosage of 10 mg and may be increased to 10 mg three times daily by the end of the first week. Many clinicians and researchers have recommended upper limits of 50 mg a day for isocarboxazid and 40 mg a day for tranylcypromine. Administration of tranylcypromine in multiple, small daily doses may reduce its hypotensive effects.

Although coadministration of MAOIs with TCAs, SSRIs, or lithium is generally contraindicated, these combinations have been used successfully and safely to treat patients with refractory depression, but they should be used with extreme caution.

Hepatic transaminase serum concentrations should be monitored periodically because of the potential for hepatotoxicity, especially with phenelzine and isocarboxazid. Elderly persons may be more sensitive to MAOI adverse effects than are younger adults. MAO activity increases with age, so that MAOI dosages for elderly persons are the same as those required for younger adults. The use of MAOIs for children has had minimal study.

Moclobemide use is initiated at 300 to 450 mg a day, divided three times per day, and may be increased to a maximum of 600 mg a day after several weeks. Dietary restrictions consist of avoidance of only large quantities of tyramine-containing foods and the administration of moclobemide after, rather than before, tyramine-containing meals. RIMAs can be used in combination with other antidepressants with somewhat less concern for hypertensive crises but still with caution.

TRANSDERMAL SELEGILINE (EMSAM)

Oral selegiline is approved only as an adjunct to levodopa or carbidopa for patients with Parkinson's disease, but some studies have found it to be effective for treating depression. Antidepressant doses are above 30 mg per day, a level that results in loss of selective inhibition of MAO_B and consequent risk of the same

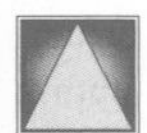

Table 36.23–3
Available Preparations and Typical Dosages of MAOIs

Generic Name	Trade Name	Preparations	Usual Daily Dose (mg)	Usual Maximal Daily Dose (mg)
Isocarboxazid[a]	Marplan	10-mg tablets	20 to 40	60
Moclobemide[b]	Manerix	100-, 150-mg tablets	300 to 600	600
Phenelzine	Nardil	15-mg tablets	30 to 60	90
Selegiline[c]	Eldepryl, Atapryl	5-mg capsules, 5-mg tablets	10	30
Tranylcypromine	Parnate	10-mg tablets	20 to 60	60

MAOIs, monoamine oxidase inhibitors.
[a] Available directly from the manufacturer.
[b] Not available in the United States.
[c] Also available as Emsam, 6-, 9-, 12- mg patch used once daily.

tyramine reactions seen with the older MAOIs. For this reason, oral selegiline is rarely used off-label as an antidepressant.

A transdermal formulation of selegiline was approved in 2006 for treating major depressive disorder. Being absorbed through the skin eliminates first-pass hepatic metabolism and, thus, alters the mix of available medication. At the lowest (6 mg) strength, transdermal selegiline delivers more selegiline to the bloodstream than does low-dose oral selegiline but without inhibiting gut MAO_A. By selectively inhibiting MAO_B, it appears to have a lower risk of potentially fatal hypertensive reaction seen with other MAOIs. The 6-mg patch provides the brain MAO_A and MAO_B inhibition necessary for an antidepressant effect while eliminating the need for dietary restrictions at this lowest dosage. At higher doses, 9 mg per day and 12 mg per day, transdermal selegiline may inhibit too much gastrointestinal MAO_A to clear tyramine from foods. The same food restrictions that apply to the older MAOIs, therefore, are necessary when prescribing transdermal selegiline at 9 or 12 mg per day.

Transdermal selegiline achieves therapeutic blood levels and reaches sustained concentration within 4 to 8 hours of administration. Compared with oral selegiline, transdermal delivery results in higher plasma selegiline concentrations (1,500 pg/mL with the 6-mg patch) with much lower exposure to metabolites.

As with oral selegiline, the transdermal patch should not be used concurrently with SSRIs, Serotonin-Norepinephrine Reuptake Inhibitors (SNRIs), tricyclic antidepressants, mirtazapine, or bupropion. Other contraindicated drugs include carbamazepine or oxcarbazepine, meperidine, tramadol, methadone, and propoxyphene, St. John's wort, cough syrups containing dextromethorphan, amphetamines, cyclobenzaprine, and drugs containing pseudoephedrine, phenylephrine, phenylpropanolamine, or ephedrine.

Because MAO inhibition persists for 2 weeks after the last dose of selegiline, requiring a 2-week "wash out" before starting a new antidepressant or stopping food restrictions in patients taking the 9-mg and 12-mg patches.

Inflammation at the application site is the most common side effect. Fair-skinned females are most at risk for this reaction. Insomnia can also occur. In clinical trials, transdermal selegiline did not impair sexual function, alter appetite, or change body weight or blood pressure compared with placebo. Transdermal selegiline was not tapered in clinical trials, yet no withdrawal symptoms were reported even after 1 year of continuous treatment.

Transdermal selegiline is started at 6 mg per day. The patch is applied to the upper torso (chest, back, or stomach) where vascularity is richer than the buttocks and legs. The patch is changed daily and is applied to a different spot each day to prevent inflammation. The dosage can be increased after 2 or 3 months if response is inadequate. Transdermal selegiline patches contain 1 mg/cm^2 of selegiline and deliver approximately 0.3 mg/cm^2 of selegiline over 24 hours. Available dosing forms are 6-, 9-, and 12-mg patches. Patches should not be cut.

References

Akhondzadah S, Tavakolian R, Davari-Ashtiani R, Arabgol F, Amini H. Selegiline in the treatment of attention deficit hyperactivity disorder in children: A double blind and randomized trial. *Prog Neuropsychopharmacol Biol Psychiatry.* 2003;27:841–845.

Bies RR, Bigos KL, Pollock BG. Gender differences in the pharmacokinetics and pharmacodynamics of antidepressants. *J Gend Specif Med.* 2003;6:12–20.

Holt A, Berry MD, Boulton AA. On the binding of monoamine oxidase inhibitors to some sites distinct from the MAO active site, and effects thereby elicited. *Neurotoxicology.* 2004;25:251–266.

Kennedy SH, Holt A, Baker GB. Monoamine oxidase inhibitors. In: Sadock BJ, Sadock VA, eds. *Kaplan & Sadock's Comprehensive Textbook of Psychiatry.* 8th ed. Vol. 2. Baltimore: Lippincott Williams & Wilkins; 2005:2854.

Patkar AA, Pae CU, Masand PS. Transdermal selegiline: The new generation of monoamine oxidase inhibitors. *CNS Spectrums.* 2006;11(5):363–375.

Rush AJ, Fava M, Wisniewski SR, Lavori PW, Trivedi MH, Sackeim HA, Thase ME, Nierenberg AA, Quitkin FM, Kashner TM, Kupfer DJ, Rosenbaum JF, Alpert J, Stewart JW, McGrath PJ, Biggs MM, Shores-Wilson K, Lebowitz BD, Ritz L, Niederehe G; STAR*D Investigators Group. Sequenced treatment alternatives to relieve depression (STAR*D): Rationale and design. *Control Clin Trials.* 2004;25:119–142.

Salsali M, Holt A, Baker GB. Inhibitory effects of the monoamine oxidase inhibitor tranylcypromine on the cytochrome P450 enzymes CYP2C19, CYP2C6, and CYP2D6. *Cell Mol Neurobiol.* 2004;24:63–76.

Youdim MBH, Edmondson D, Tipton KF. The therapeutic potential of monoamine oxidase inhibitors. *Nat Rev Neurosci.* 2006;7(4):295–309.

▲ 36.24 Nefazodone

Nefazodone (Serzone) is indicated for the treatment of major depression. It is an analog of trazodone (Desyrel). When nefazodone was introduced in 1995, expectations were that it would become widely used because it did not cause the sexual side effects and sleep disruption associated with the selective serotonin reuptake inhibitors (SSRIs). Although it was devoid of these side effects, it was nevertheless found to produce problematic sedation, nausea, dizziness, and visual disturbances. Consequently, nefazodone was never extensively adopted in clinical practice. This fact, as well as reports of rare cases of sometimes fatal hepatotoxicity, led the original manufacturer to discontinue production of branded nefazodone in 2004. Generic nefazodone remains available in the United States.

CHEMISTRY

Nefazodone is structurally related to trazodone and unrelated to the classic tricyclic and tetracyclic drugs, the monoamine oxidase inhibitors (MAOIs), SSRIs, and other currently available antidepressant drugs. Its molecular structure is shown in Figure 36.24–1.

PHARMACOLOGIC ACTIONS

Nefazodone is rapidly and completely absorbed, but is then extensively metabolized so that the bioavailability of active compounds is about 20 percent of the oral dose. Its half-life is 2 to 4 hours. Steady-state concentrations of nefazodone and its principal active metabolite, hydroxynefazodone, are achieved within 4 to 5 days. Metabolism of nefazodone in the elderly, especially women, is about half that seen in younger persons, so

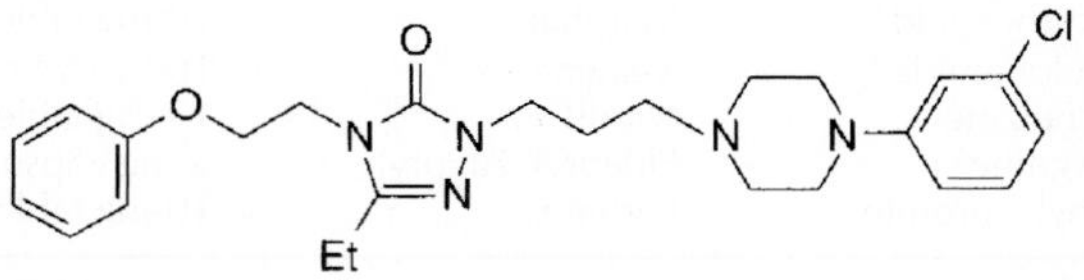

FIGURE 36.24–1
Molecular structure of nefazodone.

lowered doses are recommended for elderly persons. An important metabolite of nefazodone is meta-chlorophenylpiperazine (mCPP), which has some serotonergic effects and can cause migraine, anxiety, and weight loss.

Although nefazodone is an inhibitor of serotonin uptake and, more weakly, of norepinephrine reuptake, its antagonism of serotonin 5-HT_{2A} receptors is thought to produce its antianxiety and antidepressant effects. Nefazodone is also a mild antagonist of the α_1-adrenergic receptors, which predisposes some persons to orthostatic hypotension, but is not sufficiently potent to produce priapism.

THERAPEUTIC INDICATIONS

Nefazodone is effective for the treatment of major depression. The usual effective dose is 300 to 600 mg a day. In direct comparison with SSRIs, nefazodone is less likely to cause inhibition of orgasm or decreased sexual desire. Nefazodone is also effective for treatment of panic disorder and panic with comorbid depression or depressive symptoms, of generalized anxiety disorder, and of premenstrual dysphoric disorder, and for the management of chronic pain. It is not effective for the treatment of obsessive-compulsive disorder. Nefazodone increases rapid eye movement (REM) sleep and increases sleep continuity. Nefazodone is also of use in patients with posttraumatic stress disorder and chronic fatigue syndrome. It may also be effective in patients who have been treatment resistant to other antidepressant drugs.

PRECAUTIONS AND ADVERSE REACTIONS

The most common reasons for discontinuing nefazodone use are sedation, nausea, dizziness, insomnia, weakness, and agitation. Many patients report no specific side effect, but describe a vague sense of feeling medicated. Nefazodone also causes visual trails, where patients see an afterimage when looking at moving objects or when moving their heads quickly.

Some patients taking nefazodone may experience a drop in blood pressure (BP) that can cause episodes of postural hypotension. Nefazodone, therefore, should be used with caution by persons with underlying cardiac conditions, history of stroke or heart attack, dehydration, or hypovolemia, or by persons being treated with antihypertensive medications. Patients switched from SSRIs to nefazodone may experience an increase in side effects, possibly because nefazodone does not protect against SSRI withdrawal symptoms. One of its metabolites, mCPP, may actually intensify these discontinuation symptoms.

The effects of nefazodone on the fetus is not yet as well understood as those of the SSRIs. Nefazodone, therefore, should be used during pregnancy only if the potential benefit to the mother outweighs the potential risks to the fetus. It is not known whether nefazodone is excreted in human breast milk. Therefore, it should be used with caution by lactating mothers. The nefazodone dosage should be lowered in persons with severe hepatic disease, but no adjustment is necessary for persons with renal disease (Table 36.24–1).

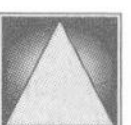

Table 36.24–1
Adverse Reactions Reported with Nefazodone (300 to 600 mg a day)

Reaction	Percentage (%)
Headache	36
Dry mouth	25
Somnolence	25
Nausea	22
Dizziness	17
Constipation	14
Insomnia	11
Weakness	11
Lightheadedness	10
Blurred vision	9
Dyspepsia	9
Infection	8
Confusion	7
Scotomata	7

DRUG INTERACTIONS AND LABORATORY INTERFERENCES

Nefazodone should not be given concomitantly with MAOIs. In addition, nefazodone has particular drug–drug interactions with the triazolobenzodiazepines triazolam (Halcion) and alprazolam (Xanax) because of the inhibition of cytochrome P450 3A4 by nefazodone. Potentially elevated levels of each of these drugs can develop after administration of nefazodone, whereas the levels of nefazodone are generally not affected. Lower the dose of triazolam by 75 percent and the dose of alprazolam by 50 percent when given concomitantly with nefazodone.

Nefazodone may slow the metabolism of digoxin; therefore, digoxin levels should be monitored carefully in persons taking both medications. Nefazodone also slows the metabolism of haloperidol (Haldol), so the dosage of haloperidol should be reduced in persons taking both medications. Addition of nefazodone may also exacerbate the adverse effects of lithium (Eskalith).

No known laboratory interferences are associated with nefazodone use.

DOSAGE AND CLINICAL GUIDELINES

Nefazodone is available in 50-, 200-, and 250-mg unscored tablets and 100- and 150-mg scored tablets. The recommended starting dosage of nefazodone is 100 mg twice a day, but 50 mg twice a day may be better tolerated, especially by elderly persons. To limit the development of adverse effects, the dosage should be slowly raised in increments of 100 to 200 mg a day at intervals of no less than 1 week per increase. The optimal dosage is 300 to 600 mg daily in two divided doses. Some studies, however, report that nefazodone is effective when taken once a day, especially at bedtime. Geriatric persons should receive dosages about two thirds of the usual nongeriatric dosages, with a maximum of 400 mg a day. Similar to other antidepressants, clinical benefit of nefazodone usually appears after 2 to 4 weeks of treatment. Patients with premenstrual syndrome are treated with a flexible dosage that averages about 250 mg a day.

References

DeVane CL, Donovan JL, Liston HL, Markowitz JS, Cheng KT, Risch SC, Willard L. Comparative CYP3A4 inhibitory effects of venlafaxine, fluoxetine, sertraline, and nefazodone in healthy volunteers. *J Clin Psychopharmacol.* 2004;24:4–10.

Gelenberg AJ, Trivedi MH, Rush AJ, Thase ME, Howland R, Klein DN, Kornstein SG, Dunner DL, Markowitz JC, Hirschfeld RM, Keitner GI, Zajecka J, Kocsis JH, Russell JM, Miller I, Manber R, Arnow B, Rothbaum B, Munsaka M, Banks P, Borian FE, Keller MB. Randomized, placebo-controlled trial of nefazodone maintenance treatment in preventing recurrence in chronic depression. *Biol Psychiatry.* 2003;54:806–817.

Khan A, Kornsten SG. Nefazodone. In: Sadock BJ, Sadock VA, eds. *Kaplan & Sadock's Comprehensive Textbook of Psychiatry.* 8th ed. Vol. 2. Baltimore: Lippincott Williams & Wilkins; 2005:2863.

Lesperance F, Frasure-Smith N, Laliberte MA, White M, Lafontaine S, Calderone A, Talajic M, Rouleau JL. An open-label study of nefazodone treatment of major depression in patients with congestive heart failure. *Can J Psychiatry.* 2003;48:695–701.

Mischoulon D, Opitz G, Kelly K, Fava M, Rosenbaum JF. A preliminary open study of the tolerability and effectiveness of nefazodone in major depressive disorder: Comparing patients who recently discontinued an SSRI with those on no recent antidepressant treatment. *Depress Anxiety.* 2004;19:43–50.

Schatzberg AF, Rush AJ, Arnow BA, Banks PLC, Blalock JA, Borian FE, Howland R, Klein DN, Kocsis JH, Kornstein SG, Manber R, Markowitz JC, Miller I, Ninan PT, Rothbaum BO, Thase ME, Trivedi MH, Keller MB. Chronic depression: Medication (nefazodone) or psychotherapy (CBASP) is effective when the other is not. *Archives of General Psychiatry.* 2005;62(5):513–520.

Taylor FB, Prather MR. The efficacy of nefazodone augmentation for treatment-resistant depression with anxiety symptoms or anxiety disorder. *Depress Anxiety.* 2003;18:83–88.

▲ 36.25 Opioid Receptor Agonists: Methadone, Buprenorphine, and Levomethadyl

The drugs discussed in this section are used to deal with opioid addiction, commonly referred to as either psychological dependence, physical dependence, or tolerance that develops after long-term abuse. Commonly abused opioids include heroin, hydromorphone (Dilaudid), codeine, meperidine (Demerol), butorphanol (Stadol), and hydrocodone (Robidone). Annually, approximately 2.6 million Americans use prescription pain relievers for nonmedical reasons and more than 3 million Americans use heroin.

The drugs discussed in this chapter include methadone (Dolophine), buprenorphine (Buprenex), and levomethadyl acetate, also called L-α-acetylmethadol (LAAM). Because of severe adverse reactions (described in the following text), LAAM was removed from the European market in 2001 and from the United States in 2003.

CHEMISTRY

The structural formulas of the synthetic opioid receptor agonists methadone, levomethadyl, and buprenorphine are shown in Figure 36.25–1.

PHARMACOLOGIC ACTIONS

Methadone, levomethadyl, and buprenorphine are absorbed rapidly from the gastrointestinal (GI) tract. Hepatic first-pass metabolism significantly affects the bioavailability of each of the drugs, but in markedly different ways. For methadone, hepatic enzymes reduce the bioavailability of an oral dosage by about half, an effect that is easily managed with dosage adjustments.

For levomethadyl, hepatic enzymes metabolize an oral dosage into normethyl-LAAM and dinormethyl-LAAM, which are actually several times more potent as μ-opioid receptor agonists than is levomethadyl itself.

For buprenorphine, in contrast, first-pass intestinal and hepatic metabolism eliminates oral bioavailability almost completely. When used in opioid detoxification, buprenorphine is given sublingually, in either a liquid or a tablet formulation.

The peak plasma concentrations of oral methadone are reached within 2 to 6 hours, and the plasma half-life initially is 4 to 6 hours in opioid-naïve persons and 24 to 36 hours after steady dosing of any type of opioid. Methadone is highly protein bound and equilibrates widely throughout the body, which ensures little postdosage variation in steady-state plasma concentrations.

The peak plasma concentrations of oral levomethadyl are reached within 1.5 to 2 hours, and the plasma half-lives of levomethadyl and its active metabolites range from 2 to 4 days.

Elimination of a sublingual dosage of buprenorphine occurs in two phases: an initial phase with a half-life of 3 to 5 hours and a terminal phase with a half-life of more than 24 hours. Buprenorphine dissociates from its receptor binding site slowly, which permits an every-other-day dosing schedule.

Methadone and levomethadyl act as pure agonists at μ-opioid receptors and have negligible agonist or antagonist activity at κ- or δ-opioid receptors. Buprenorphine is a partial agonist at μ-receptors, a potent antagonist at κ-receptors, and neither an agonist nor an antagonist at δ-receptors.

THERAPEUTIC INDICATIONS

Methadone

Methadone is used for short-term detoxification (7 to 30 days), long-term detoxification (up to 180 days), and maintenance (treatment beyond 180 days) of opioid-dependent individuals. For these purposes, it is available only through designated clinics called methadone maintenance treatment programs (MMTPs) and in hospitals and prisons. Methadone is a schedule II drug, which means that its administration is tightly governed by specific federal laws and regulations.

Enrollment in a methadone program reduces the risk of death by 70 percent reduces (1) illicit use of opioids and other substances of abuse; (2) criminal activity; (3) the risk of infectious diseases of all types, most importantly HIV and hepatitis B and C infection; and, in pregnant women, (4) the risk of fetal and neonatal morbidity and mortality. The use of methadone maintenance frequently requires lifelong treatment.

Some opioid-dependence treatment programs use a stepwise detoxification protocol in which a person addicted to heroin switches first to the strong agonist methadone, then to the weaker agonist buprenorphine, and finally to maintenance on an opioid receptor antagonist, such as naltrexone (ReVia). This approach minimizes the appearance of opioid withdrawal effects, which, if they occur, are mitigated with clonidine (Catapres). Compliance with opioid receptor antagonist treatment is poor, however, outside of settings using intensive cognitive–behavioral techniques.

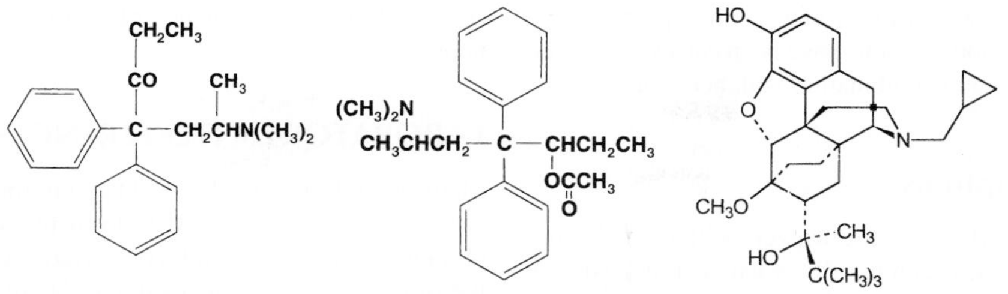

Methadone Levomethadyl Buprenorphine

FIGURE 36.25–1
Molecular structures of opioid agonists.

In contrast, noncompliance with methadone maintenance precipitates opioid withdrawal symptoms, which serve to reinforce use of methadone and make cognitive–behavioral therapy less than essential. Thus, some well-motivated, socially integrated former heroin addicts are able to use methadone for years without participation in a psychosocial support program.

Data pooled from many reports indicate that methadone is more effective when taken at dosages in excess of 60 mg a day. The analgesic effects of methadone are sometimes used in the management of chronic pain when less addictive agents are ineffective.

Pregnancy. Methadone maintenance, combined with effective psychosocial services and regular obstetric monitoring, significantly improves obstetric and neonatal outcomes for women addicted to heroin. Enrollment of a heroin-addicted pregnant woman in such a maintenance program reduces the risk of malnutrition, infection, preterm labor, spontaneous abortion, preeclampsia, eclampsia, abruptio placenta, and septic thrombophlebitis.

The dosage of methadone during pregnancy should be the lowest effective dosage, and no withdrawal to abstinence should be attempted during pregnancy. Methadone is metabolized more rapidly in the third trimester, which may necessitate higher dosages. To avoid potentially sedating postdose peak plasma concentrations, the daily dose can be administered in two divided doses during the third trimester. Methadone treatment has no known teratogenic effects.

Neonatal Methadone Withdrawal Symptoms. Withdrawal symptoms in newborns frequently include tremor, high-pitched cry, increased muscle tone and activity, poor sleep and eating, mottling, yawning, perspiration, and skin excoriation. Convulsions that require aggressive anticonvulsant therapy may also occur. Withdrawal symptoms can be delayed in onset and prolonged in neonates because of their immature hepatic metabolism. Women taking methadone are sometimes counseled to initiate breast-feeding as a means of gently weaning their infants from methadone dependence, but they should not breast-feed their babies while still taking methadone.

Levomethadyl

Levomethadyl is no longer used. It had been used only for maintenance treatment of opioid-dependent patients. It was not used for detoxification treatment or for analgesia.

Buprenorphine

Buprenorphine at a dosage of 8 to 16 mg a day appears to reduce heroin use. Buprenorphine also is effective in thrice-weekly dosing because of its slow dissociation from opioid receptors. The analgesic effects of buprenorphine are sometimes used in the management of chronic pain when less addictive agents are ineffective.

PRECAUTIONS AND ADVERSE REACTIONS

The most common adverse effects of opioid receptor agonists are lightheadedness, dizziness, sedation, nausea, constipation, vomiting, perspiration, weight gain, decreased libido, inhibition of orgasm, and insomnia or sleep irregularities. Opioid receptor agonists can induce tolerance as well as produce physiologic and psychological dependence. Other central nervous system (CNS) adverse effects include depression, sedation, euphoria, dysphoria, agitation, and seizures. Delirium has been reported in rare cases. Occasional non-CNS adverse effects include peripheral edema, urinary retention, rash, arthralgia, dry mouth, anorexia, biliary tract spasm, bradycardia, hypotension, hypoventilation, syncope, antidiuretic hormone-like activity, pruritus, urticaria, and visual disturbances. Menstrual irregularities are common in women, especially in the first 6 months of use. Various abnormal endocrine laboratory indexes of little clinical significance may also be seen.

Most persons develop tolerance to the pharmacologic adverse effects of opioid agonists during long-term maintenance, and relatively few adverse effects are experienced after the induction period.

Levomethadyl is associated with prolonged QT intervals and torsade de points, which may be fatal. As mentioned, this drug is no longer in use for these reasons.

Overdosage

The acute effects of opioid receptor agonist overdosage include sedation, hypotension, bradycardia, hypothermia, respiratory suppression, miosis, and decreased GI motility. Severe effects include coma, cardiac arrest, shock, and death. The risk of overdosage is greatest in the induction stage of treatment and in persons with slow drug metabolism because of preexisting hepatic insufficiency. Deaths have been caused during the first week of induction by methadone dosages of only 50 to 60 mg a day.

The risk of overdosage with buprenorphine appears to be lower than with methadone. Deaths have been caused, however, by use of buprenorphine in combination with benzodiazepines.

Withdrawal Symptoms

Abrupt cessation of methadone use triggers withdrawal symptoms within 3 to 4 days, which usually reach peak intensity on the 6th day. Withdrawal symptoms include weakness, anxiety, anorexia, insomnia, gastric distress, headache, sweating, and hot and cold flashes. The withdrawal symptoms usually resolve after 2 weeks. A protracted methadone abstinence syndrome is possible, however, which may include restlessness and insomnia.

The withdrawal symptoms associated with buprenorphine are similar to, but less marked than, those caused by methadone. In particular, buprenorphine is sometimes used to ease the transition from methadone to opioid receptor antagonists or abstinence, because of the relatively mild withdrawal reaction associated with discontinuation of buprenorphine.

DRUG–DRUG INTERACTIONS

Opioid receptor agonists can potentiate the CNS depressant effects of alcohol, barbiturates, benzodiazepines, other opioids, low-potency dopamine receptor antagonists, tricyclic and tetracyclic drugs, and monoamine oxidase inhibitors (MAOIs). Carbamazepine (Tegretol), phenytoin (Dilantin), barbiturates, rifampin (Rimactane, Rifadin), and heavy long-term consumption of alcohol can induce hepatic enzymes, which can lower the plasma concentration of methadone or buprenorphine and thereby precipitate withdrawal symptoms. In contrast, however, hepatic enzyme induction can raise the plasma concentration of active levomethadyl metabolites and cause toxicity.

Acute opioid withdrawal symptoms can be precipitated in persons on methadone maintenance therapy who take pure opioid receptor antagonists, such as naltrexone, nalmefene (Revex), and naloxone (Narcan); partial agonists, such as buprenorphine; or mixed agonist-antagonists, such as pentazocine (Talwin). These symptoms may be mitigated by use of clonidine, a benzodiazepine, or both.

Competitive inhibition of methadone or buprenorphine metabolism following short-term use of alcohol or administration of cimetidine (Tagamet), erythromycin, ketoconazole (Nizoral), fluoxetine (Prozac), fluvoxamine (Luvox), loratadine (Claritin), quinidine (Quinidex), and alprazolam (Xanax) can lead to higher plasma concentrations or prolonged duration of action of methadone or buprenorphine. Medications that alkalinize the urine can reduce methadone excretion.

Methadone maintenance can also increase plasma concentrations of desipramine (Norpramin, Pertofrane) and fluvoxamine. Use of methadone can increase zidovudine (Retrovir) concentrations, which increases the possibility of zidovudine toxicity at otherwise standard dosages. In vitro human liver microsome studies moreover demonstrate competitive inhibition of methadone demethylation by several protease inhibitors, including ritonavir (Norvir), indinavir (Crixivan), and saquinavir (Invirase). The clinical relevance of this finding is unknown.

Fatal drug–drug interactions with the MAOIs are associated with use of the opioids fentanyl (Sublimaze) and meperidine (Demerol) but not with use of methadone, levomethadyl, or buprenorphine.

LABORATORY INTERFERENCES

Methadone, levomethadyl, and buprenorphine can be tested for separately in urine toxicology to distinguish them from other opioids. No known laboratory interferences are associated with use of methadone, levomethadyl, or buprenorphine.

DOSAGE AND CLINICAL GUIDELINES

Methadone

Methadone is supplied in 5-, 10-, and 40-mg dispersible scored tablets; 40-mg scored wafers; 5 mg/5 mL, 10 mg/5 mL, and 10 mg/mL solutions; and a 10-mg/mL parenteral form. In maintenance programs, methadone is usually dissolved in water or juice, and dose administration is directly observed to ensure compliance. For induction of opioid detoxification, an initial methadone dose of 15 to 20 mg will usually suppress craving and withdrawal symptoms. Some individuals, however, may require up to 40 mg a day in single or divided doses. Higher dosages should be avoided during induction of treatment to reduce the risk of acute toxicity from overdosage.

Over several weeks, the dosage should be raised to at least 70 mg a day. The maximal dosage is usually 120 mg a day, and higher dosages require prior approval from regulatory agencies. Dosages above 60 mg a day are associated with much more complete abstinence from use of illicit opioids than are dosages less than 60 mg a day.

Treatment duration should not be predetermined, but should be based on response to treatment and assessment of psychosocial factors. All studies of methadone maintenance programs endorse long-term treatment (i.e., several years) as more effective than short-term programs (i.e., less than 1 year) for prevention of relapse into opioid abuse. In actual practice, however, a few programs are permitted by policy or approved by insurers to provide even 6 months of continuous maintenance treatment. Moreover, some programs actually encourage withdrawal from methadone in less than 6 months after induction. This is quite ill conceived, because more than 80 percent of persons who terminate methadone maintenance treatment eventually return to illicit drug use within 2 years. In those programs that offer both maintenance and withdrawal treatments, the overwhelming majority of participants enroll in the maintenance treatment.

Levomethadyl

Levomethadyl is no longer marketed. Because of the tendency of levomethadyl to accumulate toxic concentrations if taken daily, it was prescribed thrice weekly in doses of 60 to 90 mg.

Buprenorphine

Buprenorphine is supplied as a 0.3-mg/mL solution in 1-mL ampules. Sublingual tablet formulations of buprenorphine containing buprenorphine only or buprenorphine combined with naloxone in a 4:1 ratio are used for opioid maintenance treatment. Buprenorphine is not used for short-term opioid detoxification.

Maintenance dosages of 8 to 16 mg three times a week have effectively reduced heroin use. Physicians must be trained and certified to carry out this therapy in their private offices. A number of approved training programs are available in the United States.

References

Doran CM, Shanahan M, Mattick RP, Ali R, White J, Bell J. Buprenorphine versus methadone maintenance: A cost-effectiveness analysis. *Drug Alcohol Depend.* 2003;71:295.

Fudala PJ, Bridge P, Herbert S, Williford WO, Chiang N, Jones K, Collins J, Raisch D, Casadonte P, Goldsmith RJ, Ling W, Malkerneker U, McNicholas L, Renner J, Stine S, Tusel D. Office-based treatment of opiate addiction with a sublingual-tablet formulation of buprenorphine and naloxone. *N Engl J Med.* 2003;349:949–958.

Ling W, Wesson DR. Clinical efficacy of buprenorphine: Comparisons to methadone and placebo. *Drug Alcohol Depend.* 2003;70:S49–S57.

McRae AL, Brady KT. Opioid receptor agonists: Methadone, levomethadyl, and buprenorphine. In: Sadock BJ, Sadock VA, eds. *Kaplan & Sadock's Comprehensive Textbook of Psychiatry*. 8th ed. Vol. 2. Baltimore: Lippincott Williams & Wilkins; 2005:2870.

Rosenblum A, Joseph H, Fong C, Kipnis S, Cleland C, Portenoy RK. Prevalence and characteristics of chronic pain among chemically dependent patients in methadone maintenance and residential treatment facilities. *JAMA.* 2003;289:2370–2378.

Strain EC, Moody DE, Stoller KB, Walsh SL, Bigelow GE. Relative bioavailability of different buprenorphine formulations under chronic dosing conditions. *Drug Alcohol Depend.* 2004;74:37–43.

▲ 36.26 Opioid Receptor Antagonists: Naltrexone, Nalmefene, and Naloxone

The three opioid receptor antagonists are naltrexone (ReVia), Naloxone (Narcan), and nalmefene (Revex). Opioid receptor antagonists appear to reduce or eliminate the subjective "high" associated with consumption of opioids or alcohol, thus interrupting their reinforcing effects. Opioid receptor antagonists also reduce or eliminate the craving associated with withdrawal from chronic opioid or alcohol abuse.

Of the three opioid receptor antagonists, at present only oral naltrexone is US Food and Drug Administration (FDA)-approved for treatment of alcohol dependence and for blockade of the effects of exogenously administered opioids. Currently, the only available formulation of nalmefene and naltrexone is for intravenous (IV) administration, and both of these drugs are used to treat respiratory depression induced by opioids and to manage known or suspected overdosage of synthetic or natural opioid preparations.

CHEMISTRY

The molecular structure of naltrexone is shown in Figure 36.26–1.

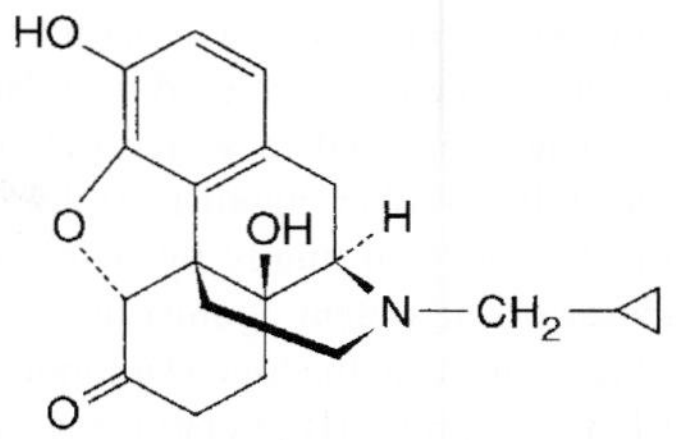

HO, O, OH, H, N—CH_2—◁, O

FIGURE 36.26–1
Molecular structure of naltrexone.

PHARMACOLOGIC ACTIONS

Oral opioid receptor antagonists are rapidly absorbed from the gastrointestinal (GI) tract, but because of first-pass hepatic metabolism, only 60 percent of a dose of naltrexone and 40 percent to 50 percent of a dose of nalmefene reach the systemic circulation unchanged. Peak concentrations of naltrexone and its active metabolite, 6-β-naltrexol, are achieved within 1 hour of ingestion. The half-life of naltrexone is 1 to 3 hours, and the half-life of 6-β-naltrexol is 13 hours. Peak concentrations of nalmefene are achieved in about 1 to 2 hours, and the half-life is 8 to 10 hours. Clinically, a single dose of naltrexone effectively blocks the rewarding effects of opioids for 72 hours. Traces of 6-β-naltrexol can linger for up to 125 hours after a single dose.

Naltrexone and nalmefene are competitive antagonists of opioid receptors. Understanding the pharmacology of opioid receptors can explain the difference in adverse effects caused by naltrexone and nalmefene. Opioid receptors in the body are typed pharmacologically as either μ, κ, or δ. Activation of the κ- and δ-receptors is thought to reinforce opioid and alcohol consumption centrally, whereas activation of μ-receptors is more closely associated with central and peripheral antiemetic effects. Because naltrexone is a relatively weak antagonist of κ- and δ-receptors and a potent μ-receptor antagonist, dosages of naltrexone that effectively reduce opioid and alcohol consumption also strongly block μ-receptors and, therefore, may cause nausea. Nalmefene, in contrast, is an equally potent antagonist of all three opioid receptor types, and dosages of nalmefene that effectively reduce opioid and alcohol consumption have no particularly increased effect on μ-receptors. Thus, nalmefene is associated clinically with few GI adverse effects.

Naloxone has the highest affinity for the μ receptor, but is a competitive antagonist at the μ, κ, and δ receptors.

Whereas the effects of opioid receptor antagonists on opioid use are easily understood in terms of competitive inhibition of opioid receptors, the effects of opioid receptor antagonists on alcohol dependence are less straightforward and probably relate to the fact that the desire for, and effects of, alcohol consumption appear to be regulated by several neurotransmitter systems, both opioid and nonopioid.

THERAPEUTIC INDICATIONS

The combination of a cognitive–behavioral program plus use of opioid receptor antagonists is more successful than either the cognitive–behavioral program or use of opioid receptor antagonists alone. Naltrexone is used as a screening test to ensure that the patient is opioid free before the induction of therapy with naltrexone (see discussion of the naloxone challenge test below).

Opioid Dependence

Patients in detoxification programs are usually weaned from potent opioid agonists such as heroin over a period of days to weeks, during which emergent adrenergic withdrawal effects are treated as needed with clonidine (Catapres). A serial protocol is sometimes used in which potent agonists are gradually replaced by weaker agonists, followed by mixed agonist–antagonists, and then finally by pure antagonists. For example, an abuser of the potent agonist heroin would switch first to the weaker agonist methadone (Dolophine), then to the partial agonist buprenorphine (Buprenex) or levomethadyl acetate (ORLAAM)—commonly called LAAM—and finally, following a 7- to 10-day washout period, to a pure antagonist, such as naltrexone or nalmefene. Even with gradual detoxification, some persons, however, continue to experience mild adverse effects or opioid withdrawal symptoms for the first several weeks of treatment with naltrexone.

As the opioid receptor agonist potency diminishes, so do the adverse consequences of discontinuing the drug. Thus, because no pharmacologic barriers exist to discontinuation of pure opioid receptor antagonists, the social environment and frequent cognitive–behavioral intervention become extremely important factors supporting continued opioid abstinence. Because of poorly tolerated adverse symptoms, most persons not simultaneously enrolled in a cognitive–behavioral program stop taking opioid receptor antagonists within 3 months. Compliance with administration of an opioid receptor antagonist regimen can also be increased with participation in a well-conceived voucher program.

Issues of medication compliance should be a central focus of treatment. If a person with a history of opioid addiction stops taking a pure opioid receptor antagonist, the person's risk of relapse into opioid abuse is exceedingly high, because reintroduction of a potent opioid agonist would yield a very rewarding subjective "high." In contrast, compliant persons do not develop tolerance to the therapeutic benefits of naltrexone, even if it is administered continuously for 1 year or longer. Individuals may undergo several relapses and remissions before achieving long-term abstinence.

Persons taking opioid receptor antagonists should also be warned that sufficiently high dosages of opioid agonists can overcome the receptor antagonism of naltrexone or nalmefene, which can lead to hazardous and unpredictable levels of receptor activation (see *Precautions and Adverse Reactions*).

Rapid Detoxification. To avoid the 7- to 10-day period of opioid abstinence generally recommended before use of opioid receptor antagonists, rapid detoxification protocols have been developed. Continuous administration of adjunct clonidine—to reduce the adrenergic withdrawal symptoms—and adjunct benzodiazepines, such as oxazepam (Serax)—to reduce muscle spasms and insomnia—can permit use of oral opioid receptor antagonists on the first day of opioid cessation. Detoxification, thus, can be completed within 48 to 72 hours, at which point opioid receptor antagonist maintenance is initiated. Moderately severe withdrawal symptoms may be experienced on the first day, but they tail off rapidly thereafter.

Because of the potential hypotensive effects of clonidine, the blood pressure (BP) of persons undergoing rapid detoxification must be closely monitored for the first 8 hours. Outpatient rapid detoxification settings, therefore, must be adequately prepared to administer emergency care.

The main advantage of rapid detoxification is that the transition from opioid abuse to maintenance treatment occurs over just 2 or 3 days. The completion of detoxification in as little time as possible minimizes the risk that the person will relapse into opioid abuse during the detoxification protocol.

Alcohol Dependence

Opioid receptor antagonists are also used as adjuncts to cognitive–behavioral programs for treatment of alcohol dependence. Opioid receptor antagonists reduce alcohol craving and alcohol consumption, and they ameliorate the severity of relapses. The risk of relapse into heavy consumption of alcohol attributable to an effective cognitive–behavioral program alone may be halved with concomitant use of opioid receptor antagonists.

The newer agent nalmefene has a number of potential pharmacologic and clinical advantages over its predecessor naltrexone for treatment of alcohol dependence. Whereas naltrexone may cause reversible transaminase elevations in persons who take dosages of 300 mg a day (which is six times the recommended dosage for treatment of alcohol and opioid dependence [50 mg a day]), nalmefene has not been associated with any hepatotoxicity. Clinically effective dosages of naltrexone are discontinued by 10 percent to 15 percent of persons because of adverse effects, most commonly nausea. In contrast, discontinuation of nalmefene because of an adverse event is rare at the clinically effective dosage of 20 mg a day and in the range of 10 percent at excessive dosages—that is, 80 mg a day. Because of its pharmacokinetic profile, a given dosage of nalmefene can also produce a more sustained opioid antagonist effect than does naltrexone.

The efficacy of opioid receptor antagonists in reducing alcohol craving can be augmented with a selective serotonin reuptake inhibitor, although data from large trials are needed to assess this potential synergistic effect more fully.

PRECAUTIONS AND ADVERSE REACTIONS

Because opioid receptor antagonists are used to maintain a drug-free state after opioid detoxification, great care must be taken to ensure that an adequate washout period elapses after the last dose of opioids and before the first dose of an opioid receptor antagonist is taken: at least 5 days for a short-acting opioid such as heroin and at least 10 days for longer-acting opioids such as methadone. The opioid-free state should be determined by self-report and urine toxicology screens. If any question persists of whether opioids are in the body despite a negative urine screen result, then a *naloxone challenge test* should be performed. Naloxone challenge is used because its opioid antagonism lasts less than 1 hour, whereas those of naltrexone and nalmefene can persist for more than 24 hours. Thus, any withdrawal effects elicited by naloxone will be relatively short-lived (see *Dosage and Clinical Guidelines*). Symptoms of acute opioid withdrawal include drug craving, feeling of temperature change, musculoskeletal pain, and GI distress. Signs of opioid withdrawal include confusion, drowsiness, vomiting, and diarrhea. Naltrexone and nalmefene should not be taken if naloxone infusion causes any signs of opioid withdrawal, except as part of a supervised rapid detoxification protocol.

A set of adverse effects, resembling a vestigial withdrawal syndrome, tends to affect up to 10 percent of persons who take opioid receptor antagonists. Up to 15 percent of persons taking naltrexone may experience abdominal pain, cramps, nausea, and vomiting, which may be limited by transiently halving the dosage or altering the time of administration. Adverse central nervous system (CNS) effects of naltrexone, experienced by up to 10 percent of persons, include headache, low energy, insomnia, anxiety, and nervousness. Joint and muscle pains may occur in up to 10 percent of persons taking naltrexone, as may rash.

Naltrexone can cause dosage-related hepatic toxicity at dosages well in excess of 50 mg a day; 20 percent of persons taking 300 mg a day of naltrexone may experience serum aminotransferase concentrations 3 to 19 times the upper limit of normal. The hepatocellular injury of naltrexone appears to be a dose-related toxic effect rather than an idiosyncratic reaction. At the lowest dosages of naltrexone required for effective opioid antagonism, hepatocellular injury is not typically observed. Naltrexone dosages as low as 50 mg a day may be hepatotoxic, however, in persons with underlying liver disease, such as persons with cirrhosis of the liver caused by chronic alcohol abuse. Serum aminotransferase concentrations should be monitored monthly for the first 6 months of naltrexone therapy and thereafter on the basis of clinical suspicion. Hepatic enzyme concentrations usually return to normal after discontinuation of naltrexone therapy.

If analgesia is required while a dose of an opioid receptor antagonist is pharmacologically active, opioid agonists should be avoided in favor of benzodiazepines or other nonopioid analgesics. Persons taking opioid receptor antagonists should be instructed that low dosages of opioids will have no effect, but larger dosages could overcome the receptor blockade and suddenly produce symptoms of profound opioid overdosage, with sedation possibly progressing to coma or death. Use of opioid receptor antagonists is contraindicated in persons who are taking opioid agonists, small amounts of which may be present in over-the-counter antiemetic and antitussive preparations; in persons with acute hepatitis or hepatic failure; and in persons who are hypersensitive to the drugs.

Because naltrexone is transported across the placenta, opioid receptor antagonists should only be taken by pregnant women if a compelling need outweighs the potential risks to the fetus. It is not known whether opioid receptor antagonists are distributed into maternal milk.

Opioid receptor antagonists are relatively safe drugs, and ingestion of high doses of them should be treated with supportive measures combined with efforts to decrease GI absorption.

DRUG INTERACTIONS

Because of its extensive hepatic metabolism, naltrexone can affect, or be affected by, other drugs that influence hepatic enzyme levels. The clinical importance of these potential interactions, however, is not known.

One potentially hepatotoxic drug that has been used in some cases with opioid receptor antagonists is disulfiram (Antabuse). Although no adverse effects were observed, frequent laboratory monitoring is indicated when such combination therapy is contemplated. Opioid receptor antagonists have been reported to potentiate the sedation associated with use of thioridazine (Mellaril), an interaction that probably applies equally to all low-potency dopamine receptor antagonists.

LABORATORY INTERFERENCES

No laboratory interferences have been described for opioid receptor antagonists, although relatively nonspecific immune-based toxicology screens for opioids could potentially yield positive results in persons taking only opioid receptor antagonists, because of their structural similarities to other opioids.

DOSAGE AND CLINICAL GUIDELINES

To avoid the possibility of precipitating an acute opioid withdrawal syndrome, several steps should be taken to ensure that the person is opioid free. Within a supervised detoxification setting, at least 5 days should elapse following the last dose of short-acting opioids, such as heroin, hydromorphone (Dilaudid), meperidine (Demerol), or morphine, and at least 10 days should elapse after the last dose of longer-acting opioids, such as methadone, before opioid antagonists are initiated. Briefer periods off opioids have been used in rapid detoxification protocols. To confirm that opioid detoxification is complete, urine toxicologic screens should demonstrate no opioid metabolites. An individual may, however, have a negative urine opioid screen result yet still be physically dependent on opioids and, thus, susceptible to antagonist-induced withdrawal effects. Therefore, once the urine screen result is negative, a naloxone challenge test is recommended, unless an adequate period of opioid abstinence can be reliably confirmed by observers (Table 36.26–1).

The initial dosage of naltrexone for treatment of opioid or alcohol dependence is 50 mg a day, which should be achieved through gradual introduction, even when the naloxone challenge test result is negative. Various authorities begin with 5, 10, 12.5, or 25 mg and titrate up to the 50-mg dosage over a period ranging from 1 hour to 2 weeks, while constantly monitoring for evidence of opioid withdrawal. Once a daily dose of 50 mg is well tolerated, it may be averaged over a week by giving 100 mg on alternate days or 150 mg every third day. Such schedules may increase compliance. The corresponding therapeutic dosage of nalmefene is 20 mg a day, divided into two equal doses. Gradual titration of nalmefene to this daily dose is probably a wise strategy, although clinical data on dosage strategies for nalmefene are not yet available.

To maximize compliance, it is recommended that ingestion of each dose be directly observed, either in a facility or by family members, and that random urine tests be taken for opioid receptor antagonists and their metabolites and for ethanol or opioid metabolites. Opioid receptor antagonists should be continued until the person is no longer considered psychologically at risk for relapse into opioid or alcohol abuse. This generally requires at least 6 months, but may take longer, particularly if there are external stresses.

Rapid Detoxification

Rapid detoxification has been standardized using naltrexone, although nalmefene would be expected to be equally effective with fewer adverse effects. In rapid detoxification protocols, the addicted person stops opioid use abruptly and begins the first

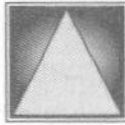

Table 36.26–1
Naloxone (Narcan) Challenge Test

The naloxone challenge test should not be performed in a patient showing clinical signs or symptoms of opioid withdrawal or in a patient whose urine contains opioids. The naloxone challenge test can be administered by either the intravenous (IV) or subcutaneous route.

Intravenous challenge: Following appropriate screening of the patient, 0.8 mg of naloxone should be drawn into a sterile syringe. If the IV route of administration is selected, 0.2 mg of naloxone should be injected, and while the needle is still in the patient's vein, the patient should be observed for 30 seconds for evidence of withdrawal signs or symptoms. If no evidence of withdrawal is seen, the remaining 0.6 mg of naloxone should be injected, and the patient observed for an additional 20 minutes for signs and symptoms of withdrawal.

Subcutaneous challenge: If the subcutaneous route is selected, 0.8 mg should be administered subcutaneously and the patient observed for signs and symptoms of withdrawal for 20 minutes.

Conditions and technique for observation of patient: During the appropriate period of observation, the patient's vital signs should be monitored, and the patient should be monitored for signs of withdrawal. It is also important to question the patient carefully. The signs and symptoms of opioid withdrawal include, but are not limited to, the following:

Withdrawal signs: Stuffiness or running nose, tearing, yawning, sweating, tremor, vomiting, or piloerection

Withdrawal symptoms: Feeling of temperature change, joint or bone and muscle pain, abdominal cramps, and formication (feeling of bugs crawling under skin)

Interpretation of the challenge: Warning—the elicitation of the enumerated signs or symptoms indicates a potential risk for the subject, and naltrexone should not be administered. If no signs or symptoms of withdrawal are observed, elicited, or reported, naltrexone may be administered. With any doubt in the observer's mind that the patient is not in an opioid-free state or is in continuing withdrawal, naltrexone should be withheld for 24 hours and the challenge repeated.

opioid-free day by taking clonidine, 0.2 mg, orally every 2 hours for nine doses, to a maximal dose of 1.8 mg, during which time BP is monitored every 30 to 60 minutes for the first 8 hours. Naltrexone, 12.5 mg, is administered 1 to 3 hours after the first dose of clonidine. To reduce muscle cramps and later insomnia, a short-acting benzodiazepine, such as oxazepam, 30 to 60 mg, is administered simultaneously with the first dose of clonidine, and half of the initial dose is readministered every 4 to 6 hours as needed. The maximal daily dosage of oxazepam should not exceed 180 mg. The person undergoing rapid detoxification should be accompanied home by a reliable escort. On the second day, similar doses of clonidine and the benzodiazepine are administered but with a single dose of naltrexone, 25 mg, taken in the morning. Relatively asymptomatic persons may return home after 3 to 4 hours. Administration of the daily maintenance dose of naltrexone, 50 mg, is begun on the third day, and the dosages of clonidine and the benzodiazepine are gradually tapered off over 5 to 10 days.

References

Dunbar JL, Turncliff RZ, Dong Q, Silverman BL, Ehrich EW, Lasseter KC. Single- and multiple-dose pharmacokinetics of long-acting injectable naltrexone. *Alcohol Clin Exp Res*. 2006;30:480.

Eguchi M. Recent advances in selective opioid receptor agonists and antagonists. *Med Res Rev*. 2003;24(2):182.

Grant JE, Kim SW, Potenza MN. Advances in the pharmacological treatment of pathological gambling. *J Gambl Stud*. 2003;19:85–109.

Krishnan-Sarin S, Rounsaville BJ, O'Malley SS. Opioid receptor antagonists: Naltrexone and nalmefene. In: Sadock BJ, Sadock VA, eds. *Kaplan & Sadock's Comprehensive Textbook of Psychiatry*. 8th ed. Vol. 2. Baltimore: Lippincott Williams & Wilkins; 2005:2875.

McGeary JE, Monti PM, Rohsenow DJ, Tidey J, Swift R, Miranda R Jr. Genetic moderators of naltrexone's effects on alcohol cue reactivity. *Alcohol Clin Exp Res*. 2006;30:1288.

▲ 36.27 Phosphodiesterase-5 Inhibitors

The introduction of the first phosphodiesterase (PDE)-5 inhibitor, sildenafil (Viagra), in 1998 revolutionized the treatment of the major sexual dysfunction affecting men—erectile disorder. Two congeners have since come on the market—vardenafil (Levitra) and tadalafil (Cialis). All have a similar method of action and have changed people's expectations of sexual functioning. Although indicated only for the treatment of male erectile dysfunction, anecdotal evidence suggests their being effective in women. They are also being misused as recreational drugs that are believed to enhance sexual performance. These drugs have been used by more than 20 million men, if not more, around the world.

CHEMISTRY

The development of sildenafil provided important information about the physiology of erection. Sexual stimulation causes the release of the neurotransmitter nitric oxide (NO), which increases the synthesis of cyclic guanosine monophosphate (cGMP), causing smooth muscle relaxation in the corpus cavernosum that allows blood to flow into the penis and that results in turgidity and tumescence. The concentration of cGMP is regulated by the enzyme PDE-5, which, when inhibited, allows cGMP to increase and enhance erectile function. Because sexual stimulation is required to cause the release of NO, PDE-5 inhibitors have no effect in the absence of such stimulation, an important point to understand when providing information to patients about their use. The congeners vardenafil and tadalafil work in the same way, by inhibiting PDE-5, thus allowing an increase in cGMP and enhancing the vasodilatory effects of NO. For this reason, these drugs are sometimes referred to as NO enhancers.

The structural formulas of sildenafil, vardenafil, and tadalafil are shown in Figure 36.27–1.

PHARMACOLOGIC ACTIONS

All three substances are fairly rapidly absorbed from the gastrointestinal (GI) tract, with maximal plasma concentrations reached in 30 to 120 minutes (median, 60 minutes) in the fasting state. Because it is lipophilic, concomitant ingestion of a high-fat meal delays the rate of absorption by up to 60 minutes and reduces the peak concentration by one quarter. These drugs are principally metabolized by the cytochrome CYP 3A4 system, which can lead to clinically significant drug–drug interactions, not all of which have been documented. Excretion of 80 percent

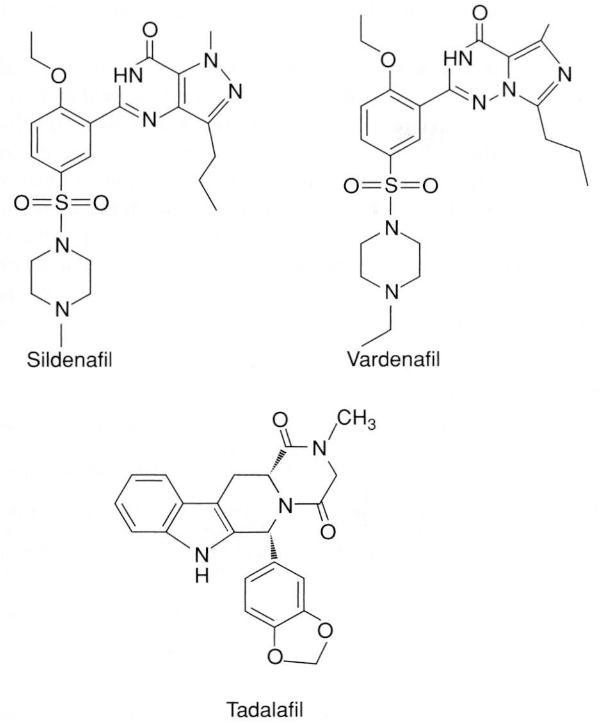

Sildenafil

Vardenafil

Tadalafil

FIGURE 36.27–1
Chemical structure of the phosphodiesterase (PDE)-5 inhibitors sildenafil, vardenafil, and tadalafil.

of the dose is via feces, and another 13 percent is eliminated in the urine. Elimination is reduced in persons over age 65 years, which results in plasma concentrations 40 percent higher than in persons aged 18 to 45 years. Elimination is also reduced in the presence of severe renal or hepatic insufficiency.

The mean half-lives of sildenafil and vardenafil are 3 to 4 hours and that of tadalafil is about 18 hours. Tadalafil can be detected in the bloodstream 5 days after ingestion, and because of its long half-life, it has been marketed as effective for up to 36 hours—the so-called weekend pill; however, more than once-a-day use can cause excessive accumulation of the drug, and the effects of inhibiting PDE for long periods of time require further investigation. The onset of sildenafil occurs about 30 minutes after ingestion on an empty stomach; tadalafil and vardenafil act somewhat more quickly.

The clinician needs to be aware of the important clinical observation that these drugs do not by themselves create an erection. Rather, the mental state of sexual arousal brought on by erotic stimulation must first lead to activity in the penile nerves which then release NO into the cavernosum, triggering the erectile cascade, the resulting erection being prolonged by the NO enhancers. Thus, full advantage may be taken of a sexually exciting stimulus, but the drug is not a substitute for foreplay and emotional arousal.

THERAPEUTIC INDICATIONS

Erectile dysfunctions have traditionally been classified as organic, psychogenic, or mixed. Over the last 20 years, the prevailing view of the cause of erectile dysfunction has shifted away from psychological causes toward organic causes. The latter include diabetes mellitus, hypertension, hypercholesterolemia, cigarette smoking, peripheral vascular disease, pelvic or spinal cord injury, pelvic or abdominal surgery (especially, prostate surgery), multiple sclerosis, peripheral neuropathy, and Parkinson's disease. Erectile dysfunction is often induced by alcohol, nicotine, and other substances of abuse and by prescription drugs.

These drugs are effective regardless of the baseline severity of erectile dysfunction, race, or age. Among those responding to sildenafil are men with coronary artery disease, hypertension, other cardiac disease, peripheral vascular disease, diabetes mellitus, depression, coronary artery bypass graft (CABG), radical prostatectomy, transurethral resection of the prostate, spina bifida, and spinal cord injury, as well as persons taking antidepressants, antipsychotics, antihypertensives, and diuretics. The response rate, however, is variable.

Sildenafil has been reported to reverse selective serotonin reuptake inhibitor (SSRI)-induced anorgasmia in men. Anecdotal reports indicate that sildenafil has a therapeutic effect on sexual inhibition in women as well.

PRECAUTIONS AND ADVERSE REACTIONS

The most important potential adverse effect associated with use of these drugs is myocardial infarction (MI). The US Food and Drug Administration (FDA) distinguished the risk of MI caused directly by these drugs from that caused by underlying conditions, such as hypertension, atherosclerotic heart disease, diabetes mellitus, and other atherogenic conditions. The FDA concluded that, when used according to the approved labeling, the drugs do not by themselves confer an increased risk of death. Increased oxygen demand and stress is placed on the cardiac muscle by sexual intercourse, however. Thus, coronary perfusion may be severely compromised and cardiac failure may occur as a result. For that reason, any person with a history of MI, stroke, renal failure, hypertension, or diabetes mellitus and any person over the age of 70 years should discuss plans to use these drugs with an internist or a cardiologist. The cardiac evaluation should specifically address exercise tolerance and the use of nitrates.

Use of PDE-5 inhibitors is contraindicated in persons who are taking organic nitrates in any form. Also, amyl nitrate (poppers), a popular substance of abuse used by gay men to enhance the intensity of orgasm, should not be used with any of the erection-enhancing drugs. The combination of organic nitrates and PDE inhibitors can cause a precipitous lowering of blood pressure (BP) and can reduce coronary perfusion to the point of causing MI and death.

Adverse effects are dose dependent, occurring at higher rates with higher dosages. The most common adverse effects are headache, flushing, and stomach pain. Other, less common adverse effects include nasal congestion, urinary tract infection, abnormal vision (colored tinge [usually blue], increased sensitivity to light, or blurred vision), diarrhea, dizziness, and rash. No cases of priapism were reported in premarketing trials. Supportive management is indicated in cases of overdosage. Tadalafil has been associated with back and muscle pain in about 10 percent of patients.

Recently there have been 50 reports and 14 verfied cases of a serious condition in men taking Sildenafil called non arteritic anterior ischemic optic neuropathy (NAION). This is an eye ailment that causes restriction of blood flow to the optic nerve and can result in permanent vision loss. The first symptoms appear within 24 hours after use of Sildenafil and include blurred vision and some degree of vision loss. The incidence of this effect is very rare—one in a million. In the reported cases, many patients had preexisting eye problems which may have increased their risk and many had a history of heart disease and diabetes which may indicate a vulnerability in these men to endothelial damage.

No data are available on the effects on human fetal growth and development or testicular morphologic or functional changes. Because these drugs are not considered an essential treatment, they should not be used during pregnancy.

DRUG INTERACTIONS

The major route of PDE-5 metabolism is through CYP450 (CYP) 3A4, and the minor route is through CYP 2C9. Inducers or inhibitors of these enzymes, therefore, will affect the plasma concentration and half-life of sildenafil. For example, 800 mg of cimetidine (Tagamet), a nonspecific CYP inhibitor, increases plasma sildenafil concentrations by 56 percent, and erythromycin (E-mycin) increases plasma sildenafil concentrations by 182 percent. Other, stronger inhibitors of CYP 3A4 include ketoconazole (Nizoral), itraconazole (Sporanox), and mibefradil (Posicor). In contrast, rifampicin (Rifadin), a CYP 3A4 inducer, decreases plasma concentrations of sildenafil.

LABORATORY INTERFERENCES

No laboratory interferences have been described.

DOSAGE AND CLINICAL GUIDELINES

Sildenafil is available as 25-, 50-, and 100-mg tablets. The recommended dose of sildenafil is 50 mg taken by mouth 1 hour prior to intercourse. Sildenafil, however, may take effect within 30 minutes. The duration of the effect is usually 4 hours, but in healthy young men, the effect may persist for 8 to 12 hours. Based on effectiveness and adverse effects, the dose should be titrated between 25 and 100 mg. Sildenafil is recommended for use no more than once a day. The dosing guidelines for use by women, an off-label use, are the same as those for men.

Increased plasma concentrations of sildenafil can occur in persons over 65 years of age and those with cirrhosis or severe renal impairment or using CYP 3A4 inhibitors. A starting dose of 25 mg should be used in these circumstances.

An investigational nasal spray formulation of sildenafil has been developed that acts within 5 to 15 minutes of administration. This formulation is highly water soluble, and it is rapidly absorbed directly into the bloodstream. Such a formulation would permit more ease of use.

Vardenafil is supplied in 2.5-, 5-, 10-, and 20-mg tablets. The initial dose is usually 10 mg taken with or without food about 1 hour before sexual activity. The dose can be increased to a maximum of 20 mg or decreased to 5 mg based on efficacy and side effects. The maximal dosing frequency is once per day. As with sildenafil, dosages may have to be adjusted in patients with hepatic impairment or in patients using certain CYP 3A4 inhibitors.

The recommended dose of tadalafil is 10 mg before sexual activity, which may be increased to 20 mg or decreased to 5 mg, depending on efficacy and side effects. Because of its long half-life, it should probably not be used more than once every 36 hours, although the manufacturer states that once-a-day use is acceptable for most patients. Similar cautions apply as mentioned earlier in patients with hepatic impairment and in those taking concomitant potent inhibitors of CYP 3A4. As with other PDE-5 inhibitors, concomitant use of nitrates in any form is contraindicated.

REFERENCES

van Ahlen H, Wahle K, Kupper W, Yassin A, Reblin T, Neureither M. Safety and efficacy of vardenafil, a selective phosphodiesterase 5 inhibitor, in patients with erectile dysfunction and arterial hypertension treated with multiple antihypertensives. *J Sex Med.* 2005;2(6):856.

Allerton CM, Barber CG, Beaumont KC, Brown DG, Cole SM, Ellis D, Lane CA, Maw GN, Mount NM, Rawson DJ, Robinson CM, Street SD, Summerhill NW. A novel series of potent and selective PDE5 inhibitors with potential for high and dose-independent oral bioavailability. *J Med Chem.* 2006;49(12):3581.

Giovannoni MP, Vergelli C, Biancalani C, Cesari N, Graziano A, Biagini P, Gracia J, Gavalda A, Dal Piaz V. Novel pyrazolopyrimidopyridazinones with potent and selective phosphodiesterase 5 (PDE5) inhibitory activity as potential agents for treatment of erectile dysfunction. *J Med Chem.* 2006;49(17):5363.

Gopalakrishnan R, Jacob KS, Kuruvilla A, Vasantharaj B, John JK. Sildenafil in the treatment of antipsychotic-induced erectile dysfunction: A randomized, double-blind, placebo-controlled, flexible-dose, two-way crossover trial. *Am J Psych.* 2006;163(3):494.

Hatzichristou D, Cuzin B, Martin-Morales A, Buvat J, Porst H, Laferriere N, Bandel TJ, Montorsi F; Vardenafil Study Group. Vardenafil improves satisfaction rates, depressive symptomatology, and self-confidence in a broad population of men with erectile dysfunction. *J Sex Med.* 2005;2(1):109.

Laties A, Sharlip I. Ocular safety in patients using sildenafil citrate therapy for erectile dysfunction. *J Sex Med.* 2006;3(1):12.

Levien TL. Phosphodiesterase inhibitors in Raynaud's phenomenon. *Ann Pharmacother.* 2006;40(7-8):1388.

Mulhall JP, McLaughlin TP, Harnett JP, Scott B, Burhani S, Russell D. Medication utilization behavior in patients receiving phosphodiesterase type 5 inhibitors for erectile dysfunction. *J Sex Med.* 2005; 2(6):848.

Seftel AD. Phosphodiesterase type 5 inhibitor differentiation based on selectivity, pharmacokinetic, and efficacy profiles. *Clin Cardiol.* 2004; 27[4 Suppl 1]: I14.

▲ 36.28 Selective Serotonin–Norepinephrine Reuptake Inhibitors

Venlafaxine (Effexor) and duloxetine (Cymbalta) are selective serotonin–norepinephrine reuptake inhibitors (SNRIs). Originally marketed as an antidepressant, venlafaxine is now also indicated for the treatment of generalized anxiety and social anxiety disorders. Duloxetine is indicated for the treatment of depression, generalized anxiety disorder, and painful diabetic neuropathy and is awaiting the indication for stress urinary incontinence.

Venlafaxine and duloxetine are not unique with respect to their dual action. Tricyclic and tetracyclic antidepressants (TCAs) also inhibit reuptake of norepinephrine and serotonin. TCAs, however, also possess numerous other receptor

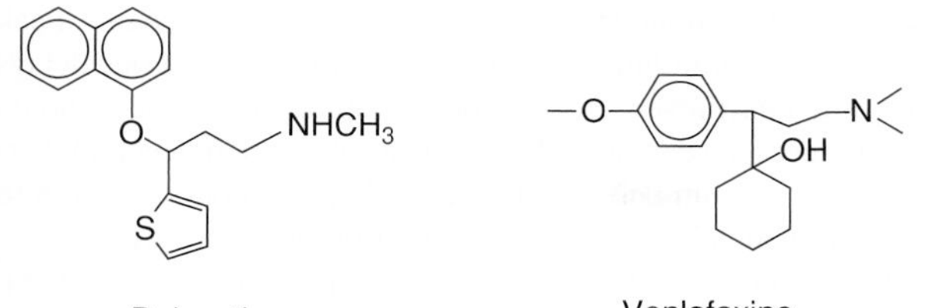

FIGURE 36.28–1
Chemical structures of the serotonin-norepinephrine reuptake inhibitors.

properties, such as muscarinic, adrenergic, and histaminergic effects, and thus are not considered selective.

CHEMISTRY

Venlafaxine and duloxetine are structurally distinct from each other and from other antidepressant drugs. The structural formulas of these agents are shown in Figure 36.28–1.

VENLAFAXINE

Pharmacologic Actions

Venlafaxine is well absorbed from the gastrointestinal (GI) tract. The extended-release formulation of venlafaxine (Effexor XR) and the metabolite *O*-desmethylvenlafaxine (ODV) reach peak plasma concentrations in 5.5 hours and 9 hours, respectively. Venlafaxine has a half-life of about 3.5 hours, and ODV has a half-life of 9 hours. It is metabolized by hepatic cytochrome P450 (CYP) 2D6. Thus, inhibitors of this isozyme, such as quinidine or paroxetine, reduce the formation of ODV. Venlafaxine is not highly bound to plasma proteins.

Venlafaxine is a potent inhibitor of serotonin and norepinephrine reuptake and a weak inhibitor of dopamine reuptake. It does not have activity at muscarinic, nicotinic, histaminergic, opioid, or adrenergic receptors, and it is not active as a monoamine oxidase inhibitor (MAOI).

Therapeutic Indications

Depression. The US Food and Drug Administration (FDA) does not recognize any class of antidepressant as being more effective than any other. This does not mean that differences do not exist, but no study to date has sufficiently demonstrated such superiority. There is some evidence to suggest that venlafaxine has a potential to induce higher rates of remission in depressed patients than do the selective serotonin reuptake inhibitors (SSRIs). This difference of the venlafaxine advantage is about 6 percent.

Generalized Anxiety Disorder. The extended-release formulation of venlafaxine is approved for treatment of generalized anxiety disorder. In clinical trials lasting 6 months, dosages of 75 to 225 mg a day were effective against insomnia, poor concentration, restlessness, irritability, and excessive muscle tension related to generalized anxiety disorder.

Social Anxiety Disorder. The extended-release formulation of venlafaxine is approved for treatment of social anxiety disorder. Its efficacy was established in 12-week studies.

Panic Disorder. The extended-release formulation of venlafaxine is also approved for treatment of panic disorder.

Other Indications. Case reports and uncontrolled studies have indicated that venlafaxine may be beneficial in the treatment of obsessive-compulsive disorder, agoraphobia, attention-deficit/hyperactivity disorder (ADHD), and in patients with a dual diagnosis of depression and cocaine dependence. It has also been used in chronic pain syndromes with good effect.

Precautions and Adverse Reactions

The frequency of specific side effects varied in studies involving different disorders. Overall, the most common adverse reactions are nausea, somnolence, dry mouth, dizziness, nervousness, constipation, asthenia, anxiety, anorexia, blurred vision, abnormal ejaculation or orgasm, erectile disturbances, and impotence. Sweating is also more common with venlafaxine than the SSRIs (and frequently treated with terazosin). The incidence of nausea can be considerably reduced by initiating treatment using 37.5-mg-per-day capsules.

Abrupt discontinuation of venlafaxine use can produce a discontinuation syndrome consisting of dizziness, anxiety, nausea, somnolence, paresthesias, and insomnia. Therefore, venlafaxine use should be tapered gradually over 2 to 4 weeks.

Venlafaxine can cause an increase in blood pressure (BP) in some persons. Diastolic hypertension was seen more often in patients treated with doses of venlafaxine greater than 300 mg per day, a dose higher than needed in most patients.

A common misconception is that risk of venlafaxine-induced hypertension is greater among persons with preexisting hypertension. It is wise periodically to monitor the BP of any patient taking venlafaxine. If a patient develops significant rise in BP, but otherwise shows a good therapeutic response, it is reasonable to consider either lowering of the dose, adding antihypertensive therapy, or both.

Venlafaxine can cause mydriasis, so patients with raised intraocular pressure or those at risk for acute narrow-angle glaucoma should be monitored during venlafaxine treatment. As in the case of SSRIs, abnormal bleeding or ecchymosis may be associated with venlafaxine use, the result of serotonin-related impairment of platelet aggregation.

The pharmacokinetic dispositions of both venlafaxine and ODV are altered in patients with hepatic cirrhosis. Venlafaxine elimination half-life is prolonged by about 30 percent and clearance decreased by about 50 percent. ODV elimination half-life is also prolonged (by about 60 percent) and its clearance decreased by about 30 percent. In patients with more severe cirrhosis, there may be a 90 percent decrease in venlafaxine clearance. Dosage adjustment, thus, is necessary in patients with liver disease.

Information concerning use of venlafaxine by pregnant and nursing women is not available at this time. Venlafaxine and ODV are excreted in human milk. Clinicians should carefully weigh the risks and benefits of venlafaxine use by pregnant and nursing women.

Drug Interactions

Cimetidine (Tagamet) appears to inhibit the first-pass hepatic metabolism of venlafaxine and to raise the levels of the unmetabolized drug. Because the metabolite is mainly responsible for the therapeutic effect, this interaction is of concern only in persons with preexisting hypertension or hepatic disease, in whom this combination should be avoided. Combined use of sustained-release bupropion (Wellbutrin SR) has been shown to increase plasma concentrations of venlafaxine. Venlafaxine may raise plasma concentrations of concurrently administered haloperidol (Haldol). As with all antidepressant medications, venlafaxine should not be used within 14 days of the use of monoamine oxidase inhibitors, and it may potentiate the sedative effects of other drugs that act on the central nervous system (CNS).

Laboratory Interferences

Data are not currently available on laboratory interferences with venlafaxine.

Dosage and Administration

Venlafaxine is available in 25-, 37.5-, 50-, 75-, and 100-mg tablets and 37.5-, 75-, and 150-mg extended-release capsules. The tablets and the extended-release capsules are equally potent, and persons stabilized with one can switch to an equivalent dosage of the other. Because the immediate-release tablets are rarely used because of their tendency to cause nausea and need for multiple daily doses, the dosage recommendations that follow refer to use of the extended-release capsules.

In depressed persons, venlafaxine demonstrates a dose-response curve. The initial therapeutic dosage is 75 mg a day, given once a day. Most persons, however, are started at a dosage of 37.5 mg for 4 to 7 days to minimize adverse effects, particularly nausea. A convenient starter kit for the drug contains a 1-week supply of both the 37.5- and 75-mg strengths. Should a rapid titration be preferred, the dosage can be raised to 150 mg per day after day 4. As a rule, the dosage can be raised in increments of 75 mg a day every 4 or more days. Although the recommended upper dosage of the extended-release preparation (Effexor XR) is 225 mg per day, it is approved by the FDA for use at dosages up to 375 mg a day. The dosage of venlafaxine should be halved in persons with significantly diminished hepatic or renal function. If discontinued, venlafaxine use should be gradually tapered over 2 to 4 weeks to avoid withdrawal symptoms.

Minor differences exist in the doses used for major depression, generalized anxiety disorder, and social anxiety disorder. In the treatment of these disorders, for example, a dose-response effect has not been found. In addition, lower mean dosages are typically used, with most patients taking 75 to 150 mg per day.

DULOXETINE

Pharmacologic Actions

Duloxetine is formulated as a delayed-release capsule to reduce the risk of severe nausea associated with the drug. It is well absorbed, but a 2-hour delay occurs before absorption begins. Peak plasma concentrations occur 6 hours after ingestion. Food delays the time to achieve maximal concentrations from 6 to 10 hours and reduces the extent of absorption by about 10 percent. Duloxetine has an elimination half-life of about 12 hours (range 8 to 17 hours). Steady-state plasma concentrations occur after 3 days. Elimination is mainly through the isozymes CYP 2D6 and CYP 1A2. Duloxetine undergoes extensive hepatic metabolism to numerous metabolites. About 70 percent of the drug appears in the urine as metabolites and about 20 percent is excreted in the feces. Duloxetine is 90 percent protein bound.

Therapeutic Indications

Depression and Generalized Anxiety Disorder (GAD). In contrast to venlafaxine, a small number of studies have compared duloxetine with SSRIs in depression. These studies are suggestive of some advantage in efficacy with duloxetine. In GAD higher doses are also used with good results.

Neuropathic Pain Associated with Diabetes and Stress Urinary Incontinence. Duloxetine is the first drug to be approved by the FDA as a treatment for neuropathic pain associated with diabetes. The drug has been studied for its effects on physical symptoms, including pain, in depressed patients, but these effects have not been compared with those seen with other widely used agents such as venlafaxine and the TCAs. Duloxetine is currently awaiting approval as a treatment for stress urinary incontinence, the inability to voluntarily control bladder voiding, which is the most frequent type of incontinence in women. The action of duloxetine in the treatment of stress urinary incontinence is associated with its effects in the sacral spinal cord, which in turn increase the activity of the striated urethral sphincter. Duloxetine will be marketed under the name Yantreve for this indication.

While duloxetine is approved for the treatment of diabetic peripheral neuropathic pain, it may worsen control of blood sugar levels. Pooled data from clinical trials show that short-term treatment with duloxetine causes an increase in fasting glucose and hemoglobin A1c levels. Body weight decreased with short-term duloxetine treatment, but increased during long-term treatment. Modest increases in cholesterol may occur during duloxetine therapy.

Precautions and Adverse Reactions

The most common adverse reactions are nausea, dry mouth, dizziness, constipation, fatigue, decreased appetite, anorexia, somnolence, and increased sweating. Nausea was the most common side effect leading to treatment discontinuation in clinical trials. The true incidence of sexual dysfunction is not known, nor are the long-term effects on body weight known. In clinical trials, treatment with duloxetine was associated with mean increases in BP averaging 2 mm Hg systolic and 0.5 mm Hg diastolic versus placebo. No studies have compared BP effects of venlafaxine and duloxetine at equivalent therapeutic doses.

Patients with substantial alcohol use should not be treated with duloxetine because of possible hepatic effects. It also should not be prescribed for patients with hepatic insufficiency and end-stage renal disease or for patients with uncontrolled narrow-angle glaucoma.

Abrupt discontinuation of duloxetine should be avoided because it can produce a discontinuation syndrome similar to that of venlafaxine. A gradual dose reduction is recommended.

Because of limited clinical experience with duloxetine, risks associated with its use by pregnant and nursing women are not available at this time. Clinicians should avoid the use of duloxetine by pregnant and nursing women unless the potential benefits justify the potential risks.

Drug Interactions

Duloxetine is a moderate inhibitor of CYP 450 enzymes.

Laboratory Interferences

Data are not currently available on laboratory interferences with duloxetine.

Dosage and Administration

Duloxetine is available in 20-, 30-, and 60-mg tablets. The recommended therapeutic, and maximal, dosage is 60 mg per day. The 20- and 30-mg doses are useful for either initial therapy or for twice-daily use as strategies to reduce side effects. In clinical trials, dosages of up to 120 mg per day were studied, but no consistent advantage in efficacy was noted at dosages higher than 60 mg per day. Duloxetine, thus, does not appear to demonstrate a dosage-response curve. Difficulties in tolerability were seen, however, with single doses above 60 mg. Accordingly, when dosages of 80 and 120 mg per day were used, they were administered as 40 or 60 mg twice daily. Because of limited clinical experience with duloxetine, it remains to be seen to what extent dosages above 60 mg per day will be necessary and whether, in fact, this will require divided doses to make the drug tolerable.

Other SNRIs

Desvenlafaxine Succinate (DVS) (Pristiq). DVS is the salt form of the isolated major active metabolite of venlafaxine, developed as separated drug. Like venlafaxine, DVS is mechanistically an SNRI. It has been developed for the treatment of depression and for the alleviation vasomotor symptoms (VMS) associated with menopause. Sympotoms of VMS include hot flashes and night sweats. There are also plans to pursue DVS indications for fibromyalgia and diabetic neuropathic pain.

As is typical of the SNRI class most common side effects of DVS are abdominal pain, asthenia, anorexia, constipation, dry mouth, nausea, vomiting, dizziness, insomnia, nervousness, somnolence, sweating, tremor, vertigo, increased blood pressure and abnormal ejaculation. The optimal dosing of DVS has not been established, but in clinical trials, doses of 200- to 300-mg were effective in treating depression, but doses up to 600 mg were needed to alleviate VMS. At these, doses no effect on the QT interval was observed.

Milnacipran. This is another SNRI that has been available in many countries as an antidepressant. It has not been studied in the United States solely as a treatment for fibromyalgia. No drugs are currently FDA-approved for use in the treatment of fibromyalgia.

Sibutramine (Meridia). This is an SNRI marketed as a short-term anti-obesity treatment. The effectiveness and safety of the drug beyond one year has not been studied. Sibutramine has not been shown to act as an antidepressant. Side effects are similar to other SNRIs and include dose-related increase in blood pressure, heart rate, and arrythmias.

References

Barkin RL, Barkin S. The role of venlafaxine and duloxetine in the treatment of depression with decremental changes in somatic symptoms of pain, chronic pain, and the pharmacokinetics and clinical considerations of duloxetine pharmacotherapy. *Am J Ther*. 2005;12(5):431.

Dell'Osso B, Nestadt G, Allen A, Hollander E. Serotonin-norepinephrine reuptake inhibitors in the treatment of obsessive-compulsive disorder: A critical review. *J Clin Psychiatry*. 2006;67(4):600.

Nemeroff CB, Entsuah AR, Willard L, Demitrack M, Thase M. Venlafaxine and SSRIs: Pooled remission analysis. *Eur Neuropsychopharmacol*. 2003;13[Suppl 4]:S255.

Raskin J, Smith TR, Wong K, Pritchett YL, D'Souza DN, Iyengar S, Wernicke JF. Duloxetine versus routine care in the long-term management of diabetic peripheral neuropathic pain. *J Palliat Med*. 2006;9(1):29.

Shelton C, Entsuah R, Padmanabhan SK, Vinall PE. Venlafaxine XR demonstrates higher rates of sustained remission compared to fluoxetine, paroxetine or placebo. *Int Clin Psychopharmacol*. 2005;20(4):233.

Thase ME. Selective serotonin-norepinephrine reuptake inhibitors. In: Sadock BJ, Sadock VA, eds. *Kaplan & Sadock's Comprehensive Textbook of Psychiatry*. 8th ed. Vol. 2. Baltimore: Lippincott Williams & Wilkins; 2005:2881.

Thase ME, Lu Y, Joliat M, Detke M. Remission rates in double-blind, placebo-controlled clinical trials of duloxetine with SSRI as a comparator. *Eur Neuropsychopharmacol*. 2003;13[Suppl 4]:S215.

Thase ME, Sloan DME. Venlafaxine. In: Schatzberg AF, Nemeroff CB, eds. *Textbook of Psychopharmacology*, 3rd ed. Washington, DC: American Psychiatric Publishing, Inc.; 2003:349–360.

Thase ME, Tran PV, Wiltse C, Pangallo BA, Mallinckrodt C, Detke MJ. Cardiovascular profile of duloxetine, a dual reuptake inhibitor of serotonin and norepinephrine. *J Clin Psychopharmacol*. 2005;25(2):132.

Wohlreich MM, Mallinckrodt CH, Watkin JG, Wilson MG, Greist JH, Delgado PL, Fava M. Immediate switching of antidepressant therapy: Results from a clinical trial of duloxetine. *Ann Clin Psychiatry*. 2005;17(4):259.

▲ 36.29 Selective Serotonin Reuptake Inhibitors

The first selective serotonin reuptake inhibitor (SSRI), fluoxetine (Prozac), which was introduced in 1987, altered attitudes about pharmacologic treatment of depression. The reasons for this included that initial side effects of fluoxetine were generally better tolerated than those of existing treatments, such as the tricyclic antidepressants (TCAs) and monoamine oxidase inhibitors (MAOIs), and the simplicity of dosing of fluoxetine.

Subsequently, other SSRIs have been introduced, all of which share the same basic properties of fluoxetine. Since 1990, the list of approved indications for drugs in the class has expanded to include not only depression, but obsessive-compulsive disorder (OCD), panic disorder, generalized anxiety disorder, premenstrual dysphoric disorder, social anxiety disorder, and eating disorders (Table 36.29–1). All SSRIs appear to be equally effective in the treatment of these disorders.

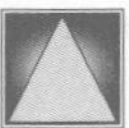

Table 36.29–1
Currently Approved Indications of the Selective Serotonin Reuptake Inhibitors in the United States for Adult and Pediatric Populations

	Citalopram (Celexa)	Escitalopram (Lexapro)	Fluoxetine (Prozac)	Fluvoxamine (Luvox)	Paroxetine (Paxil)	Sertraline (Zoloft)
Major depressive disorder	Adult	Adult	Adult[a] and pediatric	—	Adult[c]	Adult
Generalized anxiety disorder	—	Adult	—	—	Adult	—
OCD	—	—	Adult and pediatric	Adult and pediatric	Adult	Adult and pediatric
Panic disorder	—	—	Adult	—	Adult[c]	Adult
PTSD	—	—	—	—	Adult	Adult
Social anxiety disorder	—	—	—	—	Adult[c]	Adult
Bulimia nervosa	—	—	Adult	—	—	—
Premenstrual dysphoric disorder	—	—	Adult[b]	—	Adult[d]	Adult

[a] Weekly fluoxetine is approved for continuation and maintenance therapy in adults.
[b] Marketed as Sarafem.
[c] Paroxetine-and-paroxetine controlled release.
[d] Paroxetine controlled release is approved for premenstrual dysphoric disorder.
OCD, obsessive-compulsive disorder; PTSD, posttraumatic stress disorder.

CHEMISTRY

The SSRIs are each structurally and chemically distinct. Escitalopram, an isomer of citalopram (Celexa), is the only exception. This molecular diversity explains why individual responses to, and tolerability of, SSRIs are so varied. The structural formulas of escitalopram, fluoxetine, fluvoxamine, paroxetine, and sertraline are shown in Figure 36.29–1. The SSRIs possess significantly different pharmacokinetic profiles, as suggested by their diverse chemical structures.

PHARMACOLOGIC ACTIONS

Pharmacokinetics

The most significant difference among the SSRIs is their broad range of serum half-lives. Fluoxetine has the longest half-life: 4 to 6 days; its active metabolite has a half-life of 7 to 9 days. The half-life of sertraline is 26 hours, and its less active metabolite has a half-life of 3 to 5 days. The half-lives of the other three, which do not have metabolites with significant pharmacologic activity, are 35 hours for citalopram, 27 to 32 hours for escitalopram, 21 hours for paroxetine, and 15 hours for fluvoxamine. As a rule, SSRIs are well absorbed after oral administration and have their peak effects in the range of 3 to 8 hours. Absorption of sertraline may be slightly enhanced by food.

Differences in plasma protein binding percentages are also found among the SSRIs, with sertraline, fluoxetine, and paroxetine being the most highly bound and escitalopram being the least bound.

All SSRIs are metabolized in the liver by the cytochrome P450 (CYP) enzymes. Because SSRIs have such a wide therapeutic index, it is rare that other drugs produce problematic increases in SSRI concentrations. The most important drug–drug interactions involving the SSRIs occur as a result of the SSRIs inhibiting the metabolism of a coadministered medication. Each of the SSRIs possesses a potential for slowing or blocking the metabolism of many drugs (Table 36.29–2).

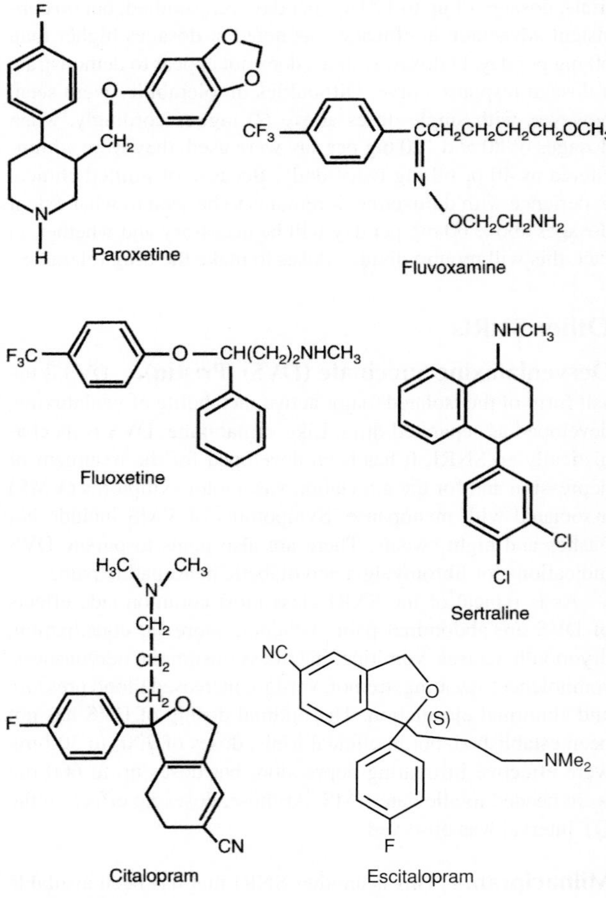

FIGURE 36.29–1
Molecular structures of selective serotonin reuptake inhibitors (SSRIs).

Table 36.29–2
Cytochrome P450 Inhibitory Potential of Commonly Prescribed Antidepressants

Relative Rank	CYP 1A2	CYP 2C	CYP 2D6	CYP 3A
Higher	Fluvoxamine (Luvox)	Fluoxetine Fluvoxamine	Bupropion Fluoxetine Paroxetine	Fluvoxamine Nefazodone Tricyclics
Moderate	Tertiary amine tricyclics Fluoxetine (Prozac)	Sertraline	Secondary amine tricyclics Citalopram (Celexa) Escitalopram (Lexapro) Sertraline	Fluoxetine Sertraline
Low or minimal	Bupropion (Wellbutrin) Mirtazapine (Remeron) Nefazodone (Serzone) Paroxetine (Paxil) Sertraline (Zoloft) Venlafaxine (Effexor)	Paroxetine Venlafaxine (Effexor)	Fluvoxamine Mirtazapine Nefazodone Venlafaxine	Citalopram Escitalopram Mirtazapine Paroxetine Venlafaxine

CYP, cytochrome P450.

Fluvoxamine is the most problematic of the drugs in this respect. It has a marked effect on several of the CYP enzymes. Examples of clinically significant interactions include fluvoxamine and theophylline (Theo-Dur) through CYP 1A2 interaction; fluvoxamine and clozapine (Clozaril) through CYP 1A2 inhibition; and fluvoxamine with alprazolam (Xanax) or clonazepam (Klonopin) through CYP 3A4 inhibition. Fluoxetine and paroxetine also possess significant effects on the CYP 2D6 isozyme, which may interfere with the efficacy of opiate analogs, such as codeine and hydrocodone, by blocking the conversion of these agents to their active form. Thus, coadministration of fluoxetine and paroxetine with an opiate interferes with its analgesic effects. Sertraline, citalopram, and escitalopram are least likely to complicate treatment because of interactions.

Pharmacodynamics

The SSRIs are believed to exert their therapeutic effects through 5-HT reuptake inhibition. They derive their name because they have little effect on reuptake of norepinephrine or dopamine. Often, adequate clinical activity, and saturation of the 5-HT transporters, are achieved at starting dosages. As a rule, higher dosages do not increase antidepressant efficacy, but may increase the risk of adverse effects.

Citalopram and escitalopram are the most selective inhibitors of serotonin reuptake, with very little inhibition of norepinephrine or dopamine reuptake and very low affinities for histamine H_1, γ-aminobutyric acid (GABA), or benzodiazepine receptors. The other SSRIs have a similar profile, except that fluoxetine weakly inhibits norepinephrine reuptake and binds to 5-HT_{2C} receptors; sertraline weakly inhibits norepinephrine and dopamine reuptake; and paroxetine has significant anticholinergic activity at higher dosages and binds to nitric oxide synthase.

A pharmacodynamic interaction appears to underlie the antidepressant effects of combined fluoxetine–olanzapine. When taken together, these drugs increase brain concentrations of norepinephrine. Concomitant use of SSRIs and drugs in the triptan class (sumatriptan [Imitrex], naratriptan [Amerge], rizatriptan [Maxalt], and zolmitriptan [Zomig]) may result in a serious pharmacodynamic interaction, the development of a serotonin syndrome (see *Precautions and Adverse Reactions*). Many people, however, use triptans while taking a low dose of an SSRI for headache prophylaxis without adverse reaction. A similar reaction may occur when SSRIs are combined with tramadol (Ultram).

THERAPEUTIC INDICATIONS

Depression

In the United States, all SSRIs other than fluvoxamine have been approved by the US Food and Drug Administration (FDA) for treatment of depression. Several studies have found that antidepressants with serotonin–norepinephrine activity, drugs such as the MAOIs, TCAs, venlafaxine, and mirtazapine, produce higher rates of remission than SSRIs in head-to-head studies. The continued role of SSRIs as first-line treatments, thus, reflects their simplicity of use, safety, and broad spectrum of action.

Direct comparisons of individual SSRIs have not revealed any to be consistently superior to another. Nevertheless, considerable diversity is seen in response to the various SSRIs among individuals. For example, more than 50 percent of people who respond poorly to one SSRI will respond favorably to another. Thus, before shifting to non-SSRI antidepressants, it is most reasonable to try other agents in the SSRI class for persons who did not respond to the first SSRI.

Some clinicians have attempted to select a particular SSRI for a specific person on the basis of the drug's unique adverse effect profile. For example, thinking that fluoxetine is an activating and stimulating SSRI, some may assume it is a better choice for an abulic person than paroxetine, which is presumed to be a sedating SSRI. These differences, however, usually vary from person to person.

Suicide. In the late 1980s, a widely publicized report suggested an association between fluoxetine use and violent acts, including suicide, but many subsequent reviews have failed to confirm this association. More recently, studies of SSRI use to treat depression in children and adolescents appeared to find a slight increase in suicidal ideation or impulses. It remains unclear whether, in fact, a cause and effect exists between SSRI use and increased risk of suicide. A few patients, however, become especially anxious and agitated when started on an SSRI. It is the appearance of these symptoms that could conceivably provoke or aggravate suicidal ideation. Thus, all depressed patients should be closely monitored during the period of maximal risk, the first few days and weeks they are taking SSRIs. It is important to keep in mind that SSRIs, as with all antidepressants, prevent potential suicides as a result of their primary action, the shortening and prevention of depressive episodes.

Depression during Pregnancy and Postpartum. Rates of relapse of major depression during pregnancy among women who discontinue, attempt to discontinue, or modify their antidepressant regimen are extremely high. Rates range from 68 percent to 100 percent of patients. Thus, many women need to continue taking their medication during pregnancy and postpartum. The impact of maternal depression on infant development is unknown. No increased risk is seen for major congenital malformations following exposure to SSRIs during pregnancy. Thus, the risk of relapse into depression when a newly pregnant mother is taken off SSRIs is several times higher than the risk to the fetus of exposure to SSRIs.

Some evidence suggests increased rates of special care nursery admissions after delivery for children of mothers taking SSRIs. Also a potential exists for a discontinuation syndrome with paroxetine. No clinically significant neonatal complications are associated with SSRI use.

Studies that have followed children into their early school years have failed to find any perinatal complications, congenital fetal anomalies, decreases in global intelligence quotient (IQ), language delays, or specific behavioral problems attributable to the use of fluoxetine during pregnancy.

Postpartum depression (with or without psychotic features) affects a small percentage of mothers. Some clinicians start administering SSRIs if the postpartum blues extend beyond a few weeks or if a woman becomes depressed during pregnancy. The head start afforded by starting SSRI administration during pregnancy if a woman is at risk for postpartum depression also protects the newborn, toward whom the woman may have harmful thoughts after parturition.

The SSRIs are secreted in breast milk, but the plasma of babies breast-feeding from mothers who are taking SSRIs is typically very low. In some cases, however, have been reported concentrations higher than average. No decision regarding the use of an SSRI is risk free. It is important to document that communication of potential risks to the patient has taken place.

Depression in the Elderly and Medically Ill. SSRIs are safe and well tolerated when used to treat the elderly and medically ill. As a class, they have little or no cardiotoxic, anticholinergic, antihistaminergic, or α-adrenergic adverse effects. Paroxetine does have some anticholinergic activity, which may lead to constipation and worsening of cognition. SSRIs can produce subtle cognitive deficits, prolonged bleeding time, and hyponatremia, all of which may have an impact on the health of this population. SSRIs are effective in poststroke depression and dramatically reduce the symptom of crying.

Depression in Children. Studies of SSRIs in depressed children and adolescents have generally failed to demonstrate the efficacy of SSRIs. Only fluoxetine has FDA approval for use as an antidepressant in this population. Given the reality that children do suffer from depression and that pharmacologic intervention is needed in many cases, many clinicians do in fact prescribe SSRIs. Reports suggest that SSRIs can increase suicidal or violent thoughts or actions in depressed children and adolescents; therefore, it is essential that treatment of children with these agents be closely monitored for the emergence of unwanted behavioral effects.

Anxiety Disorders

Obsessive-Compulsive Disorder. Fluvoxamine, paroxetine, sertraline, and fluoxetine are indicated for treatment of OCD in persons over the age of 18 years. Fluvoxamine and sertraline have also been approved for treatment of pediatric OCD (ages 6 to 17). About 50 percent of persons with OCD begin to show symptoms in childhood or adolescence, and more than half of these respond favorably to medication. Beneficial responses can be dramatic. Long-term data support the model of OCD as a genetically determined, lifelong condition that is best treated continuously with drugs and cognitive–behavioral therapy from the onset of symptoms in childhood throughout the lifespan.

The SSRI dosages for OCD may need to be higher than those required to treat depression. Although some response can be seen in the first few weeks of treatment, it may take several months for the maximal effects to become evident. Patients who fail to obtain adequate relief of their OCD symptoms with an SSRI often benefit from the addition of a small dose of risperidone (Risperdal). Apart from the extrapyramidal side effects of Risperdal, patients should be monitored for increases in prolactin levels when this combination is used. Clinically, hyperprolactinemia may manifest as gynecomastia and galactorrhea (in both men and women) and loss of menses.

A number of disorders are now considered to be within the OCD spectrum. This includes a number of conditions and symptoms characterized by nonsuicidal self-mutilation, such as trichotillomania, eyebrow-picking, nose-picking, nail-biting, compulsive picking of skin blemishes, and cutting. Patients with these behaviors benefit from treatment with SSRIs. Other spectrum disorders include compulsive gambling, compulsive shopping, hypochondriasis, and body dysmorphic disorder.

Panic Disorder. Paroxetine and sertraline are indicated for treatment of panic disorder, with or without agoraphobia. These agents work less rapidly than do the benzodiazepines alprazolam (Xanax) or clonazepam (Klonopin), but are far superior to benzodiazepines for treatment of panic disorder with comorbid depression. Citalopram, fluvoxamine, and fluoxetine also can reduce spontaneous or induced panic attacks. Because fluoxetine can initially heighten anxiety symptoms, persons with panic disorder must begin taking small dosages (5 mg a day) and raise the dosage slowly. Low doses of benzodiazepines may be given to manage this side effect.

Social Anxiety Disorder. SSRIs are effective agents in the treatment of social phobia. They reduce both symptoms and disability. The response rate is comparable to that seen with the MAOI phenelzine (Nardil), the previous standard treatment. SSRIs are safer to use than MAOIs or benzodiazepines.

Posttraumatic Stress Disorder. Pharmacotherapy for posttraumatic stress disorder (PTSD) must target specific symptoms in three clusters: reexperiencing, avoidance, and hyperarousal. For long-term treatment, SSRIs appear to have a broader spectrum of therapeutic effects on specific PTSD symptom clusters than do TCAs and MAOIs. Benzodiazepine augmentation is useful in the acute symptomatic state. SSRIs are associated with marked improvement of both intrusive and avoidant symptoms.

Generalized Anxiety Disorder. SSRIs may be useful for the treatment of specific phobias, generalized anxiety disorder, and separation anxiety disorder. A thorough, individualized evaluation is the first approach, with particular attention to identifying conditions amenable to drug therapy. In addition, cognitive–behavioral or other psychotherapies can be added for greater efficacy.

Bulimia Nervosa and Other Eating Disorders

Fluoxetine is indicated for treatment of bulimia, which is best done in the context of psychotherapy. Dosages of 60 mg a day are significantly more effective than 20 mg a day. In several well-controlled studies, fluoxetine in dosages of 60 mg a day was superior to placebo in reducing binge eating and induced vomiting. Some experts recommend an initial course of cognitive–behavioral therapy alone. If no response occurs in 3 to 6 weeks, then fluoxetine administration is added. The appropriate duration of treatment with fluoxetine and psychotherapy has not been determined.

Fluvoxamine was not effective at a statistically significant level in one double-blind, placebo-controlled trial for inpatients with bulimia.

Anorexia Nervosa. Fluoxetine has been used in inpatient treatment of anorexia nervosa to attempt to control comorbid mood disturbances and obsessive-compulsive symptoms. At least two careful studies, one of 7 months and one of 24 months, however, failed to find that fluoxetine affected the overall outcome and the maintenance of weight. Effective treatments for anorexia include cognitive–behavioral, interpersonal, psychodynamic, and family therapies in addition to a trial with SSRIs.

Obesity. Fluoxetine, in combination with a behavioral program, has been shown to be only modestly beneficial for weight loss. A significant percentage of all persons who take SSRIs, including fluoxetine, lose weight initially, but later may gain weight. All SSRIs may cause initial weight gain, however.

Premenstrual Dysphoric Disorder

Premenstrual dysphoric disorder is characterized by debilitating mood and behavioral changes in the week preceding menstruation that interfere with normal functioning. Sertraline, paroxetine, fluoxetine, and fluvoxamine have been reported to reduce the symptoms of premenstrual dysphoric disorder. Controlled trials of fluoxetine and sertraline administered either throughout the cycle or only during the luteal phase (the 2-week period between ovulation and menstruation) showed both schedules to be equally effective.

An additional observation of unclear significance was that fluoxetine was associated with changing the duration of the menstrual period by more than 4 days, either lengthening or shortening. The effects of SSRIs on menstrual cycle length are mostly unknown and may warrant careful monitoring in women of reproductive age.

Off-label Uses

Premature Ejaculation. The antiorgasmic effects of SSRIs make them useful as a treatment for men with premature ejaculation. SSRIs permit intercourse for a significantly longer period and are reported to improve sexual satisfaction in couples in which the man has premature ejaculation. Fluoxetine and sertraline have been shown to be effective for this purpose.

Paraphilias. SSRIs may reduce obsessive-compulsive behavior in people with paraphilias. SSRIs diminish the average time per day spent in unconventional sexual fantasies, urges, and activities. Evidence suggests a greater response for sexual obsessions than for paraphilic behavior.

Autism. Obsessive-compulsive behavior, poor social relatedness, and aggression are prominent autistic features that may respond to serotonergic agents such as SSRIs and clomipramine. Sertraline and fluvoxamine have been shown in controlled and open-label trials to mitigate aggressiveness, self-injurious behavior, repetitive behaviors, some degree of language delay, and, rarely, lack of social relatedness in adults with autistic spectrum disorders. Fluoxetine has been reported to be effective for features of autism in children, adolescents, and adults.

PRECAUTIONS AND ADVERSE REACTIONS

The side effects of SSRIs need to be considered in terms of their onset, duration, and severity. For example, nausea and jitteriness are early, generally mild, and time-limited side effects.

Sexual Dysfunction

All SSRIs cause sexual dysfunction, and it is the most common adverse effect of SSRIs associated with long-term treatment. It has an estimated incidence of between 50 percent and 80 percent. The most common complaints are anorgasmia, inhibited orgasm, and decreased libido. Some studies suggest that sexual dysfunction is dose related, but this has not been clearly established. Unlike most of the other adverse effects of SSRIs, sexual inhibition rarely resolves in the first few weeks of use, but usually continues as long as the drug is taken. In some cases, there may be improvement over time.

Strategies to counteract SSRI-induced sexual dysfunction are too numerous to mention, and none has been proved to be very effective. Some reports suggest decreasing the dosage or adding bupropion. Reports have described successful treatment of SSRI-induced sexual dysfunction with agents such as sildenafil (Viagra), which are used to treat erectile dysfunction. Ultimately, patients may need to be switched to antidepressants that do not interfere with sexual functioning, drugs such as mirtazapine or bupropion.

Gastrointestinal Adverse Effects

Gastrointestinal (GI) side effects, which are very common, are mediated largely through effects on the serotonin $5HT_3$ receptor. The most frequent GI complaints are nausea, diarrhea, anorexia, vomiting, flatulence, and dyspepsia. Sertraline and fluvoxamine produce the most intense GI symptoms. Delayed-release paroxetine, when compared with the immediate-release preparation of paroxetine, has less intense GI side effects during the first week of treatment. Paroxetine, because of its anticholinergic activity, frequently causes constipation, however. Nausea and loose stools are usually dose related and transient, resolving within a few weeks. Sometimes, flatulence and diarrhea persist, especially during sertraline treatment. Initial anorexia can also occur and is most common with fluoxetine. SSRI-induced appetite and weight loss begin as soon as the drug is taken and peak at 20 weeks, after which weight often returns to baseline. Up to one third of persons taking SSRIs will gain weight, sometimes more than 20 pounds. This effect is mediated through a metabolic mechanism, increase in appetite, or both. It happens gradually and is usually resistant to diet and exercise regimens. Paroxetine is associated with more frequent and more pronounced weight gain than the other SSRIs, especially among young women.

Headaches

The incidence of headache in SSRI trials was 18 percent to 20 percent, only 1 percentage point higher than the placebo rate. Fluoxetine is the SSRI most likely to cause headache. On the other hand, all SSRIs are effective prophylaxis against both migraine and tension-type headaches in many persons.

Central Nervous System Adverse Effects

Anxiety. Fluoxetine can cause anxiety, particularly in the first few weeks. These initial effects, however, usually give way to an overall reduction in anxiety after a few weeks. Increased anxiety is caused considerably less frequently by paroxetine or escitalopram, which may be a better choice if sedation is desired, as in mixed anxiety and depressive disorders.

Insomnia and Sedation. The major effect SSRIs exert in the area of insomnia and sedation is improved sleep resulting from treatment of depression and anxiety. As many as one fourth of persons taking SSRIs, however, note either trouble sleeping or excessive somnolence or overwhelming fatigue. Fluoxetine is the most SSRI likely to cause insomnia, for which reason it is often taken in the morning. Sertraline and fluvoxamine are about equally likely to cause insomnia as somnolence, and citalopram and, especially, paroxetine often cause somnolence. Escitalopram is more likely to interfere with sleep than its isomer, citalopram. Some persons benefit from taking their SSRI dose before going to bed, whereas others prefer to take it the morning. SSRI-induced insomnia can be treated with benzodiazepines, trazodone (Desyrel) (clinicians must explain the risk of priapism), or other sedating medicines. Significant SSRI-induced somnolence often requires switching to use of another SSRI or bupropion.

Other Sleep Effects. Many persons taking SSRIs report recalling extremely vivid dreams or nightmares. They describe sleep as "busy." Other sleep effects of the SSRIs include bruxism, restless legs, nocturnal myoclonus, and sweating.

Emotional Blunting. Emotional blunting is a largely overlooked but frequent side effect associated with chronic SSRI use. Patients report an inability to cry in response to emotional situations, a feeling of apathy or indifference, or a restriction in the intensity of emotional experiences. This side effect often leads to treatment discontinuation even when the drugs are providing relief from depression or anxiety.

Yawning. Close clinical observation of patients taking SSRIs reveals an increase in yawning. This side effect is not a reflection of fatigue or of poor nocturnal sleep but is the result of SSRI effects on the hypothalamus.

Seizures. Seizures have been reported in 0.1 percent to 0.2 percent of all patients treated with SSRIs, an incidence comparable to that reported with other antidepressants and not significantly different from that with placebo. Seizures are more frequent at the highest doses of SSRIs (e.g., fluoxetine 100 mg a day or higher).

Extrapyramidal Symptoms. SSRIs may rarely cause akathisia, dystonia, tremor, cogwheel rigidity, torticollis, opisthotonos, gait disorders, and bradykinesia. Rare cases of tardive dyskinesia have been reported. People with well-controlled Parkinson's disease may experience acute worsening of their motor symptoms when they take SSRIs.

Anticholinergic Effects

Paroxetine has mild anticholinergic activity that causes dry mouth, constipation, and sedation in a dose-dependent fashion. Nevertheless, most persons taking paroxetine do not experience cholinergic adverse effects. Other SSRIs are associated with dry mouth, but this effect is not mediated by muscarinic activity.

Hematologic Adverse Effects

The SSRIs can cause functional impairment of platelet aggregation, but not a reduction in platelet number. This is manifested by easy bruising and excessive or prolonged bleeding. When patients exhibit these signs, a test for bleeding time should be performed. Special monitoring is suggested when patients use SSRIs in conjunction with anticoagulants or aspirin.

Electrolyte and Glucose Disturbances

The SSRIs can acutely decrease glucose concentrations; therefore, diabetic patients should be carefully monitored. Rare cases of SSRI-associated hyponatremia and the secretion of inappropriate antidiuretic hormone (SIADH) have been seen in patients treated with diuretics who are also water deprived.

Endocrine and Allergic Reactions

The SSRIs can decrease prolactin levels and cause mammoplasia and galactorrhea in both men and women. Breast changes are reversible on discontinuation of the drug, but this can take several months to occur.

Various types of rashes appear in about 4 percent of all patients; in a small subset of these patients, the allergic reaction may generalize and involve the pulmonary system, resulting rarely in fibrotic damage and dyspnea. SSRI treatment may have to be discontinued in patients with drug-related rashes.

Serotonin Syndrome

Concurrent administration of an SSRI with an MAOI, L-tryptophan, or lithium can raise plasma serotonin concentrations to toxic levels, producing a constellation of symptoms called the *serotonin syndrome*. This serious and possibly fatal syndrome of serotonin overstimulation is composed, in order of appearance as the condition worsens, of (1) diarrhea; (2) restlessness; (3) extreme agitation, hyperreflexia, and autonomic instability with possible rapid fluctuations in vital signs; (4) myoclonus, seizures, hyperthermia, uncontrollable shivering, and rigidity; and (5) delirium, coma, status epilepticus, cardiovascular collapse, and death.

Treatment of the serotonin syndrome consists of removing the offending agents and promptly instituting comprehensive supportive care with nitroglycerine, cyproheptadine, methysergide (Sansert), cooling blankets, chlorpromazine (Thorazine), dantrolene (Dantrium), benzodiazepines, anticonvulsants, mechanical ventilation, and paralyzing agents.

Sweating

Some patients experience sweating while being treated with SSRIs. The sweating is unrelated to ambient temperature. Nocturnal sweating may drench bed sheets and require a change of night clothes. Terazosin, 1 or 2 mg per day, is often dramatically effective in counteracting sweating.

SSRI Withdrawal

The abrupt discontinuance of SSRI use, especially one with a shorter half-life (e.g., paroxetine or fluvoxamine), has been associated with a withdrawal syndrome that can include dizziness, weakness, nausea, headache, rebound depression, anxiety, insomnia, poor concentration, upper respiratory symptoms, paresthesias, and migraine-like symptoms. It usually does not appear until after at least 6 weeks of treatment and usually resolves spontaneously in 3 weeks. Persons who experienced transient adverse effects in the first weeks of taking an SSRI were more likely to experience discontinuation symptoms.

Fluoxetine is the SSRI least likely to be associated with this syndrome, because the half-life of its metabolite is more than 1 week and it effectively tapers itself. Fluoxetine, therefore, has been used in some cases to treat the discontinuation syndrome caused by termination of other SSRIs. Nevertheless, a delayed and attenuated withdrawal syndrome occurs with fluoxetine as well.

DRUG INTERACTIONS

The SSRIs do not interfere with most other drugs. A serotonin syndrome (Table 36.29–3) can develop with concurrent administration of MAOIs, tryptophan, lithium (Eskalith), or other antidepressants that inhibit reuptake of serotonin. Fluoxetine, sertraline, and paroxetine can raise plasma concentrations of tricyclic antidepressants, which can cause clinical toxicity. A number of potential pharmacokinetic interactions have been described based on in vitro analyses of the CYP enzymes, but clinically relevant interactions are rare.

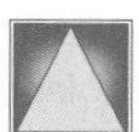

Table 36.29–3
Serotonin Syndrome

Diarrhea	Myoclonus
Diaphoresis	Hyperactive reflexes
Tremor	Disorientation
Ataxia	Lability of mood

The combination of lithium and any serotonergic drug should be used with caution because of the possibility of precipitating seizures. SSRIs, particularly fluvoxamine, should not be used with clozapine because it raises clozapine concentrations and seizures may result. SSRIs may increase the duration and severity of zolpidem (Ambien)-induced hallucinations.

Fluoxetine

Fluoxetine can be administered with tricyclic drugs, but the clinician should use low dosages of the tricyclic drug. Because it is metabolized by the hepatic enzyme CYP 2D6, fluoxetine can interfere with the metabolism of other drugs in the 7 percent of the population that has an inefficient isoform of this enzyme, the so-called *poor metabolizers*. Fluoxetine may slow the metabolism of carbamazepine (Tegretol), antineoplastic agents, diazepam (Valium), and phenytoin (Dilantin). Drug interactions have been described for fluoxetine that may affect the plasma levels of benzodiazepines, antipsychotics, and lithium. Fluoxetine has no interactions with warfarin (Coumadin), tolbutamide (Orinase), or chlorothiazide (Diuril).

Sertraline

Sertraline may displace warfarin from plasma proteins and may increase the prothrombin time. The drug interaction data on sertraline support a generally similar profile to that of fluoxetine, although sertraline does not interact as strongly with the CYP 2D6 enzyme.

Paroxetine

Paroxetine has a higher risk for drug interactions than does either fluoxetine or sertraline because it is a more potent inhibitor of the CYP 2D6 enzyme. Cimetidine (Tagamet) can increase the concentration of sertraline and paroxetine, and phenobarbital (Luminal) and phenytoin can decrease the concentration of paroxetine. Because of the potential for interference with the CYP 2D6 enzyme, the coadministration of paroxetine with other antidepressants, phenothiazines, and antiarrhythmic drugs should be undertaken with caution. Paroxetine can increase the anticoagulant effect of warfarin. Coadministration of paroxetine and tramadol (Ultram) may precipitate a serotonin syndrome in elderly persons.

Fluvoxamine

Among the SSRIs, fluvoxamine appears to present the most risk for drug–drug interactions. Fluvoxamine is metabolized by the enzyme CYP 3A4, which may be inhibited by ketoconazole (Nizoral). Fluvoxamine can increase the half-life of alprazolam (Xanax), triazolam (Halcion), and diazepam, and it should not be coadministered with these agents. Fluvoxamine can increase theophylline (Slo-bid, Theo-Dur) levels threefold and warfarin levels twofold, with important clinical consequences; thus, the serum levels of the latter drugs should be closely monitored and the doses adjusted accordingly. Fluvoxamine raises concentrations and may increase the activity of clozapine, carbamazepine, methadone (Dolophine, Methadose), propranolol (Inderal), and diltiazem (Cardizem). Fluvoxamine has no significant interactions with lorazepam (Ativan) or digoxin (Lanoxin).

Citalopram

Citalopram is not a potent inhibitor of any CYP enzymes. Concurrent administration of cimetidine increases concentrations of citalopram by about 40 percent. Citalopram does not significantly affect the metabolism of, nor is its metabolism significantly affected by, digoxin, lithium, warfarin, carbamazepine, or imipramine (Tofranil). Citalopram increases the plasma concentrations of metoprolol twofold, but this usually has no effect on blood pressure or heart rate. Data on coadministration of citalopram and potent inhibitors of CYP 3A4 or CYP 2D6 are not available.

Escitalopram

Escitalopram is a moderate inhibitor of CYP 2D6 and has been shown to significantly raise desipramine and metoprolol concentrations.

LABORATORY INTERFERENCES

The SSRIs do not interfere with any laboratory tests.

DOSAGE AND CLINICAL GUIDELINES

Fluoxetine

Fluoxetine is available in 10- and 20-mg capsules, in a scored 10-mg tablet, as a 90-mg enteric-coated capsule for once-weekly administration, and as an oral concentrate (20 mg/5 mL). Fluoxetine is also marketed as Sarafem for premenstrual dysphoric disorder. For depression, the initial dosage is usually 10 or 20 mg orally each day, usually given in the morning, because insomnia is a potential adverse effect of the drug. Fluoxetine should be taken with food to minimize the possible nausea. The long half-lives of the drug and its metabolite contribute to a 4-week period to reach steady-state concentrations. A 20 mg dose is often as effective as higher doses for treating depression. The maximal dosage recommended by the manufacturer is 80 mg a day. To minimize the early side effects of anxiety and restlessness, some clinicians initiate fluoxetine use at 5 to 10 mg a day, either with the scored 10-mg tablet or by using the liquid preparation. Alternatively, because of the long half-life of fluoxetine, its use can be initiated with an every-other-day administration schedule. The dosage of fluoxetine, and other SSRIs, that is effective in other indications may differ from the dosage generally used for depression.

Sertraline

Sertraline is available in scored 25-, 50-, and 100-mg tablets. For the initial treatment of depression, sertraline use should be initiated with a dosage of 50 mg once daily. To limit the GI effects, some clinicians begin at 25 mg a day and increase to 50 mg a day after 3 weeks. Patients who do not respond after 1 to 3 weeks may benefit from dosage increases of 50 mg every week up to a maximum of 200 mg, given once daily. Sertraline can be administered in the morning or the evening. Administration after eating may reduce the GI adverse effects. Sertraline oral concentrate (1 mL = 20 mg) has 12 percent alcohol content and must be diluted before use. When used to treat panic disorder, sertraline should be initiated at 25 mg to reduce the risk of provoking a panic attack.

Paroxetine

Immediate-release paroxetine is available in scored 20-mg tablets; in unscored 10-, 30-, and 40-mg tablets; and as an orange-flavored 10-mg/5-mL oral suspension. Paroxetine use for the treatment of depression is usually initiated at a dosage of 10 or 20 mg a day. An increase in the dosage should be considered when an adequate response is not seen in 1 to 3 weeks. At that point, the clinician can initiate upward dose titration in 10-mg increments at weekly intervals to a maximum of 50 mg a day. Persons who experience GI upset may benefit by taking the drug with food. Paroxetine can be taken initially as a single daily dose in the evening; higher dosages can be divided into two doses per day.

A delayed-release formulation of paroxetine, (Paxil CR), is available in 12.5-, 25-, and 37.5-mg tablets. The starting dosage for depression is 25 mg per day and in panic disorder 12.5 mg per day.

Paroxetine is the SSRI most likely to produce a discontinuation syndrome, because plasma concentrations drop rapidly in the absence of continuous dosing. To limit the development of symptoms of abrupt discontinuation, paroxetine use should be tapered gradually, with dosage reductions every 2 to 3 weeks.

Fluvoxamine

Fluvoxamine is available in unscored 25-mg tablets and scored 50- and 100-mg tablets. The effective daily dosage range is 50 to 300 mg a day. A usual starting dosage is 50 mg once a day at bedtime for the first week, after which the dosage can be adjusted according to the adverse effects and clinical response. Dosages above 100 mg a day can be divided into twice-daily dosing. A temporary dosage reduction or slower upward titration may be necessary if nausea develops over the first 2 weeks of therapy. Fluvoxamine can also be administered as a single evening dose to minimize its adverse effects. Tablets should be swallowed with food without chewing the tablet. Abrupt discontinuation of fluvoxamine can cause a discontinuation syndrome.

Citalopram

Citalopram is available in 20- and 40-mg scored tablets and as a liquid (10 mg/5 mL). The usual starting dosage is 20 mg a day for the first week, after which it usually is increased to 40 mg a day. For elderly persons or persons with hepatic impairment, 20 mg a day is recommended, with an increase to 40 mg a day only with no response at 20 mg a day. Tablets should be taken once daily, in either the morning or the evening, with or without food.

Escitalopram

Escitalopram is available as 10- and 20-mg scored tablets, as well as an oral solution at a concentration of 5 mg/5 mL. The recommended dosage of escitalopram is 10 mg per day. In clinical trials, no additional benefit was noted when 20 mg per day was used.

Loss of Efficacy

Some patients report a lessened response to SSRIs with recurrence of depressive symptoms after a period of time (e.g., 4 to 6 months). The exact mechanism is unknown. Potential remedies for the attenuation of response to SSRIs include increasing or decreasing the dosage; tapering drug use and then rechallenging with the same medication; switching to another SSRI or non-SSRI antidepressant; and augmenting with bupropion or another augmentation agent.

References

Dhillon S, Scott LJ, Plosker GL. Escitalopram: A review of its use in the management of anxiety disorders. *CNS Drugs*. 2006;20(9):763.

Giner L, Nichols CM, Carballo JJ, Zalsman G, Oquendo MA. Selective serotonin reuptake inhibitors in adolescent suicide. In: Merrick J, Zalsman G, eds. *Suicidal Behavior in Adolescence: An International Perspective*. London, England: Freund Publishing House; 2005:81–93.

Kelsey JE. Selective serotonin reuptake inhibitors. In: Sadock BJ, Sadock VA, eds. *Kaplan & Sadock's Comprehensive Textbook of Psychiatry*. 8th ed. Vol. 2. Baltimore: Lippincott Williams & Wilkins; 2005:2887.

Leombruni P, Amianto F, Delsedime N, Gramaglia C, Abbate-Daga G, Fassino S. Citalopram versus fluoxetine for the treatment of patients with bulimia nervosa: A single-blind randomized controlled trial. *Adv Ther*. 2006;23(3):481.

Nishawala M, Boorady RJ, Koploewicz H. Beyond the black box: Prescribing SSRIs to adolescents. *Primary Psychiatry*. 2006;13(1):51.

Thase ME, Haight BR, Richard N, Rockett CB, Mitton M, Modell JG, VanMeter S, Harriett AE, Wang Y. Remission rates following antidepressant therapy with bupropion or selective serotonin reuptake inhibitors: A meta-analysis of original data from 7 randomized controlled trials. *J Clin Psychiatry*. 2005;66(8):974.

Weintraub D, Taraborelli D, Morales KH, Duda JE, Katz IR, Stern MB. Escitalopram for major depression in Parkinson's disease: An open-label, flexible-dosage study. *J Neuropsychiatry Clin Neurosci*. 2006;18(3):377.

Williams SC. Depression—Augmentation or switch after initial SSRI treatment. *N Engl J Med*. 2006;354(24):2611.

Yuan Y, Tsoi K, Hunt RH. Selective serotonin reuptake inhibitors and risk of upper GI bleeding: Confusion or confounding? *Am J Med*. 2006;119(9):719.

▲ 36.30 Serotonin–Dopamine Antagonists: Atypical Antipsychotics

The serotonin–dopamine antagonists (SDAs) are also known as second-generation or atypical antipsychotic drugs. These drugs include risperidone (Risperdal), olanzapine (Zyprexa), quetiapine (Seroquel), clozapine (Clozaril), and ziprasidone (Geodon). They are called SDAs because they have a higher ratio of serotonin type 2 (5-HT_2) to D_2 dopamine receptor blockades than the typical, or conventional, dopamine receptor antagonists (DRAs) that previously were the mainstay of treatment. The SDAs also appear to be more specific for the mesolimbic than striatal dopamine system and, in some cases, are associated with rapid dissociation from the D_2 receptor. It is hypothesized that these properties account for the improved tolerability associated with the SDAs.

All of the SDAs share the following characteristics: (1) low D_2 receptor blocking effects when compared with DRAs, which have high D_2 receptor blockades; (2) a reduced risk of extrapyramidal side effects compared with older agents, a reduced risk that probably extends to the occurrence of tardive dyskinesia as well; (3) proved efficacy as treatments for schizophrenia; and (4) proved efficacy as treatments for acute mania. In all other respects, these agents differ markedly. All have different chemical structures, receptor affinities, and side-effect profiles. No SDA is identical in its combination of receptor affinities, and the relative contribution of each receptor interaction to the clinical effects is unknown.

Aripiprazole (Abilify), which exhibits a novel mechanism as a partial dopamine antagonist, is discussed separately below. It represents a further advance, beyond second-generation antipsychotics, in the treatment of psychotic disorders.

Although associated with a lowered but not absent risk of extrapyramidal side effects, some of the drugs in this group often produce substantial weight gain, which, in turn, increases the potential for development of diabetes mellitus. The US Food and Drug Administration (FDA) has requested that all SDAs carry a warning label that patients on the drugs be monitored closely for the development of glucose abnormalities.

Among these drugs, clozapine sits apart. It is not considered a first-line agent because of side effects and need for weekly blood tests. Although highly effective in treating both mania and depression, clozapine does not have an FDA indication for those conditions. Olanzapine is indicated for the treatment of acute and chronic manic episodes associated with bipolar I disorders; however, it is frequently used in patients who fail to respond to other interventions. The molecular structures of these compounds are shown in Figure 36.30–1.

THERAPEUTIC INDICATIONS

Although approved for the treatment of acute mania, these drugs also are useful as adjunctive therapy in treatment-resistant depression, posttraumatic stress disorder (PTSD), and behavioral disturbances associated with dementia. All these agents are considered first-line drugs, except clozapine, which causes adverse hematologic effects that require weekly blood sampling.

Schizophrenia and Schizoaffective Disorder

The SDAs are effective for treating acute and chronic psychoses, such as schizophrenia and schizoaffective disorder, in both adults and adolescents. SDAs are as good as, or better than, typical antipsychotics (DRAs) for the treatment of positive symptoms in schizophrenia and clearly superior to DRAs for the treatment of negative symptoms. Compared with persons treated with

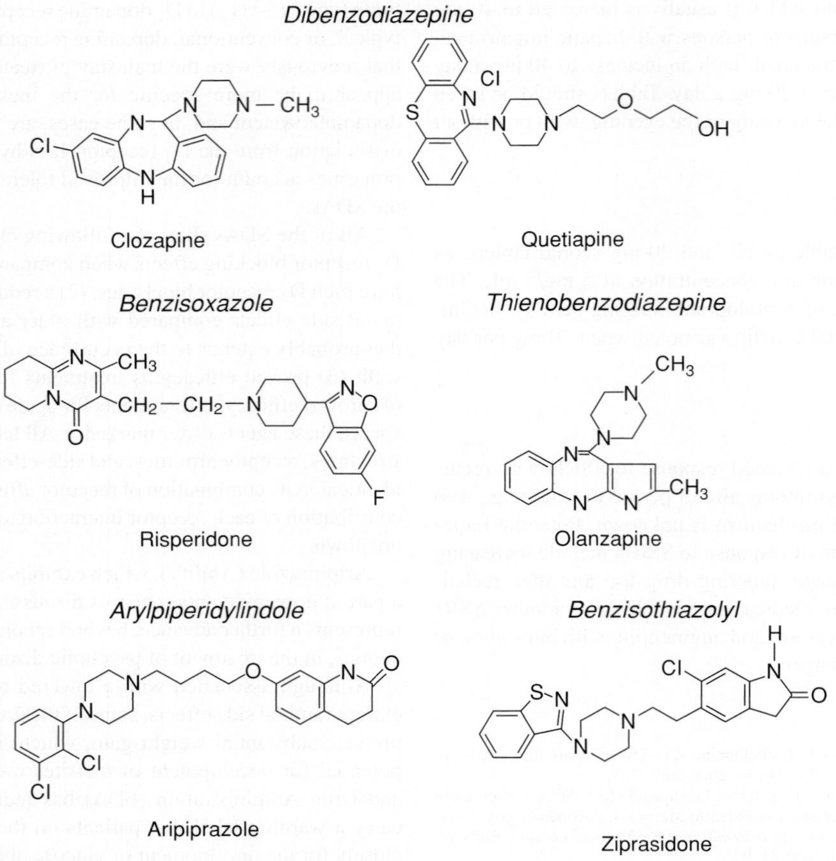

Dibenzodiazepine

Clozapine

Quetiapine

Benzisoxazole

Thienobenzodiazepine

Risperidone

Olanzapine

Arylpiperidylindole

Benzisothiazolyl

Aripiprazole

Ziprasidone

FIGURE 36.30–1
Molecular structures of serotonin–dopamine antagonists.

DRAs, persons treated with SDAs have fewer relapses and require less frequent hospitalization, fewer emergency room visits, less phone contact with mental health professionals, and less treatment in day programs.

Because clozapine has potentially life-threatening adverse effects, it is appropriate only for patients with schizophrenia that is resistant to all other antipsychotics. Other indications for clozapine include treatment of persons with severe tardive dyskinesias—which can be reversed with high dosages in some cases—and those with a low threshold for extrapyramidal symptoms. Persons who tolerate clozapine have done well on long-term therapy. The effectiveness of clozapine can be increased by augmentation with risperidone and aripiprazole which raise clozapine concentrations and sometimes results in dramatic clinical improvement.

Mood Disorders

All of the SDAs are FDA-approved for treatment of acute mania. Olanzapine is also approved for maintenance treatment of bipolar disorder. In general, however, typical antipsychotics and benzodiazepines exert calming effects in mania more rapidly than do SDAs. The SDAs improve depressive symptoms in schizophrenia, and both clinical experience and clinical trials show that all of the SDAs augment antidepressants in the acute management of major depression. A combination of SDAs and antidepressants is frequently used in treatment-resistant depression, and a fixed combination of olanzapine and fluoxetine (Symbyax) is approved by the FDA as a treatment for acute bipolar depression.

Other Indications

About 10 percent of patients with schizophrenia exhibit outwardly aggressive or violent behavior. SDAs are effective for treatment of such aggression. Other indications include acquired immunodeficiency syndrome (AIDS), autistic spectrum disorders, Tourette's disorder, Huntington's disease, and Lesch-Nyhan syndrome. Risperidone and olanzapine have been used to control aggression and self-injury in children. These drugs have also been coadministered with sympathomimetics, such as methylphenidate (Ritalin) or dextroamphetamine (Dexedrine, Dextrostat), to children with attention-deficit/hyperactivity disorder (ADHD) who are comorbid for either opposition-defiant disorder or conduct disorder. SDAs—especially olanzapine, quetiapine, and clozapine—are useful in persons who have severe tardive dyskinesia. SDA treatment suppresses the abnormal movements of tardive dyskinesia, but does not appear to worsen the movement disorder. SDAs are also effective for treating psychotic depression and for psychosis secondary to head trauma, dementia, or treatment drugs.

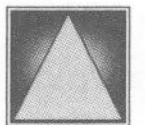

Table 36.30–1
Adverse Effects of Antipsychotic Agents[a]

Item	Conventional Antipsychotics	Clozapine	Risperidone	Olanzapine	Quetiapine	Ziprasidone
CNS						
EPS	0 to ++[b,c]	0[b]	0[b]	0[b] to +[c]	0[b]	0[b]
Tardive dyskinesia	+++	0	(+)	?	?	?
Seizures	0 to +	+++	0	+	0	0
Sedation, somnolence	+ to +++	+++	+[d]	+	+[d]	+[d]
Other						
Neuroleptic malignant syndrome	+	+	+	+	?	?
Orthostatic hypotension	+ to +++	0 to +++	+	+[d]	0[d]	0
QT_c	0 to ++	0	0 to +	0	0 to +	0 to +++
Liver transaminase increase	0 to ++	0 to +	0 to +	0 to +	0 to +	0 to +
Anticholinergic adverse effects	0 to +++	+++	0	+	0	0
Agranulocytosis	0	+++	0	0	0	0
Protactin increase	++ to +++	0	+ to ++	0[c]	0[d]	0[e]
Decreased ejaculatory volume	0 to +	0	0	0	0	0
Weight gain	0 to ++	+++	+	+++	+	0
Nasal congestion	0 to +	0 to +	0 to +	0 to +	0 to +	0

[a]0, None or not significantly different from placebo; +, mild; ++, moderate; +++, marked; ?, insufficient data.
[b]Not significantly different from placebo-treated group, which may have received conventional antipsychotic before entering the study and could have EPS carried forward into the initial weeks of the investigation.
[c]Dosage-related EPS above 6 mg per day.
[d]Transient.
[e]Dosage-related increases within the normal range.
CNS, central nervous system; EPS, extrapyramidal symptom; QTc, corrected for heart rate.
(Modified from Casey DE. Side effect profiles of new antipsychotic agents. *J Clin Psychiatry.* 1996:57[Suppl]:40, with permission.)

Treatment with SDAs decreases the risk of suicide and water intoxication in patients with schizophrenia. Patients with treatment-resistant obsessive-compulsive disorder (OCD) have responded to SDAs; however, a few persons treated with SDAs have noted treatment-emergent symptoms of OCD. Some patients with borderline personality disorder may improve with SDAs.

ADVERSE EFFECTS

The SDAs share a similar spectrum of adverse reactions, but differ considerably in terms of frequency or severity of their occurrence. Common adverse events associated with SDAs are listed in Table 36.30–1. Specific side effects that are more common with an individual SDA are emphasized in the discussion of each drug.

PHARMACOLOGY, SIDE EFFECTS, DOSAGES, AND INTERACTIONS

Risperidone

Pharmacology. Risperidone is a benzisoxazole. Risperidone undergoes extensive first-pass hepatic metabolism to 9-hydroxyrisperidone, a metabolite with equivalent antipsychotic activity. Peak plasma levels of the parent compound occur within 1 hour for the parent compound and 3 hours for the metabolite. Risperidone has a bioactivity of 70 percent. The combined half-life of risperidone and 9-hydroxyrisperidone averages 20 hours, so it is effective in once-daily dosing. Risperidone is an antagonist of the serotonin 5-HT_{2A}, dopamine D_2, α_1- and α_2-adrenergic, and histamine H_1 receptors. It has a low affinity for α-adrenergic and muscarinic cholinergic receptors. Although it is as potent an antagonist of D_2 receptors as is haloperidol (Haldol), risperidone is much less likely (except in high doses) than haloperidol to cause extrapyramidal symptoms in humans.

Side Effects. Extrapyramidal effects of risperidone are largely dosage dependent, and a trend is seen to using lower doses than initially recommended. Weight gain, anxiety, nausea and vomiting, rhinitis, erectile dysfunction, orgasmic dysfunction, and increased pigmentation are associated with risperidone use. The most common drug-related reasons for discontinuation of risperidone use are extrapyramidal symptoms, dizziness, hyperkinesias, somnolence, and nausea. Marked elevation of prolactin can occur. Weight gain occurs more commonly with risperidone use in children than in adults.

Dosages. The recommended dose range and frequency of risperidone dosing has changed since the drug first came into clinical use. Risperidone is available in 1-, 2-, 3-, and 4-mg tablets, and a 1-mg/mL oral solution and in M-tab form (rapidly dissolving). The initial dosage is usually 1 to 2 mg at night, which can then be raised to 4 mg per day. Positron emission tomography (PET) studies have shown that dosages of 1 to 4 mg per day provide the required D_2 blockade needed for a therapeutic effect. At first it was believed that because of its short elimination half-life, risperidone should be given twice a day, but studies have shown equal efficacy with once-a-day dosing. Dosages above 6 mg a day are associated with a higher incidence of adverse effects, particularly extrapyramidal symptoms. No correlation has been found between plasma concentrations and therapeutic effect.

Risperidone (Risperdal Consta) is the only SDA currently available in a depot formulation. It is given as an intramuscular (IM) injection formulation every 2 weeks. The dose may be 25, 50, or 75 mg. Oral risperidone should be coadministered with Risperdal Consta for the first 3 weeks before being discontinued.

Drug Interactions. Inhibition of CYP 2D6 by drugs such as paroxetine and fluoxetine can block the formation of risperidone's active metabolite. Risperidone is a weak inhibitor of CYP 2D6 and has little effect on other drugs. Combined use of risperidone and selective serotonin reuptake inhibitors (SSRIs) can result in significant elevation of prolactin, with associated galactorrhea and breast enlargement.

Olanzapine

Pharmacology. Approximately 85 percent of olanzapine is absorbed from the gastrointestinal (GI) tract, and about 40 percent of the dosage is inactivated by first-pass hepatic metabolism. Peak concentrations are reached in 5 hours, and the half-life averages 31 hours (range 21 to 54 hours). It is given in once-daily dosing. In addition to 5-HT_{2A} and D_2 antagonism, olanzapine is an antagonist of the D_1, D_4, α_1, 5-HT_{1A}, muscarinic M_1 through M_5, and H_1 receptors.

Side Effects. Other than clozapine, olanzapine consistently causes a greater amount and more frequent weight gain than other atypical antipsychotics which plateaus after about 10 months. This effect is not dose related and continues over time. Clinical trial data suggest it peaks after 9 months, after which it may continue to increase more slowly. Somnolence, dry mouth, dizziness, constipation, dyspepsia, increased appetite, akathisia, and tremor are associated with olanzapine use. A few patients (2 percent) may need to discontinue use of the drug because of transaminase elevation. A dose-related risk exists of extrapyramidal side effects. The manufacturer recommends "periodic" assessment of blood sugar and transaminases during treatment with olanzapine. An FDA-mandate warns about an increased risk of stroke among patients with dementia treated with olanzapine and other SDA's but this risk is small and is outweighed by improved behavioral control that treatment may produce.

Dosages. Olanzapine is available in 2.5-, 5-, 7.5-, 10-, 15- and 20-mg tablets. The initial dosage for treatment of psychosis is usually 5 or 10 mg and for treatment of acute mania is usually 10 or 15 mg, given once daily. It is also available as 5-, 10-, 15- and 20-mg orally disintegrating tablets that might be useful for patients who have difficulty swallowing pills or who "cheek" their medication. A 10 mg injection form is available for treatment of acute agitation in schizophrenia and bipolar disorder.

A starting daily dose of 5 to 10 mg is recommended. After 1 week, the dosage can be raised to 10 mg a day. Given the long half-life, 1 week must be allowed to achieve each new steady-state blood level. Dosages in clinical use ranges vary, with 5 to 20 mg a day being most commonly used, but 30 to 40 mg a day being needed in treatment-resistant patients. A word of caution, however, is that the higher dosages are associated with increased extrapyramidal and other adverse effects and doses above 20 mg a day were not studied in the pivotal trials that led to the approval of olanzapine.

Drug Interactions. Fluvoxamine (Luvox) and cimetidine (Tagamet) increase, whereas carbamazepine (Tegretol) and phenytoin decrease serum concentrations of olanzapine. Ethanol increases olanzapine absorption by more than 25 percent, leading to increased sedation. Olanzapine has little effect on the metabolism of other drugs.

Quetiapine

Pharmacology. Quetiapine is a dibenzothiazepine structurally related to clozapine, but it differs markedly from that agent in biochemical effects. It is rapidly absorbed from the GI tract, with peak plasma concentrations reached in 1 to 2 hours. Steady-state half-life is about 7 hours, and optimal dosing is two or three times per day. Quetiapine, in addition to being an antagonist of D_2 and 5-HT_2, also blocks 5-HT_6, D_1 and H_1, and α_1 and α_2 receptors. It does not block muscarinic or benzodiazepine receptors. The receptor antagonism for quetiapine is generally lower than that for other antipsychotic drugs, and it is not associated with extrapyramidal symptoms.

Side Effects. Somnolence, postural hypotension, and dizziness are the most common adverse effects of quetiapine. These are usually transient and are best managed with initial gradual upward titration of the dosage. Quetiapine is the SDA least likely to cause extrapyramidal side effects, regardless of dose. This makes it particularly useful in treating patients with Parkinson's who develop dopamine agonist-induced psychosis. Prolactin elevation is rare and both transient and mild when it occurs. Quetiapine is associated with modest weight gain in some persons, but some patients occasionally gain a considerable amount of weight. Small increases in heart rate, constipation, and a transient rise in liver transaminases can also occur. Initial concerns about cataract formation, based on animal studies, have not been borne out since the drug has been in clinical use. Nevertheless, it might be prudent to test for lens abnormalities early in treatment and periodically thereafter.

Dosages. Quetiapine is available in 25-, 100-, and 200-mg tablets. In schizophrenia a target of 400 mg a day is desired and in mania and bipolar depression 800 mg and 300 mg respectively are desired. It has become evident that the target dose can be achieved rapidly and that some patients benefit from doses of as much as 1,200 to 1,600 mg a day. Despite its short elimination half-life, quetiapine can be given once a day to many patients. This is consistent with the observation that quetiapine receptor occupancy remains even when concentrations in the blood have markedly declined. Quetiapine in doses of 25 to 300 mg at night has been used for insomnia.

Drug Interactions. The potential interactions between quetiapine and other drugs have been well studied. Other than a finding that phenytoin increases quetiapine clearance fivefold, no major pharmacokinetic interactions have been noted.

Ziprasidone

Pharmacology. Ziprasidone is a benzothiazolyl piperazine. Peak plasma concentrations of ziprasidone are reached in 2 to 6 hours. Steady-state levels ranging from 5 to 10 hours are reached between the first and third day of treatment. The mean terminal half-life at steady state ranges from 5 to 10 hours, which accounts for the recommendation that twice-daily dosing is necessary. Bioavailability doubles when ziprasidone is taken with food.

Peak serum concentrations of IM ziprasidone occur after approximately 1 hour, with a half-life of 2 to 5 hours.

Ziprasidone, as with the other SDAs, blocks 5-HT_{2A} and D_2 receptors. It is also an antagonist of 5-HT_{1D}, 5-HT_{2C}, D_3, D_4, α_1, and H_1 receptors. It has very low affinity for D_1, M_1, and α_2-receptors. Ziprasidone also has agonist activity at the serotonin 5-HT_{1A} receptors and is a serotonin reuptake inhibitor and a norepinephrine reuptake inhibitor. This is consistent with clinical reports that ziprasidone has antidepressant-like effects in nonschizophrenic patients.

Side Effects. Somnolence, headache, dizziness, nausea, and lightheadedness are the most common adverse effects in patients taking ziprasidone. It has almost no significant effects outside the central nervous system (CNS) and is associated with almost no weight gain and does not cause sustained prolactin elevation. Concerns about prolongation of the QT_c complex have deterred some clinicians from using ziprasidone as a first choice. The QT_c interval has been shown to increase by an average 4.7 to 1.4 milliseconds in patients treated with 40 and 120 mg per day, respectively. Ziprasidone is contraindicated in combination with other drugs known to prolong the QT_c interval. These include, but are not limited to, dofetilide, sotalol, quinidine, other class Ia and III antiarrhythmics, mesoridazine, thioridazine, chlorpromazine, droperidol, pimozide, sparfloxacin, gatifloxacin, moxifloxacin, halofantrine, mefloquine, pentamidine, arsenic trioxide, levomethadyl acetate, dolasetron mesylate, probucol, or tacrolimus. Ziprasidone should be avoided in patients with congenital long QT syndrome and in patients with a history of cardiac arrhythmias.

Dosages. Ziprasidone is available in 20-, 40-, 60-, and 80-mg capsules. Ziprasidone for IM use comes as a single-use 20 mg/mL vial. Oral ziprasidone dosing should be initiated at 40 mg a day, divided into two daily doses. Studies have shown efficacy in the range of 80 to 160 mg a day, divided twice daily. In clinical practice, doses as high as 240 mg a day are being used. The recommended IM dosage is 10 to 20 mg every 2 hours for the 10-mg dose and every 4 hours for the 20-mg dose. The maximal total daily dose of IM ziprasidone is 40 mg.

Other than interactions with other drugs that prolong the QT_c complex, ziprasidone appears to have low potential for clinically significant drug interactions.

Clozapine

Pharmacology. Clozapine is a dibenzodiazepine. It is rapidly absorbed, with peak plasma levels reached in about 2 hours. Steady state is achieved in less than 1 week if twice-daily dosing is used. The elimination half-life is about 12 hours. Clozapine has two major metabolites, one of which, N-dimethyl clozapine, may have some pharmacologic activity. Clozapine is an antagonist of 5-HT_{2A}, D_1, D_3, D_4, and α (especially α_1) receptors. It has relatively low potency as a D_2-receptor antagonist. Data from PET scanning show that 10 mg of haloperidol produces 80 percent occupancy of striatal D_2 receptors, whereas clinically effective dosages of clozapine occupy only 40 to 50 percent of striatal D_2 receptors. This difference in D_2 receptor occupancy is probably why clozapine does not cause extrapyramidal adverse effects. It has also been postulated that clozapine, as well as other SDAs, bind more loosely to the D_2 receptor, and as a result of this "fast dissociation," more normal dopamine neurotransmission is possible.

Special Indications. In addition to being the most effective drug treatment for patients who have failed on standard therapies, clozapine has been shown to benefit patients with severe tardive dyskinesia. Clozapine suppresses these dyskinesias, but the abnormal movements return when clozapine is discontinued. This is true despite that clozapine, on rare occasions, can cause tardive dyskinesia. Other clinical situations where clozapine can be used include the treatment of psychotic patients who are intolerant of extrapyramidal side effects caused by other agents, treatment-resistant mania, severe psychotic depression, idiopathic Parkinson's disease, Huntington's disease, and suicidal patients with schizophrenia or schizoaffective disorder. Other treatment-resistant disorders that have demonstrated response to clozapine include pervasive developmental disorder, autism of childhood, or OCD (either alone or in combination with an SSRI). Used by itself, clozapine, very rarely, induces obsessive-compulsive symptoms.

Side Effects. The most common drug-related adverse effects are sedation, dizziness, syncope, tachycardia, hypotension, electrocardiogram (ECG) changes, nausea, and vomiting. Other common adverse effects include fatigue, weight gain, various GI symptoms (most commonly, constipation), anticholinergic effects, and subjective muscle weakness. Sialorrhea, or hypersalivation, is a side effect that begins early in treatment and is most evident at night. Patients report that their pillows are drenched with saliva. This side effect is most likely the result of impairment of swallowing. Although reports suggest that clonidine or amitriptyline may help reduce hypersalivation, the most practical solution is to put a towel over the pillow.

The risk of seizures is about 4 percent in patients taking dosages above 600 mg a day. Leukopenia, granulocytopenia, agranulocytosis, and fever occur in about 1 percent of patients. During the first year of treatment, a 0.73 percent risk is seen of clozapine-induced agranulocytosis. The risk during the second year is 0.07 percent. For neutropenia, the risk is 2.32 percent and 0.69 percent during the first and second years of treatment, respectively. The only contraindications to the use of clozapine are a white blood cell (WBC) count below 3,500/mm^3cells, a previous bone marrow disorder, a history of agranulocytosis during clozapine treatment, or the use of another drug that is known to suppress the bone marrow, for example, carbamazepine.

During the first 6 months of treatment, weekly WBC counts are indicated to monitor the patient for the development of agranulocytosis. If the WBC count remains normal, the frequency of testing can be decreased to every 2 weeks. Although monitoring is expensive, early indication of agranulocytosis can prevent a fatal outcome. Clozapine should be discontinued if the WBC count is below 3,000/mm^3 cells or the granulocyte count is below 1,500/mm^3. In addition, a hematologic consultation should be obtained, and obtaining a bone marrow sample should be considered. Persons with agranulocytosis should not be reexposed to the drug. To avoid situations where a physician or patient fails to comply with the required blood tests, clozapine cannot be dispensed without proof of monitoring.

Myocarditis is also a serious risk in the use of clozapine.

Dosages. Clozapine is available in 25- and 100-mg tablets. The initial dosage is usually 25 mg one or two times daily, although a conservative initial dosage is 12.5 mg twice daily. The dosage can then be raised gradually (25 mg a day every 2 or 3 days) to 300 mg a day in divided dosages, usually two or three times daily. Dosages up to 900 mg a day can be used. Testing for blood concentrations of clozapine may be helpful in patients who fail to respond. Studies have found that plasma concentrations greater than 350 mg/mL are associated with a better likelihood of response.

Drug Interactions. Clozapine should not be used with any other drug that is associated with the development of agranulocytosis or bone marrow suppression. Such drugs include carbamazepine, phenytoin, propylthiouracil, sulfonamides, and captopril (Capoten). Lithium combined with clozapine can increase the risk of seizures, confusion, and movement disorders. Lithium should not be used in combination with clozapine by persons who have experienced an episode of neuroleptic malignant syndrome. Clomipramine (Anafranil) can increase the risk of seizure by lowering the seizure threshold and by increasing clozapine plasma concentrations. Risperidone, fluoxetine, paroxetine, and fluvoxamine increase serum concentrations of clozapine. Addition of paroxetine may precipitate clozapine-associated neutropenia.

Other SDAs

Bifeprunox. Bifeprunox, a dopamine partial agonist, is an investigational atypical antipsychotic for the treatment of schizophrenia. Although bifeprunox has been shown to have a smaller mean effect in acute psychosis, compared to other atypical antipsychotics, it may be an alternative in terms of side effects. In studies, gastrointestinal side effects were the most common adverse events. These included nausea, vomiting, constipation and abdominal discomfort. In some studies, bifeprunox was associated with a decrease in weight and improvement in the lipid profile compared to placebo.

Paliperidone (Invega). Paliperidone is the major active metabolite of the antipsychotic medication risperidone. It is a potent blocker of serotonin receptors, and partially blocks dopamine (D) 2 receptors. Published data suggest that efficacy and side effects are the same as those seen with risperidone. It is formulated to be a once-daily, extended release, oral medication. The recommended dose of paliperidone is 6 mg per day. with a dose range of 3 mg to 12 mg per day.

ARIPIPRAZOLE

As with the SDAs, aripiprazole is a potent 5-HT$_{2A}$ antagonist and is indicated for the treatment of both schizophrenia and acute mania. Unlike the SDAs, aripiprazole, however, is not a D_2 antagonist, but is a partial D_2 agonist. Partial D_2 agonists compete at D_2 receptors for endogenous dopamine, thereby producing a functional reduction of dopamine activity. Because schizophrenia and mania are disorders associated with increased dopamine activity, this reduction may account for its therapeutic effects.

Aripiprazole is usually nonsedating and has not been found to pose an increased risk of weight gain and diabetes. Aripiprazole is particularly effective in sparing, and possibly enhancing, neurocognitive functions. Use of aripiprazole is relatively new, so little off-label use has been described.

Chemistry

Aripiprazole is a quinoline derivative.

Pharmacologic Actions

Aripiprazole is well absorbed, reaching peak plasma concentrations after 3 to 5 hours. Absorption is not affected by food. The mean elimination half-life of aripiprazole is about 75 hours. It has a weakly active metabolite with a half-life of 96 hours. These relatively long half-lives make aripiprazole suitable for once-daily dosing. Clearance is reduced in the elderly. Aripiprazole exhibits linear pharmacokinetics and is primarily metabolized by CYP 3A4 and CYP 2D6 enzymes. It is 99 percent protein bound. Aripiprazole is excreted in breast milk in lactating rats.

Mechanistically, aripiprazole acts as a modulator, rather than a blocker, and acts on both postsynaptic D_2 receptors and presynaptic autoreceptors. In theory, this mechanism addresses excessive limbic dopamine (hyperdopaminergic) activity, and decreased dopamine (hypodopaminergic) activity in frontal and prefrontal areas—abnormalities that are thought to be present in schizophrenia. The absence of complete D_2 blockade in the striatal areas would be expected to minimize extrapyramidal side effects. Aripiprazole is an α_1-adrenergic receptor antagonist, which can cause some patients to experience orthostatic hypotension. As with the so-called atypical antipsychotic agents, aripiprazole is a 5-HT$_{2A}$ antagonist.

Therapeutic Indications

Schizophrenia. Short-term, 4- to 6-week studies comparing aripiprazole with haloperidol and risperidone in patients with schizophrenia and schizoaffective disorder have shown comparable efficacy. Dosages of 15, 20, and 30 mg a day were found to be effective. Long-term studies suggest that aripiprazole is effective as a maintenance treatment at a daily dose of 15 to 30 mg.

Acute Mania. Aripiprazole is useful for the initial control of agitation during a manic episode. Despite being largely devoid of sedation as a side effect, the antimanic effects of aripiprazole were evident in clinical trials as early as day 4. No studies have compared aripiprazole with lithium, divalproex, or olanzapine, other drugs that are used to treat acute mania.

Other Uses. Aripiprazole has been reported to be used successfully as an add-on to SSRIs in treatment-resistant patients with mood or anxiety disorders. Doses of 15 to 30 mg per day were used. A small study of aripiprazole as a treatment for psychotic symptoms associated with Alzheimer's disease found no clinical benefit from aripiprazole. A study of aggressive children and adolescents with oppositional defiant disorder or conduct disorder found a positive response in about 60 percent of the subjects. In this study, vomiting and somnolence led to a reduction in initial aripiprazole dosage.

Adverse Effects

The most commonly reported adverse effects of aripiprazole are headache, somnolence, agitation, dyspepsia, anxiety, and nausea. The adverse reactions listed in Table 36.30–1 reflect clinical trial findings. Although it is not a frequent cause of extrapyramidal side effects, aripiprazole does cause akathisia-like activation. Described as restlessness or agitation, it can be highly distressing and often leads to discontinuation of medication. Insomnia is another common complaint. Data so far do not indicate that weight gain or diabetes mellitus have an increased incidence with aripiprazole use. Prolactin elevation does not typically occur. Aripiprazole does not cause significant QT_c interval changes. Seizures have been reported.

Drug Interactions

Carbamazepine and valproate reduce, whereas ketoconazole, fluoxetine, paroxetine, and quinidine increase aripiprazole serum concentrations. Lithium and valproic acid, two drugs likely to be combined with aripiprazole when treating bipolar disorder, do not affect the steady-state concentrations of aripiprazole. Combined use with antihypertensives can cause hypotension. Drugs that inhibit CYP 2D6 activity reduce aripiprazole elimination.

Dosage and Clinical Guidelines

Aripiprazole is available as 5-, 10-, 15-, 20-, and 30-mg tablets. The effective dosage range is 10 to 30 mg per day. Although the starting dosage is 10 to 15 mg per day, problems with nausea, insomnia, and akathisia have led to use of lower than recommended starting dosages of aripiprazole. Many clinicians find that an initial dose of 5 mg increases tolerability. It is too early to predict optimal dosing strategy for aripiprazole in clinical practice.

CLINICAL GUIDELINES

All SDAs are appropriate for the management of an initial psychotic episode, whereas clozapine is reserved for persons refractory to all other antipsychotic drugs. If a person does not respond to the first SDA, other SDAs should be tried. Drug choice should be based on the patient's clinical status and history of response to medication. SDAs usually require 4 to 6 weeks to reach full effectiveness, and it may take up to 8 weeks for the full clinical effects of an SDA to become apparent. Much of the observed initial clinical improvement, thus, may reflect nonspecific sedation. At first glance, this would suggest that highly sedating SDAs, such as olanzapine or quetiapine, would be preferred agents for acute treatment of agitated, violent, or highly anxious patients. Interestingly, head-to-head studies do not show differences between SDAs with respect to acute effects. Nevertheless, it is acceptable practice to augment an SDA with a high-potency DRA or benzodiazepine in the first few weeks of use. Lorazepam 1 to 2 mg orally or IM can be used as needed for acute agitation. Once effective, dosages can be lowered as tolerated. Clinical improvement may take 6 months of treatment with SDAs in some particularly treatment-refractory persons.

Use of all SDAs must be initiated at low dosages and gradually tapered upward to therapeutic dosages. The gradual increase in dosage is necessitated by the potential development of adverse effects. If a person stops taking an SDA for more than 36 hours, drug use should be resumed at the initial titration schedule. After the decision to terminate olanzapine or clozapine use, dosages should be tapered whenever possible to avoid cholinergic rebound symptoms, such as diaphoresis, flushing, diarrhea, and hyperactivity.

Once a clinician has determined that a trial of an SDA is warranted for a particular person, the risks and the benefits of SDA treatment must be explained to the person and the family. In the case of clozapine, an informed consent procedure should be documented in the person's chart. The patient's history should include information about blood disorders, epilepsy, cardiovascular disease, hepatic and renal diseases, and drug abuse. The presence of a hepatic or renal disease necessitates using low starting dosages of the drug. Physical examination should include supine and standing blood pressure (BP) measurements to screen for orthostatic hypotension. The laboratory examination should include an ECG; several complete blood counts (CBCs) with WBC counts, which can then be averaged; and liver and renal function tests. Periodic monitoring of blood glucose, lipids, and body weight is recommended.

Although the transition from a DRA to an SDA may be made abruptly, it is wise to taper off the DRA slowly while titrating up the SDA. Clozapine and olanzapine both have anticholinergic effects, and the transition from one to the other can usually be accomplished with little risk of cholinergic rebound. The transition from risperidone to olanzapine is best accomplished by tapering the risperidone off over 3 weeks and simultaneously beginning olanzapine at 10 mg a day. Risperidone, quetiapine, and ziprasidone lack anticholinergic effects, and the abrupt transition from a DRA, olanzapine, or clozapine to one of these agents can cause cholinergic rebound, which consists of excessive salivation, nausea, vomiting, and diarrhea. The risk of cholinergic rebound can be mitigated by initially augmenting risperidone, quetiapine, or ziprasidone with an anticholinergic drug, which is then tapered off slowly. Any initiation and termination of SDA use should be accomplished gradually.

It is wise to overlap administration of the new drug with the old drug. Of interest, some people have a more robust clinical response while taking the two agents during the transition and then regressing on monotherapy with the newer drug. Little is known about the effectiveness and safety of a strategy of combining one SDA with another SDA or with a DRA.

Persons receiving regular injections of depot formulations of a DRA who are to switch to SDA use are given the first dose of the SDA on the day the next injection is due.

Persons who developed agranulocytosis while taking clozapine can safely switch to olanzapine use, although initiation of olanzapine use in the midst of clozapine-induced agranulocytosis can prolong the time of recovery from the usual 3 to 4 days up to 11 to 12 days. It is prudent to wait for resolution of agranulocytosis before initiating olanzapine use. Emergence or recurrence of agranulocytosis has not been reported with olanzapine, even in persons who developed it while taking clozapine.

Use of an SDA by pregnant women has not been studied, but consideration should be given to the potential of risperidone to raise prolactin concentrations, sometimes up to three to four times the upper limit of the normal range. Because the drugs can be excreted in breast milk, they should not be taken by nursing mothers.

REFERENCES

Ananth J, Parameswaran S, Gunatilake S, Burgoyne K, Sidhom T. Neuroleptic malignant syndrome and atypical antipsychotic drugs. *J Clin Psychiatry*. 2004;65:464–470.

Bowden CL. Atypical antipsychotic augmentation of mood stabilizer therapy in bipolar disorder. *J of Clin Psych*. 2005;66[Suppl 3]:12–19.

Ginsberg DL. Atomoxetine-induced mania. *Primary Psychiatry*. 2004;11(11): 25–26.

Ginsberg DL. Clozapine-induced interstitial nephritis. *Primary Psychiatry*. 2004; 11(9):24–25.

Harvey PD, Green MF, Keefe RSF, Vellgan DI. Cognitive functioning in schizophrenia: A consensus statement on its role in the definition and evaluation of effective treatments for the illness. *J Clin Psychiatry*. 2004;65:361–372.

Hirschfeld RMA, Keck PE, Kramer M, Karcher K, Canuso C, Eerdekens M, Grossman F. Rapid antimanic effect of risperidone monotherapy: A 3-week multicenter, double-blind, placebo-controlled trial. *Am J Psychiatry*. 2004;161:1057–1065.

van Kammen DP, Marder SR. Serotonin-dopamine antagonists (atypical or second-generation antipsychotics). In: Sadock BJ, Sadock VA, eds. *Kaplan & Sadock's Comprehensive Textbook of Psychiatry*. 8th ed. Vol. 2. Baltimore: Lippincott Williams & Wilkins; 2005:2914.

Kane J, Conley R, Keith S, Nasrallah H, Turner S. Guidelines for the use of long-acting injectable atypical antipsychotics. *J Clin Psychiatry*. 2004;65:120–131.

Lindenmayer JP, Czobor P, Volavka J, Lieberman JA, Citrome L, Sheitman B, McEvoy JP, Cooper TB, Chakos M. Effects of atypical antipsychotics on the syndromal profile in treatment resistant schizophrenia. *J Clin Psychiatry*. 2004;65:551–556.

McEvoy JP, Lieberman JA, Stroup TS, Davis SM, Meltzer HY, Rosenheck RA, Swartz MS, Perkins DO, Keefe RSE, Davis CE, Severe J, Hsiao JK. Effectiveness of clozapine versus olanzapine, quetiapine, and risperidone in patients with chronic schizophrenia who did not respond to prior atypical antipsychotic treatment. *Am J Psychiatry*. 2006;163:600.

Meltzer HY, Alphs L, Green AI, Altamura AC, Anand R, Bertoldi A, Bourgeois M, Chouinard G, Islam MZ, Kane J, Krishnan R, Lindenmayer JP, Potkin S; International Suicide Prevention Trial Study Group. Clozapine treatment for suicidality in schizophrenia: International Suicide Prevention Trial (InterSePT). *Arch Gen Psychiatry*. 2003;60:82–91.

Nickel MK, Muehlbacher M, Nickel C, Kettler C, Gil FP, Bachler E, Buschmann W, Rother N, Fartacek R, Egger C, Anvar J, Rother WK, Loew TH, Kaplan P. Aripiprazole in the treatment of patients with borderline personality disorder: A double-blind, placebo-controlled study. *Am J Psychiatry*. 2006;163:833.

Schneider LS, Dagerman KS, Insel P. Risk of death with atypical antipsychotic drug treatment for dementia: Meta-analysis of randomized placebo-controlled trials. *JAMA*. 2005;294:1934.

Verhoeven WMA, van der Heijden FMMA, Wijers FWHM, Tuinier S. Novel antipsychotics: Facts and fictions. *Clinical Neuropsychiatry: J of Treatment Evaluation*. 2005;2(4):212.

Volavka J, Czobor P, Cooper TB, Sheitman B, Lindenmayer JP, Citrome L, McEvoy JP, Lieberman JA. Prolactin levels in schizophrenia and schizoaffective disorder patients treated with clozapine, olanzapine, risperidone, or haloperidol. *J Clin Psychiatry*. 2004;65(1):57.

▲ 36.31 Sympathomimetics and Related Drugs

Stimulant drugs, also referred to as *psychostimulants*, mimic the effects of naturally occurring sympathomimetic amines. They increase motivation, mood, energy, and wakefulness. Psychostimulants used in psychiatry include methylphenidate (Ritalin), dexmethylphenidate (Focalin), dextroamphetamine (Dexedrine), a combination of amphetamine and dextroamphetamine (Adderall), and pemoline (Cylert), now considered a second-line agent because of rare but potentially fatal hepatic toxicity. The drugs are indicated for the treatment of attention-deficit/hyperactivity disorder (ADHD) and narcolepsy and are also effective in the treatment of depression in some patients. Both amphetamine and nonamphetamine sympathomimetics have been used as appetite suppressants. Other sympathomimetics used for appetite suppression include methamphetamine (Desoxyn), phentermine (Adipex-P, Ionamin), diethylpropion (Tenuate), and phendimetrazine (Bontril). A novel stimulant approved for treatment of narcolepsy in the United States, modafinil (Provigil), has been used as an antidepressant and a treatment for ADHD. Atomoxetine (Strattera), although not a stimulant, is indicated for use in ADHD and is included in this section.

CHEMISTRY

The molecular structures of dextroamphetamine, methylphenidate, pemoline, methamphetamine, phentermine, and modafinil are shown in Figure 36.31–1.

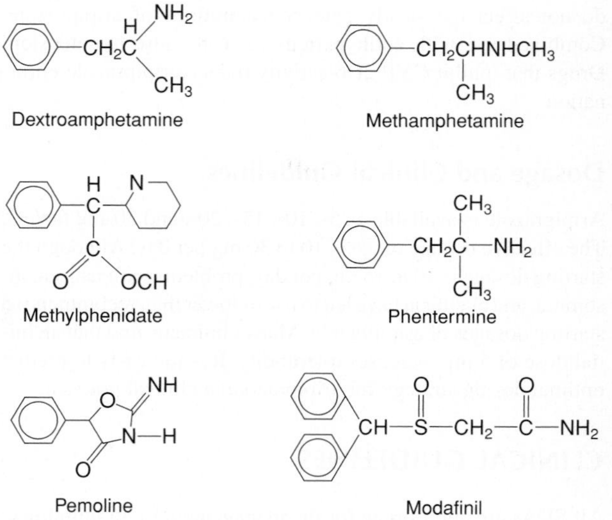

Dextroamphetamine

Methamphetamine

Methylphenidate

Phentermine

Pemoline

Modafinil

FIGURE 36.31–1
Molecular structures of selected sympathomimetics.

PHARMACOLOGIC ACTIONS

All of these drugs are well absorbed from the gastrointestinal (GI) tract. Amphetamine and dextroamphetamine reach peak plasma concentrations in 2 to 3 hours and have a half-life of about 6 hours, thereby necessitating once- or twice-daily dosing. Methylphenidate is available in immediate-release (Ritalin), sustained-release (Ritalin SR), and extended-release (Concerta) formulations. Immediate-release methylphenidate reaches peak plasma concentrations in 1 to 2 hours and has a short half-life of 2 to 3 hours, thereby necessitating multiple daily dosing. The sustained-release formulation reaches peak plasma concentrations in 4 to 5 hours and doubles the effective half-life of methylphenidate. The extended-release formulation reaches peak plasma concentrations in 6 to 8 hours and is designed to be effective for 12 hours in once-daily dosing. Dexmethylphenidate reaches peak plasma concentration in about 3 hours and is prescribed twice daily. Pemoline reaches peak plasma concentrations in 2 to 4 hours and has a half-life of about 12 hours, and modafinil reaches peak plasma concentrations in 2 to 4 hours and has a half-life of 15 hours, thereby allowing once-daily dosing of these two agents.

Methylphenidate, dextroamphetamine, and amphetamine are indirectly acting sympathomimetics, with the primary effect of causing the release of catecholamines from presynaptic neurons. Clinical effectiveness is associated with increased release of both dopamine and norepinephrine. Dextroamphetamine and methylphenidate are also weak inhibitors of catecholamine reuptake and inhibitors of monoamine oxidase. Pemoline may indirectly stimulate dopaminergic activity by a poorly understood mechanism, but it has little actual sympathomimetic activity.

The specific mechanism of action of modafinil is unknown. Narcolepsy–cataplexy results from deficiency of hypocretin, a hypothalamic neuropeptide. Hypocretin-producing neurons are activated after modafinil administration. Modafinil does not appear to work through a dopaminergic mechanism. It does have α_1-adrenergic agonist properties, which may account for its alerting effects, because the wakefulness induced by modafinil can be attenuated by prazosin, an α_1-adrenergic antagonist. Some evidence suggests that modafinil has some norepinephrine reuptake blocking effects.

THERAPEUTIC INDICATIONS

Attention-Deficit/Hyperactivity Disorder

Sympathomimetics are the first-line drugs for treatment of ADHD in children and are effective about 75 percent of the time. Methylphenidate and dextroamphetamine are equally effective and work within 15 to 30 minutes. Pemoline requires 3 to 4 weeks to reach its full efficacy; however, it is rarely used because of toxicity. Sympathomimetic drugs decrease hyperactivity, increase attentiveness, and reduce impulsivity. They may also reduce comorbid oppositional behaviors associated with ADHD. Many persons take these drugs throughout their schooling and beyond. In responsive persons, use of a sympathomimetic may be a critical determinant of scholastic success.

Sympathomimetics improve the core ADHD symptoms of hyperactivity, impulsivity, and inattentiveness and permit improved social interactions with teachers, family, other adults, and peers. The success of long-term treatment of ADHD with sympathomimetics, which are efficacious for most of the various constellations of ADHD symptoms present from childhood to adulthood, supports a model in which ADHD results from a genetically determined neurochemical imbalance that requires lifelong pharmacologic management.

Methylphenidate is the most commonly used initial agent, at a dosage of 5 to 10 mg every 3 to 4 hours. Dosages may be increased to a maximum of 20 mg four times daily or 1 mg/kg a day. Use of the 20-mg sustained-release formulation to achieve 6 hours of benefit and eliminate the need for dosing at school is supported by many experts, although other authorities feel it is less effective than the immediate-release formulation. Dextroamphetamine is about twice as potent as methylphenidate on a per milligram basis and provides 6 to 8 hours of benefit. Some 70 percent of nonresponders to one sympathomimetic may benefit from another. All the sympathomimetic drugs should be tried before switching to drugs of a different class. The previous dictum that sympathomimetics worsen tics and, therefore, should be avoided by persons with comorbid ADHD and tic disorders has been questioned. Small dosages of sympathomimetics do not appear to cause an increase in the frequency and severity of tics. Alternatives to sympathomimetics for ADHD include bupropion (Wellbutrin), venlafaxine (Effexor), guanfacine (Tenex), clonidine (Catapres), and tricyclic drugs. Further studies are needed to determine whether modafinil decreases the symptoms of ADHD.

Short-term use of the sympathomimetics induces a euphoric feeling; however, tolerance develops for both the euphoric feeling and the sympathomimetic activity. Importantly, tolerance does not develop for the therapeutic effects in ADHD.

Narcolepsy and Hypersomnolence

Narcolepsy consists of sudden sleep attacks (*narcolepsy*), sudden loss of postural tone (*cataplexy*), loss of voluntary motor control going into (hypnagogic) or coming out of (hypnopompic) sleep (*sleep paralysis*), and hypnagogic or hypnopompic *hallucinations*. Sympathomimetics reduce narcoleptic sleep attacks and also improve wakefulness in other types of hypersomnolent states. Modafinil is approved as an antisomnolence agent for treatment of narcolepsy, for people who cannot adjust to night shift work, and for those who do not sleep well because of obstructive sleep apnea.

Other sympathomimetics are also used to maintain wakefulness and accuracy of motor performance in persons subject to sleep deprivation, such as pilots and military personnel. Persons with narcolepsy, unlike persons with ADHD, may develop tolerance for the therapeutic effects of the sympathomimetics.

In direct comparison with amphetamine-like drugs, modafinil is equally effective at maintaining wakefulness, with a lower risk of excessive activation.

Depressive Disorders

Sympathomimetics can be used for treatment-resistant depressive disorders, usually as augmentation of standard antidepressant drug therapy. Possible indications for use of sympathomimetics as monotherapy include depression in the elderly, who are at increased risk for adverse effects from standard antidepressant drugs; depression in medically ill persons, especially persons with acquired immunodeficiency syndrome (AIDS); obtundation because of chronic use of opioids; and clinical situations in which a rapid response is important but for which electroconvulsive therapy (ECT) is contraindicated. Depressed patients with abulia and anergia may also benefit.

Dextroamphetamine may be useful in differentiating pseudodementia of depression from dementia. A depressed person generally responds to a 5-mg dose with increased alertness and improved cognition. Sympathomimetics are thought to provide only short-term benefit (2 to 4 weeks) for depression, because most persons rapidly develop tolerance for the antidepressant effects of the drugs. Some clinicians, however report that long-term treatment with sympathomimetics can benefit some persons.

Encephalopathy Caused by Brain Injury

Sympathomimetics increase alertness, cognition, motivation, and motor performance in persons with neurologic deficits caused by strokes, trauma, tumors, or chronic infections. Treatment with sympathomimetics may permit earlier and more robust participation in rehabilitative programs. Poststroke lethargy and apathy may respond to long-term use of sympathomimetics.

Obesity

Sympathomimetics are used in the treatment of obesity because of their anorexia-inducing effects. Because tolerance develops for the anorectic effects and because of the drugs' high abuse potential, their use for this indication is limited. Of the sympathomimetic drugs, phentermine is the most widely used for appetite suppression. Phentermine was the second half of "fen-phen," an off-label combination of fenfluramine and phentermine, widely used to promote weight loss until fenfluramine and dexfenfluramine were withdrawn from commercial availability because of an association with cardiac valvular insufficiency, primary pulmonary hypertension, and irreversible loss of cerebral serotoninergic nerve fibers. The toxicity of fenfluramine is attributed to its stimulating release of massive amounts of serotonin from nerve endings, a mechanism of action not shared by phentermine. Use of phentermine alone has not been reported to cause the same adverse effects as those caused by fenfluramine or dexfenfluramine.

Careful limitation of caloric intake and judicious exercise are at the core of any successful weight loss program. Sympathomimetic drugs facilitate loss of, at most, an additional fraction of a pound per week. Sympathomimetic drugs are effective appetite suppressants only for the first few weeks of use; then the anorexigenic effects tend to decrease.

Fatigue

Between 70 percent and 90 percent of individuals with multiple sclerosis experience fatigue. Modafinil, amphetamines, methylphenidate, and the dopamine receptor agonist amantadine (Symmetral) are sometimes effective in combating this symptom. Other causes of fatigue, such as chronic fatigue syndrome, respond to stimulants in many cases.

PRECAUTIONS AND ADVERSE REACTIONS

The most common adverse effects associated with amphetamine-like drugs are stomach pain, anxiety, irritability, insomnia, tachycardia, cardiac arrhythmias, and dysphoria. Sympathomimetics cause decreased appetite, although tolerance usually develops for this effect. The treatment of common adverse effects in children with ADHD is usually straightforward (Table 36.31–1). The drugs can also cause increases in heart rate and blood pressure (BP) and may cause palpitations. Less common adverse effects include the possible induction of movement disorders, such as tics, Tourette's disorder-like symptoms, and dyskinesias, which are often self-limited over 7 to 10 days. If a person taking a

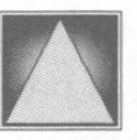

Table 36.31–1
Management of Common Stimulant-Induced Adverse Effects in Attention-Deficit/Hyperactivity Disorder

Adverse Effect	Management
Anorexia, nausea, weight loss	▸ Administer stimulant with meals. ▸ Use caloric-enhanced supplements. Discourage forcing meals. ▸ If using pemoline, check liver function tests.
Insomnia, nightmares	▸ Administer stimulants earlier in day. ▸ Change to short-acting preparations. ▸ Discontinue afternoon or evening dosing. ▸ Consider adjunctive treatment (e.g., antihistamines, clonidine, antidepressants).
Dizziness	▸ Monitor BP. ▸ Encourage fluid intake. ▸ Change to long-acting form.
Rebound phenomena	▸ Overlap stimulant dosing. ▸ Change to long-acting preparation or combine long- and short-acting preparations. ▸ Consider adjunctive or alternative treatment (e.g., clonidine, antidepressants).
Irritability	▸ Assess timing of phenomena (during peak or withdrawal phase). ▸ Evaluate comorbid symptoms. ▸ Reduce dose. ▸ Consider adjunctive or alternative treatment (e.g., lithium, antidepressants, anticonvulsants).
Dysphoria, moodiness, agitation	▸ Consider comorbid diagnosis (e.g., mood disorder). ▸ Reduce dosage or change to long-acting preparation. ▸ Consider adjunctive or alternative treatment (e.g., lithium, anticonvulsants, antidepressants).

BP, blood pressure.
(From Wilens TE, Blederman J. The stimulants. In: Shaffer, D, ed. *The Psychiatric Clinics of North America: Pediatric Psychopharmacology.* Philadelphia: WB Saunders; 1992, with permission.)

sympathomimetic develops one of these movement disorders, a correlation between the dose of the medication and the severity of the disorder must be firmly established before adjustments are made in the medication dosage. In severe cases, augmentation with risperidone (Risperdal), clonidine, or guanfacine is necessary. Methylphenidate may worsen tics in one third of persons; these persons fall into two groups: those whose methylphenidate-induced tics resolve immediately on metabolism of the dosage and a smaller group in whom methylphenidate appears to trigger tics that persist for several months, but eventually resolve spontaneously.

Longitudinal studies do not indicate that sympathomimetics cause growth suppression. Sympathomimetics can exacerbate glaucoma, hypertension, cardiovascular disorders, hyperthyroidism, anxiety disorders, psychotic disorders, and seizure disorders.

High dosages of sympathomimetics can cause dry mouth, pupillary dilation, bruxism, formication, excessive ebullience, restlessness, and emotional lability. Long-term use of high dosages can cause a delusional disorder that resembles paranoid schizophrenia. Overdosages of sympathomimetics result in hypertension, tachycardia, hyperthermia, toxic psychosis, delirium, and occasionally seizures. Overdosages of sympathomimetics can also result in death, often caused by cardiac arrhythmias. Seizures can be treated with benzodiazepines, cardiac effects with β-adrenergic receptor antagonists, fever with cooling blankets, and delirium with dopamine receptor antagonists (DRAs).

The most limiting adverse effect of sympathomimetics is their association with psychological and physical dependence. At the doses used for treatment of ADHD, psychological dependence virtually never develops. A greater concern is the presence of adolescent or adult cohabitants who might confiscate the supply of sympathomimetics for abuse or sale.

Sympathomimetic use should be avoided during pregnancy, especially during the first trimester. Dextroamphetamine and methylphenidate pass into the breast milk, and it is not known whether pemoline or modafinil do.

A review of postmarketing experience with pemoline found several cases of acute hepatic failure, some of which were in children. This prompted the US Food and Drug Administration (FDA) to change the package insert to recommend that pemoline no longer be considered first-line therapy for ADHD. It is now rarely used.

DRUG INTERACTIONS

The coadministration of sympathomimetics and tricyclic or tetracyclic antidepressants, warfarin (Coumadin), primidone (Mysoline), phenobarbital (Luminal), phenytoin (Dilantin), or phenylbutazone (Butazolidin) decreases the metabolism of these compounds, resulting in increased plasma levels. Sympathomimetics decrease the therapeutic efficacy of many antihypertensive drugs, especially guanethidine (Esimil, Ismelin). The sympathomimetics should be used with extreme caution with monoamine oxidase inhibitors (MAOIs).

LABORATORY INTERFERENCES

Dextroamphetamine can elevate plasma corticosteroid levels and interfere with some assay methods for urinary corticosteroids.

DOSAGE AND ADMINISTRATION

Many psychiatrists believe that amphetamine use has been overly regulated by governmental authorities. Amphetamines are listed as schedule II drugs by the Drug Enforcement Agency (DEA). In some states, physicians must use triplicate prescriptions for such drugs; one copy is filed with a state government agency. Such mandates worry both patients and physicians about breaches in confidentiality, and physicians are concerned that their prescribing practices may be misinterpreted by official agencies. Consequently, some physicians may withhold prescription of sympathomimetics, even from persons who may benefit from the medications.

The dosage ranges and the available preparations for sympathomimetics are presented in Table 36.31–2. Dextroamphetamine, methylphenidate, amphetamine, benzphetamine, and methamphetamine are schedule II drugs; in some states, they require triplicate prescriptions. Phendimetrazine and phenmetrazine are schedule III drugs, and modafinil, phentermine, diethylpropion, and mazindol are schedule IV drugs.

Pretreatment evaluation should include an evaluation of the person's cardiac function, with particular attention to the presence of hypertension or tachyarrhythmias. The clinician should also examine the person for the presence of movement disorders, such as tics and dyskinesia, because these conditions can be exacerbated by the administration of sympathomimetics. If tics are present, many experts will not use sympathomimetics, but will instead choose clonidine or antidepressants. Recent data, however, indicate that sympathomimetics may cause only a mild increase in motor tics and may actually suppress vocal tics. Liver function and renal function should be assessed, and dosages of sympathomimetics should be reduced for persons with impaired metabolism. In the case of pemoline, any elevation of liver enzymes is a compelling reason to discontinue the medication.

Persons with ADHD can take immediate-release methylphenidate at 8 AM, 12 noon, and 4 PM. Dextroamphetamine, sustained-release methylphenidate, or 18 mg of extended-release methylphenidate may be taken once at 8 AM. Pemoline is taken at 8 AM. The starting dose of methylphenidate ranges from 2.5 mg of regular to 20 mg of sustained-release in children and 90 mg daily in adults. If this is inadequate, the dosage may be increased to a maximal dosage of 80 mg. The dosage of dextroamphetamine is 2.5 to 40 mg a day up to 0.5 mg/kg a day. Pemoline is given in dosages of 18.75 to 112.5 mg a day. Liver function tests should be monitored when using pemoline. Although it is not clear that the routine liver screening can predict acute liver failure caused by pemoline, it is certainly necessary to stop pemoline use if screening tests give any hint of hepatic dysfunction. Children are generally more sensitive to adverse effects than are adults. Dosing for treatment of narcolepsy and depression is comparable to that for treatment of ADHD.

The starting dosage of modafinil is 200 mg in the morning in medically healthy individuals and 100 mg in the morning in persons with hepatic impairment. Some persons take a second 100- or 200-mg dose in the afternoon. The maximal recommended daily dosage is 400 mg, although dosages of 600 to 1,200 mg a day have been used safely. Adverse effects become prominent at dosages above 400 mg a day. Compared with amphetamine-like drugs, modafinil promotes wakefulness, but produces less attentiveness and less irritability. Some persons with excessive

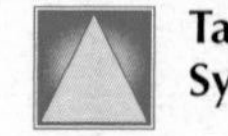

Table 36.31–2
Sympathomimetics Commonly Used in Psychiatry

Generic Name	Trade Name	Preparations	Initial Daily Dose	Usual Daily Dose for ADHD[a]	Usual Daily Dose for Narcolepsy	Maximal Daily Dose
Atomoxetine	Strattera	10-, 18-, 25-, 40-, 60-mg tablets	20 mg	40 to 80 mg	Not used	Children: 80 mg Adults: 100 mg
Amphetamine-dextroamphetamine	Adderall	5-, 10-, 20-, 30-mg tablets	5 to 10 mg	20 to 30 mg	5 to 60 mg	Children: 40 mg Adults: 60 mg
Dexmethylphenidate	Focalin	2.5-, 5-, 10-mg capsules	5 mg	5 to 20 mg	Not used	20 mg
Dextroamphetamine	Dexedrine, Dextrostat	5-, 10-, 15-mg ER capsules; 5-, 10-mg tablets	5 to 10 mg	20 to 30 mg	5 to 60 mg	Children: 40 mg Adults: 60 mg
Modafinil	Provigil	100-, 200-mg tablets	100 mg	Not used	400 mg	400 mg
Methamphetamine	Desoxyn	5-mg tablets; 5-, 10-, 15-mg ER tablets	5 to 10 mg	20 to 25 mg	Not generally used	45 mg
Methylphenidate	Ritalin, Methidate, Methylin, Attenade	5-, 10-, 20-mg tablets; 10-, 20-mg SR tablets	5 to 10 mg	5 to 60 mg	20 to 30 mg	Children: 80 mg Adults: 90 mg
	Concerta	18-, 36-mg ER tablets	18 mg	18 to 54 mg	Not yet established	54 mg
Pemoline	Cylert	18.75-, 37.5-, 75-mg tablets; 37.5 chewable tablets	37.5 mg	56.25 to 75 mg	Not used	112.5 mg

[a]For children 6 years of age or older.
ADHD, attention-deficit/hyperactivity disorder; ER, extended release; SR, sustained released.

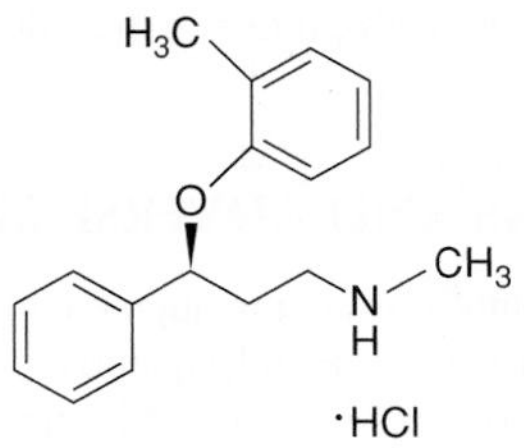

FIGURE 36.31–2
Molecular structure of atomoxetine.

daytime sleepiness extend the activity of the morning modafinil dose with an afternoon dose of methylphenidate.

ATOMOXETINE (STRATTERA)

Atomoxetine is the first nonstimulant drug to be approved by the FDA as a treatment of ADHD in children, adolescents, and adults. It is included in this chapter because it shares this indication with the stimulants described above.

Chemistry

Atomoxetine has a tricyclic-like structure but is classified as a phenylpropanolamine derivative (Fig. 36.31–2).

Pharmacologic Actions

Atomoxetine is believed to produce a therapeutic effect through selective inhibition of the presynaptic norepinephrine transporter. It is well absorbed after oral administration and is minimally affected by food. High-fat meals may decrease the rate but not the extent of absorption. Maximal plasma concentrations are reached after approximately 1 to 2 hours. At therapeutic concentrations, 98 percent of atomoxetine in plasma is bound to protein, mainly albumin. Atomoxetine has a half-life of approximately 5 hours and is metabolized principally by the cytochrome P450 (CYP) 2D6 pathway. Poor metabolizers of this compound reach a fivefold higher area under the curve and fivefold higher peak plasma concentration than normal or extensive metabolizers. This is important to consider in patients receiving medications that inhibit the CYP 2D6 enzyme. For example, the antidepressant-like pharmacology of atomoxetine has led to its use as an add-on to selective serotonin reuptake inhibitors (SSRIs) or other antidepressants. Drugs such as fluoxetine (Prozac), paroxetine (Paxil), or bupropion are CYP 2D6 inhibitors and may raise atomoxetine levels.

Therapeutic Indications

Atomoxetine is used for the treatment of ADHD. It should be considered for use in patients who find stimulants too activating or who experience other intolerable side effects. Because atomoxetine has no abuse potential, it a reasonable choice in the treatment of patients with both ADHD and substance abuse, patients who complain of ADHD symptoms but are suspected of seeking stimulant drugs, or patients who are in recovery.

Atomoxetine may enhance cognition when used to treat patients with schizophrenia. It also can be used as an alternative or add-on to antidepressants in patients who fail to respond to standard therapies.

Precautions and Adverse Reactions

Common side effects of atomoxetine include abdominal discomfort, decreased appetite with resulting weight loss, sexual dysfunction, dizziness, vertigo, irritability, and mood swings. Minor increases in BP and heart rate have also been observed. Cases have been seen of severe liver injury in a few patients taking atomoxetine. The drug should be discontinued in patients with jaundice (yellowing of the skin or whites of the eyes, itching) or laboratory evidence of liver injury. Atomoxetine should not be taken at the same time as, or within 2 weeks of taking, a MAOI or by patients with narrow-angle glaucoma.

The effects of overdose greater than twice the maximal recommended daily dose in humans are unknown. No specific information is available on the treatment of overdose with atomoxetine.

Dosage and Clinical Guidelines

Atomoxetine is available as 10-, 18-, 25-, 40-, and 60-mg capsules. In children and adolescents up to 70 kg in body weight, atomoxetine should be initiated at a total daily dose of approximately 0.5 mg/kg and increased after a minimum of 3 days to a target total daily dose of approximately 1.2 mg/kg administered either as a single daily dose in the morning or as evenly divided doses in the morning and late afternoon or early evening. The total daily dose in smaller children and adolescents should not exceed 1.4 mg/kg or 100 mg—whichever is less. Dosing of children and adolescents over 70 kg in body weight and adults should start at a total daily dose of 40 mg and then be increased after a minimum of 3 days to a target total daily dose of approximately 80 mg. The doses can be administered either as a single daily dose in the morning or as evenly divided doses in the morning and late afternoon or early evening. After 2 to 4 additional weeks, the dose may be increased to a maximum of 100 mg in patients who have not achieved an optimal response. The maximal recommended total daily dose in children and adolescents over 70 kg and adults is 100 mg.

References

Fawcett J. Sympathomimetics and dopamine receptor agonists. In: Sadock BJ, Sadock VA, eds. *Kaplan and Sadock's Comprehensive Textbook of Psychiatry.* 8th ed. Vol. 2. Baltimore: Lippincott, Williams, & Wilkins; 2005:2938.

Goldberg JF, Burdick KE, Endick CJ. Preliminary randomized, double-blind, placebo-controlled trial of pramipexole added to mood stabilizers for treatment-resistant bipolar depression. *Am J Psychiatry.* 2004;161:564–566.

Rektorova I, Rektor I, Bares M, Dostal V, Ehler E, Franfrdlova Z, Fiedler J, Klajblova H, Kulistak P, Ressner P, Svatova J, Urbanek K, Veliskova J. Pramipexole and pergolide on the treatment of depression in Parkinson's disease: A national multicentre prospective randomized study *Eur J Neurol.* 2003;10: 399–406.

▲ 36.32 Thyroid Hormones

Thyroid hormones—levothyroxine (Synthroid, Levothroid, Levoxine) and liothyronine (Cytomel)—are used in psychiatry, either alone or as augmentation to treat persons with depression or rapid-cycling bipolar I disorder. They can convert an antidepressant-nonresponsive person into an antidepressant-responsive person. Thyroid hormones are also used as

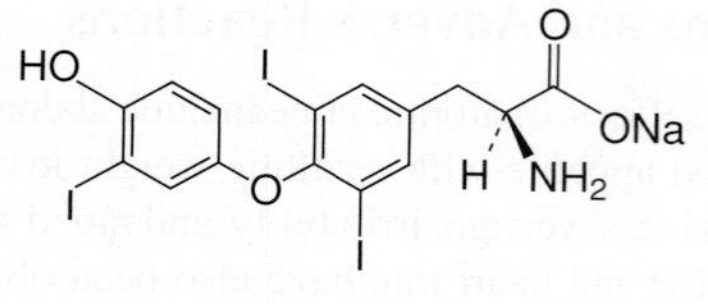

FIGURE 36.32–1

Molecular structures of liothyronine and levothyroxine.

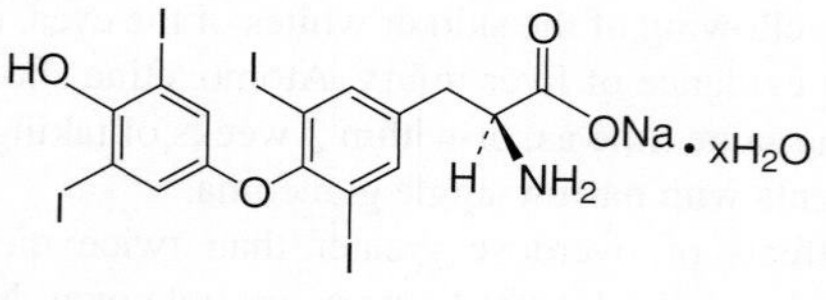

replacement therapy for persons treated with lithium (Eskalith) who have developed a hypothyroid state.

CHEMISTRY

Liothyronine and levothyroxine are the levorotatory forms of the endogenous hormones triiodothyronine (T_3) and thyroxine (T_4), respectively. The molecular structures of levothyroxine and liothyronine are shown in Figure 36.32–1.

PHARMACOLOGIC ACTIONS

Thyroid hormones are administered orally, and their absorption from the gastrointestinal (GI) tract is variable. Absorption is increased if the drug is administered on an empty stomach. In the brain, T_4 crosses the blood–brain barrier and diffuses into neurons, where it is converted into T_3, which is the physiologically active form. The half-life of T_4 is 6 to 7 days and that of T_3 is 1 to 2 days.

The mechanism of action for thyroid hormone effects on antidepressant efficacy is unknown. Thyroid hormone binds to intracellular receptors that regulate the transcription of a wide range of genes, including several receptors for neurotransmitters.

THERAPEUTIC INDICATIONS

The major indication for thyroid hormones in psychiatry is as an adjuvant to antidepressants. No clear correlation has been found between the laboratory measures of thyroid function and the response to thyroid hormone supplementation of antidepressants. If a patient has not responded to a 6-week course of antidepressants at appropriate dosages, adjuvant therapy with either lithium or a thyroid hormone is an alternative. Most clinicians use adjuvant lithium before trying a thyroid hormone. Several controlled trials have indicated that liothyronine use converts about 50 percent of antidepressant nonresponders to responders.

The dosage of liothyronine is 25 or 50 μg a day added to the patient's antidepressant regimen. Liothyronine has been used primarily as an adjuvant for tricyclic drugs; however, evidence suggests that liothyronine augments the effects of all the antidepressant drugs.

Thyroid hormones have not been shown to cause particular problems in pediatric or geriatric patients; however, the hormones should be used with caution in the elderly, who may have occult heart disease.

PRECAUTIONS AND ADVERSE REACTIONS

At the dosages usually used for augmentation—25 to 50 μg a day—adverse effects occur infrequently. The most common adverse effects associated with thyroid hormones are transient headache, weight loss, palpitations, nervousness, diarrhea, abdominal cramps, sweating, tachycardia, increased blood pressure (BP), tremors, and insomnia. Osteoporosis can also occur with long-term treatment, but this has not been found in studies involving liothyronine augmentation. Overdoses of thyroid hormones can lead to cardiac failure and death.

Thyroid hormones should not be taken by persons with cardiac disease, angina, or hypertension. The hormones are contraindicated in thyrotoxicosis and uncorrected adrenal insufficiency and in persons with acute myocardial infarctions. Thyroid hormones can be administered safely to pregnant women, provided that laboratory thyroid indexes are monitored. Thyroid hormones are minimally excreted in the breast milk and have not been shown to cause problems in nursing babies.

DRUG INTERACTIONS

Thyroid hormones can potentiate the effects of warfarin (Coumadin) and other anticoagulants by increasing the catabolism of clotting factors. They may increase the insulin requirement for diabetic persons and the digitalis requirement for persons with cardiac disease. Thyroid hormones should not be coadministered with sympathomimetics, ketamine (Ketalar), or maprotiline (Ludiomil) because of the risk of cardiac decompensation. Administration of selective serotonin reuptake inhibitors (SSRIs), tricyclic and tetracyclic drugs, lithium, or carbamazepine (Tegretol) can mildly lower serum thyroxine and raise serum thyrotropin concentrations in euthyroid persons or persons taking thyroid replacements. This interaction warrants close serum monitoring and may require an increase in the dosage or initiation of thyroid hormone supplementation.

LABORATORY INTERFERENCES

Levothyroxine has not been reported to interfere with any laboratory test other than thyroid function indexes. Liothyronine, however, suppresses the release of endogenous T_4, thereby lowering the result of any thyroid function test that depends on the measure of T_4.

THYROID FUNCTION TESTS

Several thyroid function tests are available, including tests for T_4 by competitive protein binding (T_4 [D]) and by radioimmunoassay (T_4 [RIA]) involving a specific antigen-antibody reaction. More than 90 percent of T_4 is bound to serum protein and is responsible for thyroid-stimulating hormone (TSH) secretion and cellular metabolism. Other thyroid measures include the free T_4 index (FT_4I), T_3 uptake, and total serum T_3 measured by radioimmunoassay (T_3 [RIA]). Those tests are used to rule out hypothyroidism, which can be associated with symptoms of depression. In some studies, up to 10 percent of patients complaining of depression and associated fatigue had incipient hypothyroid disease. Lithium can cause hypothyroidism and, more rarely, hyperthyroidism. Neonatal hypothyroidism results in mental retardation and is preventable if the diagnosis is made at birth.

Thyrotropin-Releasing Hormone Stimulation Test

The thyrotropin-releasing hormone (TRH) stimulation test is indicated for patients who have marginally abnormal thyroid test results with suspected subclinical hypothyroidism, which may account for clinical depression. It is also used in patients with possible lithium-induced hypothyroidism. The procedure entails an intravenous (IV) injection of 500 mg of protirelin (TRH), which produces a sharp rise in serum TSH levels, which are measured at 15, 30, 60, and 90 minutes. An increase in serum TSH of 5 to 25 mIU/mL above the baseline is normal. An increase of less than 7 mIU/mL is considered a blunted response, which may correlate with a diagnosis of depression. Of all patients with depression, 8 percent have some thyroid illness.

DOSAGE AND CLINICAL GUIDELINES

Liothyronine is available in 5-, 25-, and 50-μg tablets. Levothyroxine is available in 12.5-, 25-, 50-, 75-, 88-, 100-, 112-, 125-, 150-, 175-, 200-, and 300-μg tablets; it is also available in a 200- and 500-μg parenteral form. The dosage of liothyronine is 25 or 50 μg a day added to the person's antidepressant regimen. Liothyronine has been used as an adjuvant for all the available antidepressant drugs. An adequate trial of liothyronine supplementation should last 2 to 3 weeks. If liothyronine supplementation is successful, it should be continued for 2 months and then tapered off at the rate of 12.5 μg a day every 3 to 7 days.

References

Hume R, Simpson J, Delahunty C, Van Toor H, Wu SY, Williams F, Visser T. Human fetal and cord serum thyroid hormones: Developmental trends and interrelationships. *J Clin Endocrinol Metab.* 2004;89(8):4097–4103.

Joffe R. Thyroid hormones. In: Sadock BJ, Sadock VA, eds. *Kaplan & Sadock's Comprehensive Textbook of Psychiatry.* 8th ed. Vol. 2. Baltimore: Lippincott, Williams & Wilkins; 2005:2945.

Kikuchi M, Komuro R, Oka H, Kidani T, Hanaoka A, Koshino Y. Relationship between anxiety and thyroid function in patients with panic disorder. *Prog Neuropsychopharmacol Biol Psychiatry.* 2005;29(1):77.

Kratzsch J, Fiedler G, Leichtle A, Brügel M, Buchbinder S, Otto L, Sabri O, Matthes G, Thiery J. New reference intervals for thyrotropin and thyroid hormones based on National Academy of Clinical Biochemistry Criteria and Regular Ultrasonography of the Thyroid. *Clin Chem.* 2005;51:1480–1486.

Takser L, Mergler D, Baldwin M, de Grosbois S, Smargiassi A, Lafond J. Thyroid hormones in pregnancy in relation to environmental exposure to organochlorine compounds and mercury. *Environ Health Perspect.* 2005;113(8):1039–1045.

▲ 36.33 Trazodone

Trazodone (Desyrel) was introduced as a treatment of major depression in 1998, but never achieved widespread use in that role because many patients found it to be too sedating at therapeutic doses. It has become extensively used, however, at low doses as an alternative to hypnotic agents, particularly to counteract the frequent sleep disturbances associated with selective serotonin reuptake inhibitors (SSRIs).

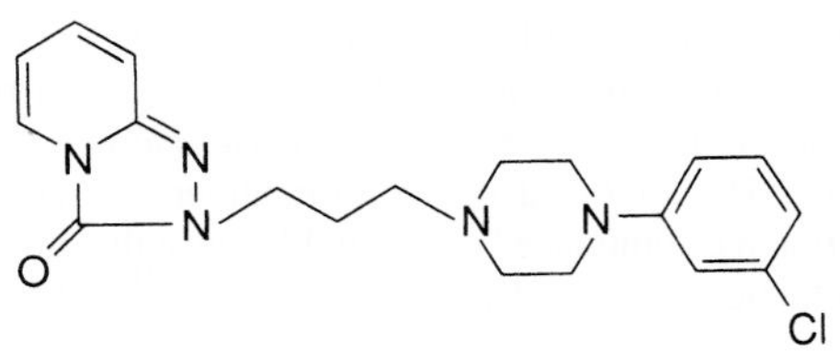

FIGURE 36.33–1
Molecular structure of trazodone.

CHEMISTRY

Trazodone is structurally related to nefazodone (Serzone) and structurally unrelated to other currently available antidepressant drugs. The structural formula of trazodone is shown in Figure 36.33–1.

PHARMACOLOGIC ACTIONS

Trazodone is readily absorbed from the gastrointestinal (GI) tract and reaches peak plasma levels in about 1 hour. It has a half-life of 5 to 9 hours. Trazodone is metabolized in the liver, and 75 percent of its metabolites are excreted in the urine.

Trazodone is a weak inhibitor of serotonin reuptake and a potent antagonist of serotonin 5-HT_{2A} and 5-HT_{2C} receptors. The active metabolite of trazodone is *m*-chlorophenylpiperazine (mCPP), which is an agonist at 5-HT_{2C} receptors and has a half-life of 14 hours. mCPP has been associated with migraine, anxiety, and weight loss. The adverse effects of trazodone are partially mediated by α_1-adrenergic receptor antagonism.

THERAPEUTIC INDICATIONS

Depressive Disorders

The main indication for the use of trazodone is major depressive disorder. A clear dose–response relationship is seen, with dosages of 250 to 600 mg a day being necessary for trazodone to have therapeutic benefit. Trazodone increases total sleep time, decreases the number and the duration of nighttime awakenings, and decreases the amount of rapid eye movement (REM) sleep. Unlike tricyclic drugs, trazodone does not decrease stage 4 sleep. Trazodone, thus, is useful for depressed persons with anxiety and insomnia.

Insomnia

Trazodone is a first-line agent for the treatment of insomnia because of its marked sedative qualities and favorable effects on sleep architecture (see above), combined with its lack of anticholinergic effects. Trazodone is effective for insomnia caused both by depression and by use of drugs. When used as a hypnotic, the usual initial dosage is 25 to 100 mg at bedtime.

Erectile Disorder

Trazodone is associated with an increased risk of priapism. Trazodone can potentiate erections resulting from sexual stimulation, thus it has been used to prolong erectile time and turgidity in some men with erectile disorder. The dosage for this indication is 150 to 200 mg a day. Trazodone-triggered priapism (an erection lasting more than 3 hours with pain) is a medical emergency. The use of trazodone for treatment of male erectile dysfunction has diminished considerably since the introduction of phosphodiesterase (PDE)-5 agents.

Other Indications

Trazodone may be useful in low dosages (50 mg a day) to control severe agitation in children with developmental disabilities and elderly persons with dementia. At dosages above 250 mg a day, trazodone reduces the tension and apprehension associated with generalized anxiety disorder. It has been used to treat depression in patients with schizophrenia. Trazodone may have a beneficial effect on insomnia and nightmares in posttraumatic stress disorder (PTSD).

PRECAUTIONS AND ADVERSE REACTIONS

The most common adverse effects associated with trazodone are sedation, orthostatic hypotension, dizziness, headache, and nausea. Some persons experience dry mouth or gastric irritation. The drug is not associated with anticholinergic adverse effects, such as urinary retention, weight gain, and constipation. A few case reports have noted an association between trazodone and arrhythmias in persons with preexisting, premature ventricular contractions or mitral valve prolapse. Neutropenia, usually not of clinical significance, can develop, which should be considered if persons have fever or sore throat.

Trazodone can cause significant orthostatic hypotension 4 to 6 hours after a dose is taken, especially if taken concurrently with antihypertensive agents or if a large dose is taken without food. Administration of trazodone with food slows absorption and reduces the peak plasma concentration, thus reducing the risk of orthostatic hypotension.

Trazodone causes priapism, prolonged erection in the absence of sexual stimuli, in 1 of every 10,000 men. Trazodone-induced priapism usually appears in the first 4 weeks of treatment, but can occur as late as 18 months into treatment. It can appear at any dose. In such cases, trazodone use should be discontinued and another antidepressant should be used. Painful erections or erections lasting more than 1 hour are warning signs that warrant immediate discontinuation of the drug and medical evaluation. The first step in the emergency management of priapism is intracavernosal injection of an α_1-adrenergic agonist pressor agent, such as metaraminol (Aramine) or epinephrine. Trazodone is less likely to precipitate mania in vulnerable persons than are other antidepressant drugs.

Trazodone use is contraindicated in pregnant and nursing women. Trazodone should be used with caution in persons with hepatic and renal diseases.

DRUG INTERACTIONS

Trazodone potentiates the central nervous system (CNS) depressant effects of other centrally acting drugs and alcohol. Concurrent use of trazodone and antihypertensives can cause hypotension. No cases of hypertensive crisis have been reported when trazodone has been used to treat monoamine oxidase inhibitor (MAOI)-associated insomnia. Trazodone can increase levels of digoxin and phenytoin. Trazodone should be used with caution in combination with warfarin. Drugs that inhibit CYP 3A4 can increase levels of trazodone's major metabolite, mCPP, leading to an increase in side effects.

LABORATORY INTERFERENCES

No known laboratory interferences are associated with the administration of trazodone.

DOSAGE AND CLINICAL GUIDELINES

Trazodone is available in 50-, 100-, 150-, and 300-mg tablets. Once-a-day dosing is as effective as divided dosing and reduces daytime sedation. The usual starting dose is 50 mg before sleep. The dosage can be increased in increments of 50 mg every 3 days if sedation or orthostatic hypotension does not become a problem. The therapeutic range for trazodone is 200 to 600 mg a day in divided doses. Some reports indicate that dosages of 400 to 600 mg a day are required for maximal therapeutic effects; other reports indicate that 250 to 400 mg a day is sufficient. The dosage can be titrated up to 300 mg a day; then, the person can be evaluated for the need for further dosage increases on the basis of the presence or the absence of signs of clinical improvement.

References

Einarson A, Bonari L, Voyer-Lavigne S, Addis A, Matsui D, Johnson Y, Koren G. A multicentre prospective controlled study to determine the safety of trazodone and nefazodone use during pregnancy. *Can J Psychiatry*. 2003;48:106–110.

Hettema J, Kornstein S. Trazodone. In: Sadock BJ, Sadock VA, eds. *Kaplan & Sadock's Comprehensive Textbook of Psychiatry*. 8th ed. Vol. 2. Baltimore: Lippincott Williams & Wilkins; 2005:2949.

James SP, Mendelson WB. The use of trazodone as a hypnotic: A critical review. *J Clin Psychiatry*. 2004;65(6):752.

Le Bon O, Murphy JR, Staner L, Hoffmann G, Kormoss N, Kentos M, Dupont P, Lion K, Pelc I, Verbanck P. Double-blind, placebo-controlled study of the efficacy of trazodone in alcohol post-withdrawal syndrome: Polysomnographic and clinical evaluations. *J Clin Psychopharmacol*. 2003;23:377–383.

Mendelson WB. A review of the evidence for the efficacy and safety of trazodone in insomnia. *J Clin Psychiatry*. 2005;66(4):469.

Saletu-Zyhlarz GM, Anderer P, Arnold O, Saletu B. Confirmation of the neurophysiologically predicted therapeutic effects of trazodone on its target symptoms depression, anxiety, and insomnia by postmarketing clinical studies with a controlled-release formulation in depressed outpatients. *Neuropsychobiology*. 2003;48:194–208.

▲ 36.34 Tricyclics and Tetracyclics

The tricyclic antidepressants and tetracyclic antidepressants (TCAs) have a long history of use in psychiatry, having become available in the mid-1950s. Introduced as antidepressants, their therapeutic indications now also include panic disorder, generalized anxiety disorder, posttraumatic stress disorder (PTSD), obsessive-compulsive disorder (OCD), and pain syndromes. The introduction of newer agents, such as the selective serotonin reuptake inhibitors (SSRIs), bupropion (Wellbutrin), venlafaxine (Effexor), and mirtazapine (Remeron), has sharply decreased prescriptions of the TCAs; nevertheless, they remain extremely useful.

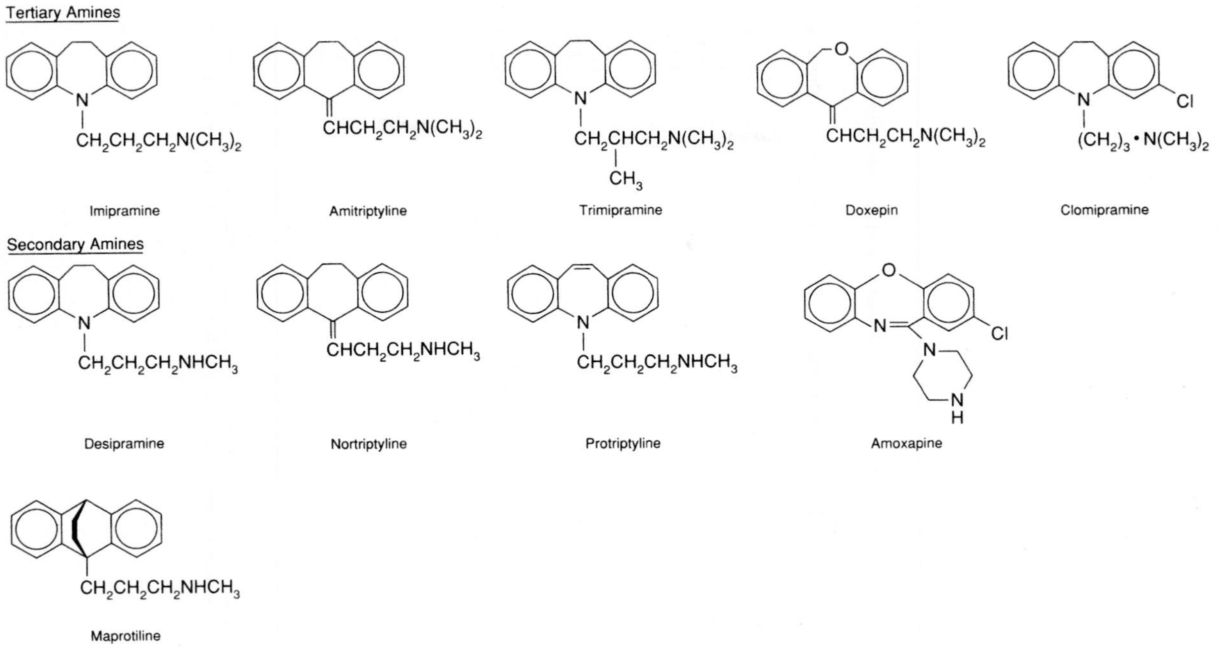

Tertiary Amines

$CH_2CH_2CH_2N(CH_3)_2$ Imipramine

$CHCH_2CH_2N(CH_3)_2$ Amitriptyline

$CH_2CHCH_2N(CH_3)_2$, CH_3 Trimipramine

$CHCH_2CH_2N(CH_3)_2$ Doxepin

$(CH_2)_3 \cdot N(CH_3)_2$, Cl Clomipramine

Secondary Amines

$CH_2CH_2CH_2NHCH_3$ Desipramine

$CHCH_2CH_2NHCH_3$ Nortriptyline

$CH_2CH_2CH_2NHCH_3$ Protriptyline

Amoxapine

$CH_2CH_2CH_2NHCH_3$ Maprotiline

FIGURE 36.34–1
Molecular structures of tricyclics and tetracyclics.

CHEMISTRY

The structural formulas of the TCAs are shown in Figure 36.34–1.

PHARMACOLOGIC ACTIONS

Absorption of most TCAs is complete after oral administration, and significant metabolism occurs from the first-pass effect. Peak plasma concentrations occur within 2 to 8 hours, and the half-lives of the TCAs vary from 10 to 70 hours; nortriptyline (Aventyl, Pamelor), maprotiline (Ludiomil), and, particularly, protriptyline (Vivactil) can have longer half-lives. The long half-lives allow all the compounds to be given once daily; 5 to 7 days are needed to reach steady-state plasma concentrations. Imipramine pamoate (Tofranil) is a depot form of the drug for intramuscular (IM) administration; indications for the use of this preparation are limited.

The TCAs undergo hepatic metabolism by the cytochrome P450 (CYP) enzyme system. Clinically relevant drug interactions can result from competition for enzyme CYP 2D6 between TCAs and quinidine, cimetidine (Tagamet), fluoxetine (Prozac), sertraline (Zoloft), paroxetine (Paxil), phenothiazines, carbamazepine (Tegretol), and the type IC antiarrhythmics propafenone (Rythmol) and flecainide (Tambocor). Concomitant administration of TCAs and these inhibitors may slow the metabolism and raise the plasma concentrations of TCAs. Additionally, genetic variations in the activity of CYP 2D6 may account for up to a 40 times difference in plasma TCA concentrations in different persons. The dosage of the TCA may need to be adjusted to correct changes in the rate of hepatic TCA metabolism.

The TCAs block the transporter site for norepinephrine and serotonin, thus increasing synaptic concentrations of these neurotransmitters. Each drug differs in its affinity for each of these transporters, with clomipramine (Anafranil) being the most serotonin selective and desipramine (Norpramin, Pertofrane) the most norepinephrine selective of the TCAs. Secondary effects of the TCAs include antagonism at the muscarinic acetylcholine, histamine H_1, and α_1- and α_2-adrenergic receptors (Table 36.34–1). It is the potency of these effects on other receptors that largely determines the side-effect profile of each drug. Amoxapine (Asendin), nortriptyline, desipramine, and maprotiline have the least anticholinergic activity; doxepin (Adapin, Sinequan) has the most antihistaminergic activity. Although they are more likely to cause constipation, sedation, dry mouth, or lightheadedness than the SSRIs, the TCAs are less likely to cause sexual dysfunction, significant long-term weight gain, and sleep disturbances than the SSRIs. The half-life and plasma clearance for most TCAs are very similar.

THERAPEUTIC INDICATIONS

Each of the following indications is also an indication for SSRIs, which have widely replaced the TCAs in clinical practice. TCAs, however, represent a reasonable alternative for persons who cannot tolerate the adverse effects of the SSRIs.

Major Depressive Disorder

The treatment of a major depressive episode and the prophylactic treatment of major depressive disorder are the principal indications for using TCAs. Whereas the TCAs are effective in the treatment of depression in persons with bipolar I disorder,

Table 36.34–1
Receptor Affinity or Potency of Cyclic Antidepressants in Human Brain

Drug	Receptor Affinity						Potency–Uptake Blockade		
	α_1	α_2	Histamine 1	Muscarinic Type 1	Serotonin Type 1	Serotonin Type 2	Serotonin	Norepinephrine	Dopamine
Tertiary tricyclic drugs									
Amitriptyline (Elavil)	3.7	0.11	91	5.6	0.53	3.4	23	2.9	0.031
Clomipramine (Anafranil)	2.6	0.03	3.2	2.7	0.01	3.7	360	2.6	0.046
Doxepin (Sinequan)	4.2	0.09	420	1.2	0.35	4.0	1.5	3.4	0.031
Imipramine (Tofranil)	1.1	0.03	9.1	1.1	0.01	1.2	71	2.7	0.012
Trimipramine (Surmontil)	4.2	0.15	370	1.7	0.01	3.1	0.67	0.041	0.026
Secondary tricyclic drugs									
Desipramine (Norpramin, Pertofrane)	0.77	0.01	0.91	0.50	0.01	0.36	5.7	120	0.031
Nortriptyline (Aventyl, Pamelor)	1.70	0.04	10.0	0.67	0.32	2.3	5.6	23	0.088
Protriptyline (Vivactil)	0.77	0.02	4.0	4.0	0.03	1.5	5.1	71	0.048
Tetracyclic drugs									
Amoxapine (Asendin)	2	0.04	4.0	0.10	0.46	170	1.7	6.3	0.023
Moprotiline (Ludiomil)	1.1	0.01	50.0	0.18	0.01	0.83	0.017	9.0	0.1
Reference compounds									
Phentolamine (Regitine)	6.7	—	—	—	—	—	—	—	—
Yohimbine (Actibine)	—	62	—	—	—	—	—	—	—
Diphenhydramine (Benadryl)	—	—	7.1	—	—	—	—	—	—
Atropine	—	—	—	42	—	—	—	—	—
Buspirone (BuSpar)	—	—	—	—	26	—	—	—	—
Methysergide (Sansert)	—	—	—	—	—	26	—	—	—

Note: Affinity and potency = $10 \times 1/K_d$ = equilibrium dissociation constant in molarity.
Uptake potency data adapted from Latsum M, Groshan K, Biakely RD, et al. Pharmacological profile of antidepressants and related compounds of human monoamine transporters. *Eur J Pharmacol.* 1997;340:249. Receptor affinity data adapted from Richeison E, Nelson A. Antagonism by antidepressants of neurotransmitter receptors of normal human brain in vitro. *J Pharmacol Exp Ther.* 1984;230:94, with permission.

they are more likely to induce mania, hypomania, or cycling than newer antidepressants, most notably the SSRIs and bupropion. Thus, it is not advised that TCAs be routinely used to treat depression associated with bipolar I or bipolar II disorder.

Melancholic features, prior major depressive episodes, and a family history of depressive disorders increase the likelihood of a therapeutic response. All available TCAs are equally effective in the treatment of depressive disorders. In the case of an individual person, however, one tricyclic or tetracyclic may be effective, whereas another one may be ineffective. The treatment of a major depressive episode with psychotic features almost always requires the coadministration of an antipsychotic drug and an antidepressant.

Although it is used worldwide as an antidepressant, clomipramine is only approved in the United States for the treatment of OCD.

Panic Disorder with Agoraphobia

Imipramine is the TCA most studied for panic disorder with agoraphobia, but other TCAs are also effective when taken at the usual antidepressant dosages. Because of the potential initial anxiogenic effects of the TCAs, starting dosages should be small, and the dosage should be titrated upward slowly. Small doses of benzodiazepines can be used initially to deal with this side effect.

Generalized Anxiety Disorder

The use of doxepin for the treatment of anxiety disorders is approved by the US Food and Drug Administration (FDA). Some research data show that imipramine may also be useful. Although rarely used anymore, a chlordiazepoxide–amitriptyline combination (Limbitrol) is available for mixed anxiety and depressive disorders.

Obsessive-Compulsive Disorder

Obsessive-compulsive disorder appears to respond specifically to clomipramine, as well as the SSRIs. Some improvement is usually seen in 2 to 4 weeks, but a further reduction in symptoms may continue for the first 4 to 5 months of treatment. None of the other TCAs appears to be nearly as effective as clomipramine for treatment of this disorder. Clomipramine may also be a drug of choice for depressed persons with marked obsessive features.

Pain

The TCAs are widely used to treat chronic neuropathic pain and in prophylaxis of migraine headache. Amitriptyline is the TCA most often used in this role. During treatment of pain, doses are generally lower than those used in depression, for example, 75 mg of amitriptyline may be effective. These effects also appear more rapidly.

Other Disorders

Childhood enuresis is often treated with imipramine. Peptic ulcer disease can be treated with doxepin, which has marked antihistaminergic effects. Other indications for TCAs are narcolepsy, nightmare disorder, and PTSD. The drugs are sometimes used for treatment of children and adolescents with attention-deficit/hyperactivity disorder (ADHD), sleepwalking disorder, separation anxiety disorder, and sleep terror disorder. Clomipramine has also been used to treat premature ejaculation, movement disorders, and compulsive behavior in children with autistic disorders; however, because TCAs have caused sudden death in several children and adolescents, their use is best avoided in this population.

PRECAUTIONS AND ADVERSE REACTIONS

The TCAs are associated with a wide range of problematic side effects, and can be lethal when taken in overdose. Table 36.34–2 lists the adverse-effect profiles of the TCAs.

Psychiatric Effects

The TCAs can induce a switch to mania or hypomania in susceptible individuals. TCAs can also exacerbate psychotic disorders in susceptible persons. At high plasma concentrations (levels

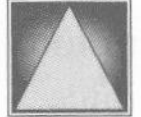

Table 36.34–2
Side Effect Profile of Tricyclic and Tetracyclic Antidepressants

	Anticholinergic Effects	Sedation	Orthostatic Hypotension	Seizures	Conduction Abnormalities
Tertiary amines					
Amitriptyline	++++	++++	+++	+++	++++
Clomipramine	++++	++++	+++	+++	++++
Doxepin	+++	++++	++	+++	++
Imipramine	+++	+++	++++	+++	++++
Trimipramine	++++	++++	+++	+++	+++++
Secondary amines					
Desipramine	++	++	+++	++	+++
Nortriptyline	+++	+++	+	++	+++
Protriptyline	+++	+	++	++	++++
Tetracyclics					
Amoxapine	+++	++	+	+++	++
Maprotiline	++	+++	++	++++	+++

++++, high; +++, moderate; ++, low; + very low.

above 300 ng/mL), the anticholinergic effects of the TCAs can cause confusion or delirium. Patients with dementia are particularly vulnerable to this development.

Anticholinergic Effects

Anticholinergic effects often limit the tolerable dosage to relatively low ranges. Some persons may develop a tolerance for the anticholinergic effects with continued treatment. Anticholinergic effects include dry mouth, constipation, blurred vision, delirium, and urinary retention. Sugarless gum, candy, or fluoride lozenges can alleviate the dry mouth. Bethanechol (Urecholine), 25 to 50 mg three or four times a day, may reduce urinary hesitancy and may be helpful in erectile dysfunction when the drug is taken 30 minutes before sexual intercourse. Narrow-angle glaucoma can also be aggravated by anticholinergic drugs, and the precipitation of glaucoma requires emergency treatment with a miotic agent. TCAs should be avoided in persons with narrow-angle glaucoma, and an SSRI should be substituted. Severe anticholinergic effects can lead to a central nervous system (CNS) anticholinergic syndrome with confusion and delirium, especially if TCAs are administered with dopamine receptor antagonists (DRAs) or anticholinergic drugs. IM or intravenous (IV) physostigmine (Antilirium, Eserine) is used to diagnose and treat anticholinergic delirium.

Cardiac Effects

When administered in their usual therapeutic dosages, the TCAs can cause tachycardia, flattened T waves, prolonged quick test (QT) intervals, and depressed ST segments in the electrocardiographic (ECG) recording. Imipramine has a quinidine-like effect at therapeutic plasma concentrations and may reduce the number of premature ventricular contractions. Because the drugs prolong conduction time, their use is contraindicated in persons with preexisting conduction defects. In persons with a history of any type of heart disease, TCAs should be used only after SSRIs or other newer antidepressants have been found ineffective, and if used, they should be introduced at low dosages, with gradual increases in dosage and monitoring of cardiac functions. All TCAs can cause tachycardia, which may persist for months and is one of the most common reasons for drug discontinuation, especially in younger persons. At high plasma concentrations, as seen in overdoses, the drugs become arrhythmogenic.

Other Autonomic Effects

Orthostatic hypotension is the most common cardiovascular autonomic adverse effect, and the most common reason TCAs are discontinued. It can result in falls and injuries in affected persons. Nortriptyline may be the drug least likely to cause this problem. Orthostatic hypotension is treated with avoidance of caffeine, intake of at least 2 L of fluid per day, and addition of salt to the diet unless the person is being treated for hypertension. In persons taking antihypertensive agents, a dosage reduction may reduce the risk of orthostatic hypotension. Other possible autonomic effects are profuse sweating, palpitations, and increased blood pressure (BP). Although some persons respond to fludrocortisone (Florinef), 0.02 to 0.05 mg twice a day, substitution of an SSRI is preferable to addition of a potentially toxic mineralocorticoid such as fludrocortisone. TCA use should be discontinued several days before elective surgery because of the occurrence of hypertensive episodes during surgery in persons receiving TCAs.

Sedation

Sedation is a common effect of TCAs and may be welcomed if sleeplessness has been a problem. The sedative effect of TCAs is a result of anticholinergic and antihistaminergic activities. Amitriptyline, trimipramine, and doxepin are the most sedating agents; imipramine, amoxapine, nortriptyline, and maprotiline are less sedating; and desipramine and protriptyline are the least sedating agents.

Neurologic Effects

A fine rapid tremor may occur. Myoclonic twitches and tremors of the tongue and the upper extremities are common. Rare effects include speech blockage, paresthesia, peroneal palsies, and ataxia.

Amoxapine is unique in causing parkinsonian symptoms, akathisia, and even dyskinesia because of the dopaminergic blocking activity of one of its metabolites. Amoxapine can also cause neuroleptic malignant syndrome in rare cases. Maprotiline can cause seizures when the dosage is increased too quickly or is kept at high levels for too long. Clomipramine and amoxapine may lower the seizure threshold more than other drugs in the class. As a class, however, the TCAs have a relatively low risk for inducing seizures, except in persons who are at risk for seizures (e.g., persons with epilepsy and those with brain lesions). Although TCAs can still be used by such persons, the initial dosages should be lower than usual, and subsequent dosage increases should be gradual.

Allergic and Hematologic Effects

Exanthematous rashes are seen in 4 percent to 5 percent of all persons treated with maprotiline. Jaundice is rare. Agranulocytosis, leukocytosis, leukopenia, and eosinophilia are rare complications of TCA treatment. A person who has a sore throat or a fever during the first few months of TCA treatment, however, should have a complete blood count (CBC) done immediately.

Hepatic Effects

Mild and self-limited rise in serum transaminase concentrations can occur and should be monitored. TCAs can also produce a fulminant acute hepatitis in 0.1 percent to 1 percent of persons. This can be life threatening and the antidepressant should be discontinued.

Other Adverse Effects

Modest weight gain is common. Amoxapine exerts a DRA effect and can cause hyperprolactinemia, impotence, galactorrhea, anorgasmia, and ejaculatory disturbances. Other TCAs have also been associated with gynecomastia and amenorrhea. Inappropriate secretion of antidiuretic hormone has also been reported with TCAs. Other effects include nausea, vomiting, and hepatitis.

Precautions

The TCAs can cause a withdrawal syndrome in newborns, consisting of tachypnea, cyanosis, irritability, and poor sucking reflex. The drugs do pass into breast milk, but at concentrations that are usually undetectable in the infant's plasma. The drugs should be used with caution in persons with hepatic and renal diseases. TCAs should not be administered during a course of electroconvulsive therapy (ECT), primarily because of the risk of serious adverse cardiac effects.

DRUG INTERACTIONS

Monoamine Oxidase Inhibitors

The TCAs should not be taken within 14 days of administration of a monoamine oxidase inhibitor (MAOI).

Antihypertensives

The TCAs block the neuronal reuptake of guanethidine (Esimil, Ismelin), which is required for antihypertensive activity. The antihypertensive effects of β-adrenergic receptor antagonists (e.g., propranolol [Inderal] and clonidine [Catapres]) can also be blocked by TCAs. The coadministration of a TCA and α-methyldopa (Aldomet) can cause behavioral agitation.

Antiarrhythmic Drugs

The antiarrhythmic properties of TCAs can be additive to those of quinidine, an effect that is further exacerbated by the inhibition of TCA metabolism by quinidine.

Dopamine Receptor Antagonists

Concurrent administration of TCAs and DRAs increases the plasma concentrations of both drugs. Desipramine plasma concentrations can rise twofold during concurrent administration with perphenazine (Trilafon). DRAs also add to the anticholinergic and sedative effects of the TCAs.

Central Nervous System Depressants

Opioids, alcohol, anxiolytics, hypnotics, and over-the-counter cold medications have additive effects by causing CNS depression when coadministered with TCAs. Persons should be advised to avoid driving or using dangerous equipment if sedated by TCAs.

Sympathomimetics

Tricyclic drug use with sympathomimetic drugs can cause serious cardiovascular effects.

Oral Contraceptives

Birth control pills can decrease TCA plasma concentrations through the induction of hepatic enzymes.

Other Drug Interactions

Nicotine can reduce TCA concentrations. Plasma concentrations can also be lowered by ascorbic acid, ammonium chloride, barbiturates, cigarette smoking, carbamazepine, chloral hydrate, lithium (Eskalith), and primidone (Mysoline). TCA plasma concentrations can be increased by concurrent use of acetazolamide (Diamox), sodium bicarbonate, acetylsalicylic acid, cimetidine, thiazide diuretics, fluoxetine, paroxetine, and fluvoxamine (Luvox). Plasma concentrations of TCAs can rise threefold to fourfold when administered concurrently with fluoxetine, fluvoxamine, and paroxetine.

LABORATORY INTERFERENCES

Laboratory interferences with the TCAs have not been reported.

DOSAGE AND CLINICAL GUIDELINES

Persons who intend to take TCAs should have a routine physical and laboratory examination, including a complete blood count (CBC), a white blood cell (WBC) count with differential, and serum electrolytes with liver function tests. An ECG should be obtained for all persons, especially women over 40 years of age and men over 30 years of age. TCAs are contraindicated in persons with a QT_c greater than 450 milliseconds. The initial dose should be small and should be raised gradually. Because of the availability of highly effective alternatives to TCAs, a newer agent should be used in the presence of any medical condition that could interact adversely with the TCAs.

The elderly and children are more sensitive to TCA adverse effects than are young adults. In children, the ECG should be regularly monitored during use of a TCA.

The available preparations of TCAs are presented in Table 36.34–3. The dosages and therapeutic blood levels for the TCAs vary among the drugs (Table 36.34–4). With the exception of protriptyline, all TCAs can be started at 25 mg a day and increased as tolerated. Divided doses at first reduce the severity of the adverse effects, although most of the dosage should be given at night to help induce sleep if a sedating drug, such as amitriptyline, is used. Eventually, the entire daily dose can be given at bedtime. A common clinical mistake is to stop increasing the dosage when the person is tolerating the drug but taking less than the maximal therapeutic dose and does not show clinical improvement. The clinician should routinely assess the person's pulse and orthostatic changes in BP while the dosage is being increased.

Nortriptyline use should be started at 25 mg a day. Most patients need only 75 mg a day to achieve a blood level of 100 mg/nL. The dosage, however, can be raised to 150 mg a day, if needed. Amoxapine can be started at 150 mg a day and raised to 400 mg a day. Protriptyline use should be started at 15 mg a day and raised to 60 mg a day. Maprotiline has been associated with an increased incidence of seizures if the dosage is raised too quickly or is maintained at too high a level. Maprotiline use should be started at 25 mg a day and increased over 4 weeks to 225 mg a day. It should be kept at that level for only 6 weeks and then be reduced to 175 to 200 mg a day.

Persons with chronic pain can be particularly sensitive to adverse effects when TCA use is started. Therefore, treatment should begin with low dosages that are raised in small increments. Persons with chronic pain may experience relief, however, on long-term low-dosage therapy, such as amitriptyline or nortriptyline at 10 to 75 mg a day.

The TCAs should be avoided in children, except as a last resort. Dosing guidelines in children for imipramine include initiation at 1.5 mg/kg a day. The dosage can be titrated to no more than 5 mg/kg a day. In enuresis, the dosage is usually 50 to

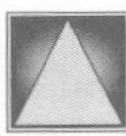

Table 36.34–3
Tricyclic and Tetracyclic Drug Preparations

Drug	Tablets	Capsules	Parenteral	Solution
Imipramine (Tofranil)	10, 25 and 50 mg	75, 100, 125, and 150 mg	12.5 mg/mL	—
Desipramine (Norpramin, Pertofrane)	10, 25, 50, 75, 100, and 150 mg	—	—	—
Trimipramine (Surmontil)	—	25, 50, and 100 mg	—	—
Amitriptyline (Elavil)	10, 25, 50, 75, 100, and 150 mg	—	10 mg/mL	—
Nortriptyline (Aventyl, Pamelor)	—	10, 25, 50, and 75 mg	—	10 mg/5 mL
Protriptyline (Vivoctil)	5 and 10 mg	—	—	—
Amoxapine (Asendin)	25, 50, 100, and 150 mg	—	—	—
Doxepin (Sinequan)	—	10, 25, 50, 75, 100, and 150 mg	—	10 mg/mL
Maprotiline (Ludiomil)	25, 50, and 75 mg	—	—	—
Clomipramine (Anafranil)	—	25, 50, and 75 mg	—	—

100 mg a day taken at bedtime. Clomipramine use can be initiated at 50 mg a day and increased to no more than 3 mg/kg a day or 200 mg a day.

When TCA treatment is discontinued, the dosage should first be decreased to three fourths the maximal dosage for a month. At that time, if no symptoms are present, drug use can be tapered by 25 mg (5 mg for protriptyline) every 4 to 7 days. Slow tapering avoids a cholinergic rebound syndrome consisting of nausea, upset stomach, sweating, headache, neck pain, and vomiting. This syndrome can be treated by reinstituting a small dosage of the drug and tapering more slowly than before. Several case reports note the appearance of rebound mania or hypomania after the abrupt discontinuation of TCA use.

Plasma Concentrations and Therapeutic Drug Monitoring

Clinical determinations of plasma concentrations should be conducted after 5 to 7 days on the same dosage of medication and 8 to 12 hours after the last dose. Because of variations in absorption and metabolism, a 30 to 50 times difference may be noted in the plasma concentrations in persons given the same dosage of a TCA (Table 36.34–4). Nortriptyline is unique in its association with a therapeutic window; that is, plasma concentrations below 50 ng/mL or above 150 ng/mL may reduce its efficacy.

Plasma concentrations can be useful in confirming compliance, assessing reasons for drug failures, and documenting effective plasma concentrations for future treatment. Clinicians should always treat the person's condition and not the plasma concentration. Some persons have adequate clinical responses with seemingly subtherapeutic plasma concentrations, and other persons only respond at supratherapeutic plasma concentrations, without experiencing adverse effects. The latter situation, however, should alert the clinician to monitor the person's condition with, for example, serial ECG recordings.

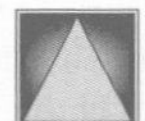

Table 36.34–4
General Information for the Tricyclic and Tetracyclic Antidepressants

Generic Name	Trade Name	Usual Adult Dosage Range (mg/day)	Therapeutic Plasma Concentrations (μg/mL)
Imipramine	Tofranil	150–300	150–300[a]
Desipramine	Norpramin, Pertobrane	150–300	150–300[a]
Trimipramine	Surmontil	150–300	?
Amitriptyline	Elavil, Endep	150–300	100–250[b]
Nortriptyline	Pamelor, Aventyl	50–150	50–150[a] (maximum)
Protriptyline	Vivactil	15–60	75–250
Amaxapine	Asendin	150–400	?
Doxepin	Adapin, Sinequan	150–300	100–250[a]
Maprotiline	Ludiomil	150–230	150–300[a]
Clomipramine	Anafranil	130–250	?

[a] Exact range may vary among laboratories.
[b] Includes parent compound and desmethyl metabolite.
? therapeutic plasma levels unknown.

Overdose Attempts

Overdose attempts with TCAs are serious and can often be fatal. Prescriptions for these drugs should be nonrefillable and for no longer than a week at a time for patients at risk for suicide. Amoxapine may be more likely than the other TCAs to result in death when taken in overdose. The newer antidepressants are safer in overdose.

Symptoms of overdose include agitation, delirium, convulsions, hyperactive deep tendon reflexes, bowel and bladder paralysis, dysregulation of BP and temperature, and mydriasis. The patient then progresses to coma and perhaps respiratory depression. Cardiac arrhythmias may not respond to treatment. Because of the long half-lives of TCAs, the patients are at risk of cardiac arrhythmias for 3 to 4 days after the overdose, so they should be monitored in an intensive care medical setting.

References

Amitai Y, Frischer H. Excess fatality from desipramine in children and adolescents. *J Am Acad Child Adolesc Psychiatry*. 2006:45(1):54–60.

Cerra D. Trimipramine for refractory panic attacks. *Am J Psychiatry*. 2006;163(3):584.

Derijks HJ, De Koning FH, Meyboom RH, Heerdink ER, Spooren PF, Egberts AC. Impaired glucose homeostasis after imipramine intake in a diabetic patient. *J Clin Psychopharmacol*. 2005;25(6):621–3.

Kirchheiner J, Muller G, Meineke I, Wernecke KD, Roots I, Brockmoller J. Effects of polymorphisms in CYP2D6, CYP2C9, and CYP2C19 on trimipramine pharmacokinetics. *J Clin Psychopharmacol*. 2003 *Oct*;23(5):459–66.

Kurpius MP, Alexander B. Rates of in vivo methylation of desipramine and nortriptyline. *Pharmacotherapy*. 2006;26(4):505–10.

Nelson J. Tricyclics and tetracyclics. In: Sadock BJ, Sadock VA, eds. *Kaplan and Sadock's Comprehensive Textbook of Psychiatry*. 8th ed. Vol. 2. Baltimore: Lippincott Williams & Wilkins; 2005:2956.

Reed BD, Caron AM, Gorenflo DW, Haefner HK. Treatment of vulvodynia with tricyclic antidepressants: efficacy and associated factors. *J Low Genit Tract Dis*. 2006;10(4):245–51.
van den Broek WW, Birkenhager TK, Mulder PG, Bruijn JA, Moleman P. Imipramine is effective in preventing relapse in electroconvulsive therapy-responsive depressed inpatients with prior pharmacotherapy treatment failure: a randomized, placebo-controlled trial. *J Clin Psychiatry*. 2006;67(2):263–8.
Walsh BT, Sysko R, Parides MK. Early response to desipramine among women with bulimia nervosa. *Int J Eat Disord*. 2006;39(1):72–5.
Watson A, Litovitz TL, Rodgers GC, Klein-Schwartz W, Youniss J, Rose SR, Borys D, May ME. 2000 annual report of the American Association of Poison Control Centers toxic surveillance system. *Am J Emerg Med*. 2003;21:353–421.

▲ 36.35 Valproate

Valproate (Depakene, Depakote), or valproic acid, is used for the treatment of acute manic or mixed episodes associated with bipolar I disorder. Other indications include seizure disorder and migraine prophylaxis.

CHEMISTRY

Valproate is a simple-chain branch carboxylic acid. It is called valproic acid because it is rapidly converted to the acid form in the stomach. The structural formula of valproate is shown in Figure 36.35–1. Multiple formulations of valproic acid are marketed. These include valproic acid (Depakene); divalproex sodium (Depakote), an enteric-coated delayed release 1:1 mixture of valproic acid and sodium valproate; and sodium valproate injection (Depacon). An extended-release preparation is also available. Each of these is therapeutically equivalent, because at physiologic pH, valproic acid dissociates into valproate ion.

PHARMACOLOGIC ACTIONS

Regardless of how it is formulated, valproate is rapidly and completely absorbed 1 to 2 hours after oral administration, with peak concentrations occurring 4 to 5 hours after oral administration. The plasma half-life of valproate is 10 to 16 hours. Valproate is highly protein bound. Protein binding becomes saturated and concentrations of therapeutically effective free valproate increase at serum concentrations above 50 to 100 μg/mL. The extended-release preparation produces lower peak concentrations and higher minimal concentrations and can be given once a day. Valproate is metabolized primarily by hepatic glucuronidation and mitochondrial β oxidation.

The biochemical basis of valproate's therapeutic effects remains poorly understood. Postulated mechanisms include enhancement of γ-aminobutyric acid (GABA) activity, modulation of voltage-sensitive sodium channels, and action on extrahypothalamic neuropeptides.

THERAPEUTIC INDICATIONS

Bipolar I Disorder

Acute Mania. About two thirds of persons with acute mania respond to valproate. Most patients with mania usually respond within 1 to 4 days after achieving valproate serum concentrations above 50 μg/mL. Antimanic response is generally associated with levels greater than 50 μg/mL, in a range of 50 to 150 μg/mL. Using gradual dosing strategies, this serum concentration can be achieved within 1 week of initiation of dosing, but newer, rapid oral loading strategies achieve therapeutic serum concentrations in 1 day and can control manic symptoms within 5 days. The short-term antimanic effects of valproate can be augmented with addition of lithium (Eskalith), carbamazepine (Tegretol), or dopamine receptor antagonists (DRAs). Because of its more favorable profile of cognitive, dermatologic, thyroid, and renal adverse effects, valproate is preferred to lithium for treatment of acute mania in children and elderly persons.

Mixed Episodes. Divalproex sodium extended-release tablets are approved for the treatment of acute manic or mixed episodes associated with bipolar disorder, with or without psychotic features. Mixed mania is a state of mind characterized by symptoms of both mania and depression. Patients often simultaneously feel agitated, angry, depressed, and irritable.

Acute Bipolar Depression. Valproate possesses some activity as a short-term treatment of depressive episodes in bipolar I disorder, but this effect is far less pronounced than for treatment of manic episodes. Among depressive symptoms, valproate is more effective for treatment of agitation than dysphoria. In clinical practice, valproate is most often used as add-on therapy to an antidepressant to prevent the development of mania or rapid cycling.

Prophylaxis. Studies suggest that valproate is effective in the prophylactic treatment of bipolar I disorder, resulting in fewer, less severe, and shorter manic episodes. In direct comparison, valproate is at least as effective as, and better tolerated than, lithium. It may be particularly effective in persons with rapid-cycling and ultrarapid-cycling bipolar disorders, dysphoric or

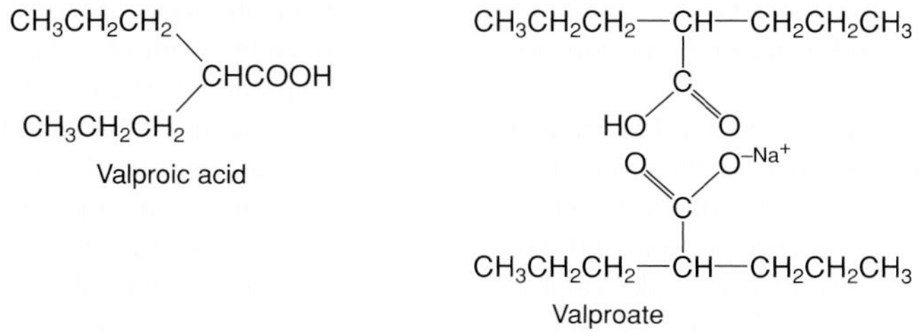

$CH_3CH_2CH_2$ / $CH_3CH_2CH_2$ > $CHCOOH$

Valproic acid

$CH_3CH_2CH_2-CH-CH_2CH_2CH_3$; C(=O)OH … O^-Na^+ C(=O); $CH_3CH_2CH_2-CH-CH_2CH_2CH_3$

Valproate

FIGURE 36.35-1
Molecular structure of valproic acid and valproate.

mixed mania, and mania due to a general medical condition as well as in persons who have comorbid substance abuse or panic attacks and in persons who have not had complete favorable responses to lithium treatment.

Schizophrenia and Schizoaffective Disorder

Valproate may accelerate response to antipsychotic therapy in patients with schizophrenia or schizoaffective disorder. Valproate alone is generally less effective in schizoaffective disorder than in bipolar I disorder. Valproate alone is ineffective for treatment of psychotic symptoms and is typically used in combination with other drugs in patients with these symptoms.

Other Mental Disorders

Valproate has been studied for possible efficacy in a broad range of psychiatric disorders. These include alcohol withdrawal and relapse prevention, panic disorder, posttraumatic stress disorder (PTSD), impulse control disorder, borderline personality disorder, and behavioral agitation and dementia. Evidence supporting use in these cases is weak, and any observed therapeutic effects may be related to treatment of comorbid bipolar disorder.

PRECAUTIONS AND ADVERSE REACTIONS

Although valproate treatment is generally well tolerated and safe, it carries quite a few black box warnings and other warnings (Table 36.35–1). The two most serious adverse effects of valproate treatment affect the pancreas and the liver. Risk factors for potentially fatal hepatotoxicity include young age (less than 3 years), concurrent use of phenobarbital, and the presence of neurologic disorders, especially inborn errors of metabolism. The rate of fatal hepatotoxicity in persons who have been treated with only valproate is 0.85 per 100,000 persons; no persons over the age of 10 years are reported to have died from hepatotoxicity. Therefore, the risk of this adverse reaction in adult psychiatric patients seems low. Nevertheless, if symptoms of lethargy, malaise, anorexia, nausea and vomiting, edema, and abdominal pain occur in a person treated with valproate, the clinician must consider the possibility of severe hepatotoxicity. A modest increase in liver function test results does not correlate with the development of serious hepatotoxicity. Rare cases of pancreatitis have been reported; they occur most often in the first 6 months of treatment, and the condition occasionally results in death. Pancreatic function can be assessed and followed with serum amylase concentrations. Other potentially serious consequences of treatment include hyperammonemia-induced encephalopathy and thrombocytopenia. Thrombocytopenia and platelet dysfunction occur most commonly at high dosages and result in the prolongation of bleeding times.

If at all possible, valproate should not be used by pregnant women. Women who require valproate therapy, therefore, should inform their physicians if they intend to become pregnant. The drug is associated with neural tube defects (e.g., spina bifida) in about 1 percent to 4 percent of all women who take valproate during the first trimester of the pregnancy. The risk of valproate-induced neural tube defects can be reduced with daily folic acid supplements (1 to 4 mg a day). All women on the drug with childbearing potential should be given folic acid supplements. Infants breast-fed by mothers taking valproate develop serum valproate concentrations 1 percent to 10 percent of maternal serum concentrations, and no data suggest that this poses a risk to the infant. Valproate is not contraindicated in nursing mothers. Clinicians should not administer the drug to persons with hepatic diseases. Valproate may be especially problematic for adolescent and young adult females. Cases of polycystic ovary disease have been reported in women using valproate. Even when the full syndromal criteria for this syndrome are not met, many of these women develop menstrual irregularities, hair loss, and hirsutism. These effects are thought to result from a metabolic syndrome that is driven by insulin resistance and hyperinsulinemia.

The common adverse effects associated with valproate (Table 36.35–2) are those affecting the gastrointestinal (GI) system, such as nausea, vomiting, dyspepsia, and diarrhea. The GI effects are generally most common in the first month of treatment, particularly if the dosage is increased rapidly. Unbuffered valproic acid (Depakene) is more likely to cause GI symptoms than are the enteric-coated "sprinkle" or the delayed-release divalproex sodium formulations. Other common adverse effects involve the nervous system, such as sedation, ataxia, dysarthria, and tremor.

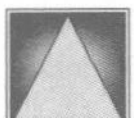

Table 36.35–1
Black Box Warnings and Other Warnings

More Serious Side Effect	Management Considerations
Hepatotoxicity	Rare, idiosyncratic event Estimated risk 1:118,000 (adults) Greatest risk profile (polypharmacy, younger than 2 yr of age, mental retardation) → 1:800
Pancreatitis	Rare, similar pattern to hepatotoxicity Incidence in clinical trials data is 2 of 2,416 (0.0008%) Postmarketing surveillance shows no increased incidence Relapse with rechallenge Asymptomatic amylase not predictive
Hyperammonemia	Rare—more common in combination with carbamazepine (Tegretol) Associated with coarse tremor and may respond to L-carnitine administration
Associated with urea cycle disorders	Discontinue valproate and protein intake Assess underlying urea cycle disorder Divalproex is contraindicated in patients with urea cycle disorders
Teratogenicity	Neural tube defect: 1% to 4% with valproate Preconceptual education and folate–vitamin B complex supplementation for all young women of child-bearing potential
Somnolence in the elderly	Slower titration than conventional doses Regular monitoring of fluid and nutritional intake
Thrombocytopenia	Decrease dose if clinically symptomatic (i.e., bruising, bleeding gums) Thrombocytopenia more likely with valproate levels ≥110 μg/mL (women) and ≥135 μg/mL (men)

(Adapted from *Physician's Desk Reference*. Oradell, NJ: Medical Economics Company; 2002, with permission.)

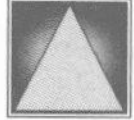

Table 36.35–2
Adverse Effects of Valproate

Common
- GI irritation
- Nausea
- Sedation
- Tremor
- Weight gain
- Hair loss

Uncommon
- Vomiting
- Diarrhea
- Ataxia
- Dysarthria
- Persistent elevation of hepatic transaminases

Rare
- Fatal hepatotoxicity (primarily in pediatric patients)
- Reversible thrombocytopenia
- Platelet dysfunction
- Coagulation disturbances
- Edema
- Hemorrhagic pancreatitis
- Agranulocytosis
- Encephalopathy and coma
- Respiratory muscle weakness and respiratory failure

GI, gastrointestinal.

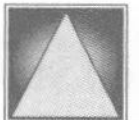

Table 36.35–3
Interactions of Valproate with Other Drugs

Drug	Interactions Reported with Valproate
Lithium	Increased tremor
Antipsychotics	Increased sedation; increased extrapyramidal effects; delirium and stupor (single report)
Clozapine	Increased sedation; confusional syndrome (single report)
Carbamazepine	Acute psychosis (single report); ataxia, nausea, lethargy (single report); can decrease valproate serum concentrations
Antidepressants	Amitriptyline and fluoxetine can increase valproate serum concentrations
Diazepam	Serum concentration increased by valproate
Clonazepam	Absence status (rare; reported only in patients with preexisting epilepsy)
Phenytoin	Serum concentration decreased by valproate
Phenobarbital	Serum concentration increased by valproate; increased sedation
Other CNS depressants	Increased sedation
Anticoagulants	Possible potentiation of effect

CNS, central nervous system.

Valproate-induced tremor may respond well to treatment with β-adrenergic receptor antagonists or gabapentin. Treatment of the other neurologic adverse effects usually requires lowering the valproate dosage.

Weight gain is a common adverse effect, especially in long-term treatment, and can best be treated by strict limitation of caloric intake. Hair loss can occur in 5 percent to 10 percent of all persons treated, and rare cases of complete loss of body hair have been reported. Some clinicians have recommended treatment of valproate-associated hair loss with vitamin supplements that contain zinc and selenium. Of persons taking valproate, 5 to 40 percent experience a persistent but clinically insignificant elevation in liver transaminases up to three times the upper limit of normal, which is usually asymptomatic and resolves after discontinuation of the drug. High dosages of valproate (above 1,000 mg a day) may rarely produce mild to moderate hyponatremia, most likely because of some degree of the syndrome of secretion of inappropriate antidiuretic hormone (SIADH), which is reversible on lowering of the dosage. Overdoses of valproate can lead to coma and death.

DRUG INTERACTIONS

Valproate is commonly prescribed as part of a regimen involving other psychotropic agents. The only consistent drug interaction with lithium, if both drugs are maintained in their respective therapeutic ranges, is the exacerbation of drug-induced tremors, which can usually be treated with β-receptor antagonists. The combination of valproate and DRAs can result in increased sedation, as can be seen when valproate is added to any central nervous system (CNS) depressant (e.g., alcohol), and increased severity of extrapyramidal symptoms, which usually respond to treatment with antiparkinsonian drugs. Valproate can usually be safely combined with carbamazepine or serotonin–dopamine antagonists. Perhaps the most worrisome interaction of valproate and a psychotropic drug involves lamotrigine. Since the approval of lamotrigine for the treatment of bipolar disorder, the likelihood that patients will be treated with both agents has increased. Valproate more than doubles lamotrigine concentrations, increasing the risk of a serious rash.

The plasma concentrations of carbamazepine, diazepam (Valium), amitriptyline (Elavil), nortriptyline (Pamelor), and phenobarbital (Luminal) can also be increased when these drugs are coadministered with valproate, and the plasma concentrations of phenytoin (Dilantin) and desipramine (Norpramin) can be decreased when they are combined with valproate. The plasma concentrations of valproate may be decreased when the drug

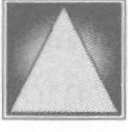

Table 36.35–4
Recommended Laboratory Tests During Valproate Therapy

Prior to treatment
- Standard chemistry screen with special attention to liver function tests
- CBC, including white cell and platelet count

During treatment
- Liver function tests at 1 month, then every 6 to 24 months if no abnormalities are found
- Complete blood work with platelet count at 1 month, then every 6 to 24 months if findings are normal

Liver function test results become abnormal
- Mild transaminase elevation (less than three times normal): monitoring every 1 to 2 weeks: if stable and patient is responding to valproate, results are monitored monthly to every 3 months
- Pronounced transaminase elevation (more than three times normal): dosage reduction or discontinuation of valproate; increase dose or rechallenge if transaminases normalize and if the patient is a valproate responder

CBC, complete blood count.

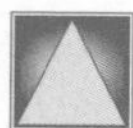

Table 36.35–5
Valproate Preparations Available in the United States

Generic Name	Trade Name, Form (doses)	Time to Peak
Valproate sodium injection	Depacon injection (100 mg valproic acid/mL)	1 hr
Valproic acid	Depakene, syrup (250 mg/5 mL)	1 to 2 hrs
	Depakene, capsules (250 mg)	1 to 2 hrs
Divalproex sodium	Depakote, delayed-released tablets (125, 250, 500 mg)	3 to 8 hrs
Divalproex sodium coated particles in capsules	Depakote, sprinkle capsules (125 mg)	Compared with divalproex tablets, divalproex sprinkle has earlier onset and slower absorption, with slightly lower peak plasma concentration

is coadministered with carbamazepine and may be increased when coadministered with guanfacine (Tenex), amitriptyline, or fluoxetine (Prozac). Valproate can be displaced from plasma proteins by carbamazepine, diazepam, and aspirin. Persons who are treated with anticoagulants (e.g., aspirin and warfarin [Coumadin]) should also be monitored when valproate use is initiated to assess the development of any undesired augmentation of the anticoagulation effects. Interactions of valproate with other drugs are listed in Table 36.35–3.

LABORATORY INTERFERENCES

Valproate can cause laboratory increase of serum free fatty acids. Valproate metabolites can produce a false-positive test result for urinary ketones as well as falsely abnormal thyroid function test results.

DOSAGE AND CLINICAL GUIDELINES

When starting valproate therapy, a baseline hepatic panel, complete blood cell (CBC) and platelet counts, and pregnancy testing should be ordered. Additional testing should include amylase and coagulation studies, if baseline pancreatic disease or coagulopathy is suspected. In addition to baseline laboratory tests, white blood cell (WBC) and platelet counts and hepatic transaminase concentrations should be obtained 1 month after initiation of therapy and every 6 to 24 months thereafter. Because even frequent monitoring may not predict serious organ toxicity, it is more prudent, however, to reinforce the need for prompt evaluation of any illnesses when reviewing the instructions with patients. Asymptomatic elevation of transaminase concentrations up to three times the upper limit of normal are common and do not require any change in dosage. Table 36.35–4 lists the recommended laboratory tests for valproate treatment.

Valproate is available in a number of formulations (Table 36.35–5). For treatment of acute mania, an oral loading strategy of initiation with 20 to 30 mg/kg a day can be used to accelerate control of symptoms. This is usually well tolerated, but can cause excessive sedation and tremor in elderly persons. Agitated behavior can be rapidly stabilized with intravenous (IV) infusion of valproate. If acute mania is absent, it is best to initiate drug treatment gradually to minimize the common adverse effects of nausea, vomiting, and sedation. The dose on the first day should be 250 mg administered with a meal. The dosage can be raised up to 250 mg orally three times daily over the course of 3 to 6 days. The plasma concentrations can be assessed in the morning before the first daily dose is administered. Therapeutic plasma concentrations for the control of seizures range between 50 and 150 μg/mL, but concentrations up to 200 μg/mL are usually well tolerated. It is reasonable to use the same range for the treatment of mental disorders; most of the controlled studies have used 50 to 125 μg/mL. Most persons attain therapeutic plasma concentrations on a dosage between 1,200 and 1,500 mg a day in divided doses. Once a person's symptoms are well controlled, the full daily dose can be taken all at once before sleep.

REFERENCES

Aichhorn W, Marksteiner J, Walch T, Zernig G, Saria A, Kemmler G. Influence of age, gender, body weight and valproate co-medication on quetiapine plasma. *Int Clin Psychopharm.* 2006;21(2):81.

Hao Y, Creson T, Zhang L, Li P, Du F, Yuan P, Gould T, Manji H, Chen G. Mood stabilizer valproate promotes ERK pathway-dependent cortical neuronal growth and neurogenesis. *J Neurosci.* 2004;24(29):6590–6599.

Nelson J. Tricyclics and tetracyclics. In: Sadock BJ, Sadock VA, eds. *Kaplan and Sadock's Comprehensive Textbook of Psychiatry.* 8th ed. Vol. 2. Baltimore: Lippincott Williams & Wilkins; 2005:2956.

Nicolson A, Appleton R, Chadwick D, Smith D. The relationship between treatment with valproate, lamotrigine, and topiramate and the prognosis of the idiopathic generalised epilepsies. *J Neurol Neurosurg Psychiatry.* 2004;75:75–79.

Salloum I, Cornelius J, Daley D, Kirisci L, Himmelhoch J, Thase M. Efficacy of valproate maintenance in patients with bipolar disorder and alcoholism. *Arch Gen Psychiatry.* 2005;62:37–45.

▲ 36.36 Yohimbine

Yohimbine (Yocon) is an α_2-adrenergic receptor antagonist that is sometimes used as a treatment for both idiopathic and medication-induced erectile disorder. Currently, sildenafil (Viagra) and its congeners (*see* Section 36.27) and alprostadil (Impulse, Caverject) are considered more efficacious for this indication than yohimbine.

CHEMISTRY

Yohimbine hydrochloride is derived from an alkaloid found in *Rubaceae* and related trees and in the *Rauwolfia serpentina* plant. Its molecular structure is shown in Figure 36.36–1.

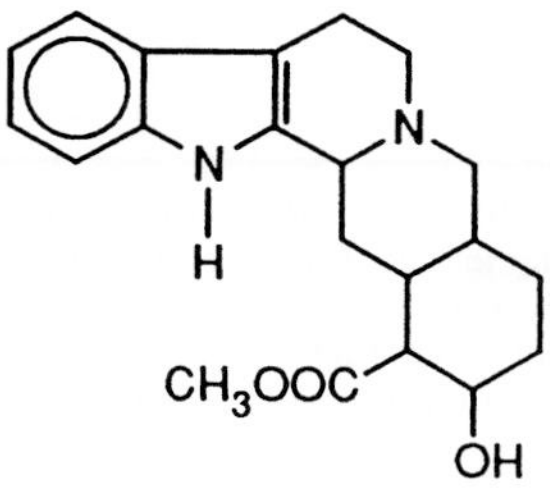

FIGURE 36.36–1
Molecular structure of yohimbine.

PHARMACOLOGIC ACTIONS

Yohimbine is erratically absorbed following oral administration, with bioavailability ranging from 7 percent to 87 percent. There is extensive hepatic first-pass metabolism. Yohimbine affects the sympathomimetic autonomic nervous system by increasing plasma concentrations of norepinephrine. The half-life of yohimbine is 0.5 to 2 hours.

Yohimbine is an antagonist of α_2-receptors located both presynaptically and postsynaptically on noradrenergic neurons. The α_2-receptors are also located on synaptic terminals of some serotonergic neurons. Stimulation of presynaptic α_2-receptors results in a decrease in the release of neurotransmitters from the neuron; therefore, blockade of the receptors results in an increase in the release of neurotransmitters. Both norepinephrine and serotonin are involved in the physiology of male sexual response. Clinically, yohimbine produces increased parasympathetic (cholinergic) tone.

THERAPEUTIC INDICATIONS

Yohimbine has been used to treat erectile dysfunction. Penile erection has been linked to cholinergic activity and to α_2-adrenergic blockade, which theoretically results in increased penile inflow of blood, decreased penile outflow of blood, or both.

Yohimbine is reported to help counteract the loss of sexual desire and the orgasmic inhibition caused by some serotonergic antidepressants (e.g., selective serotonin reuptake inhibitors). It has not been found useful in women for these indications.

PRECAUTIONS AND ADVERSE EFFECTS

The side effects of yohimbine include anxiety, elevated blood pressure (BP) and heart rate, increased psychomotor activity, irritability, tremor, headache, skin flushing, dizziness, urinary frequency, nausea, vomiting, and sweating. Patients with panic disorder show heightened sensitivity to yohimbine and experience increased anxiety, increased BP, and increased plasma 3-methoxy-4-hydroxyphenylglycol (MHPG).

Yohimbine should be used with caution in female patients and should not be used in patients with renal disease, cardiac disease, glaucoma, or a history of gastric or duodenal ulcer.

DRUG INTERACTIONS

Yohimbine blocks the effects of clonidine (Catapres), guanfacine (Tenex), and other α_2-receptor agonists.

LABORATORY INTERFERENCES

No known laboratory interferences are associated with yohimbine use.

DOSAGE AND CLINICAL GUIDELINES

Yohimbine is available in 5.4-mg tablets. The dosage of yohimbine in the treatment of erectile disorder is approximately 18 mg a day given in dosages that range from 2.7 to 5.4 mg three times a day. In the event of significant adverse effects, dosage should first be reduced, and then gradually increased again. Yohimbine should be used judiciously in psychiatric patients because it may have an adverse effect on their mental status. Because yohimbine has no consistent effect on erectile dysfunction, its use remains controversial. Phosphodiesterase-5 inhibitors are the preferred medication for this disorder.

REFERENCES

Etzel J, Rana B, Wen G, Parmer R, Schork N, O'Connor D, Insel P. Genetic variation at the human α_{2B}-adrenergic receptor locus: Role in blood pressure variation and yohimbine response. *Hypertension*. 2005;45:1207.

Sanacora G, Berman RM, Cappiello A, Oren DA, Kugaya A, Liu N, Gueorguieva R, Fasula D, Charney DS. Addition of the alpha2-antagonist yohimbine to fluoxetine: Effects on rate of antidepressant response. *Neuropsychopharmacology*. 2004;29(6):1166–1171.

Swann AC, Birnbaum D, Jagar AA, Dougherty DM, Moeller FG. Acute yohimbine increases laboratory-measured impulsivity in normal subjects. *Biol Psychiatry*. 2005;57(10):1209.

▲ 36.37 Brain Stimulation Methods

36.37.1 Electroconvulsive Therapy

Use of electroconvulsive therapy (ECT) has diminished since the middle of the 20th century: however, because ECT remains the most effective treatment for major depression and a rapidly effective treatment for life-threatening psychiatric conditions, unlike its contemporaneous somatic therapies, ECT remains in the active treatment portfolio of modern therapeutics. Its use has shifted from public to private institutions, and it is estimated that approximately 100,000 patients have received ECT annually in the United States. A limiting variable in its use has been the adverse effect of confusion and memory loss associated with the course of treatment; however, both are reversible and most of the major innovations in ECT technique over the past 20 years have sought to diminish cognitive effects while maintaining benefits. New developments in ECT technique offer the hope that this form of treatment will find better acceptance among psychiatrists and patients.

The Nobel Laureate Paul Greengard has suggested that the term *electrocortical therapy* might be used to replace the current term electroconvulsive therapy. Greengard has acknowledged that if the mechanism of action of ECT, as yet unknown, turns out to be subcortical, then the term might have limited use. Until that time, however, the authors of this text think Greengard's suggestion deserves consideration. It would

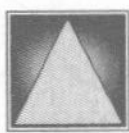

Table 36.37.1–1
Milestones in the History of Convulsive Therapy

1500s	Paracelsus induces seizures by administering camphor (by mouth) to treat psychiatric illness.
1785	First published report of the use of seizure induction to treat mania, again using camphor.
1934	Ladislaus Meduna begins the modern era of convulsive therapy using intramuscular injection of camphor for catatonic schizophrenia. Camphor is soon replaced with pentylenetetrazol.
1938	Lucio Cerletti and Ugo Bini conduct the first electrical induction of a series of seizures in a catatonic patient and produce a successful treatment response
1940	ECT is introduced to the United States.
	Curare developed for use as a muscle relaxant at ECT.
1951	Introduction of succinylcholine.
1958	First controlled study of unilateral ECT.
1960	Attenuation of seizure expression with an anticonvulsant agent (lidocaine [Dalcaine]) reduces the efficacy of ECT. Subconvulsive treatment produces only weak clinical responses; the hypothesis that seizure activity is necessary and sufficient for efficacy is upheld.
1960s	Randomized clinical trials of the efficacy of ECT versus medications in the treatment of depression yield response rates that are significantly higher with ECT.
	Comparisons of neuroleptics and ECT show that neuroleptic medication is superior for acute treatment, although ECT may be more effective in the long term.
1970	The most common electrode positioning for right unilateral ECT developed.
1976	A constant current, brief pulse ECT device, the prototype for modern devices, is developed.
1978	The American Psychiatric Association publishes the first Task Force Report on ECT with the aim of establishing standards for consent and the technical and clinical aspects of the conduct of ECT.
Late 1970s–early 1980s	Randomized, controlled trials demonstrate that ECT is more effective than sham treatment for major depression.
1985	The National Institutes of Health and National Institute of Mental Health Consensus Conference on ECT endorses a role for the use of ECT and advocates research and national standards of practice.
1987	The belief that the seizure in itself is sufficient for clinical response is challenged by H. A. Sackheim and collaborators, who report that the combination of dosage just above seizure threshold and right unilateral electrode placement, while producing a seizure of sufficient duration, is ineffective.
1988	Randomized, controlled clinical trials of ECT versus lithium (Eskalith) demonstrate them to be equally effective in mania.
2000	In controlled trials, the dose–response relationship for right unilateral ECT is validated; high-dose right unilateral and bilateral ECT show equal response rates in major depression, but right unilateral electrode placement is associated with fewer adverse cognitive effects.
	Convulsive treatment is induced with magnetic stimulation by S. H. Lisanby and colleagues.
2001	The largest modern controlled trial of relapse prevention post-ECT with continuation pharmacotherapy demonstrates a significantly better outcome for combined treatment with a tricyclic antidepressant (nortriptyline) plus lithium compared with nortriptyline alone or placebo during the first 6 months post-ECT.

ECT, electroconvulsive therapy.

help diminish the fear associated with the word convulsion and help destigmatize a very effective treatment method.

HISTORY

Electroconvulsive therapy is one of the oldest treatments for mental illness in continuous use. Table 36.37.1–1 lists the milestones in the history of convulsive therapy dating back to the 1500s when the Swiss physician Paracelsus (1493–1541) used camphor to treat mental illness.

ELECTROPHYSIOLOGY IN ELECTROCONVULSIVE THERAPY

Neurons maintain a resting potential across the plasma membrane and may propagate an action potential, which is a transient reversal of the membrane potential. Normal brain activity is desynchronized; that is, neurons fire action potentials asynchronously. A convulsion, or seizure, occurs when a large percentage of neurons fire in unison. Such rhythmical changes in the extracellular potential entrain neighboring neurons, propagate the seizure activity across the cortex and into deeper structures, and eventually engulf the entire brain in high-voltage synchronous neuronal firing. Cellular mechanisms work to contain the seizure activity and to maintain cellular homeostasis, and the seizure eventually ends. In epilepsy, any of possibly several hundred genetic defects can alter the balance in favor of unrestrained activity. In ECT, seizures are triggered in normal neurons by application through the scalp of pulses of current, under conditions that are carefully controlled to create a seizure of a particular duration over the entire brain.

The qualities of the electricity used in ECT can be described by Ohm's law, $E = IR$, or $I = E/R$, in which E is voltage, I is current, and R is resistance. The intensity or dose of electricity in ECT is measured in terms of charge (milliampere-seconds or millicoulombs) or energy (watt-seconds or joules). Resistance is synonymous with impedance and, in the case of ECT, both the electrode's contact with the body and the nature of the bodily tissues are the major determinants of resistance. The skull has a high impedance; the brain has a low impedance. Because scalp tissues are much better conductors of electricity than bone, only about 20 percent of the applied charge actually enters the skull to excite neurons. The ECT machines that are now widely used can be adjusted to administer the electricity under conditions of constant current, voltage, or energy.

MECHANISM OF ACTION

The induction of a bilateral generalized seizure is necessary for both the beneficial and the adverse effects of ECT. Although a seizure superficially seems as though it is an all-or-none event, some data indicate that not all generalized seizures involve all the neurons in deep brain structures (e.g., the basal ganglia and the thalamus); recruitment of these deep neurons may be necessary for full therapeutic benefit. After the generalized seizure, the electroencephalogram (EEG) shows about 60 to 90 seconds of postictal suppression. This period is followed by the appearance of high-voltage delta and theta waves and a return of the EEG to preseizure appearance in about 30 minutes. During the course of a series of ECT treatments, the interictal EEG is generally slower and of greater amplitude than usual, but the EEG returns to pretreatment appearance 1 month to 1 year after the end of the course of treatment.

One research approach to the mechanism of action for ECT has been to study the neurophysiological effects of treatment. Positron emission tomography (PET) studies of both cerebral blood flow and glucose use have shown that, during seizures, cerebral blood flow, use of glucose and oxygen, and permeability of the blood–brain barrier increase. After the seizure, blood flow and glucose metabolism are decreased, perhaps most markedly in the frontal lobes. Some research indicates that the degree of decrease in cerebral metabolism is correlated with therapeutic response.

Seizure foci in idiopathic epilepsy are hypometabolic during interictal periods; ECT itself acts as an anticonvulsant because its administration is associated with an increase in the seizure threshold as treatment progresses. Recent data suggest that for 1 to 2 months following a session of ECT, EEGs record a large increase in slow-wave activity located over the prefrontal cortex in patients who responded well to the ECT. High-intensity, bilateral stimulation produced the best response; low-intensity, unilateral stimulation, the weakest. These data are of unclear significance, however, because the specific EEG correlate disappeared 2 months after ECT, whereas the clinical benefit persisted.

Electroconvulsive therapy affects the cellular mechanisms of memory and mood regulation and raises the seizure threshold. The latter effect may be blocked by the opiate antagonist naloxone (Narcan).

Neurochemical research into the mechanisms of action of ECT has focused on changes in neurotransmitter receptors and, recently, changes in second-messenger systems. Virtually every neurotransmitter system is affected by ECT, but a series of ECT sessions results in downregulation of postsynaptic β-adrenergic receptors, the same receptor change observed with virtually all antidepressant treatments. The effects of ECT on serotonergic neurons remain controversial. Various research studies have reported an increase in postsynaptic serotonin receptors, no change in serotonin receptors, and a change in the presynaptic regulation of serotonin release. ECT has also been reported to effect changes in the muscarinic, cholinergic, and dopaminergic neuronal systems. In second-messenger systems, ECT has been reported to affect the coupling of G-proteins to receptors, the activity of adenylyl cyclase and phospholipase C, and the regulation of calcium entry into neurons.

INDICATIONS

Major Depressive Disorder

The most common indication for ECT is major depressive disorder, for which ECT is the fastest and most effective available therapy. ECT should be considered for use in patients who have failed medication trials, have not tolerated medications, have severe or psychotic symptoms, are acutely suicidal or homicidal, or have marked symptoms of agitation or stupor. Controlled studies have shown that up to 70 percent of patients who fail to respond to antidepressant medications may respond positively to ECT.

Electroconvulsive therapy is effective for depression in both major depressive disorder and bipolar I disorder. Delusional or psychotic depression has long been considered particularly responsive to ECT; but recent studies have indicated that major depressive episodes with psychotic features are no more responsive to ECT than nonpsychotic depressive disorders. Nevertheless, because major depressive episodes with psychotic features respond poorly to antidepressant pharmacotherapy alone, ECT should be considered much more often as the first-line treatment for patients with the disorder. Major depressive disorder with melancholic features (e.g., markedly severe symptoms, psychomotor retardation, early morning awakening, diurnal variation, decreased appetite and weight, and agitation) is considered likely to respond to ECT. ECT is particularly indicated for persons who are severely depressed, who have psychotic symptoms, who show suicidal intent, or who refuse to eat. Depressed patients less likely to respond to ECT include those with somatization disorder. Elderly patients tend to respond to ECT more slowly than do young patients. ECT is a treatment for major depressive episode and does not provide prophylaxis unless it is administered on a long-term maintenance basis.

Manic Episodes

Electroconvulsive therapy is at least equal to lithium (Eskalith) in the treatment of acute manic episodes. The pharmacological treatment of manic episodes, however, is so effective in the short term and for prophylaxis that the use of ECT to treat manic episodes is generally limited to situations with specific contraindications to all available pharmacological approaches. The relative rapidity of the ECT response indicates its usefulness for patients whose manic behavior has produced dangerous levels of exhaustion. ECT should not be used for a patient who is receiving lithium, because lithium can lower the seizure threshold and cause a prolonged seizure.

Schizophrenia

Although an effective treatment for the symptoms of acute schizophrenia, ECT is not for those of chronic schizophrenia. Patients with schizophrenia who have marked positive symptoms, catatonia, or affective symptoms are considered most likely to respond to ECT. In such patients, the efficacy of ECT is about equal to that of antipsychotics, but improvement may occur faster.

Other Indications

Small studies have found ECT effective in the treatment of catatonia, a symptom associated with mood disorders, schizophrenia, and medical and neurological disorders. ECT is also reportedly useful to treat episodic psychoses, atypical psychoses, obsessive-compulsive disorder, and delirium and such medical conditions as neuroleptic malignant syndrome, hypopituitarism, intractable seizure disorders, and the on-off phenomenon of Parkinson's disease. ECT may also be the treatment of choice for depressed suicidal pregnant women who require treatment and cannot take medication; for geriatric and medically ill patients who cannot take antidepressant drugs safely; and perhaps even for severely depressed and suicidal children and adolescents who may be less likely to respond to antidepressant drugs than are adults. ECT is not effective in somatization disorder (unless accompanied by depression), personality disorders, and anxiety disorders.

CLINICAL GUIDELINES

Patients and their families are often apprehensive about ECT; therefore, clinicians must explain both beneficial and adverse effects and alternative treatment approaches. The informed-consent process should be documented in the patients' medical records and should include a discussion of the disorder, its natural course, and the option of receiving no treatment. Printed literature and videotapes about ECT may be useful in attempting to obtain a truly informed consent. The use of involuntary ECT is rare today and should be reserved for patients who urgently need treatment and who have a legally appointed guardian who has agreed to its use. Clinicians must know local, state, and federal laws about the use of ECT.

Pretreatment Evaluation

Pretreatment evaluation should include standard physical, neurological, and preanesthesia examinations and a complete medical history. Laboratory evaluations should include blood and urine chemistries, a chest X-ray, and an electrocardiogram (ECG). A dental examination to assess the state of patients' dentition is advisable for elderly patients and patients who have had inadequate dental care. An X-ray of the spine is needed if other evidence of a spinal disorder is seen. Computed tomography (CT) or magnetic resonance imaging (MRI) should be performed if a clinician suspects the presence of a seizure disorder or a space-occupying lesion. Practitioners of ECT no longer consider even a space-occupying lesion to be an absolute contraindication to ECT, but with such patients the procedure should be performed only by experts.

Concomitant Medications. Patients' ongoing medications should be assessed for possible interactions with the induction of a seizure, for effects (both positive and negative) on the seizure threshold, and for drug interactions with the medications used during ECT. The use of tricyclic and tetracyclic drugs, monoamine oxidase inhibitors, and antipsychotics is generally considered acceptable. Benzodiazepines used for anxiety should be withdrawn because of their anticonvulsant activity; lithium (Eskalith) should be withdrawn because it can result in increased postictal delirium and can prolong seizure activity; clozapine (Clozaril) and bupropion (Wellbutrin) should be withdrawn because they are associated with the development of late-appearing seizures. Lidocaine (Xylocaine) should not be administered during ECT because it markedly increases the seizure threshold; theophylline (Theo-Dur) is contraindicated because it increases the duration of seizures. Reserpine (Serpasil) is also contraindicated because it is associated with further compromise of the respiratory and cardiovascular systems during ECT.

Premedications, Anesthetics, and Muscle Relaxants

Patients should not be given anything orally for 6 hours before treatment. Just before the procedure, the patient's mouth should be checked for dentures and other foreign objects, and an intravenous (IV) line should be established. A bite block is inserted in the mouth just before the treatment is administered to protect the patient's teeth and tongue during the seizure. Except for the brief interval of electrical stimulation, 100 percent oxygen is administered at a rate of 5 L a minute during the procedure until spontaneous respiration returns. Emergency equipment for establishing an airway should be immediately available in case it is needed.

Muscarinic Anticholinergic Drugs. Muscarinic anticholinergic drugs are administered before ECT to minimize oral and respiratory secretions and to block bradycardias and asystoles, unless the resting heart rate is above 90 beats a minute. Some ECT centers have stopped the routine use of anticholinergics as premedications, although their use is still indicated for patients taking β-adrenergic receptor antagonists and those with ventricular ectopic beats. The most commonly used drug is atropine, which can be administered 0.3 to 0.6 mg intramuscularly (IM) or subcutaneously (SC) 30 to 60 minutes before the anesthetic or 0.4 to 1.0 mg IV 2 or 3 minutes before the anesthetic. An option is to use glycopyrrolate (Robinul) (0.2 to 0.4 mg IM, IV, or SC), which is less likely to cross the blood–brain barrier and less likely to cause cognitive dysfunction and nausea, although it is thought to have less cardiovascular protective activity than does atropine.

Anesthesia. Administration of ECT requires general anesthesia and oxygenation. The depth of anesthesia should be as light as possible, not only to minimize adverse effects but also to avoid elevating the seizure threshold associated with many anesthetics. Methohexital (Brevital) (0.75 to 1.0 mg/kg IV bolus) is the most commonly used anesthetic because of its shorter duration of action and lower association with postictal arrhythmias than thiopental (Pentothal) (usual dose 2 to 3 mg/kg IV), although this difference in cardiac effects is not universally accepted. Four other anesthetic alternatives are etomidate (Amidate), ketamine (Ketalar), alfentanil (Alfenta), and propofol (Diprivan). Etomidate (0.15 to 0.3 mg/kg IV) is sometimes used because it does not increase the seizure threshold; this effect is particularly useful for elderly patients because the seizure threshold increases with age. Ketamine (6 to 10 mg/kg IM) is sometimes used because it does not increase the seizure threshold, although its use is limited by the frequent association of psychotic symptoms with emergence from anesthesia with this drug. Alfentanil (2 to 9 mg/kg

IV) is sometimes coadministered with barbiturates to allow the use of low doses of the barbiturate anesthetics and, thus, reduce the seizure threshold less than usual, although its use can be associated with an increased incidence of nausea. Propofol (0.5 to 3.5 mg/kg IV) is less useful because of its strong anticonvulsant properties.

Muscle Relaxants. After the onset of the anesthetic effect, usually within a minute, a muscle relaxant is administered to minimize the risk of bone fractures and other injuries resulting from motor activity during the seizure. The goal is to produce profound relaxation of the muscles, not necessarily to paralyze them, unless the patient has a history of osteoporosis or spinal injury or has a pacemaker and, therefore, is at risk for injury related to motor activity during the seizure. Succinylcholine, an ultrafast-acting depolarizing blocking agent, has gained virtually universal acceptance for the purpose. Succinylcholine is usually administered in a dose of 0.5 to 1 mg/kg as an IV bolus or drip. Because succinylcholine is a depolarizing agent, its action is marked by the presence of muscle fasciculations, which move in a rostrocaudal progression. The disappearance of these movements in the feet or the absence of muscle contractions after peripheral nerve stimulation indicates maximal muscle relaxation. In some patients, tubocurarine (3 mg IV) is administered to prevent myoclonus and increases in potassium and muscle enzymes; these reactions can be a problem in patients with musculoskeletal or cardiac disease. To monitor the duration of the convulsion, a blood pressure cuff may be inflated at the ankle to a pressure in excess of the systolic pressure before infusion of the muscle relaxant, to allow observation of relatively innocuous seizure activity in the foot muscles.

If a patient has a known history of pseudocholinesterase deficiency, atracurium (Tracrium) (0.5 to 1 mg/kg IV) or curare can be used instead of succinylcholine. In such a patient, the metabolism of succinylcholine is disrupted, and prolonged apnea may necessitate emergency airway management. In general, however, because of the short half-life of succinylcholine, the duration of apnea after its administration is generally shorter than the delay in regaining consciousness caused by the anesthetic and the postictal state.

Electrode Placement

Electroconvulsive therapy can be conducted with either bilaterally or unilaterally placed electrodes. Bilateral placement usually yields a more rapid therapeutic response, and unilateral placement results in less marked cognitive adverse effects in the first week or weeks after treatment, although this difference between placements is absent 2 months after treatment. In bilateral placement, which was introduced first, one stimulating electrode is placed several centimeters apart over each hemisphere of the brain. In unilateral ECT, both electrodes are placed several centimeters apart over the nondominant hemisphere, almost always the right hemisphere. Some attempts have been made to vary the location of the electrodes in unilateral ECT, but these attempts have not obtained the rapidity of response seen with bilateral ECT or have further reduced the cognitive adverse effects. The most common approach is to initiate treatment with unilateral ECT because of its more favorable adverse effect profile. If a patient does not improve after four to six unilateral

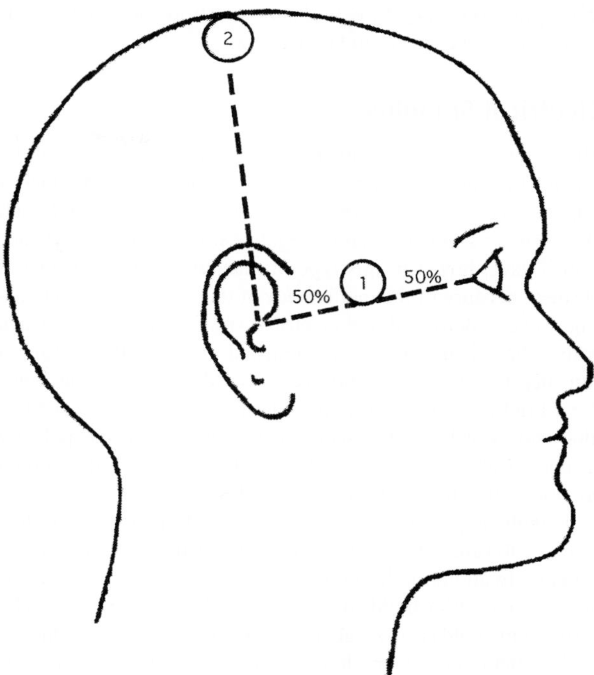

FIGURE 36.37.1–1
Electrode placements. Position 1 represents the frontotemporal position, used for both electrodes, one on each side of the head, in conducting bilateral electroconvulsive therapy (ECT). For right unilateral ECT, one electrode is in the right frontotemporal position, and the other is just to the right of the vertex at position 2. (Courtesy of American Psychiatric Association, with permission.)

treatments, bilateral placement is used. Initial bilateral placement of the electrodes may be indicated in the following situations: severe depressive symptoms, marked agitation, immediate suicide risk, manic symptoms, catatonic stupor, and treatment-resistant schizophrenia. Some patients are particularly at risk for anesthetic-related adverse effects, and these patients may also be treated with bilateral placement from the beginning to minimize the number of treatments and exposure to anesthetics.

In traditional bilateral ECT, the electrodes are placed bifrontotemporally with the center of each electrode about 1 inch above the midpoint of an imaginary line drawn from the tragus to the external canthus. With unilateral ECT, one stimulus electrode typically is placed over the nondominant frontotemporal area. Although several locations for the second stimulus electrode have been proposed, placement on the nondominant centroparietal scalp, just lateral to the midline vertex, appears to provide the most effective configuration (Fig. 36.37.1–1).

Which cerebral hemisphere is dominant can generally be determined by a simple series of performance tasks (e.g., for handedness and footedness) and stated preference. Right body responses correlate highly with left brain dominance. If the responses are mixed or if they clearly indicate left body dominance, clinicians should alternate the polarity of unilateral stimulation during successive treatments. Clinicians should also monitor the time that it takes for patients to recover consciousness and to answer simple orientation and naming questions. The side of stimulation associated with less rapid recovery and return of function is considered dominant. The left hemisphere is dominant in most persons; therefore, unilateral electrode placement is almost always over the right hemisphere.

Electrical Stimulus

The electrical stimulus must be sufficiently strong to reach the seizure threshold (the level of intensity needed to produce a seizure). The electrical stimulus is given in cycles, and each cycle contains a positive and a negative wave. Old machines use a sine wave; however, this type of machine is now considered obsolete because of the inefficiency of that wave shape. When a sine wave is delivered, the electrical stimulus in the sine wave before the seizure threshold is reached and after the seizure is activated is unnecessary and excessive. Modern ECT machines use a brief pulse waveform that administers the electrical stimulus usually in 1 to 2 milliseconds at a rate of 30 to 100 pulses a second. Machines that use an ultrabrief pulse (0.5 milliseconds) are not as effective as brief pulse machines.

Establishing a patient's seizure threshold is not straightforward. A 40 times variability in seizure thresholds occurs among patients. In addition, during the course of ECT treatment, a patient's seizure threshold may increase 25 to 200 percent. The seizure threshold is also higher in men than in women and higher in older than in younger adults. A common technique is to initiate treatment at an electrical stimulus that is thought to be below the seizure threshold for a particular patient and then to increase this intensity by 100 percent for unilateral placement and by 50 percent for bilateral placement until the seizure threshold is reached. A debate in the literature concerns whether a minimally suprathreshold dose, a moderately suprathreshold dose (one and a half times the threshold), or a high suprathreshold dose (three times the threshold) is preferable. The debate about stimulus intensity resembles the debate about electrode placement. Essentially, the data support the conclusion that doses of three times the threshold are the most rapidly effective and that minimal suprathreshold doses are associated with the fewest and least severe cognitive adverse effects.

Induced Seizures

A brief muscular contraction, usually strongest in a patient's jaw and facial muscles, is seen concurrently with the flow of stimulus current, regardless of whether a seizure occurs. The first behavioral sign of the seizure is often a plantar extension, which lasts 10 to 20 seconds and marks the tonic phase. This phase is followed by rhythmic (i.e., clonic) contractions that decrease in frequency and finally disappear. The tonic phase is marked by high-frequency, sharp EEG activity on which a higher frequency muscle artifact may be superimposed. During the clonic phase, bursts of polyspike activity occur simultaneously with the muscular contractions but usually persist for at least a few seconds after the clonic movements stop.

Monitoring Seizures. A physician must have an objective measure that a bilateral generalized seizure has occurred after the stimulation. The physician should be able to observe either some evidence of tonic-clonic movements or electrophysiological evidence of seizure activity from the EEG or electromyogram (EMG). Seizures with unilateral ECT are asymmetrical, with higher ictal EEG amplitudes over the stimulated hemisphere than over the nonstimulated hemisphere. Occasionally, unilateral seizures are induced; for this reason, at least a single pair of EEG electrodes should be placed over the contralateral hemisphere when using unilateral ECT. For a seizure to be effective in the course of ECT, it should last at least 25 seconds.

Failure to Induce Seizures. If a particular stimulus fails to cause a seizure of sufficient duration, up to four attempts at seizure induction can be tried during a course of treatment. The onset of seizure activity is sometimes delayed as long as 20 to 40 seconds after the stimulus administration. If a stimulus fails to result in a seizure, the contact between the electrodes and the skin should be checked, and the intensity of the stimulus should be increased by 25 to 100 percent. The clinician can also change the anesthetic agent to minimize increases in the seizure threshold caused by the anesthetic. Additional procedures to lower the seizure threshold include hyperventilation and administration of 500 to 2,000 mg IV of caffeine sodium benzoate 5 to 10 minutes before the stimulus.

Prolonged and Tardive Seizures. Prolonged seizures (seizures lasting more than 180 seconds) and status epilepticus can be terminated either with additional doses of the barbiturate anesthetic agent or with IV diazepam (Valium) (5 to 10 mg). Management of such complications should be accompanied by intubation, because the oral airway is insufficient to maintain adequate ventilation over an extended apneic period. Tardive seizures—that is, additional seizures appearing some time after the ECT treatment—may develop in patients with preexisting seizure disorders. Rarely, ECT precipitates the development of an epileptic disorder in patients. Such situations should be managed clinically as if they were pure epileptic disorders.

Number and Spacing of Treatments

Electroconvulsive therapy treatments are usually administered two to three times a week; twice-weekly treatments are associated with less memory impairment than thrice-weekly treatments. In general, the course of treatment of major depressive disorder can take 6 to 12 treatments (although up to 20 sessions are possible); the treatment of manic episodes can take 8 to 20 treatments; the treatment of schizophrenia can take more than 15 treatments; and the treatment of catatonia and delirium can take as few as 1 to 4 treatments. Treatment should continue until the patient achieves what is considered the maximal therapeutic response. Further treatment does not yield any therapeutic benefit, but increases the severity and duration of the adverse effects. The point of maximal improvement is usually thought to occur when a patient fails to continue to improve after two consecutive treatments. If a patient is not improving after 6 to 10 sessions, bilateral placement and high-density treatment (three times the seizure threshold) should be attempted before ECT is abandoned.

Multiple Monitored Electroconvulsive Therapy. Multiple monitored ECT (MMECT) involves giving multiple ECT stimuli during a single session, most commonly two bilateral stimuli within 2 minutes. This approach may be warranted in severely ill patients and in those at especially high risk from the anesthetic procedures. MMECT is associated with the most frequent occurrences of serious cognitive adverse effects.

Maintenance Treatment

A short-term course of ECT induces a remission in symptoms but does not, of itself, prevent a relapse. Post-ECT maintenance treatment should always be considered. Maintenance therapy is generally pharmacological, but maintenance ECT treatments (weekly, biweekly, or monthly) have been reported to be effective relapse prevention treatments, although data from large studies are lacking. Indications for maintenance ECT treatments can include rapid relapse after initial ECT, severe symptoms, psychotic symptoms, and the inability to tolerate medications. If ECT was used because a patient was unresponsive to a specific medication, then, following ECT, the patient should be given a trial of a different medication.

Failure of Electroconvulsive Therapy Trial

Patients who fail to improve after a trial of ECT should again be treated with the pharmacological agents that failed in the past. Although the data are primarily anecdotal, many reports indicate that patients who had previously failed to improve while taking an antidepressant drug do improve while taking the same drug after receiving a course of ECT treatments, even if the ECT seemed to be a therapeutic failure. Nonetheless, with the increased availability of drugs that act at diverse receptor sites, it is less often necessary to return to a drug that has failed than it was formerly.

ADVERSE EFFECTS

Contraindications

Electroconvulsive therapy has no absolute contraindications, only situations in which a patient is at increased risk and has an increased need for close monitoring. Pregnancy is not a contraindication for ECT, and fetal monitoring is generally considered unnecessary unless the pregnancy is high risk or complicated. Patients with space-occupying central nervous system lesions are at increased risk for edema and brain herniation after ECT. If the lesion is small, however, pretreatment with dexamethasone (Decadron) is given, and hypertension is controlled during the seizure, and the risk of serious complications can be minimized for these patients. Patients who have increased intracerebral pressure or are at risk for cerebral bleeding (e.g., those with cerebrovascular diseases and aneurysms) are at risk during ECT because of the increased cerebral blood flow during the seizure. This risk can be lessened, although not eliminated, by control of the patient's blood pressure during the treatment. Patients with recent myocardial infarctions are another high-risk group, although the risk is greatly diminished 2 weeks after the myocardial infarction and is even further reduced 3 months after the infarction. Patients with hypertension should be stabilized on their antihypertensive medications before ECT is administered. Propranolol (Inderal) and sublingual nitroglycerin can also be used to protect such patients during treatment.

Mortality

The mortality rate with ECT is about 0.002 percent per treatment and 0.01 percent for each patient. These numbers compare favorably with the risks associated with general anesthesia and childbirth. ECT death is usually from cardiovascular complications and is most likely to occur in patients whose cardiac status is already compromised.

Central Nervous System Effects

Common adverse effects associated with ECT are headache, confusion, and delirium shortly after the seizure while the patient is coming out of anesthesia. Marked confusion may occur in up to 10 percent of patients within 30 minutes of the seizure and can be treated with barbiturates and benzodiazepines. Delirium is usually most pronounced after the first few treatments and in patients who receive bilateral ECT or who have coexisting neurological disorders. The delirium characteristically clears within days or a few weeks at the longest.

Memory. The greatest concern about ECT is the association between ECT and memory loss. About 75 percent of all patients given ECT say that the memory impairment is the worst adverse effect. Although memory impairment during a course of treatment is almost the rule, follow-up data indicate that almost all patients are back to their cognitive baselines after 6 months. Some patients, however, complain of persistent memory difficulties. For example, a patient may not remember the events leading up to the hospitalization and ECT, and such autobiographical memories may never be recalled. The degree of cognitive impairment during treatment and the time it takes to return to baseline are related, in part, to the amount of electrical stimulation used during treatment. Memory impairment is most often reported by patients who have experienced little improvement with ECT. Despite the memory impairment, which usually resolves, no evidence indicates brain damage caused by ECT. This subject has been the focus of several brain-imaging studies, using a variety of modalities; virtually all concluded that permanent brain damage is not an adverse effect of ECT. Neurologists and epileptologists generally agree that seizures that last less than 30 minutes do not cause permanent neuronal damage.

Other Adverse Effects of Electroconvulsive Therapy

Fractures often accompanied treatments in the early days of ECT. With routine use of muscle relaxants, fractures of long bones or vertebrae should not occur. Some patients, however, may break teeth or experience back pain because of contractions during the procedure. Muscle soreness can occur in some individuals, but it often results from the effects of muscle depolarization by succinylcholine and is most likely to be particularly troublesome after the first session in a series. This soreness can be treated with mild analgesics, including nonsteroidal anti-inflammatory drugs (NSAIDs). A significant minority of patients experience nausea, vomiting, and headaches following an ECT treatment. Nausea and vomiting can be prevented by treatment with antiemetics at the time of ECT (e.g., metoclopramide [Reglan], 10 mg IV, or prochlorperazine [Compazine], 10 mg IV; ondansetron [Zofran] is an acceptable alternative if adverse effects preclude use of dopamine receptor antagonists).

Electroconvulsive therapy can be associated with headaches, although this effect is usually readily manageable. Headaches often respond to NSAIDs given in the ECT recovery period. In patients with severe headaches, pretreatment with ketorolac (Toradol) (30 to 60 mg IV), an NSAID approved for brief parenteral use, can be helpful. Acetaminophen (Tylenol), tramadol (Ultram), propoxyphene (Darvon), and more potent analgesia provided by opioids can be used individually or in various combinations (e.g., pretreatment with ketorolac and postseizure management with acetaminophen-propoxyphene) to manage more intractable headache. ECT can induce migrainous headache and related symptoms; sumatriptan (Imitrex) (6 mg SC or 25 mg orally) may be a useful addition to the agents described above. Ergot compounds can exacerbate cardiovascular changes observed during ECT and probably should not be a component of ECT pretreatment.

References

Baghai TC, di Michele F, Schule C, Eser D, Zwanzger P, Pasini A, Romeo E, Rupprecht R. Plasma concentrations of neuroactive steroids before and after electroconvulsive therapy in major depression. *Neuropsychopharmacology.* 2005;30(6):1181–1186.

Byrne P, Cassidy B, Higgins P. Knowledge and attitudes towards electroconvulsive therapy among health care professionals and students. *J ECT.* 2006;22(2):133.

Dombrovski AY, Mulsant BH, Haskett RF, Prudic J, Begley AE, Sackeim HA. Predictors of remission after electroconvulsive therapy in unipolar major depression. *J Clin Psychiatry.* 2005;66(8):1043–1049.

Gershon AA, Dannon PN, Grunhaus L. Transcranial magnetic stimulation in the treatment of depression. *Am J Psychiatry.* 2003;160:835.

Kho KH, van Vreeswijk MF, Simpson S, Zwinderman AH. A meta-analysis of electroconvulsive therapy efficacy in depression. *J ECT.* 2003;19:139.

Lisanby SH, Luber B, Schlaepfer TE, Sackheim HA. Safety and feasibility of magnetic seizure therapy (MST) in major depression: Randomized within-subject comparison with electroconvulsive therapy. *Neuropsychopharmacology.* 2003;28:1852.

Marangell LB, Silver JM, Goff DC, Yudofsky SC. Psychopharmacology and electroconvulsive therapy. In: Hales RE, Yudofsky SC, eds. *Essentials of Clinical Psychiatry.* 2nd ed. Washington DC: American Psychiatric Publishing, Inc.; 2004:783.

Munk-Olsen T, Laursen TM, Videbech P, Rosenberg R, Mortensen PB. Electroconvulsive therapy: Predictors and trends in utilization from 1976 to 2000. *J ECT.* 2006;22(2):127.

Perera TD, Luber B, Nobler MS, Prudic J, Anderson C, Sackheim HA. Seizure expression during electroconvulsive therapy: Relationships with clinical outcome and cognitive side effects. *Neuropsychopharmacology.* 2004;29:813.

Prudic J. Electroconvulsive therapy. In: Sadock BJ, Sadock VA, eds. *Kaplan & Sadock's Comprehensive Textbook of Psychiatry.* 8th ed. Vol. 2. Baltimore: Lippincott Williams & Wilkins; 2005:2968.

Prudic J, Olfson M, Marcus SC, Fuller RB, Sackheim HA. Effectiveness of electroconvulsive therapy in community settings. *Biol Psychiatry.* 2004;55:301.

Ucok A, Cakr S. Electroconvulsive therapy in first-episode schizophrenia. *J ECT.* 2006;22(1):38–42.

Vishne T, Amiaz R, Grunhaus L. Promethazine for the treatment of agitation after electroconvulsive therapy: A case series. *J of ECT.* 2005;21(2):118–121.

Warnell RL, Duk AD, Christison GW, Haviland MG. Teaching electroconvulsive therapy to medical students: Effects of instructional method on knowledge and attitudes. *Academic Psychiatry.* 2005;29(5):433–436.

36.37.2 Other Brain Stimulation Methods

In addition to electroconvulsive therapy (ECT), described in the Section 36.37.1, a variety of other techniques have been developed to modify the brain anatomically and functionally in an effort to cure mental illness. These techniques were developed to treat patients who had not responded to repeated exposures

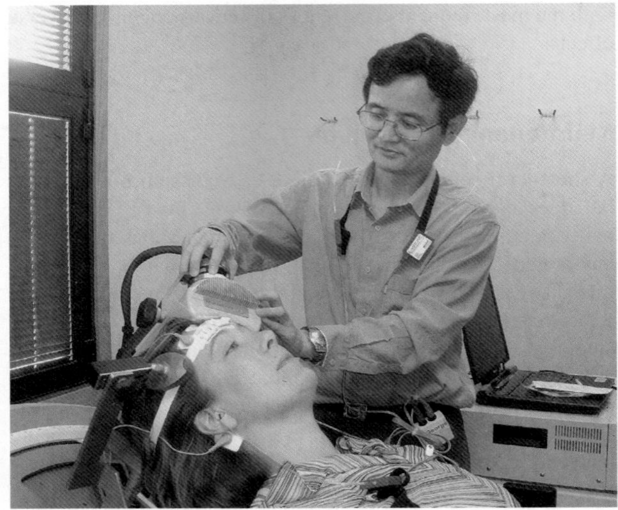

FIGURE 36.37.2–1

For TMS, the subject is awake and alert and sitting in a reclined chair. The headholder maintains the TMS coil in the correct position next to the prefrontal cortex. In antidepressant trials, patients receive TMS in this manner for about 30 minutes every weekday for several weeks. **Note**: The patient is wearing noise-cancelling earphones (as is the TMS treator). She also has the active sham system being used in the NIMH optimization of TMS for the treatment of depression clinical trial, with EEG being recorded and an active sham system. TMS, transcranial magnetic stimulation; NIMH, National Institute of Mental Health; EEG, electroencephalogram. (From George MS, Nahas Z, Li X, et al. Current status of daily repetitive transcranial magnetic stimulation for the treatment of depression. *Primary Psychiatry.* 2005:12(10), with permission.)

to conventional treatments and whose illnesses were extraordinarily severe and incapacitating. Some of these methods are described in this section.

REPEATED TRANSCRANIAL MAGNETIC STIMULATION

Repeated transcranial magnetic stimulation (rTMS) is a noninvasive technique for stimulating cells of the cerebral cortex. It creates a time-varying magnetic field in which a localized pulse magnetic field over the surface of the head depolarizes the superficial neurons. TMS uses a hand-held magnet to allow focused electrical stimulation across the scalp and cranium without the pain associated with percutaneous electrical stimulation (Fig. 36.37.2–1). If TMS pulses are delivered repetitively and rhythmically, the technique is called rTMS. rTMS was originally used to map cortical motor control and hemisphere dominance. Stimulating the motor cortex with rTMS results in a contralateral motor response. Likewise, stimulating Broca's area with rTMS has resulted in speech blockage. Currently, the potential use of rTMS for the treatment of neurological and psychiatric disorders is being explored actively.

In rTMS, a powerful electrical current is passed through a small coil applied to the scalp. This current generates a focused magnetic field of 1.5 to 2.0 T that passes through the scalp and is largely unimpeded by bone or tissue. The magnetic field, in turn, depolarizes brain cells to a depth of 2 cm from the coil. Cortical interneurons are more likely to be stimulated than are cortical output cells, because the interneurons tend to lie parallel to the brain surface. rTMS uses magnetic stimulators with multiple capacitors capable of generating rapid pulses as great as 60 Hz. Low-frequency pulses in the range of 1 Hz may have an inhibitory effect on cortical cells, whereas higher frequencies have an excitatory effect. Higher intensities of stimulation might be needed to reach the prefrontal cortex, especially in elderly patients with prefrontal atrophy. Also, the therapeutic effects of TMS take several weeks to consolidate, and, thus, the initial trials of TMS in acute depression, which have lasted 2 weeks or less, may be too short to assess efficacy.

Some psychiatric conditions, such as major depression, may be characterized by hypoactive cortical areas. Functional imaging, including positron emission tomography (PET), has revealed a relative hypofrontality in some patients with major depression. It has been proposed that rTMS stimulation of these frontal areas would relieve symptoms of depression.

A metaanalysis of 23 published comparisons for controlled TMS prefrontal antidepressant trials and noted a moderate to large antidepressant effect. In addition, recent functional imaging studies have suggested that the baseline hypofrontality associated with major depressive disorder can be reversed with active treatment but not with a sham rTMS procedure. In addition to major depressive disorder, rTMS has shown some preliminary efficacy in obsessive-compulsive disorder (OCD) and in posttraumatic stress disorder (PTSD). The procedure is considered to be safe and no cognitive, neurological or cardiovascular adverse events have been reported with its use.

The application of rTMS to psychiatric conditions has lagged behind its neurological applications. rTMS has been used to map the motor cortex, to help determine hemispheric dominance, and to probe short-term memory. In some symptoms of Parkinson's disease, including bradykinesia, diminished reaction time has improved transiently with rTMS. Finally, rTMS has been used to help elucidate the pathophysiology of migraine headache, and some patients have had temporary symptom relief with rTMS.

Transcranial magnetic stimulation appears safe, but the major serious concern is its causing a seizure. This is more probable with rTMS versus single-pulse TMS. As best as can currently be determined, TMS at moderate intensity has no clear lasting adverse effects.

The most interesting aspect of TMS or rTMS might be its ability to combine with functional imaging on directly monitoring TMS effects on the brain. This allows delineation of not only the behavioral neuropsychology of depression (and perhaps other psychiatric disorders), but also some of the pathophysiological brain circuits in the brain involved in the etiology of various psychiatric syndromes.

Studies are underway by the National Institute of Mental Health to fully evaluate this method. The neurobiological mechanisms of action require further study as does determining which patients are most likely to respond. Further work is needed.

VAGAL NERVE STIMULATION

Since 1985, a tremendous amount of work has been done on how the sensory afferent fibers from the vagal nerve cause brain changes. The vagal nerve (cranial nerve X) is a parasympathetic efferent nerve that relays information from the nucleus tractus solitarius (NTS) to many areas of the brain, including the locus ceruleus. Vagal nerve stimulation (VNS) refers to stimulation of the left vagus nerve using commercially available devices. The VNS is delivered through a bipolar pulse generator, which is multiprogrammable and implanted in the left chest wall through a bipolar lead (Fig. 36.37.2–2).

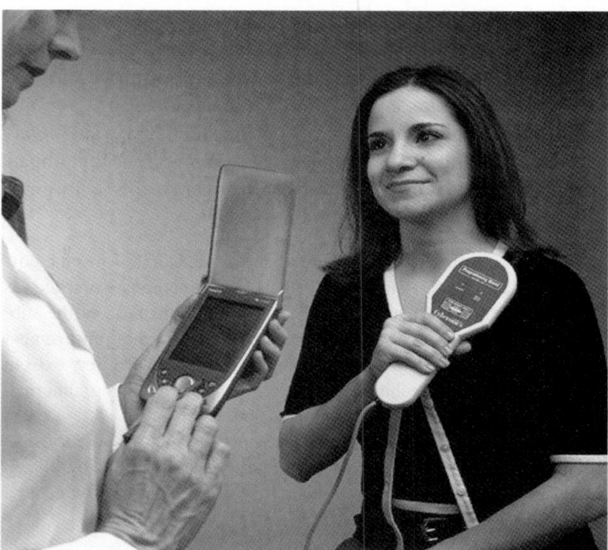

FIGURE 36.37.2–2
Demonstration of physician using a handheld computer and programming want to adjust the settings of the VNS device in an outpatient setting. VNS, vagal nerve stimulation. (From Marangell LB, Martinez M, Martinez JM, et al. Vagus nerve stimulation: A new tool for treating depression. *Primary Psychiatry.* 2005;12(10):41, with permission.)

Vagal nerve stimulation is an alternative treatment for patients with refractory epilepsy who cannot tolerate surgery for the epileptic seizures. With increasing use and knowledge of safety (minimal gastrointestinal [GI] and cardiac side effects despite VNS), it is used in the less severely ill patient. It has been estimated that VNS leads to a 50 percent reduction of seizures in approximately 30 percent of patients with seizure who are treated, with approximately 10 percent of patients becoming seizure free over long periods of time.

Observations of mood effects of VNS in patients with epilepsy have led to a possible indication for the use of VNS in depression. It has been shown through brain imaging studies that VNS affects the metabolism of limbic structures that are involved in mood stabilization, and neurochemical effects on brain monoamines are known to be involved in regulation of depressed mood.

Vagal nerve stimulation open studies in depression have noted a 50 percent response in 12 of 30 patients with treatment-resistant depression and a complete remission (Hamilton Depression [HAMD] Scale score <10) in 5 of 30 patients. An extension of this study over 6 months found response (50 percent reduction in HAMD score) in 17 of 30 patients who were described to have low to moderate treatment resistance. VNS did not seem to have any efficacy in severe treatment resistance. The VNS procedure does not seem to give adverse effects, with the exception of mild transient hoarseness in approximately 55 percent of patients.

Vagal nerve stimulation was recently approved by the US Food and Drug Administration (FDA) as an adjunctive long-term treatment for patients with recurrent or chronic major depressive disorders who have failed at least four antidepressant medication trials.

DEEP BRAIN STIMULATION

Deep brain stimulation (DBS) involves creating a small hole in the skull and passing a fine wire into selected brain regions. This wire can be excited on its terminal end by a pacemaker-like device connected subdermally and implanted in the chest wall. When the DBS is implanted, the wire stimulates at high frequencies and temporarily stops the function at that region.

Deep brain stimulation in the thalamus is approved for the treatment of Parkinson's disease. The technique involves implanting DBS at the subthalamic nucleus and the internal globus pallidus. This allows determination of motor regions that impair movements and, thus, the ability to counteract this with high-frequency DBS gives more fluid movement.

Deep brain stimulation of the internal capsule has shown some positive effects for OCD. The mood effects are sometimes worsened, as a case report noted a patient became depressed with DBS at the subthalamic nucleus. It is possible that, with respect to the improvement in Parkinson's disease, mood-enhancing effects with DBS may exist at other locations. The technique has been of use in reducing abnormal movements in patients with Tourette's disorder.

Deep brain stimulation is less invasive than ablative surgery. The device can be turned off, and wires can be removed without significant sequelae. It is under review whether it will be approved for general use.

PSYCHOSURGERY

Psychosurgery involves surgical modification of the brain with the goal of reducing the symptoms of the most severely ill psychiatric patients who have not responded adequately to less radical treatments. Psychosurgical procedures focus on lesion-specific brain regions (e.g., lobotomies and cingulotomies) or their connecting tracts (e.g., tractotomies and leukotomies). Psychosurgical techniques are also used in the treatment of neurological disorders, such as epilepsy and chronic pain disorder.

The interest in psychosurgical approaches to mental disorders has only recently been rekindled. The renewed interest is based on several factors, including much-improved techniques that allow neurosurgeons to make exact stereotactically placed lesions, improved preoperative diagnoses, and comprehensive preoperative and postoperative psychological assessments. New techniques also facilitate gathering complete follow-up data and enable a growing understanding of the neuroanatomical basis of some mental disorders.

In 1935, after C. F. Jacobsen and John F. Fulton at Yale University in New Haven, Connecticut, demonstrated that frontal lobe ablation in a monkey had a calming effect, Antonio Egas Moniz, working in Portugal, severed frontal lobe white matter in 20 psychotic patients and reported a decrease in their tension and psychotic symptoms. In 1936, Walter Freeman and James Watts at George Washington University in Washington, DC, introduced the psychosurgical technique of prefrontal lobotomy to the United States. Although early procedures required burr holes or other exposure of the brain, Freeman eventually developed the technique of transorbital leukotomy, which involved the introduction and lateral movement of a sharp instrument through the eye socket as a method of sectioning the white matter of the frontal lobes. By the late 1940s, psychosurgery was being performed worldwide, and an estimated 5,000 patients were being operated on each year. In 1949, Egas Moniz won the Nobel Prize for his work in developing psychosurgical techniques. Shortly thereafter, the introduction of antipsychotic drugs and the increasing public concern about the ethics of psychosurgery led to a near abandonment of these techniques for the treatment of psychiatric patients, although psychosurgical procedures for pain control and epilepsy continued to be used.

Stereotactic neurosurgical equipment now allows neurosurgeons to place discrete lesions in the brain. Radioactive implants, cryoprobes, electrical coagulation, proton beams, and ultrasonic waves are used to make the actual lesions.

The major indication for psychosurgery is the presence of a debilitating, chronic mental disorder that has not responded to any other treatment. A reasonable guideline is that the disorder should have been present for 5 years, during which a wide variety of alternative treatment approaches was attempted. Chronic intractable major depressive disorder and OCD are the two disorders reportedly most responsive to psychosurgery. The presence of vegetative symptoms and marked anxiety further increases the likelihood of a successful therapeutic outcome. Whether psychosurgery is a reasonable treatment for intractable and extreme aggression is still controversial. Psychosurgery is not indicated for the treatment of schizophrenia, and data about manic episodes are controversial.

When patients are carefully selected, between 50 and 70 percent have significant therapeutic improvement with psychosurgery. Fewer than 3 percent become worse. Continued improvement is often noted from 1 to 2 years after surgery, and patients often respond better to traditional pharmacological and behavioral treatment approaches than they did before psychosurgery. Postoperative seizures are present in fewer than 1 percent of patients, and these seizures are usually controlled with phenytoin (Dilantin). As measured by intelligence quotient (IQ) scores, cognitive abilities improve after surgery, probably because of patients' increased ability to attend to cognitive tasks. No undesired changes in personality have been noted with modern limited procedures.

References

Anderson SW, Booker MB Jr. Cognitive behavioral therapy versus psychosurgery for refractory obsessive-compulsive disorder. *J Neuropsychiatry Clin Neurosci*. 2006;18(1):129.

Guehl D, Edwards R, Cuny E, Burbaud P, Rougier A, Modolo J, Beuter A. Statistical determination of the optimal subthalamic nucleus stimulation site in patients with Parkinson disease. *J Neurosurg*. 2007;106(1):101–10.

Khedr EM, Rothwell JC, Shawky OA, Ahmed MA, Hamdy A. Effect of daily repetitive transcranial magnetic stimulation on motor performance in Parkinson's disease. *Mov Disord*. 2006;21(12):2201–5.

Kim YH, You SH, Ko MH, Park JW, Lee KH, Jang SH, Yoo WK, Hallett M. Repetitive transcranial magnetic stimulation-induced corticomotor excitability and associated motor skill acquisition in chronic stroke. *Stroke*. 2006;37(6):1471–6.

Kopell BH, Machado AG, Rezai AR. Not your father's lobotomy: Psychiatric surgery revisited. *Clin Neurosurg*. 2005:52:315–30.

Marrosu F, Maleci A, Cocco E, Puligheddu M, Marrosu MG. Vagal nerve stimulation effects on cerebellar tremor in multiple sclerosis. *Neurology*. 2005;65(3):490.

Pahwa R, Lyons KE, Wilkinson SB, Simpson RK Jr, Ondo WG, Tarsy D, Norregaard T, Hubble JP, Smith DA, Hauser RA, Jankovic J. Long-term evaluation of deep brain stimulation of the thalamus. *J Neurosurg*. 2006;104(4):506–12.

Peselow ED. Other pharmacological and biological therapies. In: Sadock BJ, Sadock VA, eds. *Kaplan & Sadock's Comprehensive Textbook of Psychiatry*. 8th ed. Vol 2. Baltimore: Lippincott Williams and Wilkins; 2005:2990.

Rauch SL, Greenberg BD, Cosgrove GR. Neurosurgical treatments and deep brain stimulation. In: Sadock BJ, Sadock VA, eds. *Kaplan & Sadock's Comprehensive Textbook of Psychiatry*. 8th ed. Vol 2. Baltimore: Lippincott Williams and Wilkins; 2005:2983.

Sailer A, Cunic DI, Paradiso GO, Gunraj CA, Wagle-Shukla A, Moro E, Lozano AM, Lang AE, Chen R. Subthalamic nucleus stimulation modulates afferent inhibition in Parkinson disease. *Neurology*. 2007;68(5):356–63.

37 Child Psychiatry: Assessment, Examination, and Psychological Testing

Psychiatric assessment of a child or adolescent includes identifying the reasons for referral; assessing the nature and extent of the child's psychological and behavioral difficulties; and determining family, school, social, and developmental factors that may be influencing the child's emotional well-being.

A comprehensive evaluation of a child is composed of interviews with the parents, the child, and other family members; gathering information regarding the child's current school functioning; and often, a standardized assessment of the child's intellectual level and academic achievement. In some cases, standardized measures of developmental level and neuropsychological assessments are useful. Psychiatric evaluations of children are rarely initiated by the child, so clinicians must obtain information from the family and the school to understand the reasons for the evaluation. In some cases, the court or a child protective service agency may initiate a psychiatric evaluation. Children can be excellent informants about symptoms related to mood and inner experiences, such as psychotic phenomena, sadness, fears, and anxiety, but they often have difficulty with the chronology of symptoms and are sometimes reticent about reporting behaviors that have gotten them into trouble. Very young children often cannot articulate their experiences verbally and do better showing their feelings and preoccupations in a play situation.

The first step in the comprehensive evaluation of a child or adolescent is to obtain a full description of the current concerns and a history of the child's previous psychiatric and medical problems. This is often done with the parents for school-aged children, whereas adolescents may be seen alone first, to get their perception of the situation. Direct interview and observation of the child is usually next, followed by psychological testing, when indicated.

Clinical interviews offer the most flexibility in understanding the evolution of problems and in establishing the role of environmental factors and life events, but they may not systematically cover all psychiatric diagnostic categories. To increase the breadth of information generated, the clinician may use semistructured interviews such as the *Kiddie Schedule for Affective Disorders and Schizophrenia for School-Age Children* (K-SADS); structured interviews such as the *National Institute for Mental Health Diagnostic Interview Schedule for Children Version IV* (NIMH DISC-IV); and rating scales, such as the *Child Behavior Checklist* and *Connors Parent or Teacher Rating Scale for ADHD*.

It is not uncommon for interviews from different sources, such as parents, teachers, and school counselors, to reflect different or even contradictory information about a given child. When faced with conflictual information, the clinician must determine whether apparent contradictions actually reflect an accurate picture of the child in different settings. Once a complete history is obtained from the parents, the child is examined, the child's current functioning at home and at school is assessed, and psychological testing is completed, the clinician can use all the available information to make a best-estimate diagnosis and can then make recommendations.

Once clinical information is obtained about a given child or adolescent, it is the clinician's task to determine whether criteria are met for one or more psychiatric disorder according to the text revision of the 4th edition of the *Diagnostic and Statistic Manual of Mental Disorders* (DSM-IV-TR). This most current version is a categorical classification reflecting the consensus on constellations of symptoms believed to comprise discrete and valid psychiatric disorders. Psychiatric disorders are defined by the DSM-IV-TR as a clinically significant set of symptoms that is associated with impairment in one or more areas of functioning. Whereas clinical situations requiring intervention do not always fall within the context of a given psychiatric disorder, the importance of identifying psychiatric disorders when they arise is to facilitate meaningful investigation of childhood psychopathology.

CLINICAL INTERVIEWS

To conduct a useful interview with a child of any age, clinicians must be familiar with normal development to place the child's responses in the proper perspective. For example, a young child's discomfort on separation from a parent and a school-age child's lack of clarity about the purpose of the interview are both perfectly normal and should not be misconstrued as psychiatric symptoms. Furthermore, behavior that is normal in a child at one age, such as temper tantrums in a 2-year-old, takes on a different meaning, for example, in a 17-year-old.

The interviewer's first task is to engage the child and develop a rapport so that the child is comfortable. The interviewer should inquire about the child's concept of the purpose of the interview and should ask what the parents have told the child. If the child appears to be confused about the reason for the interview, the examiner may opt to summarize the parents' concerns in a developmentally appropriate and supportive manner. During the interview with the child, the clinician seeks to learn about the child's relationships with family members and peers, academic achievement and peer relationships in school, and the child's pleasurable activities. An estimate of the child's cognitive functioning is a part of the mental status examination.

The extent of confidentiality in child assessment is correlated with the age of the child. In most cases, almost all specific information can appropriately be shared with the parents of a very young child, whereas privacy and permission of an older child or adolescent are mandated before sharing information with parents. School-age and older children are informed that if the clinician becomes concerned that any child is dangerous to himself or herself or to others, this information must be shared with parents and, at times, additional adults. As part of a psychiatric assessment of a child of any age, the clinician must determine whether that child is safe in his or her environment and must develop an index of suspicion about whether the child is a victim of abuse or neglect. Whenever there is a suspicion of child maltreatment, the local child protective service agency must be notified.

Toward the end of the interview, the child may be asked in an open-ended manner whether he or she would like to bring up anything else. Each child should be complimented for his or her cooperation and thanked for participating in the interview, and the interview should end on a positive note.

Infants and Young Children

Assessments of infants usually begin with the parents present, because very young children may be frightened by the interview situation; the interview with the parents present also allows the clinician to assess the parent–infant interaction. Infants may be referred for a variety of reasons, including high levels of irritability, difficulty being consoled, eating disturbances, poor weight gain, sleep disturbances, withdrawn behavior, lack of engagement in play, and developmental delay. The clinician assesses areas of functioning that include motor development, activity level, verbal communication, ability to engage in play, problem-solving skills, adaptation to daily routines, relationships, and social responsiveness.

The child's developmental level of functioning is determined by combining observations made during the interview with standardized developmental measures. Observations of play reveal a child's developmental level and reflect the child's emotional state and preoccupations. The examiner can interact with an infant age 18 months or younger in a playful manner by using such games as peek-a-boo. Children between the ages of 18 months and 3 years can be observed in a playroom. Children ages 2 years or older may exhibit symbolic play with toys, revealing more in this mode than through conversation. The use of puppets and dolls with children under 6 years of age is often an effective way to elicit information, especially if questions are directed to the dolls, rather than to the child.

School-Age Children

Some school-age children are at ease when conversing with an adult; others are hampered by fear, anxiety, poor verbal skills, or oppositional behavior. School-age children can usually tolerate a 45-minute session. The room should be sufficiently spacious for the child to move around, but not so large as to reduce intimate contact between the examiner and the child. Part of the interview can be reserved for unstructured play, and various toys can be made available to capture the child's interest and to elicit themes and feelings. Children in lower grades may be more interested in the toys in the room, whereas by the sixth grade, children may be more comfortable with the interview process and less likely to show spontaneous play.

The initial part of the interview explores the child's understanding of the reasons for the meeting. The clinician should confirm that the interview was not set up because the child is "in trouble" or as a punishment for "bad" behavior. Techniques that can facilitate disclosure of feelings include asking the child to draw peers, family members, a house, or anything else that comes to mind. The child can then be questioned about the drawings. Children may be asked to reveal three wishes, to describe the best and worst events of their lives, and to name a favorite person to be stranded with on a desert island. Games such as Donald W. Winnicott's "squiggle," in which the examiner draws a curved line and then the child and the examiner take turns continuing the drawing, may facilitate conversation.

Questions that are partially open-ended with some multiple choices may elicit the most complete answers from school-age children. Simple, closed (yes or no) questions may not elicit sufficient information, and completely open-ended questions can overwhelm a school-age child who cannot construct a chronological narrative. These techniques often result in a shoulder shrug from the child. The use of indirect commentary—such as, "I once knew a child who felt very sad when he moved away from all his friends"—is helpful, although the clinician must be careful not to lead the child into confirming what the child thinks the clinician wants to hear. School-age children respond well to clinicians who help them compare moods or feelings by asking them to rate feelings on a scale of 1 to 10.

Adolescents

Adolescents usually have distinct ideas about why the evaluation was initiated, and can usually give a chronological account of the recent events leading to the evaluation, although some may disagree with the need for the evaluation. The clinician should clearly communicate the value of hearing the story from an adolescent's point of view and must be careful to reserve judgment and not assign blame. Adolescents may be concerned about confidentiality, and clinicians can assure them that permission will be requested from them before any specific information is shared with parents, except situations involving danger to the adolescent or others, in which case confidentiality must be sacrificed. Adolescents can be approached in an open-ended manner; however, when silences occur during the interview, the clinician should attempt to reengage the patient. Clinicians can explore what the adolescent believes the outcome of the evaluation will be (change of school, hospitalization, removal from home, removal of privileges).

Some adolescents approach the interview with apprehension or hostility, but open up when it becomes evident that the clinician is neither punitive nor judgmental. Clinicians must be aware of their own responses to adolescents' behavior (countertransference) and stay focused on the therapeutic process even in the face of defiant, angry, or difficult teenagers. Clinicians should set appropriate limits and should postpone or discontinue an interview if they feel threatened or if patients become destructive to property or engage in self-injurious behavior. Every interview should include an exploration of suicidal thoughts, assaultive behavior, psychotic symptoms, substance use, and knowledge of safe sexual practices along with a sexual history. Once rapport has been established, many adolescents appreciate the opportunity to tell their side of the story and may reveal things that they have not disclosed to anyone else.

Family Interview

An interview with parents and the patient may take place first or may occur later in the evaluation. Sometimes, an interview with the entire family, including siblings, can be enlightening. The purpose is to observe the attitudes and behavior of the parents toward the patient and the responses of the children to their parents. The clinician's job is to maintain a nonthreatening atmosphere in which each member of the family can speak freely without feeling that the clinician is taking sides with any particular member. Although child psychiatrists generally function as advocates for the child, the clinician must validate each family member's feelings in this setting, because lack of communication often contributes to the patient's problems.

Parents

The interview with the patient's parents or caretakers is necessary to get a chronological picture of the child's growth and development. A thorough developmental history and details of any stressors or important events that have influenced the child's development must be elicited. The parents' view of the family dynamics, their marital history, and their own emotional adjustment are also elicited. The family's psychiatric history and the upbringing of the parents are pertinent. Parents are usually the best informants about the child's early development and previous psychiatric and medical illnesses. They may be better able to provide an accurate chronology of past evaluations and treatment. In some cases, especially with older children and adolescents, the parents may be unaware of significant current symptoms or social difficulties of the child. Clinicians elicit the parents' formulation of the causes and nature of their child's problems and ask about expectations about the current assessment.

DIAGNOSTIC INSTRUMENTS

The two main types of diagnostic instruments used by clinicians and researchers are diagnostic interviews and questionnaires. Diagnostic interviews are administered to either children or their parents and are often designed to elicit sufficient information on numerous aspects of functioning to determine whether criteria are met from the DSM-IV-TR.

Semistructured interviews, or "interviewer-based" interviews, such as K-SADS and the *Child and Adolescent Psychiatric Assessment* (CAPA) serve as guides for the clinician. They help the clinician clarify answers to questions about symptoms. Structured interviews, or "respondent-based" interviews, such as NIMH DISC-IV, the *Children's Interview for Psychiatric Syndromes* (ChIPS), and the *Diagnostic Interview for Children and Adolescents* (DICA), basically provide a script for the interviewer without interpretation of the subject's responses. Two other diagnostic instruments use pictures, the *Dominic-R* and the *Pictorial Instrument for Children and Adolescents* (PICA-III-R). These instruments use pictures as cues, along with an accompanying question to elicit information about symptoms, especially for young children as well as for adolescents.

Diagnostic instruments aid the collection of information in a systematic way. Diagnostic instruments, even the most comprehensive, however, cannot replace clinical interviews, because clinical interviews are superior in understanding the chronology of symptoms, the interplay between environmental stressors and emotional responses, and developmental issues. Clinicians often find it helpful to combine the data from diagnostic instruments with clinical material gathered in a comprehensive evaluation.

Questionnaires can cover a broad range of symptom areas, such as the *Achenbach Child Behavior Checklist*, or they can be focused on a particular type of symptomatology and are often called rating scales, such as the *Connors Parent Rating Scale for ADHD*.

Semistructured Diagnostic Interviews

Kiddie Schedule for Affective Disorders and Schizophrenia for School-Age Children. The K-SADS can be used for children from 6 years to 18 years of age. It presents multiple items with some space for further clarification of symptoms. It elicits information on current diagnosis and on symptoms present in the previous year. Another version can also ascertain lifetime diagnoses. It assesses diagnoses according to DSM-IV-TR. This instrument has been used extensively, especially in evaluation of mood disorders, and includes measures of impairment caused by symptoms. The schedule comes in a form for parents to give information about their child and in a version for use directly with the child. The schedule takes about 1 to 1.5 hours to administer. The interviewer should have some training in the field of child psychiatry, but need not be a psychiatrist.

Child and Adolescent Psychiatric Assessment. The CAPA is an "interviewer-based" instrument that can be used for children from 9 to 17 years of age. It comes in modular form so that certain diagnostic entities can be administered without having to give the entire interview. It covers disruptive behavior disorders, mood disorders, anxiety disorders, eating disorders, sleep disorders, elimination disorders, substance use disorders, tic disorders, schizophrenia, posttraumatic stress disorder, and somatization symptoms. It focuses on the 3 months before the interview, called the "primary period." In general, it takes about 1 hour to administer. It has a glossary to aid in decision-making regarding symptoms and provides separate ratings of presence and severity of symptoms. It can be used to determine diagnoses according to the fourth edition of DSM (DSM-IV), the revised third edition of DSM (DSM-III-R), or the tenth revision of *International Statistical Classification of Diseases and Related Health Problems* (ICD-10). Training is necessary to administer this interview, and the interviewer must be prepared to use some clinical judgment in interpreting elicited symptoms.

Structured Diagnostic Interviews

National Institute of Mental Health Interview Schedule for Children Version IV. The NIMH DISC-IV is a highly structured interview designed to assess more than 30 DSM-IV diagnostic entities administered by trained "laypersons." It is available in parallel child and parent forms. The parent form can be used for children from 6 to 17 years of age, and the direct child form of the instrument was designed for children from 9 to 17 years of age. It is applicable for a multitude of diagnoses keyed to DSM-IV-TR. A computer scoring algorithm is available. This instrument assesses the presence of diagnoses that have been present within the last 4 weeks, and also within the last year. Because it is a fully structured interview, the instructions serve as a complete guide for the questions, and the examiner need not have any knowledge of child psychiatry to administer the interview correctly.

Children's Interview for Psychiatric Syndromes. The ChIPS is a highly structured interview designed for use by trained interviewers with children from 6 to 18 years of age. It is composed of 15 sections, and it elicits information on psychiatric symptoms as well as psychosocial stressors targeting 20 psychiatric disorders, according to DSM-IV criteria. There are parent and child forms. It takes approximately 40 minutes to administer the ChIPS. Diagnoses covered include depression, mania, attention-deficit/hyperactivity disorder (ADHD), separation disorder, obsessive-compulsive disorder (OCD), conduct disorder, substance use disorder, anorexia, and bulimia. The ChIPS was designed for use as a screening instrument for clinicians and a diagnostic instrument for clinical and epidemiological research.

Diagnostic Interview for Children and Adolescents. The current version of the DICA was developed in 1997 to assess information resulting in diagnoses according to either DSM-IV or DSM-III-R. Although it was originally designed to be a highly structured interview, it can now be used in a semistructured format. This means that, although interviewers are allowed to use additional questions and probes to clarify elicited information, the method of probing is standardized so that all interviewers will follow a specific pattern. When using the interview with younger children, more flexibility is built in, allowing interviewers to deviate from written questions to ensure that the child understands the question. Parent and child interviews are expected to be used. It covers children 6 to 17 years of age and generally takes 1 to 2 hours to administer. It covers externalizing behavior disorders, anxiety disorders, depressive disorders, and substance abuse disorders, among others.

Pictorial Diagnostic Instruments

Dominic-R. The Dominic-R is a pictorial, fully structured interview designed to elicit psychiatric symptoms from children 6 to 11 years of age. The pictures illustrate abstract emotional and behavioral content of diagnostic entities according to DSM-III-R. The instrument uses a picture of a child called "Dominic" who is experiencing the symptom in question. Some symptoms have more than one picture, with a brief story that is read to the child. Along with each picture is a sentence asking about the situation being shown and asking the child if he or she has experiences similar to the one that Dominic is having. Diagnostic entities covered by the Dominic-R include separation anxiety, generalized anxiety, depression and dysthymia, ADHD, oppositional defiant disorder, conduct disorder, and specific phobia. Although symptoms of the above diagnoses can be fully elicited from the Dominic-R, no specific provision within the instrument inquires about frequency of the symptom, duration, or age of onset. The paper version of this interview takes about 20 minutes, and the computerized version of this instrument takes about 15 minutes. Trained lay-interviewers can administer this interview. Computerized versions of this interview are available with pictures of a child who is white, black, Latino, or Asian.

Pictorial Instrument for Children and Adolescents. PICA-III-R is composed of 137 pictures organized in modules and designed to cover five diagnostic categories, including disorders of anxiety, mood, psychosis, disruptive disorders, and substance use disorder. It is designed to be administered by clinicians and can be used for children and adolescents ranging from 6 to 16 years of age. It provides a categorical (diagnosis present or absent) and a dimensional (range of severity) assessment. This instrument presents pictures of a child experiencing emotional, behavioral, and cognitive symptoms. The child is asked, "How much are you like him/her?" and a five-point rating scale with pictures of a person with open arms in increasing degrees is shown to the child to help him or her identify the severity of the symptoms. It takes about 40 minutes to 1 hour to administer the interview. This instrument is currently keyed to DSM-III-R. It can be used to aid in clinical interviews and in research diagnostic protocols.

QUESTIONNAIRES AND RATING SCALES

Achenbach Child Behavior Checklist

The parent and teacher versions of the *Achenbach Child Behavior Checklist* were developed to cover a broad range of symptoms and several positive attributes related to academic and social competence. The checklist presents items related to mood, frustration tolerance, hyperactivity, oppositional behavior, anxiety, and various other behaviors. The parent version consists of 118 items to be rated 0 (not true), 1 (sometimes true), or 2 (very true). The teacher version is similar, but without the items that apply only to home life. Profiles were developed based on normal children of three different age groups (4to 5, 6 to 11, and 12 to 16).

Such a checklist identifies specific problem areas that might otherwise be overlooked, and it may point out areas in which the child's behavior deviates from that of normal children of the same age group. The checklist is not used specifically to make diagnoses.

Revised Achenbach Behavior Problem Checklist

Consisting of 150 items that cover a variety of childhood behavioral and emotional symptoms, the *Revised Achenbach Behavior Problem Checklist* discriminates between clinic-referred and nonreferred children. Separate subscales have been found to correlate in the appropriate direction with other measures of intelligence, academic achievement, clinical observations, and peer popularity. As with the other broad rating scales, this instrument can help elicit a comprehensive view of a multitude of behavioral areas, but it is not designed to make psychiatric diagnoses.

Connors Abbreviated Parent-Teacher Rating Scale for ADHD

In its original form, the *Connors Abbreviated Parent-Teacher Rating Scale for ADHD* consisted of 93 items rated on a 0 to 3 scale and was subgrouped into 25 clusters, including problems with restlessness, temper, school, stealing, eating, and sleeping. Over the years, multiple versions of this scale were developed and used to aid in systematic identification of children with ADHD. A highly abbreviated form of this rating scale, the *Connors Abbreviated Parent-Teacher Questionnaire*, was developed for use with both parents and teachers by Keith Connors in 1973. It consists of ten items that assess both hyperactivity and inattention.

Brief Impairment Scale

A newly validated 23-item instrument suitable to obtain information on children ranging from 4 years to 17 years, the *Brief Impairment Scale* (BIS) evaluates three domains of functioning: interpersonal relations, school/work functioning, and care/self-fulfillment. This scale is administered to an adult informant about his or her child, does not take long to administer, and provides a global measure of impairment along the above three dimensions. This scale cannot be used to make clinical decisions on individual patients, but it can provide information on the degree of impairment that a given child is experiencing in a certain area.

COMPONENTS OF THE CHILD PSYCHIATRIC EVALUATION

Psychiatric evaluation of a child includes a description of the reason for the referral, the child's past and present functioning, and any test results. An outline of the evaluation is given in Table 37–1.

Identifying Data

To understand the clinical problems to be evaluated, the clinician must first identify the patient and keep in mind the family constellation surrounding the child. The clinician must also pay attention to the source of the referral—that is, whether it is the child's family, school, or another agency—because this influences the family's attitude toward the evaluation. Finally, many informants contribute to the child's evaluation, and each must be identified to gain insight into the child's functioning in different settings.

History

A comprehensive history contains information about the child's current and past functioning, from the child's report, from clinical and structured interviews with the parents, and from information from teachers and previous treating clinicians. The chief complaint and the history of the present illness are generally obtained from both the child and the parents. Naturally, the child will articulate the situation according to his or her developmental level. The developmental history is more accurately obtained from the parents. Psychiatric and medical histories, current physical examination findings, and immunization histories can be augmented with reports from psychiatrists and pediatricians who have treated the child in the past. The child's report is critical in understanding the current situation regarding peer relationships and adjustment to school. Adolescents are the best informants regarding knowledge of safe sexual practices, drug or alcohol use, and suicidal ideation. The family's psychiatric and social histories, and family function are best obtained from the parents.

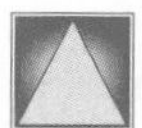

Table 37–1
Child Psychiatric Evaluation

Identifying data
- Identified patient and family members
- Source of referral
- Informants

History
- Chief complaint
- History of present illness
- Developmental history and milestones
- Psychiatric history
- Medical history, including immunizations
- Family social history and parents' marital status
- Educational history and current school functioning
- Peer relationship history
- Current family functioning
- Family psychiatric and medical histories
- Current physical examination

Mental status examination

Neuropsychiatric examination (when applicable)

Developmental, psychological, and educational testing

Formulation and summary

DSM-IV-TR diagnosis

Recommendations and treatment plan

DSM-IV-TR, text revision of the fourth edition of the *Diagnostic and Statistical Manual of Mental Disorders.*

Mental Status Examination

A detailed description of the child's current mental functioning can be obtained through observation and specific questioning. An outline of the mental status examination is presented in Table 37–2. Table 37–3 lists components of a comprehensive neuropsychiatry mental status.

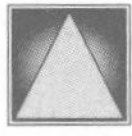

Table 37–2
Mental Status Examination for Children

1. Physical appearance
2. Parent–child interaction
3. Separation and reunion
4. Orientation to time, place, and person
5. Speech and language
6. Mood
7. Affect
8. Thought process and content
9. Social relatedness
10. Motor behavior
11. Cognition
12. Memory
13. Judgment and insight

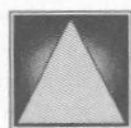

Table 37–3
Neuropsychiatric Mental Status Examination*

A. General Description
  1. General appearance and dress
  2. Level of consciousness and arousal
  3. Attention to environment
  4. Posture (standing and seated)
  5. Gait
  6. Movements of limbs, trunk, and face (spontaneous, resting, and after instruction)
  7. General demeanor (including evidence of responses to internal stimuli)
  8. Response to examiner (eye contact, cooperation, ability to focus on interview process)
  9. Native or primary language

B. Language and Speech
  1. Comprehension (words, sentences, simple and complex commands, and concepts)
  2. Output (spontaneity, rate, fluency, melody or prosody, volume, coherence, vocabulary, paraphasic errors, complexity of usage)
  3. Repetition
  4. Other aspects
    a. Object naming
    b. Color naming
    c. Body part identification
    d. Ideomotor praxis to command

C. Thought
  1. Form (coherence and connectedness)
  2. Content
    a. Ideational (preoccupations, overvalued ideas, delusions)
    b. Perceptual (hallucinations)

D. Mood and Affect
  1. Internal mood state (spontaneous and elicited; sense of humor)
  2. Future outlook
  3. Suicidal ideas and plans
  4. Demonstrated emotional status (congruence with mood)

E. Insight and Judgment
  1. Insight
    a. Self-appraisal and self-esteem
    b. Understanding of current circumstances
    c. Ability to describe personal psychological and physical status
  2. Judgment
    a. Appraisal of major social relationships
    b. Understanding of personal roles and responsibilities

F. Cognition
  1. Memory
    a. Spontaneous (as evidenced during interview)
    b. Tested (incidental, immediate repetition, delayed recall, cued recall, recognition; verbal, nonverbal; explicit, implicit)
  2. Visuospatial skills
  3. Constructional ability
  4. Mathematics
  5. Reading
  6. Writing
  7. Fine sensory function (stereognosis, graphesthesia, two-point discrimination)
  8. Finger gnosis
  9. Right-left orientation
  10. "Executive functions"
  11. Abstraction

*Questions should be adapted to the age of the child.
Courtesy of Eric D. Caine, M.D., and Jeffrey M. Lyness, M.D.

Physical Appearances. The examiner should document the child's size, grooming, nutritional state, bruising, head circumference, physical signs of anxiety, facial expressions, and mannerisms.

Parent–Child Interaction. The examiner can observe the interactions between parents and child in the waiting area before the interview and in the family session. The manner in which parents and child converse and the emotional overtones are pertinent.

Separation and Reunion. The examiner should note both the manner in which the child responds to the separation from a parent for an individual interview and the reunion behavior. Either lack of affect at separation and reunion or severe distress on separation or reunion can indicate problems in the parent–child relationship or other psychiatric disturbances.

Orientation to Time, Place, and Persons. Impairments in orientation can reflect organic damage, low intelligence, or a thought disorder. The age of the child must be kept in mind, however, because very young children are not expected to know the date, other chronological information, or the name of the interview site.

Speech and Language. The examiner should evaluate the child's speech and language acquisition. Is it appropriate for the child's age? A disparity between expressive language usage and receptive language is notable. The examiner should also note the child's rate of speech, rhythm, latency to answer, spontaneity of speech, intonation, articulation of words, and prosody. Echolalia, repetitive stereotypical phrases, and unusual syntax are important psychiatric findings. Children who do not use words by age 18 months or who do not use phrases by age 2.5 to 3 years, but who have a history of normal babbling and responding appropriately to nonverbal cues, are probably developing normally. The examiner should consider the possibility that a hearing loss is contributing to a speech and language deficit.

Mood. A child's sad expression, lack of appropriate smiling, tearfulness, anxiety, euphoria, and anger are valid indicators of mood, as are verbal admissions of feelings. Persistent themes in play and fantasy also reflect the child's mood.

Affect. The examiner should note the child's range of emotional expressivity, appropriateness of affect to thought content, ability to move smoothly from one affect to another, and sudden labile emotional shifts.

Thought Process and Content. In evaluating a thought disorder in a child, the clinician must always consider what is developmentally expected for the child's age and what is deviant for any age group. The evaluation of thought form considers loosening of associations, excessive magical thinking, perseveration, echolalia, the ability to distinguish fantasy from reality, sentence coherence, and the ability to reason logically. The evaluation of thought content considers delusions, obsessions, themes, fears, wishes, preoccupations, and interests.

Suicidal ideation is always a part of the mental status examination for children who are sufficiently verbal to understand the questions and old enough to understand the concept. Children of average intelligence more than 4 years of age usually have some understanding of what is real and what is make-believe and may be asked about suicidal ideation, although a firm concept of the permanence of death may not be present until several years later.

Aggressive thoughts and homicidal ideation are assessed here. Perceptual disturbances, such as hallucinations, are also assessed. Very young children are expected to have short attention spans and may change the topic and conversation abruptly without exhibiting a symptomatic flight of ideas. Transient visual and auditory hallucinations in very young children do not necessarily represent major psychotic illnesses, but they do deserve further investigation.

Social Relatedness. The examiner assesses the appropriateness of the child's response to the interviewer, general level of social skills, eye contact, and degree of familiarity or withdrawal in the interview process. Overly friendly or familiar behavior may be as troublesome as are extremely retiring and withdrawn responses. The examiner assesses the child's self-esteem, general and specific areas of confidence, and success with family and peer relationships.

Motor Behavior. The motor behavior part of the mental status examination includes observations of the child's coordination and activity level and ability to pay attention and carry out developmentally appropriate tasks. It also involves involuntary movements, tremors, motor hyperactivity, and any unusual focal asymmetries of muscle movement.

Cognition. The examiner assesses the child's intellectual functioning and problem-solving abilities. An approximate level of intelligence can be estimated by the child's general information, vocabulary, and comprehension. For a specific assessment of the child's cognitive abilities, the examiner can use a standardized test.

Memory. School-age children should be able to remember three objects after 5 minutes and to repeat five digits forward and three digits backward. Anxiety can interfere with the child's performance, but an obvious inability to repeat digits or to add simple numbers may reflect brain damage, mental retardation, or learning disabilities.

Judgment and Insight. The child's view of the problems, reactions to them, and suggested solutions may give the clinician a good idea of the child's judgment and insight. In addition, the child's understanding of what he or she can realistically do to help and what the clinician can do adds to the assessment of the child's judgment.

Neuropsychiatric Assessment

A neuropsychiatric assessment is appropriate for children who are suspected of having a neurological disorder, a psychiatric impairment that coexists with neurological signs, or psychiatric symptoms that may be caused by neuropathology. The neuropsychiatric evaluation combines information from neurological, physical, and mental status examinations. The neurological examination can identify asymmetrical abnormal signs (hard signs) that may indicate lesions in the brain. A physical examination can evaluate the presence of physical stigmata of particular syndromes in which neuropsychiatric symptoms or developmental aberrations play a role (e.g., fetal alcohol syndrome, Down syndrome).

An important part of the neuropsychiatric examination is the assessment of neurological soft signs and minor physical anomalies. The term *neurological soft signs* was first noted by Loretta Bender in the 1940s in reference to nondiagnostic abnormalities in the neurological examinations of children with schizophrenia. Soft signs do not indicate focal neurological disorders, but they are associated with a wide variety of developmental disabilities and occur frequently in children with low intelligence, learning disabilities, and behavioral disturbances. Soft signs may refer to both behavioral symptoms (which are sometimes associated with brain damage, such as severe impulsivity and hyperactivity), physical findings (including contralateral overflow movements), and a variety of nonfocal signs (e.g., mild choreiform movements, poor balance, mild incoordination, asymmetry of gait, nystagmus, and the persistence of infantile reflexes). Soft signs can be divided into those that are normal in a young child, but become abnormal when they persist in an older child, and those that are abnormal at any age. The *Physical and Neurological Examination for Soft Signs* (PANESS) is an instrument used with children up to the age of 15 years. It consists of 15 questions about general physical status and medical history and 43 physical tasks (e.g., touch your finger to your nose, hop on one foot to the end of the line, tap quickly with your finger). Neurological soft signs are important to note, but they are not useful in making a specific psychiatric diagnosis.

Minor physical anomalies or dysmorphic features occur with a higher than usual frequency in children with developmental disabilities, learning disabilities, speech and language disorders, and hyperactivity. As with soft signs, the documentation of minor physical anomalies is part of the neuropsychiatric assessment, but it is rarely helpful in the diagnostic process and does not imply a good or bad prognosis. Minor physical anomalies include a high-arched palate, epicanthal folds, hypertelorism, low-set ears, transverse palmar creases, multiple hair whorls, a large head, a furrowed tongue, and partial syndactyl of several toes.

When a seizure disorder is being considered in the differential diagnosis or a structural abnormality in the brain is suspected, an electroencephalogram (EEG), computed tomography (CT), or magnetic resonance imaging (MRI) may be indicated.

Developmental, Psychological, and Educational Testing

Psychological tests are not always required to assess psychiatric symptoms, but they are valuable in determining a child's developmental level, intellectual functioning, and academic difficulties. A measure of adaptive functioning (including the child's competence in communication, daily living skills, socialization, and motor skills) is a prerequisite when a diagnosis of mental retardation is being considered. Table 37–4 outlines the general categories of psychological tests.

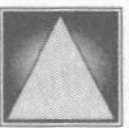

Table 37–4
Commonly Used Child and Adolescent Psychological Assessment Instruments

Test	Age/Grades	Data Generated and Comments
Intellectual ability		
Wechsler Intelligence Scale for Children—Third Edition (WISC-III-R)	6–16	Standard scores: verbal, performance and full-scale IQ; scaled subtest scores permitting specific skill assessment.
Wechsler Adult Intelligence Scale—(WAIS-III)	16–adult	Same as WISC-III-R.
Wechsler Preschool and Primary Scale of Intelligence—Revised (WPPSI-R)	3–7	Same as WISC-III-R.
Kaufman Assessment Battery for Children (K-ABC)	2.6–12.6	Well grounded in theories of cognitive psychology and neuropsychology. Allows immediate comparison of intellectual capacity with acquired knowledge. Scores: Mental Processing Composite (IQ equivalent); sequential and simultaneous processing and achievement standard scores: scaled mental processing and achievement subtest scores; age equivalents; percentiles.
Kaufman Adolescent and Adult Intelligence Test (KAIT)	11–85+	Composed of separate Crystallized and Fluid scales. Scores: Composite Intelligence Scale; Crystallized and Fluid IQ; scaled subtest scores; percentiles.
Stanford-Binet, 4th Edition (SB:FE)	2–23	Scores: IQ; verbal, abstract/visual, and quantitative reasoning; short-term memory; standard age.
Peabody Picture Vocabulary Test—III (PPVT-III)	4–adult	Measures receptive vocabulary acquisition; standard scores, percentiles, age equivalents.
Achievement		
Woodcock-Johnson Psycho-Educational Battery—Revised (W-J)	K–12	Scores: reading and mathematics (mechanics and comprehension), written language, other academic achievement; grade and age scores, standard scores, percentiles.
Wide Range Achievement Test—3, Levels 1 and 2 (WRAT-3)	Level 1: 1–5 Level 2: 12–75	Permits screening for deficits in reading, spelling, and arithmetic; grade levels, percentiles, stanines, standard scores.
Kaufman Test of Educational Achievement, Brief and Comprehensive Forms (K-TEA)	1–12	Standard scores: reading, mathematics, and spelling; grade and age equivalents, percentiles, stanines. Brief Form is sufficient for most clinical applications; Comprehensive Form allows error analysis and more detailed curriculum planning.
Wechsler Individual Achievement Test (WIAT)	K–12	Standard scores: basic reading, mathematics reasoning, spelling, reading comprehension, numerical operations, listening comprehension, oral expression, written expression. Conormal with WISC-III-R.
Adaptive behavior		
Vineland Adaptive Behavior Scales	Normal: 0–19 Retarded: All ages	Standard scores: adaptive behavior composite and communication, daily living skills, socialization and motor domains; percentiles, age equivalents, developmental age scores. Separate standardization groups for normal, visually handicapped, hearing impaired, emotionally disturbed, and retarded.
Scales of Independent Behavior—Revised	Newborn–adult	Standard scores: four adaptive (motor, social interaction, communication, personal living, community living) and three maladaptive (internalized, asocial, and externalized) areas; General Maladaptive Index and Broad Independence cluster.
Attentional capacity		
Trail Making Test	8–adult	Standard scores, standard deviations, ranges; corrections for age and education.
Wisconsin Card Sorting Test	6.6–adult	Standard scores, standard deviations, T-scores, percentiles, developmental norms for number of categories achieved, perseverative errors, and failures to maintain set; computer measures.
Behavior Assessment System for Children (BASC)	4–18	Teacher and parent rating scales and child self-report of personality permitting multireporter assessment across a variety of domains in home, school, and community. Provides validity, clinical, and adaptive scales. ADHD component avails.
Home Situations Questionnaire—Revised (HSQ-R)	6–12	Permits parents to rate child's specific problems with attention or concentration. Scores for number of problem settings, mean severity, and factor scores for compliance and leisure situations.
ADHD Rating Scale	6–12	Score for number of symptoms keyed to DSM cutoff for diagnosis of ADHD; standard scores permit derivation of clinical significance for total score and two factors (Inattentive-Hyperactive and Impulsive-Hyperactive).

(continued)

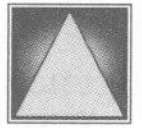

Table 37–4 (Continued)

Test	Age/Grades	Data Generated and Comments
School Situations Questionnaire (SSQ-R)	6–12	Permits teachers to rate a child's specific problems with attention or concentration. Scores for number of problem settings and mean severity.
Child Attention Profile (CAP)	6–12	Brief measure allowing teachers' weekly ratings of presence and degree of child's inattention and overactivity. Normative scores for inattention, overactivity, and total score.
Projective tests		
Rorschach Inkblots	3–adult	Special scoring systems. Most recently developed and increasingly universally accepted is John Exner's Comprehensive System (1974). Assesses perceptual accuracy, integration of affective and intellectual functioning, reality testing, and other psychological processes.
Thematic Apperception Test (TAT)	6–adult	Generates stories which are analyzed qualitatively. Assumed to provide especially rich data regarding interpersonal functioning.
Machover Draw-A-Person Test (DAP)	3–adult	Qualitative analysis and hypothesis generation, especially regarding subject's feelings about self and significant others.
Kinetic Family Drawing (KFD)	3–adult	Qualitative analysis and hypothesis generation regarding an individual's perception of family structure and sentient environment. Some objective scoring systems in existence.
Rotter Incomplete Sentences Blank	Child, adolescent, and adult forms	Primarily qualitative analysis, although some objective scoring systems have been developed.
Personality tests		
Minnesota Multiphasic Personality Inventory-Adolescent (MMPI-A)	14–18	1992 version of widely used personality measure, developed specifically for use with adolescents. Standard scores: 3 validity scales, 14 clinical scales, additional content and supplementary scales.
Million Adolescent Personality Inventory (MAPI)	13–18	Standard scores for 20 scales grouped into three categories: Personality styles; expressed concerns; behavioral correlates. Normed on adolescent population. Focuses on broad functional spectrum, not just problem areas. Measures 14 primary personality traits, including emotional stability, self-concept level, excitability, and self-assurance.
Children's Personality Questionnaire	8–12	Generates combined broad trait patterns including extraversion and anxiety.
Neuropsychological screening tests and test batteries		
Developmental Test of Visual-Motor Integration (VMI)	2–16	Screening instrument for visual motor deficits. Standard scores, age equivalents, percentiles.
Benton Visual Retention Test	6–adult	Assesses presence of deficits in visual-figure memory. Mean scores by age.
Benton Visual Motor Gestalt Test	5–adult	Assesses visual-motor deficits and visual-figural retention. Age equivalents.
Reitan-Indiana Neuropsychological Test Battery for Children	5–8	Cognitive and perceptual-motor tests for children with suspected brain damage.
Halstead-Reitan Neuropsychological Test Battery for Older Children	9–14	Same as Reitan-Indiana.
Luria-Nebraska Neuropsychological Battery: Children's Revision LNNB:C	8–12	Sensory-motor, perceptual, cognitive tests measuring 11 clinical and 2 additional domains of neuropsychological functioning. Provides standard scores.
Developmental status		
Bayley Scales of Infant Development-Second Edition	16 days–42 mos	Mental, motor, and behavior scales measuring infant, development. Provides standard scores.
Mullen Scales of Early Learning	Newborn–5 yrs	Language and visual scales for receptive and expressive ability. Yields age scores and T scores.

(Adapted from Racusin G, Moss N. Psychological assessment of children and adolescents. In: Lewis M, ed. *Child and Adolescent Psychiatry: A Comprehensive Textbook*. Baltimore: Williams & Wilkins; 1991, with permission.)

Development Tests for Infants and Preschoolers. The *Gesell Infant Scale*, the *Cattell Infant Intelligence Scale*, *Bayley Scales of Infant Development*, and the *Denver Developmental Screening Test* include developmental assessments of infants as young as 2 months of age. When used with very young infants, the tests focus on sensorimotor and social responses to a variety of objects and interactions. When these instruments are used with older infants and preschoolers, emphasis is placed on language acquisition. The *Gesell Infant Scale* measures development in four areas: motor, adaptive functioning, language, and social.

An infant's score on one of these developmental assessments is not a reliable way to predict a child's future intelligence quotient (IQ) in most cases. Infant assessments are valuable, however, in detecting developmental deviation and mental retardation and in raising suspicions of a developmental disorder. Whereas infant assessments rely heavily on sensorimotor functions, intelligence testing in older children and adolescents includes later-developing functions, including verbal, social, and abstract cognitive abilities.

Intelligence Tests for School-Age Children and Adolescents. The most widely used test of intelligence for school-age children and adolescents is the third edition of the *Wechsler Intelligence Scale for Children* (WISC-III-R). It can be given to children from 6 to 17 years of age and yields a verbal IQ, a performance IQ, and a combined full-scale IQ. The verbal subtests consist of vocabulary, information, arithmetic, similarities, comprehension, and digit span (supplemental) categories. The performance subtests include block design, picture completion, picture arrangement, object assembly, coding, mazes (supplemental), and symbol search (supplemental). The scores of the supplemental subtests are not included in the computation of IQ.

Each subcategory is scored from 1 to 19, with 10 being the average score. An average full-scale IQ is 100; 70 to 80 represents borderline intellectual function; 80 to 90 is in the low average range; 90 to 109 is average; 110 to 119 is high average; and above 120 is in the superior or very superior range. The multiple breakdowns of the performance and verbal subscales allow great flexibility in identifying specific areas of deficit and scatter in intellectual abilities. Because a large part of intelligence testing measures abilities used in academic settings, the breakdown of the WISC-III-R can also be helpful in pointing out skills in which a child is weak and may benefit from remedial education.

The *Stanford-Binet Intelligence Scale* covers an age range from 2 to 24 years. It relies on pictures, drawings, and objects for very young children and on verbal performance for older children and adolescents. This intelligence scale, the earliest version of an intelligence test of its kind, leads to a mental age score as well as an intelligence quotient.

The *McCarthy Scales of Children's Abilities* and the *Kaufman Assessment Battery for Children* are two other intelligence tests that are available for preschool and school-age children. They do not cover the adolescent age group.

LONG-TERM STABILITY OF INTELLIGENCE. Although a child's intelligence is relatively stable throughout the school-age years and adolescence, some factors can influence intelligence and a child's score on an intelligence test. The intellectual functions of children with severe mental illnesses and of those from low socioeconomic levels may decrease over time, whereas the IQs of children whose environments have been enriched may increase over time. Factors that influence a child's score on a given test of intellectual functioning and, thus, affect the accuracy of the test are motivation, emotional state, anxiety, and cultural milieu.

Perceptual and Perceptual Motor Tests. The *Bender Visual Motor Gestalt Test* can be given to children between the ages of 4 and 12 years. The test consists of a set of spatially related figures that the child is asked to copy. The scores are based on the number of errors. Although not a diagnostic test, it is useful in identifying developmentally age-inappropriate perceptual performances.

Personality Tests. Personality tests are not of much use in making diagnoses, and they are less satisfactory than intelligence tests in regard to norms, reliability, and validity, but they can be helpful in eliciting themes and fantasies.

The Rorschach test is a projective technique in which ambiguous stimuli—a set of bilaterally symmetrical inkblots—are shown to a child, who is then asked to describe what he or she sees in each. The hypothesis is that the child's interpretation of the vague stimuli reflects basic characteristics of personality. The examiner notes the themes and patterns. Two sets of norms have been established for the Rorschach test, one for children between 2 and 10 years and one for adolescents between 10 and 17 years.

A more structured projective test is the *Children's Apperception Test* (CAT), which is an adaptation of the *Thematic Apperception Test* (TAT). The CAT consists of cards with pictures of animals in scenes that are somewhat ambiguous, but are related to parent–child and sibling issues, caretaking, and other relationships. The child is asked to describe what is happening and to tell a story about the scene. Animals are used because it was hypothesized that children might respond more readily to animal images than to human figures.

Drawings, toys, and play are also applications of projective techniques that can be used during the evaluation of children. Dollhouses, dolls, and puppets have been especially helpful in allowing a child a nonconversational mode in which to express a variety of attitudes and feelings. Play materials that reflect household situations are likely to elicit a child's fears, hopes, and conflicts about the family.

Projective techniques have not fared well as standardized instruments. Rather than being considered tests, projective techniques are best considered as additional clinical modalities.

Educational Tests. Achievement tests measure the attainment of knowledge and skills in a particular academic curriculum. The *Wide-Range Achievement Test-Revised* (WRAT-R) consists of tests of knowledge and skills and timed performances of reading, spelling, and mathematics. It is used with children from 5 years of age to adulthood. The test yields a score that is compared with the average expected score for the child's chronological age and grade level.

The *Peabody Individual Achievement Test* (PIAT) includes word identification, spelling, mathematics, and reading comprehension.

The *Kaufman Test of Educational Achievement*, the *Gray Oral Reading Test-Revised* (GORT-R), and the *Sequential Tests of Educational Progress* (STEP) are achievement tests that determine whether a child has achieved the educational level expected for his or her grade level. Children with an average IQ, whose achievement is significantly lower than expected for their grade level in one or more subjects, are considered to be learning disabled. Thus, achievement testing, combined with a measure of intellectual function, can identify specific learning disabilities for which remediation is recommended. Children who do not reach their grade level according to their chronological age, but who function intellectually in the borderline range or lower, are not necessarily learning disabled unless a disparity exists between their IQs and their levels of achievement.

Biopsychosocial Formulation. The clinician's task is to integrate all of the information obtained into a formulation that takes into account the biological predisposition, psychodynamic factors, environmental stressors, and life events that have led to the child's current level of functioning. Psychiatric disorders and any specific physical, neuromotor, or developmental abnormalities must be considered in the formulation of etiologic factors for current impairment. The clinician's conclusions are an integration of clinical information along with data from standardized psychological and developmental assessments. The psychiatric formulation includes an assessment of family function as well as the appropriateness of the child's educational setting. A determination of the child's overall safety in his or her current situation is made. Any suspected maltreatment must be reported to the local child protective service agency. The child's overall well-being regarding growth, development, and academic and play activities is considered.

Diagnosis

Current evidence suggests that the use of structured and semistructured (evidence-based) assessment tools enhance a clinician's ability to make the most accurate diagnoses. These instruments, described earlier, include the K-SADS, the CAPA, and the NIMH DISC-IV interviews. The advantages of including an evidence-based instrument in the diagnostic process include decreasing potential clinician bias to make a diagnosis without all of the necessary symptoms information, and serving as guides for the clinician to consider each symptom that could contribute to a given diagnosis. These data can enable the clinician to optimize his expertise to make challenging judgments regarding child and adolescent disorders which may possess overlapping symptoms. The clinician's ultimate task includes making all appropriate diagnoses according to DSM-IV-TR. Some clinical situations do not fulfill criteria for DSM-IV-TR diagnoses, but cause impairment and require psychiatric attention and intervention. Clinicians who evaluate children are frequently in the position of determining the impact of behavior of family members on the child's well-being. In many cases, a child's level of impairment is related to factors extending beyond a psychiatric diagnosis, such as the child's adjustment to his or her family life, peer relationships, and educational placement.

RECOMMENDATIONS AND TREATMENT PLAN

The recommendations for treatment are derived by a clinician who integrates the data gathered during the evaluation into a coherent formulation of the factors that are contributing to the child's current problems, the consequences of the problems, and strategies that may ameliorate the difficulties. The recommendations can be broken down into their biological, psychological, and social components. That is, identification of a biological predisposition to a particular psychiatric disorder may be clinically relevant to inform a psychopharmacologic recommendation. As part of the formulation, an understanding of the psychodynamic interactions between family members may lead a clinician to recommend treatment that includes a family component. Educational and academic problems are addressed in the formulation and may lead to a recommendation to seek a more effective academic placement. The overall social situation of the child or adolescent is taken into account when recommendations for treatment are developed. Of course, the physical and emotional safety of a child or adolescent is of the utmost importance and always at the top of the list of recommendations.

The child or adolescent's family, school life, peer interactions, and social activities often have a direct impact on the child's success in overcoming his or her difficulties. The psychological education and cooperation of a child or adolescent's family are essential ingredients in successful application of treatment recommendations. Communications from clinicians to parents and family members that balance the observed positive qualities of the child and family with the weak areas are often perceived as more helpful than a focus only on the problem areas. Finally, the most successful treatment plans are those developed cooperatively between the clinician, child, and family members during which each member of the team perceives that he or she has been given credit for positive contributions.

References

Achenbach TM, Dumenci L, Rescorla LA. Ratings of relations between DSM-IV diagnostic categories and items of the CBCL/6-18, TRF, and YSR. Burlington, VT: University of Vermont, Research Center for Children, Youth, & Families; 2001.

Bird HR, Canino GJ, Davies M, Ramirez R, Chavez L, Duarte C, Shen S. The Brief Impairment Scale (BIS): A multidimensional scale of functional impairment for children and adolescents. *J Am Acad Child Adolesc Psychiatry*. 2005;44:699.

Doss AJ. Evidence-based diagnosis: Incorporating diagnostic instruments into clinical practice. *J Am Acad Child Adolesc Psychiatry*. 2005;44;947.

Hamilton J. Clinician's guide to evidence-based practice. *J Am Acad Child Adolesc Psychiatry*. 2005;44:494.

Hamilton J. The answerable question and a hierarchy of evidence. *J Am Acad Child Adolesc Psychiatry*. 2005;44:596.

Kestenbaum CJ. The clinical interview of the child. In: Wiener JM, Dulcan MK, eds. *The American Psychiatric Publishing Textbook of Child and Adolescent Psychiatry*. 3rd ed. Washington, DC: American Psychiatric Publishing, Inc.; 2004:103–111.

King RA, Schwab-Stone ME, Peterson BS, Thies AP. Psychiatric examination of the infant, child, and adolescent. In: Sadock BJ, Sadock VA, eds. *Kaplan & Sadock's Comprehensive Textbook of Psychiatry*. 8th ed. Vol. 2. Baltimore: Lippincott Williams & Wilkins; 2005:3044.

Lyneham HJ, Rapee RM. Evaluation and treatment of anxiety disorders in the general pediatric population: A clinician's guide. *Child Adolesc Psychiatr Clin N Am*. 2005;14(4):845.

Pataki CS. Child psychiatry: Introduction and overview. In: Sadock BJ, Sadock VA, eds. *Kaplan & Sadock's Comprehensive Textbook of Psychiatry*. 8th ed. Vol. 2. Baltimore: Lippincott Williams & Wilkins; 2005:3015.

Puig-Antich J, Orraschel H, Tabrizi MA, Chambers W. Schedule for Affective Disorders and Schizophrenia for School-Age Children-Epidemiologic Version. New York: New York State Psychiatric Institute and Yale School of Medicine; 1980.

Staller JA. Diagnostic profiles in outpatient child psychiatry. *American Journal of Orthopsychiatry*. 2006;76(1):98.

Winters NC, Collett BR, Myers KM. Ten-year review of rating scales, VII: Scales assessing functional impairment. *J Am Acad Child Adolesc Psychiatry*. 2005;44:309.

Youngstrom EA, Duax J. Evidence-based assessment of pediatric bipolar disorder. Part 1: Base rate and family history. *J Am Acad Child Adolesc Psychiatry*. 2005;44:712.

38 Mental Retardation

The conceptualization of mental retardation includes deficits in cognitive abilities as well as in behaviors required for social and personal sufficiency, known as *adaptive functioning.* Wide acceptance of this definition has led to the concensus that an assessment of both social adaptation and intelligence quotient (IQ) are necessary to determine the level of mental retardation. Measures of adaptive function assess competency in performance of everyday tasks, whereas measures of intellectual function focus on cognitive abilities. Evidence shows that individuals with a given intellectual level do not all have the same adaptive function, yet it is likely that IQ contributes an upper limit or ceiling to adaptive accomplishments.

In the mid-1800s many children with mental retardation were placed in residential educational facilities in conjunction with the belief that if these children received sufficient intensive training, they would be able to return to their families and function in society at a higher level. The original plan of educating the children so they could overcome their disabilities was not realized. Gradually, these residential programs became larger, and eventually the focus began to shift from intensive education to custodial care. These residential institutional settings for children with mental retardation received their maximal use in the mid-1900s, until public awareness of the crowded, unsanitary, and, in some cases, abusive conditions sparked the movement toward "deinstitutionalization." An important force in the deinstitutionalization of children with mental retardation was the philosophy of "normalization" in living situations and "inclusion" in educational settings. Since the late 1960s, few children with mental retardation have been placed in institutional settings, and the concepts of "normalization" and inclusion became prominent issues among advocacy groups and most citizens.

The passage of Public Law 94-142 (the Education for all Handicapped Children Act) in 1975 mandates the public school system to provision of appropriate educational service to all children with disabilities. The Individuals with Disabilities Act in 1990 extended and modified the above legislation. Currently, provision of public education for all children, including those with disabilities, "within the least restrictive environment" is mandated by law.

In addition to the educational system, advocacy groups, including the Council for Exceptional Children (CEC) and the National Association for Retarded Citizens (NARC) are well known parental lobbying organizations for children with mental retardation and were instrumental in advocating for Public Law 94-142. The most prominent advocacy organization in this field is the American Association on Mental Retardation (AAMR), which has been most influential in educating the public about mental retardation and in supporting research and legislation relating to mental retardation.

The AAMR, promotes a view of mental retardation as a functional interaction between an individual and the environment, instead of a static description of a person's limitations. Within this conceptual framework, a person is designated as needing intermittent, limited, extensive, or pervasive "environmental support" with respect to a specific set of adaptive function domains. These areas of function are communication, self-care, home living, social or interpersonal skills, use of community resources, self-direction, functional academic skills, work, leisure, health, and safety.

The AAMR promotes designating an IQ of 75, rather than 70, as the beginning level of the mild mental retardation range, thereby enabling many more persons to receive services as mentally retarded. The advantage of the AAMR view is that, instead of defining a person's degree of mental retardation by the level of cognitive and adaptive impairment, the degree of "support" necessary for functioning becomes the defining feature. The disadvantage of this nomenclature is that it is difficult to quantify the "supports" and it would be problematic to match new research with the existing body of research using an IQ cutoff of 70. The decision of the work group of the 4th edition of *Diagnostic and Statistical Manual of Mental Disorders* (DSM-IV) and its text revision (DSM-IV-TR) was that an IQ cutoff of 70 would be retained, and the adaptive function domains recommended by the AAMR would be included in the diagnostic criteria for mental retardation.

NOMENCLATURE

Accurately defining mental retardation has challenged clinicians over the centuries. In the 1800s, the notion that mental retardation was based primarily on a deficit in social or moral reasoning was promoted. Since then, the addition of intellectual deficit was added to the concept of inadequate social function. All current classification systems retain the understanding that mental retardation is based on more than intellectual deficits, that is, it also depends on a lower than expected level of adaptive function. According to DSM-IV-TR, a diagnosis of mental retardation can be made only when both the IQ, as measured by a standardized test, is subaverage and a measure of adaptive function reveals deficits in at least two of the areas of adaptive function. Mental retardation diagnoses are coded on Axis II in the DSM-IV-TR.

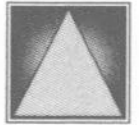

Table 38–1
Developmental Characteristics of Mentally Retarded Persons

Degree of Mental Retardation	Preschool Age (0 to 5 yrs) Maturation and Development	School Age (6 to 20 yrs) Training and Education	Adult (21 yrs and Above) Social and Vocational Adequacy
Profound	Gross retardation; minimal capacity for functioning in sensorimotor areas; needs nursing care; constant aid and supervision required	Some motor development present; may respond to minimal or limited training in self-help	Some motor and speech development; may achieve very limited self-care; needs nursing care
Severe	Poor motor development; speech minimal; generally unable to profit from training in self-help; little or no communication skills	Can talk or learn to communicate; can be trained in elemental health habits; profits from systematic habit training; unable to profit from vocational training	May contribute partially to self-maintenance under complete supervision; can develop self-protection skills to a minimal useful level in controlled environment
Moderate	Can talk or learn to communicate; poor social awareness; fair motor development; profits from training in self-help; can be managed with moderate supervision	Can profit from training in social and occupational skills; unlikely to progress beyond second-grade level in academic subjects; may learn to travel alone in familiar places	May achieve self-maintenance in unskilled or semiskilled work under sheltered conditions; needs supervision and guidance when under mild social or economic stress
Mild	Can develop social and communication skills; minimal retardation in sensorimotor areas; often not distinguished from normal until later age	Can learn academic skills up to approximately sixth-grade level by late teens; can be guided toward social conformity	Can usually achieve social and vocational skills adequate to minimal self-support, but may need guidance and assistance when under unusual social or economic stress

(Adapted from *Mental Retarded Activities of the US Department of Health, Education and Welfare*. Washington, DC: US Government Printing Office; 1989:2, with permission. DSM-IV criteria are adapted essentially from this chart.)

CLASSIFICATION

According to the DSM-IV-TR, mental retardation is defined as significantly subaverage general intellectual functioning resulting in, or associated with, concurrent impairment in adaptive behavior and manifested during the developmental period, before the age of 18. The diagnosis is made regardless of whether the person has a coexisting physical disorder or other mental disorder. Table 38–1 presents an overview of developmental levels in communication, academic functioning, and vocational skills expected of persons with various degrees of mental retardation.

General intellectual functioning is determined by the use of standardized tests of intelligence, and the term *significantly subaverage* is defined as an IQ of approximately 70 or below or two standard deviations below the mean for the particular test. Adaptive functioning can be measured by using a standardized scale, such as the *Vineland Adaptive Behavior Scale*. This scale scores communications, daily living skills, socialization, and motor skills (up to 4 years, 11 months) and generates an adaptive behavior composite that is correlated with the expected skills at a given age.

Approximately 85 percent of persons who are mentally retarded fall within the mild mental retardation category (IQ between 50 and 70). The adaptive functions of mildly retarded persons are effective in several areas, such as communications, self-care, social skills, work, leisure, and safety. Mental retardation is influenced by genetic, environmental, and psychosocial factors; previously, the development of mild retardation was often attributed to severe psychosocial deprivation. More recently, however, researchers have increasingly recognized the likely contribution of a host of subtle biological factors, including chromosomal abnormalities, subclinical lead intoxication, and prenatal exposure to drugs, alcohol, and other toxins. Furthermore, evidence is increasing that subgroups of persons who are mentally retarded, such as those with fragile X syndrome, Down syndrome, and Prader-Willi syndrome, have characteristic patterns of social, linguistic, and cognitive development and typical behavioral manifestations.

The DSM-IV-TR has included in its text on mental retardation additional information regarding the etiological factors and their association with mental retardation syndromes (e.g., fragile X syndrome).

DEGREES OF SEVERITY OF MENTAL RETARDATION

The degrees, or levels, of mental retardation are expressed in various terms. DSM-IV-TR presents four levels of mental retardation: mild, moderate, severe, and profound. The category borderline mental retardation (between one and two standard deviations below the test mean) was eliminated in 1973. Borderline intellectual functioning, according to DSM-IV-TR, is not within the diagnostic boundary of mental retardation and refers to a full-scale IQ in the 71 to 84 range that is a focus of psychiatric attention.

Mild mental retardation (IQ range, 50 to 70) represents approximately 85 percent of persons with mental retardation. In general, children with mild mental retardation are not identified until after first or second grade, when academic demands increase. By late adolescence, they often acquire academic skills at approximately a sixth grade level. Specific causes for the mental retardation are often unidentified in this group. Many adults with mild mental retardation can live independently with appropriate support and raise their own families.

Moderate mental retardation (IQ range, 35–50) represents about 10 percent of persons with mental retardation. Most children with moderate mental retardation acquire language and can communicate adequately during early childhood. They are challenged academically and often are not able to achieve academically above a second to third grade level. During adolescence, socialization difficulties often set these persons apart, and a great deal of social and vocational support is beneficial. As adults, persons with moderate mental retardation may be able to perform semiskilled work under appropriate supervision.

Severe mental retardation (IQ range, 20–35) comprises about 4 percent of individuals with mental retardation. They may be able to develop communication skills in childhood and often can learn to count as well as recognize words that are critical to functioning. In this group, the cause for the mental retardation is more likely to be identified than it is in milder forms of mental retardation. In adulthood, persons with severe mental retardation may adapt well to supervised living situations, such as group homes, and may be able to perform work-related tasks under supervision.

Profound mental retardation (IQ range below 20) constitutes approximately 1 to 2 percent of persons with mental retardation. Most individuals with profound mental retardation have identifiable causes for their condition. Children with profound mental retardation may be taught some self-care skills and learn to communicate their needs given the appropriate training.

The DSM-IV-TR lists mental retardation, severity unspecified, as a type reserved for persons who are strongly suspected of having mental retardation, but who cannot be tested by standard intelligence tests or are too impaired or uncooperative to be tested. This type may be applicable to infants whose significantly subaverage intellectual functioning is clinically judged but for whom the available tests (e.g., *Bayley Scales of Infant Development* and *Cattell Infant Scale*) do not yield numerical IQ values. This type should not be used when the intellectual level is presumed to be above 70.

EPIDEMIOLOGY

The prevalence of mental retardation at any one time is estimated to range from 1 percent to 3 percent of the population. The incidence of mental retardation is difficult to calculate because mild mental retardation sometimes goes unrecognized until middle childhood. In some cases, even when intellectual function is limited, good adaptive skills are not challenged until late childhood or early adolescence, and the diagnosis is not made until that time. The highest incidence is in school-age children, with the peak at ages 10 to 14 years. Mental retardation is about 1.5 times more common among men than among women. In older persons, prevalence is lower; those with severe or profound mental retardation have high mortality rates because of the complications of associated physical disorders.

COMORBIDITY

Prevalence

Epidemiological surveys indicate that up to two thirds of children and adults with mental retardation have comorbid mental disorders; this rate is several times higher than that in the community samples of those not mentally retarded. The prevalence of psychopathology seems to be correlated with the severity of mental retardation; the more severe the mental retardation, the higher the risk for other mental disorders. A recent epidemiological study found that 40.7 percent of intellectually disabled children between 4 and 18 years of age met criteria for at least one psychiatric disorder. The severity of retardation affected the type of psychiatric disorder. Disruptive and conduct-disorder behaviors occurred more commonly in the mildly retarded group; the more severely retarded group exhibited psychiatric problems more often associated with autistic disorder, such as self-stimulation and self-mutilation. In contrast to the epidemiology of psychopathology in children in general, age and sex did not affect the prevalence of psychiatric disorders in this study. Those with profound mental retardation were less likely to exhibit psychiatric symptoms.

The mental disorders that occur among persons who are mentally retarded appear to run the gamut of those seen in persons not mentally retarded, including mood disorders, schizophrenia, attention-deficit/hyperactivity disorder (ADHD), and conduct disorder. Those with severe mental retardation have a particularly high rate of autistic disorder and pervasive developmental disorders. About 2 to 3 percent of mentally retarded persons meet the criteria for schizophrenia; this percentage is several times higher than the rate for the general population. Up to 50 percent of mentally retarded children and adults had a mood disorder when such instruments as the *Kiddie Schedule for Affective Disorders and Schizophrenia*, the *Beck Depression Inventory*, and the *Children's Depression Inventory* were used in pilot studies, but because these instruments have not been standardized within the mentally retarded population, these findings must be considered preliminary.

Highly prevalent psychiatric symptoms that can occur in mentally retarded persons outside the context of a mental disorder include hyperactivity and short attention span, self-injurious behaviors (e.g., head-banging and self-biting), and repetitive stereotypical behaviors (hand-flapping and toe-walking). Personality styles and traits in mentally retarded persons are not unique to them, but negative self-image, low self-esteem, poor frustration tolerance, interpersonal dependence, and a rigid problem-solving style are overrepresented. Specific causal syndromes seen in mental retardation can also predispose affected persons to various types of psychopathologies.

Neurological Disorders

Comorbid psychiatric disorders are increased in individuals with mental retardation who also have known neurological conditions, such as seizure disorders. Rates of psychopathology increase with the severity of mental retardation; thus, neurological impairment increases as intellectual impairment increases. In a recent review of psychiatric disorders in children and adolescents with mental retardation and epilepsy, approximately one third also had autistic disorder or an autistic-like condition. The combination of mental retardation, active epilepsy, and autism or an autistic-like condition occurs at a rate of 0.07 percent in the general population.

Psychosocial Features

A negative self-image and poor self-esteem are common features of mildly and moderately mentally retarded persons, who are well aware of being different from others. They experience repeated failure and disappointment in not meeting their parents' and society's expectations and in falling progressively behind their peers and even their younger siblings. Communication difficulties further increase their vulnerability to feelings of ineptness and frustration. Inappropriate behaviors, such as withdrawal, are common. The perpetual sense of isolation and inadequacy has been linked to feelings of anxiety, anger, dysphoria, and depression.

ETIOLOGY

Etiological factors in mental retardation can be primarily genetic, developmental, acquired, or a combination. Genetic causes include chromosomal and inherited conditions; developmental factors include prenatal exposure to infections and toxins; and acquired syndromes include perinatal trauma (e.g., prematurity) and sociocultural factors. The severity of the resulting mental retardation is related to the timing and duration of the trauma as well as to the degree of exposure to the central nervous system (CNS). The more severe the mental retardation, the more likely it is that the cause is evident. In about three fourths of persons with severe mental retardation, the cause is known, whereas the cause is apparent in only half of those with mild mental retardation. A recent study of 100 consecutive children with mental retardation admitted to a clinical genetics unit of a university pediatric hospital reported that in 41 percent of cases, a causative diagnosis was made. In general, etiological classifications used included genetic, multifactorial, environmental, and unknown etiology. No cause is known for three fourths of persons with borderline intellectual functioning. Overall, in up to two thirds of all mentally retarded persons, the probable cause can be identified. Among chromosomal and metabolic disorders, Down syndrome, fragile X syndrome, and phenylketonuria (PKU) are the most common disorders that usually produce at least moderate mental retardation. Those with mild mental retardation sometimes have a familial pattern apparent in parents and siblings. Deprivation of nutrition, nurturance, and social stimulation can contribute to the development of mental retardation. Current knowledge suggests that genetic, environmental, biological, and psychosocial factors work additively in mental retardation.

Genetic Etiological Factors in Mental Retardation

Abnormalities in autosomal chromosomes are frequently associated with mental retardation, whereas aberrations in sex chromosomes can result in characteristic physical syndromes that do not include mental retardation (e.g., Turner's syndrome with XO and Klinefelter's syndrome with XXY, XXXY, and XXYY variations). Some children with Turner's syndrome have normal to superior intelligence. Agreement exists on a few predisposing factors for chromosomal disorders—among them, advanced maternal age, increased age of the father, and X-ray radiation.

Genetic Mental Retardation Syndromes and Behavioral Phenotypes

Many researchers in the field of mental retardation have noted specific and predictable behaviors are associated with certain genetic mental retardation syndromes. These behavioral phenotypes are defined as a syndrome of observable behaviors that occur with a greater probability than expected among those individuals with a specific genetic abnormality.

Examples of behavioral phenotypes occur in genetically determined syndromes such as fragile X syndrome, Prader-Willi syndrome, and Down syndrome in which specific behavioral manifestations can be expected (Fig. 38–1). Persons with fragile X syndrome have extremely high rates (up to three fourths of those studied) of ADHD. High rates of aberrant interpersonal behavior and language function often meet the criteria for autistic disorder and avoidant personality disorder. Prader-Willi syndrome is almost always associated with compulsive eating disturbances, hyperphagia, and obesity. Children with the syndrome have been described as oppositional and defiant. Socialization is an area of weakness, especially in coping skills. Externalizing behavior problems—such as temper tantrums, irritability, and arguing—seem to be heightened in adolescence. Researchers and clinicians are working toward developing specific questionnaires to identify behavioral phenotypes of the above, and other mental retardation syndromes.

Down Syndrome. The description of Down syndrome, first made by the English physician Langdon Down in 1866, was based on the physical characteristics associated with subnormal mental functioning. Since then, Down syndrome has been the most investigated, and most discussed, syndrome in mental retardation. Children with this syndrome were originally called *mongoloid* because of their physical characteristics of slanted eyes, epicanthal folds, and flat nose. Despite a plethora of theories and hypotheses advanced in the past 100 years, the cause of Down syndrome is still unknown.

The problem of cause is complicated even further by the recent recognition of three types of chromosomal aberrations in Down syndrome:

1. Patients with trisomy 21 (three chromosome 21, instead of the usual two) represent the overwhelming majority; they have 47 chromosomes, with an extra chromosome 21. The mothers' karyotypes are normal. A nondisjunction during meiosis, occurring for unknown reasons, is held responsible for the disorder.
2. Nondisjunction occurring after fertilization in any cell division results in mosaicism, a condition in which both normal and trisomic cells are found in various tissues.
3. In translocation, a fusion occurs of two chromosomes, usually 21 and 15, resulting in a total of 46 chromosomes, despite the presence of an extra chromosome 21. The disorder, unlike trisomy 21, is usually inherited, and the translocated chromosome may be found in unaffected parents and siblings. The asymptomatic carriers have only 45 chromosomes.

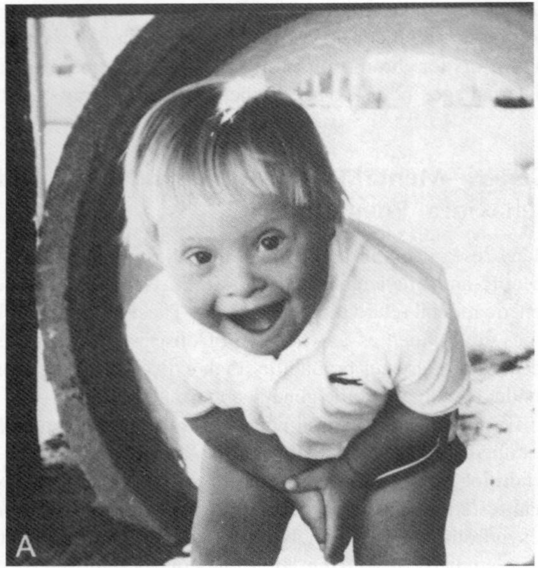

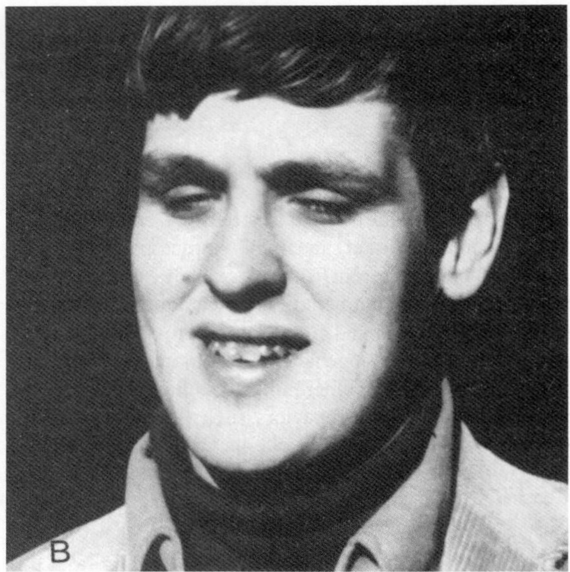

FIGURE 38–1

A. A young child with Down syndrome. **B.** A young adult with fragile X syndrome. (Courtesy of L.S. Syzmanski, M.D., and A.C. Crocker, M.D.)

The incidence of Down syndrome in the United States is about 1 in every 700 births. In his original description, Down mentioned the frequency of 10 percent among all mentally retarded patients. For a middle-aged mother (more than 32 years of age), the risk of having a child with Down syndrome with trisomy 21 is about 1 in 100 births, but when translocation is present, the risk is about 1 in 3. These facts assume special importance in genetic counseling.

Mental retardation is the overriding feature of Down syndrome. Most persons with the syndrome are moderately or severely retarded, with only a minority having an IQ above 50. Mental development seems to progress normally from birth to 6 months of age; IQ scores gradually decrease from near normal at 1 year of age to about 30 at older ages. The decline in intelligence may not be readily apparent. Infantile tests may not reveal the full extent of the defect, which may become manifest when sophisticated tests are used in early childhood. According to many sources, children with Down syndrome are placid, cheerful, and cooperative and adapt easily at home. With adolescence, the picture changes: Youngsters may experience various emotional difficulties, behavior disorders, and (rarely) psychotic disorders.

In Down syndrome, language function is a relative weakness, whereas sociability and social skills, such as interpersonal cooperation and conformity with social conventions, are relative strengths. Most studies have noted muted affect in children with Down syndrome relative to children of the same mental age who are not retarded. Those with Down syndrome also manifest deficiencies in scanning the environment; they are likely to focus on a single stimulus and have difficulty noticing environmental changes. A variety of mental disorders occurs in persons with Down syndrome, but the rates appear to be lower than those of other mental retardation syndromes, especially autistic disorder.

The diagnosis of Down syndrome is made with relative ease in an older child, but is often difficult in newborn infants. The most important signs in a newborn include general hypotonia; oblique palpebral fissures; abundant neck skin; a small, flattened skull; high cheekbones; and a protruding tongue. The hands are broad and thick, with a single palmar transversal crease, and the little fingers are short and curved inward. Moro reflex is weak or absent. More than 100 signs or stigmata are described in Down syndrome, but rarely are all found in one person. Life expectancy was once about 12 years; with the advent of antibiotics, few young patients die from Down syndrome, but many do not live beyond the age of 40. Life expectancy is increasing, however.

Persons with Down syndrome tend to exhibit marked deterioration in language, memory, self-care skills, and problem-solving in their 30s. Postmortem studies of those with Down syndrome over the age of 40 have shown a high incidence of senile plaques and neurofibrillary tangles, as seen in Alzheimer's disease. Neurofibrillary tangles are known to occur in a variety of degenerative diseases, whereas senile plaques seem to be found most often in Alzheimer's disease and in Down syndrome. Thus, the two disorders may share some pathophysiology.

Fragile X Syndrome. Fragile X syndrome is the second most common single cause of mental retardation. The syndrome results from a mutation on the X chromosome at what is known as the fragile site (Xq27.3). The fragile site is expressed in only some cells, and it may be absent in asymptomatic males and female carriers. Much variability is present in both genetic and phenotypic expression. Fragile X syndrome is believed to occur in about 1 of every 1,000 males and 1 of every 2,000 females. The typical phenotype includes a large, long head and ears, short stature, hyperextensible joints, and postpubertal macroorchidism. The mental retardation ranges from mild to severe. The behavioral profile of persons with the syndrome includes a high rate of ADHD, learning disorders, and pervasive developmental disorders, such as autism. Deficits in language function include rapid perseverative speech with abnormalities in combining words into phrases and sentences. Persons with fragile X syndrome seem to have relatively strong skills in communication and socialization; their intellectual functions seem to decline in the pubertal period. Female carriers are often less impaired than males with fragile X syndrome, but females can also manifest the typical physical characteristics and can be mildly retarded.

Prader-Willi Syndrome. Prader-Willi syndrome is postulated to result from a small deletion involving chromosome 15, usually occurring sporadically. Its prevalence is less than 1 of 10,000. Persons with the syndrome exhibit compulsive eating behavior and often obesity, mental retardation, hypogonadism, small stature, hypotonia, and small hands and feet. Children with the syndrome often have oppositional and defiant behavior.

Cat's Cry (Cri-du-Chat) Syndrome. Children with cat's cry syndrome lack part of chromosome 5. They are severely retarded and show many signs often associated with chromosomal aberrations, such as microcephaly, low-set ears, oblique palpebral fissures, hypertelorism, and micrognathia. The characteristic cat-like cry caused by laryngeal abnormalities that gave the syndrome its name gradually changes and disappears with increasing age.

Other Chromosomal Abnormalities. Other syndromes of autosomal aberrations associated with mental retardation are much less prevalent than Down syndrome.

Phenylketonuria. PKU was first described by Ivar Asbjörn Fölling in 1934 as the paradigmatic inborn error of metabolism. PKU is transmitted as a simple recessive autosomal mendelian trait and occurs in about 1 of every 10,000 to 15,000 live births. For parents who have already had a child with PKU, the chance of having another child with PKU is 1 of every 4 to 5 successive pregnancies. Although the disease is reported predominantly in persons of North European origin, a few cases have been described in blacks, Yemenite Jews, and Asians. The frequency among institutionalized retarded patients is about 1 percent. The basic metabolic defect in PKU is an inability to convert phenylalanine, an essential amino acid, to paratyrosine because of the absence or inactivity of the liver enzyme phenylalanine hydroxylase, which catalyzes the conversion. Two other types of hyperphenylalaninemia have recently been described. One is caused by a deficiency of the enzyme dihydropteridine reductase, and the other to a deficiency of a cofactor, biopterin. The first defect can be detected in fibroblasts, and biopterin can be measured in body fluids. Both these rare disorders carry a high risk of fatality.

Most patients with PKU are severely retarded, but some are reported to have borderline or normal intelligence. Eczema, vomiting, and convulsions occur in about a third of all patients. Although the clinical picture varies, typical children with PKU are hyperactive; they exhibit erratic, unpredictable behavior, and are difficult to manage. They frequently have temper tantrums and often display bizarre movements of their bodies and upper extremities, including twisting hand mannerisms; their behavior sometimes resembles that of children with autism or schizophrenia. Verbal and nonverbal communication is usually severely impaired or nonexistent. The children's coordination is poor, and they have many perceptual difficulties.

The disease was previously diagnosed on the basis of a urine test: Phenylpyruvic acid in the urine reacts with ferric chloride solution to yield a vivid green color. The test, however, has its limitations; it may not detect the presence of phenylpyruvic acid in urine before a baby is 5 or 6 weeks of age, and it may give positive responses with other aminoacidurias. Currently, a more reliable screening test, the Guthrie inhibition assay is more widely applied; it uses a bacteriological procedure to detect phenylalanine in the blood.

In the United States, newborn infants are now routinely screened for PKU. Early diagnosis is important, because a low-phenylalanine diet, in use since 1955, significantly improves both behavior and developmental progress. The best results seem to be obtained with early diagnosis and the start of dietary treatment before the child is 6 months of age. Dietary treatment, however, is not without risk. Phenylalanine is an essential amino acid, and its omission from the diet can lead to such severe complications as anemia, hypoglycemia, edema, and even death. Dietary treatment of PKU should be continued indefinitely. Children who receive a diagnosis before the age of 3 months and are placed on an optimal dietary regimen may have normal intelligence. A low-phenylalanine diet does not influence the level of mental retardation in untreated older children and adolescents with PKU, but the diet does decrease irritability and abnormal electroencephalogram (EEG) changes and does increase social responsiveness and attention span. The parents of children with PKU and some of the children's normal siblings are heterozygous carriers. The disease can be detected by a phenylalanine tolerance test, which may be important in genetic counseling of the family members.

Rett's Disorder. Rett's disorder is hypothesized to be an X-linked dominant mental retardation syndrome that is degenerative and affects only females. In 1966, Andreas Rett reported on 22 girls with a serious progressive neurological disability. Deterioration in communications skills, motor behavior, and social functioning starts at about 1 year of age. Autistic-like symptoms are common, as are ataxia, facial grimacing, teeth-grinding, and loss of speech. Intermittent hyperventilation and a disorganized breathing pattern are characteristic while the child is awake. Stereotypical hand movements, including hand-wringing, are typical. Progressive gait disturbance, scoliosis, and seizures occur. Severe spasticity is usually present by middle childhood. Cerebral atrophy occurs with decreased pigmentation of the substantia nigra, which suggests abnormalities of the dopaminergic nigrostriatal system.

Neurofibromatosis. Also called *von Recklinghausen's* disease, neurofibromatosis is the most common of the neurocutaneous syndromes caused by a single dominant gene, which may be inherited or be a new mutation. The disorder occurs in about 1 of 5,000 births and is characterized by café au lait spots on the skin and by neurofibromas, including optic gliomas and acoustic neuromas, caused by abnormal cell migration. Mild mental retardation occurs in up to one third of those with the disease.

Tuberous Sclerosis. Tuberous sclerosis is the second most common of the neurocutaneous syndromes; a progressive mental retardation occurs in up to two thirds of all affected persons. It occurs in about 1 of 15,000 persons and is inherited by autosomal dominant transmission. Seizures are present in all those who are mentally retarded and in two thirds of those who are not. Infantile spasms may occur as early as 6 months of age. The phenotypic presentation includes adenoma sebaceum and ash-leaf spots that can be identified with a slit lamp.

Lesch-Nyhan Syndrome. Lesch-Nyhan syndrome is a rare disorder caused by a deficiency of an enzyme involved in purine metabolism. The disorder is X-linked; patients have mental retardation, microcephaly, seizures, choreoathetosis, and spasticity. The syndrome is also associated with severe compulsive self-mutilation by biting the mouth and fingers. Lesch-Nyhan syndrome is another example of a genetically determined syndrome with a specific, predictable behavioral pattern.

Adrenoleukodystrophy. The most common of several disorders of sudanophilic cerebral sclerosis, adrenoleukodystrophy is characterized by diffuse demyelination of the cerebral white matter resulting in visual and intellectual impairment, seizures, spasticity, and progression to death. The cerebral degeneration in adrenoleukodystrophy is accompanied by adrenocortical insufficiency. The disorder is transmitted by a sex-linked gene located on the distal end of the long arm of the X chromosome. The clinical onset is generally between 5 and 8 years of age, with early seizures, disturbances in gait, and mild intellectual impairment. Abnormal pigmentation reflecting adrenal insufficiency sometimes precedes the neurological symptoms, and attacks of crying are common. Spastic contractures, ataxia, and swallowing disturbances are also frequent. Although the course is often rapidly progressive, some patients may have a relapsing and remitting course. The story of a child with the disorder was presented in the 1992 film *Lorenzo's Oil.*

Maple Syrup Urine Disease. The clinical symptoms of maple syrup urine disease appear during the first week of life. The infant deteriorates rapidly and has decerebrate rigidity, seizures, respiratory irregularity, and hypoglycemia. If untreated, most patients die in the first months of life, and the survivors are severely retarded. Some variants have been reported with transient ataxia and only mild retardation. Treatment follows the general principles established for PKU and consists of a diet very low in the three involved amino acids—leucine, isoleucine, and valine.

Other Enzyme Deficiency Disorders. Several enzyme deficiency disorders associated with mental retardation have been identified, and still more diseases are being added as new discoveries are made, including Hartnup disease, galactosemia, and glycogen-storage disease. Table 38–2 lists 30 important disorders with inborn errors of metabolism, hereditary transmission patterns, defective enzymes, clinical signs, and relation to mental retardation.

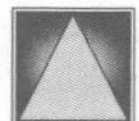

Table 38–2
Thirty Impairment Disorders with Inborn Errors of Metabolism

Disorder	Hereditary Transmission[a]	Enzyme Defect	Prenatal Diagnosis	Mental Retardation	Clinical Signs
I. LIPID METABOLISM					
Niemann-Pick disease					
Group A, infantile		Unknown			Hepatomegaly
Group B, adult	A.R.	Sphingomyelinase	+	±	Hepatosplenomegaly
Groups C and D, intermediate		Unknown	–	+	Pulmonary infiltration
Infantile Gaucher's disease	A.R.	β-Glucosidase	+	±	Hepatosplenomegaly, pseudobulbar palsy
Tay-Sachs disease	A.R.	Hexosaminidase A	+	+	Macular changes, seizures, spasticity
Generalized gangliosidosis	A.R.	β-Galactosidase	+	+	Hepatosplenomegaly, bone changes
Krabbe's disease	A.R.	Galactocerebroside β-Galactosidase	+	+	Stiffness, seizures
Metachromatic leukodystrophy	A.R.	Cerebroside sulfatase	+	+	Stiffness, developmental failure
Wolman's disease	A.R.	Acid lipase	+	–	Hepatosplenomegaly, adrenal calcification, vomiting, diarrhea
Farber's lipogranulomatosis	A.R.	Acid ceramidase	+	+	Hoarseness, arthropathy, subcutaneous nodules
Fabry's disease	X.R.	α-Galactosidase	+	–	Angiokeratomas, renal failure
II. MUCOPOLYSACCHARIDE METABOLISM					
Hurler's syndrome MPS I	A.R.	Iduronidase	+	+	?
Hurler's disease II	X.R.	Iduronate sulfatase	+	+	?
Sanfilippo's syndrome III	A.R.	Various sulfatases (types A–D)	+	+	Varying degrees of bone changes, hepatosplenomegaly, joint restriction, etc.
Morquio's disease IV	A.R.	*N*-Acetylgalactosamine-6-sulfate sulfatase	+	–	?
Maroteaux-Lamy syndrome VI	A.R.	Arylsulfatase B	+	±	?
III. OLIGOSACCHARIDE AND GLYCOPROTEIN METABOLISM					
I-cell disease	A.R.	Glycoprotein *N*-acetylglucosaminyl-phosphotransferase	+	+	Hepatomegaly, bone changes, swollen gingivae
Mannosidosis	A.R.	Mannosidase	+	+	Hepatomegaly, bone changes, facial coarsening
Fucosidosis	A.R.	Fucosidase	+	+	Same as above
IV. AMINO ACID METABOLISM					
Phenylketonuria	A.R.	Phenylalanine hydroxylase	–	+	Eczema, blonde hair, musty odor
Hemocystinuria	A.R.	Cystathionine β-synthetase	+	+	Ectopia lentis, Marfan-like phenotype, cardiovascular anomalies
Tyrosinosis	A.R.	Tyrosine amine transaminase	–	+	Hyperkeratotic skin lesions, conjunctivitis
Maple syrup urine disease	A.R.	Branched-chain ketoacid decarboxylase	+	+	Recurrent ketoacidosis
Methylmalonic acidemia	A.R.	Methylmalonyl-CoA mutase	+	+	Recurrent ketoacidosis, hepatomegaly, growth retardation

(*continued*)

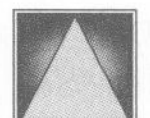

Table 38–2 (Continued)

Disorder	Hereditary Transmission[a]	Enzyme Defect	Prenatal Diagnosis	Mental Retardation	Clinical Signs
Propionic acidemia	A.R.	Propionyl-CoA carboxylase	+	+	Same as above
Nonketotic hyperglycinemia	A.R.	Glycine cleavage enzyme	+	+	Seizures
Urea cycle disorders	Mostly A.R.	Urea cycle enzymes	+	+	Recurrent acute encephalopathy, vomiting
Hartnup disease	A.R.	Renal transport disorder	–	–	None consistent
V. OTHERS					
Galactosemia	A.R.	Galactose-1-phosphate uridyltransferase	+	+	Hepatomegaly, cataracts, ovarian failure
Wilson's hepatolenticular degeneration	A.R.	Unknown factor in copper metabolism	–	±	Liver disease, Kayser-Fleischer ring, neurological problems
Menkes' kinky-hair disease	X.R.	Same as above	+	–	Abnormal hair, cerebral degeneration
Lesch-Nyhan syndrome	X.R.	Hypoxanthine guanine phosphoribosyltransferase	+	+	Behavioral abnormalities

[a]A.R., autosomal recessive transmission; X.R., X-linked recessive transmission.
(Adapted from Leroy JC. Hereditary, development, and behavior. In: Levine MD, Carey WB, Crocker AC, eds. *Developmental-Behavioral Pediatrics.* Philadelphia: WB Saunders; 1983:315, with permission.)

Acquired and Developmental Factors

Prenatal Period. Important prerequisites for the overall development of the fetus include the mother's physical, psychological, and nutritional health during pregnancy. Maternal chronic illnesses and conditions affecting the normal development of the fetus's CNS include uncontrolled diabetes, anemia, emphysema, hypertension, and long-term use of alcohol and narcotic substances. Maternal infections during pregnancy, especially viral infections, have been known to cause fetal damage and mental retardation. The extent of fetal damage depends on such variables as the type of viral infection, the gestational age of the fetus, and the severity of the illness. Although numerous infectious diseases have been reported to affect the fetus's CNS, the following medical disorders have been definitely identified as high-risk conditions for mental retardation.

Rubella (German Measles). Rubella has replaced syphilis as the major cause of congenital malformations and mental retardation caused by maternal infection. The children of affected mothers may show several abnormalities, including congenital heart disease, mental retardation, cataracts, deafness, microcephaly, and microphthalmia. Timing is crucial, because the extent and frequency of the complications are inversely related to the duration of the pregnancy at the time of maternal infection. When mothers are infected in the first trimester of pregnancy, 10 to 15 percent of the children are affected, but the incidence rises to almost 50 percent when the infection occurs in the first month of pregnancy. The situation is often complicated by subclinical forms of maternal infection that often go undetected. Maternal rubella can be prevented by immunization.

Cytomegalic Inclusion Disease. In many cases, cytomegalic inclusion disease remains dormant in the mother. Some children are stillborn, and others have jaundice, microcephaly, hepatosplenomegaly, and radiographic findings of intracerebral calcification. Children with mental retardation from the disease frequently have cerebral calcification, microcephaly, or hydrocephalus. The diagnosis is confirmed by positive findings of the virus in throat and urine cultures and the recovery of inclusion-bearing cells in the urine.

Syphilis. Syphilis in pregnant women was once the main cause of various neuropathological changes in their offspring, including mental retardation. Today, the incidence of syphilitic complications of pregnancy fluctuates with the incidence of syphilis in the general population. Some recent alarming statistics from several major cities in the United States indicate that there is still no room for complacency.

Toxoplasmosis. Toxoplasmosis can be transmitted by the mother to the fetus. It causes mild or severe mental retardation and, in severe cases, hydrocephalus, seizures, microcephaly, and chorioretinitis.

Herpes Simplex. The herpes simplex virus can be transmitted transplacentally, although the most common mode of infection is during birth. Microcephaly, mental retardation, intracranial calcification, and ocular abnormalities may result.

Acquired Immune Deficiency Syndrome (AIDS). Many fetuses of mothers with AIDS never come to term because of stillbirth or spontaneous abortion. Of infants born infected with the human immunodeficiency virus (HIV), up to half have progressive encephalopathy, mental retardation, and seizures within the first year of life. Children born with HIV infection often live only a few years; however, most babies born to HIV-infected mothers are not infected with the virus.

Fetal Alcohol Syndrome. Fetal alcohol syndrome results in mental retardation and a typical phenotypic picture of facial dysmorphism that includes hypertelorism, microcephaly, short palpebral fissures, inner epicanthal folds, and a short, turned-up nose. Often, the affected children have learning disorders and ADHD. Cardiac defects are also frequent. The entire syndrome occurs in up to 15 percent of babies born to women who regularly ingest large amounts of alcohol. Babies born to women who consume alcohol regularly during pregnancy have a high incidence of ADHD, learning disorders, and mental retardation without the facial dysmorphism.

Prenatal Drug Exposure. Prenatal exposure to opioids, such as heroin, often results in infants who are small for their gestational age, with a head circumference below the tenth percentile and withdrawal symptoms that appear within the first 2 days of life. The withdrawal symptoms of infants include irritability, hypertonia, tremor, vomiting, a high-pitched cry, and an abnormal sleep pattern. Seizures are unusual, but the withdrawal syndrome can be life threatening to infants if it is untreated. Diazepam (Valium), phenobarbital (Luminal), chlorpromazine (Thorazine), and paregoric have been used to treat neonatal opioid withdrawal. The long-term sequelae of prenatal opioid exposure are not fully known; the children's developmental milestones and intellectual functions may be within the normal range, but they have an increased risk for impulsivity and behavioral problems. Infants prenatally exposed to cocaine are at high risk for low birthweight and premature delivery. In the early neonatal period, they may have transient neurological and behavioral abnormalities, including abnormal results on EEGs, tachycardia, poor feeding patterns, irritability, and excessive drowsiness. Rather than a withdrawal reaction, the physiological and behavioral abnormalities are a response to the cocaine, which may be excreted for up to a week postnatally.

Complications of Pregnancy. Toxemia of pregnancy and uncontrolled maternal diabetes present hazards to the fetus and sometimes result in mental retardation. Maternal malnutrition during pregnancy often results in prematurity and other obstetrical complications. Vaginal hemorrhage, placenta previa, premature separation of the placenta, and prolapse of the cord can damage the fetal brain by causing anoxia. The potential teratogenic effect of pharmacological agents administered during pregnancy was widely publicized after the thalidomide tragedy (the drug produced a high percentage of deformed babies when given to pregnant women). So far, with the exception of metabolites used in cancer chemotherapy, no usual dosages of medications are known to damage the fetus's CNS, but caution and restraint in prescribing drugs to pregnant women are certainly indicated. The use of lithium during pregnancy was recently implicated in some congenital malformations, especially of the cardiovascular system (e.g., Ebstein's anomaly).

Perinatal Period. Some evidence indicates that premature infants and infants with low birthweight are at high risk for neurological and intellectual impairments that appear during their school years. Infants who sustain intracranial hemorrhages or show evidence of cerebral ischemia are especially vulnerable to cognitive abnormalities. The degree of neurodevelopmental impairment generally correlates with the severity of the intracranial hemorrhage. Recent studies have documented that, among children with very low birthweight (less than 1,000 g), 20 percent had significant disabilities, including cerebral palsy, mental retardation, autism, and low intelligence with severe learning problems. Very premature children and those who suffered intrauterine growth retardation were found to be at high risk for developing both social problems and academic difficulties. Socioeconomic deprivation can also affect the adaptive function of these vulnerable infants. Early intervention may improve their cognitive, language, and perceptual abilities.

Acquired Childhood Disorders. Occasionally, a child's developmental status changes dramatically as a result of a specific disease or physical trauma. In retrospect, it is sometimes difficult to ascertain the full picture of the child's developmental progress before the insult, but the adverse effects on the child's development or skills are apparent afterward.

Infection. The most serious infections affecting cerebral integrity are encephalitis and meningitis. Measles encephalitis has been virtually eliminated by the universal use of measles vaccine, and the incidence of other bacterial infections of the CNS has been markedly reduced with antibacterial agents. Most episodes of encephalitis are caused by viruses. Sometimes a clinician must retrospectively consider a probable encephalitic component in a previous obscure illness with high fever. Meningitis that was diagnosed late, even when followed by antibiotic treatment, can seriously affect a child's cognitive development. Thrombotic and purulent intracranial phenomena secondary to septicemia are rarely seen today except in small infants.

Head Trauma. The best-known causes of head injury in children that produces developmental handicaps, including seizures, are motor vehicle accidents, but more head injuries are caused by household accidents, such as falls from tables, from open windows, and on stairways. Child abuse is also a cause of head injury.

Other Issues. Brain damage from cardiac arrest during anesthesia is rare. One cause of complete or partial brain damage is asphyxia associated with near drowning. Long-term exposure to lead is a well-established cause of compromised intelligence and learning skills. Intracranial tumors of various types and origins, surgery, and chemotherapy can also adversely affect brain function.

Environmental and Sociocultural Factors

Mild retardation can result from significant deprivation of nutrition and nurturance. Children who have endured these conditions are subject to long-lasting damage to their physical and emotional development. Prenatal environment compromised by poor medical care and poor maternal nutrition can be contributing factors in the development of mild mental retardation. Teenage pregnancies are risk factors and they are associated with obstetrical complications, prematurity, and low birthweight. Poor postnatal medical care, malnutrition, exposure to such toxic substances as lead, and physical trauma are risk factors for mild mental retardation. Family instability, frequent moves, and multiple but inadequate caretakers may deprive an infant of necessary emotional relationships, leading to failure to thrive and potential risk to the developing brain.

An incapacitating mental disorder in a parent may interfere with appropriate child care and stimulation and cause developmental risk. Children of parents with mood disorders and schizophrenia are known to be at risk for these and related disorders. Some studies indicate a higher than expected prevalence of motor skills disorder and developmental disorders, but not necessarily mental retardation, among the children of parents with chronic mental disorders.

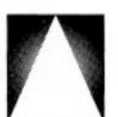

Table 38–3
DSM-IV-TR Diagnostic Criteria for Mental Retardation

A. Significantly subaverage intellectual functioning: an IQ of approximately 70 or below on an individually administered IQ test (for infants, a clinical judgment of significantly subaverage intellectual functioning).
B. Concurrent deficits or impairments in present adaptive functioning (i.e., the person's effectiveness in meeting the standards expected for his or her age by his or her cultural group) in at least two of the following areas: communication, self-care, home living, social/interpersonal skills, use of community resources, self-direction, functional academic skills, work, leisure, health, and safety.
C. The onset is before age 18 years.

Code based on degree of severity reflecting level of intellectual impairment:

Mild mental retardation:	IQ level 50–55 to approximately 70
Moderate mental retardation:	IQ level 35–40 to 50–55
Severe mental retardation:	IQ level 20–25 to 35–40
Profound mental retardation:	IQ level below 20 or 25
Mental retardation, severity unspecified:	When there is strong presumption of mental retardation but the person's intelligence is untestable by standard tests

(From American Psychiatric Association. *Diagnostic and Statistical Manual of Mental Disorders.* 4th ed. Text rev. Washington, DC: American Psychiatric Association; copyright 2000, with permission.)

DIAGNOSIS

The diagnosis of mental retardation can be made after the history, a standardized intellectual assessment, and a measure of adaptive function indicate that a child's current behavior is significantly below the expected level (Table 38–3). The diagnosis itself does not specify either the cause or the prognosis. A history and psychiatric interview are useful in obtaining a longitudinal picture of the child's development and functioning, and examination of physical signs, neurological abnormalities, and laboratory tests can be used to ascertain the cause and prognosis.

History

The history is most often obtained from the parents or the caretaker, with particular attention to the mother's pregnancy, labor, and delivery; the presence of a family history of mental retardation; consanguinity of the parents; and hereditary disorders. As part of the history, the clinician assesses the overall level of functioning and intellectual capacity of the parents and the emotional climate of the home.

Psychiatric Interview

Two factors are of paramount importance when interviewing the patient: the interviewer's attitude and manner of communicating. The interviewer should not be guided by the patient's mental age, which cannot fully characterize the person. A mildly retarded adult with a mental age of 10 is not a 10-year-old child. When addressed as if they were children, some retarded persons become justifiably insulted, angry, and uncooperative. Passive and dependent persons, alternatively, may assume the child's role that they think is expected of them. In neither case can valid diagnostic data be obtained.

The patient's verbal abilities, including receptive and expressive language, should be assessed as soon as possible by observing the communication between the caretakers and the patient and by taking the history. The clinician often finds it helpful to see the patient and the caretakers together. If the patient uses sign language, the caretaker may have to stay during the interview as an interpreter. Retarded persons often have the lifelong experience of failing in many areas, and they may be anxious about seeing an interviewer. The interviewer and the caretaker should attempt to give such patients a clear, supportive, concrete explanation of the diagnostic process, particularly patients with sufficiently receptive language. Giving patients the impression that their bad behavior is the cause of the referral should be avoided. Support and praise should be offered in language appropriate to the patient's age and understanding. Leading questions should be avoided, because retarded persons may be suggestible and wish to please others. Subtle direction, structure, and reinforcement may be necessary to keep them focused on the task or topic.

The patient's control over motility patterns should be ascertained, and clinical evidence of distractibility and distortions in perception and memory may be evaluated. The use of speech, reality testing, and the ability to generalize from experiences should be noted. The nature and maturity of the patient's defenses—particularly exaggerated or self-defeating uses of avoidance, repression, denial, introjection, and isolation—should be observed. Frustration, tolerance, and impulse control—especially over motor, aggressive, and sexual drives—should be assessed. Also important are self-image and its role in the development of self-confidence, as well as an assessment of tenacity, persistence, curiosity, and willingness to explore the unknown. In general, the psychiatric examination of a retarded person should reveal how the patient has coped with the stages of development.

Physical Examination

Various parts of the body may have certain characteristics that have prenatal causes and are commonly found in persons who are mentally retarded. For example, the configuration and the size of the head offer clues to a variety of conditions, such as microcephaly, hydrocephalus, and Down syndrome. The patient's face may have some signs of mental retardation that greatly facilitate the diagnosis, such as hypertelorism, a flat nasal bridge, prominent eyebrows, epicanthal folds, corneal opacities, retinal changes, low-set and small or misshapen ears, a protruding tongue, and a disturbance in dentition. Facial expression, such as a dull appearance, can be misleading and should not be relied on without other supporting evidence. The color and texture of the skin and hair, a high-arched palate, the size of the thyroid gland, and the size of the child and his or her trunk and extremities should also be explored. The circumference of the head should be measured as part of the clinical investigation. Dermatoglyphics may offer another diagnostic tool, because uncommon ridge patterns and flexion creases on the hand are often found in persons who are retarded. Abnormal dermatoglyphics occur in chromosomal disorders and in persons who were prenatally infected with rubella. Table 38–4 lists the multiple handicaps associated

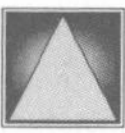

Table 38–4
Representative Sample of Mental Retardation Syndromes and Behavioral Phenotypes

Disorder	Pathophysiology	Clinical Features and Behavioral Phenotype
Down syndrome	Trisomy 21, 95% nondisjunction, approx, 4% translocation; 1/1,000 live births: 1:2,500 in women less than 30 years old, 1:80 over 40 years old, 1:32 at 45 years old; possible overproduction of β-amyloid due to defect at 21q21.1	Hypotonia, upward-slanted palpebral fissures, midface depression, flat wide nasal bridge, simian crease, short stature, increased incidence of thyroid abnormalities and congenital heart disease Passive, affable, hyperactivity in childhood, stubborn; verbal > auditory processing, increased risk of depression, and dementia of the Alzheimer type in adulthood
Fragile X syndrome	Inactivation of *FMR-1* gene at X q27.3 due to CGG base repeats, methylation; recessive; 1:1,000 male births, 1:3,000 female; accounts for 10–12% of mental retardation in males	Long face, large ears, midface hypoplasia, high arched palate, short stature, macroorchidism, mitral valve prolapse, joint laxity, strabismus Hyperactivity, inattention, anxiety, stereotypies, speech and language delays, IQ decline, gaze aversion, social avoidance, shyness, irritability, learning disorder in some females; mild mental retardation in affected females, moderate to severe in males; verbal IQ > performance IQ
Prader-Willi syndrome	Deletion in 15q12 (15q11–15q13) of paternal origin; some cases of maternal uniparental disomy; dominant 1/10,000 live births; 90% sporadic; candidate gene: small nuclear ribonucleoprotein polypeptide (SNRPN)	Hypotonia, failure to thrive in infancy, obesity, small hands and feet microorchidism, cryptorchidism, short stature, almond-shaped eyes, fair hair and light skin, flat face, scoliosis, orthopedic problems, prominent forehead and bitemporal narrowing Compulsive behavior, hyperphagia, hoarding, impulsivity, borderline to moderate mental retardation, emotional lability, tantrums, excess daytime sleepiness, skin picking, anxiety, aggression
Angelman syndrome	Deletion in 15q12 (15q11–15q13) of maternal origin; dominant; frequent deletion of γ-aminobutyric acid (GABA) B-3 receptor subunit, prevalence unknown but rare, estimated 1/20,000–1/30,000	Fair hair and blue eyes (66%); dysmorphic faces including wide smiling mouth, thin upper lip, and pointed chin; epilepsy (90%) with characteristic EEG; ataxia; small head circumference, 25% microcephalic Happy disposition, paroxysmal laughter, hand flapping, clapping; profound mental retardation; sleep disturbance with nighttime waking; possible increased incidence of autistic features; anecdotal love of water and music
Cornelia de Lange syndrome	Lack of pregnancy associated plasma protein A (PAPPA) linked to chromosome 9q33; similar phenotype associated with trisomy 5p, ring chromosome 3; rare (1/40,000–1/100,000 live births); possible association with 3q26.3	Continuous eyebrows, thin downturning upper lip, microcephaly, short stature, small hands and feet, small upturned nose, anteverted nostrils, malformed upper limbs, failure to thrive Self-injury, limited speech in severe cases, language delays, avoidance of being held, stereotypic movements, twirling, severe to profound mental retardation
Williams syndrome	1/20,000 births; hemizygous deletion that includes elastin locus chromosome 7q11–23; autosomal dominant	Short stature, unusual facial features including broad forehead, depressed nasal bridge, stellate pattern of the iris, widely spaced teeth, and full lips; elfinlike facies; renal and cardiovascular abnormalities; thyroid abnormalities; hypercalcemia Anxiety, hyperactivity, fears, outgoing, sociable, verbal skills > visual spatial skills
Cri-du-chat syndrome	Partial deletion 5p; 1/50,000; region may be 5p15.2	Round face with hypertelorism, epicanthal folds, slanting palpebral fissures, broad flat nose, low-set ears, micrognathia; prenatal growth retardation; respiratory and ear infections; congenital heart disease; gastrointestinal abnormalities Severe mental retardation, infantile catlike cry, hyperactivity, stereotypies, self-injury
Smith-Magenis syndrome	Incidence unknown, estimated 1/25,000 live births; complete or partial deletion of 17p11.2	Broad face; flat midface; short, broad hands; small toes; hoarse, deep voice Severe mental retardation; hyperactivity; severe self-injury including hand biting, head banging, and pulling out finger- and toenails; stereotyped self-hugging; attention seeking; aggression; sleep disturbance (decreased REM)
Rubinstein-Taybi syndrome	1/250,000, approx. male = female; sporadic; likely autosomal dominant; documented microdeletions in some cases at 16p13.3	Short stature and microcephaly, broad thumb and big toes, prominent nose, broad nasal bridge, hypertelorism, ptosis, frequent fractures, feeding difficulties in infancy, congenital heart disease, EEG abnormalities, seizures Poor concentration, distractible, expressive language difficulties, performance IQ > verbal IQ; anecdotally happy, loving, sociable, responsive to music, self-stimulating behavior; older patients have mood lability and temper tantrums

(*continued*)

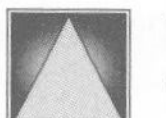

Table 38–4 (Continued)

Disorder	Pathophysiology	Clinical Features and Behavioral Phenotype
Tuberous sclerosis complex 1 and 2	Benign tumors (hamartomas) and malformations (hamartias) of central nervous system (CNS), skin, kidney, heart; dominant; 1/10,000 births; 50% TSC 1, 9q34; 50% TSC 2, 16p13	Epilepsy, autism, hyperactivity, impulsivity, aggression; spectrum of mental retardation from none (30%) to profound; self-injurious behaviors, sleep disturbances
Neurofibromatosis type 1 (NF1)	1/2,500–1/4,000; male = female; autosomal dominant; 50% new mutations; more than 90% paternal NF1 allele mutated; *NFI* gene 17q11.2; gene product is neurofibromin thought to be tumor suppressor gene	Variable manifestations; café au lait spots, cutaneous neurofibromas, Lisch nodules; short stature and macrocephaly in 30–45% Half with speech and language difficulties; 10% with moderate to profound mental retardation; verbal IQ > performance IQ; distractible, impulsive, hyperactive, anxious; possibly associated with increased incidence of mood and anxiety disorders
Lesch-Nyhan syndrome	Defect in hypoxanthine guanine phosphoribosyl-transferase with accumulation of uric acid; Xq26–27; recessive; rare (1/10,000–1/38,000)	Ataxia, chorea, kidney failure, gout Often severe self-biting behavior; aggression; anxiety; mild to moderate mental retardation
Galactosemia	Defect in galactose-1-phosphate uridyltransferase or galactokinase or empiramase; autosomal recessive; 1/62,000 births in the U.S.	Vomiting in early infancy, jaundice, hepatosplenomegaly; later cataracts, weight loss, food refusal, increased intracranial pressure and increased risk for sepsis, ovarian failure, failure to thrive, renal tubular damage Possible mental retardation even with treatment, visuospatial deficits, language disorders, reports of increased behavioral problems, anxiety, social withdrawal, and shyness
Phenylketonuria	Defect in phenylalanine hydroxylase (PAH) or cofactor (biopterin) with accumulation of phenylalanine; approximately 1/11,500 births; varies with geographical location; gene for PAH, 12q22–24.1; autosomal recessive	Symptoms absent neonatally, later development of seizures (25% generalized), fair skin, blue eyes, blond hair, rash Untreated: mild to profound mental retardation, language delay, destructiveness, self-injury, hyperactivity
Hurler's syndrome	1/100,000; deficiency in α-L- iduronidase activity; autosomal recessive	Early onset; short stature, hepatosplenomegaly; hirsutism, corneal clouding, death before age 10 years, dwarfism, coarse facial features, recurrent respiratory infections Moderate-to-severe mental retardation, anxious, fearful, rarely aggressive
Hunter's syndrome	1/100,000, X-linked recessive; iduronate sulfatase deficiency; X q28	Normal infancy; symptom onset at age 2–4 years; typical coarse faces with flat nasal bridge, flaring nostrils; hearing loss, ataxia, hernia common; enlarged liver and spleen, joint stiffness, recurrent infections, growth retardation, cardiovascular abnormality Hyperactivity, mental retardation by 2 years; speech delay; loss of speech at 8–10 years; restless, aggressive, inattentive, sleep abnormalities; apathetic, sedentary with disease progression
Fetal alcohol syndrome	Maternal alcohol consumption (trimester III>II>I); 1/3,000 live births in Western countries; 1/300 with fetal alcohol effects	Microcephaly, short stature, midface hypoplasia, short palpebral fissure, thin upper lip, retrognathia in infancy, micrognathia in adolescence, hypoplastic long or smooth philtrum Mild to moderate mental retardation, irritability, inattention, memory impairment

(Table by B. H. King, M.D., R. M. Hodapp, Ph.D., and E. M. Dykens, Ph.D.)

with various mental retardation syndromes. The clinician should bear in mind during the examination that mentally retarded children, particularly those with associated behavioral problems, are at increased risk for child abuse.

Neurological Examination

Sensory impairments occur frequently among persons who are mentally retarded; for example, up to 10 percent are hearing impaired, a rate that is four times that of the general population. Sensory disturbances can include hearing difficulties, ranging from cortical deafness to mild hearing deficits. Visual disturbances can range from blindness to disturbances of spatial concepts, design recognition, and concepts of body image. Various other neurological impairments also occur frequently in mentally retarded persons; seizure disorders occur in about 10 percent of all mentally retarded persons and in one third of those with severe retardation. When neurological abnormalities are present, their incidence and severity generally rise in direct proportion to the degree of retardation. Many severely retarded children, however, have no neurological abnormalities; conversely, about 25 percent of all children with cerebral palsy have normal intelligence.

Disturbances in motor areas are manifested in abnormalities of muscle tone (spasticity or hypotonia), reflexes (hyperreflexia), and involuntary movements (choreoathetosis). Less disability is revealed in clumsiness and poor coordination.

The infants with the poorest prognoses are those who manifest a combination of inactivity, general hypotonia, and exaggerated response to stimuli. In older children, hyperactivity, short attention span, distractibility, and a low frustration tolerance are often signs of brain damage. In general, the younger the child at the time of investigation, the more caution is indicated in predicting future ability, because the recovery potential of the infantile brain is very good. Observing the child's development at regular intervals is probably the most reliable approach.

Skull X-rays are usually taken routinely, but are illuminating in only a relatively few conditions, such as craniosynostosis, hydrocephalus, and other disorders that result in intracranial calcifications (e.g., toxoplasmosis, tuberous sclerosis, cerebral angiomatosis, and hypoparathyroidism). Computed tomography (CT) scans and magnetic resonance imaging (MRI) have become important tools for uncovering CNS pathology associated with mental retardation. Occasionally, findings are of internal hydrocephalus, cortical atrophy, or porencephaly in severely retarded, brain-damaged children. An EEG is best interpreted with caution in cases of mental retardation. The exceptions are patients with hypsarhythmia and grand mal seizures, in whom the EEG may help establish the diagnosis and suggest treatment. In most other conditions, a diffuse cerebral disorder produces nonspecific EEG changes, characterized by slow frequencies with bursts of spikes and sharp or blunt wave complexes. The confusion over the significance of the EEG in the diagnosis of mental retardation is best illustrated by the reports of frequent EEG abnormalities in Down syndrome, which are in the range of 25 percent in most patients examined.

CLINICAL FEATURES

Mild mental retardation may not be diagnosed until the affected children enter school; their social skills and communication may be adequate in the preschool years. As they get older, however, such cognitive deficits as poor ability to abstract and egocentric thinking may distinguish them from others of their age. Although mildly retarded persons can function academically at the high elementary level and their vocational skills suffice to support themselves in some cases, social assimilation can be difficult. Communication deficits, poor self-esteem, and dependence can contribute to their relative lack of social spontaneity. Some persons who are mildly retarded may fall into relationships with peers who exploit their shortcomings. In most cases, persons with mild mental retardation can achieve some social and vocational success in a supportive environment.

Moderate mental retardation is likely to be diagnosed at a younger age than mild mental retardation; communication skills develop more slowly in persons who are moderately retarded, and their social isolation may begin in the elementary school years. Although academic achievement is usually limited to the middle-elementary level, moderately retarded children benefit from individual attention focused on the development of self-help skills. Children with moderate mental retardation are aware of their deficits and often feel alienated from their peers and frustrated by their limitations. They continue to require a relatively high level of supervision but can become competent at occupational tasks in supportive settings.

Severe mental retardation is generally obvious in the preschool years; affected children's speech is minimal, and their motor development is poor. Some language development may occur in the school-age years. By adolescence, if language is poor, nonverbal forms of communication may have evolved; the inability to articulate needs fully may reinforce the physical means of communicating. Behavioral approaches can help promote some self-care, although those with severe mental retardation generally need extensive supervision.

Children with profound mental retardation require constant supervision and are severely limited in communication and motor skills. By adulthood, some speech development may be present, and simple self-help skills may be acquired. Even in adulthood, nursing care is needed.

Surveys have identified several clinical features that occur with greater frequency in persons who are mentally retarded than in the general population. These features, which can occur in isolation or as part of a mental disorder, include hyperactivity, low frustration tolerance, aggression, affective instability, repetitive and stereotypic motor behaviors, and various self-injurious behaviors. Self-injurious behaviors seem to be more frequent and more intense with increasingly severe mental retardation. It is often difficult to decide whether these clinical features are comorbid mental disorders or direct sequelae of the developmental limitations imposed by mental retardation.

Robert was a full-term infant, the last of three children born to his 38-year-old mother, a high school music teacher, and 40-year-old father, a high school science teacher. Pregnancy was unremarkable, and Robert's two older sisters were healthy and developing nicely. The family lived in a rural town in the Midwest.

Robert was an extremely fussy newborn and had extended periods of crying that the pediatrician labeled classic colic. At 2 months of age, the parents were told that Robert had a mild case of supravalvular aortic stenosis, one that warranted monitoring but no surgeries. Although Robert became slightly less fussy over time, he was a picky eater, refusing solid foods. Robert's parents also noted that he was more "high-strung" than his siblings, often quick to cry or cringe when his sisters played too loudly.

Milestones were slightly delayed, with Robert sitting unassisted at 10 months and walking at 18 months. Language was also delayed, and, although his first words appeared at 20 months, Robert had always made his wants and needs known. Although his parents were concerned that he was delayed compared with his sisters, they were reassured by the pediatrician's sense that boys often had slight delays and that he was a lively, social boy who would quickly catch up.

When Robert was 3 years of age, his parents insisted on a developmental evaluation, which showed modest delays in cognitive, linguistic, and motor functioning, with a developmental quotient (DQ) of 74. He was described as friendly and engaging, a real "charmer," with a cute face that endeared him to many. Robert was enrolled in a special kindergarten, and he remained in a combination of special education and mainstreamed classes throughout his academic career. As his mother and sisters, Robert enjoyed listening to music and singing, and he took an active interest in tinkering on the piano.

At 7 years of age, the school psychologist evaluated Robert and believed that he fit a "learning disability" profile. Robert had an overall IQ of 66, with close to average functioning in short-term memory and expressive language and pronounced deficits in long-term memory and expressive language and pronounced deficits in visual-spatial functioning. He struggled with writing tasks and arithmetic, but loved science and music and was amazingly conversant with anyone who would listen to him. Indeed, his parents feared he was "too friendly," as well as too active, and with transient, intense interests in unusual items, such as vacuum cleaners.

As he entered adolescence, Robert became increasingly anxious, so much so that he occasionally rubbed his hands or rocked, and he "fretted" about day-to-day issues and what would happen next. His long-term sensitivities to loud sounds seemed to wane slightly, but he developed fears of storm clouds and dogs and refused as well to ride on elevators. He became tearful and upset after one of his older sisters left for college and worried about her health and ability to watch the weather at college. Although Robert experienced nightmares and would occasionally pace with worry and complain of stomachaches, he attended school and had a small group of friends in the Special Olympics bowling league. Furthermore, he enjoyed singing with the high school chorus and was delighted to be routinely selected to play the piano at school concerts.

When Robert was 17 years of age, his parents happened to watch a television documentary on Williams syndrome. They were overwhelmed by the similarities between Robert and the people described in the program. They later described the experience like a "jolt." They had always accepted Robert, quirks and all, and had stopped pushing their doctors for reasons "why" when Robert was a preschooler. Nevertheless, they immediately called the informational number offered in the show, and, within 2 months, they had the genetic tests done that confirmed their strong suspicion that Robert had Williams syndrome.

Although Robert's day-to-day life did not change dramatically since his diagnosis, his parents' report a big difference in Robert's outlook. He met new Williams syndrome friends at a conference, he applied to go to a summer music camp for young adults with Williams syndrome, and he states that he feels less alone. Robert's parents report a mixture of feelings at having such a late diagnosis—disappointment in their doctors, relief in finally knowing, and twinges of guilt. They are energized by having a new community of Williams syndrome families with whom to share their feelings and worries; as their son, they also feel less alone.

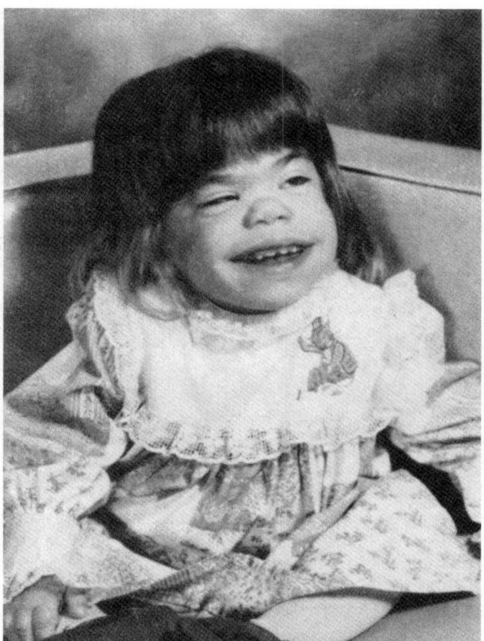

FIGURE 38–2

A 6-year-old girl with Hurler's syndrome. Her care has involved a class for seriously multihandicapped children, attention to cardiac problems, and special counseling for patients. (Courtesy of L.S. Syzmanski, M.D., and A.C. Crocker, M.D.)

LABORATORY EXAMINATION

Laboratory tests used to elucidate the causes of mental retardation, include chromosomal analysis, urine and blood testing for metabolic disorders, and neuroimaging. Chromosomal abnormalities are the single most common cause of mental retardation found in individuals for whom a cause can be identified.

Chromosome Studies

The determination of the karyotype in a genetic laboratory is considered whenever a chromosomal disorder is suspected or when the cause of the mental retardation is unknown. Amniocentesis, in which a small amount of amniotic fluid is removed from the amniotic cavity transabdominally at about the 15th week of gestation, has been useful in diagnosing prenatal chromosomal abnormalities. It is often considered when an increased fetal risk exists, such as with increased maternal age, or Down syndrome. Amniotic fluid cells, mostly fetal in origin, are cultured for cytogenetic and biochemical studies. Many serious hereditary disorders can be predicted with amniocentesis, and it should be considered by pregnant women over the age of 35.

Chronic villi sampling (CVS) is a screening technique to determine fetal chromosomal abnormalities. It is done at 8 to 10 weeks of gestation, 6 weeks earlier than amniocentesis is done. The results are available in a short time (hours or days) and, if the result is abnormal, the decision to terminate the pregnancy can be made within the first trimester. The procedure has a miscarriage risk between 2 and 5 percent; the risk in amniocentesis is lower (1 in 200).

Urine and Blood Analysis

Lesch-Nyhan syndrome, galactosemia, PKU, Hurler's syndrome (Figure 38–2), and Hunter's syndrome (Figure 38–3) are examples of disorders that include mental retardation that can be identified through assays of the appropriate enzyme or organic or amino acids. Enzymatic abnormalities in chromosomal disorders, particularly Down syndrome, promise to become useful diagnostic tools. Unexplained growth abnormality, seizure disorder, poor muscle tone, ataxia, bone or skin abnormalities, and eye abnormalities are some indications for testing metabolic function.

Electroencephalography

Electroencephalography is indicated whenever a seizure disorder is considered.

Neuroimaging

Neuroimaging studies are currently being utilized to gather data that may uncover biological mechanisms contributing to mental

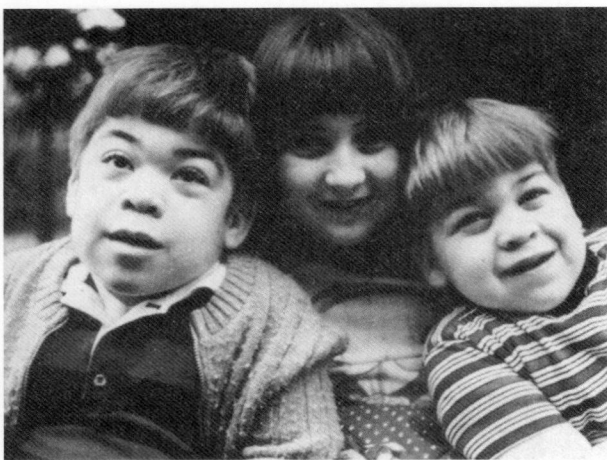

FIGURE 38–3
Two brothers, age 6 and 8 years, with Hunter's syndrome, shown with their normal older sister. They have had significant developmental delay, trouble with recurrent respiratory infection, and behavioral abnormalities. (Courtesy of L.S. Syzmanski, M.D., and A.C. Crocker, M.D.)

retardation syndromes. MRI, including structural MRI, functional MRI, and other forms of neuroimaging are currently being used by researchers seeking to identify specific etiologies of mental retardation syndromes. For example, current data suggest that individuals with fragile X syndromes who exhibit attentional deficits are also more likely to show aberrant frontal-striatal pathways seen on MRI. MRI can show abnormalities in the brain such as myelination patterns. MRI studies can also provide a baseline for comparison of a later, potentially degenerative process in the brain.

Hearing and Speech Evaluations

Hearing and speech should be evaluated routinely. Speech development may be the most reliable criterion in investigating mental retardation. Various hearing impairments often occur in persons who are mentally retarded, but in some instances impairments can simulate mental retardation. The commonly used methods of hearing and speech evaluation, however, require the patient's cooperation and, thus, are often unreliable in severely retarded persons.

Psychological Assessment

Examining clinicians can use several screening instruments for infants and toddlers. As in many areas of mental retardation, the controversy over the predictive value of infant psychological tests is heated. Some report the correlation of abnormalities during infancy with later abnormal functioning as very low, and others report it to be very high. The correlation rises in direct proportion to the age of the child at the time of the developmental examination; however, copying geometric figures, the *Goodenough Draw-a-Person Test*, the *Kohs Block Test*, and geometric puzzles all may be used as quick screening tests of visual-motor coordination. Psychological testing, performed by an experienced psychologist, is a standard part of an evaluation for mental retardation. The Gesell and Bayley scales and the *Cattell Infant Intelligence Scale* are most commonly used with infants. For children, the *Stanford-Binet Intelligence Scale* and the third edition of the *Wechsler Intelligence Scale for Children* (WISC-III) are those most widely used in the United States. Both tests have been criticized for penalizing culturally deprived children, for being culturally biased, for testing mainly the potential for academic achievement and not for adequate social functioning, and for their unreliability in children with IQs below 50. Some persons have tried to overcome the language barrier of persons who are mentally retarded by devising picture vocabulary tests, of which the *Peabody Vocabulary Test* is the one most widely used. The tests often found useful in detecting brain damage are the *Bender Gestalt Test* and the *Benton Visual Retention Test* (see Figs. 5.2–1 and 5.2–3 in Section 5.2). These tests are also useful for mildly retarded children. In addition, a psychological evaluation should assess perceptual, motor, linguistic, and cognitive abilities. Information about motivational, emotional, and interpersonal factors is also important.

COURSE AND PROGNOSIS

In most cases of mental retardation, the underlying intellectual impairment does not improve, yet the affected person's level of adaptation can be influenced positively by an enriched and supportive environment. In general, persons with mild and moderate mental retardation have the most flexibility in adapting to various environmental conditions. As in those who are not mentally retarded, the more comorbid mental disorders there are, the more guarded is the overall prognosis. When clear-cut mental disorders are superimposed on mental retardation, standard treatments for the comorbid mental disorders are often beneficial. Yet, clarity about the classification of such aberrant behaviors as hyperactivity, emotional lability, and social dysfunction is still lacking.

DIFFERENTIAL DIAGNOSIS

By definition, mental retardation must begin before the age of 18. A mentally retarded child has to cope with so many difficult social and academic situations that maladaptive patterns often complicate the diagnostic process. Children whose family life provides inadequate stimulation may manifest motor and mental retardation that can be reversed if an enriched, stimulating environment is provided in early childhood. Several sensory disabilities, especially deafness and blindness, can be mistaken for mental retardation if no compensation is allowed during testing. Speech deficits and cerebral palsy often make a child seem retarded, even in the presence of borderline or normal intelligence. Chronic, debilitating diseases of any kind can depress a child's functioning in all areas. Convulsive disorders can give an impression of mental retardation, especially in the presence of uncontrolled seizures. Chronic brain syndromes can result in isolated handicaps—failure to read (alexia), failure to write (agraphia), failure to communicate (aphasia), and several others—that can exist in a person of normal and even superior intelligence. Children with learning disorders (which can coexist with mental retardation) experience a delay or failure of development in a specific area, such as reading or mathematics, but they develop normally in other areas. In contrast, children with mental retardation show general delays in most areas of development.

Mental retardation and pervasive developmental disorders often coexist; 70 to 75 percent of those with pervasive developmental disorders have an IQ below 70. A pervasive developmental disorder results in distortion of the timing, rate, and sequence of many basic psychological functions necessary for social development. Because of their general level of functioning, children with pervasive developmental disorders have more problems with social relatedness and more deviant language than those with mental retardation. In mental retardation, generalized delays in development are present, and mentally retarded children behave in some ways as though they were passing through an earlier normal developmental stage, rather than one with completely aberrant behavior.

A most difficult differential diagnostic problem concerns children with severe mental retardation, brain damage, autistic disorder, schizophrenia with childhood onset, or, according to some, Heller's disease. The confusion stems from details of the child's early history that are often unavailable or unreliable. In addition, when the children are evaluated, many with these conditions display similar bizarre and stereotyped behavior—mutism, echolalia, or functioning on a retarded level. By the time the children are usually seen, it does not matter from a practical point of view whether their retardation is secondary to a primary early infantile autistic disorder or schizophrenia or whether the personality and behavioral distortions are secondary to brain damage or mental retardation. In a recent epidemiological study, pervasive developmental disorders (such as autistic disorder) were found in 19.8 percent of children with mental retardation.

Children under the age of 18 years who meet the diagnostic criteria for dementia and who have an IQ below 70 are given the diagnoses of dementia and mental retardation. Those whose IQs drop below 70 after the age of 18 years and who have new onsets of cognitive disorders are not given the diagnosis of mental retardation but only the diagnosis of dementia.

TREATMENT

The treatment of individuals with mental retardation is based on an assessment of social, educational, psychiatric, and environmental need. Mental retardation is associated with a variety of comorbid psychiatric disorders that often require specific treatment, in addition to psychosocial support. Of course, when preventative measures are available, optimal treatment of conditions that could lead to mental retardation include primary, secondary, and tertiary prevention.

Primary Prevention

Primary prevention concerns actions taken to eliminate or reduce the conditions that lead to development of the disorders associated with mental retardation. Such measures include education to increase the general public's knowledge and awareness of mental retardation; continuing efforts of health professionals to ensure and upgrade public health policies; legislation to provide optimal maternal and child health care; and eradication of the known disorders associated with CNS damage. Family and genetic counseling helps reduce the incidence of mental retardation in a family with a history of a genetic disorder associated with mental retardation. For the children and the mothers of low socioeconomic status, proper prenatal and postnatal medical care and various supplementary enrichment programs and social service assistance may help minimize medical and psychosocial complications.

Secondary and Tertiary Prevention

Once a disorder associated with mental retardation has been identified, the disorder should be treated to shorten the course of the illness (secondary prevention) and to minimize the sequelae or consequent disabilities (tertiary prevention). Hereditary metabolic and endocrine disorders, such as PKU and hypothyroidism, can be treated effectively in an early stage by dietary control or hormone replacement therapy. Mentally retarded children frequently have emotional and behavioral difficulties requiring psychiatric treatment. Their limited cognitive and social capabilities require modified psychiatric treatment modalities based on their level of intelligence.

Education for the Child. Educational settings for children who are mentally retarded should include a comprehensive program that addresses training in adaptive skills, social skills, and vocation. Particular attention should focus on communication and efforts to improve the quality of life. Group therapy has often been a successful format in which mentally retarded children can learn and practice hypothetical real-life situations and receive supportive feedback.

Behavioral, Cognitive, and Psychodynamic Therapies. The difficulties in adaptation among mentally retarded persons are widespread and so varied that several interventions alone or in combination may be beneficial. Behavior therapy has been used for many years to shape and enhance social behaviors and to control and minimize aggressive and destructive behaviors. Positive reinforcement for desired behaviors and benign punishment (e.g., loss of privileges) for objectionable behaviors have been helpful. Cognitive therapy, such as dispelling false beliefs and relaxation exercises with self-instruction, has also been recommended for mentally retarded persons who can follow the instructions. Psychodynamic therapy has been used with patients and their families to decrease conflicts about expectations that result in persistent anxiety, rage, and depression.

Family Education. One of the most important areas that a clinician can address is educating the family of a mentally retarded patient about ways to enhance competence and self-esteem while maintaining realistic expectations for the patient. The family often finds it difficult to balance the fostering of independence and the providing of a nurturing and supportive environment for a mentally retarded child, who is likely to experience some rejection and failure outside the family context. The parents may benefit from continuous counseling or family therapy and should be allowed opportunities to express their feelings of guilt, despair, anguish, recurring denial, and anger about their child's disorder and future. The psychiatrist should be prepared to give the parents all the basic and current medical information regarding causes, treatment, and other pertinent areas (e.g., special training and the correction of sensory defects). Table 38–5 lists some important needs of families of children with mental retardation and resources for them.

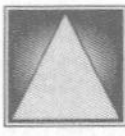

Table 38–5
Service Needs and Resources for Families of Disabled Children at Different Ages

	Needs	Resources
Age 0 to 3 years		
Child	Evaluation: physical, motor, cognitive, linguistic, social-emotional; early intervention services	Multidisciplinary evaluation, which results in an Individualized Family Service Plan (IFSP), with child and family receiving either center- or home-based early intervention services for a set number of hours per week
Mother	Emotional support, caregiving behaviors	Support groups by disability, region, and etiology; part of early intervention evaluation, intervention, and IFSP
Family	Support, financial assistance; information	Support groups; depending on problem, state of developmental disabilities or insurance payment for some services; hospitals, agencies, groups
Age 3 to 21 years		
Child	Evaluation, referral, and Individualized Educational Program (IEP)	School system: involves legal process of evaluation and placement (notification, hearings, appeals if necessary); information on transition to adult services as child nears age 21 (and school services end)
Family	Information, financial assistance, support	Local and national groups; state departments in some states; includes respite care, camps, art (Very Special Arts) or athletic activities (Special Olympics), scholarships for adolescents with some disabilities (deafness, blindness)
Above 21 years		
Offspring	Residential services, work	Both run by state developmental disability departments (parents and offspring have major say concerning whether residential or work placements are appropriate)
Family	Support, information, guardianship issues	Continuation of many of the services provided during the school years; particularly for individuals with severe disabilities, provisions for residential and work status after parents can no longer serve as legal guardians

(Adapted from Hodapp RD. *Development and Disabilities.* New York: Cambridge University Press; 1998, with permission.)

Social Intervention. One of the most prevalent problems among persons who are mentally retarded is a sense of social isolation and social skills deficits. Thus, improving the quantity and quality of social competence is a critical part of their care. Special Olympics International is the largest recreational sports program geared for this population. In addition to providing a forum to develop physical fitness, Special Olympics also enhances social interactions, friendships, and (it is hoped) general self-esteem. A recent study confirmed positive effects of the Special Olympics on the social competence of the mentally retarded adults who participated.

Pharmacology. Pharmacological approaches to the treatment of behavioral and psychological symptoms in mentally retarded patients are much the same as for those patients who are not mentally retarded. Increasing data support the use of a variety of medications for patients with mental disorders who are not mentally retarded, and some studies have focused on the use of medications for the following behavioral syndromes that are frequent among persons who are mentally retarded.

COMMON COMORBID PSYCHIATRIC DISORDERS

Attention-Deficit/Hyperactivity Disorder. Studies of methylphenidate (Ritalin) treatment in mildly retarded patients with ADHD have shown significant improvement in the ability to maintain attention and to stay focused on tasks. Methylphenidate treatment studies have not shown evidence of long-term improvement in social skills or learning. In a recent treatment study of ADHD in a group of children and adolescents with moderate mental retardation, risperidone (Risperdal) was compared with methylphenidate with respect to reduction of impulsivity and short attention span. Risperidone was found to be highly beneficial in reducing symptoms of ADHD in this population. Another large open study of 500 children with disruptive behavior disorders and mental retardation treated with risperidone at a mean dose of 1.6 mg a day for a period of 1 year showed improvement and tolerated the medication well. They concluded that adverse events at this dose of medication were mild, and the only clinically relevant laboratory test change was an increase in serum prolactin level. Although risperidone has been shown to be associated with significant symptom reduction of hyperactivity and disruptive behavior, and in general, adverse events during a year of treatment were mild, given its side effect profile compared with methylphenidate, it is still prudent to begin with a trial of a stimulant medication before the use of antipsychotic prepeparations for the treatment of ADHD.

Aggression and Self-Injurious Behavior. There are few well-controlled clinical trials to guide optimal treatment of aggression and self-injurious behavior. Some evidence from controlled and uncontrolled studies indicates that lithium (Eskalith) has been useful in decreasing aggression and self-injurious behavior. Narcotic antagonists such as naltrexone have not been systematically shown to diminish aggression or self-injurious behaviors. Anticonvulsants, such as carbamazepine (Tegretol) and valproic acid (Depakene), have been used clinically for aggressive behavior in children and adolescents. Double-blind, placebo-controlled studies in mentally retarded adults and open clinical trials in mentally retarded children and adolescents have indicated that risperidone is efficacious in decreasing aggression and

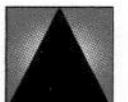

Table 38–6
ICD-10 Diagnostic Criteria for Mental Retardation

Detailed clinical diagnostic criteria that can be used internationally for research cannot be specified for mental retardation in the same way as they can for most of the other disorders in Chapter V(F) of ICD-10. This is because manifestations of the two main components of mental retardation, namely low cognitive ability and diminished social competence, are profoundly affected by social and cultural influences. Only general guidance can be given here about the most appropriate methods of assessment to use.

Level of cognitive abilities

Depending upon the cultural norms and expectations of the individuals being studied, research workers must make their own judgments as to how best to estimate the intelligence quotient (IQ) or mental age according to the bands given below:

Category	Mental retardation	IQ range	Mental age (years)
F70	Mild	50–69	9 to under 12
F71	Moderate	35–49	6 to under 9
F72	Severe	20–34	3 to under 6
F73	Profound	Below 20	Less than 3

Level of social competence

Within most European and North American cultures, the Vineland Social Maturity Scale[a] is recommended for use, if it is judged to be appropriate. Modified versions or equivalent scales should be developed for use in other cultures.

A fourth character may be used to specify the extent of associated impairment of behaviour:

No, or minimal, impairment of behaviour
Significant impairment of behaviour requiring attention or treatment
Other impairments of behaviour
Without mention of impairment of behaviour

Comments

A specially designed multi-axial system is required to do justice to the variety of personal, clinical, and social statements needed for the comprehensive assessment of the causes and consequences of mental retardation. One such system is now in preparation for this section of Chapter V(F) of ICD-10.

[a]Doll EA. *Vineland Social Maturity Scale, Condensed Manual of Directions.* Circle Pines, MN: American Guidance Service; 1965.
(From World Health Organization. *ICD-10 Classification of Mental and Behavioural Disorders: Diagnostic Criteria for Research.* Copyright, World Health Organization, Geneva, 1993, with permission.)

self-injurious behavior. Persons with mental retardation appear to be at higher risk for the development of tardive dyskinesia after use of a variety of antipsychotic medications. The atypical antipsychotics, including risperidone and clozapine (Clozaril), may provide some relief with a decreased risk of tardive dyskinesia.

Depressive Disorders. The diagnosis of depressive disorders among individuals with mental retardation may be overlooked when behavioral problems are prominent, and the need for antidepressant treatment for individuals with mental retardation may be underestimated. Some have reported disinhibition in response to serotonin reuptake inhibitors (e.g., fluoxetine [Prozac], paroxetine, sertraline [Zoloft]) in mentally retarded individuals who also have a diagnosis of pervasive developmental disorder. In general, given the relative safety of these medications, their use is indicated when a depressive disorder is diagnosed.

Stereotypical Motor Movements. Antipsychotic medications, such as haloperidol (Haldol) and chlorpromazine, decrease repetitive self-stimulatory behaviors in mentally retarded patients, but these medications have not increased adaptive behavior. Some mentally retarded children and adults (up to one third) face a high risk for tardive dyskinesia with the continued use of antipsychotic medications. Obsessive-compulsive symptoms often overlap with the repetitive stereotypical behaviors seen in mentally retarded children and adolescents and in those with mental retardation and a pervasive developmental disorder. Serotonin reuptake inhibitors, such as fluoxetine, fluvoxamine (Luvox), paroxetine, and sertraline, have been shown to have efficacy in treating obsessive-compulsive symptoms in children and adolescents and, thus, may have some efficacy for stereotyped motor movements.

Explosive Rage Behavior. β-Adrenergic receptor antagonists (beta-blockers), such as propranolol (Inderal), reportedly result in fewer explosive rages in patients with mental retardation and autistic disorder. Antipsychotic medications have also been used in the treatment of explosive rage. Systematic controlled studies are indicated to confirm the efficacy of these drugs in the treatment of rage outbursts.

ICD-10

The 10th revision of *International Statistical Classification of Diseases and Related Health Problems* (ICD-10) approaches the diagnosis of mental retardation from a somewhat different viewpoint than DSM-IV-TR. According to ICD-10, mental retardation is a condition of "arrested or incomplete development of the mind" characterized by impaired developmental skills that "contribute to the overall level of intelligence." ICD-10 offers categories for specifying the extent of behavior impairment: none or minimal; significant, requiring treatment or attention; other impairments; no mention of impairments (Table 38–6).

SERVICES AND SUPPORT FOR CHILDREN WITH MENTAL RETARDATION

Early Intervention

Early intervention programs serve individuals for the first 3 years of life. Such services are generally provided by the state and begin with a specialist visiting the home for several hours per week.

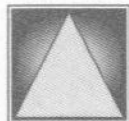

Table 38–7
Prominent Organizations in Mental Retardation

Association of Retarded Citizens of the United States (The ARC)
500 E. Border Street
Arlington, TX 76010
(817) 261–6003

American Association on Mental Retardation (AAMR)
1710 Kalorama Road, NW
Washington, DC 20009-2683
(800) 424–3688

Council for Exceptional Children (CEC)
1920 Association Drive
Reston, VA 22091–1589

American Association of University-Affiliated Programs for Persons with Developmental Disabilities
8630 Fenton Street, Suite 410
Silver Spring, MD 20910

TASH: The Association for Persons with Severe Handicaps
29 W. Susquehanna Avenue, Suite 210
Baltimore, MD 21204
(410) 828–8274

CAPP National Parent Resource Center Federation for Children with Special Needs
95 Berkeley Street, Suite 104
Boston, MA 02116

Clearinghouse on Disability Information
Office of Special Education and Rehabilitative Services
330 "C" Street SW
Room 3132, Switzer Building
Washington, DC 20202
(202) 205–8241

National Information Center for Children and Youth with Disabilities
P.O. Box 1492
Washington, DC 20013
(800) 695–0285

National Organization for Rare Disorders (NORD)
100 Route 37
P.O. Box 8923
New Fairfield, CT 06812

Alliance of Genetic Support Groups
35 Wisconsin Circle
Suite 440
Chevy Chase, MD 29815
(301) 652–5553

National Parent Network on Disabilities
1600 Prince Street
Suite 115
Alexandria, VA 22314
(703) 684–1205

Sibling Information Network
1775 Ellington Road
South Windsor, CT 07074
(203) 648–1205

Resources for Children with Special Needs, Inc.
200 Park Avenue South, Suite 816
New York, NY 10003
(212) 677–4650

Association for Children with Down Syndrome
2616 Martin Ave.
Bellmore, NY 11710
(516) 221–4700

National Down Syndrome Society
666 Broadway
New York, NY 10012
(800) 221–4602

National Down Syndrome Congress
1800 Dempster Street
Park Ridge, IL 60068
(800) 232–6372

National Fragile X Syndrome Foundation
1441 York Street, Suite 215
Denver, CO 80206

Prader-Willi Syndrome Association
6490 Excelsior Blvd., E-102
St. Louis Park, MN 55426
(612) 926–1947

Prader-Willi Syndrome International Information Forum
40 Holly Lane
Roslyn Heights, NY 11577
(800) 358–0682

The Williams Syndrome Association
P.O. Box 297
Clawson, MI 48017–0297
(810) 541–3630

Since the passage of Public Law 99-447, the Education of the Handicapped Amendments of 1986, early intervention services for the entire family are emphasized. Agencies are required to develop an Individualized Family Service Plan (IFSP) for each family identifying specific interventions to best help the family and child.

School

From the age of 3 years until 21 years of age, school is responsible by law to provide appropriate educational services to children with mental retardation. These mandates were created by the passage of Public Law 94-142, the Education for all Handicapped Children Act of 1975, and expanded with the addition of the Individuals with Disabilities Act (IDEA) of 1990. Through these two laws, public schools must develop and provide an individualized educational program for each student with mental retardation, determined at a meeting designated as the Individualized Education Plan (IEP) with school personnel and the family. The educational plan must be provided for the child in the "least restrictive environment" that will allow the child an education.

Supports

A wide variety of organized groups and services are available for children with mental retardation and their families. These include short-term respite care, allowing families a break, generally set up by state agencies. Other programs include the Special Olympics, which allows children with mental retardation to participate in team sports and in sports competitions.

Many organizations (Table 38–7) also exist for families who wish to connect with others who have children with mental retardation syndromes.

References

Bradinova I, Shopova S, Simeonov E. Mental retardation in childhood: Clinical and diagnostic profile in 100 children. *Genet Couns.* 2005;16:239.

Brosco JP, Mattingly M, Sanders LM. Impact of specific medical interventions on reducing the prevalence of mental retardation. *Arch Pediatr Adolesc Med.* 2006;160:302–309.

Correia Filho AG, Bodanase R, Silva TL, Alvarez JP, Aman M, Rohde LA. Comparison of risperidone and methylphenidate for reducing ADHD symptoms in children and adolescents with moderate mental retardation. *J Am Acad Child Adolesc Psychiatry*. 2005;44:748.

Crane L. Quality-of-life assessment of persons with mental retardation. *Assessment for Effective Intervention*. 2005;30(4):41.

Croonenberghs J, Fegert JM, Findling R, De Smedt G, Van Dongen S; the Risperidone Disruptive Behavior Study Group. Risperidone in children with disruptive behavior disorders and subaverage intelligence: A 1-year, open-label study of 504 patients. *J Am Acad Child Adolesc Psychiatry*. 2005;44:64.

de Bildt A, Sytema S, Kraijer D, Minderaa R. Prevalence of pervasive developmental disorders in children and adolescents with mental retardation. *J Child Psychol Psychiatry*. 2005;46(3):275.

Gothelf D, Furfaro JA, Penniman LC, Glover GH, Reiss AL. The contribution of novel brain imaging techniques to understanding the neurobiology of mental retardation and developmental disabilities. *Ment Retard Dev Disabil Res Rev*. 2005;11:331.

Hodapp RM, Dykens EM. Measuring behavior in genetic disorders of mental retardation. *Ment Retard Dev Disabil Res Rev*. 2005;11:340.

King BH, Hodapp RM, Dykens EM. Mental retardation. In: Sadock BJ, Sadock VA, eds. *Kaplan & Sadock's Comprehensive Textbook of Psychiatry.* 8th ed. Vol 2. Baltimore: Lippincott Williams & Wilkins; 2005: 3076.

Lemay R. Social role valorization insights into the social integration conundrum. *Ment Retard*. 2006;44(1):1.

Reinblatt SP, Rifkin A, Castellanos FX, Coffey BJ. General psychiatry residents' perceptions of specialized training in the field of mental retardation. *Psychiatr Serv.* 2004;55(3):312.

Smith TEC. Assessment of individuals with mental retardation: Introduction to special issue. *Assessment for Effective Intervention*. 2005;30(4):1.

Yeates KO, Armstrong K, Janusz J, Taylor HG, Wade S, Stancin T, Drotar D. Long-term attention problems in children with traumatic brain injury. *J Am Acad Child Adolesc Psychiatry*. 2005;44:574.

39 Learning Disorders

Learning disorders in a child or adolescent are characterized by academic underachievement in reading, written expression, or mathematics in comparison with the overall intellectual ability of the child. Children with learning disorders often find it difficult to keep up with their peers in certain academic subjects, whereas they excel in others. Learning disorders result in underachievement that is unexpected based on the child's potential as well as the opportunity to have learned more. When academic achievement testing is administered along with a measure of intellectual capability, this psychoeducational assessment can identify learning problems. Learning problems in a child or adolescent that are identified in this manner can establish eligibility for academic services through the public school system.

Learning disorders affect at least 5 percent of school-age children. This represents approximately half of all public school children who receive special education services in the United States. In 1975, Public Law 94-142 (the Education for All Handicapped Children Act) mandated all states to provide free and appropriate educational services to all children. Since that time, the number of children identified with learning disorders has increased, and a variety of definitions of learning disabilities has arisen. The term *learning disorders*, formally referred to as *academic skills disorders*, was introduced by the 4th edition of the *Diagnostic and Statistical Manual of Mental Disorders* (DSM-IV). To meet the criteria for a diagnosis of learning disorder, a child's achievement in that particular learning disorder must be significantly lower than expected and the learning problems interfere with academic achievement or activities of daily living.

The most recent revised version of the DSM-IV (DSM-IV-TR) includes four diagnostic categories of learning disorders: reading disorder, mathematics disorder, disorder of written expression, and learning disorder not otherwise specified. Children with a learning disorder, such as reading disorder, for example, can be identified in two different ways: children who read poorly compared with most other children of the same age and children whose achievement in reading is significantly lower than their overall IQ would predict. DSM-IV-TR criteria for learning disorders require a substantial IQ–achievement discrepancy and significantly poor achievement in reading compared with that of most children of the same age. Research studies have led to questions regarding inclusion of an IQ–achievement discrepancy component in the definition of a learning disorder, because current data suggest that most children with reading disorders, for example, have similar deficits in phonological processing skills, regardless of their IQ. That is, most children with reading disorders have trouble with word recognition and "sounding out" words because they cannot understand and use phonemes, the smaller bits of words that are associated with particular sounds.

Learning disorders often make it agonizing for a child to succeed in school and, in some cases, lead to eventual demoralization, low self-esteem, chronic frustration, and poor peer relationships. Learning disorders are associated with higher than average risk of a variety of comorbid disorders, including attention-deficit/hyperactivity disorder (ADHD), communication disorders, conduct disorders, and depressive disorders. Adolescents with learning disorders are about one and a half times more likely to drop out of school, approximating rates of 40 percent. Adults with learning disorders are at increased risk for difficulties in employment and social adjustment. Learning disorders can be associated with other developmental disorders, major depressive disorder, and dysthymic disorder.

Genetic predisposition, perinatal injury, and neurological and other medical conditions can contribute to the development of learning disorders, but many children and adolescents with learning disorders have no specific risk factors. Learning disorders, nevertheless, are frequently found in association with conditions such as lead poisoning, fetal alcohol syndrome, and in utero drug exposure.

READING DISORDER

Reading disorders are present in approximately 75 percent of children and adolescents with learning disorders. Students who have learning problems in other academic areas most commonly experience difficulties with reading as well.

Reading disorder is defined as reading achievement below the expected level for a child's age, education, and intelligence, with the impairment interfering significantly with academic success or the daily activities that involve reading. According to DSM-IV-TR, if a neurological condition or sensory disturbance is present, the reading disability exhibited exceeds that usually associated with the other condition.

Reading disorder is characterized by an impaired ability to recognize words, slow and inaccurate reading, and poor comprehension. In addition, children with ADHD are at high risk for reading disorder. Historically, many different labels have been used to describe reading disabilities, including word blindness, reading backward, learning disability, alexia, and developmental word blindness. The term *developmental alexia* was accepted and defined as a developmental deficit in the recognition of printed symbols. This term was simplified by adopting the term *dyslexia* in the 1960s. Dyslexia was used extensively for many years to describe a reading disability syndrome that often included speech and language deficits and right-left confusion. Reading disorder is frequently accompanied by disabilities in other academic skills, and the term dyslexia has been replaced by broader terms, such as *learning disorder*.

Epidemiology

An estimated 4 percent of school-age children in the United States have reading disorder; prevalence studies find rates ranging between 2 and 8 percent. Three to four times as many boys as girls are reported to have reading disability in clinically referred samples. Careful epidemiological studies have found closer to equal rates of reading disorder among boys and girls. Boys with reading disorder may be referred for evaluation more often than girls because of frequently associated behavior problems. No clear gender differential is seen among adults who report reading difficulties.

Comorbidity

Children with reading disorder are at higher than average risk for attentional problems, disruptive behavior disorders, and depressive disorders, particularly older children and adolescents. Data suggest that up to 25 percent of children with reading disorder also have ADHD. Conversely, it is estimated that between 15 and 30 percent of children diagnosed with ADHD have a learning disorder. Although these disorders frequently occur concurrently, they are distinct conditions and require separate interventions. Family studies indicate, however, in some cases, ADHD and reading disorder may be genetically transmitted together. That is, some common genetic factors are producing both reading disorder and attentional syndromes. Some evidence also suggests that higher than random incidence of aggressive behavior is present in young children with reading disorders. It appears that in samples of children and adolescents with conduct disorders, reading disorder was more frequent than expected. Children with reading disorders have higher than average rates of depression on self-report measures and experience higher levels of anxiety symptoms than children without learning disorders. Furthermore, children with reading disorders tend to be at increased risk for problematic peer relationships and less skill in responding to subtle social cues.

Etiology

Data from cognitive, neuroimaging and genetic studies indicate that reading disorder is most accurately described as a neurobiological disorder with a genetic origin. It is currently believed to reflect a deficiency in processing sounds of spoken language. That is, children who struggle with reading have a deficit in phonological processing skills. These children cannot identify effectively the parts of words that denote specific sounds, which leads to grave difficulty in recognizing and sounding out words. Children with reading disorders are slower than average in naming letters and numbers, even when controlling for IQ. Thus, the core deficit for children with reading disorders lies within the domain of language use.

Given that reading disorder is essentially a language deficit, the left brain has been hypothesized to be the anatomical site of the dysfunction. Several research studies using magnetic resonance imaging (MRI) studies have suggested that the planum temporale in the left brain shows less asymmetry than the same site in the right brain in children with both language and learning disorders. Positron emission tomographic (PET) studies have led some researchers to conclude that left temporal blood flow patterns during language tasks differ between children with and without learning disorders. Also, some cell analysis studies suggest that in reading-disordered persons, the visual magnocellular system (which normally contains large cells) contains more disorganized and smaller cell bodies than expected. None of the above studies provide conclusive evidence regarding brain differences between those who are reading-disordered and those who are not.

Many studies support the hypothesis that genetic factors play a major role in the presence of reading disorders. Studies indicate that 35 to 40 percent of first-degree relatives of children with reading disorder also have some reading disability. Several recent studies have suggested that phonological awareness (i.e., the ability to decode sounds and sound out words) is linked to chromosome 6. Furthermore, the ability to identify single words has been linked to chromosome 15. Impairment in reading and spelling has now been linked to susceptibility loci on multiple chromosomes, including chromosomes 1, 2, 3, 6, 15, and 18. Although a recent research study identified a locus on chromosome 18 as a strong influence on single word reading and phoneme awareness, generalist genes have also been implicated as responsible for learning disorders. Many genes associated with common learning disorders, such as reading disability, mathematics impairment, and language disorders, are believed to be generalists in the following ways. First, genes that affect common learning disorders may also influence normal variation in learning abilities. In addition, genes that affect one learning disorder are also more likely to affect other learning disorders.

Several historical hypotheses about the origin of reading disorders are now known to be untrue. The first myth is that reading disorders are primarily caused by visual-motor problems, or what has been termed *scotopic sensitivity syndrome*. No evidence indicates that children with reading disorders have visual problems or difficulties with their visual-motor system. The second theory with no supporting evidence is that allergies can cause, or contribute to, reading disabilities. Finally, unsubstantiated theories have implicated the cerebellar–vestibular system as the source of reading disorder.

Research in the fields of cognitive neuroscience and neuropsychology supports the hypothesis that encoding processes and working memory, rather than attention or long-term memory, are areas of weakness for children with reading disorder. Developmental factors have been hypothesized to play a role in reading disorders. One recent study found an association between dyslexia and birth in the months of May, June, and July, which suggests that prenatal exposure to a maternal infectious illness, such as influenza, in the winter months may contribute to reading disorder. Studies in the 1930s attempted to explain reading disorder according to the cerebral hemispheric function model, which suggested positive correlations of reading disorder with left-handedness, left-eyedness, or mixed laterality. Subsequent epidemiological studies did not find any consistent association between reading disorder and laterality of handedness or eyedness, but right-left confusion has been shown to be associated with reading difficulties.

Complications during pregnancy and prenatal and perinatal difficulties are common in the histories of children with reading disorder. Extremely low birthweight and severely premature children are at higher risk for reading disorder and other learning disorders than children who are born full term and have normal birthweight. A recent study reviewed the relationship between critical periods for brain growth and babies born significantly preterm. Children who are born very preterm who attend mainstream schools have been noted to be at increased risk of minor motor, behavioral, and learning disorders. These appear to be associated with postnatal growth, particularly of the head. Although intrauterine growth retardation may play a role in compromised intellectual capacity, interventions that aim to improve motor ability and potentially learning disorders should focus on optimal nutrition and care postnatally.

A higher than average incidence of reading disorder occurs among children of normal intelligence who have cerebral palsy, and epileptic children exhibit a slightly increased incidence of reading disorder. Children with postnatal brain lesions in the left occipital lobe, which results in right visual-field blindness, may have secondary reading disorder, as may children with lesions in the splenium of the corpus callosum that blocks transmission of visual information from the intact right hemisphere to the language areas of the left hemisphere.

Data have documented an association of developmental delays and learning disabilities in fetal alcohol syndrome. Recent evidence suggests that certain peptides, such as those derived from activity-dependent neurotrophic factor-12, may mitigate alcohol-induced fetal death and developmental learning disabilities. This demonstrates that a single treatment with a peptide may be efficacious in preventing and mitigating alcohol-induced fetal damage. Other studies suggest an association between malnutrition and subsequent reading disorder. Children who were malnourished for long periods during early childhood are at increased risk of subaverage performance in many cognitive areas, including reading. Their cognitive performances appear to be lower than those of siblings who were not subjected to the same degree of malnutrition.

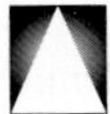

Table 39–1
DSM-IV-TR Diagnostic Criteria for Reading Disorder

A. Reading achievement, as measured by individually administered standardized tests of reading accuracy or comprehension, is substantially below that expected given the person's chronological age, measured intelligence, and age-appropriate education.

B. The disturbance in Criterion A significantly interferes with academic achievement or activities of daily living that require reading skills.

C. If a sensory deficit is present, the reading difficulties are in excess of those usually associated with it.

Coding note: If a general medical (e.g., neurological) condition or sensory deficit is present, code the condition on Axis III.

(From American Psychiatric Association. *Diagnostic and Statistical Manual of Mental Disorders*. 4th ed. Text rev. Washington, DC: American Psychiatric Association; copyright 2000, with permission.)

Diagnosis

Reading disorder is diagnosed when a child's reading achievement is significantly below that expected of a child of the same age and intellectual capacity (Table 39–1). Characteristic diagnostic features include difficulty recalling, evoking, and sequencing printed letters and words; processing sophisticated grammatical constructions; and making inferences. Clinically, a child may be first identified with a reading disorder after becoming demoralized or exhibiting symptoms of depression related to being unable to succeed in school. School failure and ensuing poor self-esteem can exacerbate the problems as the child becomes more consumed with a sense of failure and spends less time focusing on academic work. Students suspected of having reading disorders are entitled to an educational evaluation through the school district to determine eligibility for special education services. Special education classification, however, is not uniform across states or regions, and students with identical reading difficulties may be eligible for services in one region, but ineligible in another. In some cases, an evaluation is requested on the basis of disruptive behavioral problems that occur in conjunction with the reading disorder.

Clinical Features

Children who have reading disorder can usually be identified by the age of 7 years (second grade). Reading difficulty may be apparent among students in classrooms where reading skills are expected as early as the first grade. Children can sometimes compensate for reading disorder in the early elementary grades by the use of memory and inference, particularly when the disorder is associated with high intelligence. In such instances, the disorder may not be apparent until age 9 (fourth grade) or later. Children with reading disorder make many errors in their oral reading. The errors are characterized by omissions, additions, and distortions of words. Such children have difficulty in distinguishing between printed letter characters and sizes, especially those that differ only in spatial orientation and length of line. The problems in managing printed or written language can pertain to individual letters, sentences, and even a page. The child's reading speed is slow, often with minimal comprehension. Most children with reading disorder have an age-appropriate ability to copy from a written or printed text, but nearly all spell poorly.

Associated problems include language difficulties, exhibited often as impaired sound discrimination and difficulty in sequencing words properly. A child with disorders may start a word either in the middle or at the end of a printed or written sentence. At times, because of a poorly established left-right tracking sequence, such children transpose letters to be read. Failures in both memory recall and sustained elicitation result in poor recall of letter names and sounds.

Most children with reading disorder dislike and avoid reading and writing. Their anxiety is heightened when they are confronted with demands that involve printed language. Many children with the disorder who do not receive remedial education have a sense of shame and humiliation because of their continuing failure and subsequent frustration. These feelings grow more intense with time. Older children tend to be angry and depressed and exhibit poor self-esteem.

Jason, an 11-year-old boy, was referred for evaluation of increasing problems at school, including failing to complete in-class assignments and homework; failing tests in reading, spelling, and arithmetic; skipping classes; and some truancy. For the past 2 years (grades 5 and 6), he had been attending a special education class every morning in the local community school, based on placement recommendations from a prior assessment when he was in grade 2. At that time, he did not meet DSM-IV-TR criteria for any externalizing disorder, but was not doing well in school, and a specific learning disorder was queried. A subsequent psychoeducational assessment by a clinical psychologist confirmed reading problems, but he did not meet the school board's criteria for learning disorder, which was based on IQ–achievement discrepancy. Thus, he was not eligible for special education services. A change in the following year in the school board's policy regarding the need for a discrepancy-based definition of learning disorder meant that Jason was now eligible for special education, whereupon he started attending the half-day program. He was in a class with eight other students ranging from 6 to 12 years of age.

Clinical interview with his parents revealed a normal pregnancy, but a history of language delay. In preschool and kindergarten, he was reported to have had difficulty with rhyming games and showed a marked lack of interest in books and preferred to play with construction toys. In the primary grades, he had more difficulty learning to read than other boys in his class and continued to have problems pronouncing multisyllabic words (e.g., he said "aminals" for "animals" and "sblanation" for "explanation"). Family history was positive for reading disorder and ADHD. Specifically, Jason's father admitted a history of reading problems but commented that, although he still cannot read too well (and never for pleasure), he runs a successful business. The older brother, 15 years of age, had ADHD, which was responding fairly well to stimulant medication. The parents' main concern was that Jason seemed to "be getting just like his brother and not focusing on school work," and they queried whether he also had ADHD. In the clinical interview with Jason, it was noted that he rarely made eye contact with the clinician, mumbled a lot, and struggled to find the right word (e.g., manifested many false starts, hesitations, and nonspecific terms, such as "the thing that you draw . . . um . . . pencil—no . . . um . . . lines with"). He admitted to skipping class and sometimes school, adding the comment: "Reading is boring and stupid—I'd rather be cycling." He also complained about the amount of reading he had to do—even in math—and commented, "Reading takes so much time. By the time I figure out a word, I can't 'member what I just read and so have to read the stuff again."

Psychological and psychoeducational assessment included the Wechsler Intelligence Scale for Children-IV, Clinical Evaluation of Language Fundamentals-IV (CELF-IV), the Wechsler Individual Achievement Test-II, and self-ratings of anxiety, depression, and self-esteem. Results indicated low-average verbal and above average performance IQ, poor word attack and word identification skills (below 12th percentile), poor comprehension (below 9th percentile), poor spelling (below 6th percentile), weak comprehension of oral language (below 16th percentile), elevated but subthreshold scores on the Children's Depression Inventory, and low self-esteem. Although Jason manifested several marked symptoms of inattention, some restlessness, and oppositional behavior (particularly at school), he did not meet criteria for ADHD or any other internalizing or externalizing disorder. However, he did meet DSM-IV-TR criteria for reading disorder and receptive-expressive language disorders. Comparison with results from the previous psychoeducational assessment revealed that, although he had made some small gains, he had not closed the gap between his reading skills and those of his peers, despite being in special education for 2 years. Recommendations included continuation in special education plus attendance at a summer camp specializing in children with reading disorder, as well as ongoing monitoring of self-esteem and depressive traits.

At 1-year follow-up, Jason and his parents reported striking improvements in his reading, overall school performance, mood, and self-esteem, which they attributed to the specialized instruction provided during the summer camp. The program had provided one-on-one focused and explicit instruction for 1 hour a day for a total of 70 hours. Jason explained that he had been taught a set of specific decoding strategies to use in a systematic way ("like a game plan") and challenged the clinician to give him a "really tough long word to read." He demonstrated the strategies that he used to read the word "unconditionally" and also explained what it meant. To boost his fluency in reading and reading comprehension, the clinical team recommended the use of repeated reading, reading along with audio taped (unabridged) versions of his favorite books, use of graphic organizers to facilitate reading for comprehension, and further participation in the summer camp reading program. (Courtesy of Rosemary Tannock, Ph.D.)

Pathology and Laboratory Examination

No specific physical signs or laboratory measures are helpful in the diagnosis of reading disorder. Psychoeducational testing, however, is critical in determining this diagnosis. The diagnosis of reading disorder is made after collecting data from a standardized intelligence test and an educational assessment of achievement. The diagnostic battery generally includes a standardized spelling test, written composition, processing and using oral language, design copying, and judgment of the adequacy of pencil use. The reading subtests of the *Woodcock-Johnson Psycho-Educational Battery-Revised*, and the *Peabody Individual Achievement Test-Revised* are useful in identifying reading disability. A screening projective battery may include human-figure drawings, picture-story tests, and sentence completion. The evaluation should also include systematic observation of behavioral variables.

Course and Prognosis

Many children with reading disorder gain some knowledge of printed language during their first 2 years in grade school, even without any remedial assistance. By the end of the first grade, many children with reading disorder, in fact, have learned how to read a few words; however, by the time a child with a reading disorder reaches the third grade, keeping up with classmates is exceedingly difficult without remedial educational intervention. In the best circumstances, a child is recognized as being at risk for a reading disorder during the kindergarten year or early in the first grade. When remediation is instituted early, in milder cases, it is no longer necessary by the end of the first or second grade. In severe cases and depending on the pattern of deficits and strengths, remediation may be continued into the middle and high school years.

Differential Diagnosis

Reading disorder is often accompanied by comorbid disorders, such as expressive language disorder, disorder of written expression, and ADHD. A recent study indicates that children with reading disorder consistently present difficulties with linguistic abilities, whereas children with ADHD do not. Children with reading disorder who do not qualify for a diagnosis of ADHD, however, were shown to have some overlapping deficits in the area of cognitive inhibition such that they perform impulsively on continuous performance tasks. Deficits in expressive language and speech discrimination in reading disorder can be sufficiently severe to warrant the additional diagnosis of expressive language disorder or mixed receptive-expressive language disorder. Some children exhibit a discrepancy between scores on verbal and performance intelligence. Visual perceptual deficits occur in only about 10 percent of cases. Reading disorder must be differentiated from mental retardation syndromes in which reading, along with other skills, is below the achievement expected for a child's chronological age. Intellectual testing helps to differentiate global deficits from more specific reading difficulties.

Poor reading skills resulting from inadequate schooling can be detected by finding out whether other children in the same school have similarly poor reading performances on standardized reading tests. Hearing and visual impairments should be ruled out with screening tests.

Treatment

Most current remediation strategies for children with reading disorder are characterized by direct instruction of the various components of reading that focus a child's attention to the connections between speech sounds and spelling. A recent survey of the efficacy of specific word study with text reading practice or word study tutoring in first graders who scored within the lowest quartile for reading skills indicated that students exposed to either of the above instructions outperformed those who received only classroom instruction. Improvements were noted on measures of reading accuracy, reading comprehension, reading efficiency, passage reading fluency, and spelling. Many effective remediation programs begin by teaching the child to make accurate associations between letters and sounds. This approach is based on the current consensus that, in most cases, the core deficits in reading disorders are related to difficulty recognizing and remembering the associations between letters and sounds. After individual letter-sound associations have been mastered, remediation can target larger components of reading such as syllables and words. The exact focus of any reading program can be determined only after accurate assessment of a child's specific deficits and weaknesses. Positive coping strategies include small, structured reading groups that offer individual attention and make it easier for a child to ask for help.

Children and adolescents with reading disorders are entitled to an individual education program (IEP) provided by the public school system. Yet, for high school students with persistent reading disorders and ongoing difficulties with decoding and work identification, IEP services may not be sufficient to remediate their problems. A recent study of students with reading disorders in 54 schools indicated that, at the high school level, specific goals are not adequately met solely through school remediation. It is likely that high schoolers with persisting reading difficulties may have greater benefit from individualized reading remediation.

Reading instruction programs such as the Orton Gillingham and Direct Instructional System for Teaching and Remediation (DISTAR) approaches begin by concentrating on individual letters and sounds, advance to the mastery of simple phonetic units, and then blend these units into words and sentences. Thus, if children are taught to cope with graphemes, they will learn to read. Other reading remediation programs, such as the Merill program, and the *Science Research Associates, Inc. (SRA) Basic Reading Program*, begin by introducing whole words first and then teach children how to break them down and recognize the sounds of the syllables and the individual letters in the word. Another approach teaches children with reading disorders to recognize whole words through the use of visual aids and bypasses the sounding-out process. One such program is called the *Bridge Reading Program*. The Fernald method uses a multisensory approach that combines teaching whole words with a tracing technique so that the child has kinesthetic stimulation while learning to read the words.

As in psychotherapy, the therapist–patient relationship is important to a successful treatment outcome in remedial educational therapy. Children should be placed in a grade as close as possible to their social functional level and given special remedial work in reading. Coexisting emotional and behavioral problems should be treated by appropriate psychotherapeutic means. Parental counseling may also be helpful. Approximately 75 percent of children with learning disorders can be differentiated from comparison samples by lower measures of social competence. It is important, therefore, to include social skills improvement as a therapeutic component of a treatment program for children with reading disorders.

MATHEMATICS DISORDER

Children with mathematics disorder have difficulty learning and remembering numerals, cannot remember basic facts about numbers, and are slow and inaccurate in computation. Poor achievement in four groups of skills have been identified in mathematics disorder: linguistic skills (those related to understanding mathematical terms and converting written problems into mathematical symbols), perceptual skills (the ability to recognize and understand symbols and order clusters of numbers), mathematical skills (basic addition, subtraction, multiplication, division, and following sequencing of basic operations), and attentional skills (copying figures correctly and observing operational symbols correctly). A variety of terms over the years, including *dyscalculia, congenital arithmetic disorder, acalculia, Gerstmann syndrome*, and *developmental arithmetic disorder* have been used to denote the difficulties present in mathematics disorder.

Mathematics disorder can occur in isolation or in conjunction with language and reading disorders. The diagnosis of mathematics disorder consists of deficits in arithmetic skills expected for a child's intellectual capacity and educational level, as measured by standardized, individually administered tests. This lack of expected mathematics ability must interfere with school performance or daily life activities, and the difficulties must exceed impairment associated with any existing neurological or sensory deficits.

Epidemiology

Mathematics disorder alone is estimated to occur in about 1 percent of school-age children, that is, approximately 1 of every

5 children with learning disorder. Epidemiological studies have indicated that up to 6 percent of school-age children have some difficulty with mathematics. Mathematics disorder may occur with greater frequency in girls. Many studies of learning disorders in children have grouped several disorders together rather than separating them into individual disorders, which makes it more difficult to ascertain the precise prevalence of mathematics disorder.

Comorbidity

Mathematics disorder is commonly found comorbid with reading disorder and disorder of written expression. Children with mathematics disorder may also be at higher risk for expressive language disorder, mixed receptive-expressive language disorder, and developmental coordination disorder.

Etiology

Mathematics disorder, as with other learning disorders, is probably at least partly caused by genetic factors. An early theory proposed a neurological deficit in the right cerebral hemisphere, particularly in the occipital lobe areas. These regions are responsible for processing visual-spatial stimuli that, in turn, are responsible for mathematical skills. This theory, however, has received little support in subsequent neuropsychiatric studies.

Currently, the cause is thought to be multifactorial, so that maturational, cognitive, emotional, educational, and socioeconomic factors account in varying degrees and combinations for mathematics disorder. Compared with reading, arithmetic abilities seem to depend more on the amount and quality of instruction.

Diagnosis

The diagnosis of mathematics disorder is made when a child's skills in mathematics fall significantly below what is expected for that child's age, intellectual ability, and education. Many different skills are needed for mathematics proficiency. These include linguistic skills, conceptual skills, and computational skills. Linguistic skills involve being able to understand mathematical terms, understand word problems, and translate them into the proper mathematical process. Conceptual skills involve recognition of mathematical symbols and being able to use mathematical signs correctly. Computational skills include the ability to line up numbers correctly and to follow the "rules" of the mathematical operation. A definitive diagnosis can be made only after a child takes an individually administered standardized arithmetic test and scores markedly below the level expected in view of the child's schooling and intellectual capacity as measured by a standardized intelligence test. A pervasive developmental disorder and mental retardation should also be ruled out before confirming the diagnosis of mathematics disorder. The DSM-IV-TR diagnostic criteria for mathematics disorder are given in Table 39–2.

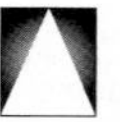

Table 39–2
DSM-IV-TR Diagnostic Criteria for Mathematics Disorder

A. Mathematical ability, as measured by individually administered standardized tests, is substantially below that expected given the person's chronological age, measured intelligence, and age-appropriate education.

B. The disturbance in Criterion A significantly interferes with academic achievement or activities of daily living that require mathematical ability.

C. If a sensory deficit is present, the difficulties in mathematical ability are in excess of those usually associated with it.

Coding note: If a general medical (e.g., neurological) condition or sensory deficit is present, code the condition on Axis III.

(From American Psychiatric Association. *Diagnostic and Statistical Manual of Mental Disorders.* 4th ed. Text rev. Washington, DC: American Psychiatric Association; copyright 2000, with permission.)

Clinical Features

Common features of mathematics disorder include difficulty with various components of mathematics, such as learning number names, remembering the signs for addition and subtraction, learning multiplication tables, translating word problems into computations, and doing calculations at the expected pace. Most children with mathematics disorder can be detected during the second and third grades in elementary school. A child with mathematics disorder generally has significant problems with concepts, such as counting and adding even one-digit numbers, compared with classmates of the same age. During the first 2 or 3 years of elementary school, a child with mathematics disorder may just get by in mathematics by relying on rote memory. But soon, as mathematics problems require discrimination and manipulation of spatial and numerical relations, a child with mathematics disorder is overwhelmed.

Some investigators have classified mathematics disorder into the following categories: difficulty learning to count meaningfully; difficulty mastering cardinal and ordinal systems; difficulty performing arithmetic operations; and difficulty envisioning clusters of objects as groups. Children with the disorder may have trouble associating auditory and visual symbols, understanding the conservation of quantity, remembering sequences of arithmetic steps, and choosing principles for problem-solving activities. Children with these problems are presumed to have good auditory and verbal abilities.

Mathematics disorder often coexists with other disorders affecting reading, expressive writing, coordination, and expressive and receptive language. Spelling problems, deficits in memory or attention, and emotional or behavioral problems may be present. Young grade-school children often first show other learning disorders and should be checked for mathematics disorder. Children with cerebral palsy may have mathematics disorder with normal overall intelligence.

The relation between mathematics disorder and other communication and learning disorders is not clear. Although children with mixed receptive-expressive language disorder and expressive language disorder are not necessarily affected by mathematics disorder, the conditions often coexist, because they are associated with impairments in both decoding and encoding processes.

K. R., an 8-year-old girl, was referred for evaluation of increasing problems in attention, behavior, and learning, which were first noted in kindergarten but were now causing difficulty at home and school. At the time of this first assessment, she was enrolled in a regular third-grade class in a local public school, which she had been attending since midway through grade 1, when the family had moved into the district.

Clinical interview with her parents revealed a normal pregnancy, but noted that she had been somewhat slow to talk (e.g., first words at approximately 20 months of age and short sentences at approximately 3 years of age), but otherwise had no major developmental concerns until kindergarten, when the teacher had raised concerns about K. R.'s inattentiveness and difficulty following instructions and mastering basic number concepts (e.g., inaccurate counting of sets of objects). A speech, language, and hearing assessment completed at the end of kindergarten revealed mild receptive and expressive language problems that did not warrant specific intervention. School reports from grade 1 noted ongoing concerns about inattention, some difficulty learning to read, difficulty mastering simple arithmetic facts, and "making careless mistakes in copying numbers from the board and in doing addition and subtraction." These problems continued through grade 2, despite some in-school accommodations (e.g., moving K. R.'s seat closer to the teacher and next to an academically strong student) and modifications (e.g., provision of printed sheets of arithmetic problems to reduce copying errors and reduction in number of assigned problems). Her parents also reported a 3-year history and current problems with losing things, twirling her hair and fiddling with anything in sight, difficulty concentrating on games and schoolwork, and forgetting to bring notes to and from school. Parents also reported that the older sibling (female) was also weak in mathematics and added the comment, "but I guess that is fairly common among girls." Psychological assessment included the Wechsler Intelligence Scale for Children-III, Clinical Evaluation of Language Fundamentals-IV, Comprehensive Test of Phonological Processing, and the Woodcock-Johnson Psychoeducational Battery–III. Results indicated average intelligence, with relatively weaker performance on tests of perceptual organization, weak phonological awareness, subclinical problems in receptive and expressive language, and reading and arithmetic abilities that were well below grade level. Parent and teacher ratings on a standardized behavior questionnaire (Conners' Rating Scales-Long Form) were above clinical threshold for DSM-IV inattention.

The clinical team formulated a diagnosis of ADHD, predominantly inattentive type, and reading disorder, based on the developmental history, clinical picture, and standardized assessment. She did not meet criteria for communication disorder, and it was speculated that her arithmetic difficulties were most likely associated with the reading disorder and ADHD. Recommendations included the following: psychoeducation (primarily bibliotherapy for ADHD and reading disorder), specific educational intervention for reading, and treatment of the marked inattentiveness with psychostimulant medication.

At 1-year follow-up, K. R. and her parents reported a marked lessening of her inattention, but ongoing problems with reading and mathematics, although she had just started to read "chapter books" with the special education teacher who was providing small-group instruction several times a week. Another follow-up appointment was recommended, but no other changes were made in treatment. Two years later, when K. R. was 11 years of age, her parents called for an "urgent reevaluation" because of increasing home and school difficulties. Clinical evaluation revealed persisting ADHD, inattentive type, that was responding well to stimulant treatment and slow but fairly accurate reading albeit with weak comprehension but marked difficulties with mathematics. The parents reported that K. R. had started lying about having mathematics homework or refused to do it, was suspended from mathematics class twice in the past 3 months because of oppositional behavior, and had failed sixth-grade mathematics. K. R. acknowledged disliking and worrying about math: "whenever the teacher starts asking questions and looks in my direction, my mind just goes blank and I feel sort of shaky—it's so bad in tests that I have to leave class to get myself together." At this point, the clinical team formulated the following diagnoses: ADHD, inattentive type; reading disorder; mathematics disorder; and also noted marked math anxiety. Recommendations were expanded to include specific educational remediation for mathematics. At follow-up, K. R. reported that the resource teacher had taught her some helpful strategies to address her anxiety about mathematics, as well as ways of classifying word problems and differentiating critical information from irrelevant information. The availability of several extended-release formulations of stimulant medication allowed a change from standard to longer-acting stimulant, which addressed K. R.'s concerns about having to go to the school office for her midday dose and difficulties concentrating on homework after school. (Courtesy of Rosemary Tannock, Ph.D.)

Pathology and Laboratory Examination

No physical signs or symptoms indicate mathematics disorder, but educational testing and standardized measurement of intellectual function are necessary to make this diagnosis. The *Keymath Diagnostic Arithmetic Test* measures several areas of mathematics including knowledge of mathematical content, function, and computation. It is used to assess ability in mathematics of children in grades 1 to 6.

Course and Prognosis

A child with a mathematics disorder can usually be identified by the age of 8 years (third grade). In some children, the disorder is apparent as early as 6 years (first grade); in others, it may not be apparent until age 10 (fifth grade) or later. Too few data are currently available from longitudinal studies to predict clear patterns of developmental and academic progress of children classified as having mathematics disorder in early school grades. On the other hand, children with a moderate mathematics disorder who do not receive intervention may have complications, including continuing academic difficulties, shame, poor self-concept, frustration, and depression. These complications can lead to reluctance to attend school, truancy, and eventual hopelessness about academic success.

Differential Diagnosis

Mathematics disorder must be differentiated from global causes of impaired functioning such as mental retardation syndromes. Arithmetic difficulties in mental retardation are accompanied by generalized impairment in overall intellectual functioning. In unusual cases of mild mental retardation, arithmetic skills may be significantly below the level expected on the basis of a person's schooling and level of mental retardation. In such cases, an additional diagnosis of mathematics disorder should be made. Treatment of the arithmetic difficulties can particularly help a child's chances for employment in adulthood. Inadequate schooling can often affect a child's poor arithmetic performance on a standardized arithmetic test. Conduct disorder or ADHD can occur with mathematics disorder and, in these cases, both diagnoses should be made.

Treatment

Mathematics difficulties for children has not been shown to be a stable disorder over time, thus, early intervention may lead to improved skills in basic computation. The presence of reading disorder along with mathematics difficulties can impede progress, yet children are responsive to remediation in early grade school. For children as early as in kindergarten, indications of mathematics disorder and the need for intervention include lack of mastery in knowledge of which digit in a pair is larger, counting abilities, identification of numbers, and poor working memory for numbers, such as difficulty with reverse digit span. Currently, the most effective treatments for mathematics disorder combine teaching mathematics concepts with continuous practice in solving math problems. Flash cards, workbooks, and computer games can be a viable part of this treatment. A recent report indicates that mathematics instruction is most helpful when the focus is on problem-solving activities, including word problems, rather than only computation. *Project MATH*, a multimedia self-instructional or group-instructional in-service training program, has been successful for some children with mathematics disorder. Computer programs can be helpful and can increase compliance with remediation efforts.

Social skills deficits can contribute to a child's hesitation in asking for help, so a child identified with a mathematics disorder may benefit from gaining positive problem-solving skills in a social arena as well as in mathematics.

DISORDER OF WRITTEN EXPRESSION

Written expression is the most complex skill acquired to convey an understanding of language and to express thoughts and ideas. Writing skills are highly correlated with reading for most children; for some children, however, reading comprehension may far surpass their ability to express complex thoughts. Written expression in some cases is a sensitive index of more subtle, although impairing, deficits in language usage that typically are not detected by standardized reading and language tests.

Disorder of written expression is characterized by writing skills that are significantly below the expected level for a child's age and intellectual capacity. These difficulties impair the child's academic performance and writing in everyday life. The many components of writing disorder include poor spelling, errors in grammar and punctuation, and poor handwriting. Spelling errors are among the most common difficulties for a child with a writing disorder. Spelling mistakes are most often phonetic errors; that is, an erroneous spelling that sounds like the correct spelling. Examples of common types of spelling errors are fone for phone, or beleeve for believe.

Historically, dysgraphia (i.e., poor writing skills) was considered to be a form of reading disorder; however, evidence indicates that disorder of written expression can occur on its own. Terms once used to describe writing disability include *spelling disorder* and *spelling dyslexia*. Writing disabilities are often associated with other learning disorders, but they may be diagnosed later because expressive writing is acquired later than language and reading.

In addition to a disorder similar to DSM-IV-TR's disorder of written expression, the 10th revision of *International Statistical Classification of Diseases and Related Health Problems* (ICD-10) includes a separate specific spelling disorder.

Epidemiology

The prevalence of disorder of written expression alone has not been studied, but as with reading disorder, it is estimated to occur in approximately 4 percent of school-age children. The gender ratio in writing disorder is believed to be similar that of reading disorder, occurring in about three times as many boys. Disorder of written expression often occurs along with reading disorder, but not always.

Comorbidity

Children with writing disorder are at higher risk for a variety of other learning and language disorders, including reading disorder, mathematics disorder, and expressive and receptive language disorders. ADHD occurs with greater frequency in children with writing disorders than in the general population. Finally, children with writing disorders are believed to be at higher risk for social skills difficulties, and some go on to develop poor self-esteem and depressive symptoms.

Etiology

Causes of writing disorders are believed to be similar to those of reading disorder, that is, a deficit in the use of the components of language related to letter sounds. It is likely that genetic factors are significant in the development of writing disorder. Writing difficulties often accompany language disorders in which a given child may have trouble understanding grammatical rules, finding words, and expressing ideas clearly. According to one hypothesis, a disorder of written expression may result from the combined effects of one or more of the following: expressive language disorder, mixed receptive-expressive language disorder, and reading disorder. Hereditary predisposition to the disorder is supported by findings that most children with disorder of written expression have first-degree relatives with the disorder. Children with limited attention spans and high levels of distractibility may find writing an arduous task.

Diagnosis

A diagnosis of disorder of written expression is based on a child's poor performance on composing written text, including handwriting and impaired ability to spell and to place words sequentially in coherent sentences, compared with most other children of the same age and intellectual ability. In addition to spelling mistakes, a child with writing disorder may have serious grammatical mistakes, such as using incorrect tenses, forgetting words in sentences, and placing words in the wrong order. Punctuation may be incorrect, and the child may have poor ability to remember which words begin with capital letters. Poor handwriting may also contribute to writing disorder, including letters that are not legible, inverted letters, and mixtures of capital and lowercase letters in a given word. Other features of writing disorders include poor organization of written stories, which lack critical elements such as "where," "when," and "who" or clear expression of the plot.

Clinical Features

Children with disorder of written expression have difficulties early in grade school in spelling words and expressing their thoughts according to age-appropriate grammatical norms. Their spoken and written sentences contain an unusually large number of grammatical errors and poor paragraph organization. During and after the second grade, these children commonly make simple grammatical errors in writing a short sentence. For example, despite constant reminders, they frequently fail to capitalize the first letter of the first word in a sentence and to end the sentence with a period. Common features of the disorder of written expression are spelling errors, grammatical errors, punctuation errors, poor paragraph organization, and poor handwriting.

As they grow older and progress into higher grades in school, such children's spoken and written sentences become more conspicuously primitive, odd, and inferior to what is expected of students at their grade level. Their word choices are erroneous and inappropriate; their paragraphs are disorganized and are not in proper sequence; and spelling correctly becomes increasingly difficult as their vocabulary becomes larger and more abstract. Associated features of disorder of written expression include refusal or reluctance to go to school and to do assigned written homework, poor academic performance in other areas (e.g., mathematics), general avoidance of school work, truancy, attention deficit, and conduct disturbance.

Many children with disorder of written expression become frustrated and angry because of feelings of inadequacy and failure in their academic performance. In severe cases, depressive disorders can result from a growing sense of isolation, estrangement, and despair. Young adults with disorder of written expression who do not receive remedial intervention continue to have difficulties in social adaptation involving writing skills and a continuing sense of incompetence, inferiority, isolation, and estrangement. Some even try to avoid writing a response letter or a simple greeting card for fear of exposing their writing incompetence.

Cole, an 11-year-old boy, was referred for evaluation of increasing problems in school over the past 2 years, including consistent failure to complete assigned schoolwork and homework, some inattention and oppositional behavior, and a pattern of deteriorating grades and test scores. At the time of assessment, he was enrolled in a regular fifth-grade class in a public school, which he had been attending since grade 1.

Clinical interview with parents revealed that Cole had a twin brother (monozygotic) and was born at term after an unremarkable pregnancy. His brother has a history of language problems for which he received speech-language therapy in the preschool years and remedial reading in the primary grades. Cole had not exhibited any difficulty in speech or language development, according to parental report and scores on standardized tests of oral language administered in the preschool years. His current and previous school reports indicate that, although Cole participated well in class discussions and had no difficulty in reading or mathematics computation, his written work was so far below grade level that he was at risk for failing the current year. Over the past 2 years, the teachers had expressed increasing concerns about Cole's unwillingness or refusal to complete written work, failure to hand in homework, daydreaming and fidgeting in class, skipping classes, and some defiant behavior. Cole admitted to an increasing dislike of school and finding writing to be an extremely tedious activity. He explained that he had lots of ideas and that school would be more fun if the teacher would simply allow him to talk about his ideas, rather than writing everything ("It's writing, writing all day long—even in math and science. I know how to do the problems and the experiments, but I hate having to write it all down—my mind just goes blank."). He also admitted to skipping class, but only when he knew that he would have to do a lot of written work ("well, he [the teacher] is always on at me, telling me that I'm lazy and haven't done enough, and that my writing is atrocious. He slings my work back at me to do over again, gives me a detention, and when I try to explain he tells me, I've got a bad attitude—so why should I go to class?"). Both Cole and his parents reported that, over the past year, he exhibited low self-esteem, increasing frustration with, and refusal to do, homework, and a few brief episodes of depressed mood.

Testing by a clinical psychologist revealed average to high-average scores on the verbal and performance scales of the Wechsler Intelligence Scale for Children-III and average scores on the reading and arithmetic subtests of the Wide Range Achievement Test-3 (WRAT-3). However, scores on the WRAT-3 spelling subtest were below the 9th percentile, which was significantly below expectations for age and ability. Examination of his spelling errors revealed that, although his spelling was typically phonologically accurate (i.e., could plausibly be pronounced to sound like the target word), it was orthographically unacceptable in that he used letter sequences that did not resemble English orthography, regardless of pronunciation (e.g., "houses" was written as "howssis," "phones" was written as "fones," and "exact" was written as "egszakt"). Further evidence of poor orthographic skills was demonstrated on a timed orthographic choice task, which required him to circle the real word in a pair of printed words that are pronounced the same (same phonological code), but spelled differently (different orthographic code; e.g., sammon and salmon). Moreover, his performance was well below age and grade on standardized tests of written expression (TOWL-3), as well as on a brief (5-minute) informal assessment of expository text generation on a favorite topic (e.g., newspaper article on recent sports event). During the 5-minute writing activity, he was observed to frequently stare out of the window, to shift positions and to chew on his pencil, to get up to sharpen his pencil and to sigh when he did put pencil to paper, and to write slowly and laboriously. At the end of 5 minutes, he had produced three short sentences without any punctuation or capitalization that were barely legible, containing several misspellings and grammatical errors, and that were not linked semantically. By contrast, later in the assessment, he described the sporting event with detail and enthusiasm. A speech-language evaluation revealed average scores on standard tests of oral language (Clinical Evaluation of Language Fundamentals-IV), but he was noted to omit sounds or syllables in a multisyllabic word in a nonword repetition test, which has been found to be sensitive to mild residual language impairments and written language impairments.

The clinical team formulated a diagnosis of disorder of written expression, based on the clinical picture of this boy's inability to compose written text, poor spelling, and grammatical errors in the absence of low intelligence, reading or mathematics disorder, or history of, or current, language impairments. He did not meet diagnostic criteria for any other DSM-IV disorder, including oppositional defiant disorder, ADHD, or mood disorder. Recommendations included the following: psychoeducation (primarily bibliotherapy), the need for educational accommodations (e.g., provision of additional time for test taking and written assignments, specific educational intervention to facilitate written expression and to teach note taking, and use of specific computer software to support written composition and spelling), and counseling or psychotherapy should his depressive episodes continue or worsen. (Courtesy of Rosemary Tannock, Ph.D.)

Pathology and Laboratory Examination

Whereas no physical stigmata of a writing disorder exist, educational testing is used in making a diagnosis of writing disorder. Diagnosis is based on a child's writing performance being markedly below his or her intellectual capacity, as confirmed by an individually administered standardized expressive writing test (Table 39–3). Currently available tests of written language include the Test of Written Language (TOWL), the DEWS, and the Test of Early Written Language (TEWL). The presence of a major disorder, such as a pervasive developmental disorder, or mental retardation may obviate the diagnosis of disorder of written expression. Other disorders to be differentiated from disorder of written expression are communication disorders, reading disorder, and impaired vision and hearing.

A child suspected of having disorder of written expression should first be given a standardized intelligence test, such as WISC-III or the revised Wechsler Adult Intelligence Scale (WAIS-R) to determine the child's overall intellectual capacity.

Course and Prognosis

Because writing, language, and reading disorders often coexist and because a child normally speaks well before learning to read and learns to read well before writing well, a child with all these disorders has expressive language disorder diagnosed first and disorder of written expression diagnosed last. In severe cases, a disorder of written expression is apparent by age 7 (second grade); in less severe cases, the disorder may not be apparent until age 10 (fifth grade) or later. Most persons with mild and moderate disorder of written expression fare well if they receive timely remedial education early in grade school. Severe disorder of written expression requires continual, extensive remedial treatment through the late part of high school and even into college.

The prognosis depends on the severity of the disorder, the age or grade when the remedial intervention is started, the length and continuity of treatment, and presence or absence of associated or secondary emotional or behavioral problems. Those who later become well compensated or who recover from disorder of written expression are often from families with high socioeconomic backgrounds.

Differential Diagnosis

It is important to determine whether another disorder, such as ADHD or a depressive disorder, is preventing a child from being able to concentrate on writing tasks in the absence of writing disorder itself. If this is the case, treatment for the other disorder should improve a child's writing performance. Disorder of written expression can also occur with a variety of other language and learning disorders. Common associated disorders are reading disorder, mixed receptive-expressive language disorder, expressive language disorder, mathematics disorder, developmental coordination disorder, and disruptive behavior disorder and ADHD.

Treatment

Remedial treatment for writing disorder includes direct practice in spelling and sentence writing as well as a review of grammatical rules. Intensive and continuous administration of individually tailored, one-on-one expressive and creative writing therapy appears to effect favorable outcome. Teachers in some special schools devote as much as 2 hours a day to such writing instruction. The effectiveness of a writing intervention largely depends on an optimal relationship between the child and the writing specialist. Success or failure in sustaining the patient's motivation greatly affects the treatment's long-term efficacy. Associated secondary emotional and behavioral problems should be given prompt attention, with appropriate psychiatric treatment and parental counseling.

LEARNING DISORDER NOT OTHERWISE SPECIFIED

Learning disorder not otherwise specified is a new category in DSM-IV-TR for disorders that do not meet the criteria for any

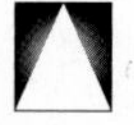

Table 39–3
DSM-IV-TR Diagnostic Criteria for Disorder of Written Expression

A. Writing skills, as measured by individually administered standardized tests (or functional assessments of writing skills), are substantially below those expected given the person's chronological age, measured intelligence, and age-appropriate education.
B. The disturbance in Criterion A significantly interferes with academic achievement or activities of daily living that require the composition of written texts (e.g., writing grammatically correct sentences and organized paragraphs).
C. If a sensory deficit is present, the difficulties in writing skills are in excess of those usually associated with it.

Coding note: If a general medical (e.g., neurological) condition or sensory deficit is present, code the condition on Axis III.

(From American Psychiatric Association. *Diagnostic and Statistical Manual of Mental Disorders.* 4th ed. Text rev. Washington, DC: American Psychiatric Association; copyright 2000, with permission.)

Table 39–4
DSM-IV-TR Diagnostic Criteria for Learning Disorder Not Otherwise Specified

This category is for disorders in learning that do not meet criteria for any specific learning disorder. This category might include problems in all three areas (reading, mathematics, written expression) that together significantly interfere with academic achievement even though performance on tests measuring each individual skill is not substantially below that expected given the person's chronological age, measured intelligence, and age-appropriate education.

(From American Psychiatric Association. *Diagnostic and Statistical Manual of Mental Disorders.* 4th ed. Text rev. Washington, DC: American Psychiatric Association; copyright 2000, with permission.)

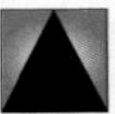

Table 39–5
ICD-10 Diagnostic Criteria for Specific Developmental Disorders of Scholastic Skills

Specific reading disorder

A. Either of the following must be present:
   (1) A score on reading accuracy and/or comprehension that is at least 2 standard errors of prediction below the level expected on the basis of the child's chronological age and general intelligence, with both reading skills and IQ assessed on an individually administered test standardized for the child's culture and educational system.
   (2) A history of serious reading difficulties, or test scores that met Criterion A(1) at an earlier age, plus a score on a spelling test that is at least 2 standard errors of prediction below the level expected on the basis of the child's chronological age and IQ.

B. The disturbance described in Criterion A significantly interferes with academic achievement or with activities of daily living that require reading skills.

C. The disorder is not the direct result of a defect in visual or hearing acuity, or of a neurological disorder.

D. School experiences are within the average expectable range (i.e., there have been no extreme inadequacies in educational experiences).

E. *Most commonly used exclusion clause*: IQ is below 70 on an individually administered standardized test.

Possible additional inclusion criterion

For some research purposes, investigators may wish to specify a history of some level of impairment during the preschool years in speech, language, sound categorization, motor coordination, visual processing, attention, or control or modulation of activity.

Comments

The above criteria would not include general reading backwardness of a type that would fall within the clinical guidelines. The research diagnostic criteria for general reading backwardness would be the same as for specific reading disorder except that Criterion A(1) would specify reading skills 2 standard errors of prediction below the level expected on the basis of chronological age (i.e., not taking IQ into account), and Criterion A(2) would follow the same principle for spelling. The validity of the differentiation between these two varieties of reading problem is not unequivocally established, but it seems that the specific type has a more specific association with language retardation (whereas general reading backwardness is associated with a wider range of developmental disabilities), and is more prevalent in boys than in girls.

There are further research differentiations that are based on analyses of the types of spelling error.

Specific spelling disorder

A. The score on a standardized spelling test is at least 2 standard errors of prediction below the level expected on the basis of the child's chronological age and general intelligence.

B. Scores on reading accuracy and comprehension and on arithmetic are within the normal range (±2 standard deviations from the mean).

C. There is no history of significant reading difficulties.

D. School experience is within the average expectable range (i.e., there have been no extreme inadequacies in educational experiences).

E. Spelling difficulties have been present from the early stages of learning to spell.

F. The disturbance described in Criterion A significantly interferes with academic achievement or with activities of daily living that require spelling skills.

G. *Most commonly used exclusion clause*: IQ is below 70 on an individually administered standardized test.

Specific disorder of arithmetical skills

A. The score on a standardized arithmetic test is at least 2 standard errors of prediction below the level expected on the basis of the child's chronological age and general intelligence.

B. Scores on reading accuracy and comprehension and on spelling are within the normal range (±2 standard deviations from the mean).

C. There is no history of significant reading or spelling difficulties.

D. School experience is within the average expectable range (i.e., there have been no extreme inadequacies in educational experiences).

E. Arithmetical difficulties have been present from the early stages of learning arithmetic.

F. The disturbance described in Criterion A significantly interferes with academic achievement or with activities of daily living that require arithmetical skills.

G. *Most commonly used exclusion clause*: IQ is below 70 on an individually administered standardized test.

Mixed disorder of scholastic skills

This is an ill-defined, inadequately conceptualized (but necessary) residual category of disorders in which both arithmetical and reading or spelling skills are significantly impaired, but in which the disorder is not solely explicable in terms of general mental retardation or inadequate schooling. It should be used for disorders meeting the criteria for specific disorder of arithmetical skills and either specific reading disorder or specific spelling disorder.

Other developmental disorders of scholastic skills

Developmental disorder of scholastic skills, unspecified

This category should be avoided as far as possible and should be used only for unspecified disorders in which there is a significant disability of learning that cannot be solely accounted for by mental retardation, visual acuity problems, or inadequate schooling.

(From World Health Organization. The *ICD-10 Classification of Mental and Behavioural Disorders: Diagnostic Criteria for Research.* Copyright, World Health Organization, Geneva; 1993, with permission.)

specific learning disorder, but cause impairment and reflect learning abilities below those expected for a person's intelligence, education, and age (Table 39–4). An example of a disability that could be placed in this category is a spelling skills deficit.

ICD-10

The ICD-10 classifies specific developmental disorders of scholastic skills learning disorders under the category disorders of psychological development, which must have an onset during infancy or childhood, must show a delay or impairment in developing functions strongly related to the biological maturation of the CNS, and must undergo a steady course without remissions and relapses typical of many mental disorders. Scholastic skills learning disorders are usually of unknown cause, but often have a family history of similar or related disorders, lending support to the probability of genetic influences. Environmental factors may play a part, but are often not identified as major factors.

Specific developmental disorders of scholastic skills include specific reading disorder; specific spelling disorder; specific disorder of arithmetic skills; mixed disorder of scholastic skills; other developmental disorders of scholastic skills; and developmental disorder of scholastic skills, unspecified (Table 39–5). Normal patterns of skill acquisition are disturbed because of abnormalities in cognitive processing that derive largely from biological dysfunction. Diagnostic difficulties can arise from the need to differentiate the disorders from normal variations and to consider developmental course, the fact that these skills must be taught and learned and are not simply a function of biological maturation, and the difficulty in distinguishing between cognitive abnormalities that cause reading problems and those that arise from reading problems.

References

Catone WV, Brady SA. The inadequacy of Individual Educational Program (IEP) goals for high school students with word-level reading difficulties. *Annals of Dyslexia*. 2005;55:53.

Cragg L, Nation K. Exploring written narrative in children with poor reading comprehension. *Educational Psychology*. 2006;26:55–72.

Endres M, Toso L, Roberson R, Park J, Abebe D, Poggi S, Spong CY. Prevention of alcohol-induced developmental delays and learning abnormalities in a model of fetal alcohol syndrome. *Am J Obstet Gynecol*. 2005;193:1028.

Fletcher JM. Predicting math outcomes: Reading predictors and comorbidity. *J Learn Disabil.* 2005;38:308.

Gersten R, Jordan NC, Flojo JR. Early identification and interventions for students with mathematics difficulties. *J Learn Disabil.* 2005;38:305

Gordon N. The "medical" investigation of specific learning disorders. *Pediatr Neurol*. 2004;2(1):3.

Jura MB, Humphrey LH. Neuropsychological and cognitive assessment of children. In: Sadock BJ, Sadock VA, eds. *Kaplan & Sadock's Comprehensive Textbook of Psychiatry.* 8th ed. Vol. 2. Philadelphia: Lippincott Williams & Wilkins; 2005;895

Meeks J, Adler A, Kunert K, Floyd L. Individual psychotherapy of the learning-disabled adolescent. In: Flaherty LT, ed. *Adolescent Psychiatry: Developmental and Clinical Studies*. Vol. 28. Hillsdale, NJ: Analytic Press; 2004:231.

Plomin R, Kovas Y. Generalist genes and learning disabilities. *Psychol Bull.* 2005;131:592.

Tannock R. Reading disorder. In: Sadock BJ, Sadock VA, eds. *Kaplan & Sadock's Comprehensive Textbook of Psychiatry.* 8th ed. Vol. 2. Baltimore: Lippincott Williams & Wilkins; 2005:3107.

Tannock R. Mathematics disorder. In: Sadock BJ, Sadock VA, eds. *Kaplan & Sadock's Comprehensive Textbook of Psychiatry.* 8th ed. Vol. 2. Baltimore: Lippincott Williams & Wilkins; 2005:3116.

Tannock R. Disorder of written expression and learning disorder not otherwise specified. In: Sadock BJ, Sadock VA, eds. *Kaplan & Sadock's Comprehensive Textbook of Psychiatry*. 8th ed. Vol. 2. Baltimore: Lippincott Williams & Wilkins; 2005:3123.

Vadasy PF, Sanders EA, Peyton JA. Relative effectiveness of reading practice or word-level instruction in supplemental tutoring: how text matters. *J Learn Disabil*. 2005; 38:364.

40 Motor Skills Disorder: Developmental Coordination Disorder

Children with developmental motor coordination struggle to perform accurately the motor activities of daily life, such as jumping, hopping, running, or catching a ball. Children with coordination problems may also agonize to use utensils correctly, tie their shoelaces, or write. A child with developmental coordination disorder may exhibit delays in achieving motor milestones, such as sitting, crawling, and walking, because of clumsiness, and yet excel at verbal skills.

Developmental coordination disorder, thus, may be characterized by either clumsy gross and/or fine motor skills, resulting in poor performance in sports and even in academic achievement because of poor writing skills. A child with developmental coordination disorder may bump into things more often than siblings or drop things. In the 1930s, the term *clumsy child syndrome* began to be used in the literature to denote a condition of awkward motor behaviors that could not be correlated with any specific neurological disorder or damage. This term continues to be used to identify imprecise or delayed gross and fine motor behavior in children, resulting in subtle motor inabilities, but often significant social rejection. Currently, certain indications are that perinatal problems, such as prematurity, low birthweight, and hypoxia may contribute to the emergence of developmental coordination disorders. Children with developmental coordination disorder are at higher risk for language and learning disorders. A strong association is seen between speech and language problems and coordination problems, as well as an association of coordination difficulties with hyperactivity, impulsivity, and poor attention span.

Children with developmental coordination disorder may resemble younger children because of their inability to master motor activities typical for their age group. For example, children with developmental coordination disorder in elementary school may not be adept at bicycle riding, skateboarding, running, skipping, or hopping. In the middle school years, children with this disorder may have trouble in team sports, such as soccer, baseball, or basketball. Fine motor skill manifestations of developmental coordination disorder typically include clumsiness using utensils and difficulty with buttons and zippers in the preschool age group. In older children, using scissors and more complex grooming skills, such as styling hair or putting on makeup, is difficult. Children with developmental coordination disorder are often ostracized by peers because of their poor skills in many sports, and they often have long-standing difficulties with peer relationships. Developmental coordination disorder is the sole disorder in the text revision of the 4th edition of the American Psychiatric Association's *Diagnostic and Statistical Manual of Mental Disorders* (DSM-IV-TR) category motor skills disorder. Gross and fine motor impairment in this disorder cannot be explained on the basis of a medical condition, such as cerebral palsy, muscular dystrophy, or any other neuromuscular disorder.

EPIDEMIOLOGY

The prevalence of developmental coordination disorder has been estimated at about 5 percent of school-age children. The male-to-female ratio in referred populations tends to show increased rates of the disorder in males, but schools refer boys more often for testing and special education evaluations. Reports in the literature of the male-to-female ratio have ranged from 2 to 1 to as much as 4 to 1. These rates may also be inflated because motor behaviors in boys are scrutinized more closely than those in girls.

COMORBIDITY

Developmental coordination disorder is strongly associated with speech and language disorders. Children with coordination difficulties have higher than expected rates of speech and language disorders, and studies of children with speech disorders report very high rates of "clumsiness." Some studies have found associations between fine motor skills in the upper arms and expressive and receptive language disorders, whereas gross motor problems and visual motor coordination problems were not associated with language disturbance. Developmental coordination disorder is also associated with reading disorders, mathematics disorder, and disorder of written expression. Higher than expected rates of attention-deficit/hyperactivity disorders (ADHD) are also associated with developmental coordination disorder. A recent study of children with developmental coordination disorder reported that, although motor ability accounts largely for accuracy in tasks that require speed, the degree of motor incoordination is not correlated with degree of inattention. Therefore, developmental coordination disorder and ADHD appear to be distinct disorders that occur concurrently with greater frequency than chance.

Secondary peer relationship problems are common among children with developmental coordination disorders, because of the rejection that occurs along with their poor performance in sports and games that require good motor skill. Adolescents with coordination problems often exhibit poor self-esteem and academic difficulties. Recent studies underscore the importance of attention to both victimization of children and adolescents with developmental motor coordination by peers and the potential resulting damage to self-worth. Children and adolescents with developmental coordination disorder who are bullied have higher rates of poor self-esteem that often deserves clinical attention.

ETIOLOGY

The causes of developmental coordination disorder are believed to include both "organic" and "developmental" factors. Risk factors postulated to contribute to this disorder include prematurity, hypoxia, perinatal malnutrition, and low birthweight. Prenatal exposure to alcohol, cocaine, and nicotine has also been hypothesized to contribute to both low birthweight and cognitive and behavioral abnormalities. Neurochemical abnormalities and parietal lobe lesions have also been suggested to contribute to coordination deficits. Developmental coordination disorder and communication disorders have strong associations, although the specific causative agents are unknown for both. Coordination problems are also more frequently found in children with hyperactivity syndromes and learning disorders. Recent studies of postural control, that is, the ability to regain balance after being in motion, indicate that children with developmental coordination disorder who do not have significant difficulties with balance when standing still, are unable accurately to correct for movement, resulting in impaired balance compared with other children. A recent study concluded that, in children with developmental coordination disorder, signals from the brain to particular muscles (including the tibialis anterior and peroneus muscles), involved in balance, are not being optimally sent or received. These findings have implicated the cerebellum as a contributing origin of dysfunction for developmental coordination disorder.

DIAGNOSIS

The diagnosis of developmental coordination disorder depends on poor performance, for a child's age and intellectual level, in activities requiring coordination. Diagnosis is based on a history of the child's delay in achieving early motor milestones, as well as on direct observation of current deficits in coordination. An informal screen for developmental coordination disorder involves asking the child to perform tasks involving gross motor coordination (e.g., hopping, jumping, and standing on one foot); fine motor coordination (e.g., finger-tapping and shoelace tying); and hand-eye coordination (e.g., catching a ball and copying letters). Judgments regarding poor performance must be based on what is expected for a child's age. A child who is mildly clumsy, but whose functioning is not impaired, does not qualify for a diagnosis of developmental coordination disorder.

The diagnosis may be associated with below-normal scores on performance subtests of standardized intelligence tests and by

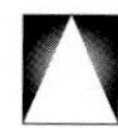

Table 40–1
DSM-IV-TR Diagnostic Criteria for Developmental Coordination Disorder

A. Performance in daily activities that require motor coordination is substantially below that expected given the person's chronological age and measured intelligence. This may be manifested by marked delays in achieving motor milestones (e.g., walking, crawling, sitting), dropping things, "clumsiness," poor performance in sports, or poor handwriting.

B. The disturbance in Criterion A significantly interferes with academic achievement or activities of daily living.

C. The disturbance is not due to a general medical condition (e.g., cerebral palsy, hemiplegia, or muscular dystrophy) and does not meet criteria for a pervasive developmental disorder.

D. If mental retardation is present, the motor difficulties are in excess of those usually associated with it.

Coding note: If a general medical (e.g., neurological) condition or sensory deficit is present, code the condition on Axis III.

(From American Psychiatric Association. *Diagnostic and Statistical Manual of Mental Disorders.* 4th ed. Text rev. Washington, DC: American Psychiatric Association; copyright 2000, with permission.)

normal or above-normal scores on verbal subtests. Specialized tests of motor coordination can be useful, such as the *Bender Visual Motor Gestalt Test*, the *Frostig Movement Skills Test Battery*, and the *Bruininks-Oseretsky Test of Motor Development.* The child's chronological age and intellectual capacity must be taken into account, and the disorder cannot be caused by a neurological or neuromuscular condition. Examination, however, may occasionally reveal slight reflex abnormalities and other soft neurological signs. The DSM-IV-TR diagnostic criteria are given in Table 40–1.

CLINICAL FEATURES

The clinical signs suggesting the existence of developmental coordination disorder are evident as early as infancy in some cases, when a child begins to attempt tasks requiring motor coordination. The essential clinical feature is significantly impaired performance in motor coordination. The difficulties in motor coordination may vary with a child's age and developmental stage (Table 40–2).

In infancy and early childhood, the disorder may be manifested by delays in developmental motor milestones, such as turning over, crawling, sitting, standing, walking, buttoning shirts, and zipping up pants. Between the ages of 2 and 4 years, clumsiness appears in almost all activities requiring motor coordination. Affected children cannot hold objects and drop them easily, their gait may be unsteady, they often trip over their own feet, and they may bump into other children while attempting to go around them. Older children may display impaired motor coordination in table games, such as putting together puzzles or building blocks, and in any type of ball game. Although no specific features are pathognomonic of developmental coordination disorder, developmental milestones are frequently delayed. Many children with the disorder also have speech and language difficulties. Older children may have secondary problems, including academic difficulties, as well as poor peer relationships

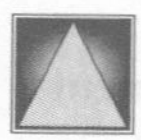

Table 40–2
Manifestations of Developmental Coordination Disorder

Gross motor manifestations
- Preschool age
  - Delays in reaching motor milestones, such as sitting, crawling, and walking
  - Balance problems: falling, getting bruised frequently, and poor toddling
  - Abnormal gait
  - Knocking over objects, bumping into things, and destructiveness
- Primary-school age
  - Difficulty with riding bikes, skipping, hopping, running, jumping, and doing somersaults
  - Awkward or abnormal gait
- Older
  - Poor at sports, throwing, catching, kicking, and hitting a ball

Fine motor manifestations
- Preschool age
  - Difficulty learning dressing skills (tying, fastening, zipping, and buttoning)
  - Difficulty learning feeding skills (handling knife, fork, or spoon)
- Primary-school age
  - Difficulty assembling jigsaw pieces, using scissors, building with blocks, drawing, or tracing
- Older
  - Difficulty with grooming (putting on makeup, blow-drying hair, and doing nails)
  - Messy or illegible writing
  - Difficulty using hand tools, sewing, and playing piano

based on social rejection. It has been reported widely that children with motor coordination problems are more likely to have problems understanding subtle social cues and are often rejected by peers. A recent study indicated that children with motor difficulties were found to perform more poorly on scales that measure recognition of static and changing facial expressions of emotion. This finding is likely to be correlated to the clinical observations that children with motor coordination have difficulties in social behavior and peer relationships.

Peter was brought for evaluation of poor coordination at 8 years of age after complaining to his parents that he was being teased by peers for being "bad" in sports, and he was always picked last for the team. His friends laughed at him, because he always dropped the ball even when he could initially catch it, and he looked "funny" while running. He was so upset about ridicule from peers that he no longer wanted to play baseball or basketball with his friends. A developmental history obtained from his parents revealed that Peter's development had been delayed for sitting, which he could not do until 10 months of age, and he was not able to walk without falling over until 24 months of age. His parents reported an awareness that he was somewhat clumsy, but they believed that he would outgrow that. On questioning about Peter's current motor function, his parents reported that, during meal times, Peter still constantly spilled his drinks and was awkward when he used a fork. His food often fell off of a fork or spoon before it reached his mouth, and he had great difficulty using a knife and a fork.

A comprehensive assessment of fine and gross motor skills yielded the following results: Peter was able to hop, but he could not skip without briefly stopping after each step. Peter could stand with both feet together, but could not stand on tiptoe. Although Peter could catch a ball, he held a ball bounced to him at chest level, and he could not catch a ball bounced to him on the ground from a distance of 15 feet. Peter's agility and coordination were measured with the Bruininks-Oseretsky Test of Motor Development, which revealed functioning levels commensurate with those of an average 6-year-old child.

Peter was referred to a neurologist for a comprehensive evaluation, because he appeared to be generally weak, and his muscles seemed floppy. Neurological evaluation was negative for diagnosable neurological disorders, and his muscle strength was actually found to be normal, despite his appearance. Based on the negative neurological examination and the finding of the Bruininks-Oseretsky Test of Motor Development, Peter was given a diagnosis of developmental coordination disorder. Peter's symptoms included mild hypotonia and fine motor clumsiness.

After the diagnosis of developmental motor coordination was made, a treatment plan was developed that included private sessions with an occupational therapist who used perceptual-motor exercises to improve his fine motor skills, targeting particularly writing and use of utensils, and a request for an individualized evaluation from the school with a goal of administering an adaptive physical education program. He was also enrolled in a treatment program using motor imagery training to reduce his clumsiness, administered by a psychologist.

Peter was relieved to be receiving help, especially for his writing and for sports activities, because these were the areas in which his peers had teased him. Over a period of 3 months of treatment, Peter showed significant improvement in the legibility of his handwriting, although he remained a slow writer. He felt much better with this improvement, because he was receiving more praise from his teachers and parents, and his classmates were teasing him less. As he began to feel better about himself, he began to play sports informally with his peers, although not competitively. He was given a modified physical education program in school, and he was not required to play on teams, but he practiced throwing and catching a ball and playing basketball.

Peter continued to have some degree of clumsiness in his fine motor skills over the next few years, but he was cooperative with the occupational therapy interventions, and he showed continual improvement. (Courtesy of Caroly Pataki, M.D. and Sarah Spence, M.D.)

DIFFERENTIAL DIAGNOSIS

The differential diagnosis includes medical conditions that produce coordination difficulties (e.g., cerebral palsy and muscular dystrophy), pervasive developmental disorders, and mental retardation. In mental retardation and in the pervasive developmental disorders, coordination usually does not stand out as a significant deficit compared with other skills. Children with neuromuscular disorders may exhibit more global muscle impairment rather than clumsiness and delayed motor milestones. Neurological examination and workups usually reveal more extensive deficits in neurological conditions than in developmental coordination disorder. Extremely hyperactive and impulsive children may be physically careless because of their high levels of motor activity. Clumsy gross and fine motor behavior and ADHD seem to be associated.

COURSE AND PROGNOSIS

Few data are available on the prospective longitudinal outcomes of both treated and untreated children with developmental coordination disorder. For the most part, although clumsiness may continue, some children can compensate by developing interests in other skills. Some studies suggest a favorable outcome for children who have an average or above-average intellectual capacity, in that they come up with strategies to develop friendships that do not depend on physical activities. Clumsiness generally persists into adolescence and adult life. One study following a group of children with developmental coordination problems over a decade found that the clumsy children remained less dexterous, showed poor balance, and continued to be physically awkward. The affected children were also more likely to have both academic problems and poor self-esteem. Commonly associated features include delays in nonmotor milestones, expressive language disorder, and mixed receptive-expressive language disorder.

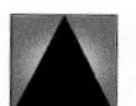

Table 40–3
ICD-10 Diagnostic Criteria for Specific Developmental Disorder of Motor Function

A. The score on a standardized test of fine or gross motor coordination is at least 2 standard deviations below the level expected for the child's chronological age.
B. The disturbance described in Criterion A significantly interferes with academic achievement or with activities of daily living.
C. There is no diagnosable neurological disorder.
D. Most commonly used exclusion clause. IQ is below 70 on an individually administered standardized test.

(From World Health Organization. The *ICD-10 Classification of Mental and Behavioural Disorders: Diagnostic Criteria for Research.* Copyright, World Health Organization, Geneva; 1993, with permission.)

TREATMENT

Interventions for children with developmental coordination disorder utilize multiple modalities, including visual, auditory, and tactile materials targeting perceptual motor training for specific motor tasks. More recently, motor imagery training has been incorporated into treatment. These approaches are visual imagery exercises using CD-ROM; they have a broad range of foci, including predictive timing for motor tasks, relaxation and mental preparation, visual modeling of fundamental motor skills, and mental rehearsal of various tasks. This type of intervention is based on the notion that improved internal representation of a movement task will improve a child's actual motor behavior. The treatment of developmental coordination disorder generally includes versions of sensory-integration programs and modified physical education. Sensory integration programs, usually administered by occupational therapists, consist of physical activities that increase awareness of motor and sensory function. For example, a child who bumps into objects often might be given the task of trying to balance on a scooter, under supervision, to improve balance and body awareness. Children who have difficulty writing letters are often given tasks to increase awareness of hand movements. School-based occupational therapies for motor coordination problems in writing include utilizing mechanisms that provide resistance or vibration during writing exercises, to improve grip, and practicing vertical writing on a chalk board to increase arm strength and stability while writing. These programs have been shown to improve legibility of student's writing, but not necessarily speed because students learn to write with greater accuracy and deliberate letter formation. Currently, many schools also allow and may even encourage children with coordination difficulties that affect writing to use computers to aid in writing reports and long papers.

Adaptive physical education programs are designed to help children enjoy exercise and physical activities without the pressures of team sports. These programs generally incorporate certain sports actions, such as kicking a soccer ball or throwing a basketball. Children with coordination disorder may also benefit from social skills groups and other prosocial interventions. The Montessori technique (developed by Maria Montessori) may promote motor skill development, especially with preschool children, because this educational program emphasizes the development of motor skills. Small studies have suggested that exercise in rhythmic coordination, practicing motor movements, and learning to use word processing keyboards may be beneficial. Parental counseling may help reduce parents' anxiety and guilt about their child's impairment, increase their awareness, and facilitate their confidence to cope with the child.

A recent investigation of children with developmental coordination disorder showed positive results using a computer game designed to improve ability to catch a ball. These children were able to improve their game score by practicing virtual catching without specific instructions on how to utilize the visual cues. This has implications for treatment in that certain types of motor task coordination can be positively influenced through the practice of specific motor tasks, even without overt instructions.

ICD-10

According to the 10th revision of *International Statistical Classification of Diseases and Related Health Problems* (ICD-10), the main feature of specific developmental disorder of motor function (sometimes called clumsy child syndrome) is a "serious impairment in the development of motor coordination that is not solely explicable in terms of general intellectual retardation or of any specific congenital or acquired neurological disorder (other than the one that may be implicit in the coordination abnormality)." The motor clumsiness is usually associated with "impaired performance on visuospatial cognitive tasks." The ICD-10 diagnostic criteria are presented in Table 40–3.

References

Bernie C, Rodger S. Cognitive strategy use in school-aged children with developmental coordination disorder. *Phys Occup Ther Pediatr*. 2004;24(4):23–45.

Cairney J, Hay JA, Faught BE, Wade TJ, Corna L, Flouris A. Developmental coordination disorder, generalized self-efficacy toward physical activity, and participation in organized and free play activities. *J Pediatr*. 2005;147(4): 515–520.

Cummins A, Pick JP, Dyck MJ. Motor coordination, empathy, and social behaviour in school-aged children. *Dev Med Child Neurol*. 2005;47:437.

Dewey D, Bottos S. Neuroimaging of developmental motor disorders. In: Dewey D, Tupper DE, eds. *Developmental Motor Disorders: A Neuropsychological perspective*. New York: Guilford Press; 2004:26.

Dewey D, Tupper DE, eds. *Developmental Motor Disorders: A Neuropsychological perspective*. New York: Guilford Press; 2004.

Geuze RH. Postural control in children with developmental coordination disorder. *Neural Plast*. 2005;12:183.

Groen SE, de Blecourt ACE, Postema K, Hadders-Algra M. General movements in early infancy predict neuromotor development at 9 to 12 years of age. *Dev Med Child Neurol*. 2005;47(11):731.

Hay JA, Hawes R, Faught BE. Evaluation of a screening instrument for developmental coordination disorder. *J Adolesc Health*. 2004;34(4):308–313.

Pataki CS, Spence SJ. Motor skills disorder: developmental coordination disorder. In: Sadock BJ, Sadock VA, eds. *Kaplan & Sadock's Comprehensive Textbook of Psychiatry*. 8th ed. Vol. 2. Baltimore: Lippincott Williams & Wilkins; 2005:3130.

Piek JP, Dyck MJ, Nieman A, Anderson M, Hay D, Smith LM, McCoy M, Hallmayer J. The relationship between motor coordination, executive functioning and attention in school aged children. *Arch Clin Neuropsychol*. 2004;19:1063.

Piek JP, Barrett NC, Allen LS, Jones A, Loise M. The relationship of bullying and self-worth in children with movement coordination problems. *Br J Educ Psychol*. 2005;75:453.

Richardson AJ, Montgomery P. The Oxford-Durham study: A randomized, controlled trial of dietary supplementation with fatty acids in children with developmental coordination disorder. *Pediatrics*. 2005;115:1360.

Wilson PH. Practitioner review: Approaches to assessment and treatment of children with DCD: An evaluative review. *J Child Psychol Psychiatry*. 2005;46:806.

41 Communication Disorders

Communication disorders are among the most common disorders in childhood. To communicate effectively, children must have a mastery of language—that is the ability to understand and express ideas—using words and speech, the manner in which words are spoken. Language disorders include expressive and mixed receptive-expressive language disorder, whereas speech disorders include phonological disorder and stuttering. Children with expressive language disorders have difficulties expressing their thoughts with words and sentences at a level of sophistication expected for their age and developmental level in other areas. These children may struggle with limited vocabularies, speak in sentences that are short or ungrammatical, and often present descriptions of situations that are disorganized, confusing, and infantile. They may be delayed in developing an understanding and a memory of words compared with others their age.

Language and speech are pragmatically intertwined, despite the distinct categories of language disorders and speech disorders within the text revision of the 4th edition of the American Psychiatric Association's *Diagnostic and Statistical Manual of Mental Disorders* (DSM-IV-TR). Language competence spans four domains: phonology, grammar, semantics, and pragmatics. *Phonology* refers to the ability to produce sounds that constitute words in a given language and the skills to discriminate the various phonemes (sounds that are made by a letter or group of letters in a language). To imitate words, a child must be able to produce the sounds of a word. *Grammar* designates the organization of words and the rules for placing words in an order that makes sense in that language. *Semantics* refers to the organization of concepts and the acquisition of words themselves. A child draws from a mental list of words to produce sentences. Children with language impairments exhibit a wide range of difficulties with semantics that include acquiring new words, storage and organization of known words, and word retrieval. Speech and language evaluations that are sufficiently broad to test all of the above skill levels will be more accurate in evaluating a child's remedial needs. *Pragmatics* has to do with skill in the actual use of language and the "rules" of conversation, including pausing so that a listener can answer a question and knowing when to change the topic when a break occurs in a conversation. By age 2 years, toddlers may know up to 200 words, and by age 3 years, most children understand the basic rules of language and can converse effectively. Table 41–1 provides an overview of typical milestones in language and nonverbal development.

EXPRESSIVE LANGUAGE DISORDER

Expressive language disorder is diagnosed when a child demonstrates a selective deficit in expressive language development relative to receptive language skills and nonverbal intelligence. Thus, a child with expressive language disorder may be identified using the *Wechsler Intelligence Scale for Children III* (WISC-III) in that verbal intellectual level may appear to be depressed compared with the child's overall intelligence quotient (IQ). A child with expressive language disorder is likely to function below the expected levels of acquired vocabulary, correct tense usage, complex sentence constructions, and word recall. Children with expressive language disorder often present verbally as younger than their age. Language disability can be acquired at any time during childhood (e.g., secondary to a trauma or a neurological disorder) or it can be developmental; it is usually congenital, without an obvious cause. Most childhood language disorders fall in the developmental category. In either case, deficits in receptive skills (language comprehension) or expressive skills (ability to use language) can occur. Expressive language disturbance often appears in the absence of comprehension difficulties, whereas receptive dysfunction generally diminishes proficiency in the expression of language. Children with expressive language disorder alone have courses and prognoses that differ from children with mixed receptive-expressive language disorder.

In DSM-IV-TR, the diagnosis of expressive language disorder can be made in the absence of receptive language disorder. Mixed receptive-expressive language disorder is diagnosed according to DSM-IV-TR when both receptive and expressive language syndromes are present, and mixed receptive-expressive language disorder is an exclusionary criterion for expressive language disorder. In general, whenever receptive skills are sufficiently impaired to warrant a diagnosis, expressive skills are also impaired. In DSM-IV-TR, expressive language disorder and mixed receptive-expressive language disorder are not limited to developmental language disabilities; acquired forms of language disturbances are included. To meet the criteria for expressive language disorder, patients must have scores on standardized measures of expressive language markedly below those of standardized nonverbal IQ subtests and standardized tests of receptive language.

Epidemiology

The prevalence of expressive language disorder is estimated to be as high as 6 percent in children between the ages of 5 and 11 years of age. Surveys have indicated rates of expressive language as high as 15 percent in children under age 3 years. In school-age children over the age of 11 years, the estimates are lower, ranging from 3 percent to 5 percent. The disorder is two to three times more common in boys than in girls and is most prevalent among

Table 41–1
Normal Development of Speech, Language, and Nonverbal Skills in Children

Speech and Language Development	Nonverbal Development
1 year	
Recognizes own name	Stands alone
Follows simple directions accompanied by gestures (e.g., bye-bye)	Takes first steps with support
Speaks one or two words	Uses common objects (e.g., spoon, cup)
Mixes words and jargon sounds	Releases objects willfully
Uses communicative gestures (e.g., showing, pointing)	Searches for object in location where last seen
2 years	
Uses 200 to 300 words	Walks up and down stairs alone, but without alternating feet
Names most common objects	Runs rhythmically, but is unable to stop or start smoothly
Uses two-word or longer phrases	Eats with a fork
Uses a few prepositions (e.g., in, on), pronouns (e.g., you, me), verb endings (e.g., -ing, -s, -ed) and plurals (-s), but not always correctly	Cooperates with adult in simple household tasks
	Follows simple commands not accompanied by gestures
Enjoys play with action toys	
3 years	
Uses 900 to 1,000 words	Rides tricycle
Creates three- to four-word sentences, usually with subject and verb but simple structure	Enjoys simple "make-believe" play
	Matches primary colors
Follows two-step commands	Balances momentarily on one foot
Repeats five- to seven-syllable sentences	Shares toys with others for short periods
Speech is usually understood by family members	
4 years	
Uses 1,500 to 1,600 words	Walks up and down stairs with alternating feet
Recounts stories and events from recent past	Hops on one foot
Understands most questions about immediate environment	Copies block letters
Uses conjunctions (e.g., if, but, because)	Role-plays with others
Speech is usually understood by strangers	Categorizes familiar objects
5 years	
Uses 2,100 to 2,300 words	Dresses self without assistance
Discusses feelings	Cuts own meat with knife
Understands most prepositions referring to space (e.g., above, beside, toward) and time (e.g., before, after, until)	Draws a recognizable person
	Plays purposefully and constructively
Follows three-step commands	Recognizes part-whole relationships
Prints own name	
6 years	
Defines words by function and attributes	Rides a bicycle
Uses a variety of well-formed complex sentences	Throws a ball well
Uses all parts of speech (e.g., verbs, nouns, adverbs, adjectives, conjunctions, prepositions)	Sustains attention to motivating tasks
	Enjoys competitive games
Understands letter-sound associations in reading	
8 years	
Reads simple books for pleasure	Understands conservation of liquid, number, length, and so forth
Enjoys riddles and jokes	
Verbalizes ideas and problems readily	Knows left and right of others
Understands indirect requests (e.g., "It's hot in here" understood as request to open window)	Knows differences and similarities
	Appreciates that others have different perspectives
Produces all speech sounds in an adult-like manner	Categorizes same object into multiple categories

(Adapted from Owens RE. *Language Development: An Introduction.* 4th ed. Needham Heights, MA: Allyn & Bacon; 1996, with permission.)

children whose relatives have a family history of phonological disorder or other communication disorders.

Comorbidity

Children with developmental language disorders, such as expressive language disorder, have above-average rates of comorbid psychiatric disorders. In one large study of children with speech and language disorders by Lorian Baker and Dennis Cantwell, the most common comorbid disorders were attention-deficit/hyperactivity disorder (ADHD) (19 percent), anxiety disorders (10 percent), oppositional defiant disorder, and conduct disorder (7 percent combined). Children with expressive language disorder are also at higher risk for a speech disorder, receptive difficulties, and other learning disorders. Many disorders—such as reading disorder, developmental coordination disorder, and other communication disorders—are associated with expressive language disorder. Children with expressive language disorder often have some receptive impairment, although not always sufficiently significant for the diagnosis of mixed receptive-expressive language disorder. Delayed motor milestones and a history of enuresis are common in children with expressive language disorder. Phonological disorder is commonly found in young children with the disorder, and neurological abnormalities have been reported in a number of children, including soft neurological signs, depressed vestibular responses, and electroencephalogram (EEG) abnormalities. On the other hand, a recent study found that boys with serious behavior problems also had high levels of unidentified expressive language disorders, thus it may be important to screen for language dysfunction in children who are extremely behavior disordered.

Etiology

The specific cause of developmental expressive language disorder is likely to be multifactorial. Subtle cerebral damage and maturational lags in cerebral development have been postulated as underlying causes. Some children with language disorders have difficulty processing information in a time-limited manner. Scant data are available on the specific brain structure of children with language disorder, but limited magnetic resonance imaging (MRI) studies suggest that language disorders are associated with a loss of the normal left-right brain asymmetry in the perisylvian and planum temporale regions. Results of one small MRI study suggested possible inversion of brain asymmetry (right > left). Left-handedness or ambilaterality appears to be associated with expressive language problems. Evidence shows that language disorders occur with higher frequency in certain families. Genetic factors have been suspected to play a role, and several studies of twins show significant concordance for monozygotic twins for developmental language disorders. A recent report described a hypothesis of specific genes at 7q11.23 that appear to be exquisitely sensitive to dosage alterations that can influence human language and visuospatial capabilities. The Williams-Beuren syndrome (WBS) locus at 7q11.23 is susceptible to recurrent chromosomal rearrangements, including the microdeletion that causes WBS. WBS typically presents as a phenotype, including characteristic cardiovascular, cognitive, and behavioral features. It is hypothesized, however, that instead of microdeletions, reciprocal duplications of the WBS could also occur and may be associated with the phenotype of language dysfunction. Some studies have found that some individuals with WBS are at an increased risk of expressive language disorder. Environmental and educational factors are also postulated to contribute to developmental language disorders. Data suggest that prenatal exposure to substances such as alcohol and cocaine, for example, are likely to be associated with both delays in language acquisition, and expressive language ability.

Diagnosis

Expressive language disorder is present when a child has a selective deficit in language skills and is functioning well in nonverbal areas and in receptive skills. Markedly below-age-level verbal or sign language, accompanied by a low score on standardized expressive verbal tests, is diagnostic of expressive language disorder (Table 41–2). The disorder is not caused by a pervasive developmental disorder, and a child with an expressive language disorder usually develops some nonverbal strategies to aid in socialization. A child with an expressive language disorder exhibits the following features: limited vocabulary, simple grammar, and variable articulation. "Inner language" or the appropriate use of toys and household objects is present. One recent assessment tool, the *Carter Neurocognitive Assessment* has the capacity to itemize and quantify skills in areas of social awareness, visual attention, auditory comprehension, and vocal communication even when there are compromised expressive language and motor skills in very young children—up to 2 years of age. Such a tool may be able to provide a more positive view of the cognitive potential of children with handicaps including expressive language. To confirm the diagnosis, a child is given standardized expressive language and nonverbal intelligence tests. Observations of children's verbal and sign language patterns in various settings (e.g., school yard, classroom, home, and playroom) and during interactions with other children help ascertain the severity and specific areas of a child's impairment and aid in early detection of behavioral and emotional complications. Family history should include the presence or absence of expressive language disorder among relatives.

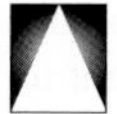

Table 41–2
DSM-IV-TR Diagnostic Criteria for Expressive Language Disorder

A. The scores obtained from standardized individually administered measures of expressive language development are substantially below those obtained from standardized measures of both nonverbal intellectual capacity and receptive language development. The disturbance may be manifest clinically by symptoms that include having a markedly limited vocabulary, making errors in tense, or having difficulty recalling words or producing sentences with developmentally appropriate length or complexity.
B. The difficulties with expressive language interfere with academic or occupational achievement or with social communication.
C. Criteria are not met for mixed receptive-expressive language disorder or a pervasive developmental disorder.
D. If mental retardation, a speech-motor or sensory deficit, or environmental deprivation is present, the language difficulties are in excess of those usually associated with these problems.

Coding note: If a speech-motor or sensory deficit or a neurological condition is present, code the condition on Axis III.

(From American Psychiatric Association. *Diagnostic and Statistical Manual of Mental Disorders*. 4th ed. Text rev. Washington, DC: American Psychiatric Association; copyright 2000, with permission.)

Clinical Features

Children with expressive language disorders may be ostracized by peers because of their poor ability to explain what they are talking about. They may appear vague when telling a story and use many filler words such as "stuff" and "things" instead of naming specific objects.

The essential feature of expressive language disorder is marked impairment in the development of age-appropriate expressive language, which results in the use of verbal or sign language markedly below the expected level in view of a child's nonverbal intellectual capacity. Language understanding (decoding) skills remain relatively intact. When severe, the disorder becomes recognizable by about the age of 18 months, when a child fails to utter spontaneously or even echo single words or sounds. Even simple words, such as "Mama" and "Dada," are absent from the child's active vocabulary, and the child points or uses gestures to indicate desires. The child seems to want to communicate, maintains eye contact, relates well to the mother, and enjoys games such as pat-a-cake and peek-a-boo. The child's vocabulary is severely limited. At 18 months, the child may be limited to pointing to common objects when they are named.

When a child with expressive language disorder begins to speak, the language impairment gradually becomes apparent. Articulation is often immature; numerous articulation errors occur but are inconsistent, particularly with such sounds as *th*, *r*, *s*, *z*, *y*, and *l*, which are either omitted or are substituted for other sounds.

By the age of 4 years, most children with expressive language disorder can speak in short phrases, but may have difficulty retaining new words. After beginning to speak, they acquire language more slowly than do most children. Their use of various grammatical structures is also markedly below the age-expected level, and their developmental milestones may be slightly delayed. Emotional problems involving poor self-image, frustration, and depression may develop in school-age children.

Josh was an alert, energetic 2-year-old, whose expressive vocabulary was limited to only four words (*mama*, *daddy*, *hi*, and *more*). He used these words one at a time in appropriate situations. He supplemented his infrequent verbal communications with pointing and other simple gestures to request desired objects or actions. He rarely communicated, however, for other purposes (e.g., commenting or protesting). Josh appeared to be developing normally in all other areas, except for expressive language. He sat, stood, and walked at the expected times. He played happily with other children, enjoying activities and toys that were appropriate for 2-year-olds. Although he had a history of frequent ear infections, a recent hearing test revealed normal hearing. Importantly, he showed age-appropriate comprehension for the names of familiar objects and actions and for simple verbal instructions (e.g., "Put that down." "Get your shirt." "Clap your hands."). Of course, at his age, comprehension testing had to be carefully conducted to ensure his attention and motivation.

Despite Josh's slow start in language development, most specialists would be reluctant to diagnose an expressive language disorder at his young age. Prospective research on the development of late talkers such Josh has demonstrated that most of them spontaneously overcome their initial slow start in language development. A parental report measure of vocabulary comprehension has shown promise as a prognostic indicator that can be used as early as 10 months of age.

Amy was a sociable, active 5-year-old, who was diagnosed with expressive language disorder. She often played with Lisa, her kindergarten classmate. During pretend play one day, each girl told the story of Little Red Riding Hood to her doll. Lisa's story began: "Little Red Riding Hood was taking a basket of food to her grandmother who was sick. A bad wolf stopped Red Riding Hood in the forest. He tried to get the basket away from her but she wouldn't give it to him."

By contrast, Amy's story illustrated her marked difficulties in verbal expression: "Riding Hood going to grandma house. Her taking food. Bad wolf in a bed. Riding Hood say, what big ears, grandma? Hear you, dear. What big eyes, grandma? See you, dear. What big mouth, grandma? Eat you all up!"

Amy's story contained many features characteristic of children with expressive disorders at her age, including short, incomplete sentences; simple sentence structures; omission of grammatical function words (e.g., *is* and *the*) and inflectional endings (e.g., possessives and present tense verbs); problems in question formation; and incorrect use of pronouns (e.g., *her* for *she*). Amy, however, performed as well as Lisa did in understanding the details and plot of the Riding Hood tale, as long as she was tested with methods that did not involve verbal responding. Amy also demonstrated adequate comprehension skills in her kindergarten classroom, where she readily followed the teacher's complex, multistep verbal instructions (e.g., "After you write your name in the top left corner of your paper, get your crayons and scissors, put your library books under your chair, and line up at the back of the room.").

Julio was a quiet, sullen 8-year-old whose expressive language problems were no longer obvious in casual, social conversations. His speech now rarely contained the incomplete sentences and grammatical errors that were so evident when he was younger. His expressive problems, however, still surfaced in tasks involving elaborate or abstract uses of language, such as those required in much of his third-grade academic work. An example was Julio's explanation of the outcome of a recent science experiment: "The teacher had stuff in some jars. He poured it, and it got pink. The other thing made it white." Although each sentence was grammatical, his explanation as a whole was difficult to follow, because key ideas and details were omitted or poorly explained. Julio also showed problems in word finding, that is, in using specific words for the concepts and actions he was describing. Instead, he relied on vague and nonspecific terms, such as *thing*, *stuff*, and *got*.

In early elementary grades, Julio had kept pace with his classmates in reading, writing, and other academic skills. By third grade, however, the increasing demands for written work began to negatively affect his overall academic standing. His written work was characterized by problems similar to those noted in his oral expression, such as poor organization and lack of specificity. Classmates also began to tease him about his difficulties, and he reacted quite aggressively, sometimes to the point of fighting. Nonetheless, Julio continued to show relatively good comprehension of spoken language, including classroom lectures concerning abstract concepts. He also comprehended sentences that were grammatically and conceptually complex (e.g., "The car the truck hit had hubcaps that were stolen. Had it been possible, she would have notified us by mail or by phone.").

Differential Diagnosis

Language disorders are associated with many other psychiatric disorders and, thus, the language disorder itself may be difficult to separate from other difficulties. In mental retardation, patients have an overall impairment in intellectual functioning, as shown by below-normal intelligence test scores in all areas, but the nonverbal intellectual capacity and functioning of children with expressive language disorder are within normal limits. In mixed receptive-expressive language disorder, language comprehension (decoding) is markedly below the expected age-appropriate level, whereas in expressive language disorder, language comprehension remains within normal limits.

In pervasive developmental disorders, in addition to the cardinal cognitive characteristics, affected children have no inner language, symbolic or imagery play, appropriate use of gesture, or capacity to form warm and meaningful social relationships. Moreover, children show little or no frustration with the inability to communicate verbally. In contrast, all these characteristics are present in children with expressive language disorder.

Children with acquired aphasia or dysphasia have a history of early normal language development; the disordered language had its onset after a head trauma or other neurological disorder (e.g., a seizure disorder). Children with selective mutism have a history of normal language development. Often these children will speak only in front of family members (e.g., mother, father, and siblings). Children affected by selective mutism are socially anxious and withdrawn outside the family.

Pathology and Laboratory Examination

Children with speech and language disorders should have an audiogram to rule out hearing loss.

Course and Prognosis

The prognosis for expressive language disorder is related to the severity of the disorder. Studies of "late talkers" concur that 50 to 80 percent of these children master language skills that are within the expected level during the preschool years. Most children who begin to talk later than average but catch up during preschool years, are not at high risk to develop further language or learning disorders. Outcome of expressive language disorder is influenced by other comorbid disorders. If children do not develop mood disorders or disruptive behavior problems, the prognosis is better. The rapidity and extent of recovery depend on the severity of the disorder, the child's motivation to participate in therapy, and the timely institution of speech and other therapeutic interventions. The presence or absence of other factors—such as moderate to severe hearing loss, mild mental retardation, and severe emotional problems—also affects the prognosis for recovery. As many as 50 percent of children with mild expressive language disorder recover spontaneously without any sign of language impairment, but children with severe expressive language disorder may later display features of mild to moderate language impairment.

Recent literature has shown that children who demonstrate poor comprehension, poor articulation, or poor academic performance tend to continue to have problems in these areas at follow-up 7 years later. An association is also seen between particular language impairment profiles and persistent mood and behavior problems. Children who have poor comprehension associated with expressive difficulties seem to be the most socially isolated and impaired with respect to peer relationships.

Expressive language level and many nonverbal and communication skills are strongly related in children with language impairment. Expressive language may be seen as an index of general development or as a marker of social and other communication skills. Especially in preschool age groups, expressive language appears to be related to social and nonverbal communication skills as much as it is simply a measure of knowledge of words.

Treatment

Controversy exists among experts whether intervention for young children with expressive language difficulties should be initiated as soon as it is noted, or whether waiting until age 4 or 5 years is the optimal time to begin treatment. Treatment for expressive language disorder is still generally not initiated unless it persists after the preschool years. Various techniques have been used to help a child improve use of such parts of speech as pronouns, correct tenses, and question forms. Direct interventions use a speech and language pathologist who works directly with the child. Mediated interventions, in which a speech and language professional teaches a child's teacher or parent how to promote therapeutic language techniques, have also been efficacious. Language therapy is often aimed at using words to improve communication strategies and social interactions as well. Such therapy consists of behaviorally reinforced exercises and practice with phonemes (sound units), vocabulary, and sentence construction. The goal is to increase the number of phrases by using block-building methods and conventional speech therapies.

Psychotherapy may be useful for children whose language impairment has affected their self-esteem, insofar as it can be used as a positive model for more effective communication and broadening social skills. Supportive parental counseling may be indicated in some cases. Parents may need help to reduce intrafamilial tensions arising from difficulties in rearing language-disordered children and to increase their awareness and understanding of the disorder.

More research is needed to establish whether early intervention for preschoolers with language deficits has long-term benefits and to develop comprehensive treatment programs that may address the direct language interventions along with interventions for common comorbid communication and learning disorders.

MIXED RECEPTIVE-EXPRESSIVE LANGUAGE DISORDER

Children with mixed receptive-expressive learning disorders exhibit impaired skills in the expression and reception (understanding and comprehension) of spoken language. The expressive difficulties in these children may be similar to those of children with only expressive language disorder, which is characterized by limited vocabulary, use of simplistic sentences, and short sentence usage. Children with receptive language difficulties may be experiencing additional deficits in basic auditory processing skills, such as discriminating between sounds, rapid sound changes, association of sounds and symbols, and the memory of sound sequences. These deficits may lead to a whole host of communication barriers for a child, including a lack of understanding of questions or directives from others, or inability to follow the conversations of peers or family members. Recognition of the disorder in children with mixed expressive-receptive language disorders may be delayed because of early misattribution of their communication by teachers and parents as a behavioral problem rather than a deficit in understanding.

The essential features of mixed receptive-expressive language disorder are shown by scores on standardized tests; both receptive (comprehension) and expressive language development scores fall substantially below those obtained from standardized measures of nonverbal intellectual capacity. Language difficulties must be sufficiently severe to impair academic achievement or daily social communication. A patient with this disorder must not meet the criteria for a pervasive developmental disorder, and the language dysfunctions must exceed those usually associated with mental retardation and other neurological and sensory-deficit syndromes.

Epidemiology

Mixed receptive-expressive language disorder is believed to occur in about 5 percent of preschoolers and to persist in approximately 3 percent of school-age children. It is less common than expressive language disorder alone. Mixed receptive-expressive language disorder is believed to be at least twice as prevalent in boys as in girls.

Comorbidity

Children with mixed receptive-expressive disorder are at high risk for additional speech and language disorders, learning disorders, and additional psychiatric disorders. About half of children with this disorder also have pronunciation difficulties leading to phonological disorder, and about half also have reading disorder. These rates are significantly higher than the comorbidity found in children with expressive language disorder alone. ADHD is present in at least one third of children with mixed receptive-expressive language disorder.

Etiology

Language disorders most likely have multiple determinants, including genetic factors, developmental brain abnormalities, environmental influences, neurodevelopmental immaturity, and auditory processing features in the brain. As with expressive language disorder alone, evidence is found of familial aggregation of mixed receptive-expressive language disorder. Genetic contribution to this disorder is implicated by twin studies, but no mode of genetic transmission has been proved. Some studies of children with various speech and language disorders have also shown cognitive deficits, particularly slower processing of tasks involving naming objects, as well as fine motor tasks. Slower myelinization of neural pathways has been hypothesized to account for the slow processing found in children with developmental language disorders. Several studies suggest an underlying impairment of auditory discrimination, because most children with the disorder are more responsive to environmental sounds than to speech sounds.

Diagnosis

Children with mixed receptive-expressive language disorder develop language more slowly than their peers and have trouble understanding conversations that peers can follow. In mixed receptive-expressive language disorder, receptive dysfunction coexists with expressive dysfunction. Therefore, standardized tests for both receptive and expressive language abilities must be given to anyone suspected of having mixed receptive-expressive language disorder.

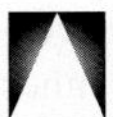

Table 41–3
DSM-IV-TR Diagnostic Criteria for Mixed Receptive-Expressive Language Disorder

A. The scores obtained from a battery of standardized individually administered measures of both receptive and expressive language development are substantially below those obtained from standardized measures of nonverbal intellectual capacity. Symptoms include those for expressive language disorder as well as difficulty understanding words, sentences, or specific types of words, such as spatial terms.
B. The difficulties with receptive and expressive language significantly interfere with academic or occupational achievement or with social communication.
C. Criteria are not met for a pervasive developmental disorder.
D. If mental retardation, a speech-motor or sensory deficit, or environmental deprivation is present, the language difficulties are in excess of those usually associated with these problems.

Coding note: If a speech-motor or sensory deficit or a neurological condition is present, code the condition on Axis III.

(From American Psychiatric Association. *Diagnostic and Statistical Manual of Mental Disorders.* 4th ed. Text rev. Washington, DC: American Psychiatric Association; copyright 2000, with permission.)

A markedly below-expected level of comprehension of verbal or sign language with intact age-appropriate nonverbal intellectual capacity, confirmation of language difficulties by standardized receptive language tests, and the absence of pervasive developmental disorders confirm the diagnosis of mixed receptive-expressive language disorder (Table 41–3).

Clinical Features

The essential clinical feature of the disorder is significant impairment in both language comprehension and language expression. In the mixed disorder, the expressive impairments are similar to those of expressive language disorder, but can be more severe. The clinical features of the receptive component of the disorder typically appear before the age of 4 years. Severe forms are apparent by the age of 2 years; mild forms may not become evident until age 7 (second grade) or older, when language becomes complex. Children with mixed receptive-expressive language disorder show markedly delayed and below-normal ability to comprehend (decode) verbal or sign language, although they have age-appropriate nonverbal intellectual capacity. In most cases of receptive dysfunction, verbal or sign expression (encoding) of language is also impaired. The clinical features of mixed receptive-expressive language disorder in children between the ages of 18 and 24 months result from a child's failure to utter a single phoneme spontaneously or to mimic another person's words.

Many children with mixed receptive-expressive language disorder have auditory sensory difficulties or cannot process visual symbols, such as explaining the meaning of a picture. They have deficits in integrating both auditory and visual symbols—for example, recognizing the basic common attributes of a toy truck and a toy passenger car. Whereas at 18 months, a child with expressive language disorder only can comprehend simple commands and can point to familiar household objects when told to do so, a child of the same age with mixed receptive-expressive language disorder cannot either point to common objects or obey simple commands. A child with mixed receptive-expressive language disorder usually appears to be deaf, but the child can hear. He or she responds normally to nonlanguage sounds from the environment, but not to spoken language. If the child later starts to speak, the speech contains numerous articulation errors, such as omissions, distortions, and substitutions of phonemes. Language acquisition is much slower for children with mixed receptive-expressive language disorder than for children without this disorder.

Children with mixed receptive-expressive language disorder have difficulty recalling early visual and auditory memories and recognizing and reproducing symbols in proper sequence. In some cases, bilateral EEG abnormalities are seen. Some children with mixed receptive-expressive language disorder have a partial hearing defect for true tones, an increased threshold of auditory arousal, and an inability to localize sound sources. Seizure disorders and reading disorder are more common among the relatives of children with mixed receptive-expressive language disorder than they are in the general population.

Most children with mixed receptive-expressive language disorder are impaired socially and in terms of nonverbal communication. This impairment causes a variety of additional difficulties and often results in poor self-esteem and feelings of inferiority that, in turn, can further prevent the child from succeeding in the usual developmental tasks.

Pathology and Laboratory Examination

An audiogram is indicated for all children thought to have mixed receptive-expressive language disorder, to rule out or confirm the presence of deafness and to determine the types of auditory deficits. A history of the child and family and observation of the child in various settings help to clarify the diagnosis.

Susan was a pleasant 2-year-old, who did not yet use any spoken words. She made her needs known with vocalizations and simple gestures (e.g., showing or pointing) such as those typically used by younger children. She seemed to understand the names for a few familiar people and objects (e.g., *mommy*, *daddy*, *cat*, *bottle*, and *cookie*). Compared with other children her age, she had a small comprehension vocabulary and showed limited understanding of simple verbal directions (e.g., "Get your doll." "Close your eyes."). Nonetheless, her hearing was normal, and her motor and play skills were developing as expected for her age. She showed interest in her environment and in the activities of the other children at her day care.

Min was a shy, reserved 5-year-old who grew up in a bilingual home. Min's parents and older siblings spoke English and Cantonese proficiently. Her grandparents, who lived in the same home, spoke only Cantonese. Min began to understand and speak both languages much later than her older siblings had. Throughout her preschool years, Min continued to develop slowly in comprehension and production. At the start of kindergarten, Min understood fewer English words for objects, actions, and relations than her classmates did. She showed difficulties in following classroom instructions, particularly those that involved words for concepts of time (e.g., *tomorrow*, *before*, or *day*) and space (e.g., *behind*, *next to*, or *under*). It was also hard for Min to match one of several pictures to a syntactically complex sentence that she had heard (e.g., "It was not the train she was waiting for." "Because he had already completed his work, he was not kept after school."). Min occasionally tried to speak with other children. These conversations usually broke down, however, because she misinterpreted what others said or could not express her own thoughts clearly. Consequently, her classmates generally ignored her, preferring instead to play with more verbally competent peers. Min's infrequent interactions further limited her opportunities to learn and to practice her already weak language skills. Min also showed limited receptive and expressive skills in Cantonese, as revealed by an assessment conducted with the assistance of a Cantonese interpreter. Nonetheless, her nonverbal cognitive and motor skills were within the normal range for her age. She showed no difficulties in solving spatial, numerical, conceptual, or analogical problems, provided they were presented nonverbally.

Fred received a diagnosis of mixed receptive-expressive language disorder when he was a preschooler. By 8 years of age, he had also received the comorbid diagnoses of reading disorder and ADHD. This combination of language, reading, and attention problems made it virtually impossible for Fred to succeed in school. His comprehension and attention difficulties limited his ability to understand and to learn important information from classroom instructions, discussions, and lectures. Because the unlearned information was critical to the understanding of future academic lessons, Fred fell further and further behind his classmates. He was also disadvantaged because he could read only a few familiar words. This meant that he could not learn other academic information that his classmates acquired by reading textbooks, library books, newspapers, and other written materials. His poor reading ability also limited his opportunities to learn the new vocabulary, complex sentence forms, and sophisticated ideas that other children absorbed from reading. Despite his academic problems, however, Fred continued to show nonverbal intellectual skills within the low normal range, although his scores were somewhat lower than those he had earned as a preschooler.

Differential Diagnosis

Children with significant mixed receptive-expressive language disorder have a deficit in language comprehension. This deficit may be overlooked at first, because the expressive language deficit may be more obvious. In expressive language disorder alone, comprehension of spoken language (decoding) remains within age norms. Children with phonological disorder or stuttering have normal expressive and receptive language competence, despite the speech impairments. Hearing impairment should be ruled out.

Most children with mixed receptive-expressive language disorder have a history of variable and inconsistent responses to sounds; they respond more often to environmental sounds than to speech sounds (Table 41–4). Mental retardation, selective mutism, acquired aphasia, and pervasive developmental disorders should also be ruled out. Hearing impairment, pervasive developmental disorders, and severe environmental deprivation can contribute significantly to language impairment.

Course and Prognosis

The overall prognosis for mixed receptive-expressive language disorder is less favorable than that for expressive language

Table 41–4
Differential Diagnosis of Language Disorders

	Hearing Impairment	Mental Retardation	Infantile Autism	Expressive Language Disorder	Mixed Receptive-Expressive Language Disorder	Selective Mutism	Phonological Disorder
Language comprehension	–	–	–	+	–	+	+
Expressive language	–	–	–	–	–	Variable	+
Audiogram	–	+	+	+	Variable	+	+
Articulation	–	–	– (Variable)	– (Variable)	– (Variable)	+	–
Inner language	+	+ (Limited)	–	+	+ (Slightly limited)	+	+
Uses gestures	+	+ (Limited)	–	+	+	+ (Variable)	+
Echoes	–	+	+ (Inappropriate)	+	+	+	+
Attends to sounds	Loud or low frequency only	+	–	+	Variable	+	+
Watches faces	+	+	–	+	+	+	+
Performance	+	–	+	+	+	+	+

+, normal; –, abnormal.
(Courtesy of Lorian Baker, Ph.D., and Dennis Cantwell, M.D.)

disorder alone. When the mixed disorder is identified in a young child, it is usually severe, and the short-term prognosis is poor. Language develops at a rapid rate in early childhood, and young children with the disorder may appear to be falling behind. In view of the likelihood of comorbid learning disorders and other mental disorders, the prognosis is guarded. Young children with severe mixed receptive-expressive language disorder are likely to have learning disorders in the future. In children with mild versions, mixed disorder may not be identified for several years, and the disruption in everyday life may be less overwhelming than that in severe forms of the disorder. Over the long run, some children with mixed receptive-expressive language disorder achieve close to normal language functions. The prognosis for children who have mixed receptive-expressive language disorder varies widely and depends on the nature and severity of the damage.

Treatment

A comprehensive speech and language evaluation is recommended for children with mixed receptive-expressive language disorder, before embarking on a speech and language remediation program. Preschoolers with mixed receptive-expressive language disorder optimally receive interventions designed to promote social communication and literacy as well as oral language. For children at the kindergarten level, optimal intervention includes direct teaching of key prereading skills as well as social skills training. An important early goal of interventions for young children with mixed receptive-expressive language disorder is the achievement of rudimentary reading skills in that these skills are protective against the academic and psychosocial ramifications of falling behind early on in reading. Some language therapists favor a low-stimuli setting, in which children are given individual linguistic instruction. Others recommend that speech and language instruction be integrated into a varied setting with several children who are taught several language structures simultaneously. Often, a child with mixed receptive-expressive language disorder will benefit from a small, special-educational setting that allows more individualized learning.

Psychotherapy may be helpful for children with mixed receptive-expressive language disorder who have associated emotional and behavioral problems. Particular attention should be paid to evaluating the child's self-image and social skills. Family counseling in which parents and children can develop more effective, less frustrating means of communicating may be beneficial.

PHONOLOGICAL DISORDER

Children with phonological disorder are unable to produce speech sounds correctly because of omissions of sounds, distortions of sounds, or atypical pronunciation. Typical speech disturbances in this disorder include omitting the last sounds of the word (e.g., saying *mou* for *mouse* or *drin* for *drink*), or substituting one sound for another (saying *bwu* instead of *blue* or *tup* for *cup*). Distortions in sounds can occur when children allow too much air to escape from the side of their mouths while saying sounds like *sh* or producing sounds like *s* or *z* with their tongue protruded. Speech sound errors can also occur in patterns because a child has an interrupted air flow instead of a steady airflow preventing the entire word to be pronounced (e.g., *pat* for *pass* or *bacuum* for *vacuum*). Children with a phonological disorder can be mistaken for younger children because of their difficulties in producing speech sounds correctly. The diagnosis of a phonological disorder is made by comparing the skills of a given child with the expected skill level of others of the same age. The disorder results in errors in whole words because of incorrect pronunciation of consonants, substitution of one sound for another, omission of entire phonemes, and, in some cases, dysarthria (slurred speech because of incoordination of speech muscles) or dyspraxia (difficulty planning and executing speech). Speech sound development is believed to be based on both linguistic and motor development that must be integrated to produce sounds. According to DSM-IV-TR, if mental retardation, a speech-motor or sensory deficit, or environmental deprivation is present, the language dysfunction must exceed that associated with those problems.

Components of phonological disorder, such as dysarthria and dyspraxia, are more likely to have a neurological basis. Developmental articulation disorder, however, is the most common phonological disorder in children. Developmental phonological disorder, characterized by frequent misarticulation, sound substitution, and speech sound omission, gives the impression of "baby talk." The developmental form of this disorder is not caused by anatomical, structural, physiological, auditory, or neurological abnormalities. It varies from mild to severe and results in speech that ranges from completely intelligible to unintelligible.

Epidemiology

Surveys indicate that the prevalence of phonological disorder is at least 3 percent in preschoolers, 2 percent in children 6 to 7 years of age, and 0.5 percent in 17-year-old adolescents. Approximately 7 to 8 percent of 5-year-old children in one large community sample had speech sound production problems of developmental, structural, or neurological origins. Another study found that up to 7.5 percent of children between the ages of 7 and 11 years had phonological disorders. Of those, 2.5 percent had speech delay (deletion and substitution errors past the age of 4 years) and 5 percent had residual articulation errors beyond the age of 8 years. Developmental phonological disorders occur much more frequently than disorders with known structural or neurological origin. The disorder is approximately two to three times more common in boys than in girls. It is also more common among first-degree relatives of patients with the disorder than in the general population. According to DSM-IV-TR, the prevalence falls to 0.5 percent by mid to late adolescence.

Comorbidity

More than half of children with developmental phonological disorder have some difficulty with expressive language. Disorders that commonly present with phonological disorder are expressive language disorder, mixed receptive-expressive language disorder, reading disorder, and developmental coordination disorder. Enuresis may also accompany the disorder. A delay in reaching speech milestones (e.g., first word and first sentence) has been reported in some children with phonological disorder, but most children with the disorder begin speaking at the appropriate age. Children with phonological disorder who also have language disorders are at greatest risk for attentional problems and learning disorders. Children with phonological disorder who do not have language dysfunction have lower risk of comorbid psychiatric or behavioral problems.

Etiology

The likely causes of phonological disturbance include multiple variables—perinatal problems, genetic factors, auditory processing problems, hearing impairment, and structural abnormalities related to speech. A developmental lag or maturational delay in the neurological process underlying speech has been postulated in some cases. The likelihood of a subtle brain abnormality is supported by the observation that children with phonological disorder are also more likely to manifest "soft neurological signs" as well as additional disorders, including receptive and expressive language difficulties and a higher-than-expected rate of reading disorder. Genetic factors are implicated by data from twin studies that show concordance rates for monozygotic twins that are higher than chance.

Articulation disorders caused by structural or mechanical problems are rare. Phonological disorders caused by neurological impairment can be divided into dysarthria and apraxia or dyspraxia. Dysarthria results from an impairment in the neural mechanisms regulating the muscular control of speech. This can occur in congenital conditions, such as cerebral palsy, muscular dystrophy, or head injury or because of infectious processes. Apraxia or dyspraxia is characterized by difficulty in the execution of speech even when no obvious paralysis or weakness of the muscles used in speech exists.

Environmental factors may play a role in developmental phonological disorder, but constitutional factors seem to make the most significant contribution. The high proportion of phonological disorder in certain families implies a genetic component in the development of this disorder. Poor motor coordination, laterality, and handedness are not associated with phonological disorder.

Diagnosis

The essential feature of phonological disorder is a child's delay or failure to produce developmentally expected speech sounds, especially consonants, resulting in sound omissions, substitutions, and distortions of phonemes. A rough guideline for clinical assessment of children's articulation is that normal 3-year-olds correctly articulate *m*, *n*, *ng*, *b*, *p*, *h*, *t*, *k*, *q*, and *d*; normal 4-year-olds correctly articulate *f*, *y*, *ch*, *sh*, and *z*; and normal 5-year-olds correctly articulate *th*, *s*, and *r*.

Phonological disorder cannot be attributed to structural or neurological abnormalities, and it is accompanied by normal language development. The DSM-IV-TR diagnostic criteria for phonological disorder are given in Table 41–5.

Clinical Features

Children with phonological disorder are delayed in, or incapable of, producing speech sounds that are expected for their age, intelligence, and dialect. The sounds are often substitutions—for example, the use of *t* instead of *k*—and omissions, such as leaving off the final consonants of words. Phonological disorder can be recognized in early childhood. In severe cases, the disorder is first recognized at about 3 years of age. In less severe cases, the disorder may not be apparent until the age of 6 years. A child's articulation is judged disordered when it is significantly behind that of most children at the same age level, intellectual level, and educational level.

In very mild cases, a single speech sound (i.e., phoneme) may be affected. When a single phoneme is affected, it is usually one that is acquired late in normal language acquisition. The speech

Table 41–5
DSM-IV-TR Diagnostic Criteria for Phonological Disorder

A. Failure to use developmentally expected speech sounds that are appropriate for age and dialect (e.g., errors in sound production, use, representation, or organization such as, but not limited to, substitutions of one sound for another [use of /t/ for target /k/ sound] or omissions of sounds such as final consonants).
B. The difficulties in speech sound production interfere with academic or occupational achievement or with social communication.
C. If mental retardation, a speech-motor or sensory deficit, or environmental deprivation is present, the speech difficulties are in excess of those usually associated with these problems.

Coding note: If a speech-motor or sensory deficit or a neurological condition is present, code the condition on Axis III.

(From American Psychiatric Association. *Diagnostic and Statistical Manual of Mental Disorders.* 4th ed. Text rev. Washington, DC: American Psychiatric Association; copyright 2000, with permission.)

sounds most frequently misarticulated are also those acquired late in the developmental sequence, including *r*, *sh*, *th*, *f*, *z*, *l*, and *ch*. In severe cases and in young children, sounds such as *b*, *m*, *t*, *d*, *n*, and *h* may be mispronounced. One or many speech sounds may be affected, but vowel sounds are not among them.

Children with phonological disorder cannot articulate certain phonemes correctly and may distort, substitute, or even omit the affected phonemes. With omissions, the phonemes are absent entirely—for example, bu for blue, ca for car, or whaa? for what's that? With substitutions, difficult phonemes are replaced with incorrect ones—for example, wabbit for rabbit, fum for thumb, or whath dat? for what's that? With distortions, the correct phoneme is approximated but is articulated incorrectly. Rarely, additions (usually of the vowel uh) occur—for example, puhretty for pretty, what's uh that uh? for what's that?

Omissions are thought to be the most serious type of misarticulation, with substitutions the next most serious, and distortions the least serious type. Omissions, which are most frequent in the speech of young children, usually occur at the ends of words or in clusters of consonants (ka for car, scisso for scissors). Distortions, which are found mainly in the speech of older children, result in a sound that is not part of the speaker's dialect. Distortions may be the last type of misarticulation remaining in the speech of children whose articulation problems have mostly remitted. The most common types of distortions are the lateral slip—in which a child pronounces *s* sounds with the airstream going across the tongue, producing a whistling effect—and the palatal or lisp—in which the *s* sound, formed with the tongue too close to the palate, produces a *ssh* sound effect.

The misarticulations of children with phonological disorder are often inconsistent and random. A phoneme may be pronounced correctly one time and incorrectly another time. Misarticulations are most common at the ends of words, in long and syntactically complex sentences, and during rapid speech.

Omissions, distortions, and substitutions also occur normally in the speech of young children learning to talk. But, whereas young, normally speaking children soon replace these misarticulations, children with phonological disorder do not. Even as children with phonological disorder grow and finally acquire the correct phoneme, they may use it only in newly acquired words and may not correct the words learned earlier that they have been mispronouncing for some time.

Most children eventually outgrow phonological disorder, usually by the third grade. After the fourth grade, however, spontaneous recovery is unlikely, and so it is important to try to remediate the disorder before the development of complications. Often, beginning kindergarten or school precipitates the improvement when recovery from phonological disorder is spontaneous. Speech therapy is clearly indicated for children who have not shown spontaneous improvement by the third or fourth grade. Speech therapy should be initiated at an early age for children whose articulation is significantly unintelligible and who are clearly troubled by their inability to speak clearly.

Children with phonological disorder may have various concomitant social, emotional, and behavioral problems, particularly when comorbid expressive language problems are present. Children with expressive language disorder and severe articulation impairment and those whose disorder is chronic and nonremitting are the ones most likely to suffer from psychiatric problems.

Ramon was a talkative, likeable 3-year-old with virtually unintelligible speech, despite his normal hearing and language comprehension skills. Ramon's level of expressive language development could not be determined, because his speech was so difficult to understand. The rhythm and melody of his speech, however, suggested that he was trying to produce multiword utterances, as would be expected at his age. Ramon produced only a few vowels (*/ee/*, */ah/*, and */oo/*), some early-developing consonants (*/m/*, */n/*, */d/*, */t/*, */p/*, */b/*, */h/*, and */w/*), and limited syllables. This reduced sound repertoire made many of his spoken words indistinguishable from one another (e.g., he said *bahbah* for *bottle*, *baby*, and *bubble*, and he used *nee* for *knee*, *need*, and *Anita* [his sister]). Moreover, he consistently omitted consonant sounds at the end of words and in consonant cluster sequences (e.g., */tr-/*, */st-/*, */-nt/*, and */-mp/*). On occasion, Ramon reacted with frustration and tantrums to his difficulties in making his needs understood.

Kent was a pleasant, cooperative 5-year-old, who had been diagnosed with a developmental phonological disorder when he was a preschooler. His hearing and language comprehension skills were within normal limits. He showed some mild expressive language problems, however, in the use of certain grammatical features (e.g., pronouns, auxiliary verbs, and past-tense word endings) and in the formulation of complex sentences. He correctly produced all vowel sounds and most of the early-developing consonants, but was inconsistent in his attempts to produce later-developing consonants (e.g., */r/*, */l/*, */s/*, */z/*, */sh/*, */th/*, and */ch/*). Sometimes, he omitted them; sometimes, he substituted other sounds for them (e.g., */w/* for */r/* or */f/* for */th/*); occasionally, he even produced them correctly. Kent had particular problems in correctly producing consonant cluster sequences and multisyllabic words. Cluster sequences had omitted or incorrect sounds (e.g., *blue* might be produced as *bue* or *bwue*, and *hearts* might be said as *hots* or *hars*). Multisyllabic words had syllables omitted (e.g., *efant* for *elephant* and *getti* for *spaghetti*) and sounds mispronounced or even transposed (e.g., *aminal* for *animal* and *lemon* for *melon*). Strangers were unable to understand

Table 41–6
Differential Diagnosis of Phonological Dysfunctions

Criteria	Phonological Dysfunction Due to Structural or Neurological Abnormalities (Dysarthria)	Phonological Dysfunction Due to Hearing Impairment	Phonological Disorder	Phonological Dysfunction Associated with Mental Retardation, Infantile Autism, Developmental Dysphasia, Acquired Aphasia, or Deafness
Language development	Within normal limits	Within normal limits unless hearing impairment is serious	Within normal limits	Not within normal limits
Examination	Possible abnormalities of lips, tongue, or palate; muscular weakness, incoordination, or disturbance of vegetative functions, such as sucking or chewing	Hearing impairment shown on audiometric testing	Normal	
Rate of speech	Slow; marked deterioration of articulation with increased rate	Normal	Normal; possible deterioration of articulation with increased rate	
Phonemes affected	Any phonemes, even vowels	*f, th, sh,* and *s*	*r, sh, th, ch, dg, j, f, v, s,* and *z* are most commonly affected	

(Courtesy of Lorian Baker, Ph.D., and Dennis Cantwell, M.D.)

approximately 80 percent of Kent's speech. Kent often spoke more slowly and clearly than usual, however, when he was asked to repeat something, as he often was.

Natasha was a shy, reserved 8-year-old, with a history of significant speech delay. During her preschool and early school years, she had overcome many of her earlier speech errors. A few late-developing sounds (/*r*/, /*l*/, and /*th*/), however, continued to pose a challenge for her. Natasha often substituted /*f*/ or /*d*/ for /*th*/ and produced /*w*/ for /*r*/ and /*l*/. Overall, her speech was easily understood, despite these minor errors. Nonetheless, she was often reluctant to speak in front of others because of the teasing she received from her classmates about her speech.

Differential Diagnosis

The differential diagnosis of phonological disorder includes a careful determination of symptoms severity and possible medical conditions that might be producing the symptoms. First, the clinician must determine that the misarticulations are sufficiently severe to be considered impairing, rather than a normative developmental process of learning to speak. Second, the clinician must determine that no physical abnormalities account for the articulation errors and must rule out neurological disorders that may cause dysarthria, hearing impairment, mental retardation, and pervasive developmental disorders. Third, the clinician must obtain an evaluation of receptive and expressive language to determine that the speech difficulty is not solely attributable to the above mentioned disorders.

Neurological, oral structural, and audiometric examinations may be necessary to rule out physical factors that cause certain types of articulation abnormalities. Children with dysarthria, a disorder caused by structural or neurological abnormalities, differ from children with developmental phonological disorder in that dysarthria is less likely to remit spontaneously and may be more difficult to remediate. Drooling, slow, or uncoordinated motor behavior; abnormal chewing or swallowing; and awkward or slow protrusion and retraction of the tongue indicate dysarthria. A slow rate of speech also indicates dysarthria (Table 41–6).

Course and Prognosis

Spontaneous remission of symptoms is common in children whose misarticulations involve only a few phonemes. Children who persist in exhibiting articulation problems after the age of 5 years may be experiencing a myriad of other speech and language impairments, so that a comprehensive evaluation may be indicated at this time. Children over the age of 5 with articulation problems are at higher risk for auditory perceptual problems. Spontaneous recovery is rare after the age of 8 years.

Treatment

Treatment is typically recommended for children with moderate to severe developmental phonological disorders. Two main approaches have been used successfully to improve phonological difficulties. The first one, the *phonological approach*, is usually chosen for children with extensive patterns of multiple speech sound errors that may include final consonant deletion, or consonant cluster reduction. Exercises in this approach to treatment focus on guided practice of specific sounds, such as final consonants, and when that skill is mastered, practice is extended to use in meaningful words and sentences. The other approach, the *traditional approach* is utilized for children who produce substitution or distortion errors in just a few sounds. In this approach, the child practices the production of the problem sound while the clinician provides immediate feedback and cues concerning the correct placement of the tongue and mouth for improved articulation. Children who have errors in articulation because of an abnormal swallowing resulting in tongue thrust and lisps are treated with exercises that improve swallowing patterns and, in turn, improve speech. Speech therapy is typically provided by a speech-language pathologist, yet parents can be taught to provide adjunctive help by practicing techniques used in the treatment. Early intervention can be helpful because, for many children with mild articulation difficulties, even several months of intervention may be helpful in early elementary school. In general, when a child's articulation and intelligibility is noticeably different than peers by the age of 8 years of age, speech deficits often lead to problems with peers, learning, and self-image, especially when the disorder is so severe that many consonants are misarticulated, and when errors involve omissions and substitutions of phonemes, rather than distortions.

Children with persistent articulation problems are likely to be teased or ostracized by peers and may become isolated and demoralized. Therefore, it is important to give support to children with phonological disorders and, whenever possible, to support prosocial activities and social interactions with peers. Parental counseling and monitoring of child–peer relationships and school behavior can help minimize the social impairment with speech and language disorder.

STUTTERING

Stuttering is a condition in which the normal flow of speech is disrupted by involuntary speech motor events. Stuttering can include a variety of specific disruptions of fluency, including sound or syllable repetitions, sound prolongations, dysrhythmic phonations, and complete blocking or unusual pauses between sounds and syllables of words. In severe cases, the stuttering may be accompanied by accessory or secondary attempts to compensate such as respiratory, abnormal voice phonations, or tongue clicks. Associated behaviors, such as eye blinks, facial grimacing, head jerks, and abnormal body movements, may be observed before or during the disrupted speech. The disorder usually originates in childhood.

Controversy is found among speech and language experts as to whether stuttering should be considered an independent entity or part of a broader speech and language disorder. Some question whether stuttering should be considered a psychiatric condition at all. Many children who stutter do endure significant psychological distress, and stuttering does cause impairment in everyday life for many children with this condition.

Epidemiology

Surveys conducted mainly in the United States and Europe indicate the prevalence of stuttering is about 1 percent in the general population. Stuttering tends to be most common in young children and has often resolved spontaneously by the time the child is older. The typical age of onset is 2 to 7 years of age with a peak at age 5 years. Estimates are that up to 3 to 4 percent of individuals may have stuttered at some time in their lives. Approximately 80 percent of young children who stutter are likely to have a spontaneous remission over time. According to DSM-IV-TR, it dips to 0.8 percent by adolescence. Stuttering affects about three to four males for every female. The disorder is significantly more common among family members of affected children than in the general population. According to DSM-IV-TR, for male persons who stutter, 20 percent of their male children and 10 percent of their female children will also stutter.

Comorbidity

Very young children who stutter typically show some delay in the development of language and articulation without additional disorders of speech and language. Preschoolers and school-age children who stutter exhibit an increased incidence of social anxiety, school refusal, and other anxiety symptoms. Older children who stutter also do not necessarily have comorbid speech and language disorders, but often manifest anxiety symptoms and disorders. When stuttering persists into adolescence, social isolation occurs at higher rates than in the general adolescent population. Stuttering is also associated with a variety of abnormal motor movements, upper body tics, and facial grimaces. Other disorders that coexist with stuttering include phonological disorder, expressive language disorder, mixed receptive-expressive language disorder, and ADHD.

Etiology

Converging evidence indicates that cause of stuttering is multifactorial, including genetic, neurophysiological, and psychological factors that predispose a child to have poor speech fluency. Although research evidence does not indicate that anxiety or conflicts cause stuttering or that persons who stutter have more psychiatric disturbances than those with other forms of speech and language disorders, stuttering can be exacerbated by certain stressful situations.

Other theories about the cause of stuttering include organic models and learning models. Organic models include those that focus on incomplete lateralization or abnormal cerebral dominance. Several studies using EEG found that stuttering males had right-hemispheric alpha suppression across stimulus words and tasks; nonstutterers had left-hemispheric suppression. Some studies of stutterers have noted an overrepresentation of left-handedness and ambidexterity. Twin studies and striking gender differences in stuttering indicate that stuttering has some genetic basis.

Learning theories about the cause of stuttering include the semantogenic theory, in which stuttering is basically a learned response to normative early childhood dysfluencies. Another learning model focuses on classic conditioning, in which the stuttering becomes conditioned to environmental factors. In the cybernetic model, speech is viewed as a process that depends on appropriate feedback for regulation; stuttering is hypothesized to occur because of a breakdown in the feedback loop. The observations that stuttering is reduced by white noise and that delayed auditory feedback produces stuttering in normal speakers lend support to the feedback theory.

The motor functioning of some children who stutter appears to be delayed or slightly abnormal. The observation of difficulties in speech planning exhibited by some children who stutter suggests that higher-level cognitive dysfunction may contribute to stuttering. Although children who stutter do not routinely exhibit other speech and language disorders, family members of these children often exhibit an increased incidence of a variety of speech and language disorders. Stuttering is most likely to be caused by a set of interacting variables that include both genetic and environmental factors.

Diagnosis

The diagnosis of stuttering is not difficult when the clinical features are apparent and well developed and each of the four phases (described in the next section) can be readily recognized. Diagnostic difficulties can arise when trying to determine the existence of stuttering in young children, because some preschool children experience transient dysfluency. It may not be clear whether the nonfluent pattern is part of normal speech and language development or whether it represents the initial stage in the development of stuttering. If incipient stuttering is suspected, referral to a speech pathologist is indicated. Table 41–7 presents the DSM-IV-TR diagnostic criteria for stuttering.

Clinical Features

Stuttering usually appears between the ages of 18 months and 9 years, with two sharp peaks of onset between the ages of 2 to 3.5 years and 5 to 7 years. Some, but not all, stutterers have other speech and language problems, such as phonological disorder and expressive language disorder. Stuttering does not begin suddenly; it typically develops over weeks or months with a repetition of initial consonants, whole words that are usually the first words of a phrase, or long words. As the disorder progresses, the repetitions become more frequent, with consistent stuttering on the most important words or phrases. Even after it develops, stuttering may be absent during oral readings, singing, and talking to pets or inanimate objects.

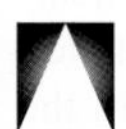

Table 41–7
DSM-IV-TR Diagnostic Criteria for Stuttering

A. Disturbance in the normal fluency and time patterning of speech (inappropriate for the individual's age), characterized by frequent occurrences of one or more of the following:
  (1) sound and syllable repetitions
  (2) sound prolongations
  (3) interjections
  (4) broken words (e.g., pauses within a word)
  (5) audible or silent blocking (filled or unfilled pauses in speech)
  (6) circumlocutions (word substitutions to avoid problematic words)
  (7) words produced with an excess of physical tension
  (8) monosyllabic whole-word repetitions (e.g., "I-I-I-I see him")

B. The disturbance in fluency interferes with academic or occupational achievement or with social communication.

C. If a speech-motor or sensory deficit is present, the speech difficulties are in excess of those usually associated with these problems.

Coding note: If a speech-motor or sensory deficit or a neurological condition is present, code the condition on Axis III.

(From American Psychiatric Association. *Diagnostic and Statistical Manual of Mental Disorders.* 4th ed. Text rev. Washington, DC: American Psychiatric Association; copyright 2000, with permission.)

Four gradually evolving phases in the development of stuttering have been identified:

- **Phase 1** occurs during the preschool period. Initially, the difficulty tends to be episodic and appears for weeks or months between long interludes of normal speech. A high percentage of recovery from these periods of stuttering occurs. During this phase, children stutter most often when excited or upset, when they seem to have a great deal to say, and under other conditions of communicative pressure.
- **Phase 2** usually occurs in the elementary school years. The disorder is chronic, with few if any intervals of normal speech. Affected children become aware of their speech difficulties and regard themselves as stutterers. In phase 2, the stuttering occurs mainly with the major parts of speech—nouns, verbs, adjectives, and adverbs.
- **Phase 3** usually appears after the age of 8 years and up to adulthood, most often in late childhood and early adolescence. During phase 3, stuttering comes and goes largely in response to specific situations, such as reciting in class, speaking to strangers, making purchases in stores, and using the telephone. Some words and sounds are regarded as more difficult than others.
- **Phase 4** typically appears in late adolescence and adulthood.

Stutterers show a vivid, fearful anticipation of stuttering. They fear words, sounds, and situations. Word substitutions and circumlocutions are common. Stutterers avoid situations requiring speech and show other evidence of fear and embarrassment.

Stutterers may have associated clinical features: vivid, fearful anticipation of stuttering, with avoidance of particular words, sounds, or situations in which stuttering is anticipated; and eye blinks, tics, and tremors of the lips or jaw. Frustration, anxiety, and depression are common among those with chronic stuttering.

Differential Diagnosis

Normal speech dysfluency in preschool years is difficult to differentiate from incipient stuttering. In stuttering occurs more nonfluencies, part-word repetitions, sound prolongations, and disruptions in voice airflow through the vocal track. Children who stutter appear to be tense and uncomfortable with their speech pattern, in contrast to young children who are nonfluent in their speech but seem to be at ease. Spastic dysphonia is a stuttering-like speech disorder distinguished from stuttering by the presence of an abnormal breathing pattern.

Cluttering is a speech disorder characterized by erratic and dysrhythmic speech patterns of rapid and jerky spurts of words and phrases. In cluttering, those affected are usually unaware of the disturbance, whereas, after the initial phase of the disorder, stutterers are aware of their speech difficulties. Cluttering is often an associated feature of expressive language disorder.

Course and Prognosis

The course of stuttering is usually long term, with some periods of partial remission lasting for weeks or months and exacerbations occurring most frequently when a stutterer is under pressure to communicate. Of all children who stutter, mostly those with mild cases, 50 to 80 percent recover spontaneously. School-age children who stutter chronically may have impaired peer relationships as a result of testing and social ostracism. The children may face academic difficulties if they avoid speaking in class. Later major complications include an affected person's limitations in occupational choice and advancement.

Treatment

Two distinct forms of intervention have been used in the treatment of stuttering. Direct speech therapy typically targets modification of the stuttering response to fluent-sounding speech by systematic steps and rules of speech mechanics that the person can practice. Another form of therapy for stuttering targets diminishing tension and anxiety during speech. These treatments utilize breathing exercises and relaxation techniques, to help children slow the rate of speaking and modulate speech volume. Until the end of the 19th century, the most common treatments for stuttering were distraction, suggestion, and relaxation. Recent approaches using distraction include teaching stutterers to talk in time to rhythmic movements of the arm, hand, or fingers. Stutterers are also advised to speak slowly in a sing-song or monotone manner. These approaches, however, remove stuttering only temporarily. Suggestion techniques, such as hypnosis, also stop stuttering but, again, only temporarily. Relaxation techniques are based on the premise that it is nearly impossible to be relaxed and stutter in the usual manner at the same time. Current interventions for stuttering use individualized combinations of behavioral distraction, relaxation techniques, and directed speech modification.

Stutterers who have poor self image, comorbid anxiety disorders or depressive disorders are likely to require additional treatments. Most modern treatments of stuttering include components that target stuttering as, in part, a learned behavior that can be modified through behavioral techniques regardless of the complexity of how they emerged. These approaches work directly with the speech difficulty to minimize stuttering responses, to modify or decrease the severity of stuttering by eliminating the secondary symptoms, and to encourage stutterers to speak, even when stuttering, in a relatively easy and effortless fashion that aims to eliminate fear and blocks.

One example of this approach is the self-therapy proposed by the Speech Foundation of America. Self-therapy is based on the premise that stuttering is not a symptom, but a behavior that can be modified. Stutterers are told that they can learn to control their difficulty partly by modifying their feelings about stuttering and attitudes toward it and partly by modifying the deviant behaviors associated with their stuttering blocks. The approach includes desensitizing; reducing the emotional reaction to, and fears of, stuttering; and substituting positive action to control the moment of stuttering.

Recently developed therapies focus on restructuring fluency. The entire speech production pattern is reshaped, with emphasis on a variety of target behaviors, including rate reduction, easy or gentle onset of voicing, and smooth transitions between sounds, syllables, and words. The approaches have met with substantial success in establishing perceptually fluent speech in adults, but fluency maintenance over long periods and relapses remain problems for all involved in adult-stuttering treatment.

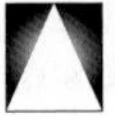

Table 41–8
DSM-IV-TR Diagnostic Criteria for Communication Disorder Not Otherwise Specified

This category is for disorders in communication that do not meet criteria for any specific communication disorder; for example, a voice disorder (i.e., an abnormality of vocal pitch, loudness, quality, tone, or resonance).

(From American Psychiatric Association. *Diagnostic and Statistical Manual of Mental Disorders.* 4th ed. Text rev. Washington, DC: American Psychiatric Association; copyright 2000, with permission.)

Psychopharmacological intervention, such as treatment with benzodiazepines (e.g., clonazepam [Klonopin]), have been used to promote relaxation; no data exist to assess the efficacy of this approach. Whichever therapeutic approach is used, individual and family assessments and supportive interventions may be helpful. A team assessment of a child or adolescent and his or her family should be made before any approaches to treatment are begun.

COMMUNICATION DISORDER NOT OTHERWISE SPECIFIED

Disorders that do not meet the diagnostic criteria for any specific communication disorder fall into the category of communication disorder not otherwise specified. An example is voice disorder, in which the patient has an abnormality in pitch, loudness, quality, tone, or resonance. To be coded as a disorder, the voice abnormality must be sufficiently severe to impair academic achievement or social communication (Table 41–8). Operationally, speech production can be broken down into five interacting subsystems, including respiration (airflow from the lungs), phonation (sound generation in the larynx), resonance (shaping of the sound quality in the pharynx and nasal cavity), articulation (modulation of the sound stream into consonant and vowel sounds with the tongue, jaw, and lips), and suprasegmentalia (speech rhythm, loudness, and intonation). Altogether, these systems work together to convey information and, as importantly, voice quality conveys information about the speaker's emotional, psychological, and physical status. Thus, voice abnormalities can cover a broad area of communication as well as indicate many different types of abnormalities.

Cluttering is not listed as a disorder in DSM-IV-TR, but it is an associated speech abnormality in which the disturbed rate and rhythm of speech impair intelligibility. Speech is erratic and dysrhythmic and consists of rapid, jerky spurts that are inconsistent with normal phrasing patterns. The disorder usually occurs in children between 2 and 8 years of age; in two thirds of cases, the patient recovers spontaneously by early adolescence. Cluttering is associated with learning disorders and other communication disorders.

J. K. was a 14-year-old boy with a repaired unilateral complete cleft lip and palate who presented at his cleft palate center for a follow-up examination. Approximately 4 years had passed since his last appointment with the cleft palate team, partly because his family had moved. J. K. was still mildly hypernasal, but did not exhibit any of the common cleft-type compensatory articulations. For the hypernasality, he was having speech-language therapy in his new hometown. It became immediately obvious during the interview that the pitch of his voice was too high. J. K. was of regular height and build for his age, and, when the clinician palpated his larynx, it had an age-appropriate size.

During the interview, the patient and his family reported that he had experienced teasing at school because of his high-pitched voice. The patient and his family attributed the voice quality to the repaired cleft lip and palate. During a brief course of diagnostic voice therapy, J. K. could immediately be stimulated to lower his pitch to a physiological level. The diagnosis of postmutational falsetto was made. This condition usually has a strong psychogenic component, so the speech-language pathologist recommended an additional psychiatric consultation as a standard procedure. The patient and his family, however, declined further psychiatric evaluations at this time. The speech-language pathologist in J. K.'s hometown was informed about the diagnosis. She was instructed to change her focus of therapy and treat the voice disorder on its own merits. When the patient came back to the cleft center 1 year later, the problem had been resolved and the patient had an age-appropriate pitch.

Because the patient and the family had refused a psychiatric evaluation, the exact causes of the postmutational falsetto could not be determined. Research shows, however, that psychopathology is not higher in persons with cleft lip and palate than in the normal population. The postmutational falsetto was probably an independent condition that was mistakenly assumed to be caused by the cleft lip and palate by the patient, as well as by professionals involved with his care.

ICD-10

The 10th revision of *International Statistical Classification of Diseases and Related Health Problems* (ICD-10) includes four disorders of speech and language as well as two residual categories (Table 41–9). ICD-10 defines cluttering as a "rapid rate of speech with breakdown in fluency, but no repetitions or hesitations, of a severity to give rise to reduced speech intelligibility. Speech is erratic and dysrhythmic, with rapid, jerky spurts that usually involve faulty phrasing patterns." The faulty speech patterns may include using groups of words unrelated to

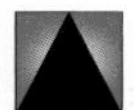

Table 41–9
ICD-10 Diagnostic Criteria for Specific Developmental Disorders of Speech and Language

Specific speech articulation disorder

Note. This disorder is also referred to as specific speech phonological disorder.

A. Articulation (phonological) skills, as assessed on standardized tests, are below the 2 standard deviations limit for the child's age.
B. Articulation (phonological) skills are at least 1 standard deviation below nonverbal IQ as assessed on standardized tests.
C. Language expression and comprehension, as assessed on standardized tests, are within the 2 standard deviations limit for the child's age.
D. There are no neurological, sensory, or physical impairments that directly affect speech sound production, nor is there a pervasive developmental disorder.
E. Most commonly used exclusion clause: Nonverbal IQ is below 70 on a standardized test.

Expressive language disorder

A. Expressive language skills, as assessed on standardized tests, are below the 2 standard deviations limit for the child's age.
B. Expressive language skills are at least 1 standard deviation below nonverbal IQ as assessed on standardized tests.
C. Receptive language skills, as assessed on standardized tests, are within the 2 standard deviations limit for the child's age.
D. Use and understanding of nonverbal communication and imaginative language functions are within the normal range.
E. There are no neurological, sensory, or physical impairments that directly affect use of spoken language, nor is there a pervasive developmental disorder.
F. Most commonly used exclusion clause: Nonverbal IQ is below 70 on a standardized test.

Receptive language disorder

Note. This disorder is also referred to as mixed receptive/expressive disorder.

A. Language comprehension, as assessed on standardized tests, is below the 2 standard deviations limit for the child's age.
B. Receptive language skills are at least 1 standard deviation below nonverbal IQ as assessed on standardized tests.
C. There are no neurological, sensory, or physical impairments that directly affect receptive language, nor is there a pervasive developmental disorder.
D. Most commonly used exclusion clause: Nonverbal IQ is below 70 on a standardized test.

Acquired aphasia with epilepsy [Landau-Kleffner syndrome]

A. Severe loss of expressive and receptive language skills occurs over a period of time not exceeding 6 months.
B. Language development was normal before the loss.
C. Paroxysmal EEG abnormalities affecting one or both temporal lobes become apparent within a time span extending from 2 years before to 2 years after the initial loss of language.
D. Hearing is within the normal range.
E. A level of nonverbal intelligence within the normal range is retained.
F. There is no diagnosable neurological condition other than that implicit in the abnormal EEG and presence of epileptic seizures (when they occur).
G. The disorder does not meet the criteria for a pervasive developmental disorder.

Other developmental disorders of speech and language

Developmental disorder of speech and language, unspecified

This category should be avoided as far as possible and should be used only for unspecified disorders in which there is significant impairment in the development of speech or language that cannot be accounted for by mental retardation, or by neurological, sensory, or physical impairments that directly affect speech or language.

(From World Health Organization. The *International Classification of Mental and Behavioural Disorders: Diagnostic Criteria for Research.* Copyright, World Health Organization, Geneva, 1993, with permission.)

the sentence's grammar. According to ICD-10, cluttering must be distinguished from stuttering. ICD-10 defines stuttering as speech "characterized by frequent repetition or prolongation of sounds or syllables or words, or by frequent hesitations or pauses that disrupt the rhythmic flow of speech." Minor stuttering is common throughout life, but persistent, severe stuttering that destroys the fluency of speech must be present for stuttering to be diagnosed. The disorder may be accompanied by movements of the face or body that coincide with speech.

References

Brackenbury T, Pye C. Semantic deficits in children with language impairments: issues for clinical assessment. *Language, Speech, and Hearing Services in Schools*. 2005;36:5.

Cone-Wessen B. Prenatal alcohol and cocaine exposure: Influences on cognition, speech, language and hearing. *J Commun Disord*. 2005;38:279.

Johnson CJ, Beitchman JH. Expressive language disorder. In: Sadock BJ, Sadock VA, eds. *Kaplan & Sadock's Comprehensive Textbook of Psychiatry*. 8th ed. Vol. 2. Philadelphia: Lippincott Williams & Wilkins; 2005:3136.

Johnson CJ, Beitchman JH. Mixed receptive-expressive language disorder. In: Sadock BJ, Sadock VA, eds. *Kaplan & Sadock's Comprehensive Textbook of Psychiatry*. 8th ed. Vol. 2. Philadelphia: Lippincott Williams & Wilkins; 2005: 3142.

Johnson CJ, Beitchman JH. Phonological disorder. In: Sadock BJ, Sadock VA, eds. *Kaplan & Sadock's Comprehensive Textbook of Psychiatry*. 8th ed. Vol. 2. Philadelphia: Lippincott Williams & Wilkins; 2005:3148.

Kroll R, Beitchman JH. Stuttering. In: Sadock BJ, Sadock VA, eds. *Kaplan & Sadock's Comprehensive Textbook of Psychiatry*. 8th ed. Vol. 2. Philadelphia: Lippincott Williams & Wilkins; 2005:3155.

Leevers HJ, Roesler CP, Flax J, Benasich AA. The Carter Neurocognitive Assessment for children with severely compromised expressive language and motor skills. *J Child Psychol Psychiatry*. 2005;46:287.

Nass RD, Trauner D. Social and affective impairments are important recovery after acquired stroke in children. *CNS Spectrums*. 2004;9(6):420.

Rvachew S, Grawburg M. Correlates of phonological awareness in preschoolers with speech sound disorders. *Journal of Speech, Language, and Hearing Research*. 2006;49:74–87.

Ripley K, Yuill N. Patterns of language impairment and behavior in boys excluded from school. *Br J Educ Psychol*. 2005;75:37.

Smith BL, Smith TD, Taylor L, Hobby M. Relationship between intelligence and vocabulary. *Percept Mot Skills*. 2005;100:101.

Somerville MJ, Mervis CB, Young EJ, Seo EJ, Del Campo M, Bamforth S, Peregrine E, Loo W, Lilley M, Perez-Jurado LA, Morris CA, Scherer SW, Osborne LR. Severe expressive-language delay related to duplication of the Williams-Beuren locus. *N Engl J Med*. 2005;353:1655.

Verhoeven L, van Balkom H, eds. *Classification of Developmental Language Disorders. Theoretical Issues and Clinical Implications*. Mahwah, NJ: Erlbaum; 2004.

42

Pervasive Developmental Disorders

Pervasive developmental disorders include several that are characterized by impaired reciprocal social interactions, aberrant language development, and restricted behavioral repertoire. Pervasive developmental disorders typically emerge in young children before the age of 3 years, and parents often become concerned about a child by 18 months as language development does not occur as expected. In about 25 percent of cases, some language develops and is subsequently lost. Some children with pervasive developmental disorders are not identified with problems until school age, because they make relatively few demands and have minimal conflicts with others owing to their infrequent social engagement. Children with pervasive developmental disorders often exhibit idiosyncratic intense interest in a narrow range of activities, resist change, and are not appropriately responsive to the social environment. These disorders affect multiple areas of development, are manifested early in life, and cause persistent dysfunction. Autistic disorder, the best known of these disorders, is characterized by sustained impairment in comprehending and responding to social cues, aberrant language development and usage, and restricted, stereotypical behavioral patterns. According to the text revision of the 4th edition of *Diagnostic and Statistical Manual of Mental Disorders* (DSM-IV-TR), to meet criteria for autistic behavior, abnormal functioning in at least one of the above areas must be present by age 3 years. More than two thirds of children with autistic disorder have mental retardation, although it is not required for the diagnosis.

The DSM-IV-TR includes five pervasive developmental disorders: autistic disorder, Rett's disorder, childhood disintegrative disorder, Asperger's disorder, and pervasive developmental disorder not otherwise specified. Rett's disorder appears to occur exclusively in girls; it is characterized by normal development for at least 6 months, stereotyped hand movements, a loss of purposeful motions, diminishing social engagement, poor coordination, and decreasing language use. In childhood disintegrative disorder, development progresses normally for the first 2 years, after which the child shows a loss of previously acquired skills in two or more of the following areas: language use, social responsiveness, play, motor skills, and bladder or bowel control. Asperger's disorder is a condition in which the child is markedly impaired in social relatedness and shows repetitive and stereotyped patterns of behavior without a delay in language development. In Asperger's disorder, a child's cognitive abilities and adaptive skills are normal. A recent survey revealed that the average age of diagnosis for children with pervasive developmental disorders was 3.1 years for children with autistic disorder, 3.9 years for pervasive developmental disorder not otherwise specified, and 7.2 years for Asperger's disorder. Children with severe language deficits received a diagnosis an average of a year earlier than other children. Children with behaviors such as hand-flapping, toe-walking, and odd play were identified with disorders at a younger age.

AUTISTIC DISORDER

Autistic disorder (historically called *early infantile autism*, *childhood autism*, or *Kanner's autism*) is characterized by symptoms from each of the following three categories: qualitative impairment in social interaction, impairment in communication, and restricted repetitive and stereotyped patterns of behavior or interests.

History

As early as 1867, Henry Maudsley, a psychiatrist, noted a group of very young children with severe mental disorders who had marked deviation, delay, and distortion in development. In that era, most serious disturbance in young children was believed to fall within the category of psychoses. In 1943 Leo Kanner, in his classic paper "Autistic Disturbances of Affective Contact," coined the term *infantile autism* and provided a clear, comprehensive account of the early childhood syndrome. He described children who exhibited extreme autistic aloneness; failure to assume an anticipatory posture; delayed or deviant language development with echolalia and pronominal reversal (using you for I); monotonous repetitions of noises or verbal utterances; excellent rote memory; limited range of spontaneous activities, stereotypies, and mannerisms; anxiously obsessive desire for the maintenance of sameness and dread of change; poor eye contact; abnormal relationships with persons; and a preference for pictures and inanimate objects. Kanner suspected that the syndrome was more frequent than it seemed and suggested that some children with this disorder had been misclassified as mentally retarded or schizophrenic. Before 1980, children with pervasive developmental disorders were generally diagnosed with childhood schizophrenia. Over time, it became evident that autistic disorder and schizophrenia were two distinct psychiatric entities. In some cases, however, a child with autistic disorder may develop a comorbid schizophrenic disorder later in childhood.

Epidemiology

Prevalence. Autistic disorder is believed to occur at a rate of about 8 cases per 10,000 children (0.08 percent). Multiple epidemiologic surveys mainly in Europe have resulted in variable rates of autistic disorder ranging from 2 to 30 cases per 10,000. By definition, the onset of autistic disorder is before the age of 3 years, although in some cases, it is not recognized until a child is much older.

Sex Distribution. Autistic disorder is four to five times more frequent in boys than in girls. Girls with autistic disorder are more likely to have more severe mental retardation.

Socioeconomic Status. Early studies suggested that a high socioeconomic status was more common in families with autistic children; however, these findings were probably based on referral bias. Over the past 25 years, no epidemiological studies have demonstrated an association between autistic disorder and any socioeconomic status.

Etiology and Pathogenesis

Genetic Factors. Current evidence supports a genetic basis for the development of autistic disorder in most cases, with a contribution of up to four or five genes. Family studies have demonstrated a 50 to 200 times increase in the rate of autism in siblings of an index child with autistic disorder. Additionally, even when not affected with autism, siblings are at increased risk for a variety of developmental disorders often related to communication and social skills. These difficulties in the nonautistic relatives of people with autistic disorder are also known by researchers as the "broad phenotype." The specific modes of inheritance are not yet clear. Hypotheses include genetic inheritance of a more general predisposition to developmental difficulties and specific genetic etiology of autistic disorder.

Current research has revealed promising leads on candidate genes likely to underlie the development of autistic disorder. Linkage analyses have demonstrated that regions of chromosomes 7, 2, 4, 15, and 19 are likely to contribute to the genetic basis of autism. It now appears that multiple genes are involved in the development of autism. Researchers hypothesize that some genetic forms of autism may be identified in the near future.

The concordance rate of autistic disorder in the two largest twin studies was 36 percent in monozygotic pairs versus 0 percent in dizygotic pairs in one study and about 96 percent in monozygotic pairs versus about 27 percent in dizygotic pairs in the second study. High rates of cognitive difficulties, even in the nonautistic twin in monozygotic twins with perinatal complications, suggest that contributions of perinatal insult along with genetic vulnerability may lead to autistic disorder.

Fragile X syndrome, a genetic disorder in which a portion of the X chromosome fractures, appears to be associated with autistic disorder. Approximately 1 percent of children with autistic disorder also have fragile X syndrome. Children with fragile X syndrome tend to show gross motor and fine motor difficulties as well as relatively poorer expressive language compared with children with autism without fragile X syndrome. Tuberous sclerosis, a genetic disorder characterized by multiple benign tumors, with autosomal dominant transmission is found with greater frequency among children with autistic disorder. Up to 2 percent of children with autistic disorder may also have tuberous sclerosis.

Recently, researchers screened the DNA of more than 150 pairs of siblings with autism. They found extremely strong evidence that two regions on chromosomes 2 and 7 contain genes involved with autism. Likely locations for autism-related genes were also found on chromosomes 16 and 17, although the strength of the correlation was somewhat weaker. Historically, Kanner, in 1943, described 11 cases of developmentally disordered people and hypothesized that their autistic features were caused by emotionally unresponsive "refrigerator" mothers, but no validity exists to this hypothesis. On the other hand, much evidence supports a biological substrate for this disorder.

Biological Factors. The high rate of mental retardation among children with autistic disorder and the higher-than-expected rates of seizure disorders further support the biological basis for autistic disorder. Approximately 70 percent of children with autistic disorder have mental retardation. About one third of these children have mild to moderate mental retardation, and close to half of these children are severely or profoundly mentally retarded. Children with autistic disorder and mental retardation typically show more marked deficits in abstract reasoning, social understanding, and verbal tasks than in performance tasks, such as block design and digit recall, in which details can be remembered without reference to the "gestalt" meaning.

Of persons with autism, 4 to 32 percent have grand mal seizures at some time, and about 20 to 25 percent show ventricular enlargement on computed tomography (CT) scans. Various electroencephalogram (EEG) abnormalities are found in 10 to 83 percent of autistic children, and although no EEG finding is specific to autistic disorder, there is some indication of failed cerebral lateralization. Recently, one magnetic resonance imaging (MRI) study revealed hypoplasia of cerebellar vermal lobules VI and VII, and another MRI study revealed cortical abnormalities, particularly polymicrogyria, in some autistic patients. Those abnormalities may reflect abnormal cell migrations in the first 6 months of gestation. An autopsy study revealed fewer Purkinje's cells, and another study found increased diffuse cortical metabolism during positron emission tomography (PET) scanning.

Autistic disorder is also associated with neurological conditions, notably congenital rubella, phenylketonuria (PKU), and tuberous sclerosis. Autistic children have higher than expected histories of perinatal complications compared with the general population and also compared with children with other psychiatric disorders. The finding that autistic children have significantly more minor congenital physical anomalies than expected suggests abnormal development within the first trimester of pregnancy.

Immunological Factors. Several reports have suggested that immunological incompatibility (i.e., maternal antibodies directed at the fetus) may contribute to autistic disorder. The lymphocytes of some autistic children react with maternal antibodies, which raises the possibility that embryonic neural or extraembryonic tissues may be damaged during gestation.

Perinatal Factors. A higher-than-expected incidence of perinatal complications seems to occur in infants who are later diagnosed with autistic disorder. Maternal bleeding after the first trimester and meconium in the amniotic fluid have been reported in the histories of autistic children more often than in the general population. In the neonatal period, autistic children have a high incidence of respiratory distress syndrome and neonatal anemia.

Males with autism, as a group, have been found to be the products of longer gestational age and were heavier at birth than babies in the general population. Females with autism are more likely to be the product of postterm pregnancies than babies in the general population.

Neuroanatomical Factors. The neuroanatomical basis of autism remains unknown; however, recent evidence suggests that enlargement of gray and white matter cerebral volumes, but not cerebellar volumes, are present in children with autistic disorder at 2 years of age. Head circumference appears normal at birth, and the increased rate of head circumference growth appears to emerge at about 12 months of age. Previous MRI studies comparing autistic subjects and normal controls revealed total brain volume was larger in those with autism, although autistic children with severe mental retardation generally have smaller heads. The greatest average percentage increase in size occurred in the occipital lobe, parietal lobe, and temporal lobe. No differences were found in the frontal lobes. Specific origins of this enlargement are unknown. The increased volume can arise from three different possible mechanisms: increased neurogenesis, decreased neuronal death, and increased production of nonneuronal brain tissue, such as glial cells or blood vessels. Brain enlargement has been suggested as a possible biological marker for autistic disorder.

The temporal lobe is believed to be one of the critical areas of brain abnormality in autistic disorder. This suggestion is based on reports of autistic-like syndromes in some persons with temporal lobe damage. When the temporal region of animals is damaged, normal social behavior is lost, and restlessness, repetitive motor behavior, and a limited behavioral repertoire are seen. Some brains of autistic individuals exhibit a decrease in cerebellar Purkinje's cells, which is believed to account potentially for abnormalities of attention, arousal, and sensory processes.

Interesting reports of differences between male and female brains are hypothesized to have possible implications for understanding autism insofar as the traits of "empathy" and "systemizing." Empathizing, the capacity to predict and respond to feelings and behavior of others by inferring their emotional states, is a stronger trait in females than in males at a population level. Males, on the other hand, at a population level, are stronger at systemizing, that is, inferring rules that govern "cause and effect" relationships of behaviors. People with pervasive developmental disorders are characterized by deficits in empathizing, and those with high intellectual capacity have been reported to have relative strengths in rule bound thinking.

Biochemical Factors. A number of studies in the last few decades have demonstrated that about one third of patients with autistic disorder have high plasma serotonin concentrations. This finding, however, is not specific to autistic disorder, and persons with mental retardation without autistic disorder also display this trait. Several studies have reported that autistic individuals without mental retardation have a high incidence of hyperserotonemia. In some autistic children, a high concentration of homovanillic acid (the major dopamine metabolite) in cerebrospinal fluid (CSF) is associated with increased withdrawal and stereotypes. Some evidence indicates that symptom severity decreases as the ratio of 5-hydroxyindoleacetic acid (5-HIAA, metabolite of serotonin) to homovanillic acid in CSF increases. The 5-HIAA concentration in CSF may be inversely proportional to blood serotonin concentrations, which are increased in one third of autistic disorder patients, a nonspecific finding that also occurs in mentally retarded persons.

Psychosocial and Family Factors. Studies comparing parents of autistic children with parents of normal children have shown no significant differences in child-rearing skills.

Children with autistic disorder, as children with other disorders, can respond with exacerbated symptoms to psychosocial stressors, including family discord, the birth of a new sibling, or a family move. Some children with autistic disorder may be excruciatingly sensitive to even small changes in their families and immediate environment.

Diagnosis and Clinical Features

The DSM-IV-TR diagnostic criteria for autistic disorder are given in Table 42–1.

Physical Characteristics. On first glance, children with autistic disorder do not show any physical signs indicating the disorder. These children do have high rates of minor physical anomalies, such as ear malformations, and others that may reflect abnormalities in fetal development of those organs along with parts of the brain.

A greater than expected number of autistic children do not show lateralization and remain ambidextrous at an age when cerebral dominance is established in most children. Autistic children also have a higher incidence of abnormal dermatoglyphics (e.g., fingerprints) than those in the general population. This finding may suggest a disturbance in neuroectodermal development.

Behavioral Characteristics

QUALITATIVE IMPAIRMENTS IN SOCIAL INTERACTION. Autistic children do not exhibit the expected level of subtle reciprocal social skills that demonstrate relatedness to parents and peers. As infants, many lack a social smile and anticipatory posture for being picked up as an adult approaches. Less frequent or poor eye contact is common. The social development of autistic children is characterized by impaired, but not usually totally absent, attachment behavior. Autistic children often do not acknowledge or differentiate the most important persons in their lives—parents, siblings, and teachers—and may show extreme anxiety when their usual routine is disrupted, but they may not react overtly to being left with a stranger. When autistic children have reached school age, their withdrawal may have diminished and be less obvious, particularly in higher-functioning children. A notable deficit is seen in ability to play with peers and to make friends; their social behavior is awkward and may be inappropriate. Cognitively, children with autistic disorder are more skilled in visual-spatial tasks than in tasks requiring skill in verbal reasoning.

One description of the cognitive style of children with autism is that they cannot infer the feelings or mental state of others around them. That is, they cannot make attributions about the motivation or intentions of others and, thus, cannot develop empathy. This lack of a "theory of mind" leaves them unable to

Table 42–1
DSM-IV-TR Diagnostic Criteria for Autistic Disorder

A. A total of six (or more) items from (1), (2), and (3), with at least two from (1), and one each from (2) and (3):
  (1) qualitative impairment in social interaction, as manifested by at least two of the following:
    (a) marked impairment in the use of multiple nonverbal behaviors such as eye-to-eye gaze, facial expression, body postures, and gestures to regulate social interaction
    (b) failure to develop peer relationships appropriate to developmental level
    (c) a lack of spontaneous seeking to share enjoyment, interests, or achievements with other people (e.g., by a lack of showing, bringing, or pointing out objects of interest)
    (d) lack of social or emotional reciprocity
  (2) qualitative impairments in communication as manifested by at least one of the following:
    (a) delay in, or total lack of, the development of spoken language (not accompanied by an attempt to compensate through alternative modes of communication such as gesture or mime)
    (b) in individuals with adequate speech, marked impairment in the ability to initiate or sustain a conversation with others
    (c) stereotyped and repetitive use of language or idiosyncratic language
    (d) lack of varied, spontaneous make-believe play or social imitative play appropriate to developmental level
  (3) restricted repetitive and stereotyped patterns of behavior, interests, and activities, as manifested by at least one of the following:
    (a) encompassing preoccupation with one or more stereotyped and restricted patterns of interest that is abnormal either in intensity or focus
    (b) apparently inflexible adherence to specific, nonfunctional routines or rituals
    (c) stereotyped and repetitive motor mannerisms (e.g., hand or finger flapping or twisting, or complex whole-body movements)
    (d) persistent preoccupation with parts of objects

B. Delays or abnormal functioning in at least one of the following areas, with onset prior to age 3 years: (1) social interaction, (2) language as used in social communication, or (3) symbolic or imaginative play.

C. The disturbance is not better accounted for by Rett's disorder or childhood disintegrative disorder.

(From American Psychiatric Association. *Diagnostic and Statistical Manual of Mental Disorders*. 4th ed. Text rev. Washington, DC: American Psychiatric Association; copyright 2000, with permission.)

interpret the social behavior of others and leads to a lack of social reciprocation.

In late adolescence, autistic persons often desire friendships, but their difficulties in responding to another's interests, emotions, and feelings are major obstacles in developing them. They are often shunned by peers and behave in awkward ways that alienate them from others. Autistic adolescents and adults experience sexual feelings, but their lack of social competence and skills prevents many of them from developing sexual relationships.

DISTURBANCES OF COMMUNICATION AND LANGUAGE. Deficits in language development and difficulty using language to communicate ideas are among the principal criteria for diagnosing autistic disorder. Autistic children are not simply reluctant to speak, and their speech abnormalities do not result from lack of motivation. Language deviance, as much as language delay, is characteristic of autistic disorder. In contrast to normal and mentally retarded children, autistic children have significant difficulty putting meaningful sentences together even when they have large vocabularies. When children with autistic disorder do learn to converse fluently, their conversations may impart information without providing a sense of acknowledging how the other person is responding. In children with autism and nonautistic children with language disorders, nonverbal communication skills may also be impaired when significant difficulty with expressive language exists.

In the first year of life, an autistic child's pattern of babbling may be minimal or abnormal. Some children emit noises—clicks, sounds, screeches, and nonsense syllables—in a stereotyped fashion, without a seeming intent of communication. Unlike normal young children, who generally have better receptive language skills than expressive ones, verbal autistic children may say more than they understand. Words and even entire sentences may drop in and out of a child's vocabulary. It is not atypical for a child with autistic disorder to use a word once and then not use it again for a week, a month, or years. Children with autistic disorder typically exhibit speech that contains echolalia, both immediate and delayed, or stereotyped phrases that seem out of context. These language patterns are frequently associated with pronoun reversals. A child with autistic disorder might say, "You want the toy" when she means that she wants it. Difficulties in articulation are also common. Many children with autistic disorder use peculiar voice quality and rhythm. About 50 percent of autistic children never develop useful speech. Some of the brightest children show a particular fascination with letters and numbers. Children with autistic disorder sometimes excel in certain tasks or have special abilities; for example, a child may learn to read fluently at preschool age (hyperlexia), often astonishingly well. Very young autistic children who can read many words, however, have little comprehension of the words read.

STEREOTYPED BEHAVIOR. In the first years of an autistic child's life, much of the expected spontaneous exploratory play is absent. Toys and objects are often manipulated in a ritualistic manner, with few symbolic features. Autistic children generally do not show imitative play or use abstract pantomime. The activities and play of these children are often rigid, repetitive, and monotonous. Ritualistic and compulsive phenomena are common in early and middle childhood. Children often spin, bang, and line up objects and may exhibit an attachment to a particular inanimate object. Many autistic children, especially those who are severely mentally retarded, exhibit movement abnormalities. Stereotypies, mannerisms, and grimacing are most frequent when a child is left alone and may decrease in a structured situation. Autistic children are generally resistant to transition and change. Moving to a new house, moving furniture in a room, or a change, such as having breakfast before a bath when the reverse was the routine, may evoke panic, fear, or temper tantrums.

INSTABILITY OF MOOD AND AFFECT. Some children with autistic disorder exhibit sudden mood changes, with bursts of laughing or crying without an obvious reason. It is difficult to learn more about these episodes if the child cannot express the thoughts related to the affect.

RESPONSE TO SENSORY STIMULI. Autistic children have been observed to overrespond to some stimuli and underrespond to other sensory stimuli (e.g., to sound and pain). It is not uncommon for a child with autistic disorder to appear deaf, at times showing little response to a normal speaking voice; on the other hand, the same child may show intent interest in the sound of a wristwatch. Some children with autistic disorder have a heightened pain threshold or an altered response to pain. Indeed, some autistic children do not respond to an injury by crying or seeking comfort. Many autistic children reportedly enjoy music. They frequently hum a tune or sing a song or commercial jingle before saying words or using speech. Some particularly enjoy vestibular stimulation—spinning, swinging, and up-and-down movements.

ASSOCIATED BEHAVIORAL SYMPTOMS. Hyperkinesis is a common behavior problem in young autistic children. Hypokinesis is less frequent; when present, it often alternates with hyperactivity. Aggression and temper tantrums are observed, often prompted by change or demands. Self-injurious behavior includes head banging, biting, scratching, and hair pulling. Short attention span, poor ability to focus on a task, insomnia, feeding and eating problems, and enuresis are also common among children with autism.

ASSOCIATED PHYSICAL ILLNESS. Young children with autistic disorder have been reported to have a higher-than-expected incidence of upper respiratory infections and other minor infections. Gastrointestinal symptoms commonly found among children with autistic disorder include excessive burping, constipation, and loose bowel movements. Also seen is an increased incidence of febrile seizures in children with autistic disorder. Some autistic children do not show temperature elevations with minor infectious illnesses and may not show the typical malaise of ill children. In some children, behavior problems and relatedness seem to improve noticeably during a minor illness, and in some, such changes are a clue to physical illness.

A standardized instrument that can be very helpful in eliciting comprehensive information regarding developmental disorders is the *Autism Diagnostic Observation Schedule-Generic* (ADOS-G).

John was the second of two children born to middle-class parents after normal pregnancy, labor, and delivery. As an infant, John appeared undemanding and relatively placid; motor development proceeded appropriately, but language development was delayed. Although his parents indicated that they were first concerned about his development when he was 18 months of age and still not speaking, in retrospect, they noted that, in comparison to their previous child, he had seemed relatively uninterested in social interaction and the social games of infancy. Stranger anxiety had never really developed, and John did not exhibit differential attachment behaviors toward his parents. Their pediatrician initially reassured John's parents that he was a "late talker," but they continued to be concerned. Although John seemed to respond to some unusual sounds, the pediatrician obtained a hearing test when John was 24 months old. Levels of hearing appeared adequate for development of speech, and John was referred for developmental evaluation. At 24 months, motor skills were age appropriate, and John exhibited some nonverbal problem-solving skills close to age level. His language and social development, however, were severely delayed, and he was noted to be resistant to changes in routine and unusually sensitive to aspects of the inanimate environment. His play skills were quite limited, and he used play materials in unusual and idiosyncratic ways. His older sister had a history of some learning difficulties, but the family history was otherwise negative. A comprehensive medical evaluation revealed a normal EEG and CT scan; genetic screening and chromosome analysis were normal as well.

John was enrolled in a special education program, in which he gradually began to speak. His speech was characterized by echolalia, extreme literalness, a monotonic voice quality, and pronoun reversal. He rarely used language in interaction and remained quite isolated. By school age, John had developed some evidence of differential attachments to family members; he also had developed a number of self-stimulatory behaviors and engaged in occasional periods of head banging. Extreme sensitivity to change continued. Intelligence testing revealed marked scatter, with a full-scale intelligence quotient (IQ) in the moderately retarded range. As an adolescent, John's behavioral functioning deteriorated, and he developed a seizure disorder. Now an adult, he lives in a group home and attends a sheltered workshop. He has a rather passive interactional style but exhibits occasional outbursts of aggression and self-abuse. (Courtesy of Fred Volkmar, M.D.)

Intellectual Functioning. About 70 to 75 percent of children with autistic disorder function in the mentally retarded range of intellectual function. About 30 percent of children function in the mild to moderate range, and about 45 to 50 percent are severely to profoundly mentally retarded. Epidemiological and clinical studies show that the risk for autistic disorder increases as the IQ decreases. About one fifth of all autistic children have a normal, nonverbal intelligence. The IQ scores of autistic children tend to reflect most severe problems with verbal sequencing and abstraction skills, with relative strengths in visuospatial or rote memory skills. This finding suggests the importance of defects in language-related functions.

Unusual or precocious cognitive or visuomotor abilities occur in some autistic children. The abilities, which may exist even in the overall retarded functioning, are referred to as *splinter functions* or *islets of precocity*. Perhaps the most striking examples are idiot or autistic savants, who have prodigious rote memories or calculating abilities, usually beyond the capabilities of their normal peers. Other precocious abilities in young autistic children include hyperlexia, an early ability to read well (although they cannot understand what they read), memorizing and reciting, and musical abilities (singing or playing tunes or recognizing musical pieces).

Differential Diagnosis

Autism must first be differentiated from one of the other pervasive developmental disorders such as Asperser's disorder and pervasive developmental disorder not otherwise specified. Further, it must be differentiated from other developmental disorders, including mental retardation syndromes and developmental language disorders. Other disorders in the differential diagnosis are schizophrenia with childhood onset, congenital deafness or severe hearing disorder, psychosocial deprivation, and disintegrative (regressive) psychoses. It is sometimes difficult to make the diagnosis of autism because of its overlapping symptoms with childhood schizophrenia, mental retardation syndromes with behavioral symptoms, mixed receptive-expressive language disorder, and hearing disorders. Because children with a pervasive

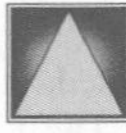

Table 42–2
Procedure for Differential Diagnosis on a Multiaxial System

1. Determine intellectual level
2. Determine level of language development
3. Consider whether child's behavior is appropriate for
   (i) chronological age
   (ii) mental age
   (iii) language age
4. If not appropriate, consider differential diagnosis of psychiatric disorder according to
   (i) pattern of social interaction
   (ii) pattern of language
   (iii) pattern of play
   (iv) other behaviors
5. Identify any relevant medical conditions
6. Consider whether there are any relevant psychosocial factors

(From Rutter M, Hersov I. *Child and Adolescent Psychiatry: Modern Approaches.* 2nd ed. Oxford: Blackwell; 1985:73, with permission.)

developmental disorder usually have many concurrent problems, Michael Rutter and Lionel Hersov suggested a stepwise approach to the differential diagnosis (Table 42–2).

Schizophrenia with Childhood Onset. Although a wealth of literature on autistic disorder is available, few data exist on children under age 12 who meet the diagnostic criteria for schizophrenia. Schizophrenia is rare in children under the age of 5. It is accompanied by hallucinations or delusions, with a lower incidence of seizures and mental retardation and a more even IQ than autistic children exhibit. Table 42–3 compares autistic disorder and schizophrenia with childhood onset.

Mental Retardation with Behavioral Symptoms. About 40 percent of autistic children are moderately, severely, or profoundly retarded, and retarded children may have behavioral symptoms that include autistic features. When both disorders are present, both should be diagnosed. The main differentiating features between autistic disorder and mental retardation are that mentally retarded children usually relate to adults and other children in accordance with their mental age, use the language they do have to communicate with others, and exhibit a relatively even profile of impairments without splinter functions.

Mixed Receptive-Expressive Language Disorder. Some children with mixed receptive-expressive language disorder have mild autistic-like features and may present a diagnostic problem. Table 42–4 summarizes the major differences between autistic disorder and mixed receptive-expressive language disorder.

Acquired Aphasia with Convulsion. Acquired aphasia with convulsion is a rare condition that is sometimes difficult to differentiate from autistic disorder and childhood disintegrative disorder. Children with the condition are normal for several years before losing both their receptive and their expressive language over a period of weeks or months. Most have a few seizures and generalized EEG abnormalities at the onset, but these signs usually do not persist. A profound language comprehension disorder then follows, characterized by deviant speech pattern and speech impairment. Some children recover, but with considerable residual language impairment.

Congenital Deafness or Severe Hearing Impairment. Because autistic children are often mute or show a selective disinterest in spoken language, they are often thought to be deaf. Differentiating factors include the following: Autistic infants may babble only infrequently, whereas deaf infants have a history of relatively normal babbling that then gradually tapers off and may stop at 6 months to 1 year of age. Deaf children respond only to loud sounds, whereas autistic children may ignore loud or normal sounds and respond to soft or low sounds. Most

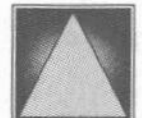

Table 42–3
Autistic Disorder versus Schizophrenia with Childhood Onset

Criteria	Autistic Disorder	Schizophrenia (with Onset before Puberty)
Age of onset	Before 38 months	Not under 5 years of age
Incidence	2 to 5 in 10,000	Unknown, possibly same or even rarer
Sex ratio (M:F)	3 to 4:1	1.67:1 (nearly equal, or slight preponderance of males)
Family history of schizophrenia	Not raised or probably not raised	Raised
Socioeconomic status (SES)	Overrepresentation of upper SES groups (artifact)	More common in lower SES groups
Prenatal and perinatal complications and cerebral dysfunction	More common in autistic disorder	Less common in schizophrenia
Behavioral characteristics	Failure to develop relatedness; absence of speech or echolalia; stereotyped phrases; language comprehension absent or poor; insistence on sameness and stereotypies	Hallucinations and delusions; thought disorder
Adaptive functioning	Usually always impaired	Deterioration in functioning
Level of intelligence	In most cases subnormal, frequently severely impaired (70%)	Usually within normal range, mostly dull normal (15% to 70%)
Pattern of IQ	Marked unevenness	More even
Grand mal seizures	4% to 32%	Absent or lower incidence

(Courtesy of Magda Campbell, M.D., and Wayne Green, M.D.)

Table 42–4
Autistic Disorder versus Mixed Receptive-Expressive Language Disorder

Criteria	Autistic Disorder	Mixed Receptive-Expressive Language Disorder
Incidence	2 to 5 of 10,000	5 of 10,000
Sex ratio (M:F)	3 to 4:1	Equal or almost equal sex ratio
Family history of speech delay or language problems	Present in about 25% of cases	Present in about 25% of cases
Associated deafness	Very infrequent	Not infrequent
Nonverbal communication (e.g., gestures.)	Absent or rudimentary	Present
Language abnormalities (e.g., echolalia, stereotyped phrases out of context)	More common	Less common
Articulatory problems	Less frequent	More frequent
Level of intelligence	Often severely impaired	Although may be impaired, less frequently severe
Patterns of intelligence quotient (IQ) tests	Uneven, lower on verbal scores than dysphasic patients, lower on comprehension subtest than dysphasic patients	More even, although verbal IQ lower than performance IQ
Autistic behaviors, impaired social life, stereotypies, and ritualistic activities	More common and more severe	Absent or, if present, less severe
Imaginative play	Absent or rudimentary	Usually present

(Adapted from Magda Campbell, M.D., and Wayne Green, M.D.)

importantly, audiogram or auditory-evoked potentials indicate significant hearing loss in deaf children. Unlike autistic children, deaf children usually relate to their parents, seek their affection, and enjoy being held as infants.

Psychosocial Deprivation. Severe disturbances in the physical and emotional environment (e.g., maternal deprivation, psychosocial dwarfism, hospitalism, and failure to thrive) can cause children to appear apathetic, withdrawn, and alienated. Language and motor skills can be delayed. Children with these signs almost always improve rapidly when placed in a favorable and enriched psychosocial environment, but such improvement is not the case with autistic children.

Course and Prognosis

Autistic disorder is generally a lifelong disorder with a guarded prognosis. Autistic children with IQs above 70 and those who use communicative language by ages 5 to 7 years tend to have the best prognoses. Recent follow-up data comparing high-IQ autistic children at the age of 5 years with their current symptomatology at ages 13 through young adulthood found that a small proportion no longer met criteria for autism, although they still exhibited some features of the disorder. Most demonstrated positive changes in communication and social domains over time.

The symptom areas that did not seem to improve over time were those related to ritualistic and repetitive behaviors. In general, adult-outcome studies indicate that about two thirds of autistic adults remain severely handicapped and live in complete dependence or semidependence, either with their relatives or in long-term institutions. Only 1 to 2 percent acquires a normal, independent status with gainful employment, and 5 to 20 percent achieve a borderline normal status. The prognosis is improved if the environment or home is supportive and capable of meeting the extensive needs of such a child. Although symptoms decrease in many cases, severe self-mutilation or aggressiveness and regression may develop in others. About 4 to 32 percent have grand mal seizures in late childhood or adolescence, and the seizures adversely affect the prognosis.

Treatment

The goals of treatment for children with autistic disorder are to target behaviors that will improve their abilities to integrate into schools, develop meaningful peer relationships, and increase the likelihood of maintaining independent living as adults. To do this, treatment interventions aim to increase socially acceptable and prosocial behavior, to decrease odd behavioral symptoms, and to improve verbal and nonverbal communication. Both language and academic remediation are often required. In addition, treatment goals generally include reduction of disruptive behaviors that may be exacerbated especially during transitions and in school. Children with mental retardation need intellectually appropriate behavioral interventions to reinforce socially acceptable behaviors and encourage self-care skills. In addition, parents, often distraught, need support and counseling. Insight-oriented individual psychotherapy has proved ineffective. Educational and behavioral interventions are currently considered the treatments of choice. Structured classroom training, in combination with behavioral methods, is the most effective treatment for many autistic children.

Well-controlled studies indicate that gains in the areas of language and cognition and decreases in maladaptive behaviors are achieved by consistent behavioral programs. Careful training of parents in the concepts and skills of behavior modification and resolution of the parents' concerns may yield considerable gains in children's language, and cognitive and social areas of behavior. These training programs, however, are rigorous and require much parental time. An autistic child requires as much structure as possible, and a daily program for as many hours as feasible is desirable.

Facilitated communication is a technique by which an autistic or a mentally retarded child with some language is aided in communication by a teacher who helps the child pick out letters on a computer or letter board. Some facilitators have reported success in eliciting language to produce messages demonstrating a child's ability to read and write, to do mathematics, to express feelings, and even to write poetry. Although these techniques are risky, because the facilitator may need to inject much interpretation to produce typical communication, some families of autistic children support this technique and continue to use it.

Current psychopharmacologic trials are under way to investigate efficacy of a variety of classes of agents on promoting social interactions and reducing disruptive behaviors in children and adolescents with autism and other pervasive developmental disorders. Currently, no specific medications with proved efficacy in the treatment of the core symptoms of autistic disorder are available; however medications have been shown to be promising in reducing hyperactivity, obsessions and compulsive behaviors, irritability, aggression, and self-injurious behaviors.

A recent open trial of escitalopram (Lexapro) in children with pervasive developmental disorders showed a trend toward improvement in 61 percent of subjects on the following subscales of the *Aberrant Behavior Checklist-Community Version* (ABC-CV) *Irritability, Lethargy, Stereotypy, Hyperactivity, and Inappropriate Speech.* Although irritability was the main outcome variable, the other domains were also rated as improved.

A recent randomized, controlled, crossover trial of methylphenidate (Ritalin) in 72 children between the ages of 5 and 14 years with pervasive developmental disorders and hyperactivity revealed that methylphenidate was superior to placebo in the treatment of hyperactivity in 49 percent of the subjects. Although this response rate is substantially lower than for children with ADHD without pervasive developmental disorders, response rate was significant in almost half of the sample. Adverse effects led to discontinuation of medication in 18 percent of the subjects, which is higher than expected for children with ADHD without pervasive developmental disorders.

The administration of antipsychotic medication has been shown to be efficacious in the reduction of aggressive and self-injurious behavior. One early study indicated that haloperidol (Haldol) reduced behavioral symptoms such as hyperactivity, stereotypies, withdrawal, fidgetiness, irritability, and labile affect and accelerated learning. Given its potentially serious adverse effects, haloperidol is no longer the antipsychotic agent of choice in the treatment of self-injurious behaviors in children with autistic disorder.

The atypical antipsychotic agents are known to have a lower risk of causing extrapyramidal adverse effects, although some sensitive individuals cannot tolerate the extrapyramidal or anticholinergic adverse effects of the atypical antipsychotic agents. The atypical antipsychotic agents include risperidone (Risperdal), olanzapine (Zyprexa), quetiapine (Seroquel), clozapine (Clozaril), and ziprasidone (Geodon).

Risperidone, a high-potency antipsychotic with combined dopamine D_2 and serotonin 5-HT_2 receptor antagonist properties, has been used to subdue aggressive or self-injurious behaviors. Several reports have suggested that risperidone is effective in diminishing aggressiveness, hyperactivity, and self-injurious behavior in children with autistic disorder. In some cases, it reportedly encouraged socially acceptable behaviors. Studies of risperidone use in the treatment of adult and adolescent psychosis indicate that a dosage up to 4 to 6 mg per day may be necessary for optional effect. For children with autism, lower dosages ranging from 0.5 to 4 mg per day are used in clinical practice. Extrapyramidal effects and akathisia have been reported adverse effects, as well as sedation, dizziness, and weight gain. A recent report on acute and long-term safety and tolerability of risperidone in children with autism documented the following side effects as moderate or higher in children on placebo versus risperidone: Somnolence (12 percent vs. 37 percent), excessive appetite (10 percent vs. 33 percent), and rhinitis (8 percent vs. 16 percent). Drooling was reported more in the risperidone group compared with the placebo group. In this sample, extrapyramidal symptoms were not reported more commonly in the risperidone group. The side effects that caused the most concern were somnolence and weight gain.

Olanzapine specifically blocks 5-HT_{2A} and D_2 receptors and also blocks muscarinic receptors. No studies provide specific guidelines regarding the use of olanzapine in children with autism. Dosages that have been used clinically to target aggression and self-injurious behaviors range from 2.5 to about 10 mg per day. Among olanzapine's most common adverse effects are sedation, orthostatic hypotension, and (over time) weight gain.

Quetiapine is an antipsychotic with more potent 5-H_2 than D_2 receptor blocking properties. Although no data on its effectiveness on aggression in children with autism exist, it is sometimes tried when risperidone and olanzapine are not efficacious or well tolerated. No guidelines exist about best dosage; it has been used in clinical practice at dosages ranging from 50 to 200 mg per day. Adverse effects include drowsiness, tachycardia, agitation, and weight gain.

Clozapine has a heterocyclic chemical structure that is related to certain conventional antipsychotics, such as loxapine (Loxitane), although clozapine carries a lower risk of extrapyramidal symptoms. It is not generally used in the treatment of aggression and self-injurious behavior unless those behaviors coexist with psychotic symptoms. Its most serious adverse effect is agranulocytosis, which necessitates monitoring white blood cell count weekly during clozapine's use. Its use is generally limited to treatment-resistant psychotic patients.

Ziprasidone has receptor-blocking properties at the 5-HT_{2A} and D_2 receptor sites and carries little risk of extrapyramidal and antihistaminic effects. No guidelines exist for its use in autistic children with aggressive and self-injurious behaviors, but it has been used clinically to treat the latter behaviors in children who are treatment resistant. In studies of its use in adults with schizophrenia, dosage ranges of 40 to 160 mg were found to be effective. Adverse effects include sedation, dizziness, and lightheadedness. An electrocardiogram (ECG) is generally obtained before use of this medication.

Lithium (Eskalith) can be administered in the treatment of aggressive or self-injurious behaviors when antipsychotic medications fail.

A recent double-blind study investigated the efficacy of amantadine (Symmetrel), which blocks *N*-methyl-D-aspartate (NMDA) receptors, in the treatment of behavioral disturbance, such as irritability, aggression, and hyperactivity in children with autism. Some have suggested that abnormalities of the glutamatergic system may contribute to the emergence of pervasive developmental disorders. High glutamate levels have been found in children with Rett's syndrome. In the amantadine study, 47 percent of children on amantadine were rated "improved" by their parents, and 37 percent of children on placebo were rated "improved" by parents in irritability and hyperactivity, although this difference was not statistically significant. Investigators rated the children on amantadine "significantly improved" with respect to hyperactivity. A double-blind, placebo-controlled study of the efficacy of the anticonvulsant lamotrigine (Lamictal) on hyperactivity in children with autism showed high rates of placebo improvement in ratings of hyperactivity.

Clomipramine (Anafranil) has been used in autistic disorders, but without positive results. Fenfluramine (Pondimin), which reduces blood serotonin levels, has also been used unsuccessfully in the treatment of autism. Improvement does not seem to be associated with a reduction in blood serotonin level. Naltrexone (ReVia), an opioid receptor antagonist, has been investigated without much success, based on the notion that blocking endogenous opioids would reduce autistic symptoms.

Tetrahydrobiopterin, a coenzyme that enhances the action of enzymes, has recently been used in a double-blind placebo-controlled crossover study of 12 children with autistic disorder and low concentrations of spinal tetrahydrobiopterin. The children received a daily dose of 3 mg tetrahydrobiopterin per kilogram during a 6-month period alternating with placebo. Results indicated small, nonsignificant changes in the total scores on the *Childhood Autism Rating Scale* after 3- and 6-month treatment. Post hoc analysis of the three core symptoms of autism—social interaction, communication, and stereotyped behaviors—revealed a significant improvement in social interaction score after 6 months of active treatment. A positive correlation was noted between social response and IQ. These results suggest that there is a possible effect of tetrahydrobiopterin on the social functioning of children with autism.

A recent case report suggested that low-dose venlafaxine (Effexor) was efficacious in three adolescents and young adults with autistic disorder with self-injurious behavior and hyperactivity. Dose of venlafaxine used was 18.75 mg per day, and efficacy was reported to be sustained over a 6-month period.

RETT'S DISORDER

In 1965, Andreas Rett, an Australian physician, identified a syndrome in 22 girls who appeared to have developed normally for at least 6-months followed by devastating developmental deterioration. Rett's disorder is a progressive condition that has its onset after some months of what appears to be normal development. Head circumference is normal at birth and developmental milestones are unremarkable in early life. Between 5 and 48 months of age, generally between 6 months and a year, head growth begins to decelerate.

Available data indicate a prevalence of 6 to 7 cases of Rett's disorder per 100,000 girls. Originally, it was believed that Rett's disorder occurred only in females, but males with the disorder or syndromes that are very close to this disorder have now been described.

Etiology

The cause of Rett's disorder is unknown, although the progressive deteriorating course after an initial normal period is compatible with a metabolic disorder. In some patients with Rett's disorder, the presence of hyperammonemia has led to postulation that an enzyme metabolizing ammonia is deficient, but hyperammonemia has not been found in most patients with Rett's disorder. It is likely that Rett's disorder has a genetic basis. It has been seen primarily in girls, and case reports so far indicate complete concordance in monozygotic twins.

Diagnosis and Clinical Features

During the first 5 months after birth, infants have age-appropriate motor skills, normal head circumference, and normal growth. Social interactions show the expected reciprocal quality. At 6 months to 2 years of age, however, these children develop progressive encephalopathy with a number of characteristic features. The signs often include the loss of purposeful hand movements, which are replaced by stereotypic motions, such as handwringing; the loss of previously acquired speech; psychomotor retardation; and ataxia. Other stereotypical hand movements may occur, such as licking or biting the fingers and tapping or slapping. The head circumference growth decelerates and produces microcephaly. All language skills are lost, and both receptive and expressive communicative and social skills seem to plateau at developmental levels between 6 months and 1 year. Poor muscle coordination and an apraxic gait with an unsteady and stiff quality develop. All of these clinical features are diagnostic criteria for the disorder (Table 42–5).

Associated features include seizures in up to 75 percent of affected children and disorganized EEGs with some epileptiform discharges in almost all young children with Rett's disorder, even in the absence of clinical seizures. An additional associated feature is irregular respiration, with episodes of hyperventilation, apnea, and breath holding. The disorganized breathing occurs in most patients while they are awake; during sleep, the breathing usually normalizes. Many patients with Rett's disorder also have scoliosis. As the disorder progresses, muscle tone seems

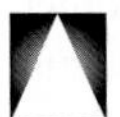

Table 42–5
DSM-IV-TR Diagnostic Criteria for Rett's Disorder

A. All of the following:
   (1) apparently normal prenatal and perinatal development
   (2) apparently normal psychomotor development through the first 5 months after birth
   (3) normal head circumference at birth
B. Onset of all of the following after the period of normal development:
   (1) deceleration of head growth between ages 5 and 48 months
   (2) loss of previously acquired purposeful hand skills between ages 5 and 30 months with the subsequent development of stereotyped hand movements (e.g., hand wringing or hand washing)
   (3) loss of social engagement early in the course (although often social interaction develops later)
   (4) appearance of poorly coordinated gait or trunk movements
   (5) severely impaired expressive and receptive language development with severe psychomotor retardation

(From American Psychiatric Association. *Diagnostic and Statistical Manual of Mental Disorders*. 4th ed. Text rev. Washington, DC: American Psychiatric Association; copyright 2000, with permission.)

to change from an initial hypotonic condition to spasticity to rigidity.

Although children with Rett's disorder may live for well over a decade after the onset of the disorder, after 10 years, many patients are wheelchair-bound, with muscle wasting, rigidity, and virtually no language ability. Long-term receptive and expressive communication and socialization abilities remain at a developmental level of less than 1 year.

Darla was born at term after an uncomplicated pregnancy. An amniocentesis had been obtained because of maternal age and was normal. At birth, Darla was in good condition; weight, height, and head circumference were all near the 50th percentile. Her development during the first months of life was within normal limits. At approximately 8 months of age, her development seemed to stagnate and her interest in the environment, including the social environment, waned. Her developmental milestones then became markedly delayed; she was just starting to walk at her second birthday and had no spoken language. Evaluation at that time revealed that head growth had decelerated. Some self-stimulatory behaviors were present. Marked cognitive and communicative delays were noted on formal testing. Darla began to lose purposeful hand movements and developed unusual hand-washing stereotyped behaviors. By age 6, her EEG was abnormal and purposeful hand movements were markedly impaired. Subsequently, she developed truncal ataxia and breath-holding spells, and motor skills deteriorated further. (Courtesy of Fred Volkmar, M.D.)

Differential Diagnosis

Some children with Rett's disorder receive initial diagnoses of autistic disorder because of the marked disability in social interactions in both disorders, but the two disorders have some predictable differences. In Rett's disorder, a child shows deterioration of developmental milestones, head circumference, and overall growth; in autistic disorder, aberrant development is usually present from early on. In Rett's disorder, specific and characteristic hand motions are always present; in autistic disorder, hand mannerisms may or may not appear. Poor coordination, ataxia, and apraxia are predictably part of Rett's disorder; many persons with autistic disorder have unremarkable gross motor function. In Rett's disorder, verbal abilities are usually lost completely; in autistic disorder, patients use characteristically aberrant language. Respiratory irregularity is characteristic of Rett's disorder, and seizures often appear early; in autistic disorder, no respiratory disorganization is seen, and seizures do not develop in most patients; when seizures do develop, they are more likely in adolescence than in childhood.

Course and Prognosis

Rett's disorder is progressive. The prognosis is not fully known, but patients who live into adulthood remain at a cognitive and social level equivalent to that in the first year of life.

Treatment

Treatment is symptomatic. Physiotherapy has been beneficial for the muscular dysfunction, and anticonvulsant treatment is usually necessary to control the seizures. Behavior therapy, along with medication, may help control self-injurious behaviors, as it does in the treatment of autistic disorder, and it may help regulate the breathing disorganization.

CHILDHOOD DISINTEGRATIVE DISORDER

Childhood disintegrative disorder is characterized by marked regression in several areas of functioning after at least 2 years of apparently normal development. Childhood disintegrative disorder, also called *Heller's syndrome* and *disintegrative psychosis*, was described in 1908 as a deterioration over several months of intellectual, social, and language function occurring in 3- and 4-year-olds with previously normal functions. After the deterioration, the children closely resembled children with autistic disorder.

Epidemiology

Epidemiological data have been complicated by the variable diagnostic criteria used, but childhood disintegrative disorder is estimated to be at least one tenth as common as autistic disorder, and the prevalence has been estimated to be about 1 case in 100,000 boys. The ratio of boys to girls is estimated to be between 4 and 8 boys to 1 girl.

Etiology

The cause of childhood disintegrative disorder is unknown, but it has been associated with other neurological conditions, including seizure disorders, tuberous sclerosis, and various metabolic disorders.

Diagnosis and Clinical Features

The diagnosis is made on the basis of features that fit a characteristic age of onset, clinical picture, and course. Cases reported have ranged in onset from ages 1 to 9 years, but in most, the onset is between 3 and 4 years; according to DSM-IV-TR, the minimum age of onset is 2 years (Table 42–6). The onset may be insidious over several months or relatively abrupt, with abilities diminishing in days or weeks. In some cases, a child displays restlessness, increased activity level, and anxiety before the loss of function. The core features of the disorder include loss of communication skills, marked regression of reciprocal interactions, and the onset of stereotyped movements and compulsive behavior. Affective symptoms are common, particularly anxiety, as is the regression of self-help skills, such as bowel and bladder control.

To receive the diagnosis, a child must exhibit loss of skills in two of the following areas: language, social or adaptive behavior; bowel or bladder control; play; and motor skills. Abnormalities must be present in at least two of the following categories: reciprocal social interaction, communication skills, and stereotyped or restricted behavior. The main neurological associated feature is seizure disorder.

Bob's early history was within normal limits. By age 2, he was speaking in sentences, and his development appeared to be proceeding appropriately. At age 40 months he abruptly exhibited a

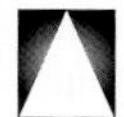

Table 42–6
DSM-IV-TR Diagnostic Criteria for Childhood Disintegrative Disorder

A. Apparently normal development for at least the first 2 years after birth as manifested by the presence of age-appropriate verbal and nonverbal communication, social relationships, play, and adaptive behavior.
B. Clinically significant loss of previously acquired skills (before age 10 years) in at least two of the following areas:
 (1) expressive or receptive language
 (2) social skills or adaptive behavior
 (3) bowel or bladder control
 (4) play
 (5) motor skills
C. Abnormalities of functioning in at least two of the following areas:
 (1) qualitative impairment in social interaction (e.g., impairment in nonverbal behaviors, failure to develop peer relationships, lack of social or emotional reciprocity)
 (2) qualitative impairments in communication (e.g., delay or lack of spoken language, inability to initiate or sustain a conversation, stereotyped and repetitive use of language, lack of varied make-believe play)
 (3) restricted, repetitive, and stereotyped patterns of behavior, interests, and activities, including motor stereotypies and mannerisms
D. The disturbance is not better accounted for by another specific pervasive developmental disorder or by schizophrenia.

(From American Psychiatric Association. *Diagnostic and Statistical Manual of Mental Disorders.* 4th ed. Text rev. Washington, DC: American Psychiatric Association; copyright 2000, with permission.)

period of marked behavioral regression shortly after the birth of a sibling. He lost previously acquired skills in communication and was no longer toilet trained. He became uninterested in social interaction, and various unusual self-stimulatory behaviors became evident. Comprehensive medical examination failed to reveal any conditions that might account for this developmental regression. Behaviorally, he exhibited features of autistic disorder. At follow-up at age 12 he spoke only an occasional single word and was severely retarded. (Courtesy of Fred Volkmar, M.D.)

Differential Diagnosis

The differential diagnosis of childhood disintegrative disorder includes autistic disorder and Rett's disorder. In many cases, the clinical features overlap with autistic disorder, but childhood disintegrative disorder is distinguished from autistic disorder by the loss of previously acquired development. Before the onset of childhood disintegrative disorder (occurring at 2 years or older), language has usually progressed to sentence formation. This skill is strikingly different from the premorbid history of even high-functioning patients with autistic disorder, in whom language generally does not exceed single words or phrases before diagnosis of the disorder. Once the disorder occurs, however, those with childhood disintegrative disorder are more likely to have no language abilities than are high-functioning patients with autistic disorder. In Rett's disorder, the deterioration occurs much earlier than in childhood disintegrative disorder, and the characteristic hand stereotypies of Rett's disorder do not occur in childhood disintegrative disorder.

Course and Prognosis

The course of childhood disintegrative disorder is variable, with a plateau reached in most cases, a progressive deteriorating course in rare cases, and some improvement in occasional cases to the point of regaining the ability to speak in sentences. Most patients are left with at least moderate mental retardation.

Treatment

Because of the clinical similarity to autistic disorder, the treatment of childhood disintegrative disorder includes the same components available in the treatment of autistic disorder.

ASPERGER'S DISORDER

Asperger's disorder is characterized by impairment and oddity of social interaction and restricted interest and behavior reminiscent of those seen in autistic disorder. Unlike autistic disorder, in Asperger's disorder no significant delays occur in language, cognitive development, or age-appropriate self-help skills. In 1944, Hans Asperger, an Austrian physician, described a syndrome that he named "autistic psychopathy." His original description of the syndrome applied to persons with normal intelligence who exhibit a qualitative impairment in reciprocal social interaction and behavioral oddities without delays in language development. Asperger's disorder occurs in a wide variety of severities, including cases in which very subtle social cues are missed, but overall social interactions are mastered.

Etiology

The cause of Asperger's disorder is unknown, but family studies suggest a possible relationship to autistic disorder. The similarity of Asperger's disorder to autistic disorder supports the presence of genetic, metabolic, infectious, and perinatal contributing factors.

Diagnosis and Clinical Features

The clinical features include at least two of the following indications of qualitative social impairment: Markedly abnormal nonverbal communicative gestures, the failure to develop peer relationships, the lack of social or emotional reciprocity, and an impaired ability to express pleasure in other persons' happiness. Restricted interests and patterns of behavior are always present, but when they are subtle, they may not be immediately identified or singled out as different from those of other children. According to DSM-IV-TR, the patient shows no language delay, clinically significant cognitive delay, or adaptive impairment (Table 42–7).

Tom was an only child. Birth, medical, and family histories were unremarkable. His motor development was somewhat delayed, but communicative milestones were within normal limits. His parents became concerned about him at age 4 when he was enrolled in a

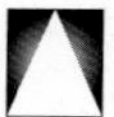

Table 42–7
DSM-IV-TR Diagnostic Criteria for Asperger's Disorder

A. Qualitative impairment in social interaction, as manifested by at least two of the following:
 (1) marked impairment in the use of multiple nonverbal behaviors such as eye-to-eye gaze, facial expression, body postures, and gestures to regulate social interaction
 (2) failure to develop peer relationships appropriate to developmental level
 (3) a lack of spontaneous seeking to share enjoyment, interests, or achievements with other people (e.g., by a lack of showing, bringing, or pointing out objects of interest to other people)
 (4) lack of social or emotional reciprocity

B. Restricted repetitive and stereotyped patterns of behavior, interests, and activities, as manifested by at least one of the following:
 (1) encompassing preoccupation with one or more stereotyped and restricted patterns of interest that is abnormal either in intensity or focus
 (2) apparently inflexible adherence to specific, nonfunctional routines or rituals
 (3) stereotyped and repetitive motor mannerisms (e.g., hand or finger flapping or twisting, or complex whole-body movements)
 (4) persistent preoccupation with parts of objects

C. The disturbance causes clinically significant impairment in social, occupational, or other important areas of functioning.

D. There is no clinically significant general delay in language (e.g., single words used by age 2 years, communicative phrases used by age 3 years).

E. There is no clinically significant delay in cognitive development or in the development of age-appropriate self-help skills, adaptive behavior (other than in social interaction), and curiosity about the environment in childhood.

F. Criteria are not met for another specific pervasive developmental disorder or schizophrenia.

(From American Psychiatric Association. *Diagnostic and Statistical Manual of Mental Disorders.* 4th ed. Text rev. Washington, DC: American Psychiatric Association; copyright 2000, with permission.)

nursery school and was noted to have marked difficulties in peer interaction that were so pronounced that he could not continue in the program. In grade school, he was enrolled in special education classes and was noted to have some learning problems. His greatest difficulties arose in peer interaction—he was viewed as markedly eccentric and had no friends. His preferred activity, watching the weather channel on television, was pursued with great interest and intensity. On examination at age 13, he had markedly circumscribed interests and exhibited pedantic and odd patterns of communication with a monotonic voice quality. Psychological testing revealed an IQ within the normal range, with marked scatter evident. Formal communication examination revealed age-appropriate skills in receptive and expressive language but marked impairment in pragmatic language skills. (Courtesy of Fred Volkmar, M.D.)

Differential Diagnosis

The differential diagnosis includes autistic disorder, pervasive developmental disorder not otherwise specified, and, in patients approaching adulthood, schizoid personality disorder. According to DSM-IV-TR, the most obvious distinctions between Asperger's disorder and autistic disorder are the absence of language delay and dysfunction. The lack of language delay and impaired use of language are requirements for Asperger's disorder, whereas language impairment is a core feature in autistic disorder. Recent studies comparing children with Asperger's disorder and autistic disorder find that children with Asperger's disorder were more likely to look for social interaction and sought more vigorously to make friends. Although significant general delay in language is an exclusionary criterion in the diagnosis of Asperger's disorder, some delay in the acquisition of language has been seen in more than one third of clinical samples.

Course and Prognosis

Although little is known about the cohort described by the DSM-IV-TR diagnostic criteria, past case reports have shown variable courses and prognoses for patients who have received diagnoses of Asperger's disorder. The factors associated with a good prognosis are a normal IQ and high-level social skills. Anecdotal reports of some adults diagnosed with Asperger's disorder as children show them to be verbal and intelligent; however, they relate in an awkward way to other adults, appear socially uncomfortable and shy, and often exhibit illogical thinking.

Treatment

Treatment of Asperger's disorder is supportive, and goals are to promote social behaviors and peer relationships. Interventions are initiated with the goal of shaping interactions so that they better match those of peers. Very often children with Asperger's disorder are highly verbal and have excellent academic achievement. The tendency of children and adolescents with Asperger's disorder to rely on rigid rules and routines can become a source of difficulty for them and be an area that requires therapeutic intervention. A comfort with routines, however, can be utilized to foster positive habits that may enhance the social life of a child with Asperger's disorder. Self-sufficiency and problem-solving techniques are often helpful for these individuals in social situations and in a work setting. Some of the same techniques

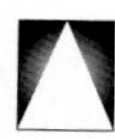

Table 42–8
DSM-IV-TR Diagnostic Criteria for Pervasive Developmental Disorder Not Otherwise Specified (Including Atypical Autism)

This category should be used when there is a severe and pervasive impairment in the development of reciprocal social interaction associated with impairment in either verbal or nonverbal communication skills or with the presence of stereotyped behavior, interests, and activities, but the criteria are not met for a specific pervasive developmental disorder, schizophrenia, schizotypal personality disorder, or avoidant personality disorder. For example, this category includes "atypical autism"—presentations that do not meet the criteria for autistic disorder because of late age at onset, atypical symptomatology, or subthreshold symptomatology, or all of these.

(From American Psychiatric Association. *Diagnostic and Statistical Manual of Mental Disorders.* 4th ed. Text rev. Washington, DC: American Psychiatric Association; copyright 2000, with permission.)

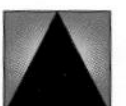

Table 42–9
ICD-10 Diagnostic Criteria for Pervasive Developmental Disorders

Childhood autism

A. Abnormal or impaired development is evident before the age of 3 years in at least one of the following areas:
(1) receptive or expressive language as used in social communication;
(2) the development of selective social attachments or of reciprocal social interaction;
(3) functional or symbolic play.

B. A total of at least six symptoms from (1), (2), and (3) must be present, with at least two from (1) and at least one from each of (2) and (3):
(1) Qualitative abnormalities in reciprocal social interaction are manifest in at least two of the following areas:
(a) failure adequately to use eye-to-eye gaze, facial expression, body posture, and gesture to regulate social interaction;
(b) failure to develop (in a manner appropriate to mental age, and despite ample opportunities) peer relationships that involve a mutual sharing of interests, activities, and emotions;
(c) lack of socioemotional reciprocity as shown by an impaired or deviant response to other people's emotions; or lack of modulation of behavior according to social context; or a weak integration of social, emotional, and communicative behaviors;
(d) lack of spontaneous seeking to share enjoyment, interests, or achievements with other people (e.g., a lack of showing, bringing, or pointing out to other people objects of interest to the individual).
(2) Qualitative abnormalities in communication are manifest in at least one of the following areas:
(a) a delay in, or total lack of, development of spoken language that is not accompanied by an attempt to compensate through the use of gesture or mime as an alternative mode of communication (often preceded by a lack of communicative babbling);
(b) relative failure to initiate or sustain conversational interchange (at whatever level of language skills is present), in which there is reciprocal responsiveness to the communications of the other person;
(c) stereotyped and repetitive use of language or idiosyncratic use of words or phrases;
(d) lack of varied spontaneous make-believe or (when young) social imitative play.
(3) Restricted, repetitive, and stereotyped patterns of behavior, interests, and activities are manifest in at least one of the following areas:
(a) an encompassing preoccupation with one or more stereotyped and restricted patterns of interest that are abnormal in content or focus; or one or more interests that are abnormal in their intensity and circumscribed nature though not in their content or focus;
(b) apparently compulsive adherence to specific, nonfunctional routines or rituals;
(c) stereotyped and repetitive motor mannerisms that involve either hand or finger flapping or twisting, or complex whole body movements;
(d) preoccupations with part-objects or nonfunctional elements of play materials (such as their odor, the feel of their surface, or the noise or vibration that they generate).

C. The clinical picture is not attributable to the other varieties of pervasive developmental disorder: specific developmental disorder of receptive language with secondary socioemotional problems; reactive attachment disorder or disinhibited attachment disorder, mental retardation with some associated emotional or behavioral disorder; schizophrenia of unusually early onset; and Rett's syndrome.

Atypical autism

A. Abnormal or impaired development is evident at or after the age of 3 years (criteria as for autism except for age of manifestation).

B. There are qualitative abnormalities in reciprocal social interaction or in communication, or restricted, repetitive, and stereotyped patterns of behavior, interests, and activities. (Criteria as for autism except that it is unnecessary to meet the criteria for number of areas of abnormality.)

C. The disorder does not meet the diagnostic criteria for autism. Autism may be atypical in either age of onset or symptomatology; the two types are differentiated with a fifth character for research purposes. Syndromes that are atypical in both respects should be coded. Atypicality in both ages of onset and symptomatology.

Atypicality in age of onset

A. The disorder does not meet Criterion A for autism; that is, abnormal or impaired development is evident only at or after the age of 3 years.

B. The disorder meets Criteria B and C for autism.

Atypicality in symptomatology

A. The disorder meets Criterion A for autism; that is, abnormal or impaired development is evident before the age of 3 years.

B. There are qualitative abnormalities in reciprocal social interactions or in communication, or restricted, repetitive, and stereotyped patterns of behavior, interests, and activities. (Criteria as for autism except that it is unnecessary to meet the criteria for number of areas of abnormality.)

C. The disorder meets Criterion C for autism.

D. The disorder does not fully meet Criterion B for autism.

Atypicality in both age of onset and symptomatology

A. The disorder does not meet Criterion A for autism; that is, abnormal or impaired development is evident only at or after the age of 3 years.

B. There are qualitative abnormalities in reciprocal social interactions or in communication, or restricted, repetitive, and stereotyped patterns of behavior, interests, and activities. (Criteria as for autism except that it is unnecessary to meet the criteria for number of areas of abnormality.)

C. The disorder meets Criterion C for autism.

D. The disorder does not fully meet Criterion B for autism.

Rett's syndrome

A. There is an apparently normal prenatal and perinatal period *and* apparently normal psychomotor development through the first 5 months *and* normal head circumference at birth.

B. There is deceleration of head growth between 5 months and 4 years *and* loss of acquired purposeful hand skills between 5 and 30 months of age that is associated with concurrent communication dysfunction and impaired social interactions and the appearance of poorly coordinated/unstable gait and/or trunk movements.

C. There is severe impairment of expressive and receptive language, together with severe psychomotor retardation.

D. There are stereotyped midline hand movements (such as hand-wringing or "hand-washing") with an onset at or after the time when purposeful hand movements are lost.

(*continued*)

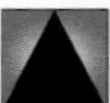

Table 42–9
(Continued)

Other childhood disintegrative disorder

A. Development is apparently normal up to the age of at least 2 years. The presence of normal age-appropriate skills in communication, social relationships, play, and adaptive behavior at age 2 years or later is required for diagnosis.

B. There is a definite loss of previously acquired skills at about the time of onset of the disorder. The diagnosis requires a clinically significant loss of skills (not just a failure to use them in certain situations) in at least two of the following areas:
(1) expressive or receptive language;
(2) play;
(3) social skills or adaptive behavior;
(4) bowel or bladder control;
(5) motor skills.

C. Qualitatively abnormal social functioning is manifest in at least two of the following areas:
(1) qualitative abnormalities in reciprocal social interaction (of the type defined for autism);
(2) qualitative abnormalities in communication (of the type defined for autism);
(3) restricted, repetitive, and stereotyped patterns of behavior, interests, and activities, including motor stereotypies and mannerisms;
(4) a general loss of interest in objects and in the environment.

D. The disorder is not attributable to the other varieties of pervasive developmental disorder; acquired aphasia with epilepsy; elective mutism; Rett's syndrome; or schizophrenia.

Overactive disorder associated with mental retardation and stereotyped movements

A. Severe motor hyperactivity is manifest by at least two of the following problems in activity and attention:
(1) continuous motor restlessness, manifest in running, jumping, and other movements of the whole body;
(2) marked difficulty in remaining seated: the child will ordinarily remain seated for a few seconds at most except when engaged in a stereotypic activity (see Criterion B);
(3) grossly excessive activity in situations where relative stillness is expected;
(4) very rapid changes of activity, so that activities generally last for less than a minute (occasional longer periods spent in highly favored activities do not exclude this, and very long periods spent in stereotypic activities can also be compatible with the presence of this problem at other times).

B. Repetitive and stereotyped patterns of behavior and activity are manifest by at least one of the following:
(1) fixed and frequently repeated motor mannerisms: these may involve either complex movements of the whole body or partial movements such as hand-flapping;
(2) excessive and nonfunctional repetition of activities that are constant in form: this may be play with a single object (e.g., running water) or a ritual of activities (either alone or involving other people);
(3) repetitive self-injury.

C. IQ is less than 50.

D. There is no social impairment of the autistic type, i.e., the child must show at least three of the following:
(1) developmentally appropriate use of eye gaze, expression, and posture to regulate social interaction;
(2) developmentally appropriate peer relationships that include sharing of interests, activities, etc.;
(3) approaches to other people, at least sometimes, for comfort and affection;
(4) ability to share other people's enjoyment at times; other forms of social impairment, e.g., a disinhibited approach to strangers, are compatible with the diagnosis.

E. The disorder does not meet diagnostic criteria for autism, childhood disintegrative disorder, or hyperkinetic disorders.

Asperger's syndrome

A. There is no clinically significant general delay in spoken or receptive language or cognitive development. Diagnosis requires that single words should have developed by 2 years of age or earlier and that communicative phrases be used by 3 years of age or earlier. Self-help skills, adaptive behavior, and curiosity about the environment during the first 3 years should be at a level consistent with normal intellectual development. However, motor milestones may be somewhat delayed and motor clumsiness is usual (although not a necessary diagnostic feature). Isolated special skills, often related to abnormal preoccupations, are common, but are not required for diagnosis.

B. There are qualitative abnormalities in reciprocal social interaction (criteria as for autism).

C. The individual exhibits an unusually intense, circumscribed interest or restricted, repetitive, and stereotyped patterns of behavior, interests, and activities (criteria as for autism; however, it would be less usual for these to include either motor mannerisms or preoccupations with part-objects or nonfunctional elements of play materials).

D. The disorder is not attributable to the other varieties of pervasive developmental disorder: simple schizophrenia; schizotypal disorder; obsessive-compulsive disorder; anakastic personality disorder; reactive and disinhibited attachment disorders of childhood.

Other pervasive developmental disorders
Pervasive developmental disorder, unspecified

This is a residual diagnostic category that should be used for disorders which fit the general description for pervasive developmental disorders but in which contradictory findings or a lack of adequate information mean that the criteria for any of the other pervasive developmental disorders codes cannot be met.

(From World Health Organization. *The ICD-10 Classification of Mental and Behavioral Disorders: Diagnostic Criteria for Research*. Copyright, World Health Organization, Geneva, 1993, with permission.)

used for autistic disorder are likely to benefit patients with Asperger's disorder with severe social impairment.

PERVASIVE DEVELOPMENTAL DISORDER NOT OTHERWISE SPECIFIED

The DSM-IV-TR defines pervasive disorder not otherwise specified as severe, pervasive impairment in communication skills or the presence of stereotyped behavior, interests, and activities with associated impairment in social interactions. The criteria for a specific pervasive developmental disorder, schizophrenia, and schizotypal and avoidant personality disorders are not met, however (Table 42–8). Some children who receive the diagnosis exhibit a markedly restricted repertoire of activities and interest. The condition usually shows a better outcome than autistic disorder.

Leslie was the oldest of two children. She had been a difficult baby who was not easy to console but whose motor and communicative development seemed appropriate. She was socially related and sometimes enjoyed interaction, but was easily overstimulated. She exhibited some hand flapping. Her parents sought evaluation when she was 4 years of age because of difficulties in nursery school. Leslie had problems with peer interaction. She was often preoccupied with possible adverse events. At evaluation she displayed both communicative and cognitive functions within the normal range. Although differential social relatedness was present, Leslie had difficulty using her parents as sources of support and comfort. She displayed behavioral rigidity and a tendency to impose routines on social skills. Subsequently, she was placed in a transitional kindergarten and did well academically although problems in peer interactions and unusual affective responses persisted. As an adolescent, she describes herself as a "loner" who has difficulties with social interaction and tends to enjoy solitary activities. (Courtesy of Fred Volkmar, M.D.)

Treatment

The treatment approach is basically the same as in autistic disorder. Mainstreaming in school may be possible. Compared with autistic children, those with pervasive developmental disorder not otherwise specified generally have better language skills and more self-awareness, so they are better candidates for psychotherapy.

ICD-10

As the description of pervasive developmental disorders in DSM-IV-TR, in the 10th revision of the *International Statistical Classification of Diseases and Related Health Problems* (ICD-10), these disorders are described as characterized by "qualitative abnormalities in reciprocal social interactions and in patterns of communications, and by a restricted, stereotyped, repetitive repertoire of interests and activities." Although cognitive impairment is frequently present, the disorders are defined in terms of behavior "that is deviant in relation to mental age (whether the individual is retarded or not)."

Among these disorders, ICD-10 includes childhood autism, atypical autism, Rett's syndrome, other childhood disintegrative disorder, overactive disorder associated with mental retardation and stereotyped movements, Asperger's syndrome, other pervasive developmental disorders, and pervasive developmental disorder, unspecified. The ICD-10 childhood autism category corresponds to autistic disorder in DSM-IV-TR. According to ICD-10, however, atypical autism differs from childhood autism in age or onset or in failure to fulfill all three sets of diagnostic criteria. It first becomes apparent only after the age of 3 years, shows fewer abnormalities in the areas required for diagnosing autism, and generally occurs in children who are profoundly retarded or who have a severe "specific developmental disorder of receptive language."

According to ICD-10, overactive disorder associated with mental retardation and stereotyped movements is "an ill-defined disorder of uncertain nosological validity." ICD-10 includes this diagnosis because children with severe mental retardation who have hyperactivity and inattention problems also frequently show stereotyped behaviors. Their overactivity tends not to benefit from stimulant drugs as does that of children with a normal IQ; in adolescents, these children tend toward underactivity. They may also display developmental delays. (In ICD-10, cases of mild retardation with hyperkinetic syndrome are classified in the category of hyperkinetic disorders.) The ICD-10 criteria are presented in Table 42–9.

References

Aman MG, Arnold MKLE, McDougle CJ, Vitiello B, Scahill L, Davies M, McCracken JT, Tierney E, Nash PL, Posey DJ, Chuang S, Martin A, Shah B, Gonzalez HM, Swiezy NB, Ritz L, Koenig K, McGough J, Ghuman JK, Lindsay RL. Acute and long-term safety and tolerability of risperidone in children with autism. *J Child Adolesc Psychopharmacol*. 2005;15:869.

Baron-Cohen S, Knickmeyer RC, Belmonte MK. Sex differences in the brain: Implications for explaining autism. *Science*. 2005;310:819.

Bishop DV, Mayberry M, Wong D, Maley A, Hallmayer J. Characteristics of the broader phenotype in autism: A study of siblings using the children's communication checklist-2. *Am J Med Genet B Neruopsychiatr Genet*. 2006;141B:117–122.

Carminati GG, Deriaz N, Bertschy G. Low-dose venlafaxine in three adolescents and young adults with autistic disorder improves self-injurious behavior and attention deficit/hyperactivity disorder (ADHD)-like symptoms. *Prog Neuropsychopharmacol Biol Psychiatry*. 2006;30:312.

Constantino JN, Lajonchere C, Lutz M, Gray T, Abbacchi A, McKenna K, Singh D, Todd RD. Autistic social impairment in the siblings of children with pervasive developmental disorders. *Am J Psychiatry*. 2006;163:294–296.

Danfors T, von Knorring AL, Hartvig P, Langstrom B, Moulder R, Stromberg B, Tortenson R, Wester U, Watanabe Y, Eeg-Olofsson O. Tetrahydrobiopterin in the treatment of children with autistic disorder: A double-blind placebo-controlled crossover study. *J Clin Psychopharmacol*. 2005;25:485.

Gadow KD, DeVincent CJ, Pomeroy J. ADHD symptom subtypes in children with pervasive developmental disorder. *J Autism Dev Disord*. 2006;36(2): 271–223.

Hazlett HC, Poe, M, Gerig C, Smith RG, Provenzale J, Ross A, Gilmore J, Piven J. Magnetic resonance imaging and head circumference study of brain size in autism: Birth through age 2 years. *Arch Gen Psychiatry*. 2005;62:1366.

Ke JY, Chen CL, Chen YJ, Chen CH, Lee LF, Chiang TM. Features of developmental functions and autistic profiles in children with fragile X syndrome. *Chang Gung Med J*. 2005;28:551.

Koyama T, Tachimori H, Osada H, Kurita H. Cognitive and symptom profiles in high-functioning pervasive developmental disorder not otherwise specified and attention-deficit/hyperactivity disorder. *J Autism Dev Disord*. 2006;36(3): 373–380.

Mandell DS, Novak MM, Zubritsky CD. Factors associated with age of diagnosis among children with autism spectrum disorders. *Pediatrics*. 2005;116:1480.

Owley T, Walton L, Salt J, Guter SJ, Winnega M, Leventhal BL, Cook EH. An open–label trial of escitalopram in pervasive developmental disorders. *J Am Acad Child Adolesc Psychiatry*. 2005;44:343.

Research Units on Pediatric Psychopharmacology Autism Network. Randomized, controlled crossover trial of methylphenidate in pervasive developmental disorders with hyperactivity. *Arch Gen Psychiatry*. 2005;62:1266.

Sugie Y, Sugie H, Fukuda T, Ito M. Neonatal factors in infants with autistic disorder and typically developing infants. *Autism*. 2005;9:487.

Volkmar FR, Klin A, Schultz RT. Pervasive developmental disorders. In: Sadock BJ, Sadock VA, eds. *Kaplan & Sadock's Comprehensive Textbook of Psychiatry*. 8th ed. Vol. 2. Baltimore: Lippincott Williams & Wilkins; 2005: 3164.

43 Attention-Deficit Disorders

ATTENTION-DEFICIT/HYPERACTIVITY DISORDER

Attention-deficit/hyperactivity disorder (ADHD) is characterized by a pattern of diminished sustained attention and higher levels of impulsivity in a child or adolescent than expected for someone of that age and developmental level. Whereas in the past, hyperactivity was believed to be the underlying impairing symptom in this disorder, the current consensus is that hyperactivity is often secondary to poor impulse control. Impulsivity and hyperactivity share one dimension in today's diagnostic criteria for ADHD. Currently, the diagnosis of ADHD is based on the consensus of experts that three observable subtypes: *inattentive*, *hyperactive/impulsive*, or *combined* are all manifestations of the same disorder. To meet the criteria for the diagnosis of ADHD, some symptoms must be present before the age of 7 years, although ADHD is not diagnosed in many children until they are older than 7 years when their behaviors cause problems in school and other places. To confirm a diagnosis of ADHD, impairment from inattention and/or hyperactivity-impulsivity must be observable in at least two settings and interfere with developmentally appropriate functioning socially, academically, or in extracurricular activities. ADHD is not diagnosed when symptoms occur in a child, adolescent, or adult with a pervasive developmental disorder, schizophrenia, or other psychotic disorder.

The disorder has been identified in the literature for many years under a variety of terms. In the early 1900s, impulsive, disinhibited, and hyperactive children—many of whom had neurological damage caused by encephalitis—were grouped under the label *hyperactive syndrome*. In the 1960s, a heterogeneous group of children with poor coordination, learning disabilities, and emotional lability, but without specific neurological damage, were described as having minimal brain damage. Since then, other hypotheses have been put forth to explain the origin of the disorder, such as genetically based condition involving abnormal arousal and poor ability to modulate emotions. This theory was initially supported by the observation that stimulant medications help produce sustained attention and improve these children's ability to focus on a given task. Currently, no single factor is believed to cause the disorder, although many environmental variables may contribute to it and many predictable clinical features are associated with it.

Epidemiology

Reports on the incidence of ADHD in the United States have varied from 2 to 20 percent of grade-school children. A conservative figure is about 3 to 7 percent of prepubertal elementary school children. In Great Britain a lower incidence is reported than in the United States, less than 1 percent. ADHD is more prevalent in boys than in girls, with the ratio ranging from 2 to 1 to as much as 9 to 1. First-degree biological relatives (e.g., siblings of probands with ADHD) are at high risk to develop it as well as to develop other disorders, including disruptive behavior disorders, anxiety disorders, and depressive disorders. Siblings of children with ADHD are also at higher risk than the general population to have learning disorders and academic difficulties. The parents of children with ADHD show an increased incidence of hyperkinesis, sociopathy, alcohol use disorders, and conversion disorder. Symptoms of ADHD are often present by age 3 years, but the diagnosis is generally not made until the child is in a structured school setting, such as preschool or kindergarten, when teacher information is available comparing the attention and impulsivity of the child in question with peers of the same age.

Etiology

Current consensus that the etiology of ADHD involves complex interactions of neuroanatomical and neurochemical systems is based on twin and adoption family genetic studies, dopamine transport gene studies, neuroimaging studies, and neurotransmitter data. Most children with ADHD have no evidence of gross structural damage in the central nervous system (CNS). Despite the lack of a specific neurophysiological or neurochemical basis for the disorder, it is predictably associated with a variety of other disorders that affect brain function, such as learning disorders. The suggested contributory factors for ADHD include prenatal toxic exposures, prematurity, and prenatal mechanical insult to the fetal nervous system. Food additives, colorings, preservatives, and sugar have also been proposed as possible causes of hyperactive behavior. No scientific evidence indicates that these factors cause ADHD.

Genetic Factors. Evidence for a genetic contribution to the emergence of ADHD includes greater concordance in monozygotic than in dizygotic twins. Also, siblings of hyperactive children have about twice the risk of having the disorder as those in the general population. One sibling may have predominantly hyperactivity symptoms, and others may have predominantly inattention symptoms. Biological parents of children with the disorder have a higher risk for ADHD than adoptive parents. Children with ADHD are at higher risk of developing conduct disorders, and alcohol use disorders and antisocial personality disorder are more common in their parents than in those in the general population.

Developmental Factors. Reports in the literature state that September is the peak month for births of children with ADHD with and without comorbid learning disorders. The implication is that prenatal exposure to winter infections during the first trimester may contribute to the emergence of ADHD symptoms in some susceptible children.

BRAIN DAMAGE. It has been speculated that some children affected by ADHD had subtle damage to the CNS and brain development during their fetal and perinatal periods. The hypothesized brain damage may potentially be associated with circulatory, toxic, metabolic, mechanical, or physical insult to the brain during early infancy caused by infection, inflammation, and trauma. Children with ADHD exhibit nonfocal (soft) neurological signs at higher rates than those in the general population.

Neurochemical Factors. Many neurotransmitters have been associated with ADHD symptoms. Animal studies have shown that the locus ceruleus, consisting of mainly noradrenergic neurons, plays a major role in attention. The noradrenergic system consists of the central system (originating in the locus ceruleus) and the peripheral sympathetic system. The peripheral noradrenergic system may be of more importance in ADHD. Thus, a dysfunction in peripheral epinephrine, which causes the hormone to accumulate peripherally, could potentially feed back to the central system and "reset" the locus ceruleus to a lower level. In part, hypotheses about the neurochemistry of the disorder have arisen from the impact of many medications that exert a positive effect on it. The most widely studied drugs in the treatment of ADHD, the stimulants, affect both dopamine and norepinephrine, leading to neurotransmitter hypotheses that include possible dysfunction in both the adrenergic and the dopaminergic systems. Stimulants increase catecholamine concentrations by promoting their release and blocking their uptake. Stimulants and some tricyclic drugs—for example, desipramine (Norpramin)—reduce levels of urinary 3-methoxy-4-hydroxyphenylglycol (MHPG), a metabolite of norepinephrine. Clonidine (Catapres), a norepinephrine agonist, has been helpful in treating hyperactivity. Other drugs that have reduced hyperactivity include tricyclic drugs and monoamine oxidase inhibitors (MAOIs). Overall, no clear-cut evidence implicates a single neurotransmitter in the development of ADHD, but many neurotransmitters may be involved in the process.

Neurophysiological Factors. The human brain normally undergoes major growth spurts at several ages: 3 to 10 months, 2 to 4 years, 6 to 8 years, 10 to 12 years, and 14 to 16 years. Some children have a maturational delay in the sequence and manifest symptoms of ADHD that appear to normalize by about age 5. A physiological correlate is the presence of a variety of nonspecific abnormal electroencephalogram (EEG) patterns that are disorganized and characteristic of young children. In some cases, the EEG findings normalize over time. A recent study of quantitative EEGs in children with ADHD, in children with undifferentiated attentional problems, and in normal controls indicates that both groups with attentional problems evince increased beta band relative percentages and decreased rare tone P3000 amplitudes. Increased beta band percentage or decreased delta band percentage is associated with increased arousal.

Computed tomographic (CT) head scans of children with ADHD show no consistent findings. Studies using positron emission tomography (PET) have found lower cerebral blood flow and metabolic rates in the frontal lobe areas of children with ADHD than in controls. PET scans have also shown that adolescent females with the disorder have globally lower glucose metabolism than both normal control females and males with the disorder. One theory explains these findings by supposing that the frontal lobes in children with ADHD are not adequately performing their inhibitory mechanism on lower structures, an effect leading to disinhibition.

Psychosocial Factors. Children in institutions are frequently overactive and have poor attention spans. These signs result from prolonged emotional deprivation, and they disappear when deprivational factors are removed, such as through adoption or placement in a foster home. Stressful psychic events, disruption of family equilibrium, and other anxiety-inducing factors contribute to the initiation or perpetuation of ADHD. Predisposing factors may include the child's temperament, genetic-familial factors, and the demands of society to adhere to a routinized way of behaving and performing. Socioeconomic status does not seem to be a predisposing factor.

Diagnosis

The principal signs of inattention, impulsivity, and hyperactivity are based on a detailed history of a child's early developmental patterns along with direct observation of the child, especially in situations that require sustained attention. Hyperactivity may be more severe in some situations (e.g., school) and less marked in others (e.g., one-on-one interviews), and it may be less obvious in pleasant structured activities (sports). The diagnosis of ADHD requires persistent, impairing symptoms of either hyperactivity/impulsivity or inattention that cause impairment in at least two different settings. For example, many children with ADHD have difficulties in school and at home. The diagnostic criteria for ADHD are outlined in Table 43–1.

Other distinguishing features of ADHD are short attention span and easy distractibility. In school, children with ADHD cannot follow instructions and often demand extra attention from their teachers. At home, they often do not comply with their parents' requests. They act impulsively, show emotional lability, and are explosive and irritable.

Children who have hyperactivity as a predominant feature are more likely to be referred for treatment than are children with primarily symptoms of attention deficit. Children with the predominantly hyperactive-impulsive type are more likely to have a stable diagnosis over time and to have concurrent conduct disorder than are children with the predominantly inattentive type without hyperactivity. Disorders involving reading, arithmetic, language, and coordination can occur in association with ADHD. A child's history may give clues to prenatal (including genetic), natal, and postnatal factors that may have affected the CNS structure or function. Rates of development, deviations in development, and parental reactions to significant or stressful behavioral transitions should be ascertained, because they may help clinicians determine the degree to which parents have contributed or reacted to a child's inefficiencies and dysfunctions.

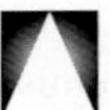

Table 43–1
DSM-IV-TR Diagnostic Criteria for Attention-Deficit/Hyperactivity Disorder

A. Either (1) or (2):
1. six (or more) of the following symptoms of inattention have persisted for at least 6 months to a degree that is maladaptive and inconsistent with developmental level:
Inattention
(a) often fails to give close attention to details or makes careless mistakes in schoolwork, work, or other activities
(b) often has difficulty sustaining attention in tasks or play activities
(c) often does not seem to listen when spoken to directly
(d) often does not follow through on instructions and fails to finish schoolwork, chores, or duties in the workplace (not due to oppositional behavior or failure to understand instructions)
(e) often has difficulty organizing tasks and activities
(f) often avoids, dislikes, or is reluctant to engage in tasks that require sustained mental effort (such as schoolwork or homework)
(g) often loses things necessary for tasks or activities (e.g., toys, school assignments, pencils, books, or tools)
(h) is often easily distracted by extraneous stimuli
(i) is often forgetful in daily activities
2. six (or more) of the following symptoms of **hyperactivity-impulsivity** have persisted for at least 6 months to a degree that is maladaptive and inconsistent with developmental level:
Hyperactivity
(a) often fidgets with hands or feet or squirms in seat
(b) often leaves seat in classroom or in other situations in which remaining seated is expected
(c) often runs about or climbs excessively in situations in which it is inappropriate (in adolescents or adults, may be limited to subjective feelings of restlessness)
(d) often has difficulty playing or engaging in leisure activities quietly
(e) is often "on the go" or often acts as if "driven by a motor"
(f) often talks excessively
Impulsivity
(g) often blurts out answers before questions have been completed
(h) often has difficulty awaiting turn
(i) often interrupts or intrudes on others (e.g., butts into conversations or games)

B. Some hyperactive-impulsive or inattentive symptoms that caused impairment were present before age 7 years.
C. Some impairment from the symptoms is present in two or more settings (e.g., at school [or work] and at home).
D. There must be clear evidence of clinically significant impairment in social, academic, or occupational functioning.
E. The symptoms do not occur exclusively during the course of a pervasive developmental disorder, schizophrenia, or other psychotic disorder and are not better accounted for by another mental disorder (e.g., mood disorder, anxiety disorder, dissociative disorder, or a personality disorder).

Code based on type:
Attention-deficit/hyperactivity disorder, combined type: if both Criteria A1 and A2 are met for the past 6 months
Attention-deficit/hyperactivity disorder, predominantly inattentive type: if Criterion A1 is met but Criterion A2 is not met for the past 6 months
Attention-deficit/hyperactivity disorder, predominantly hyperactive-impulsive type: if Criterion A2 is met but Criterion A1 is not met for the past 6 months
Coding note: For individuals (especially adolescents and adults) who currently have symptoms that no longer meet full criteria, "in partial remission" should be specified.

(From American Psychiatric Association. *Diagnostic and Statistical Manual of Mental Disorders.* 4th ed. Text rev. Washington, DC: American Psychiatric Association; copyright 2000, with permission.)

School history and teachers' reports are important in evaluating whether a child's difficulties in learning and school behavior are primarily caused by the child's inability to sustain attention or compromised understanding of the academic material. Additional school difficulties can result from attitudinal or maturational problems, social rejection, and poor self-image because of felt inadequacies. These reports may also reveal how the child has handled these problems. How the child has related to siblings, to peers, to adults, and to free and structured activities gives valuable diagnostic clues to the presence of ADHD and helps identify the complications of the disorder.

The mental status examination may show a secondarily depressed mood, but no thought disturbance, impaired reality testing, or inappropriate affect. A child may show great distractibility, perseveration, and a concrete and literal mode of thinking. Indications of visual-perceptual, auditory-perceptual, language, or cognition problems may be present. Occasionally, evidence appears of a basic, pervasive, organically based anxiety, often referred to as *body anxiety*. A neurological examination may reveal visual, motor, perceptual, or auditory discriminatory immaturity or impairments without overt signs of visual or auditory acuity disorders. Children may have problems with motor coordination and difficulty copying age-appropriate figures, rapid alternating movements, right-left discrimination, ambidexterity, reflex asymmetries, and a variety of subtle nonfocal neurological signs (soft signs).

Clinicians should obtain an EEG to recognize the child with frequent bilaterally synchronous discharges resulting in short absence spells. Such a child may react in school with hyperactivity out of sheer frustration. The child with an unrecognized temporal lobe seizure focus can have a secondary behavior disorder. In these instances, several features of ADHD are often present. Identification of the focus requires an EEG obtained during drowsiness and during sleep.

Clinical Features

Attention-deficit/hyperactivity disorder can have its onset in infancy, although it is rarely recognized until a child is at least toddler age. Infants with the disorder are unduly sensitive to stimuli and are easily upset by noise, light, temperature, and other environmental changes. At times, the reverse occurs, and the children are placid and limp, sleep much of the time, and appear to develop slowly in the first months of life. More commonly, however, infants with ADHD are active in the crib, sleep little, and cry a great deal. They are far less likely than normal children to reduce their locomotor activity when their environment is structured by social limits.

In school, children with ADHD may attack a test rapidly, but answer only the first two questions. They may be unable to wait to be called on in school and may respond before everyone else. At home, they cannot be put off for even a minute. Children with ADHD are often explosive or irritable. The irritability may be set off by relatively minor stimuli, which may puzzle and dismay the children. They are frequently emotionally labile and easily set off to laughter or to tears; their mood and performance are apt to be variable and unpredictable. Impulsiveness and an inability to delay gratification are characteristic. Children are often susceptible to accidents.

Concomitant emotional difficulties are frequent. The resulting negative self-concept and reactive hostility are worsened by the children's recognition that they have problems.

The most cited characteristics of children with ADHD, in order of frequency, are hyperactivity, perceptual motor impairment, emotional lability, general coordination deficit, attention deficit (short attention span, distractibility, perseveration, failure to finish tasks, inattention, poor concentration), impulsivity (action before thought, abrupt shifts in activity, lack of organization, jumping up in class), memory and thinking deficits, specific learning disabilities, speech and hearing deficits, and equivocal neurological signs and EEG irregularities. About 75 percent of children with ADHD show behavioral symptoms of aggression and defiance fairly consistently. But, whereas defiance and aggression are generally associated with adverse intrafamily relationships, hyperactivity is more closely related to impaired performance on cognitive tests requiring concentration.

School difficulties, both learning and behavioral, commonly coexist with ADHD. They sometimes come from concomitant communication disorders or learning disorders or from the child's distractibility and fluctuating attention, which hampers the acquisition, retention, and display of knowledge. These difficulties are noted especially on group tests. The adverse reactions of school personnel to the behavior characteristics of ADHD and the lowering of self-regard because of felt inadequacies may combine with the adverse comments of peers to make school a place of unhappy defeat. This situation can lead to acting-out antisocial behavior and self-defeating, self-punitive behaviors.

Anthony was first referred to a child psychiatric clinic at age 7. Reasons for referral included the following:

- Severe restlessness and hyperactivity since he began to walk
- Poor concentration
- Disobedient, not listening (teachers "liked" Anthony but wanted him out of the class)
- Poor speech articulation
- Repeating grade 1
- Very untidy and disorganized

Anthony's birth history was uneventful, and his EEG and neurological examination findings were normal. Anthony's *Wechsler Intelligence Scale for Children* (WISC) (Full Scale) was 115, with marked scatter. He was found to have body image and visuomotor difficulties. Psychiatric evaluation revealed a friendly, good-looking, 7-year-old boy with speech (i.e., articulation) difficulties who was restless and hyperactive. The parents stated they were happily married and there were two older sisters, both doing well. The father was a sales executive and traveled a great deal, the mother a homemaker. Their ethnic origin was Anglo-Saxon. A diagnosis of ADHD was made.

FIVE-YEAR FOLLOW-UP: 14 YEARS OF AGE

This evaluation was delayed because Anthony had been away at boarding school for 3 years, and we had to wait until he was on holiday. He had received stimulants for only a short period because he was noncompliant, because he hated the dampening effects. At 14 years, Anthony seemed very immature and was still restless and distractible. His learning difficulties made school success in a regular classroom almost impossible, but Anthony had a "happy-go-lucky" attitude about his failures. There was no stealing or other indication of antisocial behavior, but Anthony had no close friends. His mother believed he was worse because he did not accept responsibility and had no goals for the future. He was very poor at spelling and behind in reading and found schoolwork boring. Although he lacked any insight into his difficulties, he was found to be friendly and likable. Repeat WISC IQ (Full Scale) was unchanged.

TEN-YEAR FOLLOW-UP: 20 YEARS OF AGE

Anthony was seen late also for the 10-year follow-up study because his parents had moved overseas, where his father had started a business. We wrote to Anthony there, sending him numerous self-rating scales and a history for him to complete. The former included the *California Personality Inventory* (CPI), a self-rating scale that all subjects completed. We did not hear from Anthony for 2 years after the forms were mailed and gave up on him as a lost subject. One day, Anthony knocked at G. W.'s office door and announced himself and his girlfriend, Sally. He said he had come from New Zealand to see us with Sally to let us know that the CPI was a truly crazy test and there was no way that he could ever complete "500 dumb questions." When asked what he was really doing here, he said he had told us the truth, then gave a report of his past 5 years and agreed to complete the whole 10-year follow-up evaluation.

While still living with his parents overseas, Anthony had refused to continue schooling, but he had completed grade 9 in Montreal. He worked intermittently at various menial jobs and lived with his parents. (His last job was collecting stray cats and dogs for the local Society for the Prevention of Cruelty to Animals.) He believed his father looked down on this job even though he had told Anthony that any honest job is OK. "He obviously didn't mean it," Anthony added. "Anyway, I got laid off, and since I have ants in my pants, I went to New Zealand." He planned to go perhaps to find work, perhaps for a holiday. But there he met Sally, who suggested that he could try mowing people's lawns for some income. Sally and Anthony soon lived together, and she helped Anthony settle down. She encouraged him to work hard, and soon he had saved $1,500. They borrowed another $1,000 and bought a few second-hand lawnmowers. They then employed younger boys to mow lawns, and a year later had saved $5,500 and paid back the debts. "I gave up the lawnmower business because one day I just found it boring and tense, and I wanted to quit and travel. Also, I wanted to see you to show you how crazy this test that you sent me is."

Anthony appeared happy and as impulsive as ever and had great charm. He had succeeded in getting Sally a job in Montreal, which was extremely difficult at the time, by telling the immigration department that if they did not give her a work permit, he would marry her, and then they would have to give her one anyway. They would feel sorry to have made him marry so young (Sally got her work permit).

Sally turned out to be a bright, quite delightful, stable young woman who appreciated Anthony's qualities and had a strong influence on him. She made subsequent appointments for him and made sure he was on time for them. They planned to return to New Zealand after a few months in Montreal but see the world on the way back.

FIFTEEN-YEAR-FOLLOW-UP: 25 YEARS OF AGE

We could not go to New Zealand to interview Anthony, but we were able to meet with his parents, who were visiting Montreal. They had recently visited Anthony in New Zealand and were in close touch with him and with Sally. Anthony was now taking a university degree in communications. It seemed that where he ended up, he could enter university as a mature student without completing high school (he had completed only grade 9). He was pursuing his courses with some difficulties but was passing in spite of concentration problems. He was interested in what he was doing. Anthony and Sally were still living together and were planning on getting married. During this time, Sally had had a malignant lump removed from her breast. Anthony's parents stated that he and Sally "had an excellent relationship" and that they had dealt with their grief and anxiety over her diagnosis well. Sally, they stated, still takes charge of organizational family matters and helps Anthony with his writing assignments. The friends they have are made by Sally, as Anthony lets her take all the initiative with friends; however, he is well liked by them. His parents believe that in the past year, partly as a result of Sally's medical problems, Anthony has matured greatly. He was described as still impulsive, still very restless, but he listens to Sally. He still talks too much and "has a big mouth." He has occasionally lost part-time jobs because of this. The couple has no debts, and Anthony plans to start an advertising business when he receives his university degree. His father stated he would help him financially but still would not trust him to handle money responsibly. Anthony himself is not close to the friends the couple has, but he feels close to Sally. Although Sally has obviously done a great deal for Anthony, it was believed that the relationship is complementary rather than neurotic.

We asked Anthony's parents what they believed were the reasons for Anthony's good outcome because they were extremely happy about his progress. His father stated, "Even while Anthony was hyperactive and a discipline problem as a child, he was very lovable. In school, he couldn't learn because he felt so inferior. At 17 years, we sent him to Switzerland to learn a trade, but this did not work out. At 18 years, we gave him a one-way ticket to New Zealand and said to him, if you want to come back you have to earn the money for your ticket. Sally was the turning point for Anthony. She gave him what we couldn't, confidence in himself and a sense of direction. She had always loved him and even way back believed in his future when we frankly did not. Sally and Anthony are now saving to buy a house, and we send them money toward this, but we always send it to Sally. She keeps the books."

It seemed clear to us that Anthony without his fiancée would not be functioning as well as he is and would still be having many life difficulties related to the ADHD disorder. (Courtesy of G. Weiss, M.D.)

Pathology and Laboratory Examination

No specific laboratory measures are pathognomonic of ADHD. Several laboratory measures often yield nonspecific abnormal results in hyperactive children, such as a disorganized, immature result on an EEG, and PET may show decreased cerebral blood flow in the frontal regions. Cognitive testing that helps to confirm a child's inattention and impulsivity includes a continuous performance task, in which a child is asked to press a button each time a particular sequence of letters or numbers is flashed on a screen. Children with poor attention make errors of omission—that is, they fail to press the button, even when the sequence has flashed. Impulsivity is manifested by errors of commission, in which children cannot resist pushing the button, although the desired sequence has not yet appeared on the screen.

Differential Diagnosis

A temperamental constellation consisting of high activity level and short attention span but in the normal range of expectation for a child's age should be considered first. Differentiating these temperamental characteristics from the cardinal symptoms of ADHD before the age of 3 years is difficult, mainly because of the overlapping features of a normally immature nervous system and the emerging signs of visual-motor-perceptual impairments frequently seen in ADHD. Anxiety in a child needs to be evaluated. Anxiety can accompany ADHD as a secondary feature, and anxiety alone can be manifested by overactivity and easy distractibility.

It is not uncommon for a child with ADHD to become demoralized or, in some cases, to develop depressive symptoms in reaction to persistent frustration with academic difficulties and resulting low self-esteem. Mania and ADHD share many core features, such as excessive verbalization, motoric hyperactivity, and high levels of distractibility. Additionally, in children with mania, irritability seems to be more common than euphoria. Although mania and ADHD can coexist, children with bipolar I disorder exhibit more waxing and waning of symptoms than those with ADHD. Recent follow-up data for children who met the criteria for ADHD and subsequently developed bipolar disorder suggest that certain clinical features occurring during the course of ADHD predict future mania. Children with ADHD who had developed bipolar I disorder at 4-year follow-up had a greater co-occurrence of additional disorders and a greater family history of bipolar disorders and other mood disorders than children without bipolar disorder.

Frequently, conduct disorder and ADHD coexist, and both must be diagnosed. Learning disorders of various kinds must also be distinguished from ADHD; a child may be unable to read or do mathematics because of a learning disorder, rather than because of inattention. ADHD often coexists with one or more learning disorders, including reading disorder, mathematics disorder, and disorder of written expression.

Course and Prognosis

The course of ADHD is variable. Symptoms have been shown to persist into adolescence or adult life in approximately 50 percent of cases. In the remaining 50 percent, they may remit at puberty, or in early adulthood. In some cases, the hyperactivity may disappear, but the decreased attention span and impulse-control problems persist. Overactivity is usually the first symptom to remit, and distractibility is the last. ADHD does not usually remit during middle childhood. Persistence is predicted by a family history of the disorder, negative life events, and comorbidity with conduct symptoms, depression, and anxiety disorders. Remission is unlikely before the age of 12 years. When remission

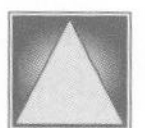

Table 43–2
Stimulant Medications in the Treatment of Attention-Deficit/Hyperactivity Disorder (ADHD)

Medication	Preparation (mg)	Approx. Duration (hr)	Recommended Dose
Methylphenidate preparations			
Ritalin	5, 10, 15, 20	3 to 4	0.3–1 mg/kg t.i.d; up to 60 mg/d
Ritalin-SR	20	8	Up to 60 mg/d
Concerta	18, 36, 54	12	Up to 54 mg/q AM
Metadate ER	10, 20	8	Up to 60 mg/d
Metadate CD	20	12	Up to 60 mg/q AM
Ritalin LA	5, 10, 15, 20	8	
Dexmethylphenidate preparation			
Focalin	2.5, 5, 10	3 to 4	Up to 10 mg
Focalin XR	5, 10, 20	6 to 8	Up to 20 mg
Dextroamphetamine preparations			
Dexedrine	5, 10	3 to 4	0.15 to 0.5 mg/kg b.i.d.; up to 40 mg/d
Dexedrine Spansule	5, 10, 15	8	Up to 40 mg/d
Dextroamphetamine and amphetamine salt preparations			
Adderall	5, 10, 20, 30	4 to 6	0.15 to 0.5 mg/kg b.i.d.; up to 40 mg/d
Adderall XR	10, 20, 30	12	Up to 40 mg q AM

t.i.d., three times daily; q, every; b.i.d., twice daily.

does occur, it is usually between the ages of 12 and 20. Remission can be accompanied by a productive adolescence and adult life, satisfying interpersonal relationships, and few significant sequelae. Most patients with the disorder, however, undergo partial remission and are vulnerable to antisocial behavior, substance use disorders, and mood disorders. Learning problems often continue throughout life.

In about 40 to 50 percent of cases, symptoms persist into adulthood. Those with the disorder may show diminished hyperactivity, but remain impulsive and accident-prone. Although their educational attainments as a group are lower than those of people without ADHD, their early employment histories do not differ from those of people with similar educations.

Children with the disorder whose symptoms persist into adolescence are at risk for developing conduct disorder. Children with both ADHD and conduct disorder are also at risk for developing a substance-related disorder. The development of substance abuse disorders during adolescence appears to be related to the presence of conduct disorder rather than to ADHD alone.

Most children with ADHD have some social difficulties. Socially dysfunctional children with ADHD have significantly higher rates of comorbid psychiatric disorders and experience more problems with behavior in school as well as with peers and family members. Overall, the outcome of ADHD in childhood seems to be related to the degree of persistent comorbid psychopathology, especially conduct disorder, social disability, and chaotic family factors. Optimal outcomes may be promoted by ameliorating children's social functioning, diminishing aggression, and improving family situations as early as possible.

Treatment

Pharmacotherapy. Pharmacologic treatment is considered to be the first line of treatment for ADHD. Central nervous system stimulants are the first choice of agents in that they have been shown to have the greatest efficacy with generally mild tolerable side effects. Although excellent safety records are documented for short- and sustained-release preparations of methylphenidate (Ritalin, Ritalin-SR, Concerta, Metadate CD, Metadate ER), dextroamphetamine (Dexedrine, Dexedrine spansules), and dextroamphetamine and amphetamine salt combinations (Adderall, Adderall XR), current strategies favor once a day sustained release preparations for their convenience and diminished rebound side effects. A newer preparation of methylphenidate, containing only the d-enantiomer, dexmethylphenidate (Focalin), was recently placed on the market, aimed at maximizing the target effects and minimizing the adverse effects in individuals with ADHD who obtain partial response from methylphenidate, or who were responsive but adequate dosing was limited by side effects. Advantages of the sustained-release preparations for children are that one dose in the morning will sustain the effects all day, and the child is no longer required to interrupt his or her school day, as well as the physiologic advantage that the medication is sustained at an approximately even level in the body throughout the day so that periods of rebound and irritability are avoided. Table 43–2 contains comparative information on the above medications. Second-line agents with evidence of efficacy for some children and adolescents with ADHD include Atomoxetine (Stratera), a norepinephrine uptake inhibitor, shown to be effective in the treatment of children with ADHD; antidepressants, such as bupropion (Wellbutrin, Wellbutrin SR), venlafaxine (Effexor, Effexor XR); and the α-adrenergic receptor agonists clonidine (Catapres), and guanfacine (Tenex). (Table 43–3 contains comparative information on the nonstimulant medications.) The US Food and Drug Administration (FDA) approved the use of dextroamphetamine in children 3 years of age and older and methylphenidate in children 6 years of age and older. These are the two most commonly used pharmacologic agents for the treatment of children with ADHD.

STIMULANT MEDICATIONS. Methylphenidate and amphetamine preparations are dopamine agonists; however, the precise mechanism of the stimulant's central action remains unknown. The idea of paradoxical response by hyperactive children is no longer accepted. Methylphenidate has been shown to be highly effective in up to three quarters of all children with

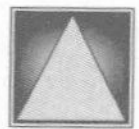

Table 43–3
Nonstimulant Medications for Attention-Deficit/Hyperactivity Disorder (ADHD)

Medication	Preparation (mg)	Recommended Dose
Atomoxetine HCL		
Strattera	10, 18, 25, 40	(0.5 to 1.8 mg/kg) 40 to 80 mg/d, may use b.i.d. dosing
Bupropion preparations		
Wellbutrin	75, 100	(3 to 6 mg/kg) 150 to 300 mg/d; up to 150 mg/dose b.i.d.
Wellbutrin SR	100, 150	(3 to 6 mg/kg) 150 to 300 mg/d; up to 150 mg q AM; >150 mg/d, use b.i.d. dosing
Venlafaxine		
Effexor	25, 37.5, 50, 75, 100	25 to 150 mg/d; use b.i.d. dosing
Effexor XR	37.5, 75, 150	37.5 to 150 mg q AM
α-Adrenergic agonists		
Clonidine (Catapres)	0.1, 0.2, 0.3	3 to 10 μg/kg/d divided t.i.d.; up to 0.1 mg t.i.d.
Guanfacine (Tenex)	1, 2	0.5 to 1.5 mg/d

b.i.d, twice daily; q, every; t.i.d., three times daily.

ADHD, with relatively few adverse effects. Methylphenidate is a short-acting medication that is generally used to be effective during school hours, so that children with the disorder can attend to tasks and remain in the classroom. The drug's most common adverse effects include headaches, stomachaches, nausea, and insomnia. Some children experience a rebound effect, in which they become mildly irritable and appear to be slightly hyperactive for a brief period when the medication wears off. In children with a history of motor tics, some caution must be used; in some cases, methylphenidate can exacerbate the tic disorder. Another common concern about methylphenidate is whether it causes some growth suppression. During periods of use, methylphenidate is associated with growth suppression, but children tend to make up the growth when they are given drug holidays in the summer or on weekends. An important question about using methylphenidate is how much it normalizes school performance. A recent study found that about 75 percent of a group of hyperactive children exhibited significant improvement in their ability to pay attention in class and on measures of academic efficiency when treated with methylphenidate. The drug has been shown to improve hyperactive children's scores on tasks of vigilance, such as the continuous performance task and paired associations. Dextroamphetamine and dextroamphetamine/amphetamine salt combinations are usually the second drugs of choice when methylphenidate is not effective. A transdermal delivery system has recently been developed for administering methylphenidate, the methylphenidate transedermal system, (MTS), designed to release methylphenidate continuously on application of the patch to the skin. Advantages of this form of administration of methylphenidate include an alternate mode of receiving the medication for children who have difficulties swallowing pills, and also that the patch continues to deliver the medication until it is removed. A recent double-blind randomized study of MTS use in children with ADHD who wore the patch for 12 hours at a time, showed efficacy of the patch preparation doses ranging from patches delivering (0.45 mg per hour) of methylphenidate, to those delivering 1.8 mg per hour of methylphenidate. The effectiveness of the patch reached a plateau without much further improvement as dose was increased, but intensive behavioral interventions were also being administered. A delay in the onset of effect of the transdermal medication was approximately an hour. Side effects were similar to oral preparations of methylphenidate. Approximately half of the children did exhibit at least minor erythematous reactions to the patch, although none of the study subjects discontinued the MTS because of severe skin reactions. It is not clear how long the effect of methylphenidate remains after the patch is removed. The MTS provides a new strategy for administering a medication well established in the treatment of ADHD that is likely to be on the market within the next year.

NONSTIMULANT MEDICATIONS. Atomoxetine HCl (Strattera) is a norepinehprhine uptake inhibitor approved by the FDA in the treatment of ADHD for children age 6 years and above. The mechanism of action is not well understood, but it is believed to involve selective inhibition of presynaptic norepinephrine transporter. Atomoxetine is well absorbed by the gastrointestinal tract and maximal plasma levels are reached in 1 to 2 hours after ingestion. It has been shown to be effective for inattention as well as impulsivity in children and in adults with ADHD. Its half-life is approximately 5 hours and it is usually administered twice daily. Most common side effects include diminished appetite, abdominal discomfort, dizziness, and irritability. In some cases, increases in blood pressure and heart rate have been reported. Atomoxetine is metabolized by the cytochrome P450 (CYP) 2D6 hepatic enzyme system. A small fraction of the population are poor metabolizers of CYP 2D6-metabolized drugs and, for those individuals, plasma concentrations of the drug may rise as much as fivefold for a given dose of medication. Drugs that inhibit CYP 2D6, including fluoxetine, paroxetine, and quinidine, may lead to increased plasma levels of this medication. Despite its short half-life, atomoxetine has been shown in a recent study to be effective in reducing symptoms of ADHD in children during the school day when administered once daily. Another recent study of a combination of atomoxetine alone and combined with fluoxetine in the treatment of 127 children with ADHD and symptoms of anxiety or depression suggested that atomoxetine alone can lead to improvements in mood and anxiety. Children who received combined atomoxetine and fluoxetine experienced greater increases in blood pressure and pulse than those who were treated with atomoxetine only.

Bupropion has been shown to be an effective antidepressant and is effective for some children and adolescents in the treatment of ADHD. A recent multisite, double-blind, placebo-controlled study confirmed the efficacy of bupropion. No further studies have compared bupropion with other stimulants. The risk of seizure development while on this drug is similar to that of other antidepressant medications when dosage does not exceed 450 mg per day. Venlafaxine has been used in clinical practice, especially for children and adolescents with combinations of ADHD and depression or anxiety features. No clear empirical evidence supports the use of venlafaxine in the treatment of ADHD. Clonidine has also been used in the treatment of ADHD with some success, according to case reports. It may be helpful when patients also have tic disorders. Few data confirm the efficacy of selective serotonin reuptake inhibitors (SSRIs) in the treatment of ADHD, but because of the comorbidity of depression and anxiety with the disorder, these drugs are sometimes considered.

Tricyclic drugs and pemoline (Cylert), previously used to treat ADHD, are no longer recommended because of potential adverse effects on liver function (pemoline) and potential cardiac arrhythmia effects (tricyclic drugs). The report of sudden death in at least four children with ADHD who were being treated with desipramine (Norpramin, Pertofrane) has made the tricyclic antidepressants a less likely choice. Why the deaths occurred is unclear, but they reinforce the need for close follow-up of any child receiving a tricyclic drug. Antipsychotics are occasionally used to treat refractory hyperactivity in children and adolescents who are severely impaired and do not respond to other treatments. Antipsychotics may be efficacious for some children with the disorder, but with the alternative medications available and the risk for tardive dyskinesia, withdrawal dyskinesia, and neuroleptic malignant syndrome, they are less desirable.

Modafinil (Provigil), another type of CNS stimulant, originally developed to reduce daytime sleepiness in patients with narcolepsy, has been tried clinically in the treatment of adults with ADHD. A recent randomized, double-blind, placebo controlled study of the efficacy and safety of modafinil film-coated tablets in approximately 250 adolescents with ADHD showed that 48 percent of those on active treatment were rated as "much" or "very much" improved compared with 17 percent of patients receiving placebo. The dosage range was from 170 to 425 mg administered once daily, titrated to optimal doses based on efficacy and tolerability. The most common side effects included insomnia, headache, and decreased appetite. This study concluded that modafinil, once daily, is a viable treatment for adolescents with ADHD based on it safety and effectiveness in this sample of adolescents. Although stimulants remain the drugs of choice in the pharmacological treatment of ADHD, a body of evidence now supports the use of nonstimulants, including atomoxetine, and modafinil.

A recent open-label report of reboxetine, a selective norepinephrine reuptake inhibitor in 31 children and adolescents with ADHD who were resistant to methylphenidate treatment suggested that this agent may have efficacy. In this open trial, reboxetine was initiated and maintained at 4 mg per day. Most common side effects included drowsiness, sedation, and gastrointestinal symptoms. Reboxetine and other new agents in this class await controlled studies to further evaluate their potential efficacy.

TREATMENT OF CNS STIMULANT SIDE EFFECTS. CNS stimulants are generally well tolerated and current consensus is that once a day dosing is preferable with regard to convenience and rebound side effects. A recent study of the long-term tolerability of once-daily mixed amphetamine salts has shown mild side effects, most commonly decreased appetite, insomnia, and headache.

Given the predictable side effects of central stimulant medications, strategies have been developed to ameliorate these problems. For example, a variety of strategies have been suggested by experts for a given a child or adolescent with ADHD who responds favorably to methylphenidate, (Concerta), but for whom insomnia has become a significant problem. Suggestions for the management of insomnia in such a case include the use of diphenhydramine (25 to 75 mg), low dose of trazodone (25 to 50 mg), or addition of an α-adrenergic agent, such as guanfacine. In some cases, insomnia may attenuate on its own after several months of treatment.

Monitoring Pharmacological Treatment

Stimulants. At baseline, the most recent American Academy of Child and Adolescent Psychiatry (AACAP) practice parameters recommend the following workup before starting use of stimulant medications:

- Physical examination
- Blood pressure
- Pulse
- Weight
- Height

It is recommended that children and adolescents being treated with stimulants have their height, weight, blood pressure, and pulse checked on a quarterly basis and have a physical examination annually.

EVALUATION OF THERAPEUTIC PROGRESS. Monitoring starts with the initiation of medication. Because school performance is most markedly affected, special attention and effort should be given to establishing and maintaining a close collaborative working relationship with a child's school personnel. In most patients, stimulants reduce overactivity, distractibility, impulsiveness, explosiveness, and irritability. No evidence indicates that medications directly improve any existing impairments in learning, although, when the attention deficits diminish, children can learn more effectively. In addition, medication can improve self-esteem when children are no longer constantly reprimanded for their behavior.

Psychosocial Interventions. Medication alone is often not sufficient to satisfy the comprehensive therapeutic needs of children with the disorder and is usually but one facet of a multimodality regimen. Social skills groups, training for parents of children with ADHD, and behavioral interventions at school and at home are often efficacious in the overall management of children with ADHD. Evaluation and treatment of coexisting learning disorders or additional psychiatric disorders is important.

Children who are prescribed medications should be taught the purpose of the medication and given the opportunity to reveal their feelings about it. Doing so helps dispel misconceptions about medication use (such as "I'm crazy") and makes it clear that the medication helps the child handle situations better than before. When children are helped to structure their environment, their anxiety diminishes. It is often beneficial for parents and teachers to work together to develop a concrete set of expectations for the child and a system of rewards for the child when the expectations are met.

A common goal of therapy is to help parents of children with ADHD recognize and promote the notion that, although the child may not "voluntarily" exhibit symptoms of ADHD, he or she is still capable of being responsible for meeting reasonable expectations. Parents should also be helped to recognize that, despite their child's difficulties, every child faces the normal tasks of maturation, including significant building of self-esteem when he or she develops a sense of mastery. Therefore, children with ADHD do not benefit from being exempted from the requirements, expectations, and planning applicable to other children. Parental training is an integral part of the psychotherapeutic interventions for ADHD. Most parental training is based on helping parents develop usable behavioral interventions with positive reinforcement that target both social and academic behaviors.

Group therapy aimed at both refining social skills and increasing self-esteem and a sense of success may be very useful for children with ADHD who have great difficulty functioning in group settings, especially in school. A recent year-long group therapy intervention in a clinical setting for boys with the disorder described the goals as helping the boys improve skills in game playing and feeling a sense of mastery with peers. The boys were first asked to do a task that was fun, in pairs, and then were gradually asked to do projects in a group. They were directed in following instructions, waiting, and paying attention and were praised for successful cooperation. This level of highly structured group therapeutic "play" is developmentally appropriate for these children, who benefit from an increased ability to participate in any group activities.

ATTENTION-DEFICIT/HYPERACTIVITY DISORDER NOT OTHERWISE SPECIFIED

The DSM-IV-TR includes ADHD not otherwise specified as a residual category for disturbances with prominent symptoms of inattention or hyperactivity that do not meet the criteria for ADHD (Table 43–4).

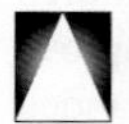

Table 43–4
DSM-IV-TR Diagnostic Criteria for Attention-Deficit/Hyperactivity Disorder Not Otherwise Specified

This category is for disorders with prominent symptoms of inattention or hyperactivity-impulsivity that do not meet criteria for attention-deficit/hyperactivity disorder. Examples include:

1. Individuals whose symptoms and impairment meet the criteria for attention-deficit/hyperactivity disorder, predominantly inattentive type but whose age at onset is 7 years or after
2. Individuals with clinically significant impairment who present with inattention and whose symptom pattern does not meet the full criteria for the disorder but have a behavioral pattern marked by sluggishness, daydreaming, and hypoactivity

(From American Psychiatric Association. *Diagnostic and Statistical Manual of Mental Disorders.* 4th ed. Text rev. Washington, DC: American Psychiatric Association; copyright 2000, with permission.)

ADULT MANIFESTATIONS OF ADHD

Attention-deficit/hyperactivity disorder was historically believed to be a childhood condition resulting in delayed development of impulse control that would be outgrown by adolescence. Only in the last few decades have adults with ADHD been identified, diagnosed, and successfully treated. Longitudinal follow-up has shown that up to 40 to 60 percent of children with ADHD have persistent impairment from symptoms into adulthood. Genetic studies, brain imaging, and neurocognitive and pharmacologic studies in adults with ADHD have virtually replicated findings demonstrated in children with ADHD. Increased public awareness and treatment studies within the last decade have led to widespread acceptance of the need for diagnosis and treatment of adults with ADHD.

Epidemiology

Among adults, evidence suggests an approximate 4 percent prevalence of ADHD in the population. ADHD in adulthood is generally diagnosed by self-report, given the lack of school information and observer information available; therefore, it is more difficult to make an accurate diagnosis.

Etiology

Currently, ADHD is believed to be largely transmitted genetically, and increasing evidence supports this hypothesis, including the genetic studies, twin studies, and family studies outlined in the child and adolescent ADHD section. Brain imaging studies have obtained data suggesting that adults with ADHD exhibit decreased prefrontal glucose metabolism on PET compared with adults without ADHD. It is unclear whether these data reflect the presence of the disorder or a secondary effect of having ADHD over a period of time. Further studies using single photon emission tomography (SPECT) have revealed increased dopamine transporter (DAT) binding densities in the striatum of the brain in samples of adults with ADHD. This finding may be understood within the context of treatment for ADHD in that standard stimulant treatment for ADHD, such as methylphenidate, acts to block DAT activity, possibly leading to a normalization of the striatal brain region in individuals with ADHD.

Factors associated with early childhood emergence of ADHD include premature birth, maternal use of nicotine during the pregnancy, and increased serum lead levels. Factors that protect against emergence of ADHD until later in childhood are not known.

Diagnosis and Clinical Features

The clinical phenomenology of ADHD in children that has evolved over the last few decades has resulted in features of inattention and manifestations of impulsivity prevailing as the core of this disorder. For adults, a leading figure in the development of criteria for adult manifestations of ADHD is Paul Wender, from the University of Utah, who began his work on adult ADHD in the 1970s. Wender developed criteria that could be applied to adults (Table 43–5). They included a retrospective diagnosis of ADHD in childhood, and evidence of current impairment from

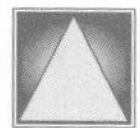

Table 43–5
Utah Criteria for Adult Attention-Deficit/ Hyperactivity Disorder (ADHD)

I. Retrospective childhood ADHD diagnosis
 A. Narrow criterion: met DSM-IV criteria in childhood by parent interview[a]
 B. Broad criterion: both (1) and (2) are met as reported by patient[b]
  1. Childhood hyperactivity
  2. Childhood attention deficits

II. Adult characteristics: five additional symptoms, including ongoing difficulties with inattentiveness and hyperactivity and at least three other symptoms:
 A. Inattentiveness
 B. Hyperactivity
 C. Mood lability
 D. Irritability and hot temper
 E. Impaired stress tolerance
 F. Disorganization
 G. Impulsivity

III. Exclusions: not diagnosed in presence of severe depression, psychosis, or severe personality disorder

[a]Parent report aided with 10-item *Parent Rating Scale of Childhood Behavior.*
[b]Patient self-report of retrospective childhood symptoms aided by *Wender Utah Rating Scale.*
DSM-IV, *Diagnostic and Statistical Manual of Mental Disorders*, 4th ed.

ADHD symptoms in adulthood. Furthermore, evidence exists of several additional symptoms that are typical of adult behavior as opposed to childhood behaviors.

In adults, residual signs of the disorder include impulsivity and attention deficit (e.g., difficulty in organizing and completing work, inability to concentrate, increased distractibility, and sudden decision-making without thought of the consequences). Many people with the disorder have a secondary depressive disorder associated with low self-esteem related to their impaired performance and which affects both occupational and social functioning.

A 24-year-old man complained of poor attention span, distractibility, and feelings of restlessness. In childhood, he had persistent problems with academic achievement and behavior. He endorsed a history of seven inattentive and nine hyperactive-impulsive DSM-IV ADHD symptoms during early grade school. He was frequently sent to the principal, and his parents were similarly frustrated at home. Although he was considered a bright student, he made average grades and had no aspirations for college. He worked in construction after graduation, but became dissatisfied with his job prospects. As a result of urging from a friend, he enlisted in the military, and, surprisingly, thrived under military discipline. After receiving an honorable discharge, he enrolled in community college, hoping to become a paralegal.

The ADHD rating scales of childhood behavior confirmed considerable difficulties with inattentive and hyperactive-impulsive symptoms. Ratings of current symptoms were notable for inattention. Clinical review of current DSM symptoms revealed impairment from six inattentive and three hyperactive symptoms. The patient was diagnosed with adult ADHD; no evidence was seen of other coexisting psychopathology.

After receiving education about the nature of ADHD, the patient agreed to a medication trial. Escalating doses of a once-a-day stimulant were titrated over several weeks. At his return visit, the physician reviewed response during the titration and determined an optimal dose. The patient experienced significant reduction of his inattentive symptoms and reported greatly improved academic functioning. He continued to take medication regularly and subsequently transferred to a 4-year university. He married his longtime girlfriend before beginning law school.

Differential Diagnosis

A diagnosis of ADHD is likely when symptoms of inattention and impulsivity are described by adults as a life-long problem, not as episodic events. The overlap of ADHD and hypomania, bipolar II disorder, and cyclothymia is controversial and difficult to sort out retrospectively. Clear-cut histories of discrete episodes of hypomania and mania, with or without periods of depression, are suggestive of a mood disorder rather than a clinical picture of ADHD; however, ADHD may have predated the emergence of a mood disorder in some individuals. In such a case, ADHD and bipolar disorder can be diagnosed as comorbid disorders. Adults with an early history of chronic school difficulties related to paying attention, activity level, and impulsive behavior are generally diagnosed with ADHD, even when a mood disorder occurs later in life. Anxiety disorders can coexist with ADHD, and are less difficult than hypomania to distinguish from it.

Course and Prognosis

The prevalence of ADHD diminishes over time, although at least half of children and adolescents may have the disorder into adulthood. Many children initially diagnosed with ADHD, combined type, exhibit fewer impulsive-hyperactive symptoms as they get older and, by the time they are adults, will meet criteria for ADHD, inattentive type. As with children, adults with ADHD demonstrate higher rates of learning disorders, anxiety disorders, mood disorders, and substance use disorder compared with the general population.

Treatment

Treatment of ADHD in adults targets pharmacotherapy similar to that used with children and adolescents with ADHD. Central nervous stimulants, including methylphenidate, amphetamine, and amphetamine salts, are the first line of treatment. Signs of a positive response are an increased attention span, decreased impulsiveness, and improved mood. Psychopharmacological therapy may be needed indefinitely. Clinicians should use standard ways to monitor drug response and patient compliance.

ICD-10

In the 10th revision of *International Statistical Classification of Diseases and Related Health Problems* (ICD-10), the category hyperkinetic disorders includes disturbance of activity and attention (which in turn encompasses attention-deficit disorder or syndrome with hyperactivity, ADHD), hyperkinetic conduct disorder, other hyperkinetic disorders, and hyperkinetic disorder, unspecified. According to ICD-10, hyperkinetic disorders are characterized by "early onset; a combination of overactive,

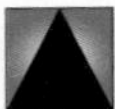

Table 43–6
ICD-10 Diagnostic Criteria for Hyperkinetic Disorders

Note: The research diagnosis of hyperkinetic disorder requires the definite presence of abnormal levels of inattention, hyperactivity, and restlessness that are pervasive across situations and persistent over time and that are not caused by other disorders such as autism or affective disorders.

G1. *Inattention.* At least six of the following symptoms of inattention have persisted for at least 6 months, to a degree that is maladaptive and inconsistent with the developmental level of the child:
(1) often fails to give close attention to details, or makes careless errors in schoolwork, work, or other activities;
(2) often fails to sustain attention in tasks or play activities;
(3) often appears not to listen to what is being said to him or her;
(4) often fails to follow through on instructions or to finish schoolwork, chores, or duties in the workplace (not because of oppositional behavior or failure to understand instructions);
(5) is often impaired in organizing tasks and activities;
(6) often avoids or strongly dislikes tasks, such as homework, that require sustained mental effort;
(7) often loses things necessary for certain tasks or activities, such as school assignments, pencils, books, toys, or tools.
(8) is often easily distracted by external stimuli;
(9) is often forgetful in the course of daily activities.

G2. *Hyperactivity.* At least three of the following symptoms of hyperactivity have persisted for at least 6 months, to a degree that is maladaptive and inconsistent with the developmental level of the child:
(1) often fidgets with hands or feet or squirms on seat;
(2) leaves seat in classroom or in other situations in which remaining seated is expected;
(3) often runs about or climbs excessively in situations in which it is inappropriate (in adolescents or adults, only feelings of restlessness may be present);
(4) is often unduly noisy in playing or has difficulty in engaging quietly in leisure activities;
(5) exhibits a persistent pattern of excessive motor activity that is not substantially modified by social context or demands.

G3. *Impulsivity.* At least one of the following symptoms of impulsivity has persisted for at least 6 months, to a degree that is maladaptive and inconsistent with the developmental level of the child:
(1) often blurts out answers before questions have been completed;
(2) often fails to wait in lines or await turns in games or group situations;
(3) often interrupts or intrudes on others (e.g., butts into others' conversations or games);
(4) often talks excessively without appropriate response to social constraints.

G4. Onset of the disorder is no later than the age of 7 years.

G5. *Pervasiveness.* The criteria should be met for more than a single situation, e.g., the combination of inattention and hyperactivity should be present both at home and at school, or at both school and another setting where children are observed, such as a clinic. (Evidence for cross-situationality will ordinarily require information from more than one source; parental reports about classroom behavior, for instance, are unlikely to be sufficient).

G6. The symptoms in G1–G3 cause clinically significant distress or impairment in social, academic, or occupational functioning.

G7. The disorder does not meet the criteria for pervasive developmental disorders, manic episode, depressive episode, or anxiety disorders.

Comments
Many authorities also recognize conditions that are subthreshold for hyperkinetic disorder. Children who meet criteria in other ways but do not show abnormalities of hyperactivity-impulsiveness may be recognized as showing *attention deficit*; conversely, children who fall short of criteria for attention problems but meet criteria in other respects may be recognized as showing *acitivity disorder.* In the same way, children who meet criteria for only one situation (e.g., only the home or only the classroom) may be regarded showing a *home-specific* or *classroom-specific disorder.* These conditions are not yet included in the main classification because of insufficient empirical predictive validation, and because many children with subthreshold disorders show other syndromes (such as oppositional defiant disorder) and should be classified in the appropriate category.

Disturbance of activity and attention
The general criteria for hyperkinetic disorder must be met, but not those for conduct disorders.

Hyperkinetic conduct disorder
The general criteria for both hyperkinetic disorder and conduct disorders must be met.

Other hyperkinetic disorders

Hyperkinetic disorder, unspecified
This residual category is not recommended and should be used only when there is a lack of differentiation between disturbance of activity and attention and hyperkinetic conduct disorder but the overall criteria for hyperkinetic disorders are fulfilled.

(From World Health Organization. *The ICD-10 Classification of Mental and Behavioural Disorders: Diagnostic Criteria for Research.* Copyright, World Health Organization, Geneva, 1993, with permission.)

poorly modulated behavior with marked inattention and lack of persistent task involvement; and pervasiveness over situations and persistence over time." The ICD-10 criteria for hyperkinetic disorders are given in Table 43–6.

References

Abikoff H, McGough J, Vitiello B, McCracken J, Davies M, Walkup J, Riddle M, Oatis M, Greenhill L, Skrobala A, March J, Gammon P, Robinson J, Lazell R, McMahon DJ, Ritz L, The RUPP ADHD/Anxiety Study Group. Sequential pharmacotherapy for children with comorbid attention-deficit/hyperactivity and anxiety disorders. *J Am Acad Child Adolesc Psychiatry*. 2005;44:418.

Ginsberg DL. Theophyllin treatment of ADHD. *Primary Psychiatry*. 2004; 11(10):28.

Hechtman, L. Attention-deficit disorders. In: Sadock BJ, Sadock VA, eds. *Kaplan & Sadock's Comprehensive Textbook of Psychiatry*. 8th ed. Vol. 2. Baltimore: Lippincott Williams & Wilkins; 2005:3183.

Kratochvil CJ, Newcorn JH, Arnold E, Duesenberg D, Emslie GJ, Quintana H, Sarkis EH, Wagner KD, Gao H, Michelson D, Biederman J. Atomoxetine alone or combined with fluoxetine for treating ADHD with comorbid depressive or anxiety symptoms. *J Am Acad Child Adolesc Psychiatry.* 2005;44:915.

Kratochvil CJ, Lake M, Pliszka SR, Walkup JT. Pharmacologic management of treatment-induced insomnia in ADHD. *J Am Acad Child Adolesc Psychiatry.* 2005;44:499.

McGough J. Adult manifestations of attention-deficit/hyperactivity disorder. In: Sadock BJ, Sadock VA, eds. *Kaplan & Sadock's Comprehensive Textbook of Psychiatry.* 8th ed. Vol. 2. Baltimore: Lippincott Williams & Wilkins; 2005:3198.

Monastra VJ. *Parenting Children with ADHD: 10 Lessons That Medicine Cannot Teach.* Washington DC: American Psychological Association; 2004.

Pelham WE, Manos MJ, Ezzell CE, Tresco KE, Gnagy EM, Hoffman MT, Onyango AN, Fabiano GA, Lopez-Williams A, Wymbs BT, Caserta D, Chronis AM, Burrows-Maclean L, Morse G. A dose-ranging study of a methylphenidate transdermal system in children with ADHD. *J Am Acad Child Adolesc Psychiatry.* 2005;44:522.

Ratner A, Laor N, Bronstein Y, Weizman A, Toren P. Six-week open-label reboxetine treatment in children and adolescents with attention-deficit/hyperactivity disorder. *J Am Acad Child Adolesc Psychiatry.* 2005;44:428.

Weiss M, Tannock R, Kratochvil C, Dunn D, Velez-Borras J, Thomason C, Tamura R, Kelsey D, Stevens L, Allen AJ. A randomized, placebo-controlled study of once-daily atomoxetine in the school setting in children with ADHD. *J Am Acad Child Adolesc Psychiatry.* 2005;44:647.

Wilens TE, Gignac M, Swezey A, Monuteaux MC, Biederman J. Characteristics of adolescents and young adults with ADHD who divert or misuse their prescribed medications. *J Am Acad Child Adolesc Psychiatry.* 2006;45(4):408–414.

44 Disruptive Behavior Disorders

Oppositional and aggressive behaviors during childhood are among the most frequent reasons that a given youth is referred for mental health evaluation. Many youth who exhibit negativistic or oppositional behaviors will find other forms of expression as they mature and will no longer demonstrate these behaviors in adulthood. Children who develop enduring patterns of aggressive behaviors that begin in early childhood and violate the basic rights of peers and family members, however, may be destined to an entrenched pattern of conduct disordered behaviors over time. Controversy has arisen whether a set of "voluntary" antisocial behaviors can be construed as a psychiatric disorder, or can be better accounted for as maladaptive responses to overly harsh or punitive parenting or as strategies that have survival value in chronically threatening environmental situations. Longitudinal studies have demonstrated that, for some youth, early patterns of disruptive behavior may become a lifelong pervasive repertoire culminating in adult antisocial personality disorder. The origin of stable patterns of disruptive behavior is widely accepted as a convergence of multiple contributing factors, including biological, temperamental, learned, and psychological conditions.

Disruptive behavior disorders can be divided into two distinct constellations of symptoms categorized as oppositional defiant disorder and conduct disorder, both of which result in impaired social or academic functioning in a child. Some defiance and refusal to comply with adult requests is developmentally appropriate and marks growth in all children, yet children with the following disorders are themselves impaired by the frequency and severity of their disruptive behaviors.

Oppositional defiant disorder is characterized by enduring patterns of negativistic, disobedient, and hostile behavior toward authority figures, as well as an inability to take responsibility for mistakes, leading to placing blame on others. Children with oppositional defiant disorder frequently argue with adults and become easily annoyed by others, leading to a state of anger and resentment. Children with oppositional defiant disorder may have difficulty in the classroom and with peer relationships, but generally do not resort to physical aggression or significantly destructive behavior.

In contrast, children with *conduct disorder* engage in severe repeated acts of aggression that can cause physical harm to themselves and others and frequently violate the rights of others. Children with conduct disorder usually have behaviors characterized by aggression to persons or animals, destruction of property, deceitfulness or theft, and multiple violations of rules, such as truancy from school. These behavior patterns cause distinct difficulties in school life as well as in peer relationships. Conduct disorder has been divided into a childhood-onset subtype, in which at least one symptom has emerged repeatedly before age 10 years, and adolescent-onset type, in which no characteristic persistent symptoms were seen until after age 10 years. Although some young children show persistent patterns of behavior consistent with violating the rights of others or destroying property, the diagnosis of conduct disorder in children appears to increase with age.

OPPOSITIONAL DEFIANT DISORDER

In oppositional defiant disorder, a child's temper outbursts, active refusal to comply with rules, and annoying behaviors exceed expectations for these behaviors for children of the same age. The disorder is an enduring pattern of negativistic, hostile, and defiant behaviors in the absence of serious violations of social norms or of the rights of others.

Epidemiology

Oppositional, negativistic behavior, in moderation, is developmentally normal in early childhood and adolescence. Epidemiological studies of negativistic traits in nonclinical populations found such behavior in 16 to 22 percent of school-age children. According to text revision of the 4th edition of the American Psychiatric Association's *Diagnostic and Statistical Manual of Mental Disorders* (DSM-IV-TR), prevalence rates for this disorder range from 2 to 16 percent. Although oppositional defiant disorder can begin as early as 3 years of age, it typically is noted by 8 years of age and usually not later than adolescence. Oppositional defiant disorder has been reported to occur at rates ranging from 2 to 16 percent. The disorder seems more prevalent in boys than in girls before puberty, and the sex ratio appears to be equal after puberty. One authority suggests that girls are classified as having oppositional disorder more frequently than boys, because boys more often receive the diagnosis of conduct disorder. No distinct family patterns have been noted, but many parents of children with the disorder are themselves overly concerned with issues of power, control, and autonomy.

Etiology

The ability of a child to communicate his or her own will and opposing others' will is crucial to normal development as a route toward establishing autonomy, forming an identity, and setting inner standards and controls. The most dramatic example of normal oppositional behavior peaks between 18 and 24 months, the "terrible twos," when toddlers behave negativistically as an expression of growing autonomy. Pathology begins when this developmental phase persists abnormally, authority figures overreact, or oppositional behavior recurs considerably more frequently than in most children of the same mental age.

Children exhibit a range of temperamental predispositions to strong will, strong preferences, or great assertiveness. Parents who model more extreme ways of expressing and enforcing their own will may contribute to the development of chronic struggles with their children that are then reenacted with other authority figures. What begins for an infant as an effort to establish self-determination may become transformed into an exaggerated behavioral pattern. In late childhood, environmental trauma, illness, or chronic incapacity, such as mental retardation, can trigger oppositionalism as a defense against helplessness, anxiety, and loss of self-esteem. Another normative oppositional stage occurs in adolescence as an expression of the need to separate from the parents and to establish an autonomous identity.

Classic psychoanalytic theory implicates unresolved conflicts as fueling aggressive behaviors targeting authority figures. Behaviorists have suggested that oppositionality is a reinforced, learned behavior through which a child exerts control over authority figures; for example, by having a temper tantrum when an undesired act is requested, a child coerces the parents to withdraw their request. In addition, increased parental attention—for example, long discussions about the behavior—can reinforce the behavior.

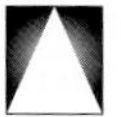

Table 44–1
DSM-IV-TR Diagnostic Criteria for Oppositional Defiant Disorder

A. A pattern of negativistic, hostile, and defiant behavior lasting at least 6 months, during which four (or more) of the following are present:
   (1) often loses temper
   (2) often argues with adults
   (3) often actively defies or refuses to comply with adults' requests or rules
   (4) often deliberately annoys people
   (5) often blames others for his or her mistakes or misbehavior
   (6) is often touchy or easily annoyed by others
   (7) is often angry and resentful
   (8) is often spiteful or vindictive

Note: Consider a criterion met only if the behavior occurs more frequently than is typically observed in individuals of comparable age and developmental level.

B. The disturbance in behavior causes clinically significant impairment in social, academic, or occupational functioning.

C. The behaviors do not occur exclusively during the course of a psychotic or mood disorder.

D. Criteria are not met for conduct disorder, and, if the individual is age 18 years or older, criteria are not met for antisocial personality disorder.

(From American Psychiatric Association. *Diagnostic and Statistical Manual of Mental Disorders.* 4th ed. Text rev. Washington, DC: American Psychiatric Association; copyright 2000, with permission.)

Diagnosis and Clinical Features

Children with oppositional defiant disorder often argue with adults, lose their temper, and are angry, resentful, and easily annoyed by others. Frequently, they actively defy adults' requests or rules and deliberately annoy other persons. They tend to blame others for their own mistakes and misbehavior. Manifestations of the disorder are almost invariably present in the home, but they may not be present at school or with other adults or peers. In some cases, features of the disorder from the beginning of the disturbance are displayed outside the home; in other cases, the behavior starts in the home, but is later displayed outside. Typically, symptoms of the disorder are most evident in interactions with adults or peers whom the child knows well. Thus, a child with the disorder is likely to show little or no sign of the disorder when examined clinically. Usually, these children do not regard themselves as oppositional or defiant, but justify their behavior as a response to unreasonable circumstances. The disorder appears to cause more distress to those around the child than to the child. Diagnostic criteria for oppositional defiant disorder from DSM-IV-TR are given in Table 44–1.

Chronic oppositional defiant disorder almost always interferes with interpersonal relationships and school performance. These children are often friendless and perceive human relationships as unsatisfactory. Despite adequate intelligence, they do poorly or fail in school, as they withhold participation, resist external demands, and insist on solving problems without others' help. Secondary to these difficulties are low self-esteem, poor frustration tolerance, depressed mood, and temper outbursts. Adolescents may abuse alcohol and illegal substances. Often, the disturbance evolves into a conduct disorder or a mood disorder.

Pathology and Laboratory Examination. No specific laboratory tests or pathological findings help diagnose oppositional defiant disorder. Because some children with the disorder become physically aggressive and violate the rights of others as they get older, they may share some of the same characteristics under investigation in violent people, such as low serotonin levels in the central nervous system (CNS).

Differential Diagnosis

Because oppositional behavior is both normal and adaptive at specific developmental stages, these periods of negativism must be distinguished from oppositional defiant disorder. Developmental-stage oppositional behavior, which is of shorter duration than oppositional defiant disorder, is neither considerably more frequent nor more intense than that seen in other children of the same mental age.

Oppositional defiant behavior occurring temporarily in reaction to a stress should be diagnosed as an adjustment disorder. When features of oppositional defiant disorder appear during the course of conduct disorder, schizophrenia, or a mood disorder, the diagnosis of oppositional defiant disorder should not be made. Oppositional and negativistic behaviors can also be present in attention-deficit/hyperactivity disorder (ADHD), cognitive disorders, and mental retardation. Whether a concomitant diagnosis of oppositional defiant disorder should be made depends on the severity, pervasiveness, and duration of such behavior. Some young children who receive a diagnosis of oppositional defiant disorder go on in several years to meet the criteria for conduct disorder. Some investigators believe that the two disorders may be developmental variants of each other, with conduct disorder being the natural progression of oppositional defiant behavior when a child matures. Most children with oppositional defiant disorder, however, do not later meet the criteria for conduct disorder, and up to one quarter of children with oppositional defiant disorder may not meet the diagnosis several years later.

The subtype of oppositional defiant disorder that tends to progress to conduct disorder is one in which aggression is prominent. Most children who have ADHD and conduct disorder develop conduct disorder before the age of 12 years. Most children who develop conduct disorder have a history of oppositional defiant disorder. Overall, the current consensus is that two subtypes of oppositional defiant disorder may exist. One type, which is likely to progress to conduct disorder, includes certain symptoms of conduct disorder (e.g., fighting, bullying). The other type, which is characterized by less aggression and fewer antisocial traits, does not progress to conduct disorder.

Jared, age 8 years, was brought to the clinic for evaluation of misbehavior by his mother. She complained that he has frequent tantrums, usually in response to limits on his behavior or not getting his way. She describes the tantrums as consisting of shouting, cursing, crying, slamming doors, and sometimes throwing books or objects on the floor. She states that these outbursts occur almost daily. She feels that sometimes it seems as though he is trying to provoke her. Recently, he was kicking his foot against his mother's chair and she asked him to stop. He looked at her and continued to kick her chair. She says that she has given up on asking him to pick up his room or help with chores, because it inevitably results in an argument. Jared appears sullen and irritable on interview. He says that it was his mother's fault and she is always after him about one thing or another. He interrupts her several times during the joint interview, saying that she was lying or giving his version of events. His grades at school are excellent, and there are no reports of any behavior problems or disobedience at school. His mother says that he does not have many friends, because he has difficulty sharing his things and tends to be bossy. He had a series of ear infections as an infant and occasionally experiences seasonal allergies, but is otherwise in good health, with normal physical development. His mother describes him as being fussy as an infant and difficult to comfort when upset. He is an only child, and his parents separated and divorced when he was 3. He has had no contact with his father since then. His mother was depressed for a year after the divorce until she sought treatment. She has always felt guilty that his father is not in his life and worries that he blames her for not having his father around. She believes his behaviors have become worse since she recently started dating again.

Course and Prognosis

The course of oppositional defiant disorder depends largely on the severity of the symptoms and the ability of the child to develop more adaptive responses to authority. The stability of oppositional defiant disorder varies over time. Persistence of oppositional defiant symptoms poses an increased risk of additional disorders, such as conduct disorder and substance use disorders. Positive outcomes are more likely for intact families who can modify their own expression of demands and give less attention to the child's argumentative behaviors.

About one quarter of all children who receive the diagnosis of oppositional defiant disorder do not continue to meet diagnostic criteria over the next several years. It is not clear in these cases whether the criteria captured children whose behavior was not developmentally abnormal or whether the disorder spontaneously remitted. Patients in whom the diagnosis persists may remain stable or go on to violate the rights of others and, thus, develop conduct disorder. Such patients should receive guarded prognoses.

An association exists between conduct disorder and later substance use disorders, as well as elevated rates of mood disorders, in children with oppositional defiant disorder, conduct disorder, and ADHD. Parental psychopathology, such as antisocial personality disorder and substance abuse, appears to be more common in families with children who have oppositional defiant disorder than in the general population, which creates additional risks for chaotic and troubled home environments. The prognosis for oppositional defiant disorder in a child depends somewhat on family functioning and the development of comorbid psychopathology.

Treatment

The primary treatment of oppositional defiant disorder is family intervention using both direct training of the parents in child management skills and careful assessment of family interactions. Behavior therapists emphasize teaching parents how to alter their behavior to discourage the child's oppositional behavior and encourage appropriate behavior. Behavior therapy focuses on selectively reinforcing and praising appropriate behavior and ignoring or not reinforcing undesired behavior.

Children with oppositional defiant behavior may also benefit from individual psychotherapy insofar as the child is exposed to a situation with an adult in which to "practice" more adaptive responses. In the therapeutic relationship, the child can learn new strategies to develop a sense of mastery and success in social situations with peers and families. In the safety of a more "neutral" relationship, children may discover that they are capable of less provocative behavior. Often, self-esteem must be restored before a child with oppositional defiant disorder can make more positive responses to external control. Parent–child conflict strongly predicts conduct problems; patterns of harsh physical and verbal punishment particularly evoke the emergence of aggression and deviance in children. Thus, it is likely that eliminating harsh, punitive parenting and increasing positive parent–child interactions may positively influence the course of oppositional and defiant behaviors.

CONDUCT DISORDER

Children with conduct disorder are likely to demonstrate behaviors in the following four categories: physical aggression or threats of harm to people, destruction of their own property or that of others, theft or acts of deceit, and frequent violation of age-appropriate rules. Conduct disorder is an enduring set of behaviors that evolves over time, usually characterized by aggression and violation of the rights of others. Conduct disorder is associated with many other psychiatric disorders including ADHD, depression, and learning disorders, and it is also associated with certain psychosocial factors, such as harsh, punitive parenting; family discord; lack of appropriate parental supervision; lack of social competence; and low socioeconomic level. The DSM-IV-TR criteria require three specific behaviors of the 15 listed, which include bullying, threatening, or intimidating others, and staying out at night despite parental prohibitions, beginning before 13 years of age. DSM-IV-TR also specifies that truancy from school must begin before 13 years of age to be considered a symptom of conduct disorder. The disorder can be diagnosed in a person older than 18 years only if the criteria for antisocial personality disorder are not met. DSM-IV-TR describes a mild level of the disorder as showing few, if any, conduct problems in excess of those needed to make the diagnosis and conduct problems that cause only minor harm to others. According to DSM-IV-TR, the severe level shows many conduct problems in excess of the minimal diagnostic criteria or conduct problems that cause considerable harm to others.

Epidemiology

Occasional rule breaking and rebellious behavior is common during childhood and adolescence, but in youth with conduct disorder, behaviors that violate the rights of others are repetitive and pervasive. Estimated rates of conduct disorder among the general population range from 1 to 10 percent, with a general population rate of approximately 5 percent. The disorder is more common among boys than girls, and the ratio ranges from 4 to 1 to as much as 12 to 1. Conduct disorder occurs with greater frequency in the children of parents with antisocial personality disorder and alcohol dependence than in the general population. The prevalence of conduct disorder and antisocial behavior is associated with socioeconomic factors.

Etiology

No single factor can fully account for a child's antisocial behavior and conduct disorder. Rather, many biopsychosocial factors contribute to development of the disorder.

Parental Factors. Harsh, punitive parenting characterized by severe physical and verbal aggression is associated with the development of children's maladaptive aggressive behaviors. Chaotic home conditions are associated with conduct disorder and delinquency. Divorce itself is considered a risk factor, but the persistence of hostility, resentment, and bitterness between divorced parents may be the more important contributor to maladaptive behavior. Parental psychopathology, child abuse, and negligence often contribute to conduct disorder. Sociopathy, alcohol dependence, and substance abuse in the parents are associated with conduct disorder in their children. Parents may be so negligent that a child's care is shared by relatives or assumed by foster parents. Many such parents were scarred by their own upbringing and tend to be abusive, negligent, or engrossed in getting their own personal needs met.

In the 1980s, particularly in urban areas, cocaine abuse and acquired immunodeficiency syndrome (AIDS) increased family dysfunction. Recent studies suggest that many parents of children with conduct disorder have serious psychopathology, including psychotic disorders. Psychodynamic hypotheses suggest that children with conduct disorder unconsciously act out their parents' antisocial wishes, however data suggests that children who exhibit a pattern of aggressive behavior have received physically or emotionally harsh parenting.

Sociocultural Factors. Socioeconomically deprived children are at higher risk for the development of conduct disorder, as are children and adolescents who grow up in urban environments. Unemployed parents, lack of a supportive social network, and lack of positive participation in community activities seem to predict conduct disorder. Associated findings that may influence the development of conduct disorder in urban areas are increased rates and prevalence of substance use. A recent survey of alcohol use and mental health in adolescents found that weekly alcohol use among adolescents is associated with increased delinquent and aggressive behavior. Significant interactions between frequent alcohol use and age indicated that those adolescents with weekly alcohol use at younger ages were most likely to exhibit aggressive behaviors and mood disorders. Although drug and alcohol use does not cause conduct disorder, it increases the risks associated with it. Drug intoxication itself can also aggravate the symptoms. Thus, all factors that increase the likelihood of regular substance use may, in fact, promote and expand the disorder.

Psychological Factors. Children brought up in chaotic, negligent conditions often express poor modulation of emotions, including anger, frustration, and sadness. Poor modeling of impulse control and the chronic lack of having their own needs met leads to a less well-developed sense of empathy.

Neurobiological Factors. Neurobiological factors in conduct disorder have been little studied, but research in ADHD yields some important findings, and this disorder often coexists with conduct disorder. In some children with conduct disorder, a low level of plasma dopamine β-hydroxylase, an enzyme that converts dopamine to norepinephrine, has been found. This finding supports a theory of decreased noradrenergic functioning in conduct disorder. Some conduct-disordered juvenile offenders have high serotonin levels in blood. Evidence indicates that blood serotonin levels correlate inversely with levels of the serotonin metabolite 5-hydroxyindoleacetic acid (5-HIAA) in the cerebrospinal fluid (CSF) and that low 5-HIAA levels in CSF correlates with aggression and violence.

Neurologic Factors. A recent Canadian study investigated the relationship between resting frontal brain electrical activity (EEG), emotional intelligence, and aggression and rule breaking in 10-year-old children. Frontal resting brain electrical activity has been hypothesized to reflect the ability to regulate emotionality. Results of this study indicate that children with higher reported externalizing behaviors had significantly greater relative right frontal EEG activity during rest compared with children with little or no reported aggressive behavior. Boys tended to show lower emotional intelligence than girls and greater aggressive behavior than girls. No relationship, however, was found between emotional intelligence and pattern of frontal EEG activation. This study suggests an association between resting pattern of EEG activation and aggressive behavior.

Child Abuse and Maltreatment. It is widely accepted that children chronically exposed to violence, especially those receiving repeated physical or sexual abuse that starts at a young age are at high risk for behaving aggressively. Children who are exposed to caregivers who are exposed to violence are also likely to demonstrate disruptive and aggressive behaviors themselves. A recent study of female caregivers' exposed to intimate partner violence revealed a strong association with offspring aggression and mood disturbance. Children exposed as witnesses to maternal abuse or recipients of abuse themselves may be reticent to verbalize their experiences because of direct threats from the abusive adult, and therefore may instead demonstrate their feelings through aggressive and destructive behaviors. Severely abused children and adolescents tend to be hypervigilant; in some cases, they misperceive benign situations as directly threatening, and respond with violence. Not all expressed physical behavior in adolescents is synonymous with conduct disorder, but children with a pattern of hypervigilance and violent responses are likely to violate the rights of others.

Comorbid Factors. ADHD, CNS dysfunction or damage, and early extremes of temperament can predispose a child to conduct disorder. Propensity to violence correlates with CNS dysfunction and signs of severe psychopathology, such as delusional tendencies. Longitudinal temperament studies suggest that many behavioral deviations are initially a straightforward response to a poor fit between a child's temperament and emotional needs, on one hand, and parental attitudes and child-rearing practices, on the other.

Diagnosis and Clinical Features

Conduct disorder does not develop overnight; instead, many symptoms evolve over time until a consistent pattern develops that involves violating the rights of others. Very young children are unlikely to meet the criteria for the disorder, because they are not developmentally able to exhibit the symptoms typical of older children with conduct disorder. A 3-year-old does not break into someone's home, steal with confrontation, force someone into sexual activity, or deliberately use a weapon that can cause serious harm. School-age children, however, can become bullies, initiate physical fights, destroy property, or set fires. The DSM-IV-TR diagnostic criteria for conduct disorder are given in Table 44–2.

The average age of onset of conduct disorder is younger in boys than in girls. Boys most commonly meet the diagnostic criteria by 10 to 12 years of age, whereas girls often reach 14 to 16 years of age before the criteria are met.

Children who meet the criteria for conduct disorder express their overt aggressive behavior in various forms. Aggressive antisocial behavior can take the form of bullying, physical aggression, and cruel behavior toward peers. Children may be hostile, verbally abusive, impudent, defiant, and negativistic toward adults. Persistent lying, frequent truancy, and vandalism are common. In severe cases, destructiveness, stealing, and physical violence often occur. Some adolescents with conduct disorder make little attempt to conceal their antisocial behavior. Sexual behavior and regular use of tobacco, liquor, or nonprescribed psychoactive substances begin unusually early for such children and adolescents. Suicidal thoughts, gestures, and acts are frequent in children and adolescents with conduct disorder who are in conflict with peers, family members, or the law and are unable to problem solve their difficulties.

Some children with aggressive behavioral patterns have impaired social attachments, as evinced by their difficulties with peer relationships. Some may befriend a much older or younger person or have superficial relationships with other antisocial youngsters. Many children with conduct problems have poor self-esteem, although they may project an image of toughness. They may lack the skills to communicate in socially acceptable ways and appear to have little regard for the feelings, wishes, and welfare of others. Children and adolescents with conduct disorders often feel guilt or remorse for some of their behaviors, but try to blame others to stay out of trouble.

Many children and adolescents with conduct disorder suffer from the deprivation of having few of their dependency needs

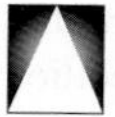

Table 44–2
DSM-IV-TR Diagnostic Criteria for Conduct Disorder

A. A repetitive and persistent pattern of behavior in which the basic rights of others or major age-appropriate societal norms or rules are violated, as manifested by the presence of three (or more) of the following criteria in the past 12 months, with at least one criterion present in the past 6 months:

Aggression to people and animals
(1) often bullies, threatens, or intimidates others
(2) often initiates physical fights
(3) has used a weapon that can cause serious physical harm to others (e.g., a bat, brick, broken bottle, knife, gun)
(4) has been physically cruel to people
(5) has been physically cruel to animals
(6) has stolen while confronting a victim (e.g., mugging, purse snatching, extortion, armed robbery)
(7) has forced someone into sexual activity

Destruction of property
(8) has deliberately engaged in fire setting with the intention of causing serious damage
(9) has deliberately destroyed others' property (other than by fire setting)

Deceitfulness or theft
(10) has broken into someone else's house, building, or car
(11) often lies to obtain goods or favors or to avoid obligations (i.e., "cons" others)
(12) has stolen items of nontrivial value without confronting a victim (e.g., shoplifting, but without breaking and entering; forgery)

Serious violations of rules
(13) often stays out at night despite parental prohibitions, beginning before age 13 years
(14) has run away from home overnight at least twice while living in parental or parental surrogate home (or once without returning for a lengthy period)
(15) is often truant from school, beginning before age 13 years

B. The disturbance in behavior causes clinically significant impairment in social, academic, or occupational functioning.

C. If the individual is age 18 years or older, criteria are not met for antisocial personality disorder.

Code based on age at onset:
Conduct disorder, childhood-onset type: onset of at least one criterion characteristic of conduct disorder prior to age 10 years
Conduct disorder, adolescent-onset type: absence of any criteria characteristic of conduct disorder prior to age 10 years
Conduct disorder, unspecified onset: age at onset is not known

Specify severity:
Mild: few if any conduct problems in excess of those required to make the diagnosis and conduct problems cause only minor harm to others
Moderate: number of conduct problems and effect on others intermediate between "mild" and "severe"
Severe: many conduct problems in excess of those required to make the diagnosis or conduct problems cause considerable harm to others

(From American Psychiatric Association. *Diagnostic and Statistical Manual of Mental Disorders.* 4th ed. Text rev. Washington, DC: American Psychiatric Association; copyright 2000, with permission.)

met and may have had either overly harsh parenting or a lack of appropriate supervision. The deficient socialization of many children and adolescents with conduct disorder can be expressed in physical violation of others and, for some, in sexual violation of others. Severe punishments for behavior in children with conduct disorder almost invariably increases their maladaptive expression of rage and frustration rather than ameliorating the problem.

In evaluation interviews, children with aggressive conduct disorders are typically uncooperative, hostile, and provocative. Some have a superficial charm and compliance until they are urged to talk about their problem behaviors. Then, they often deny any problems. If the interviewer persists, the child may attempt to justify misbehavior or become suspicious and angry about the source of the examiner's information and perhaps bolt from the room. Most often, the child becomes angry with the examiner and expresses resentment of the examination with open belligerence or sullen withdrawal. Their hostility is not limited to adult authority figures, but is expressed with equal venom toward their age-mates and younger children. In fact, they often bully those who are smaller and weaker than they. By boasting, lying, and expressing little interest in a listener's responses, such children reveal their lack of trust in adults to understand their position.

Evaluation of the family situation often reveals severe marital disharmony, which initially may center on disagreements about management of the child. Because of a tendency toward family instability, parent surrogates are often in the picture. Children with conduct disorder are more likely to be unplanned or unwanted babies. The parents of children with conduct disorder, especially the father, have higher rates of antisocial personality disorder or alcohol dependence. Aggressive children and their family show a stereotyped pattern of impulsive and unpredictable verbal and physical hostility. A child's aggressive behavior rarely seems directed toward any definable goal and offers little pleasure, success, or even sustained advantages with peers or authority figures.

In other cases, conduct disorder includes repeated truancy, vandalism, and serious physical aggression or assault against others by a gang, such as mugging, gang fighting, and beating. Children who become part of a gang usually have the skills for age-appropriate friendships. They are likely to show concern for the welfare of their friends or their own gang members and are unlikely to blame them or inform on them. In most cases, gang members have a history of adequate or even excessive conformity during early childhood that ended when the youngster became a member of the delinquent peer group, usually in preadolescence or during adolescence. Also present in the history is some evidence of early problems, such as marginal or poor school performance, mild behavior problems, anxiety, and depressive symptoms. Some family social or psychological pathology is usually evident. Patterns of paternal discipline are rarely ideal and can vary from harshness and excessive strictness to inconsistency or relative absence of supervision and control. The mother has often protected the child from the consequences of early mild misbehavior, but does not seem to encourage delinquency actively. Delinquency, also called juvenile delinquency, is most often associated with conduct disorder but can also result from other psychological or neurological disorders.

Violent Video Games and Violent Behavior. Over the last few decades violent video games have become ubiquitous in western societies, especially as frequent activities for child and adolescent males. A recent review of the literature of the effect of violent video games on children and adolescents revealed that violent video game playing is related to aggressive affect, physiologic arousal, and aggressive behaviors. It stands to reason that the degree of exposure to violent games and the more restriction of activity would be related to a greater preoccupation with violent themes.

Pathology and Laboratory Examination

No specific laboratory test or neurological pathology helps make the diagnosis of conduct disorder. Some evidence indicates that amounts of certain neurotransmitters, such as serotonin in the CNS, are low in some persons with a history of violent or aggressive behavior toward others or themselves. Whether this association is related to the cause, or is the effect, of violence or is unrelated to the violence is not clear.

Differential Diagnosis

Disturbances of conduct may be part of many childhood psychiatric conditions, ranging from mood disorders to psychotic disorders to learning disorders. Therefore, clinicians must obtain a history of the chronology of the symptoms to determine whether the conduct disturbance is a transient or reactive phenomenon or an enduring pattern. Isolated acts of antisocial behavior do not justify a diagnosis of conduct disorder; an enduring pattern must be present. The relation of conduct disorder to oppositional defiant disorder is still under debate. Historically, oppositional defiant disorder has been conceptualized as a mild precursor of conduct disorder, which is likely to be diagnosed in young children at risk for conduct disorder. Children who progress from oppositional defiant disorder to conduct disorder do maintain their oppositional characteristics, but some evidence indicates that the two disorders are independent. Many children with oppositional defiant disorder never go on to have conduct disorder, and when conduct disorder first appears in adolescence, it may be unrelated to oppositional defiant disorder. The main distinguishing clinical feature of the two disorders is that in conduct disorder, the basic rights of others are violated, whereas in oppositional defiant disorder, hostility and negativism fall short of seriously violating the rights of others.

Mood disorders are often present in children who exhibit irritability and aggressive behavior. Both major depressive disorder and bipolar disorders must be ruled out, but the full syndrome of conduct disorder can occur and be diagnosed during the onset of a mood disorder. Substantial comorbidity exists of conduct disorder and depressive disorders. A recent report concludes that the high correlation between the two disorders arises from shared risk factors for both disorders rather than a causal relation. Thus, a series of factors, including family conflict, negative life events, early history of conduct disturbance, level of parental involvement, and affiliation with delinquent peers, contribute to the development of affective disorders and conduct disorder. This is not the case with oppositional defiant disorder, which cannot be diagnosed if it occurs exclusively during a mood disorder.

Attention-deficit/hyperactivity disorder and learning disorders are commonly associated with conduct disorder. Usually, the symptoms of these disorders predate the diagnosis of conduct disorder. Substance abuse disorders are also more common in adolescents with conduct disorder than in the general population. Evidence indicates an association between fighting behaviors as a child and substance use as an adolescent. Once a pattern of drug use is formed, this pattern may interfere with the development of positive mediators, such as social skills and problem-solving, which could enhance remission of the conduct disorder. Thus, once substance abuse develops, it may promote continuation of the conduct disorder. Obsessive-compulsive disorder also frequently seems to coexist with disruptive behavior disorders. All the disorders described here should be noted when they co-occur. Children with ADHD often exhibit impulsive and aggressive behaviors that may not meet the full criteria for conduct disorder.

John, age 12 years, was referred for outpatient evaluation after being picked up by police for running away from home. He states that he just wanted to get out of the house and visit his friends. His mother says that he has been out of the home overnight on three other occasions in the past year, but usually returns the next morning. She complains that he is constantly in trouble. He has shoplifted on several occasions that she knows of, the first time at age 8 years. She suspects that he also steals from neighbors or school, because there are always items at home that he claims he found. The police have been involved only for his running away from home. He has a quick temper, and she knows he was involved in several fights over the past year in the neighborhood. He is particularly cruel to his younger brother, constantly taunting and teasing him. She stated that he lies constantly, sometimes for no apparent reason. When he was 6 years of age, he was fascinated with fire and set several small fires at home, fortunately with no serious injury or damage. She ended by saying that John is just like his no-good father and that she wished she never had him. John initially refused to answer questions but gradually began to talk. He presented a tough image with an indifferent attitude about the various problems. He denies any abuse at home, saying that he ran off because he was bored. He acknowledged his misbehaviors, but dismissed them as just having fun. He explained the fights as provoked by the others and denied the use of any weapons, although he bragged about breaking the nose of another youth. His record indicates that he was evaluated for symptoms of ADHD when he was in first grade. Methylphenidate (Ritalin) was prescribed; however, the family did not continue with treatment, and he is currently on no medication. He is currently in 6th grade special education classes, having failed and repeated 5th grade. His current grades are failing, and he may have to repeat 6th grade. He admits to truancy on several occasions this year in addition to his problems with completing schoolwork. His previous evaluation indicates that child protective services evaluated the family for possible neglect when he was 5 years of age after he and his brother were found barefoot and unkempt on the street late one evening. Apparently, the family was referred for counseling and never attended, but the case was eventually dismissed. Both of John's parents have a history of drug and alcohol abuse. His birth was unplanned, and his mother used drugs during pregnancy. His parents separated soon after his birth, and his mother returned to live with her parents briefly. He and his mother moved to live with her boyfriend when John was 3 years of age after she became pregnant with his younger brother. This relationship ended within a year, and only John, his mother, and his brother live in their apartment. She has worked several different jobs, and John thinks she still has a drinking problem.

Course and Prognosis

In general, the prognosis for children with conduct disorder is most guarded in those who have symptoms at a young age, exhibit the greatest number of symptoms, and express them most frequently. This finding is true partly because those with severe conduct disorder seem to be most vulnerable to comorbid disorders later in life, such as mood disorders and substance use disorders. It stands to reason that the more concurrent mental disorders a person has, the more troublesome life will be. A recent report found that, although assaultive behavior in childhood and parental criminality predict a high risk for incarceration later in life, the diagnosis of conduct disorder per se was not correlated with imprisonment. A good prognosis is predicted for mild conduct disorder in the absence of coexisting psychopathology and the presence of normal intellectual functioning.

Treatment

Multimodality treatment programs that use all the available family and community resources are likely to bring about the best results in efforts to control conduct-disordered behavior. Multimodal treatments can involve the use of behavioral interventions in which rewards may be earned for prosocial and nonaggressive behaviors, social skills training, family education and therapy, and pharmacologic interventions. Overall, treatment programs have been more successful in decreasing overt symptoms of conduct, such as aggression, than the covert symptoms, such as lying or stealing. Treatment strategies for young children that focus on increasing social behavior and social competence are believed to reduce aggressive behavior. A recent study of 548 third graders administered a school-based intervention instead of a regular health curriculum in several public schools in North Carolina, called *Making Choices: Social Problem Solving Skills For Children* (MC) program along with supplemental teacher and parent components. Compared with 3rd graders receiving the routine health curriculum, children exposed to the MC program were rated lower on the posttest social and overt aggression, and higher on social competence. They further scored higher on an information-processing skills posttest. These findings support the notion that school-based prevention programs have the potential to strengthen social and emotional skills and diminish aggressive behavior among normal populations of school-age children. No treatment is considered curative for the entire spectrum of behaviors that contribute to conduct disorder, but

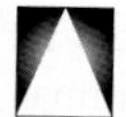

Table 44–3
DSM-IV-TR Diagnostic Criteria for Disruptive Behavior Disorder Not Otherwise Specified

This category is for disorders characterized by conduct or oppositional defiant behaviors that do not meet the criteria for conduct disorder or oppositional defiant disorder. For example, include clinical presentations that do not meet full criteria either for oppositional defiant disorder or conduct disorder, but in which there is clinically significant impairment.

(From American Psychiatric Association. *Diagnostic and Statistical Manual of Mental Disorders.* 4th ed. Text rev. Washington, DC: American Psychiatric Association; copyright 2000, with permission.)

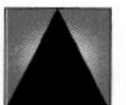

Table 44–4
ICD-10 Diagnostic Criteria for Conduct Disorders

G1. There is a repetitive and persistent pattern of behavior, in which either the basic rights of others or major age-appropriate societal norms or rules are violated, lasting at least 6 months, during which some of the following symptoms are present (see individual subcategories for rules or numbers of symptoms).

Note: The symptoms in 11, 13, 15, 16, 20, 21, and 23 need only have occurred once for the criterion to be fulfilled.

The individual:

(1) has unusually frequent or severe temper tantrums for his or her developmental level;
(2) often argues with adults;
(3) often actively refuses adults' requests or defies rules;
(4) often, apparently deliberately, does things that annoy other people;
(5) often blames others for his or her own mistakes or misbehavior;
(6) is often "touchy" or easily annoyed by others;
(7) is often angry or resentful;
(8) is often spiteful or vindictive;
(9) often lies or breaks promises to obtain goods or favors or to avoid obligations;
(10) frequently initiates physical fights (this does not include fights with siblings);
(11) has used a weapon that can cause serious physical harm to others (e.g., bat, brick, broken bottle, knife, gun);
(12) often stays out after dark despite parental prohibition (beginning before 13 years of age);
(13) exhibits physical cruelty to other people (e.g., ties up, cuts, or burns a victim);
(14) exhibits physical cruelty to animals;
(15) deliberately destroys the property of others (other than by fire-setting);
(16) deliberately sets fires with a risk or intention of causing serious damage;
(17) steals objects of nontrivial value without confronting the victim, either within the home or outside (e.g., shoplifting, burglary, forgery);
(18) is frequently truant from school, beginning before 13 years of age;
(19) has run away from parental or parental surrogate home at least twice or has run away once for more than a single night (this does not include leaving to avoid physical or sexual abuse);
(20) commits a crime involving confrontation with the victim (including purse-snatching, extortion, mugging);
(21) forces another person into sexual activity;
(22) frequently bullies others (e.g., deliberate infliction of pain or hurt, including persistent intimidation, tormenting, or molestation);
(23) breaks into someone else's house, building, or car.

G2. The disorder does not meet the criteria for dissocial personality disorder, schizophrenia, manic episode, depressive episode, pervasive developmental disorders, or hyperkinetic disorder. (If criteria for emotional disorder are met, the diagnosis should be mixed disorder of conduct and emotions.)

It is recommended that the age of onset be specified:

– *childhood-onset type:* onset of at least one conduct problem before the age of 10 years;
– *adolescent-onset type:* no conduct problems before the age of 10 years.

Specification for possible subdivisions

Authorities differ on the best way of subdividing the conduct disorders, although most agree that the disorders are heterogeneous. For determining prognosis, the severity (indexed by number of symptoms) is a better guide than the precise type of symptomatology. The best-validated distinction is that between *socialized* and *unsocialized* disorders, defined by the presence or absence of lasting peer friendships. However, it seems that disorders confined to the family context may also constitute an important variety, and a category is provided for this purpose. It is clear that further research is needed to test the validity of all proposed subdivisions of conduct disorder.

In addition to these categorizations, it is recommended that cases be described in terms of their scores on three dimensions of disturbance:

(1) hyperactivity (inattentive, restless behavior);
(2) emotional disturbance (anxiety, depression, obsessionality, hypochondriasis); and
(3) severity of conduct disorder:
  (a) *mild:* few if any conduct problems are in excess of those required to make the diagnosis, *and* conduct problems cause only minor harm to others;
  (b) *moderate:* the number of conduct problems and the effects on others are intermediate between "mild" and "severe";
  (c) *severe:* there are many conduct problems in excess of those required to make the diagnosis, *or* the conduct problems cause considerable harm to others, e.g., severe physical injury, vandalism, or theft.

Conduct disorder confined to the family context

A. The general criteria for conduct disorder must be met.
B. Three or more of the symptoms listed for criterion G1 must be present, with at least three from items (9)–(23).
C. At least one of the symptoms from items (9)–(23) must have been present for at least 6 months.
D. Conduct disturbance must be limited to the family context.

Unsocialized conduct disorder

A. The general criteria for conduct disorder must be met.
B. Three or more of the symptoms listed for conduct disorder criterion G1 must be present, with at least three from items (9)–(23).
C. At least one of the symptoms from items (9)–(23) must have been present for at least 6 months.
D. There must be definitely poor relationships with the individual's peer group, as shown by isolation, rejection, or unpopularity, and by a lack of lasting close reciprocal friendships.

Socialized conduct disorder

A. The general criteria for conduct disorder must be met.
B. Three or more of the symptoms listed for criterion G1 must be present, with at least three from items (9)–(23).
C. At least one of the symptoms from items (9)–(23) must have been present for at least 6 months.
D. Conduct disturbance must include settings outside the home or family context.
E. Peer relationships are within normal limits.

Oppositional defiant disorder

A. The general criteria for conduct disorder must be met.
B. Four or more of the symptoms listed for criterion G1 must be present, but with no more than two symptoms from items (9)–(23).
C. The symptoms in criterion B must be maladaptive and inconsistent with the developmental level.
D. At least four of the symptoms must have been present for at least 6 months.

Other conduct disorders

Conduct disorder, unspecified

This residual category is not recommended and should be used only for disoders that meet the general criteria for conduct disorder but that have not been specified as to subtype or that do not fulfill the criteria for any of the specified subtypes.

(From World Health Organization. *The ICD-10 Classification of Mental and Behavioural Disorders: Dignostic Criteria for Research.* Copyright, World Health Organization, Geneva, 1993, with permission.)

a variety of treatments may be helpful in containing symptoms and promoting prosocial behavior.

An environmental structure that provides support, along with consistent rules and expected consequences, can help control a variety of problem behaviors. The reduction of violence and aggression in schools is an important setting for interventions. A thoughtful approach to the management of threats of violence includes provision of a functioning security hierarchy, peer-participant programs, threat assessment, and crisis response initiatives. All of these strategies increase the structure necessary to maintain a safe school environment. The structure can be applied to family life in some cases, so that parents become aware of behavioral techniques and grow proficient at using them to foster appropriate behaviors. Families in which psychopathology or environmental stressors prevent parental understanding of the techniques may require parental psychiatric evaluation and treatment before making such an endeavor. When a family is abusive or chaotic, the child may have to be removed from the home to benefit from a consistent and structured environment. School settings can also use behavioral techniques to promote socially acceptable behavior toward peers and to discourage covert antisocial incidents.

Behaviorally based individual psychotherapy targeting problem-solving skills with appropriate rewards can be useful, because children with conduct disorder may have a long-standing pattern of maladaptive responses to daily situations. The age at which treatment begins is important, because the longer the maladaptive behaviors continue, the more entrenched they become.

Pharmacologic treatments for aggression have become more accepted adjunctive treatment in the context of conduct disorder. Overt explosive aggression responds to several medications. Early studies of antipsychotics, most notably haloperidol (Haldol), have reported decreased aggressive and assaultive behaviors in children with a variety of psychiatric disorders. Currently, the atypical antipsychotics risperidone (Risperdal), olanzapine (Zyprexa), quetiapine (Seroquel), ziprasidone (Geodon), and aripiprazole (Abilify) have replaced the older antipsychotics because of their comparable efficacy and improved side effect profiles. Risperidone has been shown to reduce aggression in children with disruptive behavior disorders, in placebo-controlled, randomized trials, particularly in populations with pervasive developmental disorders and aggression. Growing evidence suggests that atypical antipsychotics are efficacious in contributing to the management of aggression among children and adolescents. Long-term effects of the use of these agents are largely unknown and require further investigation. Side effects include sedation, increased prolactin levels, (with risperidone use) and extrapyriamidal symptoms, including akathisia. In general, however, the atypical antipsychotics appear to be well tolerated. A preliminary study of clozapine (Clozaril), used mainly in the treatment of refractory schizophrenia, has reported decreased aggressive behavior in a sample of treatment refractory children and adolescents with schizophrenia and aggressive behavior. Lithium (Eskalith) has been reported to have efficacy for some aggressive children with or without comorbid bipolar disorders. Although previous trials suggested that carbamazepine (Tegretol) may help control aggression, a double-blind, placebo-controlled study did not show superiority of carbamazepine over placebo in decreasing aggression. A recent pilot study found that clonidine (Catapres) may decrease aggression. The selective serotonin reuptake inhibitors (SSRIs), such as fluoxetine (Prozac), sertraline (Zoloft), paroxetine (Paxil), and citalopram (Celexa), have been used in an attempt to diminish impulsivity, irritability, and lability of mood, which often occur with conduct disorder. Conduct disorder frequently coexists with ADHD, learning disorders, and, over time, mood disorders and substance-related disorders; thus, the treatment of any concurrent disorders must also be addressed.

DISRUPTIVE BEHAVIOR DISORDER NOT OTHERWISE SPECIFIED

According to DSM-IV-TR, the category of disruptive behavior disorder not otherwise specified can be used for disorders of conduct or oppositional-defiant behaviors that do not meet the diagnostic criteria for either conduct disorder or oppositional defiant disorder, but in which there is notable impairment (Table 44–3).

ICD-10

In the 10th revision of *International Statistical Classification of Diseases and Related Health Problems* (ICD-10), conduct disorders include disorder confined to the family context, unsocialized conduct disorder, socialized conduct disorder, oppositional defiant behavior, other conduct disorders, and conduct disorder, unspecified. ICD-10 characterizes conduct disorders as repetitive and persistent patterns of "dissocial, aggressive, or defiant conduct."

In ICD-10, oppositional defiant disorder is sometimes considered a less severe variant of conduct disorder rather than a distinct type. Although, according to ICD-10, it is uncertain whether the distinction is qualitative or quantitative, findings suggest that it is distinctive "mainly or only in younger children." In older children, conduct disorders generally include behavior that is aggressive or dissocial beyond defiance, even when it was preceded by oppositional defiant behaviors. Thus, this disorder accommodates "common diagnostic practice" and facilitates "the classification of disorders occurring in younger children."

The ICD-10 criteria for conduct disorders are listed in Table 44–4. The criteria for mixed disorders of conduct and emotions are listed in Table 44–5.

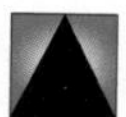

Table 44–5
ICD-10 Diagnostic Criteria for Mixed Disorders of Conduct and Emotions Depressive Conduct Disorder

A. The general criteria for conduct disorders must be met.
B. Criteria for one of the mood (affective) disorders must be met.

Other mixed disorders of conduct and emotions

A. The general criteria for conduct disorders must be met.
B. Criteria for one of the neurotic, stress-related, and somatoform disorders or childhood emotional disorders must be met.

Mixed disorder of conduct and emotions, unspecified

(From World Health Organization. The *ICD-10 Classification of Mental and Behavioural Disorders: Diagnostic Criteria for Research.* Copyright, World Health Organization, Geneva; 1993, with permission.)

References

Findling RL, Steiner H, Weller EB. Use of antipsychotics in children and adolescents. *J Clin Psychiatry*. 2005;66[Suppl 7]:29.

Fraser MW, Galinsky MJ, Smokowski PR, Day SH, Terzian MA, Rose RA, Guo S. Social information-processing skills training to promote social competence and prevent aggressive behavior in the third grades. *J Consult Clin Pychol*. 2005;73:1045.

Gentile DA, Stone W. Violent videogame effects on children and adolescents. A review of the literature. *Merva Pediatr*. 2005;57:337.

Greene MB. Reducing violence and aggression in schools. *Trauma Violence Abuse* 2005;6:236.

Hazen AL, Connelly CD, Kelleher KJ, Barth RP, Landsverk JA. Female caregivers' experiences with intimate partner violence and behavior problems in children investigated as victims of maltreatment. *Pediatrics*. 2006;117:99.

Kranzler H, Roofeh D, Gerbino-Rosen G, Dombrowski C, McMeniman M, DeThomas C, Frederickson A, Nusser L, Bienstock MD, Fisch GS, Kumra S. Clozapine: Its impact on aggressive behavior among children and adolescents with schizophrenia. *J Am Acad Child Adolesc Psychiatry*. 2005; 44:55.

LeBlanc JC, Binder CE, Armenteros JL, Aman MG, Want JS, Hew H, Kusumakar V. Risperidone reduces aggression in boys with a disruptive behavior disorder and below average intelligence quotient: Analysis of two placebo-controlled randomized trials. *Int Clin Psychopharmacol*. 2005;20:275.

Patel NC, Crismon ML, Hoagwood K, Jensen PS. Unanswered questions regarding atypical antipsychotic use in aggressive children and adolescents. *J Child Adolesc Psyychopharmacol*. 2005;15:270.

Pelletier J, Collett B, Gimpel G, Crowley S. Assessment of disruptive behaviors in preschoolers: Psychometric Properties of the Disruptive Behavior Disorders Rating Scale and School Situations Questionnaire. *Journal of Psychoeducational Assessment*. 2006;24:3–18.

Reyes M, Buitelaar J, Toren P, Augustyns I, Eerdekens M. A randomized, double-blind, placebo-controlled study of risperidone maintenance treatment in children and adolescents with disruptive behavior disorders. *Am J Psychiatry*. 2006;163:402–410.

Santesso DL, Reker DL, Schmidt LA, Segalowitz SJ. Frontal electroencephalogram activation asymmetry, emotional intelligence, and externalizing behaviors in 10-year-old children. *Child Psychiatr Hum Dev* 2006; 36:311–328.

Tse J. Research on day treatment programs for preschoolers with disruptive behavior disorders. *Psychiatr Serv*. 2006;57:477–486.

Verdurmen J, Monshouwer K, van Dorsselaer Ster Bogt T, Vollebergh W. Alcohol use and mental health in adolescents: Interactions with age and gender-findings from the Dutch 2001 Health Behaviour in School-Aged Children survey. *J Stud Alcohol* 2005;66:605–609.

45 Feeding and Eating Disorders of Infancy or Early Childhood

Feeding disorders during infancy and early childhood highlight the interactive nature between the infant and caregiver. In broad terms, feeding disorder is characterized by a variety of conditions, including food refusal, food avoidance, active attempts to reject the feeding process, or a delay in self-feeding. Feeding disorder has been an underlying process in some children who have been described as picky eaters, poor eaters, or demonstrating feeding resistances. A feeding disorder may or may not be accompanied by physical sequelae of the maladaptive eating patterns, but without well-defined criteria, the term has been used interchangeably with *failure to thrive*, which refers to inadequate weight gain based on standard growth charts. Failure to thrive syndromes, in some cases, are caused by a medical disease process; however, this term is often applied to children without medical illness who have been exposed to parental deprivation or neglect. The text revision of the 4th edition of *Diagnostic and Statistical Manual of Mental Disorders* (DSM-IV-TR) includes three distinct disorders of feeding and eating in this age group: pica, rumination disorder, and feeding disorder of infancy or early childhood. A high rate of spontaneous recovery from all of these feeding disorders occurs, although a subset of infants refuses to eat and has persistent eating problems throughout childhood. Additional maladaptive feeding patterns that cause impaired nutritional intake that are not included in the DSM-IV-TR include (1) infantile anorexia, (2) feeding disorder of caregiver–infant reciprocity, (3) sensory food aversions, and (4) posttraumatic feeding disorder.

PICA

In DSM-IV-TR, pica is described as persistent eating of nonnutritive substances for at least 1 month. The behavior must be developmentally inappropriate, not culturally sanctioned, and sufficiently severe to merit clinical attention. Pica is diagnosed even when these symptoms occur in the context of another disorder, such as autistic disorder, schizophrenia, or Kleine-Levin syndrome. Pica appears much more frequently in young children than in adults; it also occurs in persons who are mentally retarded. Among adults, certain forms of pica, including geophagia (clay eating) and amylophagia (starch eating), have been reported in pregnant women.

Epidemiology

A survey of a large clinic population reported that 75 percent of 12-month-old infants and 15 percent of 2- to 3-year-old toddlers placed nonnutritive substances in their mouth. Pica is more common among children and adolescents with mental retardation. It has been reported in up to 15 percent of persons with severe mental retardation. Pica appears to affect both sexes equally.

Etiology

Pica is most often a transient disorder that typically lasts for several months and then remits. In younger children, it is more frequently seen among children with developmental speech and social developmental delays. Among adolescents with pica, a substantial number of them exhibited depressive symptoms and use of substances. Several theories have been proposed to explain the phenomenon of pica, but none has been universally accepted. A higher than expected incidence of pica seems to occur in the relatives of persons with the symptoms. Nutritional deficiencies have been postulated as causes of pica; in particular circumstances, cravings for nonedible substances have been produced by dietary insufficiencies. For example, cravings for dirt and ice are sometimes associated with iron and zinc deficiencies, which are corrected by their administration. A high incidence of parental neglect and deprivation has been associated with cases of pica. Theories relating children's psychological deprivation and subsequent ingestion of inedible substances have suggested that pica is a compensatory mechanism to satisfy oral needs.

Diagnosis and Clinical Features

Eating nonedible substances repeatedly after 18 months of age is usually considered abnormal. The onset of pica is usually between ages 12 and 24 months, and the incidence declines with age. The specific substances ingested vary with their accessibility, and they increase with a child's mastery of locomotion and the resultant increased independence and decreased parental supervision. Typically, young children paint, plaster, string, hair, and cloth; older children with pica may ingest dirt, animal feces, stones, and paper. The clinical implications can be benign or life-threatening, depending on the objects ingested. Among the most serious complications are lead poisoning (usually from lead-based paint), intestinal parasites after ingestion of soil or feces, anemia and zinc deficiency after ingestion of clay, severe iron deficiency after ingestion of large quantities of starch, and intestinal obstruction from the ingestion of hair balls, stones, or gravel. Except in persons who are mentally retarded, pica usually remits by adolescence. Pica associated with pregnancy is usually

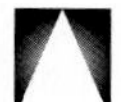

Table 45–1
DSM-IV-TR Diagnostic Criteria for Pica

A. Persistent eating of nonnutritive substances for a period of at least 1 month.
B. The eating of nonnutritive substances is inappropriate to the developmental level.
C. The eating behavior is not part of a culturally sanctioned practice.
D. If the eating behavior occurs exclusively during the course of another mental disorder (e.g., mental retardation, pervasive developmental disorder, schizophrenia), it is sufficiently severe to warrant independent clinical attention.

(From American Psychiatric Association. *Diagnostic and Statistical Manual of Mental Disorders.* 4th ed. Text rev. Washington, DC: American Psychiatric Association; copyright 2000, with permission.)

limited to the pregnancy itself. The DSM-IV-TR diagnostic criteria for pica are given in Table 45–1.

Susan was 3 years of age when her mother took her to the pediatrician because of abdominal pain and lack of appetite. The mother complained that Susan put everything in her mouth but did not want to eat regular food. The pediatrician observed that Susan looked pale, thin, and withdrawn. She sucked her thumb and quietly looked down while her mother reported that Susan liked to chew on newspapers and put plaster in her mouth.

The medical examination revealed that Susan was anemic and suffered from lead poisoning. She was admitted to the hospital for treatment, and a psychiatric consultation was obtained.

Further exploration of the history and the observation of mother and child during feeding and play revealed that the mother was overwhelmed with the care of three young children and had little affection for Susan. The mother was unmarried and lived with her three children and five other family members in a three-bedroom apartment in an old housing project. Her 4-year-old son was hyperactive and demanded almost constant supervision. The 18-month-old infant was an engaging and active little girl, whereas Susan would sit quietly, rock herself, suck her thumb, or chew on newspaper.

The treatment plan included the involvement of social services and protective services to remove any lead paint from the walls in the present apartment and to look for better living arrangements for the family. The mother was helped to enroll Susan and her brother in a preschool program that provided them with more structure and stimulation and gave the mother a few hours of relief every day. In addition, Susan was seen with her mother and her younger sister in play therapy to help the mother understand the different temperament of each child and to make her more responsive to Susan's weak attempts to engage her mother. Once the mother felt more supported and less overwhelmed by her situation, she became more empathic and understanding of Susan. When Susan put something in her mouth, the mother was able to engage her in a play activity rather than screaming at her and scolding her for whatever she was doing. Over the period of 1 year, the relationship between Susan and her mother gradually improved, and Susan seemed less in need of putting her thumb or inedible things in her mouth.

Pathology and Laboratory Examination

No single laboratory test confirms or rules out a diagnosis of pica, but several laboratory tests are useful because pica has frequently been associated with abnormal indexes. Levels of iron and zinc in serum should always be determined; in many cases of pica, these levels are low and may contribute to the development of pica. Pica may disappear when oral iron and zinc are administered. A patient's hemoglobin level should be determined; if the level is low, anemia can result. In children with pica, the lead level in serum should be determined; lead poisoning can result from ingesting lead. When a child's lead level is high, this condition must be treated.

Differential Diagnosis

The differential diagnosis of pica includes iron and zinc deficiencies. Pica also can occur in conjunction with failure to thrive and several other mental and medical disorders, including schizophrenia, autistic disorder, anorexia nervosa, and Kleine-Levin syndrome. In psychosocial dwarfism, a dramatic but reversible endocrinological and behavioral form of failure to thrive, children often show bizarre behaviors, including ingesting toilet water, garbage, and other nonnutritive substances. A recent case report presented an association of pica with hypersomnolence, lead intoxication, and precocious puberty. Precocious puberty implicates the hypothalamus as a site for at least part of the dysfunction. Lead intoxication is known to be associated with pica as well as several other neuropsychiatric abnormalities in memory and cognitive performance. A few children with autistic disorder and schizophrenia may have pica. For children who exhibit pica along with another medical disorder, both disorders should be coded according to DSM-IV-TR.

In certain regions of the world and among certain cultures, such as the Australian aborigines, rates of pica in pregnant women are reportedly high. According to DSM-IV-TR, however, if such practices are culturally accepted, the diagnostic criteria for pica are not met.

Course and Prognosis

The prognosis for pica is usually good, because in children of normal intelligence it generally remits spontaneously within several months. In childhood, pica usually resolves with increasing age; in pregnant women, pica is usually limited to the term of the pregnancy. In some adults, however, especially those who are mentally retarded, pica can continue for years. Follow-up data on these populations are too limited to permit conclusions.

Treatment

The first step in the treatment of pica is determining the cause whenever possible. When pica is associated with situations of neglect or maltreatment, these circumstances naturally need to be altered. Exposure to toxic substances, such as lead, must also be eliminated. No definitive treatment exists for pica; most treatment is aimed at education and behavior modification. Treatments emphasize psychosocial, environmental, behavioral, and family guidance approaches. An effort should be made to ameliorate any significant psychosocial stressors. When lead is present in the surroundings, it must be eliminated or rendered inaccessible or the child must be moved to new surroundings.

Several behavioral techniques have been used with some effect. The most rapidly successful technique seems to be mild aversion therapy or negative reinforcement (e.g., a mild electric shock, an unpleasant noise, or an emetic drug). Positive reinforcement, modeling, behavioral shaping, and overcorrection treatment have also been used. Increasing parental attention, stimulation, and emotional nurturance may yield positive results. One study found that pica was negatively correlated with involvement with play materials and occurred most frequently in impoverished environments. In some patients, correcting an iron or zinc deficiency has eliminated pica. Medical complications (e.g., lead poisoning) that develop secondarily to the pica must also be treated.

RUMINATION DISORDER

Rumination can be observed in developmentally normal infants who put their thumb or hand in the mouth, suck their tongue rhythmically, and arch their back to initiate regurgitation. This behavior pattern is not infrequently observed in infants who receive inadequate emotional interaction and have learned to soothe and stimulate themselves through rumination. The onset of the disorder generally occurs after 3 months of age; once the regurgitation occurs, the food may be swallowed or spit out. Infants who ruminate are observed to strain to bring the food back into their mouths and appear to find the experience pleasurable. Infants who are "experienced" ruminators are able to bring up the food through tongue movements and may not spit out the food at all, but hold it in their mouths and reswallow it. The disorder is rare in older children, adolescents, and adults. It varies in severity and is sometimes associated with medical conditions, such as hiatal hernia, that result in esophageal reflux. In its most severe form, the disorder can be fatal.

The diagnosis of rumination disorder can be made whether or not an infant has attained a normal weight for his or her age. Failure to thrive, therefore, is not a necessary criterion of this disorder, but it is sometimes a sequela. According to DSM-IV-TR, the disorder must be present for at least 1 month after a period of normal functioning, and it is not associated with gastrointestinal illness or other general medical conditions.

Rumination has been recognized for hundreds of years. An awareness of the disorder is important, so that it is correctly diagnosed and that unnecessary surgical procedures and inappropriate treatment are avoided. *Rumination* is derived from the Latin word *ruminare*, meaning "to chew the cud." The Greek equivalent is *merycism*, the act of regurgitating food from the stomach into the mouth, rechewing the food, and reswallowing it.

Epidemiology

Rumination is a rare disorder. It seems to be more common among male infants, and emerges between 3 months and 1 year of age. It persists more frequently among children and adults who are mentally retarded. Adults with rumination usually maintain a normal weight. No reliable figures on predisposing factors or familial patterns are available.

Etiology

Rumination and gastroesophageal reflux often coexist, leading to a spectrum of variable contributions from organic and psychological factors for the emergence of the disorder. In some cases, vomiting secondary to gastroesophageal reflux or an acute illness precedes a pattern of rumination that lasts for several months. It appears, for some infants, that the rumination behavior is self-soothing or produces a sense of relief, leading to a continuation of behaviors to bring it about. In those who are mentally retarded, the disorder may be attributed to self-stimulatory behavior. Psychodynamic theories hypothesize various disturbances in the mother–child relationship as a contributing factor in the development of rumination disorder. The mothers of infants with the disorder have been characterized as immature, exposing the infant to increased levels of marital conflict, leading to understimulation and inadequate emotional attention to the baby. These factors are hypothesized to result in insufficient emotional gratification and stimulation for the infant who seeks to self-stimulate. The rumination is interpreted as the infant's attempt to recreate the feeding process and to provide gratification that the mother does not.

Overstimulation and tension have also been suggested as causes of rumination. A dysfunctional autonomic nervous system may be implicated. As sophisticated and accurate investigative techniques are refined, a substantial number of children classified as ruminators are shown to have gastroesophageal reflux or hiatal hernia.

Behaviorists attribute rumination to the positive reinforcement of pleasurable self-stimulation and to the attention the baby receives from others as a consequence of the disorder.

Diagnosis and Clinical Features

The DSM-IV-TR diagnostic criteria for rumination disorder are given in Table 45–2. DSM-IV-TR notes that the essential feature of the disorder is repeated regurgitation and rechewing of food for a period of at least 1 month after a period of normal functioning. Partially digested food is brought up into the mouth without nausea, retching, disgust, or associated gastrointestinal disorder. This activity can be distinguished from vomiting by the clear, purposeful movements the infant makes to induce it. The food is then ejected from the mouth or reswallowed. A characteristic position of straining and arching of the back, with the head held back, is observed. The infant makes sucking movements with the tongue and gives the impression of gaining considerable satisfaction from the activity. Usually, the infant is irritable and hungry between episodes of rumination.

Initially, rumination may be difficult to distinguish from the regurgitation that frequently occurs in normal infants. In fully developed cases, however, the diagnosis is obvious. Food or milk is regurgitated without nausea, retching, or disgust and is subjected

Table 45–2
DSM-IV-TR Diagnostic Criteria for Rumination Disorder

A. Repeated regurgitation and rechewing of food for a period of at least 1 month following a period of normal functioning.
B. The behavior is not due to an associated gastrointestinal or other general medical condition (e.g., esophageal reflux).
C. The behavior does not occur exclusively during the course of anorexia nervosa or bulimia nervosa. If the symptoms occur exclusively during the course of mental retardation or a pervasive developmental disorder, they are sufficiently severe to warrant independent clinical attention.

(From American Psychiatric Association. *Diagnostic and Statistical Manual of Mental Disorders.* 4th ed. Text rev. Washington, DC: American Psychiatric Association; copyright 2000, with permission.)

to what appears to be innumerable pleasurable sucking and chewing movements. The food is then reswallowed or ejected from the mouth.

Although spontaneous remissions are common, severe secondary complications can develop, such as progressive malnutrition, dehydration, and lowered resistance to disease. Failure to thrive, with absence of growth and developmental delays in all areas, can occur. A mortality rate as high as 25 percent has been reported in severe cases. An additional complication is that the mother or caretaker is often discouraged by failure to feed the infant successfully and can become alienated if this is not already the case. Further alienation often occurs as the noxious odor of the regurgitated material leads to avoidance of the infant.

Justin was 9 months old when he was referred by a gastroenterologist for a psychiatric evaluation because of concerns that he continued to vomit because of rumination. Justin was born full-term and had developed nicely until he was approximately 6 weeks old, when he began to vomit increasing amounts of milk during and after feedings. He was diagnosed with gastroesophageal reflux, which was treated with thickened feedings and medication. Justin responded well to the treatment; he stopped vomiting almost completely and gained weight adequately. Because Justin was doing so well, his mother decided to go back to work when Justin was 8 months old. She transitioned his care to a young woman who would come to the house during the mother's working hours. Justin started to vomit soon after his mother left the house. The vomiting seemed to increase from day to day in frequency and in intensity, and, after 2 weeks of the mother's return to work, Justin vomited several times daily and was losing weight. He was seen by a gastroenterologist, and during the barium swallow, it was noticed that Justin put his hand in his mouth, which seemed to trigger vomiting. Justin was put back on medication for gastroesophageal reflux, but he continued to vomit with increasing frequency, which led to the psychiatric consultation.

Observation of mother and infant during feeding revealed that, as soon as Justin finished feeding, he put his hand in his mouth and vomited. When his mother restricted his hand, Justin moved his tongue back and forth in a rhythmic manner until he vomited again. This happened repeatedly, and Justin continued the rhythmic tongue movements even when he could not bring up any more milk.

Because of his poor nutritional state and moderate dehydration, Justin was admitted to the hospital, and a nasojejunal tube was inserted for feedings. When Justin was awake, a special nurse or the parents played with him and tried to distract him whenever he attempted to put his hand in his mouth or thrust his tongue rhythmically. Justin became increasingly engaged, and his ruminatory activity decreased accordingly. After 1 week in the hospital, small feedings were started; however, Justin tried to ruminate again, and the oral feedings had to be stopped. At this point, the mother decided to stop working and take Justin home to continue the treatment at home. The mother started small feedings, played with Justin after feedings, and was able to keep him from ruminating. After 4 weeks of slow increments in his feedings, Justin was able to take all his feedings by mouth without ruminating, and the nasojejunal tube could be removed.

Pathology and Laboratory Examination

No specific laboratory examination is pathognomonic of rumination disorder. Clinicians must rule out physical causes of vomiting, such as pyloric stenosis and hiatal hernia, before making the diagnosis of rumination disorder. Rumination disorder can be associated with failure to thrive and varying degrees of starvation. Thus, laboratory measures of endocrinological function (thyroid function tests, dexamethasone-suppression test), serum electrolytes, and a hematological workup help determine the severity of the effects of rumination disorder.

Differential Diagnosis

To make the diagnosis of rumination disorder, clinicians must rule out gastrointestinal congenital anomalies, infections, and other medical illnesses. Pyloric stenosis is usually associated with projectile vomiting and is generally evident before 3 months of age, when rumination has its onset. Rumination has been associated with various mental retardation syndromes in which other stereotypic behaviors and eating disturbances, such as pica, are present. Rumination disorder can occur in patients with other eating disorders, such as bulimia nervosa.

Course and Prognosis

Rumination disorder is believed to have a high rate of spontaneous remission. Indeed, many cases of rumination disorder may develop and remit without ever being diagnosed. Only limited data are available about the prognosis of rumination disorder in adults.

Treatment

The treatment of rumination disorder is often a combination of education and behavioral techniques. Sometimes, an evaluation of the mother–child relationship reveals deficits that can be influenced by offering guidance to the mother. Behavioral interventions, such as squirting lemon juice into the infant's mouth whenever rumination occurs, can be effective in diminishing the behavior. This practice appears to be the most rapidly effective treatment, with rumination reportedly eliminated in 3 to 5 days. In the aversive-conditioning reports on rumination disorder, infants were doing well at 9- or 12-month follow-up, with no recurrence of the rumination and with weight gains, increased activity levels, and increased responsiveness to persons. Rumination may be decreased by the technique of withdrawing attention from the child whenever this behavior occurs. The effectiveness of treatments is difficult to evaluate. Most reported are single-case studies; patients are not randomly assigned to controlled studies.

Treatments include improvement of the child's psychosocial environment, increased tender loving care from the mother or caretakers, and psychotherapy for the mother or both parents. When anatomical abnormalities, such as hiatal hernia, are present, surgical repair may be necessary. If an infant is malnourished and continues to lose most nutrition through rumination, a jejunal tube may need to be inserted before other treatments can be utilized.

Medications are not a standard part of the treatment of rumination. Case reports, however, cite a variety of medications that have been tried, including metoclopramide (Reglan), cimetidine (Tagamet), and antipsychotics such as haloperidol (Haldol) and thioridazine (Mellaril) have been cited to be helpful according to anecdotal reports. One study showed that when infants were allowed to eat as much as they wanted, the rate of rumination decreased.

Table 45–3
DSM-IV-TR Diagnostic Criteria for Feeding Disorder of Infancy or Early Childhood

A. Feeding disturbance as manifested by persistent failure to eat adequately with significant failure to gain weight or significant loss of weight over at least 1 month.
B. The disturbance is not due to an associated gastrointestinal or other general medical condition (e.g., esophageal reflux).
C. The disturbance is not better accounted for by another mental disorder (e.g., rumination disorder) or by lack of available food.
D. The onset is before age 6 years.

(From American Psychiatric Association. *Diagnostic and Statistical Manual of Mental Disorders*. 4th ed. Text rev. Washington, DC: American Psychiatric Association; copyright 2000, with permission.)

The treatment of adolescents with rumination disorder is often complex and includes a multidisciplinary approach consisting of individual psychotherapy, nutritional intervention, and pharmacologic treatment for the frequent comorbid anxiety and depressive symptoms.

FEEDING DISORDER OF INFANCY OR EARLY CHILDHOOD

Feeding disorder of infancy, a broadly defined maladaptive pattern of eating behaviors in infants, features the interactive process between caregiver and infant. This disorder has variable components that range from food refusal, food selectivity, eating too little, food avoidance, and delayed self-feeding. According to DSM-IV-TR, feeding disorder of infancy or early childhood is a persistent failure to eat adequately, reflected in significant failure to gain weight or in significant weight loss over 1 month. The symptoms are not better accounted for by a medical condition or by another mental disorder and are not caused by lack of food (Table 45–3). The disorder has its onset before the age of 6 years.

Children with feeding disorders have been found to display less affectionate touch, more negative touch, and more rejection of mother's touch than children without feeding problems. In addition, more rejecting maternal responses to the child's touch have also been observed, and children with feeding disorders are more often positioned out of reach of their mothers' arms. Children with feeding disorders are often withdrawn, and touch is diminished during the entire feeding process compared with other children. It is likely that patterns of proximity and touch between mothers and infants during feeding may serve as an index of risk for future feeding difficulties and potential growth failure.

Epidemiology

It is estimated that between 15 and 35 percent of infants and young children have transient feeding difficulties. A recent survey of feeding problems in nursery school children revealed a prevalence of 4.8 percent with equal gender distribution. Children with feeding problems exhibited more somatic complaints and mothers of affected infants exhibited increased risk of anxiety symptoms. Data from community samples estimate a prevalence of failure to thrive syndromes in approximately 3 percent of infants with approximately half of those infants exhibiting feeding disorders.

Differential Diagnosis

Feeding disorder of infancy must be differentiated from structural problems with the infants' gastrointestinal tract that may be contributing to discomfort during the feeding process. Because feeding disorders and organic causes of swallowing difficulties often coexist, it is important to rule out medical reasons for feeding difficulties. A recent study of videofluoroscopic evaluation of children with feeding and swallowing problems revealed that clinical evaluation was 92 percent accurate in identifying those children at increased risk of aspiration. This type of evaluation is necessary before psychotherapeutic interventions in cases where a medical contribution to feeding problems is suspected.

Course and Prognosis

Most infants with feeding disorders exhibit symptoms within the first year of life and, with appropriate recognition and intervention, do not go on to develop failure to thrive. When feeding disorders have their onset later, in children 2 to 3 years of age, growth and development can be affected when the disorder lasts for several months. It is estimated that about 70 percent of infants who persistently refuse food in the first year of life continue to have some feeding problems during childhood.

Thomas was 3 months old when he was referred for a psychiatric evaluation because of his feeding difficulties and poor weight gain since birth. His parents were college-educated, and both had pursued their professional careers until Thomas was born. Although Thomas was full-term and weighed 7 pounds at birth, he had difficulty drinking from the breast. When he was 4 weeks old, his mother had reluctantly switched him to bottle feedings because he was losing weight. Although his intake improved somewhat on bottle feedings, he gained weight very slowly and was still less than 8 pounds at 3 months of age. His mother appeared tired and described how Thomas would drink only 1, 2, or 3 ounces at a time; wiggle and cry; and refuse to continue with the feeding. But after a few hours, he might cry again as if he were hungry. However, she could not settle him to feed and he would continue to cry inconsolably. The mother described that she would attempt to feed him on an average of 10 to 15 times in a 24-hour period, that Thomas would cry a lot during the day and at night, and that everybody in the family was getting very little sleep.

The observation of mother–infant interactions during feeding and play revealed that Thomas was a very alert and wiggly baby who had difficulty settling in his mother's arms. While drinking from the bottle he would kick his feet and move around with his arms, and soon the nipple of the bottle would slip out of his mouth. This upset him, and he started crying. His mother appeared anxious and tried to restart him by changing his position in various ways, but this only agitated him more. After repeated unsuccessful attempts to continue the feeding, mother and baby appeared exhausted, and the mother gave up.

The assessment revealed that Thomas was a very active and excitable baby who had difficulty keeping calm during feedings. After reviewing the videotape with the mother, the therapist explored ways in which the mother could better facilitate calming during feedings. Using a quiet corner in the house, swaddling Thomas in a blanket,

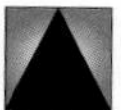

Table 45–4
ICD-10 Diagnostic Criteria for Feeding Disorder of Infancy and Childhood

A. There is persistent failure to eat adequately, or persistent rumination or regurgitation of food.
B. The child fails to gain weight, loses weight, or exhibits some other significant health problem over a period of at least 1 month. (In view of the frequency of transient eating difficulties, researchers may prefer a minimum duration of 3 months for some purposes.)
C. Onset of the disorder is before the age of 6 years.
D. The child exhibits no other mental or behavioral disorder in the ICD-10 classification (other than mental retardation).
E. There is no evidence of organic disease sufficient to account for the failure to eat.

(From World Health Organization. *The ICD-10 Classification of Mental and Behavioural Disorders: Diagnostic Criteria for Research.* Copyright, World Health Organization, Geneva, 1993, with permission.)

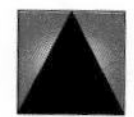

Table 45–5
ICD-10 Diagnostic Criteria for Pica of Infancy and Childhood

A. There is persistent or recurrent eating of nonnutritive substances, at least twice a week.
B. Duration of the disorder is at least 1 month. (For some purposes, researchers may prefer a minimum period of 3 months.)
C. The child exhibits no other mental or behavioral disorder in the ICD-10 classification (other than mental retardation).
D. The child's chronological and mental age is at least 2 years.
E. The eating behavior is not part of a culturally sanctioned practice.

(From World Health Organization. The *ICD-10 Classification of Mental and Behavioural Disorders: Diagnostic Criteria for Research.* Copyright, World Health Organization, Geneva, 1993, with permission.)

and singing to him before starting the feeding were the most useful suggestions. Thomas stayed calm during feedings, was able to drink larger amounts of milk, and waited longer between feedings. This, in turn, relieved the mother's anxiety and helped both to have calmer interactions.

Treatment

Treatments for feeding disorders need to be individualized and include interventions aimed at the infant, the mother, and most often targeting the interactions between the infant and mother, or caregiver.

If an infant tires before ingesting an adequate amount of nutrition, it may be necessary to begin treatment with the placement of a nasogastric tube for supplemental oral feedings. On the other hand, if the mother or caregiver is unable to participate in the intervention, it may be necessary to include additional caregivers to contribute to feeding the infant. In rare cases, an infant may require hospitalization until adequate nutrition on a daily basis is accomplished.

Most interventions for feeding disorders are aimed at optimizing the interaction between the mother and infant during feedings, and identifying any factors that can be changed to promote greater ingestion. The mother is helped to become more aware of the infant's stamina for length of individual feedings, the infant's biological regulation patterns, and when the infant is fatigued, with a goal of increasing the level of engagement between mother and infant during feeding.

A transactional model of intervention has been proposed by Irene Chatoor, M.D., a leading expert in the field, for infants who exhibit the "difficult" temperamental traits of emotional intensity, stubbornness, lack of hunger cues, irregular eating and sleeping patterns, strong will in refusing to eat a sufficient amount, and who are intensely interested in noneating exploration of their environment. The treatment includes education for the parents regarding the temperamental traits of the infant, exploration of the parents' anxieties about the infant's nutrition, and training for the parents regarding changing their behaviors to promote internal regulation of eating in the infant. Parents are encouraged to feed the infant on a regular basis at 3- to 4-hour intervals, and offer only water between meals. The parents are trained to deliver praise to the infant for any self-feeding efforts, regardless of the amount of food ingested. Furthermore, parents are guided to limit any distracting stimulation during meals and give attention and praise to positive eating behaviors rather than intense negative attention to inappropriate behavior during meals. This training process for parents is recommended to be done in an intense manner within a short period of time. Many parents are able to facilitate improved eating patterns in the infant in a short period of time.

For older children with severe feeding disorders resulting in failure-to-thrive syndromes, hospitalization and nutritional supplementation is necessary before optimal psychotherapeutic interventions. Medication is not a standard component of treatment for feeding disorders, although several anecdotal reports have suggested benefit with adjunctive pharmacologic agents. One recent case report indicated that several preadolescents with failure-to-thrive and feeding disorders who received enteral nutritional interventions and were comorbid for anxiety and mood symptoms, the addition of risperidone (Risperdal) was observed to be associated with an increase in oral intake and accelerated weight gain.

ICD-10

In the 10th revision of *International Statistical Classification of Diseases and Related Health Problems* (ICD-10), feeding disorder of infancy and childhood, which also includes rumination disorder (Table 45–4), and pica of infancy and childhood (Table 45–5) are included in the category other emotional and behavioral disorders with onset usually occurring in childhood and adolescence.

References

Araujo CL, Victora CG, Hallal PC, Gigante DP. Breastfeeding and overweight in childhood: Evidence from the Pelotas 1993 birth cohort study. *Int J Obes.* 2005;30(3):500.

Berger-Gross P, Colettoi DJ, Hirschkorn K, Terranova E, Simpser EF. The effectiveness of risperidone in the treatment of three children with feeding disorders. *J Child Adolesc Psychopharmacol.* 2004;14:621.

Chatoor I. Feeding and eating disorders of infancy or early childhood. In: Sadock BJ, Sadock VA, eds. *Kaplan & Sadock's Comprehensive Textbook of Psychiatry*. 8th ed. Vol. 2. Baltimore: Lippincott Williams & Wilkins; 2005:3217.

Cohen E, Rosen Y, Yehuda B, Iancu I. Successful multidisciplinary treatment in an adolescent case of rumination. *Isr J Psychiatry Relat Sci*. 2004;41:222.

DeMatteo C, Matovich D, Hjartarson A. Comparison of clinical and videofluoroscopic evaluation of children with feeding and swallowing difficulties. *Dev Med Child Neurol*. 2005;47:149.

Esparo G, Canals J, Ballespi S, Vinas F, Domenech E. Feeding problems in nursery children: prevalence and psychosocial factors. *Acta Pediatr* 2004;93:663.

Feldaman R, Keren M, Gross-Rozval O, Tyano S. Mother-child touch patterns in infant feeding disorders: Relation to maternal, child, and environmental factors. *J Am Acad Child Adolesc Psychiatry.* 2004;43:1089.

Hughes SO, Anderson CB, Power TG, Micheli N, Jaramillo S, Nicklas TA. Measuring feeding in low-income African-American and Hispanic parents. *Appetite*. 2006;46(2):215.

Jacobi C, Agras WS, Bryson S, Hammer LD. Behavioral validation, precursors, and concomitants of picky eating in childhood. *J Am Acad Child Adolesc Psychiatry*. 2003;42:76.

Lewinsohn PM, Holm-Denoma JM, Gau JM, Joiner TE Jr., Striegel-Moore R, Bear P, Lamoureux B. Problematic eating and feeding behaviors of 36-month-old children. *Int J Eat Disord*. 2005;38(3):208–219.

Linscheid TN. Behavioral treatments for pediatric feeding disorders. *Behav Modif*. 2006;30:6–23.

Liu YL, Malik N, Sanger GJ, Friedman MI, Andrews PL. Pica—A model of nausea? Species differences in response to cisplatin. *Physiol Behav*. 2005;85(3):271–277.

46 Tic Disorders

Tic disorders are distinguished by the type of tic symptoms, their frequency, and the pattern in which they emerge over time. Tics are abnormal movements or vocalizations that most commonly affect the muscles of the face and neck, such as eye-blinking, head-jerking, mouth-grimacing, or head-shaking. Typical vocal tics include throat-clearing, grunting, snorting, and coughing. Tics are defined as rapid and repetitive muscle contractions resulting in movements or vocalizations that are experienced as involuntary. Children and adolescents may exhibit tic behaviors that occur after a stimulus or in response to an internal urge. Tic disorders, a group of neuropsychiatric disorders, generally begin in childhood or adolescence with a stable or fluctuating course in childhood and generally wane by adolescence. Although tics are not volitional, in some individuals they may be suppressed for periods.

The most widely known and most severe tic disorder is Gilles de la Tourette syndrome, also known as Tourette's disorder. The text revision of the 4th edition of the *Diagnostic and Statistical Manual of Mental Disorders* (DSM-IV-TR) includes several other tic disorders, such as chronic motor or vocal tic disorder, transient tic disorder, and tic disorder not otherwise specified. Although tics have no particular purpose, they often consist of motions that are used in volitional movements. One half to two thirds of children with Tourette's disorder exhibit a reduction or complete remission of tic symptoms during adolescence. Obsessive-compulsive symptoms or disorder (OCD) has been found to coexist in one third to two thirds of children and adolescents with Tourette's disorder, and about one third of adults with Tourette's disorder have persistent OCD into adulthood. The obsessive-compulsive symptoms most likely to occur in those individuals with Tourette's disorder are characteristically related to ordering, symmetry, counting and repetitive touching, whereas OCD disorders in the absence of tic disorders are characterized by symptoms more often associated with fears of contamination and fears of harming others. A recent study has found that the risk of developing OCD symptoms in children with Tourette's disorder by early adulthood was significantly higher in those children with higher intellectual quotients (IQ), that is, above 120, compared with those with an average IQ of 100.

Motor and vocal tics are divided into simple and complex types. *Simple motor tics* are those composed of repetitive, rapid contractions of functionally similar muscle groups—for example, eye-blinking, neck-jerking, shoulder-shrugging, and facial-grimacing. Common *simple vocal tics* include coughing, throat-clearing, grunting, sniffing, snorting, and barking. *Complex motor tics* appear to be more purposeful and ritualistic than simple tics. Common *complex motor tics* include grooming behaviors, the smelling of objects, jumping, touching behaviors, echopraxia (imitation of observed behavior), and copropraxia (display of obscene gestures). *Complex vocal tics* include repeating words or phrases out of context, coprolalia (use of obscene words or phrases), palilalia (a person's repeating his or her words), and echolalia (repetition of the last-heard words of others).

Some persons with tic disorders can suppress the tics for minutes or hours, but others, especially young children, either are not cognizant of their tics or experience their tics as irresistible. Tics may be attenuated by sleep, relaxation, or absorption in an activity. Tics often, but not always, disappear during sleep.

TOURETTE'S DISORDER

According to DSM-IV-TR, tics in Tourette's disorder are multiple motor tics and one or more vocal tics. The tics occur many times a day for more than 1 year. Tourette's disorder causes distress or significant impairment in important areas of functioning. The disorder has an onset before the age of 18 years, and it is not caused by a substance or by a general medical condition.

Georges Gilles de la Tourette (1857–1904) first described a patient with what was later known as Tourette's disorder in 1885, while he was studying with Jean-Martin Charcot in France. De la Tourette noted a syndrome in several patients that included multiple motor tics, coprolalia, and echolalia.

Epidemiology

The lifetime prevalence of Tourette's disorder is estimated to be 4 to 5 per 10,000. More children exhibit this disorder than adults, such that 5 to 30 of 10,000 children are affected, but by adulthood, only 1 to 2 of 10,000 meet diagnostic criteria. The onset of the motor component of the disorder generally occurs by the age of 7 years; vocal tics emerge on average by the age of 11 years. Tourette's disorder occurs about three times more often in boys than in girls.

Etiology

Genetic Factors. Twin studies, adoption studies, and segregation analysis studies all support a genetic cause for Tourette's disorder. Twin studies indicate that concordance for the disorder in monozygotic twins is significantly greater than that in dizygotic twins. That Tourette's disorder and chronic motor or vocal tic disorder are likely to occur in the same families lends support to the view that the disorders are part of a genetically-determined spectrum. The sons of mothers with Tourette's disorder seem to be at the highest risk for the disorder. Evidence in some families indicates that Tourette's disorder is transmitted in an autosomal dominant fashion. Recent studies of a long family pedigree suggest that Tourette's disorder may be transmitted in a bilinear mode; that is, Tourette's disorder appears to be inherited through an autosomal pattern in some families, intermediate between dominant and recessive. A recent study of 174 unrelated probands with Tourette's disorder identified a greater than chance occurrence of a rare sequence variant in SLITRK1 believed to be a candidate gene on chromosome 13q31.

A relation is found between Tourette's disorder and attention-deficit/hyperactivity disorder (ADHD); up to half of all patients with Tourette's disorder also have ADHD. A relation also appears between Tourette's disorder and OCD; up to 40 percent of all those with Tourette's disorder also have OCD. In addition, first-degree relatives of persons with Tourette's disorder are at high risk for the development of the disorder, of chronic motor or vocal tic disorder, and of OCD. The presence of symptoms of ADHD in more than half of persons with Tourette's disorder raises questions about a genetic relation between these two disorders.

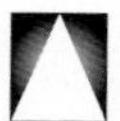

Table 46–1
DSM-IV-TR Diagnostic Criteria for Tourette's Disorder

A. Both multiple motor and one or more vocal tics have been present at some time during the illness, although not necessarily concurrently. (A tic is a sudden, rapid, recurrent, nonrhythmic, stereotyped motor movement or vocalization.)
B. The tics occur many times a day (usually in bouts) nearly every day or intermittently throughout a period of more than 1 year, and during this period there was never a tic-free period of more than 3 consecutive months.
C. The onset is before age 18 years.
D. The disturbance is not due to the direct physiological effects of a substance (e.g., stimulants) or a general medical condition (e.g., Huntington's disease or postviral encephalitis).

(From American Psychiatric Association. *Diagnostic and Statistical Manual of Mental Disorders.* 4th ed. Text rev. Washington, DC: American Psychiatric Association; copyright 2000, with permission.)

Neurochemical and Neuroanatomical Factors. Compelling, but indirect, evidence of dopamine system involvement in tic disorders includes the observations that pharmacological agents that antagonize dopamine (haloperidol [Haldol], pimozide [Orap], and fluphenazine [Prolixin]) suppress tics and that agents that increase central dopaminergic activity (methylphenidate [Ritalin], amphetamines, pemoline [Cylert], and cocaine) tend to exacerbate tics. The relation of tics to neurotransmitter systems is complex and not yet well understood; for example, in some cases, antipsychotic medications, such as haloperidol, are not effective in reducing tics and the effect of stimulants on tic disorders reportedly varies. In some cases, Tourette's disorder has emerged during treatment with antipsychotic medications.

More direct analyses of the neurochemistry of Tourette's disorder have been possible utilizing brain proton magnetic resonance spectroscopy, a method only recently used to investigate Tourette's disorder. A recent investigation examining the cellular neurochemistry of patients with Tourette's disorder utilizing magnetic resonance spectroscopy of the frontal cortex, caudate nucleus, putamen, and thalamus demonstrated that these patients had a reduced amount of choline and N-acetylaspartate in the left putamen along with reduced levels of bilaterally in the putamen. In the frontal cortex, patients with Tourette's disorder were found to have lower concentrations of N-acetylaspartate bilaterally, lower levels of creatine on the right side and reduced myoinositol on the left side. These results imply that deficits in the density of neuronal and nonneuronal cells are present in patients with Tourette's disorder.

Endogenous opioids may be involved in tic disorders and OCD. Some evidence indicates that pharmacological agents that antagonize endogenous opiates—for example, naltrexone (ReVia)—reduce tics and attention deficits in patients with Tourette's disorder. Abnormalities in the noradrenergic system have been implicated in some cases by the reduction of tics with clonidine (Catapres). This adrenergic agonist reduces the release of norepinephrine in the central nervous system and, thus, may reduce activity in the dopaminergic system. Abnormalities in the basal ganglia result in various movement disorders, such as Huntington's disease, and are implicated as possible sites of disturbance in Tourette's disorder, OCD, and ADHD.

Immunological Factors and Postinfection. An autoimmune process that is secondary to streptococcal infections is a potential mechanism for Tourette's disorder. Such a process could act synergistically with a genetic vulnerability for this disorder. Poststreptococcal syndromes have also been associated with one potential causative factor in the development of OCD in children.

Diagnosis and Clinical Features

To make a diagnosis of Tourette's disorder, clinicians must obtain a history of multiple motor tics and the emergence of at least one vocal tic at some point in the disorder. According to DSM-IV-TR, the tics must occur many times a day nearly every day or intermittently for more than 1 year. The average age of onset of tics is 7 years, but tics can occur as early as age 2 years. The onset must occur before the age of 18 years (Table 46–1).

In Tourette's disorder, the initial tics are in the face and neck. Over time, the tics tend to occur in a downward progression. The most commonly described tics are those affecting the face and head, the arms and hands, the body and lower extremities, and the respiratory and alimentary systems. In these areas, the tics take the form of grimacing; forehead puckering; eyebrow-raising; eyelid-blinking; winking; nose-wrinkling; nostril-trembling; mouth-twitching; displaying the teeth; biting the lips and other parts; tongue-extruding; protracting the lower jaw; nodding, jerking, or shaking the head; twisting the neck; looking sideways; head-rolling; hand-jerking; arm-jerking; plucking fingers; writhing fingers; fist-clenching; shoulder-shrugging; foot, knee, or toe shaking; walking peculiarly; body writhing; jumping; hiccupping; sighing; yawning; snuffing; blowing through the nostrils; whistling; belching; sucking or smacking sounds; and clearing the throat. Several assessment instruments are currently available that are useful in making diagnoses of tic disorders, including comprehensive self-report assessment tools, such as the *Tic Symptom Self Report* and the *Yale Global Tic Severity Scale,* administered by a clinician (Table 46–2).

Typically, prodromal behavioral symptoms (e.g., irritability, attention difficulties, and poor frustration tolerance) are evident before, or coincide with the onset of, tics. More than 25 percent of persons in some studies received stimulants for a diagnosis of ADHD before receiving a diagnosis of Tourette's disorder. The most frequent initial symptom is an eye-blink tic, followed by a head tic or a facial grimace. Most complex motor and vocal symptoms emerge several years after the initial symptoms. Coprolalia usually begins in early adolescence and occurs in about one third of all patients. Mental coprolalia—in which a patient thinks a sudden, intrusive, socially unacceptable thought or obscene word—can also occur. In some severe cases, physical injuries, including retinal detachment and orthopedic problems, have resulted from severe tics.

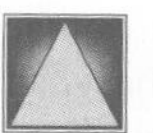

Table 46–2
Clinical Assessment Tools in Tic Disorders

Domain	Type	Reliability and Validity	Sensitive to Change
Tics			
Tic Symptom Self-Report	Parent/self	Good	Yes
Yale Global Tic Severity Scale	Clinician	Excellent	Yes
Attention-deficit/hyperactivity disorder			
Swanson, Nolan, and Pelham-IV	Parent/teacher	Excellent	Yes
Abbreviated Conners' Questionnaire	Parent/teacher	Excellent	Yes
Obsessive-compulsive disorder			
Yale-Brown Obsessive Compulsive Scale and Children's Yale-Brown Obsessive Compulsive Scale	Clinician	Excellent	Yes
National Institute of Mental Health Global	Clinician	Excellent	Yes
General			
Child Behavior Checklist	Parent/teacher	Excellent	No

Obsessions, compulsions, attention difficulties, impulsivity, and personality problems have been associated with Tourette's disorder. Attention difficulties often precede the onset of tics, whereas obsessive-compulsive symptoms often occur after their onset. Whether these problems usually develop secondarily to a patient's tics or are caused primarily by the same underlying pathological condition is still being debated. Many tics have an aggressive or sexual component that may result in serious social consequences for the patient. Phenomenologically, tics resemble a failure of censorship, both conscious and unconscious, with increased impulsivity and inability to inhibit a thought from being put into action.

CASE HISTORY

Todd, age 8 years, came to the Tourette Syndrome Clinic for an evaluation of tics, hyperactivity, and impulsive behavior. He is a third-grade student in a regular class at the local public school. Before the consultation, parent and teacher ratings, including the *Child Behavior Checklist* (CBCL), *Swanson, Nolan, and Pelham-IV* (SNAP-IV), *Conners' Parent and Teacher Questionnaires*, *Tic Symptom Self-Report* (TSSR), and medical history survey, were sent to his family (Table 46–2). His mother and the classroom teacher rated him well above the norm for hyperactivity, inattention, and impulsiveness. He was failing in school, often argued with adults, was occasionally aggressive, and had few friends. His tics were rated as mild.

Todd's mother recalls difficulties with overactivity and reckless behavior since preschool. At age 5, his kindergarten teacher encouraged the family to obtain consultation for his behavior. The family's pediatrician made a diagnosis of ADHD and recommended a trial of methylphenidate (Ritalin), which eventually occurred in the first grade. Within 2 weeks of starting medication, his behavior showed a dramatic improvement. He was able to stay in his seat and complete his work and was more able to wait his turn on the playground. The next several months went well. After a dosage increase in the spring of his first-grade year, however, he began showing motor and phonic tics consisting of head-jerking, facial movements, coughing, and grunting. The medication was immediately stopped and, although the tics subsided, they did not go away. In hindsight, Todd's mother recalled that he had shown blinking and throat-clearing before starting methylphenidate, but she had dismissed these tics as unimportant.

Off medication, the second grade did not go well, and Todd was placed in special education class. At his mother's insistence, Todd returned to the regular class for third grade. However, his adjustment to the third-grade classroom was poor. The family went back to the pediatrician, who made the referral to the Tourette Syndrome Clinic.

Todd is healthy with no history of serious illness or injuries. The pregnancy, labor, and delivery were uncomplicated, and his developmental milestones were achieved at appropriate times. Intelligence testing completed by the school psychologist revealed average intellectual ability. His appetite is good. His mother notes that Todd has long-standing trouble falling asleep but sleeps through the night. Although he is described as argumentative and easily frustrated with frequent outbursts of temper, his mood is generally upbeat.

BEHAVIORAL OBSERVATIONS

Todd is of average height and weight with no dysmorphic features. His speech is rapid in tempo but normal in tone and volume. His discourse is coherent and developmentally appropriate, and no evidence is seen of thought disorder. He does not appear depressed and denies worries about everyday issues such as friends and school performance, although he recognizes that school is not going so well. He also denies recurring worries about contamination or harm coming to him or family members, or fears of acting on unwanted impulses. Other than mild touching habits involving the need to touch objects with each hand three times or in combinations of three, he denies repetitive rituals. Several tics were observed during the evaluation session, including blinking, facial-grimacing, head-jerking, and grunting. He was restless and easily distracted throughout the session and often needed assistance with entertaining himself when not directly involved in conversation.

IMPRESSION

Given the history of enduring motor and phonic tics, which are confirmed by direct observation, Todd meets criteria for Tourette's syndrome. Based on history, he also meets criteria for ADHD, combined type.

TREATMENT PLAN

Although recent studies have shown that children with a tic disorder can tolerate stimulant medication without inducing an exacerbation in tics, some children show an increase in tics on exposure to stimulants. Thus, guanfacine (Systemic), 0.5 mg, is recommended with planned increases of 0.5 mg every 4 to 5 days as tolerated to a maximum of 3 mg per day in three divided doses. Blood pressure, pulse, sleep, appetite, energy level, and tics will be monitored every 2 weeks during the dose adjustment phase. Parent and teacher ratings will be obtained at 4 and 8 weeks to assess response.

Parents will be given educational materials about Tourette's syndrome and ADHD and referred for parent training. The parent training will focus on distinguishing between tics and oppositional behavior, how to modify disruptive behavior, and how to cultivate positive behavior. With the parents' permission, the school will be informed of the diagnosis, and a special education classification in the "other health impaired" category is likely. Although Todd may remain in the regular classroom, he may benefit from a teacher's aide to monitor his behavior and help him organize his school work. (Courtesy of L. Scahill M.S.N., Ph.D. and J.F. Leckman, M.D.)

Pathology and Laboratory Examination

No specific laboratory diagnostic test exists for Tourette's disorder, but many patients with Tourette's disorder have nonspecific abnormal electroencephalographic findings. Computed tomography (CT) and magnetic resonance imaging (MRI) scans have revealed no specific structural lesions, although about 10 percent of all patients with Tourette's disorder show some nonspecific abnormality on CT scans.

Differential Diagnosis

Tics must be differentiated from other disordered movements (e.g., dystonic, choreiform, athetoid, myoclonic, and hemiballismic movements) and the neurological diseases that they characterize (e.g., Huntington's disease, parkinsonism, Sydenham's chorea, and Wilson's disease), as listed in Table 46–3. Tremors, mannerisms, and stereotypic movement disorder (e.g., head-banging or body-rocking) must also be distinguished from tic disorders. Stereotypic movement disorders, including movements such as rocking, hand-gazing, and other self-stimulatory behaviors, seem to be voluntary and often produce a sense of comfort, in contrast to tic disorders. Although tics in children and adolescents may or may not feel controllable, they rarely produce a sense of well-being. Compulsions are sometimes difficult to distinguish from complex tics and may be on the same continuum biologically. Tic disorders also occur comorbidly with multiple behavioral and mood disturbances. In a recent survey, the greater the severity of tics, the higher the probability of both aggressive and depressive symptoms in children. Even in a given child with Tourette's disorder, it has been reported that when there is exacerbation of tic symptoms, behavior and mood also seem to deteriorate. This phenomenon occurs with children who have Tourette's disorder and ADHD and also with those who have depression or oppositional-defiant disorders. In children with Tourette's disorder and ADHD, even when the tic disorder had always been mild, a high frequency of disruptive behavior problems and mood disorder still exists. Both autistic and mentally retarded children may exhibit symptoms similar to those seen in tic disorders, including Tourette's disorder. A greater than expected occurrence of Tourette's disorder, autistic disorder, and bipolar disorder also is present.

Before instituting treatment with an antipsychotic medication, clinicians must make a baseline evaluation of preexisting abnormal movements; such medication can mask abnormal movements and, if the movements occur later, they can be mistaken for tardive dyskinesia. Stimulant medications (e.g., methylphenidate, amphetamines, and pemoline) have reportedly exacerbated preexisting tics in some cases. These effects have been reported primarily in some children and adolescents being treated for ADHD. In most, but not all cases, after the drug was discontinued, the tics remitted or returned to premedication levels. Most experts suggest that children and adolescents who experience tics while receiving stimulants are probably genetically predisposed and would have experienced tics regardless of their treatment with stimulants. Until the situation is clarified, clinicians should use great caution and should frequently monitor children at risk for tics who are given stimulants.

Course and Prognosis

Tourette's disorder is a childhood-onset neuropsychiatric disorder that includes both motor and vocal tics with a natural history leading to reduction or complete resolution of tics symptoms in most cases by adolescence. During childhood, individual tic symptoms may decrease, persist, or increase, and old symptoms may be replaced by new ones. Severely afflicted persons may have serious emotional problems, including major depressive disorder. Impairment may also be associated with the motor and vocal tic symptoms of Tourette's disorder; however, in many cases, interference in function is exacerbated by comorbid ADHD and OCD, both of which frequently coexist with the disorder. When the above three disorders are comorbid, severe social, academic, and occupational problems may ensue. Although most children with Tourette's disorder will experience a decline in the frequency and severity of tic symptoms during adolescence, at present, no clinical measures exist to predict which children may have persistent symptoms into adulthood. Previous imaging studies have provided cross-sectional data showing that Tourette's disorder is associated with reduced caudate nucleus volume. A recent prospective investigation measuring clinical symptom severity and basal ganglia volumes in 43 children over an average length of 7.5 years found that the smaller the volume of the caudate nucleus, as measured by high-resolution MRI, the more likely were tic symptoms and OCD to persist into early adulthood. Thus, caudate volumes in children with Tourette's disorder were predictive of severity and persistence of symptoms over time. Caudate volumes were not correlated, however, with the severity of symptoms in childhood when the initial magnetic resonance scans were done. Thus, the severity of childhood tics does not always predict persistence or severity of symptoms in adulthood.

Children with mild forms of Tourette's disorder often have satisfactory peer relationships, function well in school, and develop adequate self-esteem, and may not require treatment.

Treatment

Consideration of a child or adolescent's overall functioning is the first step in determining the most appropriate treatments for tic disorders. Families, teachers, and peers sometimes misinterpret tics as purposeful behaviors, and a child may be treated as if he or she has a "behavior" problem when the tics are actually experienced as involuntary. Treatment should begin with

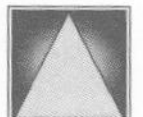

Table 46–3
Differential Diagnosis of Tic Disorders

Disease or Syndrome	Age at Onset	Associated Features	Course	Predominant Type of Movement
Hallervorden-Spatz	Childhood-adolescence	May be associated with optic atrophy, club feet, retinitis pigmentosa, dysarthria, dementia, ataxia, emotional lability, spasticity, autosomal recessive inheritance	Progressive to death in 5 to 20 years	Choreic, athetoid, myoclonic
Dystonia musculorum deformans	Childhood-adolescence	Autosomal recessive inheritance commonly, primarily among Ashkenazi Jews; a more benign autosomal dominant form also occurs	Variable course, often progressive but with rare remissions	Dystonia
Sydenham's chorea	Childhood, usually 5–15 yrs	More common in females, usually associated with rheumatic fever (carditis elevated ASLO titers)	Usually self-limited	Choreiform
Huntington's disease	Usually 30 to 50 yrs, but childhood forms are known	Autosomal dominant inheritance, dementia, caudate atrophy on CT scan	Progressive to death in 10 to 15 years after onset	Choreiform
Wilson's disease (hepatolenticular degeneration)	Usually 10 to 25 yrs	Kayser-Fleischer rings, liver dysfunction, inborn error of copper metabolism; autosomal recessive inheritance	Progressive to death without chelating therapy	Wing-beating tremor, dystonia
Hyperreflexias (including latah, myriachit, jumper disease of Maine)	Generally in childhood (dominant inheritance)	Familial; may have generalized rigidity and autosomal inheritance	Nonprogressive	Excessive startle response; may have echolalia, coprolalia, and forced obedience
Myoclonic disorders	Any age	Numerous causes, some familial, usually no vocalizations	Variable, depending on cause	Myoclonus
Myoclonic dystonia	5 to 47 yrs	Nonfamilial, no vocalizations	Nonprogressive	Torsion dystonia with myoclonic jerks
Paroxysmal myoclonic dystonia with vocalization	Childhood	Attention, hyperactive, and learning disorders; movements interfere with ongoing activity	Nonprogressive	Bursts of regular, repetitive clonic (less tonic) movements and vocalizations
Tardive Tourette's disorder syndromes	Variable (after antipsychotic medication use)	Reported to be precipitated by discontinuation or reduction of medication	May terminate after increase or decrease of dosage	Orofacial dyskinesias, choreoathetosis, tics, vocalization
Neuroacanthocytosis	Third or fourth decade	Acanthocytosis, muscle wasting, parkinsonism, autosomal recessive inheritance	Variable	Orofacial dyskinesia and limb chorea, tics, vocalization
Encephalitis lethargica	Variable	Shouting fits, bizarre behavior, psychosis, Parkinson's disease	Variable	Simple and complex motor and vocal tics, coprolalia, echolalia, echopraxia, palilalia
Gasoline inhalation	Variable	Abnormal EEG; symmetrical theta and theta bursts frontocentrally	Variable	Simple motor and vocal tics
Postangiographic complications	Variable	Emotional lability, amnestic syndrome	Variable	Simple motor and complex vocal tics, palilalia
Postinfectious	Variable	EEG: occasional asymmetrical theta bursts before movements, elevated ASLO titers	Variable	Simple motor and vocal tics, echopraxia
Posttraumatic	Variable	Asymmetrical tic distribution	Variable	Complex motor tics
Carbon monoxide poisoning	Variable	Inappropriate sexual behavior	Variable	Simple and complex motor and vocal tics, coprolalia, echolalia, palilalia

(*continued*)

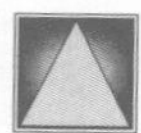

Table 46–3 (Continued)

Disease or Syndrome	Age at Onset	Associated Features	Course	Predominant Type of Movement
XYY genetic disorder	Infancy	Aggressive behavior	Static	Simple motor and vocal tics
XXY and 9_p mosaicism	Infancy	Multiple physical anomalies, mental retardation	Static	Simple motor and vocal tics
Duchenne's muscular dystrophy (X-linked recessive)	Childhood	Mild mental retardation	Progressive	Motor and vocal tics
Fragile X syndrome	Childhood	Mental retardation, facial dysmorphism, seizures, autistic features	Static	Simple motor and vocal tics, coprolalia
Developmental and perinatal disorders	Infancy, childhood	Seizures, EEG and CT abnormalities, psychosis, aggressivity, hyperactivity, Ganser's syndrome, compulsivity, torticollis	Variable	Motor and vocal tics, echolalia

ASLO, Antistreptolysin O, Serum; CT, computed tomography; EEG, electroencephalogram.

comprehensive education for families so that children are not unwittingly punished for their tic behaviors. Families must also understand the waxing and waning nature of many tic disorders. In mild cases, children with tic disorders who are functioning well socially and academically may not require treatment. In more severe cases, children with tic disorders may be ostracized by peers and have academic work compromised by the disruptive nature of tics, and a variety of treatments must be considered.

Pharmacological interventions have some efficacy in tic suppression, and behavioral interventions such as "habit reversal" techniques are being used to help children and adolescents become more aware of their tics and initiate voluntary movements that can "counter" tics. Older children, adolescents, and adults often report tics to be preceded by an unpleasant sensation denoted as a "premonitory urge." Premonitory urge phenomena may play an important role in behavioral interventions in that a patient's ability to recognize and respond to a premonitory urge can become the basis of replacing the tic behavior with a desired behavior before it emerges. A scale for premonitory urge called the *Premonitory Urge for Tics Scale* (PUTS), recently devised and examined psychometrically, was found to be internally consistent and correlated with overall tic severity in youth over 10 years of age.

Other behavioral techniques—including massed (negative) practice, self-monitoring, incompatible response training, presentation and removal of positive reinforcement, as well as habit reversal treatment—were reviewed by Stanley A. Hobbs. He reported that tic frequency was reduced in many cases, particularly with habit reversal treatment; currently, additional studies are under way to replicate the efficacy of these techniques. Behavioral techniques, including relaxation, may reduce the stress that often exacerbates Tourette's disorder. It is hypothesized that behavioral techniques and pharmacotherapy together have a synergistic effect.

Pharmacotherapy. Haloperidol (Haldol) and pimozide (Orap) are the two most well-investigated antipsychotic agents in the treatment of Tourette's disorder, although atypical antipsychotics such as risperidone (Risperadal) and olanzapine (Zyprexa) are often chosen as first-line agents due to their safer side-effect profiles. High-potency dopamine receptor antagonists (typical antipsychotics), such as haloperidol, trifluoperazine (Stelazine), and pimozide, have been shown to reduce tics significantly. Up to 80 percent of patients have some favorable response; their symptoms decrease by as much as 70 to 90 percent of baseline frequency. Follow-up studies, however, indicate that only 20 to 30 percent of these patients continue to take long-term maintenance therapy. Discontinuation is often based on the drug's adverse effects, including extrapyramidal effects and dysphoria. The initial daily haloperidol dose for adolescents is usually between 0.25 and 0.5 mg. Haloperidol is not approved for use in children younger than 3 years of age. For children between 3 and 12 years of age, the recommended total daily dose is between 0.05 and 0.075 mg/kg, administered in divided doses either two or three times a day.

The initial dosage of pimozide is usually 1 to 2 mg daily in divided doses; the dosage may be increased every other day. Most patients are maintained on less than 0.2 mg/kg a day or 10 mg a day, whichever is less. A dosage of 0.3 mg/kg a day or 20 mg a day should never be exceeded because of cardiotoxic adverse effects. Pimozide appears to be relatively safe at recommended dosages, with cardiotoxicity limited to prolonged QT wave intervals. Electrocardiography is needed at baseline and periodically during treatment. Little experience is reported in administering pimozide to children less than 12 years of age.

Clinicians must forewarn patients and families of the possibility of acute dystonic reactions and parkinsonian symptoms when use of a conventional or atypical antipsychotic medication is to be initiated. Atypical antipsychotics (serotonin-dopamine antagonists), including risperidone and olanzapine (Zyprexa), can be initiated as a treatment option instead of the conventional antipsychotics in the hope that adverse effects will be less pervasive. Risperidone has been used in the treatment of Tourette's disorder in doses ranging from 1 to 6 mg per day with some success. Adverse effects include weight gain, sedation, and extrapyramidal adverse effects. Risperidone and pimozide were found to be of equal efficacy in one study of 50 children, adolescents, and adults with Tourette's disorder. Olanzapine is generally well tolerated, although weight gain and reports of cognitive dulling have limited its use. Even with the serotonin-dopamine antagonists, diphenhydramine (Benadryl) or benztropine (Cogentin) may be required to control extrapyramidal adverse effects.

Although not presently approved by the US Food and Drug Administration (FDA) for use in Tourette's disorder, several studies reported that clonidine, an α_2-adrenergic agonist, was efficacious; 40 to 70 percent of patients benefited from the medication. In addition to the reduction in tic symptoms, patients may experience less tension and improved attention span. Another α_2-adrenergic agonist, guanfacine (Tenex), has also been used in the treatment of tic disorders. Clonidine has generally been used in dosages ranging from 0.05 mg orally thrice daily to 0.1 mg four times daily; and guanfacine is usually used in dosages ranging from 1 to 4 mg per day. When used in these dosage ranges, adverse effects of the α-adrenergic agents include drowsiness, headache, irritability, and occasional hypotension.

In view of the frequent comorbidity of tic behaviors and obsessive-compulsive symptoms or disorders, the selective serotonin reuptake inhibitors (SSRIs) have been used alone or in combination with antipsychotics in the treatment of Tourette's disorder. Some data suggest that SSRIs, such as fluoxetine (Prozac), may be helpful.

Although clinicians must weigh the risks and benefits of using stimulants in cases of severe hyperactivity and comorbid tics, a recent study reports that methylphenidate does not increase the rate or intensity of motor or vocal tics in most children with hyperactivity and tic disorders. A recent study of atomoxetine (Strattera) at doses ranging from 0.5 mg/kg to 1.5 mg/kg, in the treatment of children and adolescents with ADHD and tic disorders revealed that the atomoxetine did not exacerbate tics and may be associated with some tic reduction. One case report on the use of bupropion (Wellbutrin), an antidepressant of the aminoketone class, indicated increased tic behavior in several children being treated for Tourette's disorder and ADHD. Other antidepressants, such as imipramine (Tofranil) and desipramine (Norpramin, Pertofrane), may decrease disruptive behavior in children with Tourette's disorder, but are no longer widely used because of their potentially serious cardiac adverse effects.

CHRONIC MOTOR OR VOCAL TIC DISORDER

In DSM-IV-TR, chronic motor or vocal tic disorder is defined as the presence of either motor tics or vocal tics, but not both. The other features are the same as those of Tourette's disorder, but chronic motor or vocal tic disorder cannot be diagnosed if the criteria for Tourette's disorder have ever been met. According to DSM-IV-TR criteria, the disorder must have its onset before the age of 18 years.

Epidemiology

The rate of chronic motor or vocal tic disorder has been estimated to be from 100 to 1,000 times greater than that of Tourette's disorder. School-age boys are at highest risk, but the incidence is unknown. Although the disorder was once believed to be rare, current estimates of the prevalence of chronic motor or vocal tic disorder range from 1 to 2 percent.

Etiology

Tourette's disorder and chronic motor or vocal tic disorder aggregate in the same families. Twin studies have found a high concordance for either Tourette's disorder or chronic motor tics in monozygotic twins. This finding supports the importance of hereditary factors in the transmission of at least some tic disorders.

Diagnosis and Clinical Features

The onset of chronic motor or vocal tic disorder appears to be in early childhood. The types of tics and their locations are similar to those in transient tic disorder. Chronic vocal tics are considerably rarer than chronic motor tics. The chronic vocal tics are usually much less conspicuous than those in Tourette's disorder. The vocal tics are usually not loud or intense and are not primarily produced by the vocal cords; they consist of grunts or other noises caused by thoracic, abdominal, or diaphragmatic contractions. The DSM-IV-TR diagnostic criteria are given in Table 46–4.

Differential Diagnosis

Chronic motor tics must be differentiated from a variety of other motor movements, including choreiform movements, myoclonus, restless legs syndrome, akathisia, and dystonias. Involuntary vocal utterances can occur in certain neurological disorders, such as Huntington's disease and Parkinson's disease.

Course and Prognosis

Children whose tics start between the ages of 6 and 8 years seem to have the best outcomes. Symptoms usually last for 4 to 6 years and stop in early adolescence. Children whose tics involve the limbs or trunk tend to do less well than those with only facial tics.

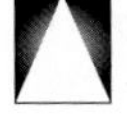

Table 46–4
DSM-IV-TR Diagnostic Criteria for Chronic Motor or Vocal Tic Disorder

A. Single or multiple motor or vocal tics (i.e., sudden, rapid, recurrent, nonrhythmic, stereotyped motor movements or vocalizations), but not both, have been present at some time during the illness.
B. The tics occur many times a day nearly every day or intermittently throughout a period of more than 1 year, and during this period there was never a tic-free period of more than 3 consecutive months.
C. The onset is before age 18 years.
D. The disturbance is not due to the direct physiological effects of a substance (e.g., stimulants) or a general medical condition (e.g., Huntington's disease or postviral encephalitis).
E. Criteria have never been met for Tourette's disorder.

(From American Psychiatric Association. *Diagnostic and Statistical Manual of Mental Disorders.* 4th ed. Text rev. Washington, DC: American Psychiatric Association; copyright 2000, with permission.)

Treatment

The treatment of chronic motor or vocal tic disorder depends on the severity and frequency of the tics; the patient's subjective distress; the effects of the tics on school or work, job performance, and socialization; and the presence of any other concomitant mental disorder. Psychotherapy may be indicated to minimize the secondary social difficulties caused by severe tics. Several studies found that behavioral techniques, particularly habit reversal treatments, were effective in treating chronic motor or vocal tic disorder. Antianxiety agents have been unsuccessful. Haloperidol has been helpful in some cases, but the risks must be weighed against the possible clinical benefits because of the drug's adverse effects, including the development of tardive dyskinesia.

TRANSIENT TIC DISORDER

In the DSM-IV-TR, transient tic disorder is defined as the presence of a single tic or multiple motor or vocal tics or both. The tics occur many times a day for at least 4 weeks but no longer than 12 months. The other features are the same as those for Tourette's disorder, but transient tic disorder cannot be diagnosed if the criteria for Tourette's disorder or chronic motor or vocal tic disorder have ever been met. According to DSM-IV-TR, the disorder must have its onset before the age of 18 years.

Epidemiology

Transient tic-like movements and nervous muscular twitches are common in children. From 5 to 24 percent of all school-age children have a history of tics. The prevalence of tics as defined here is unknown.

Etiology

Transient tic disorder probably has organic origins, with some tics-combining psychogenic contributions as well. Early-onset of tics, which are probably most likely to progress to Tourette's disorder, occur with greater frequency in children with an increased family history of tics. Tics that progress to chronic motor or vocal tic disorder are most likely to have components of both organic and psychogenic origin. Tics of all sorts are *exacerbated* by stress and anxiety, but no evidence indicates that tics are *caused* by stress or anxiety.

Diagnosis and Clinical Features

The DSM-IV-TR criteria for establishing the diagnosis of transient tic disorder are as follows: The tics are single or multiple, motor or vocal. They occur many times a day nearly every day for at least 4 weeks, but no longer than 12 consecutive months. The patient has no history of Tourette's disorder or chronic motor or vocal tic disorder. The onset is before age 18 years. The tics do not occur exclusively during substance intoxication, and they are not caused by a general medical condition. The diagnosis should specify whether a single episode or recurrent episodes are present (Table 46–5). Transient tic disorder can be distinguished from chronic motor or vocal tic disorder and Tourette's disorder only by observing the symptoms' progression over time.

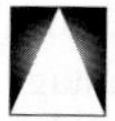

Table 46–5
DSM-IV-TR Diagnostic Criteria for Transient Tic Disorder

A. Single or multiple motor and/or vocal tics (i.e., sudden, rapid, recurrent, nonrhythmic, stereotyped motor movements or vocalizations)
B. The tics occur many times a day, nearly every day for at least 4 weeks, but for no longer than 12 consecutive months.
C. The onset is before age 18 years.
D. The disturbance is not due to the direct physiological effects of a substance (e.g., stimulants) or a general medical condition (e.g., Huntington's disease or postviral encephalitis).
E. Criteria have never been met for Tourette's Disorder or Chronic Motor or Vocal Tic Disorder.

Specify if:
Single episode or **Recurrent**

(From American Psychiatric Association. *Diagnostic and Statistical Manual of Mental Disorders.* 4th ed. Text rev. Washington, DC: American Psychiatric Association; copyright 2000, with permission.)

Course and Prognosis

Motor tics are frequent among young children and, in general, are not associated with severe impairment. Over time, tics either disappear permanently or recur during periods of special stress. Only a small percentage of those with tics develop chronic motor or vocal tic disorder or Tourette's disorder.

Treatment

Whether the tics will disappear spontaneously, progress, or become chronic is unclear at the beginning of treatment. Focusing much attention on mild or infrequent tics may serve to cause undue stress for a child, but if tics are sufficiently severe to cause impairment in social, academic, or emotional function, psychiatric and pediatric neurological examinations are recommended. Psychopharmacology is recommended when symptoms are severe and disabling. Several studies have found that behavioral techniques, particularly habit reversal treatment, are effective in treating transient tics.

TIC DISORDER NOT OTHERWISE SPECIFIED

According to DSM-IV-TR, tic disorder not otherwise specified refers to disorders characterized by tics but not otherwise meeting the criteria for a specific tic disorder (Table 46–6).

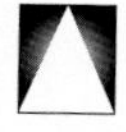

Table 46–6
DSM-IV-TR Diagnostic Criteria for Tic Disorder Not Otherwise Specified

This category is for disorders characterized by tics that do not meet criteria for a specific tic disorder. Examples include tics lasting less than 4 weeks or tics with an onset after age 18 years.

(From American Psychiatric Association. *Diagnostic and Statistical Manual of Mental Disorders.* 4th ed. Text rev. Washington, DC: American Psychiatric Association; copyright 2000, with permission.)

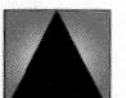

Table 46–7
ICD-10 Diagnostic Criteria for Tic Disorders

Note: A tic is an involuntary, sudden, rapid, recurrent, nonrhythmic, stereotyped motor movement or vocalization.

Transient tic disorder

A. Single or multiple motor or vocal tic(s) or both occur many times a day, on most days, over a period of at least 4 weeks.

B. Duration of the disorder is 12 months or less.

C. There is no history of Tourette's syndrome, and the disorder is not the result of physical conditions or side effects of medication.

D. Onset is before the age of 18 years.

Chronic motor or vocal tic disorder

A. Motor or vocal tics, but not both, occur many times per day, on most days, over a period of at least 12 months.

B. No period of remission during that year lasts longer than 2 months.

C. There is no history of Tourette's syndrome, and the disorder is not the result of physical conditions or side effects of medication.

D. Onset is before the age of 18 years.

Combined vocal and multiple motor tic disorder (de la Tourette's syndrome)

A. Multiple motor tics and one or more vocal tics have been present at some time during the disorder, but not necessarily concurrently.

B. The frequency of tics must be many times a day, nearly every day, for more than 1 year, with no period of remission during that year lasting longer than 2 months.

C. Onset is before the age of 18 years.

Other tic disorders

Tic disorder, unspecified

A nonrecommended residual category for a disorder that fulfills the general criteria for a tic disorder but in which the specific subcategory is not specified or in which the features do not fulfill the criteria for transient tic disorders, chronic motor or vocal tic disorder, combined vocal and multiple motor tic disorder (de la Tourette's syndrome).

(From World Health Organization. The *ICD-10 Classification of Mental and Behavioural Disorders: Diagnostic Criteria for Research.* Copyright, World Health Organization, Geneva, 1993, with permission.)

ICD-10

In the 10th revision of *International Statistical Classification of Diseases and Related Health Problems* (ICD-10), tic disorders form a category under disorders of childhood and adolescence. ICD-10 includes the same tic disorders as DSM-IV-TR and adds another, other tic disorders. Tics—motor movements or vocal productions that serve no apparent purpose and are of sudden onset—are described as the predominant manifestation in these syndromes. The severity of tics varies greatly, from near normal, with 1 in 5 or 1 in 10 children occasionally manifesting tics, to Tourette's syndrome, which is rare, severe, and incapacitating. Tic disorders are more common in boys than in girls, and a family history of tics is frequent (Table 46–7).

References

Abelson JF, Kwan KY, O'Roak BJ, Baek DY, Stillman AA, Morgan TM, Mathews CA, Pauls DL, Rasin MR, Gunel M, Davis NR, Ercan-Sencicek AG, Guez DH, Spertus JA, Leckman JF, Dure LS IV, Kurlan R, Singer HS, Gilbert DL, Farhi A, Louvi A, Lifton RP, Sestan N, State MW. Sequence variants in LSITRK1 are associated with Tourette's syndrome. *Science*. 2005;310:317.

Allen AJ, Kurlan RM, Gilbert DL, Coffey BJ, Linder SL, Lewis DW, Winner PK, Dunn DW, Dure LS, Sallee FR, Milton DR, Mintz MI, Ricardi RK, Erenberg G, Layton LL, Feldman PD, Kelsey KD, Spencer TJ. Atomoxetine treatment in children and adolescents with ADHD and comorbid tic disorders. *Neurology*. 2005;65:1941.

Bloch MH, Peterson BS, Scahill L, Otka J, Katsovich L, Zhang H, Leckman JF. Adulthood outcome of tic and obsessive-compulsive symptom severity in children with Tourette syndrome. *Arch Pediatr Adolesc Med*. 2006;160:65.

Bloch MH, Leckman JF, Zhu H, Peterson BS. Caudate volumes in childhood predict symptom severity in adults with Tourette's syndrome. *Neurology*. 2005;65:1253.

DeVito TJ, Drost DJ, Pavlovsky W, Neufeld RW, Rajakumar N, McKinlay BD, Williamson PC, Nicolson R. Brain magnetic resonance spectroscopy in Tourette's disorder. *J Am Acad Child Adolesc Psychiatry*. 2005;44:1301.

Ford R, Greenhill L. Stimulant medication in the treatment of ADHD. In: Martin A, Scahill L, Leckman JF, Charney D, eds. *Principles and Practice in Pediatric Psychopharmacology*. New York: Oxford Press; 2003.

Gilbert DL, Dure L, Sethuraman G, Raab D, Lane J, Sallee FR. Tic reduction with pergolide in a randomized controlled trial in children. *Neurology*. 2003;60:606.

King RA, Scahill L, Lombroso P, Leckman JF. Tourette syndrome: Pharmacotherapy. In: Martin A, Scahill L, Leckman JF, Charney D, eds. *Principles and Practice in Pediatric Psychopharmacology*. New York: Oxford Press; 2003.

Mathews CA, Bimson B, Lowe TL, Herrera LD, Budman CL, Erenberg G, Naarden A, Bruun RD, Freimer NB, Reus VI. Association between maternal smoking and increased symptom severity in Tourette's syndrome. *Am J Psych*. 2006;163(6):1066.

Murphy TK, Sajid M, Soto O, Shapira N, Edge P, Yang M, Lewis MH, Goodman WK. Detecting pediatric autoimmune neuropsychiatric disorders associated with streptococcus in children with obsessive-compulsive disorder and tics. *Biol Psychiatry*. 2004;55:61.

Peterson BS, Thomas P, Kane MJ, Scahill L, Zhang H, Bronen R, King RA, Leckman JF, Staib L. Basal ganglia volumes in patients with Gilles de la Tourette syndrome. *Arch Gen Psychiatry*. 2003;60:415–424.

Scahill L, Leckman JF. Tic disorders. In: Sadock BJ, Sadock VA, eds. *Kaplan & Sadock's Comprehensive Textbook of Psychiatry*. 8th ed. Vol. 2. Baltimore: Lippincott Williams & Wilkins; 2005:3228.

Storch EA, Murphy TK, Geffken GR, Sajid M, Allen P, Roberti JW, Goodman WK. Reliability and validity of the Yale Global Tic Severity Scale. *Psychol Assess*. 2005;17:486.

Woods DW, Piacentini J, Himle MB, Chang S. Premonitory urge for tics scale (PUTS): Initial psychometric results and examination of the premonitory urge phenomenon in youths with tic disorders. *J Dev Behav Pediatr*. 2005;26:397.

47 Elimination Disorders

The developmental milestones of mastering control over bowel and bladder function are complex processes that occur over a period of months for the typical toddler. Infants generally void small volumes of urine approximately every hour, commonly stimulated by feeding, and may have incomplete emptying of the bladder. As the infant matures to be a toddler, bladder capacity increases, and between 1 and 3 years of age, cortical inhibitory pathways develop allowing the child to have voluntary control over reflexes that control the bladder muscles. The ability to have muscular control over the bowel occurs even before bladder control for most toddlers, and the assessment of fecal soiling includes determining whether the clinical presentation occurs with or without chronic constipation and overflow soiling. The normal sequence of developing control over bowel and bladder functions is the development of nocturnal fecal continence, diurnal fecal continence, diurnal bladder control, and nocturnal bladder control. Bowel and bladder control develops gradually over time. Toilet training is affected by many factors, such as a child's intellectual capacity and social maturity, cultural determinants, and the psychological interactions between child and parents.

Enuresis and encopresis are the two elimination disorders described in the text revision of the 4th edition of *Diagnostic and Statistical Manual of Mental Disorders* (DSM-IV-TR). These disorders are considered after age 4 years, for encopresis, and after age 5 years for enuresis, when a child is chronologically, developmentally, and physiologically expected to be able to master these skills. Normal development encompasses a range of time in which a given child is able to devote the attention, motivation, and physiological skills to exhibit competency in elimination processes. Encopresis is defined as a pattern of passing feces in inappropriate places, such as in clothing or other places, at least once per month for 3 consecutive months, whether the passage is involuntary or intentional. The child with encopresis typically exhibits dysregulated bowel function; for example, with infrequent bowel movements, constipation, or recurrent abdominal pain and sometimes pain on defecations. Encopresis is a nonorganic condition in a child who is chronologically at least 4 years. Enuresis is the repeated voiding of urine into clothes or bed, whether the voiding is involuntary or intentional. The behavior must occur twice weekly for at least 3 months or must cause clinically significant distress or impairment socially or academically. The child's chronological or developmental age must be at least 5 years.

ENCOPRESIS

Epidemiology

Incidence rates for encopretic behavior decrease drastically with increasing age. Although the diagnosis is not made until after age 4 years, encopretic behavior is present in 8.1 percent of 3 year olds, 2.2 percent of 5 year olds, and 0.75 percent of 10 to 12 year olds. In Western cultures, bowel control is established in more than 95 percent of children by their fourth birthday and in 99 percent by the fifth birthday. Encopresis is virtually absent in youth with normal intellectual function by the age of 16. Males are found to be about six times more likely to have encopresis than females. A significant relation exists between encopresis and enuresis.

Etiology

Encopresis involves an often complicated interplay between physiological and psychological factors. Although encopresis is considered a nonorganic disorder, a typical child with encopresis may show evidence of chronic constipation, leading to infrequent defecation, withholding of bowel movements, and avoidance of defecation. Children may avoid the pain of having a bowel movement by holding in the bowel movement, which then leads to impaction and eventual overflow soiling. This pattern is observed in more than 75 percent of children with encopretic behavior. This common set of circumstances in most children with encopresis supports a behavioral intervention with a focus on ameliorating constipation while increasing appropriate toileting behavior. Inadequate training or the lack of appropriate toilet training may delay a child's attainment of continence.

Evidence indicates that some encopretic children have lifelong inefficient and ineffective sphincter control. Other children may soil involuntarily, either because of an inability to control the sphincter adequately or because of excessive fluid caused by a retentive overflow.

Encopresis has been demonstrated to occur with significantly greater frequency among children with known sexual abuse compared with a normal sample of children, and it occurs with greater frequency among children with a variety of psychiatric disturbances compared with controls. Encopresis, however, is not a specific indicator of sexual abuse, because it also occurs with increased frequency in nonabused children with other behavioral problems. Some evidence indicates that encopresis in children is associated with measures of maternal hostility, and harsh and punitive parenting. A recent study evaluating the frequency of encopresis and enuresis in children with prepubertal and early adolescent bipolar I disorder found a greater prevalence of encopresis among children with bipolar disorder compared with healthy controls; in most cases, however, the encopresis predated the onset of the affective illness.

It is evident that once a given child has developed a pattern of withholding bowel movements with resulting pain with attempts to defecate, a child's fear and resistance to changing the pattern can lead to a power struggle between child and parent over effective toileting behavior. Perpetual battles often aggravate the disorder and frequently cause secondary behavioral difficulties. Many children with encopresis who are not reported to have early behavioral problems end up being socially ostracized and rejected because of the encopresis. The social consequences of soiling can further lead to the development of psychiatric problems. On the other hand, children with encopresis who clearly can control their bowel function adequately but chronically deposit feces of relatively normal consistency in abnormal places are more likely to have a preexisting neurodevelopmental problems, easy distractibility, short attention span, low frustration tolerance, hyperactivity, or poor coordination. Occasionally, a child has a specific fear of using the toilet, leading to a phobia.

Encopresis, in some children, can be considered secondary, that is, emerging after a period of normal bowel habits in conjunction with a disruptive life event, such as the birth of a sibling or a move to a new home. When encopresis manifests after a long period of fecal continence, it may reflect a response indicative of a developmental regressive behavior; for example, based on a severe stressor, such as a parental separation, loss of a best friend, or an unexpected academic failure.

Psychogenic Megacolon. Most children with encopresis retain feces and become constipated, either voluntarily or secondarily to painful defecation. In some cases a subclinical preexisting anorectal dysfunction exists that contributes to the constipation. In either case, resulting chronic rectal distention from large, hard fecal masses can cause loss of tone in the rectal wall and desensitization to pressure. Thus, children in this situation become even less aware of the need to defecate, and overflow encopresis occurs, usually with relatively small amounts of liquid or soft stool leaking out.

Anecdotal reports indicate that children whose parenting has been harsh and punitive and who have been severely punished for "accidents" during toilet training are at greater risk of developing encopresis.

Diagnosis and Clinical Features

According to DSM-IV-TR, encopresis is diagnosed when feces are passed into inappropriate places on a regular basis (at least once a month) for 3 months (Table 47–1). Encopresis may be present in children who have bowel control and intentionally deposit feces in their clothes or other places for a variety of emotional reasons. Anecdotal reports have suggested that occasionally encopresis is attributable to an expression of anger or rage in a child whose parents have been punitive or of hostility at a parent. In a case such as this, once a child develops this inappropriate repetitive behavior eliciting negative attention, it is difficult to break the cycle of continuous negative attention. In other children, sporadic episodes of encopresis can occur during times of stress—for example, proximal to the birth of a new sibling—but in such cases, the behavior is usually transient and does not fulfill the diagnostic criteria for the disorder.

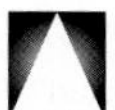

Table 47–1
DSM-IV-TR Diagnostic Criteria for Encopresis

A. Repeated passage of feces into inappropriate places (e.g., clothing or floor) whether involuntary or intentional.
B. At least one such event a month for at least 3 months.
C. Chronological age is at least 4 years (or equivalent developmental level).
D. The behavior is not due exclusively to the direct physiological effects of a substance (e.g., laxatives) or a general medical condition except through a mechanism involving constipation.

Code as follows:
With constipation and overflow incontinence
Without constipation and overflow incontinence

(From American Psychiatric Association. *Diagnostic and Statistical Manual of Mental Disorders*. 4th ed. Text rev. Washington, DC: American Psychiatric Association; copyright 2000, with permission.)

Encopresis can also be present on an involuntary basis in the absence of physiological abnormalities. In these cases, a child may not exhibit adequate control over the sphincter muscles, either because the child is absorbed in another activity or because he or she is unaware of the process. The feces may be of normal, near-normal, or liquid consistency. Some involuntary soiling occurs from chronic retaining of stool, which results in liquid overflow. In rare cases, the involuntary overflow of stool results from psychological causes of diarrhea or anxiety disorder symptoms.

The DSM-IV-TR breaks down the types of encopresis into *with* constipation and overflow incontinence and *without* constipation and overflow incontinence. To receive a diagnosis of encopresis, a child must have a developmental or chronological level of at least 4 years. If the fecal incontinence is directly related to a medical condition, encopresis is not diagnosed.

Studies have indicated that children with encopresis who do not have gastrointestinal illnesses have high rates of abnormal anal sphincter contractions. This finding is particularly prevalent among children with encopresis with constipation and overflow incontinence who have difficulty relaxing their anal sphincter muscles when trying to defecate. Children with constipation who have difficulties with sphincter relaxation are not likely to respond well to laxatives in the treatment of their encopresis. Children with encopresis without abnormal sphincter tone are likely to improve over a short period.

Jack was a 9-year-old boy with daily encopresis, enuresis, and a history of hoarding behaviors, along with hiding the feces around the house. He resided with his adoptive parents having been removed from his biological parents at age 3 years because of neglect, and physical and sexual abuse. He was reported to be cocaine addicted at birth, but was otherwise healthy. His mother was a known drug and alcohol user, and his father had spent time in jail for drug sales. Jack has always been enuretic at night, and when he was younger he had a history of daytime enuresis as well. Jack had a short attention span, was highly impulsive and had great difficulty staying in his seat at school and remaining on task. He had reading difficulties and was placed in a contained special education classroom because of his disruptive behavior as well as his academic difficulties. Jack also qualified for a diagnosis of oppositional-defiant disorder. Despite experiencing physical and sexual abuse, he has not experienced flashbacks or other symptoms indicating the presence of posttraumatic stress disorder. Jack is being treated for attention-deficit/hyperactivity disorder (ADHD) and is responding to methylphenidate (Concerta 36 mg per day).

Jack's adoptive family resided in an urban area that had access to a university hospital with an outpatient program that had expertise in the behavioral treatment of encopresis. This program coupled the bowel training method with a psychoeducational component and psychotherapy. It was determined that Jack's encopresis was not of the retentive-overflow type, and the feces were always well formed. Much to the surprise of the psychiatric consultant, several-week outpatient bowel training course coupled with the psychoeducational component and psychotherapy resulted in significant improvement in the frequency of the encopresis. Jack was proud and gave his therapist a diagram of the functioning of the digestive system that was part of the psychoeducational program. In retrospect, it appeared that although there were symbolic aspects to Jack's encopretic behavior, the soiling was ego-dystonic, and he was motivated to change the behavior. (Courtesy of Edwin J. Mikkelsen, M.D. and Caroly Pataki, M.D.)

Pathology and Laboratory Examination

Although no specific test indicates a diagnosis of encopresis, clinicians must rule out medical illnesses, such as Hirschsprung's disease, before making a diagnosis. If it is unclear whether fecal retention is responsible for encopresis with constipation and overflow incontinence, a physical examination of the abdomen is indicated, and an abdominal X-ray can help determine the degree of constipation present. Sophisticated tests to determine whether sphincter tone is abnormal are generally not conducted in simple cases of encopresis.

Differential Diagnosis

In encopresis with constipation and overflow incontinence, constipation can begin as early as the child's first year and can peak between the second and fourth years. Soiling usually begins at age 4. Frequent liquid stools and hard fecal masses are found in the colon and the rectum on abdominal palpation and rectal examination. Complications include impaction, megacolon, and anal fissures.

Encopresis with constipation and overflow incontinence can be caused by faulty nutrition; structural disease of the anus, rectum, and colon; medicinal adverse effects; or nongastrointestinal medical (endocrine or neurological) disorders. The chief differential problem is aganglionic megacolon or Hirschsprung's disease, in which a patient may have an empty rectum and no desire to defecate, but may still have an overflow of feces. The disorder occurs in 1 in 5,000 children; signs appear shortly after birth.

Given the frequency of comorbid psychiatric disorders and increased incidence of encopresis among children who have been sexually abused, it is imperative to investigate the possibility of sexual and physical abuse during the evaluation of encopresis.

Course and Prognosis

The outcome of encopresis depends on the cause, the chronicity of the symptoms, and coexisting behavioral problems. In many cases, encopresis is self-limiting, and it rarely continues beyond middle adolescence. Encopresis in children who have contributing physiological factors, such as poor gastric motility and an inability to relax the anal sphincter muscles, is more difficult to treat than that in those with constipation but normal sphincter tone.

Encopresis is a particularly repugnant disorder to most persons, including family members; thus, family tension is often high. The child's peers are also sensitive to the developmentally inappropriate behavior and often ostracize the child. A child with encopresis is often scapegoated by peers and shunned by adults. Many of these children have abysmally low self-esteem and are aware of their constant rejection. Psychologically, the child may appear blunted toward the symptoms or may be entrenched in a pattern of encopresis as a mode of expressing anger. The outcome of cases of encopresis is affected by the family's willingness and ability to participate in treatment without being overly punitive and by the child's awareness of when the passage of feces is about to occur.

Treatment

The treatment plan for encopresis cannot be established until a medical assessment of bowel function is completed as well as a full psychiatric assessment. A typical treatment plan for a child with encopresis includes an initial medical plan to address constipation, in most cases, as well as an ongoing behavioral intervention to enhance appropriate bowel behavior and diminish anxiety related to bowel movement. By the time a child is brought for treatment, considerable family discord and distress are common. Family tensions about the symptom must be reduced, and a nonpunitive atmosphere established. Similar efforts should be made to reduce the child's embarrassment at school. Many changes of underwear with a minimum of fuss should be arranged. Education of the family and correction of misperceptions that a family may have about soiling must occur before treatment. A useful physiological approach involves a combination of daily laxatives or mineral oil along with a behavioral intervention in which the child sits on the toilet for timed intervals daily and is rewarded for successful defecation. Laxatives are not necessary for children who are not constipated and do have good bowel control, but regular, timed intervals on the toilet may be useful with these children as well.

A recent report confirms the success of an interactive parent–child family guidance intervention for young children with encopresis based on psychological and behavioral interventions for children under the age of 9 years.

Supportive psychotherapy and relaxation techniques may be useful in treating the anxieties and other sequelae of children with encopresis, such as low self-esteem and social isolation. Family interventions can be helpful for children who have bowel control but continue to deposit their feces in inappropriate locations. A good outcome occurs when a child feels in control of life events.

Coexisting behavior problems predict a poorer outcome. In all cases, proper bowel habits may need to be taught. In some cases, biofeedback techniques have been of benefit.

ENURESIS

Epidemiology

The prevalence of enuresis decreases with increasing age. The diagnosis of enuresis is not made until the chronologic and developmental age of 5 years, but enuretic behavior nocturnally and during the daytime is common, with reported prevalence from 2 percent to 5 percent among school-aged children. Enuretic behavior is considered developmentally appropriate among young toddlers, precluding diagnoses of enuresis; however, enuretic behavior occurs in 82 percent of 2-year-olds, 49 percent of 3-year-olds, 26 percent of 4-year-olds, and 7 percent of 5-year-olds on a regular basis. Prevalence rates vary, however, on the basis of the population studied and the tolerance for the symptoms in various cultures and socioeconomic groups.

The Isle of Wight study reported that 15.2 percent of 7-year-old boys were enuretic occasionally and that 6.7 percent of them were enuretic at least once a week. The study reported that 3.3 percent of girls at the age of 7 years were enuretic at least once a week. By age 10, the overall prevalence of enuresis was reported to be 3 percent. The rate drops drastically for teenagers; a prevalence of 1.5 percent has been reported for 14-year-olds. Enuresis affects about 1 percent of adults.

Although most children with enuresis do not have a comorbid psychiatric disorder, children with enuresis are at higher risk for the development of a variety of developmental and behavioral disturbances compared with children without enuresis.

Nocturnal enuresis is about 50 percent more common in boys and accounts for about 80 percent of children with enuresis. Diurnal enuresis is also more often seen in boys who often delay voiding until it is too late. A spontaneous resolution of nocturnal enuresis is about 15 percent per year. Nocturnal enuresis consists of a normal volume of voided urine, whereas, when small volumes of urine are voided at night, other medical causes may be present.

Etiology

Most children with nocturnal enuresis do not exhibit neurological conditions that account for the symptoms. Voiding dysfunction in the absence of a specific neurogenic cause is believed to originate from behavioral factors that affect normal voiding habits and inhibit the maturation of normal voluntary control.

The most severe form of dysfunctional voiding is called Hinman's syndrome, and is thought of as a non-neurogenic neurogenic bladder resulting from habitual, voluntary tightening of the external sphincter during urges to urinate. The pattern may be set in a young child who may start out with a normal or overactive detrusor muscle in the bladder, but in any case, repeatedly attempts to prevent leaking or urination when there is an urge to void. Over time, the sensation of the urge to urinate is diminished and the bladder does not empty regularly, leading to enuresis at night when the bladder is relaxed and can empty without resistance. This immature pattern of urinating can account for some cases of enuresis, especially when the pattern has been in place since early childhood. Most children are not enuretic by intention or even with awareness until after they are wet. Physiological factors often play a role in the development of enuresis, and behavioral patterns are likely to maintain the maladaptive urination. Normal bladder control, which is acquired gradually, is influenced by neuromuscular and cognitive development, socioemotional factors, toilet training, and genetic factors. Difficulties in one or more of these areas can delay urinary continence.

Genetic factors are believed to play a role in the expression of enuresis, given that the emergence of enuresis has been found to be significantly greater in first-degree relatives. A longitudinal study of child development found that children with enuresis were about twice as likely to have concomitant developmental delays as those who did not have enuresis. About 75 percent of children with enuresis have a first-degree relative who has or has had enuresis. A child's risk for enuresis has been found to be more than seven times greater if the father was enuretic. The concordance rate is higher in monozygotic twins than in dizygotic twins. A strong genetic component is suggested, and much can be accounted for by tolerance for enuresis in some families and by other psychosocial factors.

Studies indicate that children with enuresis with a normal anatomic bladder capacity report urge to void with less urine in the bladder than children without enuresis. Other studies report that nocturnal enuresis occurs when the bladder is full because of lower than expected levels of nighttime antidiuretic hormone. This could lead to a higher-than-usual urine output. Enuresis does not appear to be related to a specific stage of sleep or time of night; rather, bed-wetting appears randomly. In most cases, the quality of sleep is normal. Little evidence indicates that children with enuresis sleep more soundly than other children.

Psychosocial stressors appear to precipitate enuresis in a subgroup of children with the disorder. In young children, the disorder has been particularly associated with the birth of a sibling, hospitalization between the ages of 2 and 4, the start of school, the breakup of a family because of divorce or death, and a move to a new home.

Diagnosis and Clinical Features

Enuresis is the repeated voiding of urine into a child's clothes or bed; the voiding may be involuntary or intentional. For the diagnosis to be made, a child must exhibit a developmental or chronological age of at least 5 years. According to DSM-IV-TR, the behavior must occur twice weekly for a period of at least 3 months or must cause distress and impairment in functioning to meet the diagnostic criteria. Enuresis is diagnosed only if the behavior is not caused by a medical condition. Children with enuresis are at higher risk for ADHD compared with the general population. They are also more likely to have comorbid encopresis. DSM-IV-TR and the 10th revision of *International Statistical Classification of Diseases and Related Health Problems* (ICD-10) break down the disorder into three types: nocturnal only, diurnal only, and nocturnal and diurnal (Table 47–2).

Pathology and Laboratory Examination

No single laboratory finding is pathognomonic of enuresis; but clinicians must rule out organic factors, such as the presence of

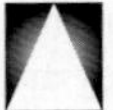

Table 47–2
DSM-IV-TR Diagnostic Criteria for Enuresis

A. Repeated voiding of urine into bed or clothes (whether involuntary or intentional).
B. The behavior is clinically significant as manifested by either a frequency of twice a week for at least 3 consecutive months or the presence of clinically significant distress or impairment in social, academic (occupational), or other important areas of functioning.
C. Chronological age is at least 5 years (or equivalent developmental level).
D. The behavior is not due exclusively to the direct physiological effect of a substance (e.g., a diuretic) or a general medical condition (e.g., diabetes, spina bifida, a seizure disorder).

Specify type:
Nocturnal only
Diurnal only
Nocturnal and diurnal

(From American Psychiatric Association. *Diagnostic and Statistical Manual of Mental Disorders.* 4th ed. Text rev. Washington, DC: American Psychiatric Association; copyright 2002, with permission.)

urinary tract infections, that may predispose a child to enuresis. Structural obstructive abnormalities may be present in up to 3 percent of children with apparent enuresis. Sophisticated radiographic studies are usually deferred in simple cases of enuresis with no signs of repeated infections or other medical problems.

Differential Diagnosis

To make the diagnosis of enuresis, organic causes of bladder dysfunction must be investigated and ruled out. Organic syndromes, such as urinary tract infections, obstructions, or anatomical conditions, are found most often in children who experience both nocturnal and diurnal enuresis combined with urinary frequency and urgency. The organic features include genitourinary pathology—structural, neurological, and infectious—such as obstructive uropathy, spina bifida occulta, and cystitis; other organic disorders that can cause polyuria and enuresis, such as diabetes mellitus and diabetes insipidus; disturbances of consciousness and sleep, such as seizures, intoxication, and sleepwalking disorder, during which a child urinates; and adverse effects from treatment with antipsychotics (e.g., thioridazine [Mellaril]).

Course and Prognosis

Enuresis is often self-limited, and a child with enuresis may have a spontaneous remission without psychological sequelae. Most such children find their symptoms ego-dystonic and enjoy enhanced self-esteem and improved social confidence when they become continent. About 80 percent of affected children have never achieved a year-long period of dryness. Enuresis after at least one dry year usually begins between the ages of 5 and 8 years; if it occurs much later, especially during adulthood, organic causes must be investigated. Some evidence indicates that late onset of enuresis in children is more frequently associated with a concomitant psychiatric difficulty than is enuresis without at least one dry year. Relapses occur in children with enuresis who are becoming dry spontaneously and in those who are being treated. The significant emotional and social difficulties of these children usually include poor self-image, decreased self-esteem, social embarrassment and restriction, and intrafamilial conflict. The course of children with enuresis may be influenced by whether they receive appropriate evaluation and treatment for common comorbid disorders such as ADHD.

Treatment

A treatment plan for typical enuresis can be developed after organic causes of urinary dysfunction have been ruled out. Modalities that have been used successfully for enuresis include both behavioral and pharmacological interventions. A relatively high rate of spontaneous remission over long periods also occurs. The first step in any treatment plan is to review appropriate toilet training. If toilet training was not attempted, the parents and the patient should be guided in this undertaking. Record-keeping is helpful in determining a baseline and following the child's progress and may itself be a reinforcer. A star chart may be particularly helpful. Other useful techniques include restricting fluids before bed and night lifting to toilet train the child. Another basic intervention for those children with enuresis and bowel dysfunction is to assess whether chronic constipation is contributing to urinary dysfunction, and consider increasing dietary fiber to diminish constipation.

Behavioral Therapy. Classic conditioning with the bell (or buzzer) and pad apparatus is generally the most effective treatment for enuresis, with dryness resulting in more than 50 percent of cases. The treatment is equally effective in children with and without concomitant mental disorders, and no evidence suggests symptom substitution. Difficulties may include child and family noncompliance, improper use of the apparatus, and relapse. Bladder training—encouragement or reward for delaying micturition for increasing times during waking hours—has also been used. Although sometimes effective, this method is decidedly inferior to the bell and pad.

Pharmacotherapy. Medication is considered when enuresis is causing impairment in social, family, and school function and behavioral, dietary, and fluid restriction have not been efficacious. When the problem interferes significantly with a child's functioning, several medications can be considered, although the problem often recurs as soon as medications are withdrawn.

Imipramine (Tofranil) is efficacious and has been approved for use in treating childhood enuresis, primarily on a short-term basis. Initially, up to 30 percent of patients with enuresis stay dry, and up to 85 percent wet less frequently than before treatment. The success often does not last, however, and tolerance can develop after 6 weeks of therapy. Once the drug is discontinued, relapse and enuresis at former frequencies usually occur within a few months. The drug's adverse effects, which include cardiotoxicity, are also a serious problem.

The tricyclic drugs are not currently used frequently for enuresis because of their risks and reports of sudden death in several children with ADHD who were taking desipramine (Norpramin, Pertofrane). Desmopressin (DDAVP), an antidiuretic compound that is available as an intranasal spray, has shown some initial success in reducing enuresis. Reduction of enuresis

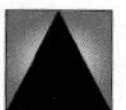

Table 47–3
ICD-10 Diagnostic Criteria for Nonorganic Encopresis

A. The child repeatedly passes feces in places that are inappropriate for the purpose (e.g., clothing, floor), either involuntarily or intentionally. (The disorder may involve overflow incontinence secondary to functional fecal retention.)
B. The child's chronological and mental age is at least 4 years.
C. There is at least one encopretic event per month.
D. Duration of the disorder is at least 6 months.
E. There is no organic condition that constitutes a sufficient cause for the encopretic events.

(From World Health Organization. The *ICD-10 Classification of Mental and Behavioural Disorders: Diagnostic Criteria for Research.* Copyright, World Health Organization, Geneva, 1993, with permission.)

has varied from 10 to 90 percent with the use of desmopressin. In most studies, enuresis recurred shortly after discontinuation of this medication. Adverse effects that can occur with desmopressin include headache, nasal congestion, epistaxis, and stomachache. The most serious adverse effect reported with the use of desmopressin to treat enuresis was a hyponatremic seizure experienced by a child.

Reboxetine (Edronax, Vestra), a norepinephrine reuptake inhibitor with a noncardiotoxic side effect profile has recently been investigated as a safer alternative to imipramine in the treatment of childhood enuresis. A trial in which 22 children with socially handicapping enuresis who had not responded to an enuresis alarm, desmopressin, or anticholinergics were administered 4 to 8 mg of reboxetine at bedtime. Of the 22 children, 13 (59 percent) in this open trial achieved complete dryness with reboxetine alone, or in combination with desmopressin. Side effects were minimal and did not lead to discontinuation of the medication in this trial. Future placebo-controlled trials are indicated to determine the efficacy of this promising medication in the treatment of enuresis.

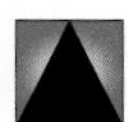

Table 47–4
ICD-10 Diagnostic Criteria for Nonorganic Enuresis

A. The child's chronological and mental age is at least 5 years.
B. Involuntary or intentional voiding of urine into bed or clothes occurs at least twice a month in children aged under 7 years, and at least once a month in children aged 7 years or more.
C. The enuresis is not a consequence of epileptic attacks or of neurological incontinence, and not a direct consequence of structural abnormalities of the urinary tract or any other nonpsychiatric medical condition.
D. There is no evidence of any other psychiatric disorder that meets the criteria for other ICD-10 categories.
E. Duration of the disorder is at least 3 months.

(From World Health Organization. The *ICD-10 Classification of Mental and Behavioural Disorders: Diagnostic Criteria for Research.* Copyright, World Health Organization, Geneva, 1993, with permission.)

Psychotherapy. Psychotherapy may be useful in dealing with the coexisting psychiatric problems and the emotional and family difficulties that arise secondary to chronic enuresis. Although many psychological and psychoanalytic theories regarding enuresis have been advanced, controlled studies have found that psychotherapy alone is not effective in the short-term treatment of enuresis.

ICD-10

In the revision of *International Statistical Classification of Diseases and Related Health Problems* (ICD-10), nonorganic encopresis (Table 47–3) and nonorganic enuresis (Table 47–4) are classified as other behavioral and emotional disorders with onset usually occurring in childhood or adolescence.

References

Baeyens D, Roeyers H, D'Haese L, Pieters F, Hoebeke P, Vande Walle J. The prevalence of ADHD in children with enuresis: Comparison between a tertiary and non-tertiary care sample. *Acta Paediatr.* 2006;95:347.

Bahar RJ, Reid H. Treatment of encopresis and chronic constipation in young children: Clinical results from interactive parent-child guidance. *Clin Pediatr.* 2006;45:157.

Benninga MA, Voskuijl WP, Akkerhius GW, Taminiau JA, Buller HA. Colonic transit times and behaviour profiles in children with defecation disorders. *Arch Dis Child.* 2004;89:13.

Di Lorenzo C, Benninga MA. Pathophysiology of pediatric fecal incontinence. *Gastroenterology.* 2004;126[Suppl 1]:S533.

Feldman AS, Bauer SB. Diagnosis and management of dysfunctional voiding. *Curr Opin Pediatr.* 2006;18:139.

Fitzgerald MP, Thom DH, Wassel-Fyr C, Subak L, Brubaker L, Van Den Deden SK, Brown JS. Childhood urinary symptoms predict adult overactive bladder symptoms. *J Urol.* 2006;175:989.

Kajiwara M, Inoue K, Kato M, Usui A, Kurihara M, Usui T. Nocturnal enuresis and overactive bladder in children: An epidemiological study. *Int J Urol.* 2006;13:36.

Klages T, Geller B, Tillman R, Bolhofner K, Zimerman B. Controlled study of encopresis and enuresis in children with a prepubertal and early adolescent bipolar-I disorder phenotype. *J Am Acad Child Adolesc Psychiatry.* 2005;44:1050.

Landgraf JM, Abidari J, Cilento BG Jr., Cooper CS, Schulman SL, Ortenberg J. Coping, commitment, and attitude: Quantifying the everyday burden of enuresis on children and their families. *Pediatrics.* 2004;113:334.

Mellon MW, Whiteside SP, Friedrich WN. The relevance of fecal soiling as an indicator of child sexual abuse: A preliminary analysis. *J Dev Behav Pediatr.* 2006;27:25.

Mikkelsen EJ. Elimination disorders. In: Sadock BJ, Sadock VA, eds. *Kaplan & Sadock's Comprehensive Textbook of Psychiatry.* 8th ed. Vol. 2. Baltimore: Lippincott Williams & Wilkins; 2005:3237.

Nevus T. Reboxetine in therapy-resistant enuresis: results and pathogenetic implications. *Scand J Urol Nephrol.* 2006;40:31.

Pennesi M, Pitter M, Borduga A, Minisini S, Peratoner L. Behavioral therapy for primary nocturnal enuresis. *J Urol.* 2004;171:408.

Von Gontard A, Hollmann E. Comorbidity of functional urinary incontinence and encopresis: somatic and behavioral associations. *J Urology.* 2004;171:2644.

48 Other Disorders of Infancy, Childhood, and Adolescence

▲ 48.1 Reactive Attachment Disorder of Infancy or Early Childhood

Reactive attachment disorder (RAD) is a clinical disorder characterized by aberrant social behaviors in a young child reflecting an environment of maltreatment that interfered with the development of normal attachment behavior. Unlike most disorders in the text revision of the 4th edition of the *Diagnostic and Statistical Manual of Mental Disorders* (DSM-IV-TR), a diagnosis of RAD is based on the presumption that the etiology is directly linked to environmental deprivation experienced by the child. The diagnosis of RAD is a relatively recent entity, added to the third edition of the DSM (DSM-III) in 1980. The formation of this diagnosis is largely based on the building blocks of attachment theory, which describes the quality of a child's generalized affective relationship with primary caregivers, usually parents. This basic relationship is the product of a young child's need for protection, nurturance, and comfort and the interaction of the parents and child in fulfilling these needs.

Based on observations of a young child and parents during a brief separation and reunion, designated the "strange situation procedure" pioneered by Mary Ainsworth and colleagues, researchers have designated a child's basic pattern of attachment to be characterized as secure, insecure, or disorganized. Children who exhibit secure attachment behavior are believed to experience their caregivers as emotionally available and appear to be more exploratory and well adjusted than children who exhibit insecure or disorganized attachment behavior. Insecure attachment is believed to result from a young child's perception that the caregiver is not consistently available, whereas a child with disorganized attachment behavior is believed to be experiencing the need for proximity to the caregiver with apprehension in approaching the caregiver. These early patterns of attachment are believed to influence a child's future complex capacities for affect regulation, self-soothing, and relationship building. According to DSM-IV-TR, RAD of infancy or early childhood is marked by an inappropriate social relatedness that occurs in most contexts. The disorder appears before the age of 5 years and is associated with "grossly pathological care." It is not accounted for solely by a developmental delay and does not meet the criteria for pervasive developmental disorder. The pattern of care may exhibit lasting disregard for a child's emotional or physical needs or repeated changes of caregivers as when a child is frequently relocated during foster care. The pathological care pattern is believed to cause the disturbance in social relatedness.

The disorder has two subtypes: the *inhibited* type, in which the disturbance takes the form of constantly failing to initiate and respond to most social interactions in a developmentally normal way; and the *disinhibited* type, in which the disturbance takes the form of undifferentiated, unselective social relatedness. These developmentally inappropriate behaviors are presumed to be caused mostly by pathogenic caregiving, but less severe disturbances in parenting may also be associated with infants who exhibit the disorder.

The disorder may result in a picture of failure to thrive, in which an infant shows physical signs of malnourishment and does not exhibit the expected developmental motor and verbal milestones. When this is the case, the failure to thrive is coded on Axis III.

EPIDEMIOLOGY

Few data exist on the prevalence, sex ratio, or familial pattern of RAD. It has been estimated to occur in less than 1 percent of the population. Studies have used selected high-risk populations. In a retrospective report of children in one county of the United States who were removed from their homes because of neglect or abuse before the age of 4 years, 38 percent exhibited signs of emotionally withdrawn or indiscriminate RAD. A study in 2004 established the reliability of the diagnosis by reviewing videotaped assessments of children at risk interacting with caregivers along with a structured interview with caregivers. Given that pathogenic care, including maltreatment, occurs more frequently in the presence of general psychosocial risk factors, such as poverty, disrupted families, and mental illness among caregivers, these circumstances are likely to increase the risk of RAD. In unusual circumstances, however, a caregiver may be fully satisfactory for one child, whereas another child in the same household is maltreated and develops RAD.

ETIOLOGY

The essence of RAD is the malformation of normal attachment behaviors. The inability of a young child to develop normative social interactions that culminate in aberrant attachment behaviors in RAD is inherent in the disorder's definition. RAD is linked to maltreatment, including emotional neglect, physical abuse, or both as well. Grossly pathogenic care of an infant or young child by the caregiver presumably causes the markedly disturbed social relatedness that is usually evident. The emphasis is on the unidirectional cause; that is, the caregiver does something inimical or neglects to do something essential for the infant or child. In evaluating a patient for whom such a diagnosis is appropriate, however, clinicians should consider the contributions of each member of the caregiver-dyad and their interactions. Clinicians should weigh such things as infant or child temperament, deficient or defective bonding, a developmentally disabled or sensorially impaired child, and a particular caregiver–child mismatch. The likelihood of neglect increases with parental mental retardation; lack of parenting skills because of personal upbringing, social isolation, or deprivation and lack of opportunities to learn about caregiving behavior; and premature parenthood (during early and middle adolescence), in which parents are unable to respond to, and care for, an infant's needs and in which the parents' own needs take precedence over their infant's or child's needs. Frequent changes of the primary caregiver—as may occur in institutionalization, repeated lengthy hospitalizations, and multiple foster care placements—may also cause a reactive attachment disorder of infancy or early childhood.

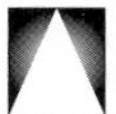

Table 48.1–1
DSM-IV-TR Diagnostic Criteria for Reactive Attachment Disorder of Infancy or Early Childhood

A. Markedly disturbed and developmentally inappropriate social relatedness in most contexts, beginning before age 5 years, as evidenced by either (1) or (2):
  (1) persistent failure to initiate or respond in a developmentally appropriate fashion to most social interactions, as manifest by excessively inhibited, hypervigilant, or highly ambivalent and contradictory responses (e.g., the child may respond to caregivers with a mixture of approach, avoidance, and resistance to comforting, or may exhibit frozen watchfulness)
  (2) diffuse attachments as manifest by indiscriminate sociability with marked inability to exhibit appropriate selective attachments (e.g., excessive familiarity with relative strangers or lack of selectivity in choice of attachment figures)

B. The disturbance in Criterion A is not accounted for solely by developmental delay (as in mental retardation) and does not meet criteria for a pervasive developmental disorder.

C. Pathogenic care as evidenced by at least one of the following:
  (1) persistent disregard of the child's basic emotional needs for comfort, stimulation, and affection
  (2) persistent disregard of the child's basic physical needs
  (3) repeated changes of primary caregiver that prevent formation of stable attachments (e.g., frequent changes in foster care)

D. There is a presumption that the care in Criterion C is responsible for the disturbed behavior in Criterion A (e.g., the disturbances in Criterion A began following the pathogenic care in Criterion C).

Specify type:
  Inhibited type: if Criterion A1 predominates in the clinical presentation
  Disinhibited type: if Criterion A2 predominates in the clinical presentation

(From American Psychiatric Association. *Diagnostic and Statistical Manual of Mental Disorders.* 4th ed. Text rev. Washington, DC: American Psychiatric Association; copyright 2000, with permission.)

DIAGNOSIS AND CLINICAL FEATURES

Children with RAD may initially be identified by a preschool teacher or by a pediatrician based on direct observation of the child's inappropriate social responses. The diagnosis of RAD is based on documenting evidence of pervasive disturbance of attachment leading to inappropriate social behaviors present before the age of 5 years. The clinical picture varies greatly, depending on a child's chronological and mental ages, but expected social interaction and liveliness are not present. Often, the child is not progressing developmentally or is frankly malnourished. Perhaps the most typical clinical picture of an infant with one form of RAD is the nonorganic failure to thrive. Such infants usually exhibit hypokinesis, dullness, listlessness, and apathy with a poverty of spontaneous activity. Infants look sad, joyless, and miserable. Some infants also appear frightened and watchful, with a radar-like gaze. Nevertheless, they may exhibit delayed responsiveness to a stimulus that would elicit fright or withdrawal from a normal infant (Table 48.1–1). Infants with failure to thrive and RAD appear significantly malnourished, and many have protruding abdomens. Occasionally, foul-smelling, celiac-like stools are reported. In unusually severe cases, a clinical picture of marasmus appears.

The infant's weight is often below the third percentile and markedly below the appropriate weight for his or her height. If serial weights are available, the weight percentiles may have decreased progressively because of an actual weight loss or a failure to gain weight as height increases. Head circumference is usually normal for the infant's age. Muscle tone may be poor. The skin may be colder and paler or more mottled than skin of a normal child. Laboratory findings are usually within normal limits, except for abnormal findings coincident with any malnutrition, dehydration, or concurrent illness. Bone age is usually retarded. Growth hormone levels are usually normal or elevated, a finding suggesting that growth failure in these children is secondary to caloric deprivation and malnutrition. The children improve physically and gain weight rapidly after they are hospitalized.

Socially, the infants usually show little spontaneous activity and a marked diminution of both initiative toward others and reciprocity in response to the caregiving adult or examiner. Both mother and infant may be indifferent to separation on hospitalization or to termination of subsequent hospital visits. The infants frequently show none of the normal upset, fretting, or protest about hospitalization. Older infants usually show little interest in their environment. They may not play with toys, even if encouraged; however, they rapidly or gradually take an interest in, and relate to, their caregivers in the hospital.

Classic psychosocial dwarfism or psychosocially determined short stature is a syndrome that usually is first manifest in children 2 to 3 years of age. The children are typically unusually short and have frequent growth hormone abnormalities and severe behavioral disturbances. All of these symptoms result from an inimical caregiver–child relationship. The affectionless character may appear when there is a failure, or lack of opportunity, to form attachments before the age of 2 to 3 years. Children cannot form lasting relationships, and their inability is sometimes accompanied by a lack of guilt, an inability to obey rules, and a need for attention and affection. Some children are indiscriminately friendly.

A 6-year-old boy was referred by his adoptive parents because of hyperactivity and disruptive behavior at school. He had been adopted at 5 years of age, after living most of his life in a Romanian orphanage in which he received care from a rotating shift of caregivers. Although he had been below the 5th percentile for height and weight on arrival, he quickly approached the 10th percentile in his new home. However, both of his adoptive parents were frustrated by their inability to "reach him." They had initially worried about a hearing disturbance, although testing and his capacity to engage many adults and children verbally suggested otherwise. He showed interest in anyone and would often follow strangers willingly. He showed little empathy when others were hurt and blandly resisted redirection in school. He was frequently injured because of seemingly reckless behavior, although he had an extremely high tolerance for pain. Intensive intervention focused on problem behaviors at home decreased his self-endangering behavior, although he remained oddly overfriendly and nonempathic at home and in school. The boy was diagnosed with reactive attachment disorder, disinhibited type. (Courtesy of Neil W. Boris, M.D. and Charles H. Zeanah, Jr., M.D.)

PATHOLOGY AND LABORATORY EXAMINATION

Although no single specific laboratory test is used to make a diagnosis, many children with RAD have disturbances of growth and development. Thus, establishing a growth curve and examining the progression of developmental milestones may be helpful in determining whether associated phenomena, such as failure to thrive, are present.

DIFFERENTIAL DIAGNOSIS

The differential diagnosis of RAD must consider other psychiatric disorders that are more likely to arise in conjunction with conditions of maltreatment, including posttraumatic stress disorders, developmental language disorders, and mental retardation syndromes. Metabolic disorders, pervasive developmental disorders, mental retardation, various neurological abnormalities, and psychosocial dwarfism are also considerations in the differential diagnosis. Children with autistic disorder are typically well nourished and of age-appropriate size and weight; they are generally alert and active, despite their impairments in reciprocal social interactions. Moderate, severe, or profound mental retardation is present in about 50 percent of children with autistic disorder, whereas when mental retardation is comorbid with RAD, it is generally in milder forms. Unlike most children with RAD, children with autistic disorder do not improve rapidly if they are removed from their homes and placed in a hospital or other favorable environment. Mentally retarded children may show delays in all social skills. Such children, unlike children with RAD, are usually adequately nourished, their social relatedness is appropriate to their mental age, and they show a sequence of development similar to that seen in normal children.

COURSE AND PROGNOSIS

Most of the data available on the natural course of children with RAD come from follow-up studies of institutionalized children with histories of serious neglect. Findings from these studies suggest that in children with the inhibited patterns of RAD who are adopted into more normative caring environments, the quality of attachment behaviors tends to become more normalized over time. Children with the indiscriminate sociability and disinhibited forms of RAD appear to persist in behavioral patterns of children for years even when they appear to be attached to new caregivers. Children with indiscriminate social behavior tend to exhibit poor peer relationships over time. The prognosis for children with reactive attachment disorders is influenced by the duration and severity of the neglectful and pathogenic parenting and on associated complications, such as failure to thrive. Constitutional and nutritional factors interact in children, who may either respond resiliently to treatment or continue to fail to thrive. Outcomes range from the extremes of death to the developmentally healthy child. In general, the longer a child remains in the adverse environment without adequate intervention, the more the physical and emotional damage and the worse the prognosis. After the pathological environmental situation has been recognized, the amount of treatment and rehabilitation that the family receives affects the child who returns to this family. Children who have multiple problems stemming from pathogenic caregiving may recover physically faster and more completely than they do emotionally.

TREATMENT

Recommendations in the management of RAD must begin with a comprehensive assessment of the current level of safety and adequate caregiving. Thus, the first consideration in treating the disorder is a child's safety. With suspicion of maltreatment currently persisting in the home, the first decision is often whether to hospitalize the child or to attempt treatment while the child remains in the home. If neglect, or emotional, physical, or sexual abuse is suspected, legally, such must be reported to the appropriate law enforcement and child protective services in the area. The child's physical and emotional state and the level of pathological caregiving determine the therapeutic strategy. A determination must be made regarding the nutritional status of the child and the presence of ongoing physical abuse or threat. Hospitalization is necessary for children with malnourishment. Along with an assessment of the child's physical well-being, an evaluation of the child's emotional condition is important. Immediate intervention must address the parents' awareness and capacity to participate in altering the injurious patterns that have ensued. The treatment team must begin to alter the unsatisfactory relationship between the caregiver and child, which usually requires extensive and intensive intervention and education with the mother or with both parents when possible.

The caregiver–child relationship is the basis of the assessment of RAD symptoms, and the substrate from which to modify attachment behaviors. Structured observations allow a clinician to determine the range of attachment behaviors established with various family members. The clinician's first task in the treatment of RAD is to advocate for providing the child with a caregiver who is emotionally available and committed to developing a positive attachment to the child. This may necessitate placement in a foster care situation when no relatives are available to fill this role. The clinician may work closely with the caregiver and the child to facilitate greater sensitivity in their

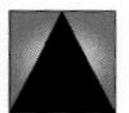

Table 48.1–2
ICD-10 Diagnostic Criteria for Disorders of Social Functioning with Onset Specific to Childhood or Adolescence

Elective mutism

Note. Thid disorder is also referred to as selective mutism.

A. Language expression and comprehension, as assessed on individually administreted standardized tests, is within the 2 standard deviations limit for the child's age.
B. There is demonstrable evidence of a consistent failure to speak in specific social situations in which the child would be expected to speak (e.g., in school), despite speaking in other situations.
C. Duration of the elective mutism exeeds 4 weeks.
D. There is no pervasive developmental disorder.
E. The disorder is not accounted for by a lack of knowledge of the spoken language required in the social situation in which there is a failure to speak.

Reactive attachment disorder of childhood

A. Onset is before the age of 5 years.
B. The child exhibits strongly contradictory or ambivalent social responses that extend across social situations (but that may show variability from relationship to relationship).
C. Emotional disturbance is shown by lack of emotional responsiveness, withdrawal reactions, aggressive responses to the child's own or other's distress, and/or fearful hypervigilance.
D. Some capacity for social reciprocity and responsiveness is evident in interactions with normal adults.
E. The criteria for pervasive developmental disorders are not met.

Disinhibited attachment disorder of childhood

A. Diffuse attachments are a persistent feature during the first 5 years of life (but do not necessarily persist into middle childhood). Diagnosis requires a relative failure to show selective social attachments manifest by:
   (1) a normal tendency to seek comfort from others when distressed and
   (2) an abnormal (relative) lack of selectivity in the people from whom comfort is sought
B. Social interactions with unfamiliar people are poorly modulated.
C. At least one of the following must be present:
   (1) generally clinging behavior in infancy
   (2) attention-seeking and indiscriminately friendly behavior in early or middle childhood
D. The general lack of situation-specificity in the above features must be clear. Diagnosis requires that the symptoms in Criteria A and B above are manifest across the range of social contacts experienced by the child.

Other childhood disorders of social functioning
Childhood disorder of social functioning, unspecified

(From World Health Organization. The *ICD-10 Classification of Mental and Behavioural Disorders: Diagnostic Criteria for Research.* Copyright, World Health Organization, Geneva; 1993, with permission.)

interactions. Three basic psychotherapeutic modalities are helpful in promoting positive bonds between children and caregiver. First, a clinician can target the caregiver to promote positive interaction with a child who does not yet have the repertoire to respond positively. Second, a clinician can work with the child and the caregiver together as a dyad to advocate for practicing appropriate positive reinforcement for each other, and through the use of videotapes, the interactions can then be viewed and modifications can be suggested to increase the positive engagement. The third modality for clinical intervention is through individual work with the child. Working with the child and caregiver together is often more effective in producing more emotionally meaningful exchanges.

Psychosocial interventions for families in which a child has RAD include (1) psychosocial support services, including hiring a homemaker, improving the physical condition of the apartment, or obtaining more adequate housing; improving the family's financial status; and decreasing the family's isolation; (2) psychotherapeutic interventions, including individual psychotherapy, psychotropic medications, and family or marital therapy; (3) educational counseling services, including mother–infant or mother–toddler groups, and counseling to increase awareness and understanding of the child's needs and to increase parenting skills; and (4) provisions for close monitoring of the progression of the patient's emotional and physical well-being. Sometimes, separating a child from the stressful home environment temporarily, as in hospitalization, allows the child to break out of the accustomed pattern. A neutral setting, such as the hospital, is the best place to start with families who are genuinely available emotionally and physically for intervention. If interventions are unfeasible or inadequate or if they fail, placement with relatives or in foster care, adoption, or a group home or residential treatment facility must be considered.

ICD-10

The 10th revision of *International Statistical Classification of Diseases and Related Health Problems* (ICD-10) includes a category for disorders of social functioning. This category includes reactive attachment disorders of childhood, disinhibited attachment disorder of childhood, elective mutism, and two residual categories (Table 48.1–2).

The ICD-10 describes the disorders of social functioning with onset specific to childhood and adolescence as a heterogeneous group that shares common abnormalities in social functioning arising during the developmental period, but that is not mainly characterized by social incapacity or deficit impairing all areas of functioning. Severe environmental "distortions or privations are commonly associated and are thought to play a crucial etiological role in many instances." Although the disorders are well known, they are not clearly defined diagnostically, and workers disagree about the appropriate classifications.

References

Boris NW, Zeanah CH. Reactive attachment disorder of infancy and early childhood. In: Sadock BJ, Sadock VA, eds. *Kaplan & Sadock's Comprehensive Textbook of Psychiatry.* 8th ed. Vol. 2. Baltimore: Lippincott Williams & Wilkins; 2005:3248.

Chaffin M, Hanson R, Saunders BE, Nichols T, Barnett D, Zeanah C, Berliner L, Egeland B, Newman E, Lyon T, LeTourneau E, Miller-Perrin C. Report of the APSAC task force on attachment therapy, reactive attachment disorder, and attachment problems. *Child Maltreat.* 2006;11:76.

Heller SS, Boris NW, Fuselier SH, Pate T, Koren-Karie N, Miron D. Reactive attachment disorder in maltreated twins follow-up: From 18 months to 8 years. *Attach Hum Dev.* 2006;8:63.

O'Connor TG, Marvin RS, Rutter M, Olrick J, Britner PA. The ERA Study Team. Child–parent attachment following early institutional deprivation. *Dev Psychopathol.* 2003;15:19–38.

O'Connor TG, Zeanah CH. Attachment disorders: Assessment strategies and treatment approaches. *Attach Hum Dev.* 2003;5:223–244.

Practice Parameter for the Assessment and Treatment of Children and Adolescents with Reactive Attachment Disorder of Infancy and Early Childhood. *J Am Acad Child Adolesc Psychiatry.* 2005;44:1206.

Task Force on Research Diagnostic Criteria: Infancy and preschool: Research diagnostic criteria for infants and preschool children. *J Am Acad Child Adolesc Psychiatry.* 2003;42:1504.
Zeanah CH, Scheeringa MS, Boris NW, Heller SS, Smyke AT, Trapani J. Reactive attachment disorder in maltreated toddlers. *Child Abuse Negl.* 2004; 28:877.
Zeanah CH, Smyke T, Dumitrescu A. Attachment disturbances in young children II: Indiscriminate behavior and institutional care. *J Am Acad Child Adolesc Psychiatry.* 2002;41:983.
Zilberstein K. Clarifying core characteristics of attachment disorders: A review of current research and theory. *Am J Orthopsychiatry.* 2006;76:55.

▲ 48.2 Stereotypic Movement Disorder and Disorder of Infancy, Childhood, or Adolescence Not Otherwise Specified

STEREOTYPIC MOVEMENT DISORDER

Stereotypic movements are repetitive voluntary, often rhythmic movements, that occur in normal children, and with increased frequency in children who have received a diagnosis of pervasive developmental disorder and mental retardation syndromes. These movements appear to be purposeless, but in some cases, such as body rocking, head rocking, or hand flapping, they may be either self-soothing or self-stimulating. In other cases, stereotypic movements, such as head banging, face slapping, eye poking, or hand biting, can cause significant self-harm. Nail-biting, thumb-sucking, and nose-picking are generally not included as symptoms of stereotypic movement disorder because they rarely cause impairment.

According to the text revision of the 4th edition of *Diagnostic and Statistical Manual of Mental Disorders* (DSM-IV-TR), stereotypic movement disorder is repetitive, nonfunctional motor behavior that seems to be compulsive. The behavior significantly interferes with normal activities or produces self-inflicted bodily injuries sufficiently severe to require medical care unless the child is protected. For children with mental retardation, the injurious behavior is sufficiently dangerous to become the focus of treatment.

Epidemiology

The incidence of transient stereotypic habits is reported to be about 7 percent in the normal pediatric populations, with a prevalence of about 15 to 20 percent in children under the age of 6 years. After age 6 years, the rates of stereotypic movements in the normal population are unknown, but believed to be negligible. The prevalence of self-injurious behaviors, however, has been estimated to be in the range of 2 to 3 percent among children and adolescents with mental retardation.

Behaviors such as nail-biting are common and affect as many as one half of all school-age children; behaviors such as thumb-sucking and rocking are normal in young children, but are often maladaptive in older children and adolescents. These behaviors usually do not constitute a stereotypic movement disorder; most children who bite their nails function in daily activities without impairment or self-injury. In one pediatric clinic, as many as 20 percent of children had a history of rocking, head-banging, or swaying in one form or another.

Deciding which cases are sufficiently severe to confirm a diagnosis of stereotypic movement disorder may be difficult. The diagnosis is a compilation of many symptoms, and various behaviors must be studied separately to obtain data about prevalence, sex ratio, and familial patterns. It is clear, however, that stereotypic movement disorder is more prevalent in boys than in girls. Stereotypic behaviors are common among children who are mentally retarded; 10 to 20 percent are affected. Self-injurious behaviors occur in some genetic syndromes, such as Lesch-Nyhan syndrome, and also in some patients with Tourette's disorder. Self-injurious stereotypic behaviors are increasingly common in persons with severe mental retardation. Stereotypic behaviors are also common in children with sensory impairments, such as blindness and deafness.

Etiology

The causes of stereotypic movement disorder can be considered from the standpoint of behavioral factors, developmental factors, and functional and neurobiological perspectives. Some stereotypic behaviors in young children can be associated with normal development; for example, up to 80 percent of all normal children show rhythmic activities that phase out by 4 years of age. These rhythmic patterns seem to be purposeful, to provide sensorimotor stimulation and tension release, and to be satisfying and pleasurable to the children. The movements may increase at times of frustration, boredom, and tension.

The progression from early expressions of stereotyped behavior in toddlers to stereotypic movement disorder in older children often reflects disordered development, as in mental retardation or a pervasive developmental disorder. Genetic factors likely play a role in some stereotypic movements, such as the X-linked recessive deficiency of enzymes leading to Lesch-Nyhan syndrome, which has predictable features including mental retardation, hyperuricemia, spasticity, and self-injurious behaviors. Other stereotypic movements (e.g., nail-biting), although often causing minimal or no impairment, seem to run in families. Some stereotypic behaviors seem to emerge or become exaggerated in situations of neglect or deprivation; such behaviors as head-banging have been associated with psychosocial deprivation.

Stereotypic movements seem to be associated with dopamine activity. Neurobiological factors may contribute to the development of stereotypic movement disorders. Dopamine agonists induce or increase stereotypic behaviors, whereas dopamine antagonists decrease them. In one report, four children with attention-deficit/hyperactivity disorder (ADHD) who were treated with a stimulant medication began to bite their nails and fingertips. The nail-biting ceased when the medication was eliminated. Endogenous opioids also have been implicated in producing self-injurious behaviors.

Diagnosis and Clinical Features

The presence of multiple repetitive stereotyped symptoms tends to occur among those most severely afflicted with mental retardation or a pervasive developmental disorder. Patients with

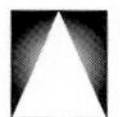

Table 48.2–1
DSM-IV-TR Diagnostic Criteria for Stereotypic Movement Disorder

A. Repetitive, seemingly driven, and nonfunctional motor behavior (e.g., hand shaking or waving, body rocking, head banging, mouthing of objects, self-biting, picking at skin or bodily orifices, hitting own body).
B. The behavior markedly interferes with normal activities or results in self-inflicted bodily injury that requires medical treatment (or would result in an injury if preventive measures were not used).
C. If mental retardation is present, the stereotypic or self-injurious behavior is of sufficient severity to become a focus of treatment.
D. The behavior is not better accounted for by a compulsion (as in obsessive-compulsive disorder), a tic (as in tic disorder), a stereotypy that is part of a pervasive developmental disorder, or hair pulling (as in trichotillomania).
E. The behavior is not due to the direct physiological effects of a substance or a general medical condition.
F. The behavior persists for 4 weeks or longer.

Specify if:
With self-injurious behavior: if the behavior results in bodily damage that requires specific treatment (or that would result in bodily damage if protective measures were not used)

(From American Psychiatric Association. *Diagnostic and Statistical Manual of Mental Disorders.* 4th ed. Text rev. Washington, DC: American Psychiatric Association; copyright 2000, with permission.)

multiple stereotyped movements frequently have other significant mental disorders, including disruptive behavior disorders. In extreme cases, severe mutilation and life-threatening injuries can result, and secondary infection and septicemia may follow self-inflicted trauma. The DSM-IV-TR diagnostic criteria for stereotypic movement disorder are listed in Table 48.2–1.

Head Banging. Head banging exemplifies a stereotypic movement disorder that can result in functional impairment. According to the DSM-IV-TR, the male-to-female ratio is 3 to 1. Typically, head-banging begins during infancy, between 6 and 12 months of age. Infants strike their heads with a definite rhythmic and monotonous continuity against the crib or another hard surface. They seem to be absorbed in the activity, which can persist until they become exhausted and fall asleep. The head-banging is often transitory, but sometimes persists into middle childhood. Head-banging that is a component of temper tantrums differs from stereotypic head-banging and ceases after the tantrums and their secondary gains have been controlled.

Nail Biting. Nail biting begins as early as 1 year of age and increases in incidence until age 12. All nails are usually bitten. Most cases are not sufficiently severe to meet the DSM-IV-TR diagnostic criteria. In other cases, children cause physical damage to the fingers themselves, usually by associated biting of the cuticles, which leads to secondary infections of the fingers and nail beds. Nail-biting seems to occur or increase in intensity when a person is either anxious or bored. Some of the most severe nail-biting occurs in those who are severely and profoundly mentally retarded and some patients with paranoid schizophrenia; however, some nail-biters have no obvious emotional disturbance.

Pathology and Laboratory Examination

No specific laboratory measures are helpful in the diagnosis of stereotypic movement disorder.

Victor, a legally blind 14-year-old boy with severe mental retardation, was evaluated when he transferred to a new residential school for children with multiple disabilities. Observed in his classroom, he was noted to be a small boy who appeared younger than his age. He held his hands in his pockets and spun around in place. Periodically, he approached his teacher, kissed her, positioned himself to receive a return kiss, and clearly enjoyed the contact with her. When offered a toy (which had to be held close to his eyes), he took it and manipulated it for awhile. When he was prompted to engage in various tasks that required that he take his hands out of his pockets, he began hitting his head with his hands. If his hands were held by the teacher, he hit his head with his knees. He was adept in contorting himself, so that he could hit or kick himself in almost any position, even while walking. Soon, his face and forehead were covered with black-and-blue marks.

Only sketchy personal history was available. He was a premature baby, with birthweight of 2 pounds. Retinopathy of prematurity and severe mental retardation were diagnosed early in life. His development was delayed in all spheres, and he never developed language. Comprehensive studies did not disclose the etiology of Victor's developmental disabilities other than prematurity. He lived at home and attended a special educational program. His self-injurious behaviors developed early in life, and, when his parents tried to stop him, he became aggressive. Gradually, he became too difficult for them to manage, and, at 3 years of age, he was placed in a special school. The self-abusive and self-restraining (i.e., holding his hands in his pockets) behavior was present throughout his stay there, and, virtually all of the time, he was on one antipsychotic medication or another. He carried a diagnosis of *cerebral dysfunction.* Although the psychiatrist's notes mentioned improvement in his self-injurious behavior, other notes described it as continuing and fluctuating. He was transferred to the new school because of lack of progress and difficulties in managing him as he became bigger and stronger. His intellectual functioning was within the 34 to 40 intelligence quotient (IQ) range. His adaptive skills were poor. He required full assistance in self-care, could not provide even for his own simple needs, and required constant supervision for his safety.

In a few months, Victor settled into the routine in his new school. His self-injurious behavior fluctuated. It was reduced or even absent when he restrained himself by holding his hands in his pockets or inside his shirt or even by manipulating some object with his hands. If left to himself, he could contort himself, while holding his hands inside his shirt, to such degree that he was nicknamed Pretzel. Because the stereotypic self-injurious and self-restraining behavior interfered with his daily activities and education, it became a primary focus of a behavior modification program. For a few months, he did well, especially when he developed a good relationship with a new teacher, who was firm, consistent, and nurturing. With him, Victor could engage in some school tasks. When the teacher left, Victor regressed. To prevent injuries, the staff started blocking his self-hitting with a pillow. He was offered activities that he liked and in which he could engage without resorting to self-injury. After several months, his antipsychotic medication was slowly discontinued, over a period of 11 months, without any behavioral deterioration. (Courtesy of Bhavik Shah, M.D.)

Differential Diagnosis

The differential diagnosis of stereotypic movement disorder includes obsessive-compulsive disorder (OCD) and tic disorders, both of which are exclusionary criteria in DSM-IV-TR. Although stereotypic movements are voluntary and not spasmodic, it is difficult to differentiate these features from tics in all cases. A recent study of stereotyped movements compared with tics found that stereotyped movements tended to be longer in duration, and displayed more rhythmic qualities than tics. Tics seemed to occur more when a child was in an "alone" condition, rather than when the child was in a play condition, whereas stereotypic movements occurred with the same frequency in these two different conditions. Stereotypic movements are likely to be self-soothing, whereas tics are often associated with distress. In OCD, the compulsions must be ego-dystonic, although this, too, is difficult to discern in young children.

Differentiating dyskinetic movements from stereotypic movements can be difficult. Because antipsychotic medications can suppress stereotypic movements, clinicians must note any stereotypic movements before initiating treatment with an antipsychotic agent. Stereotypic movement disorder may be diagnosed concurrently with substance-related disorders (e.g., amphetamine use disorders), severe sensory impairments, central nervous system and degenerative disorders (e.g., Lesch-Nyhan syndrome), and severe schizophrenia.

Course and Prognosis

The duration and course of stereotypic movement disorder vary, and the symptoms may wax and wane. As many as 80 percent of normal children show rhythmic activities that seem purposeful and comforting and tend to disappear by 4 years of age. When stereotypic movements are present or emerge more severely later in childhood or in a noncomforting manner, they range from brief episodes occurring under stress to an ongoing pattern in the context of a chronic condition, such as mental retardation or a pervasive developmental disorder. Even in chronic conditions, stereotypic behaviors may come and go. In some cases, stereotypic movements are prominent in early childhood and diminish as a child gets older.

The severity of the dysfunction caused by stereotypic movements also varies with the associated frequency, amount, and degree of self-injury. Children who exhibit frequent, severe, self-injurious stereotypic behaviors have the poorest prognosis. Repetitive episodes of head-banging, self-biting, and eye-poking can be difficult to control without physical restraints. Most nail-biting is benign and often does not meet the diagnostic criteria for stereotypic movement disorder. In severe cases in which the nail beds are repetitively damaged, bacterial and fungal infections can occur. Although chronic stereotypic movement disorders can severely impair daily functioning, several treatments help control the symptoms.

Treatment

Treatment modalities yielding the most promising effects include behavioral techniques, such as habit reversal and differential reinforcement of other behavior, as well as pharmacological interventions. A recent report on utilizing both habit reversal (in which the child is trained to replace the undesired repetitive behavior with a more acceptable behavior) and reinforcement for reducing the unwanted behavior indicated that these treatments had efficacy among 12 nonautistic children between 6 and 14 years.

Pharmacologic interventions have been used in clinical practice to minimize self-injury in children whose stereotyped movements caused significant harm to their bodies. In the past, typical antipsychotics were utilized; more recently, however, atypical antipsychotics are favored. Small open-label studies have reported benefit of atypical antipsychotics, and case reports have indicated use of serotonin reuptake inhibitor agents in the management of self-injurious stereotypies. Valproic acid has been used clinically, although no current controlled trial supports its use.

The dopamine antagonists have been the commonly used medications for treating stereotypic movements and self-injurious behavior. Phenothiazines have been the most frequently used drugs. Opiate antagonists have reduced self-injurious behaviors in some patients without exposing them to tardive dyskinesia or impaired cognition. Additional pharmacological agents that have been tried in the treatment of stereotypic movement disorder include fenfluramine (Pondimin), clomipramine (Anafranil), and fluoxetine (Prozac). In some reports, fenfluramine diminished stereotypic behaviors in children with autistic disorder; in other studies, the results were less encouraging. Open trials indicate that both clomipramine and fluoxetine may decrease self-injurious behaviors and other stereotypic movements in some patients. Trazodone (Desyrel) and buspirone (BuSpar) have also been tried, with unclear results.

DISORDER OF INFANCY, CHILDHOOD, OR ADOLESCENCE NOT OTHERWISE SPECIFIED

The DSM-IV-TR describes disorder of infancy, childhood, or adolescence not otherwise specified as a category that includes disorders with onset in infancy, childhood, or adolescence that do not meet the criteria for any specific disorder. The DSM-IV-TR diagnostic criteria are shown in Table 48.2–2. The following two case histories exemplify children who have disorder of regulation and attachment, respectively, that cause impairment but do not fit neatly into any of the other developmental disorders of infancy.

A 3-year, 2-month-old boy was brought to the infant and preschool clinic by his mother, who was concerned about his extreme and chronic irritability, fussiness, and difficulty adapting to any environmental change. He was described as a difficult infant, the product of an uncomplicated full-term pregnancy, who was slow to develop a stable eating and sleeping cycle and was difficult to soothe. His mother was finding it increasingly difficult to leave him

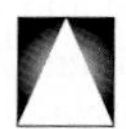

Table 48.2–2
DSM-IV-TR Diagnostic Criteria for Disorder of Infancy, Childhood, or Adolescence Not Otherwise Specified

This category is a residual category for disorders with onset in infancy, childhood, or adolescence that do not meet criteria for any specific disorder in the classification.

(From American Psychiatric Association. *Diagnostic and Statistical Manual of Mental Disorders.* 4th ed. Text rev. Washington, DC: American Psychiatric Association; copyright 2000, with permission.)

with alternate caretakers (i.e., baby-sitters) owing to the severe and extended tantrums that would result, and she was becoming anxious about his ability to transition into preschool. On further interview, it was revealed that the child was extremely rigid in a number of areas with which the family had unwittingly complied (and therefore barely recognized as symptoms on interview). The child had a small repertoire of food that he would eat that appeared to be largely limited by texture and temperature. He refused to eat anything that was too warm or too cold: All foods had to be room temperature, and his mother had taken significant care to ensure that this was the case at each meal.

Similarly, the child was extremely sensitive to tactile stimuli as well, tolerating only cotton fabrics and preferring not to wear clothing at all. He had the inclination to take off his clothes while at home, independent of the season. He routinely comforted himself by stroking a soft lambskin blanket, which he found soothing. Strikingly, he was drawn to articles of clothing with a restricted range of colors. Family vacations were nearly impossible, because the child would become extremely irritable and would have a tantrum when faced with the need to sleep in an unfamiliar bed. In particular, he was highly sensitive to the smell and texture of unfamiliar sheets and pillows. He openly expressed his discomfort with the unusual smell of the new setting of the hotel room and was unable to enjoy himself, appearing distressed and whining throughout the trip. The child's verbal skills were within normal limits for his chronological age, and no core impairment in interpersonal relatedness was present. He was interested in same-age peers and expressed a desire to play with them but insisted on doing this at his own home. After a four-session dyadic evaluation, the diagnosis of a regulatory disorder was made, and the conclusion was that his behavioral dysregulation (e.g., tantrums) was precipitated by his extreme hypersensitivity. Previous clinicians had suggested the diagnosis of pervasive developmental disorder not otherwise specified (NOS); however, his parents felt strongly that he was simply a child with an extremely difficult temperament. (Courtesy of Joan Luby, M.D.)

K. S. was a 3-year-old Romanian girl who was adopted by her parents and brought to the United States from a Romanian orphanage at 8 months of age. No details of her biological family history or perinatal development were known. However, it was clear that conditions in the orphanage were not optimal and that K. S. had spent significant amounts of time in a crib in a room without windows and with little social stimulation. Although she displayed language and motor delays (some growth retardation) at the time of adoption, she made rapid developmental gains during the first 12 months in her new home. Although she appeared to be functioning well in her preschool overall, her parents had become concerned about her lack of spontaneous eye contact, extreme sensitivity, and hypervigilance to potentially frightening noises or events (e.g., sirens and thunderstorms), and the concern that she was not engaging in peer relationships in an age-appropriate manner. Both parents reported that she understood their roles as special caregivers; however, she was unusually friendly to strangers and would become highly engaging with every unfamiliar service person who came to the home.

During two play observations with each parent, it was noted that the child had a tendency to play alone and failed to engage spontaneously either parent in play, although she was responsive to parental overtures. Although she did seem open to, and was not avoidant of, physical contact (or displays of physical affection) with each parent, she did not spontaneously seek physical proximity. She demonstrated no apparent anxiety in engaging with the unfamiliar examiner and was no more inclined to engage a parent in play or to request assistance from a parent than from the examiner. Despite her adequate functioning in the preschool setting, her lack of significant social withdrawal, and the lack of extreme disinhibition (which prevent her from meeting criteria for a DSM-IV-TR reactive attachment disorder), it was determined that she had a clinically significant (but relatively less severe) form of an attachment disorder that was classified using the NOS category, which did require formal psychotherapeutic intervention. (Courtesy of Joan Luby, M.D.)

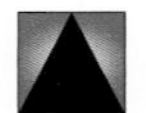

Table 48.2–3
ICD-10 Diagnostic Criteria for Stereotyped Movement Disorders

A. The child exhibits stereotyped movements to an extent that either causes physical injury or markedly interferes with normal activities.
B. Duration of the disorder is at least 1 month.
C. The child exhibits no other mental or behavioral disorder in the ICD-10 classification (other than mental retardation).

(Reprinted with permission from World Health Organization. The *ICD-10 Classification of Mental and Behavioural Disorders: Diagnostic Criteria for Research.* Copyright, World Health Organization, Geneva, 1993.)

ICD-10

The criteria for stereotyped movement disorders from the 10th revision of *International Statistical Classification of Diseases and Related Health Problems* (ICD-10) are listed in Table 48.2-3. ICD-10 also includes two residual categories for childhood mental disorders: (1) other specified behavioral and emotional disorders with onset usually occurring in childhood and adolescence and (2) unspecified behavioral and emotional disorders with onset usually occurring in childhood and adolescence.

References

Boris N, Hinshaw-Fuselier SS, Smyke AT, Scheeringa MS, Heller SS, Zeanah CH. Comparing criteria for attachment disorders: Establishing reliability and validity in high-risk samples. *J Am Acad Child Adolesc Psychiatry.* 2004;43:568.

Crosland KA, Zarcone JR, Schroeder S, Zarcone T, Fowler S. Use of an antecedent analysis and a force sensitive platform to compare stereotyped movements and motor tics. *Am J Ment Retard.* 2005;110:181.

Fernandez AE. Primary versus secondary stereotypic movements. *Rev Neurol.* 2004;38[Suppl 1]:21.

Luby JL. Disorders of infancy and early childhood not otherwise specified. In: Sadock BJ, Sadock VA, eds. *Kaplan & Sadock's Comprehensive Textbook of Psychiatry.* 8th ed. Vol. 2. Baltimore: Lippincott Williams & Wilkins; 2005: 3257.

Mahone EM, Bridges D, Prahme C, Singer HS. Repetitive arm and hand movements (complex motor stereotypies) in children. *J Pediatr.* 2004;145:391.

Melnick SM, Dow-Edwards DL. Correlating brain metabolism with sterotypic and locomotor behavior. *Behav Res Methods Instrum Comput.* 2003;35:452.

Miller JM, Singer HS, Bridges DD, Waranch HR. Behavioral therapy for treatment of stereotypic movements in nonautistic children. *J Child Neurol.* 2006;21: 119.

Presti MF, Watson CJ, Kennedy RT, Yang M, Lewis MH. Behavior-related alterations of striatal neurochemistry in a mouse model of stereotyped movement disorder. *Pharmacol Biochem Behav.* 2004;77:501.

Shah BG. Stereotypic movement disorder of infancy. In: Sadock BJ, Sadock VA, eds. *Kaplan & Sadock's Comprehensive Textbook of Psychiatry.* 8th ed. Vol. 2. Baltimore: Lippincott Williams & Wilkins; 2005:3254.

Tang JC, Patterson TG, Kennedy CH. Identifying specific sensory modalities maintaining the stereotypy of students with multiple profound disabilities. *Res Dev Disabil.* 2003;24:433.

Zeanah CH, Keyes A, Settles L. Attachment relationship experiences and childhood psychopathology. *Ann NY Acad Sci.* 2003;1008:22.

49 Mood Disorders and Suicide in Children and Adolescents

▲ 49.1 Depressive Disorders and Suicide in Children and Adolescents

Depressive disorders occur in children of all ages, but are much more prevalent with increasing age. Children and adolescents with depressive disorders often display irritability, withdrawal from family and peers, and deterioration in academic investment, leading to devastating social isolation. The core features of major depressive disorder have striking similarities in children, adolescents, and adults, although developmental factors influence its clinical presentation.

Although suicidal thoughts and behaviors can occur in the context of a depressive disorder, most youth who contemplate, attempt, or complete suicide are not in the midst of a major depression. Most children and adolescents with depressive disorders do not exhibit suicidal behaviors. Thus, it is not clear that optimal treatments for depression mitigate the risks of suicidality among youth in general.

Mood disorders among children and adolescents have been increasingly recognized over the last three decades, and evidence suggests that combined treatment modalities, including medication and cognitive-behavioral strategies, may have the greatest efficacy. Although clinicians and parents have readily acknowledged transient sadness and despair, among youth, it has become clear that the full criteria of persistent disorders of mood can occur even in prepubertal children. Two criteria for mood disorders in childhood and adolescence are a disturbance of mood, such as depression or elation, and irritability.

Although diagnostic criteria for mood disorders in the text revision of the 4th edition of *Diagnostic and Statistical Manual of Mental Disorders* (DSM-IV-TR) are almost identical across all age groups, the expression of disturbed mood varies in children according to their age. Young, depressed children commonly show symptoms that appear less often as they grow older, including mood-congruent auditory hallucinations, somatic complaints, withdrawn and sad appearance, and poor self-esteem. Symptoms that are more common among depressed youngsters in late adolescence than in young childhood are pervasive anhedonia, severe psychomotor retardation, delusions, and a sense of hopelessness. Symptoms that appear with the same frequency, regardless of age and developmental status, include suicidal ideation, depressed or irritable mood, insomnia, and diminished ability to concentrate.

Developmental issues, however, influence the expression of all symptoms. For example, unhappy young children who exhibit recurrent suicidal ideation are rarely able to propose a realistic suicide plan or to carry out such a plan. Children's moods are especially vulnerable to the influences of severe social stressors, such as chronic family discord, abuse and neglect, and academic failure. Most young children with major depressive disorder have histories of abuse or neglect. Children with depressive disorders in the midst of toxic environments may have remission of some or many depressive symptoms when the stressors diminish or when the children are removed from the stressful environment. Bereavement often becomes a focus of psychiatric treatment when children have lost a loved one, even when a depressive disorder is not present.

Depressive disorders are generally episodic, although their onset may be insidious and remain unidentified until impairment in peer relationships, deterioration in academic function, or withdrawal from sports activities emerges. Attention-deficit/hyperactivity disorder (ADHD), oppositional defiant disorder, and conduct disorder can occur among children who later experience depression. In some cases, conduct disturbances or disorders occur in the context of a major depressive episode and resolve with the resolution of the depressive episode. Clinicians must clarify the chronology of the symptoms to determine whether a given behavior (e.g., poor concentration, defiance, or temper tantrums) was present before the depressive episode and is unrelated to it or whether the behavior is occurring for the first time and is related to the depressive episode.

EPIDEMIOLOGY

Depressive disorders increase in frequency with increasing age, in the general population. Mood disorders among preschool-age children are extremely rare; the rate of major depressive disorder in preschoolers is estimated to be about 0.3 percent in the community and 0.9 percent in a clinic setting. Among prepubertal school-age children in the community, the point prevalence is approximately 1 percent. Depression, in referred samples of school-age children, is about the same in boys as in girls, with some surveys indicating a slightly increased rate among boys. Among adolescents, reported rates of major depression range from 1 percent to about 6 percent in community samples, and the rate of depression among adolescent females is double the rate in adolescent males. Estimates of cumulative prevalence of depression among older adolescents range between 14 and 25 percent. Reported rates of dysthymic disorder are generally lower than those of major depressive disorder, with rates of 5 of 100,000 in prepubertal children compared with 1 percent for major depressive disorder. School-age children with dysthymic disorder have a high likelihood of developing major depressive disorder at some point after 1 year of the dysthymic disorder. In adolescents, as in adults, dysthymic disorder is reported to occur in about 5 of 1,000 adolescents compared with about 5 percent for major depressive disorder.

Among hospitalized children and adolescents, the rates of major depressive disorder are much higher than in the general community; of these, as many as 20 percent of children and 40 percent of adolescents are depressed

ETIOLOGY

Considerable evidence indicates that the mood disorders in childhood are the same fundamental diseases experienced by adults.

Molecular Genetic Studies

Two genes have been identified as incurring vulnerability for depressive disorder. The first one, the MAOA gene, is responsible for the functioning of monoamine oxidase, and the second is the serotonin transporter gene (5-HTT). The serotonin transporter gene which is involved in the process of making serotonin available, is present in homozygous long alleles, a heterozygous one long and one short allele pair, and homozygous short alleles. A large longitudinal study in New Zealand found a relationship of early environmental stress and subsequent depression in children with one or two short alleles, but not in those children in the sample with two long alleles. Because the short alleles are less efficient in transcription, this finding suggests that the availability of the transporter gene may provide a marker for vulnerability to depression. Thus, a stress-diathesis model for the emergence of depression may best fit with the above data.

Familiality. Mood disorders in children, adolescents, and adult patients tend to cluster in the same families. An increased incidence of mood disorders is generally found among children of parents with mood disorders and relatives of children with mood disorders; having one depressed parent probably doubles the risk for offspring. Having two depressed parents probably quadruples the risk of a child having a mood disorder before age 18 compared with the risk for children with two unaffected parents. Some evidence indicates that the number of recurrences of parental depression increases the likelihood that the children will be affected, but this increase may be only partly related to the affective loading of the parent's own family tree. Similarly, children with the largest number of severe episodes have shown much evidence of dense and deep familial aggregation for major depressive disorder.

Biological Factors. Studies of prepubertal major depressive disorder and adolescent mood disorder have revealed a variety of biological abnormalities. For example, prepubertal children in an episode of depressive disorder secrete significantly more growth hormone during sleep than do normal children and those with nondepressed mental disorders. These children also secrete significantly less growth hormone in response to insulin-induced hypoglycemia than do nondepressed patients. Both abnormalities persist for at least 4 months of full, sustained clinical response, with the last month in a drug-free state. In contrast, the data conflict regarding cortisol hypersecretion during major depressive disorder; some workers report hypersecretion, and others report normal secretion.

Sleep studies are inconclusive in depressed children and adolescents. Polysomnography shows either no change or changes characteristic of adults with major depressive disorder: reduced rapid eye movement (REM) latency and an increased number of REM periods.

Magnetic Resonance Imaging. Magnetic resonance imaging (MRI) scans in more than 100 psychiatrically hospitalized children with mood disturbances report a low frontal lobe volume and a high ventricular volume. These results are consistent with MRI findings in adults with major depression insofar as postmortem studies of depressed adults have demonstrated selective loss of frontal lobe cells and frontal lobe serotonin. Damage to the frontal lobes has also been associated with depressive symptoms in patients after stroke. The frontal lobes seem to have multiple connections with the basal ganglia and the limbic system and are also believed to be involved in the neuropathology of depressive symptomatology.

Endocrine Studies. Thyroid hormone studies have found lower free total thyroxine (FT4) levels in depressed adolescents than in a matched control group. These values were associated with normal thyroid-stimulating hormone (TSH). This finding suggests that, although values of thyroid function remain in the normative range, FT4 levels have been shifted downward. These downward shifts in thyroid hormone possibly contribute to the clinical manifestations of depression. Some data suggest that the addition of exogenous thyroid hormone can potentiate the effects of antidepressant medication in adults with depression. Impairment in mood and cognitive function in adults with subclinical hypothyroidism has been found to be corrected with exogenous thyroid hormone.

Social Factors

The finding that identical twins do not have 100 percent concordance suggests a role for nongenetic factors in the emergence of major depressive disorder. Despite a lack of definitive evidence, given the stress-diathesis hypotheses of depression, genetic vulnerability in combination with a variety of social factors, including level of family conflict, abuse or neglect, conflict, family socioeconomic status, parental separation or divorce, may play a significant role in the emergence of depressive disorders in children. Evidence indicates that boys whose fathers died before they were 13 years of age are at greater risk than controls to develop depression.

The psychosocial impairment that characterizes depressed children lingers far after recovery from the index episode of depression. These deficits can be compounded by the relatively long duration of at least 1 year for a dysthymic episode and an average of 9 months to a year for a depressive episode in a child or adolescent. For an adolescent, a major depressive episode significantly interferes with social and academic skills which are poorly accomplished or unaccomplished during the episode. Among preschoolers with depressive clinical presentations, the role of environmental influences is likely to have a significant impact on the course and recovery of the young child.

DIAGNOSIS AND CLINICAL FEATURES

Major Depressive Disorder

Major depressive disorder in children is diagnosed most easily when it is acute and occurs in a child without previous psychiatric symptoms. Often, however, the onset is insidious, and the disorder occurs in a child who has had several years of difficulties with hyperactivity, separation anxiety disorder, or intermittent depressive symptoms.

According to the DSM-IV-TR diagnostic criteria for major depressive episode, at least five symptoms must be present for a period of 2 weeks, and there must be a change from previous functioning. Among the necessary symptoms is either a depressed or irritable mood or a loss of interest or pleasure. Other symptoms from which the other four diagnostic criteria are drawn include a child's failure to make expected weight gains, daily insomnia or hypersomnia, psychomotor agitation or retardation, daily fatigue or loss of energy, feelings of worthlessness or inappropriate guilt, diminished ability to think or concentrate, and recurrent thoughts of death. These symptoms must produce social or academic impairment. To meet the diagnostic criteria for major depressive disorder, the symptoms cannot be the direct effects of a substance (e.g., alcohol) or a general medical condition. A diagnosis of major depressive disorder is not made within 2 months of the loss of a loved one, except when marked functional impairment, morbid preoccupation with worthlessness, suicidal ideation, psychotic symptoms, or psychomotor retardation is present.

A major depressive episode in a prepubertal child is likely to be manifest by somatic complaints, psychomotor agitation, and mood-congruent hallucinations. Anhedonia is also frequent, but anhedonia, as well as hopelessness, psychomotor retardation, and delusions, are more common in adolescent and adult major depressive episodes than in those of young children. Adults have more problems with sleep and appetite than depressed children and adolescents. In adolescence, negativistic or frankly antisocial behavior and the use of alcohol or illicit substances can occur and may justify the additional diagnoses of oppositional defiant disorder, conduct disorder, and substance abuse or dependence. Feelings of restlessness, grouchiness, aggression, sulkiness, reluctance to cooperate in family ventures, withdrawal from social activities, and a desire to leave home are all common in adolescent depression. School difficulties are likely. Adolescents may be inattentive to personal appearance and show increased emotionality, with particular sensitivity to rejection in love relationships.

Children can be reliable reporters about their own behavior, emotions, relationships, and difficulties in psychosocial functions. They may, however, refer to their feelings by many names. Clinicians, therefore, must ask children about feeling sad, empty, low, down, blue, or very unhappy; about feeling like crying or about having a bad feeling that is present most of the time. Depressed children usually identify one or more of these terms as their persistent feeling. Clinicians should assess the duration and periodicity of the depressive mood to differentiate relatively universal, short-lived, and sometimes frequent periods of sadness, usually after a frustrating event, from a true, persistent depressive mood. The younger the child, the more imprecise his or her time estimates are likely to be.

Mood disorders tend to be chronic if they begin early. Childhood onset may be the most severe form of mood disorder and tends to appear in families with a high incidence of mood disorders and alcohol abuse. The children are likely to have such secondary complications as conduct disorder, alcohol and other substance abuse, and antisocial behavior. Functional impairment associated with a depressive disorder in childhood extends to practically all areas of a child's psychosocial world; school performance and behavior, peer relationships, and family relationships all suffer. Only highly intelligent and academically oriented children with no more than a moderate depression can compensate for their difficulties in learning by substantially increasing their time and effort. Otherwise, school performance is invariably affected by a combination of difficulty concentrating, slowed thinking, lack of interest and motivation, fatigue, sleepiness, depressive ruminations, and preoccupations. Depression in a child may be misdiagnosed as a learning disorder. Learning problems secondary to depression, even when long-standing, are corrected rapidly after a child's recovery from the depressive episode.

Children and adolescents with major depressive disorder may have hallucinations and delusions. Usually, these psychotic symptoms are thematically consistent with the depressed mood, occur with the depressive episode (usually at its worst), and do not include certain types of hallucinations (such as conversing voices and a commenting voice, which are specific to schizophrenia). Depressive hallucinations usually consist of a single voice speaking to the person from outside his or her head, with derogatory or suicidal content. Depressive delusions center on themes of guilt, physical disease, death, nihilism, deserved punishment, personal inadequacy, and (sometimes) persecution. These delusions are rare in prepuberty, probably because of cognitive immaturity, but are present in about one half of psychotically depressed adolescents.

Adolescent onset of a mood disorder can be difficult to diagnose when first seen if the adolescent has attempted self-medication with alcohol or other illicit substances. In a recent study, 17 percent of young persons with a mood disorder first received medical attention because of substance abuse. Only after detoxification could the psychiatric symptoms be assessed properly and the mood disorder diagnosed correctly.

Dysthymic Disorder

Dysthymic disorder in children and adolescents consists of a depressed or irritable mood for most of the day, for more days than not, over a period of at least 1 year. DSM-IV-TR notes that in children and adolescents, irritable mood can replace the depressed mood criterion for adults and that the duration criterion is not 2 years but 1 year for children and adolescents. According to the DSM-IV-TR diagnostic criteria, at least three of the following symptoms must accompany the depressed or irritable mood: poor self-esteem, pessimism or hopelessness, loss of interest, social withdrawal, chronic fatigue, feelings of guilt or brooding about the past, irritability or excessive anger, decreased activity or productivity, and poor concentration or memory. During the year of the disturbance, these symptoms do not resolve for more than 2 months at a time. In addition, the diagnostic criteria for dysthymic disorder specify that during the first year, no major depressive episode emerges. To meet the DSM-IV-TR diagnostic criteria for dysthymic disorder, a child must not have a history of a manic or hypomanic episode. Dysthymic disorder is also not diagnosed if the symptoms occur exclusively during a chronic psychotic disorder or if they are the direct effects of a substance or a general medical condition. DSM-IV-TR provides for specification of early onset (before 21 years of age) or late onset (after 21 years of age).

A child or adolescent with dysthymic disorder may have had a major depressive episode before developing a dysthymic disorder, but it is much more common for a child with dysthymic disorder for more than 1 year to have major depressive episode. In this case, both depressive diagnoses are given (double depression). Dysthymic disorder in children is known to have an average age of onset that is several years earlier than the age of onset of major depressive disorder. Controversy still exists among clinicians and researchers to whether dysthymic disorder is best categorized as a chronic, insidious version of major depressive disorder or represents a separate disorder. Occasionally, young persons fulfill the criteria for dysthymic disorder, except that their episodes last only 2 weeks to several months, with symptom-free intervals lasting for 2 to 3 months. These minor mood presentations in children are likely to indicate severe mood disorder episodes in the future. Current knowledge suggests that the longer, the more recurrent, the more frequent, and perhaps the less related to social stress these episodes are, the greater the likelihood of a severe mood disorder in the future. When minor depressive episodes follow a significant stressful life event by less than 3 months, it is often part of an adjustment disorder.

Cyclothymic Disorder

The only difference in the DSM-IV-TR diagnostic criteria for child or adolescent cyclothymic disorder is that a period of 1 year of numerous mood swings is necessary instead of the adult criterion of 2 years. Some adolescents with cyclothymic disorder probably experience bipolar I disorder.

Schizoaffective Disorder

The criteria for schizoaffective disorder in children and adolescents are identical to those in adults. Although some adolescents and probably some children do fit the criteria for schizoaffective disorder, little is known about the natural course of their illness, family history, psychobiology, and treatment. In DSM-IV-TR, schizoaffective disorder in children is classified as a psychotic disorder.

Bereavement

Bereavement is a state of grief related to the death of a loved one, which can occur with symptoms characteristic of a major depressive episode. Typical depressive symptoms associated with bereavement include feelings of sadness, insomnia, diminished appetite, and, in some cases, weight loss. Grieving children may become withdrawn and appear sad, and they are not easily drawn into even favorite activities.

In DSM-IV-TR, bereavement is not a mental disorder but is in the category of additional conditions that may be a focus of clinical attention. Children in the midst of a typical bereavement period may also meet the criteria for major depressive disorder when the symptoms persist longer than 2 months after the loss. In some instances, severe depressive symptoms within 2 months of the loss are considered to be beyond the scope of normal grieving, and a diagnosis of major depressive disorder is warranted. Symptoms indicating major depressive disorder exceeding usual bereavement include guilt related to issues beyond those surrounding the death of the loved one, preoccupation with death other than thoughts about being dead to be with the deceased person, morbid preoccupation with worthlessness, marked psychomotor retardation, prolonged serious functional impairment, and hallucinations other than transient perceptions of the voice of the deceased person.

The duration of a normal period of bereavement varies; in children, the duration may depend partly on the support system in place. For example, a child who must be removed from home because of the death of the only parent in the home may feel devastated and abandoned for a long time. Children who lose loved ones may feel that the death occurred because they were bad or did not perform as expected. The reaction to the loss of a loved one can be partly influenced by the child's being prepared for the death because of chronic illness.

PATHOLOGY AND LABORATORY EXAMINATION

No single laboratory test is useful in making a diagnosis of a mood disorder. A screening test for thyroid function can rule out the possibility of an endocrinological contribution to a mood disorder. Dexamethasone-suppression tests may be performed serially in cases of major depressive disorder to document whether an initial nonsuppressor becomes a suppressor with treatment or with resolution of the symptoms.

DIFFERENTIAL DIAGNOSIS

Substance-induced mood disorder can sometimes be differentiated from other mood disorders only after detoxification. Anxiety symptoms and conduct-disordered behavior can coexist with depressive disorders and frequently can pose problems in differentiating those disorders from nondepressed emotional and conduct disorders.

Of particular importance is the distinction between agitated depressive or manic episodes and ADHD, in which the persistent excessive activity and restlessness can cause confusion. Prepubertal children do not show classic forms of agitated depression, such as hand-wringing and pacing. Instead, an inability to sit still and frequent temper tantrums are the most common symptoms. Sometimes, the correct diagnosis becomes evident only after remission of the depressive episode. If a child has no difficulty concentrating, is not hyperactive when recovered from a depressive episode, and is in a drug-free state, ADHD probably is not present.

COURSE AND PROGNOSIS

The course and prognosis of mood disorders in children and adolescents depend on the age of onset, episode severity, and the presence of comorbid disorders. In most cases, the younger the age of onset, recurrent episodes, and comorbid disorders predict a poorer prognosis. The mean length of an episode of major depression in children and adolescents is about 9 months; the cumulative probability of recurrence is 40 percent by 2 years and 70 percent by 5 years. Reportedly, depressed children who live in families with high levels of chronic conflict are more likely to have relapses. Follow-up studies have found that in 20 to 40 percent of adolescents who have a major depression, bipolar I disorder will develop in a period of 5 years after the index depression. Clinical characteristics of the depressive episode that suggest the highest risk of developing bipolar I disorder include delusionality and psychomotor retardation in addition to a family history of bipolar illness. Depressive disorders are associated with short-term and long-term peer relationship difficulties and complications, poor academic achievement, and persistently poor self-esteem. Dysthymic disorder has an even more protracted recovery than major depression; the mean episode length is about 4 years. Early-onset dysthymic disorder is associated with significant risks of comorbidity with major depression (70 percent), bipolar disorder (13 percent), and eventual substance abuse (15 percent). The risk of suicide, which represents 12 percent of mortalities in the adolescent age range, is significant among adolescents with depressive disorders.

TREATMENT

Hospitalization

Safety is the most immediate consideration in evaluating a child or adolescent with major depression, and determining whether hospitalization is indicated to keep the child or adolescent safe becomes the first decision point. Children and adolescents who are depressed and express suicidal thoughts or behaviors are in need of an extended evaluation in the hospital to provide maximal protection against the patient's own self-destructive impulses and behavior. Hospitalization also may be needed when a child or adolescent has coexisting substance abuse or dependence.

Evidence-Based Treatments

A current body of published literature reflects evidence of efficacy of various treatments for childhood and adolescent depression based on randomized placebo-controlled trials (RCTs) with various pharmacologic agents, RCTs comparing cognitive-behavioral therapy (CBT) with other psychosocial interventions, and one large multicenter trial that assessed the efficacy of combined CBT and a serotonin reuptake inhibitor with each above treatment strategy alone. This recent investigation, Treatment for Adolescents with Depression Study (TADS) Team (2004) divided the 439 adolescents, between the ages of 12 and 17 years, into three treatment groups of 12 weeks, composed of either fluoxetine (Prozac) alone (10 to 40 mg per day), fluoxetine with the same dose range in combination with CBT, or CBT alone. Based on ratings of the *Children's Depression Rating Scale-Revised* (CDRS-R) and clinical global ratings, the group of depressed adolescents receiving the combination treatment had significantly superior response rates compared with either treatment alone. Based on clinical global improvement, rates of much or very much improvement were 71 percent for the group that received the combined treatment, 61 percent for the group that received fluoxetine, and 43 percent for the CBT alone. The placebo group had a 35 percent response rate. Thus, based on this large study, combination treatment appears to be the optimal strategy in the treatment of depression among youth.

Psychotherapy

Cognitive-behavioral therapy is widely recognized as an efficacious intervention for the treatment of moderately severe depression in children and adolescents. Cognitive-behavioral therapy aims to challenge maladaptive beliefs and enhance problem-solving abilities and social competence. A recent review of controlled cognitive-behavioral studies in children and adolescents revealed that, as with adults, both children and adolescents showed consistent improvement with these methods. Other "active" treatments, including relaxation techniques, were also shown to be helpful as adjunctive treatment for mild to moderate depression. Findings from one large controlled study comparing cognitive-behavioral interventions with nondirective supportive psychotherapy and systemic behavioral family therapy showed that 70 percent of adolescents had some improvement with each of the interventions; cognitive-behavioral intervention had the most rapid effect. Another controlled study comparing a brief course of CBT with relaxation therapy favored the cognitive-behavioral intervention. At a 3- to 6-month follow-up, however, no significant differences existed between the two treatment groups. This effect resulted from relapse in the cognitive-behavioral group, along with continued recovery in some patients in the relaxation group. Factors that seem to interfere with treatment responsiveness include the presence of comorbid anxiety disorder that probably was present before the depressive episode.

Family education and participation are necessary treatment components for children with depression, especially to promote more effective conflict resolution. As depressed children's psychosocial function can remain impaired for long periods, even after the depressive episode has remitted, long-term social support from families and (in some cases) social skills interventions are helpful. Modeling and role-playing techniques can be useful in fostering good problem-solving skills.

Pharmacotherapy

Pharmacologic agents from among the selective serotonin reuptake inhibitors (SSRIs) are widely accepted as first-line pharmacological intervention for moderate to severe depressive disorders in children and adolescents. Currently, acute randomized clinical trials have demonstrated efficacy of fluoxetine, citalopram (Celexa), and sertraline (Zoloft) compared with placebo in the treatment of major depression in children and adolescents. In September, 2004, the US Food and Drug Administration (FDA) received information from their Psychopharmacologic Drug and Pediatric advisory committee indicating, based on their review of reported suicidal thoughts and behavior among depressed children and adolescents who participated in randomized clinical trials with nine different antidepressants, an increased risk of suicidality in those children on active antidepressant medications. Although no suicides were reported, the rates of suicidal thinking and behaviors were 2 percent for patients on placebo, versus 4 percent among patients on antidepressant medications. The FDA, in accordance with the recommendation of their advisory committees, instituted a "black-box" warning to the health professional label of all antidepressant medication indicating the increased risk of suicidal thoughts and behaviors in children and adolescents being treated with antidepressant medications, and the need for close monitoring for these symptoms.

Fluoxetine is currently the only antidepressant that has FDA approval in the treatment of depression in children and adolescents. Three RCTs with fluoxetine demonstrate its efficacy. Common side effects observed with fluoxetine include headache, gastrointestinal symptoms, sedation, and insomnia.

Sertraline has been shown to provide efficacy in two multicenter, double-blind, placebo-controlled trials of 376 children and adolescents who were treated with sertraline at doses that ranged from 50 mg to 200 mg a day, or placebo. Response rates greater than 40 percent decrease in depression rating scale scores were found to be 69 percent in the patients treated with sertraline, compared with 56 percent in the placebo group. Most common side effects are anorexia, vomiting, diarrhea, and agitation.

Citalopram has been demonstrated in one RCT in the United States to be efficacious in 174 children and adolescents treated with citalopram at doses of 20 to 40 mg a day or placebo for 8 weeks. Significantly more of the group on citalopram showed improvement compared with placebo on the depression rating scale (CDRS-R). A significantly increased response rate (response defined as less than 28 on CDRS-R) of 35 percent was found in the citalopram group, compared with 24 percent of the placebo group. Common side effects that emerged included headache, nausea, insomnia, rhinitis, abdominal pain, dizziness fatigue, and flu-like symptoms.

Similar to the literature for adult depression, as many negative as positive study findings have emerged in RCTs of the treatment of childhood and adolescent depression. RCTs to date that have not shown efficacy on primary outcome measures include those using paroxetine (Paxil), escitalopram (Lexapro), venlafaxine (Effexor), mirtazapine (Remeron), nefazodone (Serzone), and tricyclic antidepressants.

Buproprion (Wellbutrin) has demonstrated efficacy in adult depressed populations, but has not been studied in a randomized placebo-controlled trial of depression among children and adolescents. Starting doses of SSRIs for prepubertal children are lower than doses recommended for adults, and adolescents are generally treated at the same dosages recommended for adults.

When first-line SSRI medications have not led to improvement, other antidepressant agents are used clinically, although without proved efficacy. For example, Bupropion has stimulant properties as well as antidepressant efficacy and has been used for youth with both ADHD and depression. It has few anticholinergic properties or other adverse effects such as sedation. Venlafaxine, which blocks both serotonin and norepinephrine uptake has been used clinically in the treatment of depression in adolescents. Adverse effects are usually mild, and include agitation, nervousness, and nausea. Mirtazapine is also a serotonin and norepinephrine uptake inhibitor with a relatively safe adverse-effect profile, but it has not been used as frequently because of its adverse effect of sedation.

Tricyclic antidepressants are not generally recommended for the treatment of depression in children and adolescents because of the lack of proved efficacy along with the potential risk of cardiac arrhythmia associated with their use.

One possible outcome of treating a depressed child or adolescent with an antidepressant agent is the emergence of behavioral activation, or induction of hypomanic symptoms. In these cases, the medication should be discontinued to determine whether the activation resolves with discontinuation of the medication, or evolves into a hypomanic or manic episode. Hypomanic symptom responses to antidepressants, however, do not necessarily predict that bipolar disorder has emerged.

Duration of Treatment

Based on available longitudinal data and the natural history of major depression in children and adolescents, current recommendations include maintaining antidepressant treatment for 1 year in a depressed child who has achieved a good response, and then discontinue the medication at a time of relatively low stress for a medication-free period.

Pharmacologic Treatment Strategies for Resistant Depression

Given the available data, the current pharmacologic recommendations, taking into account a consensus panel for the Texas Children's Medication Algorithm Project (TMAP) are to treat first with one of the SSRIs alone and, if no response occurs within a reasonable amount of time—perhaps, up to 3 months, —change to another SSRI medication. If a child is not responsive to the second SSRI medication, then either a combination of antidepressants or augmentation strategies may be reasonable choices as well as an antidepressant from another class of medications.

Electroconvulsive Therapy. Electroconvulsive therapy (ECT) has been used for a variety of psychiatric illnesses in adults, primarily severe depressive and manic mood disorders and catatonia. ECT rarely is used for adolescents, although published case reports indicate its efficacy in adolescents with depression and mania. Currently, case reports suggest that ECT may be a relatively safe and useful treatment for adolescents who have persistent severe affective disorders, particularly with psychotic features, catatonic symptoms, or persistent suicidality.

SUICIDE

In the United States, suicide is the third leading cause of death among adolescents, topped by accidental death and homicide. In all countries, suicide rarely occurs in children who have not reached puberty. In the last 15 years, the rates of both completed suicide and suicidal ideation rates have decreased among adolescents. This decrease appears to coincide with the increase in

SSRI medications prescribed to adolescents with mood and behavioral disturbance. Suicidal ideation, gestures, and attempts are frequently, but not always, associated with depressive disorders. Reports indicate that as many as half of suicidal individuals express suicidal intentions to a friend or a relative within 24 hours before enacting suicidal behavior.

Suicidal ideation occurs in all age groups and with greatest frequency in children and adolescents with severe mood disorders. More than 12,000 children and adolescents are hospitalized in the United States each year because of suicidal threats or behavior, but completed suicide is rare in children younger than 12 years of age. A young child is hardly capable of designing and carrying out a realistic suicide plan. Cognitive immaturity seems to play a protective role in preventing even children who wish they were dead from committing suicide. Completed suicide occurs about five times more often in adolescent boys than in girls, although the rate of suicide attempts is at least three times higher among adolescent girls than among boys. Suicidal ideation is not a static phenomenon; it can wax and wane with time. The decision to engage in suicidal behavior may be made impulsively without much forethought or the decision may be the culmination of prolonged rumination.

The method of the suicide attempt influences the morbidity and completion rates, independent of the severity of the intent to die at the time of the suicidal behavior. The most common method of completed suicide in children and adolescents is the use of firearms, which accounts for about two thirds of all suicides in boys and almost one half of suicides in girls. The second most common method of suicide in boys, occurring in about one fourth of all cases, is hanging; in girls, about one fourth commit suicide through ingestion of toxic substances. Carbon monoxide poisoning is the next most common method of suicide in boys, but it occurs in less than 10 percent; suicide by hanging and carbon monoxide poisoning are equally frequent among girls and account for about 10 percent each. Additional risk factors in suicide include a family history of suicidal behavior, exposure to family violence, impulsivity, substance abuse, and availability of lethal methods.

Epidemiology

Suicide rates in 2000 among boys and girls 10 to 14 years of age were 2.3 and 0.6 per 100,000, whereas among late adolescent boys and girls the rates increased to 13.2 and 2.8 per 100,000. Large surveys indicate that, although up to 20 percent of high school students in the United States have experienced suicidal ideation, and 10 percent have exhibited suicidal behaviors, only about 2 percent of adolescents who attempt suicide come to medical attention. In the last 15 years, the rates of both completed suicide and suicidal ideation rates have decreased.

The rates for suicide depend on age, and they increase significantly after puberty. Whereas less than 1 per 100,000 completed suicide occurs in persons younger than 14 years of age, about 10 per 100,000 completed suicides occur in adolescents between 15 and 19 years of age. In adolescents younger than 14 years of age, suicide attempts are at least 50 times more common than suicide completions. Between 15 and 19 years of age, however, the rate of suicide attempts is about 15 times greater than the rate of suicide completions. The number of adolescent suicides over the past several decades has tripled or quadrupled.

Etiology

Universal features in adolescents who resort to suicidal behaviors are the inability to synthesize viable solutions to ongoing problems and the lack of coping strategies to deal with immediate crises. Therefore, a narrow view of the options available to deal with recurrent family discord, rejection, or failure contributes to a decision to commit suicide.

Genetic Factors. Completed suicide and suicidal behavior is two to four times more likely to occur in individuals with a first-degree family member with similar behavior. Evidence of a genetic contribution to suicidal behavior is based on family suicide risk studies and the higher concordance for suicide among monozygotic twins than dizygotic twins.

Biological Factors. Recent studies have documented a reduction in the density of serotonin transporter receptors in the prefrontal cortex, and serotonin receptors among individuals with suicidal behaviors. Neurochemical findings show some overlap between persons with aggressive, impulsive behaviors and those who complete suicide. Low levels of serotonin and its major metabolite, 5-hydroxyindoleacetic acid (5-HIAA), have been found postmortem in the brains of persons who completed suicide. Low levels of 5-HIAA have been found in the cerebrospinal fluid of depressed persons who attempted suicide by violent methods. Alcohol and other psychoactive substances may lower 5-HIAA levels, perhaps by increasing the vulnerability for suicidal behavior in an already predisposed person. Low serotonin may turn out to be a marker, rather than a cause, of aggression and suicidal propensity, influencing behavioral responses to stress.

Psychosocial Factors. Although major depressive illness is the most significant risk factor for suicide, increasing its risk by 20 percent, many severely depressed individuals are not suicidal. Various features, including a sense of hopelessness, impulsivity, recurrent substance use, and a history of aggressive behavior, have been associated with an increase risk of suicide. A wide range of psychopathological symptoms can result from exposure to violent and abusive homes. Aggressive, self-destructive, and suicidal behaviors seem to occur with greatest frequency among youth who have endured chronically stressful family lives. Large community studies have provided data suggesting that sexual orientation is a risk factor, with increased rates of suicidal behavior of two to six times among youth who identify themselves as gay, lesbian, or bisexual. The mechanisms of this correlation are unknown; however this population of adolescents has higher rates of depressive disorders as well as substance use disorders, which may contribute to this relationship.

Diagnosis and Clinical Features

The characteristics of adolescents who attempt suicide and those who complete suicides are similar and as many as 40 percent of suicidal persons have made a previous attempt. Direct questioning of children and adolescents about suicidal thoughts is necessary, because studies have consistently shown that parents are frequently unaware of such ideas in their children. Suicidal thoughts (i.e., children talking about wanting to harm themselves) and suicidal threats (e.g., children stating that they want to jump in front of a car) are more common than suicide completion.

Most suicidal youth meet diagnostic criteria for one or more psychiatric disorders, which often include major depressive disorder, manic episodes, and psychotic disorders. Those with mood disorders in combination with substance abuse and a history of aggressive behavior are particularly at high risk. Those without mood disorders who are violent, aggressive, and impulsive may be susceptible to suicide during family or peer conflicts. High levels of hopelessness, poor problem-solving skills, and a history of aggressive behavior are risk factors for suicide. Depression alone is a more serious risk factor for suicide in girls than in boys, but boys often have more severe psychopathology than girls who commit suicide. The profile of an adolescent who commits suicide is occasionally one of high achievement and perfectionistic character traits; such an adolescent may have been humiliated recently by a perceived failure, such as diminished academic performance.

In psychiatrically disturbed and vulnerable adolescents, suicide attempts typically are related to recent stressors. The precipitants of suicidal behavior include conflicts and arguments with family members and boyfriends or girlfriends. Alcohol and other substance use can further predispose an already vulnerable adolescent to suicidal behavior. In other cases, an adolescent attempts suicide in anticipation of punishment after being caught by the police or other authority figures for a forbidden behavior.

About 40 percent of youthful persons who complete suicide had previous psychiatric treatment, and about 40 percent had made a previous suicide attempt. A child who has lost a parent by any means before age 13 is at high risk for mood disorders and suicide. The precipitating factors include loss of face with peers, a broken romance, school difficulties, unemployment, bereavement, separation, and rejection. Clusters of suicides among adolescents who know one another and go to the same school have been reported. Suicidal behavior can precipitate other such attempts within a peer group through identification—so-called copycat suicides. Some studies have found an increase in adolescent suicide after television programs in which the main theme was the suicide of a teenager. In general, however, many other factors are involved, including a necessary substrate of psychopathology.

One recent study investigated two clusters of teenage suicide in Texas. The researchers found that indirect exposure to suicide through the media was not significantly associated with suicide. Factors that were associated included previous suicidal threats or attempts, self-injury, exposure to someone who had died violently, recent romantic breakups, and a high frequency of moves and changes in schools attended and parental figures lived with.

The tendency of disturbed young persons to imitate highly publicized suicides has been called the *Werther syndrome*, after the protagonist in Johann Wolfgang von Goethe's novel, *The Sorrows of Young Werther*. The novel, in which the hero kills himself, was banned in some European countries after its publication more than 200 years ago because of a rash of suicides by young men who read it; some dressed like Werther before killing themselves or left the book open at the passage describing his death. In general, although imitation may play a role in the timing of suicide attempts by vulnerable adolescents, the overall suicide rate does not seem to increase when media exposure increases.

Treatment

The prognostic significance of suicidal behavior among adolescents ranges from relatively benign to heralding a grave risk of completed suicide. Adolescents who come to medical attention because of suicidal attempts must be evaluated before determining whether hospitalization is necessary. Those who fall into high-risk groups should be hospitalized until the acute suicidality is no longer present. Persons at high risk include those who have made previous suicide attempts; boys older than 12 years of age with histories of aggressive behavior or substance abuse; those who have made an attempt with a lethal method, such as a gun or a toxic ingested substance; those with major depressive disorder characterized by social withdrawal, hopelessness, and a lack of energy; girls who have run away from home, are pregnant, or have made an attempt with a method other than ingesting a toxic substance; and any person who exhibits persistent suicidal ideation. A child or an adolescent with suicidal ideation must be hospitalized if a clinician has any doubt about the family's ability to supervise the child or to cooperate with treatment in an outpatient setting. In such a situation, child protective services must be involved before the child can be discharged. When adolescents with suicidal ideation report that they are no longer suicidal, discharge can be considered only after a complete discharge plan is in place.

Relatively few adolescents evaluated for suicidal behavior in a hospital emergency room subsequently engage in ongoing psychiatric treatment. Factors that may increase the probability of psychiatric interventions include initiating psychoeducation for the family in the emergency room, diffusing acute family conflict, and setting up an outpatient follow-up during the emergency room visit. Frequent emergency room discharge plans include a written contract with the adolescent, outlining the adolescent's agreement not to engage in suicidal behavior and providing an alternative if suicidal ideation reoccurs, and a telephone hot-line number provided to the adolescent and the family in case suicidal ideation reappears.

Scant data exist to evaluate the efficacy of psychotherapy in reducing suicidal behavior among adolescents. Cognitive-behavioral therapy has been shown to be effective in the treatment of depression among adolescents; however, no evidence is available to assess its efficacy in preventing suicidal behavior per se. Dialectical behavior therapy (DBT) a long-term behavioral intervention that can be applied to individuals or groups of patients, has been shown to reduce suicidal behavior in adults, and has yet to be investigated in adolescents. Components of DBT include mindfulness training to improve self-acceptance, assertiveness training, instruction on avoiding situations that may trigger self-destructive behavior, and increasing the ability to tolerate psychological distress. This approach warrants investigation among adolescents.

Pharmacologic efficacy in the treatment of suicidal behavior has been shown in adults with depression and cluster B personality with SSRI antidepressants, and in suicidal adults with bipolar disorder using lithium.

In children and adolescents with major depression, fluoxetine, citalopram and sertraline have all been shown to have efficacy through randomized clinical trials; however, pharmacologic interventions targeting suicidal behavior has not been investigated in this population. Given the reduction in completed suicide among adolescents over the last decade during the same period in which SSRI antidepressants treatment in this population has markedly risen, it is possible that SSRI antidepressants have been instrumental in this effect. Given the data concluding an increased rate of suicidality among depressed children and adolescents in randomized clinical trials on antidepressant medications (leading to the "black-box" warning for all antidepressants use in children), as well as anecdotal reports suggesting potential induction of suicidality shortly after introducing antidepressant treatment in depressed children, close monitoring for suicidality is mandatory for any child or adolescent being treated with antidepressants.

References

Emslie GJ, Hughes CW, Crimson ML, Lopez M, Pliszka S, Toprac MG, Boemer C. A feasibility study of the childhood depression medication algorithm: The Texas Children's Medication Algorithm Project (CMAP). *J Am Acad Child Adolesc Psychiatry*. 2004;43:519.

Gould MS, Greenberg T, Velting DM, Shaffer D. Youth suicide risk and preventive interventions: A review of the past ten years. *J Am Acad Child Adolesc Psychiatry*. 2003;42:386.

Hall WD. How have the SSRI antidepressants affected suicide risk? *Lancet*. 2006; 367(9527):1959.

Heiligenstein JH, Hoog SL, Wagner KD, Findling RL, Galil N, Kaplan S, Busner J, Nilsson ME, Brown EB, Jacobson JG. Fluoxetine 40–60 mg versus fluoxetine 20 mg in the treatment of children and adolescents with a less-than-complete response to nine-week treatment with fluoxetine 10–20 mg: A pilot study. *J Child Adolesc Psychopharmacology*. 2006;1/2:207.

Olfson M, Shaffer D, Marcus SC, Greenberg T. Relationship between antidepressant medication treatment and suicide in adolescents. *Arch Gen Psychiatry*. 2003; 60:978.

Rosso IM, Cintron CM, Steingard RJ, Renshaw PF, Young AD, Yurgelun-Todd DA. Amygdala and hippocampus volumes in pediatric major depression. *Biol Psychiatry*. 2005;57(1):21.

Shaffer D. Depressive disorders and suicide in children and adolescents. In: Sadock BJ, Sadock VA, eds. *Kaplan & Sadock's Comprehensive Textbook of Psychiatry*. 8th ed. Vol. 2. Baltimore: Lippincott Williams & Wilkins; 2005: 3262.

Von Knorring AL, Olsson GI, Thomson PH, Lemming OM, Hulten A. A randomized, double-blind, placebo-controlled study of citalopram in adolescents with major depressive disorder. *J Clin Psychopharmacology*. 2006;26:311.

Wagner KD. Pharmacotherapy for major depression in children and adolescents. *Prog Neuropsychopharmacol Biol Psychiatry*. 2005;29:819.

Whittington CJ, Kendall T, Fonagy P, Cotrell D, Cotgrove A, Boddington E. Selective serotonin reuptake inhibitors in childhood depression: Systematic review of published versus unpublished data. *Lancet*. 2004;363:1341.

▲ 49.2 Early-Onset Bipolar Disorders

Bipolar I disorder is being diagnosed with increasing frequency in prepubertal children, with the caveat that "classic" manic episodes are uncommon in this age group, even when depressive symptoms have already appeared. Because few prepubertal children with features of depression and mania or hypomania exhibit discrete mood "cycles," that these children satisfy diagnostic criteria for bipolar disorder remains controversial. These "atypical" manic episodes among prepubertal children are sometimes associated with family histories of classic bipolar I disorder. Features of the mood and behavior disturbances among prepubertal children who are currently diagnosed with bipolar disorder by some clinicians include extreme mood variability, intermittent aggressive behavior, high levels of distractibility, and poor attention span. This constellation of mood and behavior disturbance is often not clearly episodic, but fluctuating and appears to be less responsive to mood-stabilizing agents than classic episodes of depression or mania in older adolescents and adults. Children with atypical hypomanic episodes often have past histories of severe attention-deficit/hyperactivity disorder (ADHD), making the diagnosis of bipolar disorder even more complicated. In general, families with many relatives with ADHD do not have family histories with an increased rate of bipolar I disorder. Children with atypical bipolar disorder function poorly, often require hospitalization, exhibit symptoms of depression, and often have a history of ADHD. How many of these children will develop discrete mood cycling as they mature or whether their clinical pictures will remain consistent over time remains under investigation.

Among adults and older adolescents, a major depressive episode typically precedes a manic episode in the natural evolution of bipolar I disorder. A classic manic episode in an adolescent emerges as a distinct departure from a preexisting state often characterized by grandiose and paranoid delusions and hallucinatory phenomena. According to the text revision of the 4th edition of *Diagnostic and Statistical Manual of Mental Disorders* (DSM-IV-TR), the diagnostic criteria for a manic episode are the same for children and adolescents as for adults (*see* Table 15.1–6). The diagnostic criteria for a manic episode include a distinct period of an abnormally elevated, expansive, or irritable mood that lasts at least 1 week or for any duration if hospitalization is necessary. In addition, during periods of mood disturbance, at least three of the following significant and persistent symptoms must be present: inflated self-esteem or grandiosity, decreased need for sleep, pressure to talk, flight of ideas or racing thoughts, distractibility, an increase in goal-directed activity, and excessive involvement in pleasurable activities that may result in painful consequences. The mood disturbance suffices to cause marked impairment, and it is not caused by the direct effect of a substance or a general medical condition. Thus, manic states precipitated by somatic medications (e.g., antidepressants) cannot be interpreted as indicating a diagnosis of bipolar I disorder.

When mania appears in an adolescent, there is a higher incidence of psychotic features than occurs in adults, and hospitalization is often necessary. Delusions and hallucinations of adolescents may involve grandiose notions about their power, worth, knowledge, family, or relationships. Persecutory delusions and flight of ideas are common. Overall, gross impairment of reality testing is common in adolescent manic episodes. In adolescents with major depressive disorder destined for bipolar I disorder, those at highest risk have family histories of bipolar I disorder and exhibit acute, severe depressive episodes with psychosis, hypersomnia, and psychomotor retardation.

EPIDEMIOLOGY

The prevalence of early-onset bipolar disorder is rare based on the diagnostic criteria within the DSM-IV-TR. Epidemiologic studies in older adolescents have reported lifetime prevalence of bipolar I and II disorders to be approximately 1 percent. A recent epidemiologic survey of current illness in children under 13 years of age found no cases of classic bipolar illness.

The most valid diagnosis for prepubertal children with mood lability, extreme irritability, or rapid mood cycling remains controversial. Among adults with bipolar disorder, the 20 to 30 percent who exhibit "mixed mania," are most likely to have a chronic course, absence of discrete episodes, higher risk of suicidal behavior, onset of the disorder in childhood and adolescence, neuropsychological features similar to children with ADHD, and show a poorer response to treatment. These phenomenological features appear to be similar to the clinical presentation of the prepubertal children who are more frequently being described as having atypical bipolar disorders. Longitudinal studies are warranted to determine if children with early-onset atypical bipolar disorders become adults with bipolar disorders with mixed mania.

ETIOLOGY

Genetic Factors

Family studies consistently demonstrate that offspring of a parent with bipolar I disorder have a 25 percent chance of having a mood disorder, and offspring of two parents with bipolar disorder have a 50 to 75 percent risk of developing a mood disorder. The high rates of comorbid ADHD among children with early-onset bipolar disorder has led to questions regarding the co-transmission of these disorders in family members. Offspring of parents with bipolar disorder have been found to have higher rates of ADHD compared with controls. In first-degree relatives of children with bipolar disorder, ADHD occurs with the same rate as in first-degree relatives of children with ADHD only. The combination of ADHD and bipolar disorder was not found as frequently in relatives of children with ADHD only, however, compared with first-degree relatives of children with the combination. These results suggest that childhood bipolar disorder may be distinguished as a subtype of bipolar disorder that emerges in children whose family histories are heavily loaded for bipolar disorder and psychiatric comorbidities, such as ADHD.

Neurobiological Factors

The neurobiology of early-onset bipolar disorder is in its infancy, although an area of current investigation. Although brain volume reaches about 90 percent of its adult size by age 6 years, according to work done by J. N. Giedd, increasing white matter over the next 20 years has been shown using magnetic resonance imaging (MRI). The few studies with children with bipolar disorder suggest a dysfunction in neural circuitry in the amygdala, striatal, thalamic, and prefrontal structures of the brain.

Neuropsychological Studies

A growing body of evidence suggests that children and adolescents with bipolar disorder make a greater number of emotion recognition errors compared with controls. Their over reporting of faces as "angry" occurred when they were presented with adult faces, whereas these errors did not occur when they were shown children's faces. Impaired perception of facial expression has also been reported in studies of adults with bipolar disorder. Preliminary data suggest that, on tasks of working memory, processing speed, and attention, children and adolescents with comorbid bipolar disorder and ADHD demonstrated more pronounced impairments compared with those without ADHD. Very preliminary findings suggest similarities between neuropsychological profiles of child, adolescent, and adult bipolar disorder.

DIAGNOSIS AND CLINICAL FEATURES

Early-onset bipolar disorder is characterized by extreme irritability that is severe and persistent and may include aggressive outbursts and violent behavior. In between outbursts, children with this syndrome may continue to be angry or dysphoric. Occasionally, a child with early-onset bipolar disorder may exhibit grandiose thoughts or euphoric mood; for the most part, children with this disorder are predominantly intensely emotional with a fluctuating but overriding negative mood. Current diagnostic criteria for bipolar disorders in children and adolescents in DSM-IV-TR are the same as those used in adults. The clinical picture of early-onset bipolar disorder, however, is complicated by the prevalent comorbid psychiatric disorders.

Comorbidity with ADHD

One of the main sources of diagnostic confusion regarding children with early-onset bipolar disorder is the comorbid ADHD, which is present in 60 to 90 percent of them. One of the reasons for the vast concurrence of these two disorders is that they share many diagnostic criteria, including distractibility, hyperactivity, and talkativeness. Even when the overlapping symptoms are removed from the diagnostic count, 89 percent of children with bipolar disorder continued to meet the full criteria for ADHD. This implies that both disorders with their own distinct features are present in many cases.

Comorbidity with Conduct Disorder

Rates of comorbid conduct disorder have been found to range from 48 to 69 percent among children and adolescents with bipolar disorder. J. Biederman found that the two manic symptoms more common in the comorbid group than the bipolar only group were *physical restlessness* and *poor judgment*.

Comorbidity with Anxiety Disorders

Children and adolescents with bipolar disorder have been reported to have higher than expected rates of panic and other anxiety disorders. Lifetime prevalence of panic disorder was found to be 21 percent among subjects with bipolar disorder compared with 0.8 percent in those without mood disorders. Patients with bipolar disorder with high levels of anxiety symptoms were reported to abuse alcohol and exhibit suicidal behavior.

PATHOLOGY AND LABORATORY EXAMINATION

No specific laboratory indices are currently helpful in making the diagnosis of bipolar disorders among children and adolescents.

DIFFERENTIAL DIAGNOSIS

A consensus of research studies in children diagnosed with early-onset bipolar disorder suggests that between 80 and 90 percent also meet diagnostic criteria for ADHD. Among youth with adolescent-onset of mania, rates of ADHD have been found to be 60 percent, a rate that is still markedly increased compared with controls. Although childhood ADHD tends to have its onset earlier than pediatric mania, current evidence from family studies supports the presence of ADHD and bipolar disorders as highly comorbid in children, and the concurrence is not because of the overlapping symptoms that the two disorders share. In a recent study by S. Faraone and colleagues of more than 300 children and adolescents who attended a psychopharmacology clinic and received a diagnosis of ADHD, bipolar disorder was also evident in almost one third of those children with ADHD who had combined–type and hyperactive-types, and occurred with much less frequency (i.e., in less than 10 percent) in children with ADHD, inattentive-type.

COURSE AND PROGNOSIS

Presently, it is not known if early-onset bipolar disorders have the same natural history over time as bipolar disorders with an onset during adolescence or early adulthood. Current investigations of the course of early-onset bipolar disorder have focused on rates of recovery, recurrence, changes in symptoms over time, and predictors of outcome. A recent longitudinal study of 263 child and adolescent inpatients and outpatients with bipolar disorders followed for an average of 2 years found that approximately 70 percent recovered from their index episode within that period. Half of these patients had at least one recurrence of a mood disorder during this time, more frequently a depressive episode than a mania. No differences were found in the rates of recovery for children and adolescents whose diagnosis was bipolar I disorder, bipolar II disorder, or bipolar disorder not otherwise specified; however, those youth whose diagnosis was bipolar disorder not otherwise specified had a significant longer duration of illness before recovery, with less frequent recurrences once they recovered. About 19 percent of patients changed polarity once per year or less, 61 percent shifted 5 or more times per year, about half cycled more than 10 times per year, and about one third cycled more than 20 times per year. Predictors of more rapid cycling included lower socioeconomic status (SES), presence of lifetime psychosis, and bipolar disorder not otherwise specified diagnosis. Over the follow-up period, about 20 percent of subjects who were diagnosed with bipolar II disorder converted to bipolar I disorder, and 25 percent of the bipolar disorder not otherwise specified subjects developed bipolar I disorder or bipolar II disorder during the follow-up period. Similar to the literature depicting the natural history of bipolar disorders in adults, the youth followed in this study had a wide range of symptom severity in manic and depressed episodes. The more frequent diagnostic conversion from bipolar II disorder to bipolar I disorder among the youth in this study and other investigations of bipolar disorders among children and adolescents, compared with the adult literature highlights the lack of stability of the bipolar II disorder diagnosis in youth. This is also the case in this study with respect to conversion from bipolar disorder not otherwise specified to other bipolar disorders.

All of the existing longitudinal literature on bipolar disorders in early childhood has found that when the illness emerges in young children, recovery rates are lower. Also, a greater likelihood is seen of mixed states and rapid cycling, and higher rates of polarity changes compared with those who develop bipolar disorders in late adolescence or early adulthood. Further investigations are needed to understand the mechanisms by which low SES, psychosis, and less well-defined mood episodes predict more changes in polarity and a poorer prognosis.

TREATMENT

Few randomized, placebo controlled treatment trials have been conducted with youth diagnosed with early-onset bipolar disorder. Therefore, current clinical strategies for youth diagnosed with bipolar disorders continue to include downward extensions of the literature from older adolescent and adult treatment studies of bipolar disorders.

Mood stabilizing agents, particularly lithium has been demonstrated to be an effective treatment for adults with bipolar disorder for acute mania, and bipolar depressive states, and has been shown to offer prophylactive properties in bipolar disorders. In childhood, controlled trials have provided evidence suggesting that lithium is efficacious in the management of aggression behavior disorders.

Open trials and retrospective chart reviews of children with early-onset bipolar disorder suggest that valproate (Depacon) is efficacious in the treatment of mania in childhood.

A recent randomized clinical trial comparing divalproex (Depakote) and quetiapine, (Seroquel) an atypical antipsychotic in the treatment of 50 adolescent patients with mania suggested that quetiapine is at least as effective as divalproex in the treatment of acute manic symptoms and quetiapine may work more quickly. Placebo-controlled trials will be necessary to determine if quetiapine is an effective monotherapy for child and adolescent mania.

An open-label trial of lamotrigine (Lamictal) in the treatment of bipolar depression among youth provides preliminary support for its use in children and adolescents. Given the 8-week trial with 20 adolescents, whose mean final dose of lamotrigine was approximately 130 mg a day, no significant weight changes, rash, or other adverse events were seen during the trial.

Open trials using atypical antipsychotics including risperidone (Risperdal) and others using risperidone in combination with either lithium or valproate suggest that these combinations may be efficacious in controlling symptoms of mania.

An open trial of olanzapine monotherapy in the treatment of childhood bipolar disorder found improvements in measures of both mania and depression after 8 weeks of treatment at doses ranging from 2.5 mg to 20 mg per day.

Psychosocial treatment intervention studies for bipolar disorder among youth include a pilot study by D. J. Miklowitz using an adjunctive family-focused psychoeducational treatment (FFT-A) modified for children and adolescents which had been shown to reduce relapse rate when used in adult bipolar patients. Results of this pilot investigation in children and adolescents treated with mood-stabilizing agents in addition to the psychosocial intervention included improvement in depressive symptoms, manic symptoms, and behavioral disturbance over 1 year.

In addition to managing manic and depressive symptoms in early-onset bipolar disorder, most children with bipolar disorder are likely to need treatment for comorbid ADHD. Chart reviews indicate that treatment of ADHD is significantly more successfully achieved after mood stabilization is accomplished.

More investigation is needed to determine the most efficacious treatments for early-onset bipolar disorder and its frequent comorbidities.

References

Biederman J. Early-onset bipolar disorders In: Sadock BJ, Sadock VA, eds. *Kaplan & Sadock's Comprehensive Textbook of Psychiatry*. 8th ed. Vol. 2. Baltimore: Lippincott Williams & Wilkins; 2005:3274.

Birmaher B, Axelson D, Strober M, Gill MK, Valeri S, Chiapetta L, Ryan N, Leonard H, Hunt J, Iyengar S, Keller M. Clinical course of children and adolescents with bipolar spectrum disorders. *Arch Gen Psychiatry*. 2006;63:175.

DelBello MP, Kowatch RA, Adler CM, Stanford KE, Welge JA, Barzman DH, Nelson E, Strakowski SM. A double-blind randomized pilot study comparing quetiapine and divalproex for adolescent mania. *J Am Acad Child Adolesc Psychiatry*. 2006;45:305.

DelBello MP, Adler CM, Strakowski SM. The neurophysiology of childhood and adolescent bipolar disorder. *Central Nervous System Spectr*. 2006;11:298.

Chang K, Saxene K, Howe M. An open-label study of lamotrigine adjunct or monotherapy for the treatment of adolescents with bipolar depression. *J Am Acad Child Adolesc Psychiatry*. 2006;45:298.

Giedd JN. Structural magnetic resonance imaging of the adolescent brain. *Ann N Y Acad Sci*. 2004;1021:77.

Kowatch RA, Fristad MA, Birmaher B, Wagner KD, Findling RL, Hallards M, Bipolar Disorder Work Group. Treatment guidelines for children and adolescents with bipolar disorders. *J Am Acad Child Adolesc Psychiatry*. 2005;44: 213.

Kyet ZA, Carlson GA, Goodyer IM. Clinical and neuropsychological characteristics of child and adolescent bipolar disorder. *Psychol Med*. 2006;1.

Masi G, Perugi G, Toni C, Millipiedi S, Mucci M, Bertini N, Akiskal H. The clinical phenotypes of juvenile bipolar disorder: Toward a validation of the episodic-chronic distinction. *Biol Psychiatry*. 2006;59:603.

Miklowitz DJ, George EL, Axelson DS, Kim EY, Birmaher B, Schneck C, Beresford C, Craighead WE, Brent DA. Family-focused treatment for adolescents with bipolar disorder. *J Affect Disord*. 2004;82(S1):S113–S128.

Pavuluri MN, Henry DB, Carbray JA, Sampson GA, Naylor MW, Janicak PG. Open label prospective trial of risperidone in combination with lithium or divalproex sodium in pediatric mania. *J Affective Dis*. 2004;82(S1):S103–S111.

Pavulari MN, Schenkel LS, Aryal S, Harral E, Hill S, Herbener ES, Sweeney JA. Neurocognitive function in undedicated and medicated euthymic pediatric bipolar patients. *Am J Psychiatry*. 2006;163:286.

50 Anxiety Disorders of Infancy, Childhood, and Adolescence

▲ 50.1 Obsessive-Compulsive Disorder of Infancy, Childhood, and Adolescence

Obsessive-compulsive disorder (OCD) is characterized by the presence of recurrent intrusive thoughts associated with anxiety or tension and/or repetitive purposeful mental or physical actions aimed at reducing fears and tensions caused by obsessions. It has become increasingly evident that the majority of cases of OCD begin in childhood or adolescence. The clinical presentation of OCD in childhood and adolescence is similar to that in adults and the only alteration in diagnostic criteria in the text revision of the fourth edition of *Diagnostic and Statistical Manual of Mental Disorders* (DSM-IV-TR) for children is that they do not necessarily demonstrate awareness that their thoughts or behaviors are unreasonable. Pediatric OCD has been investigated with respect to treatment with placebo-controlled trials of pharmacologic agents and cognitive-behavioral therapy (CBT) and to date, it is the only childhood anxiety disorder with data showing optimal treatment to include a combination of serotoninergic agents and CBT treatment.

EPIDEMIOLOGY

Obsessive-compulsive disorder is common among children and adolescence with a point prevalence of about 0.5 percent and a lifetime rate of 1 percent to 3 percent. The rate of OCD rises exponentially with increasing age among youth, with rates of 0.3 percent in children between the ages of 5 years and 7 years, rising to rates of 0.6 percent among teens. Rates of OCD among adolescents are greater than rates for disorders such as schizophrenia or bipolar disorder. Among young children with OCD there appears to be a slight male predominance which diminishes with age.

ETIOLOGY

Genetic Factors

OCD is a heterogeneous disorder that has been recognized for decades to run in families. Family studies have documented an increased risk of at least fourfold in first- degree relatives of early-onset OCD. In addition, the presence of subclinical symptom constellations in family members appears to breed true. Molecular genetic studies have suggested linkage to regions of chromosomes 2 and 9, in certain pedigrees with multiple members exhibiting early-onset OCD. Candidate gene studies have been inconclusive thus far. Family studies have pointed to a relationship between OCD, tic disorders such as Tourette's syndrome. OCD and tic disorders are believed to share susceptibility factors along with the concept of a broader "obsessive-compulsive spectrum" including as eating disorders, and somatoform disorders may account for expression of repetitive and stereotyped symptoms.

Neuroimmunology

The association of emergence of OCD syndromes following a documented exposure to or infection with group A β-hemolytic streptococcus in a subgroup of children and adolescents has led to the studies of immune responses in OCD. Cases of infection triggered OCD have been termed pediatric autoimmune neuropsychiatric disorders associated with streptococcus (PANDAS) and believed to signify an autoimmune process such as that of Sydenham's chorea during rheumatic fever. It is hypothesized that exposure to streptococcal bacteria activates the immune system leading to inflammation of the basal ganglia and resulting disruption of the cortical-striatal-thalamo-cortical function. MRI has documented a proportional relationship between the size of the basal ganglia and the severity of OCD symptoms. The presentation of OCD in children and adolescence due to acute exposure to group A beta hemolytic streptococcus represents a minority of OCD cases in this population.

Neurochemistry

Involvement of several neurotransmitter systems including the serotonin system, and the dopamine system have been postulated to contribute to the emergence of OCD. The observation that serotonin reuptake inhibitors (SSRIs) diminish symptoms of OCD, along with the findings of altered sensitivity to the acute administration of 5-hydroxytryptamine (5-HT) agonists support the likelihood that the serotonin system plays a role in OCD. In addition, the dopamine system is believed to be influential in this disorder, especially in light of the frequent comorbidity of

OCD with tic disorders in children. Clinical observations have indicated that obsessions and compulsions may be exacerbated during treatment of ADHD (another frequent comorbidity) with stimulant agents. Dopamine antagonists administered along with SSRIs may augment effectiveness of SSRIs in the treatment of OCD. It is most likely that multiple neurotransmitter systems may play a role in OCD.

Neuroimaging

Both computed tomography (CT) and magnetic resonance imaging (MRI) of untreated children and adults with OCD have revealed smaller volumes of basal ganglia segments compared to normal controls. In children, there is a suggestion that thalamic volume is increased. Adult studies have provided evidence of hypermetabolism of frontal cortical-striatal-thalamo-cortical networks in untreated individual with OCD. Interestingly, imaging studies of before and after treatment have revealed that both medication and behavioral interventions lead to a reduction of orbit frontal and caudate metabolic rates in children and adults with OCD.

DIAGNOSIS AND CLINICAL FEATURES

Children and adolescents with obsessions or compulsions are often referred for treatment due to the excessive time that they devote to their intrusive thoughts and repetitive rituals. For some children their compulsive rituals are perceived as reasonable response to their extreme fears and anxieties. Nevertheless, they are aware of their discomfort and inability to carry out usual daily activities in a timely manner due to the compulsions, such as getting ready to leave their homes to go to school each morning.

The most commonly reported obsessions in children and adolescents include extreme fears of contamination, exposure to dirt, germs or disease, followed by worries related to harm befalling themselves, family members, or fear of harming others due to losing control over aggressive impulses. Also commonly reported are obsessional need for symmetry or exactness, hoarding, and excessive religious or moral concerns. Typical compulsive rituals among children and adolescents involve cleaning, checking, counting, repeating behaviors or arranging items. Associated features in children and adolescents with OCD include avoidance, indecision, doubt and a slowness to complete tasks. In most cases of OCD among youth, obsessions and compulsions are present. According to DSM-IV-TR, diagnosis of OCD is identical to that of adults with the modification that children are not required as are adults to recognize that their obsessions or compulsions are excessive or irrational. Table 50.1–1 designates DSM-IV-TR diagnostic criteria for OCD.

The majority of children who develop OCD will have an insidious presentation and may hide their symptoms when possible, while a minority of children, particularly males with early onset may have a rapid unfolding of multiple symptoms within a few months. OCD is commonly found to be comorbid with other psychiatric disorders, especially other anxiety disorders. There are also higher than expected rates of attention-deficit/hyperactivity disorder (ADHD) and tic disorders, including Tourette's syndrome, among children and adolescents with OCD. Children with comorbid OCD and tic disorders are more likely to exhibit counting, arranging, or ordering compulsions and less likely to manifest excessive washing and cleaning compulsions. The high comorbidity of OCD, Tourette's syndrome, and ADHD has led investigators to postulate a common genetic vulnerability to all three of these disorders. It is important to search for comorbidity in children and adolescents with OCD so that optimal treatments can be administered.

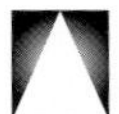

Table 50.1–1
DSM-IV-TR Diagnostic Criteria for Obsessive-Compulsive Disorder

A. Either obsessions or compulsions:
Obsessions as defined by (1), (2), (3), and (4):
(1) Recurrent and persistent thoughts, impulses, or images that are experienced, at some time during the disturbance, as intrusive and inappropriate and that cause marked anxiety or distress
(2) The thoughts, impulses, or images are not simply excessive worries about real-life problems
(3) The person attempts to ignore or suppress such thoughts, impulses, or images, or to neutralize them with some other thought or action
(4) The person recognizes that the obsessional thoughts, impulses, or images are a product of his or her own mind (not imposed from without as in thought insertion)
Compulsions as defined by (1) and (2):
(1) Repetitive behaviors (e.g., hand washing, ordering, checking) or mental acts (e.g., praying, counting, repeating words silently) that the person feels driven to perform in response to an obsession, or according to rules that must be applied rigidly
(2) The behaviors or mental acts are aimed at preventing or reducing distress or preventing some dreaded event or situation; however, these behaviors or mental acts either are not connected in a realistic way with what they are designed to neutralize or prevent or are clearly excessive

B. At some point during the course of the disorder, the person has recognized that the obsessions or compulsions are excessive or unreasonable. **Note:** This does not apply to children.

C. The obsessions or compulsions cause marked distress, are time consuming (take more than 1 hour a day), or significantly interfere with the person's normal routine, occupational (or academic) functioning, or usual social activities or relationships.

D. If another Axis I disorder is present, the content of the obsessions or compulsions is not restricted to it (e.g., preoccupation with food in the presence of an eating disorder; hair pulling in the presence of trichotillomania; concern with appearance in the presence of body dysmorphic disorder; preoccupation with drugs in the presence of a substance use disorder; preoccupation with having a serious illness in the presence of hypochondriasis; preoccupation with sexual urges or fantasies in the presence of a paraphilia; or guilty ruminations in the presence of major depressive disorder).

E. The disturbance is not due to the direct physiological effects of a substance (e.g., a drug of abuse, a medication) or a general medical condition.

Specify if:
With poor insight: if, for most of the time during the current episode, the person does not recognize that the obsessions and compulsions are excessive or unreasonable

From American Psychiatric Association. Diagnostic and Statistical Manual of Mental Disorders. 4th ed. Text rev. Washington, DC: American Psychiatric Association; copyright 2000, with permission.

John, a 9-year-old boy in the third grade, was brought for evaluation by his parents, who expressed concerns over his repeated questioning and anxious and sad moods. The parents described John as a previously happy and well-adjusted boy who abruptly developed unusual behaviors approximately 2 to 3 months before the evaluation. These behaviors included John's concern about contracting illness, washing rituals, uncertainty over his own behavior, needing reassurance, repeating rituals, and avoidance.

Specifically, John had begun to express the worry that he may have been exposed to human immunodeficiency virus (HIV) whenever he would observe another person in public who he believed may be suffering with acquired immune deficiency syndrome (AIDS). For example, while riding in the car, if John saw someone who appeared to him to be poor or ill-kempt, he would begin asking his parents if they thought it possible that he may have been exposed to germs even from quite a distance. Although his parents' reassurances had some effect, John usually insisted on vigorously washing himself once home. John also had begun to express doubts over his control of his own behavior. He would often ask his parents, "Did I use the s__ word? Did I use the f__ word?" Reassurance was only temporarily calming. Of much concern to John was his new-found difficulty with schoolwork. Reading passages from assigned materials, John would frequently get to the end of a sentence, only to question whether he might have missed a word or content of the sentence and need to reread the material. Completing a page could take up to 15 to 30 minutes. Over several weeks, he was less and less capable of completing assignments, and as a result he was very distressed over his dropping grades.

Examination of the family history suggested that John's older sister may have had similar traits but with less interference in functioning, and she had never received any treatment for those behaviors.

At the intake interview, John appeared as a quiet and sad boy who was cooperative with questioning. He did not volunteer as much information as his parents regarding the nature and extent of his symptoms but did not deny what his parents reported. He acknowledged that he felt his mind was "tricking" him and that it led to his need to ask for reassurance from his parents. John met full criteria for OCD. Some symptoms of depression were present but not sufficient for major depressive disorder.

An initial attempt at cognitive-behavioral therapy (CBT) was attempted, but John continued to feel overwhelmed and discouraged by these behaviors. He began to try to refuse school, apparently due to his increasing distress associated with reading. Given limited progress during the first 2 months of cognitive-behavioral therapy, fluoxetine (Prozac) was added and increased up to 40 mg per day, with good improvement. After three more months of CBT and SSRI treatment, John was able to stop cognitive-behavioral therapy and maintain substantial improvement. Follow-up over the next year showed John to be able to retain all of his gains from initial treatment and to show minimal interference from occasional OCD symptoms. (Courtesy of James T. McCracken, M.D.)

Pathology and Laboratory Examination

No specific laboratory measures are useful in the diagnosis of obsessive-compulsive disorder.

When the onset of obsessions or compulsions is believed to be associated with an exposure to or recent infection with group A beta hemolytic streptococcus, antigens and antibodies to the bacteria can be obtained, though a diagnosis of OCD can not be confirmed on the basis of positive results.

DIFFERENTIAL DIAGNOSIS

Developmentally appropriate rituals in the play and behavior of young children must be differentiated from obsessive-compulsive disorder in that age group. Preschoolers often engage in ritualistic play and request a predictable routine such as bathing, reading stories or selecting the same stuffed animal at bedtime, to promote a sense of security and comfort. These routines allay developmentally normal fears and lead to reasonable completion of daily activities, contrary to obsessions or compulsions which are driven by extreme fears and interfere with normative daily function due to the excessive time that they consume and the extreme distress when not fully completed. The rituals of preschoolers generally become less rigid by the time they enter grade school and school aged children usually do not have a surge of anxiety when they encounter small changes in their routine.

Children and adolescents with anxiety disorders such as generalized anxiety disorder, separation anxiety disorder or social phobia experience more intense worries than children without any anxiety disorders, and may express their concerns repeatedly but these are differentiated from typical obsessions by their more mundane content, whereas obsessions are so excessive that they approach seeming bizarre. A child with generalized anxiety disorder might worry repeatedly about their performance on academic examinations, whereas a child with OCD is likely to have intrusive concerns that he may lose control and harm someone he loves. The compulsions of OCD are not exhibited in other anxiety disorders, but children and adolescents with pervasive developmental disorders often display repetitive behaviors that resemble those of OCD. In contrast with the rituals of OCD, however, the children with pervasive developmental disorder are not responding to anxiety, but are more often manifesting stereotyped behaviors which are self-stimulating or self–comforting.

Children and adolescents with tic disorders such as Tourette's syndrome, may exhibit complex repetitive compulsive behaviors which are similar to the compulsions seen in OCD. In fact, children and adolescents with tic disorders are at higher risk for the development of concurrent OCD.

In severe cases of OCD, it may be difficult to differentiate whether psychosis is present, given the extreme and bizarre nature that obsessions and compulsions can possess. In adults and often in children and adolescents with OCD, despite the inability to control the obsessions or the irresistible drive to complete the compulsions, insight about their lack of reasonableness is preserved. When insight is present, and underlying anxiety can be described, even in the face of significant dysfunction due to bizarre obsessions and compulsion, the diagnosis of OCD is suspect.

COURSE AND PROGNOSIS

OCD with an onset in childhood and adolescence is characterized as a chronic, though waxing and waning disorder with a great variation in severity and outcome. Follow-up studies suggest that up to 50 percent of children and adolescence affected experience recovery from OCD with minimal remaining symptoms. In a recent study of childhood OCD, treatment with sertraline resulted in close to 50 percent of subjects experiencing complete remission and partial remission in another 25 percent with a follow-up time of one year. Predictors of the best outcome were in those children and adolescents without comorbid disorders including tic disorders and ADHD. Overall, the prognosis is hopeful for most children and adolescents with mild to moderate OCD. In a minority of cases, however, the OCD diagnosis may be considered a prodrome of a psychotic disorder which has been found to emerge in up to 10 percent in some samples of children and adolescents with OCD. In children with subthreshold symptoms of OCD, there is a high risk of the development of the full OCD disorder within a period of two years. In the majority of studies of childhood OCD, available treatments result in improvement if not complete remission in the majority of cases.

TREATMENT

Results from multiple randomized placebo-controlled trials of both medication and Cognitive-behavioral interventions in children and adolescents with OCD have confirmed the most evidence for successful treatment of this disorder compared to any of the other anxiety disorders of childhood. A recent multi-site National Institute of Health funded investigation of sertraline and cognitive-behavioral therapy each alone, and in combination for the treatment of childhood onset OCD, the Pediatric OCD Treatment Study (POTS) revealed that the combination was superior to either treatment alone. Each treatment alone also provided encouraging levels of response. Mean daily dose of sertraline was 133 mg/day in the group administered the combination treatment, and 170 mg/day for the sertraline alone group.

A meta-analysis of 13 studies of SSRIs, including sertraline, fluvoxamine, fluoxetine and paroxetine have provided evidence of efficacy of SSRI medications with a moderate effect size. There have been no apparent differences in the rate of response for the individual SSRIs.

Currently, three SSRIs : sertraline (at least 6 yrs), fluoxetine (at least 7 years), and fluvoxamine (at least 8 years) have now received US Federal Drug Administration (FDA) approval for the treatment of OCD. The black box warning for antidepressants used in children for any disorder, including OCD is applicable so that close monitoring for suicidal ideation or behavior is mandated when these agents are used in the treatment of childhood OCD.

Typical side effects that emerge with the use of SSRI agents include insomnia, nausea, agitation, tremor, and fatigue. Dosage ranges for the various SSRIs found to have efficacy in randomized clinical trials are Fluoxetine (20 mg to 60 mg), sertraline (50 mg to 200 mg), fluvoxamine (up to 200 mg), and paroxetine (up to 50 mg).

Clomipramine was the first SSRI studied in the treatment of OCD in childhood and the only tricyclic antidepressant that has a US FDA approval for the treatment of anxiety disorders in childhood. Clomipramine was found to be efficacious in doses up to 200 mg, or 3 mg/kg, whichever is less, and may be chosen for children or adolescents who can not tolerate other SSRIs due to insomnia, significant appetite suppression or activation. Nevertheless, clomipramine is not recommended as a first line treatment due to its greater potential risks compared to other SSRI agents, including cardiovascular risk of hypotension and arrhythmia, and seizure risk.

Cognitive-behavioral therapy (CBT) geared toward children of varying ages is based on the principle of developmentally appropriate exposure to the feared stimuli coupled with response prevention, leading to diminishing anxiety over time experienced upon exposure to feared situations. CBT manuals have been developed to ensure that developmentally appropriate interventions are made and that comprehensive education is provided to the child and parents.

Most treatment guidelines for children and adolescents with mild to moderate OCD recommend a trial of cognitive-behavioral therapy prior to initiating medication, though there is evidence from one large investigation (POTS) that optimal treatment includes the combination of SSRI medication and CBT. In terms of pharmacologic interventions, acute treatment of childhood OCD has been shown to occur within 8 to 12 weeks of treatment. The vast majority of children and adolescents who experienced a remission with acute treatment using SSRIs were still responsive over a period of a year. Given the lack of data on discontinuation, recommendations for maintaining medication include stabilization, education about relapse risk, and tapering medication during the summer is likely to be advised in order to minimize academic compromise in case of relapse. For children and adolescents with more severe or multiple episodes of significant exacerbation of symptoms, treatment for a longer period of time, more than a year is recommended.

Augmentation strategies enhancing serotonergic effects, such as atypical antipsychotics such as risperidone have demonstrated increased response when partial response has been achieved with SSRI agents.

Overall, efficacy of treatment for children and adolescents with OCD is high with choices of SSRI agents and CBT therapy.

REFERENCES

Barrett P, Healy-Farrell L, March J. Cognitive-behavioral family treatment of childhood obsessive-compulsive disorder: A controlled trial. *J of the Am Acad Child Adolesc Psych.* 2004;43(1):46–62.

Geller DA, Wagner KD, Emslie G, et al. Paroxetine treatment in children and adolescents with obsessive-compulsive disorder: a randomized, multicenter, double-blind, placebo-controlled trial. *J Am Cad Child Adolesc Psychiatry.* 2004;43: 1387.

Geller D, Biederman J, Stewart S, Mullin B, Martin A, Spencer T, Faraone S. Which SSRI? A meta-analysis of pharmacotherapy trials in pediatric obsessive-compulsive disorder. *Am J Psychiatry.* 2003;160:11.

McCracken J. Obsessive-compulsive Disorder in children. In: Sadock BJ, Sadock VA, eds. *Kaplan & Sadock's Comprehensive Textbook of Psychiatry* 8th edition. Vol 2. Baltimore:. Lippincott Williams & Wilkins; 2005:3280.

Miguel EC, Leckman JF, Rauch S et al. Obsessive-compulsive disorder phenotypes: implications for genetic studies. *Mol Psychiatry.* 2005;10:258.

Pediatric OCD Treatment Study Team. Cognitive-behavior therapy, sertraline, and their combination for children and adolescents with obsessive-compulsive disorder: the Pediatric OCD Treatment Study (POTS) randomized controlled trial. *JAMA.* 2004;292:1969.

Piacentini J, Bergman R, Jacobs C, McCracken J, Kretchman J. Open trial of cognitive behavior therapy for childhood onset obsessive-compulsive disorder. *J Anxiety Disord.* 2002;16:207.

Reinblatt SP, Walkup JT. Psychopharmacologic treatment of pediatric anxiety disorders. *Child Adolesc Psychiatric Clin N Am.* 2005;14:877.

Stewart Se, Geller DA, Jenike M. et al. Long-term outcome of pediatric obsessive-compulsive disorder: a meta-analysis and qualitative review of the literature. *Acta Psychiatr Scand.* 2004;110:4.

Szeszko PR, MacMillan S, McMeniman M, Chen S, Baribault K, Lim KO, Ivey J, Rose M, Banerjee SP, Bhandari R, Moore GJ, Rosenberg DR. Brain Structural Abnormalities in Psychotropic Drug-Naive Pediatric Patients With Obsessive-Compulsive Disorder. *Am J Psychiatry.* 2004;161:1049–1056.

Waslick B. Psychopharmacology intervention for pediatric anxiety disorders: a research update. *Child Adolesc Psychiatr Clin N Am.* 2006;1:51.

▲ 50.2 Posttraumatic Stress Disorder of Infancy, Childhood, and Adolescence

Posttraumatic stress disorder (PTSD) is characterized by a set of symptoms such as reexperiencing symptoms, distressing recollections, persistent avoidance, and hyperarousal in response to exposure to one or more traumatic events. PTSD is the only disorder described in the text revision of the fourth edition of the *Diagnostic and Statistical Manual of Mental Disorders* (DSM-IV-TR) in which the etiologic factors, exposure to an extreme traumatic stressor either directly or as a witness is the first diagnostic criterion of the disorder. Many children and adolescents are exposed to traumatic events, ranging from direct experiences with physical or sexual abuse, domestic violence, motor vehicle accidents, severe medical illnesses, or natural or human created disasters, leading to full-blown PTSD in some, and at least some PTSD symptoms in many others. Although the presence of posttraumatic stress symptoms has been described among adults for more than a century, it was first officially recognized as a psychiatric disorder in 1980 with the publication of the third edition of DSM (DSM-III) Recognition of its frequent emergence in children and adolescence has broadened over the last decade. PTSD occurs frequently in children and adolescents with up to 6 percent of youth meeting criteria for this diagnosis at some point. Developmental factors strongly influence the manifestations of symptoms, many of which reflect internal states that are identified mainly through verbal articulation by the patient. In children and adolescents reexperiencing of a traumatic event is often observed through play, recurrent nightmares without recall of the traumatic events, and behaviors that reenact the traumatic situation, along with agitation, fear, or disorganization.

EPIDEMIOLOGY

Epidemiologic studies have reported lifetime prevalence rates of PTSD ranging from 1.3 to 8 percent in adults in the United States. A recent epidemiologic survey of preschoolers aged 4 to 5 years found a rate of 1.3 percent of PTSD, whereas among children of 2 to 3 years of age, the full criteria for PTSD were not met. Epidemiologic studies of children from 9 to 17 years of age have found 3-month prevalence rates of PTSD ranging from 0.5 to 4 percent. Among trauma-exposed samples of persons not referred for treatment, a wide range of 25 percent to 90 percent of them have been reported to exhibit the full diagnosis of PTSD. Children exposed chronically to trauma, such as child abuse, or other traumas resulting in the dissolution of the family and ongoing exposure to broader disruption of entire communities, such as war, result in the greatest risk for the development of PTSD. In addition to the staggering rate of the full-blown disorder of PTSD among youth, several studies indicate that most children exposed to severe or chronic trauma develop PTSD symptoms sufficiently severe to disrupt functioning, even in the absence of the full diagnosis.

ETIOLOGY

Biological Factors

Given that some children who are exposed to significant traumatic events do not develop PTSD, investigations have documented that risk factors in children for developing PTSD include preexisting anxiety disorders. This suggests that a genetic predisposition for anxiety disorders, as well as a family history with increased risk of depressive disorders, may also predispose a trauma-exposed child to develop PTSD. Children with PTSD have been found to exhibit increased excretion of adrenergic and dopaminergic metabolites, smaller intracranial volume and corpus callosum, memory deficits, and lower intelligence quotients (IQs) compared with age-matched controls. Adults with PTSD have been found to have overactive amygdale regions of the brain and decreased hippocampal volume. What is unclear at the present time, because the above findings were retrospective, is whether these findings are sequelae of PTSD or markers of vulnerability to the disorder.

Psychological Factors

Although the exposure to trauma is the initial etiologic factor in the development of PTSD, the enduring symptoms typical of PTSD, such as avoidance of the place where the trauma occurred, can be conceptualized, in part, as the result of both classic and operant conditioning. The extreme physiological responses that accompany fear of a given traumatic event, such as an adolescent who was terrorized by an attack by a group of students near school, who then develops an extreme negative physiologic reaction each time he or she is near the school. This is an example of classic conditioning in that a neutral cue (the school) has become paired with an intensely fearful past event. Operant conditioning occurs when a child learns to avoid traumatic reminders to prevent distressing feelings from arising. For example, if a child was in a motor vehicle accident, the child may then refuse to ride in cars altogether to prevent negative physiologic reactions and fear from occurring.

Another conceptualization in developing and maintaining symptoms of PTSD is through the mechanism of modeling, which is a form of learning. For example, when parents and children are exposed to traumatic events, such as natural disasters, children may emulate parental responses, such as avoidance, withdrawal, or extreme expressions of fear, and "learn" to respond to their own memories of the traumatic event in the same manner.

Social Factors

Family support and reactions to traumatic events in children may play a significant role in the development of PTSD, in that adverse parental emotional reactions to a child's abuse may increase that child's risk of developing PTSD. Lack of parental support, psychopathology among parents—especially maternal depression—has been identified as a risk factor in the development of PTSD after a child has been exposed to a traumatic event.

DIAGNOSIS AND CLINICAL FEATURES

For PTSD to ensue, exposure to a traumatic event consisting of either a direct personal experience or witnessing an event

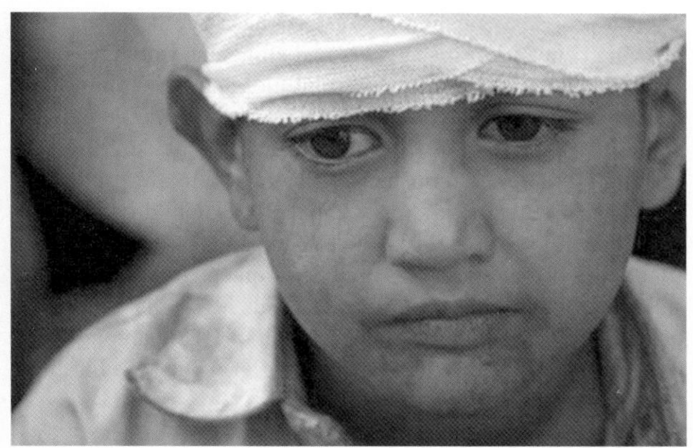

FIGURE 50.2–1
The face of a boy in Pakistan shortly after a 7.6 magnitude earthquake hit South Asia leaving millions homeless. (Courtesy of Samoon Ahmad, M.D.)

involving the threat of death, serious injury, or serious harm must occur. Most common traumatic exposures for children and adolescents include physical or sexual abuse; domestic, school or community violence; being kidnapped; terrorist attacks; motor vehicle or household accidents; or disasters, such as floods, hurricanes, tornadoes, fires, explosions, or airline crashes. The child's response must involve intense fear, terror, helplessness, horror, or disorganized or agitated behavior (Fig. 50.2–1).

Symptoms of PTSD include *reexperiencing* the traumatic event in at least one of the following ways. Children may have intrusive thoughts that they perceive as recurrently coming into their head, memories, images, or body sensations that remind them of the event. In very young children, it is common to observe play that includes elements of the traumatic event, or behaviors, such as sexual behaviors that are not developmentally expected. Children may experience periods during which they either act or feel that the event is taking place presently, which is a dissociative event usually described by adults as "flashbacks."

Another critical symptom characteristic of PTSD is *avoidance and numbing*. Children with PTSD exhibit avoidance, either by making active physical efforts to avoid the places that would present traumatic reminders to them of the event, or they may be unable to recall important aspects of the traumatic event. The inability to remember parts of a traumatic event is termed *psychological amnesia*. After a traumatic event, children may experience a sense of detachment from their usual play activities ("psychological numbing)" or a diminished capacity to feel emotions, whereas older adolescents may express a fear that they anticipate that they will die young (sense of foreshortened future).

Other typical responses to traumatic events include symptoms of hyperarousal that were not present before the traumatic exposure, such as difficulty falling asleep or staying asleep; hypervigilance regarding safety and increased checking that doors are locked; or exaggerated startle reaction. In some children, hyperarousal can present as a generalized inability to relax with increased irritability, outbursts, and impaired ability to concentrate.

To meet the diagnostic criteria for PTSD, according to the DSM-IV-TR, the symptoms must be present for at least 1 month, and cause distress and impairment in important functional areas of life. When all of the diagnostic symptoms of PTSD are met, but they resolve within 3 months, acute PTSD is diagnosed. When the full syndrome of PTSD persists beyond 3 months, it becomes designated as chronic PTSD. In some cases, the PTSD symptoms increase over time, and it is not until more than 6 months have elapsed after the exposure to the trauma that the whole syndrome emerges; in that case, the diagnosis is PTSD, delayed onset. DSM-IV-TR criteria are described in Table 50.2–1.

It is not uncommon for children and adolescents with PTSD to experience feelings of guilt, especially if they have survived the trauma and others in the situation did not. They may blame themselves for the demise of the others and may go on to develop a comorbid depressive episode. Childhood PTSD is also associated with increased rates of other anxiety disorders in addition to depressive episodes, substance use disorders, and attentional difficulties.

Pathology and Laboratory Examination

Although reports indicate some alterations in both neurophysiologic and neuroimaging studies of children and adolescents with PTSD, no current laboratory tests can help in making this diagnosis.

Differential Diagnosis

A number of overlapping symptoms are seen between childhood presentations of anxiety disorders, such as obsessive-compulsive disorder (OCD) or social phobia, in which occur recurrent intrusive thoughts and avoidance, in the case of social phobia of situations in which the given child may experience anxiety. Children with depressive disorders often exhibit withdrawal and a sense of isolation from peers as well as guilt about life events over which they realistically have no control. Irritability, poor concentration, sleep disturbance, and decreased interest in usual activities can also be observed in both PTSD and major depressive disorder.

Children who have lost a loved one in a traumatic event may go on to experience both PTSD and a major depressive disorder when bereavement persists beyond its expected course. Children with PTSD may also be confused with children who have disruptive behavior disorders, because they often show poor concentration, inattention, and irritability. It is critical to elicit a history of traumatic exposure and evaluate the chronology of the trauma and the onset of the symptoms to make an accurate diagnosis of PTSD.

Course and Prognosis

Many studies have documented the presence of both partial PTSD syndromes and the full syndrome in children who have been exposed to traumatic events. A wide range of outcomes exists, depending on the severity and intensity of the trauma and the preexisting emotional and psychiatric state of the child. For many children and adolescents with milder forms of PTSD, symptoms may persist for 1 to 2 years after which they diminish and attenuate. In more severe circumstances, however, PTSD syndromes persist for many years or decades in children and adolescents, with spontaneous remission in only a portion of them.

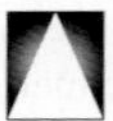

Table 50.2–1
DSM-IV-TR Diagnostic Criteria for Posttraumatic Stress Disorder

A. The person has been exposed to a traumatic event in which both of the following were present:
 (1) the person experienced, witnessed, or was confronted with an event or events that involved actual or threatened death or serious injury, or a threat to the physical integrity of self or others
 (2) the person's response involved intense fear, helplessness, or horror. **Note**: In children, this may be expressed instead by disorganized or agitated behavior.

B. The traumatic event is persistently reexperienced in one (or more) of the following ways:
 (1) recurrent and intrusive distressing recollections of the event, including images, thoughts, or perceptions. **Note**: In young children, repetitive play may occur in which themes or aspects of the trauma are expressed.
 (2) recurrent distressing dreams of the event. **Note**: In children, there may be frightening dreams without recognizable content.
 (3) acting or feeling as if the traumatic event were recurring (includes a sense of reliving the experience, illusions, hallucinations, and dissociative flashback episodes, including those that occur on awakening or when intoxicated). **Note**: In young children, trauma-specific reenactment may occur.
 (4) intense psychological distress at exposure to internal or external cues that symbolize or resemble an aspect of the traumatic event
 (5) physiological reactivity on exposure to internal or external cues that symbolize or resemble an aspect of the traumatic event

C. Persistent avoidance of stimuli associated with the trauma and numbing of general responsiveness (not present before the trauma), as indicated by three (or more) of the following:
 (1) efforts to avoid thoughts, feelings, or conversations associated with the trauma
 (2) efforts to avoid activities, places, or people that arouse recollections of the trauma
 (3) inability to recall an important aspect of the trauma
 (4) markedly diminished interest or participation in significant activities
 (5) feeling of detachment or estrangement from others
 (6) restricted range of affect (e.g., unable to have loving feelings)
 (7) sense of a foreshortened future (e.g., does not expect to have a career, marriage, children, or a normal life span)

D. Persistent symptoms of increased arousal (not present before the trauma), as indicated by two (or more) of the following:
 (1) difficulty falling or staying asleep
 (2) irritability or outbursts of anger
 (3) difficulty concentrating
 (4) hypervigilance
 (5) exaggerated startle response

E. Duration of the disturbance (symptoms in Criteria B, C, and D) is more than 1 month.

F. The disturbance causes clinically significant distress or impairment in social, occupational, or other important areas of functioning.

Specify if:
Acute: if duration of symptoms is less than 3 months
Chronic: if duration of symptoms is 3 months or more
Specify if:
With delayed onset: if onset of symptoms is at least 6 months after the stressor

(From American Psychiatric Association. *Diagnostic and Statistical Manual of Mental Disorders.* 4th ed. Text rev. Washington, DC: American Psychiatric Association; copyright 2000, with permission.)

The prognosis of untreated PTSD has become an issue of growing concern for researchers and clinicians who have documented a variety of serious comorbidities and psychobiological abnormalities associated with PTSD. In one study, children and adolescents with severe PTSD were at risk for decreased intracranial volume, diminished corpus callosum area and lower IQs. compared with children without PTSD. Children and adolescents with histories of physical and sexual abuse have been found to exhibit higher rates of depression and suicidality themselves and in their offspring as well. This highlights the importance of early recognition and treatment of PTSD among youth that may significantly improve the long-term outcome for them.

TREATMENT

Trauma-Focused Cognitive-Behavior Therapy

Several randomized clinical trials have provided evidence for the efficacy of trauma-focused cognitive-behavior therapy (CBT) in the treatment of PTSD in children and adolescents. This treatment is generally administered over 10 to 16 treatment sessions, including a number of components. The first component of trauma-focused CBT is *psychoeducation* regarding the nature of typical emotional and physiological reactions to traumatic events and PTSD. Next, *stress inoculation* in which children are guided to utilize muscle relaxation, focused breathing, affective modulation, thought-stopping, and cognitive coping techniques to diminish feelings of helplessness and distress. *Gradual exposure* may then be introduced as a technique for a child to recall, first in small segments and then in increasing amounts, the details of the traumatic exposure and describe the thoughts, feelings, and physical sensations experienced during the trauma as well as in the retelling of the event. *Cognitive processing* is the next step in identifying those associated thoughts, feelings, and ideas that may be inaccurate and serving to cause additional impairment to the victim, so that reframing of the thoughts and feelings can help them alleviate the sense of being incapacitated by them. At this time, during the cognitive processing, a *parental treatment component* is added that provides parent management strategies for the parent to use to enhance the child's ability to communicate proactively and elicit support from the parents. This set of therapeutic strategies is designated by experts as the currently accepted first line of treatment of PTSD symptoms. They can be adapted for use in group settings in school, with entire families who have been traumatized, and in groups of adolescents.

A variant of trauma-focused CBT for PTSD is called *eye movement desensitization and reprocessing* (EMDR) in which an exposure and cognitive reprocessing interventions are paired with directed eye movements. This technique is not as well accepted as the more extensive trauma-focused CBT detailed above.

Crisis Intervention/Psychological Debriefing

Crisis intervention/psychological debriefing typically consists of several sessions immediately after an exposure to a traumatic event in which a traumatized child or adolescent is encouraged to describe the traumatic event in the context of a supportive environment. Psychoeducation is provided and guidance about the management of initial emotional reactions may be provided.

Anecdotal reports suggest that this intervention may be helpful, but no controlled studies have yet provided evidence that this intervention leads to a more positive outcome.

Psychopharmacologic Treatment

Serotonin reuptake inhibitors (SSRIs) are frequently used in children with PTSD in the absence of evidence demonstrating efficacy. Citalopram (Celexa) from 20 mg to 40 mg has been reported to be helpful in the management of PTSD in children and adolescents according to results of an open trial over an 8 week period. Most of the SSRI efficacy data have been obtained through open trials with adults suggesting that they are beneficial.

In adults clonidine (Catapres) and propranolol (Inderal) have been used to treat PTSD, especially nightmares and exaggerated startle response, with a suggestion of improvement. One report of propranolol treatment in 11 pediatric patients with PTSD, based on sexual or physical abuse, with a mean age of 8.5 years who exhibited agitation and hyperarousal indicated some decrease in symptoms in 8 of the 11 children studied. Another open study of transdermal clonidine treatment of preschoolers with PTSD suggests that clonidine may be efficacious in this population in decreasing activation and hyperarousal. An additional open trial of oral clonidine with dosage ranges of 0.05 to 0.1 mg twice daily similarly suggests that this medication may provide some relief for the symptoms of hyperarousal, impulsivity and agitation in young children with PTSD.

One open study utilized imipramine (Tofranil) in the treatment of acute stress disorder symptoms in 25 children with burns suggests that possibility that this medication provided benefit for sleep. A case report indicated that guanfacine (Tenex) treated PTSD nightmares in a child.

Currently no randomized placebo-controlled trials of medication for youth in the treatment of PTSD have been conducted and, in general, extrapolation from adult studies points to the likelihood that SSRI medications may provide relief for some symptoms of PTSD among youth.

References

Barakat LP, Alderfer MA, Kazak AE. Posttraumatic growth in adolescent survivors of cancer and their mothers and fathers. *J Pediatr Psychol*. 2006;31(4):413–419.

Cohen JA. Posttraumatic stress disorder in children and adolescents. In: Sadock BJ, Sadock VA, eds. *Kaplan & Sadock's Comprehensive Textbook of Psychiatry*. 8th ed. Vol 2. Baltimore: Lippincott Williams and Wilkins; 2005:3286.

Cohen JA. Deblinger E, Mannarino AP, Steer R. A multisite randomized controlled trial for children with sexual abuse-related PTSD symptoms. *J Am Acad Child Adolesc Psychiatry*. 2004;42:393.

Cohen JA, Perel JM, DeBellis MD, Friedman MJ, Putnam FW. Treating traumatized children: clinical implications of the psychobiology of PTSD. *TVA: A Review Journal*. 2002;3:91.

DeBellis MD, Van Dillen T. Childhood post-traumatic stress disorder: An overview. *Child Adolesc Psychiatr Clin N Am*. 2005;14(4):745–772.

Reinblatt SP, Walkup JT. Psychopharmacologic treatment of pediatric anxiety disorders. *Child Adolesc Psychiatric Clin N Am*. 2005;14:877.

Scheeringa MS, Wright MJ, Hunt JP, Zeanah CH. Factors affecting the diagnosis and prediction of PTSD symptomatology in children and adolescents. *Am J Psychiatry*. 2006;163(4):644–651.

Scheeringa MS, Zeanah CH, Myers L, Putnam FW. Predictive validity in a prospective follow-up of PTSD in preschool children. *J Am Acad Child Adolesc Psychiatry*. 2005;44(9):899–906.

Seedat S, Stein DJ, Ziervogel C, et al. Comparison of response to a selective serotonin reuptake inhibitor in children, adolescents, and adults with posttraumatic stress disorder. *J Child Adolesc Psychopharmacol*. 2002;12:37.

Waslick B. Psychopharmacology intervention for pediatric anxiety disorders: A research update. *Child Adolesc Psychiatr Clin N Am*. 2006;1:51.

▲ 50.3 Separation Anxiety Disorder, Generalized Anxiety Disorder, and Social Phobia

Anxiety disorders are among the most common disorders in youth, affecting more than 10 percent of children and adolescents at some point in their development. Separation anxiety is a universal human developmental phenomenon emerging in infants less than 1 year of age and marking a child's awareness of a separation from his or her mother or primary caregiver. Normative separation anxiety peaks between 9 months and 18 months and diminishes by about 2.5 years of age, enabling young children to develop a sense of comfort away from their parents in preschool. Separation anxiety or stranger anxiety as it has been termed most likely evolved as a human response that has survival value. The expression of transient separation anxiety is also normal in young children entering school for the first time. Approximately 15 percent of young children display intense and persistent fear, shyness, and social withdrawal when faced with unfamiliar settings and people. Young children with this pattern of behavioral inhibition are at higher risk for the development of separation anxiety disorder, generalized anxiety disorder, and social phobia. Behaviorally inhibited children, as a group, exhibit characteristic physiologic traits, including higher than average resting heart rates, higher morning cortisol levels than average, and low heart rate variability. Separation anxiety disorder is diagnosed when developmentally inappropriate and excessive anxiety emerges related to separation from the major attachment figure. According to the text revision of the fourth edition of *Diagnostic and Statistical Manual of Mental Disorders* (DSM-IV-TR), separation anxiety disorder requires the presence of at least three symptoms related to excessive worry about separation from the major attachment figures. The worries may take the form of refusal to go to school, fears and distress on separation, repeated complaints of such physical symptoms as headaches and stomachaches when separation is anticipated, and nightmares related to separation issues.

Separation anxiety disorder, along with *selective mutism* are the two anxiety disorders currently found in the child and adolescent section of DSM-IV-TR, although childhood onset of all of the anxiety disorders is frequent. Children who exhibit recurrent excessive worries pertaining to their performance in school and social settings and experience at least one physiologic symptom, such as restlessness, poor concentration, or irritability related to their fears, may be diagnosed with generalized anxiety disorder. Children with generalized anxiety disorder tend to feel fearful in multiple settings, and expect more negative outcomes when faced with academic or social challenges compared with peers. Children who experience recurrent extreme anxiety and avoid social situations in which they fear scrutiny or humiliation may meet the DSM-IV-TR diagnostic criteria for *social phobia*, a disorder that also occurs in adolescents and adults. Children with social phobia experience distress and discomfort in the presence of peers as well as adults. Separation anxiety disorder, generalized anxiety, and social phobia in children are often considered together in a differential diagnosis and in developing treatment strategies because they are highly comorbid, and have overlapping symptoms. A child with separation anxiety disorder, generalized anxiety disorder, or social phobia has a 60 percent chance of having at least one of the other two disorders as well. Of children with one of the above anxiety disorders, 30 percent have all three of them. Children and adolescents may also have other anxiety disorders described among the adult disorders of DSM-IV-TR, including specific phobia, panic disorder, obsessive-compulsive disorder (OCD), and posttraumatic stress disorder (PTSD).

EPIDEMIOLOGY

The prevalence of anxiety disorders has varied with the age group of the children surveyed and the diagnostic instruments used. Lifetime prevalence of any anxiety disorder in children and adolescents ranges from 8.3 percent to 27 percent. A recent epidemiologic survey using the *Preschool Age Psychiatric Assessment* (PAPA) found that 9.5 percent of preschoolers met DSM-IV-TR criteria for any anxiety disorder, with 6.5 percent exhibiting generalized anxiety disorder, 2.4 percent meeting criteria for separation anxiety disorder, and 2.2 percent meeting criteria for social phobia. Separation anxiety disorder is estimated to be about 4 percent in children and young adolescents. Separation anxiety disorder is more common in young children than in adolescents and has been reported to occur equally in boys and girls. The onset may occur during preschool years, but is most common in children 7 to 8 years of age. The rate of generalized anxiety disorder in school-age children is estimated to be approximately 3 percent, the rate of social phobia is 1 percent, and the rate of simple phobias is 2.4 percent. In adolescents, lifetime prevalence for panic disorder was found to be 0.6 percent; the prevalence for generalized anxiety disorder was 3.7 percent.

ETIOLOGY

Biopsychosocial Factors

In very young children, psychosocial factors in conjunction with temperament may influence the degree of separation anxiety that emerges in situations of brief separation and exposure to unfamiliar environments. The relation between temperamental traits and the predisposition to develop anxiety symptoms has been investigated. The temperamental tendency to be unusually shy or to withdraw in unfamiliar situations seems to be an enduring response pattern, and young children with this propensity are at higher risk of developing separation anxiety disorder, generalized anxiety disorder, social anxiety disorders, or all three during their next few years of life.

Neurophysiological correlation is found with behavioral inhibition (extreme shyness); children with this constellation are shown to have a higher resting heart rate and an acceleration of heart rate with tasks requiring cognitive concentration. Additional physiological correlates of behavioral inhibition include elevated salivary cortisol levels, elevated urinary catecholamine levels, and greater papillary dilation during cognitive tasks. The quality of maternal attachment also appears to play a role in the development of anxiety disorder in children. Mothers with anxiety disorders who are observed to show insecure attachment to their children tend to have children with higher rates of anxiety disorders. It is difficult to separate the contribution of the relationship between mother and child from the mother's potential genetic contribution to anxiety. Families in which a child manifests separation anxiety disorder may be close-knit and caring, and the children often seem to be the objects of parental overconcern. External life stresses often coincide with development of the disorder. The death of a relative, a child's illness, a change in a child's environment, or a move to a new neighborhood or school is frequently noted in the histories of children with separation anxiety disorder. In a vulnerable child, these changes probably intensify anxiety.

Social Learning Factors

Fear, in response to a variety of unfamiliar or unexpected situations, may be unwittingly communicated from parents to children by direct modeling. If a parent is fearful, the child will probably have a phobic adaptation to new situations, especially to a school environment. Some parents appear to teach their children to be anxious by overprotecting them from expected dangers or by exaggerating the dangers. For example, a parent who cringes in a room during a lightning storm teaches a child to do the same. A parent who is afraid of mice or insects conveys the affect of fright to a child. Conversely, a parent who becomes angry with a child when the child expresses fear of a given situation, for example when exposed to animals, may promote a phobic concern in the child by exposing the child to the intensity of the anger expressed by the parent. Social learning factors in the development of anxiety reactions are magnified when parents have anxiety disorders themselves. These factors may be pertinent in the development of separation anxiety disorder as well as in generalized anxiety disorder and social phobia. In a recent study of adverse psychosocial events, such as ongoing family conflict, no association, however, was found between psychosocial hardships and behavioral inhibition among young children. It appears that temperamental predisposition to anxiety disorders emerges as a highly heritable constellation of traits, and is not created by psychosocial stressor.

Genetic Factors

Genetic studies of families suggest that genes account for at least one third of the variance in the development of anxiety disorders in children. Thus, temperamental constellation of behavioral inhibition, excessive shyness, the tendency to withdraw from unfamiliar situations, and the eventual emergence of anxiety disorders have a genetic contribution; however, approximately two thirds of young children with behavioral inhibition do not appear to go on to develop anxiety disorders. Family studies have shown that the biological offspring of adults with anxiety disorders are susceptible to parents with panic disorder with agoraphobia who appear to have an increased risk of having a child with separation anxiety disorder. Separation anxiety disorder and depression in children overlap, and the presence of an anxiety disorder increases the risk of a future episode of a depressive disorder. Current consensus on the genetics of anxiety disorders suggests that what is inherited is a general predisposition toward anxiety, with resulting heightened levels of arousability, emotional reactivity, and increased negative affect, all of which increase the risk for the development of separation anxiety disorder, generalized anxiety disorder, and social phobia.

DIAGNOSIS AND CLINICAL FEATURES

Separation anxiety disorder, generalized anxiety disorder, and social phobia are highly related in children and adolescence because, in most children, if one occurs, another is present as well. Generalized anxiety disorder is the most common anxiety disorder in childhood, but in 30 percent of cases, a child with generalized anxiety disorder also exhibits the other two disorders. Separation anxiety disorder and selective mutism are the two anxiety disorders contained in the childhood section of the DSM-IV-TR, however most anxiety disorders originate in childhood or adolescence. Diagnostic criteria for separation anxiety disorder, according to DSM-IV-TR, include three of the following symptoms for at least 4 weeks: persistent and excessive worry about losing, or possible harm befalling, major attachment figures; persistent and excessive worry that an untoward event can lead to separation from a major attachment figure; persistent reluctance or refusal to go to school or elsewhere because of fear of separation; persistent and excessive fear or reluctance to be alone or without major attachment figures at home or without significant adults in other settings; persistent reluctance or refusal to go to sleep without being near a major attachment figure or to sleep away from home; repeated nightmares involving the theme of separation; repeated complaints of physical symptoms, including headaches and stomachaches, when separation from major attachment figures is anticipated; and recurrent excessive distress when separation from home or major attachment figures is anticipated or involved (Tables 50.3–1 through 50.3–3).

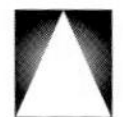

Table 50.3–1
DSM-IV-TR Diagnostic Criteria for Separation Anxiety Disorder

A. Developmentally inappropriate and excessive anxiety concerning separation from home or from those to whom the individual is attached, as evidenced by three (or more) of the following:
 (1) recurrent excessive distress when separation from home or major attachment figures occurs or is anticipated
 (2) persistent and excessive worry about losing, or about possible harm befalling, major attachment figures
 (3) persistent and excessive worry that an untoward event will lead to separation from a major attachment figure (e.g., getting lost or being kidnapped)
 (4) persistent reluctance or refusal to go to school or elsewhere because of fear of separation
 (5) persistently and excessively fearful or reluctant to be alone or without major attachment figures at home or without significant adults in other settings
 (6) persistent reluctance or refusal to go to sleep without being near a major attachment figure or to sleep away from home
 (7) repeated nightmares involving the theme of separation
 (8) repeated complaints of physical symptoms (such as headaches, stomachaches, nausea, or vomiting) when separation from major attachment figures occurs or is anticipated

B. The duration of the disturbance is at least 4 weeks.

C. The onset is before age 18 years.

D. The disturbance causes clinically significant distress or impairment in social, academic (occupational), or other important areas of functioning.

E. The disturbance does not occur exclusively during the course of a pervasive developmental disorder, schizophrenia, or other psychotic disorder and, in adolescents and adults, is not better accounted for by panic disorder with agoraphobia.

Specify if:
Early onset: if onset occurs before age 6 years

(From American Psychiatric Association. *Diagnostic and Statistical Manual of Mental Disorders.* 4th ed. Text rev. Washington, DC: American Psychiatric Association; copyright 2000, with permission.)

Alan W, was an 8-year-old boy referred for outpatient evaluation by his family physician. He was having trouble sleeping in his room alone at night and was refusing to go to school. Alan expressed recurrent fears that something bad would happen to his mother. He worried that she would get into a car accident or that there would be a fire at home and his mother would be killed. Developmental history showed Alan was anxious and irritable as an infant and toddler. He had trouble adjusting to baby-sitters in the preschool years. There was a history of panic disorder, with agoraphobia in the mother and major depression in the father.

Nighttime was a particularly difficult time at home. While Mrs. W would read to her son and talk with him before bedtime, Alan would often whine and cry, asking to have mother lie in bed with him until he fell asleep. He also expected his mother to be in the master bedroom across the hall from his room throughout the evening. Mrs. W reported that some evenings her son would get up and peek through the crack in the master bedroom door, as frequently as every 10 minutes, to be certain that she was still there. Alan reported frequent bad dreams that his parents were killed or that monsters caught him and took him away from his family forever.

During the daytime, he would shadow his mother around the house. Alan would agree to play a game with his sister in the lower level of the house only if his mother was close by. When Mrs. W went upstairs, he would interrupt the game and follow her upstairs. He was reluctant to sleep at a friend's house; a couple of times he attempted to do this. However, as the evening progressed, he described a queasy sensation in his stomach, a feeling of sadness, and missing his mother. Subsequently Alan would call home and his parents would pick him up.

On school days, Alan had stomachaches and tried to stay home. He appeared quite distressed and panicky when it was time to separate from his mother. Once at school, he seemed calmer and less anxious, but occasionally was seen in the nurse's office, complaining of nausea and seeking to be sent home. (Courtesy of Gail A. Bernstein, M.D. and Anne E. Layne, Ph.D.)

The essential feature of separation anxiety disorder is extreme anxiety precipitated by separation from parents, home, or other familiar surroundings, whereas in generalized anxiety disorder, fears are extended to negative outcomes for all kinds of events, including academic, peer relationship, and family activities. In generalized anxiety disorder, a child or adolescent experiences at least one recurrent physiologic symptom, such as restlessness, poor concentration, irritability, or muscle tension. In social phobia, the child's fears peak during performance situations involving exposure to unfamiliar people or situations. Children and adolescents with social phobia have extreme concerns about being embarrassed, humiliated, or negatively judged.

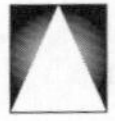

Table 50.3–2
DSM-IV-TR Diagnostic Criteria for Generalized Anxiety Disorder

A. Excessive anxiety and worry (apprehensive expectation), occurring more days than not for at least 6 months, about a number of events or activities (such as work or school performance).
B. The person finds it difficult to control the worry.
C. The anxiety and worry are associated with three (or more) of the following six symptoms (with at least some symptoms present for more days than not for the past 6 months). **Note:** Only one item is required in children.
   (1) Restlessness or feeling keyed up or on edge
   (2) Being easily fatigued
   (3) Difficulty concentrating or mind going blank
   (4) Irritability
   (5) Muscle tension
   (6) Sleep disturbance (difficulty falling or staying asleep, or restless unsatisfying sleep)
D. The focus of the anxiety and worry is not confined to features of an Axis I disorder, e.g., the anxiety or worry is not about having a panic attack (as in panic disorder), being embarrassed in public (as in social phobia), being contaminated (as in obsessive-compulsive disorder), being away from home or close relatives (as in separation anxiety disorder), gaining weight (as in anorexia nervosa), having multiple physical complaints (as in somatization disorder), or having a serious illness (as in hypochondriasis), and the anxiety and worry do not occur exclusively during posttraumatic stress disorder.
E. The anxiety, worry, or physical symptoms cause clinically significant distress or impairment in social, occupational, or other important areas of functioning.
F. The disturbance is not due to the direct physiological effects of a substance (e.g., a drug of abuse, a medication) or a general medical condition (e.g., hyperthyroidism) and does not occur exclusively during a mood disorder, psychotic disorder, or a pervasive developmental disorder.

(From American Psychiatric Association. *Diagnostic and Statistical Manual of Mental Disorders.* 4th ed. Text rev. Washington, DC: American Psychiatric Association; 2000, with permission.)

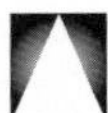

Table 50.3–3
DSM-IV-TR Diagnostic Criteria for Social Phobia

A. A marked and persistent fear of one or more social or performance situations in which the person is exposed to unfamiliar people or to possible scrutiny by others. The individual fears that he or she will act in a way (or show anxiety symptoms) that will be humiliating or embarrassing. **Note**: In children, there must be evidence of capacity for age-appropriate social relationships with familiar people and the anxiety must occur in peer settings, not just in interactions with adults.
B. Exposure to the feared social situation almost invariably provokes anxiety, which may take the form of a situationally bound or situationally predisposed panic attack. **Note**: In children, the anxiety may be expressed by crying, tantrums, freezing, or shrinking from social situations with unfamiliar people.
C. The person recognizes that the fear is excessive or unreasonable. **Note**: In children, this feature may be absent.
D. The feared social or performance situations are avoided, or else endured with intense anxiety or distress.
E. The avoidance, anxious anticipation, or distress in the feared social or performance situation(s) interferes significantly with the person's normal routine, occupational (academic) functioning, or social activities or relationships with others, or there is marked distress about having the phobia.
F. In individuals under age 18 years, the duration is at least 6 months.
G. The fear or avoidance is not due to the direct physiological effects of a substance (e.g., a drug of abuse, a medication) or a general medical condition, and is not better accounted for by another mental disorder (e.g., panic disorder with or without agoraphobia, separation anxiety disorder, body dysmorphic disorder, a pervasive developmental disorder, or schizoid personality disorder).
H. If a general medical condition or other mental disorder is present, the fear in Criterion A is unrelated to it, (e.g., the fear is not of stuttering, trembling in Parkinson's disease, or exhibiting abnormal eating behavior in anorexia nervosa or bulimia nervosa).

Specify if:
Generalized: If the fears include most social situations (also consider the additional diagnosis of avoidant personality disorder).

(From American Psychiatric Association. *Diagnostic and Statistical Manual of Mental Disorders.* 4th ed. Text rev. Washington, DC: American Psychiatric Association; 2000, with permission.)

In each of the above anxiety disorders, the child's experience can approach terror or panic. The distress is greater than that normally expected for the child's developmental level and cannot be explained by any other disorder. Morbid fears, preoccupations, and ruminations characterize separation anxiety disorder. Children with anxiety disorders overestimate the probability of danger and the likelihood of negative outcome. Children with separation anxiety disorder and generalized anxiety disorder become overly fearful that someone close to them will be hurt or that something terrible will happen to them or their families, especially when they are away from important caring figures. Many children with anxiety disorders are preoccupied with health and worry that their families or friends will become ill. Fears of getting lost, being kidnapped, and losing the ability to be in contact with their families are predominant among children with separation anxiety disorder.

Adolescents with anxiety disorders may not directly express their worries however; their behavior patterns often reflect either separation anxiety or other anxiety if they exhibit discomfort about leaving home, engage in solitary activities because of fears about how they will perform in front of peers, or have distress when away from their families. Separation anxiety disorder in children is often manifested at the thought of travel or in the course of travel away from home. Children may refuse to go to camp, a new school, or even a friend's house. Frequently, a continuum exists between mild anticipatory anxiety before separation from an important figure and pervasive anxiety after the separation has occurred. Premonitory signs include irritability, difficulty eating, whining, staying in a room alone, clinging to parents, and following a parent everywhere. Often, when a family moves, a child displays separation anxiety by intense clinging to the mother figure. Sometimes, geographical relocation anxiety is expressed in feelings of acute homesickness or psychophysiological symptoms that break out when the child is away from home or is going to a new country. The child yearns to return home and becomes preoccupied with fantasies of how much better the old home was. Integration into the new life situation

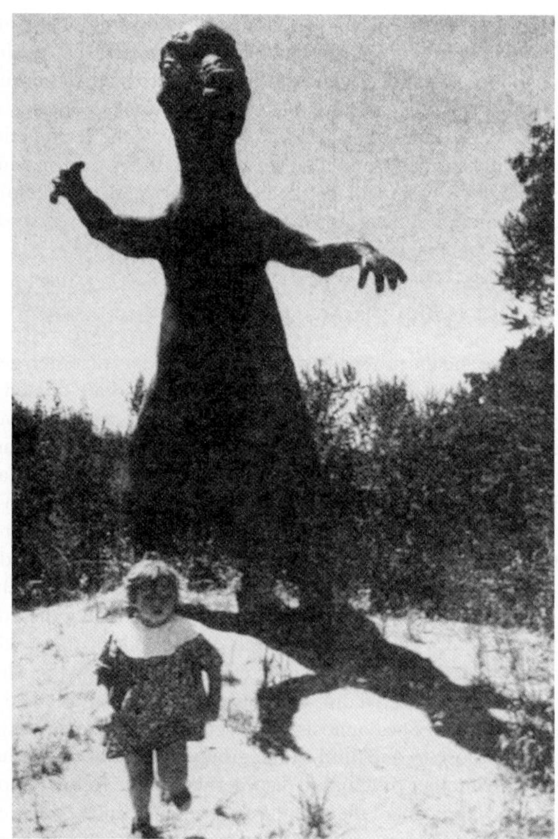

FIGURE 50.3–1
This surrealistic photograph symbolically represents the anxiety in a childhood nightmare. (Courtesy of Arthur Tress for Magnum Photos, Inc.)

may become extremely difficult. Children with anxiety disorders may retreat from social or group activities and express feelings of loneliness because of their self-imposed isolation.

Sleep difficulties are frequent in children and adolescents with any anxiety disorder or in severe separation anxiety; a child or adolescent may require having someone remain with him or her until he or she falls asleep. An anxious child may awaken and go to a parent's bed or even sleep at the parents' door in an effort to diminish anxiety. Nightmares and morbid fears may be expressions of anxiety (Fig. 50.3–1).

Associated features of anxiety disorders include fear of the dark and imaginary, bizarre worries. Children may have the feeling that eyes are staring at them and monsters reaching out for them in their bedrooms. Children with anxiety disorders often complain of somatic symptoms and are very sensitive to changes in their bodies. They are often more sensitive than peers and more easily brought to tears. Frequent somatic complaints include gastrointestinal symptoms, nausea, vomiting, and stomachaches; unexplained pain in various parts of the body; sore throats; and flu-like symptoms. Older children typically complain of somatic experiences classically reported by adults with anxiety, such as cardiovascular and respiratory symptoms—palpitations, dizziness, faintness, and feelings of strangulation. Physiologic signs of anxiety are a part of the diagnostic criteria for generalized anxiety disorder, but they are more often also experienced by children with separation anxiety and social phobia than the general population. The most common anxiety disorder that coexists with separation anxiety disorder is specific phobia, which occurs in about one third of referred cases of separation anxiety disorder.

Julie T was an 11-year-old girl referred for an evaluation by her pediatrician based on concern that the source of her chronic gastrointestinal complaints was anxiety. On interview, Julie was meek but responsive to questions. She endorsed a number of worries that included concerns about her health, her parents' safety, her school performance, and her peer relationships. Julie's greatest worries were related to threats to her health and safety. Julie's mother, Mrs. T, reported that Julie had recently been very reluctant to play outside, because she feared she would contract Lyme disease from a tick bite or West Nile virus from a mosquito bite. Mrs. T reported that Julie was also very distressed by news reports about negative events locally and around the world (e.g., kidnapping, crime, terrorism) and that they no longer have the news on when Julie is home. Mrs. T described her as overly conscientious about her schoolwork and as often being concerned about adult matters (e.g., finances, parents' job security). Symptoms that accompanied Julie's worries primarily involved stomach pain and problems falling asleep. Julie's mother stated that, when worrying about something, Julie tended to be quite perseverative; worrying even after reassurance was given. Julie said that she worried often and could not "turn off" her worried thoughts.

Julie was the product of a normal pregnancy and delivery. Her medical history was unremarkable, with the exception of frequent gastrointestinal pain since kindergarten. Julie was described as irritable and difficult to soothe as an infant. Developmental milestones were met within normal limits. She was described as very obedient and had no history of externalizing behavior problems. She was very concerned about her academic performance from an early age and earned A's with an occasional B. Julie was somewhat shy in social situations but well liked by her peers. Family history included depression in her maternal grandmother and a maternal history of separation anxiety disorder as a child. Julie had two younger siblings who were high functioning and without notable problems. (Courtesy of Gail A. Bernstein, M.D., and Ann E. Layne, Ph.D.)

Tina is an 11-year-old 6th grader who lives with her biological parents and two sisters, age 9 and 14 years. Tina is a very articulate girl who has always been a good student, although she never volunteers answers in school unless she is called on by her teacher. She gets along well with her sisters when at home, but since she entered middle school this school year, she has declined invitations to go to friend's homes, has turned down opportunities to go to parties, and has even stopped going on outings with her sisters to the neighborhood mall and the movies. Tina reports that she gets too nervous, and blushes when she is with friends outside of the classroom at school because she can't think of anything to say to them. She reports that she is embarrassed to go shopping or to the movies with her sisters because they often run into neighborhood peers along the way, stop to chat, and this makes her feel "stupid" because she does not say anything, and believes that her sisters' friends will laugh at her shyness. Recently, one of her best friends from the 5th grade confronted her about why she had stopped "hanging out" with her and their other friends. Tina stopped eating lunch with her friends in school because she felt humiliated when they would talk about their weekend plans and even when they invited her to join, she would just look the other way and ignore the conversation. Tina was becoming more isolated, even in school, and admitted to her sister that she was lonely. Tina was brought for an evaluation after her older sister told her mother that Tina was spending all of her time alone whenever her sisters saw their friends, and that she looked sad and stressed out whenever she was around peers. Tina was in good spirits and had fun whenever her sisters stayed home and played with her, but this was becoming rarer because both of her sisters liked being with their own friends. On various occasions Tina's older sister had offered to accompany Tina to parties or to friend's homes, but Tina had declined and burst into tears.

Tina was evaluated by a child psychiatrist who made the diagnosis of social phobia and described a range of treatment options, including cognitive-behavioral therapy (CBT) and a trial of a serotonin reuptake inhibitor agent such as fluvoxamine (Luvox). Tina and her family discussed the options and decided to try the medication. Tina was started on 50 mg of fluvoxamine and over the next month was titrated to a dose of 200 mg. By the third week of the medication trial, Tina was noticeably less resistant to going out with her sisters to places where they were likely to encounter peers. Her sisters noticed that she did not seem as stressed, and started to eat lunch with her friends in the school cafeteria. She stated that she did not feel as self-conscious as she used to in class and was willing to go to a friend's house. She still declined to go to a birthday party of a classmate that she didn't know very well. Tina continued on this dose of medication and within 2 months, she was significantly less anxious in social situations. She complained occasionally of a stomachache, but overall tolerated the medication well. Her family was impressed when she requested they plan a large birthday party for her 12th birthday and decided to invite 25 peers.

Pathology and Laboratory Examination

No specific laboratory measures help in the diagnosis of separation anxiety disorder.

DIFFERENTIAL DIAGNOSIS

Because some degree of separation anxiety is a normal phenomenon in a very young child, clinical judgment must be used in distinguishing normal anxiety from separation anxiety disorder in this age group. In older school-age children, it is apparent when a child is experiencing more than normal distress when school is refused on a regular basis. For children who resist school, it is important to distinguish whether fear of separation, general worry about performance, or more specific fears of humiliation in front of peers or the teacher are driving the resistance. In many cases in which anxiety is the primary obstacle, all three of the above feared scenarios come into play. In generalized anxiety disorder, anxiety is not focused on separation. In pervasive developmental disorders and schizophrenia, anxiety about separation may occur but is viewed as caused by these conditions rather than being a separate disorder. When depressive disorders occur in children, the comorbid diagnosis of separation anxiety disorder should also be made when the criteria for both disorders are met; the two diagnoses often coexist. Panic disorder with agoraphobia is uncommon before 18 years of age; the fear is of being incapacitated by a panic attack rather than of separation from parental figures. In some adult cases, however, many symptoms of separation anxiety disorder may be present. In conduct disorder, truancy is common, but children stay away from home and do not have anxiety about separation. School refusal is a frequent symptom in separation anxiety disorder, but is not pathognomonic of it. Children with other diagnoses, such as simple phobias, social phobias, or fear of failure in school because of learning disorder, also evince school refusal. When school refusal occurs in an adolescent, the severity of the dysfunction is generally greater than when separation anxiety emerges in a young child. Similar and distinguishing characteristics of childhood separation anxiety disorder, generalized anxiety disorder and social phobia are presented in Table 50.3–4.

COURSE AND PROGNOSIS

The course and the prognosis of separation anxiety disorder, generalized anxiety, and social phobia are varied and are related to the age of onset, the duration of the symptoms, and the development of comorbid anxiety and depressive disorders. Young children who can maintain attendance in school, after-school activities, and peer relationships generally have a better prognosis than children or adolescents who refuse to attend school or drop out of social activities. A follow-up study of children and adolescents with anxiety disorders over a 3-year period reported that up to 82 percent no longer met criteria for the anxiety disorder at follow-up. Of the group followed, 96 percent of those with separation anxiety disorder had a remission at follow-up. Most children who recovered did so within the first year. Early age of onset and later age at diagnosis were factors that predicted slower recovery. Close to one third of the group studied, however, had developed another psychiatric disorder within the follow-up period, and 50 percent of these children developed another anxiety disorder. Reports have indicated a significant overlap of separation anxiety disorder and depressive disorders. In these complicated cases, the prognosis is guarded. Most follow-up studies have methodological problems and are limited to hospitalized, school-phobic children, not children with separation anxiety disorder per se. Little is reported about the outcome of mild cases, whether children are seen in outpatient treatment or receive no treatment. Notwithstanding the limitations of the studies, reports indicate that some children with severe school phobia continue to resist attending school for many years.

During the 1970s, it was reported that many adult women with agoraphobia had suffered from separation anxiety disorder in childhood. Research indicates that children with anxiety disorders are at increased risk for adult anxiety disorders, although the specific link between separation anxiety disorder in childhood and agoraphobia in adulthood has not been established clearly. Studies do indicate that anxious parents are at increased risk of having children with anxiety disorders. In recent years, some cases of children with both panic disorder and separation anxiety disorder have been reported.

TREATMENT

The treatment of separation anxiety disorder, generalized anxiety disorder, and social phobia are often considered together, given the frequent comorbidity and overlapping symptomatology of these disorders. A multimodal comprehensive treatment approach may include CBT, family education, family psychosocial intervention, and pharmacologic interventions. A trial of CBT may be applied first, if available, when a child is able to function sufficiently well to engage in daily activities while obtaining

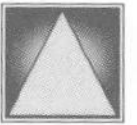

Table 50.3–4
Common Characteristics of Selected Anxiety Disorders That Occur in Children

Criteria	Separation Anxiety Disorder	Social Phobia	Generalized Anxiety Disorder
Minimal duration to establish diagnosis	At least 4 weeks	No minimum	At least 6 months
Age of onset	Preschool to 18 years	Not specified	Not specified
Precipitating stresses	Separation from significant parental figures, other losses, travel	Pressure for social participation with peers	Unusual pressure for performance, damage to self-esteem, feelings of lack of competence
Peer relationships	Good when no separation is involved	Tentative, overly inhibited	Overly eager to please, peers sought out and dependent relationships established
Sleep	Reluctance or refusal to go to sleep, fear of dark, nightmares	Difficulty in falling asleep at times	Difficulty in falling asleep
Psychophysiological symptoms	Complaints of stomachaches, nausea, vomiting, flu-like symptoms, headaches, palpitations, dizziness, faintness	Blushing, body tension	Stomachaches, nausea, vomiting, lump in the throat, shortness of breath, dizziness, palpitations
Differential diagnosis	Generalized anxiety disorder, schizophrenia, depressive disorders, conduct disorder, pervasive developmental disorders, major depressive disorder, panic disorder with agoraphobia	Adjustment disorder with depressed mood, generalized anxiety disorder, separation anxiety disorder, major depressive disorder, dysthymic disorder, avoidant personality disorder, borderline personality disorder	Separation anxiety disorder, attention-deficit/hyperactivity disorder, social phobia, adjustment disorder with anxiety, obsessive-compulsive disorder, psychotic disorders, mood disorders

Adapted from Sidney Werkman, M.D.

this treatment. At the present time, evidence from a recent large mutisite National Institute of Mental Health investigation (Research Units in Pediatric Psychopharmacology [RUPP]) confirms the safety and efficacy of fluvoxamine (Luvox) in the treatment of childhood separation anxiety disorder, generalized anxiety disorder, and social phobia. This double-blind, placebo controlled study of 128 children and adolescents revealed 76 percent of children in the group treated with fluvoxamine showed significant improvement compared with 29 percent of those in the placebo group. Response to medication was noticeable after as little as 2 weeks of treatment. Fluvoxamine dosages ranged from 50 mg to 250 mg per day in children and up to 300 mg per day in adolescents. Children and adolescents with less comorbid depressive symptoms had the best response. Children and adolescents who responded to this medication were continued on fluvoxamine for a period of 6 months and almost all of them continued to be responders at the 6-month mark. Several other randomized clinical trials have also supported the efficacy of selective serotonin reuptake inhibitor (SSRI) medications in the treatment of child and adolescent anxiety disorders. A recent trial showed fluoxetine, at a dose of 20 mg per day, to be safe and effective for children with these disorders, with minor side effects, including gastrointestinal distress, headache, and drowsiness. Additionally, a randomized clinical trial for the treatment of generalized anxiety disorder in children lends support for the efficacy of sertraline (Zoloft). Finally, a large industry randomized clinical trial of paroxetine (Paxil) in the treatment of children with social phobia found that paroxetine was associated with response in 78 percent of children treated. Paroxetine was utilized at a dosage range of 10 mg per day to 50 mg per day. The US Food and Drug Administration (FDA) has placed a "black box" warning on antidepressants, including all of the SSRI agents, used in the treatment of any childhood disorder, because of concerns about increased suicidality; however, no individual childhood anxiety study has found a statistically significant increase in suicidal thoughts or behaviors. Clearly, SSRI medications have been shown to be both safe and efficacious in the treatment of childhood anxiety disorders, yet the evidence is not yet in whether the optimal treatment approach is to administer CBT first, medication first, or both simultaneously. An ongoing National Institute of Mental Health (NIMH)-funded Child/Adolescent Anxiety Multimodal Treatment Study (CAMS) is investigating these questions. This double-blind, placebo controlled study, in progress now, includes over 300 children and adolescents with separation anxiety disorder, generalized anxiety disorder, or social phobia who are being treated with either sertraline alone, CBT alone, both CBT and medication, or placebo. This is the first large scale study to investigate the combination of therapeutic interventions compared with each condition alone in the treatment of child and adolescent anxiety disorders. The data from this study will be available within the next few years so that optimal treatment strategies can be designed for anxiety disorders in childhood. Without evidence to support clinical decisions, pharmacological interventions have historically been recommended as second-line treatments when psychosocial strategies have not been effective. Cognitive-behavioral therapy is currently widely accepted as a first-line treatment for a variety of anxiety disorders for children, including separation anxiety disorder, social phobia, and selective mutism. Specific cognitive strategies and relaxation

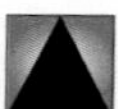

Table 50.3–5
ICD-10 Diagnostic Criteria for Emotional Disorders with Onset Specific to Childhood

Note. Phobic anxiety disorder of childhood, social anxiety disorder of childhood, and general anxiety disorder of childhood have obvious similarities to some of the disorders in neurotic, stress-related and somatoform disorders, but current evidence and opinion suggest that there are sufficient differences in the ways that anxiety disorders present in children for additional categories to be provided. Further studies should show whether descriptions and definitions can be developed that can be used satisfactorily for both adults and children, or whether the present distinction should be preserved.

Separation anxiety disorder of childhood

A. At least three of the following must be present:
  (1) unrealistic and persistent worry about possible harm befalling major attachment figures or about the loss of such figures (e.g., fear that they will leave and not return or that the child will not see them again), or persistent concerns about the death of attachment figures;
  (2) unrealistic and persistent worry that some untoward event will separate the child from a major attachment figure (e.g., the child getting lost, being kidnapped, admitted to hospital, or killed);
  (3) persistent reluctance or refusal to go to school because of fear over separation from a major attachment figure or in order to stay at home (rather than for other reasons such as fear over events at school);
  (4) difficulty in separating at night, as manifested by any of the following:
    (a) persistent reluctance or refusal to go to sleep without being near an attachment figure;
    (b) getting up frequently during the night to check on, or to sleep near, an attachment figure;
    (c) persistent reluctance or refusal to sleep away from home
  (5) persistent inappropriate fear of being alone, or otherwise without the major attachment figure, at home during the day;
  (6) repeated nightmares involving themes of separation;
  (7) repeated occurrence of physical symptoms (such as nausea, stomachache, headache, or vomiting) on occasions that involve separation from a major attachment figure, such as leaving home to go to school or on other occasions involving separation (holidays, camps, etc.).
  (8) excessive, recurrent distress in anticipation of, during, or immediately after separation from a major attachment figure (as shown by: anxiety, crying, tantrums; persistent reluctance to go away from home; excessive need to talk with parents or desire to return home; misery, apathy, or social withdrawal).

B. The criteria for generalized anxiety disorder of childhood are not met.
C. Onset is before the age of 6 years.
D. The disorder does not occur as part of a broader disturbance of emotions, conduct, or personality or of a pervasive developmental disorder, psychotic disorder, or psychoactive substance use disorder.
E. Duration of the disorder is at least 4 weeks.

Phobic anxiety disorder of childhood

A. The individual manifests a persistent or recurrent fear (phobia) that is developmentally phase-appropriate (or was so at the time of onset) but that is abnormal in degree and is associated with significant social impairment.
B. The criteria for generalized anxiety disorder of childhood are not met.
C. The disorder does not occur as part of a broader disturbance of emotions, conduct, or personality or of a pervasive developmental disorder, psychotic disorder, or psychoactive substance use disorder.
D. Duration of the disorder is at least 4 weeks.

Social anxiety disorder of childhood

A. Persistent anxiety in social situations in which the child is exposed to unfamiliar people, including peers, is manifested by socially avoidant behavior.
B. The child exhibits self-consciousness, embarrassment, or over-concern about the appropriateness of his or her behavior when interacting with unfamiliar figures.
C. There is significant interference with social (including peer) relationships, which are consequently restricted; when new or forced social situations are experienced, they cause marked distress and discomfort as manifested by crying, lack of spontaneous speech, or withdrawal from the social situation.
D. The child has satisfying social relationships with familiar figures (family members or peers that he or she knows well).
E. Onset of the disorder generally coincides with a developmental phase in which these anxiety reactions are considered appropriate. The abnormal degree, persistence over time, and associated impairment must be manifest before the age of 6 years.
F. The criteria for generalized anxiety disorder of childhood are not met.
G. The disorder does not occur as part of broader disturbances of emotions, conduct, or personality or of a pervasive developmental disorder, psychotic disorder, or psychoactive substance use disorder.
H. Duration of the disorder is at least 4 weeks.

Sibling rivalry disorder

A. The child has abnormally intense negative feelings toward an immediately younger sibling.
B. Emotional disturbance is shown by regression, tantrums, dysphoria, sleep difficulties, oppositional behavior, or attention-seeking behavior with one or both parents (two or more of these must be present).
C. Onset is within 6 months of the birth of an immediately younger sibling.
D. Duration of the disorder is at least 4 weeks.

Other childhood emotional disorders

Generalized anxiety disorder of childhood

Note: In children and adolescents, the range of complaints by which the general anxiety is manifest is often more limited than in adults (see Generalized anxiety disorder), and the specific symptoms of autonomic arousal are often less prominent. For these individuals, the following alternative set of criteria can be used if preferred:

A. Extensive anxiety and worry (apprehensive expectation) occur on at least half of the total number of days over a period of at least 6 months, the anxiety and worry referring to at least several events or activities (such as work or school performance).
B. The individual finds it difficult to control the worry.
C. The anxiety and worry are associated with at least three of the following symptoms (with at least two symptoms present on at least half of the total number of days):
  (1) restlessness, feeling "keyed up" or "on edge" (as shown, for example, by feelings of mental tension combined with an inability to relax);
  (2) feeling tired, "worn out," or easily fatigued because of worry or anxiety;
  (3) difficulty in concentrating or mind "going blank";
  (4) irritability;
  (5) muscle tension;
  (6) sleep disturbance (difficulty in falling or staying asleep, or restless, unsatisfying sleep) because of worry or anxiety.

(*continued*)

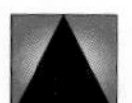

Table 50.3–5 (Continued)

D. The multiple anxieties and worries occur across at least two situations, activities, contexts, or circumstances. Generalized anxiety does not present as discrete paroxysmal episodes (as in panic disorder), nor are the main worries confined to a single, major theme (as in separation anxiety disorder or phobic disorder of childhood). (When more focused anxiety is identified in the broader context of a generalized anxiety, generalized anxiety disorder takes precedence over other anxiety disorders.)
E. Onset occurs in childhood or adolescence (before the age of 18 years).
F. The anxiety, worry, or physical symptoms cause clinically significant distress or impairment in social, occupational, or other important areas of functioning.
G. The disorder is not due to the direct effects of a substance (e.g., psychoactive substances, medication) or a general medical condition (e.g., hperthyroidism) and does not occur exclusively during a mood disorder, psyhotic disorder, or pervasive developmental disorder.

Childhood emotional disorder, unspecified

(From World Health Organization. *The ICD-10 Classification of Mental and Behavioural Disorders: Diagnostic Criteria for Research*. Copyright, World Health Organization, Geneva, 1993, with permission.)

exercises may also be added components of treatment for some children as self-contained strategies to control their own anxiety. Family interventions are also frequently critical in the management of separation anxiety disorder, especially in children who refuse to attend school, so that firm encouragement of school attendance is maintained while appropriate support is also provided.

Pharmacologic management of childhood anxiety disorders in clinical practice often includes the use of agents even when no evidence base exists for such management. Current widely recommended SSRIs include fluoxetine, fluvoxamine, sertraline, paroxetine, and citalopram (Celexa). Tricyclic drugs are not currently recommended due to their potentially serious cardiac adverse effects. β-adrenergic receptor antagonists, such as propranolol (Inderal), and buspirone (BuSpar) have been used clinically in children with anxiety disorders, but currently no data support their efficacy. Diphenhydramine (Benadryl) may be used in the short term to control sleep disturbances in children with anxiety disorders. Open trials and one double-blind, placebo-controlled study suggested that alprazolam (Xanax), a benzodiazepine, may help to control anxiety symptoms in separation anxiety disorder. Clonazepam (Klonopin) has been studied in open trials and may be useful in controlling symptoms of panic and other anxiety symptoms.

School refusal associated with separation anxiety disorder can be viewed as a psychiatric emergency. A comprehensive treatment plan involves the child, the parents, and the child's peers and school. The child should be encouraged to attend school, but when a return to a full school day is overwhelming, a program should be arranged so the child can progressively increase the time spent at school. Graded contact with an object of anxiety is a form of behavior modification that can be applied to any type of separation anxiety. Some severe cases of school refusal require hospitalization. Cognitive-behavioral modalities include exposure to feared separations and cognitive strategies, such as coping self-statements aimed at increasing a sense of autonomy and mastery.

ICD-10

The 10th revision of *International Statistical Classification of Diseases and Related Health Problems* (ICD-10) includes a category for emotional disorders with onset specific to childhood. This category contains five specific childhood-onset anxiety disorders and one residual diagnosis (Table 50.3–5). According to ICD-10, several reasons exist for traditionally differentiating emotional disorders specific to childhood and adolescence from those of adulthood. First, research has consistently shown that most children with emotional disorders become normal adults and that many adult emotional disorders have an onset in adult life and lack precursors in childhood. Second, many emotional disorders of childhood appear to be exaggerations of normal developmental trends rather than abnormalities. Third, the mental mechanisms of childhood emotional disorders are believed often to differ from those of adult disorders; this point, however, has not been verified empirically. Finally, childhood emotional disorders are less clearly separated into specific categories, such as phobic or obsessional disorders, but epidemiological data suggest that this distinction is only relative because it is often difficult to differentiate adult disorders as well. Thus, the second feature, developmental appropriateness, is the key factor in diagnosing differences between disorders with specific childhood onset and the neurotic disorders in general; some empirical evidence supports this hypothesis.

References

Angold A, Egger HL. Psychiatric diagnosis in preschool children. In: DelCarmen-Wiggins R, Carter A, eds. *Handbook of Infant, Toddler, and Preschool Mental Health Assessment*. New York: Oxford University Press; 2004;123.

Birmaher B, Axelson DA, Monk K, Kalas C, Clark DB, Ehmann M, Bridge J, Heo J, Brent DA. Fluvoxamine for the treatment of childhood anxiety disorders. *J Am Acad Child Adolesc Psychiatry*. 2003;42:415.

Clark DT, Birmaher B, Axelson D, Monk K, Kalas C, Ehmann M, Bridge J, Wood DS, Muthen B, Brent D. Fluoxetine for the treatment of childhood anxiety disorders: Open-label, long-term, extension to a controlled trial. *J Am Acad Child Adolesc Psychiatry*. 2005;44:1263.

Costello EJ, Egger HL, Angold A. The developmental epidemiology of anxiety disorders: phenomenology, prevalence, and comorbidity. *Child Adolesc Psychiatric Clin N Am*. 2005;14:631.

Gibbons RD, Jur K, Bhaumik DK, Mann JJ. The relationship between antidepressant medication use and rate of suicide. *Arch Gen Psychiatry*. 2005;62:165.

Hanna GL, Fischer DJ, Fluent TE. Separation anxiety disorder and school refusal in children and adolescents. *Pediatr Rev*. 2006;27:56–63.

Hudson JL, Deveney C, Taylor L. Nature, assessment, and treatment of generalized anxiety disorder in children. *Pediatr Ann*. 2005;34(2):97–106.

Kearney CA. *Social Anxiety and Social Phobia in Youth: Characteristics, Assessment, and Psychological Treatment*. New York : Springer; 2005.

Reinblatt SP, Walkup JT. Psychopharmacologic treatment of pediatric anxiety disorders. *Child Adolesc Psychiatric Clin N Am*. 2005;14:877.

Vanderwerker LC, Jacobs SC, Parkes CM, Prigerson HG. An exploration of associations between separation anxiety in childhood and complicated grief in later life. *J Nerv Ment Dis*. 2006;194(2):121–123.

Wagner KD, Berard R, Stein MB, Wetherhold E, Carpenter DJ, Perera P, Gee M, Davy K, Machin A. A multicenter, randomized, double-blind, placebo controlled

trial of paroxetine in children and adolescents with social anxiety disorder. *Arch Gen Psychiatry*. 2004;61:1153.
Waslick B. Psychopharmacology intervention for pediatric anxiety disorders: a research update. *Child Adolesc Psychiatr Clin Am*. 2006;1:51.

▲ 50.4 Selective Mutism

Selective mutism is characterized in a child by persistent failure to speak in one or more specific social situations, most typically including the school setting. A child with selective mutism may remain completely silent or near silent, in some cases whispering instead of speaking out loud. The most recent conceptualization of selective mutism highlights the relationship between underlying social anxiety and the resulting failure to speak. Most children with the disorder are completely silent during the stressful situations, whereas some may verbalize almost inaudibly single-syllable words. Children with selective mutism are fully capable of speaking competently when not in a socially anxiety-producing situation. Some children with the disorder communicate with eye contact or nonverbal gestures. These children speak fluently in other situations, such as at home and in certain familiar settings. Selective mutism is believed to be an expression of social phobia because of its expression in selective social situations.

EPIDEMIOLOGY

The prevalence of selective mutism varies with age, with younger children at increased risk for the disorder. One epidemiologic study utilizing text revision of the fourth edition of *Diagnostic and Statistical Manual of Mental Disorders* (DSM-IV-TR) criteria reported a rate of selective mutism in preschoolers to be 0.6 percent. Another large epidemiologic survey in the United Kingdom reported a prevalence rate of selective mutism to be 0.69 percent in children 4 to 5 years of age, which dropped to 0.8 percent near the end of the same academic year. Another survey in the United Kingdom identified 0.06 percent of 7-year-olds as having selective mutism. Selective mutism has been estimated to range between 3 and 8 per 10,000 children. Some surveys indicate that it may occur in up to 0.5 percent of schoolchildren in the community. Young children are more vulnerable to the disorder than older ones. Selective mutism appears to be more common in girls than in boys.

ETIOLOGY

Genetic Contribution

Over the last two decades the conceptualization of selective mutism has evolved from one that focused on oppositionality or childhood trauma as possible contributing factors to current consensus that it has the same etiologic factors leading to the emergence of social phobia. Those, which include genetic factors leading to social phobia and other comorbid anxiety disorders, have histories of delayed onset of speech or speech abnormalities that may be contributory. In a recent survey, 90 percent of children with selective mutism met diagnostic criteria for social phobia. These children showed high levels of social anxiety without notable psychopathology in other areas, according to parent and teacher ratings. Thus, selective mutism may not represent a distinct disorder, but may be better conceptualized as a subtype of social phobia. Similar to families with children who exhibit other anxiety disorders, maternal anxiety, depression, and heightened dependence needs are often noted in families of children with selective mutism.

Parental Interactions

Given the likely higher levels of anxiety disorders in parents of children with selective mutism, anxiety tinged interpersonal interactions between parents and child may unwittingly serve to promote social anxiety in children with selective mutism. Maternal overprotection and an overly close, but ambivalent, relationship between parents and a selectively mute child may promote symptoms. Children with selective mutism usually speak freely at home; and only exhibit symptoms when under social pressure either in school or other social situations. Some children seem predisposed to selective mutism after early emotional or physical trauma; thus, some clinicians refer to the phenomenon as *traumatic mutism* rather than selective mutism.

Speech and Language Factors

Selective mutism is a psychologically determined inhibition or refusal to speak, yet a higher than expected proportion of children with the disorder have a history of speech delay. An interesting finding suggests that children with selective mutism are at higher risk for a disturbance in auditory processing, which may interfere with efficient processing of incoming sounds. For the most part, however, speech and language problems in children with selective mutism are subtle and are exclusionary criteria for the diagnosis of selective mutism.

DIAGNOSIS AND CLINICAL FEATURES

The diagnostic criteria from DSM-IV-TR appear in Table 50.4–1. The diagnosis of selective mutism is not difficult to make after it is clear that a child has adequate language skills

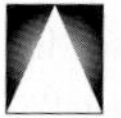

Table 50.4–1
DSM-IV-TR Diagnostic Criteria for Selective Mutism

A. Consistent failure to speak in specific social situations (in which there is an expectation for speaking, e.g., at school) despite speaking in other situations.
B. The disturbance interferes with educational or occupational achievement or with social communication.
C. The duration of the disturbance is at least 1 month (not limited to the first month of school).
D. The failure to speak is not due to a lack of knowledge of, or comfort with, the spoken language required in the social situation.
E. The disturbance is not better accounted for by a communication disorder (e.g., stuttering) and does not occur exclusively during the course of a pervasive developmental disorder, schizophrenia, or other psychotic disorder.

(From American Psychiatric Association. *Diagnostic and Statistical Manual of Mental Disorders*. 4th ed. Text rev. Washington, DC: American Psychiatric Association; copyright 2000, with permission.)

in some environments but not in others. The mutism may have developed gradually or suddenly after a disturbing experience. The age of onset can range from 4 to 8 years. Mute periods are most commonly manifested in school or outside the home; in rare cases, a child is mute at home but not in school. Children who exhibit selective mutism may also have symptoms of separation anxiety disorder, school refusal, and delayed language acquisition. Because social anxiety is almost always present in children with selective mutism, behavioral disturbances, such as temper tantrums and oppositional behaviors, may also occur in the home.

Beth is a 5-year-old Vietnamese-American girl who lives with her biological mother, father, and siblings. Beth's parents reported a 2-year history of not speaking at school (preschool) or to any children or adults outside of her family, despite speaking normally at home. At home, she reportedly is animated and quite talkative with her immediate family and a few young cousins as well. Although she speaks to adult relatives outside of her immediate family, her communication is often limited to one-word responses to their questions. By her parents' report, Beth also exhibits extreme social anxiety, to the point of "freezing" in certain situations when attention is focused on her. At the time of her evaluation, Beth had not received prior treatment for selective mutism or any other emotional or behavioral disorders. Beth speaks fluent English, as well as Vietnamese, and, according to her parents, met all developmental milestones on time and appears to have above-average intelligence. They also reported that Beth enjoys dancing, singing, and imaginative play with her sisters.

During initial evaluation, Beth failed to make eye contact or respond in any way to the intake clinician. Beth's parents reported that this behavior is typical of her when in a new situation with new people but that she communicates nonverbally and makes eye contact with most people once she "gets to know them." On request, Beth's parents provided a videotaped recording of Beth playing at home with her sisters. In this video, Beth appeared animated and was speaking spontaneously and fluently without obvious impairment. Beth received diagnoses of selective mutism (severe) and social phobia (moderately severe). Behavioral treatment was recommended at this time.

Behavioral treatment was initiated after the intake evaluation. Initially, the therapist instructed Beth and her mother to come up with lists of easy, medium, and hard speaking situations and lists of small, medium, and large rewards. These lists then became the basis for assignments (and reinforcement) for speaking tasks that gradually increased in difficulty. In general, sessions included time with Beth and her mother together to review past and future assignments and time with Beth and the therapist alone.

When treatment began, Beth did not communicate at all verbally or nonverbally with the therapist. The therapist gradually increased rapport (via unstructured play) while having Beth try increasingly difficult tasks, such as first whispering to her mother with the therapist in the corner, then nodding yes or no, pointing, whispering to a stuffed animal, whispering to her mother while facing the therapist, and then subsequently responding to the therapist directly. A successful technique in working with Beth was the use of pretend play; the therapist often used several puppets as additional "participants" in the treatment. Talking to, for, or about these animals in the context of pretend play provided Beth with a good "warm-up" period and facilitated talking. After three sessions, Beth consistently and spontaneously talked to the therapist. Beth received stickers for completing each speaking assignment, and, after filling up sticker charts, she received rewards (small toy or treat from reward list).

Beth was also given assignments that involved her teacher and classmates. These were implemented in gradual fashion and included waving to the teacher, playing an audiotape of her saying "hello" to the teacher, whispering "hello" to the teacher, speaking "hello" to the teacher in a regular voice, and so on. After approximately 14 sessions, Beth spoke a complete sentence in front of the class when called on and spoke to her teacher in front of several other students.

During the last few sessions, which were tapered over several weeks, Beth's mother took an increasingly primary role in assigning and following up on speaking assignments. Beth entered kindergarten and, after only a few days, began regularly speaking to her teacher (both privately and in front of peers) and to most peers in class. After completion of therapy, the mother continued to monitor Beth's speaking behaviors and to promote speaking in new situations by encouraging (and rewarding) Beth's gradual successes with novel people and situations. (Courtesy of R. Lindsey Bergman, Ph.D. and John Piacentini, Ph.D.)

Pathology and Laboratory Examination

No specific laboratory measures are useful in the diagnosis or treatment of selective mutism.

DIFFERENTIAL DIAGNOSIS

Differential diagnosis of children who are silent in social situations emphasizes ruling out pervasive developmental disorders, such as autism. Once it is confirmed that the child is fully capable of speaking in certain situations which are comfortable, but not in school and other social situations, an anxiety-related disorder comes to mind. Shy children may exhibit a transient muteness in new, anxiety-provoking situations. These children often have histories of not speaking in the presence of strangers and of clinging to their mothers. Most children who are mute on entering school improve spontaneously and may be described as having transient adaptational shyness. Selective mutism must also be distinguished from mental retardation, pervasive developmental disorders, and expressive language disorder. In these disorders, the symptoms are widespread, and no one situation exists in which the child communicates normally; the child may have an inability, rather than a refusal, to speak. In mutism secondary to conversion disorder, the mutism is pervasive. Children introduced into an environment in which a different language is spoken may be reticent to begin using the new language. Selective mutism should be diagnosed only when children also refuse to converse in their native language and when they have gained communicative competence in the new language but refuse to speak it.

COURSE AND PROGNOSIS

Many very young children with early symptoms of selective mutism in the transitional period when entering preschool may have a spontaneous improvement over a number of months and never fulfill criteria for the full disorder. Children with selective mutism are often abnormally shy during preschool years, but the onset of the full disorder is usually not until age 5 or 6 years. The most common pattern is that children speak almost exclusively at home with the nuclear family but not elsewhere, especially not at school. Consequently, they may have academic difficulties and even failure. Children with selective mutism are generally shy, anxious, and vulnerable to the development of depression. Most children with mild forms of anxiety disorder, including selective mutism, remit with or without treatment. With recent data suggesting that fluoxetine (Prozac) may influence the course of selective mutism, recovery may be enhanced. Children in whom the disorder persists often have difficulty forming social relationships. Teasing and scapegoating by peers may cause them to refuse to go to school. Some children with this severe social phobia are characterized by rigidity, compulsive traits, negativism, temper tantrums, and oppositional and aggressive behavior at home. Other children with the disorder tolerate the feared situation better by communicating with gestures, such as nodding, shaking the head, and saying "Uh-huh" or "No." Most cases last for only a few weeks or months, but some cases persist for years. In one follow-up study, about one half of the children improved within 5 to 10 years. Children who do not improve by age 10 years appear to have a long-term course and a worse prognosis than those who do improve by age 10. As many as one third of children with selective mutism, with or without treatment, may develop other psychiatric disorders, particularly other anxiety disorders and depression.

TREATMENT

Published data on the successful treatment of children with selective mutism is very scant, yet solid evidence indicates that children with social phobia respond to various selective serotonin reuptake inhibitor agents (SSRIs) and, currently, cognitive behavior treatments are under investigation in a multisite, randomized placebo-controlled trial of children with anxiety disorders.

In the absence of data to support an approach utilizing therapy or medication alone or in combination, a multimodal approach using psychoeducation for the family, cognitive-behavioral therapy, and SSRI medication as needed, is recommended. Preschool children may also benefit from a therapeutic nursery. For school-age children, individual cognitive-behavioral therapy is recommended as a first-line treatment. Family education and cooperation are beneficial. SSRI medication is now an accepted component of treatment when psychosocial interventions do not suffice to manage symptoms.

A recent report of 21 children with selective mutism treated in an open trial with fluoxetine suggested that this medication may be effective for childhood selective mutism. Reports have confirmed the efficacy of fluoxetine in the treatment of adult social phobia and in at least one double-blind, placebo-controlled study using fluoxetine with children with mutism. A large National Institute of Mental Health-funded study of anxiety disorders in children and adolescents, including social phobia, Research Units in Pediatric Psychopharmacology (RUPP) has shown distinct superiority of fluvoxamine over placebo in the treatment of childhood anxiety. Children with selective mutism may benefit similarly to those with social phobia given the current belief that it is a subgroup of social phobia. SSRI medications that have been shown in randomized, placebo-controlled trials to have benefit in the treatment of children with social phobia include fluoxetine (20 mg to 60 mg per day), fluvoxamine (Luvox) (50 mg to 300 mg per day), sertraline (Zoloft) (25 mg to 200 mg per day), and paroxetine (Paxil) (10 mg to 50 mg per day).

Other medications such as phenelzine (Nardil) reportedly improve symptoms of social phobia in adults, but are rarely recommended for mutism in school-age children, given the choice of multiple SSRI agents with significantly safer side effect profiles.

ICD-10

The 10th revision of *International Statistical Classification of Diseases and Related Health Problems* (ICD-10) contains the diagnosis elective mutism for children who fail to speak in specific situations. In ICD-10, elective mutism is classified with the attachment disorders (*see* Table 48.1–2).

References

Bergman RL, Piacentini J. Selective mutism. In: Sadock BJ, Sadock VA, eds. *Kaplan & Sadock's Comprehensive Textbook of Psychiatry*. 8th ed. Vol. 2. Baltimore: Lippincott Williams & Wilkins; 2005:3302.

Birmaher B, Axelson DA, Monk K, Kalas C, Clark DB, Ehmann M, Bridge J, Heo J, Brent DA. Fluvoxamine for the treatment of childhood anxiety disorders. *J Am Acad Child Adolesc Psychiatry*. 2003;42:415.

Costello EJ, Egger HL, Angold A. The developmental epidemiology of anxiety disorders: Phenomenology, prevalence, and comorbidity. *Child Adolesc Psychiatric Clin N Am*. 2005;14:631.

Kehle TJ, Bray MA, Theodore LA. Selective mutism. In: Bear GG, Minke KM, eds. *Children's needs III: Development, Prevention, and Intervention*. Washington DC: National Association of School Psychologists; 2006:293.

McInnes A, Fung D, Manassis K, Fiksenbaum L, Tannock R. Narrative skills in children with selective mutism: An exploratory study. *American Journal of Speech-Language Pathology*. 2004;13:304–315.

Morris TL, March JS. *Anxiety Disorders in Children and Adolescents*. 2nd ed. New York: The Guilford Press; 2004.

Reinblatt SP, Walkup JT. Psychopharmacologic treatment of pediatric anxiety disorders. *Child Adolesc Psychiatric Clin N Am*. 2005;14:877.

Schwartz RH, Freedy AS, Sheridan MJ. Selective mutism: Are primary care physicians missing the silence? *Clin Pediatr (Phila)*. 2006;45:43–48.

Toppelberg CO, Tabors P, Coggins A, Lum K, Burger C. Differential diagnosis of selective mutism in bilingual children. *J Am Acad Child & Adolescent Psychiatry*. 2005;44(6):592–595.

Wagner KD, Berard R, Stein MB, Wetherhold E, Carpenter DJ, Perera P, Gee M, Davy K, Machin A. A multicenter, randomized, double-blind, placebo controlled trial of paroxetine in children and adolescents with social anxiety disorder. *Arch Gen Psychiatry*. 2004;61:1153.

Waslick B. Psychopharmacology intervention for pediatric anxiety disorders: A research update. *Child Adolesc Psychiatr Clin N Am*. 2006;1:51.

Yeganeh R, Beidel DC, Turner SM. Selective mutism: More than social anxiety? *Depress Anxiety*. 2006;23(3):117.

51 Early-Onset Schizophrenia

Childhood-onset schizophrenia (COS) is a rare and severe form of schizophrenia characterized by an onset of psychotic symptoms by age 12 years, believed to represent a subgroup of affected individuals with an increased heritable etiology. Children diagnosed with childhood onset schizophrenia have high rates of premorbid developmental abnormalities that appear to be nonspecific markers of severe early impaired neurodevelopment. Recent imaging studies have provided data to suggest that children with COS have decreased anterior cingulated gyrus (ACG) volumes with age, unlike controls, and an absence of the normal decreased left to right ACG volume asymmetry. These structural differences are hypothesized to be related to abnormal neurodevelopment influencing attention and emotion regulation, which are characteristic of some cognitive impairments in psychosis. The frequency of COS is reported to be less than 1 case in 10,000 children, whereas among adolescents between the ages of 13 and 18 years, the frequency of schizophrenia is markedly increased. Schizophrenia with childhood onset has the same core phenomenological features as schizophrenia in adolescence and adulthood; however, extremely high rates are seen of comorbid psychiatric disorders, including attention-deficit/hyperactivity disorder (ADHD), depressive disorders, and separation anxiety disorder in children and adolescents with COS.

Psychosocial stressors are known to influence the course of schizophrenia, and the same stressors may possibly interact with biological risk factors in the emergence of the disorder, given that children who are diagnosed with COS have marked neuropsychological deficits in a wide range of brain functions, including attention, working memory, and executive functions. Similar defects have been demonstrated in adolescents and adults with schizophrenia; however, children with schizophrenia have been shown to have more significant deficits in measures of intelligence quotient (IQ), memory, and tests of perceptuomotor skills compared with adolescent onset of schizophrenia and adolescents had greater deficits in these areas than adults with schizophrenia. Differences in these cognitive measures of IQ, memory, and perceptuomotor skills in persons with schizophrenia of different ages of onset suggests that these deficits may not be a sequelae of the disorder, but are markers of brain dysfunction even before the onset of the illness. Further, the brain dysfunction in schizophrenia occurs on a continuum with COS, reflecting the most severe neuropsychological deficits. In addition, a study comparing the severity of cognitive deficits between adolescents and adults early in the course of schizophrenia concluded that, although greater cognitive deficits are seen in earlier onset schizophrenia, a waning may occur of the development of certain cognitive domains influencing working memory and attention following the onset of schizophrenia in adolescent patients. The clinical presentation of schizophrenia, however, taking into consideration developmental level of the child, remains remarkably similar across the ages. Schizophrenia in prepubertal children includes the presence of at least two of the following: hallucinations, delusions, grossly disorganized speech or behavior, and severe withdrawal for at least 1 month. Social or academic dysfunction must be present, and continuous signs of the disturbance must persist for at least 6 months. The diagnostic criteria for schizophrenia in children are identical to the criteria for the adult form, except that instead of showing deteriorating functioning, children may fail to achieve their expected levels of social and academic functioning.

Before the 1960s, the term *childhood psychosis* was applied to a heterogeneous group of pervasive developmental disorders without hallucinations and delusions. In the 1960s and 1970s, children with evidence of a profound psychotic disturbance early in life often were observed to be mentally retarded, socially dysfunctional with severe communication and language impairments, and without a family history of schizophrenia. In children with psychoses that emerged after the age of 5, however, auditory hallucinations, delusions, inappropriate affects, thought disorder, and normal intelligence were manifest, and these children often had a family history of schizophrenia; they were viewed as exhibiting schizophrenia, whereas the younger children were identified as having an entirely different disorder, either autistic disorder or a pervasive developmental disorder.

In the 1980s, schizophrenia with childhood onset was formally separated from autistic disorder. This change reflected evidence accrued during the 1960s and 1970s that the clinical picture, family history, age of onset, and course of the two disorders differed. After the separation of the disorders, two controversies ensued. First, a few researchers remained of the opinion that a subgroup of autistic children will eventually have schizophrenia, as evidence shows for a small group. The diagnosis of schizophrenia is specifically differentiated from autistic disorder (*see* Table 42–1). Many children with early onset schizophrenia have neurodevelopmental abnormalities, some of which are also evident in children with autistic disorder. Children with autistic disorder are impaired in multiple areas of adaptive functioning from early life onward. The onset is almost always before 3 years of age, whereas the onset of childhood schizophrenia occurs before early adolescence but often is not apparent in children until after the age of 3 years. COS is more rare than onset in adolescence or young adulthood, and practically no reports are found of an onset of schizophrenia before 5 years of age. According to the text revision of the fourth edition of *Diagnostic and Statistical*

Manual of Mental Disorders (DSM-IV-TR), schizophrenia can be diagnosed in the presence of autistic disorder.

One of the challenges in applying adult diagnostic criteria COS is that some very young children who report hallucinations and apparent thought disorders in conjunction with developmental immaturities in language and in the concepts of differentiating reality from fantasy may be manifesting phenomena that are better accounted for by immaturity than psychosis.

EPIDEMIOLOGY

Schizophrenia in prepubertal children is exceedingly rare; it is estimated to occur in less than 1 of 10,000 children. In adolescents, the prevalence of schizophrenia is estimated to be 50 times that in younger children, with probable rates of 1 to 2 per 1,000. Boys seem to have a slight preponderance among children diagnosed with schizophrenia, with an estimated ratio of about 1.67 boys to 1 girl. Boys often become identified at a younger age than girls. It has been estimated that 0.1 to 1 percent present before age 10 years with 4 percent before 15 years of age. The rate of onset increases sharply during adolescence. Schizophrenia rarely is diagnosed in children younger than 5 years of age. Psychotic symptoms usually emerge insidiously, and the diagnostic criteria are met gradually over time. Occasionally, the onset of schizophrenia is sudden and occurs in a previously well-functioning child. Schizophrenia also may be diagnosed in a child who has had chronic difficulties and then experiences a significant exacerbation. The prevalence of schizophrenia among the parents of children with schizophrenia is about 8 percent, which is close to twice the prevalence in the parents of patients with adult-onset schizophrenia.

Schizotypal personality disorder is similar to schizophrenia in its inappropriate affects, excessive magical thinking, odd beliefs, social isolation, ideas of reference, and unusual perceptual experiences, such as illusions. Schizotypal personality disorder, however, does not have psychotic features; still, the disorder seems to aggregate in families with adult-onset schizophrenia. Therefore, the relation between the two disorders is unclear.

ETIOLOGY

The etiology of COS has multiple contributing factors, and estimates of its heritability are as high as 80 percent. COS is a severe form of schizophrenia which may increase its likelihood of heritability to among the highest of estimates. Genetic studies provide substantial evidence for a significant genetic basis in the development of schizophrenia. The precise mechanisms of transmission of schizophrenia are still not well understood. Schizophrenia is known to be up to eight times more prevalent among first-degree relatives of those with schizophrenia than in the general population. Adoption studies of patients with adult-onset schizophrenia have shown that schizophrenia occurs in the biological relatives, not the adoptive relatives. Additional genetic evidence is supported by higher concordance rates for schizophrenia in monozygotic twins than in dizygotic twins. Higher rates of schizophrenia have been established among relatives of those with childhood-onset schizophrenia than in the relatives of those with adult-onset schizophrenia. A recent case report identified a rare genetic occurrence in which an offspring receives two chromosome homologues from the same parent (uniparental isodisomy) of chromosome 5, already implicated in several linkage studies to be associated with schizophrenia in a child with COS.

Currently, no reliable method can identify persons at the highest risk for schizophrenia in a given family. Neurodevelopmental abnormalities and higher-than-expected rates of neurological soft signs and impairments in sustaining attention and in strategies for information processing appear among children at high risk. Increased rates of disturbed communication styles are found in families with a member with schizophrenia. Recent reports have documented marked neuropsychological deficits in attention, working memory, and premorbid IQ among children who develop schizophrenia and its spectrum disorders. High expressed emotion, characterized by overly critical responses in families, has been shown to be correlated with increased relapse rates among patients with schizophrenia.

Recent studies have documented gray matter loss in the brains of children with COS that started in the parietal region and proceeded frontally to dorsolateral prefrontal and temporal cortices, including superior temporal gyri. Magnetic resonance imaging (MRI) studies of 12 children with COS at baseline and at follow-up 5 years later were compared with normal controls. Children with COS showed severe bilateral frontal gray matter loss over the 5-year period that occurred in a dorsal-to-ventral pattern across the medial hemispheres. Frontal regions were most affected, whereas cingulated-limbic regions were less vulnerable, which correlates with the brain areas responsible for the cognitive and metabolic dysfunction typically observed in schizophrenia. Children and adolescents with schizophrenia are more likely to have a premorbid history of social rejection, poor peer relationships, clingy withdrawn behavior, and academic trouble than those with adult-onset schizophrenia. Some children with schizophrenia first seen in middle childhood have early histories of motor milestones and delayed language acquisition that are similar to some symptoms of autistic disorder. The mechanisms of biological vulnerability and environmental influences producing manifestations of schizophrenia remain under investigation.

DIAGNOSIS AND CLINICAL FEATURES

All of the symptoms included in adult-onset schizophrenia may be manifest in children with the disorder. The onset is frequently insidious; after first exhibiting inappropriate affects of unusual behavior, a child may take months or years to meet all of the diagnostic criteria for schizophrenia. Children who eventually meet the criteria often are socially rejected and clingy and have limited social skills. They may have histories of delayed motor and verbal milestones and do poorly in school, despite normal intelligence. Although children with schizophrenia and autistic disorder may be similar in their early histories, children with schizophrenia have normal intelligence and do not meet the criteria for a pervasive developmental disorder.

According to DSM-IV-TR, a child with schizophrenia may experience deterioration of function, along with the emergence of psychotic symptoms, or the child may never achieve the expected level of functioning (*see* Table 13–4). Auditory hallucinations commonly occur in children with schizophrenia. They may hear several voices making an ongoing critical commentary, or command hallucinations may tell children to kill themselves or others. The voices may be bizarre, identified as "a computer in my head," Martians, or the voice of someone familiar, such as a relative. Visual hallucinations are experienced by a significant number of children with schizophrenia and often are frightening; the children may see the devil, skeletons, scary faces, or space creatures. Transient phobic visual hallucinations also occur in traumatized children who do not eventually have a major psychotic disorder.

Delusions are present in more than one half of children with schizophrenia; the delusions take various forms, including persecutory, grandiose, and religious. Delusions increase in frequency with increased age. Blunted or inappropriate affects appear almost universally in children with schizophrenia. Children with schizophrenia may giggle inappropriately or cry without being able to explain why. Formal thought disorders, including loosening of associations and thought blocking, are common features among children with schizophrenia. Illogical thinking and poverty of thought are also often present. Unlike adults with schizophrenia, children with schizophrenia do not have poverty of speech content, but they speak less than other children of the same intelligence and are ambiguous in the way they refer to persons, objects, and events. The communication deficits observable in children with schizophrenia include unpredictably changing the topic of conversation without introducing the new topic to the listener (loose associations). Children with schizophrenia also exhibit illogical thinking and speaking and tend to underuse self-initiated repair strategies to aid in their communication. When an utterance is unclear or vague, normal children attempt to clarify their communication with repetitions, revision, and more detail. Children with schizophrenia, on the other hand, fail to aid communication with revision, fillers, or starting over. These deficits may be conceptualized as negative symptoms in childhood schizophrenia.

The core phenomena for schizophrenia seem to be the same among various age groups, but a child's developmental level influences the presentation of the symptoms. Delusions of young children are less complex, therefore, than those of older children. Age-appropriate content, such as animal imagery and monsters, is likely to be a source of delusional fear in children. Other features that seem to occur frequently in children with schizophrenia are poor motor functioning, visuospatial impairments, and attention deficits.

In the DSM-IV-TR are delineated five types of schizophrenia: paranoid, disorganized, catatonic, undifferentiated, and residual.

A 12-year-old boy developed concerns that his parents might be poisoning his food. Over the next year, his symptoms progressed with increased fearfulness, preoccupation with food, and beliefs that Satan and voices from the radio and television were sending him bad thoughts. During this time, his parents also observed bizarre behaviors, including talking and yelling to himself, perseverating about devils and demons, assaulting family members because he thought they were evil, and attempting to hurt himself because he believed it would please God. No predominant mood symptoms or any history of substance abuse were found.

Developmentally, he was the product of a full-term pregnancy complicated by a difficult labor and forceps delivery. His early motor and speech milestones were normal. As a younger child, he tended to be quiet and socially awkward. His intelligence was felt to be in the normal range, but academic testing was consistently below grade level.

He has had no significant medical problems. An organic workup included normal serum chemistries, thyroid functions, toxicology screen, ceruloplasmin, and brain MRI. His family psychiatric history was significant for depression in a maternal aunt and a completed suicide in a maternal great-grandparent. His symptoms have not significantly improved in the 5 years subsequent to the onset of his illness. He has been hospitalized nine times, including placement in a long-term residential program. He has been on numerous antipsychotic medications, both traditional neuroleptics and atypical agents, and numerous other agents, including selective serotonin reuptake inhibitors (SSRIs) and mood stabilizers. His mental status examination continued to display tangential and disorganized thinking, paranoid delusions, loose associations, perseverative speech patterns, and a flat, at times inappropriate, affect. His time has generally been spent pacing and muttering to himself, with no social interaction with others unless initiated by adults. Some improvement was finally noted with clozapine (Clozaril) therapy, although he remained symptomatic. (Courtesy of Jon M. McClellan, M.D.)

PATHOLOGY AND LABORATORY EXAMINATIONS

No specific laboratory tests are diagnostically specific for COS. Although neuroimaging studies are converging to suggest that children with COS have decreased ACG volumes with age, and an absence of the normal decreased left-to-right ACG volume asymmetry, this research cannot be used as an index for diagnosis. High incidences of pregnancy and birth complications have been reported in the histories of children with schizophrenia, but presently, no specificity has been found in these risks for childhood schizophrenia. Electroencephalogram (EEG) studies have not been helpful in distinguishing children with schizophrenia from other children. Although data exist to suggest that hypoprolinemia is associated with the risk of schizoaffective disorder because of an alteration on chromosome 22q11, no association has been found of hyperporlinemia with childhood onset schizophrenia.

DIFFERENTIAL DIAGNOSIS

The differential diagnosis of COS includes autistic disorder, bipolar disorders, depressive psychotic disorders, multicomplex developmental syndromes, *Asberger's* syndrome, drug-induced psychosis, and psychotic states caused by organic disorders. Children with COS have been shown to have multiple frequently occurring concurrent disorders, including ADHD, oppositional defiant disorder, and depression. Children with schizotypal personality disorder have some traits in common with children who meet diagnostic criteria for schizophrenia. Blunted affect, social isolation, eccentric thoughts, ideas of reference, and bizarre behavior can be seen in both disorders; however, in schizophrenia, overt psychotic symptoms, such as hallucinations, delusions, and incoherence, must be present at some point. When they are present, they exclude a diagnosis of schizotypal personality disorder. Hallucinations alone, however, are not evidence of schizophrenia; patients must show either a deterioration of function or an inability to meet an expected developmental level to warrant the diagnosis of schizophrenia. Auditory and visual hallucinations can appear as self-limited events in nonpsychotic young children who are faced with extreme psychosocial stressors, such as the breakup of their parents, and in children experiencing a major loss or significant change in lifestyle.

Psychotic phenomena are common among children with major depressive disorder, in which both hallucinations and, less commonly, delusions may occur. The congruence of mood with psychotic features is most pronounced in depressed children, although children with schizophrenia may also seem sad. The hallucinations and delusions of schizophrenia are more likely to have a bizarre quality than those of children with depressive disorders. In children and adolescents with bipolar I disorder, it often is difficult to distinguish a first episode of mania with psychotic features from schizophrenia if the child has no history of previous depressions. Grandiose delusions and hallucinations are typical of manic episodes, but clinicians often must follow the natural history of the disorder to confirm the presence of a mood disorder. Pervasive developmental disorders, including autistic disorder with normal intelligence, often share some features with schizophrenia. Most notably, difficulty with social relationships, an early history of delayed language acquisition, and ongoing communication deviance occur in both disorders; however, hallucinations, delusions, and formal thought disorder are core features of schizophrenia and are not expected features of pervasive developmental disorders. Pervasive developmental disorders usually are diagnosed by 3 years of age, but schizophrenia with childhood onset can rarely be diagnosed before 5 years of age.

Alcohol and other substance abuse sometimes can result in a deterioration of function, psychotic symptoms, and paranoid delusions. Amphetamines, lysergic acid diethylamide (LSD), and phencyclidine (PCP) may lead to a psychotic state. A sudden, flagrant onset of paranoid psychosis is more suggestive of substance-induced psychotic disorder than an insidious onset. Medical conditions that can induce psychotic features include thyroid disease, systemic lupus erythematosus, and temporal lobe disease.

COURSE AND PROGNOSIS

Important predictors of the course and outcome of early-onset schizophrenia include the child's level of functioning before the onset of schizophrenia, the age of onset, IQ, response to pharmacologic interventions, how much functioning the child regained after the first episode, and the amount of support available from the family. Children with developmental delays, learning disorders, lower IQ, and premorbid behavioral disorders, such as ADHD and conduct disorder, seem to respond less well to medication treatment of schizophrenia and are likely to have the most guarded prognoses. In a long-term outcome study of patients with schizophrenia with onset before 14 years of age, the worst prognoses occurred in children with schizophrenia that was diagnosed before they were 10 years of age and who had preexisting personality disorders.

An additional issue in outcome studies is the stability of the diagnosis of schizophrenia. In one study, one third of children who received a diagnosis of schizophrenia were diagnosed with bipolar disorder in adolescence. Children and adolescents with bipolar I disorder may have a better long-term prognosis than children and adolescents with schizophrenia. In adult-onset schizophrenia, family interactions, such as high expressed emotion, may be associated with increased relapse rates. No clear-cut data are available regarding childhood schizophrenia, but the degree of supportiveness, as opposed to critical and overinvolved family responses, probably influences the prognosis.

Childhood-onset schizophrenia appears to be a more malignant type of schizophrenia which presents a greater challenge to treat with pharmacology and psychosocial interventions. It seems to respond less to medication than schizophrenia with adult onset or adolescent onset, and the prognosis may be poorer. Positive symptoms—that is, hallucinations and delusions—are likely to be more responsive to medication than negative symptoms such as withdrawal. In a recent report of 38 children with schizophrenia who had been hospitalized, two thirds required placement in residential facilities, and only one third improved sufficiently to return home.

TREATMENT

The treatment of COS requires a multimodal approach, including pharmacologic interventions, family education, social skills interventions, and appropriate educational placement. Current research suggests that, in adolescents and young adults, early interventions during the prodrome of schizophrenia with atypical antipsychotics and psychosocial support may improve symptoms and delay or prevent progression to full blown schizophrenia. Investigation is needed on the recognition of prodromal states of COS to assess the benefits of very early interventions. Current treatments for COS are based on very limited data. Antipsychotic medications are indicated, given the degree of impairment in both social relationships and academic function exhibited by children with schizophrenia. Children with COS may have less robust responses to antipsychotic medications than adolescents and adults with the same disorder. Family education and ongoing family interventions are critical to maximize the level of support that the family can give the patient. The proper educational setting for the child is also important, because social skills deficits, attention deficits, and academic difficulties often accompany childhood schizophrenia.

Pharmacotherapy

Atypical antipsychotics, serotonin-dopamine antagonists are current first-line treatment for children and adolescents with schizophrenia, having replaced the dopamine receptor antagonists because of their more favorable side effect profiles. The serotonin-dopamine agonists, including risperidone (Risperdal), olanzapine (Zyprexa), and clozapine (Clozaril) differ from the conventional antipsychotics in that they act as serotonin receptor antagonists with some dopamine (D2) activity, but without a predominance of D2 receptor antagonism. They are hypothesized to be more effective in reducing positive and negative symptoms of schizophrenia, and incur less risk of causing extrapyramidal adverse effects. Additional atypical antipsychotics, such as quetiapine (Seroquel), ziprasidone (Geodon), and aripiprazole (Abilify), are also serotonin-dopamine antagonists that are used in clinical practice for children and adolescents with psychotic disorders who do not respond to other atypical antipsychotics. A limited evidence base exists to inform the treatment of COS with the atypical antipsychotics and a need is seen for randomized clinical trials in this patient population.

A recent double-blind, randomized 8-week controlled trial compared the efficacy and safety of olanzapine to clozapine in COS. Children with COS who were resistant to at least two previous treatments with antipsychotics were randomized to treatment for 8 weeks with either olanzapine or clozapine followed by a 2-year open-label follow-up. Using the *Clinical Global Impression of Severity of Symptoms Scale and Schedule for the Assessment of Negative/Positive Symptoms*, clozapine was found to be associated with a significant reduction in all outcome measures, whereas olanzapine showed improvement on some measures but not on all. The only statistically significant measure in which clozapine was superior to olanzapine was in alleviating negative symptoms, compared with baseline. Clozapine was associated with more adverse events, such as lipid abnormalities and a seizure in one patient.

Several recent studies have provided evidence that risperidone, a benzisoxazole derivative, is as effective as the older high-potency conventional antipsychotics, such as haloperidol (Haldol), and causes less frequent severe side effects, in the treatment of schizophrenia in older adolescents and adults. Published case reports and limited larger controlled studies have supported the efficacy of risperidone in the treatment of psychosis in children and adolescents. Risperidone has been reported to cause weight gain and dystonic reactions and other extrapyramidal adverse effects in children and adolescents. Olanzapine is generally well tolerated with respect to extrapyramidal adverse effects compared with conventional antipsychotics and risperidone but is associated with moderate sedation and significant weight gain.

High-potency conventional antipsychotics, such as haloperidol and trifluoperazine (Stelazine), are available as second-line treatments; however, lower potency antipsychotics, such as chlorpromazine (Thorazine) may be preferable for young children because of their decreased risk of dystonic reaction. Acute dystonic reactions do occur in children, and 1 to 2 mg a day of benztropine (Cogentin) usually is sufficient to treat the extrapyramidal adverse effects.

Children and adolescents who are treated with antipsychotic medications are at risk for withdrawal dyskinesia when the medication is withdrawn. The long-term adverse effects, including tardive dyskinesia, are perpetual risks for any patients treated with an antipsychotic medication.

Psychotherapy

Psychosocial interventions aimed at family education, and patient and family support are recognized as critical component of the treatment plan for COS. Psychotherapists who work with children with schizophrenia must take into account a child's developmental level. They must continually support the child's good reality testing and be sensitive to the child's sense of self. Long-term intensive and supportive psychotherapy combined with pharmacotherapy is the most effective approach to this disorder.

References

Biswas P, Malhotra S, Malhotra A, Gupta N. Comparative study of neuropsychological correlates in schizophrenia with childhood onset, adolescence and adulthood. *Eur Child Adolesc Psychiatry*. 2006;15:360.

Fagerlund B, Pagsberg AK, Hemmingsen RP. Cognitive deficits and levels of IQ in adolescent onset schizophrenia and other psychotic disorders. *Schizophr Res*. 2006;85(1–3):30.

Jacquet H, Rapoport JL, Hecketsweiler B, Bobb A, Thibaut F, Frebourg T, Campion D. Hyperprolinemia is not associate with childhood onset schizophrenia. *Am J Med Genet B Neuropsychiatr Genet*. 2006;141:192.

Kester HM, Sevy S, Yechiam E, Burdick KE, Cervellione KL, Kumra S. Decision-making impairment in adolescents with early-onset schizophrenia. *Schizophr Res*. 2006;85(1–3):113.

Marquardt RK, Levitt JG, Blanton RE, Caplan R, Asarnow R, Siddarth P, Fadale D, McCracken JT, Toga AW. Abnormal development of the anterior cingulated in childhood-onset schizophrenia: a preliminary quantitative MRI study. *Psychiatry Res*. 2005;138:221.

McClennan JM. Early-onset schizophrenia. In: Sadock BJ, Sadock VA, eds. *Kaplan & Sadock's Comprehensive Textbook of Psychiatry*. 8th ed. Vol. 2. Baltimore: Lippincott Williams & Wilkins; 2005:3307.

Reichenberg A, Weiser M, Caspi A, Knobler HY, Lubin G, Harvey PD, Rabinowitz J, Davidson M. Premorbid intellectual functioning and risk of schizophrenia and spectrum disorders. *J Clin Exp Neuropsychol*. 2006;28:193.

Remschmidt H, Theisen FM. Schizophrenia and related disorders in children and adolescents. *J Neural Transm Suppl*. 2005;69:121.

Rhinewine JP, Lencz T, Thaden EP, Cervellione KL, Burdick KE, Henderson I, Bhaskar S, Keehlisen L, Kane J, Kohn N, Fisch GS, Bilder RM, Kumra S. Neurocognitive profile in adolescents with early-onset schizophrenia: Clinical correlates. *Biol Psychiatry*. 2005;58(9):705.

Ross RG, Heinlein S, Tregllas H. High rates of comorbidity are found in childhood-onset schizophrenia. *Schizophr Res*. 2006;88(1):90–95.

Rutter M, Kim-Cohen J, Maughan B. Continuities and discontinuities in psychopathology between childhood and adult life. *J Child Psychol Psychiatry*. 2006;47:276.

Seal JL, Gornick MC, Gotgay N, Shaw P, Greenstein DK, Coffee M, Gochman PA, Stromberg T, Chen Z, Merriman B, Nelson SF, Brooks J, Arepalli S, Wavrant-De Vrieze F, Hardy J, Rapoport JL, Addington AM. Segmental uniparental isodisomy on 5q32-qter in a patient with childhood-onset schizophrenia. *J Med Genet*. 2006;43(11):887–892.

Taylor JL, Blanton RE, Levitt JG, Caplan R, Nobel D, Toga AW. Superior temporal gyrus differences in childhood-onset schizophrenia. *Schizophr Res*. 2005; 73:235.

Thomas LE, Woods SW. The schizophrenia prodrome L a developmentally informed review and update for psychopharmacological treatment. *Child Adolesc Pscyhiatr Clin N Am*. 2006;15:109.

Vidal CN, Rapoport JL, Hayashi KM, Geaga JA, Sui Y, McLemore LE, Alaghband Y, Giedd JN, Gochman P, Blumenthal J, Gogtay N, Nicolson R, Toga AW, Thompson PM. Dynamically spreading frontal and cingulated deficits mapped in adolescents with schizophrenia. *Arch Gen Psychiatry*. 2006;63:25.

White T, Ho BC, Ward J, O'Leary D, Andreasen NC. Neuropsychological performance in first-episode adolescents with schizophrenia: A comparison with first-episode adults and adolescent control subjects. *Biol Psychiatry*. 2006;60:463.

52 Adolescent Substance Abuse

Adolescent substance use and abuse includes a wide range of substances, such as alcohol, marijuana, nicotine, cocaine, heroin, inhalants, phencyclidine (PCP), lysergic acid diethylamide (LSD), dextromorphan, anabolic steroids and various club drugs, 3,4-methylenedioxymethamphetamine (MDMA or Ecstasy), flunitrazepam (Rohypnol), gamma-hydroxybutyrate (GHB), and ketamine (Ketalar). It is estimated that approximately 20 percent of 8th graders in the United States have tried illicit drugs and about 30 percent of 10th through 12th graders have used an illicit substance. Alcohol remains the most common substance used and abused by adolescents. Binge drinking occurs in about 6 percent of adolescents, and teens with alcohol use disorders are at greater risk of problems with other substances as well.

Many risk and protective factors influence the age of onset and severity of substance use among adolescents. Psychosocial risk factors mediating the development of substance use disorders include parent modeling of substance use, family conflict, lack of parental supervision, peer relationships, and individual stressful life events. Protective factors that mitigate substance use among adolescents include variables such as a stable family life, strong parent–child bond, consistent parental supervision investment in academic achievement, and a peer group who model prosocial family and school behaviors. Interventions that diminish risk factors are likely to mitigate substance use.

Approximately one of five adolescents has used marijuana or hashish. Approximately one third of adolescents have used cigarettes by age 17 years. Studies of alcohol use among adolescents in the United States have shown that by 13 years of age, one third of boys and almost one fourth of girls have tried alcohol. By 18 years of age, 92 percent of males and 73 percent of females reported trying alcohol, and 4 percent reported using alcohol daily. Of high school seniors, 41 percent reported using marijuana; 2 percent reported using the drug daily. Emergency room visits for heroin use among those 18 to 25 years of age increased over 50 percent from 1997 to 2000.

Drinking among adolescents follows adult demographic drinking patterns: The highest proportion of alcohol use occurs among adolescents in the northeast; whites are more likely to drink than are other groups; among whites, Roman Catholics are the least likely nondrinkers. The four most common causes of death in persons between the ages of 10 and 24 years are motor vehicle accidents (37 percent), homicide (14 percent), suicide (12 percent), and other injuries or accidents (12 percent). Of adolescents treated in pediatric trauma centers, more than one third are treated for alcohol or drug use.

Studies considering alcohol and illicit drug use by adolescents as psychiatric disorders have demonstrated a greater prevalence of substance use, particularly alcoholism, among biological children of alcoholics than among adopted youngsters. This finding is supported by family studies of genetic contributions, by adoption studies, and by observing children of substance users reared outside the biological home.

Numerous risk factors influence the emergence of adolescent substance abuse. These include parental belief in the harmlessness of substances, lack of anger control in families of substance abusers, lack of closeness and involvement of parents with children's activities, maternal passivity, academic difficulties, comorbid psychiatric disorders such as conduct disorder and depression, parental and peer substance use, impulsivity, and early onset of cigarette smoking. The greater the number of risk factors, the more likely it is that an adolescent will be a substance user.

EPIDEMIOLOGY

Alcohol

A recent survey showed that drinking was a significant problem for 10 to 20 percent of adolescents. In the age range of 13 to 17 years, in the United States, are 3 million problem drinkers and 300,000 adolescents with alcohol dependence. The gap between male and female alcohol consumers is narrowing. Drinking was reported by 70 percent of 8th grade students: 54 percent reported drinking within the past year, 27 percent reported having gotten drunk at least once, and 13 percent reported binge drinking in the 2 weeks before the survey. By the 12th grade, 88 percent of high school students reported drinking, and 77 percent drank within the past year; 5 percent of 8th grade students, 1.3 percent of 10th grade students, and 3.6 percent of 12th grade students reported daily alcohol use.

Marijuana

Marijuana is the most widely used illicit drug among high school students. It has been termed a "gateway drug," because the strongest predictor of future cocaine use is frequent marijuana use during adolescence. Of 8th grade, 10th grade, and 12th grade students, 10, 23, and 36 percent, respectively, report using marijuana, a slight decrease from the year preceding the survey. Of 8th grade, 10th grade, and 12th grade students, 0.2, 0.8, and 2 percent, respectively, report daily marijuana use. Prevalence rates for marijuana are highest among Native American males and females; these rates are nearly as high in white males and females and Mexican American males. The lowest annual rates are reported by Latin American females, African American females, and Asian American males and females. Among juvenile arrests for illicit drug use in 2000, marijuana was the most commonly used drug by both males (55 percent) and females (60 percent).

Cocaine

The annual cocaine use reported by high school seniors decreased more than 30 percent between 1990 and 2000. Currently, about 0.5 percent of 8th grade students, 1 percent of 10th grade students, and 2 percent of 12th grade students are estimated to have used cocaine. The prevalence rates for crack cocaine use, however, is increasing and is most common among those between the ages of 18 and 25.

Crystal Methamphetamine

Crystal methamphetamine, or "ice", was at a relative low level of use in adolescence about one decade ago of 0.5 percent and has steadily increased to a recent rate of 1.5 percent among 12th graders.

Lysergic Acid Diethylamide (LSD)

Lysergic acid diethylamide is reportedly used by 2.7 percent of 8th grade students, 5.6 percent of 10th grade students, and 8.8 percent of 12th grade students. Of 12th grade students, 0.1 percent report daily use. The current LSD rates are lower than rates of LSD use during the past two decades.

3,4-Methylenedioxymethamphetamine (MDMA)

The popularity of MDMA has increased over the past decade and current rates of usage in the United States are in the range of about 5 percent for 10th graders and 8 percent of 12th graders, despite that the perceived harmfulness of this drug has increased over the last decade to almost 50 percent among 12th graders. Accidental adolescent deaths have been associated with the use of MDMA.

Gamma-Hydroxybutyrate

Gamma-hydroxybutyrate, a club drug, has been found in surveys to have a annual prevalence rate of 1.1 percent for 8th graders, 1.0 percent rate for 10 graders, and a 1.6 percent rate of use for 12th graders.

Ketamine (Ketalar)

Ketamine, another club drug, recently was found to have a rate of 1.3 percent annual prevalence for 8th graders, 2.1 percent for 10th graders, and 2.5 percent rate for 12th graders.

Flunitrazepam (Rohypnol)

Flunitrazepam (Rohypnol), a third club drug, has been found to have an annual prevalence rate of about 1 percent for all high school grades combined.

Anabolic Steroids

Despite reported knowledge of the risks of anabolic steroids among high school students, surveys over the last 5 years found rates of anabolic steroid use to be 1.6 percent among 8th graders and 2.1 percent among 10th graders. Up to 45 percent of 10th and 12th graders reported knowledge of the risks of anabolic steroids; however, over the last decade it appears that seniors reported less disapproval of their use.

Inhalants

The use of inhalants in the form of glue, aerosols, and gasoline is relatively more common among younger than older adolescents. Among 8th grade, 10th grade, and 12th grade students, 17.6, 15.7, and 17.6 percent, respectively, report using inhalants; 0.2 percent of 8th grade students, 0.1 percent of 10th grade students, and 0.2 percent of 12th grade students report daily use of inhalants.

Multiple Substance Use

Among adolescents enrolled in substance abuse treatment programs, 96 percent are polydrug users; 97 percent of adolescents who abuse drugs also use alcohol. (See Chapter 12, *Substance-Related Disorders*, for a thorough overview of the epidemiologic data for illicit drug use.)

ETIOLOGY

Genetic Factors

The concordance for alcoholism is reportedly higher among monozygotic than dizygotic twins. Considerably fewer studies have been conducted of families of drug abusers. One twin study of drug users showed that the drug abuse concordance for male monozygotic twins was twice that for dizygotic twins. Studies of children of alcoholics reared away from their biological homes have shown that these children have about a 25 percent chance of becoming alcoholics.

Psychosocial Factors

A recent study concluded that children in families with the lowest measures of parental supervision and monitoring initiated alcohol, tobacco, and other drug use earlier than children from families with more supervision. The risk was greatest for children below 11 years of age. With more rigorous parental monitoring, young adolescents might be delayed in, or prevented from, initiating drug and alcohol use. Furthermore, increased supervision during middle childhood years may diminish drug and alcohol sampling and ultimately diminish the risk of using marijuana, cocaine, or inhalants in the future.

Comorbidity

Rates of alcohol and drug use are reportedly higher in relatives of children with depression and bipolar disorders. On the other hand, mood disorders are common among those with alcoholism. Evidence indicates a strong link between early antisocial behavior, conduct disorder, and substance abuse. Substance abuse can be viewed as one form of behavioral deviance that, unsurprisingly, is associated with other forms of social and behavioral deviance. Early intervention with children who show early signs of social deviance and antisocial behavior may conceivably impede the processes that contribute to later substance abuse.

Comorbidity, the occurrence of more than one substance use disorder or the combination of a substance use disorder and another psychiatric disorder, is common. It is important to know about all comorbid disorders, which may show differential responses to treatment. Surveys of adolescents with alcoholism show rates of 50 percent or higher for additional psychiatric disorders, especially mood disorders. A recent survey of adolescents who used alcohol found that more than 80 percent met criteria for another disorder. The disorders most frequently present were depressive disorders, disruptive behavior disorders, and drug use disorders. These rates of comorbidity are even higher than those for adults. The diagnosis of alcohol abuse or dependence was likely to follow, rather than precede, other disorders; that a large proportion of adolescents with alcoholism have a previous childhood disorder may have both etiological and treatment implications. In this survey, the onset of alcohol disorders did not systematically precede drug abuse or dependence. In 50 percent of cases, alcohol use followed drug use. Alcohol use may be a gateway to drug use, but is not in most cases. The presence of other psychiatric disorders was associated with an earlier onset of alcohol disorder, but it did not seem to indicate a more protracted course of alcoholism.

DIAGNOSIS AND CLINICAL FEATURES

According to the text revision of the fourth edition of *Diagnostic and Statistical Manual of Mental Disorders* (DSM-IV-TR), substance-related disorders include substance dependence, substance abuse, substance intoxication, substance withdrawal, and various substance-induced disorders (e.g., alcohol-induced anxiety disorder). Substance dependence refers to a cluster of cognitive, behavioral, and physiological symptoms indicating that a person continues the use of a substance, despite significant substance-related problems. A pattern of repeated self-administration can result in tolerance, withdrawal, and compulsive drug-taking behavior. Dependence can be applied to every substance, with the exception of caffeine. It requires the presence of at least three symptoms of the maladaptive pattern, which can occur at any time during the same 12-month period. Symptoms of dependence can include tolerance, withdrawal, heavier use of the substance than was intended, an unsuccessful desire to cut down or control use, and reduction of social or occupational activities because of substance use. In addition, the user knows that the substance causes significant impairment, but does not give it up. Physiological dependence (evidence of tolerance or withdrawal) may or may not be present.

Substance abuse refers to a maladaptive pattern of substance use leading to clinically significant impairment or distress, manifest by one or more of the following symptoms within a 12-month period: recurrent substance use in situations that cause physical danger to the user, recurrent substance use in the face of obvious impairment in school or work situations, recurrent substance use despite resulting legal problems, or recurrent substance use despite social or interpersonal problems. To meet the criteria for substance abuse, the symptoms must never have met the criteria for substance dependence for this class of substance.

Substance intoxication refers to the development of a reversible, substance-specific syndrome caused by use of a substance. Clinically significant maladaptive behavioral or psychological changes must be present.

Substance withdrawal refers to a substance-specific syndrome caused by the cessation of, or reduction in, prolonged substance use. The substance-specific syndrome causes clinically significant distress or impairs social or occupational functioning.

The diagnosis of alcohol or drug use in adolescents is made through careful interview, observations, laboratory findings, and history provided by reliable sources. Many nonspecific signs may point to alcohol or drug use, and clinicians must be careful to corroborate hunches before jumping to conclusions. Substance use can be viewed on a continuum with experimentation (the mildest use), regular use without obvious impairment, abuse, and finally, dependence. Changes in academic performance, nonspecific physical ailments, changes in relationships with family members, changes in peer group, unexplained phone calls, or changes in personal hygiene may indicate substance use in an adolescent. Many of these indicators, however, also can be consistent with the onset of depression, adjustment to school, or the prodrome of a psychotic illness. It is important, therefore, to keep the channels of communication with an adolescent open when substance use is suspected.

Nicotine

Nicotine is one of the most addictive substances known, involving cholinergic receptors, and enhancing acetylcholine, serotonin and β-endorphin release. Young teens who smoke cigarettes are also exposed to other drugs more frequently than nonsmoking peers.

Alcohol

Alcohol use in adolescents rarely results in the sequelae observed in adults with chronic abuse of alcohol, such as withdrawal seizures, Korsakoff's syndrome, Wernicke's aphasia, or cirrhosis of the liver. R. DeBellis, however, has reported that adolescent exposure to alcohol may result in diminished hippocampal brain volume. Because the hippocampus is involved with attention, it is conceivable that adolescent alcohol use could result in compromised cognitive function, especially with respect to attention.

Marijuana

The short-term effects of the active ingredient in marijuana, tetrahydrocannabinol (THC), include impairment in memory and learning, distorted perception, diminished problem-solving ability, loss of coordination, increased heart rate, anxiety, and panic attacks. Abrupt cessation of heavy marijuana use by adolescents has been reported to result in a withdrawal syndrome characterized by insomnia, irritability, restlessness, drug craving, depressed mood, and nervousness followed by anxiety, tremors, nausea, muscle twitches, increased sweating, myalgia, and general malaise. Typically, the withdrawal syndrome begins 24 hours after the last use, peaks at 2 to 4 days, and diminishes after 2 weeks.

Cocaine

Cocaine can be sniffed or snorted, injected, or smoked. *Crack* is the term given to cocaine after it has been changed to a free base for smoking. Cocaine's effects include constriction of peripheral blood vessels, dilated pupils, hyperthermia, increased heart rate, and hypertension. High doses or prolonged use of cocaine can induce paranoid thinking. The immediate risk of death can occur secondary to cardiac arrest or from seizures followed by respiratory arrest. In contrast to stimulants used to treat attention-deficit/hyperactivity disorder (ADHD), such as methylphenidate, cocaine quickly crosses the blood–brain barrier and moves off the dopamine transporter within 20 minutes, unlike methylphenidate, which remains bound to dopamine for long periods of time.

Heroin

Heroin, a derivative of morphine, is produced from a poppy plant. Heroin usually appears as a white or brown powder that can be snorted, but more commonly is used intravenously. Withdrawal symptoms include restlessness, muscle and bone pain, insomnia, diarrhea and vomiting, cold flashes with goose bumps, and kicking movements. Withdrawal occurs within a few hours after use and symptoms peak between 48 and 72 hours later, and remit within about a week.

Club Drugs

Adolescents who frequent nightclubs, raves, bars, or music clubs also frequently use MDMA, GHB, Rohypnol, and ketamine. GHB, Rohypnol (a benzodiazepine) and ketamine (an anesthetic) are primarily depressants and can be added to drinks without detection because they are often colorless, tasteless, and odorless. The Drug-Induced Rape Prevention and Punishment Act of 1996 was passed after these were found to be associated with date rape. MDMA is a derivative of methamphetamine, a synthetic with both stimulant and hallucinogenic properties. MDMA can inhibit serotonin and dopamine reuptake. MDMA can result in dry mouth, increased heart rate, fatigue, muscle spasm, and hyperthermia.

Lysergic Acid Diethylamide

Lysergic acid diethylamide is odorless, colorless, and has a slightly bitter taste. Higher doses of LSD can produce visual hallucinations and delusions and, in some cases, panic. The sensations experienced after ingestion of LSD usually diminishes after 12 hours. Flashbacks can occur up to 1 year after use. LSD can produce tolerance; that is, after multiple uses, more is needed to provide the same degree of intoxication.

Substance use is related to a variety of high-risk behaviors, including an early sexual experimentation, risky driving, destruction of property, stealing, "heavy metal" or alternative music, and, occasionally, preoccupation with cults or Satanism. Although none of these behaviors necessarily predicts substance use, at the extreme, these behaviors reflect alienation from the mainstream of developmentally expected social behavior. Adolescents with inadequate social skills may use a substance as a modality to join a peer group. In some cases, adolescents begin their substance use at home with their parents, who also use substances to enhance their social interactions. Although no evidence indicates what determines a typical adolescent user of alcohol or drugs, many substance users seem to have underlying social skills deficits, academic difficulties, and less than optimal peer relationships.

TREATMENT

Treatment of substance use disorders in adolescents is designed to directly prevent the substance use behaviors and to provide education for the patient and family and to address cognitive, emotional, and psychiatric factors that influence the substance use in a variety of settings such as a residential milieu, group, and individual psychosocial session.

A validated instrument used as a guide for clinicians in the treatment of adolescent substance use designates levels of care appropriate for the symptoms. This instrument called the *Child and Adolescent Levels of Care Utilization Services* (CALOCUS) outlines 6 levels of care:

- Level 0: Basic services (prevention)
- Level 1: Recovery maintenance (relapse prevention)
- Level 2: Outpatient (once per week visits)
- Level 3: Intensive Outpatient (2 or more visits per week)
- Level 4: Intensive integrated services (day treatment, partial hospitalization, wraparound services)
- Level 5: Nonsecure, 24-hour medically monitored service (group home, residential treatment facility)
- Level 6: Secure 24-hour medical management (inpatient psychiatric or highly programmed residential facility)

Treatment settings that serve adolescents with alcohol or drug use disorders include inpatient units, residential treatment facilities, halfway houses, group homes, partial hospital programs, and outpatient settings. Basic components of adolescent alcohol or drug use treatment include individual psychotherapy, drug-specific counseling, self-help groups (Alcoholics Anonymous [AA], Narcotics Anonymous [NA], Alateen, Al-Anon), substance abuse education and relapse prevention programs, and random urine drug testing. Family therapy and psychopharmacological intervention may be added.

Before deciding on the most appropriate treatment setting for a particular adolescent, a screening process must take place in which structured and unstructured interviews help to determine the types of substances being used and their quantities and frequencies. Determining coexisting psychiatric disorders is also critical. Rating scales are typically used to document pretreatment and posttreatment severity of abuse. The *Teen Addiction Severity Index* (T-ASI), the *Adolescent Drug and Alcohol Diagnostic Assessment* (ADAD), and the *Adolescent Problem Severity Index* (APSI) are several severity-oriented rating scales. The T-ASI is broken down into dimensions that include a family function, school or employment status, psychiatric status, peer social relationships, and legal status.

After most of the information about substance use and the patient's overall psychiatric status has been obtained, a treatment strategy must be chosen and an appropriate setting must be determined. Two very different approaches to the treatment of substance abuse are embodied in the Minnesota model and the multidisciplinary professional model. The Minnesota model is based on the premise of AA; it is an intensive 12-step program with a counselor who functions as the primary therapist. The program uses self-help participation and group processes. Inherent in this treatment strategy is the need for adolescents to admit that substance use is problematic and that help is necessary. Furthermore, they must be willing to work toward altering their lifestyle to eradicate substance use. The multidisciplinary professional model consists of a team of mental health professionals that usually is led by a physician. Following a case-management model, each member of the team has specific areas of treatment for which he or she is responsible. Interventions may include cognitive-behavioral therapy, family therapy, and pharmacological intervention. This approach usually is suited for adolescents with comorbid psychiatric diagnoses.

Cognitive-behavioral approaches to psychotherapy for adolescents with substance use generally require that adolescents be motivated to participate in treatment and refrain from further substance use. The therapy focuses on relapse prevention and maintaining abstinence.

Psychopharmacological interventions for adolescent alcohol and drug users are still in their early stages. The presence of mood disorders clearly indicates the need for antidepressants, and generally, the selective serotonin reuptake inhibitors are the first line of treatment. In the past, some pharmacological interventions have been aimed at aiding the abstinence process. For example, disulfiram (Antabuse) has been used in alcoholism to cause an aversive reaction if alcohol is ingested. In certain instances, administration of a medication has been used to block the reinforcing effect of the illicit drug, for instance, giving naltrexone (ReVia) for opioid or alcohol abuse. Some medications mitigate the craving or withdrawal symptoms for a drug that is no longer being used. Clonidine (Catapres) has been used transiently during heroin withdrawal. Occasionally, an intervention is made to substitute the illicit drug with another drug that is more amenable to the treatment situation; for example, using methadone instead of heroin. Adolescents are required to have two documented attempts at detoxification and consent from an adult before they can enter such a treatment program.

Fred, a 16-year-old male, was admitted to substance abuse treatment for the second time, following a relapse and threats of suicide. He was initially admitted to an inpatient program following a serious suicide attempt. He reported a long history of disruptive behavior and academic failure since childhood. He was increasingly truant and difficult for his family to control. During his first treatment episode, he reported an onset of substance use at age 11 years, rapid progression in substance involvement since age 13 years, then current use of marijuana on a daily basis, drinking alcohol up to several times a week, frequent trips on LSD, and experimentation with a variety of substances. Fred attended group sessions focusing on his initial denial of a substance use problem and then learned the process of recovery while attending other groups and AA and NA meetings. Family group sessions showed him and his parents the need for better communication and more adaptive interactions. Fred gradually responded to the structure of the treatment program, although he had frequent problems with anger control when confronted by peers or staff or when frustrated. Depressive symptoms failed to remit following 2 weeks of abstinence, and Fred was given fluoxetine (Prozac). He showed rapid improvement in mood and treatment compliance. On discharge, he was attending NA meetings and outpatient therapy. Family conflict soon recurred, however, and Fred became noncompliant with outpatient treatment, medication, and meetings. He resumed old relationships with deviant peers and relapsed into daily marijuana use and occasional alcohol use. (Courtesy of Oscar G. Bukstein, M.D.)

Efficacious treatments for cigarette smoking cessation include nicotine-containing gum, patches, or nasal spray or inhaler. Bupropion (Zyban) aids in diminishing cravings for nicotine and is beneficial in the treatment of smoking cessation.

Because comorbidity influences treatment outcome, it is important to pay attention to other disorders, such as mood disorders, anxiety disorders, conduct disorder, or ADHD during the treatment of substance use disorders.

References

Bukstein OG, Bernet W, Arnold V, Beitchman J, Shaw J, Benson RS, Kinlan J, McClellan J, Stock S, Ptakowski KK. Work Group on Quality Issues. Practice parameter for the assessment and treatment of children and adolescents with substance use disorders. *J Am Acad Child Adolesc Psychiatry*. 2005;44:609.

Bukstein OG, Cornelius J, Trunzo AC, Kelly Tm, Wood DS. Clinical predictors of treatment in a population of adolescents with alcohol use disorders. *Addict Behav*. 2005;30:1663.

Collins CC, Moolchan ET. Shorter time to first cigarette of the day in menthol adolescent cigarette smokers. *Addict Behav*. 2006;31(8):1460.

Cornelius JR, Clark DB, Bukstein OG, Salloum IM. Treatment of co-occurring alcohol, drug and psychiatric disorders. *Recent Dev Alcohol*. 2005;17:349.

Cornelius JR, Clark DB, Bukstein OG, Birmaher B, Salloum IM, Brown SA. Acute phase and five-year follow-up study of fluoxetine in adolescents with major depression and a comorbid substance use disorder: A review. *Addict Behav*. 2005; 30:1824.

Crowley TJ. Adolescents and substance-related disorders: research agenda to guide decisions on Diagnostic and Statistical Manual of Mental Disorders, 5th edition (DSM-V). *Addiction*. 2006;101[Suppl 1]:115.

Deas D. Adolescent substance abuse and psychiatric comorbidities. *J Clin Psychiatry*. 2006;67[Suppl 7]:18.

Elek E, Miller-Day M, Hecht ML. Influences of personal, injunctive, and descriptive norms on early adolescent substance abuse. *Journal of Drug Issues*. 2006; 36(1):147.

Fournier ME, Levy S. Recent trends in adolescent substance use, primary care screening and updates in treatment options. *Curr Opin. Pediatr*. 2006;18:352.

Harrow BS, Tompkins CP, Mitchell PD, Smith KW, Soldz S, Kasten L, Fleming K. The impact of publicly funded managed care on adolescent substance abuse treatment outcomes. *Am J Drug Alcohol Abuse*. 2006;32(3):379.

Nation M, Heflinger CA. Risk factors for serious alcohol and drug use: The psychosocial variables in predicting the frequency of substance use among adolescents. *Am J Drug Alcohol Abuse*. 2006;32:415.

Radin SM, Neighbors C, Walker PS, Walker RD, Marlatt GA, Larimer M. The changing influences of self-worth and peer deviance on drinking problems in urban American Indian adolescents. *Psychol Addict Behav*. 2006;20(2):161.

Samuolis J, Hogue A, Dauber S, Liddle HA. Autonomy and relatedness in inner-city families of substance abusing adolescents. *Journal of Child & Adolescent Substance Abuse*. 2005;15(2):53.

Simkin D. Adolescent substance abuse. In: Sadock BJ, Sadock VA, eds. *Kaplan & Sadock's Comprehensive Textbook of Psychiatry*. 8th ed. Vol. 2. Baltimore: Lippincott Williams & Wilkins; 2005:3470.

Young SE, Rhee SH, Stallings MC, Corley RP, Hewitt JK. Genetic and environmental vulnerabilities underlying adolescent substance use and problem use: General or specific? *Behav Genet*. 2006;36(4):603.

53 Child Psychiatry: Additional Conditions That May Be a Focus of Clinical Attention

BORDERLINE INTELLECTUAL FUNCTIONING

Intellectual functioning of a child or adolescent is influenced by multiple factors, including birth history of full-term gestation, neonatal head circumference, learning, nutritional status, and brain development after birth. Brain parameters, parental head circumference, and prenatal nutrition are most correlated to the head circumference of the newborn. In a sample of Chilean school-age children, those born with small head circumference of at least 2 standard deviations below the mean (microcephalic) were most likely to present with lower overall brain volume, compromised intellectual and scholastic functions, and poor nutrition. Although intellectual quotients (IQ) are generally believed to be stable over time, in some cases, a single measurement of intellectual functioning does not accurately predict intellectual function in all areas over the long term. For example, a follow-up study conducted to investigate the stability of IQ measurement in a group of dyslexia adolescents and young adults who were tested at age 12 years and retested after a mean interval of 6.5 years found the following differences over time. Compared with first IQ tests, for the teens and young adults, the retests showed a significant relative decrease in verbal IQ (VIQ), which was interpreted as either poor reliability of the test or a loss of ability based on diminished experience with reading and writing compared with same age peers over time. Performance IQ (PIQ), however, was found to be significantly increased, leading to the hypothesis that a compensatory process had been naturally developed by these children with dyslexia, such as a more visual or creative way to process information leading to greater success on performance test items. The conclusion was that a single IQ test in childhood may not be a fully accurate predictor of later abilities and that potential interventions to help children with disabilities such as dyslexia keep up academically with peers may have implications for final IQ and intellectual functioning.

Borderline intellectual functioning, according to the text revision of the 4th edition of the American Psychiatric Association's *Diagnostic and Statistical Manual of Mental Disorders* (DSM-IV-TR), is a category that can be used when the focus of clinical attention is on a child or adolescent's IQ in the 71 to 84 range. The intellectual functioning of children plays a major role in their adjustment to school, social relationships, and family function. Children who cannot quite understand class work and may also be slow in understanding rules of games and the "social" rules of their peer group are often bitterly rejected. Some children with borderline intellectual functioning can mingle socially better than they can keep up academically in class. In these cases, the strengths of these children may be peer relationships, especially if they excel at sports, but eventually, their academic struggles will take a toll on self-esteem, if they are not appropriately remediated.

Impaired adaptive functioning , which is diagnosed when difficulties in academic, social, or vocational areas pertaining to borderline intellectual functioning, which accompanies borderline intellectual functioning, become the focus of clinical attention.

Clinicians must assess a patient's intellectual level and current and past levels of adaptive functioning to diagnose borderline intellectual functioning. In patients with major mental disorders whose current level of adaptive functioning has deteriorated, the diagnosis of borderline intellectual functioning may not be clearly evident. In such situations, clinicians must evaluate the patient's history to determine whether the level of adaptive functioning was compromised even before the onset of the mental disorder.

Only about 6 to 7 percent of the population has a borderline IQ as determined by the Stanford-Binet test or the Wechsler scales. The premise behind the inclusion of borderline intellectual functioning in DSM-IV-TR is that persons may experience difficulties in their adaptive capacities as a result of the intellectual deficits and, thus, may require attention. In the absence of specific intrapsychic conflicts, developmental traumas, biochemical abnormalities, and other factors linked to any other mental disorder, such persons may experience severe emotional distress. Frustration and embarrassment over their difficulties may shape their life choices and lead to circumstances warranting psychiatric intervention.

Etiology

Genetic factors are increasingly found to play a role in intellectual deficits. Environmental deprivation and infectious and toxic exposures can also contribute to cognitive impairment. Twin and adoption studies support hypotheses that many genes contribute to the development of a particular IQ. Specific infectious processes (e.g., congenital rubella), prenatal exposures (e.g., fetal alcohol syndrome), and specific chromosomal abnormalities (e.g., fragile X syndrome) result in mental retardation.

Diagnosis

The DSM-IV-TR contains the following statement about borderline intellectual functioning:

> This category can be used when the focus of clinical attention is associated with borderline intellectual functioning, that is, an IQ in the 71 to 84 range. Differential diagnosis between Borderline Intellectual Functioning and Mental Retardation (an IQ of 70 or below) is especially difficult when the coexistence of certain mental disorders (e.g., Schizophrenia) is involved. Coding note: This is categorized on a V Code.

A 13-year-old boy was referred to a partial hospital program because of anger outbursts, temper tantrums, and moodiness in the home. He was in a regular classroom setting, and his grades were marginal. He appeared passive, but, when given adult attention and guidance in school and at home, his overall demeanor and performance brightened. In addition to the psychiatric assessment, evaluation included a pediatric medical examination, blood tests, and urine screening for illicit drugs. School psychological testing was reviewed. Results were generally unremarkable.

There were no medical problems. However, verbal IQ was 75, performance IQ was 80, and adaptive skills proficiency was several years below that expected for his age. A primary diagnosis of borderline intellectual functioning was made. Treatment included heavy emphasis on special help with resource room and accommodations in school, psychoeducation for the family, and brief individual, group, and behavior modification for the patient. Mood and behavior at home significantly improved, self-esteem was enhanced, and school performance—academically and socially—strengthened. (Courtesy of Frank John Ninivaggi, M.D.)

Treatment

The goals of treatment are to maximize educational and vocational placements so that individuals can develop the most optimal practical adaptive skills, social skills, and self-esteem. The goal is to improve the match between the person's capabilities and lifestyle. After the underlying problem becomes known to the therapist, psychiatric treatment can be useful. Many persons with borderline intellectual functioning can function at a superior level in some areas while being markedly deficient in others. By directing such persons to appropriate areas of endeavor, by pointing out socially acceptable behavior, and by teaching them living skills, the therapist can help improve their self-esteem.

ACADEMIC PROBLEM

Academic difficulties in children and adolescents can accompany a wide range of psychosocial conditions related to family life, the environment, mood and behavioral problems, and connection with certain peer groups. In the absence of a specific learning disorder or a direct result of a psychiatric disorder, academic function is related to scholastic strengths, motivation, and ability to apply oneself to the work, and stressful life events. A recent investigation of the effects of students' perception of support from parents, teachers, and peers showed a correlation with adolescent academic achievement. That is, adolescents' perception of support from their teachers and parents was directly related to their academic achievement, whereas perceived peer support was indirectly related to actual academic achievement, it contributed to an adolescent's overall perception of support, which was correlated to achievement.

Behavioral choices and life events can also exacerbate academic problems in the absence of learning disorder and can interfere with lessening academic failures. For example, once a student perceives that he or she is falling behind academically, a greater temptation is to replace academic pursuits with other activities, such as drug use. A recent study assessed the level of, and deterioration in, academic achievement in relation to initiation of marijuana use among young teens. In a sample of rural teens, 36 percent of boys and 23 percent of girls initiated use of marijuana by the end of the 9th grade and that deteriorating academic performance was a significant predictor of initiating marijuana use. The hypothesis remaining to be tested is whether timely intervention to improve academic standing would lower the risk of beginning drug use.

The DSM-IV-TR refers to an academic problem as a problem that is not caused by a mental disorder or, if caused by a mental disorder, is sufficiently severe to warrant clinical attention. This diagnostic category is used when a child or adolescent is having significant academic difficulties that are not deemed to be caused by a specific learning disorder or communication disorder or directly related to a psychiatric disorder. Nevertheless, intervention is necessary because the child's achievement in school is significantly impaired. A child or adolescent of normal intelligence and is free of a learning disorder or a communication disorder, but is failing in school or doing poorly, falls into this category.

Etiology

Many psychological factors contribute to a child's confidence, competence, and academic success. In the absence of a specific learning disorder to account for the academic difficulty or primary psychiatric disorder responsible for the academic compromise, subclinical states of anxiety or depression, peer and family stressors such as divorce, marital discord, abuse, or mental illness in a family member, may interrupt academic production. Children who are troubled by social isolation, identity issues, preoccupation with sexuality, or extreme shyness may withdraw from full participation in academic activities. Academic problems may be the result of a confluence of multiple contributing factors and may occur in adolescents who were previously high academic achievers. School is the main social and educational venue for children and adolescents. Success and acceptance in the school setting depend on children's physical, cognitive, social, and emotional adjustment. Children's general coping mechanisms in many developmental tasks usually are reflected in their academic and social success in school. Boys and girls must cope with the process of separation from parents, adjustment to new environments, adaptation to social contacts, competition, assertion, intimacy, and exposure to unfamiliar attitudes. A corresponding relation often exists between school performance and how well these tasks are mastered.

Anxiety can play a major role in interfering with children's academic performances. Anxiety can hamper their abilities to perform well on tests, to speak in public, and to ask questions when they do not understand something. Some children are so concerned about the way others view them that they cannot attend to their academic tasks. For some children, conflicts about success and fears of the consequences imagined to accompany the attainment of success can hamper academic success. Sigmund Freud described persons with such conflicts as "those wrecked by success." For example, an adolescent girl may be unable to succeed in school because she fears social rejection or the loss of femininity, or both, and she perceives success as being involved with aggression and competition with boys.

Depressed children also may withdraw from academic pursuits; they require specific interventions to improve their academic performances and to treat their depression. Children who do not have major depressive disorder, but who are consumed by family problems, such as financial troubles, marital discord in their parents, and mental illness in family members, may be distracted and unable to attend to academic tasks. Children who receive mixed messages from their parents about accepting criticism and redirection from their teachers can become confused and unable to perform well in school. The loss of the parents as the primary and predominant teachers in a child's life can result in identity conflicts for some children. Some students lack a stable sense of self and cannot identify goals for themselves, a situation that leads to a sense of boredom or futility.

Cultural and economic background can play a role in how well accepted a child feels in school and can affect the child's academic achievement. Familial socioeconomic level, parental education, race, religion, and family functioning can influence a child's sense of fitting in and can affect preparation to meet school demands.

Schools, teachers, and clinicians can share insights about how to foster productive and cooperative environments for all students in a classroom. Teachers' expectations about their students' performance influence these performances. Teachers serve as agents whose varying expectations can shape the differential development of students' skills and abilities. Such conditioning early in school, especially when negative, can disturb academic performance. A teacher's affective response to a child, therefore, can prompt the appearance of an academic problem. Most important is a teacher's humane approach to students at all levels of education, including medical school.

Diagnosis

The DSM-IV-TR contains the following statement about academic problem:

> This category can be used when the focus of clinical attention is an academic problem that is not due to a mental disorder or, if due to a mental disorder, is sufficiently severe to warrant independent clinical attention. An example is a pattern of failing grades or of significant underachievement in a person with adequate intellectual capacity in the absence of a learning or a communication disorder or any other mental disorder that would account for the problem.

A 15-year-old boy was admitted to an intensive outpatient program for evaluation of insidiously declining grades at school, isolative behavior, and anhedonia occurring for the first time over the course of the last semester at high school. The patient had no previous psychiatric history and was in good health. School reports showed his full-scale IQ to be 100 and revealed no previous behavior or academic problems. Interviews with family and patient revealed that the boy had an intact family with no apparent or unusual conflicts noted and that his mother found evidence of drug paraphernalia—cigarette papers, small pipe, matches, and a suspicious-looking dried substance in his bedroom. When confronted, the patient revealed a 6-month use of marijuana. A primary diagnosis of cannabis abuse, in addition to academic problem, was made. Referral to a therapeutic drug and alcohol program was immediately implemented. (Courtesy of Frank John Ninivaggi, M.D.)

Treatment

The initial step in determining a useful intervention for an academic problem is a comprehensive diagnostic evaluation. Identifying and addressing family-, school-, and peer-related stressors are critical. Substance use disorders must be carefully ruled out, as well as concurrent psychiatric disorders that may require treatment before improvement in academic function. An individualized educational plan evaluation and meeting may be requested in writing to the school so that specific educational testing can be integrated into the assessment of the overall academic problem, and educational accommodations can be considered.

Psychosocial intervention may be applied successfully for scholastic difficulties related to poor motivation, poor self-concept, and underachievement. Early efforts to relieve the problem are critical: Sustained problems in learning and school performance frequently are compounded and precipitate severe difficulties. Feelings of anger, frustration, shame, loss of self-respect, and helplessness—emotions that most often accompany school failures—damage self-esteem emotionally and cognitively, disabling future performance and clouding expectations for success. Generally, children with academic problems require either school-based intervention or individual attention.

Tutoring is an effective technique for dealing with academic problems and should be considered in most cases. Tutoring has proved of value in preparing for objective multiple choice examinations, such as the *Scholastic Aptitude Test* (SAT) and *Medical College Aptitude Test* (MCAT). Taking such examinations repetitively and using relaxation skills are two behavioral techniques of great value in diminishing anxiety.

CHILDHOOD OR ADOLESCENT ANTISOCIAL BEHAVIOR

Antisocial behaviors are the most common reason for a child or adolescent to be referred for a psychiatric evaluation. Antisocial behaviors, however, are so varied in severity and frequency and occur in children and adolescents of a wide range of ages and developmental levels that it would be difficult to identify a single etiology. Prospective studies of youth at risk for antisocial behavior have shown that meaningful subtypes exist of antisocial behavior. One way to classify these behaviors is by separating them into authority-defying behaviors, overt and covert antisocial acts. Less serious antisocial behaviors in childhood tend to be characterized as defiance, or defying authority figures. Covert antisocial behaviors, such as stealing, typically occur in later childhood, whereas the most severe overt antisocial acts, such as violent behaviors, do not usually emerge until adolescence. Youth with the poorest prognoses tend to exhibit overt antisocial acts at younger ages, and display a pattern of overt, covert, and authority-defying behaviors over time.

Some of the most striking displays of antisocial behavior among youth in recent times have been the shootings of students and staff at Columbine High School in Colorado, and Santana High School in California. The relationship of antisocial behavior to psychopathology is complex in so far as a given act of violence is not always equitably directly related to a specific psychiatric disorder. Current data on the etiology of antisocial behavior fit best into a cumulative risk factor model in which the likelihood of antisocial acts increases as the risks accumulate.

This complex mechanism seems to perpetuate itself in the following way. A vulnerable child interacts with his or her immediate family, environment, and peer group to develop a pattern of impulsivity, aggression, and a disregard for the feelings and rights of others. When children with these negative behavioral patterns and cognitions then develop a second tier of negative interactions through rejection by peers, teachers, and parents, and especially when additional adverse life events or losses occur, even more negative behaviors ensue. A recent investigation by the US Secret Service and Department of Education found that youth who perpetrate attacks in schools were often shunned by peer groups, were poorly coping with personal losses, and experiencing academic and other failures. An additional typical factor in the profile is the regular access in their home environments to weapons. So, although no clear profile can predict who specifically may turn out to be a violent threat to a school, the data found that youth who have committed violent acts in schools were generally characterized as socially isolated, were exhibiting signs and symptoms of social and emotional stress, and had access to weapons, mainly guns.

According to DSM-IV-TR, child or adolescent antisocial behavior refers to behavior that is not caused by a mental disorder and includes isolated antisocial acts, not a pattern of behavior. This category covers many acts by children and adolescents that violate the rights of others, such as overt acts of aggression and violence, and covert acts of lying, stealing, truancy, and running away from home. Certain antisocial acts, such as fire-setting, possession of a weapon, or a severe act of aggression toward another child, require intervention for even a single occurrence. Sometimes, children without a pattern of recurrent aggression or antisocial behavior become involved in occasional less severe behaviors that nevertheless require some intervention. The DSM-IV-TR definition of conduct disorder requires a repetitive pattern of at least three antisocial behaviors for at least 6 months, but childhood or adolescent antisocial behavior may consist of isolated events that do not constitute a mental disorder but do become the focus of clinical attention. The emergence of occasional antisocial symptoms is common among children who have a variety of mental disorders, including psychotic disorders, depressive disorders, impulse-control disorders, disruptive behavior, and attention-deficit disorders, such as attention-deficit/hyperactivity disorder (ADHD) and oppositional defiant disorder.

A child's age and developmental level affect the manifestations of disturbed conduct and influence the child's likelihood to meet the diagnostic criteria for a conduct disorder, as opposed to childhood antisocial behavior. Therefore, a child of 5 or 6 years of age is not likely to meet the criteria for three antisocial symptoms—for example, physical confrontations, the use of weapons, and forcing someone into sexual activity—but a single symptom, such as initiating fights, is common in children 5 to 6 years of age. The term *juvenile delinquent* is defined by the legal system as a youth who has violated the law in some way, but the term does not imply that the youth meets the criteria for a mental disorder.

Epidemiology

Estimates of antisocial behavior range from 5 to 15 percent of the general population and somewhat less among children and adolescents. Reports have documented a higher frequency of antisocial behaviors in urban settings than in rural areas. In one report, the risk of coming into contact with the police for antisocial behavior was estimated to be 20 percent for teenage boys and 4 percent for teenage girls.

Etiology

Antisocial behaviors can occur in the context of a mental disorder or in its absence. Antisocial behavior is multidetermined and occurs most frequently in children or adolescents with many risk factors. Among the most common risk factors are harsh and physically abusive parenting, parental criminality, and a child's tendency toward impulsive and hyperactive behavior. Protective factors can attenuate the risk of antisocial behaviors by exerting an independent influence on strengthening core aspects of functioning and thereby decreasing risk. Protective factors can include high intelligence, an easy or self-directed temperament, high levels of social skill, competence in school or in other domains of artistic or athletic skill, and finally, a strong bond with at least one parent. Additional associated features of children and adolescents with antisocial behavior are low IQ, academic failure, and low levels of adult supervision. (See Chapter 33 for a discussion of genetic and social factors as causes of adult antisocial behavior.)

Psychological Factors. If their parenting is poor, children experience emotional deprivation, which leads to low self-esteem and unconscious anger. When children are not given any limits, their consciences are deficient because they have not internalized parental prohibitions that account for superego formation. Therefore, they have so-called *superego lacunae*, which allow them to commit antisocial acts without guilt. At times, such children's antisocial behavior is a vicarious source of pleasure and gratification for parents who act out their own forbidden wishes and impulses through their children. A consistent finding in persons who perform repeated acts of violent behavior is a history of physical abuse.

Diagnosis and Clinical Features

The DSM-IV-TR contains the following statement about childhood or adolescent antisocial behavior:

> This category can be used when the focus of clinical attention is antisocial behavior in a child or adolescent that is not due to a mental disorder (e.g., Conduct Disorder or an Impulse-Control Disorder). Examples include isolated antisocial acts of children or adolescents (not a pattern of antisocial behavior).

The childhood behaviors most associated with antisocial behavior are theft, incorrigibility, arrests, school problems, impulsiveness, promiscuity, oppositional behavior, lying, suicide attempts, substance abuse, truancy, running away, associating with undesirable persons, and staying out late at night. The more symptoms present in childhood, the greater the probability of adult antisocial behavior; however, the presence of many symptoms also indicates the development of other mental disorders in adult life.

Differential Diagnosis

Substance-related disorders (including alcohol, cannabis, and cocaine use disorders), bipolar I disorder, and schizophrenia in childhood often manifest themselves as antisocial behavior.

A 9-year-old child was arrested by police for breaking into a local hardware store. He was accompanied by two friends. The three had ridden their bikes in a suburban neighborhood until after dark and engaged in a play of "cops and robbers," taking turns in pursuing and being pursued. To make the game more lifelike, one of the three suggested that they actually break into this store, whose owner was a somewhat gruff and intimidating man. The three decided that such an adventure would be quite exciting and proceeded to smash in the glass door with a brick. Shortly after the glass broke, the police arrived and arrested them. Parents were called to come and to collect their children. None of the three had any previous contact with the police or any social service agency. Although they previously engaged in some mischief in the neighborhood, such as throwing toilet paper on people's houses and egging cars, none of the three had any serious infractions of societal rules, and none of the three boys had any more of these events cluster in the past few months. One of them had a history of ADHD and some learning difficulties at school, whereas the other two boys had no particular risk factors for the persistence of antisocial behavior. The antisocial activities of the child with ADHD progressed to the point of fulfilling conduct disorder criteria in early adolescence. Much of his future acting out consisted of drug-related offenses, that is, the use and sales of drugs, stealing, and other covert delinquent activities. The two boys without risks proceeded to develop through a normative, turbulent, and lively adolescence without any further legal involvement. (Courtesy of Hans Steiner, M.D., and Niranjan Karnik, M.D., Ph.D.)

Treatment

Antisocial behavior does not specifically represent a corresponding psychiatric disorder; therefore, a comprehensive psychiatric assessment and the context in which the antisocial behavior emerged must be conducted to delineate the place of the antisocial behavior with respect to any comorbid psychopathology.

Disturbances of conduct frequently accompany the onset of various other psychiatric disorders. The first step in determining the appropriate treatment for a child or an adolescent who is manifesting antisocial behavior is to evaluate the need to treat any coexisting mental disorder, such as bipolar I disorder, a psychotic disorder, or a depressive disorder, that may be contributing to the antisocial behavior. The treatment of antisocial behavior usually involves behavioral management, which is most effective when the patient is in a controlled environment in a structured day or residential setting. In less severe situations, the child's family members are able to manage the symptoms in collaboration with the clinician by utilizing a cooperative behavioral program.

In some cases, special educational settings are necessary to provide the essential monitoring and feedback necessary to diminish the undesired behaviors. In some cases, even regular school classroom teachers can help modify antisocial behavior in the classroom. Rewards for prosocial behaviors and positive reinforcement for the control of unwanted behaviors have merit.

Medications generally are not used in patients with rare or occasional antisocial behaviors, especially when no comorbid psychiatric disorders exist. Medications have been used with some success when repetitive episodes of explosive behavior, aggression, or violent outbursts ensue. Lithium (Eskalith), divalproex (Depakote) and atypical antipsychotics such as risperidone (Risperdal), olanzapine (Zyprexa), quetiapine (Seroquel), ziprasidone (Geodon), or aripiprazole (Abilify) may reduce explosive behavior and rage outbursts. For young children who are sensitive to the extrapyramidal side effects of antipsychotics, chlorpromazine (Thorazine), despite its sedating properties, may be better tolerated and more efficacious in managing acute aggression. The use of diphenhydramine (Benadryl) or lorazepam (Ativan) may be helpful as adjunctive medications in the short-term control of aggressive behavior. When symptoms of ADHD, such as hyperactivity and impulsivity, are contributing factors, short- or long-acting methylphenidate agents (Ritalin, Concerta), or short- or long-acting amphetamine and amphetamine salts (Adderall, Adderall XR) may help to reduce impulsivity and decrease aggression.

It is more difficult to treat children and adolescents who exhibit long-term patterns of antisocial behavior, particularly covert behaviors, such as stealing and lying. Group therapy in the context of residential treatment centers has been used for these behaviors, and cognitive problem-solving approaches are potentially helpful.

IDENTITY PROBLEM

The conceptualization of identity encompasses cognitive, psychodynamic, psychosexual, neurobiological, and cultural development. The developmentalist Erik Erikson proposed, in his writings "Identity and the Life Cycle," that the central task of adolescence is to achieve a sense of selfsameness and continuity in time. The normative developmental process for an adolescent was conceptualized by Erikson as an adolescent crisis of identity. The transition between a childhood identity and the process of accepting a more mature sense of self is the resolution of the "crisis." The notion of an identity crisis in adolescence gained widespread attention by clinicians and the popular media during the late 1960s and early 1970s when many adolescents displayed rejection of mainstream cultural values and ideas and demonstrated alternate lifestyles. The concept of *identity disorder* as a psychiatric diagnosis was embraced in the 1980s when the DMS-III was devised, as a disorder usually first evident in childhood. It was meant to include adolescents who presented with "severe subjective distress regarding uncertainty about a variety of issues relating to identity" to the point where they became impaired. So, according to DSM-IV-TR, identity problem refers to uncertainty about issues, such as goals, career choice, friendships, sexual behavior, moral values, and group loyalties. An identity problem can cause severe distress for a young person and can lead a person to seek psychotherapy or guidance. Identity problem, however, is not recognized as a mental disorder in DSM-IV-TR. It sometimes manifests in the context of such mental disorders as mood disorders, psychotic disorders, and borderline personality disorder.

Epidemiology

No reliable information is available regarding predisposing factors, familial pattern, sex ratio, or prevalence, but problems with identity formation seem to be a result of life in modern society. Today, children and adolescents often experience great instability in family life, problems with identity formation, conflicts between adolescent peer values and the values of parents and society, and exposure through the media and education to various moral, behavioral, and lifestyle possibilities.

Etiology

The causes of identity problems often are multifactorial and include the pressures of a highly dysfunctional family and the influences of coexisting mental disorders. In general, adolescents with major depressive disorder, psychotic disorders, and other mental disorders report feeling alienated from family members and experience some turmoil. Children who have had difficulty mastering expected developmental tasks all along are likely to have difficulty with the pressure to establish a well-defined identity during adolescence. Erikson used the term *identity versus role diffusion* to describe the developmental and psychosocial tasks challenging adolescents to incorporate past experiences and present goals into a coherent sense of self.

Diagnosis and Clinical Features

The DSM-IV-TR contains the following statement about identity problem:

> This category can be used when the focus of clinical attention is uncertainty about multiple issues relating to identity such as long-term goals, career choice, friendship patterns, sexual orientation and behavior, moral values, and group loyalties.

The essential features of identity problem seem to revolve around the question, "Who am I?" Conflicts are experienced as irreconcilable aspects of the self that the adolescent cannot integrate into a coherent identity. As Erikson described identity problem, youth manifests severe doubting and an inability to make decisions, a sense of isolation, inner emptiness, a growing inability to relate to others, disturbed sexual functioning, a distorted time perspective, a sense of urgency, and the assumption of a negative identity. The associated features frequently include marked discrepancy between the adolescent's self-perception and the views that others have of the adolescent; moderate anxiety and depression that are usually related to inner preoccupation, rather than external realities; and self-doubt and uncertainty about the future, with either difficulty making choices or impulsive experiments in an attempt to establish an independent identity. Some persons with identity problem join cult-like groups.

Differential Diagnosis

Identity problem must be differentiated from a mental disorder (e.g., borderline personality disorder, schizophreniform disorder, schizophrenia, or a mood disorder). At times, what initially seems to be an identity problem may be the prodromal manifestations of one of these disorders. Intense, but normal, conflicts associated with maturing, such as adolescent turmoil and midlife crisis, may be confusing, but they usually are not associated with marked deterioration in school, in vocational or social functioning, or with severe subjective distress. Considerable evidence indicates that adolescent turmoil often is not a phase that is outgrown but an indication of true psychopathology.

Course and Prognosis

The onset of identity problem most frequently occurs in late adolescence, as teenagers separate from the nuclear family and attempt to establish an independent identity and value system. The onset usually is characterized by a gradual increase in anxiety, depression, regressive phenomena (e.g., loss of interest in friends, school, and activities), irritability, sleep difficulties, and changes in eating habits. The course usually is relatively brief, as developmental lags respond to support, acceptance, and the provision of a psychosocial moratorium.

Extensive prolongation of adolescence with continued identity problem can lead to the chronic state of role diffusion, which may indicate a disturbance of early developmental stages and the presence of borderline personality disorder, a mood disorder, or schizophrenia. An identity problem usually resolves by the mid-20s. If it persists, the person with the identity problem may be unable to make career commitments or lasting attachments.

Cory, an 8-year-old girl, was adopted in Taiwan at 10 months of age by a white midwestern couple. As she grew, her vulnerability to separations became increasingly more pronounced. Even the possibility that her adoptive mother would leave her for the day triggered what appeared to be dramatic disruptions in Cory's reality contact, as well as outbursts of rage and misbehavior in school. She pleaded with her mother to care for the many aches and pains that plagued her. If her mother stayed with her, they could both enjoy the girl's favorite game—the mother playing the part of an Asian queen, with Cory as her beloved princess. Yet, the girl's demands, including the requirements of "royalty," were so exhausting that, at times, the mother would seek relief at her own mother's home in a nearby town.

Such "abandonment" would more than perturb the idyllic fantasy of the queen and her princess. Without the love, protection, and presence of the queen, Cory herself changed, turning into a "Chinese bitch." Later, in therapy, she discussed how a vivid fantasy would come to her at times of separation. In this fantasy, a witch, a vicious vixen of mixed Caucasian and Asian features, taunted Cory and threatened to drag her down into a bottomless pit.

Cory hated this witch nearly as much as she hated the "Chinese bitch" she herself became. She hated, in particular, the rage and anguish that overwhelmed her. To punish the "bitch," she would hit herself and poke at her skin until it bled.

By the time she reached adolescence, Cory's self-mutilating behavior was firmly established. She responded to frustration, separations, or perceived threats of abandonment by cutting herself or burning herself with cigarette lighters. Eventually, she was able to verbalize the multiple functions that self-injury served for her. It forced others to respond to her instead of ignoring her; it allowed her to "stick it" to others without having to take responsibility for her aggression; it produced in her feelings that countered the sense of deadness and emptiness that came on her when she felt desperate; and, last, but certainly not least, it created for her the illusion that she could control hope and healing, as she could literally see the healing taking place in her skin after she had wounded it, rather than waiting for someone else to hurt her or depending on others to provide her with a sense of hope. (Courtesy of Efrain Bleiberg, M.D.)

Treatment

Considerable concensus exists among clinicians, in the absence of an evidence base, that adolescents experiencing identity problems may respond to brief psychosocial intervention. Individual psychotherapy directed toward encouraging growth and development usually is considered the therapy of choice. Adolescents with identity problems often feel developmentally unprepared to deal with the increasing demands for social, emotional, and sexual independence. Issues of separation and individuation from their families can be challenging and overwhelming. Treatment is aimed at helping these adolescents develop a sense of competence and mastery about necessary social and vocational choices. A therapist's empathic acknowledgment of an adolescent's struggle can be helpful in the process.

References

Bambauer KZ, Connor DF. Characteristics of aggression in clinically referred children. *CNS Spectrums*. 2005;10(9):709.

Bleiberg E. Identity problem and borderline disorders in children and adolescents In: Sadock BJ, Sadock VA, eds. *Kaplan & Sadock's Comprehensive Textbook of Psychiatry*. 8th ed. Vol. 2. Baltimore: Lippincott Williams & Wilkins; 2005: 3457.

Chabrol H, Leichsenring F. Borderline personality organization and psychopathic traits in nonclinical adolescents: Relationship of identity diffusion, primitive defense mechanism and reality testing with callousness and impulsivity traits. *Bull Menninger Clin*. 2006;70:160.

Chen JJ. Relation of academic support from parents, teachers and peers to Hong Kong adolescents' academic achievement: The mediating role of academic engagement. *Genet Soc Gen Psychol Monogr*. 2005;131:77.

Erikson EH. Identity and the life cycle: Selected papers. *Psychol Issues*. 1959;1:1.

Henry KL, Smith EA, Caldwell LL. Deterioration of academic achievement and marijuana use onset among rural adolescents. *Health Educ Res*. 2006;(ahead of pub).

Ingesson SG. Stability of IQ measures in teenagers and young adults with developmental dyslexia. *Dyslexia*. 2006;12:81.

Ivanovic DM, Leiva BP, Perez HT, Olivares MG, Diaz NS, Urrutia MS, Almagia AF, Toro TD, Miller PT, Bosch EO, Larrain CG. Head size and intelligence, learning, nutritional status and brain development. Head, IQ, learning, nutrition and brain. *Neuropsychologica*. 2004;42:1118.

Ninivaggi FJ. Borderline intellectual functioning and academic problem. In: Sadock BJ, Sadock VA, eds. *Kaplan & Sadock's Comprehensive Textbook of Psychiatry*. 8th ed. Vol. 2. Baltimore: Lippincott Williams & Wilkins; 2005:2272.

Steiner H, Karnik N. Child or adolescent antisocial behavior. In: Sadock BJ, Sadock VA, eds. *Kaplan & Sadock's Comprehensive Textbook of Psychiatry*. 8th ed. Vol. 2. Lippincott Williams & Wilkins; 2005:3441.

Sukhodolsky DG, Ruchkin V. Juvenile justice. *Child Adolescent Psychiatr Clin N Am*. 2006:15(2):501–16.

54 Psychiatric Treatment of Children and Adolescents

▲ 54.1 Individual Psychotherapy

Individual psychotherapy for children and adolescents can take many forms, including short- and long-term approaches within a variety of conceptual frameworks, such as cognitive-behavioral, behavioral, psychodynamic, supportive, interpersonal, and "eclectic" mixtures of these techniques. In recent years, randomized clinical trials have provided data to support the efficacy of cognitive-behavioral interventions for a wide range of childhood psychiatric disorders including obsessive-compulsive disorder (OCD), anxiety disorders, and depressive disorders. The initial goal of any psychotherapeutic strategy is to establish a working relationship with the child or adolescent. In general, successful individual psychotherapeutic interventions with children also require establishing a therapeutic rapport with parents. To approach a child therapeutically, requires a sense of normal development of a child of a given age as well as an understanding of the context in which particular symptoms emerged. Individual psychotherapy with children focuses on improving children's adaptive skills as well as diminishing specific symptomatology. Treatment reflects an understanding of children's developmental levels and shows cultural sensitivity toward families and environments in which children live. Most children do not seek psychiatric treatment; they are taken to a psychotherapist because of a disturbance noted by a family member, a schoolteacher, or a pediatrician. Children often believe that they are being taken for treatment because of their *misbehavior* or as a punishment for *wrongdoing*.

Children and adolescents are the most accurate informants of their own thoughts, feelings, moods, and perceptual experiences; external behavior problems are often identified by others, however, yet children's internal experiences may be largely unknown. Children often can describe their feelings in a particular situation, but cannot execute therapeutic changes without an advocate's help. Thus, child psychotherapists function as advocates for their child patients in interactions with schools, legal agencies, and community organizations. Child psychotherapists may be called on to make recommendations that affect various aspects of children's lives.

THEORIES AND TECHNIQUES

Emotional, social, and academic issues of children of varying ages and developmental levels can be addressed by clinicians utilizing a working knowledge of diverse psychotherapeutic techniques and their applications in childhood. Psychodynamic approaches are generally mixed with supportive components and behavioral management techniques to build a comprehensive treatment plan for a child. Individual psychotherapy with a child frequently takes place in conjunction with family therapy, group therapy, and, when indicated, psychopharmacology. Several theoretical systems underlie psychotherapeutic approaches with children, including psychoanalytic theories, behavioral theories, family systems theories, and developmental theories.

Psychoanalytic Theories

In classic psychoanalytic theory, exploratory psychotherapy applies to patients of all ages by reversing the evolution of psychopathological processes. A principal difference noted with advancing age is a sharpening distinction between psychogenetic and psychodynamic factors. The younger the child, the more the genetic and dynamic forces are intertwined. The development of these pathological processes generally is believed to begin with experiences that have proved to be particularly significant to children and to have affected them adversely. Although in one sense the experiences were real, in another sense, they may have been misinterpreted or imagined. In any event, to children, these were traumatic experiences that caused unconscious complexes. Being inaccessible to conscious awareness, the unconscious elements readily escape rational adaptive maneuvers and are subject to pathological misuse of adaptive and defensive mechanisms. The result is the development of conflicts leading to distressing symptoms, character attitudes, or patterns of behavior that constitute the emotional disturbance.

The psychoanalytic view of emotional disturbances in children has increasingly assumed a developmental orientation. Thus, the maladaptive defensive functioning is directed against conflicts between impulses that characterize a specific developmental phase and environmental influences or a child's internalized representations of environment. In this framework, disorders result from environmental interference with maturational timetables or conflicts with the environment engendered by developmental progress. The result is difficulty achieving or resolving developmental tasks and fulfilling capacities that are specific to later phases of development. These developmental stages can be expressed in various ways, from Anna Freud's lines of development to Erik Erikson's concept of sequential psychosocial capacities.

The goal of therapy is to help develop good conflict-resolution skills in children so they can function at their appropriate developmental levels. Therapy may again be necessary as children face the challenges of subsequent developmental periods.

Psychoanalytic psychotherapy, a modified form of psychotherapy, is expressive and exploratory and endeavors to reverse the evolution of emotional disturbance through reenacting and desensitizing traumatic events by freely expressing thoughts and feelings in an interview-play situation. Ultimately, therapists help patients understand the warded-off feelings, fears, and wishes that have beset them.

Whereas the psychoanalytic psychotherapeutic approach seeks improvement by exposure and resolution of buried conflicts, suppressive-supportive-educative psychotherapy works in the opposite fashion by aiming to facilitate repression. Therapists, capitalizing on patients' desire to please, encourage them to substitute new adaptive and defensive mechanisms. In this therapy, clinicians use interpretations minimally; instead, they emphasize suggestion, persuasion, exhortation, operant reinforcement, counseling, education, direction, advice, abreaction, environmental manipulation, intellectual review, gratification of the patient's current dependent needs, and similar techniques.

Behavioral Theories

All behavior, whether adaptive or maladaptive, is a consequence of the same basic principles of behavior acquisition and maintenance. Behavior is either learned or unlearned. What renders behavior abnormal or disturbed is its social significance. Although theories and their derivative therapeutic intervention techniques have become increasingly complex over the years, all learning can be subsumed in two global basic mechanisms. One is classic *respondent conditioning*, akin to Ivan Pavlov's famous experiments, and the second is *operant instrumental learning*, which is associated with B. F. Skinner, although it is basic to both Edward Thorndike's law of effect, which is about the influence of reinforcing consequences of behavior, and to Sigmund Freud's pain-pleasure principle. Both of these basic mechanisms assign the highest priority to the immediate precipitants of behavior and deemphasize remote underlying causal determinants that are important in the psychoanalytic tradition.

The respondent conditioning theory asserts that only two types of abnormal behavior exist: behavioral deficits that result from a failure to learn and deviant maladaptive behavior that is a consequence of learning inappropriate things. Such concepts have always been an implicit part of the rationale underlying all child psychotherapy. Intervention strategies derive much of their success, particularly with children, from rewarding previously unnoticed good behavior, thereby highlighting it, and making it occur more frequently than in the past.

Family Systems Theories

Although families have long been an interest of child psychotherapists, the understanding of transactional family processes has been greatly enhanced by conceptual contributions from cybernetics, systems theory, communications theory, object relations theory, social role theory, ethology, and ecology. The bedrock premise entails the idea of a family functioning as a self-regulating, open system that possesses its own unique history and structure. This structure is constantly evolving as a consequence of dynamic interaction between the family's mutually interdependent systems and persons who share a complementarity of needs. From this conceptual foundation, a wealth of ideas has emerged under rubrics such as family development, life cycle, homeostasis, functions, identity, values, goals, congruence, symmetry, myths, rules; roles, such as spokesperson, symptoms-bearer, scapegoat, affect barometer, pet, persecutor, victim, arbitrator, distractor, saboteur, rescuer, breadwinner, disciplinarian, nurturer; structure, such as boundaries, splits, pairings, alliances, coalitions, enmeshed, disengaged; and double bind, scapegoating, pseudomutuality, and mystification. Increasingly, appreciation of the family system sometimes explains why a minute therapeutic input at a critical junction may result in far-reaching changes, whereas in other situations, huge amounts of therapeutic effort seem to be absorbed with minimal evidence of change.

Developmental Theories

Underlying child psychotherapy is the assumption that, in the absence of unusual interference, children mature in basically orderly, predictable ways that can be codified in a variety of interrelated psychosociobiological sequential systematizations. The central, overriding role of a developmental frame of reference in child psychotherapy distinguishes it from adult psychotherapy. A therapist's orientation should entail more than a knowledge of age-appropriate behavior derived from such studies as Arnold Gesell's description of the morphology of behavior. It should encompass more than psychosexual development with ego psychological and sociocultural amendments, exemplified by Erikson's epigenetic schema. It extends beyond familiarity with Jean Piaget's sequence of intellectual evolution as a basis for knowing the level of abstraction at which children of various ages may be expected to function or for assessing their capacities for moral orientation.

TYPES OF PSYCHOTHERAPIES

Developing a psychotherapeutic intervention for a particular child includes evaluation of the child's age, developmental level, type of problem, and communication style. Whichever style or combination of techniques a therapist chooses to use in psychotherapy, the relationship between child and therapist is a critical element. The relationship itself often is the primary, if not the sole, ingredient in psychotherapy. The therapist provides a safe space in which to listen, empathize, and solve problems with the child.

John, a bright 14-year-old, was treated with brief (25 sessions) psychotherapy. The initial complaint was that his grades had dropped during the academic year; he had withdrawn from sports, was anhedonic, had difficulty relating to his peers, and whined a lot. His parents divorced when John was 7 years old. He had two younger sisters, ages 12 and 9. John "hated" his father; therefore, he missed many visitations with him, pretending that he was sick or too busy to see him. His sisters kept close contact with the father. His mother had a live-in boyfriend who moved in the year that John became symptomatic. John also "hated" the boyfriend. He felt miserable and reproached everyone in his environment. During the first two therapy sessions, two issues to be addressed were delineated: John feeling rejected by his father and mother (who had found another man) and his issues with rivalry. During the following treatment sessions, an empathetic and supportive therapist helped John acquire insight into his feelings through interpretation of his defenses, transferential manifestations, and clarifications. John and the therapist discussed strategies and activities to be carried out during the treatment period to alleviate his discomfort. By session 16, John had reestablished regular contact with his father and was able to tolerate his mother's boyfriend. The termination phase included the integration of what had been discussed, learned, and practiced, and gave John the ability to understand his internal conflicts and find more appropriate ways of managing them. His rivalry issues had diminished, as he was also able to share his father with his sisters. His biological parents and his mother's boyfriend were seen in parallel. The sessions consisted of psychoeducational approaches concerning John's developmental level of functioning and the way he perceived and experienced his environment. His parents were helped to recognize and handle John's problems, as well their own conflicts, and strategies were proposed for facilitating John's development. At termination, it was agreed that John would return to see the therapist for one follow-up session every 3 months in the first year and every 6 months in the following 2 years. At the 2-year follow-up, it was apparent that John had improved academically and had resumed his outside activities, such as sports. He remained sensitive to rejection, but he was able to use the skills he had learned to manage those feelings. (Courtesy of Euthymia D. Hibbs, Ph.D.)

Cognitive-behavioral therapy (CBT) is an amalgam of behavioral therapy and cognitive psychology. It emphasizes how children may use thinking processes and cognitive modalities to reframe, restructure, and solve problems. A child's distortions are addressed by generating alternative ways of dealing with problematic situations. Cognitive-behavioral strategies have been shown in multiple studies to be effective in the treatment of child and adolescent mood disorders, OCD, and anxiety disorders. A recent study compared a family-focused CBT: the "Building Confidence Program" with traditional child-focused CBT with minimal family involvement for children with anxiety disorders. Both interventions included coping skills training and in vivo exposure, but the family CBT intervention also included parent communication training. Compared with the child-focused CBT, family CBT was associated with greater improvement on independent evaluators' ratings and parent reports of child anxiety, but not on children's self-reports of improvement. Family-focused CBT has also been used in the treatment of pediatric bipolar disorder with promising success.

One of the limiting factors in providing CBT to children with OCD, anxiety disorders, and depressive disorders is the lack of sufficient numbers of trained child and adolescent cognitive-behavioral therapists, and a recent study addressed the issue of the feasibility of combining a CBT via clinic-plus-internet condition. Children who received the clinic-plus internet condition showed significantly greater reductions in anxiety from pre- to posttreatment condition and maintained gains for a period of 12 months compared with children who received no active treatment, but were on a wait-list condition. The internet treatment was acceptable to families and dropout rate was minimal.

A recent study of a CBT in conjunction with an attachment-based family therapy (ABFT) used in adolescents with anxiety disorders and their families showed significant improvements utilizing individual CBT along with a family therapy condition. Participants followed at 6 to 9 months after the treatment showed significant decreases in anxiety and depressive symptoms. Cognitive behavior therapy has now been shown in multiple randomized clinical trials to demonstrate efficacy in the treatment of anxiety disorders in children and adolescents. Using a variety of components, including behavioral exposure, cognitive restructuring, and psychoeducation, CBT has been shown to be adaptable to a variety of formats, including individual, family, and group treatment.

Michael was a 16-year-old boy from an intact middle-class family enrolled in the 11th grade of a public school. He sought evaluation and treatment for a long-standing history of shyness and anxiety in social situations. Evaluation revealed social phobia as the primary disorder. Michael was motivated for treatment and reported that he wished to feel more comfortable with other people and in social situations with peers. Consequently, Michael was treated with cognitive-behavioral group treatment for adolescents with social phobia, a 16-session course of treatment combining education, cognitive restructuring, behavioral exposure, relapse prevention, and four sessions of parent involvement. As treatment progressed, Michael increased his visibility at school-sponsored social events such that he caught the attention of a female classmate and was asked to attend the prom with her. The therapists designed several prom exposures whereby the various things that could happen at a dance or on a date were presented to Michael, including being offered alcohol or drugs, having a good time dancing, being left alone or ignored by his date, having an argument with the date, and having other girls ask him to dance. As it turned out, Michael's date did, in fact, ignore him and leave him at the dance. Michael, prepared for this less-than-desired outcome by the group experience, asked other girls to dance and interacted with other peers. He considered the evening a success and subsequently went on to other social events with friends made at the prom. In this case study, the importance of exposing youth to the range of potential outcomes for a given social situation was crucial to Michael's trust in the therapy and therapists and a belief in the credibility of treatment. Moreover, he was appropriately prepared through behavioral exposure and practice to handle what could have been an awkward and discouraging situation. (Courtesy of Anne Marie Albano, Ph.D.)

Freddy was a 3-year-old boy from an intact lower-income family, referred by his preschool teacher because of selective mutism. Freddy was the product of a normal, full-term pregnancy and vaginal delivery and attained all developmental milestones either as expected or early. However, temperamentally, he was a shy baby and toddler and reticent to explore surroundings on his own or to stay with adults other than his parents. Freddy spoke in full sentences and spontaneously up until 3 months before the referral, when he ceased speaking to anyone, including his parents. According to his parents, Freddy was left with a 16-year-old cousin for baby-sitting, but the cousin left the child alone in the apartment. Freddy let himself out of the apartment and was found wandering the street by the police. Subsequently, Freddy was taken into protective custody and spent a night in a foster placement, until his parents were able to rectify the situation with the authorities. Freddy stopped speaking from the moment of being taken by the police. He did not speak to his parents, but he did cry on their reunion. After his return home, Freddy did not speak to his parents for the first week, but then began asking for things and responding to his parents with simple one- or two-word sentences. He refused to speak to anyone else, however.

Freddy had begun preschool shortly before the incident and was speaking then but stopped after the incident. Although he was observed constantly, he was never "caught" speaking to peers. He was described as an overly obedient and pleasant child who smiled and played with others and followed requests without problem, but just stared at a speaker and offered no reply or nonverbal communication. During evaluation, it was revealed that Freddy enjoyed eating Froot Loops in a favorite cup as a treat. Treatment was designed to provide incentive for speaking through the delivery of a contingent reinforcer of high value, the Froot Loops. Hence, Froot Loops became available only in the preschool and the therapist's office and, temporarily, were not available in his home. The therapist enacted a process of graduated shaping of communication behaviors—first nonverbal and then vocal noises—and trained the preschool teacher to do the same. Froot Loop boxes were kept in full view of Freddy at all times during the initial phase of treatment and, when he was "caught" gazing at the box, the therapist or teacher would prompt Freddy for acknowledgment that he wanted the treat. Pointing, looking, and nodding in their direction resulted in receiving four Froot Loops. Next, Freddy was asked to make a sound or ask for the Froot Loop to receive the reward. This step was accomplished as he grunted and eventually said, "Loop." Finally, prompts to ask for the Froot Loops in a sentence were enacted, and Freddy complied with this demand. This phase of treatment took 2 days at the preschool and 2 hours of therapy to accomplish. Eventually, the boxes of Froot Loops were removed from the environments, but the teacher kept the cereal with her to deliver four Loops whenever Freddy made sounds or spoke in school. This shaping procedure took an additional 3 days to result in Freddy speaking to the teacher and peers, albeit in short sentences. The treat was faded—that is, delivered on a variable ratio schedule of every three to eight times that he spoke, to promote further speaking and decrease the association with the treat. By the end of the second week of training, Freddy was speaking at the rate and level that he had before the incident. His parents were instructed to provide the treat in the home as was usual. Moreover, they were cautioned to allow or prompt Freddy to speak for himself in social situations (e.g., order his own food at a restaurant, say hello to others, make his own requests before providing a treat) as a way of relapse prevention. (Courtesy of Anne Marie Albano, Ph.D.)

Maryanne was a 12-year-old girl with a family history of anxiety and mood disorders. Her parents brought her to treatment because of recurrent obsessions involving contamination and germs, with corresponding compulsions whereby she had her parents check her food and washed her hands repeatedly to the point of their becoming raw and bleeding. Evaluation revealed a fear that, unless her parents checked her food for bugs or germs, the meal was contaminated. Hence, her parents had to physically pull apart her food and examine it to her satisfaction, which could take upward of 1 hour for each meal. This caused much distress and discord between Maryanne and her family. In addition, Maryanne washed her hands constantly—after opening a door, reading a book, using a pencil, or touching any object that she deemed dirty. The process of exposure and response prevention was used whereby a hierarchy of her obsessions and compulsions was constructed, from the least upsetting (checking food prepared by her mother) to the most upsetting (touching something that was wet or slimy and then touching her mouth). Systematically, the therapist had Maryanne first engage in imaginal exposure to a scene (e.g., you take a bite of hamburger and something tastes gritty to you and you realize that your mom did not check the burger) until her anxiety dropped to minimal levels. This usually occurred after 25 minutes. Next, the scene was enacted in vivo, whereby foods were introduced with "contaminants" in them (e.g., putting pieces of uncooked rice into the burger to mimic "grit"), and Maryanne ate the food without having her parents check. As treatment progressed, Maryanne learned that her feared consequence of becoming sick was not likely to occur. Similarly, washing rituals were addressed by having her touch items with various substances coating them and then touching her face and mouth. Treatment occurred over a 14-session program with her parents taught to assist her with these exposures in the home. The parents were also instructed to refrain from engaging in her rituals. Relapse prevention plans were enacted to expand her range of food choices and situational contexts (cafeterias, food stands, restaurants) for exposure. By the end of treatment, Maryanne was eating without the need for checking and with minimal to no anxiety. Moreover, she was engaging in a wide range of activity without the need to wash after touching various objects. (Courtesy of Anne Marie Albano, Ph.D.)

Remedial, educational, and patterning psychotherapy is focused on teaching new attitudes and patterns of behavior to children who persist in using immature and inefficient patterns that are often presumed to be caused by a maturational lag. Supportive psychotherapy is particularly helpful in enabling a well-adjusted youngster to cope with emotional turmoil engendered by a crisis. It also is used with disturbed youngsters whose less-than-adequate ego functioning may be seriously disrupted by an expressive-exploratory mode or by other forms of therapeutic intervention.

At the beginning of most psychotherapy, regardless of a patient's age and the nature of the therapeutic interventions, the principal therapeutic elements perceived by patients tend to be supportive as a consequence of therapists' universal efforts to be reliably and sensitively responsive. In fact, some therapy may never proceed beyond the supportive level, whereas other therapy develops an expressive-exploratory or behavioral modification flavor on top of the supportive foundation.

Preschool-age children are sometimes treated through the parents, a process called *filial therapy*. Therapists using the strategy should be alert to the possibility that apparently successful filial treatment can obscure a significant diagnosis because patients are not treated directly. The first case of filial therapy was that of Little Hans, reported by Freud in 1905. Hans was a 5-year-old phobic child who was treated by his father under Freud's supervision.

While historically psychotherapy had its roots in psychodynamic theories, current evidence has shown that cognitive-behavioral therapeutic techniques are efficacious in the treatment of anxiety disorders and mood disorders in youth. Children generally are unaware of these unreal dangers, their fear of them, and the psychological defenses they use to avoid both the danger and the fear. With the awareness that is facilitated, patients can evaluate the usefulness of their defensive maneuvers and can relinquish unnecessary maneuvers that constitute the symptoms of their emotional disturbance.

A 10-year-old girl was seen in twice-weekly psychodynamic psychotherapy. As the child left her sessions, her mother would ask each time, "How is she doing?" The therapist made a separate appointment with the parents to discuss these concerns further, while also exploring how the child felt about this meeting. The girl had concerns about "what they are going to say about me," but acceded with support and understanding from the therapist. After discussion with the parents, it was agreed that the therapist would meet with the parents once every month to discuss the child's progress and current functioning, provide support and guidance to the parents, and monitor the parents' anxiety. Once this plan was initiated, the mother's anxiety seemed to lessen, and she no longer waited expectantly after the sessions with her daughter. (Courtesy of David L. Kaye, M.D.)

A 6-year-old boy was brought for treatment because of longstanding severe aggression and destructiveness. In addition to an evaluation for medication, the child was seen in twice-weekly psychoanalytically oriented psychotherapy. The beginning sessions were marked by the repeated need to set limits and contain the child's aggressive behaviors. Two months into treatment, he began to pump himself up, roar, and announce that he was "the Incredible Hulk." He would then proceed to stomp around the play therapy room, attempting to destroy the toys. The therapist then said, "You know you can't really *be* the Hulk. You can *pretend* that you are the Hulk, and then maybe we can play this together." After a number of similar exchanges, the child gradually and increasingly became able to play the part without becoming it. (Courtesy of David L. Kaye, M.D.)

Child psychoanalysis, an intensive, uncommon form of psychoanalytic psychotherapy, works on unconscious resistance and defenses during three to four sessions a week. Under these circumstances, therapists anticipate unconscious resistance and allow transference manifestations to mature to a full transference neurosis, through which neurotic conflicts are resolved. Interpretations of dynamically relevant conflicts are emphasized in psychoanalytic descriptions, and elements that are predominant in other types of psychotherapies are not overlooked. Indeed, in all psychotherapy, children should derive support from the consistently understanding and accepting relationship with their therapists. Remedial educational guidance is provided when necessary.

Probably the most vivid examples of the integration of psychodynamic and behavioral approaches, although they are not always explicitly conceptualized as such, appear in the milieu of child and adolescent psychiatric therapy in inpatient, residential, and day treatment facilities. Behavioral change is initiated in these settings, and its repercussions are explored concurrently in individual psychotherapeutic sessions, so that the action in one arena and the information stemming from it augment and illuminate what transpires in the other arena.

DIFFERENCES BETWEEN CHILDREN AND ADULTS

Logic suggests that psychotherapy with children, who generally are more flexible than adults and who have simpler defenses and other mental mechanisms, should consume less time than comparable treatment of adults. Experience usually does not confirm this expectation, because children usually lack some elements that contribute to successful treatment. A child, for example, typically does not seek help. As a consequence, one of a therapist's first tasks is to stimulate a child's motivation for treatment. Children commonly begin therapy involuntarily, often without the benefit of true parental support. Although parents may want their children to be helped or changed, the desire often is generated by frustrated anger toward the children. Typically, the anger is accompanied by relative insensitivity to what therapists perceive as the children's need and the basis for a therapeutic alliance. Therefore, whereas adult patients frequently perceive advantages in getting well, children may envision therapeutic change as nothing more than conforming to a disagreeable reality, an attitude that heightens the likelihood of their perceiving a therapist as the parent's punitive agent. This is hardly the most fertile soil in which to nurture a therapeutic alliance.

Children have a limited capacity for self-observation, with the notable exception of some obsessive children who resemble adults in this ability. Such obsessive children, however, usually isolate the vital emotional components. In exploratory-interpretative psychotherapies, the development of a capacity for ego splitting—that is, simultaneous emotional involvement and self-observation—is most helpful. Only by identifying with a trusted adult and in alliance with this adult can children approach such an ideal. A therapist's gender and the relatively superficial aspects of the therapist's demeanor may be important elements in the development of a trusting relationship with a child.

Recognition of the importance of play constituted a major forward stride in these efforts.

PLAYROOM

The structure, design, and furnishing of the playroom are important. Some therapists maintain that the toys should be few, simple, and carefully selected to facilitate the communication of fantasy. Other therapists suggest that a wide variety of playthings should be available to increase the range of feelings that children can express. These contrasting recommendations have been attributed to differences in therapeutic methods. Some therapists tend to avoid interpretation, even of conscious ideas, whereas others recommend the interpretation of unconscious content directly and quickly.

Therapists tend to change their preferences in equipment as they accumulate experience and develop confidence in their abilities. Although special equipment—such as genital dolls, amputation dolls, and see-through anatomically complete (except for genitalia) models—has been used in therapy, many therapists have observed that the unusual nature of such items risks making children wary and suspicious of a therapist's motives. Until dolls available to children in their own homes include genitalia, the psychological content that special dolls are designed to elicit may be more available at the appropriate time with conventional dolls.

Although the choices of play materials vary among therapists, the following equipment can constitute a well-balanced playroom or play area: multigenerational families of flexible, but sturdy dolls of various races; additional dolls representing special roles and feelings, such as police officer, doctor, and soldier; dollhouse furnishings with or without a dollhouse; toy animals; puppets; paper, crayons, paint, and blunt-ended scissors; a sponge-like ball; clay or something comparable; tools such as rubber hammers, rubber knives, and guns; building blocks, cars, trucks, and airplanes; and eating utensils. The toys should enable children to communicate through play. Therapists should avoid toys and materials that are fragile or break easily, that can result in physical injury to a child, or that can increase a child's guilt.

INITIAL APPROACH

Various approaches are associated with each therapist's individual style and perception of children's needs, from approaches in which a therapist endeavors to direct children's thought content and activity (release therapy, some behavior therapy, and certain educational patterning techniques) to exploratory methods in which a therapist endeavors to follow children's leads. Although children determine the focus, therapists structure the situation. Encouraging children to say whatever they wish and to play freely, as in exploratory psychotherapy, establishes a definite structure. Therapists create an atmosphere in which they get to know all about a child—the good side as well as the bad side, as children would put it. A therapist may communicate to a child that the child's response elicits neither anger nor pleasure, but only understanding from the therapist. Such an assertion does not imply that therapists have no emotions, but it assures the young patient that the therapist's personal feelings and standards are subordinate to understanding the youngster.

THERAPEUTIC INTERVENTIONS

Psychotherapy with children and adolescents generally is more directed and active than it often is with adults. Children usually cannot synthesize histories of their own lives, but they are excellent reporters of their current internal states. Even with adolescents, a therapist often takes an active role, is somewhat less open-ended than with adults, and offers more direction and advocacy than with adults. A child or adolescent therapist often makes exclamations and expresses confrontations in which attention is directed to data of which patients are cognizant. A therapist may use interpretations, designed to expand patients' conscious awareness of themselves, by making explicit the elements that have previously been expressed implicitly in the patients' thoughts, feelings, and behavior. Beyond interpretation, therapists may educatively offer new information to which patients have not been exposed previously. At the most active end of the continuum are advising, counseling, and directing, which are designed to help patients adopt a course of action or a conscious attitude.

Nurturing and maintaining a therapeutic alliance may require educating children about the process of therapy. Another educational intervention may entail assigning labels to affects that have not been part of a youngster's experience. Rarely, does therapy have to compensate for a real absence of education about acceptable decorum and playing games. Children usually are not in therapy because they have never been exposed to educational efforts, but because repeated educational efforts have failed. Therefore, therapy generally need not include additional teaching efforts, despite the frequent temptation to offer them.

The temptation for therapists to offer themselves as a model for identification may also stem from helpful educational attitudes toward children. Although this may sometimes be an appropriate therapeutic strategy, therapists should not lose sight of the pitfalls of this apparently innocuous maneuver.

PARENTS

Psychotherapy with children requires parental involvement, which does not necessarily reflect parental culpability for a youngster's emotional difficulties, but is a reality of a child's dependent state.

Parents are involved in child psychotherapy to varying degrees. For preschool-age children, the entire therapeutic effort may be directed toward the parents, without any direct treatment of the child. At the other extreme, children can be treated in psychotherapy without any parental involvement beyond the payment of fees and perhaps transporting the child to the therapy sessions. Most practitioners, however, prefer to maintain an informative alliance with parents to obtain additional information about the child.

Probably the most frequent parental arrangements are those developed in child guidance clinics—that is, parent guidance focused on the child or the parent–child interaction and therapy for the parents' own individual needs concurrent with the child's therapy. Parents may be seen by their child's therapist or by someone else. Recently, increasing efforts have been made to shift the focus from the child as the primary patient to the child as the family's emissary to the clinic. In such family therapy, all or selected members of the family are treated simultaneously as a family group. Although the preferences of specific clinics and practitioners for either an individual or a family therapeutic approach may be unavoidable, the final decision regarding which therapeutic strategy or combination to use should be derived from the clinical assessment.

CONFIDENTIALITY

The issue of confidentiality takes on greater meaning as children grow older. Very young children are unlikely to be as concerned about this issue as are adolescents. Confidentiality usually is preserved unless a child is believed to be in danger or to be a danger to someone else. In other situations, a child's permission usually is sought before a specific issue is raised with parents. Advantages exist to creating an atmosphere in which children can feel that all words and actions are viewed by therapists as simultaneously both serious and tentative. In other words, children's communications do not bind therapists to a commitment; nevertheless, they are too important to be communicated to a third party without a patient's permission. Although such an attitude may be implied, sometimes therapists should explicitly discuss confidentiality with children. Most of what children do and say in psychotherapy is common knowledge to the parents.

The therapist should try to enlist parents' cooperation in respecting the privacy of children's therapeutic sessions. The respect is not always readily honored, because parents are naturally curious about what transpires, and they may be threatened by a therapist's apparently privileged position.

Routinely reporting to a child the essence of communications with third parties about the child underscores the therapist's reliability and respect for the child's autonomy. In certain treatments, the report can be combined with soliciting the child's guesses about these transactions. A therapist also may find it fruitful to invite children, particularly older children, to participate in discussions about them with third parties.

A 13-year-old boy was noted by his parents to be extremely worried about contracting germs from his surroundings. He insisted on washing his hands more than 25 times a day and would often spend more than an hour a day making sure that his body and hands were clean and "free of contamination." After evaluation, the diagnosis of OCD was made, and the boy and his parents opted for CBT. The therapist started by helping the boy to rank his fears on a scale of 1 to 10, with 10 assigned to objects that he believed were most germ-laden, and 1 assigned to those objects that were of little or no concern. The boy was then taught both relaxation techniques and how to engage in thought interruption, and he used these techniques in a step-wise fashion to overcome first the more benign elements on his list, followed by the most severe. Eventually, he was able to modify his behavior by combining his understanding of what worried him most with his capacity to master and eventually overcome his fears. (Courtesy of Eugene V. Beresin, M.D. and Steven C. Scholozman, M.D.)

INDICATIONS

Psychotherapy usually is indicated for children with emotional disorders that seem to be sufficiently permanent to impede maturational and developmental forces. Psychotherapy also may be indicated when a child's development is not impeded, but is inducing reactions in the environment that are considered pathogenic. Such disharmonies ordinarily are dealt with by the child with parental assistance; however, when these efforts are persistently inadequate, psychotherapeutic interventions may be indicated.

Psychotherapy should be limited to instances in which positive indicators point to its potential usefulness. For a child to benefit from psychotherapy, the home situation must provide a certain amount of nurturance, stability, and motivation for therapy. A child must have adequate cognitive resources to participate in the process and profit from it. Psychotherapy must be judged with common sense. If a psychotherapy situation is not effective, it is important to determine whether the therapist and patient are poorly matched, whether the type of psychotherapy is inappropriate to the nature of the problems, and whether the child is cognitively inappropriate for the treatment.

References

Albano AM. Cognitive-behavioral psychotherapy for children and adolescents. In: Sadock BJ, Sadock VA, eds. *Kaplan & Sadock's Comprehensive Textbook of Psychiatry*. 8th ed. Vol. 2. Baltimore: Lippincott Williams & Wilkins; 2005: 3332.

Beresin EB, Schlozman S. Psychiatric treatment of adolescents. In: Sadock BJ, Sadock VA, eds. *Kaplan & Sadock's Comprehensive Textbook of Psychiatry*. 8th ed. Vol. 2. Baltimore: Lippincott Williams & Wilkins; 2005:3395.

Berg B. Cognitive-behavioral interventions for bullies, victims, and bystanders. In: Gallo-Lopez L, Schaefer CE, eds. *Play Therapy with Adolescents*. Lanham, MD: Jason Aronson; 2005:267.

Hibbs ED. Child psychiatry: Short-term psychotherapy. In: Sadock BJ, Sadock VA, eds. *Kaplan & Sadock's Comprehensive Textbook of Psychiatry*. 8th ed. Vol. 2. Baltimore: Lippincott Williams & Wilkins; 2005:3322.

Kaye DL. Individual psychodynamic psychotherapy. In: Sadock BJ, Sadock VA, eds. *Kaplan & Sadock's Comprehensive Textbook of Psychiatry*. 8th ed. Vol. 2. Baltimore: Lippincott Williams & Wilkins; 2005:3315.

Pavulari MN, Graczyk PA, Henrey DB, Carbray JA, Heidenrich J, Miklowitz. Child and family-focused cognitive-behavioral therapy for pediatric bipolar disorder: Development and preliminary results. *J Am Acad Child Adolesc Psychiatry*. 2004;43:528.

Roblek T, Piacentini J. Cognitive-behavior therapy for childhood anxiety disorders. *Child Adolesc Psychaitr Clin N Am*. 2005;14:863.

Siqueland L, Rynn M, Diamond GS. Cognitive behavioral and attachment based family therapy for anxious adolescents: Phase I and II studies. *J Anxiety Disord*. 2005;19:361.

Spence SH, Holmes JM, March S, Lipp OV. The feasibility and outcome of clinic plus internet delivery of cognitive-behavior therapy for childhood anxiety. *J Consult Clin Pscyhol*. 2006;74:614.

Wood JJ, Piacentini JC, Southam-Cerow M, Chu BC, Sigman M. Family cognitive behavioral therapy for child anxiety disorders. *J Am Acad Child Adolesc Psychiatry*. 2006;45:314.

▲ 54.2 Group Psychotherapy

Group formats have been demonstrated to be useful in randomized clinical trials using cognitive-behavioral techniques to treat childhood anxiety disorders. Groups have been used for a wide range of clinical situations, including anger-management for aggressive adolescents, social skills improvement, survivors of childhood sexual abuse and other traumatic events such as the trauma of the September 11th World Trade Center tragedy, adolescents with social phobia and obsessive compulsive disorder (OCD), children with psychotic disorders, interventions for adolescents with substance abuse, and for children and adolescents with learning disorders. A recent study formed a psychotherapy group for adolescent survivors of homicide victims. Group therapy can be done with children of all ages using developmentally appropriate formats. Group therapy can be structured to address a variety of communication skills, including issues of interpersonal competence, peer relationships, and social skill. Group psychotherapy can be modified to suit groups of children of various ages and can focus on behavioral, educational, and social skills and psychodynamic issues. The mode in which the group functions depends on children's developmental levels, intelligence, and problems to be addressed. In behaviorally and cognitive-behavioral groups, the group leader is a directive, active participant who facilitates prosocial interactions and desired behaviors. In groups using psychodynamic approaches, the leader may monitor interpersonal interactions less actively than in behavior therapy groups.

Gathering children and adolescents into groups may lead to greater psychological impact than treating them individually. A number of factors, described by Irving Yalom, may contribute to the effectiveness of groups. These factors include the following theoretical components:

Hope: Hope may be generated by gathering with others who are experiencing similar difficulties and by observing others actively mastering the problems.

Universality: Children and adolescents with psychiatric disorders often feel isolated and alienated from peers. Working together in groups may diffuse the isolation and help children and adolescents view their disorder as only a small part of their overall identity.

Imparting Information: Children and adolescents are familiar with a format of gaining new information in a group setting, such as in school. The group therapy format provides an opportunity to reinforce learning when the child or adolescent "helps" or demonstrates what he or she has learned to peers.

Altruism: Helping other peers in a group setting by supporting them and identifying with their struggles can improve a child or adolescent's self-esteem and help them gain a sense of mastery over their own issues.

Improved Social Skills: Group therapy is a safe format in which children and adolescents with poor social skills can improve their interpersonal and communication abilities under the supervision of a leader and with peers who also benefit from the practice scenarios.

Groups can be highly effective modalities to provide peer feedback and support to children who are either socially isolated or unaware of their effects on their peers. Groups with very young children generally are highly structured by the leader and use imagination and play to foster socially acceptable peer relationships and positive behavior. Therapists must be keenly aware of the level of children's attention span and the need for consistency and limit setting. Leaders of preschool-age groups can model supportive adult behavior in meaningful ways for children who have been deprived or neglected. School-age children's groups can be single sex or include both boys and girls. School-age children are more sophisticated in verbalizing their feelings than preschoolers, but they also benefit from structured therapeutic games. Children of school age need frequent reminders about rules, and they are quick to point out infractions of the rules to each other. Interpersonal skills can be addressed nicely in group settings with school-age children.

Same-sex groups are often used among early adolescents. Physiological changes in early adolescence and the new demands of high school lead to stress that may be ameliorated when groups of same-age peers compare and share. In older adolescence, groups more often include both boys and girls. Even with older adolescents, the leader often uses structure and direct intervention to maximize the therapeutic value of the group. Adolescents who are feeling dejected or alienated may find a special sense of belonging in a therapy group.

Johnny was a high-functioning, 14-year-old boy diagnosed with autistic disorder. He had been in individual and family therapy for several months before he was considered ready for group therapy. Johnny was an awkward-looking adolescent who looked and acted younger than his chronological age. His academic level was above average, but his social development was very limited. A supercilious, hypermoralistic attitude of more recent development contributed considerably to his social isolation, particularly after starting 7th grade. He was assigned to an established group of early adolescents with a mixture of clinical conditions, meeting once weekly for 75 minutes. Initially, Johnny limited his participation to monosyllabic answers to direct questions, then he would go back to reading a book on the history of Napoleon, his favorite subject and object of fascination. Group members chose to ignore him after a while. Over a period of several weeks, his interest in the book seemed to abate. Johnny brought it, but it remained unopened on his lap. He would make an occasional remark, mostly to criticize another group member for his "vulgarity." The group laughed at his remarks, but scapegoating could be avoided. They seemed to respect his "differentness." Two months later, Peter, a very shy schizoid 13-year-old boy joined the group. After a few sessions Johnny developed an unexpected interest in Peter and sat by him and encouraged him to interact with the group. Soon Johnny was not bringing a book any longer and was more actively involved with group members. He responded to social cues in a more age-typical and appropriate manner, and although he continued having morbid preoccupations with power and a fascination with Napoleon, the intensity was considerably diminished. Johnny's growing interest in people was clinically evident. Group therapy was used in combination with individual and family therapy and psychotropic medication over 18 months. Although the group experience was only one component of the treatment plan, it became a most significant tool to help Johnny with his interpersonal deficits. (Courtesy of Alberto C. Serrano, M.D.)

PRESCHOOL-AGE AND EARLY SCHOOL-AGE GROUPS

Work with a preschool-age group usually is structured by a therapist through the use of a particular technique, such as puppets or artwork, or is couched in terms of a permissive play atmosphere. In therapy with puppets, children project their fantasies onto the puppets in a way not unlike ordinary play. The main value lies in the cathexis afforded children, especially if they show difficulty expressing their feelings. Here, the group aids the child less by interaction with other members than by action with the puppets.

In play group therapy, the emphasis rests on children's interactional qualities with each other and with the therapist in the permissive playroom setting. A therapist should be a person who can allow children to produce fantasies verbally and in play but who can also use active restraint when children undergo excessive tension. The toys are the traditional ones used in individual play therapy. The children use the toys to act out aggressive impulses and to relive their home difficulties with group members and with the therapist. The children selected for group treatment have a common social hunger and need to be like their peers and be accepted by them. Selected children usually include those with phobias, effeminate boys, shy and withdrawn children, and children with disruptive behavior disorders.

Modifications of these criteria have been used in group psychotherapy for autistic children, parent group therapy, and art therapy. A modification of group psychotherapy has been used for toddlers with physical disabilities who show speech and language delays. The experience of twice-weekly group activities involves mothers and children in a mutual teaching-learning setting. This experience has proved effective for mothers who received supportive psychotherapy in the group experience; their formerly hidden fantasies about their children emerged and were dealt with therapeutically.

SCHOOL-AGE GROUPS

Activity group psychotherapy is based on the idea that poor, divergent experiences have led to deficits in children's appropriate personality development; therefore, corrective experiences in a therapeutically conditioned environment modify them. Because some latency-age children have deep disturbances involving fears, high anxiety levels, and guilt, a modification of activity-interview group psychotherapy has evolved. The format uses interview techniques, verbal explanations of fantasies, group play, work, and other communications. In this type of group psychotherapy, children verbalize in a problem-oriented manner, with the awareness that problems brought them together and that the group aims to change them. They report dreams, fantasies, daydreams, and traumatic and unpleasant experiences. Open discussion includes both the experiences and the group behavior.

Therapists vary in their use of time, cotherapists, food, and materials. Most groups meet after school for at least 1 hour, although other group leaders prefer a 90-minute session. Some therapists serve food during the last 10 minutes; others prefer serving times when the children are together for talking. Food, however, does not become a major feature and is never central to the group's activities.

PUBERTAL AND ADOLESCENT GROUPS

Group therapy methods similar to those used in younger-age groups can be modified to apply to pubertal children, who are often grouped monosexually. Their problems resemble those of late latency-age children, but they (especially the girls) are also beginning to feel the effects and pressures of early adolescence. Groups offer help during a transitional period; they seem to satisfy the social appetite of preadolescents, who compensate for feelings of inferiority and self-doubt by forming groups. This therapy takes advantage of the influence of the socialization process during these years. Because pubertal children experience difficulties in conceptualizing, pubertal therapy groups tend to use play, drawing, psychodrama, and other nonverbal modes of expression. The therapist's role is active and directive.

Activity group psychotherapy has been the recommended group therapy for pubertal children who do not have significantly disturbed personality patterns. The children, usually of the same sex and in groups of not more than eight, freely engage in activities in a setting especially designed and planned for its physical and environmental characteristics. Samuel Slavson, a pioneer in group psychotherapy, pictured the group as a substitute family in which the passive, neutral therapist becomes the surrogate for parents. The therapist assumes various roles, mostly in a nonverbal manner, as each child interacts with the therapist and other group members. Currently, however, therapists tend to see the group as a form of peer group, with its attendant socializing processes, rather than a reenactment of the family.

Late adolescents, 16 years of age and older, often may be included in groups of adults. Group therapy has been useful in the treatment of substance-related disorders. Combined therapy (the use of group and individual therapy) also has been used successfully with adolescents.

OTHER GROUP SITUATIONS

Groups are also helpful in more focused treatments, such as specific social skills training for children with attention-deficit/hyperactivity disorder (ADHD), cognitive-behavioral group interventions for depressed children and for children with bereavement problems or eating disorders. In these more specialized groups, the issues are more specific, and actual tasks (as in social skills groups) can be practiced within the group. Some residential and day treatment units use group psychotherapy techniques. Group psychotherapy in schools for underachievers and children from low socioeconomic levels has relied on reinforcement and on modeling theory, in addition to traditional techniques, and has been supplemented by parent groups.

In controlled conditions, residential treatment units have been used for specific studies in group psychotherapy, such as behavioral contracting. Behavioral contracting with reward-punishment reinforcement provides positive reinforcements among preadolescent boys with severe concerns in basic trust, low self-esteem, and dependence conflicts. Somewhat akin to formal residential treatment units are social group work homes. For children who undergo many psychological assaults before placement, supportive group psychotherapy offers ventilation and catharsis, but more often it succeeds in letting children become aware of the enjoyment of sharing activities and developing skills.

Public schools—also a structured environment, although not usually considered the best site for group psychotherapy—have been used by several workers. Group psychotherapy as group counseling readily lends itself to school settings. One such group used gender- and problem-homogeneous selection for groups of six to eight students, who met once a week during school hours over 2 to 3 years.

INDICATIONS

Many indications exist for the use of group psychotherapy as a treatment modality. Some indications are situational; a therapist may work in a reformatory setting, in which group psychotherapy seems to reach adolescents better than individual treatment does. Another indication is time economics; more patients can be reached in a given time by the use of groups than by individual therapy. Group therapy best helps a child at a given age and developmental stage and with a given type of problem. In young age groups, children's social hunger and their potential need for peer acceptance help determine their suitability for group therapy. Criteria for unsuitability are controversial and have been loosened progressively.

PARENT GROUPS

In group psychotherapy, as in most treatment procedures for children, parental difficulties can present obstacles. Sometimes, uncooperative parents refuse to bring a child or to participate in their own therapy. The extreme of this situation reveals itself when severely disturbed parents use a child as their channel of communication to work out their own needs. In such circumstances, a child is in the unfortunate position of receiving positive group experiences that seem to create havoc at home.

Parent groups, therefore, can be a valuable aid to group psychotherapy for their children. A recent study of a cognitive-behavioral group intervention for parents to learn how to utilize therapeutic interventions with their anxiety disordered children suggested that parent groups to teach these skills can be successfully utilized with their children. Parents of children in therapy often have difficulty understanding their children's ailments, discerning the line of demarcation between normal and pathological behavior, relating to the medical establishment, and coping with feelings of guilt. Parent groups assist in these areas and help members formulate guidelines for action.

REFERENCES

Baer S, Garland EJ. Pilot study of community-based cognitive behavioral group therapy for adolescents with social phobia. *J Am Acad Child Adolesc Psychiatry*. 2005;44:258.

Eggers CH. Treatment of acute and chronic psychoses in childhood and adolescence. *MMW Fortschr Med*. 2005;147:43.

Haen C. Rebuilding security: Group therapy with children affected by September 11. *Int J Group Psychother*. 2005;55:391.

Kaminer Y. Cognitive group therapy for aggressive boys. *J Am Acad Child Adolesc Psychiatry*. 2004;43:1478.

Kreidler M. Group therapy for survivors of childhood sexual abuse who have chronic mental illness. *Arch Psychiatr Nurs*. 2005:19:176.

Liddle HA, Rowe CL, Dakof GA, Ungaro RA, Henderson CE. Early intervention for adolescent substance abuse: Pretreatment to posttreatment outcomes of a randomized clinical trial comparing multidimensional family therapy and peer group treatment. *J Psychoactive Drugs*. 2004;36:49.

Manassis K , Mendlowitz SL, Scapillato D, Avery D, Fiksenbaum L, Freire M, Monga S, Owens M. Group and individual cognitive-behavioral therapy for childhood anxiety disorders: A randomized trial. *J Am Acad Child Adolesc Psychiatry*. 2002:41:14243.

Mishna F, Muskat B. "I'm not the only one!" Group therapy with older children and adolescents who have learning disabilities. *Int J Group Psychother*. 2004;54:455.

Muris P, Meesters C, van Melick M. Treatment of childhood anxiety disorders: A preliminary comparison between cognitive-behavioral group therapy and a psychological placebo intervention. *J Behav Ther Exp Psychiatry*. 2002;33:143.

Thienemann ML. Child psychiatry: Group psychotherapy. In: Sadock BJ, Sadock VA, eds. *Kaplan & Sadock's Comprehensive Textbook of Psychiatry*. 8th ed. Vol. 2. Baltimore: Lippincott Williams & Wilkins; 2005:2813.

Thienemann M, Moore P, Tompkins K. A parent-only intervention for children with anxiety disorders: Pilot study. *J Am Acad Child Adolesc Psychiatry*. 2006; 45:37.

▲ 54.3 Residential, Day, and Hospital Treatment

Current national trends in available treatment and delivery systems for children and adolescents with psychiatric disorders indicate a significant decline in the availability of child and adolescent inpatient beds. Given that just under 10 million children and adolescents with psychiatric disorders exist, questions arise as to the most effective ways of providing psychiatric care to these individuals. Given the paucity of psychiatric inpatient units for children and adolescents, those children with severe psychiatric conditions may turn to residential treatment centers and various types of intensive outpatient programs or partial hospital treatment programs. Residential treatment centers and facilities are appropriate settings for children and adolescents with mental disorders who require a highly structured and supervised setting for a substantial time. Such settings have the advantage of providing a stable, consistent environment with a high level of psychiatric monitoring but less intensive than in a hospital. Children and adolescents with serious psychiatric disturbances often end up in residential facilities because of difficulties managing their own psychiatric problems and because of family situations in which appropriate supervision and parenting are impossible. Residential settings offer many treatments, including behavioral management, psychotherapy, medication, special education, and the therapeutic milieu itself. Children and adolescents who benefit from residential settings have a wide variety of psychiatric problems and commonly have difficulty with impulse control and structuring their own time. Many residents of such programs also have families with serious psychiatric, financial, and parenting difficulties. Given the multitude of treatment modalities now available for children and adolescents with psychiatric disorders, including cognitive-behavioral and interpersonal individual therapies, social skills and cognitive-behavioral group therapies, family education and therapy, psychopharmacology, special educational services, and therapeutic recreational therapies, residential facilities are even more critical in providing the setting in which to conduct the evidence-based research for the above interventions.

Partial hospitalization has been used more frequently with the advent of managed care as an alternative to hospitalization to provide short-term crisis stabilization, or as a step-down from inpatient treatment for children and adolescents with psychiatric disorders. Day treatment programs, sometimes used interchangeably with the term *partial hospitalization*, are designed to serve the needs of children and adolescents with severe disorders who require interventions focused on improved level of function, but who do not meet criteria of medical necessity to be in the hospital. A variety of intensive outpatient programming constitutes a day treatment program. One of the key ingredients of a day treatment program is the provision of a therapeutic day that optimally includes an educational component. Day treatment programs are excellent alternatives for children and adolescents who require more intensive support, monitoring, and supervision than is available in the community, but who can live successfully at home if they receive the proper level of intervention. In most cases, children and adolescents who attend day hospital programs have serious mental disorders and might warrant psychiatric hospitalization without the program's support. Family therapy, group and individual psychotherapy, psychopharmacology, behavioral management programs, and special education are integral parts of these programs.

Tammy, age 13, was first seen in a pediatric emergency department on a Saturday morning by a psychiatry resident who determined that, although she had continued suicidal ideation, she did not have a specific plan and could be treated without hospitalization. Over the weekend, the resident contacted Tammy and her family twice by phone and arranged for her to be admitted to a partial hospital program on Monday morning. During her first few days in the program, she was monitored closely by the staff, and her suicide potential was evaluated at the end of each day by the medical director. During the first week, her suicidal ideation resolved in response to the support and structure of the program. At the end of her second week in the partial hospital program, she was stabilized, started on antidepressant medication, and transitioned to outpatient family and group therapy after stated commitments to follow up by the patient and her parents. The use of partial hospitalization prevented a psychiatric inpatient admission for this acutely symptomatic adolescent. (Courtesy of Laurel J. Kiser, Ph.D., M.B.A., Jerry Heston M.D., and David Pruitt, M.D.)

During a hospitalization for a life-threatening suicide attempt, Jamie's family's managed care company decertified his admission, saying he was no longer at acute risk for suicide. Because of continued serious depressive symptoms and chronic family dysfunction, he was determined to be inappropriate for routine outpatient management. He was admitted to a day program with a strong family systems orientation. Over the course of his 8-week treatment, he was able to develop a therapeutic alliance with his individual therapist, and significant family restructuring was accomplished. The consulting child and adolescent psychiatrist was able to manage Jamie's medication and regularly monitor his suicide potential. At the end of 8 weeks, his depressive symptoms were decreased to the extent that he could transition to outpatient therapy and return to school successfully. This use of the ambulatory behavioral continuum allowed for prompt discharge from the hospital with continued consolidation of progress in a highly structured system. (Courtesy of Laurel J. Kiser, Ph.D., M.B.A., Jerry Heston M.D., and David Pruitt, M.D.)

Eric was a 7-year-old boy referred to a rural community mental health center for services. Eric presented with a family history of schizophrenia, extreme irritability, labile mood, noncompliance, tantrums, and physical violence toward his peers and adults. He had received multiple school suspensions and was at risk for expulsion. On intake to services, the clinician recommended participation in a newly established day treatment program housed at Eric's elementary school. The clinician also recommended individual therapy, family therapy, case management, psychiatric evaluation, and nursing services.

During Eric's 6-month participation in the day treatment program, his academic program was infused with daily mental health services in the classroom setting. His daily goals included increasing compliance, decreasing anger outbursts, and decreasing physical aggression. He was able to improve peer relations while receiving immediate feedback and direct instruction on social skills by a master's-level clinician, teacher, and teacher's assistant. Each of the adult staff was able to consistently apply behavior management principles in their domain areas. Eric's parents actively participated in parent conferences, as well as in family therapy sessions. After initial reluctance, they agreed to schedule a psychiatric evaluation, after which Eric was further stabilized on medication. Eric was gradually transitioned to a regular classroom setting, where he is being maintained successfully. He continues with outpatient services. (Courtesy of Laurel J. Kiser, Ph.D., M.B.A., Jerry Heston, M.D., and David Pruitt, M.D.)

HOSPITALIZATION

Psychiatric hospitalization is needed when a child or adolescent exhibits dangerous behavior, is contemplating suicide, or is experiencing an exacerbation of a psychotic disorder or another serious mental disorder. Safety, stabilization, and effective treatment are the goals of hospitalization. Recently, the length of stay for child and adolescent psychiatric patients has decreased because of financial pressures and increased availability of day treatment programs. Psychiatric hospitalization may be some children's first opportunity to experience a stable, safe environment. Hospitals often are the most appropriate places to start use of new medications, and they provide an around-the-clock setting in which to observe a child's behavior. Children may show remission of some symptoms by virtue of their removal from a stressful or abusive environment. After a child has been observed for several weeks, the best treatment and disposition may become clear.

RESIDENTIAL TREATMENT

More than 20,000 emotionally disturbed children are in residential treatment centers in the United States, and this number is increasing. Deteriorating social conditions, particularly in cities, often make it impossible for a child with a serious mental disorder to live at home. In these cases, residential treatment centers serve a real need. They provide a structured living environment in which children may form strong attachments to, and receive commitments from, staff members. The purpose of the center is to provide treatment and special education for children and their families.

Staff and Setting

Staffing patterns include various combinations of child-care workers, teachers, social workers, psychiatrists, pediatricians, nurses, and psychologists; therefore, residential treatment can be very expensive. The Joint Commission on the Mental Health of Children made the following structural and setting recommendations:

> In addition to space for therapy programs, there should be facilities for a first-rate school and a rich evening activity program, and there should be ample space for play, both indoors and out. Facilities should be small, seldom exceeding 60 patients in capacity with a limit of 100 patients, and they should make provisions for children to live in small groups. The centers should be located near the families they serve and should be readily accessible by public transportation. They should be located for ready access to special medical and educational services and to various community resources, including consultants. The centers should be open institutions whenever possible; locked buildings, wards, or rooms should be required only rarely. In designing residential programs, the guiding principle should be that children should be removed from their normal life settings the least possible distance in space, in time, and in the psychological texture of the experience.

Indications

Most children who are referred for residential treatment have had multiple evaluations by professionals, such as school psychologists, outpatient psychotherapists, juvenile court officials, or state welfare agency staff. Attempts at outpatient treatment and foster home placement usually precede residential treatment. Sometimes, the severity of a child's problems or the inability of a family to provide for the child's needs prohibits sending a child home. Many children sent to residential treatment centers have disruptive behavior problems in addition to other problems, including mood disorders and psychotic disorders. In some cases, serious psychosocial problems, such as physical or sexual abuse, neglect, indigence, or homelessness, necessitate out-of-home placement. The age range of the children varies among institutions, but most children are between 5 and 15 years of age. Boys are referred more frequently than girls.

An initial review of data enables the intake staff to determine whether a particular child is likely to benefit from the treatment program; often, for every child accepted for admission, three are rejected. The next step usually is interviews with the child and the parents by various staff members, such as a therapist, a group-living worker, and a teacher. Psychological testing and neurological examinations are given, when indicated, if they have not already been performed. The child and parents should be prepared for these interviews.

Group Living

Most of a child's time in a residential treatment setting is spent in group living. The group-living staff consists of child-care workers who offer a structured environment that forms a therapeutic milieu; the environment places boundaries and limitations on the children. Tasks are defined within the limits of children's abilities; incentives, such as additional privileges, encourage them to progress rather than regress. In milieu therapy, the environment is structured, limits are set, and a therapeutic atmosphere is maintained.

The children often select one or more staff members with whom to form a relationship; through this relationship, they

Table 54.3–1
Education Process in Residential Treatment

Preentry Assessment →	Intervention Program Planning ↔		Evaluation and Reevaluation →	Educational Placement →	Follow-up
Nature of emotional conflict	Educational skill development	Anxiety reduction program	Weekly staff meetings	Regular school	
Nature of learning difficulties	Remedial reading	Supportive adult relationships	Interdisciplinary meetings and conferences	Special class	
	Basic skill development	Stable, trusted models			
	Perceptual motor and impulse-control teaching	Life-space interviewing	Daily teacher reports	Private school	
	Arts and crafts skills	Individual psychotherapy	Psychological testing	State institution	
	Music skills	Removal from classroom area	Continuous criterion testing		
	Total group project	Guidance room standardized	Semiannual educational testing		
	Academic skills built on six instructional cycles of 25 days in which assessment diagnosis, individual objectives and prescription, and new objectives or alternatives are planned	Quiet room safety in unit	Semiannual total staff evaluation		

(Courtesy of Melvin Lewis, M.B., B.S. [London], F.R.C.Psych., D.C.H.)

express, consciously and unconsciously, many of their feelings about their parents. The child-care staff should be trained to recognize such transference reactions and to respond to them in a way that differs from the children's expectations, which are based on their previous or even current relationships with their parents.

To maintain consistency and balance, the group-living staff members must communicate freely and regularly with each other and with the other professional and administrative staff members of the residential setting, particularly the children's teachers and therapists. The child-care staff members must recognize any tendencies toward becoming the good (or bad) parent in response to a child's splitting behavior. This tendency may be manifest as a pattern of blaming other staff members for a child's disruptive behavior. Similarly, the child-care staff must recognize and avoid such individual and group countertransference reactions as sadomasochistic and punitive behavior toward a child.

The structured setting should offer a corrective emotional experience and opportunities for facilitating and improving children's adaptive behavior, particularly when such problems as speech and language deficits, intellectual retardation, inadequate peer relationships, bed-wetting, poor feeding habits, and attention deficits are present. Some attention deficits are the basis of a child's poor academic performance and unsocialized behavior, including temper tantrums, fighting, and withdrawal.

Behavior modification principles also have been used, particularly in group work with children. Behavior therapy is part of a residential center's total therapeutic effort.

Education

Children in residential treatment frequently have severe learning disorders, disruptive behavior, and attention-deficit disorders (ADHD). Usually, the children cannot function in a regular community school and consequently need a special on-grounds school. A major goal of the on-grounds school is to motivate children to learn. The educational process in residential treatment is complex; Table 54.3–1 shows some of its components.

Therapy

Most residential facilities use a basic behavior modification program to set guidelines and to give the residents a concrete sense of how to earn privileges. These behavioral programs range in detail and intensity. Some programs operate with level systems that are associated with privileges and responsibilities. Some programs use a token economy system in which residents earn points for appropriate behavior and for meeting specific goals. Most programs include basic tasks of living as well as specific therapeutic goals for the residents.

Psychotherapy offered in these programs generally is supportive and oriented toward reunion with the family when possible. Insight-oriented psychotherapy is included when it can be used by a resident.

Parents

Concomitant work with parents is essential. Children usually have a strong tie to at least one parent, no matter how disturbed the parent may be. Sometimes, a child idealizes the parent, who repeatedly fails the child. Other times, the parent has an ambivalent or unrealistic expectation that the child will return home. In some instances, the parent must be helped to enable the child to live in another setting when it is in the child's best interest. Most residential treatment centers offer individual or group therapy for parents, couples or marital therapy, and in some cases, conjoint family therapy.

DAY TREATMENT

The concept of daily comprehensive therapeutic experiences that do not require removing children from their homes or families is derived partly from experiences with a therapeutic nursery school. Day hospital programs for children were then developed, and the number of programs continues to grow. The main advantages of day treatment are that children remain with their families and the families can be more involved in day treatment than they are in residential or hospital treatment. Day treatment also is much less expensive than residential treatment. At the same time, the risks of day treatment are a child's social isolation and confinement to a narrow band of social contacts in the program's disturbed peer population.

Indications

The primary indication for day treatment is the need for a more structured, intensive, and specialized treatment program than can be provided on an outpatient basis. At the same time, the home in which the child is living should be able to provide an environment that is at least not destructive to the child's development. Children who are likely to benefit from day treatment may have a wide range of diagnoses, including autistic disorder, conduct disorder, ADHD, and mental retardation. Exclusion symptoms include behavior that is likely to be destructive to the children themselves or to others under the treatment conditions. Therefore, some children who threaten to run away, set fires, attempt suicide, hurt others, or significantly disrupt the lives of their families while they are at home may not be suitable for day treatment.

Programs

The same ingredients that lead to a successful residential treatment program apply to day treatment. These ingredients include clear administrative leadership, team collaboration, open communication, and an understanding of children's behavior. Indeed, having a single agency offer both residential and day treatment has advantages.

A major function of child-care staff in day treatment for psychiatrically disturbed children is to provide positive experiences and a structure that enables the children and their families to internalize controls and to function better than in the past regarding themselves and the outside world. Again, the methods used are essentially similar to those in full residential treatment programs.

Because the ages, needs, and range of diagnoses of children who may benefit from some form of day treatment vary, many day treatment programs have been developed. Some programs specialize in special educational and structured environmental needs of mentally retarded children. Others offer special therapeutic efforts required to treat children with autism and schizophrenia. Still other programs provide the total spectrum of treatment usually found in full residential treatment, of which they may be a part. Children may move from one part of the program to another and may be in residential treatment or day treatment according to their needs. The school program always is a major component of day treatment, and psychiatric treatment varies according to a child's needs and diagnosis.

Results

Recently, attempts have been made to analyze the treatment outcome of day treatment and partial hospitalization. Many different dimensions exist to analyzing overall benefits of such programs. Assessment of level of improvement in clinical status, academic progress, peer relationships, community interactions (legal difficulties), and family relationships are some pertinent areas to measure. In a recent follow-up 1 year after discharge from a partial hospital program, comparison of patients at admission and 1 year postdischarge showed statistically significant improvement in clinical symptoms on each subscale of the *Child Behavior Checklist*, except for sex problems. These improvements were in mood symptoms, somatic complaints, attention problems, thought problems, delinquent behavior, and aggressive behavior. The assessment of long-term effectiveness of day treatment is fraught with difficulties, from the point of view of a child's maintenance of gains, a therapist's view of psychological gains, or cost-to-benefit ratios.

At the same time, the advantage of day treatment has encouraged further development of programs. Moreover, the lessons learned from day treatment programs have moved mental health disciplines toward having services follow children, rather than perpetuating discontinuities of care. The experiences of day treatment for psychiatric conditions of children and adolescents have also encouraged pediatric hospitals and departments to adopt a model that promotes continuity of care for the medical treatment of children with chronic physical illnesses.

References

DeAntonio M. Child psychiatry: Residential and inpatient treatment. In: Sadock BJ, Sadock VA, eds. *Kaplan & Sadock's Comprehensive Textbook of Psychiatry*. 8th ed. Vol. 2. Baltimore: Lippincott Williams & Wilkins; 2005:3384.

Epstein RA Jr. Inpatient and residential treatment effects for children and adolescents: A review and critique. *Child Adolesc Psychiatr Clin N Am*. 2004;13:411.

Geller JL, Biebel K. The premature demise of public child and adolescent inpatient beds: Part I: Overview and current conditions. *Psychiatric Q*. 2006;77:251.

Geller JL, Biebel K. The premature demise of public child and adolescent inpatient beds: Part II: Challenges and implications. *Psychiatr Q*. 2006; Winter; 77(4): 273–91.

Kiser LJ, Heston JD, Pruitt DB. Partial hospital and ambulatory behavioral health services. In: Sadock BJ, Sadock VA, eds. *Kaplan & Sadock's Comprehensive Textbook of Psychiatry*. 8th ed. Vol. 2. Baltimore: Lippincott Williams & Wilkins; 2005:3376.

▲ 54.4 Biological Therapies

PHARMACOTHERAPY

During the last decade, significant accomplishments have been made with respect to knowledge of efficacy and safety of psychopharmacologic agents in the treatment of child and adolescent psychiatric disorders. Placebo-controlled trials have been undertaken to ascertain short-term efficacy for fluoxetine (Prozac), sertraline (Zoloft), paroxetine (Paxil), escitalopram (Lexapro), nefazodone, quetiapine (Seroquel), olanzapine (Zyprexa), risperidone (Risperdal), mirtazapine (Remeron), and venlafaxine (Effexor). Published data support the efficacy and safety of fluoxetine, sertraline, and escitalopram for the treatment of depression in children and adolescents, and paroxetine in the treatment of childhood obsessive-compulsive disorders (OCDs).

Additional contributions in psychopharmacologic research have been in the area of attention-deficity/hyperactivity disorder (ADHD), for which long-acting stimulant medications, including methylphenidate preparations (Concerta) and amphetamine and amphetamine salt preparations (Adderall XR) have been tested and simplified efficacious treatment of childhood ADHD so that a once-a-day treatment strategy is now accepted.

Perhaps the most significant contributions in the last decade have been the publicly funded research studies comparing combinations of pharmacologic interventions with psychosocial treatments alone and in combination for several childhood disorders, including OCD and major depressive disorders. Both the Pediatric OCD Treatment Study (POTS) (2004) and the Treatment for Adolescents with Depression Study (2004) found the combination of cognitive-behavioral psychotherapy in combination with selective serotonin reuptake inhibitor (SSRI) medications to have advantages over either treatment alone. Current trials are in progress investigating the combination of cognitive-behavior therapy (CBT) alone and in combination with SSRIs for childhood anxiety disorders.

Another area of progress is in testing medication efficacy and safety in younger age groups. For example, the publicly funded Preschooler with ADHD Treatment Study (PATS) was the first multisite study of preschool children with ADHD treated first with a parent training component and, for most whose symptoms were still problematic, with methylphenidate effectively.

Over the last decade, advances in the pharmacotherapy of psychiatric disorders in childhood, support the efficacy of SSRIs in the treatment of depressive disorders, OCDs, and anxiety disorders. Double-blind, placebo-controlled studies have provided evidence for the efficacy of fluoxetine, sertraline, and citalopram, treatment for depressive disorders in youth, and efficacy of fluoxetine, sertraline, and fluvoxamine for the treatment of OCD in youth. The tricyclic drugs have rarely been recommended since SSRIs appeared on the market, because of their more favorable adverse-effect profiles.

In 2004, the US Food and Drug Administration (FDA) released a statement on the recommendation of the Psychopharmacologic Drugs and Pediatric Advisory Committees of a "black-box" warning relating to an increased risk for suicidality in pediatric patients for all antidepressant medications. The advisory committees came to the conclusion that an increased risk of suicidal behaviors existed, although no suicides completed among the data reviewed. All of the antidepressant medications are included in the black box warning for pediatric patients regardless of whether they have been studied in pediatric populations, or are being used to treat depression. The antidepressants include clomipramine (Anafranil), nortriptyline (Pamelor, Aventyl), citalopram, trazodone (Desyrel), venlafaxine, amitriptyline (Elavil, Endep), escitalopram, maprotiline (Ludiomil), chlordiazepoxide, fluvoxamine, phenelzine, desipramine, paroxetine, sertraline, fluoxetine, mirtazepine, imipramine (Tofranil), bupropion (Wellbutrin) and others.

Currently, the serotonin-dopamine antagonists (SDAs) have generally replaced the conventional antipsychotics (dopamine receptor antagonists) in the treatment of psychotic disorders and aggressive behavior management.

Therapeutic Considerations

As psychopharmacologic interventions for childhood psychiatric disorders have gained an evidence base, establishing a therapeutic alliance, identifying and monitoring target symptoms, and promoting medication compliance are important components of successful clinical outcomes. Teamwork between the child, parents, and psychiatrist is critical in successful treatment of childhood disorders with psychopharmacologic agents.

Table 54.4–1
Diagnostic Processes of Biological Therapy

1. Diagnostic evaluation
2. Symptom measurement
3. Risk-benefit ratio analysis
4. Periodic reevaluation
5. Termination and tapered drug withdrawal

An evaluation for psychopharmacotherapy must first include an assessment of a child's psychopathology and physical condition to rule out any predisposition for side effects (Table 54.4–1). An assessment of the child's caregivers focuses on their ability to provide a safe, consistent environment in which a clinician can conduct a drug trial. The physician must consider the risk-to-benefit ratio and must explain it to the patient, if he or she is old enough, and to the child's caregivers and others (e.g., child welfare workers) who may be involved in the decision to medicate.

The clinician must obtain baseline ratings before medicating. Behavioral rating scales help objectify the child's response to medication. The physician generally starts at a low dose and titrates upward on the basis of the child's response and the appearance of adverse effects. Optimal drug trials cannot be rushed (e.g., by insurance-imposed, inadequately short hospital stays or by infrequent outpatient visits), nor can drug trials be prolonged by the physician's insufficient contact with the patient and the caregivers. The success of drug trials often hinges on the physician's daily accessibility.

Childhood Pharmacokinetics

Compared with adults, children have greater hepatic capacity, more glomerular filtration, and less fatty tissue. Thus, stimulants, antipsychotics, and tricyclic drugs are eliminated more rapidly by children than by adults; lithium (Eskalith) may also be eliminated more rapidly, and children may be less able to store drugs in their fat. Because of children's quick elimination, the half-lives of many medications may be shorter in children than in adults.

Little evidence indicates that clinicians can predict a child's blood level from the dosage or a treatment response from the plasma level. Relatively low serum levels of haloperidol seem to be adequate to treat Tourette's disorder in children. No correlation is seen between the methylphenidate (Ritalin) serum level and a child's response. The data are incomplete and conflicting about major depressive disorder and serum levels of tricyclic drugs. Serum level is related to response for tricyclic drugs in the treatment of enuresis.

With lithium therapy, a ratio of lithium concentration in saliva to that in serum can be established for a child by averaging three to four individual ratios. The average ratio can then be used to convert subsequent saliva levels to serum levels and, thus, avoid some venipuncture in children who are stressed by blood tests. As with serum levels, regular clinical monitoring for adverse effects is necessary. Table 54.4–2 lists representative drugs and their indications, dosages, adverse reactions, and monitoring requirements.

Indications

Attention-Deficit/Hyperactivity Disorder. Pharmacotherapy remains the primary treatment for ADHD in children,

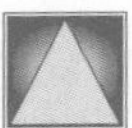

Table 54.4–2
Common Psychoactive Drugs in Childhood and Adolescence

Drug	Indications	Dosage	Adverse Reactions and Monitoring
Antipsychotics—also known as *major tranquilizers, neuroleptics* Divided into (1) high-potency, low-dosage e.g., haloperidol (Haldol), pimozide (Orap), trifluoperazine (Stelazine), thiothixene (Navane); (2) low-potency high-dosage (more sedating) e.g., chlorpromazine (Thorazine); and (3) atypicals (e.g., risperidone (Risperdal), olanzapine (Zyprexa), quetiapine (Seroquel), and clozapine (Clozaril)	Psychoses; agitated self-injurious behaviors in MR, PDDs, CD, and Tourette's disorder—haloperidol and pimozide Clozapine—refractory schizophrenia in adolescence	All can be given in two to four divided doses or combined into one dose after gradual buildup Haloperidol—child 0.5–6 mg/d, adolescent 0.5–16 mg/d Clozapine—dosage not determined in children; <600 mg/d in adolescents Risperidone—1–3 mg/d Olanzapine—2.5–10 mg/d Quetiapine—25–500 mg/d	Sedation, weight gain, hypotension, lowered seizure threshold, constipation, extrapyramidal symptoms, jaundice, agranulocytosis, dystonic reaction, tardive dyskinesia Hyperprolactinemia with atypicals except quetiapine Monitor blood pressure, CBC count, LFTs and prolactin if indicated; with thioridazine, pigmentary retinopathy is rare but dictates ceiling of 800 mg in adults and proportionally lower in children; with clozapine, weekly WBC counts for development of agranulocytosis and EEG monitoring because of lowering of seizure threshold
Stimulants			
Dextroamphetamine (Dexedrine) and amphetamine-dextroamphetamine (Adderall) FDA-approved for children 3 years and older Methylphenidate (Ritalin, Concerta) and pemoline (Cylert)—FDA-approved for children 6 years and older	In ADHD for hyperactivity, impulsivity, and inattentiveness Narcolepsy	Dextroamphetamine and methylphenidate are generally given at 8 AM and noon Dextroamphetamine—about half the dosage of methylphenidate Methylphenidate—10–60 mg/d or up to about 0.5 mg/kg per dose Adderall—about half the dosage of methylphenidate	Insomnia, anorexia, weight loss (possibly growth delay), rebound hyperactivity, headache, tachycardia, precipitation or exacerbation of tic disorders With pemoline, monitor LFTs, as hepatotoxicity and liver failure are possible
Daytrana patch	ADHD	15 mg, 20 mg, 30 mg Wear for 9 hours per day	Skin irritation
Non-stimulants			
Atomoxetine (Straterra)	ADHD	Begin with 0.5 mg/kg Up to 1.8 mg/kg	Abdominal pain Loss of appetite
Mood stabilizers			
Lithium—considered an antimanic drug; also has antiaggression properties	Studies support use in MR and CD for aggressive and self-injurious behaviors; can be used for same in PDD; also indicated for early-onset bipolar disorder	600–2,100 mg in two or three divided doses; keep blood levels to 0.4–1.2 mEq/L	Nausea, vomiting, polyuria, headache, tremor, weight gain, hypothyroidism Experience with adults suggests renal function monitoring
Divalproex (Depakote)	Bipolar disorder, aggression	Up to about 20 mg/kg per day; therapeutic blood level range appears to be 50–100 μg/mL	Monitor CBC count and LFTs for possible blood dyscrasias and hepatotoxicity Nausea, vomiting, sedation, hair loss, weight gain, possibly polycystic ovaries
Carbamazepine (Tegretol)—an anticonvulsant	Aggression or dyscontrol in MR or CD Bipolar disorder	Start with 10 mg/kg per day, can build to 20–30 mg/kg per day; therapeutic blood-level range appears to be 4–12 mg per day	Drowsiness, nausea, rash, vertigo, irritability Monitor CBC count and LFTs for possible blood dyscrasias and hepatotoxicity; must obtain blood concentrations

(continued)

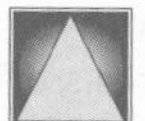

Table 54.4–2 (Continued)

Drug	Indications	Dosage	Adverse Reactions and Monitoring
Antidepressants			
Tricyclic antidepressants—imipramine (Tofranil), nortriptyline (Pamelor), clomipramine (Anafranil)	Major depressive disorder, separation anxiety disorder, bulimia nervosa, enuresis; sometimes used in ADHD, sleepwalking disorder, and sleep terror disorder Clomipramine is effective in childhood OCD and sometimes in PDD	Imipramine—start with divided doses totaling about 1.5 mg/kg per day; can build up to not more than 5 mg/kg per day and eventually combine in one dose, which is usually 50–100 mg before sleep Clomipramine—start at 50 mg/d; can raise to not more than 3 mg/kg per day or 200 mg/d	Dry mouth, constipation, tachycardia, arrhythmia
Selective serotonin reuptake inhibitors— fluoxetine (Prozac), sertraline (Zoloft), fluvoxamine (Luvox), paroxetine (Paxil), citalopram (Celexa)	OCD; may be useful in major depressive disorder, anorexia nervosa, bulimia nervosa, repetitive behaviors in MR or PDD	Less than adult dosages	Nausea, headache, nervousness, insomnia, dry mouth, diarrhea, drowsiness, disinhibition
Bupropion (Wellbutrin)	ADHD	Start low and titrate up to between 100 and 250 mg/d	Disinhibition, insomnia, dry mouth, gastrointestinal problems, tremor, seizures
Anxiolytics			
Benzodiazepines			
Clonazepam (Klonopin)	Panic disorder, generalized anxiety disorder	0.5–2.0 mg/d	Drowsiness, disinhibition
Alprazolam (Xanax)	Separation anxiety disorder	Up to 1.5 mg/d	Drowsiness, disinhibition
Buspirone (BuSpar)	Various anxiety disorders	15–90 mg/d	Dizziness, upset stomach
α_2-Adrenergic receptor agonists			
Clonidine (Catapres)	ADHD, Tourette's disorder, aggression	Up to 0.4 mg/d	Bradycardia, arrhythmia, hypertension, withdrawal hypotension
Guanfacine (Tenex)	ADHD	0.5–3.0 mg/d	Same as with clonidine plus headache, stomachache
β-Adrenergic receptor antagonist (beta blocker)			
Propranolol (Inderal)	Explosive aggression	Start at 20–30 mg/d and titrate	Monitor for bradycardia, hypotension, bronchoconstriction Contraindicated in asthma and diabetes
Other agents			
Naltrexone (ReVia)	Hyperactivity or self-injurious behavior in autism or MR	0.5–1.0 mg/kg per day	Drowsiness, vomiting, anorexia, headache, nasal congestion, hyponatremic seizures
Desmopressin (DDAVP)	Nocturnal enuresis	20–40 μg intranasally	Headache, nasal congestion, hyponatremic seizures (rare)

MR, mental retardation; PDD, pervasive development disorder; CD, conduct disorder; CBC, complete blood count; LFT, liver function test; WBC, white blood cell; ADHD, attention-deficit/hyperactivity disorder; OCD, obsessive-compulsive disorder.

adolescents, and adults. Multiple studies support the efficacy of stimulant medications for ADHD. Current practice is leaning toward more use of once-a-day, long-acting preparations of stimulants such as methylphenidate, amphetamine and amphetamine salts, and dex-methylphenidate (Focalin LA). The most frequently researched and used stimulant is methylphenidate. Dextroamphetamine (Dexedrine) has comparable efficacy and, unlike methylphenidate, is approved by the FDA for children 3 years of age and older; the starting age for methylphenidate is 6 years. The amphetamine, Adderall, combines dextroamphetamine and amphetamine salts. The extended-release preparations, such as Concerta and Adderall XR, have the advantages of coverage of symptoms throughout the school day without the necessity of taking another dose, as well as a more continuous delivery of medication. Stimulants reduce hyperactivity, inattentiveness, and impulsivity in about 75 percent of children with ADHD. The effects are not paradoxical, because normal children respond similarly. The dose-related adverse effects of stimulants are listed in Table 54.4–3.

The methylphenidate transdermal patch (Daytrana) has recently been approved by the FDA in the treatment of ADHD in children age 6 to 12 years. Daytrana comes in patches that can

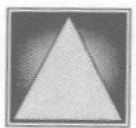

Table 54.4–3
Common Dose-Related Side Effects of Stimulants

Insomnia
Decreased appetite
Irritability or nervousness
Weight loss

deliver 15 mg, 20 mg, and 30 mg when worn for 9 hours per day. The medication begins to have its effects on the target symptoms of ADHD approximately 2 hours after the patch is placed, and continues to deliver medication throughout the wear time. Given that its active ingredient is methylphenidate, the side effects are generally the same as those for methylphenidate, except for the potential skin irritation that may emerge from wearing the patch. The patch should not be worn in the presence of a heating pad or electric blanket because heat increases the rate of methylphenidate delivery into the skin. Patients with glaucoma or known hypersensitivity to methylphenidate products should not begin treatment with Daytrana. Daytrana has the advantages of being able to deliver medication until the patch is removed and, for children who are unable to swallow pills, Daytrana offers a unique administration option.

Recent studies support the use of atomoxetine (Strattera), a norepinephrine reuptake inhibitor, as an efficacious nonstimulant treatment for ADHD in children and adolescents. Atomoxetine is well absorbed after ingestion and reaches its maximal plasma concentration after about 1 to 2 hours. Common side effects of atomoxetine include abdominal discomfort, decreased appetite, dizziness, and irritability. Rarely, minor increases in blood pressure and heart rate have been noted. Atomoxetine is metabolized by the cytochrome P450 (CYP) 2D6 hepatic enzyme system and a fraction of the population (about 7 percent of Caucasians and 2 percent of African Americans) are poor metabolizers, which may increase the plasma half-life by about fivefold. When combined with other medications that inhibit CYP 2D6, such as fluoxetine and paroxetine, diminished metabolism of atomoxetine can occur and the dose may need to be decreased. Atomoxetine is generally initiated at 0.5 mg/kg given once per day and increased to a therapeutic dose ranging between 1.4 mg/kg and 1.8 mg/kg either in one dose or in two divided dosages.

Autistic Disorder. No specific pharmacotherapy exists for the core symptoms of autistic disorder; however, it is not uncommon for a child with autistic disorder to exhibit symptoms of impulsivity and inattention, compulsive and ritualistic behaviors, irritability, temper outbursts with or without self-injurious behaviors, and anxiety symptoms. Pharmacologic agents currently receiving the most attention in the treatment of autistic disorder are atypical antipsychotics, such as risperidone, olanzapine, and aripiprazole, glutaminergic agents, and SSRI antidepressants. A large multisite study is underway to gain evidence for optimal treatments for autistic disorders.

The behavioral problems of children with autistic disorder range from mild to very severe. In past studies, antipsychotic agents, including risperidone and haloperidol, have been used with varying degrees of success in reducing temper tantrums, aggression, stereotypies, self-injurious behavior, and hyperactivity. Haloperidol is much less frequently chosen compared with the atypical antipsychotic agents because of the increased risks of extrapyramidal symptoms and, withdrawal dyskinesia. SSRIs, including fluoxetine, and citalopram have been studied in autistic disorder, because of the association between the compulsive behaviors in OCD and stereotypic behaviors common in children with autism. To date, clomipramine (Anafranil) and fluoxetine have shown promise in ending stereotypies and other behaviors in autistic children and adults.

The opioid antagonists naloxone (Narcan) and naltrexone have not proved effective in diminishing self-injurious behavior in children with autistic disorder. A variety of agents, including β-adrenergic receptor antagonists (beta blockers), lithium, and anticonvulsants are used in clinical practice to ameliorate the multiple symptoms seen in children with pervasive disorder. Stimulants are often tried to reduce hyperactivity and inattentiveness in children with autism.

Attention-deficit/hyperactivity disorder often coexists with oppositional defiant disorder or conduct disorder. With concurrent externalizing psychiatric disorders, the risks of aggressive behaviors, including impulsive or reckless behavior, may emerge. Stimulants have been found to reduce aggression in children with ADHD who are impulsive, but it is not a first-line treatment for dangerous, repeated episodes of assaultive or explosive outbursts. Atomoxetine (Strattera) is typically the second line of pharmacologic therapy for ADHD in children who do not respond to stimulants. Bupropion has been shown to be effective in some children with ADHD who either cannot tolerate stimulants or atomoxetine because of side effects or for whom other agents are ineffective. A few studies have shown that clonidine (Catapres), an α-adrenergic agonist agent, has some success in ADHD. Guanfacine (Tenex), another α-adrenergic agonist, has also been used in clinical practice for children and adolescents with ADHD who do not respond to the stimulants. Antipsychotics are not indicated in the treatment of ADHD, unless accompanied by psychosis, given the risks of sedation and tardive dyskinesia. ADHD often precedes and coexists with tic disorders.

The dietary management of hyperactivity has historically received public attention, but controlled studies have not substantiated its benefit.

Conduct Disorder. The explosive and assaultive behaviors associated with some forms of conduct disorder continue to be treated with pharmacotherapy. Atypical antipsychotics, such as risperidone, olanzapine, quetiapine (Seroquel) and aripiprazole (Abilify), lead to hope of effective behavioral improvement with fewer long-term adverse effects. Lithium has been shown in multiple investigations to reduce aggression in conduct disorder, and propranolol (Inderal) has been chosen as an agent to control aggression in open trials, although no evidence supports its use in children and adolescents. Carbamazepine (Tegretol) has not been shown to be effective in controlling aggression in child and adolescent conduct disorders.

When conduct disorder is associated with ADHD, a trial of a stimulant is indicated; stimulants are faster acting than atypical antipsychotics or mood stabilizing agents used in clinical practice to control dangerously aggressive behaviors.

The management of severe aggression, disruptive behavior, and ADHD remains a challenge. Combinations of antipsychotics with mood-stabilizing agents or stimulants are sometimes used in treatment-resistant cases, although few studies attest to the efficacy or safety of drug combinations. Newer "atypical" antipsychotic medications—SDAs—such as risperidone, olanzapine, clozapine (Clozaril), ziprasidone (Geodon), and aripiprazole have enabled a wider range of treatment-resistant patients to benefit from neuroleptic treatment. The SDAs are believed to relieve both the positive and negative symptoms of schizophrenia and to produce less risk of extrapyramidal adverse effects and less potential for the development of tardive dyskinesia. Nevertheless, all antipsychotics pose some risk of extrapyramidal adverse effects and tardive dyskinesia. One challenge in obtaining optimal pharmacological treatment for children is to decrease maladaptive behaviors and promote productive academic functioning. To this end, clinicians must consider medication adverse effects that result in cognitive "dulling." Certain pharmacological agents used in pediatric populations are associated with a specific disorder or with target symptoms that appear in several disorders. For example, haloperidol was shown in past studies to be effective in the treatment of Tourette's disorder, but it has also been used to control severe aggression.

Tourette's Disorder. The high-potency antipsychotics haloperidol and pimozide (Orap) still have the greatest body of evidence as effective medications for Tourette's disorder, although they also have considerable drawbacks. Pimozide prolongs the QT interval and, thus, requires electrocardiographic (ECG) monitoring. Clonidine, a presynaptic α-adrenergic blocking agent, is less effective than either of the above antipsychotics, but has the advantage of avoiding the risk for tardive dyskinesia; sedation is a frequent side effect of clonidine.

Tic disorders often coexist with ADHD in children and adolescents. Stimulant use is controversial; it can precipitate tics and should be avoided in these patients, although recent studies indicate that the prohibition may not be totally warranted. Clonidine reduces tics in both ADHD and the comorbid cases. A small study supports the use of nortriptyline (Pamelor).

Enuresis. Before initiating psychopharmacotherapy for treating enuresis, clinicians must consider the merits of waiting for a possible spontaneous remission and of using behavioral techniques; bell-and-pad conditioning (a bell awakens the child when the mattress becomes wet), perhaps the most elaborate behavioral treatment, seems to be more successful than medication.

Desmopressin (DDAVP) is effective in about 50 percent of patients, and has largely replaced prior use of imipramine, a tricyclic antidepressant, because of its increased safety profile. Improvement ranges from complete cessation of wetting to continued wetting, but with less urine volume. Desmopressin has been used intranasally in dosages of 10 to 40 mg a day. When used over months, nasal discomfort can occur, and water retention is potentially a problem. Patients who respond with full dryness should continue to take the medication for several months to prevent relapses. Desmopressin is now available in oral tablets, and a controlled multicenter study found equal efficacy between intranasal and oral administration of desmopressin in the treatment of enuresis. A dosage of 400 mg of oral desmopressin was the study condition associated with greater effectiveness than the lower, 200 mg used.

Separation Anxiety Disorder, Generalized Anxiety Disorder, and Social Phobia. A substantial evidence base exists for the efficacy of SSRI medications in the treatment of separation anxiety, generalized anxiety disorder, and social phobia in children and adolescents. Randomized clinical trials have confirmed efficacy of fluoxetine, fluvoxamine, sertraline, and paroxetine in the treatment of these anxiety disorders. Thus, SSRIs are currently recommended as first-line medications in the treatment of childhood anxiety. Separation anxiety disorder, generalized anxiety disorder, and social phobia are often studied together because they so commonly coexist. A given child with one of the above anxiety disorders has a 60 percent chance of having a second one and, in 30 percent of cases, all three are comorbid. Several randomized clinical trials have provided data to support the use of sertraline, fluoxetine, and fluvoxamine. Alprazolam (Xanax) may be helpful in separation anxiety disorder, but randomized clinical trials are still needed. CBT has been shown to be an effective intervention in childhood anxiety disorders.

Schizophrenia. The atypical antipsychotic agents represent a major advance in the pharmacologic treatment for schizophrenia in children and adolescents, as well as in adults. The atypical antipsychotic agents have largely replaced traditional antipsychotics because of their more favorable side-effect profiles, greater effectiveness for negative symptomatology, and mood stabilizing effects. Although the atypical agents are generally recommended currently as first-line agents in the treatment of psychotic disorders in children and adolescents, only one published controlled National Institute of Mental Health (NIMH) trial has been conducted using an atypical agent in the treatment of schizophrenia for youth. The NIMH study for clozapine provided evidence of its superiority to haloperidol (clozapine mean doses of 176 mg per day) for treating positive and negative symptoms of schizophrenia in 21 youth. The serious drawbacks of clozapine, however, limit it as a first line agent for this disorder. In the NIMH trial, five youth developed significant neutropenia, and two of them experienced seizures. Clozapine is chosen for treatment-resistant schizophrenia.

Open label trials in schizophrenic youth have suggested efficacy of other atypical antipsychotic agents such as olanzapine, risperidone, and quetiapine. Case reports have suggested that ziprasidone is effective. One of the main side effects of the atypical antipsychotic agents is significant weight gain. A newer atypical agent, aripiprazole awaits clinical trials to confirm its potential to be an efficacious and more weight neutral agent for the treatment of childhood psychoses. Although conventional antipsychotics, such as haloperidol, loxapine (Loxitane), and thioridazine (Mellaril) have been shown to be significantly superior to placebo in the treatment of psychosis in youth, given their side effect profiles they are typically chosen as first-line treatments. Schizophrenia with onset in late adolescence is treated as is adult-onset schizophrenia.

Mood Disorders. Randomized clinical trials have provided evidence for the efficacy and safety of fluoxetine, sertraline, and citalopram (Celexa) in the treatment of major depression in children and adolescents. The SSRIs currently are the drugs of choice in the pharmacological treatment of depressive disorders in children and adolescents. Given the FDA placement of the "black-box" warning in 2004 on all antidepressants used in children and adolescents because of the slightly increased risk of suicidal behaviors, it is imperative that close monitoring of suicidal ideation and behavior is achieved by all clinicians who prescribe these medications. Tricyclic drugs have not been shown to be superior to placebo in double-blind, placebo-controlled studies of children and adolescents with major depressive disorder and have been largely replaced by the SSRIs in the treatment of childhood mood disorders. The SSRIs are favored because of their apparent efficacy, mild adverse-effect profile, and lower risk in overdose. Although most side effects of SSRIs are tolerable, anecdotal recent reports indicate occasional SSRI-induced apathy in children and adolescents treated with SSRIs.

Manic episodes in childhood and adolescence are treated as they are in adulthood. Use of lithium in treating adolescent mania, has been supported in many open trials. Divalproex is currently used frequently to treat bipolar disorder in children and adolescents. A recent double-blind, randomized pilot study comparing quetiapine (400 to 600 mg a day) or divalproex (serum level 80 to 120 mg/mL) in a trial lasting approximately 1 month, found that quetiapine is at least as effective as divalproex in treating acute manic symptoms. Reduction of symptoms occurred more quickly with quetiapine compared with divalproex.

Obsessive-Compulsive Disorder. Current literature has provided evidence from randomized clinical trials of efficacy and safety of fluoxetine, fluvoxamine, and sertraline as first-line agents for children and adolescents with OCD. The POTS of CBT, sertraline, and their combination for children and adolescents with OCD has shown that CBT combined with sertraline resulted in the best outcome for children and adolescents with OCD compared with medication or therapy alone. Previously, clomipramine was proved effective in diminishing obsessions and compulsions in children and adolescents, but although clomipramine is often well tolerated, the SSRIs have a more favorable adverse-effect profile and appear to be as effective as clomipramine.

Eating Disorders. The treatment of anorexia nervosa does not focus primarily on pharmacological interventions, but drugs can be important adjuncts in many cases. The SSRIs are not used uncommonly in this population; the target symptoms are obsessions and compulsions and high levels of anxiety and depressive symptoms. Cyproheptadine (Periactin) was used historically and reported to benefit some patients with anorexia, and antidepressants may benefit those with comorbid depressive disorders. The compromised metabolism of many patients with anorexia can put them at high risk for cardiac arrhythmias, however, if tricyclic drugs are administered.

Evidence from controlled studies indicates that high-dosage SSRI treatment (fluoxetine at doses of approximately 60 mg per day) can reduce binge eating and purging in bulimia nervosa. Bupropion must be used with care in patients with bulimia nervosa because of the risk of seizures.

Mental Retardation. No pharmacotherapy exists that is specifically designed for mental retardation; however, children and adolescents with mental retardation are at higher risk for comorbid psychiatric disorders. The psychopharmacotherapy for youth with mental retardation most often addresses behavioral problems, especially aggression, and the coexistence of other mental disorders. For severe aggression, antipsychotics are most commonly used, and cognitive dulling can best be avoided with high-potency drugs. β-adrenergic receptor antagonists have reduced aggression in uncontrolled studies of adults and children with mental retardation. Lithium and anticonvulsants such as carbamazepine may also be tried. Antipsychotics have the advantage of a fast onset of action and little need for laboratory monitoring of their adverse effects, but the use of other drugs eliminates the risk for tardive dyskinesia.

The endogenous opioid antagonists, such as naltrexone (ReVia), and the SSRIs, such as fluoxetine, have been prescribed in an attempt to diminish self-injurious behavior in patients with mental retardation. When ADHD coexists with mental retardation, methylphenidate often is effective.

Recently, attempts have been made to treat the behavioral problems associated with fragile X syndrome with folic acid supplements. Some prepubescent children experienced less active or less aggressive behavior and concentrated better when they took folic acid than they did before treatment.

Learning Disorders. No pharmacological agent significantly improves any learning disorder, but many children with other mental disorders also have learning disorders, and many who have learning disorders also have behavioral problems. These associations and the importance of school and learning in children's lives raise questions about the cognitive effects of psychotropics. Table 54.4–4 summarizes the effects of drugs on cognitive tests of learning functions. In children with learning disorders who have attention problems, even in the absence of meeting full criteria for ADHD, methylphenidate facilitates performance on several standard cognitive, psycholinguistic, memory, and vigilance tests, but does not improve children's academic achievement ratings or teacher ratings. Cognitive impairment from psychotropic drugs, especially antipsychotics, may be an even greater problem for persons who are mentally retarded than for those with learning disorders.

Sleep Terror Disorder and Sleepwalking Disorder. Sleep terror disorder and sleepwalking disorder occur in the transition from deep delta-wave sleep (stages 3 and 4) to light sleep. Benzodiazepines and tricyclics are effective in these disorders. They work by reducing both delta-wave sleep and arousals between sleep stages. The medications should be used temporarily and only in severe cases, because tolerance to the medications develops. Cessation of these medications can lead to severe rebound worsening of the disorders, and reducing delta sleep in children may have deleterious effects; thus, behavioral approaches are preferred for these disorders.

Patients with early-onset panic disorder and panic attacks have benefited from clonazepam (Klonopin) in several open trials.

Adverse Effects and Complications

Antidepressants. Adverse effects related to antidepressants have been diminished significantly since SSRI antidepressants

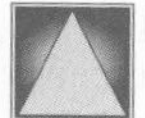

Table 54.4–4
Effects of Psychotropic Drugs on Cognitive Tests of Learning Functions[a]

			Test Function			
Drug Class	**Continuous Performance Test (Attention)**	**Matching Familiar Figures (Impulsivity)**	**Paired Associates (Verbal Learning)**	**Porteus Maze (Planning Capacity)**	**Short-Term Memory[a]**	**WISC (Intelligence)**
Stimulant	↑	↑	↑	↑	↑	↑
Antidepressant	↑	0	0	0	0	0
Antipsychotic	↑↓	0	↓	↓	↓	0

↑, Improved; ↑↓, inconsistent; ↓, worse; 0, no effect.
[a]Various tests, digit span, word recall, etc.
(Adapted from Amar MG. Drugs, learning and the psychotherapies. In: Werry JS, ed. *Pediatric Psychopharmacology: The Use of Behavior Modifying Drugs in Children*. New York: Brunner/Mazel; 1978:356, with permission.)

have been widely accepted as first-line treatments for depressive disorders in children and adolescents. Tricyclics are rarely recommended because of the significant risks of dangerous adverse effects. The adverse effects of tricyclics for children usually are similar to those for adults and result from the drugs' anticholinergic properties. The adverse effects include dry mouth, constipation, palpitations, tachycardia, loss of accommodation, and sweating. The most serious adverse effects are cardiovascular; in children, diastolic hypertension is more common and postural hypotension occurs more rarely than in adults. ECG changes are most likely seen in children receiving high dosages. Slowed cardiac conduction (PR interval greater than 0.20 seconds or QRS interval greater than 0.12) may necessitate lowering the dosage. FDA guidelines limit dosages to a maximum of 5 mg/kg a day. The drugs can be toxic in an overdose and, in small children, ingestion of 200 to 400 mg can be fatal. When the dosage is lowered too rapidly, withdrawal effects occur, mainly gastrointestinal symptoms—cramping, nausea, and vomiting—and sometimes apathy and weakness. Treatment is tapering the dosage more slowly.

Antipsychotics. The SDAs have generally replaced the conventional antipsychotics as first-line agents in the treatment of all psychotic disorders in children and adolescents. Historically, the best-studied antipsychotics given to pediatric age groups are chlorpromazine (Thorazine) and haloperidol. High-potency and low-potency antipsychotics are believed to differ in their adverse-effect profiles. The phenothiazine derivatives (chlorpromazine and thioridazine) have the most pronounced sedative and atropinic actions, whereas the high-potency antipsychotics are commonly believed to be associated with extrapyramidal reactions, such as parkinsonian symptoms, akathisia, and acute dystonias. The risk of tardive dyskinesia in relation to antipsychotics leads to caution in the use of drugs. Tardive dyskinesia, which is characterized by persistent abnormal involuntary movements of the tongue, face, mouth, or jaw and sometimes the extremities, is a known hazard when giving antipsychotics to patients of all age groups. No known treatment is effective. Tardive dyskinesia has not been reported in patients taking less than 375 to 400 g of chlorpromazine equivalents. Because nonpersistent choreiform movements of the extremities and trunk are common after abrupt discontinuation of antipsychotics, clinicians must distinguish these symptoms from persistent dyskinesia.

OTHER BIOLOGICAL THERAPIES

Electroconvulsive therapy (ECT) is rarely initiated in childhood and adolescence. In cases of catatonia, treatment-resistant mania, and severe depression, however, suggestion is that it is efficacious.

Psychosurgery for severe and intransigent OCD is virtually absent from the literature in children and adolescents.

No controlled studies provide evidence that food allergies or sensitivities play a role in childhood mental disorders. Diets that eliminate food additives, colorings, and sugar are difficult to maintain and usually have no effect. Megavitamin therapy has not been shown to influence behavioral disorders (unless the child has a frank vitamin deficiency) and can cause serious adverse effects.

Significant advances have been made in scientific studies assessing the efficacy and safety of pharmacologic agents in the treatment of childhood psychiatric disorders and, given the trend of increased use of psychotropic medications in the treatment of childhood disorders, future large multisite studies are needed to confirm optimal pharmacologic treatments and combinations of psychosocial and pharmacologic treatments.

REFERENCES

Delbello MP, Kowatch RA, Adler CM, Stanford K, Welge JA, Barzman DH, Nelson E, Strakowski S. A double-blind randomized pilot comparing quetiapine and divalproex for adolescent mania. *J Am Acad Child Adolesc Psychiatry*. 2006;45:305.

Geller DA, Wagner KD, Emslie G, Murphy T, Carpenter D, Wetherhold E, Perera P, Machin A, Gardiner C. Paroxetine treatment in children and adolescents with obsessive-compulsive disorder: A randomized, multicenter, double-blind, placebo-controlled trial. *J Am Acad Child Adolesc Psychiatry*. 2004;43:1387.

Greenhill LL, Abikoff H, Chuang S, Cooper T, Cunningham C, Davies M, Ghuman J, Kollins S, McCracken J, McGough J, Posner K, Riddle MA, Skrobala A, Swanson A, Vitiello B, Wigal S, Wigal T. Efficacy and safety of immediate-release methylphenidate treatment for preschoolers with ADHD. *J Am Acad Child Adolesc Psychiatry*. 2006;45:11.

Joshi SV. Teamwork: the therapeutic alliance in pediatric pharmacotherapy. *Child Adolesc Psychiatr Clin N Am*. 2006;12:239.

King BH, Bostic JQ. An update on pharmacologic treatments for autism spectrum disorders. *Child Adolesc Psychiatr Clin N Am*. 2006;15:161.

Pavuluri MN, Birmaher B, Nayulor MW. Pediatric bipolar disorder: a review of the past 10 years. *J Am Acad Child Adolesc Psychiatry*. 2005;44:846.

Pediatric OCD Treatment Study (POTS) Team Cognitive-behavior therapy, sertraline, and their combination for children and adolescents with obsessive-compulsive disorder: The Pediatric OCD Treatment Study (POTS) randomized controlled trial. *JAMA*. 2004;292:1969.

Reinblatt SP, Riddle MA. Selective serotonin reuptake inhibitor-induced apathy: A pediatric case series. *J Child Adolesc Psychopharmacol*. 2006;16:227.

Swanson JM, Wigal SB, Wigal T, Sonuga-Barke E, Greenhill LL, Biederman J, Kollins S, Nguyen AS, DeCory HH, Hirshe Dirksen SJ, Hatch SJ; COMACS Study Group. A comparison of once-daily extended-release methylphenidate formulations in children with attention-deficit/hyperactivity disorder in the laboratory school (the CONACS study). *Pediatrics*. 2004;113:e206.

TADS Team. The Treatment of Adolescents with Depression Study (TADS): short-term effectiveness and safety outcomes. *JAMA* 2004;292:807.

Vitiello B. Research in child and adolescent psychopharmacology: recent accomplishments and new challenges. *Psychopharmacology*. 2007;19:5.

Vitiello B. An update on publicly funded multisite trials in pediatric psychopharmacology. *Child Adolesc. Psychiatr Clin N Am*. 2006;15:1.

Wagner DK. Pharmacotherapy for major depression in children and adolescents. *Prog Neuropsychopharmacol Biol Psychiatry*. 2005;29:819.

Wagner KD, Ambrosini P, Rynn M, Wohlberg C, Yang R, Greenbaum MS et al. Efficacy of sertraline in the treatment of children and adolescents with major depressive disorder: two randomized controlled trials. *JAMA*. 2003;290:033.

Wagner KD, Robb AS, Findling RL, Jin J, Gutierrez MM, Heydorn WE. A randomized, placebo-controlled trial of citalopram for the treatment of major depression in children and adolescents. *Am J Psychiatry*. 2004;161:1079.

Wagner KD, Berard R, Stein MB, Wetherhold E, Carpenter DJ, Perera P, Gee M, Davy K, Machin A. A multicenter, randomized, double-blind, placebo controlled trial of paroxetine in children and adolescents with social anxiety disorder. *Arch Gen Psychiatry*. 2004;61:1153.

Waslick B. Psychopharmacology interventions for pediatric anxiety disorders: a research update. *Child Adolesc Psychiatr Clin N Am*. 2006;15:51.

▲ 54.5 Psychiatric Treatment of Adolescents

Psychiatric treatment is indicated for an adolescent in whom is found a disturbance of thought, affect, or behavior to the point that it disrupts normal functioning. For adolescents, this includes influences on eating, sleeping, and school function, as well as relationships with family and peers. A variety of serious psychiatric disorders, including schizophrenia, bipolar disorder, eating disorders, and substance abuse typically have their onset during adolescence. In addition, the risk for completed suicide drastically increases in adolescence. Although some stress is virtually universal in adolescence, most teenagers without mental disorders can cope well with the environmental demands. Teenagers with preexisting mental disorders may experience exacerbations during adolescence and may become frustrated, alienated, and demoralized.

Clinicians and parents must be sensitive to adolescents' perceptions of themselves. A range of emotional maturity exists in a group of teenagers of the same age. Issues that are specific to adolescents are related to their new evolving identities, the development of sexual activity, and their plans to meet future life goals.

DIAGNOSIS

Adolescents can be assessed in both their specific stage-appropriate functions and their general progress in accomplishing the tasks of adolescence. For almost all adolescents in today's culture, at least until their late teens, school performance and peer relationships are the primary barometers of healthy functioning. Intellectually normal adolescents who are not functioning satisfactorily academically, or teens who are isolated from peers have significant psychological problems whose nature and causes should be identified.

Questions to be asked regarding adolescents' stage-specific tasks are the following: What degree of separation from their parents have they achieved? What sort of identities are evolving? How do they perceive their past? Do they perceive themselves as responsible for their own development or only the passive recipients of their parents' influences? How do they perceive themselves with regard to the future, and how do they anticipate their future responsibilities for themselves and others? Can they think about the varying consequences of different ways of living? How do they express their sexual and affectionate interests? These tasks occupy all adolescents and normally are performed at varying times.

Adolescents' family and peer relationships must be evaluated. Do they perceive and accept both good and bad qualities in their parents? Do they see their peers and boyfriends or girlfriends as separate persons with needs and identities of their own, or do others exist only for the adolescents' own needs?

A respect for, and (if possible) some actual understanding of, an adolescent's subcultural and ethnic background are essential. For example, in some groups, depression is acceptable; in other groups, overt depression is a sign of weakness and is masked by antisocial acts, substance misuse, and self-destructive risks. A psychiatrist need not be of the same race or group identity as an adolescent to treat him or her effectively. Respect and knowledgeable concern are human qualities and are not group restricted.

INTERVIEWS

Whenever circumstances permit, both an adolescent patient and his or her parents should be interviewed. Other family members also may be included, depending on their involvement in the teenager's life and difficulties. Clinicians should see the adolescent first, however; preferential treatment helps avoid the appearance of being the parents' agent. In psychotherapy with an older adolescent, the therapist and the parents usually have little contact after the initial part of the therapy, because ongoing contact inhibits the adolescent's desire to open up.

Interview Techniques

All patients' test and mistrust therapists, but adolescents often manifest these reactions crudely, intensely, provocatively, and for prolonged periods. Clinicians must establish themselves as trustworthy and helpful adults to promote a therapeutic alliance. They should encourage adolescents to tell their own stories, without interrupting to check discrepancies; such a tactic seems as though correcting and expressing disbelief. Clinicians should ask patients for explanations and theories about what happened. Why did these behaviors or feelings occur? When did things change? What caused the identified problems to begin when they did?

Sessions with adolescents generally follow the adult model; the therapist sits across from the patient. In early adolescence, however, board games (e.g., checkers) may help to stimulate conversation in an otherwise quiet, anxious patient.

Language is crucial. Even when a teenager and a clinician come from the same socioeconomic group, their languages are seldom the same. Psychiatrists should use their own language, explain any specialized terms or concepts, and ask for an explanation of unfamiliar in-group jargon or slang. Many adolescents do not talk spontaneously about illicit substances and suicidal tendencies but do respond honestly to a therapist's questions. A therapist may need to ask specifically about each substance and the amount and frequency of its use.

The sexual histories and current sexual activities of adolescents are increasingly important pieces of information for adequate evaluation. The nature of adolescents' sexual behaviors often is a vignette of their whole personality structures and ego development, but a long time may elapse in therapy before adolescents begin to talk about their sexual behavior.

The parents of a 13-year-old boy noted that it was difficult for him to get up in the morning. He seemed as though he was not sleeping. When asked about his sleep, he was reluctant to answer and simply indicated that he was having "a little trouble" falling asleep at night. His parents began watching him and found that he was up until 2 or 3 AM. He was getting up out of bed numerous times. They also found that he took longer and longer time in the bathroom. In school, he often missed classes and was found in the bathroom. When confronted, he disclosed that he had developed a number of bedtime rituals that took longer and longer to complete because if he did them incorrectly, he had to repeat them. They included checking the locks on the windows and doors, placing objects in the "right" places on his dresser, and repeating a prayer 16 times. He also revealed that when in the bathroom, he had to wash his hands a certain way and dry them "just so," or he feared something terrible would happen. His psychiatric evaluation revealed significant obsessive-compulsive disorder (OCD) and social phobia. Treatment was initiated, including use of a selective serotonin reuptake inhibitor (SSRI), cognitive-behavioral therapy (CBT), and problem-solving family therapy. Over the course of 6 months, his OCD responded well to the combination of medications and CBT, and the family learned ways of helping him both at home and in school. (Courtesy of Eugene V. Beresin, M.D. and Steven C. Schlozman, M.D.)

A 14-year-old girl gymnast began increasing her daily exercise and restricting her diet. She had never achieved menses because of her low weight. She became fixated on the size of her thighs and belly and lost so much weight that her coach and pediatrician did not allow her to participate in athletics. She became increasingly terrified of getting fat and secretly exercised any chance she could. She was a perfectionist in academics as well as in gymnastics. Because of excessive weight loss, she was hospitalized, and the diagnosis of anorexia nervosa, nonpurging type, was established without comorbid disorders. After hospitalization with modest weight gain, an outpatient plan was initiated, including regular meetings with her pediatrician for monitoring of vital signs, weekly meetings with a nutritionist, weekly family therapy, and individual psychodynamic psychotherapy. In her psychotherapy, over the course of 2 years, she was able to understand that her perfectionism was a defense against low self-esteem, that she was very angry with her mother, who lived vicariously through her gymnastics and did not validate who she really was, and that she was, as an only child, the focus in her family, holding her parents' marriage together. Over time, she was able to understand the function of her anorexia as a way to avoid her maturation as a woman, as a dysfunctional means of developing some kind of identity, and as a passive-aggressive attack on her parents. With time, her weight increased, and she was able to resume her athletics and developed close friends. (Courtesy of Eugene V. Beresin, M.D. and Steven C. Schlozman, M.D.)

TREATMENT

Psychiatric treatment of an adolescent can occur in numerous venues and modalities. Treatment can focus on individual or group settings, and can include interventions that are pharmacologic (when indicated), psychosocial, and from an environmental perspective. The best choices for treatment of psychiatric disorders in adolescents must take into account the characteristics of the individual adolescent and the family or social milieu. Adolescents' striving for autonomy may complicate problems of compliance with therapy and may result in the need for stabilization in inpatient settings, whereas this level of care may not be necessary at a different stage of life. Therefore, the following discussion is less a set of guidelines than a brief summary of what each treatment modality can or should offer.

Individual Psychotherapy

Individual psychosocial modalities with an evidence base for efficacy with adolescents include cognitive-behavioral treatments for psychiatric disorders, such as anxiety disorders, mood disorders, and OCD. Interpersonal therapy is a technique that has been applied to mood disorders in adolescents. Few adolescent patients are trusting or open without considerable time and testing, and it is helpful to anticipate the testing period by letting patients know that it is to be expected and is natural and healthy. Pointing out the likelihood of therapeutic problems—for instance, impatience and disappointment with the psychiatrist, with the therapy, with the time required, and with the often intangible results—may help keep problems under control. Therapeutic goals should be stated in terms that adolescents understand and value. Although they may not see the point in exercising self-control, enduring dysphoric emotions, or forgoing impulsive gratification, they may value feeling more confident than in the past and gaining more control over their lives and the events that affect them.

Typical adolescent patients need a real relationship with a therapist they can perceive as a real person. The therapist becomes another parent, because adolescents still need appropriate parenting or reparenting. Thus, a professional who is impersonal and anonymous is a less useful model than one who can accept and respond rationally to an angry challenge or confrontation without fear or false conciliation—one that can impose limits and controls when adolescents cannot, can admit mistakes and ignorance, and can openly express the gamut of human emotions. Adolescents perceive as indifference or collusion a failure to take a stand about self-damaging and self-destructive behavior or to respond actively to manipulative and dishonest behavior.

Countertransference reactions can be intense in psychotherapeutic work with adolescents, and therapists must be aware of them. An adolescent often expresses hostile feelings toward adults, such as parents and teachers. A therapist may react with over identification with the adolescent or with the parents. Such reactions are determined, at least in part, by a therapist's own experiences during adolescence or, when applicable, the therapist's own experiences as a parent.

Individual outpatient therapy is appropriate for adolescents whose problems are manifest in conflicted emotions and nondangerous behavior, who are not too disorganized to be maintained outside a structured setting, and whose families or other living environments are not sufficiently disturbed to negate the influence of therapy. Such therapy characteristically focuses on intrapsychic conflicts and inhibitions; on the meanings of emotions, attitudes, and behavior; and on the influence of the past and the present. Antianxiety agents can be considered in adolescents whose anxiety may be high at certain times during psychotherapy, but adolescents' potential for abusing these drugs must be weighed carefully.

Psychopharmacotherapy and Combined Therapy

Randomized clinical trials have provided evidence of the superiority of CBT in combination with SSRI medication in the treatment of mood disorders, OCD, and, most likely, anxiety disorders in adolescents.

Attention-deficit/hyperactivity disorder (ADHD) has not been studied systematically with regard to effectiveness in treating adolescents with ADHD in combination with CBT. In the Mutimodal Treatment Study of Children with ADHD (MTA), psychosocial interventions did not add to the efficacy of the stimulant treatments for the core symptoms of ADHD. Other outcome measures of psychosocial improvements are needed, however, in future studies of combination treatment. Psychostimulants, such as methylphenidate (Ritalin, Concerta), dextroamphetamine (Dexedrine) and amphetamine salts (Adderall, Adderall XR), however, have been found to be efficacious in adolescents in the treatment of ADHD.

Advances in drug development have widened the choice of medications to treat mood disorders (e.g., SSRIs) and schizophrenia (e.g., serotonin-dopamine antagonists [SDAs], including risperidone [Risperdal], olanzapine [Zyprexa], and clozapine [Clozaril]). Although these medications have been used to treat adolescent disorders, systematic research is required to determine the efficacy and safety profiles of these medications for treatment of adolescent psychopathology.

A comprehensive workup is needed before starting psychopharmacotherapy with adolescents, including a physical examination; blood tests to evaluate hematological, kidney, liver, thyroid, and other physiological functions; and an electrocardiogram (ECG) to measure cardiac function. Neurological assessment with an electroencephalogram (EEG) is necessary if seizure disorder is suspected or if the medication is likely to lower the seizure threshold.

A 17-year-old girl complained of episodes of rapid heartbeat, sweating, trembling, and fears of going out alone to the shopping mall. She had entered her senior year in high school, was considering her choice of colleges, and was planning to take her college entrance examination. Her parents wanted her to maintain the family tradition and go to the college from which her mother graduated. Psychoanalytically oriented outpatient treatment and treatment with an SSRI were instituted to alleviate the panic disorder symptoms. The psychotherapy focused on the patient's conflicts with her parents, highlighting her chronic concern that she could not meet parental expectations and fears of her independence. Medication appeared to reduce symptoms of tachycardia, tremulousness, and preoccupation with lack of competence. Psychotherapy was maintained for 8 months during her last year in high school. (Courtesy of Cynthia R. Pfeffer, M.D.)

Group Psychotherapy

In many ways, group psychotherapy is a natural setting for adolescents. Most teenagers are more comfortable with peers than with adults. A group diminishes the sense of unequal power between the adult therapist and the adolescent patient. Participation varies, depending on an adolescent's readiness. Not all interpretations and confrontations should come from the parent-figure therapist; group members often are adept at noticing symptomatic behavior in each other, and adolescents may find it easier to hear and consider critical or challenging comments from their peers.

Group psychotherapy usually addresses interpersonal and current life issues. Some adolescents, however, are too fragile for group psychotherapy or have symptoms or social traits that are too likely to elicit peer group ridicule; they need individual therapy to attain sufficient ego strength to struggle with peer relationships. Conversely, other adolescents must resolve interpersonal issues in a group before they can tackle intrapsychic issues in the intensity of one-on-one therapy.

Family Therapy

Family therapy is the primary modality when adolescents' difficulties mainly reflect a dysfunctional family (e.g., teenagers with school refusal, runaways). The same may be true when developmental issues, such as adolescent sexuality and striving for autonomy, trigger family conflicts or when family pathology is severe, as in cases of incest and child abuse. In these instances, adolescents usually need individual therapy as well, but family therapy is mandatory if an adolescent is to remain in the home or return to it. Serious character pathology, such as that underlying antisocial and borderline personality disorders, often develops from highly pathogenic early parenting. Family therapy is strongly indicated whenever possible for such disorders, but most authorities consider it adjunctive to intensive individual psychotherapy when individual psychopathology has become so internalized that it persists regardless of the current family status.

Inpatient Treatment

Residential treatment schools often are preferable for long-term therapy, but hospitals are more suitable for emergencies, although some adolescent inpatient hospital units also provide educational, recreational, and occupational facilities for long-term patients. Adolescents whose families are too disturbed or incompetent, who are dangerous to themselves or others, who are out of control in ways that preclude further healthy development, or who are seriously disorganized require, at least temporarily, the external controls of a structured environment.

Long-term inpatient therapy is the treatment of choice for severe disorders that are considered wholly or largely psychogenic in origin, such as major ego deficits that are caused by early massive deprivation and that respond poorly or not at all to medication. Severe borderline personality disorder, for example, regardless of the behavioral symptoms, requires a full-time corrective environment in which regression is possible and safe and in which ego development can take place. Psychotic disorders in adolescence often require hospitalization, but psychotic adolescents often respond to appropriate medication so that therapy usually is feasible in an outpatient setting, except during exacerbation. Adolescent patients with schizophrenia who exhibit a long-term deteriorating course may require hospitalization periodically.

Day Hospitals

In day hospitals, which have become increasingly popular, adolescents spend the day in class, individual and group psychotherapy, and other programs, but they go home in the evenings. Day hospitals are less expensive than full hospitalization and usually are preferred by patients.

CLINICAL PROBLEMS

Atypical Puberty

Pubertal changes that occur 2.5 years earlier or later than the average age are within the normal range. Body image is so important to adolescents, however, that extremes of the norm may be distressing to some, either because markedly early maturation subjects them to social and sexual pressures for which they are unready or because late maturation makes them feel inferior and excludes them from some peer activities. Medical reassurance, even if based on examination and testing to rule out pathophysiology, may not suffice. An adolescent's distress may show as sexual or delinquent acting out, withdrawal, or problems at school that are sufficiently serious to warrant therapeutic intervention. Therapy also may be prompted by similar disturbances in some adolescents who fail to achieve peer-valued stereotypes of physical development despite normal pubertal physiology.

Substance-Related Disorders

Some experimentation with psychoactive substances is almost ubiquitous among adolescents, especially if this category of behavior includes alcohol use. Most adolescents, however, do not become abusers, particularly of prescription drugs and illegal substances. Any regular substance abuse represents disturbance. Substance abuse sometimes is self-medication against depression or schizophrenic deterioration and sometimes it signals a character disorder in teenagers whose ego deficits render them unequal to the stresses of puberty and the tasks of adolescence. Some substances, including cocaine, have a physiologically reinforcing action that acts independently of preexisting psychopathology. When substance abuse covers an underlying illness or is a maladaptive response to current stresses or disturbed family dynamics, treatment of the underlying cause may diminish the substance use; in most cases of significant abuse, however, the drug-taking behavior typically requires intervention. Substance abuse treatments typically include a 12-step program with behavioral monitoring to accomplish sobriety as well as the ability to verbalize regarding the motivations for substance use. These philosophies are adapted to inpatient, intensive outpatient, and once-a-week outpatient treatment.

Suicide

Suicide is currently the second leading cause of death among adolescents. Many hospital admissions of adolescents result from suicidal ideation or behavior. Among adolescents who are not psychotic, the highest suicidal risks occur in those who have a history of parental suicide, who are unable to form stable attachments, who display impulsive behavior, and who abuse alcohol or other substances. Many adolescents who complete suicide have backgrounds that include long-standing family conflict and social problems since early childhood and the escalation of subjective distress under the pressure of a sudden perceived conflict or loss. Early childhood loss of parents, of childhood—also can increase the risk of depression in adolescence. The adolescents who are susceptible to rapid and extreme mood swings and a history of impulsive behavior are at greater risk to respond to despair with impulsive suicide attempts. And alcohol and other substances are known added risks for suicidal behavior in adolescents with suicidal ideations. The developmentally predictable "omnipotent" attitudes of adolescents may cloud the immediate sense of permanence of death that result in impulsive self-destructive behavior in adolescents.

During a psychiatric evaluation of an adolescent with suicidal thoughts, plans, and past attempts must be discussed directly when the concern arises and information is not volunteered. Recurring suicidal thoughts should be taken seriously, and a clinician must evaluate the imminent clinical danger requiring inpatient hospitalization versus an adolescent's ability to engage in an agreement or contract mandating that the adolescent will seek help before engaging in self-destructive behavior. Adolescents typically are honest in their refusal of such agreements, and, in such cases, hospitalization is indicated. Hospitalization of a suicidal adolescent by a clinician is an act of serious, protective concern. See Section 49.1 for a more complete discussion of suicide in adolescents.

References

Beresin EV, Schlozman SC. Psychiatric treatment of adolescents. In: Sadock BJ, Sadock VA, eds. *Kaplan & Sadock's Comprehensive Textbook of Psychiatry*. 8th ed. Vol. 2. Baltimore: Lippincott Williams & Wilkins; 2005:3395.

Connor DF, McLaughlin TJ, Jeffers-Terry M, O'Brien WH, Stille CJ, Young LM, Antonelli RC. Targeted child psychiatric services: A new model of pediatric primary clinician–child psychiatry collaborative care. *Clin Pediatr (Phila)*. 2006;45:423.

Mufson L, Dorta KP, Wickramaratne P, Nomura Y, Olfson M, Weissman MM. A randomized effectiveness trial of interpersonal psychotherapy for depressed adolescents. *Arch Gen Psychiatry*. 2004;61(6):577.

Olfson M, Marcus SC, Shaffer D. Antidepressant drug therapy and suicide in severely depressed children and adolescents: A case-control study. *Arch Gen Psychiatry*. 2006;63:865.

Romano E, Zoccolillo M, Paquette D. Histories of child maltreatment and psychiatric disorder in pregnant adolescents. *J Am Acad Child Adolesc Psychiatry*. 2006;45:329.

Seidman LJ. Neuropsychological functioning in people with ADHD across the lifespan. *Clin Psychol Rev*. 2006;26:466.

55 Child Psychiatry: Special Areas of Interest

▲ 55.1 Forensic Issues in Child Psychiatry

Forensic child and adolescent psychiatry is a subspecialty of psychiatry involving the relationships between psychiatry and the law. Currently, board certification in forensic psychiatry is based on a 1-year fellowship that is not specifically geared to children and adoelscents; however, many programs offer exposure to child and adolescent cases. Traditionally, forensic child and adolescent psychiatrists have dealt largely with custody evaluation and recommendations, and with the ramifications of child abuse and neglect. Child and adolescent psychiatrists are increasingly being sought out by patients and attorneys for evaluations and expert opinions related to child sexual and physical abuse, to criminal behaviors perpetrated by minors, and to evaluate the relations between traumatic life events and the emergence of psychiatric symptoms in children and adolescents. As more youth enter the juvenile justice system, an increasing need exists for forensic psychiatrists with expertise in evaluation and treatment for detainees and committed youths. The American Academy of Child and Adolescent Psychiatry (AACAP) provided *Practice Parameters for the Forensic Evaluation of Children and Adolescents Who May Have Been Physically or Sexually Abused;* for custody evaluations and for children with posttraumatic stress disorder (PTSD). Throughout the fields in medicine, ethical principles have alluded to moral obligations as a guide for acceptable as behavior that physicians follow; the Hippocratic oath summarizing the main ethical values of a physician. During the past few decades, however, more complex ethical and moral dilemmas have arisen with the greater sophistication of medical technology. For example, a patient may be kept alive for long periods while in a coma or a pregnant woman's life may be saved by aborting her fetus.

Society's view of children and their rights has evolved dramatically in the 20th century. The institution of a juvenile court system about 100 years ago was an acknowledgment that children must be protected and provided for differently than adults. In 1980, the AACAP published a code of ethics that was developed to publicly endorse the ethical standards of this discipline. The code is based on the assumption that children are vulnerable and unable to take adequate care of themselves; as they mature, however, their capacity to make judgments of, and choices about, their well-being develop as well. The code has several caveats: From the standpoint of child and adolescent psychiatrists, issues of consent, confidentiality, and professional responsibility must be seen in the context of overlapping and potentially conflicting rights of children, parents, and society.

Confidentiality, or intensive trust, refers to the relationship between two persons with respect to the "entrustment of secrets." Until the 1970s, little attention was paid to issues of confidentiality pertaining to minors. In 1980, among the items in the *AACAP Code of Ethics*, six principles were related to confidentiality. Breaches and limits of confidentiality can be obtained in cases of child abuse or maltreatment or for purposes of appropriate education. Although unnecessary with a child or adolescent, consent for disclosure should be obtained when possible. In 1979, the American Psychiatric Association (APA) stated that a child 12 years of age could give consent for disclosure of confidential information and, with the exception of safety issues, a minor's consent is required for disclosure of information to others, including the child's parents. According to the *AACAP Code of Ethics*, the consent of a minor is not required for disclosure of confidential information. Specific ages for consent are not addressed in the code. Child and adolescent psychiatrists often face the dilemma of weighing the potential benefits and possible harm in sharing information obtained confidentially from a child with the child's parents. Although the smoothest transition occurs when the child and the physician agree that certain information can be shared, in many situations that border on "dangerousness to the child or others," the child or adolescent does not agree to share the information with a parent or another responsible adult. Among adolescents, these secrets that are sometimes shared with a psychiatrist may involve drug or alcohol use, unsafe sex practices, or a thrill-seeking act that places the adolescent in danger. A psychiatrist may choose to work with the child or adolescent toward agreeing to share confidential information when it is determined by the treating psychiatrist that the probable outcome would be beneficial. The initial treatment contract, however, limits confidentiality to situations of "danger" to the child or others.

Other arenas that can pose confidentiality dilemmas include educational and scientific settings, research activities, and third-party agencies. Professional settings, such as annual psychiatric conventions, often include individual case presentations. In the context of a clinical symposium, doctors should realize that confidentiality means more than changing or dropping a patient's name; other information in a case study may pose a threat to a patient's privacy. Research projects sometimes are impeded by laws designed to protect the privacy of children and their families. In some cases, long-term follow-up studies may no longer be "legal" because of a time limitation on a written consent for study. Third-party payers are requiring more and more confidential information before they consider reimbursement of psychiatric services. Information disclosed to insurance companies often is shared with many reviewers in the company, which also places it in danger of being merged into a database in a computer system that is neither highly restricted nor confidential.

In general, no way exists to simplify the many difficult, complex confidentiality issues that may emerge in treating children and adolescents. Child and adolescent psychiatrists function as advocates for their patients and must always remain aware of minors' vulnerabilities and of the importance of maintaining trust in the treatment relationship.

CHILD CUSTODY

Child custody evaluations by child and adolescent psychiatrists may be initiated by divorcing parents who cannot come to an agreement regarding custody of their children, or can be requested by an attorney. Attorneys are most likely to seek child custody evaluations when allegations are made of parental incompetence, or issues of alleged physical or sexual abuse arise. Comprehensive custody evaluations by mental health professionals may play a significant role in successful negotiations of custody by parents without the necessity of proceeding to a trial.

The evolution of child custody decision-making has been influenced by increasing awareness and recognition of the rights of children and women, as well as by a broadening perspective on the developmental and psychological needs of the children involved. Historically, children were considered to be their fathers' property. At the beginning of the 20th century, the "tender years" doctrine became the standard for determining child custody. According to this doctrine, the relationship between mother and infant, later generalized to mother and child, is responsible for the optimal emotional development of the child; the doctrine thus supported custody decisions in the mother's favor in most cases. With this doctrine as its guide, psychological issues in developing children became an acceptable dimension to consider in the determination of custody. In controversial and unclear cases, psychological expert testimony began to be accepted as a valuable part of child custody decision-making.

The "best interest of the child" standard replaced the "tender years" doctrine and expanded considerations of the optimal parent to include assessing issues of emotional climate, safety, and educational and social opportunities for the children. The "best interest of the child" grew from the movement to support legislation about the rights of children in the areas of compulsory education, child labor laws, and child abuse and neglect protection laws. Therefore, although "best interest" standards have broadened the dimensions considered in evaluating which parent is best able to serve the best interest of the child, how to measure these qualities in a parent remains vague. In view of the lack of clarity regarding what specific parameters in a parent best correspond to the interest of the child, child and adolescent psychiatrists have increasingly been asked to help make decisions by defining relevant psychological conditions in parents and in the relationships between parents and children.

Psychiatric evaluators may be asked to give an opinion about child custody at various points during the separation and divorce process. Sometimes, a psychiatric evaluation is requested by the parents before any legal action occurs. When the parents and an evaluator can agree on custody decisions before the legal process, a court is likely to go along with these decisions rather than launch an additional investigation. A psychiatric evaluation may be ordered by the court or by the attorneys representing the feuding parents. In such cases, an evaluator is faced with two disgruntled parents who often are consumed by their mutual conflict to the point that neither is willing to compromise, even in the child's interest. The advantage in such cases, however, is that evaluators represent the court and can act as advocate for the child without the same pressures that an evaluator hired by only one parent faces. A psychiatric evaluation also may be initiated by a *guardian ad litem,* an attorney who is appointed by the court to represent the child. Psychiatric evaluators also may be requested to give an opinion about custody during a mediation process. Mediation is a legal process that usually involves one attorney and one evaluator. Because mediation can occur outside the judicial system, some families may prefer it to going through a trial. In addition to custody, psychiatric evaluators often are asked to give opinions about visitation.

In undertaking a custody evaluation, an evaluator is expected to determine the best interests of the child while keeping in mind the standard elements that the court considers. These considerations include the wishes of the parents and the child; relationships with significant others in the child's life; the child's adjustment to the current home, school, and community; the psychiatric and physical health of all parties; and the level of conflict and potential danger to the child under the care of either parent. A psychiatric evaluator must maintain his or her role as an advocate for the best interest of the child and does not consider the fairest outcome for parents. The psychiatric evaluator conducts a series of interviews, often including at least one separate interview with each parent and the child alone and one interview with the child and both parents. The evaluator may obtain a written waiver of confidentiality from all parties because he or she may have made disclosures to opposing attorneys and in court before the judge. The evaluator uses direct questioning as well as observations of the relationships between the child and each parent. The age and developmental needs of the child are considered in making a judgment regarding which parent may better serve the child's interests. As part of the psychiatric assessment of the child custody evaluation, the evaluator determines the need for psychiatric treatment of any of the parties involved.

The child custody evaluation generally is provided in a written report. This document is not confidential and can be used in court. The report contains a description of the relationship between the child and parents, the capabilities of the parents, and finally, the custody recommendations. In view of data supporting the importance of continuing a relationship with both parents in most cases, it is recommended that joint custody be considered before other options. When sufficient cooperation exists to negotiate for joint custody, the best interests of the child often are served. Joint custody may not be the best option for a child when the relationship of the child with either parent is jeopardized and undermined by the other. The next most frequent choice when joint custody is not advisable is full custody by one parent with visitation rights for the other parent. The parent awarded full custody should be able to support the visitations and relationship with the noncustodial parent. In custody disputes involving a biological parent and a nonbiological parent, the biological parent generally has the right to custody unless he or she is shown to be unable to provide for the child. After the custody evaluation has been submitted in writing, the results must be communicated to the parents, the child, and possibly their respective attorneys. The evaluator may be called on to testify in court, and the parties can use the custody evaluation to mediate other areas of their dispute.

Many complications can occur in an ongoing bitter dispute between divorcing or divorced parents. Both true and false allegations of psychiatric illness, drug or alcohol abuse, or sexual or physical abuse are not uncommon during custody battles. The evaluator must be prepared to verify any allegations and to carefully discuss their effects on custody and visitation. Evidence suggests that markedly elevated numbers of unfounded allegations of child sexual abuse occur during the course of custody disputes.

Joey, age 8 years, has been in a therapeutic foster home for 2 years, having been removed from his home along with his younger sister (who was subsequently returned home) owing to profound neglect, as well as abuse. Although he is receiving appropriate services, he remains volatile, with extensive developmental problems; and typically becomes more aggressive and regressed after weekly supervised visits with his family. Joey's guardian *ad litem* requests that Dr. Jacobs perform a forensic evaluation to determine whether visits should continue. She reviews extensive records, evaluates each parent, obtains history from them and the foster parent, and then observes a visit. Joey's little sister totally dominates the visit, and the parents are at a loss to control her aggressive and hyperactive behavior. Joey is passive and not very engaged with either parent. According to the visitation supervisor, this is a fairly typical visit. When Dr. Jacobs meets individually with Joey, Joey expresses concerns that his sister is still being abused at home, and his need to check on her seems to be the only reason he wants to continue the visits. Dr. Jacobs tells Joey that both parents are getting help and doing better with their parenting, but he remains unconvinced. Joey evidences a positive relationship with his foster father and, in contrast, has little to say about his parents. Dr. Jacobs recommends a psychiatric evaluation of the sister, but Joey's parents do not follow through with one. She further recommends cutting visits back to monthly, but Joey's anxiety and aggressive behavior persist around these limited visits. It also becomes apparent that the parents are not up to the demands of caring for two special-needs children. She recommends ceasing efforts at parental reunification but maintaining some contact between Joey and his sister. (Courtesy of Diane H. Schetky, M.D.)

JUVENILE OFFENDERS

The creation of a separate juvenile court system in the United States occurred by statute in the state of Illinois in the late 1800s. Its mandate was to rehabilitate rather than to punish. Despite the protective intentions of the legal sytem, children and adolescents involved in the juvenile justice system are at high risk for multiple psychiatric disorders and suicidal thoughts and behavior. A recent survey of 991 youth at an initial juvenile justice intake revealed high levels of suicidal ideation with recent attempts more comon in females, and youth with major depression or substance use disorders, and those who were violent offenders. The omission of various constitutional safeguards, such as the rights to counsel, confrontation, and cross-examination of an accuser, eventually led to criticism and disillusionment with this system. Juvenile offenders of small and significant crimes often were sent to state-run residential programs that were criticized for being overcrowded, neglectful, and frankly abusive. Despite the strong sentiment to increase due process protection for juveniles rather than pretrial, trial, and sentencing, the juvenile court system includes intake, adjudication, and disposition. The intake is a determination of whether probable cause exists that the youth committed a crime. A youth who confesses may be diverted from the court system altogether at this time, and appropriate plans for rehabilitation can be made in a community setting. For more serious crimes or when juveniles deny perpetrating a crime, the process continues. Juveniles must be represented by counsel, and an attorney is provided if the family cannot afford to provide its own.

Unlike adult court, in juvenile court guilt or innocence is determined by a judge, not a jury. The case is argued by a prosecuting attorney and a defense attorney, and the judge is bound by the same standards as in adult court; that is, a judgment of delinquency requires proof beyond a reasonable doubt. When the charge is substantiated and the judgment is for delinquency, the juvenile is an "adjudicated delinquent." Disposition must next be determined. Dispositions include a wide range of options, from placement in youth correctional facilities, to residential treatment settings, to psychiatric hospitalizations for further evaluation. *Delinquent acts* refer to ordinary crimes committed by juveniles; *status offenses* refer to behaviors that would not be criminal if perpetrated by adults, such as truancy, running away, or drinking alcohol. Sometimes, youths who are believed to have committed a serious crime are turned over (receive a waiver) to adult criminal court.

A psychiatrist may be asked to evaluate a juvenile to make recommendations about appropriate diversion plans. Psychiatric evaluation can be sought for adjudicated delinquents to determine whether treatment for a psychiatric illness would work in favor of preventing future delinquent acts and, if so, in what setting. Psychiatric evaluations also may be requested when the court is considering a waiver to adult court. In some states, such decisions are based, in part, on the juvenile's psychiatric history and current mental status.

MENTAL HEALTH NEEDS OF YOUTH IN THE JUVENILE JUSTICE SYSTEM

Youth in the juvenile justice system are at extremely high risk for psychiatric disturbance and unmet mental health needs have reached such high proportions that they are of public health concern. Adolescents in juvenile justice residential facilities not only have higher rates of psychiatric disorders, including depression, substance use, and suicidal behavior, but they are also significantly more likely to have been victims of physical and sexual abuse, educational failure, and family conflict. Few studies have documented the needs of juveniles in residential facilities and the medical and psychiatric care available. A recent study collected data from the US Department of Justice censuses of all public and private juvenile justice facilities in the United States: The Juvenile Residential Facilities Census (JRFC) and the Census of Juveniles in Residential Placement (CJRP) investigated data on death rates of youth under the age of 21 years who had been charged with, or adjudicated for, an offense and are housed in that facility because of the offense. In the 2-year period covered by the 2000 and 2002 statistics, a total of 62 deaths of youth occurred. The leading cause of death was from suicide (20 cases), followed by accidents (17 cases), illness (14 cases), and homicides by nonresidents (6 cases). No deaths resulted from acquired immunodeficiency syndrome (AIDS), homicide by another resident, or an injury that occurred before placement. The risk for death of youth in juvenile justice facilities was found to be 8 percent higher than the death rate for the general population of adolescents aged 15 to 19 years. Above all, the risk for suicide is clearly increased in the juvenile justice facility compared with the general population, indicating a significant need for increased mental health evaluation and treatment in this population.

ADVERSE LIFE EVENTS AND PSYCHIATRIC SYMPTOMS

Child and adolescent psychiatrists are frequently sought out to evaluate children or adolescents who have been exposed to a traumatic or adverse life event and are exhibiting a variety of psychiatric symptoms. The child and adolescent psychiatrist may be asked to determine whether a child or adolescent is experiencing posttraumatic stress disorder or whether a given set of symptoms is likely to have been caused by exposure to the adverse life event. A recent report by William Bernet M.D. and David Corwin M.D. detail an evidence-based approach to estimate present and future damages from a traumatic event, such as sexual abuse. This requires the child and adolescent psychiatrist to carefully interview the patient and family as well as review the published literature on the aspects of childhood sexual abuse that would help to render opinions that are based on individual and systematic approaches to similar situations. Thus, the first question asked was whether the child was injured by the sexual abuse. Given the clinical case history of the child in question, it was clear that intrusive painful memories, depressed mood, suicidal ideation, poorly controlled rage, and substance abuse following the sexual abuse were reasonable indicators of harm. The question of whether the child who has been sexually abused is at increased risk of future psychiatric problems was reasonably ascertained by reviewing the literature of multiple children who were sexually abused and found to have rates of psychiatric disorders two to three times higher than would otherwise be expected. Regarding the efficacy of treatment, the psychiatrist was able to extrapolate from the published literature that the child would likely be better off with a psychosocial intervention after abuse than with none. Thus, the principles of evidenced-base approaches to forensic evaluations can increase the validity and usefulness of the recommendations.

Another common request to a child and adolescent psychiatrist is to render an expert opinion regarding whether, for example, a child diagnosed with autistic disorder is likely to have been at greater risk for the disorder because of a particular treatment given to the mother during pregnancy. It is much easier for a child and adolescent psychiatrist to verify the presence of a psychiatric disorder in a child than to determine its exact cause. Evaluations requiring a psychiatrist to make a judgment identifying a single cause of a complex psychiatric disorder are generally difficult or impossible because of the lack of data linking psychiatric disorders to single causes.

Dr. Abibi is called by a defense attorney to review discovery material in a case that alleges permanent harm and suffering in 6-year-old Tony, who is alleged to have been sexually abused at age 3 in his day care center. Dr. Green, the forensic expert for the plaintiff, has evaluated the child and performed psychological testing of him and concluded that the boy's conduct problems are all related to the alleged abuse, which the child has difficulty recalling. His early history on the boy is cursory, however, and he has little information about the mother, who is a single parent, and did not review medical records. In her thorough review of discovery material, Dr. Abibi learns that Tony has witnessed extensive domestic violence and his mother's rape, shown signs of hyperactivity since age 2, and has exhibited much anxiety related to his mother's safety and several separations from her at times when she was unable to care for him owing to depression. Tony also has had delayed language development. Dr. Green, at the time of his deposition, was asked why he had not asked about these matters. He said he considered the mother's personal life a private matter and did not see its relevance to the litigation. Dr. Abibi, when deposed, points out that many other factors beside the alleged abuse might account for Tony's behavioral problems. (Courtesy of Diane H. Schetky, M.D.)

References

Barrett B, Byford S, Chitsabesan P, Kenning C. Mental health provision for young offenders: Service use and cost. *Br J Psychiatry*. 2006;188:541.

Bernet W, Corwin D. An evidence-based approach for estimating present and future damages from child sexual abuse. *J Am Acad Pscyhiatry Law*. 2006;34:224.

Gallagher CA, Dobrin AD. Deaths in juvenile justice residential facilities. *J Adolesc Health*. 2006;38:662.

Haynes K. Principles and practice of child and adolescent forensic psychiatry. *Psychiatr Serv*. 2003;54(10):1416.

Leverette JS. Enhancing the learning curve in child and adolescent forensic psychiatry: Inter-professional relationships, resource and policy development. *Curr Opin Psychiatry*. 2004;17(5):391.

Lewis A. A career in forensic child and adolescent psychiatry. *BMJ*. 2003;326 (7398):167.

Schetky DH. Forensic child and adolescent psychiatry. In: Sadock BJ, Sadock VA, eds. *Kaplan & Sadock's Comprehensive Textbook of Psychiatry*. 8th ed. Vol. 2. Baltimore: Lippincott Williams & Wilkins; 2005:3490.

Waller EM, Daniel AE. Purpose and utility of child custody evaluations: The attorney's perspective. *J Am Acad Psychiatry Law*. 2005;33:199.

Wasserman GA, McReynolds LS. Suicide risk at juvenil justice intake. *Suicide Life Threat Behav*. 2006;36:239.

▲ 55.2 Adoption and Foster Care

As many as 500,000 to 700,000 children are in foster care each year in the United States. Foster care caseloads more than doubled in the last two decades. In recent years, child abuse and neglect and abandonment, often in conjunction with parental substance abuse and psychiatric illness, have emerged as significant reasons for placement. Foster care is intended to be temporary out-of-home care provided by the welfare system for children and adolescents whose immediate families are unable to care for them. Given the severity of the vulnerable parents, however, care is often needed for many months and years. In 1997, President Clinton signed the Adoption and Safe Families Act (PL-105-89), a law designed to improve provisions for child safety, to decrease the length of time that a child remains in foster care without long-term planning, and to limit the amount of time in which a biological parent has to to undergo rehabilitation to 12 months. An additional law, PL 99-272, was added to allocate federal funds for independent living assistance for adolescents and young adults 16 to 21 years of age who leave foster care to assist them in transitioning to independent living.

EPIDEMIOLOGY AND DEMOGRAPHICS OF FOSTER CARE

Minority children are overrepresented in the foster care population. Approximately 38 percent are African Americans, more than three times the representation in the general population. Whites make up approximately 48 percent, and Hispanics make up almost 15 percent. Of foster children, 55 to 69 percent are girls, and 83.4 percent enter foster care at a mean age of 3 years. Children placed in care as infants are more likely to stay in care. Those younger than 5 years of age currently comprise the fastest growing segment of the foster care population. Studies reveal that as many as 62 percent of foster children had prenatal drug exposure. A 1989 Department of Health and Human Services (HHS) study revealed that 30 to 50 percent of all drug-exposed children entered foster care; among African Americans, parental drug use precipitated almost 80 percent of foster care placements. Parental drug use is positively correlated with maltreatment, with approximately 89 percent of maltreatment cases involving drug abuse. In one California study, 89 percent of maltreated infants tested positive for drugs at birth—cocaine being the drug identified in 85 percent of those who were positive for drug use.

Needs of Foster Care Children

Children entering foster care have enormous mental health needs; more than 80 percent of them have developmental, emotional, or behavioral problems. Growth abnormalities (including failure to thrive), neurological abnormalities, neuromuscular disorders, language disorders, cognitive delays, and asthma are prevalent. Their health care needs cost six to ten times as much as matched non-foster care peers. Among children 0 to 5 years of age, approximately 25 percent are seriously emotionally damaged. Attachment disorders are increasingly diagnosed. Foster care children use the full range of mental health services: outpatient, acute inpatient, day treatment, partial hospitalization, and residential treatment. Adolescents in foster care are at increased risk for substance abuse, teenage pregnancies, and sexually transmitted diseases, including human immunodeficiency virus (HIV). With public health care increasingly adopting a managed health care system, which is designed to limit care, grave concern exists that the provision and delivery of services to this medically and psychiatrically vulnerable population can be seriously compromised.

Kinship Care for Foster Children

More states are recognizing kinship care as an alternative placement option and are authorizing licensing and reimbursement to kinship caregivers who are generally female (mostly maternal grandmothers), of low income, of low education, and of minority status. Currently, nationwide, approximately 23 percent of African American children are in foster kinship care. It is unknown just how many children are in informal kinship care within the African American population, which has had a long cultural tradition of taking in children of family members who are unable to care for their offspring. The few studies available indicate that outcomes, although mixed, are somewhat more positive than for those children in nonkinship care. Children reportedly receive more positive regard from caregivers in kinship care, and a consistent outcome, when it works, is that it provides more stability than nonrelative foster care. Most foster children have consistently said that they would rather be with a family member than stay in the system. When foster children feel embraced by their families of origin, and the latter can provide appropriate nurturance and access to good therapeutic services, the foster children's sense of identity and belonging is less disrupted. As best as can be determined, however, no demonstrable difference is seen in the need for mental health, medical, and special educational services for these children. Research on kinship care is ongoing and should be providing increasingly reliable data. Initial data from Robert B. Clyman and associates on outcomes from kinship care are not favorable, but should be interpreted cautiously and within the context of that particular research design.

THERAPEUTIC FOSTER CARE

Therapeutic foster care (TFC) has emerged as a cost-effective alternative to the more restrictive *residential treatment center* (RTC). Therapeutic effectiveness is mixed. TFC is designed to provide nurturing family-based care with specialized treatment interventions from an interdisciplinary treatment team. Therapeutic foster parents are supposed to be the agents of therapeutic change, functioning as *extenders* of the clinical treatment team. Because of the children's special needs, therapeutic foster parents must have more extensive training, receive a higher reimbursement, and receive more intensive monitoring, supervision, and support from the foster care agency. Although the concept of TFC is promising, good outcome data do not show consistent success. Several models exist, but implementation that shows fidelity to empirically tested models is often spotty. Some models, although efficacious in the research setting, have proved too expensive and complicated to implement in the real-world setting. The concept of professional therapeutic parents, who are actually paid competitive full-time wages to care for special needs foster children, has been gaining increasing interest and definitely holds some promise as an alternative to current prevailing practice. Clinical practice demonstrates that, when adequate and appropriate intensive in-home services, with good case management, can be provided in a well-managed foster care setting, children can show significant gains.

Cultural Competence

Anna McPhatter defines *cultural competence* as the ability to use knowledge and cultural awareness to design psychosocial interventions that support and sustain healthy client–system functioning within a cultural context that is meaningful to the client. Because the American society is still significantly encumbered by racial conflicts, some children have been denied placement with families of a different race, and they ended up in long-term foster care rather than in a permanent adoption placement. The Association of Black Social Workers went on record as opposing transracial placement of African American children. In 1978, the Indian Child Welfare Act (PL 95-608) transferred to Tribal Courts the power to make placement decisions about Native American children to reverse the practice of placement in non-Native American homes. Adoption studies have shown that it is not inherently harmful for children to be cross-racially adopted. Congress has passed legislation, the Multiethnic Placement Act of 1994, facilitating transracial adoptions, while maintaining the language of cultural awareness in placement decisions. The need for cultural sensitivity, respect, and a capacity to facilitate a foster child's cultural development and identity are well acknowledged. These issues must be addressed in training providers of foster care services. Although it is now common practice to include *cultural competence* as a requirement in the implementation of child welfare programs, no rigorous research, however, has yet identified the essential variables that make for success in cultural competency.

PSYCHOLOGICAL ISSUES IN FOSTER CARE CHILDREN

As previously, foster care children are overrepresented in psychiatric populations. Among those who return home, 40 percent reenter the foster care system. These children struggle with issues of abandonment, neglect, rejection, and physical, emotional, and sexual maltreatment. The child's age, home environment, and the specific reasons for going into placement affect the emotional issues that he or she must handle. Early abandonment and neglect can lead to anaclitic depression. Attachment issues are prevalent in this young population, because they have not had an opportunity to form secure attachments with consistent nurturing figures in early life.

Foster children are often unprepared for separations, which can be abrupt and repeated in the current foster care climate. Early separation from the primary caretaker is considered a major trauma for the child and sets the stage for a vulnerability to subsequent trauma. Those children who bounce from foster home to foster home have their capacity to form enduring emotional attachments compromised; trust becomes a lifelong challenge. Defense mechanisms tend to be primitive, that is, denial, splitting, projection, and introjection. Characterological problems are common in adulthood. Not surprisingly, children who have never had their narcissistic needs appropriately met may become unempathetic adults with pathological narcissism, which is associated with criminality.

Children who have experienced traumatic physical and sexual abuse often become mistrustful, hypervigilant, aggressive, impulsive, oppositional, and avoidant as they attempt to negotiate a world that they experience as threatening, hostile, and uncaring. When children are raised in a psychosocial environment of trauma, aggression, and lack of empathy from adults, the psychological seeds are sown for later violence against the self and others. The range of psychopathology of foster care children covers several psychiatric diagnostic categories. Attention-deficit/hyperactivity disorder (ADHD), attachment disorders, oppositional defiant disorder, conduct disorders, impulse-control disorders, posttraumatic stress disorder (PTSD), dissociative disorders, mood and anxiety disorders, sleep disorders, and developmental disorders are some that are frequently diagnosed. A pervasive problem is one of dysregulation: dysregulation of behavior, emotions and affect, attention, and sleep. In reviewing the empirical data on the neurobiology of maltreatment on the developing brain, it is clear that stress hormones play an important role in adaptation and coping, and that these capacities are compromised in varying degrees of severity in abused and neglected children. The data also show that, because of the developmental plasticity of the brain, if appropriate early intervention can be done, hope exists for remediation and repair at the neurobiological level.

A boy was placed in care because of maternal drug involvement. When seen for a psychiatric evaluation, it was noted that all of his primary teeth were full of dental caries. The foster mother was asked about dental care, and she responded that the dentist had said that he would wait until the teeth had fallen out, because they were his first set of teeth and did not require intervention. This response aroused suspicion about neglect as being the cause of the behavioral (encopresis and smearing) and emotional problems with which this youngster presented. A neglect report was made and the investigation revealed that the boy was not only neglected, but was also being physically abused in that foster care placement. Subsequent to removal and placement with a good foster family, this boy has shown considerable emotional stabilization, does well academically and socially, and is now being adopted by that family. (Courtesy of Marilyn B. Benoit, M.D., Steven L. Nickman, M.D., and Alvin Rosenfeld, M.D.)

FAMILY PRESERVATION

Family preservation has come under increasing scrutiny in the last decade. Estimates on the percentage of children who are reportedly reunited vary from 66 to 90 percent. Philosophically, family reunification appears to be the right thing to do, yet approximately 40 percent of reunified children reenter out-of-home care. The field needs discriminating criteria that would identify psychosocial profiles of families that could best benefit from family preservation services. In 1996, the Child Welfare League of America (CWLA) acknowledged the failure of family preservation efforts and requested that child welfare policy makers rethink the current use of intensive family preservation. Recent research has validated poor outcomes with family preservation. Hopes are that the Adoption and Safe Families Act of 1997 (PL 105-89) will give child welfare agencies the opportunity to step back from the myopic view of family preservation and to consider seriously the needs of the child as the major priority. The American Academy of Child and Adolescent Psychiatry (AACAP) and the CWLA jointly launched a national effort to address the mental health needs of children in foster care. This effort is supported by a broad-based coalition of agencies that are all stakeholders in foster care. The coalition proposes that the foster care system be child focused, but inclusive of the biological and foster families in intervention planning on the child's behalf if families are to be preserved. Another area of concern regarding improving family preservation is that of substance abuse as a major contributing factor to families' dysfunction. The data are clear that this is the single major contributor to children going into care. The high incidence of comorbid mental illness in the biological parent population makes rehabilitation a challenging endeavor that requires more comprehensive interventions than are currently provided.

One case of a 7-year-old boy who was in foster care for 2 years is illustrative of why some family preservation efforts fail. When he was returned to his biological mother, she was in a new marriage with a new baby. Her husband was new to parenting. The family was financially strapped and lived under harsh conditions. The mother did the required parenting course for resuming custody of her child, but no supports were put in place to assist this young couple financially or with any family therapy, psychoeducation, or case management interventions. Frequent and increasingly urgent calls to the child welfare family reunification services were of no avail. The outcome for this youngster was that he was reabused and had to reenter the foster care system.

This outcome represents a failure of the system, but also translates into a fractured and debilitated family, with everyone internalizing a profound sense of failure and impotence. (Courtesy of Marilyn B. Benoit, M.D., Steven L. Nickman, M.D., and Alvin Rosenfeld, M.D.)

FOSTER CARE OUTCOMES AND RESEARCH INITIATIVES

The overall quality of available outcome studies is poor. Some patterns, however, recur across studies. Several studies reveal that 15 to 39 percent of the homeless are foster care graduates, who are also overrepresented among adult substance abusers and clients in the criminal justice system. It is likely that the reasons that initially precipitated the child's foster care placement contributed to the negative adult outcomes. Studies indicate that children entering care who have been victimized, who have substance-abusing parents or parents with major mental illness or high criminality, or both, and who come from homes with a high degree of domestic violence are at greater risk of having poor outcomes. Research on early maltreatment indicates that the influence of maltreatment on brain development can be profound over the life span. Developmental disabilities occur in more than 50 percent of the foster care population. Children returned to their families of origin typically have fared worse than those who have remained in long-term placement.

Several studies report findings indicating that multiple placements and poor parental involvement consistently lead to negative outcomes. Federal mandate (PL 96-272) requires states to maintain a tracking system for children in foster care. New reporting systems, the Adoption and Foster Care Analysis and Reporting System (AFCARS) and the Statewide Automated Child Welfare Information System (SACWIS), are available nationwide. States are being monitored for compliance with their use, and continued federal funds are contingent on the implementation of these information systems. Because foster care placement is the result of psychosocial environmental failure, fixing the existing system requires more than good information systems. Integration of sound, theory-driven, child-focused, family-centered services, collaboratively funded by multiple governmental agencies, is essential. Through the use of longitudinal, research-based performance measures, reliable data are emerging. The National Institutes of Mental Health (NIH) has funded some research focusing on foster care children and youth. Some examples of such research initiatives include preventive interventions for foster care youths to reduce problem behaviors and to improve prosocial development, tailoring services to foster infants' needs, improving casework and collaboration across agencies, and examining the use of mental health services by youths leaving care. The complexity of the impact of ever-changing psychosocial variables makes this type of research challenging. Despite that, it must be done if welfare dollars are to be spent doing the right thing for needy children and their families. In 2004, in a groundbreaking study, the Pew Commission on Children in Foster Care made sweeping recommendations to overhaul the system, stating that "children deserve more from our child welfare system."

HISTORY OF ADOPTION

Adoption has existed in different forms throughout history. In ancient Babylonia, it provided for the transmission of property or artisan's skills, whereas, in the Roman Empire, it was often used to elevate the status of an adult protégé. In some Pacific islands, adoption of young children formed part of an exchange system between related clans. Concerns expressed by adopted persons about not knowing their roots are as ancient as they are contemporary. Euripides' *Ion* contains a touching dialogue between a woman in search of the child she had given up years before and a young priest of Apollo, who does not know that he is the woman's son and says that the only mother he knows is Apollo's priestess.

In the 19th century, the newly established social work profession took on the task of adoption placement, facilitated by legislation that enabled children to become legal members of families, although, in some cases, the child was not entitled to an inheritance. Because of concerns about the possibility of children having undesirable inherited traits, they were kept and observed in hospitals for as long as a year to ensure desirability. With a change in focus to addressing the needs of children as a priority, infant placements are encouraged to take place as soon as possible to promote secure attachment.

After World War II, European children were placed in the United States, and, after the Korean War, Korean children were placed in American homes. Continuing transracial and transcultural (domestic and international) adoptive placements have raised some controversy, having opponents and proponents of the practice.

Historically, *closed adoptions* were common practice. That was done to ensure the sealed identities of birth and adoptive parents and was believed to be in the best interests of adopted children. That practice is now considered flawed, and contemporary, although still controversial, thinking is that most adoptees should grow up knowing of their adoption status, as well as the identities of their birth parents. Currently, adoptees, as well as many birth parents and adoptive parents, increasingly have shared interests in legislation that affects the open or closed status of birth records and the placement of children in families. The phrase *adoption triad* has come to stand for these shared interests, represented by the American Adoption Congress and other organizations. In addition, other organizations represent each of these three groups, and those organizations often have divergent agendas. Since the 1980s, adoption practice has been profoundly affected by federal legislation.

EPIDEMIOLOGY OF ADOPTION

From 1.5 to 2.0 percent of children grow up in nonrelated adoptive placements, whereas another 1.5 percent are adopted by relatives or stepparents. Figures from the National Adoption Information Clearinghouse (NAIC) for 1992 indicate that, in 1992, 127,441 adoptions were finalized in the United States. Of these, 42 percent were by stepparents or relatives, and 58 percent were unrelated adoptions. Of the unrelated adoptions, 27 percent were conducted by public agencies (i.e., adoptions from the foster care system); 8 percent were from other countries, with the largest numbers from Korea; and 64 percent were arranged by a private agency or were independent adoptions, in approximately equal numbers. The number of completed adoptions from the US foster care system does not give a full picture of the numbers of waiting children—primarily, minority children in the public child welfare system. The NAIC estimates that, as of March 1998, approximately 500,000 children were currently in foster care in the United States. Of these, 110,000 (just more than 20 percent) were eligible for adoption. Some are legally free for adoption and waiting in not yet legalized adoptive homes, whereas others are still waiting to be placed in adoptive families. Other children not yet legally free for adoption live in preadoptive foster placements, but most remain in traditional foster homes or residential facilities. The pattern of international adoptions by American families varies with world events: wars, internal conflicts, and policy changes. A sense of this can be seen by comparing the rank-order list of countries sending the most children to the United States in 1991 and 2001: China ranked 17th in 1991 but first in 2001; Russia does not appear on the 1991 list but is second in 2001; whereas Colombia, in fourth place in 1991, descends to 12th place 10 years later.

INTERNATIONAL ADOPTION

Each year more than 20,000 children are adopted from overseas and many of these are transracial adoptions. More than 17,000 children were adopted from Guatemala, for example, in the last two decades. In the Guatamalan adoptees, the mean age was 1.5 years and the children had previously resided in orphanages, foster homes, or mixed-care settings. Investigation of the health records of children who were evaluated after arrival in the United States in an international adoption specialty clinic revealed that younger children at time of adoption have better growth, language development, cognitive skills, and activities of daily living compared with children who were older at time of adoption. Among children matched for age, gender, and time from adoption to evaluation, those who were previously living in foster care were observed to have higher cognitive scores and improved growth compared with children who had resided in orphanages. These findings support the priority of adoptive placement at younger ages and that foster care has benefits over orphanage care.

EARLY CHILDHOOD VS LATE ADOPTION

Data suggest that earlier age adoption predicts better outcome than adoption in middle or late childhood. A recent prospective study examined factors related to successful outcome in public adoption of children ranging in age from 5 to 11 years of age. Prospective data were collected from domestic adoptions in the United Kingdom at 1 year, and 6 years later on 108 adoptees who were placed primarily because of situations involving childhood abuse and neglect. Outcome was assessed by the disruption rate and measures of psychological adaptation. At the adolescent follow-up, 23 percent of the adoption placements had been disrupted, 49 percent were continuing with positive adaptations, and 28 percent were ongoing but with significant conflicts. Four factors contributed independently to the risk of disruptions: older age at placement, report of being singled out and rejected by siblings, time in care, and greater degree of behavioral problems. Given that almost half of the placements were ongoing, later childhood age of adoption can be successful; however, the constellation of families, and assessment of behavioral problems may determine the likelihood of positive outcome for school-aged child adoptees.

BIRTH PARENTS: SEARCH AND REUNION

The increasing trend toward open adoption allows the opportunity for adoptees to more easily search and successfully find their birth parents. Many adoptive parents choose open adoptions so that they can experience a greater connection with the child if they have some relationship with the birth mother. Some adoptees want to develop an ongoing relationship with birth parents, but many who search are satisfied to meet birth parents without further correspondence. Outcomes of reunions with birth parents vary widely and, in some cases, especially when the birth parents are well functioning and welcoming toward their child, the adoptee may experience a sense of relief and joy in knowing that their birth mother is no longer vulnerable.

References

Benoit MB, Nickman SL, Rosenfield A. Adoption and foster care. In: Sadock BJ, Sadock VA, eds. *Kaplan & Sadock's Comprehensive Textbook of Psychiatry*. 8th ed. Vol. 2. Baltimore: Lippincott Williams & Wilkins; 2005:3406.

Brenner E, Freundlich M. Enhancing the safety of children in foster care and family support programs: Automated critical incident reporting. *Child Welfare*. 2006;85:611.

Hansen ME, Hansen BA. The economics of adoption of children from foster care. *Child Welfare*. 2006;85:559.

Harden BJ. Safety and stability for foster chidren: A developmental perspective. *Future Child*. 2004;14:31.

Maynard J. Permanancy mediation: A path to open adoption for children in out-of-home care. *Child Welfare*. 2005;84:507.

McGuinness TM, Dyer JG. International adoption as a natural experiment. *J Pedatr Nusrs*. 2006;21:276.

McWey LM, Henderson TL, Tice SN. Mental health issues and the foster care system: An examination of the impact of the Adoption and Safe Families Act. *J Marital Fam Ther*. 2006;32:195.

Miller L, Chan W, Comfort K, Tirella L. Health of children adopted from Guatemala: Comparison of orphanage and foster care. *Pediatrics*. 2005;115: e710.

The Pew Commission on Children in Foster Care. Fostering the Future: Safety Permanence and Well-Being for Children in Foster Care. Washington, DC; 2004.

Rushton A, Dacne C. The adoption of children from public care: A prospective study of outcome in adolescence. *J Am Acad Child Adolesc Psychiatry*. 2006;45: 877

Swann CA, Sylvester MS. The foster care crisis: What caused caseloads to grow? *Demography*. 2006;43:309.

Wilcox BL, Weisz, Miller MK. Practical guidelines for educating policy makers: The family impact seminar as an approach to advancing the interests of children and families in the policy arena. *J Clin Child Adolesc Psychol*. 2005;34:638.

▲ 55.3 Child Maltreatment and Abuse

Child and adolescent maltreatment and abuse is prevalent and its long-term consequences multiple. Estimates of children maltreated in the United States each year is close to 1 million, and the annual number of deaths caused by abuse or neglect has been estimated to be nearly 1,500.

The National Longitudinal Study of Adolescent Health, a prospective study following a national sample of adolescents, recently investigated the prevalence, risk factors, and health consequences in adolescents who reported retrospective child maltreatment. The most common forms of maltreatment reported were being left home alone as a child, indicating potential supervision neglect (reported by 41.5 percent), physical assault (reported by 28.4 percent), then physical neglect (reported by 11.8 percent), and sexual abuse (reported by 4.5 percent). Each type of maltreatment was associated with at least eight of the ten adolescent health risks examined, including self-report of depression, regular alcohol use, binge drinking, marijuana use, overweight status, generally "poor" health, inhalant use, and violent behaviors, including fighting and hurting others. Clearly, the effects of self-reported maltreatment had far ranging and long-lasting associations with multiple detrimental consequences.

The identification, management, and treatments for child maltreatment require cooperative efforts between multiple professionals, including primary care physicians, emergency room staff, law enforcement, attorneys, social service staff, and mental health professionals. Perpetrators typically deny abuse or neglect and maltreated children often fear disclosure of their abuse or neglect.

DEFINITIONS

DSM-IV-TR

The somewhat terse classification system provided by the revised 4th edition of the *Diagnostic and Statistical Manual of Mental Disorders* (DSM-IV-TR) lists *physical abuse of child, sexual abuse of child*, and *neglect of child*. The three classifications appear in the chapter "Other Conditions That May Be a Focus of Clinical Attention" and in the section "Problems Related to Abuse or Neglect." These categories should be used when the focus of clinical attention is severe mistreatment of one individual by another. These conditions and problems are coded on Axis I.

The DSM-IV-TR does not include detailed definitions or criteria for diagnosis. Circumstances in which the focus of attention is on the perpetrator of child abuse or neglect or on the relational unit in which it occurs have one code. Three different codes cover situations in which the focus of attention is on the victim (for neglect of child, for physical abuse of child, or for sexual abuse of child).

Federal Law

The Child Abuse Prevention and Treatment Act was passed in 1974 and has been amended several times, most recently in 2003. In federal law, *child abuse* and *neglect* mean, as a minimum, any recent act or failure to act on the part of a parent or caretaker that results in death, serious physical or emotional harm, or sexual abuse or exploitation. It also includes an act or failure to act that presents an imminent risk of serious harm. In federal law, *sexual abuse* means the employment, use, persuasion, inducement, enticement, or coercion of any child to engage in or to assist any other person to engage in any sexually explicit conduct (or simulation of such conduct for the purpose of producing a visual depiction of such conduct) or the rape (and in cases of caretaker or interfamilial relationships, statutory rape), molestation, prostitution, or other forms of sexual exploitation of children or incest with children.

State Law

A large mass of legal definitions and guidelines exists at the state level. The legal definitions of terms related to the maltreatment of children vary from one jurisdiction to another, so clinicians should be aware of the definitions used in their own locale. The following generic definitions are used in this section.

Neglect

Neglect, the most prevalent form of child maltreatment, is the failure to provide adequate care and protection for children. Children can be harmed by malicious or ignorant withholding of physical, emotional, and educational necessities. Neglect includes failure to feed children adequately and to protect them from danger. Physical neglect includes abandonment, expulsion from home, disruptive custodial care, inadequate supervision, and reckless disregard for a child's safety and welfare. Medical neglect includes refusal, delay, or failure to provide medical care. Educational neglect includes failure to enroll a child in school and allowing chronic truancy.

Physical Abuse

Physical abuse can be defined as any act that results in a nonaccidental physical injury, such as beating, punching, kicking, biting, burning, and poisoning. Some physical abuse is the result of unreasonably severe corporal punishment or unjustifiable punishment. Physical abuse can be organized by damage to the site of injury: skin and surface tissue, the head, internal organs, and skeletal.

Emotional Abuse

Emotional or *psychological abuse* occurs when a person conveys to children that they are worthless, flawed, unloved, unwanted, or endangered. The perpetrator may spurn, terrorize, ignore, isolate, or berate the child. Emotional abuse includes verbal assaults (e.g., belittling, screaming, threats, blaming, or sarcasm), exposing the child to domestic violence, overpressuring through excessively advanced expectations, and encouraging or instructing the child to engage in antisocial activities. The severity of emotional abuse depends on (1) whether the perpetrator actually intends to inflict harm on the child and (2) whether the abusive behaviors are likely to cause harm to the child. Some authors believe that the terms *emotional* or *psychological abuse* should not be used and that *verbal abuse* more accurately describes the pathological behavior of the caregiver.

Sexual Abuse

Sexual abuse of children refers to sexual behavior between a child and an adult or between two children when one of them is significantly older or uses coercion. The perpetrator and the victim may be of the same sex or the opposite sex. The sexual behaviors include touching breasts, buttocks, and genitals, whether the victim is dressed or undressed; exhibitionism; fellatio; cunnilingus; and penetration of the vagina or anus with sexual organs or objects. Sexual abuse can involve behavior over an extended time or a single incident. Developmental factors must be considered in assessing whether sexual activities between two children are abusive or normative. In addition to the forms of inappropriate sexual touching, *sexual abuse* also refers to sexual exploitation of children, for instance, conduct or activities related to pornography depicting minors and promoting or trafficking in prostitution of minors.

Ritual Abuse

Cult-based *ritual abuse*, which includes satanic ritual abuse, is physical, sexual, or psychological abuse that involves bizarre or ceremonial activity that is religiously or spiritually motivated. Typically, multiple perpetrators abuse multiple victims over an extended period of time. Ritual abuse is a controversial concept; some professionals believed in the 1990s that ritual abuse was a common, horrible phenomenon in society, whereas others were skeptical about most allegations and descriptions of ritual abuse.

Perpetrators of Abuse

Some lack of consistency is seen in who may be defined as an *abuse perpetrator*. Usually, a person must be a parent or designated caregiver to be charged with neglect, physical abuse, or emotional abuse. Another adult (e.g., a stranger) who injures a child would be charged with battery, not with child abuse. On the other hand, a caretaker or any other person could be charged with child sexual abuse. State laws vary in this regard.

COMPARATIVE NOSOLOGY

Neither the 1st edition (DSM-I) nor the 2nd edition of the DSM (DSM-II) (1968) mentioned child maltreatment. The Group for the Advancement of Psychiatry (1974) mentioned child maltreatment among the pathogenic factors of childhood mental disorders: "The deleterious effects . . . of open rejection or neglect, occasionally involving willful injury or inadequate feeding, are well documented." The Group for the Advancement of Psychiatry, however, did not include child maltreatment in their proposed system of classification.

When the 3rd edition of the DSM (DSM-III) (1980) was published, the American Psychiatric Association Task Force on Nomenclature and Statistics introduced a chapter called "V Codes for Conditions Not Attributable to a Mental Disorder That Are a Focus of Attention or Treatment." The V Codes, which were modeled on the practice in the 9th edition, clinical modification, of the *International Classification of Diseases* (ICD-9-CM), did not include specific categories for child maltreatment. It was intended, however, that child abuse would be coded as a *parent–child problem*, the category used "when a focus of attention or treatment is a parent–child problem that is apparently not due to a mental disorder of the individual (parent or child) who is being evaluated." DSM-III specifically stated that "an example (of parent–child problem) is child abuse not attributable to a mental disorder of the parent." The emphasis of *parent–child problem* was apparently on identifying perpetrators of abuse, not the child victims of abuse.

The revised 3rd edition of the DSM (DSM-III-R) (1987) provided a similar definition for *parent–child problem*: "This category can be used for either a parent or a child when the focus of attention or treatment is a parent–child problem that is apparently not due to a mental disorder of the person who is being evaluated." The example involving child abuse was replaced, however, by "conflict between a mentally healthy adolescent and her parents about her choice of friends."

In the 4th edition of the DSM (DSM-IV) (1994), the name of the chapter changed to "Other Conditions That May Be a Focus of Clinical Attention." Also, a specific section was introduced, "Problems Related to Abuse or Neglect," which included terms related to child maltreatment. The editors noted that this category was "included because of the clinical and public health significance of these conditions." For the first time, it was possible to diagnose clearly *physical abuse of child*, *sexual abuse of child*, and *neglect of child*. Furthermore, DSM-IV made it possible to distinguish whether the person being evaluated is the perpetrator of abuse or the victim of abuse.

The terminology regarding child maltreatment in DSM-IV-TR (2000) is the same as that in DSM-IV. DSM-IV and DSM-IV-TR terminology are the same as that in the tenth edition of the ICD (ICD-10); only the codes differ.

EPIDEMIOLOGY

Each year, the Children's Bureau, an agency within the Department of Health and Human Services, collects data on child maltreatment. The results are published in an annual document called *Child Maltreatment*. The agency estimated that, in 2002, approximately 3 million alleged victims were reported to child protective services. Of those reports, approximately 896,000 were substantiated; this represents 12.3 of every 1,000 children. The substantiated cases were distributed as follows: neglect, 60 percent; physical abuse, 20 percent; sexual abuse, 10 percent; and emotional abuse, 7 percent. The Children's Bureau estimated that 1,400 children died as the result of maltreatment in 2002. Approximately 41 percent of these deaths were children younger than 1 year of age.

The data were analyzed for patterns of maltreatment by the sex and age of victims. Rates of many types of maltreatment were similar for male and female children, but the sexual abuse rate for female children was higher than the sexual abuse rate for male children. Examining the age distribution of victims of abuse, the age group from 0 to 3 years of age had the highest victimization rate, and the rate of victimization declined as the age of the victims increased. For example, the rate for infants (0 to 3 years of age) was 16 per 1,000, whereas the rate for adolescents (16 to 17 years of age) was 6 per 1,000. Regarding the perpetrators of abuse, it was reported that, overall, 58 percent were female, and 42 percent were male.

All of these figures are approximations, because the actual number of cases of abuse is unclear. The reporting of abuse and the annual victimization rate increased during the 1980s and reached a high in 1993 (when the victimization rate was 15.2 per 1,000 children in the population). This increase resulted from greater public awareness and willingness to report child abuse, improvement in data collection techniques by individual states, and local economic conditions that placed a larger number of families under stress. The victimization rate has fallen after 1993 and reached a low in 1999 (when the victimization rate was 11.8 per 1,000 children).

ETIOLOGY

Physical Abuse

Although child abuse occurs at all socioeconomic levels, it is highly associated with poverty and psychosocial stress, especially financial stress. Child maltreatment is strongly correlated with less parental education, underemployment, poor housing, welfare reliance, and single parenting. Child abuse tends to occur in multiproblem families, that is, families characterized by domestic violence, social isolation, parental mental illness, and parental substance abuse, especially alcoholism. The probability of maltreatment may be increased by risk factors such as prematurity, mental retardation, and physical handicap. Also, the risk of child abuse increases in families with many children.

Sexual Abuse

Social, cultural, physiological, and psychological factors all contribute to the breakdown of the incest taboo. Incestuous behavior has been associated with alcohol abuse, overcrowding, increased physical proximity, and rural isolation that prevents adequate extrafamilial contacts. Some communities may be more tolerant of incestuous behavior. Major mental disorders and intellectual deficiency have been described in some perpetrators of incest and sexual abuse.

DIAGNOSIS AND CLINICAL FEATURES

Abused children manifest a variety of emotional, behavioral, and somatic reactions. These psychological symptoms are neither specific nor pathognomonic: The same symptoms can occur without any history of abuse. The psychological symptoms manifested by abused children and the behaviors of abusive parents can be organized into clinical patterns. Although it may be helpful to note whether a particular case falls into one of these patterns, that in itself is not diagnostic of child abuse.

Physically Abused Children

In many cases, the physical examination and radiological evaluation show evidence of repeated suspicious injuries. Abused children display behaviors that should arouse the suspicions of the health professional. For example, these children may be unusually fearful, docile, distrustful, and guarded. On the other hand, they may be disruptive and aggressive. They may be wary of physical contact and show no expectation of being comforted by adults, they may be on the alert for danger and continually size up the environment, and they may be afraid to go home.

The literature regarding the psychological consequences of physical abuse and neglect indicates a wide range of effects: affect dysregulation, insecure and atypical attachment patterns, impaired peer relationships involving increased aggression or social withdrawal, and academic underachievement. Physically abused children exhibit a range of psychopathology, including depression, conduct disorder, attention-deficit/hyperactivity disorder (ADHD), oppositional defiant disorder, dissociation, and posttraumatic stress disorder (PTSD).

Physically Abusive Parents

Abusive parents typically delay seeking help for the injuries. The history given by the parents is implausible or incompatible with the physical findings. The parents blame a sibling or claim that the children injured themselves. The characteristics of abusive parents include a history of abuse in their own early lives, a lack of empathy for the child, unrealistic expectations of the child, and an impaired parent–child attachment, especially to babies who are defective in some way.

Carol, 4 years of age, had a change in her behavior at preschool approximately 3 months after the birth of her sister. Her teacher saw Carol push other children and hit a classmate with a wooden block, causing a laceration of the child's lip. When Carol's teacher took her aside to talk about her behavior, she noticed what seemed to be belt marks on Carol's abdomen and forehead. The teacher reported possible child abuse to protective services. Also, the family was referred for psychiatric evaluation.

Carol's baby sister was colicky and slept only for short periods of time throughout the day and night. She stopped crying only when her mother held her. Her mother, therefore, had little time for Carol, and Carol's father took over her care on evenings after day care and on weekends. He began to drink more than usual and became increasingly irritable. The parents argued over the mother's attention to the infant and the requirement that the father take care of Carol. Carol, who was a bright, curious, and talkative child, constantly asked questions and often asked to carry the baby. When refused, she would lie on the floor and have a tantrum. She also began to have difficulty falling asleep and awoke repeatedly during the night. Carol's father was unable to cope with her requests for attention and often told her to shut up and slapped her when she continued her demands. On many occasions, he responded to her tantrums or repeated questions by hitting her with his belt.

While protective services monitored the situation, Carol and her parents began a family therapy program that included parenting training and behavioral therapy for Carol, which was coordinated with the preschool. Carol's father attended Alcoholics Anonymous (AA) meetings and stopped drinking. He was able to control his anger at his daughter. Six months later, Carol's aggressive behavior ceased. She was doing well with peers, was sleeping through the night, and stopped having temper tantrums. (Courtesy of William Bernet, M.D.)

Sexually Abused Children

A variety of symptoms, behavioral changes, and diagnoses sometimes occur in sexually abused children: anxiety symptoms, dissociative reactions and hysterical symptoms, depression, disturbances in sexual behaviors, and somatic complaints.

Anxiety Symptoms. Anxiety symptoms include fearfulness, phobias, insomnia, nightmares that directly portray the abuse, somatic complaints, and PTSD.

Dissociative Reactions and Hysterical Symptoms. The child may exhibit periods of amnesia, daydreaming, trance-like states, hysterical seizures, and symptoms of dissociative identity disorder.

Depression. Depression may be manifested by low self-esteem and suicidal and self-mutilative behaviors.

Disturbances in Sexual Behaviors. Some sexual behaviors are particularly suggestive of abuse, such as masturbating with an object, imitating intercourse, and inserting objects into the vagina or anus. Sexually abused children may display sexually aggressive behavior toward others. Other sexual behaviors are less specific, such as showing genitals to other children and touching the genitals of others. A younger child may manifest age-inappropriate sexual knowledge. In contrast to these overly sexualized behaviors, the child may avoid sexual stimuli through phobias and inhibitions.

Somatic Complaints. Somatic complaints include enuresis, encopresis, anal and vaginal itching, anorexia, bulimia, obesity, headache, and stomachache.

These symptoms are not pathognomonic. Nonabused children may exhibit any of these symptoms and behaviors. For example, normal, nonabused children commonly exhibit sexual behaviors, such as masturbating, displaying their genitals, and trying to look at people who are undressing.

Approximately one third of sexually abused children have no apparent symptoms. Most adults who were abused as children have no significant abuse-related symptoms. On the other hand, the following factors tend to be associated with more severe symptoms in the victims of sexual abuse: greater frequency and duration of abuse, sexual abuse that involved force or penetration, and sexual abuse perpetrated by the child's father or stepfather. Other factors associated with poorer prognosis are the child's perception of being less believed, family dysfunction, and lack of maternal support. Also, multiple investigatory interviews appear to increase symptoms.

Intrafamilial Sexual Abuse

Incest can be defined strictly as sexual relations between close blood relatives, that is, between a child and the father, uncle, or sibling. Because of increased reporting, sibling incest is an area of growing concern. In its broader sense, incest includes sexual intercourse between a child and a stepparent or stepsibling. Although father–daughter incest is the most common form, incest can also involve father and son, mother and daughter, and mother and son.

Intrafamilial sexual abuse and other sexual abuse that occurs over a period of time is characterized by a particular pattern or sequence of steps. Victims of sexual abuse recount a gradual progression of boundary violations by the perpetrator, starting with tiny invasions and escalating to serious, overwhelming intrusions. Healthy, self-confident children rebuff the intrusions directly (via temper tantrums and verbal disagreements) or indirectly (through silence and distancing maneuvers) or by adopting any strategy that causes the offender to refrain.

Sexual abuse that occurs over a period of time evolves through five phases: engagement, sexual interaction, secrecy, disclosure, and suppression.

Engagement Phase. The perpetrator induces the child into a special relationship. The daughter in father–daughter incest has frequently had a close relationship with her father throughout her childhood and may be pleased at first when he approaches her sexually.

Sexual Interaction Phase. The sexual behaviors progress from less to more intrusive forms of abuse. As the behavior continues, the abused daughter becomes confused and frightened, because she never knows whether her father will be parental or sexual. If the victim tells her mother about the abuse, the mother may not be supportive. The mother often refuses to believe her daughter's reports or refuses to confront her husband with her suspicions. Because the father provides special attention to a particular daughter, her brothers and sisters may distance themselves from her.

Secrecy Phase. The perpetrator threatens the victim not to tell. The father, fearful that his daughter may expose their relationship and often jealously possessive of her, interferes with the girl's development of normal peer relationships.

Disclosure Phase. The abuse is discovered accidentally (when another person walks in the room and sees it), through the child's reporting it to a responsible adult, or when the child is brought for medical attention and an alert clinician asks the right questions.

Suppression Phase. The child often retracts the statements of the disclosure because of family pressure or because of the child's own mental processes. That is, the child may perceive that violent or intrusive attention is synonymous with interest or affection. Many incest survivors rally around their perpetrators, seeking to capture any modicum of tenderness or interest. At times, affection for the perpetrator outweighs the facts of abuse, and children recant their statements about sexual assault, regardless of substantiated evidence of molestation.

Financially comfortable parents lived in a pleasant, clean house in a nice neighborhood, but they had no friends. Their four teenagers never had visitors. One day, the oldest girl, 17 years of age, went to the police and told them that she had a baby at home and that her own father was the father of the baby. The girl said that her father had been having sexual relations with her for more than 4 years and that he was now doing the same with her younger sisters. The mother admitted knowing about the situation for years, but she had not reported it to the authorities for fear of losing her husband. (Courtesy of William Bernet, M.D.)

Extrafamilial Sexual Abuse

Of course, sexual abuse is not limited to incest. Children can be abducted and sexually abused by strangers. A perpetrator may observe a playground and may identify a child who is not closely supervised. A pedophile may molest this child and hundreds of other children before he or she is apprehended. For the child, this is usually a single, isolated experience.

On the other hand, children can be repeatedly abused by trusted adults, such as teachers, counselors, family friends, and clergy. In this scenario, the pedophilic perpetrator grooms the child over a period of time. He or she gains the friendship of children through enjoyable activities and gifts, introduces sexual activities that may seem innocent and even pleasurable, and progresses to more intrusive activities. The pedophile encourages secrecy.

A solo sex ring is a form of child sexual abuse that involves one adult perpetrator and multiple child victims, who may know about each other's sexual activities with the perpetrator. A sex ring may also involve multiple perpetrators and multiple victims.

Neurobiological Consequences of Child Maltreatment

Severe physical abuse and repeated sexual abuse cause changes in the child's developing brain that persist into adulthood. Adult survivors of abuse are more likely to have abnormalities of their electroencephalograms (EEGs) that indicate limbic irritability. They are more likely to have abnormalities on magnetic resonance imaging (MRI) of the brain that indicate reduced size of the adult hippocampus. These abnormalities are more pronounced on the left side of the brain. Deficient integration exists between the left and right hemispheres, manifested by reduced size of the corpus callosum. These neurobiological effects of child maltreatment probably mediate the behavioral and psychological symptoms that follow abuse, such as increased aggressiveness, heightened autonomic arousal, depression, and memory problems.

EVALUATION PROCESS

The evaluation of a child or adolescent who may have been physically or sexually abused depends on its circumstances and context. Practitioners must consider whether they are conducting a forensic evaluation, which has legal implications and may ultimately be used in court, or a clinical evaluation, which is done for a therapeutic purpose. A forensic evaluation emphasizes collecting accurate and complete data to determine—as objectively as possible—what happened to the child. Was the injury an accident, was it self-inflicted, or was it a result of parental abuse? Was the child actually sexually abused, or was he or she indoctrinated to believe that he or she was abused? The data collected in a forensic evaluation must be preserved in a reliable manner through audiotape, videotape, or detailed notes. The results of the forensic evaluation are organized into a report that is read by attorneys, a judge, and others. On the other hand, the emphasis in a therapeutic evaluation is to assess psychological strengths and weaknesses, to make a clinical diagnosis, to develop a treatment plan, and to lay the foundation for continuing psychotherapy. The clinician may also be interested in determining what happened to the child, but it is not so essential to distinguish facts from fantasies. Compared with the forensic evaluation, the psychotherapist does not need to keep such detailed records and ordinarily does not prepare a report for court.

In addition to distinguishing a forensic examination from a therapy meeting, a number of factors can affect the evaluation of a child who was abused or may have been abused: whether one is a pediatrician in an emergency department or a child psychiatrist in an office, whether a parent or another person is suspected of the abuse, the severity of the abuse and the victim's relationship to the perpetrator, whether physical signs of abuse are obvious or absent, the age and gender of the child, and the degree of anxiety, defensiveness, anger, or mental disorganization that the child exhibits. Often, the examiner must be creative and persistent.

From the psychiatric perspective, the interview is usually the primary source of information, and the physical examination is secondary. In practice, children who may have been neglected or sexually abused are interviewed first and are later given a physical examination and other tests. A child who has been physically abused is more likely to have a physical examination that may be followed by a psychiatric interview.

Parent Interviews

The evaluator obtains a history from the parents (separately, in most cases) and other pertinent informants, as well as from the child. The emphasis of the interview depends on the circumstances.

Suspected Physical Abuse. The examiner should consider the possibility that the parents are not telling the truth. The physician becomes a detective, because the parents who bring the injured child to the emergency department may also be perpetrators of the abuse. To obtain treatment, the caregivers lie about how the injury occurred.

When the child is brought to the emergency room, a detailed and spontaneous account of the injury should be obtained promptly from parents or other caregivers before secondary details and rationalizations cloud the information provided. The interviewer should allow the caregiver to explain, to expound, to derail, or to detour the story line. An abuser or codependent parent may claim to have happened on the injured child in a coma or bleeding from some unknown trauma or to have noticed significant bruising, burns, or a crooked extremity while bathing the child. Comparing the parents' histories can provide valuable insight into how power is wielded in the family unit.

> A 30-day-old girl was transferred from a rural hospital to a university medical center because of supposed near sudden infant death syndrome (SIDS). The child was unresponsive and required mechanical ventilation. A brain scan revealed bilateral subdural hematomas, subarachnoid hemorrhage, and hemorrhage in the parenchyma of the brain. An X-ray skeletal survey showed two posterior rib fractures. An ophthalmologist observed extensive retinal hemorrhages. After the child was admitted to the Pediatric Intensive Care Unit, the child abuse consultant interviewed the parents separately. The mother, 28 years of age, said that she had recently started a new job. The baby was perfectly fine when she left her in the care of her live-in boyfriend, the child's biological father. The father, 24 years of age, said that when he checked on the baby, he found her not breathing, blue, and unresponsive. He ran to report this to a neighbor and then called 911. The child abuse consultant told the father that the child must have been injured in some way and asked whether the father had any explanation for this injury. The father said, "I shook the baby after I found her not breathing." The consultant concluded that severe child abuse had occurred in the form of shaken baby syndrome. The consultant notified child protective services and the local police department, so that they could initiate and coordinate their investigation. (Courtesy of William Bernet, M.D.)

Suspected Sexual Abuse. The examiner should consider the possibility that the parents are not telling the truth. This situation is more complex, however, than suspected physical abuse. For example, the mother may wish to avoid the discovery of father–daughter incest by blaming the child's genital injury on another child or a stranger. In another scenario, the mother may concoct an allegation of incest when the child had never been abused at all. The first version protects a father who is guilty; the second version implicates a father who is innocent.

The examiner should determine how the allegation originally arose and what subsequent statements were made. Determine the emotional tone of the first disclosure (e.g., whether the disclosure arose in the context of a high level of suspicion of abuse). Determine the sequence of previous examinations, the techniques used, and what was reported. Try to determine whether the previous interviews likely distorted the child's recollections. If possible, review transcripts, audiotapes, and videotapes of earlier interviews. Seek a history of overstimulation, prior abuse, or other traumas. Consider other stressors that could account for the child's symptoms. The examiner should also ask about exposure to other possible male and female perpetrators.

In Either Case. Whether physical or sexual abuse is involved, a pertinent psychosocial history should be collected and organized, including the following:

1. Symptoms and behavioral changes that sometimes occur in abused children
2. Confounding variables, such as psychiatric disorder or cognitive impairment, that may need to be considered
3. Family's attitude toward discipline, sex, and modesty
4. Developmental history from birth through periods of possible trauma to the present
5. Family history, such as earlier abuse of the parents, substance abuse by the parents, spouse abuse, and psychiatric disorder in the parents
6. Underlying motivation and possible psychopathology of adults involved

Collateral Information

The evaluator should consider requesting collateral information from the following, after obtaining authorizations: protective services, school personnel, other caregivers (e.g., babysitters), other family members (e.g., siblings), the pediatrician, and police reports.

Child Interview

Several structured and semistructured interview protocols have been introduced that were designed to maximize the amount of accurate information and to minimize mistaken or false information provided by children. These approaches include the *Cognitive Interview*, which encourages witnesses to search their memories in various ways, such as recalling events forward and then backward. The *Step-Wise Interview* is a funnel approach that starts with open-ended questions and, if necessary, moves to more specific questions. The interview protocol developed at the National Institute of Child Health and Human Development (NICHD) includes a series of phases and makes use of detailed interview scripts.

Although these protocols may be particularly important in a forensic context, experienced clinicians endorse flexibility and consistent good-hearted behavior by the interviewer. As when seeing any patient, the evaluator must size up the situation and use techniques that are likely to help the youngster become comfortable and communicative. One victim might need a favorite object (e.g., a teddy bear or a toy truck); another might need to have a particular person included in the interview. Some children are comfortable talking; others prefer to draw pictures. An unrelated joke, a shared cookie, or a picture on the evaluator's wall may lead to a disclosure of abuse. Important comments might be made while chatting during the break time, instead of during the structured interviews.

CULTURAL CONSIDERATIONS IN CHILD MALTREATMENT

Parenting practices vary widely in American society and the cultural context of alleged abuse must be understood to facilitate helpful communication with families regarding discipline practices that contain characteristics of abuse. A recent study of the characteristics of child abuse among immigrant Korean families in Los Angeles who had active files with the Los Angeles County Department of Children and Family Services (LAC-DCFS) found that immigrant Korean families are more likely to be charged with phyiscal abuse (49.4 percent) and less likely to be charged with neglect (20.6 percent) compared with all other groups with active DCFS files in Los Angeles. That is, the circumstances under which physical abuse occurred most frequently was corporal punishment used by parents with an intention to discipline their children. The context of emotional abuse occurred most often among Korean families in which children witnessed domestic violence. A culturally sensitive approach is suggested to achieve effective child abuse prevention and interventions that will be accepted by Korean families.

GENOTYPE AND MALTREATMENT: RISKS FOR VIOLENT BEHAVIOR

Two recent studies of caucasian males have provided evidence that particular genotypes with high levels of monoamine oxidase A (MAOA) seem to protect against the malignant impact of childhood maltreatment on the development of conduct disorder and antisocial behavioral patterns. Subjects in a prospective cohort design involving court-substantiated cases of child abuse and neglect and matched comparison groups were followed into adulthood. A composite index of violent and antisocial behavior (VASB) was created based on arrest record, self-report and diagnostic information. Genotypes associated with high levels of MAOA activity were correlated with less risk of violent and antisocial behavior in later life for caucasians, but this effect was not found for non-caucasians. This result was not replicated in a group of adolescents with respect to the development of adolescent conduct disorder. Further studies are needed to understand the possible links between genotypes of high levels of MAOA and potential behavioral outcomes.

TREATMENT AND PREVENTION STRATEGIES

The immediate strategic intervention is to ensure the child's safety, which may require the child's removal from an abusive or neglectful home environment. Physicians are among a group of professionals who are mandated by law to report suspected child abuse or neglect to the local protective services agency.

Children who have been maltreated are at increased risk for further maltreatment according to studies of child victims of abuse and maltreatment. Studies have shown that four factors were most consistently identified as predictors of future maltreatment: number of previous episodes of maltreatment; neglect as the form of maltreatment; parental conflict; and parental psychiatric illness. Maltreated children were found to be about six times more likely to experience recurrent maltreatment, and the risk of recurrence was highest within 30 days of the index experience. This underscores the importance of a careful examination of the protective factors in the home environment. Investigation has recently shown that even less striking forms of maltreatment, such as verbal aggression by parents, contribute to the malignant effects of child maltreatment.

Once a literal safe place is established for a maltreated child, a multimodal treatment strategy may begin utilizing components of psychoeducation, anxiety management, exposure related to the feared experiences, and cognitive-behavioral interventions. Given the multiple long-term effects of maltreatment, children may require monitoring and support for long periods of time after the abuse has ended.

References

Bernet W. Child maltreatment. In Sadock BJ, Sadock VA, eds. *Kaplan & Sadock's Comprehensive Textbook of Psychiatry*. 8th ed. Vol. 2. Baltimore: Lippincott Williams & Wilkins; 2005:3406.

Bernet W, Corwin D. An evidence-based appropach for estimating present and future damages from child sexual abuse. *J Am Acad Psychiatry Law*. 2006;34:224.

Chang J, Rhee S, Weaver D. Characteristics of child abuse in immigrant Korean families and correlates of placement decisions. *Child Abuse Negl*. 2006;30:881.

Freisthler B, Merritt DH, LaScala EA. Understanding the ecology of child maltreatment: A review of the literature and directions for future research. *Child Maltreat*. 2006;11:263.

Heyman RE, Smith Slep AM. Creating and field-testing diagnostic criteria for partner and child maltreatment. *J Fam Psychol*. 2006;20:397.

Hinkdley N, Ramchandani PG, Jones DP. Risk factors for recurrence of maltreatment: A systematic review. *Arch Dis Child*. 2006;91:744.

Hussey JM, Chang JJ, Kotch JB. Child maltreatment in the United States: Prevalence, risk factors and adolescent health consequences. *Pediatrics*. 2006;118:933.

Teicher MH, Samson JA, Polcari A, McGreenery CE. Sticks, stones, and hurtful words: Relative effects of various forms of maltreatment. *Am J Psychiatry*. 2006;163:993.

Teicher MH, Tomoda A, Andersen SL. Neurobiological consequences of early stress and childhood maltreatment: are results from human and animal studies comparable? *Ann NY Acad Sci*. 2006;1071:313.

US Department of Health and Human Services, Administration on Children, Youth and Families. Child Maltreatment 2004. Washington, DC: US Government Printing Office; 2006.

Widom CS, Brzustowicz LM. MAOA and the "cycle of violence:" Childhood abuse and neglect, MAOA genotype, and risk for violent and antisocial behavior. *Biol Psychiatry*. 2006;60:684.

Young SE, Smolen A, Hewitt JK, Haberstick BC, Stallings MC, Corley RP, Crowley TJ. Interaction between MAO-A genotype and maltreatment in the risk for conduct disorder: Failure to confirm in adolescent patients. *Am J Psychiatry.* 2006;163:951.

▲ 55.4 Impact of Terrorism on Children

Over the last decade, children and adolescents in the United States have experienced large-scale domestic terrorist attacks, such as the September 11, 2001 attack on the World Trade Center in New York City, attacks against Americans in other parts of the world, and devastating violence toward peers in school shootings.

The United States has launched a series of initiatives in response to the threats and consequences of terrorism in the form of an act of Congress in 2002 called the Public Health Security and Bioterrorism Preparedness and Response Act. Despite these global US actions, children and adolescents continue to view frequent media exposure to terrorist events throughout the world that perpetuates a sense of danger.

The concept of terrorist acts is characterized by three distinct features: (1) They produce a societal atmosphere of extreme danger and fear, (2) they inflict significant personal harm and destruction, and (3) they undermine the implicit social contract between citizens and the perception that the state is able to protect them.

Child and adolescent reactions to exposure to terrorism is mediated by numerous factors, including personal appraisal of persisting danger, the likelihood of recurrent attack, and the perception of the relative safety of one's family and close friends. Children's responses to terrorist exposure is influenced by how their parents cope with the trauma and resulting turmoil and how well they understood the situation. Posttraumatic stress disorder (PTSD) has been studied in adolescents, with and without learning disabilities, who have been exposed to terror attacks. Findings from this study revealed that personal exposure to terror, past personal life-threatening events, and history of anxiety all contributed to the development of posttraumatic stress reactions. In addition, adolescents with learning disabilities who had difficulties in cognitively processing the traumatic events were at higher risk of developing PTSD when this was combined with the other high risk factors, such as being personally exposed to the traumatic events.

Table 55.4–1 identifies the relationship between objective features of danger and subjective features related to exposure to terrorist acts.

The following summarizes data collected after the terrorist attack of the World Trade Center on September 11, 2001.

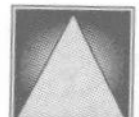

Table 55.4–1
Experience of Danger Consequent to Terrorist Acts

Objective Features	Subjective Features
Actualized threat Realistic threats False alarms Hoaxes	Disruption of protective shield Appraisals of threat Fears of recurrence Living with uncertainty Ongoing worries about significant others
Official risk communication, media coverage, and personal exchanges of information	Modulation of information exposure
Heightened security	Safety and protective behaviors
Mobilization of prevention and response capabilities	Anxious and restrictive behaviors Aggressive and reckless behaviors
Attribution of responsibility	Categorization over discrimination of threat—risk of intolerance
Evacuation and rescue efforts	Themes of heroism and patriotism
Military mobilization	Political ideology
War	—
Additional dangers, terrorist acts, and personal tragedies	Changes in spiritual schema Parental demoralization

(Courtesy of Robert S. Pynoos, M.D. M.P.H., Merritt D. Schreiber, Ph.D., Alan M. Steinberg Ph.D., and Betty Pfefferbaum, M.D., J.D.)

September 11, 2001 Attacks

The US Department of Education, through Project SERV, supported the New York City Board of Education in conducting a needs assessment of New York City schoolchildren. Christine W. Hoven and colleagues surveyed more than 8,000 randomly selected students 6 months after the September 11, 2001 attacks. Striking differences were seen in direct exposure among students in the vicinity of Ground Zero as compared with students in the rest of the city, in exposure to smoke and dust, fleeing for safety, problems getting home, and smelling smoke in the days and weeks after September 11. Approximately 70 percent of all children, however, were exposed to one of these factors. Interpersonal exposure through direct victimization of a family member was greater among children attending schools outside the Ground Zero vicinity as compared with those attending school in this area. Media exposure was extensive and prolonged. Signs of heightened security were visible throughout the city.

The study used several of the *Diagnostic Interview Schedule for Children* (DISC) predictive scales. In contrast to most disaster studies among children, which have used continuous scale instruments, the abbreviated PTSD self-report diagnostic instrument used a yes/no response format that overly emphasizes category C (avoidance) as the diagnostic discriminatory symptom. As a result, no age-, sex-, or exposure-related full symptom profiles were obtainable to more fully inform understanding of the nature, severity, and course of children's reactions to terrorism and public mental health response planning. In addition, higher estimated rates of PTSD (up to 20 percent among 4th- and 5th-graders) were found among school-age children, who are well documented to be the age group at most risk for avoidant behavior, than for high school students (6 percent), who, in pilot screenings in lower Manhattan, had low rates of avoidance and higher rates of irritability. No exposure-related differences were found in the rates of PTSD among high school students. Extremely high rates (52 percent) were found, however, among children who lost a parent or sibling, although no reported analysis was done of the contribution of symptoms of traumatic bereavement to this finding. Three sets of findings stand out from this study. First, similar to the findings by Armen K. Goenjian and colleagues after the catastrophic 1988 Spitak earthquake in Armenia, a significant degree of persistent separation anxiety was seen, especially among school-age children, but also among adolescents. Second, reflecting an age-related vulnerability to incident-specific new fears (e.g., subways and buses) and avoidant behavior of school-age children, a nearly 25 percent rate of agoraphobia was reported among 4th- and 5th-graders. Care must be taken, however, not to misrepresent *incident-specific new fears* as agoraphobia, because the course of recovery and intervention strategies may differ. Third, an enormous reservoir of prior traumatic experiences (more than one half of the total sample) was associated with severity of current PTSD symptoms, emphasizing the need to attend to prior trauma in conducting needs assessments, surveillance, and intervention strategies. Other risk factors, in addition to younger age, included female gender and Hispanic ethnicity. The finding of age-related increases in rates of conduct disorder also needs to be interpreted in light of adolescent response to an ecology of danger in which overly aggressive, reckless, and risk-taking behaviors are well documented and associated with posttraumatic stress reactions. A major strength of this study was the inclusion of self-reported impairment as well as symptoms, setting an important standard for future studies.

J. Stuber and colleagues conducted a telephone survey of a random sample of adult residents of Manhattan 1 to 2 months after the September 11th attacks. The sample included more than 100 parents who were asked to describe the experiences and reactions of their children. Not surprisingly, given the time of the incident, most children were at school or day care when the disaster occurred. Many of the parents recalled concern about their children's safety at the time, and most were not reunited with their children for more than 4 hours. More than 20 percent of the parents studied reported that their children had received counseling related to the disaster. Receiving counseling was associated with male gender, parental posttraumatic stress, and having at least one sibling living in the household.

Also using parent report in a New York City telephone survey, Gerry Fairbrother and colleagues assessed predictors of posttraumatic stress reactions in children between the ages of 4 and 17 years, 4 to 5 months after the attacks. Almost 20 percent of children were reported by their parents to have experienced severe or very severe posttraumatic stress reactions, and approximately two thirds had moderate posttraumatic stress reactions. Parental reactions and viewing three or more graphic images of the disaster on television were associated with severe or very severe posttraumatic stress reactions in children.

More recently, Fairbrother and colleagues reported that 27 percent of children with severe or very severe posttraumatic stress reactions received some mental health care 4 to 5 months after September 11th.

Exploring behavior problems in New York City children, Stuber and colleagues compared data from three cross-sectional telephone surveys of representative samples of adults. Two surveys were conducted after the September 11th attacks, the first between 4 and 5 months and the second between 6 and 9 months after the attacks. Behavior problems were related to the child's race or ethnicity, family income, living in a single-parent household, disaster event experiences, and parental reactions to the attacks. The results of these surveys were examined in light of findings from a representative survey conducted before September 11th. The rate of behavior problems was lower in the first post-September 11th survey (4 to 6 months after the attacks) than rates in the pre-September 11th survey, but problems returned to pre-September 11th levels by the second post-September 11th study (6 to 9 months after the attacks). Consistent with findings in studies of Hurricane Andrew, these results suggest that behavior problems may actually decrease in the months after a disaster or that parents may be insensitive to them, but that they return to predisaster levels over time.

Media coverage of the September 11th attacks brought renewed debate about its impact, especially on children, even children with no direct exposure. Mark A. Schuster and colleagues reported extensive exposure to television coverage in children throughout the nation by using a representative survey of adults conducted in the first days after the attacks. Approximately one third of the parents surveyed attempted to limit or to prevent their children's viewing, but, among those whose parents made no attempt to restrict viewing, the number of hours of disaster coverage watched was related to the number of reported stress symptoms.

Using a Web-based, nationally representative sample of adults, William E. Schlenger and colleagues examined distress in children 1 to 2 months after the attacks by asking parents if their children were upset by the events. Considering the children perceived as most upset, 20 percent had trouble sleeping, 30 percent were irritable or easily upset, and 27 percent feared separation from their parents. The mean age of children perceived as most upset was 11 years, with no statistically significant gender differences. The proportion of parents reporting at least one child upset did not differ by community in analysis of data from the New York City metropolitan area, Washington, DC, other major metropolitan areas, and the rest of the country.

A strength of these surveys was their examination of representative samples, but earlier work points to concern about assessing children by interviewing their parents. Furthermore, as with the Oklahoma City studies, the samples were composed mainly of indirectly exposed children, and the clinical significance of the findings is unclear.

Seven-year-old J survived the traumatic loss of two grandparents on the first plane into the World Trade Center. He was first seen in treatment 2 weeks after September 11, 2001. J's grandparents were on board American Airlines Flight No. 11 enroute to take care of J and his younger siblings. J and his siblings were preparing to leave for school when the family learned the news, and J observed the profound distress of his parents as they confirmed the presence of his grandparents aboard the aircraft. He observed the famous video segments of the second plane crashing into the second tower several times that morning before television access was limited. J was the first grandchild in his extended family, and he lived with his grandparents for the first 3 years of his life; thereafter, his grandparents spent approximately one half of the year with him and his family on the West Coast. They had enjoyed an exceptionally close relationship since his birth, and he participated in many activities (such as karate) solely with them until September 11th.

Almost immediately after the terrorist attacks, his parents became worried that J was taking the loss of his grandparents extremely hard, and they became increasingly concerned that he was preoccupied with the grisly nature of their deaths. He was becoming increasingly agitated as he talked about the gruesome aspects of their deaths. In treatment, he began to ask a continual series of questions about the nature of their deaths, including aspects of burning, fragmentation, pain, blood, and the exact moment of their deaths in comparison with what he had initially observed on television. This became the theme for the early phase of his care, which dealt with the questions about the nature of their deaths (i.e., whether they were intact or "blown up in a thousand pieces" and the sequence of fire, burning, pain, and death). J developed nightmares within days in which he awakened and called for his parents on the average of three times a night. J felt that he could not discuss the content of his dreams with his parents, given his observations of their own distress. He began to express fears that the "hijackers" would hurt his parents and other family members. He became focused on the concept that "half our freedom is gone," and he was concerned that one half of New York City was destroyed. His play centered on repetitively creating the World Trade Center with blocks and then crashing them down. Although he was able to resume sleeping through the night, he reported new troubling dreams with themes of ghosts "popping out" and "everyone is killed, and then I'm killed." This worsened after the onset of the war in Afghanistan, and he sought to reassure himself by repeatedly saying the "war is not here" (California) and by hoping that American forces would kill many.

He developed an intervention fantasy in which the therapist would have a time machine like "Jimmy Neutrino" and that he and the therapist could be transported back in time on board his grandparents' flight before it crashed. While his father (a former military pilot) flew the plane, he and the therapist overpowered the "hijackers" and threw them off the plane, and then his father landed the plane safely in Boston or at his home. After landing, his grandparents and their fellow passengers tell him "thank you," and they continue with their planned visit to see him. After expressing his wish verbally, he initiated play and used the same blocks to create the World Trade Center and then repeatedly had his "grandparents' plane" narrowly avoid the twin towers, as he and the therapist took control of the hijackers while his father deftly landed the plane safely. This appeared to be soothing and satisfying, and he began to recall many positive activities with his grandparents and a series of happy, highly detailed memories of himself and his grandparents, with profound sadness at the realization that these would be no more. While playing Candyland, he landed on a square that reminded him of his grandmother baking for him and the affectionate nicknames that they called him and that he called them, and he said "a piece of my heart is gone" and "I want them back."

He later expressed that they were more than grandparents, and he recalled living with them for a time in their home as both of his parents worked. At several phases, he alternately expressed rage and anger and confusion about the actions of "Osama Bin Laden." He acted out danger, aggression, and defense, repetitively using chess pieces to build a wall of protection between the opposing colors. This led to anxiety about his "plotting again" and concern for the safety of his parents. Around the Jewish holiday of Passover, J expressed to his family and friends that Passover was a celebration of "dead people" and "this night we have a cake, everyone eats a cake that represents people who died, it's sort of like a birthday party with special foods . . . they take a picture with a candle, and they can scan the image of the person lost." (Courtesy of Robert S. Pynoos, M.D. M.P.H., Merritt D. Schreiber, Ph.D., Alan M . Steinberg Ph.D., Betty Pfefferbaum, M.D., J.D.)

Recently, Avraham Bleichman and colleagues, using a telephone survey of 512 Israeli citizens, found that 60 percent of the population reported that they believed that their lives were in danger. Approximately 38 percent of the sample of adults reported at least one symptom of traumatic stress, and more than one half reported feeling depressed, with 28 percent reporting being very depressed.

To respond to the mental health needs of children and adolecents who have been exposed to terrorism either through personal experience or through exposure to media depicting world-wide terrorism, the adverse psychological reactions listed in Table 55.4–2 must be considered.

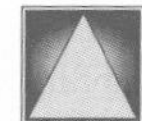

Table 55.4–2
Psychological Disorders Associated with Terrorism

Acute stress disorder
PTSD
Depression
Anxiety
Separation anxiety disorder
Agoraphobia
Phobic disorders
Bereavement
Somatization
Irritability
Dissociative reactions
Sleep disturbances
Diminished self-esteem
Deterioration in school performance
Distress when exposed to traumatic reminders
Substance abuse

COMPONENTS OF MECHANISMS FOR RECOVERY FROM EXPOSURE TO TERRORISM

Perception of Safety

The notion of perceived safety is an important protective factor as well as a component of recovery for a child, adolescent, or adult who has been exposed to terrorism. A recent report of symptoms of PTSD, depression, and perceived safety in disaster workers 2 weeks after the September 11th terrorist attacks found that lower perceived safety was associated with increased symptoms of hyperarousal and intrusive fearful thoughts, but not avoidance. An expected diminished sense of safety was found in those individuals who had personally been in greater physical danger, or who had worked with dead bodies compared with others who were physically less exposed. To regain a sense of security, reestablishment of a perception of safety is a necessary first step.

Reestablishment or Maintenance of Daily Routines

Although it is clearly not always possible to maintain usual daily routines amidst war or exposure to terrorism, a study of Israeli adolescents found that those whose families were able to maintain their usual activities, such as attending school and family functions, were at lower risk for the development of posttraumatic reactions. On the other hand, adolescents' perceptions of family maintaining routine activities was a predictor of higher levels of avoidance and of posttraumatic reactions.

Proactive Interventions to Enhance Resilience

Perceived personal resilience has been shown in studies to be protective against symptoms of posttraumatic stress development. Proactive interventions aimed at enhancing a sense of personal resilience and an ability to cope with the stressful situation may serve to decrease the risk of psychiatric symptoms after exposure to terrorism. Interventions may include regaining a sense of perceived safety through reestablishing routines, altruistic tasks, family preparedness planning, and parental expression of security.

References

Committee on Environmental Health; Committee on Infectious Diseases; Michale WS, Julia AM. Chemical-biological terrorism and its impact on children. *Pediatrics.* 2006;118:1267.

Demaria T, Barrett M, Kerasiotis B, Rohlih J, Chemtob C. Bio-psycho-social assessment of 9/11-bereaved chidlren. *Ann NY Acad Sci.* 1006;1071:481.

Duarte CS, Hoven CW, Wu P, Bin F, Cotel S, Mandell DJ, Nagasawa M, Balaban V, Wernikoff L, Markenson D. Posttraumatic stress in children with first responders in their families. *J Trauma Stress.* 2006;19:301.

Finzi-Dottan R, Dekel R, Lavi T, Su'ali T. Posttraumatic stress disorder reactions among children with learning disabilities exposed to terror attacks. *Compr Psychiatry.* 2006;47:144.

Fremont WP, Pataki C, Beresin EV. The impact of terrorism on children and adolescents: Terror in the skies, terror on television. *Child Adolesc Psychiatr Clin N Am.* 2005:14:429.

Fullerton CS, Ursano RJ, Reeves J, Shigemura J, Grieger T. Perceived safety in disaster workers following 9/11. *J Nerv Mental Dis.* 2006;194:61.

Laor N, Wolmer L, Alon M, Siev J, Samuel E, Toren P. Risk and protective factors mediating psychological symptoms and ideological commitment of adolescents facing continuous terrorism. *J Nerv Ment Dis.* 2006;194:279.

Martin SD, Bush AC, Lynch JA. A national survey of terrorism preparedness training among pediatric, family practice, and emergency medicine program. *Pediatrics.* 2006;118:e620.

Pat-Horenczyk R, Schiff M, Coppelt O. Maintaining routine despite ongoing exposure to terrorism: A healthy strategy for adolescents? *J Adolesc Health.* 2006; 39:199.

Pfefferbaum B, Stuber J, Galea S., Fairbrother G. Panic reacitons to terrorist attacks and probable posttraumatic stress disorder in adolescents. *J Trauma Stress.* 2006;19:217.

Pynoos RS, Schrieber MD, Steinberg AM, Pfefferbaum BJ. Impact of terrorism on children. In: Sadock BJ, Sadock VA, eds. *Kaplan & Sadock's Comprehensive Textbook of Psychiatry.* 8th ed. Vol. 2. Baltimore: Lippincott Williams & Wilkins; 2005:3551.

Schiff M, Benbenishty R, McKay M, Devoe E, Liu X, Hasin D. Exposure to terrorism and Israeli youths' psychological distress and alcohol use: An exploratory study. *Am J Addict.* 2006;15:220.

Stephens RD, Feinberg T. Managing America's schools in an age of terrorism, war and civil unrest. *Int J Emerg Ment Health.* 2006;8:111.

Willilams R. The psychosocial consequences for chidren and young people who are exposed to terrorism, war, conflict and natural disasters. *Curr Opin Psychiatry.* 2006;19:337.

Wilson AL. Going down the drain: When children's fears become real—Responding to chidren when disaster strikes. *S D Med.* 2006;59:58.

56 Geriatric Psychiatry

Old age is not a disease. It is a phase of the life cycle characterized by its own developmental issues, many of which are concerned with loss of physical agility, and mental acuity, friends and loved ones, and status and power. At the same time, old age is associated with the accumulation of wisdom and the opportunity to pass that on to future generations, one of the tasks that informs Erik Erikson's view of healthy old age as a time of integrity and not a time of despair. In contrast to this group of the well-old, there are the sick-old, persons with mental or physical disorders, or both, that impair their ability to function or even survive. This group is the concern of geriatric psychiatry, which deals with preventing, diagnosing, and treating psychological disorders in older adults. The American Board of Psychiatry and Neurology established geropsychiatry (from the Greek *geros* ["old age"] and *iatros* ["physical"]) as a subspecialty in 1991, and today geriatric psychiatry is one of the fastest growing fields in psychiatry.

SCOPE OF THE PROBLEM

Advances in medical technology have contributed to what has been described as an age revolution, essentially, a rapid growth in the proportion of the population in the upper age groups. This older segment of the US population will continue to grow (Table 56–1). Although their expansion slowed slightly during the 1990s, because relatively fewer babies were born during the Great Depression of the 1930s, the generation of so-called *baby boomers* is now rapidly approaching middle age and beyond, leading to an ever increasing number of people 65 years of age and older. In the year 2005, 35 million people were in this age group, and this figure will double to approximately 70 million by 2030 and will reach 82 million by 2050. By that time, the projected proportion of older adults will be 35.7 percent, compared with 17 percent in 2005.

The most rapidly growing segment of the population is the age group 85 years and older, the group with the highest morbidity and the highest rate of psychiatric and medical comorbidities. This age group grew 40-fold, from 100,000 in 1900 to more than 4 million in 2005, and is projected to reach 19.4 million by 2050 (Table 56-1).

Prevalence data for mental disorders in elderly persons vary widely, but a conservatively estimated 25 percent have significant psychiatric symptoms. The number of mentally ill elderly persons was estimated to be about 9 million in the year 2005. That figure is expected to rise to 20 million by the middle of the century.

STRESSORS

High-ranking stresses of aging include acute and chronic medical illnesses (Table 56–2), the concomitant use of therapeutic drugs, and the complicating drug–drug and drug–disease interactions. Thus, geriatric psychiatrists must be able to recognize the physical and mental ills of their patients, as well as have skills in the social sciences, knowledge of the health care delivery system, and information about the availability of financial and social supports, especially nursing homes. Moreover, self-assessment of health is associated with income. The loss of one's job, including voluntary and involuntary retirement, carries with it the loss of financial resources, social status, and much of the person's social network; the loss of contemporaries through death, illness, and migration brings both psychological deprivation of an intimate love object and a void that usually remains unfilled; forming new relationships that result in marriage is difficult in old age. In part, because of their greater life expectancy, older women are more likely to live alone than older men. Physical limitations and the loss of friends are frequently associated with restricted mobility, which leads to further social isolation and increased difficulty in pursuing the tasks of daily living, such as procuring food and clothing and maintaining one's shelter. Often, homes are lost because of financial strains and the inability to perform home upkeep. Many middle class widows, for example, have had to move from the five- to ten-room family homes, which they occupied for most of their lives, to one-half of a room in a residential extended-care facility for the elderly. In addition to losing most of their worldly possessions and social support, they also lose their privacy and their sense of self-worth.

A technological development that may militate against such isolation is greater access to computers and the Internet, which provide older persons an opportunity to remain socially connected to family and friends. Older adults trail all other age groups with respect to computer ownership (25.8 percent) and Internet access (14.6 percent). By contrast, households in the middle-age groups (35 to 55 years of age) lead all other age groups in personal computer penetration (nearly 55 percent) and Internet access (more than 34 percent). Although data show lower levels of access for older persons than for the general population, it is encouraging that many older adults are beginning to maintain social connections through the Internet.

Poverty in the Aged

A strong correlation exists between poverty and increased rates of mental and physical illness in the elderly. For workers 65 years and older, the median earned income in 2005 was $15,000. Although the overall rate of poverty is relatively low, it remains

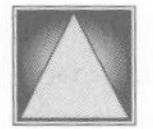

Table 56–1
Aging Population of the United States: 1900–2050

			Population, in Millions and As a Percentage of Total Population				
			All Ages	65 yrs and Older		85 yrs and Older	
Year	Median Age	Mean Age	(N)	(N)	(%)	(N)	(%)
1900	—	—	76.0	3.1	4.1	0.1	0.1
1950	—	—	150.1	12.3	8.2	0.6	0.4
1990	—	—	248.7	31.1	12.5	3.0	1.2
2000	35.8	36.5	275.3	34.8	12.6	4.3	1.6
2010	37.4	37.9	299.9	39.7	13.2	5.8	1.9
2030	38.9	40.2	351.1	70.3	20.0	8.9	2.5
2050	38.8	40.7	403.7	82.0	20.3	19.4	4.8

(Adapted from Population: U.S. Bureau of the Census: Current Population Reports, Special Studies, P23–190, 65+ in the United States. Washington, DC: U.S. Government Printing Office; 1996; and Projections of the Total Resident Population by 5-Year Age Groups and Sex with Special Age Categories: Middle Series, 1999 to 2100 (NP-T3). U.S. Census Bureau, Population Division, Population Projections Branch; August 2, 2002; with permission.)

high for women, minorities, the less-educated, and those older than 80. Of Americans 65 or older, 28 percent had incomes of less than $10,000 in 2005, whereas 10 percent had incomes of $50,000 or more. Earnings from work continue to be an important source of income for older Americans, especially those under age 70. Although a trend was seen toward earlier retirement from about 1960 to 1985, over the past 20 years more Americans have continued to work at older ages. In 2005, median earnings for individuals age 55 to 61 who worked were $34,000, whereas median earned income for workers age 62 to 64 was $27,000.

PSYCHIATRIC EXAMINATION OF THE OLDER PATIENT

Psychiatric history-taking and the mental status examination of older adults follow the same format as those of younger adults; however, because of the high prevalence of cognitive disorders in older persons, psychiatrists must determine whether a patient understands the nature and purpose of the examination. When a patient is cognitively impaired, an independent history should be obtained from a family member or caretaker. The patient still should be seen alone—even in cases of clear evidence of impairment—to preserve the privacy of the doctor–patient relationship and to elicit any suicidal thoughts or paranoid ideation, which may not be voiced in the presence of a relative or nurse.

When approaching the examination of the older patient, it is important to remember that older adults differ markedly from one another. The approach to examining the older patient must take into account whether the person is a healthy 75-year-old who recently retired from a second career or a frail 96-year-old who just lost the only surviving relative with the death of the 75-year-old caregiving daughter.

Psychiatric History

A complete psychiatric history includes preliminary identification (name, age, sex, marital status), chief complaint, history of the present illness, history of previous illnesses, personal history, and family history. A review of medications (including over-the-counter medications) that the patient is currently using or has used in the recent past is also important.

Patients older than age 65 often have subjective complaints of minor memory impairments, such as forgetting persons' names and misplacing objects. Minor cognitive problems also can occur because of anxiety in the interview situation. These age-associated memory impairments are of no

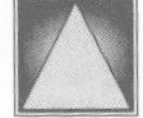

Table 56–2
Top Ten Chronic Conditions for Persons 65 Years of Age and Older, by Age and Race: 1996 (Number per 1,000 Persons)

	Age (yrs)				Race (65 yrs of Age and Older)	
Condition	45–64	65+	65–74	75+	White	Black
Arthritis	240.1	482.7	453.1	523.6	477.6	538.4
Hypertension	214.1	363.5	356.0	373.8	348.1	487.0
Hearing impairment	131.5	303.4	255.2	369.8	320.3	155.4
Heart disease	116.4	268.7	238.2	310.7	278.2	150.5
Cataracts	23.3	171.5	151.9	198.6	174.8	157.7
Deformity or orthopedic impairment	177.8	157.6	175.1	133.5	161.9	134.4
Chronic sinusitis	174.1	117.1	127.0	103.5	118.3	121.7
Diabetes	58.2	100.0	98.4	102.3	87.5	199.1
Tinnitus[a]	59.6	87.7	95.0	76.2	90.7	55.1
Visual impairment	48.3	84.2	69.6	104.3	86.1	81.9

[a]The 1989 survey order was the same except for tinnitus, which replaced visual impairment as number nine, and varicose veins was dropped from the list.
(From National Center for Health Statistics: Current Estimates. National Health Interview Survey, 1996. (PHS) 99–1528. Government Printing Office stock number 017-01471-8, with permission.)

significance; the term *benign senescent forgetfulness* has been used to describe them.

A patient's childhood and adolescent history can provide information about personality organization and give important clues about coping strategies and defense mechanisms used under stress. A history of learning disability or minimal cerebral dysfunction is significant. The psychiatrist should inquire about friends, sports, hobbies, social activity, and work. The occupational history should include the patient's feelings about work, relationships with peers, problems with authority, and attitudes toward retirement. The patient also should be questioned about plans for the future. What are the patient's hopes and fears?

The family history should include a patient's description of parents' attitudes and adaptation to their old age and, if applicable, information about the causes of their deaths. Alzheimer's disease is transmitted as an autosomal-dominant trait in 10 to 30 percent of the offspring of parents with Alzheimer's disease; depression and alcohol dependence also run in families. The patient's current social situation should be evaluated. Who cares for the patient? Does the patient have children? What are the characteristics of the patient's parent–child relationships? A financial history helps the psychiatrist evaluate the role of economic hardship in the patient's illness and to make realistic treatment recommendations.

The marital history includes a description of the spouse and the characteristics of the relationship. If the patient is a widow or a widower, the psychiatrist should explore how grieving was handled. If the loss of the spouse occurred within the past year, the patient is at high risk for an adverse physical or psychological event.

The patient's sexual history includes sexual activity, orientation, libido, masturbation, extramarital affairs, and sexual symptoms (e.g., impotence and anorgasmia). Young clinicians may have to overcome their own biases about taking a sexual history: Sexuality is an area of concern for many geriatric patients, who welcome the chance to talk about their sexual feelings and attitudes.

Mental Status Examination

The mental status examination offers a cross-sectional view of how a patient thinks, feels, and behaves during the examination. With older adults, a psychiatrist may not be able to rely on a single examination to answer all of the diagnostic questions. Repeat mental status examinations may be needed because of fluctuating changes in the patient's family.

General Description. A general description of the patient includes appearance, psychomotor activity, attitude toward the examiner, and speech activity.

Motor disturbances (e.g., shuffling gait, stooped posture, "pill rolling" movements of the fingers, tremors, and body asymmetry) should be noted. Involuntary movements of the mouth or tongue may be adverse effects of phenothiazine medication. Many depressed patients seem to be slow in speech and movement. A mask-like facies occurs in Parkinson's disease.

The patient's speech may be pressured in agitated, manic, and anxious states. Tearfulness and overt crying occur in depressive and cognitive disorders, especially if the patient feels frustrated about being unable to answer one of the examiner's questions. The presence of a hearing aid or another indication that the patient has a hearing problem (e.g., requesting repetition of questions) should be noted.

The patient's attitude toward the examiner—cooperative, suspicious, guarded, ingratiating—can give clues about possible transference reactions. Because of transference, older adults can react to younger physicians as if the physicians were parent figures, despite the age difference.

Functional Assessment. Patients older than 65 years of age should be evaluated for their capacity to maintain independence and to perform the activities of daily life, which include toileting, preparing meals, dressing, grooming, and eating. The degree of functional competence in their everyday behaviors is an important consideration in formulating a treatment plan for these patients.

Mood, Feelings, and Affect. Suicide is a leading cause of death of older persons, and an evaluation of a patient's suicidal ideation is essential. Loneliness is the most common reason cited by older adults who consider suicide. Feelings of loneliness, worthlessness, helplessness, and hopelessness are symptoms of depression, which carries a high risk for suicide. Nearly 75 percent of all suicide victims suffer from depression, alcohol abuse, or both. The examiner should specifically ask the patient about any thoughts of suicide: Does the patient feel life is no longer worth living? Does the patient think he or she would be better off dead or, when dead, would no longer be a burden to others? Such thoughts—especially when associated with alcohol abuse, living alone, recent death of a spouse, physical illness, and somatic pain—indicate a high suicidal risk.

Disturbances in mood states, most notably depression and anxiety, can interfere with memory functioning. An expansive or euphoric mood may indicate a manic episode or may signal a dementing disorder. Frontal lobe dysfunction often produces witzelsucht, which is the tendency to make puns and jokes and then laugh aloud at them.

The patient's affect may be flat, blunted, constricted, shallow, or inappropriate, all of which can indicate a depressive disorder, schizophrenia, or brain dysfunction. Such affects are important abnormal findings, although they are not pathognomonic of a specific disorder. Dominant lobe dysfunction causes dysprosody, an inability to express emotional feelings through speech intonation.

Perceptual Disturbances. Hallucinations and illusions by older adults can be transitory phenomena resulting from decreased sensory acuity. The examiner should note whether the patient is confused about time or place during the hallucinatory episode; confusion points to an organic condition. It is particularly important to ask the patient about distorted body perceptions. Because hallucinations can be caused by brain tumors and other focal pathology, a diagnostic workup may be indicated. Brain diseases cause perceptive impairments; agnosia, the inability to recognize and interpret the significance of sensory impressions, is associated with organic brain diseases. The examiner should note the type of agnosia—the denial of illness (anosognosia), the denial of a body part (atopognosia), or the inability to recognize objects (visual agnosia) or faces (prosopagnosia).

Language Output. The language output category of the geriatric mental status examination covers the aphasias, which are disorders of language output related to organic lesions of the brain. The best described are nonfluent or Broca's aphasia, fluent or Wernicke's aphasia, and global aphasia, a combination of fluent and nonfluent aphasias. In nonfluent or Broca's aphasia, the patient's understanding remains intact, but the ability to speak is impaired. The patient cannot pronounce "Methodist Episcopalian." Words are generally mispronounced and speech may be telegraphic. A simple test for Wernicke's aphasia is to point to some common objects—such as a pen or a pencil, a doorknob, and a light switch—and ask the patient to name them. The patient also may be unable to demonstrate the use of simple objects, such as a key and a match (ideomotor apraxia).

Visuospatial Functioning. Some decline in visuospatial capability is normal with aging. Asking a patient to copy figures or a drawing may be helpful in assessing the function. A neuropsychological assessment should be performed when visuospatial functioning is obviously impaired.

Thought. Disturbances in thinking include neologisms, word salad, circumstantiality, tangentiality, loosening of associations, flight of ideas, clang associations, and blocking. The loss of the ability to appreciate nuances of meaning (abstract thinking) may be an early sign of dementia. Thinking is then described as concrete or literal.

Thought content should be examined for phobias, obsessions, somatic preoccupations, and compulsions. Ideas about suicide or homicide should be discussed. The examiner should determine whether delusions are present and how such delusions affect the patient's life. Delusions may be present in nursing home patients and may have been a reason for admission. Ideas of reference or of influence should be described. Patients who are hard of hearing can be classified mistakenly as paranoid or suspicious.

Sensorium and Cognition. *Sensorium* concerns the functioning of the special senses; *cognition* concerns information processing and intellect. The survey of both areas, known as the neuropsychiatric examination, consists of the clinician's assessment and a comprehensive battery of psychological tests.

CONSCIOUSNESS. A sensitive indicator of brain dysfunction is an altered state of consciousness in which the patient does not seem to be alert, shows fluctuations in levels of awareness, or seems to be lethargic. In severe cases, the patient is somnolescent or stuporous.

ORIENTATION. Impairment in orientation to time, place, and person is associated with cognitive disorders. Cognitive impairment often is observed in mood disorders, anxiety disorders, factitious disorders, conversion disorder, and personality disorders, especially during periods of severe physical or environmental stress. The examiner should test for orientation to place by asking the patient to describe his or her present location. Orientation to person may be approached in two ways: Does the patient know his or her own name, and are nurses and doctors identified as such? Time is tested by asking the patient the date, the year, the month, and the day of the week. The patient also should be asked about the length of time spent in a hospital, during what season of the year, and how the patient knows these facts. Greater significance is given to difficulties concerning person than to difficulties of time and place, and more significance is given to orientation to place than to orientation to time.

MEMORY. Memory usually is evaluated in terms of immediate, recent, and remote memory. Immediate retention and recall are tested by giving the patient six digits to repeat forward and backward. The examiner should record the result of the patient's capacity to remember. Persons with unimpaired memory usually can recall six digits forward and five or six digits backward. The clinician should be aware that the ability to do well on digit-span tests is impaired in extremely anxious patients. Remote memory can be tested by asking for the patient's place and date of birth, the patient's mother's name before she was married, and names and birthdays of the patient's children.

In cognitive disorders, recent memory deteriorates first. Recent memory assessment can be approached in several ways. Some examiners give the patient the names of three items early in the interview and ask for recall later. Others prefer to tell a brief story and ask the patient to repeat it verbatim. Memory of the recent past also can be tested by asking for the patient's place of residence, including the street number; the method of transportation to the hospital; and some current events. If the patient has a memory deficit, such as amnesia, careful testing should be performed to determine whether it is retrograde amnesia (loss of memory before an event) or anterograde amnesia (loss of memory after the event). Retention and recall also can be tested by having the patient retell a simple story. Patients who confabulate make up new material in retelling the story.

INTELLECTUAL TASKS, INFORMATION, AND INTELLIGENCE. Various intellectual tasks can be presented to estimate the patient's fund of general knowledge and intellectual functioning. Counting and calculation can be tested by asking the patient to subtract 7 from 100 and to continue subtracting 7 from the result until the number 2 is reached. The examiner records the responses as a baseline for future testing. The examiner can also ask the patient to count backward from 20 to 1, and can record the time necessary to complete the exercise. The patient also can be asked to do simple arithmetic—for example, to state the number of nickels in $1.35.

The patient's fund of general knowledge is related to intelligence. The patient can be asked to name the president of the United States, to name the three largest cities in the United States, to give the population of the United States, and to give the distance from New York to Paris. The examiner must take into account the patient's educational level, socioeconomic status, and general life experience in assessing the results of some of these tests.

READING AND WRITING. It may be important for the clinician to examine the patient's reading and writing and to determine whether the patient has a specific speech deficit. The examiner may have the patient read a simple story aloud or write a short sentence to test for a reading or writing disorder. Whether the patient is right-handed or left-handed should be noted.

Judgment. Judgment is the capacity to act appropriately in various situations. Does the patient show impaired judgment? What would the patient do on finding a stamped, sealed, addressed envelope in the street? What would the patient do if he or she smelled smoke in a theater? Can the patient discriminate? What is the difference between a dwarf and a boy? Why are couples required to get a marriage license?

Neuropsychological Evaluation

A thorough neuropsychological examination includes a comprehensive battery of tests that can be replicated by various examiners and can be repeated over time to assess the course of a specific illness. The most widely used test of current cognitive functioning is the *Mini-Mental State Examination* (MMSE), which assesses orientation, attention, calculation, immediate and short-term recall, language, and the ability to follow simple commands (*see* Table 5.2–3). The MMSE is used to detect impairments, follow the course of an illness, and monitor the patient's treatment responses. It is not used to make a formal diagnosis. The maximal MMSE score is 30. Age and educational level influence cognitive performance as measured by the MMSE.

The assessment of intellectual abilities is performed with the *Wechsler Adult Intelligence Scale-Revised* (WAIS-R), which gives verbal, performance, and full-scale intelligence quotient (IQ) scores. Some test results, such as those of vocabulary tests, hold up as aging progresses; results of other tests, such as tests of similarities and digit-symbol substitution, do not. The performance part of the WAIS-R is a more sensitive indicator of brain damage than the verbal part.

Visuospatial functions are sensitive to the normal aging process. The *Bender Gestalt Test* is one of a large number of instruments used to test visuospatial functions; another is the *Halstead-Reitan Battery*, which is the most complex battery of tests covering the entire spectrum of information processing and cognition. Depression, even in the absence of dementia, often impairs psychomotor performance, especially visuospatial functioning and timed motor performance. The *Geriatric Depression Scale* is a useful screening instrument that excludes somatic complaints from its list of items. The presence of somatic complaints on a rating scale tends to confound the diagnosis of a depressive disorder.

Medical History. Elderly patients have more concomitant, chronic, and multiple medical problems and take more medications than younger adults; many of these medications can influence their mental status. The medical history includes all major illnesses, traumata, hospitalizations, and treatment interventions. The psychiatrist should also be alert to underlying medical illness. Infections, metabolic and electrolyte disturbances, and myocardial infarction and stroke may first be manifested by psychiatric symptoms. Depressed mood, delusions, and hallucinations may precede other symptoms of Parkinson's disease by many months. On the other hand, a psychiatric disorder can also cause such somatic symptoms as weight loss, malnutrition, and inanition of severe depression.

Careful review of medications (including over-the-counter medications, laxatives, vitamins, tonics, and lotions) and even substances recently discontinued is extremely important. Drug effects can be long lasting and may induce depression (e.g., antihypertensives), cognitive impairment (e.g., sedatives), delirium (e.g., anticholinergics), and seizures (e.g., neuroleptics). The review of medications must include sufficient detail to identify misuse (overdose, underuse) and relate medication use to special diets. A dietary history is also important; deficiencies and excesses (e.g., protein, vitamins) can influence physiological function and mental status.

EARLY DETECTION AND PREVENTION STRATEGIES

Many age-related illnesses develop insidiously and gradually progress over the years. The most common cause of late-life cognitive impairment, Alzheimer's disease, is characterized neuropathologically by a gradual accumulation of neuritic plaques and neurofibrillary tangles in the brain. Clinically, a progression of cognitive decline is seen, which begins with mild memory loss and ends with severe cognitive and behavioral deterioration.

Because it will likely be easier to prevent neural damage than to repair it once it occurs, investigators are developing strategies for early detection and prevention of age-related illnesses, such as Alzheimer's disease. Considerable progress has been made in the detection component of this strategy, using brain imaging technologies, such as positron emission tomography (PET) and functional magnetic resonance imaging (fMRI), in combination with genetic risk measures. With these approaches, subtle brain changes can now be detected that progress and can be followed over time. Such surrogate markers allow clinical scientists to track disease progression and to test novel treatments designed to decelerate brain aging. Clinical trials of cholinesterase inhibitor drugs, anticholesterol drugs, anti-inflammatory drugs, and others (e.g., vitamin E) are in progress to determine if such treatments delay the onset of Alzheimer's disease or the progression of brain metabolic or cognitive decline.

Novel approaches to measuring the physical evidence of Alzheimer's disease, the plaques and tangles in the cerebral cortex, have been successful in initial studies and will likely facilitate the testing of innovative treatments designed to rid the brain of these pathognomonic lesions. Scientists may not be able to cure Alzheimer's disease in its advanced stages, but they may be able to delay its onset effectively, thus helping patients live longer without the debilitating manifestations of the disease, including cognitive decline.

MENTAL DISORDERS OF OLD AGE

The National Institute of Mental Health's Epidemiologic Catchment Area (ECA) program has found that the most common mental disorders of old age are depressive disorders, cognitive disorders, phobias, and alcohol use disorders. Older adults also have a high risk for suicide and drug-induced psychiatric symptoms. Many mental disorders of old age can be prevented, ameliorated, or even reversed. Of special importance are the reversible causes of delirium and dementia; if not diagnosed accurately and treated in a timely fashion, however, these conditions can progress to an irreversible state requiring a patient's institutionalization. Table 56–3 lists the general cognitive domains assessed in a neuropsychological evaluation, with the tests used to measure that skill and a description of the specific behaviors measured by each

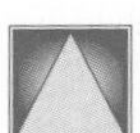

Table 56–3
Cognitive Domains

Gross cognitive functioning
Mini-Mental State Examination: *orientation, repetition, following commands, naming, constructional skill, written expression, memory, mental flexibility, and calculations*

Intelligence
Wechsler Adult Intelligence Scale-Revised (WAIS-R) or Wechsler Intelligence Scale-III (WAIS-III): *verbal and nonverbal intelligence*

Basic attention
WAIS-R or WAIS-III Digit Span: *repetition of digits forward and backward*

Information-processing speed
WAIS-R or WAIS-III Digit Symbol: *rapid graphomotor tracking*
Trailmaking Part A: *rapid graphomotor tracking*
Stroop A and B: *rapid word reading and color naming*

Motor dexterity
Finger tapping: *right and left index finger dexterity*

Language
Boston Naming Test: *word retrieval*
WAIS-R or WAIS-III Vocabulary: *vocabulary range*

Visual perceptual/spatial
WAIS-R or WAIS-III Picture Completion: *visual perception*
WAIS-R or WAIS-III Block Design: *constructional ability*
Rey-Osterrieth Complex Figure: *paper-and-pencil copy of complex design*
Beery Developmental Test of Visual Motor Integration: *paper-and-pencil copy of simple-to-complex designs*

Learning and memory
An 8- to 10-item word list learning task: *learning and recall of rote verbal information*
Wechsler Memory Scale-Revised (WMS-R) or Wechsler Memory Scale-III (WMS-III)
- Logical Memory subtest: *immediate and delayed recall of paragraph information*
- Visual Reproduction subtest: *immediate and delayed recall of visual designs*

Rey-Osterrieth Complex Figure 3-minute delayed recall: *delayed recall of complex design*

Executive functions
Trailmaking Part B: *rapid alternation between tasks*
Stroop C: *inhibition of an overlearned response*
Wisconsin Card Sorting Test: *categorization and mental flexibility*
Verbal fluency (FAS and category): *rapid word generation*
Design fluency: *rapid generation of novel designs*

(Courtesy of Kyle Brauer Boone, Ph.D.)

test. The tests listed in the table constitute a comprehensive test battery generally appropriate for use with a geriatric population. Use of a comprehensive battery is preferable for confident determination of presence and type of dementia or other cognitive disorder in elderly persons; in some circumstances, however, administering a several-hour battery is not possible. Tests marked with an asterisk are the core tests that are most sensitive for detection of a dementia.

Several psychosocial risk factors also predispose older persons to mental disorders. These risk factors include loss of social roles, loss of autonomy, the deaths of friends and relatives, declining health, increased isolation, financial constraints, and decreased cognitive functioning.

Many drugs can cause psychiatric symptoms in older adults. These symptoms can result from age-related alterations in drug absorption, a prescribed dosage that is too large, not following instructions and taking too large a dose, sensitivity to the medication, and conflicting regimens presented by several physicians. Almost the entire spectrum of mental disorders can be caused by drugs.

Dementing Disorders

Only arthritis is a more common cause of disability among adults age 65 and older than dementia, a generally progressive and irreversible impairment of the intellect, the prevalence of which increases with age. About 5 percent of persons in the United States older than age 65 have severe dementia, and 15 percent have mild dementia. Of persons older than age 80, about 20 percent have severe dementia. Known risk factors for dementia are age, family history, and female sex.

In contrast to mental retardation, the intellectual impairment of dementia develops over time—that is, previously achieved mental functions are lost gradually. The characteristic changes of dementia involve cognition, memory, language, and visuospatial functions, but behavioral disturbances are common as well and include agitation, restlessness, wandering, rage, violence, shouting, social and sexual disinhibition, impulsiveness, sleep disturbances, and delusions. Delusions and hallucinations occur during the course of the dementias in nearly 75 percent of patients.

Cognition is impaired by many conditions, including brain injuries, cerebral tumors, acquired immune deficiency syndrome (AIDS), alcohol, medications, infections, chronic pulmonary diseases, and inflammatory diseases. Although dementias associated with advanced age typically are caused by primary degenerative central nervous system (CNS) disease and vascular disease, many factors contribute to cognitive impairment; in older persons, mixed causes of dementia are common. Cognitive disorders including dementia and delirium are covered in Chapter 10.

About 10 to 15 percent of all patients who exhibit symptoms of dementia have potentially treatable conditions. The treatable conditions include systemic disorders, such as heart disease, renal disease, and congestive heart failure; endocrine disorders, such as hypothyroidism; vitamin deficiency; medication misuse; and primary mental disorders, most notably depressive disorders.

Depending on the site of the cerebral lesion, dementias are classified as cortical and subcortical. A subcortical dementia occurs in Huntington's disease, Parkinson's disease, normal pressure hydrocephalus, vascular dementia, and Wilson's disease. The subcortical dementias are associated with movement disorders, gait apraxia, psychomotor retardation, apathy, and akinetic mutism, which can be confused with catatonia. Table 56–4 lists some potentially reversible conditions that may resemble dementia. The cortical dementias occur in dementias of the Alzheimer's type, Creutzfeldt-Jakob disease (CJD), and Pick's disease, which frequently manifest aphasia, agnosia, and apraxia. In clinical practice, the two types of dementias overlap and, in most cases, an accurate diagnosis can be made only by autopsy. Human prion diseases result from coding mutations in the prion protein gene (PRNP) and may be inherited, acquired, or sporadic. They include familial CJD, Gerstmann-Sträussler-Scheinker syndrome, and fatal familial insomnia. These are inherited as autosomal-dominant mutations. The acquired diseases include kuru and iatrogenic CJD. Kuru was an epidemic prion disease of the Fore people of Papua, New Guinea, caused by cannibalistic funeral rituals, which peaked in incidence in the 1950s. Iatrogenic disease is rare and is caused, for example, by the use of contaminated dura mater and corneal grafts and treatment with human cadaveric pituitary-derived growth hormone and gonadotropin. Sporadic CJD accounts for 85 percent of the human prion diseases and occurs worldwide, with a uniform distribution and an incidence of about 1 in 1 million per annum, with a mean age at onset of 65 years. It is exceedingly rare in individuals under 30 years of age. (Additional information on dementia and prion disease is contained in Chapter 10, Section 10.3.)

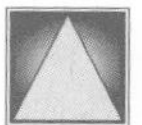

Table 56–4
Some Potentially Reversible Conditions That May Resemble Dementia

Substance
Anticholinergic agents
Antihypertensives
Antipsychotics
Corticosteroids
Digitalis
Narcotics
Nonsteroidal anti-inflammatory agents
Phenytoin
Polypharmacotherapy
Sedative hypnotics
Psychiatric Disorders
Anxiety
Depression
Mania
Delusional (paranoid) disorders
Metabolic and Endocrine Disorders
Addison's disease
Cushing's syndrome
Hepatic failure
Hypercarbia (chronic obstructive pulmonary disease)
Hypernatremia
Hyperparathyroidism
Hyperthyroidism
Hypoglycemia
Hyponatremia
Hypothyroidism
Renal failure
Volume depletion
Miscellaneous Conditions
Fecal impaction
Hospitalization
Impaired hearing or vision

(Courtesy of Gary W. Small, M.D.)

Depressive Disorders

Depressive symptoms are present in about 15 percent of all older adult community residents and nursing home patients. Age itself is not a risk factor for the development of depression, but being widowed and having a chronic medical illness are associated

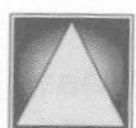

Table 56–5
Geriatric Depression Scale (Short Version)

Answers indicating depression are boldfaced. Each answer counts one point; scores greater than 5 indicate probable depression.

1. Are you basically satisfied with your life?	Yes/No
2. Have you dropped many of your activities and interests?	Yes/No
3. Do you feel that your life is empty?	Yes/No
4. Do you often get bored?	Yes/No
5. Are you in good spirits most of the time?	Yes/No
6. Are you afraid that something bad is going to happen to you?	Yes/No
7. Do you feel happy most of the time?	Yes/No
8. Do you often feel helpless?	Yes/No
9. Do you prefer to stay at home, rather than going out and doing new things?	Yes/No
10. Do you feel you have more problems with memory than most?	Yes/No
11. Do you think it is wonderful to be alive now?	Yes/No
12. Do you feel pretty worthless the way you are now?	Yes/No
13. Do you feel full of energy?	Yes/No
14. Do you feel that your situation is hopeless?	Yes/No
15. Do you think that most people are better off than you are?	Yes/No

Special Instructions. The scale can be used as a self-rating or observer-rated metric. It has also been used as an observer-rated scale in mildly demented subjects.

(From Yesavage JA. Geriatric Depression Scale. *Psychopharmacol Bull.* 1988;24:709, with permission.)

with vulnerability to depressive disorders. Late-onset depression is characterized by high rates of recurrence.

The common signs and symptoms of depressive disorders include reduced energy and concentration, sleep problems (especially early morning awakening and multiple awakenings), decreased appetite, weight loss, and somatic complaints. The presenting symptoms may be different in older depressed patients from those seen in younger adults because of an increased emphasis on somatic complaints in older persons. Older persons are particularly vulnerable to major depressive episodes with melancholic features, characterized by depression, hypochondriasis, low self-esteem, feelings of worthlessness, and self-accusatory trends (especially about sex and sinfulness) with paranoid and suicidal ideation. A geriatric depression scale is shown in Table 56–5.

Cognitive impairment in depressed geriatric patients is referred to as the *dementia syndrome of depression* (pseudodementia), which can be confused easily with true dementia. In true dementia, intellectual performance usually is global, and impairment is consistently poor; in pseudodementia, deficits in attention and concentration are variable. Compared with patients who have true dementia, patients with pseudodementia are less likely to have language impairment and to confabulate; when uncertain, they are more likely to say "I don't know"; and their memory difficulties are more limited to free recall than to recognition on cued recall tests. Pseudodementia occurs in about 15 percent of depressed older patients, and 25 to 50 percent of patients with dementia are depressed. Depression and bipolar disorder are covered in Section 15.1.

Schizophrenia

Schizophrenia usually begins in late adolescence or young adulthood and persists throughout life. Although first episodes diagnosed after age 65 are rare, a late-onset type beginning after age 45 has been described. Women are more likely to have a late onset of schizophrenia than men. Another difference between early-onset and late-onset schizophrenia is the greater prevalence of paranoid schizophrenia in the late-onset type. About 20 percent of persons with schizophrenia show no active symptoms by age 65; 80 percent show varying degrees of impairment. Psychopathology becomes less marked as patients age.

The residual type of schizophrenia occurs in about 30 percent of persons with schizophrenia. Its signs and symptoms include emotional blunting, social withdrawal, eccentric behavior, and illogical thinking. Delusions and hallucinations are uncommon. Because most persons with residual schizophrenia cannot care for themselves, long-term hospitalization is required.

Older persons with schizophrenic symptoms respond well to antipsychotic drugs. Medication must be administered judiciously, and lower-than-usual dosages often are effective for older adults. Schizophrenia is covered in Chapter 13.

Delusional Disorder

The age of onset of delusional disorder usually is between ages 40 and 55, but it can occur at any time during the geriatric period. Delusions can take many forms; the most common are persecutory—patients believe that they are being spied on, followed, poisoned, or harassed in some way. Persons with delusional disorder may become violent toward their supposed persecutors. Some persons lock themselves in their rooms and live reclusive lives. Somatic delusions, in which persons believe they have a fatal illness, also can occur in older persons. In one study of persons older than 65 years of age, pervasive persecutory ideation was present in 4 percent of persons sampled.

Among those who are vulnerable, delusional disorder can occur under physical or psychological stress and can be precipitated by the death of a spouse, loss of a job, retirement, social isolation, adverse financial circumstances, debilitating medical illness or surgery, visual impairment, and deafness. Delusions also can accompany other disorders—such as dementia of the Alzheimer's type, alcohol use disorders, schizophrenia, depressive disorders, and bipolar I disorder—which need to be ruled out. Delusional syndromes also can result from prescribed medications or be early signs of a brain tumor. The prognosis is fair to good in most cases; best results are achieved through a combination of psychotherapy and pharmacotherapy.

A late-onset delusional disorder called *paraphrenia* is characterized by persecutory delusions. It develops over several years and is not associated with dementia. Some workers believe that the disorder is a variant of schizophrenia that first becomes manifest after age 60. Patients with a family history of schizophrenia show an increased rate of paraphrenia. Delusional disorders are covered in Section 14.3.

Anxiety Disorders

The anxiety disorders include panic disorder, phobias, obsessive-compulsive disorder (OCD), generalized anxiety disorder, acute stress disorder, and posttraumatic stress disorder (PTSD). Anxiety disorders begin in early or middle adulthood, but some appear for the first time after age 60. An initial onset of panic disorder in older persons is rare, but can occur. The ECA study determined that the 1-month prevalence of anxiety disorders in persons age 65 and older is 5.5 percent. By far the most common disorders are phobias (4 to 8 percent). The rate for panic disorder is 1 percent.

The signs and symptoms of phobia in older adults are less severe than those that occur in younger persons, but the effects are equally, if not more, debilitating for older patients. Existential theories help explain anxiety when no specifically identifiable stimulus exists for a chronically anxious feeling. Older persons must come to grips with death. The person may deal with the thought of death with a sense of despair and anxiety, rather than with equanimity and Erikson's "sense of integrity." The fragility of the autonomic nervous system in older persons may account for the development of anxiety after a major stressor. Because of concurrent physical disability, older persons react more severely to PTSD than younger persons.

Obsessions and compulsions may appear for the first time in older adults, although older adults with OCD usually had demonstrated evidence of the disorder (e.g., being orderly, perfectionistic, punctual, and parsimonious) when they were younger. When symptomatic, patients become excessive in their desire for orderliness, rituals, and sameness. They may become generally inflexible and rigid and have compulsions to check things again and again. OCD (in contrast to obsessive-compulsive personality disorder) is characterized by ego-dystonic rituals and obsessions and may begin late in life. Anxiety disorders are covered in Chapter 16.

Somatoform Disorders

Somatoform disorders, characterized by physical symptoms resembling medical diseases, are relevant to geriatric psychiatry because somatic complaints are common among older adults. More than 80 percent of persons over 65 years of age have at least one chronic disease—usually arthritis or cardiovascular problems. After age 75, 20 percent have diabetes and an average of four diagnosable chronic illnesses that require medical attention.

Hypochondriasis is common in persons over 60 years of age, although the peak incidence is in those 40 to 50 years of age. The disorder usually is chronic, and the prognosis guarded. Repeated physical examinations help reassure patients that they do not have a fatal illness, but invasive and high-risk diagnostic procedures should be avoided unless medically indicated.

Telling patients that their symptoms are imaginary is counterproductive and usually engenders resentment. Clinicians should acknowledge that the complaint is real, that the pain is really there and perceived as such by the patient, and that a psychological or pharmacological approach to the problem is indicated.

Alcohol and Other Substance Use Disorder

Older adults with alcohol dependence usually give a history of excessive drinking that began in young or middle adulthood. They usually are medically ill, primarily with liver disease, and are either divorced, widowed, or are men who never married. Many have arrest records and are numbered among homeless persons. A large number have chronic dementing illness, such as Wernicke's encephalopathy and Korsakoff's syndrome. Of nursing home patients, 20 percent have alcohol dependence.

Over all, alcohol and other substance use disorders account for 10 percent of all emotional problems in older persons, and dependence on such substances as hypnotics, anxiolytics, and narcotics is more common in old age than is generally recognized. Substance-seeking behavior characterized by crime, manipulativeness, and antisocial behavior is rarer in older than in younger adults. Older patients may abuse anxiolytics to allay chronic anxiety or to ensure sleep. The maintenance of chronically ill cancer patients with narcotics prescribed by a physician produces dependence, but the need to provide pain relief takes precedence over the possibility of narcotic dependence and is entirely justified.

The clinical presentation of older patients with alcohol and other substance use disorders varies and includes confusion, poor personal hygiene, depression, malnutrition, and the effects of exposure and falls. The sudden onset of delirium in older persons hospitalized for medical illness is most often caused by alcohol withdrawal. Alcohol abuse also should be considered in older adults with chronic gastrointestinal problems.

Older persons may misuse over-the-counter substances, including nicotine and caffeine. Over-the-counter analgesics are used by 35 percent of older persons and 30 percent use laxatives. Unexplained gastrointestinal, psychological, and metabolic problems should alert clinicians to over-the-counter substance abuse.

Sleep Disorders

Advanced age is the single most important factor associated with the increased prevalence of sleep disorders. Sleep-related phenomena reported more frequently by older than by younger adults are sleeping problems, daytime sleepiness, daytime napping, and the use of hypnotic drugs. Clinically, older persons experience higher rates of breathing-related sleep disorder and medication-induced movement disorders than younger adults.

In addition to altered regulatory and physiological systems, the causes of sleep disturbances in older persons include primary sleep disorders, other mental disorders, general medical disorders, and social and environmental factors. Among the primary sleep disorders, dyssomnias are the most frequent, especially primary insomnia, nocturnal myoclonus, restless legs syndrome, and sleep apnea. Of the parasomnias, rapid eye movement (REM) sleep behavior disorder occurs almost exclusively among elderly men. The conditions that commonly interfere with sleep in older adults also include pain, nocturia, dyspnea, and heartburn. The lack of a daily structure and of social or vocational responsibilities contributes to poor sleep.

As a result of the decreased length of their daily sleep–wake cycle, older persons without daily routines, especially patients in nursing homes, may experience an advanced sleep phase, in which they go to sleep early and awaken during the night.

Even modest amounts of alcohol can interfere with the quality of sleep and can cause sleep fragmentation and early morning awakening. Alcohol can also precipitate or aggravate obstructive sleep apnea. Many older persons use alcohol, hypnotics, and other CNS depressants to help them fall asleep, but data show that these persons experience more early morning awakening than trouble falling asleep. When prescribing sedative-hypnotic drugs for older persons, clinicians must monitor the patients for unwanted cognitive, behavioral, and psychomotor effects, including memory impairment (anterograde amnesia), residual sedation, rebound insomnia, daytime withdrawal, and unsteady gait.

Changes in sleep structure among persons over 65 years of age involve both REM sleep and non-rapid eye movement (NREM) sleep. The REM changes include the redistribution of REM sleep throughout the night, more REM episodes, shorter REM episodes, and less total REM sleep. The NREM changes include the decreased amplitude of delta waves, a lower percentage of stages 3 and 4 sleep, and a higher percentage of stages 1 and 2 sleep. In addition, older persons experience increased awakening after sleep onset.

Much of the observed deterioration in the quality of sleep in older persons is caused by the altered timing and consolidation of sleep. For example, with advanced age, persons have a lower amplitude of circadian rhythms, a 12-hour sleep-propensity rhythm, and shorter circadian cycles.

SUICIDE RISK

Elderly persons have a higher risk for suicide than any other population. The suicide rate for white men over the age of 65 is five times higher than that of the general population. One third of elderly persons report loneliness as the principal reason for considering suicide. Approximately 10 percent of elderly individuals with suicidal ideation report financial problems, poor medical health, or depression as reasons for suicidal thoughts. Suicide victims differ demographically from individuals who attempt suicide. About 60 percent of those who commit suicide are men; 75 percent of those who attempt suicide are women. Suicide victims, as a rule, use guns or hang themselves, whereas 70 percent of suicide attempters take a drug overdose, and 20 percent cut or slash themselves. Psychological autopsy studies suggest that most elderly persons who commit suicide have had a psychiatric disorder, most commonly depression. Psychiatric disorders of suicide victims, however, often do not receive medical or psychiatric attention. More elderly suicide victims are widowed and fewer are single, separated, or divorced than is true of younger adults. Violent methods of suicide are more common in the elderly, and alcohol use and psychiatric histories appear to be less frequent. The most common precipitants of suicide in older individuals are physical illness and loss, whereas problems with employment, finances, and family relationships are more frequent precipitants in younger adults. Most elderly persons who commit suicide communicate their suicidal thoughts to family or friends before the act of suicide.

Older patients with major medical illnesses or a recent loss should be evaluated for depressive symptomatology and suicidal ideation or plans. Thoughts and fantasies about the meaning of suicide and life after death may reveal information that the patient cannot share directly. There should be no reluctance to question patients about suicide, because no evidence indicates that such questions increase the likelihood of suicidal behavior.

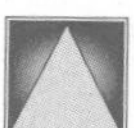

Table 56–6
Causes of Syncope

Cardiac Disorders
- Anatomical/valvular
  - Aortic stenosis
  - Mitral prolapse and regurgitation
  - Hypertrophic cardiomyopathy
  - Myxoma
- Electrical
  - Tachyarrhythmia
  - Bradyarrhythmia
  - Heart block
  - Sick sinus syndrome
- Functional
  - Ischemia and infarct

Situational Hypotension
- Dehydration (diarrhea, fasting)
- Orthostatic hypotension
- Postprandial hypotension
- Micturition, defecation, coughing, swallowing

Abnormal Cardiovascular Reflexes
- Carotid sinus syndrome
- Vasovagal syncope

Drugs
- Vasodilators
- Calcium channel blockers
- Diuretics
- Beta blockers

Central Nervous System Abnormalities
- Cerebrovascular insufficiency
- Seizures

Metabolic Abnormalities
- Hypoxemia
- Hypoglycemia or hyperglycemia
- Anemia

Pulmonary Disorders
- Chronic obstructive pulmonary disease
- Pneumonia
- Pulmonary embolus

OTHER CONDITIONS OF OLD AGE

Vertigo

Feelings of vertigo or dizziness, a common complaint of older adults, cause many older adults to become inactive because they fear falling. The causes of vertigo vary and include anemia, hypotension, cardiac arrhythmia, cerebrovascular disease, basilar artery insufficiency, middle ear disease, acoustic neuroma, and Ménière's disease. Most cases of vertigo have a strong psychological component, and clinicians should ascertain any secondary gain from the symptom. The overuse of anxiolytics can cause dizziness and daytime somnolence. Treatment with meclizine (Antivert), 25 to 100 mg daily, has been successful in many patients with vertigo.

Syncope

The sudden loss of consciousness associated with syncope results from a reduction of cerebral blood flow and brain hypoxia. A thorough medical workup is required to rule out the various causes listed in Table 56–6.

Hearing Loss

About 30 percent of persons over age 65 have significant hearing loss (presbycusis). After age 75, that figure rises to 50 percent. Causes vary. Clinicians should be sensitive to hearing loss in patients who complain they can hear but cannot understand what is being said or who ask that questions be repeated. Most elderly persons with hearing loss can be treated with hearing aids.

Elder Abuse

An estimated 10 percent of persons above 65 years of age are abused. Elder abuse is defined by the American Medical Association as "an act or omission which results in harm or threatened harm to the health or welfare of an elderly person." Mistreatment includes abuse and neglect—physically, psychologically, financially, and materially. Sexual abuse does occur. Acts of omission include withholding food, medicine, clothing, and other necessities.

Family conflicts and other problems often underlie elder abuse. The victims tend to be very old and frail. They often live with their assailants, who may be financially dependent on the victims. Both the victim and the perpetrator tend to deny or minimize the presence of abuse. Interventions include providing legal services, housing, and medical, psychiatric, and social services.

SPOUSAL BEREAVEMENT

Demographic data suggest that 51 percent of women and 14 percent of men over the age of 65 will be widowed at least once. Spousal loss is among the most stressful of all life experiences. As a group, older adults appear to have a more favorable outcome than expected following the death of a spouse. Depressive symptoms peak within the first few months after a death, but decline significantly within a year. A relationship exists between spousal loss and subsequent mortality. Elderly survivors of spouses who committed suicide are especially vulnerable, as are those with psychiatric illness.

PSYCHOPHARMACOLOGICAL TREATMENT OF GERIATRIC DISORDERS

Certain guidelines should be followed regarding the use of all drugs in older adults. A pretreatment medical evaluation is essential, including an electrocardiogram (ECG). It is especially useful to have the patient or a family member bring in all currently used medications, because multiple drug use could be contributing to the symptoms.

Most psychotropic drugs should be given in equally divided doses three or four times over a 24-hour period. Older patients may not be able to tolerate a sudden rise in drug blood level resulting from one large daily dose. Any changes in blood pressure and pulse rate and other side effects should be watched. For patients with insomnia, however, giving the major portion of an antipsychotic or antidepressant at bedtime takes advantage of its sedating and soporific effects. Liquid preparations are useful for older patients who cannot, or will not, swallow tablets. Clinicians should frequently reassess all patients to determine the need for maintenance medication, changes in dosage, and development of adverse effects. If a patient is taking psychotropic drugs at the time of the evaluation, the clinician should discontinue these medications, if possible, and, after a washout period, reevaluate the patient during a drug-free baseline state.

Adults over 65 years of age use the greatest number of medications of any age group; 25 percent of all prescriptions are written for them. Adverse drug reactions caused by medications result in the hospitalization of nearly 250,000 persons in the United States each year. Psychotropic drugs are among the most commonly prescribed, along with cardiovascular and diuretic medications; 40 percent of all hypnotics dispensed in the United States each year are to those older than 75 years of age, and 70 percent of older persons use over-the-counter medications, compared with only 10 percent of young adults. (Chapter 36 presents a comprehensive survey of the psychopharmacological agents.)

Principles

The major goals of the pharmacological treatment of older persons are to improve the quality of life, maintain persons in the community, and delay or avoid their placement in nursing homes. Individualization of dosage is the basic tenet of geriatric psychopharmacology.

Alterations in drug dosages are required because of the physiological changes that occur as persons age. Renal disease is associated with decreased renal clearance of drugs; liver disease results in a decreased ability to metabolize drugs; cardiovascular disease and reduced cardiac output can affect both renal and hepatic drug clearance; and gastrointestinal disease and decreased gastric acid secretion influence drug absorption. As a person ages, the ratio of lean to fat body mass also changes. With normal aging, lean body mass decreases and body fat increases. Changes in the ratio of lean to fat body mass that accompany aging affect the distribution of drugs. Many lipid-soluble psychotropic drugs are distributed more widely in fat than in lean tissue, so a drug's action can be unexpectedly prolonged in older persons. Similarly, changes in end-organ or receptor-site sensitivity must be taken into account. In older persons, the increased risk of orthostatic hypotension from psychotropic drugs is related to reduced functioning of blood pressure-regulating mechanisms.

As a general rule, the lowest possible dose should be used to achieve the desired therapeutic response. Clinicians must know the pharmacodynamics, pharmacokinetics, and biotransformation of each drug prescribed and the effects of the interaction of the drug with other drugs that a patient is taking.

PSYCHOTHERAPY FOR GERIATRIC PATIENTS

The standard psychotherapeutic interventions—such as insight-oriented psychotherapy, supportive psychotherapy, cognitive therapy, group therapy, and family therapy—should be available to geriatric patients. According to Sigmund Freud, persons older than 50 years are not suited for psychoanalysis because their mental processes lack elasticity. In the view of many who followed Freud, however, psychoanalysis is possible after age 50. Advanced age certainly limits plasticity of the personality, but as Otto Fenichel stated, "It does so in varying degrees and at very different ages so that no general rule can be given." Insight-oriented psychotherapy may help remove a specific symptom, even in older persons. It is of most benefit when patients have possibilities for libidinal and narcissistic gratification, but it is contraindicated if it would bring only the insight that life has been a failure and that the patient has no opportunity to make up for it.

Common age-related issues in therapy involve the need to adapt to recurrent and diverse losses (e.g., the deaths of friends and loved ones), the need to assume new roles (e.g., the adjustment to retirement and the disengagement from previously defined roles), and the need to accept mortality. Psychotherapy helps older persons to deal with these issues and the emotional problems surrounding them and to understand their behavior and the effects of their behavior on others. In addition to improving interpersonal relationships, psychotherapy increases self-esteem and self-confidence, decreases feelings of helplessness and anger, and improves the quality of life. As described by Alvin Goldfarb, geriatric psychotherapy has the general aim of assisting older adults to have minimal complaints, to help them make and keep friends of both sexes, and to have sexual relations when they have interest and capacity.

Psychotherapy helps relieve tensions of biological and cultural origins and helps older persons work and play within the limits of their functional status and as determined by their past training, activities, and self-concept in society. In patients with impaired cognition, psychotherapy can produce remarkable gains in both physical and mental symptoms. In one study conducted in an old-age home, 43 percent of the patients receiving psychotherapy showed less urinary incontinence, improved gait, greater mental alertness, improved memory, and better hearing than before psychotherapy.

Therapists must be more active, supportive, and flexible in conducting therapy with older than with younger adults, and they must be prepared to act decisively at the first sign of an incapacity that requires the active involvement of another physician, such as an internist, or that requires consulting with, or enlisting the aid of, a family member.

Older persons usually seek therapy for a therapist's unqualified and unlimited support, reassurance, and approval. Patients often expect a therapist to be all powerful, all knowing, and able to effect a magical cure. Most patients eventually recognize that the therapist is human and that they are engaged in a collaborative effort. In some cases, however, the therapist may have to assume the idealized role, especially when the patient is unable or unwilling to test reality effectively. With the help of the therapist, the patient deals with problems that had been avoided previously. As the therapist offers direct encouragement, reassurance, and advice, the patient's self-confidence increases as conflicts are resolved.

Goldfarb has described a brief, supportive therapy technique for institutionalized, cognitively impaired patients. The therapist promotes patients' foundering self-esteem, sense of control, and safety by permitting them to develop an apparent special relationship with the therapist, who is perceived as a benevolent and powerful figure. The patients believe they have some control over the benevolent physician. This is accomplished in small, subtle ways. For example, the physician elicits the patient's preferences for the frequency of sessions, daily timetables, diet, or socializing and then acquiesces to the patient's wishes, while maintaining a quiet caution about being unduly manipulative. The technique includes weekly, short (15 minutes) visits and gratifying the patient's realistic requests when possible.

Life Review or Reminiscence Therapy

Robert Butler and others have noted the universal tendency of the aging person to reflect on, and reminisce about, the past. Reminiscence is characterized by the progressive return of memories of past experiences, especially those that were meaningful and conflictual. To varying degrees, elderly patients in therapy reminisce about the past, search for meaning in their lives, and strive for some resolution of past interpersonal and intrapsychic conflicts. Life review therapy systematically enhances this reminiscing process and makes it more conscious and deliberate. The therapist may guide the process by encouraging the patient to write or tape a biography with review of special events and turning points. Techniques include reunions with family and good friends and looking through memorabilia, such as scrapbooks or picture albums. This technique has been reported to resolve old problems, increase tolerance of conflict, relieve guilt and fears, and enhance self-esteem, creativity, generosity, and acceptance of the present.

References

Ancoli-Israel S, Ayalon L. Diagnosis and treatment of sleep disorders in older adults. *Am J Geriatr Psychiatry*. 2006;14:95–103.

Conner KR, Conwell Y, Duberstein PR, Eberly S. Aggression in suicide among adults age 50 and over. *Am J Geriatr Psychiatry*. 2004;12:37–42.

Depp CA, Jeste DV. Definitions and predictors of successful aging: A comprehensive review of larger quantitative studies. *Am J Geriatr Psychiatry*. 2006;14:6–20.

Jarvik LF, Small GW. Geriatric psychiatry: Introduction and overview. In: Sadock BJ, Sadock VA, eds. *Kaplan & Sadock's Comprehensive Textbook of Psychiatry*. 8th ed. Vol. 2. Baltimore: Lippincott Williams & Wilkins; 2005:3587.

Jeary K. Sexual abuse and sexual offending against elderly people: A focus on perpetrators and victims. *Journal of Forensic Psychiatry and Psychology*. 2005;16(2):328–343.

Kales HC, Maixner DF, Mellow AM. Cerebrovascular disease and late-life depression. *Am J Geriatr Psychiatry*. 2005;13:88–98.

Leentjens AFG. Depression in Parkinson's disease: Conceptual issues and clinical challenges. *J Geriatr Psychiatry Neurol*. 2004;17(3):120–126.

Mast BT, Neufeld S, MacNeill SE, Lichtenberg PA. Longitudinal support for the relationship between vascular risk factors and late-life depressive symptoms. *Am J Geriatr Psychiatry*. 2004;12:93–101.

Mueller TI, Kohn R, Leventhal N, Leon AC, Solomon D, Coryell W, Endicott J, Alexopoulos GS, Keller MB. The course of depression in elderly patients. *Am J Geriatr Psychiatry*. 2004;12:22–29.

Reynolds CF III, Dew MA, Pollock BG, Mulsant BH, Frank E, Miller MD, Houck PR, Mazumdar S, Butters MA, Stack JA, Schlernitzauer MA, Whyte EM, Gildengers A, Karp J, Lenze E, Szanto K, Bensasi S, Kupfer DJ. Maintenance treatment of major depression in old age. *N Engl J Med*. 2006;354:1130–1138.

Sadavoy J, Jarvik LF, Grossberg GT, Meyers BS, eds. *Comprehensive Textbook of Geriatric Psychiatry*. 3rd ed. New York: Norton; 2004.

Takeshita J, Ahmed I. Culture and geriatric psychiatry. In: Tseng W-S, Streltzer J, eds. *Cultural Competence in Clinical Psychiatry*. Washington, DC: American Psychiatric Publishing, Inc.; 2004:147–161.

57 End of Life Care and Palliative Medicine

▲ 57.1 Palliative Medicine and Pain Management

Marguerite S. Lederberg M.D. at Memorial Sloan-Kettering Cancer Center in New York makes the following observation:

> A dying human being whose physical, social, emotional, and spiritual needs are being effectively attended to seldom demands to be helped to commit suicide, and the family members—given proper help and support—derive a deep sense of peace from having helped their loved one to die feeling loved and secure.

This section deals with ensuring that those needs are attended to with effective palliative care so all patients in extremis experience a peaceful death and most importantly, a painless one.

CARING FOR THE DYING PATIENT

One of the most important tasks for a physician caring for a dying patient is to determine when the time for curative care has ceased. It is only then that palliative care can begin. Some physicians are so upset by death that they are reluctant to use palliative methods; rather, they continue to treat the patient knowing that efforts are futile. Or, they resort to using so-called heroic methods that do not prevent death and that may produce needless suffering. Ideally, physicians should strive to extend life and decrease suffering; at the same time, they must accept death as a defining characteristic of life. Some physicians, however, have developed dysfunctional attitudes about death, which have been reinforced throughout their lives by their experiences and training. It has been postulated that doctors are more frightened of death than members of other professional group and that many enter the study of medicine so that they may gain control of their own mortality using the defense mechanism of intellectualization. Risk factors that can interfere with a physician's ability to care optimally for the dying patient are listed in Table 57.1–1. These factors range from over-identifying with the patient to being fearful of death as mentioned above.

Physicians able to deal with death and dying are able to communicate effectively in several areas: diagnosis and prognosis; the nature of terminal illness; advance directives about life-sustaining treatment; hospice care; legal and ethical issues; grief and bereavement; and psychiatric care. Each of these areas is covered below. Palliative care physicians must be skilled in pain management, especially in the use of powerful opioids—the gold standard of drugs used for pain relief. In 1991 the American Board of Pain Medicine was established to ensure that physicians treating patients in pain were both qualified to do so and were kept up to date on the latest advances in the field.

COMMUNICATION

After a diagnosis and prognosis have been made, physicians need to talk to the patient and the patient's family. Formerly, doctors subscribed to a conspiracy of silence, believing that their patient's chances for recovery would improve if they knew less, because news of impending death might bring despair. The current practice is now one of honesty and openness toward patients; in fact, the question is not whether to tell the patient, but when and how. The American Hospital Association in 1972 drafted the Patient's Bill of Rights, declaring that patients have the "right to obtain complete, current information regarding diagnosis, treatment and prognosis in terms the patient can be reasonably expected to understand."

Breaking Bad News

When breaking news of impending death to the patient, as when relating any bad news, diplomacy and compassion should be guiding principles. Often, bad news is not completely related during one meeting, but rather is absorbed gradually over a series of separate conversations. Advance preparations, including scheduling sufficient time for the visit, researching pertinent information, such as test results and facts about the case, and even arranging furniture appropriately can only make the patient feel more comfortable.

If possible, these conversations should take place in a private, suitable space with the patient on equal terms with the physician (i.e., the patient dressed and the physician seated). If it is possible and desired by the patient, the patient's spouse or partner should be present. The treating physician should explain the current situation to the patient in clear, simple language, even when speaking to highly educated patients. Information may need to be repeated or additional meetings may be necessary to communicate all of the information. A gentle, sensible approach will help modulate the patient's own denial and acceptance. At no time should physicians take their patient's angry comments personally, and they should never criticize the patient's response to the bad news.

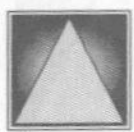

Table 57.1–1
Risk Factors for the Development of Aversive Reactions in Physicians

The physician:
- Identifies with the patient: looks, profession, age, character, etc.
- Identifies the patient with someone in his own life.
- Is currently dealing with a sick family member.
- Is recently bereaved or dealing with unresolved loss or grief issues.
- Feels professionally insecure.
- Is fearful of death and disability.
- Is unconsciously reflecting feelings felt or expressed by the patient or family.
- Cannot tolerate high and protracted levels of ambiguity or uncertainty.
- Carries a psychiatric diagnosis, such as depression or substance abuse.

(Adapted from Meier: The inner life of physicians and care of the seriously ill. *JAMA.* 2001;286:3007–3014, with permission.)

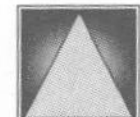

Table 57.1–2
Some Difficult Questions from Patients

"Why me?"
"Why didn't you catch this earlier? Did you make a mistake?"
"How long do I have?"
"What would you do in my shoes?"
"Should I try experimental therapy?"
"Should I go to a 'medical mecca' for treatment or a second opinion?"
"If my suffering gets really bad, will you help me die?"
"Will you work with me all the way through to my death, no matter what?"

(From Quill TF. Initiating end-of-life discussions with seriously ill patients. *JAMA.* 2000;284:2502, with permission.)

Physicians can signal their availability for honest communication by encouraging and answering questions from patients. Estimates on how long a patient has to live are usually inaccurate and, thus, should not be given or given with that caveat. Also, physicians should make it clear to their patients that they are willing to see them through until death occurs. Ultimately, physicians must choose how much information to give and when on the basis of each patient's needs and capacities.

The same general approaches apply as physicians seek to comfort members of the patient's family. Helping family members deal with feelings about the patient's illness can be just as important as comforting the patient, because family members are often the main source of emotional support for patients.

Telling the Truth

Tactful honesty is the doctor's most important aid. Honesty, however, need not preclude hope or guarded optimism. It is important to be aware that if 85 percent of patients with a particular disease die in 5 years, 15 percent are still alive after that time. The principles of doing good and not doing harm inform the decision of whether to tell the patient the truth. In general, most patients want to know the truth about their condition. Various studies of patients with malignancies show that 80 to 90 percent want to know their diagnosis.

Doctors, however, should ask patients how much they want to know because some persons do not want to know all the facts about their illness. Such patients, if told the truth, deny that they ever were told, and they cannot participate in end-of-life decisions, such as the use of life-sustaining equipment. The patients who openly request that they not be given "bad news" are often those who most fear death. Physicians should deal with these fears directly, but if the patient still cannot bear to hear the truth, someone closely related to the patient must be informed.

Informed Consent

In the United States, informed consent is legally required for both conventional and experimental treatment. Patients must be given sufficient information about their diagnosis, prognosis, and treatment options to make a knowledgeable decision. This includes discussion of potential risks and benefits, available alternative treatments, and the results of not receiving treatment. This approach may come at some psychological cost; severe anxiety and occasional psychiatric decompensation can occur when patients feel overburdened by demands to make decisions. Nevertheless, patients respond best to doctors who explain the various options in detail. Physicians must be prepared to deal with these and other difficult questions posed by patients. Some of them are listed in Table 57.1–2.

End-of-life discussions are challenging, especially because they can influence how patients make informed choices. Table 57.1–3 lists representative questions that doctors can ask their patients to initiate the discussion of such end-of-life issues as do not resuscitate (DNR) orders, pain management, and advance directives.

TERMINAL CARE DECISIONS

Modern society is poorly equipped to cope with the life-and-death decisions spawned by technology. When it first emerged, cardiopulmonary resuscitation was enthusiastically supported by the medical profession. It was endowed with magical power and eventually became a ritualized rite, rather than an optional medical treatment. That practice played into the therapeutic activism characteristic of many physicians. By the end of the 20th century, however, a countermovement began. First, the right to refuse treatment was established, largely because of synergy between the consumer movement and the bioethics movement with its emphasis on patient autonomy. Next, the legality of DNR orders and the moral equivalence of stopping and not starting treatment were established. The medical profession was less enthusiastic than the public about these changes, perhaps because practitioners know too well the emotional ambiguities that surround death and must repeatedly experience them.

Brain Death and Persistent Vegetative State

In an attempt to deal with these ambiguities, the concept of brain death emerged. Brain death is associated with the loss of higher brain functions (e.g., cognition) and all brain stem function (e.g., pupillary and reflex eye movement), respiration, and gag and corneal reflexes. Determination of brain death is generally accepted criterion for death. Some clinicians advocate an absence

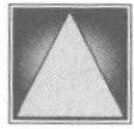

Table 57.1–3
Representative Questions for Initiating the Discussion about End-of-Life Issues

Domain	Representative Questions[a]
Goals	Given the severity of your illness, what is most important for you to achieve? What do you think about balancing quality of life with length of life in terms of your treatment? What are your most important hopes? What are your biggest fears?
Values	What makes life most worth living for you? Would there be any circumstances under which you would find life not worth living? What do you consider your quality of life to be like now? Have you seen or been with someone who had a particularly good death or particularly difficult death?
Advance directives	If with future progression of your illness you are not able to speak for yourself, who would be best able to represent your views and values? (health care proxy) Have you given any thought to what kind of treatment you would want (and not want) if you become unable to speak for yourself in the future? (living will)
Do-not-resuscitate order	If you were to die suddenly, that is, you stopped breathing or your heart stopped, we could try to revive you by using cardiopulmonary resuscitation (CPR). Are you familiar with CPR? Have you given thought as to whether you would want it? Given the severity of your illness, CPR would in all likelihood be ineffective. I would recommend that you choose not to have it, but that we continue all potentially effective treatments. What do you think?
Palliative care (pain and other symptoms)	Have you ever heard of hospice (palliative care)? What has been your experience with it? Tell me about your pain. Can you rate it on a 10-point scale? What is your breathing like when you feel at your best? How about when you are having trouble?
Palliative care ("unfinished business")	If you were to die sooner rather than later, what would be left undone? How is your family handling your illness? What are their reactions? Has religion been an important part of your life? Are there any spiritual issues you are concerned about at this point?

[a]Physicians should give the patient an opportunity to respond to each question. Base follow-up questions and responses on careful listening to the patient, using his or her own words whenever possible.
(From Quill TE. Initiating end-of-life discussions with seriously ill patients. *JAMA*. 2000;284:2502, with permission.)

of brain waves on electroencephalography (EEG) to confirm the diagnosis.

Persistent vegetative state was defined by the American Academy of Neurology as a condition in which exists no awareness of self or environment associated with severe neurological damage (Table 57.1–4). Medical treatment provides no benefits to patients in a persistent vegetative state and once the diagnosis is established DNR and do not intubate (DNI) orders can be followed and life-sustaining methods (e.g., feeding tubes, ventilators) can be removed.

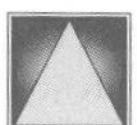

Table 57.1–4
Persistent Vegetative State

No evidence of awareness of self or environment; no interaction with others
No meaningful response to stimuli
No receptive or expressive language
Return of sleep–wake cycles, arousal, even smiling, frowning, yawning
Preserved brainstem or hypothalamic autonomic functions to permit survival
Bowel and bladder incontinence
Variably preserved cranial nerve and spinal reflexes

In 1976, the case of Karen Quinlan made international headlines when her parents sought the assistance of a judge to discontinue the use of a ventilator in their daughter, who was in a persistent vegetative state. Ms. Quinlan's physician had refused her parents' request to remove the ventilator because, they said, they feared that they might be held civilly or even criminally liable for her death. The New Jersey Supreme Court ruled that competent persons have a right to refuse life-sustaining treatment and that this right should not be lost when a person becomes incompetent. Because the Court believed that the physicians were unwilling to withdraw the ventilator because of the fear of legal liability, not precepts of medical ethics, it devised a mechanism to grant the physicians prospective legal immunity for taking this action. Specifically, the New Jersey Supreme Court ruled that after a prognosis, confirmed by a hospital ethics committee, that "no reasonable possibility of a patient returning to a cognitive, sapient state," exists, life-sustaining treatment can be removed and no one involved, including the physicians, can be held civilly or criminally responsible for the death.

The publicity surrounding the Quinlan case motivated two independent developments: It encouraged states to enact "living will" legislation that provided legal immunity to physicians who honored patients' written "advance directives" specifying how they would want to be treated if they ever became incompetent; and it encouraged hospitals to establish ethics committees that could attempt to resolve similar treatment disputes without going to court. (Annas GJ. "Culture of life" Politics at the bedside. *N Eng J Med*. 2005;352:16.)

Advance Directives

Advance directives are wishes and choices about medical intervention when the patient's condition is considered terminal. Advance directives, which are legally binding in all 50 states, include three types: living will, health care proxy, and DNR and DNI orders.

Living Will. In a living will, a patient who is mentally competent gives specific instructions that doctors must follow when the patient cannot communicate them because of illness. These instructions may include rejection of feeding tubes, artificial airways, or any other measures to prolong life.

Health Care Proxy. Also known as *durable power of attorney*, the health care proxy gives another person the power to make medical decisions if the patient cannot do so. That person, also known as the surrogate, is empowered to make all decisions about terminal care on the basis of what he or she thinks the patient would want.

Do Not Resuscitate and Do Not Intubate Orders. These orders prohibit doctors from attempting to resuscitate (DNR) or intubate (DNI) the patient who is in extremis. DNR and DNI orders are made by the patient who is competent to do so. They can be made part of the living will or expressed by the health care proxy. A sample advance directive that incorporates both a living will and a health care proxy is given in Table 57.1–5.

The *Uniform Rights of the Terminally Ill Act*, drafted by the National Conference on Uniform State Laws, was approved and recommended for enactment in all states. This act authorizes an adult to control the decisions regarding the administration of life-sustaining treatment by executing a declaration instructing a physician to withhold or to withdraw life-sustaining treatment if the person is in a terminal condition and cannot participate in medical treatment decisions. In 1991 the *Federal Patients Self-Determination Act* became law in the United States and required that all health care facilities (1) provide each patient admitted to a hospital with written information about the right to refuse treatment, (2) ask about advance directives, and (3) keep written records of whether the patient has an advance directive or has designated a health care proxy.

Today, patients who have left no advance directives or who are legally incompetent to do so have access to hospital ethics committees that hold active legal and ethical debates about these issues. These ethics committees are also of help to doctors, who can gain both legal and moral support when recommending that no further treatment occur. It is much easier for all parties, however, if the patient has advance directives or a proxy. Ideally, physicians should initiate discussions with patients about advance directives and proxies early, even while the patient is healthy. The patient should be reminded that these early formulations can be modified, but that even having preliminary

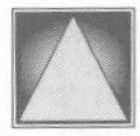

Table 57.1–5
Advance Directive Living Will and Health Care Proxy

Death is a part of life. It is a reality like birth, growth, and aging. I am using this advance directive to convey my wishes about medical care to my doctors and other people looking after me at the end of my life. It is called an advance directive because it gives instructions in advance about what I want to happen to me in the future. It expresses my wishes about medical treatment that might keep me alive. I want this to be legally binding.

If I cannot make or communicate decisions about my medical care, those around me should rely on this document for instructions about measures that could keep me alive.

I do not want medical treatment (including feeding and water by tube) that will keep me alive if:

- I am unconscious and there is no reasonable prospect that I will ever be conscious again (even if I am not going to die soon in my medical condition), or
- I am near death from an illness or injury with no reasonable prospect of recovery.

I do want medicine and other care to make me more comfortable and to take care of pain and suffering. I want this even if the pain medicine makes me die sooner.

I want to give some extra instructions: [*Here list any special instructions, e.g., some people fear being kept alive after a debilitating stroke. If you have wishes about this, or any other condition, please write them here.*]

The legal language in the box that follows is a health care proxy. It gives another person the power to make medical decisions for me.

I name____________________.
who lives at____________________,
phone number________________, to make medical decisions for me if I cannot make them myself. This person is called a health care "surrogate," "agent," "proxy," or "attorney in fact." This power of attorney shall become effective when I become incapable of making or communicating decisions about my medical care. This means that this document stays legal when and if I lose the power to speak for myself, for instance, if I am in a coma or have Alzheimer's disease.

My health care proxy has power to tell others what my advance directive means. This person also has power to make decisions for me based either on what I would have wanted, or, if this is not known, on what he or she thinks is best for me.

If my first choice health care proxy cannot or decides not to act for me, I name____________________,
address____________________,
phone number________________, as my second choice.

I have discussed my wishes with my health care proxy, and with my second choice if I have chosen to appoint a second person. My proxy(ies) has(have) agreed to act for me.

I have thought about this advance directive carefully. I know what it means and want to sign it. I have chosen two witnesses, neither of whom is a member of my family, nor will inherit from me when I die. My witnesses are not the same people as those I named as my health care proxies. I understand that this form should be notarized if I use the box to name (a) health care proxy(ies).

Signature____________________
Date____________________
Address____________________
Witness's signature____________________
Witness's printed name____________________
Address____________________
Witness's signature____________________
Witness's printed name____________________
Address____________________
Notary [to be used if proxy is appointed]____________________

(From Choice in Dying, Inc.—the National Council for the Right to Die, with permission.) [Choice in Dying is a national not-for-profit organization that works for the rights of patients at the end of life. In addition to this generic advance directive, Choice in Dying distributes advance directives that conform to each state's specific legal requirements and maintains a national Living Will Registry for completed documents.]

advance directives will ensure that treating physicians observe the patient's wishes in the event of an emergency.

CARING FOR THE FAMILY

Family members play an important role as caregivers to the terminally ill and have needs of their own that often go unrecognized. Their responsibilities can be overwhelming, especially if only one family member is available or if family members themselves are infirm or elderly. Table 57.1–6 lists some family caregiving tasks. Many of these tasks require long hours of work or supervision that can lead to physical and emotional fatigue. One study of caregivers reports that 25 to 30 percent lost their jobs and more than half moved to lower-paying jobs to accommodate the need for flexibility. The highest stress level was found in families who cared for a terminally ill patient at home, especially when death occurs in the home, and realized in retrospect that they would have preferred an environment in which death occurs in the presence of skilled caretakers.

Dying at Home

Depending on the patient's wishes and the nature of his or her disease, the choice to die at home is one that should be explored. Although it is more burdensome on a family than dying in a hospital or hospice, death at home can be a welcome alternative for the patient and family seeking to spend quality time together. A home care team can assess a home for its suitability and suggest ways to facilitate activities of daily living, including modifications to furniture, hospital bed leasing, and installation of assistive devices, such as handrails and commodes. The family's care can be supplemented with house calls by physicians, nurses, therapists, and chaplains. In any case, the family must know what their responsibilities are and must be well prepared to care for the patient. Recently, hospice home care was approved by Medicare and is being more widely used.

Family therapy sessions allow family members to explore feelings about death and dying. They serve as a forum in which anticipatory grief and mourning can take place. The ability to share feelings can be cathartic, especially if guilt is involved. Family members often have to deal with feelings of guilt about past interactions with the dying patient.

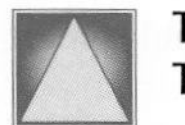

Table 57.1–6
Tasks of Family Members

1. Administering medications
2. Dealing with adverse effects of medications
3. Providing help with, or actually performing, activities of daily living (ADLs)
4. Changing wound dressing
5. Managing ambulatory infusion pumps or other equipment
6. Providing symptom management (e.g., for pain, nausea and vomiting, shortness of breath, seizures, and terminal agitation)
7. Notifying the nurse or doctor when they are needed
8. Shopping for needed items and picking up prescriptions
9. Providing a presence and companionship
10. Attending to spiritual and religious needs
11. Carrying out advance directives
12. Managing financial matters

Family sessions also help to achieve consensus about the patient's advance directives. If family members disagree about the patient's wishes, the medical staff may be unable to act. In such cases, legal action may be needed to resolve family disputes about what course of action to pursue.

PALLIATIVE CARE

Palliative care is the most important part of end-of-life care. It refers to providing relief from the suffering caused by pain or other symptoms of terminal disease. Although this is most commonly associated with analgesic drug administration, many other medical interventions and surgical procedures fall under the umbrella of palliative care because they can make the patient more comfortable. Monitors and their alarms, peripheral and central lines, phlebotomy, measurement of signs, and even supplemental oxygen are usually discontinued to allow the patient to die peacefully. Relocating the patient to a quiet, private room (as opposed to an intensive care unit) and allowing family members to be present is another very important palliative care modality.

The shift from active, curative treatment to palliative care is sometimes the first tangible sign that the patient will die, a transition that is emotionally difficult for everyone concerned about the patient to accept. The discontinuation of machines and measurements, which up until this point have been an integral part of the hospital experience, can be extremely disconcerting to the patient, family members, and even other physicians. Indeed, if these parties are not active in planning this transition, it can easily seem that persons have given up on the patient.

Because of this difficulty, palliative care is sometimes avoided altogether (i.e., curative treatment is continued until the patient dies). This approach is likely to cause problems if it is adopted merely to avoid the reality of impending death. A well-negotiated transition to palliative care often decreases anxiety after the patient and family go through an appropriate anticipatory grief reaction. Furthermore, a positive emotional outcome is much more likely if the physician and staff project a conviction that palliative care will be an active, involved process, without hint of withdrawal or abandonment. When this does not occur or when the family cannot tolerate the transition, the ensuing stress frequently results in a need for psychiatric consultation.

A 36-year-old physician with end-stage leukemia was seen in psychiatric consultation because he reported seeing the "angel of death" at the foot of his hospital bed. He described the experience as frightening and inexplicable. The consultant asked the patient, "Are you afraid that you are going to die?" That was the first time anyone had mentioned death or dying in any context to the patient. He welcomed the opportunity to talk openly about his fears to the medical staff and to his family and eventually died a peaceful death.

Psychiatric consultation is indicated for patients who become severely anxious, suicidal, depressed, or overtly psychotic. In each instance, appropriate psychiatric medication can be prescribed to provide relief. Patients who are suicidal do not always have to be transferred to a psychiatric service. An attendant or nurse can be assigned to the patient on a 24-hour basis (one-on-one coverage). In such instances, the relationship that develops between the observer and the patient may have therapeutic overtones, especially with patients whose depression is related to a sense of abandonment. Patients who are terminal and who are at high risk for suicide are usually in pain. When pain is relieved, suicidal ideation is likely to diminish. A careful evaluation of suicide potential is required for all patients. A premorbid history of past suicide attempts is a high risk factor for suicide in terminally ill patients. In patients who become psychotic, impaired cognitive function secondary to metastatic lesions to the brain must always be considered. Such patients respond to antipsychotic medications, and psychotherapy may also be of use.

PAIN MANAGEMENT

Types of Pain

Dying patients are subject to several different kinds of pain, summarized in Table 57.1–7. The distinctions are important because they call for different treatment strategies; somatic and visceral pain are responsive to opiates, whereas neuropathic and sympathetically maintained pain may require adjuvant medications in addition to opiates. Most patients with advanced cancer, for example, have more than one kind of pain and require complex treatment regimens.

Treatment of Pain

It cannot be overemphasized that pain management should be aggressive, and treatment should be multimodal. In fact, a good pain regimen may require several drugs or the same drug used in different ways and administered via different routes. For example, intravenous morphine can be supplemented by self-administered oral "rescue" doses, or a continuous epidural drip can be supplemented by bolus intravenous doses. Transdermal patches may provide baseline concentrations in patients for whom intravenous or oral intake is difficult. Patient-controlled analgesia systems for intravenous opiate administration result in better pain relief with lower amounts dispensed than in staff-administered dosing.

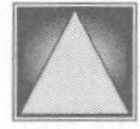

Table 57.1–7
Types of Pain

Nociceptive pain	
Somatic pain	Usually, but not always constant, aching, gnawing, and well localized (e.g., bone metastases)
Visceral pain	Usually, but not always constant, deep, squeezing, poorly localized, with possible cutaneous referral (e.g., pleural effusion leading to [1] deep chest pain, [2] diaphragmatic irritation referred to shoulder)
Neuropathic pain	Burning dysesthetic pain with shock-like paroxysms associated with direct damage to peripheral receptors, afferent fibers, or central nervous system (CNS), leading to loss of central inhibitory modulation and spontaneous firing (e.g., phantom limb pain; can involve sympathetic somatic afferents)
Psychogenic pain	Variable characteristics, secondary to psychological factors in the absence of medical factors; rare as a pure phenomenon in patients with cancer, but often an additional factor in the presence of organic pain

(Courtesy of Marguerite S. Lederberg, M.D., and Jimmie C. Holland, M.D.)

Opioids commonly cause delirium and hallucinations. A frequent mechanism of psychotoxicity is the accumulation of drugs or metabolites whose duration of analgesia is shorter than their plasma half-life (morphine, levorphanol [Levo-Dromoran], and methadone [Dolophine]). Use of drugs such as hydromorphone (Dilaudid), which have half-lives closer to their analgesic duration, can relieve the problem without loss of pain control. Cross-tolerance is incomplete between opiates; hence, several should be tried in any patient with the dosage lowered when switching drugs. Table 57.1–8 lists opioid analgesics.

The benefits of maintenance analgesia administration in terminally ill patients compared with as-needed administration cannot be overemphasized. Maintenance dosing improves pain control, increases drug efficiency, and relieves patient anxiety, whereas as-needed orders allow pain to increase while waiting for the drug to be given. Moreover, as-needed analgesia administration perversely sets up the patient for staff complaints about drug-seeking behavior. Even when maintenance treatment is used, extra doses of medication should be available for breakthrough pain, and repeated use of these medications should signal the need to raise the maintenance dose. Depending on their previous experiences with opioid analgesics and their weight, it is not unusual for some patients to require 2 g or more of morphine per day for relief of symptoms.

Knowing doses of different drugs and different routes of administration is important to avoid accidental undermedication. For example, when changing a patient from intramuscular to oral morphine use, the intramuscular dose must be multiplied by 6 to avoid causing the patient pain and provoking drug-seeking behavior. Many adjuvant drugs used for pain are psychotropics with which psychiatrists are familiar, but in some cases, their analgesic effect is separate from their primary psychotropic effect. Commonly used adjuvants include antidepressants, mood stabilizers (e.g., gabapentin) phenothiazines, butyrophenones, antihistamines, amphetamines, and steroids. They are particularly important in neuropathic and sympathetically maintained pain, for which they can be the mainstay of treatment.

Other developments in pain management include more intrusive procedures, such as nerve blocks or the use of continuous epidural infusions. Additionally, radiation therapy, chemotherapy, and even surgical resection can be considered as pain management modalities in palliative care. Short courses of radiotherapy or chemotherapy can be used to shrink tumors or manage metastatic lesions that cause pain or impairment. In patients with end-stage Hodgkin's disease, for example, systemic chemotherapy can improve the patient's quality of life by decreasing tumor burden. Surgical resection of invasive tumors, most notably breast carcinomas, can be useful for the same reason.

PALLIATION OF OTHER SYMPTOMS

Symptom management is a high priority in palliative care. Patients are often more concerned about the day-to-day distress of their symptoms than they are about their impending death, which may not be as real to them. Table 57.1–9 lists common end-of-life symptoms. A comprehensive approach to palliation involves attending to these end-of-life symptoms as well as pain. Sources of distress include psychiatric symptoms, such as anxiety, and physical symptoms. Foremost among physical symptoms are those involving the gastrointestinal system, including diarrhea, constipation, anorexia, nausea, vomiting, and bowel obstruction. Other important symptoms include insomnia, confusion, mouth

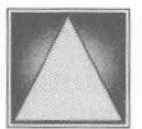

Table 57.1–8
Opioid Analgesics for Management of Pain

Drug and Equianalgesic Dose Relative Potency	Dose (mg IM or oral)	Plasma Half-Life (hr)[a]	Starting Oral Dose[b] (mg)	Available Commercial Preparations
Morphine	10 IM 60 oral	3–4	30–60	Oral: tablet, liquid, slow-release tablet Rectal: 5–30 mg Injectable: SC, IM, IV, epidural, intrathecal
Hydromorphone	1.5 IM 7.5 oral	2–3	2–18	Oral: tablets: 1, 2, 4 mg Injectable: SC, IM, IV 2 mg/mL, 3 mg/mL, and 10 mg/mL
Methadone	10 IM 20 oral	12–24	5–10	Oral: tablets, liquid Injectable: SC, IM, IV
Levorphanol	2 IM 4 oral	12–16	2–4	Oral: tablets Injectable: SC, IM, IV
Oxymorphone	1	2–3	NA	Rectal: 10 mg Injectable: SC, IM, IV
Heroin	5 IM 60 oral	3–4	NA	NA
Meperidine	75 IM 300 oral	3–4 (normeperidine 12–16)	75	Oral: tablets Injectable: SC, IM, IV
Codeine	130 oral 200 oral	3–4	60	Oral: tablets and combination with acetylsalicylic acid, acetaminophen, liquid
Oxycodone[c]	15 oral 30 oral	—	5	Oral: tablets, liquid, oral formulation in combination with acetaminophen (tablet and liquid) and aspirin (tablet)

[a]The time of peak analgesia in nontolerant patients ranges from ½ hour to 1 hour, and the duration from 4 to 6 hours. The peak analgesic effect is delayed, and the duration is prolonged after oral administration.
[b]Recommended starting IM doses; the optimal dose for each patient is determined by titration, and the maximal dose is limited by adverse effects.
[c]A long-acting sustained-release form of oxycodone (Oxycontin) has been abused by drug addicts and its use has been criticized because of this; however, it is a very useful preparation available in 10-, 20-, 40-, and 160-mg doses that need to be taken once every 12 hours. It is used as a maintenance therapy for severe persistent pain.
(Adapted from Foley K. Management of cancer pain. In: DeVita VT, Hellman S, Rosenberg SA, eds. *Cancer: Principles and Practice of Oncology.* 4th ed. Philadelphia: JB Lippincott; 1993:936, with permission.)
SC, subcutaneous; IM, intramuscular; IV, intravenous; NA, not applicable.

sores, dyspnea, cough, pruritus, decubitus ulcers, and urinary frequency or incontinence. Caretakers should follow these symptoms closely and establish appropriate early and aggressive care for these symptoms before they become burdensome.

An effective treatment for nausea and vomiting associated with chemotherapy is the use of Δ-tetrahydrocannabinol (THC), the active ingredient of marijuana. Oral synthetic cannabinoid, dronabinol (Marinol) is used in 1- to 2-mg doses every 8 hours. The use of marijuana cigarettes to deliver THC is believed to be more effective than pills. Proponents say that its absorption is faster and antiemetic properties are more potent via the pulmonary system. Repeated attempts to legalize marijuana cigarettes for medical use have met with only limited success in this country.

> A 47-year-old man with incurable lung cancer who had been treated unsuccessfully with chemotherapy and radiotherapy had been suffering from intractable dyspnea for 1 week. His family, nursing, and other staff were increasingly upset by his difficulty breathing and his pleas for relief. The attending physician refused to prescribe anything stronger than codeine. The palliative care team at the hospital intervened at the family's request. Relief was obtained with the use of 5 to 10 mg of intravenous bolus of morphine every 15 minutes. When the patient became comfortable, a continuous drip of intravenous morphine was instituted, complemented by subcutaneous morphine as needed.

The American Medical Association supports the position that patients with a terminal condition require substantial doses of opioids on a regular basis and should not be denied drugs for fear of producing physical dependence. A similar view is endorsed in *Goodman and Gilman's the Pharmacological Basis of Therapeutics* as follows:

> The physician should not wait until the pain becomes agonizing; no patient should ever wish for death because of a physician's reluctance to use adequate amounts of effective opioids. Accordingly, physicians who treat the terminally ill should not be intimidated by legal oversight.

This is especially important because the Drug Enforcement Administration (DEA) is considering examining the prescribing practices of physicians who care for terminally ill patients. In a strongly worded editorial (*New England Journal of Medicine*, January 5, 2006), the DEA was criticized for its involvement into what constitutes acceptable medical practice for dying patients because the DEA's federal mandate is limited to combating criminal substance abuse, not monitoring the care of dying patients. Physicians must be vigilant and forceful in protecting their rights to administer opioids to treat patients for intractable pain.

HOSPICE CARE

In 1967 the founding of St. Christopher's Hospice in England by Cicely Saunders launched the modern hospice movement. Several factors in the 1960s propelled the development of hospices, including concerns about inadequately trained physicians, inept terminal care, gross inequities in health care, and neglect of the elderly. Life expectancy had increased, and heart disease and

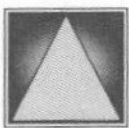

Table 57.1–9
Common End-of-Life Symptoms/Signs

Symptom Sign	Comments
Delusions	Occur in 90% of all terminal patients; can be reversed if cause is treatable, e.g., pain, medication; respond to antipsychotic medication
Fatigue or weakness	Most common occurrence in terminal illness; psychostimulants can be used for short-term relief
Dysphagia	Common in neurological disease end states, e.g., multiple sclerosis, amyotrophic lateral sclerosis
Incontinence	May follow pelvic radiation, which can produce fistulas; use indwelling or condom catheter
Dyspnea or cough	Produces severe anxiety with fear of suffocation; occurs in 80% of terminal lung cancer patients; opioids, bronchodilators of use
Nausea or vomiting	Adverse effect of radiation and chemotherapy; antiemetics, e.g., metoclopramide, prochlorperazine, of use; marijuana cigarettes of use in selected patients
Anorexia	All terminal disease states are associated with cachexia secondary to anorexia and dehydration; feeding tubes do not prevent aspiration
Loss of skin integrity	Decubiti most common on weight-bearing areas, e.g., hips, sacrum, outer ankle; important to turn body frequently; elbow and hip pads of use
Anxiety or depression	Psychological factors, e.g., fear of death, abandonment; physiological factors, e.g., pain, hypoxia; antianxiety and antidepressant medication of use; opioids have strong antianxiety effects

(From Mitka M. Suggestions for help when the end is near. *JAMA* 2000; 284:2441; adapted from National Coalition on Health Care (NCHC) and the Institute for Health Care Improvement (IHI). Promises to Keep: Changing the Way We Provide Care at the End of Life, release, October 12, 2000, with permission.)

cancer were becoming more common. Saunders emphasized an interdisciplinary approach to symptom control, care of the patient and family as a unit, the use of volunteers, continuity of care (including home care), and follow-up with family members after a patient's death. The first hospice in the United States, Connecticut Hospice, opened in 1974. By 2000, more than 3,000 hospices were open in the United States. Round-the-clock pain control with opioids is an essential component of hospice management. In 1983, Medicare began reimbursing hospice care. Medicare hospice guidelines emphasize home care, with benefits provided for a broad spectrum of physician, nursing, psychosocial, and spiritual services at home or, if necessary, in a hospital or nursing home. To be eligible, the patient must be physician certified as having 6 months or less to live. By electing hospice care, patients agree to receive palliative rather than curative treatment. Many hospice programs are hospital-based, sometimes in separate units and sometimes in the form of hospice beds interspersed throughout the facility. Other program models include free-standing hospices and programs, hospital-affiliated hospices, nursing home hospice care, and home care programs.

Nursing homes are the site of death for many elderly patients with incurable chronic illness, yet dying nursing home residents have limited access to palliative and hospice care. For example, in 1997, 3 percent of hospice enrollees were in nursing homes, whereas 87 percent were in private homes. Families generally express satisfaction with their personal involvement in hospice care. Savings with hospice care vary, but home care programs generally cost less than conventional institutional care, particularly in the final months of life. Hospice patients are less likely to receive diagnostic studies or such intensive therapy as surgery or chemotherapy; however a new trend is to allow treatment programs to continue while the patient remains in the hospice. Hospice care is a proved, viable alternative for patients who elect a palliative approach to terminal care. In addition, hospice goals of dignified, comfortable death for the terminally ill and care for patient and family together have been increasingly adopted into mainstream medicine.

NEONATAL AND INFANT END-OF-LIFE CARE

Advances in reproductive medicine have increased the number of infants born prematurely as well as the number of multiple births. These advances have increased the need for life-sustaining methods of care and have made decisions about when to use palliative care more complex. Some bioethicists believe that withholding life-sustaining interventions is appropriate under certain circumstances; others maintain that life-sustaining methods should not be used at all. An extensive study of attitudes among neonatologists about end-of-life decisions found no consensus about if and when to terminate life.

Most decisions to forego life-sustaining procedures for newborns concern those whose death is imminent. Even if their future quality of life is determined to be bleak, most physicians feel that some life is better than no life at all. Those physicians who support withholding intensive care consider the following quality-of-life issues: (1) extent of bodily damage (e.g., severe neurological impairment), (2) the burden that a disabled child will place on the family, and (3) the ability of the child to derive some pleasure from existence (e.g., having an awareness of being alive and being able to form relationships).

The American Academy of Pediatrics permits nontreatment decisions for newborns when the infant is irreversibly comatose or when treatment would be futile and only prolong the process of dying. These standards do not permit the parents to have any input into the decision-making process. In a well-publicized case in England in 2000, it was decided to surgically separate conjoined twins knowing that one would die as a result of the procedure and despite the objections of the parents, who believed that nature should take its course even if that led to the death of both infants. Neonatal end-of-life decisions remain in a state of limbo. No clear-cut criteria exist about which patients should receive intensive care and which should receive palliative care.

CHILD END-OF-LIFE CARE

After accidents, cancer is the second most common cause of death in children. Although many childhood cancers are treatable, palliative care is necessary for children with cancers that are not. Children require more support than adults in coping with death. On average, a child does not view death as permanent until the age of about 10; before that, death is viewed as a sleep or separation. Therefore, children should be told only what they can understand; if they are capable, they should be involved in the decision-making process about treatment plans. Assurances that patients are pain-free and physically comfortable are just as important for children as they are for adults.

A unique aspect of end-of-life care in children involves addressing their fear of being separated from their parents. It is helpful to have parents participate in end-of-life care tasks within their capacities. Family sessions with the child in attendance allow feelings to emerge and questions to be answered.

SPIRITUAL ISSUES

The inclusion of a section on religious or spiritual problems in the text revision of the 4th edition of *Diagnostic and Statistical Manual of Mental Disorders* (DSM-IV-TR) is but one sign of increasing awareness of the importance of this area to patients, families, and many staff members as well. Several studies have shown that religious beliefs are often associated with mature and active coping methods, and the field of psychological and spiritual interfaces in terminally ill patients is spawning a whole new area of psychological research within the traditional medical establishment. The psychiatric consultant should inquire about faith, its meaning, associated religious practices, and impact on the coping response. It can be a source of strength or guilt at all stages of the disease, ranging from the earliest "What did I do to cause this?" through "Will God give me only what I can carry?" to the poignant life review of the late stage. It is often a primary factor in the reactions to suicidality and in attitudes toward terminal care decisions. Mental health professionals should deal with these areas in an unself-conscious and noncondescending manner and work to help patients fully integrate this aspect of their personality into their current crisis. The professional should also work in harmony with the patient's spiritual guide, if one is available. Sometimes, an experienced, effective chaplain working with the appropriate patient can achieve positive results more directly than any psychotherapy. The following case exemplifies how creative pastoral care can relieve suffering.

A young woman was admitted to a hospice in a terminal state. She was experiencing a severe depression, which she attributed to not being able to see her oldest daughter receive her first communion. Arrangements were made for a ceremonial communion for her daughter to take place at the hospice. After the ceremony, the patient's mood improved markedly as one of her fears was alleviated and a religious need was satisfied. As her mood improved, she was able to address other unresolved issues and have quality visits with her children in her remaining days. (From O'Neil MT. Pastoral care. In: Cimino JE, Brescia MJ, eds. *Calvary Hospital Model for Palliative Care in Advanced Cancer*. Bronx: Palliative Care Institute; 1998, with permission.)

ALTERNATIVE AND COMPLEMENTARY MEDICINE

Many patients, once they are told they are terminally ill, seek alternative treatments, ranging from innocuous programs aimed at enhancing general health to more aggressive, harmful, or fraudulent regimens. Although most patients combine the alternative and the traditional, a substantial number favor complementary medicine as the only treatment for their disease.

Complementary methods to cure terminal illness, especially cancer, emphasize a holistic approach, involving purification of the body, detoxification through internal cleansing, and attention to nutritional and emotional well-being. Despite their widespread appeal, not one of these methods has been demonstrated to cure cancer or prolong life, yet all have strong followings bolstered by anecdotal accounts of their efficacy. The popular metabolic therapy attributes cancer and other potentially fatal illnesses to toxins and waste materials accumulating in the body; treatment is based on reversing this process by diet, vitamins, minerals, enzymes, and colonic irrigations. Another approach includes macrobiotic diets or megavitamins to enhance the body's capacity to destroy malignancy. In 1987, the National Research Council recommended minimizing carcinogenic substances and fat in the diet and increasing whole-grain, fruit, and vegetable consumption as preventive guidelines. Psychological approaches cite maladaptive personality and coping styles as contributors to fatal diseases; treatment consists of shaping a positive attitude. Spiritual approaches aim at achieving harmony between the patient and nature. Some groups use spirituality as a way to ward off illness, which is sometimes seen as an external evil to be exorcised. Immunotherapies have gained popularity in recent years; cancer is attributed to a defective immune system, and restoration of immunocompetency is seen as the cure. Many patients find increased strength to endure the suffering of terminal illness with the help of alternative medicine, even though the course of the disease may not be affected. (For a further discussion of alternative medicine, see Chapter 29.)

References

Fins JJ. *Palliative Ethic of Care: Clinical Wisdom at Life's End*. Sudbury, Mass: Jones and Bartlett; 2006.

Han PKJ. Palliative care services, patient abandonment, and the scope of physicians' responsibilities in end-of-life care. *J Palliat Med*. 2005;8(6):1238–1245.

Himelstein BP, Hilden JM, Boldt AM, Weissman D. Pediatric palliative care. *N Eng J Med*. 2004;350(17):1752–1762.

Hulbert NJ, Morrison VL. A preliminary study into stress in palliative care: Optimism, self-efficacy and social support. *Psychology, Health & Medicine*. 2006;11(2):246.

Kelly B, Burnett P, Badger S, Pelusi D, Varghese FT, Robertson M. *Psycho-Oncology*. 2003;12(4):375–384.

Lo B, Rubenfeld G. Palliative sedation in dying patients: "We turn to it when everything else hasn't worked". *JAMA*. 2005;294(14):1810–1816.

O'Leary N, Flynn J, MacCallion A, Walsh E, McQuillan R. Pediatric palliative care delivered by an adult palliative care service. *Palliat Med*. 2006; 20(4):433.

Payne A, Kelleher MJ, Hayes Y, O'Brien T. Liaison psychiatry in palliative care. *Irish Journal of Psychological Medicine*. 2004;21(1):25–27.

Perry JE, Churchill LR, Kirshner HS. The Terri Shiavo case: Legal ethical and medical perspectives. *Ann Intern Med*. 2005;143:744.

Quill TE, Meier DE. The big chill—Inserting the DEA with end-of-live care. *N Eng J Med*. 2006;1:354.

Schofield P, Carey M, Love A, Nehill C, Wein S. "Would you like to talk about your future treatment options?" Discussing the transition from curative cancer treatment to palliative care. *Palliat Med*. 2006;20(4):397.

Tan A, Zimmermann C, Rodin G. Interpersonal processes in palliative care: An attachment perspective on the patient–clinician relationship. *Palliat Med*. 2005;19(2):143–150.

Wessel EM, Rutledge DN. Home care and hospice nurses' attitudes toward death and caring for the dying: Effects of palliative care education. *Journal of Hospice & Palliative Nursing*. 2005;7(4):212–218.

Woodruff R. *Palliative Medicine: Evidence-Based Symptomatic and Supportive Care for Patients with Advanced Cancer.* New York: Oxford University Press; 2004.

▲ 57.2 Euthanasia and Physician-Assisted Suicide

EUTHANASIA

From the Greek term for good death, euthanasia means compassionately allowing, hastening, or causing the death of another. Generally, someone resorts to euthanasia to relieve suffering, maintain dignity, and shorten the course of dying when death is inevitable. Euthanasia can be *voluntary* if the patient has requested it or *involuntary* if the decision is made against the patient's wishes or without the patient's consent. Euthanasia can be *passive*—simply withholding heroic lifesaving measures—or *active*—deliberately taking a person's life. Euthanasia assumes that the intent of the physician is to aid and abet the patient's wish to die.

Arguments for euthanasia revolve around patient autonomy and dignified dying. One of the most dramatic ways patients can exercise their right to self-determination is by asking that life-sustaining treatment to be withdrawn. If the patient is mentally competent, physicians must respect such wishes. Proponents of active, voluntary euthanasia argue that the same rights should be extended to patients who are not on life-sustaining treatment, but also choose to have their physicians help them die.

Opponents of euthanasia also provide strong ethical and medical justification for their position. First, active euthanasia, even if the patient voluntarily requests it, is a form of killing, and should never be sanctioned. Second, many patients who request aid in dying may be suffering from depression which, when treated, will change the patient's mind about wanting to die.

Most medical, religious, and legal groups in the United States are against euthanasia. Both the American Psychiatric Association (APA) and the American Medical Association (AMA) condemn active euthanasia as illegal and contrary to medical ethics; however, few individuals have been convicted of euthanasia. Most physicians and medical groups in other parts of the world also oppose legalizing euthanasia. In the United Kingdom, for example, the British Medical Association believes that euthanasia is "alien to the traditional ethos and moral focus of medicine" and, if legalized, "would irrevocably change the context of health care for everyone, but especially for the most vulnerable."

The World Medical Association issued the following declaration on euthanasia in October 1987:

> "Euthanasia, that is, the act of deliberately ending the life of a patient, even at his own request or at the request of his close relatives, is unethical. This does not prevent the physician from respecting the will of a patient to allow the natural process of death to follow its course in the terminal phase of sickness."

Again, in 2002, the World Medical Association reissued a resolution condemning euthanasia as "unethical" and urging all doctors and medical associations to refrain from the practice.

Similarly, the New York State Committee on Bioethical Issues issued a statement declaring its opposition to euthanasia. The committee stated that the physician's obligation to relieve pain and suffering and to promote the dignity and autonomy of dying patients in their care, includings providing effective palliative treatment, even though it may occasionally hasten death. Physicians, however, should not perform active euthanasia or participate in assisted suicide. The Committee felt that support, comfort, respect for patient autonomy, good communication, and adequate pain control would dramatically decrease the demand for euthanasia and assisted suicide. They argued that the societal risks of involving physicians in medical interventions to cause a patient's death were too great to condone active euthanasia or physician-assisted suicide. In response to shifting public opinion and lobbying groups with different views, state laws that banned physician-assisted death in Washington State and New York were sent to the United States Supreme Court, challenging the constitutionality of these prohibitions. In June 1997, the Court unanimously held that terminally ill patients do not have the right to physician aid in dying. The ruling, however, left room for continuing debate and future policy initiates at the state level.

PHYSICIAN-ASSISTED SUICIDE

In the United States, most of the debate centers on physician-assisted suicide rather than on euthanasia. Some have argued that physician-assisted suicide is a humane alternative to active euthanasia in that the patient maintains more autonomy, remains the actual agent of death, and may be less likely to be coerced. Others feel that the distinctions are capricious in that the intent in both cases is to bring about a patient's death. Indeed, it may be difficult to justify providing a lethal dose of medication to a terminally ill patient (physician-assisted suicide) while ignoring the desperate pleas of another patient who may be even more ill and distressed, but who cannot complete the act because of problems with swallowing, dexterity, or strength.

Several degrees are seen to which a physician may assist the suicidal patient to end his or her life. Physician-assisted suicide can involve providing information on ways of committing suicide, supplying a prescription for a lethal dose of medication, or a means of inhaling a lethal amount of carbon monoxide, or, perhaps, even providing a suicide device that the patient can operate.

The controversy over physician-suicide came to national attention surrounding the activities of retired pathologist Jack Kevorkian, who, in 1989, provided his suicide machine to a 54-year-old woman with probable Alzheimer's disease. After the woman killed herself with his device, Kevorkian was charged with first-degree murder. The charges were later dismissed because Michigan had no law against physician-assisted suicide. Since that first case, Kevorkian has assisted in several more suicides, often for persons he met on only a few occasions, and frequently for persons who did not have a terminal illness. Claiming to have helped more than 130 people take their lives, Kevorkian was sent to prison in 1999 and was released in 2006. His attorneys and followers applaud his courage in easing pain and suffering; his detractors counter that he is a serial mercy killer. Opponents of Kevorkian's methods charge that, without safeguards, consultations, and thorough psychiatric evaluations, patients may search out suicide not because of terminal illness or intractable pain, but because of untreated depressive disorders. They argue that suicide rarely occurs in the absence of psychiatric illness. Finding more effective treatments for pain and depression, rather than inventing more sophisticated devices to help desperate patients kill themselves, defines compassionate and effective physician care.

In 1994, Oregon passed a ballot initiative legalizing physician-assisted suicide (Death with Dignity Act), making Oregon the first state in the United States to permit assisted suicides (Table 57.2–1). An assessment of the first 4 years revealed the following: Patients dying from physician-assisted suicide represent approximately 8 of 10,000 deaths. The most common underlying illnesses were cancer, amyotrophic lateral sclerosis, and chronic lower respiratory disease. The three most common end-of-life concerns were loss of autonomy (85 percent), a decreasing ability to participate in activities that made life enjoyable (77 percent), and losing control of bodily functions (63 percent). Eighty percent of the patients were enrolled in hospice programs, and 91 percent died at home. The prescribing physician was present in 52 percent of the cases.

In 2001, attorney general John Ashcroft attempted to prosecute Oregon doctors who helped terminally ill patients die

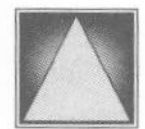

Table 57.2–1
Oregon's Assisted Suicide Law

The patient must be terminally ill and expected to die within 6 mos; mentally competent; fully informed about his or her diagnosis, prognosis, risks, and alternatives, such as comfort care; and be making a voluntary choice.
A second doctor must agree that the patient is terminally ill, acting on his or her own free will, fully informed, and capable of making health care decisions.
If either doctor thinks that the patient is suffering from any form of mental illness that could affect his or her judgment, they must refer the patient for counseling.
The patient must make one written request and two spoken requests.
The doctor must ask the patient to tell the next of kin, but the patient may decide not to do so.
The patient is free to change his or her mind at any time.
There is a 15-day waiting period between the patient making the request and the doctor writing the prescription.
All information must be written down in the medical records.
Only people who normally live in Oregon may use the Act.
Mercy killing, lethal injection, and active euthanasia are not permitted.
Pharmacists must be told of the prescribed medication's ultimate use.
Physicians, pharmacists, and health care systems are under no obligation to participate in the Death with Dignity Act.

claiming that doctor-assisted suicide is not a legitimate medical purpose. The case was brought to the Supreme Court, who in 2006 supported the Oregon law and said the "authority claimed by the attorney general is both beyond his expertise and incongruous with the statutory purposes and design."

Despite the abhorrence that many physicians and medical ethicists express regarding physician-assisted suicide, poll after poll shows that as many as two thirds of Americans favor the legalization of physician-assisted suicide in certain circumstances and evidence even indicates that the formerly uniform opposition to physician-assisted suicide within the medical community has eroded. Consistent with their positions on active euthanasia, the AMA, APA, and American Bar Association, however, continue to oppose physician-assisted suicide. Recently, the American College of Physicians–American Society of Internal Medicine (ACP-ASIM) expressed its commitment to improving care for patients at the end of life, while recommending against legalization of physician-assisted suicide. The ACP-ASIM feels physician-assisted suicide raises serious ethical concerns, undermines the physician–patient relationship and the trust necessary to sustain it, alters the medical profession's role in society, and endangers the values American society places on life, especially on the lives of disabled, incompetent, and vulnerable individuals.

The American Association of Suicidology in its 1996 *Report of the Committee on Physician-Assisted Suicide and Euthanasia* concluded that involuntary euthanasia can never be condoned; the report also stated, however, that "intolerable, prolonged suffering of persons in extremis should never be insisted upon, against their wishes, in single-minded efforts to preserve life at all cost." This position acknowledges that patients can die as a result of treatment given to them for the explicit purpose of relieving suffering; but death associated with palliative care differs greatly from physician-assisted suicide in that death is not the goal of treatment and is not intentional.

How to Deal with Requests for Suicide

To help guide clinicians facing requests for physician-assisted suicide, the AMA's Institute for Ethics has proposed the following eight-step clinical protocol:

1. Evaluation of the patient for depression or other psychiatric conditions that could cause disordered thought
2. Evaluation of the patient's "decision-making competence"
3. Discussion with the patient about his or her goals for care
4. Evaluation and response to the patient's "physical, mental, social, and spiritual suffering"
5. Discussion with the patient about the full range of treatment and care options
6. Consultation by the attending physician with other professional colleagues
7. Assurance that care plans chosen by the patient are being followed, including removal of unwanted treatment and the provision of adequate pain and symptom relief
8. Discussion with the patient explaining why physician-assisted suicide is to be avoided and why it is not compatible with the principled nature of the care protocol

Psychiatrists view suicide as an irrational act that is the product of mental illness, usually depression. In almost every case in which a patient asks to be put to death, a triad exists of depression associated with an incurable medical condition that causes the patient intolerable pain. In these instances, every effort should be made to provide antidepressants or psychostimulants for depression and opioids for pain. Psychotherapy, spiritual counseling, or both, may also be needed. In addition, family therapy to help with the stress of dealing with a dying patient may be necessary. Family therapy is also useful because some patients may ask to be put to death because they do not wish to be a burden to their families; others may feel coerced by their families into believing that they are, or will be, a burden and may choose death as a result. Currently, no professional codes countenance euthanasia or assisted suicide in the United States. Therefore, psychiatrists must stand on the side of responsible rescue and treatment.

A distinction also is needed between major depression and suffering. The nature of suffering has not been sufficiently studied by psychiatrists. It remains the province of theologians and philosophers. Suffering is a complex mix of spiritual, emotional, and physical factors that transcends pain and other symptoms of terminal illness. Physicians are more skilled at dealing with depression than with suffering. Anatole Broyard, who chronicled his own death in his book *Intoxicated by My Illness*, wrote the following:

> I see no reason or need for my doctor to love me nor would I expect him to suffer with me. I wouldn't demand a lot of my doctor's time; I just wish he would brood on my situation for perhaps five minutes, that he would give me his whole mind just once, be bonded with me for a brief space, survey my soul as well as my flesh, to get at my illness, for each man is ill in his own way.

FUTURE DIRECTIONS

Advances in technology bring more complex medical, legal, moral, and ethical controversies regarding life, death, euthanasia, and physician-assisted suicide. Some forms of euthanasia have found a place in modern medicine, and expansion of the boundaries of patients' rights and their ability to choose the way they live and die are inevitable. Both patients and physicians need to be better educated about depression, pain management, palliative care, and quality of life. Medical schools and residency training programs need to give the topics of death, dying, and palliative care the attention they deserve. Society must ensure that economics, ageism, and racism do not get in the way of adequate and humane management of patients with a chronic terminal illness. Finally, national health care policy must provide adequate insurance coverage, home care, and hospice services to all appropriate patients. If these mandates are followed, the argument for physician assistance in dying will lose much of its impact.

References

Battin MP. *Ending Life: Ethics and the Way We Die*. New York: Oxford University Press; 2005.

Groenewoud JH, Van Der Heide A, Tholen AJ, Schudel WJ, Hengeveld MW, Onwuteaka-Philipsen BD, Van Der Maas PJ, Van Der Wal G. Psychiatric consultation with regard to requests for euthanasia or physician-assisted suicide. *Gen Hosp Psychiatry*. 2004;26(4):323–330.

Jansen-van der Weide MC, Onwuteaka-Philipsen BD, van der Wal G. Granted, undecided, withdrawn, and refused requests for euthanasia and physician-assisted suicide. *Arch Intern Med.* 2005;165:1698–1704.

Johansen S, Hølen JC, Kaasa S, Loge JH, Materstvedt LJ. Attitudes towards, and wishes for, euthanasia in advanced cancer patients at a palliative medicine unit. *Palliat Med.* 2005;19(6):454–460.

Lavi SJ. *The Modern Art of Dying: A History of Euthanasia in the United States*. Princeton, NJ: Princeton University Press; 2005.

Loewy EH. Euthanasia, physician assisted suicide and other methods of helping along death. *Health Care Analysis*. 2004;12(3):181–193.

Mak YY, Elwyn G. Voices of the terminally ill: Uncovering the meaning of desire for euthanasia. *Palliat Med.* 2005;19(4):343–350.

Marcoux I, Onwuteaka-Philipsen BD, Jansen-van der Weide MC, van der Wal G. Withdrawing an explicit request for euthanasia or physician-assisted suicide: A retrospective study on the influence of mental health status and other patient characteristics. *Psychol Med.* 2005;35(9):1265–1274.

Materstvedt LJ. Euthanasia and letting die. *Palliat Med.* 2006;20(1):49–50.

Okie S. Physician-assisted suicide—Oregon and beyond. *N Engl J Med.* 2005; 352:1627–1630.

Pearlman RA, Hsu C, Starks H, Back AL, Gordon JR, Bharucha AJ, Koenig BA, Battin MP. Motivations for physician-assisted suicide. *J Gen Intern Med.* 2005; 20(3):234–239.

Quill TE, Battin MP, eds. *Physician-Assisted Dying: The Case for Palliative Care and Patient Choice*. Baltimore: Johns Hopkins University Press; 2004.

Rurup ML, Muller MT, Onwuteaka-Philipsen BD, Van Der Heide A, Van Der Wal G, Van Der Maas PJ. Requests for euthanasia or physician-assisted suicide from older persons who do not have a severe disease: An interview study. *Psychol Med.* 2005;35(5):665–671.

Shalowitz D, Emanuel E. Euthanasia and physician-assisted suicide: Implications for physicians. *J Clin Ethics*. 2004;15(3):232–236.

Van der Lee ML, van der Bom JG, Swarte NB, Heintz APM, de Graeff A, van den Bout J. Euthanasia and depression: A prospective cohort study among terminally ill cancer patients. *J Clin Oncol*. 2005;23(27):6607–6612.

58

Clinical-Legal Issues in Psychiatry

Psychiatric practice is influenced by four major factors: (1) the psychiatrist's professional, ethical, and legal duties to provide competent care to patients; (2) the patients' rights of self-determination to receive or refuse treatment; (3) court decisions, legislative directives, governmental regulatory agencies, and licensure boards; and (4) the ethical codes and practice guidelines of professional organizations. All of these issues fall within the realm of forensic psychiatry. The word forensic means belonging to the courts of law and at various times psychiatry and the law converge.

Medical Malpractice

Medical malpractice is a tort, or civil wrong. It is a wrong resulting from a physician's negligence. Simply put, negligence means doing something that a physician with a duty to care for the patient should not have done or failing to do something that should have been done as defined by current medical practice. Usually, the standard of care in malpractice cases is established by expert witnesses. The standard of care is also determined by reference to journal articles, professional textbooks, such as the *Comprehensive Textbook of Psychiatry*, professional practice guidelines, and ethical practices promulgated by professional organizations.

To prove malpractice, the plaintiff (e.g., patient, family, or estate) must establish by a preponderance of evidence that (1) a doctor–patient relationship existed that created a *duty* of care, (2) a *deviation* from the standard of care occurred, (3) the patient was *damaged*, and (4) the deviation *directly* caused the damage.

These elements of a malpractice claim are sometimes referred to as the *4 Ds* (duty, deviation, damage, direct causation).

Each of the four elements of a malpractice claim must be present or there can be no finding of liability. For example, a psychiatrist whose negligence is the direct cause of harm to an individual (physical, psychological, or both) is not liable for malpractice if no doctor–patient relationship existed to create a duty of care. Psychiatrists are not likely to be sued successfully if they give advice on a radio program that is harmful to a caller, particularly if a caveat was given to the caller that no doctor–patient relationship was being created. No malpractice claim will be sustained against a psychiatrist if a patient's worsening condition is unrelated to negligent care. Not every bad outcome is the result of negligence. Psychiatrists cannot guarantee correct diagnoses and treatments. When the psychiatrist provides due care, mistakes may be made without necessarily incurring liability. Most psychiatric cases are complicated. Psychiatrists make judgment calls when selecting a particular treatment course among the many options that may exist. In hindsight, the decision may prove wrong, but not be a deviation in the standard of care.

In addition to negligence suits, psychiatrists can be sued for the intentional torts of assault, battery, false imprisonment, defamation, fraud or misrepresentation, invasion of privacy, and intentional infliction of emotional distress. In an intentional tort, wrongdoers are motivated by the intent to harm another person or realize, or should have realized, that such harm is likely to result from their actions. For example, telling a patient that sex with the therapist is therapeutic perpetrates a fraud. Most malpractice policies do not provide coverage for intentional torts.

Negligent Prescription Practices

Negligent prescription practices usually include exceeding recommended dosages and then failing to adjust the medication level to therapeutic levels, unreasonable mixing of drugs, prescribing medication that is not indicated, prescribing too many drugs at one time, and failing to disclose medication effects. Elderly patients frequently take a variety of drugs prescribed by different physicians. Multiple psychotropic medications must be prescribed with special care because of possible harmful interactions and adverse effects.

Psychiatrists who prescribe medications must explain the diagnosis, risks, and benefits of the drug within reason and as circumstances permit (Table 58–1). Obtaining competent informed consent can be problematic if a psychiatric patient has diminished cognitive capacity because of mental illness or chronic brain impairment; a substitute health care decision maker may need to provide consent.

Informed consent should be obtained each time a medication is changed and a new drug is introduced. If patients are injured because they were not properly informed of the risks and consequences of taking a medication, sufficient grounds may exist for a malpractice action.

The question is often asked: How frequently should patients be seen for medication follow-up? The answer is that patients should be seen according to their clinical needs. No stock answer about the frequency of visits can be given. The longer the time interval between visits, however, the greater the likelihood of adverse drug reactions and clinical developments. Patients taking medications should probably not go beyond 6 months for follow-up visits. Managed care policies that do not reimburse for frequent follow-up appointments can result in a psychiatrist prescribing large amounts of medications. The psychiatrist is duty bound to provide appropriate treatment to the patient, quite apart from managed care or other payment policies.

Other areas of negligence involving medication that have resulted in malpractice actions include failure to treat adverse effects that have, or should have, been recognized; failure to monitor a patient's compliance with prescription limits; failure to prescribe medication or appropriate levels of medication according to the treatment needs of the patient; prescribing addictive drugs to vulnerable patients; failure to refer a patient for consultation or treatment by a specialist; and negligent withdrawal of medication treatment.

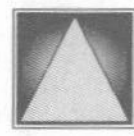

Table 58–1
Informed Consent: Reasonable Information to Be Disclosed

Although there exists no consistently accepted standard for information disclosure for any given medical or psychiatric situation, as a rule of thumb, five areas of information are generally provided:

1. Diagnosis—description of the condition or problem
2. Treatment—nature and purpose of proposed treatment
3. Consequences—risks and benefits of the proposed treatment
4. Alternatives—viable alternatives to the proposed treatment including risks and benefits
5. Prognosis—projected outcome with and without treatment

(From Simon RI. *Clinical Psychiatry and the Law.* 2nd ed. Washington, DC: American Psychiatric Press; 1992, with permission.)

Split Treatment

In split treatment, the psychiatrist provides medication and a nonmedical therapist conducts the psychotherapy. The following vignette illustrates a possible complication.

A psychiatrist provided medications for a depressed 43-year-old woman. A master's level counselor saw the patient for outpatient psychotherapy. The psychiatrist saw the patient for 20 minutes during the initial evaluation and prescribed a tricyclic drug, and the patient was prescribed sufficient drugs for follow-up in 3 months. The psychiatrist's initial diagnosis was recurrent major depression. The patient denied suicidal ideation. Appetite and sleep were markedly diminished. The patient had a long history of recurrent depression with suicide attempts. No further discussions were held between the psychiatrist and the counselor, who saw the patient once a week for 30 minutes in psychotherapy. Within 3 weeks, after a failed romantic relationship, the patient stopped taking her antidepressant medication, started to drink heavily, and committed suicide with an overdose of alcohol and antidepressant drugs. The counselor and psychiatrist were sued for negligent diagnosis and treatment.

Psychiatrists must do an adequate evaluation, obtain prior medical records, and understand that no such thing as a partial patient exists. Split treatments are potential malpractice traps because patients can "fall between the cracks" of fragmented care. The psychiatrist retains full responsibility for the patient's care in a split treatment situation. This does not preempt the responsibility of the other mental health professionals involved in the patient's treatment. Section V, annotation 3 of the *Principles of Medical Ethics with Annotations Especially Applicable to Psychiatry* states: "When the psychiatrist assumes a collaborative or supervisory role with another mental health worker, he/she must expend sufficient time to assure that proper care is given."

In managed care or other settings, a marginalized role of merely prescribing medication apart from a working doctor–patient relationship does not meet generally accepted standards of good clinical care. The psychiatrist must be more than just a medication technician. Fragmented care in which the psychiatrist only dispenses medication while remaining uninformed about the patient's overall clinical status constitutes substandard treatment that may lead to a malpractice action. At a minimum, such a practice diminishes the efficacy of the drug treatment itself or may even lead to the patient's failure to take the prescribed medication.

Split-treatment situations require that the psychiatrist remain fully informed of the patient's clinical status as well as the nature and quality of treatment the patient is receiving from the nonmedical therapist. In a collaborative relationship, the responsibility for the patient's care is shared according to the qualifications and limitations of each discipline. The responsibilities of each discipline do not diminish those of the other disciplines. Patients should be informed of the separate responsibilities of each discipline. The psychiatrist and the nonmedical therapist must periodically evaluate the patient's clinical condition and requirements to determine whether the collaboration should continue. On termination of the collaborative relationship, both parties treating the patient should inform the patient either separately or jointly. In split treatments, if the nonmedical therapist is sued, the collaborating psychiatrist will likely be sued, and vice versa.

Psychiatrists who prescribe medications in a split-treatment arrangement should be able to hospitalize a patient, if that should become necessary. If the psychiatrist does not have admitting privileges, prearrangements should be made with other psychiatrists who can hospitalize patients if emergencies arise. Split treatment is increasingly used by managed care companies and is a potential malpractice minefield.

PRIVILEGE AND CONFIDENTIALITY

Privilege

Privilege is the right to maintain secrecy or confidentiality in the face of a subpoena. Privileged communications are statements made by certain persons within a relationship—such as husband–wife, priest–penitent, or doctor–patient—that the law protects from forced disclosure on the witness stand. The right of privilege belongs to the patient, not to the physician, and so the patient can waive the right.

Psychiatrists, who are licensed to practice medicine, may claim medical privilege, but privilege has some qualifications. For example, privilege does not exist at all in military courts, regardless of whether the physician is military or civilian and whether the privilege is recognized in the state in which the court martial takes place.

In 1996, the United States Supreme Court recognized a psychotherapist–patient privilege in Jaffee v. Redmon. Emphasizing the important public and private interests served by the psychotherapist–patient privilege, the Court wrote:

> Because we agree with the judgment of the state legislatures and the Advisory Committee that a psychotherapist-patient privilege will serve a "public good transcending the normal predominant principle utilizing all rational means for ascertaining truth"... we hold that confidential communications between a licensed psychotherapist and her patients in the course of diagnosis or treatment are protected from compelled disclosure under Rule 501 of the Federal Rules of Evidence.

Confidentiality

A long-held premise of medical ethics binds physicians to hold secret all information given by patients. This professional obligation is called *confidentiality*. Confidentiality applies to certain populations and not to others; a group that is within the circle of confidentiality shares information without receiving specific permission from a patient. Such groups include, in addition to the physician, other staff members treating the patient, clinical supervisors, and consultants.

A subpoena can force a psychiatrist to breach confidentiality, and courts must be able to compel witnesses to testify for the law to function adequately. A subpoena ("under penalty") is an order to appear as a witness in court or at a deposition. Physicians usually are served with a *subpoena duces tecum*, which requires that they also produce their relevant records and documents. Although the power to issue subpoenas belongs to a judge, they are routinely issued at the request of an attorney representing a party to an action.

In bona fide emergencies, information may be released in as limited a way as feasible to carry out necessary interventions. Sound clinical practice holds that a psychiatrist should make the effort, time allowing, to obtain the patient's permission anyway and should debrief the patient after the emergency.

As a rule, clinical information may be shared with the patient's permission—preferably written permission, although oral permission suffices with proper documentation. Each release is good for only one piece of information, and permission should be reobtained for each subsequent release, even to the same party. Permission overcomes only the legal barrier, not the clinical one; the release is permission, not obligation. If a clinician believes that the information may be destructive, the matter should be discussed, and the release may be refused, with some exceptions.

Third-Party Payers and Supervision. Increased insurance coverage for health care is precipitating a concern about confidentiality and the conceptual model of psychiatric practice. Today, insurance covers about 70 percent of all health care bills; to provide coverage, an insurance carrier must be able to obtain information with which it can assess the administration and costs of various programs.

Quality control of care necessitates that confidentiality not be absolute; it also requires a review of individual patients and therapists. The therapist in training must breach a patient's confidence by discussing the case with a supervisor. Institutionalized patients who have been ordered by a court to get treatment must have their individualized treatment programs submitted to a mental health board.

Discussions about Patients. In general, psychiatrists have multiple loyalties: to patients, to society, and to the profession. Through their writings, teaching, and seminars, they can share their acquired knowledge and experience and provide information that may be valuable to other professionals and to the public. It is not easy to write or talk about a psychiatric patient, however, without breaching the confidentiality of the relationship. Unlike physical ailments, which can be discussed without anyone's recognizing the patient, a psychiatric history usually entails a discussion of distinguishing characteristics. Psychiatrists have an obligation not to disclose identifiable patient information (and, perhaps, any descriptive patient information) without appropriate informed consent. Failure to obtain informed consent could result in a claim based on breach of privacy, defamation, or both.

Child Abuse. In many states, all physicians are legally required to take a course on child abuse for medical licensure. All states now legally require that psychiatrists, among others, who have reason to believe that a child has been the victim of physical or sexual abuse, make an immediate report to an appropriate agency. In this situation, confidentiality is decisively limited by legal statute on the ground that potential or actual harm to vulnerable children outweighs the value of confidentiality in a psychiatric setting. Although many complex psychodynamic nuances accompany the required reporting of suspected child abuse, such reports generally are considered ethically justified.

HIGH-RISK CLINICAL SITUATIONS

Tardive Dyskinesia

It is estimated that at least 10 to 20 percent of patients and perhaps as high as 50 percent of patients treated with neuroleptic drugs for more than 1 year exhibit some tardive dyskinesia. These figures are even higher for elderly patients. Despite the possibility for many tardive dyskinesia-related suits, relatively few psychiatrists have been sued. In addition, patients who develop tardive dyskinesia may not have the physical energy and psychological motivation to pursue litigation. Allegations of negligence involving tardive dyskinesia are based on a failure to evaluate a patient properly, a failure to obtain informed consent, a negligent diagnosis of a patient's condition, and a failure to monitor.

Suicidal Patients

Psychiatrists may be sued when their patients commit suicide, particularly when psychiatric inpatients kill themselves. Psychiatrists are assumed to have more control over inpatients, making the suicide preventable.

The evaluation of suicide risk is one of the most complex, dauntingly difficult clinical tasks in psychiatry. Suicide is a rare event. In our current state of knowledge, clinicians cannot accurately predict when or if a patient will commit suicide. No professional standards exist for predicting who will or will not commit suicide. Professional standards do exist for assessing suicide risk, but at best, only the degree of suicide risk can be judged clinically following a comprehensive psychiatric assessment.

A review of the case law on suicide reveals that certain affirmative precautions should be taken with a suspected or confirmed suicidal patient. For example, failing to perform a reasonable assessment of a suicidal patient's risk for suicide or implement an appropriate precautionary plan will likely render a practitioner liable. The law tends to assume that suicide is preventable if it is foreseeable. Courts closely scrutinize suicide cases to determine if a patient's suicide was foreseeable. Foreseeability is a deliberately vague legal term that has no comparable clinical counterpart, a common-sense rather than a scientific construct. It does not (and should not) imply that clinicians can predict suicide. Foreseeability should not be confused with preventability, however. In hindsight, many suicides seem preventable that were clearly not foreseeable.

Violent Patients

Psychiatrists who treat violent or potentially violent patients may be sued for failure to control aggressive outpatients and for the discharge of violent inpatients. Psychiatrists can be sued for failing to protect society from the violent acts of their patients if it was reasonable for the psychiatrist to have known about the patient's violent tendencies and if the psychiatrist could have done something that could have safeguarded the public. In the landmark case *Tarasoff v. Regents of the University of California*, the California Supreme Court ruled that mental health professionals have a duty to protect identifiable, endangered third parties from imminent threats of serious harm made by their outpatients. Since then, courts and state legislatures have increasingly held psychiatrists to a fictional standard of having to predict the future behavior (dangerousness) of their potentially violent patients. Research has consistently demonstrated that psychiatrists cannot predict future violence with any dependable accuracy.

The duty to protect patients and endangered third parties should be considered primarily a professional and moral obligation and, only secondarily, a legal duty. Most psychiatrists acted to protect both their patients and others threatened by violence long before *Tarasoff*.

If a patient threatens harm to another person, most states require that the psychiatrist perform some intervention that might prevent the harm from occurring. In states with duty-to-warn statutes, the options available to psychiatrists and psychotherapists are defined by law. In states offering no such guidance, health care providers are required to use their clinical judgment and act to protect endangered third persons. Typically, a variety of options to warn and protect are clinically and legally available, including voluntary hospitalization, involuntary hospitalization (if civil commitment requirements are met), warning the intended victim of the threat, notifying the police, adjusting medication, and seeing the patient more frequently. Warning others of danger, by itself, is usually insufficient. Psychiatrists should consider the *Tarasoff* duty to be a national standard of care, even if they practice in states that do not have a duty to warn and protect.

Tarasoff I. This issue was raised in 1976 in the case of *Tarasoff v. Regents of University of California* (now known as *Tarasoff I*). In this case, Prosenjiit Poddar, a student and a voluntary outpatient at the mental health clinic of the University of California, told his therapist that he intended to kill a student readily identified as Tatiana Tarasoff. Realizing the seriousness of the intention, the therapist, with the concurrence of a colleague, concluded that Poddar should be committed for observation under a 72-hour emergency psychiatric detention provision of the California commitment law. The therapist notified the campus police, both orally and in writing, that Poddar was dangerous and should be committed.

Concerned about the breach of confidentiality, the therapist's supervisor vetoed the recommendation and ordered all records relating to Poddar's treatment destroyed. At the same time, the campus police temporarily detained Poddar, but released him on his assurance that he would "stay away from that girl." Poddar stopped going to the clinic when he learned from the police about his therapist's recommendation to commit him. Two months later, he carried out his previously announced threat to kill Tatiana. The young woman's parents thereupon sued the university for negligence.

As a consequence, the California Supreme Court, which deliberated the case for the unprecedented time of about 14 months, ruled that a physician or a psychotherapist who has reason to believe that a patient may injure or kill someone warn the potential victim.

The discharge of the duty imposed on the therapist to warn intended victims against danger may take one or more forms, depending on the case. Therefore, stated the court, it may call for the therapist to notify the intended victim or others likely to notify the victim of the danger, to notify the police, or to take whatever other steps are reasonably necessary under the circumstances.

The *Tarasoff I* ruling does not require therapists to report a patient's fantasies; instead, it requires them to report an intended homicide, and it is the therapist's duty to exercise good judgment.

Tarasoff II. In 1982, the California Supreme Court issued a second ruling in the case of *Tarasoff v. Regents of University of California* (now known as *Tarasoff II*), which broadened its earlier ruling extending the duty to warn to include the duty to protect.

The *Tarasoff II* ruling has stimulated intense debates in the medicolegal field. Lawyers, judges, and expert witnesses argue the definition of protection, the nature of the relationship between the therapist and the patient, and the balance between public safety and individual privacy.

Clinicians argue that the duty to protect hinders treatment because a patient may not trust a doctor if confidentiality is not maintained. Furthermore, because it is not easy to determine whether a patient is sufficiently dangerous to justify long-term incarceration, unnecessary involuntary hospitalization may occur because of a therapist's defensive practices.

As a result of such debates in the medicolegal field, since 1976, the state courts have not made a uniform interpretation of the *Tarasoff II* ruling (the duty to protect). Generally, clinicians should note whether a specific identifiable victim seems to be in imminent and probable danger from the threat of an action contemplated by a mentally ill patient; the harm, in addition to being imminent, should be potentially serious or severe. Usually, the patient must be a danger to another person and not to property; the therapist should take clinically reasonable action.

HOSPITALIZATION

All states provide for some form of involuntary hospitalization. Such action usually is taken when psychiatric patients present a danger to themselves or others in their environment to the extent that their urgent need for treatment in a closed institution is evident. Certain states allow involuntary hospitalization when patients are unable to care for themselves adequately.

The doctrine of *parens patriae* allows the state to intervene and to act as a surrogate parent for those who are unable to care for themselves or who may harm themselves. In English common law, *parens patriae* ("father of his country") dates to the time of King Edward I and originally referred to a monarch's duty to protect the people. In US common law, the doctrine has been transformed into a paternalism in which the state acts for persons who are mentally ill and for minors.

The statutes governing hospitalization of persons who are mentally ill generally have been designated commitment laws, but psychiatrists have long considered the term to be undesirable. *Commitment* legally means a warrant for imprisonment. The American Bar Association and the American Psychiatric Association have recommended that the term *commitment* be replaced by the less offensive and more accurate term *hospitalization*, which most states have adopted. Although this change in terminology does not correct the punitive attitudes of the past, the emphasis on hospitalization is in keeping with psychiatrists' views of treatment rather than punishment.

Procedures of Admission

Four procedures of admission to psychiatric facilities have been endorsed by the American Bar Association to safeguard civil liberties and to make sure that no person is railroaded into a mental hospital. Although each of the 50 states has the power to enact its own laws on psychiatric hospitalization, the procedures outlined here are gaining much acceptance.

Informal Admission. Informal admission operates on the general hospital model, in which a patient is admitted to a psychiatric unit of a general hospital in the same way that a medical or surgical patient is admitted. Under such circumstances, the ordinary doctor–patient relationship applies, with the patient free to enter and to leave, even against medical advice.

Voluntary Admission. In cases of voluntary admission, patients apply in writing for admission to a psychiatric hospital. They may come to the hospital on the advice of a personal physician, or they may seek help on their own. In either case, patients are admitted if an examination reveals the need for hospital treatment. The patient is free to leave, even against medical advice.

Temporary Admission. Temporary admission is used for patients who are so senile or so confused that they require hospitalization and are not able to make decisions on their own and for patients who are so acutely disturbed that they must be admitted immediately to a psychiatric hospital on an emergency basis. Under the procedure, a person is admitted to the hospital on the written recommendation of one physician. Once the patient has been admitted, the need for hospitalization must be confirmed by a psychiatrist on the hospital staff. The procedure is temporary because patients cannot be hospitalized against their will for more than 15 days.

Involuntary Admission. Involuntary admission involves the question of whether patients are suicidal and, thus, a danger to themselves or homicidal and, thus, a danger to others. Because these persons do not recognize their need for hospital care, the application for admission to a hospital may be made by a relative or a friend. Once the application is made, the patient must be examined by two physicians, and if both physicians confirm the need for hospitalization, the patient can then be admitted.

Involuntary hospitalization involves an established procedure for written notification of the next of kin. Furthermore, the patients have access at any time to legal counsel, who can bring the case before a judge. If the judge does not think that hospitalization is indicated, the patient's release can be ordered.

Involuntary admission allows a patient to be hospitalized for 60 days. After this time, if the patient is to remain hospitalized, the case must be reviewed periodically by a board consisting of psychiatrists, nonpsychiatric physicians, lawyers, and other citizens not connected with the institution. In New York State, the board is called the Mental Health Information Service.

Persons who have been hospitalized involuntarily and who believe that they should be released have the right to file a petition for a writ of habeas corpus. Under law, a writ of habeas corpus can be proclaimed by those who believe that they have been illegally deprived of liberty. The legal procedure asks a court to decide whether a patient has been hospitalized without due process of law. The case must be heard by a court at once, regardless of the manner or the form in which the motion is filed. Hospitals are obligated to submit the petitions to the court immediately.

RIGHT TO TREATMENT

Among the rights of patients, the right to the standard quality of care is fundamental. This right has been litigated in highly publicized cases in recent years under the slogan of "right to treatment."

In 1966, Judge David Bazelon, speaking for the District of Columbia Court of Appeals in *Rouse v. Cameron*, noted that the purpose of involuntary hospitalization is treatment and concluded that the absence of treatment draws into question the constitutionality of the confinement. Treatment in exchange for liberty is the logic of the ruling. In this case, the patient was discharged on a writ of habeas corpus, the basic legal remedy to ensure liberty. Judge Bazelon further held that, if alternative treatments that infringe less on personal liberty are available, involuntary hospitalization cannot take place.

Alabama Federal Court Judge Frank Johnson was more venturesome in the decree he rendered in 1971 in *Wyatt v. Stickney*. The *Wyatt* case was a class-action proceeding brought under newly developed rules that sought not release but treatment. Judge Johnson ruled that persons civilly committed to a mental institution have a constitutional right to receive such individual treatment as will give them a reasonable opportunity to be cured or to have their mental condition improved. Judge Johnson set out minimal requirements for staffing, specified physical facilities and nutritional standards, and required individualized treatment plans.

The new codes, more detailed than the old ones, include the right to be free from excessive or unnecessary medication; the right to privacy and dignity; the right to the least restrictive environment; the unrestricted right to be visited by attorneys, clergy, and private physicians; and the right not to be subjected to lobotomies, electroconvulsive treatments, and other procedures without fully informed consent. Patients can be required to perform therapeutic tasks, but not hospital chores, unless they volunteer for them and are paid the federal minimum wage. This requirement is an attempt to eliminate the practice of peonage, in which psychiatric patients were forced to work at menial tasks, without payment, for the benefit of the state.

In a number of states today, medication or electroconvulsive therapy cannot be forcibly administered to a patient without first obtaining court approval, which may take as long as 10 days.

RIGHT TO REFUSE TREATMENT

The right to refuse treatment is a legal doctrine that holds that, except in emergencies, persons cannot be forced to accept treatment against their will. An emergency is defined as a condition in clinical practice that requires immediate intervention to prevent death or serious harm to the patient or another person or to prevent deterioration of the patient's clinical state.

In the 1976 case of *O'Connor v. Donaldson*, the Supreme Court of the United States ruled that harmless mentally ill patients cannot be confined against their will without treatment if they can survive outside. According to the Court, a finding of mental illness alone cannot justify a state's confining persons in a hospital against their will. Instead, involuntarily confined patients must be considered dangerous to themselves or others or possibly so unable to care for themselves that they cannot survive outside. As a result of the 1979 case of *Rennie v. Klein*, patients have the right to refuse treatment and to use an appeal process. As a result of the 1981 case of *Roger v. Oken*, patients have an absolute right to refuse treatment, but a guardian may authorize treatment.

Questions have been raised about psychiatrists' ability to accurately predict dangerousness to self or others and about the risk to psychiatrists, who may be sued for monetary damages if persons who are involuntarily hospitalized are thereby deprived of their civil rights.

CIVIL RIGHTS OF PATIENTS

Because of several clinical, public, and legal movements, criteria for the civil rights of persons who are mentally ill, apart from their rights as patients, have been both established and affirmed.

Least Restrictive Alternative

The principle holds that patients have the right to receive the least restrictive means of treatment for the requisite clinical effect. Therefore, if a patient can be treated as an outpatient, commitment should not be used; if a patient can be treated on an open ward, seclusion should not be used.

Although apparently fairly straightforward on first reading, difficulty arises when clinicians attempt to apply the concept to choose among involuntary medication, seclusion, and restraint as the intervention of choice. Distinguishing among these interventions on the basis of restrictiveness proves to be a purely subjective exercise fraught with personal bias. Moreover, each of these three interventions is both more and less restrictive than each of the other two. Nevertheless, the effort should be made to think in terms of restrictiveness when deciding how to treat patients.

Visitation Rights

Patients have the right to receive visitors and to do so at reasonable hours (customary hospital visiting hours). Allowance must be made for the possibility that, at certain times, a patient's clinical condition may not permit visits. This fact should be clearly documented, however, because such rights must not be suspended without good reason.

Certain categories of visitors are not limited to the regular visiting hours; these include a patient's attorney, private physician, and members of the clergy—all of whom, broadly speaking, have unrestricted access to the patient, including the right to privacy in their discussions. Even here, a bona fide emergency may delay such visits. Again, the patient's needs come first. Under similar reasoning, certain noxious visits may be curtailed (e.g., a patient's relative bringing drugs into the ward).

Communication Rights

Patients should generally have free and open communication with the outside world by telephone or mail, but this right varies regionally to some degree. Some jurisdictions charge the hospital administration with a responsibility for monitoring the communications of patients. In some areas, hospitals are expected to make available reasonable supplies of paper, envelopes, and stamps for patient's use.

Specific circumstances affect communication rights. A patient who is hospitalized in relation to a criminal charge of making harassing or threatening phone calls should not be given unrestricted access to the telephone, and similar considerations apply to mail. As a rule, however, patients should be allowed private telephone calls, and their incoming and outgoing mail should not be opened by hospital staff members.

Private Rights

Patients have several rights to privacy. In addition to confidentiality, they are allowed private bathroom and shower space, secure storage space for clothing and other belongings, and adequate floor space per person. They also have the right to wear their own clothes and to carry their own money.

Economic Rights

Apart from special considerations related to incompetence, psychiatric patients generally are permitted to manage their own financial affairs. One feature of this fiscal right is the requirement that patients be paid if they work in the institution (e.g., gardening or preparing food). This right often creates tension between the valid therapeutic need for activity, including jobs, and exploitative labor. A consequence of this tension is that valuable occupational, vocational, and rehabilitative therapeutic programs may have to be eliminated because of the failure of legislatures to supply the funding to pay wages to patients who participate in these programs.

SECLUSION AND RESTRAINT

Seclusion and restraint raise complex psychiatric legal issues. Seclusion and restraint have both indications and contraindications (Table 58–2). Seclusion and restraint have become increasingly regulated over the past decade.

Legal challenges to the use of restraints and seclusion have been brought on behalf of institutionalized mentally ill and mentally retarded persons. Typically, these lawsuits do not stand alone but are part of a challenge to a wide range of alleged abuses.

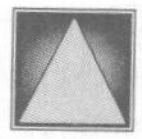

Table 58–2
Indications and Contraindications for Seclusion and Restraint

Indications
Prevent clear, imminent harm to the patient or others
Prevent significant disruption to treatment program or physical surroundings
Assist in treatment as part of ongoing behavior therapy
Decrease sensory overstimulation[a]
Patient's voluntary reasonable request

Contraindications
Extremely unstable medical and psychiatric conditions[b]
Delirious or demented patients who are unable to tolerate decreased stimulation[b]
Overtly suicidal patients[b]
Patients with severe drug reactions or overdoses or who require close monitoring of drug dosages[b]
For punishment or convenience of staff

[a]Seclusion only.
[b]Unless close supervision and direct observation are provided.
(Adapted from American Psychiatric Association. *The Psychiatric Uses of Seclusion and Restraint (Task Force Report No. 22)*. Washington, DC: American Psychiatric Association; 1985, with permission.)

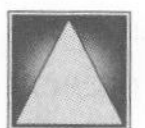

Table 58–3
Restrictions for Seclusion and Restraint

Restraints and seclusion can be implemented only when a patient creates a risk of harm to self or others and no less restrictive alternative is available.
Restraint and seclusion can only be implemented by a written order from an appropriate medical official.
Orders are to be confined to specific, time-limited periods.
A patient's condition must be regularly reviewed and documented.
Any extension of an original order must be reviewed and reauthorized

Generally, courts hold, or consent decrees provide, that restraints and seclusion be implemented only when a patient creates a risk of harm to self or others and no less restrictive alternative is available. Table 58–3 lists additional restrictions.

INFORMED CONSENT

Lawyers representing an injured claimant now invariably add to a claim of negligent performance of procedures (malpractice) an informed consent claim as another possible area of liability. Ironically, this is one claim under which the requirement of expert testimony may be avoided. The usual claim of medical malpractice requires the litigant to produce an expert to establish that the defendant physician departed from accepted medical practice. But in a case in which the physician did not obtain informed consent, the fact that the treatment was technically well performed, was in accord with the generally accepted standard of care, and effected a complete cure is immaterial. As a practical matter, however, unless the treatment had adverse consequences, a complainant will not get far with a jury in an action based solely on an allegation that the treatment was performed without consent.

In the case of minors, the parent or guardian is legally empowered to give consent to medical treatment. By statute, most states, however, list specific diseases and conditions that a minor can consent to have treated—including venereal disease, pregnancy, substance dependence, alcohol abuse, and contagious diseases. In an emergency, a physician can treat a minor without parental consent. The trend is to adopt the so-called mature minor rule, which allows minors to consent to treatment under ordinary circumstances. As a result of the Supreme Court's 1967 *Gault* decision, all juveniles must now be represented by counsel, must be able to confront witnesses, and must be given proper notice of any charges. Emancipated minors have the rights of an adult when it can be shown that they are living as adults with control over their own lives.

Consent Form

The basic elements of a consent form should include a fair explanation of the procedures to be followed and their purposes, including identification of any procedures that are experimental; a description of any attendant discomforts and risks reasonably to be expected; a description of any benefits reasonably to be expected; a disclosure of any appropriate alternative procedures that may be advantageous to the patient; an offer to answer any inquiries concerning the procedures; and an instruction that the patient is free to withdraw patient consent and to discontinue participation in the project or activity at any time without prejudice.

Some theorists have suggested that the form can be replaced by a standardized discussion that covers the issues noted above and a progress note that documents that the issues were discussed.

CHILD CUSTODY

The action of a court in a child-custody dispute is now predicated on the child's best interests. The maxim reflects the idea that a natural parent does not have an inherent right to be named a custodial parent, but the presumption, although a bit eroded, remains in favor of the mother in the case of young children. As a rule, the courts presume that the welfare of a child of tender years generally is best served by maternal custody when the mother is a good and fit parent. The best interest of the mother may be served by naming her as the custodial parent, because a mother may never resolve the effects of the loss of a child, but her best interest is not to be equated ipso facto with the best interest of the child. Care and protection proceedings are the court's interventions in the welfare of a child when the parents are unable to care for the child.

More fathers are asserting custodial claims. In about 5 percent of all cases, fathers are named custodians. The movement supporting women's rights also is enhancing the chances of paternal custody. With more women going to work outside the home, the traditional rationale for maternal custody has less force today than it did in the past.

Currently, every state has a statute allowing a court, usually a juvenile court, to assume jurisdiction over a neglected or abused child and to remove the child from parental custody. It usually orders that the care and custody of the child be supervised by the welfare or probation department.

TESTAMENTARY AND CONTRACTUAL CAPACITY AND COMPETENCE

Psychiatrists may be asked to evaluate patients' testamentary capacities or their competence to make a will. Three psychological abilities are necessary to prove this competence. Patients must know the nature and the extent of their bounty (property), the fact that they are making a bequest, and the identities of their natural beneficiaries (spouse, children, and other relatives).

When a will is being probated, one of the heirs or another person may challenge its validity. A judgment in such cases must be based on a reconstruction, using data from documents and from expert psychiatric testimony, of the testator's mental state at the time the will was written. When a person is unable to, or does not exercise the right to, make a will, the law in all states provides for the distribution of property to the heirs. If there are no heirs, the estate goes to the public treasury.

Witnesses at the signing of a will, who might include a psychiatrist, may attest that the testator was rational at the time the will was executed. In unusual cases, a lawyer may videotape the signing to safeguard the will from attack. Ideally, persons who are thinking of making a will and believe that questions might be raised about their testamentary competence hire a forensic psychiatrist to perform a dispassionate examination antemortem to validate and record their capacity.

An incompetence proceeding and the appointment of a guardian may be considered necessary when a family member is spending the family's assets and the property is in danger of dissipation, as in the case of aged, retarded, alcohol-dependent, and psychotic persons. At issue is whether such persons are capable of managing their own affairs. A guardian appointed to take control of the property of one deemed incompetent, however, cannot make a will for the ward (the incompetent person).

Competence is determined on the basis of a person's ability to make a sound judgment—to weigh, to reason, and to make reasonable decisions. Competence is task specific, not general; the capacity to weigh decision-making factors (competence) often is best demonstrated by a person's ability to ask pertinent and knowledgeable questions after the risks and the benefits have been explained. Although physicians (especially psychiatrists) often give opinions on competence, only a judge's ruling converts the opinion into a finding; a patient is not competent or incompetent until the court so rules. The diagnosis of a mental disorder is not, in itself, sufficient to warrant a finding of incompetence. Instead, the mental disorder must cause an impairment in judgment for the specific issues involved. After they have been declared incompetent, persons are deprived of certain rights: they cannot make contracts, marry, start a divorce action, drive a vehicle, handle their own property, or practice their professions. Incompetence is decided at a formal courtroom proceeding, and the court usually appoints a guardian who will best serve a patient's interests. Another hearing is necessary to declare a patient competent. Admission to a mental hospital does not automatically mean that a person is incompetent.

Competence also is essential in contracts, because a contract is an agreement between parties to do a specific act. A contract is declared invalid, if, when it was signed, one of the parties was unable to comprehend the nature and effect of his or her act. The marriage contract is subject to the same standard and, thus, can be voided if either party did not understand the nature, duties, obligations, and other characteristics entailed at the time of the marriage. In general, however, the courts are unwilling to declare a marriage void on the basis of incompetence.

Whether competence is related to wills, contracts, or the making or breaking of marriages, the fundamental concern is a person's state of awareness and capacity to comprehend the significance of the particular commitment made.

Durable Power of Attorney

A modern development that permits persons to make provisions for their own anticipated loss of decision-making capacity is called a *durable power of attorney*. The document permits the advance selection of a substitute decision maker who can act without the necessity of court proceedings when the signatory becomes incompetent through illness or progressive dementia.

CRIMINAL LAW

Competence to Stand Trial

The Supreme Court of the United States stated that the prohibition against trying someone who is mentally incompetent is fundamental to the US system of justice. Accordingly, the Court, in *Dusky v. United States*, approved a test of competence that seeks to ascertain whether a criminal defendant "has sufficient present ability to consult with his lawyer with a reasonable degree of rational understanding—and whether he has a rational as well as factual understanding of the proceedings against him."

Competence to Be Executed

One of the new areas of competence to emerge in the interface between psychiatry and the law is the question of a person's competence to be executed. The requirement for competence in this area is believed to rest on three general principles. First, a person's awareness of what is happening is supposed to heighten the retributive element of the punishment. Punishment is meaningless unless the person is aware of it and knows the punishment's purpose. Second, a competent person who is about to be executed is believed to be in the best position to make whatever peace is appropriate with religious beliefs, including confession and absolution. Third, a competent person who is about to be executed preserves, until the end, the possibility (admittedly slight) of recalling a forgotten detail of the events or the crime that may prove exonerating.

The need to preserve competence was supported recently in the Supreme Court case of *Ford v. Wainwright*. But no matter the outcome of legal struggles with this question, most medical bodies have gravitated toward the position that it is unethical for any clinician to participate, no matter how remotely, in state-mandated executions; a physician's duty to preserve life transcends all other competing requirements. Major medical societies, such as the American Medical Association (AMA) believe that doctors should not participate in the death penalty. A psychiatrist who agrees to examine a patient slated for execution may find the person incompetent on the basis of a mental disorder and may recommend a treatment plan, which, if implemented, would ensure the person's fitness to be executed. Although room exists for a difference of opinion regarding whether or not a psychiatrist should become involved, the authors of this text believe such involvement to be wrong.

Criminal Responsibility

According to criminal law, committing an act that is socially harmful is not the sole criterion of whether a crime has been committed. Instead, the objectionable act must have two components: voluntary conduct (*actus reus*) and evil intent (*mens rea*). An evil intent cannot exist when an offender's mental status is so deficient, so abnormal, or so diseased to have deprived the offender of the capacity for rational intent. The law can be invoked only when an illegal intent is implemented. Neither behavior, however harmful, nor the intent to do harm is, in itself, a ground for criminal action.

M'Naghten Rule. The precedent for determining legal responsibility was established in 1843 in the British courts. The so-called M'Naghten rule, which, until recently, has determined criminal responsibility in most of the United States, holds that persons are not guilty by reason of insanity if they labored under a mental disease such that they were unaware of the nature, the quality, and the consequences of their acts or if they were incapable of realizing that their acts were wrong. Moreover, to

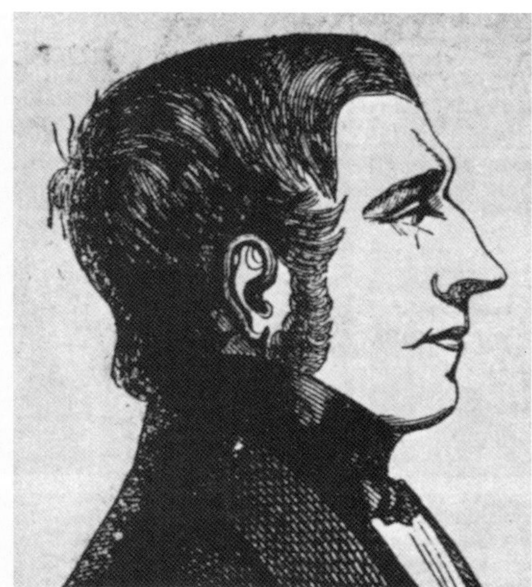

FIGURE 58–1
Daniel M'Naghten. His 1843 murder trial led to the establishment of rules still generally observed in legal insanity pleas. (Courtesy of Culver Pictures.)

absolve persons from punishment, a delusion used as evidence must be one that, if true, would be an adequate defense. If the delusional idea does not justify the crime, such persons are presumably held responsible, guilty, and punishable. The M'Naghten rule is known commonly as the right-wrong test.

The M'Naghten rule derives from the famous M'Naghten case of 1843 (Fig. 58–1). When Daniel M'Naghten murdered Edward Drummond, the private secretary of Robert Peel, M'Naghten had been suffering from delusions of persecution for several years, had complained to many persons about his "persecutors," and finally had decided to correct the situation by murdering Robert Peel. When Drummond came out of Peel's home, M'Naghten shot Drummond, mistaking him for Peel. The jury, as instructed under the prevailing law, found M'Naghten not guilty by reason of insanity. In response to questions about what guidelines could be used to determine whether a person could plead insanity as a defense against criminal responsibility, the English chief judge wrote:

1. To establish a defense on the ground of insanity, it must be clearly proved that, at the time of committing the act, the party accused was laboring under such a defect of reason, from disease of the mind, as not to know the nature and quality of the act he was doing, or if he did know it, he did not know he was doing what was wrong.
2. Where a person labors under partial delusions only and is not in other respects insane and as a result commits an offense, he must be considered in the same situation regarding responsibility as if the facts with respect to which the delusion exists were real.

According to the M'Naghten rule, the question is not whether the accused knows the difference between right and wrong in general, it is whether the defendant understood the nature and the quality of the act and whether the defendant knew the difference between right and wrong with respect to the act—that is, specifically whether the defendant knew the act was wrong or perhaps thought the act was correct, a delusion causing the defendant to act in legitimate self-defense.

Jeffery Dahmer (Fig. 58–2) killed 17 young men and boys between June 1978 and July 1991. Most of his victims were either homosexual or bisexual. He would meet and select his prey at gay bars or bathhouses and then lure them by offering them money for posing for photographs or simply to enjoy some beer and videos. Then he would drug them, strangle them, masturbate on the body or have sex with the corpse, dismember the body and dispose of it. Sometimes, he would keep the skull or other body parts as souvenirs.

On July 13, 1992, Dahmer changed his plea to guilty by means of insanity. That Dahmer could plan his murders and systematically dispose of the bodies convinced the jury, however, that he was able to control his behavior. All of the testimony bolstered the notion that, as with most serial killers, Dahmer knew what he was doing and knew right from wrong. Finally, the jury did not accept the defense that Dahmer experienced a mental illness to the degree that it had disabled his thinking or behavioral controls. Dahmer was sentenced to 15 consecutive life terms or a total of 957 years in prison. He was killed by an inmate on November 28, 1994.

Irresistible Impulse. In 1922, a committee of jurists in England reexamined the M'Naghten rule. The committee suggested broadening the concept of insanity in criminal cases to include the irresistible impulse test, which rules that a person charged with a criminal offense is not responsible for an act if the act was committed under an impulse that the person was unable to resist because of mental disease. The courts have chosen to interpret this concept in such a way that it has been called the *policeman-at-the-elbow law*. In other words, the court grants an impulse to be irresistible only when it can be determined that the accused would have committed the act even if a policeman had been at the accused's elbow. To most psychiatrists, this interpretation is unsatisfactory, because it covers only a small, special group of those who are mentally ill.

Durham Rule. In the case of *Durham v. United States*, Judge Bazelon handed down a decision in 1954 in the District of Columbia Court of Appeals. The decision resulted in the product rule of criminal responsibility, namely that an accused is not criminally responsible if his or her unlawful act was the product of mental disease or mental defect. In the Durham case, Judge Bazelon expressly stated that the purpose of the rule was to get good and complete psychiatric testimony. He sought to release the criminal law from the theoretical straitjacket of the M'Naghten rule, but judges and juries in cases using the *Durham* rule became mired in confusion over the terms "product," "disease," and "defect." In 1972, some 18 years after the rule's adoption, the Court of Appeals for the District of Columbia, in *United States v. Brawner*, discarded the rule. The court—all nine members, including Judge Bazelon—decided in a 143-page opinion to throw out its *Durham* rule and to adopt in its place the test recommended in 1962 by the American Law Institute in its model penal code, which is the law in the federal courts today.

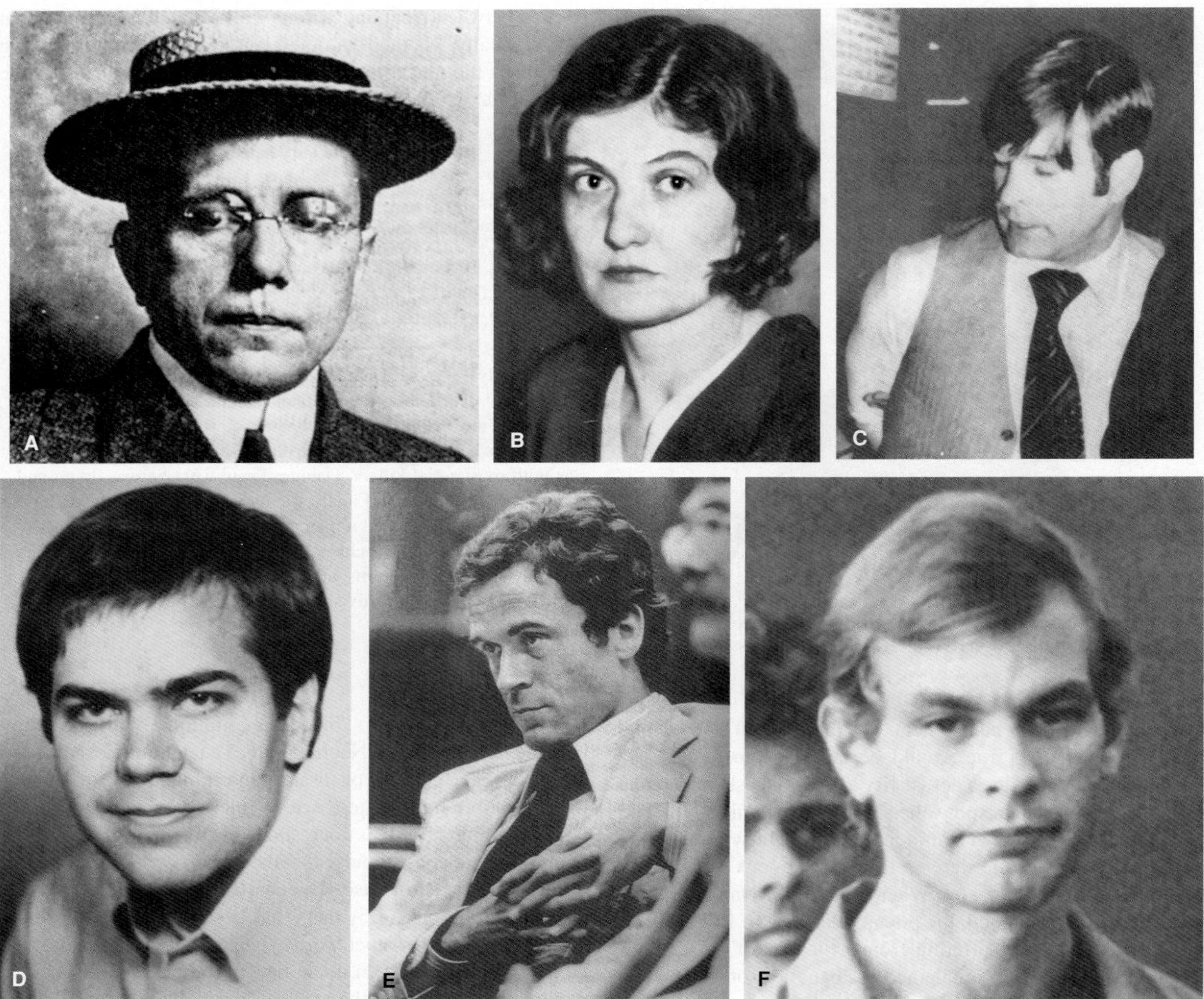

FIGURE 58–2
Cases of persons in the legal system. **A.** Harry K. Thaw. In 1908 Thaw, a millionaire playboy, was convicted of killing architect Stanford White at Madison Square Garden in New York City. He was found legally insane and sent to a mental institution from which he was ultimately released in 1924. He died in Florida in 1947 at the age of 76. **B.** Winnie Ruth Judd. Known as the "trunk murderess" of the early 1930's, Judd was saved from execution by a sanity hearing. She was committed in an Arizona state hospital from which she made her seventh escape in 1962. She was found in 1969 working as a receptionist. An Arizona Board of Pardons and Parole recommended her freedom in 1971. She died in 1998 at age 93. **C.** Dan White. The former San Francisco supervisor killed San Francisco mayor George Moscone and supervisor Harvey Milk at City Hall in 1978. White's "Twinkie defense" helped reduce his crime from murder to manslaughter, for which he served 5 years. White committed suicide a few days after he was released from prison. **D.** John Hinckley, Jr., who attempted to assassinate President Ronald Reagan in 1981, was declared not guilty by reason of insanity. He is currently a patient in a mental hospital in Washington, DC. **E.** Serial killer Ted Bundy exhibited antisocial behavior at its most extreme and dangerous. Bundy was executed in Florida in 1989 after confessing, without showing any remorse, to the murder of 36 women (some authorities estimate the number was probably closer to 100). **F.** Jeffrey Dahmer. His murder trail for the deaths of 17 young men and boys gained widespread notoriety after accusations of cannibalistic practices were made. Dahmer was killed in prison by a psychotic inmate in 1994. (Figure A, courtesy of United Press International, Inc.; Figures B-F courtesy of World Wide Photos.)

Model Penal Code. In its model penal code, the American Law Institute recommended the following test of criminal responsibility: Persons are not responsible for criminal conduct if, at the time of such conduct, as a result of mental disease or defect, they lacked substantial capacity either to appreciate the criminality (wrongfulness) of their conduct or to conform their conduct to the requirement of the law. The term *mental disease or defect* does not include an abnormality manifest only by repeated criminal or otherwise antisocial conduct.

Subsection 1 of the American Law Institute rule contains five operative concepts: mental disease or defect, lack of substantial capacity, appreciation, wrongfulness, and conformity of conduct to the requirements of law. The rule's second subsection, stating that repeated criminal or antisocial conduct is not, of itself, to be taken as mental disease or defect, aims to keep the sociopath or psychopath within the scope of criminal responsibility.

Guilty but Mentally Ill. Some states have established an alternative verdict of guilty but mentally ill. Under guilty but mentally ill statutes, this alternative verdict is available to the jury if the defendant pleads not guilty by reason of insanity. Under an insanity plea, four outcomes are possible: not guilty, not guilty by reason of insanity, guilty but mentally ill, and guilty.

The problem with guilty but mentally ill is that it is an alternative verdict without a difference. It is basically the same as finding the defendant just plain guilty. The court must still impose a sentence on the convicted person. Although the convicted person supposedly receives psychiatric treatment, if necessary, this treatment provision is available to all prisoners.

Some famous cases of persons declared not guilty by reason of insanity are illustrated in Figure 58–2.

OTHER AREAS OF FORENSIC PSYCHIATRY

Emotional Damage and Distress

A rapidly rising trend in recent years is to sue for psychological and emotional damage, both secondary to physical injury or as a consequence of witnessing a stressful act and from the suffering endured under the stress of such circumstances as concentration camp experiences. The German government heard many of these claims from persons detained in Nazi camps during World War II. In the United States, the courts have moved from a conservative to a liberal position in awarding damages for such claims. Psychiatric examinations and testimony are sought in these cases, often by both the plaintiffs and the defendants.

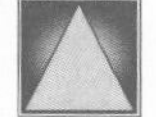

Table 58–4
Risk Management Principles for Cases of Recovered Memories of Abuse in Psychotherapy

1. Maintain therapist neutrality: Do not suggest abuse.
2. Stay clinically focused: Provide adequate evaluation and treatment for patients presenting problems and symptoms.
3. Carefully document the memory recovery process.
4. Manage personal bias and countertransference.
5. Avoid mixing treater and expert witness roles.
6. Closely monitor supervisory and collaborative therapy relationships.
7. Clarify nontreatment roles with family members.
8. Avoid special techniques (e.g., hypnosis or sodium amobarbital [Amytal]) unless clearly indicated; obtain consultation first.
9. Stay within professional competence: Do not take cases that you cannot handle.
10. Distinguish between narrative truth and historical truth.
11. Obtain consultation in problematic cases.
12. Foster patient autonomy and self-determination: Do not suggest lawsuits.
13. In managed care settings, inform patients with recovered memories that more than brief therapy may be required.
14. When making public statements, distinguish personal opinions from scientifically established facts.
15. Stop and refer, if uncomfortable with a patient who is recovering memories of childhood abuse.
16. Do not be afraid to ask about abuse as part of a competent psychiatric evaluation.

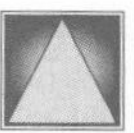

Table 58–5
Sexual Exploitation: Legal and Ethical Consequences

Civil lawsuit
  Negligence
  Loss of consortium
Breach-of-contract action
Criminal sanctions (e.g., statutory, adultery, sexual assault, rape)
Civil action for intentional tort (e.g., battery, fraud)
License revocation
Ethical sanctions
Dismissal from professional organizations

(From Simon RI. *Clinical Psychiatry and the Law.* 2nd ed. Washington, DC: American Psychiatric Press; 1992, with permission.)

Recovered Memories

Patients alleging recovered memories of abuse have sued parents and other alleged perpetrators. In a number of instances, the alleged victimizers have sued therapists who, they claim, negligently induced false memories of sexual abuse. In an about-face, some patients have recanted and joined forces with others (usually their parents) to sue therapists.

Courts have handed down multimillion dollar judgments against mental health practitioners. A fundamental allegation in these cases is that the therapist abandoned a position of neutrality to suggest, to persuade, to coerce, and to implant false memories of childhood sexual abuse. The guiding principle of clinical risk management in recovered memory cases is maintenance of therapist neutrality and establishment of sound treatment boundaries. Table 58–4 lists the risk management principles that should be considered when evaluating or treating a patient who recovers memories of abuse in psychotherapy.

Worker's Compensation

The stresses of employment can cause or accentuate mental illness. Patients are entitled to be compensated for their job-related disabilities or to receive disability retirement benefits. A psychiatrist is often called on to evaluate such situations.

Civil Liability

Psychiatrists who sexually exploit their patients are subject to civil and criminal actions in addition to ethical and professional licensure revocation proceedings. Malpractice is the most common legal action (Table 58–5).

References

Adshead G. Evidence-based medicine and medicine-based evidence: The expert witness in cases of factitious disorder by proxy. *J Am Acad Psychiatry Law.* 2005;33:99–105.

Arboleda-Florez JE. The ethics of forensic psychiatry. *Current Opinion in Psych.* 2006;19(5):544.

Baker T. *The Medical Malpractice Myth.* Chicago: University of Chicago Press; 2005.

Billick SB, Ciric SJ. Role of the psychiatric evaluator in child custody disputes. In: Rosner R, ed. *Principles and Practice of Forensic Psychiatry,* 2nd ed. New York: Chapman & Hall; 2003.

Meyer DJ, Price M. Forensic psychiatric assessments of behaviorally disruptive physicians. *J Am Acad Psychiatry Law.* 2006;34:1:72–81.

Reid WH. Forensic practice: A day in the life. *Journal of Psychiatric Practice.* 2006;12(1):50.

Rogers R, Shuman DW. *Fundamentals of Forensic Practice: Mental Health and Criminal Law.* New York: Springer Science + Business Media; 2005.

Rosner R, ed. *Principles and Practice of Forensic Psychiatry.* 2nd ed. New York: Chapman & Hall; 2003.

Simon RI. Clinical-legal issues in psychiatry. In: Sadock BJ, Sadock VA, eds.

Kaplan & Sadock's Comprehensive Textbook of Psychiatry. 8th ed. Vol. 2. Baltimore: Lippincott Williams & Wilkins; 2005:3969.

Simon RI, ed. *Posttraumatic Stress Disorder in Litigation.* 2nd ed. Washington, DC: American Psychiatric Publishing, Inc; 2003.

Simon RI, Gold LH. *The American Psychiatric Publishing Textbook of Forensic Psychiatry.* Washington, DC: American Psychiatric Publishing; 2004.

Studdert DM, Mello MM, Gawande AA, Gandhi TK, Kachalia A, Yoon C, Puopolo AL, Brennan TA. Claims, errors, and compensation payments in medical malpractice litigation. *N Engl J Med.* 2006;354(19):2024–2033.

Wecht CH. The history of legal medicine. *J Am Acad Psychiatry Law*. 2005; 33(2): 245.

59 Ethics in Psychiatry

Ethical guidelines and a knowledge of ethical principles help psychiatrists avoid *ethical conflicts* (which can be defined as tension between what one wants to do and what is ethically right to do) and think through *ethical dilemmas* (conflicts between ethical perspectives or values).

Ethics deal with the relations between people in different groups and often entail balancing rights. *Professional ethics* refer to the appropriate way to act when in a professional role. Professional ethics derive from a combination of morality, social norms, and the parameters of the relationship people have agreed to have.

PROFESSIONAL CODES

Most professional organizations and many business groups have codes of ethics that reflect a consensus about the general standards of appropriate professional conduct. The American Medical Association's *Principles of Medical Ethics* and the American Psychiatric Association's (APA) *Principles of Medical Ethics with Annotations Especially Applicable to Psychiatry* articulate ideal standards of practice and professional virtues of practitioners. These codes include exhortations to use skillful and scientific techniques, to self-regulate misconduct within the profession, and to respect the rights and needs of patients, families, colleagues, and society. A summary of these principles is provided in Table 59–1.

BASIC ETHICAL PRINCIPLES

Four ethical principles that psychiatrists ought to weigh in their work are respect for autonomy, beneficence, nonmaleficence, and justice. At times, they are in conflict, and decisions must be made concerning how to balance them.

Respect for Autonomy

Autonomy requires that a person act intentionally after being given sufficient information and time to understand the benefits, risks, and costs of all reasonable options. It may mean honoring an individual's right not to hear every detail and even choosing someone else (e.g., family or doctor) to decide the best course of treatment.

Psychiatrists need to provide patients with a rational understanding of their disorder and options for treatment. Patients need conceptual understanding; the psychiatrist should not simply state isolated facts. Patients also need time to think and to talk with friends and family about their decision. Finally, if a patient is not in a state of mind to make decisions for himself or herself, the psychiatrist should consider mechanisms for alternative decision-making, such as guardianship, conservators, and health care proxy.

A young adult experienced a schizophrenic episode in which his religious fervor turned into psychotic delusions. After being involuntarily hospitalized because he became suicidal, he insistently refused medication, claiming that his physicians were trying to poison him. His psychiatrist decided to respect his refusal of medication as long as his suicidal tendencies could be controlled. As his mental suffering became more intense, in 1 week, the patient changed his mind about medication and agreed to try it. The therapeutic relationship with his psychiatrist deepened, and the patient left the hospital willing to continue with both antipsychotic medication and psychotherapy. Although not all cases work out so well, this one illustrates the benefits of negotiation about treatment even when hopitalization is involuntary.

Beneficence

The requirement for psychiatrists to act with beneficence derives from their fiduciary relationship with patients and the profession's belief that they also have an obligation to society. As a result of the role obligation of trust, psychiatrists must heed their patients' interests, even to the neglect of their own.

The expression of the principle is paternalism, the use of the psychiatrist's judgment about the best course of action for the patient or research subject. *Weak paternalism* is acting beneficently when the patient's impaired faculties prevent an autonomous choice. *Strong paternalism* is acting beneficently, despite the patient's intact autonomy.

Guidelines have been proposed for permitting beneficence to overrule patient autonomy; when the patient faces substantial harm or risk of harm, the paternalistic act is chosen that ensures the optimal combination of maximal harm reduction, low added risk, and minimal necessary infringement on patient autonomy.

Nonmaleficence

To adhere to the principle of nonmaleficence (*primum non nocere* or *first do no harm*), psychiatrists must be careful in their decisions and actions and must ensure that they have had adequate training for what they do. They also need to be open to

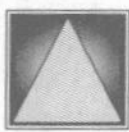

Table 59–1
The Principles of Medical Ethics with Annotations Especially Applicable to Psychiatry

Each of the AMA principles of medical ethics printed separately (in italics) along with annotations especially applicable to psychiatry.

Preamble

The medical profession has long subscribed to a body of ethical statements developed primarily for the benefit of the patient. As a member of this profession, a physician must recognize responsibility not only to patients but also to society, to other health professionals, and to self. The following Principles, adopted by the American Medical Association, are not laws but standards of conduct, which define the essentials of honorable behavior for the physician.

Section 1

A physician shall be dedicated to providing competent medical service with compassion and respect for human dignity.[a]

1. A psychiatrist shall not gratify his/her own needs by exploiting a patient. The psychiatrist shall be ever vigilant about the impact that his/her conduct has upon the boundaries of the doctor–patient relationship and thus upon the well-being of the patient. These requirements become particularly important because of the essentially private, highly personal, and sometimes intensely emotional nature of the relationship with the psychiatrist.
2. A psychiatrist should not be a party to any type of policy that excludes, segregates, or demeans the dignity of any patient because of ethnic origin, race, sex, creed, age, socioeconomic status, or sexual orientation.
3. In accord with the requirements of law and accepted medical practice, it is ethical for a physician to submit his/her work to peer review and to the ultimate authority of the medical staff executive body and the hospital administration and its governing body.
4. A psychiatrist should not be a participant in a legally authorized execution.

Section 2

A physician shall deal honestly with patients and colleagues, and strive to expose those physicians deficient in character or competence, or who engage in fraud or deception.

1. The requirement that the physician conduct himself/herself with propriety in his/her profession and in all the actions of his/her life is especially important for the psychiatrist because the patient tends to model his/her behavior on that of his/her psychiatrist by identification. Further, the necessary intensity of the treatment relationship may tend to activate sexual and other needs and fantasies of both patient and psychiatrist, while weakening the objectivity necessary for control. Additionally, the inherent inequality in the doctor–patient relationship may lead to exploitation of the patient. Sexual activity with a current or former patient is unethical.
2. The psychiatrist should diligently guard against exploiting information furnished by the patient and should not use the unique position of power afforded by the psychotherapeutic situation to influence patients in any way not directly relevant to the treatment goals.
3. A psychiatrist who regularly practices outside his/her area of professional competence should be considered unethical. Determination of professional competence should be made by peer review boards or other appropriate bodies.
4. Special consideration should be given to psychiatrists who, due to illness, jeopardize the welfare of their patients and their own reputations and practices. It is ethical, even encouraged, for another psychiatrist to intercede in such situations.
5. Psychiatric services, like all medical services, are dispensed in the context of a contractual arrangement between the patient and the treating physician. The provisions of the contractual arrangement, which are binding on both the physician and the patient, should be explicitly established.
6. It is ethical for a psychiatrist to make a charge for a missed appointment when it falls within the terms of the specific contractual agreement with the patient. Charging for a missed appointment or for one not canceled 24 hours in advance need not, in itself, be considered unethical if a patient is fully advised that the physician will make such a charge. The practice, however, should be resorted to infrequently and always with the utmost consideration for the patient and his/her circumstances.
7. An arrangement in which a psychiatrist provides supervision or administration to other physicians or nonmedical persons for a percentage of their fees or gross income is not acceptable; this would constitute fee splitting.

Section 3

A physician shall respect the law and also recognize a responsibility to seek changes in those requirements which are contrary to the best interests of the patient.

1. It would seem self-evident that a psychiatrist who is a law-breaker might be ethically unsuited to practice his/her profession. When such illegal activities bear directly upon his/her practice, this would obviously be the case. However, in other instances, illegal activities such as those concerning the right to protest social injustices might not bear on either the image of the psychiatrist or the ability of the specific psychiatrist to treat his/her patient ethically and well.

Section 4

A physician shall respect the rights of patients, of colleagues, and of other health professionals, and shall safeguard patient confidences within the constraints of the law.

1. Psychiatric records, including even the identification of a person as a patient, must be protected with extreme care. Confidentiality is essential to psychiatric treatment. This is based in part on the special nature of psychiatric therapy as well as on the traditional ethical relationship between physician and patient. Growing concern regarding the civil rights of patients and the possible adverse effects of computerization, duplication equipment, and data banks make the dissemination of confidential information an increasing hazard. Because of the sensitive and private nature of the information with which the psychiatrist deals, he/she must be circumspect in the information that he/she chooses to disclose to others about a patient. The welfare of the patient must be a continuing consideration.
2. A psychiatrist may release confidential information only with the authorization of the patient or under proper legal compulsion. The continuing duty of the psychiatrist to protect patients includes fully apprising him/her of the connotations of waiving the privilege of privacy. This may become an issue when the patient is being investigated by a government agency, is applying for a position, or is involved in legal action. The same principles apply to the release of information concerning treatment to medical departments of government agencies, business organizations, labor unions, and insurance companies. Information gained in confidence about patients seen in student health services should not be released without the students' explicit permission.
3. Clinical and other materials used in teaching and writing must be adequately disguised to preserve the anonymity of the individuals involved.
4. The ethical responsibility of maintaining confidentiality holds equally for consultations in which the patient may not have been present and in which the consultee was not a physician. In such instances, the physician consultant should alert the consultee to his/her duty of confidentiality.
5. Ethically, the psychiatrist may disclose only the information that is relevant to a given situation. He/she should avoid offering speculation as fact. Sensitive information such as an individual's sexual orientation or fantasy material is usually unnecessary.
6. Psychiatrists are often asked to examine individuals for security purposes, to determine suitability for various jobs, and to determine legal competence. The psychiatrist must fully describe the nature, purpose, and lack of confidentiality of the examination to the examinee at the beginning of the examination.

(*continued*)

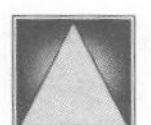

Table 59–1 (Continued)

7. Careful judgment must be exercised by the psychiatrist to include, when appropriate, the parents or guardian in the treatment of a minor. At the same time, the psychiatrist must assure the minor proper confidentiality.
8. When in the clinical judgment of the treating psychiatrist the risk of danger is deemed to be significant, the psychiatrist may reveal confidential information disclosed by the patient.
9. When the psychiatrist is ordered by the court to reveal the confidences entrusted to him/her by patients, he/she may comply or he/she may ethically hold the right to dissent within the framework of the law. When a psychiatrist is in doubt, the right of the patient to confidentiality and, by extension, to unimpaired treatment, should be given priority. The psychiatrist should reserve the right to raise the question of adequate need for disclosure. In the event the necessity for legal disclosure is demonstrated by the court, the psychiatrist may request the right to disclose only that information which is relevant to the legal question at hand.
10. With regard for the person's dignity and privacy and with truly informed consent, it is ethical to present a patient to a scientific gathering if the confidentiality of the presentation is understood and accepted by the audience.
11. When involved in funded research, the ethical psychiatrist advises human subjects of the funding source, retains his/her freedom to reveal data and results, and follows all appropriate and current guidelines relative to human subject protection.
12. Ethical considerations in medical practice preclude the psychiatric evaluation of any person charged with criminal acts prior to access to, or availability of, legal council. The only exception is rendering care to the person for the sole purpose of medical treatment.
13. Sexual involvement between a faculty member or supervisor and a trainee or student, in situations in which an abuse of power can occur, often takes advantage of inequalities in the working relationship and may be unethical because (a) any treatment of a patient being supervised may be deleteriously affected; (b) it may damage the trust relationship between teacher and student; and (c) teachers are important professional role models for their trainees and affect their trainees' future professional behavior.

Section 5

A physician shall continue to study, apply, and advance scientific knowledge, make relevant information available to patients, colleagues, and the public, obtain consultation, and use the talents of other health professionals when indicated.

1. Psychiatrists are responsible for their own continuing education and should remember that theirs must be a lifetime of learning.
2. In the practice of their specialty, the psychiatrists consult, associate, collaborate, or integrate their work with that of many professionals, including psychologists, psychometricians, social workers, alcoholism counselors, marriage counselors, and public health nurses. Furthermore, the nature of modern psychiatric practice extends the psychiatrist's contacts to such people as teachers, juvenile and adult probation officers, attorneys, welfare workers, agency volunteers, and neighborhood aides. Psychiatrists should ensure that the allied professionals or paraprofessionals with whom they are dealing and who refer patients for treatment, counseling, or rehabilitation are recognized members of their own discipline and are competent to carry out the therapeutic task required. Psychiatrists should have the same altitude toward members of the medical profession to whom they refer patients. Psychiatrists should not refer patients whenever they have reason to doubt the training, skill, or ethical qualifications of the allied professional.
3. When psychiatrists assume a collaborative or supervisory role with another mental health worker, they must expend sufficient time to ensure that proper care is given. It is contrary to the interests of the patient and to patient care if they allow themselves to be used as a figurehead.
4. In relationships between psychiatrists and practicing licensed psychologists, physicians should not delegate to the psychologist or, in fact, to any nonmedical person any matter requiring the exercise of professional medical judgment.
5. Psychiatrists should agree to the request of a patient for consultation or to such a request from the family of an incompetent or minor patient. Psychiatrists may suggest possible consultants, but the patient or family should be given free choice of the consultant. If psychiatrists disapprove of the professional qualifications of the consultant or if they cannot resolve difference of opinion they may, after suitable notice, withdraw from the case. If this disagreement occurs within an institution or agency framework, the differences should be resolved by mediation or arbitration by higher professional authority within the institution or agency.

Section 6

A physician shall, in the provision of appropriate patient care, except in emergencies, be free to choose whom to serve, with whom to associate, and the environment in which to provide medical services.

1. Physicians generally agree that the doctor–patient relationship is such a vital factor in effective treatment of the patient that preservation of optimal conditions for development of a sound working relationship between the doctors and their patient should take precedence over all other considerations.

Section 7

A physician shall recognize a responsibility to participate in activities contributing to an improved community.

1. Psychiatrists should foster the cooperation of those legitimately concerned with the medical, psychological, social, and legal aspects of mental health and illness. Psychiatrists are encouraged to serve society by advising and consulting with the executive, legislative, and judiciary branches of the government. Psychiatrists should clarify whether they speak as an individual or as a representative of an organization. Furthermore, psychiatrists should avoid cloaking their public statements with the authority of the profession (e.g., "Psychiatrists know that....")
2. Psychiatrists may interpret and share with the public their expertise in the various psychosocial issues that may affect mental health and illness. Psychiatrists should always be mindful of their separate roles as dedicated citizens and as experts in psychological medicine.
3. On occasion psychiatrists are asked for an opinion about individuals who are in the light of public attention or who have disclosed information about themselves through public media. In such circumstance, psychiatrists may share their expertise about psychiatric issues in general with the public. However, it is unethical for psychiatrists to offer a professional opinion about a specific individual unless they have conducted an examination and have been granted proper authorization for such a statement.
4. Psychiatrists may permit their certification to be used for the involuntary treatment of any person only after their personal examination of that person. To do so, they must find that the person, because of mental illness, cannot form a judgment about what is in his/her own best interests and that without such treatment, substantial impairment is likely to occur to that person or others.

[a]Statements in italics are taken directly from the American Medical Association's Principles of Medical Ethics. Reprinted with permission from American Psychiatric Association. *The Principles of Medical Ethics with Annotations Especially Applicable to Psychiatry.* Washington, DC: American Psychiatric Association; 2001.

seeking second opinions and consultations. They need to avoid creating risks for patients by an action or inaction.

Justice

The concept of justice concerns the issues of reward and punishment and the equitable distribution of social benefits. Relevant issues include whether resources should be distributed equally to those in greatest need, whether they should go to where they can have the greatest impact on the well-being of each individual served, or to where they will ultimately have the greatest impact on society.

SPECIFIC ISSUES

From a practical point of view, several specific issues most frequently involve psychiatrists. These include (1) sexual boundary violations, (2) nonsexual boundary violations, (3) violations of confidentiality, (4) mistreatment of the patient (incompetence, double agentry), and (5) illegal activities (insurance, billing, insider stock trading).

Sexual Boundary Violations

For a psychiatrist to engage a patient in a sexual relationship is clearly unethical. Furthermore, legal sanctions against such behavior make the ethical question moot. Various criminal law statutes have been used against psychiatrists who violate this ethical principle. Rape charges may be, and have been, brought against such psychiatrists; sexual assault and battery charges also have been used to convict psychiatrists.

In addition, patients who have been victimized sexually by psychiatrists and other physicians have won damages in malpractice suits. Insurance carriers for the APA and the American Medical Association (AMA) no longer insure against patient–therapist sexual relations, and the carriers exclude liability for any such sexual activity.

The issue of whether sexual relations between an ex-patient and a therapist violate an ethical principle, however, remains controversial. Proponents of the view, "Once a patient, always a patient," insist that any involvement with an ex-patient—even one that leads to marriage—should be prohibited. They maintain that a transferential reaction that always exists between the patient and the therapist prevents a rational decision about their emotional or sexual union. Others insist that, if a transferential reaction still exists, the therapy is incomplete and that as autonomous human beings, ex-patients should not be subjected to paternalistic moralizing by physicians. Accordingly, they believe that no sanctions should prohibit emotional or sexual involvements by ex-patients and their psychiatrists. Some psychiatrists maintain that a reasonable time should elapse before such a liaison. The length of the "reasonable" period remains controversial: Some have suggested 2 years. Other psychiatrists maintain that any period of prohibited involvement with an ex-patient is an unnecessary restriction. *The Principles,* however, states: "Sexual activity with a current or *former* patient is unethical."

Although not spelled out in *The Principles*, sexual activity with a patient's family member is also unethical. This is most important when the psychiatrist is treating a child or adolescent. Most training programs in child and adolescent psychiatry emphasize that the parents are patients too and that the ethical and legal proscriptions apply to parents (or parent surrogates) as well as to the child. Nevertheless, some psychiatrists misunderstand this concept. Sexual activity between a doctor and a patient's family member is also unethical.

An egregious example of a sexual boundary violation was reported in the *Medical Board of California Action Report (July 2006)* of a psychiatrist who had a 7-year affair with a patient who was schizophrenic. The doctor not only had sex with the patient but had her procure prostitutes with whom he and the patient would have group sex. He paid for their services by providing them with prescriptions for controlled substances and went so far as to bill Medi-Cal for these encounters as group therapy. The physician's license was revoked and he was also criminally convicted of fraud.

Nonsexual Boundary Violations

The relationship between a doctor and a patient for the purposes of providing and obtaining treatment is what is usually called the *doctor–patient relationship*. That relationship has both boundaries around it and boundaries within it. Either person may cross the boundary.

Not all boundary crossings are boundary violations. For example, a patient may say to a doctor at the end of an hour "I have left my money at home and I need a dollar to get my car out of the garage. Will you lend me a dollar until next time?" The patient has invited the doctor to cross the doctor–patient boundary and set up a lender–borrower relationship as well. Depending on the doctor's theoretical orientation, the clinical situation with the patient, and other factors, the doctor may elect to cross the boundary. Whether the boundary crossing is also a boundary violation is debatable. A *boundary violation* is a boundary crossing that is exploitative. It gratifies the doctor's needs at the expense of the patient. The doctor is responsible for preserving the boundary and for ensuring that boundary crossings are held to a minimum and that exploitation does not occur.

A resident in psychiatry was admonished by her psychotherapy supervisor to never, under any circumstances, accept a gift from a patient. In the course of treating a young girl with schizophrenia, she was offered a Christmas gift (a cotton scarf), which she refused to accept, explaining as gently as possible that it was not permitted by the "rules of the hospital." The next day the patient attempted suicide. She experienced the resident's refusal to accept the gift as a profound rejection (to which patients with schizophrenia are exquisitely sensitive), which she could not tolerate. The case illustrates the need to understand the dynamics of gift-giving and the transferential meaning to the patients of rejecting (or accepting) the gift.

The story (possibly apocryphal) is told of how Freud, who was an inveterate cigar smoker, was offered a box of difficult-to-find Havana cigars by a patient during the course of his analysis. Freud accepted the cigars and then proceeded to ask his patient to explore his motivations in offering the gift. Freud's reasons for accepting the cigars are more obvious than the patient's unconscious motivation for giving them, about which no information is available.

Harm to the patient is not a component of a boundary violation. For example, using information supplied by the patient (e.g., a stock tip) is an unethical boundary violation, although no obvious harm may come to the patient. For purposes of discussion, nonsexual boundary violations may be grouped into several arbitrary (overlapping and not mutually exclusive) categories.

Business. Almost any business relationship with a former patient is problematic, and almost any business relationship with a current patient is unethical. Naturally, the circumstance and location may play a significant role in this admonition. In a rural area or a small community, a doctor might be treating the only pharmacist (or plumber or couch upholsterer) in town; then when doing business with the pharmacist–patient, the doctor tries to keep boundaries in check. Ethical psychiatrists try to avoid doing business with a patient or a patient's family member or asking a patient to hire one of their family members. Ethical psychiatrists avoid investing in a patient's business or collaborating with a patient in a business deal.

Ideological Issues. Ideological issues can cloud judgment and may lead to ethical lapses. Any clinical decision should be based on what is best for the patient; the psychiatrist's ideology should play as little a part as possible in such a decision. A psychiatrist who is consulted by a patient with an illness should tell the patient what forms of treatment are available to treat the illness and allow the patient to decide on a course of treatment. Naturally, psychiatrists should recommend the treatment that they feel is in the best interest of the patient, but ultimately, the patient should be free to choose.

Social. The particular locale and circumstances must be considered in any discussion of the behavior of an ethical psychiatrist in social situations. The overarching principle is that the boundaries of the psychiatrist–patient relationship should be respected. Further, if options exist, they should be exercised in favor of the patient. Problems often arise in treatment situations when friendships develop between the psychiatrist and the patient. Objectivity is compromised, therapeutic neutrality is impaired, and factors outside the consciousness of either party may play a destructive role. Such friendship should be avoided during treatment. Similarly, psychiatrists should not treat their social friends for the same set of reasons. Obviously, in an emergency, a person does what a person must.

Financial. For psychiatrists who practice in the private sector, dealing with the patient about money is a part of treatment. Issues surrounding setting the fee, collecting the fee, and other financial matters are grist for the mill. Even so, ethical concerns must be observed. *The Principles* advises the doctor on such matters as charging for missed appointments and other contractual problems. Ethics complaints against doctors are frequently precipitated by financial issues; thus, the doctor must recognize the power that these issues have in the therapeutic relationship. Because the psychotherapeutic relationship is so much like a social relationship—the office looks like a living room, the doctor wears regular clothes, some patients might, without recognizing it, assume that a friendship exists that forgives payment of a fee. When the bill is presented, feelings, even though they are unconscious, are ruffled. The idea that psychiatric services are dispensed in a contractual context cannot be sufficiently emphasized. Early in their careers, psychiatrists are often reluctant to discuss fees openly out of a sense of embarrassment over discussing money or a sense of protecting the patient.

How an ethical psychiatrist handles the situation when a patient temporarily or permanently runs out of money is important. Many options are available—some more problematic than others. The psychiatrist can certainly lower the fee, but caution is needed because a fee lowered to the point where the treatment is not somehow being compensated may evoke countertransference resentment. The number of patients being seen at a reduced fee is a similar consideration. Running up a bill can also be a problem. Is there an expectation of eventually being paid? Is the hypertrophic bill a sham? The frequency of sessions may have to be altered. Any psychiatrist who sees private patients will definitely face these problems.

Confidentiality

Confidentiality refers to the therapist's responsibility not to release information learned in the course of treatment to third parties. *Privilege* refers to the patient's right to prevent disclosure of information from treatment in judicial hearings. Psychiatrists must maintain confidentiality because it is an essential ingredient of psychiatric care, as it is a prerequisite for patients to be willing to speak freely to therapists. Violating confidentiality by gossiping embarrasses people and violates nonmaleficence. Violation of confidentiality also breaks the promise that a psychiatrist has explicitly or implicitly made to keep material confidential.

Confidentiality must also give way to the responsibility to protect others when a patient makes a credible threat to harm someone. The situation becomes complicated when the risk is not to a particular individual, such as when a doctor is impaired or someone's mental state adversely affects his or her performance of a dangerous job, such as police work, firefighting, or use of dangerous machinery. Erosion has also arisen from the demands of an insurance company for detailed information. Patients must be told that information may be released to insurance companies, but they do not need to be warned that information concerning abuse of a child or threat to themselves or others needs to be reported.

Various settings exist in which patient data can be used to some degree. The general rule for doing so is to disclose only that information that is truly necessary. In teaching, research, and supervision, patients' names or information that might allow others to identify them should not be unnecessarily released. In ward rounds and case conferences, in which patient material is presented, attendees should be reminded that what they hear should not be repeated.

Confidentiality endures after death, with the ethical obligation to withhold information unless the next of kin provides consent. A subpoena is not automatic license to release the entire record. A psychiatrist can petition the judge for an in-camera (private) review to define what precise information must be disclosed.

Ethics in Managed Care

Psychiatrists have certain responsibilities toward patients treated in managed care settings, including the responsibilities to disclose all treatment options, to exercise appeal rights, to continue emergency treatment, and to cooperate reasonably with utilization reviewers.

Responsibility to Disclose. Psychiatrists have a continuing responsibility to the patient to obtain informed consent for treatments or procedures. All treatment options should be fully disclosed, even those not covered under the terms of a managed care plan. Most states have enacted legislation making gag rules illegal that limit information about treatment provided to patients under managed care.

Responsibility to Appeal. The AMA Council on Ethical and Judicial Affairs states that physicians have an ethical obligation to advocate for any care that they believe will materially benefit their patients, regardless of any allocation guidelines or gatekeeper directives.

Responsibility to Treat. Physicians are liable for failure to treat their patients within the defined standard of care. The treating physician has sole responsibility to determine what is medically necessary. Psychiatrists must be careful not to discharge suicidal or violent patients prematurely merely because continued coverage of benefits is not approved by a managed care company.

Responsibility to Cooperate with Utilization Review. The psychiatrist should cooperate with utilization reviewers' requests for information on proper authorization from the patient. When benefits are denied, it is important to understand and follow grievance procedures carefully, return telephone calls from review agencies, and provide documented, solid justification for continued treatment.

With the advent of managed care and the need to send periodic progress reports and documentation of signs and symptoms to third-party reviewers to pay for treatment, some psychiatrists may diminish or exaggerate symptomatology. The following case report and discussion illustrates the ethical difficulties psychiatrists face in dealing with managed care.

Mrs. P admitted herself to the hospital because she was afraid she might kill herself. She was experiencing a major depressive episode, but she improved markedly during the first weeks on Dr. A's ward. Although Dr. A believed that Mrs. P was no longer suicidal, he thought she would benefit greatly from continued hospitalization. Because he knew that Mrs. P could not afford to pay for hospitalization and that the insurance company would pay only if the patient was suicidally depressed, he decided not to document Mrs. P's improvement. He noted in the chart that "the patient continues to have a risk of suicide."

Does Dr. A engage in a form of deception? Yes, he intentionally misleads by what he writes and what he omits writing in the chart. Although what he writes is true in some literal sense, his statement is misleading in the context of treatment. Mrs. P is not suicidally depressed in the way that she was.

What Dr. A omits from the chart is also deceptive. Whether a particular omission is deceptive depends, in part, on the roles and expectations of the people involved. Not telling a colleague that one dislikes his tie is not a deception. It is simply tact, unless the role or relationship involves the expectation that one offers a candid opinion. Dr. A's case is different. His professional role is to document the patient's course, and the expectation is that he will note any significant improvement. Thus, his failure to document Mrs. P's progress accurately is a kind of deception.

The second and more difficult question is whether deception is justified in this instance. The answer to that question depends on the reasons for the deception, the reasons against it, and the alternatives available. The reasons for this deception are obvious. Dr. A's aim and primary obligation is to help the patient. He believes that Mrs. P would benefit greatly from continued hospitalization that she cannot afford. He may also believe that it is unfair for the insurance company to refuse to pay for inpatient treatment of nonsuicidal depression and that his deception rectifies that unfair practice.

Important reasons also exist against this deception. The first concerns honesty and social trust. It is a good thing if people can rely on what others say and write. Without some honesty and trust, many social exchanges and practices would be impossible. Deception, even for beneficent purposes, has real potential to damage social trust. A risk exists that deception may damage people's trust in the profession of psychiatry and even patients' trust in their psychiatrists. Damage to trust may, in turn, compromise treatment.

The second reason concerns future medical treatment. If Mrs. P seeks medical treatment in the future, the physicians who attend her will read the misleading notes. If they believe that the notes are an accurate account of the previous treatment, they may suggest an inappropriate treatment for the present problem. Even if they have doubts about the accuracy of the notes in her chart, they are deprived of an accurate history and report. In either case, the prior deception can hinder treatment.

The third reason concerns obligations and coverage policies. Dr. A seems to ignore the obligation that he has to the population that is covered by the insurance policy. He shifts a burden onto this population by forcing the insurance company to pay for treatment that it did not agree to cover. Perhaps the insurance company should pay for inpatient treatment in cases such as Mrs. P's; perhaps its policies are unreasonable and unfair. However, Dr. A's deception does not challenge the insurance company and pressure it to change its policy, nor does his deception encourage patients and their families to contest the company's policies. The use of deception simply circumvents, in an ad hoc way, a policy that should be challenged and discussed.

Dr. A also seems to ignore his obligation to future patients. By introducing an inaccuracy into the chart, he compromises the value of medical records research. His deception works, in a small way, to deprive future patients of the benefit of research that relies on medical records.

Whether the deception is justified depends on both the weight of the reasons for and against the deception and the available alternatives. One alternative is to tailor the chart. Another alternative is to describe Mrs. P's response accurately and to discharge her to outpatient care. However, a third alternative exists. Dr. A can accurately document the patient's course and can recommend continued hospitalization. He can petition the insurance company for coverage. If the insurance company decides not to approve further inpatient care for the patient, Dr. A can appeal that decision. This alternative is more time consuming, and nothing guarantees that it will succeed, but it avoids all the problems associated with the use of deception.

Impaired Physicians

A physician may become impaired as the result of psychiatric or medical disorders or the use of mind-altering and habit-forming substances (e.g., alcohol and drugs). Many organic illnesses can interfere with the cognitive and motor skills required to provide competent medical care. Although the legal responsibility to report an impaired physician varies, depending on the state, the ethical responsibility remains universal. An incapacitated physician should be reported to an appropriate authority, and the reporting physician is required to follow specific hospital, state, and legal procedures. A physician who treats an impaired physician should not be required to monitor the impaired physician's progress or fitness to return to work. This monitoring should be performed by an independent physician or group of physicians who have no conflicts of interest.

The Office of Professional Medical Conduct (OPMC) in New York State regulates the practice of medicine by investigating illegal or unethical practice by physicians and other health professionals, such as physician assistants. Similar regulatory agencies exist in other states. Professional misconduct in New York State is defined as one of the following:

1. Practicing fraudulently and with gross negligence or incompetence.
2. Practicing while the ability to practice is impaired.
3. Being habitually drunk or being dependent on, or a habitual user of, narcotics or a habitual user of other drugs having similar effects.
4. Immoral conduct in the practice of the profession.
5. Permitting, aiding, or abetting an unlicensed person to perform activities requiring a license.
6. Refusing a client or patient service because of creed, color, or national origin.
7. Practicing beyond the scope of practice permitted by law.
8. Being convicted of a crime or being the subject of disciplinary action in another jurisdiction.

Professional misconduct complaints derive mainly from the public in addition to insurance companies, law enforcement agencies, and doctors, among others.

Physicians in Training

It is unethical to delegate authority for patient care to anyone who is not appropriately qualified and experienced, such as a medical student or a resident, without adequate supervision from an attending physician. Residents are physicians in training and, as such, must provide a good deal of patient care. Within a healthy, ethical teaching environment, residents and medical students may be involved with, and responsible for, the day-to-day care of many ill patients, but they are supervised, supported, and directed by highly trained and experienced physicians. Patients have the right to know the level of training of their care providers and should be informed about the resident's or medical student's level of training. Residents and medical students should know and acknowledge their limitations and should ask for supervision from experienced colleagues as necessary.

Physician Charter of Professionalism

In 2001, a movement to clarify the concept of "professionalism" was begun by the American Board of Internal Medicine. A set of principles called the *Physician Charter of Professionalism* was developed, which describes what it means for physicians to perform at their highest and most ethical level. Table 59–2 lists the principles and commitments of professional behaviors in the *Physician Charter of Professionalism* to which all physicians (including psychiatrists) are expected to adhere.

A summary of ethical issues discussed in this section is presented in a question-and-answer format in Table 59–3.

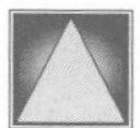

Table 59–2
Physician Charter of Professionalism

Fundamental Principles

- **Primacy of patient welfare.** Altruism contributes to the trust central to doctor–patient relationships. Market forces, societal pressures, and administrative exigencies must not compromise this principle.
- **Patient autonomy.** Physicians must be honest with patients and empower them to make informed decisions about treatment.
- **Social justice.** Physicians should work actively to eliminate discrimination in health care, whether based on race, gender, socioeconomic status, ethnicity, religion, or any other social category.

A Set of Commitments

- **Professional competence.** Physicians must be committed to life-long learning. The profession, as a whole, must strive to see that all of its members are competent.
- **Honesty with patients.** Physicians must ensure that patients are completely and honestly informed before consenting to a treatment; they must be empowered to decide about the course of therapy. Physicians should also acknowledge that medical errors that injure patients sometimes occur. If a patient is injured through error, he or she should be informed promptly, because failure to do so seriously compromises patient and societal trust.
- **Patient confidentiality.** Fulfilling the commitment to confidentiality is more pressing now than ever before, given the widespread use of electronic information systems for compiling patient data.
- **Maintaining appropriate relations with patients.** Physicians should never exploit patients for any sexual advantage, personal financial gain, or other private purpose.
- **Improving quality of care.** This commitment entails both maintaining clinical competence and working collaboratively with other professionals to reduce medical error, increase patient safety, minimize overuse of health care resources, and optimize the outcomes of care.
- **Improving access to care.** Physicians must individually and collectively strive to reduce barriers to equitable health care.
- **Just distribution of finite resources.** Physicians should be committed to working with other physicians, hospitals, and payers to develop guidelines for cost-effective care. The physician's professional responsibility for appropriate allocation of resources requires scrupulous avoidance of superfluous tests and procedures.
- **Scientific knowledge.** Physicians have a duty to uphold scientific standards, to promote research, and to create new knowledge and ensure its appropriate use.
- **Maintaining trust by managing conflicts of interest.** Physicians have an obligation to recognize, disclose to the general public, and address conflicts of interest. Relationships between industry and opinion leaders should be disclosed.
- **Professional responsibilities.** Physicians are expected to participate in the process of self-regulation, including remediation and discipline of members who have failed to meet professional standards.

Military Psychiatry

Psychiatrists in the military face unique ethical problems, because confidentiality does not exist under the military code of conduct.

A 19-year-old, white, single man, new to military service, presented with a history of periodic episodes of anxiety when taking showers in groups with other men. He identified himself as gay and recognized that his anxiety was related to his fear of acting out his sexual impulses, thus risking court-martial and dishonorable discharge, should he ever be discovered. The psychiatrist was

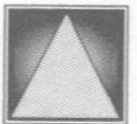

Table 59–3
Ethical Questions and Answers

Topic	Question	Answer
Abandonment	How can psychiatrists avoid being charged with patient abandonment on retirement?	Retiring psychiatrists are not abandoning patients if they provide their patients with sufficient notice and make every reasonable effort to find follow-up care for the patients.
	Is it ethical to provide only outpatient care to a seriously ill patient, who may require hospitalization?	This could constitute abandonment unless the outpatient practitioner or agency arranges for their patients to receive inpatient care from another provider.
Bequests	A dying patient bequeaths his or her estate to his or her treating psychiatrist. Is this ethical?	No. Accepting the bequest seems improper and exploitational of the therapeutic relationship. However, it may be ethical to accept a token bequest from a deceased patient who named his or her psychiatrist in the will without that psychiatrist's knowledge.
Competency	Is it ethical for psychiatrists to perform vaginal exams? Hospital physicals?	Psychiatrists may provide nonpsychiatric medical procedures if they are competent to do so and if the procedures do not preclude effective psychiatric treatment by distorting the transference. Pelvic exams carry a high risk of distorting the transference and would be better performed by another clinician.
	Can ethics committees review issues of physician competency?	Yes. Incompetency is an ethical issue.
Confidentiality	Must confidentiality be maintained after the death of a patient?	Yes. Ethically, confidences survive a patient's death. Exceptions include protecting others from imminent harm or proper legal compulsions.
	Is it ethical to release information about a patient to an insurance company?	Yes, if the information provided is limited to that which is needed to process the insurance claim.
	Can a videotaped segment of a therapy session be used at a workshop for professionals?	Yes, if informed, uncoerced consent has been obtained, anonymity is maintained, the audience is advised that editing makes this an incomplete session, and the patient knows the purpose of the videotape.
	Should a physician report mere suspicion of child abuse in a state requiring reporting of child abuse?	No. A physician must make several assessments before deciding whether to report suspected abuse. One must consider whether abuse is ongoing, whether abuse is responsive to treatment, and whether reporting will cause potential harm. Check specific statutes. Make safety for potential victims the top priority.
Conflict of interest	Is there a potential ethical conflict if a psychiatrist has both psychotherapeutic and administrative duties in dealing with students or trainees?	Yes. You must define your role in advance to the trainees or students. Administrative opinions should be obtained from a psychiatrist who is not involved in a treatment relationship with the trainee or student.
Diagnosis without examination	Is it ethical to offer a diagnosis based only upon review of records to determine, for insurance purposes, if suicide was the result of illness?	Yes.
	Is it ethical for a supervising psychiatrist to sign a diagnosis on an insurance form for services provided by a supervisee when the psychiatrist has not examined the patient?	Yes, if the psychiatrist ensures that proper care is given and the insurance form clearly indicates the role of supervisor and supervisee.
Exploitation (also see Bequests)	What constitutes exploitation of the therapeutic relationship?	Exploitation occurs when the psychiatrist uses the therapeutic relationship for personal gain. This includes adopting or hiring a patient as well as sexual or financial relationships.
Fee splitting	What is fee splitting?	Fee splitting occurs when one physician pays another for a patient referral. This would also apply to lawyers giving a forensic psychiatrist referrals in exchange for a percentage of the fee. Fee splitting may occur in an office setting if the psychiatrist takes a percentage of his or her office-mates' fees for supervision or expenses. Costs for such items or services must be arranged separately. Otherwise, it would appear that the office owner could benefit from referring patients to a colleague in the office. Fee splitting is illegal.
Informed consent	Is it ethical to refuse to divulge information about a patient who has agreed to give this information to those requesting it?	No. It is the patient's decision, not the therapist's.
	Is informed consent needed when presenting or writing about case material?	Not if the patient is aware of the supervisory/teaching process and confidentiality is preserved.
Moonlighting	Can psychiatric residents ethically "moonlight"?	They can if their duties are not beyond their ability, if they are properly supervised, and if the moonlighting does not interfere with their residency training.

(continued)

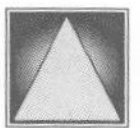

Table 59–3 (Continued)

Topic	Question	Answer
Reporting	Should psychiatrists expose or report unethical behavior of a colleague or colleagues? Can a spouse bring an ethical complaint?	Psychiatrists are obligated to report colleagues' unethical behavior. A spouse with knowledge of unethical behavior can bring an ethical complaint as well.
Research	How can ethical research be performed with subjects who cannot give informed consent?	Consent can be given by a legal guardian or via a living will. Incompetent persons have the right to withdraw from the research project at any time.
Retirement	See Abandonment.	
Supervision	What are the ethical requirements when a psychiatrist supervises other mental health professionals?	The psychiatrist must spend sufficient time to ensure that proper care is given and that the supervisee is not providing services that are outside the scope of his or her training. It is ethical to charge a fee for supervision.
Taping and recording	Can videotapes of patient interviews be used for training purposes on a national level (e.g., workshops, board exam preparation)?	Appropriate and explicit informed consent must be obtained. The purpose and scope of exposure of the tape must be emphasized in addition to the resulting loss of confidentiality.

Table by Eugene Rubin, M.D. (Data derived from American Psychiatric Association. *Opinions of the Ethics Committee on the Principles of Medical Ethics with Annotations Especially Applicable to Psychiatry.* Washington, DC: American Psychiatric Association; 2001.)

faced with a dilemma: whether to report the soldier to his commanding officer (as he was obliged to do under the military code) or to protect the soldier from acting on his impulses that would place him in danger (in keeping with the medical ethic to do no harm). After discussing various options, he and the patient agreed on the latter option. A diagnosis of anxiety disorder was made, which allowed the patient to receive an honorable discharge on medical grounds, based on a recognized psychiatric disorder. No record of his homosexual orientation was made.

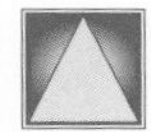

Table 59–4
Patient's Rights under the Privacy Rule

Physicians must give the patient a written notice of his or her privacy rights, the privacy policies of the practice, and how patient information is used, kept, and disclosed. A written acknowledgment should be taken from the patient verifying that they have seen such notice.

Patients should be able to obtain copies of their medical records and to request revisions to those records within a stated amount of time (usually 30 days). Patients do not have the right to see psychotherapy notes.

Physicians must provide the patient with a history of most disclosures of their medical history on request. Some exceptions exist. The APA Committee on Confidentiality has developed a model document for this requirement.

Physicians must obtain authorization from the patient for disclosure of information other than for treatment, payment, and health care operations (these three are considered to be routine uses, for which consent is not required). The APA Committee on Confidentiality has developed a model document for this requirement.

Patients may request another means of communication of their protected information (i.e., request that the physician contact them at a specific phone number or address).

Physicians cannot generally limit treatment to obtaining patient authorization for disclosure of their information for nonroutine uses.

Patients have the right to complain about Privacy Rule violations to the physician, their health plan, or to the Secretary of HHS.

APA, American Psychiatric Association; HHS, Department of Health and Human Services.

Health Insurance Portability and Accountability Act

The Health Insurance Portability and Accountability Act (HIPAA) was passed in 1996 to address the medical delivery system's mounting complexity and its rising dependence on electronic communication. The act orders that the federal Department of Health and Human Services (HHS) develop rules protecting the transmission and confidentiality of patient information, and all units under HIPAA must comply with such rules.

The Privacy Rule, administered by the Office of Civil Rights (OCR) at HHS, protects the confidentiality of patient information (Table 59–4).

References

AMA Guidelines on Gifts to Physicians from Drug Industry. Available at: http://www.ama-assn.org/ama/pub/category/4263.html. Accessed June 10, 2004.

Belmont Report: Ethical Principles and Guidelines for the Protection of Human Subjects of Research. Federal Register Document 79-12065. Available at: http://history.nih.gov/history/laws/belmont.html. Accessed June 10, 2004.

Blass DM, Rye RM, Robbins BM, Miner MM, Handel S, Carroll JL Jr., Rabins PV. Ethical issues in mobile psychiatric treatment with homebound elderly patients: The Psychogeriatric Assessment and Treatment in City Housing Experience. *J Am Geriatr Soc*. 2006;54(5):843.

DuVal G. Ethics in psychiatric research: Study design issues. *Can J Psychiatry*. 2004;49(1):55–59.

Fleischman AR, Wood EB. Ethical issues in research involving victims of terror. *J Urban Health Bull N Y Acad Med.* 2002;79:315–321.

Green SA. The ethical commitments of academic faculty in psychiatric education. *Academic Psychology*. 2006;30(1):48.

Kaldjian LC, Weir RF, Duffy TP. A clinician's approach to clinical ethical reasoning. *J Gen Intern Med*. 2005;20:306.

Kipnis K. Gender, sex, and professional ethics in child and adolescent psychiatry. *Child Adolesc Psychiatr Clin North Am*. 2004;13(3):695–708.

Lubit RH, Ladds B, Eth S. Ethics in psychiatry. In: Sadock BJ, Sadock VA, eds. *Kaplan & Sadock's Comprehensive Textbook of Psychiatry*. 8th ed. Vol. 2. Baltimore: Lippincott Williams & Wilkins; 2005:3988.

Merlino JP. Psychoanalysis and ethics-relevant then, essential now. *J Am Acad Psychoanal Dyn Psychiatry*. 2006;34(2):231–247.

Parker MJ. Judging capacity: Paternalism and the risk-related standard. *J Law Med*. 2004;11(4):482–491.

Roberts LW. Ethical philanthropy in academic psychiatry. *Am J Psychiatry*. 2006; 163(5):772.

Schneider PL, Bramstedt KA. When psychiatry and bioethics disagree about patient decision making capacity (DMC). *J Med Ethics* 2006;32:90–93.

Simon L. Psychotherapy as civics: The patient and therapists as citizens. *Ethical Human Psychology and Psychiatry*. 2005;7(1):57.

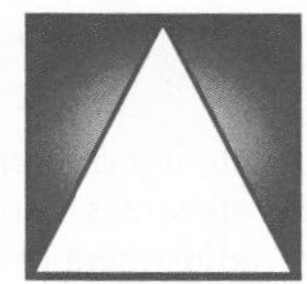

Index

Page numbers followed by *f* indicate figures, page numbers followed by *t* indicated tables, and page numbers in **boldface** indicate main discussions.